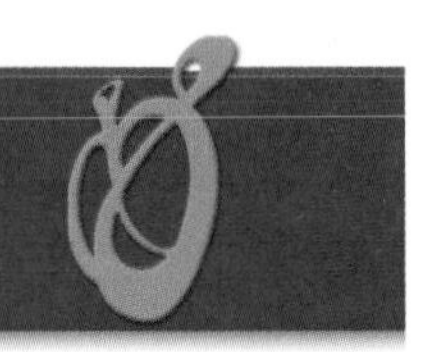

Heart Failure

A Companion to Braunwald's Heart Disease

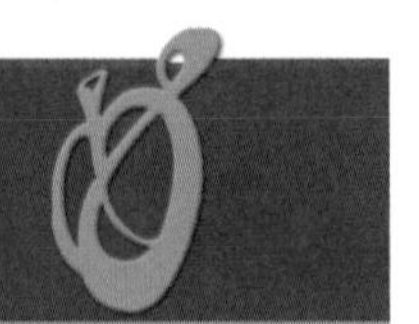

Heart Failure

A Companion to Braunwald's Heart Disease

Second Edition

Douglas L. Mann, MD, FACC
Lewin Professor and Chief
Cardiovascular Division
Washington University School of Medicine;
Cardiologist-in-Chief
Barnes Jewish Hospital
St. Louis, Missouri

ELSEVIER
SAUNDERS

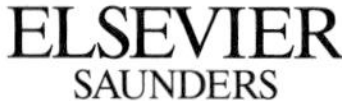

ELSEVIER
SAUNDERS

3251 Riverport Lane
St. Louis, Missouri 63043

HEART FAILURE: A COMPANION TO BRAUNWALD'S HEART DISEASE, SECOND EDITION ISBN: 978-1-4160-5895-3

Notices

Knowledge and best practice in this field are constantly changing. As new research and experience broaden our understanding, changes in research methods, professional practices, or medical treatment may become necessary.

Practitioners and researchers must always rely on their own experience and knowledge in evaluating and using any information, methods, compounds, or experiments described herein. In using such information or methods they should be mindful of their own safety and the safety of others, including parties for whom they have a professional responsibility.

With respect to any drug or pharmaceutical products identified, readers are advised to check the most current information provided (i) on procedures featured or (ii) by the manufacturer of each product to be administered, to verify the recommended dose or formula, the method and duration of administration, and contraindications. It is the responsibility of practitioners, relying on their own experience and knowledge of their patients, to make diagnoses, to determine dosages and the best treatment for each individual patient, and to take all appropriate safety precautions.

To the fullest extent of the law, neither the Publisher nor the authors, contributors, or editors, assume any liability for any injury and/or damage to persons or property as a matter of products liability, negligence or otherwise, or from any use or operation of any methods, products, instructions, or ideas contained in the material herein.

Library of Congress Cataloging-in-Publication Data
Heart failure : a companion to Braunwald's heart disease / [edited by] Douglas L. Mann. -- 2nd ed.
p. ; cm
Companion v. to: Braunwald's heart disease / edited by Peter Libby ... [et al.]. 8th ed. c2008.
Includes bibliographical references and index.
ISBN 978-1-4160-5895-3
1. Heart failure. I. Mann, Douglas L. II. Braunwald's heart disease.
[DNLM: 1. Heart Failure. WG 370 H43618 2010]
RC685.C53H426 2010
616.1'2--dc22 2010010218

Executive Publisher: Natasha Andjelkovic
Developmental Editor: Brad McIlwain
Publishing Services Manager: Catherine Jackson
Project Manager: Janaki Srinivasan Kumar
Design Direction: Steven Stave

Printed in United States of America

Last digit is the print number: 9 8 7 6 5 4 3 2 1

To my teachers and mentors, for their enduring encouragement and support,
especially Dr. James W. Covell, whom I have never thanked enough,
and Dr. Andrew I. Schafer, whom I can never thank enough.

Douglas L. Mann, MD, FACC

Contributors

Michael Acker, MD
Professor of Surgery, Cardiothoracic Surgery Division, Department of Surgery, University of Pennsylvania School of Medicine, Philadelphia, Pennsylvania

Kirkwood F. Adams, Jr., MD
Professor of Medicine, Departments of Medicine and Radiology, University of North Carolina at Chapel Hill, Chapel Hill, North Carolina

Inder S. Anand, MD, FRCP, DPhil (Oxon)
Professor of Medicine, Division of Cardiology, University of Minnesota Medical School; Director of Heart Failure Clinic, Veterans Affairs Medical Center, Minneapolis, Minnesota

Stefan D. Anker, MD, PhD
Professor of Medicine, Applied Cachexia Research, Department of Cardiology, Charité Medical School, Campus Virchow-Klinikum, Berlin, Germany; Centre for Clinical and Basic Research, IRCCS San Raffaele, Rome, Italy

Piero Anversa, MD
Professor of Medicine and Anesthesia, Departments of Anesthesia and Medicine, Cardiovascular Division, Brigham and Women's Hospital, Harvard Medical School, Boston, Massachusetts

Catalin F. Baicu, PhD
Research Assistant Professor of Medicine, The Ralph H. Johnson Department of Veterans Affairs Medical Center, Charleston, South Carolina

Kenneth M. Baker, MD
Professor and Vice Chair, Department of Medicine, Division of Molecular Cardiology; Director, Mayborn Chair in Cardiovascular Research, Texas A&M Health Science Center, Temple, Texas

Rob S. Beanlands, MD
Chief, Cardiac Imaging, University of Ottawa Heart Institute, Ottawa, Ontario, Canada

Kerstin Bethmann, PhD
Department of Cardiology and Angiology, Hannover Medical School, Hannover, Germany

Courtney L. Bickford, PharmD, BCSPS
Division of Pharmacy, University of Texas M.D. Anderson Cancer Center, Houston, Texas

Guido Boerrigter, MD
Cardiorenal Research Laboratory, Division of Cardiovascular Diseases, Mayo Heart and Lung Research Center, Mayo Clinic and Mayo Clinic College of Medicine, Rochester, Minnesota

Roberta C. Bogaev, MD
Cardiopulmonary Transplant Service, Texas Heart Institute, Houston, Texas

Robert O. Bonow, MD
Max and Lilly Goldberg Distinguished Professor of Cardiology, Northwestern University Feinberg School of Medicine; Co-Director, Bluhm Cardiovascular Institute, Northwestern Memorial Hospital, Chicago, Illinois

Julian Booker, MD
Department of Cardiology, Baylor College of Medicine, Houston, Texas

Biykem Bozkurt, MD, PhD
Professor of Medicine, Cardiology Section, Michael E. DeBakey Veterans Affairs Medical Center, Winters Center for Heart Failure Research, Baylor College of Medicine, Houston, Texas

Michael R. Bristow, MD, PhD
Professor of Medicine, Deparment of Medicine, Division of Cardiology, University of Colorado Health Sciences Center, Aurora, Colorado

John C. Burnett, Jr., MD
Professor of Medicine, Cardiorenal Research Laboratory, Division of Cardiovascular Diseases, Mayo Heart and Lung Research Center, Mayo Clinic and Mayo Clinic College of Medicine, Rochester, Minnesota

Daniel J. Cantillon, MD
Professor of Medicine, Cleveland Clinic Lerner College of Medicine, Case Western Reserve University, Cleveland, Ohio

Blase A. Carabello, MD, FACC
Professor of Medicine and Vice Chairman, Department of Medicine, Baylor College of Medicine; Medical Care Line Executive, Houston Veterans Affairs Medical Center, Houston, Texas

Jay N. Cohn, MD
Professor of Medicine, Director, Rasmussen Center for Cardiovascular Disease Prevention, Cardiovascular Division, University of Minnesota Medical School, Minneapolis, Minnesota

Wilson S. Colucci, MD
Professor of Medicine, Cardiovascular Medicine Section, Department of Medicine, Boston University Medical Center, Boston, Massachusetts

Leslie T. Cooper, Jr., MD
Professor of Medicine, Division of Cardiovascular Diseases, Mayo Clinic, Rochester, Minnesota

Lisa Costello-Boerrigter, MD, PhD
Cardiorenal Research Laboratory, Division of Cardiovascular Diseases, Mayo Heart and Lung Research Center, Mayo Clinic and Mayo Clinic College of Medicine, Rochester, Minnesota

Lori B. Daniels, MD
Division of Cardiology, University of California, San Diego, San Diego, California

Reynolds M. Delgado III, MD
Cardiopulmonary Transplant Service, Texas Heart Institute, Houston, Texas

Anita Deswal, MD, MPH
Associate Professor of Medicine, Section of Cardiology, Michael E. DeBakey Veterans Affairs Medical Center and Winters Center for Heart Failure Research, Baylor College of Medicine, Houston, Texas

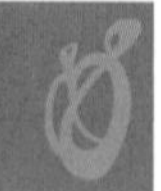

Abhinav Diwan, MBBS
Assistant Professor of Medicine, Center for Pharmacogenomics and Cardiovascular Division, Department of Internal Medicine, Washington University and St. Louis Veterans Affairs Medical Center, St. Louis, Missouri

Wolfram Doehner, MD, PhD
Professor of Medicine, Center for Stroke Research, Applied Cachexia Research, Department of Cardiology, Charité University Medical School, Campus Virchow-Klinikum, Berlin, Germany

Hisham Dokainish, MD
Department of Medicine, Baylor College of Medicine, Houston, Texas

Gerald W. Dorn II, MD
Professor of Medicine, Center for Pharmacogenomics and Cardiovascular Division, Department of Internal Medicine, Washington University,
St. Louis, Missouri

Helmut Drexler, MD
Professor of Cardiology, Department of Cardiology and Angiology, Hannover Medical School, Hannover, Germany

Arthur M. Feldman, MD, PhD
Magee Professor and Chairman, Department of Medicine, Jefferson Medical College, Philadelphia, Pennsylvania

G. Michael Felker, MD, MHS
Associate Professor of Medicine, Division of Cardiology, Duke Clinical Research Institute, Duke University Medical Center, Durham, North Carolina

James D. Flaherty, MD
Assistant Professor of Medicine, Interventional Cardiology, Northwestern University Feinberg School of Medicine, Chicago, Illinois

John S. Floras, MD, DPhil, FRCPC, FACC, FAHA
Professor of Medicine, Mount Sinai Hospital, University Health Network, Division of Cardiology, The University of Toronto, Toronto, Ontario, Canada

Viorel G. Florea, MD, PhD, DSc, FACC
Assistant Professor of Medicine, University of Minnesota Medical School, Veteran's Affairs Medical Center, Minneapolis, Minnesota

Gary S. Francis, MD
Professor of Medicine, Cardiovascular Division, University of Minnesota, Minneapolis, Minnesota

Wayne Franklin, MD
Assistant Professor of Medicine; Medical Director, Texas Adult Congenital Heart Disease Center, Baylor College of Medicine, Houston, Texas

O. H. Frazier, MD
Cardiopulmonary Transplant Service, Texas Heart Institute, Houston, Texas

Matthias Freidrich, MD
The Libin Cardiovascular Institute, Calgary, Alberta, Canada

Ronald S. Freudenberger, MD
Director, Center for Advanced Heart Failure, Lehigh Valley Hospital and Health Network, Allentown, Pennsylvania; Professor of Medicine, Pennsylvania State University College of Medicine, State College, Pennsylvania

Mihai Gheorghiade, MD, FACC
Professor of Medicine and Surgery; Associate Chief, Division of Cardiology; Chief, Cardiology Clinical Service, Director, Telemetry Unit, Northwestern University Feinberg School of Medicine, Chicago, Illinois

Thomas D. Giles, MD
Professor of Medicine, Heart and Vascular Institute, Tulane University Health Sciences Center, New Orleans, Louisiana

Stephen Gottlieb, MD
Professor of Medicine, University of Maryland School of Medicine, Baltimore, Maryland

Yusuf Hassan, MD
Division of Cardiology, The University of Texas Houston Health Science Center, Houston, Texas

Edward P. Havranek, MD
Professor of Medicine, Denver Health Medical Center, University of Colorado Denver School of Medicine, Denver, Colorado

Shunichi Homma, MD
Associate Chief, Division of Cardiology; Director, Cardiovascular Ultrasound Laboratories, Professor of Medicine, Margaret Milliken Hatch Professor of Medicine, New York Presbyterian Hospital, New York, New York

Burkhard Hornig, MD
Department of Cardiology and Angiology, Hannover Medical School, Hannover, Germany

Steven R. Houser, PhD, FAHA
Professor of Phys, Cardiovascular Research Center, Molecular and Cellular Cardiology Laboratories, Department of Physiology, Temple University School of Medicine, Philadelphia, Pennsylvania

Joanne S. Ingwall, PhD
Professor of Medicine (Physiology), Brigham and Women's Hospital, Harvard Medical School, Boston, Massachusetts

Shahrokh Javaheri, MD
Emeritus Professor of Medicine, University of Cincinnati, College of Medicine; Medical Director, Sleepcare Diagnostics, Cincinnati, Ohio

John Lynn Jefferies, MD, MPH
Assistant Professor of Pediatrics, Department of Pediatrics, Baylor College of Medicine, Texas Children's Hospital, Houston, Texas

Mariell Jessup, MD
Professor of Medicine, Cardiovascular Division, Department of Medicine, University of Pennsylvania School of Medicine, Philadelphia, Pennsylvania

Saurabh Jha, MBBS
Assistant Professor of Radiology, Hospital at the University of Pennsylvania, Philadelphia, Pennsylvania

Jan Kajstura, PhD
Department of Anesthesia, Brigham and Women's Hospital, Harvard Medical School, Boston, Massachusetts

David A. Kass, MD
Abraham and Virginia Weiss Professor of Cardiology; Professor of Medicine; Professor of Biomedical Engineering, Institute of Molecular Cardiobiology, Division of Cardiology, Johns Hopkins Medical Institutions, Baltimore, Maryland

Arnold M. Katz, MD, DMed (Hon)
Professor of Medicine Emeritus, University of Connecticut School of Medicine, Farmington, Connecticut; Visiting Professor of Medicine and Physiology, Dartmouth Medical School, Hanover, New Hampshire

Richard N. Kitsis, MD
Professor of Medicine, Department of Medicine, Albert Einstein College of Medicine, Bronx, New York

Marvin A. Konstam, MD
Professor of Medicine, Tufts University School of Medicine; Director, Cardiovascular Center, Tufts Medical Center, Boston, Massachusetts

Varda Konstam, PhD
University of Massachusetts, Boston, Massachusetts

William E. Kraus, MD
Professor of Medicine, Duke University School of Medicine, Durham, North Carolina

Rajesh Kumar, PhD
Assistant Professor, Department of Internal Medicine, Division of Molecular Cardiology, Texas A&M Health Science Center, College of Medicine, Temple, Texas

Ulf Landmesser, MD
Assistant Professor of Medicine, Department of Cardiology and Angiology, Hannover Medical School, Hannover, Germany

Thierry H. Le Jemtel, MD
Henderson Chair and Professor of Medicine; Director, Heart Failure and Cardiac Transplantation Program, Tulane University, New Orleans, Louisiana

Ilana Lehmann, PhD
University of Massachusetts, Boston, Massachusetts

Annarosa Leri, MD
Associate Professor, Department of Anesthesia, Brigham and Women's Hospital, Harvard Medical School, Boston, Massachusetts

Martin M. LeWinter, MD
Professor of Medicine and Molecular Physiology and Biophysics, University of Vermont College of Medicine, Burlington, Vermont

Chang-Seng Liang, MD, PhD
Professor of Medicine, Cardiovascular Medicine Section, Department of Medicine, Boston University Medical Center, Boston, Massachusetts

Alan S. Maisel, MD
Professor of Medicine, Division of Cardiology, University of California–San Diego, Veterans Affairs Medical Center, San Diego, California

Donna M. Mancini, MD
Professor of Medicine, Columbia-Presbyterian Medical Center, New York, New York

Douglas L. Mann, MD, FACC
Lewin Professor and Chief, Cardiovascular Division, Washington University School of Medicine; Cardiologist-in-Chief, Barnes Jewish Hospital, St. Louis, Missouri

Kenneth B. Margulies, MD
Professor of Medicine, Cardiovascular Institute, Department of Medicine, University of Pennsylvania School of Medicine, Philadelphia, Pennsylvania

Ali J. Marian, MD
Professor of Molecular Medicine and Internal Medicine (Cardiology); Director, Center for Cardiovascular Genetic Research, The Brown Foundation Institute of Molecular Medicine, The University of Texas Health Science Center, Texas Heart Institute at St. Luke's Episcopal Hospital, Houston, Texas

Mathew Maurer, MD
Assistant Professor of Clinical Medicine, Columbia University College of Physicians and Surgeons, New York, New York

Dennis M. McNamara, MD, MSc
Professor of Medicine, Director, Heart Failure/Transplantation Program, University of Pittsburgh Medical Center, Pittsburgh, Pennsylvania

Mandeep R. Mehra, MBBS, FACC, FACP
Professor of Medicine, Herbert Berger Professor and Head of Cardiology, University of Maryland School of Medicine, Baltimore, Maryland

Gustavo F. Méndez Machado, MD, MSc, FESC
Consultant Cardiologist, Department of Research, IMSS Adolfo Ruiz Cortines National Medical Center, Veracruz, Mexico

Marco Metra, MD
Division of Cardiology, Department of Experimental and Applied Medicine, University of Brescia, Brescia, Italy

Debra K. Moser, DNSc, RN, FAAN
Professor and Gill Endowed Chair of Nursing, University of Kentucky, College of Nursing, Lexington, Kentucky

Wilfried Mullens, MD
Heart and Vascular Institute, Cleveland Clinic, Cleveland, Ohio

Ashleigh A. Owen, MD
Medical University of South Carolina, Ralph H. Johnson Veterans Affairs Medical Center, Charleston, South Carolina

Jing Pan, MD, PhD
Assistant Professor, Department of Internal Medicine, Division of Molecular Cardiology, Texas A&M Health Science Center, College of Medicine, Temple, Texas

Richard D. Patten, MD, FACC
Assistant Professor of Medicine, Catholic Medical Center, New England Heart Institute, Manchester, New Hampshire

Naveen Pereira, MD
Division of Cardiovascular Diseases, Mayo Clinic, Rochester, Minnesota

Linda R. Peterson, MD, FACC, FAHA, FASE
Associate Professor of Medicine and Radiology, Cardiovascular Division, Division of Geriatrics and Nutritional Sciences, Washington University School of Medicine, St. Louis, Missouri

Ileana L. Piña, MD
Professor of Medicine, Case Western Reserve University, Louis Stokes Cleveland Veterans Affairs Medical Center, Cleveland, Ohio

Philip J. Podrid, MD
Professor of Medicine and Associate Professor of Pharmacology, Boston University School of Medicine, Boston, Massachusetts

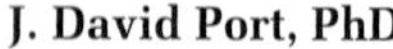

J. David Port, PhD
Deparment of Medicine, Division of Cardiology, Department of Pharmacology, University of Colorado Health Sciences Center, Aurora, Colorado

Kumudha Ramasubbu, MD
Assistant Professor of Medicine, Winters Center for Heart Failure Research, Department of Medicine, Michael E. DeBakey Veterans Affairs Medical Center, Houston, Texas

Barbara Riegel, DNSc, RN, FAAN
Professor, University of Pennsylvania, School of Nursing, Philadelphia, Pennsylvania

Gary E. Sander
Professor of Medicine, Heart and Vascular Institute, Tulane University Health Sciences Center, New Orleans, Louisiana

Douglas B. Sawyer, MD, PhD
Professor of Medicine, Cardiovascular Medicine Section, Department of Medicine, Vanderbilt University Medical Center, Nashville, Tennessee

Joel Schilling, MD, PhD
Instructor in Medicine, Cardiovascular Division, Washington University School of Medicine, St. Louis, Missouri

Leo Slavin, MD
Research Physician, Division of Cardiology, University of California–San Diego, San Diego, California

Francis G. Spinale, MD, PhD
Professor of Surgery, Medical University of South Carolina, Ralph H. Johnson Veterans Affairs Medical Center, Charleston, South Carolina

Randall C. Starling, MD, MPH
Professor of Medicine, Department of Cardiovascular Medicine, Section of Heart Failure and Cardiac Transplant Medicine, Kaufman Center for Heart Failure, Heart and Vascular Institute, Cleveland Clinic, Cleveland, Ohio

Lynne Warner Stevenson, MD
Professor of Medicine, Brigham and Women's Hospital, Harvard Medical School, Boston, Massachusetts

Carmen Sucharov, PhD
Assistant Professor of Medicine, Department of Medicine, Division of Cardiology, University of Colorado Health Sciences Center, Aurora, Colorado

Heinrich Taegtmeyer, MD, DPhil
Professor of Medicine, Department of Internal Medicine, Division of Cardiology, The University of Texas–Houston Medical School, Houston, Texas

W. H. Wilson Tang, MD
Professor of Medicine, Department of Cardiovascular Medicine, Heart and Vascular Institute, Cleveland Clinic, Cleveland, Ohio

Anne L. Taylor, MD
Professor of Medicine, Columbia University College of Physicians and Surgeons, New York, New York

John R. Teerlink, MD
Professor of Clinical Medicine, Section of Cardiology, San Francisco Veterans Affairs Medical Center, University of California–San Francisco, San Francisco, California

Veli K. Topkara, MD
Center for Cardiovascular Research, Division of Cardiology, Department of Medicine, Washington University School of Medicine, St. Louis, Missouri

Jeffrey A. Towbin, MD
Professor of Pediatrics, The Heart Institute, Department of Pediatrics, Cincinnati Children's Hospital Medical Center, Cincinnati, Ohio

Patricia A. Uber, PharmD
Assistant Professor of Medicine, Division of Cardiology, University of Maryland School of Medicine, Baltimore, Maryland

Peter VanBuren, MD
Associate Professor of Medicine and Molecular Physiology and Biophysics, University of Vermont College of Medicine, Burlington, Vermont

Ramachandran S. Vasan, MD
Section Chief, Preventive Medicine, The Preventative Medicine and Cardiology Sections, Boston University School of Medicine, Boston, Massachusetts

Raghava S. Velagaleti, MD
The National Heart, Lung and Blood Institute's Framingham Heart Study, Framingham, Massachusetts

Stephan von Haehling, MD
Applied Cachexia Research, Department of Cardiology, Charité University Medical School, Campus Virchow-Klinikum, Berlin, Germany

Bruce L. Wilkoff, MD
Director of Cardiac Pacing and Tachyarrhythmia Devices, Section of Cardiac Pacemakers and Electrophysiology, Robert and Suzanne Tomsich Department of Cardiovascular Medicine, Cleveland Clinic; Professor of Medicine, Cleveland Clinic Lerner College of Medicine, Case Western Reserve University, Cleveland, Ohio

Kai C. Wollert, MD
Professor of Cardiology, Department of Cardiology and Angiology, Hannover Medical School, Hannover, Germany

Edward T. H. Yeh, MD
Professor of Medicine, Department of Cardiology, The University of Texas M.D. Anderson Cancer Center, Houston, Texas

James B. Young, MD
Professor of Medicine and Executive Dean, Cleveland Clinic Lerner College of Medicine, Case Western Reserve University, Cleveland, Ohio

Maria C. Ziadi, MD
University of Ottawa Heart Institute, Ottawa, Ontario, Canada

Michael R. Zile, MD
Professor of Medicine, Division of Cardiology, Department of Medicine, Medical University of South Carolina, The Gazes Cardiac Research Institute, Charleston, South Carolina

Foreword

In what seems on the surface to be a paradox, the prevalence, incidence, and mortality of heart failure are steadily climbing despite phenomenal progress in the diagnosis and treatment of all forms of cardiac disease. As we successfully manage—yet not cure—patients with heart disease, the damage to their cardiac muscles persists and sometimes progresses as adaptive compensatory mechanisms become maladaptive. With steadily increasing life spans and the growing "epidemics" of diabetes, obesity, and atrial fibrillation in the elderly, the stage is now set for a large increase in the number of heart failure cases. Thus we are facing great challenges in our quest to control cardiac disease.

How are we going to win this battle? Surely not with a single magic bullet, whether it is a gene, device, or drug. We believe Douglas Mann's excellent book, *Heart Failure,* details the right plan. As with any battle, we must understand the terrain on which it will be fought. The first three sections of *Heart Failure* do just that. Section I delves into the basic underlying mechanisms on genetic, molecular, tissue, organ, and organismal levels, whereas Section II describes the pathophysiology of disease progression. These discussions involve not only the heart but also the vascular bed, neurohormonal systems, kidneys, and lungs. The most common etiologies of heart failure are described in Section III.

Section IV provides a detailed description of the clinical manifestations and laboratory features of heart failure. Finally, the current armamentaria in the treatment of heart failure—drugs, devices, and surgery—and how each of these (and their combinations) can be optimally deployed are described in Section V.

A leader in the fight against one of humankind's most stubborn enemies, Dr. Mann should be congratulated on selecting the right topics and the best authors to write about them. His skillful editing pulled everything together, making this book much greater than simply the sum of the excellent individual chapters.

This second edition builds on the first, which was warmly received. Fully one third of the chapters are new. Many chapters that appeared in the last edition have new authors and all have been updated to include the most current data and research.

Special thanks are due the authors, all distinguished investigators or clinicians, for their fine contributions. This splendid second edition of *Heart Failure* will be enormously useful to cardiovascular specialists who care for the growing number of patients with heart failure; it will be equally useful to those who are training to deliver this care, as well as to their teachers. However, the ultimate beneficiaries of this book will be the millions of patients with heart failure worldwide.

We are proud that this second edition of *Heart Failure* is a valued and indispensable companion to *Heart Disease: A Textbook of Cardiovascular Disease.*

Eugene Braunwald
Boston, Massachusetts

Robert Bonow
Chicago, Illinois

Peter Libby
Boston, Massachusetts

Douglas P. Zipes
Indianapolis, Indiana

Preface

The observation that several of the topics discussed as emerging therapies in the first edition of *Heart Failure: A Companion to Braunwald's Heart Disease* have now become either the standard of care (e.g., cardiac resynchronization) or are being tested in multicenter, multinational clinical trials (e.g., stem cell therapy) could be viewed as the major justification for publishing a second edition of the *Heart Failure Companion*. Beyond updating the chapters covered in the first edition, the vision for the second edition was to provide an extremely broad educational platform that would serve to foster a more complete understanding and appreciation of the clinical syndrome of heart failure.

To that end, the second edition contains 20 entirely new chapters that were not included in the first edition. Particular emphasis has been given to the sections on clinical assessment and treatment of heart failure (see below), which have been expanded by 75% compared to the first edition. As with the first edition, the goal in organizing this text was to provide trainees, scientists, and practicing clinicians with a resource that would present a complete bench-to-bedside overview of the field of heart failure that could be read from start to finish, or section by section. The second edition retains the same organization as the first edition and is divided into five sections that progress logically from basic molecular and cellular mechanisms that underlie heart failure (Section 1), to the mechanisms that lead to disease progression in heart failure (Section 2), to the etiologic basis for heart failure (Section 3), and finally to the clinical assessment (Section 4) and treatment of heart failure (Section 5).

As with the first edition, many of the chapters were designed to parallel one another, which should allow readers to focus on the aspects of heart failure that they find most interesting. For example, the second edition features chapters that cover the basic and clinical aspects of heart failure with a preserved ejection fraction as well as basic and clinical aspects of stem cell therapy and myocardial regeneration. The second edition also includes new chapters that reflect the overall growth in the field (e.g., biomarkers, cardiac devices, cardiac imaging, pharmacogenomics, palliative care in heart failure), as well as increased depth of understanding in the field (e.g., myocardial recovery, diabetic cardiomyopathy, heart failure as a consequence of chemotherapy, heart failure in special populations). In addition, this edition features several unique chapters that have not heretofore been covered in traditional textbooks on heart failure, including the important topic of heart failure in developing countries, the emerging issue of meaningfully measuring quality of outcomes in heart failure, and the neglected area of cognition in heart failure.

The extent to which the second edition of *Heart Failure: A Companion to Braunwald's Heart Disease* provides readers with a comprehensive bench-to-bedside overview of the field of heart failure reflects the extraordinary expertise and scholarship of the authors who contributed their professional time and efforts to this undertaking. It has been a great pleasure to work with them and it has been my great fortune to learn from them. Although every attempt was made to make the content of individual chapters as up-to-date as possible and include all the changes that were occurring in the field while this text was in development, we recognize the challenge of capturing all the essential elements of a field that is evolving rapidly. Accordingly, this second edition will be accessible online as well as in print, on the same Expert Consult platform that houses the parent text, *Braunwald's Heart Disease,* which features regular content updates.

Douglas L. Mann, MD, FACC

In Memoriam – Helmut Drexler

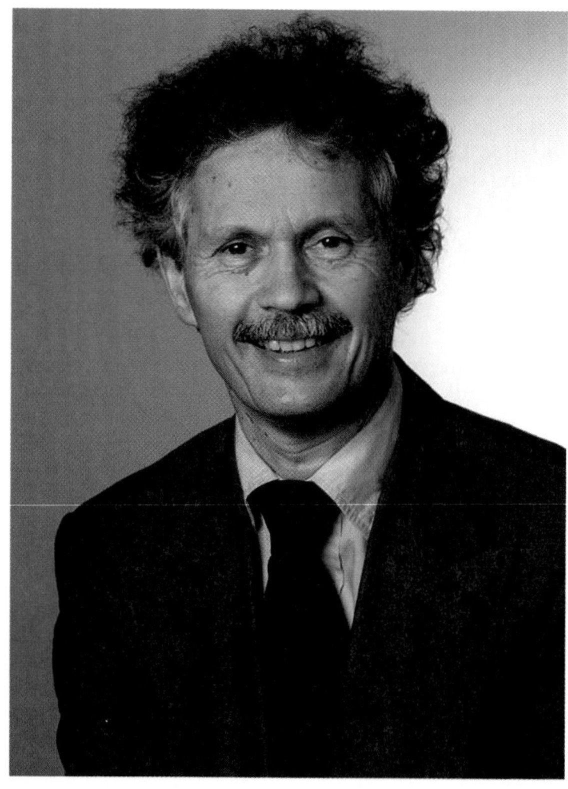

I first met Helmut Drexler in December 1996 at a symposium at the European Heart House in Sophia Antipolis, France. Helmut was in the audience listening to a presentation that I was giving. After the presentation was finished, Helmut stood up and began asking a series of challenging and incredibly insightful questions. Although I did my best to answer his questions, he must not have been satisfied because he waited until I stepped down from the podium and continued to ask me even more challenging questions. He was absolutely relentless. Thus began my friendship with Helmut Drexler that lasted up until his untimely death on September 13, 2009.

Helmut was a critical thinker who took nothing for granted. He was a classic epistemologist, who questioned everything because he wanted to understand the nature of things at their most fundamental level. His passion for understanding the basic mechanisms of heart failure was unending and his energy for translating this knowledge to the bedside was boundless. Over the span of his career he made seminal contributions to our understanding of the role of endothelial dysfunction, the renin angiotensin system, and inflammation in heart failure. He was the first to direct a randomized clinical trial of transcoronary bone marrow cell therapy for patients with acute myocardial infarction, as well as the first to highlight the shortcomings of this trial. His most significant work, which came shortly before his death, focused on the molecular mechanisms of postpartum cardiomyopathy and has paved the way for developing a potential new treatment for patients with this orphan disease. Despite all of his success Helmut's foremost priorities were always his family and friends, as well as his faculty, many of whom have gone on to have successful independent academic careers, such as Denise Hilfiker-Kleiner, Kai Wollert, Bernhard Schieffer, and Ulf Landmesser, among others. He is survived by his beautiful wife Krista and daughter Beatrice, who has recently completed medical school.

The last time I saw Helmut we had dinner together. After updating each other on our scientific pursuits and sharing our mutual passion for family, friends, and red wine, I told him that I was thinking of moving to a different city to assume a new academic position. Helmut raised his eyes from the table and was genuinely excited for me, but then mentioned that moving was difficult because it was hard to establish strong friendships as one became older. As I learned during the years that I knew Helmut, he was generally right about most things. With his death, I have lost a good friend who cannot be replaced at any age.

Douglas L. Mann, MD, FACC

Acknowledgments

Any clinical reference work of the size and complexity of *Heart Failure: A Companion to Braunwald's Heart Disease* does not occur in a vacuum. I would like to begin, first and foremost, by thanking Dr. Eugene Braunwald for giving me the opportunity to edit the companion volume focusing on heart failure. I would also like to thank Drs. Bonow, Libby, and Zipes, who taught me the art of editing during my apprenticeship on the eighth edition of *Braunwald's Heart Disease*. The extent to which the second edition of the heart failure companion is improved over the first is attributable to what I learned from my senior co-editors. I also want to thank the incredibly supportive staff at Elsevier, who enabled me to make a myriad of improvements to the content and visual design of the text as it was being developed. In particular, I would like to thank the following members of the Elsevier staff for their forbearance and indefatigable assistance: developmental editor Marla Sussman, project manager Janaki Srinivasan, executive publisher Natasha Andjelkovic, and her editorial assistant Brad McIlwain. I would also like to thank my administrative assistant, Ms. Mary Wingate, who remained unflappable no matter how many times I asked her to re-edit, re-format, or redo the same chapter. Lastly, I would be completely remiss if I did not thank my incredibly supportive wife, Laura, who tolerated both my presence and absence throughout the process of editing and writing for the second edition of *Heart Failure: A Companion to Braunwald's Heart Disease.*

Douglas L. Mann, MD, FACC

Contents

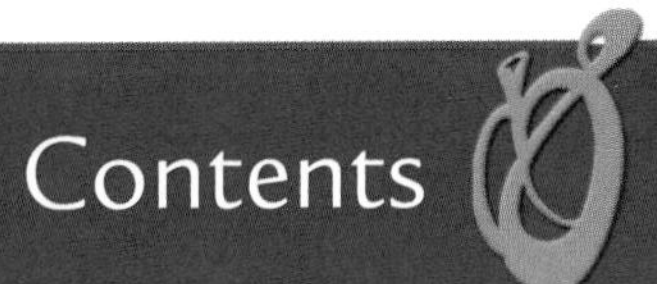

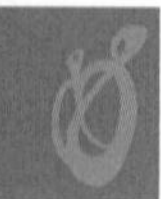

SECTION V: Therapy for Heart Failure

LOOK FOR THESE OTHER TITLES IN THE BRAUNWALD'S HEART DISEASE FAMILY!

Theroux: Acute Coronary Syndromes, 2nd Edition
Taylor: Atlas of Cardiac Computed Tomography
Kramer and Hundley: Atlas of Cardiac Magnetic Resonance
Lilly: Heart Disease Review & Assessment
Otto and Bonow: Valvular Heart Disease, 3rd Edition
Issa: Clinical Arrhythmology and Lipidology
Ballantyne: Clinical Lipidology
Antman: Cardiovascular Therapeutics, 3rd Edition
Black and Elliott: Hypertension
Creager, Loscalzo and Dzau: Vascular Medicine
Moser and Riegel: Cardiac Nursing

CHAPTER 1

Evolving Concepts in the Pathophysiology of Heart Failure

Arnold M. Katz

We have achieved our current understanding of heart failure through a remarkable evolution of ideas that, for Western medicine, extends back more than 2500 years.[1–2] Since the fifth century BCE, physicians and scientists have viewed this clinical syndrome in at least nine different ways (Table 1-1).[3] Improved understanding of this syndrome has been made possible by an interplay between basic and clinical sciences that is narrowing the gap between bench and bedside, between basic science and clinical medicine.[4] This iterative process has used new knowledge of pathophysiology to improve patient care while at the same time clinical validation of new therapeutic approaches has added to our knowledge of basic physiology.

HEART FAILURE AS A CLINICAL SYNDROME

The clinical texts attributed to Hippocrates, most of which were written between the fifth and third centuries BCE, describe patients with shortness of breath, edema, and anasarca.[5] However, as these are not specific, many of these patients probably suffered from conditions other than heart failure. The major reason why diagnosis is difficult, and often impossible, is that these texts lack a foundation in pathophysiology. Palpitation and shortness of breath, for example, were commonly attributed to the passage of phlegm, a cold humor generated by the brain, into the chest.

During the third century BCE, the center of medical science shifted to Alexandria, Egypt, where Herophilus and Erasistratus carried out human dissection and physiological experiments. Although the Alexandrian physiologists recognized that the heart contracts and understood the function of the semilunar valves, their efforts had no impact on understanding heart failure because they did not realize that the heart is a pump that circulates the blood. Their views did, however, have a major influence on Galen, a Greek physician who lived in the Roman Empire during the second century and whose writings were to dominate western thinking for more than 1500 years. Galen also knew that ventricular volume decreases during systole and understood the function of the heart's valves, but viewed the heart as a source of heat rather than a pump (Figure 1-1). Galen palpated the arterial pulse and described what almost certainly represents atrial fibrillation when he noted "complete irregularity or unevenness [of the pulse], both in the single beat and in the succession of beats";[6] however, he believed that the pulse is transmitted along the walls of the arteries, rather than by pulsatile blood flow through their lumens.[7]

Failure to understand the pathophysiology of heart failure made it impossible to appreciate the causes of the signs and symptoms of this syndrome and precluded any rational therapy. This provided a background for treatments of dyspnea and dropsy that include "take scabwort and grind and squeeze its juice through a cloth, collect in an eggshell and temper with honeycomb; give the patient daily a full shell of the juice, do this for eleven days when the moon is waning because also man wanes in his abdomen."[8]

HEART FAILURE AS A CIRCULATORY DISORDER

Correlations between clinical manifestations and cardiac abnormalities became possible at the beginning of the sixteenth century, when physicians began to perform autopsies to identify causes of illness.[9] However, there was no way to define mechanistic relationships between the clinical and autopsy findings in patients with heart failure until 1628, when William Harvey (Figure 1-2) described the circulation:

"I am obliged to conclude that in animals the blood is driven round a circuit with an unceasing, circular sort of movement that this is an activity or function of the heart which it carries out by virtue of its pulsation, and that in sum it constitutes the sole reason for that heart's pulsatile movement."[10]

During the following century, physicians began to use Harvey's discovery to understand the pathophysiology of heart failure (Figure 1-3). The first description of the hemodynamic basis of this syndrome cannot be credited to a single individual in part because medical advances in the seventeenth and eighteenth centuries were

TABLE 1–1	Changing Views of Heart Failure*
I. A clinical syndrome	
II. A circulatory disorder	
III. Altered architecture of failing hearts	
IV. Abnormal hemodynamics	
V. Disordered fluid balance	
VI. Biochemical abnormalities Energy starvation Depressed contractility Neurohumoral stimulation	
VII. Maladaptive hypertrophy	
VIII. Genomics	
IX. Epigenetics	

*Modified from Reference 1.

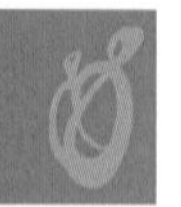

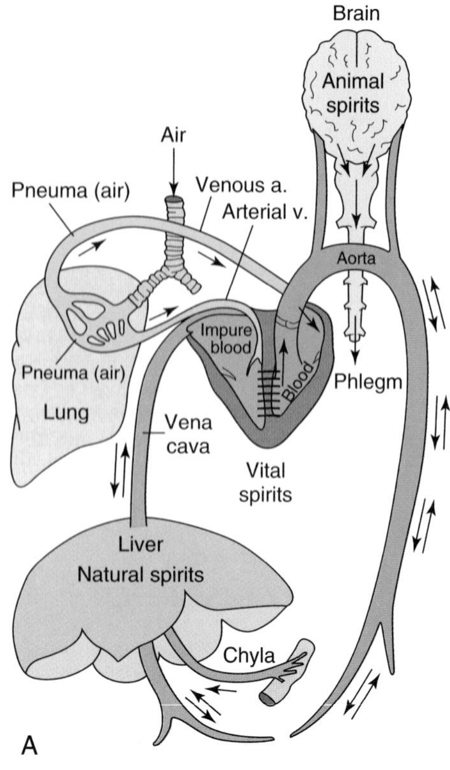

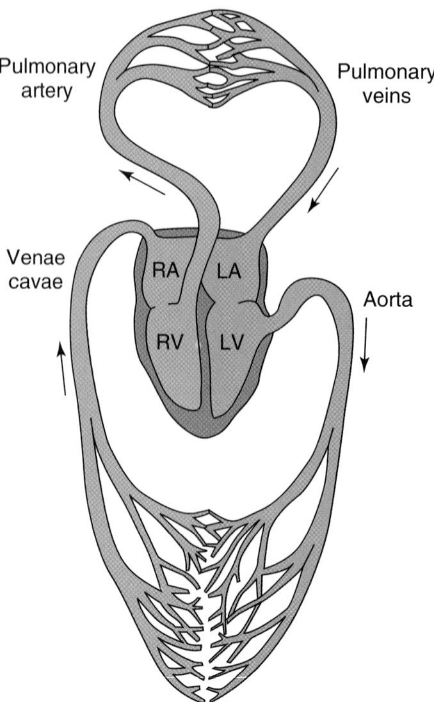

FIGURE 1–1 Two views of the circulation. **A,** Galen's view. Pneuma derived from air reaches the heart from the lungs via the venous artery (pulmonary artery) and arterial vein (pulmonary veins). Natural spirits that enter the heart from the liver, along with vital spirits (heat) generated in the left ventricle, are distributed throughout the body by an ebb and flow in the arteries. Animal spirits transported from the brain through nerves as phlegm contribute to the formation of pleural effusions. **B,** The view after Harvey. Deoxygenated blood is darkly shaded, oxygenated blood is lightly shaded. Modified from Katz AM, Konstam MA. *Heart failure: pathophysiology, molecular biology, clinical management*, ed 2, Philadelphia, Lippincott/Williams (2009).[73]

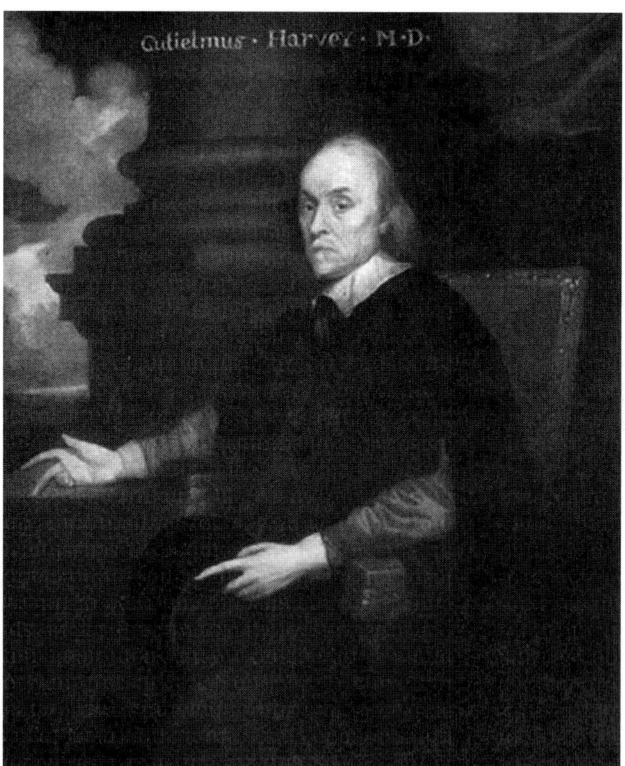

FIGURE 1–2 William Harvey. State portrait at the Royal College of Physicians, painted when Harvey was in his late 60s.

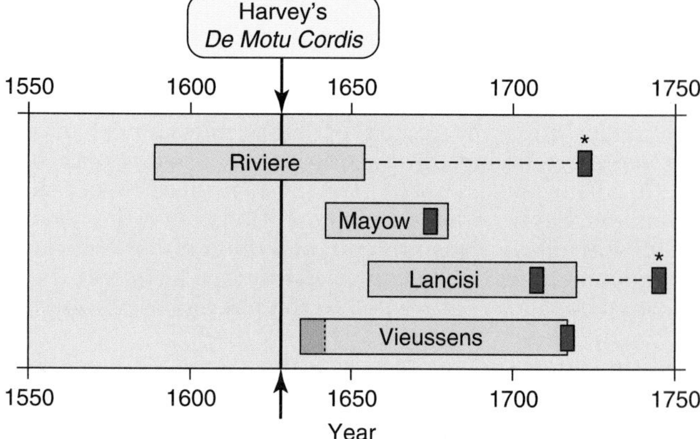

FIGURE 1–3 Time lines showing events following the publication of Harvey's *De Motu Cordis* in 1628 (*vertical dotted line*), and the birth and death of Rivière, Mayow, Lancisi, and Vieussens (*rectangles*; the shaded area for Vieussens reflects uncertainty regarding the date of his birth). Dates of key publications are shown by the thick vertical rectangles; posthumous publications are indicated by asterisks. Modified from Katz AM. Raymond Vieussens and the "first" pathophysiological description of heart failure. *Dialog Cardiovasc Med* 2004;9:179–182.[74]

widely discussed among authorities and there were few publications, many of which appeared after the author's death. Among the first to relate the clinical features of heart failure to abnormal hemodynamics were Rivière,[11] Mayow,[12] Lancisi,[13] and Vieussens.[14] The latter (Figure 1-4), in his *Traité nouveau de la structure et des causes du movement naturel du coeur*, published in 1715 (the year he died), integrated a superb case history, a detailed autopsy, and a surprisingly modern discussion of pathophysiology to describe the hemodynamic basis for the dyspnea and pleural effusions in a patient with rheumatic mitral stenosis.

ALTERED ARCHITECTURE OF FAILING HEARTS

Efforts to understand heart failure shifted to the architecture of diseased hearts at the beginning of the eighteenth century. Lancisi, in 1707, distinguished between "dilation," where cavity size is increased, and "hypertrophy," where wall thickness is increased,[13] and in 1759 Morgagni described the causal

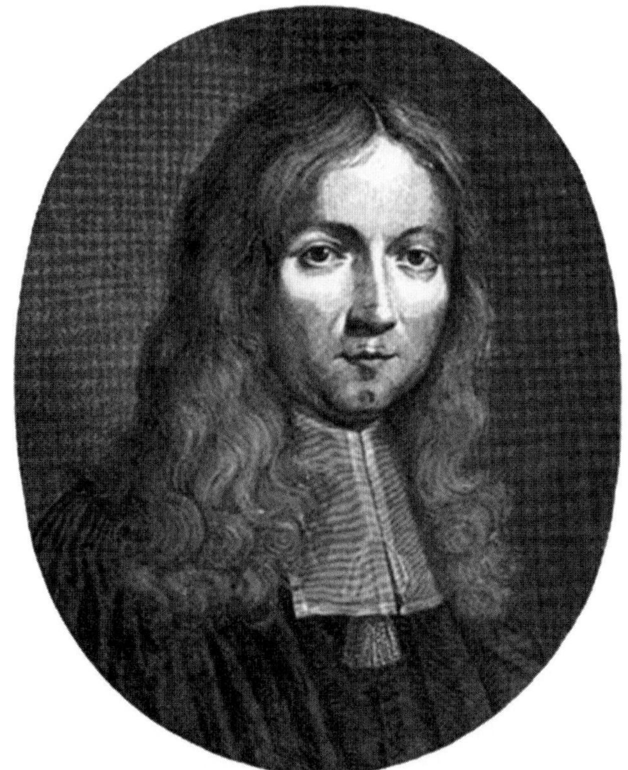

FIGURE 1–4 Vieussens as a young man. Reproduced from Fishman AP, Richards DW. *Circulation of the blood: men and ideas*, New York, 1964, Oxford University Press.[75]

link between hemodynamic overload and cardiac hypertrophy.[15] These observations were followed by more than a century of discovery that focused on architectural changes in the failing heart. Corvisart's observation that dilation (eccentric hypertrophy) of the left ventricle has a worse prognosis than concentric hypertrophy[16] led Flint to suggest that hypertrophy is an adaptive response that protects the patient from the adverse effects of dilation.[17] By the end of the nineteenth century, however, it had become apparent to Osler[18] and others that hypertrophy itself is deleterious.

Abnormal Hemodynamics

Many nineteenth century physiologists had been aware that a physiological increase in diastolic volume leads to an increase in cardiac output,[19] whereas physicians had viewed the effects of increased cavity size in terms of evidence that pathological dilation is associated with a poor prognosis (see previous discussion). Starling's description of the Law of the Heart that bears his name, which demonstrated that physiological increases in end-diastolic volume increase cardiac output,[20] was confusing to clinicians because it seemed to contradict the nineteenth century view that dilation weakens the heart. Furthermore, for the next 60 years it was commonly taught that failing hearts operate on the descending limb of the Starling curve, where increasing chamber volume decreases the heart's ability to eject.[21] This erroneous view became untenable when, in 1965, I pointed out that it is impossible for a heart operating on the descending limb of the Starling curve to function at a steady state.[22]

Hemodynamics remained central for understanding heart failure throughout the first half of the twentieth century, when most patients with heart disease had structural abnormalities caused by rheumatic fever, syphilis, and congenital anomalies. However, the work of Starling, Wiggers, and others who studied cardiac hemodynamics had little impact on patient care until the early 1940s, when Cournand and Richards brought cardiac catheterization to the bedside.[23] Subsequent developments in cardiac surgery[24] made it possible to palliate many forms of structural heart disease, both rheumatic and congenital, but did not solve the challenges posed by heart failure because ischemic heart disease, dilated cardiomyopathies, and diastolic heart failure were emerging as the major causes of this syndrome.

Disordered Fluid Balance

Dyspnea and anasarca, which had dominated the clinical picture in heart failure since the time of Hippocrates, gave rise to horrible suffering that is virtually unknown today. Although fluid retention had been proposed as a cause of dropsy as early as the sixteenth century, there had been no safe way to get rid of the excess salt and water until 1920, when Saxl and Heilig accidentally observed the diuretic properties of an organic mercurial that had been given to treat syphilitic heart disease.[25] Subsequent efforts to develop powerful diuretics that could be administered orally shifted the focus in heart failure research to renal physiology. This effort ended successfully in the 1950s and 1960s with the introduction of the thiazides, and subsequently of loop diuretics. Although these and other drugs can usually cause a diuresis so effective as to eliminate congestion, albeit sometimes at the expense of causing a low output state, they do little to alter the underlying causes of this syndrome. For this reason, the focus in heart failure research returned to the heart.

Biochemical Abnormalities

Three areas of biochemistry began to have a major impact on cardiology during the 1950s. The first was energetics, which had influenced thinking in muscle physiology since the beginning of the nineteenth century (see Chapter 7). The second, elucidation of the mechanisms responsible for muscle contraction, relaxation, and excitation-contraction coupling, became part of cardiology when the role of changing myocardial contractility was recognized as a key to an understanding how hearts failed (see Chapter 3 and 13). The third area, the biochemistry of ligand-receptor interactions and the intracellular signal transduction pathways responsible for the neurohumoral response to reduced cardiac output, led in the 1980s to the first major advances in treating this syndrome since the introduction of mercurial diuretics (see Chapter 2).

Energy Starvation

Muscle thermodynamics had been studied since 1848 when Helmholtz, who described the First Law of Thermodynamics, published records of energy release by muscle as work and heat. Between the 1920s and 1950s, several groups studied the mechanical efficiency of failing hearts, but most experimental studies at that time had little pathophysiological resemblance to clinical heart failure because they used either mammalian heart-lung preparations that had deteriorated when particulates in the perfusates occluded the coronary microcirculation, or a model of heart failure caused by pulmonary stenosis and tricuspid insufficiency. More recently, NMR spectroscopy and other analytic methods demonstrated that myocardial ATP and phosphocreatine levels are significantly reduced in failing hearts,[26–27] and so made it clear that energy starvation plays an important role in heart failure (see Chapter 7 and 20).

Depressed Contractility

In 1955, Sarnoff's demonstration that the heart can shift from one Starling curve to another clarified the role of *myocardial contractility* in regulating cardiac performance.[28] Although

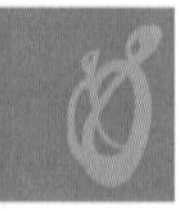

characterization of this regulatory mechanism in patients was hampered by difficulties in measuring myocardial contractility, in the late 1960s Braunwald's group was able to show that contractility is reduced in patients with chronic heart failure.[29] This emphasis on myocardial contractility occurred at a time when muscle biochemists had found that calcium delivery to the cytosol and its binding to troponin, a regulatory protein in the myofilaments, are major determinants of contractility.[30] The widely held view that powerful inotropic agents would benefit patients with failing hearts, along with discoveries regarding mechanisms that depress contractility, stimulated efforts to develop new inotropic drugs. However, clinical trials showed that long-term inotropic therapy with β-agonists and phosphodiesterase inhibitors does more harm than good.[31–32]

The importance of impaired filling in the pathogenesis of heart failure was not widely recognized until the 1980s, when echocardiography and nuclear cardiology made it possible to document lusitropic abnormalities in clinical heart failure. Unfortunately, efforts to improve ventricular filling and prognosis in patients with heart failure and preserved left ventricular ejection fraction have had little success (see Chapter 48).

Neurohumoral Stimulation

The importance of a third type of biochemical abnormality in failing hearts was described in 1983, when Harris[33] pointed out the adverse effects of the neurohumoral responses to reduced cardiac output. Although these responses, the most important of which are vasoconstriction, salt and water retention, and adrenergic stimulation, had evolved to maintain cardiac output during exercise and support the circulation when cardiac output falls after hemorrhage, they become harmful when they are sustained in chronic heart failure.[34]

The ability of vasoconstriction to increase cardiac energy expenditure[35] and reduce cardiac output[36] led Cohn and others to examine the effects of vasodilators on long-term prognosis in patients with heart failure.[37–38] V-HeFT and subsequent trials made it clear that although afterload reduction causes a short-term hemodynamic improvement, not all vasodilators prolong survival and some worsen long-term prognosis.[39] The dramatic benefit of angiotensin II–converting enzyme (ACE) inhibitors, which was first documented in the CONSENSUS I trial,[40] suggested that beneficial effects of ACE inhibitors are due to factors other than their ability to reduce afterload (see later discussion).

MALADAPTIVE HYPERTROPHY

By the late 1980s, therapy for heart failure had become so effective that it was often assumed that the judicious use of diuretics, vasodilators, and inotropes could solve most of the problems in these patients. At that time, before clinical trials had documented the poor prognosis in heart failure, many experts denied that this was a progressive syndrome. However, the view that heart failure is simply a hemodynamic disorder complicated by fluid retention was challenged when long-term trials showed that direct-acting vasodilators can worsen prognosis, and a central role for depressed contractility became untenable when inotropes were found to shorten survival in these patients (see previous discussion). Explanations for these apparently counterintuitive clinical findings began to emerge in the 1990s, when new data from the expanding fields of molecular biology rekindled interest in the deleterious effects of cardiac hypertrophy.

The emphasis on cardiac hypertrophy a century earlier (see previous discussion) had not been entirely forgotten; Meerson, who in the 1950s used modern methods to study the hypertrophic response to hemodynamic overload in animals, observed, as had Osler more than 50 years earlier,[18] that overload-induced hypertrophy is both beneficial and deleterious.[41] The beneficial effects of this growth response were shown clearly in the 1960s and 1970s when left ventricular hypertrophy was found to normalize wall stress in compensated aortic stenosis.[42–44] These findings, which also demonstrated that deterioration of failing hearts is not simply a consequence of sustained overload, suggested that the hypertrophic response itself might play a central role in causing maladaptive hypertrophy.[45]

Evidence that changes in the molecular composition of failing hearts play a role in this syndrome was published in the 1950s, when the molecular weight of myosins isolated from failing hearts was reported to increase.[46] However, the inability of several other groups to reproduce these findings[47] provoked a fierce controversy that was resolved when the original physicochemical data were shown to have been technically flawed.[48] A more durable line of evidence stemmed from early findings that changes in myosin ATPase activity represent a "tonic" mechanism that regulates myocardial contractility, which differs fundamentally from the "phasic" mechanisms mediated by changes in calcium binding to the contractile proteins (see previous discussion).[49]

The modern era in understanding the pathophysiology of heart failure began in 1962, when Alpert and Gordon reported that ATPase activity is reduced in myofibrils isolated from failing human hearts.[50] The molecular basis for this abnormality was identified in 1976 by Hoh et al,[51] who found that differences in the rate of energy release by myosin are the result of expression of different myosin isoforms. Scheuer and Penpargkul, in collaboration with my group, found that overload not only decreases energy turnover by the contractile proteins, but also slows calcium transport by the sarcoplasmic reticulum.[52] Izumo, Nadal-Ginard, and others[53–54] subsequently demonstrated that increased expression of the low ATPase β-myosin heavy chain isoform in failing hearts is part of a reversion to the fetal phenotype. The importance of these molecular changes was highlighted by the finding that *opposite* changes occur in training-induced physiological hypertrophy (the "athlete's heart"), where increased expression of the high ATPase α-myosin heavy chain isoform increases ATPase activity and contractility.[55]

The practical importance of maladaptive hypertrophy became apparent in 1985 when Janis Pfeffer, Mark Pfeffer, and Braunwald reported that ACE inhibitors slow the progressive cavity enlargement, which they called *remodeling*, that follows experimental myocardial infarction (see Chapter 15).[56] At the same time, evidence began to appear suggesting that these drugs are not only vasodilators, but also modify proliferative signaling.[57] These observations, along with evidence that overload causes the heart to deteriorate (see previous discussion), indicates that the hypertrophic response can, depending on the specific signaling mechanisms that are activated, be either adaptive or maladaptive.[58–62]

GENOMICS

Shortly after molecular biology moved to center stage in cardiology in the late 1980s,[63] the Seidman laboratory described the first molecular cause of a familial cardiomyopathy, a missense mutation in the cardiac β-myosin heavy chain gene.[64] This molecular abnormality was subsequently shown to represent only one of a growing number of mutations involving additional proteins that cause both hypertrophic and dilated cardiomyopathies (see Chapter 27).[65] The possibility of modifying the signal pathways controlled by these mutations to activate adaptive cardiac myocyte growth and inhibit maladaptive hypertrophy represents one of today's most promising lines of investigation.[58–61]

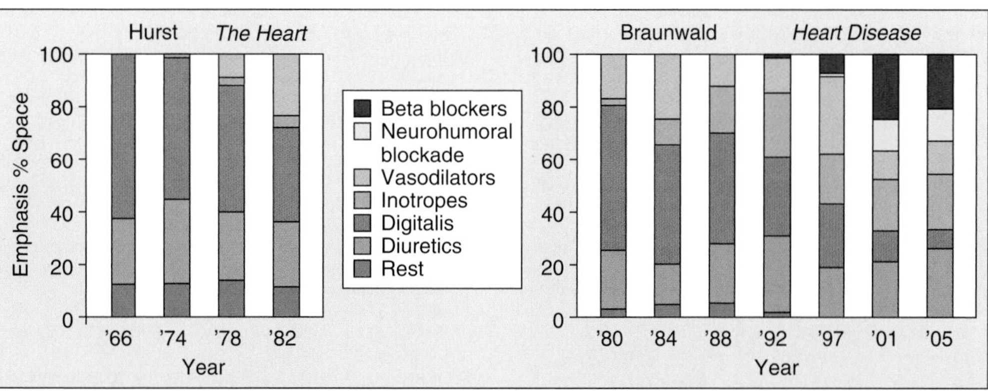

FIGURE 1-5 Changing management of heart failure over the past 40 years as documented by the number of pages devoted to various treatments in several editions of Hurst's *The Heart* and Braunwald's *Heart Disease*. (Electronic and mechanical devices and surgical therapies are not included.) From Katz AM, Konstam MA. *Heart failure: pathophysiology, molecular biology, clinical management*, ed 2, Philadelphia, Lippincott/Williams (in press).[73]

EPIGENETICS

A newly discovered type of regulation, referred to as *epigenetics*,[66] has recently been found to operate in heart failure. Epigenetic regulation differs from the more familiar genomic mechanisms, whose primary targets include transcription factors that interact with DNA and alternative splicing that allows synthesis of different protein isoforms by rearranging the information encoded in the exons of genomic DNA. Epigenetic mechanisms modify proliferative signaling by methylation of cytosine in genomic DNA, acetylation of histone, and inhibition of RNA translation by small RNA sequences called microRNAs. Cytosine methylation has been implicated in some familial cardiomyopathies,[67–68] while histone acetylation can modify overload-induced cardiac hypertrophy.[69–70] Evidence that microRNAs regulate cardiac hypertrophy[71–72] is of potential therapeutic importance because short RNA segments, called small interfering (si)RNAs, can silence specific genes. The ability of (si)RNAs, which are readily synthesized commercially to block specific proliferative pathways, promise additional approaches slowing deterioration of failing hearts by inhibiting maladaptive hypertrophy.

CONCLUSIONS AND FUTURE DIRECTIONS

The growing impact of the discoveries summarized in this chapter on patient care are apparent when discussions of therapy for heart failure in recent cardiology textbooks are compared (Figure 1-5). The first edition of Hurst and Logue's *Heart Disease*, published in 1966, devotes almost two thirds of the discussion to cardiac glycosides and their toxicity; the remainder describes diuretics and rest. The relative lengths of the discussions of rest, diuretics, and digitalis in this text differ little from those in White's 1931 textbook *Heart Disease*. Looking back even farther, to 1908, the description of therapy for heart failure in Mackenzie's *Diseases of the Heart* devotes more than 11 pages to the actions and toxicity of the cardiac glycosides; a half page each to nitroglycerin and amyl nitrite, which are described as "vaso-dilators"; two pages to the appropriate level of activity; three to diet; care of the bowels and the "mental factor" receive a half page each; and there is virtually nothing about diuretics.

Textbook discussions of heart failure therapy have been changing dramatically since the 1970s. The space allocated to diuretics has remained about the same, but recommendations for rest have virtually disappeared and discussions of digitalis have decreased remarkably. The latter is due in part to a decrease in the frequency of digitalis toxicity because cardiac glycosides, once viewed as among the few effective forms of therapy, were commonly given at very high doses in severely ill patients. Discussion of nonglycoside inotropes appeared in the 1970s, as did the short-term benefits of vasodilators. Neurohumoral blockade and β-blockers received separate discussions in the 2001 edition of Braunwald's *Heart Disease: A Textbook of Cardiovascular Medicine*. Even more striking are recent advances in device therapy, which are not included in Figure 1-5.

The evolution of our understanding of the pathophysiology and treatment of heart failure described in this chapter represents one of the major successes in biomedical research. This remarkable progress, which has been made possible by increasingly effective interactions between basic science and clinical investigation, continues a tradition that began when Harvey described the circulation. The growing impact of molecular biology, coupled with better understanding of the benefits and side effects of therapy offers considerable promise for future gains in our ability to manage patients with heart failure.

REFERENCES

1. Katz, A. M. (1997). Evolving concepts of heart failure: cooling furnace, malfunctioning pump, enlarging muscle. Part I. Heart failure as a disorder of the cardiac pump. *J Cardiac Fail*, *3*, 319–334.
2. Katz, A. M. (1998). Evolving concepts of heart failure: cooling furnace, malfunctioning pump, enlarging muscle. Part II. Hypertrophy and dilatation of the failing heart. *J Cardiac Fail*, *4*, 67–81.
3. Katz, A. M. (2008). The "modern" view of heart failure: how did we get here?. *Circ Heart Fail*, *1*, 63–71.
4. Katz, A. M. (2008). The "gap" between bench and bedside: widening or narrowing. *J Cardiac Fail*, *14*, 91–94.
5. Katz, A. M., & Katz, P. B. (1962). Diseases of the heart in the works of Hippocrates. *Brit Heart J*, *24*, 257–264.
6. Siegel, R. E. (1968). *Galen's system of physiology and medicine*. Basel, Switzerland: Karger.
7. Harris, C. R. S. (1973). *The heart and vascular system in ancient Greek medicine*. Oxford, UK: Oxford University Press.
8. Singer, C. (1988). The fasciculus medicinae of Johannes de Ketha. *Birmingham Ala*, Classics of Medicine.
9. White, P. D. (1957). The evolution of our knowledge about the heart and its diseases since 1628. *Circulation*, *15*, 915–923.
10. Harvey, W. (1628). *Exercitatio Anatomica de Moto Cordis et Sanguinis in Animalibus*. Frankfurt, Germany: William Fitzer.
11. Major, R. H. (1945). *Classic descriptions of disease* (3rd ed.). Springfield Ill: CC Thomas.
12. Mayow, J. (1674). *Tractus Quinque Medico-Physici.in Medico-Physical Works*, Edinburgh, UK: The Alembic Club; 1907.
13. Lancisi, G. M. Aneurysmatibus. Opus posthumam, Rome, 1745, Palladis (Translated by W. C. Wright, New York, 1952, Macmillan).
14. Jarcho, S. (1980). *The concept of heart failure. From Avicenna to Albertini*. Cambridge Mass: Harvard University Press.
15. Morgagni, J. B. (1769). *The seats and causes of diseases investigated by anatomy: in five books*. London: Millar and Cadell (Translated by B. Alexander).
16. Corvisart, J. N. (1812). *An essay on the organic diseases and lesions of the heart and great vessels*. Boston: Bradford & Read (Translated by J. Gates).
17. Flint, A. (1870). *Diseases of the heart* (ed 2). Philadelphia: HC Lea.

18. Osler, W. (1892). *The principles and practice of medicine.* New York: Appleton.
19. Katz, A. M. (2002). Ernest Henry Starling, his predecessors, and the "law of the heart.". *Circulation, 106,* 2986–2992.
20. Starling, E. H. (1918). *The Linacre lecture on the law of the heart.* London: Longmans Green.
21. McMichael, J. (1950). *Pharmacology of the failing heart.* Springfield Ill: CC Thomas.
22. Katz, A. M. (1965). The descending limb of the Starling curve and the failing heart. *Circulation, 32,* 871–875.
23. Cournand, A. (1975). Cardiac catheterization. Development of the technique, its contributions to experimental medicine, and its initial application in man. *Acta Med Scand Suppl, 579,* 3–32.
24. Comroe, J. H., Jr., & Dripps, R. D. (1974). Ben Franklin and open heart surgery. *Circ Res, 35,* 661–669.
25. Saxl, P., & Heilig, R. (1920). Über die diuretiche Wirkung von Novasurol und anderen Quecksilberinjektionen. *Wien Klin Wochenschr, 33,* 943–944.
26. Ingwall, J. S. (2002). *ATP and the heart.* Norwell Mass: Kluwer.
27. Neubauer, S. (2007). The failing heart - an engine out of fuel. *N Engl J Med, 356,* 1140–1151.
28. Sarnoff, S. J. (1955). Myocardial contractility as described by ventricle function curves: observations on Starling's law of the heart. *Physiol Rev, 35,* 107–122.
29. Gault, J. H., Ross, J., Jr., & Braunwald, E. (1968). Contractile state of the left ventricle in man: instantaneous tension-velocity-length relations in patients with and without disease of the left ventricular myocardium. *Circ Res, 22,* 451–463.
30. Katz, A. M. (1967). Regulation of cardiac muscle contractility. *J Gen Physiol, 50,* 185–196.
31. Yusef, S., & Teo, K. (1990). Inotropic agents increase mortality in patients with congestive heart failure. *Circulation, 82*(suppl III), III-673 (abstract).
32. Felker, G. M., & O'Connor, C. M. (2001). Inotropic therapy for heart failure: an evidence-based approach. *Am Heart J, 142,* 393–401.
33. Harris, P. (1983). Evolution and the cardiac patient. *Cardiovasc Res, 17,* 313–319, 373–378, 437–445.
34. Francis, G. S., Goldsmith, S. R., Levine, T. B., et al. (1984). The neurohumoral axis in congestive heart failure. *Ann Intern Med, 101,* 370–377.
35. Evans, C. L., & Matsuoka, Y. (1915). The effect of various mechanical conditions on the gaseous metabolism and efficiency of the mammalian heart. *J Physiol (Lond), 49,* 378–405.
36. Ross, J., Jr. (1976). Afterload mismatch and preload reserve: a conceptual framework for the analysis of ventricular function. *Prog Cardiovasc Dis, 18,* 255–264.
37. Cohn, J. N., & Franciosa, J. A. (1977). Vasodilator therapy of cardiac failure. *N Engl J Med, 297,* 27–31, 254–258.
38. Cohn, J. N., Archibald, D. G., Ziesche, S., et al. (1986). Effect of vasodilator therapy on mortality in chronic congestive heart failure. Results of a Veterans Administration cooperative study (V-HeFT). *N Engl J Med, 314,* 1547–1552.
39. Francis, G. S. (2001). Pathophysiology of chronic heart failure. *Am J Med, 110*(suppl 7A), 37S–46S.
40. CONSENSUS Trial Study Group. (1987). Effects of enalapril on mortality in severe congestive heart failure. Results of the cooperative North Scandinavian enalapril survival study. *N Engl J Med, 316,* 1429–1434.
41. Meerson, F. Z. (1961). On the mechanism of compensatory hyperfunction and insufficiency of the heart. *Cor Vasa, 3,* 161–177.
42. Sandler, H., & Dodge, H. T. (1963). Left ventricular tension and stress in man. *Circ Res, 13,* 91–104.
43. Hood, W. P., Jr., Rackley, C. E., & Rolett, E. L. (1968). Wall stress in the normal and hypertrophied human left ventricle. *Am J Cardiol, 22,* 5550–5558.
44. Grossman, W., Jones, D., & McLaurin, L. P. (1975). Wall stress and patterns of hypertrophy in the human left ventricle. *J Clin Invest, 56,* 56–64.
45. Katz, A. M. (1990). Cardiomyopathy of overload. A major determinant of prognosis in congestive heart failure. *N Engl J Med, 322,* 100–110.
46. Olson, R. E., Ellenbogen, E., & Iyengar, R. (1961). Cardiac myosin and congestive heart failure in the dog. *Circulation, 24,* 471–482.
47. Katz, A. M. (1970). Contractile proteins of the heart. *Physiol Rev, 50,* 63–158.
48. Mueller, H., Franzen, J., Rice, R. V., et al. (1964). Characterization of cardiac myosin from the dog. *J Biol Chem, 239,* 1447–1456.
49. Katz, A. M. (1976). Tonic and phasic mechanisms in the regulation of myocardial contractility. *Basic Res Cardiol, 71,* 447–455.
50. Alpert, N. R., & Gordon, M. S. (1962). Myofibrillar adenosine triphosphatase activity in congestive heart failure. *Am J Physiol, 202,* 940–946.
51. Hoh, J. Y., McGrath, P. A., & White, R. I. (1976). Electrophoretic analysis of multiple forms of myosin in fast-twitch and slow-twitch muscles of the chick. *Biochem J, 157,* 87–95.
52. Penpargkul, S., Repke, D. I., Katz, A. M., et al. (1977). Effect of physical training on calcium transport by rat cardiac sarcoplasmic reticulum. *Circ Res, 40,* 134–138.
53. Izumo, S., Lompré, A. M., Matsuoka, R., et al. (1987). Myosin heavy chain messenger RNA and protein isoform transitions during cardiac hypertrophy. Interaction between hemodynamic and thyroid hormone-induced signals. *J Clin Invest, 79,* 970–977.
54. Izumo, S., Nadal-Ginard, B., & Mahdavi, V. (1988). Protooncogene induction and reprogramming of cardiac gene expression produced by pressure overload. *Proc Natl Acad Sci U S A, 85,* 339–343.
55. Scheuer, j., Buttrick, P. (1985). The cardiac hypertrophic responses to pathologic and physiologic loads. *Circulation, 75*(part 2):1, 63–I–68.
56. Pfeffer, J. M., Pfeffer, M. A., & Braunwald, E. (1985). Influence of chronic captopril therapy on the infarcted left ventricle of the rat. *Circ Res, 57,* 84–95.
57. Katz, A. M. (1990). Angiotensin II: hemodynamic regulator or growth factor?. *J Mol Cell Cardiol, 22,* 739–747.
58. McKinsey, T. A., & Olson, E. N. (2005). Toward transcriptional therapies of the failing heart: chemical screens to modulate genes. *J Clin Invest, 115,* 538–546.
59. Bock, G., & Goode, J. (Eds.). (2006). *Heart failure: molecules, mechanisms, and therapeutic targets* Chichester, UK: Wiley.
60. Selvetella, G., Hirsch, E., Notte, A., et al. (2004). Adaptive and maladaptive hypertrophic pathways: points of convergence and divergence. *Cardiovasc Res, 63,* 373–380.
61. Dorn, G. W., II, & Force, T. (2005). Protein kinase cascades in the regulation of cardiac hypertrophy. *J Clin Invest, 115,* 527–537.
62. Hill, J. A., & Olson, E. N. (2008). Cardiac plasticity. *N Engl J Med, 358,* 1370–1380.
63. Katz, A. M. (1988). Molecular biology in cardiology, a paradigmatic shift. *J Mol Cell Cardiol, 20,* 355–366.
64. Geisterfer-Lowrance, A. A. T., Kass, S., Tanigawa, G., et al. (1990). A molecular basis for familial hypertrophic cardiomyopathy: a β-cardiac myosin heavy chain gene missense mutation. *Cell, 62,* 999–1006.
65. Ho, C. Y., & Seidman, C. E. (2006). A contemporary approach to hypertrophic cardiomyopathy. *Circulation, 113,* 858–862.
66. Goldberg, A. D., Allis, C. D., & Bernstein, W. (2007). Epigenetics: a landscape takes shape. *Cell, 128,* 635–638.
67. Robertson, K. D. (2005). DNA methylation and human disease. *Nat Rev Genet, 6,* 597–610.
68. Rodenhiser, D., & Mann, M. (2007). Epigenetics and human disease: translating basic biology into clinical applications. *CMAJ, 174,* 341–348.
69. Backs, J., & Olson, E. N. (2006). Control of cardiac growth by histone acetylation/deacetylation. *Circ Res, 98,* 15–24.
70. Trivedi, C. M., Luo, Y., Yin, Z., et al. (2007). Hdac2 regulates the cardiac hypertrophic response by modulating Gsk3 beta activity. *Nat Med, 13,* 324–331.
71. Chien, K. R. (2007). MicroRNAs and the tell-tale heart. *Nature, 447,* 389–390.
72. van Rooij, E., & Olson, E. N. (2007). MicroRNAs: powerful new regulators of heart disease and provocative therapeutic targets. *J Clin Invest, 117,* 2369–2376.
73. Katz, A. M., Konstam, M. A. (2009). *Heart failure: pathophysiology, molecular biology, clinical management,* ed 2, Philadelphia, Lippincott/Williams.
74. Katz, A. M. (2004). Raymond Vieussens and the "first" pathophysiological description of heart failure. *Dialog Cardiovasc Med, 9,* 179–182.
75. Fishman, A. P., & Richards, D. W. (1964). *Circulation of the blood: men and ideas.* New York: Oxford University Press.

CHAPTER 2

Molecular Basis for Heart Failure

Abhinav Diwan and Gerald W. Dorn II

Heart failure begins after an initial index event produces a decline in pumping capacity of the ventricle. At the cellular level, heart failure is caused by changes in the biology of the cardiac myocyte (see Chapter 3) as well as through progressive loss of cardiac myocytes (see Chapter 6). The loss of myocytes may be focal (e.g., myocardial infarction), or diffuse (e.g., viral infection, hemodynamic overload, genetic abnormalities). Thus heart failure is the common clinical syndrome caused by any of a diverse group of injurious stimuli sufficient to produce myocardial insufficiency. The specific characteristics and clinical course of heart failure may be determined more by the myocardial response to injury and its accompanying hemodynamic overload than by the specific nature of the primary insult. With cardiac injury or hemodynamic stress, a multitude of signaling pathways are activated that may be predominantly compensatory or maladaptive. Accordingly, molecular surveys performed over the past 3 decades have defined biochemical and transcriptional signatures of failing myocardium, and reductionist experimentation has delineated responsible mechanisms of functional adaptation and decompensation.

Accumulated data reveal that molecular signaling of heart failure is complex and involves activation of multiple pathways exhibiting cross-talk inhibition and potentiation, functional redundancy, and feedback or feedforward regulation. Clinically important pathophysiological linkages have been established between molecular determinants of cardiomyocyte contractility, cardiomyocyte growth, and cardiomyocyte death. Thus the themes of heart failure pathophysiology have transitioned from a primary focus on mechanical to molecular factors. As a consequence, the field has moved away from early therapeutics that stimulated neurohormone pathways in attempts to enhance pump function by increasing cardiac myocyte inotropy (catecholamines, phosphodiesterase inhibitors) or by decreasing hemodynamic loading (arterial and venous vasodilators, diuretics).[1,2] The current approach for treating end-stage heart failure combines pharmacological inhibition of maladaptive molecular signaling pathways (β-adrenergic blockers, angiotensin-converting enzyme inhibitors) with "bionic" measures aimed at resting, restoring, and recovering failing myocardium (ventricular assist devices), or correcting electromechanical cardiac dysfunction (resynchronization therapy).[3-5] Ongoing and future clinical trials of gene- and cell-based therapies are building upon fresh molecular insights to develop novel targets and approaches for heart failure (see Chapter 50).[6]

INVESTIGATIVE TECHNIQUES AND MOLECULAR MODELING

The explosion of molecular information on the pathophysiology of heart failure is the result of reductionist experimentation using advanced molecular and physiological modeling in genetically manipulated systems, and a more integrated approach that takes advantage of recently developed high-throughput platforms for genetic analysis of small clinical specimens in human heart failure. The overall paradigm is that of an extrinsic biomechanical stimulus that activates molecular signaling pathways. The cardiomyocyte responds with altered gene expression that changes the protein makeup of the cell, and ultimately the structure and function of the heart. Experimental models for dissecting out and identifying important molecular events have therefore tended to genetically and physiologically perturb a hypertrophy stimulus (e.g., transgenic overexpression of Gαq[7] and induction of pressure overload by microsurgical creation of a transverse aortic constriction[8]). Experimental manipulation of signaling pathways has largely transitioned away from pharmacological activators and inhibitors and toward creating gain-of-function and loss-of-function mutant organisms with complementary perturbations of the candidate factor specifically in the specific cell type of interest (cardiomyocyte). To enhance appreciation of the following detailed discussion of molecular pathways for hypertrophy and heart failure, here we briefly review some general techniques and approaches used in these types of studies.

Molecular investigation of cardiac hypertrophy began with development by Paul Simpson of an in vitro model system using neonatal rat cardiac myocytes.[9] In contrast to adult cardiac myocytes, neonatal rat myocytes are relatively easy to prepare and can be maintained in tissue culture for weeks. Under serum-free conditions, cardiomyocytes stimulated with Gq-coupled neurohormones such as phenylephrine, angiotensin, and endothelin undergo cellular hypertrophy with many characteristics of in vivo cardiomyocyte hypertrophy: Cells enlarge, protein synthesis is accelerated, and hypertrophy-associated genes are increased in expression, including atrial natriuretic factor (ANF)[10] and α-skeletal actin.[11] Even when the stimulus is simple mechanical stretching, neonatal rat cardiac myocytes exhibit a characteristic hypertrophic gene program mimicking pathological hypertrophy.[12] Neonatal cardiac myocytes are less useful for studies of excitation-contraction coupling due to incompletely developed sarcomeres and sarcoplasmic reticulum network. Thus techniques were developed to isolate calcium-tolerant adult cardiac myocytes from multiple vertebrate species including mice, the predominant species used for genetic manipulation.[13,14] Isolated individual field-paced adult cardiac myocytes are now routinely used to

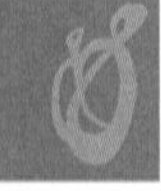

measure the effects of experimental manipulations on contraction, relaxation, and calcium transients.

A major limitation of cultured and isolated cardiac myocyte studies is that the impact of the experiment on integrated cardiac and cardiovascular function cannot be determined. This requires perturbation and analysis in an intact organism with sufficient similarity to man for conclusions to have relevance to the human condition. An additional requirement is the ability to perform specific genetic manipulations in the organism, which permits specificity of molecular perturbation and tissue targeting that is typically not possible using pharmacological agents. Although important basic information has derived from studies of fruit flies and zebra fish, the genetically modified (transgenic or knockout) and physiologically modeled mouse has become the dominant experimental system for in vivo examination of the molecular event mediating cardiac hypertrophy and heart failure.

Transgenic *gain-of-function* approaches are typically employed to evaluate whether a particular gene and its protein product are, by virtue of the protein's functional involvement in a particular pathway, *sufficient* to provoke a particular outcome. Cardiomyocyte-specific expression is conventionally achieved by driving cDNA expression using cardiac-specific promoters such as Mlc2v and aMHC.[15,16] These promoters drive high-level gene expression in the early embryonic heart (Mlc2v) or shortly after birth (αMHC) and thereafter. For genes with deleterious effects on fetal or postnatal cardiac development that confound the experimental interpretation or can be lethal,[17] conditional expression systems permit transgene expression under temporally defined conditions by administering tetracycline or mifepristone.[18-20]

Loss-of-function approaches are helpful to determine whether a certain gene (or its protein product) is *necessary* for a given outcome. There are several ways to decrease gene function, such as transgenic expression of dominant inhibitory mutants and transgenic or adenoviral/AAV-mediated expression of specific short interfering RNAs (siRNAs). Because of specificity and stability issues with siRNAs, the potential for unanticipated effects of mutant inhibitory proteins, and the possibility that forced expression itself can induce pathology,[21] targeted gene ablation is considered the gold standard for loss of function.[22] Limitations of germ line gene ablation relating to noncardiac effects have been addressed by tissue-specific ablation using Cre-Lox technology and cardiomyocyte-expressed Cre.[23,24]

Although genetic manipulations can produce cardiac phenotypes permitting mechanistic insight, frequently the consequences of an overexpressed or ablated gene are further interrogated through surgical or pharmacological intervention. Mouse cardiac surgery was not performed when genetic manipulation of the mouse first came of age. The development of microsurgical modeling for pressure overload, volume overload, heterotopic transplantation, infarction, and ischemia-reperfusion, together with advances in microanalytical techniques for invasive hemodynamic or electrophysiological studies and sophisticated noninvasive echocardiographic and magnetic resonance imaging, has completed the investigational "tool kit" for in vivo studies of genetically and physiologically modeled mice.[7,25-27]

Molecular Ontogeny is Recapitulated by Cardiac Hypertrophy

Cardiac hypertrophy and heart failure in the adult are characterized by reexpression of fetal cardiac genes.[28-30] Here, we explore the reasons for this prototypical feature. Since cardiac failure results from loss of functioning myocardium, the optimal compensatory response to cardiac insufficiency is myocardial repair or regeneration. Indeed, the universal response to myocardial insufficiency is cardiac hypertrophy. Hypertrophy is measured at the organ level using electrocardiographic, echocardiographic, or magnetic resonance imaging indices of myocardial mass and cardiac size, and is reflected by cardiomyocyte enlargement in the short axis (pressure overload) or long axis (volume overload).[31] Although there are many similarities in gene and protein content between developing embryonic hearts and hypertrophying adult hearts, a critical difference is the inability of adult cardiac myocytes to increase in number through mitosis and cytokinesis after the early postnatal period.[32,33] Accumulating evidence supports the presence of pluripotent resident and immigrant cardiac progenitor cells in the adult myocardium,[34,35] but the regenerative potential of these cells is not yet known; and these cells are not currently believed to contribute in a major way to cardiomyocyte renewal and repopulation under typical circumstances.

A hallmark of pathological hypertrophy in the adult heart is reexpression of embryonic cardiac genes (and the proteins they encode), often referred to as the "fetal gene program." This is the clearest example of how the cardiac response to stress or injury recapitulates aspects of cardiac development. As might be expected for a coordinated program of expressed genes, the earliest detectable change (within hours after pressure overloading hearts or stimulating cultured cardiomyocytes to hypertrophy) is induction of regulatory transcription factors, *c-fos, c-jun, jun-B, c-myc,* and *egr-1/nur77*, and heat shock protein (HSP) 70.[8] These changes are typical of cell cycle entry.[36] Induction of these and other transcription factors, called "early response genes," drives the expression of downstream genes in the fetal program (Figure 2-1). Atrial natriuretic factor (ANF) is the prototypical fetal cardiac gene, expressed early during heart development through the coordinated interactions of the Nkx2.5, GATA-4, and PTX transcription factors.[37]

GATA4, a zinc finger DNA binding protein, is essential for embryogenesis and formation of the linear heart tube[38] and is also expressed in the adult heart. GATA4 binding sites are found on the promoters of various cardiac expressed genes as ANF, BNP, ET-1, α-skeletal actin, αMHC, βMHC, cardiac troponin c, and AT1R and regulates transcription of multiple genes in response to pressure overload and neurohormonal signaling. Forced expression of GATA4 at low levels causes mild hypertrophy with increased fibrosis, whereas cardiomyocyte-specific deletion of GATA4 diminished exercise-induced and pressure-overload hypertrophy, with no effect on normal cardiac growth.[39] Antihypertrophic signaling mediated by GSK3β, a kinase downstream of the IGF-1-PI3K-Akt axis that regulates normal cardiac growth (see later discussion), is transduced in part by GSK3β-induced phosphorylation and suppression of GATA4 transcriptional activity. GATA4 also complexes with other transcription factors such as Nkx2.5, MEF2, coactivator p300, SRF, and NFAT to affect cardiac gene expression (see Figure 2-1).[40]

SRF (serum response factor), a cardiac-enriched transcription factor, [41] was identified as a transcriptional regulator that associated with the serum response element (SRE) with characteristic recognition sequences (CArG boxes) in the *c-fos* gene promoter. SRF is essential for sarcomerogenesis based on its coordinated interaction with other transcription factors, such as SMAD1/3, Nkx2-5, and GATA4. Conditional cardiac-specific gene ablation of SRF resulted in embryonic lethality due to cardiac insufficiency during chamber maturation, associated with cardiomyocyte apoptosis.[42] Confirmatory evidence for a critical role of SRF in normal cardiac and cardiomyocyte homeostasis came from conditional cardiomyocyte gene ablation in the adult mouse, which demonstrated progressive development of cardiomyopathy with disorganization of the sarcomeres leading to heart failure.[43] Myocardin is a cardiac and smooth muscle–specific co-activator of SRF.

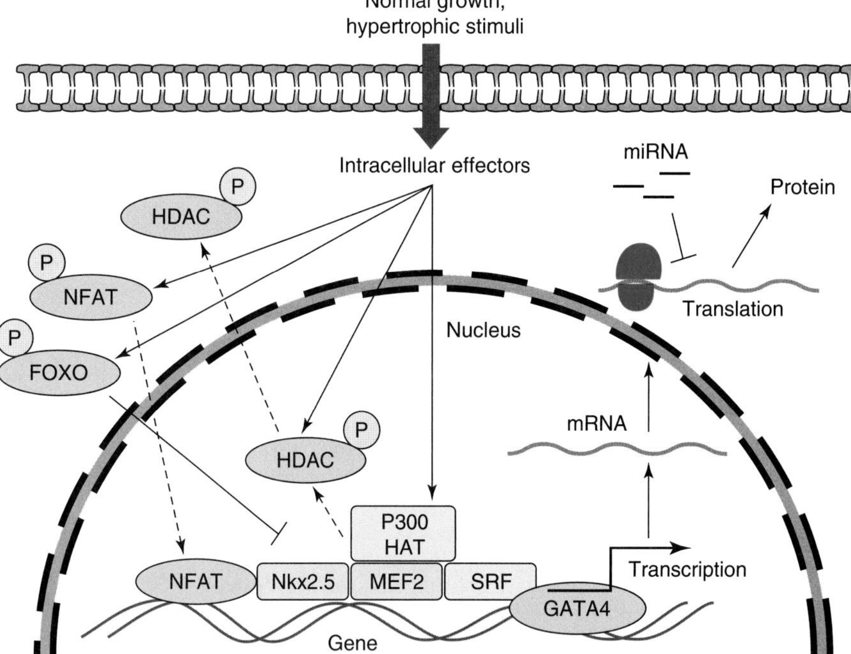

FIGURE 2–1 Regulation of gene expression in normal growth and pathological hypertrophy. A common set of transcription factors determine normal cardiac growth and pathological hypertrophy, such as GATA4, Nkx2.5, SRF, MEF2, and NFATs. Hypertrophy signaling pathways result in phosphorylation of histone deacetylases (HDACs) with export out of the nucleus, permitting histone acetylation by histone acetyl transferases (HATs), with activation of gene transcription to generate messenger RNA (mRNA). mRNA is spliced to yield a mature form, which recruits the protein synthesis machinery leading to protein translation. MicroRNAs (miRNAs) inhibit mRNA translation and/or enhance mRNA degradation to negatively regulate translation. The FoxO3 family and Wnt transcription factors (not shown) negatively regulate hypertrophic growth.

Its expression is induced by phenylephrine (PE) in vitro and it binds to SRF and induces ANF transcription. Accordingly, forced cardiac expression of myocardin causes pathologic in vivo hypertrophy with fetal gene expression.[44]

The consequences of altered cardiac gene expression on myocardial function are varied: (1) Ventricular ANF (and related brain natriuretic peptide [BNP]) expression is robust in pathological hypertrophy and heart failure, and the increase in BNP secretion from the heart forms the basis for a widely used clinical biomarker assay of heart failure.[45] (2) Because of differences in ATPase activity, and therefore efficiency, it has been suggested that increased β-MHC could impair myocardial contractility,[46,47] but there is little direct supportive evidence.[48] (3) Downregulation of the gene encoding the sarcoplasmic reticulum Ca^{2+} ATPase (SERCA), the Ca^{2+} pump responsible for rapid reuptake of calcium into the sarcoplasmic reticulum,[49] appears to be responsible for the characteristic calcium signaling abnormalities observed in experimental and human heart failure.[50,51] Experimental gene therapies for heart failure are therefore targeting SERCA and its endogenous inhibitor phospholamban.[52]

In addition to the classic five reported fetal genes (*βMHC, α-skeletal actin, ANF, BNP,* and *SERCA*), transcriptome analysis using high-throughput microarrays in failing human and mouse hearts have identified hundreds of upregulated and downregulated genes in cardiac hypertrophy and failure[53-55] (a comprehensive database of these gene expression changes is now available at cardiogenomics.org). In addition to providing mechanistic insight into heart failure, myocardial mRNA signatures may be prognostic biomarkers or therapeutic guides.[56-59]

An exciting new prospect is the potential for microRNAs to provide incremental information on the molecular status of the myocardium.[60] MicroRNAs (miRNAs) are small (~22 nucleotide) naturally occurring RNAs that negatively regulate gene expression by promoting degradation of mRNAs and/or inhibiting mRNA translation,[61] thereby suppressing protein synthesis (Figure 2-1). Myocardial miRNA expression is altered in hypertrophic and failing myocardium,[60,62,63] suggesting that stress-induced regulation of miRNA contributes to reprogramming of myocardial genes in pathological hypertrophy and heart failure.

Molecular Signaling of Normal Heart Growth and Physiological Cardiac Hypertrophy

Cardiac hypertrophy is frequently classified as either "physiological" (i.e., normal postnatal growth and the cardiac enlargement that results from physical conditioning) or "pathological" (i.e., reactive hypertrophy in response to hemodynamic overload and myocardial injury).[31,64,65] Descriptive terms such as "physiological" or "pathological" hypertrophy indicate the probable outcome of the hypertrophy and the nature of the inciting stimulus and signaling pathway. Physiological stimuli such as exercise and pregnancy produce physiological hypertrophy, whereas cardiac pathologies such as hemodynamic overload, myocardial infarction, or toxic and infectious myocardial damage produce pathological hypertrophy. The stimulus-response relationship was clearly defined in a recent study that used advanced microsurgical techniques to produce intermittent pressure overload, which induced quantitatively less severe hypertrophy with minimal fibrosis and fetal gene reexpression, but with the key pathological characteristics of traditional reactive pressure overload hypertrophy.[66]

Physiological hypertrophy of the adult heart shares important traits with normal cardiac growth that distinguish physiological from pathological hypertrophy: The extent of physiological hypertrophy in athletes and during pregnancy is typically not sufficient to impede normal cardiac mechanical function, myocardial collagen deposition is not observed, capillary density increases in proportion to the increase in myocardial mass, bioenergetic alterations enhancing fatty acid metabolism and mitochondrial biogenesis are favorable, and physiological hypertrophy regresses without permanent sequelae upon interruption of the inciting stimulus.[65] A likely determinant of these favorable characteristics is the absence of the hallmark fetal gene program seen in pathological hypertrophy.[67] Because of the generally beneficial effects of physiological hypertrophy, exercise[68] and molecular manipulation of cardiac growth signaling pathways[69] have been investigated to prevent or ameliorate the effects of pathological hypertrophy and heart failure.

Both normal cardiac growth and physiological hypertrophy are mediated via the peptide growth factor, IGF-1.[70]

Growth hormone released from the pituitary gland stimulates IGF-1 synthesis in various tissues, primarily the liver. Likewise, development of physiological cardiac hypertrophy in response to exercise is also triggered by IGF-1, levels of which are increased in trained athletes and in cardiomyocytes in response to hemodynamic stress.[71] The direct effects of IGF-1 stimulation are beneficial, including decreased cardiomyocyte apoptosis in response to noxious stimuli in vitro and in vivo, and prevention of adverse remodeling with preservation of systolic function in vivo.[72] IGF-1 does not seem to be necessary for pathological hypertrophy, however, because knockout mice lacking IGF-1 exhibit a normal hypertrophic response to pressure overload. Thus the cardiomyocyte autonomous effects of IGF-1 appear to be stimulation of normal and physiological growth.

IGF-1, insulin, and other peptide growth factors activate membrane receptors with intrinsic tyrosine kinase activity (Figure 2-2). IGF-1 or transgenic expression of IGF-1 receptor causes physiological hypertrophy,[73,74] whereas ablation of insulin receptors and/or IGFR1 depresses normal myocardial growth.[75,76] PI3Kα is recruited to activated IGF-1 receptors (see Figure 2-2). Genomic ablation of PI3K p110α is embryonic lethal at day 9.5 of gestation,[77] but dominant negative expression of p110α in the postnatal heart reduces adult heart size and prevents development of swimming-induced hypertrophy[78]; and forced cardiac expression of p110α stimulates physiological growth.[79] PI3K p110α maintains ventricular function via membrane recruitment of protein kinase B/Akt (see Figure 2-2): IGFR-mediated translocation of the p110α subunit to the cell membrane facilitates phosphorylation of membrane phosphatidylinositols at the 3′ location, resulting in binding of Akt and its activator PDK1 via pleckstrin homology (PH) domains. Ablation of Akt1 and/or Akt2, and PDK1, reduces cardiac mass.[80,81]

Although IGF-1 and its downstream effectors clearly produce physiological hypertrophy, IGF-1 mediated hypertrophy evolves over time into pathological hypertrophy, with fibrosis and systolic dysfunction.[82] This transitional phenotype is similar to that observed with forced expression of Akt, in which inadequate angiogenesis contributes to the transition from hypertrophy to cardiac failure.[83] The hypothesis is that cardiomyocyte growth beyond a certain physical limit, whether initially physiological or pathological, exceeds the capacity for oxygen and nutrient delivery due to lack of concordant angiogenesis needed to meet the demands of the hypertrophied myocyte.[84] Thus there may be pathological consequences to excessive physiological hypertrophy that could explain the relatively rare occurrences of irreversible ventricular hypertrophy and dilation in endurance sports athletes.[85]

PATHOLOGICAL HYPERTROPHY: THE CARDIOMYOCYTE GROWTH/DEATH CONNECTION

Pathological cardiac hypertrophy is an independent risk factor for cardiac death (see Chapter 22)[86] and classically exhibits progression from a compensated or nonfailing state to failing dilated cardiomyopathy.[87,88] At the cellular level, massive

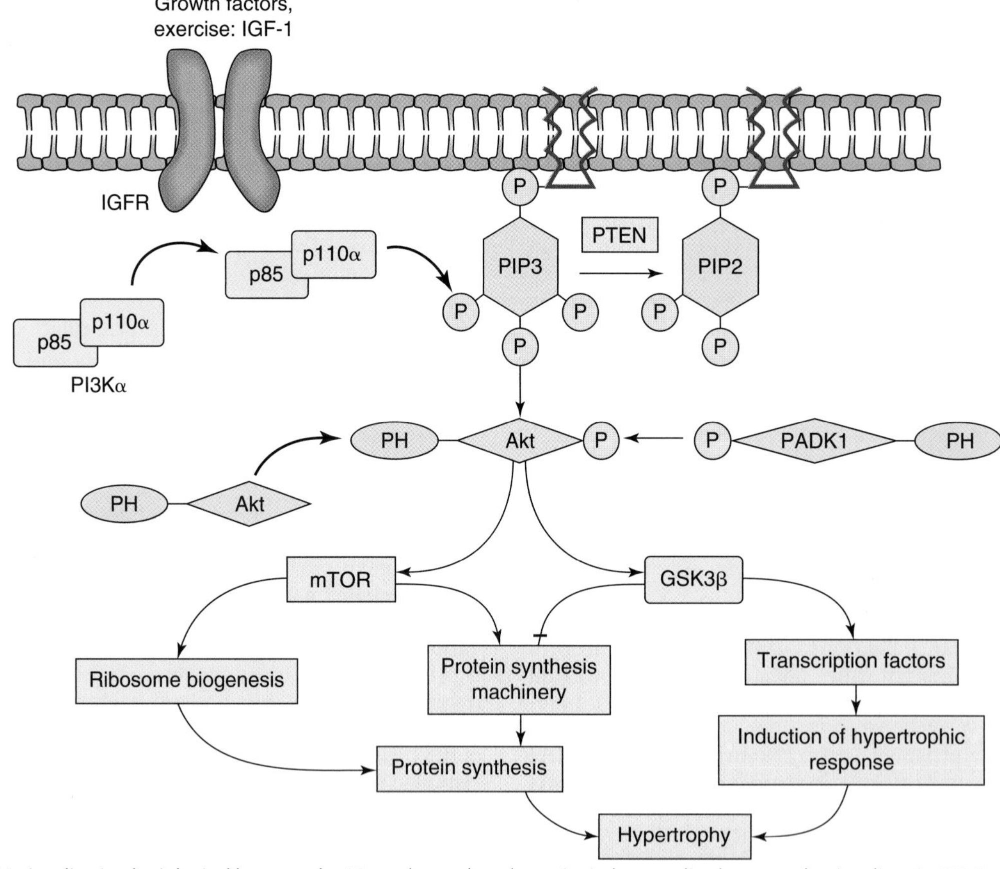

FIGURE 2–2 IGF-1 signaling in physiological hypertrophy. Normal growth and exercise induce cardiac hypertrophy signaling via IGF-1 release. IGF-1 binds to the membrane-bound IGF receptor (IGFR), leading to autophosphorylation and recruitment of PI3K isoform, p110α to the cell membrane. PI3Kα phosphorylates phosphatidylinositols in the membrane at the 3' position in the inositol ring, generating phosphatidylinositol triphosphate (PIP3). Protein kinase B (Akt) and its activator, PDK1, associate with PIP3, resulting in Akt activation, which also requires phosphorylation by PDK2 for full activity (not shown). Activated Akt phosphorylates and activated mTOR, resulting in ribosome biogenesis and stimulation of protein synthesis. Akt also phosphorylates GSK3 (both α and β isoforms), resulting in repression of its antihypertrophic signaling. The phosphatase PTEN dephosphorylates PIP3 to generate PIP2 and shut off the signaling pathway.

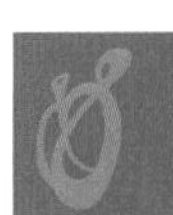

cardiomyocyte hypertrophy is almost always observed in dilated cardiomyopathies. Thus hypertrophy both contributes to, and is a consequence of, heart failure. The essential feature of cardiac hypertrophy is increased cardiomyocyte size/volume. Other myocardial alterations, such as fibroblast hyperplasia, deposition of extracellular matrix, and a relative decrease in vascular smooth muscle and capillary density[89,90] also contribute to the progression from hypertrophy to heart failure (reviewed in Chapter 6).

Conventional wisdom has long held that the primary change in ventricular geometry in reactive pressure overload hypertrophy (i.e., wall thickening)[91] is helpful in postponing the inevitable functional decompensation and adverse remodeling (wall thinning and chamber dilation[92]) because ventricular systolic wall stress is normalized.[87] This relationship is described by the Laplace equation, $s = Pr/2h$, where s is wall stress (force per unit of cross-sectional area), which is synonymous with afterload and is directly proportional to P (intraventricular pressure) and r (ventricular radius), and is inversely proportional to h (ventricular wall thickness). Accordingly, an increase in ventricular h to r ratio in pressure overload (concentric) hypertrophy decreases wall stress for a given intracavitary pressure. The physics of ventricular remodeling are not disputed, but there is accumulating evidence that the quantity of myocardium may be a less important determinant of left ventricular ejection performance than the quality of myocardium.[88] Indeed, because of pathological upregulation of fetal cardiac genes[29,30] and increased programmed cardiomyocyte death,[93,94] it has been suggested that reactive hypertrophy may be entirely dispensable to functional compensation after hemodynamic overloading.[95,96]

Cardiomyocyte death or degeneration is a seminal feature of failing hearts, and is also detectable in pathological hypertrophy before the development of cardiomyopathy. Cardiomyocyte death may be programmed (cell suicide by necrosis, apoptosis, or autophagy) or nonelective (conventional necrosis),[97] and there is evidence for all three forms of death in end-stage human cardiomyopathy.[98]

Apoptosis

Apoptosis (see Chapter 6), derived from the Greek expression for "the deciduous autumnal falling of leaves" (*apo* means away from, and *ptosis* means falling),[99] is an orderly and highly regulated energy requiring process that, in many tissues, provides for targeted removal of individual cells without provoking an immune response that could produce more extensive, collateral tissue damage.[100]

Geographically localized apoptosis is essential to normal development of the heart and ventricular outflow tract.[101] Apoptotic indices (number of TUNEL-positive nuclei/total nuclei) are highest in the outflow tract (~50%),[102] intermediate in the endocardial cushions that are sites of valve formation and left ventricular myocardium (10% to 20%),[103] and lowest in the right ventricular myocardium (~0.1% at birth).[104] Cardiomyocyte apoptosis parallels cardiomyocyte mitosis and therefore decreases toward the end of embryonic development, and apoptotic cardiomyocytes are extremely rare in normal adult myocardium (1 apoptotic cell per 10,000 to 100,000 cardiomyocytes).[33] Abnormal persistence of apoptosis in right ventricular myocardium may contribute to the pathogenesis of arrhythmogenic right ventricular dysplasia,[105] a disorder caused by mutations of the plakoglobin and desmoplakin genes and disorder of Wnt signaling, and that is characterized by right ventricular–specific apoptosis and fibrofatty replacement associated with arrhythmias and sudden death.[106] The prevalence of cardiomyocyte apoptosis is markedly increased in chronic cardiomyopathies.[107,108] Likewise, myocardial ischemia and reperfusion injury induce acute cardiomyocyte apoptosis in human disease[109] and experimental animal models,[110] and in the subacute period following the infarction, wherein it contributes to ventricular remodeling.[111] Apoptotic cardiomyocyte death likely also plays a role in the transition of pressure overload hypertrophy to dilated cardiomyopathy.[93,112]

A powerful stimulus for cardiomyocyte apoptosis in heart failure is high levels of circulating cytokines.[113] Sustained experimental pressure overload is sufficient to induce expression of the prototypical death-promoting cytokine, TNF-α,[114] and TNF signaling via the TNFR1 receptor is both negatively inotropic and stimulates cardiomyocyte hypertrophy and apoptosis.[115,116] A causal role for this cytokine in heart failure is suggested by elevated TNF-α plasma levels that are correlated with the degree of cardiac cachexia,[117] and by studies where TNF-α infusion or forced cardiac expression of the cytokine created myocardial hypertrophy with increased cardiomyocyte apoptosis, adverse ventricular remodeling, and systolic dysfunction in rodent models.[118,119]

TNF binds to the TNFR1 receptor homotrimer to trigger death receptor signaling (Figure 2-3). This results in formation of death inducing signaling complex (DISC) with recruitment of the adaptor protein FADD and activation of caspase 8, an upstream member of a family of executioner cysteine proteases (see Figure 2-3).[120] Activated caspase 8 cleaves caspase 3, the effector caspase, which activates a nuclear DNAse (CAD—caspase activated DNAse), resulting in internucleosomal cleavage of DNA and chromatin condensation. Caspase 8 also cleaves Bid, a proapoptotic Bcl-2 family protein. Generation of truncated (*t*Bid) links the extrinsic and intrinsic pathways (see Figure 2-3), leading to their simultaneous activation in TNF-induced cardiomyocyte apoptosis.[119]

Whereas TNF-α receptors activate cardiomyocyte death pathways[113] cell survival signaling is stimulated by the IL-6 family of cytokines, including IL-6, cardiotrophin, and LIF. A shared membrane receptor for IL-6 family cytokines is glycoprotein (gp) 130 that, as with all cytokine and peptide growth factor receptors, has intrinsic tyrosine kinase activity. Binding of IL-6 or cardiotrophin induces gp130 homodimerization or oligomerization with α-subunits of other cytokine receptors, stimulating autophosphorylation on receptor cytoplasmic tails and activating intrinsic tyrosine kinase activity (Figure 2-4). Receptor tyrosine phosphorylation permits binding of adaptor proteins Grb2 and Shc to SH2 binding domains, upon which multiple signaling effectors assemble for activation of the following signaling pathways (see Figure 2-4): (1) Janus kinases (JAKs) that phosphorylate STAT transcription factors, which then migrate to the nucleus as active dimers to regulate gene expression[121]; (2) SH2 domain-containing cytoplasmic protein tyrosine phosphatase (SHP2), which activates the MEK/ERK pathway; and (3) the Ras/mitogen-activated protein kinase that activates MAPK and extracellular signal-regulated kinase (ERK) signaling. These signaling pathways are inhibited by SOCS family proteins,[122] and transcriptional upregulation of SOCS proteins via STAT signaling providing for feedback inhibition of JAK/STAT pathways (see Figure 2-4).

Consistent with important roles in cardiac development and homeostasis during periods of stress, cardiotrophin 1 and related IL-6 family member cytokines are expressed in embryonic and adult myocardium and stimulate increases in cardiomyocyte size and protein synthesis.[123] Gp130 signaling is essential for embryonic cardiac development since germline deletion in mice is lethal at embryonic day 12.5 and the mice exhibit myocardial abnormalities[124] (although this does not appear to be a cell-autonomous requirement[125]). Gp130 signaling is sufficient to provoke hypertrophy in the adult heart,[126] whereas expression of dominant negative gp130 attenuates pressure overload hypertrophy.[127]

The gp130 signaling axis plays a critical role in cardiomyocyte survival after stress. Mice with cardiomyocyte-specific deletion of gp130 develop massive cardiomyocyte

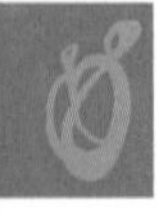

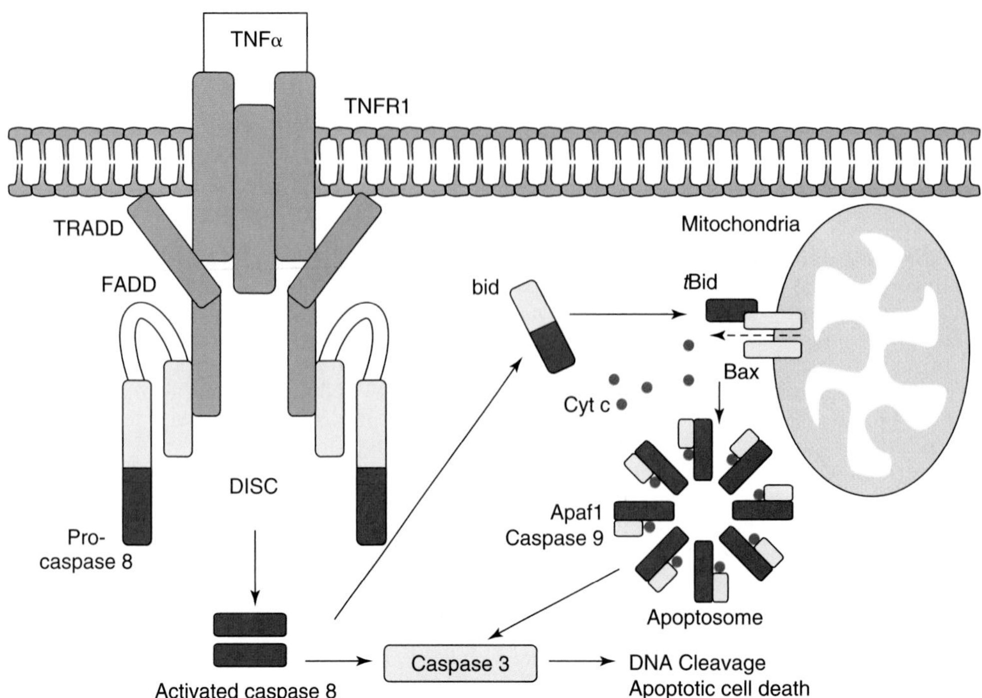

FIGURE 2–3 TNF-induced death signaling in heart failure: TNF-α binds to TNF receptor 1 (TNFR1) homotrimer, resulting in recruitment of proteins via death domains, namely TRADD and FADD; and procaspase 8 and assembly of DISC (death-inducing signaling complex). This causes cleavage activation of caspase 8, which cleaves and activates the effector caspase: caspase 3. Activated caspase 3 proteolyzes cellular substrates, causing cell death. This pathway is amplified by caspase 8-induced cleavage of Bid, a BH3 domain only Bcl-2 family protein, the truncated form of which, *t*Bid, interacts with multidomain proapoptotic Bcl-2 proteins Bax and Bak (not shown). This results in mitochondrial outer membrane permeabilization and release of cytochrome c (cyt c), which associates with adapter protein Apaf-1, ATP, and procaspase 9, forming the apoptosome, with activation of caspase 9. Activated caspase 9 activates caspase 3. This process is opposed by Bcl-2 and Bcl-xl (not shown), and inhibitor protein XIAP. Smac/DIABLO and Omi/HtrA2 are released during mitochondrial permeabilization (not shown) and bind to XIAP, relieving its inhibitory effect. Also released are DNAses: AIF (apoptosis-inducing factor) and endoG, which cause DNA cleavage.

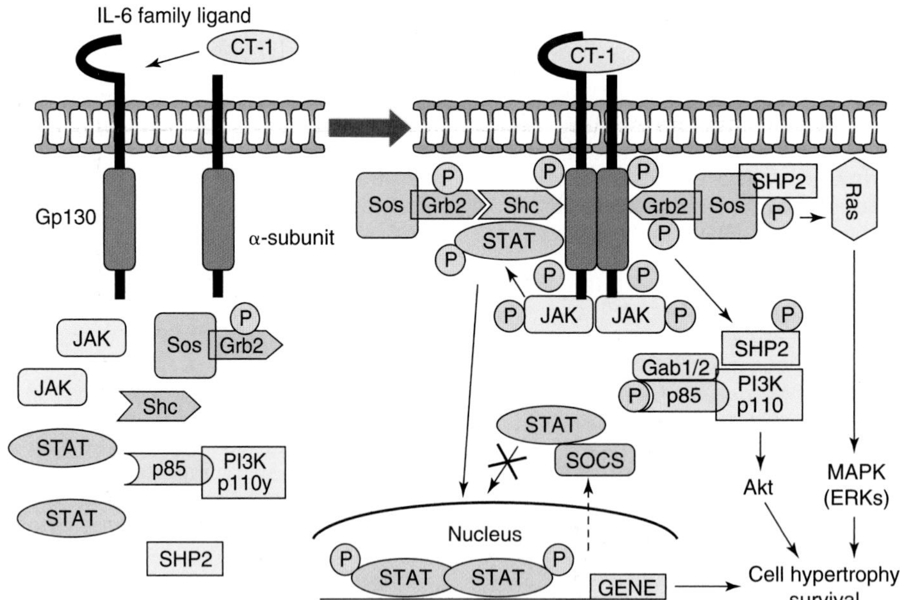

FIGURE 2–4 Gp130-mediated survival signaling in heart failure: Ligand-induced homodimerization of Gp130, a transmembrane receptor protein, or heterodimerization with α-receptor subunits for IL-6 cytokine family members such as CT-1, LIF, or oncostatin M, causes tyrosine autophosphorylation and recruitment and activation of JAK1/2. Subsequently, two major intracellular signaling cascades are triggered: (1) Signal transducer and activator of transcription (STAT)-1/3 pathway, with STAT dimerization and translocation to the nucleus with activation of gene transcription. This pathway is opposed by induction of SOCS proteins, which bind to and prevent STAT translocation. (2) SH2-domain containing cytoplasmic protein phosphatase (SHP2)/MEK/Extracellular signal-regulated kinase (ERK) pathway. Additionally, Grb2 binding with Gab1/2 causes PI3K mediated Akt activation. These pathways signal to promote cardiomyocyte hypertrophy and survival.

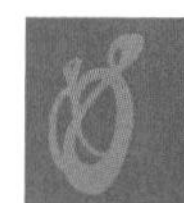

apoptosis and rapid cardiomyopathic decompensation after induction of surgical pressure overload.[125] Gp130 activation is only transiently observed after pressure overload and the pathway is deactivated during the transition to failure.[128] A mechanism for the transition to failure in pressure overload stress-induced hypertrophy may be interruption of gp130-JAK-STAT signaling by stress-induced SOCS3 and resulting suppression of STAT3 signaling.[129] Accordingly, adenoviral-mediated transduction of SOCS3 prevents prohypertrophic and antiapoptotic signaling of cardiomyocyte gp130 receptors by inhibiting JAK2-STAT3/MEK1-ERK1/Akt activation. Signaling through gp130 also protects against viral myocarditis by accelerating viral clearance, whereas cardiomyocyte-specific gp130 gene ablation, or expression of the gp130 inhibitor, SOCS3, accelerates the myocarditis.[130]

Autophagy (see Chapter 6)

Autophagy (in Greek *auto* means "self" and *phagein* means "to eat") is a normal cellular response to starvation and has been implicated in cell survival and cell death, depending upon the developmental stage, level of induction, and chronicity of the inciting stimulus.[131] Autophagic degradation of cellular proteins plays an important role in supplying the energy needs of newborns at birth, when a state of starvation occurs between separation from placental nutrients and not feeding. Accordingly, mice deficient in the important component of autophagy, ATG5, cannot upregulate the autophagic response and are prone to death during this period.[132]

Foci of degenerated cardiomyocytes with autophagic vacuoles are observed in human dilated cardiomyopathy and aortic stenosis.[133] Likewise, acute pressure overloading in mice causes rapid appearance of autophagic markers that persist during functional decompensation and the transition to dilated cardiomyopathy.[134] In this experimental model, induction of autophagy is clearly maladaptive because suppression of autophagy prevents ventricular remodeling and cardiomyopathic decompensation. However, the role of autophagy in hypertrophy development and decompensation is unclear at this time. Decreased autophagy is observed in pressure overloaded and catecholamine challenged myocardium,[135] but inhibition of autophagy that is induced in ischemic myocardium (a normal "starvation" response) increases cardiomyocyte death.[136] Autophagy increases with reperfusion, but autophagy inhibition protects against reperfusion injury.[136] Finally, inhibition of cardiomyocyte autophagy by conditional *ATG5* ablation early in mouse cardiac development does not affect normal developmental cardiac growth or pressure overload hypertrophy, but is associated with accelerated heart failure.[137] Available data suggest a multifaceted role for autophagy, which can be pathological, but may be necessary to prevent cardiomyopathic decompensation after cardiac injury or stress by eliminating misfolded or degraded proteins.

Necrosis (see Chapter 6)

The theme of capillary/myocardial mismatch as a causative factor in progression from hypertrophy to dilated cardiomyopathy has been advanced over the past few years as a general mechanism for decompensation of pathological hypertrophy. An adequate blood supply for growing myocardium is necessary for normal cardiac function. Accordingly, capillary density is closely coupled to myocardial growth during development.[138] Cardiac hypertrophy, on the other hand, is associated with decreased capillary density and coronary flow reserve, and increased diffusion distance to myocytes.[139] Capillary density is increased during the compensated phase of pathological hypertrophy, but decreases and is associated with cardiomyocyte "dropout" during decompensation.[140] GATA4-mediated regulation of angiogenic VEGF and angiopoietin play an important role in hypertrophy-associated capillary/myocardial mismatch.[39,83,141,142]

Catecholamine Cardiomyopathy: The Cardiomyocyte Contractility/Death Connection

Activation of the sympathetic nervous system in heart failure happens early after stress to maintain cardiac function (see Chapter 10). Persistent sympathetic activation, however, becomes progressively maladaptive over time. Catecholamines are toxic to cardiomyocytes in vitro and persistent activation of catecholamine signaling pathways causes cardiomyopathies associated with cardiomyocyte loss.[143,144] These are largely β_1-receptor-mediated effects, and can be blocked by pharmacological inhibition of the L-type calcium channel.

There are nine subtypes of adrenergic receptors (three each of α_1, α_2, and β), of which β_1-receptors are the most abundant in the myocardium.[145] Catecholamine signaling via cardiomyocyte β-adrenoreceptors increases myocardial contractility by stimulatory G protein (Gαs)-mediated activation of adenyl cyclase, resulting in cyclic AMP production that activates protein kinase A (Figure 2-5). β_2-adrenoreceptors couple to both Gαs and the inhibitory G protein Gαi, which can inhibit adenyl cyclase and downregulate c-AMP levels. In normal myocardium, the β_1-receptors represent 70% to 80% of all the β-adrenoreceptors. In heart failure, preferential downregulation of β_1-receptors proportionately increases inhibitory Gαi signaling.[146]

An important mechanism by which β_1-adrenoreceptor/Gsα/PKA signaling increases contractility is PKA-mediated phosphorylation of phospholamban (see Figure 2-5) (see Chapter 3). In its unphosphorylated state, phospholamban inhibits SERCA to decrease diastolic calcium uptake into the sarcoplasmic reticulum (SR). Phosphorylation of phospholamban relieves the inhibition of SERCA, resulting in increased SR calcium loading and larger systolic calcium transients, which augments contractility. PKA also phosphorylates L-type calcium channels to enhance calcium entry and ryanodine receptors to enhance calcium release.[147] The mechanism by which catecholamines are toxic to cardiomyocytes has been addressed by genetic manipulation of signaling receptors and effectors. Forced expression of low levels of β_2 (60 times normal) enhances cardiac function and rescues genetic cardiomyopathy[148-150] without pathological consequences. However, forced expression of low levels of β_1- or high levels of β_2-adrenoreceptors caused a dilated and fibrotic cardiomyopathy.[148,151] Likewise, transgenic expression of the β_1-adrenoreceptor effector Gsα causes myocardial hypertrophy that progresses to an apoptotic and fibrotic cardiomyopathy.[152]

Gαs-coupled β_1-receptors (but not the β_2-receptors) stimulate cell death via reactive oxygen species and activation of the JNK family of MAPKinases, leading to mitochondrial cytochrome *c* release and mitochondrial permeability transition pore formation.[153] β_1-adrenoreceptor signaling leads to increased SR calcium load via increased L-type calcium channel-mediated calcium influx and disinhibition of SERCA. There is increasing evidence that increased SR calcium levels may enhance contractility at the expense of increasing programmed cell death. The initial observation that intracellular calcium overload can trigger necrosis in cardiac myocytes was made more than 3 decades ago.[154] Intracellular calcium overload may trigger programmed cell death via opening of the mitochondrial permeability transition pore.[155] In transgenic mice with inducible cardiac expression of the $\beta_2\alpha$ subunit of the L-type calcium channel, increased intracellular and SR calcium provoked widespread cardiomyocyte necrosis with cardiomyopathic decompensation,[156] which could be prevented by L-type calcium channel inhibition by transgene suppression, calcium channel blockade, or ablation of cyclophilin D, a critical component of the mitochondrial permeability transition pore.[157] Increased calcium influx via the L-type calcium channel in response to β_1-adrenergic stimulation also activates calcium/calmodulin kinase (CaMKII), which

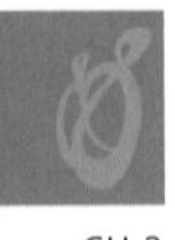

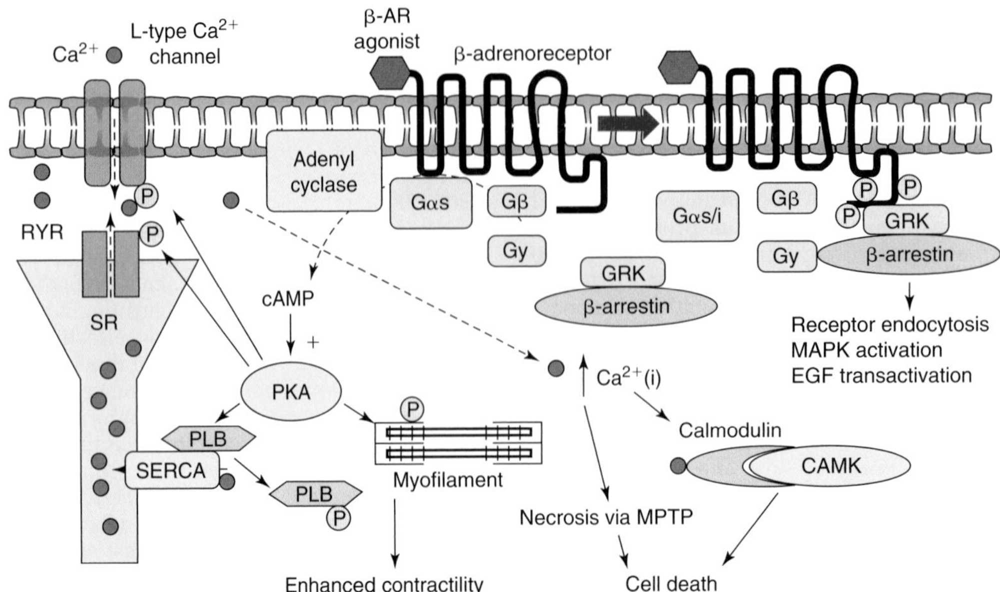

FIGURE 2–5 β-adrenoreceptor signaling in heart failure: Catecholamine binding to the seven transmembrane myocardial β_1-adrenoreceptors activates Gsα, with displacement of bound GDP by GTP. This causes cyclic AMP generation via stimulation of adenyl cyclase, which activates PKA. PKA phosphorylates the L-type calcium channel, enhancing Ca^{2+} entry, and phosphorylates RyR, enhancing calcium release from the SR, increasing intracellular calcium (Ca^{2+}(i)) available for excitation contraction coupling. PKA phosphorylates phospholamban (PLB) de-repressing SERCA activity with enhanced SR Ca^{2+} reuptake; and phosphorylates troponin on the myofilaments, with the net effect of enhancing contractility. Termination of G protein signaling occurs with GTPase activity of Gsα, causing GTP hydrolysis and cAMP degradation by phosphodiesterases (not shown). Additionally, activated β-adrenoreceptors are phosphorylated at their cytoplasmic tails by G-protein receptor kinases (GRK), causing receptor endocytosis. Increased Ca^{2+}(i) with chronic adrenoreceptor signaling causes necrotic cell death via calmodulin-mediated CaMK activation and mitochondrial permeability transition pore formation (MPTP) (see text). β_2-adrenoreceptor activation stimulates Gαi with inhibition of adenylcyclase (not shown). A delayed phase of signaling downstream of the β_1-adrenoreceptor is activated by GRK-mediated recruitment of β-arrestin with transactivation of EGF with enhanced survival signaling (see text).

phosphorylates phospholamban, thereby inhibiting its activity further and increasing the SR calcium load, and causing cardiomyocyte apoptosis in vitro.[158] Inhibition of CaMKII by forced expression of a dominant negative peptide in the heart results in decreased SR calcium stores, which attenuates cardiomyocyte apoptosis[159] and protects against development of catecholamine-induced cardiomyopathy.[160]

β_2-receptors can signal both via Gs and Gi, and at physiological levels, primarily mediate cell survival in the heart.[161,162] β_2-adrenoreceptor signaling switches from the stimulatory Gsα pathway to the inhibitory Giα signaling upon phosphorylation of the receptor by PKA activation downstream of the Gsα subunit.[163] This causes dissociation of the Gβγ subunit from Giα, resulting in activation of the PI3K-Akt survival pathway. In vitro studies employing selective expression of each β-receptor in cardiac myocytes from mice with combinatorial deletion of both β_1- and β_2-receptors revealed a proapoptotic effect for β_1-signaling and an antiapoptotic PI3K-Akt mediated signaling cascade downstream of the β_2-receptor.[162] Indeed, the Giα pathway appears to protect against cell death after ischemic reperfusion injury in vivo.[164]

The application of insights from experimental mouse models to the human condition is supported by the clinical effects of single nucleotide polymorphisms in genes encoding adrenoreceptor signaling factors. Increased adrenergic signaling downstream of β_1-receptors in individuals carrying an activating polymorphism in the β_1-receptor (β_1Arg389), combined with an inhibitory polymorphism in the presynaptic α2c receptor (α_2CDel322-325), increases the risk of heart failure.[165] Likewise, the gain-of-function polymorphism of the β_1-receptor may alter the response to β-blockers in heart failure.[166]

β-adrenoreceptor signaling is downregulated in heart failure due to receptor phosphorylation by G-protein receptor kinases (GRK) (see Figure 2-5). GRK-phosphorylated receptors attract β-arrestins 1 and 2, which terminate the receptor Gα subunit interaction. GRK2 (a.k.a. β-ARK), 5, and 6 are expressed in the myocardium. Forced cardiac expression of GRK2 and GRK5 blunts the attenuated isoproterenol-mediated increase in contractility, whereas cardiac ablation or dominant negative inhibition enhances the contractile response, suggesting that GRK2 plays an essential role in modulating cardiac function.[24,167] The consequences of GRK2-mediated β_1-adrenoreceptor downregulation in heart failure are not entirely clear. Whereas a GRK2-dominant negative protein (β-ARKct) has improved some genetic and most physiological models of cardiomyopathy,[168,169] cardiac-specific ablation of GRK2 worsened catecholamine-mediated cardiomyopathy[24] but improved cardiac function after myocardial infarction.[170]

Human heart failure is characterized by sympathetic activation with increased circulating catecholamine levels associated with desensitization and downregulation of β-adrenoreceptors.[146] β_1-adrenoreceptors are markedly downregulated and both β_1- and β_2-adrenoreceptors are uncoupled, with elevated myocardial levels of GRK2. β-adrenergic blockers reverse these changes in heart failure and are associated with improved survival and reversal of adverse structural and functional remodeling parameters.[171]

A novel survival pathway may also be triggered downstream from β_1-adrenoreceptor signaling via *EGF receptor transactivation* (see Figure 2-5). β-arrestin coupled with GRK5 and 6 activates a nonreceptor tyrosine kinase, Src, which activates a membrane-bound metalloproteinase, leading to cleavage of a heparin-binding EGF ligand (see later discussion under growth factors) and EGF receptor activation that is protective against catecholamine-induced cardiomyopathy by enhancing survival signaling.[172] Indeed, interindividual differences in β-blocker efficacy may be due to different abilities to activate signaling through this alternate pathway (biased antagonism).[173] These studies are particularly intriguing in the context of genetic studies revealing that a gain-of-function polymorphism in GRK5 is protective in heart failure.[174] Whether the beneficial effects are due to enhanced β-adrenoreceptor desensitization or to increased EGF receptor transactivation is not known.

Integrins Are Biomechanical Sensors for Hypertrophy

A major stimulus for hypertrophy after myocardial injury is increased load sensed by individual myocytes and surrounding myocardial fibroblasts. Attempts to isolate the biomechanical sensor of cellular load focused on mechanical deformation or "cell stretch." Passively stretching cardiomyocytes cultured on deformable substrates provokes reactive hypertrophy with upregulation of early response and fetal genes.[12] One of the mechanisms by which stretch is transduced into a biochemical signal for hypertrophy is activation of integrins, a diverse family of cell surface receptors that link the extracellular milieu to intracellular signaling scaffolds called focal adhesion complexes.[175] Integrins consist of two subunits α and β in various combinations, each with an extracellular domain to interact with extracellular matrix proteins, a transmembrane part that anchors them, and a short cytoplasmic tail (Figure 2-6). Integrin cytoplasmic tails interact with the cytoskeleton at the focal adhesion complex and serve as adaptors for multiple prohypertrophic signaling proteins (see Figure 2-6): (1) Focal adhesion kinase (FAK), a tyrosine kinase; (2) Srcs, a membrane-bound SH2 domain containing tyrosine kinase; (3) Grb2-associated binder (Gab) family proteins, which are scaffolding proteins that transduce signals downstream of growth factor and cytokine receptors; (4) integrin-linked kinase (ILK), a serine-threonine kinase; and (5) adaptor proteins, such as melusin and vinculin, that link integrins to the cytoskeleton at the focal adhesion complex.

Integrin signaling activated by pressure overload recruits c-Src and FAK leading to activation of ERK1/2 kinases with prohypertrophic signaling.[176] Cardiomyocyte-specific ablation of FAK prevents induction of ANF in response to transverse aortic constriction, without altering the late development of fibrosis and cardiomyopathy.[177] Inhibiting FAK with siRNA prevents and reverses pressure overload hypertrophy and preserves contractile function.[178] The β_1 subunit of integrins activates ILK, small GTPases, and prohypertrophic PI3K and ERK-MAPKinase pathways.[179] Forced expression of ILK causes compensated cardiac hypertrophy in mice, and dominant negative ILK prevents the hypertrophic response to angiotensin stimulation.[179] Cardiac-specific deletion of β_1-integrin or ILK causes spontaneous development of cardiomyopathy.[180]

Other proteins that interact with the cytoplasmic tail of integrins, such as melusin and vinculin, also appear to be essential for mechanotransduction. Ablation of melusin, a striated muscle-specific protein, prevents the myocardial hypertrophic response in response to pressure overload but not neurohormonal infusion, suggesting a specific role for melusin in integrin-mediated mechanotransduction.[181] Cardiac-specific ablation of vinculin, a ubiquitously expressed protein that connects the actin cytoskeleton to the cell membrane, causes progressive development of cardiomyopathy by 6 months of age in mice.[182] Indeed, the β_1-integrin vinculin interface may have a critical homeostatic role in cardiomyocytes as ablation of β_1-integrin causes cardiac defects and periimplantation mortality, and ablation of β_3-integrin causes spontaneous cardiac hypertrophy that was exacerbated with pressure overload.[183]

Another putative mechanical stretch sensor is at the Z-disk, wherein the small LIM-domain protein MLP (muscle LIM protein) is anchored and transduces stress stimuli via interaction with a complex of transducing proteins.[184] Titin, a giant sarcomeric protein component of the thin filament that anchors the Z-disk at one end and extends to the M line at the other, is another candidate, postulated to function as a molecular spring providing passive stiffness to the cell and acting as a biomechanical sensor.[185]

Autocrine/Paracrine Effects of Neurohormones and Growth Factors. Mechanical stretch can transduce hypertrophy via autocrine and paracrine release of neurohormones, and activation of respective seven-transmembrane spanning G protein-coupled receptors. Cardiomyocyte deformation induces autocrine secretion of angiotensin II, endothelin 1,

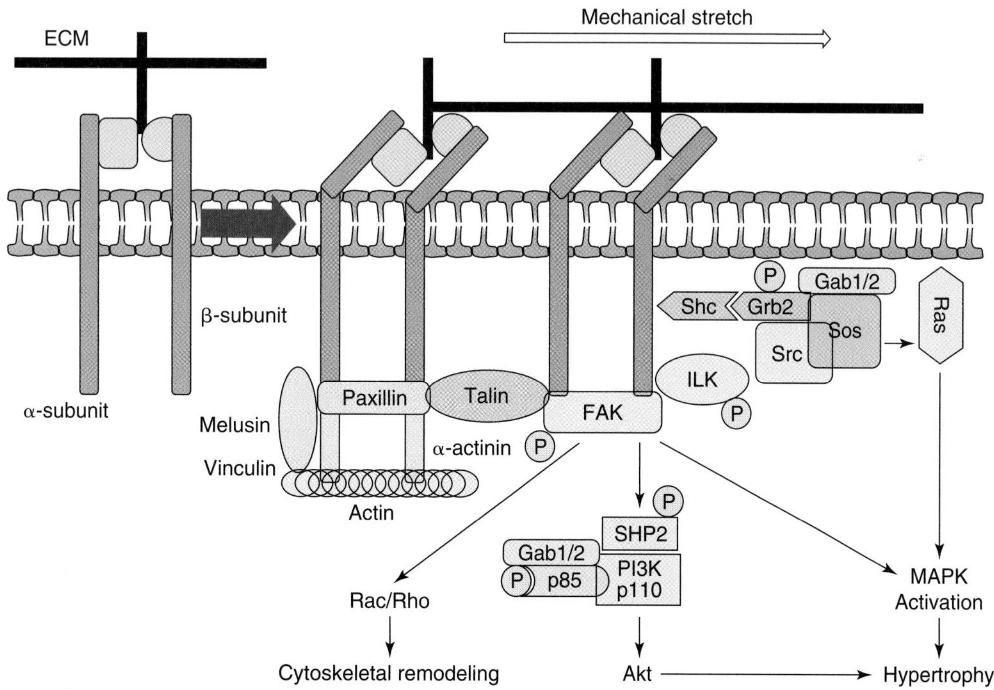

FIGURE 2–6 Integrin-mediated transduction of biomechanical stress: Integrins are heterodimeric proteins formed by the association of various combinations of single-transmembrane α and β subunits, which are attached to the extracellular matrix proteins such as laminin and fibronectin. Biomechanical stress induces change in conformation and integrin clustering, resulting in assembly of the focal adhesion complex consisting of the kinases FAK, Src, and ILK, along with adaptor proteins vinculin, paxillin, talin, α-actinin, and melusin that connect the integrins to the cytoskeletal elements (actin). Stretch-mediated phosphorylation and activation of FAK and ILK causes MAPK (ERK) activation and Akt activation via the SHP2/PI3K pathway, resulting in hypertrophic signaling. Additionally FAK activates small G proteins Rac and Rho (see later discussion), which transduce cytoskeletal reorganization in hypertrophy. Integrin signaling also activates Ras via Shc/Grb2/Gab1/2-mediated Src kinase activation, which transduces hypertrophy signaling via MAPK (ERK) activation.

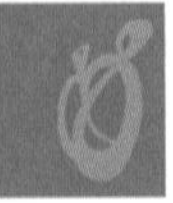

and peptide growth factors such as FGF.[186] Integrins can also transduce hypertrophic stimuli in part via upregulation of angiotensin II.[187] Interestingly, angiotensin may not be essential for hypertrophy transduced by stretch-induced activation of AT1R.[188] Paracrine release of neurohormones, growth factors, and cytokines by nonmyocytes in the mechanically overloaded heart also leads to cardiac fibroblast proliferation,[189] acting as an amplification loop to increase neurohormonal effects on cardiomyocytes. Evidence for simultaneous involvement of multiple growth factors in stretch-induced hypertrophy is consistent with the notion that signaling pathways converge through various neurohormonal receptors.[186]

Neurohormonal Activation of Hypertrophy Signaling

Norepinephrine, angiotensin II, and endothelin signal via heptahelical transmembrane receptors coupled to the Gq heterotrimeric G protein. G proteins consist of three polypeptide chains—α, β, and γ (Figure 2-7). The α-subunits are primarily responsible for determining activation of downstream signaling effectors and are organized into four groups: Gαs, Gαi, Gαq, and Gα12. Inactive Gα subunits bind to GDP (guanosine diphosphate) and Gβγ subunits. Upon recruitment to a ligand occupied transmembrane receptor, GTP is exchanged for GDP, resulting in dissociation of the Gα-GTP subunit from the βγ subunit and activation of downstream signaling cascades. Hydrolysis of GTP by intrinsic GTPase activity (that is augmented by regulators of G protein signaling (RGS) proteins) terminates the signal. Gαq-coupled receptors activate phospholipase C, which catalyzes the hydrolysis of phosphatidylinositol 4,5 bisphosphate (PIP_2) into inositol 1,4,5 triphosphate (IP_3) and diacylglycerol (DAG). DAG activates the PKC family of growth-stimulating serine-threonine kinases (see Figure 2-7) and IP3 causes intracellular Ca^{2+} release that can activate signaling through calcium-dependent PKCs, calcium-calmodulin dependent kinases (CaMKs), and calcineurin. Another arm of signaling is initiated by the free Gβγ subunits, which recruit PI3Kγ to the sarcolemma and facilitate interaction with phosphoinositides. This PI3K signaling differs from the activation of the PI3Kα isoform in adaptive hypertrophic signaling, which was discussed earlier.

Heart failure causes systemic and myocardial release of catecholamines, leading to Gαq activation via α_1-adrenergic receptors. There are three receptor subtypes: α_1A/C, α_1B, and α_1D, the first two of which are implicated in transducing catecholamine-induced hypertrophy signaling in the heart. In the adult human myocardium, the α_1A receptor subtype predominates over α_1B. Norepinephrine and phenylephrine treatment of cardiomyocytes stimulates hypertrophy in vitro with reactivation of the fetal gene program, increased cardiomyocyte size, and protein synthesis.[9] Forced cardiac expression of α_1B receptors provokes a cardiomyopathy and downregulated β-receptor signaling, but forced expression of α_1A receptors enhances systolic function without stimulating hypertrophy.[190] Gene ablation of α_1A/C or α_1B receptors suggests a role in blood pressure modulation without an effect on cardiac hypertrophy. Combinatorial deletion of both subtypes revealed a modest effect of α_1-receptor signaling in normal cardiac growth because the double knockout hearts were approximately 13% smaller than wild types.[191] In response to pressure overload, double α_1-receptor knockout mice developed a cardiomyopathy, with decreased survival, increased cell death, and markedly decreased upregulation of "fetal genes,"[192] likely related to the absence of prosurvival ERK signaling transduced by these receptors.[193] These results indicate that α_1-receptors signal in normal cardiac growth and cardiomyocyte survival in response to stress and are redundant in the transduction of pressure overload hypertrophy.

Angiotensin II (Ang II), a powerful vasoconstrictor, is a potent inducer of cardiac growth via the AT_1 and AT_2 receptors. There are two AT_1R subtypes: $AT_{1a}R$ and $AT_{1b}R$, which are both coupled to Gαq signaling. Forced cardiac expression of $AT_{1a}R$ causes cardiac hypertrophy progressing to adverse

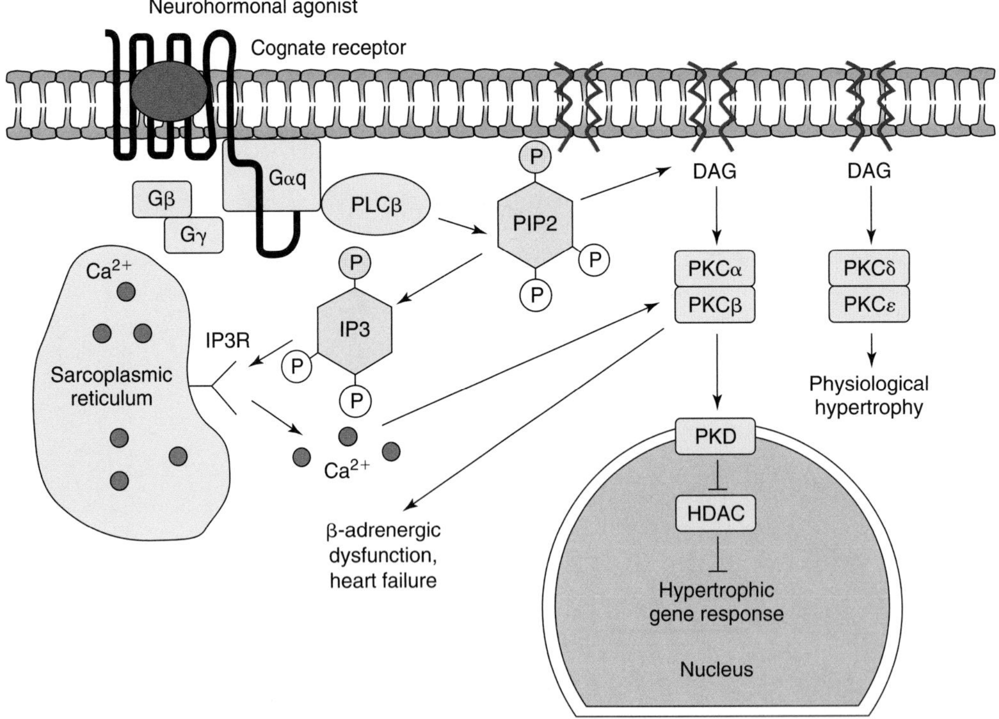

FIGURE 2–7 Neurohormonal signaling via Gαq in pathological myocardial hypertrophy. Binding of neurohormones to the cognate neurohormonal receptor causes GTP exchange and activation of the Gαq subunit, with dissociation from the Gβγ subunits and recruitment of PLCβ to the cell membrane. PLCβ causes hydrolysis of PIP2 with generation of IP3 and DAG. IP3 binds to IP3 receptors (IP3Rs) on the sarcoplasmic/endoplasmic reticulum causing Ca^{2+} release, which causes PKC activation along with DAG for classical PKCs (α and β). Novel PKCs (δ and ε) are activated by DAG alone. See text for details of PKC signaling in heart failure. Classical PKCs activate PKD, which phosphorylates class II HDACs (5 and 9) resulting in export from the nucleus and de-repression of hypertrophy gene transcription.

remodeling and dysfunction[194] and mice lacking $AT_{1a}R$ demonstrate attenuated myocardial hypertrophy in response to pressure overload with preserved systolic function.[195] Angiotensin receptor antagonism attenuates hypertrophy in vitro and when given therapeutically to humans with heart failure.[196] However, in vivo, there is no critical requirement for AT_1R signaling in transducing pressure overload hypertrophy, likely due to angiotensin signaling via $AT_{1b}R$ (which is not present in humans) or redundancy in signaling with other neurohormones.[197]

Endothelin-1 (ET-1) is a 21–amino acid polypeptide cleaved from a larger precursor by endothelin converting enzyme. ET-1 is predominantly produced by endothelial cells, although cardiomyocytes and fibroblasts also produce small amounts. ET-1 signals via the $ET1_A$ and $ET1_B$ receptors, which are both coupled to Gα. ET-1 appears to be a part of the autoregulatory loop with Ang II because ET-1 is produced in response to Ang II stimulation, and the ET-1 receptor blockade antagonizes Ang II-mediated hypertrophy.[198] Endothelin receptor blockade delays, but does not prevent, development of hypertrophy and pathological decompensation in response to pressure overload.[199] Cardiomyocyte-specific deletion of $ET\text{-}1_A$ did not prevent hypertrophy due to Ang II and phenylephrine infusion in vivo,[200] implying that ET-1-induced signaling is redundant in transducing pathological hypertrophy.

Gq/Phospholipase/Protein Kinase C. Redundancy in signal transduction at the receptor level in transduction of pathological hypertrophy signals led researchers to look for nodal signaling points that could be inhibited to prevent pathological hypertrophy.[201] The heterotrimeric G proteins, Gαq and G_{11}, transduce signals from angiotensin, endothelin, norepinephrine, and other neurohormones.[145] Gαq/G_{11} signaling is essential in embryonic cardiac growth because combined ablation of Gq (*gnaq*) and G_{11} (*gna11*) causes embryonic lethality at day 11 with cardiac hypoplasia and failure of ventricular septation.[202] In vivo, unabated Gαq signaling by forced cardiac expression was the first nodal signaling molecule shown to recapitulate pathological hypertrophy.[7] Superimposed pressure overload or the hemodynamic stress of pregnancy provokes rapid cardiomyopathic decompensation caused by widespread cardiomyocyte apoptosis.[203,204] Indeed, dominant negative inhibition of Gαq,[205] inhibition of Gαq signaling by forced expression of inhibitory RGS4,[206] or combined cardiomyocyte-specific ablation of Gαq and G_{11}, all prevent pressure overload hypertrophy, establishing a critical role for neurohormonal activation of Gαq in transducing the pressure overload stimulus.[207] Polymorphisms in the *gnaq* (Gαq) gene promoter that affect Gαq expression have been associated with changes in human hypertrophy and heart failure. A common single base pair change from GC to TT at position −694/−695 in the *gnaq* gene promoter eliminates SP-1 transcription factor binding[208,209] and increases Gαq promoter activity, which is associated with increased prevalence of left ventricular hypertrophy in normal subjects[209] and increased mortality in African American patients with heart failure.[208]

Phospholipase Cβ (PLCβ) is the downstream effector of Gαq (see Figure 2-7). Of the four isoforms, $PLC\beta_1$ and β_3 are expressed in the heart. An essential role for either of these isoforms has not been evaluated for pathological cardiac hypertrophy signaling because the $PLC\beta_1$ knockout mice develop epilepsy and increased mortality beginning at 3 weeks of age,[210] and $PLC\beta_3$ knockout mice demonstrate a normal life span with abnormalities in neutrophil chemotaxis and skin ulcers, but no apparent abnormalities in cardiac development.[211] PLCε is another cardiac expressed phospholipase, levels of which are increased in human dilated cardiomyopathy and in response to experimental isoproterenol treatment or pressure overload.[212] PLCε is downstream of Ras and regulates β-adrenergic responsiveness in cardiomyopathy. Germline ablation of PLCε is associated with reduced ventricular systolic function and diminished β-adrenergic responsiveness and exaggerated hypertrophy and cardiomyopathic decompensation in response to isoproterenol.[212]

Protein kinase C (PKC) is downstream of Gαq/PLCβ and has emerged as a key mediator of altered myocardial contractility and cardiomyocyte survival in pathological hypertrophy (see Figure 2-7). The heart expresses four functionally important PKC isoforms: PKC α and β ("conventional group," activated by DAG with a requirement for Ca^{2+}) and PKC δ and ε ("novel" PKCs, activated by DAG without a requirement for Ca^{2+}).[201] PKCs translocate to specific subcellular locations upon activation: PKCα to the membrane from the cytosol, PKCβ from the cytoplasm to the nucleus, PKCε from the cytoplasm and nucleus to the myofibrils, and PKCδ redistributes to the mitochondria and to a perinuclear location.

PKCα is upregulated in rodent pressure overload hypertrophy[7,213] and human heart failure.[214] Treatment of neonatal rat ventricular myocytes with phorbol ester, a nonspecific activator of PKC signaling, causes hypertrophy resembling that of PE and Ang II. Because PKC activation requires translocation to the membrane and binding to specific anchoring proteins (RACKs), studies have interrogated specific PKC effects by transgenic expression of peptides that either facilitate or inhibit PKC translocation, conventional overexpression, or gene ablation. PKCα activation negatively regulates myocardial contractility but not hypertrophy.[215,216] Indeed, inhibition of PKCα prevents contractile dysfunction in pathological hypertrophy.[215,217] PKCβ overexpression is sufficient to cause myocardial hypertrophy,[218] but it is not necessary since pressure overload hypertrophy is unaltered in PKCβ knockout mice.[219] PKCδ appears to be a critical modifier of cell death in response to ischemic injury, without affecting myocardial hypertrophy,[220] whereas PKCε is both activated in, and sufficient to cause, hypertrophy.[203,221] An additional clue to the adaptive nature of PKCε-mediated hypertrophy comes from its ability to reduce Gαq-mediated pathological hypertrophy and decompensation when activated, and markedly worsen Gαq-mediated cardiomyopathic decompensation when inhibited.[222]

Ca^{2+}-dependent, nonconventional PKCs also activate protein kinase D (PKD). Protein kinase D directly phosphorylates class II HDACs (histone deacetylases; see Figure 2-7) resulting in their export from the nucleus and de-repression of transcription. Constitutively active PKD1 causes hypertrophy progressing to cardiomyopathy and siRNA-mediated knockdown of PKD1 prevents hypertrophic cardiomyocyte growth by agonists that signal via Gαq and Rho GTPase.[223] Cardiomyocyte-specific deletion of PKD1 renders the myocardium insensitive to pressure overload, angiotensin II, and isoproterenol treatment, with preserved cardiac function and prevention of remodeling,[224] secondary to their role in phosphorylating class II HDACs.

Mitogen Activated Protein Kinases (MAPKs)

Activated G protein-coupled receptors activate mitogen activated protein kinases (MAPKs) via the free Gβγ subunits, either directly or indirectly through cross talk with small Raslike G proteins (Figure 2-8). Multiple other signaling pathways such as receptor tyrosine kinases, receptor serine/threonine kinases (transforming growth factor β [TGF-β]), Janus-activated kinases (JAKs via cardiotrophin-1 [gp130 receptor]), and stress stimuli, such as stretch, also activate mitogen-activated protein kinases (MAPKs) in the heart.[225] MAPK pathways are activated in a cascade manner (see Figure 2-8). There are three major groups of MAPKs: extracellular signal regulated kinases (ERK), JNKs, and p38. Specific MAPKKs activate each MAPK: MAPK1/2 for ERK1/2, MAPK3/6 for p38, and MAPK4/7 for JNK. At the next tier, each MAPKKK can activate different MAPKK-MAPK pathways, providing a mechanism for integration of upstream signaling.

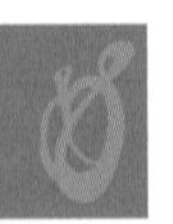

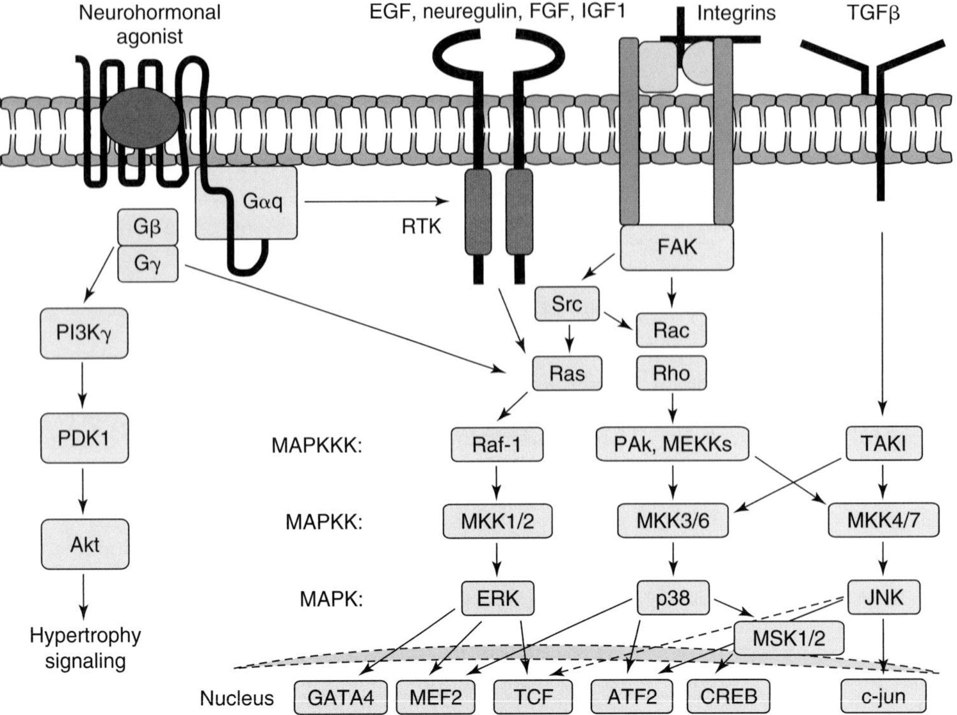

FIGURE 2–8 Activation of MAPK signaling in pathological hypertrophy. Activated Gαq protein activates small G proteins such as Ras either directly via the released Gβγ subunits or via cross-talk with receptor tyrosine kinases (RTKs), which are activated by growth factors such as EGF, neuregulin, FGF, and IGF-1 (see discussion in text). This leads to stimulation of the mitogen-activated protein kinase (MAPK) signaling cascades. MAPKs are also activated by integrin signaling and TGF receptor-mediated activation of TAK1. MAPK cascades are organized into three tiers: MAPKinase kinase kinases (MAPKKKs) that activate MAPKinase kinases (MAPKKs), which subsequently activate MAPKinases. MAPKs signal redundantly via multiple transcription factors (see details in text). Gβγ subunits of the Gαq signaling complex also activate PI3Kγ, resulting in Akt activation and hypertrophy signaling.

The top tier of MAPK pathway consists of the MAPKKKinases (see Figure 2-8). One such MAPKKK is Mst1, forced expression of which causes an apoptotic cardiomyopathy.[226] Subsequent stepwise activation of kinases (see Figure 2-8) serially culminates in the activation of the effector kinases. ERK1/2 are activated via Gαq-coupled agonists in response to hypertrophic agonists in vitro as Ang II, PE, ET-1, and stretch and in vivo by pressure overload.[227] Gαq signaling in response to pressure overload is essential for ERK activation because expression of a truncated Gαq peptide blocks aortic banding-induced ERK activation.[227]

Available evidence suggests a role for the ERK signaling axis in promoting hypertrophy, and p38 and JNK in regulating cell survival and fibrosis. Forced expression of MEK1-ERK1 causes concentric hypertrophy via activation of the calcineurin-NFAT pathway[228] without adverse ventricular remodeling. A critical role for this pathway in hypertrophic signaling is not established because gene ablation either causes no cardiac defects (*Erk1–/–*);[229] or has not yet been pursued in a conditional cardiac-specific manner (*Erk2–/–* mice are embryonic lethal with lack of trophoblast development).[230] ERK 5 is related to ERK1/2 with a similar activation motif, and is activated in the heart in response to gp130 signaling (by LIF or cardiotrophin 1). Similar to ERK1/2, forced cardiac expression of MEK5 (activator of ERK5, a.k.a. big ERK) causes eccentric cardiac hypertrophy associated with the addition of sarcomeres in series within individual cardiomyocytes,[231] and gene ablation of ERK5 affects embryonic survival.[232]

MAPKs phosphorylate multiple substrates, including enzymes and transcription factors with overlapping specificity that regulate cardiac gene expression ("immediate early response" factors), cell survival, mRNA translation (eIF4E), and mRNA stability.[225] Specificity for downstream substrates is primarily determined via docking interactions. For example, p90RSKs are phosphorylated primarily by ERK1/2, whereas MAPKAPK2 is phosphorylated by p38-MAPK; and Msk1/2 may be phosphorylated by either ERK1/2 or p38-MAPK. Transcription factors activated by MAPKs are nuclear localized, which suggests that MAPKs or downstream kinases translocate into the nucleus to influence gene expression. The differential effects of MAPK signaling on hypertrophy and/or survival responses may also be related to the timing and duration of the signal and integration with other signaling cascades that crosstalk with MAPK signaling.

P38 and JNK kinases were originally discovered as "stress-responsive kinases" due to their rapid activation in response to stressful stimuli. Of the four genes encoding for p38, p38α is the most abundant in the heart, with minimal p38β detected. P38 and JNK transduce their signals by activating transcription factors c-jun, ATF2, ATF6, Elk-1, p53, and NFAT4. Activation of p38 signaling by forced expression of MKK3 and MKK6 causes early cardiac failure with ventricular fibrosis, whereas forced expression of dominant negative proteins (MKK3, MKK6, p38α, or p38β) and *p38α* gene ablation reveal an antihypertrophic role for p38 in cardiomyocytes.[233] This antihypertrophic effect appears to be mediated via suppression of Akt and calcineurin-NFAT signaling. The effects of p38 activation on cardiomyocyte survival are unclear because nonspecific pharmacological inhibition of p38 inhibits pressure overload and ischemia–reperfusion-induced apoptotic cell death, whereas p38α ablation protects against pressure-overload-induced cardiomyocyte apoptosis.[233] Similarly, JNK signaling (c-Jun N-terminal kinases) appears to be antihypertrophic because mice with either dominant negative inhibition or combined ablation of *JNK1* and *2* show basal and pressure-overload-induced hypertrophy with de-repressed calcineurin-NFAT signaling.[234] Pharmacological inhibition of JNK1 attenuates ischemia–reperfusion-induced cardiomyocyte apoptosis, whereas combinatorial ablation *JNK1,2,* and *3* increases cardiomyocyte apoptosis in response to pressure overload and ischemic reperfusion injury.[233]

Ask-1 is a MAPKKinase, which is upregulated in the myocardium by angiotensin stimulation via AT1R-induced oxidative stress and NF κB activation. *Ask-1* ablation attenuates cardiomyocyte apoptosis and cardiomyopathic decompensation induced by angiotensin infusion[235] in response to pressure overload and coronary artery ligation without an effect on hypertrophy.[236]

IP3-induced Ca^{2+}-mediated Signaling. Gαq signaling causes IP3 production, which interacts with IP3 receptors to cause intracellular release of Ca^{2+} (see Figures 2-7 and 2-9). In cardiac myocytes, IP3-induced Ca^{2+} fluxes are localized

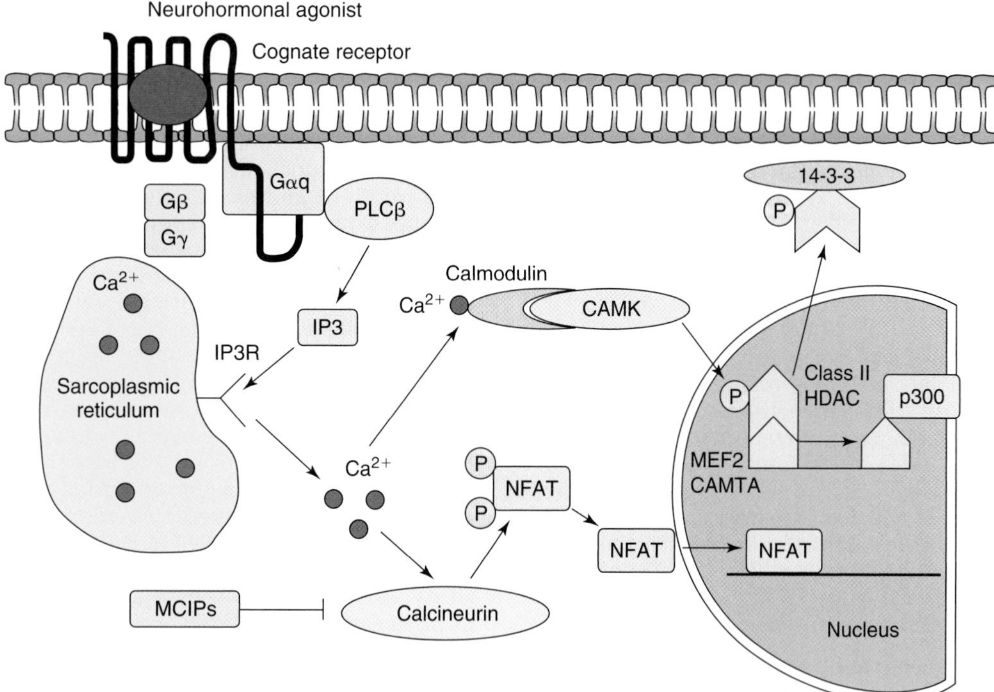

FIGURE 2–9 Neurohormonal activation of calcineurin and CaMK signaling. Gq/G_{11}-mediated production of IP3 via PLCβ causes release of intracellular Ca^{2+} via the IP3Rs, leading to activation of the protein phosphatase calcineurin. Calcineurin dephosphorylates NFAT transcription factor, resulting in its nuclear translocation and activation of hypertrophy gene transcription. MCIPs are endogenous inhibitors of calcineurin activity. The increased cytoplasmic calcium concentration (Ca^{2+} (i)) also causes activation of CaMKs via interaction with calmodulin. CaMKs phosphorylate class II HDACs, resulting in HDAC translocation out of the nucleus and binding to 14-3-3 protein in the cytoplasm. This allows histone acetylation by HAT p300, de-repressing hypertrophic gene transcription mediated by transcription factors such as MEF2 and CAMTA.

to microdomains, in effect compartmentalizing the Ca^{2+}-induced signaling and segregating the signaling effects of local Ca^{2}+ from the global calcium of excitation–contraction coupling. For example, β_2-adrenergic receptors are associated with caveolin-3 protein within caveolar microdomains on cardiomyocytes, and this allows for the regulation of L-type calcium channel activity with β_2-dependent activation, which is prevented by disruption of the caveolar architecture.[237] Other examples of spatially localized IP3-induced Ca^{2+} release affecting signaling are calsarcin-mediated regulation of Ca^{2+}-induced activation of prohypertrophic phosphatase calcineurin at the Z-disk and perinuclear CaMK signaling to influence gene transcription via export of HDACs.[238]

Calcineurin

IP3-mediated release of intracellular calcium activates calcineurin and calcium/calmodulin-dependent kinase (CaMK) pathways that regulate cardiac growth (Figure 2-9).[30] Calcineurin (Cn), a serine-threonine phosphatase also known as protein phosphatase (PP2B), is stimulated by Ca^{2+} binding to calmodulin and dephosphorylates the transcription factor Nuclear Factor of Activated T cells (NFAT) at the N-terminal serine residue, allowing its translocation to the nucleus. The functional calcineurin protein is a dimer consisting of two subunits A and B, and is encoded by five genes (CnA by α, β, and γ and CnB by CnB1 and B2), of which the mammalian heart expresses CnAα, CnAβ, and CnB1. In vitro stimulation of cardiomyocytes with hypertrophic stimuli activates calcineurin[239] and calcineurin activity is increased in human compensated hypertrophy and heart failure.[240] Calcineurin activity is also increased in animal models of pressure-overload-induced and exercise-induced cardiac hypertrophy. Forced expression of calcineurin causes myocardial hypertrophy that progresses to heart failure[239] without inducing cardiomyocyte apoptosis.[241] Studies with pharmacological inhibition of calcineurin activity with FK506 and cyclosporine have suggested that calcineurin transduces pathological hypertrophy signaling in response to PE, Ang II, and ET-1 in vitro, and pressure-overload hypertrophy in vivo (reviewed in Heineke et al[30,242]). Forced expression of dominant negative calcineurin[243] and gene ablation of CnAβ decrease cardiomyocyte hypertrophy in response to pressure-overload stimulus and neurohormones.

Calcineurin is localized at the Z-disk in a complex with calsarcins. Ablation of calsarcin-1 increases calcineurin signaling in pressure overload, resulting in rapid progression to heart failure.[244] Ablation of NFATc1[245] and Nfatc2/c3/c4[246] causes cardiac defects. Forced cardiac expression of constitutively active NFATc4 causes massive cardiac hypertrophy.[239] Ablation of NFATc2 and NFATc3 attenuate pathological hypertrophic by transgenic calcineurin and protect against pressure-overload–and angiotensin-induced hypertrophy without affecting the development of exercise-induced adaptive hypertrophy.[247,248]

Calcineurin signaling is restrained by modulatory calcineurin inhibitory proteins (MCIP) (see Figure 2-9),[249] which bind to calcineurin and inhibit its activity. *MCIP1* gene transcription is activated in the heart by calcineurin-mediated NFAT activation, providing a negative feedback loop for calcineurin signaling, whereas *MCIP2* expression is induced by thyroid hormone signaling.[250] Forced expression of *MCIP1* reduces unstressed heart weight (by 5% to 10%), attenuates calcineurin and swimming-induced hypertrophy, and prevents ventricular remodeling after pressure overload. *MCIP1* overexpression likewise attenuates development of pathological hypertrophy, ventricular remodeling, and cardiomyopathic decompensation after myocardial infarction, suggesting a beneficial effect of preventing pathological hypertrophy in the surviving myocardium.[251] Thus *MCIP1* appears to be antihypertrophic in many forms of cardiac growth.

MCIP1 gene ablation does not result in cardiac abnormalities, indicating that *MCIP1* does not regulate cardiac developmental growth.[252] However, *MCIP1* ablation sensitizes the heart to calcineurin signaling, resulting in accelerated heart failure in calcineurin transgenic mice, but paradoxically reduces hypertrophy in response to pressure overload and isoproterenol.[252] Indeed, a recent study suggested that MCIPs can act as facilitators of calcineurin activity, thereby having dual functions in hypertrophy signaling.[253]

Calmodulin-dependent Protein Kinase (CaMK)

Increased cytosolic Ca^{2+} activates CaMKs, a family of regulatory enzymes that phosphorylate multiple proteins that modulate myocardial contractility,[254] hypertrophy, and survival signaling (see Figure 2-9). All four CaMKs, I-IV, activate MEF2-mediated transcription of fetal genes[255] that causes cardiomyocyte hypertrophy. Forced cardiac expression of CaMKIV causes eccentric hypertrophy with contractile impairment,[255] but CaMKIV knockout mice develop pressure overload hypertrophy, suggesting that other CaMK isoforms primarily transduce pathological hypertrophy.[256] Indeed, CaMKII is the predominant cardiac isoform[254] and forced expression of CaMKIIδb (nuclear isoform) or CaMKIIδC (cytosolic isoform) in cardiomyocytes causes pathological hypertrophy.[257,258] Expression of dominant negative CaMKIIδb blocks PE-induced cardiomyocyte hypertrophy and pathological gene expression in vitro.[259]

HAT/HDAC-mediated Transcriptional Regulation via MEF2/CAMTA

CaMKIIδ isoforms bind to and phosphorylate HDAC4, a class II histone deactylase. The process of histone acetylation-deacetylation controls access of transcription factors, such as MEF2 and CAMTA to the chromatin machinery. Histones are nuclear proteins that constitute the nucleosome, a compact structure of chromatin genomic DNA tightly coiled around histone octamers that prevents access of transcription factors to DNA and represses gene expression. Histone acetyltransferases (HATs) acetylate conserved lysine residues in histone tails, which neutralizes the positive charge, and destabilizes histone-histone and histone-DNA interactions. Thus HATs stimulate gene expression. In contrast, histone deacetylases (HDACs) counter this effect, which promotes chromatin condensation and represses transcription (see Figure 2-9).

HATs belong to five families, and p300 and CREB binding protein (CBP) are the most abundant HAT family members in the cardiac muscle.[260] The HAT activity of p300 appears to play a critical role in cardiac development because targeted gene ablation is lethal between embryonic day 9.5 and 11.5, with failure to develop cardiac trabeculation and upregulate muscle-specific genes such as βMHC and α-actinin.[261] P300 binds to and acts as a transcriptional coactivator of GATA4, MEF2, and SRF. Activation of p300 and CBP by ERK phosphorylation is required for expression of ANF and βMHC.[262] Forced cardiac expression of these proteins stimulates hypertrophic signaling by facilitating GATA4 acetylation[262] and causes adverse remodeling after myocardial infarction.[263] Dominant negative p300 prevents acetylation and coactivation of GATA-4, which is associated with development of cardiomyopathy.[262] Inhibition of p300 HAT activity by curcumin (a polyphenol abundant in the spice, turmeric) prevents hypertrophy and cardiomyopathic decompensation and regresses established pressure overload.[264]

The HDACs are classified into three categories based on the homology with the yeast HDACs. Class I HDACs primarily consist of a catalytic domain, whereas class II HDACs have phosphorylation sites that serve as targets for signaling pathways, and interact with transcription factors. Class III HDACs require NAD for activity. Class I HDACs (HDAC 1 and 2) stimulate cardiac growth. Forced cardiac expression of HDAC2 causes hypertrophy and HDAC2 null mice are resistant to hypertrophic stimuli.[265] Resistance to hypertrophy in HDAC2 knockout mice is associated with increased expression of the gene encoding for inositol polyphosphate-5-phosphatase f (Inpp5f), which activates the antihypertrophic kinase GSK3β (see later discussion).

In contrast to class I HDACs, class II HDACs (HDAC4, HDAC5, HDAC7, and HDAC9) inhibit cardiac growth. Forced expression of HDAC5 and HDAC9 prevents hypertrophy in vitro in response to PE and serum, whereas *HDAC5* and *HDAC9* knockout hearts develop spontaneous cardiac hypertrophy[266] and exaggerated hypertrophy in response to pressure overload.[267] In contrast, their response to swimming-induced hypertrophy is not altered, suggesting these HDACs suppress only pathological hypertrophy. Class II HDACs are commonly associated with the MEF2 proteins in the nucleoplasm. MEF2 (myocyte enhancer factor 2) family transcription factors are essential for myogenesis and cardiac development. There are four MEF2 isoforms that bind DNA through a MADS DNA binding domain found on promoters of many cardiac expressed genes as SERCA, aMHC, and MLC2v. MEF2A and MEF2D are the predominant cardiac-expressed transcripts that regulate stress-induced gene expression.[268] MEF2 activity is restrained by binding to class II histone deacetylases (HDAC4, 5, and 7), and this repression is relieved by phosphorylation of HDACs by CaMKs, which induced HDAC nuclear export (see Figure 2-9),[269] and allows p300 to associate with MEF2, promoting gene transcription. By this mechanism, multiple hypertrophy signaling pathways (MAPKs, calcineurin, CaMKII, and protein kinase D) converge on MEF2 activation by class II HDAC export and relieve the transcriptional repression (see Figures 2-1, 2-7, and 2-9). *MEF2D* ablation prevents hypertrophy, ventricular remodeling, and gene dysregulation in response to pressure overload.[270]

Pharmacological inhibition of histone deacetylases inhibits hypertrophy.[271] Treatment of aortic-banded mice subjected with Trichostatin A and Scriptaid (two broad spectrum HDAC inhibitors), or SK7041 (a specific class I HDAC inhibitor),[272] improves survival and myocardial and cardiomyocyte hypertrophy and preserves systolic function. HDAC inhibition also regresses established cardiac hypertrophy and prevents cardiomyocyte apoptosis and myocardial fibrosis in pressure-overloaded animals, accompanied by reversion to the adult myosin gene expression pattern (αMHC predominant).

Class III HDACs, such as the Sir2 family, regulate life span.[273] Deacetylation by class III HDACs requires NAD+ and produces 2′-O-acetyl-ADP-ribose (O-AADPR) and nicotinamide. Sirt1 is one of the seven Sir2 kinases or Sirtuins, and can be activated pharmacologically by resveratrol (a component of red wine, consumption of which is associated with cardiovascular benefits). Forced expression of moderate levels of Sirt1 in the heart decreases aging-associated hypertrophy, fibrosis, and diastolic function, associated with reduced oxidative stress,[274] in contrast to higher levels of forced expression, which cause cardiomyopathy.

CaMK signaling also activate calmodulin binding transcription activator (CAMTA) transcription factors. CAMTA2 was discovered as an essential coactivator with Nkx2.5 of ANF gene transcription in cardiomyocytes. CAMTA2 activity is normally repressed by interaction with a class II HDAC (HDAC5). Gαq-mediated activation of PKCε and PKD phosphorylates HDAC5 resulting in export from the nucleus, de-repression of CAMTA2,[275] and activation of hypertrophic signaling. Forced expression of CAMTA2 provokes myocardial hypertrophy, which is enhanced by *HDAC5* gene ablation. *CAMTA2* knockout mice exhibit attenuated hypertrophic response to pressure overload, angiotension, and phenylephrine.[276]

Cross Talk Between Gαq and PI3K/Akt Hypertrophy Signaling Pathways

Gαq/phospholipase C pathways cross talk with PI3K/Akt signaling axis in transducing pathological hypertrophy signals. Gαq-coupled receptors activate PI3Kγ, which is distinct from the α-isoform activated in physiological hypertrophy signaling. Whereas PI3Kα is activated by receptor-mediated tyrosine phosphorylation, PI3Kγ binds to dissociated Gβγ, providing access to membrane phosphoinositides (see Figures 2-8 and 2-10).[277] PI3Kγ (p110γ) signaling is processed through Akt, which transduces both physiological and pathological cardiac growth (see Figure 2-10), depending upon the duration of activation.[278] There is transient activation of p110α by exercise, but in pressure-overload/Gαq–mediated signaling, sustained activation of PI3Kγ occurs with recruitment of additional signaling pathways in the phospholipase Cβ and calcineurin/NFAT axis.

Akt signaling by Gβγ/PI3Kγ is divergent (see Figure 2-10), which may also contribute to whether the hypertrophy is adaptive or maladaptive. One pathway involves activation of mTOR (mammalian target of rapamycin) and induction of protein synthesis. mTOR exists in two complexes (mTORCs)[279]: mTORC1 with Raptor, which is rapamycin sensitive and is the predominant mass-regulating complex downstream of Akt signaling; and mTORC2 with Rictor and Sin, which controls the actin cytoskeleton and determines cell shape. Pharmacological inhibition of mTOR with rapamycin prevents and regresses hypertrophy.[280] The mechanism by which mTOR stimulates protein synthesis is phosphorylation of S6 kinases that induce phosphorylation of ribosomal S6 protein, which recruits eukaryotic elongation factor 4E (eIF4E).[281] Forced expression of S6 kinase 1 (p70/85) causes cardiac hypertrophy.[282] However, combinatorial ablation of S6 kinase 1 (p70/85) and 2 (p54/56) does not alter the degree of hypertrophy in response to pressure overload, swimming, exercise, or transgenic IGFR1 expression, suggesting that activation of the S6 kinase pathway is not absolutely required for induction of protein synthesis in cardiac hypertrophy.[282]

A second Akt pathway leads to phosphorylation and suppression of glycogen synthase kinase (GSK3β, see Figure 2-10), and disinhibition of hypertrophy signaling. GSK3β is tonically active in the heart and its phosphorylation by Akt relieves antihypertrophic signaling. In vivo, pressure overload causes rapid phosphorylation of GSK3β within 10 minutes after transverse aortic constriction is applied, suggesting early recruitment of the kinase in the hypertrophic response.[181] Forced cardiac expression of GSK3β suppresses normal growth and causes cardiomyocyte dysfunction[283] and prevents isoproterenol- and pressure-overload–induced hypertrophy.[284] GSK3β phosphorylates and negatively regulates the translation initiation factor e1F2B.[285] GSK3β also counter-regulates the calcineurin NFAT signaling axis by phosphorylating the NFAT residues that are dephosphorylated by calcineurin (see Figure 2-10).[284] GSK3β is also phosphorylated by protein kinase A (PKA) activation and G protein-PKC-ERK-p90 ribosomal S6 kinase-based signaling, de-repressing downstream hypertrophic signaling (see Figure 2-10).

Like GSK3β, GSK3α signaling is also antihypertrophic, and its forced expression reduces cardiac mass, while siRNA-based knockdown prevents development of hypertrophy in response to pressure overload by inhibiting ERKs.[286] Forced expression of dominant negative GSK3β increases resting heart size, enhances contractility, and prevents decompensation of pressure overload hypertrophy.[287]

Antihypertrophic effects of GSK3β signaling are transduced in part through the canonical Wnt signaling axis (see Figure 2-10). Wnts are extracellular proteins that signal either cell to cell as membrane-bound proteins or as secreted proteins via heptahelical frizzled receptors and single transmembrane-pass coreceptors known as low-density lipoprotein receptor-related proteins (LRPs).[288] Tonic activity of GSK3β phosphorylates β-catenin, a transcription factor in the Wnt pathway, which targets it for degradation by the ubiquitin-proteosome system.[289] When Wnts signal via the frizzled LRP receptors, the entire complex gets recruited to the receptor with the scaffolding protein Dishevelled, resulting

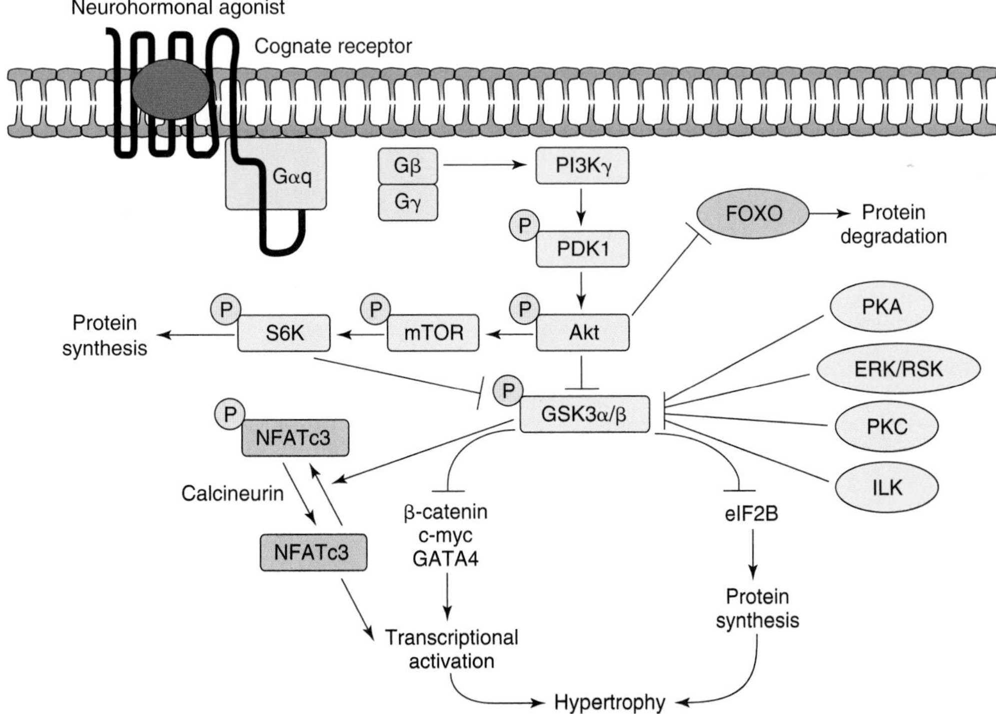

FIGURE 2–10 Neurohormonal regulation of hypertrophy via Akt/mTOR/GSK3β signaling. Gβγ-mediated PI3Kγ activation leads to Akt activation and stimulation of protein synthesis via mTOR and suppression of antihypertrophic signaling via GSK3β. Akt also phosphorylates and causes export of FOXO transcription factors from the nucleus, suppressing ubiquitin-proteosome-mediated protein degradation. GSK3α/β exerts a tonic inhibition on multiple prohypertrophic transcription factors and its phosphorylation relieves this inhibition, resulting in hypertrophy signaling. Inhibition of GSK3 is a nodal point for convergence of hypertrophy signaling pathways and also occurs via phosphorylation by PKA (via Gsα), PKCs (via Gαq), ERK/ribosomal S6 kinases (downstream of small G protein signaling), and ILK (downstream of integrin signaling).

in phosphorylation of LRP and Dishevelled, which inhibits GSK3β and prevents GSK3β-mediated phosphorylation of β-catenin. β-catenin therefore accumulates in the nucleus and complexes with a transcription factor TCF/LEF1 (T-cell-specific transcription factor/lymphoid enhancer binding factor 1) by displacing its binding protein Groucho, facilitating gene transcription. The Wnt-β-catenin signaling pathway is antihypertrophic in the heart.[290] Cardiomyocyte-specific deletion of β-catenin mildly increases cardiac mass and the cardiomyocyte cross-sectional area and upregulates hypertrophy gene expression.[291] In contrast, β-catenin stabilization decreases cardiomyocyte area, upregulates the atrophy-related protein IGFBP5, and attenuates Ang II-induced hypertrophy.[291] In this instance, the attenuated hypertrophy was associated with cardiomyopathic decompensation, suggesting that the Wnt pathway suppresses adaptive hypertrophy.

Akt also suppresses protein degradation via the ubiquitin-proteosome system. Akt phosphorylates FoxO (O family of forkhead/winged-helix) transcription factors, which suppresses their transcriptional activity by facilitating interaction with 14-3-3 proteins, leading to export out of the nucleus and targeting for ubiquitin-proteasome degradation (see Figures 2-1 and 2-10). Akt-mediated suppression of FoxO signaling downregulates multiple atrophy-related genes or atrogins.[292] Atrogin-1 is a cardiac- and skeletal muscle-specific F-box protein that regulates skeletal muscle atrophy by binding to Skp1, Cul1, and Roc1, the common components of SCF ubiquitin ligase complexes.[293] Since antihypertrophic FoxO-Atroxin signaling works in opposition to prohypertrophic pathways, in vivo adenoviral transduction of FoxO3 in mice reduces cardiac cell size,[294] and forced cardiac expression of Atrogin-1 suppresses Akt-mediated adaptive hypertrophy signaling[294] and targets calcineurin for proteasome degradation.[295]

Non-IGF Growth Factors in Hypertrophy. Cardiac myocytes elaborate peptide growth factors in response to stress. The role of signaling downstream of two prototypical growth factors, neuregulin, and TGF-β are reviewed here in detail.

Neuregulin is a member of the epidermal growth factor (EGF) signaling pathway. As with other growth factors, neuregulins cause dimerization of tyrosine kinase receptors (ErbB2, ErbB3, and ErbB4), leading to tyrosine autophosphorylation and recruitment of downstream signaling effectors[296] (Figure 2-11). Neuregulin is produced in the heart primarily by the endothelial cells and therefore functions as a paracrine growth factor. All three isoforms of neuregulin are cleaved by membrane-bound metalloproteinases, producing an activated fragment that is released and associates with EGF receptor (juxtacrine signaling) (see Figure 2-11). Neuregulin-mediated EGF receptor signaling is activated by neurohormonal stimuli via β-arrestin-mediated transactivation of the β-adrenergic receptors.[297] Neuregulin is induced by pressure overload paralleling the development of concentric hypertrophy[298] and its levels decline along with those of ErbB2 and ErbB4 receptors during transition to dilated cardiomyopathy.[299] Ablation of neuregulin 1 or ErbB2 and ErbB4 receptors causes cardiac hypoplasia and loss of trabeculation.[296] Neuregulin signaling via Erb receptors primarily regulates cardiomyocyte survival and not hypertrophy as cardiomyocyte-specific ablation of ErbB2 receptor causes spontaneous development of apoptotic cardiomyopathy,[300,301] which is rescued by adenoviral transduction of the antiapoptotic protein BXL-xl. Also, cardiomyocyte-specific ablation of the ErbB2 receptor markedly increases mortality after pressure overload and decreases cardiomyocyte survival with anthracycline exposure.[301] Exogenously administered recombinant neuregulin improves survival, improves LV function, and retards cardiomyopathic changes in experimental cardiomyopathy.[302] The importance of ErbB2 signaling in provoking cardiac pathology was unexpectedly established when an antibody against ErbB2 (a.k.a. "her2"), which is effective against metastatic breast cancer, caused a high incidence of dilated cardiomyopathy.[303]

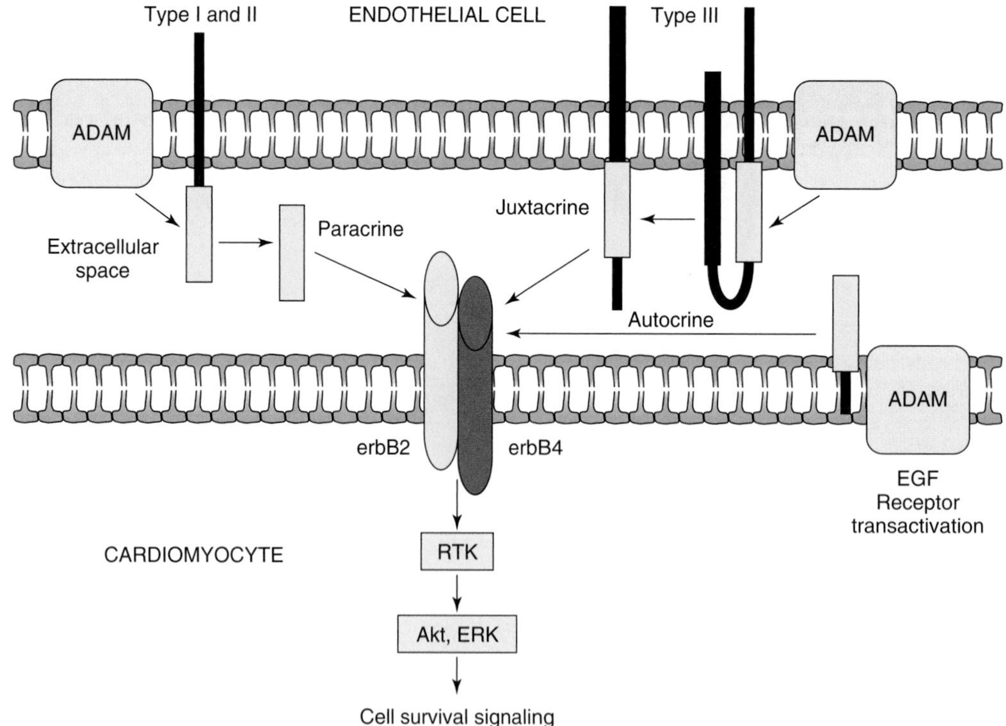

FIGURE 2–11 Neuregulin/EGF signaling in hypertrophy. Neuregulins are transmembrane proteins of the EGF family, present mainly on endothelial cells as three different types (I, II, and III). Proteolytic cleavage by ADAM (a disintegrin and metalloproteinase) family enzyme causes exposure of an EGF-like signaling domain, which interacts with erbB2 and erbB4 receptors resulting in receptor tyrosine kinase activation. EGF signaling is also activated by GRK-β-arrestin–mediated EGF cleavage by ligand-occupied seven-transmembrane neurohormonal receptors. Neuregulin/EGF activates Akt and ERK signaling pathways to promote cell survival in the heart.

The transforming growth factor family is a large group of polypeptide growth factors divided into two groups: the TGF/activin subfamily and the bone morphogenic proteins (reviewed in Xiao[304]). TGF-β_1 is secreted in a latent form and is tethered to the extracellular matrix, whereupon its stimulus-mediated proteolytic cleavage allows interactions with its serine-threonine kinase receptors, TGF-βRI and TGF-βRII. TGF-β is transcriptionally induced during the transition from compensated hypertrophy to failure in the spontaneously hypertensive rat model of pathological hypertrophy. Forced expression of TGF-β_1 in the heart induces mild hypertrophy,[305] and absence of TGF-β_1 markedly attenuates hypertrophy but preserves myocardial function in response to Ang II infusion.[306] TGF-β signaling activates MAPKs, such as the TAK1 (TGF-activated kinase)-MEK4-JNK1 and TAK1-MEK3/6-p38 axes (see Figure 2-8), and tyrosine kinase pathways, such as Ras/extracellular signal-regulated kinase (ERK) and RhoA/p160 Rho-associated kinase (ROCK).[307] Increased TAK1 activity is detected in pressure-overload hypertrophy, and forced cardiac expression of TAK1 causes cardiomyocyte hypertrophy with cardiomyopathic decompensation with increased mortality because of heart failure.[308]

Smad 4 is the canonical effector of TGF-β, and cardiomyocyte-specific ablation of Smad 4 causes cardiac hypertrophy with reexpression of fetal genes and the activation of the MEK1-ERK1/2 pathway.[309] Thus Smad4 acts in opposition to TGF-β-induced MAPK activation. Smad 2 activation is induced by growth differentiation factor 15 (GDF15), a TGF-β family member induced by pressure overload[310] and facilitates antihypertrophic signaling. Forced cardiac expression of GDF15 attenuates pressure-overload hypertrophy, without affecting the fetal gene expression program[310] and *GDF15* ablation exaggerates hypertrophy, leading to rapid cardiomyopathic decompensation after pressure overload.

Small G Proteins

Peptide growth factors and G protein–coupled receptors also transduce neurohormone and stretch-induced hypertrophy by nonreceptor tyrosine kinases such as Src, Ras, and Raf.[311] Ras, a member of the small G protein family (along with Rac, Rho, Rab, Ran, and ADP ribosylation factors) is the prototypical signaling molecule downstream of receptor tyrosine kinases (RTKs) that exist bound to GDP in the inactive state (see Figure 2-8). Upon stimulation, the GDP is exchanged for GTP and followed by a conformational change resulting in stimulation of mitogen-activated protein kinase (MAPK) cascade. Intrinsic GTPase activity then turns the signal off, returning the G protein to its basal state. GEFs are proteins that facilitate GTP exchange, and GAPs promote inactivation by activating the GTPase activity. There are four Ras proteins identified in the mammalian myocardium of which H-Ras has been the most carefully studied. Expression of constitutively active Ras promotes and dominant negative Ras inhibits cardiomyocyte hypertrophy in vitro in response to α-adrenergic agonists. Forced expression of H-Ras induces cardiomyocyte hypertrophy in vivo with preserved systolic function, myofibrillar disarray, and increased fibrosis with a unique gene expression profile consisting of ANF and BNP upregulation without upregulation of MHC or α-skeletal actin. Ras signaling also activates multiple MAPK pathways (both ERK and JNK mediated), with the combinatorial effect of its overexpression resulting in cardiomyopathic decompensation.

The Rho family of kinases is constituted by at least 14 members grouped into Rho, Rac, and cdc42 subfamilies. RhoA and Rac1 are activated by Gαq signaling,[312] and this in turn activates Rho kinases, ROCK1 and ROCK2. The Rho signaling pathway does not affect development of hypertrophy but has deleterious effects in pathological hypertrophic signaling. Mice with forced cardiac expression of Rho A develop fatal cardiomyopathy with conduction abnormalities and severe atrial enlargement.[313] Pharmacological Rho kinase inhibition prevents ventricular dilation and development of fibrosis in response to pressure overload hypertrophy in rats[314] and *ROCK1* deletion markedly reduces fibrosis in mice subjected to pressure overload.[315] Forced expression of constitutively activated Rac1, another Rho family member, causes lethal cardiomyopathy. Rac1 interacts with gp91(phox) and p67(phox) components of NAPDH oxidase, and its activation causes increased generation of reactive oxygen species.[316] Cardiomyocyte-specific gene ablation for Rac1[316] attenuates myocardial oxidative stress and hypertrophy in response to Ang II infusion.

Raf kinases are a family of three serine/threonine-specific kinases (A-Raf, B-Raf, and Raf-1) ubiquitously expressed throughout embryonic development. Raf is downstream of Ras signaling and activates the MEK1-ERK axis, with enhanced hypertrophic and prosurvival effects.[317] Cardiac specific ablation of Raf causes apoptotic cardiomyopathy, which is rescued by inhibition of Ask-1 (apoptosis signal–regulating kinase-1),[318] which physically interacts with Raf.

FUTURE DIRECTIONS

Much of the information described in this chapter has been generated through relatively recent techniques of molecular manipulation in cell-based and murine systems that engendered a revolution in reductionist experimentation (i.e., molecular dissection of pathophysiological processes). As a consequence, the past two decades have produced a literal encyclopedia of individual factors and their functional consequences in hypertrophy and heart failure. Yet, with all this new information, no magic bullet has been identified that prevents or cures heart failure, and a major conclusion from this work seems to be that molecular cross talk and functional redundancy between signaling factors and pathways is so prevalent that achieving a magic bullet is unlikely, if not impossible. It is interesting that two of the current foci of investigational therapeutics—targeting neurohormonal pathways[166,173] and correcting calcium abnormalities[156,159,319]—are the same as when the senior author was a medical student approximately 30 years ago.[146,320-323]

Targeted gain- and loss-of-function approaches that teased out possible roles for individual components of complex biological pathways have helped us develop an essential informational framework describing molecular processes and players in the heart. Now, the reductionist revolution of experimental molecular manipulation may be waning, and the future seems to be bright for integrated molecular studies of the human condition. Aside from the critical need to apply molecular information to human disease, there have been recent technical developments that position the field for a reorientation of approach. One is the availability of experimental platforms permitting high-throughput analysis of massive numbers of endpoints using specimens obtained from individual patients. Examples of currently available and clinically applicable large-scale molecular readouts include comprehensive mRNA and microRNA signatures from cardiac tissue and detailed personal gene polymorphism profiles. Proteomic profiling and analysis of individual exomes and genomes with a resolution down to single nucleotides is within reach in the next few years. The surprising degree of interindividual variability observed in our genetic code[324,325] undoubtedly contributes to observed heterogeneity in cardiac disease and response to therapy. Molecular epidemiology and a systems approach combining clinical investigation and bioinformatics, supported by basic studies, will be needed to determine how differences in gene product expression or function relate to the pathological interplay between factors and pathways.

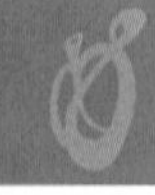

A second example of the need for an integrated approach to pathway analysis is the promise of regenerative cardiology (see Chapter 4). This is a very new field whose foundation is cell, developmental, and molecular biology. It is obvious that success in rebuilding myocardium from cardiac scar requires creation not just of cardiac myocytes, but also the tissue infrastructure that is essential for myocyte maintenance and function (i.e., cardiac interstitium, myocardial vasculature, intermyocyte physical and electrical connectivity). This is a monumental challenge, and will likely require a highly refined understanding of the interplay between myocyte and vascular growth, death, and contractile signaling. Fortunately, such an understanding is forthcoming.

REFERENCES

1. Packer, M. (1995). Evolution of the neurohormonal hypothesis to explain the progression of chronic heart failure. *Eur Heart J, 16*(suppl F), 4–6.
2. Adams, K. F., Jr., Lindenfeld, J., Arnold, J. M. O., et al. (2006). Executive summary: HFSA 2006 comprehensive heart failure practice guideline. *J Cardiac Fail, 12*(1), 10–38.
3. Mudd, J. O., & Kass, D. A. (2008). Tackling heart failure in the twenty-first century. *Nature, 451*, 919–928.
4. Baughman, K. L., & Jarcho, J. A. (2007). Bridge to life-cardiac mechanical support. *N Engl J Med, 357*(9), 846–849.
5. McAlister, F. A., Ezekowitz, J., Hooton, N., et al. (2007). Cardiac resynchronization therapy for patients with left ventricular systolic dysfunction: a systematic review. *JAMA, 297*(22), 2502–2514.
6. Rosamond, W., Flegal, K., Furie, K., et al. (2008). Heart disease and stroke statistics 2008 update. A report from the American Heart Association statistics committee and stroke statistics subcommittee. *Circulation, 117*(4), e25–e146.
7. D'Angelo, D. D., Sakata, Y., Lorenz, J. N., et al. (1997). Transgenic G-alphaq overexpression induces cardiac contractile failure in mice. *Proc Natl Acad Sci U S A, 94*(15), 8121–8126.
8. Rockman, H. A., Ross, R. S., Harris, A. N., et al. (1991). Segregation of atrial-specific and inducible expression of an atrial natriuretic factor transgene in an in vivo murine model of cardiac hypertrophy. *Proc Natl Acad Sci U S A, 88*(18), 8277–8281.
9. Simpson, P., McGrath, A., & Savion, S. (1982). Myocyte hypertrophy in neonatal rat heart cultures and its regulation by serum and by catecholamines. *Circ Res, 51*(6), 787–801.
10. Day, M. L., Schwartz, D., Wiegand, R. C., et al. (1987). Ventricular atriopeptin. Unmasking of messenger RNA and peptide synthesis by hypertrophy or dexamethasone. *Hypertension, 9*(5), 485–491.
11. Bishopric, N. H., Simpson, P. C., & Ordahl, C. P. (1987). Induction of the skeletal alpha-actin gene in alpha 1-adrenoceptor-mediated hypertrophy of rat cardiac myocytes. *J Clin Invest, 80*(4), 1194–1199.
12. Sadoshima, J., Jahn, L., Takahashi, T., et al. (1992). Molecular characterization of the stretch-induced adaptation of cultured cardiac cells. *J Biol Chem, 267*(15), 10551–10560.
13. Dorn, G. W., II, Robbins, J., Ball, N., et al. (1994). Myosin heavy chain regulation and myocyte contractile depression after LV hypertrophy in aortic-banded mice. *Am J Physiol, 267*(1 pt 2), H400–H405.
14. O'Connell, T. D., Rodrigo, M. C., & Simpson, P. C. (2007). Isolation and culture of adult mouse cardiac myocytes. *Methods Mol Biol, 357*, 271–296.
15. Hunter, J. J., Tanaka, N., Rockman, H. A., et al. (1995). Ventricular expression of a MLC-2v-ras fusion gene induces cardiac hypertrophy and selective diastolic dysfunction in transgenic mice. *J Biol Chem, 270*(39), 23173–23178.
16. Subramanian, A., Jones, W. K., Gulick, J., et al. (1991). Tissue-specific regulation of the alpha-myosin heavy chain gene promoter in transgenic mice. *J Biol Chem, 266*(36), 24613–24620.
17. Yussman, M. G., Toyokawa, T., Odley, A., et al. (2002). Mitochondrial death protein Nix is induced in cardiac hypertrophy and triggers apoptotic cardiomyopathy. *Nat Med, 8*(7), 725–730.
18. Sanbe, A., Gulick, J., Hanks, M. C., et al. (2003). Reengineering inducible cardiac-specific transgenesis with an attenuated myosin heavy chain promoter. *Circ Res, 92*(6), 609–616.
19. Bo, J., Yu, W., Zhang, Y. M., et al. (2005). Cardiac-specific and ligand-inducible target gene expression in transgenic mice. *J Mol Cell Cardiol, 38*(4), 685–691.
20. Syed, F., Odley, A., Hahn, H. S., et al. (2004). Physiological growth synergizes with pathological genes in experimental cardiomyopathy. *Circ Res, 95*(12), 1200–1206.
21. Huang, W. Y., Aramburu, J., Douglas, P. S., et al. (2000). Transgenic expression of green fluorescence protein can cause dilated cardiomyopathy. *Nat Med, 6*(5), 482–483.
22. Capecchi, M. R. (2005). Gene targeting in mice: functional analysis of the mammalian genome for the twenty-first century. *Nat Rev Genet, 6*(6), 507–512.
23. Moses, K. A., DeMayo, F., Braun, R. M., et al. (2001). Embryonic expression of an Nkx2-5/Cre gene using ROSA26 reporter mice. *Genesis, 31*(4), 176–180.
24. Matkovich, S. J., Diwan, A., Klanke, J. L., et al. (2006). Cardiac-specific ablation of G-protein receptor kinase 2 redefines its roles in heart development and beta-adrenergic signaling. *Circ Res, 99*(9), 996–1003.
25. Rockman, H. A., Ono, S., Ross, R. S., et al. (1994). Molecular and physiological alterations in murine ventricular dysfunction. *Proc Natl Acad Sci U S A, 91*(7), 2694–2698.
26. Michael, L. H., Entman, M. L., Hartley, C. J., et al. (1995). Myocardial ischemia and reperfusion: a murine model. *Am J Physiol, 269*, H2147–H2154.
27. Diwan, A., Krenz, M., Syed, F. M., et al. (2007). Inhibition of ischemic cardiomyocyte apoptosis through targeted ablation of Bnip3 restrains postinfarction remodeling in mice. *J Clin Invest, 117*(10), 2825–2833.
28. Rajabi, M., Kassiotis, C., Razeghi, P., et al. (2007). Return to the fetal gene program protects the stressed heart: a strong hypothesis. *Heart Fail Rev, 12*(3–4), 331–343.
29. Dorn, G. W., II (2005). Physiologic growth and pathologic genes in cardiac development and cardiomyopathy. *Trends Cardiovasc Med, 15*(5), 185–189.
30. Heineke, J., & Molkentin, J. D. (2006). Regulation of cardiac hypertrophy by intracellular signaling pathways. *Nat Rev Mol Cell Biol, 7*(8), 589–600.
31. Dorn, G. W., II, Robbins, J., & Sugden, P. H. (2003). Phenotyping hypertrophy: eschew obfuscation. *Circ Res, 92*(11), 1171–1175.
32. Li, F., Wang, X., Capasso, J. M., et al. (1996). Rapid transition of cardiac myocytes from hyperplasia to hypertrophy during postnatal development. *J Mol Cell Cardiol, 28*(8), 1737–1746.
33. Soonpaa, M. H., & Field, L. J. (1998). Survey of studies examining mammalian cardiomyocyte DNA synthesis. *Circ Res, 83*(1), 15–26.
34. Jackson, K. A., Majka, S. M., Wang, H., et al. (2001). Regeneration of ischemic cardiac muscle and vascular endothelium by adult stem cells. *J Clin Invest, 107*(11), 1395–1402.
35. Beltrami, A. P., Barlucchi, L., Torella, D., et al. (2003). Adult cardiac stem cells are multipotent and support myocardial regeneration. *Cell, 114*(6), 763–776.
36. Makino, R., Hayashi, K., & Sugimura, T. (1984). C-myc transcript is induced in rat liver at a very early stage of regeneration or by cycloheximide treatment. *Nature, 310*(5979), 697–698.
37. Chien, K. R., Knowlton, K. U., Zhu, H., et al. (1991). Regulation of cardiac gene expression during myocardial growth and hypertrophy: molecular studies of an adaptive physiologic response. *FASEB J, 5*(15), 3037–3046.
38. Pu, W. T., Ishiwata, T., Juraszek, A. L., et al. (2004). GATA4 is a dosage-sensitive regulator of cardiac morphogenesis. *Dev Biol, 275*(1), 235–244.
39. Oka, T., Maillet, M., Watt, A. J., et al. (2006). Cardiac-specific deletion of Gata4 reveals its requirement for hypertrophy, compensation, and myocyte viability. *Circ Res, 98*(6), 837–845.
40. Oka, T., Xu, J., & Molkentin, J. D. (2007). Re-employment of developmental transcription factors in adult heart disease. *Semin Cell Dev Biol, 18*(1), 117–131.
41. Niu, Z., Li, A., Zhang, S. X., et al. (2007). Serum response factor micromanaging cardiogenesis. *Curr Opin Cell Biol, 19*(6), 618–627.
42. Niu, Z., Yu, W., Zhang, S. X., et al. (2005). Conditional mutagenesis of the murine serum response factor gene blocks cardiogenesis and the transcription of downstream gene targets. *J Biol Chem, 280*(37), 32531–32538.
43. Parlakian, A., Charvet, C., Escoubet, B., et al. (2005). Temporally controlled onset of dilated cardiomyopathy through disruption of the SRF gene in adult heart. *Circulation, 112*(19), 2930–2939.
44. Xing, W., Zhang, T. C., Cao, D., et al. (2006). Myocardin induces cardiomyocyte hypertrophy. *Circ Res, 98*(8), 1089–1097.
45. Braunwald, E. (2008). Biomarkers in heart failure. *N Engl J Med, 358*(20), 2148–2159.
46. Tardiff, J. C., Hewett, T. E., Factor, S. M., et al. (2000). Expression of the beta (slow)-isoform of MHC in the adult mouse heart causes dominant-negative functional effects. *Am J Physiol Heart Circ Physiol, 278*(2), H412–H419.
47. Fielitz, J., Kim, M. S., Shelton, J. M., et al. (2007). Myosin accumulation and striated muscle myopathy result from the loss of muscle RING finger 1 and 3. *J Clin Invest, 117*(9), 2486–2495.
48. James, J., Martin, L., Krenz, M., et al. (2005). Forced expression of alpha-myosin heavy chain in the rabbit ventricle results in cardioprotection under cardiomyopathic conditions. *Circulation, 111*(18), 2339–2346.
49. Komuro, I., Kurabayashi, M., Shibazaki, Y., et al. (1989). Molecular cloning and characterization of a Ca^{2+} + Mg^{2+}-dependent adenosine triphosphatase from rat cardiac sarcoplasmic reticulum. Regulation of its expression by pressure overload and developmental stage. *J Clin Invest, 83*(4), 1102–1108.
50. Mercadier, J. J., Lompre, A. M., Duc, P., et al. (1990). Altered sarcoplasmic reticulum Ca^{2+}-ATPase gene expression in the human ventricle during end-stage heart failure. *J Clin Invest, 85*, 305–309.
51. Bers, D. M. (2006). Altered cardiac myocyte Ca regulation in heart failure. *Physiology (Bethesda), 21*, 380–387.
52. Ly, H., Kawase, Y., Yoneyama, R., et al. (2007). Gene therapy in the treatment of heart failure. *Physiology (Bethesda), 22*, 81–96.
53. Hwang, J. J., Allen, P. D., Tseng, G. C., et al. (2002). Microarray gene expression profiles in dilated and hypertrophic cardiomyopathic end-stage heart failure. *Physiol Genomics, 10*, 31–44.
54. Margulies, K. B., Matiwala, S., Cornejo, C., et al. (2005). Mixed messages: transcription patterns in failing and recovering human myocardium. *Circ Res, 96*(5), 592–599.
55. Aronow, B. J., Toyokawa, T., Canning, A., et al. (2001). Divergent transcriptional responses to independent genetic causes of cardiac hypertrophy. *Physiol Genomics, 6*(1), 19–28.
56. Dorn, G. W., II, & Matkovich, S. J. (2008). Put your chips on transcriptomics. *Circulation, 118*(3), 216–218.
57. Barth, A. S., & Hare, J. M. (2006). The potential for the transcriptome to serve as a clinical biomarker for cardiovascular diseases. *Circ Res, 98*(12), 1459–1461.
58. Kittleson, M. M., Ye, S. Q., Irizarry, R. A., et al. (2004). Identification of a gene expression profile that differentiates between ischemic and nonischemic cardiomyopathy. *Circulation, 110*(22), 3444–3451.
59. Heidecker, B., Kasper, E. K., Wittstein, I. S., et al. (2008). Transcriptomic biomarkers for individual risk assessment in new-onset heart failure. *Circulation, 118*(3), 238–246.
60. van Rooij, E., Sutherland, L. B., Liu, N., et al. (2006). A signature pattern of stress-responsive microRNAs that can evoke cardiac hypertrophy and heart failure. *Proc Natl Acad Sci U S A, 103*(48), 18255–18260.
61. Bartel, D. P. (2004). MicroRNAs: genomics, biogenesis, mechanism, and function. *Cell, 116*(2), 281–297.

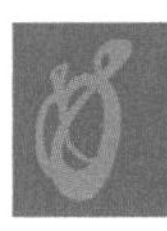

62. Thum, T., Galuppo, P., Wolf, C., et al. (2007). MicroRNAs in the human heart: a clue to fetal gene reprogramming in heart failure. *Circulation, 116*(3), 258–267.
63. Carè, A., Catalucci, D., Felicetti, F., et al. (2007). MicroRNA-133 controls cardiac hypertrophy. *Nat Med, 13*(5), 613–618.
64. Bishop, S. P. (1990). The myocardial cell: normal growth, cardiac hypertrophy and response to injury. *Toxicol Pathol, 18*(4 pt 1), 438–453.
65. Dorn, G. W., II (2007). The fuzzy logic of physiological cardiac hypertrophy. *Hypertension, 49*(5), 962–970.
66. Perrino, C., Prasad, S. V., Mao, L., et al. (2006). Intermittent pressure overload triggers hypertrophy-independent cardiac dysfunction and vascular rarefaction. *J Clin Invest, 116*(6), 1547–1560.
67. Eghbali, M., Deva, R., Alioua, A., et al. (2005). Molecular and functional signature of heart hypertrophy during pregnancy. *Circ Res, 96*(11), 1208–1216.
68. Scheuer, J., Malhotra, A., Hirsch, C., et al. (1982). Physiologic cardiac hypertrophy corrects contractile protein abnormalities associated with pathologic hypertrophy in rats. *J Clin Invest, 70*(6), 1300–1305.
69. McMullen, J. R., Amirahmadi, F., Woodcock, E. A., et al. (2007). Protective effects of exercise and phosphoinositide 3-kinase(p110alpha) signaling in dilated and hypertrophic cardiomyopathy. *Proc Natl Acad Sci U S A, 104*(2), 612–617.
70. Lupu, F., Terwilliger, J. D., Lee, K., et al. (2001). Roles of growth hormone and insulin-like growth factor 1 in mouse postnatal growth. *Dev Biol, 229*(1), 141–162.
71. Gastone, G., Serneri, N., Boddi, M., et al. (2001). Increased cardiac sympathetic activity and insulin-like growth factor-1 formation are associated with physiological hypertrophy in athletes. *Circ Res, 89*, 977–982.
72. Li, Q., Li, B., Wang, X., et al. (1997). Overexpression of insulin-like growth factor-1 in mice protects from myocyte death after infarction, attenuating ventricular dilation, wall stress, and cardiac hypertrophy. *J Clin Invest, 100*(8), 1991–1999.
73. Duerr, R. L., Huang, S., Miraliakbar, H. R., et al. (1995). Insulin-like growth factor-1 enhances ventricular hypertrophy and function during the onset of experimental cardiac failure. *J Clin Invest, 95*(2), 619–627.
74. McMullen, J. R., Shioi, T., Huang, W. Y., et al. (2004). The insulin-like growth factor 1 receptor induces physiological heart growth via the phosphoinositide-3-kinase(p110alpha) pathway. *J Biol Chem, 279*(6), 4782–4793.
75. Belke, D. D., Betuing, S., Tuttle, M. J., et al. (2002). Insulin signaling coordinately regulates cardiac size, metabolism, and contractile protein isoform expression. *J Clin Invest, 109*(5), 629–639.
76. Laustsen, P. G., Russell, S. J., Cui, L., et al. (2007). Essential role of insulin and insulin-like growth factor 1 receptor signaling in cardiac development and function. *Mol Cell Biol, 27*(5), 1649–1664.
77. Bi, L., Okabe, I., Bernard, D. J., et al. (1999). Proliferative defect and embryonic lethality in mice homozygous for a deletion in the p110alpha subunit of phosphoinositide 3-kinase. *J Biol Chem, 274*(16), 10963–10968.
78. McMullen, J. R., Shioi, T., Zhang, L., et al. (2003). Phosphoinositide 3-kinase(p110alpha) plays a critical role for the induction of physiological, but not pathological, cardiac hypertrophy. *Proc Natl Acad Sci U S A, 100*(21), 12355–12360.
79. Shioi, T., Kang, P. M., Douglas, P. S., et al. (2000). The conserved phosphoinositide 3-kinase pathway determines heart size in mice. *EMBO J, 19*(11), 2537–2548.
80. Mora, A., Davies, A. M., Bertrand, L., et al. (2003). Deficiency of PDK1 in cardiac muscle results in heart failure and increased sensitivity to hypoxia. *EMBO J, 22*(18), 4666–4676.
81. Cho, H., Thorvaldsen, J. L., Chu, Q., et al. (2001). Akt1/PKBalpha is required for normal growth but dispensable for maintenance of glucose homeostasis in mice. *J Biol Chem, 276*(42), 38349–38352.
82. Delaughter, M. C., Taffet, G. E., Florotto, M. L., et al. (1999). Local insulin-like growth factor 1 expression induces physiologic, then pathologic, cardiac hypertrophy in transgenic mice. *FASEB J, 13*(14), 1923–1929.
83. Shiojima, I., Sato, K., Izumiya, Y., et al. (2005). Disruption of coordinated cardiac hypertrophy and angiogenesis contributes to the transition to heart failure. *J Clin Invest, 115*(8), 2108–2118.
84. Vatner, S. F. (1988). Reduced subendocardial myocardial perfusion as one mechanism for congestive heart failure. *Am J Cardiol, 62*(8), 94E–98E.
85. Pelliccia, A., Maron, B. J., De Luca, R., et al. (2002). Remodeling of left ventricular hypertrophy in elite athletes after long-term deconditioning. *Circulation, 105*(8), 944–949.
86. Levy, D., Garrison, R. J., Savage, D. D., et al. (1990). Prognostic implications of echocardiographically determined left ventricular mass in the Framingham heart study. *N Engl J Med, 322*(22), 1561–1566.
87. Grossman, W., Jones, D., & McLaurin, L. P. (1975). Wall stress and patterns of hypertrophy in the human left ventricle. *J Clin Invest, 56*(1), 56–64.
88. Katz, A. M. (1991). The cardiomyopathy of overload: a hypothesis. *J Cardiovasc Pharmacol, 18*(suppl 2), S68–S71.
89. Scholz, D. G., Kitzman, D. W., Hagen, P. T., et al. (1988). Age-related changes in normal human hearts during the first 10 decades of life. Part 1 (growth): a quantitative anatomic study of 200 specimens from subjects from birth to 19 years old. *Mayo Clin Proc, 63*(2), 126–136.
90. Diez, J., González, A., López, B., et al. (2005). Mechanisms of disease: pathologic structural remodeling is more than adaptive hypertrophy in hypertensive heart disease. *Nat Clin Pract Cardiovasc Med, 2*(4), 209–216.
91. Lorell, B. H., & Carabello, B. A. (2000). Left ventricular hypertrophy: pathogenesis, detection, and prognosis. *Circulation, 102*(4), 470–479.
92. Opie, L. H., Commerford, P. J., Gersh, B. J., et al. (2006). Controversies in ventricular remodelling. *Lancet, 367*(9507), 356–367.
93. Teiger, E., Than, V. D., Richard, L., et al. (1996). Apoptosis in pressure overload-induced heart hypertrophy in the rat. *J Clin Invest, 97*(12), 2891–2897.
94. Dorn, G. W., II, & Hahn, H. S. (2004). Genetic factors in cardiac hypertrophy. *Ann N Y Acad Sci, 1015*, 225–237.
95. Esposito, G., Rapacciuolo, A., Naga Prasad, S. V., et al. (2002). Genetic alterations that inhibit in vivo pressure-overload hypertrophy prevent cardiac dysfunction despite increased wall stress. *Circulation, 105*(1), 85–92.
96. Hill, J. A., Rothermel, B., Yoo, K. D., et al. (2002). Targeted inhibition of calcineurin in pressure-overload cardiac hypertrophy. Preservation of systolic function. *J Biol Chem, 277*(12), 10251–10255.
97. Majno, G., & Joris, I. (1995). Apoptosis, oncosis, and necrosis. An overview of cell death. *Am J Pathol, 146*(1), 3–15.
98. Hein, S., Arnon, E., Kostin, S., et al. (2003). Progression from compensated hypertrophy to failure in the pressure-overloaded human heart: structural deterioration and compensatory mechanisms. *Circulation, 107*(7), 984–991.
99. Kerr, J. F. R., & Harmon, B. V. (1991). Definition and incidence of apoptosis: an historical perspective. In L. D. Tomei & F. O. Cope (Eds.). *Apoptosis: the molecular basis of cell death.* New York: Cold Spring Harbor Laboratory Press.
100. Lockshin, R. A., & Zakeri, Z. (2001). Programmed cell death and apoptosis: origins of the theory. *Nat Rev Mol Cell Biol, 2*(7), 545–550.
101. Fisher, S. A., Langille, B. L., & Srivastava, D. (2000). Apoptosis during cardiovascular development. *Circ Res, 87*(10), 856–864.
102. Watanabe, M., Choudhry, A., Berlan, M., et al. (1998). Developmental remodeling and shortening of the cardiac outflow tract involves myocyte programmed cell death. *Development, 125*(19), 3809–3820.
103. Zhao, Z., & Rivkees, S. A. (2000). Programmed cell death in the developing heart: regulation by BMP4 adn FSG2. *Dev Dyn, 217*(4), 388–400.
104. Kajstura, J., Mansukhani, M., Cheng, W., et al. (1995). Programmed cell death and expression of the protooncogene bcl-2 in myocytes during postnatal maturation of the heart. *Exp Cell Res, 219*(1), 110–121.
105. Mallat, Z., Tedgui, A., Fontaliran, F., et al. (1996). Evidence of apoptosis in arrhythmogenic right ventricular dysplasia. *N Engl J Med, 335*(16), 1190–1196.
106. Garcia-Gras, E., Lombardi, R., Giocondo, M. J., et al. (2006). Suppression of canonical Wnt/beta-catenin signaling by nuclear plakoglobin recapitulates phenotype of arrhythmogenic right ventricular cardiomyopathy. *J Clin Invest, 116*(7), 2012–2021.
107. Narula, J., Haider, N., Virmani, R., et al. (1996). Apoptosis in myocytes in end-stage heart failure. *N Engl J Med, 335*(16), 1182–1189.
108. Olivetti, G., Abbi, R., Quaini, F., et al. (1997). Apoptosis in the failing human heart. *N Engl J Med, 336*(16), 1131–1141.
109. Saraste, A., Pulkki, K., Kallajoki, M., et al. (1997). Apoptosis in human acute myocardial infarction. *Circulation, 95*(2), 320–323.
110. Gottlieb, R. A., Burleson, K. O., Kloner, R. A., et al. (1994). Reperfusion injury induces apoptosis in rabbit cardiomyocytes. *J Clin Invest, 94*(4), 1621–1628.
111. Dorn, G. W., II, & Diwan, A. (2008). The rationale for cardiomyocyte resuscitation in myocardial salvage. *J Mol Med.*
112. Diwan, A., & Dorn, G. W. (2007). Decompensation of cardiac hypertrophy: cellular mechanisms and novel therapeutic targets. *Physiology (Bethesda), 22*, 56–64.
113. Mann, D. L. (2003). Stress-activated cytokines and the heart: from adaptation to maladaptation. *Annu Rev Physiol, 65*, 81–101.
114. Baumgarten, G., Knuefermann, P., Kalra, D., et al. (2002). Load-dependent and -independent regulation of proinflammatory cytokine and cytokine receptor gene expression in the adult mammalian heart. *Circulation, 105*(18), 2192–2197.
115. Oral, H., Dorn, G. W., & Mann, D. L. (1997). Sphingosine mediates the immediate negative inotropic effects of tumor necrosis factor-alpha in the adult mammalian cardiac myocyte. *J Biol Chem, 272*(8), 4836–4842.
116. Yokoyama, T., Nakano, M., Bednarczyk, J. L., et al. (1997). Tumor necrosis factor-α provokes a hypertrophic growth response in adult cardiac myocytes. *Circulation, 95*(5), 1247–1252.
117. Levine, B., Kalman, J., Mayer, L., et al. (1990). Elevated circulating levels of tumor necrosis factor in severe chronic heart failure. *N Engl J Med, 323*(4), 236–241.
118. Sivasubramanian, N., Coker, M. L., Kurrelmeyer, K. M., et al. (2001). Left ventricular remodeling in transgenic mice with cardiac restricted overexpression of tumor necrosis factor. *Circulation, 104*(7), 826–831.
119. Haudek, S. B., Taffet, G. E., Schneider, M. D., et al. (2007). TNF provokes cardiomyocyte apoptosis and cardiac remodeling through activation of multiple cell death pathways. *J Clin Invest, 117*(9), 2692–2701.
120. Crow, M. T., Mani, K., Nam, Y. J., et al. (2004). The mitochondrial death pathway and cardiac myocyte apoptosis. *Circ Res, 95*(10), 957–970.
121. Aaronson, D. S., & Horvath, C. M. (2002). A road map for those who don't know JAK-STAT. *Science, 296*(5573), 1653–1655.
122. Yoshimura, A., Naka, T., & Kubo, M. (2007). SOCS proteins, cytokine signalling and immune regulation. *Nat Rev Immunol, 7*(6), 454–465.
123. Fischer, P., & Hilfiker-Kleiner, D. (2008). Role of gp130-mediated signalling pathways in the heart and its impact on potential therapeutic aspects. *Br J Pharmacol, 153*(suppl 1), S414–S427.
124. Yoshida, K., Taga, T., Saito, M., et al. (1996). Targeted disruption of gp130, a common signal transducer for the interleukin 6 family of cytokines, leads to myocardial and hematological disorders. *Proc Natl Acad Sci U S A, 93*(1), 407–411.
125. Hirota, H., Chen, J., Betz, U. A., et al. (1999). Loss of a gp130 cardiac muscle cell survival pathway is a critical event in the onset of heart failure during biomechanical stress. *Cell, 97*(2), 189–198.
126. Hirota, H., Yoshida, K., Kishimoto, T., et al. (1995). Continuous activation of gp130, a signal-transducing receptor component for interleukin 6-related cytokines, causes myocardial hypertrophy in mice. *Proc Natl Acad Sci U S A, 92*(11), 4862–4866.
127. Uozumi, H., Hiroi, Y., Zou, Y., et al. (2001). gp130 plays a critical role in pressure overload-induced cardiac hypertrophy. *J Biol Chem, 276*(25), 23115–23119.
128. Pan, J., Fukuda, K., Saito, M., et al. (1999). Mechanical stretch activates the JAK/STAT pathway in rat cardiomyocytes. *Circ Res, 84*(10), 1127–1136.
129. Yasukawa, H., Hoshijima, M., Gu, Y., et al. (2001). Suppressor of cytokine signaling-3 is a biomechanical stress-inducible gene that suppresses gp130-mediated cardiac myocyte hypertrophy and survival pathways. *J Clin Invest, 108*(10), 1459–1467.
130. Yajima, T., Yasukawa, H., Jeon, E. S., et al. (2006). Innate defense mechanism against virus infection within the cardiac myocyte requiring gp130-STAT3 signaling. *Circulation, 114*, 2364–2373.

131. Mizushima, N., Levine, B., Cuervo, A. M., et al. (2008). Autophagy fights disease through cellular self-digestion. *Nature, 451*(7182), 1069–1075.
132. Kuma, A., Hatano, M., Matsui, M., et al. (2004). The role of autophagy during the early neonatal starvation period. *Nature, 432*(7020), 1032–1036.
133. Schaper, J., Froede, R., Hein, S., et al. (1991). Impairment of the myocardial ultrastructure and changes of the cytoskeleton in dilated cardiomyopathy. *Circulation, 83*(2), 504–514.
134. Zhu, H., Tannous, P., Johnstone, J. L., et al. (2007). Cardiac autophagy is a maladaptive response to hemodynamic stress. *J Clin Invest, 117*(7), 1782–1793.
135. Dammrich, J., & Pfeifer, U. (1983). Cardiac hypertrophy in rats after supravalvular aortic constriction. II. Inhibition of cellular autophagy in hypertrophying cardiomyocytes. *Virchows Arch B Cell Pathol Incl Mol Pathol, 43*(3), 287–307.
136. Matsui, Y., Takagi, H., Qu, X., et al. (2007). Distinct roles of autophagy in the heart during ischemia and reperfusion: roles of AMP-activated protein kinase and Beclin 1 in mediating autophagy. *Circ Res, 100*(6), 914–922.
137. Nakai, A., Yamaguchi, O., Takeda, T., et al. (2007). The role of autophagy in cardiomyocytes in the basal state and in response to hemodynamic stress. *Nat Med, 13*(5), 619–624.
138. Tomanek, R. J. (1992). Age as a modulator of coronary capillary angiogenesis. *Circulation, 86*(1), 320–321.
139. Anversa, P., & Capasso, J. M. (1991). Loss of intermediate-sized coronary arteries and capillary proliferation after left ventricular failure in rats. *Am J Phys, 260*(5 pt 2), H1552–H1560.
140. Walsh, K., & Shiojima, I. (2007). Cardiac growth and angiogenesis coordinated by intertissue interactions. *J Clin Invest, 117*(11), 3176–3179.
141. Heineke, J., Auger-Messier, M., Xu, J., et al. (2007). Cardiomyocyte GATA4 function as a stress-responsive regulator of angiogenesis in the murine heart. *J Clin Invest, 117*(11), 3198–3210.
142. Sano, M., Minamino, T., Toko, H., et al. (2007). p53-induced inhibition of Hif-1 causes cardiac dysfunction during pressure overload. *Nature, 446*(7134), 444–448.
143. Mann, D. L., Kent, R. L., Parsons, B., et al. (1992). Adrenergic effects on the biology of the adult mammalian cardiocyte. *Circulation, 85*(2), 790–804.
144. Shizukuda, Y., Buttrick, P. M., Geenen, D. L., et al. (1998). β-adrenergic stimulation causes cardiocyte apoptosis: influence of tachycardia and hypertrophy. *Am J Phys, 275*(3 pt 2), H961–H968.
145. Rockman, H. A., Koch, W. J., & Lefkowitz, R. J. (2002). Seven-transmembrane-spanning receptors and heart function. *Nature, 415*(6868), 206–212.
146. Bristow, M. R., Ginsburg, R., Minobe, W., et al. (1982). Decreased catecholamine sensitivity and beta-adrenergic-receptor density in failing human hearts. *N Engl J Med, 307*(4), 205–211.
147. Bers, D. M. (2008). Calcium cycling and signaling in cardiac myocytes. *Annu Rev Physiol, 70*, 23–49.
148. Liggett, S. B., Tepe, N. M., Lorenz, J. N., et al. (2000). Early and delayed consequences of beta(2)-adrenergic receptor overexpression in mouse hearts: critical role for expression level. *Circulation, 101*(14), 1707–1714.
149. Milano, C. A., Allen, L. F., Rockman, H. A., et al. (1994). Enhanced myocardial function in transgenic mice overexpressing the beta 2-adrenergic receptor. *Science, 264*(5158), 582–586.
150. Dorn, G. W., II, Tepe, N. M., Lorenz, J. N., et al. (1999). Low- and high-level transgenic expression of beta2-adrenergic receptors differentially affect cardiac hypertrophy and function in Galphaq-overexpressing mice. *Proc Natl Acad Sci U S A, 96*(11), 6400–6405.
151. Engelhardt, S., Hein, L., Wiesmann, F., et al. (1999). Progressive hypertrophy and heart failure in beta1-adrenergic receptor transgenic mice. *Proc Natl Acad Sci U S A, 96*(12), 7059–7064.
152. Iwase, M., Bishop, S. P., Uechi, M., et al. (1996). Adverse effects of chronic endogenous sympathetic drive induced by cardiac GS alpha overexpression. *Circ Res, 78*(4), 517–524.
153. Communal, C., Singh, K., Sawyer, D. B., et al. (1999). Opposing effects of β(1)- and β(2)-adrenergic receptors on cardiac myocyte apoptosis: role of a pertussis toxin-sensitive G protein. *Circulation, 100*(22), 2210–2212.
154. Fleckenstein, A., Janke, J., Doring, H. J., et al. (1974). Myocardial fiber necrosis due to intracellular Ca overload—a new principle in cardiac pathophysiology. *Recent Adv Stud Cardiac Struct Metab, 4*, 563–580.
155. Danial, N. N., & Korsmeyer, S. J. (2004). Cell death: critical control points. *Cell, 116*(2), 205–219.
156. Nakayama, H., Chen, X., Baines, C. P., et al. (2007). Ca^{2+}- and mitochondrial-dependent cardiomyocyte necrosis as a primary mediator of heart failure. *J Clin Invest, 117*(9), 2431–2444.
157. Baines, C. P., Kaiser, R. A., Purcell, N. H., et al. (2005). Loss of cyclophilin D reveals a critical role for mitochondrial permeability transition in cell death. *Nature, 434*(7033), 658–662.
158. Zhu, W. Z., Wang, S. Q., Chakir, K., et al. (2003). Linkage of β1-adrenergic stimulation to apoptotic heart cell death through protein kinase A-independent activation of Ca^{2+}/calmodulin kinase II. *J Clin Invest, 111*(5), 617–625.
159. Yang, Y., Zhu, W. Z., Joiner, M. L., et al. (2006). Calmodulin kinase II inhibition protects against myocardial cell apoptosis in vivo. *Am J Physiol Heart Circ Physiol, 291*(6), H3065–H3075.
160. Zhang, R., Khoo, M. S., Wu, Y., et al. (2005). Calmodulin kinase II inhibition protects against structural heart disease. *Nat Med, 11*(4), 409–417.
161. Xiao, R. P. (2001). β-adrenergic signaling in the heart: dual coupling of the β2-adrenergic receptor to G(s) and G(i) proteins. *Sci STKE, 104*, RE15.
162. Zhu, W. Z., Zheng, M., Koch, W. J., et al. (2001). Dual modulation of cell survival and cell death by β(2)-adrenergic signaling in adult mouse cardiac myocytes. *Proc Natl Acad Sci U S A, 98*(4), 1607–1612.
163. Daaka, Y., Luttrell, L. M., & Lefkowitz, R. J. (1997). Switching of the coupling of the β1-adrenergic receptor to different G proteins by protein kinase A. *Nature, 390*(6655), 88–91.
164. DeGeorge, B. R., Jr., Gao, E., Boucher, M., et al. (2008). Targeted inhibition of cardiomyocyte Gi signaling enhances susceptibility to apoptotic cell death in response to ischemic stress. *Circulation, 117*(11), 1378–1387.
165. Small, K. M., Wagoner, L. E., Levin, A. M., et al. (2002). Synergistic polymorphisms of beta1- and alpha2C-adrenergic receptors and the risk of congestive heart failure. *N Engl J Med, 347*(15), 1135–1142.
166. Liggett, S. B., Mialet-Perez, J., Thaneemit-Chen, S., et al. (2006). A polymorphism within a conserved beta(1)-adrenergic receptor motif alters cardiac function and beta-blocker response in human heart failure. *Proc Natl Acad Sci U S A, 103*(30), 11288–11293.
167. Koch, W. J., Rockman, H. A., Samama, P., et al. (1995). Cardiac function in mice overexpressing the β-adrenergic receptor kinase or a βARK inhibitor. *Science, 268*(5215), 1350–1353.
168. Rockman, H. A., Chien, K. R., Choi, D. J., et al. (1998). Expression of a β-adrenergic receptor kinase 1 inhibitor prevents the development of myocardial failure in gene-targeted mice. *Proc Natl Acad Sci U S A, 95*(12), 7000–7005.
169. Harding, V. B., Jones, L. R., Lefkowitz, R. J., et al. (2001). Cardiac beta ARK1 inhibition prolongs survival and augments beta blocker therapy in a mouse model of severe heart failure. *Proc Natl Acad Sci U S A, 98*(10), 5809–5814.
170. Raake, P. W., Vinge, L. E., Gao, E., et al. (2008). G protein-coupled receptor kinase 2 ablation in cardiac myocytes before or after myocardial infarction prevents heart failure. *Circ Res.*
171. Lowes, B. D., Gilbert, E. M., Abraham, W. T., et al. (2002). Myocardial gene expression in dilated cardiomyopathy treated with β-blocking agents. *N Engl J Med, 346*(18), 1357–1365.
172. Noma, T., Lemaire, A., Naga Prasad, S. V., et al. (2007). β-arrestin-mediated β1-adrenergic receptor transactivation of the EGFR confers cardioprotection. *J Clin Invest, 117*(9), 2445–2458.
173. Wisler, J. W., DeWire, S. M., Whalen, E. J., et al. (2007). A unique mechanism of β-blocker action: carvedilol stimulates β-arrestin signaling. *Proc Natl Acad Sci U S A, 104*(42), 16657–16662.
174. Liggett, S. B., Cresci, S., Kelly, R. J., et al. (2008). A GRK5 polymorphism that inhibits β-adrenergic receptor signaling is protective in heart failure. *Nat Med, 14*(5), 510–517.
175. Barki-Harrington, L., & Rockman, H. A. (2003). Sensing heart stress. *Nat Med, 9*(1), 19–20.
176. Laser, M., Willey, C. D., Jiang, W., et al. (2000). Integrin activation and focal complex formation in cardiac hypertrophy. *J Biol Chem, 275*(45), 35624–35630.
177. Dimichele, L. A., Doherty, J. T., Rojas, M., et al. (2006). Myocyte-restricted focal adhesion kinase deletion attenuates pressure overload-induced hypertrophy. *Circ Res, 99*(6), 636–645.
178. Clemente, C. F., Tornatore, T. F., Theizen, T. H., et al. (2007). Targeting focal adhesion kinase with small interfering RNA prevents and reverses load-induced cardiac hypertrophy in mice. *Circ Res, 101*(12), 1339–1348.
179. Lu, H., Fedak, P. W., Dai, X., et al. (2006). Integrin-linked kinase expression is elevated in human cardiac hypertrophy and induces hypertrophy in transgenic mice. *Circulation, 114*(21), 2271–2279.
180. Hannigan, G. E., Coles, J. G., & Dedhar, S. (2007). Integrin-linked kinase at the heart of cardiac contractility, repair, and disease. *Circ Res, 100*(10), 1408–1414.
181. Brancaccio, M., Fratta, L., Notte, A., et al. (2003). Melusin, a muscle-specific integrin beta1-interacting protein, is required to prevent cardiac failure in response to chronic pressure overload. *Nat Med, 9*(1), 68–75.
182. Zemlijic-Harpf, A. E., Miller, J. C., Henderson, S. A., et al. (2007). Cardiac-myocyte-specific excision of the vinculin gene disrupts cellular junctions, causing sudden death or dilated cardiomyopathy. *Mol Cell Biol, 27*(21), 7522–7537.
183. Ren, J., Avery, J., Zhao, H., et al. (2007). β3 integrin deficiency promotes cardiac hypertrophy and inflammation. *J Mol Cell Cardiol, 42*(2), 367–377.
184. Knöll, R., Hoshijima, M., Hoffman, H. M., et al. (2002). The cardiac mechanical stretch sensor machinery involves a Z disc complex that is defective in a subset of human dilated cardiomyopathy. *Cell, 111*(7), 943–955.
185. Granzier, H. L., & Labeit, S. (2004). The giant protein titin: a major player in myocardial mechanics, signaling, and disease. *Circ Res, 94*(3), 284–295.
186. Lammerding, J., Kamm, R. D., & Lee, R. T. (2004). Mechanotransduction in cardiac myocytes. *Ann N Y Acad Sci, 1015*, 53–70.
187. Sadoshima, J., Xu, Y., Slayter, H. S., et al. (1993). Autocrine release of angiotensin II mediates stretch-induced hypertrophy of cardiac myocytes in vitro. *Cell, 75*(5), 977–984.
188. Zou, Y., Akazawa, H., Qin, Y., et al. (2004). Mechanical stress activates angiotensin II type 1 receptor without the involvement of angiotensin II. *Nat Cell Biol, 6*(6), 499–506.
189. Kim, N. N., Villarreal, F. J., Printz, M. P., et al. (1995). Trophic effects of angiotensin II on neonatal rat cardiac myocytes are mediated by cardiac fibroblasts. *Am J Physiol Endocrinol Metab, 269*, E426–E437.
190. Woodcock, E. A. (2007). Roles of a1A- and a1B-adrenoceptors in heart: insights from studies of genetically modified mice. *Clin Exp Pharmacol Physiol, 34*(9), 884–888.
191. O'Connell, T. D., Ishizaka, S., Nakamura, A., et al. (2003). The alpha(1A/C)- and alpha(1B)-adrenergic receptors are required for physiological cardiac hypertrophy in the double-knockout mouse. *J Clin Invest, 111*(11), 1783–1791.
192. O'Connell, T. D., Swigart, P. M., Rodrigo, M. C., et al. (2006). α1-adrenergic receptors prevent a maladaptive cardiac response to pressure overload. *J Clin Invest, 116*(4), 1005–1015.
193. Huang, Y., Wright, C. D., Merkwan, C. L., et al. (2007). An α1A-adrenergic-extracellular signal-related kinase survival signaling pathway in cardiac myocytes. *Circulation, 115*(6), 763–772.
194. Paradis, P., Dali-Youcef, N., Paradis, F. W., et al. (2000). Overexpression of angiotensin II type 1 receptor in cardiomyocytes induces cardiac hypertrophy and remodeling. *Proc Natl Acad Sci U S A, 97*(2), 931–936.
195. Harada, K., Sugaya, T., Murakami, K., et al. (1999). Angiotensin II type 1A receptor knockout mice display less left ventricular remodeling and improved survival after myocardial infarction. *Circulation, 100*(20), 2093–2099.

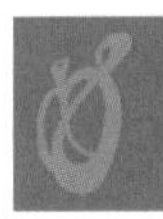

196. Granger, C. B., McMurray, J. J., Yusuf, S., et al. (2003). Effects of candesartan in patients with chronic heart failure and reduced left-ventricular systolic function intolerant to angiotensin-converting-enzyme inhibitors: the CHARM-alternative trial. *Lancet, 362*(9386), 772–776.
197. Salazar, N. C., Chen, J., & Rockman, H. A. (2007). Cardiac GPCRs: GPCR signaling in healthy and failing hearts. *Biochim Biophys Acta, 1768*(4), 1006–1018.
198. Ito, H., Hirata, Y., Adachi, S., et al. (1993). Endothelin-1 is an autocrine/paracrine factor in the mechanisms of angiotensin II-induced hypertrophy in cultured rat cardiomyocytes. *J Clin Invest, 92*(1), 398–403.
199. Ito, H., Hiroe, M., Hirata, Y., et al. (1994). Endothelin ETA receptor antagonist blocks cardiac hypertrophy provoked by hemodynamic overload. *Circulation, 89*(5), 2198–2203.
200. Kedzierski, R. M., Grayburn, P. A., Kisanuki, Y. Y., et al. (2003). Cardiomyocyte-specific endothelin A receptor knockout mice have normal cardiac function and an unaltered hypertrophic response to angiotensin II and isoproterenol. *Mol Cell Biol, 23*(22), 8226–8232.
201. Dorn, G. W., II, & Force, T. (2005). Protein kinase cascades in the regulation of cardiac hypertrophy. *J Clin Invest, 115*(3), 527–537.
202. Offermanns, S., Zhao, L. P., Gohla, A., et al. (1998). Embryonic cardiomyocyte hypoplasia and craniofacial defects in G alpha q/G alpha 11-mutant mice. *EMBO J, 17*(15), 4304–4312.
203. Adams, J. W., Sakata, Y., Davis, M. G., et al. (1998). Enhanced Galphaq signaling: a common pathway mediates cardiac hypertrophy and apoptotic heart failure. *Proc Natl Acad Sci U S A, 95*(17), 10140–10145.
204. Sakata, Y., Hoit, B. D., Liggett, S. B., et al. (1998). Decompensation of pressure-overload hypertrophy in G alpha q-overexpressing mice. *Circulation, 97*(15), 1488–1495.
205. Akhter, S. A., Luttrell, L. M., Rockman, H. A., et al. (1998). Targeting the receptor-Gq interface to inhibit in vivo pressure overload myocardial hypertrophy. *Science, 280*(5363), 574–577.
206. Rogers, J. H., Tamirisa, P., Kovacs, A., et al. (1999). RGS4 causes increased mortality and reduced cardiac hypertrophy in response to pressure overload. *J Clin Invest, 104*(5), 567–576.
207. Wettschureck, N., Rutten, H., Zywietz, A., et al. (2001). Absence of pressure overload induced myocardial hypertrophy after conditional inactivation of Galphaq/Galpha11 in cardiomyocytes. *Nat Med, 7*(11), 1236–1240.
208. Liggett, S. B., Kelly, R. J., Parekh, R. R., et al. (2007). A functional polymorphism of the Galphaq (GNAQ) gene is associated with accelerated mortality in African-American heart failure. *Hum Mol Genet, 16*(22), 2740–2750.
209. Frey, U. H., Lieb, W., Erdmann, J., et al. (2008). Characterization of the GNAQ promoter and association of increased Gq expression with cardiac hypertrophy in humans. *Eur Heart J, 29*(7), 888–897.
210. Kim, D., Jun, K. S., Lee, S. B., et al. (1997). Phospholipase C isozymes selectively couple to specific neurotransmitter receptors. *Nature, 389*(6648), 290–293.
211. Li, Z., Jiang, H., Xie, W., et al. (2000). Roles of PGC-β2 and -β3 and P13Kγ in chemoattractant-mediated signal transduction. *Science, 287*(5455), 1046–1049.
212. Wang, H., Oestreich, E. A., Maekawa, N., et al. (2005). Phospholipase C epsilon modulates β-adrenergic receptor-dependent cardiac contraction and inhibits cardiac hypertrophy. *Circ Res, 97*(12), 1305–1313.
213. Dorn, G. W., II, Tepe, N. M., Wu, G., et al. (2000). Mechanisms of impaired beta-adrenergic receptor signaling in G(alphaq)-mediated cardiac hypertrophy and ventricular dysfunction. *Mol Pharmacol, 57*(2), 278–287.
214. Bowling, N., Walsh, R. A., Song, G., et al. (1999). Increased protein kinase C activity and expression of $Ca2^+$-sensitive isoforms in the failing human heart. *Circulation, 99*(3), 384–391.
215. Braz, J. C., Gregory, K., Pathak, A., et al. (2004). PKC-alpha regulates cardiac contractility and propensity toward heart failure. *Nat Med, 10*(3), 248–254.
216. Hahn, H. S., Marreez, Y., Odley, A., et al. (2003). Protein kinase Ca negatively regulates systolic and diastolic function in pathological hypertrophy. *Circ Res, 93*(11), 1111–1119.
217. Hambleton, M., Hahn, H., Pleger, S. T., et al. (2006). Pharmacological and gene therapy-based inhibition of protein kinase Ca/b enhances cardiac contractility and attenuates heart failure. *Circulation, 114*(6), 574–582.
218. Wakasaki, H., Koya, D., Schoen, F. J., et al. (1997). Targeted overexpression of protein kinase C beta2 isoform in myocardium causes cardiomyopathy. *Proc Natl Acad Sci U S A, 94*(17), 9320–9325.
219. Roman, B. B., Geenen, D. L., Leitges, M., et al. (2001). PKC-beta is not necessary for cardiac hypertrophy. *Am J Physiol Heart Circ Physiol, 280*(5), H2264–H2270.
220. Chen, L., Hahn, H., Wu, G., et al. (2001). Opposing cardioprotective actions and parallel hypertrophic effects of delta PKC and epsilon PKC.. *Proc Natl Acad Sci U S A, 98*(20), 11114–11119.
221. Mochly-Rosen, D., Wu, G., Hahn, H., et al. (2000). Cardiotrophic effects of protein kinase C epsilon: analysis by in vivo modulation of PKCepsilon translocation. *Circ Res, 86*(11), 1173–1179.
222. Wu, G., Toyokawa, T., Hahn, H., et al. (2000). Epsilon protein kinase C in pathological myocardial hypertrophy. Analysis by combined transgenic expression of translocation modifiers and Galphaq. *J Biol Chem, 275*(39), 29927–29930.
223. Harrison, B. C., Kim, M. S., van Rooij, E., et al. (2006). Regulation of cardiac stress signaling by protein kinase D1. *Mol Cell Biol, 26*(10), 3875–3888.
224. Fielitz, J., Kim, M. S., Shelton, J. M., et al. (2008). Requirement of protein kinase D1 for pathological cardiac remodeling. *Proc Natl Acad Sci U S A, 105*(8), 3059–3063.
225. Clerk, A., Cullingford, T. E., Fuller, S. J., et al. (2007). Signaling pathways mediating cardiac myocyte gene expression in physiological and stress responses. *J Cell Physiol, 212*(2), 311–322.
226. Yamamoto, S., Yang, G., Zablocki, D., et al. (2003). Activation of Mst1 causes dilated cardiomyopathy by stimulating apoptosis without compensatory ventricular myocyte hypertrophy. *J Clin Invest, 111*(10), 1463–1474.
227. Esposito, G., Prasad, S. V., Rapacciuolo, A., et al. (2001). Cardiac overexpression of a G(q) inhibitor blocks induction of extracellular signal-regulated kinase and c-Jun NH(2)-terminal kinase activity in in vivo pressure overload. *Circulation, 103*(10), 1453–1458.
228. Sanna, B., Bueno, O. F., Dai, Y. S., et al. (2005). Direct and indirect interactions between calcineurin-NFAT and MEK1-extracellular signal-regulated kinase1/2 signaling pathways regulate cardiac gene expression and cellular growth. *Mol Cell Biol, 25*(3), 865–878.
229. Pagès, G., Guérin, S., Grall, D., et al. (1999). Defective thymocyte maturation in p44 MAP kinase (Erk 1) knockout mice. *Science, 286*(5443), 1374–1377.
230. Saba-El-Leil, M. K., Vella, F. D., Vernay, B., et al. (2003). An essential function of the mitogen-activated protein kinase Erk2 in mouse trophoblast development. *EMBO Rep, 4*(10), 964–968.
231. Nicol, R. L., Frey, N., Pearson, G., et al. (2001). Activated MEK5 induces serial assembly of sarcomeres and eccentric cardiac hypertrophy. *EMBO J, 20*(11), 2757–2767.
232. Wang, X., Merritt, A. J., Seyfried, J., et al. (2005). Targeted deletion of mek5 causes early embryonic death and defects in the extracellular signal-regulated kinase 5/myocyte enhancer factor 2 cell survival pathway. *Mol Cell Biol, 25*(1), 336–345.
233. Wang, Y. (2007). Mitogen-activated protein kinase in heart development and diseases. *Circulation, 116*(12), 1413–1423.
234. Liang, Q., Bueno, O. F., Wilkins, B. J., et al. (2003). c-Jun N-terminal kinases (JNK) antagonize cardiac growth through cross-talk with calcineurin-NFAT signaling. *EMBO J, 22*(19), 5079–5089.
235. Izumiya, Y., Kim, S., Izumi, Y., et al. (2003). Apoptosis signal-regulating kinase 1 plays a pivotal role in angiotensin II-induced cardiac hypertrophy and remodeling. *Circ Res, 93*(9), 874–883.
236. Yamaguchi, O., Higuchi, Y., Hirotani, S., et al. (2003). Targeted deletion of apoptosis signal-regulating kinase 1 attenuates left ventricular remodeling. *Proc Natl Acad Sci U S A, 100*(26), 15883–15888.
237. Balijepalli, R. C., Foell, J. D., Hall, D. D., et al. (2006). Localization of cardiac L-type Ca (2+) channels to a caveolar macromolecular signaling complex is required for β(2)-adrenergic regulation. *Proc Natl Acad Sci U S A, 103*(19), 7500–7505.
238. Wu, X., Zhang, T., Bossuyt, J., et al. (2006). Local InsP3-dependent perinuclear Ca^{2+} signaling in cardiac myocyte excitation-transcription coupling. *J Clin Invest, 116*(3), 675–682.
239. Molkentin, J. D., Lu, J. R., Antos, C. L., et al. (1998). A calcineurin-dependent transcriptional pathway for cardiac hypertrophy. *Cell, 93*(2), 215–228.
240. Haq, S., Choukroun, G., Lim, H., et al. (2001). Differential activation of signal transduction pathways in human hearts with hypertrophy versus advanced heart failure. *Circulation, 103*(5), 670–677.
241. De Windt, L. J., Lim, H. W., Taigen, T., et al. (2000). Calcineurin-mediated hypertrophy protects cardiomyocytes from apoptosis in vitro and in vivo: an apoptosis-independent model of dilated heart failure. *Circ Res, 86*(3), 255–263.
242. Dorn, G. W., II, & Molkentin, J. D. (2004). Manipulating cardiac contractility in heart failure: data from mice and men. *Circulation, 109*(2), 150–158.
243. Zou, Y., Hiroi, Y., Uozumi, H., et al. (2001). Calcineurin plays a critical role in the development of pressure overload-induced cardiac hypertrophy. *Circulation, 104*(1), 97–101.
244. Frey, N., Barrientos, T., Shelton, J. M., et al. (2004). Mice lacking calsarcin-1 are sensitized to calcineurin signaling and show accelerated cardiomyopathy in response to pathological biomechanical stress. *Nat Med, 10*(12), 1336–1343.
245. de la Pompa, J. L., Timmerman, L. A., Takimoto, H., et al. (1998). Role of the NF-ATc transcription factor in morphogenesis of cardiac valves and septum. *Nature, 392*(6672), 182–186.
246. Chang, C. P., Neilson, J. R., Bayle, J. H., et al. (2004). A field of myocardial-endocardial NFAT signaling underlies heart valve morphogenesis. *Cell, 118*(5), 649–663.
247. Bourajjaj, M., Armand, A. S., da Costa Martins, P. A., et al. (2008). NFATc2 is a necessary mediator of calcineurin-dependent cardiac hypertrophy and heart failure. *J Biol Chem.*
248. Wilkins, B. J., De Windt, L. J., Bueno, O. F., et al. (2002). Targeted disruption of NFATc3, but not NFATc4, reveals an intrinsic defect in calcineurin-mediated cardiac hypertrophic growth. *Mol Cell Biol, 22*(21), 7603–7613.
249. Rothermel, B. A., Vega, R. B., & Williams, R. S. (2003). The role of modulatory calcineurin-interacting proteins in calcineurin signaling. *Trends Cardiovasc Med, 13*(1), 15–21.
250. Yang, J., Rothermel, B., Vega, R. B., et al. (2000). Independent signals control expression of the calcineurin inhibitory proteins MCIP1 and MCIP2 in striated muscles. *Circ Res, 87*(12), E61–E68.
251. van Rooij, E., Doevendans, P. A., Crijns, H. J., et al. (2004). MCIP1 overexpression suppresses left ventricular remodeling and sustains cardiac function after myocardial infarction. *Circ Res, 94*(3), e18–e26.
252. Vega, R. B., Rothermel, B. A., Weinheimer, C. J., et al. (2003). Dual roles of modulatory calcineurin-interacting protein 1 in cardiac hypertrophy. *Proc Natl Acad Sci U S A, 100*(2), 669–674.
253. Sanna, B., Brandt, E. B., Kaiser, R. A., et al. (2006). Modulatory calcineurin-interacting proteins 1 and 2 function as calcineurin facilitators in vivo. *Proc Natl Acad Sci U S A, 103*(19), 7327–7332.
254. Couchonnal, L. F., & Anderson, M. E. (2008). The role of calmodulin kinase II in myocardial physiology and disease. *Physiology (Bethesda), 23*, 151–159.
255. Passier, R., Zeng, H., Frey, N., et al. (2000). CaM kinase signaling induces cardiac hypertrophy and activates the MEF2 transcription factor in vivo. *J Clin Invest, 105*(10), 1395–1406.
256. Colomer, J. M., Mao, L., Rockman, H. A., et al. (2003). Pressure overload selectively up-regulates Ca^{2+}/calmodulin-dependent protein kinase II in vivo. *Mol Endocrinol, 17*(2), 183–192.
257. Zhang, T., Johnson, E. N., Gu, Y., et al. (2002). The cardiac-specific nuclear d_B isoform of Ca^{2+}/calmodulin-dependent protein kinase II induces hypertrophy and dilated cardiomyopathy associated with increased protein phosphatase 2A activity. *J Biol Chem, 277*(2), 1261–1267.
258. Maier, L. S., Zhang, T., Chen, L., et al. (2003). Transgenic CaMKIIdeltaC overexpression uniquely alters cardiac myocyte Ca^{2+} handling: reduced SR Ca^{2+} load and activated SR Ca^{2+} release. *Circ Res, 92*(8), 904–911.
259. Backs, J., Song, K., Bezprozvannaya, S., et al. (2006). CaM kinase Ii selectively signals to histone deacetylase 4 during cardiomyocyte hypertrophy. *J Clin Invest, 116*(7), 1853–1864.

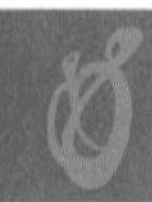

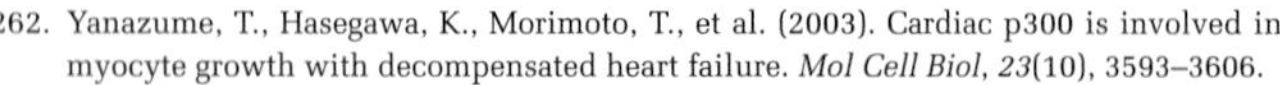

260. Epstein, J. A. (2008). Currying favor for the heart. *J Clin Invest, 118*(3), 850–852.
261. Shikama, N., Lutz, W., Kretzschmar, R., et al. (2003). Essential function of p300 acetyltransferase activity in heart, lung and small intestine formation. *EMBO J, 22*(19), 5175–5185.
262. Yanazume, T., Hasegawa, K., Morimoto, T., et al. (2003). Cardiac p300 is involved in myocyte growth with decompensated heart failure. *Mol Cell Biol, 23*(10), 3593–3606.
263. Miyamoto, S., Kawamura, T., Morimoto, T., et al. (2006). Histone acetyltransferase activity of p300 is required for the promotion of left ventricular remodeling after myocardial infarction in adult mice in vivo. *Circulation, 113*(5), 679–690.
264. Li, H. L., Liu, C., de Couto, G., et al. (2008). Curcumin prevents and reverses murine cardiac hypertrophy. *J Clin Invest, 118*(3), 879–893.
265. Trivedi, C. M., Luo, Y., Yin, Z., et al. (2007). Hdac2 regulates the cardiac hypertrophic response by modulating Gsk3 b activity. *Nat Med, 13*(3), 324–331.
266. Zhang, C. L., McKinsey, T. A., Chang, S., et al. (2002). Class II histone deacetylases act as signal-responsive repressors of cardiac hypertrophy. *Cell, 110*(4), 479–488.
267. Chang, S., McKinsey, T. A., Zhang, C. L., et al. (2004). Histone deacetylases 5 and 9 govern responsiveness of the heart to a subset of stress signals and play redundant roles in heart development. *Mol Cell Biol, 24*(19), 8467–8476.
268. McKinsey, T. A., & Olson, E. N. (2005). Toward transcriptional therapies for the failing heart: chemical screens to modulate genes. *J Clin Invest, 115*(3), 538–546.
269. Olson, E. N., Backs, J., & McKinsey, T. A. (2006). Control of cardiac hypertrophy and heart failure by histone acetylation/deacetylation. *Novartis Found Symp, 274*, 3–12.
270. Kim, Y., Phan, D., van Rooij, E., et al. (2008). The MEF2D transcription factor mediates stress-dependent cardiac remodeling in mice. *J Clin Invest, 118*(1), 124–132.
271. Kook, H., Lepore, J. J., Gitler, A. D., et al. (2003). Cardiac hypertrophy and histone deacetylase-dependent transcriptional repression mediated by the atypical homeodomain protein Hop. *J Clin Invest, 112*(6), 863–871.
272. Kee, H. J., Sohn, I. S., Nam, K. I., et al. (2006). Inhibition of histone deacetylation blocks cardiac hypertrophy induced by angiotensin II infusion and aortic banding. *Circulation, 113*(1), 51–59.
273. Hsu, C. P., Odewale, I., Alcendor, R. R., et al. (2008). Sirt1 protects the heart from aging and stress. *J Biol Chem, 389*(3), 221–231.
274. Alcendor, R. R., Gao, S., Zhai, P., et al. (2007). Sirt1 regulates aging and resistance to oxidative stress in the heart. *Circ Res, 100*(10), 1512–1521.
275. Vega, R. B., Harrison, B. C., Meadows, E., et al. (2004). Protein kinases C and D mediate agonist-dependent cardiac hypertrophy through nuclear export of histone deacetylase 5. *Mol Cell Biol, 24*(19), 8374–8385.
276. Song, K., Backs, J., McAnally, J., et al. (2006). The transcriptional coactivator CAMTA2 stimulates cardiac growth by opposing class II histone deacetylases. *Cell, 125*(3), 453–466.
277. Crackower, M. A., Oudit, G. Y., Kozieradzki, I., et al. (2002). Regulation of myocardial contractility and cell size by distinct PI3K-PTEN signaling pathways. *Cell, 110*(6), 737–749.
278. Patrucco, E., Notte, A., Barberis, L., et al. (2004). PI3Kgamma modulates the cardiac response to chronic pressure overload by distinct kinase-dependent and -independent effects. *Cell, 118*(3), 375–387.
279. Wullschleger, S., Loewith, R., & Hall, M. N. (2006). TOR signaling in growth and metabolism. *Cell, 124*(3), 471–484.
280. McMullen, J. R., Sherwood, M. C., Tarnavski, O., et al. (2004). Inhibition of mTOR signaling with rapamycin regresses established cardiac hypertrophy induced by pressure overload. *Circulation, 109*(24), 3050–3055.
281. Fingar, D. C., Richardson, C. J., Tee, A. R., et al. (2004). mTOR controls cell cycle progression through its cell growth effectors S6K1 and 4E-BP1/eukaryotic translation initiation factor 4E. *Mol Cell Biol, 24*(1), 200–216.
282. McMullen, J. R., Shioi, T., Zhang, L., et al. (2004). Deletion of ribosomal S6 kinases does not attenuate pathological, physiological, or insulin-like growth factor 1 receptor-phosphoinositide 3-kinase-induced cardiac hypertrophy. *Mol Cell Biol, 24*(14), 6231–6240.
283. Michael, A., Haq, S., Chen, X., et al. (2004). Glycogen synthase kinase-3β regulates growth, calcium homeostasis, and diastolic function in the heart. *J Biol Chem, 279*(20), 21383–21393.
284. Antos, C. L., McKinsey, T. A., Frey, N., et al. (2002). Activated glycogen synthase-3 beta suppresses cardiac hypertrophy in vivo. *Proc Natl Acad Sci U S A, 99*(2), 907–912.
285. Proud, C. G. (2004). Ras, PI3-kinase and mTOR signaling in cardiac hypertrophy. *Cardiovasc Res, 63*(3), 403–413.
286. Zhai, P., Gao, S., Holle, E., et al. (2007). Glycogen synthase kinase-3α reduces cardiac growth and pressure overload-induced cardiac hypertrophy by inhibition of extracellular signal-regulated kinases. *J Biol Chem, 282*(45), 33181–33191.
287. Hirotani, S., Zhai, P., Tomita, H., et al. (2007). Inhibition of glycogen synthase kinase 3β during heart failure is protective. *Circ Res, 101*(11), 1164–1174.
288. Gordon, M. D., & Nusse, R. (2006). Wnt signaling: multiple pathways, multiple receptors, and multiple transcription factors. *J Biol Chem, 281*(32), 22429–22433.
289. Sugden, P. H., Fuller, S. J., Weiss, S. C., et al. (2008). Glycogen synthase kinase 3 (GSK3) in the heart: a point of integration in hypertrophic signalling and a therapeutic target? A critical analysis. *Br J Pharmacol, 153*(suppl 1), S137–S153.
290. Zelarayan, L., Gehrke, C., & Bergmann, M. W. (2007). Role of β-catenin in adult cardiac remodeling. *Cell Cycle, 6*(17), 2120–2126.
291. Baurand, A., Zelarayan, L., Betney, R., et al. (2007). β-catenin downregulation is required for adaptive cardiac remodeling. *Circ Res, 100*(9), 1353–1362.
292. Skurk, C., Izumiya, Y., Maatz, H., et al. (2005). The FOXO3a transcription factor regulates cardiac myocyte size downstream of AKT signaling. *J Biol Chem, 280*(21), 20814–20823.
293. Sandri, M., Sandri, C., Gilbert, A., et al. (2004). Foxo transcription factors induce the atrophy-related ubiquitin ligase atrogin-1 and cause skeletal muscle atrophy. *Cell, 117*(3), 399–412.
294. Li, H. H., Willis, M. S., Lockyer, P., et al. (2007). Atrogin-1 inhibits Akt-dependent cardiac hypertrophy in mice via ubiquitin-dependent coactivation of Forkhead proteins. *J Clin Invest, 117*(11), 3211–3223.
295. Li, H. H., Kedar, V., Zhang, C., et al. (2004). Atrogin-1/muscle atrophy F-box inhibits calcineurin-dependent cardiac hypertrophy by participating in an SCF ubiquitin ligase complex. *J Clin Invest, 114*(8), 1058–1071.
296. Lemmens, K., Doggen, K., & De Keulenaer, G. W. (2007). Role of neuregulin-1/ErbB signalling in cardiovascular physiology and disease: implications for therapy of heart failure. *Circulation, 116*(8), 954–960.
297. Gschwind, A., Zwick, E., Prenzel, N., et al. (2001). Cell communication networks: epidermal growth factor receptor transactivation as the paradigm for interreceptor signal transmission. *Oncogene, 20*(13), 1594–1600.
298. Lemmens, K., Segers, V. F., Demolder, M., et al. (2006). Role of neuregulin-1/ErbB2 signaling in endothelium-cardiomyocyte cross-talk. *J Biol Chem, 281*(28), 19469–19477.
299. Rohrbach, S., Yan, X., Weinberg, E. O., et al. (1999). Neuregulin in cardiac hypertrophy in rats with aortic stenosis. Differential expression of erbB2 and erbB4 receptors. *Circulation, 100*(4), 407–412.
300. Ozcelik, C., Erdmann, B., Pilz, B., et al. (2002). Conditional mutation of the ErbB2 (HER2) receptor in cardiomyocytes leads to dilated cardiomyopathy. *Proc Natl Acad Sci U S A, 99*(13), 8880–8885.
301. Crone, S. A., Zhao, Y. Y., Fan, L., et al. (2002). ErbB2 is essential in the prevention of dilated cardiomyopathy. *Nat Med, 8*(5), 459–465.
302. Liu, X., Gu, X., Li, Z., et al. (2006). Neuregulin-1/erbB-activation improves cardiac function and survival in models of ischemic, dilated, and viral cardiomyopathy. *J Am Coll Cardiol, 48*(7), 1438–1447.
303. Slamon, D. J., Leyland-Jones, B., Shak, S., et al. (2001). Use of chemotherapy plus a monoclonal antibody against HER2 for metastatic breast cancer that overexpresses HER2. *N Engl J Med, 344*(11), 783–792.
304. Xiao, H., & Zhang, Y. Y. (2008). Understanding the role of transforming growth factor-β signalling in the heart: overview of studies using genetic mouse models. *Clin Exp Pharmacol Physiol, 35*(3), 335–341.
305. Nakajima, H., Nakajima, H. O., Salcher, O., et al. (2000). Atrial but not ventricular fibrosis in mice expressing a mutant transforming growth factor-b(1) transgene in the heart. *Circ Res, 86*(5), 571–579.
306. Schultz, J. J., Witt, S. A., Glascock, B. J., et al. (2002). TGF-β1 mediates the hypertrophic cardiomyocyte growth induced by angiotensin II. *J Clin Invest, 109*(6), 787–796.
307. Derynck, R., & Zhang, Y. E. (2003). Smad-dependent and Smad-independent pathways in TGF-β family signalling. *Nature, 425*(6958), 577–584.
308. Zhang, D., Gaussin, V., Taffet, G. E., et al. (2000). TAK1 is activated in the myocardium after pressure overload and is sufficient to provoke heart failure in transgenic mice. *Nat Med, 6*(5), 556–563.
309. Wang, J., Xu, N., Feng, X., et al. (2005). Targeted disruption of Smad4 in cardiomyocytes results in cardiac hypertrophy and heart failure. *Circ Res, 97*(8), 821–828.
310. Xu, J., Kimball, T. R., Lorenz, J. N., et al. (2006). GDF15/MIC-1 function as a protective and antihypertrophic factor released from the myocardium in association with SMAD protein activation. *Circ Res, 98*(3), 342–350.
311. Clerk, A., & Sugden, P. H. (2006). Ras: the stress and the strain. *J Mol Cell Cardiol, 41*(4), 595–600.
312. Brown, J. H., Del Re, D. P., & Sussman, M. A. (2006). The Rac and Rho hall of fame: a decade of hypertrophic signalling hits. *Circ Res, 98*(6), 730–742.
313. Sah, V. P., Minamisawa, S., Tam, S. P., et al. (1999). Cardiac-specific overexpression of RhoA results in sinus and atrioventricular nodal dysfunction and contractile failure. *J Clin Invest, 103*(12), 1627–1634.
314. Kontaridis, M. I., Yang, W., Bence, K. K., et al. (2008). Deletion of Ptpn11 (Shp2) in cardiomyocytes causes dilated cardiomyopathy via effects on the extracellular signal regulated kinase/mitogen-activated protein kinase and RhoA signaling pathways. *Circulation, 117*, 1423–1435.
315. Zhang, Y. M., Bo, J., Taffet, G. E., et al. (2006). Targeted deletion of ROCK1 protects the heart against pressure overload by inhibiting reactive fibrosis. *FASEB J, 20*(7), 916–925.
316. Satoh, M., Ogita, H., Takeshita, K., et al. (2006). Requirement of Rac1 in the development of cardiac hypertrophy. *Proc Natl Acad Sci U S A, 103*(19), 7432–7437.
317. Harris, I. S., Zhang, S., Treskov, I., et al. (2004). Raf-1 kinase is required for cardiac hypertrophy and cardiomyocyte survival in response to pressure overload. *Circulation, 110*(6), 718–723.
318. Yamaguchi, O., Watanabe, T., Nishida, K., et al. (2004). Cardiac-specific disruption of the c-raf-1 gene induces cardiac dysfunction and apoptosis. *J Clin Invest, 114*(7), 937–943.
319. Miyamoto, M. I., del Monte, F., Schmidt, U., et al. (2000). Adenoviral gene transfer of SERCA2a improves left-ventricular function in aortic-banded rats in transition to heart failure. *Proc Natl Acad Sci U S A, 97*(2), 793–798.
320. Sack, D. W., Cooper, G., & Harrison, C. E. (1977). The role of Ca^{++} ions in the hypertrophied myocardium. *Basic Res Cardiol, 72*(2–3), 268–273.
321. Fowler, M. B., & Bristow, M. R. (1985). Rationale for beta-adrenergic blocking drugs in cardiomyopathy. *Am J Cardiol, 55*(10), 120D–124D.
322. Gwathmey, J. K., Copelas, L., MacKinnon, R., et al. (1987). Abnormal intracellular calcium handling in myocardium from patients with end-stage heart failure. *Circ Res, 61*(1), 70–76.
323. Nagai, R., Zarain-Herzberg, A., Brandl, C., et al. (1989). Regulation of myocardial Ca^{2+}-ATPase and phospholamban mRNA expression in response to pressure overload and thyroid hormone. *Proc Natl Acad Sci U S A, 86*(8), 2966–2970.
324. Levy, S., Sutton, G., Ng, P. C., et al. (2007). The diploid genome sequence of an individual human. *PLoS Biol, 5*(10), e254.
325. Wheeler, D. A., Srinivasan, M., Egholm, M., et al. (2008). The complete genome of an individual by massively parallel DNA sequencing. *Nature, 452*(7189), 872–876.

Abbreviations Used in This Chapter

Abbreviation	Name	Note
Ang II	Angiotensin II	Hypertrophic agonist
AMPK	Adenosine monophosphate kinase	
ANF	Atrial natriuretic factor	Early response gene
AP-1	Activator protein 1	Transcription factor
$AT_{1a}R$, $AT_{1b}R$	Angiotensin II receptor type Ia or Ib	
Ask-1	Apoptosis signal regulating kinase 1	MAP kinase kinase
ATF-1	Activating transcription factor 1	
β-ARK (GRK2)	β-adrenergic receptor kinase (G-protein receptor kinase 2)	Gβγ dependent, phosphorylates β-adrenergic receptors
BMP	Bone morphogenic proteins	
BNP	Brain natriuretic peptide	TGF-β super family ligands
CAD	Caspase associated DNAase	
CaMK	Ca^{2+} calmodulin-dependent kinase	
cAMP	Cyclic adenosine monophosphate	
cAMP kinase	Cyclic 3′,5′-adenosine monophosphate kinase	
CREB	cAMP response element-binding protein	cAMP responsive transcription factor
CT-1	Cardiotrophin-1	IL-6 family cytokine
DAG	Diacylglycerol	Endogenous PKC agonist
DISC	Death induced signaling complex	Signaling complex downstream of death receptor
4E-BP	4E-binding protein	
EGF	Epidermal growth factor	
egr-1	Early growth response gene 1	Transcription factor
eIF4F	Eukaryotic initiation factor 4F	Stimulates initiation of translation at a subset of transcripts
ErbB2-4	EGF family tyrosine kinase receptors	Receptors for neuregulins
ET-1	Endothelin 1	
ET_A, ET_B	Endothelin receptors A, B	
ECM	Extracellular matrix	
EGF	Epidermal growth factor	
Elk-1	TCF family transcription factor	
Ets1	TCF family transcription factor	
ERK	Extracellular receptor kinase	MAP kinase
FAK	Focal adhesion kinase	Nonreceptor tyrosine kinase
FGF	Fibroblast growth factor	Growth factor
c-fos	c-fos oncogene	Component of transcription factor AP-1
Gα, Gβγ	Subunits of heterotrimeric G proteins	
GAP	GTPase activating proteins	
GATA4	GATA binding protein 4	
GDP	Guanosine diphosphate	
GDF15	Growth differentiation factor 15	TGF-β family protein
GEF	Guanine exchange factor	Activators of small G proteins
gp130	Glycoprotein 130	Receptor for IL-6 family cytokines
GPCR	Heterotrimeric G protein-coupled receptor	
Grb2	Growth factor receptor bound protein 2	Adaptor protein linking RTKs and Ras

Continued

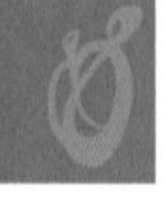

Abbreviations Used in This Chapter—cont'd

Abbreviation	Name	Note
GRK	G protein receptor kinase	Inhibits G protein signaling and recruits adaptor proteins to stimulate alternate pathways
GSK3β	Glycogen synthase kinase 3β	Kinase downregulated by hypertrophic stimuli
GTP	Guanosine triphosphate	
HB-EGF	Heparin-binding EGF-like growth factor	
HAT	Histone acetyltransferase	Induces histone acetylation with activation of transcription
HDAC	Histone deacetylase	Represses transcription by inducing histone deacetylation
IGF-1	Insulin-like growth factor	Growth factor
IL-6	Interleukin-6	Cytokine
IP3	Inositol 1,4,5 triphosphate	
ILK	Integrin linked kinase	Serine threonine kinase associated with β-integrin
JAK	Janus activating kinase	Tyrosine kinase activated by gp130
JNK	Jun N terminal kinase	MAP kinase
c-jun	*jun* oncogene	Component of AP-1 transcription factor
LIF	Leukemia inhibitory factor	IL-6 cytokine
MADS domain	DNA binding motif	Present in SRF and MEF2 transcription factors
MAPK	Mitogen-activated protein kinase	
MAPKK	MAPK kinase	Also known as MEK or MK
MAPKKK	MAPK kinase kinase	Also known as MEKK or MKK
MEF2	Myocyte enhancer factor 2	Transcription factor
MEK-1	MAP kinase kinase 1	Activator of ERK MAPKs
MCIP	Modularity calcineurin-inhibitory proteins	Endogenous inhibitor of calcineurin
MHC	Myosin heavy chain	
miRNAs	MicroRNAs	Endogenous RNAs that inhibit mRNA translation/enhance degradation
MLC	Myosin light chain	
MLP	Muscle LIM protein	
mTOR	Mammalian target of rapamycin	Kinase involved in regulation of protein synthesis
c-myc	*myc* oncogene	Transcription factor
NE	Norepinephrine	Catecholamine
NFAT	Nuclear factor of activated T cells	Transcription factor
PDK1	Phosphoinositide-dependent kinase 1	Downstream effector of PI3K
PE	Phenylephrine	α-adrenergic agonist
PI3K	Phosphoinositide 3-kinase	
PIP2	Phosphatidyl inositol 4,5-bisphosphate	
PIP3	Phosphatidyl inositol 3,4,5-triphosphate	
PKA	Protein kinase A	
PKB	Protein kinase B	Also known as Akt
PKC	Protein kinase C	
PKD	Protein kinase D	
PLC	Phospholipase C	
PMA	Phorbol 12-myristate 13-acetate	PKC agonist
p53	Tumor suppressor gene	Transcription factor
p70S6K	Ribosomal p70 S6 kinase	Protein kinase involved in protein synthesis
Ras	*Ras* oncogene	Small G protein

Continued

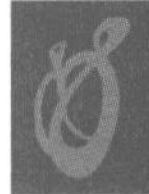

Abbreviations Used in This Chapter—cont'd

Abbreviation	Name	Note
RTK	Receptor tyrosine kinase	
ROCK	Rho kinases	
RyR	Ryanodine receptor	
SERCA	Sarcoplasmic reticulum Ca^{2+} ATPase	Pumps Ca^{2+} from cytoplasm to sarcoplasmic reticulum
SH2	Src homology domain 2	Binds phosphotyrosine residues
SHP2	SH2 domain-containing cytoplasmic protein tyrosine phosphatase	
siRNAs	Short interfering RNAs	Inhibit mRNA translation
SOCS	Suppressors of cytokine signaling	Endogenous repressor of STATs
c-Src	*Src* oncogene	Nonreceptor tyrosine kinase
SRF	Serum response factor	Transcription factor
STAT	Signal transducer and activator of transcription	Transcription factor regulated by JAKs
TCF	Ternary complex factor	Transcription factor regulated by MAPKs
TAK1	TGF-β activated kinase 1	MAPKK activated by TGF-β
TGF-β	Transforming growth factor β	Cytokine
TNF-α	Tumor necrosis factor α	Cytokine
VEGF	Vascular endothelial growth factor	Angiogenic cytokine

CHAPTER 3

Cellular Basis for Heart Failure

Kenneth B. Margulies and Steven R. Houser

Congestive heart failure (CHF) is a syndrome characterized by deterioration of cardiac pump function. Progressive alterations in the processes that regulate contractility of single ventricular myocytes are thought to be the important contributors to this pump degeneration (see Chapter 2). Those findings that have enhanced our understanding of abnormal electrophysiology, excitation-contraction coupling, Ca^{2+} handling, and contractile proteins in relation to the deterioration of ventricular myocyte contractility in the failing heart are the topic of this chapter.

CHARACTERISTIC ELECTROMECHANICAL ABNORMALITIES OF FAILING MYOCYTES

Prolongation of the action potential duration, a depressed force generating capacity, and slowed contraction and relaxation rates are the hallmark functional changes of the failing human heart. The action potential abnormalities cause prolongation of the surface electrocardiogram (acquired long QT syndrome),[1] which renders the heart prone to arrhythmias and contributes to sudden death.[2] The mechanical abnormalities of the failing heart contribute to its poor pump performance and limit its ability to increase function during daily routine activities.

The cellular and molecular bases of CHF electromechanical abnormalities have been studied both in human tissues and cells and in animal models of human disease. Animal models of human disease have been useful for those studies seeking to identify the potential causes and therapies for the cardiac dysfunction seen in hypertrophy and CHF. These animal models in large part mimic human heart disease by increasing hemodynamic loading conditions (pressure and volume overload, interrupting myocardial blood flow (infarction), and by altering the heart rate (rapid pacing or atrioventricular [AV] block). Increasingly, genetically induced deletion or overexpression of specific cardiac myocyte proteins have been used to gain novel insights into the fundamental causes and potential cures of CHF. Chamber remodeling, including increased myocardial mass and left ventricular (LV) chamber dilation, is a common feature of CHF with dilation increasing with CHF severity.[3] Dilation induces increases in systolic wall stress so that muscle cells in the failing heart must develop greater than normal force to develop the pressures required to support a normal blood pressure.

The consensus from most studies performed to date is that mild to moderate cardiac insults are usually followed by a compensatory response that involves hypertrophy and some LV chamber remodeling (see Chapter 15).[4] In these compensatory stages, myocyte function appears to be near normal and may even be increased, which would help the heart maintain pump function in the face of increased hemodynamic demands. As the cardiac insult becomes more severe, CHF with LV (LV) dilation and deterioration of pump, muscle, and myocyte performance are induced. The factors that precipitate the transition from compensated to depressed myocyte and pump function are discussed later, as are those issues that are still unresolved and deserving of additional study.

In Vivo Cardiac Function Versus In Vitro Muscle and Myocyte Contractility

In CHF, the dilated heart has a reduced ejection fraction and ejects blood slowly. These derangements are signs of markedly increased hemodynamic loading (systolic wall stress). Under these conditions the failing heart struggles to maintain blood pressure and cardiac output. Clinical studies have documented that systolic wall stress is increased in the failing heart and is a strong predictor of heart failure severity. This parameter is also inversely related to clinical outcome.[5,6] These clinical data show that the myocytes surrounding the failing ventricle must develop high force (pathologically increased systolic wall stress) to produce ejection. Persistent activation of sympathetic and renin-angiotensin signaling cascades are needed to support this contractile function.[7,8] It is imperative to keep in mind that the in vitro studies performed with muscles or myocytes removed from failing hearts (human or animal models) have largely been conducted in the absence of the altered inotropic environment of the failing heart. As we discuss later, when studied under these conditions many investigators have found that the basal contractile properties of the heart are depressed.[9,10] Collectively these studies show that the poor pump function of the failing heart results from two factors, excessive loading conditions (systolic wall stress) and inherent defects in myocyte contractility. Fixing these structural and functional abnormalities has been a major therapeutic challenge.

CHF has many different causes and yet changes in functional characteristics of the failing heart muscle are surprisingly consistent. Slowing of contraction and relaxation rates and prolongation of the action potential duration have consistently been the first changes observed in the early stages of CHF.[11,12] Reduced force production and shortening magnitude and decreases rather than increases in contractility as the heart rate increases (positive versus negative force-frequency relationships) are observed in more advanced CHF.[13]

An important finding of many in vitro studies is that nonfailing and failing human myocytes have similar contractile characteristics at low workloads (slow pacing rates, low bath Ca^{2+}, absence of catecholamine stimulation).[13] Peak developed force (or shortening) is not significantly different in nonfailing versus failing human left ventricle muscles or in myocytes paced at slow frequencies (<30/min) and the rates of force development (muscles) or shortening (myocytes) are only modestly slower than normal in failing muscles. Changes in heart rate, Ca^{2+} influx, or catecholamine exposure all bring out significant differences between nonfailing and failing myocardium and myocytes. Increasing the pacing rate into the physiological range causes contractility to increase in nonfailing myocytes (positive force-frequency) but causes contractility to decrease (or remains constant) in HF myocytes (negative force-frequency relationship). Therefore, at physiological heart rates, the contractility of the failing heart is depressed.

The contractile enhancing effects of high bath $[Ca^{2+}]$ and β-adrenergic agonists are also significantly blunted in failing myocytes.[14,15] These results suggest that the phenotypical adaptations of failing myocytes cause preservation of contractility at low workloads (rates) but at the cost of blunted contractile reserve. If a cellular and molecular alteration contributes to the CHF contractile phenotype, it must contribute to these prototypical contractile alterations.

CALCIUM-DEPENDENT CAUSES OF ELECTROMECHANICAL DYSFUNCTION IN THE FAILING HEART

Morgan and colleagues were the first to observe alterations in the Ca^{2+} transient of failing human ventricular muscle.[16] These early studies stimulated a large body of research on the role of deranged Ca^{2+} homeostasis in the mechanical abnormalities of the failing heart. Fairly consistent changes in Ca^{2+} handling have been observed in studies using large- and small-animal model CHF and in failing human heart muscles and myocytes, as previously reviewed in Houser et al.[9,10]

As mentioned previously, increasing the beating rate of normal human ventricular myocytes causes an increase in the size of the Ca^{2+} transient and the force of contraction (positive force-frequency relationship). In myocytes with mild to moderate hypertrophy without CHF, the peak systolic Ca^{2+} is normal in the basal state and only becomes depressed when conditions that increase cellular Ca^{2+} loading are imposed (faster pacing rates, high bath $[Ca^{2+}]$ or catecholamine exposure). As the severity of the inciting hypertrophic stimulus increases and ventricular function begins to change, Ca^{2+} transient and contractile abnormalities are found at progressively slower rates of stimulation and in normal bath $[Ca^{2+}]$. When CHF is severe, such as in end-stage human heart failure, peak systolic Ca^{2+} and force (or shortening) are both close to normal only at very slow pacing rates. As the beating rate is increased, there is either no change or a decrease in peak systolic Ca^{2+} and force of contraction (negative force-frequency relationship) in the failing heart.[15,16] In addition, as CHF progresses, there is an associated increase in diastolic Ca^{2+} with increased heart rate.[15] These results strongly support the hypothesis that changes in cellular Ca^{2+} handling are a final common pathway for progressive deterioration of cardiac pump function in CHF. The changes in Ca^{2+} handling are also likely to be critically involved in the arrhythmias,[7,17] metabolic disturbances, and activation of cell death pathways[18-21] and hypertrophy[22] that develop during this time. This hypothesis is also strongly supported by studies in animal models that show that the transition from compensated hypertrophy to CHF coincides with the time that myocytes first lose their ability to normally maintain physiological levels of systolic and diastolic Ca^{2+}.[23]

The cellular and molecular bases of the altered Ca^{2+} homeostasis of the failing cardiac myocytes have been studied in some detail. Studies performed over the past decade show that changes in the abundance and regulatory state (phosphorylation, nitrosylation, etc.) of critical Ca^{2+} regulatory proteins are largely responsible for abnormal Ca^{2+} regulation.[24]

In normal myocytes the systolic Ca^{2+} transient (rise in cytosolic $[Ca^{2+}]$) determines the rate and magnitude of contraction. The Ca^{2+} transient is derived from two sources: Ca^{2+} influx through L-type Ca^{2+} channels and Ca^{2+} release from the sarcoplasmic reticulum (SR). L-type Ca^{2+} channels in the transverse tubules are activated during the early portion of the cardiac action potential. Ca^{2+} enters myocytes through these channels and accumulates in diffusion limiting spaces between the T-tubules and the junctional SR. Ca^{2+} in this space binds to the cytoplasmic face of the Ca^{2+} release channel (ryanodine receptor, RyR), causing it to open. Ca^{2+} then moves out of the SR into the cytoplasm. Collectively these processes increase cytoplasmic Ca^{2+} and activate contraction. The Ca^{2+} transient is terminated when the Ca^{2+} entry and release channels close and Ca^{2+} efflux (Na/Ca^{2+} exchange) and SR reuptake by the SR Ca^{2+} ATPase (SERCA2) reestablish steady-state conditions. The amplitude and duration of the Ca^{2+} transient is regulated to modulate the rate, magnitude, and duration of contraction. SR Ca^{2+} release is induced and graded by Ca^{2+} influx through L-type Ca^{2+} channels.[25] The magnitude of SR Ca^{2+} release is also determined by the amount of Ca^{2+} stored in the SR.[26,27] Alterations in the abundance or activity (by abnormal phosphorylation) of any or all of these Ca^{2+} regulatory proteins have been shown to play a role in the abnormal Ca^{2+} transients in the failing heart (Figure 3-1). Most studies show that the amount of Ca^{2+} released from the SR of failing human (and most animal models) myocytes is smaller than normal and that this difference is accentuated at rapid heart rates.[27,28] The molecular bases of the abnormal Ca^{2+} transient are discussed next.

L-Type Ca^{2+} Channel

The L-type Ca^{2+} channel opens when the membrane potential depolarizes during the upstroke of the cardiac action potential. The subsequent Ca^{2+} influx ($I_{Ca,L}$) contributes to the plateau phase of the action potential, directly elevates cytoplasmic $[Ca^{2+}]$, and induces SR Ca^{2+} release[29] (see Figure 3-1). Ca^{2+} influx via the L-type Ca^{2+} current is also an important source of Ca^{2+} to maintain and modify the amount of Ca^{2+} stored in the SR.[30] Reductions in the number of these Ca^{2+} channels, abnormal localization, or abnormal activity could explain many aspects of disrupted Ca^{2+} homeostasis in CHF. Reduced $I_{Ca,L}$ density,[31] slow inactivation,[32] and reduced β-adrenergic regulation[33] have all been reported in animal models, but these changes have not been consistently observed in failing human myocytes.[34] An interesting study in failing canine myocytes suggested that the density of L-type Ca^{2+} channels is reduced but $I_{Ca,L}$ density is maintained.[35] We have shown that the density of the L-type Ca^{2+} channel is reduced in failing human myocytes but the Ca^{2+} current is maintained by increased PKA-mediated phosphorylation of the channels, which increase their activity.[36] Since the channels are largely phosphorylated in the basal state, sympathetic agonists had little ability to increase the current further. Therefore, blunted adrenergic effects on myocyte contractility are likely to involve a failure to increase Ca^{2+} influx and increase SR Ca^{2+} loading. These ideas are supported by experiments by

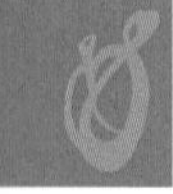

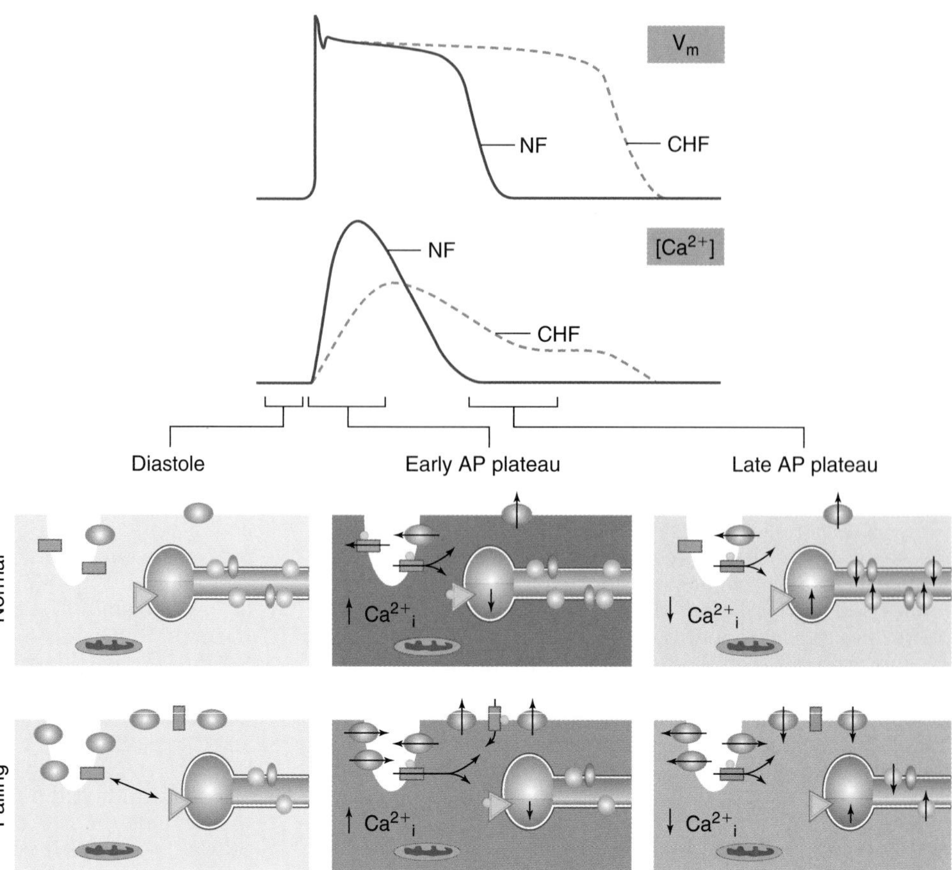

FIGURE 3–1 The upper panel depicts the differences in the action potential (AP) wave shape and cytosolic free Ca^{2+} $[Ca^{2+}]_i$ between normal (N) and failing (CHF) human ventricular myocytes. The lower panels depict the potential subcellular alterations in CHF that cause abnormal $[Ca^{2+}]_i$ transients. The gray level represents the $[Ca^{2+}]_i$. In diastole the $[Ca^{2+}]_i$ is similar in N and CHF myocytes. However, SR Ca^{2+} loading (depicted by the blue level in the SR) is smaller in the failing myocyte. Also note the difference in the density and location of Ca^{2+} regulatory proteins in the N versus CHF myocytes. Peak systolic $[Ca^{2+}]_i$ during the early AP plateau phase is lower than normal in the failing myocyte because SR Ca^{2+} release is smaller and Ca^{2+}efflux via forward mode NCX is greater than normal. SR Ca^{2+} release is also reduced in the failing myocyte because of defective EC coupling. During the late phase of the AP plateau $[Ca^{2+}]_i$ is greater than normal in the failing myocyte because the prolonged AP duration promotes reverse-mode NCX (Ca^{2+} influx) and SR uptake is slower than normal. Repolarization of the membrane potential is required for full recovery of diastolic Ca^{2+} in failing myocytes. See text for further discussion.

others in which the open probability of single Ca^{2+} channels from failing human ventricular myocytes was shown to be increased, consistent with increased phosphorylation.[37] It is also important to keep in mind that most studies of $I_{Ca,L}$ in failing myocytes have been performed at slow pacing rates where differences in inactivation properties would not have an impact on Ca^{2+} homeostasis. One study has shown that $I_{Ca,L}$ decreases more in failing than in normal myocytes when the beating frequency is increased.[38] These results also suggest that rate-related reduction of $I_{Ca,L}$ may be an important component of disrupted rate-dependent regulation of contractility in CHF.

Important questions regarding $I_{Ca,L}$ in heart failure that still need to be resolved include (1) whether or not CaMKII-mediated regulation of Ca^{2+} channels is altered in human CHF, (2) if restoring Ca^{2+} influx in CHF improves pump function or induces cell death by promoting SR Ca^{2+} overload and exacerbated pump dysfunction, (3) if L-type Ca^{2+} channels are appropriately targeted to junctional regions of the T-tubules where EC coupling occurs, and (4) if changes in Ca^{2+} influx are involved in abnormal hypertrophic signaling and structural remodeling.

Abnormalities in the triggered release of Ca^{2+} from the SR may contribute to contractility defects and arrhythmias in heart failure. Ca^{2+} influx through the L-type Ca^{2+} channel during the early portions of the action potential is now known to be the exclusive trigger for the release of Ca^{2+} from the SR by activating the Ca^{2+} release channel (ryanodine receptor, RyR).[39] There is evidence for the hypothesis that $I_{Ca,L}$ is a less effective trigger of SR Ca^{2+} release in hypertrophied and failing (rat ventricular) myocytes (decreased EC coupling "gain").[40] This defective signaling can be rescued in hypertrophied but not failing myocytes by exposure to β-agonists. These studies support the idea that the reduced size of the Ca^{2+} transient in failing rat myocytes results from a decrease in the fractional SR Ca^{2+} release rather than from a reduction in SR Ca^{2+} loading as has been observed in failing human ventricular myocytes.[41] The idea that EC coupling "gain" is reduced in CHF is not supported by our studies in failing human myocytes.[42,43] Our results suggest that the triggered release of Ca^{2+} from the SR is reduced in failing human myocytes because SR Ca^{2+} stores are depleted rather than because EC coupling is deranged.[43] In addition, a fixed defect in EC coupling "gain" does not adequately explain the fact that Ca^{2+} transients are similar in normal and failing human myocytes at slow pacing rates and only become significantly different when the heart rate increases. A frequency-dependent decrease in $I_{Ca,L}$ and reduced SR Ca^{2+} loading are more likely contributors to the associated reduction in SR Ca^{2+} release in failing human myocytes at physiologically relevant heart rates.[38]

Pieske et al[28] have shown that the flattened (or negative) force-frequency relationship of failing human ventricular myocytes results from the fact that SR Ca^{2+} loading does not increase normally with stimulation rate.[26] These authors suggest that SR Ca^{2+} release decreases at higher stimulation rates in the failing myocardium because the smaller than normal increase in SR Ca^{2+} loading cannot offset frequency-dependent EC coupling refractoriness. These findings suggest that abnormal SR Ca^{2+} loading and changes in the effectiveness of $I_{Ca,L}$ as a trigger for SR Ca release are centrally involved in the depressed contractility of failing human myocytes.[28] Since publication this study a number of others have shown that decreased SR Ca^{2+} loading is a central feature of deranged Ca^{2+} handling in CHF.[10,24]

Ryanodine Receptor

Ca^{2+}-induced opening of RyR allows Ca^{2+} to be released from the SR with each heart beat. The Marks laboratory has pioneered the idea that abnormal RyR function is involved in dysregulated Ca^{2+} in human heart failure.[44] This laboratory has published extensively on the idea that PKA-mediated hyperphosphorylation of RyR at serine 2808 increases

Ca^{2+}-induced channel opening, thereby inducing what has been termed SR Ca^{2+} leak. The idea that RyR behaves abnormally in CHF and can produce a diastolic leak of SR Ca^{2+} has been studied extensively by a number of groups.[45-47] While most have been unable to confirm an exclusive role for PKA-mediated phosphorylation,[48] most have shown RyR dysfunction in CHF, and a number of studies have provided very strong new evidence that CaMKII-mediated phosphorylation of RyR at serine 2814 is critical for RyR dysfunction.[49] Important unresolved issues are the precise factors that cause RyR dysfunction in CHF, the specific role of these RyR functional changes in contractile abnormalities, and the role of RyR dysregulation in arrhythmias.

The Sarcoplasmic Reticulum

The small size and slow decay rate of the Ca^{2+} transient in the failing heart is likely to involve slowed Ca^{2+} transport by SERCA2. This idea has been examined in numerous studies. SERCA mRNA, protein, and function (in vesicular preparations) have been measured in many models of hypertrophy and failure and in tissue samples from failing human hearts (Table 3-1). Most of these studies have shown that SERCA mRNA and/or protein are reduced in the end-stage failing human heart. However, the few studies that have failed to observe reduced SERCA protein abundance or Ca^{2+} uptake rates in failing human hearts[50,51] suggest that the routinely observed derangements in cellular Ca^{2+} handling in human myocytes are not always caused by a reduction in the abundance of SERCA protein. In this regard, the activity of the SERCA protein is inhibited by an associated protein, phospholamban (PLN). When PLN is phosphorylated (primarily by PKA-mediated pathways), it disassociates from SERCA and the associated inhibition is relieved. Increases in the PLN/SERCA stoichiometry or reduced PLN phosphorylation could both cause deranged SR Ca^{2+} transport without involving a change in SERCA abundance. There is support in the literature for both of these possibilities.[52] These are important issues in light of the in vitro studies showing that the contractility of failing human myocytes is improved when SERCA expression is increased and that heart failure in transgenic ($MLP^{-/-}$) mice can be prevented by eliminating PLN expression and thereby increasing SERCA function.[40] These results suggest that SERCA may be an important therapeutic target in CHF. Most studies have found that the SR Ca^{2+} uptake rate is slowed in heart failure and this can lead to increased diastolic Ca^{2+} (diastolic dysfunction) and reduced SR Ca^{2+} storage (reduced systolic performance). Therefore, improving SR Ca^{2+} uptake might normalize abnormal diastolic and systolic Ca^{2+} abnormalities. An ongoing clinical trial[53] in which SERCA2 expression is increased in the failing heart via gene therapy should directly test this idea.

The idea that depressed SR function and reduced SR Ca^{2+} storage is linked to cardiac decompensation is supported by animal studies showing that increasing SERCA expression (with adenoviral infection techniques) improves the function of the hypertrophied or senescent[54,55] rat hearts and presumably delays the onset of CHF (see Chapter 50). This hypothesis is also supported by recent observations in genetically modified $MLP^{-/-}$ mice that develop CHF.[4] When these mice are crossed with either the phospholamban knockout mouse ($PLN^{-/-}$) or a β-ARK-CT mouse, in which downregulation of β-adrenergic signaling is eliminated, the CHF phenotype does not develop over its normal time course.[56,57] The $PLB^{-/-}$ and β-ARK-CT mouse hearts and the SERCA-infected rat hearts cause their physiological effects via different Ca^{2+} regulatory proteins. However, all have enhanced SR function and improved contractility as their common phenotypical features. These studies suggest that an inability of the SR to take up and store Ca^{2+} is a critical factor in heart failure induction and progression.

TABLE 3–1 Calcium Regulatory Protein Levels in End-Stage Human Heart Failure

Molecule	Assay	Quantity	Reference
Calsequestrin (CSQ)			
mRNA	Northern blot	No difference	(125)
Protein	Western blot	No difference	(126-128)
Dihydropyridine Receptor (DHP)/L-type Calcium Channel ($I_{Ca,L}$)			
mRNA	Northern blot	Decreased	(128)
Protein	Western blot	No difference	(128)
	Ligand binding	Decreased	(129)
Density	Patch clamp	No difference	(130,131)
		Decreased	(132)
Phospholamban (PLB)			
mRNA	Northern blot	~ANF	(57)
	Northern blot	Decreased	(40,56)
Protein	Western blot	Decreased	(42)
Regulation	Amino acid phosphorylation states		(61,62)
Ryanodine Receptor (RyR2)			
mRNA	Northern blot	~ANF	(125)
	Northern blot	Decreased	(133) (ICM)
	Northern blot	No difference	(133) (DCM)
	Northern blot	Decreased	(134)
Protein	Western blot	No difference	(126,135)
	Ligand binding	Decreased	(134)
Regulation	Amino acid phosphorylation states		(136)
SR Ca^{2+}-ATPase (SERCA2a)			
mRNA	Northern blot	~ANF	(125)
	Northern blot	Decreased	(127,137-139)
Protein	Western blot	No difference	(127,138-140)
	Western blot	Decreased	(52,126)
Activity	Vesicular preparation	No difference	(141)
		Decreased	(140)
Sodium-Calcium Exchanger (NCX)			
mRNA	Northern blot	Increased	(142,143)
Protein		No difference	(142)
	Western blot	Increased	(142)
	Western blot	No difference	(144)
Activity	Vesicular preparation	Increased	(23,143,145)

Phospholamban

PLN is an SR protein that associates with SERCA[51] and inhibits its Ca^{2+} transport rate. Phosphorylation of PLN by either protein kinase A at serine 16 or Ca^{2+}-calmodulin dependent protein kinase at threonine 17[58] causes PLN to disassociate from SERCA and its inhibitory effect is removed. The enhanced SR Ca^{2+} transport increases the rate of decay of the Ca^{2+} transient and the amount of Ca^{2+} stored in the SR. These effects are centrally involved in the increased cardiac function needed to support aerobic exercise and other physiological activities

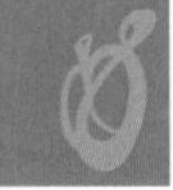

that require an increase in cardiac output. Alterations in either the abundance of PLN,[23] the PLN/SERCA stoichiometry,[59] reduced basal PLN phosphorylation[60] or a reduced ability of β-adrenergic signaling to phosphorylate PLN[61] could all contribute to the slow Ca^{2+} uptake and reduced SR Ca^{2+} load in CHF. In mouse studies, elimination of PLN, which will increase SR Ca^{2+} uptake, prevents the appearance of CHF in the $MLP^{-/-}$ mouse[56] and in some other mouse CHF models. These studies suggest that eliminating the PLN inhibitory effects on SERCA prevents and might even reverse CHF contractile effects. However, recent observations in humans with PLN mutations that reduce the inhibitory effects of PLN on SERCA suggest that in humans these changes cause cardiac dysfunction and premature death.[62] Therefore, at the present time it seems that PLN is a better heart failure therapeutic target in mice than in humans. Future work will need to explore why eliminating PLNs inhibitory effect on SERCA induces fundamentally different effects on the hearts of large and small animals.

The Sodium-Calcium Exchanger

Under normal conditions, Ca^{2+} enters myocytes from the extracellular space down a large, inwardly directed electrochemical gradient. At the normal resting potential of −80 mV and with normal concentrations of intracellular Na^+ there is sufficient energy in the Na^+ electrochemical gradient to remove Ca^{2+} from the cell via NCX (termed *forward-mode NCX*). This indirect, energy-utilizing active transport is the principal mechanism for Ca^{2+} efflux in cardiac myocytes.[10] When the membrane potential is depolarized and/or intracellular Na increases, the energy in the Ca^{2+} electrochemical gradient can be sufficient to produce Ca^{2+} entry coupled to Na^+ efflux via reverse-mode NCX.[63] This aspect of Ca^{2+} transport via the exchanger has been largely ignored in previous studies of Ca^{2+} homeostasis in diseased cardiac myocytes.

Increases in the abundance and activity of the NCX in CHF are associated with altered Ca^{2+} homeostasis.[64] Some have suggested that the increased NCX activity in CHF is a compensation for the associated reduction in SERCA function.[65] This seems unlikely in myocytes from large mammals (like humans) because SR Ca^{2+} release and reuptake occur while the membrane potential is depolarized (during the plateau phase of the action potential) and depolarization reduces and may even eliminate forward-mode NCX activity.[66] Therefore, forward mode NCX and SERCA are unlikely to work in concert to lower cytosolic Ca^{2+} in human myocytes. In small mammals such as rats and mice, forward-mode NCX and SERCA function in concert to produce the decay of the Ca^{2+} transient because the AP duration in these species is much shorter than that of the Ca^{2+} transient.[67] It is also noteworthy that in these species the SERCA/NCX transport rate is large and Ca^{2+} efflux via NCX makes a very small contribution to the decay of the Ca^{2+} transient, even when the NCX is overexpressed.[68] These fundamental differences in normal Ca^{2+} transport mechanisms in large and small mammals point out that extrapolation of finding from one species to another must be done cautiously.

Our studies in human myocytes show that increased Ca^{2+} entry via reverse-mode NCX activity contributes to abnormal Ca^{2+} handling in failing human ventricular myocytes.[25] It appears that in failing human myocytes Ca^{2+} entry via the NCX during the plateau phase of the AP contributes to the slow decay of the Ca^{2+} transient and also is the preferential source of Ca^{2+} (in place of $I_{Ca,L}$) to load the SR (Figure 3-2). These results show that the increased NCX abundance in human CHF actually contributes to the slow decay of the Ca^{2+} transient by adding Ca^{2+} to the bulk cytoplasm during systole. Our data suggest that Ca^{2+} homeostasis is abnormal in

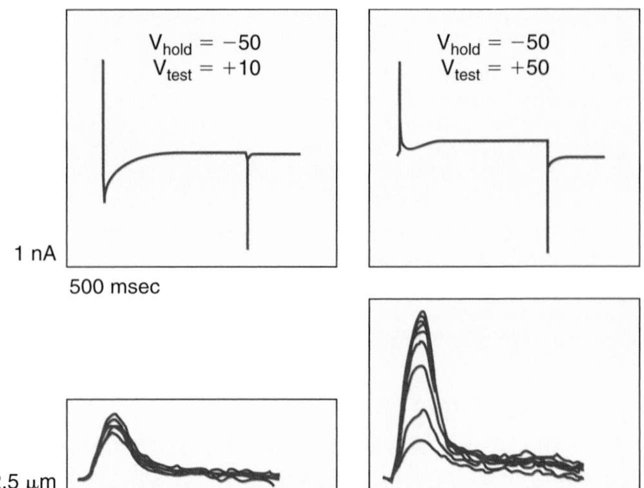

FIGURE 3–2 Contribution of the L-type Ca^{2+} channel and reverse-mode Na^+/Ca^{2+} exchange to sarcoplasmic reticulum Ca^{2+} loading: voltage clamp experiments on a failing ventricular myocyte at 37° C in Tyrode solution with 1 mM Ca^{2+}. Multiple steps from a holding potential (V_{hold}) of −50 mV to a test potential (V_{test}) after a 1-minute rest period are shown. The left panel shows the steps to +10-mV-activated Ca^{2+} influx and small contractions with very little contractile staircase. The right panel shows the steps to +50-mV activated larger reverse-mode exchange current, smaller Ca^{2+} influx, and larger contractile staircase.

CHF because of a shift in the balance of activity of SERCA and NCX (a decrease in the SERCA/NCX transport capacities). This hypothesis predicts that changes in either the abundance or activity of either of these two Ca^{2+} transporters would lead to imbalances in Ca^{2+} homeostasis. These ideas are supported by the fact that decreases in the SERCA/NCX abundance are associated with reduced SR Ca^{2+} loading, slow decay of the Ca^{2+} transient, and a negative force-frequency relationship in the failing human heart.[69] We suggest that when this activity ratio is decreased, the peak systolic Ca^{2+} will be blunted because forward-mode NCX will eliminate Ca^{2+} from the cytoplasm.[60] This imbalance of SERCA and NCX transport would also produce a persistent unloading of SR Ca^{2+} stores that would further reduce the peak level of activator Ca^{2+} (Figure 3-3). The resulting lower levels of systolic Ca^{2+} coupled with the prolonged AP duration of the failing myocytes would promote reverse-mode NCX activity during the late phases of the AP plateau.[25] These changes slow the decay of the Ca^{2+} transient and produce elevated cytosolic Ca^{2+} during the terminal phases of the AP, thereby contributing to diastolic dysfunction. Our "balance of activity" hypothesis predicts that there can be many causes for dysfunctional Ca^{2+} regulation in CHF (see Figure 3-3) and that there will be multiple unique pharmacological and molecular targets that can prevent or rescue these defects. The ongoing clinical trial with SERCA2[53] should give some insight into these issues. New studies in large animal models of human CHF in which the relative activities of NCX and SERCA are manipulated would also provide important new insights.

Deranged Ca^{2+} Metabolism may not be Due to a Change in the Abundance of Ca^{2+} Regulatory Proteins

The studies summarized previously support the idea that abnormal Ca^{2+} handling is a central player in the progressive deterioration of myocyte function in CHF. However, the idea that a change in the abundance of one specific Ca^{2+} regulatory protein causes the deranged Ca^{2+} metabolism of CHF is not well supported by the literature. There is more support for the idea that changes in the interaction of the Ca^{2+} regulatory proteins

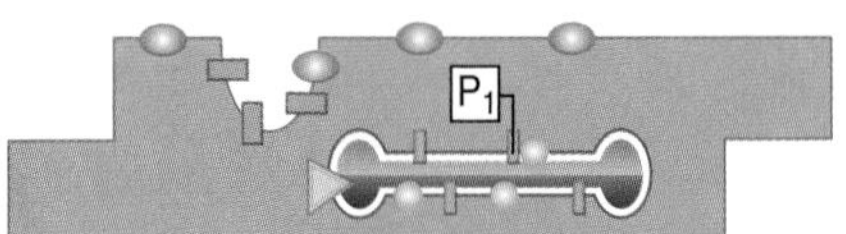

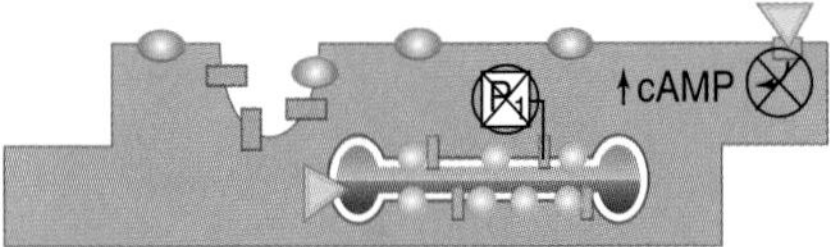

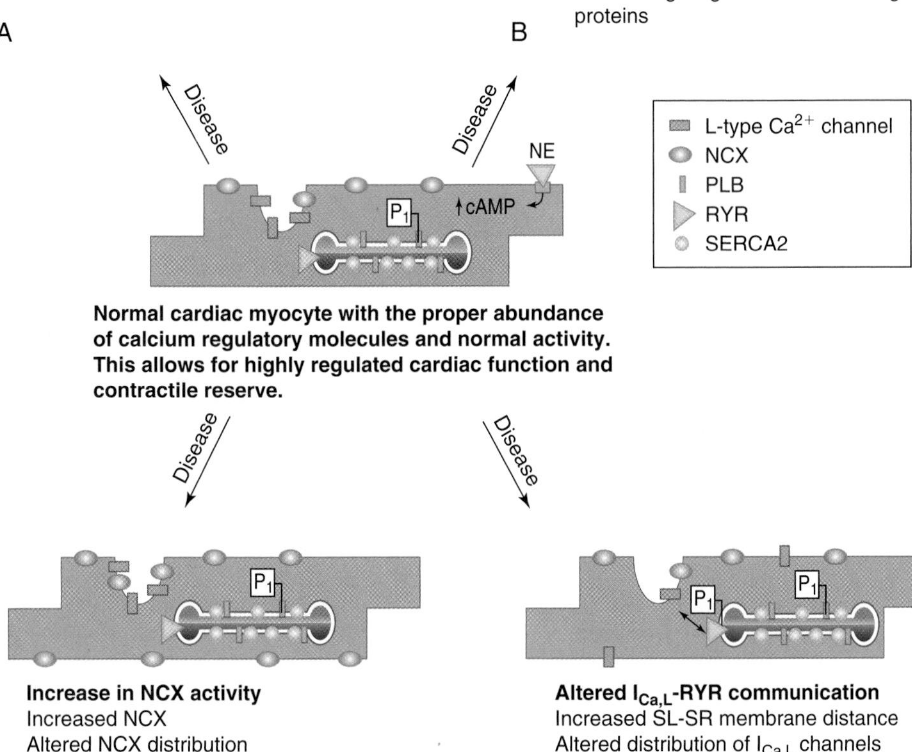

FIGURE 3–3 Potential contributors to deranged Ca^{2+} homeostasis in congestive heart failure. **A,** Decreased abundance of SERCA2 protein could explain reduced SR Ca^{2+} loading and slow decay of the Ca^{2+} transient in CHF. Alterations in SERCA2 protein due to phosphorylation or other modifications needs to be explored. **B,** SR function could be depressed in CHF because of increased expression of PLB (which could inhibit SERCA2) or from abnormal phosphorylation of PLB (which relieves the inhibition). **C,** Increased abundance of NCX (activity) could increase Ca^{2+} efflux during early phases of the Ca^{2+} transient and deplete SR calcium stores. Slow decay of the calcium transient could involve Ca^{2+} influx via reverse-mode NCX. NCX function in CHF could also be abnormal because of increased $[Na^+]_i$ or changes in the transporter distribution in surface and t-tubular membranes. **D,** Reduced SR Ca^{2+} release in CHF could result from altered junctional microarchitecture, changes in L-type Ca^{2+} channel distribution, or dysfunctional phosphorylation of the RyR release channels.

that work together to produce and modulate the size and shape of the Ca^{2+} transient cause the dysfunctional Ca^{2+} handling of the failing human myocyte. Recent studies clearly show that changes in the phosphorylation or other unrecognized modifications of Ca^{2+} handling proteins, rather than from a simple change in protein abundance, are likely causes of deranged contractility.[70] Future studies with proteomic (and other) approaches should provide new insights into these issues.

Is Dysregulated Ca^{2+} the Cause or the Effect of Heart Failure?

Ca^{2+} handling is abnormal in the failing heart and the severity of the derangements increase with the severity of CHF. As heart failure progresses and the heart dilates, systolic wall stress increases and, in turn, increases the demand for contractile activity in the myocyte. Is the generalized blunting of Ca^{2+} handling in CHF a myocyte reactive response that helps reduce Ca^{2+} overload and the associated activation of cell death signaling or are these changes primary to the progression of the syndrome? The model systems to address many of these issues have recently been developed and should provide us with novel insights in the future.

Alterations in myocyte Ca^{2+} handling are centrally involved in the dysfunctional characteristics of the failing heart. The abundance, phosphorylation, and localization of almost all important Ca^{2+} handling proteins contribute to these defects. No one molecule is uniquely responsible. A major unanswered question is still whether restoring normal Ca^{2+} handling in the context of the CHF environment will be beneficial or will enhance CHF progression by inducing myocyte death from Ca^{2+} overload, or cause sudden death via lethal ventricular arrhythmias.

THE ROLE OF CONTRACTILE PROTEINS IN REGULATING CARDIAC PERFORMANCE

In addition to abnormalities in myocyte calcium cycling, alterations in cardiac myofilament dynamics can contribute to reduced cardiac pump function in the setting of pathological cardiac hypertrophy and heart failure. Accordingly, the remainder of this chapter will highlight the involvement of contractile proteins and related molecules as key determinants of myocyte contractility and the abnormalities observed in failing myocytes. After an overview of basic features of sarcomeric architecture, actin-myosin cross-bridge dynamics, and length-dependent modulation of contractile performance, we will consider several sarcomeric proteins that have emerged as functionally important regulators of normal and abnormal myocyte contractility. In this context, we will elucidate how naturally occurring mutations, transgenic manipulations, and disease-associated modifications to sarcomeric proteins continue to reveal their physiological and pathophysiological importance. These discussions will highlight the ways in which posttranslational regulation of myofilament activity via phosphorylation of key proteins has increasingly emerged as a critical regulator of cardiac performance in the setting of acute and chronic cardiac insults. Where evidence exists, defects observed in failing human hearts will be highlighted.

At the same time, one must recognize that contractile protein physiology cannot be completely dissociated from cellular Ca^{2+} homeostasis. Specifically, it is the cytosolic Ca^{2+} transient that triggers actin-myosin cross-bridge cycling that is the fundamental event of cellular shortening. Thus the cellular processes regulating action potential shape, excitation-contraction coupling, and the size and shape of the resulting Ca^{2+} transient, as discussed previously, clearly impact responses at the level of the contractile proteins. Conversely, because the contractile proteins themselves are by far the largest Ca^{2+} buffer in the cardiac myocyte, changes in the effective calcium sensitivity (affinity) of contractile proteins unavoidably affect the shape of the calcium transient and the ionic fluxes that affect the action potential. Finally, as illustrated by sarcomeric protein mutations, defects in contractile proteins often trigger cardiac hypertrophy and its attendant abnormalities in cardiac electrophysiology, calcium cycling, and neurohumoral regulation.

Normal Contractile Protein Structure and Function

A large body of research has helped elucidate the intricate and truly exquisite molecular dynamics that contribute to the conformational and biochemical changes that ultimately produce actin-myosin cross-bridge cycling. Though space does not permit detailed review of these molecular dynamics, which are reviewed elsewhere,[71] an understanding of the abnormalities observed in failing hearts requires an overview of the major molecules that constitute and regulate the myocyte contractile proteins and their interactions under normal circumstances.

Within each sarcomere, there are two major contractile elements: the thick filament, consisting mainly of myosin and associated proteins, and the thin filament containing actin, tropomyosin, and the troponin complex, as illustrated in Figure 3-4. The thick filament protruding from the *M*-line consists of myosin, titin, and myosin-binding protein-C (MyBP-C), and myosin consists of the constituent proteins myosin heavy chain (MHC), essential light chain (ELC or MLC-1), and regulatory light chain (RLC or MLC-2). The hexagonal cross section of the thick filament is ideally suited for its interaction with six neighboring thin filaments. Filamentous actin (F-actin) is formed by polymerization of actin monomers. Two tropomyosin (Tm) strands and the troponin complex together regulate the affinity of F-actin for the myosin heads that drive the power stroke for sarcomere shortening. Actomyosin ATPase is the key enzyme driving cross-bridge cycling and this enzyme is regulated by the troponin complex. The troponin complex, in turn, is a heterotrimer composed of the following distinct gene products: troponin C (TnC), the Ca^{2+} receptor; troponin I (TnI), an inhibitor of the actin-myosin interaction that shuttles between tight binding to actin and tight binding to the Ca^{2+}-bound TnC; and troponin T (TnT) a tropomyosin binding component. The position of tropomyosin, as regulated by TnT, is ultimately the major determinant of the actin-myosin cross-bridge interaction. In systole, increased Ca^{2+} binding to TnC leads to conformational changes, including a movement of tropomyosin away from the F-actin groove toward a more peripheral location that exposes the myosin binding site and permits cross-bridge formation. During diastole, decreases in cytosolic Ca^{2+} reverse the conformational changes of systole resulting in marked reductions in, and a weakening of, actin-myosin cross-bridges.[71]

As shown in Figure 3-5, the normal relationship between the Ca^{2+} concentration and the force generated through cross-bridge interaction is sigmoidal. The relatively steep slope within the middle of this relationship reflects the cooperative nature of the interactions between attached cross-bridges and new thin filament binding of cross-bridges. Even in the absence of calcium, such cooperative binding can be demonstrated in vitro between reconstituted thin filaments and the globular region of myosin.[72] The maximal slope of the Ca^{2+}-force relationship is often referred to as the Hill coefficient. Changes in the cooperativity of cross-bridge dynamics are reflected by a change in the Hill coefficient. Recent studies have demonstrated that motifs within the C-terminal region of

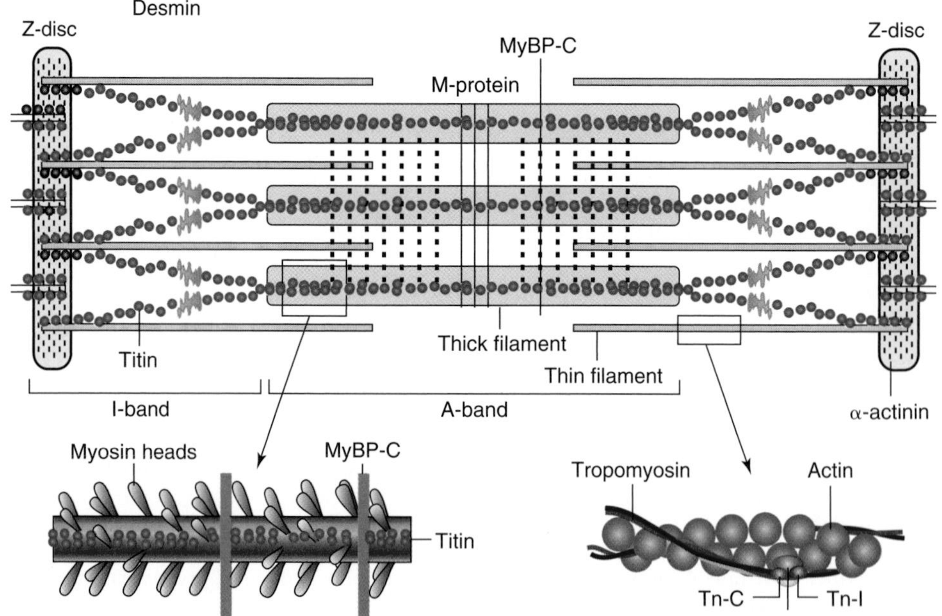

FIGURE 3–4 Diagram of the myocyte sarcomeric proteins. *MyBP-C,* myocyte binding protein-C; *Tn-C,* Troponin C; *TnI,* Troponin I; *Tn-T,* Troponin T. (Courtesy Granzier H.)

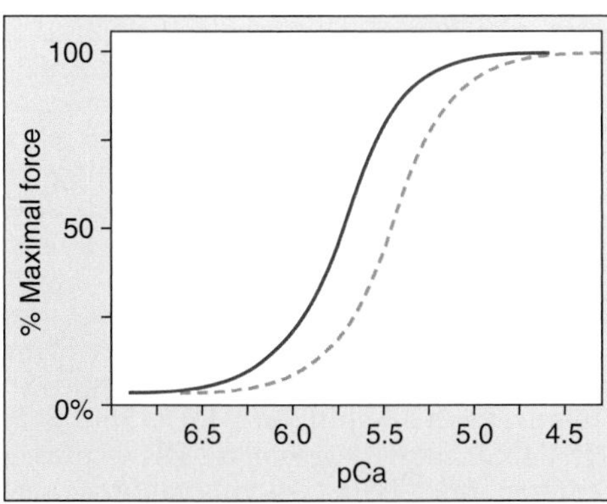

FIGURE 3–5 Typical force-calcium relationship in an isolated cardiac muscle strip preparation. The dotted line represents a *decrease* in myofilament $[Ca^{2+}]_i$ sensitivity such that higher $[Ca^{2+}]_i$ levels are required to achieve an equivalent tension.

cTnI play a central role in negatively regulating cooperativity such that either natural mutations or purposeful deletions in this region induce increases in cooperative binding between the myosin head and the thin filament.[73] Decreases in myofilament calcium sensitivity are reflected by a shift to the right while increases in calcium sensitivity are reflected by a shift to the left. The main modulators of myofilament calcium sensitivity are sarcomere length and the phosphorylation states of key sarcomeric proteins. Actin-myosin interactions are further regulated by other contractile proteins, such as the myosin light chains and myosin-binding protein C in addition to the large elastic protein titin, as will be discussed later. For both the troponin complex and these other sarcomere-associated proteins, increasing evidence indicates that the balance of kinase-mediated phosphorylation and phosphatase-mediated dephosphorylation represents the major factor regulating myofilament calcium sensitivity in health and disease. Moreover, recently revised models of the spatial limitations within the sarcomere lattice indicate that the interaction between myosin and actin under basal physiological conditions is limited to only one cross-bridge for every seven actin molecules.[74] Accordingly, modulation of myofilament responses above basal conditions represents a source of contractile reserve available to meet increases in hemodynamic demands.

Length Dependence of Contractility

Normal cardiac muscle exhibits increased contractile performance as preload or resting sarcomere length is increased. This phenomenon, often referred to as the length dependence of cardiac contractility, is the basis for the Frank-Starling relationship and represents one of the most important physiological mechanisms regulating cardiac pump function in vivo. Early studies in mammalian heart muscle demonstrated that alterations in muscle length modulate both the intracellular calcium transient[75] and myofilament Ca^{2+} sensitivity.[76] While these initial observations have been confirmed repeatedly, the mechanisms underlying the length dependence of calcium sensitivity have been controversial. One proposed mechanism is that the number of interacting cross-bridges is related to the degree of overlap of thick and thin filaments. However, the large increases in force observed with relatively small length changes suggest that other mechanisms are quantitatively more important.[77] A related geometric consideration is that *decreases* in lateral spacing between the thin and thick filaments during cell lengthening lead to enhanced cross-bridge interactions and improvements in contractile performance. However, studies by Konhilas et al indicate that changes in the lateral spacing between myofilaments can be dissociated from length-dependent alterations in force.[78] Other studies had supported a potential role for titin, the giant elastic protein within each sarcomere in converting altered passive tension to changes in Ca^{2+} sensitivity.[79] Cazola et al demonstrated reduced length-dependent augmentation in force in mice with targeted deletion of myosin-binding protein; however, the augmented Ca^{2+} sensitivity at baseline may account for the reduced effect on increased sarcomere length in these in the MBP ablated animals.[80] Most recently, studies have suggested that the inhibitory region on TnI that includes the PKC phosphorylation site (Thr-144) is pivotal for determining the degree of length-dependent augmentation of contractility in cardiac sarcomeres in that replacement of this site with a proline (as in slow skeletal TnI) effectively eliminates myofilament length dependency.[81] Together, these findings suggest that signaling pathways involving troponin, myosin-binding protein and actin, rather than simply spatial relationships between actin and myosin, have a predominating influence on the magnitude of increased force generation in response to increases in sarcomere length.

In contrast to the defects in frequency-dependent increases in contractility and adrenergic responses characteristic of failing hearts, length dependence of contractility and the Frank-Starling mechanism are relatively intact in the failing heart. Beyond animal models supporting this assertion, several studies have used severely failing human hearts, available through cardiac transplantation, to examine the length dependence of contraction. Specifically, in studies using both intact hearts and isolated cardiac muscle strips, Holubarsch et al observed intact preload dependence of contractility in failing human hearts obtained at the time of cardiac transplantation.[82] These investigators and others further demonstrated length-dependent changes in calcium sensitivity in severely failing human hearts. The balance of this chapter will describe the current understanding of the ways in which alterations in sarcomeric proteins contribute to the pathophysiology of heart failure. On a general level, sarcomeric protein mutations, isoform switches, and posttranslational modifications have each emerged as functionally relevant and clinically important factors that can cause and/or contribute to contractile abnormalities observed in failing hearts. While each of these pathophysiological mechanisms will be discussed separately, it is all but certain that interactions among these mechanisms can and do occur in diseased hearts. Indeed, in the midst of substantial new revelations about functionally, significant pathophysiological mechanisms, defining the relative contributions of multiple simultaneous pathological adaptations represent a daunting investigative challenge.

HEART FAILURE DUE TO MUTATIONS OF SARCOMERIC PROTEINS

A growing number of rare mutations have been shown to produce heritable cardiomyopathies. As discussed in Chapter 27, elucidation of a genetic cause is most frequent for hypertrophic cardiomyopathies with more than 450 different heritable mutations identified as capable of inducing increases in wall thickness in the absence of increased hemodynamic load.[83] Interestingly, most of these mutations involve a single nucleotide within the coding region of a cardiac myocyte sarcomeric protein and exhibit autosomal dominant inheritance with variable penetrance. A primary genetic cause has also been inferred, and sometimes identified, in cases of arrhythmogenic right ventricular dysplasia and LV noncompaction cardiomyopathy. Even in dilated cardiomyopathies with less distinctive morphologies, recent analyses suggest that more than 30% of cases are directly caused by single gene mutations; these are often related to cytoskeletal or metabolic function, with less than 20% linked to sarcomeric protein mutations.[84] The mutations of sarcomeric proteins identified to date in human myocardium are listed in Table 3-2. One interesting observation from this list is that the

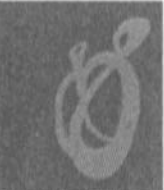

TABLE 3–2 Sarcomeric Protein Mutations Associated with Heritable Cardiomyopathy

Mutations Associated with a Familial Hypertrophic Cardiomyopathy[85]
• Cardiac troponin I (cTnI) • Cardiac troponin T (cTnT) • Cardiac troponin C (cTnC) • Cardiac β-myosin heavy chain • Cardiac α-myosin heavy chain • Essential myosin light chain • Regulatory myosin light chain • α-tropomyosin • Titin • Actin
Mutations Associated with a Familial Dilated Cardiomyopathy[84,146]
• Cardiac troponin T (cTnT) • Cardiac troponin I (cTnI) • Cardiac β-myosin heavy chain • Cardiac myosin-binding protein C (cMBP-C) • α-tropomyosin • Actin

morphological and functional phenotype of hearts with distinct mutations involving different sarcomeric protein can be quite similar. For example, defects involving at least 11 different sarcomeric proteins can produce a primary hypertrophic cardiomyopathy in humans.[85] Conversely, alternative point mutations within a single sarcomeric protein such as TnT can be associated with very different phenotypical features depending on the exact location of the mutation.[84] For example, cardiac troponin T, titin, myosin-binding protein C, and tropomyosin mutations can be observed with either hypertrophic or dilated cardiomyopathies. As will be discussed for specific sarcomeric proteins, the ability to create an animal model analogue of mutations producing human genetic cardiomyopathies has increasingly empowered investigations defining how particular sarcomeric protein domains regulate myocyte contractility. Analogously, site-directed mutagenesis in experimental animal models also permits insights into the role of specific coding sequences that have not yet been associated with spontaneous mutations.

The composite body of knowledge from such careful observational and experimental studies is growing rapidly and already permits several interesting and important generalizations about heritable cardiomyopathies. For example, there is a gene-dosage effect for sarcomeric protein mutations such that the phenotypical manifestations can be correlated with the magnitude of pathological gene expression. Finally, it is clear that the full morphological and functional impact of a particular allelic mutation is clearly the result of secondary adaptations to the initial mutation.[84] For example, one specific mutation affecting myofilament Ca^{2+} sensitivity may trigger a compensatory concentric hypertrophy and be associated with a primary diastolic abnormality, while another mutation affecting cross-bridge cycling may alter force transmission and be manifested as a dilated cardiomyopathy phenotype with systolic dysfunction. These stereotyped secondary adaptations to sarcomeric mutations likely explain why there are relatively few distinct phenotypes associated with a wide variety of single gene mutations.

SARCOMERIC PROTEIN ISOFORM SWITCHES IN FAILING HEARTS

Independent of either total or relative myofibrillar protein abundance in failing human hearts, several studies have also reported changes in contractile protein isoforms, some of which are analogous to isoform shifts observed in animal models of heart failure. For example, normal adult rat hearts express almost entirely the α-isoform of myosin heavy chain (α-MHC), while rats with experimental hypothyroidism or heart failure develop an almost complete conversion to β-MHC.[86] In failing human hearts, multiple studies have reported qualitatively similar, but quantitatively lesser, shifts with α-MHC expression decreasing from 5% to 15% in the normal myocardium to values up to 2% in the failing human myocardium.[87] Other studies using animals with experimental hypothyroidism and in vitro constructs have demonstrated that such relatively small shifts in α-MHC abundance can be functionally significant with greater α-MHC expression allowing faster contraction.[88] Using a similar approach, Metzger et al also showed that increased β-MHC was associated with a decrease in myofilament calcium sensitivity.[89] From a mechanistic standpoint, recent studies demonstrated that a highly conserved miRNA (miR-208) encoded by an intron of an α-myosin heavy chain (MHC) gene plays a pivotal role in regulating the balance of α- and β-MHC experimental hypothyroidism and pressure overload.[90] Interestingly, miRNA-208 knockout mice unable to upregulate β-MHC were resistant to hypertrophy and fibrosis during chronic pressure overload, but developed age-dependent defects in sarcomere structure and cardiac performance. These studies demonstrate a functionally significant role for a cardiac-specific miRNA in the elegant coordination of contractile protein expression in normal and stressed hearts and also suggest that the pathological α- to β-MHC isoform switch might have an adaptive role in the setting of sustained hemodynamic overload.

Analogous shifts to fetal isoforms during heart failure have also been observed for other contractile proteins. For example, smooth muscle α-actin is normally expressed during cardiac myogenesis, but is absent in the normal adult mammalian heart that expresses only the skeletal and cardiac actin isoforms. However, during cardiac hypertrophy triggered by pressure overload in rats or dilated cardiomyopathy in humans, smooth muscle α-actin is reexpressed in the heart.[91] Similar pathological expression of an atrial isoform of the cardiac myosin essential light chain (cMLC-1) has been reported in failing human hearts with congenital heart disease.[92] In the latter case, the magnitude of atrial MLC expression in the right ventricular myocardium of patients with tetralogy of Fallot was positively correlated with shortening velocity at a variety of different afterloads.[92] Investigators from the Morano laboratory have also observed a similar correlation between myocardial atrial MLC content and both in vitro and in vivo measures of contractility among patients with hypertrophic cardiomyopathy.[93] Moreover, in these studies investigators demonstrated a gene-dose response in human myocardium with greater "pathological" ventricular expression of the atrial MLC-1 expression associated with faster rates of contraction, suggesting that some isoform switches in failing hearts may be adaptive. More recently, developmental isoform switches have also been observed for titin, the large elastic filament that plays a prominent role in regulating myocyte passive tension. In the developing heart, the longer, more compliant titin isoform (N2BA) predominates in cardiac myocytes.[94] After birth, there is a transition to greater representation of the stiffer N2B isoform, which ultimately becomes the dominant isoform in the left ventricle. In the setting of advanced systolic heart failure with a severely reduced ejection fraction, there is a relative increase in the N2BA isoform associated with increased myofibrillar compliance.[95] On the other hand, in patients with heart failure and preserved ejection fraction, sometimes called diastolic heart failure, a lower ratio N2BA:N2B has been reported in association with a relative increase in stiffness,[96] as shown in Figure 3-6. Despite these compelling results, a challenge to interpreting the overall functional significance of isoform switches in human myocardium derives from the fact that multiple isoform shifts typically occur concurrently in the same muscle preparation.

PHOSPHORYLATION-DEPENDENT REGULATION OF SARCOMERIC PROTEINS

Some of the most important and dynamic ways in which sarcomeric protein function is regulated in normal and failing hearts are via posttranslational modifications. In particular, it has been increasingly evident that the regulation of contractile protein function and interactions by the phosphorylation state of several key molecules is as important as the regulation of Ca^{2+} cycling dynamics in regulating contractility. Indeed, coordinated regulation of both Ca^{2+} cycling and Ca^{2+} sensitivity is a defining feature of physiological signaling while distortions in both processes conspire to produce the characteristic defects observed in myocytes from diseased hearts. Further complicating the situation is the fact that multiple different signaling pathways and kinases are involved in phosphorylation of sarcomeric proteins and at least two of these proteins (cTnI and titin) are phosphorylated via more than one kinase. Table 3-3 summarizes the current understanding of the types and functional effects of sarcomeric protein phosphorylation in normal hearts and the alterations observed in failing mammalian hearts.

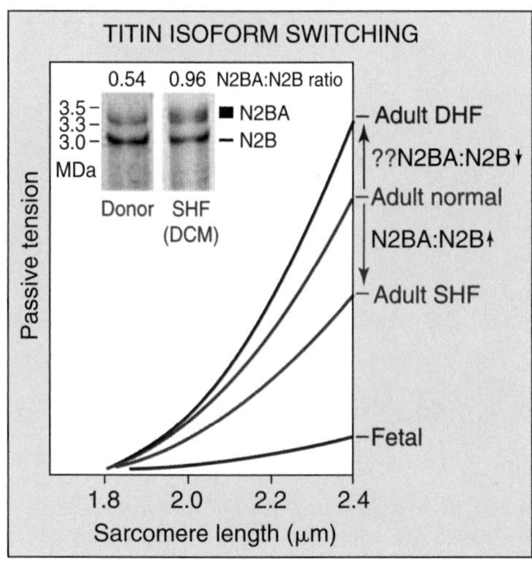

FIGURE 3-6 Functional impact of titin isoform switching. Shown are exemplary passive sarcomere length-tension relationships of cardiac myofibrils. *SHF,* systolic heart failure; *DHF,* diastolic heart failure; *DCM,* dilated cardiomyopathy. (From Kruger M, Linke WA. Titin-based mechanical signaling in normal and failing myocardium. *J Mol Cell Cardiol* 2009;46:490-498.)

PKA-mediated Phosphorylation

Myocardial contractile performance is augmented when β-adrenergic receptors are stimulated by catecholamines, resulting in activation of protein kinase A (PKA) and PKA-mediated phosphorylation of several myocyte proteins. Specifically, combined with phosphorylation of the L-type calcium channel, the ryanodine receptor, and phospholamban, PKA-mediated phosphorylation of key myofibrillar proteins permits the inotropy and faster relaxation required for achievement of enhanced stroke volume and faster heart rates required during physiological stress. It is well established that PKA-dependent phosphorylation of three molecules, cardiac TnI, myosin-binding protein C, and titin, can affect myofilament calcium sensitivity, cross-bridge dynamics, passive stiffness, and overall contractile performance.

Under normal circumstances, increased adrenergic stimulation leads to *decreased* myofibrillar calcium sensitivity via PKA-dependent phosphorylation of cTnI and cMBP-C.[80,97] PKA-dependent stimulation of cTnI involves phosphorylation of two serine residues in the N-terminal region of cardiac TnI,[98] which lowers the affinity of TnC for Ca^{2+}. PKA-dependent stimulation of cMBP-C involves phosphorylation of three separate serine residues resulting in greater interaction between the thick filament and actin and enhanced force generation.[99] PKA-dependent phosphorylation of cMBP-C also accelerates actin-myosin cross-bridge kinetics and augments in vivo myocardial contractile performance both in vitro and in vivo.[100] Under loaded conditions, the net effect of cTnI and cMBP-C phosphorylation via PKA is increased force-generating capacity and increased absolute power output, likely reflecting a predominating effect of cMBP-C on cross-bridge cycling.[101,102]

Recognizing that the syndrome of heart failure is characterized by chronic increases in cardiac adrenergic stimulation (see Chapter 10), several groups have examined the state of PKA-mediated regulation of myofibrillar function in failing human hearts and animal models of heart failure. Despite the potential effect of increased cTnI phosphorylation to decrease Ca^{2+} sensitivity, greater myofibrillar Ca^{2+} sensitivity has been reported in failing mouse, rat, dog, pig, and human hearts compared with nonfailing controls,[103] as shown in Figure 3-7. In each of these models, there was an intact or enhanced response to direct (receptor-independent) PKA stimulation in vitro and a decreased level of in vivo cTnI phosphorylation despite increased ambient adrenergic tone, suggesting uncoupling of the adrenergic stimulation cascade. In interspecies comparisons, it is particularly noteworthy that the greatest degree of enhanced Ca^{2+} sensitivity and uncoupling was observed in failing human myocardium, with rodent models of heart failure tending to substantially underestimate the defects. These

TABLE 3-3 Summary of Sarcomeric Protein Phosphorylation in Mammalian Hearts

Sarcomeric Protein	Kinase	No. of Sites	Normal Phosphorylation Effect	HF Abnormality
Troponin I (cTnI)	PKA	2	Reduces Ca sensitivity and increases cross-bridge kinetics[147]	Reduced phosphorylation[103]
	PKC	1	Reduces Ca sensitivity[148]	Increased phosphorylation[112]
Troponin T (cTnT)	PKC	4	Reduces Ca sensitivity and slows cross-bridge kinetics[109]	Increased phosphorylation[110]
Myosin-binding protein C (cMBP-C)	PKA	3	Speeds force activation and force decay[100]	Reduced phosphorylation [80]
Myosin essential light chain (cMLC1)	MLCK	2	Reduces contractility[149]	Unknown
Myosin regulatory light chain (cMLC2)	MLCK	2	Increases peak force and Ca sensitivity, slows rate of force decay[150]	Reduced phosphorylation[151]
Titin	PKA	1	Decreases passive stiffness[113]	Reduced phosphorylation[116]
	PKG	1	Decreases passive stiffness[114]	Reduced phosphorylation[114]

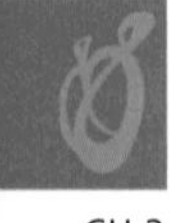

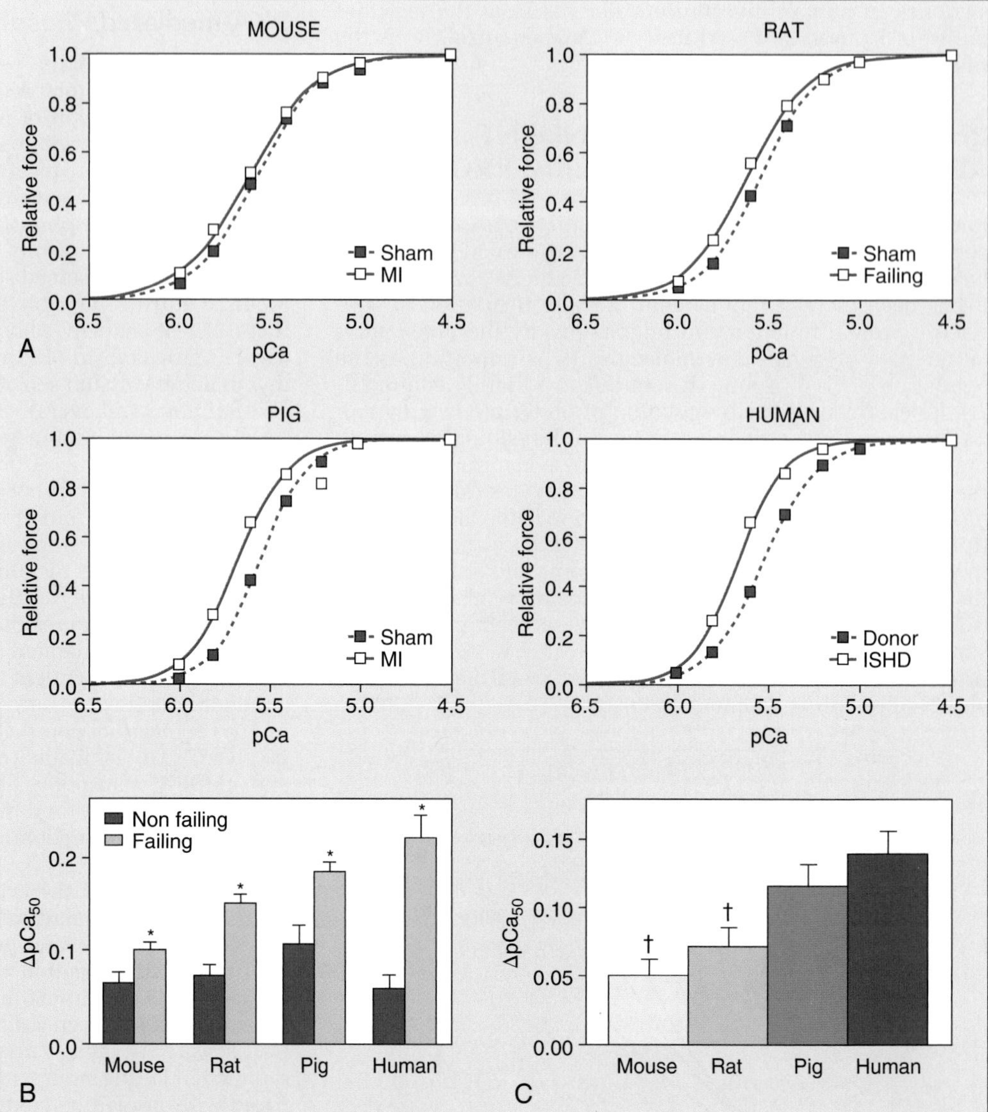

FIGURE 3–7 Ca^{2+}-sensitivity of myofilaments in different species. **A,** Ca^{2+}-sensitivity of the myofilaments was significantly higher in failing compared with nonfailing controls in all studies. **B,** A reduction in maximal force generating capacity was observed in postinfarct remodeled myocardium. $P < .05$, animal versus human in Bonferroni posttest analysis. **C,** Force measurements in cardiomyocytes from human catheter biopsies revealed enhanced cardiomyocyte stiffness in heart failure patients with reduced left ventricular ejection fraction (HFREF) compared with controls. *$P < .05$, failing versus nonfailing in unpaired Student *t*-test; #$P < .05$, effect of PKA in paired Student *t*-test. (From Hamdani N, de Waard M, Messer AE, et al. Myofilament dysfunction in cardiac disease from mice to men. *J Muscle Res Cell Motil* 2008;29:189-201.)

differences could reflect the relatively small dynamic range of adrenergic responses in rodents,[103] or the fact that failing human tissue is typically obtained from profoundly diseased hearts at the time of cardiac transplantation. Complementing these findings, several investigators have demonstrated reduced baseline phosphorylation of cTnI and cMBP-C in failing human hearts compared with nonfailing controls.[103,104]

PKC-mediated Phosphorylation

Analogous to PKA-dependent phosphorylation involved with adrenergic stimulation, it is well established that many of cellular actions of vasoactive peptides like angiotensin II and endothelin are mediated via PKC-dependent signaling processes. Gwathmey and Hajjar demonstrated that PKC-dependent phosphorylation can modulate the Ca^{2+}/force relationship in both failing and nonfailing human myocardium.[105] Specifically, these investigators observed that phorbol ester reduces the peak force development and the slope of the Ca^{2+}/force relationship, consistent with PKC-mediated reductions in Ca^{2+} sensitivity. These findings were complemented by studies demonstrating that phosphorylation of both cTnI and/or cTnT by direct PKC stimulation causes inhibition of Mg ATPase activity.[106] Moreover, studies using transgenic mutants lacking sites for PKC-mediated phosphorylation of troponins have defined the relative roles of these regulatory molecules. In this manner, Noland et al have demonstrated that phosphorylation of cardiac cTnI at Ser-43/Ser-45 is responsible for PKC-mediated decreases in Ca^{2+} sensitivity while cTnI phosphorylation at Ser-23/Ser-24 is responsible for regulation of actomyosin MgATPase.[107] In addition, PKC-dependent phosphorylation of cardiac cTnT may amplify the myofilament desensitization induced by PKC-mediated phosphorylation of cTnI.[108] Other studies demonstrate that the Thr-206 phosphorylation site on cTnT is capable of reducing maximum Ca^{2+}-saturated force, myofilament Ca^{2+} sensitivity, and the rate of cross-bridge cycling.[109]

Recent studies indicate that increased PKC-dependent phosphorylation of myofilament target proteins contributes to altered contractility in failing hearts. For example, Noguchi et al linked PKC phosphorylation of thin filaments from failing human hearts to decreased maximal force development despite increased shortening velocity.[110] In isolated cardiac myocytes from human hearts, van der Velden et al reported a PKC-mediated decrease in Ca(2+) sensitivity with minimal effects on peak force development.[111] By examining PKC-mediated effects with and without antecedent PKA activation, these studies demonstrated that intact PKC-dependent phosphorylation of both cTnI and cTnT may serve to improve diastolic function in failing human myocardium in which PKA-mediated TnI phosphorylation is decreased. These studies also implicated specific upregulation of PKCα and PKCβ isoforms as contributors to increased PKC-dependent activity in heart failure with reduced expression of these isoforms observed after LVAD-support. Complementary studies by Belin et al also demonstrated significant increases in PKCα content and activity in severely failing hearts following either myocardial infarction or pressure-overload hypertrophy in rats, but observed no change in PKCα activity in animals with compensated hypertrophy.[112] By demonstrating that PKCα stimulation had an enhanced effect on normal myocardium while dephosphorylation via protein phosphatase 1A had an enhanced effect on failing myocardium (Figure 3-8), these studies support a functionally important role for PKC-dependent hyperphosphorylation of myofilament proteins in severely failing hearts.

Titin Phosphorylation and Passive Properties of Myocytes

Although preload-dependent modulation of contractility is relatively intact in failing hearts, a key potential regulator of preload-dependent contractility in vivo is the passive stiffness of the myocardium. In multicellular preparations from failing human hearts, a greater increase in resting tension is typically required to achieve any given increment in muscle length (increased stiffness) so that the ratio of increased developed force to increased passive force is somewhat decreased. Though not excluding an additional role for extracellular matrix components in causing increased passive stiffness, recent studies demonstrate that increased passive stiffness of cardiac myocytes themselves is a characteristic of hearts with severely reduced systolic dysfunction.[103]

Recent studies demonstrate that titin phosphorylation via either a cAMP/PKA-dependent mechanism[113] or cGMP/PKG-dependent signaling[114] may alter this sarcomeric protein's contribution to cardiac myocyte passive stiffness in failing hearts. In contrast to the titin isoform switches discussed previously, these adaptations can occur on a beat-to-beat basis. Under normal circumstances, the decrease in passive tension induced by titin phosphorylation is greater following PKA phosphorylation than following PKG phosphorylation[115] as illustrated in Figure 3-9. In this context, the observation that increased myocyte passive stiffness with systolic dysfunction can be abrogated by direct PKA activation supports a role for impaired adrenergic signaling as an underlying mechanism for this pathophysiological defect.[103] Other studies suggest that defects in adrenergic signaling contribute even more to increased myocyte passive stiffness in failing hearts with preserved systolic function that is often referred to as "diastolic function").[96,116]

Defects in PKG-mediated titin phosphorylation, as is activated by nitric oxide or natriuretic peptide signaling, have likewise been implicated as contributing to increased myocyte passive stiffness in failing human and canine hearts.[114] In these studies, reductions in both PKA- and PKG-dependent titin phosphorylations were observed in failing hearts compared with nonfailing controls. These studies raise the therapeutic possibility that pathological increases in myocardial stiffness could be abrogated by interventions that enhance PKA- or PKG-dependent signaling in failing hearts. Supporting this possibility, two separate groups have demonstrated that sustained inhibition of cGMP proteolysis via phosphodiesterase 5 inhibition improves indices of LV diastolic function in murine hearts.[117,118]

LIMITED PROTEOLYSIS OF CONTRACTILE PROTEINS

Another potentially important posttranslational modification of contractile proteins contributing to contractile dysfunction is proteolysis of myofilaments themselves or key regulatory proteins. Using explanted human heart tissue, studies by Hein et al have demonstrated that contractile proteins manifest clear-cut structural changes by immunohistochemistry after only 10 minutes of ex vivo warm ischemia.[119] In this

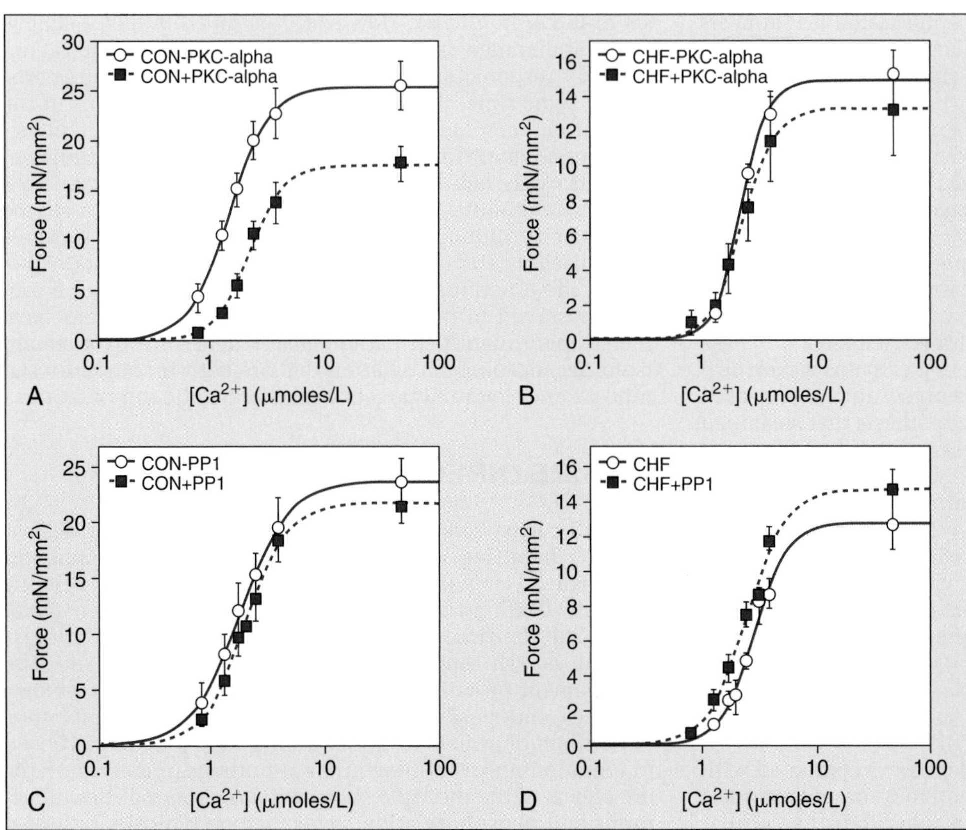

FIGURE 3–8 Functional effects of PKC phosphorylation in isolated myocytes. **A,** Average force-[Ca^{2+}] relations for control (CON) myocytes (n = 10) before (CON-PKC) and after (CON+PKC) incubation with recombinant PKC-. **B,** Average force-[Ca^{2+}] relations for CHF myocytes (n = 7) before (CHF-PKC) and after (CHF+PKC) incubation with recombinant PKC-. **C,** Average force-[Ca^{2+}] relations for control (CON) myocytes (n = 9) before (CON-PP1) and after (CON+PP1) incubation with the catalytic subunit of protein PP1 (0.15 U/mL). **D,** Average force-[Ca^{2+}] relations for CHF myocytes (n = 8) before (CHF-PP1) and after (CHF+PP1) incubation with the catalytic subunit of protein PP1 (0.15 U/mL). (From Belin RJ, Sumandea MP, Allen EJ, et al. Augmented protein kinase C-alpha-induced myofilament protein phosphorylation contributes to myofilament dysfunction in experimental congestive heart failure. *Circ Res* 2007;101:195-204.)

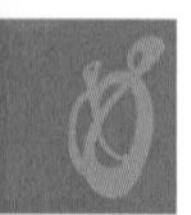

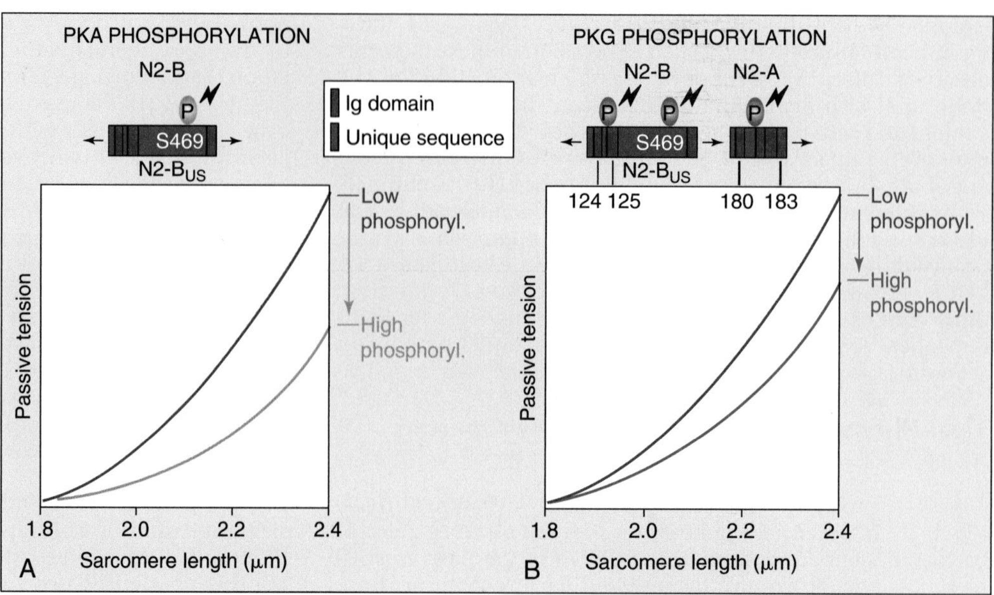

FIGURE 3–9 Functional impact of titin phosphorylation. Shown are exemplary passive sarcomere length-tension relationships of cardiac myofibrils. *N2-B$_{us}$,* unique sequence of the cardiac N2-B titin domain; *S469,* serine residue 469 of the human N2-B$_{us}$; 124, 125, 180, 183, I-band titin Ig-domains. (From Kruger M, Linke WA. Titin-based mechanical signalling in normal and failing myocardium. *J Mol Cell Cardiol* 2009;46:490-498.)

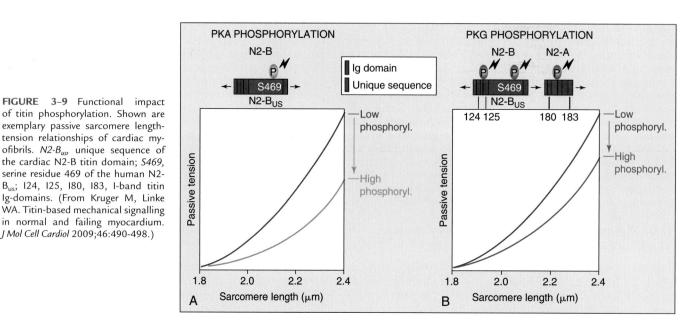

context, a growing body of literature has demonstrated that limited proteolysis of contractile proteins plays a pivotal role in the pathophysiology of myocardial stunning, a phenomenon in which a transient ischemic insult, followed by reperfusion, produces a sustained decrease in contractile dysfunction. In one representative study, Gao et al reported that rat cardiac trabeculae exposed to 20 minutes of ischemia and reperfusion before isolation exhibited relatively intact cytosolic Ca^{2+} transients in association with a severe contractile defect, suggesting decreased thin filament Ca^{2+} sensitivity.[120] Subsequent studies by McDonough et al correlated thin filament dysfunction with stepwise degradation of cTnI during progressive increases in the duration of transient cardiac ischemia.[121] With more severe ischemia, there is release of TnI fragments (e.g., $TnI_{1\text{-}193}$) from myocytes enabling detection of myonecrosis by plasma assays. Interestingly, a subpopulation of phosphorylated TnI appears to be more resistant to ischemia-induced proteolysis demonstrating one of many interactions among posttranslational modifications of contractile proteins.

Building on these observations, some investigators have suggested that limited proteolysis of myofibrils with associated changes in Ca^{2+} sensitivity and force generation could be an important initiating or propagating pathophysiological process within the failing heart.[122] In this context, Feng et al demonstrated that increased preload during transient ischemia is a key factor mediating limited proteolysis and that significantly elevated preload can induce limited TnI proteolysis even in the absence of frank ischemia.[123] These studies further implicated activation of μ-calpains as key degradative enzymes mediating TnI proteolysis during increased preload. These findings suggest the hypothesis that sustained increases in LV end-diastolic pressure, as are often observed among patients with advanced heart failure, could contribute to contractile dysfunction via thin filament proteolysis. Potential therapeutic opportunities related to these mechanisms are suggested by recent studies demonstrating that heat shock protein 27 (Hsp27) activation via overexpression protects cTnI, cTnT, and other sarcomeric proteins against proteolysis during transient ischemia or acute calcium overload.[124]

CONCLUSIONS

Advanced physiological and molecular assays combined with a rapidly increasing array of informative transgenic models have accelerated the pace of new insights into the cellular basis of myocardial contractile dysfunction. Although these new insights have helped define the mechanisms behind many previously unexplained physiological and pathological phenomena, they have also highlighted previously unanticipated levels of complexity relevant to cardiac myocyte signaling and biophysics. These complexities include varied mechanisms of control and interaction that raise many new and important questions concerning the heirarchy pathological mechanisms operating within cardiac myocytes from failing human hearts.

Alterations in myocyte Ca^{2+} handling appear to be centrally involved in the dysfunctional characteristics of the failing heart. Indeed, the literature suggests that changes in the abundance or activity of almost all of the important Ca^{2+} regulatory molecules contribute to deranged Ca^{2+} homeostasis in the failing heart. However, it is unlikely that a change in the abundance of a single Ca^{2+} regulatory molecule is consistently responsible for contractile defects in failing hearts. At the same time, there is little doubt that alterations at the level of the sarcomeric proteins contribute to the pathophysiology of advanced heart failure in humans. While studies of patients with familial cardiomyopathies demonstrate how single allelic mutations affecting sarcomeric proteins can be sufficient to induce profound phenotypical manifestations, such disease-causing mutations represent only a small fraction of the functionally important changes in sarcomeric proteins observed in failing hearts. Indeed, recent studies have increasingly identified pathological changes in myofilament isoforms and phosphorylation that are both functionally significant and potential targets with therapeutic interventions.

FUTURE DIRECTIONS

A major unanswered question is still whether restoring normal Ca^{2+} handling in the context of the CHF environment will be beneficial or will enhance CHF progression by inducing myocyte death from Ca^{2+} overload or cause sudden death via lethal ventricular arrhythmias. Likewise, as we address current gaps in our knowledge of pathological changes in myofilament proteins, we will need to define which isoform switches and posttranslational modifications are adaptive, rather than detrimental. In addition, future studies will need to include improved integration of findings to determine the net effects of the multiple simultaneous abnormalities of isoforms and phosphorylation states that are typically observed in failing hearts. These and other studies characterizing HF-associated defects, particularly those examining human hearts, must move beyond the most extreme comparisons of end-stage hearts with nonfailing hearts to better reflect the full spectrum of abnormalities, including hearts with mild and moderate systolic dysfunction and failing hearts with preserved systolic ejection. In this regard, the clinical impact of new information will be particularly enhanced by studies clarifying whether particular cellular targets of therapy are relevant across a wide spectrum of disease or only applicable to a particular etiology or disease stage. Though not usually an initial step, such therapeutic interventions should ultimately be examined in the context of established clinical pharmacotherapy. For example, to what extent do β-blockers obviate the need for targeting abnormalities of PKA-dependent signaling observed at the level of Ca^{2+} cycling and myofilament proteins?

REFERENCES

1. Harding, J. D., Piacentino, V., III, Gaughan, J. P., et al. (2001). Electrophysiological alterations after mechanical circulatory support in patients with advanced cardiac failure. *Circulation, 104*, 1241–1247.
2. Davey, P. (2000). QT interval and mortality from coronary artery disease. *Prog Cardiovasc Dis, 42*, 359–384.
3. Katz, A. M. (2002). Maladaptive growth in the failing heart: the cardiomyopathy of overload. *Cardiovasc Drugs Ther, 16*, 245–249.
4. Shorofsky, S. R., Aggarwal, R., Corretti, M., et al. (1999). Cellular mechanisms of altered contractility in the hypertrophied heart: big hearts, big sparks. *Circ Res, 84*, 424–434.
5. Walsh, T. F., Dall'Armellina, E., Chughtai, H., et al. (2009). Adverse effect of increased left ventricular wall thickness on five year outcomes of patients with negative dobutamine stress. *J Cardiovasc Magn Reson, 11*, 25.
6. Teerlink, J. R. (2005). Overview of randomized clinical trials in acute heart failure syndromes. *Am J Cardiol, 96*, 59G–67G.
7. Desantiago, J., Ai, X., Islam, M., et al. (2008). Arrhythmogenic effects of beta2-adrenergic stimulation in the failing heart are attributable to enhanced sarcoplasmic reticulum Ca load. *Circ Res, 102*, 1389–1397.
8. Sipido, K. R. (2007). CaM or cAMP: linking beta-adrenergic stimulation to "leaky" RyRs. *Circ Res, 100*, 296–298.
9. Houser, S. R., & Margulies, K. B. (2003). Is depressed myocyte contractility centrally involved in heart failure?. *Circ Res, 92*, 350–358.
10. Bers, D. M. (2006). Altered cardiac myocyte Ca regulation in heart failure. *Physiology (Bethesda), 21*, 380–387.
11. Nuss, H. B., & Houser, S. R. (1994). Effect of duration of depolarisation on contraction of normal and hypertrophied feline ventricular myocytes. *Cardiovasc Res, 28*, 1482–1489.
12. Maier, L. S., Brandes, R., Pieske, B., et al. (1998). Effects of left ventricular hypertrophy on force and Ca^{2+} handling in isolated rat myocardium. *Am J Physiol, 274*, H1361–H1370.
13. Rossman, E. I., Petre, R. E., Chaudhary, K. W., et al. (2004). Abnormal frequency-dependent responses represent the pathophysiologic signature of contractile failure in human myocardium. *J Mol Cell Cardiol, 36*, 33–42.
14. Harding, S. E., Jones, S. M., O'Gara, P., et al. (1992). Isolated ventricular myocytes from failing and non-failing human heart: the relation of age and clinical status of patients to isoproterenol response. *J Mol Cell Cardiol, 24*, 549–564.
15. Davies, C. H., Davia, K., Bennett, J. G., et al. (1995). Reduced contraction and altered frequency response of isolated ventricular myocytes from patients with heart failure. *Circulation, 92*, 2540–2549.
16. Gwathmey, J. K., Copelas, L., MacKinnon, R., et al. (1987). Abnormal intracellular calcium handling in myocardium from patients with end-stage heart failure. *Circ Res, 61*, 70–76.
17. Antoons, G., Oros, A., Bito, V., et al. (2007). Cellular basis for triggered ventricular arrhythmias that occur in the setting of compensated hypertrophy and heart failure: considerations for diagnosis and treatment. *J Electrocardiol, 40*, S8–S14.
18. Chakir, K., Daya, S. K., Tunin, R. S., et al. (2008). Reversal of global apoptosis and regional stress kinase activation by cardiac resynchronization. *Circulation, 117*, 1369–1377.
19. Chen, X., Zhang, X., Kubo, H., et al. (2005). Ca^{2+} influx-induced sarcoplasmic reticulum Ca^{2+} overload causes mitochondrial-dependent apoptosis in ventricular myocytes. *Circ Res, 97*, 1009–1017.
20. Diwan, A., Matkovich, S. J., Yuan, Q., et al. (2009). Endoplasmic reticulum-mitochondria crosstalk in NIX-mediated murine cell death. *J Clin Invest, 119*, 203–212.
21. Nakayama, H., Chen, X., Baines, C. P., et al. (2007). Ca^{2+}- and mitochondrial-dependent cardiomyocyte necrosis as a primary mediator of heart failure. *J Clin Invest, 117*, 2431–2444.
22. Molkentin, J. D. (2006). Dichotomy of Ca^{2+} in the heart: contraction versus intracellular signaling. *J Clin Invest, 116*, 623–626.
23. Kiss, E., Ball, N. A., Kranias, E. G., et al. (1995). Differential changes in cardiac phospholamban and sarcoplasmic reticular Ca(2+)-ATPase protein levels. Effects on Ca^{2+} transport and mechanics in compensated pressure-overload hypertrophy and congestive heart failure. *Circ Res, 77*, 759–764.
24. Kranias, E. G., & Bers, D. M. (2007). Calcium and cardiomyopathies. *Subcell Biochem, 45*, 523–537.
25. Mattiello, J. A., Margulies, K. B., Jeevanandam, V., et al. (1998). Contribution of reverse-mode sodium-calcium exchange to contractions in failing human left ventricular myocytes. *Cardiovasc Res, 37*, 424–431.
26. Bassani, J. W., Yuan, W., & Bers, D. M. (1995). Fractional SR Ca release is regulated by trigger Ca and SR Ca content in cardiac myocytes. *Am J Physiol, 268*, C1313–C1319.
27. Quaile, M. P., Rossman, E. I., Berretta, R. M., et al. (2007). Reduced sarcoplasmic reticulum Ca(2+) load mediates impaired contractile reserve in right ventricular pressure overload. *J Mol Cell Cardiol, 43*, 552–563.
28. Pieske, B., Maier, L. S., Bers, D. M., et al. (1999). Ca^{2+} handling and sarcoplasmic reticulum Ca^{2+} content in isolated failing and nonfailing human myocardium. *Circ Res, 85*, 38–46.
29. Weber, C. R., Piacentino, V., III, Ginsburg, K. S., et al. (2002). Na(+)-Ca(2+) exchange current and submembrane [Ca(2+)] during the cardiac action potential. *Circ Res, 90*, 182–189.
30. Weber, C. R., Piacentino, V., III, Margulies, K. B., et al. (2002). Calcium influx via I(NCX) is favored in failing human ventricular myocytes. *Ann N Y Acad Sci, 976*, 478–479.
31. Nuss, H. B., & Houser, S. R. (1991). Voltage dependence of contraction and calcium current in severely hypertrophied feline ventricular myocytes. *J Mol Cell Cardiol, 23*, 717–726.
32. Kleiman, R. B., & Houser, S. R. (1988). Calcium currents in normal and hypertrophied isolated feline ventricular myocytes. *Am J Physiol, 255*, H1434–H1442.
33. Mukherjee, R., Hewett, K. W., Walker, J. D., et al. (1998). Changes in L-type calcium channel abundance and function during the transition to pacing-induced congestive heart failure. *Cardiovasc Res, 37*, 432–444.
34. Li, S., Margulies, K. B., Cheng, H., et al. (1999). Calcium current and calcium transients are depressed in failing human ventricular myocytes and recover in patients supported with left ventricular assist devices (abstract). *Circulation, 100*, I60.
35. He, J., Conklin, M. W., Foell, J. D., et al. (2001). Reduction in density of transverse tubules and L-type Ca(2+) channels in canine tachycardia-induced heart failure. *Cardiovasc Res, 49*, 298–307.
36. Chen, X., Piacentino, V., III, Furukawa, S., et al. (2002). L-type Ca^{2+} channel density and regulation are altered in failing human ventricular myocytes and recover after support with mechanical assist devices. *Circ Res, 91*, 517–524.
37. Schroder, F., Handrock, R., Beuckelmann, D. J., et al. (1998). Increased availability and open probability of single L-type calcium channels from failing compared with nonfailing human ventricle. *Circulation, 98*, 969–976.
38. Sipido, K. R., Stankovicova, T., Flameng, W., et al. (1998). Frequency dependence of Ca^{2+} release from the sarcoplasmic reticulum in human ventricular myocytes from end-stage heart failure. *Cardiovasc Res, 37*, 478–488.
39. Piacentino, V., III, Dipla, K., Gaughan, J. P., et al. (2000). Voltage-dependent Ca^{2+} release from the SR of feline ventricular myocytes is explained by Ca^{2+}-induced Ca^{2+} release. *J Physiol, 523*(pt 3), 533–548.
40. Gomez, A. M., Valdivia, H. H., Cheng, H., et al. (1997). Defective excitation-contraction coupling in experimental cardiac hypertrophy and heart failure. *Science, 276*, 800–806.
41. Lindner, M., Erdmann, E., & Beuckelmann, D. J. (1998). Calcium content of the sarcoplasmic reticulum in isolated ventricular myocytes from patients with terminal heart failure. *J Mol Cell Cardiol, 30*, 743–749.
42. Li, S., Margulies, K. B., Cheng, H., et al. (1999). Calcium current and calcium transients are depressed in failing human ventricular myocytes and recover in patients supported with left ventricular assist devices (abstract). *Circulation, 100*, I60.
43. Piacentino, V., III, Weber, C. R., Chen, X., et al. (2003). Cellular basis of abnormal calcium transients of failing human ventricular myocytes. *Circ Res, 92*, 651–658.
44. Marx, S. O., Reiken, S., Hisamatsu, Y., et al. (2000). PKA phosphorylation dissociates FKBP12.6 from the calcium release channel (ryanodine receptor): defective regulation in failing hearts. *Cell, 101*, 365–376.
45. Wehrens, X. H., Lehnart, S. E., Reiken, S., et al. (2006). Ryanodine receptor/calcium release channel PKA phosphorylation: a critical mediator of heart failure progression. *Proc Natl Acad Sci U S A, 103*, 511–518.
46. Eisner, D. A., Kashimura, T., O'Neill, S. C., et al. (2009). What role does modulation of the ryanodine receptor play in cardiac inotropy and arrhythmogenesis? *J Mol Cell Cardiol, 46*, 474–481.
47. Tateishi, H., Yano, M., Mochizuki, M., et al. (2009). Defective domain-domain interactions within the ryanodine receptor as a critical cause of diastolic Ca^{2+} leak in failing hearts. *Cardiovasc Res, 81*, 536–545.
48. Li, Y., Kranias, E. G., Mignery, G. A., et al. (2002). Protein kinase A phosphorylation of the ryanodine receptor does not affect calcium sparks in mouse ventricular myocytes. *Circ Res, 90*, 309–316.
49. Chelu, M. G., Sarma, S., Sood, S., et al. (2009). Calmodulin kinase II-mediated sarcoplasmic reticulum Ca^{2+} leak promotes atrial fibrillation in mice. *J Clin Invest, 119*, 1940–1951.
50. Schwinger, R. H., Bohm, M., Schmidt, U., et al. (1995). Unchanged protein levels of SERCA II and phospholamban but reduced Ca^{2+} uptake and Ca^{2+}-ATPase activity of cardiac sarcoplasmic reticulum from dilated cardiomyopathy patients compared with patients with nonfailing hearts. *Circulation, 92*, 3220–3228.
51. Movsesian, M. A., Bristow, M. R., & Krall, J. (1989). Ca^{2+} uptake by cardiac sarcoplasmic reticulum from patients with idiopathic dilated cardiomyopathy. *Circ Res, 65*, 1141–1144.
52. Kubo, H., Margulies, K. B., Piacentino, V., III, et al. (2001). Patients with end-stage congestive heart failure treated with beta-adrenergic receptor antagonists have improved ventricular myocyte calcium regulatory protein abundance. *Circulation, 104*, 1012–1018.
53. Hajjar, R. J., Zsebo, K., Deckelbaum, L., et al. (2008). Design of a phase 1/2 trial of intracoronary administration of AAV1/SERCA2a in patients with heart failure. *J Card Fail, 14*, 355–367.
54. Miyamoto, M. I., del Monte, F., Schmidt, U., et al. (2000). Adenoviral gene transfer of SERCA2a improves left-ventricular function in aortic-banded rats in transition to heart failure. *Proc Natl Acad Sci U S A, 97*, 793–798.

55. Schmidt, U., del Monte, F., Miyamoto, M. I., et al. (2000). Restoration of diastolic function in senescent rat hearts through adenoviral gene transfer of sarcoplasmic reticulum Ca^{2+}-ATPase. *Circulation, 1*, 790–796.
56. Minamisawa, S., Hoshijima, M., Chu, G., et al. (1999). Chronic phospholamban-sarcoplasmic reticulum calcium ATPase interaction is the critical calcium cycling defect in dilated cardiomyopathy. *Cell, 99*, 313–322.
57. Rockman, H. A., Chien, K. R., Choi, D. J., et al. (1998). Expression of a beta-adrenergic receptor kinase 1 inhibitor prevents the development of myocardial failure in gene-targeted mice. *Proc Natl Acad Sci U S A, 95*, 7000–7005.
58. Kirchberger, M. A., Tada, M., & Katz, A. M. (1974). Adenosine 3′:5′-monophosphate-dependent protein kinase-catalyzed phosphorylation reaction and its relationship to calcium transport in cardiac sarcoplasmic reticulum. *J Biol Chem, 249*, 6166–6173.
59. Meyer, M., Bluhm, W. F., He, H., et al. (1999). Phospholamban-to-SERCA2 ratio controls the force-frequency relationship. *Am J Physiol, 276*, H779–H785.
60. Schmidt, U., Hajjar, R. J., Kim, C. S., et al. (1999). Human heart failure: cAMP stimulation of SR Ca(2+)-ATPase activity and phosphorylation level of phospholamban. *Am J Physiol, 277*, H474–H480.
61. Huang, B., Wang, S., Qin, D., et al. (1999). Diminished basal phosphorylation level of phospholamban in the postinfarction remodeled rat ventricle: role of beta-adrenergic pathway, Gi protein, phosphodiesterase, and phosphatases. *Circ Res, 85*, 848–855.
62. DeWitt, M. M., MacLeod, H. M., Soliven, B., et al. (2006). Phospholamban R14 deletion results in late-onset, mild, hereditary dilated cardiomyopathy. *J Am Coll Cardiol, 48*, 1396–1398.
63. Eisner, D. A., Lederer, W. J., & Vaughan-Jones, R. D. (1984). The quantitative relationship between twitch tension and intracellular sodium activity in sheep cardiac Purkinje fibres. *J Physiol, 355*, 251–266.
64. Chaudhary, K. W., Rossman, E. I., Piacentino, V., III, et al. (2004). Altered myocardial Ca^{2+} cycling after left ventricular assist device support in the failing human heart. *J Am Coll Cardiol, 44*, 837–845.
65. Hasenfuss, G., Meyer, M., Schillinger, W., et al. (1997). Calcium handling proteins in the failing human heart. *Basic Res Cardiol, 92*(suppl 1), 87–93.
66. Bers, D. M., & Bridge, J. H. (1989). Relaxation of rabbit ventricular muscle by Na-Ca exchange and sarcoplasmic reticulum calcium pump. Ryanodine and voltage sensitivity. *Circ Res, 65*, 334–342.
67. Bridge, J. H., Ershler, P. R., & Cannell, M. B. (1999). Properties of Ca^{2+} sparks evoked by action potentials in mouse ventricular myocytes. *J Physiol, 518*, 469–478.
68. Yao, A., Su, Z., Nonaka, A., et al. (1998). Effects of overexpression of the Na^{+}-Ca^{2+} exchanger on Ca^{2+} i transients in murine ventricular myocytes. *Circ Res, 82*, 657–665.
69. Hasenfuss, G., Reinecke, H., Studer, R., et al. (1994). Relation between myocardial function and expression of sarcoplasmic reticulum Ca^{2+}-ATPase in failing and nonfailing human myocardium. *Circ Res, 75*, 434–442.
70. Murphy, A. M., Kögler, H., Georgakopoulos, D., et al. (2000). Transgenic mouse model of stunned myocardium. *Science, 287*, 488–491.
71. Solaro, R. J., & Rarick, H. M. (1998). Troponin and tropomyosin: proteins that switch on and tune in the activity of cardiac myofilaments. *Circ Res, 83*, 471–480.
72. Greene, L. E., & Eisenberg, E. (1980). Cooperative binding of myosin subfragment-1 to the actin-troponin-tropomyosin complex. *Proc Natl Acad Sci U S A, 77*, 2616–2620.
73. Engel, P. L., Kobayashi, T., Biesiadecki, B., et al. (2007). Identification of a region of troponin I important in signaling cross-bridge-dependent activation of cardiac myofilaments. *J Biol Chem, 282*, 183–193.
74. Rice, J. J., Wang, F., Bers, D. M., et al. (2008). Approximate model of cooperative activation and crossbridge cycling in cardiac muscle using ordinary differential equations. *Biophys J, 95*, 2368–2390.
75. Allen, D. G., & Kurihara, S. (1982). The effects of muscle length on intracellular calcium transients in mammalian cardiac muscle. *J Physiol, 327*, 79–94.
76. Hibberd, M. G., & Jewell, B. R. (1982). Calcium- and length-dependent force production in rat ventricular muscle. *J Physiol, 329*, 527–540.
77. Allen, D. G., & Kentish, J. C. (1985). The cellular basis of the length-tension relation in cardiac muscle. *J Mol Cell Cardiol, 17*, 821–840.
78. Konhilas, J. P., Irving, T. C., & de Tombe, P. P. (2002). Myofilament calcium sensitivity in skinned rat cardiac trabeculae: role of interfilament spacing. *Circ Res, 90*, 59–65.
79. Cazorla, O., Wu, Y., Irving, T. C., et al. (2001). Titin-based modulation of calcium sensitivity of active tension in mouse skinned cardiac myocytes. *Circ Res, 88*, 1028–1035.
80. Cazorla, O., Szilagyi, S., Vignier, N., et al. (2006). Length and protein kinase A modulations of myocytes in cardiac myosin binding protein C-deficient mice. *Cardiovasc Res, 69*, 370–380.
81. Tachampa, K., Wang, H., Farman, G. P., et al. (2007). Cardiac troponin I threonine 144: role in myofilament length dependent activation. *Circ Res, 101*, 1081–1083.
82. Holubarsch, C., Ruf, T., Goldstein, D. J., et al. (1996). Existence of the Frank-Starling mechanism in the failing human heart. Investigations on the organ, tissue, and sarcomere levels. *Circulation, 94*, 683–689.
83. Alcalai, R., Seidman, J. G., & Seidman, C. E. (2008). Genetic basis of hypertrophic cardiomyopathy: from bench to the clinics. *J Cardiovasc Electrophysiol, 19*, 104–110.
84. Kamisago, M., Sharma, S. D., DePalma, S. R., et al. (2000). Mutations in sarcomere protein genes as a cause of dilated cardiomyopathy. *N Engl J Med, 343*, 1688–1696.
85. Soor, G. S., Luk, A., Ahn, E., et al. (2009). Hypertrophic cardiomyopathy: current understanding and treatment objectives. *J Clin Pathol, 62*, 226–235.
86. Ojamaa, K., Samarel, A. M., Kupfer, J. M., et al. (1992). Thyroid hormone effects on cardiac gene expression independent of cardiac growth and protein synthesis. *Am J Physiol, 263*, E534–E540.
87. Miyata, S., Minobe, W., Bristow, M. R., et al. (2000). Myosin heavy chain isoform expression in the failing and nonfailing human heart. *Circ Res, 86*, 386–390.
88. Korte, F. S., Herron, T. J., Rovetto, M. J., et al. (2005). Power output is linearly related to MyHC content in rat skinned myocytes and isolated working hearts. *Am J Physiol Heart Circ Physiol, 289*, H801–H812.
89. Metzger, J. M., Wahr, P. A., Michele, D. E., et al. (1999). Effects of myosin heavy chain isoform switching on Ca^{2+}-activated tension development in single adult cardiac myocytes. *Circ Res, 84*, 1310–1317.
90. van Rooij, E., Sutherland, L. B., Qi, X., et al. (2007). Control of stress-dependent cardiac growth and gene expression by a microRNA. *Science, 316*, 575–579.
91. Adachi, S., Ito, H., Tamamori, M., et al. (1998). Skeletal and smooth muscle alpha-actin mRNA in endomyocardial biopsy samples of dilated cardiomyopathy patients. *Life Sci, 63*, 1779–1791.
92. Morano, M., Zacharzowski, U., Maier, M., et al. (1996). Regulation of human heart contractility by essential myosin light chain isoforms. *J Clin Invest, 98*, 467–473.
93. Ritter, O., Luther, H. P., Haase, H., et al. (1999). Expression of atrial myosin light chains but not alpha-myosin heavy chains is correlated in vivo with increased ventricular function in patients with hypertrophic obstructive cardiomyopathy. *J Mol Med, 77*, 677–685.
94. Lahmers, S., Wu, Y., Call, D. R., et al. (2004). Developmental control of titin isoform expression and passive stiffness in fetal and neonatal myocardium. *Circ Res, 94*, 505–513.
95. Makarenko, I., Opitz, C. A., Leake, M. C., et al. (2004). Passive stiffness changes caused by upregulation of compliant titin isoforms in human dilated cardiomyopathy hearts. *Circ Res, 95*, 708–716.
96. van Heerebeek, L., Borbely, A., Niessen, H. W., et al. (2006). Myocardial structure and function differ in systolic and diastolic heart failure. *Circulation, 113*, 1966–1973.
97. Wolff, M. R., Buck, S. H., Stoker, S. W., et al. (1996). Myofibrillar calcium sensitivity of isometric tension is increased in human dilated cardiomyopathies: role of altered beta-adrenergically mediated protein phosphorylation. *J Clin Invest, 98*, 167–176.
98. Kentish, J. C., McCloskey, D. T., Layland, J., et al. (2001). Phosphorylation of troponin I by protein kinase A accelerates relaxation and crossbridge cycle kinetics in mouse ventricular muscle. *Circ Res, 88*, 1059–1065.
99. Kulikovskaya, I., McClellan, G., Flavigny, J., et al. (2003). Effect of MyBP-C binding to actin on contractility in heart muscle. *J Gen Physiol, 122*, 761–774.
100. Tong, C. W., Stelzer, J. E., Greaser, M. L., et al. (2008). Acceleration of crossbridge kinetics by protein kinase A phosphorylation of cardiac myosin binding protein C modulates cardiac function. *Circ Res, 103*, 974–982.
101. Stelzer, J. E., Patel, J. R., Walker, J. W., et al. (2007). Differential roles of cardiac myosin-binding protein C and cardiac troponin I in the myofibrillar force responses to protein kinase A phosphorylation. *Circ Res, 101*, 503–511.
102. Herron, T. J., Korte, F. S., & McDonald, K. S. (2001). Power output is increased after phosphorylation of myofibrillar proteins in rat skinned cardiac myocytes. *Circ Res, 89*, 1184–1190.
103. Hamdani, N., de Waard, M., Messer, A. E., et al. (2008). Myofilament dysfunction in cardiac disease from mice to men. *J Muscle Res Cell Motil, 29*, 189–201.
104. Zakhary, D. R., Moravec, C. S., Stewart, R. W., et al. (1999). Protein kinase A (PKA)-dependent troponin-I phosphorylation and PKA regulatory subunits are decreased in human dilated cardiomyopathy. *Circulation, 99*, 505–510.
105. Gwathmey, J. K., & Hajjar, R. J. (1990). Effect of protein kinase C activation on sarcoplasmic reticulum function and apparent myofibrillar Ca^{2+} sensitivity in intact and skinned muscles from normal and diseased human myocardium. *Circ Res, 67*, 744–752.
106. Noland, T. A., Jr., Raynor, R. L., & Kuo, J. F. (1989). Identification of sites phosphorylated in bovine cardiac troponin I and troponin T by protein kinase C and comparative substrate activity of synthetic peptides containing the phosphorylation sites. *J Biol Chem, 264*, 20778–20785.
107. Noland, T. A., Jr., Guo, X., Raynor, R. L., et al. (1995). Cardiac troponin I mutants. Phosphorylation by protein kinases C and A and regulation of Ca(2+)-stimulated MgATPase of reconstituted actomyosin S-1. *J Biol Chem, 270*, 25445–25454.
108. Montgomery, D. E., Chandra, M., Huang, Q., et al. (2001). Transgenic incorporation of skeletal TnT into cardiac myofilaments blunts PKC-mediated depression of force. *Am J Physiol Heart Circ Physiol, 280*, H1011–H1018.
109. Sumandea, M. P., Pyle, W. G., Kobayashi, T., et al. (2003). Identification of a functionally critical protein kinase C phosphorylation residue of cardiac troponin T. *J Biol Chem, 278*, 35135–35144.
110. Noguchi, T., Hunlich, M., Camp, P. C., et al. (2004). Thin-filament-based modulation of contractile performance in human heart failure. *Circulation, 110*, 982–987.
111. van der Velden, J., Narolska, N. A., Lamberts, R. R., et al. (2006). Functional effects of protein kinase C-mediated myofilament phosphorylation in human myocardium. *Cardiovasc Res, 69*, 876–887.
112. Belin, R. J., Sumandea, M. P., Allen, E. J., et al. (2007). Augmented protein kinase C-alpha-induced myofilament protein phosphorylation contributes to myofilament dysfunction in experimental congestive heart failure. *Circ Res, 101*, 195–204.
113. Yamasaki, R., Wu, Y., McNabb, M., et al. (2002). Protein kinase A phosphorylates titin's cardiac-specific N2B domain and reduces passive tension in rat cardiac myocytes. *Circ Res, 90*, 1181–1188.
114. Kruger, M., Kotter, S., Grutzner, A., et al. (2009). Protein kinase G modulates human myocardial passive stiffness by phosphorylation of the titin springs. *Circ Res, 104*, 87–94.
115. Kruger, M., & Linke, W. A. (2009). Titin-based mechanical signalling in normal and failing myocardium. *J Mol Cell Cardiol, 46*, 490–498.
116. Borbely, A., van der Velden, J., Papp, Z., et al. (2005). Cardiomyocyte stiffness in diastolic heart failure. *Circulation, 111*, 774–781.
117. Takimoto, E., Champion, H. C., Li, M., et al. (2005). Chronic inhibition of cyclic GMP phosphodiesterase 5A prevents and reverses cardiac hypertrophy. *Nat Med, 11*, 214–222.
118. Salloum, F. N., Abbate, A., Das, A., et al. (2008). Sildenafil (Viagra) attenuates ischemic cardiomyopathy and improves left ventricular function in mice. *Am J Physiol Heart Circ Physiol, 294*, H1398–H1406.

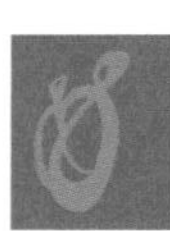

119. Hein, S., Scheffold, T., & Schaper, J. (1995). Ischemia induces early changes to cytoskeletal and contractile proteins in diseased human myocardium. *J Thorac Cardiovasc Surg, 110*, 89–98.
120. Gao, W. D., Atar, D., Backx, P. H., et al. (1995). Relationship between intracellular calcium and contractile force in stunned myocardium. Direct evidence for decreased myofilament Ca^{2+} responsiveness and altered diastolic function in intact ventricular muscle. *Circ Res, 76*, 1036–1048.
121. McDonough, J. L., Arrell, D. K., & Van Eyk, J. E. (1999). Troponin I degradation and covalent complex formation accompanies myocardial ischemia/reperfusion injury. *Circ Res, 84*, 9–20.
122. Murphy, A. M. (2006). Heart failure, myocardial stunning, and troponin: a key regulator of the cardiac myofilament. *Congest Heart Fail, 12*, 32–38, quiz 39–40.
123. Feng, J., Schaus, B. J., Fallavollita, J. A., et al. (2001). Preload induces troponin I degradation independently of myocardial ischemia. *Circulation, 103*, 2035–2037.
124. Lu, X. Y., Chen, L., Cai, X. L., et al. (2008). Overexpression of heat shock protein 27 protects against ischaemia/reperfusion-induced cardiac dysfunction via stabilization of troponin I and T. *Cardiovasc Res, 79*, 500–508.
125. Arai, M., Alpert, N. R., MacLennan, D. H., et al. (1993). Alterations in sarcoplasmic reticulum gene expression in human heart failure. A possible mechanism for alterations in systolic and diastolic properties of the failing myocardium. *Circ Res, 72*, 463–469.
126. Meyer, M., Bluhm, W. F., He, H., et al. (1995). Alterations of sarcoplasmic reticulum proteins in failing human dilated cardiomyopathy. *Circulation, 92*, 778–784.
127. Movsesian, M. A., Kirimi, M., Green, K., et al. (1994). Ca^{2+} transporting ATPase, phospholamban and calsequestrin levels in nonfailing and failing human myocardium. *Circulation, 90*, 653–657.
128. Takahashi, T., Allen, P. D., Lacro, R. V., et al. (1992). Expression of dihydropyridine receptor (Ca^{2+} channel) and calsequestrin genes in the myocardium of patients with end-stage heart failure. *J Clin Invest, 90*, 927–935.
129. Rasmussen, R. P., Minobe, W., & Bristow, M. R. (1990). Calcium antagonist binding sites in failing and nonfailing human ventricular myocardium. *Biochem Pharmacol, 39*, 691–696.
130. Mewes, T., & Ravens, U. (1994). L-type calcium currents of human myocytes from ventricle of non-failing and failing hearts and from atrium. *J Mol Cell Cardiol, 26*, 1307–1320.
131. Beuckelmann, D. J., & Erdmann, E. (1992). Ca^{2+}-currents and intracellular Ca^{2+} i-transients in single ventricular myocytes isolated from terminally failing human myocardium. *Basic Res Cardiol, 87*(suppl 1), 235–243.
132. Li, S., Margulies, K. B., Cheng, H., et al. (1999). Calcium current and calcium transients are depressed in failing human ventricular myocytes and recover in patients supported with left ventricular assist devices (abstract). *Circulation, 100*, I60.
133. Brillantes, A. M., Allen, P., & Takahash, I. T. (1992). Differences in cardiac calcium release channel (ryanodine receptor) expression in myocardium from patients with end-stage heart failure caused by ischemic versus dilated cardiomyopathy. *Circ Res, 71*, 18–26.
134. Go, L. O., Moschella, M. C., Watras, J., et al. (1995). Differential regulation of two types of intracellular calcium release channels during end-stage heart failure. *J Clin Invest, 95*, 888–894.
135. Schillinger, W., Meyer, M., Kuwajima, G., et al. (1996). Unaltered ryanodine receptor protein levels in ischemic cardiomyopathy. *Mol Cell Biochem*, 160–161, 297–302.
136. Marx, S. O., Reiken, S., Hisamatsu, Y., et al. (2000). PKA phosphorylation dissociates FKBP12.6 from the calcium release channel (ryanodine receptor): defective regulation in failing hearts. *Cell, 101*, 365–376.
137. Mercadier, J. J., Lonpre, A. M., Duc, P., et al. (1990). Altered sarcoplasmic reticulum Ca^{2+}-ATPase gene expression in the human ventricle during end-stage heart failure. *J Clin Invest, 85*(1), 305–309.
138. Schwinger, R. H., Wang, J., Frank, K., et al. (1995). Unchanged protein levels of SERCA II and phospholamban but reduced Ca^{2+} uptake and Ca^{2+}-ATPase activity of cardiac sarcoplasmic reticulum from dilated cardiomyopathy patients compared with patients with nonfailing hearts. *Circulation, 92*, 3220–3228.
139. Linck, B. B., Oknik, P., Eschenhagen, T., et al. (1996). Messenger RNA expression and immunological quantification of phospholamban and SR-Ca^{2+}ATPase in failing and nonfailing human hearts. *Cardiovasc Res, 31*, 625–632.
140. Schmidt, U., Hajjar, R. J., Helm, P. A., et al. (1998). Contribution of abnormal sarcoplasmic reticulum ATPase activity to systolic and diastolic dysfunction in human heart failure. *J Mol Cell Cardiol, 30*, 1929–1937.
141. Movsesian, M. A., Bristow, M. R., & Krall, J. (1989). Ca^{2+} uptake by cardiac sarcoplasmic reticulum from patients with idiopathic dilated cardiomyopathy. *Circ Res, 65*, 1141–1144.
142. Studer, R., Reinecke, H., Bilger, J., et al. (1994). Gene expression of the cardiac Na^+-Ca^{2+} exchanger in end-stage human heart failure. *Circ Res, 75*, 443–453.
143. Flesch, M., Schwinger, R. H., Schiffer, F., et al. (1996). Evidence for functional relevance of an enhanced expression of the Na^+-Ca^{2+} exchanger in failing human myocardium. *Circulation, 94*, 992–1002.
144. Schwinger, R. H., Munch, G., Bolck, B., et al. (1999). Reduced sodium pump alpha1, alpha3, and beta1-isoform protein levels and Na^+-K^+-ATPase activity but unchanged Na^+-Ca^{2+} exchanger protein levels in human heart failure. *Circulation, 99*, 2105–2112.
145. Kavaler, F., & Morad, M. (1966). Paradoxical effects of epinephrine on excitation-contraction coupling in cardiac muscle. *Circ Res, 18*, 492–501.
146. Zeller, R., Ivandic, B. T., Ehlermann, P., et al. (2006). Large-scale mutation screening in patients with dilated or hypertrophic cardiomyopathy: a pilot study using DGGE. *J Mol Med, 84*, 682–691.
147. Solaro, R. J., Moir, A. J., & Perry, S. V. (1976). Phosphorylation of troponin I and the inotropic effect of adrenaline in the perfused rabbit heart. *Nature, 262*, 615–617.
148. Wang, H., Grant, J. E., Doede, C. M., et al. (2006). PKC-betaII sensitizes cardiac myofilaments to Ca^{2+} by phosphorylating troponin I on threonine-144. *J Mol Cell Cardiol, 41*, 823–833.
149. Meder, B., Laufer, C., Hassel, D., et al. (2009). A single serine in the carboxyl terminus of cardiac essential myosin light chain-1 controls cardiomyocyte contractility in vivo. *Circ Res, 104*, 650–659.
150. Olsson, M. C., Patel, J. R., Fitzsimons, D. P., et al. (2004). Basal myosin light chain phosphorylation is a determinant of Ca^{2+} sensitivity of force and activation dependence of the kinetics of myocardial force development. *Am J Physiol Heart Circ Physiol, 287*, H2712–H2718.
151. Jacques, A. M., Briceno, N., Messer, A. E., et al. (2008). The molecular phenotype of human cardiac myosin associated with hypertrophic obstructive cardiomyopathy. *Cardiovasc Res, 79*, 481–491.

CHAPTER 4

Cellular Basis for Myocardial Repair and Regeneration

Piero Anversa, Jan Kajstura, and Annarosa Leri

The regenerative capacity of organs is a property of particular significance in organisms with a long life span. Preservation of the components of each tissue and their functional integration is essential for survival. Damage creates a barrier to *restitutio ad integrum* and promotes the initiation of a repair process that leads to the development of a scar. Scar formation is crucial for rapid handling and seclusion of the lesion from healthy tissue, preventing a cascade of uncontrolled deleterious events. However, the scar does not possess the properties of the uninjured tissue and therefore negatively affects the overall performance of the organ. Despite the presence of resident adult stem cells in several organs, tissue repair involves scar formation.[1-3] Tissue repair in embryos is rapid, efficient, and scar-free.[4-7] Skin wounds in the early mammalian embryo heal with *restitutio ad integrum,* whereas wounds in adults result in scarring. The most important difference between these two conditions involves the inflammatory response. In embryonic wounds, a lower number of less differentiated inflammatory cells is present in the damaged region and the growth factors that accumulate at the site of healing are different from those in the adult.[4,7,8] Therefore, modulation of the inflammatory response may improve repair in adult organs but the removal of these extrinsic signals may interfere with long-term regeneration. Resident stem cells or exogenous progenitor cells administered in proximity of the lesion can modify the microenvironment by secreting cytokines that favor cell homing, growth, and differentiation.[9-12] Enhancement of intrinsic growth by resident or nonresident stem cells constitutes the basis of myocardial regeneration. Although 11 independent laboratories have identified cardiac progenitor cells (CPCs) in the adult heart,[13-25] the controversy concerning myocyte regeneration has not been resolved yet.[26-28] Questions continue to be posed regarding CPC function and the mechanisms modulating myocyte turnover with aging and cardiac repair in the presence of pathological states. Similarly, the plasticity of bone marrow–derived progenitor cells (BMPCs) and in particular their ability to transdifferentiate and acquire the myocyte lineage has been challenged and data in favor[12,29-36] or against[37-44] this possibility continue to appear in the literature (for review see Leri[45]).

CELL THERAPY

Endothelial progenitor cells, mononuclear bone marrow cells, and CD34-positive cells have been administered to patients affected by acute myocardial infarction, chronic ischemic heart failure, and refractory angina.[46-62] These interventions have had positive outcomes documenting not only the feasibility and safety of this therapeutic approach but also beneficial effects on cardiac function.[63-65] While patients are currently enrolled in large clinical trials (see Chapter 51), the documentation of cardiac-specific adult progenitor cells has created great expectations concerning the use of this new cell for the management of human disease. Theoretically, the most logic and potentially powerful cell to be employed for cardiac repair is the CPC.[66-68] It is intuitively apparent that if the adult heart possesses a pool of primitive, undifferentiated, multipotent cells, these cells must be tested first before more complex and unknown cells are explored. The attraction of this approach is its simplicity. Cardiac regeneration would be accomplished by enhancing the normal turnover of myocardial cells. However, difficulties exist in the acquisition of myocardial samples in humans, and in the isolation and expansion of CPCs in quantities that can be employed therapeutically. Conversely, BMPCs constitute an appealing form of cell intervention; BMPCs can be easily collected from bone marrow aspirates or the peripheral blood upon their mobilization from the bone marrow with cytokines.[32] At present, it is unknown whether CPCs and BMPCs are similarly effective in reconstituting necrotic myocardium after infarction or limitations exist in CPC growth and BMPC transdifferentiation resulting in inadequate restoration of lost tissue. Also, BMPCs may constitute a necessary initial form of intervention for the infarcted heart, whereas CPCs might be employed later during the chronic evolution of the cardiac myopathy.[45,53-65] Thus a fundamental question that remains to be addressed initially experimentally and later clinically is whether BMPCs are superior, equal, or inferior to CPCs for the regeneration of cardiomyocytes and coronary vessels in ischemic heart failure (Figure 4-1).

Cardiac repair after infarction is mediated by several factors including (1) number of cells to be administered, (2) cell death and survival in the hostile milieu of the infarct and periinfarcted region, (3) cell engraftment, and (4) cell growth and differentiation. An additional variable of BMPCs is their level of plasticity, which is dictated by their ability to acquire the myocyte, and vascular smooth muscle (SMC) and endothelial cell (EC) lineages. In an identical manner, CPCs have to promote the formation of a proportional number of parenchymal cells and coronary vessels. Moreover, the injected CPCs and BMPCs can contribute indirectly to cardiac regeneration by releasing a variety of peptides that exert a paracrine action on the myocardium and its resident CPCs.[12,69-74] These mechanisms are not mutually exclusive and both progenitor cell populations may participate directly and indirectly in the repair process. In all cases, progenitor cells have to engage themselves in homing into the myocardium to perform specific functions. These biological processes depend on a successful interaction between progenitor cell classes and tissue microenvironment.

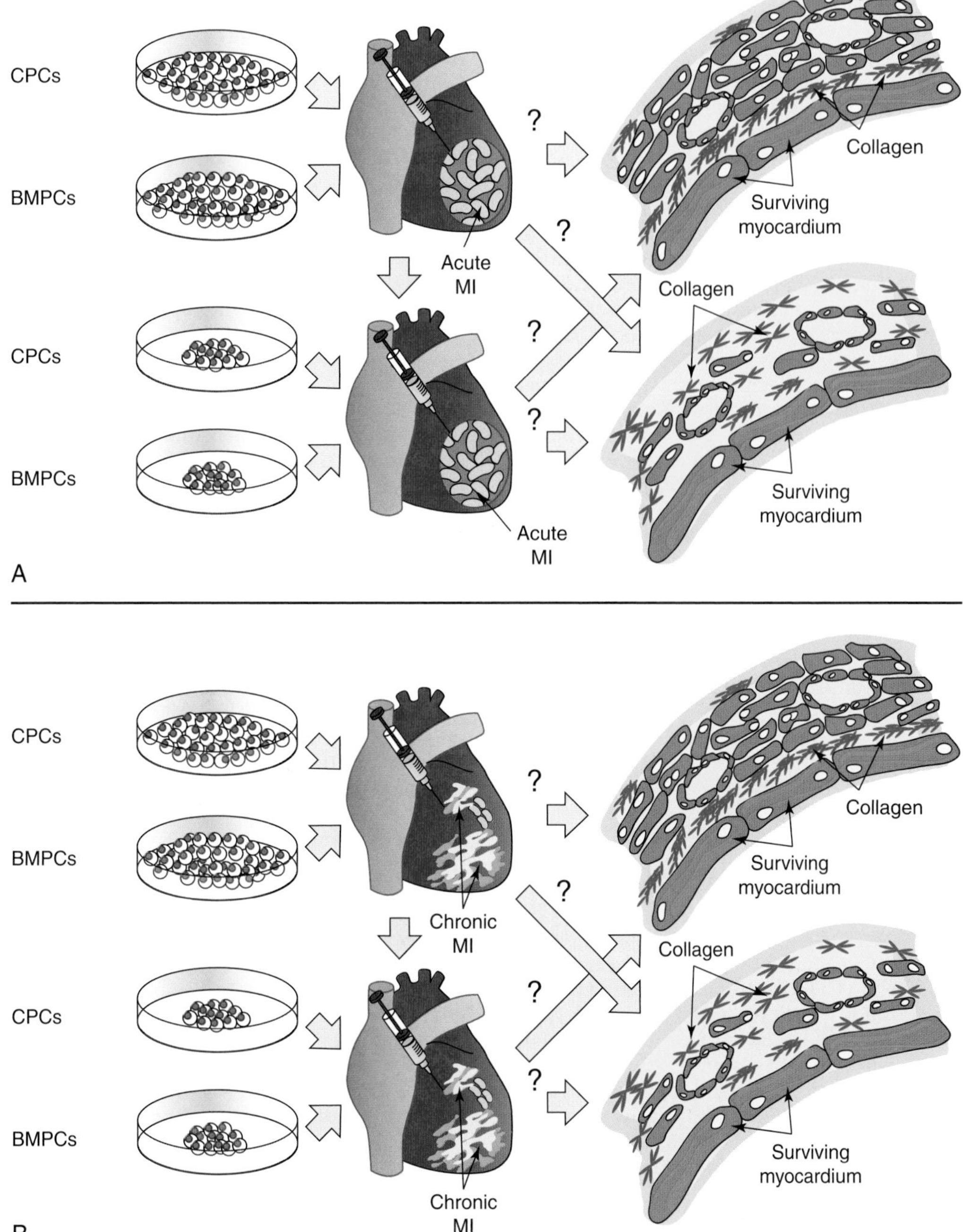

FIGURE 4–1 CPCs, BMPCs, and myocardial regeneration. **A** and **B,** The positive or negative outcome of myocardial regeneration mediated by the injection of human CPCs and BMPCs with distinct growth and/or differentiation potential is illustrated schematically in a model of acute **(A)** and chronic **(B)** myocardial infarction in immunodeficient animals. *MI,* myocardial infarction.

Importantly, the unfavorable microenvironment of the infarct varies with time and infarct healing. Apoptotic myocytes and vascular cells are replaced by diffuse cell necrosis, inflammation, and myocardial scarring. These evolving characteristics of the dead myocardium may have different consequences on CPC and BMPC homing, survival, growth, and differentiation. Cardiac repair may be severely blunted in chronic postinfarct heart failure with both BMPCs and CPCs, or one cell type might be less powerful than the other. The continuous debate in the field in terms of variety of cells being implemented and the difficulty in defining the destiny of the delivered cells has not favored a common effort in the scientific community; these critical questions have not been addressed in a collaborative, comprehensive manner. Dissimilarities in experimental designs, cell characteristics, and modality of delivery, together with substantial differences in the method of analysis of the myocardium, have further clouded understanding of the actual effects of the injected cells on the structure and function of the damaged heart. Very positive results are contrasted by completely negative findings, adding a significant level of confusion to an already rather complex and confusing new area of research and therapy.[34,41,43,67]

The Controversy

The possibility that cardiomyocytes and coronary vessels are formed by endogenous and/or exogenous progenitor cells has promoted a profound shift in paradigm of the heart, which has been viewed for decades as a terminally differentiated

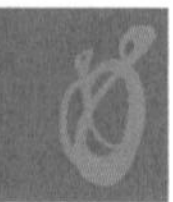

postmitotic organ. This dramatic change in understanding of cardiac behavior and function originated from observations made in the 1940s, which have continued to accumulate over the years.[75,76] However, the disagreement that persists among the members of the scientific community today was present then and has continued for nearly 70 years. The reason for the controversy is unclear, but it seems to reflect unshakable positions based on preconceived beliefs more than on careful analysis and proper consideration of published results.[66,67,75] In the course of the controversy, recurrent statements have been made to undermine the technical protocols used in studies supporting the existence of cardiac regeneration. Consistently, the data in favor of myocardial regeneration are claimed to be the product of methodological artifacts,[41,76-79] which precludes any constructive interaction among laboratories with divergent results.

Unfortunately, the old dogma has profoundly conditioned basic and clinical research in cardiology for the past 35 years.[45,66] The premise of this work is that cardiomyocytes undergo cellular hypertrophy only and cannot be replaced either by the entry into the cell cycle of a subpopulation of nonterminally differentiated myocytes or by the activation of a pool of primitive cells that become committed to the myocyte lineage. However, the efforts made to introduce a highly dynamic perspective of the heart has led to the identification and characterization of a resident pool of stem cells that can generate myocytes and ECs and SMCs organized in coronary vessels.[14] This discovery has created a new heated dispute concerning the implementation of adult cardiac stem cells in the treatment of heart failure of ischemic and nonischemic origin. Collectively, the substrate that governs the debate involves the inability of BMPCs to transdifferentiate and the limited therapeutic potential of adult CPCs for myocardial regeneration.

CELL THERAPY AND MYOCARDIAL INFARCTION

Results from our laboratory* and others† have documented that autologous BMPCs and CPCs promote cardiac repair after acute myocardial infarction, suggesting that both cell types may have important clinical implications for the management of the human disease. The stem cell antigen c-kit is expressed in a population of BMPCs that are capable of differentiating into cardiomyocytes, SMCs, and ECs restoring in large part myocardial infarcts and ventricular performance.[29,30,33,35] Similarly, c-kit is present in resident CPCs that are self-renewing, clonogenic, and multipotent in vitro and replace dead tissue with functional myocardium in vivo.[14,25,80-83] Therefore the stem cell epitope c-kit has been employed to isolate progenitor cells from the bone marrow and the heart; c-kit provides a uniform reference point for comparison between BMPCs and CPCs. The presence of the stem cell antigen c-kit has previously been found to be associated with comparable functional behavior of progenitor cells whether they derive from the heart or bone marrow. Although this approach allows us to obtain a reasonably homogeneous preparation of progenitor cells, it has limitations related to the uncommitted or early committed state of the cells, their quiescent or cycling condition, and their migratory properties. However, the collection of progenitor cell classes by stem cell antigens remains the most reasonable and sensitive strategy to date.

The mechanisms that guide stem cell homing in the myocardium are not completely understood. Cardiac injury may be necessary for migration and long-term engraftment of stem cells in the myocardium. In the absence of tissue damage, the implanted stem cells are at a growth disadvantage with respect to the endogenous stem cells. The ischemic myocardium provides a microenvironment that is particularly rich in cytokines, favoring seeding, survival, and growth of progenitor cells. The binding of SDF-1 to its receptor CXCR4 is critical in promoting homing of BMPCs to the bone marrow and distant organs,[88-98] although IGF-1 and HGF may be crucial in opposing death signals and facilitating migration, respectively.[80,81,99] SDF-1, IGF-1, and HGF are upregulated in the border zone acutely after infarction and may enhance BMPC and CPC viability, translocation, and homing (Figure 4-2).[92,100-102]

How unfavorable the scarred myocardium becomes for cell seeding is unknown and an important question. Engraftment of CPCs and BMPCs necessitates the formation of adherens and gap junctions with resident myocytes and fibroblasts, which are the supporting cells in the niches and anchor the injected cells to the host myocardium (Figure 4-3).[25,35,82,83,103] Interaction between integrin receptors on progenitor cells and extracellular matrix proteins is fundamental for cell lodging, division, and maturation.[103,104] CPCs may be better equipped than BMPCs to colonize the heart, but BMPCs may possess a high degree of plasticity adapting rapidly their phenotype to the cardiac microenvironment. Scarring may modify in an unpredictable way the possibility of cardiac regeneration. The process of transdifferentiation may alter the growth behavior of BMPCs, which may lose in part their ability to divide after the acquisition of the myocyte phenotype. Similarly, myocytes derived from BMPCs may possess inherent limitations in the acquisition of the adult phenotype. BMPCs may have a growth potential, which is superior to CPCs but transdifferentiation could affect this characteristic and CPCs may constitute a more powerful form of therapy for cardiac repair. The opposite may also be true and BMPCs may retain even after transdifferentiation a stronger regenerative capacity than CPCs representing the most appropriate cells for the damaged heart. These are all critical issues in need of resolution, which have only been partially investigated so far.

Later sections summarize current information on the growth properties of BMPCs and derived myocytes and CPCs and myocyte progeny to establish the efficacy of these progenitor cell classes for cardiac repair after infarction. A direct comparison between these two cell populations for myocardial regeneration has not been performed yet but significant knowledge has been acquired regarding their ability to engraft and form cardiomyocytes that are integrated structurally and functionally with the recipient myocardium. Additionally, limitations in the capacity of BMPCs and CPCs to differentiate and acquire the adult cardiomyocyte phenotype have been identified, pointing to crucial new areas of investigation to understand the fundamental biological processes that regulate progenitor cell function.

Progenitor Cell Homing

The movement of hematopoietic stem cells (HSCs) from the peripheral blood to the bone marrow is termed homing and is characterized by the active translocation of HSCs across the blood/bone marrow endothelial barrier and their lodging into bone marrow niches.[105-113] Following homing, engraftment occurs.[91,93,107,112] Although homing and engraftment are regulated by common mechanisms, engraftment is a long-term process that requires cell division and commitment of the stem cell progeny.[93,112] Here, homing does not refer to migration of cells from the blood and across the coronary endothelium to the myocardium, but to the migration of the delivered cells within the tissue through interstitial tunnels by the interaction of integrin receptors with extracellular matrix proteins (Figure 4-4).[80,83] This process conditions the fraction of progenitor cells that ultimately lodge within the heart and lead to

---

*References 14, 25, 29, 30, 33, 35, 80-83.
†References 12, 13, 15-23, 69-71, 73, 84-87.

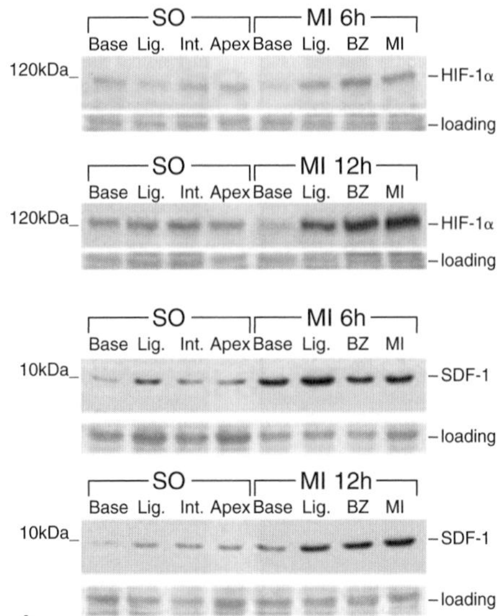

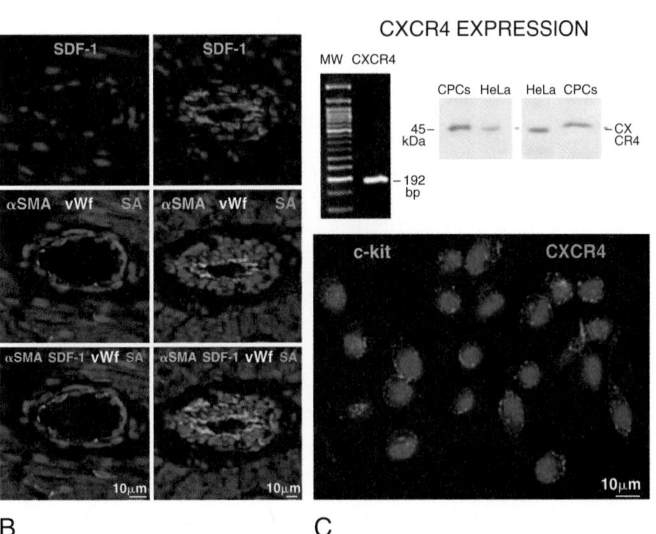

FIGURE 4–2 Myocardial ischemia and the HIF-1α-SDF-1 pathway. **A,** With respect to sham-operated rats (SO), the expression of HIF-1α and SDF-1 is enhanced in the ischemic myocardium at 6 and 12 hours after infarction. *MI,* myocardial infarct. **B,** In a model of permanent occlusion of the left anterior descending coronary artery, SDF-1 (green) was negligible in resistance arterioles located above the ligature (*left panels*), but was highly expressed in arterioles below the ligature (*right panels*). Central panels show myocytes (α-sarcomeric actin, red), ECs (von Willebrand factor, white), and SMCs (α-smooth muscle actin, magenta). **C,** CPCs express CXCR4 at the mRNA and protein levels. The presence of CXCR4 (red) in c-kit-positive (green) CPCs was confirmed by immunocytochemistry.

myocardial regeneration. Importantly, engraftment requires the expression of surface proteins involved in cell-to-cell contact and the connection between the delivered cells and the interstitial compartment.[93,103,112,114,115] Cell homing is characterized by the formation of adherens junctions (N-cadherin, E-cadherin) and gap junctions (connexin 43, connexin 45) between progenitor cells and supporting cells.

The heart typically shows discrete structures in the interstitium where CPCs are clustered together forming cardiac niches. The documentation that stem cell niches are present in the adult myocardium has been based on the identification of pockets of CPCs and the detection of cell-to-cell contact between CPCs and myocytes and fibroblasts. In the heart and in other self-renewing organs, stem cells are connected structurally and functionally to the supporting cells by junctional and adhesion proteins represented by connexins and cadherins.[108,114-117] Connexins are gap junction channel proteins that mediate passage of small molecules involved in cell-to-cell communication.[116,117] Cadherins are calcium-dependent transmembrane adhesion molecules, which have a dual function; they anchor stem cells to the microenvironment and promote a cross talk between stem cells and between stem cells and supporting cells.[108,114,115] Cardiac niches create the necessary permissive milieu for the long-term residence, survival and growth of CPCs.[103] The arrangement of CPCs and supporting cells in the cardiac niches is similar to that found in the bone marrow[109-111,113,118,119] and the brain,[120-122] providing elements of analogy for these organs. In the bone marrow, osteoblasts and stromal cells function as supporting cells.[109,111] They can be considered the equivalent of myocytes and fibroblasts found in the heart.

To date, the hematopoietic stem cell appears to be the most versatile stem cell in crossing lineage boundaries and the most prone to break the law of tissue fidelity.[123] Early studies on c-kit-positive BMPC differentiation into myocardium have generated great enthusiasm[29,30] but other observations have rejected the initial positive results[38-40] and promoted a wave of skepticism about the therapeutic potential of BMPCs

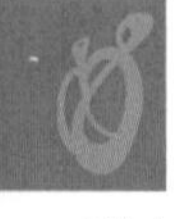

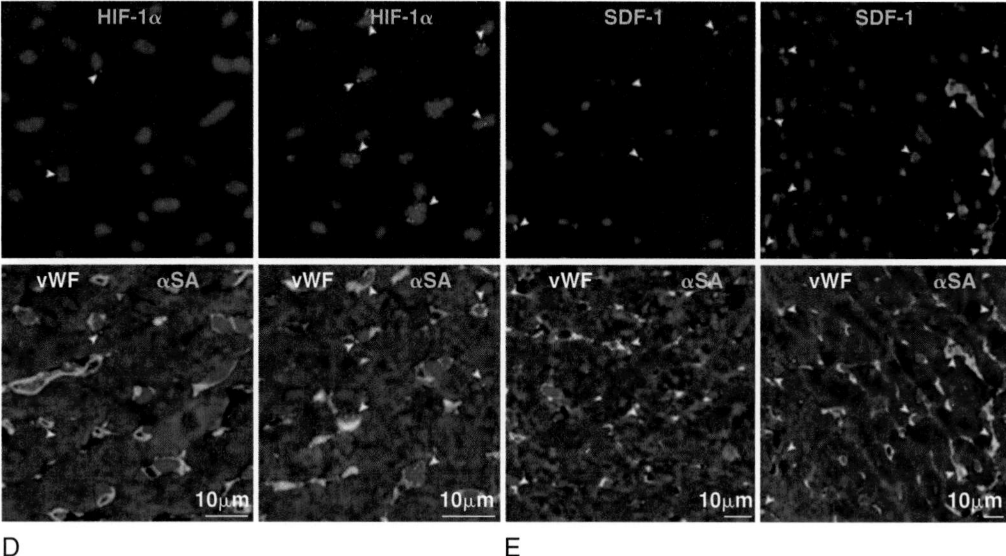

FIGURE 4–2, cont'd **D,** By immunolabeling, HIF-1α (*upper panels*; green, *arrowheads*) was detected rarely above the ligature (*left panel*) and in numerous nuclei below the ligature (*right panel*). HIF-1α is expressed in nuclei of ECs (von Willebrand factor, white) and myocytes (α-sarcomeric actin, red) (*lower panels*). **E,** SDF-1 (green, *arrowheads*) was restricted to coronary vessels; it was minimally detectable above the ligature (*left panel*) but was apparent in the border zone at 6 hours after infarction (*right panel*). Lower panels show SDF-1 together with ECs and myocytes. (From Tillmanns J, Rota M, Hosoda T, et al. Formation of large coronary arteries by cardiac progenitor cells. *Proc Natl Acad Sci U S A* 2008;105:1668–1673.)

for the injured heart. The center of the controversy is the lack of unequivocal evidence in favor of myocardial regeneration by the injection of bone marrow cells in the infarcted heart. Because of the great interest in cell-based therapy for heart failure, several approaches including gene reporter assay, genetic tagging, cell genotyping, PCR-based detection of donor genes, and direct immunofluorescence with quantum dots have recently been employed to prove or disprove bone marrow cell transdifferentiation into functionally competent myocardium after permanent coronary occlusion. To demonstrate reproducibility of results, four laboratories with complementary expertise decided to undertake a series of joined experiments to acquire unequivocal information on the plasticity of BMPCs and their therapeutic potential for the infarcted heart.[35]

A necessary premise of BMPC transdifferentiation with acquisition of the cardiogenic fate involves the engraftment of the donor cells within the host myocardium. Shortly after cell implantation, donor BMPCs seed within the viable myocardium of the border zone and integrate structurally within the surrounding tissue (Figure 4-5). Junctional and adhesion complexes form between BMPCs and between BMPCs and adjacent myocytes and fibroblasts.[35] In the absence of engraftment, BMPCs die by apoptosis; cell death is restricted to BMPCs that fail to express connexin 43 and N-cadherin and are unable to take residence in the host myocardium. This aspect of cell death is termed anoikis and is triggered by the lack of cell-to-cell contact.[124-126] This is one of the aspects of programmed cell death initiated by the inability of cells to make proper interconnections with adjacent cells; *anoikis* is a Greek word that means "homelessness." Conversely, at 48 hours, most engrafted BMPCs are proliferating. There is a time-dependent decrease in the rate of cell death and a time-dependent increase in the rate of cell division of the injected BMPCs. Because of these two variables, approximately 25% of the injected BMPCs are present in the border zone at 2 days. Importantly, similar results have been obtained following the intramyocardial injection of CPCs.[25,82,83]

Thus, adult BMPCs implanted in the infarcted heart integrate within the host myocardium by establishing temporary niches, which create the microenvironment necessary for the engrafted cells to lose the hematopoietic fate, adopt the cardiac destiny, and form de novo myocardium. By this mechanism, the engrafted cells can then exert a regenerative effect, a paracrine effect, or both. Similarly, adult CPCs engraft, survive, and grow within the myocardium, forming junctional complexes with resident myocytes and fibroblasts; they lose their primitive undifferentiated phenotype and commit to cardiac cell lineages.

Formation of Temporary Niches

As discussed and documented previously, the surviving myocardium after infarction contains niches that can host BMPCs and CPCs, but putative new niches may be formed within the thin layer of viable myocytes—interstitium surrounding the infarct. Clustering of engrafted prelabeled CPCs or BMPCs together with unlabeled recipient progenitor cells joined together by adherens junctions and gap junctions has allowed us to define expanded niches while pockets of labeled progenitor cells and labeled early committed cells have reflected the generation of putative new niches within the remaining noninfarcted myocardium. These mechanisms of CPC or BMPC engraftment may not be operative in the normal intact heart. Because of the absence of damage and need to regenerate dead myocardium, BMPCs and CPCs delivered to control intact hearts are expected to undergo apoptosis. A few cells may persist shortly after injection but they are at a growth disadvantage and subsequently die without dividing or differentiating.[82,83] Competitive repopulation studies with HSCs from different mouse strains have shown in a bone marrow transplantation protocol the behavior postulated for CPCs and BMPCs. In nonmyeloablated C57BL/6 recipients, DBA/2 HSCs become quiescent and do not show clonal growth or contribute to hematopoiesis.[127,128]

The spared myocardium after infarction contains functional niches and despite the apparent structural integrity, it is not a "normal" tissue, particularly the region bordering the infarct.[129-131] The increased wall stress and functional demand trigger myocyte hypertrophy and regeneration together with activation of interstitial fibroblasts, collagen accumulation, and capillary formation.[132] Acutely and chronically after infarction, the distant myocardium is less affected by these abnormalities creating a gradient in the reaction of the heart to ischemic damage.[133] The tissue response, however, does

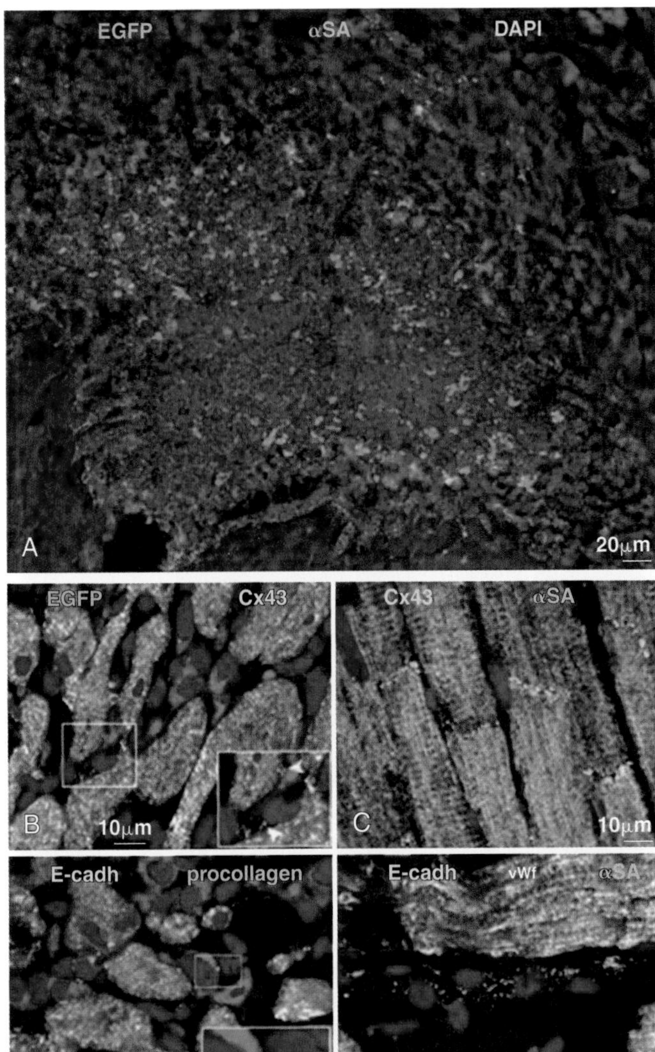

FIGURE 4-3 Engraftment of CPCs injected in proximity of the occluded coronary artery in infarcted rats. **A,** Site of injection of EGFP-positive CPCs (green) 24 hours after infarction. **B-E,** Connexin 43 (Cx43, yellow) and E-cadherin (E-cadh, yellow) are expressed between the injected CPCs (EGFP, green) and the recipient myocytes (B, α-sarcomeric actin; white) and fibroblasts (D, procollagen; red). Gap and adherens junctions are shown at higher magnifications in the insets (*arrowheads*). Cardiomyocytes and coronary vessels were employed as positive controls for connexin 43 and E-cadherin labeling. (From Tillmanns J, Rota M, Hosoda T, et al. Formation of large coronary arteries by cardiac progenitor cells. *Proc Natl Acad Sci U S A* 2008;105:1668–1673.)

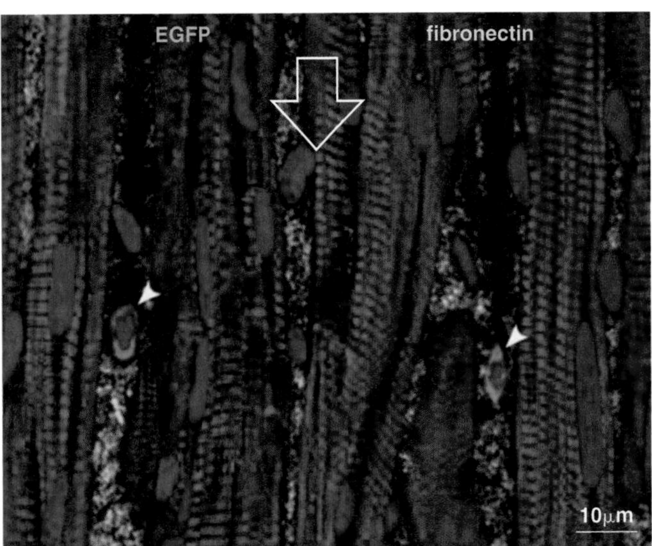

FIGURE 4-4 CPC migration towards a chemotactic gradient. Hepatocyte growth factor (HGF) was injected in the border zone of a myocardial infarct 5 hours after coronary artery ligation. EGFP-positive cells (green, *arrowheads*) translocate within interstitial tunnels made of fibronectin (yellow). The large open arrow indicates the direction of migration. (From Urbanek K, Rota M, Cascapera S. Cardiac stem cells possess growth factor-receptor systems that after activation regenerate the infarcted myocardium, improving ventricular function and long-term survival. *Circ Res* 2005;97:663–673.)

not counteract the loss in muscle mass; ventricular dilation, wall thinning, myocyte death, and inadequate vascular growth supervene, leading to a severely decompensated myopathy.[134] These alterations in combination with local accumulation of growth factors and cytokines may favor a similar gradient in engraftment of BMPCs and CPCs. However, BMPCs and CPCs may not behave in a comparable manner and may have a different capacity to lodge within the infarcted hearts, conditioning distinct degrees of myocardial regeneration and tissue repair.

To document the formation of cardiac niches, we have performed studies in which EGFP-positive–c-kit-positive CPCs were injected in proximity of the border zone after infarction (Figure 4-6). Cells homed to this region and occasionally to the remote myocardium. Cells were distributed in the interstitium as doublets or triplets and continued to express c-kit. CPCs engrafted within preexisting pockets of CPCs; cadherins and connexins were present between EGFP-positive–c-kit-positive CPCs and fibroblasts or myocytes, which are the supporting cells of the cardiac niches.[103] A different phenomenon occurs when, shortly after coronary artery ligation, progenitor cells are injected locally within the myocardium at the base of the heart, far away from the border zone and the infarct. The lack of injury together with a relatively intact microenvironment appears to act against CPC homing and engraftment activating predominantly the apoptotic pathway.[124-126] These heterogeneous myocardial environments allow comparing distinct regions of the infarcted heart and identify substrates favoring homing and engraftment of implanted CPCs and BMPCs or activating the cell death pathway. Whether CPCs and BMPCs similarly adapt to these variable conditions of the myocardium is unknown and critically relevant to stem cell therapy. Currently, there is no systematic analysis of the ability of BMPCs and CPCs to expand or create niche structures within the infarcted heart.

Engraftment of BMPCs and CPCs locally within the myocardium is mediated by SDF-1. The hypoxia-inducible factor-1 (HIF-1) is a transcriptional regulator of the SDF-1 chemokine.[94,135,136] HIF-1 and SDF-1 are upregulated with ischemia and correlate with the oxygen gradient within the tissue.[136] This myocardial response may create a gradient in which hypoxia increases progressively from the border zone to the apex of the infarcted ventricle. Such distribution of oxygen may be seen in longitudinal sections of the infarcted heart (Figure 4-7). Ischemia activates a rapid response characterized by upregulation of HIF-1 protein in vascular ECs coupled with SDF-1 synthesis and accumulation in the interstitium. CPCs and BMPCs express CXCR4,[82,90,96,137,138] the receptor of SDF-1 suggesting that progenitor cell engraftment may be triggered by the local formation of SDF-1 followed by the activation of CXCR4 receptors on progenitor cells.[139-141] SDF-1 binding to CXCR4 is required for successful engraftment of CPCs or BMPCs into the myocardium (see Figure 4-2);[35,82,83] this may lead to the generation of temporary niches, the expansion of existing niches or both, before the acquisition of specific cell phenotypes and the formation of functionally competent cardiac cells.

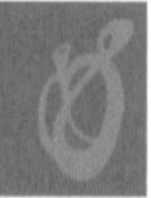

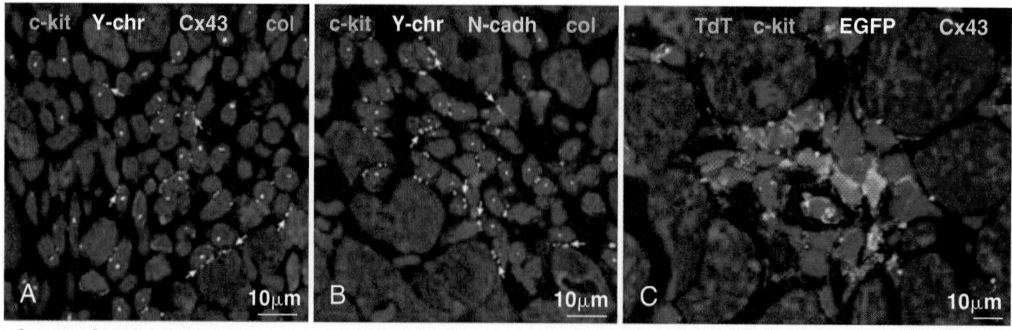

FIGURE 4–5 Engraftment of BMPCs in the acutely infarcted heart. EGFP-positive male BMPCs were injected in the border zone shortly after coronary occlusion. **A** and **B,** Within 12 to 24 hours, clusters of BMPCs engraft within the recipient myocardium. BMPCs are c-kit-positive (green) and carry the Y chromosome (Y-chr, white dots). Connexin 43 (A, Cx43; yellow dots) and N-cadherin (B, N-cadh; yellow dots) are present between male BMPCs (*arrows*), and between male BMPCs and Y-chromosome-negative female myocytes (α-sarcomeric-actin, red; *arrows*) and fibroblasts (procollagen, col, magenta; *arrows*). **C,** Apoptosis (TdT, magenta) involves exclusively nonengrafted EGFP-positive (white) BMPCs (c-kit, green). Connexin 43 (Cx43, yellow dots) is absent in apoptotic BMPCs. (From Rota M, Kajstura J, Hosoda T. Bone marrow cells adopt the cardiomyogenic fate in vivo. *Proc Natl Acad Sci U S A* 2007;104:17783–17788.)

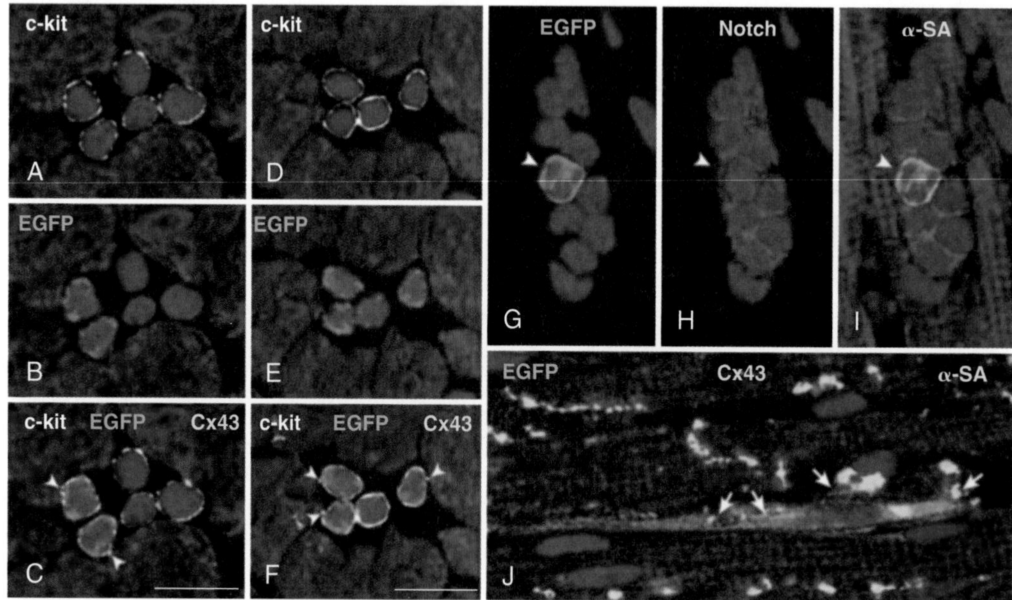

FIGURE 4–6 Formation of niches in the viable myocardium after infarction. Following injection in the border zone, EGFP-positive c-kit-positive CPCs can engraft within preexisting niches (A-C, G-I, expanded niches) or form new niches (D-F). **A-C,** Five c-kit-positive CPCs (A, C, white), two of which are EGFP-positive (B, C, green) are present in the same niche. **D-F,** Four c-kit-positive CPCs (D, F, white), which are all EGFP-positive (E, F, green) are present in the same niche. **G-I,** One EGFP-positive CPC (G, I, green) lodged into a cluster of CPCs expressing the Notch1 receptor (H, I, red). **J,** One EGFP-positive CPC engrafted and differentiated into a myocyte. Note the presence of connexin 43 (yellow dots, *arrows*) between the EGFP-positive and EGFP-negative myocytes.

Regulation of Progenitor Cell Growth

A critical aspect of cell therapy involves the characterization of the growth properties of the cells to be administered. It is rather surprising that this fundamental factor of cell function with great clinical import has been largely neglected. Comments in this regard are frequently made but, with some exceptions,[68] no specific protocols have been defined or proposed. Proliferation of CPCs and BMPCs is regulated by telomerase activity and telomeric length.[142-146] Replicative senescence corresponds to G1 growth arrest triggered by shortening of telomeres beyond a critical length.[147-150] Currently, it is unknown whether in the same organism BMPCs and CPCs have similar telomerase activity and telomeric length and, thereby, similar growth reserve.

Defects in hematopoiesis[151-154] and cardiomyogenesis[155] are present in telomerase null mice but a direct comparison between BMPC and CPC growth remains to be performed. For effective cardiac repair, BMPCs have to engraft and commit to the myocyte phenotype and this process requires transdifferentiation of BMPCs to a lineage distinct from the organ of origin.[45,123,156] Defects in telomerase activity and telomere length oppose lodging of progenitor cells.[154,157] Also the transdifferentiated progeny could have a limited capacity to divide and form functionally competent cardiomyocytes. Importantly, telomere dysfunction can occur by abnormalities in the expression and/or DNA-binding properties of telomere-related proteins.[158-160] We have found that defects in TRF1, TRF2, DNAPKcs, Ku86, Ku70, and PARP develop together with telomeric shortening and the expression of the senescent proteins[147-150,160-162] p53 and $p16^{INK4a}$ in CPCs and amplifying myocytes with heart failure in animal models and humans (Figure 4-8).[99,163-166] Therefore measurements of telomerase activity and telomere integrity and function are crucial for the recognition of the potential therapeutic efficacy of BMPCs and CPCs before their injection within the myocardium. This baseline information has to be complemented with in situ measurements of the cell cycle and telomeric length in engrafted cells to define cell division and telomere length at the single cell level. Additionally, the distribution of these parameters needs to be integrated with the assessment of cellular senescence by detection of p53 and

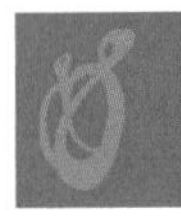

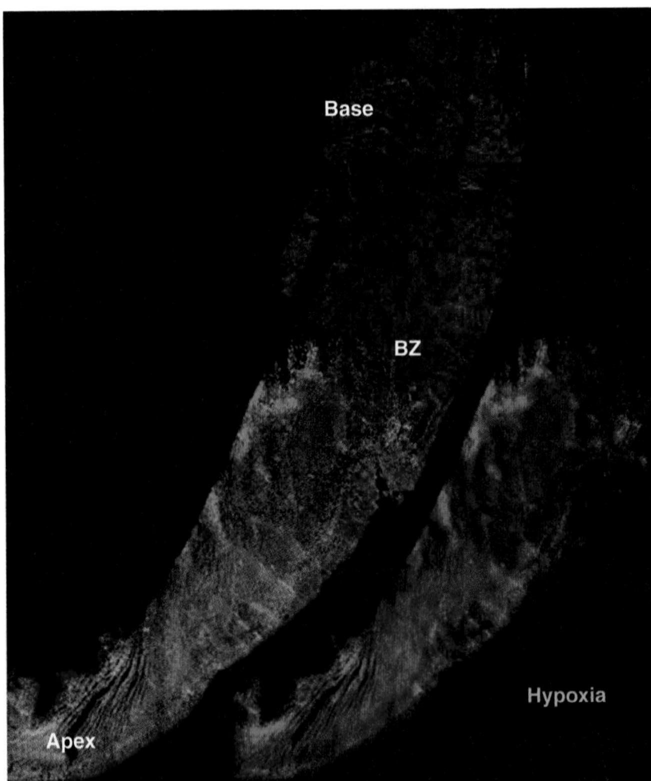

FIGURE 4–7 Hypoxia in the infarcted heart. After coronary artery ligation, a gradient is formed in which hypoxia increases progressively from the border zone to the apex of the ventricle. The distribution of oxygen is shown in longitudinal sections of the infarcted heart 12 hours after the injection of a pimonidazole probe. Ischemic areas are depicted in green and fluorescence intensity corresponds to the degree of hypoxia. *BZ,* Border zone.

p16^{INK4a}.[155,163-166] Similar analyses have to be done in the population of amplifying myocytes to establish the reparative potential of progenitor cell categories and their committed progeny (see Figure 4-8).

By this integrated approach, the therapeutic efficacy of BMPCs and CPCs can be determined before their delivery to the myocardium. These parameters condition the outcome of the treatment and may be employed to vary the number of cells to be administered in each patient to optimize cell therapy. The relevance of the telomerase-telomere axis and cellular senescence of progenitor cells for understanding cell turnover and regeneration in the normal and diseased heart has recently been emphasized.[68,167,168]

Fate of the Engrafted Cells

Successful engraftment of CPCs and BMPCs in proximity or within the infarct is the initial fundamental process of tissue repair. However, this is only the first part of the complex and long journey of progenitor cells. In proximity of the infarct, the engrafted cells have to survive within the myocardium and migrate from the seeding site to the border of the damaged area, invade the infarct, and ultimately grow and differentiate. The concentration of HGF and IGF-1 increases after infarction and this mimics the response of HIF-1 and SDF-1, suggesting that the local levels of HGF and IGF-1 may play a critical role in the ability of progenitor cells to counteract death signals and translocate to the infarct or remain viable within the dead tissue.[80,81] Myocardial reconstitution necessitates the generation of a cardiomyocyte compartment and a well-balanced coronary vasculature. Myocytes alone in the absence of adequate blood supply cannot perform their function and generate force, and coronary vessels alone without muscle mass cannot restore ventricular performance.[45,169] The question is whether commitment of engrafted progenitor cells leads to a coordinated growth response in which cardiomyocytes, resistance arterioles, and capillary profiles are concurrently developed to engender functionally competent myocardium. Coronary blood flow is regulated by resistance to coronary arterioles,[170] while oxygen availability and diffusion are controlled by the capillary network.[133,171,172] The effects that CXCR4-SDF-1, c-Met-HGF, and IGF-1R-IGF-1 growth factor systems have on CPC and BMPC engraftment, survival, growth, and differentiation have only been partially elucidated.[80,81,137-140,173-175]

Results obtained in our laboratory suggest that local activation of resident CPCs by growth factors acutely after infarction results in a significant recovery of muscle mass and approximately 20% of the regenerated myocytes acquire the adult phenotype over a period of 4 months.[80] Shorter intervals lead to the formation of a minimal number of myocytes with volumes comparable to those present in the adult heart. Similarly, the intramyocardial injection of CPCs induces a substantial recovery of the infarcted myocardium but also in this case, the regenerated myocytes are small and resemble fetal-neonatal cells.[14] Whether this is a time-dependent process or constitutes an intrinsic biological defect in CPC differentiation is unknown. This problem is even more apparent when BMPCs are employed for myocardial repair. The mobilization of BMPCs with cytokines[30] or the direct implantation of BMPCs in proximity of the infarcted myocardium[29,33,35] is not associated with the development of adult myocytes. And this phenomenon persists up to 3 months with either treatment. The possible superior efficacy of resident CPCs has also been suggested by their ability to rescue animals with infarcts commonly incompatible with life in rodents,[80] a phenomenon that was not observed with BMPCs.[29,30,33,35] However, it is difficult to make appropriate comparisons between CPCs and BMPCs with available work. None of the experiments was designed to analyze the therapeutic impact of CPCs versus BMPCs. The number of injected or activated cells was not controlled in the two conditions, and parallel studies were not performed. This is of crucial import because if BMPCs and CPCs have similar beneficial effects on cardiac repair and myocyte differentiation, BMPCs may become the most appropriate form of cell therapy for the infarcted heart. BMPCs have been well characterized biologically[176] and, most importantly, have been employed clinically for nearly 3 decades.[177,178] They are easy to obtain, they are safe, and they do not generate malignant neoplasms when injected in the systemic circulation.

To establish whether CPCs and BMPCs have comparable or dissimilar efficacy in cardiac repair after infarction, the number and phenotypic properties of generated myocytes will have to be characterized. If we assume that the physiological postnatal maturation of the heart[132,143,179] represents the gold standard paradigm for effective and successful myocardial regeneration, several criteria will have to be met: (1) Shortly after engraftment, progenitor cells would be expected to generate a large number of myocytes resembling neonatal cells, approximately 1000 μm^3 in volume;[*] (2) myocyte proliferation should decrease rapidly and cellular enlargement should become the predominant form of expansion of muscle mass, reaching the adult phenotype approximately 20,000 to 25,000 μm^3;[†] (3) myocyte apoptosis should be relatively high in the early phases of cardiac repair and minimal when the myocytes have fully matured[‡];(4) because of the small size of cardiomyocytes, there should be approximately one capillary every 10 to 15 myocytes early during regeneration, but a ratio of nearly one capillary to one myocyte should be reached in a

*References 14, 29, 30, 33, 35, 80, 81.
†References 14, 29, 30, 33, 35, 80, 81.
‡References 14, 29, 30, 33, 35, 80, 81.

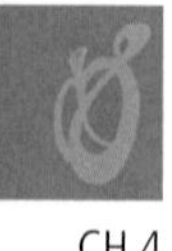

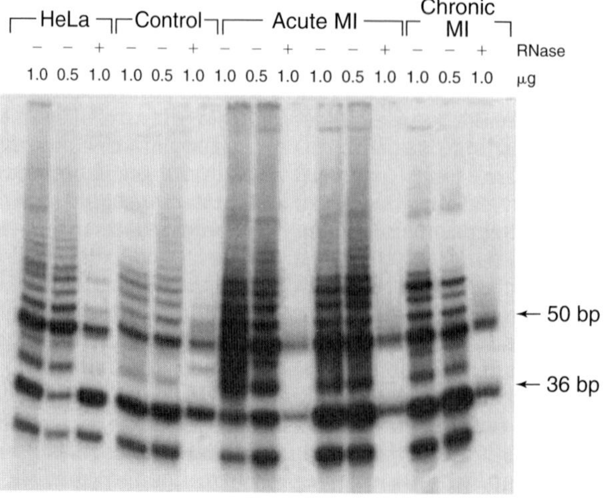

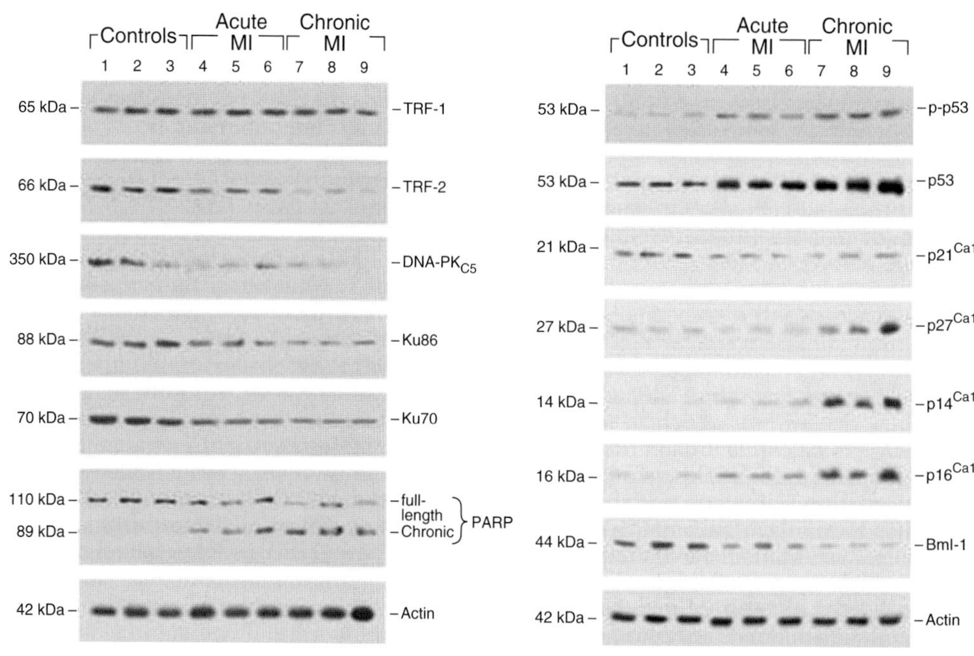

FIGURE 4–8 Heart failure and CPCs. **A,** Telomerase activity was measured by the telomeric repeat amplification protocol assay in control human hearts and in human hearts affected by acute (acute MI) and chronic (chronic MI) ischemic cardiomyopathy. Products of telomerase activity start at 50 bp and display a 6-bp periodicity. Samples treated with RNase (+) were used as a negative control and HeLa cells as a positive control. Serial dilutions of proteins (0.5 and 1.0 µg) were used to confirm the specificity of the reaction. The band at 36 bp corresponds to an internal control for PCR efficiency. **B,** Expression of the telomere-related proteins, TRF-1, TRF-2, and DNA-PK (DNA-PKcs, Ku86, and Ku70), and full-length and cleaved poly (ADP-ribose) polymerase. The expression of cell cycle inhibitors and markers of cellular senescence was also measured.

period of 4 to 6 weeks;[§] and (5) numerous coronary resistance arterioles should develop to decrease coronary resistance, and promote the integration of the new coronary vasculature with the remaining coronary circulation.[‖]

Local hypoxia is commonly present during organogenesis and in adult tissues where it induces the formation of niches that protect and preserve the biological properties of stem cells in an unfavorable environment.[92,97,180-182] Hypoxia in vitro promotes survival and growth, and maintains multipotentiality of hematopoietic and neural progenitor cells.[183-185] Hypoxia also inhibits myogenesis of skeletal muscle satellite cells.[186] If myocardial regeneration recapitulates the fetal program, inadequate oxygenation of the forming myocardium may favor myocyte replication rather than differentiation. This seems to be the case since there are only a few capillaries within the regenerating myocardium and HIF-1 is upregulated in the developing myocyte nuclei and interstitial cell nuclei (Figure 4-9). In the embryonic heart, activation of the Notch receptor affects cardiomyogenesis,[187-191] pointing to the Notch pathway as a modulator of progenitor cell fate, a condition which might be mimicked in the forming myocardium. And hypoxia-induced HIF-1 expression may result in increased stability of the intracellular domain of Notch, NICD, and expression of RBP-Jk.[192]

The components of the Notch pathway, which include Notch receptors, NICD, and RBP-Jk, are present in BMPCs and in CPCs as well.[193,194] Notch interferes with BMPC maturation[195] and skeletal myogenesis[196] but favors muscle regeneration with aging.[197-199] Our recent results indicate

§References 14, 29, 30, 33, 35, 80, 81, 132, 143.

‖References 14, 29, 30, 33, 35, 80, 81.

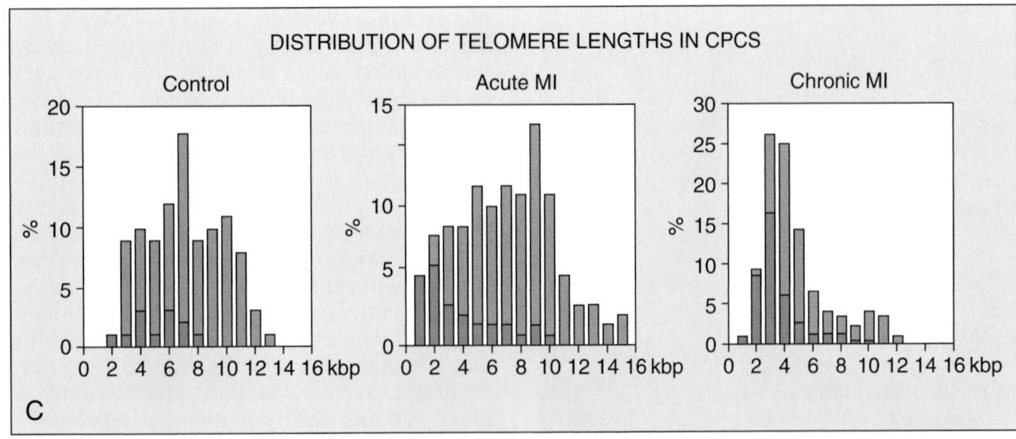

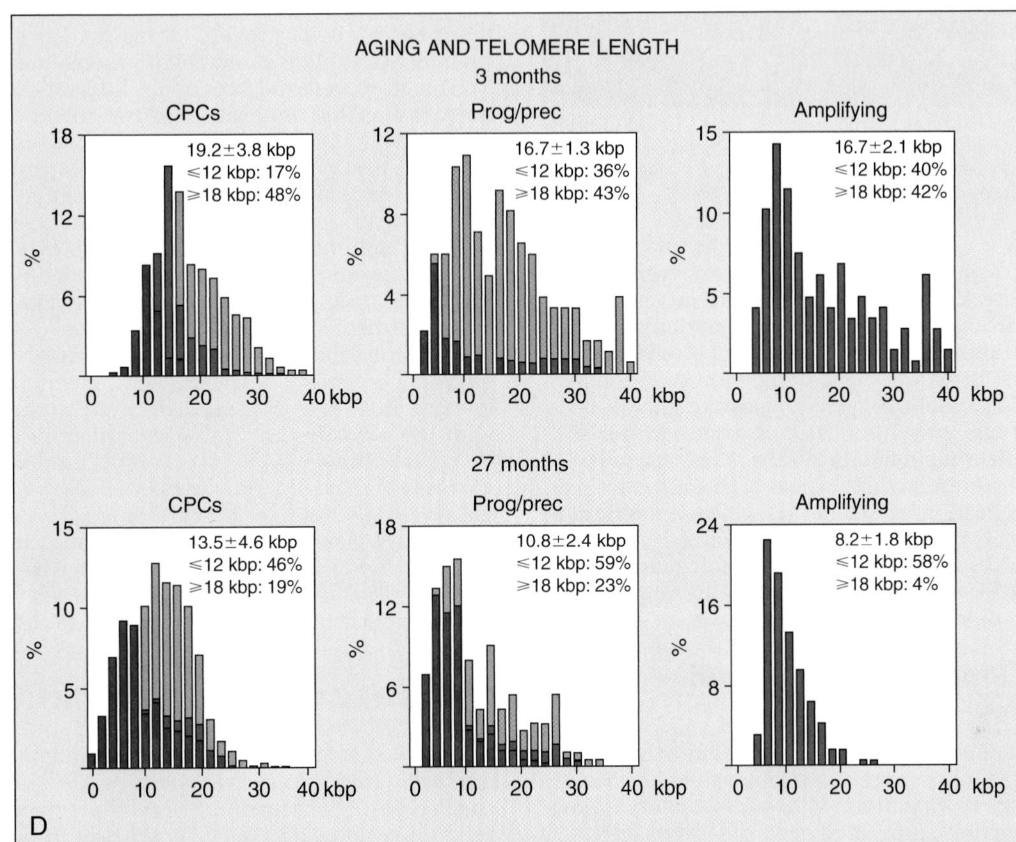

FIGURE 4–8, cont'd **C,** Telomere length in hCPCs is shifted to the left to shorter telomeres in chronic MI. The filled portion of the bars corresponds to p16^{INK4a} and/or p53-positive CPCs; they increase in acute and chronic infarcts but more dramatically in chronic infarcts. **D,** Telomere length was measured in lineage negative CPCs, myocyte progenitors-precursors, and amplifying myocytes in young (*upper panels*) and old (*lower panels*) rat hearts. Average telomere length is listed together with the percentage of cells with telomeres ≤ 12 kbp and ≥ 18 kbp. Green solid bars correspond to the fractions of cycling Ki-67-positive cells while red solid bars indicate the fractions of senescent p16^{INK4a}-positive-cells. (From Gonzalez A, Rota M, Nurzynska D. Activation of cardiac progenitor cells reverses the failing heart senescent phenotype and prolongs life span. *Circ Res* 2008;102:597-606; and Urbanek K, Torella D, Sheikh RF. Myocardial regeneration by activation of multipotent cardiac stem cells in ischemic heart failure. *Proc Natl Acad Sci U S A* 2005;102:8692-8697.)

that Notch is operative in early myocyte differentiation.[194] In the search for the molecular control of CPC differentiation, we have found that a perfect consensus site for RBP-Jk is present in the promoter region of Nkx2.5, suggesting that Nkx2.5 is a novel target gene of Notch1; band-shift assays and chromatin immunoprecipitation experiments are consistent with this possibility (Figure 4-10). Reporter gene assays have documented that the physical interaction between RBP-Jk protein and Nkx2.5 DNA leads to upregulation of Nkx2.5 function.

Importantly, Nkx2.5 recruits GATA4 to the promoter regions of several genes that are essential for the progression of myocyte growth from the early stages of myocyte differentiation to the acquisition of the adult myocyte phenotype.[200] Complete null mutation of Nkx2.5 in the mouse does not abolish myocyte formation and initial heart looping. Nkx2.5 is required for late myocyte differentiation and Nkx2.5 deletion results in the arrest of heart development at 10 days pc.[200] GATA4 expression appears to follow the attenuation in Nkx2.5 mRNA, suggesting that the transcriptional regulation of Notch and Nkx2.5 is linked to the preservation of the pool of highly dividing amplifying myocytes while GATA4 promotes their further differentiation.[194]

Collectively, these observations suggest that HIF-1 may lead to a prolonged activation of Nkx2.5 Notch in CPCs and BMPCs, sustaining their early committed state. Myocyte

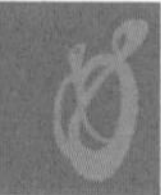

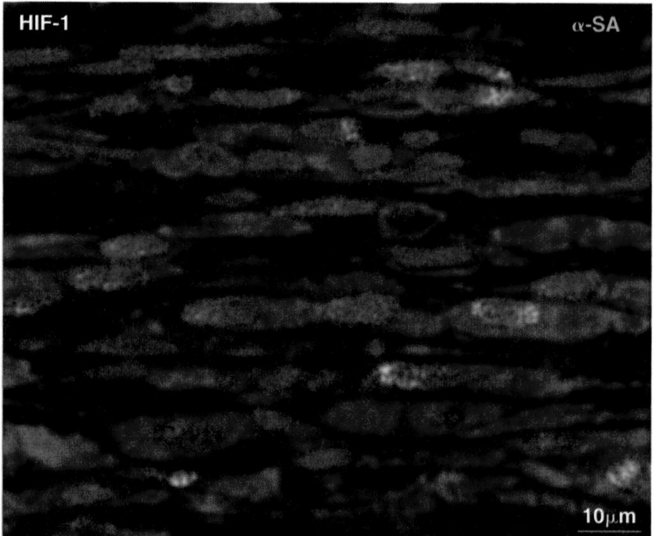

FIGURE 4–9 Properties of regenerated myocytes. Newly formed myocytes in the regenerating myocardium 3 weeks after CPC implantation are small in size and express HIF-1 (white) in their nuclei. Myocytes are recognized by the red fluorescence of α-sarcomeric actin.

maturation may be a time-dependent process regulated by oxygen availability to the forming cells. When vasculogenesis provides sufficient coronary blood flow, normoxia is reestablished, inhibition of differentiation may be relieved, and myocytes acquire the adult phenotype. However, whether CPCs and BMPCs are both capable of generating adult myocytes or whether one progenitor cell possesses a higher and/or faster differentiation potential than the other remains to be determined. This unresolved biological problem has tremendous clinical implications; it defines the efficacy and limit of these two forms of cell therapy for the infarcted heart. The forthcoming clinical implementation of autologous CPCs in patients affected by ischemic cardiomyopathy imposes the resolution of this dilemma.

Mechanics of Progenitor Cells Derived Cardiomyocytes

A relevant aspect of BMPC and CPC differentiation is whether the formed myocytes are functionally competent electrically and mechanically.* Work performed in our laboratory following the injection of these progenitor cell classes has addressed this issue. Because of the controversy in the field, we are illustrating data collected with the intramyocardial delivery of BMPCs.[35] Shortly after treatment, cells positive for the stem cell antigen c-kit or the reporter gene EGFP have been identified, but these cells fail to show electrical properties of developing myocytes and to contract in response to electrical stimulation. At 15 to 30 days after infarction and cell implantation, small new myocytes have been found and these cells exhibit membrane currents similar to those of mature cells. However, regenerated myocytes show a prolongation of the action potential and enhanced cell shortening (Figure 4-11).

The recognition that BMPCs differentiate into myocytes that contract in vitro raised the question whether these new cells are integrated structurally and functionally in vivo participating in ventricular performance. In this regard, connexin 43 has been detected between spared and developing myocytes, documenting the structural integration between these two cell populations (see Figure 4-11). Additionally, synchronicity in calcium transients between new and resident myocytes has been documented by an ex vivo preparation and two-photon microscopy (see Figure 4-11). Collectively, these observations provide strong evidence in favor of the functional coupling of old and regenerated cardiomyocytes.

The structural and functional integration of the restored myocardium has multiple positive effects on the anatomical characteristics and hemodynamic performance of the infarcted heart. The injection of BMPCs restores in part the loss of contraction in the infarcted region of the ventricular wall (Figure 4-12). Moreover, cardiac repair decreases chamber volume and increases the wall thickness-to-chamber radius ratio and the ventricular mass-to-chamber volume ratio (see Figure 4-12). Hemodynamically, infarcted untreated hearts show a marked increase in left ventricular end-diastolic pressure (LVEDP) and a decrease in LVDP and ±dP/dt. Conversely, myocardial regeneration attenuates the increase in LVEDP and improves LVDP and ±dP/dt. Together with the reduction in ventricular dilation, the amelioration in cardiac function by cell therapy produces a significant decrease in diastolic wall stress (see Figure 4-12). Thus, c-kit-positive-BMPCs adopt the cardiomyogenic fate structurally, electrically, and mechanically, improving the performance of the infarcted heart. Similar findings have been obtained with CPCs,[14,25,80-83] although we do not know yet whether one progenitor cell is superior to the other.

CELL THERAPY AND CHRONIC INFARCT

The use of progenitor cell therapy acutely after infarction has been introduced in several small clinical trials (see chapter 51).[62-64] Ischemic heart failure in humans is typically characterized by segmental losses of myocardium with scar formation and collagen accumulation in the interstitial compartment.[45] Although areas of spontaneous regeneration have been found,[166,201] these regions are minute and do not reduce significantly infarct size. Myocyte formation occurs acutely[201] and chronically[166] but the addition of new cells is mostly restricted to the viable myocardium. If we consider the evolution of the postinfarcted heart, the size of the infarct is not an infallible predictor of the short-, mid-,

*References 14, 25, 29, 30, 33-35, 45, 80-83, 169.

FIGURE 4–10, cont'd *Nkx2.5* is a target gene of Notch1 in CPCs. **A,** With respect to control nontreated (C) cells, the expression of Hes1 increases significantly in Jagged1-treated (Jag1) CPCs. N1ICD and RBP-Jk generate a complex in Jagged1-treated CPCs, which is fourfold greater than in untreated cells. The RBP-Jk band detected in the supernatant (SN) of nontreated CPCs corresponds to RBP-Jk not bound to N1ICD. *IP,* immunoprecipitation; *K,* kidney (positive control). **B,** Band shift assay in nuclear extracts of P19 cells nontransfected (NT) and transfected (T) with an RBP-Jk expression vector. Shifted bands correspond to the RBP-Jk/oligonucleotide complex (arrow); the band is supershifted (*arrowhead*) in the presence of RBP-Jk antibody (Ab). Nkx2.5, oligonucleotide probe in the absence of nuclear extracts; *Co,* specific competitor; *NS-Co,* nonspecific competitor. **C,** ChIP assay in P19 cells was performed with primers for sequences associated with the genes for Nkx2.5, Hes1 (positive control), and MEF2C (negative control). The amount of DNA in each sample (input) is shown. Immunoprecipitation was performed without primary antibody (no Ab) and with anti-RBP-Jk antibody (RBP-Jk Ab). Arrows indicate the amplified bands obtained with primers that recognize Nkx2.5 (Nkx2.5) and Hes1 (Hes1) promoters. *IgG,* isotype control. **D,** ChIP in CPCs was performed with the same protocol used for P19 cells. **E,** Nkx2.5 promoter activity measured by luciferase assay in CPCs after transfection with reporter plasmids carrying wild-type Nkx2.5 promoter or Nkx2.5 promoter containing a mutated RBP-Jk binding site. (From Boni A, Urbanek K, Nascimbene A. Notch1 regulates the fate of cardiac progenitor cells. *Proc Natl Acad Sci U S A* 2008;105:15529–15534.)

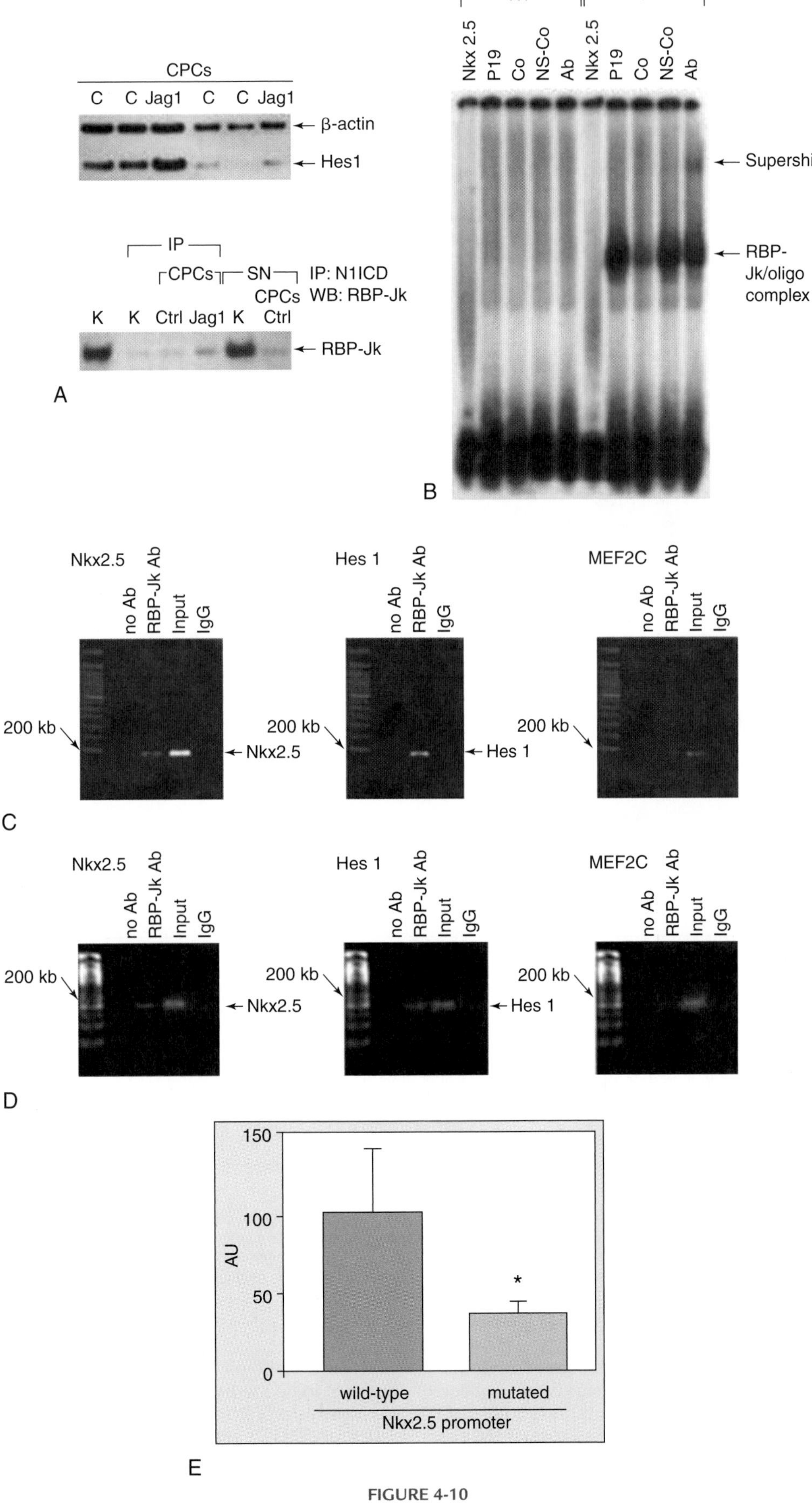
CPCs
C C Jag1 C C Jag1
β-actin
Hes1
IP
CPCs
SN
IP: N1ICD
CPCs WB: RBP-Jk
K K Ctrl Jag1 K Ctrl
RBP-Jk
A
NT
T
Nkx 2.5
P19
Co
NS-Co
Ab
Supershift
RBP-Jk/oligo complex
B
Nkx2.5
Hes 1
MEF2C
no Ab
RBP-Jk Ab
Input
IgG
200 kb
C
D
150
100
50
0
AU
wild-type
mutated
Nkx2.5 promoter
E

FIGURE 4-10

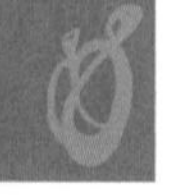

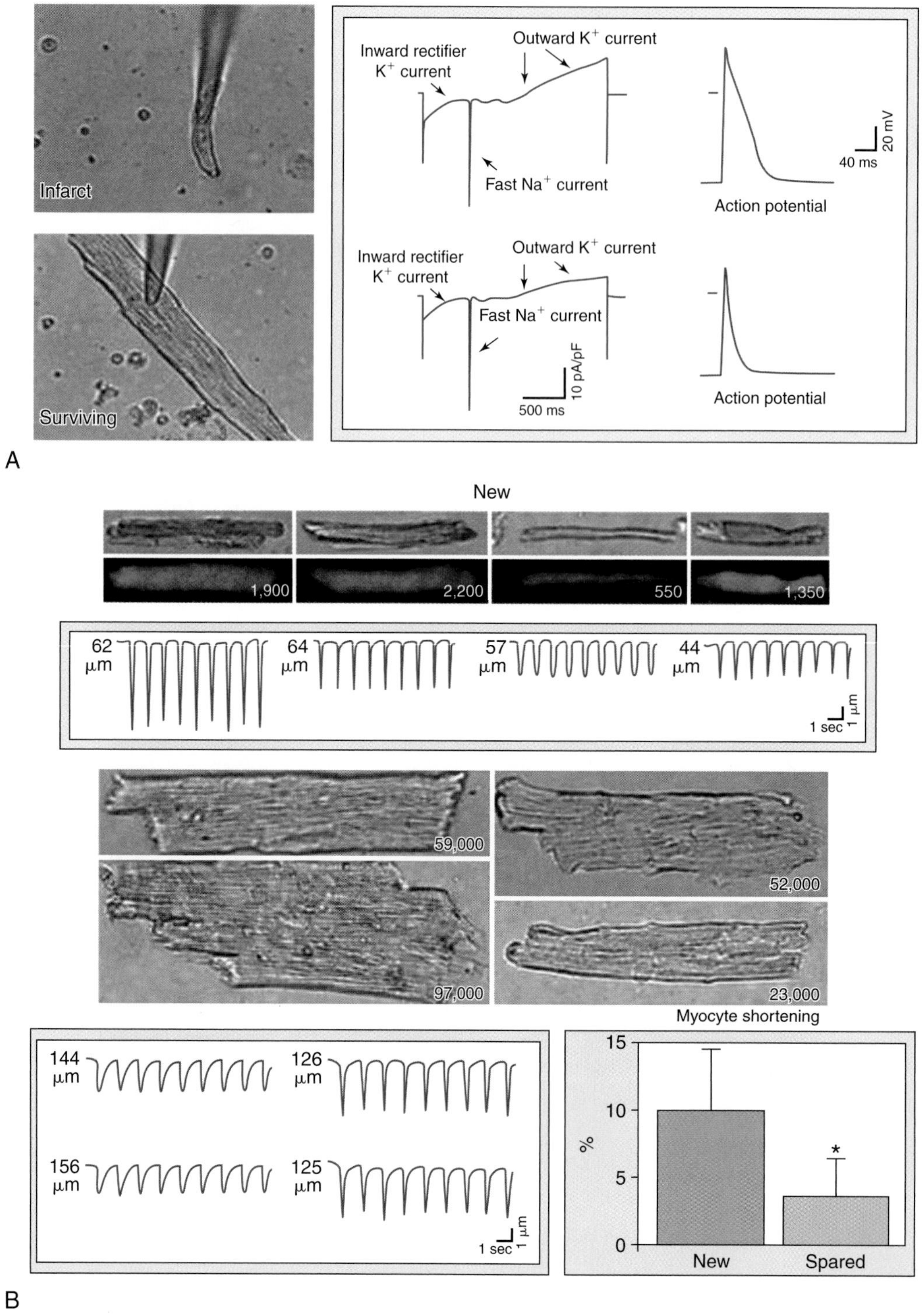

FIGURE 4–11 BMPCs differentiate into functionally competent cardiomyocytes. At 15 to 30 days after myocardial infarction and BMPC injection, small EGFP-positive myocytes are found in the infarcted area. **A,** Electrical properties of BMPC-derived and spared myocytes. BMPC-derived myocytes exhibit electrical characteristics similar to spared myocytes but show a prolongation of the action potential. **B,** Newly formed EGFP-positive myocytes are electrically excitable. BMPC-derived myocytes show enhanced cell shortening while spared myocytes have depressed fractional shortening. Values are mean ± SD. *, $P < .05$ versus new myocytes.

and long-term outcome of the disease.[133] Negative remodeling and accumulation of damage in the surviving myocardium may become the critical determinants of the onset of cardiac deterioration and its progression to terminal failure. The number of acute events differs in the patient population, and by the nature of the damage the chronically postinfarcted heart necessitates therapeutic approaches that are by far more complex than those required by acute infarcts. Recent observations in humans suggest that BMPCs may be effective in long-term ischemic heart disease and this beneficial impact appears to be mediated by reduction of the originally scarred myocardium.[53,56] In this regard, it is relevant to determine whether BMPCs and CPCs can replace regions of scarring with functionally competent myocardium and whether the mechanisms postulated to be involved in acute infarcts are operative in the chronic disease.

Although data on BMPCs are not currently available in terms of the ability of these cells to invade and replace the

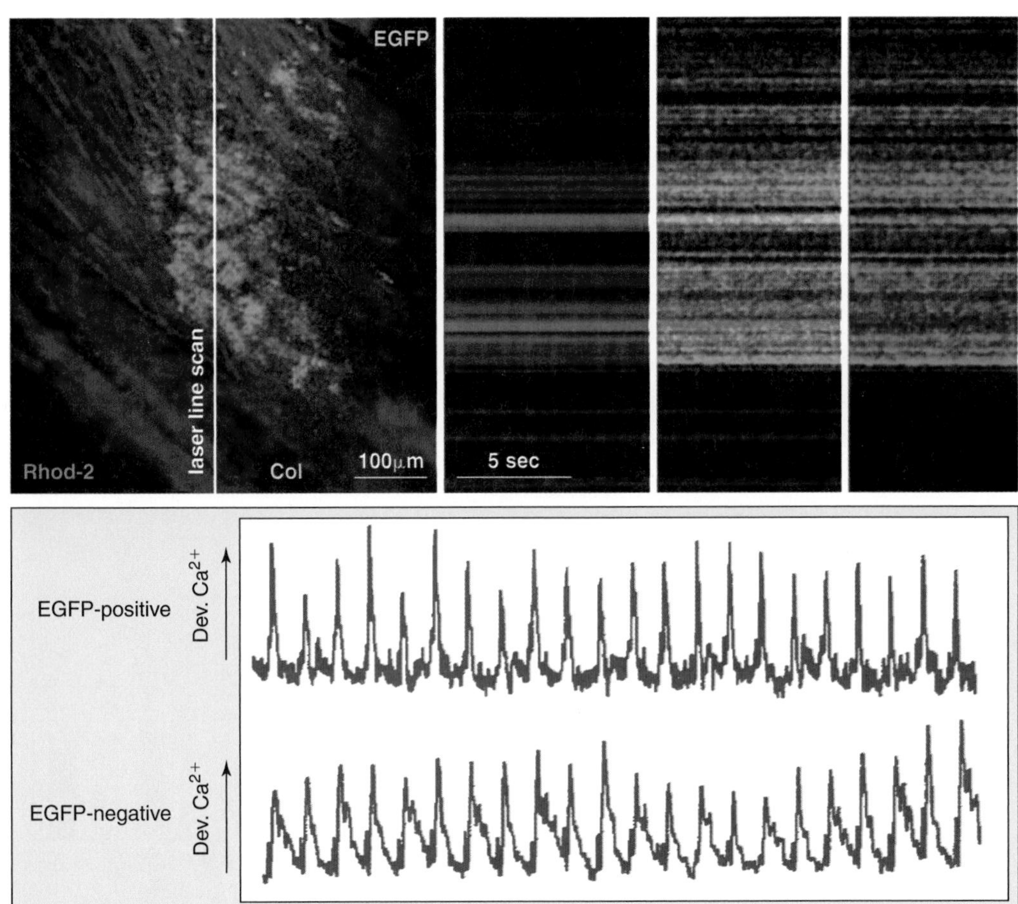

FIGURE 4–11, cont'd **C,** The functional integration of regenerated EGFP-positive-myocytes with the surrounding myocardium has been documented by an ex vivo preparation and two-photon microscopy in hearts at 1 month after coronary artery ligation. The heart is perfused retrogradely through the aorta with an oxygenated Tyrode solution containing the calcium indicator Rhod-2 and then stimulated at 1 Hz. Calcium transient is detected in EGFP-positive BMPC-derived myocytes and EGFP-negative mouse myocytes. The synchronicity in calcium transients between these two myocyte populations provides strong evidence in favor of the functional coupling of old and new myocytes. (From Rota M, Kajstura J, Hosoda T. Bone marrow cells adopt the cardiomyogenic fate in vivo. *Proc Natl Acad Sci U S A* 2007;104:17783–17788.)

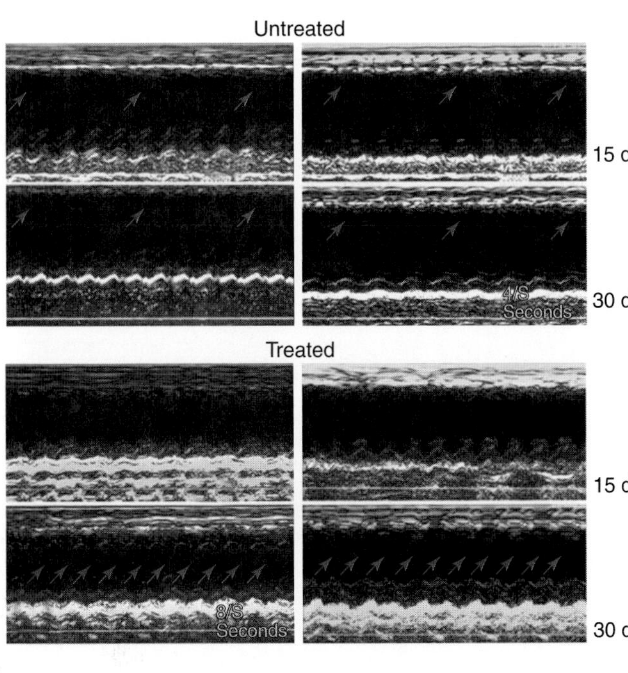

FIGURE 4–12 BMPCs and the infarcted heart. **A,** M-mode echocardiography shows lack of contraction in untreated-infarcted hearts (*upper*). Contraction reappears in the infarcted region of the wall in infarcted hearts treated with BMPCs (*lower*).

Continued

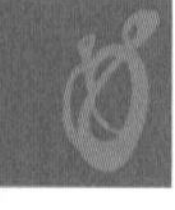

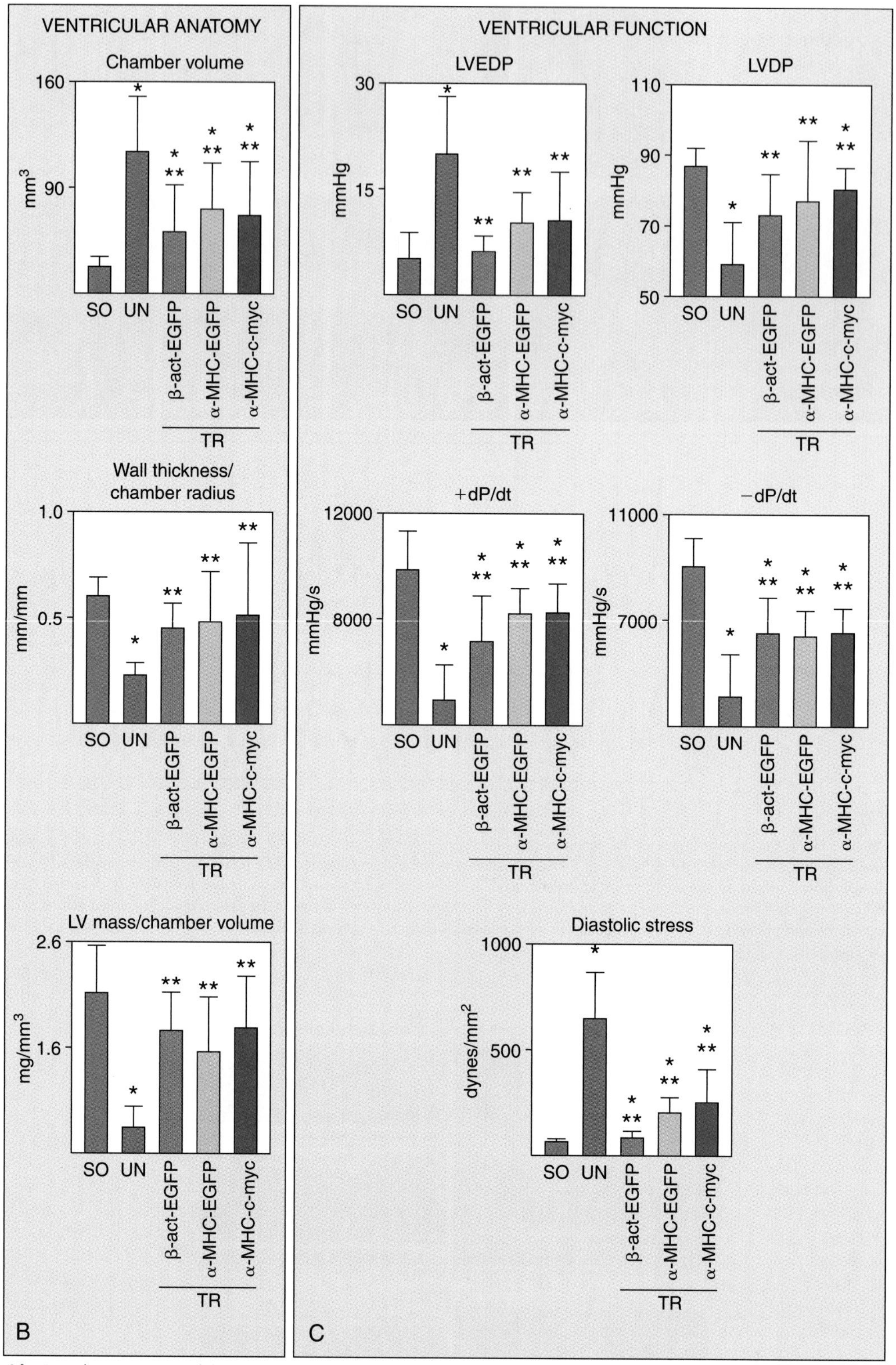

FIGURE 4–12, cont'd **B** and **C,** Anatomical **(B)** and functional **(C)** characteristics of the infarcted heart at 30 days. BMPCs for myocardial regeneration were obtained from three transgenic mice. In the first, EGFP was driven by the ubiquitous β-actin promoter (β-act-EGFP); in the second, EGFP was driven by the cardiac-specific α-myosin heavy chain promoter (α-MHC-EGFP); and in the third, a *c-myc*-tagged nuclear-targeted-Akt transgene was driven by the α-MHC-promoter (α-MHC-*c-myc*). Values are mean ± SD. *, *P* <.05 versus sham-operated (SO); **,*P* <.05 versus untreated infarcted hearts (UN). *TR,* treated infarcted hearts; *LVEDP,* left ventricular end diastolic pressure; *LVDP,* left ventricular developed pressure. (From Rota M, Kajstura J, Hosoda T. Bone marrow cells adopt the cardiomyogenic fate in vivo. *Proc Natl Acad Sci USA* 2007;104:17783–17788.)

scarred tissue with mechanically active myocardium, recent results have been obtained in our laboratory concerning the therapeutic efficacy of CPCs in healed infarcts in rodents.[83] In this study, rats with a healed myocardial infarct were treated with implantation of CPCs or with intramyocardial delivery of HGF and IGF-1. These growth factors (GFs) were employed because CPCs express c-Met and IGF-1 receptors and HGF is a powerful chemoattractant of CPCs while IGF-1 promotes their division and survival.[80,81]

Resident CPCs locally activated by GFs or injected directly in proximity of a healed infarct can rescue nearly 45% of the infarct by replacing fibrotic tissue with functionally competent myocardium.[83] Myocardial regeneration protects the infarcted heart from the progressive increase in cavitary dilation, decrease in wall thickness, and deterioration in ventricular function with time. Together with observations in the acutely infarcted heart,[14,25,80-82,202-204] these findings strongly suggest that CPCs are a powerful form of cell therapy for ischemic cardiomyopathy. CPCs are effective whether administered intramyocardially[14,25] via the coronary route[202] or activated in situ with HGF and IGF-1, which trigger their growth and mobilization shortly after an ischemic event[80,81] and chronically at the completion of healing. CPCs migrate through the myocardial interstitium, reaching areas of necrotic and scarred myocardium where they home, divide, and differentiate into myocytes and vascular structures. From a clinical perspective, CPCs appear to represent an ideal candidate for cardiac repair in patients with chronic heart failure in which discrete areas of damage are present in combination with multiple foci of replacement fibrosis across the ventricular wall.[45] Potentially, CPCs may be isolated from endomyocardial biopsy or surgical samples and, following their expansion in vitro, administrated back to patients avoiding the inevitable and threatening adverse effects of rejection and other complications with nonautologous transplantation. Alternatively, GFs can be delivered locally to stimulate resident CPCs and promote myocardial regeneration. Importantly, these strategies may be repeated to reduce further myocardial scarring and expand the working myocardium.

Myocardial scarring interferes with the migration and engraftment of locally injected or GF-activated CPCs. Acute infarcts are more amenable to CPC translocation and homing, providing a milieu in which CPCs rapidly accumulate and generate a committed progeny (Figure 4-13).[80] Despite the less favorable environment dictated by collagen deposition chronically after infarction, CPCs retained the ability to infiltrate the scar, digest part of the connective tissue, and form cardiomyocytes and coronary vessels. The comparable effects on myocardial regeneration obtained by local CPC-delivery and GF-activation of resident CPCs may be explained by the pattern of migration of these cells within the scar; the higher number of cells found with intramyocardial injection of CPCs was compensated by the faster speed of migration of GF-activated CPCs. When these two variables are considered, i.e., speed and cell number, the accumulation of cells under these conditions is remarkably similar.[83] However, this was not the case in acute infarcts in which cell infiltration was more efficient following CPC-implantation than after CPC-activation by GFs (see Figure 4-13).

The invasion of the scarred tissue by CPCs appeared to be mediated by enhanced activity of MMP-9 and possibly MMP-14. MMP-9 is critical for the recruitment of bone marrow stem cells and their mobilization from quiescent to proliferative niches,[205] and a similar mechanism may be operative in the translocation to the chronically infarcted heart of GF-treated resident CPCs or delivered CPCs. The upregulation of MMP-9 expression and activity in CPCs is dependent on HGF.[80,81,99] Additionally, SDF-1, which is highly expressed in myocytes and endothelial cells after ischemic injury, acts on MMP-9 and promotes the differentiation of CPCs into vascular cells and cardiomyocytes.[82] The lack of increase in MMP-2 activity observed here may favor the stability of SDF-1, which is degraded by this protease.[206]

Importantly, with respect to the intact heart, the content of cytokines and growth factors differed in the scarred myocardium (Figure 4-14).[83] The enhanced expression of the chemotactic factors sICAM-1, CXCL7, and bFGF in chronic infarcts may have created a condition facilitating migration and homing of CPCs.[207] Additionally, the presence of sICAM-1, CXCL7, and TIMP-1 in the scar could have promoted CPC mobilization, EC migration and differentiation, and vessel formation.[208] The increases in CXCL7 and TIMP-1 were restricted to chronic infarcts. As expected, the acutely infarcted myocardium displayed a cytokine profile that reflected an inflammatory response and tissue reaction to acute injury (see Figure 4-14). However, the higher levels of sICAM-1 and bFGF within the scar are particularly relevant for myocardial regeneration since sICAM-1 may have created a niche structure that supported the engraftment of CPCs and bFGF is critical for the differentiation of resident CPCs into myocytes.[21]

The analysis of cytokine and growth factor expression in acute and chronic infarcted hearts[83] offers the possibility to establish whether the delivery of CPCs participates in the synthesis and secretion of soluble proteins, which exert an autocrine or paracrine effect on myocardial regeneration. The presence of CPCs in the scar attenuates, at least in part, the differences in cytokine profile with acute infarcts by increasing the quantities of LIX that are involved in stem cell maintenance and proliferation[209] and IP-10 that modulates vessel homeostasis and growth.[210] Thus acute and chronic myocardial damage leads to the expression of genes that create a microenvironment that conditions the activation, migration, and growth of CPCs, ultimately controlling the regenerative response of the pathological heart.

Whether these results have implications for the treatment of chronic human heart failure is difficult to predict. Risk factors such as aging and diabetes are frequently present in patients with ischemic cardiomyopathy, and they have profound negative consequences on the number and function of CPCs.[68] However, functionally competent human CPCs have been isolated from a variety of patients undergoing open heart surgery[25] or endomyocardial biopsy[23] and the activation of CPCs by GFs in senescent rats with severe ventricular decompensation reverses the cardiac phenotype and prolongs lifespan.[99]

Progenitor Cells and Fusion Events

In all studies performed so far in our laboratory with BMPCs or CPCs,* the collected data indicate that progenitor cells undergo lineage commitment and give rise to myocytes and coronary vessels within the acutely and chronically infarcted myocardium in the absence of cell fusion. Heart homeostasis is modulated by CPCs that continuously differentiate into new younger cells replacing old dying cells. This mechanism of cardiac cell turnover is operative in animals[14,16,19,81] and humans[25] and does not involve cell fusion. Similarly, BMPCs acquire cardiac cell lineages independent of cell fusion.[33,35]

However, the generation of cardiomyocytes by CPCs[15] or BMPCs[40] has been postulated to be largely the product of cell fusion. If this were to occur, the process of cell fusion would require the merging of a CPC or BMPC with a terminally differentiated, binucleated myocyte, approximately 25,000 μm^3 in volume or larger. Thus, a trinucleated heterokaryon, a binucleated hyperploid synkaryon, restricted to one of the two nuclei, or a binucleated hyperploid synkaryon with a proportional partition of the DNA of the BMPC to each of the myocyte nuclei would be formed.[45,123] The unusual trinucleated myocyte heterokaryon will be no longer terminally

*References 14, 25, 29, 30, 33-35, 45, 80-83, 169.

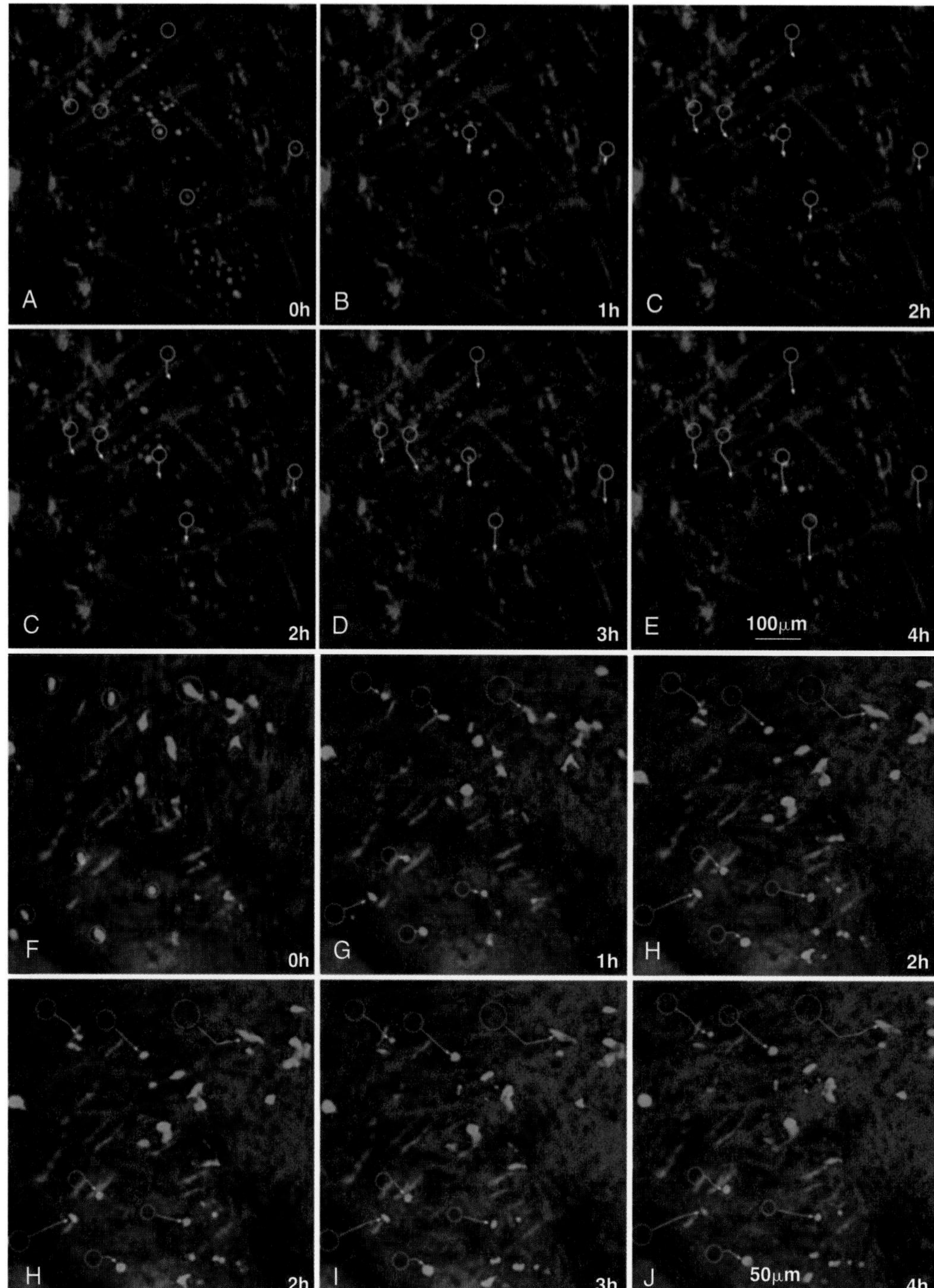

FIGURE 4–13 Migration of CPCs in the infarct. **A-E,** Translocation of EGFP-positive CPCs at 24 hours after cell implantation in an acute infarct. The same field, examined at 1-hour intervals is illustrated. Green: EGFP-positive cells; red: coronary vasculature perfused with rhodamine-labeled-dextran. Blue: collagen. White circles in A indicate the position of selected cells at the beginning of observation. White arrows reflect the direction of migration and the distance covered by the cells in 1 to 4 hours. **F-J,** Translocation of EGFP-positive CPCs at 24 hours after cell implantation in a chronic infarct. The movement of cells is illustrated as described above. (From Rota M, Padin-Iruegas E, Misao Y, et al. Local activation or implantation of cardiac progenitor cells rescues scarred infarcted myocardium improving cardiac function. *Circ Res.* 2008;103:107-116.)

differentiated; it will reenter the cell cycle, become approximately 50,000 μm^3 in volume, and then divide, creating two trinucleated daughter cells, approximately 25,000 μm^3 each. When cell fusion is accompanied by nuclear fusion, the high DNA content leads to genetic instability and minimal or null replicative potential.[211] However, the replicating and nonreplicating myocytes originated from BMPCs or CPCs are predominantly mononucleated, at times binucleated and never trinucleated. Nearly 80% of these cells vary from 500 μm^3 to 3000 μm^3; only a minimal fraction reaches a volume of 10,000 μm^3 or larger. All cells have a 2n karyotype, and possess two sex chromosomes.[25,33,35]

Surprisingly, the differentiation of CPCs into myocytes and the possibility of a phenotype conversion of adult BMPCs have been challenged in favor of the complex mechanism of cell fusion.[212] This rather unrealistic model of myocyte biology has been claimed to be operative based on results obtained with the Cre-Lox genetic system, which has been accepted at face value and viewed today as the gold standard for studies of myocardial regeneration and BMPC

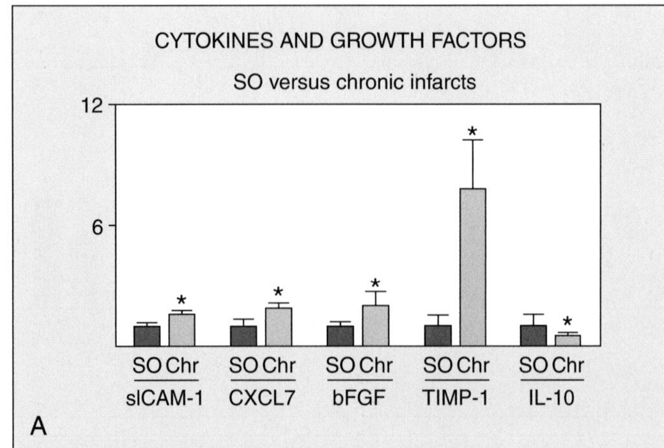

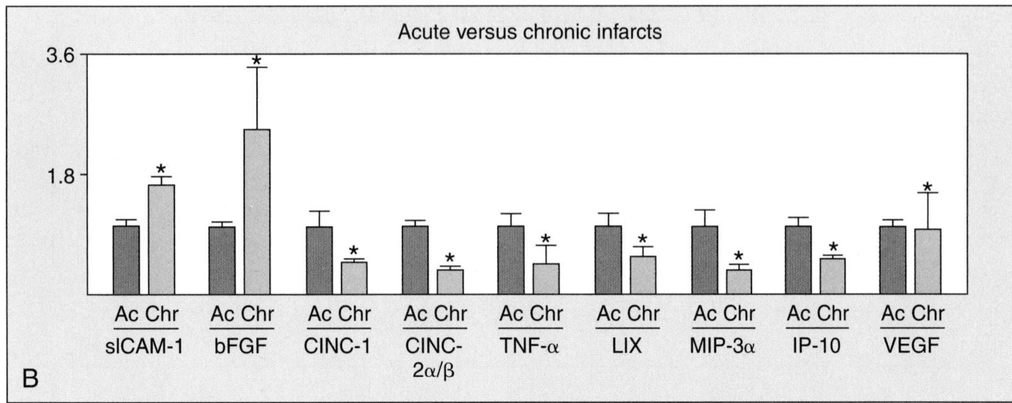

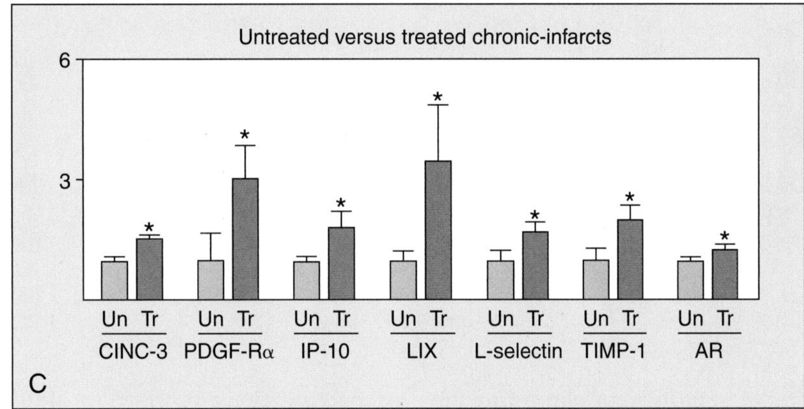

FIGURE 4–14 Cytokines and growth factors regulate homing of CPCs in the infarct. A cytokine and growth factor array was performed to identify the signals involved in the migration and engraftment of CPCs in the acute and chronic infarcted heart. The content of cytokines and growth factors was analyzed in myocardial tissue samples. The different expression profile in acute and chronic infarcts indicates that distinct environmental cues characterize the cardiac milieu in the two conditions. **A-E,** Fold changes in protein quantities. Data are means ±SD. *P <.05. *sICAM-1,* Soluble intercellular adhesion molecule-1; *CXCL7,* C-X-C motif chemokine 7; *bFGF,* basic fibroblast growth factor; *TIMP-1,* tissue inhibitor of metalloproteinases-1; *IL,* interleukin; *CINC,* cytokine-induced neutrophil chemoattractant; *TNF,* tumor necrosis factor; *LIX,* LPS-induced CXC chemokine; *MIP,* macrophage inflammatory protein; *IP-10,* interferon-γ-inducible protein-10; *VEGF,* vascular endothelial growth factor; *PDGF-R,* platelet-derived growth factor receptor; *AR,* amphiregulin; *G-CSF,* granulocyte/colony-stimulating factor; IL-1Ra, interleukin-1 receptor antagonist; *TGF-β,* transforming GF-β; *MIG,* migration-inducing protein. (From Rota M, Padin-Iruegas E, Misao Y, et al. Local activation or implantation of cardiac progenitor cells rescues scarred infarcted myocardium improving cardiac function. *Circ Res.* 2008;103:107-116.)

Continued

transdifferentiation.[15,40,212] Cre is a recombinase enzyme that cuts DNA segments flanked by binding sequences termed LoxP sites. The *Cre* recombinase gene is driven by a cell-specific promoter, such as the α-myosin heavy chain. The *LoxP* sequences flank the stop codon, which is located between the *LacZ* or *EGFP* gene and its promoter, repressing the expression of *LacZ* or *EGFP* (*LoxP* mouse). When cells that contain this construct fuse with cells carrying the *Cre* recombinase gene, the *LoxP* and stop codon sequences are recognized and excised by the Cre recombinase. Therefore, the *LacZ* or *EGFP* gene is expressed in the fused cells and β-Gal or EGFP is synthesized under the control of the cell-specific promoter.

Unfortunately, the Cre-Lox model is not perfect. The unmodified Cre-recombinase present in progenitor cells can cross the membrane of the recipient cell,[213] mimicking fusion events. Also, the formation of nanotubules[214] may lead to the transfer of Cre recombinase to the cell carrying the *LacZ* gene, resulting in a β-Gal positive cell in the absence of cell fusion.[45] Fusion of a CPC or BMPC with a mature myocyte cannot trigger the division of the recipient terminally differentiated cell.

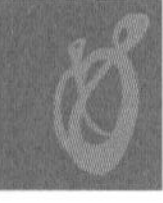

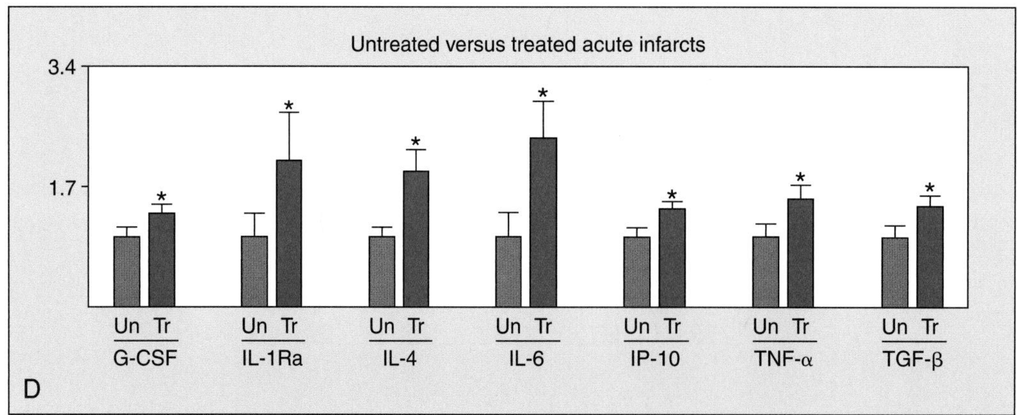

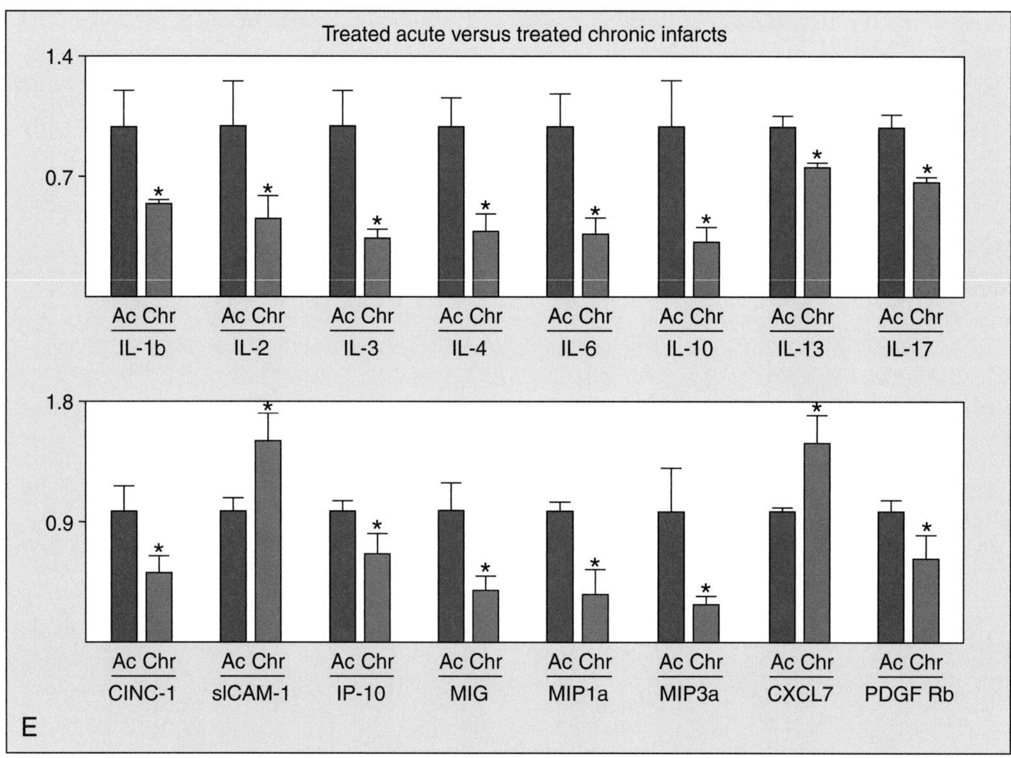

FIGURE 4–14, cont'd.

The hybrid cell loses the ability to proliferate, abrogating the fundamental role of CPCs or BMPCs. The generation of nanotubules between BMPCs[214] strongly suggests that expression of an enzyme cannot be interpreted as proof of cell fusion. The recognition that nanotubules are formed between cells explains the translocation of enzymes between adjacent cells and the migration of organelles from one cell to the neighboring cell. By inference, the cross talk between cells is not limited to membrane-to-membrane interaction but involves a more sophisticated network of structural and functional bridges. Therefore, cell fusion has to be studied by analyzing DNA content together with the number of sex chromosomes in nuclei of newly formed myocytes (Figure 4-15). So far, the collected findings challenge cell fusion as a mechanism of myocardial regeneration by differentiation of CPCs and BMPCs.[34,45,67,123]

FUTURE DIRECTIONS

The field of cardiac stem cell biology is in its infancy and we have little understanding of the mechanisms involved in the homeostasis and repair of the adult human heart. Historically, the foundations for the view of the heart as a terminally differentiated postmitotic organ incapable of regeneration can be traced back to the mid-1920s.[215] The dogma was established that the postnatal heart is composed of a fixed number of myocytes and that, if myocytes die, they are permanently lost and the myocardium must maintain its vital role with a reduced number of cells. The remaining myocytes cannot be triggered into the replicating phase;[216] they continue to perform their physiological function, undergo cellular hypertrophy, and ultimately die.[217] Based on this paradigm, the age of myocytes, the organ, and organism were assumed to coincide, implying that myocytes in humans may have a life span that exceeds 100 years.[167] For several decades, no effort was made to reexamine this rather unusual view of the biology of the heart and cardiac homeostasis. Remarkably, there is not a single piece of evidence that demonstrates the inability of the heart to replace its dying myocytes. It seems rather extravagant that cardiomyocytes can contract 70 times per minute over 100 years and continue to be functional. During this period, they would have contracted 3.7 billion times and still be operative. If this were to be the case, adult myocytes would be essentially immortal cells. This unrealistic view of the heart forms the basis of our limited knowledge on the

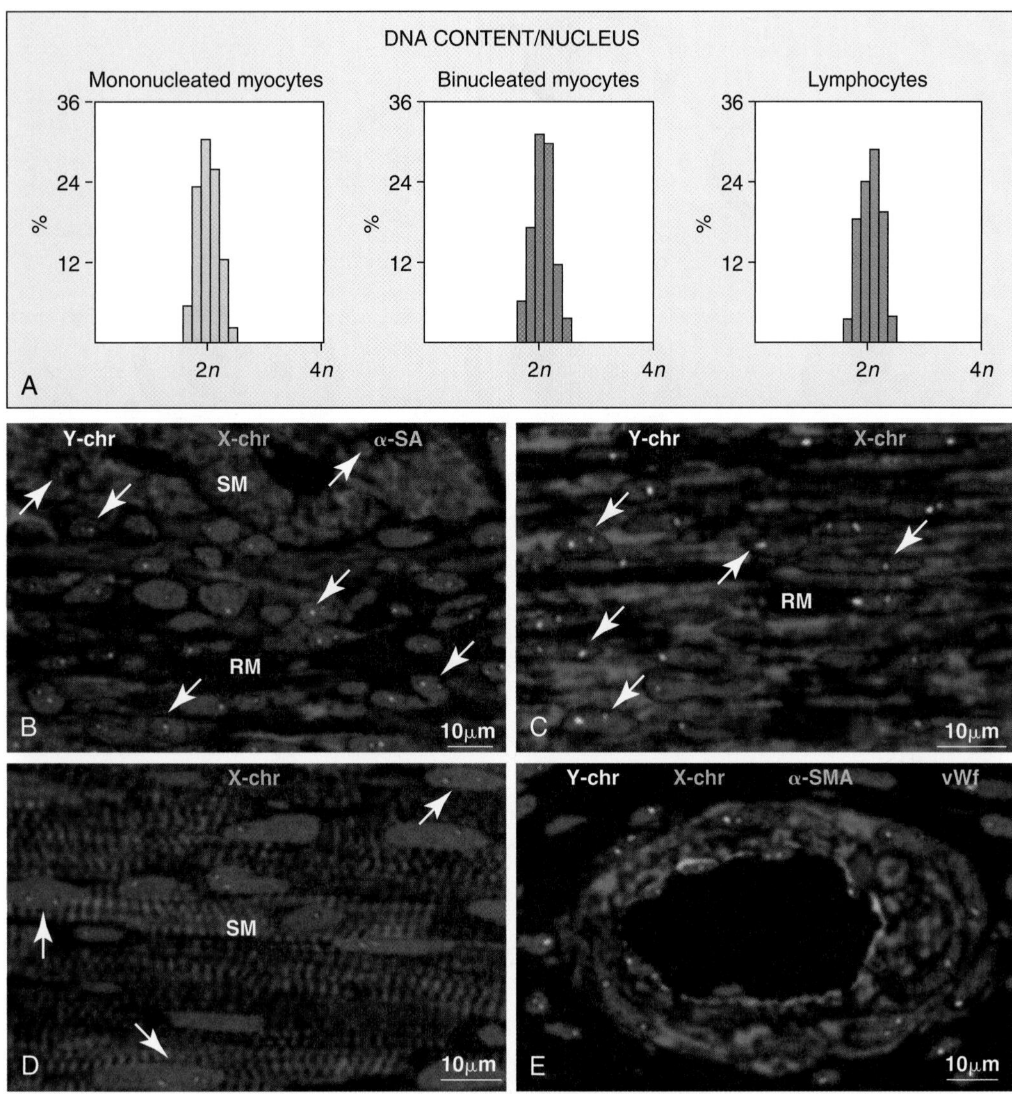

FIGURE 4–15 Cell fusion. **A,** A 2n DNA content per nucleus was found in newly formed myocytes, ECs, and SMCs originated from BMPCs injected in the border zone of an acute infarct. Lymphocytes were used as control. **B-D,** Sections illustrating the interface between the surviving (SM) and regenerated myocardium (RM) at low **(B)** and higher **(C** and **D)** magnification. At 30 days, newly formed myocytes (*arrows*) have at most one Y-chr (white) and one X-chr (green), indicating their diploid male genotype. Spared myocytes (*arrowheads*) showed, at most, two X-chr, indicating their diploid female genotype. **E,** SMCs in a regenerated arteriole possess, at most, one Y-chr and one X-chr, documenting their diploid male genotype. (From Rota M, Kajstura J, Hosoda T. Bone marrow cells adopt the cardiomyogenic fate in vivo. *Proc Natl Acad Sci.USA* 2007;104:17783–17788.)

function of resident human CPCs and their potential role in cardiac cell turnover and regeneration.

Human myocytes larger than 30,000 μm³ cannot reenter the cell cycle and proliferate.[163] Cycling myocytes are small and mononucleated. It would be inefficient for large myocytes to divide once or at most twice to expand the cardiac mass. Heart weight in humans can increase nearly threefold, reaching values of 1000 g or larger.[218-221] Heart failure typically shows increases in myocyte number that vary from 20% to 100% or more.[218-223] This phenomenon is not affected by age; in an analysis of 7112 human hearts, from birth to 110 years of age, Linzbach has shown that extreme forms of organ hypertrophy are detectable up to the ninth decade of life, and heart weights of 500 and 600 g are present in patients at 100 years of age and older.[224] Collectively, these observations point to the CPC as the controlling cells of cardiac homeostasis and repair. Surprisingly, despite the fact that the controversy on myocardial regeneration persists, several distinct types of CPCs have been claimed by different laboratories with values that would transform the heart from a postmitotic organ to the most self-renewing organ in the organism. These uncertainties strengthen the need for the acquisition of fundamental knowledge on the growth and differentiation of CPCs.

Understanding CPC function is critical for the implementation of CPCs in the daily treatment of the chronically decompensated human heart. In fact, the heart now belongs to the group of constantly renewing organs, where the capacity to replace cells depends on the persistence of a stem cell compartment.[109,110,225-231] Regeneration conforms to a hierarchical archetype in which slowly dividing stem cells give rise to proliferating, lineage-restricted progenitor-precursor cells, which then become highly dividing amplifying cells, which eventually reach terminal differentiation and growth arrest.[231-234] Stem cells have a high propensity for cell division and this property is maintained throughout the life span of the organ and organism.[227,228,230,233,234] In contrast, the less primitive, transient amplifying cells represent a group of dividing cells that have a limited proliferation capacity. Amplifying cells divide and concurrently differentiate,[225,228,235-237] and when complete differentiation is reached, the ability to replicate is permanently lost. This forms the foundation of a new

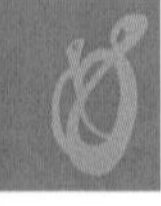

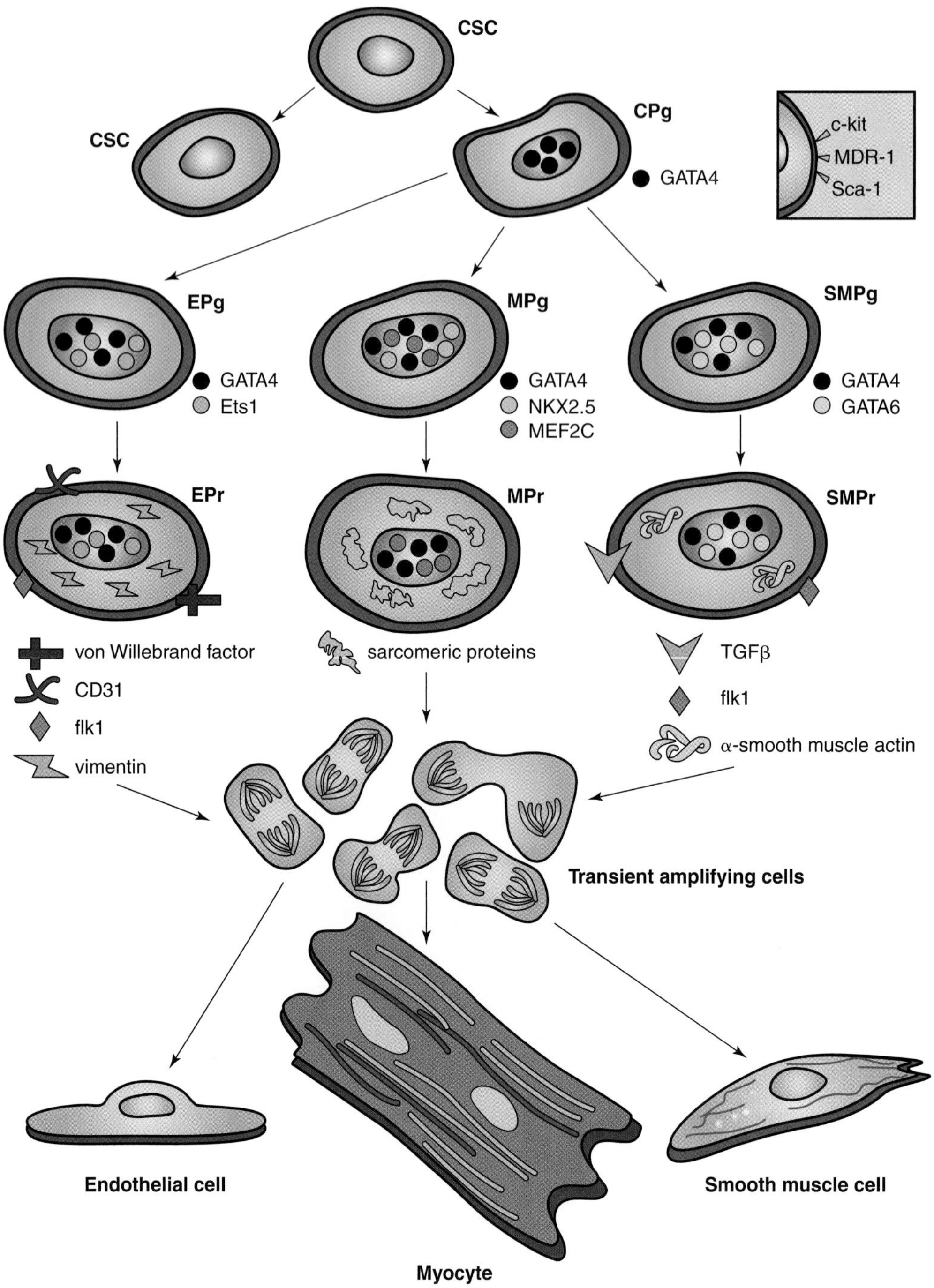

FIGURE 4–16 Hierarchy of cardiac stem cell (CSC) growth and differentiation. Asymmetrical division of a CSC into a daughter CSC and a daughter cardiac progenitor (CPg). CPg gives rise to myocyte progenitor (MPg) and precursor (MPr), EC progenitor (EPg) and precursor (EPr), and SMC progenitor (SMPg) and precursor (SMPr). Precursors become transient amplifying cells, which divide and differentiate into mature myocytes, ECs, and SMCs. CSCs are lineage-negative cells that express only c-kit, MDR1, or Sca-1. Progenitors express stem cell antigens and transcription factors of cardiac cells but do not exhibit specific cytoplasmic proteins. Precursors possess stem cell antigens, transcription factors, and membrane and cytoplasmic proteins typical of myocytes, ECs, and SMCs. Amplifying cells have nuclear, cytoplasmic, and membrane proteins of cardiac cell lineages but are negative for stem cell antigens. TGF-β, transforming growth factor β-receptor. (From Anversa P, Kajstura J, Leri A, et al. Life and death of cardiac stem cells: a paradigm shift in cardiac biology. *Circulation* 2006;113:1451–1463.)

paradigm of the heart in which multipotent resident CPCs are implicated in the constant turnover of myocytes, ECs, SMCs, and fibroblasts (Figure 4-16). The recognition that activated CPCs translocate to areas of need where they grow and differentiate makes the possibility of myocardial regeneration a feasible reality. Theoretically, in a manner comparable to HSCs that repopulate and completely reconstitute the ablated bone marrow,[238,239] CPCs may be capable of rebuilding the damaged myocardium and converting a severely diseased heart into a physiologically functional heart.

The recognition that the adult atrial and ventricular myocardium contains a pool of CPC that are self-renewing, clonogenic, and multipotent in vitro and regenerate cardiomyocytes and coronary vessels in vivo has raised the unprecedented opportunity to repair the diseased heart.[13-25] Hypothetically, CPCs can be isolated from biopsy samples and, following their expansion, can be implanted within regions of damage where they reconstitute the lost myocardium.[25] Alternatively, portions of infarcted or injured myocardium can be restored by cytokine activation of resident CPCs, which

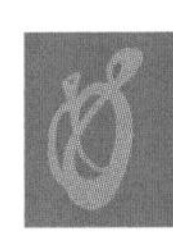

migrate to the site of injury where subsequently they form myocytes and vascular structures.[80,81] At last, the injured tissue is replaced by new functionally competent myocardium. These two forms of therapy are not mutually exclusive and in fact complement each other. In a heart severely depleted of its CPC compartment, the identification and expansion of the remaining CPCs may be a preferable option while, in the presence of a relatively intact CPC pool, the administration of cytokines may be as effective as direct cell implantation. Collectively, the findings in small and large animals are encouraging but have left unanswered the question whether the cells currently available for myocardial regeneration possess the inherent property to mature into adult myocytes and form the vascular framework necessary for the oxygenation of the developing myocardium. These important issues constitute the target of future research, which aims at the identification of novel strategies for the treatment of chronic heart failure of ischemic and nonischemic origin.

REFERENCES

1. Lopez, L. R., Shocket, A. L., Stanford, R. E., et al. (1980). Gastrointestinal involvement in leukocytoclastic vasculitis and polyarteritis nodosa. *J Rheumatol, 7*, 677–684.
2. Saegusa, M., Takano, Y., & Okudaira, M. (1993). Human hepatic infarction: histopathological and postmortem angiological studies. *Liver, 1993*, 239–245.
3. Watanabe, K., Abe, H., Mishima, T., et al. (2003). Polyangiitis overlap syndrome: a fatal case combined with adult Henoch-Schönlein purpura and polyarteritis nodosa. *Pathol Int, 53*, 569–573.
4. Adzick, N. S., & Lorenz, H. P. (1994). Cells, matrix, growth factors and the surgeon. The biology of scarless fetal wound repair. *Ann Surg, 220*, 10–18.
5. Mackool, R. J., Gittes, G. K., & Longaker, M. T. (1998). Scarless healing: the fetal wound. *Clin Plast Surg, 25*, 357–361.
6. Ferguson, M. W., & O'Kane, S. (2004). Scar-free healing: from embryonic mechanisms to adult therapeutic intervention. *Philos Trans R Soc Lond B Biol Sci, 359*, 839–850.
7. Chen, W., Fu, X., Ge, S., et al. (2005). Ontogeny of expression of transforming growth factor-β and its receptors and their possible relationship with scarless healing in human fetal skin. *Wound Repair Regen, 13*, 68–75.
8. Beddington, R. S., & Robertson, E. J. (1989). An assessment of the developmental potential of embryonic stem cells in the midgestation mouse embryo. *Development, 105*, 733–737.
9. Wollert, K. C., Meyer, G. P., Lotz, J., et al. (2004). Intra-coronary autologous bone-marrow cell transfer after myocardial infarction: the BOOST randomized controlled clinical trial. *Lancet, 364*, 141–148.
10. Kinnaird, T., Stabile, E., Burnett, M. S., et al. (2004). Bone-marrow-derived cells for enhancing collateral development: mechanisms, animal data, and initial clinical experiences. *Circ Res, 95*, 354–363.
11. Kinnaird, T., Stabile, E., Burnett, M. S., et al. (2004). Marrow-derived stromal cells express genes encoding a broad spectrum of arteriogenic cytokines and promote in vitro and in vivo arteriogenesis through paracrine mechanisms. *Circ Res, 94*, 678–685.
12. Yoon, Y. S., Wecker, A., Heyd, L., et al. (2005). Clonally expanded novel multipotent stem cells from human bone marrow regenerate myocardium after myocardial infarction. *J Clin Invest, 115*, 326–338.
13. Hierlihy, A. M., Seale, P., Lobe, C. G., et al. (2002). The post-natal heart contains a myocardial stem cell population. *FEBS Lett, 530*, 239–243.
14. Beltrami, A. P., Barlucchi, L., Torella, D., et al. (2003). Adult cardiac stem cells are multipotent and support myocardial regeneration. *Cell, 114*, 763–766.
15. Oh, H., Bradfute, S. B., Gallardo, T. D., et al. (2003). Cardiac progenitor cells from adult myocardium: homing, differentiation, and fusion after infarction. *Proc Natl Acad Sci U S A, 100*, 12313–12318.
16. Matsuura, K., Nagai, T., Nishigaki, N., et al. (2004). Adult cardiac Sea-1-positive cells differentiate into beating cardiomyocytes. *J Biol Chem, 279*, 11384–11391.
17. Martin, C. M., Meeson, A. P., Robertson, S. M., et al. (2004). Persistent expression of the ATP-binding cassette transporter. Abcg2 identifies cardiac SP cells in the developing and adult heart. *Dev Biol, 265*, 262–275.
18. Messina, E., De Angelis, L., Frati, G., et al. (2004). Isolation and expansion of adult cardiac stem cells from human and murine heart. *Circ Res, 95*, 911–921.
19. Pfister, O., Mouquet, F., Jain, M., et al. (2005). CD31- but not CD31+ cardiac side population cells exhibit functional cardiomyogenic differentiation. *Circ Res, 97*, 52–61.
20. Laugwitz, K. L., Moretti, A., Lam, J., et al. (2005). Postnatal isl1+cardioblasts enter fully differentiated cardiomyocyte lineages. *Nature, 433*, 585–587.
21. Rosenblatt-Velin, N., Lepore, M. G., Cartoni, C., et al. (2005). FGF-2 controls the differentiation of resident cardiac precursors into functional cardiomyocytes. *J Clin Invest, 115*, 1724–1733.
22. Tomita, Y., Matsumura, K., Wakamtsu, Y., et al. (2005). Cardiac neural crest cells contribute to the dormant multipotent stem cell in the mammalian heart. *J Cell Biol, 170*, 1135–1146.
23. Smith, R. R., Barile, L., Cho, H. C., et al. (2007). Regenerative potential of cardiosphere-derived cells expanded from percutaneous endomyocardial biopsy specimens. *Circulation, 115*, 896–908.
24. Anversa, P., Kajstura, J., & Leri, A. (2007). If I can stop one heart from breaking. *Circulation, 115*, 829–832.
25. Bearzi, C., Rota, M., Hosoda, T., et al. (2007). Human cardiac stem cells. *Proc Natl Acad Sci U S A, 104*, 14068–14073.
26. Pasumarthi, K. B., & Field, L. J. (2002). Cardiomyocyte cell cycle regulation. *Circ Res, 90*, 1044–1054.
27. Nakajima, H., Nakajima, H. O., Dembowsky, K., et al. (2006). Cardiomyocyte cell cycle activation ameliorates fibrosis in the atrium. *Circ Res, 98*, 141–148.
28. Rubart, M., & Field, L. J. (2006). Cardiac regeneration: repopulating the heart. *Annu Rev Physiol, 68*, 29–49.
29. Orlic, D., Kajstura, J., Chimenti, S., et al. (2001). Bone marrow cells regenerate infarcted myocardium. *Nature, 410*, 701–705.
30. Orlic, D., Kajstura, J., Chimenti, S., et al. (2001). Mobilized bone marrow cells repair in infarcted heart, improving function and survival. *Proc Natl Acad Sci U S A, 98*, 10344–10349.
31. Kawada, H., Fujita, J., Kinjo, K., et al. (2004). Nonhematopoietic mesenchymal stem cells can be mobilized and differentiate into cardio myocytes after myocardial infarction. *Blood, 104*, 3581–3587.
32. Anversa, P., Sussman, M. A., & Bolli, R. (2004). Molecular genetic advances in cardiovascular medicine: focus on the myocyte. *Circulation, 109*, 2832–2838.
33. Kajstura, J., Rota, M., Whang, B., et al. (2005). Bone marrow cells differentiate in cardiac cell lineages after infarction independently of cell fusion. *Circ Res, 96*, 127–137.
34. Anversa, P., Leri, A., & Kajstura, J. (2006). Cardiac regeneration. *J Am Coll Cardiol, 47*, 1769–1776.
35. Rota, M., Kajstura, J., Hosoda, T., et al. (2007). Bone marrow cells adopt the cardiomyogenic fate in vivo. *Proc Natl Acad Sci U S A, 104*, 17783–17788.
36. Sussman, M. A., & Murry, C. E. (2008). Bones of contention: marrow-derived cells in myocardial regeneration. *J Mol Cell Cardiol, 44*, 950–953.
37. Wagers, A. J., Sherwood, R. I., Christensen, J. L., et al. (2002). Little evidence for developmental plasticity of adult hematopoietic stem cells. *Science, 297*, 2256–2259.
38. Murry, C. E., Soonpaa, M. H., Reinecke, H., et al. (2004). Haematopoietic stem cells do not transdifferentiate into cardiac myocytes in myocardial infarcts. *Nature, 428*, 664–668.
39. Balsam, L. B., Wagers, A. J., Christensen, J. L., et al. (2004). Haematopoietic stem cells adopt mature haematopoietic fates in ischaemic myocardium. *Nature, 428*, 668–673.
40. Nygren, J. M., Jovinge, S., Breitbach, M., et al. (2004). Bone marrow-derived hematopoietic cells generate cardiomyocytes at a low frequency through cell fusion. *Nat Med, 10*, 494–501.
41. Laflamme, M. A., & Murry, C. E. (2005). Regenerating the heart. *Nat Biotechnol, 23*, 845–856.
42. Murry, C. E., Reinecke, H., & Pabon, L. M. (2006). Regeneration gaps: observations on stem cells and cardiac repair. *J Am Coll Cardiol, 47*, 1777–1785.
43. Reinecke, H., Minami, E., Zhu, W. Z., et al. (2008). Cardiogenic differentiation and transdifferentiation of progenitor cells. *Circ Res, 103*, 1058–1071.
44. Scherschel, J. A., Soonpaa, M. H., Srour, E. F., et al. (2008). Adult bone marrow-derived cells do not acquire functional attributes of cardiomyocytes when transplanted into peri-infarct myocardium. *Mol Ther, 16*, 1129–1137.
45. Leri, A., Kajstura, J., & Anversa, P. (2005). Cardiac stem cells and mechanisms of myocardial regeneration. *Physiol Rev, 85*, 1373–1416.
46. Strauer, B. E., Brehm, M., Zeus, T., et al. (2002). Repair of infarcted myocardium by autologous intracoronary mononuclear bone marrow cell transplantation in humans. *Circulation, 106*, 1913–1918.
47. Assmus, B., Schachinger, V., Teupe, C., et al. (2002). Transplantation of progenitor cells and regeneration enhancement in acute myocardial infarction (TOPCARE-AMI). *Circulation, 106*, 3009–3017.
48. Britten, M. B., Abolmaali, N. D., Asmus, B., et al. (2003). Infarct remodeling after intracoronary progenitor cell treatment in patients with acute myocardial infarction (TOPCARE-AMI): mechanistic insights from serial contrast-enhanced magnetic resonance imaging. *Circulation, 108*, 2212–2218.
49. Perin, E. X., Dohmann, H. F., Borojevic, R., et al. (2003). Transendocardial, autologous bone marrow cell transplantation for severe, chronic ischemic heart failure. *Circulation, 107*, 2294–2302.
50. Schachinger, V., Assmus, B., Britten, M. B., et al. (2004). Transplantation of progenitor cells and regeneration enhancement in acute myocardial infarction: final one-year results of the TOPCARE-AMI trial. *J Am Coll Cardiol, 44*, 1690–1699.
51. Wollert, K. C., Meyer, G. P., Lotz, J., et al. (2004). Intracoronary autologous bone-marrow cell transfer after myocardial infarction: the BOOST randomized controlled clinical trial. *Lancet, 364*, 141–148.
52. Dohmann, H. F., Perin, E. C., Takya, C. M., et al. (2005). Transendocardial autologous bone marrow mononuclear cell injection in ischemic heart failure: postmortem anatomopathologic and immunohistochemical findings. *Circulation, 112*, 521–526.
53. Strauer, B. E., Brehm, M., Zeus, T., et al. (2005). Regeneration of human infarcted heart muscle by intracoronary autologous bone marrow cell transplantation in chronic coronary artery disease: the IACT study. *J Am Coll Cardiol, 46*, 1651–1658.
54. Erbs, S., Linke, A., Adams, V., et al. (2005). Transplantation of blood-derived progenitor cells after recanalization of chronic coronary artery occlusion: first randomized and placebo-controlled study. *Circ Res, 97*, 756–762.
55. Meyer, G. P., Wollert, K. C., Lotz, J., et al. (2006). Intracoronary bone marrow cell transfer after myocardial infarction: eighteen months' follow-up data from the randomized, controlled BOOST (BOne marrOw transfer to enhance ST-elevation infarct regeneration) trial. *Circulation, 113*, 1287–1294.
56. Assmus, B., Honold, J., Schächinger, V., et al. (2006). Transcoronary transplantation of progenitor cells after myocardial infarction. *N Engl J Med, 355*, 1222–1232.
57. Schächinger, V., Erbs, S., Elsässer, A., et al. (2006). Intracoronary bone marrow-derived progenitor cells in acute myocardial infarction. *N Engl J Med, 355*, 1210–1221.
58. Meluzín, J., Mayer, J., Groch, L., et al. (2006). Autologous transplantation of mononuclear bone marrow cells in patients with acute myocardial infarction: the effect of the dose of transplanted cells on myocardial function. *Am Heart J, 152*, 975, 975.e15.
59. Assmus, B., Walter, D. H., Lehmann, R., et al. (2006). Intracoronary infusion of progenitor cells is not associated with aggravated restenosis development or atheroscle-

rotic disease progression in patients with acute myocardial infarction. *Eur Heart J, 27*, 2989–2995.

60. Schächinger, V., Erbs, S., Elsässer, A., et al. (2006). Improved clinical outcome after intracoronary administration of bone-marrow-derived progenitor cells in acute myocardial infarction: final 1-year results of the REPAIR-AMI trial. *Eur Heart J, 27*, 2775–2783.
61. Losordo, D. W., Schatz, R. A., White, C. J., et al. (2007). Intramyocardial transplantation of autologous CD34+ stem cells for intractable angina: a phase I/IIa double-blind, randomized controlled trial. *Circulation, 115*, 3165–3172.
62. Martin-Rendon, E., Brunskill, S. J., Hyde, C. J., et al. (2008). Autologous bone marrow stem cells to treat acute myocardial infarction: a systematic review. *Eur Heart J, 29*, 1807–1818.
63. Abdel-Latif, A., Bolli, R., Tleyjeh, I. M., et al. (2007). Adult bone marrow-derived cells for cardiac repair: a systematic review and meta-analysis. *Arch Intern Med, 167*, 989–997.
64. Kang, S., Yang, Y. J., Li, C. J., et al. (2008). Effects of intracoronary autologous bone marrow cells on left ventricular function in acute myocardial infarction: a systematic review and meta-analysis for randomized controlled trials. *Coron Artery Dis, 19*, 327–335.
65. Herbots, L., D'hooge, J., Eroglu, E., et al. (2008). Improved regional function after autologous bone marrow-derived stem cell transfer in patients with acute myocardial infarction: a randomized, double-blind strain rate imaging study. *Eur Heart J* (Epub ahead of print).
66. Anversa, P., Kajstura, J., Leri, A., et al. (2006). Life and death of cardiac stem cells: a paradigm shift in cardiac biology. *Circulation, 113*, 1451–1463.
67. Anversa, P., Leri, A., Rota, M., et al. (2007). Concise review: stem cells, myocardial regeneration, and methodological artifacts. *Stem Cells, 25*, 589–601.
68. Dimmeler, S., & Leri, A. (2008). Aging and disease as modifiers of efficacy of cell therapy. *Circ Res, 102*, 1319–1330.
69. Mangi, A. A., Noiseux, N., Kong, D., et al. (2003). Mesenchymal stem cells modified with Akt prevent remodeling and restore performance of infarcted hearts. *Nat Med, 9*, 1195–1201.
70. Gnecchi, M., He, H., Liang, O. D., et al. (2005). Paracrine action accounts for marked protection of ischemic heart by Akt-modified mesenchymal stem cells. *Nat Med, 11*, 367–368.
71. Mirotsou, M., Zhang, Z., Deb, A., et al. (2007). Secreted frizzled related protein 2 (Sfrp2) is the key Akt-mesenchymal stem cell-released paracrine factor mediating myocardial survival and repair. *Proc Natl Acad Sci U S A, 104*, 1643–1648.
72. Phinney, D. G., & Prockop, D. J. (2007). Concise review: mesenchymal stem/multipotent stromal cells: the state of transdifferentiation and modes of tissue repair—current views. *Stem Cells, 25*, 2896–2902.
73. Cho, H. J., Lee, N., Lee, J. Y., et al. (2007). Role of host tissues for sustained humoral effects after endothelial progenitor cell transplantation into the ischemic heart. *J Exp Med, 204*, 3257–3269.
74. Gnecchi, M., Zhang, Z., Ni, A., et al. (2008). Paracrine mechanisms in adult stem cell signaling and therapy. *Circ Res, 103*, 1204–1219.
75. Anversa, P., & Kajstura, J. (1998). Ventricular myocytes are not terminally differentiated in the adult mammalian heart. *Circ Res, 83*, 1–14.
76. Soonpaa, M. H., & Field, L. J. (1998). Survey of studies examining mammalian cardiomyocyte DNA synthesis. *Circ Res, 83*, 15–26.
77. Wagers, A. J., & Weissman, I. L. (2004). Plasticity of adult stem cells. *Cell, 116*, 639–648.
78. Murry, C. E., Field, L. J., & Menasché, P. (2005). Cell-based cardiac repair: reflections at the 10-year point. *Circulation, 112*, 3174–3183.
79. Rubart, M., & Field, L. J. (2006). Cardiac regeneration: repopulating the heart. *Annu Rev Physiol, 68*, 29–49.
80. Urbanek, K., Rota, M., Cascapera, S., et al. (2005). Cardiac stem cells possess growth factor-receptor systems that after activation regenerate the infarcted myocardium, improving ventricular function and long-term survival. *Circ Res, 97*, 663–673.
81. Linke, A., Muller, P., Nurzynska, D., et al. (2005). Stem cells in the dog heart are self-renewing, clonogenic, and multipotent and regenerate infarcted myocardium, improving cardiac function. *Proc Natl Acad Sci U S A, 102*, 8966–8971.
82. Tillmanns, J., Rota, M., Hosoda, T., et al. (2008). Formation of large coronary arteries by cardiac progenitor cells. *Proc Natl Acad Sci U S A, 105*, 1668–1673.
83. Rota, M., Padin-Iruegas, M. E., Misao, Y., et al. (2008). Local activation or implantation of cardiac progenitor cells rescues scarred infarcted myocardium improving cardiac function. *Circ Res, 103*, 107–116.
84. Murasawa, S., Kawamoto, A., Horii, M., et al. (2005). Niche-dependent translineage commitment of endothelial progenitor cells, not cell fusion in general, into myocardial lineage cells. *Arterioscler Thromb Vasc Biol, 25*, 1388–1394.
85. Iwasaki, H., Kawamoto, A., Ishikawa, M., et al. (2006). Dose-dependent contribution of CD34-positive cell transplantation to concurrent vasculogenesis and cardiomyogenesis for functional regenerative recovery after myocardial infarction. *Circulation, 113*, 1311–1325.
86. Kawamoto, A., Iwasaki, H., Kusano, K., et al. (2006). CD34-positive cells exhibit increased potency and safety for therapeutic neovascularization after myocardial infarction compared with total mononuclear cells. *Circulation, 114*, 2163–2169.
87. Tamaki, T., Akatsuka, A., Okada, Y., et al. (2008). Cardiomyocyte formation by skeletal muscle-derived multi-myogenic stem cells after transplantation into infarcted myocardium. *PLoS One, 3*, e1789.
88. Dutt, P., Wang, J. F., & Groopman, J. E. (1998). Stromal cell-derived factor-1 alpha and stem cell factor/kit ligand share signaling pathways in hemopoietic progenitors: a potential mechanism for cooperative induction of chemotaxis. *J Immunol, 161*, 3652–3658.
89. Shen, H., Cheng, T., Olszak, I., et al. (2001). CXCR-4 desensitization is associated with tissue localization of hemopoietic progenitor cells. *J Immunol, 166*, 5027–5033.
90. Epstein, R. J. (2004). The CXCL12-CXCR4 chemotactic pathway as a target of adjuvant breast cancer therapies. *Nat Rev Cancer, 4*, 901–909.
91. Avigdor, A., Goichberg, P., Shivtiel, S., et al. (2004). CD44 and hyaluronic acid cooperate with SDF-1 in the trafficking of human CD34+ stem progenitor cells to bone marrow. *Blood, 103*, 2981–2990.
92. Ceradini, D. J., Kulkarni, A. R., Callaghan, M. J., et al. (2004). Progenitor cell trafficking is regulated by hypoxic gradients through HIF-1 induction of SDF-1. *Nat Med, 10*, 858–864.
93. Quesenberry, P. J., Colvin, G., & Abedi, M. (2005). Perspective: fundamental and clinical concepts on stem cell homing and engraftment: a journey to niches and beyond. *Exp Hematol, 33*, 9–19.
94. Kucia, M., Reca, R., Miekus, K., et al. (2005). Trafficking of normal stem cells and metastasis of cancer stem cells involve similar mechanisms: pivotal role of the SDF-1-CXCR4 axis. *Stem Cells, 23*, 879–894.
95. Zagzag, D., Krishnamachary, B., Yee, H., et al. (2005). Stromal cell-derived factor-1 alpha and CXCR4 expression in hemangioblastoma and clear cell-renal cell carcinoma: von Hippel-Lindau loss-of-function induces expression of a ligand and its receptor. *Cancer Res, 65*, 6178–6188.
96. Foudi, A., Jarrier, P., Zhang, Y., et al. (2006). Reduced retention of radioprotective hematopoietic cells within the bone marrow microenvironment in CXCR4$^{-/-}$ chimeric mice. *Blood, 107*, 2243–2251.
97. Ceradini, D. J., & Gurtner, G. C. (2005). Homing to hypoxia: HIF-1 as a mediator of progenitor cell recruitment to injured tissue. *Trends Cardiovasc Med, 15*, 57–63.
98. Scharner, D., Rössig, L., Carmona, G., et al. (2009). Caspase-8 is involved in neovascularization-promoting progenitor cell functions. *Arterioscler Thromb Vasc Biol*, Epub ahead of print.
99. Gonzalez, A., Rota, M., Nurzynska, D., et al. (2008). Activation of cardiac progenitor cells reverses the failing heart senescent phenotype and prolongs lifespan. *Circ Res, 102*, 597–606.
100. Cheng, W., Reiss, K., Li, P., et al. (1996). Aging does not affect the activation of the myocyte insulin-like growth factor-1 autocrine system after infarction and ventricular failure in Fischer 344 rats. *Circ Res, 78*, 536–546.
101. Abbott, J. D., Huang, Y., Liu, D., et al. (2004). Stromal cell-derived factor-1alpha plays a critical role in stem cell recruitment to the heart after myocardial infarction but is not sufficient to induce homing in the absence of injury. *Circulation, 110*, 3300–3305.
102. Gude, N. A., Emmanuel, G., Wu, W., et al. (2008). Activation of Notch-mediated protective signaling in the myocardium. *Circ Res, 102*, 1025–1035.
103. Urbanek, K., Cesselli, D., Rota, M., et al. (2006). Cardiac stem cell niches control cardiomyogenesis in the adult mouse heart. *Proc Natl Acad Sci U S A, 103*, 9226–9231.
104. Qin, G., Ii, M., Silver, M., et al. (2006). Functional disruption of alpha4 integrin mobilizes bone marrow-derived endothelial progenitors and augments ischemic neovascularization. *J Exp Med, 203*, 153–163.
105. Whetton, A. D., & Graham, G. J. (1999). Homing and mobilization in the stem cell niche. *Trends Cell Biol, 9*, 233–238.
106. Imai, K., Kobayashi, M., Wang, J., et al. (1999). Selective transendothelial migration of hematopoietic progenitor cells: a role in homing of progenitor cells. *Blood, 93*, 149–156.
107. Szilvassy, S. J., Meyerrose, T. E., Ragland, P. L., et al. (2001). Differential homing and engraftment properties of hematopoietic progenitor cells from murine bone marrow, mobilized peripheral blood, and fetal liver. *Blood, 98*, 2108–2115.
108. Lapidot, T., & Petie, I. (2002). Current understanding of stem cell mobilization: the roles of chemokines, proteolytic enzymes, adhesion molecules, cytokines, and stromal cells. *Exp Hematol, 30*, 973–981.
109. Calvi, L. M., Adams, G. B., Weibrecht, K. W., et al. (2003). Osteoblastic cells regulate the haematopoietic stem cell niches. *Nature, 23*, 841–846.
110. Moore, K. A., & Lemischka, I. R. (2004). "Tie-ing" down the hematopoietic niche. *Cell, 118*, 139–140.
111. Arai, F., Hirao, A., Ohmura, M., et al. (2004). Tie2/angiopoietin-1 signaling regulates hematopoietic stem cell quiescence in the bone marrow niche. *Cell, 118*, 149–161.
112. Lapidot, T., Dar, A., & Kollet, O. (2005). How do stem cells find their way home? *Blood, 106*, 1901–1910.
113. Adams, G. B., Chabner, K. T., Alley, I. R., et al. (2006). Stem cell engraftment at the endosteal niche is specified by the calcium-sensing receptor. *Nature, 439*, 599–603.
114. Song, X., Zhu, C. H., Doan, C., et al. (2002). Germline stem cells anchored by adherens junctions in the Drosophila ovary niches. *Science, 296*, 1855–1857.
115. Perez-Moreno, M., Jamora, C., & Fuchs, E. (2003). Sticky business: orchestrating cellular signals at adherens junctions. *Cell, 112*, 535–548.
116. Cancelas, J. A., Koevoet, W. L., de Koning, A. E., et al. (2000). Connexin-43 gap junctions are involved in multiconnexin-expressing stromal support of hemopoietic progenitors and stem cells. *Blood, 96*, 498–505.
117. Presley, C. A., Lee, A. W., Kastl, B., et al. (2005). Bone marrow connexin-43 expression is critical for hematopoietic regeneration after chemotherapy. *Cell Commun Adhes, 12*, 307–317.
118. Yin, T., & Li, L. (2006). The stem cell niches in bone. *J Clin Invest, 116*, 1195–1201.
119. Kiel, M. J., & Morrison, S. J. (2008). Uncertainty in the niches that maintain haematopoietic stem cells. *Nat Rev Immunol, 8*, 290–301.
120. Doetsch, F. (2003). A niche for adult neural stem cells. *Curr Opin Genet Dev, 13*, 543–550.
121. Ma, D. K., Ming, G. L., & Song, H. (2005). Glial influences on neural stem cell development: cellular niches for adult neurogenesis. *Curr Opin Neurobiol, 15*, 514–520.
122. Tavazoie, M., Van der Veken, L., Silva-Vargas, V., et al. (2008). A specialized vascular niche for adult neural stem cells. *Cell Stem Cell, 3*, 279–288.
123. Leri, A., Kajstura, J., & Anversa, P. (2005). Identity deception: not a crime for a stem cell. *Physiology (Bethesda), 20*, 162–168.
124. Frisch, S. M., & Screaton, R. A. (2001). Anoikis mechanisms. *Curr Opin Cell Biol, 13*, 555–562.
125. Reddig, P. J., & Juliano, R. L. (2005). Clinging to life: cell to matrix adhesion and cell survival. *Cancer Metastasis Rev, 24*, 425–439.

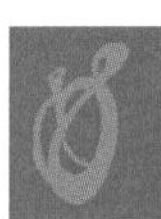

126. Chiarugi, P., & Giannoni, E. (2008). Anoikis: a necessary death program for anchorage-dependent cells. *Biochem Pharmacol, 76*, 1352–1364.
127. Geiger, H., & Van Zant, G. (2002). The aging of lympho-hematopoietic stem cells. *Nat Immunol, 3*, 329–333.
128. Roeder, I., Kamminga, L. M., Braesel, K., et al. (2005). Competitive clonal hematopoiesis in mouse chimeras explained by a stochastic model of stem cell organization. *Blood, 106*, 609–616.
129. Pfeffer, M. A., & Braunwald, E. (1990). Ventricular remodeling after myocardial infarction. Experimental observations and clinical implications. *Circulation, 81*, 1161–1172.
130. Braunwald, E. (2008). Biomarkers in heart failure. *N Engl J Med, 358*, 2148–2159.
131. Braunwald, E. (2008). The management of heart failure: the past, the present, and the future. *Circ Heart Fail, 1*, 58–62.
132. Anversa, P., Leri, A., Beltrami, C. A., et al. (1998). Myocyte death and growth in the failing heart. *Lab Invest, 78*, 767–786.
133. Anversa, P., & Olivetti, G. (2002). In E. Page, H. A. Fozzard, & R. J. Solaro (Eds.). *Handbook of physiology, section 2: the cardiovascular system: the heart cellular basis of physiological and pathological myocardial growth* (vol. 1). New York: Oxford University Press.
134. Nadal-Ginard, B., Kajstura, J., Leri, A., et al. (2003). Myocyte death, growth and regeneration in cardiac hypertrophy and failure. *Circ Res, 92*, 139–150.
135. Hitchon, C., Wong, K., Ma, G., et al. (2002). Hypoxia-induced production of stromal cell-derived factor 1 (CXCL12) and vascular endothelial growth factor by synovial fibroblasts. *Arthritis Rheum, 46*, 2587–2597.
136. Greijer, A. E., van der Groep, P., Kemming, D., et al. (2005). Up-regulation of gene expression by hypoxia is mediated predominantly by hypoxia-inducible factor 1 (HIF-1). *J Pathol, 206*, 291–304.
137. Zhang, G., Nakamura, Y., Wang, X., et al. (2007). Controlled release of stromal cell-derived factor-1 alpha in situ increases c-kit+ cell homing to the infarcted heart. *Tissue Eng, 13*, 2063–2071.
138. Burger, J. A., & Peled, A. (2009). CXCR4 antagonists: targeting the microenvironment in leukemia and other cancers. *Leukemia, 23*, 43–52.
139. Urbich, C., & Dimmeler, S. (2004). Endothelial progenitor cells: characterization and role in vascular biology. *Circ Res, 95*, 343–353.
140. Walter, D. H., Haendeler, J., Reinhold, J., et al. (2005). Impaired CXCR4 signaling contributes to the reduced neovascularization capacity of endothelial progenitor cells from patients with coronary artery disease. *Circ Res, 97*, 1142–1151.
141. Grunewald, M., Avraham, I., Dor, Y., et al. (2006). VEGF-induced adult neovascularization: recruitment, retention, and role of accessory cells. *Cell, 124*, 175–189.
142. Morrison, S. J., Prowse, K. R., Ho, P., et al. (1996). Telomerase activity in hematopoietic cells is associated with self-renewal potential. *Immunity, 5*, 207–216.
143. Allsopp, R. C., Morin, G. B., DePinho, R., et al. (2003). Telomerase is required to slow telomere shortening and extend replicative lifespan of HSCs during serial transplantation. *Blood, 102*, 517–520.
144. Lansdorp, P. M. (2005). Role of telomerase in hematopoietic stem cells. *Ann N Y Acad Sci, 1044*, 220–227.
145. Lansdorp, P. M. (2008). Telomeres, stem cells, and hematology. *Blood, 111*, 1759–1766.
146. Aubert, G., & Lansdorp, P. M. (2008). Telomeres and aging. *Physiol Rev, 88*, 557–579.
147. Kim, S. H., Kaminker, P., & Campisi, J. (2002). Telomeres, aging and cancer: in search of a happy ending. *Oncogene, 21*, 503–511.
148. Campisi, J. (2005). Senescent cells, tumor suppression, and organismal aging: good citizens, bad neighbors. *Cell, 120*, 513–522.
149. Finkel, T., Serrano, M., & Blasco, M. A. (2007). The common biology of cancer and ageing. *Nature, 448*, 767–774.
150. Serrano, M., & Blasco, M. A. (2007). Cancer and ageing: convergent and divergent mechanisms. *Nat Rev Mol Cell Biol, 8*, 715–722.
151. Lee, H. W., Blasco, M. A., Gottlieb, G. J., et al. (1998). Essential role of mouse telomerase in highly proliferative organs. *Nature, 392*, 569–574.
152. Samper, E., Fernandez, P., Eguia, R., et al. (2002). Long-term repopulating ability of telomerase-deficient murine hematopoietic stem cells. *Blood, 99*, 2767–2775.
153. Hao, L. Y., Armanios, M., Strong, M. A., et al. (2005). Short telomeres, even in the presence of telomerase, limit tissue renewal capacity. *Cell, 123*, 1121–1131.
154. Ju, Z., Jiang, H., Jaworski, M., et al. (2007). Telomere dysfunction induces environmental alterations limiting hematopoietic stem cell function and engraftment. *Nat Med, 13*, 742–747.
155. Leri, A., Franco, S., Zacheo, A., et al. (2003). Ablation of telomerase and telomere loss leads to cardiac dilatation and heart failure associated with p53 upregulation. *EMBO J, 22*, 131–139.
156. Leri, A., Kajstura, J., Nadal-Ginard, B., et al. (2004). Some like it plastic. *Circ Res, 94*, 132–134.
157. Flores, I., Cayuela, M. L., & Blasco, M. A. (2005). Effects of telomerase and telomere length on epidermal stem cell behavior. *Science, 309*, 1253–1256.
158. Greenwood, M. J., & Lansdorp, P. M. (2003). Telomeres, telomerase, and hematopoietic stem cell biology. *Arch Med Res, 34*, 489–495.
159. de Lange, T. (2004). T-loops and the origin of telomeres. *Nat Rev Mol Cell Biol, 5*, 323–329.
160. Blasco, M. A. (2005). Telomeres and human disease: ageing, cancer and beyond. *Nat Rev Genet, 6*, 611–622.
161. Campisi, J. (2002). Cancer and aging: yin, yang, and p53. *Sci Aging Knowledge Environ, 2002*, pe1.
162. Sharpless, N. E., & DePinho, R. A. (2004). Telomeres, stem cells, senescence, and cancer. *J Clin Invest, 113*, 160–168.
163. Urbanek, K., Quaini, F., Tasca, G., et al. (2003). Intense myocyte formation from cardiac stem cells in human cardiac hypertrophy. *Proc Natl Acad Sci U S A, 100*, 10440–10445.
164. Chimenti, C., Kajstura, J., Torella, D., et al. (2003). Senescence and death of primitive cells and myocytes lead to premature cardiac aging and heart failure. *Circ Res, 93*, 604–613.
165. Torella, D., Rota, M., Nurzynska, D., et al. (2004). Cardiac stem cell and myocyte aging, heart failure, and insulin-like growth factor-1 overexpression. *Circ Res, 94*, 514–524.
166. Urbanek, K., Torella, D., Sheikh, R. F., et al. (2005). Myocardial regeneration by activation of multipotent cardiac stem cells in ischemic heart failure. *Proc Natl Acad Sci U S A, 102*, 8692–8697.
167. Anversa, P., Rota, M., Urbanek, K., et al. (2005). Myocardial aging—a stem cell problem. *Basic Res Cardiol, 100*, 482–493.
168. Kajstura, J., Rota, M., Urbanek, K., et al. (2006). The telomere-telomerase axis and the heart. *Antioxid Redox Signal, 8*, 2125–2141.
169. Leri, A., Kajstura, J., Anversa, P., et al. (2008). Myocardial regeneration and stem cell repair. *Curr Probl Cardiol, 33*, 91–153.
170. Vitullo, J. C., Penn, M. S., Rakusan, K., et al. (1993). Effects of hypertension and aging on coronary arteriolar density. *Hypertension, 21*, 406–414.
171. Rakusan, K., & Turek, Z. (1985). The effect of heterogeneity of capillary spacing and O_2 consumption-blood flow mismatching on myocardial oxygenation. *Adv Exp Med Biol, 191*, 257–262.
172. Anversa, P., Capasso, J. M., Ricci, R., et al. (1989). Morphometric analysis of coronary capillaries during physiologic myocardial growth and induced cardiac hypertrophy: a review. *Int J Microcirc Clin Exp, 8*, 353–363.
173. Pietrzkowski, Z., Wernicke, D., Porcu, P., et al. (1992). Inhibition of cellular proliferation by peptide analogues of insulin-like growth factor 1. *Cancer Res, 52*, 6447–6451.
174. Matsumoto, K., & Nakamura, T. (2005). Mechanisms and significance of bifunctional NK4 in cancer treatment. *Biochem Biophys Res Commun, 333*, 316–327.
175. Larochelle, A., Krouse, A., Metzger, M., et al. (2006). AMD3100 mobilizes hematopoietic stem cells with long-term repopulating capacity in non-human primates. *Blood, 107*, 3772–3778.
176. Martinez-Agosto, J. A., Mikkola, H. K., Hartenstein, V., et al. (2007). The hematopoietic stem cell and its niche: a comparative view. *Genes Dev, 21*, 3044–3060.
177. Goldman, J. M., & Horowitz, M. M. (2002). The international bone marrow transplant registry. *Int J Hematol, 76*(suppl 1), 393–397.
178. Karanes, C., Nelson, G. O., Chitphakdithai, P., et al. (2008). Twenty years of unrelated donor hematopoietic cell transplantation for adult recipients facilitated by the National Marrow Donor Program. *Biol Blood Marrow Transplant, 14*, 8–15.
179. Dorn, G. W., II (2005). Physiologic growth and pathologic genes in cardiac development and cardiomyopathy. *Trends Cardiovasc Med, 15*, 185–189.
180. Maltepe, E., & Simon, M. C. (1998). Oxygen, genes, and development: an analysis of the role of hypoxic gene regulation during murine vascular development. *J Mol Med, 76*, 391–401.
181. Gebb, S. A., & Jones, P. L. (2003). Hypoxia and lung branching morphogenesis. *Adv Exp Med Biol, 28*, 133–137.
182. Tepper, O. M., Capla, J. M., Galiano, R. D., et al. (2005). Adult vasculogenesis occurs through in situ recruitment, proliferation, and tubulization of circulating bone marrow-derived cells. *Blood, 105*, 1068–1077.
183. Pennathur-Das, R., & Levitt, L. (1987). Augmentation of in vitro human marrow erythropoiesis under physiological oxygen tensions is mediated by monocytes and T lymphocytes. *Blood, 69*, 899–907.
184. Scortegagna, M., Morris, M. A., Oktay, Y., et al. (2003). The HIF family member EPAS1/HIF-2alpha is required for normal hematopoiesis in mice. *Blood, 102*, 1634–1640.
185. Tomita, S., Ueno, M., Sakamoto, M., et al. (2003). Defective brain development in mice lacking the Hif-1alpha gene in neural cells. *Mol Cell Biol, 23*, 6739–6749.
186. Germani, A., DiCarlo, A., Mangoni, A., et al. (2003). Vascular endothelial growth factor modulates skeletal myoblast function. *Am J Pathol, 163*, 1417–1428.
187. Loomes, K. M., Underkoffler, L. A., Morabito, J., et al. (1999). The expression of Jagged1 in the developing mammalian heart correlates with cardiovascular disease in Alagille syndrome. *Hum Mol Genet, 8*, 2443–2449.
188. Schroeder, T., Fraser, S. T., Ogawa, M., et al. (2003). Recombination signal sequence-binding protein Jkappa alters mesodermal cell fate decisions by suppressing cardiomyogenesis. *Proc Natl Acad Sci U S A, 100*, 4018–4023.
189. Timmerman, L. A., Grego-Bessa, J., Raya, A., et al. (2004). Notch promotes epithelial-mesenchymal transition during cardiac development and oncogenic transformation. *Genes Dev, 18*, 99–115.
190. Fischer, A., Klattig, J., Kneitz, B., et al. (2005). Hey basic helix-loop-helix transcription factors are repressors of GATA4 and GATA6 and restrict expression of the GATA target gene ANF in fetal hearts. *Mol Cell Biol, 25*, 8960–8970.
191. Grego-Bessa, J., Luna-Zurita, L., del Monte, G., et al. (2007). Notch signaling is essential for ventricular chamber development. *Dev Cell, 12*, 415–429.
192. Gustafsson, M. V., Zheng, X., Pereira, T., et al. (2005). Hypoxia requires notch signaling to maintain the undifferentiated cell state. *Dev Cell, 9*, 575–576.
193. Bray, S. J. (2006). Notch signalling: a simple pathway becomes complex. *Nat Rev Mol Cell Biol, 7*, 678–689.
194. Boni, A., Urbanek, K., Nascimbene, A., et al. (2008). Notch1 regulates the fate of cardiac progenitor cells. *Proc Natl Acad Sci U S A, 105*, 15529–15534.
195. Tanigaki, K., & Honjo, T. (2007). Regulation of lymphocyte development by Notch signaling. *Nat Immunol, 8*, 451–456.
196. Kitamura, T., Kitamura, Y. I., Funahashi, Y., et al. (2007). A Foxo/Notch pathway controls myogenic differentiation and fiber type specification. *J Clin Invest, 117*, 2477–2485.
197. Conboy, I. M., & Rando, T. A. (2002). The regulation of Notch signaling controls satellite cell activation and cell fate determination in postnatal myogenesis. *Dev Cell, 3*, 397–409.
198. Conboy, I. M., Conboy, M. J., Smythe, G. M., et al. (2003). Notch-mediated restoration of regenerative potential to aged muscle. *Science, 302*, 1575–1577.
199. Carlson, M. E., Hsu, M., & Conboy, I. M. (2008). Imbalance between pSmad3 and Notch induces CDK inhibitors in old muscle stem cells. *Nature, 454*, 528–532.
200. Tanaka, M., Chen, Z., Bartunkova, S., et al. (1999). The cardiac homeobox gene Csx/Nkx2.5 lies genetically upstream of multiple genes essential for heart development. *Development, 126*, 1269–1280.

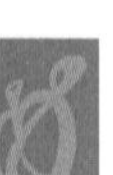

201. Beltrami, A. P., Urbanek, K., Kajstura, J., et al. (2001). Evidence that human cardiac myocytes divide after myocardial infarction. *N Engl J Med, 344*, 1750–1757.
202. Dawn, B., Stein, A. B., Urbanek, K., et al. (2005). Cardiac stem cells delivered intravascularly traverse the vessel barrier, regenerate infarcted myocardium, and improve cardiac function. *Proc Natl Acad Sci U S A, 102*, 3766–3771.
203. Zuba-Surma, E. K., Kucia, M., Dawn, B., et al. (2008). Bone marrow-derived pluripotent very small embryonic-like stem cells (VSELs) are mobilized after acute myocardial infarction. *J Mol Cell Cardiol, 44*, 865–873.
204. Dawn, B., Tiwari, S., Kucia, M. J., et al. (2008). Transplantation of bone marrow-derived very small embryonic-like stem cells attenuates left ventricular dysfunction and remodeling after myocardial infarction. *Stem Cells, 26*, 1646–1655.
205. Heissig, B., Hattori, K., Dias, S., et al. (2002). Recruitment of stem and progenitor cells from the bone marrow niche requires MMP-9 mediated release of kit-ligand. *Cell, 109*, 625–637.
206. Segers, V. F., Tokunou, T., Higgins, L. J., et al. (2007). Local delivery of protease-resistant stromal cell derived factor-1 for stem cell recruitment after myocardial infarction. *Circulation, 116*, 1683–1692.
207. Schmidt, A., Ladage, D., Schinköthe, T., et al. (2006). Basic fibroblast growth factor controls migration in human mesenchymal stem cells. *Stem Cells, 24*, 1750–1758.
208. Gho, Y. S., Kim, P. N., Li, H. C., et al. (2001). Stimulation of tumor growth by human soluble intercellular adhesion molecule-1. *Cancer Res, 61*, 4253–4257.
209. Choong, M. L., Yong, Y. P., Tan, A. C., et al. (2004). LIX: a chemokine with a role in hematopoietic stem cells maintenance. *Cytokine, 25*, 239–245.
210. Rosenkilde, M. M., & Schwartz, T. W. (2004). The chemokine system—a major regulator of angiogenesis in health and disease. *APMIS, 112*, 481–495.
211. Pomerantz, J., & Blau, H. M. (2004). Nuclear reprogramming: a key to stem cell function in regenerative medicine. *Nat Cell Biol, 6*, 810–816.
212. Vieyra, D. S., Jackson, K. A., & Goodell, M. A. (2005). Plasticity and tissue regenerative potential of bone marrow-derived cells. *Stem Cell Rev, 1*, 65–69.
213. Will, E., Klump, H., Heffner, N., et al. (2002). Unmodified Cre recombinase crosses the membrane. *Nucleic Acids Res, 30*, e59.
214. Koyanagi, M., Brandes, R. P., Haendeler, J., et al. (2005). Cell-to-cell connection of endothelial progenitor cells with cardiac myocytes by nanotubes: a novel mechanism for cell fate changes? *Circ Res, 96*, 1039–1041.
215. Karsner, H. T., Saphir, O., & Todd, T. W. (1925). The state of the cardiac muscle in hypertrophy and atrophy. *Am J Pathol, 1*, 351–371.
216. Nakamura, T., & Schneider, M. D. (2003). The way to a human's heart is through the stomach: visceral endoderm-like cells drive human embryonic stem cells to a cardiac fate. *Circulation, 107*, 2638–2639.
217. MacLellan, W. R., & Schneider, M. D. (2000). Genetic dissection of cardiac growth control pathways. *Annu Rev Physiol, 62*, 289–319.
218. Linzbach, A. J. (1947). Mikrometrische und histologische Analyse hypertopher menschlicher Herzen. *Virchows Arch Pathol Anat Physiol Klin Med, 314*, 534–594.
219. Linzbach, A. J. (1960). Heart failure from the point of view of quantitative anatomy. *Am J Cardiol, 5*, 370–382.
220. Astorri, E., Bolognesi, R., Colla, B., et al. (1977). Left ventricular hypertrophy: a cytometric study on 42 human hearts. *J Mol Cell Cardiol, 9*, 763–775.
221. Olivetti, G., Cigola, E., Maestri, R., et al. (1996). Aging, cardiac hypertrophy and ischemic cardiomyopathy do not affect the proportion of mononucleated and multinucleated myocytes in the human heart. *J Mol Cell Cardiol, 28*, 1463–1477.
222. Adler, C. P., & Costabel, U. (1975). Cell number in human heart in atrophy, hypertrophy, and under the influence of cytostatics. In A. Fleckenstein & G. Roma (Eds.). *Recent advances in studies on cardiac structure and metabolism: pathophysiology and morphology of myocardial cell alteration.* Baltimore: University Park Press.
223. Grajek, S., Lesiak, M., Pyda, M., et al. (1993). Hypertrophy or hyperplasia in cardiac muscle. Post-mortem human morphometric study. *Eur Heart J, 14*, 40–47.
224. Lizbach, A. M., & Akuamao-Boateng, E. (1973). Die Alternsveranderungen des menschlichen Herzens I. Die Herzgewicht im Alter. *Klin Wochenschr, 51*, 156–163.
225. Jones, P. H., & Watt, F. M. (1993). Separation of human epidermal stem cells from transit amplifying cells on the basis of differences in integrin function and expression. *Cell, 73*, 713–724.
226. Watt, F. M., & Hogan, B. L. M. (2000). Out of Eden: stem cells and their niches. *Science, 287*, 1427–1438.
227. Taylor, G., Lehrer, M. S., Jensen, P. J., et al. (2000). Involvement of follicular stem cells in forming not only the follicle but also the epidermis. *Cell, 102*, 451–461.
228. Wright, N. A. (2000). Epithelial stem cell repertoire in the gut: clues to the origin of cell lineages, proliferative units and cancer. *Int J Exp Pathol, 81*, 117–143.
229. Shinohara, T., Orwig, K. E., Avarbock, M. R., et al. (2001). Remodeling of the postnatal mouse testis is accompanied by dramatic changes in stem cell number and niche accessibility. *Proc Natl Acad Sci U S A, 98*, 6186–6191.
230. Lie, D. C., Song, H., Colamarino, S. A., et al. (2004). Neurogenesis in the adult brain: new strategies for central nervous system diseases. *Annu Rev Pharmacol Toxicol, 44*, 399–421.
231. Yin, T., & Li, L. (2006). The stem cell niches in bone. *J Clin Invest, 116*, 1195–1201.
232. Flickinger, R. A. (1999). Hierarchical differentiation of multipotent progenitor cells. *Bioessays, 21*, 333–338.
233. Quesenberry, P. J., Colvin, G. A., Abedi, M., et al. (2005). The stem cell continuum. *Ann N Y Acad Sci, 1044*, 228–235.
234. Götz, M., & Huttner, W. B. (2005). The cell biology of neurogenesis. *Nat Rev Mol Cell Biol, 6*, 777–788.
235. Watt, F. M. (1998). Epidermal stem cells: markers, patterning and the control of stem cell fate. *Philos Trans R Soc Lond B Biol Sci, 353*, 831–837.
236. Kaur, P. (2006). Interfollicular epidermal stem cells: identification, challenges, potential. *J Invest Dermatol, 126*, 1450–1458.
237. Díaz-Flores, L., Jr., Madrid, J. F., Gutiérrez, R., et al. (2006). Adult stem and transit-amplifying cell location. *Histol Histopathol, 21*, 995–1027.
238. Kondo, M., Wagers, A. J., Manz, M. G., et al. (2003). Biology of hematopoietic stem cells and progenitors: implications for clinical application. *Annu Rev Immunol, 21*, 759–806.
239. Shizuru, J. A., Negrin, R. S., & Weissman, I. L. (2005). Hematopoietic stem and progenitor cells: clinical and preclinical regeneration of the hematolymphoid system. *Annu Rev Med, 56*, 509–538.

CHAPTER 5

Myocardial Basis for Heart Failure: Role of the Cardiac Interstitium

Ashleigh A. Owen and Francis G. Spinale

With a prolonged cardiovascular stress or pathophysiological stimuli, a cascade of compensatory structural events occurs within the myocardium. This process occurs as a continuum and has been defined as myocardial remodeling (see Chapter 15). This remodeling process has been demonstrated within the myocardial compartment following myocardial infarction (MI), with hypertrophy, or cardiomyopathic disease. A commonly employed index of the left ventricular (LV) remodeling process is quantitation of chamber volumes.[1-5] Progressive LV dilation in patients with chronic heart failure (CHF) is associated with a greater incidence of morbidity and mortality.[3,4] Furthermore, pharmacological treatments that provide a beneficial effect on survival in CHF patients are very often associated with an attenuation in the rate and extent of LV dilation.[1-7] These observational data suggest that interventions that directly alter the LV myocardial remodeling process hold therapeutic promise in the setting of CHF. A number of cellular and extracellular factors likely contribute to the complex process of myocardial remodeling. For example, myocardial remodeling following MI includes changes in coronary vascular structure and function, myocyte loss, hypertrophy of remaining myocytes, and increased size and number of nonmyocyte cells, all of which result in nonuniform changes in LV myocardial wall geometry. While myocardial remodeling is accompanied by changes in the cellular constituents of the LV myocardium, significant alterations in the structure and composition of the extracellular matrix (ECM) occurs.[8-12] Moreover, it has become increasingly evident that the myocardial ECM is not a static structure, but rather a dynamic entity that may play a fundamental role in myocardial adaptation to a pathological stress and thereby facilitate the remodeling process.[8-27] A greater appreciation for the highly complex and dynamic nature of the ECM can be realized by myocardial imaging and direct interrogation of the interstitium.[28-30] An example of the complexity of the ECM and the tight interface with respect to tissue structure and function is exemplified by the freeze-etched electron microscopic studies illustrated in Figure 5-1.[31] These imaging studies underscore how the ECM environment is tightly coupled to the cell membrane and intracellular structures. In both human and animal studies, it has been reported that alterations in the collagen interface, both in structure and composition, occur within the LV myocardium, which in turn may influence LV geometry.[14-28,32-36] Therefore, identification and understanding of the biological systems responsible for ECM synthesis and degradation within the myocardium hold particular relevance in the progression of CHF. Accordingly, the purpose of this chapter is fourfold. First, present a brief overview of myocardial ECM structure and biosynthesis. Second, briefly demonstrate how the ECM is altered in important disease states that cause CHF: MI, hypertension, and cardiomyopathy. Third, discuss how increased activation of an interstitial proteolytic system likely contributes to ECM remodeling in CHF. Fourth, define signaling and cellular pathways that may be potential therapeutic targets for modulating ECM structure and function in the context of CHF.

MYOCARDIAL EXTRACELLULAR MATRIX STRUCTURE AND COMPOSITION

The myocardial ECM contains a fibrillar collagen network, a basement membrane, proteoglycans, and glycosaminoglycans, and bioactive signaling molecules. The myocardial fibrillar collagens such as collagen types I and III ensure structural integrity of adjoining myocytes, provide the means by which myocyte shortening is translated into overall LV pump function, and is essential for maintaining alignment of myofibrils within the myocyte through a collagen-integrin-cytoskeletal-myofibril relation.[8,10,32-36] While the fibrillar collagen matrix was initially considered to form a relatively static complex, it is now recognized that these structural proteins can undergo rapid degradation and fairly rapid turnover. The complex fibrillar collagen weave, which surrounds individual myocytes within the myocardium, is demonstrated in Figure 5-1. Collagen fibril formation entails posttranslational modification. The carboxyterminal of the procollagen fibril is cleaved by a proteolytic reaction, which results in a conformational change necessary for collagen fibril cross-linking and triple helix formation.[37] A critical step in the proper formation and structural orientation of the fibrillar collagen matrix is collagen cross-linking. Interruption of collagen cross-linking has been clearly demonstrated to alter myocardial ECM structure and in turn LV geometry and function.[38-40] Furthermore, alterations in fibrillar collagen cross-linking have been identified in myocardial samples taken from patients with end-stage CHF.[15] While the newly formed, uncross-linked collagen fibrils are vulnerable to degradation, the triple helical collagen fiber is resistant to nonspecific proteolysis and further degradation requires specific enzymatic cleavage. During collagen cross-link formation, the carboxyterminal peptide is released into the vascular space.[41-43] Collagen type I

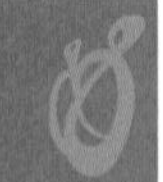

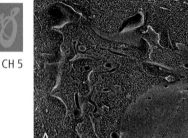

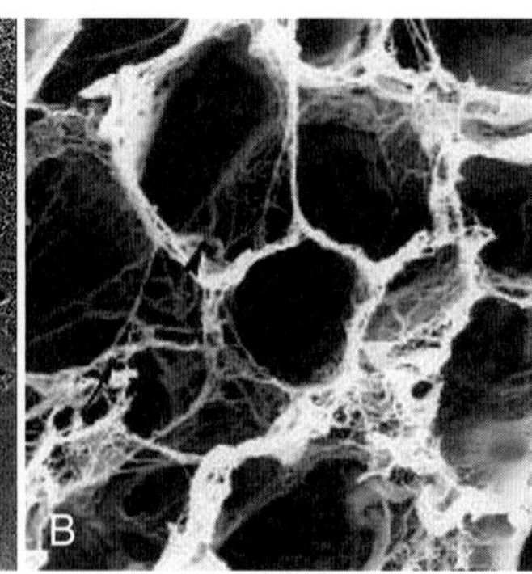

FIGURE 5–1 **A,** An example of the complex nature of the ECM and the tightly coupled interrelationship to the cell membrane and intracellular structures is exemplified in this micrograph of a chondrocyte and the ECM obtained by quick-freeze, deep-etched microscopy.[31] The ECM is densely filled with a highly structured architecture that directly interfaces with the plasma membrane (PM), and in turn the intracellular (IN) space. The nuclear pores are evident on the nuclear membrane (NM) and emphasize the tightly coupled arrangement between the nucleus to the ECM. This image reinforces the concept that changes in ECM structure and function will directly affect cellular processes. **B,** Sections of myocardium were perfusion fixed and then subjected to maceration digestion and scanning electron microscopy to remove cellular constituents and provide a greater relief of the fibrillar collagen matrix.[179] The fibrillar collagen weave surrounding individual myocyte profiles and the degree of complexity regarding the 3-dimensional ECM network can be readily appreciated through this process. (**A,** Image courtesy of Dr. Robert Mecham, Washington University School of Medicine. **B,** Reproduced from Rossi MA. Connective tissue skeleton in the normal left ventricle and in hypertensive left ventricular hypertrophy and chronic chagasic myocarditis. *Med Sci Monit* 2001;7:820–832.)

fiber formation results in the release of a 100-kDa procollagen type I carboxyterminal propeptide (PIP).[43-45] Similarly, the formation of mature collagen III fibers results in the release of a 42 kDa procollagen peptide (PIIIP).[43,44]

The integrins are a family of transmembrane proteins that serve multiple functions with respect to myocardial structure and function.[32-34] Integrins form the binding interface with proteins comprising the basement membrane and therefore directly influence myocyte growth and geometry. Moreover, the integrins coalesce at important structural sites within the myocyte called costameres, which are composed of cytoskeletal proteins such as α-actinin and vinculin which form a key intracellular support network for contractile protein assembly and maintaining sarcomeric alignment.[32-34,46,47] The myocyte costamere is also where the integrins appear to cluster and interdigitate with an intracellular signaling cascade system such as focal adhesion kinase. Thus disruption of normal integrin-ECM interactions will likely result in significant changes in myocyte structure and function.

There are a number of extracellular proteins that comprise the basement membrane, such as collagen IV, fibronectin, and laminin. It is the basement membrane that forms the anchoring points for the fibrillar matrix and contact points for other proteoglycans such as chondroitin sulfate within the ECM. For example, the abundant binding of negatively charged unbranched glycosaminoglycans within chondroitin sulfate results in a molecule with a very high osmotic activity.[48] Accordingly, changes in the content and distribution of these proteoglycans will affect hydration within the extracellular space and in turn directly influence myocardial compliance characteristics. Moreover, these highly charged molecules within the ECM result in the formation of a hydrated gel, which serves as a reservoir for signaling molecules and bioactive peptides. Therefore, the ECM is an important determinant of extracellular receptor-ligand interactions. Another important function of the myocardial ECM is that it serves as a reservoir for critical biological signaling molecules that regulate myocardial structure and function. For example, tumor necrosis factor α (TNF-α) is initially a membrane-bound molecule that requires proteolytic processing and release into the interstitial space to form ligand complexes with cognate receptors.[49-51] Also, transforming growth factor β (TGF-β) exists in a latent form bound to the ECM and requires proteolytic processing within the myocardial interstitium to become a competent signaling molecule.[52-54] TGF signaling produces multiple cellular responses—most importantly, the stimulation of ECM protein synthesis.[55-57] Thus while this chapter will primarily focus upon the collagen fibrillar network, it is becoming recognized that the myocardial interstitium is a complex environment that contains structural and signaling molecules that directly affect overall myocardial form and function.

MYOCARDIAL EXTRACELLULAR MATRIX REMODELING IN CHRONIC HEART FAILURE

The myocardium is a highly organized structure that contains a vascular network, nonmyocyte cells such as fibroblasts and macrophages, and cardiac myocytes. The ECM forms a continuum between these cell types within the myocardium and provides a structural supporting network to maintain myocardial geometry during the cardiac cycle. Significant changes in myocardial ECM structure and composition have been identified in cardiac disease states that give rise to the clinical manifestation of CHF.

Myocardial Extracellular Matrix Remodeling in Myocardial Infarction

It is now recognized that a number of architectural events occur following acute MI that involve both the infarcted and noninfarcted regions.[3-5,7,10-12] The LV remodeling process, which occurs in the post-MI period, can be considered in two phases: the acute healing phase and the chronic adaptive phase. The acute phase of MI healing involves myocyte necrosis and replacement fibrosis (see Chapter 15). In the chronic adaptive phase, changes within the MI region and in the noninfarcted region occur. Within the MI region, fibroblasts proliferate and form an extracellular matrix that provides a support structure for infarct scar maturation. This extracellular matrix within the MI region also provides a means to tether viable myocyte fascicles and thereby forms a substrate to resist deformation from the intracavitary stresses generated during the cardiac cycle. Failure of this extracellular support has been associated with LV wall thinning and slippage of myocyte fascicles.[3-5,8-12] This adverse remodeling process has been termed "infarct expansion" and occurs in the absence of additional myocyte injury or alterations in LV loading conditions. Studies performed over the past decade have clearly demonstrated that alterations within the myocardial matrix contributes to the LV remodeling process post-MI.[1-10,19,20,23,24] A number of clinical studies have clearly demonstrated an increased risk for the development of heart failure and mortality in those patients with MI-expansion and regional dilation.[1,3,7] In fact, the extent of infarct expansion that occurs post-MI and the subsequent myocardial remodeling of the left ventricle are the strongest predictors for the development of CHF.[6,7] In addition to CHF, impaired ECM formation within the MI region has been associated with LV rupture.[23] In contrast to the MI region, it has been postulated that an acceleration of ECM degradation occurs within the myocardium surrounding the MI (border zone) and may facilitate the infarct expansion process. These events within the myocardial ECM occur in a time- and region-dependent manner following MI. Thus different patterns of ECM remodeling are taking place simultaneously in the post-MI period; enhanced ECM accumulation occurs within the MI region while increased degradation occurs within the border zone. Therapeutic strategies that are targeted at minimizing the degree of infarct expansion must take into account the absolute requirement to maximize ECM stability within the MI region. Animal studies demonstrated that modulating ECM degradation in the early post-MI period reduced the relative degree of infarct expansion; however, it also impaired the wound healing response within the MI.[23,24] Past studies have also clearly demonstrated that therapeutic strategies targeted at the inflammatory response in the early post-MI period are not associated with favorable outcomes.[3,4] The mechanisms and stimuli that determine the balance between ECM synthesis and degradation are likely to be different within each region of the left ventricle following MI. Thus elucidating the molecular mechanisms that locally control ECM synthesis and degradation in the post-MI period will likely yield specific therapeutic strategies that will facilitate the wound healing response, while also attenuating the adverse myocardial remodeling that gives rise to infarct expansion and LV failure.

Myocardial Extracellular Matrix Remodeling in Left Ventricular Hypertrophy

The hallmark of myocardial structural remodeling with pressure overload hypertrophy (POH), such as hypertension or aortic stenosis, is ECM accumulation.[58-63] Specifically, prolonged POH is associated with significantly increased collagen accumulation between individual myocytes and myocyte fascicles. The extent and degree of ECM remodeling with POH are clearly exemplified by the landmark studies of Weber and Janicki.[47,48] As shown in Figure 5-2, these studies demonstrated thickening of the collagen weave and overall increased relative content between myocytes in a nonhuman primate model of POH. While the accumulation of ECM with POH is not exclusive to collagen, these initial structural studies gave rise to the generic term myocardial fibrosis to describe this extracellular remodeling process. In POH, the accumulation of ECM and eventual myocardial fibrosis significantly contributes to LV function. With POH, the highly organized architecture of the ECM is replaced with a thickened, poorly organized ECM. Thus initial degradation of the normal ECM is likely followed by decreased capacity for ECM degradation and turnover in the later stages of POH.[43-45,60-71] Increased plasma levels of PIP and PIIIP occur in hypertension and imply that significant ECM synthesis and remodeling occur, which may be associated with the LV remodeling process.[45-47] In particular, enhanced synthesis and deposition of myocardial ECM is directly associated with increased properties of LV myocardial stiffness, which in turn causes poor filling characteristics during diastole.[64-71] Indeed, recent clinical evidence suggests that progressive ECM accumulation and diastolic dysfunction are important underlying pathophysiological mechanisms for heart failure in patients with POH.[60,61,69-72] Moreover, serial studies in patients with AS have shown that the significant changes in myocardial ECM structure and composition that occur during the progression of POH may not be readily reversible.[73-75] Thus an emerging concept supported by both basic and clinical studies is that dynamic changes in myocardial ECM structure and composition occur in POH, and can contribute to certain manifestations of diastolic dysfunction and ultimately CHF. A chapter contained within this text by Zile et al discusses in greater detail the factors that contribute to diastolic dysfunction and eventually CHF.[76]

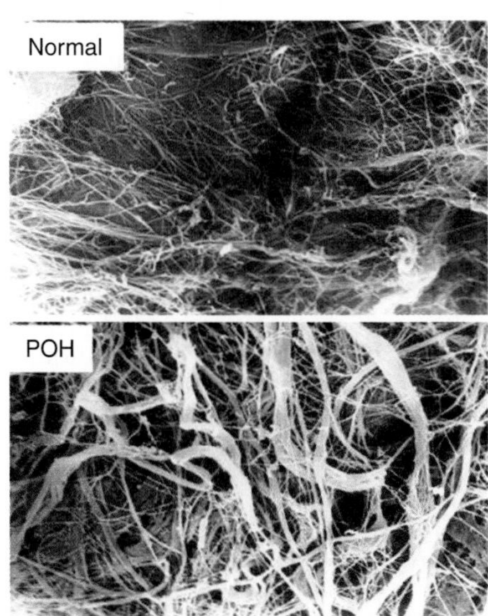

FIGURE 5-2 Scanning electron micrographs taken from normal nonhuman primate LV myocardium and following the induction of pressure overload hypertrophy (POH). These microscopic studies demonstrated thickening of the collagen weave and overall increased relative content between myocytes with POH. (Figures reproduced from Abrahams C, Janicki JS, Weber KT. Myocardial hypertrophy in *Macaca fascicularis*. Structural remodeling of the collagen matrix. *Lab Invest* 1987;56:676–683.)

Myocardial Extracellular Matrix Remodeling in Cardiomyopathy

The dilated cardiomyopathies are a classification of primary myocardial disease states that constitute a significant proportion of patients with heart failure. While the causes for dilated cardiomyopathy are diverse, a general pathophysiological classification scheme has been developed and termed ischemic, idiopathic (nonischemic), or infectious. The pathophysiology of dilated cardiomyopathy involves an increase in LV ventricular chamber radius compared with wall thickness. This increased ratio is accompanied by increased myocardial wall stress, which can in turn promote further dilation. In patients with rapidly progressive LV remodeling and dilation, morbidity and mortality are increased.[77,78] At the myocardial level, significant changes in the myocardial ECM occur in patients with cardiomyopathic disease and likely facilitate this remodeling process.[8,9,13-16] For example, a loss of the normal fibrillar collagen weave surrounding myocytes and diminished fibrillar collagen cross-linking have been reported in patients with DCM.[8,15]

EXTRACELLULAR MATRIX PROTEOLYTIC DEGRADATION: THE MATRIX METALLOPROTEINASES

The matrix metalloproteinases (MMPs) are a family of zinc-dependent proteases that play a role in a number of tissue remodeling processes.[11,12,77-84] Currently, more than 25 distinct human MMPs have been identified and characterized. MMPs have been shown to be responsible for matrix remodeling in a number of physiological processes, such as bone growth and wound healing along with pathological processes such as inflammation, tumor invasion, and metastasis.[77-84] While initially thought to only cause ECM proteolysis, the MMPs likely possess a large portfolio of biological functions.[85-87] Analysis of MMP protein structure has revealed four well-conserved modular regions. The signal peptide and propeptide sequences constitute the NH_2-terminal domain. The catalytic domain contains the zinc (Zn^{2+}) binding region and is responsible for proteolytic activity. The hemopexin/vitronectin domain is found in all MMPs except MMP-7, and confers substrate specificity. For MMP activation to occur, a sequence of proteolytic events must take place. In the latent state, the MMP catalytic domain is concealed by

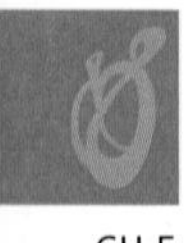

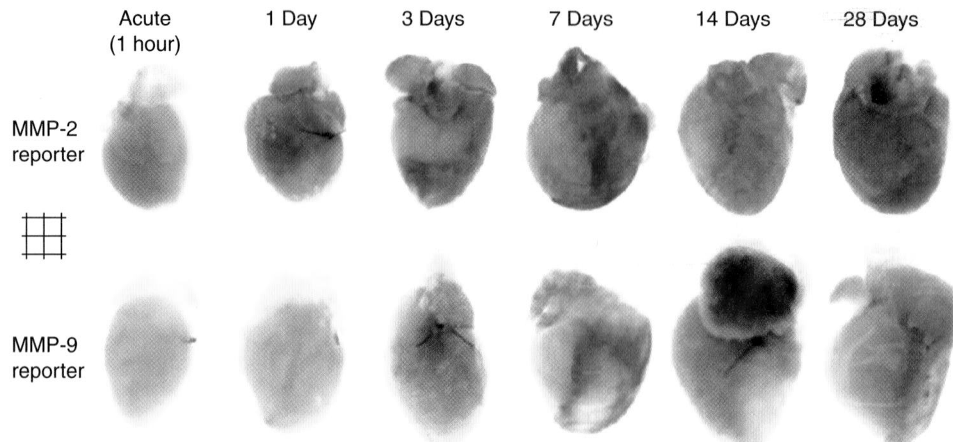

FIGURE 5–3 The full-length MMP-2 or MMP-9 promoter was ligated to the β-galactosidase reporter and fused into mice, thereby providing an in vivo index of selective MMP promoter activity. An MI was induced in these transgenic constructs and reporter levels visualized at 1 to 28 days post-MI. MMP-2 promoter activity could be readily observed by 3 days post-MI and MMP-9 promoter activity by 7 days post-MI. MMP-2 promoter activity was initially localized to the MI region but later extended to the border and remote regions as time passed post-MI. Similarly intense MMP-9 promoter activity could be observed within the area surrounding the MI (border region) that then extended into the remote regions with longer post-MI periods. Scale bar 2 mm × 2 mm square. (Figure reproduced from Mukherjee R, Mingoia JT, Bruce JA, et al. Selective spatiotemporal induction of matrix metalloproteinase-2 and matrix metalloproteinase-9 transcription after myocardial infarction. *Am J Physiol Heart Circ Physiol* 2006;291(5):H2216–H2228.)

the propeptide mediated by a cysteine-Zn^{2+} interaction.[83,88] This biochemical interaction of concealing the catalytic site with subsequent activation is known as the cysteine switch. The MMPs were historically classified into subgroups based upon substrate specificity and/or structure, and an informal nomenclature for some of the individual MMPs arose from these initial substrate studies. However, there is significant overlap in MMP proteolytic substrates and a more rigid numerical classification is now used. Important MMPs in the context of this review include the collagenases such as MMP-1 and MMP-13, the stromelysins/matrilysins MMP-3/MMP-7, the gelatinases MMP-9 and MMP-2, and the membrane-type MMPs (MT-MMPs). Once activated, the MMPs can work synergistically to degrade the entire extracellular matrix component. For this reason it is important that their activity is kept under tight control.

Transcriptional Regulation

The control of gene expression through changes in transcription is an important determinant of MMP tissue levels.[85-93] Characterization of MMP gene promoters has provided some insight into possible mechanisms that regulate MMP gene expression. Studies have identified several consensus sequences for nuclear binding proteins on MMP genes.[85,86] These elements include the tumor response element (TRE), activator protein-1 (AP-1) binding sites, and the polyoma virus enhancer A–binding protein-3 (PEA-3) sites. The AP-1 and TRE sites bind the dimers of Fos and Jun families, while the members of the Ets family of transcription factors bind to the PEA-3 sites. Although there are similarities among MMP promoters, the promoter of MMP-2 is notably distinct from other members of the MMP family.[85,86,91] Although most MMP genes contain similar promoter elements, the position of the elements relative to the transcription start site differs between different MMPs, which may partly account for different expression patterns. A clear example of differential MMP transcriptional regulation within the myocardium has been achieved using MMP promoter-reporter constructs.[94,95] Specifically, the full-length MMP promoter is fused to a reporter and placed into the mouse genome.[94,95] Through this approach, MMP-type specific promoter activity can be examined from a spatial and temporal aspect following a pathological stimulus such as MI. Representative whole heart mounts for MMP-9 and MMP-2 promoter activity are shown in Figure 5-3. The promoter activity of MMP-9 and MMP-2 were readily appreciated following the induction of MI in the transgenic mice, but the spatial-temporal patterns were different. These studies clearly demonstrate that regulation of MMP promoter activity constitutes an important focus for selective MMP induction within the myocardium.

Matrix Metalloproteinase Gene Polymorphisms

The potential importance of MMP gene/transcriptional regulation can also be shown from clinical studies identifying variant forms of DNA sequences and polymorphisms for several of the MMP subtypes.[96-109] The polymorphisms that have been identified thus far often affect the promoter region of the MMP gene, and thereby influence critical steps in the binding of transcription factors and the overall efficiency of transcription. An overview of some of the major polymorphisms reported with respect to MMP-9, -2, -3, and MMP-1 and the potential consequences of these alterations in DNA sequences are summarized in Table 5-1. The most intensely studied to date are polymorphisms that occur within the promoter region for MMP-9 and MMP-3.[96-103,107,109] With respect to MMP-9, a gene variant has been observed within the promoter region located at position −1562 relative to the transcription start site. This MMP-9 variant is a single base substitution where a transition between cytosine(C) and thymidine(T) occurs. The *T* allele results in a higher relative level of promoter activity when compared with the *C* allele.[96-98] In turn, presence of the *MMP-9 1562(T)* allele has been associated with increased plasma levels of MMP-9 protein.[96] A naturally occurring variant in the MMP-3 promoter region is the *5A* and *6A* alleles that signify a 5 or 6 adenine sequence, respectively. The *5A* allele has been associated with increased MMP-3 promoter activity, and in turn increased relative MMP-3 protein levels.[99-103] In contrast, the *6A* allele has been associated with reduced MMP-3 promoter activity. In a study performed in more than 2800 Japanese patients, the 5A polymorphism was associated with increased risk of MI in women.[101] Mizon-Gerad et al have also reported that homozygosity for the *5A* allele in patients with nonischemic cardiomyopathy was associated with a reduced survival rate.[98] One preliminary clinical study showed that the addition of guanine within the MMP-1 promoter region (−1607 1G/2G) is associated with the

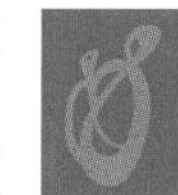

TABLE 5–1 Polymorphisms in Matrix Metalloproteinase Promoter Sequences

Polymorphism	Biological Effect	Clinical Association	Reference
MMP-9			
−1562 C/T	↑Promoter activity	↑Risk of post-MI remodeling	96, 97
		↑Remodeling in DCM	98
−279 R/Q	↑Catalytic activity	↑Remodeling in DCM	98, 109
MMP-2			
−1306 C/T	↑Promoter activity	Unknown	108
−790 G/T	↑Transcription factor binding	↑Coronary artery disease	108
MMP-3			
1171-5A/6A	↑Promoter activity	↑Risk of post-MI remodeling	99, 100, 101, 102, 107
		↑Remodeling in DCM	98
MMP-1			
−1607 1G/2G	↑Transcription factor binding	↑Risk of post-MI remodeling	104, 105
−519-340 A/G-C/T	↓Promoter activity	↓Risk of post-MI remodeling	106

acceleration of adverse LV myocardial remodeling in patients post-MI.[104,105] In another study, certain single nucleotide polymorphisms within the MMP-1 promoter that are believed to reduce MMP-1 transcriptional activity were identified and associated with reduced risk of MI.[106] While it is likely that additional MMP polymorphisms will be identified, it must be recognized that these MMP genotyping approaches do not provide a clear cause-effect relationship between the MMP system and myocardial matrix remodeling. Another consideration is that these MMP polymorphisms may not occur as independent events but rather are associated with other polymorphisms in the genome. However, it is intriguing to speculate that these MMP polymorphisms may be able to identify those patients who are more vulnerable to adverse matrix myocardial remodeling and therefore are likely to experience a more rapid progression of CHF.

Neurohormones, Cytokines, and Intracellular Activation

MMP mRNA expression can be influenced by a variety of biological signaling molecules, such as neurohormones, corticosteroids, and cytokines (see Chapter 11).* For example, cytokines such as TNF have been demonstrated to influence MMP gene expression by activating and modulating response elements on MMP gene promoters in several cell systems.[90,92,111-113] While the mechanisms of MMP induction by these factors can be complex, one common pathway appears to involve the AP-1 site.[89,90] Other factors such as retinoids, TGF, and glucocorticoids are thought to inhibit MMP gene expression by several mechanisms, which include sequestering unbound AP-1 proteins.[114] Transcription of MMPs is not only dependent upon a specific portfolio of transcription factors, but it may also be determined by a cell-specific response. For example, interleukin-1 induces expression of MMP-1 and MMP-3 in fibroblasts but not in keratinocytes, and transforming growth factor β suppresses MMP-9 production in fibroblasts but induces its production in keratinocytes.[115] Another potentially important promoter binding site located on MMPs, such as the one on MMP-9, is the nuclear factor κB site.[110,111] Exposure of human fibroblasts to inflammatory cytokines, which induce nuclear factor κB, have been shown to cause an upregulation of MMP-9.[116,117] In several cell systems, exposure to phorbol esters, which activates the protein kinase C (PKC) intracellular pathway, also increases MMP mRNA transcription.[111] Finally, past studies have identified a transmembrane protein that induces the expression of specific MMPs in vitro; the extracellular matrix metalloproteinase inducer protein (EMMPRIN).[118-121] The most active area of EMMPRIN investigation has been with respect to tumor invasion where increased EMMPRIN expression has been localized to areas with intense remodeling activity or highly invasive tumors.[119] In this pathological tissue remodeling process, it is likely that EMMPRIN is a contributory factor in the stimulation of MMPs required for tumor invasion and metastasis. A recent clinical study has clearly demonstrated an upregulation of EMMPRIN in platelets following MI.[121] Moreover, increased EMMPRIN levels have been identified in patients with DCM.[14] For these reasons EMMPRIN may also be an important contributory factor in the upregulation of various MMPs in the context of myocardial remodeling.

Matrix Metalloproteinase Activation

While the level of MMP synthesis is an important determinant of matrix degradation, the true degradative capacity of the MMPs is dependent upon the activation of the MMP proenzyme. After being synthesized in a latent, pro-enzyme, or zymogen form, the MMPs are secreted into the extracellular space. For MMP zymogen activation to occur, a sequence of proteolytic events must take place. Thus an important control point of MMP activity is proteolytic cleavage by other enzymes (e.g., serine proteases and other MMP species), or exposure to certain physical and chemical effectors.[83,84,88] For MMP activation to occur, the NH_2 terminal sequence of the propeptide domain must be cleaved, resulting in the exposure of the zinc binding site of the catalytic domain. It has been demonstrated serine proteases such as plasmin can generate active MMPs. In addition, MMP activation can also occur at the cell surface involving the MT-MMPs.[122-128] At the cell membrane, MT-MMP is already in an active state such that it can then activate other MMP species at the cell surface. It has been clearly established that MT1-MMP activates MMP-2, and in fact may be the predominant pathway for MMP-2 activation.[123-128] Moreover, it appears that a very wide proteolytic portfolio for MT1-MMP exists, which would imply that this MMP type may participate in a number of enzymatic and signaling cascades within the myocardial ECM.[85-87] This is likely to hold particular relevance since robust levels of MT1-MMP have been identified within both experimental and clinical forms of CHF.[14,25,30,129-131]

Endogenous Matrix Metalloproteinase Inhibition

Another important control point of MMP activity is in the inhibition of the activated enzyme by action of a group of specific MMP inhibitors termed tissue inhibitors of matrix metalloproteinases (TIMPs).[11,12,81-84] There are four known TIMP species of which TIMP-1 and TIMP-2 are the best characterized. The TIMPs are low molecular weight proteins that can complex noncovalently with high efficiency to MMPs in a 1:1 molar ratio. Therefore, these inhibitory proteins are an

*References.11, 51, 82, 88, 89, 92, 110, 111.

important endogenous system for regulating MMP activity in vivo. While the TIMPs are expressed in a variety of cells, TIMP-4 shows a high level of expression in cardiovascular tissue.[132,133] While it is believed that the predominant role of TIMPs is the inhibition of active enzymes, this is likely to be an oversimplistic view of the function of these proteins. For example, studies have demonstrated TIMPs to be involved in the process of MMP activation, to exhibit growth factor–like properties, and to participate in apoptosis.[134-137] In one study the overexpression of TIMP-1, -2, -3, -4 was induced in murine myocardial fibroblasts by adenoviral-mediated transduction.[135] Many differential biological consequences were observed after the induction of TIMPs, including effects on collagen synthesis and apoptosis. These differences were not secondary to MMP inhibition since past studies involving pharmacological MMP inhibition did not recapitulate these effects, thus indicating a direct action of TIMPs on fibroblast function. Moreover, TIMP-specific effects were also observed; TIMP-2 caused a robust increase in collagen synthesis whereas TIMP-3 accelerated fibroblast apoptosis. These results underscore the highly diverse and complex nature of the proteins existing within the myocardial interstitium.

Matrix Metalloproteinases and Myocardial Remodeling

Matrix Metalloproteinases and Myocardial Infarction

While dependent upon the severity and duration of the ischemic insult, alterations in LV myocardial collagen structure can occur following MI that would implicate changes in MMP activity within the myocardial interstitium.[8-12] Several clinical studies have provided data to demonstrate that increased plasma levels of MMPs occur in patients in the early post-MI period.[138-141] As discussed in a subsequent section, a time-dependent change in plasma MMP and TIMP profiles occurs in patients post-MI. However, the specificity of this MMP release with respect to myocardial MMP activation and the relationship to clinical outcomes remains an area of active investigation.

Experimental studies have provided mechanistic evidence that increased expression and activation of MMPs contribute to the post-MI remodeling process.[19,20,22-24,29,129-131] For example, it has been demonstrated that manipulating MMP expression in transgenic mice can alter tissue remodeling within the MI region and influence the degree of post-MI remodeling.[22-24,27] These past studies have demonstrated that MMPs may play an operative role in several phases of the evolving MI. First, early activation of MMPs may be essential for degradation of the extracellular interface between the ischemic and nonischemic regions and thereby provide an egress for inflammatory cells into the MI region. Second, activation of MMPs within the MI region may facilitate the extracellular protein degradation necessary for proper scar formation and angiogenesis. Third, prolonged activation or an acceleration of MMP expression within the viable post-MI myocardium may contribute to the process of infarct expansion. A common event following myocardial ischemia and subsequent reperfusion is an influx of inflammatory cells into the ischemic region, which results in the release and activation of a number of proteolytic enzymes. Neutrophils have been demonstrated to release several species of MMPs, including MMP-8 and MMP-9.[79-84] Fibroblasts and smooth muscle cells also synthesize a complement of MMPs including MMP-9. Past studies have demonstrated that MMPs, particularly MMP-2 and MMP-9, can be synthesized by myocytes.[11,12] Thus the induction of MMP-9 following MI is likely the result of liberated MMP-9 from endogenous and exogenous cell types. The putative role for MMP-9 induction to contribute to the post-MI remodeling process has been exemplified in transgenic mouse studies.[24] However, it is unlikely that a single MMP type is responsible for the adverse post-MI remodeling process. For example, gene deletion of MMP-2 has also been demonstrated to cause favorable effects on LV geometry and function in the early post-MI period.[22]

In addition to the induction of a large portfolio of MMPs in the post-MI period, a loss of MMP inhibitory control also appears to play an important role in the adverse LV remodeling process. First, pharmacological MMP inhibition deployed in various animal models of MI have invariably demonstrated a favorable effect on the early post-MI remodeling process.[23,130,131] Second, the induction of MMPs within the myocardium post-MI is not paralleled by an induction of TIMPs.[129,130] Finally, gene deletion of TIMPs, such as TIMP-1 or TIMP-3, have been shown to cause accelerated post-MI LV remodeling.[20,142] These findings suggest that increased MMP expression and activation coupled with a loss of endogenous MMP inhibitory control occurs early in the post-MI period and contributes to post-MI remodeling.

Matrix Metalloproteinases in Hypertrophy

LV hypertrophy occurs in response to a persistent increase in either pressure or volume overload. These chronic overload states result in two very different patterns of LV remodeling and changes in the extracellular matrix.[11,12,58-76] In states of chronic pressure overload, a common observation is the accumulation of myocardial fibrillar collagen secondary to an increase in collagen synthesis and deposition combined with a decrease in collagen degradation.[1,111] For example, chronic hypertension is associated with a relative reduction in the plasma levels of collagen telopeptides, which may also suggest a reduction in the proteolytic activity of MMPs.[43-45] In pressure overload secondary to aortic stenosis, the significant myocardial collagen accumulation was associated with a concomitant increase in relative myocardial TIMP levels.[60,63] In addition, reduced plasma MMP levels and increased TIMP levels have been reported in patients with systemic hypertension and LV hypertrophy.[64-70] For example, as shown in Figure 5-4, increased plasma levels of TIMP-1 are directly associated with the presence of LV hypertrophy, and TIMP-1 levels continue to increase with the presence of heart failure.[70] Experimental studies support the concept that diminished myocardial MMP activity can facilitate collagen

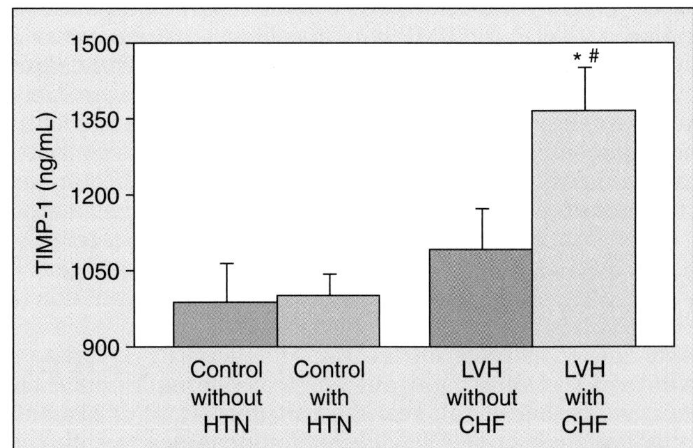

FIGURE 5–4 Plasma TIMP-1 levels were quantified in age-matched patients with no history of hypertension (control, *n* = 39), patients with hypertension (HTN) but no LV hypertrophy (*n* = 14), patients with LV hypertrophy (LVH) but without symptoms of heart failure (*n* = 23), and in patients with LVH and congestive heart failure (CHF, *n* = 26). TIMP-1 levels appeared to increase incrementally as a function of the natural history of hypertensive heart disease, with a significant increase in patients with LVH and CHF (*P <.05 vs. control, #P <.05 vs. LVH with no CHF). (Figure reproduced from Ahmed SH, Clark LL, Pennington WR, et al. Matrix metalloproteinases/tissue inhibitors of metalloproteinases: relationship between changes in proteolytic determinants of matrix composition and structural, functional, and clinical manifestations of hypertensive heart disease. *Circulation* 2006;113(17):2089–2096.)

accumulation in developing hypertrophy.[143-146] In the spontaneously hypertensive rat, the development of compensated hypertrophy is associated with increased myocardial TIMP levels, which would imply reduced MMP activity.[145,146] The changes in myocardial MMP activation are likely to be time dependent and may not be constant throughout the development of pressure overload hypertrophy. In support of this postulate, studies completed by this laboratory demonstrate time-dependent changes in myocardial MMP levels following an acute and prolonged pressure overload stimulus.[62] Furthermore, using a microdialysis method to directly measure MMP interstitial activity, it was demonstrated that MMP activity was reduced as a function of LV afterload.[28]

In contrast to chronic pressure overload, a disruption of the normal myocardial fibrillar collagen weave has been reported in chronic volume overload states such as mitral regurgitation or aorto-caval fistula. This disruption is associated with increased myocardial MMP levels and zymographic activity. [11,12,62,143,144] For example, in a rat model of volume overload, increased myocardial MMP zymographic activity was associated with changes in LV volumes and mass.[144] These studies would suggest that the early induction of myocardial MMP activity occurs with an overload stimulus that in turn alters extracellular myocyte support. These changes in extracellular fibrillar support and architecture in turn facilitate alterations in myocyte size and geometry, which is the structural basis of hypertrophy.

Matrix Metalloproteinases and Dilated Cardiomyopathy

There are several animal models of dilated cardiomyopathy (DCM) that have identified increased MMPs within the myocardium.[18,21,25] A model of CHF reporting a relationship between LV remodeling and MMP activity is the pacing-induced heart failure model.[17,18,21] In this pacing protocol, MMP activity as measured by an in vitro assay was increased. This study demonstrated that increased abundance of several species of MMPs within the myocardium coincided with the onset of LV remodeling and dilation. Moreover, these changes in MMP myocardial levels and LV geometry preceded significant alterations in cardiomyocyte contractile function, suggesting that the induction of myocardial MMPs is an early event in the progression of the heart failure process. In several rodent models of a dilated LV phenotype, a correlation between increased MMP expression and the myocardial remodeling process has also been established.[25,143,144] More definitive cause-effect relationships between LV myocardial remodeling and MMP induction have been shown through the use of pharmacological MMP inhibitors.[18,25] For example, MMP inhibition in the pacing model of heart failure attenuated the degree of LV dilation and dysfunction.[18] In the canine model of ischemic DCM, pharmacological MMP inhibition attenuated the progression of LV dilation and systolic dysfunction.[147] Thus a contributory mechanism for LV remodeling in experimentally provoked DCM is MMP induction and heightened MMP activity within the LV myocardium.

A number of studies have examined relative MMP and TIMP expression in DCM and have uniformly demonstrated an increase in certain MMP species in end-stage human heart failure.[13-17] One of the first studies was by Gunja-Smith et al in which increased myocardial MMP gelatinolytic activity was reported in DCM.[15] Using immunoblotting procedures, subsequent studies identified several MMP species that were increased in LV myocardial extracts taken from patients with end-stage DCM.[13,14] Specifically, increased MMP-3 and MMP-9 levels were observed in the DCM myocardial extracts compared with normal myocardium. In addition, MMP-13 was barely detected in the normal myocardium, while a robust immunoreactive signal for MMP-13 was observed in DCM myocardium.[14] These past observations may hold relevance for several reasons. First, MMP-13 has been associated with pathological remodeling states such as breast carcinomas.[148,149] Second, MMP-13 is activated by MT1-MMP whereas MMP-1 is not.[85-88] Therefore the emergence of this virulent form of interstitial collagenase as the predominant collagenase within the DCM myocardium may contribute to increased degradation of the myocardial fibrillar collagen network. In addition to increased MMP-13 levels with DCM, the most robust change in MMP types was the increased levels of MT1-MMP.[14] Moreover, the increased levels of MT1-MMP appeared to be due to an induction within LV myocytes and fibroblasts. Specifically, a robust signal for MT1-MMP has been localized to the LV myocyte sarcolemma.[14] Furthermore, recent studies have shown that a persistent induction and expression of MT1-MMP occurred in DCM fibroblasts when compared with myocardial fibroblasts harvested from nonfailing patients (Figure 5-5).[150] The increased levels of MT1-MMP along the myocyte and fibroblast interface form a localized site for MMP activation and a persistent induction of MMP proteolytic activity within the myocardial interstitium of DCM patients.

One potential mechanism for increased myocardial MMP activity associated with myocardial remodeling is a loss of endogenous TIMP inhibitory control.[13,14,16] Li et al provided evidence to suggest that changes in the MMP/TIMP stoichiometric ratio occurred with end-stage DCM disease.[16] Specifically, TIMP-1 and TIMP-3 levels were reduced in the DCM samples, whereas TIMP-2 levels were unchanged when compared with nonfailing samples. Additionally, in both ischemic and nonischemic DCM, an absolute reduction in MMP-1/TIMP-1 complex formation has been observed.[14] In a transgenic model of TIMP-3 deletion, a DCM phenotype was reported as a function of age.[151] Taken together, these results suggest that reduced MMP/TIMP complex formation may occur in cardiomyopathic disease states, which in turn contribute to increased myocardial MMP activity and ECM remodeling.

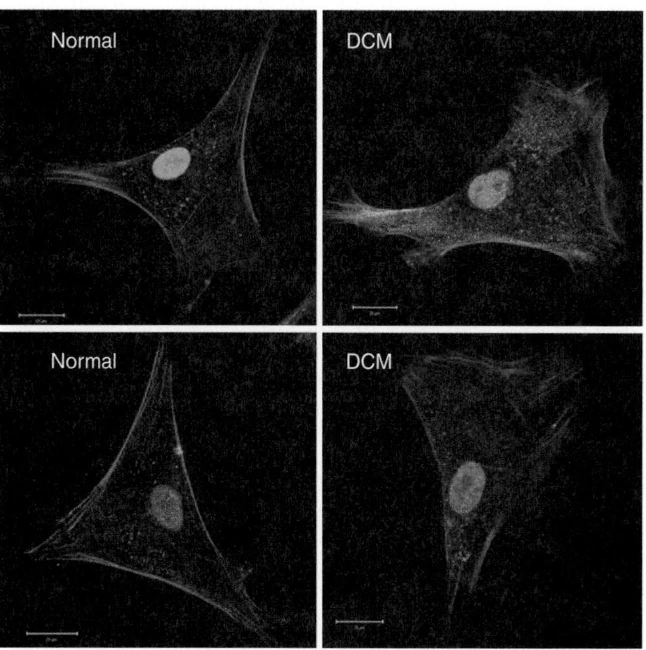

FIGURE 5–5 Representative high-power confocal images of normal (*left panels*) and DCM (*right panels*) human myocardial fibroblasts that were stained for MT1-MMP, DNA, and cytoskeletal actin. A more robust cytoplasmic staining for MT1-MMP was observed in DCM fibroblasts that appeared to coalesce near the actin filaments. (Reproduced from Spruill LS, Lowry AS, Stroud RE, et al. Membrane-type-1 matrix metalloproteinase transcription and translation in myocardial fibroblasts from patients with normal left ventricular function and from patients with cardiomyopathy. *Am J Physiol Cell Physiol* 2007;293(4):C1362-C1373.)

The cellular and molecular events that likely trigger the induction of MMPs with DCM are likely to be multifactorial. Increased neurohormonal activation and increased levels of cytokines are biological hallmarks of the DCM process. Thus it would be a reasonable assumption that these signaling molecules produce transcription factors that lead to the induction of MMP. As discussed in an earlier section, MMP genes contain response elements that bind members of the AP-1 protein family. Bioactive peptides and cytokines, such as TNF, can induce transcription factors that bind to AP-1 promoter elements found on several MMP genes.[50,89-92,111,112] Clinical evidence to support a relationship between TNF receptor activation and MMP induction was demonstrated through simultaneous measurement of soluble TNF receptors and plasma MMP levels in patients with CHF.[152,153] Physical stimuli, such as stress and strain, also likely induce MMP expression within the failing myocardium.[26,62] In DCM patients, chronic unloading of the left ventricle through the use of ventricular assist devices was associated with a reduction in LV chamber dilation and myocardial MMP levels.[26] These clinical observations suggest that the persistently elevated LV myocardial wall stress common to DCM can augment MMP levels.

MODULATION OF MYOCARDIAL EXTRACELLULAR MATRIX REMODELING: DIAGNOSTIC AND THERAPEUTIC TARGETS

One diagnostic/prognostic potential is to monitor ECM remodeling through profiling determinants of myocardial interstitial synthesis and degradation. As detailed in a previous section, several studies have demonstrated that profiling collagen peptide and TIMP levels in patients with pressure overload hypertrophy provides insight into the rate of ECM synthesis and predictive value with respect to identifying patients with diastolic dysfunction and CHF.[43,44,64-70] In large survey studies, plasma levels of MMPs and TIMPs have provided clear prognostic information with respect to cardiovascular events and mortality.[71,153-156] Perhaps the most actively studied cardiovascular disease state with respect to plasma profiling MMPs/TIMPs is in coronary artery disease and subsequent MI.[138-141] For example, relative TIMP-1 levels do not match the increase in MMP-9 levels post-MI, resulting in an elevated MMP-9/TIMP-1 ratio.[138,140] The temporal pattern for TIMP-4, which is preferentially expressed within the cardiovascular system, was examined in patients up to 6 months following MI.[140] In this study, a large increase in plasma MMP-9 accompanied by a relative reduction in TIMP-4 was observed early in the post-MI period. One potential net effect of the relative reduction in MMP inhibition during the post-MI period would be an increase in overall matrix degradation. Indeed, unique profiles of plasma MMP levels during the post-MI period are emerging as an independent predictor of adverse LV remodeling and probability of progression to CHF.[140,141,157] For example, a study by Wagner et al showed that an early increase in MMP-9 concentration was associated with an increased risk of developing heart failure in the future (odds ratio of 6.5).[157] Taking these studies together, a specific MMP/TIMP profile is emerging with respect to patients with coronary artery disease at risk for an acute coronary syndrome, and in patients post-MI.[158-168] This profile is summarized in Table 5-2. However, the degree in which modifying the changes in plasma MMP/TIMP profiles during the post-MI period may beneficially alter the course of LV remodeling and progression to CHF remains to be established.

With respect to therapeutic interventions, modulating ECM biosynthesis may provide novel strategies. For example, the importance of posttranslational processing with respect to collagen cross-linking has been demonstrated.[37-41,68,69] Thus strategies that alter collagen fibril stability may provide a unique

TABLE 5-2 Proteolytic profiles in ischemic heart disease

	CORONARY ARTERY DISEASE		*ACUTE CORONARY SYNDROME/MYOCARDIAL INFARCTION*	
	Directional Change	**References**	**Directional Change**	**References**
MMP-1	→	158	→	140, 165
MMP-2	→	159	↑Early ↓late	138, 164, 166, 141, 167
MMP-3	→	158-159	→	158, 107
MMP-7			→	
MMP-8	↑	160	↑↑	140
MMP-9	↑	161, 162, 138, 163	↑↑↑	159, 138, 140, 165, 166, 141, 157, 168
MMP-12	→	164	NS	
MMP-13			→	
TIMP-1	→↑	154	↓Early ↑late	140, 166
TIMP-2	→	159, 161		

Plasma profiling in patients with established coronary artery disease (left columns) and following an acute coronary syndrome/MI (right columns). A specific MMP/TIMP portfolio emerges when compared with baseline or referent control values. For example, MMP-8 and MMP-9 levels are increased in patients with stable coronary disease and continue to markedly increase during and following an MI. In contrast, TIMP levels do not parallel these changes in MMP levels, which would favor a heightened proteolytic state. Data extracted and summarized from the references shown (Key: arrows indicate changes from baseline/referent controls)

approach in modulating ECM myocardial structure and function. Due to the fact that MMPs play a prominent role in tissue remodeling processes, a large effort was made to develop pharmacological MMP inhibitors. These were initially constructed around a hydroxamate structure.[169,172] A significant and somewhat paradoxical systemic side effect was termed the musculoskeletal syndrome (MSS) or the "frozen joint" syndrome.[169,173-175] While the mechanisms and pathways responsible for this adverse effect remained unknown, the use of hydroxymate-based MMP inhibitors was for the most part abandoned. Accordingly, a number of nonhydroxymate MMP inhibitors were subsequently developed.* These MMP inhibitors exhibited inhibitory effects across a wide range of MMP types, and therefore were generically termed "broad spectrum" MMP inhibitors. Preclinical studies of the broad spectrum MMP inhibitors were successfully performed in several animal models and beneficial effects were uniformly provided regarding LV remodeling and the slowing of CHF progression.† However, concern arose whether and to what degree these broad spectrum MMP inhibitors may affect closely related proteases. Moreover, it was postulated that the inhibition of certain MMPs, such as MMP-1, may significantly contribute to the development of MSS. Accordingly, more selective MMP inhibitors were developed that could be pharmacologically titrated to prevent inhibition of certain MMP types; particularly MMP-1. The most advanced of these "selective" MMP inhibitors in terms of cardiovascular disease was PG11680.[131,147,176,177] This MMP inhibitor was evaluated in several animal models of myocardial remodeling and eventually advanced to a clinical study. In this study (Prevention of Myocardial Infarction Early Remodeling, PREMIER), 253 post-MI patients primarily

*References 18, 19, 22, 23, 25, 131, 147, 169, 170-176.

†References 11, 12, 18, 19, 22, 23, 25, 130, 144.

from international study centers were enrolled. Initially the study design called for a 200-mg dose to be given orally twice daily for the entire study interval of 180 days. However, due to historical concerns regarding the risk of MSS, the dosing regimen was altered following initiation of the study.[177] Specifically, patients randomized to PG116800 were treated initially with 200 mg once per day for the study period. The major endpoint of this study was echocardiographic indices of LV size. As a composite, LV end-diastolic volumes increased slightly from baseline (~10%) at 90 days. The relative degree of LV dilation, as a function of baseline values, was 8.4% in the PG11680 group and 10.3% in the placebo group. This did not reach statistical significance by *t*-test. The reasons for the neutral result of this MMP inhibitor are likely to be multifactorial and include an inadequate dosing regimen, a minimal change in the primary response variable, and experimental design issues. With respect to the dosing regimen, it is unlikely that this study achieved significant therapeutic efficacy of PG11680 in a large number of patients. Specifically, using published and available pharmacokinetic data,[147,176] the predicted plasma levels for PG11680 given as a single oral 200-mg dose fell well below an effective inhibitory concentration of any MMP type for durations of approximately 12 hours each day. The initial outfall from this clinical study was the closure of a number of development programs for MMP inhibitors. The longer term consequences from this initial clinical study are yet to be fully realized, but the near future for developing pharmacological strategies for MMP inhibition in the clinical context of cardiovascular disease is certainly in question. However, there are some important lessons that can be learned from this initial clinical MMP inhibitor study. First, these results underscore the complexity of translating basic studies into clinical therapeutics in general. Second, this study emphasizes the complexity and diversity of the MMP system.

Clinical and experimental studies suggest that MMP upregulation in developing CHF is far from a nonselective, nonspecific process. Thus a specific cassette of MMPs may be responsible for the pathological progression of myocardial ECM remodeling in CHF. An important future direction would be to define the specific portfolio of MMPs that are expressed within the failing myocardium and develop selective targeting strategies to inhibit these MMP species. The biophysical stimuli that contribute to the local expression of myocardial MMPs is likely to be a complex and dynamic process determined by the summation of a number of extracellular signals. While a number of therapeutic interventions are likely to be developed that will directly modulate the myocardial extracellular environment, it is important to recognize that the temporal sequence and pattern of myocardial ECM remodeling are distinctly different post-MI, with overload-induced hypertrophy or in cardiomyopathic disease states. For example, inhibiting ECM degradation may be desirable in rapidly progressive cardiomyopathies, but may actually exacerbate LV function in hypertrophy. Early induction and activation of MMPs may be essential for the wound healing response post-MI and exogenous MMP pharmacological inhibition may actually worsen myocardial viability in the acute MI period. However, persistently increased myocardial MMP activation following an established MI may contribute to the maladaptive process of infarct expansion. Thus interventional strategies targeted at modulating the myocardial ECM must be time and disease specific. Further advancements in directly interrogating the myocardial ECM,[28,30] and directly imaging MMP activity within the myocardium,[29] are likely to provide the necessary tools to address this complex issue.

From the first report of the importance of collagenase by Gross et al[178] regarding the reabsorption of a tadpole tail, it is now clearly recognized that ECM remodeling plays a critical role in tissue structure and function. The myocardial ECM is not a passive entity, but rather a complex and dynamic microenvironment that represents an important structural and signaling system within the myocardium. Future translational and clinical research focused upon the molecular and cellular mechanisms that regulate ECM structure and function will likely contribute to an improved understanding of the LV remodeling process in CHF and yield novel therapeutic targets.

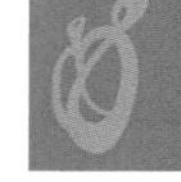

ACKNOWLEDGMENTS

The authors wish to recognize the significant contributions of past MUSC medical and graduate students who participated in the cardiothoracic research program that eventually made this chapter possible.

REFERENCES

1. Konstam, M., Kronenberg, M., Rousseau, M., et al. (1993). Effects of angiotensin converting enzyme on the long-term progression of left ventricular dilation in patients with asymptomatic systolic dysfunction. *Circulation, 88*(1), 2277–2283.
2. Greenberg, B., Quinones, M. A., Kollpillai, C., et al. (1995). Effects of long term enalapril therapy on cardiac structure and function in patients with left ventricular dysfunction. *Circulation, 91*, 2573–2581.
3. Erlebacher, J. A., Weiss, J. L., Weisfeldt, J. L., et al. (1984). Early dilation of the infarcted segment in acute transmural myocardial infarction: role of infarct expansion in acute left ventricular enlargement. *J Am Coll Cardiol, 4*(2), 201–208.
4. Pfeffer, M. A., & Braunwald, E. (1990). Ventricular remodeling after myocardial infarction. Experimental observations and clinical implications. *Circulation, 81*, 1161–1172.
5. Sutton, M. G., & Sharpe, N. (2000). Left ventricular remodeling after myocardial infarction: pathophysiology and therapy. *Circulation, 101*(25), 2981–2988.
6. Doughty, R. N., Whalley, G. A., Gamble, G., et al. (1997). Left ventricular remodeling with carvedilol in patients with congestive heart failure due to ischemic heart disease. *J Am Coll Cardiol, 29*, 1060–1066.
7. St John Sutton, M., Pfeffer, M. A., Plappert, T., et al. (1994). Quantitative two-dimensional echocardiographic measurements are major predictors of adverse cardiovascular events after myocardial infarction. The protective effects of captopril. *Circulation, 89*, 68–75.
8. Burlew, B. S., & Weber, K. T. (2000). Connective tissue and the heart, functional significance and regulatory mechanisms. *Cardiol Clin, 18*(3), 435–442.
9. Weber, K. T., Pick, R., Janicki, J. S., et al. (1988). Inadequate collagen tethers in dilated cardiomyopathy. *Am Heart J, 116*, 1641–1646.
10. Cluetjens, J. P. M., Verluyten, M. J. A., Smits, J. F. M., et al. (1995). Collagen remodeling after myocardial infarction in the rat heart. *Am J Pathol, 147*(2), 325–338.
11. Spinale, F. G. (2007). Matrix remodeling and the matrix metalloproteinases: influence on cardiac form and function. *Physiol Rev, 87*(4), 1285–1342.
12. Chapman, R. E., & Spinale, F. G. (2004). Extracellular protease activation and unraveling of the myocardial interstitium: critical steps toward clinical applications. *Am J Physiol, 286*(1), H1–H10.
13. Thomas, C. V., Coker, M. L., Zellner, J. L., et al. (1998). Increased matrix metalloproteinase activity and selective upregulation in LV myocardium from patients with end-stage dilated cardiomyopathy. *Circulation, 97*, 1708–1715.
14. Spinale, F. G., Coker, M. L., Heung, L. J., et al. (2000). A matrix metalloproteinase induction/activation system exists in the human left ventricular myocardium and is upregulated in heart failure. *Circulation, 102*, 1944–1949.
15. Gunja-Smith, Z., Morales, A. R., Romanelli, R., et al. (1996). Remodeling of human myocardial collagen in idiopathic dilated cardiomyopathy: role of metalloproteinases and pyridinoline cross links. *Am J Pathol, 148*, 1639–1648.
16. Li, Y. Y., Feldman, A. M., Sun, Y., et al. (1998). Differential expression of tissue inhibitors of metalloproteinases in the failing human heart. *Circulation, 98*, 1728–1734.
17. Spinale, F. G., Coker, M. L., Thomas, C. V., et al. (1998). Time dependent changes in matrix metalloproteinase activity and expression during the progression of congestive heart failure: relation to ventricular and myocyte function. *Circ Res, 82*, 482–495.
18. Spinale, F. G., Krombach, R. S., Coker, M. L., et al. (1999). Matrix metalloproteinase inhibition during developing congestive heart failure in pigs: effects on left ventricular geometry and function. *Circ Res, 85*, 364–376.
19. Rohde, L. E., Ducharme, A., Arroyo, L. H., et al. (1999). Matrix metalloproteinase inhibition attenuates early left ventricular enlargement after experimental myocardial infarction in mice. *Circulation, 99*, 3063–3070.
20. Creemers, E., Davis, J. N., Parkhurst, A. M., et al. (2003). Deficiency of the tissue inhibitor of matrix metalloproteinase-1 gene exacerbates LV remodeling following myocardial infarction in mice. *Am J Physiol, 284*(1), H364–H371.
21. Coker, M. L., Thomas, C. V., Clair, M. J., et al. (1998). Myocardial matrix metalloproteinase activity and abundance with congestive heart failure. *Am J Physiol, 274*(43), H1516–H1523.
22. Matsumura, S., Iwanaga, S., Mochizuki, S., et al. (2005). Targeted deletion or pharmacological inhibition of MMP-2 prevents cardiac rupture after myocardial infarction in mice. *J Clin Invest, 115*(3), 599–609.
23. Heymans, S., Luttun, A., Nuyens, D., et al. (1999). Inhibition of plasminogen activators or matrix metalloproteinases prevents cardiac rupture but impairs therapeutic angiogenesis and causes cardiac failure. *Nat Med, 5*, 1135–1142.

24. Ducharme, A., Frantz, S., Aikawa, M., et al. (2000). Targeted deletion of matrix metalloproteinase-9 attenuates left ventricular enlargement and collagen accumulation after experimental myocardial infarction. *J Clin Invest*, *106*, 55–62.
25. Peterson, J. T., Hallak, H., Johnson, L., et al. (2001). Matrix metalloproteinase inhibition attenuates left ventricular remodeling and dysfunction in a rat model of progressive heart failure. *Circulation*, *103*, 2303–2309.
26. Li, Y. Y., Feng, Y., McTiernan, C. F., et al. (2001). Downregulation of matrix metalloproteinases and reduction in collagen damage in the failing human heart after support with left ventricular assist devices. *Circulation*, *104*, 1147–1152.
27. Kim, H. E., Dalal, S. S., Young, E., et al. (2000). Disruption of the myocardial extracellular matrix leads to cardiac dysfunction. *J Clin Invest*, *106*, 857–866.
28. Deschamps, A. M., Apple, K. A., Hardin, A. E., et al. (2005). Myocardial interstitial matrix metalloproteinase activity is altered by mechanical changes in LV load: interaction with the angiotensin type 1 receptor. *Circ Res*, *96*(10), 1110–1118.
29. Su, H., Spinale, F. G., Dobrucki, L. W., et al. (2005). Noninvasive targeted imaging of matrix metalloproteinase activation in a murine model of postinfarction remodeling. *Circulation*, *112*(20), 3157–3167.
30. Deschamps, A. M., Yarbrough, W. M., Squires, C. E., et al. (2005). Trafficking of the membrane type-1 matrix metalloproteinase (MT1-MMP) in ischemia and reperfusion: relation to interstitial MT1-MMP activity. *Circulation*, *111*(9), 1166–1174.
31. Mecham, R. P., & Heuser, J. (1990). Three-dimensional organization of extracellular matrix in elastic cartilage as viewed by quick freeze, deep etch electron microscopy. *Connect Tissue Res*, *24*(2), 83–93.
32. Ross, R. S., & Borg, T. K. (2001). Integrins and the myocardium. *Circ Res*, *88 (11)*, 1112–1119, 8.
33. Keller, R. S., Shai, S. Y., Babbitt, C. J., et al. (2001). Disruption of integrin function in the murine myocardium leads to perinatal lethality, fibrosis, and abnormal cardiac performance. *Am J Pathol*, *158*, 1079–1090.
34. Hornberger, L. K., Singhroy, S., Cavalle-Garrido, T., et al. (2000). Synthesis of extracellular matrix and adhesion through beta(1) integrins are critical for fetal ventricular myocyte proliferation. *Circ Res*, *87*, 508–515.
35. Spinale, F. G., Tomita, M., Zellner, J. L., et al. (1991). Collagen remodeling and changes in LV function during the development and recovery from supraventricular tachycardia. *Am J Physiol*, *261*, H308–H318.
36. Stroud, J. D., Baicu, C. F., Barnes, M. A., et al. (2002). Viscoelastic properties of pressure overload hypertrophied myocardium: effects of treatment with a serine protease treatment. *Am J Physiol Heart Circ Physiol*, *282*(6), H232–H235.
37. Nimni, M. E. (1993). Fibrillar collagens: their biosynthesis, molecular structure, and mode of assembly. In M. A. Zern & L. M. Reid (Eds.). *Extracellular matrix*. New York: Marcel Dekker.
38. Asif, M., Egan, J., Vasan, S., et al. (2000). An advanced glycation endproduct cross-link breaker can reverse age related increases in myocardial stiffness. *Proc Natl Acad Sci U S A*, *97*(6), 2809–2813.
39. Kato, S., Spinale, F. G., Tanaka, R., et al. (1995). Inhibition of collagen cross-linking: effects on fibrillar collagen and left ventricular diastolic function. *Am J Physiol*, *269*(38), H863–H868.
40. Cooper, M. E. (2004). Importance of advanced glycation end products in diabetes-associated cardiovascular and renal disease. *Am J Hypertens*, *17*(12 pt 2), 31S–38S.
41. Risteli, L., & Risteli, J. (1990). Noninvasive methods for detection of organ fibrosis. In M. Rojkind (Ed.). *Focus on connective tissue in health and disease*. Boca Raton, FL: CRC Press.
42. Schuppan, D. (1991). Connective tissue polypeptides in serum as parameters to monitor antifibrotic treatment in hepatic fibrogenesis. *J Hepatol*, *13*(suppl 3), S17–S25.
43. Diez, J., & Laviades, C. (1997). Monitoring fibrillar collagen turnover in hypertensive heart disease. *Cardiovasc Res*, *35*, 202–205.
44. Diez, J., Laviades, C., Mayor, G., et al. (1995). Increased serum concentrations of procollagen peptides in essential hypertension. Relation to cardiac alterations. *Circulation*, *91*, 1450–1456.
45. Diez, J., Panizo, A., Gil, M. J., et al. (1996). Serum markers of collagen type I metabolism in spontaneously hypertensive rats. Relation to myocardial fibrosis. *Circulation*, *93*, 1026–1032.
46. Borg, T. K., Goldsmith, E. C., & Price, R. (2000). et. Specialization of the Z line of cardiac myocytes. *Cardiovasc Res*, *46*, 277–285.
47. Pham, C. G., Harpf, A. E., Keller, R. S., et al. (2000). Striated muscle specific beta(1D) integrin and FAK are involved in cardiac myocyte hypertrophic response pathway. *Am J Physiol*, *279*(6), H2916–H2926.
48. Kuettner, K. E., & Kimuar, J. H. (1985). Proteoglycans: an overview. *J Cell Biochem*, *27*, 327–336.
49. Sivasubramanian, N., Coker, M. L., Kurrelmeyer, K. M., et al. (2001). Left ventricular remodeling in transgenic mice with cardiac restricted overexpression of tumor necrosis factor. *Circulation*, *104*(7), 826–831.
50. Bradham, W. S., Bozkurt, B., Gunasinghe, H., et al. (2002). Tumor necrosis factor-alpha and myocardial remodeling in progression of heart failure: a current perspective. *Cardiovasc Res*, *53*(4), 822–830.
51. Fowlkes, J. L., & Winkler, M. K. (2002). Exploring the interface between metalloproteinase activity and growth factor and cytokine bioavailability. *Cytokine Growth Factor Rev*, *13*(3), 277–287.
52. Annes, J. P., Munger, J. S., & Rifkin, D. B. (2003). Making sense of latent TGFbeta activation. *J Cell Sci*, *116*(pt 2), 217–224.
53. Isogai, Z., Ono, R. N., Ushiro, S., et al. (2003). Latent transforming growth factor beta-binding protein 1 interacts with fibrillin and is a microfibril-associated protein. *J Biol Chem*, *278*(4), 2750–2757.
54. Rifkin, D. B. (2005). Latent transforming growth factor-beta (TGF-beta) binding proteins: orchestrators of TGF-beta availability. *J Biol Chem*, *280*(9), 7409–7412.
55. Bobik, A. (2006). Transforming growth factor-betas and vascular disorders. *Arterioscler Thromb Vasc Biol*, *26*(8), 1712–1720.
56. Roberts, A. B., Sporn, M. B., Assoian, R. K., et al. (1986). Transforming growth factor type beta: rapid induction of fibrosis and angiogenesis in vivo and stimulation of collagen formation in vitro. *Proc Natl Acad Sci U S A*, *83*(12), 4167–4171.
57. Leask, A., & Abraham, D. J. (2004). TGF-beta signaling and the fibrotic response. *FASEB J*, *18*(7), 816–827.
58. Weber, K. T., Janicki, J. S., Shroff, S. G., et al. (1988). Collagen remodeling of the pressure-overloaded, hypertrophied nonhuman primate myocardium. *Circ Res*, *62*, 757–765.
59. Abrahams, C., Janicki, J. S., & Weber, K. T. (1987). Myocardial hypertrophy in *Macaca fascicularis*. Structural remodeling of the collagen matrix. *Lab Invest*, *56*, 676–683.
60. Fielitz, J., Leuschner, M., Zurbrugg, H. R., et al. (2004). Regulation of matrix metalloproteinases and their inhibitors in the left ventricular myocardium of patients with aortic stenosis. *J Mol Med*, *82*, 809–820.
61. Polyakova, V., Hein, S., Kostin, S., et al. (2004). Matrix metalloproteinases and their tissue inhibitors in pressure-overloaded human myocardium during heart failure progression. *J Am Coll Cardiol*, *44*, 1609–1618.
62. Nagatomo, Y., Carabello, B. A., Coker, M. L., et al. (2000). Differential effects of pressure or volume overload on myocardial MMP levels and inhibitory control. *Am J Physiol Heart Circ Physiol*, *278*, H151–H161.
63. Heymans, S., Schroen, B., Vermeersch, P., et al. (2005). Increased cardiac expression of tissue inhibitor of metalloproteinase-1 and tissue inhibitor of metalloproteinase-2 is related to cardiac fibrosis and dysfunction in the chronic pressure-overloaded human heart. *Circulation*, *112*, 1136–1144.
64. Lindsay, M. M., Maxwell, P., & Dunn, F. G. (2002). TIMP-1: a marker of left ventricular diastolic dysfunction and fibrosis in hypertension. *Hypertension*, *40*(2), 136–141.
65. Tayebjee, M. H., MacFadyen, R. J., & Lip, G. Y. (2003). Extracellular matrix biology: a new frontier in linking the pathology and therapy of hypertension? *J Hypertens*, *21*(12), 2211–2218.
66. Tayebjee, M. H., Karalis, I., Nadar, S. K., et al. (2005). Circulating matrix metalloproteinase-9 and tissue inhibitors of metalloproteinases-1 and -2 levels in gestational hypertension. *Am J Hypertens*, *18*(3), 325–329.
67. Tayebjee, M. H., Lim, H. S., Nadar, S., et al. (2005). Tissue inhibitor of metalloprotein ase-1 is a marker of diastolic dysfunction using tissue Doppler in patients with type 2 diabetes and hypertension. *Eur J Clin Invest*, *35*(1), 8–12.
68. López, B., González, A., Querejeta, R., et al. (2006). Alterations in the pattern of collagen deposition may contribute to the deterioration of systolic function in hypertensive patients with heart failure. *J Am Coll Cardiol*, *48*(1), 89–96.
69. Martos, R., Baugh, J., Ledwidge, M., et al. (2007). Diastolic heart failure: evidence of increased myocardial collagen turnover linked to diastolic dysfunction. *Circulation*, *115*(7), 888–895.
70. Ahmed, S. H., Clark, L. L., Pennington, W. R., et al. (2006). Matrix metalloproteinases/tissue inhibitors of metalloproteinases: relationship between changes in proteolytic determinants of matrix composition and structural, functional, and clinical manifestations of hypertensive heart disease. *Circulation*, *113*(17), 2089–2096.
71. Elmas, E., Lang, S., Dempfle, C. E., et al. (2007). High plasma levels of tissue inhibitor of metalloproteinase-1 (TIMP-1) and interleukin-8 (IL-8) characterize patients prone to ventricular fibrillation complicating myocardial infarction. *Clin Chem Lab Med*, *45*(10), 1360–1365.
72. Hess, O. M., Villari, B., & Krayenbuehl, H. P. (1993). Diastolic dysfunction in aortic stenosis. *Circulation*, *87*(suppl 5), IV73–IV76.
73. Krayenbuehl, H. P., Hess, O. M., Monrad, E. S., et al. (1989). Left ventricular myocardial structure in aortic valve disease before, intermediate, and late after aortic valve replacement. *Circulation*, *79*(4), 744–755.
74. Monrad, E. S., Hess, O. M., Murakami, T., et al. (1988). Time course of regression of left ventricular hypertrophy after aortic valve replacement. *Circulation*, *77*(6), 1345–1355.
75. Lund, O., Emmertsen, K., Dørup, I., et al. (2003). Regression of left ventricular hypertrophy during 10 years after valve replacement for aortic stenosis is related to the preoperative risk profile. *Eur Heart J*, *24*(15), 1437–1446.
76. Zile, M. R., Baicu, C. F., Alterations in ventricular function: diastolic heart failure. In Mann DL, editor. *Heart failure: a companion to Braunwald's heart disease*.
77. Poole-Wilson, P. A. (1993). Relation of pathophysiological mechanisms to outcome in heart failure. *J Am Coll Cardiol*, *22*, 22A–29A.
78. Douglas, P. S., Morrow, R., Joli, A., et al. (1989). Left ventricular shape, afterload, and survival in idiopathic dilated cardiomyopathy. *J Am Coll Cardiol*, *13*, 311–315.
79. Stetler-Stevenson, W. G. (2008). The tumor microenvironment: regulation by MMP-independent effects of tissue inhibitor of metalloproteinases-2. *Cancer Metastasis Rev*, *27*(1), 57–66.
80. Catania, J. M., Chen, G., & Parrish, A. R. (2007). Role of matrix metalloproteinases in renal pathophysiologies. *Am J Physiol Renal Physiol*, *292*(3), F905–F911.
81. Verstappen, J., & Von den Hoff, J. W. (2006). Tissue inhibitors of metalloproteinases (TIMPs): their biological functions and involvement in oral disease. *J Dent Res*, *85*(12), 1074–1084.
82. Varghese, S. (2006). Matrix metalloproteinases and their inhibitors in bone: an overview of regulation and functions. *Front Biosci*, *11*, 2949–2966.
83. Nagase, H., Visse, R., & Murphy, G. (2006). Structure and function of matrix metalloproteinases and TIMPs. *Cardiovasc Res*, *69*(3), 562–573.
84. Malemud, C. J. (2006). Matrix metalloproteinases (MMPs) in health and disease: an overview. *Front Biosci*, *11*, 1696–1701.
85. Hwang, I. K., Park, S. M., Kim, S. Y., et al. (2004). A proteomic approach to identify substrates of matrix metalloproteinase-14 in human plasma. *Biochim Biophys Acta*, *1702*, 79–87.
86. Overall, C. M., Tam, E. M., Kappelhoff, R., et al. (2004). Protease degradomics: mass spectrometry discovery of protease substrates and the CLIP-CHIP, a dedicated DNA microarray of all human proteases and inhibitors. *Biol Chem*, *385*, 493–504.
87. Woessner, J. F., Jr., & Nagase, H. (2000). Protein substrates of the MMPs. In *Matrix metalloproteinases and TIMPs*. New York: Oxford University Press.

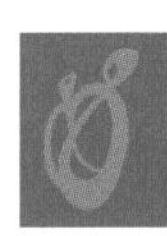

88. Woessner, J. F., Jr., & Nagase, H. (2000). Activation of the zymogen forms of MMPs. In *Matrix metalloproteinases and TIMPs*. New York: Oxford University Press.
89. Vincenti, M. P. (2001). The matrix metalloproteinase (MMP) and tissue inhibitor of metalloproteinase (TIMP) genes. In I. Clark (Ed.). *Matrix metalloproteinase protocols*. Totowa, NJ: Humana Press.
90. Vincenti, M. P., & Brinckerhoff, C. E. (2002). Transcriptional regulation of collagenase (MMP-1, MMP-13) genes in arthritis: integration of complex signaling pathways for the recruitment of gene-specific transcription factors. *Arthritis Res*, *4*, 157–164.
91. Bergman, M. R., Cheng, S., Honbo, N., et al. (2003). A functional activating protein 1 (AP-1) site regulates matrix metalloproteinase 2 (MMP-2) transcription by cardiac cells through interactions with JunB-Fra1 and JunB-FosB heterodimers. *Biochem J*, *369*, 485–496.
92. Siwik, D. A., Chang, D. L., & Colucci, W. S. (2000). Interleukin-1beta and tumor necrosis factor-alpha decrease collagen synthesis and increase matrix metalloproteinase activity in cardiac fibroblasts in vitro. *Circ Res*, *86*, 1259–1265.
93. Rangaswami, H., Bulbule, A., & Kundu, G. C. (2004). Nuclear factor-inducing kinase plays a crucial role in osteopontin-induced MAPK/IkappaBalpha kinase-dependent nuclear factor kappaB-mediated promatrix metalloproteinase-9 activation. *J Biol Chem*, *279*, 38921–38935.
94. Alfonso-Jaume, M. A., Bergman, M. R., Mahimkar, R., et al. (2006). Cardiac ischemia-reperfusion injury induces matrix metalloproteinase-2 expression through the AP-1 components FosB and JunB. *Am J Physiol Heart Circ Physiol*, *291*(4), H1838–H1846.
95. Mukherjee, R., Mingoia, J. T., Bruce, J. A., et al. (2006). Selective spatiotemporal induction of matrix metalloproteinase-2 and matrix metalloproteinase-9 transcription after myocardial infarction. *Am J Physiol Heart Circ Physiol*, *291*(5), H2216–H2228.
96. Blankenberg, S., Rupprecht, H. J., Poirier, O., et al. (2003). Plasma concentrations and genetic variation of matrix metalloproteinase 9 and prognosis of patients with cardiovascular disease. *Circulation*, *107*, 1579–1585.
97. Zhang, B., Ye, S., Herrmann, S. M., et al. (1999). Functional polymorphism in the regulatory region of gelatinase B gene in relation to severity of coronary atherosclerosis. *Circulation*, *99*(14), 1788–1794.
98. Mizon-Gérard, F., de Groote, P., Lamblin, N., et al. (2004). Prognostic impact of matrix metalloproteinase gene polymorphisms in patients with heart failure according to the aetiology of left ventricular systolic dysfunction. *Eur Heart J*, *25*(8), 688–693.
99. Liu, P. Y., Chen, J. H., Li, Y. H., et al. (2003). Synergistic effect of stromelysin-1 (matrix metallo-proteinase-3) promoter 5A/6A polymorphism with smoking on the onset of young acute myocardial infarction. *Thromb Haemost*, *90*, 132–139.
100. Terashima, M., Akita, H., Kanazawa, K., et al. (1999). Stromelysin promoter 5A/6A polymorphism is associated with acute myocardial infarction. *Circulation*, *99*(21), 2717–2719.
101. Yamada, Y., Ohno, Y., Nakashima, Y., et al. (2002). Prediction and assessment of extrapyramidal side effects induced by risperidone based on dopamine D(2) receptor occupancy. *Synapse*, *46*(1), 32–37.
102. Beyzade, S., Zhang, S., Wong, Y. K., et al. (2003). Influences of matrix metalloproteinase-3 gene variation on extent of coronary atherosclerosis and risk of myocardial infarction. *J Am Coll Cardiol*, *41*, 2130–2137.
103. Hirashiki, A., Yamada, Y., Murase, Y., et al. (2003). Association of gene polymorphisms with coronary artery disease in low- or high-risk subjects defined by conventional risk factors. *J Am Coll Cardiol*, *42*(8), 1429–1437.
104. Nojiri, T., Morita, H., Imai, Y., et al. (2003). Genetic variations of matrix metalloproteinase-1 and -3 promoter regions and their associations with susceptibility to myocardial infarction in Japanese. *Int J Cardiol*, *92*(2-3), 181–186.
105. Martin, T. N., Penney, D. E., Smith, J. A., et al. (2004). Matrix metalloproteinase-1 promoter polymorphisms and changes in left ventricular volume following acute myocardial infarction. *Am J Cardiol*, *94*(8), 1044–1046.
106. Pearce, E., Tregouet, D. A., Samnegård, A., et al. (2005). Haplotype effect of the matrix metalloproteinase-1 gene on risk of myocardial infarction. *Circ Res*, *97*(10), 1070–1076.
107. Samnegård, A., Silveira, A., Lundman, P., et al. (2005). Serum matrix metalloproteinase-3 concentration is influenced by MMP-3-1612 5A/6A promoter genotype and associated with myocardial infarction. *J Intern Med*, *258*(5), 411–419.
108. Vasku, A., Goldbergová, M., Izakovicová Hollá, L., et al. (2004). A haplotype constituted of four MMP-2 promoter polymorphisms (-1575G/A, -1306C/T, -790T/G and -735C/T) is associated with coronary triple-vessel disease. *Matrix Biol*, *22*(7), 585–591.
109. Horne, B. D., Camp, N. J., Carlquist, J. F., et al. (2007). Multiple-polymorphism associations of 7 matrix metalloproteinase and tissue inhibitor metalloproteinase genes with myocardial infarction and angiographic coronary artery disease. *Am Heart J*, *154*(4), 751–758.
110. Vincenti, M. P., & Brinckerhoff, C. E. (2007). Signal transduction and cell-type specific regulation of matrix metalloproteinase gene expression: can MMPs be good for you? *J Cell Physiol*, *213*(2), 355–364.
111. Deschamps, A. M., & Spinale, F. G. (2006). Spotlight review: pathways of matrix metalloproteinase induction in heart failure: bioactive molecules and transcriptional regulation. *Cardiovasc Res*, *69*(3), 666–676.
112. Mauviel, A. (1993). Cytokine regulation of metalloproteinase gene expression. *J Cell Biochem*, *53*, 288–295.
113. MacNaul, K. L., Chartrain, N., Lark, M., et al. (1990). Discoordinate expression of stromelysin, collagenase, and tissue inhibitor of metalloproteinases-1 in rheumatoid human synovial fibroblasts: synergistic effects of interleukin-1 and tumor necrosis factor-α on stromelysin expression. *J Biol Chem*, *265*, 17238–17245.
114. Schroen, D. J., & Brincherhoff, C. E. (1996). Nuclear hormone receptors inhibit matrix metalloproteinase (MMP) gene expression through diverse mechanisms. *Gene Expr*, *6*(4), 197–207.
115. Ries, C., & Petrides, P. E. (1995). Cytokine regulation of matrix metalloproteinase activity and regulatory dysfunction in disease. *Biol Chem*, *376*, 345–355.
116. Bond, M., Fabunmi, R. P., Baker, A. H., et al. (1998). Synergistic upregulation of metalloproteinase-9 by growth factors and inflammatory cytokines: an absolute requirement for transcription factor NF-kappa B. *FEBS Lett*, *435*(1), 29–34.
117. Kida, Y., Kobayashi, M., Suzuki, T., et al. (2005). Interleukin-1 stimulates cytokines, prostaglandin E2 and matrix metalloproteinase-1 production via activation of MAPK/AP-1 and NF-kappaB in human gingival fibroblasts. *Cytokine*, *29*, 159–168.
118. Biswas, C., Zhang, Y., DeCastro, R., et al. (1995). The human tumor cell-derived collagenase stimulatory factor (renamed EMMPRIN) is a member of the immunoglobulin superfamily. *Cancer Res*, *55*, 434–439.
119. Toole, B. P. (2003). Emmprin (CD147), a cell surface regulator of matrix metalloproteinase production and function. *Curr Top Dev Biol*, *54*, 371–389.
120. Guo, H., Zucker, S., Gordon, M. K., et al. (1997). Stimulation of matrix metalloproteinase production by recombinant extracellular matrix metalloproteinase inducer from transfected Chinese hamster ovary cells. *J Biol Chem*, *272*, 24–27.
121. Schmidt, R., Bultmann, A., Ungerer, M., et al. (2006). Extracellular matrix metalloproteinase inducer regulates matrix metalloproteinase activity in cardiovascular cells: implications in acute myocardial infarction. *Circulation*, *113*, 834–841.
122. Sato, H., Takino, T., Okada, Y., et al. (1994). A matrix metalloproteinase expressed on the surface of invasive tumour cells. *Nature*, *370*, 61–65.
123. Osenkowski, P., Toth, M., & Fridman, R. (2004). Processing, shedding, and endocytosis of membrane type 1-matrix metalloproteinase (MT1-MMP). *J Cell Physiol*, *200*, 2–10.
124. Lehti, K., Valtanen, H., Wickstrom, S. A., et al. (2000). Regulation of membrane-type-1 matrix metalloproteinase activity by its cytoplasmic domain. *J Biol Chem*, *275*, 15006–15013.
125. Remacle, A. G., Rozanov, D. V., Baciu, P. C., et al. (2005). The transmembrane domain is essential for the microtubular trafficking of membrane type-1 matrix metalloproteinase (MT1-MMP). *J Cell Sci*, *118*, 4975–4984.
126. Pavlaki, M., Cao, J., Hymowitz, M., et al. (2002). A conserved sequence within the propeptide domain of membrane type 1 matrix metalloproteinase is critical for function as an intramolecular chaperone. *J Biol Chem*, *277*, 2740–2749.
127. Guo, C., & Piacentini, L. (2003). Type I collagen-induced MMP-2 activation coincides with up-regulation of membrane type 1-matrix metalloproteinase and TIMP-2 in cardiac fibroblasts. *J Biol Chem*, *278*, 46699–46708.
128. Stawowy, P., Meyborg, H., Stibenz, D., et al. (2005). Furin-like proprotein convertases are central regulators of the membrane type matrix metalloproteinase-pro-matrix metalloproteinase-2 proteolytic cascade in atherosclerosis. *Circulation*, *111*, 2820–2827.
129. Wilson, E. M., Moainie, S. L., Baskin, J. M., et al. (2003). Region- and type-specific induction of matrix metalloproteinases in post-myocardial infarction remodeling. *Circulation*, *107*, 2857–2863.
130. Mukherjee, R., Brinsa, T. A., Dowdy, K. B., et al. (2003). Myocardial infarct expansion and matrix metalloproteinase inhibition. *Circulation*, *107*, 618–625.
131. Yarbrough, W. M., Mukherjee, R., Escobar, G. P., et al. (2003). Selective targeting and timing of matrix metalloproteinase inhibition in post-myocardial infarction remodeling. *Circulation*, *108*, 1753–1759.
132. Greene, J., Wang, M., Liu, Y. E., et al. (1996). Molecular cloning and characterization of human tissue inhibitor of metalloproteinase 4. *J Biol Chem*, *271*, 30375–30380.
133. Liu, Y. E., Wang, M., Greene, J., et al. (1997). Preparation and characterization of recombinant tissue inhibitor of metalloproteinase 4 (TIMP-4). *J Biol Chem*, *272*, 20479–20483.
134. Tummalapalli, C. M., Heath, B. J., & Tyagi, S. C. (2001). Tissue inhibitor of metalloproteinase-4 instigates apoptosis in transformed cardiac fibroblasts. *J Cell Biochem*, *80*, 512–521.
135. Lovelock, J. D., Baker, A. H., Gao, F., et al. (2005). Heterogeneous effects of tissue inhibitors of matrix metalloproteinases on cardiac fibroblasts. *Am J Physiol Heart Circ Physiol*, *288*, H461–H468.
136. Oelmann, E., Herbst, H., Zuhlsdorf, M., et al. (2002). Tissue inhibitor of metalloproteinases 1 is an autocrine and paracrine survival factor, with additional immune-regulatory functions, expressed by Hodgkin/Reed-Sternberg cells. *Blood*, *99*, 258–267.
137. Guedez, L., Stetler-Stevenson, W. G., Wolff, L., et al. (1998). In vitro suppression of programmed cell death of B cells by tissue inhibitor of metalloproteinases-1. *J Clin Invest*, *102*, 2002–2010.
138. Kai, H., Ikeda, H., Yusakawa, H., et al. (1998). Peripheral blood levels of matrix metalloproteinases-2 and -9 are elevated in patients with acute coronary syndromes. *J Am Coll Cardiol*, *32*, 368–372.
139. Hojo, Y., Ikeda, U., Ueno, S., et al. (2001). Expression of matrix metalloproteinases in patients with acute myocardial infarction. *Jpn Circ J*, *65*, 71–75.
140. Webb, C. S., Bonnema, D. D., Ahmed, S. H., et al. (2006). Specific temporal profile of matrix metalloproteinase release occurs in patients after myocardial infarction: relation to left ventricular remodeling. *Circulation*, *114*(10), 1020–1027.
141. Orn, S., Manhenke, C., Squire, I. B., et al. (2007). Plasma MMP-2, MMP-9 and N-BNP in long-term survivors following complicated myocardial infarction: relation to cardiac magnetic resonance imaging measures of left ventricular structure and function. *J Card Fail*, *13*(10), 843–849.
142. Tian, H., Cimini, M., Fedak, P. W., et al. (2007). TIMP deficiency accelerates cardiac remodeling after myocardial infarction. *J Mol Cell Cardiol*, *43*(6), 733–743.
143. Brower, G. L., Chancey, A. L., Thanigaraj, S., et al. (2002). Cause and effect relationship between myocardial mast cell number and matrix metalloproteinase activity. *Am J Physiol Heart Circ Physiol*, *283*(2), H518–H525.
144. Chancey, A. L., Brower, G. L., Peterson, J. T., et al. (2002). Effects of matrix metalloproteinase inhibition on ventricular remodeling due to volume overload. *Circulation*, *105*(16), 1983–1988.
145. Mujumdar, V. S., & Tyagi, S. C. (1999). Temporal regulation of extracellular matrix components in transition from compensatory hypertrophy to decompensatory heart failure. *J Hypertens*, *17*, 261–270.

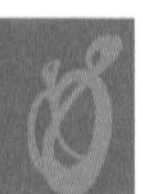

146. Li, H., Simon, H., Bocan, T. M., et al. (2000). MMP/TIMP expression in spontaneously hypertensive heart failure rats; the effect of ACE and MMP inhibition. *Cardiovasc Res*, *46*, 298–306.
147. Morita, H., Khanal, S., Rastogi, S., et al. (2006). Selective matrix metalloproteinase inhibition attenuates progression of left ventricular dysfunction and remodeling in dogs with chronic heart failure. *Am J Physiol Heart Circ Physiol*, *290*(6), H2522–H2527.
148. Leeman, M. F., Curran, S., & Murray, G. I. (2002). The structure, regulation, and function of human matrix metalloproteinase-13. *Crit Rev Biochem Mol Biol*, *37*(3), 149–166.
149. Brinckerhoff, C. E., Rutter, J. L., & Benbow, U. (2000). Interstitial collagenases as markers of tumor progression. *Clin Cancer Res*, *6*(12), 4823–4830.
150. Spruill, L. S., Lowry, A. S., Stroud, R. E., et al. (2007). Membrane-type-1 matrix metalloproteinase transcription and translation in myocardial fibroblasts from patients with normal left ventricular function and from patients with cardiomyopathy. *Am J Physiol Cell Physiol*, *293*(4), C1362–C1373.
151. Fedak, P. W., Smookler, D. S., Kassiri, Z., et al. (2004). TIMP-3 deficiency leads to dilated cardiomyopathy. *Circulation*, *110*(16), 2401–2409.
152. Yan, A. T., Yan, R. T., Spinale, F. G., et al. (2008). Relationships between plasma levels of matrix metalloproteinases and neurohormonal profile in patients with heart failure. *Eur J Heart Fail*, *10*(2), 125–128.
153. Yan, A. T., Yan, R. T., Spinale, F. G., et al. (2006). Plasma matrix metalloproteinase-9 level is correlated with left ventricular volumes and ejection fraction in patients with heart failure. *J Card Fail*, *12*(7), 514–519.
154. Cavusoglu, E., Ruwende, C., Chopra, V., et al. (2006). Tissue inhibitor of metalloproteinase-1 (TIMP-1) is an independent predictor of all-cause mortality, cardiac mortality, and myocardial infarction. *Am Heart J*, *151*, e1101–e1108.
155. Sundstrom, J., Evans, J. C., Benjamin, E. J., et al. (2004). Relations of plasma matrix metalloproteinase-9 to clinical cardiovascular risk factors and echocardiographic left ventricular measures: the Framingham Heart Study. *Circulation*, *109*, 2850–2856.
156. Sundstrom, J., Evans, J. C., Benjamin, E. J., et al. (2004). Relations of plasma total TIMP-1 levels to cardiovascular risk factors and echocardiographic measures: the Framingham Heart Study. *Eur Heart J*, *25*, 1509–1516.
157. Wagner, D. R., Delagardelle, C., Ernens, I., et al. (2006). Matrix metalloproteinase-9 is a marker of heart failure after acute myocardial infarction. *J Card Fail*, *12*, 66–72.
158. Inoue, T., Kato, T., Takayanagi, K., et al. (2003). Circulating matrix metalloproteinase-1 and -3 in patients with an acute coronary syndrome. *Am J Cardiol*, *92*(12), 1461–1464.
159. Nanni, S., Melandri, G., Hanemaaijer, R., et al. (2007). Matrix metalloproteinases in premature coronary atherosclerosis: influence of inhibitors, inflammation, and genetic polymorphisms. *Transl Res*, *149*(3), 137–144.
160. Tuomainen, A. M., Nyyssönen, K., Laukkanen, J. A., et al. (2007). Serum matrix metalloproteinase-8 concentrations are associated with cardiovascular outcome in men. *Arterioscler Thromb Vasc Biol*, *27*(12), 2722–2728.
161. Tayebjee, M. H., Lip, G. Y., Tan, K. T., et al. (2005). Plasma matrix metalloproteinase-9, tissue inhibitor of metalloproteinase-2, and CD40 ligand levels in patients with stable coronary artery disease. *Am J Cardiol*, *96*(3), 339–345.
162. Blankenberg, S., Rupprecht, H. J., Poirier, O., et al. (2003). Plasma concentrations and genetic variation of matrix metalloproteinase 9 and prognosis of patients with cardiovascular disease. *Circulation*, *107*(12), 1579–1585.
163. Giansante, C., Fiotti, N., Di Chiara, A., et al. (2007). In-hospital outcome of patients with acute coronary syndrome: relationship with inflammation and remodeling markers. *J Cardiovasc Med (Hagerstown)*, *8*(8), 602–607.
164. Jguirim-Souissi, I., Jelassi, A., Addad, F., et al. (2007). Plasma metalloproteinase-12 and tissue inhibitor of metalloproteinase-1 levels and presence, severity, and outcome of coronary artery disease. *Am J Cardiol*, *100*(1), 23–27.
165. Fukuda, D., Shimada, K., Tanaka, A., et al. (2006). Comparison of levels of serum matrix metalloproteinase-9 in patients with acute myocardial infarction versus unstable angina pectoris versus stable angina pectoris. *Am J Cardiol*, *97*(2), 175–180.
166. Squire, I. B., Evans, J., Ng, L. L., et al. (2004). Plasma MMP-9 and MMP-2 following acute myocardial infarction in man: correlation with echocardiographic and neurohumoral parameters of left ventricular dysfunction. *J Card Fail*, *10*(4), 328–333.
167. Hlatky, M. A., Ashley, E., Quertermous, T., et al. (2007). Matrix metalloproteinase circulating levels, genetic polymorphisms, and susceptibility to acute myocardial infarction among patients with coronary artery disease. *Am Heart J*, *154*(6), 1043–1051.
168. Manginas, A., Bei, E., Chaidaroglou, A., et al. (2005). Peripheral levels of matrix metalloproteinase-9, interleukin-6, and C-reactive protein are elevated in patients with acute coronary syndromes: correlations with serum troponin I. *Clin Cardiol*, *28*(4), 182–186.
169. Peterson, J. T. (2006). The importance of estimating the therapeutic index in the development of matrix metalloproteinase inhibitors. *Cardiovasc Res*, *69*, 677–687.
170. Yip, D., Ahmad, A., Karapetis, C. S., et al. (1999). Matrix metalloproteinase inhibitors: applications in oncology. *Invest New Drugs*, *17*, 387–399.
171. Tierney, G. M., Griffin, N. R., Stuart, R. C., et al. (1999). A pilot study of the safety and effects of the matrix metalloproteinase inhibitor marimastat in gastric cancer. *Eur J Cancer*, *35*, 563–568.
172. Rosemurgy, A., Harris, J., Langleben, A., et al. (1999). Marimastat in patients with advanced pancreatic cancer: a dose-finding study. *Am J Clin Oncol*, *22*, 247–252.
173. Renkiewicz, R., Qiu, L., Lesch, C., et al. (2003). Broad-spectrum matrix metalloproteinase inhibitor marimastat-induced musculoskeletal side effects in rats. *Arthritis Rheum*, *48*, 1742–1749.
174. Matter, H., & Schudok, M. (2004). Recent advances in the design of matrix metalloprotease inhibitors. *Curr Opin Drug Discov Devel*, *7*, 513–535.
175. Overall, C. M., & Lopez-Otin, C. (2002). Strategies for MMP inhibition in cancer: innovations for the post-trial era. *Nat Rev Cancer*, *2*, 657–672.
176. King, M. K., Coker, M. L., Goldberg, A., et al. (2003). Selective matrix metalloproteinase inhibition with developing heart failure: effects on left ventricular function and structure. *Circ Res*, *92*, 177–185.
177. Hudson, M. P., Armstrong, P. W., Ruzyllo, W., et al. (2006). Effects of selective matrix metalloproteinase inhibitor (PG-116800) to prevent ventricular remodeling after myocardial infarction: results of the PREMIER (prevention of myocardial infarction early remodeling) trial. *J Am Coll Cardiol*, *48*, 15–20.
178. Gross, J., & Lapiere, C. M. (1962). Collagenolytic activity in amphibian tissues: a tissue culture assay. *Proc Natl Acad Sci U S A*, *48*, 1014–1022.
179. Rossi, M. A. (2001). Connective tissue skeleton in the normal left ventricle and in hypertensive left ventricular hypertrophy and chronic chagasic myocarditis. *Med Sci Monit*, *7*, 820–832.

CHAPTER 6

Myocardial Basis for Heart Failure: Role of Cell Death

Saurabh Jha and Richard N. Kitsis

In advanced heart failure, the myocardium is unable to pump sufficient blood to meet the requirements of the body. Traditionally, the pathogenesis of this syndrome is thought to result from multiple structural and functional abnormalities in the myocardium including cardiac myocytes, nonmyocytes, and the interstitium.[1] Inciting triggers include increases in hemodynamic load, inflammatory cytokines, renin-angiotensin-aldosterone signaling, and catecholamines. The resulting abnormalities within cardiac myocytes include alterations in multiple intracellular signaling pathways, including adrenergic desensitization, abnormalities of intracellular Ca^{2+} handling, dysregulation of excitation-contraction coupling, myofibrillar and cytoskeletal remodeling, and alterations in mitochondrial function and energetics. These mechanisms, which are discussed elsewhere in this volume, are indeed important in the pathogenesis of heart failure.

In contrast to the previously mentioned processes, which induce dysfunction in living cells, recent work has highlighted a critical role for cardiac myocyte death in the pathogenesis of heart failure.[2] In some cases, cardiac myocyte death is triggered by the same stimuli that elicit cardiac myocyte dysfunction, although it remains unclear in most situations as to whether cellular dysfunction and death are causally linked. Most commonly, however, the underlying precipitant of cardiac myocyte death is multifactorial. The absolute rate of cardiac myocyte death in failing hearts is quite low, but as discussed later, is 10-fold to 100-fold higher than that of control hearts. Moreover, as heart failure is a chronic condition, a modest increase in the rate of cell death can result in a substantial cumulative loss of cells over the course of the disease. While regeneration of cardiac myocytes from progenitor cells[3] and/or through self-replication[4] may mitigate some of these losses, the magnitude of this response, at least under basal conditions, appears inadequate to compensate. Loss of cardiac myocytes causes pathological remodeling and systolic dysfunction, although detailed mechanisms have not been delineated.

CELL DEATH OVERVIEW

Cell death has classically been viewed as passive and unregulated, the one exception being some instances of cell death during development, where the highly reproducible temporo-spatial pattern of cell demise suggests that these events are somehow "programmed." In the mid-1980s, H. Robert Horvitz et al proved this was the case by identifying a small network of genes that regulates cell death in the developing nematode (round worm) *Caenorhabditis elegans*[5] (Figure 6-1, *A*). This work was groundbreaking in that it provided the first definitive proof that cell death could be a regulated process that was carried out by the cell itself. The term "programmed cell death" was used to describe these developmental cell deaths, and later was applied more loosely to describe any type of regulated cell death. It is important to note, however, that "programmed" does not imply that the signals to die need to originate exclusively within the cell. In fact, the cellular death machinery may be triggered by cues both within and outside the cell.

A second big surprise came in the 1990s when orthologs of the genes identified by Horvitz were recognized to regulate a type of mammalian cell death termed "apoptosis" (see Figure 6-1, *B*, and discussed later). These observations demonstrate a basic commonality in the regulation of developmental cell death in the worm and apoptosis in mammals. Moreover, they demonstrate a high degree of conservation of this cell death mechanism over 600 million years of evolution.

Apoptosis is one of three major forms of cell death, the others being necrosis and autophagic cell death (Table 6-1). Pending a more complete understanding of molecular mechanisms, this classification is based upon morphological characteristics (Table 6-2). Apoptosis is a highly regulated process, and many of the underlying mechanisms and pathways have been delineated over the past 2 decades.

In contrast to apoptosis, necrosis has traditionally been seen as the major example of unregulated cell death. Recent data have mandated a shift in that view.[6-9] At least a portion, if not more, of necrotic deaths are regulated. Although our understanding of the molecular basis of necrosis remains primitive, this field is progressing quickly with two key pathways identified to date.

Autophagy is a normal intracellular process in which organelles, proteins, and lipids are catabolized in the lysosome to provide energy and substrates.[10] Autophagy serves as a means of quality control for proteins and organelles, and functions as a survival mechanism during cellular starvation and stress. Cell death has been described in association with autophagy in some contexts. This has raised several questions including: (1) Does autophagy cause cell death or is it merely associated with it? (2) If autophagy causes cell death, does it kill using its own death machinery or via that of necrosis or apoptosis? (3) If autophagy causes cell death, what converts its survival function to a death function? The amount of autophagy? Other factors? These questions notwithstanding, autophagy and autophagic cell death—and apoptosis and necrosis—are found in the failing heart.

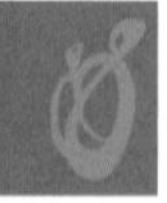

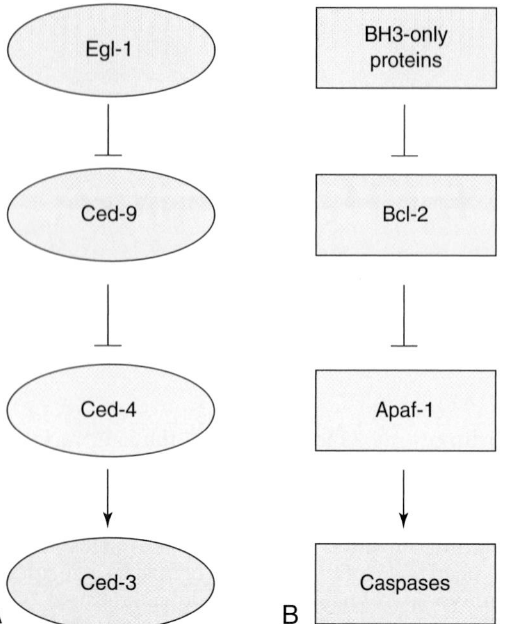

FIGURE 6–1 Evolutionary conservation of apoptosis pathways. **A,** Programmed cell death during *Caenorhabditis elegans* development. Precisely 131 cells (out of the 1090 somatic cells in the adult hermaphrodite) die at specific times during nematode development. Mutagenesis studies have revealed genes that regulate these deaths.[170] These genes are termed *cell death* abnormal, or *ced*, and include *ced-3* and *ced-4*, which promote death, and *ced-9*, which inhibits death. Loss-of-function mutations of *ced-9* result in widespread death, which can be rescued by loss-of-function mutations of either *ced-4* or *ced-3*. Thus *ced-9* is upstream of and inhibits *ced-4* and *ced-3*. The relationship between *ced-4* and *ced-3* was elucidated in studies in which *ced-4* killing was shown to require *ced-3*.[171] **B,** Mammalian apoptosis. Although apoptosis in worms and mammals differs in some respects, the genetic blueprint has been conserved over 600 million years of evolution from worms to mammals. The ortholog of Ced-3 is the caspase family of cysteine proteases. Ced-4 is represented by a single protein, Apaf-1, which functions as an adaptor in the apoptosome. Orthologs of Ced-9 are the antiapoptotic branch of the Bcl-2 family. The mammalian Bcl-2 family also contains two subfamilies of proapoptotic proteins, one of which, the BH3-only branch, is present in *C. elegans*. The worm BH3-only protein Egl-1 (Egg laying defective-1) inhibits Ced-9 to promote apoptosis. The equivalent step in mammals is the inhibition of Bcl-2 by various BH3-only proteins. Mammalian BH3-only proteins may also induce apoptosis through additional mechanisms. (Reprinted with permission from the Annual Review of Physiology, Volume 72 (c) 2010 by Annual Reviews www.annualreviews.org.)

TABLE 6–1 Cell Death

Process	Evolutionary Conservation	What Is It?
Apoptosis	Metazoans	Regulated cell suicide
Necrosis	Metazoans More ancient?	Traditionally considered unregulated, but regulated in at least some cases
Autophagic cell death	Unicellular eukaryotes and metazoans	Autophagy—normal survival process Death process caused by autophagy? Triggers not defined?

Cell death is essential for normal life in metazoan organisms. For example, apoptosis is needed for normal embryonic development and viability in the mouse.[11] Necrosis also occurs during development, but its role has not yet been defined. An important developmental role for autophagic "degeneration" has been clearly demonstrated in *Drosophila*.[12] Apoptosis also plays critical homeostatic functions in postnatal life. By regulating cell number, it maintains the composition of complex tissues. In addition, apoptosis is a major means of disposal for transformed and damaged cells.

TABLE 6–2 Morphology of Apoptosis and Necrosis

Apoptosis	Necrosis
Cell shrinkage	Cell swelling
Plasma membrane blebbing	Plasma membrane loss of integrity
Chromatin condensation (classically against nuclear membrane) Nuclear fragmentation	Sometimes chromatin condensation
Cytoplasmic organelles: grossly intact Sometimes mild mitochondrial changes	Mitochondria grossly swollen
Fragmentation of cell and nucleus into membrane-enclosed apoptotic bodies. These get phagocytosed by macrophages and/or neighboring cells.	Lysis of cell with release of intracellular contents into the extracellular space
Classically, single cells affected, but sometimes more diffuse	Groups of cells affected
No inflammation	Inflammation

Given these fundamental functions, it is not surprising that dysregulation of cell death (too little, too much, or mislocalized) often results in disease. For example, defects in apoptosis characterize most, if not all, cancers. The burst of cell death during acute myocardial infarction and stroke occurs through both apoptosis and necrosis.[2,7,8] Similarly, both apoptosis and necrosis are causal factors in the pathogenesis of heart failure.[2,13] Again, the possible role of autophagic cell death in these processes is more controversial and will be discussed later.

The notion that cell death can be both regulated and a causal factor in the pathogenesis of human disease has raised hopes of pharmacologically manipulating cell death to therapeutic advantage. In fact, this has already been realized with ABT-737[14] (Abbott Pharmaceuticals), a small molecule "BH3-only-mimetic" (see later discussion) that induces apoptosis and which is currently in trials for human cancer. Conversely, it may be possible to devise new therapies for myocardial infarction, stroke, heart failure, diabetes, and certain neurodegenerative disorders based around the concept of inhibiting cell death.

This chapter will review the fundamental basis of cell death and its relationship to the pathogenesis of advanced heart failure. Interplay among the various forms of cell death will be considered. When possible, death mechanisms will be placed within the context of the traditional pathophysiology of heart failure. Finally, we will summarize challenges related to the development of novel therapies based on inhibiting cell death.

APOPTOSIS

The quintessential morphological features of apoptosis include cytoplasmic shrinkage, chromatin condensation, and margination against the inner aspect of the nuclear membrane; budding of the plasma membrane; and fragmentation of the cytoplasm and nucleus into membrane-enclosed apoptotic bodies[15] (see Table 6-2). The latter get phagocytosed by macrophages or neighboring cells. Plasma membrane integrity is maintained until late in the process, thereby not eliciting an inflammatory response. In contrast to apoptosis, necrosis involves early loss of plasma membrane integrity and loss of intracellular contents into interstitium, leading to inflammation.

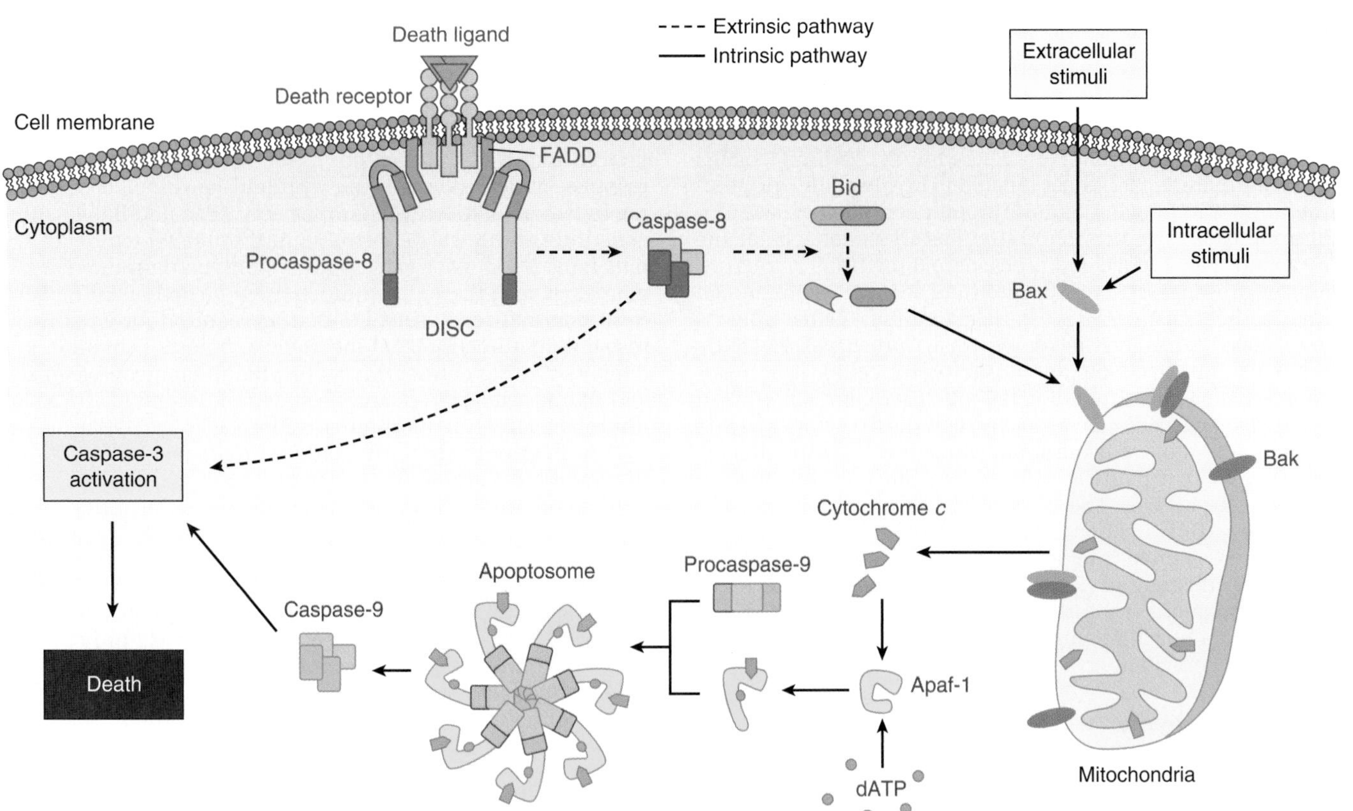

FIGURE 6–2 Apoptosis pathways. Apoptosis is mediated by an extrinsic pathway involving cell surface death receptors and by an intrinsic pathway that uses the mitochondria and endoplasmic reticulum. The extrinsic pathway is activated by binding of the death ligand to its receptor, which triggers formation of the DISC. Caspase 8 is activated by forced proximity within the DISC and then cleaves and activates downstream procaspases. Caspase 8 can also cleave the BH3-only protein Bid, the carboxyl portion of which translocates to the mitochondria to trigger apoptotic mitochondrial events. The intrinsic pathway is activated by diverse biological, chemical, and physical stimuli. These signals are transduced to the mitochondria and ER (not shown) by proapoptotic Bcl-2 proteins: Bax (a multidomain protein) and BH3-only proteins. These death signals trigger the release of apoptogens from the mitochondria into the cytosol, one of which, cytochrome *c*, is depicted here. Cytosolic cytochrome *c* triggers the formation of a second multiprotein complex, the apoptosome, in which procaspase 9 undergoes activation. Caspase 9 then cleaves and activates downstream procaspases. Downstream caspases cleave several hundred cellular proteins to bring about the apoptotic death of the cell. (Reprinted with permission from the Annual Review of Physiology, Volume 72 (c) 2010 by Annual Reviews www.annualreviews.org)

Although defined by the previously mentioned morphological criteria, the main functional characteristic of apoptosis is its regulated nature. The apoptotic machinery is part of the cell itself. In most cases, the relevant proteins are present constitutively and need only to be triggered to assemble into specific multiprotein complexes that bring about cell death (see later discussion). The death stimuli themselves can originate inside (e.g., oxidative stress, misfolded proteins) or outside (e.g., cytokines, nutrient deprivation) the cell. Apoptosis is mediated by two interconnected, evolutionarily conserved pathways: the extrinsic (or death receptor) pathway and the intrinsic (or mitochondrial/endoplasmic reticulum [ER]) pathway (Figure 6-2). The immediate objective of these pathways is to activate caspases.

Caspases

Caspases are a family of cysteine proteases that cleave proteins following aspartic acid residues.[16] These proteases exist in a hierarchy with upstream caspases 2, 8, 9, and 10 and downstream caspases 3, 6, and 7. Caspases are synthesized as largely inactive procaspases. Upstream procaspases, which are normally monomeric, become activated when forced to dimerize[17] following recruitment into multiprotein complexes, such as the death-inducing signaling complex (DISC) or apoptosome. Once activated, upstream caspases undergo autocleavage, but dimerization rather than autocleavage is the primary activating event. Activated upstream caspases then cleave downstream procaspases. In contrast to upstream procaspases, downstream procaspases already exist as dimers. Instead, the activating event for downstream procaspases is cleavage,[18] which separates the procaspase into three parts: prodomain, p20 subunit, and p10 subunit. The activated downstream caspase is formed by the noncovalent reassembly of two p20 and two p10 subunits. The major role of downstream caspases is to cleave up to several hundred cellular proteins, structural and regulatory, to bring about cell death. The precise mechanisms by which this proteolytic cascade deconstructs the cell are incompletely understood. Downstream caspases also accelerate cell killing by cleaving and activating other key proapoptotic proteins.[19,20]

Extrinsic Pathway

The extrinsic (or death receptor) pathway relays signals from a variety of specialized death ligands.[21] Some of these are soluble (e.g., tumor necrosis factor α [TNF-α]), while others are located on the plasma membranes of other cells (Fas ligand). When death ligands bind their cognate death receptors (e.g., TNF receptor 1 or 2 [TNFR1 or TNFR2] or Fas), formation of the DISC is triggered.[22] This will be described for Fas signaling. The more complex events involved in TNF-α signaling will be considered in the discussion of necrosis.

The binding of the Fas ligand to Fas is thought to trigger a conformational change in the intracellular domain of Fas, which results in recruitment of FADD (Fas-associated

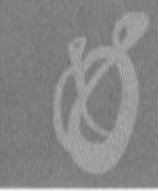

via death domain) through an interaction mediated by death domains (DD) in each of these proteins. FADD, in turn, recruits procaspase 8 or 10, the binding in this case mediated by death effector domains (DED) in each protein. DDs, DEDs, and Caspase Recruitment Domains (CARDs) are members of the death-fold superfamily.[23] These motifs, which consist of six antiparallel α-helices, mediate many of the protein-protein interactions in the multiprotein complexes that carry out apoptosis. At a minimum, the Fas DISC consists of the Fas ligand, Fas, FADD, and procaspase 8 (or 10). The recruitment of procaspase 8 (or 10) into the DISC causes its forced dimerization, resulting in caspase activation. Caspase 8 goes on to cleave and activate downstream procaspases. While this alone could activate apoptosis (type I cells), it is insufficient in most cells (type II cells) to trigger large amounts of downstream caspase activation and cell death.[24] For extrinsic pathway activators to bring about efficient cell killing, signals from the extrinsic pathway must be amplified by activation of the intrinsic pathway. The key molecule connecting these two pathways is Bid (BH3 [Bcl-2 (B cell leukemia/lymphoma-2) homology domain 3]-interacting domain death agonist).[20] Bid is a direct substrate of caspase 8. Following cleavage, its C-terminal fragment (truncated Bid [*t*Bid]) translocates to the outer mitochondrial membrane and triggers events to be discussed that contribute to activation of the intrinsic pathway.

Intrinsic Pathway

Premitochondrial/Endoplasmic Reticulum Events

The intrinsic (or mitochondrial/ER) pathway transduces a wide spectrum of death signals that originate both inside and outside the cell. These include deficiency of survival factors, deficiency and/or excess of nutrients, hypoxia, oxidative/nitrosative stress, radiation, drugs, DNA damage, and misfolded proteins. These stimuli are transduced to the mitochondria and/or ER by a variety of proapoptotic Bcl-2 (B cell leukemia/lymphoma-2) proteins. These events stimulate the release of mitochondrial apoptogens (e.g., cytochrome *c*[25,26]) and ER Ca^{2+}[27,28] into the cytosol. Once cytosolic, cytochrome *c* triggers the formation of the apoptosome,[29,30] which leads to caspase activation. Other mitochondrial apoptogens relieve the inhibition of already activated caspases.[31-34] Ca^{2+} released by the ER is taken up by the mitochondria, resulting in cell death as will be discussed later.

The Bcl-2 proteins regulate the integrity of the outer mitochondrial membrane (OMM) and therefore the release of mitochondrial apoptogens.[26,35] Antiapoptotic Bcl-2 proteins inhibit OMM permeabilization and apoptogen release, while proapoptotic Bcl-2 proteins promote these events. Bcl-2 proteins possess one or more Bcl-2 homology (BH) domains.[36] Members of the antiapoptotic branch, typified by Bcl-2 and Bcl-x_L (Bcl-x, long isoform), contain multiple domains. Proceeding from the amino to the carboxyl end of the protein, these include BH4 (found only in antiapoptotic family members), BH3, BH1, and BH2. The proapoptotic branch of the family is divided into two classes. The first includes the multidomain proapoptotics, such as Bax (Bcl-2-associated X protein) and Bak (Bcl-2 homologous antagonist/killer), each of which possesses BH3, BH1, and BH2 domains. The second proapoptotic class is composed of the BH3-only proteins.

Under normal conditions, Bax resides primarily in the cytosol in an inactive conformation. In response to intrinsic pathway stimuli, it undergoes conformational activation, which in part involves exposure of a C-terminal transmembrane domain.[37] Although several proteins that bind Bax and influence its conformational activation have been identified, the precise regulatory events and the pathways connecting them with death stimuli remain incompletely understood.[38,39] Bax conformational activation is linked to its translocation to the mitochondria and ER, although key mechanistic details are lacking. Once at the mitochondria, Bax inserts into the OMM through its transmembrane domain. Bak, the other major multidomain proapoptotic Bcl-2 protein, resides constitutively at the OMM and ER membrane. Under normal conditions, Bak is maintained in an inactive conformation at the mitochondria through its interactions with several proteins.[40,41] In response to death signals, these proteins are displaced, resulting in Bak activation. Most importantly, Bax and Bak together constitute an obligate control point through which death signals must pass to activate apoptotic mitochondrial events. In many systems, there is redundancy in the actions of Bax and Bak such that the absence of both is required for a cell to be resistant to mitochondrial-mediated apoptosis.[42] In other systems, including cardiac myocytes, redundancy between Bax and Bak appears significantly less complete, and loss of either diminishes the full apoptotic response.[43]

The BH3-only proteins play a critical role in facilitating the apoptotic mitochondrial events mediated by the multidomain proapoptotic proteins. In contrast to the multidomain proapoptotics, which provide a universal gateway to mitochondrial apoptotic events, each BH3-only protein transduces signals from only a subset of apoptotic stimuli.[36] In addition, these signals activate BH3-only proteins through a diversity of molecular mechanisms. For example, the BH3-only protein Bad is important in sensing deficiencies of growth/survival factors. Inadequate IGF-1 results in dephosphorylation of Bad, leading to its release from the 14-3-3 protein. Bad subsequently translocates to the mitochondria and contributes to apoptogen release. BH3-only proteins Noxa and PUMA (p53-upregulated modulator of apoptosis), on the other hand, undergo transcriptional activation by p53, which itself is activated by a variety of noxious insults. Bid, which we have already discussed as a link between extrinsic and intrinsic apoptotic pathways, is a BH3-only protein that is activated by caspase 8 cleavage.

How the BH3-only proteins work to promote apoptosis is a matter of debate and reflects larger questions as to the biochemical relationships among the antiapoptotic, multidomain proapoptotic, and BH3-only Bcl-2 proteins. One model holds that some BH3-only proteins (*t*Bid, PUMA, and Bim [Bcl-2-interacting mediator of cell death]) directly interact with and activate Bax and Bak.[44] Conversely, antiapoptotic Bcl-2 proteins inhibit apoptosis by binding *t*Bid, PUMA, and Bim, rather than by directly inhibiting Bax and Bak. Other BH3-only proteins promote apoptosis by displacing *t*Bid, Bim, and PUMA from antiapoptotic Bcl-2 proteins, thereby making *t*Bid, Bim, and PUMA available to activate Bax and Bak. Thus, in this model, certain BH3-only proteins activate the multidomain proapoptotics. According to a competing model, Bax and Bak are constitutively inhibited by antiapoptotic Bcl-2 proteins. BH3-only proteins do not interact with Bax or Bak, but instead bind antiapoptotic Bcl-2 proteins and, thereby, disinhibit Bax and Bak.[45]

Mitochondrial Events

Although it is clear that Bax and Bak promote OMM permeabilization, the molecular/physical basis for this event is unclear. It is known that activation of the intrinsic pathway stimulates a complex pattern of Bax/Bak homo-oligomerization and hetero-oligomerization,[46,47] which may be facilitated by BH3-only proteins such as Bid.[48] Although these higher ordered complexes correlate with OMM permeabilization, a mechanism remains obscure. Bax and Bak are known to form channels in artificial lipid bilayers, but the existence of such channels in cells is debatable. Other theories focus on the possibility that Bax and Bak regulate a yet to be identified protein or lipid, modulate OMM topology, or induce mitochondrial fission.[49] It is important to emphasize, however, that OMM permeabilization during apoptosis is distinct from OMM rupture that sometimes occurs in necrosis (see later discussion).

Bax/Bak-dependent OMM permeabilization is critical for the release of mitochondrial apoptogens, which reside in the intermembrane space (between the OMM and inner mitochondrial membrane [IMM]) and/or are loosely attached to the IMM itself. The efficient release of some mitochondrial apoptogens, however, also involves additional events.[50] For example, remodeling of mitochondrial cristae junctions is required to mobilize a large portion of cytochrome *c* from within cristae to the intermembrane space for subsequent release. Interestingly, remodeling of cristae may involve cyclophilin D,[50] a matrix protein that is a critical regulator of necrosis (discussed later), suggesting one potential point of convergence between apoptosis and necrosis signaling.

Mitochondrial apoptogens are proteins that are released into the cytosol and directly or indirectly promote apoptosis. These proteins include cytochrome *c*,[25,26] Smac/DIABLO (second mitochondria-derived activator of caspase/direct IAP-binding protein with low PI),[31,32] Omi/HtrA2 (Omi/high temperature requirement protein A2),[33,34] AIF (apoptosis inducing factor),[51] and EndoG (Endonuclease G).[52] In contrast to their death-promoting properties in the cytosol, mitochondrial apoptogens are thought to carry out important physiological functions within the mitochondria of normal cells. This is best exemplified by cytochrome *c*, which is essential for electron transport during respiration.

Postmitochondrial Events

The release of apoptogens into the cytosol brings about a series of events that are critical for the induction of apoptosis via the intrinsic pathway. Cytochrome *c* in the cytosol is the trigger for apoptosome formation.[29] The apoptosome is a multiprotein complex, which provides a dimerization interface for the activation of upstream procaspase 9. The binding of cytochrome *c* and dATP (which is already present in the cytosol) to Apaf-1 (apoptotic protease activating factor-1) stimulates Apaf-1 oligomerization and its subsequent recruitment of procaspase 9 (through CARD-CARD interactions). The resulting apoptosome consists of a heptad of Apaf-1, cytochrome *c*, dATP, and procaspase 9 in a wheel-and-spoke arrangement.[30] Procaspase 9 is activated by forced dimerization, following which it cleaves and activates downstream procaspases.

Other mitochondrial apoptogens have different roles. Smac/DIABLO and Omi/HtrA2 counteract apoptosis inhibitors, and discussion of their functions will be deferred to the section on apoptosis inhibitors. Following its release from mitochondria, AIF translocates to the nucleus where it may contribute to the large-scale (200 kb to 50 kb) DNA cleavage during apoptosis, presumably through a yet to be identified endonuclease.[51] These actions of AIF do not require caspases, and AIF-induced cell death is often described as caspase-independent. This term may not be completely accurate, however, as in some contexts, caspases appear necessary for AIF release and/or translocation.[53,54] Subsequent cleavage of DNA into oligonucleosomal fragments is carried out by EndoG[52] and CAD (caspase-activated deoxyribonuclease), whose functions appear to be redundant.

ER Stress-induced Apoptosis

In addition to its physiological roles in protein folding and posttranslational modifications, lipid biosynthesis, and Ca^{2+} homeostasis, the ER is a critical mediator of cell death. Important death signals include misfolded proteins, oxidative stress, and certain lipids.[28] Although a unifying mechanism for ER stress-induced apoptosis remains elusive, some critical components have been delineated.

Improperly folded proteins can cause severe cellular stress, dysfunction, or even death. The unfolded protein response (UPR) is a normal cellular mechanism in which the recognition of unfolded proteins is transduced into a transcriptional response, the goal of which is to temporarily halt further translation and refold denatured proteins.[55] The UPR is initiated when unfolded proteins in the ER lumen recruit BiP/GRP78 (immunoglobulin heavy chain binding protein/glucose-regulated protein 78) away from PERK (double-stranded RNA-dependent protein kinase R [PKR]-like ER kinase), IRE1α (inositol-requiring enzyme 1α), and ATF6 (activating transcription factor 6), which are integral ER membrane proteins that control the three arms of the UPR. Dissociation of BiP/GRP78 leads to activation of PERK, IRE1α, and ATF6, which initiates a complex network of transcriptional events to correct misfolding and restore cellular homeostasis. When the UPR is severe and prolonged, however, apoptosis can result. Although the factors that convert this compensatory response to a death response are not understood, some of the proteins that mediate apoptosis have been identified. One key molecule is the transcription factor CHOP (C/EBP [CCAAT/enhancer-binding protein]-homologous protein), which is downstream of PERK, IRE1α, and ATF6. CHOP activates genes that mediate not only the UPR, but also apoptosis including DR5 (death receptor 5), TRB3 (tribbles-related protein 3), Bim, and GADD34 (growth arrest and DNA damage-inducible protein 34).

A second mechanism of ER stress-induced apoptosis involves the release of Ca^{2+} from the ER lumen into the cytosol.[28] This mechanism appears particularly relevant to ER stress-induced apoptosis triggered by oxidative stimuli and certain lipids (e.g., arachidonic acid). The basic schema is that a death stimulus triggers the release of a Ca^{2+} bolus into the cytosol followed by its subsequent uptake into the mitochondria. It is not clear how mitochondrial Ca^{2+} overload stimulates cell death in this context. Possibilities include triggering of mitochondrial permeability transition pore (MPTP) opening, a seminal event in necrosis (see later discussion), and classic apoptosis with apoptogen release, although the mechanism is unclear.

The magnitude of the Ca^{2+} bolus elicited by an apoptotic stimulus is determined by the resting ER luminal Ca^{2+} concentration. Resting ER luminal Ca^{2+} concentration is determined by an interplay between Bax/Bak and Bcl-2 proteins.[28] As with the mitochondria, Bak and Bcl-2 reside at the ER membrane. Moreover, Bax can translocate from cytosol to ER in response to an apoptotic signal. Bcl-2 interacts with IP3R-1 (inositol 1,4,5-triphosphate receptor-1) to induce a baseline Ca^{2+} "leak" into the cytosol. This leak is cytoprotective because by decreasing basal ER luminal Ca^{2+} concentrations, it diminishes the magnitude of the Ca^{2+} bolus that can be induced by a subsequent death stimulus. In contrast, the presence of Bax and Bak decreases the interaction of Bcl-2 with IP3R-1, thereby opposing the Bcl-2-induced IP3R-1 Ca^{2+} leak. Bax and Bak therefore increase the resting ER luminal Ca^{2+} concentration, ensuring that a subsequent death stimulus will result in a larger bolus of Ca^{2+} release. Thus, by regulating the baseline ER luminal Ca^{2+} concentration, Bcl-2 proteins influence the magnitude of Ca^{2+} released by an ER death stimulus.

ER death pathways may also interface with the extrinsic pathway. Bap31 (B-cell receptor-associated protein 31), an integral ER membrane protein, can be cleaved by caspase 8 activated at the DISC or by the procaspase 8L isoform, which is recruited and activated in complex with Bap31.[27,56] Bap31 cleavage triggers the release of ER Ca^{2+} and mitochondrial cytochrome *c* (through unclear mechanisms), and cell death. This pathway appears to represent an amplification mechanism for the extrinsic pathway using the ER, similar to the Bid-mediated mechanism by which the extrinsic pathway is amplified using the mitochondria. This amplification mechanism may be self-reinforcing as recent work shows that procaspase 8 is activated by ER stress and critical for ER stress-induced cell death.[57]

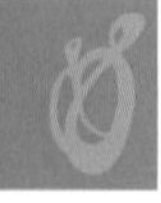

Although procaspase 12 has been considered to be a mediator of ER stress-induced apoptosis, critical examination of the data raises serious doubts about its role. While the initial knockout mouse provided strong evidence that procaspase 12 is critical for ER stress-induced apoptosis,[58] an independent knockout indicates that it is dispensable.[59] Moreover, full-length, functional procaspase 12 protein is absent from most humans due to genetic variation.[60] While there is some evidence that procaspase 12 may modulate activation of procaspase 1 and inflammation/sepsis, the role of procaspase 12 in ER stress-induced cell death is questionable.

Inhibitors of Apoptosis

Because of the potentially profound and irreversible consequences of initiating apoptosis, key activating molecules are opposed by a variety of endogenous inhibitors. c-FLIP (FLICE [FADD-like interleukin-1β converting enzyme]-inhibitory protein), an important inhibitor of the extrinsic pathway, inhibits formation of the DISC.[61] c-FLIP exists as two isoforms that arise from alternative splicing. The long isoform ($FLIP_L$) is homologous to procaspase 8, but enzymatically inactive due to mutation of the catalytic cysteine. The short isoform ($FLIP_S$) contains only two DEDs. $FLIP_S$ blocks DISC assembly probably by binding the DEDs on FADD and procaspase 8, thereby preventing FADD from recruiting procaspase 8. In contrast, low concentrations of $FLIP_L$ can promote the recruitment and activation of procaspase 8, while high concentrations are inhibitory.

Bcl-2 and Bcl-x_L, which oppose OMM permeabilization and the release of mitochondrial apoptogens into the cytosol, are key inhibitors of the intrinsic pathway. Models for their mechanisms of action have been discussed previously.[44,45]

The IAP (inhibitor of apoptosis) family of proteins (e.g., XIAP [X-linked inhibitor of apoptosis protein] and cIAP 1 and 2 [cellular inhibitor of apoptosis 1 and 2]) antagonize the postmitochondrial intrinsic pathway. IAPs bind to and inhibit already activated downstream caspases 3 and 7 by blocking the access of substrate to the caspase active site.[18,62,63] In addition, IAPs bind to and inhibit the activation of procaspase 9 in the apoptosome.[64] IAPs also contain E3-ubiquitin ligase activity. Consistent with their role as apoptosis inhibitors, the E3 ligase activity promotes the degradation of downstream caspases.[65] However, IAPs can also promote their own degradation,[66] perhaps to limit their window of activity. As will be discussed later in the necrosis section, the E3-ubiquitin ligase activities of cIAP 1 and 2 also promote survival through K63 polyubiquitination of RIP1 and TRAF2.[67-69]

Having introduced the IAP family of apoptosis inhibitors, we can now consider the two remaining mitochondrial apoptogens, Smac/DIABLO[31,32] and Omi/HtrA2,[33,34] which promote apoptosis by neutralizing IAPs. Smac/DIABLO and Omi/HtrA2 bind directly to IAPs, thereby displacing the active caspases bound by IAPs. Thus, Smac/DIABLO and Omi/HtrA2 relieve IAP-mediated inhibition of caspases. Furthermore, Omi/HtrA2 possesses a serine protease activity that inactivates IAPs irreversibly through cleavage.[70] These mechanisms underscore that efficient cell killing requires not only activation of proapoptotic molecules but also inactivation of inhibitors.

Most endogenous inhibitors of apoptosis target circumscribed steps in either the extrinsic or intrinsic pathway. By contrast, ARC (apoptosis repressor with CARD [caspase recruitment domain]) antagonizes both the extrinsic and intrinsic pathways through a variety of mechanisms.[71] The extrinsic pathway is inhibited by the direct interaction of ARC with Fas, FADD, and procaspase 8, which prevents DISC assembly as required for extrinsic pathway activation.[71] ARC inhibits the intrinsic pathway through several mechanisms. It binds directly to Bax, which inhibits Bax conformational activation and translocation to the mitochondria.[71,72] In addition, ARC neutralizes p53, a transcription factor that activates multiple proapoptotic genes.[73] The mechanism involves direct binding between ARC and p53 in the nucleus. This inhibits p53 tetramerization, which both cripples p53 function as a transcription factor and reveals a nuclear export signal in the p53 molecule that relocates p53 to the cytoplasm. These events markedly decrease p53-dependent transcription.

NECROSIS

Necrosis is characterized by severe cellular ATP depletion and the early loss of plasma membrane integrity. Decreases in ATP levels reflect severe mitochondrial dysfunction, while the cause of plasma membrane dysfunction is not yet understood. Moreover, it is unclear whether ATP depletion or plasma membrane dysfunction or neither is the primary insult. The most characteristic morphological feature of necrosis is cellular swelling, reflecting loss of plasma membrane integrity (see Table 6-2). In contrast, apoptotic cells are shrunken. Loss of plasma membrane integrity in necrosis results in the release of the intracellular contents into the extracellular space, which often engenders a marked inflammatory response. In contrast, apoptotic cells maintain plasma membrane integrity, even after fragmenting into apoptotic bodies, so long as phagocytosis is carried out in a timely manner. Thus apoptosis takes place without inflammation, resulting in the silent deletion of cells.

Although necrosis has long been considered an unregulated death process, a body of work over the past decade indicates that at least a portion of necrotic cell deaths is actively mediated and highly regulated. While the precise proportions of necrotic cell deaths that are regulated versus unregulated is not known, regulated necrosis has been shown to be a significant component of the cell death in myocardial infarction,[7,8] heart failure,[13] and stroke.[9] Current understanding of the mechanisms that mediate necrosis is incomplete—especially in comparison to the detailed apoptotic pathways that have been delineated over the past 20 years. Nevertheless, two necrosis pathways have been identified to date (Figure 6-3). As in apoptosis, one involves cell surface receptors (death receptor/RIP pathway) and the other the mitochondria (cyclophilin D/MPTP pathway). Beyond these superficial similarities, however, these necrosis pathways are different biochemically and functionally from those that mediate apoptosis.

Death Receptor/RIP Pathway

In addition to their role in apoptosis described previously, death receptors also signal cellular survival, proliferation, and necrosis.[6] This has been most extensively studied in the case of TNFR1. TNF kills most cells inefficiently because it activates death and survival pathways simultaneously. The ability of TNF to kill is unmasked when survival mechanisms are inhibited. TNF can induce apoptosis. But when apoptosis is inhibited, TNF killing occurs by necrosis.

These pleiotropic effects are mediated by two multiprotein complexes.[74] Complex 1 signals survival. Its assembly at the plasma membrane is triggered by the binding of TNF to TNFR1, which stimulates the recruitment of TRADD (TNFRSF1A [TNF receptor superfamily 1A]-associated via death domain), RIP1 (receptor interacting protein 1, a serine/threonine kinase), TRAF2 (TNF receptor-associated factor 2), and cellular inhibitor of apoptosis proteins cIAP1 and 2 (which, as noted previously, possess E3-ubiquitin ligase activity). cIAP1 and 2, along with TRAF2, promote the K63-polyubiquitination of RIP1 and TRAF2.[67-69] Once polyubiquitinated, RIP1 and TRAF2 recruit TAB 2/3 (TAK1 [TGF-β-activated kinase 1]-binding protein 2/30), leading to the activation of TAK1, a MAPKKK (mitogen-activated protein

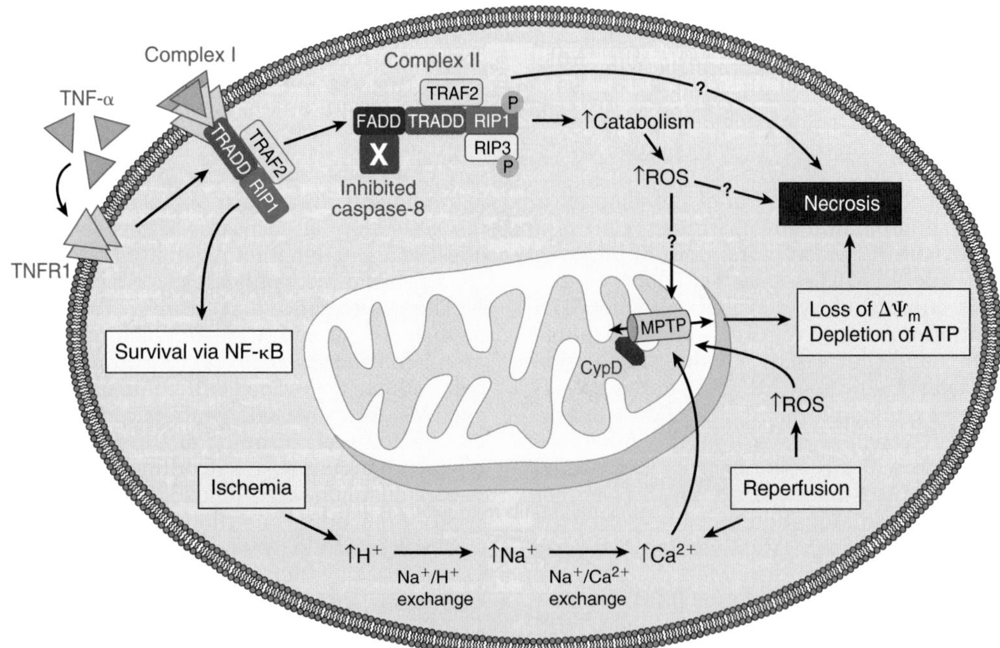

FIGURE 6–3 Necrosis pathways. Information about necrosis signaling is currently limited to two pathways. The first involves death receptors, as exemplified by TNFR1 (tumor necrosis factor α receptor 1). Depending on context, activation of TNFR1 can promote cell survival or either apoptotic or necrotic cell death. These choices are mediated by multiprotein complexes I and II. The binding of TNF-α to TNFR1 stimulates formation of complex I, which contains TNFR1, TRADD, RIP1, TRAF2, and cIAP1/2. The exact relationships among these proteins have not yet been defined, but one model postulates that TNFR1-TRADD-RIP1 proteins are linked through their respective death domains (DDs). RIP1 and TRAF2 undergo K63 polyubiquitination by cIAP1/2 in conjunction with TRAF2 (not shown). Polyubiquitinated RIP1 and TRAF2 recruit TAK1, which activates NF κB, thereby stimulating transcription of survival genes (see text for details). Death effects of TNFR1 signaling are mediated via complex II, which forms following endocytosis of complex I, the dissociation of TNFR1, and the deubiquitination of RIP1 by CYLD and A20 (not shown). TRADD recruits FADD (DD-DD interactions), and FADD recruits procaspase 8 (DED-DED interactions). Unless inhibited, procaspase 8 undergoes activation and cleaves RIP1, rendering RIP1 unable to signal either survival or necrosis. Caspase 8 also activates downstream caspases inducing apoptosis. In contrast, if procaspase 8 is inhibited (genetically or pharmacologically), RIP1 is not cleaved and instead recruits RIP3. RIP1 and RIP3 undergo a complex set of phosphorylation events, and necrosis ensues through unclear mechanisms. One potential mechanism may involve the activation of catabolic pathways and ROS production as shown. A second necrosis pathway involves the mitochondrial permeability transition pore (MPTP) in the inner mitochondrial membrane and its regulation by cyclophilin D (CypD). This pore may be opened by increased Ca^{2+}, oxidative stress, decreased ATP, and other stimuli that operate during ischemia/reperfusion and heart failure. Ischemia/reperfusion can lead to increased Ca^{2+} and ROS as depicted. MPTP opening results in profound alterations in mitochondrial structure and function as described in text, which results in decreased ATP. No definitive connections have been delineated between death receptor and mitochondrial necrosis pathways. A possible connection is RIP3-induced ROS generation. (Reprinted with permission from the Annual Review of Physiology, Volume 72 (c) 2010 by Annual Reviews www.annualreviews.org)

kinase kinase kinase).[67,68] Activated TAK1 phosphorylates the IKK (IkB [inhibitor of κB] kinase) complex, leading to activation of NF κB (nuclear factor κ light-chain enhancer of activated B cells).[67] NF κB transcriptionally activates multiple genes encoding survival proteins including c-FLIP. The net result is TNF-induced survival.

In contrast to complex 1, complex 2 mediates the killing functions (apoptosis and necrosis) of TNF. Complex 2 is thought to form from complex 1. This involves endocytosis of complex 1, dissociation of TNFR1, deubiquitination of RIP1 by CYLD (cylindromatosis) and A20, and recruitment of FADD and procaspase 8.[74-76] Recruitment to complex 2 activates procaspase 8 and initiates apoptosis. One important caspase 8 substrate in complex 2 is RIP1, which as described later is critical for necrosis. The cleavage of RIP1 by caspase 8 abrogates the ability of RIP1 to promote necrosis[77] and its previously described survival functions.[78] Furthermore, the C-terminal RIP1 fragment resulting from caspase 8 cleavage enforces further caspase 8 activation and apoptosis.[78]

Under conditions in which procaspase 8 activation/caspase 8 activity is inhibited, however, RIP1 remains intact and recruits RIP3 into complex 2.[79,80] RIP1 and RIP3 undergo a complex series of phosphorylation events that trigger necrosis. While the kinase activity of RIP1 is not required for its survival functions in complex 1, the kinase activities of both RIP1 and RIP3 are critical for necrosis.[6,79] In one mechanism, RIP3 binds and activates several metabolic enzymes, resulting in the generation of reactive oxygen species that presumably contribute to necrosis.[81] It is likely that other yet to be identified RIP1/RIP3 targets are also involved in necrosis signaling.

The physiological significance of the death receptor/RIP pathway has not been fully delineated. The fact that necrosis was revealed only when caspase 8 was inhibited has suggested that necrosis serves as a default pathway when apoptosis is unavailable. This scenario may be relevant to certain cancer cells that induce molecules such as c-FLIP, which inhibit procaspase 8 activation, or infection with certain viruses that encode caspase inhibitors.[82] Further work will be needed to determine the general applicability of the notion that necrosis is a default to apoptosis. As will be discussed later, suppression of apoptosis does not appear to be a prerequisite for induction of necrosis via the cyclophilin D/MPTP pathway.

Cyclophilin D/MPTP Pathway

Mitochondrial dysfunction is a hallmark of both apoptosis and necrosis. For example, during apoptosis, the release to the cytosol of cytochrome *c* and perhaps other mitochondrial apoptogens can lead to defects in mitochondrial function. However, gross alterations in mitochondrial morphology are uncommon in apoptosis until late in the process. In contrast, necrosis is characterized by marked swelling of mitochondria, decreases in ATP formation, and increases in the generation of reactive oxygen species.

A major event underlying these mitochondrial abnormalities is mitochondrial permeability transition (MPT) caused by opening of the MPTP in the IMM.[83] The MPTP is a nonselective channel that can accommodate molecules less than 1.5 kDa. A variety of proteins have been hypothesized to be components of the pore including adenine nucleotide translocase (IMM), cyclophilin D (matrix), voltage-dependent anion channel (OMM), peripheral benzodiazepine receptor (OMM), mitochondrial phosphate carrier (IMM), and others. Current opinion, however, is that the composition of the channel is not known with any certainty. Moreover, while cyclophilin D may or may not be part of the structural pore, it plays an important regulatory role, as will be discussed later.

MPTP opening is stimulated by elevated mitochondrial matrix Ca^{2+} concentration, oxidative stress, elevated phosphate concentration, and decreased adenine nucleotide concentration. The consequences of MPTP opening are (1) Redistribution of water and solutes across the IMM. In particular, there is a massive entry of water from the mitochondrial intermembrane space (IMS) to the matrix. This occurs because the osmolality of the matrix is significantly higher than that of the IMS. This redistribution of water causes the matrix to swell and expands the IMM. Since the IMM has considerably more surface area than the OMM, this swelling outstrips the ability of the OMM to contain the IMM. Rupture of the OMM can ensue. (2) Loss of the electrical potential difference across the IMM ($\Delta\psi_m$). Electron transport generates an electrical potential difference ($\Delta\psi_m$) across the IMM, in which the matrix is markedly negative in relation to the IMS. Opening of MPTP causes loss of $\Delta\psi_m$, which is the electromotive force coupled to the phosphorylation of ADP to ATP. Thus, ATP production plummets. (3) Increased ROS production due to electron transport chain dysfunction and electron leakage.

Cyclophilin D is a peptidyl-prolyl *cis-trans* isomerase encoded by the *ppif* gene. The endogenous substrates of its enzymatic activity are not known with certainty, although it is clear that this enzymatic activity is needed for MPTP opening. Overexpression of cyclophilin D in transgenic mice causes mitochondrial swelling and cell death. Conversely, mitochondria derived from cyclophilin D knockout mice are resistant to swelling induced by Ca^{2+} (an MPTP opener), but remain sensitive to cytochrome *c* release in response to Bax and *t*Bid (classic apoptotic stimuli). Similarly, primary cells isolated from cyclophilin D knockout mice are resistant to killing by Ca^{2+} and oxidative stress while remaining sensitive to Bax-induced death. Taken together, cyclophilin D does not appear to mediate apoptosis, but rather regulates a death process with several key features of necrosis.[7-9]

It is instructive to consider differences between mitochondrial events in apoptosis and necrosis. The major mitochondrial event in apoptosis is permeabilization of the OMM resulting in apoptogen release. In contrast, the most important mitochondrial event in necrosis is opening of the MPTP in the IMM. As noted, mitochondrial swelling resulting from MPTP opening, however, can lead to OMM rupture. This, in turn, can permit the release of apoptogens, although their importance in cell killing, as compared with the catastrophic IMM events during necrosis, is not clear. At one time, it was thought that OMM permeabilization during apoptosis was caused by OMM rupture resulting from IMM events (e.g., MPTP opening and loss of $\Delta\psi_m$). It is now known, however, that OMM permeabilization during apoptosis is distinct from OMM rupture during necrosis. In fact, IMM events, such as loss of $\Delta\psi_m$, which sometimes occur during apoptosis, are not required for OMM permeabilization and usually occur after OMM permeabilization.[50,84] To summarize, OMM permeabilization during apoptosis is a Bax/Bak-dependent process, while OMM rupture during necrosis results from cyclophilin D–dependent MPTP opening in the IMM. There may be areas of functional overlap, however. For example, as previously noted, remodeling of the IMM to "open" cristae and free cytochrome *c* stores for release during apoptosis may involve cyclophilin D.[50]

Ca^{2+}/Proteases

A proteolytic cascade mediated by caspases is a critical feature of apoptotic cell death. Indeed, a major goal of both the extrinsic and intrinsic apoptosis pathways is to bring about the activation of caspases. These observations have raised questions as to whether necrosis is also mediated by a hierarchy of executioner proteases.

There is evidence that orthologs of calpains and cathepsins mediate necrosis in *C. elegans*. Gain-of-function mutations in *mec-4* (*mechanosensory 4*), encoding a Ca^{2+} and Na^+ channel, induce necrotic death in neurons.[85,86] *mec-4*-induced necrosis is decreased by mutation or knockdown of *unc-68* (encoding an ortholog of the ryanodine receptor, a Ca^{2+} release channel), *itr-1* (encoding an ortholog of IP3R, a Ca^{2+} release channel), *crt-1* (encoding an ortholog of calreticulin), or *cnx-1* (encoding an ortholog of calnexin). Thapsigargin (an inhibitor of SERCA [sarcoplasmic/endoplasmic reticulum Ca^{2+}-ATPase], which pumps Ca^{2+} from the cytoplasm into the ER lumen) antagonizes the rescue of *mec-4*-induced necrosis by *crt-1* mutation. Taken together, these data suggest that increases in cytoplasmic Ca^{2+} may mediate necrosis, perhaps related to the role of Ca^{2+} in MPTP opening.

As shown previously, gain-of-function mutations in Ca^{2+} and Na^+ channels that induce necrosis in worms are associated with high cytoplasmic Ca^{2+} levels. Calpains are Ca^{2+}-activated noncaspase cysteine proteases. Loss-of-function mutations in *clp-1* or *tra-3* (encoding calpain orthologs) ameliorate necrosis induced by gain-of-function mutations in Ca^{2+} or Na^+ channels.[87] Taken together, these data suggest that calpain orthologs mediate necrosis in the worm. Cathepsins, another family of proteases that reside in lysosomes, may be released during cellular stress. Loss-of-function mutations in *asp-3* and *asp-4* (encoding cathepsin orthologs) also suppress necrosis due to Ca^{2+} or Na^+ channels,[87] suggesting that cathepsin orthologs are also involved in necrosis in the worm.

The involvement of calpains, cathepsins, and other proteases in mammalian necrosis is less clear. There is evidence that calpains play important signaling roles in apoptosis. Calpain-cleavage can promote apoptosis by activating Bid and Bax, inactivating Bcl-2 and Bcl-x_L, and generating a fragment of Atg5 (autophagy-related 5 homolog, discussed later) that translocates to mitochondria where it binds Bcl-x_L.[88] In contrast, calpain-mediated cleavage of caspases can inhibit apoptosis. Its role in signaling aside, there is currently no compelling evidence that calpains or other proteases play a central proteolytic role in necrosis.

Some Unresolved Questions

We have discussed two emerging pathways that mediate necrosis: the death receptor/RIP pathway and cyclophilin D/MPTP pathway. These pathways affirm that necrosis, at least in some situations, is an actively mediated and regulated process. While these pathways are almost certainly interconnected, there has been little work thus far to define their genetic or mechanistic relationships. Preliminary evidence that the two pathways are connected in the myocardium is suggested by ischemia-reperfusion experiments showing that necrostatin-1 (which inhibits RIP1 kinase activity[89]) does not augment cardioprotection resulting from cyclophilin D ablation.[90] One likely molecular connection between the pathways is RIP3-generated ROS, which may play a role in MPTP opening.[81] Finally, there are likely to be additional necrosis pathways based on genomewide siRNA screens[76] that have revealed unexpected mediators of necrosis such as Bmf (Bcl-2 modifying factor), a BH3-only protein with a well-established proapoptotic role.

The most essential necrosis phenotypes are ATP depletion and plasma membrane disruption. ATP depletion is due, in large part, to MPTP opening. However, additional mechanisms may operate. For example, PARP (poly [ADP-ribose] polymerase), which is activated in certain instances of necrosis (e.g., DNA damage from alkylating agents), adds ADP-ribose to histones and, in so doing, consumes NAD^+ and depletes ATP.[91] In contrast, the basis for loss of plasma membrane integrity in necrosis is poorly understood.

AUTOPHAGIC CELL DEATH

Autophagy

Before considering autophagic cell death, we will discuss autophagy,[92] which is a normal cellular survival process. There are three types of autophagy, but this discussion will be restricted to macroautophagy, referred to hereafter as autophagy. Autophagy (meaning "self-eating") is a process in which organelles, proteins, and lipids are transported in double membrane vesicles, called autophagosomes, for catabolism in lysosomes to provide the cell with amino acids, free fatty acids, and energy during times of starvation or stress. In addition, autophagy is one of the major pathways in the cell for regulating protein degradation. Finally, autophagy provides a critical quality control mechanism for proteins and organelles and regulates organelle abundance.

The macromolecules and organelles destined for degradation are first surrounded by a double membrane vesicle termed the *autophagosome*. This process, which is regulated by evolutionarily conserved *atg* (*autophagy-related*) genes, begins with vesicle nucleation involving Beclin-1, UVRAG (UV radiation resistance-associated gene), Vps34 (vacuolar protein sorting 34), IP3R, and others.[92] Next, vesicle elongation is directed by Atg12 and Atg8 conjugation pathways. Finally, the autophagosome fuses with the lysosome to create the autophagolysosome, and lysosomal enzymes degrade its contents.

Autophagy is regulated by mTOR (mammalian target of rapamycin), which under normal nutrient conditions, phosphorylates and inactivates Atg proteins to inhibit autophagy. In contrast, deficiency of nutrients decreases the activity of the class I PI3K (phosphatidylinositol 3-kinase)-Akt axis, decreasing mTOR activity, and inducing autophagy. A second pathway involves Beclin-1, which binds Vps34, a class III PI3K, to promote autophagosome formation. Interestingly, Beclin-1 possesses a BH3 domain,[93] a motif discussed previously in connection with Bcl-2 proteins. Antiapoptotic Bcl-2 proteins, such as Bcl-2 and Bcl-x_L, interact with Beclin-1 through the Beclin-1 BH3 domain. Moreover, the binding of Bcl-2 and Bcl-x_L to Beclin-1 inhibits starvation-induced autophagy in the myocardium.[94] On the other hand, the binding of Beclin-1 does not abrogate the antiapoptotic effects of Bcl-2 and Bcl-x_L.[95]

Autophagic Cell Death

Because autophagic morphology (e.g., autophagosomes) can be observed in association with damaged/dying cells, the possibility has been raised that autophagic cell death may be an independent form of cell demise. The most pressing question is whether autophagy causes the resulting cell death versus merely being associated with it. The strongest evidence to date in support of a causal connection between autophagy and cell death comes from studies of salivary gland degradation during development in *Drosophila* showing that both apoptosis and autophagy play important roles.[12] A second critical question is whether specific death machinery carries out autophagic cell death and, if so, whether it is that used in apoptosis, necrosis, or novel. A third important question is what converts autophagy as a survival mechanism to autophagic cell death. One hypothesis is that too much autophagy begets autophagic cell death, while another is that the switch is unrelated to the intensity of autophagy. Clearly, further work is needed to resolve this question.

A general problem in the field of autophagic cell death research is that, in contrast to autophagy, there are no markers for autophagic cell death. The only way to diagnose autophagic cell death is by electron microscopy showing autophagosomes or autophagolysosomes in a degenerating cell. Although this is the gold standard, it presents several problems including not knowing for sure whether the cell is dead, and more importantly, not knowing whether autophagy is contributing to or ameliorating cell death. In many studies, electron microscopy is not carried out. Rather, autophagy is manipulated genetically, and changes in autophagy (not autophagic cell death) are correlated with a downstream functional readout.

PUTTING CELL DEATH TOGETHER

It is possible that different regulated death processes coexist in the same cell. We already know that, despite their distinct morphological features, the various forms of cell death share important mechanistic and functional connections. Mechanistic connections may take the form of common mediators such as Ca^{2+} (necrosis[83] and apoptosis[88]), Bcl-2 (apoptosis[26,35] and autophagy[94]), and others. Other potential connections between death processes may result from common or closely situated sites of action. For example, the IMM is central to MPTP opening in necrosis,[83] but is also involved in remodeling of cristae during apoptosis.[50] There are likely to be additional, more direct connections. For example, caspase 3 activated during apoptosis can cleave NDUFS1 (NADH dehydrogenase [ubiquinone] Fe-S protein 1), a component of respiratory complex 1 in the IMM to trigger a necrotic phenotype.[96] Presumably, caspase 3 gains access to this protein through the previously permeabilized OMM. Conversely, as described previously, rupture of the OMM during necrosis can allow the release of mitochondrial apoptogens,[7] although their contribution to the demise of the necrotic cell is unclear. Although not yet tested, these situations may place different death programs in series with one another, in addition to their conventional parallel relationships. These concepts raise the possibility of new relationships among death programs (see Whelan[97] for a more in-depth consideration).

LESSONS FROM MYOCARDIAL INFARCTION

Although the focus of this chapter is the role of cell death in heart failure, we will review the larger body of information pertaining to the regulation of cardiac myocyte death in models of myocardial infarction (for a more detailed discussion, see Foo[2] and Whelan,[97] and references therein). These models have been studied extensively both for their clinical relevance and because the large magnitude and limited time frame of cell death provides a more robust readout than the heart failure models. Rodent myocardial infarction models include (1) permanent surgical occlusion of the left coronary artery and (2) prolonged, but transient, surgical occlusion of the left coronary artery followed by reperfusion (I/R). Ischemia in either model subjects the myocardium to severe deficits of oxygen, nutrients, and survival factors and the buildup of H^+ and waste products. Reperfusion is the standard therapy for ST-segment elevation myocardial infarction because it results in net salvage of myocardium.[98] Despite this, reperfusion is accompanied by potentially toxic effects including oxidative stress from the sudden reintroduction of oxygenated blood; increased cytosolic and mitochondrial

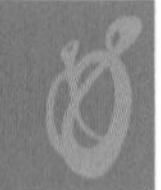

Ca^{2+}; too rapid normalization of intracellular acidosis, which can trigger MPTP opening; and inflammation.[99] Although the timing and proportions of apoptosis and necrosis vary with the model, both permanent coronary occlusion and I/R result in both forms of cell death in the infarct zone itself.[100-102] Autophagy also occurs during permanent coronary occlusion and I/R,[103,104] but data are lacking on autophagic cell death.

Myocardial I/R activates both the intrinsic and extrinsic apoptosis pathways. Mutations causing decreased abundance or function of multiple mediators in these pathways (e.g., Fas,[105] PUMA,[106] and Bax[107]) decrease cardiac myocyte apoptosis and infarct size and, when measured, lessen cardiac dysfunction in vivo. Similar results are obtained with overexpression of apoptosis inhibitors (Bcl-2,[108,109] ARC,[110] and c-IAP2[111]) and pharmacological inhibitors of caspases[112-115] or the serine protease of Omi/HtrA2.[116,117] These data indicate that the intrinsic and extrinsic apoptosis pathways mediate the death of cardiac myocytes during I/R.

In addition to apoptosis, I/R also elicits substantial amounts of cardiac myocyte necrosis. Deletion of cyclophilin D decreases necrotic death and lessens infarct size following I/R.[7,8] As previously discussed, similar results are obtained with necrostatin-1, an RIP1 kinase inhibitor.[90] These studies show that both the death receptor/RIP and cyclophilin D/MPTP necrosis pathways are important in myocardial infarction.

Autophagy is induced during permanent occlusion and I/R.[103,104] During permanent occlusion, increases in autophagy are mediated by AMPK (5′adenosine monophosphate-activated protein kinase), a negative regulator of mTOR. Overexpression of dominant negative AMPK inhibits induction of autophagy, and this is accompanied by increased infarct size.[104] These data suggest that autophagy plays a protective role during permanent occlusion, although pleiotropic effects of AMPK on metabolism and apoptosis must also be considered. Induction of autophagy during I/R is mediated by increases in Beclin-1 levels. Heterozygous deletion of Beclin-1 decreases infarct size during I/R, suggesting that autophagy is pathogenic in this setting,[103] although other data suggest a beneficial role for autophagy in this setting.[118] Thus the role of autophagy in I/R is currently unresolved. Note that the variable under study in these experiments is autophagy, not autophagic cell death.

Taken together, these data demonstrate that regulated cardiac myocyte death plays a critical causal role in the genesis of myocardial infarction during I/R. An important issue relates to the possible connections among death programs that were discussed previously. If the programs are connected in a substantial way, the interpretation of studies that perturb a given death program will need to be reinterpreted in light of their effects on other programs (i.e., while each of the genetic or pharmacological manipulations discussed previously clearly modulates infarct size, the question is through which death programs). Future experiments to assess connections among death programs will be critical in understanding the effect of mutations in one program on the others and on overall cell loss.

CELL DEATH AND HEART FAILURE

Various underlying diseases (e.g., prior myocardial infarction[s], hypertension, etc.) set into motion a complex series of molecular, cellular, and mechanical events that lead to heart failure.[1] The initial response is usually compensated cardiac hypertrophy, characterized by increased myocyte volume (primarily increases in cell width), addition of sarcomeres in parallel, increased wall thickness with normalization of wall stress, normal or reduced chamber volume, normal systolic function, and reversion to a "fetal program" of gene expression. Eventually, however, there is a transition to overt heart failure, characterized by chamber dilation, wall thinning, and deterioration of systolic function. Myocytes exhibit increased length with sarcomeres arranged in a series. Moreover, there is evidence of myocyte loss, which may occur by apoptosis, necrosis, and autophagic cell death.[119,120] The molecular and cellular basis of the transition from compensated hypertrophy to heart failure is not understood. As previously noted, multiple processes have been implicated including derangements in signaling, Ca^{2+}/excitation-contraction coupling, energetics, contractile proteins, and cytoskeleton, inflammation, and cell death.

In this section, we will focus on cardiac myocyte death as a causal component for both myocardial remodeling and failure. While the central events of cell death described previously are common to most death signals, the upstream pathways are usually stimulus-specific. Accordingly, we will first discuss connections between stimuli of clinical relevance to heart failure and cell death. Second, we will consider genetic and pharmacological models that attempt to isolate the critical issue of whether cell death is playing a causal role in the pathogenesis of heart failure.

Stimuli and Pathways That Mediate Cardiac Myocyte Death in Heart Failure

Stretch

As shown in rats, chronic pressure overload induces cardiac hypertrophy accompanied by myocyte apoptosis.[121] Pressure overload is mediated by a complex interplay of mechanical and humoral factors. While the exact signaling events are unclear, some data link mechanical stretch with cell death. First, stretch can induce myocyte apoptosis in isolated rat papillary muscles accompanied by increased ROS.[122] Second, cardiac myocyte in vivo can lead to anoikis, disruption of cellular anchorage seen in apoptotic death.[123] Third, stretch of isolated rat cardiac myocytes elicits the release of angiotensin II, resulting in both cardiac hypertrophy[124] and apoptosis.[125] As will be discussed later, survival signals appear important in suppressing mouse cardiac myocyte apoptosis in response to hemodynamic overload.[126] In summary, stretch induces cardiac myocyte apoptosis through incompletely defined signaling pathways in association with the transition to heart failure.

Adrenergic Signaling

Levels of plasma norepinephrine correlate directly with the severity of heart failure[127] and mortality in humans.[128] Cardiac-specific overexpression of the β_1-adrenergic receptor (β_1AR) leads to hypertrophy with enhanced function in younger mice, but chamber dilation and dysfunction accompanied by increased cardiac myocyte apoptosis in older mice.[129,130] Most of the harmful effects of β-adrenergic receptor activation, including cardiac myocyte apoptosis, are mediated by the β_1-isoform.[131] In contrast, the β_2-isoform inhibits apoptosis.[132] For example, inhibition of the β_1-isoform and activation of the β_2-isoform attenuate myocyte apoptosis in a rodent model of postinfarct remodeling.[133] As the β_1-isoform is most abundant in the myocardium, the net effect of catecholamines is induction of apoptosis.

Although the mechanism by which β_1AR activation causes cardiac myocyte apoptosis is not well understood, calcium/calmodulin-dependent protein kinase II (CaMKII) has been shown in mouse cells to play an important role.[134] Interestingly, the classic cAMP-protein kinase A pathway does not appear to be critical. β_1AR activation increases CaMKII activity.[134] Moreover, transgenic cardiac-specific overexpression of CaMKII-δ, the predominant isoform, exacerbates isoproterenol-induced cardiac myocyte apoptosis[134] and precipitates lethal heart failure.[135] Conversely, general inhibition or CaMKII or deletion of CaMKII-δ ameliorates cardiac myocyte apoptosis induced by isoproterenol or prior myocardial infarction[134,136] and blunts the

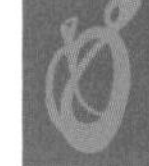

development of hypertrophy or failure in response to hemodynamic overload in mice.[137,138] Thus CaMKII-δ mediates β_1AR-induced cardiac myocyte death. Identification of relevant CaMKII-δ substrates will likely extend our understanding of this pathway.

Renin-Angiotensin-Aldosterone System

The renin-angiotensin-aldosterone system is one of the major neurohumoral pathways in heart failure. Interruption of this axis ameliorates cardiac remodeling and dysfunction, and improves morbidity and mortality in a variety of pathological contexts in humans.[139] Renin-angiotensin-aldosterone signaling can affect cardiac myocytes directly or indirectly through alteration of systemic hemodynamics. In addition, cardiac myocytes possess an intrinsic "local" renin-angiotensin system that acts in an autocrine/paracrine manner. This complexity makes it difficult to identify precise mechanisms responsible for the striking clinical benefits noted previously. These caveats notwithstanding, angiotensin II and aldosterone each induce apoptosis in isolated rat cardiac myocytes through activation of the angiotensin II type 1 (AT_1) and mineralocorticoid receptors, respectively.[140,141] Knockout or pharmacological blockade of AT_1 lessens cardiac myocyte apoptosis induced by doxorubicin or diabetes in rodents in vivo.[142,143] Similarly, blockade of the mineralocorticoid receptor attenuates postinfarct remodeling and periinfarct apoptosis in rats.[144] The mechanism by which AT_1 activation brings about apoptosis is incompletely understood. AT_1 can signal through Gαq to transcriptionally activate Nix, a BH3-only-like protein that stimulates cardiac myocyte apoptosis in mice.[145] AT_1 may also induce myocyte apoptosis through NADPH oxidase (nicotinamide adenine dinucleotide phosphate-oxidase) and ASK1 (apoptosis signal-regulating kinase 1).[146,147] Additional evidence suggests a positive feedback loop in which AT_1 activates p53, whose target genes may include angiotensinogen and AT_1.[146]

Proinflammatory Cytokines

Proinflammatory cytokines play an important role in heart failure via their effects on myocyte contractility, inflammation, and cell death and endothelial function. The cytokines most relevant to heart failure are TNF, interleukin (IL)-1, and IL-6. In the Framingham Heart Study, elevated levels of TNF and IL-6 were associated with increased risk of heart failure in asymptomatic patients without prior myocardial infarction.[148] Among other effects, IL-1 and TNF can induce apoptosis in isolated rat cardiac myocytes.[149,150] As discussed previously, however, TNF activates survival and death pathways simultaneously under many conditions and, therefore, does not kill efficiently.[74,75] IL-6 is believed to be antiapoptotic.

Cardiac-specific overexpression of TNF in mice causes cardiac hypertrophy, dilation, and dysfunction accompanied by induction of cardiac myocyte apoptosis via the extrinsic and intrinsic pathways.[151,152] Deletion of TNFR1 blunts heart failure and improves survival in TNF overexpressors, while deletion of TNFR2 does the opposite.[152] Moreover, TNFR1 promotes, and TNFR2 inhibits, cardiac myocyte apoptosis during postinfarction remodeling.[153] Thus, it appears that TNFR1 mediates the deleterious effects of excess TNF on postinfarct remodeling, while TNFR2 is protective. In contrast, infarct size following permanent occlusion is unaffected by deletion of either TNFR1 or TNFR2, but rather is increased significantly by deletion of both, and this is accompanied by increased apoptosis but not necrosis.[154] Thus, both TNFR1 and TNFR2 seem to exert a protective role during acute infarction. These data underscore divergent roles played by TNF receptor subtypes in different contexts.

The ability of TNF antagonism to improve heart failure in humans has been assessed in three clinical trials. RENAISSANCE (Randomized Etanercept North American Strategy to Study AntagoNism of CytokinEs)[155] and RECOVER (Research into Etanercept CytOkine antagonism in VEntriculaR dysfunction)[155] used etanercept, a soluble TNFR2 fusion protein, while ATTACH (Anti-TNFα Therapy Against Congestive Heart failure)[156] used infliximab, a mouse-human chimeric monoclonal antibody that specifically and potently binds to and neutralizes soluble TNF homotrimer. These clinical trials failed to demonstrate any beneficial role of TNF inhibition in heart failure. Possible explanations include inadequate dosing or duration of treatment, upregulation of endogenous TNF (not measured), redundancy of other proinflammatory cytokines in heart failure pathogenesis, and complexities of TNF signaling including possibly opposing effects of the receptor subtypes. Regarding the latter, the treatment strategy in these trials may have abrogated beneficial, as well as deleterious, effects.

Heart Failure and Apoptosis

In contrast to the large but brief burst of apoptosis during myocardial infarction, heart failure is characterized by a modest—but clearly elevated—level of cardiac myocyte apoptosis that can persist for months. This is illustrated by patients with end-stage dilated cardiomyopathy who exhibit rates of cardiac myocyte apoptosis of 0.08% to 0.25% compared with 0.001% to 0.002% in controls.[157-159] Many studies have assessed the role of cardiac myocyte apoptosis in the pathogenesis of heart failure. We will review several that have been particularly illustrative of key points.

Although clearly higher than controls, the modest rates of apoptosis in failing hearts call into question a role for cell death in heart failure. On the other hand, heart failure is a protracted syndrome, opening up the possibility that even moderately elevated levels of cell death could result in substantial cell loss over time. To resolve this question, transgenic mice were created with cardiac-specific expression of a caspase 8 allele that exhibits low levels of activation at baseline (Figure 6-4).[160] These mice develop a lethal dilated cardiomyopathy over 2 to 6 months. In contrast, nontransgenic mice and mice expressing an enzymatically-dead caspase 8 at similar levels are normal. Control mice exhibit apoptotic rates of 0.001% to 0.002%. In contrast, rates of cardiac myocyte apoptosis in mice expressing the activated caspase 8 allele were 0.023%, or tenfold higher. Notably, these rates of apoptosis are threefold to tenfold lower than the rates in patients with dilated cardiomyopathy as specified previously. Thus this transgenic model illustrates that a modest, although elevated, rate of cardiac myocyte apoptosis is sufficient to cause a lethal dilated cardiomyopathy over time. To test whether cardiac myocyte apoptosis in this model is causally linked with heart failure, a caspase inhibitor was administered chronically before the development of cardiomyopathy. The caspase inhibitor decreased cardiac myocyte apoptosis (as expected) and markedly attenuated development of left ventricular dilation and dysfunction over time. These data demonstrate a causal connection between modest levels of cardiac myocyte apoptosis and heart failure.

While the caspase 8 transgenic mice are informative with respect to one of the most critical questions, this gain-of-function model is ultimately artificial. Accordingly, the goal of the next level of inquiry was to assess the effect of inhibiting cardiac myocyte apoptosis in models of heart failure. Gαq transduces hypertrophic signals from the AT_1, endothelin, and α_1-adrenergic receptors. Accordingly, transgenic cardiac-specific overexpression of Gαq results in hypertrophy. This transitions to heart failure accompanied by cardiac myocyte apoptosis.[161] In addition, a high proportion of pregnant Gαq transgenic females die from fulminant cardiomyopathy accompanied by high rates of cardiac myocyte apoptosis.[162] Transcriptional profiling of the hearts of Gαq transgenic mice

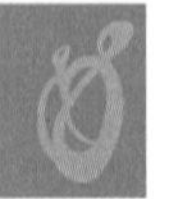

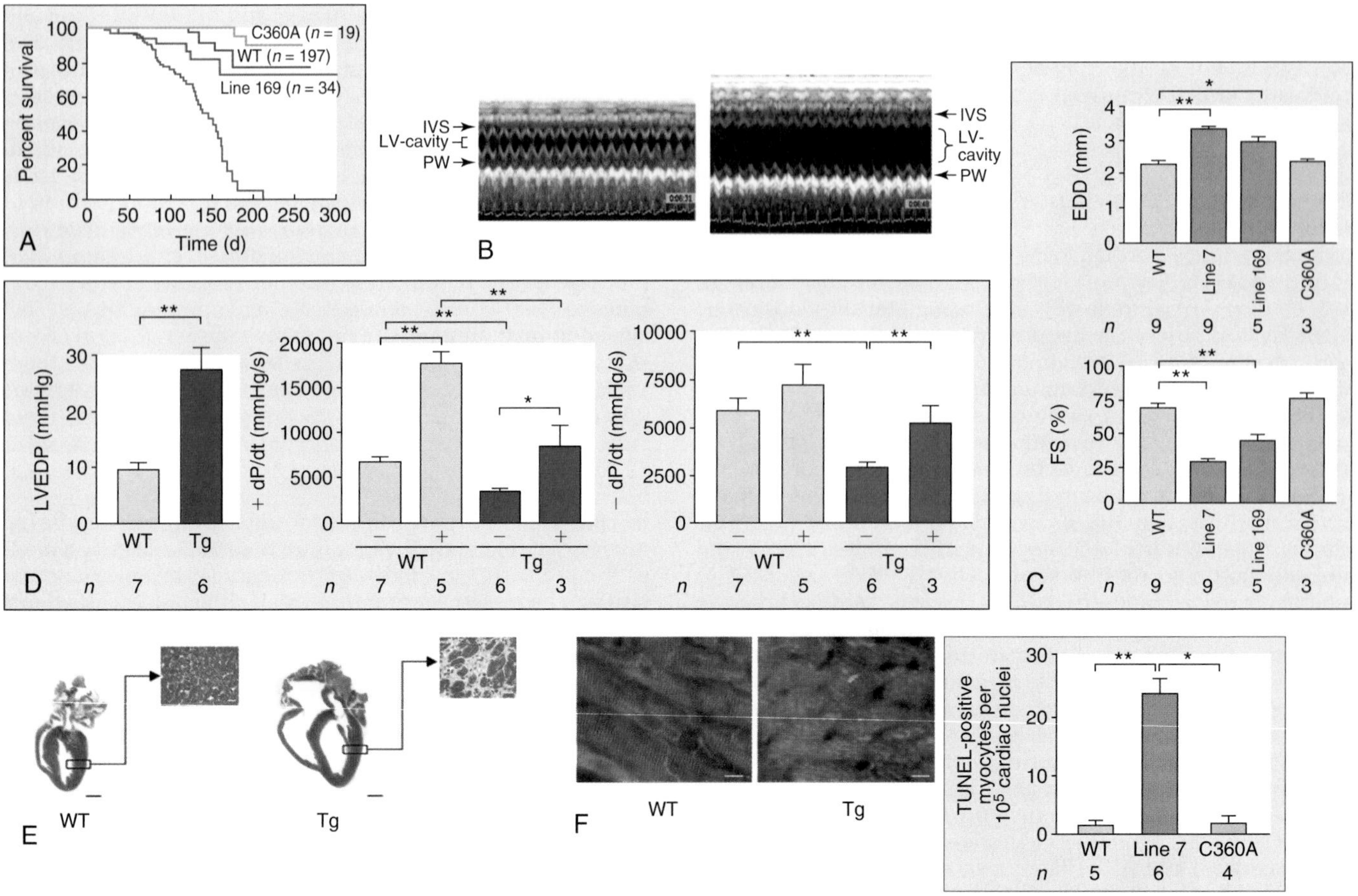

FIGURE 6-4 Very low levels of cardiac myocyte apoptosis are sufficient to induce a lethal, dilated cardiomyopathy.[160] Mice with cardiac-specific transgenic overexpression of a modified caspase 8 allele exhibited chronic low, but abnormal, levels of cardiac myocyte apoptosis, cardiomyopathy, and premature death. The transgene protein consisted of the p20 and p10 catalytic subunits of human procaspase 8 fused to a trimer of the FK binding protein (FKBP) and a myristoylation signal to target the protein to the plasma membrane. Not shown here: Administration of the dimeric FKBP ligand, FK1012H2, triggers forced dimerization and activation of the caspase 8 transgene protein leading to rapid destruction of the heart and death of the mouse (see Figure 1 in Wencker[160]). However, even in the absence of FK1012H2, chronic, low-level activation of the caspase 8 transgene protein results in modest, but abnormal, levels of cardiac myocyte apoptosis, cardiomyopathy, and organismal death over 6 months. **A,** Kaplan-Meier survival curve showing increased mortality in line 7 mice that express the caspase 8 transgene at higher levels. In contrast, mortality is normal in line 169 mice that express the caspase 8 transgene at lower levels and in line C360A, which expresses high levels of a catalytically inactive caspase 8 mutant. $P < .0001$ for line 7 vs. wild type (WT), line C360A, or line 169. **B** and **C,** Representative echocardiograms and quantification demonstrating left ventricular dilation and markedly decreased fractional shortening in lines 7 and 169. *EDD,* left ventricular end-diastolic dimension; *FS,* fractional shortening. $^{*}P < .01$, $^{**}P < .001$. **D,** Left ventricular hemodynamics showing that line 7 transgenics exhibit increased left ventricular end-diastolic pressure (LVEDP) and decreased +dP/dt and −dP/dt at baseline (−) and in response to isoproterenol (+). $^{*}P < .02$, $^{**}P < .002$. **E,** Hematoxylin and eosin staining of coronal heart sections (bar 1 mm) and Masson trichrome staining in boxed insets (bar 25 μm) illustrate cardiomegaly and fibrosis, respectively, in transgenic hearts. **F,** Increased cardiac myocyte apoptosis in caspase 8 transgenic mice. Left panels: Double staining for TUNEL (*green*) and desmin (*red,* to identify myocytes) in hearts of WT and transgenic line 7 (bar 10 μm). Right panel: Quantification of TUNEL-positive cardiac myocytes per 10^5 nuclei in WT, transgenic line 7, and C360A mice. $^{*}P < .002$, $^{**}P < .0003$. Note that rates of cardiac myocyte apoptosis as low as 23 per 10^5 (compared with 1 to 2 per 10^5 in WT) were sufficient to beget a lethal, dilated cardiomyopathy. (Reproduced with permission from Wencker D, Chandra M, Nguyen K, et al. A mechanistic role for cardiac myocyte apoptosis in heart failure. *J Clin Invest* 2003;111(10):1497-1504.)

revealed induction in the expression of Nix/Bnip3L (Nip3 [19 kDa interacting protein-3]-like protein X/Bcl-2/adenovirus E1B), a BH3-only-like protein.[145] Transgenic expression of Nix/Bnip3L in mice is accompanied by dramatic cardiac myocyte apoptosis and increased mortality.[145] In contrast, transgenic expression of sNix, a dominant negative splice variant of Nix/Bnip3L, attenuates cardiac myocyte apoptosis, cardiac dysfunction, and mortality in the peripartum cardiomyopathy of Gαq transgenic mice.[145] Similarly, caspase inhibition rescues the Gαq peripartum cardiomyopathy.[163] Thus, overexpression of Gαq leads to transcriptional activation of Nix/Bnip3L expression, which triggers apoptosis. From the perspective of the pathogenesis of heart failure, the most important conclusion from these experiments is that cardiac myocyte apoptosis is a critical component of heart failure.

The next set of experiments examines the role of cardiac myocyte apoptosis in postinfarct remodeling (Figure 6-5). Bnip3 (Bcl-2/adenovirus E1B 19 kDa interacting protein 3) is a BH3-only-like protein that is induced in cardiac myocytes by hypoxia and heart failure. Generalized knockout of Bnip3 in the mouse does not affect infarct size in response to I/R, perhaps because the time window for hypoxic induction is too narrow. In contrast, Bnip3 deletion attenuates cardiac myocyte apoptosis in the periinfarct and remote myocardium, and lessens postinfarct remodeling and cardiac dysfunction.[164] Viral transduction of the antiapoptotic Bcl-2 into rabbit myocardium results in similar findings.[165] These data indicate an important role for cardiac myocyte apoptosis in postinfarct remodeling.

Endogenous survival mechanisms often function to help cells withstand stressful stimuli. If stimuli are too noxious or prolonged, the endogenous survival mechanism is often inactivated, allowing the cell to die. Cardiac myocytes are subjected to ongoing biomechanical stress. The next set of experiments suggests that the gp130 pathway may provide a survival mechanism that allows cardiac myocytes to withstand not only basal stress but also increased biomechanical

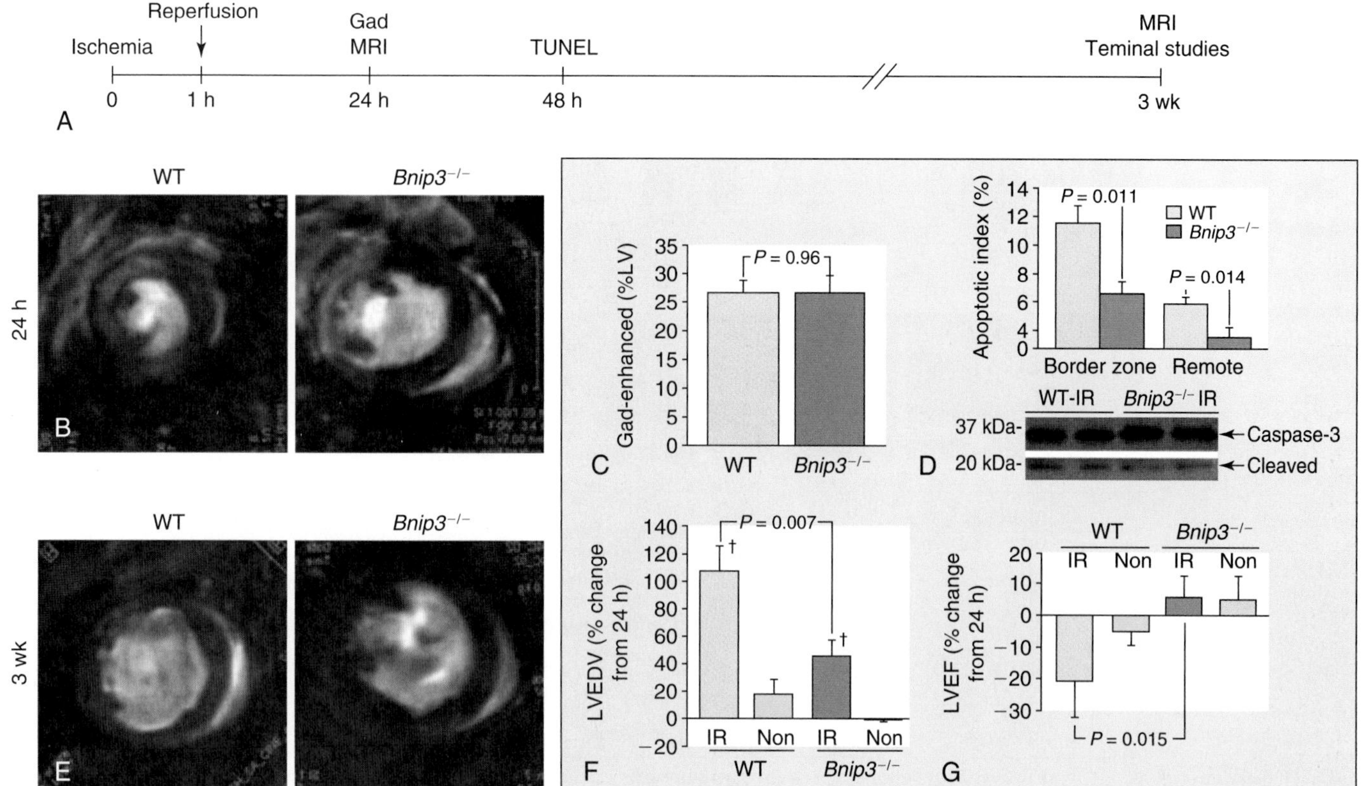

FIGURE 6–5 Effects of Bnip3 ablation on postinfarct remodeling.[164] **A,** Schematic depiction of experimental design for in vivo I/R studies. *Gad,* gadolinium. **B** and **C,** Representative gadolinium-enhanced (*white*) MRI midventricle end-diastolic images 24 hours after I/R showing no significant difference in infarct size in WT and Bnip3−/− mice. **D,** TUNEL and caspase 3 activation 48 hours after I/R. The number of TUNEL-positive cells is decreased significantly in the border zone and remote myocardium of Bnip3−/− mice 48 hours postinfarct. **E-G,** Representative midventricle end-diastolic MRI images 3 weeks after I/R and quantitative analysis of MRI-derived LV end-diastolic volume (LVEDV) and LV ejection fraction (LVEF) as compared with these parameters at 24 hours. Deletion of Bnip3 attenuates post-I/R abnormalities in both LVEDV and LVEF. This study shows that the proapoptotic BH3-only-like protein Bnip3 plays a role in postinfarct remodeling following I/R. The absence of an effect of Bnip3 on infarct size may be due to inadequate time for its induction by hypoxia following I/R. (Reproduced with permission from Diwan A, Krenz M, Syed FM, et al. Inhibition of ischemic cardiomyocyte apoptosis through targeted ablation of Bnip3 restrains postinfarction remodeling in mice. *J Clin Invest* 2007;117(10):2825-2833.)

stress during hemodynamic overload. gp130 is a subunit of the receptors that bind several prosurvival cytokines of the IL-6 family, including cardiotrophin-1 (which mediates cardiac hypertrophy), LIF (leukemia inhibitory factor), IL-6, and oncostatin M. Cardiac-specific deletion of gp130 in the mouse results in no baseline cardiac abnormalities. The imposition of hemodynamic overload from transverse aortic constriction, however, precipitates massive cardiac myocyte apoptosis and fulminant cardiomyopathy.[126] Absence of gp130 abrogates hemodynamic overload-induced phosphorylation of STAT3 (signal transducer and activator of transcription 3), which in turn prevents activation of the transcription of antiapoptotic Bcl-x_L. These results suggest that the gp130 pathway provides an endogenous survival mechanism that suppresses hemodynamic overload-induced cardiac myocyte apoptosis and heart failure.

Heart Failure and Necrosis

Rates of necrosis are increased in human heart failure.[119,120] The recent recognition that necrosis can be regulated and that regulated necrosis is critical to myocardial damage during I/R has suggested the possibility that necrosis is also important for the pathogenesis of heart failure.[6-9,74] Of note, this idea has been previously suggested.[119,120,157] To assess the role of necrosis in heart failure, this death process was inhibited genetically (Figure 6-6). For these experiments, a new model was created in which Ca^{2+} overload from transgenic overexpression of the β_2a subunit of the L-type Ca^{2+} channel triggers progressive cardiac myocyte necrosis, heart failure, and mortality.[13] These abnormalities were attenuated by deletion of cyclophilin D, which abrogates necrosis. Interestingly, overexpression of the antiapoptotic Bcl-2 had no effect on this phenotype. Cyclophilin D deletion also lessened heart failure in a model of doxorubicin-induced cardiomyopathy. These data provide the initial proof of concept that cardiac myocyte necrosis plays a crucial role in the pathogenesis of heart failure. It will be important to retest this hypothesis in additional clinically relevant models of heart failure, such as those resulting from hemodynamic overload and myocardial infarction.

Heart Failure and Autophagy

Rates of cardiac myocyte autophagic cell death, determined by electron microscopy, have been reported to be increased in human heart failure.[119,120,166] Experiments have assessed the role of autophagy, but not autophagic cell death per se, in heart failure. In the first set of studies, autophagy was inhibited in the hearts of adult mice by cardiac-specific deletion of Atg5.[167] Loss of autophagy in the baseline state precipitated severe heart failure accompanied by increased abundance of ubiquitinated proteins and cardiac myocyte apoptosis, the latter possibly due to proteotoxic ER stress. In contrast, when Atg5 was deleted at embryonic day 8.0, no abnormalities were evident at birth, probably due to compensation. When these animals were stressed with transverse aortic constriction, however, mice lacking Atg5 went into heart failure, while

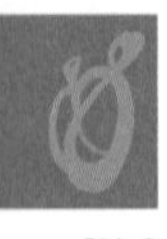

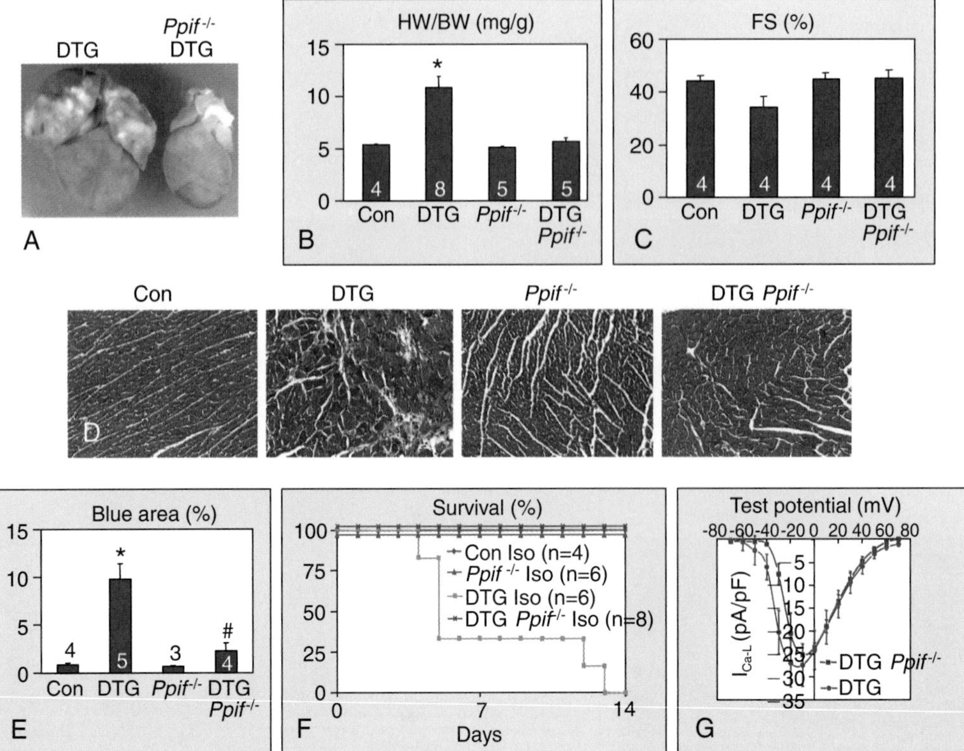

FIGURE 6–6 Loss of cyclophilin D rescues cardiomyopathy in transgenic mice with Ca^{2+} overload.[13] Transgenic mice with cardiac-specific, inducible overexpression of the β_2a subunit of the L-type Ca^{2+} channel (LTCC) were generated, resulting in enhanced Ca^{2+} currents in cardiac myocytes, cardiac myocyte necrosis, and cardiomyopathy. This figure shows that simultaneous deletion of cyclophilin D, which regulates MPTP opening, significantly rescues this cardiomyopathy. Necrosis is normally thought of as a mechanism of ischemic death. The importance of this work is that it implicates necrosis as a mechanism of heart failure. Although the model employed is artificial, the paper also suggests that necrosis may play a role in doxorubicin-induced cardiomyopathy. In this figure, DTG (double transgenic) denotes mice that overexpress the β_2a subunit of the LTCC in cardiac myocytes in the absence of doxycycline. (Note: doxycycline is absent in the experiments depicted here.) The gene encoding cyclophilin D is called *ppif*, and *ppif*–/– denotes a knockout of both alleles of this gene. **A,** Gross morphology of hearts from a DTG mouse and a DTG mouse lacking *ppif*. Note the decrease in size of the DTG, *ppif*–/– heart. **B,** Heart weight normalized to body weight measurements showing that deletion of *ppif* decreases the hypertrophy of DTG hearts. **C,** Echocardiographic measurements of fractional shortening showing that deletion of *ppif* in DTG mice trends toward preservation of function (not significant). **D** and **E,** Masson trichrome staining of cardiac sections showing increased fibrosis in DTG and rescued by deletion of *ppif*. **F,** The drug isoproterenol synergizes with transgenic β_2a overexpression to cause Ca^{2+} overload. Accordingly, mortality was scored during a 14-day infusion of isoproterenol. Mortality of DTG mice was markedly increased. In contrast, deletion of *ppif* in the context of DTG resulted in zero mortality. **G,** This is a control panel showing that deletion of *ppif* does not affect Ca^{2+} currents at different test potentials. **P* <.05 versus control; #*P* <.05 versus DTG. (Reproduced with permission from Nakayama H, Chen X, Baines CP, et al. Ca^{2+} - and mitochondrial-dependent cardiomyocyte necrosis as a primary mediator of heart failure. *J Clin Invest* 2007;117(9):2431-2444).

wild-type mice did not.[167] Of note, both genotypes exhibited similar degrees of cardiac hypertrophy. These data suggest that (1) basal levels of autophagy are critical for maintaining normal cardiac myocyte structure, function, and survival and (2) autophagy is required during hemodynamic overload to avoid transitioning into heart failure. Taken together, this set of experiments suggests that autophagy is a compensatory mechanism in heart failure.

The role of autophagy in hemodynamic overload-induced heart failure was also assessed by using Beclin-$1^{+/-}$ mice to inhibit autophagy.[168] When subjected to transverse aortic constriction, Beclin-$1^{+/-}$ mice exhibit reduced autophagy, pathological cardiac remodeling, and cardiac dysfunction as compared with wild-type mice. The degree of hypertrophy was similar to wild-type mice, however. Conversely, transgenic overexpression of Beclin-1 augmented autophagy and pathological remodeling in response to transverse aortic constriction. These data suggest that autophagy plays a pathological role in heart failure due to hemodynamic overload.

The Atg$5^{-/-}$ and Beclin-$1^{+/-}$ studies yielded opposite conclusions regarding the role of autophagy in hemodynamic overload-induced heart failure. Although an explanation is not evident, there are differences between the studies. First, the genetic manipulations differ. Second, the degree of inhibition of autophagy differs in that both alleles were inactivated in the case of *Atg5,* while only a single *Beclin-1* allele was inactivated. Third, the transverse aortic constriction model was probably more severe in the Beclin-$1^{+/-}$ study. Although it is difficult to know how these differences may account for the opposing conclusions, one possibility is that autophagy is protective early in the disease process and pathological later. If the mice in the Beclin-$1^{+/-}$ study were at a later stage of the disease, perhaps inhibition of autophagy at this stage would reveal a pathological role. Further work is needed to explore these and other possibilities.

The role of autophagy was also examined in a model of desmin-related cardiomyopathy (transgenic mice expressing R120G mutation of αB crystallin).[169] Inhibition of autophagy by deleting one allele of *beclin-1* increased polyubiquitinated proteins and aggregates, fibrosis, cardiac dysfunction, heart failure, and mortality. Thus autophagy plays an adaptive/protective function in this model of desmin-related cardiomyopathy.

The previous two studies, both using Beclin-$1^{+/-}$ mice, conclude that autophagy plays opposite roles in heart failure induced by hemodynamic overload versus desmin-related cardiomyopathy. While the manipulated gene and gene dosage are identical, the studies differ markedly with respect to the stimulus for heart failure. The key stimulus in desmin-related cardiomyopathy is proteotoxicity, which will induce

ER stress and possibly cell death. Autophagy would be expected to mitigate proteotoxic stress, consistent with the adaptive role reported previously. Hemodynamic overload, on the other hand, involves a number of mechanical and humoral stimuli, oxidative stress, and abnormalities in myocardial energetics. Many of these stimuli potentially interface with autophagy pathways, although it is difficult to predict which would dominate. Future efforts to delineate how various component stimuli impact differentially on autophagy will provide insights into the roles of autophagy in heart failure of various causes.

As previously mentioned, an important caveat regarding the previously noted studies is that autophagy, not autophagic cell death, was perturbed, measured, and correlated with a downstream readout. Thus, the only conclusion that can be drawn at this time pertains to the effects of changes in autophagy itself—not autophagic cell death—on heart failure.

CELL DEATH IN HEART DISEASE: THE BIG PICTURE

Apoptosis, necrosis, and autophagic cell death take place during myocardial infarction and heart failure and impact on pathogenesis in the ways discussed previously. Despite this, little is known about the *relative* contributions of each type of cell death to either syndrome. A temporal and spatial map of the number of cell deaths attributable to each death program is needed for each syndrome. This information has not been easy to acquire, however, due to technical and conceptual issues.

The technical issues have to do with molecular markers used to identify the various forms of cell death. While reasonable markers exist for apoptosis, there are far fewer for necrosis, especially when assessing intact tissues. Moreover, as discussed previously, markers for autophagic cell death (as opposed to autophagy) are lacking. In addition, the utility of any marker is limited by its temporal window of sensitivity, the complexity of which is magnified when attempting to use markers to quantify several forms of cell death. While labor intensive, electron microscopy can simultaneously detect apoptosis, necrosis, and perhaps autophagic cell death and, thereby, address some of these concerns.

The conceptual issue has to do with the aforementioned possibility that different forms of cell death are linked. It should be emphasized that this is only a theoretical consideration at present. Cross talk between parallel death pathways has already been demonstrated. If death programs are also linked (e.g., in series), dying cells may exhibit hybrid morphologies and markers. These issues will require reexamination pending a better understanding of the relationships among the death programs (see Whelan[97] for a more detailed discussion).

These holes in knowledge aside, we will consider the current best assessment as to the types of cell death that occur during myocardial infarction and heart failure. Myocytes in the infarct zone appear to die by both necrosis and apoptosis during myocardial infarction (whether infarction is induced by I/R or permanent coronary occlusion).[100,101] In the case of I/R, manipulations that decrease either necrosis or apoptosis reduce infarct size, consistent with the notion that both necrosis and apoptosis causally contribute to generation of the infarct. Autophagy also occurs during myocardial infarction,[103,104] but as discussed previously, its role in myocardial damage appears to vary. It may be protective in permanent coronary occlusion, and perhaps detrimental in I/R, although this result remains controversial.

Cardiac myocytes die by apoptosis and necrosis during heart failure, and genetic manipulation of each of these death programs can limit pathological remodeling and deterioration of cardiac function. At this point, apoptosis has been studied in a wider variety of models than has necrosis. Thus, the importance of necrosis in heart failure remains to be determined. Results are presently inconclusive concerning a role for autophagy in heart failure.

TRANSLATION INTO THERAPEUTICS

Work in rodent models has provided strong evidence that cardiac myocyte death is a critical mechanism in the pathogenesis of heart failure. Whether these conclusions translate to humans remains to be assessed. In addition, it is crucial to note that cardiac myocyte death is not the only important factor in heart failure. Indeed, dysfunction of individual cardiac myocytes, resulting from mechanisms that will be discussed elsewhere in this volume, are also important factors. Nevertheless, there has been intense interest in devising ways to inhibit cardiac myocyte death because cell death is irreversible once completed. Given the existence of a substantial body of information concerning apoptosis and a promising start to understanding necrosis, it is tempting to consider the possibility of novel heart failure therapies directed at inhibiting cardiac myocyte death. In fact, some current therapies (β_1AR blockers, angiotensin II converting enzyme inhibitors, and angiotensin II type 1 receptor blockers) inhibit myocyte apoptosis, although the importance of this antiapoptotic effect in their overall actions is not clear.

Multiple antiapoptotic and antinecrotic agents have been tested for their abilities to inhibit cardiac myocyte death in rodent models of I/R. Promising small molecules include polycaspase inhibitors, UCF-101 (inhibits the serine protease activity of Omi/HtrA2), cyclosporine A (inhibits MPTP opening), and necrostatin-1 (inhibits kinase activity of RIP1). We have recently reviewed these[97] and other[2] potential therapies. In contrast to I/R, there has been minimal evaluation of cell death inhibitors in heart failure models. One exception is that caspase inhibition has been shown to improve cardiac function and/or mortality in the caspase 8 transgenic heart failure model[160] and the Gαq transgenic peripartum cardiomyopathy model,[163] discussed previously.

Beyond the question of which specific anti–cell death therapy may work is the larger question of safety. In contrast to ischemia-reperfusion where one can envision inhibiting cell death for 8 to 24 hours, inhibition of cell death as a treatment for heart failure would potentially be chronic. If administered systemically, cancer would be a likely complication, which some patients might find unacceptable. On the other hand, advanced heart failure is a lethal disease with limited treatment options for most. If an effective anti–cell death therapy existed for heart failure, an informed patient with advanced heart failure may deem the risk of cancer to be acceptable, just as a patient treated with certain chemotherapeutic agents accepts the risk of cardiomyopathy.

This discussion leads to a consideration of whether anti–cell death therapy could be administered locally to the heart, where it would hopefully eliminate or minimize the risk of cancer. There are at least two obvious approaches. The first is cardiac gene therapy. Given the chronic nature of heart failure, this may be one of the few instances in which there is adequate time to contemplate this approach. While a discussion of technical details is beyond the scope of this chapter, presumably the gene of interest would be driven by a cardiac myocyte-specific promoter and enhancer sequences (e.g., α-cardiac myosin heavy chain promoter). With gene therapy, the repertoire of anti–cell death approaches would be expanded to large molecules. For example, one could employ Bcl-2 (or a stable mutant of Bcl-2). Of course, this approach may still entail various issues that have beset gene therapy to date, including delivery of the vector, efficiency of transduction, duration of expression, safety of the vector, and expressed gene. A second local approach could be based on materials science/nanotechnology. This would involve the long-term deployment of small molecules or viral vectors in the myocardium. Further thought is needed if anti–cell death therapy is to become a reality for heart failure.

SUMMARY

Heart failure is accompanied by chronic low levels of cardiac myocyte death, which are 10-fold to 100-fold higher than those seen in nonfailing hearts. Cardiac myocytes die by apoptosis, necrosis, and perhaps autophagic cell death. Inhibition of apoptosis or necrosis in rodent models diminishes pathological cardiac remodeling, cardiac dysfunction, and in some cases, mortality. The recognition that much of cardiac myocyte death (apoptosis and necrosis) is actively mediated begs the question as to whether anti–cell death therapies for human heart failure could be developed.

ACKNOWLEDGMENTS

We thank Gerald Dorn and Jeffery Molkentin for use of published figures. We thank Vladimir Kaplinskiy for critical reading of the manuscript. RNK was supported by NIH grants R01HL60665, P01HL078825, and P60DK020541, a New York State Stem Cell Initiative grant, The Dr. Gerald and Myra Dorros Chair in Cardiovascular Disease, and the David Himelberg Foundation. We are very grateful for the generous support of the Wilf Family Cardiovascular Research Institute.

REFERENCES

1. Mudd, J. O., & Kass, D. A. (2008). Tackling heart failure in the twenty-first century. *Nature, 451*(7181), 919–928.
2. Foo, R. S., Mani, K., & Kitsis, R. N. (2005). Death begets failure in the heart. *J Clin Invest, 115*(3), 565–571.
3. Kubo, H., Jaleel, N., Kumarapeli, A., et al. (2008). Increased cardiac myocyte progenitors in failing human hearts. *Circulation, 118*(6), 649–657.
4. Bersell, K., Arab, S., Haring, B., et al. (2009). Neuregulin1/ErbB4 signaling induces cardiomyocyte proliferation and repair of heart injury. *Cell, 138*(2), 257–270.
5. Ellis, H. M., & Horvitz, H. R. (1986). Genetic control of programmed cell death in the nematode C. elegans. *Cell, 44*(6), 817–829.
6. Holler, N., Zaru, R., Micheau, O., et al. (2000). Fas triggers an alternative, caspase-8-independent cell death pathway using the kinase RIP as effector molecule. *Nat Immunol, 1*(6), 489–495.
7. Baines, C. P., Kaiser, R. A., Purcell, N. H., et al. (2005). Loss of cyclophilin D reveals a critical role for mitochondrial permeability transition in cell death. *Nature, 434*(7033), 658–662.
8. Nakagawa, T., Shimizu, S., Watanabe, T., et al. (2005). Cyclophilin D-dependent mitochondrial permeability transition regulates some necrotic but not apoptotic cell death. *Nature, 434*(7033), 652–658.
9. Schinzel, A. C., Takeuchi, O., Huang, Z., et al. (2005). Cyclophilin D is a component of mitochondrial permeability transition and mediates neuronal cell death after focal cerebral ischemia. *Proc Natl Acad Sci U S A, 102*(34), 12005–12010.
10. Mizushima, N., Levine, B., Cuervo, A. M., et al. (2008). Autophagy fights disease through cellular self-digestion. *Nature, 451*(7182), 1069–1075.
11. Yoshida, H., Kong, Y. Y., Yoshida, R., et al. (1998). Apaf1 is required for mitochondrial pathways of apoptosis and brain development. *Cell, 94*(6), 739–750.
12. Berry, D. L., & Baehrecke, E. H. (2007). Growth arrest and autophagy are required for salivary gland cell degradation in *Drosophila. Cell, 131*(6), 1137–1148.
13. Nakayama, H., Chen, X., Baines, C. P., et al. (2007). $Ca^{2+/-}$ and mitochondrial-dependent cardiomyocyte necrosis as a primary mediator of heart failure. *J Clin Invest, 117*(9), 2431–2444.
14. Oltersdorf, T., Elmore, S. W., Shoemaker, A. R., et al. (2005). An inhibitor of Bcl-2 family proteins induces regression of solid tumours. *Nature, 435*(7042), 677–681.
15. Kerr, J. F., Wyllie, A. H., & Currie, A. R. (1972). Apoptosis: a basic biological phenomenon with wide-ranging implications in tissue kinetics. *Br J Cancer, 26*(4), 239–257.
16. Pop, C., & Salvesen, G. S. (2009). Human caspases: activation, specificity, and regulation. *J Biol Chem, 284*(33), 21777–21781.
17. Boatright, K. M., Renatus, M., Scott, F. L., et al. (2003). A unified model for apical caspase activation. *Mol Cell, 11*(2), 529–541.
18. Chai, J., Wu, Q., Shiozaki, E., et al. (2001). Crystal structure of a procaspase-7 zymogen: mechanisms of activation and substrate binding. *Cell, 107*(3), 399–407.
19. Cardone, M. H., Salvesen, G. S., Widmann, C., et al. (1997). The regulation of anoikis: MEKK-1 activation requires cleavage by caspases. *Cell, 90*(2), 315–323.
20. Li, H., Zhu, H., Xu, C. J., et al. (1998). Cleavage of BID by caspase 8 mediates the mitochondrial damage in the Fas pathway of apoptosis. *Cell, 94*(4), 491–501.
21. Peter, M. E., & Krammer, P. H. (2003). The CD95(APO-1/Fas) DISC and beyond. *Cell Death Differ, 10*(1), 26–35.
22. Kischkel, F. C., Hellbardt, S., Behrmann, I., et al. (1995). Cytotoxicity-dependent APO-1 (Fas/CD95)-associated proteins form a death-inducing signaling complex (DISC) with the receptor. *EMBO J, 14*(22), 5579–5588.
23. Park, H. H., Lo, Y. C., Lin, S. C., et al. (2007). The death domain superfamily in intracellular signaling of apoptosis and inflammation. *Annu Rev Immunol, 25*, 561–586.
24. Scaffidi, C., Schmitz, I., Zha, J., et al. (1999). Differential modulation of apoptosis sensitivity in CD95 type I and type II cells. *J Biol Chem, 274*(32), 22532–22538.
25. Liu, X., Kim, C. N., Yang, J., et al. (1996). Induction of apoptotic program in cell-free extracts: requirement for dATP and cytochrome c. *Cell, 86*(1), 147–157.
26. Kluck, R. M., Bossy-Wetzel, E., Green, D. R., et al. (1997). The release of cytochrome c from mitochondria: a primary site for Bcl-2 regulation of apoptosis. *Science, 275*(5303), 1132–1136.
27. Nguyen, M., Breckenridge, D. G., Ducret, A., et al. (2000). Caspase-resistant BAP31 inhibits fas-mediated apoptotic membrane fragmentation and release of cytochrome c from mitochondria. *Mol Cell Biol, 20*(18), 6731–6740.
28. Scorrano, L., Oakes, S. A., Opferman, J. T., et al. (2003). BAX and BAK regulation of endoplasmic reticulum Ca^{2+}: a control point for apoptosis. *Science, 300*(5616), 135–139.
29. Li, P., Nijhawan, D., Budihardjo, I., et al. (1997). Cytochrome c and dATP-dependent formation of Apaf-1/caspase-9 complex initiates an apoptotic protease cascade. *Cell, 91*(4), 479–489.
30. Acehan, D., Jiang, X., Morgan, D. G., et al. (2002). Three-dimensional structure of the apoptosome: implications for assembly, procaspase-9 binding, and activation. *Mol Cell, 9*(2), 423–432.
31. Du, C., Fang, M., Li, Y., et al. (2000). Smac, a mitochondrial protein that promotes cytochrome c-dependent caspase activation by eliminating IAP inhibition. *Cell, 102*(1), 33–42.
32. Verhagen, A. M., Ekert, P. G., Pakusch, M., et al. (2000). Identification of DIABLO, a mammalian protein that promotes apoptosis by binding to and antagonizing IAP proteins. *Cell, 102*(1), 43–53.
33. Faccio, L., Fusco, C., Chen, A., et al. (2000). Characterization of a novel human serine protease that has extensive homology to bacterial heat shock endoprotease HtrA and is regulated by kidney ischemia. *J Biol Chem, 275*(4), 2581–2588.
34. Suzuki, Y., Imai, Y., Nakayama, H., et al. (2001). A serine protease, HtrA2, is released from the mitochondria and interacts with XIAP, inducing cell death. *Mol Cell, 8*(3), 613–621.
35. Kharbanda, S., Pandey, P., Schofield, L., et al. (1997). Role for Bcl-xL as an inhibitor of cytosolic cytochrome C accumulation in DNA damage-induced apoptosis. *Proc Natl Acad Sci U S A, 94*(13), 6939–6942.
36. Youle, R. J., & Strasser, A. (2008). The BCL-2 protein family: opposing activities that mediate cell death. *Nat Rev Mol Cell Biol, 9*(1), 47–59.
37. Nechushtan, A., Smith, C. L., Hsu, Y. T., et al. (1999). Conformation of the Bax C-terminus regulates subcellular location and cell death. *EMBO J, 18*(9), 2330–2341.
38. Suzuki, M., Youle, R. J., & Tjandra, N. (2000). Structure of Bax: coregulation of dimer formation and intracellular localization. *Cell, 103*(4), 645–654.
39. Gavathiotis, E., Suzuki, M., Davis, M. L., et al. (2008). BAX activation is initiated at a novel interaction site. *Nature, 455*(7216), 1076–1081.
40. Cheng, E. H., Sheiko, T. V., Fisher, J. K., et al. (2003). VDAC2 inhibits BAK activation and mitochondrial apoptosis. *Science, 301*(5632), 513–517.
41. Leu, J. I., Dumont, P., Hafey, M., et al. (2004). Mitochondrial p53 activates Bak and causes disruption of a Bak-Mcl1 complex. *Nat Cell Biol, 6*(5), 443–450.
42. Wei, M. C., Zong, W. X., Cheng, E. H., et al. (2001). Proapoptotic BAX and BAK: a requisite gateway to mitochondrial dysfunction and death. *Science, 292*(5517), 727–730.
43. Hochhauser, E., Cheporko, Y., Yasovich, N., et al. (2007). Bax deficiency reduces infarct size and improves long-term function after myocardial infarction. *Cell Biochem Biophys, 47*(1), 11–20.
44. Kim, H., Rafiuddin-Shah, M., Tu, H. C., et al. (2006). Hierarchical regulation of mitochondrion-dependent apoptosis by BCL-2 subfamilies. *Nat Cell Biol, 8*(12), 1348–1358.
45. Willis, S. N., Fletcher, J. I., Kaufmann, T., et al. (2007). Apoptosis initiated when BH3 ligands engage multiple Bcl-2 homologs, not Bax or Bak. *Science, 315*(5813), 856–859.
46. Antonsson, B., Montessuit, S., Sanchez, B., et al. (2001). Bax is present as a high molecular weight oligomer/complex in the mitochondrial membrane of apoptotic cells. *J Biol Chem, 276*(15), 11615–11623.
47. Mikhailov, V., Mikhailova, M., Degenhardt, K., et al. (2003). Association of Bax and Bak homo-oligomers in mitochondria. Bax requirement for Bak reorganization and cytochrome c release. *J Biol Chem, 278*(7), 5367–5376.
48. Wei, M. C., Lindsten, T., Mootha, V. K., et al. (2000). tBID, a membrane-targeted death ligand, oligomerizes BAK to release cytochrome c. *Genes Dev, 14*(16), 2060–2071.
49. Antignani, A., & Youle, R. J. (2006). How do Bax and Bak lead to permeabilization of the outer mitochondrial membrane? *Curr Opin Cell Biol, 18*(6), 685–689.
50. Scorrano, L., Ashiya, M., Buttle, K., et al. (2002). A distinct pathway remodels mitochondrial cristae and mobilizes cytochrome c during apoptosis. *Dev Cell, 2*(1), 55–67.
51. Susin, S. A., Lorenzo, H. K., Zamzami, N., et al. (1999). Molecular characterization of mitochondrial apoptosis-inducing factor. *Nature, 397*(6718), 441–446.
52. Li, L. Y., Luo, X., & Wang, X. (2001). Endonuclease G is an apoptotic DNase when released from mitochondria. *Nature, 412*(6842), 95–99.
53. Arnoult, D., Gaume, B., Karbowski, M., et al. (2003). Mitochondrial release of AIF and EndoG requires caspase activation downstream of Bax/Bak-mediated permeabilization. *EMBO J, 22*(17), 4385–4399.
54. Lakhani, S. A., Masud, A., Kuida, K., et al. (2006). Caspases 3 and 7: key mediators of mitochondrial events of apoptosis. *Science, 311*(5762), 847–851.
55. Zhang, K., & Kaufman, R. J. (2008). From endoplasmic-reticulum stress to the inflammatory response. *Nature, 454*(7203), 455–462.

56. Breckenridge, D. G., Nguyen, M., Kuppig, S., et al. (2002). The procaspase-8 isoform, procaspase-8L, recruited to the BAP31 complex at the endoplasmic reticulum. *Proc Natl Acad Sci U S A, 99*(7), 4331–4336.
57. Chen, L. H., Jiang, C. C., Watts, R., et al. (2008). Inhibition of endoplasmic reticulum stress-induced apoptosis of melanoma cells by the ARC protein. *Cancer Res, 68*(3), 834–842.
58. Nakagawa, T., Zhu, H., Morishima, N., et al. (2000). Caspase-12 mediates endoplasmic-reticulum-specific apoptosis and cytotoxicity by amyloid-beta. *Nature, 403*(6765), 98–103.
59. Saleh, M., Mathison, J. C., Wolinski, M. K., et al. (2006). Enhanced bacterial clearance and sepsis resistance in caspase-12-deficient mice. *Nature, 440*(7087), 1064–1068.
60. Saleh, M., Vaillancourt, J. P., Graham, R. K., et al. (2004). Differential modulation of endotoxin responsiveness by human caspase-12 polymorphisms. *Nature, 429*(6987), 75–79.
61. Peter, M. E. (2004). The flip side of FLIP. *Biochem J, 382*(pt 2), e1–e3.
62. Riedl, S. J., Renatus, M., Schwarzenbacher, R., et al. (2001). Structural basis for the inhibition of caspase-3 by XIAP. *Cell, 104*(5), 791–800.
63. Huang, Y., Park, Y. C., Rich, R. L., et al. (2001). Structural basis of caspase inhibition by XIAP: differential roles of the linker versus the BIR domain. *Cell, 104*(5), 781–790.
64. Shiozaki, E. N., Chai, J., Rigotti, D. J., et al. (2003). Mechanism of XIAP-mediated inhibition of caspase-9. *Mol Cell, 11*(2), 519–527.
65. Suzuki, Y., Nakabayashi, Y., & Takahashi, R. (2001). Ubiquitin-protein ligase activity of X-linked inhibitor of apoptosis protein promotes proteasomal degradation of caspase-3 and enhances its anti-apoptotic effect in Fas-induced cell death. *Proc Natl Acad Sci U S A, 98*(15), 8662–8667.
66. Yang, Y., Fang, S., Jensen, J. P., et al. (2000). Ubiquitin protein ligase activity of IAPs and their degradation in proteasomes in response to apoptotic stimuli. *Science, 288*(5467), 874–877.
67. Ea, C. K., Deng, L., Xia, Z. P., et al. (2006). Activation of IKK by TNFalpha requires site-specific ubiquitination of RIP1 and polyubiquitin binding by NEMO. *Mol Cell, 22*(2), 245–257.
68. Mahoney, D. J., Cheung, H. H., Mrad, R. L., et al. (2008). Both cIAP1 and cIAP2 regulate TNFalpha-mediated NF-kappaB activation. *Proc Natl Acad Sci U S A, 105*(33), 11778–11783.
69. Varfolomeev, E., Goncharov, T., Fedorova, A. V., et al. (2008). c-IAP1 and c-IAP2 are critical mediators of tumor necrosis factor alpha (TNFalpha)-induced NF-kappaB activation. *J Biol Chem, 283*(36), 24295–24299.
70. Yang, Q. H., Church-Hajduk, R., Ren, J., et al. (2003). Omi/HtrA2 catalytic cleavage of inhibitor of apoptosis (IAP) irreversibly inactivates IAPs and facilitates caspase activity in apoptosis. *Genes Dev, 17*(12), 1487–1496.
71. Nam, Y. J., Mani, K., Ashton, A. W., et al. (2004). Inhibition of both the extrinsic and intrinsic death pathways through nonhomotypic death-fold interactions. *Mol Cell, 15*(6), 901–912.
72. Gustafsson, A. B., Tsai, J. G., Logue, S. E., et al. (2004). Apoptosis repressor with caspase recruitment domain protects against cell death by interfering with Bax activation. *J Biol Chem, 279*(20), 21233–21238.
73. Foo, R. S., Nam, Y. J., Ostreicher, M. J., et al. (2007). Regulation of p53 tetramerization and nuclear export by ARC. *Proc Natl Acad Sci U S A, 104*(52), 20826–20831.
74. Micheau, O., & Tschopp, J. (2003). Induction of TNF receptor I-mediated apoptosis via two sequential signaling complexes. *Cell, 114*(2), 181–190.
75. Wang, L., Du, F., & Wang, X. (2008). TNF-alpha induces two distinct caspase-8 activation pathways. *Cell, 133*(4), 693–703.
76. Hitomi, J., Christofferson, D. E., Ng, A., et al. (2008). Identification of a molecular signaling network that regulates a cellular necrotic cell death pathway. *Cell, 135*(7), 1311–1323.
77. Chan, F. K., Shisler, J., Bixby, J. G., et al. (2003). A role for tumor necrosis factor receptor-2 and receptor-interacting protein in programmed necrosis and antiviral responses. *J Biol Chem, 278*(51), 51613–51621.
78. Lin, Y., Devin, A., Rodriguez, Y., et al. (1999). Cleavage of the death domain kinase RIP by caspase-8 prompts TNF-induced apoptosis. *Genes Dev, 13*(19), 2514–2526.
79. He, S., Wang, L., Miao, L., et al. (2009). Receptor interacting protein kinase-3 determines cellular necrotic response to TNF-alpha. *Cell, 137*(6), 1100–1111.
80. Cho, Y. S., Challa, S., Moquin, D., et al. (2009). Phosphorylation-driven assembly of the RIP1-RIP3 complex regulates programmed necrosis and virus-induced inflammation. *Cell, 137*(6), 1112–1123.
81. Zhang, D. W., Shao, J., Lin, J., et al. (2009). RIP3, an energy metabolism regulator that switches TNF-induced cell death from apoptosis to necrosis. *Science, 325*(5938), 332–336.
82. Zhou, Q., Snipas, S., Orth, K., et al. (1997). Target protease specificity of the viral serpin CrmA. Analysis of five caspases. *J Biol Chem, 272*(12), 7797–7800.
83. Halestrap, A. P. (2009). What is the mitochondrial permeability transition pore? *J Mol Cell Cardiol, 46*(6), 821–831.
84. Bossy-Wetzel, E., Newmeyer, D. D., & Green, D. R. (1998). Mitochondrial cytochrome c release in apoptosis occurs upstream of DEVD-specific caspase activation and independently of mitochondrial transmembrane depolarization. *EMBO J, 17*(1), 37–49.
85. Xu, K., Tavernarakis, N., & Driscoll, M. (2001). Necrotic cell death in *C. elegans* requires the function of calreticulin and regulators of Ca(2+) release from the endoplasmic reticulum. *Neuron, 31*(6), 957–971.
86. Bianchi, L., Gerstbrein, B., Frokjaer-Jensen, C., et al. (2004). The neurotoxic MEC-4(d) DEG/ENaC sodium channel conducts calcium: implications for necrosis initiation. *Nat Neurosci, 7*(12), 1337–1344.
87. Syntichaki, P., Xu, K., Driscoll, M., et al. (2002). Specific aspartyl and calpain proteases are required for neurodegeneration in *C. elegans*. *Nature, 419*(6910), 939–944.
88. Orrenius, S., Zhivotovsky, B., & Nicotera, P. (2003). Regulation of cell death: the calcium-apoptosis link. *Nat Rev Mol Cell Biol, 4*(7), 552–565.
89. Degterev, A., Hitomi, J., Germscheid, M., et al. (2008). Identification of RIP1 kinase as a specific cellular target of necrostatins. *Nat Chem Biol, 4*(5), 313–321.
90. Lim, S. Y., Davidson, S. M., Mocanu, M. M., et al. (2007). The cardioprotective effect of necrostatin requires the cyclophilin-D component of the mitochondrial permeability transition pore. *Cardiovasc Drugs Ther, 21*(6), 467–469.
91. Zong, W. X., Ditsworth, D., Bauer, D. E., et al. (2004). Alkylating DNA damage stimulates a regulated form of necrotic cell death. *Genes Dev, 18*(11), 1272–1282.
92. He, C., & Klionsky, D. J. (Aug 4, 2009). Regulation mechanisms and signaling pathways of autophagy. *Annu Rev Genet*, Epub ahead of print.
93. Oberstein, A., Jeffrey, P. D., & Shi, Y. (2007). Crystal structure of the Bcl-XL-Beclin 1 peptide complex: Beclin 1 is a novel BH3-only protein. *J Biol Chem, 282*(17), 13123–13132.
94. Pattingre, S., Tassa, A., Qu, X., et al. (2005). Bcl-2 antiapoptotic proteins inhibit Beclin 1-dependent autophagy. *Cell, 122*(6), 927–939.
95. Ciechomska, I. A., Goemans, G. C., Skepper, J. N., et al. (2009). Bcl-2 complexed with Beclin-1 maintains full anti-apoptotic function. *Oncogene, 28*(21), 2128–2141.
96. Ricci, J. E., Munoz-Pinedo, C., Fitzgerald, P., et al. (2004). Disruption of mitochondrial function during apoptosis is mediated by caspase cleavage of the p75 subunit of complex I of the electron transport chain. *Cell, 117*(6), 773–786.
97. Whelan, R. S., Kaplinskiy, V., & Kitsis, R. N. (2010). Cell death in the pathogenesis of heart disease: mechanisms and significance. *Annu Rev Physiol, 72*, in press.
98. Reimer, K. A., & Jennings, R. B. (1979). The "wavefront phenomenon" of myocardial ischemic cell death. II. Transmural progression of necrosis within the framework of ischemic bed size (myocardium at risk) and collateral flow. *Lab Invest, 40*(6), 633–644.
99. Yellon, D. M., & Hausenloy, D. J. (2007). Myocardial reperfusion injury. *N Engl J Med, 357*(11), 1121–1135.
100. Gottlieb, R. A., Burleson, K. O., Kloner, R. A., et al. (1994). Reperfusion injury induces apoptosis in rabbit cardiomyocytes. *J Clin Invest, 94*(4), 1621–1628.
101. Kajstura, J., Cheng, W., Reiss, K., et al. (1996). Apoptotic and necrotic myocyte cell deaths are independent contributing variables of infarct size in rats. *Lab Invest, 74*(1), 86–107.
102. Fliss, H., & Gattinger, D. (1996). Apoptosis in ischemic and reperfused rat myocardium. *Circ Res, 79*(5), 949–956.
103. Matsui, Y., Takagi, H., Qu, X., et al. (2007). Distinct roles of autophagy in the heart during ischemia and reperfusion: roles of AMP-activated protein kinase and Beclin 1 in mediating autophagy. *Circ Res, 100*(6), 914–922.
104. Takagi, H., Matsui, Y., Hirotani, S., et al. (2007). AMPK mediates autophagy during myocardial ischemia in vivo. *Autophagy, 3*(4), 405–407.
105. Lee, P., Sata, M., Lefer, D. J., et al. (2003). Fas pathway is a critical mediator of cardiac myocyte death and MI during ischemia-reperfusion in vivo. *Am J Physiol, 284*(2), H456–H463.
106. Toth, A., Jeffers, J. R., Nickson, P., et al. (2006). Targeted deletion of Puma attenuates cardiomyocyte death and improves cardiac function during ischemia-reperfusion. *Am J Physiol, 291*(1), H52–H60.
107. Hochhauser, E., Kivity, S., Offen, D., et al. (2003). Bax ablation protects against myocardial ischemia-reperfusion injury in transgenic mice. *Am J Physiol, 284*(6), H2351–H2359.
108. Brocheriou, V., Hagege, A. A., Oubenaissa, A., et al. (2000). Cardiac functional improvement by a human Bcl-2 transgene in a mouse model of ischemia/reperfusion injury. *J Gene Med, 2*(5), 326–333.
109. Chen, Z., Chua, C. C., Ho, Y. S., et al. (2001). Overexpression of Bcl-2 attenuates apoptosis and protects against myocardial I/R injury in transgenic mice. *Am J Physiol, 280*(5), H2313–H2320.
110. Pyo, J. O., Nah, J., Kim, H. J., et al. (2008). Protection of cardiomyocytes from ischemic/hypoxic cell death via Drbp1 and pMe2GlyDH in cardio-specific ARC transgenic mice. *J Biol Chem, 283*(45), 30707–30714.
111. Chua, C. C., Gao, J., Ho, Y. S., et al. (2007). Overexpression of IAP-2 attenuates apoptosis and protects against myocardial ischemia/reperfusion injury in transgenic mice. *Biochim Biophys Acta, 1773*(4), 577–583.
112. Yaoita, H., Ogawa, K., Maehara, K., et al. (1998). Attenuation of ischemia/reperfusion injury in rats by a caspase inhibitor. *Circulation, 97*(3), 276–281.
113. Holly, T. A., Drincic, A., Byun, Y., et al. (1999). Caspase inhibition reduces myocyte cell death induced by myocardial ischemia and reperfusion in vivo. *J Mol Cell Cardiol, 31*(9), 1709–1715.
114. Huang, J. Q., Radinovic, S., Rezaiefar, P., et al. (2000). In vivo myocardial infarct size reduction by a caspase inhibitor administered after the onset of ischemia. *Eur J Pharmacol, 402*(1–2), 139–142.
115. Yang, W., Guastella, J., Huang, J. C., et al. (2003). MX1013, a dipeptide caspase inhibitor with potent in vivo antiapoptotic activity. *Br J Pharmacol, 140*(2), 402–412.
116. Liu, H. R., Gao, E., Hu, A., et al. (2005). Role of Omi/HtrA2 in apoptotic cell death after myocardial ischemia and reperfusion. *Circulation, 111*(1), 90–96.
117. Bhuiyan, M. S., & Fukunaga, K. (2007). Inhibition of HtrA2/Omi ameliorates heart dysfunction following ischemia/reperfusion injury in rat heart in vivo. *Eur J Pharmacol, 557*(2–3), 168–177.
118. Hamacher-Brady, A., Brady, N. R., & Gottlieb, R. A. (2006). Enhancing macroautophagy protects against ischemia/reperfusion injury in cardiac myocytes. *J Biol Chem, 281*(40), 29776–29787.
119. Kostin, S., Pool, L., Elsasser, A., et al. (2003). Myocytes die by multiple mechanisms in failing human hearts. *Circ Res, 92*(7), 715–724.
120. Hein, S., Arnon, E., Kostin, S., et al. (2003). Progression from compensated hypertrophy to failure in the pressure-overloaded human heart: structural deterioration and compensatory mechanisms. *Circulation, 107*(7), 984–991.
121. Condorelli, G., Morisco, C., Stassi, G., et al. (1999). Increased cardiomyocyte apoptosis and changes in proapoptotic and antiapoptotic genes bax and bcl-2 during left ventricular adaptations to chronic pressure overload in the rat. *Circulation, 99*(23), 3071–3078.
122. Cheng, W., Li, B., Kajstura, J., et al. (1995). Stretch-induced programmed myocyte cell death. *J Clin Invest, 96*(5), 2247–2259.

123. Ding, B., Price, R. L., Goldsmith, E. C., et al. (2000). Left ventricular hypertrophy in ascending aortic stenosis mice: anoikis and the progression to early failure. *Circulation, 101*(24), 2854–2862.
124. Sadoshima, J., Xu, Y., Slayter, H. S., et al. (1993). Autocrine release of angiotensin II mediates stretch-induced hypertrophy of cardiac myocytes in vitro. *Cell, 75*(5), 977–984.
125. Leri, A., Claudio, P. P., Li, Q., et al. (1998). Stretch-mediated release of angiotensin II induces myocyte apoptosis by activating p53 that enhances the local renin-angiotensin system and decreases the Bcl-2-to-Bax protein ratio in the cell. *J Clin Invest, 101*(7), 1326–1342.
126. Hirota, H., Chen, J., Betz, U. A., et al. (1999). Loss of a gp130 cardiac muscle cell survival pathway is a critical event in the onset of heart failure during biomechanical stress. *Cell, 97*(2), 189–198.
127. Francis, G. S., Benedict, C., Johnstone, D. E., et al. (1990). Comparison of neuroendocrine activation in patients with left ventricular dysfunction with and without congestive heart failure. A substudy of the studies of left ventricular dysfunction (SOLVD). *Circulation, 82*(5), 1724–1729.
128. Cohn, J. N., Levine, T. B., Olivari, M. T., et al. (1984). Plasma norepinephrine as a guide to prognosis in patients with chronic congestive heart failure. *N Engl J Med, 311*(13), 819–823.
129. Engelhardt, S., Hein, L., Wiesmann, F., et al. (1999). Progressive hypertrophy and heart failure in beta1-adrenergic receptor transgenic mice. *Proc Natl Acad Sci U S A, 96*(12), 7059–7064.
130. Bisognano, J. D., Weinberger, H. D., Bohlmeyer, T. J., et al. (2000). Myocardial-directed overexpression of the human beta(1)-adrenergic receptor in transgenic mice. *J Mol Cell Cardiol, 32*(5), 817–830.
131. Mann, D. L., & Bristow, M. R. (2005). Mechanisms and models in heart failure: the biomechanical model and beyond. *Circulation, 111*(21), 2837–2849.
132. Communal, C., Singh, K., Sawyer, D. B., et al. (1999). Opposing effects of beta(1)- and beta(2)-adrenergic receptors on cardiac myocyte apoptosis: role of a pertussis toxin-sensitive G protein. *Circulation, 100*(22), 2210–2212.
133. Ahmet, I., Krawczyk, M., Heller, P., et al. (2004). Beneficial effects of chronic pharmacological manipulation of beta-adrenoreceptor subtype signaling in rodent dilated ischemic cardiomyopathy. *Circulation, 110*(9), 1083–1090.
134. Zhu, W. Z., Wang, S. Q., Chakir, K., et al. (2003). Linkage of beta1-adrenergic stimulation to apoptotic heart cell death through protein kinase A-independent activation of Ca^{2+}/calmodulin kinase II. *J Clin Invest, 111*(5), 617–625.
135. Zhang, T., Maier, L. S., Dalton, N. D., et al. (2003). The deltaC isoform of CaMKII is activated in cardiac hypertrophy and induces dilated cardiomyopathy and heart failure. *Circ Res, 92*(8), 912–919.
136. Yang, Y., Zhu, W. Z., Joiner, M. L., et al. (2006). Calmodulin kinase II inhibition protects against myocardial cell apoptosis in vivo. *Am J Physiol, 291*(6), H3065–H3075.
137. Backs, J., Backs, T., Neef, S., et al. (2009). The delta isoform of CaM kinase II is required for pathological cardiac hypertrophy and remodeling after pressure overload. *Proc Natl Acad Sci U S A, 106*(7), 2342–2347.
138. Ling, H., Zhang, T., Pereira, L., et al. (2009). Requirement for Ca^{2+}/calmodulin-dependent kinase II in the transition from pressure overload-induced cardiac hypertrophy to heart failure in mice. *J Clin Invest, 119*(5), 1230–1240.
139. Mann, D. L., Deswal, A., Bozkurt, B., et al. (2002). New therapeutics for chronic heart failure. *Annu Rev Med, 53*, 59–74.
140. Kajstura, J., Cigola, E., Malhotra, A., et al. (1997). Angiotensin II induces apoptosis of adult ventricular myocytes in vitro. *J Mol Cell Cardiol, 29*(3), 859–870.
141. De Angelis, N., Fiordaliso, F., Latini, R., et al. (2002). Appraisal of the role of angiotensin II and aldosterone in ventricular myocyte apoptosis in adult normotensive rat. *J Mol Cell Cardiol, 34*(12), 1655–1665.
142. Toko, H., Oka, T., Zou, Y., et al. (2002). Angiotensin II type 1a receptor mediates doxorubicin-induced cardiomyopathy. *Hypertens Res, 25*(4), 597–603.
143. Fiordaliso, F., Li, B., Latini, R., et al. (2000). Myocyte death in streptozotocin-induced diabetes in rats is angiotensin II-dependent. *Lab Invest, 80*(4), 513–527.
144. Takeda, M., Tatsumi, T., Matsunaga, S., et al. (2007). Spironolactone modulates expressions of cardiac mineralocorticoid receptor and 11beta-hydroxysteroid dehydrogenase 2 and prevents ventricular remodeling in post-infarct rat hearts. *Hypertens Res, 30*(5), 427–437.
145. Yussman, M. G., Toyokawa, T., Odley, A., et al. (2002). Mitochondrial death protein Nix is induced in cardiac hypertrophy and triggers apoptotic cardiomyopathy. *Nat Med, 8*(7), 725–730.
146. Kajstura, J., Bolli, R., Sonnenblick, E. H., et al. (2006). Cause of death: suicide. *J Mol Cell Cardiol, 40*(4), 425–437.
147. Izumiya, Y., Kim, S., Izumi, Y., et al. (2003). Apoptosis signal-regulating kinase 1 plays a pivotal role in angiotensin II-induced cardiac hypertrophy and remodeling. *Circ Res, 93*(9), 874–883.
148. Vasan, R. S., Sullivan, L. M., Roubenoff, R., et al. (2003). Inflammatory markers and risk of heart failure in elderly subjects without prior myocardial infarction: the Framingham Heart Study. *Circulation, 107*(11), 1486–1491.
149. Krown, K. A., Page, M. T., Nguyen, C., et al. (1996). Tumor necrosis factor alpha-induced apoptosis in cardiac myocytes. Involvement of the sphingolipid signaling cascade in cardiac cell death. *J Clin Invest, 98*(12), 2854–2865.
150. Ing, D. J., Zang, J., Dzau, V. J., et al. (1999). Modulation of cytokine-induced cardiac myocyte apoptosis by nitric oxide, Bak, and Bcl-x. *Circ Res, 84*(1), 21–33.
151. Haudek, S. B., Taffet, G. E., Schneider, M. D., et al. (2007). TNF provokes cardiomyocyte apoptosis and cardiac remodeling through activation of multiple cell death pathways. *J Clin Invest, 117*(9), 2692–2701.
152. Higuchi, Y., McTiernan, C. F., Frye, C. B., et al. (2004). Tumor necrosis factor receptors 1 and 2 differentially regulate survival, cardiac dysfunction, and remodeling in transgenic mice with tumor necrosis factor-alpha-induced cardiomyopathy. *Circulation, 109*(15), 1892–1897.
153. Hamid, T., Gu, Y., Ortines, R. V., et al. (2009). Divergent tumor necrosis factor receptor-related remodeling responses in heart failure: role of nuclear factor-kappaB and inflammatory activation. *Circulation, 119*(10), 1386–1397.
154. Kurrelmeyer, K. M., Michael, L. H., Baumgarten, G., et al. (2000). Endogenous tumor necrosis factor protects the adult cardiac myocyte against ischemic-induced apoptosis in a murine model of acute myocardial infarction. *Proc Natl Acad Sci U S A, 97*(10), 5456–5461.
155. Mann, D. L., McMurray, J. J., Packer, M., et al. (2004). Targeted anticytokine therapy in patients with chronic heart failure: results of the randomized etanercept worldwide evaluation (RENEWAL). *Circulation, 109*(13), 1594–1602.
156. Chung, E. S., Packer, M., Lo, K. H., et al. (2003). Randomized, double-blind, placebo-controlled, pilot trial of infliximab, a chimeric monoclonal antibody to tumor necrosis factor-alpha, in patients with moderate-to-severe heart failure: results of the anti-TNF therapy against congestive heart failure (ATTACH) trial. *Circulation, 107*(25), 3133–3140.
157. Guerra, S., Leri, A., Wang, X., et al. (1999). Myocyte death in the failing human heart is gender dependent. *Circ Res, 85*(9), 856–866.
158. Olivetti, G., Abbi, R., Quaini, F., et al. (1997). Apoptosis in the failing human heart. *N Engl J Med, 336*(16), 1131–1141.
159. Saraste, A., Pulkki, K., Kallajoki, M., et al. (1999). Cardiomyocyte apoptosis and progression of heart failure to transplantation. *Eur J Clin Invest, 29*(5), 380–386.
160. Wencker, D., Chandra, M., Nguyen, K., et al. (2003). A mechanistic role for cardiac myocyte apoptosis in heart failure. *J Clin Invest, 111*(10), 1497–1504.
161. D'Angelo, D. D., Sakata, Y., Lorenz, J. N., et al. (1997). Transgenic Galphaq overexpression induces cardiac contractile failure in mice. *Proc Natl Acad Sci U S A, 94*(15), 8121–8126.
162. Adams, J. W., Sakata, Y., Davis, M. G., et al. (1998). Enhanced Galphaq signaling: a common pathway mediates cardiac hypertrophy and apoptotic heart failure. *Proc Natl Acad Sci U S A, 95*(17), 10140–10145.
163. Hayakawa, Y., Chandra, M., Miao, W., et al. (2003). Inhibition of cardiac myocyte apoptosis improves cardiac function and abolishes mortality in the peripartum cardiomyopathy of Galpha(q) transgenic mice. *Circulation, 108*(24), 3036–3041.
164. Diwan, A., Krenz, M., Syed, F. M., et al. (2007). Inhibition of ischemic cardiomyocyte apoptosis through targeted ablation of Bnip3 restrains postinfarction remodeling in mice. *J Clin Invest, 117*(10), 2825–2833.
165. Chatterjee, S., Stewart, A. S., Bish, L. T., et al. (2002). Viral gene transfer of the anti-apoptotic factor Bcl-2 protects against chronic postischemic heart failure. *Circulation, 106*(12 suppl. 1), 1212–1217.
166. Knaapen, M. W., Davies, M. J., De Bie, M., et al. (2001). Apoptotic versus autophagic cell death in heart failure. *Cardiovasc Res, 51*(2), 304–312.
167. Nakai, A., Yamaguchi, O., Takeda, T., et al. (2007). The role of autophagy in cardiomyocytes in the basal state and in response to hemodynamic stress. *Nat Med, 13*(5), 619–624.
168. Zhu, H., Tannous, P., Johnstone, J. L., et al. (2007). Cardiac autophagy is a maladaptive response to hemodynamic stress. *J Clin Invest, 117*(7), 1782–1793.
169. Tannous, P., Zhu, H., Johnstone, J. L., et al. (2008). Autophagy is an adaptive response in desmin-related cardiomyopathy. *Proc Natl Acad Sci U S A, 105*(28), 9745–9750.
170. Ellis, R. E., Yuan, J. Y., & Horvitz, H. R. (1991). Mechanisms and functions of cell death. *Annu Rev Cell Biol, 7*, 663–698.
171. Shaham, S., & Horvitz, H. R. (1996). Developing *Caenorhabditis elegans* neurons may contain both cell-death protective and killer activities. *Genes Dev, 10*(5), 578–591.

CHAPTER 7

Energetic Basis for Heart Failure

Joanne S. Ingwall

Shown by investigators using many different tools studying human myocardium and a wide variety of animal models of heart failure, it is now known that one characteristic of the failing heart is a progressive loss of ATP. Given that the requirement for ATP for all metabolic processes and for cell viability is absolute, the biochemistry of ATP is now a major focus of research in cardiac metabolism. Questions now being asked are: what mechanisms explain the fall in [ATP], what are the consequences of decreased [ATP], can metabolism be manipulated to restore a normal ATP supply, and does increasing energy supply have physiological consequences (i.e., does it lead to improved contractile performance in the failing heart)? Here, we address each of these questions from two points of view: using what we know about the basic biochemistry of ATP and what we are learning from new analyses of the human heart and of animal models of heart failure. Demonstrating renewed interest in this subject, there have been many reviews published over the past few years relevant to the energetics of the heart.[1-23]

ENERGETICS OF THE NORMAL HEART

The normal mammalian cardiomyocyte maintains the average cytosolic [ATP] at a constant level of approximately 10 mM, enough ATP to support only a few beats. To supply enough ATP to meet beat-to-beat variations in ATP demand, the terminal phosphoryl group of ATP turns over as much as 10,000 times a day. Thus the rates of ATP synthesis and use in the heart are extraordinarily large. Energy metabolism is designed so that the rate of ATP synthesis via rephosphorylation of ADP closely matches the varying rate of ATP use by myosin, ion pumps, synthesis, and degradation of large and small molecules, etc. (Figure 7-1). The primary driver is ATP demand, and the myosin ATPase reaction is the main ATP consumer. The primary source of ATP resynthesis from ADP is via fatty acid oxidation (FAO) in the mitochondria; the contribution from glycolysis is quantitatively small. In addition to glucose and FA, other metabolites can be used for ATP synthesis as well, including glycogen, lactate, and certain amino acids. Phosphoryl transfer between sites of ATP production and use occurs by means of metabolic relays via creatine kinase (CK), adenylate kinase (AK), and glycolysis.

The relative contribution of the different metabolic pathways to overall ATP synthesis constantly changes even in the normal myocardium. The different pathways for ATP supply have different rates of ATP synthesis: phosphoryl transfer via CK is approximately 10- times faster than ATP synthesis in mitochondria, which is approximately 20- times faster than glycolysis. By summing reactions with varying rates of ATP synthesis, [ATP] is maintained high and constant on a beat-to-beat basis. Fluxes through existing pathways for ATP synthesis change rapidly in response to changes in fuel supply, hormonal and neural signals, and the availability of substrates and inhibitors of specific enzyme reactions, and also by chemical modification of regulating proteins. Thus during acute increases in work in the normal myocardium, the *sum* of increased rates of ATP synthesis by the mitochondria, by glycolysis and glycogenolysis, and by the phosphotransferase reactions matches the increase in the total rate of ATP use. The increases in glycolysis and phosphotransferase rates are not due to a limitation in either O_2 supply or due to inadequate capacity of the mitochondria to support substrate oxidation. Rather, these biochemical pathways are designed to rapidly mobilize substrates such as glycogen to influx more glucose, to use phosphocreatine (PCr) to support acute demands for high ATP, and to salvage ADP via CK and AK to replenish ATP. Metabolism is designed so that during increased demand for ATP, inhibition of glycolysis by metabolic sensors coupling high FA use with low glucose use is partially relieved.

ATP synthesis pathways not only function to supply large amounts of ATP needed for beat-to-beat variations in cardiac work, but they also function to maintain a high ratio of [ATP] to the products of ATP hydrolysis [ADP] and [Pi] on the same time scale. The ratio, [ATP][ADP][Pi], known as the phosphorylation potential, determines the free energy available from ATP hydrolysis, $|\Delta G_{\sim ATP}|$ that is used to drive ATP-requiring reactions. Without the energy supplied from the hydrolysis of ATP, myosin heads would not move, ions could not move against their concentration gradients, and most biological reactions simply would not proceed. ATP hydrolysis provides the chemical driving force for the unfavorable reactions required for excitation, contraction, and the basic workings of the myocyte. Maintaining a high chemical driving force to support the ATPase reactions during variations in work output is so important that the heart has several energy reserve systems, namely, CK and AK, that function to minimize large fluctuations in the chemical driving force.

ATP Synthesis in Mitochondria

The heart derives as much as 90% of its energy from the oxidation of carbon-based fuels in the mitochondria. The capacity for oxidative phosphorylation (OXPHOS) in the heart is very large; the fraction of the

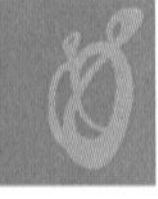

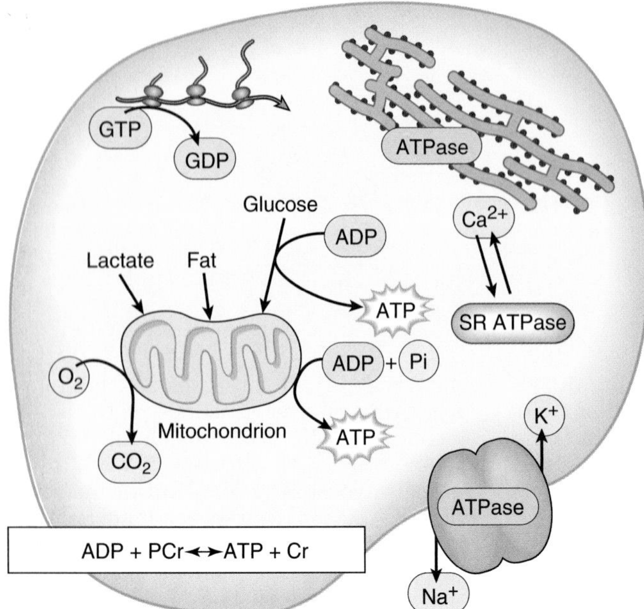

FIGURE 7–1 Cartoon summarizing the integration of the ATP synthesizing and using pathways.[117] The primary ATP using reactions (shown on the right) are actomyosin ATPase in the myofibril, the Ca^{2+}-ATPase in the sarcoplasmic reticulum and the Na^+, K^+-ATPase in the sarcolemma. Also shown is a polypeptide chain representing the requirement of ATP for macromolecular synthesis (in the form of GTP for protein synthesis). The primary ATP synthesizing pathways (*left*) are oxidative phosphorylation in the mitochondria and the glycolytic pathway. Also shown (*bottom*) is the creatine kinase (CK) reaction, representing the kinases that supply ATP via rapid phosphoryl transfer. (Redrawn with permission from Ingwall JS. (2002). *ATP and the heart.* Boston: Kluwer Academic, Norwell, MA.)[28]

adult mammalian cardiomyocyte occupied by mitochondria is approximately 0.35. High capacity and high turnover rates are illustrated in experiments simultaneously measuring indices of work and O_2 consumed (MVO_2). For example, in a small animal heart, the relationship between work and MVO_2 is linear over a fivefold range.[24] [ATP] remained constant, showing that ATP synthesis rates by O_2-dependent reactions matched ATP use rates.

Figure 7-2 shows the major steps for oxidizing FA and pyruvate (made by glycolysis) in the mitochondria (see Chapter 20). OXPHOS is the process whereby ATP is formed as electrons are transferred from NADH or $FADH_2$ made in the tricarboxylic acid (TCA) cycle to molecular O_2 by a series of electron carriers. This is why MVO_2 is a good measure of the ATP synthesis rate. The amount of ATP produced from FAO is much greater than the yield from oxidation of glucose because FAs supply many acetyl-CoA molecules (1 acetyl-CoA for each 2-carbon unit in the FA chain) while the same number of glucose molecules yields only two acetyl-CoA molecules. Although the efficiency of ATP production from the oxidation per mole of O_2 reduced is slightly greater for glucose (P:O ~3.05 for glucose vs. <2.9 for fatty acids), on a molar basis, the amount of ATP produced from FAO is many-fold higher than for glucose oxidation. For example, for the equivalent number of moles, 129 ATPs are made from oxidation of palmitate versus 38 ATPs from oxidation of glucose. FAs are the predominant fuel for energy production in adult hearts whereas glucose and lactate are the major carbon sources for fetal and neonatal hearts and when O_2 is limiting as in the ischemic myocardium.

Mitochondrial respiration is controlled by availability of ADP, Pi, NADH, H^+, Ca^{2+}, and O_2. Relatively new information supporting the role of Ca^{2+} in regulating rates of respiration suggests that Ca^{2+} is the most likely candidate for *rapid* control of respiration.[14] Which metabolite or signaling ion is the primary regulator supplying ATP to meet demand at any given time is likely to depend on the workload on the heart, the type and amount of carbon-based fuels available, and the extent of any molecular reprogramming that may have occurred. The existence of multiple regulators minimizes fluctuations in [ATP] and maintains a high phosphorylation potential in the cytosol. The importance of efficiently coupling ATP synthesis and use reactions by the same metabolic and ionic regulators for normal contraction cannot be overemphasized.

ATP Synthesis by Glycolysis

In the normal heart, the amount of ATP produced via glycolysis is a small fraction of the amount made as a result of the oxidation of glucose: 2 versus 38 ATPs. Nonetheless, glucose and glycogen are important sources of ATP during rapid transitions to increased work or in other acute ATP supply/demand mismatches. Figure 7-3 shows the major steps in glucose metabolism.

ATP Synthesis by Phosphotransfer Reactions

The primary phosphoryl transferase reactions in muscle are catalyzed by CK and AK. Both enzymes are highly abundant in muscle cells and exist as families of isozymes that change in development and in disease states. The physical association of CK and AK with energy-producing and energy-using proteins provides the basis for the energy-transfer or relay properties attributed to these enzymes. These physical complexes also create microenvironments whereby phosphoryl groups can be supplied to ATPases without exchange with bulk cytosolic pools, improving the efficiency of ATP supply.[3,9,25]

Under conditions when ATP demand exceeds ATP supply, as in acute pump failure in ischemia and in acute and chronic conditions of high wall stress, use of PCr via the CK reaction (PCr + ADP + H^+ ↔ Cr + ATP) is one way that the heart maintains high [ATP] and low [ADP]. Thus the CK reaction has two main functions: to supply ATP rapidly (~10 times faster than ATP resynthesis by mitochondria) and to maximize the chemical driving force for ATPase reactions. Most (but not all) reports of high work states in both cardiac and skeletal muscles of large and small animals report decreases in [PCr] and concomitant increases in [ADP] and [Pi].[24,26,27] AK also functions to maintain high levels of ATP by transferring phosphoryl groups among the adenine nucleotides: 2ADP ↔ ATP + AMP. To know whether ATP-requiring reactions may be limited because of an insufficient chemical driving force, we need to know [ADP] and [Pi] along with [ATP]. The cytosolic concentrations of [ATP], [ADP], and [Pi] in normal ventricular tissue are approximately 10 mM, less than 50 μM, and less than 1 mM, respectively. Figure 7-4 illustrates the coupling of the CK reaction to myosin ATPase to supply ATP and, using metabolite concentrations calculated from ^{31}P NMR spectroscopy experiments, shows how variations in [ATP], [ADP], and [Pi] caused by acute inotropic challenge change the value of $\Delta G_{\sim ATP}$. In this example, the value of $\Delta G_{\sim ATP}$ changed by approximately 4 kJ/mol. This is a large fraction, 4/7, of the range of $\Delta G_{\sim ATP}$ observed for the well-oxygenated beating heart: −54 to −61 kJ/mol. See Ingwall[28] for more discussion.

ATP AND THE FAILING HEART

The ability of the metabolic machinery to use a variety of fuels for ATP synthesis ensures that ATP supply matches ATP demand and that the chemical driving force for ATP-requiring reactions remains high on a beat-to-beat basis. We now know that the integration of ATP synthesizing and using reactions changes in the hypertrophied and failing myocardium. The cellular machinery designed to make and use ATP remodels

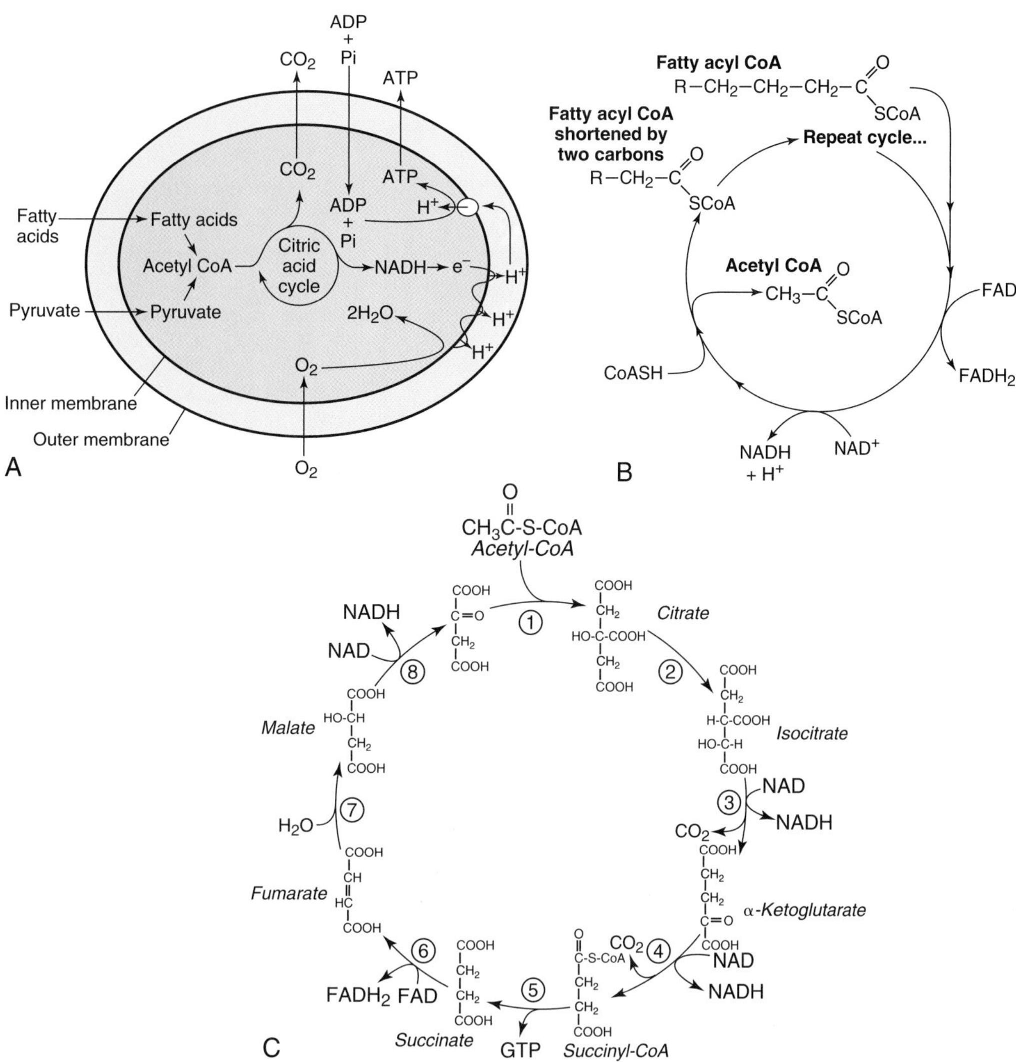

FIGURE 7–2 **A,** Overall strategy for making ATP in mitochondria. **B,** Processing of fatty acids via β-oxidation to form acetyl-CoA; **C,** TCA cycle using acetyl-CoA to make molecules needed in the electron transport chain.

There are six basic steps in the pathway whereby fuels are converted into molecules that efficiently couple ATP synthesis to the reduction of O_2. Known changes in the failing myocardium are in ***italics***.

1. The first step is to ***transport*** fatty acids (FA) of different lengths or pyruvate into the mitochondrial matrix **(A)**. *Long-chain FA carrier carnitine palmitoyl transferase-I is decreased.*
2. Once in the matrix, these substrates are ***converted into acetyl-CoA*** to fuel the citric acid cycle. Pyruvate is converted to acetyl-CoA by pyruvate dehydrogenase; fatty acids are converted to acetyl-CoA by β-oxidation **(B)**. *A smaller fraction of PDH exists in the active form.*
3. ***The citric acid (TCA) cycle***: Each acetyl-CoA that enters the citric acid cycle yields 1 GTP, 1 $FADH_2$, and 3 NADH; each GTP, $FADH_2$, and NADH ultimately yields 1, 2, or 3 ATPs, respectively. TCA cycle flux matches work output of the heart. *Citrate synthase activity is close to normal, suggesting that flux, not amount, is lower in the failing heart.*
4. $FADH_2$ and NADH are used in the electron transport chain. NADH and $FADH_2$ are the obligatory intermediary molecules that transfer electrons to O_2. The transfer of electrons is energetically driven by the dissipation of a proton gradient across the inner mitochondrial membrane. The number of mitochondrial-encoded and nuclear-encoded gene transcripts for respiratory chain proteins *decrease.*
5. The flow of electrons provides the energy needed to phosphorylate ADP to form ATP via the ***F_1, F_0-ATPase***. *Both activity and mRNA levels decrease.*
6. Mitochondrial ATP is then exchanged for cytosolic ADP via the ***adenine nucleotide transporter*** (ANT). *ANT1 isozyme falls in failing hearts. Pattern of ANT isozyme shifts is cardiomyopathy-specific.* (Redrawn with permission from Ingwall JS. (2002). *ATP and the heart.* Boston: Kluwer Academic, Norwel, MA.)[28]

(Figure 7-5). The remodeling is not random, but is controlled by energy sensors that produce changes in phosphorylation state (and many other chemical modifications) of many proteins leading to short-term preservation of ATP and by activation of transcription factors that coordinately control long-term remodeling of ATP synthesis and using pathways. There is consensus that in compensated hypertrophy, in addition to a long-recognized decreased capacity for phosphotransferase reactions,[29-31] glucose use increases while FAO either remains the same[32,33] or decreases.[34] In uncompensated hypertrophy, FAO is decreased; the increases in glucose uptake and use are not sufficient to compensate for overall decreases in ATP supply.[17,35,36]

Here we begin by describing the change in [ATP] and, the proximal mechanisms for the loss of [ATP] and then describe how and why the ATP synthesis pathways change in the failing heart. We will then do the same for Cr. For both ATP and Cr, we will discuss the physiological consequences of these changes and attempts to manipulate metabolism to rescue the failing myocardium. We conclude with a brief comment on clinical implications and future directions for research in this emerging area. Space does not allow discussion of either the energetics of the ATP-using reactions in the failing heart or the energetics of the diabetic heart; some of this was presented in the first edition of this monograph.

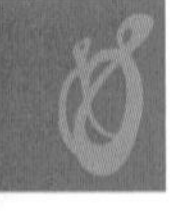

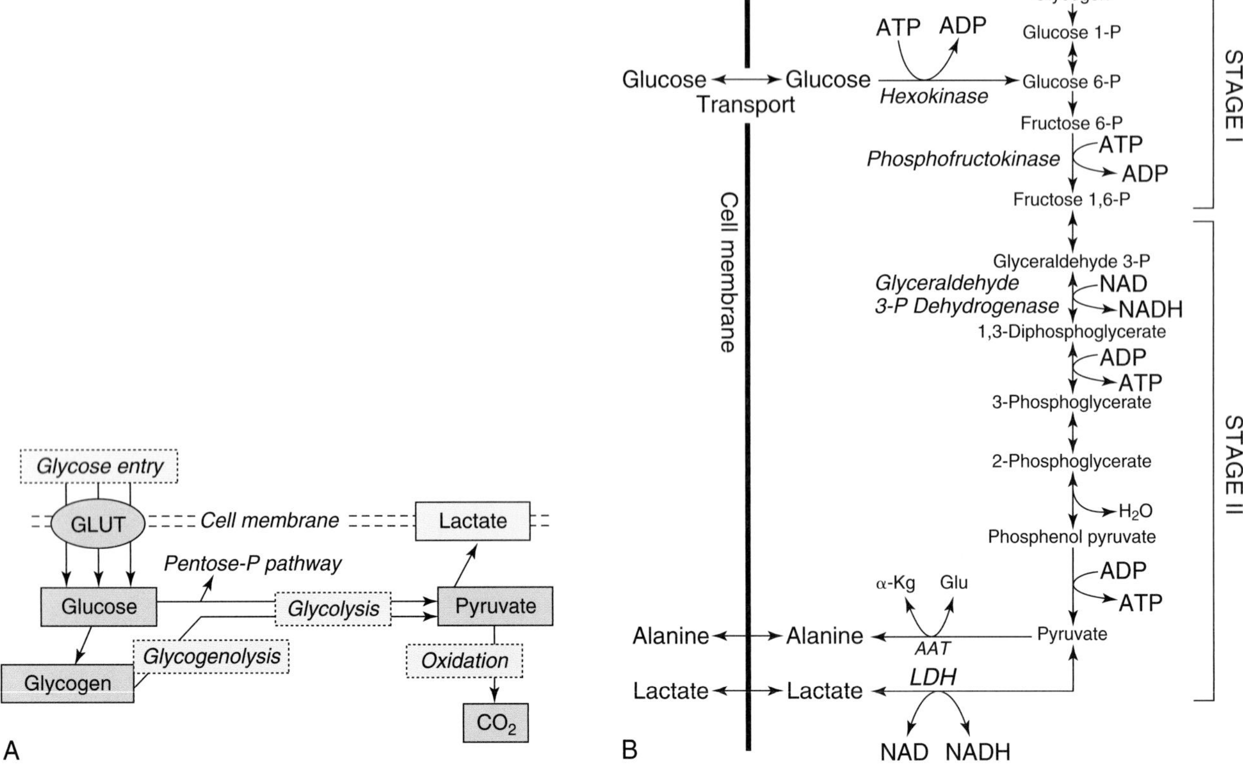

FIGURE 7–3 **A,** Overall pathway for glycolysis. **B,** Details of glycolytic pathway.
The overall strategy of glycolysis is:
Step 1: transport glucose into the cell. *Increase in LVH/failure.*
Step 2: add phosphoryl groups to glucose.
Step 3: convert phosphorylated metabolites to compounds with high phosphoryl-transfer capacity.
Step 4: couple the metabolism of these compounds to the formation of ATP. *Increase in LVH /failure.*
The overall reaction of the breakdown of glucose to pyruvate is:
glucose + 2 NAD^+ + 2 Pi + 2 ADP → 2 pyruvate + 2 NADH + 2 H^+ + 2 ATP + 2 H_2O. Two ATPs are made via glycolysis for every glucose transported into the cell that directly enters glycolysis. If the glucose is transiently stored as glycogen, the yield is 3 ATPs. If the pyruvate made from glucose enters the mitochondrion and is oxidized, the total yield is 38 ATPs per mole glucose. (Redrawn with permission from Ingwall JS. (2002). *ATP and the heart.* Boston: Kluwer Academic, Norwell, MA.)[28]

ATP Progressively Falls in the Failing Heart

In the severely failing human myocardium and in hearts of animal models of severe failure, [ATP] is approximately 30% lower than in normal myocardium (Table 7-1). Importantly the fall in [ATP] occurs in both left and right ventricular myocardium, in widely different species, and due to a variety of causes. Emphasizing the universality of this endpoint for the severely failing myocardium caused by widely different demands for ATP, a fall in [ATP] has even been shown in hearts of birds selected for ultrarapid growth. The energy requirements for exceptionally rapid macromolecular synthesis needed to support ultrarapid growth led to heart failure and a fall in myocardial [ATP].[37]

The rate of ATP loss is progressive.[38] In a longitudinal study of heart failure using the pacing-induced canine heart failure model, the rate of fall was approximately 0.12 nmol/mg protein per day or 0.35% of the total ATP pool per day. Thus making a quantitatively reliable measurement for the fall in ATP is possible only in severe failure, explaining the apparently conflicting results in the literature on this point.

The Proximal Mechanism

The proximal mechanism explaining the loss of ATP is the loss of the adenine nucleotide pool. The primary pathway for ATP degradation is ATP→ADP→AMP→adenosine→inosine→hypoxanthine. Phosphorylated metabolites do not readily cross the cell wall, but nucleosides and bases readily diffuse to the extracellular space down their concentration gradients. Nucleosides and bases do not accumulate in the hypertrophied or failing myocardium (blood flow is not limiting), and the fall in the sum of [ATP+ADP+AMP] parallels the fall in [ATP].[38] Activation of cytosolic AMP-dependent 5′-nucleotidase (5′-NT), which converts [AMP] to adenosine, is sufficient to explain the decrease in the [ATP] in the failing heart. In the normal myocardium, the small loss of purine that constantly occurs is matched by *de novo* purine synthesis from glycine, glutamine, aspartate, and formate at a rate of approximately 1.5 nM/sec.[39] To put this into perspective, *de novo* purine synthesis is approximately 10^6 times slower than ATP synthesis from OXPHOS. Experiments determining whether the rate of *de novo* purine synthesis changes in the failing myocardium remain to be made.

It is not known what prevents [ATP] and the total adenine nucleotide pool (TAN) from falling to values less than approximately 70% of normal. A recent report describing a mathematical model of cardiac energetics that successfully recapitulated the quantitative fall in [ATP] and [TAN] in the failing heart suggests that this is an emergent or intrinsic property of cardiac metabolism and referred to this value as a critical tipping point beyond which the heart would be severely compromised.[40] This is reminiscent of the comparison of [ATP] and [TAN] in trivial, moderate, and severe ischemia in the canine myocardium showing sustained [ATP] and [TAN] for moderate ischemia (TAN ~73%

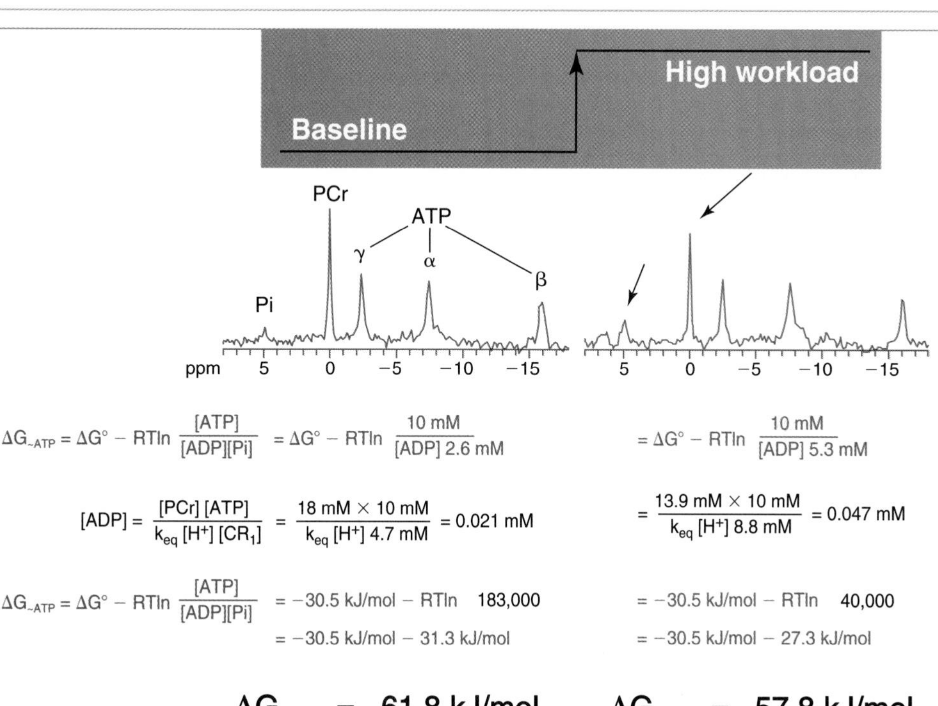

FIGURE 7–4 Crash course in energetics. Coupling of the CK and ATPase reactions provide chemical driving force, $\Delta G_{\sim ATP}$, needed to drive the ATPase reactions. The chemical driving force changes in response to work. $|\Delta G_{\sim ATP}|$ is calculated from the constant value for ATP hydrolysis under standard conditions, $\Delta Go\sim_{ATP}$, corrected for the actual concentrations of ATP, ADP, and Pi in the cytosol. The only terms in this equation that can change are the concentrations of the reactants in the *ln* term. To change $\Delta G\sim_{ATP}$ even by 4 kJ/mol as shown here, there must be large changes in the concentrations of ATP, ADP, and/or Pi. Classical biochemical tools used to analyze extracts of even carefully freeze-clamped tissue cannot provide accurate measures of [ADP] and [Pi]. For example, estimates for [ADP] in tissue extracts are in the 1 to 2 mM range, whereas the size of the metabolically active pool of ADP is 10 to 50 μM (i.e., about two orders of magnitude lower. [Pi] is also overestimated, by as much as tenfold. It is now possible to measure [ATP] and [Pi] and to obtain good estimates for [ADP] (using the CK equilibrium expression as shown) using ^{31}P NMR spectroscopy for human hearts and hearts of animal models of heart failure.

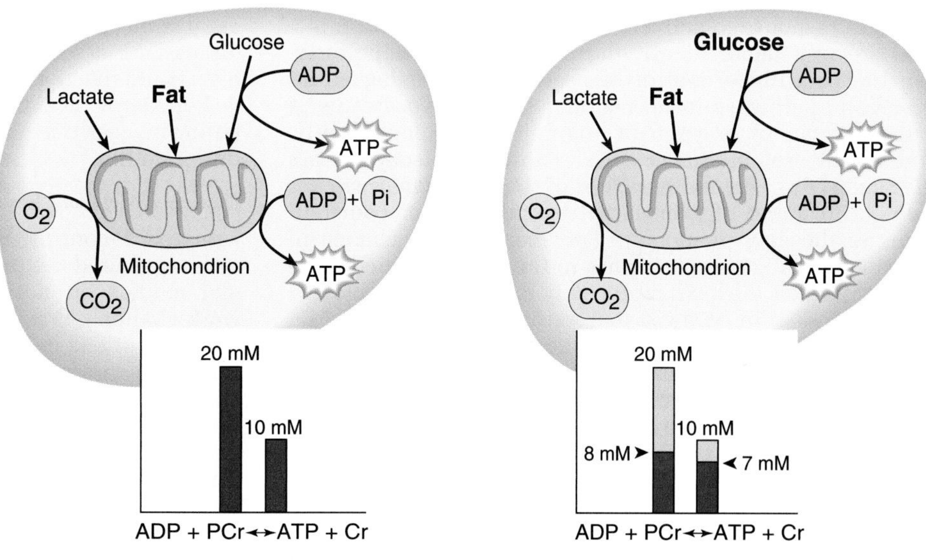

FIGURE 7–5 Summary of the major changes in metabolic regulation in the failing heart. The normal heart *(left)* uses primarily fatty acids for adenosine triphosphate (ATP) synthesis and, by the integration of ATP-synthesis and ATP-use pathways, maintains [ATP] and phosphocreatine ([PCr]) concentrations at approximately 10 and 20 mM, respectively. In the severely failing heart (right), fatty oxidation decreases while glucose use (and probably lactate as well) increases. The capacity of the phosphotransferase reaction catalyzed by creatine kinase decreases. The net result is lower [ATP] and [PCr]. *ADP,* adenosine diphosphate; *Cr,* creatine; *Pi,* inorganic phosphate.

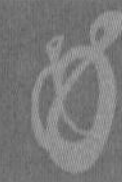

TABLE 7–1 Cytosolic Purine Nucleotide Concentrations in Normal, Compensated Hypertrophied, and Failing Myocardium*

	ATP(mM) →	ADP(μM) →	AMP(μM)
Animal Models			
Control rat[48]	10	11	0.02
50% LVH due to aortic banding	9	41	0.21 ↑
Control rat[114]	28†		
65% RVH due to monocrotaline supply	18[b]		
Control dog[38]	10	64	0.42
Pacing induced HF	8.0	49	0.34 ↓
Nonfailing TO-2 hamster[31]	8.7	74	0.60
Failing TO-2 hamster	6.4	36	0.20 ↓
Control turkey[116]	8.5	47	0.25
Furazolidone DCM	6.5	23	0.08 ↓
Broiler chicken—no HF[37]	1.6‡		
Broiler—HF	1.1[c]		
Human Myocardium			
Control[30]	10	43	0.17
Failing	7.6	31	0.14 ↓

*LV except where indicated. *LVH,* Left ventricular hypertrophy; *RVH,* right ventricular hypertrophy; *HF,* heart failure; *DCM,* dilated cardiomyopathy.
†μmol/g dry weight
‡μg/mg tissue

of normal at 30 minutes and 59% at 5 hours) but not severe ischemia (TAN ~66% of normal at 30 minutes falling to 14% at 5 hours).[41] The similarity in the tipping points for both severe ischemia and severe heart supports the notion that this is an emergent or intrinsic property of cardiac metabolism.

The Long-Term Mechanisms

Metabolism remodels in hypertrophied and failing myocardium: the mix of oxidizable substrates transported across the sarcolemma changes, proteins are modified leading to their short-term (in)activation, and new mRNA transcripts made in response to activation of certain transcription factors are translated. Identifying the mechanisms underlying the coordinate control of proteins comprising entire metabolic pathways in normal and failing myocardium is a major focus of research in this field today. Importantly, individual proteins that exist as families of isozymes are also subject to remodeling. Some of these *isozyme switches* (which are rarely if ever complete) make major contributions to the new phenotype. For example, the change in lactate dehydrogenase isozymes in the hypertrophied myocardium makes the heart more likely to metabolize lactate.[42] The decreases in MM-CK and sarcomeric mitochondrial CK (sMtCK) isozymes decrease phosphoryl transfer at specific sites where CK isozymes colocalize with ATP-using and ATP-synthesizing reactions.[3,43] The species-specific "switch" in myosin heavy chain (MyHC) isozymes alters the intrinsic myosin ATPase activity, which determines the maximal force and speed of contraction of the heart.[44] Changes in titin isozymes contribute to the greater stiffness of the failing heart.[45]

Changes in Glucose Uptake and Use

There appears to be universal agreement studying animal models and patients with cardiac hypertrophy and failure that glucose uptake rate and glycolysis increase (see chapter 20).[46-52] Increased glucose supply and use in the setting of chronic ATP demand is important because increased glycolysis could at least partially compensate for decreased ATP synthesis by other pathways. As several experimental studies of compensated hypertrophy have observed increased glycolysis with no change in FA use,[32,53] it seems likely that decreased FAO occurs later in the evolution of uncompensated hypertrophy (see later discussion).

The increase in glucose uptake is explained by increased expression of the basal insulin-independent glucose transporter GLUT1; expression of the dominant insulin-regulated glucose transporter GLUT4 is decreased or remains the same.

One mechanism explaining increased glucose uptake and use in the hypertrophied myocardium is triggered, at least in part, by the demand for more ATP (Figure 7-6). In chronic pressure-overload hypertrophy in the rat, decreases in [PCr] without a concomitant fall in total [Cr] lead to increases in [ADP], [AMP], and [Pi]. The increase in [AMP] activates the "low-on-fuel" sensor AMP-activated protein kinase (AMPK).[46,54] The consequences of activating AMPK are to activate proteins in ATP-synthesis pathways (increasing ATP) and to decrease the activity of proteins in ATP-consuming pathways (conserving ATP). Key among these are GLUT1 and phosphofructokinase-2 (PFK-2), leading to production of fructose-2,6-Pi_2, a potent allosteric activator of the rate-limiting protein for glycolysis, PFK (see Figures 7-4 and 7-6). In this model of compensated cardiac hypertrophy, both cytosolic [AMP] and fructose-2,6-Pi_2 increased by approximately tenfold, sufficient to explain the approximately threefold increase in the rate of glucose uptake, and approximately twofold increase in the rate of glycolysis for the same amount of O_2 consumed.[48] These results suggest that increased ATP demand (manifest as decreased PCr) in the hypertrophied heart signals an increase in glycolytic flux by several coordinate mechanisms: increasing glucose transport (thereby increasing substrate supply) and activating PFK (thereby increasing use) both via AMPK-dependent processes and via classic substrate control.

Unless AMPK can be activated by AMP-independent mechanisms,[46] however, it seems unlikely that AMPK remains activated in the failing myocardium for two reasons. First, cytosolic [AMP] decreases in severely failing myocardium (see Table 7-1). Second, activating AMPK is known to stimulate translocation of FA transporters to the sarcolemma and promote FA use for ATP synthesis; however, FA uptake and oxidation have been shown to be decreased, not increased, in a variety of experimental models of failing myocardium and in heart failure patients (see later discussion). It seems likely that an AMPK-dependent mechanism could function only as long as there is increased [AMP].

Long-term regulation of glycolysis in hypertrophied and failing myocardium is under transcriptional control (see later discussion).

Decreased Metabolic Reserve via Glycolysis

Unlike for control hearts, glucose uptake and glycolytic rates measured in the hypertrophied myocardium of animal models do not increase substantially *further* during work challenge[47,50] (but see later discussion for an analysis of contributions to oxidative metabolism).[36] Importantly, the limitation in metabolic reserve for glycolysis has also been observed in a group of Class I/II patients with dilated cardiomyopathy (DCM).[49] The approximately twofold increase in glucose uptake observed for DCM myocardium at baseline did not increase further when the heart rate increased, whereas it doubled in normal subjects. In terms of absolute values, glucose uptake was as high at baseline for DCM

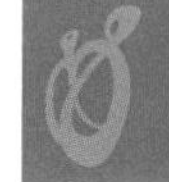

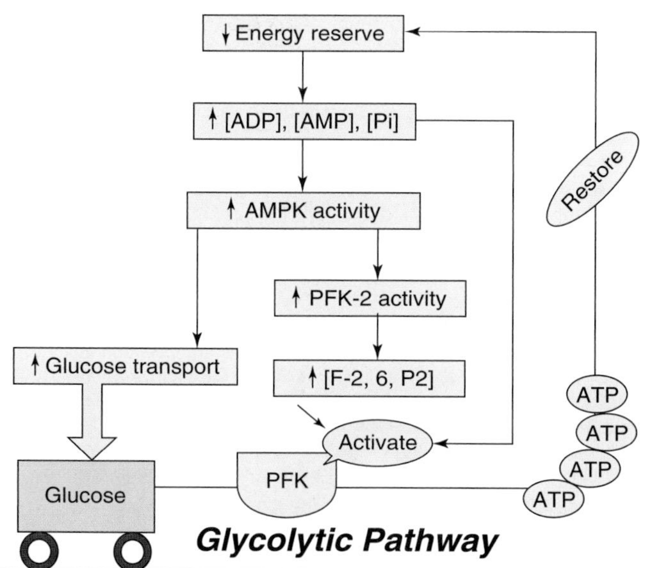

FIGURE 7–6 In chronic pressure-overload cardiac hypertrophy in the rat, increased ATP demand (signaled as decreased PCr) leads to an increase in glycolytic flux by two coordinate mechanisms: increasing glucose transport (increasing substrate supply) and activating PFK in the glycolytic pathway (increasing use), both mediated by AMPK. See text for more explanation. (Reprinted with permission from Nascimben, L., Ingwall, J., Lorell, B., et al. (2004) Mechanism for increased glycolysis in the hypertrophied rat heart. *Hypertension*. 44, 662-667.)[48]

myocardium as it was for normal myocardium with pacing, suggesting that there is an upper limit for glucose uptake in the DCM myocardium. FA uptake and oxidation, lower in DCM hearts, remained low. The authors described the inability of the DCM myocardium to meet increased ATP demand by increasing glucose uptake as "metabolic rigidity." These results are important because they support that hypothesis that any increase in glycolysis in developing and compensated hypertrophy (presumably adaptive) is not sufficient to meet the ATP demand in uncompensated hypertrophy. In this scenario, ATP use would exceed supply, contributing the inexorable loss of ATP in the failing heart.

Rescuing the failing heart by manipulating glucose metabolism

Genetic strategies testing whether the glycolytic reserve of the hypertrophied heart is sufficient to support increased contractile demand and if it can be manipulated to improve survival rates merit highlighting here.

One example used mouse hearts deficient (see Chapter 50) in the transcriptional activator peroxisome proliferator activated receptor α (PPARα), which have a threefold decrease in FAO and threefold increase in carbohydrate use, properties characteristic of the failing heart.[55] Isolated perfused PPARα null mouse hearts are able to sustain baseline function, but not high workloads. PPARα null mouse hearts had higher than normal MVO_2, yet produced less ATP, and [ATP] fell with inotropic challenge. Importantly, increasing glucose uptake and use *further* by crossing the PPARα null mouse with a transgenic mouse with cardiac-specific overexpression of GLUT1 rescued the PPARα phenotype. Hearts with augmented glucose uptake via GLUT1 were able to sustain increased work without losing [ATP], and MVO_2 and ATP synthesis rates returned to near normal. Another experiment found that increasing glucose availability in this way rendered hypertrophied hearts more tolerant to chronic hemodynamic overload and improved survival.[56] These genetic studies suggest that increasing ATP synthesis in the failing heart, in this case by substantially increasing glucose availability, can alter the natural history of heart failure. Achieving this in the failing human heart remains to be accomplished.

Changes in Mitochondrial ATP Synthesis

Genomic and proteomic studies,[57] and measures of specific enzyme activities, have shown that many proteins involved in FA transport and use are downregulated in failing hearts, contributing to the overall decrease in mitochondrial ATP synthesis rate.

Decreased Oxidative Capacity

Based on NMR experiments measuring desaturation of myoglobin in large animal hearts as an index of O_2 supply relative to O_2 use, it was shown that O_2 is not limiting in the failing heart.[58] The failing myocardium is not ischemic.[27]

Although O_2 is not limiting and does not prevent increases in cardiac performance in response to inotropic stimulation, it is likely that the failing myocardium operates near its maximum in oxidative capacity. In a study comparing compensated hypertrophy and failure caused by pressure overload in swine,[27] both hypertrophied and failing myocardium increased MVO_2 with catecholamine stimulation. PCr/ATP fell in the normal and hypertrophied myocardium but did not fall further in the failing hearts. However, when mitochondria were chemically uncoupled during inotropic stimulation to provide a measure of maximal oxidative capacity, the failing but not the compensated hypertrophied hearts were found to be functioning at their limit. Experiments using isolated mitochondria, skinned fibers, and isolated hearts[59,60] all support the conclusions that oxidative capacity of mitochondria is reduced in the failing myocardium and that mitochondria in a failing heart are at least partially uncoupled, leading to decreased cardiac efficiency.[38] Increased uncoupling proteins (UCPs)[59] and increases in reactive O_2 species and NO likely contribute.[20,60,61]

Changes in Substrate Selection for Oxidation Characteristic of the Heart Failure Phenotype Can Be Manipulated

Consistent with animal studies, patients with DCM have lower FA uptake (see Chapter 20).[49] Transplanted hearts from heart failure patients due to a variety of causes have lower total carnitine and total CPT (carnitine palmitoyltransferase) activities required for transport of long chain FA across the inner mitochondrial membrane for subsequent oxidation.[62] Analogous to increasing glucose supply to promote ATP synthesis, one approach to overcoming decreases in FA uptake is to increase FA supply. It has long been thought that supplying FA to hearts leads to lipotoxic effects, making this an unlikely strategy for rescuing the failing heart. This has recently been revisited, however, using a regimen that did not produce dysfunction on the heart.[63]

The kind of FA being oxidized is important.[46] Rates of FAO, glucose oxidation and glycolysis were compared in hypertrophied rat hearts supplied with either medium chain FA (octanoate) plus long chain FA (palmitate) or only longchain FA. With the mixture, FAO increased and, glycolysis fell to normal rates while glucose oxidation was unaltered in the hypertrophied hearts. Importantly, decreased cardiac performance of the hypertrophied heart revealed that perfusion with only long chain FA was normalized with the supply of both medium and long chain FAs. These results suggest differences in the capacity to use different classes of FAs in the hypertrophied myocardium.

^{13}C NMR spectroscopy studies of the aortic banded rat model of early heart failure have been used to define the relative contributions of endogenous triacyglycerides, exogenous FAs, glucose, and glycogen to mitochondrial ATP synthesis at baseline and when challenged to increase work.[36] At baseline levels of work, the relative contributions from glycogen, glucose, and palmitate to mitochondrial ATP production were essentially the same (±10%) as for sham hearts; the reason for this unexpected result was an absence of any contribution from endogenous triacyglycerides in the failing heart.

At high work for the failing heart, the contribution from glycogen and glucose increased by approximately 30% while that from palmitate decreased only slightly. Despite the increase in oxidation of glucose and glycogen, FAO was still the dominant source for ATP synthesis (60% for failing vs. 70% for sham hearts).

TCA cycle flux is closely matched to the amount of O_2 consumed to make ATP (see Figure 7-2), and thus plays a key role in setting the efficiency of the heart. A recent report[34] has shown that, at least in the hypertrophied myocardium, an unexpected mechanism contributes to maintaining a high TCA cycle flux needed to meet ATP demand. In response to pressure overload hypertrophy in the rat, PCr/ATP fell by 30% as expected, glycolysis was increased without an apparent increase in glucose oxidation, carnitine palmitoyltransferase (CPT-1) activity and FAO were reduced, yet MVO_2 and rate-pressure product were about the same. How were normal TCA cycle flux and MVO_2 sustained? The normal fate of pyruvate made by glycolysis in the cytosol is to be converted to acetyl-CoA for use by the TCA cycle by the pyruvate dehydrogenase complex (see Figure 7-3, *A*). That did not happen here. Instead, TCA cycle flux was sustained by use of glycolytically derived pyruvate through anaplerosis, a pathway that uses pyruvate to supply oxaloacetate downstream from acetyl-CoA in the TCA cycle (at 11 o'clock in Figure 7-4, *C*). The increase in anaplerosis is due to increased cytosolic malic enzyme in the hypertrophied myocardium, thereby increasing substrate competition for pyruvate between malic enzyme and PDH in favor of malic enzyme.[64] Activating PDH pharmacologically led to a decrease in malate, decreasing anaplerosis; importantly, triacylglylceride levels were restored and cardiac dysfunction was partially restored (improved dP/dt).[64]

There are at least three important implications of these observations. The first is that the apparent mismatch between glycolytic rate and glucose oxidation in hypertrophied myocardium is only apparent: pyruvate was used, just not to produce acetyl-CoA. Second, because conversion of pyruvate to oxaloacetate via anaplerosis consumes an ATP, this is a less efficient use of pyruvate. The increased in energy cost is unlikely to be sustainable; what appeared to be adaptive (maintaining TCA cycle flux via increased anaplerosis) is more likely maladaptive. This could be one step in the transition from compensatory hypertrophy to failure. Third, taken together, the results presented in this section show that the substrate supply for mitochondrial ATP production in the remodeled hypertrophied/early failing myocardium can be manipulated and that this can improve contractile performance.

Transcriptional Control of ATP Metabolism

The past decade has witnessed an explosion of information identifying the molecular links between physiological and metabolic stimuli and the regulation of gene expression in the heart. Not only have the metabolic targets of specific nuclear receptors and DNA-binding transcriptional activators been identified, but we are also beginning to learn how their signals are amplified and sustained (see Chapter 20).

Transcription is activated when transcriptional activators including PPARs, estrogen receptors (ERRs), retinoid receptors (RXRs), nuclear respiratory factors (NRFs), and MEF2 complex with proteins called PPARγ co-activators, PGC-1α and β, tethering it to DNA (Figure 7-7). When complexed with transcriptional activators, PGC-1s activate genes encoding proteins comprising entire metabolic pathways that control both ATP synthesis in mitochondria, phosphoryl transfer, and glucose uptake, and also ATP use. The different families of transcriptional factors bound to PGC-1 confer specificity for targets, although substantial overlap exists. PGC-1s in turn are regulated. Of particular interest here are Cdk 9 and 7, cyclin-dependent kinases that function to phosphorylate RNA polymerase II so that transcriptional elongation and mRNA capping can occur. Cdks had been thought to function to support all transcription, but recent work suggests that Cdk 7 and 9 may well target PGC-1s, thereby conferring specificity for the transcriptional control of ATP synthesizing and using reactions. Other known regulators of PGC-1s in striated muscle include p38 MAPK, calcineurin A/CaMKII, possibly AMPK,[65] and the circulating factors endothelin-1 and aldosterone.[66] The number of players in this complex hierarchical network (see Figure 7-7) increases yearly.

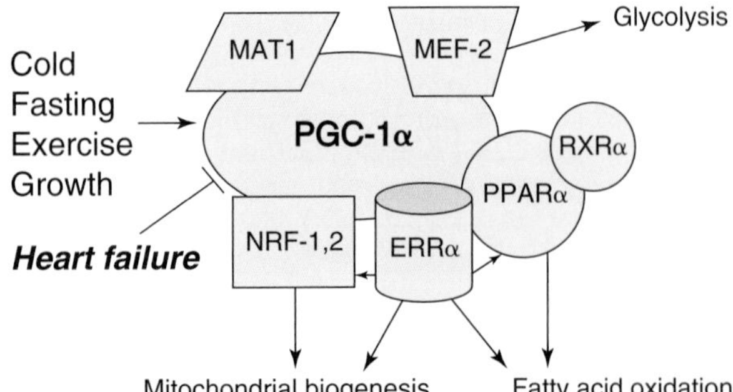

FIGURE 7-7 Schema showing transcriptional activators and coactivators important for long-term molecular remodeling of glycolysis and fatty acid metabolism in the hypertrophied and failing myocardium. Normal growth, cold and fasting all activate PGC-1α; but PGC-1α is lower in the failing heart, leading to impaired mitochondrial ATP synthesis. (Redrawn from Ingwall JS. Energetics of the failing heart: new insights using genetic modification in the mouse. 2006; *Arch des Maladies du Coeur et des Vaisseaux* 99(9):839-847.)

Important for the topic of this chapter, when measured, the failing heart has lower levels of transcriptional and coactivator factors[22,67,68] and higher levels of Cdk7 and 9.[69,70] Using loss-of-function and gain-of-function approaches in engineered mice, information has been obtained about the role of these factors in cardiac development and heart failure. A few examples will be given here.

PPARs exist as a family of FA-activated nuclear receptors abundant in the heart. PPARα is known to decrease in heart failure, and, as we have seen, loss-of-function in the bioengineered mouse heart recapitulates the heart failure phenotype of decreased FAO and increased glucose use. Gain-of-function studies using mouse hearts with PPARα, PPARβ/δ, or PPARγ overexpression suggest pathway-specific regulation of each PPAR for glucose and FA use.[71,72] Overexpressing PPARα led to decreased glucose uptake and use rates, increased FAO rates (as expected, the opposite of the heart failure metabolic phenotype) and increased triacylglyceride accumulation, leading to cardiomyopathy. Overexpressing PPARβ/δ had a different consequence: increased glucose uptake (via GLUT4) and use rates with no lipid accumulation and no cardiomyopathy. Overexpressing PPARγ led to increased FAO with no change in glucose metabolism and a dilated cardiomyopathy. While the exaggerated levels of expression of these transcriptional factors all lead to some form of cardiomyopathy that may have little to do with heart failure caused by pressure overload hypertrophy or secondary to myocardial infarction, they do help us identify how entire pathways for glucose and FA use may be regulated by PPARs: PPARβ/δ directs glucose metabolism while PPARα and PPARγ directs FAO and, via classic feedback control, indirectly should reduce glucose use.

Estrogen-related receptors (ERRs) are not activated by estrogen but instead are activated by PGC-1α and the closely related coactivator PGC-1β. ERRs may function to provide a long-term signal coupling the physiological response to hypertrophy (which can be short lived) and transcription. Using ERRα null mouse hearts at baseline and stressed by pressure overload hypertrophy,[68] it has been shown that the ERRα/PGC-1α complex targets a set of promoters common to genes encoding a wide spectrum of energy-producing (FA and glucose uptake, β-oxidation, OXPHOS, TCA cycle, electron transport chain), transferring (sMtCK and adenine nucleotide transporter), and utilizing proteins. Genes for ATP synthesis and transfer were all decreased while genes encoding the stress protein CK-B were increased. These experiments support the notion that normal ERRα/PGC-1α complex is required to blunt the loss of capacity for ATP synthesis in pressure-overload hypertrophy.

ERRγ and ERRα target a common set of promoters of genes involved in energy synthesis, transfer, and use in the adult heart.[73] In addition to the genes encoding proteins in ATP synthesis pathways, contractile protein isoforms and sarcoplasmic reticulum proteins were also identified as targets in ERRγ. In separate work,[74] ERRγ null mice exhibited newborn mortality, conduction abnormalities, and a complex energetic phenotype in the heart characterized by inability to fully metabolize pyruvate, disruption of the normal stoichiometry of the electron transport chain proteins, and decreased FAO. This phenotype suggests that ERRγ plays a major role in the metabolic shift from carbohydrate metabolism to oxidative metabolism in the postnatal heart. The partial reversal to a nonoxidative phenotype in the hypertrophied and failing heart is likely under its control as well.

Using Transgenesis to Define the Consequences of Decreased Capacity for ATP Synthesis

Although there is no doubt that decreasing ATP synthesis rates lead to decreased contractile performance in acute settings such as hypoxia and ischemia, testing whether a chronic mismatch between ATP supply and demand as occurs in the failing heart leads to contractile dysfunction is more difficult. So many changes occur in the hypertrophied and failing myocardium that it is difficult to prove cause, but it is possible to define downstream consequences of a specific change. The use of genetically modified mouse hearts in which a single change has been made has been critical in advancing our understanding of the consequences of decreased capacity for ATP synthesis. Here we present some additional examples where [ATP] and contractile performance have both been directly measured. Note that mice with genetically deleted transcription activators described previously all develop cardiomyopathy and/or demonstrate inability to sustain chronic hemodynamic load consistent with their importance in the molecular remodeling of ATP metabolism.

Modeling the observation that PGC-1α is downregulated in a hypertrophied and failing heart,[67] PGC-1α null mice have been used to define the consequences of reduced PGC-1α on ATP synthesis and contractile reserve.[75,76] The absence of PGC-1α not only led to reduced gene expression for proteins required for FAO and OXPHOS, but their enzyme activities were reduced. Importantly, [ATP] was decreased by approximately 20% (Figure 7-8), a surprisingly large decrease not unlike decreases observed in end-stage failing hearts caused by a variety of physiological stresses (see Table 7-1). This was also the case despite the presence of PGC-1β, which has many overlapping targets with PGC-1α. Central to defining the consequences of reduced ATP synthesis, PGC-1α null hearts had reduced contractile reserve (see Figure 7-8). Perhaps suggesting that PGC-1α null hearts have greater reliance on glucose, contractile reserve (although decreased) was greater in PGC-1α null hearts supplied with high concentrations of glucose and pyruvate for ATP synthesis than a mixture of substrates mimicking plasma levels of oxidizable substrates containing lower levels of glucose (see Figure 7-8). Consistent with these defects, PGC-1α null mice subjected to pressure overload progress to failure more rapidly than wild-type hearts.[77]

Cdk9 is a cyclin-activated kinase necessary for myocyte growth. Experiments in which Cdk9 was activated in myocytes showed cell enlargement with decreased PGC-1 mRNA and protein levels that could be reversed by restoring PGC-1 levels.[70] mRNAs for proteins involved in β-oxidation of FA, TCA cycle, respiratory chain, subunits of F_1,F_o-ATPase, and phosphoryl transfer by sMtCK were all observed targets. Activation of CDK9 promotes growth but suppresses genes for mitochondrial function by inhibiting PGC-1 promoter activity and, with mechanical stress, develop cardiomyopathy.

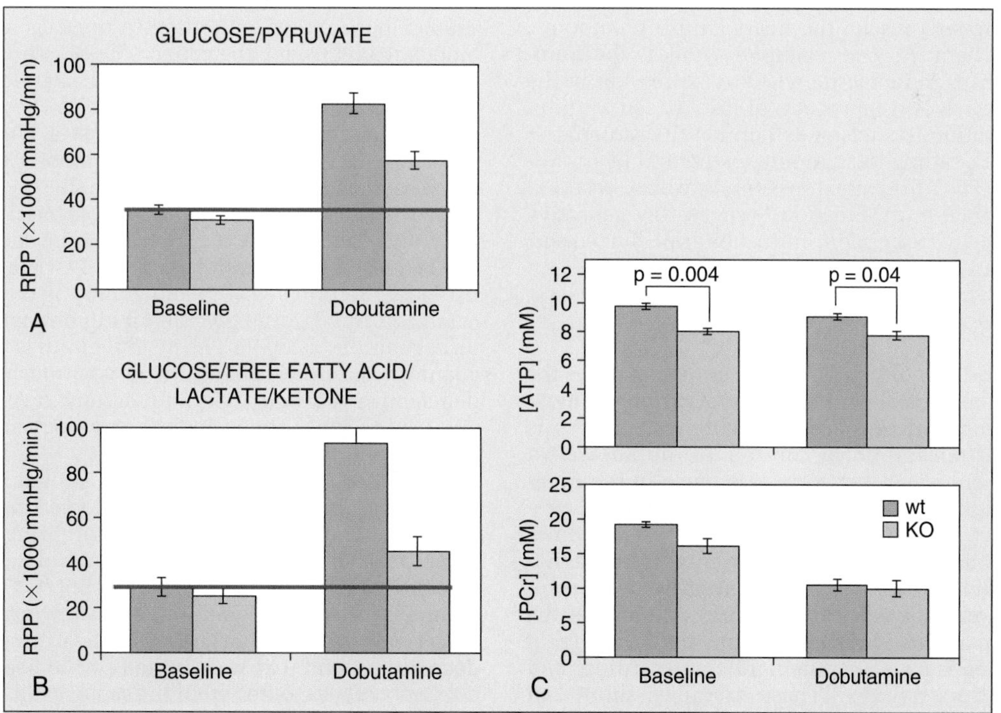

FIGURE 7–8 Mimicking what is observed in heart failure, PGC-1α null mouse hearts demonstrated increased contractile reserve, especially with glucose as the primary source of fuel for ATP synthesis (compare A vs. B) and decreased [ATP] similar to the failing heart. (Redrawn from Arany, Z., He, H., Lin, J., et al. (2005). Transcriptional coactivator PGC-1α controls the energy state and contractile function of cardiac muscle. *Cell Metab, 1,* 259-271.)[75]

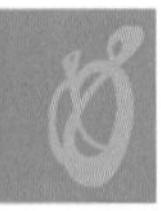

The Cdk7/cyclin H/MAT1 complex binds to PGC-1 where Cdk7 activates PGC-1 by phosphorylation. MAT1 null mouse hearts had lower mRNA and protein levels of PGC-1 and, as a result of reducing PGC-1 function, the ERRα-dependent program controlling energy metabolism was disrupted. Hearts developed mitochondrial dysfunction, impaired systolic function, and cardiomyopathy.[69] As these cyclins are activated in hypertrophy and end-stage heart failure, discovery of their role in regulating PGC-1s may make them major players in metabolic reprogramming of ATP synthesis and use pathways and the progression to failure.

Genetic manipulation in the mouse has identified many other players in the control of ATP production. For example, mouse hearts deficient in the mitochondrial transcription factor A (Tfam) gene develop progressive and rapid mitochondrial dysfunction and have a life span of only 10 to 12 weeks.[78] These hearts demonstrated an *early* shift in metabolism characterized by downregulation of genes encoding FAO proteins and, importantly, decreased activities of mitochondrial proteins. The late increase in mitochondrial mass and upregulation of genes important for glycolysis failed to compensate for these respiratory chain defects. Importantly, this metabolic remodeling took place early, suggesting cause and consequence. Lending further support to the essential role of ATP production to the failing heart, ablating muscle LIM protein in mice led to regional decreases in mitochondrial density and decreases in PGC-1α.[79] Finally, the consequences of a decrease in energy reserve via CK on contractile performance have been studied using a variety of approaches, all of which have shown that loss of the energy reserve system leads to abnormal energetics with decreased rate of ATP synthesis via CK, increased free [ADP] (correlated with loss of sMtCK[80,81]), and a lower $|\Delta G_{\sim ATP}|$.

Rescuing the Heart by Regulating Gene Expression

In addition to using loss-of-function approaches to establish cause and effect, gain-of-function strategies are important in testing whether loss of metabolic reserve contributes to contractile dysfunction. This approach has proven to be technically difficult due to the robust nature of the promoter most widely used to overexpress genes encoding cardiac proteins in attempts to rescue the heart failure phenotype, α-myosin heavy chain. A good example of this is the unintended consequences of increasing PGC-1α expression in the mouse heart. Massive overexpression of PGC-1α led to mitochondrial proliferation to such an extent that the sarcomeres became displaced, leading to cardiomyopathy and heart failure.[82] Short-term PGC-1α overexpression, however, resulted in reversible contractile dysfunction,[83] suggesting causative links among PGC-1α expression, mitochondrial biogenesis, ATP synthesis, and contractile performance.

Posttranscriptional Control of ATP Metabolism

Unlike the impressive progress made understanding the genomic events that control normal and hypertrophic growth and the development of cardiac dysfunction, much less is known about posttranscriptional control. We do know that the notion that there is a 1-to-1 correspondence in the number of mRNA transcripts and the number of functional proteins is not correct. A relevant example is the observation of a decrease in number of transcripts but an increase in activities of acyl-CoA dehydrogenases for rodent hearts with coronary artery ligation-induced heart failure.[63] Another is the mismatch among mRNA, protein amount, and activity of the CK-B and CK-M isozymes in the failing myocardium and during recovery from failure.[84] These examples show that protein activity is under posttranscriptional control and transcriptional control. As the relationships among the number of transcripts and enzyme activity and flux through metabolic pathways can be and are different for every protein, care must be taken when extrapolating both genomic and proteomic results to protein function. Another caveat is that it is not obvious whether any change in protein activity is large enough to translate into altered flux through metabolic pathways. This is an important point because enzymes in most metabolic pathways have high capacity (Vmax); moreover, and flux is usually low compared with capacity and to overall flux through the pathway. Because of this redundancy in design, decreases of even 50% to 70% in the activity of one enzyme need not affect flux through the entire pathway.[85,86] The challenges for understanding metabolism in the failing heart are immense.

CREATINE AND THE FAILING HEART

Cr Progressively Falls in the Failing Heart

It has been known since the early 1930s that [Cr] (and therefore [PCr]) falls in hypertrophied and failing myocardium.[87] This observation has been rediscovered about every 20 years.[88,89] Most recently, ^{31}P and ^{1}H NMR spectroscopy has been used to show decreased PCr/ATP and decreased absolute levels of Cr, PCr, and ATP in hypertrophied and failing human myocardium due to a wide variety of causes, in complete accord with the large number of large and small animal studies.[10,15] Since [ATP] also falls in the failing myocardium, note that the fall in PCr/ATP underestimates the fall in [PCr]. The decrease in [Cr] occurs earlier, is faster, and occurs to a greater extent than the fall in [ATP].[38] Whereas the fall in [ATP] is not more than approximately 30%, the decrease in [Cr] can be as much as 50% to 70% in severely failing myocardium.[10]

Mechanisms for Cr Uptake

In the myocardium, total [Cr] (i.e., the sum of free Cr + PCr), is 30 to 45 mM,s of which 20 to 24 mM,s is phosphorylated by CK to PCr. [PCr]/[ATP] is approximately 2 in normal mammalian myocardium, making PCr the major high-energy phosphate compound in the heart. Cr is not made in excitable tissues, but rather is supplied to muscles and brain via the bloodstream through the action of the electrogenic transporter belonging to a superfamily of Na^+, Cl^--coupled transporters of neurotransmitters, and amino acids. The Cr transporter (CrT) in the sarcolemma moves Cr against a large concentration gradient and is saturated at typical blood Cr levels. The primary sources for blood-borne Cr are dietary (meat) and from a two-step biosynthesis that occurs primarily in the kidney, liver, and pancreas. Figure 7-9 shows the steps for Cr biosynthesis and the structure of PCr. Briefly, Cr, a β-amino acid, is made by the transfer of glycine onto the arginine side chain catalyzed by arginine:glycine amidinotransferase (AGAT) to form guanidinoacetate. The methyl group is transferred to the guanidino group via guanidino methyltransferase (GAMT). Cr deficiency syndrome due to mutations in AGAT, GAMT, and CrT lead to severe neurological pathology and epilepsy with no apparent muscle involvement.[90]

Decreases in blood [Cr] cannot explain the decrease in myocardial Cr accumulation in hypertrophy and failure as skeletal muscle from heart failure animals has normal [Cr].[31] Instead, Cr transport and accumulation into the myocyte are well explained by the amount of CrT on the sarcolemma. While the original report[91] showing that the amount of CrT was decreased in the failing heart in proportion to the decrease in total [Cr] was limited by the use of a nonspecific antibody, other studies yield the same result. In a rat model of chronic heart failure, the 30% decrease in total [Cr] was well matched to the 26% decrease in the rate of Cr uptake.[92] Thus the recent report that human and rat myocardium expresses

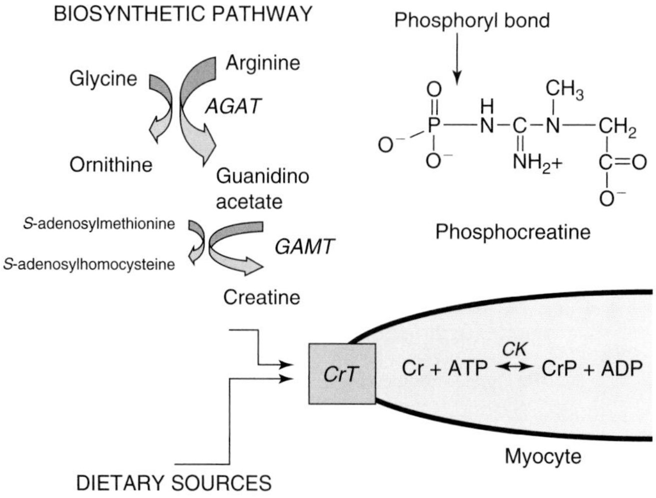

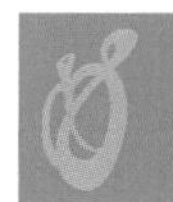

FIGURE 7–9 The primary sources for blood-borne creatine (Cr) are dietary (meat) and from a two-step biosynthesis that occurs primarily in the kidney, liver, and pancreas. Briefly, Cr, a b-amino acid, is made by the transfer of glycine onto the arginine side chain catalyzed by arginine:glycine amidinotransferase (AGAT) to form guanidinoacetate. The methyl group is transferred to the guanidino group via guanidino methyltransferase (GAMT). Cr accumulates in muscles and brain through the action of the Cr transporter (CrT) in the sarcolemma. Cr is trapped by phosphorylation to phosphocreatine (PCr, see structure) by creatine kinase (CK). (Redrawn with permission from Ingwall JS. On the hypothesis that the failing heart is energy starved: lessons learned from the metabolism of ATP and creatine. *Curr Hypertens Rep* 2006;8(6):457-464.)[11]

AGAT and that expression is reversibly elevated in heart failure was unexpected.[93] Whether the heart is capable of local Cr synthesis as suggested in this report or whether AGAT is localized in the vessel wall as suggested by a developmental study[94] remains to be determined.

The amount of CrT on the plasma membrane is regulated in two ways. First, it is regulated by the amount of plasma [Cr], with less CrT protein on the membrane when plasma [Cr] is high and vice versa.[95] Second, trafficking of CrT to the plasma membrane is regulated by a cascade initiated by stress, insulin, growth factors, and mTOR. These agents activate the serum and glucocorticoid-inducible kinase, SGK1, which phosphorylates and thereby activates phosphatidylinositol-3-phosphate-5-kinase, leading to greater formation of the metabolite phosphatidylinositol-3,5-phosphate. The increase in phosphatidylinositol-3,5-phosphate increases CrT trafficking to the plasma membrane.[96] SGK1 is known to modify the activity and abundance of many ion channels in the plasma membrane, such as the Na,H-exchanger, and other transporters such as GLUT4. The unexplained observation that total Cr was higher in transgenic mice overexpressing GLUT4[97] may now be explained by recognizing that CrT and GLUT 4 trafficking to the plasma membrane are regulated in the same way. As the calcineurin inhibitor cyclosporine A also changes the fraction of CrT on the membrane,[98] the observation that Cr was higher in calcineurin-overexpressing hearts[99] is likely explained by increased CrT trafficking. These results open a new line of research on the regulation of CrT and [Cr] in the heart. Long-term regulation of CrT synthesis remains to be defined.

Decreased Metabolic Reserve via Creatine Kinase

Because the velocity of the CK reaction is proportional to the product of [Cr] and Vmax (or maximum activity), the decrease in [Cr] coupled with the known decrease in CK (primarily MM-CK and sMtCK) activity combine to limit this energy reserve system in the hypertrophied and failing heart. In animal models of severe heart failure, approximately 30% and approximately 60% decreases in Vmax and [Cr], respectively, combine to reduce the velocity of the CK reaction by approximately 70%. Direct measure of the unidirectional CK reaction velocity using saturation transfer NMR in failing human myocardium demonstrate lower CK flux, by 50%,[100] as predicted from analysis of the CK system in human myocardium[30] and observed for experimental models.[10]

Manipulating [Cr]

Genetic modification in the mouse designed to manipulate the size of the myocardial Cr pool has expanded our understanding of the relationship between energy reserve via the CK system and contractile performance. Loss of function in the mouse was accomplished by replacing the Cr pool with its precursor guanidinoacetate by ablating GAMT in the pancreas and by taking care to ensure that Cr was not ingested by the mice (see Figure 7-9).[101] Hearts of these mice had undetectable levels of Cr and hence no PCr. As observed for hearts with low CK activity caused by a variety of maneuvers,[10] hearts from GAMT null mice had normal contractile performance at baseline but reduced contractile reserve when challenged with an inotropic agent and increased susceptibility to ischemic injury. Thus recapitulating the hypertrophied and failing heart, decreased energy reserve caused by decreasing the Cr pool led to decreased contractile reserve.

A gain-of-function strategy was used to test whether increasing CrT protein increased the cytosolic Cr pool in the mouse heart.[102] The myocardial Cr pool increased on average twofold but, unexpectedly, the fraction of Cr that was phosphorylated was lower by approximately 50%, despite normal CK activity. As a consequence of the lower PCr to Cr ratio, cytosolic [ADP] increased and the driving force for ATPase reactions, $|\Delta G_{\sim ATP}|$, was lower. Importantly, these hearts developed left ventricular hypertrophy, dilation, and dysfunction. While this experiment supports a causal relationship between decreased energy reserve and contractile dysfunction, a longitudinal analysis defining the temporal sequence of these changes remains to be done. This experiment demonstrates that it is possible to manipulate cytosolic [Cr], suggesting a new experimental approach to the study of the energetics of the heart.

A different gain-of-function strategy is to create a model of recovery from heart failure to determine whether [Cr] returns toward control and whether this correlates with improved contractile function. Such models are rare, but recently, these measurements were made in myocardium obtained during recovery from pacing-induced heart failure in the dog. [Cr] and CK activity and contractile performance all returned toward normal.[84] While this positive result is correlative and not proof, a negative result would have argued against the importance of energy reserve in supporting contractile performance.

The consequences of decreasing PCr/Cr on contractile performance may be more profound than decreasing CK activity alone. In contrast to the experiments described above, CK-MM, CK-MtCK, and CK-MM/CK-MtCK null mouse hearts did not exhibit cardiac hypertrophy or failure.[81,103-105] CK-MM/CK-MtCK null mouse hearts had elevated [ADP] and hence a lower chemical driving force for ATPases; the cost of contraction was higher. Mitochondrial biology in these hearts was abnormal.[22]

Loss of Cr: Adaptive or Maladaptive?

The observations that increased free Cr leads to contractile dysfunction, hypertrophy, and dilation[102] raises the question of whether the loss of Cr in the failing heart is compensatory

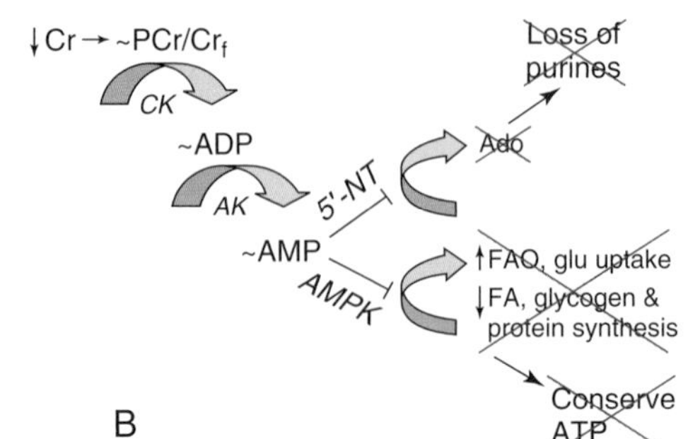

FIGURE 7–10 A question of balance. **A,** In response to an acute stress, [PCr] falls. As consequences of CK and AK near equilibrium, [ADP] and [AMP] increase. Two consequences of increased [AMP] are activation of AMPK, the "low-on-fuel" sensor leading to increased glucose uptake and FAO and decreased ATP consuming reactions, and activation of 5′-nucleotidase leading to loss of purines. **B,** As [Cr] falls, [ADP] and [AMP] normalize, slowing the loss of purines (adaptive) but also metabolic remodeling (maladaptive?). Depending on the balance between these processes, metabolic remodeling may not support contractile function. (Redrawn from Ingwall JS. Energetics of the failing heart: new insights using genetic modification in the mouse. 2006; *Arch des Maladies du Coeur et des Vaisseaux* 99(9):839-847.)

or deleterious.[38] The notion that loss of Cr could be compensatory may seem counterintuitive. Loss of Cr reduces the velocity of the CK reaction, and thus reduces the primary energy buffer in the heart at a time when overall energy supply is compromised. However, loss of Cr also minimizes the increase in free [ADP] and hence maintains a near normal $|\Delta G_{\sim ATP}|$. Maintaining low cytosolic [ADP] also keeps free [AMP] low, reducing the loss of purines. This is quantitatively important because cytosolic [AMP] calculated using the AK equilibrium expression increases with the square of [ADP]. This schema is a direct consequence of the near equilibrium of the CK and AK reactions; unless the reaction mechanisms for these enzymes change due to chemical modification or binding to other proteins, it is unlikely that this scenario would be substantially modified. The model of cardiac energy metabolism identifying the tipping point for [ATP] referred to previously suggests that both lower and higher than normal [Cr] would lead to a lower driving force for ATPase reactions.[40]

It is worthwhile discussing the likely sequence of events that occurs as the acutely stressed heart transitions to the chronically stressed heart (Figure 7-10). In response to an acute increase in stress, [PCr] decreases, initially leading to increases in free [Cr], [ADP], [AMP], and [Pi]. The immediate consequences include (1) a decrease in CK reaction velocity, the major phosphoryl transferase; (2) a decrease in the phosphorylation ratio [ATP]/[ADP][Pi] and hence in $|\Delta G_{\sim ATP}|$, the driving force for myosin and ion pumps; (3) activation of cytosolic 5′-nucleotidase by increased [AMP], leading to a loss of purines; and (4) activation of AMPK by increased [AMP], a low-on-fuel sensor, leading to rapid reprogramming of metabolic pathways including increasing glucose uptake and use. With time, the progressive loss of Cr leads to reversal or normalization of points (2), (3) and (4), and (1) worsens. This analysis shows that the timing and magnitude of any change in [PCr]/[Cr] is critically important for understanding the metabolic remodeling that occurs during hypertrophy and failure, and ultimately the fate of ATP. It also suggests that whether loss of the ATP pool is attenuated or exacerbated depends on the balance between 5′-NT and AMPK activities. Surprisingly little is known about the time courses of the activation/deactivation of 5′-NT and AMPK in hypertrophy progressing to failure. The signals connecting physiological stresses and long-term metabolic remodeling by transcriptional activators and coactivators and how they fit into this schema remain to be defined. These are important areas for future studies.

ON CAUSES AND CONSEQUENCES: ENERGETICS AND CONTRACTILE PERFORMANCE

Identifying "causes and consequences" of any molecular change characterizing the heart failure phenotype is a daunting task. Changes even in critically important proteins involved in energetics can usually be tolerated by the myocyte because the cell is designed to compensate for the loss of any important enzyme or pathway. As shown here, redundancy in the design of energy metabolism minimizes fluctuations in ATP and chemical driving forces and provides high capacity for tolerating increased ATP demand in the normal heart and in compensated hypertrophy. When this strategy fails, the heart can no longer recruit its contractile reserve and failure ensues. The major consequence of the molecular reprogramming of the pathways for ATP synthesis in the failing heart described in this chapter is that the total capacity for ATP synthesis decreases, demand for ATP outstrips supply, and [ATP] and [PCr] fall. The heart failure phenotype results from a significant and substantial change in normal metabolic regulation. As we have seen from the examples cited for the transcriptional activators, the heart failure phenotype can be elicited by many different molecular defects. It is a common endpoint phenotype. In this section, we will describe some examples of different kinds of *causes and consequences* with a focus on contractile performance.

The idea that sustained hemodynamic load causes changes in gene expression in some but not all proteins is well supported by studies showing that the decreases in MM-CK and sMtCK isozymes, but not in MB-CK, were reversed in heart failure patients given a ventricular assist device[106] and in an animal model of recovery from severe heart failure.[84] Myocyte size, their location in the heart, hemodynamic factors, and the ability to adapt to stress all play important roles leading to altered gene expression in the failing heart. This is illustrated by an early study in which cell size and enzyme activities of several proteins known to change in cardiac hypertrophy and failure were measured in myocytes isolated from different regions of hypertensive and nonhypertensive hypertrophied rat hearts.[107] The activities of some proteins increased in proportion to myocyte size while others were relatively diluted and still others increased out of proportion to myocyte size. This myocyte study also showed that gene expression changes in response to sustained hemodynamic load.

Diastolic dysfunction occurs in many forms of heart failure, often in the absence of systolic failure. It is the most common phenotype of hearts bearing missense mutations in sarcomeric proteins associated with FHC. Of the many ways that diastolic dysfunction can occur, one of them is increased cost of contraction manifest as increased [ADP] and decreased $|\Delta G_{\sim ATP}|$. Increased [ADP] is known to slow cross-bridge dissociation in skeletal muscle. Can the increase in [ADP] and consequent decrease in $|\Delta G_{\sim ATP}|$ characteristic of the hypertrophied and failing heart cause diastolic dysfunction? Recall that $|\Delta G_{\sim ATP}|$ is lower than normal when [ATP] falls, [ADP] increases, [Pi] increases, or any combination of these changes occurs (see Figure 7-4). The possibility that increasing cytosolic [ADP] is sufficient to slow dissociation of the cross-bridges enough to slow relaxation in the intact heart has been tested.[85,86] Cytosolic [ADP] was manipulated in whole heart preparations without substantially altering any of the other known regulators of contraction, namely, ATP, Pi, H^+, or Ca^{2+}; the rate of ATP synthesis from glycolysis was also constant. In the normal heart, this was accomplished by chemically inhibiting CK to varying degrees, thereby altering cytosolic [ADP]. In the heart hypertrophied due to aortic banding, the changes were the result of the perturbations in the CK-PCr system, which occur during hypertrophy and failure. In both settings, a monotonic relationship between increased LV end-diastolic pressure and increased [ADP] was found (Figure 7-11). Taken together, these studies demonstrate that increases in the average cytosolic [ADP] in the absence of changes in any of the other known regulators of myofilament function are sufficient to slow cross-bridge cycling and impair diastolic function. Thus the increases in [ADP] secondary to a decrease in [PCr] observed in many forms of hypertrophy and heart failure may be sufficient to slow cross-bridge cycling and thereby contribute to diastolic dysfunction. Similarly, the increased cost of contraction in hearts with FHC mutations likely explains, in part, diastolic dysfunction characterizing its phenotype.

Decreased capacity for phosphoryl transfer to resupply ATP via CK and AK increases the cost of mechanical work. Increasing work in mouse hearts deficient in MM-CK and sMtCK is more energy costly than for control hearts.[80,81] Studies using otherwise normal mouse hearts deficient in AK have shown that, even though flux through the CK reaction and glycolysis increased to compensate for the loss in AK, more ATP per contraction was used in AK-deficient muscle.[108] A consequence of the disruption of energy transfer relay via CK within the myocyte is well illustrated by increased electrical vulnerability of the heart caused by failure to supply ATP via CK to the K_{ATP} channel in MM-CK null mouse hearts.[43]

Another consequence is illustrated by decreased contractile reserve in hearts with less than 2% CK activity. The relationship between energy reserve and contractile reserve was defined for the normal heart in which the energy reserve was acutely decreased by chemically inhibiting CK activity.[109] Hearts with very low levels of CK activity have less free energy from ATP hydrolysis available to support an increase in work, have lower contractile reserve, and use more free energy from ATP hydrolysis to support a smaller increase in work upon inotropic challenge. Based on experiments such as these in the normal heart and in animal models of heart failure showing a relationship between energy reserve via the CK system and contractile reserve of the heart, it seems likely that the decreased energy reserve of the human failing heart has a similar functional correlate. The failing heart is "energy starved" with respect to its capacity to rapidly resynthesize ATP. The energy-poor heart cannot recruit its contractile reserve without expending a disproportionate amount of energy.

A consequence of decreased capacity to increase ATP synthesis, regardless of cause, is high risk of acute mechanical failure during an abrupt increase in work state, a hypoxic

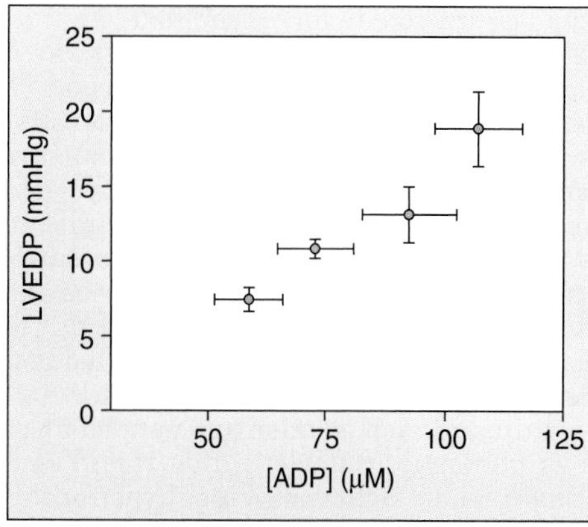

FIGURE 7-11 Relationship between the increase in the concentration of adenosine diphosphate ([ADP]) and the increase in left ventricular end-diastolic pressure (LVEDP) in isolated perfused rat hearts in which [ADP] was altered by inhibiting creatine kinase to varying extents.[69] Because all other known regulators of end-diastolic pressure were held constant, these results show that increased [ADP] is sufficient to slow cross-bridge cycling in the heart.[85]

or ischemic insult, or an arrhythmia. One demonstration of the greater susceptibility of the energy-poor heart to acute stress is the faster rate of loss of systolic performance during zero-flow ischemia in isolated mouse hearts deficient in the MM- and sMtCK genes.[110] Another example is shown by studies of myocardial infarction in the rat.[111] Myocardial [PCr] and CK reaction velocity were decreased by approximately 90% and [ATP] by 18% (a profile not unlike the heart failure phenotype) in rats by feeding them with the Cr analog β-guanidinopropionic acid, a competitive inhibitor of CrT and the CK reaction. Unlike control rat hearts that survived acute myocardial infarction, the 24-hour mortality of rats with a severely compromised CK-PCr system was 100%.

INTERVENTIONS DESIGNED TO ALTER ENERGETICS IN THE FAILING HEART: NEW STRATEGIES FOR THERAPY

There are two important lessons to be learned from this analysis of the energetics of the failing heart useful for guiding drug treatment of the decompensated heart. The first lesson is that the failing heart has limited energy reserve, and while it can increase work output, it does so at a higher cost of contraction. This increases susceptibility to arrhythmia and ischemic injury. The clinical observations that patients treated with drugs that increase ATP use to support acute increases in hemodynamics have poor long-term outcomes is most simply explained by the lack of energy reserve to support chronic increased ATP use.[1,112] Examples are positive inotropes such as digoxin (increased Na pump activity), dobutamine (increased contractility), and moxonidine (increased FA use). Research into ways of increasing systolic performance or reducing diastolic dysfunction by manipulating sarcomere function without increasing tension cost merits support. Studies of skinned fibers isolated from explanted hearts from patients with idiopathic dilated cardiomyopathy (IDCM) treated with either carvedilol or metoprolol illustrate this point.[112] Carvedilol treatment decreased tension-dependent ATP use, whereas metoprolol did not improve economy of contraction. Developing myosin activators that do not increase cost of contraction is a logical metabolic strategy.

Another pharmacological approach aims to take advantage of the small increase in the ratio of ATP production to O_2 consumed for glucose. Drugs that shift metabolism away from FAO and toward glucose metabolism improve the efficiency of ATP production. Drugs that target 3-ketoacyl CoA thiolase

(3-KAT), the last enzyme involved in β-oxidation (see Figure 7-2) such as trimetazidine, shift metabolism away from FAO and have shown promise in preserving ATP and PCr during ischemia (see Chapter 50).[5] Agents that target CPT-1, which transports FA across the inner mitochondrial membrane—such as etomoxir, perhexiline, and oxfenicine—all increase glucose use. A corollary would seem to be that decreasing plasma levels of FA and increasing glucose supply would be cardioprotective. However, this may not be the case. In patients with IDCM, acute FA depletion did not downregulate OXPHOS and efficiency fell, suggesting that both glucose and FA are required even for the failing heart.[113]

Direct manipulation of adenine nucleotide or Cr pools has been elusive clinically. Notable in this regard is the report studying experimental right ventricular hypertrophy[114] showing that folate treatment protected against loss of adenine nucleotides and diastolic dysfunction. The underlying mechanism is undefined. As folate is both readily available and inexpensive, strategies such as this may be useful in slowing the progression to failure. Beneficial effects of supplying D-ribose, a precursor of ATP, have also been reported.[115]

In any rational strategy, care should be taken to match intervention with the stage of disease. The different pathways for ATP synthesis are compromised at different times in the evolution of compensated to uncompensated hypertrophy. Loss of the energy reserve system supported by CK occurs first, and triggers an increase in glycolysis. As some models of hypertrophy show no decrease in FAO when glucose use increases, it seems likely that decreased ATP synthesis via FAO is last in this trio to change. Ideally, interventions designed to alter metabolic pathways must be matched to *stage of metabolic dysfunction*, analogous to NYHA classes.

Much more research needs to be done to test whether the metabolic remodeling of the failing heart is stable or worsens with advanced heart failure, whether the increase in glucose use (or the insufficient increase in glucose use) or decrease in fatty acid use is primary, whether there is a common molecular endpoint for all types of heart failure, and whether novel strategies based on informed knowledge of metabolic remodeling can rescue the failing human myocardium. Remodeling the "remodeled metabolome" in the failing heart would have significant clinical impact.

ACKNOWLEDGMENTS

The author wishes to thank Linda Johnson for her work preparing this manuscript, particularly the illustrations. This work was supported in part by research funds from the Department of Medicine, Brigham and Women's Hospital, and the National Institutes of Health.

REFERENCES

1. deGoma, E. M., Vagelos, R. H., Fowler, M. B., et al. (2006). Emerging therapies for the management of decompensated heart failure: From bench to bedside. *J Am Coll Cardiol, 48*, 2397–2409.
2. Dyck, J. R. B., & Lopaschuk, G. D. (2006). AMPK alterations in cardiac physiology and pathology: enemy or ally?. *J Physiol, 574*(1), 95–112.
3. Dzeja, P. P., Chung, S., & Terzic, A. (2007). Integration of adenylate kinase, glycolytic and glycogenolytic circuits in cellular energetics. In V. Saks (Ed.). *Molecular system bioenergetics: energy for life*. Weinheim, Germany: Wiley-VCH.
4. Finck, B. N., & Kelly, D. P. (2006). PGC-1 coactivators: inducible regulators of energy metabolism in health and disease. *J Clin Invest, 116*(3), 615–622.
5. Fragasso, G. (2007). Inhibition of free fatty acids metabolism as a therapeutic target in patients with heart failure. *J Clin Pract, 61*(4), 603–610.
6. Gustafsson, A. B., & Gottlieb, R. A. (2007). Heart mitochondria: gates of life and death. *Cardiovasc Res, 77*, 334–343.
7. Huss, J. M., & Kelly, D. P. (2004). Nuclear receptor signaling and cardiac energetics. *Circ Res, 95*(6), 568–578.
8. Huss, J. M., & Kelly, D. P. (2005). Mitochondrial energy metabolism in heart failure: a question of balance. *J Clin Invest, 115*(3), 547–555.
9. Ingwall, J. S. (2006). Energetics of the failing heart: new insights using genetic modification in the mouse. *Archives Des Maladies Du Coeur Et Des vaisseaux, 99*(9), 839–847.
10. Ingwall, J. S., & Weiss, R. G. (2004). Is the failing heart energy starved? *Circ Res, 95*(2), 135–145.
11. Ingwall, J. S. (2006). On the hypothesis that the failing heart is energy starved: lessons learned from the metabolism of ATP and creatine. *Curr Hypertens Rep, 8*(6), 457–464.
12. Kodde, I. F., van der Stok, J., Smolenski, R. T., et al. (2006). Metabolic and genetic regulation of cardiac energy substrate preference. *Comp Biochem Physiol A Mol Integr Physiol, 146*, 26–39.
13. Liu, T., & O'Rourke, B. (2009). Regulation of mitochondrial Ca^{2+} and its effects on energetics and redox balance in normal and failing heart. *J Bioener Biomembr, 41*(2), 127–132.
14. Maack, C., & O'Rourke, B. (2007). Excitation-contraction coupling and mitochondrial energetics. *Basic Res Cardiol, 102*, 369–392.
15. Marin-Garcia, J., & Goldenthal, M. J. (2008). Mitochondrial centrality in heart failure. *Heart Fail Rev, 13*, 137–150.
16. Neubauer, S. (2007). The failing heart—an engine out of fuel. *N Engl J Med, 356*(11), 1140–1151.
17. Stanley, W. C., Recchia, F. A., & Lopaschuk, G. D. (2005). Myocardial substrate metabolism in the normal and failing heart. *Physiol Rev, 85*(3), 1093–1129.
18. Taegtmeyer, H., Wilson, C. R., Razeghi, P., et al. (2005). Metabolic energetics and genetics in the heart. *Ann N Y Acad Sci, 1047*, 208–218.
19. Taha, M., & Lopaschuk, G. D. (2007). Alterations in energy metabolism in cardiomyopathies. *Ann Med, 39*(8), 594–607.
20. Tsutsui, H. (2006). Mitochondrial oxidative stress and heart failure. *Intern Med, 45*(13), 809–813.
21. van Bilsen, M., Smeets, P. J., Gilde, A. J., et al. (2004). Metabolic remodelling of the failing heart: the cardiac burn-out syndrome? *Cardiovasc Res, 61*(2), 218–226.
22. Ventura-Clapier, R. F., Garnier, A., & Veksler, V. (2004). Energy metabolism in heart failure. *J Physiol, 555*, 1–15.
23. Young, L. H., Li, J., Baron, S. J., et al. (2005). AMP-activated protein kinase: a key stress signaling pathway in the heart. *Trends Cardiovasc Med, 15*(3), 110–118.
24. Bittl, J. A., & Ingwall, J. S. (1985). Reaction rates of creatine kinase and ATP synthesis in the isolated rat heart. A ^{31}P NMR magnetization transfer study. *J Biol Chem, 260*(6), 3512–3517.
25. De Sousa, E., Veksler, V., Minajeva, A., et al. (1999). Subcellular creatine kinase alterations. Implications in heart failure. *Circ Res, 85*(1), 68–76.
26. Balaban, R. S., Kantor, H. L., Katz, L. A., et al. (1986). Relation between work and phosphate metabolite in the in vivo paced mammalian heart. *Science, 232*(4754), 1121–1123.
27. Gong, G., Liu, J., Liang, P., et al. (2003). Oxidative capacity in failing hearts. *Am J Physiol Heart Circ Physiol, 285*, 541–548.
28. Ingwall, J. S. (2002). *ATP and the heart.* Boston: Kluwer Academic, Norwell MA.
29. Ingwall, J. S., Kramer, M. F., Fifer, M. A., et al. (1985). The creatine kinase system in normal and diseased human myocardium. *N Engl J Med, 313*(17), 1050–1054.
30. Nascimben, L., Ingwall, J. S., Pauletto, P., et al. (1996). Creatine kinase system in failing and nonfailing human myocardium. *Circulation, 94*(8), 1894–1901.
31. Tian, R., Nascimben, L., Kaddurah-Daouk, R., et al. (1996). Depletion of energy reserve via the creatine kinase reaction during the evolution of heart failure in cardiomyopathic hamsters. *J Mol Cell Cardiol, 28*(4), 755–765.
32. Degens, H., de Brouwer, K. F., Gilde, A. J., et al. (2006). Cardiac fatty acid metabolism is preserved in the compensated hypertrophic rat heart. *Basic Res Cardiol, 101*(1), 17–26.
33. Lei, B., Lionetti, V., Young, M. E., et al. (2004). Paradoxical downregulation of the glucose oxidation pathway despite enhanced flux in severe heart failure. *J Mol Cell Cardiol, 36*(4), 567–576.
34. Sorokina, N., O'Donnell, J. M., McKinney, R. D., et al. (2007). Recruitment of compensatory pathways to sustain oxidative flux with reduced carnitine palmitoyltransferase I activity characterizes inefficiency in energy metabolism in hypertrophied hearts. *Circulation, 115*, 2033–2041.
35. Osorio, J. C., Stanley, W. C., Linke, A., et al. (2002). Impaired myocardial fatty acid oxidation and reduced protein expression of retinoid X receptor-alpha in pacing-induced heart failure. *Circulation, 106*(5), 606–612.
36. O'Donnell, J. M., Fields, A. D., Sorokina, N., et al. (2008). The absence of endogenous lipid oxidation in early stage heart failure exposes limits in lipid storage and turnover. *J Mol Cell Cardiol, 44*(2), 315–322.
37. Nain, S., Ling, B., Alcorn, J., et al. (2008). Biochemical factors limiting myocardial energy in a chicken genotype selected for rapid growth. *Comp Biochem Physiol, 149*(1), 36–43.
38. Shen, W., Asai, K., Uechi, M., et al. (1999). Progressive loss of myocardial ATP due to a loss of total purines during the development of heart failure in dogs: a compensatory role for the parallel loss of creatine. *Circulation, 100*, 2113–2118.
39. Zimmer, H. G., Trendelenburg, C., Kammermeier, H., et al. (1973). De novo synthesis of myocardial adenine nucleotides in the rat. Acceleration during recovery from oxygen deficiency. *Circ Res, 32*(5), 635–642.
40. Wu, F., Zhang, J., & Beard, D. A. (2009). Experimentally observed phenomena on cardiac energetics in heart failure emerge from simulations of cardiac metabolism. *Proc Natl Acad Sci U S A, 106*(17), 7143–7148.
41. Neill, W. A., & Ingwall, J. S. (1986). Stabilization of a derangement in adenosine triphosphate metabolism during sustained, partial ischemia in the dog heart. *J Am Coll Cardiol, 8*(4), 894–900.
42. Bishop, S. P., & Altschuld, R. A. (1970). Increased glycolytic metabolism in cardiac hypertrophy and congestive failure. *Am J Physiol, 218*(1), 153–159.
43. Abraham, M. R., Selivanov, V. A., Hodgson, D. M., et al. (2002). Coupling of cell energetics with membrane metabolic sensing. Integrative signaling through creatine kinase phosphotransfer disrupted by M-CK gene knock-out. *J Biol Chem, 277*(27), 24427–24434.

44. Hoyer, K., Krenz, M., Robbins, J., et al. (2007). Shifts in the myosin heavy chain isozymes in the mouse heart result in increased energy efficiency. *J Mol Cell Cardiol, 42*(1), 214–221.
45. Radke, M. H., Peng, J., Wu, Y., et al. (2007). Targeted deletion of titin N2B region leads to diastolic dysfunction and cardiac atrophy. *Proc Natl Acad Sci U S A, 104*(9), 3444–3449.
46. Allard, M. F., Parsons, H. L., Saeedi, R., et al. (2007). AMPK and metabolic adaptation by the heart to pressure overload. *Am J Physiol Heart Circ Physiol, 292*, 140–148.
47. Allard, M. F., Schonekess, B. O., Henning, S. L., et al. (1994). Contribution of oxidative metabolism and glycolysis to ATP production in hypertrophied hearts. *Am J Physiol, 267*(2 pt 2), H742–H750.
48. Nascimben, L., Ingwall, J., Lorell, B., et al. (2004). Mechanisms for increased glycolysis in the hypertrophied rat heart. *Hypertension, 44*, 662–667.
49. Neglia, D., De Caterina, A., Marraccini, P., et al. (2007). Impaired myocardial metabolic reserve and substrate selection flexibility during stress in patients with idiopathic dilated cardiomyopathy. *Am J Physiol Heart Circ Physiol, 293*, H3270–H3278.
50. Tian, R., & Abel, E. D. (2001). Responses of GLUT4-deficient hearts to ischemia underscore the importance of glycolysis. *Circulation, 103*(24), 2961–2966.
51. Zhang, J., Duncker, D. J., Ya, X., et al. (1995). Effect of left ventricular hypertrophy secondary to chronic pressure overload on transmural myocardial 2-deoxyglucose uptake. A ^{31}P NMR spectroscopic study. *Circulation, 92*, 1274–1283.
52. Zhang, J., Wilke, N., Wang, Y., et al. (1996). Functional and bioenergetic consequences of postinfarction left ventricular remodeling in a new porcine model MRI and ^{31}P-MRS study. *Circulation, 94*(5), 1089–1100.
53. Chandler, M. P., Kerner, J., Huang, H., et al. (2004). Moderate severity heart failure does not involve a downregulation of myocardial fatty acid oxidation. *Am J Physiol Heart Circ Physiol, 287*(4), H1538–H1543.
54. Tian, R., Musi, N., D'Agostino, J., et al. (2001). Increased adenosine monophosphate-activated protein kinase activity in rat hearts with pressure-overload hypertrophy. *Circulation, 104*(14), 1664–1669.
55. Luptak, I., Balschi, J. A., Xing, Y., et al. (2005). Decreased contractile and metabolic reserve in peroxisome proliferator-activated receptor-alpha-null hearts can be rescued by increasing glucose transport and utilization. *Circulation, 112*(15), 2339–2346.
56. Liao, R., Jain, M., Cui, L., et al. (2002). Cardiac-specific overexpression of GLUT1 prevents the development of heart failure due to pressure-overload in mice. *Circulation, 106*, 2125–2131.
57. Kong, S. W., Bodyak, N., Yue, P., et al. (2005). Genetic expression profiles during physiological and pathological cardiac hypertrophy and heart failure in rats. *Physiol Genomics, 21*, 31–42.
58. Murakami, Y., Zhang, Y., Cho, Y. K., et al. (1999). Myocardial oxygenation during high work states in hearts with postinfarction remodeling. *Circulation, 99*(7), 942–948.
59. Murray, A. J., Cole, M. A., Lygate, C. A., et al. (2008). Increased mitochondrial uncoupling proteins, respiratory uncoupling and decreased efficiency in the chronically infarcted rat heart. *J Mol Cell Cardiol, 44*, 694–700.
60. Murray, A. J., Edwards, L. M., & Clarke, K. (2007). Mitochondria and heart failure. *Curr Opin Clin Nutr Metab Care, 10*, 704–711.
61. Sheeran, F. L., & Pepe, S. (2006). Energy deficiency in the failing heart: linking increased reactive oxygen species and disruption of oxidative phosphorylation rate. *Biochim Biophys Acta, 1757*, 543–552.
62. Martin, M., Gomez, M. A., Guillen, F., et al. (2000). Myocardial carnitine and carnitine palmitoyltransferase deficiencies in patients with severe heart failure. *Biochim Biophys Acta, 1502*, 330–336.
63. Rennison, J. H., McElfresh, T. A., Okere, I. C., et al. (2008). Enhanced acyl-CoA dehydrogenase activity is associated with improved mitochondrial and contractile function in heart failure. *Cardiovasc Res, 79*, 331–340.
64. Pound, K. M., Sorokina, N., Ballal, K., et al. (2009). Substrate-enzyme competition attenuates upregulated anaplerotic flux through malic enzyme in hypertrophied rat heart and restores triacylglyceride content: attenuating upregulated anaplerosis in hypertrophy. *Circ Res, 104*(6), 805–812.
65. Puigserver, P., & Spiegelman, B. M. (2003). Peroxisome proliferator-activated receptor-gamma coactivator 1 alpha (PGC-1 alpha): transcriptional coactivator and metabolic regulator. *Endocr Rev, 24*(1), 78–90.
66. Garnier, A. Z. J., Fortin, D., N'Guessan, B., et al. (2009). Control by circulating factors of mitochondrial function and transcription cascade in heart failure. A role for endothelin-1 and angiotensin-II. *Circ Heart Fail*, (in press).
67. Garnier, A., Fortin, D., Delomenie, C., et al. (2003). Depressed mitochondrial transcription factors and oxidative capacity in rat failing cardiac and skeletal muscles. *J Physiol, 551*(pt 2), 491–501.
68. Huss, J. M., Imahashi, K., Dufour, C. R., et al. (2007). The nuclear receptor ERRα is required for the bioenergetic and functional adaptation to cardiac pressure overload. *Cell Metab, 6*, 25–37.
69. Sano, M., Izumi, Y., Helenius, K., et al. (2007). Ménage à trois 1 is critical for the transcriptional function of PPARγ coactivator 1. *Cell Metab, 5*, 129–142.
70. Sano, M., Wang, S. C., Shirai, M., et al. (2004). Activation of cardiac Cdk9 represses PGC-1 and confers a predisposition to heart failure. *EMBO J, 23*(17), 3559–3569.
71. Burkart, E. M., Sambandam, N., Han, X., et al. (2007). Nuclear receptors PPARβ/α and PPARα direct distinct metabolic regulatory programs in the mouse heart. *J Clin Invest, 117*(12), 3930–3939.
72. Son, N. H., Park, T. S., Yamashita, H., et al. (2007). Cardiomyocyte expression of PPARγ leads to cardiac dysfunction in mice. *J Clin Invest, 117*(10), 2791–2801.
73. Dufour, C. R., Wilson, B. J., Huss, J. M., et al. (2007). Genome-wide orchestration of cardiac function by the orphan nuclear receptors ERRα and γ. *Cell Metab, 5*, 345–356.
74. Alaynick, W. A., Kondo, R. P., Xie, W., et al. (2007). ERRγ directs and maintains the transition to oxidative metabolism in the postnatal heart. *Cell Metab, 6*, 13–24.
75. Arany, Z., He, H., Lin, J., et al. (2005). Transcriptional coactivator PGC-1α controls the energy state and contractile function of cardiac muscle. *Cell Metab, 1*, 259–271.
76. Lehman, J. J., Boudina, S., Banke, N. H., et al. (2008). The transcriptional coactivator PGC-1α is essential for maximal and efficient cardiac mitochondrial fatty acid oxidation and lipid homeostasis. *Am J Physiol Heart Circ Physiol, 295*(1), H185–H196.
77. Arany, Z., Novikov, M., Chin, S., et al. (2006). Transverse aortic constriction leads to accelerated heart failure in mice lacking PPARγ coactivator 1α. *Proc Natl Acad Sci U S A, 103*(26), 10086–10091.
78. Hansson, A., Hance, N., Dufour, E., et al. (2004). A switch in metabolism precedes increased mitochondrial biogenesis in respiratory chain-deficient mouse hearts. *Proc Natl Acad Sci U S A, 101*(9), 3136–3141.
79. van den Bosch, B. J., van den Burg, C. M., Schoonderwoerd, K., et al. (2005). Regional absence of mitochondria causing energy depletion in the myocardium of muscle LIM protein knockout mice. *Cardiovasc Res, 65*(2), 411–418.
80. Saupe, K. W., Spindler, M., Hopkins, J. C., et al. (2000). Kinetic, thermodynamic, and developmental consequences of deleting creatine kinase isoenzymes from the heart. Reaction kinetics of the creatine kinase isoenzymes in the intact heart. *J Biol Chem, 275*(26), 19742–19746.
81. Saupe, K. W., Spindler, M., Tian, R., et al. (1998). Impaired cardiac energetics in mice lacking muscle-specific isoenzymes of creatine kinase. *Circ Res, 82*(8), 898–907.
82. Lehman, J. J., Barger, P. M., Kovacs, A., et al. (2000). Peroxisome proliferator-activated receptor gamma coactivator-1 promotes cardiac mitochondrial biogenesis. *J Clin Invest, 106*(7), 847–856.
83. Russell, L. K., Mansfield, C. M., Lehman, J. J., et al. (2004). Cardiac-specific induction of the transcriptional coactivator peroxisome proliferator-activated receptor gamma coactivator-1α promotes mitochondrial biogenesis and reversible cardiomyopathy in a developmental stage-dependent manner. *Circ Res, 94*(4), 525–533.
84. Shen, W., Spindler, M., Higgins, M., et al. (2005). The fall in creatine levels and creatine kinase isozyme changes in the failing heart are reversible: complex post-transcriptional regulation of the components of the CK system. *J Mol Cell Cardiol, 39*(3), 537–544.
85. Tian, R., Christe, M. E., Spindler, M., et al. (1997). Role of MgADP in the development of diastolic dysfunction in the intact beating rat heart. *J Clin Invest, 99*(4), 745–751.
86. Tian, R., Nascimben, L., Ingwall, J. S., et al. (1997). Failure to maintain a low ADP concentration impairs diastolic function in hypertrophied rat hearts. *Circulation, 96*(4), 1313–1319.
87. Herrmann, G., & Decherd, M. (1939). The chemical nature of heart failure. *Ann Intern Med, 12*, 1233–1244.
88. Pool, P. E., Spann, J. F., Jr., Buccino, R. A., et al. (1967). Myocardial high energy phosphate stores in cardiac hypertrophy and heart failure. *Circ Res, 21*(3), 365–373.
89. Ingwall, J. S. (1984). The hypertrophied myocardium accumulates the MB-creatine kinase isozyme. *Eur Heart J, 5*(suppl. F), 129–139.
90. Sykut-Cegielska, J., Gradowska, W., Mercimek-Mahmutoglu, S., et al. (2004). Biochemical and clinical characteristics of creatine deficiency syndromes. *Acta Biochim Pol, 51*(4), 875–882.
91. Neubauer, S., Remkes, H., Spindler, M., et al. (1999). Down regulation of the Na(+)-creatine co-transporter in failing human myocardium and in experimental heart failure. *Circulation, 100*, 1847–1850.
92. Ten Hove, M., Chan, S., Lygate, C., et al. (2005). Mechanisms of creatine depletion in chronically failing rat heart. *J Mol Cell Cardiol, 38*(2), 309–313.
93. Cullen, M. E., Yuen, A. H., Felkin, L. E., et al. (2006). Myocardial expression of the arginine:glycine amidinotransferase gene is elevated in heart failure and normalized after recovery: potential implications for local creatine synthesis. *Circulation, 114*(suppl. 1), I16–I20.
94. Braissant, O., Henry, H., Villard, A. M., et al. (2005). Creatine synthesis and transport during rat embryogenesis: spatiotemporal expression of AGAT, GAMT and CT1. *BMC Dev Biol, 5*(1), 9.
95. Boehm, E., Chan, S., Monfared, M., et al. (2003). Creatine transporter activity and content in the rat heart supplemented by and depleted of creatine. *Am J Physiol Endocrinol Metab, 284*(2), E399–E406.
96. Strutz-Seebohm, N., Shojaiefard, M., Christie, D., et al. (2007). PIKfyve in the SGK1 mediated regulation of the creatine transporter SLC6A8. *Cell Physiol Biochem, 20*(6), 729–734.
97. Weiss, R. G., Chatham, J. C., Georgakopolous, D., et al. (2002). An increase in the myocardial PCr/ATP ratio in GLUT4 null mice. *FASEB J, 16*(6), 613–615.
98. Tran, T. T., Dai, W., & Sarkar, H. K. (2000). Cyclosporin A inhibits creatine uptake by altering surface expression of the creatine transporter. *J Biol Chem, 275*(46), 35708–35714.
99. Pinz, I., Ostroy, S. E., Hoyer, K., et al. (2008). Calcineurin-induced energy wasting in a transgenic mouse model of heart failure. *Am J Physiol Heart Circ Physiol, 294*(3), H1459–H1466.
100. Weiss, R. G., Gerstenblith, G., & Bottomley, P. A. (2005). ATP flux through creatine kinase in the normal, stressed, and failing human heart. *Proc Natl Acad Sci U S A, 102*(3), 808–813.
101. ten Hove, M., Lygate, C. A., Fischer, A., et al. (2005). Reduced inotropic reserve and increased susceptibility to cardiac ischemia/reperfusion injury in phosphocreatine-deficient guanidinoacetate-N-methyltransferase-knockout mice. *Circulation, 111*(19), 2477–2485.
102. Wallis, J., Lygate, C. A., Fischer, A., et al. (2005). Supranormal myocardial creatine and phosphocreatine concentrations lead to cardiac hypertrophy and heart failure: insights from creatine transporter-overexpressing transgenic mice. *Circulation, 112*(20), 3131–3139.
103. Crozatier, B., Badoual, T., Boehm, E., et al. (2002). Role of creatine kinase in cardiac excitation-contraction coupling: studies in creatine kinase-deficient mice. *FASEB J, 16*(7), 653–660.
104. Nahrendorf, M., Streif, J. U., Hiller, K. H., et al. (2006). Multimodal functional cardiac MRI in creatine kinase-deficient mice reveals subtle abnormalities in myocardial perfusion and mechanics. *Am J Physiol Heart Circ Physiol, 290*(6), H2516–H2521.

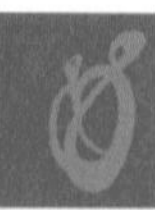

105. Lygate, C. A., Hunyor, I., Medway, D., et al. (2009). Cardiac phenotype of mitochondrial creatine kinase knockout mice is modified on a pure C57BL/6 genetic background. *J Mol Cell Cardiol, 46*(1), 93–99.
106. Park, S. J., Zhang, J., Ye, Y., et al. (2002). Myocardial creatine kinase expression after left ventricular assist device support. *J Am Coll Cardiol, 39*(11), 1773–1779.
107. Smith, S. H., Kramer, M. F., Reis, I., et al. (1990). Regional changes in creatine kinase and myocyte size in hypertensive and nonhypertensive cardiac hypertrophy. *Circ Res, 67*(6), 1334–1344.
108. Janssen, E., Dzeja, P. P., Oerlemans, F., et al. (2000). Adenylate kinase 1 gene deletion disrupts muscle energetic economy despite metabolic rearrangement. *EMBO J, 19*(23), 6371–6381.
109. Tian, R., & Ingwall, J. S. (1996). Energetic basis for reduced contractile reserve in isolated rat hearts. *Am J Physiol, 270*(4 pt 2), H1207–H1216.
110. Hopkins, J., Miao, W., & Ingwall, J. (1998). Paradoxical effects of creatine kinase deletion on systolic and diastolic function in ischemia. *Circulation, 98*(17), I–758.
111. Horn, M., Remkes, H., Stromer, H., et al. (2001). Chronic phosphocreatine depletion by the creatine analogue beta-guanidinopropionate is associated with increased mortality and loss of ATP in rats after myocardial infarction. *Circulation, 104*(15), 1844–1849.
112. Brixius, K., Lu, R., Boelck, B., et al. (2007). Chronic treatment with carvedilol improves Ca(2+)-dependent ATP consumption in triton X-skinned fiber preparations of human myocardium. *J Pharmacol Exp Ther, 322*(1), 222–227.
113. Tuunanen, H., Engblom, E., Naum, A., et al. (2006). Free fatty acid depletion acutely decreases cardiac work and efficiency in cardiomyopathic heart failure. *Circulation, 114*(20), 2130–2137.
114. Lamberts, R. R., Caldenhoven, E., Lansink, M., et al. (2007). Preservation of diastolic function in monocrotaline-induced right ventricular hypertrophy in rats. *Am J Physiol Heart Circ Physiol, 293*(3), H1869–H1876.
115. Maccarter, D., Vijay, N., Washam, M., et al. (2008). D-ribose aids advanced ischemic heart failure patients. *Int J Cardiol,* 137, 79-80.
116. Liao, R., Nascimben, L., Friedrich, J., et al. (1996). Decreased energy reserve in an animal model of dilated cardiomyopathy. Relationship to contractile performance. *Circ Res, 78*(5), 893–902.
117. Ingwall, J. S. (2002). *ATP and the heart: an overview. ATP and the heart.* Norwell, Mass: Kluwer Academic.

CHAPTER 8

Molecular and Cellular Mechanisms for Myocardial Recovery

Veli K. Topkara and Douglas L. Mann

Clinical studies have shown that medical and device therapies that reduce heart failure morbidity and mortality also lead to a recovery of the failing myocardium (Box 8-1), which is characterized anatomically by a return in left ventricular (LV) volume and mass toward normal values (see Chapter 15), and a shift in the LV end-diastolic pressure-volume relationship to the left (Figure 8-1). For want of a better term, the process of myocardial recovery, which encompasses a myriad of changes at the molecular, cellular, tissue, and organ level, has been referred to as "reverse remodeling."[1,2] Although the precise cellular and molecular mechanisms that are responsible for the remarkable return toward normal LV size and shape are not completely understood, there is a fairly consistent biological theme with respect to the parameters that return toward the baseline following pharmacological or device therapy. The importance of understanding these changes at a basic molecular level is that they may lead to the identification of novel therapeutic targets for treating/reversing heart failure.

In the 1980s and early 1990s, it was generally believed that once the heart became markedly dilated, no form of therapy could reverse this process in a meaningful manner, which led to the generally held concept of irreversible, end-stage cardiomyopathy. The concept of reverse remodeling emerged in the early 1990s based on anecdotal case reports of patients exhibiting substantial recovery of the ventricular function following mechanical unloading with left ventricular assist devices (LVAD).[3,4] Subsequent studies that showed that the end-diastolic pressure-volume relationship were gradually shifted leftward when compared in patients undergoing a cardiac myoplasty,[1] and in explanted hearts from patients who had undergone LVAD support,[2] implying that the heart was not simply unloaded, but rather that there were fundamental changes in the biological properties of the heart that allowed the ventricle to return toward normal size and shape. These early observations with devices were then mirrored by studies in heart failure patients who were treated with angiotensin-converting enzyme (ACE) inhibitors and β-blockers, in whom there were significant decreases in LV end-diastolic volume, in comparison to patients who received a placebo.[5-7] These unexpected observations with cardiac circulatory assist devices and medical therapy challenged the dogma that heart failure is an irreversible process that culminates invariably in death or cardiac transplantation, and fostered a greater interest in understanding the biological processes that are responsible for the restoration of normal cardiac structure and function.

It is now recognized that "reverse remodeling" or myocardial recovery can be recognized and defined by a series of changes that occur within the cardiocytes (i.e., resident cardiac cells, including cardiac myocytes, fibroblasts, endothelial cells), in the composition of the LV myocardium and in the geometry of the left ventricle (Box 8-2).[8] These changes may ultimately lead to improvement in ventricular function and even sustained clinical recovery from heart failure in select cases. However, it bears emphasis that many of the cellular and molecular changes that occur during the process of myocardial recovery occur in the absence of sustained clinical recovery of the patient. The reasons for this observation are unknown, but may relate to an inadequate mass of cardiac myocytes that are necessary to sustain adequate LV pump function. Although considerable research time and effort have been expended on understanding the basic mechanisms that promote LV remodeling (see Chapter 15), it is not clear whether a simple reversal of these same mechanisms will allow the heart to revert back to its normal size and shape. Accordingly, this chapter will focus only on those cellular and molecular changes that occur during reverse remodeling, as opposed to focusing on the cellular and molecular changes that occur when LV remodeling is prevented. Because of the paucity of the animal models to study myocardial recovery, the majority of our current knowledge with respect to the reverse remodeling process is derived from the clinical studies of patients undergoing heart failure therapies that improve LV structure and prolong survival.

CHANGES IN THE BIOLOGY OF THE CARDIAC MYOCYTE DURING MYOCARDIAL RECOVERY

Numerous studies have suggested that failing human cardiac myocytes undergo a number of important changes that might be expected to lead to a progressive loss of contractile function, including decreased α-myosin heavy chain gene expression with a concomitant increase in β-myosin heavy chain expression,[9] progressive loss of myofilaments in cardiac myocytes,[10] alterations in cytoskeletal proteins,[10] alterations in excitation-contraction coupling,[11] and desensitization of β-adrenergic signaling.[12] And indeed, when the contractile performance of isolated failing human myocytes has been examined under very simple experimental conditions, investigators have found that there is an approximately 50% decrease in cell shortening in failing human cardiac myocytes when compared with nonfailing human myocytes.[13] Moreover, this defect in cell shortening has a number of important components, which may act combinatorially to produce the observed phenotype of cellular contractile dysfunction. Thus the contractile dysfunction that develops within myocytes during the process of LV remodeling is likely to involve ensembles of genes, including those that regulate calcium handling, sarcomerogenesis, β-adrenergic signaling, and the cytoskeleton, all of which may interact in an exceedingly complex manner within the cardiac myocyte to produce contractile dysfunction. In the section that follows, we will review the experimental and clinical literature, which suggests that alterations in the biology and the contractility of the failing cardiac myocyte are reversible following conventional pharmacological therapies and/or treatment with cardiac devices, including LVADs, cardiac resynchronization therapy (CRT), and cardiac support devices (Table 8-1).

BOX 8–1 Pharmacological, Device, and Surgical Methods That Lead to Reverse Remodeling

Pharmacological Reverse Remodeling
β-blockers*
ACE inhibitors*
Angiotensin receptor blockers*
Aldosterone antagonists*
Hydralazine/isosorbide*

Device-based Reverse Remodeling
Mechanical circulatory assist devices
- Pulsatile*
- Continuous*

Cardiac resynchronization therapy*
Cardiac support devices

Surgical Reverse Remodeling
Myocardial revascularization
Partial ventriculectomy
Surgical ventricular reconstruction (SVR)
Mitral valve repair

*Denotes therapies that have been shown to reduce heart failure morbidity and mortality.

Cardiac Myocyte Hypertrophy

One of the essential components of the LV remodeling process is the development of cardiac myocyte hypertrophy, which is characterized morphologically by the addition of sarcomeres in series or parallel in response to hemodynamic overload, leading to the development of eccentric or concentric hypertrophy, respectively (Figure 8-2).[14] Several lines of experimental evidence suggest that cardiac myocyte hypertrophy is a dynamic process that is reversible following removal of hemodynamic pressure or volume overloading.[15] Although information is limited, there is evidence that the regression of myocyte hypertrophy that occurs following hemodynamic unloading is accompanied by changes in the activation and/or activity levels of protein kinases that are linked to cell growth, including extracellular regulated kinase-1 (ERK-1) and ERK-2, p38 (Figure 8-3),[16] Akt and GSK-3β (a negative regulator of hypertrophy), and transcription factors (GATA4) that are linked to hypertrophic growth.[17] Additional support for the concept of the reversibility of cardiac myocyte hypertrophy has been demonstrated repeatedly in pharmacological intervention studies in animal models of heart failure, which have shown that angiotensin-converting enzyme inhibitors and β-blockers can reverse cardiac myocyte hypertrophy in remodeled hearts.[18,19,20] The use of LVADs in patients with end-stage heart failure has greatly expanded our understanding of the reverse remodeling process at the cellular level in humans with heart failure (see also Chapter 56). Clinical studies from patients undergoing LVAD implantation have consistently shown a regression of myocyte hypertrophy with mechanical circulatory support (Figure 8-4),[17,21-25] although one study demonstrated a slight increase in myocyte diameter.[26] Similarly, treatment with cardiac support devices significantly reduced cardiac myocyte hypertrophy in animal models of heart failure.[27] In a prospective clinical study, cardiac resynchronization for 3 months was shown to attenuate the growth in cardiac myocytes in some patients with heart failure.[28]

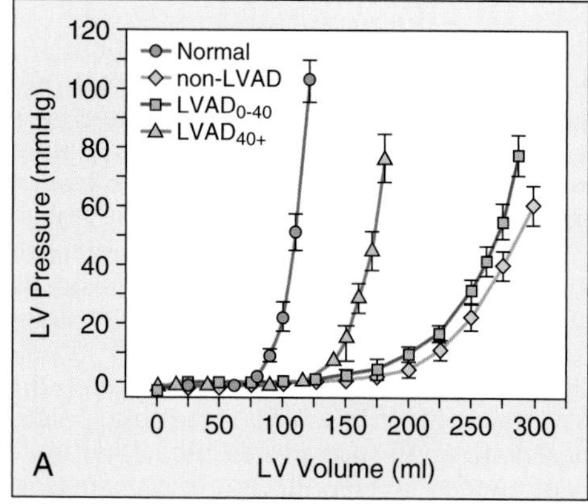

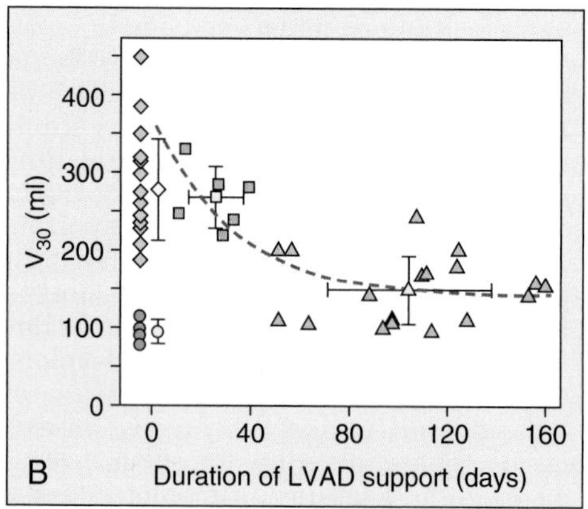

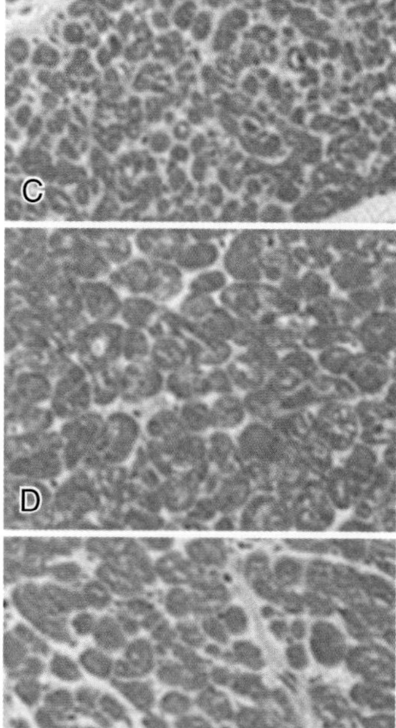

FIGURE 8–1 The ventricular end-diastolic pressure-volume relation, initially shifted far rightward in heart failure, shifts, over time, back toward normal. **A,** Average end-diastolic pressure volume relationships from normal human hearts, from failing hearts not supported with LVAD, hearts supported with an LVAD for less than 40 days, and hearts supported with an LVAD for more than 40 days. **B,** Heart size, indexed by V30, the volume required to achieve an end-diastolic pressure of 30 mm Hg as a function of the duration of LVAD support from individual hearts (see insert for symbol key). Also shown are values from normal hearts and from failing hearts not supported by LVAD. Underlying the reduction in heart size is regression of cellular hypertrophy. **C,** Cross-section of normal human myocardium. **D,** In chronic heart failure the myocytes are markedly hypertrophic. **E,** After LVAD support, LV myocardial hypertrophy regresses (individual myocyte cross-sectional area reduced). Increased interstitial fibrosis is also noted. All myocardial samples used for C-E were fixed in an unloaded state. (From Madigan JD, Barbone A, Choudhri AF, et al. Time course of reverse remodeling of the left ventricle during support with a left ventricular assist device. *J Thorac Cardiovasc Surg* 2001;121:902-908.)

MicroRNAs (miRNAs) are noncoding RNAs that regulate gene expression at the posttranscription level by promoting mRNA degradation or by inhibiting the translation of proteins from mRNA. Recent studies have identified a potentially important role for miRNAs in terms of modulating cardiac hypertrophic growth in the heart.[29] It is therefore of interest that in both rat models of mechanical unloading and in human hearts that have been supported with LVADs that there is a return in the level of expression of miRNAs toward normal values.[30,31] Matkovich et al showed that hearts that had been mechanically unloaded with an LVAD significantly had decreased expression of miR-195 when compared with patients with end-stage heart failure.[31] Given that overexpression of miR-195 in vitro was capable of inducing hypertrophic growth in neonatal ventricular cardiomyocytes, and that transgenic mice with cardiac restricted overexpression of miR-195 had a dramatic increase in the myocyte size compared with normal mice,[32] miR-195 may contribute to reversal of the heart failure phenotype. Taken together, the aggregate experimental and clinical data suggest that the cardiac myocyte hypertrophy that occurs in heart failure is a reversible process, which has given rise to the concept of the "plasticity" of the hypertrophied/failing cardiac myocyte phenotype (reviewed in Swynghedauw[33]).

BOX 8–2 Overview of the Reverse Remodeling Process

Reversal of the Myocyte Defects
Hypertrophy
Fetal gene expression
β-adrenergic desensitization
Myocytolysis
Excitation-contraction coupling
Cytoskeletal proteins

Reversal of the Myocardial Defects
Alterations in extracellular matrix
- Matrix degradation
- Replacement fibrosis
- Angiogenesis

Reversal of Abnormal LV Geometry
LV dilation
LV wall thinning
Mitral valve incompetence

Myocyte Gene Expression

The morphological changes that occur in a hypertrophied cardiac myocyte are accompanied by a series of changes in the biology of the myocyte that are secondary to reactivation of portfolios of genes, including atrial or B-type natriuretic peptides (ANP, BNP), β-myosin heavy chain (β-MHC), and α-skeletal actin (α-SKA) that are normally not expressed postnatally. The reactivation of these fetal genes, the so-called fetal gene program, is also accompanied by downregulation of a number of genes, most notably sarcoendoplastic reticulum Ca^{2+} ATPase (SERCA) and α-MHC, that are normally expressed in the adult heart. The extant literature suggests that many of the changes in gene expression are reversible with pharmacological therapies that have been shown to improve patient outcomes. Treatment with ACE inhibitors or ARBs were associated with an increase in α-MHC and a decrease in β-MHC at the transcriptional level in experimental models of heart failure.[34,35] In patients with dilated cardiomyopathy, β-blockade by metoprolol (selective β_1-blocker) or carvedilol (β_1-, β_2-, and α_1-blocker) inhibited expression of ANP and β-MHC and restored that of SERCA and α-MHC at the mRNA level (Figure 8-5).[36]

Changes in the abnormal gene expression have also been observed with the use of mechanical circulatory assist devices (Table 8-2). For example, when gene expression profiling was performed in bridge-to-transplantation patients before and after LVAD support, there was a significant downregulation of β-MHC, α-SKA, and BNP in patients with nonischemic cardiomyopathy who received LVAD support, whereas no differences were observed in patients with ischemic cardiomyopathy.[37] In a similar study that employed a proprietary gene array platform, there was a global increase in the expression of a variety of sarcomeric genes in the hearts of LVAD-supported ischemic and nonischemic cardiomyopathy patients, whereas β-MHC mRNA expression was downregulated, consistent with the previous reports.[38] In a select cohort

TABLE 8–1 Cellular and Molecular Determinants of Myocardial Recovery

	β-blocker	ACE Inhibitor	ARB	Aldosterone Antagonists	LVAD	CRT	CSD
Myocyte Defects							
Hypertrophy	Decreased	Decreased	Decreased	Decreased	Decreased	Decreased	Decreased
Fetal gene expression	Decreased	Decreased	Decreased	ND	Decreased	Decreased	Decreased
Myocytolysis	Decreased	ND	ND	ND	Decreased	ND	ND
β-adrenergic desensitization	Increased	Decreased	Decreased	ND	Decreased	Decreased	Decreased
EC coupling	ND	Increased	Increased	ND	Increased	Increased	Increased
Cytoskeletal proteins	Decreased	ND	ND	Increased	Increased	ND	Increased
Myocardial Defects							
Myocyte apoptosis	Decreased	Decreased	Decreased	ND	Decreased	Decreased	Decreased
MMP activation	Decreased	Decreased	Decreased	Decreased	Decreased	Decreased	Decreased
Fibrosis	Decreased	Decreased	Decreased	Decreased	Increased*	Decreased	Decreased
Angiogenesis	Increased	Increased	Increased	Increased	Decreased	Increased	Increased
LV Dilation	Decreased	Stabilized	Stabilized	Stabilized	Decreased	Decreased	Decreased

*With prolonged mechanical support.

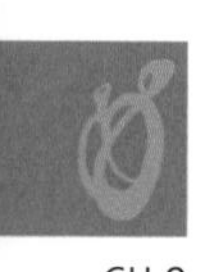

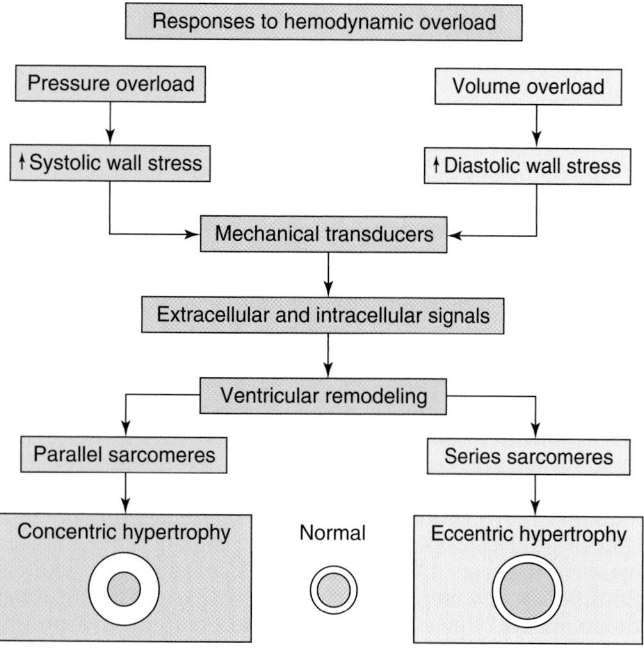

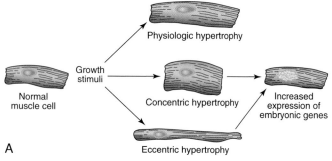

FIGURE 8–2 Patterns of cardiac myocyte hypertrophy. **A,** Morphology of cardiac myocytes in response to hemodynamic pressure and volume overloading. Phenotypically distinct changes in the morphology of myocyte occur in response to the type of hemodynamic overload that is superimposed. When the overload is predominantly due to an increase in pressure, the increase in systolic wall stress leads to the parallel addition of sarcomeres and widening of the cardiac myocytes. When the overload is predominantly due to an increase in ventricular volume, the increase in diastolic wall stress leads to the series addition of sarcomeres, and thus lengthening of cardiac myocytes. **B,** The pattern of cardiac remodeling that occurs in response to hemodynamic overloading depends on the nature of the inciting stimulus. When the overload is predominantly due to an increase in pressure (e.g., with systemic hypertension or aortic stenosis), the increase in systolic wall stress leads to the parallel addition of sarcomeres and widening of the cardiac myocytes, resulting in concentric cardiac hypertrophy. When the overload is predominantly due to an increase in ventricular volume, the increase in diastolic wall stress leads to the series addition of sarcomeres, lengthening of cardiac myocytes, and LV dilation, which is referred to as eccentric chamber hypertrophy. (Modified from Hunter JJ, Chien KR. Signaling pathways for cardiac hypertrophy and failure. *N Engl J Med* 1999;341:1276; and Colucci WS, editor. *Heart failure: cardiac function and dysfunction*, ed 2, Philadelphia, 1999, Current Medicine; and modified from Mann DL. Pathophysiology of heart failure. In Libby PL, Bonow RO, Mann DL, et al, editors. *Braunwald's heart disease*, ed 8, Philadelphia, 2004, Elsevier.)

of LVAD patients with clinical myocardial recovery leading to device explantation, mechanical unloading resulted in increased protein expression of myosin heavy and light chains, tropomyosin, and troponins I, C, and T.[39] Moreover, chronic hemodynamic unloading with an LVAD significantly reduced the expression of ANP, BNP, and natriuretic peptide receptor-C mRNA in patients with end-stage heart failure.[40] Left ventricular endomyocardial biopsies obtained from heart failure patients who underwent cardiac resynchronization therapy (CRT) revealed a significant increase in α-MHC and a nonsignificant decrease in β-MHC mRNA levels using quantitative real-time PCR.[41] Vayderheyden et al have demonstrated that CRT resulted in increased expression of α-MHC and BNP mRNA levels, and reduced the expression of β-MHC mRNA in patients who improved clinically.[42] Changes in fetal gene expression were not seen in "nonresponders," defined as failure to improve greater than 1 NYHA functional class score and a less than 25% relative increase in EF after 4 months of therapy. In a dog model of heart failure induced by intracoronary microembolization, therapy with cardiac support device resulted in a return in β-MHC, α-MHC, ANP, and BNP toward values observed in sham-operated animals.[43] Taken together, these data suggest that both drug and device therapies contribute to reversal of the fetal gene program that has been associated with abnormal contractile function of the cardiac myocyte. However, what is not clear from the extant literature is which of the previous changes is/are necessary and/or essential for myocardial recovery.

β-Adrenergic Desensitization

One of the signatures of advancing heart failure is a reduction in β_1-adrenergic receptor density, isoproterenol-mediated adenylate cyclase stimulation, and isoproterenol-stimulated muscle contraction.[12] This process of agonist-induced β-AR desensitization requires phosphorylation of the agonist-occupied receptor by the cytosolic enzyme β-adrenergic receptor kinase 1 (β-ARK1). As will be discussed later, β-AR desensitization can be reversed with pharmacological and device therapies that have been shown to improve patient outcomes.

In a substudy of MDC (the Metoprolol in Dilated Cardiomyopathy) trial, treatment with selective β_1-blocker metoprolol resulted in significantly increased total β-receptor density in the heart. Interestingly, carvedilol had no effect on β-adrenergic receptor (β-AR) density despite the fact that it was associated with a marked improvement in myocardial function and a reduction in cardiac adrenergic activity.[44] In a randomized, double-blind, placebo-controlled study, the use of the ACE inhibitor lisinopril resulted in a significant increase in myocardial β-AR density in a subset of heart failure patients with high baseline cardiac adrenergic activity.[45]

Normalization of reduced β-adrenergic receptor density and enhanced inotropic responsiveness to isoproterenol have been demonstrated consistently in LVAD-supported failing hearts.[46-48] The enhanced β-adrenergic responsiveness with LVAD support was associated with a decrease in GRK2 protein levels and total GRK activity, but no significant change in GRK5 protein and mRNA levels.[49] Similar findings have been observed following CRT therapy. After 4 months of CRT, β1-adrenergic receptor expression was significantly upregulated at the transcriptional level in heart failure patients.[50] Treatment with a cardiac support device resulted in increased inotropic responsiveness in a canine model of heart failure.[51]

Excitation-Contraction Coupling

Alterations in Ca^{2+} cycling have been closely linked to myocardial contractile dysfunction in heart failure. As discussed in Chapter 3, changes in the abundance of critical Ca^{2+} regulatory proteins including sarcoplasmic endoreticular Ca^{2+} ATPase (SERCA), ryanodine receptor (RyR), L-type calcium channel (LTCC), and sarcolemmal Na^+/Ca^{2+} exchanger (NCX) likely play an important role in the contractile dysfunction of the failing cardiac myocyte. In a transgenic mouse model of heart failure overexpressing tropomodulin, treatment with β-blockers resulted in normalization of SERCA and NCX

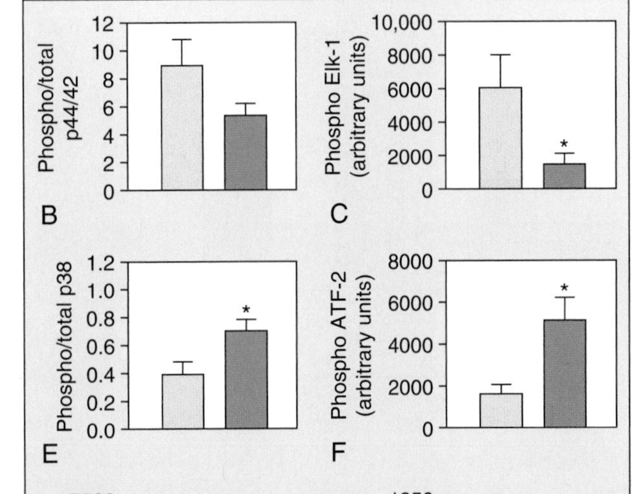
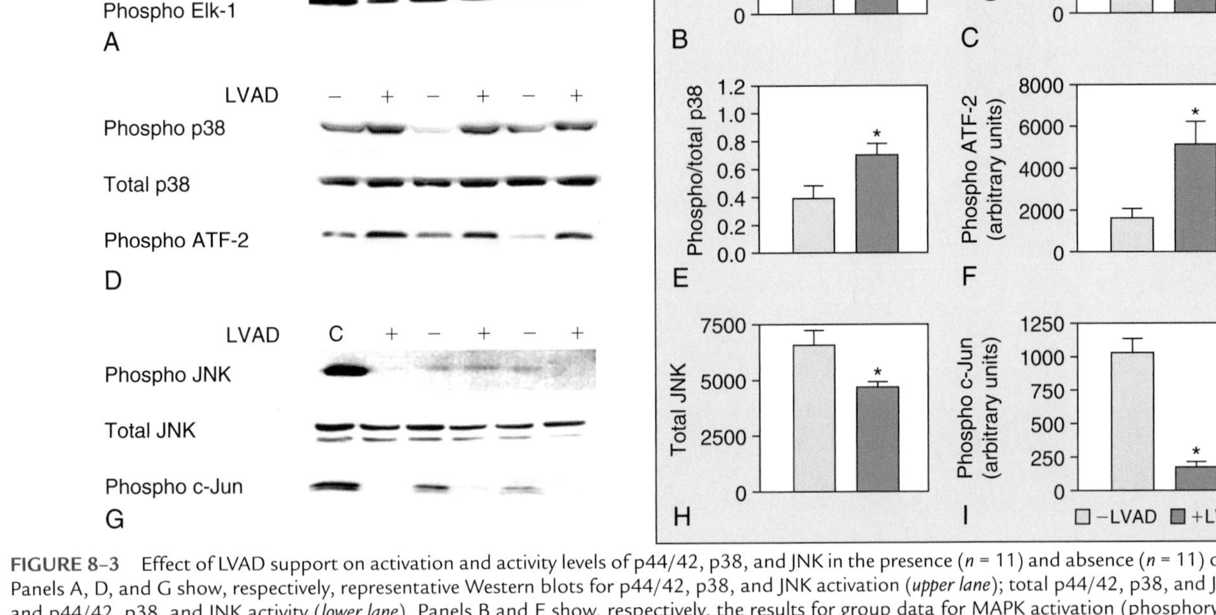

FIGURE 8–3 Effect of LVAD support on activation and activity levels of p44/42, p38, and JNK in the presence (n = 11) and absence (n = 11) of LVAD support. Panels A, D, and G show, respectively, representative Western blots for p44/42, p38, and JNK activation (*upper lane*); total p44/42, p38, and JNK (*middle lane*); and p44/42, p38, and JNK activity (*lower lane*). Panels B and E show, respectively, the results for group data for MAPK activation (phosphorylation), which is expressed as the ratio of the intensity of the bands corresponding to phosphorylated p44/42 and p38 divided by the intensity of the bands corresponding to total p44/42 and p38. Panel H shows the results for group data for total JNK before and after LVAD. Panels C, F, and I show, respectively, the results for group data for p44/42, p38, and JNK activity levels. Data were quantified by laser scanning densitometry and expressed as arbitrary units. (Key: + = LVAD; − = no LVAD; C = HeLa-cells treated with 200 U/mL TNF for 15 min (used as a positive control) (* denotes P <.05 compared to no LVAD support) (From Flesch M, Margulies KB, Mochmann HC, et al. Differential regulation of mitogen-activated protein kinases in the failing human heart in response to mechanical unloading. *Circulation* 2001;104(19):2273-2276.)

protein levels and LTCC density and function.[52] RyR phosphorylation was unchanged by treatment with β-blockers in this transgenic model. Clinical studies have shown that treatment with β-blockers results in increased myocardial SERCA mRNA and protein content (see Figure 8-5),[36,53] a trend toward a decrease in myocardial PLB and NCX protein content,[53] and reduced PKA-mediated hyperphosphorlyation of RyR.[54] Similarly, administration of ACE inhibitors or ARBs in a post-MI rat model of heart failure significantly attenuates the reduction in myocardial SERCA, RyR, and PLB mRNA and protein levels.[55,56] Collectively, these changes in gene expression would result in increased Ca^{2+} that was available for activation of the actin and myosin cross-bridges, and hence improved myocyte contractility.

Mechanical unloading with LVAD support has provided the clearest insight into the importance of changes in excitation-contraction coupling during myocardial recovery. Perhaps the clearest evidence in support of this statement is the observation that there is increased shortening, faster time to peak concentration, and reduced time to 50% relaxation in cardiac myocytes that have been isolated from LVAD supported hearts.[57] As shown in Figure 8-6 the return of contractile function in failing hearts following LVAD-induced unloading is associated with altered gene expression of key Ca^{2+} regulatory proteins, including NCX, SERCA2a, RyR, and changes in calcium cycling.[58,59] Moreover, protein kinase A-mediated hyperphosphorylation of RyR was restored to normal in failing hearts following LVAD support.[60] Nonetheless, the significance of some of the reported changes in gene expression is uncertain insofar as only SERCA2 protein levels increased, whereas protein levels of the RyR and NCX were unchanged following LVAD support (Figure 8-7).[61] Cardiac resynchronization therapy significantly increased mRNA expression for SERCA2a, RyR, and SERCA/NCX mRNA in heart failure patients.[50] Importantly, improvement in SERCA expression occurred only in patients who clinically responded to CRT.[42] Although treatment with a cardiac support device did not result in changes in SERCA2a and phospholamban expression, treatment with a cardiac support device resulted in increased sarcoplasmic reticular Ca^{+2} uptake in an experimental model.[27]

Cytoskeletal Proteins

The cytoskeleton of cardiac myocytes (see Chapter 27) consists of actin, the intermediate filament desmin, the sarcomeric protein titin, and α- and β-tubulin, which form the microtubules by polymerization. Vinculin, talin, dystrophin, and spectrin represent a separate group of membrane-associated proteins. In numerous experimental studies, the role of cytoskeletal and/or membrane-associated proteins has been implicated in the pathogenesis of heart failure, insofar as loss of integrity of the cytoskeleton and its linkage of the sarcomere to the sarcolemma and extracellular matrix would be expected to lead to contractile dysfunction at the myocyte level, and at the myocardial level.

Mechanical unloading with LVAD support also results in restoration of cytoskeletal organization. Vatta et al reported that there was loss of the N-terminal region of dystrophin (which links to the sarcomere through actin) in patients with both ischemic and dilated cardiomyopathy, and that mechanical unloading resulted in an increased N-terminal dystrophin expression (Figure 8-8).[62] The change in the level of expression of dystrophin was comparable in the right ventricle and the left ventricle after mechanical unloading; however, a greater degree of normalization was achieved in patients

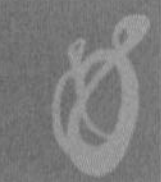

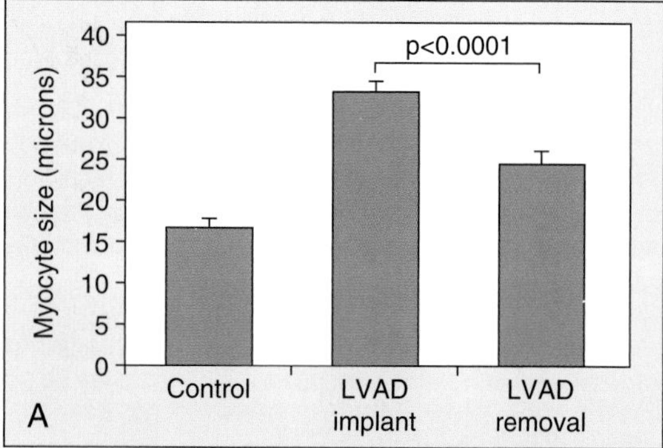

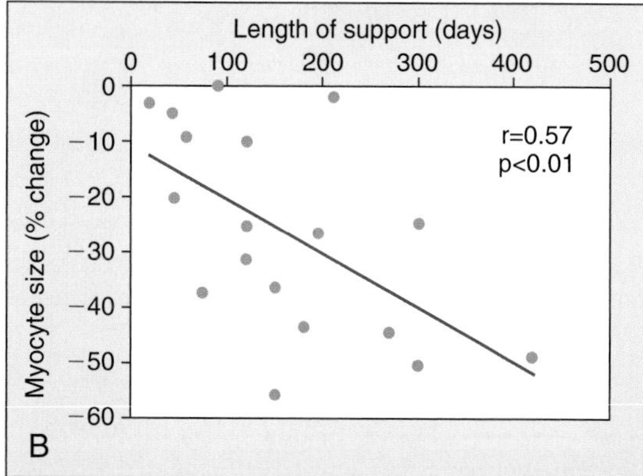

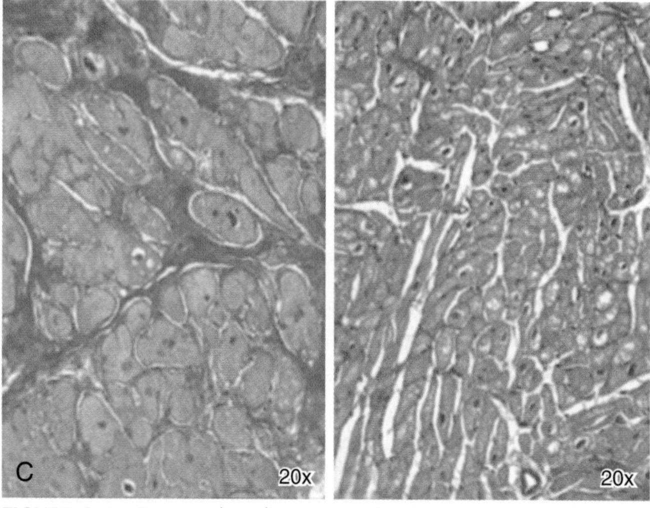

FIGURE 8–4 Decreased cardiac myocyte hypertrophy in LVAD supported hearts. **A,** Myocyte size was determined in control subjects without heart failure, failing hearts at the time of LVAD implant, and LVAD removal. After LVAD support (mean duration of 159 ± 25 days), there was a significant reduction in myocyte cell size. However, while myocyte cell size decreased in all patients following LVAD implantation, the cell size post-LVAD removal was still larger than in controls. **B,** Relation of percent reduction in myocyte size and the length of LVAD support. **C,** A representative hematoxylin eosin stain of myocardial samples obtained at the time of LVAD implant and removal from an individual patient. (Modified from Bruckner BA, Stetson SJ, Perez-Verdia A, et al. Regression of fibrosis and hypertrophy in failing myocardium following mechanical circulatory support. *J Heart Lung Transplant* 2001;20(4):457-464.)

treated with pulsatile-flow LVADs than among those treated with continuous-flow LVADs.[63] Mechanical support with an LVAD has been reported to increase immunostaining for major sarcomeric proteins including actin, troponin C, troponin T, tropomyosin, and titin, with a small, nonsignificant decrease in myosin[64]; changes in the intracellular distribution of desmin, vinculin, and tubulin; and an increase in desmin protein content, with no change in the content or distribution of α-actinin.[65] Interestingly, in one small study there was a specific pattern of changes in mRNA expression levels for both sarcomeric and nonsarcomeric cytoskeletal proteins in the myocardium (increased β-actin, α-tropomyosin, α_1-actinin, α-filamin A, with decreased troponin T_3, α_2-actinin, and vinculin) in patients who were bridged to recovery when compared with heart failure patients who were not supported, suggesting that alterations in cytoskeletal structure might play an important role in and serve as a marker of myocardial recovery.[66] Of note, myocardial titin, α- and β-tubulin mRNA expression were shown to return to normal levels following 3 months of therapy with a cardiac support device (CorCap) in a dog model of chronic heart failure.[43]

Myocytolysis

Myocytolysis refers to the degenerative loss (often reversible) of myofibrils that occurs in cardiac myocytes that have been subjected to increased myocardial stretch/strain, ischemia, and/or neurohormonal stimulation. The characteristic histopathological appearance of myocytolysis is cellular vacuolization with loss of actin and myosin myofibers. The experimental literature suggests that β-adrenergic blockade restores cardiac myocyte contractility, and that this improvement in myocyte contractility has been linked to an increase in the density of myofilaments within the failing myocytes.[67] Several reports from patients who have been supported with LVADs also suggest that myocytolysis is reversible.[68,69] However, in some reports there has been persistent disruption of sarcomeres and disoriented mitochondria in mechanically unloaded hearts, suggesting that there may not be complete recovery of the myocyte at the ultrastructural level with LVADs.

CHANGES IN THE MYOCARDIUM DURING MYOCARDIAL RECOVERY

The unfavorable alterations that occur in the failing myocardium may be categorized broadly into those that occur in the volume of cardiac myocytes, changes that occur in the volume and composition of the extracellular matrix, and changes that occur in angiogenesis. With respect to the changes that occur in cardiac myocyte component of the myocardium there is increasing evidence to suggest that progressive myocyte loss, through both necrotic and apoptotic cell death, may contribute to progressive cardiac dysfunction and LV remodeling (see Chapters 6 and 15). Insofar as prevention of loss of cardiac myocytes is more likely to play an important role in preventing disease progression than in myocardial recovery, this topic will not be discussed further in this chapter. The topic of myocardial regeneration, which can contribute to the process of myocardial recovery, is reviewed in Chapter 4. As will be discussed later, there is evidence that changes in the volume and composition of the extracellular matrix may contribute to myocardial recovery and changes in angiogenesis.

Myocardial Fibrosis

Studies in the failing human heart have shown that there is a quantitative increase in collagens I, III, VI, and IV, fibronectin, laminin, and vimentin, and that the ratio of type I collagen to type III collagen is decreased in patients with ischemic cardiomyopathy.[70] Moreover, progressive loss of cross-linking of collagen has been demonstrated in the failing myocardium. Disruption of the extracellular matrix would be expected to lead to LV dilation as a result of mural realignment ("slippage") of myocyte bundles and/or individual myocytes within the LV wall,[71] and LV dysfunction as

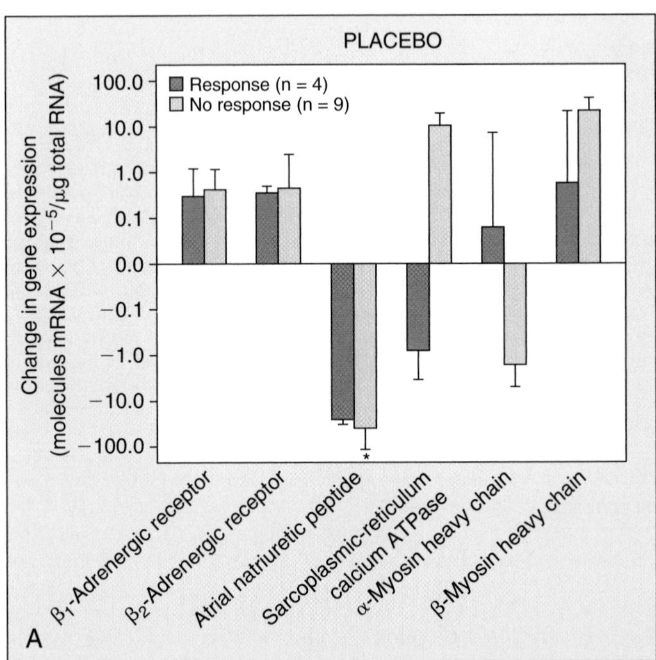

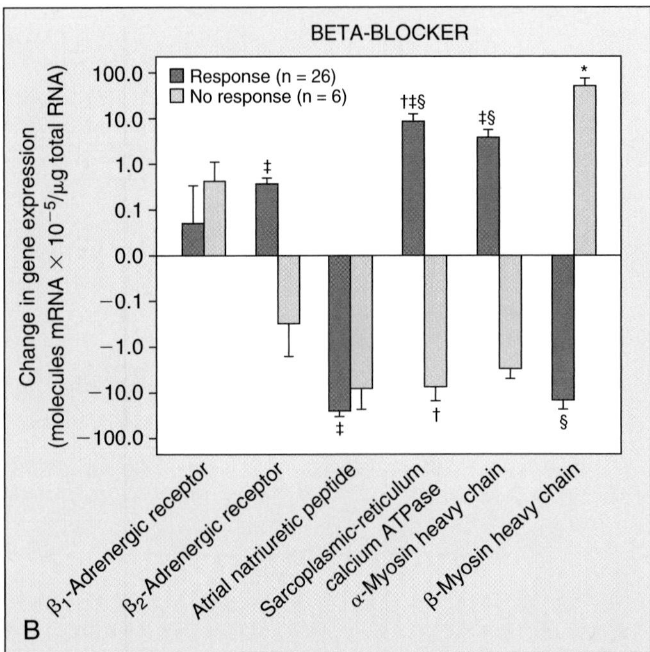

FIGURE 8-5 Changes in fetal gene expression in patients who received β-blockers. **A** and **B,** Changes between baseline and the end of the 6-month study in the abundance of myocardial mRNA for six contractility-regulating or hypertrophy-regulating proteins in patients who received a placebo or β-blocker. The changes in patients who had an improvement in left ventricular ejection fraction by at least five ejection fraction [EF] units were compared with the changes in patients who did not have such a response. Gene expression is shown as molecules of mRNA per microgram of total RNA on a logarithmic scale. The asterisk indicates $P < .10$ for the change between the baseline value and the value measured at 6 months by the paired *t*-test, the daggers $P < .05$ for the comparison with the placebo group by the test for interaction, the double daggers $P < .05$ for the change between the baseline value and the value measured at 6 months by the paired *t*-test, and the section marks $P < .05$ for the comparison with patients who did not have a response. Each panel shows the results for patients with complete data for the indicated mRNA and receptor protein measurements. (Modified from Lowes BD, Gilbert EM, Abraham WT, et al. Myocardial gene expression in dilated cardiomyopathy treated with β-blocking agents. *N Engl J Med* 2002;346:1357; and Mann DL. Management of patients with a reduced ejection fraction. In Libby PL, Bonow RO, Mann DL, et al, editors. *Braunwald's heart disease*, ed 8, Philadelphia, 2004, Elsevier.)

TABLE 8–2 Alterations in Gene Expression Patterns During LVAD Therapy

Author	Nonfailing – Failing – Post-LVAD (n)	Duration of LVAD Support (days)	ICM/NICM	Chip Platform	Criteria	Gene Alterations in Myocardial Recovery	Major Findings
Blaxall et al—2003[37]	0-6-6	~60	3/3	Affymetrix HuGene (6800 genes)	$P < .05$	↑ 295 genes ↓ 235 genes	Distinct pattern of gene expression in ischemic vs. nonischemic patients
Chen Y et al—2003[118]	0-7-7	194 ± 58	0/7	Affymetrix U133A (22,283 genes)	$P < .05$ FC >1.5	↑ 130 genes ↓ 43 genes	Significant alteration in expression of transcription factors
Chen MM et al—2003[119]	0-11-11	110 ± 92	4/7	Agilent Human 1 Catalog (12,814 clones)	FDR 0.05 Using SAM	↑ 85 genes ↓ 13 genes	LVAD therapy upregulates Apelin—angiotensin receptor-like 1 signaling
Hall et al—2004[94]	0-19-19	159 ± 40	8/11	Affymetrix U133A (22,283 genes)	FC >1.2	↑ 85 genes ↓ 22 genes	Alteration in expression of genes governing vascular organization, ↓GATA4 expression
Margulies et al—2005[120]	14-157-28	Not reported	Not reported	Affymetrix U133A A 22,242 genes B 22,577 genes	FC >1.2 (paired)	↑1544 genes ↓ 924 genes	LVAD-associated persistence of pathological dysregulation is much more common than recovery
Rodrigue-Way et al—2005[38]	4-19-12	60 ± 36	14/5	Custom array (2700 clones)	FC >1.2 $P < .05$	211 genes	Calcium handling and sarcomeric genes are upregulated by LVAD support
Hall et al—2007[121]	0-6-6	366 ± 168	0/6	Affymetrix U133A (22,283 genes)	$P < .01$	↑ 124 genes ↓ 139 genes	Upregulation of integrin pathway signaling and downregulation of cAMP pathway signaling in myocardial recovery
Matkovich et al—2009[31]	6-13-4	Not reported	7/10	Affymetrix HuEx 1.0 (21,980)	$P < .001$ FC >1.3 FDR 0.03	Not reported	Only 7% of the heart failure genes normalize with the LVAD support. MicroRNA profiling may have superior potential for diagnosis and prognosis of myocardial recovery

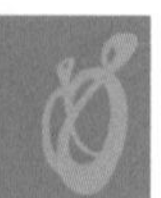

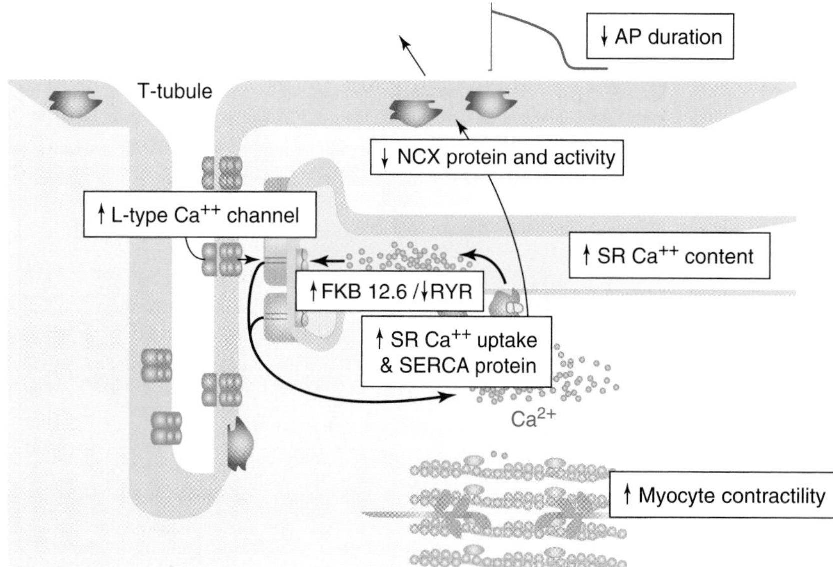

FIGURE 8–6 Summary of changes in excitation-contraction coupling in cardiac myocytes from hearts that have been supported with a left ventricular assist device. As shown there is an increase in the inward Ca^{++} current through the L-type Ca^{++} channel, a decrease in the levels and activity of the sodium-calcium exchanger (NCX), increased Ca^{++} content of the sarcoplasmic reticulum (SR), decreased activity of the ryanodine receptor (RyR), and increases in FKB 12.6 levels (a regulatory protein that prevents Ca^{++} release from the RyR). Collectively these changes would be expected to lead to improved myocyte contractility. (Key: the arrows indicate increases (↑) or decrease (↓) in various parameters) (Modified from Soppa GK, Barton PJ, Terracciano CM, et al. Left ventricular assist device-induced molecular changes in the failing myocardium. *Curr Opin Cardiol* 2008;23:206-218.)

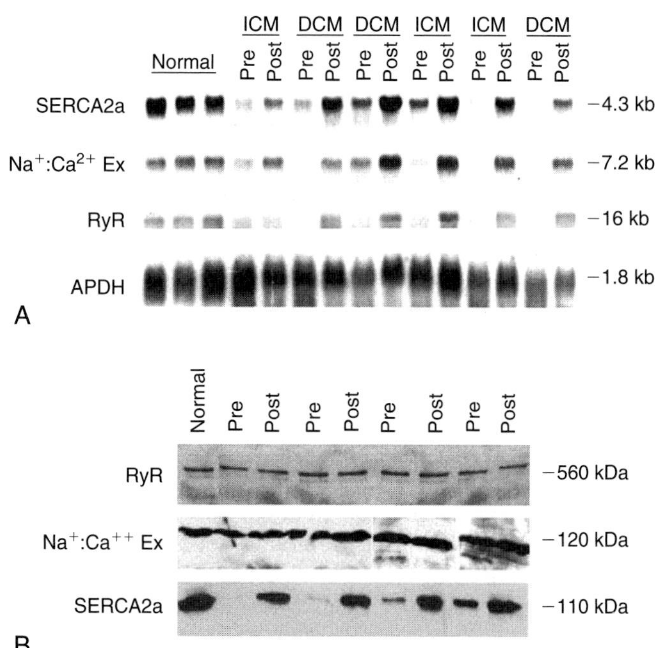

FIGURE 8–7 **A,** Representative Northern blot depicting three nonfailing hearts (normal) and six individual hearts before and after LVAD support. **B,** Representative Western blot depicting SERCA2a, RyR, and Na^+/Ca^{2+} exchanger (NCX) protein in nonfailing (normal) heart along with samples obtained from individual failing hearts before and after LVAD support. Semi-quantitative densitometric analysis of Western blots with values demonstrated no change in protein levels for RyR and NCX, with a significant increase in SERCA2a following LVAD support. (Modified from Heerdt PM, Holmes JW, et al. Chronic unloading by left ventricular assist device reverses contractile dysfunction and alters gene expression in end-stage heart failure. *Circulation* 2000;102:2713-2719.)

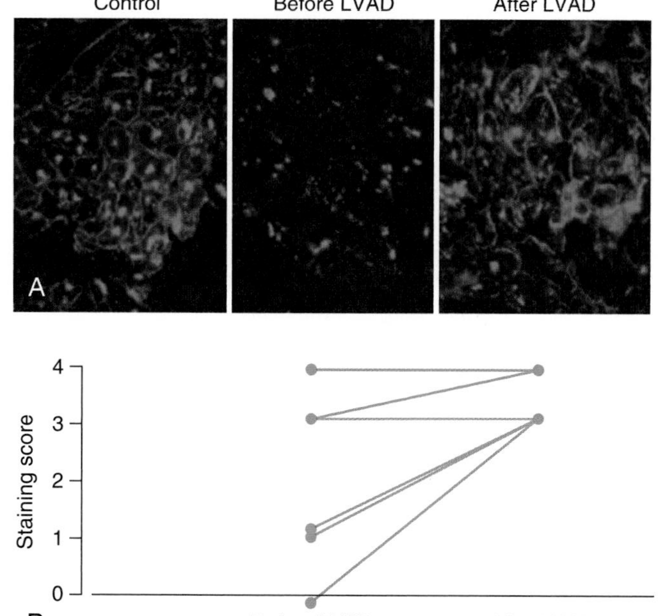

FIGURE 8–8 Effect of LVAD support on dystrophin levels in failing hearts. **A,** Immunohistochemical staining with the N-terminal-specific antibody of myocardial sections from a control sample (*left*), and paired samples from patients with end-stage cardiomyopathy before (*middle*) and after (*right*) LVAD support. Immunostaining for the N-terminal portion of dystrophin was present on the myocyte cell membranes of control hearts, absent in cell membranes from cardiomyopathy, and restored in cardiomyopathic hearts following LVAD support. **B,** Semiquantitative staining scores for N-terminal dystrophin in paired samples before and after LVAD support. (Modified from Vatta M, Stetson SJ, Perez-Verdia A, et al. Molecular remodelling of dystrophin in patients with end-stage cardiomyopathies and reversal in patients on assistance-device therapy. *Lancet* 2002;359:936-941.)

a result of dyssynchronous contraction of the left ventricle, thereby engendering LV dysfunction. Thus, both the amount and the organization of the collagen are important determinants of myocardial structure and function in the failing heart. β-blockade with metoprolol significantly decreased replacement fibrosis in a dog model of heart failure.[19] Consistent with this finding, treating patients with dilated cardiomyopathy with β-blockers for 4 months resulted in decreased myocardial collagen type I and III mRNA expression in paired myocardial RV biopsy samples.[72] Experimental studies suggest that ACE inhibitors reduce collagen deposition in the failing myocardium in various models of heart failure, and this salutary effect is mediated, at least in part, by kinins.[73,74] Similarly, treatment of patients with ischemic cardiomyopathy with captopril resulted in

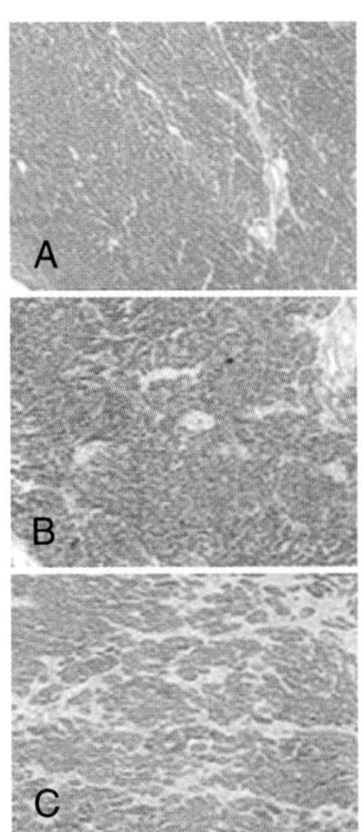

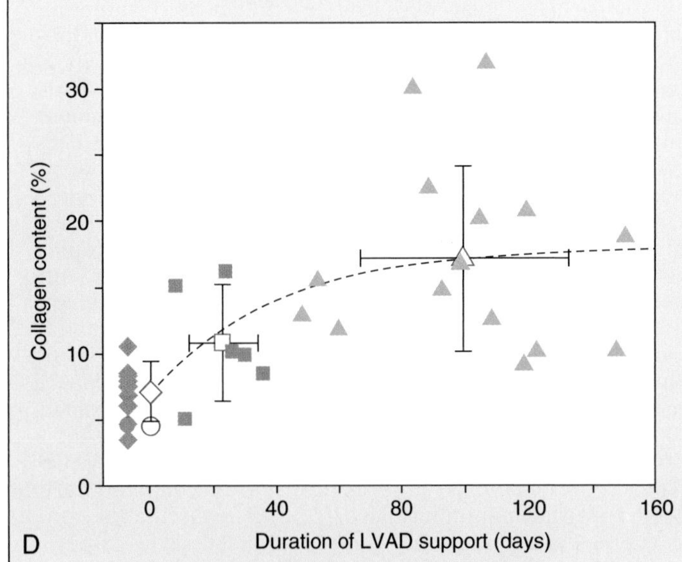

FIGURE 8-9 Effect of the duration of LVAD support on myocardial collagen content. Trichrome-stained sections of LV free wall demonstrating relative myocardial collagen content for **(A)** normal, **(B)** non-LVAD, and **(C)** $LVAD_{40+day}$ groups. **D,** Relative myocardial collagen content versus duration of LVAD support (*squares,* $LVAD_{0\text{-}40\ days}$; *triangles,* $LVAD_{40+day}$; *diamonds,* non-LVAD; *circles,* normal; *dashed line*). (Modified from Madigan JD, Barbone A, Choudhri AF, et al. Time course of reverse remodeling of the left ventricle during support with a left ventricular assist device. *J Thorac Cardiovasc Surg* 2001;121(5):902-908.)

decreased total collagen content, decreased collagen type III levels, and normalization of the collagen type I:III ratio, when compared with untreated heart failure patients.[75] Angiotensin receptor type I (AT_1) receptor blockers also reduce myocardial collagen content in experimental heart failure models; however, this decrease was not attenuated by blockade of the bradykinin B_2-receptor, suggesting that antagonism of the renin-angiotensin system alone is sufficient to reverse myocardial fibrosis.[74] Treatment with eplerenone in a dog model of heart failure significantly attenuated LV collage volume fraction by reducing both interstitial and replacement fibrosis[76] and normalized mRNA and protein expression of MMPs 1, 2, and 9, but had no effect on mRNA levels of TIMP-1,2.[77]

Mechanical circulatory support with LVADs also leads to important changes in the extracellular matrix and myocardial fibrillar content and organization. There are conflicting reports on the effect of LVAD support on LV myocardial collagen content, with several reports showing increased myocardial collagen content relative to levels observed in failing hearts that have not been supported with LVADs,[26,78-81] while other reports suggest that the collagen volume fraction decreases.[82,83] Although the reason(s) for this discrepancy is not known, it may be related to difference in heart failure cause and, differences in the degree of inotropic and/or pharmacological support and the duration of LVAD support. Of note, one report suggests that a longer duration of LVAD support results in increased myocardial collagen volume fraction in a time-dependent manner (Figure 8-9).[23] The biological basis for these changes is suggested by two studies which show that LVAD support resulted in decreased levels of MMP 1, 9 and increased expression of TIMP-1,2, resulting in decreased MMP-1/TIMP-1 ratio (favoring collagen accumulation), and an increase in the ratio of insoluble to total soluble collagen (a measure of collagen cross-linking).[78,79] Moreover, these changes were partially abrogated by concomitant therapy with ACE inhibitors during the period of LVAD support.[84] Serial myocardial biopsies from heart failure patients revealed a significant reduction in the collagen volume fraction following CRT,[28,85] with a significant decrease in MMP-9 levels in the group of patients who underwent reverse remodeling (i.e., "responders").[86] Passive cardiac restraint has been shown to reduce collagen volume fraction and to preserve the integrity of the collagen cross-links between cardiomyocytes (Figure 8-10).[87]

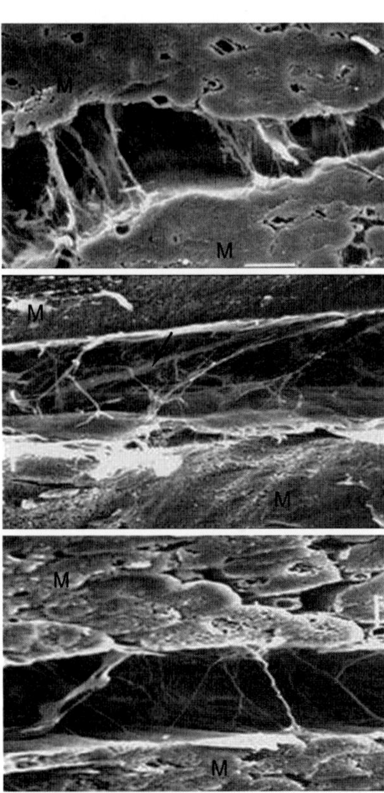

FIGURE 8-10 Scanning electron micrographs of the interstitial space between two adjacent myocytes (M) from left ventricular myocardium of a normal dog (*top*), a dog with heart failure that was not treated (*middle*), and a dog with heart failure treated for 3 months with the cardiac support device. Note the tangential or oblique orientation (*arrow*) of the matrix cross-links in the untreated heart failure dog compared with the normal suggestive slippage and the restoration of near normal cross-linking integrity following CSD therapy. (Modified from Sharov VG, Todor AV, Sabbah HN. Left ventricular histomorphometric findings in dogs with heart failure treated with the Acorn Cardiac Support Device. *Heart Fail Rev* 2005;10:141-147.)

Angiogenesis

Cardiac hypertrophy and angiogenesis are coordinately regulated during physiological cardiac growth.[88] Disruption of this coordinated growth stress following hemodynamic overload and/or cardiac injury may lead to contractile dysfunction and cell death, both of which may contribute to the development of heart failure. Of note, myocardial capillary density is reduced in patients with dilated cardiomyopathy.[89,90] Thus impaired capillary growth may contribute to the development and/or progression of heart failure. Experimental studies suggest that myocardial capillary density is restored toward normal values following treatment with pharmacological therapies that have been shown to improve patient outcomes in heart failure.[19,74,76] Moreover, some of these same therapies also lead to improved myocardial blood flow in patients with heart failure.[91-93] Whether the improved myocardial blood flow is related to increased angiogenesis, altered hemodynamic loading conditions, or both is not known. Analysis of changes in gene expression before and after LVAD support revealed significant alterations in genes that are involved in the regulation of vascular networks, including upregulation of Sprouty-1 and downregulation of neurophilin (VEGF receptor), stromal derived factor-1, FGF9, and endomucin.[94] Sprouty-1 was immunolocalized to the microvasculature, and the upregulation of Sprouty-1 in endothelial cells was associated with a decrease in VEGF-induced endothelial proliferation, which suggests that Sprouty-1 may serve as an intrinsic mediator of cardiac remodeling by regulating angiogenesis.[94] Studies in heart failure patients who underwent CRT revealed increased myocardial capillary density and an improvement in the distribution pattern of myocardial blood flow.[85,95] Sabbah et al have demonstrated enhancement of capillary density, and upregulation of angiogenetic factors bFGF and VEGF mRNA following treatment with a cardiac support device in a canine model of heart failure.[96,97]

CHANGES IN LEFT VENTRICULAR GEOMETRY DURING MYOCARDIAL RECOVERY

As noted previously, clinical studies with ACE inhibitors, β-blockers, aldosterone antagonists, LVADs, and CRT have shown that these treatment modalities lead to return of cardiac myocyte biology toward normal, and to changes in the extracellular matrix that favor increased structural integrity of the heart and reverse remodeling (Figure 8-11). In the following section, we will review the literature that shows that drugs and devices that favorably impact clinical outcomes are accompanied by reverse LV remodeling. As shown in Figure 8-12, *A*, treatment with ACE inhibitors prevented worsening LV remodeling but did not lead to reverse remodeling in a substudy of SOLVD,[6] whereas treatment with β-blockers resulted in decreased LV end-diastolic volumes when compared with a placebo (diuretics and ACE inhibitors) in a substudy of the ANZ (Australia New Zealand) trial (see Figure 8-12, *B*).[98] In an echocardiographic substudy of the Val-HeFT (Valsartan in Heart Failure) trial, treatment with valsartan added to an ACE inhibitor and/or β-blocker significantly resulted in decreased LV internal diastolic diameter (LVIDd)/body surface area from 4 months to more than 24 months (see Figure 8-12, *C*).[99] Similarly, the addition of spironolactone to

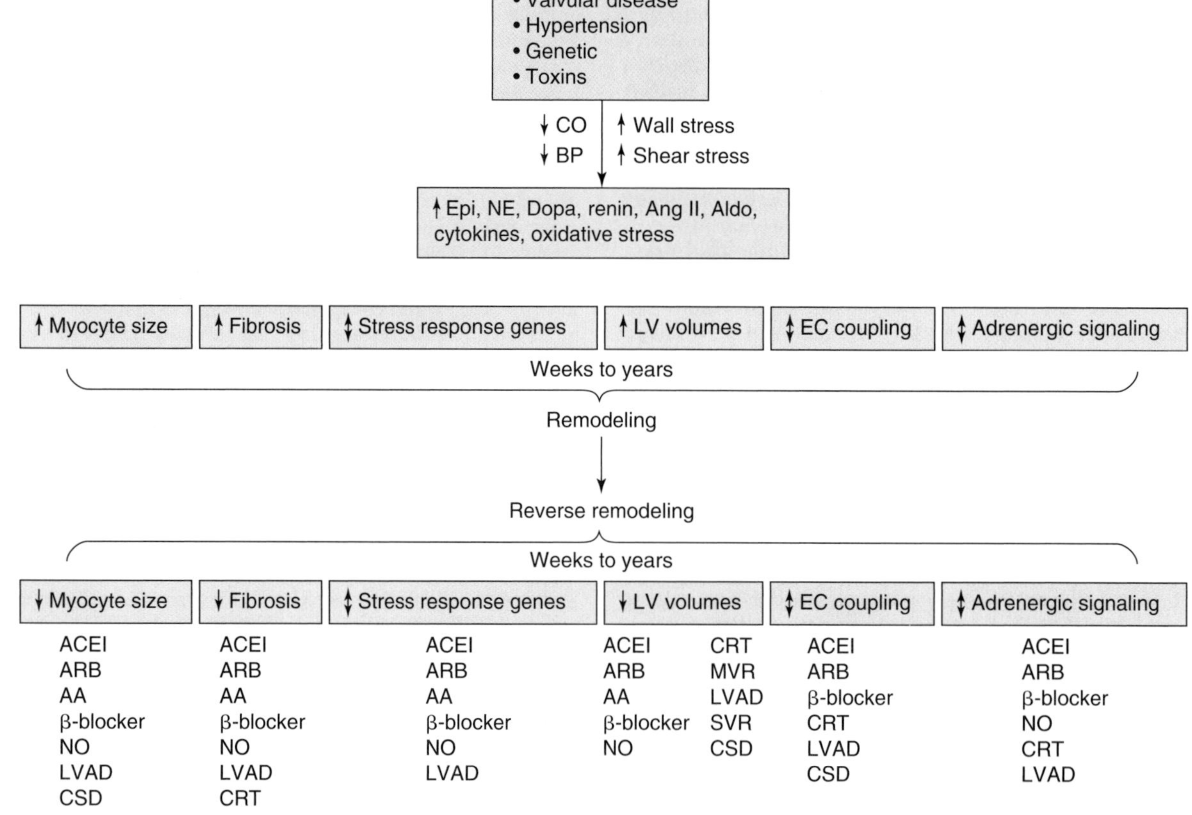

FIGURE 8-11 Structural, molecular, and cellular changes after cardiac injury leading to remodeling and those therapies that have been shown to contribute to reverse remodeling. Therapies that have been shown in humans to alter the specific reverse remodeling subheadings are bold and italicized. (Key: *AA,* aldosterone antagonists; *ALB,* angiotensin-converting enzyme inhibitor, *Aldo,* aldosterone; *Ang II,* angiotensin II; *ARB,* angiotensin receptor blocker; *BP,* blood pressure; *CO,* cardiac output; *CRT,* cardiac resynchronization; *CSD,* cardiac support device; *Dopa,* dopamine; *EC,* excitation-contraction; *Epi,* epinephrine; *LVADL,* left ventricular assist device; *MVR,* mitral valve repair; *NE,* norepinephrine; *NO,* nitric oxide; *SVR,* surgical ventricular restoration). (From Mudd JO, Kass DA. Reversing chronic remodeling in heart failure. *Expert Rev Cardiovasc Ther* 2007;5:585-598.)

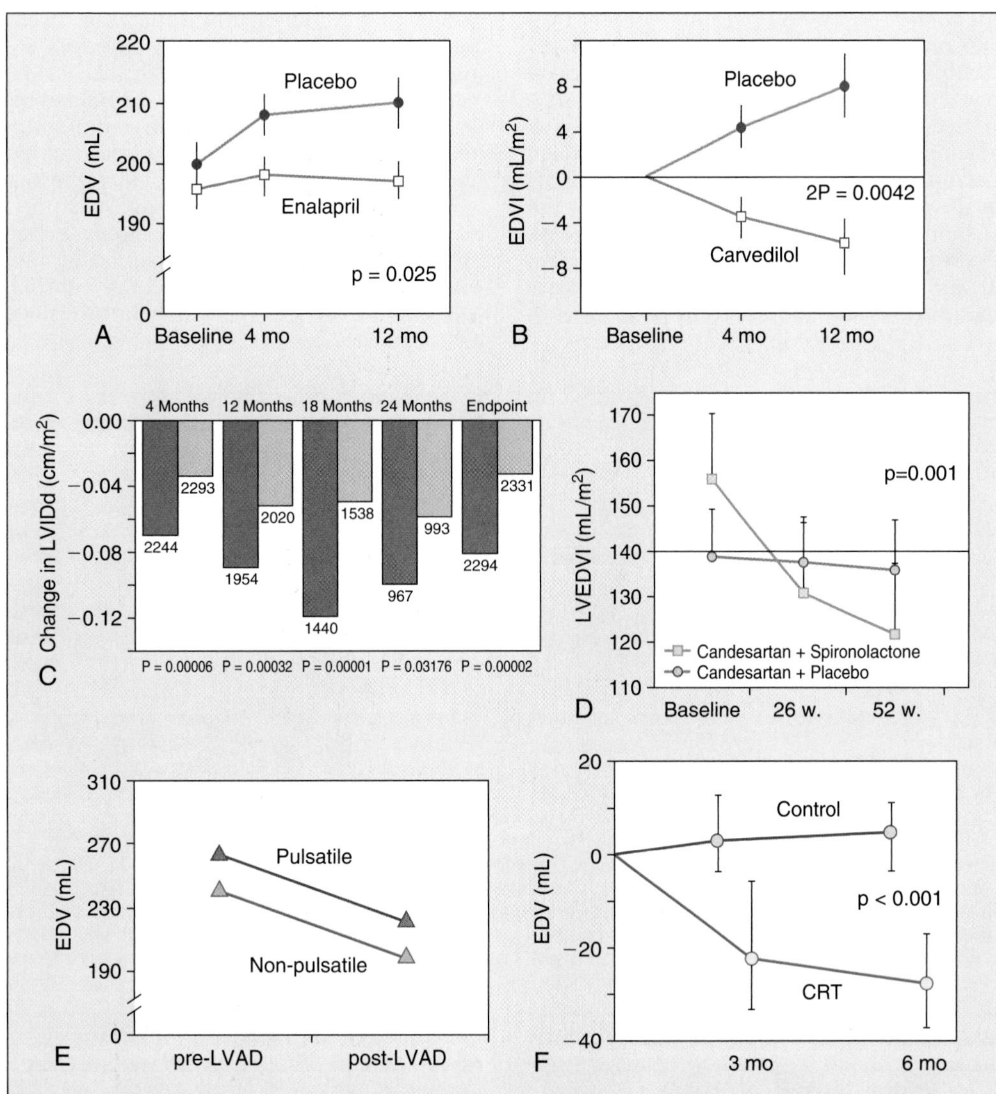

FIGURE 8–12 Reverse cardiac remodeling following pharmacological and device therapies in patients with heart failure. **A,** Changes in LV end-diastolic volume in placebo- and enalapril-treated patients in SOLVD compared with a placebo. **B,** Changes in LV volume index from baseline during the 12-month follow-up period in the ANZ trial compared with a placebo. **C,** Changes in LV end-diastolic dimension in patients treated with valsartan added to an ACE inhibitor and/or β-blocker significantly resulted in decreased LV internal diastolic diameter (normalized to body surface area [BSA]). **D,** Changes in LV volume index in patients treated with spironolactone and candesartan compared with candesartan alone. **E,** Changes in LV end-diastolic volume in pulsatile versus continuous flow LVADs. **F,** Change in LVEDV at 3 and 6 months after CRT compared with the control group in the MIRACLE trial. (A-F modified, respectfully, from Greenberg B, Quinones MA, Koilpillai C, et al. *Circulation* 1995;91:2573-2581; Doughty RN, Whalley GA, Gamble G, et al. Left ventricular remodeling with carvedilol in patients with congestive heart failure due to ischemic heart disease. *J Am Coll Cardiol* 1997;29:1060-1066; Wong M, Staszewsky L, Latini R, et al. Valsartan benefits left ventricular structure and function in heart failure: Val-HeFT echocardiographic study. *J Am Coll Cardiol* 2002;40:970-975; Chan AK, Sanderson JE, Wang T, et al. Aldosterone receptor antagonism induces reverse remodeling when added to angiotensin receptor blockade in chronic heart failure. *J Am Coll Cardiol* 2007;50:591-596; Klotz S, Deng MC, Stypmann J, et al. Left ventricular pressure and volume unloading during pulsatile versus nonpulsatile left ventricular assist device support. *Ann Thorac Surg* 2004;77:143-149; modified from St John Sutton MG, Plappert T, Abraham WT, et al. Effect of cardiac resynchronization therapy on left ventricular size and function in chronic heart failure. *Circulation* 2003;107:1985-1990.)

candesartan resulted in a significant decrease in the LV volume index at 1 year when compared with candesartan alone (see Figure 8-12, *D*).[100]

Device therapies also lead to reverse remodeling of the ventricle. Although pulsatile-flow devices provide a greater degree of ventricular unloading than continuous-flow devices,[101] the continuous-flow LVADs appear to be as effective as pulsatile-flow LVADs with regard to the degree of LV reverse remodeling (see Figure 8-12, *E*).[101,102] As noted previously, the initial clinical experience with mechanical assist devices demonstrated that there were varying degrees of structural and functional recovery of myocyte and myocardial recovery that are associated with reverse remodeling. The improvement in LV function was sufficient to allow explantation of the device in approximately 5% to 9% of explanted patients.[103,104] However, although cardiac function improves significantly after device implantation, and although there is cellular recovery and favorable remodeling of the extracellular matrix, the degree of clinical recovery is insufficient for device explantation in most patients with chronic heart failure. In the MIRACLE (Multicenter In-Synch Randomized Clinical Evaluation) trial, CRT led to improvements in LVEF, mitral regurgitant area, and LV end-diastolic diameter at 6 months in patients with moderate to severe heart failure and prolonged QRS (see Chapter 47).[105] Similar findings have been reported in the MUSTIC (Multisite Stimulation in Cardiomyopathy) and CARE-HF (Cardiac Resynchronization in Heart Failure) studies, which employed a longer follow-up period (see also Chapter 47).[106,107] Passive cardiac restraint in the Acorn Randomized Trial showed that there was a significant reduction in LV end-diastolic volume over the 12-month course of the study,[108] which was sustained at 3 years in patients with and without concomitant mitral valve surgery.[109]

In addition to the drugs and devices discussed previously, a variety of surgical techniques have been introduced to reverse the maladaptive ventricular remodeling in patients with heart failure. As discussed in Chapter 23, myocardial revascularization should be considered in patients with evidence of myocardial viability and depressed LV dysfunction. Clinical studies have demonstrated an increase in EF and a decrease in LV volume indices in patients with ischemic cardiomyopathy following coronary artery bypass surgery.[110,111] Partial left ventriculectomy, which was a technique developed by Batista in the early 1990s, involves surgical removal of part of the left ventricle to reduce LV volumes. While an interesting hypothesis, studies ultimately found this technique was ineffective,[112] suggesting that changes in volume alone are not sufficient to allow the heart to recover. One additional explanation that has been provided for the lack of efficacy or partial ventriculectomy is that acute reductions in LV mass result are accompanied by unfavorable changes in the diastolic properties of the ventricle (i.e., increased stiffness [Figure 8-13]), which in turn negatively affects the

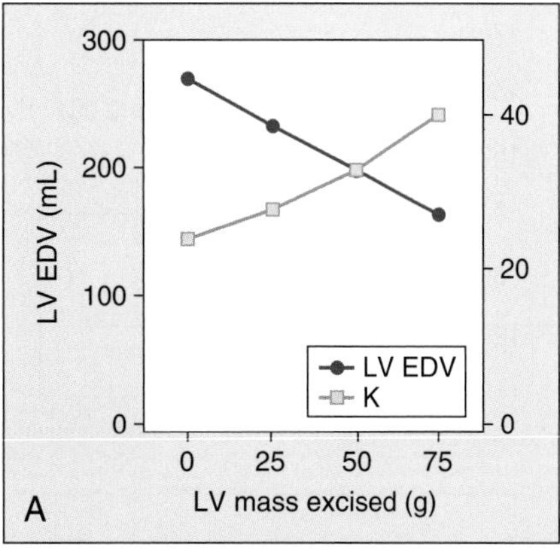

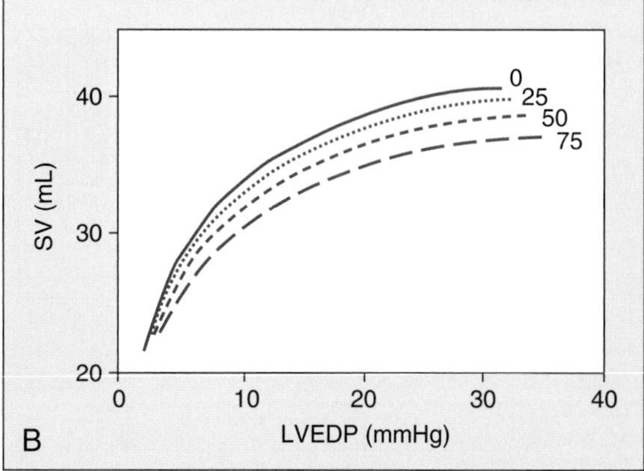

FIGURE 8–13 Effects of excision of LV mass from 0 to 75 g on LV diastolic distensibility and LV function. **A,** LV end-diastolic volume (LV EDV; *filled circles*) and the LV stiffness coefficient of the end-diastolic pressure-volume relation (K; *open squares*) as a function of LV mass excised. This measurement reflects the decrease in chamber compliance associated with LV mass reduction. **B,** Frank-Starling relationship relating stroke volume to LVEDP at the four mass reduction conditions (0 to 75 g of tissue excision). Notice that mass reduction is associated with a downward shift of the Frank-Starling curves, indicating a reduction in pump function. (From Dickstein ML, Spotnitz HM, Rose EA, et al. Heart reduction surgery: an analysis of the impact on cardiac function. *J Thorac Cardiovasc Surg* 1997;113:1032-1040.)

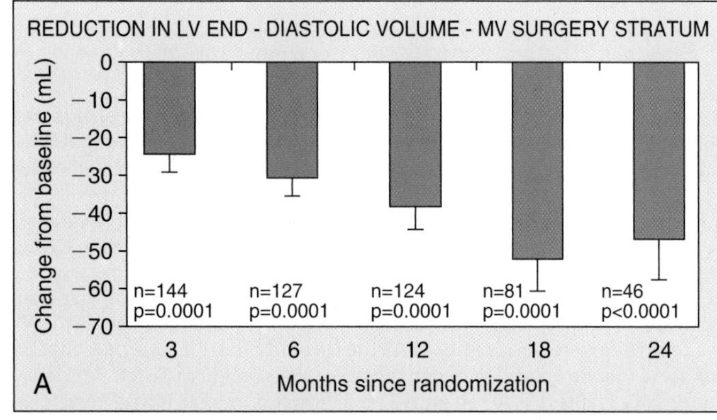

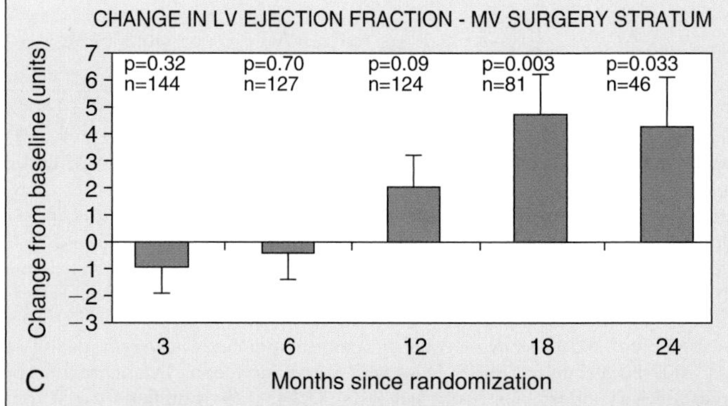

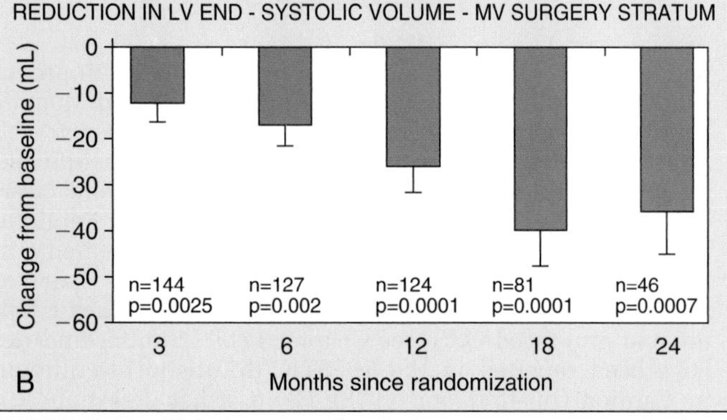

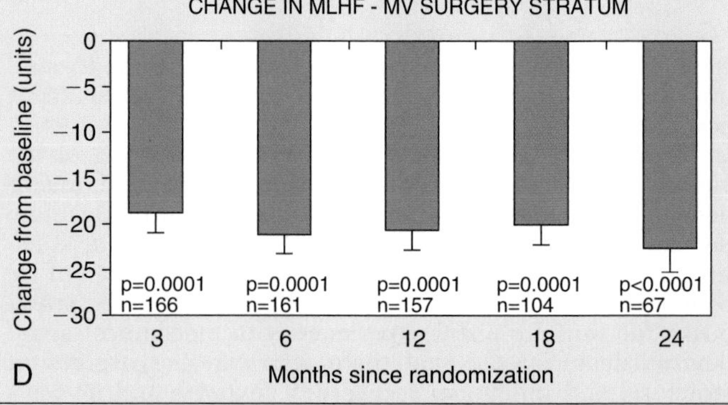

FIGURE 8–14 Clinical outcomes in mitral surgery treatment arm in the Acorn Trial. **A,** Change in LV end-diastolic volumes; **B,** change in LV end-systolic volumes; **C,** change in LVEF; **D,** change in Minnesota Living with Heart Failure (MLHF) score. (From Acker MA, Bolling S, Shemin R, et al. Mitral valve surgery in heart failure: insights from the Acorn clinical trial. *J Thorac Cardiovasc Surg* 2006;132:568-577.)

Frank-Starling relationship (see Figure 8-13, *B*).[113] Surgical ventricular reconstruction of the left ventricle (SVR) is a specific surgical procedure that was developed for the treatment of LV dysfunction in patients with large akinetic areas of nonviable myocardium secondary to coronary artery disease (see Chapter 55). Despite encouraging early results in nonrandomized studies, which showed that SVR could improve patient symptoms and reduce end-diastolic volumes,[114] the NIH sponsored STICH trial (Surgical Treatment for Ischemic Heart failure) that compared coronary artery bypass grafting (CABG) versus CABG with SVR, failed to show an improvement in patient symptoms or exercise tolerance or a reduction in the rate of death or hospitalization for cardiac causes.[111] Various explanations have been provided for the failure of SVR to improve clinical outcomes in STICH, including inappropriate patient selection, lack of a standardized surgical approach, and decreased diastolic distensibility from undersizing the left ventricle. Correction of functional mitral regurgitation in patients with ischemic cardiomyopathy was first described by Bolling et al to treat the functional regurgitation that develops in patients with heart failure (Chapter 55). Subsequent studies by this group demonstrated that there were improvements in LV volumes, EF, and the sphericity index as assessed over 1 year by echocardiography.[115] And indeed, similar findings were observed in the Acorn trial (Figure 8-14).[116] However, although mitral valve repair is technically feasible, and has been associated with improved patient quality of life (see Figure 8-14, *D*), long-term outcomes have not been shown to confer a mortality benefit for mitral valve annuloplasty as a primary treatment for patients with LV dysfunction.[117]

SUMMARY AND FUTURE DIRECTIONS

Currently available medical and device therapies for heart failure have consistently demonstrated the reversibility of the abnormal biology of the failing cardiac myocyte, reversibility of the unfavorable changes in the composition of the extracellular matrix, and the adverse geometry of the failing heart, indicating that the heart failure phenotype exhibits remarkable "plasticity" (see Figure 8-11). This statement notwithstanding, it bears emphasis that although the various components of the phenomenon of reverse remodeling have been studied carefully and characterized meticulously in experimental and clinical studies, it is unclear how these changes contribute to restoration of normal LV structure and function. That is, we simply do not understand what the essential biological "drivers" of reverse remodeling are, nor do we understand how they are coordinated. For example, it is not known whether changes in the biology of the myocyte precede, follow, or occur *pari passu* with changes in the extracellular matrix as the end-diastolic pressure volume curve shifts leftward and LV volume decreases. Moreover, it is unclear which of the changes in the biology of the myocyte is essential for the return of function in isolated failing cardiac myocytes and which of the changes is unrelated to recovery. Another question is why the heart failure phenotype is reversible at the level of the cell, the tissue, and the intact failing heart following mechanical circulatory support, and yet the number of patients who undergo sustained myocardial recovery following withdrawal of LVAD support is less than 10%. As noted previously, the reasons for this observation are unclear, but may be related to an inadequate volume of remaining functional myocytes to sustain pump function. Alternatively, there may be a degree of "hysteresis" during the process of reverse remodeling, such that the reverse remodeled ventricle is less able to withstand the same degree of hemodynamic overloading as a ventricle that has never undergone remodeling. The quest for the answers to these important questions extends well beyond simple intellectual curiosity about the biology of heart failure. Indeed, the answers to these questions may allow for the development of therapies that directly target myocardial recovery, rather than continuing to target signaling pathways that attenuate remodeling (see Chapter 15). Given the complexities of the biology of reverse remodeling outlined in the foregoing chapter, it is likely that the learning curve will be extremely steep, now and for the foreseeable future.

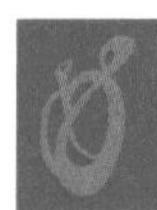

REFERENCES

1. Kass, D. A., Baughman, K. L., Pak, P. H., et al. (1995). Reverse remodeling from cardiomyoplasty in human heart failure. External constraint versus active assist. *Circulation, 91*, 2314–2318.
2. Levin, H. R., Oz, M. C., Chen, J. M., et al. (1995). Reversal of chronic ventricular dilation in patients with end-stage cardiomyopathy by prolonged mechanical unloading. *Circulation, 91*, 2717–2720.
3. Frazier, O. H. (1994). First use of an untethered, vented electric left ventricular assist device for long-term support. *Circulation, 89*, 2908–2914.
4. Levin, H. R., Oz, M. C., Catanese, K. A., et al. (1996). Transient normalization of systolic and diastolic function after support with a left ventricular assist device in a patient with dilated cardiomyopathy. *J Heart Lung Transplant, 15*, 840–842.
5. Konstam, M. A., Kronenberg, M. W., Rousseau, M. F., et al. (1993). Effects of the angiotensin converting enzyme inhibitor enalapril on the long-term progression of left ventricular dilatation in patients with asymptomatic systolic dysfunction. SOLVD (studies of left ventricular dysfunction) investigators. *Circulation, 88*, 2277–2283.
6. Greenberg, B., Quinones, M. A., Koilpillai, C., et al. (1995). Effects of long-term enalapril therapy on cardiac structure and function in patients with left ventricular dysfunction: results of the SOLVD echocardiography substudy. *Circulation, 91*, 2573–2581.
7. Australia/New Zealand Heart Failure Research Collaborative Group (1997). Randomised, placebo-controlled trial of carvedilol in patients with congestive heart failure due to ischaemic heart disease. *Lancet, 349*, 375–380.
8. Mann, D. L., & Willerson, J. T. (1998). Left ventricular assist devices and the failing heart: a bridge to recovery, a permanent assist device, or a bridge too far? *Circulation, 98*, 2367–2369.
9. Lowes, B. D., Minobe, W., Abraham, W. T., et al. (1997). Changes in gene expression in the intact human heart. Downregulation of α-myosin heavy chain in hypertrophied, failing ventricular myocardium. *J Clin Invest, 100*, 2315–2324.
10. Schaper, J., Froede, R., St., Hein, et al. (1991). Impairment of the myocardial ultrastructure and changes of the cytoskeleton in dilated cardiomyopathy. *Circulation, 83*, 504–514.
11. Beuckelmann, D. J., Nabauer, M., & Erdmann, E. (1992). Intracellular calcium handling in isolated ventricular myocytes from patients with terminal heart failure. *Circulation, 85*, 1046–1055.
12. Bristow, M. R., Ginsburg, R., Minobe, W., et al. (1982). Decreased catecholamine sensitivity and β-adrenergic-receptor density in failing human hearts. *N Engl J Med, 307*, 205–211.
13. Davies, C. H., Davia, K., Bennett, J. G., et al. (1995). Reduced contraction and altered frequency response of isolated ventricular myocytes from patients with heart failure. *Circulation, 92*, 2540–2549.
14. Hunter, J. J., & Chien, K. R. (1999). Signaling pathways for cardiac hypertrophy and failure. *N Engl J Med, 341*, 1276–1283.
15. Gerdes, A. M., Clark, L. C., & Capasso, J. M. (1995). Regression of cardiac hypertrophy after closing an aortocaval fistula in rats. *Am J Physiol, 268*, H2345–H2351.
16. Flesch, M., Margulies, K. B., Mochmann, H. C., et al. (2001). Differential regulation of mitogen-activated kinases in the failing human heart in response to mechanical unloading. *Circulation*, 104, 2273–2276.
17. Razeghi, P., Bruckner, B. A., Sharma, S., et al. (2003). Mechanical unloading of the failing human heart fails to activate the protein kinase B/Akt/glycogen synthase kinase-3beta survival pathway. *Cardiology, 100*, 17–22.
18. Weinberg, E. O., Schoen, F. J., George, D., et al. (1994). Angiotensin converting enzyme inhibition prolongs survival and modifies the transition to heart failure in rats with pressure overload hypertrophy due to ascending aortic stenosis. *Circulation, 90*, 1410–1422.
19. Morita, H., Suzuki, G., Mishima, T., et al. (2002). Effects of long-term monotherapy with metoprolol CR/XL on the progression of left ventricular dysfunction and remodeling in dogs with chronic heart failure. *Cardiovasc Drugs Ther, 16*, 443–449.
20. Goldstein, S., Sharov, V. G., Cook, J. M., et al. (1995). Ventricular remodeling: insights from pharmacologic interventions with angiotensin-converting enzyme inhibitors. *Mol Cell Biochem, 147*, 51–55.
21. Zafeiridis, A., Jeevanandam, V., Houser, S. R., et al. (1998). Regression of cellular hypertrophy after left ventricular assist device support. *Circulation, 98*, 656–662.
22. Baba, H. A., Grabellus, F., August, C., et al. (2000). Reversal of metallothionein expression is different throughout the human myocardium after prolonged left-ventricular mechanical support. *J Heart Lung Transplant, 19*, 668–674.
23. Madigan, J. D., Barbone, A., Choudhri, A. F., et al. (2001). Time course of reverse remodeling of the left ventricle during support with a left ventricular assist device. *J Thorac Cardiovasc Surg, 121*, 902–908.
24. Bruckner, B. A., Stetson, S. J., Perez-Verdia, A., et al. (2001). Regression of fibrosis and hypertrophy in failing myocardium following mechanical circulatory support. *J Heart Lung Transplant, 20*, 457–464.
25. Rivello, H. G., Meckert, P. C., Vigliano, C., et al. (2001). Cardiac myocyte nuclear size and ploidy status decrease after mechanical support. *Cardiovasc Pathol, 10*, 53–57.
26. McCarthy, P. M., Nakatani, S., Vargo, R., et al. (1995). Structural and left ventricular histologic changes after implantable LVAD insertion. *Ann Thorac Surg, 59*, 609–613.
27. Sabbah, H. N., Sharov, V. G., Gupta, R. C., et al. (2003). Reversal of chronic molecular and cellular abnormalities due to heart failure by passive mechanical ventricular containment. *Circ Res, 93*, 1095–1101.

28. Wang, J., Oliveira, G., Koerner, M. M., et al. (2006). Cardiac resynchronization therapy induces cellular reverse remodelling in failing human hearts. *Circulation, 114*(suppl II), 718, abstract.
29. Divakaran, V., & Mann, D. L. (2008). The emerging role of microRNAs in cardiac remodeling and heart failure. *Circ Res, 103*, 1072–1083.
30. Wang, J., Xu, R., Lin, F., et al. (2008). MicroRNA: novel regulators involved in the remodeling and reverse remodeling of the heart. *Cardiology, 113*, 81–88.
31. Matkovich, S. J., Van Booven, D. J., Youker, K. A., et al. (2009). Reciprocal regulation of myocardial microRNAs and messenger RNA in human cardiomyopathy and reversal of the microRNA signature by biomechanical support. *Circulation, 119*, 1263–1271.
32. van Rooij, E., Sutherland, L. B., Liu, N., et al. (2006). A signature pattern of stress-responsive microRNAs that can evoke cardiac hypertrophy and heart failure. *Proc Natl Acad Sci U S A, 103*, 18255–18260.
33. Swynghedauw, B. (2006). Phenotypic plasticity of adult myocardium: molecular mechanisms. *J Exp Biol, 209*, 2320–2327.
34. Brooks, W. W., Bing, O. H., Conrad, C. H., et al. (1997). Captopril modifies gene expression in hypertrophied and failing hearts of aged spontaneously hypertensive rats. *Hypertension, 30*, 1362–1368.
35. Wang, J., Guo, X., & Dhalla, N. S. (2004). Modification of myosin protein and gene expression in failing hearts due to myocardial infarction by enalapril or losartan. *Biochim Biophys Acta, 1690*, 177–184.
36. Lowes, B. D., Gilbert, E. M., Abraham, W. T., et al. (2002). Myocardial gene expression in dilated cardiomyopathy treated with beta-blocking agents. *N Engl J Med, 346*, 1357–1365.
37. Blaxall, B. C., Tschannen-Moran, B. M., Milano, C. A., et al. (2003). Differential gene expression and genomic patient stratification following left ventricular assist device support. *J Am Coll Cardiol, 41*, 1096–1106.
38. Rodrigue-Way, A., Burkhoff, D., Geesaman, B. J., et al. (2005). Sarcomeric genes involved in reverse remodeling of the heart during left ventricular assist device support. *J Heart Lung Transplant, 24*, 73–80.
39. Latif, N., Yacoub, M. H., George, R., et al. (2007). Changes in sarcomeric and non-sarcomeric cytoskeletal proteins and focal adhesion molecules during clinical myocardial recovery after left ventricular assist device support. *J Heart Lung Transplant, 26*, 230–235.
40. Kuhn, M., Voss, M., Mitko, D., et al. (2004). Left ventricular assist device support reverses altered cardiac expression and function of natriuretic peptides and receptors in end-stage heart failure. *Cardiovasc Res, 64*, 308–314.
41. Iyengar, S., Haas, G., Lamba, S., et al. (2007). Effect of cardiac resynchronization therapy on myocardial gene expression in patients with nonischemic dilated cardiomyopathy. *J Card Fail, 13*, 304–311.
42. Vanderheyden, M., Mullens, W., Delrue, L., et al. (2008). Myocardial gene expression in heart failure patients treated with cardiac resynchronization therapy responders versus nonresponders. *J Am Coll Cardiol, 51*, 129–136.
43. Rastogi, S., Mishra, S., Gupta, R. C., et al. (2005). Reversal of maladaptive gene program in left ventricular myocardium of dogs with heart failure following long-term therapy with the Acorn Cardiac Support Device. *Heart Fail Rev, 10*, 157–163.
44. Gilbert, E. M., Abraham, W. T., Olsen, S., et al. (1996). Comparative hemodynamic, left ventricular functional, and antiadrenergic effects of chronic treatment with metoprolol versus carvedilol in the failing heart. *Circulation, 94*, 2817–2825.
45. Gilbert, E. M., Sandoval, A., Larrabee, P., et al. (1993). Lisinopril lowers cardiac adrenergic drive and increases beta-receptor density in the failing human heart. *Circulation, 88*, 472–480.
46. Ogletree-Hughes, M. L., Stull, L. B., Sweet, W. E., et al. (2001). Mechanical unloading restores beta-adrenergic responsiveness and reverses receptor downregulation in the failing human heart. *Circulation, 104*, 881–886.
47. Schnee, P. M., Shah, N., Bergheim, M., et al. (2008). Location and density of alpha- and beta-adrenoreceptor sub-types in myocardium after mechanical left ventricular unloading. *J Heart Lung Transplant, 27*, 710–717.
48. Klotz, S., Barbone, A., Reiken, S., et al. (2005). Left ventricular assist device support normalizes left and right ventricular beta-adrenergic pathway properties. *J Am Coll Cardiol, 45*, 668–676.
49. Hata, J. A., Williams, M. L., Schroder, J. N., et al. (2006). Lymphocyte levels of GRK2 (betaARK1) mirror changes in the LVAD-supported failing human heart: lower GRK2 associated with improved beta-adrenergic signaling after mechanical unloading. *J Card Fail, 12*, 360–368.
50. Mullens, W., Bartunek, J., Wilson Tang, W. H., et al. (2008). Early and late effects of cardiac resynchronization therapy on force-frequency relation and contractility regulating gene expression in heart failure patients. *Heart Rhythm, 5*, 52–59.
51. Saavedra, W. F., Tunin, R. S., Paolocci, N., et al. (2002). Reverse remodeling and enhanced adrenergic reserve from passive external support in experimental dilated heart failure. *J Am Coll Cardiol, 39*, 2069–2076.
52. Plank, D. M., Yatani, A., Ritsu, H., et al. (2003). Calcium dynamics in the failing heart: restoration by beta-adrenergic receptor blockade. *Am J Physiol Heart Circ Physiol, 285*, H305–H315.
53. Kubo, H., Margulies, K. B., Piacentino, V., III, et al. (2001). Patients with end-stage congestive heart failure treated with beta-adrenergic receptor antagonists have improved ventricular myocyte calcium regulatory protein abundance. *Circulation, 104*, 1012–1018.
54. Reiken, S., Wehrens, X. H., Vest, J. A., et al. (2003). Beta-blockers restore calcium release channel function and improve cardiac muscle performance in human heart failure. *Circulation, 107*, 2459–2466.
55. Guo, X., Chapman, D., & Dhalla, N. S. (2003). Partial prevention of changes in SR gene expression in congestive heart failure due to myocardial infarction by enalapril or losartan. *Mol Cell Biochem, 254*, 163–172.
56. Shao, Q., Ren, B., Saini, H. K., et al. (2005). Sarcoplasmic reticulum Ca^{2+} transport and gene expression in congestive heart failure are modified by imidapril treatment. *Am J Physiol Heart Circ Physiol, 288*, H1674–H1682.
57. Dipla, K., Mattiello, J. A., Jeevanandam, V., et al. (1998). Myocyte recovery after mechanical circulatory support in humans with end-stage heart failure. *Circulation, 97*, 2316–2322.
58. Soppa, G. K., Barton, P. J., Terracciano, C. M., et al. (2008). Left ventricular assist device-induced molecular changes in the failing myocardium. *Curr Opin Cardiol, 23*, 206–218.
59. Chen, X., Piacentino, V., III, Furukawa, S., et al. (2002). L-type Ca^{2+} channel density and regulation are altered in failing human ventricular myocytes and recover after support with mechanical assist devices. *Circ Res, 91*, 517–524.
60. Marx, S. O., Reiken, S., Hisamatsu, Y., et al. (2000). PKA phosphorylation dissociates FKBP12.6 from the calcium release channel (ryanodine receptor): defective regulation in failing hearts. *Cell, 101*, 365–376.
61. Heerdt, P. M., Holmes, J. W., Cai, B., et al. (2000). Chronic unloading by left ventricular assist device reverses contractile dysfunction and alters gene expression in end-stage heart failure. *Circulation, 102*, 2713–2719.
62. Vatta, M., Stetson, S. J., Perez-Verdia, A., et al. (2002). Molecular remodelling of dystrophin in patients with end-stage cardiomyopathies and reversal in patients on assistance-device therapy. *Lancet, 359*, 936–941.
63. Vatta, M., Stetson, S. J., Jimenez, S., et al. (2004). Molecular normalization of dystrophin in the failing left and right ventricle of patients treated with either pulsatile or continuous flow-type ventricular assist devices. *J Am Coll Cardiol, 43*, 811–817.
64. de Jonge, N., van Wichen, D. F., Schipper, M. E., et al. (2002). Left ventricular assist device in end-stage heart failure: persistence of structural myocyte damage after unloading. An immunohistochemical analysis of the contractile myofilaments. *J Am Coll Cardiol, 39*, 963–969.
65. Aquila, L. A., McCarthy, P. M., Smedira, N. G., et al. (2004). Cytoskeletal structure and recovery in single human cardiac myocytes. *J Heart Lung Transplant, 23*, 954–963.
66. Birks, E. J., Hall, J. L., Barton, P. J., et al. (2005). Gene profiling changes in cytoskeletal proteins during clinical recovery after left ventricular-assist device support. *Circulation, 112*, I57–I64.
67. Tsutsui, H., Spinale, F. G., Nagatsu, M., et al. (1994). Effects of chronic β-adrenergic blockade on the left ventricular and cardiocyte abnormalities of chronic canine mitral regurgitation. *J Clin Invest, 93*, 2639–2648.
68. Frazier, O. H. (1999). Left ventricular assist device as a bridge to partial left ventriculectomy. *Eur J Cardiothorac Surg, 15*(suppl. 1), S20–S25.
69. Rose, A. G., & Park, S. J. (2005). Pathology in patients with ventricular assist devices: a study of 21 autopsies, 24 ventricular apical core biopsies and 24 explanted hearts. *Cardiovasc Pathol, 14*, 19–23.
70. Schaper, J., & Speiser, B. (1992). The extracellular matrix in the failing human heart. *Basic Res Cardiol, 87*(suppl. 1), 303–309.
71. Weber, K. T. (1989). Cardiac interstitium in health and disease: the fibrillar collagen network. *J Am Coll Cardiol, 13*(7), 1637–1652.
72. Shigeyama, J., Yasumura, Y., Sakamoto, A., et al. (2005). Increased gene expression of collagen types I and III is inhibited by beta-receptor blockade in patients with dilated cardiomyopathy. *Eur Heart J, 26*, 2698–2705.
73. Milanez, M. C., Gomes, M. G., Vassallo, D. V., et al. (1997). Effects of captopril on interstitial collagen in the myocardium after infarction in rats. *J Card Fail, 3*, 189–197.
74. Liu, Y. H., Yang, X. P., Sharov, V. G., et al. (1997). Effects of angiotensin-converting enzyme inhibitors and angiotensin II type 1 receptor antagonists in rats with heart failure. Role of kinins and angiotensin II type 2 receptors. *J Clin Invest, 99*, 1926–1935.
75. Mukherjee, D., & Sen, S. (1991). Alteration of collagen phenotypes in ischemic cardiomyopathy. *J Clin Invest, 88*, 1141–1146.
76. Suzuki, G., Morita, H., Mishima, T., et al. (2002). Effects of long-term monotherapy with eplerenone, a novel aldosterone blocker, on progression of left ventricular dysfunction and remodeling in dogs with heart failure. *Circulation, 106*, 2967–2972.
77. Rastogi, S., Mishra, S., Zaca, V., et al. (2007). Effect of long-term monotherapy with the aldosterone receptor blocker eplerenone on cytoskeletal proteins and matrix metalloproteinases in dogs with heart failure. *Cardiovasc Drugs Ther, 21*, 415–422.
78. Li, Y. Y., Feng, Y., McTiernan, C. F., et al. (2001). Downregulation of matrix metalloproteinases and reduction in collagen damage in the failing human heart after support with left ventricular assist devices. *Circulation, 104*, 1147–1152.
79. Klotz, S., Foronjy, R. F., Dickstein, M. L., et al. (2005). Mechanical unloading during left ventricular assist device support increases left ventricular collagen cross-linking and myocardial stiffness. *Circulation, 112*, 364–374.
80. Matsumiya, G., Monta, O., Fukushima, N., et al. (2005). Who would be a candidate for bridge to recovery during prolonged mechanical left ventricular support in idiopathic dilated cardiomyopathy? *J Thorac Cardiovasc Surg, 130*, 699–704.
81. Bruggink, A. H., van Oosterhout, M. F., de Jonge, N., et al. (2006). Reverse remodeling of the myocardial extracellular matrix after prolonged left ventricular assist device support follows a biphasic pattern. *J Heart Lung Transplant, 25*, 1091–1098.
82. Bruckner, B. A., Stetson, S. J., Farmer, J. A., et al. (2000). The implications for cardiac recovery of left ventricular assist device support on myocardial collagen content. *Am J Surg, 180*, 498–501.
83. Thohan, V., Stetson, S. J., Nagueh, S. F., et al. (2005). Cellular and hemodynamics responses of failing myocardium to continuous flow mechanical circulatory support using the DeBakey-Noon left ventricular assist device: a comparative analysis with pulsatile-type devices. *J Heart Lung Transplant, 24*, 566–575.
84. Klotz, S., Danser, A. H., Foronjy, R. F., et al. (2007). The impact of angiotensin-converting enzyme inhibitor therapy on the extracellular collagen matrix during left ventricular assist device support in patients with end-stage heart failure. *J Am Coll Cardiol, 49*, 1166–1174.
85. D'Ascia, C., Cittadini, A., Monti, M. G., et al. (2006). Effects of biventricular pacing on interstitial remodelling, tumor necrosis factor-alpha expression, and apoptotic death in failing human myocardium. *Eur Heart J, 27*, 201–206.
86. Hessel, M. H., Bleeker, G. B., Bax, J. J., et al. (2007). Reverse ventricular remodelling after cardiac resynchronization therapy is associated with a reduction in serum tenascin-C and plasma matrix metalloproteinase-9 levels. *Eur J Heart Fail, 9*, 1058–1063.

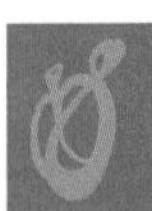

87. Sabbah, H. N. (2004). Effects of cardiac support device on reverse remodeling: molecular, biochemical, and structural mechanisms. *J Card Fail, 10*, S207–S214.
88. Hudlicka, O., Brown, M., & Egginton, S. (1992). Angiogenesis in skeletal and cardiac muscle. *Physiol Rev, 72*, 369–417.
89. Karch, R., Neumann, F., Ullrich, R., et al. (2005). The spatial pattern of coronary capillaries in patients with dilated, ischemic, or inflammatory cardiomyopathy. *Cardiovasc Pathol, 14*, 135–144.
90. Abraham, D., Hofbauer, R., Schafer, R., et al. (2000). Selective downregulation of VEGF-A(165), VEGF-R(1), and decreased capillary density in patients with dilative but not ischemic cardiomyopathy. *Circ Res, 87*, 644–647.
91. Hara, Y., Inoue, K., Ogimoto, A., et al. (2005). Effect of beta-blocker therapy on myocardial perfusion defects in thallium-201 scintigraphy in patients with dilated cardiomyopathy. *Cardiology, 104*, 16–21.
92. Akinboboye, O. O., Chou, R. L., & Bergmann, S. R. (2002). Augmentation of myocardial blood flow in hypertensive heart disease by angiotensin antagonists: a comparison of lisinopril and losartan. *J Am Coll Cardiol, 40*, 703–709.
93. de Boer, R. A., Siebelink, H. J., Tio, R. A., et al. (2001). Carvedilol increases plasma vascular endothelial growth factor (VEGF) in patients with chronic heart failure 1. *Eur J Heart Fail, 3*, 331–333.
94. Hall, J. L., Grindle, S., Han, X., et al. (2004). Genomic profiling of the human heart before and after mechanical support with a ventricular assist device reveals alterations in vascular signaling networks. *Physiol Genomics, 17*, 283–291.
95. Knaapen, P., van Campen, L. M., de Cock, C. C., et al. (2004). Effects of cardiac resynchronization therapy on myocardial perfusion reserve. *Circulation, 110*, 646–651.
96. Rastogi, S., Gupta, R. C., Mishra, S., et al. (2005). Long-term therapy with the Acorn Cardiac Support Device normalizes gene expression of growth factors and gelatinases in dogs with heart failure. *J Heart Lung Transplant, 24*, 1619–1625.
97. Chaudhry, P. A., Mishima, T., Sharov, V. G., et al. (2000). Passive epicardial containment prevents ventricular remodeling in heart failure. *Ann Thorac Surg, 70*, 1275–1280.
98. Doughty, R. N., Whalley, G. A., Gamble, G., et al. (1997). Left ventricular remodeling with carvedilol in patients with congestive heart failure due to ischemic heart disease. *J Am Coll Cardiol, 29*, 1060–1066.
99. Wong, M., Staszewsky, L., Latini, R., et al. (2002). Valsartan benefits left ventricular structure and function in heart failure: Val-HeFT echocardiographic study. *J Am Coll Cardiol, 40*, 970–975.
100. Chan, A. K., Sanderson, J. E., Wang, T., et al. (2007). Aldosterone receptor antagonism induces reverse remodeling when added to angiotensin receptor blockade in chronic heart failure. *J Am Coll Cardiol, 50*, 591–596.
101. Klotz, S., Deng, M. C., Stypmann, J., et al. (2004). Left ventricular pressure and volume unloading during pulsatile versus nonpulsatile left ventricular assist device support. *Ann Thorac Surg, 77*, 143–149.
102. Garcia, S., Kandar, F., Boyle, A., et al. (2008). Effects of pulsatile- and continuous-flow left ventricular assist devices on left ventricular unloading. *J Heart Lung Transplant, 27*, 261–267.
103. Mancini, D. M., Beniaminovitz, A., Levin, H., et al. (1998). Low incidence of myocardial recovery after left ventricular assist device implantation in patients with chronic heart failure. *Circulation, 98*, 2383–2389.
104. Maybaum, S., Mancini, D., Xydas, S., et al. (2007). Cardiac improvement during mechanical circulatory support: a prospective multicenter study of the LVAD working group. *Circulation, 115*, 2497–2505.
105. St John Sutton, M. G., Plappert, T., Abraham, W. T., et al. (2003). Effect of cardiac resynchronization therapy on left ventricular size and function in chronic heart failure. *Circulation, 107*, 1985–1990.
106. Naismith, J. H., Devine, T. Q., Brandhuber, B. J., et al. (1995). Crystallographic evidence for dimerization of unliganded tumor necrosis factor receptor. *J Biol Chem, 270*, 13303–13307.
107. Linde, C., Leclercq, C., Rex, S., et al. (2002). Long-term benefits of biventricular pacing in congestive heart failure: results from the MUltisite STimulation in cardiomyopathy (MUSTIC) study. *J Am Coll Cardiol, 40*, 111–118.
108. Mann, D. L., Acker, M. A., Jessup, M., et al. (2007). Clinical evaluation of the CorCap Cardiac Support Device in patients with dilated cardiomyopathy. *Ann Thorac Surg, 84*, 1226–1235.
109. Starling, R. C., Jessup, M., Oh, J. K., et al. (2007). Sustained benefits of the CorCap Cardiac Support Device on left ventricular remodeling: three year follow-up results from the Acorn clinical trial. *Ann Thorac Surg, 84*, 1236–1242.
110. Bouchart, F., Tabley, A., Litzler, P. Y., et al. (2001). Myocardial revascularization in patients with severe ischemic left ventricular dysfunction. Long term follow-up in 141 patients. *Eur J Cardiothorac Surg, 20*, 1157–1162.
111. Jones, R. H., Velazquez, E. J., Michler, R. E., et al. (2009). Coronary bypass surgery with or without surgical ventricular reconstruction. *N Engl J Med, 360*, 1705–1717.
112. Starling, R. C., McCarthy, P. M., Buda, T., et al. (2000). Results of partial left ventriculectomy for dilated cardiomyopathy: hemodynamic, clinical and echocardiographic observations. *J Am Coll Cardiol, 36*, 2098–2103.
113. Dickstein, M. L., Spotnitz, H. M., Rose, E. A., et al. (1997). Heart reduction surgery: an analysis of the impact on cardiac function. *J Thorac Cardiovasc Surg, 113*, 1032–1040.
114. Athanasuleas, C. L., Buckberg, G. D., Stanley, A. W., et al. (2004). Surgical ventricular restoration in the treatment of congestive heart failure due to post-infarction ventricular dilation. *J Am Coll Cardiol, 44*, 1439–1445.
115. Bach, D. S., & Bolling, S. F. (1996). Improvement following correction of secondary mitral regurgitation in end-stage cardiomyopathy with mitral annuloplasty. *Am J Cardiol, 78*, 966–969.
116. Acker, M. A., Bolling, S., Shemin, R., et al. (2006). Mitral valve surgery in heart failure: insights from the Acorn clinical trial. *J Thorac Cardiovasc Surg, 132*, 568–577.
117. Wu, A. H., Aaronson, K. D., Bolling, S. F., et al. (2005). Impact of mitral valve annuloplasty on mortality risk in patients with mitral regurgitation and left ventricular systolic dysfunction. *J Am Coll Cardiol, 45*, 381–387.
118. Chen, Y., Park, S., Li, Y., et al. (2003). Alterations of gene expression in failing myocardium following left ventricular assist device support. *Physiol Genomics, 14*, 251–260.
119. Chen, M. M., Ashley, E. A., Deng, D. X., et al. (2003). Novel role for the potent endogenous inotrope apelin in human cardiac dysfunction. *Circulation, 108*, 1432–1439.
120. Margulies, K. B., Matiwala, S., Cornejo, C., et al. (2005). Mixed messages: transcription patterns in failing and recovering human myocardium. *Circ Res, 96*, 592–599.
121. Hall, J. L., Birks, E. J., Grindle, S., et al. (2007). Molecular signature of recovery following combination left ventricular assist device (LVAD) support and pharmacologic therapy. *Eur Heart J, 28*, 613–627.

CHAPTER 9

Activation of the Renin-Angiotensin System in Heart Failure

Rajesh Kumar, Kenneth M. Baker, and Jing Pan

THE RENIN-ANGIOTENSIN SYSTEM

The renin-angiotensin system (RAS) is a major determinant of cardiovascular and renal function. RAS inhibitors often provide the first line of treatment for hypertension, afterload reduction, and prevention and treatment of heart failure (see Chapter 45).[1] In the simplest form, the RAS consists of a cascade of enzymatic reactions involving three components: angiotensinogen (Ao), renin, and angiotensin-converting enzyme (ACE), which generate angiotensin (Ang) II as the biologically active product. Ang II binds to two types of specific receptors, angiotensin type-1 (AT_1R) and type-2 (AT_2R). Both receptors belong to the family of seven transmembrane domain, heterotrimeric G protein–coupled receptors (GPCR). The majority of the deleterious actions of Ang II have been attributed to interaction with the AT_1 receptor, which is the predominant receptor in adult tissues, while AT_2 generally produces beneficial effects.[2] Several classes of drugs have been developed to block the RAS, either at the level of Ang II synthesis, by inhibiting the enzymatic reactions catalyzed by renin or ACE, or by preventing Ang II interaction with the AT_1R.

The most proximal component of the RAS, renin, was identified more than 100 years ago by Tigerstedt and Bergman.[3] Discoveries in the past 2 decades have resulted in characterization of the RAS, as both systemic and local or tissue systems.[4] The relative contribution of the systemic versus a local RAS to various cardiovascular pathologies, such as hypertension and heart failure, is still being debated.[5] In addition to categorization, several new aspects of the RAS have been identified, which include novel angiotensin peptides, enzymes that catalyze synthesis of these peptides, receptors for these novel peptides, and new roles for renin and prorenin.[6-9]

THE SYSTEMIC RAS

The systemic RAS is also known as the classical, circulatory, or endocrine RAS, with Ao and renin secreted into the circulation from the liver and kidneys (juxtaglomerular apparatus), respectively, and the final step of Ang II synthesis occurring in the circulation by the action of ACE (membrane bound on endothelial cells), which results in conversion of the decapeptide Ang I to Ang II (Figure 9-1). Circulating Ao and renin appear to contribute to Ang II synthesis locally at tissue sites, blurring the distinction between the systemic and local systems.[10] The circulating RAS is mainly involved in acute responses to maintain plasma volume and electrolyte homeostasis. These include vasoconstriction, a direct effect on tubular sodium reabsorption and aldosterone secretion. Though some of the previously described effects could be attributed to the local RAS in kidneys, recent studies have addressed this issue using tissue–specific knockout of AT_1R. It appears that while both renal and vascular AT_1R contribute equally toward the maintenance of normal blood pressure, the hypertensive effects of Ang II require AT_1R in the kidney.[11]

Angiotensinogen

Ao is a 485–amino acid protein with an N-terminal signal peptide, which is cotranslationally removed to yield the 452–amino acid mature protein, the only known substrate for renin. Though Ao is expressed in multiple tissues, plasma Ao levels are determined primarily by the rate of production by hepatocytes, which constitutively secrete Ao.[12] Circulating levels of Ao are close to the Michaelis constant for renin; thus a small increase in Ao will increase Ang II synthesis and blood pressure.[13] Several studies in genetically modified mice and rats have demonstrated hypertensive effects of increasing Ao gene copy number or overexpression.[14,15] Ao occurs in unglycosylated and multiple glycosylated forms, the significance of which is not entirely known.[16] A variety of stimuli regulate circulating levels of Ao, including glucocorticoids, estrogens, thyroid hormone, insulin, and several cytokines.[17,18] Ang II exerts positive feedback regulation on Ao expression through the AT_1R.[19-21] Polymorphisms in the Ao gene have been reported, which affect transcriptional regulation of the gene and may provide a genetic mechanism for hypertension.[22]

Renin

Juxtaglomerular cells, in the terminal afferent arteriole of the kidneys, are the major source of circulating renin. Renin is synthesized as pre-prorenin, which is converted into prorenin after removal of the signal peptide during transfer to the endoplasmic reticulum. Prorenin, which is enzymatically inactive, is proteolytically activated by removal of the 43–amino acid prosegment to produce renin. The prosegment can also be displaced nonproteolytically by low pH or binding to a newly discovered specific receptor[23] to expose the catalytic site. Juxtaglomerular cells constitutively secrete the majority of prorenin, with the remainder targeted at dense core secretory granules, where the prosegment is removed and renin is released in a regulated manner.

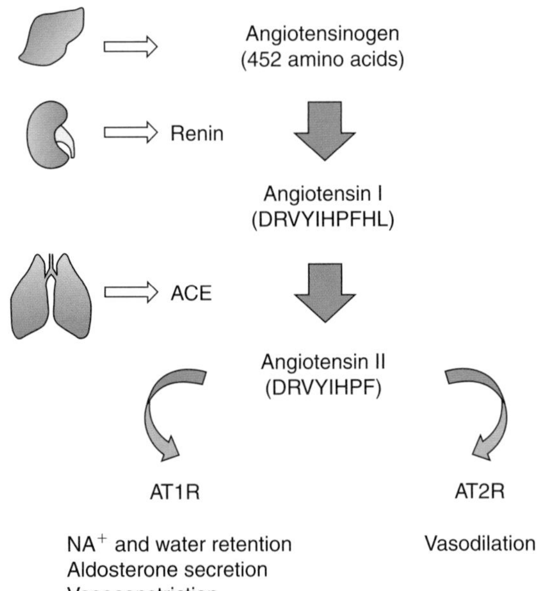

FIGURE 9-1 The systemic renin-angiotensin system. The systemic RAS is comprised of liver-derived Ao, kidney-derived renin, and endothelium-derived ACE. The latter is particularly abundant in pulmonary endothelial cells. The sequential action of renin and ACE on Ao produces the octapeptide Ang II in the circulation. Ang II acts via binding to AT_1R and AT_2R, which generally produce opposite effects. AT_1R is the predominant receptor in adult tissues. The systemic RAS is involved in acute effects to maintain salt and water homeostasis and blood pressure.

Recent evidence suggests that collecting ducts, in addition to juxtaglomerular cells, are an important source of circulating prorenin in diabetes.[24] Pregnant women have high levels of circulating prorenin, which is largely from the ovaries.[25] There is no evidence of extrarenal proteolytic conversion of prorenin to renin; thus the physiological role of circulating prorenin has been uncertain until the recent discovery of the (pro)renin receptor,[23] which will be described later.

Renin synthesis and secretion are promoted by low blood pressure, sympathetic stimuli, and prostaglandins, and are inhibited by high blood pressure, salt, and volume overload.[26] Ang II also exerts a negative feedback on renin production by the juxtaglomerular cells,[27] which is the reason for the observed reactive rise in renin with RAS blockade.

Angiotensin-Converting Enzyme

ACE is a dicarboxypeptidyl peptidase of 150 to 180 kDa, which cleaves the two terminal amino acids off of the decapeptide angiotensin I (Ang I), a product of the Ao and renin reaction, to form the octapeptide Ang II. Unlike renin, ACE is not specific to a single substrate but cleaves several peptides such as bradykinin, substance P, and the tetrapeptide *N*-acetyl-Ser-Asp-Lys-Pro (Ac-SDKP).[28] Some of the beneficial effects of ACE inhibitors have been attributed to prevention of bradykinin and Ac-SDKP degradation. In addition to vascular endothelial cells of lung, retina, and brain, ACE is also highly expressed on the proximal tubular brush border of epithelial cells in the kidneys.[29] While most ACE is anchored to the cell membrane by a C-terminus hydrophobic region, shedding of ACE releases active enzyme into various body fluids. The extracellular region of ACE contains two homologous and independent catalytic domains termed N- and C-domains. An isoform of ACE that contains only the C-domain is expressed in the testis, resulting in categorization of ACE as somatic and testis ACE. A recent study in genetically modified mice has shown that the C-domain of ACE is the predominant site of Ang I cleavage in vivo.[30] Localization of ACE on endothelial cell membranes generates Ang II in close proximity to vascular smooth muscle, which is important for vasoconstrictive effects of the peptide. ACE knockout mice have low blood pressure, with hematopoietic and developmental defects.[31]

THE LOCAL RAS

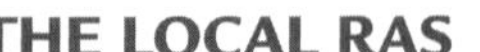

In the past 2 decades, it has become evident that several tissues, other than those that contribute to the circulating RAS, express all components of the RAS and generate Ang II locally at tissue sites. This has been most clearly demonstrated in the brain, where circulating components cannot enter due to the blood-brain barrier. The benefits of RAS inhibitors, which cannot be explained solely on the basis of blood pressure reduction, strengthened the concept of local generation and effects of Ang II. Advancements in research technology, due to the availability of transgenic and knockout animal models (of RAS components), further confirmed the significance of the local RAS in various pathologies. Local RASs have tissue–specific roles and are regulated independently of the circulating system. The major controversy associated with local RASs is regarding the expression of renin in extrarenal tissues, particularly the heart. However, this has not really undermined the concept of a local RAS, as alternative enzymes, such as cathepsins and chymase, have been identified in several tissues, and which are involved in the conversion of Ao to Ang II. A local RAS has convincingly been demonstrated in the brain, heart, vasculature, kidneys, eyes, pancreas, reproductive organs, and lymphatic and adipose tissues.[4] Recent evidence has indicated that while the circulating RAS exerts acute hemodynamic effects, the tissue RASs are involved in long-term effects of chronic RAS activation associated with target organ damage, such as renal failure and cardiac remodeling.[4] Local system functions of the RAS include cell growth and remodeling in the heart, regulation of blood pressure, central effects on food and water intake, and hormone secretion in the pancreas.[32]

The Cardiac RAS

Most evidence supports cardiac Ang II as being synthesized in situ and not originating by uptake from the circulation (Figure 9-2). A quantitative study using radiolabeled Ao infusion has shown that more than 90% of cardiac Ang I and 75% of cardiac Ang II are synthesized at cardiac sites.[33] The RAS precursor components for Ang II biosynthesis are present in both cardiac myocytes and fibroblasts.[34] The interstitial concentration of Ang II in the heart is about 100-fold more than that of plasma, though the myocardial concentration of renin and Ao is only 1% to 4% that of plasma.[35,36] There is debate as to which and in what amount RAS components are synthesized locally or are taken up from the plasma. Much of the controversy surrounds the source of renin in the heart.[10] Active uptake from the plasma by endothelial cells, cardiomyocytes, and fibroblasts, in addition to de novo synthesis, has been proposed.[37-39] Two uptake mechanisms have been described: one that is mediated by the mannose-6-phosphate receptor and another that is not.[40] The former mainly represents a clearance mechanism of circulating glycosylated prorenin by heart cells, while the latter involves uptake of nonglycosylated prorenin and results in intracellular generation of angiotensin peptides.[41] Emerging evidence suggests that under specific conditions renin is synthesized in cardiovascular tissues. Renin mRNA has been detected in cardiac atria, ventricles, and primary cultures of neonatal and adult rat ventricular myocytes.[34,42] Increased cardiac levels of renin mRNA have been reported in patients following myocardial infarction and in the ventricles of animals with experimental

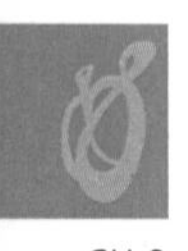

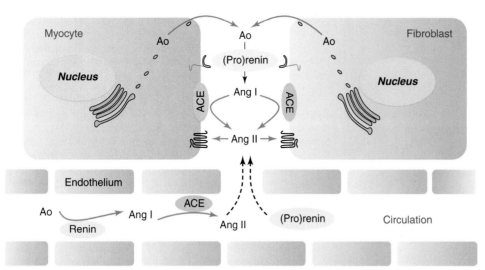

FIGURE 9-2 The cardiac renin-angiotensin system. The cardiac RAS is defined by interstitial Ang II synthesis and direct actions in the heart. A small contribution of circulatory Ang II may also be relevant in addition to the locally synthesized pool. Cardiac cells may also sequester (pro)renin from the circulation. The latter would bind to specific (pro)renin receptors on cardiac cells and convert locally produced Ao to Ang I, which is further cleaved to form Ang II by the actions of membrane-bound ACE. Both types of angiotensin receptors, AT_1 and AT_2, are expressed on cardiac cells. The major effects of Ang II in the heart include cardiac myocyte hypertrophy, cardiac fibroblast proliferation, oxidative stress, and extracellular matrix deposition.

models of infarction.[43] Renin mRNA and protein have been detected in canine cardiac myocytes, the levels of which are upregulated by ventricular-pacing-induced cardiac failure.[44] A second renin transcript, lacking the coding region for the secretory signal peptide and termed Exon 1A renin, has been detected in the brain, adrenal glands, and heart.[45] Interestingly, Exon 1A renin is the only transcript of renin expressed in the heart. The latter observation may help to explain the discrepancy in the literature regarding cardiac renin expression. Methods used in studies with negative results might not have detected this newly identified transcript. Interestingly, this potentially intracellular renin coding mRNA is upregulated in the left ventricle following myocardial infarction.[45] Thus the possibility of two cardiac RASs has been suggested, one the intracardiac RAS, and another an intracellular RAS driven by Exon 1A renin.[41]

The local production of Ao and ACE is less controversial. Ao mRNA and protein have been detected in human, dog, and rat heart, and in rat cardiac myocytes and fibroblasts in primary cell culture.[34] Upregulation of the Ao gene in the heart, in an experimental model of pressure overload, has been reported.[46] ACE has been detected in the human and rat heart, with higher amounts in atria compared with the ventricles.[47,48] Endothelial cells and fibroblasts appear to be the major cell types of the heart that express ACE. ACE has also been detected in primary cultures of adult and neonatal cardiac myocytes.[42,49] There also exist other enzymes such as cathepsins and chymase that can substitute for renin and ACE in the processing of Ao in the heart. Cathepsin D has been shown to increase in cardiac myocytes from failing, paced canine hearts, and cathepsin G was increased in mast cells of failing hearts in humans.[44,50] The role of cathepsin D involvement in Ang II generation is evident in VSMC, where cathepsin D is the predominant aspartic proteinase.[51] Cathepsin D participates in enhanced Ang II synthesis in response to high glucose or a change in VSMC, from the contractile to a synthetic phenotype.[52,53] Cathepsin D cleaves Ao into Ang I and chymase converts Ang I to Ang II. Chymase is highly specific for Ang I and does not degrade bradykinin and vasoactive intestinal peptide. In myocardial extracts from human and dog, chymase accounted for approximately 90% of Ang II forming activity; however, the contribution in intact tissue is not clear.[54,55] Dual pathways of Ang II generation, by chymase and ACE, were demonstrated to have an important role in cardiac remodeling, in pressure-overloaded hamster hearts, and in transgenic mice overexpressing human chymase in the heart.[56,57] Using an ACE-resistant Ang I peptide, a role for chymase-mediated Ang II generation in vasoconstriction in human dorsal hand veins has been demonstrated.[58] In addition to Ang II formation, chymase can produce Ang II–independent effects through conversion of latent TGF-β to active TGF-β and type-1 procollagen to collagen.[59] Consistent with an active role of chymase in cardiac remodeling, specific chymase inhibitors have been shown to have protective effects in animal models of myocardial infarction, cardiomyopathy, and tachycardia-induced heart failure.[60] Thus alternative pathways of Ang II synthesis are present in the heart; though it remains unclear in which situations renin-independent or ACE-independent Ang II synthesis occurs.

Cardiac RAS activity is under the control of tissue-specific regulatory influences and differs from that of the systemic RAS. For example, an increase in left ventricular mass produced by abdominal aortic constriction can be prevented by an ACE inhibitor with no change in afterload.[61] The activity of the cardiac RAS is influenced by several pathophysiological conditions. Volume overload is associated with increased expression of renin and ACE, while pressure overload increases the expression of Ao and AT_1.[34] Mechanical stretch of cardiac myocytes increases Ang II release from cells.[62] Ao gene expression is increased in the heart by cardiotrophin-1, glucocorticoids, estrogen, and thyroid hormone.[34,63] Ang II stimulates the production of atrial natriuretic peptide, which in turn regulates renin and Ao mRNA levels.[34] Ang II has a differential effect on renin and Ao expression in cardiac myocytes and fibroblasts, positively regulating the former, while negatively regulating the latter.[62,64] Together, these observations suggest that the cardiac RAS represents a self-sustaining paracrine/autocrine loop, involving both cardiac myocytes and fibroblasts.[65]

The Intracellular Cardiac RAS

In addition to the systemic and local RAS, recent studies have provided evidence of a complete, functional RAS within cells, described as an "intracrine" or intracellular RAS (Figure 9-3).[7] The intracellular RAS is characterized by the presence of the components inside the cell, synthesis of Ang II intracellularly, and actions of Ang II originating from the intracellular location. As alluded to earlier, Ao and renin are generally secreted from the cells in which synthesis occurs, making the concept of the intracellular synthesis of Ang II seem implausible. However, recent studies have demonstrated that under certain conditions, cells redistribute Ao and renin, resulting in intracellular synthesis and retention of Ang II.[66] Alternative enzymes, such as cathepsin D and chymase, may also substitute for renin and ACE, respectively,

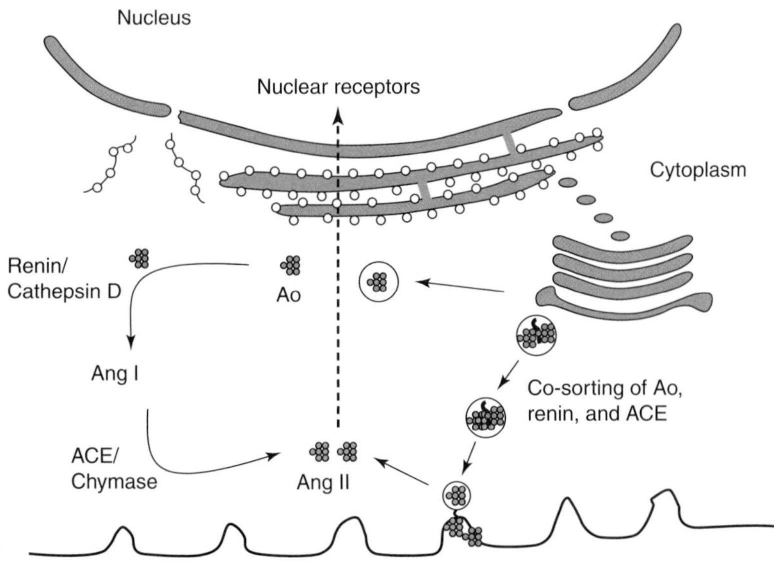

FIGURE 9–3 The intracellular renin-angiotensin system. The intracellular RAS is defined by the synthesis and resultant actions of Ang II inside a cell. The precise intracellular sites of Ang II synthesis and actions are not known. Current evidence suggests that synthesis of Ang II occurs either in secretory vesicles or other cytoplasmic locations, depending on the cell type and nature of the stimulus. Intracellular Ang II likely acts through AT_1-like receptors on the nuclear envelope, direct chromatin binding, or through unidentified intracellular receptors. Ang II can also likely freely enter the nucleus, owing to the small size (8 amino acids). The effects of intracellular Ang II include cell growth, gene expression, extracellular matrix production, and cardiac hypertrophy.

in an intracellular system.[53] Studies have shown that participation of alternative mechanisms for Ang II synthesis may depend on the stimulus and cell type.[67] Several cells, such as cardiac myocytes, fibroblasts, renal mesangial, and vascular smooth muscle cells (VSMC), have been shown to synthesize intracellular Ang II under hyperglycemic conditions.[53,66,67] Diabetic patients have also been reported to have higher cardiac levels of intracellular Ang II, which are further increased in association with hypertension.[68] In addition to Ang II synthesis, functional intracellular Ang II binding sites have been demonstrated on renal and hepatocyte nuclei and on chromatin.[69-72] Though nuclear Ang II binding sites are AT_1R-like, the nature of chromatin binding is not known. Coupling of chromatin and nuclear membrane Ang II receptors to increased RNA synthesis and gene transcription of Ao, renin, and platelet-derived growth factor (PDGF) has been demonstrated.[73]

Intracellular actions of Ang II have been termed "intracrine" actions.[74] Intracellular production of Ang II in cultured cardiac myocytes and in the mouse heart using a specific promoter resulted in hypertrophic cell growth and biventricular hypertrophy, respectively.[75] The in vivo model was accompanied by an increase in gene expression, but without any change in blood pressure. Microinjection of Ang II into rat VSMC has been shown to increase cytosolic and nuclear Ca^{2+} ($[Ca^{2+}]_i$), which was secondary to an influx of extracellular Ca^{2+}.[76] In addition, intracellular Ang II participates in diabetes-induced oxidative stress and cardiac fibrosis in rat hearts. Studies on cultured neonatal rat cardiac myocytes have shown that intracellular Ang II upregulates Ao, renin, and AT_1R receptor through a positive feedback mechanism.[66] Several of the intracrine effects of Ang II are not blocked by angiotensin receptor blockers (ARBs) due either to limited cell penetration of these drugs or to possible AT_1R-independent mechanisms.[75,77]

The pathophysiological significance of the intracellular cardiac RAS remains to be determined in the general clinical population.[78] Diabetes is a major stimulus for the activation of the intracellular RAS. Since cardiac myocyte Ang II synthesis in diabetes is chymase dependent and intracellular Ang II effects are not blocked by ARBs, therapeutic modalities, other than ARBs and ACE inhibitors, that would block intracellular synthesis or intracrine effects of Ang II, might provide a better outcome in diabetic patients, by reducing end organ damage.

NOVEL ASPECTS OF THE RAS

Ang II has traditionally been considered the biologically active end product of the RAS. Recent evidence indicates that additional shorter chain angiotensins also serve as effector peptides in this system (Figure 9-4). These shorter chain peptides include Ang (1-7), a heptapeptide that lacks the C-terminal phenylalanine of Ang II; Ang III, a heptapeptide lacking the N-terminal aspartate residue; and Ang IV, a hexapeptide, lacking the two N-terminal amino acids. Modulation of the peptide levels and the enzymes that generate these peptides has been associated with cardiovascular regulation, as discussed in the following section. In addition to these peptides, new functions of (pro)renin have been described that will likely have a significant impact on our therapeutic approaches to cardiovascular diseases.

Ang (1-7) and ACE2

Ang (1-7) is formed either by the action of neutral endopeptidase on Ang I or by the recently discovered monocarboxypeptidase, angiotensin-converting enzyme 2 (ACE2), on Ang II. Ang (1-7) elicits cardiovascular responses, such as antihypertensive, antihypertrophic, antifibrotic, and antithrombotic, that are generally opposite to those mediated by Ang II. The effects of Ang (1-7) may be mediated through direct signaling as a result of binding to the G protein–coupled Mas receptor, a product of the Mas oncogene, or by the modulation of AT_1-receptor signaling, as a result of heterodimerization of Mas and AT_1 receptors.[79,80] ACE2 affects Ang II levels by converting Ang I into Ang (1-9) and Ang II into Ang (1-7), though the latter is the preferred pathway. Local generation of Ang (1-7) in the myocardium of dogs and elevation of Ang (1-7) in cardiac myocytes during development of heart failure subsequent to coronary artery ligation have been reported.[81,82] In addition, intravenous infusion of Ang (1-7) attenuates the development of heart failure after myocardial infarction, suggesting a role for this peptide in cardiac remodeling.[83] ACE2 gene expression is significantly increased in the failing human heart.[84] ACE2-knockout mice have left ventricular dysfunction and wall thinning, along with increased Ang II levels. The ACE and ACE2 double-knockout completely prevents cardiac abnormalities and the increase in Ang II production.[85] Lentiviral-mediated ACE2 overexpression has amelioratory effects on blood pressure

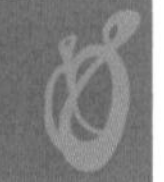

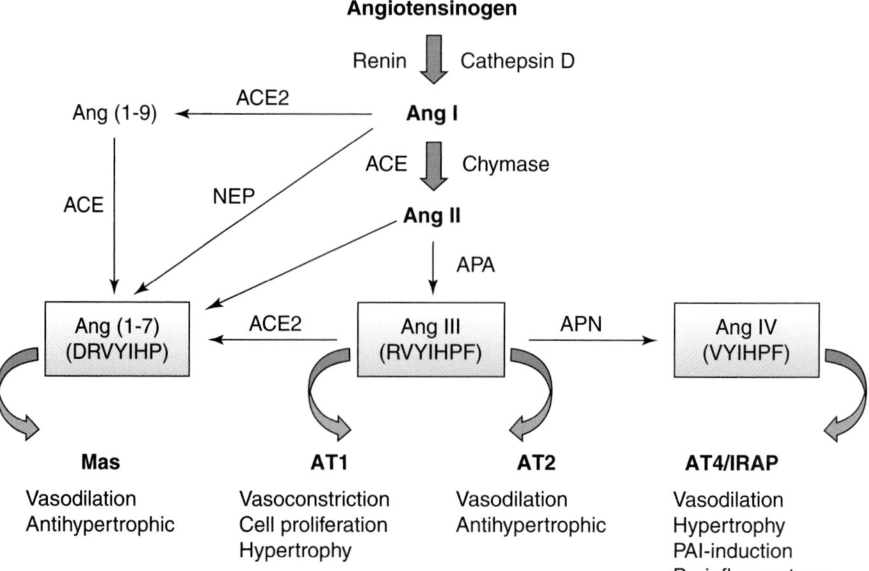

FIGURE 9-4 Novel components of the renin-angiotensin system. The major reactions of Ao to Ang II conversion may also be catalyzed by alternative enzymes, such as cathepsin D and chymase. In addition, Ang I may be converted to Ang (1-9) by an isoform of ACE, known as ACE2. Ang (1-9) can be converted to Ang (1-7) by ACE. Alternatively, Ang (1-7) can be formed by a direct action of NEP on Ang I. Ang (1-7) is a biologically active peptide that binds to a specific receptor, which is a product of the Mas oncogene. The effects of Ang (1-7) are beneficial to the cardiovascular system. Ang II can also be further cleaved by APA to produce Ang III, which binds to the same receptors as Ang II and produces similar effects. Some of the renal and brain effects, which were initially thought to be produced by Ang II, require conversion of Ang II to Ang III. Ang III can be further cleaved by APN to form Ang IV, which binds to a specific receptor that has been identified as insulin-regulated aminopeptidase (IRAP).

and cardiac fibrosis in spontaneously hypertensive rats. Similarly, there is a protective effect on the heart through preservation of cardiac function, left ventricular wall motion and contractility, in a myocardial infarction model.[86] However, transgenic mice with increased cardiac ACE2 expression show a high incidence of sudden death due to ventricular tachycardia and fibrillation as a result of gap junction remodeling.[87] ACE2 can effectively alter the balance between vasoconstrictive and the cell proliferating effects of Ang II and the vasodilatory and antiproliferating effects of Ang (1-7).[88] The age-dependent cardiomyopathy in ACE2 null mice was related to increased Ang II–mediated oxidative stress and neutrophilic infiltration in the absence of ACE2.[89] Structure-based screening of therapeutic compounds in development identified candidates that enhanced ACE2 activity in vitro and reduced blood pressure in spontaneously hypertensive rats.[90] In addition, improvement in cardiac function and reversal of myocardial, perivascular, and renal fibrosis was observed with these compounds.

Ang III

Ang III, also called Ang-(2-8), is generated from Ang II by aminopeptidase A (APA), which cleaves the Asp[1]-Arg[2] bond in Ang II. The major physiological role of Ang III is in the brain, where it has been shown to be more important than Ang II, in the central regulation of hypertension and vasopressin release.[91] Ang III has affinity for AT_1R and AT_2R receptors that is comparable to that of Ang II.[91] APA is also highly expressed in the kidneys. It was recently shown that renal conversion of Ang II to Ang III is critical for AT_2R-mediated natriuresis and may have a significant role in disorders characterized by Na^+ and fluid retention, such as hypertension and congestive heart failure.[92] Ang III, APA, and aminopeptidase N (APN) could provide a putative central therapeutic target for the treatment of hypertension.[93]

Ang IV

Ang III is metabolized to angiotensin IV (Ang IV) by APN. Ang IV mediates physiological functions in the central nervous system, including blood flow regulation, learning, and memory.[94] Ang IV binds to a type II integral membrane protein, termed AT_4, which was recently identified as insulin-regulated aminopeptidase (IRAP).[95] AT_4/IRAP is expressed in multiple tissues, including brain, kidneys, blood vessels, and heart. Actions of Ang IV, mediated through the AT_4 receptor, may be related to the activation of several intracellular signaling pathways or by inhibition of the enzymatic activity of IRAP, the physiological substrates of which include vasopressin.[96] Several studies have suggested a role for Ang IV in cardiovascular diseases in that Ang IV enhances cell growth in cardiac fibroblasts, endothelium, and VSMC.[94] In VSMC, Ang IV activates the proinflammatory transcription factor NF κB, which regulates expression of several genes involved in atherogenesis and thrombosis.[97]

Pro(renin) Receptor

Pro(renin), the inactive precursor of renin, has reported levels in blood that are up to tenfold higher than renin, particularly in diabetes.[24,98] Interestingly, no extrarenal activation site of prorenin is known, which had led to the speculation that prorenin does not have any significant physiological role. However, recent identification of a specific (pro)renin receptor has changed our understanding about the roles of (pro)renin in pathophysiological processes.[23] The (pro)renin receptor is a 350–amino acid protein, with a single transmembrane domain that is expressed in multiple tissues, including the heart. The (pro)renin receptor specifically binds both renin and prorenin. Following binding to the receptor, a conformational change makes prorenin catalytically active, which can produce Ang II locally and therefore available to bind to Ang II receptors.[99] Thus circulating prorenin might contribute significantly to tissue Ang II production.[23] The catalytic efficiency of renin for Ang II generation is also enhanced when bound to this receptor. In addition to providing an enhanced capability of local Ang II generation, the (pro)renin receptor mediates intracellular signaling events, which likely contribute to the pathological effects of RAS activation.[100] When bound to the (pro)renin receptor, renin and prorenin activate extracellular signal-related MAPKs (ERK1/2), induce DNA synthesis, and stimulate release of TGF-β and plasminogen activator inhibitor-type 1 (PAI-1) in mesangial cells, which may contribute to renal fibrotic disease, particularly when therapeutic Ang II blockade elevates levels of plasma renin.[23,101,102] It has been shown that prorenin stimulates ERK phosphorylation in VSMC, through receptor-mediated activation of tyrosine kinase and subsequently MEK, independent of the generation of Ang II or the activation of AT_1R.[103] It has also been

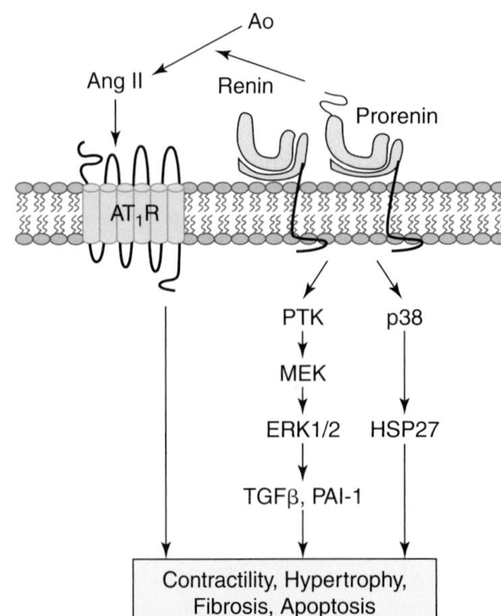

FIGURE 9–5 Intracellular effects of (Pro)renin receptors. Binding of renin and/or prorenin to the renin/prorenin receptor leads to activation of the enzymatic action of prorenin and enhancement of catalytic activity, resulting in elevated concentrations of Ang II in proximity to the cell surface. Renin and prorenin also independently activate intracellular signaling pathways. Pro(renin) receptor-mediated activation of the MEK/ERK1/2 cascade through tyrosine kinases leads to generation of transforming growth factor β (TGF-β) and plasminogen activator inhibitor-type 1 (PAI-1), resulting in hypertrophic growth and fibrosis. Pro(renin) receptor-induced activation of p38 MAPK leads to activation of heat shock protein 27 (Hsp27), which is associated with abnormal actin filament dynamics. Activation of these latter pathways is independent of Ang II.

reported that prorenin exerts angiotensin-independent effects in cardiomyocytes.[100] Prorenin also induced stimulation of the p38 MAPK/HSP27 pathway, resulting in alterations in actin filament dynamics that may underlie the severe cardiac hypertrophy described in rats with hepatic prorenin overexpression.[104] Interestingly, these effects occurred without production of Ang II or stimulation of AT_1. A direct functional role of the renin/prorenin receptor might contribute to disease processes such as hypertension, heart failure, and diabetes mellitus–induced cardiovascular complications.[105] In conclusion, the pro(renin) receptor may serve as a new treatment target (receptor blockers), which prevents both Ang II generation at tissue sites and prorenin-induced, Ang II–independent effects (Figure 9-5).

ANGIOTENSIN II–MEDIATED SIGNALING PATHWAYS IN HEART FAILURE (see Chapter 45)

Angiotensin II Receptors

Ang II, the major bioactive peptide of the renin-angiotensin system, has a critical role in controlling cardiovascular homeostasis. It is important in various cardiovascular diseases, such as hypertension, atherosclerosis, restenosis after angioplasty, and congestive heart failure.[106-108] The multiple actions of Ang II are mediated via specific, highly complex, intracellular signaling pathways that are stimulated following initial binding of the peptide to specific receptors. In mammalian cells, Ang II mediates effects via (at least) two high-affinity plasma membrane receptors: AT_1 and AT_2. Both receptor subtypes have been cloned and pharmacologically characterized.[109,110] The two receptors, which belong to the superfamily of G protein–coupled receptors (GPCR), have different signaling pathways and functions.[111,112] The AT_1 receptor (AT_1R) subtype is expressed ubiquitously and is involved in most of the well-known biological actions of Ang II. The AT_1R was first cloned in 1991[109,113] and consists of 359 amino acids with a molecular mass of 41 kDa. Two AT_1R subtypes have been described in rodents, AT_{1a} and AT_{1b}, with greater than 94% amino acid sequence identity[114] and which have similar pharmacological properties and tissue distribution. The human AT_1 gene has been mapped to chromosome 3.[115] The AT_1R is a glycoprotein containing extracellular glycosylation sites at the amino terminus (Asn^4) and the second extracellular loop (Asp^{176} and Asn^{188}). The transmembrane domain at the amino-terminal extension and segments in the first and third extracellular loops are responsible for G protein interactions with the receptor.[116] AT_1R interacts with various heterotrimeric G proteins, including Gq/11, Gi/o, Gα12, and Gα13, which couple to distinct signaling cascades. The AT_1R transactivates growth pathways and mediates the major effects of Ang II, such as vasoconstriction, aldosterone secretion, increased cardiac contractility, renal tubular sodium reabsorption, cell proliferation, vascular and cardiac hypertrophy, inflammatory responses, and oxidative stress.[117] Like most GPCR, AT_1R is also subject to internalization when stimulated by Ang II, a process dependent on specific residues located on the cytoplasmic tail.[118] Internalization of GPCR involves receptor phosphorylation, which may be mediated in part via caveola.[119] Studies have shown that a serine/threonine-rich segment of the carboxy terminus is essential for phosphorylation and internalization of the receptor[120] and that G protein receptor kinase (GRK)-mediated serine phosphorylation of AT_1R has an important role in desensitization of the agonist-occupied receptor.[121]

In contrast to AT_1R, the physiological role of AT_2R has been less well characterized. AT_2R is distinct from AT_1R in genomic organization, tissue-specific expression, and in signaling mechanisms. The AT_2R is characterized by a high affinity for the nonpeptide receptor antagonists PD123319, PD123177, and CGP42112, and a very low affinity for losartan and candesartan (selective AT_1R antagonists).[117] Ang II binds to the AT_2R with similar affinity as to the AT_1R.[122] AT_2R has been cloned in a variety of species, including humans, rats, and mice. [110,123,124] The AT_2R is a seven-transmembrane domain receptor, encoded by a 363–amino acid protein with a molecular mass of 41 kDa, but it shares only 34% sequence identity with the AT_1R.[124] Interestingly, the gene coding for AT_2R is located on chromosome X. Stimulation of AT_2R by Ang II, in contrast to AT_1R, is not followed by interaction of the activated receptor with β-arrestins and subsequent internalization,[125] suggesting that classical, β-arrestin-mediated mechanisms do not participate in the homologous desensitization of the AT_2R, and that its regulation is different from the AT_1R and most other GPCR. AT_2R is highly expressed in fetal tissues, with expression dramatically decreasing after birth, and being restricted to only a few organs, including the cardiovascular system. The AT_2R are reexpressed in the adult animal following cardiac and vascular injury and during wound healing, suggesting a role for this receptor in tissue remodeling, growth, and/or development. The AT_2R often induces opposite responses to the AT_1R, including vasodilation, antigrowth, antihypertrophic, and cardioprotective effects.[126-128] AT_2 exerts antiproliferative and apoptotic effects in VSMC and decreases neointimal formation in response to injury by counteracting Ang II actions mediated by the AT_1R.[129] In the heart, AT_2 expression is upregulated in pathological states, inhibiting growth and remodeling, and inducing vasodilation.[130] After myocardial infarction (MI), AT_2R overexpression assists in preservation of left ventricular (LV) function, indicating a beneficial role for AT_2 in postmyocardial infarction remodeling.[127,131] Overexpression of AT_2R in the left ventricle of pressure-overloaded rats reduces myocardial fibrosis and myocyte diameter, indicating that AT_2R overexpression in cardiac myocytes alters the pathological response to aortic banding-induced ventricular hypertrophy.[132] Using AT_2R knockout mice, it has been demonstrated that AT_2R mediates antiproliferative and antifibrotic effects in DOCA-salt or L-NAME–induced hypertensive rats[133] and has a significant role in the protection against early development of LV dilation and in decreasing the early mortality after MI. The cardioprotective effects of AT_1R antagonists in post-MI remodeling are likely related in part to Ang II–mediated responses via the AT_2R.[127,128]

Two other Ang II receptors have been described: AT_3 and AT_4. The AT_3R is peptide-specific, recognizing mainly Ang II. This subtype does not bind nonpeptide ligands, such as losartan or PD123319 (selective AT_2R antagonist), and has only been observed in cell lines. The AT_4R, which is distributed in heart, lung, kidney, brain, and liver, binds to Ang IV,[134] but not losartan or PD123319. AT_4R was identified in 1992 as a specific high-affinity binding site for the hexapeptide Ang IV (VYIHPF),[135] an insulin-regulated aminopeptidase.[95,136] AT_4 and AT_1/AT_2 receptors are distinct entities with different ligand specificities and differential tissue distributions.[134] Ang IV induces vasorelaxation in various vascular beds, enhances endothelial intracellular calcium release, and increases endothelial nitric oxide synthase (eNOS) activity.[137-140] Ang IV also stimulates phosphatidylinositol-3 kinase (PI3K) and phosphatidylinositol-dependent kinase 1 (PDK1) activity and induces phosphorylation of protein kinase B and ERK1/2.[141] These multiple kinase pathways are thought to regulate the cellular proliferative effects of the peptide. Ang IV induced plasminogen activator inhibitor 1 expression in endothelial cells, suggesting a role for Ang IV in fibrinolysis.[142] Ang IV also activates the NF κB pathway and increases proinflammatory genes in VSMC.[97] The AT_4R has also been characterized in the heart, where Ang IV stimulates protein synthesis in cardiac fibroblasts[143] and reduces left ventricular pressure generation and ejection fraction and the expression of the immediate early genes *c-fos* and *egr-1* in the isolated heart.[144,145] These data suggest that this Ang II degradation peptide could participate in the pathogenesis of cardiovascular diseases. However, the overall importance of AT_4R-mediated signaling in cardiovascular diseases needs to be further clarified. In this chapter, our primary focus will be on the signaling pathways mediated by AT_1 and AT_2.

AT_1-Mediated Intracellular Signaling

Classical G Protein–dependent Signaling Pathways. Like other seven membrane spanning domain receptor family members, agonist binding to the AT_1R initiates a multitude of intracellular events. AT_1R couples to the Gq/11 protein, which stimulates phospholipase C (PLC) to generate the second messengers diacylglycerol (DAG) and inositol triphosphate (IP3). DAG activates protein kinase C (PKC) and IP3 binds to its receptor on the sarcoplasmic reticulum, opening a channel that allows calcium efflux into the cytoplasm. Ang II–induced phospholipase D (PLD) activation results in hydrolysis of phosphatidylcholine to choline and phosphatidic acid (PA). PA is rapidly converted to DAG, leading to sustained activation of PKC. Both PKC- and calcium-mediated signaling are involved in vasoconstriction and cardiac hypertrophy.[146-149] Ang II has been shown to phosphorylate and activate phospholipase A_2 (PLA_2), which leads to production of arachidonic acid (AA), the precursor molecule for the generation of prostaglandins, and which is involved in the Ang II–induced growth of VSMC and cardiac hypertrophy.[150] AT_1R also couples to $G_{i/o}$, inhibiting adenylyl cyclase in several target tissues, thereby attenuating the production of the second messenger cAMP.[151] When production of this latter vasodilator is decreased due to AT_1 activation, there is resulting vasoconstriction. AT_1 is also involved in the opening of Ca^{2+} channels and an influx of extracellular Ca^{2+} into cells.[152,153] The activation of L-type Ca^{2+} channels is mediated by AT_1R coupled to $G_{12/13}$ proteins (Figure 9-6).[154]

AT_1-mediated Tyrosine Phosphorylation. Ang II induces actions through activation of tyrosine kinases, which in turn phosphorylate many downstream targets, which are associated with cellular growth and apoptosis, differentiation, transformation, and vascular contraction. Tyrosine kinases activated by Ang II/AT_1R include many receptor tyrosine kinases (RTK), such as epidermal growth factor receptor (EGFR), platelet-derived growth factor receptor (PDGFR), and insulin-like growth factor receptor (IGFR), and nonreceptor tyrosine kinases such as the Src family kinases, Janus kinases (JAKs), focal adhesion kinase (FAK), Ca^{2+}-dependent tyrosine kinases (e.g., Pyk2), p130Cas, and PI3K (Figure 9-7).[150,155-157] Ang II stimulation of cellular growth has been described in cardiac myocytes and VSMC. These effects are associated with increased tyrosine phosphorylation and activation of MAPKs and related pathways, which result in increased expression of early response genes, such as c-*fos*, c-*jun*, and c-*myc*, thereby controlling cellular proliferation and growth.[155] These actions have been linked to cardiovascular diseases, including hypertension, cardiac hypertrophy, heart failure, and atherosclerosis. The role of tyrosine kinases in Ang II–mediated signaling has been extensively reviewed in Touyz et al[150,156,158] and only recent developments will be discussed here.

Receptor Tyrosine Kinases. In recent years, it has become apparent that transactivation of RTKs by GPCR agonists is a general phenomenon that has been demonstrated for many unrelated GPCRs and RTKs.[159,160] The mitogenic effects of Ang II can be mediated through transactivation of RTKs. AT_1R-mediated transactivation has been demonstrated for EGFR, PDGFR, and IGFR.[161] The EGFR is endogenously expressed in numerous cell types and is an important receptor in the control of many fundamental cellular processes.[162] Transactivation is mediated by several intermediary signaling molecules, including Ca^{2+}, PKC, Pyk2, Src, reactive oxygen species (ROS), and metalloproteinases that generate EGF-like ligands.[161,163-165] Blocking EGFR kinase activity abolishes Ang II–mediated downstream signaling, such as activation of ERK1/2 in VSMC and cardiac myocytes,[161,166] suggesting that transactivation of EGFR accounts for the majority of growth-promoting responses induced by Ang II. Studies have demonstrated that EGFR activation is involved in Ang II–induced vascular contraction, cell growth, cardiac hypertrophy, and hypertension.[167] It has recently been shown that Ang II–induced transactivation of the IGF-1 receptor is a critical mediator of PI3K activation by Ang II.[168,169] In contrast to EGFR transactivation, Ang II–induced PDGFR transactivation may be ligand independent, requiring an ROS-sensitive kinase distinct from Src or JAK2.[170] Ang II–induced transactivation of the PDGFR has also been shown to contribute to cardiac hypertrophy and vascular remodeling.[171-173]

Nonreceptor Tyrosine Kinases

Src Family Kinases. Studies have demonstrated that Src family kinases, such as *c-Src*, have an important role in regulation of growth responses induced by Ang II.[174,175] The Src kinase family consists of at least 14 members, of which the 60-kDa *c-Src* is a prototype of the cellular members of the Src family kinases (Src, Fyn, Yes, Fgr, Lck, Lyn, Hck, Blk, and Yrk). All Src family members share common functional domains, including an N-terminal myristoylation sequence for membrane targeting, SH2 and SH3 domains for protein binding, and a kinase domain and C-terminal noncatalytic domain.[176] *c-Src* is abundantly expressed in VSMC and cardiomyocytes

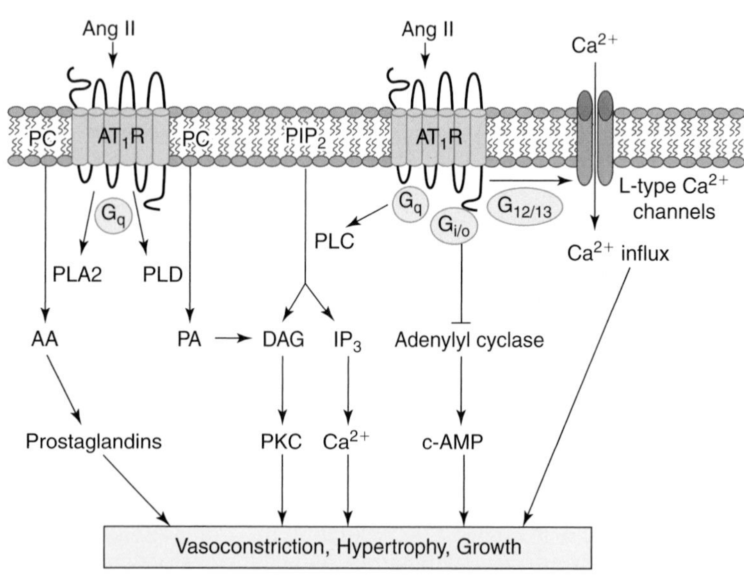

FIGURE 9–6 Classical signal transduction pathways mediated by AT_1R. Binding of Ang II to AT_1 leads to G protein–coupled activation of PLC (phospholipase C) via Gq, resulting in phosphatidylinositol hydrolysis and formation of IP_3 (inositol triphosphate) and DAG (diacylglycerol) accumulation. IP_3 mobilizes Ca^{2+} from sarcoplasmic reticular stores and DAG activates PKC (protein kinase C). Both PKC- and calcium-mediated signaling are involved in vasoconstriction and cardiac hypertrophy. AT_1R couple to $G_{i/o}$, resulting in inhibition of adenylyl cyclase and attenuation of cAMP production, leading to vasoconstriction. Activation of phospholipase A_2 (PLA_2) leads to production of arachidonic acid (AA) and the generation of prostaglandins. AT_1R coupling to $G_{12/13}$ results in the opening of L-type Ca^{2+} channels and increases the influx of extracellular Ca^{2+}.

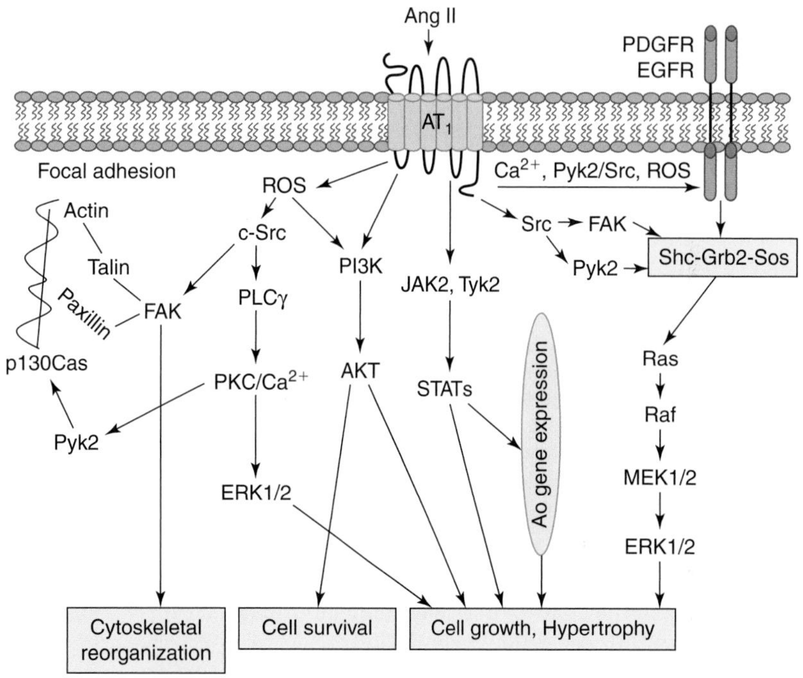

FIGURE 9–7 Ang II induces activation of tyrosine kinases through AT_1R. Ang II influences the activity of receptor tyrosine kinases, such as EGFR (epidermal growth factor receptor) and PDGFR (platelet-derived growth factor receptor). The transactivation event is mediated by several intermediary signaling molecules, including Ca^{2+}, PKC, Pyk2, Src, and reactive oxygen species (ROS). The transactivated EGFR serves as a scaffold for downstream adapters, leading to activation of MAPKs. Ang II also phosphorylates multiple nonreceptor tyrosine kinases, such as JAK-STAT, FAK, Pyk2, p130Cas, and PI3K. Activated tyrosine kinases phosphorylate many downstream targets, which regulate Ang II-induced cellular effects.

and rapidly activated by Ang II.[177] It has been shown that *c-Src* is activated by Gβγ in an ROS-dependent manner and is involved in activation of a variety of downstream pathways. Src-induced activation of PLCγ, which is a substrate for members of the Src kinase family, promotes release of Ca^{2+} from intracellular stores. Src is also required for Ang II–induced activation of ERK1/2, Pyk2, and several downstream proteins including FAK, paxillin, JAK2, STAT1, caveolin, and the adapter protein Shc,[178] indicating that activation of Src has a pivotal role in Ang II–mediated cytoskeletal reorganization, focal adhesion formation, cell migration, and growth. Increased activation of Src by Ang II may be an important mediator of cardiac hypertrophy and vascular remodeling.

FAK and PYK2 Activation. FAK and PYK2, also referred to as cell adhesion kinase, related adhesion focal tyrosine kinase, or calcium-dependent protein tyrosine kinase,[179] are localized prominently within focal adhesions, and have a signaling role in regulating cell behavior resulting from integrin interaction with the extracellular matrix. Previous studies have demonstrated that activation of FAK and PYK2 have been implicated in the progression of cardiomyocyte hypertrophy and have an important role in Ang II–mediated cellular effects.[180-183] As a consequence of association with *c-Src,* FAK undergoes further tyrosine phosphorylation, resulting in FAK binding to Grb2, Sos, and Ras, leading to ERK1/2 activation.[179] Ang II rapidly induces tyrosine phosphorylation of FAK, allowing for cell adhesion to the extracellular matrix and activation of cytoskeletal proteins, including p130Cas, Pyk2, paxillin, and talin, all of which interact to regulate cell shape and movement.[158] It has also been shown that the interaction between p130Cas, Pyk2, and PI3K activates ribosomal $p70^{S6}$ kinase, which has an important role in Ang II–mediated protein synthesis. Pyk2, a FAK homologue, is activated by AT_1 and is dependent on increased intracellular Ca^{2+} and PKC.[184,185] Since Pyk2 is a candidate to regulate *c-Src* and links G protein–coupled vasoconstrictor receptors with protein tyrosine kinase–mediated contractile, migratory, and growth responses, it may represent a point of convergence

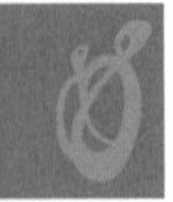

between Ca^{2+}-dependent signaling pathways and protein tyrosine kinase pathways in cardiovascular cells.

p130Cas. p130Cas was initially characterized as a phosphotyrosine-containing protein in v-Crk- and v-Src-transformed cells,[186] serving as an adapter molecule, the proline-rich sequences and SH3 domain of which allow for an interaction with Pyk2 in the presence of Ang II and provides binding motifs for the SH2 domains of Crk and Src.[187] p130Cas is important for integrin-mediated cell adhesion through recruitment of cytoskeletal signaling molecules, such as FAK, paxillin, and tensin to focal adhesions.[188] The phosphorylation of p130Cas is dependent on Ca^{2+}, *c-Src,* and PKC and requires an intact cytoskeletal network. Other studies have reported that Ang II–induced activation of p130Cas is Ca^{2+} and PKC independent.[189] Ang II–induced tyrosine phosphorylation of Src and p130Cas has been shown to be essential in Ang II–stimulated migration of VSMC through activation of ERK1/2 and JNK.[190] Though the exact functional significance of Ang II–induced activation of p130Cas is unclear, it may contribute to the regulation of α-actin expression, cellular proliferation, migration, and cell adhesion.

JAK/STAT Activation. The Janus kinase (JAK)-signal transducer and activator of transcription (STAT) pathway is involved in a wide range of distinct cellular processes, including inflammation, apoptosis, cell-cycle regulation, and development.[191,192] There are four JAK proteins in mammalian cells: JAK1, JAK2, JAK3, and TYK2.[193] JAK proteins, named after the Roman two-faced mythical god Janus, function as cytosolic tyrosine kinases and induce a cascade of phosphorylation steps that result in the activation of STAT proteins. Tyrosine phosphorylation of STATs leads to STAT homodimerization and heterodimerization. STAT dimers are rapidly transported from the cytoplasm to the nucleus, where they activate gene transcription. AT_1 activates JAK2 and Tyk2 in the cardiovascular system.[194] In VSMC, JAKs apparently phosphorylate the STAT proteins p91/84 (STAT1a/β), p113 (STAT2), and p92 (STAT3) in response to Ang II, suggesting a role for this pathway in the activation of early growth response genes by Ang II. The JAK-STAT signaling pathway activates early growth response genes, which may be a mechanism for Ang II–mediated vascular and cardiac growth, remodeling, and repair.[195,196] It has been demonstrated that STATs have an important role in angiotensinogen gene expression in the heart. Ischemia-reperfusion or myocardial infarction–induced activation of STAT5A and STAT6 promotes the binding of STATs to the St-domain of angiotensinogen, resulting in increases in the gene expression of angiotensinogen.[197,198] Blockade of AT_1R signaling or inhibition of JAK2 activation suppresses formation of the STATs/ST-domain complex and reduces the gene expression of angiotensinogen. These studies support a role for an Ang II autocrine loop in JAK-STAT signaling and cardiac injury. Ang II–induced activation of JAK2 is also an important step in the development of diabetic vascular complications.[199]

Phosphoinositide 3-OH Kinase. PI3Ks are a family of lipid and protein kinases responsible for the phosphorylation of PtdIns at position D3 of the inositol ring. These molecules act as secondary messengers and influence a variety of cellular responses, including proliferation, survival, cytoskeletal remodeling, and have recently also been identified as having an important role in the regulation of cardiomyocyte and VSMC growth.[200-202] PI3Ks are classified by substrate specificity and subunit organization.[203] Class I enzymes produce PtdIns(3,4,5)P_3 in vivo. Class IA PI3Ks are heterodimeric proteins, each of which consists of a catalytic subunit of 110 to 120 kDa (p110α, β, and δ) and an associated regulatory subunit (p85α and β) that are essential for interaction of these PI3Ks with receptor tyrosine kinases. The class IB PI3K (PI3Kγ) is activated by heterotrimeric G protein subunits and associates with a p101 adaptor required for full responsiveness to Gβγ heterodimers. Class II PI3Ks do not produce PtdIns(3,4,5)P_3, but appear to produce both PtdIns(3,4)P_2 and PtdIns3P in vivo. Class II PI3Ks are distinguished by a carboxy-terminal C2 domain, which is not found in other PI3Ks. Class III PI3K, Vps34, only produces PtdIns3P.[204] PI3Kα, which is activated by RTK, appears to have a critical role in the induction of physiological cardiac growth, but not pathological growth, and appears essential for maintaining contractile function in response to pathological stimuli.[205] PI3Kγ appears to negatively control cardiac contractility through different signaling mechanisms and as a key mediator of NADPH oxidase activation in response to Ang II.[89,206,207] Ang II–induced ERK1/2 phosphorylation is augmented by PI3K, in SHR VSMC, indicating a role of PI3K in Ang II–induced vascular remodeling.[208] Akt/PKB has been identified as an important downstream target of PI3K, in Ang II–activated cardiomyocytes, and VSMC.[209] It regulates protein synthesis by activating p70 S6-kinase and modulates Ang II–mediated Ca^{2+} responses by stimulating Ca^{2+} channel currents. Akt/PKB has also been implicated in promoting cell survival by influencing Bcl-2 and *c-myc* expression and inhibiting caspases. Though the exact role of PI3K in Ang II signaling has not been established, it is possible that this complex pathway may control the balance between mitogenesis and apoptosis.

Mitogen-activated Protein Kinases. Mitogen-activated protein kinase (MAPK) consists of a series of successively acting kinases that function as central regulators of cell growth, differentiation, and transformation. All of the MAPK members are catalytically inactive in resting cells and are activated in response to the appropriate stimulus, by phosphorylation on both threonine and tyrosine residues that appear in a threonine-X-tyrosine motif, close to the active site. This phosphorylation is regulated through a dual specificity MAPKK (MAP kinase kinase), which in turn is activated through phosphorylation by a MAPKKK (MAP kinase kinase kinase).[210] Once activated, these terminal effector kinases directly phosphorylate a diverse array of cytoplasmic, nuclear, and mitochondrial proteins to modulate gene expression, cellular metabolism, cellular physiology, and cell death.[211] At least four distinctly regulated groups of MAPKs are expressed in mammals, extracellular signal-related kinases (ERK)-1/2, *c-Jun* N-terminal kinases (JNK1/2/3), p38 proteins (p38α/β/γ/δ), and ERK5, all of which are activated by specific MKKs: MEK1/2 for ERK1/2, MKK3/6 for p38, MKK4/7 for the JNKs, and MEK5 for ERK5 (Figure 9-8). Each MKK can be activated by more than one MEKK, increasing the complexity and diversity of MAPK signaling.[212] Ang II induces phosphorylation of Ras, Raf, and Shc, leading to the activation of MEKKs and MEKs, resulting in tyrosine and threonine phosphorylation of ERK1/2, JNK2, and p38.[213] Ang II–induced activation of ERK1/2 is associated with increased expression of the early response genes *c-fos, c-myc,* and *c-jun;* DNA/protein synthesis; cell growth and differentiation; and cytoskeletal organization in cardiovascular cells.[214] Recent data have demonstrated that the ERK1/2 signaling pathway has an important role in mediating the effects of the brain RAS on sympathetic nerve activity in heart failure, suggesting that manipulating brain ERK1/2 signaling could ameliorate the adverse effects of the brain RAS on cardiovascular and renal function during the progression of heart failure.[215] In addition to ERKs, Ang II activates JNKs, which regulate cardiomyocyte and VSMC growth.[216,217] Ang II induces activation of JNK via p21-activated kinase (PAK), which is dependent on intracellular Ca^{2+} mobilization and PKC activation.[218] In the heart, activation of p38 MAPK has been observed in pressure-overload or MI-induced cardiac hypertrophy and heart failure in both human and animal models.[219-221] Cardiac-specific activation of p38 MAPK markedly attenuated cardiac contractility.[222] In addition, inhibition of p38 MAPK protected the heart against ischemic injury, attenuated cardiac remodeling, and improved cardiac

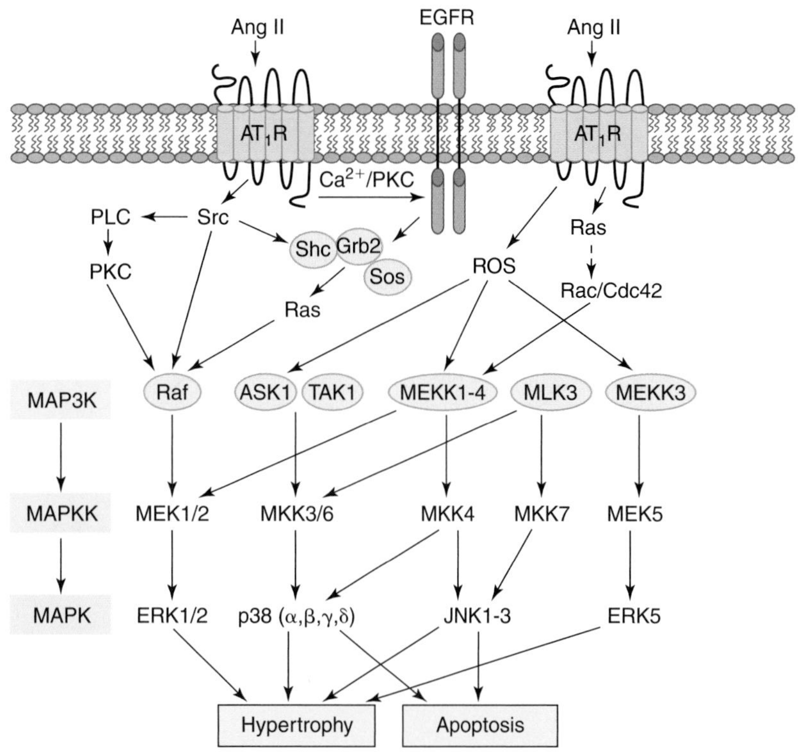

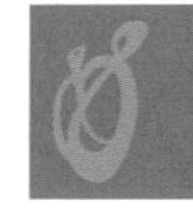

FIGURE 9–8 Schematic diagram of the major MAPK cascades stimulated by AT_1R. The MAKP pathway is a three-module cascade of phosphorylating kinases: MEKK(MAP3K)(MEK)(MAPKK)(MAPK). This pathway consists of several subfamilies among which are the ERK, JNK, and p38 MAPK pathways. Each is activated by heterotrimeric G proteins coupled to AT_1R; by Ang II–induced transactivation of EGFR; by small G proteins (such as Ras, cdc42, Rac); by protein kinases (such as Src); by PKC, via activation of PLC; and by ROS.

function in mice with heart failure after myocardial infarction.[223] Studies have also demonstrated that p38 activation is preferentially associated with the direct effects of Ang II on cardiac cells, whereas stimulation of ERK and JNK occurs in association with Ang II–induced mechanical stress.[224] These results suggest that MAPKs may provide a novel therapeutic approach to the Ang II–dependent pathophysiology that accompanies progression of heart failure.

Small GTP-binding Proteins. The small GTP-binding protein (small G protein) superfamily comprises a multitude of monomeric proteins (more than 150 members in humans), with relative molecular masses of λ 21 kDa, that regulate a wide variety of cellular processes, such as cell division, migration, and differentiation. They are structurally classified into at least five families, including the following: Ras (e.g., Ras, Rap, and Ral); Rho (RhoA, Rac1, and cdc42); Rab; Sar1/Arf; and Ran.[225] Small G proteins cycle between a GDP-bound inactive form and a GTP-bound active form, a process regulated by guanine nucleotide exchange factors (GEFs), which catalyze the exchange of GDP for GTP; GTPase activating proteins, which stimulate hydrolysis of GTP to GDP; and guanine nucleotide dissociation inhibitors (GDIs), which inhibit the dissociation of GDP and maintain small G proteins in inactive states (Figure 9-9).[226] Activated Ras proteins interact with multiple downstream effectors (Raf/MEK1/2/ERK1/2 and PI3K)[225] to regulate gene expression, cell proliferation, differentiation, and survival; the Rho GTPases (RhoA/Rac1/cdc42) regulate cytoskeletal reorganization and gene expression; the Rab and Sar1/Arf families regulate vesicle trafficking; and the Ran family regulates nucleocytoplasmic transport and microtubule organization.[227] It has been shown that small G proteins (Ras, RhoA, and Rac1) have an important role in cardiac hypertrophy and heart failure.[225,228] Transgenic mice with temporally regulated V12Ras induction in the adult heart developed ventricular hypertrophy and arrhythmias, which accompanied electrophysiological remodeling.[229] Ang II–induced activation of p21 Ras is regulated through activation of the Src family kinases and tyrosine phosphorylation of the adapter protein Shc, with subsequent recruitment of the Grb2-Sos1 complex to the membrane fraction (see Figure 9-9).[230] It has been demonstrated that Rho/Rho kinase–mediated signaling is involved in AT_1R-stimulated cardiovascular cell growth, remodeling, atherosclerosis, and vascular contraction.[231,232] Inhibition of Rho/Rho kinase attenuates Ang II–induced hypertrophy of cardiomyocytes and VSMC and expression of plasminogen activator inhibitor protein-1.[233] Rho A is also involved in Ang II–induced activation of NF κB, which controls the expression of inducible cytokines, chemokines, cell adhesion molecules, and vasoactive and antiapoptotic proteins important in the cellular stress response.[234,235] Ang II also activates Rac1, another Rho GTPase, which is an upstream regulator of p21-activated kinase (PAK) and JNK. Rac1 participates in cytoskeletal organization, cell growth, inflammation, and cardiac hypertrophy.[236,237] Recent data have shown that the Ang II/Rac1/STAT3 pathway is important in the atrial myocardium, mediating structural remodeling, and atrial fibrillation.[238] It has been demonstrated that Rac-derived superoxide in the cardiovascular system has a diverse array of functions.[239] Rac1 controls intracellular superoxide production by regulating the activity of NADPH oxidase. NADPH oxidase-produced superoxide is an essential mediator of the hypertensive and hypertrophic responses to Ang II.[240,241] These results indicate that Rac1 is critical for the progression of cardiac remodeling and suggest that therapies which target myocardial Rac1 may be beneficial in the treatment of cardiac hypertrophy and heart failure.

Generation of Reactive Oxygen Species. Accumulating evidence suggests that production of ROS and activation of reduction-oxidation (redox)-dependent signaling cascades are critically involved in Ang II–induced actions[242,243] and have an important role in the development and progression of heart failure regardless of cause.[244,245] ROS function as important intracellular and intercellular second messengers to modulate downstream signaling molecules (Figure 9-10), such as protein tyrosine phosphatases, protein tyrosine kinases, transcription factors, MAPKs, and ion channels, and have a physiological role in vascular tone and cell growth and a pathophysiological role in inflammation, ischemia-reperfusion, hypertension, and atherosclerosis.[246,247] All

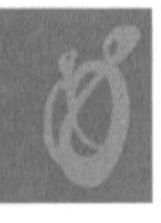

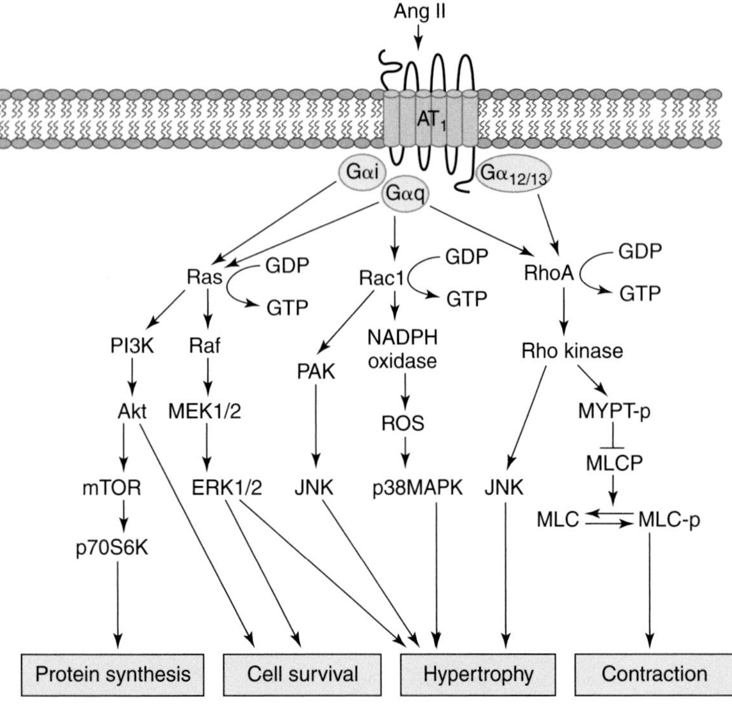

FIGURE 9–9 Regulation of Ang II–induced cellular responses through activation of small GTPases. Ang II stimulates Ras, RhoA, and Rac1 through a process dependent upon activation of a G protein–coupled receptor at the plasma membrane. Small GTPases cycle between a GDP-bound inactive form and a GTP-bound active form. Activated Ras mediated by Gq and Gi regulates the activation of PI3K (phosphatidylinositol-3 kinase) and Raf, the latter being one of the earliest components in the ERK MAPK cascade, which regulates cell survival and cardiac hypertrophy. PI3K modulates cell survival and protein synthesis through Akt and p70S6K. Rac1 activates NADPH oxidase, which in turn regulates generation of ROS. Rac1 also induces the activation of the JNK pathway, through PAK. RhoA regulates cytoskeleton- and hypertrophy-related gene expression, through Rho kinase.

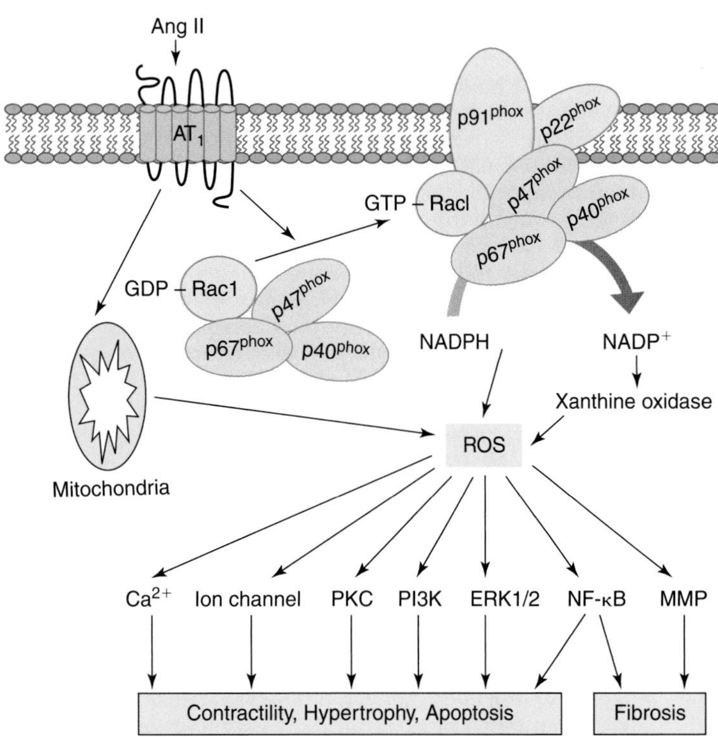

FIGURE 9–10 ROS-mediated signaling in Ang II–induced cardiac remodeling. Major enzymatic sources for intracellular ROS generation in response to Ang II are mitochondria, xanthine oxidases, and the nonphagocytic NADPH oxidases (Noxs). NADPH oxidase is a multisubunit enzyme, comprised of gp91phox, p22phox, p47phox, p67phox, and p40phox, that is regulated by Rac1, via AT_1R. Intracellular ROS modify the activity of protein tyrosine kinases (PTK), such as Src, Ras, JAK2, Pyk2, PI3K, and EGFR, and MAPKs. ROS also influence gene and protein expression by activating transcription factors, such as NF κB and activator protein-1 (AP-1). ROS stimulate ion channels, such as plasma membrane Ca^{2+} and K^+ channels, leading to changes in cation concentrations. Activation of these redox-sensitive pathways results in numerous cellular responses, which if uncontrolled, could contribute to the Ang II–induced cardiovascular remodeling process, including cardiac hypertrophy, fibrosis, apoptosis, and impaired heart function.

cardiovascular cell types are capable of producing ROS, and the major enzymatic sources in heart failure are mitochondria, xanthine oxidases, and the nonphagocytic NADPH oxidases (Noxs). A markedly increased myocardial activity of the NAD(P)H oxidase has been observed in human failing, as compared with nonfailing hearts, suggesting the importance of this enzyme system for LV remodeling and dysfunction after MI.[248] Deficiency of the NAD(P)H oxidase subunit $p47^{phox}$ prevented LV remodeling and dysfunction after MI and reduced cardiomyocyte hypertrophy, apoptosis, and interstitial fibrosis, and was associated with improved survival. NAD(P)H oxidase activity is significantly enhanced and involved in Ang II–induced cardiac and vascular remodeling.[249-251] Studies have demonstrated that mitochondria are the predominant source of ROS in failing hearts (see Chapter 12).[252,253] Chronic increases in free oxygen radical production in mitochondria can lead to a catastrophic cycle of mitochondrial DNA damage and functional decline, resulting in oxygen radical generation and cellular injury.[254,255] Inhibition of mitochondrial oxidative stress and DNA damage may provide an effective treatment strategy for heart failure. Ang II–induced mitochondrial oxidative damage has been implicated in the dysfunction of endothelial cells and VSMC.[256,257] An elevation of xanthine oxidase expression

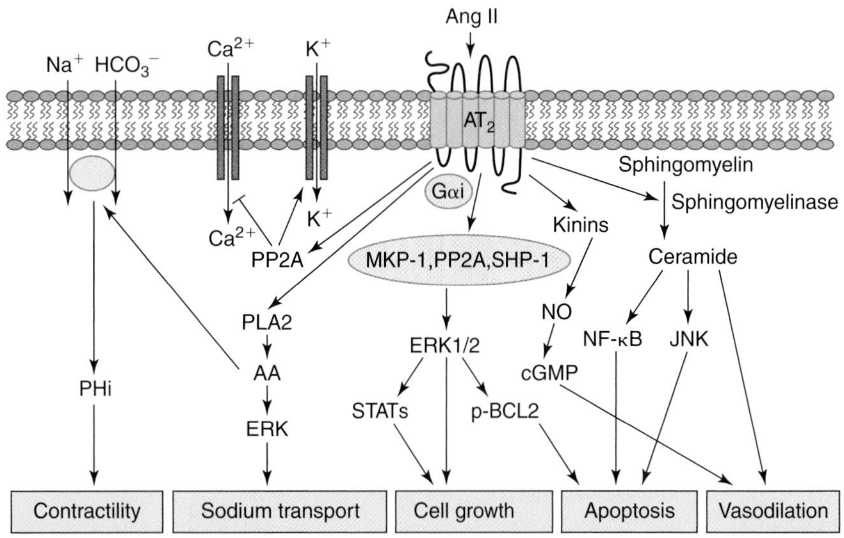

FIGURE 9–11 Signal transduction pathways and physiological effects of the AT_2R. AT_2R signaling pathways include activation of protein phosphatases such as MKP-1, PP2A, and SHP1, which result in dephosphorylation and inactivation of ERK1/2 and STATs; the NO-cGMP system; and activation of PLA2 (phospholipase A2), which mediates the release of arachidonic acid and contributes to the activation of the Na^+/HCO_3^- symporter system and regulation of intracellular pH. PP2A activation also results in the opening of potassium channels and inhibition of T-type Ca^{2+} channels. AT_2R associated apoptosis is regulated by ceramide-mediated signaling.

and activity has also been documented in end-stage human heart failure.[258,259] Recently, chronic treatment with allopurinol (xanthine oxidase inhibitor) was reported to significantly reduce adverse LV remodeling following experimental MI,[260,261] implying an involvement of xanthine oxidase in this process. Activation of xanthine oxidase is also involved in Ang II–induced endothelial oxidant stress.[262] Thus an improved understanding of the specific roles of different ROS sources in redox signaling processes involved in the development of heart failure may result in the development of new therapeutic strategies.

AT_2R-mediated Intracellular Signaling

Although structurally related to G protein–coupled receptors, the AT_2R displays atypical signal transduction and G protein–coupling mechanisms, which are distinct from AT_1R signaling. The intracellular signaling pathways of AT_2R have been studied extensively; however, only a few have been well characterized.[2,263] We will focus on several signaling pathways through which AT_2R mediates cardiovascular actions (Figure 9-11).

G Proteins. Studies have shown that AT_2R couples to intracellular signaling pathways through the pertussis toxin (PTX)-sensitive G protein G_i.[264,265] The G_i protein involved in transducing AT_2R-mediated signals is via interaction with $G_i\alpha_2$ and $G_i\alpha_3$ in rat fetal tissue and in AT_2R-mediated stimulation of Kv current in neurons. The PTX-sensitive G protein G_i is also involved in AT_2R-mediated stimulation of serine/threonine phosphatase 2A (PP2A) activity and the resulting decrease in ERK1/2 activity.[266,267]

Activation of Protein Phosphatases and Protein Dephosphorylation. Numerous studies have shown that activation of AT_2R rapidly induces activation of protein tyrosine phosphatase (PTPase) and serine/threonine phosphatases, resulting in dephosphorylation and inactivation of corresponding tyrosine kinases.[268] AT_2R stimulation results in activation of MAPK phosphatase 1 (MKP-1), SH2 domain-containing phosphatase 1 (SHP1) and PP2A, thereby inhibiting AT_1R-mediated MAP kinase activation. In vivo and in vitro studies have indicated that ERK inactivation by AT_2 may have a physiological role in vivo in relation to cardiac and vascular growth.[269-271] Recent studies indicate that MAPKs are not the only protein kinases that are modulated by AT_2R activation. It has also been demonstrated that stimulation of AT_2R in adult VSMC inhibits AT_1R-mediated tyrosine phosphorylation of STAT1, STAT2, and STAT3, via inhibiting the activation of ERK1/2.[272] AT_2R-stimulated tyrosine and serine/threonine phosphatases serve to reverse, or counterregulate, the cell proliferative and growth-promoting effects mediated by the various protein kinases in response to AT_1R activation.

The Nitric Oxide–Cyclic GMP System. Recent studies have shown that activation of AT_2R by Ang II results in a bradykinin-dependent stimulation of aortic NO release, with subsequent generation of cGMP.[273,274] The connection between AT_2R and cGMP/NO has also been made through in vivo studies in cardiovascular tissues. Inhibition of cardiac AT_2R in the hypertrophied heart amplifies the AT_1R-mediated left ventricular growth response via suppression of cGMP.[275] In the stroke-prone spontaneously hypertensive rat, the AT_2R-mediated increase in aortic cGMP was mediated by activation of bradykinin BK2 receptors, which in turn activated NO synthase, leading to NO production.[276] These studies suggest that AT_2R stimulate production of NO, resulting in an increased formation of the second messenger cGMP. cGMP, in turn, mediates many of the biological actions of NO, such as vasodilation, natriuresis, and antigrowth, by activating a cGMP-dependent protein kinase. These effects also contribute to the beneficial actions of AT_1R blockers in the treatment of hypertension.[277]

Stimulation of Phospholipase A2 and Release of Arachidonic Acid. It has been reported that AT_2R activation is related to Na^+ transport, through activation of PLA2 and release of arachidonic acid (AA) and the cytochrome P450–dependent metabolites in renal proximal tubule epithelial cells. This pathway leads to MAPK activation and p21 ras activation via the tyrosine kinase-Shc-Grb2-Sos pathway.[278,279] AT_2R have also been reported to mediate sustained AA release in cardiomyocytes, contributing to activation of the Na+/HCO$^-$ symporter system and regulation of intracellular pH, and indicating that AT_2R is also important for the regulation of intracellular acidosis, following injury.[280] These studies provide evidence for an AT_2 signaling pathway, mediated through lipid second messengers.

Sphingolipid-derived Ceramide. Ceramide belongs to a family of lipids known as sphingolipids, characterized by a sphingoid backbone and distinct head groups.[281] The AT_2R-activated signal transduction pathway associated with apoptosis involves ceramide.[282,283] Ceramide can induce apoptosis by activating stress kinases or caspases.[284,285] Moreover, ceramide is generated by sphingomyelin breakdown–mediated TNF-α and NF κB activation.[286] Providing that the AT_2R induces NF κB activation, ceramide could serve as a potential mediator of an AT_2R/NF κB signaling pathway. Studies have also implicated ceramide as a possible vasodilatory second messenger.[287] In vitro and in vivo studies have shown that ceramide inhibits VSMC proliferation.[288,289]

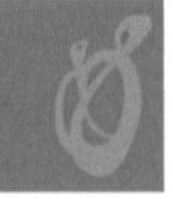

TABLE 9–1 Abbreviations

Abbreviation	Full Name	Abbreviation	Full Name
Ang	Angiotensin	MKP	Mitogen-activated protein kinase phosphatase
Ao	Angiotensinogen	MMP	Matrix metallopeptidase
AA	Arachidonic acid	mTOR	Mammalian target of rapamycin
ACE	Angiotensin-converting enzyme	MYPT	Myosin phosphatase
Ac-SDKP	*N*-acetyl-Ser-Asp-Lys-Pro tetrapeptide	NADPH	Nicotinamide adenine dinucleotide phosphate
Akt(PKB)	Protein kinase B	NEP	Neutral endopeptidase
APA	Aminopeptidase A	NF κB	Nuclear factor kappa B
APN	Aminopeptidase N	NO	Nitric oxide
ARBs	Angiotensin receptor blockers	PA	Phosphatidic acid
ASK	Apoptosis signal-regulating kinase	PAI-1	Plasminogen activator inhibitor-1
AT_1R	Angiotensin II type 1 receptor	PAK	P21-activated kinases
AT_2R	Angiotensin II type 2 receptor	PC	Phosphatidylcholine
BCL-2	B-cell lymphoma 2	PDGF	Platelet-derived growth factor
c-AMP	Cyclic adenosine monophosphate	PDGFR	Platelet-derived growth factor receptor
c-GMP	Cyclic guanosine monophosphate	PDK1	Phosphoinositide-dependent kinase 1
DAG	Diacylglycerol	PI3K	Phosphoinositide 3-kinase
EGFR	Epidermal growth factor receptor	PIP2	Phosphatidylinositol bisphosphate
ERK	Extracellular signal-regulated kinases	PLA2	Phospholipase A2
FAK	Focal adhesion kinase	PLCγ	Phospholipase C
Grb2	Growth factor receptor-bound protein 2	PLD	Phospholipase D
GPCR	G protein–coupled receptors	PKC	Protein kinase C
GEF	Guanine nucleotide exchange factor	PP2A	Protein phosphatase 2A
GDI	Guanosine nucleotide dissociation inhibitor	Pyk2	Proline-rich tyrosine kinase 2
HSP27	Heat shock protein 27	p38 MAPK	p38 mitogen-activated protein kinase
IGFR	Insulin-like growth factor receptor	p70S6K	p70 ribosomal protein S6 kinase
IP_3	Inositol 1,4,5-triphosphate	p130Cas	Crk-associated substrate, 130 kDa
IRAP	Insulin-regulated aminopeptidase	PTK	Protein tyrosine kinase
JAK	Janus kinase	RAS	Renin-angiotensin system
JNK	*c-jun N*-terminal kinases	Rho A	Ras homolog gene family, member A
LV	Left ventricle	ROS	Reactive oxygen species
MAPK	Mitogen-activated protein kinase	Shc	Src homology 2 domain containing transforming protein
MEK	MAP kinase kinase	SHP-1	SH2 domain-containing protein tyrosine phosphatase 1
MEKK	MAP kinase kinase kinase	Sos	Son of sevenless
MI	Myocardial infarction	STAT	Signal transducers and activator of transcription
MLC	Myosin light chain	TAK1	Transforming growth factor β-activated kinase 1
MLK	Mixed-lineage kinase	TGF-β	Transforming growth factor β
M6P-R	Mannose-6-phosphate receptor	VSMC	Vascular smooth muscle cells

These studies represent the initial observations that may lead to the use of ceramide signaling components as a therapeutic intervention for cardiovascular disease.

Although AT_2R can couple to multiple signaling molecules, in a fashion similar to many other hormone/neurotransmitter G protein–coupled receptors, it is apparent that much additional effort will be necessary to fully establish the various intracellular pathways that are coupled to AT_2R.

SUMMARY AND FUTURE DIRECTIONS

The RAS is a hormonal cascade that regulates cardiovascular, renal, and adrenal function. The circulatory system is important for regulation of fluid and electrolyte homeostasis and arterial pressure and plays an important role in the development and progression of heart failure (see Chapter 45). The RAS has also been more recently characterized as the local, self-contained, paracrine, autocrine, and intracrine systems. Tissue RASs are likely important in normal physiological responses, and in pathophysiological states such as hypertension, cardiac hypertrophy, congestive heart failure, and remodeling following myocardial infarction. The intracellular RAS likely does not represent an independent entity but an extension or alternative form of a local RAS, which may be manifested only under select pathophysiological conditions. This suggests a unique evolutionary role for the intracellular RAS. What remains to be determined are the mechanisms of regulation and actions and a more precise understanding of the role of the intracellular RAS in (patho)physiology. Several novel components of the RAS, such as ACE2, Ang (1-7), Ang IV, and (pro)renin receptor, have an important role in cardiovascular pathophysiology. Future research will likely target these new components for the development of therapeutic interventions. Though major progress has been made in our understanding of the physiology and pathophysiology of the circulating RAS, it will be important to elucidate more completely the role of tissue RASs in normal physiology and in the pathophysiology of cardiovascular diseases.

REFERENCES

1. Schmieder, R. E., Hilgers, K. F., Schlaich, M. P., et al. (2007). Renin-angiotensin system and cardiovascular risk. *Lancet, 369*, 1208–1219.
2. Steckelings, U. M., Kaschina, E., & Unger, T. (2005). The AT2 receptor—a matter of love and hate. *Peptides, 26*, 1401–1409.
3. Tigerstedt, R., & Bergman, P. (1898). Niere und Kreislauf. *Skand Arch Physiol, 8*, 223–271.
4. Paul, M., Poyan Mehr, A., & Kreutz, R. (2006). Physiology of local renin-angiotensin systems. *Physiol Rev, 86*, 747–803.
5. Reudelhuber, T. L., Bernstein, K. E., & Delafontaine, P. (2007). Is angiotensin II a direct mediator of left ventricular hypertrophy? Time for another look. *Hypertension, 49*, 1196–1201.
6. Carey, R. M., & Siragy, H. M. (2003). Newly recognized components of the renin-angiotensin system: potential roles in cardiovascular and renal regulation. *Endocr Rev, 24*, 261–271.
7. Kumar, R., Singh, V. P., & Baker, K. M. (2007). The intracellular renin-angiotensin system: a new paradigm. *Trends Endocrinol Metab, 18*, 208–214.
8. Nguyen, G., & Contrepas, A. (2008). Physiology and pharmacology of the (pro)renin receptor. *Curr Opin Pharmacol, 8*, 127–132.
9. Lambert, D. W., Hooper, N. M., & Turner, A. J. (2008). Angiotensin-converting enzyme 2 and new insights into the renin-angiotensin system. *Biochem Pharmacol, 75*, 781–786.
10. Danser, A. H. (2003). Local renin-angiotensin systems: the unanswered questions. *Int J Biochem Cell Biol, 35*, 759–768.
11. Crowley, S. D., Gurley, S. B., & Coffman, T. M. (2007). AT(1) receptors and control of blood pressure: the kidney and more. *Trends Cardiovasc Med, 17*, 30–34.

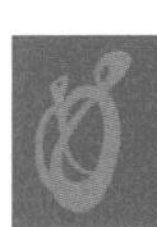

12. Stec, D. E., Davisson, R. L., Haskell, R. E., et al. (1999). Efficient liver-specific deletion of a floxed human angiotensinogen transgene by adenoviral delivery of Cre recombinase in vivo. *J Biol Chem, 274*, 21285–21290.
13. Gould, A. B., & Green, D. (1971). Kinetics of the human renin and human substrate reaction. *Cardiovasc Res, 5*, 86–89.
14. Kim, H. S., Krege, J. H., Kluckman, K. D., et al. (1995). Genetic control of blood pressure and the angiotensinogen locus. *Proc Natl Acad Sci U S A, 92*, 2735–2739.
15. Merrill, D. C., Thompson, M. W., Carney, C. L., et al. (1996). Chronic hypertension and altered baroreflex responses in transgenic mice containing the human renin and human angiotensinogen genes. *J Clin Invest, 97*, 1047–1055.
16. Campbell, D. J., Bouhnik, J., Coezy, E., et al. (1985). Characterization of precursor and secreted forms of human angiotensinogen. *J Clin Invest, 75*, 1880–1893.
17. Brasier, A. R., Han, Y., & Sherman, C. T. (1999). Transcriptional regulation of angiotensinogen gene expression. *Vitam Horm, 57*, 217–247.
18. Clauser, E., Gaillard, I., Wei, L., et al. (1989). Regulation of angiotensinogen gene. *Am J Hypertens, 2*, 403–410.
19. Herrmann, H. C., & Dzau, V. J. (1983). The feedback regulation of angiotensinogen production by components of the renin-angiotensin system. *Circ Res, 52*, 328–334.
20. Lu, H., Boustany-Kari, C. M., Daugherty, A., et al. (2007). Angiotensin II increases adipose angiotensinogen expression. *Am J Physiol Endocrinol Metab, 292*, E1280–E1287.
21. Satou, R., Gonzalez-Villalobos, R. A., Miyata, K., et al. (2008). Costimulation with angiotensin II and interleukin 6 augments angiotensinogen expression in cultured human renal proximal tubular cells. *Am J Physiol Renal Physiol, 295*, F283–F289.
22. Dickson, M. E., & Sigmund, C. D. (2006). Genetic basis of hypertension: revisiting angiotensinogen. *Hypertension, 48*, 14–20.
23. Nguyen, G., Delarue, F., Burckle, C., et al. (2002). Pivotal role of the renin/prorenin receptor in angiotensin II production and cellular responses to renin. *J Clin Invest, 109*, 1417–1427.
24. Kang, J. J., Toma, I., Sipos, A., et al. (2008). The collecting duct is the major source of prorenin in diabetes. *Hypertension, 51*, 1597–1604.
25. Sealey, J. E., Glorioso, N., Itskovitz, J., et al. (1987). Ovarian prorenin. *Clin Exp Hypertens A, 9*, 1435–1454.
26. Hackenthal, E., Paul, M., Ganten, D., et al. (1990). Morphology, physiology, and molecular biology of renin secretion. *Physiol Rev, 70*, 1067–1116.
27. Bader, M., & Ganten, D. (2000). Regulation of renin: new evidence from cultured cells and genetically modified mice. *J Mol Med, 78*, 130–139.
28. Michaud, A., Williams, T. A., Chauvet, M. T., et al. (1997). Substrate dependence of angiotensin I-converting enzyme inhibition: captopril displays a partial selectivity for inhibition of N-acetyl-seryl-aspartyl-lysyl-proline hydrolysis compared with that of angiotensin I. *Mol Pharmacol, 51*, 1070–1076.
29. Largo, R., Gomez-Garre, D., Soto, K., et al. (1999). Angiotensin-converting enzyme is upregulated in the proximal tubules of rats with intense proteinuria. *Hypertension, 33*, 732–739.
30. Fuchs, S., Xiao, H. D., Hubert, C., et al. (2008). Angiotensin-converting enzyme C-terminal catalytic domain is the main site of angiotensin I cleavage in vivo. *Hypertension, 51*, 267–274.
31. Bernstein, K. E., Xiao, H. D., Frenzel, K., et al. (2005). Six truisms concerning ACE and the renin-angiotensin system educed from the genetic analysis of mice. *Circ Res, 96*, 1135–1144.
32. Re, R. N. (2004). Tissue renin angiotensin systems. *Med Clin North Am, 88*, 19–38.
33. van Kats, J. P., Danser, A. H. J., van Maegen, J., et al. (1998). Angiotensin production in the heart: a quantitative study with use of radiolabelled angiotensin infusions. *Circulation, 98*, 73–81.
34. Dostal, D. E., & Baker, K. M. (1999). The cardiac renin-angiotensin system: conceptual, or a regulator of cardiac function? *Circ Res, 85*, 643–650.
35. Dell'Italia, L. J., Meng, Q. C., Balcells, E., et al. (1997). Compartmentalization of angiotensin II generation in the dog heart. Evidence for independent mechanisms in intravascular and interstitial spaces. *J Clin Invest, 100*, 253–258.
36. Heller, L. J., Opsahl, J. A., Wernsing, S. E., et al. (1998). Myocardial and plasma renin-angiotensinogen dynamics during pressure-induced cardiac hypertrophy. *Am J Physiol, 274*, R849–R856.
37. Catanzaro, D. F. (2005). Physiological relevance of renin/prorenin binding and uptake. *Hypertens Res, 28*, 97–105.
38. Muller, D. N., Fischli, W., Clozel, J. P., et al. (1998). Local angiotensin II generation in the rat heart: role of renin uptake. *Circ Res, 82*, 13–20.
39. Peters, J. (2008). Secretory and cytosolic (pro)renin in kidney, heart, and adrenal gland. *J Mol Med, 86*, 711–714.
40. Peters, J., Farrenkopf, R., Clausmeyer, S., et al. (2002). Functional significance of prorenin internalization in the rat heart. *Circ Res, 90*, 1135–1141.
41. Peters, J., & Clausmeyer, S. (2002). Intracellular sorting of renin: cell type specific differences and their consequences. *J Mol Cell Cardiol, 34*, 1561–1568.
42. Zhang, X., Dostal, D. E., Reiss, K., et al. (1995). Identification and activation of autocrine renin-angiotensin system in adult ventricular myocytes. *Am J Physiol, 269*, H1791–H1802.
43. Sun, Y., Zhang, J., Zhang, J. Q., et al. (2001). Renin expression at sites of repair in the infarcted rat heart. *J Mol Cell Cardiol, 33*, 995–1003.
44. Barlucchi, L., Leri, A., Dostal, D. E., et al. (2001). Canine ventricular myocytes possess a renin-angiotensin system that is upregulated with heart failure. *Circ Res, 88*, 298–304.
45. Clausmeyer, S., Reinecke, A., Farrenkopf, R., et al. (2000). Tissue-specific expression of a rat renin transcript lacking the coding sequence for the prefragment and its stimulation by myocardial infarction. *Endocrinology, 141*, 2963–2970.
46. Baker, K. M., Chernin, M. I., Wixson, S. K., et al. (1990). Renin-angiotensin system involvement in pressure-overload cardiac hypertrophy in rats. *Am J Physiol, 259*, H324–H332.
47. Hokimoto, S., Yasue, H., Fujimoto, K., et al. (1995). Increased angiotensin converting enzyme activity in left ventricular aneurysm of patients after myocardial infarction. *Cardiovasc Res, 29*, 664–669.
48. Diez, J., Panizo, A., Hernandez, M., et al. (1997). Cardiomyocyte apoptosis and cardiac angiotensin-converting enzyme in spontaneously hypertensive rats. *Hypertension, 30*, 1029–1034.
49. Dostal, D. E., Rothblum, K. N., Conrad, K. M., et al. (1992). Detection of angiotensin I and II in cultured rat cardiac myocytes and fibroblasts. *Am J Physiol, 263*, C851–C863.
50. Jahanyar, J., Youker, K. A., Loebe, M., et al. (2007). Mast cell-derived cathepsin g: a possible role in the adverse remodeling of the failing human heart. *J Surg Res, 140*, 199–203.
51. Holycross, B. J., Saye, J., Harrison, J. K., et al. (1992). Polymerase chain reaction analysis of renin in rat aortic smooth muscle. *Hypertension, 19*, 697–701.
52. Hu, W. Y., Fukuda, N., Satoh, C., et al. (2000). Phenotypic modulation by fibronectin enhances the angiotensin II-generating system in cultured vascular smooth muscle cells. *Arterioscler Thromb Vasc Biol, 20*, 1500–1505.
53. Lavrentyev, E. N., Estes, A. M., & Malik, K. U. (2007). Mechanism of high glucose induced angiotensin II production in rat vascular smooth muscle cells. *Circ Res, 101*, 455–464.
54. Balcells, E., Meng, Q. C., Johnson, W. H., Jr., et al. (1997). Angiotensin II formation from ACE and chymase in human and animal hearts: methods and species considerations. *Am J Physiol, 273*, H1769–H1774.
55. Wolny, A., Clozel, J. P., Rein, J., et al. (1997). Functional and biochemical analysis of angiotensin II-forming pathways in the human heart. *Circ Res, 80*, 219–227.
56. Li, P., Chen, P. M., Wang, S. W., et al. (2002). Time-dependent expression of chymase and angiotensin converting enzyme in the hamster heart under pressure overload. *Hypertens Res, 25*, 757–762.
57. Chen, L. Y., Li, P., He, Q., et al. (2002). Transgenic study of the function of chymase in heart remodeling. *J Hypertens, 20*, 2047–2055.
58. McDonald, J. E., Padmanabhan, N., Petrie, M. C., et al. (2001). Vasoconstrictor effect of the angiotensin-converting enzyme-resistant, chymase-specific substrate (Pro(11)(D)-Ala(12)) angiotensin I in human dorsal hand veins: in vivo demonstration of non-ace production of angiotensin II in humans. *Circulation, 104*, 1805–1808.
59. Kokkonen, J. O., Lindstedt, K. A., & Kovanen, P. T. (2003). Role for chymase in heart failure: angiotensin II-dependent or -independent mechanisms? *Circulation, 107*, 2522–2544.
60. Doggrell, S. A., & Wanstall, J. C. (2005). Cardiac chymase: pathophysiological role and therapeutic potential of chymase inhibitors. *Can J Physiol Pharmacol, 83*, 123–130.
61. Baker, K.M., Chernin, M.I., Wixson, S.K., Aceto, J.F. (1990). Renin-angiotensin system involvement in pressure-overload cardiac hypertrophy in rats. *Am J Physiol Heart Circ Physiol*, 259, H324-H332.
62. Malhotra, R., Sadoshima, J., Brosius, F. C., III, et al. (1999). Mechanical stretch and angiotensin II differentially upregulate the renin-angiotensin system in cardiac myocytes in vitro. *Circ Res, 85*, 137–146.
63. Fukuzawa, J., Booz, G. W., Hunt, R. A., et al. (2000). Cardiotrophin-1 increases angiotensinogen mRNA in rat cardiac myocytes through STAT3: an autocrine loop for hypertrophy. *Hypertension, 35*, 1191–1196.
64. Dostal, D. E., Booz, G. W., & Baker, K. M. (2000). Regulation of angiotensinogen gene expression and protein in neonatal rat cardiac fibroblasts by glucocorticoid and beta-adrenergic stimulation. *Basic Res Cardiol, 95*, 485–490.
65. Booz, G. W., & Baker, K. M. (2004). *Intracellular signaling and the cardiac renin angiotensin system.* West Sussex, UK: John Wiley & Sons.
66. Singh, V. P., Le, B., Bhat, V. B., et al. (2007). High glucose induced regulation of intracellular angiotensin II synthesis and nuclear redistribution in cardiac myocytes. *Am J Physiol Heart Circ Physiol, 293*, H939–H948.
67. Singh, V. P., Baker, K. M., & Kumar, R. (2008). Activation of the intracellular renin-angiotensin system in cardiac fibroblasts by high glucose: role in extracellular matrix production. *Am J Physiol Heart Circ Physiol, 294*, H1675–H1684.
68. Frustaci, A., Kajstura, J., Chimenti, C., et al. (2000). Myocardial cell death in human diabetes. *Circ Res, 87*, 1123–1132.
69. Booz, G. W., Conrad, K. M., Hess, A. L., et al. (1992). Angiotensin-II-binding sites on hepatocyte nuclei. *Endocrinology, 130*, 3641–3649.
70. Re, R. N., Vizard, D. L., Brown, J., et al. (1984). Angiotensin II receptors in chromatin fragments generated by micrococcal nuclease. *Biochem Biophys Res Commun, 119*, 220–227.
71. Tang, S. S., Rogg, H., Schumacher, R., et al. (1992). Characterization of nuclear angiotensin-II-binding sites in rat liver and comparison with plasma membrane receptors. *Endocrinology, 131*, 374–380.
72. Pendergrass, K. D., Averill, D. B., Ferrario, C. M., et al. (2006). Differential expression of nuclear AT_1 receptors and angiotensin II within the kidney of the male congenic mRen2.Lewis rat. *Am J Physiol Renal Physiol, 290*, F1497–F1506.
73. Eggena, P., Zhu, J. H., Clegg, K., et al. (1993). Nuclear angiotensin receptors induce transcription of renin and angiotensinogen mRNA. *Hypertension, 22*, 496–501.
74. Re, R. N. (2007). The intracellular renin angiotensin system: the tip of the intracrine physiology iceberg. *Am J Physiol Heart Circ Physiol, 293*, H905–H906.
75. Baker, K. M., Chernin, M. I., Schreiber, T., et al. (2004). Evidence of a novel intracrine mechanism in angiotensin II-induced cardiac hypertrophy. *Regul Pept, 120*, 5–13.
76. Haller, H., Lindschau, C., Erdmann, B., et al. (1996). Effects of intracellular angiotensin II in vascular smooth muscle cells. *Circ Res, 79*, 765–772.
77. Baker, K. M., & Kumar, R. (2006). Intracellular angiotensin II induces cell proliferation independent of AT_1 receptor. *Am J Physiol Cell Physiol, 291*, C995–C1001.
78. Kumar, R., Singh, V. P., & Baker, K. M. (2008). The intracellular renin-angiotensin system—implications in cardiovascular remodeling. *Curr Opin Nephrol Hypertens, 17*, 168–173.
79. Castro, C. H., Santos, R. A., Ferreira, A. J., et al. (2005). Evidence for a functional interaction of the angiotensin-(1-7) receptor Mas with AT_1 and AT_2 receptors in the mouse heart. *Hypertension, 46*, 937–942.
80. Kostenis, E., Milligan, G., Christopoulos, A., et al. (2005). G-protein-coupled receptor Mas is a physiological antagonist of the angiotensin II type 1 receptor. *Circulation, 111*, 1806–1813.

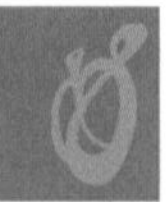

81. Averill, D. B., Ishiyama, Y., Chappell, M. C., et al. (2003). Cardiac angiotensin-(1-7) in ischemic cardiomyopathy. *Circulation, 108*, 2141–2146.
82. Wei, C. C., Ferrario, C. M., Brosnihan, K. B., et al. (2002). Angiotensin peptides modulate bradykinin levels in the interstitium of the dog heart in vivo. *J Pharmacol Exp Ther, 300*, 324–329.
83. Loot, A. E., Roks, A. J., Henning, R. H., et al. (2002). Angiotensin-(1-7) attenuates the development of heart failure after myocardial infarction in rats. *Circulation, 105*, 1548–1550.
84. Zisman, L. S., Keller, R. S., Weaver, B., et al. (2003). Increased angiotensin-(1-7)-forming activity in failing human heart ventricles: evidence for upregulation of the angiotensin-converting enzyme homologue ACE2. *Circulation, 108*, 1707–1712.
85. Crackower, M. A., Sarao, R., Oudit, G. Y., et al. (2002). Angiotensin-converting enzyme 2 is an essential regulator of heart function. *Nature, 417*, 822–828.
86. Der Sarkissian, S., Grobe, J. L., Yuan, L., et al. (2008). Cardiac overexpression of angiotensin converting enzyme 2 protects the heart from ischemia-induced pathophysiology. *Hypertension, 51*, 712–718.
87. Donoghue, M., Wakimoto, H., Maguire, C. T., et al. (2003). Heart block, ventricular tachycardia, and sudden death in ACE2 transgenic mice with downregulated connexins. *J Mol Cell Cardiol, 35*, 1043–1053.
88. Trask, A. J., Averill, D. B., Ganten, D., et al. (2007). Primary role of angiotensin-converting enzyme-2 in cardiac production of angiotensin-(1-7) in transgenic Ren-2 hypertensive rats. *Am J Physiol Heart Circ Physiol, 292*, H3019–H3024.
89. Oudit, G. Y., Kassiri, Z., Patel, M. P., et al. (2007). Angiotensin II-mediated oxidative stress and inflammation mediate the age-dependent cardiomyopathy in ACE2 null mice. *Cardiovasc Res, 75*, 29–39.
90. Hernandez Prada, J. A., Ferreira, A. J., Katovich, M. J., et al. (2008). Structure-based identification of small-molecule angiotensin-converting enzyme 2 activators as novel antihypertensive agents. *Hypertension, 51*, 1312–1317.
91. Reaux, A., Fournie-Zaluski, M. C., & Llorens-Cortes, C. (2001). Angiotensin III: a central regulator of vasopressin release and blood pressure. *Trends Endocrinol Metab, 12*, 157–162.
92. Padia, S. H., Kemp, B. A., Howell, N. L., et al. (2008). Conversion of renal angiotensin II to angiotensin III is critical for AT_2 receptor-mediated natriuresis in rats. *Hypertension, 51*, 460–465.
93. Bodineau, L., Frugiere, A., Marc, Y., et al. (2008). Orally active aminopeptidase A inhibitors reduce blood pressure: a new strategy for treating hypertension. *Hypertension, 51*, 1318–1325.
94. Ruiz-Ortega, M., Esteban, V., & Egido, J. (2007). The regulation of the inflammatory response through nuclear factor-kappaB pathway by angiotensin IV extends the role of the renin angiotensin system in cardiovascular diseases. *Trends Cardiovasc Med, 17*, 19–25.
95. Albiston, A. L., McDowall, S. G., Matsacos, D., et al. (2001). Evidence that the angiotensin IV (AT[4]) receptor is the enzyme insulin-regulated aminopeptidase. *J Biol Chem, 276*, 48623–48626.
96. Wallis, M. G., Lankford, M. F., & Keller, S. R. (2007). Vasopressin is a physiological substrate for the insulin-regulated aminopeptidase IRAP. *Am J Physiol Endocrinol Metab, 293*, E1092–E1102.
97. Esteban, V., Ruperez, M., Sanchez-Lopez, E., et al. (2005). Angiotensin IV activates the nuclear transcription factor-kappaB and related proinflammatory genes in vascular smooth muscle cells. *Circ Res, 96*, 965–973.
98. Franken, A. A., Derkx, F. H., Man in't Veld, A. J., et al. (1990). High plasma prorenin in diabetes mellitus and its correlation with some complications. *J Clin Endocrinol Metab, 71*, 1008–1015.
99. Nguyen, G. (2006). Renin/prorenin receptors. *Kidney Int, 69*, 1503–1506.
100. Saris, J. J., 'tHoen, P. A., Garrelds, I. M., et al. (2006). Prorenin induces intracellular signaling in cardiomyocytes independently of angiotensin II. *Hypertension, 48*, 564–571.
101. Nguyen, G., Delarue, F., Berrou, J., et al. (1996). Specific receptor binding of renin on human mesangial cells in culture increases plasminogen activator inhibitor-1 antigen. *Kidney Int, 50*, 1897–1903.
102. Huang, Y., Noble, N. A., Zhang, J., et al. (2007). Renin-stimulated TGF-beta1 expression is regulated by a mitogen-activated protein kinase in mesangial cells. *Kidney Int, 72*, 45–52.
103. Sakoda, M., Ichihara, A., Kaneshiro, Y., et al. (2007). (Pro)renin receptor-mediated activation of mitogen-activated protein kinases in human vascular smooth muscle cells. *Hypertens Res, 30*, 1139–1146.
104. Veniant, M., Menard, J., Bruneval, P., et al. (1996). Vascular damage without hypertension in transgenic rats expressing prorenin exclusively in the liver. *J Clin Invest, 98*, 1966–1970.
105. Campbell, D. J. (2008). Critical review of prorenin and (pro)renin receptor research. *Hypertension, 51*, 1259–1264.
106. Cohn, J. N. (2007). Reducing cardiovascular risk by blockade of the renin-angiotensin-aldosterone system. *Adv Ther, 24*, 1290–1304.
107. Marchesi, C., Paradis, P., & Schiffrin, E. L. (2008). Role of the renin-angiotensin system in vascular inflammation. *Trends Pharmacol Sci, 29*, 367–374.
108. Unger, T., Jakobsen, A., Heroys, J., et al. (2008). Targeting cardiovascular protection: the concept of dual renin-angiotensin system control. *Medscape J Med, 10*(suppl), S4.
109. Murphy, T. J., Alexander, R. W., Griendling, K. K., et al. (1991). Isolation of a cDNA encoding the vascular type-1 angiotensin II receptor. *Nature, 351*, 233–236.
110. Nakajima, M., Mukoyama, M., Pratt, R. E., et al. (1993). Cloning of cDNA and analysis of the gene for mouse angiotensin II type 2 receptor. *Biochem Biophys Res Commun, 197*, 393–399.
111. Horiuchi, M., Akishita, M., & Dzau, V. J. (1999). Recent progress in angiotensin II type 2 receptor research in the cardiovascular system. *Hypertension, 33*, 613–621.
112. Dinh, D. T., Frauman, A. G., Johnston, C. I., et al. (2001). Angiotensin receptors: distribution, signalling and function. *Clin Sci (Lond), 100*, 481–492.
113. Sasaki, K., Yamano, Y., Bardhan, S., et al. (1991). Cloning and expression of a complementary DNA encoding a bovine adrenal angiotensin II type-1 receptor. *Nature, 351*, 230–233.
114. Iwai, N., & Inagami, T. (1992). Identification of two subtypes in the rat type I angiotensin II receptor. *FEBS Lett, 298*, 257–260.
115. Guo, D. F., Furuta, H., Mizukoshi, M., et al. (1994). The genomic organization of human angiotensin II type 1 receptor. *Biochem Biophys Res Commun, 200*, 313–319.
116. Hjorth, S. A., Schambye, H. T., Greenlee, W. J., et al. (1994). Identification of peptide binding residues in the extracellular domains of the AT_1 receptor. *J Biol Chem, 269*, 30953–30959.
117. Timmermans, P. B., Wong, P. C., Chiu, A. T., et al. (1993). Angiotensin II receptors and angiotensin II receptor antagonists. *Pharmacol Rev, 45*, 205–251.
118. Thekkumkara, T. J., Thomas, W. G., Motel, T. J., et al. (1998). Functional role for the angiotensin II receptor (AT_{1A}) 3'-untranslated region in determining cellular responses to agonist: evidence for recognition by RNA binding proteins. *Biochem J, 329*(pt 2), 255–264.
119. Hunyady, L., Catt, K. J., Clark, A. J., et al. (2000). Mechanisms and functions of AT(1) angiotensin receptor internalization. *Regul Pept, 91*, 29–44.
120. Thomas, W. G., Motel, T. J., Kule, C. E., et al. (1998). Phosphorylation of the angiotensin II (AT_{1A}) receptor carboxyl terminus: a role in receptor endocytosis. *Mol Endocrinol, 12*, 1513–1524.
121. Ribas, C., Penela, P., Murga, C., et al. (2007). The G protein-coupled receptor kinase (GRK) interactome: role of GRKs in GPCR regulation and signaling. *Biochim Biophys Acta, 1768*, 913–922.
122. de Gasparo, M., Husain, A., Alexander, W., et al. (1995). Proposed update of angiotensin receptor nomenclature. *Hypertension, 25*, 924–927.
123. Koike, G., Horiuchi, M., Yamada, T., et al. (1994). Human type 2 angiotensin II receptor gene: cloned, mapped to the X chromosome, and its mRNA is expressed in the human lung. *Biochem Biophys Res Commun, 203*, 1842–1850.
124. Mukoyama, M., Nakajima, M., Horiuchi, M., et al. (1993). Expression cloning of type 2 angiotensin II receptor reveals a unique class of seven-transmembrane receptors. *J Biol Chem, 268*, 24539–24542.
125. Turu, G., Szidonya, L., Gaborik, Z., et al. (2006). Differential beta-arrestin binding of AT_1 and AT_2 angiotensin receptors. *FEBS Lett, 580*, 41–45.
126. Siragy, H. M. (2000). The role of the AT_2 receptor in hypertension. *Am J Hypertens, 13*, 62S–67S.
127. Oishi, Y., Ozono, R., Yano, Y., et al. (2003). Cardioprotective role of AT_2 receptor in postinfarction left ventricular remodeling. *Hypertension, 41*, 814–818.
128. Oishi, Y., Ozono, R., Yoshizumi, M., et al. (2006). AT_2 receptor mediates the cardioprotective effects of AT_1 receptor antagonist in post-myocardial infarction remodeling. *Life Sci, 80*, 82–88.
129. Suzuki, J., Iwai, M., Nakagami, H., et al. (2002). Role of angiotensin II-regulated apoptosis through distinct AT_1 and AT_2 receptors in neointimal formation. *Circulation, 106*, 847–853.
130. Schneider, M. D., & Lorell, B. H. (2001). AT(2), judgment day: which angiotensin receptor is the culprit in cardiac hypertrophy? *Circulation, 104*, 247–248.
131. Yang, Z., Bove, C. M., French, B. A., et al. (2002). Angiotensin II type 2 receptor overexpression preserves left ventricular function after myocardial infarction. *Circulation, 106*, 106–111.
132. Yan, X., Schuldt, A. J., Price, R. L., et al. (2008). Pressure overload-induced hypertrophy in transgenic mice selectively overexpressing AT_2 receptors in ventricular myocytes. *Am J Physiol Heart Circ Physiol, 294*, H1274–H1281.
133. Gross, V., Obst, M., & Luft, F. C. (2004). Insights into angiotensin II receptor function through AT_2 receptor knockout mice. *Acta Physiol Scand, 181*, 487–494.
134. Harding, J. W., Wright, J. W., Swanson, G. N., et al. (1994). AT_4 receptors: specificity and distribution. *Kidney Int, 46*, 1510–1512.
135. Swanson, G. N., Hanesworth, J. M., Sardinia, M. F., et al. (1992). Discovery of a distinct binding site for angiotensin II (3-8), a putative angiotensin IV receptor. *Regul Pept, 40*, 409–419.
136. Albiston, A. L., Mustafa, T., McDowall, S. G., et al. (2003). AT_4 receptor is insulin-regulated membrane aminopeptidase: potential mechanisms of memory enhancement. *Trends Endocrinol Metab, 14*, 72–77.
137. Hamilton, T. A., Handa, R. K., Harding, J. W., et al. (2001). A role for the angiotensin IV/AT_4 system in mediating natriuresis in the rat. *Peptides, 22*, 935–944.
138. Kramar, E. A., Krishnan, R., Harding, J. W., et al. (1998). Role of nitric oxide in angiotensin IV-induced increases in cerebral blood flow. *Regul Pept, 74*, 185–192.
139. Chen, S., Patel, J. M., & Block, E. R. (2000). Angiotensin IV-mediated pulmonary artery vasorelaxation is due to endothelial intracellular calcium release. *Am J Physiol Lung Cell Mol Physiol, 279*, L849–L856.
140. Patel, J. M., Martens, J. R., Li, Y. D., et al. (1998). Angiotensin IV receptor-mediated activation of lung endothelial NOS is associated with vasorelaxation. *Am J Physiol, 275*, L1061–L1068.
141. Li, Y. D., Block, E. R., & Patel, J. M. (2002). Activation of multiple signaling modules is critical in angiotensin IV-induced lung endothelial cell proliferation. *Am J Physiol Lung Cell Mol Physiol, 283*, L707–L716.
142. Mehta, J. L., Li, D. Y., Yang, H., et al. (2002). Angiotensin II and IV stimulate expression and release of plasminogen activator inhibitor-1 in cultured human coronary artery endothelial cells. *J Cardiovasc Pharmacol, 39*, 789–794.
143. Wang, L., Eberhard, M., & Erne, P. (1995). Stimulation of DNA and RNA synthesis in cultured rabbit cardiac fibroblasts by angiotensin IV. *Clin Sci (Lond), 88*, 557–562.
144. Yang, Q., Hanesworth, J. M., Harding, J. W., et al. (1997). The AT_4 receptor agonist (Nle1)-angiotensin IV reduces mechanically induced immediate-early gene expression in the isolated rabbit heart. *Regul Pept, 71*, 175–183.
145. Slinker, B. K., Wu, Y., Brennan, A. J., et al. (1999). Angiotensin IV has mixed effects on left ventricle systolic function and speeds relaxation. *Cardiovasc Res, 42*, 660–669.
146. Griendling, K. K., Ushio-Fukai, M., Lassegue, B., et al. (1997). Angiotensin II signaling in vascular smooth muscle. New concepts. *Hypertension, 29*, 366–373.
147. Capponi, A. M. (1996). Distribution and signal transduction of angiotensin II AT_1 and AT_2 receptors. *Blood Press Suppl, 2*, 41–46.

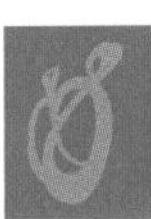

148. Ruan, X., & Arendshorst, W. J. (1996). Role of protein kinase C in angiotensin II-induced renal vasoconstriction in genetically hypertensive rats. *Am J Physiol, 270*, F945–F952.
149. Booz, G. W., Dostal, D. E., Singer, H. A., et al. (1994). Involvement of protein kinase C and Ca^{2+} in angiotensin II-induced mitogenesis of cardiac fibroblasts. *Am J Physiol, 267*, C1308–C1318.
150. Touyz, R. M., & Berry, C. (2002). Recent advances in angiotensin II signaling. *Braz J Med Biol Res, 35*, 1001–1015.
151. Anand-Srivastava, M. B. (1983). Angiotensin II receptors negatively coupled to adenylate cyclase in rat aorta. *Biochem Biophys Res Commun, 117*, 420–428.
152. Kem, D. C., Johnson, E. I., Capponi, A. M., et al. (1991). Effect of angiotensin II on cytosolic free calcium in neonatal rat cardiomyocytes. *Am J Physiol, 261*, C77–C85.
153. Iversen, B. M., & Arendshorst, W. J. (1999). AT_1 calcium signaling in renal vascular smooth muscle cells. *J Am Soc Nephrol, 10*(suppl. 11), S84–S89.
154. Macrez, N., Morel, J. L., Kalkbrenner, F., et al. (1997). A betagamma dimer derived from G13 transduces the angiotensin AT_1 receptor signal to stimulation of Ca^{2+} channels in rat portal vein myocytes. *J Biol Chem, 272*, 23180–23185.
155. Kim, S., & Iwao, H. (2000). Molecular and cellular mechanisms of angiotensin II-mediated cardiovascular and renal diseases. *Pharmacol Rev, 52*, 11–34.
156. Yin, G., Yan, C., & Berk, B. C. (2003). Angiotensin II signaling pathways mediated by tyrosine kinases. *Int J Biochem Cell Biol, 35*, 780–783.
157. Haendeler, J., & Berk, B. C. (2000). Angiotensin II mediated signal transduction. Important role of tyrosine kinases. *Regul Pept, 95*, 1–7.
158. Mehta, P. K., & Griendling, K. K. (2007). Angiotensin II cell signaling: physiological and pathological effects in the cardiovascular system. *Am J Physiol Cell Physiol, 292*, C82–C97.
159. Delcourt, N., Bockaert, J., & Marin, P. (2007). GPCR-jacking: from a new route in RTK signalling to a new concept in GPCR activation. *Trends Pharmacol Sci, 28*, 602–607.
160. Natarajan, K., & Berk, B. C. (2006). Crosstalk coregulation mechanisms of G protein-coupled receptors and receptor tyrosine kinases. *Methods Mol Biol, 332*, 51–77.
161. Saito, Y., & Berk, B. C. (2001). Transactivation: a novel signaling pathway from angiotensin II to tyrosine kinase receptors. *J Mol Cell Cardiol, 33*, 3–7.
162. Zwick, E., Bange, J., & Ullrich, A. (2002). Receptor tyrosine kinases as targets for anticancer drugs. *Trends Mol Med, 8*, 17–23.
163. Eguchi, S., Dempsey, P. J., Frank, G. D., et al. (2001). Activation of MAPKs by angiotensin II in vascular smooth muscle cells. Metalloprotease-dependent EGF receptor activation is required for activation of ERK and p38 MAPK but not for JNK. *J Biol Chem, 276*, 7957–7962.
164. Mifune, M., Ohtsu, H., Suzuki, H., et al. (2005). G protein coupling and second messenger generation are indispensable for metalloprotease-dependent, heparin-binding epidermal growth factor shedding through angiotensin II type-1 receptor. *J Biol Chem, 280*, 26592–26599.
165. Suzuki, H., Motley, E. D., Frank, G. D., et al. (2005). Recent progress in signal transduction research of the angiotensin II type-1 receptor: protein kinases, vascular dysfunction and structural requirement. *Curr Med Chem Cardiovasc Hematol Agents, 3*, 305–322.
166. Eguchi, S., & Inagami, T. (2000). Signal transduction of angiotensin II type 1 receptor through receptor tyrosine kinase. *Regul Pept, 91*, 13–20.
167. Shah, B. H., & Catt, K. J. (2003). A central role of EGF receptor transactivation in angiotensin II-induced cardiac hypertrophy. *Trends Pharmacol Sci, 24*, 239–244.
168. Zahradka, P., Litchie, B., Storie, B., et al. (2004). Transactivation of the insulin-like growth factor-I receptor by angiotensin II mediates downstream signaling from the angiotensin II type 1 receptor to phosphatidylinositol 3-kinase. *Endocrinology, 145*, 2978–2987.
169. Azar, Z. M., Mehdi, M. Z., & Srivastava, A. K. (2007). Insulin-like growth factor type-1 receptor transactivation in vasoactive peptide and oxidant-induced signaling pathways in vascular smooth muscle cells. *Can J Physiol Pharmacol, 85*, 105–111.
170. Saito, S., Frank, G. D., Mifune, M., et al. (2002). Ligand-independent trans-activation of the platelet-derived growth factor receptor by reactive oxygen species requires protein kinase C-delta and c-Src. *J Biol Chem, 277*, 44695–44700.
171. Kelly, D. J., Cox, A. J., Gow, R. M., et al. (2004). Platelet-derived growth factor receptor transactivation mediates the trophic effects of angiotensin II in vivo. *Hypertension, 44*, 195–202.
172. Kim, S., Zhan, Y., Izumi, Y., et al. (2000). In vivo activation of rat aortic platelet-derived growth factor and epidermal growth factor receptors by angiotensin II and hypertension. *Arterioscler Thromb Vasc Biol, 20*, 2539–2545.
173. Wang, C., Wu, L. L., Liu, J., et al. (2008). Crosstalk between angiotensin II and platelet derived growth factor-BB mediated signal pathways in cardiomyocytes. *Chin Med J (Engl), 121*, 236–240.
174. Godeny, M. D., & Sayeski, P. P. (2006). ANG II-induced cell proliferation is dually mediated by c-Src/Yes/Fyn-regulated ERK1/2 activation in the cytoplasm and PKC-zeta-controlled ERK1/2 activity within the nucleus. *Am J Physiol Cell Physiol, 291*, C1297–C1307.
175. Touyz, R. M., He, G., Wu, X. H., et al. (2001). Src is an important mediator of extracellular signal-regulated kinase 1/2-dependent growth signaling by angiotensin II in smooth muscle cells from resistance arteries of hypertensive patients. *Hypertension, 38*, 56–64.
176. Tatosyan, A. G., & Mizenina, O. A. (2000). Kinases of the Src family: structure and functions. *Biochemistry (Mosc), 65*, 49–58.
177. Thomas, S. M., & Brugge, J. S. (1997). Cellular functions regulated by Src family kinases. *Annu Rev Cell Dev Biol, 13*, 513–609.
178. Erpel, T., & Courtneidge, S. A. (1995). Src family protein tyrosine kinases and cellular signal transduction pathways. *Curr Opin Cell Biol, 7*, 176–182.
179. Parsons, J. T. (2003). Focal adhesion kinase: the first ten years. *J Cell Sci, 116*, 1409–1416.
180. Rocic, P., Griffin, T. M., McRae, C. N., et al. (2002). Altered PYK2 phosphorylation by ANG II in hypertensive vascular smooth muscle. *Am J Physiol Heart Circ Physiol, 282*, H457–H465.
181. Qin, J., & Liu, Z. X. (2006). FAK-related nonkinase attenuates hypertrophy induced by angiotensin-II in cultured neonatal rat cardiac myocytes. *Acta Pharmacol Sin, 27*, 1159–1164.
182. Govindarajan, G., Eble, D. M., Lucchesi, P. A., et al. (2000). Focal adhesion kinase is involved in angiotensin II-mediated protein synthesis in cultured vascular smooth muscle cells. *Circ Res, 87*, 710–716.
183. Rocic, P., Govindarajan, G., Sabri, A., et al. (2001). A role for PYK2 in regulation of ERK1/2 MAP kinases and PI 3-kinase by ANG II in vascular smooth muscle. *Am J Physiol Cell Physiol, 280*, C90–C99.
184. Guan, J. L. (1997). Role of focal adhesion kinase in integrin signaling. *Int J Biochem Cell Biol, 29*, 1085–1096.
185. Sabri, A., Govindarajan, G., Griffin, T. M., et al. (1998). Calcium- and protein kinase C-dependent activation of the tyrosine kinase PYK2 by angiotensin II in vascular smooth muscle. *Circ Res, 83*, 841–851.
186. Matsuda, M., Mayer, B. J., Fukui, Y., et al. (1990). Binding of transforming protein, P47gag-crk, to a broad range of phosphotyrosine-containing proteins. *Science, 248*, 1537–1539.
187. Defilippi, P., Di Stefano, P., & Cabodi, S. (2006). p130Cas: a versatile scaffold in signaling networks. *Trends Cell Biol, 16*, 257–263.
188. O'Neill, G. M., Fashena, S. J., & Golemis, E. A. (2000). Integrin signalling: a new Cas(t) of characters enters the stage. *Trends Cell Biol, 10*, 111–119.
189. Takahashi, T., Kawahara, Y., Taniguchi, T., et al. (1998). Tyrosine phosphorylation and association of p130Cas and c-Crk II by ANG II in vascular smooth muscle cells. *Am J Physiol, 274*, H1059–H1065.
190. Kyaw, M., Yoshizumi, M., Tsuchiya, K., et al. (2004). Src and Cas are essentially but differentially involved in angiotensin II-stimulated migration of vascular smooth muscle cells via extracellular signal-regulated kinase 1/2 and c-Jun NH2-terminal kinase activation. *Mol Pharmacol, 65*, 832–841.
191. Schindler, C., Levy, D. E., & Decker, T. (2007). JAK-STAT signaling: from interferons to cytokines. *J Biol Chem, 282*, 20059–20063.
192. Murray, P. J. (2007). The JAK-STAT signaling pathway: input and output integration. *J Immunol, 178*, 2623–2629.
193. Aaronson, D. S., & Horvath, C. M. (2002). A road map for those who don't know JAK-STAT. *Science, 296*, 1653–1655.
194. Booz, G. W., Day, J. N., & Baker, K. M. (2002). Interplay between the cardiac renin angiotensin system and JAK-STAT signaling: role in cardiac hypertrophy, ischemia/reperfusion dysfunction, and heart failure. *J Mol Cell Cardiol, 34*, 1443–1453.
195. Bolli, R., Dawn, B., & Xuan, Y. T. (2003). Role of the JAK-STAT pathway in protection against myocardial ischemia/reperfusion injury. *Trends Cardiovasc Med, 13*, 72–79.
196. Mascareno, E., & Siddiqui, M. A. (2000). The role of JAK/STAT signaling in heart tissue renin-angiotensin system. *Mol Cell Biochem, 212*, 171–175.
197. El-Adawi, H., Deng, L., Tramontano, A., et al. (2003). The functional role of the JAK-STAT pathway in post-infarction remodeling. *Cardiovasc Res, 57*, 129–138.
198. Mascareno, E., El-Shafei, M., Maulik, N., et al. (2001). JAK/STAT signaling is associated with cardiac dysfunction during ischemia and reperfusion. *Circulation, 104*, 325–329.
199. Banes-Berceli, A. K., Ketsawatsomkron, P., Ogbi, S., et al. (2007). Angiotensin II and endothelin-1 augment the vascular complications of diabetes via JAK2 activation. *Am J Physiol Heart Circ Physiol, 293*, H1291–H1299.
200. Prasad, S. V., Perrino, C., & Rockman, H. A. (2003). Role of phosphoinositide 3-kinase in cardiac function and heart failure. *Trends Cardiovasc Med, 13*, 206–212.
201. Saward, L., & Zahradka, P. (1997). Angiotensin II activates phosphatidylinositol 3-kinase in vascular smooth muscle cells. *Circ Res, 81*, 249–257.
202. Oudit, G. Y., Sun, H., Kerfant, B. G., et al. (2004). The role of phosphoinositide-3 kinase and PTEN in cardiovascular physiology and disease. *J Mol Cell Cardiol, 37*, 449–471.
203. Walker, E. H., Perisic, O., Ried, C., et al. (1999). Structural insights into phosphoinositide 3-kinase catalysis and signalling. *Nature, 402*, 313–320.
204. Fruman, D. A., Meyers, R. E., & Cantley, L. C. (1998). Phosphoinositide kinases. *Annu Rev Biochem, 67*, 481–507.
205. McMullen, J. R., Shioi, T., Zhang, L., et al. (2003). Phosphoinositide 3-kinase(p110alpha) plays a critical role for the induction of physiological, but not pathological, cardiac hypertrophy. *Proc Natl Acad Sci U S A, 100*, 12355–12360.
206. Alloatti, G., Montrucchio, G., Lembo, G., et al. (2004). Phosphoinositide 3-kinase gamma: kinase-dependent and -independent activities in cardiovascular function and disease. *Biochem Soc Trans, 32*, 383–386.
207. Kerfant, B. G., Rose, R. A., Sun, H., et al. (2006). Phosphoinositide 3-kinase gamma regulates cardiac contractility by locally controlling cyclic adenosine monophosphate levels. *Trends Cardiovasc Med, 16*, 250–256.
208. El Mabrouk, M., Touyz, R. M., & Schiffrin, E. L. (2001). Differential ANG II-induced growth activation pathways in mesenteric artery smooth muscle cells from SHR. *Am J Physiol Heart Circ Physiol, 281*, H30–H39.
209. Chen, Q. M., Tu, V. C., Purdon, S., et al. (2001). Molecular mechanisms of cardiac hypertrophy induced by toxicants. *Cardiovasc Toxicol, 1*, 267–283.
210. Pimienta, G., & Pascual, J. (2007). Canonical and alternative MAPK signaling. *Cell Cycle, 6*, 2628–2632.
211. Strniskova, M., Barancik, M., & Ravingerova, T. (2002). Mitogen-activated protein kinases and their role in regulation of cellular processes. *Gen Physiol Biophys, 21*, 231–255.
212. Chang, L., & Karin, M. (2001). Mammalian MAP kinase signalling cascades. *Nature, 410*, 37–40.
213. Kim, S., & Iwao, H. (1999). Activation of mitogen-activated protein kinases in cardiovascular hypertrophy and remodeling. *Jpn J Pharmacol, 80*, 97–102.
214. Ravingerova, T., Barancik, M., & Strniskova, M. (2003). Mitogen-activated protein kinases: a new therapeutic target in cardiac pathology. *Mol Cell Biochem, 247*, 127–138.
215. Wei, S. G., Yu, Y., Zhang, Z. H., et al. (2008). Angiotensin II-triggered p44/42 mitogen-activated protein kinase mediates sympathetic excitation in heart failure rats. *Hypertension*, 342–350.

216. Kim, S., & Iwao, H. (2003). Stress and vascular responses: mitogen-activated protein kinases and activator protein-1 as promising therapeutic targets of vascular remodeling. *J Pharmacol Sci, 91*, 177–181.
217. Wang, Y., Su, B., Sah, V. P., et al. (1998). Cardiac hypertrophy induced by mitogen-activated protein kinase kinase 7, a specific activator for c-Jun NH2-terminal kinase in ventricular muscle cells. *J Biol Chem, 273*, 5423–5426.
218. Schmitz, U., Ishida, T., Ishida, M., et al. (1998). Angiotensin II stimulates p21-activated kinase in vascular smooth muscle cells: role in activation of JNK. *Circ Res, 82*, 1272–1278.
219. Wang, Y., Huang, S., Sah, V. P., et al. (1998). Cardiac muscle cell hypertrophy and apoptosis induced by distinct members of the p38 mitogen-activated protein kinase family. *J Biol Chem, 273*, 2161–2168.
220. Hayashida, W., Kihara, Y., Yasaka, A., et al. (2001). Stage-specific differential activation of mitogen-activated protein kinases in hypertrophied and failing rat hearts. *J Mol Cell Cardiol, 33*, 733–744.
221. Haq, S., Choukroun, G., Lim, H., et al. (2001). Differential activation of signal transduction pathways in human hearts with hypertrophy versus advanced heart failure. *Circulation, 103*, 670–677.
222. Liao, P., Georgakopoulos, D., Kovacs, A., et al. (2001). The in vivo role of p38 MAP kinases in cardiac remodeling and restrictive cardiomyopathy. *Proc Natl Acad Sci U S A, 98*, 12283–12288.
223. Liu, Y. H., Wang, D., Rhaleb, N. E., et al. (2005). Inhibition of p38 mitogen-activated protein kinase protects the heart against cardiac remodeling in mice with heart failure resulting from myocardial infarction. *J Card Fail, 11*, 74–81.
224. Pellieux, C., Sauthier, T., Aubert, J. F., et al. (2000). Angiotensin II-induced cardiac hypertrophy is associated with different mitogen-activated protein kinase activation in normotensive and hypertensive mice. *J Hypertens, 18*, 1307–1317.
225. Lezoualc'h, F., Metrich, M., Hmitou, I., et al. (2008). Small GTP-binding proteins and their regulators in cardiac hypertrophy. *J Mol Cell Cardiol, 44*, 623–632.
226. Clerk, A., & Sugden, P. H. (2000). Small guanine nucleotide-binding proteins and myocardial hypertrophy. *Circ Res, 86*, 1019–1023.
227. Bhattacharya, M., Babwah, A. V., & Ferguson, S. S. (2004). Small GTP-binding protein-coupled receptors. *Biochem Soc Trans, 32*, 1040–1044.
228. Vahebi, S., & Solaro, R. J. (2005). Cardiac sarcomeric function, small G-protein signaling, and heart failure. *Panminerva Med, 47*, 133–142.
229. Ruan, H., Mitchell, S., Vainoriene, M., et al. (2007). Gi alpha 1-mediated cardiac electrophysiological remodeling and arrhythmia in hypertrophic cardiomyopathy. *Circulation, 116*, 596–605.
230. Sadoshima, J., & Izumo, S. (1996). The heterotrimeric G q protein-coupled angiotensin II receptor activates p21 ras via the tyrosine kinase-Shc-Grb2-Sos pathway in cardiac myocytes. *EMBO J, 15*, 775–787.
231. Yamakawa, T., Tanaka, S., Numaguchi, K., et al. (2000). Involvement of Rho-kinase in angiotensin II-induced hypertrophy of rat vascular smooth muscle cells. *Hypertension, 35*, 313–318.
232. Jalil, J., Lavandero, S., Chiong, M., et al. (2005). Rho/Rho kinase signal transduction pathway in cardiovascular disease and cardiovascular remodeling. *Rev Esp Cardiol, 58*, 951–961.
233. Aikawa, R., Komuro, I., Nagai, R., et al. (2000). Rho plays an important role in angiotensin II-induced hypertrophic responses in cardiac myocytes. *Mol Cell Biochem, 212*, 177–182.
234. Choudhary, S., Lu, M., Cui, R., et al. (2007). Involvement of a novel Rac/RhoA guanosine triphosphatase-nuclear factor-kappaB inducing kinase signaling pathway mediating angiotensin II-induced RelA transactivation. *Mol Endocrinol, 21*, 2203–2217.
235. Cui, R., Tieu, B., Recinos, A., et al. (2006). RhoA mediates angiotensin II-induced phospho-Ser536 nuclear factor kappaB/RelA subunit exchange on the interleukin-6 promoter in VSMCs. *Circ Res, 99*, 723–730.
236. Laufs, U., & Liao, J. K. (2000). Targeting Rho in cardiovascular disease. *Circ Res, 87*, 526–528.
237. Satoh, M., Ogita, H., Takeshita, K., et al. (2006). Requirement of Rac1 in the development of cardiac hypertrophy. *Proc Natl Acad Sci U S A, 103*, 7432–7437.
238. Tsai, C. T., Lai, L. P., Kuo, K. T., et al. (2008). Angiotensin II activates signal transducer and activators of transcription 3 via Rac1 in atrial myocytes and fibroblasts: implication for the therapeutic effect of statin in atrial structural remodeling. *Circulation, 117*, 344–355.
239. Gregg, D., Rauscher, F. M., & Goldschmidt-Clermont, P. J. (2003). Rac regulates cardiovascular superoxide through diverse molecular interactions: more than a binary GTP switch. *Am J Physiol Cell Physiol, 285*, C723–C734.
240. Harrison, D. G., Cai, H., Landmesser, U., et al. (2003). Interactions of angiotensin II with NAD(P)H oxidase, oxidant stress and cardiovascular disease. *J Renin Angiotensin Aldosterone Syst, 4*, 51–61.
241. Nakagami, H., Takemoto, M., & Liao, J. K. (2003). NADPH oxidase-derived superoxide anion mediates angiotensin II-induced cardiac hypertrophy. *J Mol Cell Cardiol, 35*, 851–859.
242. Griendling, K. K., Sorescu, D., & Ushio-Fukai, M. (2000). NAD(P)H oxidase: role in cardiovascular biology and disease. *Circ Res, 86*, 494–501.
243. Griendling, K. K., & Ushio-Fukai, M. (2000). Reactive oxygen species as mediators of angiotensin II signaling. *Regul Pept, 91*, 21–27.
244. Zhang, M., & Shah, A. M. (2007). Role of reactive oxygen species in myocardial remodeling. *Curr Heart Fail Rep, 4*, 26–30.
245. Seddon, M., Looi, Y. H., & Shah, A. M. (2007). Oxidative stress and redox signalling in cardiac hypertrophy and heart failure. *Heart, 93*, 903–907.
246. Hanna, I. R., Taniyama, Y., Szocs, K., et al. (2002). NAD(P)H oxidase-derived reactive oxygen species as mediators of angiotensin II signaling. *Antioxid Redox Signal, 4*, 899–914.
247. Cai, H., Griendling, K. K., & Harrison, D. G. (2003). The vascular NAD(P)H oxidases as therapeutic targets in cardiovascular diseases. *Trends Pharmacol Sci, 24*, 471–478.
248. Heymes, C., Bendall, J. K., Ratajczak, P., et al. (2003). Increased myocardial NADPH oxidase activity in human heart failure. *J Am Coll Cardiol, 41*, 2164–2171.
249. Li, J. M., & Shah, A. M. (2003). Mechanism of endothelial cell NADPH oxidase activation by angiotensin II. Role of the p47phox subunit. *J Biol Chem, 278*, 12094–12100.
250. Touyz, R. M., Chen, X., Tabet, F., et al. (2002). Expression of a functionally active gp91phox-containing neutrophil-type NAD(P)H oxidase in smooth muscle cells from human resistance arteries: regulation by angiotensin II. *Circ Res, 90*, 1205–1213.
251. Landmesser, U., Cai, H., Dikalov, S., et al. (2002). Role of p47(phox) in vascular oxidative stress and hypertension caused by angiotensin II. *Hypertension, 40*, 511–515.
252. Tsutsui, H., Ide, T., & Kinugawa, S. (2006). Mitochondrial oxidative stress, DNA damage, and heart failure. *Antioxid Redox Signal, 8*, 1737–1744.
253. Sawyer, D. B., & Colucci, W. S. (2000). Mitochondrial oxidative stress in heart failure: "oxygen wastage" revisited. *Circ Res, 86*, 119–120.
254. Ikeuchi, M., Matsusaka, H., Kang, D., et al. (2005). Overexpression of mitochondrial transcription factor a ameliorates mitochondrial deficiencies and cardiac failure after myocardial infarction. *Circulation, 112*, 683–690.
255. Ricci, C., Pastukh, V., Leonard, J., et al. (2008). Mitochondrial DNA damage triggers mitochondrial-superoxide generation and apoptosis. *Am J Physiol Cell Physiol, 294*, C413–C422.
256. Doughan, A. K., Harrison, D. G., & Dikalov, S. I. (2008). Molecular mechanisms of angiotensin II-mediated mitochondrial dysfunction: linking mitochondrial oxidative damage and vascular endothelial dysfunction. *Circ Res, 102*, 488–496.
257. Kimura, S., Zhang, G. X., Nishiyama, A., et al. (2005). Mitochondria-derived reactive oxygen species and vascular MAP kinases: comparison of angiotensin II and diazoxide. *Hypertension, 45*, 438–444.
258. Cappola, T. P., Kass, D. A., Nelson, G. S., et al. (2001). Allopurinol improves myocardial efficiency in patients with idiopathic dilated cardiomyopathy. *Circulation, 104*, 2407–2411.
259. Landmesser, U., Spiekermann, S., Dikalov, S., et al. (2002). Vascular oxidative stress and endothelial dysfunction in patients with chronic heart failure: role of xanthine-oxidase and extracellular superoxide dismutase. *Circulation, 106*, 3073–3078.
260. Engberding, N., Spiekermann, S., Schaefer, A., et al. (2004). Allopurinol attenuates left ventricular remodeling and dysfunction after experimental myocardial infarction: a new action for an old drug? *Circulation, 110*, 2175–2179.
261. Minhas, K. M., Saraiva, R. M., Schuleri, K. H., et al. (2006). Xanthine oxidoreductase inhibition causes reverse remodeling in rats with dilated cardiomyopathy. *Circ Res, 98*, 271–279.
262. Landmesser, U., Spiekermann, S., Preuss, C., et al. (2007). Angiotensin II induces endothelial xanthine oxidase activation: role for endothelial dysfunction in patients with coronary disease. *Arterioscler Thromb Vasc Biol, 27*, 943–948.
263. Nouet, S., & Nahmias, C. (2000). Signal transduction from the angiotensin II AT_2 receptor. *Trends Endocrinol Metab, 11*, 1–6.
264. Kang, J., Posner, P., & Sumners, C. (1994). Angiotensin II type 2 receptor stimulation of neuronal K^+ currents involves an inhibitory GTP binding protein. *Am J Physiol, 267*, C1389–C1397.
265. Zhang, J., & Pratt, R. E. (1996). The AT_2 receptor selectively associates with Gialpha2 and Gialpha3 in the rat fetus. *J Biol Chem, 271*, 15026–15033.
266. Huang, X. C., Richards, E. M., & Sumners, C. (1995). Angiotensin II type 2 receptor-mediated stimulation of protein phosphatase 2A in rat hypothalamic/brainstem neuronal cocultures. *J Neurochem, 65*, 2131–2137.
267. Huang, X. C., Sumners, C., & Richards, E. M. (1996). Angiotensin II stimulates protein phosphatase 2A activity in cultured neuronal cells via type 2 receptors in a pertussis toxin sensitive fashion. *Adv Exp Med Biol, 396*, 209–215.
268. Bottari, S. P., King, I. N., Reichlin, S., et al. (1992). The angiotensin AT_2 receptor stimulates protein tyrosine phosphatase activity and mediates inhibition of particulate guanylate cyclase. *Biochem Biophys Res Commun, 183*, 206–211.
269. Masaki, H., Kurihara, T., Yamaki, A., et al. (1998). Cardiac-specific overexpression of angiotensin II AT_2 receptor causes attenuated response to AT_1 receptor-mediated pressor and chronotropic effects. *J Clin Invest, 101*, 527–535.
270. Akishita, M., Ito, M., Lehtonen, J. Y., et al. (1999). Expression of the AT_2 receptor developmentally programs extracellular signal-regulated kinase activity and influences fetal vascular growth. *J Clin Invest, 103*, 63–71.
271. Nakajima, M., Hutchinson, H. G., Fujinaga, M., et al. (1995). The angiotensin II type 2 (AT_2) receptor antagonizes the growth effects of the AT_1 receptor: gain-of-function study using gene transfer. *Proc Natl Acad Sci U S A, 92*, 10663–10667.
272. Horiuchi, M., Hayashida, W., Akishita, M., et al. (1999). Stimulation of different subtypes of angiotensin II receptors, AT_1 and AT_2 receptors, regulates STAT activation by negative crosstalk. *Circ Res, 84*, 876–882.
273. Searles, C. D., & Harrison, D. G. (1999). The interaction of nitric oxide, bradykinin, and the angiotensin II type 2 receptor: lessons learned from transgenic mice. *J Clin Invest, 104*, 1013–1014.
274. Moore, A. F., Heiderstadt, N. T., Huang, E., et al. (2001). Selective inhibition of the renal angiotensin type 2 receptor increases blood pressure in conscious rats. *Hypertension, 37*, 1285–1291.
275. Bartunek, J., Weinberg, E. O., Tajima, M., et al. (1999). Angiotensin II type 2 receptor blockade amplifies the early signals of cardiac growth response to angiotensin II in hypertrophied hearts. *Circulation, 99*, 22–25.
276. Gohlke, P., Pees, C., & Unger, T. (1998). AT_2 receptor stimulation increases aortic cyclic GMP in SHRSP by a kinin-dependent mechanism. *Hypertension, 31*, 349–355.
277. Savoia, C., Ebrahimian, T., He, Y., et al. (2006). Angiotensin II/AT_2 receptor-induced vasodilation in stroke-prone spontaneously hypertensive rats involves nitric oxide and cGMP-dependent protein kinase. *J Hypertens, 24*, 2417–2422.
278. Jiao, H., Cui, X. L., Torti, M., et al. (1998). Arachidonic acid mediates angiotensin II effects on p21ras in renal proximal tubular cells via the tyrosine kinase-Shc-Grb2-Sos pathway. *Proc Natl Acad Sci U S A, 95*, 7417–7421.

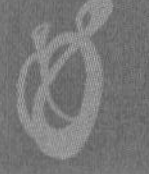

279. Dulin, N. O., Alexander, L. D., Harwalkar, S., et al. (1998). Phospholipase A2-mediated activation of mitogen-activated protein kinase by angiotensin II. *Proc Natl Acad Sci U S A, 95*, 8098–8102.
280. Kohout, T. A., & Rogers, T. B. (1995). Angiotensin II activates the $Na^+/HCO3^-$ symport through a phosphoinositide-independent mechanism in cardiac cells. *J Biol Chem, 270*, 20432–20438.
281. Hannun, Y. A., & Bell, R. M. (1989). Functions of sphingolipids and sphingolipid breakdown products in cellular regulation. *Science, 243*, 500–507.
282. Lehtonen, J. Y., Horiuchi, M., Daviet, L., et al. (1999). Activation of the de novo biosynthesis of sphingolipids mediates angiotensin II type 2 receptor-induced apoptosis. *J Biol Chem, 274*, 16901–16906.
283. Gallinat, S., Busche, S., Schutze, S., et al. (1999). AT_2 receptor stimulation induces generation of ceramides in PC12W cells. *FEBS Lett, 443*, 75–79.
284. Wang, J., Zhen, L., Klug, M. G., et al. (2000). Involvement of caspase 3- and 8-like proteases in ceramide-induced apoptosis of cardiomyocytes. *J Card Fail, 6*, 243–249.
285. Gulbins, E. (2003). Regulation of death receptor signaling and apoptosis by ceramide. *Pharmacol Res, 47*, 393–399.
286. Schutze, S., Potthoff, K., Machleidt, T., et al. (1992). TNF activates NF-kappa B by phosphatidylcholine-specific phospholipase C-induced "acidic" sphingomyelin breakdown. *Cell, 71*, 765–776.
287. Johns, D. G., Osborn, H., & Webb, R. C. (1997). Ceramide: a novel cell signaling mechanism for vasodilation. *Biochem Biophys Res Commun, 237*, 95–97.
288. Johns, D. G., Webb, R. C., & Charpie, J. R. (2001). Impaired ceramide signalling in spontaneously hypertensive rat vascular smooth muscle: a possible mechanism for augmented cell proliferation. *J Hypertens, 19*, 63–70.
289. Charles, R., Sandirasegarane, L., Yun, J., et al. (2000). Ceramide-coated balloon catheters limit neointimal hyperplasia after stretch injury in carotid arteries. *Circ Res, 87*, 282–288.

CHAPTER 10

Activation of the Adrenergic Nervous System in Heart Failure

J. David Port, Carmen Sucharov, and Michael R. Bristow

In response to a variety of physiological and pathophysiological stresses, the need for increased cardiac myocardial performance is met by a commensurate increase in cardiac adrenergic drive. To facilitate this increase, norepinephrine (NE), the primary neurotransmitter of the adrenergic system, is released from sympathetic nerve endings in the heart. Upon binding to adrenergic receptors, multiple signaling pathways are activated resulting in increases in heart rate and force of contraction and relaxation, the result being an almost immediate increase in cardiac output. In the setting of acute heart failure, adrenergic activation initially occurs in response to hemodynamic overload and/or to an intrinsic reduction in pump function. However, in the setting of chronic heart failure, a response that is normally physiological and transient must instead be sustained in an attempt to maintain myocardial performance at a homeostatic level. Under these conditions, an initially beneficial mechanism becomes maladaptive, contributing directly to the progressive natural history of heart failure.

In this chapter the long-term consequences of sustained adrenergic activation in the context of chronic heart failure (CHF) will be reviewed. Particular emphasis will be placed on the alterations in β-adrenergic signal transduction and gene expression patterns that occur in the failing human heart and the impact of these changes on myocardial disease progression. Adrenergic receptor pharmacology relevant to heart failure and recent data from transgenic animals and model systems that demonstrate the myopathic potential of individual components of the adrenergic signaling cascade will also be reviewed.

ROLE OF INCREASED ADRENERGIC DRIVE IN THE NATURAL HISTORY OF HEART FAILURE

In patients with CHF, the adrenergic nervous system is critical to the support of myocardial function. However, its chronic activation contributes concomitantly to progressive myocardial dysfunction. Regardless of cause, an intrinsic decrease in myocardial function results in cardiac adrenergic nerves releasing more norepinephrine (NE).[1,2] This increase in adrenergic signaling activates β-adrenergic receptors (β-ARs), increasing the heart rate and myocardial contractile function. The increase in contractile function favorably affects both systolic and diastolic function and, through the Frank-Starling relationship, increases cardiac output. As heart failure worsens, adrenergic drive continues to increase in an attempt to compensate for the progressive loss of cardiac function[1] (Figure 10-1). Unfortunately, long-term exposure to high levels of NE has profound adverse effects on myocardial and cardiac myocyte biology, and on the β-AR signal transduction systems themselves.[3,4] Repercussions from these effects are further increases in adrenergic drive, progressive myocardial dysfunction, and worsening heart failure, a cycle requiring therapeutic intervention. Known inhibitors of adrenergic signaling that have demonstrated favorable effects on heart failure natural history include β-blocking agents (see chapter 46) and inhibitors of the renin-angiotensin system (see chapter 45), which indirectly lower adrenergic drive (Figure 10-2).

Although the "cardiotoxic" effects of catecholamines and, in particular, NE have been recognized for almost a century,[5] we are only just beginning to understand the detailed molecular mechanisms by which they occur. Treatment of isolated cardiac myocytes with concentrations of NE present in the failing human heart can cause dramatic changes in cell morphology, and, within a matter of days, up to a 60% loss of myocyte viability.[6] This effect can be mimicked by exposing myocytes to varying concentrations of the nonselective β-agonist isoproterenol, an effect that is inhibited pharmacologically by propranolol, suggesting that the acute toxic effects of NE are mediated almost exclusively through β-ARs rather than through α-ARs.[7]

Elevated plasma concentrations of NE are a well-recognized hallmark of CHF.[8,9] Cardiac NE stores, the increased release of which is stimulated in the early stages of heart failure, are eventually depleted as adrenergic activation persists.[10] Eventually, other tissue sources of catecholamines (i.e., the adrenal medulla) are also stimulated, leading to generalized sympathetic activation and spillover of cardiac-derived NE into the systemic circulation.[4,11] As plasma NE levels increase, so does mortality in patients with heart failure,[2,9,12] illustrating the profoundly injurious effects of excess adrenergic drive on the heart. These observations have been validated further by evidence from numerous clinical trials of β-blocker therapy, demonstrating enhanced systolic function and improved survival in patients with heart failure who receive β-blocker therapy long-term.[13-18] A recent realization is that insufficient adrenergic drive in individuals with CHF can also increase mortality.[13,19] More specifically, in contrast to β-blocking agents, sympatholytic agents can actually increase mortality, presumably via excessive withdrawal of adrenergic support to the failing heart. In contrast, β-blocking agents are pharmacologically reversible, mass-action agents, and in their presence, adrenergic support to the failing heart can be accessed if needed simply by increasing cardiac adrenergic drive.

Historical studies suggested that one underlying mechanism of NE toxicity involves cAMP-mediated increases in intracellular calcium.[6] More specifically, increased formation of the second messenger cAMP leads to activation of protein kinase A (PKA), which in turn phosphorylates a variety of target proteins involved in regulating intracellular calcium, including two key targets, phospholamban (PLB) and L-type calcium channels (Figure 10-3). Enhanced phosphorylation of calcium channels in turn leads to an increased flux of extracellular calcium into the cell-activating downstream effectors including proteases, kinases, and phosphatases. Activation of the β_1-AR subtype also appears to promote increased calcium influx via cAMP-independent mechanisms.[20] β_1-ARs are also cAMP-independent activators of calcium/calmodulin-dependent kinase II (CaMKII),[21,22] which, as described later, can be a particularly adverse signaling pathway in cardiac myocytes. Regardless of the exact mechanism(s) invoked, excessive β-AR stimulation results in oxidative stress and calcium overload, conditions promoting cell death through a number of mechanisms, including necrosis and apoptosis.

In addition to the effects described previously, long-term adrenergic activation has been shown to cause changes in the gene expression profile of cardiac myocytes, the canonical response being activation of the fetal gene program (see Chapter 2).[23,24]

In the failing heart, β-ARs and certain downstream effectors in the β-adrenergic signaling cascade undergo time-dependent downregulation and desensitization, presumably in an attempt to protect the heart from an excess of deleterious signaling. These changes result in a marked attenuation of the failing heart's ability to respond to catecholamines. In other words, the amount of cAMP that is generated in response to a given amount of adrenergic stimulation is significantly decreased in chronic heart failure. Evidence for this has been provided through experiments using isolated, denervated preparations of human heart tissue revealing that failing hearts have a reduced cAMP content compared with nonfailing controls.[25] From a clinical standpoint, reduced responsiveness to catecholamines translates into a decrease in myocardial reserve, which is most commonly manifested as an impaired ability to exercise. In more severe heart failure, reduced myocardial function as a result of β-AR desensitization may also be apparent at rest.

In summary, the role of increased adrenergic drive in the natural history of heart failure is a paradoxical one. On the one hand, adrenergic activation is essential to maintain myocardial function in the failing heart; on the other hand, chronic adrenergic stimulation is a major contributor to progressive myocardial dysfunction and remodeling that characterizes heart failure.

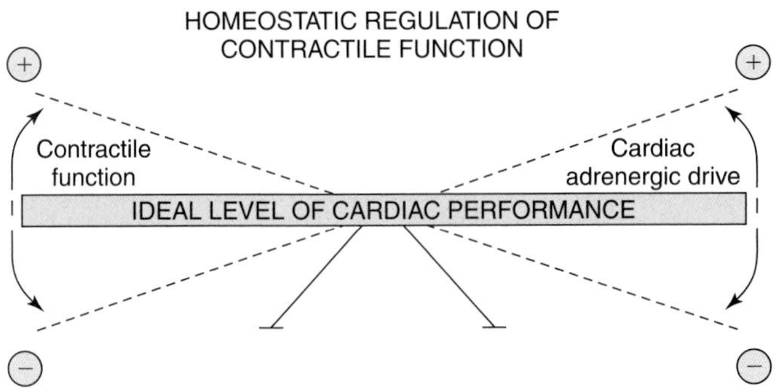

HOMEOSTATIC REGULATION OF CONTRACTILE FUNCTION

+ +

Contractile function

Cardiac adrenergic drive

IDEAL LEVEL OF CARDIAC PERFORMANCE

− −

FIGURE 10–1 Homeostatic regulation of contractile function. Adrenergic drive acts as a servo-control regulator of normal cardiac contractile function. When cardiac contractile function is adequate to sustain normal homeostasis, adrenergic drive is low or reduced. In contrast, when contractile function is inadequate to support homeostasis, cardiac adrenergic drive increases to a commensurate degree. (Adapted with permission from Port JD, Bristow MR. Altered β-adrenergic receptor gene regulation and signaling in chronic heart failure. *J Mol Cell Cardiol* 2001;33:887-905.)

ADRENERGIC RECEPTOR PHARMACOLOGY

As far back as the 1940s, Ahlquist et al[26] recognized that adrenergic receptors could be subdivided into two major classes, α-ARs and β-ARs, both of which are binding sites for the endogenous catecholamines: epinephrine and norepinephrine. In turn, each of these broad classes is subdivided further into a number of different receptor subtypes encoded by distinct gene products. Based on the groundbreaking work of Khorana et al,[27] subsequent work by Lefkowitz et al[28-30] described the molecular cloning of a number of G protein–coupled receptors, including the α- and β-ARs. More than any previous advance, this knowledge has permitted the analysis of adrenergic receptor biology in exquisite detail and allowed for an appreciation of the true complexity of adrenergic receptor signaling including the definition of a multitude of gene regulatory motifs and the recognition of highly organized multiprotein signaling complexes.

Relevant to the human heart, there are two major subclasses of α-ARs: α_1 and α_2. α_1-ARs, of which there are several subtypes,[31] are coupled to the Gq/G11-family of G proteins. The Gq pathway is linked to stimulation of phospholipase C (PL-C) that promotes phosphoinositide (PIP_2) turnover. The two primary products of this reaction are inositol triphosphate (IP_3), which stimulates the release of intracellular

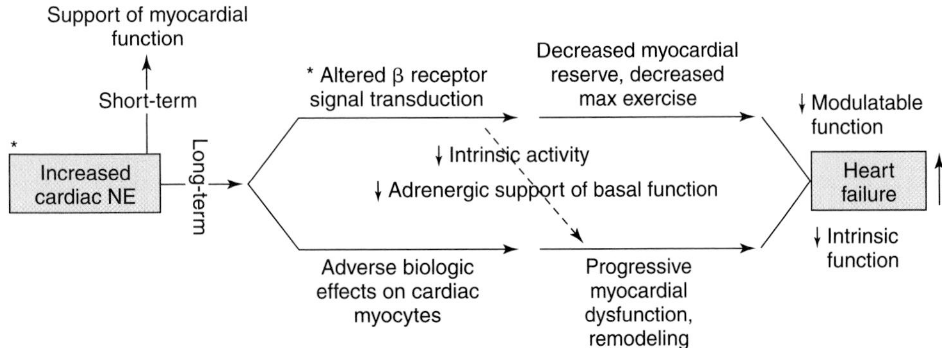

FIGURE 10–2 Role of increased adrenergic drive in the natural history of heart failure. A primary maladaptive response to chronic heart failure is a net increase in cardiac interstitial norepinephrine (NE) concentration, resulting from increased release and/or decreased reuptake. Increased NE results in a second maladaptive response to heart failure, that of altered β-AR signaling. These changes, in combination with the direct adverse biological effects of catecholamines, results in decreased myocardial reserve and progressive myocardial dysfunction, the ultimate result being decreases in both "modulatable" and intrinsic myocardial function.

calcium, and diacylglycerol (DAG), which stimulates protein kinase C (PKC) activity. Increases in intracellular calcium and PKC-mediated phosphorylation of target proteins both activate signaling pathways and gene expression patterns which, depending on the PKC subtype, ultimately result in a hypertrophic myocardial phenotype and vasoconstriction.[32] Examples of other Gq-coupled receptors whose stimulation also results in a hypertrophic phenotype are angiotensin II AT_1 receptors and endothelin-1 receptors. Each of these receptor pathways represents pharmacological targets central to the management of heart failure and/or its precursors, such as systemic or pulmonary hypertension.

In contrast to α_1-ARs, α_2-ARs are generally considered to be inhibitory presynaptic or prejunctional neuronal receptors functioning to suppress the release of NE. The potential importance of this function in the setting of heart failure has been contextualized by Small et al,[33] where a naturally occurring "loss-of-function" polymorphism of the α_{2c}-AR, when present in combination with a "gain-of-function" polymorphism of the β_1-AR, produces a significantly increased risk of heart failure in certain populations. These and other β-AR polymorphisms and their relevance to chronic heart failure are discussed in greater detail later.

β-ARs are also subdivided, with three distinct receptor subtypes—β_1-, β_2-, and β_3-ARs—having been described first by pharmacological response[34,35] and then by molecular cloning.[28,29,36] β_3-ARs are generally associated with regulation of metabolic rate and, to a much lesser degree, with changes in cardiac contractility. In distinct contrast, β_1- and β_2-ARs have clear functional significance to myocardial performance, and both are expressed at a significant abundance in the human heart.[37-39] The biochemical and pharmacological differences between these two receptors have been investigated extensively. Pharmacologically, β_1- and β_2-ARs, which respond equally well to the full agonist isoproterenol, are distinguished primarily by their affinity for NE (β_1-AR has a tenfold to thirtyfold greater affinity than β_2-AR),[35,40] and, more distinctly, by the relative affinity of highly selective receptor antagonists. In the context of heart failure, the most clinically relevant compounds distinguishing these receptors are the β_1-AR-selective antagonists metoprolol and bisoprolol. Additional functional and biochemical differences in β_1- and β_2-AR signaling are discussed in detail later.

ALTERED β-AR SIGNAL TRANSDUCTION IN THE FAILING HEART

Downregulation and desensitization of β-AR receptor signaling are major contributing factors in the contractile dysfunction of the failing human heart.[38] In response to heightened adrenergic activation, alterations in gene expression and/or catalytic activity have been demonstrated to occur at a number of levels including that of β_1- and β_2-ARs themselves,[37,38,41,42] the inhibitory G protein (Gi),[43] the effector enzyme, adenylyl cyclase,[44] and the regulatory enzyme, β-adrenergic receptor kinase (β-ARK1, also known as GRK2).[45] In the nonfailing, nonaged human heart, β_1-ARs constitute approximately 70% to 80% of all β-ARs. However, in individuals with heart failure, the β_1-AR is selectively downregulated, resulting in an approximate 60:40 ratio of β_1- to β_2-ARs.[38,41,46] In the failing heart, both receptor subtypes are distinctly uncoupled from their signaling pathways, as has been made evident in the clinical setting, by the increased concentrations of the minimally β_1-AR-selective agonist (dobutamine) necessary to evoke a stimulatory response.[47] These effects are due to downregulation of the β_1-AR but more generally to receptor desensitization secondary to phosphorylation of both receptor subtypes by specific kinases (Figure 10-4). The most relevant of these kinases are members of the GRK family, specifically GRK2 (β-ARK1), which phosphorylates both receptor subtypes in an agonist occupancy-dependent manner,[48] and GRK5,[49] a kinase of considerable importance linking β_1-ARs to epidermal growth factor receptor (EGFR) transactivation and cardioprotective effects.[50,51] β-ARs can also be phosphorylated and desensitized by other kinases including PKA and PKC.[52]

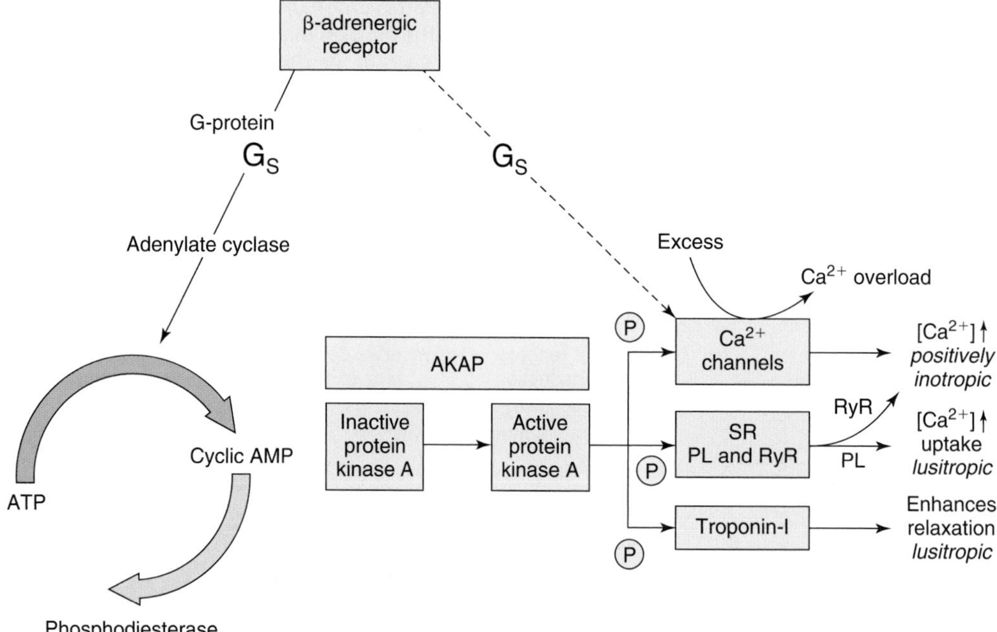

FIGURE 10-3 Key role of protein kinase A in the β-adrenergic response. The major intracellular effects of β-agonist catecholamines are by formation of cyclic AMP, which increases the activity of the cAMP-dependent protein kinase A (PKA). The latter achieves its optimal intracellular site by localizing to the scaffolding protein, A-Kinase Anchoring Protein (AKAP), whereupon PKA phosphorylates various proteins concerned with contraction and relaxation. *SR,* sarcoplasmic reticulum; *PL,* phospholamban; *RyR,* ryanodine receptor. (From Opie LH. *Heart physiology, from cell to circulation,* Philadelphia, 2004, Lippincott Williams & Wilkins. Figure copyright LH Opie, 2004; and Opie LH. Mechanisms of cardiac contraction and relaxation. In Libby P, Bonow RO, Mann DL, et al, editors. *Braunwald's heart disease,* Philadelphia, 2008, Elsevier.)

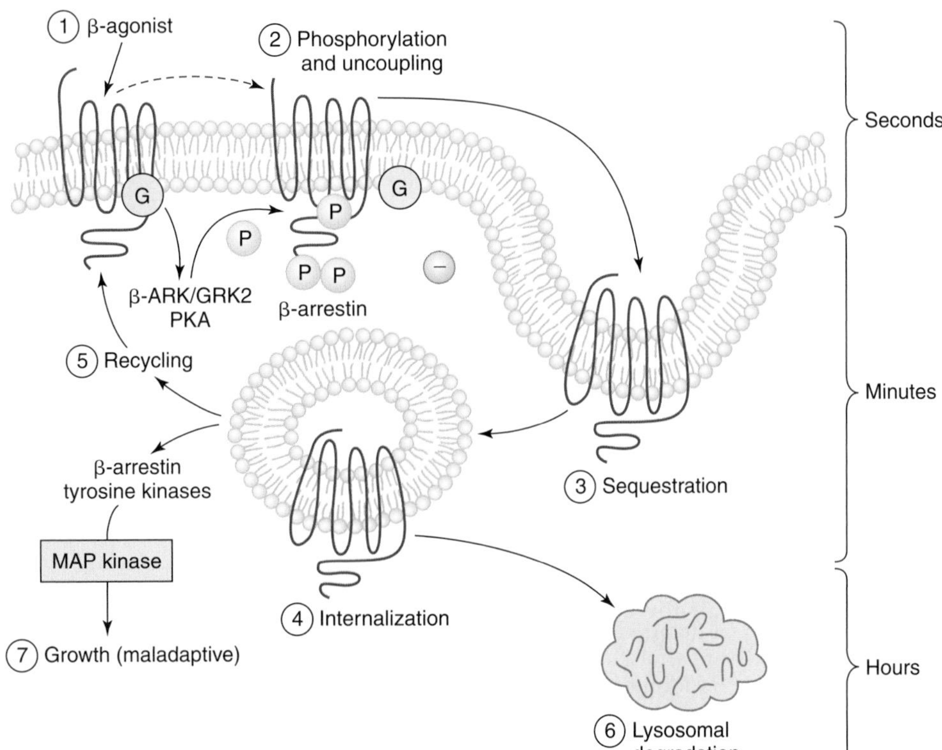

FIGURE 10–4 Mechanisms of β-adrenergic receptor desensitization and internalization. Note links between the internalized receptor complex with growth stimulation via mitogen-activated protein (MAP) kinase. *β-ARK, GRK2,* β-agonist receptor kinase or G-coupled receptor kinase; *PKA,* protein kinase A. (Modified from Hein L, Kobilka BK. Adrenergic receptors. From molecular structures to in vivo function. *Trends Cardiovasc Med* 1997;7:137-145; and Opie LH. Mechanisms of cardiac contraction and relaxation. In Libby P, Bonow RO, Mann DL, et al, editors. *Braunwald's heart disease*, Philadelphia, 2008, Elsevier.)

The major consequence of β-AR downregulation and desensitization is that for a given level of adrenergic activation, less of the second messenger cAMP is produced. Decreased formation of cAMP, in turn, leads to diminished activation of PKA. However, decreased PKA activity does not necessarily translate into decreased phosphorylation of all putative PKA substrates in the failing heart. Two of the more noteworthy targets are (a) the cardiac ryanodine receptor (RyR), a calcium release channel localized to the sarcoplasmic reticulum (SR); and the target of calcium-induced calcium release initiated by L-type calcium channels, and b) phospholamban (PLB), a small pentapeptide negative regulator of the sarcoplasmic reticulum (SR) ATP-dependent Ca^{++} pump, SERCA2. Related to the previous discussion, although PKA activity is decreased in heart failure, cardiac RyR2s have been shown to be hyperphosphorylated.[53] The net phosphorylation "state" of the RyR and PLB, and thus their activities, is due to the balance between kinase and phosphatase activities and other constituents of their respective intracellular microdomains, such as phosphodiesterases. Specifically, there is evidence for the downregulation of phosphatases (PP1 and PP2A) associated with the RyR2 and to changes in PKA activity.[53-55] Alternatively, recent studies have shown that RyR2 can be phosphorylated by CaMKII,[56-58] an activity that is in fact increased in the failing heart. Similarly, and perhaps counterintuitively, PKA-mediated phosphorylation of PLB appears to be unchanged in CHF.[25] However, PLB phosphorylation appears to be decreased in the failing heart, presumably due to the activation of the phosphatase, PP1,[59] which in a complex regulatory paradigm is regulated by protein phosphatase inhibitor I, PPI-1, a protein whose abundance is itself downregulated in heart failure.[60-62] The reduced phospholamban phosphorylation results in a greater inhibition of SERCA II, resulting in an impaired ability of the heart to relax.[63] In contrast, hyperphosphorylation of the RyR results in defective channel function during excitation-contraction coupling (see chapter 3).[64] Together, these changes result in decreased contractility in response to adrenergic stimulation.

Substantial evidence from model systems points to significant differences between β_1- and β_2-ARs and their ability to stimulate apoptosis in cardiomyocytes[7,65] with stimulation of the β_1- but not the β_2-AR pathway, resulting in an increased rate of cardiomyocyte apoptosis.[7] However, disruption of β_2-AR coupling to Gi by treatment with pertussis toxin can abrogate the potential protective, antiapoptotic signaling pathways rendering the β_2-AR pro-apoptotic.[66] Chesley et al,[67] have provided evidence to support the supposition that the antiapoptotic effects of β_2-AR are mediated in part by the stimulation of the PI3K and the Akt-PKD pathways.

In addition to the mechanisms described previously, the proapoptotic effect of the β_1-AR pathway may also be due to increased CaMKII activity. Zhu et al[68] have shown that β_1-AR stimulation results in myocyte apoptosis that is independent of PKA activation, but dependent on CaMKII activation, suggesting that β_1-AR stimulation may selectively result in CaMKII activation independent of effects on PKA. These studies demonstrate that inhibition of CaMKII, L-type calcium channel phosphorylation, or buffering of intracellular Ca^{2+}, results in an attenuation of β_1-AR-mediated apoptosis; conversely, overexpression of CaMKIIδ_c induces apoptosis. More recently, Yoo et al,[22] using transgenic mice with knockouts of β-AR subtypes, have demonstrated convincingly that postinfarct, isoproterenol-mediated increases in CaMKII signaling and apoptosis are dependent on the β_1-AR only.

In addition to mediating cardiac myocyte apoptotic effects, excessive β_1-AR signaling also activates the fetal gene program.[21,24] The change in myosin heavy chain isoform expression (see Chapter 2) to favor the lower ATPase activity, slow

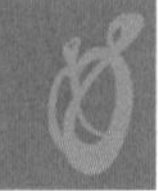

contracting β-isoform would be expected to decrease contractile function, as would the downregulation in SERCA II, another adult gene that is considered part of the adult-fetal program. Although the signaling cascades responsible for this activation are complex, CaMKII appears to play a prominent role,[21] and the altered expression of so-called fetal and adult genes is mediated by β_1- and not β_2-AR stimulation.[21,24] CaMKII activity is upregulated in the failing human heart,[69,70] suggesting that despite the desensitization that occurs in more proximal β_1-receptor signaling steps, adverse signaling through CaMKII may be maintained or even enhanced.

MOLECULAR BASIS OF β-ADRENERGIC RECEPTOR SIGNALING

Canonically, β_1- and the β_2-ARs couple to stimulatory G proteins, Gs, which are composed of two subunits, an α subunit, and a βγ-heterodimeric subunit, (Figure 10-5). Both the α and βγ subunits are competent to signal independently. Gαs is a member of the much larger class of G protein α subunits, of which there are approximately 20 subtypes. Their heterogeneity is a central basis of specificity for G protein–coupled receptor signaling, a subject reviewed in detail elsewhere.[71] Additional layers of signaling diversity are afforded by combinatorial permutations of various βγ-heterodimeric subunits (5 β-subtypes and 11 γ-subtypes) with the α subunits.

As a result of agonist stimulation, G protein α and βγ subunits dissociate with the free αs subunit acting to stimulate adenylyl cyclases (AC), for which there are multiple isoforms.[72] In cardiac tissues, the most abundant isoforms are AC V and VI, with the activities of each being feedback inhibited by increases in cytosolic calcium. Adenylyl cyclase stimulation increases production of cAMP, which in turn binds to the regulatory subunits of PKA heterotetramer. Binding causes the dissociation of the regulatory and catalytic subunits of PKA, with the catalytic subunits proceeding to phosphorylate consensus serine (S) and threonine (T) residues on a broad spectrum of intracellular target proteins.

In a number of tissues including cardiac, PKA and its targets are in close approximation because of A-kinase anchoring proteins or AKAPs.[73] An association between the β_2-AR and AKAP79 has been described.[74,75] Additionally, there is recent clarity as to the scaffolding proteins that interact with β_1-ARs in cardiac tissues.[76] Thus unique interactions between β_1- and β_2-ARs and specific AKAPs and/or other anchoring proteins would support the building "microdomain" concept of receptor subtype-specific signaling discussed in greater detail later.

Via the traditional Gαs/adenylyl cyclase pathway, β-AR stimulation results in the phosphorylation by PKA of a number of proteins including L-type calcium channels[75] and PLB, the primary modulator of the SR-associated ATP-dependent calcium pump, SERCA II, and modulatory proteins associated with regulation of the contractile apparatus (e.g., troponin I [TnI]). More directly, however, PKA phosphorylates β-ARs,[77] and other G protein–coupled receptors, resulting in partial uncoupling and desensitization of receptors to further agonist stimulation. Changes in the phosphorylation state of L-type calcium channels and PLB uniformly results in increased $[Ca^{++}]i$ and enhanced rates of myocardial contractility and relaxation. However, the increases in intracellular calcium have a number of other effects beyond enhanced contractility including the activation of calcium sensitive enzymes (e.g., Ca^{++}/calmodulin and calcineurin [phosphatase PP2B]).[78] On a more global level, changes in $[Ca^{++}]i$ can result in profound changes in gene expression patterns.

Various studies suggest that CaMKII may be involved in many of the detrimental effects of chronic β_1-AR stimulation. In support of this view, a transgenic mouse model of CaMKII inhibition was developed.[79] These mice express an inhibitory

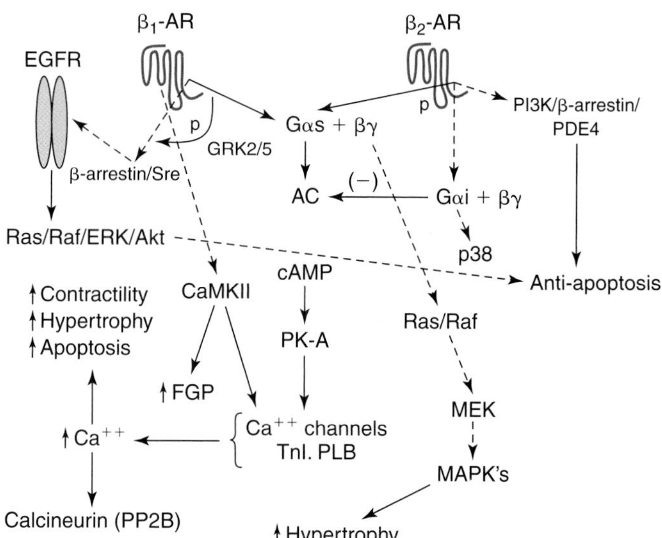

FIGURE 10–5 Signal transduction pathways stimulated by β-ARs. Canonically, both β_1- and β_2-ARs signal via the stimulatory G protein, Gαs, to stimulate adenylyl cyclase (AC) activity, increasing cAMP production and activating PKA. Downstream targets of PKA include L-type Ca^{++} channels, contractile proteins (e.g., TnI), and the regulator of sarcoplasmic reticulum calcium uptake, phospholamban (PLB). Increased $[Ca^{++}]i$ results in increased contractility and, if persistent, apoptosis. The β_1-AR activates at least two other pathways: CaMKII and the epidermal growth factor receptor (EGFR). Increased CaMKII activity results in increased $[Ca^{++}]i$ and calcineurin phosphatase activity, which activates pro-hypertrophic transcription factors causing the reexpression of the fetal gene program (FGP); it also accelerates the rate of myocyte apoptosis. In contrast, β_1-AR mediated stimulation of the EGFR is a cardioprotective, antiapoptotic pathway. The β_2-AR can also couple to the inhibitory G protein, Gi, resulting in a direct inhibition of AC activity and activation of pro-hypertrophic MAPKs and antiapoptotic pathways. (Adapted with permission from Port JD, Bristow MR. Altered β-adrenergic receptor gene regulation and signaling in chronic heart failure. *J Mol Cell Cardiol* 2001;33:887-905.)

peptide targeted to a conserved region of the CaMKII regulatory domain. Mice expressing the inhibitory peptide are resistant to pathological changes related to β-AR stimulation, and do not exhibit decreases in fractional shortening, increases in heart/body weight, or decreases in left ventricular (LV) internal diameter. Moreover, results in single cell experiments and *in vivo* models indicate that CaMKII can serve as a proarrhythmic signaling molecule.[80] These results suggest that the pathological effects of β_1-AR stimulation are mediated by CaMKII and not by PKA.

For some time, β_1- and β_2-ARs have been known to differ in the efficacy of coupling to adenylyl cyclase and to cAMP production, with the β_2-AR subtype being more efficiently coupled to cAMP production than is the β_1-AR.[39] In trabeculae isolated from the human heart, selective stimulation of contraction by either receptor pathway generally correlates well with receptor abundance.[38,81] Thus the fact that the β_2-AR produces more cAMP per unit of stimulus does not correlate with a greater inotropic potential for β_2-ARs. Overall, these data favor an argument that there is distinct intracellular compartmentalization of cAMP pools produced by β-ARs,[82] with the existence of discrete microdomains of high cAMP concentration in cardiomyocytes. Specifically, in neonatal cardiomyocytes, high concentrations of cAMP are found in the proximity of T tubules and the junctional SR. An argument is also made that diffusion of cAMP outside of these microdomains is quickly curtailed by the action of phosphodiesterases. Support for this notion is the finding that there appears to be close coordination between agonist-stimulated recruitment of phosphodiesterases to the β_2-AR, a process facilitated by interaction with β-arrestins, and the attenuation of signaling. Recent data indicates that the differential signaling and architecture of β_1- and β_2-ARs appears to be defined in part by a differential association with phosphodiesterases

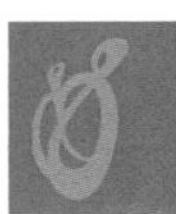

(PDEs),[83] with PDE4 activity preferentially targeting cAMP produced by the β_1-AR, whereas cAMP produced by the β_2-AR is being targeted by multiple subtypes of PDEs.[84] Perhaps counterintuitive to the highly localized responses of β-ARs being dictated by scaffolding proteins is the recent study by Nikolaev et al[84] demonstrating in transgenic mice that isoproterenol-mediated increases in cAMP in cardiac tissues leads to "far-reaching" cAMP signals for the β_1-AR, whereas β_2-AR- generated cAMP appears to remain locally confined.

It is becoming increasingly clear that both the β_1-AR and the β_2-AR pathways couple to signaling pathways beyond the "traditional" Gαs/adenylyl cyclase pathway.[85] Perhaps the best example of this diversity of signaling is the finding that the β_2-AR can interact with the inhibitory G protein, Gαi. This is of interest in the setting of CHF for two reasons. As described earlier, increased circulating NE concentrations result in chronic activation of β-ARs. This, in turn, results in increased β-ARK activity and an increased phosphorylation state of β-ARs, resulting ultimately in the uncoupling of the receptor from the stimulatory Gαs signaling pathway. It is this phosphorylated form of the β_2-AR that has an increased propensity to couple to the inhibitory Gαi pathway[86] and its downstream effectors, including inhibition of AC and activation of MAPKs. Amplifying this effect is the finding that the abundance of Gαi proteins is significantly elevated in the failing human heart.[87] Thus the increased phosphorylation state of the β_2-AR and the increased abundance of Gαi protein both facilitate increased trafficking of β_2-AR signaling via Gαi-associated pathways. The ramifications of this are potentially significant, particularly in regard to protective, antiapoptotic effects and to myocardial growth regulatory effects.

The β_1-AR, although currently thought to be less promiscuous than the β_2-AR in its ability to couple to pathways other than to Gαs, nonetheless does exhibit signaling via additional pathways, in particular the CaMKII pathway. At least in part, this extra-Gαs coupling, much like that of the β_2-AR, appears to be facilitated by the specificity of the carboxy-terminus PDZ (PSD-95/Dlg/ZO-1) domain of the receptor peptide, which drives the interaction with proteins containing specific PDZ recognition motifs. An excellent review on the general topic of regulation of β-AR signaling by scaffolding proteins has been published by Hall and Lefkowitz.[88] Examples of β_1-AR interacting proteins are PSD-95, MAGI-2, the endophilins (SH3p4/p8/p13), and CNrasGEF, all of which appear to have unique downstream roles. The association of the β_1-AR with PSD-95, which is a neuronal-associated protein, distinctly places the β_1-AR in the proximity of the synapse,[89] a location perhaps even driven by sympathetic innervation. Here, PSD-95 appears to inhibit the internalization of the β_1-AR,[90] an effect that is modulated by the kinase GRK5. Conversely, interaction of the β_1-AR with endophilins appears to negatively modulate Gαs coupling and to promote β_1-AR internalization.[91] Recently, a more detailed picture of the β_1-AR SAP97-AKAP79 scaffold at its PSD-95/DLG/ZO1 motif has been demonstrated to be necessary for both PKA-mediated phosphorylation of the β_1-AR and for receptor recycling.[76] This is in contrast to the findings describing the association of the β_1-AR with CNrasGEF (PDZ-GEF1), an effector molecule that activates Ras, and thus growth pathways. In this case, the mechanism of Ras activation is rather unique given that it appears to be via Gαs rather than the well-documented Gβγ signaling pathway (see Figure 10-3).

Additional evidence for the importance of PDZ-mediated interactions has been described by Xiang et al.[92] Specifically, mutation of the PDZ motif by disruption of the carboxy-terminus renders the β_1-AR significantly more sensitive to agonist-mediated cell surface downregulation. Further, this deletion of C-terminal amino acids renders the β_1-AR more β_2-AR-like in that it becomes capable of interacting with Gi. Thus, even though the β_1-AR[90] and β_2-AR[93] both contain PDZ motifs, the interacting proteins that each couple via these motifs are unique and are important basis of different regulatory and signaling properties. To expand this concept, the β_2-AR has been shown to modulate signaling independent of its interactions with G proteins. For example, the β_2-AR appears to couple to at least three other pathways: (1) NHERF, which in turn regulates the function of the Na^+/H^+ exchanger; (2) to a non-PKA-dependent interaction with L-type calcium channels[20,85]; and (3) the phosphatidylinositol 3′-kinase pathway (PI3K), a pathway associated with the inhibition of apoptosis,[94] and to the PI3K-PTEN pathway, which is relevant to the regulation of both myocardial contractility and cell size and shape.[95]

As alluded to previously, β-AR stimulation results in the dissociation of the stimulatory G protein, Gs, into α and βγ subunits, each of which are signaling entities. A major function of the βγ heterodimer is to recruit β-ARKs in proximity to the receptor. By virtue of the lipid-modified (isoprenylation) of the γ subunit, which promotes localization of the βγ subunit to the sarcolemmal membrane, the heterodimer is in position to orchestrate the colocalization of the β-AR with β-ARK. Protein/protein interaction of the βγ subunit with β-ARK occurs via a pleckstrin homology (PH) domain.[96] In this way, agonist-dependent β-ARK-mediated phosphorylation of β-ARs is the dominant mode of β-AR desensitization.[48] In addition to playing a scaffolding role, βγ subunits are also signaling molecules in their own right. Downstream targets of signaling include subsets of adenylyl cyclases, PI3K, K^+ channels, and Ras/Raf/MEK/MAPK pathway(s) (see Figure 10-3).

Recently, significant attention has been paid to the specifics of β-AR localization and receptor trafficking. Differential targeting of β-AR subtypes to specific intracellular compartments has been described.[97] Of note is the apparent caveolar colocalization of the β_2-ARs with the inhibitory protein, Gαi, and with PKA subunits and with GRK2. What is now becoming clear is that the localization of the β_2-AR to the caveolar compartment is an essential component of its signaling capabilities.[98] In contrast, β_1-ARs, and a number of other proteins including Gαs, and ACs V and VI, are not specifically associated with caveolea; instead, these proteins have a more generalized distribution.

Although there is no doubt that constitutive stimulation of the β_1-AR can cause significant myocardial damage, an important and newly emergent concept of β-AR signaling is that of the connection between β_1-AR signaling with the cardioprotective effects of the epidermal growth factor receptor (EGFR) pathway. Work from Rockman et al[50,51,99] has shown that GRK5/6-mediated phosphorylation of the β_1-AR targets the association of β-arrestin to the receptor, which, in addition to activating MAP kinases, facilitates the activation of matrix metalloproteinases, causing the release of heparin-bound EGF which then activates the EGFR. Activation of the EGFR leads to activation of Ras/Raf/ERK/Akt and subsequent antiapoptotic, cardioprotective effects (see Figure 10-5).

REGULATION OF β-AR GENE EXPRESSION

Genes encoding β-ARs are regulated at virtually every level, including transcriptional and posttranscriptional regulation, as well as translational and posttranslational regulation. Much like protooncogenes and cytokines, β-ARs can profoundly affect a number of cellular functions affecting cell viability, thus the need for stringent, rapid, and redundant regulatory mechanisms. β-AR expression, at both the level of mRNA and protein, is the result of a number of independently regulated processes.

At the level of transcriptional regulation, both positive and negative transcriptional regulatory elements exist within the 5′-untranslated regions (UTRs) of β-ARs. Cell culture model systems have provided significant evidence regarding the effects of a number of transcriptional regulatory pathways, starting with the most obvious, that of the direct effects of β-AR stimulation. Increases in cAMP can lead to a transient upregulation of β-AR mRNA via a cAMP-responsive element (CRE)-mediated transcriptional effect. However, it is recognized that in heart failure, at least for the β_1-AR, mRNA and protein are unequivocally downregulated.[41] Therefore, CRE-mediated upregulatory effects are unlikely to be important in the chronic setting. Conversely, β-AR genes have the potential to be negatively regulated by the transcriptional suppressor, ICER (inducible cAMP early repressor). Recent evidence points to a role for ICER in a pathophysiological feedback loop with its upregulation causing a persistent downregulation of PDE3A, a finding associated with increased isoproterenol-mediated cardiomyocyte apoptosis.[100]

In the cardiac context, a number of other transcriptional regulators of β-AR genes are also known to be important. Most notably, transcriptional regulation of β-AR genes by glucocorticoid-and thyroid hormone–responsive elements can have significant effects via their respective consensus DNA binding elements (e.g., GREs and TREs).[101,102] In general, glucocorticoids have been associated with causing an upregulation of β_2-ARs and a reciprocal downregulation of β_1-ARs,[101,103] whereas thyroid hormone has been uniformly associated with upregulation of β-AR expression.[102]

It is currently well recognized that like a number of protooncogenes, cytokines, and a number of other G protein–coupled receptors, β-ARs undergo posttranscription regulation at the level of mRNA stability. For β-ARs expressed in myocardial tissues, the relationship between mRNA and protein appears to be well preserved.[104] Thus mechanisms regulating β-AR mRNA abundance likely impacts β-AR protein expression. To this end, nucleic acid motifs known as A+U-rich elements (AREs), found within the 3′UTRs of several β-ARs, are known to be the target for a number of mRNA-binding proteins associated with changes in mRNA turnover. Previous evidence has confirmed a relationship between agonist-mediated stimulation of β-ARs, production of cAMP, and destabilization of β-AR mRNA, resulting in reduced mRNA and ultimately protein abundance.[105] Increasing evidence points to the role of MAPK pathways as critical regulators of the stability of ARE containing mRNAs including those encoding β-ARs.[106] In particular, several proteins associated with mRNA changes in mRNA turnover have been demonstrated to bind to β-AR AREs. These include AUF1/hnRNP D, which is associated with increased mRNA turnover[107,108]; HuR, which is associated with stabilization of numerous ARE containing mRNAs[109]; KSRP, which increases turnover of ARE containing mRNAs, drives muscle cell differentiation and modulates Wnt/β-catenin and PI3K/Akt signaling[110]; and tristetraprolin (TTP), which is associated with turnover of TNF-α mRNA.[111] How each of these proteins specifically affects β-AR mRNA turnover in the myocardial tissues remains to be explored. However, given the evidence that the homozygous deletion of TTP in transgenic mice results in a dramatic upregulation of TNF-α and a subsequence cardiomyopathy,[112] there is little doubt that these mechanisms are in play.

MYOPATHIC POTENTIAL OF INDIVIDUAL COMPONENTS OF ADRENERGIC RECEPTOR PATHWAYS

The development and study of transgenic animal models has provided a wealth of information with regard to understanding the role of adrenergic receptor signaling in CHF. This section will summarize a few of the more relevant findings obtained from animal models containing cardiac-targeted overexpression or deletion of various components of adrenergic receptor pathways. The impact of these changes on the development or prevention of cardiomyopathy is discussed.

Adrenergic Receptors

The idea that significant differences exist between β_1- and β_2-AR signaling in the heart has been reinforced in recent years by data from a number of transgenic mouse models. One of the more notable initial observations was that overexpression of each receptor subtype can result in strikingly different cardiac phenotypes. As originally reported by Milano et al,[113] overexpression of the wild-type β_2-AR in mice, at relatively high abundance (~50- to 200-fold), was associated with increased basal AC activity, enhanced contractility, and elevated LV function. Interestingly, no pathology was apparent in animals up to 4 months of age. In a longer-term study, Liggett et al[114] reported comparable effects of increased β_2-AR on the myocardium (i.e., enhanced cardiac function from birth); however, this group also noted linear gene dose–dependence with regard to the development of cardiomyopathy. Animals expressing more than 60 times the background β-AR concentration maintained their hyperdynamic state for more than 1 year without an apparent increase in mortality. In contrast, overexpression of the β_2-AR at approximately 100-fold resulted in progressive cardiac enlargement, the development of heart failure, and premature death occurring at close to 1 year of age. At approximately 350 times the level of wild-type expression, the β_2-AR produced a cardiomyopathy, resulting in premature death in 50% of animals as early as week 25.[114]

Compared to the unusually high levels of β_2-AR expression required to produce myopathic results, wild-type β_1-AR overexpression at relatively low abundance (~twentyfold to fortyfold) can lead to markedly decreased contractility and LV function and increased hypertrophy and fibrosis, resulting in progressive myocardial failure and premature death.[115,116] The pathophysiological mechanism(s) responsible for the detrimental effects of β_1-AR overexpression in these animals are only partially understood. Chronic increases in PKA activity is likely to be a component of the pathology associated with β_1-AR overexpression as overexpression of the catalytic subunit of PKA is, in its own right, cardiomyopathic.[117] However, in the failing heart, cAMP abundance and, therefore, PKA activity is generally decreased.[25] Thus it is possible or perhaps even likely that β_1-AR-mediated CaMKII activity, which is increased in CHF, underlies the observed pathology.

Initial studies reported an increase in systolic function in young animals overexpressing the β_1-AR, with a progressive decline in LV function occurring with age.[115,116] Interestingly, this appears to occur before any structural alterations, such as fibrosis, which do not become apparent until at least 4 months, depending on the level of expression. In this same study, the mechanism of contractile dysfunction was found to involve impaired Ca^{2+} handling in cardiac myocytes, characterized by marked prolongation of intracellular Ca^{2+} transients. Subsequent examination of the expression levels of various sarcoplasmic reticulum (SR) proteins involved in Ca^{2+} release and uptake revealed a modest increase in the expression of SERCA protein in animals at 2 months of age, and increased phosphorylation of phospholamban at Ser16, a critical regulatory site, was also detected. Collectively, these results indicate that impaired Ca^{2+} handling is likely a major causal factor in producing early contractile dysfunction in β_1-AR overexpression, with these changes occurring before the appearance of mice interstitial fibrosis or other structural alterations.

It is worth noting that overexpression of genetic variants of the β_1-AR have different phenotypes. As described later, the gain-of-function Arg389 variant of the β_1-AR produced a much more marked and rapid cardiac pathology than does the Gly389 variant.[118]

Transgenic animal models that overexpress other adrenergic receptors have also been described. Overexpression of wild-type α_1-AR subtypes has been observed to cause increases in cardiac contractility,[119] with variable effects of hypertrophy present in an α_{1b}-AR model,[120] but not in an α_{1a}-AR model.[121] However, overexpression of the wild-type α_{1b}-AR, when coupled with chronic α_1-AR stimulation by phenylephrine, results in severe myocardial hypertrophy in conjunction with high levels of β-ARK1 activity and increased mortality.[122] Similarly, overexpression of a constitutively active mutant of the α_{1b}-AR has been shown to cause a mildly hypertrophic phenotype, with evidence of upregulation of hypertrophy-related genes and β-ARK1.[113] Thus overexpression of either α_1- or β_2-ARs, mimicking increased adrenergic drive, generally recapitulates the hypertrophic phenotype, but not necessarily the heart failure phenotype, evoked by high catecholamine concentrations. This conclusion is of course gene-dose dependent.

G Proteins and Adenylyl Cyclase

As described previously, the G proteins involved in adrenergic signaling are several, including Gs and Gi, which modulate AC activity, and Gq, which is linked to activation of PLC. Similar to that observed with the β-ARs, overexpression of each of these downstream signaling components results in a variety of cardiac phenotypes. Transgenic mice overexpressing wild-type Gαs have been described as having a chronically increased heart rate, enhanced chronotropic and inotropic responses to an agonist, altered β-AR density, and an increased frequency of cardiac arrhythmias.[123] Over time, myocardial performance in Gαs overexpressing animals declines, and LV dilation is observed. Likewise, myocyte hypertrophy, apoptosis, and fibrosis become evident with age, and animals die prematurely. In addition, there is evidence that overexpression of Gαs is associated with an increase in L-type Ca^{2+} currents, an effect which appears to be independent of cAMP and AC activation. From these data, it has been suggested that Gαs may directly regulate the activity of L-type calcium channels. Interestingly, much like transgenic models of β-AR overexpression,[118] the pathophysiological changes observed with Gαs overexpression can be prevented and survival improved through treatment with β-blockers.[124]

Transgenic mice that overexpress Gαq also exhibit a myopathic phenotype characterized by marked myocyte hypertrophy, increased expression of hypertrophy-related genes, and increased fibrosis, ultimately resulting in decreased myocardial contractility.[125] The mechanism of cardiomyopathy appears to involve, at least in part, cross regulation to β-AR signaling pathways by Gαq or its downstream effectors.[126] Mice that overexpress Gαq exhibit decreased AC activity in response to an agonist, which is apparently due to impaired functional coupling of β-ARs to AC, since β-AR density is unchanged when compared with wild-type expression levels. In addition, β-AR stimulation of L-type Ca^{2+} channels is depressed in Gαq overexpressors, and expression levels of Gi are increased, as is PKC activity. In this model, inhibition of Gαi unexpectedly caused sudden death, suggesting that the change in Gαi expression may be a compensatory mechanism to counteract other detrimental signaling caused by the Gq pathway.

Cardiac-targeted overexpression of a modified Gi-coupled receptor has been reported.[127] Mice that contain this modified receptor reportedly exhibited significant ventricular conduction delays, which can be attenuated by treatment with pertussis toxin, suggesting strongly a Gi-dependent mechanism. Moreover, these animals developed a pronounced dilated cardiomyopathy, resulting in death by 15 weeks of age. These results were the first to suggest a potential causal role for increased Gi signaling in the development and progression of heart failure,[127] and stand in distinction to the notion that the Gi pathway is simply protective, acting to abrogate the deleterious stimulatory effects of the Gαs pathway. In fact, overexpression of the carboxy-terminus of Gαi (GiCT), a peptide construct that inhibits Gi signaling, has been demonstrated to enhance apoptosis associated with ischemia.[128]

In contrast to the previous discussion, overexpression of more distal components of the Gs signaling pathways, specifically ACs V or VI, does not appear to cause any form of cardiomyopathy.[129] Agonist-stimulated AC activity is higher in this model, and basal and stimulated PKA activities are also increased; however, these effects translate into modestly enhanced inotropic, lusitropic, or chronotropic function. Further, no long-term histopathological sequelae or deleterious changes in cardiac function have been noted with AC overexpression.[129] Based on this profile, gene therapy trials using adenovirus-mediated gene transfer of adenylyl cyclases are under consideration.

ADRENERGIC RECEPTOR POLYMORPHISMS IN HEART FAILURE

It has become an accepted paradigm that polymorphisms of many genes, including a number of components of adrenergic receptor signaling pathways and the renin-angiotensin system, can markedly influence the progression of cardiovascular disease and/or response to individual therapeutic agents (see Chapter 42). Depending on the genetic variant and the endpoint assessed, variable response may be generalized either to a class of agents (i.e., β-blockers) or delimited to an individual agent.

In groundbreaking work performed in large part by Liggett et al, the polymorphic variants of α- and β-ARs have been demonstrated to have profound effects on not only receptor signaling and sensitivity to pharmacological agents but also to clinical outcomes. For more detailed information on the subject, several overviews of adrenergic receptor polymorphisms have been published.[130-132] As with many genes, a number of haplotypes have been described.[133,134] Further, allele frequencies and combinations of complex haplotypes are not uniform across ethnic and geographical populations.[130,133]

Of particular importance, two major polymorphic loci have been identified for the human β_1-AR gene: variations at nucleotides 145 and 1165 encode either a serine (Ser) or glycine (Gly) variant amino acid position 49 or a Gly or arginine (Arg) variant at amino acid position 389. Data indicate that the Gly49 variant is significantly more susceptible to agonist-induced downregulation than is the Ser49 variant,[135] even though the two variants do not appear to be different in terms of their ability to couple to stimulation of adenylyl cyclase and production of cAMP. In contrast, the Arg389 variant of the β_1-AR is much more efficiently coupled to adenylyl cyclase stimulation than is the Gly389 variant.[136] For historical reasons, the Gly389 variant has been considered to be the "wild-type" allele as it was the first to be cloned[29]; however, its frequency in the Caucasian and African American populations being approximately 0.27 and 0.42, respectively,[132,137] establishes the fact that it is not the most common allele.

As a follow-up to cell-based studies, transgenic mouse studies where the β_1-AR Arg389Gly-receptor variants have been overexpressed clearly demonstrate that Arg389 is markedly more pathological.[118] Additionally, Arg389 mice are more responsive to β-blocker therapy, a notion that fits with the increased function receptor variant being able to be pharmacologically suppressed to a greater degree.

Over the past several years, a number of clinical studies, almost exclusively retrospective, have attempted to correlate clinical outcome to the β_1-AR 389Arg/Gly genotype (see Chapter 42). An example of a study demonstrating differential efficacy for carvedilol in patients with β_1-AR 389Arg/Gly variants, the endpoint being increased ejection fraction, was recently published by Chen et al.[138] Conversely, Sehnert et al[139] recently demonstrated no effect of β_1-AR 389Arg/Gly variants on the clinical endpoint of transplant-free survival for heart failure patients receiving either carvedilol or metoprolol. However, Liggett et al demonstrated an effect of β_1-AR 389Arg/Gly variants on mortality and other endpoints for the investigational β-blocker, bucindolol.[140] Thus, for the mortality endpoint, a variable effect for the β_1-AR 389Arg/Gly polymorphism may be agent dependent. It is probably fair to say that the heterogeneity of outcome for this and other polymorphisms is due to a combination of variations in populations, including complex genetic traits, environmental factors, variable endpoints (e.g., EF% vs. mortality), cause of heart failure, and intent of the study (i.e., progression of disease vs. response to therapy).

Related to disease progression, a previous study by Small et al[33] investigated the potential synergism between β_1-AR and α_{2C}-AR polymorphisms and uncovered a significant increased risk of progression to heart failure, particularly in African American subjects, when the gain-of-function (increased signaling) Arg398 allele β_1-AR is present in conjunction with the loss of function (decreased inhibition of prejunctional NE release) α_{2C}-AR deletion allele.[33] What is of particular interest is that the β_1-AR Arg389 allele does not appear to be a risk factor in and of itself; however, its presence increases considerably the risk associated with the α_{2C}-AR deletion allele.

A number of polymorphisms have also been described for the human β_2-AR, the best characterized of which is the presence of either a threonine (Thr) or isoleucine (Ile) at amino acid position 164.[141] The allele frequency of the 164 Ile, minor allele is quite low (<5%), and only 5% of the population is heterozygous Thr/Ile. Remarkably, no homozygous Ile/Ile subjects have been identified, possibly because of the myocardial dysfunction associated with this loss-of-function polymorphism. Similar to the β_1-AR Arg389 variant, the Thr164 β_2-AR is much more efficiently coupled to adenylyl cyclase activation than is the Ile164 variant. The presence of the *Ile164* allele is associated with reduced exercise capacity and reduced transplant-free survival. In a transgenic mouse model system, overexpression of the human β_2-AR Ile164 leads to impaired cardiac function,[142] a finding that recapitulates the observation that this allele is associated with reduced exercise capacity and reduced survival in patients with heart failure.[143]

As described previously, one of the major regulators of β-AR signaling are the GRKs. Interestingly, a Gln>Leu41 variant of GRK5 has been shown to be protective against heart failure–associated death or transplantation in an African American population[144] where the *Leu* allele is approximately 20 times more frequent than in Caucasian populations. The authors speculate that the increased agonist-mediated uncoupling of the β-AR by GRK5-Leu41 is, in essence, the equivalent of "genetic β-blockade."[131,145]

There would seem a high likelihood that beyond what has already been described,[146] other polymorphic variants of adrenergic receptors, other G protein–coupled receptors, and any number of downstream effectors will eventually be described. A significant question that remains to be addressed is whether or not the presence of specific polymorphisms, alone or in combination, are primary factors in the predisposition to, or in the rate of progression of, heart failure.

SUMMARY

Adrenergic mechanisms are markedly altered in chronic heart failure, and these alterations exert major effects on the natural history of this clinical syndrome. Adrenergic abnormalities can be classified into two major groups: those that produce a sustained increase in adrenergic drive and those that cause defects in β-AR signal transduction. Within each category there is the potential for benefit and harm, and successful therapeutic intervention involves interfering with the harmful components without compromising the beneficial aspects.

It should be clear from the scope of this review that adrenergic receptor signaling is far more complex than our naïve supposition that the binding of catecholamines to receptors simply increases the abundance of the second messengers, cAMP and Ca^{++}, thereby affecting an increase in myocardial contractility and heart rate. Although the importance of these functions has not been diminished, adrenergic receptors are now recognized to be important effectors in any number of cellular processes important to cardiomyocyte biology. Undoubtedly, the diversity and complexity of these signaling paradigms will continue to unfold. It is hoped that an increased appreciation of these processes, and the recognition that genetic variation is important to both disease progression and to therapeutic response, will lead to advances in heart failure therapeutics.

REFERENCES

1. Rundqvist, B., Elam, M., Bergmann-Sverrisdottir, Y., et al. (1997). Increased cardiac adrenergic drive precedes generalized sympathetic activation in human heart failure. *Circulation, 95*(1), 169–175.
2. Esler, M., Kaye. D., Lambert, G., et al. (1997). Adrenergic nervous system in heart failure. *Am J Cardiol, 80*(11A), 7L–14L.
3. Eichhorn, E. J., & Bristow, M. R. (1996). Medical therapy can improve the biological properties of the chronically failing heart. A new era in the treatment of heart failure. *Circulation, 94*(9), 2285–2296.
4. Mann, D. L. (1998). Basic mechanisms of disease progression in the failing heart: the role of excessive adrenergic drive. *Prog Cardiovasc Dis, 41*(Suppl. 1), 1–8.
5. Ziegler, K. (1905). Uber die Wirkung intravenoser adrenalin-injektion auf das Gefafssystem und ihre Beziehung zur Arteriosklerose. *Beitr Pathol Anat, 38*, 229–254.
6. Mann, D., Kent, R., Parsons, B., et al. (1992). Adrenergic effects on the biology of the adult mammalian cardiocyte. *Circulation, 85*, 790–804.
7. Communal, C., Singh, K., Sawyer, D. B., et al. (1999). Opposing effects of beta(1)- and beta(2)-adrenergic receptors on cardiac myocyte apoptosis: role of a pertussis toxin-sensitive G protein. *Circulation, 100*(22), 2210–2212.
8. Swedberg, K., Viquerat, C., Rouleau, J. L., et al. (1984). Comparison of myocardial catecholamine balance in chronic congestive heart failure and in angina pectoris without failure. *Am J Cardiol, 54*, 783–786.
9. Cohn, J. N., Levine, T. B., & Olivari, M. T. (1984). Plasma norepinephrine as a guide to prognosis in patients with chronic congestive heart failure. *N Engl J Med, 311*, 819–823.
10. Chidsey, C. A., Braunwald, E., Morrow, A. G., et al. (1963). Myocardial norepinephrine concentrations in man: effects of reserpine and of congestive heart failure. *N Engl J Med, 269*, 653–659.
11. Hasking, G. J., Esler, M. D., Jennings, G. L., et al. (1986). Norepinephrine spillover to plasma in patients with congestive heart failure: evidence of increased overall and cardiorenal sympathetic nervous activity. *Circulation, 73*(4), 615–621.
12. Swedberg, K., Eneroth, P., Kjekshus, J., et al. (1990). Hormones regulating cardiovascular function in patients with severe congestive heart failure and their relation to mortality. CONSENSUS trial study group. *Circulation, 82*(5), 1730–1736.
13. BEST. (2001). A trial of the beta-blocker bucindolol in patients with advanced chronic heart failure. *N Engl J Med, 344*(22), 1659–1667.
14. CIBIS. (1994). A randomized trial of beta-blockade in heart failure. The cardiac insufficiency bisoprolol study (CIBIS). CIBIS investigators and committees. *Circulation, 90*(4), 1765–1773.
15. CIBISII. (1999). The cardiac insufficiency bisoprolol study II (CIBIS-II): a randomised trial (see comments). *Lancet, 353*(9146), 9–13.
16. MERIT. (1999). Effect of metoprolol CR/XL in chronic heart failure: metoprolol CR/XL randomised intervention trial in congestive heart failure (MERIT-HF) (see comments). *Lancet, 353*(9169), 2001–2007.
17. Packer, M., Bristow, M. R., Cohn, J. N., et al. (1996). The effect of carvedilol on morbidity and mortality in patients with chronic heart failure. U.S. carvedilol heart failure study group. *N Engl J Med, 334*(21), 1349–1355.
18. COPERNICUS Study Group. (2001). Primary results of COPERNICUS, a pivotal landmark study (carvedilol prospective randomised cumulative survival trial). *Cardiovasc J S Afr, 12*(1), 57.
19. Swedberg, K., Bergh, C. H., Dickstein, K., et al. (2000). The effects of moxonidine, a novel imidazoline, on plasma norepinephrine in patients with congestive heart failure. Moxonidine investigators. *J Am Coll Cardiol, 35*(2), 398–404.
20. Lader, A. S., Xiao, Y. F., Ishikawa, Y., et al. (1998). Cardiac Gsalpha overexpression enhances L-type calcium channels through an adenylyl cyclase independent pathway. *Proc Natl Acad Sci USA, 95*(16), 9669–9674.
21. Sucharov, C. C., Mariner, P. D., Nunley, K. R., et al. (2006). A beta1-adrenergic receptor CaM kinase II-dependent pathway mediates cardiac myocyte fetal gene induction. *Am J Physiol Heart Circ Physiol, 291*(3), H1299–H1308.

22. Yoo, B., Lemaire, A., Mangmool, S., et al. (2009). Beta1-adrenergic receptors stimulate cardiac contractility and CaMKII activation in vivo and enhance cardiac dysfunction following myocardial infarction. *Am J Physiol Heart Circ Physiol*, in press.
23. Tan, F. L., Moravec, C. S., Li, J., et al. (2002). The gene expression fingerprint of human heart failure. *Proc Natl Acad Sci U S A*, *99*(17), 11387–11392.
24. Lowes, B. D., Gilbert, E. M., Abraham, W. T., et al. (2002). Myocardial gene expression in dilated cardiomyopathy treated with beta-blocking agents. *N Engl J Med*, *346*(18), 1357–1365.
25. Bohm, M., Reiger, B., Schwinger, R. H., et al. (1994). cAMP concentrations, cAMP dependent protein kinase activity, and phospholamban in non-failing and failing myocardium. *Cardiovasc Res*, *28*(11), 1713–1719.
26. Ahlquist, R. (1948). A study of the adrenotropic receptors. *Am J Physiol*, *153*, 586–600.
27. Dunn, R., McCoy, J., Simsek, M., et al. (1981). The bacteriorhodopsin gene. *Proc Natl Acad Sci U S A*, *78*(11), 6744–6748.
28. Dixon, R. A., Kobilka, B. K., Strader, D. J., et al. (1986). Cloning of the gene and cDNA for mammalian beta-adrenergic receptor and homology with rhodopsin. *Nature*, *321*(6065), 75–79.
29. Frielle, T., Collins, S., Daniel, K. W., et al. (1987). Cloning of the cDNA for the human beta 1-adrenergic receptor. *Proc Natl Acad Sci U S A*, *84*(22), 7920–7924.
30. Cotecchia, S., Schwinn, D. A., Randall, R. R., et al. (1988). Molecular cloning and expression of the cDNA for the hamster alpha 1-adrenergic receptor. *Proc Natl Acad Sci U S A*, *85*(19), 7159–7163.
31. Rohde, S., Sabri, A., Kamasamudran, R., et al. (2000). The alpha(1)-adrenoceptor subtype- and protein kinase C isoform-dependence of norepinephrine's actions in cardiomyocytes. *J Mol Cell Cardiol*, *32*(7), 1193–1209.
32. Bowman, J. C., Steinberg, S. F., Jiang, T., et al. (1997). Expression of protein kinase Cb in the heart causes hypertrophy in adult mice and sudden death in neonates. *J Clin Invest*, *100*, 2189–2195.
33. Small, K. M., Wagoner, L. E., Levin, A. M., et al. (2002). Synergistic polymorphisms of (beta)1- and (alpha)2c-adrenergic receptors and the risk of congestive heart failure. *N Engl J Med*, *347*(15), 1135–1142.
34. Bristow, M., & Green, R. D. (1970). A quantitative study of beta-adrenergic receptors in rabbit atria. *Eur J Pharmacol*, *12*(1), 120–123.
35. Lands, A. M., Arnold, A., McAuliff, P., et al. (1967). Differentiation of receptor systems activated by sympathomimetic amines. *Nature*, *214*, 597–598.
36. Emorine, L. J., Marullo, S., Briend-Sutren, M. M., et al. (1989). Molecular characterization of the human beta 3-adrenergic receptor. *Science*, *245*(4922), 1118–1121.
37. Bristow, M. R. (1984). Myocardial beta-adrenergic receptor downregulation in heart failure. *Int J Cardiol*, *5*(5), 648–652.
38. Bristow, M. R., Ginsburg, R., Umans, V., et al. (1986). Beta 1- and beta 2-adrenergic-receptor subpopulations in nonfailing and failing human ventricular myocardium: coupling of both receptor subtypes to muscle contraction and selective beta 1-receptor down-regulation in heart failure. *Circ Res*, *59*(3), 297–309.
39. Bristow, M. R., Hershberger, R. E., Port, J. D., et al. (1989). Beta 1- and beta 2-adrenergic receptor-mediated adenylate cyclase stimulation in nonfailing and failing human ventricular myocardium. *Mol Pharmacol*, *35*(3), 295–303.
40. Bristow, M. R., Feldman, A. M., Adams, K. F., Jr., et al. (2003). Selective versus nonselective beta-blockade for heart failure therapy: are there lessons to be learned from the COMET trial? *J Card Fail*, *9*(6), 444–453.
41. Bristow, M., Durham, C., Klien, J., et al. (1991). Down-regulation of b-adrenergic receptors and receptor mRNA in heart cells chronically exposed to norepinephrine. *Clin Res*, *39*, 256A.
42. Bohm, M., & Lohse, M. J. (1994). Quantification of beta-adrenoceptors and beta-adrenoceptor kinase on protein and mRNA levels in heart failure. *Eur Heart J*, *15*(Suppl. D), 30–34.
43. Feldman, A. M., Cates, A. E., Veazey, W. B., et al. (1988). Increase of the 40,000-mol wt pertussis toxin substrate (G protein) in the failing human heart. *J Clin Invest*, *82*(1), 189–197.
44. Bristow, M. R., & Feldman, A. M. (1992). Changes in the receptor-G protein-adenylyl cyclase system in heart failure from various types of heart muscle disease. *Basic Res Cardiol*, *87*(Suppl 1), 15–35.
45. Benovic, J. L., Strasser, R. H., Caron, M. G., et al. (1986). Beta-adrenergic receptor kinase: identification of a novel protein kinase that phosphorylates the agonist-occupied form of the receptor. *Proc Natl Acad Sci U S A*, *83*(9), 2797–2801.
46. Bristow, M. R., Hershberger, R. E., Port, J. D., et al. (1990). Beta-adrenergic pathways in nonfailing and failing human ventricular myocardium. *Circulation*, *82*(Suppl 2), I12–I25.
47. Colucci, W. S. (1989). Observations on the intracoronary administration of milrinone and dobutamine to patients with congestive heart failure. *Am J Cardiol*, *63*(2), 17A–22A.
48. Pitcher, J. A., Freedman, N. J., & Lefkowitz, R. J. (1998). G protein-coupled receptor kinases. *Annu Rev Biochem*, *67*, 653–692.
49. Hu, L. A., Chen, W., Premont, R. T., et al. (2002). G protein-coupled receptor kinase 5 regulates beta 1-adrenergic receptor association with PSD-95. *J Biol Chem*, *277*(2), 1607–1613.
50. Noma, T., Lemaire, A., Naga Prasad, S. V., et al. (2007). Beta-arrestin-mediated beta1-adrenergic receptor transactivation of the EGFR confers cardioprotection. *J Clin Invest*, *117*(9), 2445–2558.
51. Tilley, D. G., Kim, I. M., Patel, P. A., et al. (2009). Beta-arrestin mediates beta1-adrenergic receptor-epidermal growth factor receptor interaction and downstream signaling. *J Biol Chem*, *284*(30), 20375–20386.
52. Hausdorff, W., Caron, M., & Lefkowitz, R. (1990). Turning off the signal: desensitization of b-adrenergic receptor function. *FASEB J*, *4*, 2881–2889.
53. Marx, S. O., Reiken, S., Hisamatsu, Y., et al. (2000). PKA phosphorylation dissociates FKBP12.6 from the calcium release channel (ryanodine receptor): defective regulation in failing hearts. *Cell*, *101*(4), 365–376.
54. Marks, A. R., Marx, S. O., & Reiken, S. (2002). Regulation of ryanodine receptors via macromolecular complexes: a novel role for leucine/isoleucine zippers. *Trends Cardiovasc Med*, *12*(4), 166–170.
55. Reiken, S., Gaburjakova, M., Guatimosim, S., et al. (2002). Protein kinase A phosphorylation of the cardiac calcium release channel (ryanodine receptor) in normal and failing hearts. Role of phosphatases and response to isoproterenol. *J Biol Chem*, *278*(1), 444–453.
56. Wehrens, X. H., Lehnart, S. E., Reiken, S. R., et al. (2004). Ca^{2+}/calmodulin-dependent protein kinase II phosphorylation regulates the cardiac ryanodine receptor. *Circ Res*, *94*(6), e61–e70.
57. Yang, D., Zhu, W. Z., Xiao, B., et al. (2007). Ca^{2+}/calmodulin kinase II-dependent phosphorylation of ryanodine receptors suppresses Ca^{2+} sparks and Ca^{2+} waves in cardiac myocytes. *Circ Res*, *100*(3), 399–407.
58. Ling, H., Zhang, T., Pereira, L., et al. (2009). Requirement for Ca^{2+}/calmodulin-dependent kinase II in the transition from pressure overload-induced cardiac hypertrophy to heart failure in mice. *J Clin Invest*, *119*(5), 1230–1240.
59. Schwinger, R. H., Munch, G., Bolck, B., et al. (1999). Reduced Ca(2+)-sensitivity of SERCA 2a in failing human myocardium due to reduced serine-16 phospholamban phosphorylation. *J Mol Cell Cardiol*, *31*(3), 479–491.
60. El-Armouche, A., Bednorz, A., Pamminger, T., et al. (2006). Role of calcineurin and protein phosphatase-2A in the regulation of phosphatase inhibitor-1 in cardiac myocytes. *Biochem Biophys Res Commun*, *346*(3), 700–706.
61. El-Armouche, A., Gocht, F., Jaeckel, E., et al. (2007). Long-term beta-adrenergic stimulation leads to downregulation of protein phosphatase inhibitor-1 in the heart. *Eur J Heart Fail*, *9*(11), 1077–1080.
62. Nicolaou, P., Hajjar, R. J., & Kranias, E. G. (2009). Role of protein phosphatase-1 inhibitor-1 in cardiac physiology and pathophysiology. *J Mol Cell Cardiol*, *47*(3), 365–371.
63. Koss, K. L., & Kranias, E. G. (1996). Phospholamban: a prominent regulator of myocardial contractility. *Circ Res*, *79*(6), 1059–1063.
64. Marks, A. R. (2001). Ryanodine receptors/calcium release channels in heart failure and sudden cardiac death. *J Mol Cell Cardiol*, *33*(4), 615–624.
65. Communal, C., Colucci, W. S., Remondino, A., et al. (2002). Reciprocal modulation of mitogen-activated protein kinases and mitogen-activated protein kinase phosphatase 1 and 2 in failing human myocardium. *J Card Fail*, *8*(2), 86–92.
66. Communal, C., Singh, K., & Colucci, W. (1998). Gi protein protects adult rat ventricular myocytes, from b-adrenergic receptor-stimulated apoptosis in vitro. *Circulation*, *98*(17), I-742.
67. Chesley, A., Lundberg, M. S., Asai, T., et al. (2000). The (beta)2-adrenergic receptor delivers an antiapoptotic signal to cardiac myocytes through gi-dependent coupling to phosphatidylinositol 3'-kinase. *Circ Res*, *87*(12), 1172–1179.
68. Zhu, W. Z., Wang, S. Q., Chakir, K., et al. (2003). Linkage of (beta)1-adrenergic stimulation to apoptotic heart cell death through protein kinase A-independent activation of Ca^{2+}/calmodulin kinase II. *J Clin Invest*, *111*(5), 617–625.
69. Kirchhefer, U., Schmitz, W., Scholz, H., et al. (1999). Activity of cAMP-dependent protein kinase and Ca 2+/calmodulin-dependent protein kinase in failing and nonfailing human hearts. *Cardiovasc Res*, *42*(1), 254–261.
70. Calalb, M. B., McKinsey, T. A., Newkirk, S., et al. (2009). Increased phosphorylation-dependent nuclear export of class II histone deacetylases in failing human heart. *Clin Transl Sci*, in press.
71. Morris, A. J., & Malbon, C. C. (1999). Physiological regulation of G protein-linked signaling. *Physiol Rev*, *79*(4), 1373–1430.
72. Defer, N., Best-Belpomme, M., & Hanoune, J. (2000). Tissue specificity and physiological relevance of various isoforms of adenylyl cyclase. *Am J Physiol*, *279*(3), F400–F416.
73. Colledge, M., & Scott, J. D. (1999). AKAPs: from structure to function. *Trends Cell Biol*, *9*(6), 216–221.
74. Fraser, I. D., Cong, M., Kim, J., et al. (2000). Assembly of an A kinase-anchoring protein-beta(2)-adrenergic receptor complex facilitates receptor phosphorylation and signaling. *Curr Biol*, *10*(7), 409–412.
75. Gao, T., Yatani, A., Dell'Acqua, M. L., et al. (1997). cAMP-dependent regulation of cardiac L-type Ca^{2+} channels requires membrane targeting of PKA and phosphorylation of channel subunits. *Neuron*, *19*(1), 185–196.
76. Gardner, L. A., Naren, A. P., & Bahouth, S. W. (2007). Assembly of an SAP97-AKAP79-cAMP-dependent protein kinase scaffold at the type 1 PSD-95/DLG/ZO1 motif of the human beta(1)-adrenergic receptor generates a receptosome involved in receptor recycling and networking. *J Biol Chem*, *282*(7), 5085–5099.
77. Benovic, J. L., Pike, L. J., Cerione, R. A., et al. (1985). Phosphorylation of the mammalian beta-adrenergic receptor by cyclic AMP-dependent protein kinase. Regulation of the rate of receptor phosphorylation and dephosphorylation by agonist occupancy and effects on coupling of the receptor to the stimulatory guanine nucleotide regulatory protein. *J Biol Chem*, *260*(11), 7094–7101.
78. Taigen, T., De Windt, L. J., Lim, H. W., et al. (2000). Targeted inhibition of calcineurin prevents agonist-induced cardiomyocyte hypertrophy. *Proc Natl Acad Sci U S A*, *97*(3), 1196–1201.
79. Zhang, R., Khoo, M. S., Wu, Y., et al. (2005). Calmodulin kinase II inhibition protects against structural heart disease. *Nat Med*, *11*(4), 409–417.
80. Maier, L. S., Bers, D. M., & Brown, J. H. (2007). Calmodulin and Ca^{2+}/calmodulin kinases in the heart—physiology and pathophysiology. *Cardiovasc Res*, *73*(4), 629–630.
81. Bristow, M. R., Anderson, F. L., Port, J. D., et al. (1991). Differences in beta-adrenergic neuroeffector mechanisms in ischemic versus idiopathic dilated cardiomyopathy. *Circulation*, *84*(3), 1024–1039.
82. Zaccolo, M., & Pozzan, T. (2002). Discrete microdomains with high concentration of cAMP in stimulated rat neonatal cardiac myocytes. *Science*, *295*(5560), 1711–1715.
83. Richter, W., Day, P., Agrawal, R., et al. (2008). Signaling from beta1- and beta2-adrenergic receptors is defined by differential interactions with PDE4. *EMBO J*, *27*(2), 384–393.
84. Nikolaev, V. O., Bunemann, M., Schmitteckert, E., et al. (2006). Cyclic AMP imaging in adult cardiac myocytes reveals far-reaching beta1-adrenergic but locally confined beta2-adrenergic receptor-mediated signaling. *Circ Res*, *99*(10), 1084–1091.
85. Steinberg, S. F. (1999). The molecular basis for distinct beta-adrenergic receptor subtype actions in cardiomyocytes. *Circ Res*, *85*(11), 1101–1111.

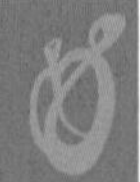

86. Daaka, Y., Luttrell, L. M., & Lefkowitz, R. J. (1997). Switching of the coupling of the beta2-adrenergic receptor to different G proteins by protein kinase A. *Nature, 390*(6655), 88–91.
87. Bohm, M., Gierschik, P., Jakobs, K. H., et al. (1990). Increase of Gi alpha in human hearts with dilated but not ischemic cardiomyopathy. *Circulation, 82*(4), 1249–1265.
88. Hall, R. A., & Lefkowitz, R. J. (2002). Regulation of G protein-coupled receptor signaling by scaffold proteins. *Circ Res, 91*(8), 672–680.
89. Shcherbakova, O. G., Hurt, C. M., Xiang, Y., et al. (2007). Organization of beta-adrenoceptor signaling compartments by sympathetic innervation of cardiac myocytes. *J Cell Biol, 176*(4), 521–533.
90. Hu, L. A., Tang, Y., Miller, W. E., et al. (2000). Beta 1-adrenergic receptor association with PSD-95. Inhibition of receptor internalization and facilitation of beta 1-adrenergic receptor interaction with N-methyl-D-aspartate receptors. *J Biol Chem, 275*(49), 38659–38666.
91. Tang, Y., Hu, L. A., Miller, W. E., et al. (1999). Identification of the endophilins (SH3p4/p8/p13) as novel binding partners for the beta1-adrenergic receptor. *Proc Natl Acad Sci U S A, 96*(22), 12559–12564.
92. Xiang, Y., Devic, E., & Kobilka, B. (2002). The PDZ binding motif of the beta 1 adrenergic receptor modulates receptor trafficking and signaling in cardiac myocytes. *J Biol Chem, 277*(37), 33783–33790.
93. Cao, T. T., Deacon, H. W., Reczek, D., et al. (1999). A kinase-regulated PDZ-domain interaction controls endocytic sorting of the beta2-adrenergic receptor. *Nature, 401*(6750), 286–290.
94. Hall, R. A., Premont, R. T., Chow, C. W., et al. (1998). The beta2-adrenergic receptor interacts with the Na^+/H^+-exchanger regulatory factor to control Na^+/H^+ exchange. *Nature, 392*(6676), 626–630.
95. Crackower, M. A., Oudit, G. Y., Kozieradzki, I., et al. (2002). Regulation of myocardial contractility and cell size by distinct PI3K-PTEN signaling pathways. *Cell, 110*(6), 737–749.
96. Pitcher, J. A., Touhara, K., Payne, E. S., et al. (1995). Pleckstrin homology domain-mediated membrane association and activation of the beta-adrenergic receptor kinase requires coordinate interaction with G beta gamma subunits and lipid. *J Biol Chem, 270*(20), 11707–11710.
97. Rybin, V. O., Xu, X., Lisanti, M. P., et al. (2000). Differential targeting of beta-adrenergic receptor subtypes and adenylyl cyclase to cardiomyocyte caveolae. A mechanism to functionally regulate the cAMP signaling pathway. *J Biol Chem, 275*(52), 41447–41457.
98. Xiang, Y., Rybin, V. O., Steinberg, S. F., et al. (2002). Caveolar localization dictates physiologic signaling of beta 2-adrenoceptors in neonatal cardiac myocytes. *J Biol Chem, 277*(37), 34280–34286.
99. Patel, P. A., Tilley, D. G., & Rockman, H. A. (2009). Physiologic and cardiac roles of beta-arrestins. *J Mol Cell Cardiol, 46*(3), 300–308.
100. Yan, C., Ding, B., Shishido, T., et al. (2007). Activation of extracellular signal-regulated kinase 5 reduces cardiac apoptosis and dysfunction via inhibition of a phosphodiesterase 3A/inducible cAMP early repressor feedback loop. *Circ Res, 100*(4), 510–509.
101. Kiely, J., Hadcock, J. R., Bahouth, S. W., et al. (1994). Glucocorticoids down-regulate beta 1-adrenergic-receptor expression by suppressing transcription of the receptor gene. *Biochem J, 302*(pt 2), 397–403.
102. Bahouth, S. W., Cui, X., Beauchamp, M. J., et al. (1997). Thyroid hormone induces beta1-adrenergic receptor gene transcription through a direct repeat separated by five nucleotides. *J Mol Cell Cardiol, 29*(12), 3223–3237.
103. Cornett, L. E., Hiller, F. C., Jacobi, S. E., et al. (1998). Identification of a glucocorticoid response element in the rat beta2-adrenergic receptor gene. *Mol Pharmacol, 54*(6), 1016–1023.
104. Bristow, M., Minobe, W., Raynolds, M., et al. (1993). Reduced b1 receptor messenger RNA abundance in the failing human heart. *J Clin Invest, 92*, 2737–2745.
105. Mitchusson, K. D., Blaxall, B. C., Pende, A., et al. (1998). Agonist-mediated destabilization of human beta1-adrenergic receptor mRNA: role of the 3' untranslated translated region. *Biochem Biophys Res Commun, 252*(2), 357–362.
106. Headley, V. V., Tanveer, R., Greene, S. M., et al. (2004). Reciprocal regulation of beta-adrenergic receptor mRNA stability by mitogen activated protein kinase activation and inhibition. *Mol Cell Biochem, 258*(1-2), 109–119.
107. DeMaria, C. T., & Brewer, G. (1996). AUF1 binding affinity to A+U-rich elements correlates with rapid mRNA degradation. *J Biol Chem, 271*(21), 12179–12184.
108. Pende, A., Tremmel, K. D., DeMaria, C. T., et al. (1996). Regulation of the mRNA-binding protein AUF1 by activation of the beta-adrenergic receptor signal transduction pathway. *J Biol Chem, 271*(14), 8493–8501.
109. Ma, W. J., Cheng, S., Campbell, C., et al. (1996). Cloning and characterization of HuR, a ubiquitously expressed elav-like protein. *J Biol Chem, 271*, 8144–8151.
110. Gherzi, R., Trabucchi, M., Ponassi, M., et al. (2006). The RNA-binding protein KSRP promotes decay of beta-catenin mRNA and is inactivated by PI3K-AKT signaling. *PLoS Biol, 5*(1), e5.
111. Lai, W. S., Carballo, E., Strum, J. R., et al. (1999). Evidence that tristetraprolin binds to AU-rich elements and promotes the deadenylation and destabilization of tumor necrosis factor alpha mRNA. *Mol Cell Biol, 19*(6), 4311–4323.
112. Taylor, G. A., Carballo, E., Lee, D. M., et al. (1996). A pathogenetic role for TNF alpha in the syndrome of cachexia, arthritis, and autoimmunity resulting from tristetraprolin (TTP) deficiency. *Immunity, 4*(5), 445–454.
113. Milano, C. A., Allen, L. F., Rockman, H. A., et al. (1994). Enhanced myocardial function in transgenic mice overexpressing the beta 2-adrenergic receptor. *Science, 264*(5158), 582–586.
114. Liggett, S. B., Tepe, N. M., Lorenz, J. N., et al. (2000). Early and delayed consequences of beta(2)-adrenergic receptor overexpression in mouse hearts: critical role for expression level. *Circulation, 101*(14), 1707–1714.
115. Engelhardt, S., Hein, L., Wiesmann, F., et al. (1999). Progressive hypertrophy and heart failure in beta1-adrenergic receptor transgenic mice. *Proc Natl Acad Sci U S A, 96*(12), 7059–7064.
116. Bisognano, J. D., Weinberger, H. D., Bohlmeyer, T. J., et al. (2000). Myocardial-directed overexpression of the human beta(1)-adrenergic receptor in transgenic mice. *J Mol Cell Cardiol, 32*(5), 817–830.
117. Antos, C. L., Frey, N., Marx, S. O., et al. (2001). Dilated cardiomyopathy and sudden death resulting from constitutive activation of protein kinase A. *Circ Res, 89*(11), 997–1004.
118. Mialet Perez, J., Rathz, D. A., Petrashevskaya, N. N., et al. (2003). Beta 1-adrenergic receptor polymorphisms confer differential function and predisposition to heart failure. *Nat Med, 9*(10), 1300–1305.
119. Akhter, S. A., Milano, C. A., Shotwell, K. F., et al. (1997). Transgenic mice with cardiac overexpression of alpha1β-adrenergic receptors. In vivo alpha1-adrenergic receptor-mediated regulation of β-adrenergic signaling. *J Biol Chem, 272*(34), 21253–21259.
120. Milano, C. A., Dolber, P. C., Rockman, H. A., et al. (1994). Myocardial expression of a constitutively active alpha 1β-adrenergic receptor in transgenic mice induces cardiac hypertrophy. *Proc Natl Acad Sci U S A, 91*(21), 10109–10113.
121. Lin, F., Owens, W. A., Chen, S., et al. (2001). Targeted (alpha)1A-adrenergic receptor overexpression induces enhanced cardiac contractility but not hypertrophy. *Circ Res, 89*(4), 343–350.
122. Iaccarino, G., Keys, J. R., Rapacciuolo, A., et al. (2001). Regulation of myocardial betaARK1 expression in catecholamine-induced cardiac hypertrophy in transgenic mice overexpressing alpha1β-adrenergic receptors. *J Am Coll Cardiol, 38*(2), 534–540.
123. Gaudin, C., Ishikawa, Y., Wight, D. C., et al. (1995). Overexpression of Gs alpha protein in the hearts of transgenic mice. *J Clin Invest, 95*(4), 1676–1683.
124. Asai, K., Yang, G. P., Geng, Y. J., et al. (1999). Beta-adrenergic receptor blockade arrests myocyte damage and preserves cardiac function in the transgenic G(s alpha) mouse. *J Clin Invest, 104*(5), 551–558.
125. D'Angelo, D. D., Sakata, Y., Lorenz, J. N., et al. (1997). Transgenic Galphaq overexpression induces cardiac contractile failure in mice. *Proc Natl Acad Sci U S A, 94*(15), 8121–8126.
126. Dorn, G. W., II, Tepe, N. M., Wu, G., et al. (2000). Mechanisms of impaired beta-adrenergic receptor signaling in G(alphaq)-mediated cardiac hypertrophy and ventricular dysfunction. *Mol Pharmacol, 57*(2), 278–287.
127. Redfern, C. H., Degtyarev, M. Y., Kwa, A. T., et al. (2000). Conditional expression of a Gi-coupled receptor causes ventricular conduction delay and a lethal cardiomyopathy. *Proc Natl Acad Sci U S A, 97*(9), 4826–4831.
128. DeGeorge, B. R., Jr., Gao, E., Boucher, M., et al. (2008). Targeted inhibition of cardiomyocyte Gi signaling enhances susceptibility to apoptotic cell death in response to ischemic stress. *Circulation, 117*(11), 1378–1387.
129. Gao, M. H., Lai, N. C., Roth, D. M., et al. (1999). Adenylylcyclase increases responsiveness to catecholamine stimulation in transgenic mice. *Circulation, 99*(12), 1618–1622.
130. Small, K. M., McGraw, D. W., & Liggett, S. B. (2003). Pharmacology and physiology of human adrenergic receptor polymorphisms. *Annu Rev Pharmacol Toxicol, 43*, 381–411.
131. Dorn, G. W., & Liggett, S. B. (2009). Mechanisms of pharmacogenomic effects of genetic variation of the cardiac adrenergic network in heart failure. *Mol Pharmacol*, mol.109.056572.
132. Liggett, S. B. (2000). Pharmacogenetics of beta-1- and beta-2-adrenergic receptors. *Pharmacology, 61*(3), 167–173.
133. Small, K. M., Mialet-Perez, J., & Liggett, S. B. (2008). Genetic variation within the beta1-adrenergic receptor gene results in haplotype-specific expression phenotypes. *J Cardiovasc Pharmacol, 51*(1), 106–110.
134. Small, K. M., Mialet-Perez, J., Seman, C. A., et al. (2004). Polymorphisms of cardiac presynaptic alpha2C adrenergic receptors: diverse intragenic variability with haplotype-specific functional effects. *Proc Natl Acad Sci U S A, 101*(35), 13020–10325.
135. Rathz, D. A., Brown, K. M., Kramer, L. A., et al. (2002). Amino acid 49 polymorphisms of the human beta1-adrenergic receptor affect agonist-promoted trafficking. *J Cardiovasc Pharmacol, 39*(2), 155–160.
136. Mason, D. A., Moore, J. D., Green, S. A., et al. (1999). A gain-of-function polymorphism in a G-protein coupling domain of the human beta1-adrenergic receptor. *J Biol Chem, 274*(18), 12670–12674.
137. Moore, J. D., Mason, D. A., Green, S. A., et al. (1999). Racial differences in the frequencies of cardiac beta(1)-adrenergic receptor polymorphisms: analysis of c145A>G and c1165G>. *C. Hum Mutat (serial online), 14*(3), 271.
138. Chen, L., Meyers, D., Javorsky, G., et al. (2007). Arg389Gly-beta1-adrenergic receptors determine improvement in left ventricular systolic function in nonischemic cardiomyopathy patients with heart failure after chronic treatment with carvedilol. *Pharmacogenet Genomics, 17*(11), 941–949.
139. Sehnert, A. J., Daniels, S. E., Elashoff, M., et al. (2008). Lack of association between adrenergic receptor genotypes and survival in heart failure patients treated with carvedilol or metoprolol. *J Am Coll Cardiol, 52*(8), 644–651.
140. Liggett, S. B., Mialet-Perez, J., Thaneemit-Chen, S., et al. (2006). A polymorphism within a conserved beta(1)-adrenergic receptor motif alters cardiac function and beta-blocker response in human heart failure. *Proc Natl Acad Sci U S A, 103*(30), 11288–11293.
141. Liggett, S. B., Wagoner, L. E., Craft, L. L., et al. (1998). The Ile164 beta2-adrenergic receptor polymorphism adversely affects the outcome of congestive heart failure. *J Clin Invest, 102*(8), 1534–1539.
142. Turki, J., Lorenz, J. N., Green, S. A., et al. (1996). Myocardial signaling defects and impaired cardiac function of a human beta 2-adrenergic receptor polymorphism expressed in transgenic mice. *Proc Natl Acad Sci U S A, 93*(19), 10483–10488.
143. Wagoner, L. E., Craft, L. L., Singh, B., et al. (2000). Polymorphisms of the beta(2)-adrenergic receptor determine exercise capacity in patients with heart failure. *Circ Res, 86*(8), 834–840.
144. Liggett, S. B., Cresci, S., Kelly, R. J., et al. (2008). A GRK5 polymorphism that inhibits beta-adrenergic receptor signaling is protective in heart failure (see comment). *Nat Med, 14*(5), 510–517.
145. Cresci, S., Reagan, J. K., Cappora, T. P., et al. (2009). Clinical and genetic modifiers of long-term survival in heart failure. *J Am Coll Cardiol, 54*, 432–444.
146. Schonberger, J., & Seidman, C. E. (2001). Many roads lead to a broken heart: the genetics of dilated cardiomyopathy. *Am J Hum Genet, 69*(2), 249–260.

CHAPTER 11

Activation of Inflammatory Mediators in Heart Failure

Douglas L. Mann

Although clinicians have recognized the pathophysiological importance of inflammatory mediators in the heart as early as 1669,[1] the formal recognition that inflammatory mediators were activated in the setting of heart failure did not occur for another three centuries. Since the sentinel description of inflammatory cytokines in patients with heart failure in 1990,[2] there has been a growing interest in the role that these molecules play in regulating cardiac structure and function, particularly with regard to their potential role in disease progression in heart failure. Accordingly, in the present chapter we will summarize the recent growth of knowledge that has taken place in this field, with a particular emphasis on the potential role that proinflammatory cytokines play as mediators of disease progression in the failing human heart. We will also summarize the results of clinical trials that have employed antiinflammatory strategies in patients with heart failure.

THE BIOLOGY OF PROINFLAMMATORY INFLAMMATORY CYTOKINES AND THEIR RECEPTORS

Cytokines are relatively small molecular weight protein molecules (generally 15 to 30 kDa) that are secreted by cells in response to a variety of different inducing stimuli. Whereas "proinflammatory cytokines" have traditionally been thought to be produced by the immune system, one of the more recent intriguing observations is that virtually all nucleated cell types within the myocardium, including cardiac myocytes themselves, are capable of synthesizing a portfolio of proinflammatory cytokines in response to various forms of cardiac injury (Box 11-1). Thus, from a conceptual standpoint, these molecules should be envisioned as proteins that are produced locally within the myocardium by "cardiocytes" (i.e., cells that reside within the myocardium), in response to one or more different forms of environmental stress. In the section that follows, we will review the biological properties of several important proinflammatory cytokines, including members of the tumor necrosis factor (TNF) family (including the recently described member TWEAK),[3] members of the IL-1 family (including the recently described members IL-18 and IL-33[4,5]), and the IL-6 family of cytokines.

Tumor Necrosis Factor (TNF) Superfamily

Tumor Necrosis Factor. Although TNF was originally defined by its antitumor activity in vitro and in vivo, TNF is now recognized as a cytokine with pleiotropic biological capacities. Besides its cytostatic and cytotoxic effects on certain tumor cells, it influences growth, differentiation, and/or function of virtually every cell type investigated, including cardiac myocytes.[6] In most cell types studied, TNF is initially synthesized as a nonglycosylated transmembrane protein of approximately 25 kDa. A 17-kDa fragment is proteolytically cleaved off the plasma membrane of the cell by a membrane-bound enzyme termed "TACE" (*T*NF-*a* *c*onvertas*e* [ADAM17]) to produce the "secreted form," which circulates as a stable 51-kDa TNF homotrimer (Figure 11-1).

The effects of TNF are initiated by binding to a lower affinity ($K_d = 2 - 10 \times 10^{-10}$) 55-kDa "type 1 receptor" (also called TNFR1) and/or a higher affinity ($K_d = 2 - 10 \times 10^{-11}$) 75-kDa "type 2 receptor" (also called TNFR2); intracellular signaling occurs as a result of TNF-induced oligomerization of the receptors. Both TNFR1 and TNFR2 share homology in their extracellular domains, which each contain a characteristic repeated cysteine consensus motif. In contrast, the intracellular domains of TNFR1 and TNFR2 differ, suggesting that each receptor has distinct modes of signaling and cellular function (see Figure 11-1). Previous studies have identified the presence of both types of TNF receptors in nonfailing[7] and failing human myocardium.[8] Both TNF receptor subtypes have been immunolocalized to the adult human cardiac myocyte, thus providing a potential basis for beginning to understand the signaling pathways that are used by TNF. Although the exact functional significance of TNFR1 and TNFR2 in the heart is not known at present, the majority of the deleterious effects of TNF are coupled to activation of TNFR1,[9] whereas activation of TNFR2 appears to exert protective effects in the heart. One interesting aspect of the biology of TNF receptors is that mammalian cells appear to "shed" TNF receptors following a variety of different stimuli, including exposure to TNF, lipopolysaccharide, okadaic acid, or phorbol esters.[10] Previous studies have shown that once the type 1 (TNFR1) and type 2 (TNFR2) TNF receptors are proteolytically cleaved from the cell membrane, they exist in the circulation as circulating "soluble" receptors (referred to as sTNFR1 and sTNFR2, respectively). Both of these soluble receptors retain their ability to bind ligand and to inhibit the cytotoxic activities of TNF in cell culture. Of interest, elevated levels of sTNFR1 and sTNFR2 have been shown to be strong independent predictors of adverse clinical outcome in hospitalized heart failure patients (Figure 11-2).[11]

Tumor Necrosis Factorlike Weak Inducer of Apoptosis (TWEAK). TNF-like weak inducer of apoptosis (TWEAK), a member of the TNF superfamily of ligands, is first synthesized as a type II transmembrane protein that is cleaved from the membrane. TWEAK functions primarily as a soluble cytokine with diverse biological roles, including proinflammatory activity, angiogenesis, regulation of cell survival, and myoblast differentiation/proliferation.[12] TWEAK induces apoptosis indirectly through secondary activation of the TNF/TNFR1 pathway. The expression of TWEAK is relatively low in normal tissues, including the heart, but undergoes dramatic upregulation in the setting of tissue injury. For example, TWEAK is expressed in the border zone of infarcted myocardium, wherein increased

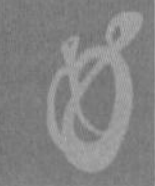

BOX 11–1 Cardiac Pathophysiological Conditions Associated with Activation of Inflammatory Mediators

Acute viral myocarditis
Cardiac allograft rejection
Myocardial infarction
Unstable angina
Myocardial reperfusion injury
Hypertrophic cardiomyopathy*
Heart failure*
Cardiopulmonary bypass*
Magnesium deficiency*
Pressure overload*

*Indicates conditions not traditionally associated with immunologically mediated inflammation.

angiogenesis is observed, and in the nonischemic myocardium remote from the infarct area.[12] Recent studies have suggested that sustained elevated circulating levels of TWEAK, induced via transgenic or adenoviral-mediated overexpression of soluble TWEAK, were sufficient to provoke LV dilation, LV fibrosis, LV dysfunction, and increased mortality in mice.[13] Moreover, circulating levels of TWEAK are elevated in patients with nonischemic cardiomyopathy compared with patients with ischemic cardiomyopathy and/or normal controls.[13]

The receptor for TWEAK, Fn14 (fibroblast growth factor-inducible 14), is the smallest member of the TNF-receptor family. Fn14 is a type 1 transmembrane protein (102 aa) that is expressed both constitutively and in an inducible manner in many tissues including the brain, the kidney, the liver, and the heart.[12] Fn14 is highly upregulated in the border zone of the heart following LAD ligation.[12] Both norepinephrine and angiotensin II also strongly upregulate Fn14 in isolated neonatal cardiomyocytes.[12] Fn14 contains sequence motifs within the cytoplasmic domain that promote aggregation of a family of adaptor proteins termed "TRAF1, 2, and 3" (TNF-receptor-associated factor), which in turn activate intracellular signal transduction cascades, including nuclear factor κB (NF κB), and the mitogen-activated protein kinases JNK, p38, and ERK.

The Interleukin-1 Superfamily

Interleukin-1 (IL-1). There are three members of the IL-1 gene family: IL-lα, IL-1β, and IL-1 receptor antagonist (IL-1Ra).[14] As will be discussed later, IL-18 and IL-33 are related family members. IL-1α and IL-1β are agonists, and IL-1Ra is a specific receptor antagonist. IL-1α and IL-1β are synthesized within mammalian cells as precursors without leader sequences. The molecular weight of each precursor is 31 kDa. Processing of IL-1α or IL-1β to "mature" forms of 17 kDa requires specific intracellular cellular proteases. In contrast, IL-1Ra has a signal peptide and is readily transported out of the cells and is then referred to as secreted IL-1Ra (sIL-1Ra). IL-1α and IL-1ß both bind to common receptors, which explains the similarity of effects of the two molecules. For the most part, IL-1α remains intracellular or is retained on the cell membrane, and is therefore not detected in the circulation in most disease states. Unlike IL-1α, the inactive or proform of IL-1ß is only marginally active. However, once the proform of IL-1ß is processed by an intracellular protease termed "ICE" (*i*nterleukin *c*onverting *e*nzyme), mature IL-1ß is rapidly secreted from the cell. The actions of IL-1α and IL-1ß can be competitively inhibited by IL-1Ra, which has a high degree of affinity for the type 1 IL-1 receptor, but lacks the ability to activate this receptor.[14] Similar to TNF, IL-1ß appears to be synthesized

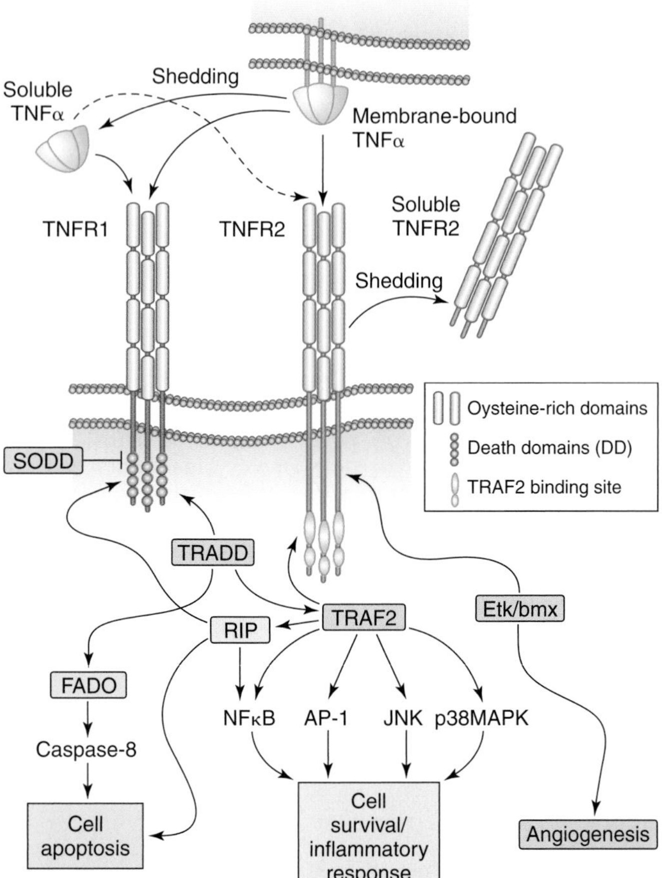

FIGURE 11–1 Overview of TNF signaling. TNF is initially expressed as a functional 26-kDa homotrimeric transmembrane that may be cleaved by a metalloproteinase termed "TACE," (TNF-α-converting enzyme [ADAM-17]). Once TNF is cleaved, it is released into the circulation as a 17-kDa protein that assembles as a functional 60-kDa homotrimer. The function of TNF is relayed by two structurally distinct receptors, termed "tumor necrosis factor receptor 1" (TNFR1; TNFRSF1A, p55, CD120a) and "tumor necrosis factor receptor 2" (TNFR2, TNFRSF1B, p75, CD120b). The TNFRs belong to the TNF receptor superfamily, a group of type I transmembrane glycoproteins that are characterized by a conserved homologous cysteine-rich domain in their extracellular region. Both TNFRs can be "shed" (cleaved) from the cell membrane, and are retained in the circulation as circulating "soluble" receptors (referred to as sTNFR1 and sTNFR2, respectively). Both of these soluble receptors retain their ability to bind ligand and to inhibit the biological activities of TNF. The main structural difference between TNFR1 and TNFR2 is the presence of a death domain (DD) in the cytoplasmic domain of TNFR1. The binding of TNF allows TRADD (TNF receptor-associated death domain protein) to interact with the DD. TRADD is an essential partner of TNFR1 for signal transduction that recruits the downstream adapter molecule FADD (fas-associated death domain), which initiates the caspase pathway responsible for apoptotic cell death. TRADD can also interact directly with RIP (receptor interacting protein) and TRAF2 (TNF receptor-associated factor 2 protein), which can activate downstream signaling pathways, such as NF κB, AP-1, c-Jun N-terminal kinase stress kinases (JNK), and p38MAPK.

within the myocardium in response to stressful environmental stimuli.[15]

Early work on the IL-1 receptor (IL-1R) suggested that there was a single receptor; however, subsequent cross-linking studies have suggested the presence of a low affinity (80 kDa; IL-1RI) receptor and a higher affinity receptor (68 kDa, IL-1RII), each coded for by a single gene product.[16] Interestingly, the type I receptor (IL-1RI) transduces a signal, whereas the type II receptor (IL-1RII) binds IL-1 but does not transduce a signal. Indeed, IL-1RII acts as a sink for IL-1 and has been termed a "decoy" receptor. When IL-1 binds to IL-1RI, a complex is formed that then recruits an accessory protein,

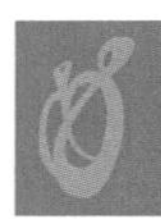

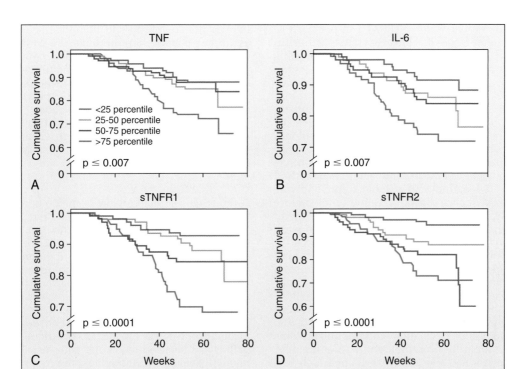

FIGURE 11–2 Kaplan-Meier survival analysis of inflammatory mediators in the VEST trial. The circulating levels of TNF (6A), IL-6 (6B), sTNFR1 (6C), and sTNFR2 (6D) were examined in relation to patient survival during follow-up (mean duration = 55 weeks; maximum duration = 78 weeks). For this analysis the circulating levels of cytokines and cytokine receptors were arbitrarily divided into quartiles. (From Deswal A, Petersen NJ, Feldman AM, et al. Cytokines and cytokine receptors in advanced heart failure: an analysis of the cytokine database from the vesnarinone trial (VEST). *Circulation* 2001;103:2055-2059.)

IL-1R-AcP. It is likely that the heterodimerization of the cytosolic domains of IL-1 RI and IL-1R-AcP trigger IL-1 signal transduction. Although IL-1Ra can bind to IL-1R1, it does not recruit IL-1R-AcP to the complex, and is thus incapable of signaling. The extracellular domains of the interleukin receptors or "soluble" portions of the IL-1RI (IL-1sRI) and IL-1RII (IL-1SRII) circulate in health and disease, and function as natural "buffers" that are capable of binding to IL-la, IL-1ß, or to IL-1Ra.[14]

Interleukin-18. Interleukin-18 (IL-18) is a member of the IL-1 superfamily.[17] Similar to IL-1ß, IL-18 is synthesized as an inactive precursor and is cleaved to its active form by caspase-1. Although IL-18 was initially recognized for its ability to induce interferon-γ (IFN-γ) and its capacity to induce T-helper 1 (Th1) responses, IL-18 was subsequently found to play an important role in LPS-induced hepatotoxicity, which stimulated further study of the role of IL-18 in other settings. Relevant to the present discussion is the recent observation that IL-18 had been shown to be produced in the heart during ischemia reperfusion injury and endotoxemia.[18] Importantly, IL-18 activates NF-κB, which is a transcriptional regulator of many proinflammatory cytokines and cellular adhesion molecules in the heart. In vitro studies have shown that IL-18 increases the production of TNF and IL-1ß in murine macrophages and human monocytes and also induces the expression of ICAM-1 and VCAM-1 on endothelial cells and monocytes.[17] In vivo studies have shown specific blockade of IL-18 using IL-18-binding protein improves contractile function in human atrial tissue following ischemia reperfusion injury,[4] and lipolysaccharide-induced LV dysfunction in experimental animals.[4]

The IL-18 receptor (IL-18R) is related to the IL-1 family of receptors, and is composed of a ligand-binding subunit, I-1Rrp1, and an accessory subunit, AcPL, both of which share sequence homology to the IL-1R family.[19] Moreover, the signal transduction pathways used by IL-1ß and IL-18 are similar. In addition, there is a third receptor-like chain, the IL-18 binding protein (IL-18BP), that lacks a transmembrane domain and thus does not signal. IL-18BP is produced constitutively and is secreted, and thus acts as a potent inhibitor of IL-18 activity.

Interleukin-33 (IL-33). As noted previously, IL-33 belongs to the IL-1 superfamily. IL-33 was identified in a search for the ligand for the ST2 receptor (see later discussion). IL-33 induces helper T cells, mast cells, eosinophils, and basophils to produce type 2 cytokines. The mode by which IL-33 exerts its effect has not been fully established but it probably acts similarly to other members of the IL-1 family. That is, precursor IL-33 is cleaved by caspases and is then released into the interstitium as an active cytokine, where it stimulates signaling in target cells.[20] In the heart, IL-33 is produced by cardiac fibroblasts in response to biomechanical strain. In vitro studies have shown that IL-33 markedly antagonizes angiotensin II and phenylephrine-induced cardiomyocyte hypertrophy; moreover, recombinant IL-33 reduced hypertrophy and fibrosis and improved survival after pressure overload in mice.[5] Thus IL-33 appears to activate a cardioprotective program in the heart.

ST2 is the cognate receptor for IL-33. There are four isoforms of ST2 (sST2 (soluble), ST2L (membrane bound), ST2V, and ST2LV. The overall structure of ST2L is similar to the structure of the type I IL-1 receptors, which consist of an extracellular domain of three linked immunoglobulin-like motifs, a transmembrane segment, and a TIR (Toll-like interleukin domain) cytoplasmic domain. sST2 lacks a transmembrane and cytoplasmic domains contained within the structure of ST2L and includes a unique 9–aminoacid C-terminal sequence.[20] Whereas ST2L is constitutively expressed primarily in hematopoietic cells, sST2 expression is largely inducible in a variety of cell types, including cells that reside in the heart. Interestingly, high baseline ST2 levels are a significant predictor of cardiovascular death and heart failure independent of baseline characteristics and NT-proBNP in patients with an ST-segment myocardial infarction.[21] The signaling pathways that are downstream from IL-33/ST2 signaling are still unclear, but may include phosphorylation of extracellular signal-regulated kinase (ERK) 1/2, p38 MAPK, JNKs, and activation of NF-κB. However, the relationship between ST2L and NF-κB activation is a matter of ongoing debate.[20]

Interleukin-6 (IL-6)

IL-6 is another multifunctional cytokine that mediates inflammatory responses. Until IL-6 was cloned and sequenced, its diverse biological roles had led to a variety of different names for this molecule, including 26K factor, B-cell stimulatory factor 2, hepatocyte stimulating factor, and β_2-interferon.[22] Human IL-6 is produced as a 212–amino acid precursor and is processed to a 184–amino acid soluble form following cleavage of a signal sequence during secretion of the mature protein.[22] The mature protein is a 26-kDa glycoprotein[23] with a number of alternative N- and O-linked glycosylation sites. IL-6 can be detected in the circulation following gram-negative bacterial infection or TNF infusion, and following myocardial stunning[24] and appears to be secreted in direct response to TNF or IL-1, which are thought to induce IL-6 gene expression by releasing a nuclear-binding protein termed "NF-κB".[22] Recently, IL-6 has been shown to exist in the circulation in "chaperoned" complexes of molecular mass 400 to 500, 150 to 200, and 25 to 35 kDa in association with binding proteins that can include soluble IL-6 receptor, anti-IL-6 antibodies, and anti-sIL-6R antibodies, and others. Sustained high levels of different particular IL-6 complexes are observed in the human circulation in cancer patients subjected to particular active anticancer immunotherapy regimens. However, "chaperoned" IL-6 complexes have not yet been reported in heart failure.[25] Recently two other cytokines that use the gp130 signaling pathway have been identified in heart failure: leukemia inhibitory factor and cardiotrophin-1.[26,27] However, the functional significance of these latter two cytokines in heart failure remains unknown at the time of this writing.

The human IL-6 receptor is a glycoprotein with a molecular mass of 80 kDa. In contrast to the receptors for IL-1 and TNF, the cytoplasmic domain of IL-6 is not necessary for intracellular signaling to occur. Moreover, when bound to its receptor, IL-6 is known to associate with a second membrane glycoprotein with a molecular mass of 130 kDa (gp130). Thus the current evidence suggests that the IL-6R system is composed of two functional chains: an 80-kDa IL-6 binding protein, termed "IL-6R," and a 130-kDa "docking protein," termed "gp130," which transmits the intracellular signal.[22] Although the presence of IL-6 receptors has not yet been identified in the adult heart,[28] it is of considerable interest that genetic mice that are deficient in gp130 are embryonic lethal because their hearts do not develop.[29] Moreover, double transgenic mice that have been genetically engineered to overexpress both IL-6 and IL-6R develop substantial concentric hypertrophy.[28] Thus the gp130 family of receptors may play an important role in normal growth and development of the heart.

Chemokines

Chemokines are a distinct family of cytokines that regulate biological processes such as chemotaxis, collagen turnover, angiogenesis, and apoptosis. The chemokine superfamily is divided into four groups (CXC, CX3C, CC, and C) according to the relative positioning of the first two closely paired cysteines of their amino acid sequence. Chemokines exert their effects by interacting with G protein–linked transmembrane receptors, referred to as "chemokine receptors", which are found on the surfaces of their target cells. A major role of chemokines is the recruitment and activation of specific subpopulations of leukocytes that play a pivotal role in the immune response and inflammation. While chemokine-dependent functions are essential for the control of infection, wound healing, and hematopoiesis, excessive chemokine activation may result in inappropriate inflammation leading to cell death and tissue damage. Studies have shown that circulating levels of CC chemokines are elevated in patients with ischemic and nonischemic heart failure, including macrophage chemoattractant protein-1 (MCP-1), macrophage inflammatory protein-1α (MIP-1α), and RANTES (regulated on activation normally T-cell expressed and secreted). The highest levels of these chemokines were noted in patients with NYHA class IV heart failure.[30] Given that these chemokines can attract inflammatory cells to the heart, they may contribute to disease progression in heart failure.

Innate Immunity

Although a complete review of innate immunity in the heart is beyond the intended scope of this chapter, this topic will be reviewed briefly herein for the sake of completeness (please see references 31 and 32 for complete reviews of the subject). Traditionally, the immune system has been divided into innate and adaptive components, each of which has a different role in helping the host to differentiate self from nonself. The innate immune system is activated by a family of "pattern recognition receptors" that reside in a variety of cell types, including cardiac myocytes. These pattern recognition receptors recognize invariant patterns (so-called pathogen-associated molecular patterns) shared by groups of microorganisms but not by host tissues. Typical examples of pathogen-associated molecular patterns include the lipopolysaccharides (LPS) of gram-negative organisms, the teichoic acids of gram-positive organisms, the glycolipids of mycobacterium, the mannans of yeast, and the double-stranded RNAs of viruses. These pathogen-associated molecular patterns are unique to these pathogens and in some cases are required for their virulence. Thus one of the quintessential features of the innate immune system is that it serves as an "early warning system" that enables the host to accurately and rapidly discriminate self from nonself. Recent studies have shown that the heart possesses a functionally intact innate immune system, and that the cardiac innate immune system is activated nonspecifically in response to all forms of acute myocardial injury, especially during ischemia/reperfusion injury (reviewed in Mann[33]). Cardiac myocytes express at least five classical receptors that belong to the innate immune system (so-called pattern recognition receptors), including CD14, the soluble pattern recognition receptor for lipopolysaccharide,[34] and Toll-like receptors -2, 3, 4, and 6 (TLR-2, TLR-3, TLR-4, and TLR-6, respectively).[35]

As shown in Figure 11-3, *A*, the signaling pathway that is used by the TLR family of receptors is highly homologous to that of the IL-1 receptor (IL-1R) family. Both TLR and IL-1R interact with an adaptor protein termed "myeloid differentiation factor 88" (MyD88) via their Toll interleukin receptor (TIR) domains. When stimulated, MyD88 recruits IL-1 receptor–associated kinase (IRAK) to the receptor. IRAK is then activated by phosphorylation and associates with tumor necrosis receptor-associated factor 6 (TRAF6), leading to NF- κB activation through the classical *N*F-κB *i*nducing *k*inase (NIK) → IKK → IκBα dependent pathway depicted in Figure 11-3, *B*.[36] Recent studies from this and other laboratories have shown that TLR-4 is critical for upregulating the expression of TNF, IL-1β, IL-6, and NOS2 in the heart following stimulation with lipopolysaccharide (LPS),[37,38] and that CD-14 and TLR-4 are essential for LPS-mediated LV dysfunction.[39,40] The role of TLR activation in heart disease is not confined to LPS-induced signaling, insofar as TLR2 and TLR4 knockout mice are protected from ischemia-reperfusion injury following reperfusion.[41,42] Moreover, both LV dilation and mortality are attenuated in TLR2 and TL4 knockout mice following acute ligation of the left anterior descending artery.[43,44] Thus the extant literature suggests that TLR signaling may contribute to myocardial inflammation and LV remodeling following cardiac injury.

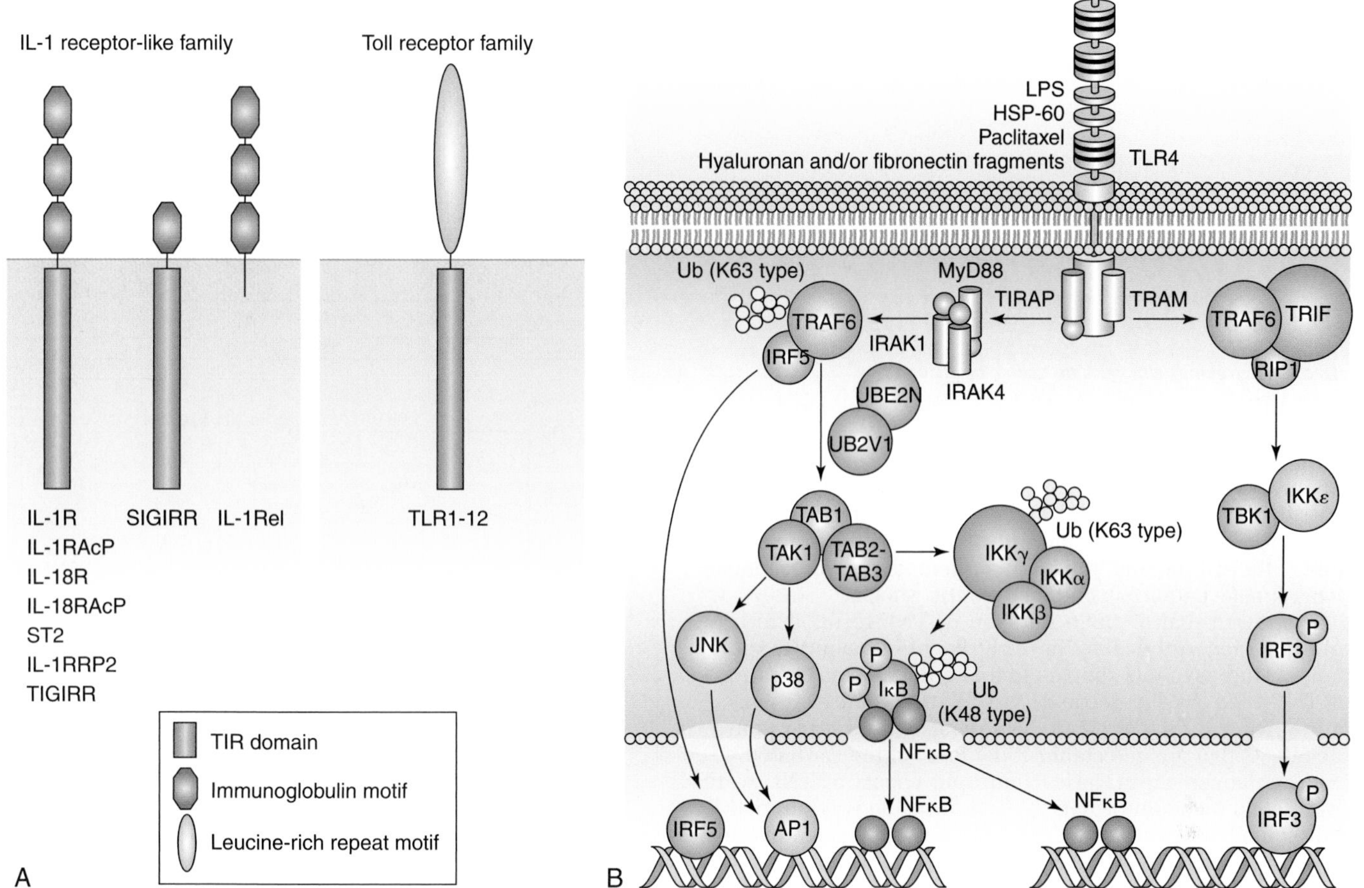

FIGURE 11–3 The Toll-like/interleukin-1 (IL-1) receptor superfamily. **A,** The Toll-like/interleukin-1 (IL-1) receptor superfamily members share a Toll/interleukin-1 receptor (TIR) sequence. The TIR domain mediates the interaction between members of the superfamily, specifically receptor-receptor, adaptor-adaptor, and receptor-adaptor protein dimerization. The Toll-like/IL-1 receptor superfamily can be further subdivided into the IL-1 receptor-like family, the Toll receptor family, and the TIR-containing adaptor protein family (*left-hand panel*). The IL-1 receptor-like subfamily shares the common feature of linked immunoglobulin motifs within the extracellular domain. Members of this family include the type I and II IL-1 receptor (IL-1R1 and IL-1R2), the IL-18 receptor (IL-18R), their accessory proteins IL-1RAcP and IL-18RAcP, and ST2 and others. The Toll receptor subfamily members are type-1 transmembrane proteins characterized by extracellular leucine-rich repeat motifs linked to an intracellular TIR containing domain (*right-hand panel*). The founding member of this family, Toll, was identified in the fruitfly and noted to be necessary for dorso-ventral polarity during embryonic development.
B, The Toll-like receptor signaling pathway. (Key: *AP-1,* activator protein 1; *HSP-60,* heat shock protein 60; *IκB,* inhibitor of nuclear factor κB; *IKKα,* inhibitor of nuclear factor κB kinase α; *IKKβ,* inhibitor of nuclear factor κB kinase-β; *IKKε,* inhibitor of nuclear factor κB kinase ε; *IKKγ,* inhibitor of nuclear factor κB kinase γ; *IRAK1,* interleukin-1 receptor-associated kinase 1; *IRAK4,* interleukin-1 receptor-associated kinase 4; *IRF3,* interferon regulatory factor 3; *IRF5,* interferon regulatory factor 5; *JNK, c-jun* N-terminal kinase; *LPS,* lipopolysaccharide; *MyD88,* myeloid differentiation primary response protein; *NF κB,* nuclear factor κB; *RIP1,* receptor-interacting protein 1; *TAB1,* TAK1-binding protein 1; *TAB2–TAB3,* TAK1 -binding proteins 2 and 3; *TAK1 (M3K7),* transforming growth factor β-activated kinase 1; *TBK1,* serine–threonine-protein kinase; *TIRAP,* TIR domain-containing adaptor protein; *TLR4,* Toll-like receptor 4; *TRAF6,* tumor necrosis factor receptor-associated factor 6; *TRAM,* TRIF-related adaptor molecule; *TRIF,* TIR-domain-containing adaptor inducing interferon β; *Ub,* ubiquitin; *UB2V1,* ubiquitin-conjugating enzyme E2 variant 1; *UBE2N,* ubiquitin-conjugating enzyme E2N (A, Modified from Kakkar R, Lee RT. The IL-33/ST2 pathway: therapeutic target and novel biomarker. *Nat Rev Drug Discov* 2008;7:827-840. B, From Frantz S, Ertl G, Bauersachs J. Mechanisms of disease: toll-like receptors in cardiovascular disease. *Nat Clin Pract Cardiovasc Med* 2007;4:444-454.)

Rationale for Studying Inflammatory Mediators in Heart Failure

The interest in understanding the role of inflammatory mediators in heart failure arises from the observation that many aspects of the syndrome of heart failure can be explained by the known biological effects of proinflammatory cytokines (Box 11-2). That is, when expressed at sufficiently high concentrations, such as those that are observed in heart failure, cytokines are sufficient to mimic some aspects of the so-called heart failure phenotype, including (but not limited to) progressive left ventricular (LV) dysfunction, pulmonary edema, LV remodeling, fetal gene expression and cardiomyopathy.[45] Thus the "cytokine hypothesis[46]" for heart failure holds that heart failure progresses, at least in part, as a result of the toxic effects exerted by endogenous cytokine cascades on the heart and the peripheral circulation. It bears emphasis that the cytokine hypothesis does not imply that cytokines cause "heart failure" per se, but rather that the overexpression of cytokine cascades contributes to disease progression of heart failure. Much like the elaboration of neurohormones, the elaboration of cytokines may represent a biological mechanism that is responsible for worsening heart failure. Although the deleterious effects of cytokines on myocardial function have received the most attention thus far, it bears emphasis that cytokines may also produce deleterious effects on LV structure (remodeling) and endothelial function. Accordingly, in the following section, we will discuss the studies that form the scientific basis for studying the role of proinflammatory mediators in the failing heart.

BOX 11–2 Deleterious Effects of Inflammatory Mediators in Heart Failure

Left Ventricular Dysfunction
Pulmonary edema in humans
Cardiomyopathy in humans
Reduced skeletal muscle blood flow
Endothelial dysfunction
Anorexia and cachexia
Receptor uncoupling from adenylate cyclase experimentally
Activation of the fetal gene program experimentally
Cardiac myocyte apoptosis experimentally

Effects of Cytokines on Left Ventricular Function

One of the signatures of proinflammatory cytokines is their ability to depress LV function. The original observation that proinflammatory cytokines were capable of modulating LV function was reported in experimental studies that showed that direct injections of TNF produced hypotension, metabolic acidosis, hemoconcentration, and death within minutes, thus mimicking the cardiac/hemodynamic response seen during endotoxin-induced septic shock.[47] Studies in dogs showed that a single infusion of TNF resulted in systolic function within the first 24 hours of infusion.[48] Experimental studies in rats showed that circulating concentrations of TNF that overlap those observed in patients with heart failure were sufficient to produce persistent negative inotropic effects that are detectable at the level of the cardiac myocyte; moreover, the negative inotropic effects of TNF were completely reversible when the TNF infusion was stopped.[45] Subsequent studies in transgenic mice with targeted overexpression of TNF in the cardiac compartment demonstrated that targeted overexpression of TNF results in depressed LV ejection performance that is dependent on TNF "gene dosage."[49,50] At the cellular level, studies in isolated contracting myocytes showed that the negative inotropic effects of TNF were the direct result of alterations in intracellular calcium homeostasis.[51] Treatment with more than 50 U.mL^{-1} TNF produced a 20% to 30% decrease in the extent of cell shortening (Figure 11-4, *A*) and a 40% decrease in peak levels of intracellular calcium (see Figure 11-4, *B*). Moreover, whole cell patch-clamp studies suggested that the decrease in intracellular calcium was not the result of changes in the voltage-sensitive inward calcium current, suggesting that TNF- induced changes in intracellular calcium homeostasis were secondary to alterations in sarcoplasmic reticular handling of calcium.[51]

Signaling Pathways for the Negative Inotropic Effects of Inflammatory Mediators. With respect to the potential mechanisms for the deleterious effects of TNF on LV function, the literature suggests that TNF modulates myocardial function through at least two different pathways: that is, an immediate pathway that is manifest within minutes and is mediated by activation of the neutral sphingomyelinase pathway,[52] and a delayed pathway that requires hours to days to develop, and is mediated by nitric oxide.[6,53] It has also been suggested recently that TNF and IL-1 produce negative inotropic effects *indirectly* through activation and/or release of IL-18, which is a recently described member of the IL-1 family of cytokines.[17] Relevant to the present discussion is the observation that specific blockade of IL-18 using the neutralizing IL-18 antibody resulted in a decrease in infarct size in rats subjected to ischemia reperfusion injury.[54] Although the signaling pathways that are responsible for the IL-18-induced negative inotropic effects have not been delineated, it is likely that they will overlap those for IL-1, given that the IL-18 receptor complex uses components of the IL-1 signaling chain, including

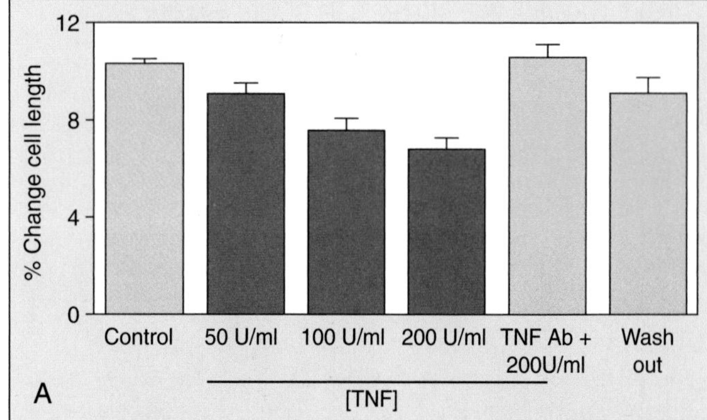

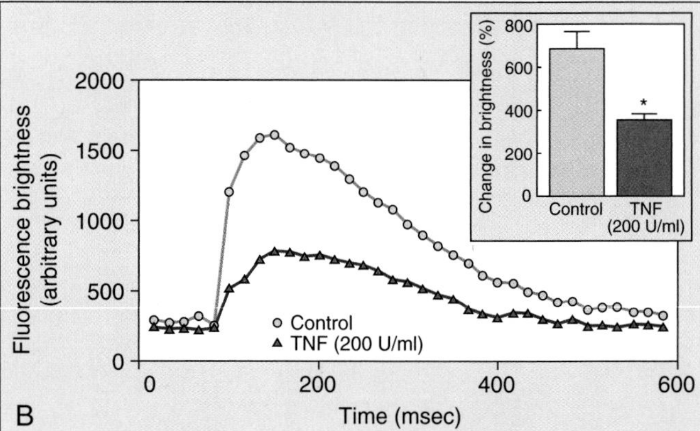

FIGURE 11–4 Effect of TNF on contractility of adult cardiac myocytes. **A,** Shows that in comparison with control (open bar) cells, cardiac myocytes treated with TNF (closed bars) developed a concentration-dependent decrease in cell shortening. Pretreatment with a neutralizing anti-TNF antibody (hatched bar) completely attenuated the effects of 200 U/mL TNF on cell shortening. When the cells were washed free of 200 U/mL TNF and allowed to recover for 45 minutes, the effects of TNF were completely reversible (*hatched bar*). **B,** Shows a typical time-intensity curve for fluorescence brightness in isolated cardiac myocytes treated with diluent (*open circles*) and 200 U/mL TNF-treated (*closed triangles*). As shown, the peak level of intracellular fluorescence brightness was reduced strikingly for the cells treated with 200 U/mL TNF. The inset of this figure, which depicts values obtained for group data, shows that there was an approximately 40% decrease in the percent change in peak intensity of fluorescence brightness for the TNF-treated cells. Taken together, panels A and B suggest that TNF produces negative inotropic effects in isolated cardiac myocytes by producing an alteration in intracellular calcium homeostasis. (Reproduced with permission from Yokoyama T, Vaca L, Rossen RD, et al. Cellular basis for the negative inotropic effects of tumor necrosis factor-alpha in the adult mammalian heart. *J Clin Invest* 1993;92:2303-2312.)

IL-1R-activating kinase (IRAK) and TNF receptor–associated factor-6 (TRAF-6).[17]

Mechanism for the Delayed Negative Inotropic Effects of Cytokines. The observation that proinflammatory cytokines increase the expression of nitric oxide (NO) through augmented transcription of nitric oxide synthase,[55] and that both the inducible (NOS2) and constitutive (NOS3) forms of NOS are expressed in rat cardiac myocytes[53,56] and in human myocardial tissue,[57] combined with the observation that NO is sufficient to depress myocardial function,[53,56] suggested that NOS/NO were responsible for the negative inotropic effects of cytokines. By way of review, NOS1 and NOS3 are calcium/calmodulin dependent, and release NO for short periods of time in direct response to changes in intracellular concentrations of calcium. Both NOS1 and NOS3 are expressed constitutively in a broad variety of cell types, and are activated by receptor and/or physical stimulation.[58] However, while combinations of cytokines may increase

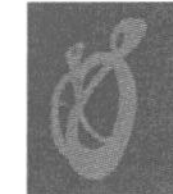

NOS1/NOS3 activity indirectly over 24 hours by increasing the synthesis of NOS cofactors,[59] cytokine-induced calcium-dependent NOS activity has not been observed thus far.[60] In contrast to the constitutive isoforms of NOS, NOS2 is inducible and is calcium independent. Moreover, NOS2 levels are directly upregulated by cytokines.[61] What is perhaps less readily appreciated, however, is that the cytokine-mediated increase in NOS2 expression requires a lag period of hours to days before NO is produced and released. Thus although an increase in NOS2 expression may explain the delayed onset of cytokine-mediated functional effects, cytokine-mediated NOS2 expression does not readily explain the more immediate negative inotropic effects that have been reported for TNF, IL-2, and IL-6.[51] The signaling mechanisms that are responsible for the negative inotropic effects of NO are complex, and include guanylyl cyclase (cGMP)-mediated alterations in calcium homeostasis,[62,63] and NO-mediated blunting of ß-adrenergic-stimulated generation of cAMP. Treatment of adult cardiac myocytes (>24 hr) with culture medium "conditioned" by activated macrophages produced an NO-mediated defect in isoproterenol-stimulated contractile function.[53] Although the mechanism for the NO-mediated defect in isoproterenol-stimulated contractile function is not known, it is interesting to note that earlier reports in neonatal cardiac myocytes suggested that TNF and IL-1 stimulation lead to a G protein–mediated defect in ß-adrenergic signal transduction.[6]

Mechanism for the Immediate Negative Inotropic Effects of Cytokines. With respect to the mechanism for the immediate negative inotropic effects of TNF, IL-2, and IL-6, one study provided indirect evidence in support of the point of view that TNF-, IL-2-, and IL-6-induced contractile dysfunction resulted from "enhanced activity of a constitutive nitric oxide synthase (NOS2) in the myocardium."[64] However, these findings with respect to induction of NOS2 activity by cytokines have not been confirmed by all laboratories.[51] There is, however, evidence that TNF-mediated activation of the neutral sphingomyelinase pathway may play an important role in mediating the immediate negative inotropic effects of cytokines.[52] Activation of the neutral sphingomyelinase pathway by a variety of ligands, including TNF and IL-1, has been shown to lead to hydrolysis of membrane-bound sphingomyelin, with the resultant generation of ceramide, which can then be deacylated to sphingosine by the enzyme ceramidase.[65] The importance of sphingosine, which is present in both skeletal and cardiac muscle,[66] is that at sufficiently high concentrations this molecule can block calcium release from the ryanodine receptor,[67] which might provide an explanation for a prior observation that TNF-induced alterations in intracellular calcium homeostasis are secondary to alterations in sarcoplasmic reticular handling of calcium.[51] Indeed, the concentrations of sphingosine that were induced by TNF in contracting cardiac myocytes were sufficient to produce negative inotropic effects and alterations of intracellular calcium homeostasis that were qualitatively and quantitatively similar to those observed with TNF alone.[52]

Effects of Cytokines on Left Ventricular Structure

Cardiac remodeling contributes to the development and progression of heart failure (see Chapters 8 and 15). However, the mechanisms that contribute to the structural changes that underlie progressive cardiac remodeling are only partially understood. As shown in Box 11-3, inflammatory mediators have a number of important effects that may play an important role in the process of LV remodeling, including myocyte hypertrophy,[68] alterations in fetal gene expression,[49] degradation of the extracellular matrix,[45,69] and progressive myocyte loss through apoptosis.[70] When concentrations of TNF that overlap those observed in patients with heart failure were infused continuously in rats, there was a time-dependent change in LV dimension that was accompanied by progressive degradation of the extracellular matrix.[45] Second, recent studies in transgenic mice with targeted overexpression of TNF have shown that these mice develop progressive LV dilation. For example, Sivasubramanian et al showed that a transgenic mouse line that overexpressed TNF in the cardiac compartment segued from a concentric LV hypertrophy phenotype to a dilated LV phenotype over a 12-week period of observation (Figure 11-5).[69] Similar findings have also been reported by Kubota et al[49] and Bryant et al,[71] who observed identical findings with respect to LV dysfunction and LV dilation in transgenic mice with targeted overexpression of TNF in the heart. With respect to the mechanisms that are involved in TNF-induced LV dilation, it has been suggested that TNF-induced activation of matrix metalloproteinases are responsible for this effect.[69] As shown in Figure 11-6 there was progressive loss of fibrillar collagen in the hearts of the transgenic mice overexpressing TNF in the cardiac compartment. Subsequent studies suggested that the loss of fibrillar collagen was secondary to increased activation of MMPs. The dissolution of the fibrillar collagen weave that surrounds the individual cardiac myocytes and links the myocytes together would be expected to allow for rearrangement ("slippage") of myofibrillar bundles within the ventricular wall.[72] In addition to TNF, the related superfamily member TWEAK has been shown to have important effects of cardiac remodeling. In a recent study, elevated circulating levels of TWEAK induced via transgenic or adenoviral-mediated gene expression in mice resulted in progressive LV remodeling with subsequent severe cardiac dysfunction (Figure 11-7) that was independent of TNF signaling. Although the mechanisms for TWEAK-mediated LV dilation have not been fully elucidated, TWEAK was shown to activate NF κB, activate the fetal gene program, and provoke cardiac myocyte hypertrophy through an FN14-dependent mechanism.

Cardiac-restricted overexpression of TNF has been shown to lead to progressive cardiac myocyte apoptosis (Figure 11-8) and LV wall thinning (see Figure 11-5, *C*).[73] Mechanistic studies showed that sustained TNF signaling resulted in activation of the intrinsic cell death pathway, leading to increased cytosolic levels of cytochrome *c*, Smac/DIABLO, and Omi/HtrA2, and activation of caspases 3 and 9. Targeted overexpression of Bcl-2 blunted activation of the intrinsic pathway and prevented LV wall thinning; however, Bcl-2 only partially attenuated cardiac myocyte apoptosis. Subsequent studies showed that caspase 8 was activated and that Bid was cleaved to *t*Bid, suggesting that the extrinsic pathway was activated concurrently.[74] Thus sustained myocardial inflammation leads to activation of multiple cell death pathways that contribute to progressive cardiac myocyte apoptosis and adverse cardiac remodeling in mice with cardiac restricted overexpression of TNF.[74] Antagonism of IL-1 signaling by administering anakinra, a recombinant-human IL-1 receptor

BOX 11–3 Effects of Inflammatory Mediators on Left Ventricular Remodeling

Alterations in the Biology of the Myocyte
- Myocyte hypertrophy
- Contractile abnormalities
- Fetal gene expression

Alteration in the Extracellular Matrix
- MMP activation
- Degradation of the matrix
- Fibrosis

Progressive Myocyte Loss
- Necrosis
- Apoptosis

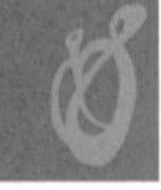

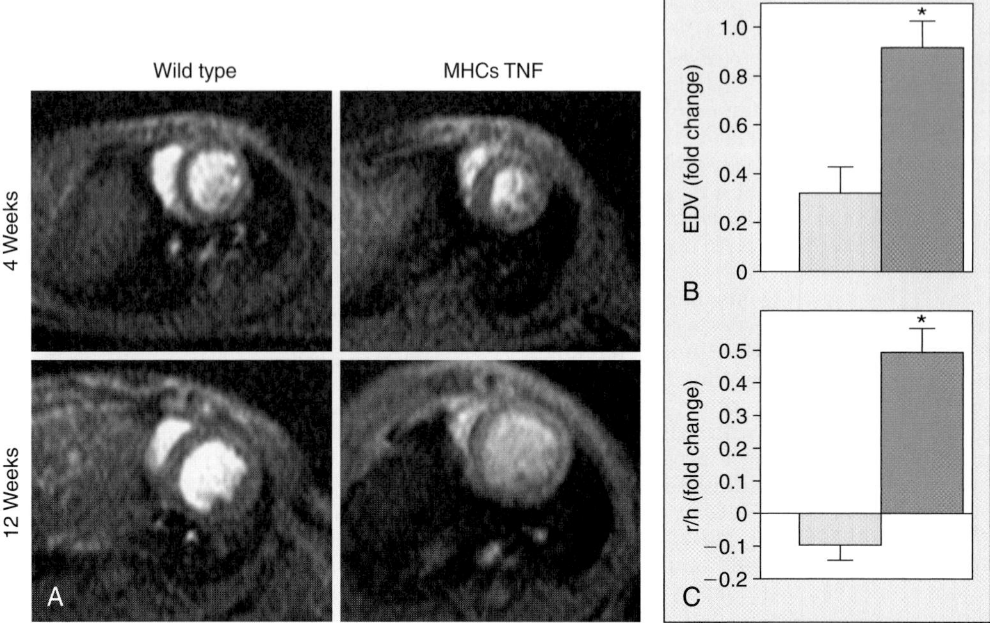

FIGURE 11–5 LV remodeling in the littermate control and TNF transgenic mice. **A,** Representative short-axis MRI images of the littermate control and TNF transgenic mice at 4 and 12 weeks. **B,** Group data for fold-change in LV end-diastolic volume (EDV) from 4 to 12 weeks. **C,** Group data for the fold-change in the LV radius to LV wall at ages 4, 8, and 12 weeks (* = $P < 0.05$). (From Engel D, Peshock R, Armstrong RC, et al. Cardiac myocyte apoptosis provokes adverse cardiac remodeling in transgenic mice with targeted TNF overexpression. *Am J Physiol Heart Circ Physiol* 2004;287:H1303-H1311.)

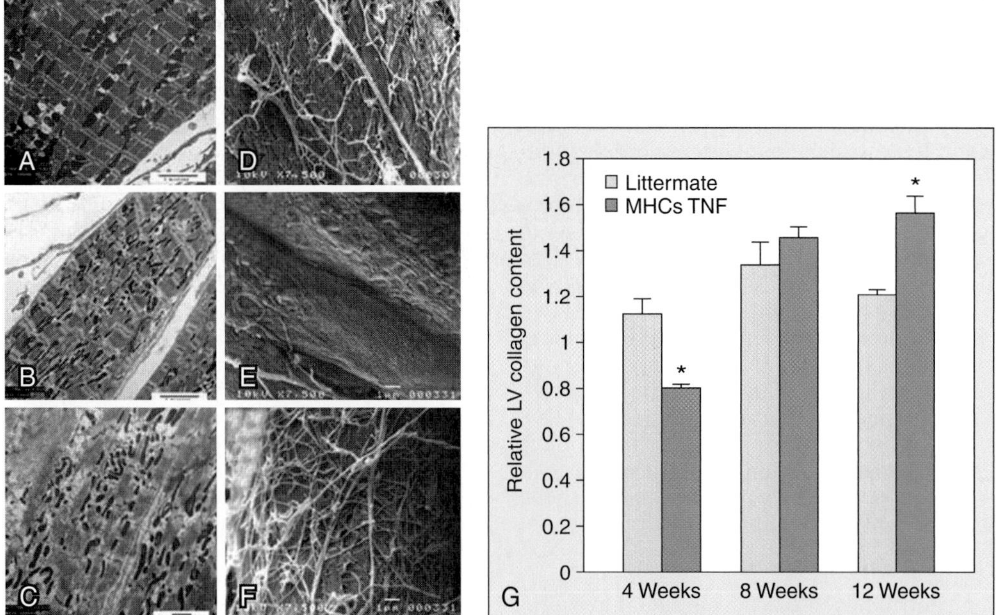

FIGURE 11–6 Effects of sustained proinflammatory cytokine expression on myocardial ultrastructure and collagen content. Panels A-C show representative transmission electron micrographs in littermate controls **(A)** and the TNF transgenic mice at 4 **(B)** and 8 weeks of age **(C)**. The transmission electron micrographs from the littermate control mice at 4 weeks (A) revealed a characteristic linear array of sarcomere and myofibril. In contrast, the myofibril in the 4-week-old TNF transgenic mice were less organized, with loss of sarcomeric registration observed in many of the sections (Figure 11-3, *B*). The ultrastructural abnormalities in the TNF transgenic mice were further exaggerated in the 12-week-old TNF transgenic mice, which showed a significant loss of sarcomere registration and myofibril disarray (C). Panels D-F show representative scanning electron micrographs in littermate controls **(D)** and the TNF transgenic mice at 4 **(E)** and 8 weeks of age **(F)**. Panel E shows that there was a significant loss of fibrillar collagen in the TNF transgenic mice at 4 weeks of age when compared with age-matched littermate controls (D). However, as the TNF transgenic mice aged (12 weeks), there was an obvious increase in myocardial fibrillar collagen content. **G,** illustrates the myocardial collagen content as determined by picro Sirius red staining. There was a loss of myocardial collagen content at 4 weeks of age in the TNF transgenic mice that was later followed by a progressive increase in myocardial collagen content at 8 and 12 weeks of age. (From Sivasubramanian N, Coker ML, Kurrelmeyer K, et al. Left ventricular remodeling in transgenic mice with cardiac restricted overexpression of tumor necrosis factor. *Circulation* 2001;104:826-831.)

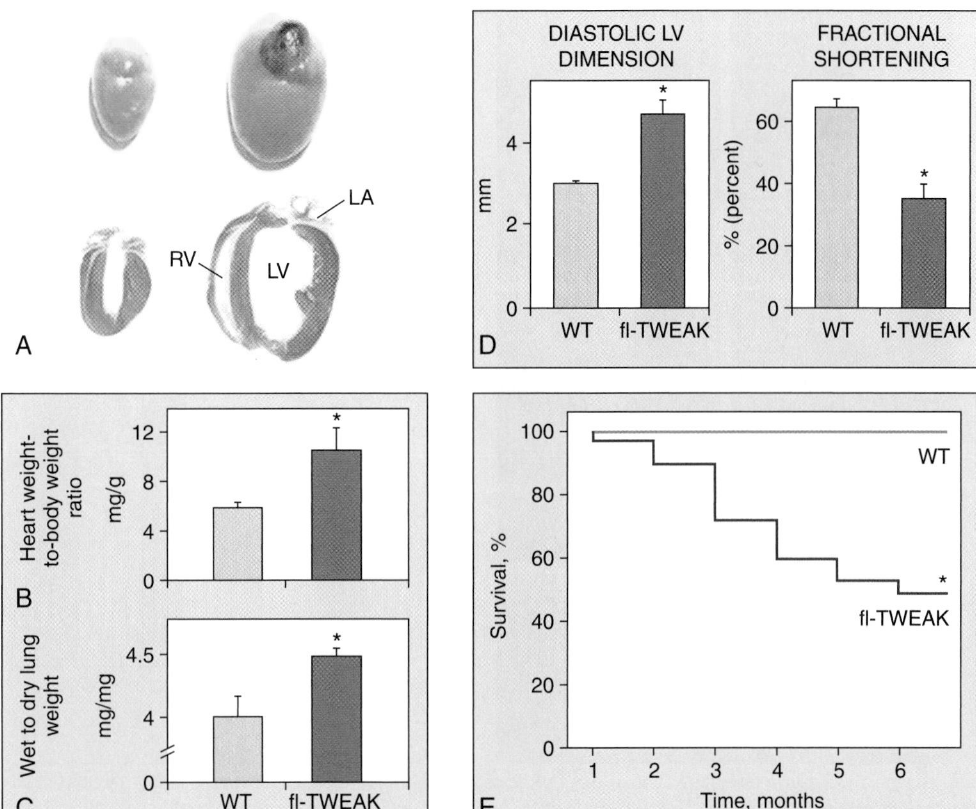

FIGURE 11–7 Effects of TWEAK on LV structure and function. **A,** Representative whole hearts and trichrome-stained longitudinal sections from wild-type and transgenic mice overexpressing a full length TWEAK construct (fl-TWEAK) (Key: *LV,* left ventricle; *RV,* right ventricular; *LA,* left atrium). **B,** Increased heart weight-to-body weight ratios in fl-TWEAK mice compared with wild-type (WT) mice. **C,** Increased wet-to-dry lung weights in fl-TWEAK mice compared with WT mice. **D,** LV end-diastolic dimension and fractional shortening in WT and fl-TWEAK mice. **E,** Kaplan Meier survival curves for WT and fl-TWEAK mice demonstrating increased mortality in the fl-TWEAK mice. (* = $P < 0.01$) (Modified from Jain M, Jakubowski A, Cui L, et al. A novel role for tumor necrosis factor-like weak inducer of apoptosis (TWEAK) in the development of cardiac dysfunction and failure. *Circulation* 2009;119:2058-2068.)

antagonist has also resulted in decreased cardiac myocyte apoptosis, decreased LV remodeling, and improved LV function in a rat infarct model.[75] In vitro studies in rat cardiac myocytes demonstrated that anakinra inhibited caspase 1 and 9 activity, and prevented apoptosis in a simulated model of ischemia.[75] From a pathophysiological standpoint, the increase in LV wall thinning that attends progressive cardiac myocyte apoptosis would be expected to contribute to increased LV wall stress (i.e., afterload mismatch), and hence sustained unfavorable loading conditions of the heart, thereby contributing to progressive cardiac decompensation. Thus excessive activation of proinflammatory cytokines may contribute to LV remodeling through a variety of different mechanisms that involve both the myocyte and nonmyocyte components of the myocardium.

Interactions Between the Renin-angiotensin System and Proinflammatory Cytokines in Adverse Cardiac Remodeling. Although neurohormonal and cytokine systems have been regarded as functionally distinct biological systems, recent studies suggest that these two systems can cross regulate each other, with the result that neurohormonal and cytokine systems may participate in positive feed forward loops that contribute to adverse cardiac remodeling. Whereas angiotensin II was traditionally viewed as a circulating neurohormone that stimulated the constriction of vascular smooth muscle cells, aldosterone release from the adrenal gland, sodium reabsorption in the renal tubule, and/or as a stimulus for growth of cardiac myocytes or fibroblasts,[76] it is becoming increasingly apparent that angiotensin II provokes inflammatory responses in a variety of different cell and tissue types. For example, angiotensin II activates NF κB, [77] which is critical for initiating the coordinated expression of classical components of the myocardial inflammatory response, including increased expression of proinflammatory cytokines, nitric oxide, chemokines, and cell adhesion molecules.[78] Pathophysiologically relevant concentrations of angiotensin II are sufficient to provoke TNF mRNA and protein synthesis in the adult heart through a NF κB dependent pathway.[79] Figure 11-10 shows that treatment with angiotensin II resulted in a rapid increase in TNF mRNA (see Figure 11-10, *A*) and protein synthesis (see Figure 11-10, *B*) in isolated buffer perfused hearts. Stimulation of isolated adult cardiac myocytes with angiotensin II resulted in an approximately threefold increase in TNF protein biosynthesis within 1 hour, and an approximately fifteenfold increase in TNF protein biosynthesis within 24 hours, suggesting that the increase in TNF biosynthesis in the intact heart was mediated, at least in part, at the level of the cardiac myocyte. The effects of angiotensin II on TNF mRNA and protein synthesis were mediated exclusively through the angiotensin type 1 receptor, insofar as pretreatment with the angiotensin type 1 receptor antagonist losartan completely abolished the effects of angiotensin II on TNF biosynthesis, whereas pretreatment with the angiotensin type 2 receptor antagonist PD123319 had no effect on angiotensin II-induced TNF biosynthesis (see Figure 11-10, *B*). This study further showed that the effects of angiotensin II on TNF myocardial biosynthesis were dependent upon protein kinase C-mediated activation of NF κB.[79]

There is also increasing evidence that inflammatory mediators are capable of upregulating various components of the renin-angiotensin system in a variety of mammalian tissues,

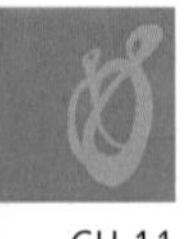

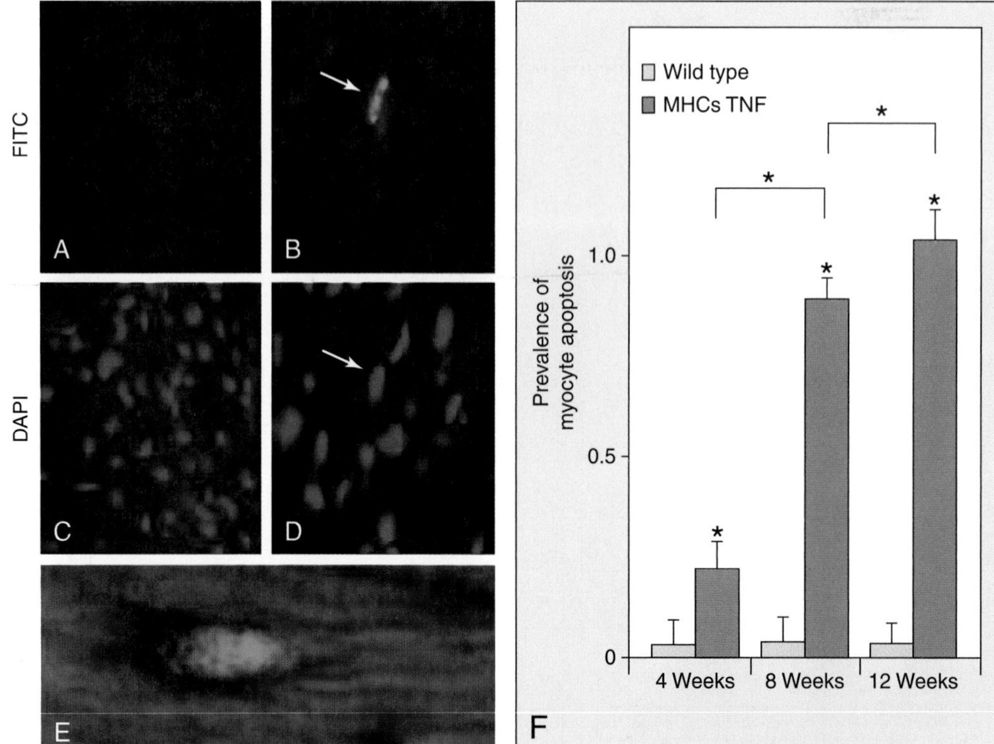

FIGURE 11–8 Cardiac myocyte apoptosis in littermate control and TNF transgenic mice. **A,** Representative myocardial sections (200× magnification) showing DNA ligase staining in a littermate control and **(B)** TNF transgenic mice. Apoptotic nuclei are shown by the bright green nuclear fluorescence (*arrow*). DAPI staining was used to identify the total number of cell nuclei in littermate control **(C)** and TNF transgenic mice **(D)**. **E,** An apoptotic nucleus stained by the ligase technique in (600× magnification) in the presence of antidesmin immunostaining. **F,** Prevalence cardiac myocyte apoptosis in littermate control and TNF transgenic mice at 4, 8, and 12 weeks (* = $P < .05$). (From Engel D, Peshock R, Armstong RC, et al. Cardiac myocyte apoptosis provokes adverse cardiac remodeling in transgenic mice with targeted TNF overexpression. *Am J Physiol Heart Circ Physiol* 2004;287:H1303-H1311.)

including the heart. As one recent example, studies using transgenic mice with cardiac-restricted overexpression of TNF have shown that targeted overexpression of TNF leads to an increase in angiotensin II peptide levels in the heart.[80] This study serially examined several components of the renin-angiotensin system, including angiotensinogen, renin, angiotensin-converting enzyme (ACE), and angiotensin I and II peptide levels in a transgenic mouse line with cardiac-restricted overexpression of TNF. There was a significant increase in ACE mRNA levels (Figures 11-11, *A*, and 11-11, *B*) and ACE activity (see Figure 11-11, *C*), and increased angiotensin II peptide levels (see Figure 11-11, *D*) in the hearts of the TNF transgenic mice relative to littermate controls. Importantly, the expression of renin and angiotensinogen was not increased in the TNF transgenic mice compared with littermate controls. Thus this study suggested that the increased levels of angiotensin II peptide levels in the TNF transgenic mice was principally the result of increased ACE activity, as opposed to increased activation of the more proximal components of the renin-angiotensin system, namely renin and angiotensinogen. This study also showed that activation of the renin-angiotensin system was functionally significant in the TNF transgenic mice. That is, treatment of the TNF transgenic mice from 4 to 8 weeks of age with losartan significantly attenuated cardiac hypertrophy, myocardial fibrosis, and cardiac myocyte apoptosis in the TNF transgenic mice.[80] Taken together, these observations suggest that interactions between the renin-angiotensin system and inflammatory mediators may contribute to adverse cardiac remodeling.

Effects of Proinflammatory Mediators on Endothelial Function

In addition to the effects of inflammatory mediators on cardiac structure and function, there is growing evidence that the concentrations of inflammatory mediators that exist in heart failure are sufficient to contribute to endothelial dysfunction. The functional role of TNF in modulating endothelial function was suggested in studies by Agnoletti et al, who demonstrated that the serum of patients with heart failure induced apoptosis and downregulated endothelial constitutive nitric oxide synthase in human umbilical vein endothelial cells.[81] The importance of TNF in their studies was suggested by experiments in which an anti-TNF antibody partially antagonized the effects of heart failure sera on endothelial cell apoptosis.[81] The role of TNF-induced endothelial dysfunction is further supported by studies by Anker et al,[82] who showed that circulating TNF levels correlated inversely with peak blood flow in heart failure patients, independently of age, ejection fraction, peak oxygen consumption, and NYHA association class, thus suggesting that TNF might contribute to peripheral skeletal muscle weakness/fatigue in patients with heart failure. Finally, in a recent clinical study that used a soluble TNF antagonist (etanercept) to neutralize TNF, there was a short-term improvement in forearm-mediated blood flow that was fully reversible following the cessation of therapy.[83]

Clinical Trials Targeting Inflammatory Mediators in Heart Failure

Given that elevated levels of proinflammatory cytokines mimic many aspects of the heart failure phenotype and that the deleterious effects of inflammatory mediators are potentially reversible once inflammation subsides, investigators have used a variety of different approaches to antagonize inflammatory mediators in heart failure (Table 11-1). As shown in Figure 11-11, the biological effects of proinflammatory mediators can be antagonized through transcriptional or translational approaches, or by so-called biological response modifiers that bind and/or neutralize soluble mediators (e.g., TNF or IL-1ß). In addition, there are several novel "immunomodulatory strategies" that alter the levels of inflammatory

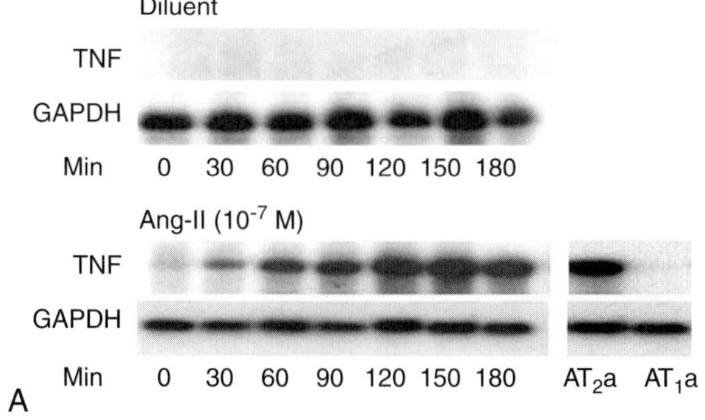

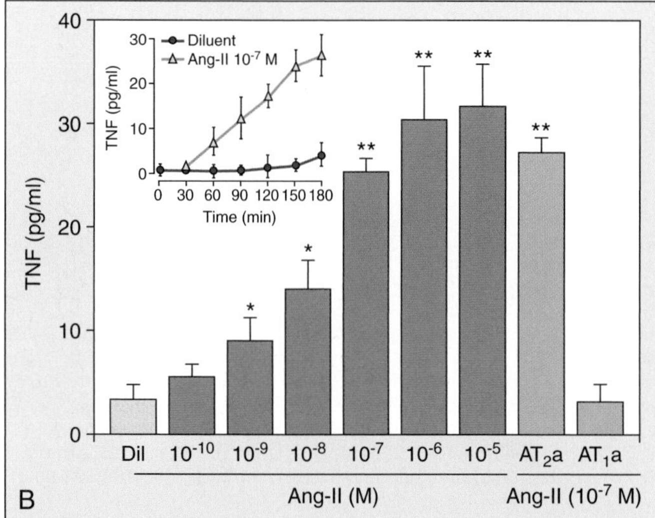

FIGURE 11–9 Angiotensin II–induced myocardial TNF biosynthesis in the adult heart. **A,** TNF mRNA expression (RNase protection assay) was assessed ex vivo in diluent and angiotensin II (10^{-7} M)–treated (up to 180 min) buffer perfused Langendorff hearts, in the presence or absence of 10^{-6} M PD123319, an AT_2 receptor antagonist (AT_2a) or 10^{-6} M losartan, an AT_1 receptor antagonist (AT_1a). **B,** Myocardial TNF protein production was assessed in the superfusates of the angiotensin II–treated hearts using ELISA in the presence or absence of PD123319 (10^{-6} M) or losartan (10^{-6} M) pretreatment. The main panel of Figure 11-1, *B*,shows the dose-dependent effects of angiotensin II (10^{-10} M to 10^{-5} M), whereas the inset shows the time course (up to 180 min) for TNF protein synthesis following stimulation with either diluent (*solid circles*) or 10^{-7} M Ang-II (*open triangles*). (Key: AT_1a = AT_1 receptor antagonist [losartan]; AT_2a = AT_2 receptor antagonist [PD123319]) (* = P <.05 and ** = P <.01 compared with diluent treated hearts). (From Kalra D, Sivasubramanian N, Mann DL. Angiotensin II induces tumor necrosis factor biosynthesis in the adult mammalian heart through a protein kinase C-dependent pathway. *Circulation* 2002;105:2198-2205.)

mediators through multiple mechanisms. In the section that follows, we will review the clinical trials that have targeted inflammatory mediators in heart failure.

Transcriptional Suppression of Proinflammatory Cytokines. Experimental studies have shown that agents that raise cAMP levels prevent TNF mRNA accumulation, largely by blocking the transcriptional activation of TNF.[84] Pentoxifylline is a xanthine-derived agent that is known to inhibit TNF transcription and translation. Thus far, 144 heart failure patients have been treated with pentoxifylline in randomized clinical trials.[85-88] As shown in Table 11-1, two studies in patients with dilated cardiomyopathy examined patients with NYHA class II and III heart failure,[85,86] whereas a third study examined patients with NYHA class IV heart failure.[88] Pentoxifylline has also been used in NYHA class I-IV patients with ischemic heart disease.[88] The use of pentoxifylline was associated with significant improvement in NYHA functional class and/or LV ejection fraction in all studies. Notably, the beneficial effects were seen in all NYHA classes of heart failure, in patients with ischemic and nonischemic cardiomyopathy, and in patients treated with ACE inhibitors and β-blockers. Relevant to the present discussion, the beneficial effects on cardiac function in some of the studies were accompanied by decreased circulating plasma levels of TNF.[89] However, it is important to recognize that pentoxifylline is a nonspecific inhibitor of phosphodiesterases and that the salutary effects of these agents might be unrelated to the immunomodulatory properties of this drug.

Thalidomide (α-N-phthalimidoglutarimide) is another class of drug that may be useful in suppressing TNF production. Thalidomide selectively inhibits TNF production in monocytes,[90] but has no effect on the production of IL-1β, IL-6, or granulocyte/macrophage colony-stimulating factor (GM-CSF). Thalidomide appears to reduce TNF levels by enhancing mRNA degradation;[91] however, the mechanisms of action of thalidomide remain unclear, and contradictory results have been reported regarding its effects on cytokine levels in vivo. Based on its immunomodulatory properties, thalidomide has been studied in heart failure. In an open-label dose escalation study, thalidomide was safe and potentially effective when used at lower doses.[92] However, dose-limiting toxicity was observed in two patients (50 and 200 mg/day). There was a significant increase in the 6-minute walk distance and a trend (P = .16) toward improvement in left ventricular ejection fraction and quality of life after 12 weeks of maintenance therapy with thalidomide.[92] In a larger placebo-controlled study of 56 patients with NYHA class II-III heart failure secondary to an ischemic or nonischemic cardiomyopathy with an LV ejection fraction less than 40%, treatment with up to 200 mg/day of thalidomide for 12 weeks resulted in an increase in LV ejection fraction and a decrease in LV end-diastolic volume.[93] These salutary changes were accompanied by a decrease in circulating levels of matrix metalloproteinase 2, but an increase in circulating levels of TNF. The effect of thalidomide on LV ejection fraction was observed to a greater degree in patients with dilated cardiomyopathy, who were able to tolerate higher doses of thalidomide.[93]

Translational Suppression of Proinflammatory Cytokines. Dexamethasone, which is thought to primarily suppress TNF biosynthesis at the translational level, may also block TNF biosynthesis at the transcriptional level.[94] One of the earliest studies to use this type of approach was performed by Parrillo et al,[95] who randomized 102 patients to treatment with prednisone (60 mg per day) or placebo. Following 3 months of therapy, they observed an increase in ejection fraction of more than 5% in 53% of the patients receiving prednisone, whereas only 27% of the controls had a significant improvement in ejection fraction (P = .005). Overall, the mean ejection fraction increased 4.3% ± 1.5% in the prednisone group, as compared with 2.1% ± 0.8% in the control group (P = .054). The patients were then categorized prospectively into two separately randomized subgroups. "Reactive" patients had fibroblastic or lymphocytic infiltration or immunoglobulin deposition on endomyocardial biopsy, a positive gallium scan, or an elevated erythrocyte sedimentation rate, and "nonreactive" patients, had none of these features. At 3 months, 67% of the reactive patients who received prednisone had improvement in LV function, as compared with 28% of the reactive controls (P = .004). In contrast, nonreactive patients did not improve significantly with prednisone (P = .51). Although specific cytokine levels were not measured in this study, their data suggest that patients with idiopathic dilated cardiomyopathy may have some improvement when given a high dose of prednisone daily.

Targeted Anticytokine Approaches Using "Biological Response Modifiers." Two different targeted approaches have been taken to selectively antagonize proinflammatory

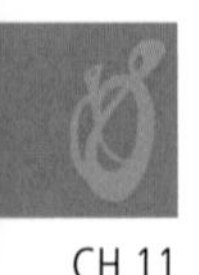

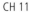

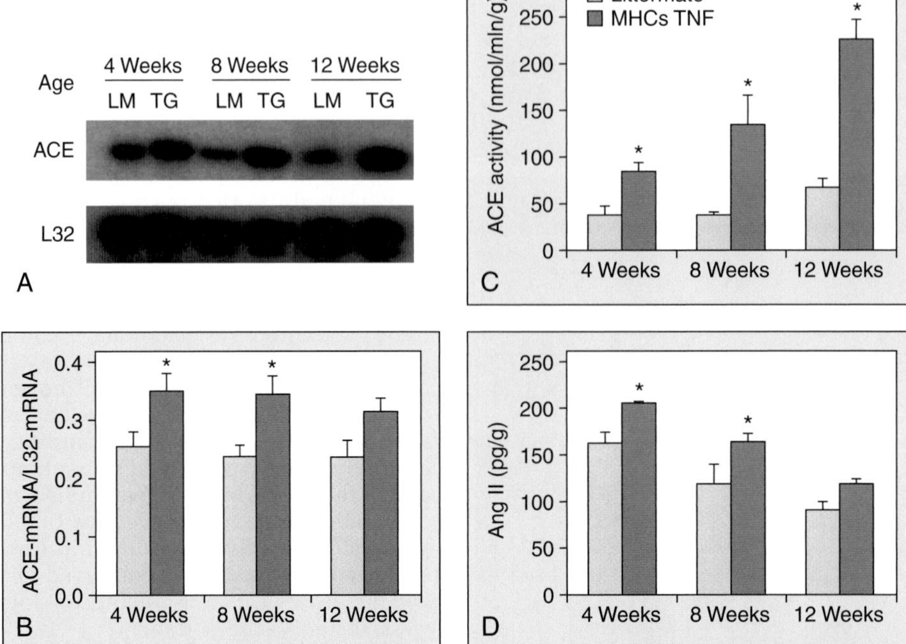

FIGURE 11–10 ACE mRNA, ACE activity, and angiotensin II peptide levels in mice with targeted overexpression of TNF and littermate control mice. **A,** Ribonuclease protection assay for ACE mRNA in the hearts of the 4-, 8-, and 12-week-old TNF transgenic mice and littermate control mice (LM) mice. **B,** Group data in hearts from 4-, 8-, and 12-week-old TNF transgenic mice (n = 7 hearts/time) and 4-, 8-, and 12-week-old littermate control mice (n = 7 hearts/time). **C,** ACE activity in the hearts from 4-, 8-, and 12-week-old TNF transgenic mice and the 4-, 8-, and 12-week-old littermate control mice. **D,** Group data for angiotensin II peptide levels in the hearts of the TNF transgenic mice and littermate control mice at 4, 8, and 12 weeks of age. (Key: *LM,* littermate control; *TG,* transgenic) (* = $P < .05$ vs. age-matched control group by Tukey test). (Reproduced with permission from Flesch M, Hoper A, Dell'Italia L, et al. Activation and functional significance of the renin-angiotensin system in mice with cardiac restricted overexpression of tumor necrosis factor. *Circulation* 2003;108:598-604.)

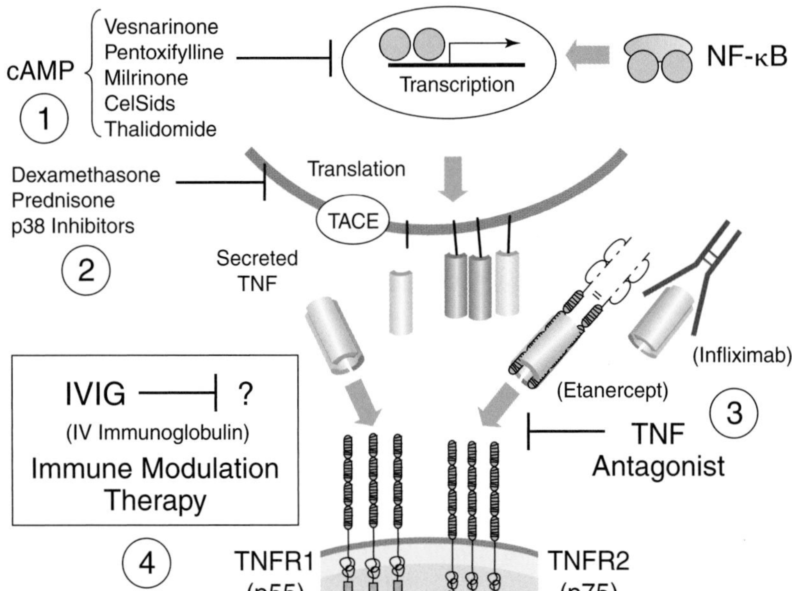

FIGURE 11–11 Therapeutic strategies for antagonizing proinflammatory mediators. TNF gene transcription is mediated, in part, by activation of NF κB. Agents that increase intracellular levels of cAMP (1) such as vesnarinone, pentoxifylline, milrinone, thalidomide, and thalidomide analogs (CelSids) decrease the level of inflammatory mediators through transcriptional blockade of inflammatory gene expression. Agents such as dexamethasone and prednisone and some p38 inhibitors suppress inflammation by blocking the translation of inflammatory mediators (2). Secreted TNF can be neutralized (3) by soluble TNF antagonists (etanercept) or by neutralizing antibodies (infliximab) that prevent TNF from binding to its cognate type 1 (p55) and type 2 (p75) TNF receptors. In addition to these targeted approaches, broad-based immodulatory strategies have been employed (4) using intravenous immunoglobulin (IVIG), statins, and irradiated (oxidized) whole blood (Celacade therapy). (Modified from Mann DL. Inflammatory mediators and the failing heart: past, present, and the foreseeable future. *Circ Res* 2002;91:988-998.)

cytokines in heart failure patients (Table 11-1). In the first approach, investigators used a recombinant human TNF receptor that acts as a "decoy" and prevents TNF from binding to its cognate receptors on target cells. The second approach that was employed was a chimeric monoclonal antibody that binds to and neutralizes circulating TNF.

Soluble TNF Receptors. Etanercept (Enbrel) is a genetically engineered, dimerized, fusion protein composed of two TNF p75 receptors and an IgG_1:Fc portion. Based on early preclinical studies that showed that etanercept was sufficient to reverse the deleterious negative inotropic effects of TNF in vitro[96] and in vivo,[45] a series of phase I clinical studies were performed in patients with moderate to advanced heart failure. These early short-term studies in small numbers of patients showed improvements in quality of life, 6-minute walk distance, and LV ejection performance following treatment with etanercept for up to 3 months.[97,98] Following this, two multicenter clinical trials were initiated using etanercept in patients with NYHA class II-IV heart failure. The trial in North America, entitled *R*andomized *E*tanercept *N*orth *A*mer*I*can Strategy

TABLE 11–1 Randomized Clinical Trials That Have Inflammation in Heart Failure

Study	Number of Patients	NYHA Class	Agent	Targeted Category	Follow-up (months)	Mean Age	Mean LVEF	% ACE-ARB/BB	Primary Endpoint	Outcome
ACCLAIM[114]	2426	II-IV	Celacade	DCM, IHD	10.2	64	23	94/87	Death or CV hospitalization	No effect on death, or CV hospitalization
ATTACH[101]	150	II-IV III, IV	Infliximab	DCM, IHD	7	61	24	100/73	Clinical composite score	High dose had adverse effect on clinical outcomes
CORONA[119]	5011	II-IV	Rosuvastatin	IHD	32.8	73	ns	91/75	CV death, nonfatal MI, and stroke	No effect on CV death, nonfatal MI and stroke, decreased HF hospitalizations
GISSI-HF[120]	4574	II-IV	Rosuvastatin	DCM, IHD	46.8	68	33*	95/62	Death and CV hospitalization	No effect on death, death and CV hospitalization
Gullestad et al[108]	40	II-IV	IVIG	DCM, IHD	6	61	27	100/75	NYHA class and LVEF	Improved clinical status and LVEF
Gullestad et al[93]	56	II, III	Thalidomide	DCM, IHD	3	66	25	100/91	LVEF, LV volumes, symptoms	Improved LVEF and LV remodeling
IMAC[109]	62/RCT	I-IV	IVIG	DCM	12	43	25	90/18	LVEF and symptoms	No effect
Parillo et al[95]	102/RCT	ns	Prednisone	DCM	3	43	17	na/na	LVEF	Improved LVEF
RECOVER/ RENAISSANCE/ RECOVER[100]	1500	II-IV	Etanercept	DCM, IHD	5.7/12.9	63	23	98/62	Clinical composite score/death, or heart failure hospitalization	No effect on clinical status, death, or heart failure hospitalization
Skudicky et al[86]	39	II, III	Pentoxifylline	DCM	6	49	24	100/100	NYHA class, exercise tolerance, and LVEF	Improved symptoms and LVEF
Sliwa et al[85]	28	II, III	Pentoxifylline	DCM	6	53	24	100/na	NYHA class and LVEF	Improved symptoms and LVEF
Sliwa et al[125]	18	IV	Pentoxifylline	DCM	1	46	15	100/na	Symptoms, cytokines, and LVEF	Improved symptoms and LVEF
Sliwa et al[88]	38	I-IV	Pentoxifylline	IHD	6	55	25	100/100	NYHA class and LVEF	Improved symptoms and LVEF
UNIVERSE[118]	87	II-IV	Rosuvastatin	DCM, IHD	6.5	62	29	98/85	LVEF	No effect on LVEF

Modified from Aukrust P, Yndestad A, Ueland T et al. Anti-inflammatory trials in chronic heart failure. *Heart Fail Monit* 2006;5:2-9.

*10% of the patients in GISSI-HF has an EF >40%.

Note: ACE, Angiotensin-converting enzyme; *ARB,* angiotensin II receptor blocker; *BB,* β-adrenergic receptor blocker; *IVIG,* intravenous immunoglobulin; *LVEF,* left ventricular ejection fraction; *mo,* months; *na,* not available; *ns,* not specified, *NYHA,* New York Heart Association; *QoL;* quality of life.

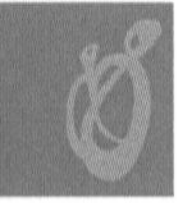

to *S*tudy *A*ntago*N*ism of *C*ytokin*E*s (RENAISSANCE; *n* = 900), and the trial in Europe and Australia entitled *R*esearch into *E*tanercept *C*yt*o*kine Antagonism in *Ve*ntricula*r* Dysfunction (RECOVER; *n* = 900), were both quality of life trials that used a clinical composite assessed at 24 weeks as the primary endpoint. The clinical composite score classifies patients as better, worse, or the same after a clinical intervention based on the patient and the physician's assessment at the end of the study.[99] Both trials had parallel study designs, but differed in the doses of etanercept that were used in the two studies; that is, RENAISSANCE employed doses of 25 mg twice a week and 25 mg three times a week, whereas RECOVER employed doses of 25 mg once a week and 25 mg twice a week). A third trial, which used the pooled data from the RENAISSANCE (twice a week and three times a week dosing) and RECOVER (twice a week dosing only), termed *R*andomized *E*tanercept *W*orldwide Eva*l*uation (RENEWAL; *n* = 1500), had a composite primary endpoint of all cause mortality and hospitalization for heart failure. On the basis of prespecified stopping rules, both trials were terminated prematurely owing to a lack of benefit: There was no significant difference between placebo and etanercept with respect to change in the clinical composite score in both RENAISSANCE ($P = .17$) and RECOVER ($P = .34$) (Figure 11-12, *A*). Moreover, in the prespecified pooled analysis in RENEWAL, there was no effect of etanercept on the primary endpoint (see Figure 11-12, *B*) of death or chronic heart failure hospitalization (hazard ratio = 1.1, 95% CI 0.91 to 1.33, $P = .33$).[100] However, in a posthoc analysis of hazard ratios for death/worsening heart failure, patients taking the twice a week dose of etanercept appeared to fare slightly better than patients taking the once a week dose of etanercept in RECOVER, with hazard ratios for death/heart failure hospitalization of 0.87 ($P = .45$) and 1.01 ($P = .97$), respectively. In contrast, RENAISSANCE patients receiving twice a week etanercept experienced an increased 1.21 ($P = .17$) risk of death/heart failure hospitalization compared with placebo, while patients receiving the three times a week dose had a slightly worse hazard ratio of 1.23 ($P = .13$). Analysis of the components of the clinical composite score in the RENAISSANCE trial showed that there was a significantly greater proportion of etanercept-treated patients (29%, $P < .04$) who were in the worsened category at 24 weeks when compared with a placebo group (20%); however, this difference was not observed in the RECOVER trial. The disparity in clinical outcomes between RECOVER and RENAISSANCE may relate, at least in part, to the different length of follow-up in the two trials. Patients in RECOVER received etanercept for a median time of 5.7 months, whereas patients in RENAISSANCE received etanercept for 12.7 months. It bears emphasis that these studies were stopped prematurely; had they been allowed to continue to completion, the hazard ratios may have been worse. On the basis of these findings, the prescribing information for etanercept has been updated and now suggests that physicians exercise caution in the use of etanercept in patients with heart failure.

Monoclonal Antibodies. Infliximab (Remicade) is a chimeric monoclonal antibody consisting of a genetically engineered murine Fab fragment (that binds human TNF) fused to a human FC portion of human IgG_1. Although infliximab had been shown to be effective in Crohn disease and rheumatoid arthritis, there were no preclinical, nor early phase I clinical studies to support the use of this agent in heart failure. The *A*nti-*T*NF-α *T*herapy *A*gainst *CH*F (ATTACH) trial was a phase II study in 150 patients with moderate to advanced heart failure (NYHA class III, IV).[101] The primary endpoint of the ATTACH trial was the clinical composite score described previously.[99] Patients were randomized to receive three separate intravenous infusions of infliximab (5 mg/kg or 10 mg/kg) at baseline and at 2 and 4 weeks, followed by an assessment of the clinical composite at 14 and 28 weeks. Although this trial went to completion, analysis of the aggregate data revealed

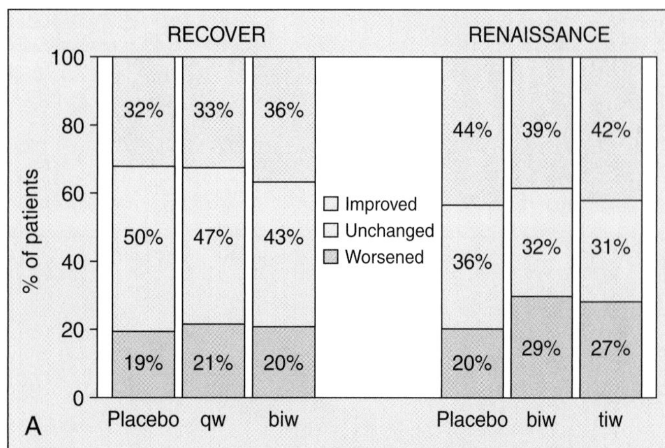

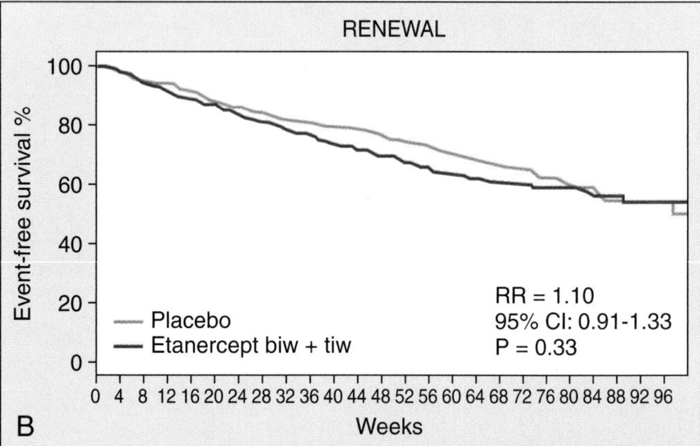

FIGURE 11–12 Results of the RENAISSANCE, RECOVER, and RENEWAL trials. **A,** Analysis of the "clinical status" composite score for the RECOVER and RENAISSANCE trials in the placebo and etanercept groups. **B,** Kaplan-Meier analysis of the time to death or heart failure hospitalizations in the placebo and etanercept group (twice a week and three times a week) in the RENEWAL analysis. (From Mann DL, McMurray JJV, Packer M, et al. Targeted anti-cytokine therapy in patients with chronic heart failure: results of the randomized etanercept worldwide evaluation (RENEWAL). *Circulation* 2004;109:1594-1602.)

increased rates of mortality and heart failure hospitalization, particularly in the group who was receiving the highest dose of infliximab (Figure 11-13). By 38 weeks of follow-up, nine infliximab patients had died (two in the 5-mg/kg group and seven in the 10-mg/kg group) compared with just one death in the placebo group. On the basis of these findings, the prescribing information for infliximab has been changed and it is now recommended that treatment with infliximab be discontinued in patients with worsening heart failure and that treatment with infliximab should not be initiated in patients with heart failure.

Why Have Targeted Anti-TNF Therapies Failed in Heart Failure Trials? Given the wealth of preclinical data and early clinical studies that suggested a role for TNF antagonism in heart failure, the negative results of the clinical trials have been discouraging. This statement notwithstanding, analysis of the aggregate clinical trial data permits some insight into the potential reasons for why these studies have been negative. It is important to recognize that neither the trials with etanercept nor the trial with infliximab was neutral (i.e., no effect): that is, in both trials there was evidence for dose- and time-dependent worsening of heart failure and/or worsening outcomes. This in turn suggests that the biological agents used in the trials either had intrinsic effects themselves, or alternatively that TNF antagonism has untoward effects in the setting of heart failure. With respect to the

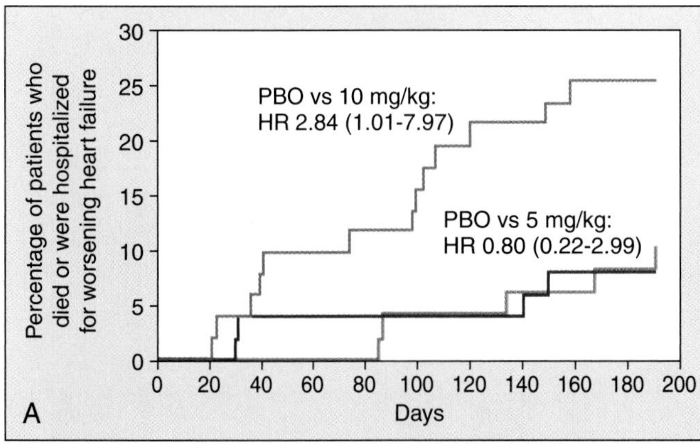

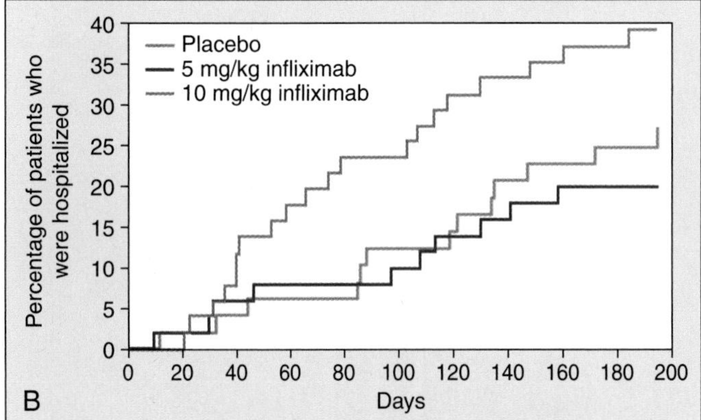

FIGURE 11–13 Results of the ATTACH trial. **A,** Kaplan-Meier rates of death and hospitalization for heart failure. **B,** Kaplan-Meier rates of hospitalization for any reason. (Key: *PBO,* placebo; *HR,* hazard ratio). (From Chung ES, Packer M, Lo KH, et al. Randomized, double-blind, placebo-controlled, pilot trial of infliximab, a chimeric monoclonal antibody to tumor necrosis factor-α, in patients with moderate-to-severe heart failure: results of the anti-TNF therapy against congestive heart failure (ATTACH) trial. *Circulation* 2003;107:3133-3140.)

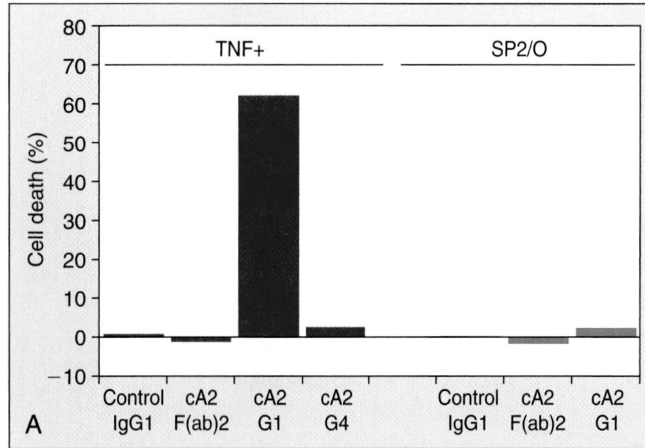

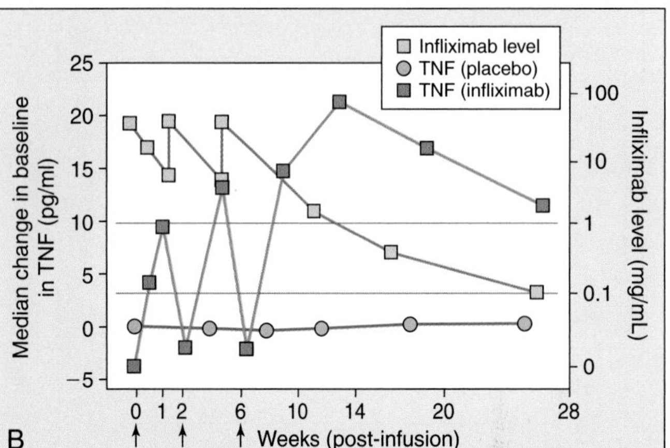

FIGURE 11–14 Biological properties of infliximab. **A,** Infliximab (cA2 G1) is cytotoxic for cells that express TNF on their cell membranes (TNF+), whereas it is not cytotoxic for cells that do not express TNF on their membranes (SP_2/O). The mechanism for the cytotoxic effects of infliximab was demonstrated using F(ab)2 fragments of infliximab, which lack the Fc domain and therefore cannot fix complement. As shown the F(ab)2 fragment of infliximab was not cytotoxic for TNF+ cells. **B,** Levels of immunoreactive TNF in patients who received a placebo and infliximab (10 mg/kg) are displayed in relation to the circulating levels of infliximab (data are redrawn from Figures 2 and 4[101]). The dotted horizontal lines depict the upper and lower limits of the therapeutic window for infliximab. (A, Modified from Scallon BJ, Moore MA, Trinh H, et al. Chimeric anti-TNF-alpha monoclonal antibody cA2 binds recombinant transmembrane TNF-alpha and activates immune effector functions. *Cytokine* 1995;7:251-259. B, Modified from Chung ES, Packer M, Lo KH, et al. Randomized, double-blind, placebo-controlled, pilot trial of infliximab, a chimeric monoclonal antibody to tumor necrosis factor-α, in patients with moderate-to-severe heart failure: results of the anti-TNF therapy against congestive heart failure (ATTACH) trial. *Circulation* 2003;107:3133-3140.)

first explanation, it bears emphasis that infliximab exerts its effects, at least in part, by fixing the complement in cells that express TNF on the membrane. As shown in Figure 11-14, *A*, infliximab is directly cytotoxic to cells expressing TNF on the membrane. Whereas this type of biological action may be beneficial in eliminating activated T cells in Crohn disease, it is likely to be overtly deleterious in the setting of heart failure, wherein failing myocytes express TNF on cell membranes.[8] Indeed complement fixation in the heart leads to sustained myocarditis, and cardiac myocyte lysis mediated by the complement membrane attack complex.[102] Analysis of the data presented in the ATTACH trial supports the point of view that infliximab was overtly deleterious. As shown in Figure 11-14, *B*, there was an increase in the plasma levels of immunoreactive TNF at the time of treatment with infliximab at 2 and 6 weeks, and after the last dose in infliximab at 6 weeks. Although the investigators attributed the increase in TNF levels to infliximab binding to TNF in the circulation, this explanation does not explain the striking twenty-fivefold increase in TNF levels from 10 to 28 weeks, when the infliximab levels were declining below detectable levels. An alternative explanation for the increase in TNF levels after infliximab was that there was ongoing tissue injury secondary to complement activation in the heart, and that the twenty-fivefold increase in TNF levels was in response to increased cardiac injury and that the increase in TNF levels and/or increased tissue damage were responsible for the increase in heart failure hospitalizations and deaths in the infliximab-treated group.

Cytokine binding proteins such as etanercept also have intrinsic biological activity and, in certain settings, can act as agonists for the cytokine that they bind.[103] As a case in point, in human studies etanercept acts as a carrier protein that stabilizes TNF and results in the accumulation of high concentrations of immunoreactive TNF in the peripheral circulation of etanercept-treated patients with heart failure (Figure 11-15, *A*).[104] As shown in Figure 11-15, *B*, TNF complexed to etanercept does not remain tightly bound, but rather dissociates with an extremely fast off-rate (~620 msec).[105] The increase in circulating levels of TNF bound to etanercept combined with the rapid off-rates of TNF from etanercept can lead to an increase in TNF bioactivity, as depicted in Figure 11-15, *C*.[104] This increase in TNF bioactivity that has been observed experimentally and may be secondary to a shift in the equilibrium between TNF monomers, dimers, and trimers in favor of more biologically active TNF homotrimers by virtue of the ability of etanercept to stabilize TNF in its functionally active

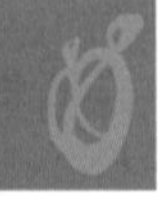

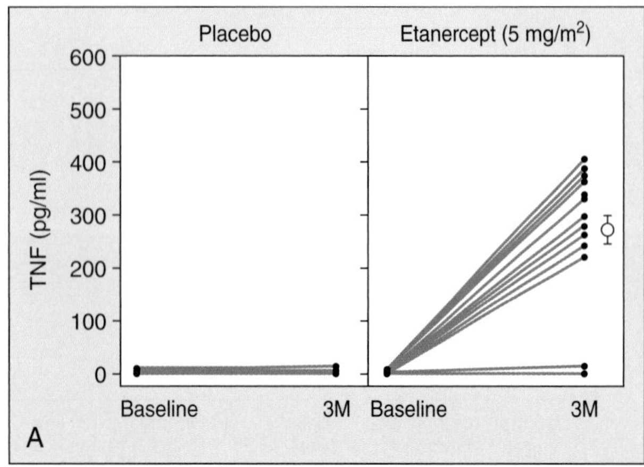

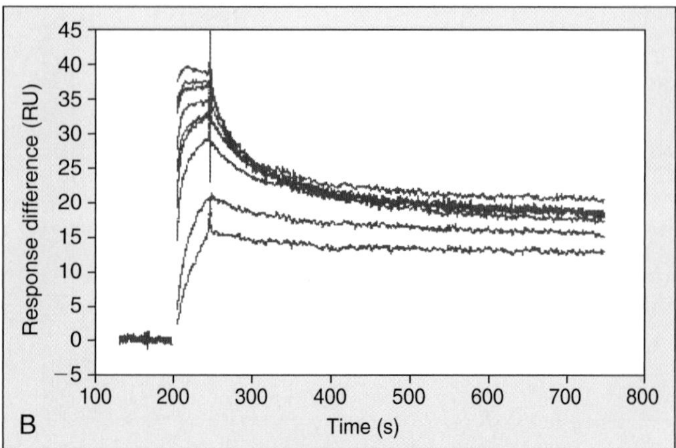

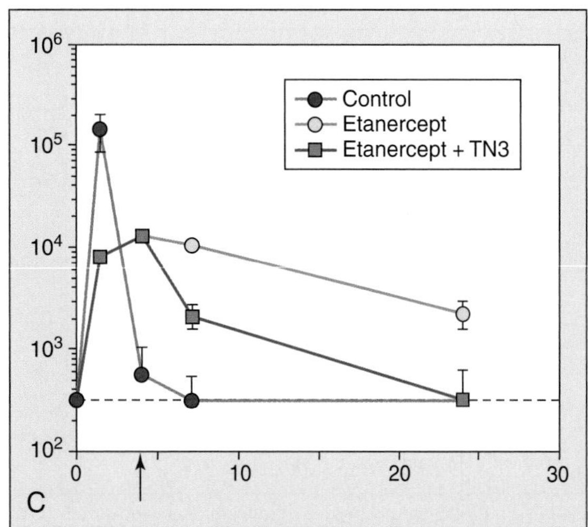

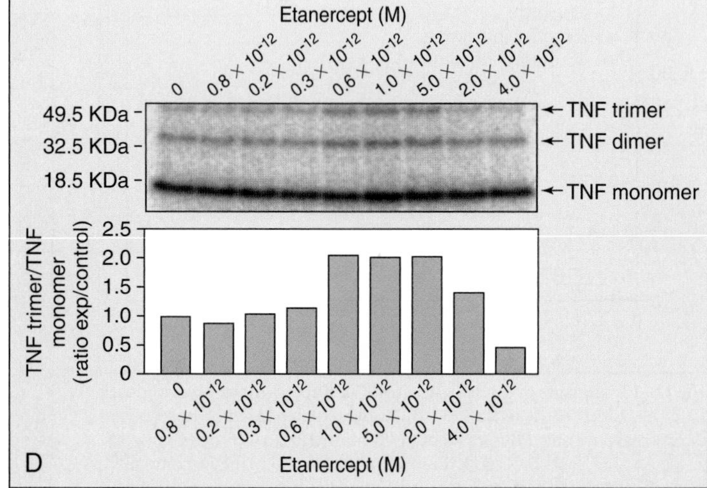

FIGURE 11–15 Biological properties of etanercept. **A,** Etanercept (5 mg/m^2) increases the circulating levels of immunoreactive TNF in heart failure patients. **B,** Kinetic analysis of TNF binding to etanercept using surface plasmon resonance biosensor technology (BIAcore assay[124]). Etanercept was exposed to 1000, 500, 250, 125, 62.5, 31.25, 16.63, 3.90, and 1.95 nM of TNF, and the kinetics of TNF binding was determined by the decay of the light signal after peak binding to etanercept. The off-rate of TNF from etanercept was determined to be 620 msec. **C,** Etanercept increases TNF bioactivity. Animals were inoculated with bacteria and levels of TNF bioactivity measured at the indicated time points. TNF bioactivity peaked at 90 min after bacterial inoculation, but was undetectable at later time points. Mice treated with etanercept after bacterial inoculation showed a significant reduction in the level of peak TNF bioactivity; however, as shown TNF bioactivity was significantly prolonged by etanercept. Mice that received etanercept after bacterial inoculation followed by an anti-TNF neutralizing antibody (TN3), had a shorter duration of TNF bioactivity. The arrow indicates the timing of the administration of the neutralizing anti-TNF antibody. **D,** Effects of etanercept on TNF stability. *Upper panel*: a fixed concentration of ^{125}I-TNF was incubated with increasing concentrations of etanercept (8 × 10^{-14} M - 6.25 × 10^{-10} M) or diluent, followed by cross-linking and autoradiography. The arrows depict TNF monomers, dimers, and trimers. Note that etanercept increases the mass of homotrimeric TNF. *Lower panel*: Group data were expressed as the ratio of trimeric to monomeric TNF, and the results displayed as the fold-change in this ratio relative to diluent treated cells. (**A,** Modified from Mann DL, Bozkurt **B,** Torre-Amione G, et al. Effect of the soluble TNF-antagonist etanercept on tumor necrosis factor bioactivity and stability. *Clin Transl Sci* 2008;1:142-145. B, Reproduced with permission from Frishman JI, Edwards CK III, Sonnenberg MG, et al. Tumor necrosis factor (TNF)-alpha-induced interleukin-8 in human blood cultures discriminates neutralization by the p55 and p75 TNF soluble receptors. *J Infect Dis* 2000;182:1722-1730. **C,** Modified from Evans TJ, Moyes D, Carpenter A, et al. Protective effect of 55- but not 75-kDa soluble tumor necrosis factor receptor-immunoglobulin G fusion proteins in an animal model of gram-negative sepsis. *J Exp Med* 1994;180:2173-2179. Copyright ©The Rockefeller University Press. **D,** Modified from Mann DL, Bozkurt B, Torre-Amione G, et al. Effect of the soluble TNF-antagonist etanercept on tumor necrosis factor bioactivity and stability. *Clin Transl Sci* 2008;1:142-145.)

homotrimeric form (Figure 11-15, *D*). Thus panels *A* to *D* in Figure 11-15 show that etanercept can, in certain settings, act as a "stimulating antagonist.[103]" While the aforementioned biological effects of etanercept might not be problematic in rheumatoid arthritis, wherein TNF is encapsulated within a joint space and peripheral circulating TNF levels are relatively low (compared with heart failure) or are nonexistent,[106] an increase in the circulating levels of biologically active TNF in a patient with heart failure might be expected to produce worsening heart failure, for all of the reasons articulated at the outset of this chapter (see Box 11-2).

Immunomodulatory Strategies. An alternative approach to targeting specific components of the inflammatory cascade is to employ strategies that dampen the various components' systemic inflammatory response. Thus far, two different approaches have been employed in heart failure studies: intravenous immunoglobulin and immune modulation therapy (IMT). The topic of immunoadsorption is reviewed in Chapter 24 (see Aukrust et al[107] for a recent review).

Intravenous Immunoglobulin. Therapy with intravenous immunoglobulin (IVIG) has been tried in a wide range of immune-mediated disorders, such as Kawasaki syndrome, dermatomyositis, multiple sclerosis, and most recently dilated cardiomyopathy (Chapter 24), wherein the initial results have been encouraging. In a double-blind, placebo-controlled study of 20 ischemic and nonischemic NYHA class II-IV heart failure patients with an LV ejection fraction less than 40%, monthly IVIG treatment for 6 months resulted in a significant increase in LV ejection fraction from 26% to 31%, independent of heart failure cause.[108] These improvements in functional class and LV function were accompanied by an increase in the antiinflammatory mediators IL-10, IL-1 receptor antagonist (IL-1Ra), and soluble TNF receptors, and a slight decrease in plasma TNF, suggesting that IVIG evoked a net antiinflammatory effect. In contrast to these encouraging results, induction therapy with IVIG in the IMAC (Intravenous in Myocarditis and Acute Cardiomyopathy) trial in patients with recent-onset cardiomyopathy (<6 months) and an LV ejection fraction less than 40% demonstrated no significant effect on LV ejection fraction when compared with a placebo.[109] However, it bears emphasis that there was also an increase in LV ejection fraction from 23% to 42% in the placebo arm, which would have made it difficult to show a statistically significant increase in LV ejection fraction in the treatment arm. Moreover, there were important differences in the IVIG dosing strategies in IMAC and the study by Gullestad et al. That is, while both studies used induction therapy (a total of 2 g/kg IVIG), in the study by Gullestad et al maintenance therapy (monthly infusions [0.4 g/kg] for a total of 5 months) was also given. Thus one possible reason for the different outcomes in these two studies is that IVIG maintenance therapy is required for an extended period of time, as has been observed in other chronic inflammatory disorders.

Immune Modulation Therapy (IMT). Immune modulation therapy (IMT; Celacade; Vasogen, Inc.) uses a medical device (the VC7000 Blood Treatment System) to expose a sample of blood to a combination of physiochemical stressors ex vivo. The treated blood sample is then administered intramuscularly along with local anesthetic into the same patient from whom the sample is obtained. The physiochemical stresses to which the autologous blood sample is subjected are known to initiate or facilitate apoptotic cell death. The uptake of apoptotic cells by macrophages results in a downregulation of proinflammatory cytokines, including TNF, IL-1β, and IL-8, and an increase in production of the antiinflammatory cytokines, including TGF-β and IL-10.[110] Recent studies have shown that IMT leads to a decrease in the production of proinflammatory cytokines and a corresponding increase in antiinflammatory cytokines in human subjects.[111] Given that an imbalance exists between proinflammatory and antiinflammatory cytokines in patients with heart failure,[112] IMT may restore this balance more towards normal. In a recent trial employing Celacade in 73 patients with moderate heart failure, the investigators noted that, compared with the placebo group, the group receiving Celacade experienced significantly fewer hospitalizations or deaths. The decrease in the event rate in the treatment arm was also supported by improvements in quality of life and NYHA clinical classification.[113] Based on the encouraging results of the early studies, the ACCLAIM (*Advance Chronic Heart Failure Clinical Assessment of Immune Modification*) pivotal study was conducted in 2426 patients with NYHA class II-IV heart failure patients with ischemic and nonischemic dilated cardiomyopathy.[114] Patients were randomly assigned to receive Celacade (n = 1213) or placebo (n = 1213) by intragluteal injection on days 1, 2, 14, and every 28 days thereafter. The primary endpoint in this event-driven trial was the composite of time to death from any cause or first hospitalization for cardiovascular reasons. As shown in Figure 11-16, *A*, there was no significant difference between the Celacade- and placebo- treated patients with respect to the primary endpoint of the trial, which was death from any cause or cardiovascular hospitalization (hazard ratio 0.92; 95% CI 0.80 to 1.05; P = .22). However, in a prespecified subgroup of patients with NYHA II heart failure (see Figure 11-16, *B*), and in those without a history of previous myocardial infarction (see Figure 11-16, *C*) Celacade was associated with a 39% (0.61; 95% CI 0.46 to 0.80; P = .0003) and 26% (0.74; 0.57 to 0.95; P = .02) reduction in the risk of primary endpoint events, respectively, suggesting that IMT may have a role as a potential treatment for selected patients without a history of myocardial infarction (NYHA class II-IV) and/or patients with milder heart failure (NYHA class II).

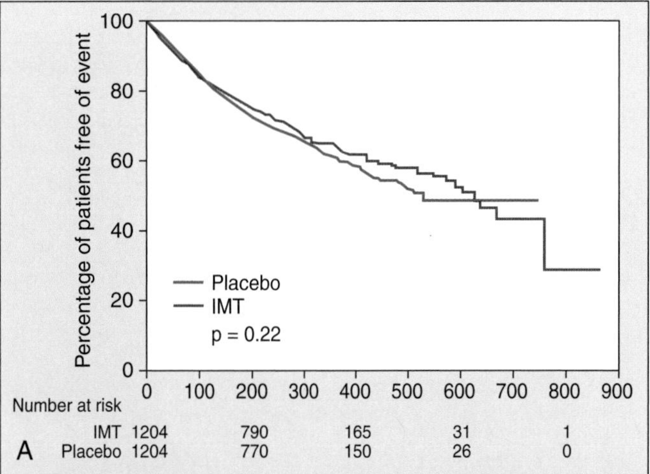

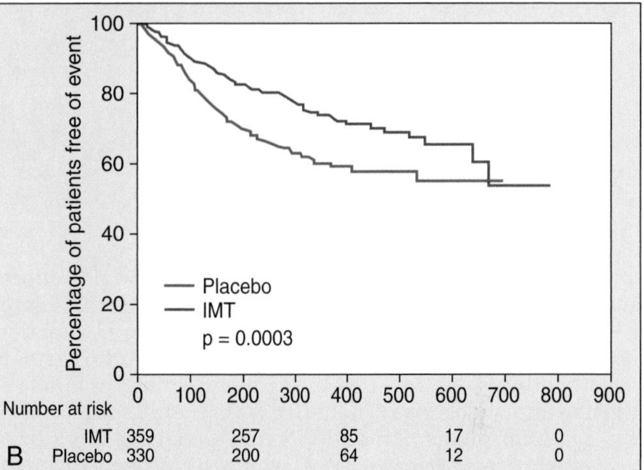

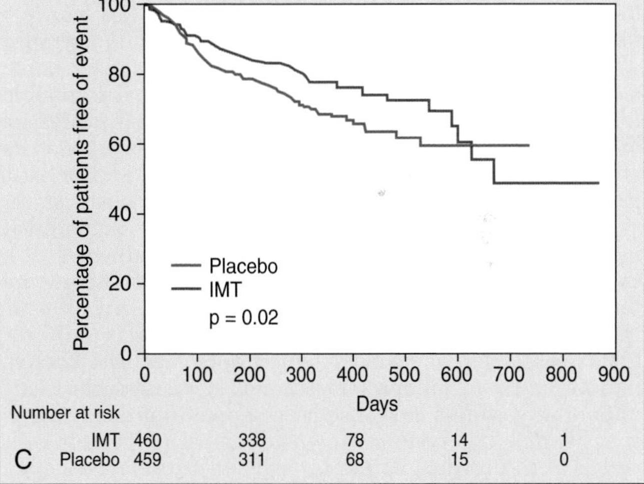

FIGURE 11–16 Results of the ACCLAIM trial. **A,** Kaplan-Meier estimates of time to primary endpoint of time to death from any cause or first hospitalization for cardiovascular reasons in all patients. **B,** Kaplan-Meier estimates of time to death from any cause or first hospitalization for cardiovascular reasons in patients with NYHA class II heart failure. **C,** Kaplan-Meier estimates of time to death from any cause or first hospitalization for cardiovascular reasons in patients with nonischemic cardiomyopathy. (Modified from Torre-Amione G, Anker SD, Bourge RC, et al. Results of a nonspecific immunomodulation therapy in chronic heart failure (ACCLAIM trial): a placebo-controlled randomized trial. *Lancet* 2008;371:228-236.)

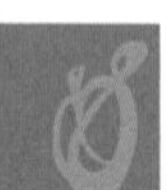

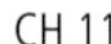

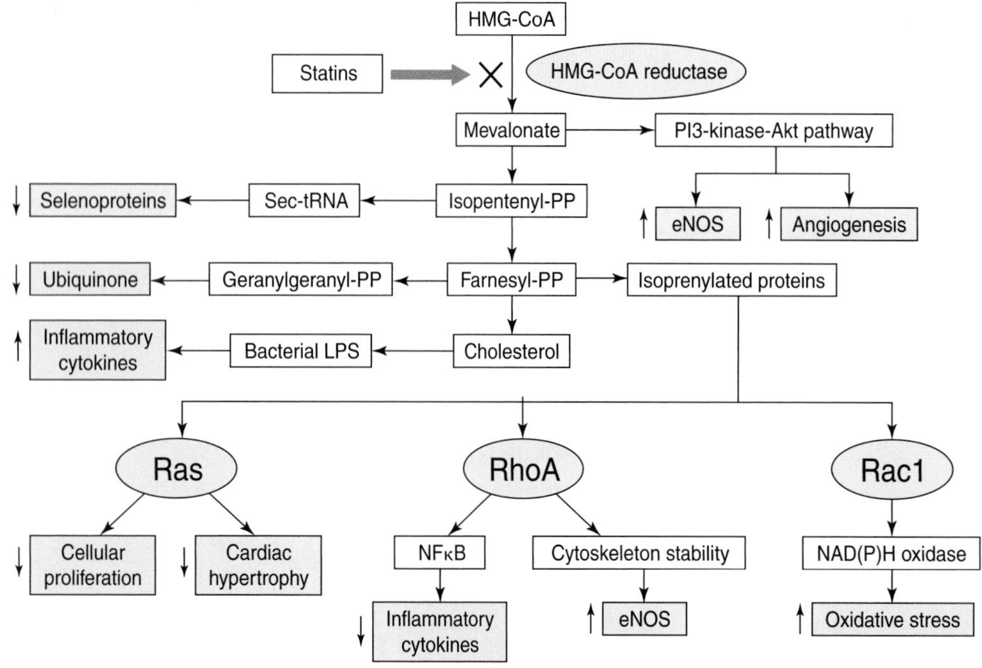

FIGURE 11–17 Cholesterol biosynthesis and the beneficial (gray background) and adverse (checked background) downstream effects of statin treatment. *eNOS,* endothelial nitric oxide synthase; *HMG-CoA,* 3-hydroxy-3-methylglutaryl coenzyme A; *LPS,* lipopolysaccharide; *NF κβ,* nuclear factor kappa B; *PI3,* phosphatidylinositol-3; *PP,* pyrophosphate. (From Ramasubbu K, Estep J, White DL, Deswal A, Mann DL. Experimental and clinical basis for the use of statins in patients with ischemic and nonischemic cardiomyopathy. *J Am Coll Cardiol* 2008;51:415-426.)

Statins. Stains have a variety of pleiotropic effects, including inhibition of inflammatory responses, increased nitric oxide bioavailability, improved endothelial function, and antioxidant properties. In addition to inhibiting cholesterol synthesis, statins also lower intermediate products in the mevalonate pathway including isoprenoids such as farnesyl pyrophosphate (farnesyl-PP) and geranylgeranyl pyrophosphate (geranylgeranyl-PP), which have been linked to activation of downstream signaling pathways mediated by Ras and Rho, respectively (Figure 11-17). The Ras family of proteins is responsible for cell proliferation and hypertrophy, whereas the Rho family of proteins is important for superoxide generation, inflammation, and cytoskeletal formation. Rho inhibition has also been linked to increased expression of endothelial nitric oxide synthesis, which has a beneficial effect on endothelial function through increased nitric oxide production. Although the mechanism is less clear, statins also activate the phosphatidylinositol 3′-kinase/Akt pathway, which is coupled to cytoprotective signaling pathways.[115] In experimental models, statins attenuated LV remodeling and improved LV ejection performance without directly affecting infarct size. The attenuation in LV remodeling was attributed to decreased cardiac myocyte hypertrophy, decreased activation of matrix metalloproteinases, and decreased fibrosis.[115] Importantly, statins have also been shown to promote angiogenesis, mobilize bone-marrow endothelial progenitor cells, and lead to downregulation of angiotensin type 1 receptor, any or all of which may have an additional beneficial effect(s) on cardiac remodeling.[115]

Several retrospective analyses of clinical trials or observational databases have suggested that the use of statins in patients with coronary artery disease has either decreased the incidence of heart failure or reduced mortality in patients with known heart failure. Given the known salutary effects of statins on outcomes in coronary artery disease, and the high prevalence of ischemic heart disease in heart failure trials, these findings are perhaps not that surprising. Nonetheless, a prespecified posthoc analysis of the TNT (Treating to New Targets), in which patients with coronary heart disease were randomized to 10 mg/day or 80 mg/day of atorvastatin and then followed for a mean of 4.9 years for traditional coronary events (death, nonfatal myocardial infarction, or stroke), showed that heart failure hospitalization rates were significantly lower in patients with a prior history of heart failure who were treated with 80 mg/day of atorvastatin when compared with the group treated with 10 mg/day (hazard ratio, 0.87; 95% confidence interval, 0.64 to 1.16; P = .34). The decrease in heart failure hospitalizations was unlikely secondary to a reduction in interim coronary events, insofar as one third of patients hospitalized for heart failure had evidence of preceding angina or myocardial infarction during the study period.[116] In addition to these retrospective trials, several small prospective trials assessing the effects of statins on nonmortality clinical endpoints and other surrogate endpoints (echocardiographic parameters and biomarkers of inflammation) also support the beneficial effects of statins in heart failure (reviewed in Ramasubbu et al[117]).

Based on the results of these promising studies, several large clinical trials were performed with rosuvastatin in patients with heart failure. The *R*osuvastatin *I*mpact *on V*entricular *R*emodeling *C*ytokines *and N*eurohormones (UNIVERSE) trial examined the of effects of rosuvastatin (40 mg/day) on LV remodeling in patients with ischemic and nonischemic dilated cardiomypathy.[118] Compared with a placebo, rosuvastatin was associated with significant reduction of low-density lipoprotein cholesterol, but had no effects on LV dimension, LV ejection fraction, or neurohormones. Similar findings were reported in the *Controlled Rosuvastatin Multinational Trial in Heart Failure* (CORONA) trial, in which 5011 patients (>60 years of age) with NYHA functional class II-IV heart failure of ischemic cause were randomized to 10 mg/day of rosuvastatin versus placebo.[119] In CORONA, treatment with rosuvastatin did not confer a significant benefit with respect to the primary endpoint (Figure 11-18, *A*), which was a composite of death from cardiovascular causes, nonfatal myocardial infarction, or nonfatal stroke (HR 0.92, 95% CI 0.83 to 1.02; P = .12). Further, there were no significant differences in several of the secondary endpoints including all-cause mortality (HR 0.95; 95% CI 0.86 to 1.05; P = .31) and coronary events (HR 0.92; 95% CI 0.82 to 1.04; P = .18), despite a significant decrease in circulating levels of low-density lipoprotein cholesterol and C-reactive protein (CRP). These results were surprising considering the known salutary effects of statins on coronary events in patients with coronary artery disease. However, it

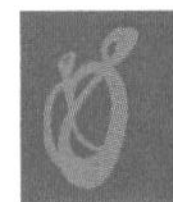

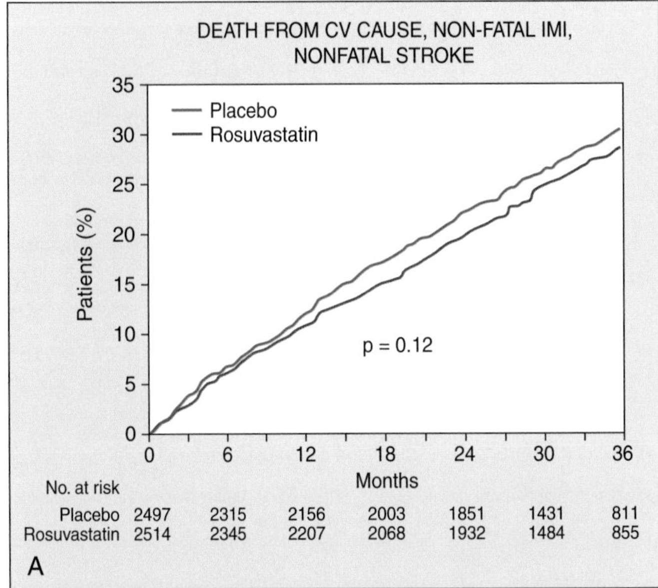

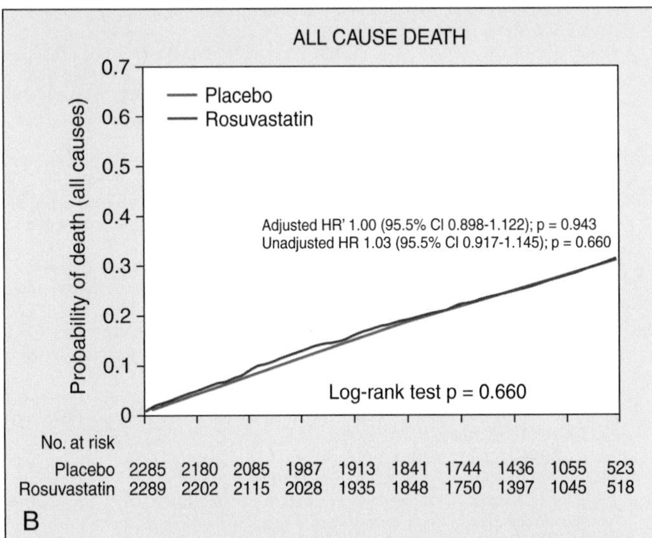

FIGURE 11–18 Results of the CORONA and GISSI-HF trials. **A,** Kaplan-Meier estimates of a composite of death from cardiovascular causes, nonfatal myocardial infarction, or nonfatal stroke in the CORONA trial. **B,** Kaplan-Meier estimates of all causes of death in the GISSI-HF trial. (A, From Kjekshus J, Apetrei E, Barrios V, et al. Rosuvastatin in older patients with systolic heart failure. *N Engl J Med* 2007;357:2248-2261. B, From Gissi-HF Investigators. Effect of rosuvastatin in patients with chronic heart failure (the GISSI-HF trial): a randomized, double-blind, placebo-controlled trial. *Lancet* 2008;372:1231-1239.)

is worth noting that the rate of atherothrombotic events was relatively low in the CORONA study, and that the majority of deaths were caused by sudden death or worsening heart failure, which reflects the fact that the patient population consisted of patients with symptomatic heart failure rather than symptomatic coronary artery disease. Thus the primary composite endpoint of the CORONA study may not have captured the beneficial effects of rosuvastatin in this elderly group of patients with advanced heart failure. And indeed, treatment with rosuvastatin resulted in a significant decrease in heart failure hospitalizations, which was a prespecified secondary endpoint in the CORONA study, thus ending speculation that treatment with statins might lead to worsening heart failure. The Gruppo Italiano per lo Studio della Sopravvivenza nell'Insuffi cienza cardiaca-Heart Failure (GISSI-HF) investigated the efficacy and safety of rosuvastatin in patients with NYHA class II-IV heart failure, irrespective of cause and/or LV ejection fraction.[120] Patients were randomly assigned to rosuvastatin 10 mg daily (n = 2285) or a placebo (n = 2289), and followed up for a median of 3.9 years. The primary endpoints of the trial were time to death or admission to hospital for cardiovascular reasons. As shown in Figure 11-18, *B*, there was no significant difference in the probability of all-cause death in patients who were treated with rosuvastatin when compared with the placebo group (adjusted HR 1.00, 95.5% CI 0.898 to 1.122, P = .943). Further, there was no significant difference in the composite endpoint of death or admission to the hospital for cardiovascular reasons (adjusted HR 1.01, 99% CI 0.908 to 1.112, P = .903). Of note, 10% of the total population in GISSI-HF had an LV ejection fraction greater than 40%. Although this subgroup was too small to draw definite conclusions about the effects of statins in heart failure with a preserved EF, there were no differences in outcomes between this subgroup when compared with the results for the overall group. In a parallel arm of the GISSI-HF study, randomized NYHA class II-IV heart failure patients received n-3 polyunsaturated fatty acids (PUFA) or a placebo (see Chapter 24). This arm of GISSI-HF showed that there was a small but statistically significant decrease in all-cause death in the n-3 PUFA-treated group when compared with the placebo group (adjusted HR 0.91, 95.5% CI 0.833 to 0.998], P = .041). There was also a reduction in the number of hospitalizations for cardiovascular reasons (adjusted HR 0.92, 99% CI 0.849 to 0.999, P = .009), raising the possibility that dietary supplementation with polyunsaturated fatty acids may benefit patients with heart failure.[121] Thus, taken together, the results of the randomized trials with rosuvastatin do not support a primary role for treating heart failure patients with statins. Whether the negative results of these studies are secondary to the hydrophilic properties of rosuvastatin or a true lack of treatment benefit of statins in heart failure patients cannot be addressed at present. Accordingly, statins should not be used as a primary treatment for patients with heart failure outside of the current practice guidelines for the treatment of coronary artery disease.

Summary and Future Perspectives

In the present review we have focused on recent clinical and experimental evidence that suggests that inflammatory mediators play a role in disease progression in heart failure by virtue of the deleterious effects that these molecules exert on the heart and the peripheral circulation. As discussed, pathophysiologically relevant concentrations of these molecules mimic many aspects of the so-called heart failure phenotype in experimental animals, including LV dysfunction, LV dilation, activation of fetal gene expression, cardiac myocyte hypertrophy, and cardiac myocyte apoptosis (see Box 11-2). Thus analogous to the proposed role for neurohormones, proinflammatory cytokines would appear to represent another distinct class of biologically active molecules that can contribute to heart failure progression. Nonetheless, the early attempts to translate this information to the bedside have not only been disappointing, but have in many instances led to worsening heart failure. While one interpretation of these findings is that inflammatory mediators are not viable targets in heart failure, based on the arguments delineated previously, the countervailing point of view is that we simply have not targeted proinflammatory mediators with agents that can be used safely in the context of heart failure, or alternatively, that targeting a single component of the inflammatory cascade is not sufficient in a disease as complex as heart failure. Moreover, it is important to recognize that all currently approved therapies for chronic heart failure, including cardiac resynchronization therapy (see Chapter 47), have a net beneficial effect on the elaboration of inflammatory mediators.[122] Accordingly, in future studies it may be necessary to use biomarkers to select heart failure patients who have ongoing inflammation despite optimal medical therapy. Indeed a recent consensus statement from the Translation Research Committee of the Heart Failure Association of the European Society of Cardiology suggested that there may not be a common inflammatory pathway that characterizes all of the different forms of heart failure, and that going forward it would be important to design specific antiinflammatory approaches for different types and stages of heart failure, and to determine the specific inflammatory pathways that are activated in different forms of heart failure.[123] Thus despite the inauspicious beginning with targeted antiinflammatory approaches, strategies that use small molecules that have a broad spectrum of antiinflammatory properties and/or immunomodulatory strategies that restore the balance of proinflammatory and antiinflammatory gene networks are currently being evaluated (e.g., pentraxins, PI3Kγ inhibitors, mannose binding lectins [reviewed in Heymans et al[123]]). As with all therapeutic approaches in heart failure, the only way to really answer the question of whether these types of antiinflammatory strategies will have any added value in heart failure is through well-designed clinical trials.

REFERENCES

1. Lower, R. (1669). *Tractatus de corde: de motu & colore sagnuinus et chyli in eum tranfitu.* London: Jacobi Alleftry.
2. Levine, B., Kalman, J., Mayer, L., et al. (1990). Elevated circulating levels of tumor necrosis factor in severe chronic heart failure. *N Engl J Med, 223,* 236–241.
3. Wiley, S. R., & Winkles, J. A. (2003). TWEAK, a member of the TNF superfamily, is a multifunctional cytokine that binds the TweakR/Fn14 receptor. *Cytokine Growth Factor Rev, 14,* 241–249.
4. Pomerantz, B. J., Reznikov, L. L., Harken, A. H., et al. (2001). Inhibition of caspase 1 reduces human myocardial ischemic dysfunction via inhibition of IL-18 and IL-1beta. *Proc Natl Acad Sci U S A, 98,* 2871–2876.
5. Sanada, S., Hakuno, D., Higgins, L. J., et al. (2007). IL-33 and ST2 comprise a critical biomechanically induced and cardioprotective signaling system. *J Clin Invest, 117,* 1538–1549.
6. Gulick, T. S., Chung, M. K., Pieper, S. J., et al. (1989). Interleukin 1 and tumor necrosis factor inhibit cardiac myocyte β-adrenergic responsiveness. *Proc Natl Acad Sci U S A, 86,* 6753–6757.
7. Torre-Amione, G., Kapadia, S., Lee, J., et al. (1995). Expression and functional significance of tumor necrosis factor receptors in human myocardium. *Circulation, 92,* 1487–1493.
8. Torre-Amione, G., Kapadia, S., Lee, J., et al. (1996). Tumor necrosis factor-α and tumor necrosis factor receptors in the failing human heart. *Circulation, 93,* 704–711.
9. Ramani, R., Mathier, M., Wang, P., et al. (2004). Inhibition of tumor necrosis factor receptor-1-mediated pathways has beneficial effects in a murine model of postischemic remodeling. *Am J Physiol Heart Circ Physiol, 287,* H1369–H1377.
10. Olsson, I., Lantz, M., Nilsson, E., et al. (1989). Isolation and characterization of a tumor necrosis factor binding protein from urine. *Eur J Haematol, 42,* 270–275.
11. Deswal, A., Petersen, N. J., Feldman, A. M., et al. (2001). Cytokines and cytokine receptors in advanced heart failure: an analysis of the cytokine database from the vesnarinone trial (VEST). *Circulation, 103,* 2055–2059.
12. Chorianopoulos, E., Heger, T., Lutz, M., et al. (2010). FGF-inducible 14-kDa protein (Fn14) is regulated via the RhoA/ROCK kinase pathway in cardiomyocytes and mediates nuclear factor-kappaB activation by TWEAK. *Basic Res Cardiol* 105; 301-313.
13. Jain, M., Jakubowski, A., Cui, L., et al. (2009). A novel role for tumor necrosis factor-like weak inducer of apoptosis (TWEAK) in the development of cardiac dysfunction and failure. *Circulation, 119,* 2058–2068.
14. Dinarello, C. A. (1996). Biological basis for interleukin-1 in disease. *Blood, 87,* 2095–2147.
15. Francis, S. E., Holden, H., Holt, C. M., et al. (1998). Interleukin-1 in myocardium and coronary arteries of patients with dilated cardiomyopathy. *J Mol Cell Cardiol, 30,* 215–223.
16. Dinarello, C. A. (1991). Interleukin-1. In A. Thomson (Ed.), *The cytokine handbook.* Boston: Academic Press.
17. Dinarello, C. A. (1999). Interleukin-18. *Methods, 19,* 121–132.
18. Raeburn, C. D., Dinarello, C. A., Zimmerman, M. A., et al. (2002). Neutralization of IL-18 attenuates lipopolysaccharide-induced myocardial dysfunction. *Am J Physiol Heart Circ Physiol, 283,* H650–H657.
19. Born, T. L., Thomassen, E., Bird, T. A., et al. (1998). Cloning of a novel receptor subunit, AcPL, required for interleukin-18 signaling. *J Biol Chem, 273,* 29445–29450.
20. Kakkar, R., & Lee, R. T. (2008). The IL-33/ST2 pathway: therapeutic target and novel biomarker. *Nat Rev Drug Discov, 7,* 827–840.
21. Sabatine, M. S., Morrow, D. A., Higgins, L. J., et al. (2008). Complementary roles for biomarkers of biomechanical strain ST2 and N-terminal prohormone B-type natriuretic peptide in patients with ST-elevation myocardial infarction. *Circulation, 117,* 1936–1944.
22. Hirano, T. (1991). Interleukin-6. In A. Thomson (Ed.), *The cytokine handbook.* Boston: Academic Press.
23. Hirano, T., Yasukawa, K., Harada, H., et al. (1986). Complementary DNA for a novel human interleukin (BSF-2) that induces B lymphocytes to produce immunoglobulin. *Nature, 324,* 73–78.
24. Finkel, M. S., Hoffman, R. A., Shen, L., et al. (1993). Interleukin-6 (IL-6) as a mediator of stunned myocardium. *Am J Cardiol, 71,* 1231–1232.
25. Sehgal, P. B. (1996). Interleukin-6 type cytokines in vivo: regulated bioavailability. *Proc Soc Exp Biol Med, 213,* 238–247.
26. Eiken, H. G., Oie, E., Damas, J. K., et al. (2001). Myocardial gene expression of leukaemia inhibitory factor, interleukin-6 and glycoprotein 130 in end-stage human heart failure. *Eur J Clin Invest, 31,* 389–397.
27. Talwar, S., Squire, I. B., Downie, P. F., et al. (2000). Elevated circulating cardiotrophin-1 in heart failure: relationship with parameters of left ventricular systolic dysfunction. *Clin Sci (Lond), 99,* 83–88.
28. Hirota, H., Yoshida, K., Kishimoto, T., et al. (1995). Continuous activation of gp130, a signal-transducing receptor component for interleukin 6-related cytokines, causes myocardial hypertrophy in mice. *Proc Natl Acad Sci U S A, 92,* 4862–4866.
29. Yoshida, K., Taga, T., Saito, M., et al. (1996). Targeted disruption of gp130, a common signal transducer for the interleukin 6 family of cytokines, leads to myocardial and hematological disorders. *Proc Natl Acad Sci U S A, 93,* 407–411.
30. Aukrust, P., Ueland, T., Muller, F., et al. (1998). Elevated circulating levels of C-C chemokines in patients with congestive heart failure. *Circulation, 97,* 1136–1143.
31. Frantz, S., Ertl, G., & Bauersachs, J. (2008). Toll-like receptor signaling in the ischemic heart. *Front Biosci, 13,* 5772–5779.
32. Chao, W. (2009). Toll-like receptor signaling: a critical modulator of cell survival and ischemic injury in the heart. *Am J Physiol Heart Circ Physiol, 296,* H1–H12.
33. Mann, D. L. (2001). Tumor necrosis factor and viral myocarditis: the fine line between innate and inappropriate immune responses in the heart. *Circulation, 103,* 626–629.
34. Cowan, D. B., Poutias, D. N., del Nido, P. J., et al. (2000). CD14-independent activation of cardiomyocyte signal transduction by bacterial endotoxin. *Am J Physiol Heart Circ Physiol, 279,* H619–H629.
35. Frantz, S., Kelly, R. A., & Bourcier, T. (2001). Role of TLR-2 in the activation of nuclear factor-kappa B by oxidative stress in cardiac myocytes. *J Biol Chem, 276,* 5197–5203.
36. Li, M., Carpio, D. F., Zheng, Y., et al. (2001). An essential role of the NF-kappa B/toll-like receptor pathway in induction of inflammatory and tissue-repair gene expression by necrotic cells. *J Immunol, 166,* 7128–7135.
37. Frantz, S., Kobzik, L., Kim, Y. D., et al. (1999). Toll4 (TLR4) expression in cardiac myocytes in normal and failing myocardium. *J Clin Invest, 104,* 271–280.
38. Baumgarten, G., Knuefermann, P., Nozaki, N., et al. (2001). In vivo expression of proinflammatory mediators in the adult heart after endotoxin administration: the role of toll-like receptor-4. *J Infect Dis, 183,* 1617–1624.
39. Nemoto, S., Vallejo, J. G., Knuefermann, P., et al. (2002). *Escherichia coli* lipopolysaccharide-induced left ventricular dysfunction: the role of toll-like receptor-4 in the adult mammalian heart. *Am J Physiol, 282,* H2316–H2323.
40. Knuefermann, P., Nemoto, S., Misra, A., et al. (2002). CD14-deficient mice are protected against lipopolysaccharide-induced cardiac inflammation and left ventricular dysfunction. *Circulation, 106,* 2608–2615.
41. Sakata, Y., Dong, J. W., Vallejo, J. G., et al. (2007). Toll-like receptor 2 modulates left ventricular function following ischemia-reperfusion injury. *Am J Physiol Heart Circ Physiol, 292,* H503–H509.
42. Oyama, J., Blais, C., Jr., Liu, X., et al. (2004). Reduced myocardial ischemia-reperfusion injury in toll-like receptor 4-deficient mice. *Circulation, 109,* 784–789.
43. Shishido, T., Nozaki, N., Yamaguchi, S., et al. (2003). Toll-like receptor-2 modulates ventricular remodeling after myocardial infarction. *Circulation, 108,* 2905–2910.
44. Riad, A., Jager, S., Sobirey, M., et al. (2008). Toll-like receptor-4 modulates survival by induction of left ventricular remodeling after myocardial infarction in mice. *J Immunol, 180,* 6954–6961.
45. Bozkurt, B., Kribbs, S., Clubb, F. J., Jr., et al. (1998). Pathophysiologically relevant concentrations of tumor necrosis factor-α promote progressive left ventricular dysfunction and remodeling in rats. *Circulation, 97,* 1382–1391.
46. Seta, Y., Shan, K., Bozkurt, B., et al. (1996). Basic mechanisms in heart failure: the cytokine hypothesis. *J Card Fail, 2,* 243–249.
47. Tracey, K. J., Beutler, B., Lowry, S. F., et al. (1986). Shock and tissue injury induced by recombinant human cachectin. *Science, 234,* 470–474.
48. Natanson, C., Eichenholz, P. W., Danner, R. L., et al. (1989). Endotoxin and tumor necrosis factor challenges in dogs simulate the cardiovascular profile of human septic shock. *J Exp Med, 169,* 823–832.
49. Kubota, T., McTiernan, C. F., Frye, C. S., et al. (1997). Dilated cardiomyopathy in transgenic mice with cardiac specific overexpression of tumor necrosis factor-alpha. *Circ Res, 81,* 627–635.
50. Franco, F., Thomas, G. D., Giroir, B. P., et al. (1999). Magnetic resonance imaging and invasive evaluation of development of heart failure in transgenic mice with myocardial expression of tumor necrosis factor-alpha. *Circulation, 99,* 448–454.
51. Yokoyama, T., Vaca, L., Rossen, R. D., et al. (1993). Cellular basis for the negative inotropic effects of tumor necrosis factor-alpha in the adult mammalian heart. *J Clin Invest, 92,* 2303–2312.
52. Oral, H., Dorn, G. W., II, & Mann, D. L. (1997). Sphingosine mediates the immediate negative inotropic effects of tumor necrosis factor-alpha in the adult mammalian cardiac myocyte. *J Biol Chem, 272,* 4836–4842.
53. Balligand, J. L., Ungureanu, D., Kelly, R. A., et al. (1993). Abnormal contractile function due to induction of nitric oxide synthesis in rat cardiac myocytes follows exposure to activated macrophage-conditioned medium. *J Clin Invest, 91,* 2314–2319.
54. Mallat, Z., Heymes, C., Corbaz, A., et al. (2004). Evidence for altered interleukin 18 (IL)-18 pathway in human heart failure. *FASEB J, 18,* 1752–1754.
55. Schulz, R., Nava, E., & Moncada, S. (1992). Induction and potential biological relevance of a Ca^{2+}-independent nitric oxide synthase in the myocardium. *Brit J Pharmacol, 105,* 575–580.

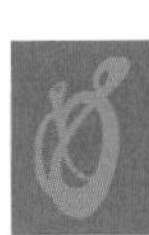

56. Balligand, J. L., Kelly, R. A., Marsden, P. A., et al. (1993). Control of cardiac muscle cell function by an endogenous nitric oxide signaling system. *Proc Natl Acad Sci U S A, 90*, 347–351.
57. De Belder, A. J., Radomski, M. W., Why, H. J. F., et al. (1993). Nitric oxide synthase activities in human myocardium. *Lancet, 341*, 84–86.
58. Kelly, R. A., Ballingand, J. L., & Smith, T. W. (1996). Nitric oxide and cardiac function. *Circ Res, 79*, 363–380.
59. Rosenkranz-Weiss, P., Sessa, W. C., Milstien, S., et al. (1994). Regulation of nitric oxide synthesis by proinflammatory cytokines in human umbilical vein endothelial cells. *J Clin Invest, 223*, 2236–2243.
60. Roberts, A. B., Vodovotz, Y., Roche, N. S., et al. (1992). Role of nitric oxide in antagonistic effects of transforming growth factor-b and interleukin-1b on the beating rate of cultured myocytes. *Mol Endocrinol, 6*, 1921–1930.
61. Stuehr, D. J., Cho, H. J., Kwon, N. S., et al. (1991). Purification and characterization of the cytokine-induced macrophage nitric oxide synthase: an FAD- and FMN-containing flavoprotein. *Proc Natl Acad Sci U S A, 88*, 7773–7777.
62. Mery, P. F., Pavoine, C., Belhasses, L., et al. (1993). Nitric oxide regulates Ca^{2+} current. *J Biol Chem, 268*, 26286–26295.
63. Shah, A. M., Lewis, M. J., & Henderson, A. H. (1991). Effects of 8-bromo-GMP on contraction and on inotropic response of ferret cardiac muscle. *J Mol Cell Cardiol, 23*, 55–64.
64. Finkel, M. S., Oddis, C. V., Jacob, T. D., et al. (1992). Negative inotropic effects of cytokines on the heart mediated by nitric oxide. *Science, 257*, 387–389.
65. Kolesnick, R. N. (1991). Sphingomyelin and derivatives as cellular signals. *Prog Lipid Res, 30*, 1–38.
66. Sabbadini, R. A., Mcnutt, W., Jenkins, G., et al. (1993). Sphingosine is endogenous to cardiac and skeletal muscle. *Biochem Biophys Res Commun, 193*, 752–758.
67. Sabbadini, R. A., Betto, R., Teresi, A., et al. (1992). The effects of sphingosine on sarcoplasmic reticulum membrane calcium release. *J Biol Chem, 267*, 15475–15484.
68. Yokoyama, T., Nakano, M., Bednarczyk, J. L., et al. (1997). Tumor necrosis factor-α provokes a hypertrophic growth response in adult cardiac myocytes. *Circulation, 95*, 1247–1252.
69. Sivasubramanian, N., Coker, M. L., Kurrelmeyer, K., et al. (2001). Left ventricular remodeling in transgenic mice with cardiac restricted overexpression of tumor necrosis factor. *Circulation, 104*, 826–831.
70. Krown, K. A., Page, M. T., Nguyen, C., et al. (1996). Tumor necrosis factor alpha-induced apoptosis in cardiac myocytes: involvement of the sphingolipid signaling cascade in cardiac cell death. *J Clin Invest, 98*, 2854–2865.
71. Bryant, D., Becker, L., Richardson, J., et al. (1998). Cardiac failure in transgenic mice with myocardial expression of tumor necrosis factor-α (TNF). *Circulation, 97*, 1375–1381.
72. Weber, K. T. (1989). Cardiac interstitium in health and disease: the fibrillar collagen network. *J Am Coll Cardiol, 13*(7), 1637–1652.
73. Engel, D., Peshock, R., Armstrong, R. C., et al. (2004). Cardiac myocyte apoptosis provokes adverse cardiac remodeling in transgenic mice with targeted TNF overexpression. *Am J Physiol Heart Circ Physiol, 287*, H1303–H1311.
74. Haudek, S. B., Taffet, G. E., Schneider, M. D., et al. (2007). TNF provokes cardiomyocyte apoptosis and cardiac remodeling through activation of multiple cell death pathways. *J Clin Invest, 117*, 2692–2701.
75. Abbate, A., Salloum, F. N., Vecile, E., et al. (2008). Anakinra, a recombinant human interleukin-1 receptor antagonist, inhibits apoptosis in experimental acute myocardial infarction. *Circulation, 117*, 2670–2683.
76. Dostal, D. E., & Baker, K. M. (1999). The cardiac renin-angiotensin system: conceptual, or a regulator of cardiac function? *Circ Res, 85*, 643–650.
77. Brasier, A. R., Jamaluddin, M., Han, Y., et al. (2000). Angiotensin II induces gene transcription through cell-type-dependent effects on the nuclear factor-kappaB (NF-kappaB) transcription factor. *Mol Cell Biochem, 212*, 155–169.
78. Luft, F. C. (2001). Workshop: mechanisms and cardiovascular damage in hypertension. *Hypertension, 37*, 594–598.
79. Kalra, D., Baumgarten, G., Dibbs, Z., et al. (2000). Nitric oxide provokes tumor necrosis factor-alpha expression in adult feline myocardium through a cgmp-dependent pathway. *Circulation, 102*, 1302–1307.
80. Flesch, M., Hoper, A., Dell'Italia, L., et al. (2003). Activation and functional significance of the renin-angiotensin system in mice with cardiac restricted overexpression of tumor necrosis factor. *Circulation, 108*, 598–604.
81. Ferrari, R., Bachetti, T., Confortini, R., et al. (1995). Tumor necrosis factor soluble receptors in patients with various degrees of congestive failure. *Circulation, 92*, 1479–1486.
82. Anker, S. D., Volterrnani, M., Egerer, K. R., et al. (1998). TNF-α as predictor of peak leg blood flow in chronic heart failure. *Q J Med, 91*, 199–203.
83. Fichtlscherer, S., Rossig, L., Breuer, S., et al. (2001). Tumor necrosis factor antagonism with etanercept improves systemic endothelial vasoreactivity in patients with advanced heart failure. *Circulation, 104*, 3023–3025.
84. Zabel, P., Schade, F. U., & Schlaak, M. (1993). Inhibition of endogenous TNF formation by pentoxifylline. *Immunbiol, 187*, 447–463.
85. Sliwa, K., Skudicky, D., Candy, G., et al. (1998). Randomized investigation of effects of pentoxifylline on left ventricular performance in idiopathic dilated cardiomyopathy. *Lancet, 351*, 1091–1093.
86. Skudicky, D., Bergemann, A., Sliwa, K., et al. (2001). Beneficial effects of pentoxifylline in patients with idiopathic dilated cardiomyopathy treated with angiotensin-converting enzyme inhibitors and carvedilol: results of a randomized study. *Circulation, 103*, 1083–1088.
87. Sliwa, K., Woodiwiss, A., Candy, G., et al. (2002). Effects of pentoxifylline on cytokine profiles and left ventricular performance in patients with decompensated congestive heart failure secondary to idiopathic dilated cardiomyopathy. *Am J Cardiol, 90*, 1118–1122.
88. Sliwa, K., Woodiwiss, A., Kone, V. N., et al. (2004). Therapy of ischemic cardiomyopathy with the immunomodulating agent pentoxifylline: results of a randomized study. *Circulation, 109*, 750–755.
89. Skudicky, D., Sliwa, K., Bergemann, A., et al. (2000). Reduction in Fas/APO-1 plasma concentrations correlates with improvement in left ventricular function in patients with idiopathic dilated cardiomyopathy treated with pentoxifylline. *Heart, 84*, 438–439.
90. Sampaio, E. P., Sarno, E. N., Galilly, R., et al. (1991). Thalidomide selectively inhibits tumor necrosis factor alpha production by stimulated human monocytes. *J Exp Med, 173*, 699–703.
91. Moreira, A. L., Sampaio, E. P., Zmuidzinas, A., et al. (1993). Thalidomide exerts its inhibitory action on tumor necrosis factor-alpha by enhancing messenger RNA degradation. *J Exp Med, 177*, 1675–1680.
92. Agoston, I., Dibbs, Z. I., Wang, F., et al. (2002). Preclinical and clinical assessment of the safety and potential efficacy of thalidomide in heart failure. *J Card Fail, 8*, 306–314.
93. Gullestad, L., Ueland, T., Fjeld, J. G., et al. (2005). Effect of thalidomide on cardiac remodeling in chronic heart failure: results of a double-blind, placebo-controlled study. *Circulation, 112*, 3408–3414.
94. Remick, D. G., Strieter, R. M., Lynch, I. J. P., et al. (1989). In vivo dynamics of murine tumor necrosis factor-α gene expression. Kinetics of dexamethasone-induced suppression. *Lab Invest, 60*, 766–771.
95. Parrillo, J. E., Cunnion, R. E., Epstein, S. E., et al. (1989). A prospective randomized controlled trial of prednisone for dilated cardiomyopathy. *N Engl J Med, 321*, 1061–1068.
96. Kapadia, S., Torre-Amione, G., Yokoyama, T., et al. (1995). Soluble tumor necrosis factor binding proteins modulate the negative inotropic effects of TNF-α in vitro. *Am J Physiol, 37*, H517–H525.
97. Deswal, A., Bozkurt, B., Seta, Y., et al. (1999). A phase I trial of tumor necrosis factor receptor (p75) fusion protein (TNFR: Fc) in patients with advanced heart failure. *Circulation, 99*, 3224–3226.
98. Bozkurt, B., Torre-Amione, G., Warren, M. S., et al. (2001). Results of targeted anti-tumor necrosis factor therapy with etanercept (ENBREL) in patients with advanced heart failure. *Circulation, 103*, 1044–1047.
99. Packer, M. (2001). Proposal for a new clinical end point to evaluate the efficacy of drugs and devices in the treatment of chronic heart failure. *J Card Fail, 7*, 176–182.
100. Mann, D. L., McMurray, J. J. V., Packer, M., et al. (2004). Targeted anti-cytokine therapy in patients with chronic heart failure: results of the randomized etanercept worldwide evaluation (RENEWAL). *Circulation, 109*, 1594–1602.
101. Chung, E. S., Packer, M., Lo, K. H., et al. (2003). Randomized, double-blind, placebo-controlled, pilot trial of infliximab, a chimeric monoclonal antibody to tumor necrosis factor-(alpha), in patients with moderate-to-severe heart failure: results of the anti-TNF therapy against congestive heart failure (ATTACH) trial. *Circulation, 107*, 3133–3140.
102. Homeister, J. W., & Lucchesi, B. R. (1994). Complement activation and inhibition in myocardial ischemia and reperfusion injury. *Annu Rev Pharmacol Toxicol, 34*, 17–40.
103. Klein, B., & Brailly, H. (1995). Cytokine-binding proteins: stimulating antagonists. *Immunol Today, 16*, 216–220.
104. Mann, D. L., Bozkurt, B., Torre-Amione, G., et al. (2008). Effect of the soluble TNF-antagonist etanercept on tumor necrosis factor bioactivity and stability. *Clin Transl Sci, 1*, 142–145.
105. Frishman, J. I., Edwards, C. K., III, Sonnenberg, M. G., et al. (2000). Tumor necrosis factor (TNF)-alpha-induced interleukin-8 in human blood cultures discriminates neutralization by the p55 and p75 TNF soluble receptors. *J Infect Dis, 182*, 1722–1730.
106. Maury, C. P., & Teppo, A. M. (1989). Cachectin/tumour necrosis factor-alpha in the circulation of patients with rheumatic disease. *Int J Tissue React, 11*, 189–193.
107. Aukrust, P., Yndestad, A., Damas, J. K., et al. (2007). Potential mechanisms of benefit with thalidomide in chronic heart failure. *Am J Cardiovasc Drugs, 7*, 127–134.
108. Gullestad, L., Aass, H., Fjeld, J. G., et al. (2001). Immunomodulating therapy with intravenous immunoglobulin in patients with chronic heart failure. *Circulation, 103*, 220–225.
109. McNamara, D. M., Holubkov, R., Starling, R. C., et al. (2001). Controlled trial of intravenous immune globulin in recent-onset dilated cardiomyopathy. *Circulation, 103*, 2254–2259.
110. Fadok, V. A., Bratton, D. L., Konowal, A., et al. (1998). Macrophages that have ingested apoptotic cells in vitro inhibit proinflammatory cytokine production through autocrine/paracrine mechanisms involving TGF-beta, PGE2, and PAF. *J Clin Invest, 101*, 890–898.
111. Babaei, S., Stewart, D. J., Picard, P., et al. (2002). Effects of VasoCare therapy on the initiation and progression of atherosclerosis. *Atherosclerosis, 162*, 45–53.
112. Aukrust, P., Ueland, T., Lien, E., et al. (1999). Cytokine network in congestive heart failure secondary to ischemic or idiopathic dilated cardiomyopathy. *Am J Cardiol, 83*, 376–382.
113. Torre-Amione, G., Sestier, F., Radovancevic, B., et al. (2004). Effects of a novel immune modulation therapy in patients with advanced chronic heart failure: results of a randomized, controlled, phase II trial. *J Am Coll Cardiol, 44*, 1181–1186.
114. Torre-Amione, G., Anker, S. D., Bourge, R. C., et al. (2008). Results of a non-specific immunomodulation therapy in chronic heart failure (ACCLAIM trial): a placebo-controlled randomised trial. *Lancet, 371*, 228–236.
115. Ramasubbu, K., & Mann, D. L. (2006). The emerging role of statins in the treatment of heart failure. *J Am Coll Cardiol, 47*, 342–344.
116. Khush, K. K., Waters, D. D., Bittner, V., et al. (2007). Effect of high-dose atorvastatin on hospitalizations for heart failure: subgroup analysis of the treating to new targets (TNT) study. *Circulation, 115*, 576–583.
117. Ramasubbu, K., Estep, J., White, D. L., et al. (2008). Experimental and clinical basis for the use of statins in patients with ischemic and nonischemic cardiomyopathy. *J Am Coll Cardiol, 51*, 415–426.
118. Krum, H., Ashton, E., Reid, C., et al. (2007). Double-blind, randomized, placebo-controlled study of high-dose HMG CoA reductase inhibitor therapy on ventricular remodeling, pro-inflammatory cytokines and neurohormonal parameters in patients with chronic systolic heart failure. *J Card Fail, 13*, 1–7.

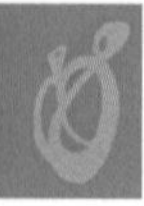

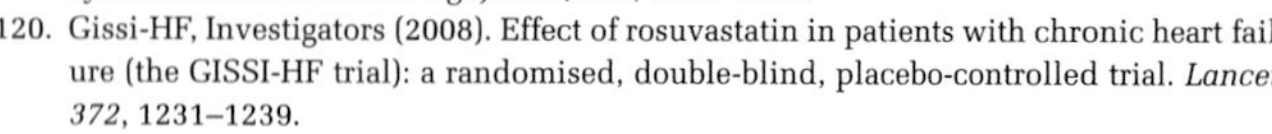

119. Kjekshus, J., Apetrei, E., Barrios, V., et al. (2007). Rosuvastatin in older patients with systolic heart failure. *N Engl J Med*, *357*, 2248–2261.

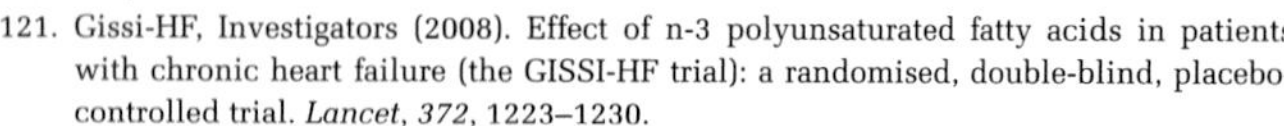

120. Gissi-HF, Investigators (2008). Effect of rosuvastatin in patients with chronic heart failure (the GISSI-HF trial): a randomised, double-blind, placebo-controlled trial. *Lancet*, *372*, 1231–1239.
121. Gissi-HF, Investigators (2008). Effect of n-3 polyunsaturated fatty acids in patients with chronic heart failure (the GISSI-HF trial): a randomised, double-blind, placebo-controlled trial. *Lancet*, *372*, 1223–1230.
122. Mann, D. L. (2002). Inflammatory mediators and the failing heart: past, present, and the foreseeable future. *Circ Res*, *91*, 988–998.
123. Heymans, S., Hirsch, E., Anker, S. D., et al. (2009). Inflammation as a therapeutic target in heart failure? A scientific statement from the translational research committee of the Heart Failure Association of the European Society of Cardiology. *Eur J Heart Fail*, *11*, 119–129.
124. Weinberger, S. R., Morris, T. S., & Pawlak, M. (2000). Recent trends in protein biochip technology. *Pharmacogenomics*, *1*, 395–416.
125. Gordon, S. (2002). Pattern recognition receptors. Doubling up for the innate immune response. *Cell*, *111*, 927–930.

CHAPTER 12

Oxidative and Nitrosative Stress in Heart Failure

Douglas B. Sawyer, Chang-seng Liang, and Wilson S. Colucci

There is now evidence that oxidative stress is increased in heart failure, and experimental studies suggest that this may contribute to the structural and functional changes leading to disease progression. Our understanding of the role of oxidative stress in myocardial dysfunction, though largely incomplete, continues to grow. In this chapter, we will review the evidence for increased oxidative stress in heart failure, in vivo evidence suggesting a role for oxidative stress in the pathogenesis of heart failure, and recent in vitro studies that suggest potential mechanisms by which reactive oxygen species (ROS) (see Chapter 15) might mediate myocardial remodeling and contractile dysfunction (see Chapter 13).

REACTIVE OXYGEN SPECIES, ANTIOXIDANT SYSTEMS, AND OXIDATIVE STRESS

Reactive oxygen species (ROS) are a byproduct of aerobic metabolism, and so the highly metabolically active myocardium is rich in ROS. As in all tissues, ROS are handled in the myocardium by both soluble and enzymatic antioxidant systems. "Oxidative stress" occurs when the production of ROS exceeds the capacity of antioxidant defense systems. ROS cascades begin with the formation of superoxide anion (O_2^-) by either enzymatic or nonenzymatic one electron reduction of molecular oxygen (Figure 12-1). The unpaired electron in O_2^- is an unstable free radical that reacts with itself and other oxygen-containing species, and directly or indirectly with organic molecules including lipids, nucleic acids, and proteins, ultimately leading to disruption of cellular functions. All aerobic organisms, from bacteria to man, have evolved a complex antioxidant defense system of enzymatic and nonenzymatic components to defend against the unavoidable formation of ROS.[1] In parallel there has been the evolution of specific ROS-generating systems that are used both in the immune system, where the toxicity of ROS is exploited to fight infectious organisms[2] and in all cell types where ROS act as signaling intermediates for the purpose of triggering specific intracellular changes in cell biology.

Primary antioxidant enzymes (defined here as those that directly interact with ROS) including superoxide dismutases (SOD), catalase, and peroxidases work in parallel with nonenzymatic antioxidants to protect cells and tissues from ROS. The mitochondrial enzymes manganese superoxide dismutase (MnSOD) and glutathione peroxidase (GPx) appear to be the most important in controlling myocardial levels of O_2^- and H_2O_2. Approximately 70% of the SOD activity in the heart, and 90% of that in the cardiac myocyte, is attributable to MnSOD (SOD2).[3] The remainder consists of cytosolic Cu/ZnSOD (SOD1), with less than 1% contributed by extracellular-SOD (ECSOD, SOD3).[4] This is in contrast to other organs, where Cu/ZnSOD plays a greater role. The relative importance of MnSOD in the regulation of oxidative stress in the myocardium is highlighted by the demonstration that homozygous knockout mice deficient in MnSOD develop normally in utero, but die soon after birth with dilated cardiomyopathy.[5] In contrast, mice deficient in CuZnSOD or ECSOD grow normally and have no overt myocardial phenotype.[4] As the only SOD located in the mitochondria, MnSOD plays a critical role in the control of mitochondrial ROS generated during normal oxidative phosphorylation (see later discussion). The phenotype of the MnSOD knockout mouse therefore also underscores the importance of the mitochondria as a source of ROS in the myocardium.

H_2O_2, the product of SOD, is handled by one of several glutathione peroxidases (GPx) and/or catalase. GPx are selenium-containing enzymes that catalyze the removal of H_2O_2 through oxidation of reduced glutathione (GSH), which is recycled from oxidized glutathione (GSSG) by the NADPH-dependent glutathione reductase (GRed). The activity of GPx requires stoichiometric quantities of GSH, and therefore low levels of GSH reduce the activity of GPx. GRed requires NAD(P)H as a reductant to recycle GSSG to GSH. In this context, enzymes in the pentose phosphate pathway and glucose-6-phosphate dehydrogenase (G6PD), the rate-limiting enzyme in this pathway, can be thought of as ancillary antioxidant enzymes that are critical to cellular antioxidant defenses.[6] Other ancillary antioxidant enzymes are emerging that work through distinct mechanisms, such as heme oxygenase-I, which is induced by oxidative stress and serves a cytoprotective function through the breakdown of pro-oxidant heme into equimolar amounts of carbon monoxide, biliverdin/bilirubin, and free ferrous iron. Carbon monoxide[7] and bilirubin[8] have been shown to exert direct cardioprotective effects via their respective antiinflammatory and antioxidant actions. Cardioselective overexpression of heme oxygenase-1 also has been shown to reduce infarct size, and inflammatory and oxidative damage, and attenuate postinfarct cardiac remodeling in animals after coronary artery occlusion and reperfusion injury.[9,10]

GPx-1, like MnSOD, is encoded on the nuclear genome but localizes to the mitochondria. Mice deficient in GPx-1 have no overt abnormality in myocardial function. GPx are selenium-containing enzymes,[11] and dietary deficiency of selenium, as occurs in some areas of China, is associated with a dilated cardiomyopathy and heart failure. There is evidence of increased oxidative stress in selenium-deficient people

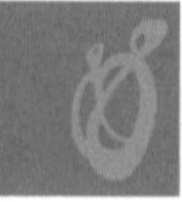

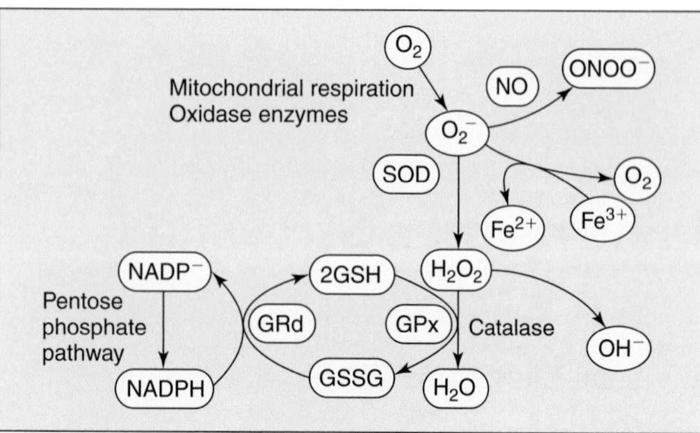

FIGURE 12–1 Reactive oxygen species (ROS) and antioxidant enzyme systems: Enzymatic or nonenzymatic formation of superoxide anion leads to the formation of other ROS (*shown in bold*). Potentially toxic ROS are removed by the enzymes superoxide dismutase (SOD), glutathione peroxidase (GPx), and catalase. The presence of Fe^{+2} or nitric oxide (NO) can allow the formation of hydoxyl radical ($OH^·$) and peroxynitrate ($ONOO^-$), respectively. These latter reactions are favored when the activity of SOD is decreased. O_2^- can increase the formation of $OH^·$ by reducing Fe^{3+} to Fe^{2+}. Glutathione plays a central role in cellular antioxidant defenses not only as a reducing agent for the action of GPx, but also through direct reactions with ROS. Glutathione is recycled by the enzyme glutathione reductase, which requires NAD(P)H. Thus indirectly, the pentose phosphate pathway, by supplying NAD(P)H, also plays an important role in antioxidant defenses.

and animals.[12] However, it appears that the effect of selenium deficiency on the heart are not due to direct effects of this oxidative stress, but perhaps due to cardiotropic viral infections evolving rapidly toward virulent strains in a selenium-deficient heart.[13] A similar phenomenon may occur in people suffering from AIDS, where selenium deficiency is a risk factor for the development of heart failure.[14]

Glutathione is an important cellular antioxidant (see Figure 12-1), both as a cofactor for GPx and a direct scavenger of reactive oxygen and nitrogen species. Cells replenish GSH both through the action of glutathione reductase on GSSG and by de novo GSH synthesis. Increased oxidative stress lowers the GSH/GSSG ratio, which may thus be used as a measure of myocardial oxidative stress.[15] Unlike the levels of lipid peroxidation products, which can reflect oxidative stress inside and/or outside of the cell, the GSH/GSSG ratio specifically measures intracellular oxidative stress. Other thiol containing proteins, such as the metal binding metallothionein, also have significant antioxidant functions through direct scavenging of ROS, and may also play a role in the control of oxidative stress in the failing heart.[16] Overexpression of metallothionein also has been shown to suppress mitochondrial oxidative stress, cardiac apoptosis, and the development of diabetic cardiomyopathy.[17]

Thioredoxin is also a thio-containing protein. It belongs to the thioredoxin system, which consists of thioredoxin reductase, thioredoxin, peroxiredoxin, and NADPH.[18] Like glutathione *S* transferase, heme oxygenase-1, and NAD(P)H oxidoreductase, this system is inducible by a variety of oxidative stresses and thioredoxin levels are increased in the myocardium of patients with cardiomyopathies,[19] and in the circulating blood of congestive heart failure (CHF) patients.[20] Thioredoxin is multifunctional. It not only exerts an antioxidant effect through thioredoxin peroxidase by scavenging ROS, but also interacts with multiple cellular signal transduction pathways, including downregulation of p38 mitogen-activated protein kinase and apoptosis signal-regulating kinase (ASK)-1, to exert an antiapoptotic effect. Part of its cardioprotective action is also mediated via activation of heme oxygenase-1 and the antiapoptotic Bcl-2 pathway.[21] Like metallothionein, induction of thioredoxin has been shown to exert a cardioprotective effect in animals after chronic myocardial infarction[21] or Adriamycin-induced cardiomyopathy.[18]

Vitamin antioxidants also play a major role in the control of ROS cascades and the prevention of free radical chain reactions. In particular, α-tocopherol and ascorbic acid, vitamins E and C, respectively, can act synergistically to prevent lipid peroxidation and membrane breakdown. α-Tocopherol is a fat-soluble vitamin that concentrates in cellular membranes. Through the aromatic ring headgroup attached to its hydrocarbon chain, α-tocopherol is able to form a "stable" tocopheryl radical when it reacts with ROS and lipid peroxy radicals. Ascorbic acid reacts with tocopheryl radicals, thereby converting them back to tocopherol. Circulating and tissue levels of α-tocopherol have been used as measures of both antioxidant capacity and oxidative stress.[15] In addition, α-tocopherol has been used as a therapeutic intervention in animal models of heart failure.[22,23]

OXIDATIVE STRESS IN HUMAN HEART FAILURE

Oxidation products of several organic molecules including lipids, proteins, and nucleic acids have been used to demonstrate oxidative stress in many diseases including heart failure (Table 12-1). While these methods can individually be criticized for their relative nonspecificity, collectively the data support the conclusion that there is increased systemic and myocardial oxidative stress in patients with heart failure. Several studies have shown that the lipid peroxidation products such as malondialdehyde (MDA)[24] and 4-hydroxynonenal[25] are increased and total thiol levels are decreased in patients with ischemic and nonischemic cardiomyopathy compared with subjects without heart failure.[26] Myeloperoxidase, a peroxidase enzyme present abundantly in granulocytes, is increased in the circulating blood of patients with heart failure (HF). Increased plasma myeloperoxidase is associated with a higher likelihood of more advanced HF patients.[27] Moreover, oxidative stress markers may have some prognostic value, as they correlate with worsening NYHA functional class, chronicity of disease,[24] cardiac dysfunction,[27] and circulating levels of other markers with prognostic value such as the soluble tumor necrosis factor α receptor.[28] Plasma myeloperoxidase also appears to be an independent predictor of death, heart transplantation, or HF hospitalization.[27] Levels of exhaled pentane, a volatile lipid peroxidation product, are also increased in patients with heart failure.[29] However, while pentane levels normalized in patients taking captopril, they did not normalize with other angiotensin-converting enzyme inhibitors (ACEI) that lack a thiol moiety. Given the apparent class benefit of ACE inhibitors in heart failure, it is hard to argue that this antioxidant effect is important therapeutically. Along a similar line, Ghatak et al showed that circulating markers of oxidative stress normalized in patients with heart failure after 4 weeks of vitamin E therapy,[30] although to date there has been no demonstrable benefit of therapy with vitamin E for up to 12 weeks.[31] Thus the prognostic value of these measures of oxidative stress remains unclear at this time.

Increased myocardial oxidative stress in heart failure has been demonstrated by measurements of 8-iso-prostaglandin $F_2α$ (8-isoprostanes). 8-Isoprostanes are a family of prostaglandin $F_2α$ isomers formed by the peroxidation of arachidonic acid through a noncyclooxygenase-mediated reaction catalyzed by free radicals.[32] In contrast to reactive aldehydes, lipid hydroperoxides, and conjugated dienes, 8-isoprostanes are more stable products of lipid peroxidation and thus have been proposed to be a more accurate indicator of oxidative stress in vivo.[33] 8-Isoprostanes are elevated in tissue subjected to increased oxidative stress, and can be extracted and measured quantitatively using several methods including

TABLE 12–1 Studies of Oxidative Stress Markers in Human Heart Failure

Markers	Studies	Findings
MDA, Thiols, SOD, GPx	McMurray et al[143]	Increased plasma MDA, decreased plasma thiols in patients with CAD and LV dysfunction.
	Belch et al[144]	Increased plasma MDA, decreased plasma thiols in patients with CHF. Weak correlation between decreasing thiols and worsening LV function.
	McMurray et al[26]	Increased MDA, decreased plasma thiols in both CAD and non-CAD patients with HF.
	Ghatak et al[30]	Increased MDA, and reduced erythrocyte SOD and GPx activities in CHF. Weak correlation with LV function. Improved by vitamin E administration.
	Diaz-Velez et al[24]	Increased MDA in CHF. No correlation with LV function. Some correlation between MDA and chronicity of illness.
	Keith et al[145]	Correlated oxidative stress with NYHA clinical class and levels of soluble TNF receptor levels as marker of prognosis.
	Maks et al[25]	Plasma unsaturated aldehydes including 4-OH-nonenal were elevated in association with impaired LV contractile function in HF patients.
	Polidori et al[146]	Plasma MDA was higher in patients with severe CHF than those with moderate disease.
	Campolo et al[147]	Reduced cysteine and MDA were increased in CHF patients.
Myeloperoxidase	Tang et al[27]	Associated with an increased likelihood of more advanced HF, and predictive of worse long-term clinical outcomes.
Breath pentane	Sobotka et al[29]	Increased exhaled pentane in CHF compared with controls. Pentane levels reduced by captopril therapy.
8-isoprostanes	Mallat et al[34]	Pericardial 8-isoprostanes in patients undergoing open-heart surgery correlated with preoperative NYHA functional class.
	Kameda et al[35]	Pericardial 8-isoprostanes correlated with LV end-diastolic volume, and activities of MMP-2 and MMP-9 and gelatinolysis in CAD patients.
	Polidori et al[36]	Plasma F2 isoprostanes correlated with antioxidant status and NYHA class.
	Nonaka-Sakukawa et al[148]	Urinary 15-Ft-isoprostanes increased in proportion to the severity of CHF, and correlated with plasma BNP and serum IL-6.
Pentosidine	Koyama et al[37]	Serum pentosidine was an independent risk factor for cardiac events in patients with HF.
Plasma carboxyls	Amir et al[38]	Serum oxidative stress levels increased with NYHA functional class and were associated with higher CRP and BNP.
8-hydroxy-2′-deoxyguanosine	Watanabe et al[42]	Correlated with NYHA functional class, left atrial diameter, LV end-diastolic diameters, LV end-systolic diameters, and plasma BNP.
	Kono et al[41]	Increased in both the serum and myocardium of patients with HF. Reduced with carvedilol therapy.
	Pignatelli et al[149]	Serum levels increased in CHF, progressively from Class I-II to Class III-IV. Correlated with TNF-α and sCD40L.
Uric acid	Cicoira et al[150]	Elevated serum uric acid levels correlated with parameters of diastolic dysfunction in HF.
	Anker et al[47]	Uric acid predicted mortality in patients with moderate to severe CHF.
	Kojima et al[45]	Correlated with Killip's classification and mortality in patients with acute MI.
	Sakai et al[43]	Positive transcardiac gradient of uric acid increased with the severity of HF and inversely correlated with LVEF.
	Kittleson et al[44]	High uric acid was associated with increased cardiac filling pressures and reduced cardiac index. Correlated with NT-proBNP.
	Ioachimescu et al[48]	An independent predictor of death in patients at high risk of cardiovascular disease.
Biopyrrins	Hokamaki et al[50]	Urinary biopyrrin levels were elevated and correlated with blood BNP and severity of HF.

Abbreviations: BNP, brain-natriuretic peptide; CAD, coronary artery disease; CHF, congestive heart failure; CRP, C-reactive peptide; IL-6, interlukin-6; GPx, glutathione peroxidase; LV, left ventricle; MDA, malonyldialdehyde; NYHA, New York Heart Association; SOD, superoxide dismutase; TNF, tumor necrosis factor.

an enzyme-linked immunoassay. Mallat et al measured 8-isoprostanes in the pericardial fluid of patients with NYHA functional Class I-III HF undergoing open heart surgery for ischemic or valvular disease.[34] They found that the level of 8-isoprostanes correlated with increasing NYHA functional class in patients preoperatively, consistent with the concept that worsening heart failure is associated with increased myocardial oxidative stress. Elevated pericardial 8-isoprostanes also correlate with left ventricular (LV) end-diastolic volume, and activities of matrix metalloproteases and gelanolysis[35] in CAD patients. Plasma and urinary isoprostanes also correlate with the severity of clinical HF, antioxidant status, and blood BNP and IL-6.[36]

In addition to the lipid peroxidation products, oxidation products of glycoproteins, proteins, and nuclear DNAs are increased in HF, indicative of increased oxidative stress. Serum pentosidine, an advanced glycation end product, is an independent risk factor for cardiac events in patients with HF.[37] Plasma carboxyls are also increased in patients with more symptomatic HF, and associated with higher C-reactive protein (CRP) and Brain Natriuretic Peptide (BNP).[38] More recently, 8-hydroxy-2′-deoxyguanosine (8-OHdG), which is formed when DNA is oxidatively damaged by ROS, has been found to be one of the most sensitive biomarkers for oxidative stress, and can be measured in plasma, urine, and tissue. Myocardial 8-OHdG is increased in animals with cardiac hypertrophy[39] and tachycardia-induced cardiomyopathy.[40] 8-OHdG is increased in both the serum and myocardium of patients with HF.[41] Plasma levels of 8-OHdG correlate with NYHA functional class, cardiac function, and several HF biochemical markers such as plasma BNP, TNF-α, and sCD40L.[42]

Uric acid, produced by the ubiquitous ROS-generating xanthine oxidase (see later discussion), has been considered as a marker for oxidative stress in the cardiovascular system. It is released from the failing human heart, with an inverse correlation between the positive transcardiac gradient of uric acid and LV ejection fraction.[43] Increased serum uric acid levels are associated with increased cardiac filling pressure and reduced cardiac index in HF,[44] and correlates with Killip's classification in acute MI,[45] plasma NT-proBNP in HF,[44] and parameters of diastolic dysfunction.[46] Uric acid is also a strong independent predictor of mortality in patients with moderate to severe HF[47] and patients at high risk of cardiovascular disease.[48] This association, however, is only significant when hyperuricemia is a marker of increased xanthine oxidase activity but not when hyperuricemia is caused by impaired renal elimination of uric acid.[49]

Biopyrrins are oxidized metabolites of bilirubin, which are increased in HF, probably secondary to hepatic dysfunction due to venous congestion and/or increased heme oxygenase-1 activity. Urinary biopyrrin levels are elevated and correlate with blood BNP and severity of HF.[50]

OXIDATIVE STRESS AND ANTIOXIDANT THERAPY IN ANIMAL MODELS OF HEART FAILURE

Although there are no positive large-scale clinical trials of antioxidant therapy in heart failure to date, there are multiple studies of oxidative stress and antioxidant therapy in animal models of heart failure. Singal et al, working with several animal models of heart failure, have characterized changes in myocardial oxidative stress and antioxidant capacity in both myocardial hypertrophy and the transition to failure. In a model of stable myocardial hypertrophy after abdominal aortic banding they found an increase in the activity of SOD and GPx.[51] However, in a model of pressure-overload leading to failure in the guinea pig, both SOD and GPx activity fell during the failure stage in association with a decreased ratio of GSH/GSSG, consistent with an increase in myocardial oxidative stress.[52]

Singal et al have also found similar changes in antioxidant capacity and oxidative stress in the rat late after myocardial infarction (MI).[15] As in the setting of pressure overload, there was a small increase in antioxidant enzyme activity early after MI. However, also like the banding model, late after MI there was evidence for increased oxidative stress. During the period from 4 to 16 weeks after MI there was a progressive decrease in LV systolic function and an increase in end-diastolic pressure. These changes in ventricular function were accompanied by (1) a progressive decline in GPx and catalase activities, (2) an increase in myocardial lipid peroxidation, (3) a decrease in the GSH/GSSG ratio, and (4) decreased levels of vitamin E. SOD activity was decreased only at the latest time point examined. Thus in both the pressure overload and post-MI models of myocardial remodeling leading to heart failure in rodents, there is evidence for increased oxidative stress and a maladaptive decrease in antioxidant enzyme capacity that correlates in time with declining ventricular function. Similar observations were made in a large animal model of volume overload-induced heart failure secondary to mitral regurgitation in which there was also evidence of increased myocardial levels of lipid peroxidation products, decreased antioxidant enzyme capacity, and depletion of vitamin E.[53]

The extent to which changes in antioxidant enzyme activity occur in the failing human heart is controversial. Two studies have reported no decrease in SOD or GPx activity in pathological samples from explanted human hearts at the time of cardiac transplant as compared with nonfailing controls.[54,55] In contrast, MnSOD activity has been found to be reduced in the failing human heart.[56] This appears to occur at a posttranscriptional level, as mRNA expression of MnSOD is increased in the same failing samples when compared with the nonfailing specimens. The discrepancy among these studies in failing human heart tissue may reflect differences in the "control" hearts, where variable degrees of pathological and pharmacological stress may be important confounding factors. Nevertheless, it remains unclear whether the decreased expression of antioxidant enzymes seen in rodent models of heart failure (i.e., decreases in SOD and GPx) contributes to the oxidative stress in the end-stage failing human heart. In the face of increased ROS production, however, the lack of an increase in antioxidant capacity in the failing human heart does most likely reflect a state of relative inadequate antioxidant capacity.

Several animal studies have now demonstrated benefits of pharmacological antioxidants with regard to the development of heart failure in the setting of hemodynamic overload (Table 12-2). Interestingly, the benefits vary depending on the model and the antioxidant used. In dogs with surgically induced mitral regurgitation, administration of vitamin E prevented in part the decline in ventricular function over a 4-month study.[53] While the administration of vitamin E partially prevented the downregulation of GPx and catalase activity and the increase in MDA, the decrease in SOD activity was not prevented. Vitamin E administration also has beneficial effects in the aortic banding model of pressure overload in the guinea pig.[22] In animals treated with implanted tablets of α-tocopherol, there was a measurable increase in myocardial α-tocopherol levels. There was no difference in the compensatory hypertrophy that occurs at early time points after banding. However at late time points, α-tocopherol administration prevented the transition to heart failure, as evidenced by improved LV peak developed pressure.

In pacing-induced rabbit cardiomyopathy, antioxidant vitamins reduced the tissue GSSG/GSH and 8-OHdG levels, and attenuated the associated cardiac dysfunction and β-receptor downregulation.[40] Vitamin E supplement also improved LV function and significantly reduced myocardial 8-isoprostanes and oxidized glutathione accumulation in rodents with diabetes and cardiac dysfunction.[23] However, vitamin E supplementation has not been shown to have any significant effects in human heart failure. In a 12-week placebo-controlled study, vitamin E supplement did not reduce plasma MDA or isoprostane levels.[31] Nor did it reduce

TABLE 12–2 Antioxidants with Therapeutic Effects in the Failing Heart

Antioxidant	Cardiomyopathy Setting	Observations (Species)
Antioxidant vitamins	Surgical mitral insufficiency	Vitamin E improved left ventricular (LV) function (dog).[53]
	Pressure overload	Vitamin E improved contractile function. Reduced dilation (rat).[22]
	Tachy-pacing cardiomyopathy	Vitamin E, C, and beta carotene increased cardiac oxidative stress and attenuated the associated systolic dysfunction, and β-AR downregulation (rabbit).[40]
	Diabetic cardiomyopathy	Vitamin E supplementation improved LV function and significantly attenuated myocardial 8-iso-prostanes and oxidized glutathione accumulation (rat).[23]
Probucol	Myocardial infarction	Improved survival and LV function; reduced cytokine expression and myocyte death (rat).[151]
Dimethylthiourea (DMTU)	Myocardial infarction	DMTU reduced LV dilation; improved systolic function (mouse).[59]

blood BNP, TNF-α, or norepinephrine, or improve the quality of life questionnaire scores in the subjects. Long-term vitamin E supplementation also produced no effects on primary prevention of cardiovascular events in humans.[57]

In a study of post-MI remodeling in the rat, administration of probucol decreased the levels of myocardial oxidative stress, preserved myocardial systolic function, and improved animal survival.[58] While the probucol-treated animals had increased wall thickness of the scarred myocardium, there was no effect of probucol on ventricular dilation. In contrast, the ROS scavenger DMTU prevented chamber dilation and pump dysfunction in the mouse post-MI.[59] The reason for the differences between the effects of probucol and DMTU in the post-MI setting remains to be determined, but is likely due to their relative abilities to reach intracellular compartments and scavenge specific ROS. In any case, it appears that chronically elevated oxidative stress in the myocardium may play a central role in the process of myocardial remodeling leading to heart failure. Collectively these and other studies (see Table 12-2) suggest that deficits in antioxidant capacity in the remodeling myocardium contribute to increased oxidative stress and the progression to heart failure.

THE CELLULAR SOURCES OF OXIDATIVE STRESS IN HEART FAILURE

There are many potential sources of O_2^- and other ROS in all eukaryotic cells, and several of these appear to be important in the failing myocardium (Figure 12-2). Several enzyme systems that generate O_2^- are present in the myocardium and some of these may produce pathophysiological amounts of O_2^- in the failing heart. Xanthine oxidoreductase, a member of the molybdoenzyme family, is a major source of ROS in human cardiovascular diseases. This enzyme system consists of two interconvertible forms: xanthine dehydrogenase and xanthine oxidase; both are involved in the conversion of hypoxanthine and xanthine to uric acid. The constitutive xanthine dehydrogenase uses NAD^+ primarily as an electron acceptor, whereas the inducible xanthine oxidase transfers electrons to molecular oxygen, yielding 4 units of ROS per unit of transformed substrate. In addition, xanthine oxidoreductase can generate superoxide via NADH oxidase activity and produce nitric acid via nitrate and nitritic reductase activities.[60] Thus activation of xanthine oxidoreductase is expected to cause both oxidative and nitrosative stresses. The gene expression of xanthine oxidase is regulated by oxygen tension, cytokines, and glucocorticoids, and it is increased in the failing heart of dilated cardiomyopathic patients[61] and in rats with heart failure produced by either monocrotaline or coronary artery occlusion.[62,63]

To study the functional importance of xanthine oxidase-induced production of ROS in heart failure, xanthine oxidase inhibitors (allopurinol, oxypurinol, and febuxostat) have been studied extensively in experimental cardiomyopathies. These agents uniformly reduce myocardial xanthine oxidase expression and activity, and attenuate the production of ROS in the failing heart. They also improve cardiac function, LV size, β-adrenergic receptor sensitivity, and myocardial mechanoenergetic coupling (e.g., see Ekelund et al[64,65]). Also, alterations in fetal gene expression (see Chapter 2) and Ca^{2+} handling pathway (see Chapter 3) seen in hypertrophied and failing heart are reduced by oxypurinol.[66] The improvements in cardiac structure and function by xanthine oxidase inhibitors are consistent with attenuation of cardiac remodeling in HF. In small mechanistic studies in human heart failure, allopurinol reduced plasma MDA, improved endothelium-dependent flow-mediated response,[67,68] reduced myocardial oxygen consumption, and improved myocardial efficiency.[61] Also, in acute and short-term studies, oxypurinol increased LV ejection fraction and

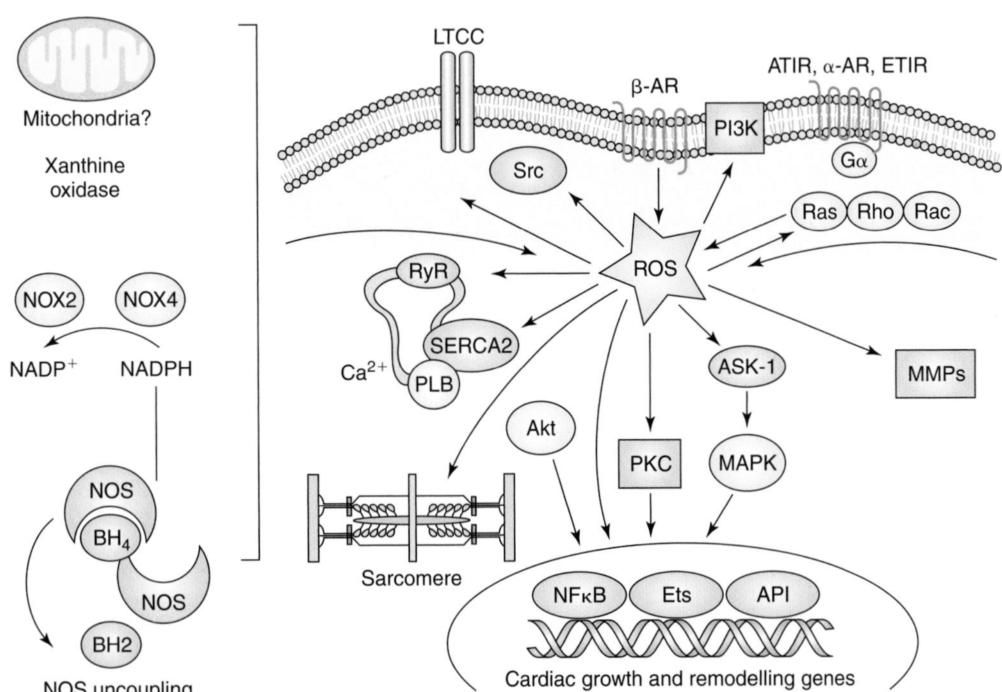

FIGURE 12–2 Cellular sources of reactive oxygen species (ROS) and ROS signaling in cardiac hypertrophy. ROS-generating systems are shown on the left and include xanthine oxidase, NADPH oxidases (NOX2, NOX4), nitric oxide synthase (NOS), and mitochondrial complexes. ROS activation has protean effects on calcium handling, myofilament function, matrix activation, kinase and phosphatase stimulation, and transcriptional regulation. Metalloproteinases (Key: *NF κB,* nuclear factor-kappaB; *PKC,* protein kinase C; *PI3K,* phosphatidylinositol 3 kinase; *PLB,* phospholamban; *RyR,* ryanodine receptor; *SERCA2,* sarcoplasmic reticular ATPase 2) (Modified from McKinsey TA, Kass DA. Small-molecule therapies for cardiac hypertrophy: moving beneath the cell surface. *Nat Rev Drug Discov* 2007;6:617-635.)

reduced LV end-diastolic volume.[69] However, the xanthine oxidase inhibitor did not improve a primary composite OPT-CHF, endpoint (mortality, HF morbidity, or quality of life) in a long-term study of symptomatic systolic HF patients.[70] In subgroup analysis, the authors noted that clinical improvements were seen in patients with elevated uric acid, and that degree of serum uric acid reduction over the course of study correlated with clinical outcomes. The magnitude of improvement in cardiac function by oxypurinol in pressure-overload heart failure also depends on the initial level of xanthine oxidase activity.[71] Thus it is possible that xanthine oxidase inhibitors may exert a beneficial effect in patients with elevated serum uric acid or if larger doses of xanthine oxidase inhibitors are employed to produce greater xanthine oxidase inhibition. Additional studies are needed.

NAD(P)H oxidase is a plasmalemmal enzyme that mediates the ROS-dependent effects of angiotensin in vascular smooth muscle cells.[72] The activation of NAD(P)H oxidase results in increased generation of O_2^- in the cytosol. This enzyme complex was first described in the neutrophil, where it is responsible for the oxidative burst which produces large amounts of cytotoxic ROS. However, NAD(P)H oxidases in other cell types appear to be capable of producing much lower levels of ROS that can act as signaling intermediates in growth pathways.[73] Recent studies have implicated this oxidase in the hypertrophic response of ventricular myocytes (see later discussion).[74,75]

Nonenzymatic autoxidation reactions of several organic molecules, including neurohormones, may also contribute to the formation of ROS in vivo. Oxidation of norepinephrine and epinephrine to adrenochrome and O_2^- has been proposed as a mechanism for myocardial injury in the presence of chronic adrenergic stimulation.[76] As small amounts of ascorbic acid can completely prevent this reaction, and there are clearly direct adrenergic receptor-mediated deleterious effects of adrenergic stimulation,[77] it is unclear whether adrenochrome-mediated injury contributes to heart failure. In addition, thiol compounds including cysteine and GSH can autoxidize to form O_2^-, particularly in the presence of transition metals such as iron. The cardiotoxicity of iron overload is likely a combination of this plus the catalysis of Fenton chemistry to generate hydroxyl radicals. Myoglobin can also autoxidize from oxymyoglobin to metmyoglobin with the release of O_2^-, and this may be another source of ROS given the high concentration of myoglobin in the ventricular myocyte.[78]

Growing evidence supports the mitochondria as an important source of myocardial ROS in the failing heart (for review see Tsutsui, 79). Some small fraction of electrons entering the mitochondrial electron transport chain "leak" to molecular oxygen to form O_2^- (Figure 12-3). Because of the density of mitochondria in cardiac myocytes this can result in a high flux of O_2^-. Ide et al have found convincing evidence of increased mitochondrial formation of ROS in the myocardium of dogs with rapid-pacing-induced heart failure.[80] As in other models of heart failure, lipid peroxidation levels were increased in the myocardium of the failing animals compared with controls. In a mitochondrial fraction form, they examined the formation of O_2^- using electroparamagnetic resonance (EPR) with the O_2^- spin-trap 5,5′-dimethyl-1-pyrroline-N-oxide (DMPO). The DMPO spin signal, which is directly proportional to the rate of formation of ROS, was 2.8-fold higher in mitochondria from failing hearts compared with nonfailing controls. This was associated with an approximately 50% decrease in the activity of mitochondrial electron transport complex I, suggesting a functional uncoupling of the mitochondria that may have contributed to the increase in ROS formation. Thus at least in this heart failure model there is evidence of oxidative stress which is due, at least in part, to increased mitochondrial formation of O_2^-.

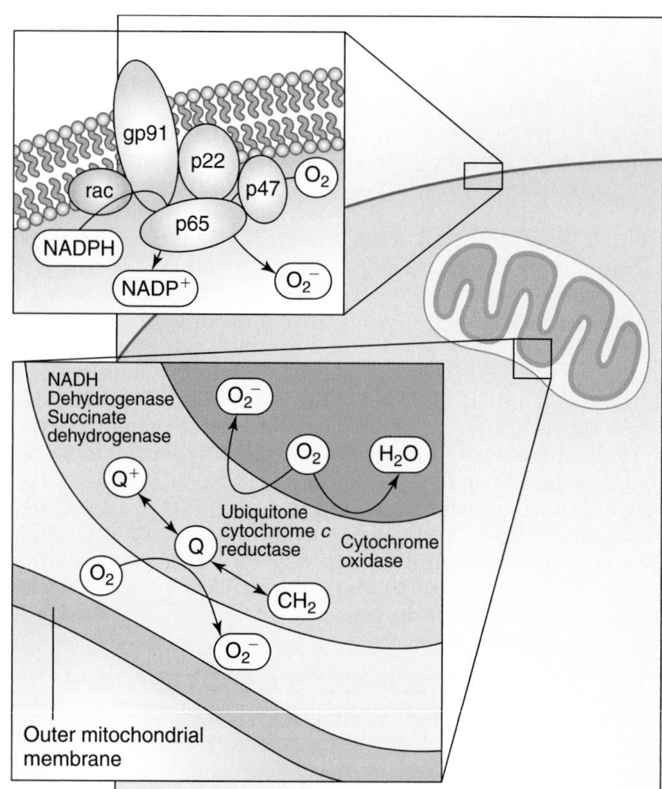

FIGURE 12–3 NAD(P)H oxidases and mitochondria as sources of ROS in the heart. An NAD(P)H oxidase is expressed in cardiac myocytes similar to that found in neutrophils and vascular cells. The oxidase is composed of at least five subunits, with two membrane proteins that comprise the oxidase activity and three cytoplasmic proteins that serve regulatory functions. The complex catalyzes the one electron reduction of O_2 to O_2^- with NADPH or NADH as a reducing cofactor. The mitochondrial electron transport chain creates a proton-motive force through the transfer of electrons from NADH dehydrogenase (complex I) and succinate dehydrogenase (complex II) to ubiquinone (Q), thereby forming reduced ubiquinone (QH_2). Partially reduced ubiquinone (Q·) is a radical that can reduce O_2 to O_2^-. This oxygen "leakage" is a potentially large source of ROS, and has been implicated in the increased oxidative stress in heart failure (see text).

EFFECTS OF OXIDATIVE STRESS ON MYOCARDIAL STRUCTURE AND FUNCTION

Role of ROS in Myocardial Remodeling

One consequence of myocardial oxidative stress may be the promotion of myocardial remodeling (see chapter15). Following an injury such as myocardial infarction there is progressive "remodeling" of the remaining, viable myocardium, a process characterized by chamber enlargement, myocardial thinning and pump dysfunction. Multiple mechanisms contribute to myocardial remodeling including myocyte hypertrophy, myocyte slippage, myocyte apoptosis and/or alterations in the turnover and properties of the extracellular matrix (see Chapter 5). The stimuli for ventricular remodeling includes increased wall stress, inflammatory cytokines (see Chapter 11), and neurohormones including catecholamines and angiotensin II. In vitro and in vivo experimental studies have shown that oxidative stress can cause myocardial remodeling, and mediate many of the effects of remodeling stimuli, raising the possibility that ROS may play a central role in the process of ventricular remodeling.

ROS regulate growth pathways in many cell types, including the cardiovascular system (see Figure 12-2). As discussed previously, the effect of angiotensin II on vascular smooth muscle cell hypertrophy depends on increased production of O_2^- via NADPH oxidase.[81] Likewise, the growth effects of stimuli that act via the small GTP-binding protein *ras* appear to be mediated by increases in O_2^-.[82] ROS appear to mediate similar growth responses in ventricular myocytes. For example, small alterations in cellular oxidative stress in cardiac myocytes in vitro can lead to changes in myocyte hypertrophy. The copper chelator diethyldithiocarbamic acid (DDC) inhibits the activity of CuZnSOD in a concentration-dependent manner leading to measurable increases in cellular O_2^- levels as assessed by lucigenin chemiluminescence or nitro-blue tetrazolium (NBT) reduction.[83] Exposure to low concentrations of DDC (1 to 10 μM) for 24 hours caused myocyte growth with increases in protein synthesis and cell size, and associated with increased expression of ANF mRNA and decreased expression of SERCA2 mRNA. All of the effects of DDC were inhibited by antioxidants, and thus support the conclusion that small increases in intracellular oxidative stress can cause typical myocyte hypertrophy.

ROS appear to mediate the hypertrophic effect of mechanical strain,[84] a well-known stimulus for myocyte hypertrophy. Low- (5%) and high- (25%) amplitude strain of cardiac myocytes causes amplitude-dependent increases in both ROS formation and myocyte hypertrophy, and the hypertrophic effect was inhibited by an SOD-mimetic. Unlike high-amplitude strain (as discussed later), there was no effect of low-amplitude strain on the frequency of apoptosis as measured by TUNEL or DNA laddering. Similarly, myocyte hypertrophy stimulated by angiotensin II or TNF-α is mediated by ROS.[85] Both TNF-α and angiotensin II increase the formation of ROS, and the hypertrophic effects of these stimuli are inhibited by concomitant treatment with soluble antioxidants including vitamin E. As formation of both angiotensin II and TNF-α have been demonstrated in myocytes subjected to mechanical strain,[86] these observations may be related to the similar observations made with mechanical strain (see previous discussion). α-Adrenergic receptor stimulation also induces myocyte ROS formation and stimulates myocyte hypertrophy through an ROS-dependent pathways.[74] Likewise, endothelin modulates myocyte early response gene expression through ROS-dependent activation of *ras*[87] and ouabain causes hypertrophy via ROS-dependent activation of a pathway involving both *ras* and mitogen-activated protein kinases (MAPK).[88]

While the details of how these agonists increase myocyte ROS formation remains to be elucidated, a growing literature suggests that a NAD(P)H oxidase is involved (see Figures 12-3 and 12-4). For example, in isolated adult rat ventricular myocytes the NAD(P)H oxidase inhibitor diphenylene iodonium completely prevents α_1-adrenergic- and endothelin-stimulated activation of the MAPKs extracellular-signal regulated kinase 1 and 2 (ERK1/2).[74] In contrast, inhibition of the mitochondrial respiratory chain with rotenone had no effect on the α_1-adrenergic receptor-stimulated activation of ERK1/2.

The neutrophil NAD(P)H oxidase is a complex consisting of at least four major subunits, including two membrane-spanning components (p22phox and gp91phox), and two cytosolic components (p67phox and p47phox) (for review see Griendling[81]). A similar oxidase system has been identified in many cell types in the cardiovascular system.[89] Although the cardiovascular NAD(P)H oxidases retain a similar enzyme complex structure to neutrophil oxidase with four subunits, their component structures and biochemical characteristics are considerably different. Using reverse transcriptase-polymerase chain reactions (RT-PCR) and Northern blot analysis, expression of the four major subunits of NAD(P)H oxidase (p22phox, gp91phox, p67phox, and p47phox) has been identified in rat cardiac myocytes.[74] The gp91phox knockout mouse has been studied in the setting of angiotensin II infusion, with results supporting a role for an NAD(P)H oxidase in both vascular and myocardial hypertrophy.[75,90]

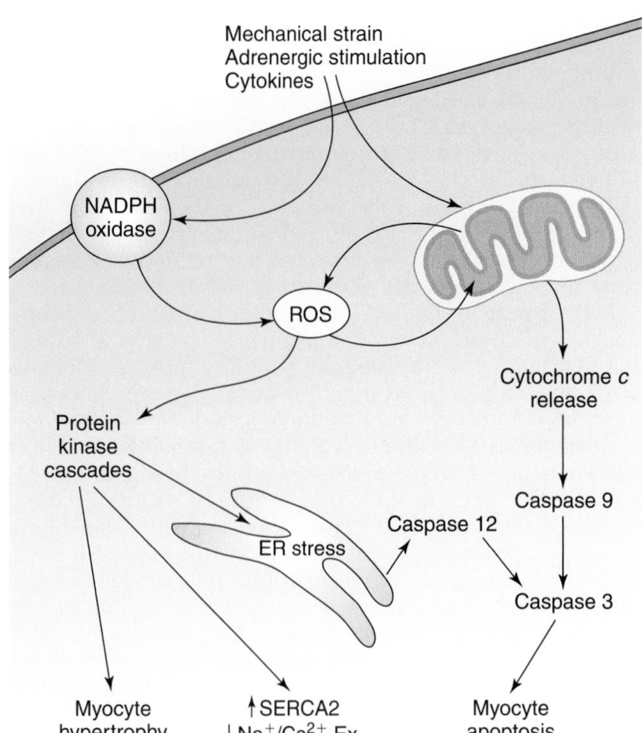

FIGURE 12–4 Schematic presentation of the effects of ROS on myocyte phenotype. Through activation of kinase cascades such as MAPK, ROS can induce myocyte hypertrophy. ROS can also alter the activity and expression of Ca^{2+} handling proteins, including SERCA2 and the Na^+/Ca^{2+} exchanger, to alter myocardial contractility. Mitochondrial ROS may be particularly prone to induce apoptosis by stimulating the mitochondrial release of cytochrome *c*, which is necessary for the activation of caspase cascades. The endoplasmic reticulum (ER) is also a source of ROS production. Under stress, the ER-resident molecular chaperone, glucose-regulated protein-78, is upregulated and leads to the transcriptional induction of ER stress response genes and the activation of caspase 12. Translational arrest decreases the workload on the ER, essential for cell recovery and survival. However, when the ER is overwhelmed by the stress, caspase 12 is released and activates caspase 3 and the final programmed cell death pathway.

Suppressor doses of angiotensin II administered subcutaneously for 2 weeks caused cardiac hypertrophy that was associated with increased myocardial expression of a fetal gene program, increased myocyte cross-sectional area, and increased myocardial collagen content in wild-type, but not gp91phox, knockout mice. Thus NADPH oxidase appears to play a central role in the cardiac hypertrophic response to several neurohormones and peptides (see Figure 12-4).

In contrast to the growth effects of low levels of ROS generated by specific oxidases and acting via specific signaling systems, higher levels of ROS-induced myocyte cell death, which may also be important in the pathophysiology of heart failure. For example, high concentrations of DDC leading to approximately 50% inhibition of SOD activity in neonatal rat ventricular myocytes induce myocyte apoptosis as assessed by nuclear morphology and TUNEL staining for DNA fragmentation.[83] At apoptotic concentrations, but not at hypertrophic concentrations, DDC increased myocyte expression of Bax, a pro-apoptotic member of the Bcl-2 family. Like the hypertrophic effect of low concentrations of DDC, the apoptotic effect of higher concentrations of DDC was prevented by antioxidants. Thus higher levels of intracellular oxidative stress cause ROS-dependent apoptosis in myocytes.

Direct addition of ROS to cardiac myocytes in culture also causes apoptosis.[91] Similarly, the cardiotoxic anthracyclines

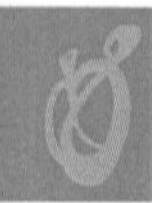

are well known to generate intracellular ROS[92] and induce both myocyte apoptosis and necrosis in a dose-dependent manner (see Chapter 58). The apoptosis, but not necrosis, could be inhibited by the addition of the iron chelator dexrazoxane, which is used clinically in the prevention of anthracycline cardiotoxicity.[93] These results implicate hydroxyl radicals formed via the Fenton reaction in anthracycline-induced apoptosis. Although not specifically examined, hydroxyl radicals may also account for the apoptotic effect of extracellular O_2^- or H_2O_2 in isolated ventricular myocytes. Thus multiple studies have shown that oxidative stress can cause myocyte apoptosis in vitro.

ROS appear to mediate the apoptotic effect of high-level mechanical strain on cardiac myocytes. Cheng et al showed that ROS formation increases in papillary muscles subjected to oxidative stress in vitro, and is associated with increased myocyte apoptosis.[94] Application of a static mechanical load (approximately sixfold the estimated normal end-diastolic wall stress) for 4 hours increased both the production of O_2^- and the frequency of apoptosis. Addition of an NO donor decreased the level of ROS formation and the frequency of apoptosis, thus suggesting a mechanistic role for ROS in strain apoptosis. More direct evidence for ROS-dependent apoptosis in the setting of increased mechanical load comes from studies in isolated ventricular myocytes. Cyclic mechanical stretch in isolated cardiac myocytes increases ROS production,[84] and when cells are stretched at a high amplitude there is an increase in the number of apoptotic myocytes, associated with an increase in Bax expression. Treatment of myocytes with an SOD-mimetic prevents stretch-induced apoptosis. Thus ROS appear to mediate both growth and death responses in cardiac myocytes.

Mechanisms of ROS-induced Phenotype in Cardiac Myocytes

The mechanism by which increases in ROS lead to myocyte hypertrophy and apoptosis appear to involve activation of one or more stress-responsive protein kinases of the MAPK superfamily,[95] which is known to respond to ROS, and activate both hypertrophy and apoptosis in myocytes in vitro (see Chapter 2). This family of protein kinases includes ERKs and two stress-responsive MAPK subfamilies (SR-MAPKs), the p38-kinases and the c-Jun *N*-terminal kinases (JNKs). The ERKs consist of p42 (ERK-1) and p44 (ERK-2). The p38-kinases consist of at least six isoforms (α_1, α_2, β_1, β_2, γ, and δ), with the α and β isoforms appearing to predominate in cardiac myocytes. The JNKs consist of 46-kDa or 54-kDa proteins.

ROS activate SR-MAPKs in the cardiovascular system. H_2O_2 activates p38-kinase, JNKs, and ERKs in neonatal rat ventricular myocytes.[96] In perfused rat hearts, H_2O_2 activated SR-MAPKs, with minimal activation of ERKs. Ischemia and ischemia/reperfusion selectively activated SR-MAPKs: p38-kinase was activated by both ischemia and ischemia/reperfusion, whereas JNKs were activated by ischemia/reperfusion, and neither stimulus activated ERKs.[97] An O_2^- scavenger inhibited p38-kinase activation, whereas a $OH^{\cdot}$ scavenger prevented activation of both p38-kinases and JNKs during ischemia/reperfusion, raising the possibility that specific ROS differentially activate specific SR-MAPKs.

The possibility that SR-MAPKs mediate the effects of oxidative stress on myocyte growth is supported by in vitro and in vivo overexpression studies using molecular constructs of specific kinases or activators, and examining the effect on myocyte growth. For example, in neonatal rat ventricular myocytes, overexpression of constitutively active p38 kinase(β) or JNKs causes a hypertrophic response, whereas constitutively active p38-kinase(α) causes apoptosis.[98] Other studies have used pharmacological inhibitors. For example, an inhibitor of ERK activation decreases the hypertrophic response of ventricular myocytes to α-adrenergic stimulation,[99] and this pathway appears to be activated by ROS generated by an NAD(P)H oxidase (see previous discussion). Inhibition of ERK activation also increases the apoptotic response to ROS, suggesting that ERKs may also exert a prosurvival effect.[91]

Apoptosis induced by oxidative stress appears to involve the activation of JNKs (see Chapter 6). In the H9C2 cardiac cell line, oxidative stress-induced apoptosis is associated with activation of JNKs, and transfection of a dominant negative JNK markedly diminishes the extent of apoptosis.[100] Similarly, ischemia/reperfusion-induced myocardial injury is associated with JNK activation and myocyte apoptosis is inhibited by the antioxidant/β-blocker carvedilol,[101] again supporting a role for JNK in ROS-induced myocyte injury. Similar mechanisms have been proposed for the beneficial effects of β-receptor blockade in chronic heart failure, although these speculations remain unproven.

Mitochondria are involved at an early step in the regulation of apoptosis in general, and appear to be involved in oxidative stress-induced apoptosis in the heart through the release of cytochrome *c* from the intermembrane space (see Chapter 6). Cytochrome *c* release activates caspase 9 and caspase 3 and appears to potentiate mitochondrial generation of ROS, possibly through effects on electron transport.[102] The process of cytochrome *c* release is modulated by the Bcl-2 family of proteins (for review see Reed[103]). Proapoptotic members of the Bcl-2 family (Bax, Bad, and Bak) interact with the outer mitochondrial membrane and allow for cytochrome *c* release and dissipation of the membrane potential through what has been termed the "mitochondrial permeability pore transition". Antiapoptotic members of the family (e.g., Bcl-2 and Bcl-xL) inhibit Bax-mediated cytochrome *c* release, caspase 3 activation, and the generation of ROS. In myocytes treated with direct addition of ROS, p53 activity increases in association with translocation of Bax and Bad from the cytosol to the mitochondrial fraction, with associated release of cytochrome *c*.[104] Interestingly, it appears that exogenous O_2^- induces apoptosis by a pathway distinct from H_2O_2. While treatment with H_2O_2 induced mitochondrial release of cytochrome *c* and activation of caspase 3, treatment with xanthine and xanthine oxidase (in the presence of catalase) as a source of O_2^- induced apoptosis without either cytochrome *c* release or activation of caspase 3. In contrast, O_2^--induced apoptosis involved activation of the laminase Mch2α, and was inhibited by the pancaspase inhibitor Z-VAD-fmk. In contrast, increasing intracellular O_2^- by inhibition of superoxide dismutase does increase Bax expression, suggesting that a mitochondrial pathway may be involved. Together these data suggest that extracellular and intracellular O_2^- may trigger apoptosis via distinct pathways. This would not be surprising, as extracellular O_2^- should enter the cell minimally given its negative charge and the negative resting membrane potential. Extracellular O_2^- might trigger apoptosis via changes in matrix/integrin interactions. The effect of extracellular xanthine/xanthine oxidase on myocyte detachment in tissue culture suggests such a mechanism.[83]

In addition to actions on the cell membrane death receptors (extrinsic pathway) and release of proapoptotic factors from the mitochondria (intrinsic pathway), ROS may exert its apoptotic effects via stress at the endoplasmic reticulum (ER) (for review see Lee[105]). The ER is a multifunctional cellular organelle responsible for posttranslational processing of newly synthesized secretary and membrane proteins, maintenance of calcium homeostasis, and production and storage of glycogen, steroids, and other macromolecules. When the cell is exposed to obnoxious stimuli, such as hypoxia, ischemia, gene mutation, oxidative insult, or unglycosylation that increase misfolded proteins or perturb intracellular Ca^{2+} homeostasis in the ER, an adaptive process that couples the ER protein load with the ER protein folding capacity occurs.[106]

This process, known as unfolded protein response (UPR), is characterized by upregulation of ER chaperones such as glucose-regulated protein 78 (GRP78), release and activation of three key transmembrane proteins (protein kinase R–like ER kinase, inositol-requiring enzyme-1, and activating transcription factor 6) to promote the transcription of UPR genes, and removal of the unfolded proteins to the ubiquitin proteasome for degradation, aiming at restoring cellular homeostasis.[107] However, if ER stimuli overwhelm the capacity of UPR to remove the unfolded proteins from the ER, a maladaptive ER overload response (EOR) occurs. EOR is associated with transcriptional induction of C/EBP homologous protein (CHOP), cleavage of the ER-resident procaspase 12 to active caspase 12, and eventual programmed cell death through the activation of caspase 9 and 3. It has now been demonstrated that UPR and EOR are activated not only in acute myocardial ischemia/reperfusion but also in cardiac hypertrophy and failure.[107-109] Dilated cardiomyopathy also has been shown to occur in transgenic mice overexpressing a mutant KDEL receptor for ER chaperones that sensitizes the cells to ER stress.[110] The ER stress is functionally linked to β-adrenergic receptor-mediated activation of Ca^{++}/calmodulin-dependent protein kinase II and p-38 MAPK.[109] It has been shown to be activated by norepinephrine and an anti-β_1-adrenoceptor antibody in an autoimmune cardiomyopathy.[111] Evidence has now accumulated that UPR and ROS production are closely linked,[112] and that ROS generation my occur both upstream and downstream to UPR signaling targets, including depolarization of the inner mitochondrial membrane following Ca^{2+} release.[113] It is also recognized that the phosphatidylinositol-3 kinase/Akt pathway and Bcl-2 family proteins are involved in the control of ER stress-induced apoptosis. Cardiac overexpression of metallothionein prevented both the inactivation of Akt and induction of ER stress in alcoholic cardiomyopathy.[114] Likewise, darbepoetin alfa treatment enhanced the activation of the phosphatidylinositol-3-kinase/Akt pathway, and reduced ER stress-related apoptosis in β-receptor peptide-induced autoimmune cardiomyopathy.[109] Akt phosphorylation is antiapoptotic; its inactivation is associated with reduction of prosurvival Bcl proteins. It is known that the Bcl-2 homolog domain-3-only protein bimakalim (Bim), which is sequestered by the prosurvival Bcl protein in healthy cells, may be freed when the level of Bcl protein is reduced, and translocates to the ER membrane to activate caspase 12[115] and ER stress-induced apoptosis by both protein phosphatase 2A-mediated dephosphorylation and CHOP-mediated direct transcription induction.[116] In contrast, in animals overexpressing Bcl-xL, ER stress is reduced as the antiapoptotic protein binds to Bim and inhibits its translocation to the ER. PUMA (p53-upregulated modulator of apoptosis) is another proapoptotic homolog domain-3-only member of the Bcl-2 protein family, which has been demonstrated to be critical for cardiomyocyte apoptosis induced by ER stress.[117]

ROS-induced Changes in Calcium Handling

Myocytes isolated from the failing heart show markedly abnormal intracellular Ca^{+2} transients along with alterations in the expression and/or activity of Ca^{+2} handling proteins,[118] and these changes may be due in part to oxidative stress. The contribution of the Ca^{+2} handling proteins to contractile dysfunction in the failing heart are discussed in detail in Chapter 3. Of note, the downregulation of sarcoplasmic reticulum Ca^{+2} ATPase (SERCA2) expression and activity in the failing heart appear to contribute to contractile dysfunction in heart failure. The mechanism by which ROS leads to decreased SERCA2 activity may involve decreases in protein expression, as in primary cultures of cardiac myocytes exposed to increased levels of ROS[83] and/or alterations in protein function due to oxidative posttranslational modifications (OPTM). In vascular smooth muscle, peroxynitrite (ONOO) causes OPTM of SERCA.[119] Low ONOO levels increase enzyme activity via a reversible glutathiolation at cysteine 674, whereas higher levels of ONOO decrease enzyme activity via irreversible sulfonylation at the same site.

There are other effects of ROS on myocyte Ca^{+2} handling that can result in changes in contractile function. ROS alter Ca^{+2} transients and excitation-contraction coupling in isolated myocytes by increasing the activity of the Na^+/Ca^{+2} exchanger, which in some situations may lead to Ca^{+2} overload.[120] A similar increase in Na^+/Ca^{+2} exchanger activity can be seen in some models of heart failure. For example, late after MI in the rabbit heart there is increased Na^+/Ca^{+2} exchanger activity together with a depressed force-frequency relationship.[121] Electrophysiological studies in isolated myocytes have also shown direct effects of reactive oxygen and nitrogen species on the voltage-dependent Ca^{2+} channel and the calcium release channel.[122,123] It remains to be seen whether these direct effects of ROS on Ca^{+2} handling proteins in vitro contribute to abnormal excitation-contraction coupling and contractility in the chronically failing heart.

ROS Regulation of Interstitial Matrix Turnover by Cardiac Fibroblasts

As discussed in Chapter 5, one mechanism for ventricular chamber dilation is via alterations in the interstitial matrix of the myocardium. Individual ventricular myocytes are mechanically coupled to other cells via interstitial matrix proteins that connect to the sarcomere via integrins and intermediate filaments. Like intracellular proteins, there is a regular turnover of interstitial matrix proteins that is regulated by proteases and the protein synthetic machinery of the cardiac cells. Collagen is the major component of the interstitium that contributes to the structural integrity of the myocardium. Myocardial collagen content is regulated by the balance between synthesis and degradation, the latter primarily due to the action of matrix metalloproteinases (MMPs).[124]

Both cardiac fibroblast collagen synthesis and MMP activity are regulated in part by oxidative stress.[125] Fibroblasts from adult or neonatal rats grown in primary culture respond to both intracellular and extracellular oxidative stress with decreases in procollagen mRNA expression and collagen synthesis. Moreover, oxidative stress increases fibroblast MMP activity as measured by in-gel zymography. It is possible that such actions would result in myocyte slippage and chamber dilation, and impaired cell-cell mechanical coupling, and thereby contribute to abnormalities in both systolic and diastolic function. A role for oxidative stress in the regulation of interstitial matrix was recently defined in the mouse heart. Early after MI there was increased expression and activity of MMPs, and treatment with an antioxidant (DMTU) reduced the extent of ventricular dilation and suppressed MMP activity.[59] These results were similar to the effect of a pharmacological inhibitor of MMPs, and suggest that antioxidant strategies may be useful in preventing ventricular dilation in heart failure.

NITRIC OXIDE AND ITS INTERACTION WITH ROS

Nitric oxide (NO) is also a free radical and can modify the myocardial response to oxidative stress both directly and indirectly. NO is synthesized in the conversion of L-arginine to L-citrulline by a family of nitric oxide synthases (NOS). NO, a free radical gas, is buffered in the cell by reactions with glutathione and reacts reversibly with sulfhydryl groups of proteins forming *S*-nitrosothiols leading to alterations in protein function.[126] Through chemical reactions with ROS, NO

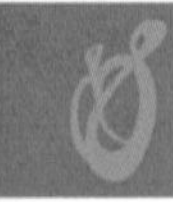

can either *decrease* or *increase* the oxidative stress in a cell or tissue. Under normal circumstances, myocardial NO is produced at low levels by NOS3. NOS3 is present in virtually all cell types in the myocardium including myocytes, fibroblasts, and endothelial cells, and is regulated by a calcium-sensitive interaction with calmodulin.[127] Inducible nitric oxide synthase (NOS2) is not regulated by Ca^{+2}, and when expressed is capable of producing high levels of cellular NO. Though NOS2 is expressed minimally in the normal myocardium, it is induced by exposure to cytokines, hypoxia, and other stimuli in both myocytes and nonmyocytes because of activation of specific transcription factors and leads to a marked increase in the production of NO.[128] Of note, there is evidence for increased expression and activity of the NOS2 in the myocardium of patients with both idiopathic and ischemic dilated cardiomyopathies.[129]

Low levels of NO, as are formed by NOS3, may reduce the level of oxidative stress by decreasing the production of O_2^- through inhibition of oxidative enzymes.[130] Indirectly, low levels of NO may also exert beneficial effects on myocardial remodeling. NO through the activation of guanylate cyclase can inhibit signaling and transcription factors that regulate cardiac hypertrophy. NO may also be able to promote cell survival by regulating steps in the apoptotic cascade including proteases.[131] Mice lacking NOS3 have worse ventricular function late after MI,[132] consistent with the notion that NOS3-derived NO is beneficial for the failing result in nitrosative heart.

Higher levels of NO may increase oxidative stress by reacting with O_2^- to generate peroxynitrite ($ONOO^-$), a free radical which is toxic and longer-lived than either NO or O_2^-.[133] $ONOO^-$ can react with many cell constituents including tyrosine residues of susceptible proteins such as MnSOD, causing irreversible inactivation.[134] Based on the relative rate constants for the reaction of O_2^- with superoxide dismutase (SOD) and NO, the formation of $ONOO^-$ is favored when the levels of O_2^- or NO are high, or the level of SOD is low. Interestingly, Xia and associates have shown that NOS2 is also capable of catalyzing the formation of O_2^-,[135] particularly in the setting of arginine depletion. Thus expression of NOS2 may contribute directly to the formation of ROS (for review see Zimmet[136]).

Multiple experimental studies have shown that high concentrations of NO can have direct toxic effects on cardiac myocytes in vitro. The cytotoxic effect of cytokines on adult rat ventricular myocytes in culture is inhibited by the NOS inhibitor L-NMMA.[137] Similarly, in neonatal rat ventricular myocytes, cytokines induce cell death via NO-dependent apoptosis.[138] Cytokine-induced apoptosis can be prevented by either an inhibitor of NOS2 or an SOD-mimetic, thus implicating $ONOO^-$. Moreover, NOS2 appears to contribute to the myocyte apoptosis that occurs in the setting of myocardial failure in vivo. In the failing mouse heart, late after MI, NOS2 expression is increased in the remote myocardium and in NOS2 knockout mice there is less myocyte apoptosis, improved contractile function, and increased animal survival, as compared with wild-type mice with MI of identical size.[139]

Animal models of autoimmune and viral myocarditis (see chapter 31) have also implicated a direct toxic effect of NO and $ONOO^-$ in vivo. In these models there is massive inflammation in the myocardium that results in overt myocyte necrosis. The amount of necrotic myocardium and the elevation of serum CK in rats with experimental autoimmune myocarditis was reduced by aminoguanidine, an inhibitor of NOS2.[140] Interestingly, treatment with aminoguanidine also decreased the amount of O_2^- anion formed. This latter effect could occur either through NOS2-dependent O_2^- production in this system or the inactivation of MnSOD by $ONOO^-$.[141]

Both good and bad aspects of NO were revealed in a model of viral myocarditis when L-NAME was used to treat mice with viral myocarditis.[142] Mice were infected with coxsackievirus B3 in the presence of increasing doses of L-NAME. At the highest dose of L-NAME, there was decreased mouse survival. At a low dose, however, L-NAME improved survival, and the severity of heart failure and extent of myocardial necrosis. The exact mechanism that determines the "optimal" NO concentration remains to be determined. Interestingly, as discussed previously, stretch-induced myocyte apoptosis was inhibited by the addition of an NO donor.[94] Coincident with the decrease in apoptosis was a decrease in the level of O_2^-. There are several potential mechanisms for this beneficial effect of NO. At low levels, NO can reduce apoptosis by inhibiting specific enzymes in the programmed cell death pathway.[131] Another possibility is that the NO donor decreased production of mitochondrial ROS production. As mentioned previously, NO decreases mitochondrial respiration and myocardial oxygen consumption and thus indirectly controls the rate of ROS production.[130]

SUMMARY

Oxidative and nitrosative stress are elevated systemically and in the myocardium of patients with chronic myocardial failure. The cause of increased ROS in this setting is still incompletely understood, but is clearly multifactorial including increased production of ROS due to increased metabolic activity, stimulated production by mechanical strain, neurohormonal activation, inflammatory cytokines, and decreased antioxidant activity. Based on both in vitro and in vivo studies, it appears likely that increases in oxidative and nitrositive stress contribute to the ventricular remodeling and contractile dysfunction in the failing heart.

Oxidative stress has many effects on myocardial structure and function. It is clear that oxidative stress can trigger a range of responses in myocytes in vitro, and that similar responses may occur in vivo in situations leading to myocardial dysfunction. As in other tissues, oxidative stress can stimulate both growth and death of cells. The mechanism by which various ROS activate cell signaling pathways remains an area of active investigation and promises to offer new therapeutic targets for pharmacological antioxidants.

There remain many unanswered questions about the role of oxidative stress in myocardial failure. In addition, the results of applying preclinical observations to develop therapeutic strategies for patients with heart failure have been disappointing. Further work is clearly needed. In developing therapeutic strategies targeted specifically at oxidative stress, we will need to understand in more detail (1) the relative contributions of decreased antioxidant activity versus increased formation of ROS; (2) the situations in which oxidative and/or nitrosative stress contribute to the pathogenesis of myocardial dysfunction in vivo; (3) the precise ROS involved; and (4) the optimal place in ROS cascades to intervene to prevent adverse effects of ROS on myocardial structure and function. Advances in our understanding of antioxidant enzymes and the technology for manipulation of these genes, and the development of animal models for acute and chronic myocardial injury, are likely to provide new insight into the potential therapeutic value of antioxidants in the treatment and prevention of myocardial dysfunction.

REFERENCES

1. McCord, J. M., & Fridovich, I. (1969). Superoxide dismutase. An enzymic function for erythrocuprein (hemocuprein). *J Biol Chem, 244*, 6049–6055.
2. Dale, D. C., Boxer, L., & Liles, W. C. (2008). The phagocytes: neutrophils and monocytes. *Blood, 112*, 935–945.
3. Assem, M., Teyssier, J. R., Benderitter, M., et al. (1997). Pattern of superoxide dismutase enzymatic activity and RNA changes in rat heart ventricles after myocardial infarction. *Am J Pathol, 151*, 549–555.
4. Carlsson, L. M., Jonsson, J., Edlund, T., et al. (1995). Mice lacking extracellular superoxide dismutase are more sensitive to hyperoxia. *Proc Natl Acad Sci U S A, 92*, 6264–6268.

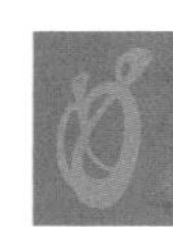

5. Li, Y., Huang, T. T., Carlson, E. J., et al. (1995). Dilated cardiomyopathy and neonatal lethality in mutant mice lacking manganese superoxide dismutase. *Nat Genet, 11*, 376–381.
6. Pandolfi, P. P., Sonati, F., Rivi, R., et al. (1995). Targeted disruption of the housekeeping gene encoding glucose 6-phosphate dehydrogenase (G6PD): G6PD is dispensable for pentose synthesis but essential for defense against oxidative stress. *EMBO J, 14*, 5209–5215.
7. Motterlini, R., Gonzales, A., Foresti, R., et al. (1998). Heme oxygenase-1-derived carbon monoxide contributes to the suppression of acute hypertensive responses in vivo. *Circ Res, 83*, 568–577.
8. Clark, J. E., Foresti, R., Sarathchandra, P., et al. (2000). Heme oxygenase-1-derived bilirubin ameliorates postischemic myocardial dysfunction. *Am J Physiol Heart Circ Physiol, 278*, H643–H651.
9. Vulapalli, S. R., Chen, Z., Chua, B. H., et al. (2002). Cardioselective overexpression of HO-1 prevents I/R-induced cardiac dysfunction and apoptosis. *Am J Physiol Heart Circ Physiol, 283*, H688–H694.
10. Liu, X., Pachori, A. S., Ward, C. A., et al. (2006). Heme oxygenase-1 (HO-1) inhibits postmyocardial infarct remodeling and restores ventricular function. *FASEB J, 20*, 207–216.
11. Rotruck, J. T., Pope, A. L., Ganther, H. E., et al. (1973). Selenium: biochemical role as a component of glutathione peroxidase. *Science, 179*, 588–590.
12. Wu, J., & Xu, G. L. (1987). Plasma selenium content, platelet glutathione peroxidase and superoxide dismutase activity of residents in Kashin-Beck disease affected area in China. *J Trace Elem Electrolytes Health Dis, 1*, 39–43.
13. Beck, M. A., Shi, Q., Morris, V. C., et al. (1995). Rapid genomic evolution of a non-virulent coxsackievirus B3 in selenium-deficient mice results in selection of identical virulent isolates. *Nat Med, 1*, 433–436.
14. Kavanaugh-McHugh, A. L., Ruff, A., Perlman, E., et al. (1991). Selenium deficiency and cardiomyopathy in acquired immunodeficiency syndrome. *JPEN J Parenter Enteral Nutr, 15*, 347–349.
15. Hill, M. F., & Singal, P. K. (1996). Antioxidant and oxidative stress changes during heart failure subsequent to myocardial infarction in rats. *Am J Pathol, 148*, 291–300.
16. Sato, M., Sasaki, M., & Hojo, H. (1995). Antioxidative roles of metallothionein and manganese superoxide dismutase induced by tumor necrosis factor-alpha and interleukin-6. *Arch Biochem Biophys, 316*, 738–744.
17. Cai, L. (2007). Diabetic cardiomyopathy and its prevention by metallothionein: experimental evidence, possible mechanisms and clinical implications. *Curr Med Chem, 14*, 2193–2203.
18. Shioji, K., Nakamura, H., Masutani, H., et al. (2003). Redox regulation by thioredoxin in cardiovascular diseases. *Antioxid Redox Signal, 5*, 795–802.
19. Nimata, M., Kishimoto, C., Shioji, K., et al. (2003). Upregulation of redox-regulating protein, thioredoxin, in endomyocardial biopsy samples of patients with myocarditis and cardiomyopathies. *Mol Cell Biochem, 248*, 193–196.
20. Jekell, A., Hossain, A., Alehagen, U., et al. (2004). Elevated circulating levels of thioredoxin and stress in chronic heart failure. *Eur J Heart Fail, 6*, 883–890.
21. Koneru, S., Penumathsa, S. V., Thirunavukkarasu, M., et al. (2009). Thioredoxin-1 gene delivery induces heme oxygenase-1 mediated myocardial preservation after chronic infarction in hypertensive rats. *Am J Hypertens, 22*, 183–190.
22. Dhalla, A. K., Hill, M. F., & Singal, P. K. (1996). Role of oxidative stress in transition of hypertrophy to heart failure. *J Am Coll Cardiol, 28*, 506–514.
23. Hamblin, M., Smith, H. M., & Hill, M. F. (2007). Dietary supplementation with vitamin E ameliorates cardiac failure in type I diabetic cardiomyopathy by suppressing myocardial generation of 8-iso-prostaglandin F2alpha and oxidized glutathione. *J Card Fail, 13*, 884–892.
24. Diaz-Velez, C. R., Garcia-Castineiras, S., Mendoza-Ramos, E., et al. (1996). Increased malondialdehyde in peripheral blood of patients with congestive heart failure. *Am Heart J, 131*, 146–152.
25. Mak, S., Lehotay, D. C., Yazdanpanah, M., et al. (2000). Unsaturated aldehydes including 4-OH-nonenal are elevated in patients with congestive heart failure. *J Card Fail, 6*, 108–114.
26. McMurray, J., Chopra, M., Abdullah, I., et al. (1993). Evidence of oxidative stress in chronic heart failure in humans. *Eur Heart J, 14*, 1493–1498.
27. Tang, W. H., Brennan, M. L., Philip, K., et al. (2006). Plasma myeloperoxidase levels in patients with chronic heart failure. *Am J Cardiol, 98*, 796–799.
28. Ferrari, R., Bachetti, T., Confortini, R., et al. (1995). Tumor necrosis factor soluble receptors in patients with various degrees of congestive heart failure. *Circulation, 92*, 1479–1486.
29. Sobotka, P. A., Brottman, M. D., Weitz, Z., et al. (1993). Elevated breath pentane in heart failure reduced by free radical scavenger. *Free Radic Biol Med, 14*, 643–647.
30. Ghatak, A., Brar, M. J., Agarwal, A., et al. (1996). Oxy free radical system in heart failure and therapeutic role of oral vitamin E. *Int J Cardiol, 57*, 119–127.
31. Keith, M. E., Jeejeebhoy, K. N., Langer, A., et al. (2001). A controlled clinical trial of vitamin E supplementation in patients with congestive heart failure. *Am J Clin Nutr, 73*, 219–224.
32. Liu, T. Z., Stern, A., & Morrow, J. D. (1998). The isoprostanes: unique bioactive products of lipid peroxidation. An overview. *J Biomed Sci, 5*, 415–420.
33. Moore, K., & Roberts, L. J., II (1998). Measurement of lipid peroxidation. *Free Radic Res, 28*, 659–671.
34. Mallat, Z., Philip, I., Lebret, M., et al. (1998). Elevated levels of 8-iso-prostaglandin F2alpha in pericardial fluid of patients with heart failure: a potential role for in vivo oxidant stress in ventricular dilatation and progression to heart failure. *Circulation, 97*, 1536–1539.
35. Kameda, K., Matsunaga, T., Abe, N., et al. (2003). Correlation of oxidative stress with activity of matrix metalloproteinase in patients with coronary artery disease. Possible role for left ventricular remodelling. *Eur Heart J, 24*, 2180–2185.
36. Polidori, M. C., Pratico, D., Savino, K., et al. (2004). Increased F2 isoprostane plasma levels in patients with congestive heart failure are correlated with antioxidant status and disease severity. *J Card Fail, 10*, 334–338.
37. Koyama, Y., Takeishi, Y., Arimoto, T., et al. (2007). High serum level of pentosidine, an advanced glycation end product (AGE), is a risk factor of patients with heart failure. *J Card Fail, 13*, 199–206.
38. Amir, O., Paz, H., Rogowski, O., et al. (2009). Serum oxidative stress level correlates with clinical parameters in chronic systolic heart failure patients. *Clin Cardiol, 32*, 199–203.
39. Yamamoto, M., Yang, G., Hong, C., et al. (2003). Inhibition of endogenous thioredoxin in the heart increases oxidative stress and cardiac hypertrophy. *J Clin Invest, 112*, 1395–1406.
40. Shite, J., Qin, F., Mao, W., et al. (2001). Antioxidant vitamins attenuate oxidative stress and cardiac dysfunction in tachycardia-induced cardiomyopathy. *J Am Coll Cardiol, 38*, 1734–1740.
41. Kono, Y., Nakamura, K., Kimura, H., et al. (2006). Elevated levels of oxidative DNA damage in serum and myocardium of patients with heart failure. *Circ J, 70*, 1001–1005.
42. Watanabe, E., Matsuda, N., Shiga, T., et al. (2006). Significance of 8-hydroxy-2'-deoxyguanosine levels in patients with idiopathic dilated cardiomyopathy. *J Card Fail, 12*, 527–532.
43. Sakai, H., Tsutamoto, T., Tsutsui, T., et al. (2006). Serum level of uric acid, partly secreted from the failing heart, is a prognostic marker in patients with congestive heart failure. *Circ J, 70*, 1006–1011.
44. Kittleson, M. M., St John, M. E., Bead, V., et al. (2007). Increased levels of uric acid predict haemodynamic compromise in patients with heart failure independently of B-type natriuretic peptide levels. *Heart, 93*, 365–367.
45. Kojima, S., Sakamoto, T., Ishihara, M., et al. (2005). Prognostic usefulness of serum uric acid after acute myocardial infarction (the Japanese acute coronary syndrome study). *Am J Cardiol, 96*, 489–495.
46. Bergamini, C., Cicoira, M., Rossi, A., et al. (2009). Oxidative stress and hyperuricaemia: pathophysiology, clinical relevance, and therapeutic implications in chronic heart failure. *Eur J Heart Fail, 11*, 444–452.
47. Anker, S. D., Doehner, W., Rauchhaus, M., et al. (2003). Uric acid and survival in chronic heart failure: validation and application in metabolic, functional, and hemodynamic staging. *Circulation, 107*, 1991–1997.
48. Ioachimescu, A. G., Brennan, D. M., Hoar, B. M., et al. (2008). Serum uric acid is an independent predictor of all-cause mortality in patients at high risk of cardiovascular disease: a preventive cardiology information system (PreCIS) database cohort study. *Arthritis Rheum, 58*, 623–630.
49. Ekundayo, O. J., Dell'italia, L. J., Sanders, P. W., et al. (2009). Association between hyperuricemia and incident heart failure among older adults: a propensity-matched study. *Int J Cardiol*, (Epub ahead of print).
50. Hokamaki, J., Kawano, H., Yoshimura, M., et al. (2004). Urinary biopyrrins levels are elevated in relation to severity of heart failure. *J Am Coll Cardiol, 43*, 1880–1885.
51. Gupta, M., & Singal, P. K. (1989). Higher antioxidative capacity during a chronic stable heart hypertrophy. *Circ Res, 64*, 398–406.
52. Dhalla, A. K., & Singal, P. K. (1994). Antioxidant changes in hypertrophied and failing guinea pig hearts. *Am J Physiol, 266*, H1280–H1285.
53. Prasad, K., Gupta, J. B., Kalra, J., et al. (1996). Oxidative stress as a mechanism of cardiac failure in chronic volume overload in canine model. *J Mol Cell Cardiol, 28*, 375–385.
54. Baumer, A. T., Flesch, M., Wang, X., et al. (2000). Antioxidative enzymes in human hearts with idiopathic dilated cardiomyopathy. *J Mol Cell Cardiol, 32*, 121–130.
55. Dieterich, S., Bieligk, U., Beulich, K., et al. (2000). Gene expression of antioxidative enzymes in the human heart: increased expression of catalase in the end-stage failing heart. *Circulation, 101*, 33–39.
56. Sam, F., Kerstetter, D. L., Pimental, D. R., et al. (2005). Increased reactive oxygen species production and functional alterations in antioxidant enzymes in human failing myocardium. *J Card Fail, 11*, 473–480.
57. Lonn, E., Bosch, J., Yusuf, S., et al. (2005). Effects of long-term vitamin E supplementation on cardiovascular events and cancer: a randomized controlled trial. *JAMA, 293*, 1338–1347.
58. Sia, Y. T., Parker, T. G., Liu, P., et al. (2002). Improved post-myocardial infarction survival with probucol in rats: effects on left ventricular function, morphology, cardiac oxidative stress and cytokine expression. *J Am Coll Cardiol, 39*, 148–156.
59. Kinugawa, S., Tsutsui, H., Hayashidani, S., et al. (2000). Treatment with dimethylthiourea prevents left ventricular remodeling and failure after experimental myocardial infarction in mice: role of oxidative stress. *Circ Res, 87*, 392–398.
60. Berry, C. E., & Hare, J. M. (2004). Xanthine oxidoreductase and cardiovascular disease: molecular mechanisms and pathophysiological implications. *J Physiol, 555*, 589–606.
61. Cappola, T. P., Kass, D. A., Nelson, G. S., et al. (2001). Allopurinol improves myocardial efficiency in patients with idiopathic dilated cardiomyopathy. *Circulation, 104*, 2407–2411.
62. de Jong, J. W., Schoemaker, R. G., de Jonge, R., et al. (2000). Enhanced expression and activity of xanthine oxidoreductase in the failing heart. *J Mol Cell Cardiol, 32*, 2083–2089.
63. Engberding, N., Spiekermann, S., Schaefer, A., et al. (2004). Allopurinol attenuates left ventricular remodeling and dysfunction after experimental myocardial infarction: a new action for an old drug? *Circulation, 110*, 2175–2179.
64. Ekelund, U. E., Harrison, R. W., Shokek, O., et al. (1999). Intravenous allopurinol decreases myocardial oxygen consumption and increases mechanical efficiency in dogs with pacing-induced heart failure. *Circ Res, 85*, 437–445.
65. Amado, L. C., Saliaris, A. P., Raju, S. V., et al. (2005). Xanthine oxidase inhibition ameliorates cardiovascular dysfunction in dogs with pacing-induced heart failure. *J Mol Cell Cardiol, 39*, 531–536.
66. Minhas, K. M., Saraiva, R. M., Schuleri, K. H., et al. (2006). Xanthine oxidoreductase inhibition causes reverse remodeling in rats with dilated cardiomyopathy. *Circ Res, 98*, 271–279.
67. Doehner, W., Schoene, N., Rauchhaus, M., et al. (2002). Effects of xanthine oxidase inhibition with allopurinol on endothelial function and peripheral blood flow in hyperuricemic patients with chronic heart failure: results from 2 placebo-controlled studies. *Circulation, 105*, 2619–2624.

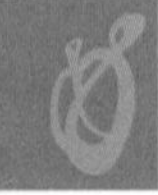

68. Farquharson, C. A., Butler, R., Hill, A., et al. (2002). Allopurinol improves endothelial dysfunction in chronic heart failure. *Circulation, 106*, 221–226.
69. Cingolani, H. E., Plastino, J. A., Escudero, E. M., et al. (2006). The effect of xanthine oxidase inhibition upon ejection fraction in heart failure patients: La Plata study. *J Card Fail, 12*, 491–498.
70. Hare, J. M., Mangal, B., Brown, J., et al. (2008). Impact of oxypurinol in patients with symptomatic heart failure. Results of the OPT-CHF study. *J Am Coll Cardiol, 51*, 2301–2309.
71. Kogler, H., Fraser, H., McCune, S., et al. (2003). Disproportionate enhancement of myocardial contractility by the xanthine oxidase inhibitor oxypurinol in failing rat myocardium. *Cardiovasc Res, 59*, 582–592.
72. Griendling, K. K., Minieri, C. A., Ollerenshaw, J. D., et al. (1994). Angiotensin II stimulates NADH and NADPH oxidase activity in cultured vascular smooth muscle cells. *Circ Res, 74*, 1141–1148.
73. Griendling, K. K., & Ushio-Fukai, M. (1998). Redox control of vascular smooth muscle proliferation. *J Lab Clin Med, 132*, 9–15.
74. Xiao, L., Pimentel, D. R., Wang, J., et al. (2002). Role of reactive oxygen species and NAD(P)H oxidase in alpha(1)-adrenoceptor signaling in adult rat cardiac myocytes. *Am J Physiol Cell Physiol, 282*, C926–C934.
75. Bendall, J. K., Cave, A. C., Heymes, C., et al. (2002). Pivotal role of a gp91(phox)-containing NADPH oxidase in angiotensin II-induced cardiac hypertrophy in mice. *Circulation, 105*, 293–296.
76. Singal, P. K., Dhillon, K. S., Beamish, R. E., et al. (1982). Myocardial cell damage and cardiovascular changes due to i.v. infusion of adrenochrome in rats. *Br J Exp Pathol, 63*, 167–176.
77. Singh, K., Communal, C., Sawyer, D. B., et al. (2000). Adrenergic regulation of myocardial apoptosis. *Cardiovasc Res, 45*, 713–719.
78. Goto, T., & Shikama, K. (1974). Autoxidation of native oxymyoglobin from bovine heart muscle. *Arch Biochem Biophys, 163*, 476–481.
79. Tsutsui, H., Kinugawa, S., & Matsushima, S. (2009). Mitochondrial oxidative stress and dysfunction in myocardial remodelling. *Cardiovasc Res, 81*, 449–456.
80. Ide, T., Tsutsui, H., Kinugawa, S., et al. (1999). Mitochondrial electron transport complex I is a potential source of oxygen free radicals in the failing myocardium. *Circ Res, 85*, 357–363.
81. Griendling, K. K., Sorescu, D., & Ushio-Fukai, M. (2000). NAD(P)H oxidase: role in cardiovascular biology and disease. *Circ Res, 86*, 494–501.
82. Irani, K., Xia, Y., Zweier, J. L., et al. (1997). Mitogenic signaling mediated by oxidants in Ras-transformed fibroblasts. *Science, 275*, 1649–1652.
83. Siwik, D. A., Tzortzis, J. D., Pimental, D. R., et al. (1999). Inhibition of copper-zinc superoxide dismutase induces cell growth, hypertrophic phenotype, and apoptosis in neonatal rat cardiac myocytes in vitro. *Circ Res, 85*, 147–153.
84. Pimentel, D. R., Amin, J. K., Xiao, L., et al. (2001). Reactive oxygen species mediate amplitude-dependent hypertrophic and apoptotic responses to mechanical stretch in cardiac myocytes. *Circ Res, 89*, 453–460.
85. Nakamura, K., Fushimi, K., Kouchi, H., et al. (1998). Inhibitory effects of antioxidants on neonatal rat cardiac myocyte hypertrophy induced by tumor necrosis factor-alpha and angiotensin II. *Circulation, 98*, 794–799.
86. Leri, A., Claudio, P. P., Li, Q., et al. (1998). Stretch-mediated release of angiotensin II induces myocyte apoptosis by activating p53 that enhances the local renin-angiotensin system and decreases the Bcl-2-to-Bax protein ratio in the cell. *J Clin Invest, 101*, 1326–1342.
87. Cheng, T. H., Shih, N. L., Chen, S. Y., et al. (1999). Reactive oxygen species modulate endothelin-I-induced c-fos gene expression in cardiomyocytes. *Cardiovasc Res, 41*, 654–662.
88. Kometiani, P., Li, J., Gnudi, L., et al. (1998). Multiple signal transduction pathways link Na^+/K^+-ATPase to growth-related genes in cardiac myocytes. The roles of Ras and mitogen-activated protein kinases. *J Biol Chem, 273*, 15249–15256.
89. Bedard, K., & Krause, K. H. (2007). The NOX family of ROS-generating NADPH oxidases: physiology and pathophysiology. *Physiol Rev, 87*, 245–313.
90. Wang, H. D., Xu, S., Johns, D. G., et al. (2001). Role of NADPH oxidase in the vascular hypertrophic and oxidative stress response to angiotensin II in mice. *Circ Res, 88*, 947–953.
91. Aikawa, R., Komuro, I., Yamazaki, T., et al. (1997). Oxidative stress activates extracellular signal-regulated kinases through Src and Ras in cultured cardiac myocytes of neonatal rats. *J Clin Invest, 100*, 1813–1821.
92. Sawyer, D. B., Fukazawa, R., Arstall, M. A., et al. (1999). Daunorubicin-induced apoptosis in rat cardiac myocytes is inhibited by dexrazoxane. *Circ Res, 84*, 257–265.
93. Speyer, J. L., Green, M. D., Kramer, E., et al. (1988). Protective effect of the bispiperazinedione ICRF-187 against doxorubicin-induced cardiac toxicity in women with advanced breast cancer. *N Engl J Med, 319*, 745–752.
94. Cheng, W., Li, B., Kajstura, J., et al. (1995). Stretch-induced programmed myocyte cell death. *J Clin Invest, 96*, 2247–2259.
95. Sugden, P. H., & Clerk, A. (1998). "Stress-responsive" mitogen-activated protein kinases (c-Jun N-terminal kinases and p38 mitogen-activated protein kinases) in the myocardium. *Circ Res, 83*, 345–352.
96. Clerk, A., Michael, A., & Sugden, P. H. (1998). Stimulation of multiple mitogen-activated protein kinase sub-families by oxidative stress and phosphorylation of the small heat shock protein, HSP25/27, in neonatal ventricular myocytes. *Biochem J, 333*, 581–589.
97. Clerk, A., Fuller, S. J., Michael, A., et al. (1998). Stimulation of "stress-regulated" mitogen-activated protein kinases (stress-activated protein kinases/c-Jun N-terminal kinases and p38-mitogen-activated protein kinases) in perfused rat hearts by oxidative and other stresses. *J Biol Chem, 273*, 7228–7234.
98. Wang, Y., Su, B., Sah, V. P., et al. (1998). Cardiac hypertrophy induced by mitogen-activated protein kinase kinase 7, a specific activator for c-Jun NH2-terminal kinase in ventricular muscle cells. *J Biol Chem, 273*, 5423–5426.
99. Xiao, L., Pimental, D. R., Amin, J. K., et al. (2001). MEK1/2-ERK1/2 mediates alpha1-adrenergic receptor-stimulated hypertrophy in adult rat ventricular myocytes. *Am J Physiol, 33*, 779–787.
100. Turner, N. A., Xia, F., Azhar, G., et al. (1998). Oxidative stress induces DNA fragmentation and caspase activation via the c-Jun NH2-terminal kinase pathway in H9c2 cardiac muscle cells. *J Mol Cell Cardiol, 30*, 1789–1801.
101. Yue, T. L., Ma, X. L., Gu, J. L., et al. (1998). Carvedilol inhibits activation of stress-activated protein kinase and reduces reperfusion injury in perfused rabbit heart. *Eur J Pharmacol, 345*, 61–65.
102. Reed, J. C. (1997). Cytochrome c: can't live with it—can't live without it. *Cell, 91*, 559–562.
103. Reed, J. C., Jurgensmeier, J. M., & Matsuyama, S. (1998). Bcl-2 family proteins and mitochondria. *Biochim Biophys Acta, 1366*, 127–137.
104. von Harsdorf, R., Li, P. F., & Dietz, R. (1999). Signaling pathways in reactive oxygen species-induced cardiomyocyte apoptosis. *Circulation, 99*, 2934–2941.
105. Lee, Y., & Gustafsson, A. B. (2009). Role of apoptosis in cardiovascular disease. *Apoptosis, 14*, 536–548.
106. Kaufman, R. J. (2002). Orchestrating the unfolded protein response in health and disease. *J Clin Invest, 110*, 1389–1398.
107. Glembotski, C. C. (2008). The role of the unfolded protein response in the heart. *J Mol Cell Cardiol, 44*, 453–459.
108. Okada, K., Minamino, T., Tsukamoto, Y., et al. (2004). Prolonged endoplasmic reticulum stress in hypertrophic and failing heart after aortic constriction: possible contribution of endoplasmic reticulum stress to cardiac myocyte apoptosis. *Circulation, 110*, 705–712.
109. Mao, W., Fukuoka, S., Iwai, C., et al. (2007). Cardiomyocyte apoptosis in autoimmune cardiomyopathy: mediated via endoplasmic reticulum stress and exaggerated by norepinephrine. *Am J Physiol Heart Circ Physiol, 293*, H1636–H1645.
110. Hamada, H., Suzuki, M., Yuasa, S., et al. (2004). Dilated cardiomyopathy caused by aberrant endoplasmic reticulum quality control in mutant KDEL receptor transgenic mice. *Mol Cell Biol, 24*, 8007–8017.
111. Liu, J., Mao, W., Iwai, C., et al. (2008). Adoptive passive transfer of rabbit beta1-adrenoceptor peptide immune cardiomyopathy into the Rag2-/- mouse: participation of the ER stress. *J Mol Cell Cardiol, 44*, 304–314.
112. Guo, R., Ma, H., Gao, F., et al. (2009). Metallothionein alleviates oxidative stress-induced endoplasmic reticulum stress and myocardial dysfunction. *J Mol Cell Cardiol, 47*, 228–237.
113. Malhotra, J. D., & Kaufman, R. J. (2007). Endoplasmic reticulum stress and oxidative stress: a vicious cycle or a double-edged sword? *Antioxid Redox Signal, 9*, 2277–2293.
114. Li, Q., & Ren, J. (2006). Cardiac overexpression of metallothionein rescues chronic alcohol intake-induced cardiomyocyte dysfunction: role of Akt, mammalian target of rapamycin and ribosomal p70s6 kinase. *Alcohol, 41*, 585–592.
115. Morishima, N., Nakanishi, K., Tsuchiya, K., et al. (2004). Translocation of Bim to the endoplasmic reticulum (ER) mediates ER stress signaling for activation of caspase-12 during ER stress-induced apoptosis. *J Biol Chem, 279*, 50375–50381.
116. Puthalakath, H., O'Reilly, L. A., Gunn, P., et al. (2007). ER stress triggers apoptosis by activating BH3-only protein Bim. *Cell, 129*, 1337–1349.
117. Nickson, P., Toth, A., & Erhardt, P. (2007). PUMA is critical for neonatal cardiomyocyte apoptosis induced by endoplasmic reticulum stress. *Cardiovasc Res, 73*, 48–56.
118. Arai, M., Alpert, N. R., MacLennan, D. H., et al. (1993). Alterations in sarcoplasmic reticulum gene expression in human heart failure. A possible mechanism for alterations in systolic and diastolic properties of the failing myocardium. *Circ Res, 72*, 463–469.
119. Cohen, R. A., & Adachi, T. (2006). Nitric-oxide-induced vasodilatation: regulation by physiologic s-glutathiolation and pathologic oxidation of the sarcoplasmic endoplasmic reticulum calcium ATPase. *Trends Cardiovasc Med, 16*, 109–114.
120. Goldhaber, J. I., & Qayyum, M. S. (2000). Oxygen free radicals and excitation-contraction coupling. *Antioxid Redox Signal, 2*, 55–64.
121. Litwin, S. E., & Bridge, J. H. (1997). Enhanced Na(+)-Ca^{2+} exchange in the infarcted heart. Implications for excitation-contraction coupling. *Circ Res, 81*, 1083–1093.
122. Campbell, D. L., Stamler, J. S., & Strauss, H. C. (1996). Redox modulation of L-type calcium channels in ferret ventricular myocytes. Dual mechanism regulation by nitric oxide and S-nitrosothiols. *J Gen Physiol, 108*, 277–293.
123. Xu, L., Eu, J. P., Meissner, G., et al. (1998). Activation of the cardiac calcium release channel (ryanodine receptor) by poly-S-nitrosylation. *Science, 279*, 234–237.
124. Spinale, F. G., Coker, M. L., Bond, B. R., et al. (2000). Myocardial matrix degradation and metalloproteinase activation in the failing heart: a potential therapeutic target. *Cardiovasc Res, 46*, 225–238.
125. Siwik, D. A., Pagano, P. J., & Colucci, W. S. (2001). Oxidative stress regulates collagen synthesis and matrix metalloproteinase activity in cardiac fibroblasts. *Am J Physiol Cell Physiol, 280*, C53–C60.
126. Stamler, J. S., Simon, D. I., Osborne, J. A., et al. (1992). S-nitrosylation of proteins with nitric oxide: synthesis and characterization of biologically active compounds. *Proc Natl Acad Sci U S A, 89*, 444–448.
127. Michel, J. B., Feron, O., Sacks, D., et al. (1997). Reciprocal regulation of endothelial nitric-oxide synthase by Ca^{2+}-calmodulin and caveolin. *J Biol Chem, 272*, 15583–15586.
128. Singh, K., Balligand, J. L., Fischer, T. A., et al. (1996). Regulation of cytokine-inducible nitric oxide synthase in cardiac myocytes and microvascular endothelial cells. Role of extracellular signal-regulated kinases 1 and 2 (ERK1/ERK2) and STAT1 alpha. *J Biol Chem, 271*, 1111–1117.
129. Haywood, G. A., Tsao, P. S., von der Leyen, H. E., et al. (1996). Expression of inducible nitric oxide synthase in human heart failure. *Circulation, 93*, 1087–1094.
130. Palacios-Callender, M., Quintero, M., Hollis, V. S., et al. (2004). Endogenous NO regulates superoxide production at low oxygen concentrations by modifying the redox state of cytochrome c oxidase. *Proc Natl Acad Sci U S A, 101*, 7630–7635.
131. Mannick, J. B., Miao, X. Q., & Stamler, J. S. (1997). Nitric oxide inhibits Fas-induced apoptosis. *J Biol Chem, 272*, 24125–24128.
132. Feng, Q., Song, W., Lu, X., et al. (2002). Development of heart failure and congenital septal defects in mice lacking endothelial nitric oxide synthase. *Circulation, 106*, 873–879.

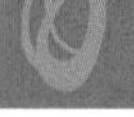

133. Pacher, P., Beckman, J. S., & Liaudet, L. (2007). Nitric oxide and peroxynitrite in health and disease. *Physiol Rev*, *87*, 315–424.
134. Ischiropoulos, H., Zhu, L., Chen, J., et al. (1992). Peroxynitrite-mediated tyrosine nitration catalyzed by superoxide dismutase. *Arch Biochem Biophys*, *298*, 431–437.
135. Xia, Y., Roman, L. J., Masters, B. S., et al. (1998). Inducible nitric-oxide synthase generates superoxide from the reductase domain. *J Biol Chem*, *273*, 22635–22639.
136. Zimmet, J. M., & Hare, J. M. (2006). Nitroso-redox interactions in the cardiovascular system. *Circulation*, *114*, 1531–1544.
137. Pinsky, D. J., Cai, B., Yang, X., et al. (1995). The lethal effects of cytokine-induced nitric oxide on cardiac myocytes are blocked by nitric oxide synthase antagonism or transforming growth factor beta. *J Clin Invest*, *95*, 677–685.
138. Arstall, M. A., Sawyer, D. B., Fukazawa, R., et al. (1999). Cytokine-mediated apoptosis in cardiac myocytes: the role of inducible nitric oxide synthase induction and peroxynitrite generation. *Circ Res*, *85*, 829–840.
139. Sam, F., Sawyer, D. B., Xie, Z., et al. (2001). Mice lacking inducible nitric oxide synthase have improved left ventricular contractile function and reduced apoptotic cell death late after myocardial infarction. *Circ Res*, *89*, 351–356.
140. Ishiyama, S., Hiroe, M., Nishikawa, T., et al. (1997). Nitric oxide contributes to the progression of myocardial damage in experimental autoimmune myocarditis in rats. *Circulation*, *95*, 489–496.
141. MacMillan-Crow, L. A., Crow, J. P., Kerby, J. D., et al. (1996). Nitration and inactivation of manganese superoxide dismutase in chronic rejection of human renal allografts. *Proc Natl Acad Sci U S A*, *93*, 11853–11858.
142. Mikami, S., Kawashima, S., Kanazawa, K., et al. (1997). Low-dose N omega-nitro-L-arginine methyl ester treatment improves survival rate and decreases myocardial injury in a murine model of viral myocarditis induced by coxsackievirus B3. *Circ Res*, *81*, 504–511.
143. McMurray, J., McLay, J., Chopra, M., et al. (1990). Evidence for enhanced free radical activity in chronic congestive heart failure secondary to coronary artery disease. *Am J Cardiol*, *65*, 1261–1262.
144. Belch, J. J., Bridges, A. B., Scott, N., et al. (1991). Oxygen free radicals and congestive heart failure. *Br Heart J*, *65*, 245–248.
145. Keith, M., Geranmayegan, A., Sole, M. J., et al. (1998). Increased oxidative stress in patients with congestive heart failure. *J Am Coll Cardiol*, *31*, 1352–1356.
146. Polidori, M. C., Savino, K., Alunni, G., et al. (2002). Plasma lipophilic antioxidants and malondialdehyde in congestive heart failure patients: relationship to disease severity. *Free Radic Biol Med*, *32*, 148–152.
147. Campolo, J., De Maria, R., Caruso, R., et al. (2007). Blood glutathione as independent marker of lipid peroxidation in heart failure. *Int J Cardiol*, *117*, 45–50.
148. Nonaka-Sarukawa, M., Yamamoto, K., Aoki, H., et al. (2003). Increased urinary 15-F2t-isoprostane concentrations in patients with non-ischaemic congestive heart failure: a marker of oxidative stress. *Heart*, *89*, 871–874.
149. Pignatelli, P., Cangemi, R., Celestini, A., et al. (2008). Tumour necrosis factor alpha upregulates platelet CD40L in patients with heart failure. *Cardiovasc Res*, *78*, 515–522.
150. Cicoira, M., Zanolla, L., Rossi, A., et al. (2002). Elevated serum uric acid levels are associated with diastolic dysfunction in patients with dilated cardiomyopathy. *Am Heart J*, *143*, 1107–1111.
151. Sia, Y. T., Lapointe, N., Parker, T. G., et al. (2002). Beneficial effects of long-term use of the antioxidant probucol in heart failure in the rat. *Circulation*, *105*, 2549–2555.

CHAPTER 13

Alterations in Ventricular Function: Systolic Heart Failure

David A. Kass

Systolic cardiac depression is a hallmark of many patients with heart failure. It reflects a fundamental weakness of the pump and thus its inability to deliver sufficient cardiac output at an adequate mean arterial pressure. The failing heart often exhibits both major decrements in resting systolic function and also limitations of systolic reserve required for individuals to perform normal activities of daily living and exercise. The underlying mechanisms for systolic dysfunction are numerous, ranging from posttranslational changes in myofilament proteins depressing force development and calcium interaction, depressed calcium cycling (see Chapter 3) into and out of the sarcoplasmic reticulum, altered ion channel function, mitochondrial and metabolism abnormalities, molecular and structural remodeling including cell death (see Chapter 6) and loss, and altered membrane receptor signaling[1-3] (Figure 13-1). In addition, interactions between the myocytes and the vasculature are providing sufficient nutrients and matching angiogenesis to organomegaly is considered important for maintaining function.[4,5] Lastly, there is tight communication between the myocyte and the matrix environment, involving key signaling in both directions that alters the collagen weave and activates molecular cascades in the muscle cells.[6]

Direct demonstration of abnormal myocyte function in failing hearts has been achieved using isolated myocytes where sarcomere shortening is generally measured in unloaded cells, and muscle preparations where developed force and length are both measured. Intact and chemically membrane-disrupted (skinned) preparations are used, the latter to assess changes in myofilament calcium dependence. Results of these studies obtained in a variety of experimental models of heart failure and human disease are discussed elsewhere in Chapter 3. In intact hearts, the quantitation and analysis of systolic dysfunction is more complex, given the dependence of most measures on the complex structure of the chamber, and on ambient loading conditions that are imposed on the heart and often abnormal themselves in the heart failure state. For example, the most common measure—ejection fraction—is determined not only by the properties of the muscle wall, but also by chamber remodeling, and by the stresses imposed by the arterial system and volume loading from the venous circuit.

The ambiguities associated with many common assessments of chamber systolic function are not solely of academic interest because they may themselves have contributed to a disappointing history of efforts to improve systolic function in the failing heart. Ejection fraction is neither very specific nor particularly sensitive to changes in underlying contractile function.[7] Thus dosing pharmaceuticals to achieve a given change in EF may risk biasing trials toward testing higher doses of medications that ultimately prove disappointing. Furthermore, classification of heart failure based on a parameter such as EF may introduce ambiguities. The interpretation of an EF less than 30% in an NYHA class I patient following a myocardial infarction is quite different from that of an individual with class III symptoms associated with dilated cardiomyopathy. Both EF declines largely reflect chamber remodeling dilation that increases the end-diastolic volume despite a relatively preserved stroke volume. However, in one instance, infarct remodeling dominates this decline and the residual myocardium could be quite normal and capable of providing adequate cardiac reserve. In the other example, the myopathy is diffuse, and there is little reserve capacity. These two situations may look similar when assessed by conventional parameters such as blood pressure, cardiac output, or EF, yet be very different when viewed by alternative approaches such as pressure-volume relations.[8]

The purpose of this chapter is to review the current understanding of the mechanisms underlying systolic depression in cardiac failure, the relationship between properties determined by the muscle and dysfunction assessed in the intact chamber, methods to assess systolic function and the impact of various loading influences on these measures, the interaction of systolic function with the arterial loading system or ventricular/arterial interaction, new approaches to therapeutic targeting of systolic dysfunction, and the contribution of contractile synchrony and effects of artificial resynchronization on systolic function.

CELLULAR AND MOLECULAR DETERMINANTS: A VIEW FROM 30,000 FEET

The greatest advances in understanding of heart failure over the past decade have come from new understandings of the molecular signaling involved and its impact on cellular and organ level pathobiology. Full justice to this topic is a book in its own right, but the reader is referred to Chapter 2 for a more comprehensive review in the current volume. Here, I want to provide a brief overview of key components that are involved with systolic failure. Systolic force generation starts at the level of the actin-myosin cross-bridge, which in turn is coupled via structural proteins to the surface membrane to transduce deformation to net chamber contraction. The contractile proteins themselves can play a central role in systolic depression both because of genetic mutations that depress the function of the molecular motors,[9-11] and by posttranslational changes particularly of regulatory thin filament proteins that modify contraction.[12,13] Mouse models recapitulating myosin mutations associated with dilated cardiomyopathy have shown weakened power generation and general loss of function in the actin-myosin cross-bridge.[14] Mutations in myosin-binding protein C (MyBP-C) are the most common cause of hypertrophic cardiomyopathy, though

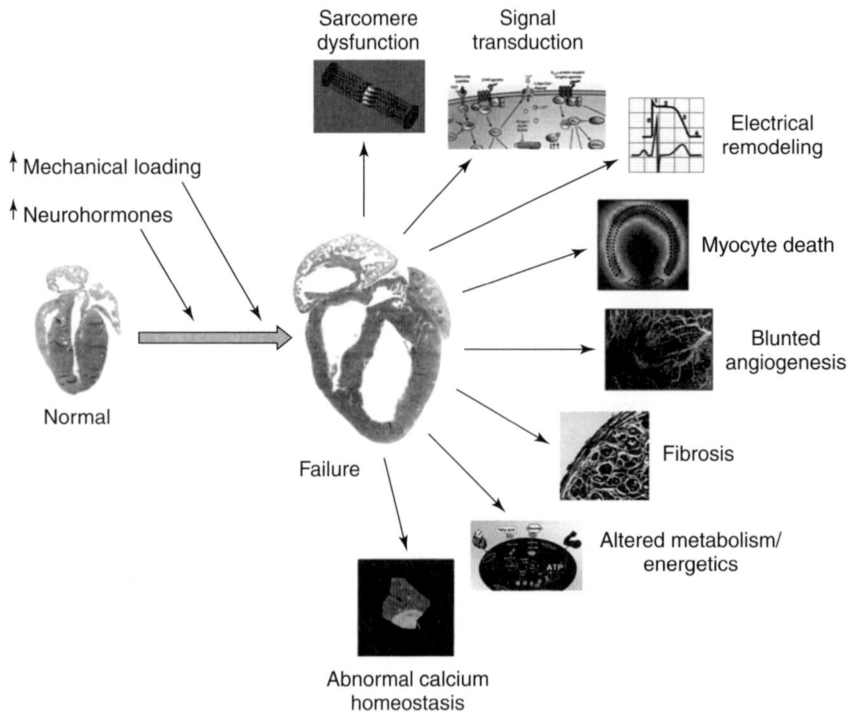

↑ Mechanical loading
↑ Neurohormones
Normal
Failure
Sarcomere dysfunction
Signal transduction
Electrical remodeling
Myocyte death
Blunted angiogenesis
Fibrosis
Altered metabolism/ energetics
Abnormal calcium homeostasis

FIGURE 13–1 Contributors to systolic dysfunction include a wide range of abnormalities and are not solely reflective of myocyte contractile protein and calcium handling changes. Other major factors include a substantial array of altered molecular signaling influencing myocyte mechanics and EC coupling, electro-physiological changes that alter conduction and regional contraction, cell survival signaling, extracellular matrix and vascular abnormalities, mitochondrial function, and bioenergetics. Importantly, these are increasingly being targeted as therapeutic options with the goal not only to suppress maladaptive heart failure remodeling, but to improve systolic performance in a way that is beneficial in the long term.

loss of function of this protein results in a dilated myopathy associated with a reduced capacity of the muscle to sustain systolic contraction.[15,16] Equally important are changes in regulatory proteins that can involve phosphorylation, redox modulation, or enzymatic cleavage (see Chapter 3). Growing evidence supports changes in troponin I and troponin T phosphorylation in mediating systolic dysfunction in the failing heart because of a loss of normal muscle response to calcium. TnI can also undergo proteolytic truncation associated with the protease calpain. This was first reported in postischemic stunned myocardium, and by itself induces a heart with depressed systolic function and chamber dilation.[17] The MyBP-C phosphorylation state also impacts systolic function, and reduction in this phosphorylation in animal models and human heart failure may also contribute to depressed sarcomere function.[16,18] Indeed, while long ignored, the role of the sarcomere as a signal-transduction target of various kinases and phosphatases, and for other posttranslational changes because of oxidation, nitration, nitrosylation, and glycosylation, is a rapidly evolving area of research.

Critical changes also occur in proteins linking the myofibrils to the cell membrane to transduce shortening. Abnormalities in muscle limb protein (MLP), sarcoglycan, desmin, dystrophin, vinculin, metavinculin, laminin, and lamin have been coupled to a dilated depressed ventricle in humans.[19-24] Murine models involving these proteins have been associated with morphogenic abnormalities, congenital defects, and dilated cardiomyopathy.

Systolic dysfunction is also critically dependent upon abnormalities of calcium homeostasis (see Chapter 3).[25-27] Changes have been described from the level of the voltage-gated calcium channels and sodium-calcium exchanger to altered expression and function of major sarcoplasmic reticular proteins involved with calcium cycling, such as phospholamban and the SR calcium ATPase. Changes in these and related proteins are presently being explored as potential new therapeutic avenues. A related signaling pathway is the phosphatase inhibitor I-1, which inactivates PP1.[28] I-1 levels decline in heart failure, enhancing PP1 dephosphorylation of phospholamban, contributing to systolic depression. Protein kinase A activates I-1, and downregulation of this pathway in the failing heart may contribute further to this change. Opposite effects occur from protein kinase Cα (e.g., inhibition of I-1, leading to greater dephosphorylation (inactivation) of phospholamban), and upregulation of PKGα in heart failure is another proposed mechanism of systolic dysfunction.[29] Changes in calcium release from the SR have been associated with sustained upregulation of calcium-calmodulin–dependent kinase IIδ and PKA-dependent phosphorylation of the ryanodine receptor to enhance SR calcium leak.[30-32] While prior focus was on the expression levels of key calcium handling proteins, more and more evidence also supports key changes at the posttranslational level involving more than just phosphorylation.[33-35] This has tightly linked excitation-contraction coupling with signal transduction mediated by stress response kinases, phosphatases, and transcription factors. These and other changes in calcium handling are reviewed more extensively elsewhere in this volume.

The molecular signaling changes observed in the failing heart are vast, and as more and more are manipulated by selective genetic gain- and loss-of-function studies, their role in contractile failure is being revealed. As a result, new approaches to treat depressed pump function are now focusing beneath the cell surface to more directly target enzyme and/or gene transcription programs. This work has been recently reviewed elsewhere and will not be further discussed in this chapter.[1,2,36] Two other major contributors to systolic dysfunction that are gaining more and more attention are energetics and metabolism. Abnormalities in mitochondrial function and ATP generation and changes in glucose and fatty acid metabolism in the failing heart have been mechanistically linked to chamber dilation and dysfunction.[37] A prime example is the impact of reduced levels of the transcription factor PGC1α, which serves as a master energy regulator.[38,39]

Systolic dysfunction also evolves from changes outside the myocyte, in particular from coupling of the cell to the extracellular matrix and to the vascular supply that surrounds each muscle cell. Signaling via proteins such as p53[4] and various growth factor signaling cascades[5] are thought to be important in maintaining adequate vasculogenesis to match the increased work and hypertrophy demands in the failing heart, and inadequacy of this matching results in depressed performance.

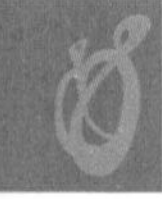

Recent studies have found changes in heart function can occur by gene-targeted manipulation of fibroblasts and vice versa—indicating strong signaling communication between systems.[40] Chamber dilation accompanying the activation of metalloproteinases (see Chapter 5), with its consequent remodeling of the extracellular matrix, is a highly active process and potently contributes to systolic dysfunction.[41-43] Myocyte geometry is also altered (longer-thinner) and likely plays a role as well.[44] Reversal of chronic dilation and myocyte geometric remodeling with a variety of therapies is often coupled with improved systolic function, though precise cause and effect cannot be determined from these studies.[45-47]

MEASURING SYSTOLIC FUNCTION BY PRESSURE-VOLUME RELATIONS

There are many ways that systolic dysfunction can be assessed, the most common being declines in fractional shortening or ejection fraction. Other parameters include the ability of the heart to generate maximal power (pressure × flow), the peak rate of rise of pressure, the capacity of the heart to generate external work for a given end-diastolic volume, etc.[7] Development of such analytic measures was a major focus of physiology in the late 1970s and early 1980s, and the tools that ultimately evolved have largely remained the same since. Among the more powerful tools was the depiction of cardiac contractility by means of simultaneous pressure-volume loops and relations.[48] This framework is now widely used in genetically engineered mouse studies[49] and other experimental models, and has been used to define the pathophysiology of human heart failure and therapy advances for several decades.[50,51]

A central concept that initially drove the analysis of cardiac systolic function by pressure-volume relations was the notion that cardiac systolic muscle activation involved a change in its material properties that are reflected by its stiffness. As the contractile proteins interact, the muscle changes from a relaxed state in diastole to one that is quite stiff due to development of actively bound cross-bridges and compression of the intrasarcomeric molecular spring titin. If one fixed cardiac trabecula is at a constant length, this stiffening was directly proportional to changes in force during contraction. Stiffness can also be measured in an intact heart, but now the property was reflected in chamber elastance (inverse of compliance). This concept and its measurement are shown in Figure 13-2, *A*. Cardiac contraction is depicted by simultaneous plots of left ventricular chamber volume (*x*-axis) and pressure (*y*-axis), with each cycle generating a pressure-volume loop (loops advance counterclockwise with contraction). The set of lines fanning from the origin reflect isochrones (i.e., connecting points on each of the loops at the same instantaneous time in contraction). The slope of each line defines the elastance (stiffness) of the chamber at that time, and this gradually rises from diastole to peak systole.

The time course of stiffening or time-varying elastance from human subjects with normal and diseased hearts is shown in Figure 13-2, *B*. Data are shown normalized to the maximal stiffness generated and time to achieve this (adjusting for differences in underlying contractility and heart rate). The curves define the activation and deactivation process in the heart, and the striking similarity among disease conditions suggests this is a fundamental property of the ventricle.[52] Stiffening occurs rapidly at the start of systole during the period of isovolumetric contraction. When the aortic valve opens, the rate of ongoing stiffening during ejection declines but remains largely at a constant rate until the peak is achieved. As a result, about 60% of net cardiac muscle stiffening develops during the process of blood ejection. This time course is remarkably similar between species as well—as shown in Figure 13-2, *C*, with a comparison between human and the mouse data.[53] The data were again normalized to peak magnitude and time scale adjusting for the tenfold difference in heart rate and greater than a 4000-fold difference in heart weight between species. This time course appears to depend in part on the function of MyBP-C, a protein linking myosin to actin and titin, and thought to control rates of cross-bridge attachment/detachment. Genetic MyBP-C deletion models are accompanied by an abbreviation of this time course during ejection, so that most all of stiffening occurs during the isovolumic period.[16,54]

Pressure-volume analysis began being applied to human studies of heart disease in the mid-1980s, and has more recently become widely used for assessing cardiac systolic function in basic science investigations conducted in genetically engineered mice.[49,55,56] By this approach, one can derive more accurate and specific quantitations of heart performance than are possible from standard clinical data. Figure 13-3, *A*, displays human left ventricular (LV) pressure-volume data obtained at rest and during transient reduction of preload volume. The bold loop represents the resting condition, and the labeling depicts end-diastole (point A), isovolumic contraction (point A-B), opening of the aortic valve (point B), ejection (point B-C), isovolumic relaxation (point C-D), opening of the mitral valve and initiation of diastolic filling (point D), and diastolic filling (point D-A). The loop width is stroke volume, the ratio of width to end-diastolic volume is EF, the loop area is external (or stroke) work. When ventricular preload is acutely reduced in the heart, there is a decline in stroke volume and peak pressures per beat (Frank-Starling dependence). Indeed, this set of data could be easily used to generate Frank-Starling curves plotting end-diastolic pressure versus stroke volume or cardiac output. However, one can also determine the ventricular end-systolic elastance by determining the slope of the upper left boundary defined by these loops. This occurs near end-ejection, and the locus of points comprises the end-systolic PV relation (ESPVR). The position and slope of this relation are used to define systolic function. An important feature of the ESPVR was its relative insensitivity to changes in cardiac vascular loading—either preload (sarcomere length or chamber volume) or afterload (force applied to the muscle or cell, or arterial impedance load). In work first conduced in the 1970s and 1980s, isolated and intact hearts demonstrated the utility of the ESPVR for this purpose.[48,57]

Figure 13-3, *A*, also shows another line—slanted upward from right to left as a diagonal across each pressure-volume loop. This depicts what is termed the "effective arterial elastance (Ea)".[58-60] Ea is a lumped parameter that indicates the net arterial load on the ventricle. Ea equals the ratio of end-systolic pressure/stroke volume. It is not synonymous with vascular stiffness; indeed its numeric value is mostly influenced by mean arterial resistance ($Ea = ESP/SV - R \times HR$). However, it serves as a useful metric of net ventricular loading—both mean and pulsatile—and importantly, unlike arterial pressure, the fact that these diagonal lines shown in Figure 13-3, *A*, are all parallel indicates that the value of this ratio is not varying despite the change in cardiac preload. Studies have used this parameter in conjunction with PV relations and Ees to determine mechanisms of drug effects (e.g., inodilator drugs such as OPC-18790,[61] population studies of heart disease and aging.[62,63]

Recent studies have demonstrated very similar behavior in intact single myocytes, in which individual cell sarcomere length and force are measured and controlled to generate pseudo force-length loops.[64] As shown in Figure 13-3, *B*, a picture very similar to that first generated in intact canine and human hearts is revealed, again with a linear peak elastance defined by the upper left corners of these data. As shown in this study, myocyte end-systolic stiffening is also rather

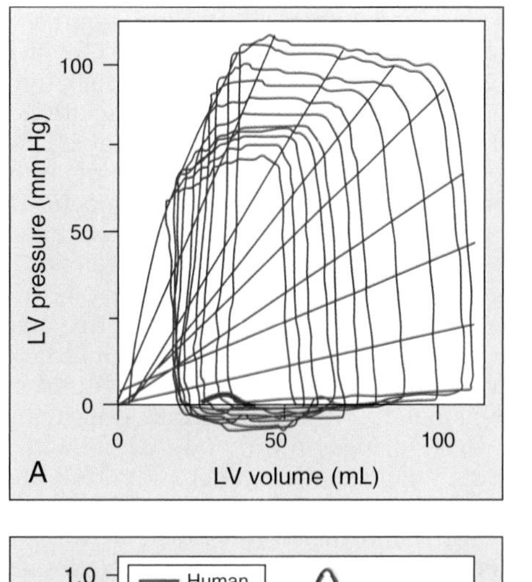

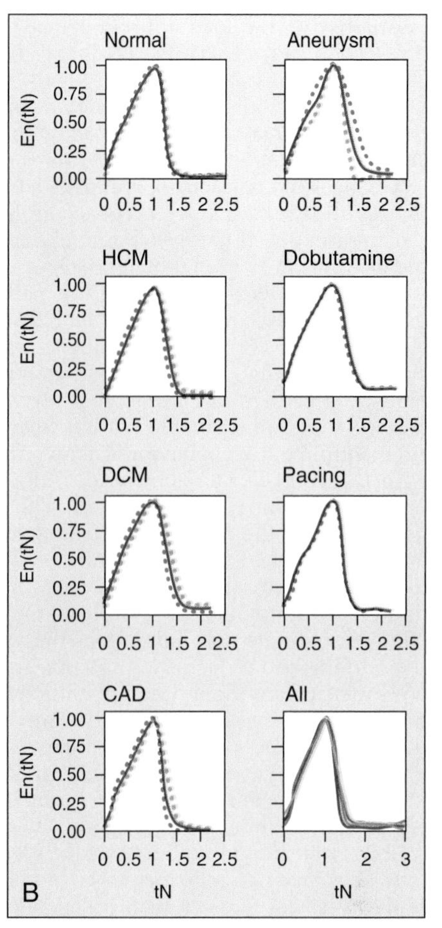

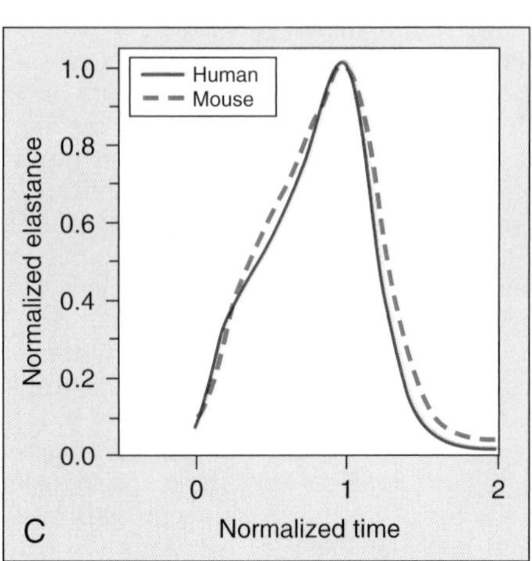

FIGURE 13-2 Time-varying elastance in the human heart. **A,** Generation of time-varying elastance from multiple cardiac cycles. Linear spokes represent isochrones (connecting points on each loop at the same time), and their slope reflects the instantaneous chamber stiffness or elastance achieved at that point in the cycle (Elastance = Pressure/(Volume−Vo)). The time-varying elastance is the change in this slope throughout the heartbeat (E(t)). **B,** E(t) curves shown normalized to both peak amplitude and time to peak amplitude from human subjects with varying cardiac diseases or with normal hearts. There is remarkable consistency in their shape as shown by the superimposed data *(lower right)*. **C,** The E(t) waveform is also similar across mammalian species. Shown here is superimposed mean data for normal human and mouse hearts. (**B,** From Senzaki H, Chen CH, Kass DA. Single beat estimation of end-systolic pressure-volume relation in humans: a new method with the potential for non-invasive application. *Circulation* 1996;94:2497-2506.)[52]

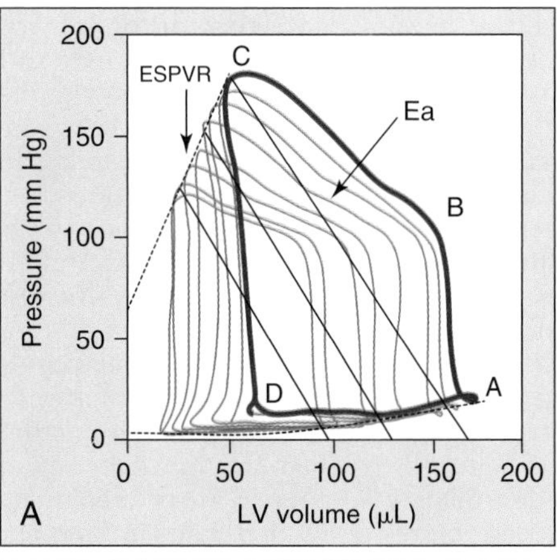

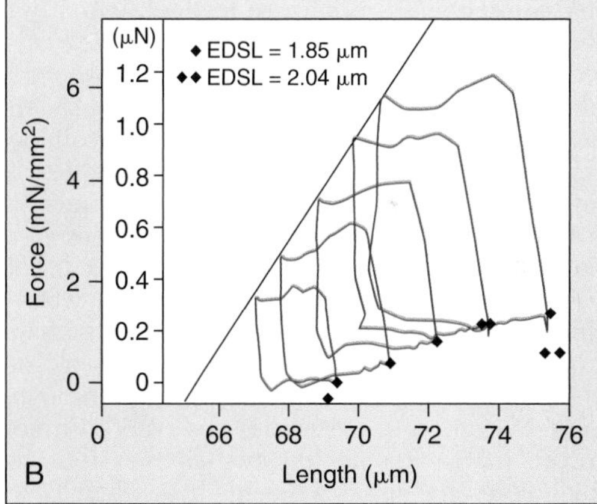

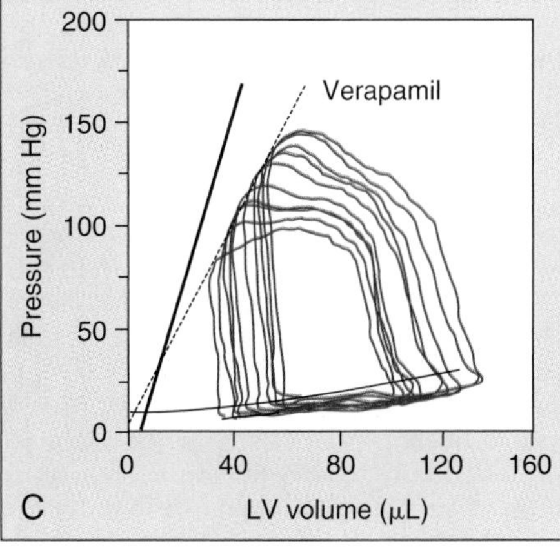

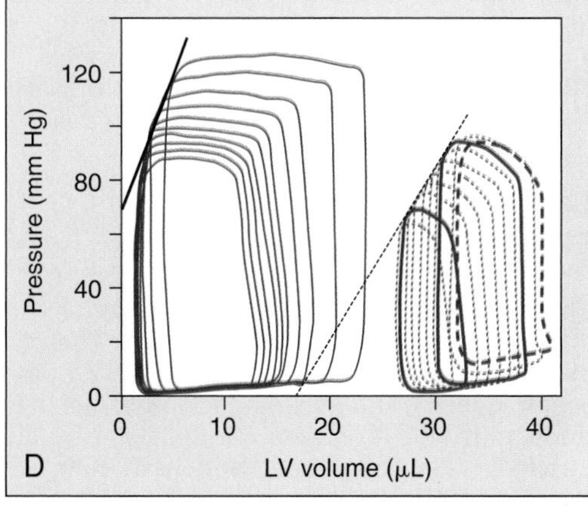

FIGURE 13-3 Pressure-volume (PV) analysis of cardiac function. **A,** Resting *(dark solid loop)* PV loop and multiple cycles derived by varying preload in human subjects. Cycle loop moves counterclockwise; (a) end diastole, (b) ejection onset, (c) end systole, (d) onset of diastolic filling. The upper left corners of the set of loops define the end-systolic PV relation, a valuable measure of chamber systolic function. The group of diagonal lines drawn within several of the beats denotes the arterial load, indexed by Ea = end-systolic pressure/stroke volume. This is similar to the decline in preload (arterial impedance is not significantly preload dependent), and thus useful as a measure of ventricular afterload. **B,** Similar types of data but obtained from a single cardiac myocyte, with force and sarcomere length measured and controlled to generate "loops." As in the intact heart, there is a time-varying stiffening of the myocyte, and a linear end-systolic force-length dependence. Thus this behavior is intrinsic to the cardiac myocyte. **C,** Prototypical response of ESPVR to a change in contractile state. Data shown are due to acute IV verapamil injection in human subjects.[65] **D,** Example of ventricular remodeling and cardiac systolic depression with sustained cardiac failure. Data are generated using a mouse model of disease (MKK3 overexpression, activating p38 MAP kinase). (B, With permission from Iribe G, Helmes M, Kohl P. Force-length relations in isolated intact cardiomyocytes subjected to dynamic changes in mechanical load. *Am J Physiol Heart Circ Physiol* 2007;292:H1487–H1497.)[64]

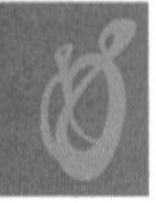

insensitive to the load applied before or during the contraction—so this is not simply a chamber-level phenomenon. This figure also shows a sort of Ea index (end-systolic force/end-diastolic sarcomere length), which as in the human example, reflects the effective load imposed by the servo system, and is also independent of preload (i.e., lines are parallel).

Changes in contractility are easily assessed by PV relations. This is shown by the prototype example in Figure 13-3, *C*, in a patient exposed to the calcium channel blocker verapamil. Indeed, the study from which this figure was taken was among the first to show the impact of this calcium channel blocker on human heart contractility, and the decline in maximal elastance (ESPVR slope shifts downward) was clear.[65] In this acute setting, the rise in end-systolic volume is not accompanied by a change in cardiac geometry. However, changes in systolic function typical of chronic heart failure involve both. An example of this behavior is shown from a study in mice,[66] with the control data shown in solid and heart failure data with dotted lines Figure 13-3, *D*. The latter display both a depression of the maximal stiffening generated by the heart, but also a marked rightward shift of the entire set of data that indicates structural remodeling/dilation. Patients with diffuse dilated cardiomyopathy typically display both components. In contrast, patients with infarctions that may result in chamber remodeling and a decline in ejection fraction but have otherwise relatively normal function of the residual wall will often display similar peak elastance but only the rightward shift of the relationship. Geometric formulas can be used to convert pressure-volume into myofibrillar stress and strain[67] to provide a less geometry-dependent parameter (i.e., assess muscle rather than chamber stiffness.

It is important to note that while acute changes in end-systolic elastance can reflect changes in contractile function, this property is not entirely load independent and may not itself be the primary reflector of systolic change. The entire relation linking end-systolic pressure-volume points (ESPVR) is rarely linear in the intact heart, but more often concave downward to the volume axis, giving rise to the frequently observed negative volume-axis intercept of the ESPVR.[68] This means higher slopes (end-systolic elastance, Ees) at reduced pressure loads, but lower ones at higher loads. Inotropic stimulation often enhances pressures and lowers systolic volumes, and this can result in apparent minimal change in Ees despite considerable leftward shifting of the relation itself. Secondly, systolic stiffening does not solely reflect contractile properties of the ventricle, but is also influenced by structural (matrix, fibroblasts, etc.) and vascular components in the myocardial wall. Chronic elevation of Ees does not automatically reflect enhanced contractile function of myocytes, but can be due to stiffening from other components of the heart. One likely example of such changes is the elevation of Ees that is observed with normal aging.[63,69] In this instance, other parameters of systolic function display negligible change, and the age-dependent Ees increase correlates with that in diastolic passive stiffness. Cardiac remodeling associated with chamber hypertrophy is also coupled with a rise in ventricular end-systolic elastance.[70] Whether this reflects intrinsic myocyte properties as opposed to more integrated myocardial/chamber properties remains unclear.

BEAT-TO-BEAT REGULATION OF SYSTOLIC FUNCTION

Three mechanisms are thought to regulate beat-to-beat systolic performance of cardiac muscle. These can be defined by the dependencies of systolic force on sarcomere length, beat frequency, and tension during systole. In the intact heart, these translate to chamber end-diastolic volume, afterload impedance or wall stress, and heart rate. All impact integrated systolic function.

The dependence of force generation upon muscle length is thought to be principally related to changes in myofilament calcium sensitivity as a function of sarcomere length.[71,72] While thick-thin filament overlap differences may contribute in skeletal muscle, this model is not easily reconciled with the operational sarcomere lengths (1.8 to 2.2 μm) of the cardiomyocyte. Despite nearly 30 years of investigations, a precise mechanism to explain length-dependent changes in calcium sensitivity remains elusive. Studies have hypothesized that greater length resulted in a reciprocal reduction of lattice spacing between the thick and thin filaments, which would be coupled to a greater probability of forming a tightly bound cross-bridge to increase force.[73-75] However, studies employing x-ray diffraction analysis of lattice spacing and models with mutations of thin-filament regulation have not supported this hypothesis.[76] Other studies have coupled length-dependent force generation to muscle LIM protein located in the z-disk[77] and to the molecular spring titin,[78] though precise mechanisms remain unknown. This further impacts our understanding of how and/or whether this fundamental mechanism is altered in heart failure.

Another rapid modulator of muscle function that impacts myofilament cycling rates and the cooperative generation of cross-bridges is shortening velocity. Maximal unloaded shortening velocity (V_{max}) depends on internal cellular viscous loading likely related to macromolecules such as titin[53] and microfilaments. Cooper et al reported that myocyte microtubular content profoundly alters unloaded cell shortening (the typical measure of systolic function in the cell, and myocyte correlate of V_{max}), which may contribute to diminished shortening in hypertrophied failing myocytes.[79-81] Cell shape may impact on cytoskeletal linkage proteins[82] (e.g., as α-actinin) to alter cross-bridge behavior as a function of shortening velocity. Another controller of actin-myosin interaction rate is MyBP-C, and in particular the phosphorylation state of this protein. In its nonphosphorylated state, early rates of cardiac contraction are slowed (revealed by lower early rates of pressure rise, dP/dt_{max}), whereas increasing phosphorylation of the protein appears to be a major factor in why dP/dt_{max} is augmented by sympathetic stimulation.

The relation between force and velocity can be transformed at the whole chamber into velocity of fiber shortening (V_{cf})—wall stress relations.[83,84] This is analogous to the midportion of a muscle force-velocity curve and has been employed to assess cardiac contractile performance in many studies. The relation is preload and heart rate dependent[85] (systolic stress is preload dependent in the intact heart). The integral under a force-velocity relation is power (force × velocity), and for the intact chamber, power is the product of pressure and flow. While preload dependent, maximal power can be adjusted to take this into account, and the resulting index provides a useful and fairly specific measure of systolic function.[86,87]

In isolated muscle, sudden perturbations of systolic load during a twitch also influence the subsequently developed tension and rate of relaxation.[88,89] Load reduction and ensuing more rapid myofiber shortening leads to cross-bridge detachment and magnifies internal viscous effects to lower force.[90-92] In the intact ventricle, such load changes often occur in late systole because of enhanced systolic wave reflections. Wave reflections result from a rapid return of the pulse to the central vasculature due to artery stiffening,[93] and this can be particularly important in the elderly and in failing hearts.[94-96] Sudden changes in systolic load are also observed regionally in hearts rendered discoordinate because of ischemia/infarction or abnormal electrical conduction. This mechanical stretch applied in midsystole can negatively impact myocyte systolic performance.

Lastly, systolic function of cardiac muscle is very sensitive to acute changes in beat frequency. This results from enhanced Ca^{2+} entry into the myocyte and enhanced uptake into the sarcoplasmic reticulum, which becomes available

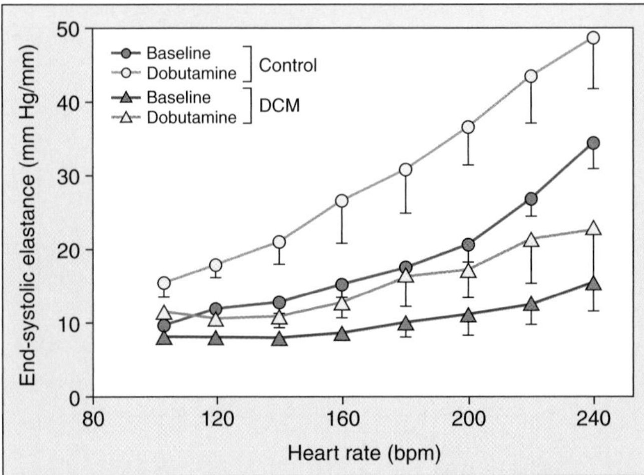

FIGURE 13-4 Force-frequency dependence in intact heart from conscious dog with and without cardiac failure (DCM). The relation is depressed in cardiac failure. Furthermore, there is an augmentation in the dependence with β-adrenergic stimulation provided by dobutamine in normal hearts, consistent with an interaction between enhanced calcium cycling dependent on PKA signaling, and because of the beat frequency. This too is blunted by cardiac failure. Data are the percent increase relative to the resting heart rate. (From Senzaki H, Isoda T, Paolocci N, et al. Improved mechanoenergetics and cardiac rest and reserve function of in vivo failing heart by calcium sensitizer EMD-57033. *Circulation* 2000;101:1040-1048.)[102]

for release to increase contraction strength.[97] There is a large body of evidence supporting an important role of this mechanism in regulating systolic function in intact mammals and man.[51,98,99] Demonstration of the effect in in vivo hearts requires an analysis of systolic function that is itself insensitive to the loading changes occurring with altered heart rate. Using end-systolic elastance or other load-insensitive parameters, intact canine, human, and murine hearts have been shown to display a force-frequency dependence. In humans, contractile function rises nearly twofold for a heart rate increase from 70 to 150 min^{-1}.[51] This is markedly blunted in cardiac failure, a primary manifestation of abnormal SR calcium handling (see Chapter 3).[27,100,101] Figure 13-4 shows this phenomenon in an intact canine model of dilated heart failure.[102] Two sets of relations are depicted: at rest and after stimulation with the β-adrenergic agonist dobutamine. Contractility was indexed by end-systolic elastance based on pressure-volume analysis. The normal positive dependence of contractility on beat frequency and its marked depression in heart failure are shown by the solid circles and triangles, respectively. When stimulated by dobutamine, the contractility-frequency dependence is further augmented in the normal hearts, but very little altered in the failing ones. In controls, the enhanced phosphorylation of the L-type Ca^{2+} channel and phospholamban (among other proteins) results in greater calcium loading, and this in turn is further augmented by frequency to provide even more trigger Ca^{2+} to the myofilaments.[103] However, in failing hearts, there is downregulation of the β-adrenergic pathway and SR function, so the augmentation is minimal.[22,80,104] During exercise, both stimulation pathways are relevant, and these data highlight the impact of their loss on contractile reserve in the failing heart.

INTEGRATIVE MEASURES OF SYSTOLIC FUNCTION

At the chamber level, analysis of systolic function generally relies on indirect measures of performance. As already noted, the ability to stiffen assessed by end-systolic elastance is very useful but not commonly employed. Many other parameters have been developed and these can be conveniently divided into early isovolumic phase parameters (e.g., dP/dt_{max}, isovolumic contraction time); early midsystolic-ejection phase parameters (e.g., maximal ventricular power, acceleration, velocity of shortening-stress relations); late systolic parameters (e.g., stroke work indexes, end-systolic elastance). To some extent, all are influenced by both intrinsic systolic properties of the sarcomere, by organization of the sarcomere, and muscle fiber into the chamber, and by the loading system to which they are coupled. In this regard, there is no direct measure of contractility—a term which itself remains conceptual rather than physical. Furthermore, not all measures of chamber function index the identical behavior, and there can be striking discrepancies among the measurements. This is less true of human myopathy, but it has been observed in various mouse models with gene targeting.

Chamber systole begins with isovolumetric contraction, and the earliest behavior that can be quantified is the rate of pressure (or force) development by the heart. The maximal rate (dP/dt_{max}) is among the most common and historically used measures of chamber systolic function. Ironically, it is also among the least directly related to physiologically relevant function —i.e., amount of net ejection or work provided during ejection. dP/dt_{max} is depressed in cardiomyopathy, and the absolute level observed in human heart failure is remarkably consistent, being near 1000 mm Hg/sec (normal being near 1600 to 1800 mm Hg/sec). As an index, it has witnessed a remarkable renaissance with the dominance of genetically engineered murine models for studying cardiovascular pathophysiology.

dP/dt_{max} is preload dependent in humans and other mammals. This is particularly so in the mouse where changes of even 2 to 3 microliters of end-diastolic volume (10% decline) often result in marked reductions in dP/dt_{max}[105,106] (Figure 13-5, *A*). This preload dependence can be minimized by regression of multiple values of dP/dt_{max} versus end-diastolic volume from variably loaded cardiac cycles.[107] While the latter is rarely clinically used because of its complexity, it remains a valuable method to minimize load sensitivity of dP/dt_{max}. dP/dt_{max} is also influenced by internal loading (such as reflected by microfilaments, perhaps titin), extracellular matrix loading (i.e., edema, inflammation, collagen dysregulation), phosphorylation state of MyBP-C, myocyte contractile depression, and the coordination of the chamber walls. Discoordinate contraction associated with bundle branch block depresses dP/dt_{max} acutely even without any primary change in contractile function of the myocytes. This is due to the effect of having part of the wall contract early against a still relaxed portion of the chamber. Pressure rises more slowly as force from one side is dissipated into stretch of the other. Acute increases in dP/dt_{max} associated with biventricular stimulation of a dyssynchronous failing heart occur within a single beat, and similarly do not indicate a change in underlying contractile function, but rather chamber-level consequences of improved coordination of wall contraction.[108,109]

Early midsystolic-ejection parameters are widely used to assess systolic function of the intact chamber. These have been briefly mentioned in the previous section with respect to their derivation from force-velocity behavior. The two most common approaches are preload-adjusted maximal power and stress/rate adjusted circumferential shortening velocity. Maximal power can be assessed from noninvasive-derived aortic flow and arterial pressure data.[110] The latter is measured by tonometer or other methods for noninvasive waveform reconstruction.[111] Once obtained, maximal power is normalized to chamber end-diastolic volume (or EDV^2 in dilated failing hearts) to obtain a parameter with relatively little preload and afterload dependence.[86,87] Importantly, its reliability depends upon a relatively high (i.e., arterial level) of afterload and the lack of notable changes in afterload. This limitation can preclude use in the right heart, for example.[112]

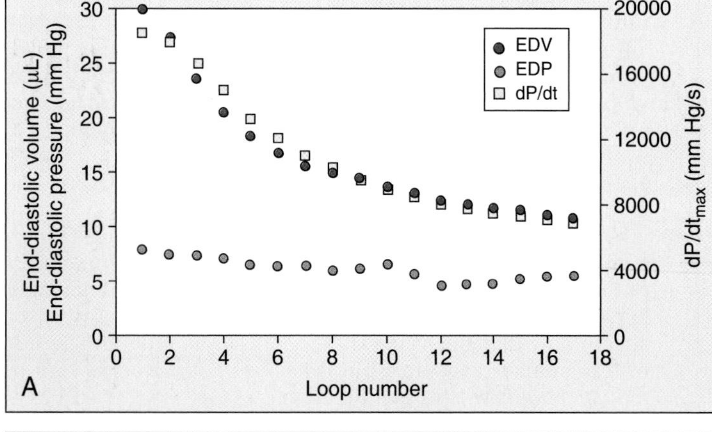

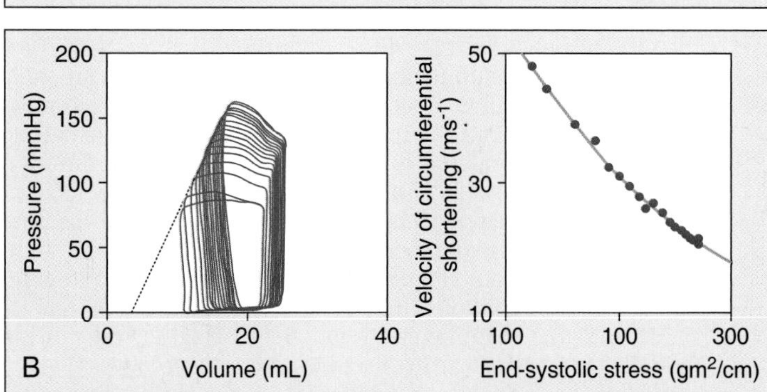

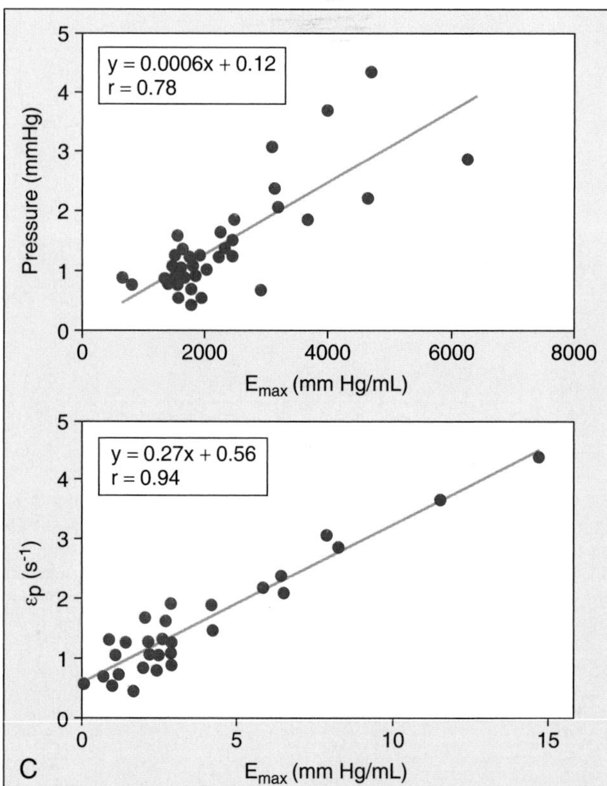

FIGURE 13-5 Indices of contractility. **A,** Preload dependence of dP/dt_{max} in mouse. Data are from a series of cycles at varying preload; beat 0 is at high preload, beat 17 at low preload. While there is negligible change in end-diastolic pressure for these cycles, preload volume (EDV) declines in direct correlation with dP/dt_{max}. **B,** Generation of velocity of shortening-stress relations from pressure-volume data at varying afterloads. **C,** Correlation of myocardial strain rate (εp; *y*-axis) to chamber dP/dt_{max} and maximal systolic elastance (E_{max}). (With permission from Greenberg NL, Firstenberg MS, Castro PL, et al. Doppler-derived myocardial systolic strain rate is a strong index of left ventricular contractility. *Circulation* 2002;105:99–105.)[114]

This index has been applied in a number of clinical studies, including during exercise testing where it displays far more marked sensitivity to contractile function than does the EF.[89] Its advantage in this regard is its simplicity and capacity to be recorded during stress procedures such as exercise. Low levels of reserve power have been shown to predict adverse outcome (need for urgent transplantation or death) in heart failure patients.[113]

The rate-adjusted Vcf-stress relation has also been widely used to index systolic function in animal and human studies. An example of this relation derived from a sequence of variably afterloaded contractions is shown in Figure 13-5, *B*. Vcf is obtained derived from 2-D midchamber level, short axis echocardiographic data, while stress is estimated based on cuff (or invasively measured pressures) and chamber long and short axis dimensions and thickness. While many studies have reported individual patient data as a single point—with stress plot on the *x*-axis, and Vcf on the *y*-axis, the actual dependence of each variable on the other depends on chamber preload as well. Furthermore, the stress estimates generally assume homogeneous material wall properties, and may not discriminate between myocyte and extracellular matrix–dependent geometric changes. Still, among parameters, this is relatively unique in attempting to incorporate chamber geometry and derive myocardial properties from chamber-level data.

More recent developments in tissue Doppler imaging have given rise to strain and strain-rate analysis.[114-117] These approaches essentially quantify myocardial wall motion—much as might be derived from MRI-based tissue tagging methods.[118] Actual regional stresses remain unknown, and can influence measured strains and strain rates. Nonetheless, strain rate has been found to correlate with dP/dt_{max} and indices derived from end-systolic pressure-volume relations (Figure 13-5, *C*),[114] and clearly is prominently influenced by chamber systolic function. In genetic models of hypertrophic cardiomyopathy, tissue Doppler has been used to define early abnormalities of chamber function that precede the evolution of cardiac hypertrophy.[119] Tissue Doppler has been widely employed to index contractile discoordination in patients with cardiac failure and conduction delay.[120,121]

The most commonly used late-systolic parameter is ejection fraction—the chamber translation of fractional shortening. EF is easy to measure, its value is independent of calibration errors of absolute volume assessment (i.e., it is dimensionless), it is moderately sensitive to inotropic changes, and it is rather insensitive to pure alterations in cardiac filling volume (preload). However, EF is highly dependent on arterial impedance load, and so declines can easily reflect both a decrement in underlying myocyte function and reduced shortening because of higher load. This is particularly important in failing hearts where the depressed heart is coupled to high arterial impedance. EF is also heart rate dependent, declining at faster rates. This effect is likely important to the enhancement of EF with chronic β-blockade therapy—in addition to any primary augmentation of underlying systolic function because of the treatment. EF also reflects chamber dilation/remodeling since the denominator (EDV) is increased in such ventricles while the numerator is often near normal range short of severe cardiodepression or restrictive filling. In this sense, the pathophysiological implication of an acutely reduced EF, which is a strong correlate of other parameters—such as end-systolic elastance or even dP/dt_{max}—may not be present if the mechanism involves chronic chamber remodeling and myocyte depression. Lastly, EF is not the most sensitive parameter to contractile change.[7]

The Frank-Starling curve remains an important element of systolic analysis, but it is limited because of strong afterload and heart rate dependencies, and ambiguities associated with the use of end-diastolic filling pressure to index preload. The latter is discussed in more detail in a subsequent section. An alternative approach has been to assess relations between cardiac stroke work and preload (preload-recruitable stroke work)—the latter indexed by end-diastolic volume rather than pressure.[122] Stroke work is less afterload dependent than stroke volume, as it incorporates pressure as well, and the SW-EDV relation is both linear and minimally influenced by chamber load, while still reflecting systolic function. A further advantage is that it has units of force, and is therefore chamber-size independent. Values for the slope of this relation are typically between 75 and 90 mm Hg and are very similar between rat, mouse, canine, porcine, and human, and other mammalian ventricles. As with Ees, methods to assess PRSW from single-beat data and noninvasive analysis have been reported.[123]

IMPACT OF PERICARDIAL LOADING ON SYSTOLIC FUNCTION

The intact chamber not only imposes complex filling and ejection loads on the heart during systole to modify its function, but also contains the chambers by a pericardial membrane that couples filling pressures from one chamber to another. While the influence of the pericardium on cardiac diastolic function is long well recognized, its impact on systolic function relations such as the Frank-Starling relation, has remained underappreciated.[124] However, studies have shown the importance of this interaction for generating the apparent descending limb of the Frank-Starling relation. While increased length and thus sarcomere stretch over 2.4 μ has been suggested to explain a decline in force generated by skeletal muscle because of reduced myofilament overlap, cardiac tissue cannot be stretched to this extent because of the extracellular matrix and cytoskeletal membrane proteins within the myocyte. Yet, cardiac output is often observed to decline with high preloads or conversely increase with preload reduction—leading to the presumption of operation along a descending limb in the failure state. The more likely explanation has been demonstrated by Tyberg et al, and relates to the importance of transmural pressure (not absolute chamber pressure) for determining the net stretch on the heart.[125,126] In patients with DCM, increased end-diastolic pressures may not be associated with elevated transmural pressure because of concomitantly higher extrinsic (pericardial) pressures. With a reduction in preload volume, actual transmural distending pressures have been shown to rise, so that real myocyte stretch is actually increasing rather than declining with the fall in EDP. Plots of CO versus EDP can appear biphasic, whereas those between CO and EDV are linear. This affects any relationship in which filing pressure is used to index the level of chamber preload.

VENTRICULAR-ARTERIAL INTERACTION

An important feature of systolic cardiac function is its dependence on the arterial loading system into which the heart must eject. The interaction of both components ultimately determines systemic variables such as cardiac output, ejection fraction, external work, mechanical efficiency, systolic pressure, and so forth. Depending upon the matching of cardiac and vascular properties, these variables can be optimized or compromised. Furthermore, the interaction of properties of the systolic ventricle and vascular system play a critical role in determining the cardiac output and blood pressure response of the heart failure patient to commonly used therapeutic interventions, such as vasodilators, diuretics, and inotropes. This interaction is also important for understanding the syndrome of cardiac failure with preserved EF. Thus it is useful to both understand how coupling can be studied and the implications for ventricular-arterial interaction in cardiac failure.

Among the more successful methods used to assess ventricular-vascular coupling is the pressure-volume framework, employing the ESPVR and a parameter used to index arterial properties, termed the "effective arterial elastance" (E_a).[59,60,127] As already noted in Figure 13-2, E_a is the ratio of end-systolic pressure to stroke volume and its value is dominated by mean arterial resistance and heart rate. It is also influenced by reactive loading properties of the arterial system—i.e., characteristic impedance and arterial compliance. In this description, coupling is generally expressed by a ratio of E_a to the ESPVR slope (i.e., E_a/E_{es}) (Figure 13-6, *A*).

Prior studies have shown that when the E_a/E_{es} ratio is near 1.0, there is optimal transfer of energy or work (power or SW) from the heart to arterial system.[128-130] Data obtained in isolated canine hearts first displayed this dependence for both work and cardiac efficiency, and subsequent studies have confirmed similar relations in intact hearts.[131] In normal individuals, the coupling ratio is near 0.8, matching ventricular and arterial properties to yield maximal power, efficiency, and external work. Importantly, this optimally matched condition is maintained during exercise,[129] and may relate to an evolutionary process designed to maintain a minimum relative cardiac/body size ratio.[132]

Work or power output is far from optimal, however, in hearts with depressed contractility and increased vascular loading, typical of the failing dilated heart. Asanoi et al[133] first reported coupling ratios in patients with normal, moderate, and severely depressed LV function. In the patients with reduced EF, ratios rise greater than 3 (Figure 13-6, *B*), consistent with a decline in cardiac efficiency and effective external work. This relation between heart and artery can play a major role in determining whether a given pharmaceutical intervention will improve chamber function or diminish it. In this example, the DCM patient with high systemic resistance was administered a bolus of intravenous nitroglycerin. The resulting beat-to-beat decline in arterial resistance led to an increase in the width of the pressure-volume loop—increasing stroke volume (and thus cardiac output) by nearly 50% and improving power output. The same intervention in a normal subject would largely reduce work or power output if basal coupling were already near optimal.

Coupling between heart and arterial effective elastance is also central to understanding whether a given intervention is more likely to enhance cardiac output or alternatively influence blood pressures. Dilated cardiomyopathy is typically associated with a depressed maximal chamber elastance (reduced Ees), and this predicts that for any decline in arterial afterload, the heart will behave principally as a pressure source, providing similar levels of systemic pressure by varying markedly the ejected volume. In contrast, hearts with increased systolic elastance—often observed in hypertrophied syndromes—behave as flow sources, providing similar levels of cardiac output despite changes in afterload (or preload), but inducing marked changes in systemic pressures. The latter behavior may play an important role in the syndrome of cardiac failure with preserved EF, often referred to as "diastolic heart failure."

Nearly half of patients over age 65 who present with symptoms of cardiac failure have apparent preservation of ejection fraction (HFpEF). While this is generally taken to mean that systolic function is itself normal, that is not necessarily the case. Differences in wall geometry, such as smaller cavities with ventricular hypertrophy, might otherwise lead to elevated EFs so that an EF of 50% is not in fact normal. Another feature of these individuals is that they can develop

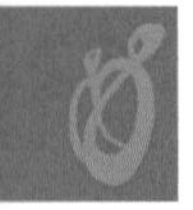

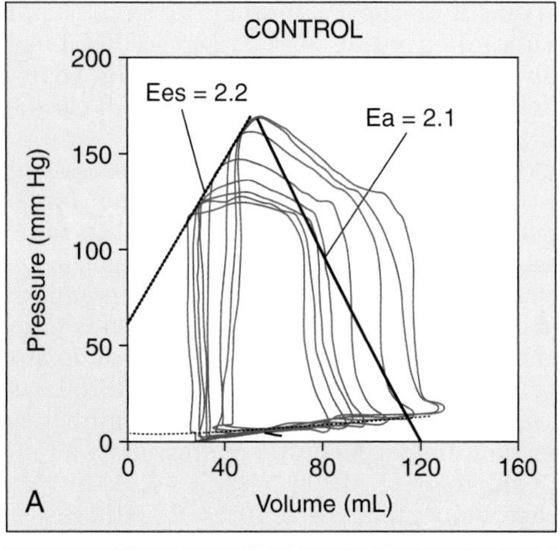

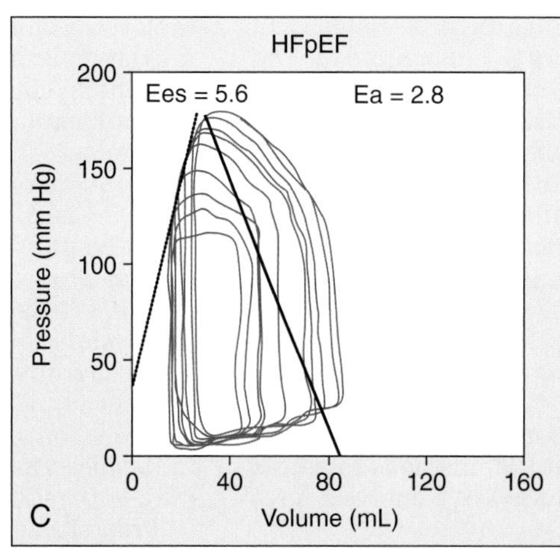

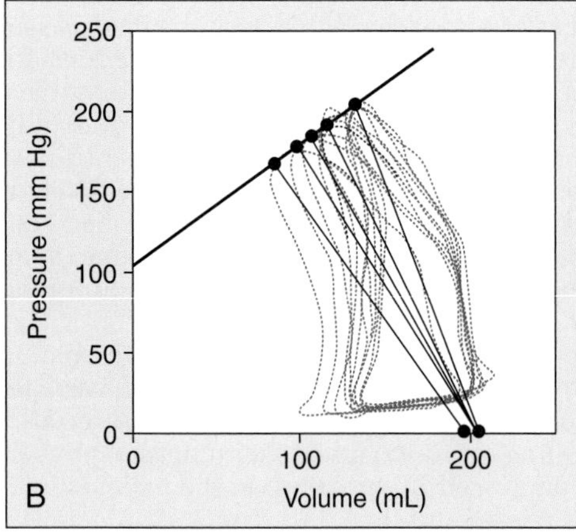

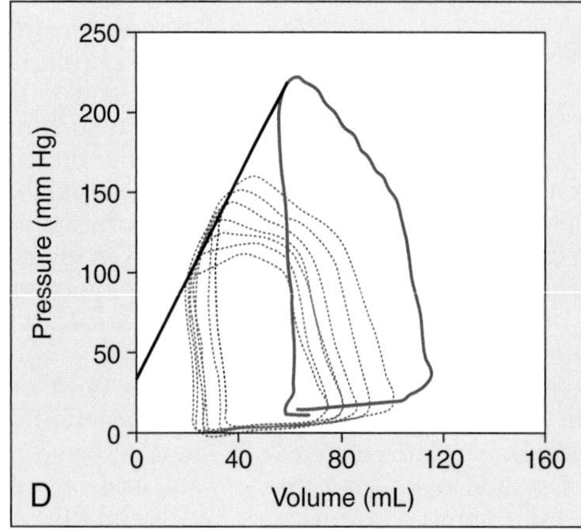

FIGURE 13-6 Ventricular-arterial coupling. **A,** Resting human PV relations showing normal matching between end-systolic elastance (Ees) and arterial elastance (Ea). This matching results in optimized cardiac function and efficiency. **B,** In contrast, the failing heart displays a reduced Ees (depressed systolic function) and elevated Ea (higher afterload) yielding a decline in chamber power output and metabolic efficiency. **C,** Subject with CHF and preserved ejection fraction. In such patients, Ees appears elevated over age/pressure-matched controls, and is accompanied by a further rise in arterial elastance because of reduced vascular distensibility. **D,** This pathophysiology can explain marked increases in blood pressure and cardiac workload with exertion. Shown here is an example subject during isometric hand exercise, with the resting PV loops (*dotted lines*) and stress-response loop as solid. (From Kawaguchi M, Hay I, Fetics B, et al. Combined ventricular systolic and arterial stiffening in patients with heart failure and preserved ejection fraction: implications for systolic and diastolic reserve limitations. *Circulation* 2003;107:714–720.)[134]

exacerbated ventricular end-systolic stiffening—beyond that observed with aging and/or hypertension. Studies in asymptomatic patients of varying ages have revealed that Ees (chamber systolic stiffening) increases in tandem with age-related arterial stiffening.[69] This was recently demonstrated in a large population study, and intriguingly women developed greater age-dependent increases in both Ees and Ea than men.[63] This may play a contributing role to the higher prevalence of HFpEF in elderly women. Combined increases in Ees and Ea can potently influence the pressures developed by the heart in response to changes in chamber filling and arterial load. Increased ventricular systolic stiffening means that even small increases or decreases in preload will amplify into marked changes in systolic pressure. This may contribute to the increased diuretic and orthostatic sensitivity in the elderly. In patients with cardiac failure symptoms yet EF greater than 50%, such stiffening is increased further[134]—though studies have shown this is likely related to the presence of systolic hypertension and ventricular hypertrophy, both common features of HFpEF patients.[62,135] The hemodynamic consequence is greater sensitivity of the heart to altered loading, exacerbated blood pressure lability, and potentially increased energetic demand to deliver reserve cardiac output.[134]

Figure 13-6, *C,* shows an example of a patient with heart failure and preserved EF, demonstrating the greatly increased stiffening of the ventricle during systole, and increased vascular stiffening. EF may appear normal in such individuals, but this does not necessarily mean that systolic function is normal and the problem resides solely with diastolic abnormalities. Increased chamber systolic stiffening and its impact on ventricular-arterial interaction may play an important pathophysiological role in symptom lability and hypertension and dysfunction during stress (Figure 13-6, *D*). Such abnormalities are consistent with the paroxysmal nature of this disorder, frequent flash pulmonary edema associated with hypertension, and sensitivity to preload reduction (diuretics). In this respect, enhanced (as with the more traditional diminished) systolic elastance may be similarly a valuable target for therapeutic intervention.

TREATING SYSTOLIC DYSFUNCTION

Despite a defining role in heart failure for many patients, the amelioration of systolic dysfunction by pharmacotherapy has generally not been a successful therapeutic approach to date (see Chapter 43). The oldest known treatment is digitalis, though the magnitude of contractile stimulation achieved by this agent in human heart failure remains essentially unknown, and it is not potent in experimental models. Acute human treatment has relied on cAMP generation either by stimulation of the β-adrenergic pathway (e.g., dobutamine) or by inhibition of a primary cAMP-targeted phosphodiesterase type 3 (e.g., milrinone). Both ultimately stimulate contraction by cAMP-dependent activation of protein kinase A, targeting calcium handling, and myofilament proteins among other key pathways involved with contractile force generation. Central to this effect is the rise in intracellular calcium involved with contraction. While useful for acute modulation, chronic effects are detrimental,[136] and this has stymied efforts in developing approaches targeting this signaling.[137]

The generation of genetically engineered mice revealed that stimulation of components of this signaling pathway can yield beneficial rather then worsening heart failure outcome. Many of these are now targets for early clinical trials using small molecules and/or gene transfer approaches. One prime example is inhibition of the β-receptor kinase GRK-2, which phosphorylates the β-receptor to suppress signaling and

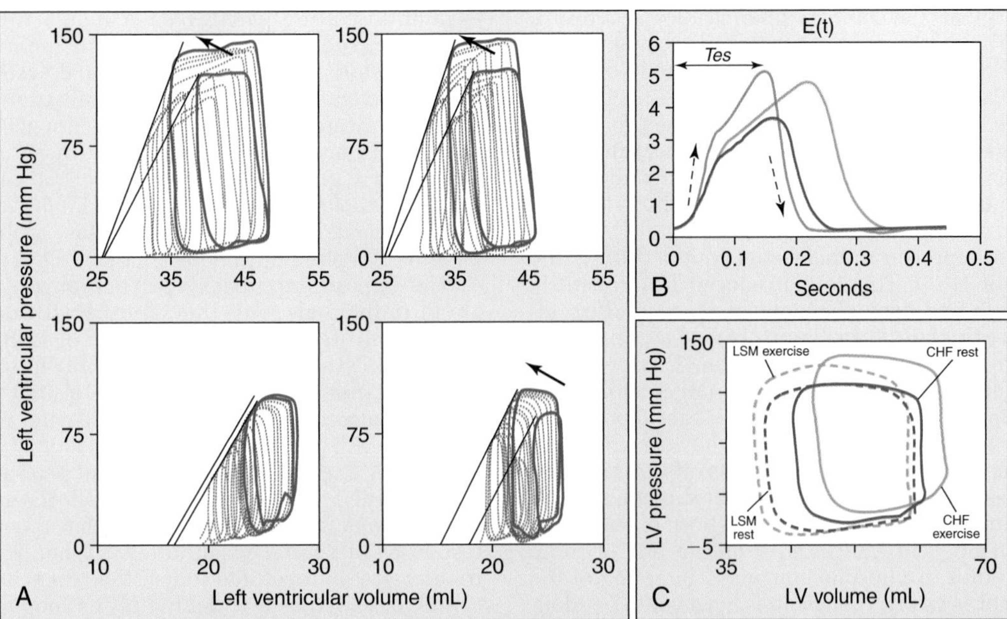

FIGURE 13-7 **A,** Influence of dobutamine versus a calcium sensitizer (EMD-57033) on contractile reserve in normal versus failing hearts. In the control hearts, both drugs stimulate contractility almost identically, reflected by the leftward shift and slope increase in the end-systolic PV relation. However, in failing hearts, the response to dobutamine is markedly depressed, whereas the contractile response to the sensitizer is maintained, consistent with its more distal site of action, directly on the myofilaments. **B,** Comparison of the time course of ventricular stiffening (Elastance, E(t)) as modified by a prototypical β-adrenergic stimulation mechanism coupled with PKA phosphorylation, versus a direct calcium sensitizer. The adrenergic agonist stimulates the kinetics of contraction both early and late in systole, abbreviating the time to peak elastance. In contrast, the sensitizer prolongs systole (greater sensitivity to trigger calcium), leaving the kinetics of early contraction and often relaxation little altered. dP/dt_{max} is not a useful index of changes with such drugs. **C,** Enhanced effectiveness from a calcium sensitizer on systolic function during exercise in a canine model of heart failure. The improvement in function reflected by the left shift of the PV loop and increase in its width (stroke volume) is modest in the heart when at rest, but potentiated during exercise. (A, From Senzaki H, Isoda T, Paolocci N, et al. Improved mechanoenergetics and cardiac rest and reserve function of in vivo failing heart by calcium sensitizer EMD-57033. *Circulation* 2000;101:1040–1048.)[102] C, With permission from Tachibana H, Cheng HJ, Ukai T, et al. Levosimendan improves LV systolic and diastolic performance at rest and during exercise after heart failure. *Am J Physiol Heart Circ Physiol* 2005;288:H914–H922.)[146]

stimulate receptor internalization and desensitization (see Chapter 10). Mutant versions of GRK-2 that lack this kinase activity have been successful in ameliorating various models of heart failure and myocardial infarction in rodents and large mammals.[138-140] Another approach is to target adenylate cyclase. Blockade of AC type 5 is associated with reduced heart failure[141] and improved longevity,[142] though upregulation of the other major isoform, AC-6, has been suggested to ameliorate heart failure.[143] This suggests where and how cAMP is generated is critical and compartmentation of this signaling central to the nature of long-term effects. Many have focused on deficiencies of the SR proteins such as phospholamban, SERCA2a, and I-1. Gene and/or small molecule clinical studies are under development to test whether upregulation of SERCA2a, for example, can ameliorate systolic dysfunction as it has clearly done in many different experimental animal models.[144,145]

Another major area of investigation is in agents that more directly influence the myofilaments to augment their response to a given level of trigger calcium. Referred to as a group as calcium sensitizers, this class can have many different targeting mechanisms such as modifying calcium–troponin C interactions or enhancing the myofibrillar ATPase. The theoretical advantages of such agents are several. First, by bypassing the adrenergic system and directly targeting the myofilaments, these drugs should work similarly well in failing as in normal hearts. An example of this behavior is shown in Figure 13-7, *A*. In this canine model of heart failure,[102] the dobutamine-stimulated contraction is markedly depressed compared with the normal control response, whereas the response to the sensitizer, EMD-57033, which is thought to target the myosin head to enhance actin attachment, is similar in both conditions. Another feature of these agents is that they can enhance contraction without requiring the level of energy use needed when this occurs via a cAMP-dependent pathway. In this sense, pure sensitizers should improve cardiac efficiency. Third, their effects on the kinetics of contraction differ from traditional cAMP/PKA-dependent inotropes, in that they have little impact on early rates of contraction (i.e., dP/dt_{max}), but more impact on later phases of systolic function such as net work, end-systolic elastance, and the duration of systole. This is demonstrated in Figure 13-7, *B*, where three time-varying elastance curves are depicted. Dobutamine results in a more rapid contraction, earlier peaking systolic stiffness, and faster relaxation. In contrast, the Ca^{2+}-sensitizer results in little change in the early phase of contraction, and a similar overall rate of stiffening that occurs for a longer period so net ejection is also enhanced. Relaxation rates can be similar or even improved based on the ability of the heart to eject to smaller end-systolic volumes. Lastly, increasing calcium sensitivity means that the impact on systolic function will itself vary with the stimulation of calcium by other means. At rest, calcium activation is reduced, so the impact on rest contractility of the sensitizer is commensurately less. However, with exercise, there are the catecholamine-and heart rate–triggered changes that, even while depressed, can still enhance the calcium trigger and thus increase the inotropic effect from the sensitizer. This was nicely demonstrated in an animal study of levosimendan[146] (Figure 13-7, *C*). Improved systolic function assessed by pressure-volume relations was modest at rest, but much more marked in animals doing treadmill exercise.

The most widely studied example of a sensitizer is levosimendan, which was originally identified by its interaction with TnC and capacity to enhance myofilament force generation. However, the drug was also shown active in inhibiting phosphodiesterase type 3, which explained some calcium dependence to its effects, and ATP-sensitive potassium channels that likely contributed to systemic vasodilation.[147] While early trials were promising, larger controlled studies were ultimately disappointing.[148] Still, this was not a real test of

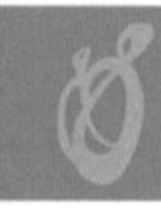

a pure sensitizer given the complex pharmacology involved. However, several other agents are currently being tested, including a small molecule identified to specifically enhance myofibrillar ATPase activity. This drug, CK-1827452, prolongs the systolic period due to its increasing the probability that a cross-bridge will be in the active force generating state. It does not appear to have any effects on cAMP signaling, and in this sense is one of the purer "calcium-sensitizing" types of agents yet tested. Clinical trials are ongoing.

Another novel approach to increasing contractility is the use of nitroxyl, or HNO. This is the reduced form of nitric oxide coupled with hydrogen; the molecule does not dissociate but attaches to thiolates (negatively charged cysteine residues) on selective proteins to modify function.[149] The reaction is reversibly controlled by redox state, in that enhancing reducing conditions can block it. HNO was first reported to enhance systolic function in the intact canine heart model of HF,[150] and later cellular mechanisms for this effect have been revealed.[151] These include demonstration of direct enhancement of SR calcium uptake and release, the former related to HNO targeting of C674 in SERCA2a,[152] and at one or more of the three cysteines in phospholamban.[153] Targeting of the ryanodine receptor is likely, though sites have yet to be identified, and there is also a calcium-sensitizing effect that may be linked to HNO modification of regulatory thin filament proteins. A clinical HNO donor has been developed and trials were initiated in class II HF patients in the spring of 2009.

SYSTOLIC EFFECTS OF DYSSYNCHRONY AND RESYNCHRONIZATION (see Chapter 47)

It has long been recognized that discoordinate cardiac contraction itself reduces the systolic performance of the chamber, and recent developments in therapies to resynchronize contraction have shown this to be a valuable target for heart failure treatment. Conduction disease at or above the AV node affects chronotropic competence and effective preload (and left atrial pressure). Both short and excessively long AV delays reduce net LV filling.[154,155] Infranodal conduction delay—commonly left-bundle-branch block pattern—induces discoordinate contraction.[156-159] DCM hearts with an LBBB display early activation of the septal wall with lateral prestretch, followed by markedly delayed lateral contraction with late systolic septal stretch towards the RV. Cardiac discoordination induced by LBBB or RV-ventricular pacing depresses systolic function, increasing the end-systolic volumes at a given pressure (rightward shift of the ESPVR), prolongs isovolumic relaxation,[160-162] and has been coupled to widening of the QRS complex.[160] The energetic cost of contraction can increase relative to effective ejection, since the early activated myocardium largely serves to increase preload on the lateral freewall, leaving the late activated wall to contract at higher stress while wasting work by stretching the more pliable early activated territory.[163-165]

These mechanical effects of discoordinate contraction were the impetus for studies performed over a decade ago in which right ventricular preexcitation was used to treat patients with hypertrophic cardiomyopathy.[166,167] In such patients, the institution of RV-apex pacing increased end-systolic volumes, reduced dP/dt_{max} and other parameters of systolic function, and importantly in this instance, resulted in a decline in hyperdynamic ejection and thus cavity obliteration. Importantly, this effect did not depend upon the presence of asymmetric hypertrophy—but was equally if not more effective in individuals with concentric LVH associated with symptoms of cardiac failure.[168] Figure 13-8, *A*, shows time tracings of apical segmental volume in a patient with hypertrophic cardiomyopathy subjected to acute RV apical pacing. While the original data shows normal timing of systolic ejection and filling, pacing results in premature contraction of the region, and later restretch (volume increase) during what is still systole. This results in residual systolic volume that is not ejected, so the end-systolic pressure-volume relation shifts rightward (Figure 13-8, *B*).[70] Though therapeutic generation of ventricular dyssynchrony in patients with septal hypertrophy proved less effective,[169,170] a small single center trial in patients with concentric LVH and cavity obliteration found benefits from reducing systolic contraction in these patients. Larger controlled trials remain to be done.

The opposite approach—resynchronizing the left ventricle in individuals with dilated cardiomyopathy and underlying basal discoordination because of LBBB—has been far more successful (see Chapter 47). Biventricular pacing or univentricular pacing of the LV lateral free wall can recoordinate contraction and is associated with systolic improvement.[108,171-174] Cardiac resynchronization effects manifest abruptly (i.e., rise in dP/dt_{max}, arterial pressures, Figure 13-8, *C*) occurring within one beat, and reflects increased systolic flow. Chronic noninvasive studies have reported sustained responses of similar magnitude.[121] When displayed as ventricular pressure-volume loops, the resynchronization effect can be observed as a widening of the loop (enhanced stroke volume), decline in end-systolic wall stress (left shift of end-systolic pressure-volume point), and increased cardiac work (Figure 13-8, *D*). Importantly, the latter is not accompanied by increases in energy consumption, but to the contrary, has been shown to be coupled with a decline in energy consumption.[175] Studies have not demonstrated major effects on diastolic function to date, although there is evidence of reverse cardiac remodeling associated with this therapy.

These initial studies established improvement in systolic function at the chamber level—though as with acute dyssynchrony, this was likely because of the coordination of contraction and not a primary improvement in myocardial contractility. However, chronic cardiac resynchronization therapy (CRT) treatment enhances rest and systolic reserve function, demonstrated by exercise capacity and the response to heart rate increases. This has been coupled to upregulation in myocardial gene expression of β_1-receptors, phospholamban, and SERCA2a, among other genes.[176-178] Importantly, new data from animal models of dyssynchronous heart failure and CRT have revealed improvement in resting myocyte function and adrenergic reserve. Myocyte results from canine hearts subjected to either 6 weeks of rapid atrial pacing in the presence of an LBBB (dyssynchronous failure, DHF) or 3 weeks of this mode followed by 3 weeks of rapid biventricular pacing (CRT) are displayed in Figure 13-8, *E*.[179] Both models involve 6 weeks of tachypacing, a method to induce dilated failure in the mammalian heart. While some global improvement with CRT was observed, overall both groups displayed features of dilated HF. Yet, while rest and isoproterenol stimulated sarcomere shortening and calcium transient responses in DHF myocytes were markedly depressed compared with normal controls, myocytes from CRT hearts displayed improvement in both variables under both conditions. The mechanisms include reversal of several abnormalities of cycling regulation, and improved adrenergic signaling cascades including enhanced suppression of inhibitory G protein and upregulation of both β_1-receptor-coupled signaling and adenylate cyclase activation.[179] Thus chronic CRT does enhance systolic function by means of direct myocyte benefits.

SUMMARY

Advances in noninvasive techniques and availability of new systems to directly assess cardiac systolic function have advanced our understanding of its presence and modification by therapies in advanced heart failure. While central to much

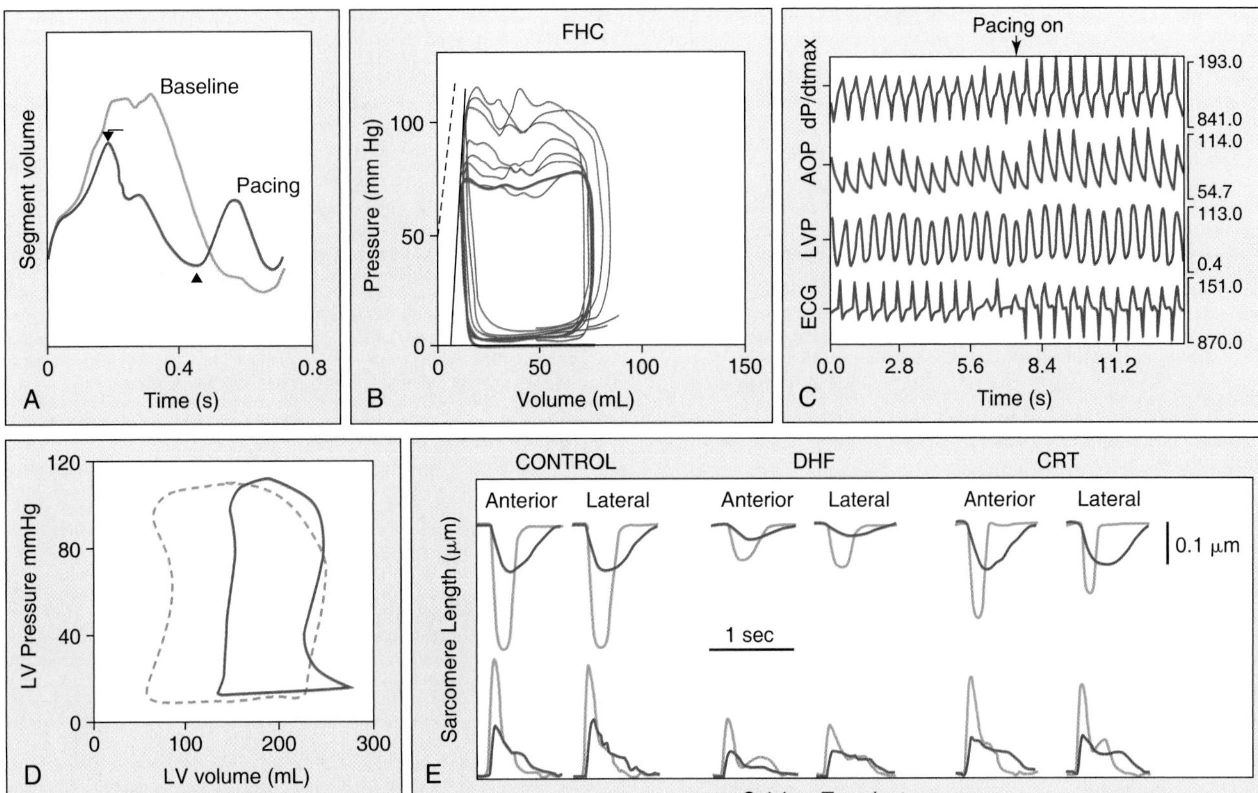

FIGURE 13-8 Impact of ventricular discoordination and resynchronization on chamber systolic function. **A,** Dyssynchrony generated by RV apex pacing in the human ventricle. The resting condition (baseline) shows normal timing of systolic ejection. With pacing, the region shortens early, and then is stretched late in what would be late systole for the rest of the heart. **B,** Global PV relations during RV apex pacing are compared with sinus controls (dashed ESPVRs). Dyssynchrony results in an increase in end-systolic volume and decline in effective systolic function. **C,** Resynchronization in human DCM patient with LBBB. Acute LV or biventricular stimulation enhances dP/dt_{max}, aortic pulse pressure, and peak LV pressure as shown after the arrow. This effect is very rapid. **D,** Example of pressure-volume loops with resynchronization (*dashed line*) showing enhanced function, increased loop width, and left shift of end-systolic point. This is the opposite to the effect observed in panel B with dyssynchrony induced by RV-apex pacing. **E,** Myocyte contraction and calcium transients from hearts with normal function, dyssynchronous heart failure (DHF), or resynchronized heart failure (CRT). DHF cells display markedly depressed function and transients with and without isoproterenol (ISO) stimulation, whereas CRT cells display improvements in both responses. These changes were demonstrated from cells obtained from both the early- and late-activated region. (B, From Pak PH, Maughan WL, Baughman KL, et al. Mechanism of acute mechanical benefit from VDD pacing in hypertrophied heart: similarity of responses in hypertrophic cardiomyopathy and hypertensive heart disease. *Circulation* 1998;98:242–248.)[70]

heart failure, systolic dysfunction has been difficult to therapeutically target thus far. However, the recent data on cardiac resynchronization showing chronic benefits on function, symptoms, and mortality for a therapy that improves systolic function, suggests optimism is warranted. Understanding how CRT functions at the molecular level may indeed provide insights into heart failure in general. Similar optimism stems from recent successes in animal models where systolic function is enhanced by gene manipulation of signaling and/or calcium handing distal to the adrenergic receptor. After nearly 15 years of relative inactivity on the inotropy front, new trials now under way may change the way we view improving systole for the failing heart. As these approaches are developed, the assessment of systolic function and its response to therapy should again become an important focus for heart failure researchers and practitioners.

REFERENCES

1. Mudd, J. O., & Kass, D. A. (2008). Tackling heart failure in the twenty-first century. *Nature*, *451*, 919–928.
2. Heineke, J., & Molkentin, J. D. (2006). Regulation of cardiac hypertrophy by intracellular signalling pathways. *Nat Rev Mol Cell Biol*, *7*, 589–600.
3. Dorn, G. W., & Force, T. (2005). Protein kinase cascades in the regulation of cardiac hypertrophy. *J Clin Invest*, *115*, 527–537.
4. Sano, M., Minamino, T., Toko, H., et al. (2007). p53-induced inhibition of Hif-1 causes cardiac dysfunction during pressure overload. *Nature*, *446*, 444–448.
5. Shiojima, I., Sato, K., Izumiya, Y., et al. (2005). Disruption of coordinated cardiac hypertrophy and angiogenesis contributes to the transition to heart failure. *J Clin Invest*, *115*, 2108–2118.
6. Manso, A. M., Elsherif, L., Kang, S. M., et al. (2006). Integrins, membrane-type matrix metalloproteinases and ADAMs: potential implications for cardiac remodeling. *Cardiovasc Res*, *69*, 574–584.
7. Kass, D. A., Maughan, W. L., Guo, Z. M., et al. (1987). Comparative influence of load versus inotropic states on indexes of ventricular contractility: experimental and theoretical analysis based on pressure-volume relationships. *Circulation*, *76*, 1422–1436.
8. Kass, D. A., & Maughan, W. L. (1988). From "Emax" to pressure-volume relations: a broader view. *Circulation*, *77*, 1203–1212.
9. Kamisago, M., Sharma, S. D., DePalma, S. R., et al. (2000). Mutations in sarcomere protein genes as a cause of dilated cardiomyopathy. *N Engl J Med*, *343*, 1688–1696.
10. Morita, H., Seidman, J., & Seidman, C. E. (2005). Genetic causes of human heart failure. *J Clin Invest*, *115*, 518–526.
11. Chang, A. N., & Potter, J. D. (2005). Sarcomeric protein mutations in dilated cardiomyopathy. *Heart Fail Rev*, *10*, 225–235.
12. Belin, R. J., Sumandea, M. P., Allen, E. J., et al. (2007). Augmented protein kinase C-alpha-induced myofilament protein phosphorylation contributes to myofilament dysfunction in experimental congestive heart failure. *Circ Res*, *101*, 195–204.
13. Kobayashi, T., Jin, L., & de Tombe, P. P. (2008). Cardiac thin filament regulation. *Pflugers Arch*, *457*, 37–46.
14. Schmitt, J. P., Debold, E. P., Ahmad, F., et al. (2006). Cardiac myosin missense mutations cause dilated cardiomyopathy in mouse models and depress molecular motor function. *Proc Natl Acad Sci U S A*, *103*, 14525–14530.
15. McConnell, B. K., Jones, K. A., Fatkin, D., et al. (1999). Dilated cardiomyopathy in homozygous myosin-binding protein-C mutant mice. *J Clin Invest*, *104*, 1235–1244.
16. Nagayama, T., Takimoto, E., Sadayappan, S., et al. (2007). Control of in vivo left ventricular contraction/relaxation kinetics by myosin binding protein C: protein kinase A phosphorylation dependent and independent regulation. *Circulation*, *116*, 2399–2408.
17. Murphy, A. M., Kogler, H., Georgakopoulos, D., et al. (2000). Transgenic mouse model of stunned myocardium. *Science*, *287*, 488–491.
18. Sadayappan, S., Gulick, J., Osinska, H., et al. (2005). Cardiac myosin-binding protein-C phosphorylation and cardiac function. *Circ Res*, *97*, 1156–1163.
19. Zolk, O., Caroni, P., & Bohm, M. (2000). Decreased expression of the cardiac LIM domain protein MLP in chronic human heart failure. *Circulation*, *101*, 2674–2677.

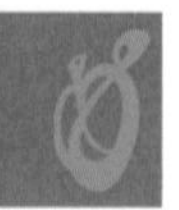

20. Arber, S., Hunter, J. J., Ross, J., Jr., et al. (1997). MLP-deficient mice exhibit a disruption of cardiac cytoarchitectural organization, dilated cardiomyopathy, and heart failure. *Cell, 88*, 393–403.
21. Heydemann, A., & McNally, E. M. (2007). Consequences of disrupting the dystrophin-sarcoglycan complex in cardiac and skeletal myopathy. *Trends Cardiovasc Med, 17*, 55–59.
22. McNally, E., Allikian, M., Wheeler, M. T., et al. (2003). Cytoskeletal defects in cardiomyopathy. *J Mol Cell Cardiol, 35*, 231–241.
23. Vatta, M., Stetson, S. J., Perez-Verdia, A., et al. (2002). Molecular remodelling of dystrophin in patients with end-stage cardiomyopathies and reversal in patients on assistance-device therapy. *Lancet, 359*, 936–941.
24. Towbin, J. A., & Bowles, N. E. (2001). Molecular genetics of left ventricular dysfunction. *Curr Mol Med, 1*, 81–90.
25. Bers, D. M. (2008). Calcium cycling and signaling in cardiac myocytes. *Annu Rev Physiol, 70*, 23–49.
26. Houser, S. R., Piacentino, V., III, & Weisser, J. (2000). Abnormalities of calcium cycling in the hypertrophied and failing heart. *J Mol Cell Cardiol, 32*, 1595–1607.
27. Bers, D. M. (2006). Altered cardiac myocyte Ca regulation in heart failure. *Physiology (Bethesda), 21*, 380–387.
28. Pathak, A., del Monte, F., Zhao, W., et al. (2005). Enhancement of cardiac function and suppression of heart failure progression by inhibition of protein phosphatase 1. *Circ Res, 96*, 756–766.
29. Braz, J. C., Gregory, K., Pathak, A., et al. (2004). PKC-alpha regulates cardiac contractility and propensity toward heart failure. *Nat Med, 10*, 248–254.
30. Marx, S. O., Reiken, S., Hisamatsu, Y., et al. (2000). PKA phosphorylation dissociates FKBP12.6 from the calcium release channel (ryanodine receptor): defective regulation in failing hearts. *Cell, 101*, 365–376.
31. Zhang, T., Maier, L. S., Dalton, N. D., et al. (2003). The deltaC isoform of CaMKII is activated in cardiac hypertrophy and induces dilated cardiomyopathy and heart failure. *Circ Res, 92*, 912–919.
32. Marks, A. R. (2002). Ryanodine receptors, FKBP12, and heart failure. *Front Biosci, 7*, d970–d977.
33. Goldhaber, J. I., & Qayyum, M. S. (2000). Oxygen free radicals and excitation-contraction coupling. *Antioxid Redox Signal, 2*, 55–64.
34. Lim, G., Venetucci, L., Eisner, D. A., et al. (2008). Does nitric oxide modulate cardiac ryanodine receptor function? Implications for excitation-contraction coupling. *Cardiovasc Res, 77*, 256–264.
35. Terentyev, D., Gyorke, I., Belevych, A. E., et al. (2008). Redox modification of ryanodine receptors contributes to sarcoplasmic reticulum Ca^{2+} leak in chronic heart failure. *Circ Res, 103*, 1466–1472.
36. Hill, J. A., & Olson, E. N. (2008). Cardiac plasticity. *N Engl J Med, 358*, 1370–1380.
37. Kelly, D. P., & Scarpulla, R. C. (2004). Transcriptional regulatory circuits controlling mitochondrial biogenesis and function. *Genes Dev, 18*, 357–368.
38. Finck, B. N., & Kelly, D. P. (2007). Peroxisome proliferator-activated receptor gamma coactivator-1 (PGC-1) regulatory cascade in cardiac physiology and disease. *Circulation, 115*, 2540–2548.
39. Finck, B. N., & Kelly, D. P. (2006). PGC-1 coactivators: inducible regulators of energy metabolism in health and disease. *J Clin Invest, 116*, 615–622.
40. Thum, T., Gross, C., Fiedler, J., et al. (2008). MicroRNA-21 contributes to myocardial disease by stimulating MAP kinase signalling in fibroblasts. *Nature, 456*, 980–984.
41. Spinale, F. G., Coker, M. L., Krombach, S. R., et al. (1999). Matrix metalloproteinase inhibition during the development of congestive heart failure: effects on left ventricular dimensions and function. *Circ Res, 85*, 364–376.
42. Spinale, F. G. (2007). Myocardial matrix remodeling and the matrix metalloproteinases: influence on cardiac form and function. *Physiol Rev, 87*, 1285–1342.
43. Spinale, F. G. (2002). Matrix metalloproteinases: regulation and dysregulation in the failing heart. *Circ Res, 90*, 520–530.
44. Gerdes, A. M., & Capasso, J. M. (1995). Structural remodeling and mechanical dysfunction of cardiac myocytes in heart failure. *J Mol Cell Cardiol, 27*, 849–856.
45. Margulies, K. B. (2000). Ventricular unloading and myocyte recovery: insight gained into the pathophysiology of congestive heart failure. *Curr Cardiol Rep, 2*, 181–188.
46. Barbone, A., Holmes, J. W., Heerdt, P. M., et al. (2001). Comparison of right and left ventricular responses to left ventricular assist device support in patients with severe heart failure: a primary role of mechanical unloading underlying reverse remodeling. *Circulation, 104*, 670–675.
47. Zafeiridis, A., Jeevanandam, V., Houser, S. R., et al. (1998). Regression of cellular hypertrophy after left ventricular assist device support. *Circulation, 98*, 656–662.
48. Suga, H., & Sagawa, K. (1974). Instantaneous pressure-volume relationships and their ratio in the excised, supported canine left ventricle. *Circ Res, 35*, 117–128.
49. Pacher, P., Nagayama, T., Mukhopadhyay, P., et al. (2008). Measurement of cardiac function using pressure-volume conductance catheter technique in mice and rats. *Nat Protoc, 3*, 1422–1434.
50. Kass, D. A., Midei, M., Graves, W., et al. (1988). Use of a conductance (volume) catheter and transient inferior vena caval occlusion for rapid determination of pressure-volume relationships in man. *Cathet Cardiovasc Diagn, 15*, 192–202.
51. Liu, C. P., Ting, C. T., Lawrence, W., et al. (1993). Diminished contractile response to increased heart rate in intact human left ventricular hypertrophy: systolic versus diastolic determinants. *Circulation, 88*(pt 1), 1893–1906.
52. Senzaki, H., Chen, C. H., & Kass, D. A. (1996). Single beat estimation of end-systolic pressure-volume relation in humans: a new method with the potential for non-invasive application. *Circulation, 94*, 2497–2506.
53. Georgakopoulos, D., Mitzner, W. A., Chen, C. H., et al. (1998). In vivo murine left ventricular pressure-volume relations by miniaturized conductance micromanometry. *Am J Physiol, 274*, H1416–H1422.
54. Palmer, B. M., Georgakopoulos, D., Janssen, P. M., et al. (2004). Role of cardiac myosin binding protein C in sustaining left ventricular systolic stiffening. *Circ Res, 94*, 1249–1255.
55. Georgakopoulos, D., Mitzner, W. A., Chen, C. H., et al. (1998). In vivo murine left ventricular pressure-volume relations by miniaturized conductance micromanometry. *Am J Physiol, 274*, H1416–H1422.
56. Georgakopoulos, D., Christe, M. E., Giewat, M., et al. (1999). The pathogenesis of familial hypertrophic cardiomyopathy: early and evolving effects from an alpha-cardiac myosin heavy chain missense mutation. *Nat Med, 5*, 327–330.
57. Kass, D. A., Yamazaki, T., Burkhoff, D., et al. (1986). Determination of left ventricular end-systolic pressure-volume relationships by the conductance (volume) catheter technique. *Circulation, 73*, 586–595.
58. Kass, D. A., & Kelly, R. P. (1992). Ventriculo-arterial coupling: concepts, assumptions, and applications. *Ann Biomed Eng, 20*, 41–62.
59. Kelly, R. P., Ting, C. T., Yang, T. M., et al. (1992). Effective arterial elastance as index of arterial vascular load in humans. *Circulation, 86*, 513–521.
60. Sunagawa, K., Maughan, W. L., Burkhoff, D., et al. (1983). Left ventricular interaction with arterial load studied in isolated canine ventricle. *Am J Physiol, 245*, H773–H780.
61. Feldman, M. D., Pak, P. H., Wu, C. C., et al. (1996). Acute cardiovascular effects of OPC-18790 in patients with congestive heart failure. Time- and dose-dependence analysis based on pressure-volume relations. *Circulation, 93*, 474–483.
62. Lam, C. S., Roger, V. L., Rodeheffer, R. J., et al. (2007). Cardiac structure and ventricular-vascular function in persons with heart failure and preserved ejection fraction from Olmsted County, Minnesota. *Circulation, 115*, 1982–1990.
63. Redfield, M. M., Jacobsen, S. J., Borlaug, B. A., et al. (2005). Age- and gender-related ventricular-vascular stiffening: a community-based study. *Circulation, 112*, 2254–2262.
64. Iribe, G., Helmes, M., & Kohl, P. (2007). Force-length relations in isolated intact cardiomyocytes subjected to dynamic changes in mechanical load. *Am J Physiol Heart Circ Physiol, 292*, H1487–H1497.
65. Kass, D. A., Wolff, M. R., Ting, C. T., et al. (1993). Diastolic compliance of hypertrophied ventricle is not acutely altered by pharmacologic agents influencing active processes. *Ann Intern Med, 119*, 466–473.
66. Liao, P., Georgakopoulos, D., Kovacs, A., et al. (2001). The in vivo role of p38 MAP kinases in cardiac remodeling and restrictive cardiomyopathy. *Proc Natl Acad Sci U S A, 98*, 12283–12288.
67. Arts, T., Bovendeerd, P. H. M., Prinzen, F. W., et al. (1991). Relation between left ventricular cavity pressure and volume and systolic fiber stress and strain in the wall. *Biophys J, 59*, 93–102.
68. Kass, D. A., Beyar, R., Lankford, E., et al. (1989). Influence of contractile state on curvilinearity of the in situ end-systolic pressure-volume relations. *Circulation, 79*, 167–178.
69. Chen, C. H., Nakayama, M., Nevo, E., et al. (1998). Coupled systolic-ventricular and vascular stiffening with age: implications for pressure regulation and cardiac reserve in the elderly. *J Am Coll Cardiol, 32*, 1221–1227.
70. Pak, P. H., Maughan, W. L., Baughman, K. L., et al. (1998). Mechanism of acute mechanical benefit from VDD pacing in hypertrophied heart: similarity of responses in hypertrophic cardiomyopathy and hypertensive heart disease. *Circulation, 98*, 242–248.
71. Allen, D. G., & Kentish, J. C. (1985). The cellular basis of the length-tension relation in cardiac muscle. *J Mol Cell Cardiol, 17*, 821–840.
72. Kentish, J. C., ter Keurs, H. E., Ricciardi, L., et al. (1986). Comparison between the sarcomere length-force relations of intact and skinned trabeculae from rat right ventricle. Influence of calcium concentrations on these relations. *Circ Res, 58*, 755–768.
73. McDonald, K. S., & Moss, R. L. (1995). Osmotic compression of single cardiac myocytes eliminates the reduction in Ca^{2+} sensitivity of tension at short sarcomere length. *Circ Res, 77*, 199–205.
74. Smith, L., Tainter, C., Regnier, M., et al. (2009). Cooperative cross-bridge activation of thin filaments contributes to the Frank-Starling mechanism in cardiac muscle. *Biophys J, 96*, 3692–3702.
75. Fitzsimons, D. P., & Moss, R. L. (1998). Strong binding of myosin modulates length-dependent Ca^{2+} activation of rat ventricular myocytes. *Circ Res, 83*, 602–607.
76. Konhilas, J. P., Irving, T. C., & de Tombe, P. P. (2002). Myofilament calcium sensitivity in skinned rat cardiac trabeculae: role of interfilament spacing. *Circ Res, 90*, 59–65.
77. Knoll, R., Hoshijima, M., Hoffman, H. M., et al. (2002). The cardiac mechanical stretch sensor machinery involves a Z disc complex that is defective in a subset of human dilated cardiomyopathy. *Cell, 111*, 943–955.
78. Fukuda, N., & Granzier, H. (2004). Role of the giant elastic protein titin in the Frank-Starling mechanism of the heart. *Curr Vasc Pharmacol, 2*, 135–139.
79. Zile, M. R., Green, G. R., Schuyler, G. T., et al. (2001). Cardiocyte cytoskeleton in patients with left ventricular pressure overload hypertrophy. *J Am Coll Cardiol, 37*, 1080–1084.
80. Tsutsui, H., Ishihara, K., & Cooper, G. (1993). Cytoskeletal role in the contractile dysfunction of hypertrophied myocardium. *Science, 260*, 682–687.
81. Koide, M., Hamawaki, M., Narishige, T., et al. (2000). Microtubule depolymerization normalizes in vivo myocardial contractile function in dogs with pressure-overload left ventricular hypertrophy. *Circulation, 102*, 1045–1052.
82. Ingber, D. E. (2002). Mechanical signaling and the cellular response to extracellular matrix in angiogenesis and cardiovascular physiology. *Circ Res, 91*, 877–887.
83. Colan, S. D., Borow, K. M., & Neumann, A. (1984). Left ventricular end-systolic wall stress-velocity of fiber shortening relation: a load-independent index of myocardial contractility. *J Am Coll Cardiol, 4*, 715–724.
84. Quinones, M. A., Gaasch, W. H., Cole, J. S., et al. (1975). Echocardiographic determination of left ventricular stress-velocity relations. *Circulation, 51*, 689–700.
85. Mirsky, I., Aoyagi, T., Crocker, V. M., et al. (1990). Preload dependence of fiber shortening rate in conscious dogs with left ventricular hypertrophy. *J Am Coll Cardiol, 15*, 899.
86. Sharir, T., van Anden, E., Marmor, A., et al. (1992). Non-invasive assessment of drug induced load versus inotropic change by maximal ventricular power/EDV^2 in humans. *Circulation, 86*, I-1834 (abstract).
87. Nakayama, M., Chen, C. H., Nevo, E., et al. (1998). Optimal preload-adjustment of maximal ventricular power index varies with cardiac chamber size. *Am Heart J, 136*, 281–288.

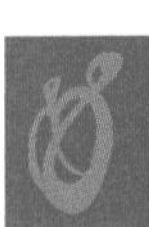

88. Brutsaert, D. L., & Sys, S. U. (1989). Relaxation and diastole of the heart. *Physiol Rev, 69*, 1228–1315.
89. Gillebert, T. C., Sys, S. U., & Brutsaert, D. L. (1989). Influence of loading patterns on peak length-tension relation and on relaxation in cardiac muscle. *J Am Coll Cardiol, 13*, 483–490.
90. Brutsaert, D. L., Claes, V. A., & Sonnenblick, E. H. (1971). Velocity of shortening of unloaded heart muscle and the length-tension relation. *Circ Res, 29*, 63–75.
91. Leach, J. K., Priola, D. V., Grimes, L. A., et al. (1999). Shortening deactivation of cardiac muscle: physiological mechanisms and clinical implications. *J Med Invest, 47*, 369–377.
92. Crozatier, B. (1996). Stretch-induced modifications of myocardial performance: from ventricular function to cellular and molecular mechanisms. *Cardiovasc Res, 32*, 25–37.
93. O'Rourke, M. F., & Kelly, R. P. (1993). Wave reflection in the systemic circulation and its implications in ventricular function. *J Hypertens, 11*, 327–337.
94. Dart, A., & Kingwell, B. (2001). Pulse pressure - a review of mechanisms and clinical relevance. *J Am Coll Cardiol, 37*, 975–984.
95. O'Rourke, M. F., Staessen, J. A., Vlachopoulos, C., et al. (2002). Clinical applications of arterial stiffness; definitions and reference values. *Am J Hypertens, 15*, 426–444.
96. Westerhof, N., & O'Rourke, M. F. (1995). Haemodynamic basis for the development of left ventricular failure in systolic hypertension and for its logical therapy. *J Hypertens, 13*, 943–952.
97. Yue, D. T., Marban, E., & Wier, G. (1986). Relationship between force and intracellular Ca^{2+} in tetanized mammalian heart muscle. *J Gen Physiol, 87*, 223–242.
98. Somura, F., Izawa, H., Iwase, M., et al. (2001). Reduced myocardial sarcoplasmic reticulum Ca(2+)-ATPase mRNA expression and biphasic force-frequency relations in patients with hypertrophic cardiomyopathy. *Circulation, 104*, 658–663.
99. Pieske, B., Maier, L. S., Bers, D. M., et al. (1999). Ca^{2+} handling and sarcoplasmic reticulum Ca^{2+} content in isolated failing and nonfailing human myocardium. *Circ Res, 85*, 38–46.
100. Maier, L. S., & Bers, D. M. (2002). Calcium, calmodulin, and calcium-calmodulin kinase II: heartbeat to heartbeat and beyond. *J Mol Cell Cardiol, 34*, 919–939.
101. Weber, C. R., Piacentino, V., III, Houser, S. R., et al. (2003). Dynamic regulation of sodium/calcium exchange function in human heart failure. *Circulation, 108*, 2224–2229.
102. Senzaki, H., Isoda, T., Paolocci, N., et al. (2000). Improved mechanoenergetics and cardiac rest and reserve function of in vivo failing heart by calcium sensitizer EMD-57033. *Circulation, 101*, 1040–1048.
103. Miura, T., Miyazaki, S., Guth, B. D., et al. (1992). Influence of the force-frequency relation on left ventricular function during exercise in conscious dogs. *Circulation, 86*, 563–571.
104. Hajjar, R. J., Schmidt, U., Kang, J. X., et al. (1997). Adenoviral gene transfer of phospholamban in isolated rat cardiomyocytes. Rescue effects by concomitant gene transfer of sarcoplasmic reticulum Ca(2+)-ATPase. *Circ Res, 81*, 145–153.
105. Kass, D. A., Hare, J. M., & Georgakopoulos, D. (1998). Murine cardiac function: a cautionary tail. *Circ Res, 82*, 519–522.
106. Georgakopoulos, D., & Kass, D. (2001). Minimal force-frequency modulation of inotropy and relaxation of in situ murine heart. *J Physiol, 534*, 535–545.
107. Little, W. C. (1985). The left ventricular dP/dt max-end diastolic volume relation in closed-chest dogs. *Circ Res, 56*, 808–815.
108. Kass, D. A., Chen, C. H., Curry, C., et al. (1999). Improved left ventricular mechanics from acute VDD pacing in patients with dilated cardiomyopathy and ventricular conduction delay. *Circulation, 99*, 1567–1573.
109. Auricchio, A., Stellbrink, C., Block, M., et al. (1999). Effect of pacing chamber and atrioventricular delay on acute systolic function of paced patients with congestive heart failure. *Circulation, 99*, 2993–3001.
110. Mandarino, W. A., Pinsky, M. R., & Gorcsan, J., III (1998). Assessment of left ventricular contractile state by preload-adjusted maximal power using echocardiographic automated border detection. *J Am Coll Cardiol, 31*, 861–868.
111. Sharir, T., Marmor, A., Ting, C. T., et al. (1993). Validation of a method for noninvasive measurement of central arterial pressure. *Hypertension, 21*, 74–82.
112. Leather, H. A., Segers, P., Sun, Y. Y., et al. (2002). The limitations of preload-adjusted maximal power as an index of right ventricular contractility. *Anesth Analg, 95*, 798–804, table.
113. Marmor, A., & Schneeweiss, A. (1997). Prognostic value of noninvasively obtained left ventricular contractile reserve in patients with severe heart failure. *J Am Coll Cardiol, 29*, 422–428.
114. Greenberg, N. L., Firstenberg, M. S., Castro, P. L., et al. (2002). Doppler-derived myocardial systolic strain rate is a strong index of left ventricular contractility. *Circulation, 105*, 99–105.
115. Suffoletto, M. S., Dohi, K., Cannesson, M., et al. (2006). Novel speckle-tracking radial strain from routine black-and-white echocardiographic images to quantify dyssynchrony and predict response to cardiac resynchronization therapy. *Circulation, 113*, 960–968.
116. Bank, A. J., & Kelly, A. S. (2006). Tissue Doppler imaging and left ventricular dyssynchrony in heart failure. *J Card Fail, 12*, 154–162.
117. Armstrong, G., Pasquet, A., Fukamachi, K., et al. (2000). Use of peak systolic strain as an index of regional left ventricular function: comparison with tissue Doppler velocity during dobutamine stress and myocardial ischemia. *J Am Soc Echocardiogr, 13*, 731–737.
118. Ozturk, C., & McVeigh, E. R. (2000). Four-dimensional B-spline based motion analysis of tagged MR images: introduction and in vivo validation. *Phys Med Biol, 45*, 1683–1702.
119. Nagueh, S. F., Kopelen, H. A., Lim, D. S., et al. (2000). Tissue Doppler imaging consistently detects myocardial contraction and relaxation abnormalities, irrespective of cardiac hypertrophy, in a transgenic rabbit model of human hypertrophic cardiomyopathy. *Circulation, 102*, 1346–1350.
120. Sogaard, P., Egeblad, H., Kim, W. Y., et al. (2002). Tissue Doppler imaging predicts improved systolic performance and reversed left ventricular remodeling during long-term cardiac resynchronization therapy. *J Am Coll Cardiol, 40*, 723–730.
121. Yu, C. M., Chau, E., Sanderson, J. E., et al. (2002). Tissue Doppler echocardiographic evidence of reverse remodeling and improved synchronicity by simultaneously delaying regional contraction after biventricular pacing therapy in heart failure. *Circulation, 105*, 438–445.
122. Glower, D. D., Spratt, J. A., Snow, N. D., et al. (1985). Linearity of the Frank-Starling relationship in the intact heart: the concept of preload recruitable stroke work. *Circulation, 71*, 994–1009.
123. Karunanithi, M. K., & Feneley, M. P. (2000). Single-beat determination of preload recruitable stroke work relationship: derivation and evaluation in conscious dogs. *J Am Coll Cardiol, 35*, 502–513.
124. Dauterman, K., Pak, P. H., Nussbacher, A., et al. (1995). Contribution of external forces to left ventricle diastolic pressure: implications for the clinical use of the Frank-Starling Law. *Ann Intern Med, 122*, 737–742.
125. Moore, T. D., Frenneaux, M. P., Sas, R., et al. (2001). Ventricular interaction and external constraint account for decreased stroke work during volume loading in CHF. *Am J Physiol Heart Circ Physiol, 281*, H2385–H2391.
126. Grant, D. A., Fauchere, J. C., Eede, K. J., et al. (2001). Left ventricular stroke volume in the fetal sheep is limited by extracardiac constraint and arterial pressure. *J Physiol, 535*, 231–239.
127. Sunagawa, K., Maughan, W. L., & Sagawa, K. (1985). Optimal arterial resistance for the maximal stroke work studied in isolated canine left ventricle. *Circ Res, 56*, 586.
128. Burkhoff, D., & Sagawa, K. (1986). Ventricular efficiency predicted by an analytical model. *Am J Physiol, 250*, R1021–R1027.
129. Little, W. C., & Cheng, C. P. (1991). Left ventricular-arterial coupling in conscious dogs. *Am J Physiol, 261*, H70–H76.
130. Starling, M. R. (1993). Left ventricular-arterial coupling relations in the normal human heart. *Am Heart J, 125*, 1659–1666.
131. de Tombe, P. P., Jones, S., Burkhoff, D., et al. (1993). Ventricular stroke work and efficiency both remain nearly optimal despite altered vascular loading. *Am J Physiol, 264*, H1817–H1824.
132. Elzinga, G., & Westerhof, N. (1991). Matching between ventricle and arterial load. An evolutionary process. *Circ Res, 68*, 1495–1500.
133. Asanoi, H., Sasayama, S., & Kameyama, T. (1989). Ventriculoarterial coupling in normal and failing heart in humans. *Circ Res, 65*, 483–493.
134. Kawaguchi, M., Hay, I., Fetics, B., et al. (2003). Combined ventricular systolic and arterial stiffening in patients with heart failure and preserved ejection fraction: implications for systolic and diastolic reserve limitations. *Circulation, 107*, 714–720.
135. Melenovsky, V., Borlaug, B. A., Rosen, B., et al. (2007). Cardiovascular features of heart failure with preserved ejection fraction versus nonfailing hypertensive left ventricular hypertrophy in the urban Baltimore community: the role of atrial remodeling/dysfunction. *J Am Coll Cardiol, 49*, 198–207.
136. Packer, M., Carver, J. R., Rodeheffer, R. J., et al. (1991). Effect of oral milrinone on mortality in severe chronic heart failure. The PROMISE study research group. *N Engl J Med, 325*, 1468–1475.
137. Kass, D. A. (2009). Rescuing a failing heart: putting on the squeeze. *Nat Med, 15*, 24–25.
138. Matkovich, S. J., Diwan, A., Klanke, J. L., et al. (2006). Cardiac-specific ablation of G-protein receptor kinase 2 redefines its roles in heart development and beta-adrenergic signaling. *Circ Res, 99*, 996–1003.
139. Pleger, S. T., Boucher, M., Most, P., et al. (2007). Targeting myocardial beta-adrenergic receptor signaling and calcium cycling for heart failure gene therapy. *J Card Fail, 13*, 401–414.
140. Raake, P. W., Vinge, L. E., Gao, E., et al. (2008). G protein-coupled receptor kinase 2 ablation in cardiac myocytes before or after myocardial infarction prevents heart failure. *Circ Res, 103*, 413–422.
141. Okumura, S., Takagi, G., Kawabe, J., et al. (2003). Disruption of type 5 adenylyl cyclase gene preserves cardiac function against pressure overload. *Proc Natl Acad Sci U S A, 100*, 9986–9990.
142. Yan, L., Vatner, D. E., O'Connor, J. P., et al. (2007). Type 5 adenylyl cyclase disruption increases longevity and protects against stress. *Cell, 130*, 247–258.
143. Phan, H. M., Gao, M. H., Lai, N. C., et al. (2007). New signaling pathways associated with increased cardiac adenylyl cyclase 6 expression: implications for possible congestive heart failure therapy. *Trends Cardiovasc Med, 17*, 215–221.
144. Kawase, Y., Ly, H. Q., Prunier, F., et al. (2008). Reversal of cardiac dysfunction after long-term expression of SERCA2a by gene transfer in a pre-clinical model of heart failure. *J Am Coll Cardiol, 51*, 1112–1119.
145. Miyamoto, M. I., del Monte, F., Schmidt, U., et al. (2000). Adenoviral gene transfer of SERCA2a improves left-ventricular function in aortic-banded rats in transition to heart failure. *Proc Natl Acad Sci U S A, 97*, 793–798.
146. Tachibana, H., Cheng, H. J., Ukai, T., et al. (2005). Levosimendan improves LV systolic and diastolic performance at rest and during exercise after heart failure. *Am J Physiol Heart Circ Physiol, 288*, H914–H922.
147. Ng, T. M. (2004). Levosimendan, a new calcium-sensitizing inotrope for heart failure. *Pharmacotherapy, 24*, 1366–1384.
148. Mebazaa, A., Nieminen, M. S., Packer, M., et al. (2007). Levosimendan vs dobutamine for patients with acute decompensated heart failure: the SURVIVE randomized trial. *JAMA, 297*, 1883–1891.
149. Paolocci, N., Jackson, M. I., Lopez, B. E., et al. (2007). The pharmacology of nitroxyl (HNO) and its therapeutic potential: not just the Janus face of NO. *Pharmacol Ther, 113*, 442–458.
150. Paolocci, N., Katori, T., Champion, H. C., et al. (2003). Positive inotropic and lusitropic effects of HNO/NO- in failing hearts: independence from beta-adrenergic signaling. *Proc Natl Acad Sci U S A, 100*, 5537–5542.
151. Tocchetti, C. G., Wang, W., Froehlich, J. P., et al. (2007). Nitroxyl improves cellular heart function by directly enhancing cardiac sarcoplasmic reticulum Ca^{2+} cycling. *Circ Res, 100*, 96–104.
152. Lancel, S., Zhang, J., Evangelista, A., et al. (2009). Nitroxyl activates SERCA in cardiac myocytes via glutathiolation of cysteine 674. *Circ Res, 104*, 720–723.

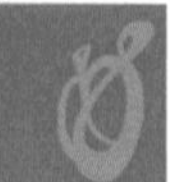

153. Froehlich, J. P., Mahaney, J. E., Keceli, G., et al. (2008). Phospholamban thiols play a central role in activation of the cardiac muscle sarcoplasmic reticulum calcium pump by nitroxyl. *Biochemistry, 47*, 13150–13152.
154. Meisner, J. S., McQueen, D. M., Ishida, Y., et al. (1985). Effects of timing of atrial systole on LV filling and mitral valve closure: computer and dog studies. *Am J Physiol, 249*, H604–H619.
155. Brecker, S. J., Xiao, H. B., Sparrow, J., et al. (1992). Effects of dual-chamber pacing with short atrioventricular delay in dilated cardiomyopathy. *Lancet, 340*, 1308–1312.
156. Prinzen, F. W., Hunter, W. C., Wyman, B. T., et al. (1999). Mapping of regional myocardial strain and work during ventricular pacing: experimental study using magnetic resonance imaging tagging. *J Am Coll Cardiol, 33*, 1735–1742.
157. Wyman, B. T., Hunter, W. C., Prinzen, F. W., et al. (1999). Mapping propagation of mechanical activation in the paced heart with MRI tagging. *Am J Physiol, 276*, H881–H891.
158. Curry, C. C., Nelson, G. S., Wyman, B. T., et al. (2000). Mechanical dyssynchrony in dilated cardiomyopathy with intraventricular conduction delay as depicted by 3-D tagged magnetic resonance imaging. *Circulation, 101*, E2.
159. McVeigh, E. R., Prinzen, F. W., Wyman, B. T., et al. (1998). Imaging asynchronous mechanical activation of the paced heart with tagged MRI. *Magn Reson Med, 39*, 507–513.
160. Burkhoff, D., Oikawa, R. Y., & Sagawa, K. (1986). Influence of pacing site on canine left ventricular contraction. *Am J Physiol, 251*, H428–H435.
161. Park, R. C., Little, W. C., & O'Rourke, R. A. (1985). Effect of alteration of the left ventricular activation sequence on the left ventricular end-systolic pressure-volume relation in closed-chest dogs. *Circ Res, 57*, 706–717.
162. Liu, L., Tockman, B., Girouard, S., et al. (2002). Left ventricular resynchronization therapy in a canine model of left bundle branch block. *Am J Physiol Heart Circ Physiol, 282*, H2238–H2244.
163. Baller, D., Wolpers, H. G., Zipfel, J., et al. (1988). Comparison of the effects of right atrial, right ventricular apex and atrioventricular sequential pacing on myocardial oxygen consumption and cardiac efficiency: a laboratory investigation. *Pacing Clin Electrophysiol, 11*, 394–403.
164. Owen, C. H., Esposito, D. J., Davis, J. W., et al. (1998). The effects of ventricular pacing on left ventricular geometry, function, myocardial oxygen consumption, and efficiency of contraction in conscious dogs. *Pacing Clin Electrophysiol, 21*, 1417–1429.
165. Prinzen, F. W., Augustijn, C. H., Arts, T., et al. (1990). Redistribution of myocardial fiber strain and blood flow by asynchronous activation. *Am J Physiol, 259*, H300–H308.
166. Fananapazir, L., Cannon, R. O. I., Tripodi, D., et al. (1992). Impact of dual-chamber permanent pacing in patients with obstructive hypertrophic cardiomyopathy with symptoms refractory to verapamil and β-adrenergic blocker therapy. *Circulation, 85*, 2149–2161.
167. Cannon, R. O. I., Tripodi, D., Dilsizian, V., et al. (1994). Results of permanent dual-chamber pacing in symptomatic nonobstructive hypertrophic cardiomyopathy. *Am J Cardiol, 73*, 571–576.
168. Kass, D. A., Chen, C. H., Talbot, M. W., et al. (1999). Ventricular pacing with premature excitation for treatment of hypertensive-cardiac hypertrophy with cavity-obliteration (see comments). *Circulation, 100*, 807–812.
169. Maron, B. J., Nishimura, R. A., McKenna, W. J., et al. (1999). Assessment of permanent dual-chamber pacing as a treatment for drug-refractory symptomatic patients with obstructive hypertrophic cardiomyopathy. A randomized, double-blind, crossover study (M-PATHY). *Circulation, 99*, 2927–2933.
170. Nishimura, R. A., Trusty, J. M., Hayes, D. L., et al. (1997). Dual-chamber pacing for hypertrophic cardiomyopathy: a randomized, double-blind, crossover trial. *J Am Coll Cardiol, 29*, 435–441.
171. Blanc, J. J., Etienne, Y., Gilard, M., et al. (1997). Evaluation of different ventricular pacing sites in patients with severe heart failure: results of an acute hemodynamic study. *Circulation, 96*, 3273–3277.
172. Leclercq, C., Cazeau, S., Le Breton, H., et al. (1998). Acute hemodynamic effects of biventricular DDD pacing in patients with end-stage heart failure. *J Am Coll Cardiol, 32*, 1825–1831.
173. Auricchio, A., Stellbrink, C., Block, M., et al. (1999). Effect of pacing chamber and atrioventricular delay on acute systolic function of paced patients with congestive heart failure. The pacing therapies for congestive heart failure study group. The guidant congestive heart failure research group. *Circulation, 99*, 2993–3001.
174. Nelson, G. S., Curry, C. W., Wyman, B. T., et al. (2000). Predictors of systolic augmentation from left ventricular preexcitation in patients with dilated cardiomyopathy and intraventricular conduction delay. *Circulation, 101*, 2703–2709.
175. Nelson, G. S., Berger, R. D., Fetics, B. J., et al. (2000). Left ventricular or biventricular pacing improves cardiac function at diminished energy cost in patients with dilated cardiomyopathy and left bundle-branch block. *Circulation, 102*, 3053–3059.
176. Vanderheyden, M., Mullens, W., Delrue, L., et al. (2008). Endomyocardial upregulation of beta1 adrenoreceptor gene expression and myocardial contractile reserve following cardiac resynchronization therapy. *J Card Fail, 14*, 172–178.
177. Vanderheyden, M., Mullens, W., Delrue, L., et al. (2008). Myocardial gene expression in heart failure patients treated with cardiac resynchronization therapy responders versus nonresponders. *J Am Coll Cardiol, 51*, 129–136.
178. Iyengar, S., Haas, G., Lamba, S., et al. (2007). Effect of cardiac resynchronization therapy on myocardial gene expression in patients with nonischemic dilated cardiomyopathy. *J Card Fail, 13*, 304–311.
179. Chakir, K., Daya, S. K., Aiba, T., et al. (2009). Mechanisms of enhanced beta-adrenergic reserve from cardiac resynchronization therapy. *Circulation, 119*, 1231–1240.

CHAPTER 14

Alterations in Ventricular Function: Diastolic Heart Failure

Michael R. Zile and Catalin F. Baicu

Approximately half of all patients with chronic heart failure have a normal or near-normal (i.e., "preserved") left ventricular ejection fraction (HFPEF).[1-7] Because the dominant abnormality present in patients with HFPEF is abnormal diastolic function, this clinical syndrome is called "diastolic heart failure" (DHF). By contrast, the dominant abnormality present in patients with heart failure and a reduced ejection fraction (HFREF) is abnormal systolic function. This clinical syndrome is called "systolic heart failure" (SHF). In the context of this chapter, we will use the terms SHF and DHF unless otherwise specified.

The demographic characteristics present in patients with DHF differ significantly from those with SHF. Patients with DHF are older, are more often female, more often have hypertensive heart disease, and less often have ischemic heart disease than patients with SHF.[1-7] Morbidity and mortality rates in both SHF and DHF are extremely high; in patients with DHF rehospitalization rate for heart failure is 50% in 6 months, and annual mortality rate is 10% to 15%/year. (Detailed discussion of epidemiology of DHF can be found in Chapter 48).

Over the past 30 years, a multitude of randomized clinical trials (RCTs) in patients with SHF have demonstrated that a variety of pharmaceutical and device treatments have successfully lowered both morbidity and mortality in these patients. Unfortunately, the five RCTs that have examined a significant number of patients with DHF have failed to demonstrate efficacy of any management strategy.[8-12] (Detailed discussion of treatment of DHF can be found in Chapter 48).

The neutral results of the RCTs in DHF have left an enormous unmet need in at least half of all patients with chronic heart failure. Why have these RCTs failed to provide effective therapy? One possible reason may be that the mechanisms targeted by the therapies were not appropriate. If the underlying mechanisms causing the development of DHF differ from those that cause SHF, then it is likely that new management strategies must be developed that target mechanisms specific to patients with DHF. The purpose of this chapter is to describe the alterations in left ventricular and myocardial structure and function that occur in patients with DHF, define the mechanisms that underlie these functional abnormalities, and suggest how knowledge of these mechanisms can lead to the development of novel and effective treatments to correct diastolic dysfunction and decrease morbidity and mortality in patients with DHF.

DEFINITIONS

Differentiating Diastolic Dysfunction from Diastolic Heart Failure

Diastolic heart failure is a clinical syndrome characterized by symptoms and signs of increased tissue/organ water, and decreased tissue/organ perfusion. Standardized criteria to diagnose heart failure have been developed, perhaps the best validated of which came from the Framingham Study[13] (Table 14-1). Defining the mechanisms that cause this clinical syndrome requires measurement of both systolic and diastolic function. When heart failure is accompanied by a dominant abnormality in diastolic function, this clinical syndrome is called DHF (or HFPEF). From a conceptual perspective, diastolic heart failure occurs when the ventricular chamber is unable to accept an adequate volume of blood during diastole, do this at normal diastolic pressures, and at volumes sufficient to maintain an appropriate stroke volume and do this both at rest and during exercise. The functional abnormalities that result in DHF include abnormal ventricular relaxation and filling, decreased left ventricular (LV) suction, and/or an increase in ventricular stiffness. Diastolic heart failure can produce symptoms that occur at rest (NYHA Class IV), symptoms that occur with less than ordinary physical activity (NYHA Class III), or symptoms that occur with ordinary physical activity (NYHA Class II).

Diastolic dysfunction refers to a condition in which abnormalities in mechanical function are present during diastole. Abnormalities in diastolic function can occur in the presence or absence of a clinical syndrome of heart failure and with normal or abnormal systolic function. Therefore, whereas diastolic dysfunction describes an abnormal mechanical property, diastolic heart failure describes a clinical syndrome. Conceptually, diastole encompasses the time period during which the myocardium loses its ability to generate force and shorten, and returns to an unstressed length and force. By extension, diastolic dysfunction occurs when these processes are prolonged, slowed, or incomplete. Whether this time period is defined using the classical concepts of Wiggers or the constructs of Brutsaert, the measurements that reflect changes in this normal function generally depend on the onset, rate, and extent of left ventricular pressure decline and filling, and the relationship between pressure and volume or stress and strain during the period of diastole.[14] Moreover, if diastolic function is truly normal, these measurements must remain normal both at rest and during the stress of a variable heart rate, stroke volume, end-diastolic volume, and blood pressure.

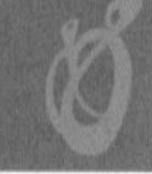

TABLE 14–1 Diagnostic Criteria for Diastolic Congestive Heart Failure

Required Criteria

1. Clinical evidence of left heart failure
   Framingham* or Boston criteria
   Plasma BNP and/or chest x-ray
   Cardiopulmonary exercise testing
2. Normal EF (≥50%)
3. Exclude nonmyocardial disease

Confirmatory Evidence

1. LVH or concentric remodeling
2. Left atrial enlargement (in absence of AF)
3. Doppler or catheterization evidence of LV diastolic dysfunction

Major	Minor
PND or orthopnea	Ankle edema
JVD or venous pressure >16 mm Hg	Nocturnal cough
Rales or acute pulmonary edema	Exertional dyspnea
Cardiomegaly	Pleural effusion
Hepatojugular reflex	Vital capacity <2/3 normal
Circulation time >25 sec	Hepatomegaly
Response to treatment (weight loss >4.5 kg/5 days) bpm	Tachycardia >120 bpm

*Framingham criteria: Two major or one major and two minor criteria must be present.

Heart Failure with a Preserved Ejection Fraction Versus Diastolic Heart Failure

HFPEF is a clinical syndrome characterized by symptoms and signs of heart failure, a preserved ejection fraction, and abnormal diastolic function. The term "preserved" EF refers to EFs that are normal or very near normal. "Normal" EF is a somewhat controversial notion. The average EF for a standard adult population is 60% to 65% with a lower boundary (2 standard deviations less than the mean) that approaches 50% to 55%. While some authors believe that 50% may be abnormal, an EF between 35% and 50% is clearly abnormal. EFs greater than 35% are often referred to as "preserved" in relation to EFs less than 35%. Most authors reserve the term "diastolic heart failure" for patients with an EF of 50% and clear evidence of diastolic dysfunction.

The use of the term HFPEF became necessary to describe heart failure populations studied in recent RCTs in which various lower limit boundaries for EF were allowed (between 35% and 50%)[8-12] (Figure 14-1). The focus of these studies was heart failure patients with an unmet need (i.e., those with no evidenced-based treatment to lower morbidity and mortality. These studies therefore broadened inclusion criteria to include patients with heart failure and an EF greater than 35% or greater than 40% or greater than 45%, all of which have now been grouped in HFPEF. These populations should be thought of as different from patients with heart failure and an EF of 50% (i.e., patients with DHF). Data from recent studies suggest that the epidemiology, natural history, and response to treatment in patients with heart failure and an EF between 35% and 50% are different from patients with heart failure and an EF of 50%.[8-12] In fact, it is becoming clearer that patients with heart failure and an EF between 35% and 50% share many or most characteristics with patients with heart failure and an EF less than 35%. Therefore, it may be more reasonable to group patients with EFs 35% to 50% into the HFREF group and conceptualize patients with CHF into two groups: SHF defined as heart failure with EF less than 50% and DHF defined as heart failure with EF of 50%.

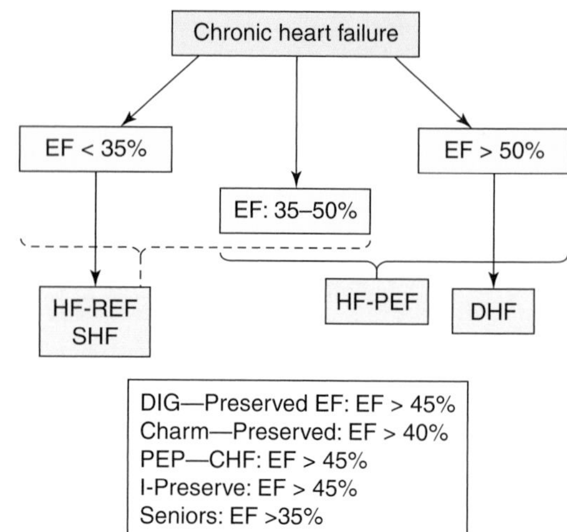

FIGURE 14–1 Ejection fraction (EF) determinants of heart failure categorizations. *HPEF,* heart failure with preserved EF; *HFREF,* heart failure with reduced EF; *SHF,* systolic heart failure; *DHF,* diastolic heart failure. Dig—Preserved,[9] Charm—Preserved,[8] PEP-CHF,[10, 11] seniors.[12]

DIAGNOSIS

European Society of Cardiology Diagnostic Criteria

The European Society of Cardiology recently published the following recommendations for DHF diagnostic criteria. The diagnosis of DHF requires the following conditions to be satisfied: (1) signs and symptoms of heart failure; (2) normal or mildly abnormal LV ejection fraction; (3) normal LV volume; and (4) evidence of diastolic LV dysfunction. Normal or mildly abnormal EF is an EF greater than 50% and a normal LV end-diastolic volume index (LVEDVI) is an LVEDVI less than 97 mL/m^2. Diagnostic evidence of diastolic LV dysfunction can be obtained invasively (LV end-diastolic pressure >16 mm Hg or mean pulmonary capillary wedge pressure >12 mm Hg) or noninvasively by Doppler (propagation velocity, transmitral flow velocity, pulmonary vein flow velocity) and tissue Doppler (mitral annular velocity, myocardial strain, or strain rate). Among the most common and well-validated indices of abnormal diastolic function is the ratio of early diastolic transmitral flow velocity (E) to early diastolic myocardial tissue Doppler velocity (E′). The E/E′ ratio serves as a good index of pulmonary capillary wedge pressure (PCWPP) with an E/E′ greater than 15 indicating a PCWP greater than 20 mm Hg (see also Chapter 36). If the E/E′ ratio is suggestive of diastolic LV dysfunction (E/E′ 8-15), additional noninvasive investigations are recommended for diagnostic evidence of diastolic LV dysfunction. These can consist of other Doppler measures of diastolic function, echo measures of LV mass index or left atrial volume index, electrocardiographic evidence of atrial fibrillation, or plasma levels of natriuretic peptides (BNP or NT-proBNP). If plasma levels of natriuretic peptides are elevated, additional confirmatory diagnostic evidence of diastolic LV dysfunction is recommended.

Lahey Clinic Criteria

Table 14-1 presents a pragmatic set of diagnostic criteria representing a synthesis of all existing guidelines.[16] To make the diagnosis of DHF, clear clinical evidence of heart failure must be present. This includes both signs and symptoms of heart failure (e.g., the Framingham or Boston criteria). The presence of clinical heart failure can be supported by elevated levels of plasma brain natriuretic peptide or specific abnormalities on the chest x-ray. Exercise limitation can be quantified by performing cardiopulmonary exercise testing. In addition to definite clinical evidence of heart failure, a normal ejection fraction is required. An EF lower limit cutoff value of greater than 50% is recommended. Evidence that confirms the diagnosis includes structural changes such as left ventricular hypertrophy or concentric remodeling. In addition, left atrial enlargement in the absence of atrial fibrillation or mitral valve disease is suggestive of increased LV diastolic pressures. Finally, echo Doppler or catheterization evidence of diastolic dysfunction can be used. Any one of these three confirms the diagnosis. Nonmyocardial diseases such as chronic obstructive lung disease must be excluded.

Natriuretic Peptides (see also Chapter 37)

A number of studies have suggested that brain natriuretic peptide (BNP or NT-ProBNP) could be used as a serum marker of increased diastolic pressures, abnormal diastolic function as evidenced by an abnormal echo-Doppler filling pattern, and the presence of diastolic heart failure.[17-22] To date, the evidence suggests that there is a good correlation between left ventricular diastolic, left atrial diastolic, and pulmonary venous pressures and the level of BNPs in patients with diastolic heart failure. However, the time course of change in BNP is not definitively known from the incident diastolic heart failure episode to a compensated convalescent condition. In addition, a clear discriminatory cutoff value with acceptable sensitivity, specificity, and predictive accuracy has not been firmly established. Nonetheless, BNP may prove to be useful as a serum marker indicating the presence of diastolic dysfunction, diastolic heart failure, or both. However, brain natriuretic peptide must be interpreted in the contexts that cause false-positive and false-negative. DHF may be absent in patients with an increased brain natriuretic peptide under the following circumstances: advanced age, renal insufficiency, atrial fibrillation, chronic lung disease, pulmonary embolism, and LVH. BNP levels are often higher in women than men. DHF may be present in patients with a normal brain natriuretic peptide under the following circumstances: obesity, after adequate treatment of DHF sufficient to normalize diastolic filling pressures. Future studies will examine the diagnostic potential of other plasma proteins, peptides, and microRNA.

MEASUREMENT OF DIASTOLIC FUNCTION IN PATIENTS WITH DHF

The dominant functional abnormality in patients with DHF is abnormal diastolic function. These functional abnormalities are associated with and may be causally related to chamber, cellular, and extracellular structural remodeling. In fact, differences in structural and functional remodeling have been used to characterize patients with DHF versus those with SHF (Table 14-2). Each of these differences is highlighted in this chapter.

Measurements of diastolic function can be divided into those that reflect the process of active relaxation and those that reflect passive stiffness. This division is in some ways arbitrary because structures and processes that alter relaxation and recoil can also result in measurable abnormalities in stiffness. However, this division is pragmatic and provides a necessary scaffold on which to develop methods of measurement. Measurements that reflect active relaxation and passive stiffness can be made both in vivo, using clinically applicable methods to examine the intact left ventricle, or in vitro, using experimental methods to examine isolated cardiomyocytes and isolated cardiac muscles. These in vitro measurements are important because they provide the methods by which the underlying basic mechanisms responsible for altering diastolic function can be defined. In this chapter, both in vivo and in vitro methods will be discussed.

TABLE 14–2 LV Structure and Function in Chronic Heart Failure

	Systolic Failure	Diastolic Failure
Remodeling		
End-diastolic volume	↑	Normal
End-systolic volume	↑	Normal
Mass	↑	↑
Geometry	Eccentric	Concentric
Cardiomyocyte	↑ Length	↑ Diameter
Extracellular matrix	↓ Collagen	↑ Collagen
LV Systolic Properties		
Performance		
Stroke volume	↓ (or normal)	Normal (or ↓)
Stroke work	↓	Normal
Function		
PR stroke work	↓	Normal
Ejection fraction	↓	Normal
Contractility		
(+)dP/dt	↓	Normal
End-systolic elastance	↓	Normal (or ↑)
Stress shortening	↓	Normal
Preload reserve	Exhausted	Limited
LV Diastolic Properties		
EDP	↑	↑
Tau	↑	↑
Chamber stiffness	↓	↑
Myocardial stiffness	Normal (or ↑)	↑

In Vivo Quantitation of Left Ventricle Chamber Diastolic Function

Relaxation

Diastole encompasses the time period during which the myocardium loses its ability to generate force and shorten and then returns to resting force and length. Relaxation occurs in a series of energy-consuming steps beginning with the release of calcium from troponin C, detachment of the actin-myosin cross-bridge, phosphorylation of phospholamban, sarcoplasmic reticulum calcium ATPase–induced calcium sequestration into the sarcoplasmic reticulum, sodium/calcium exchanger–induced extrusion of calcium from the cytoplasm, slowing of cross-bridge cycling rate, and extension of the sarcomere to rest length.[23-27] Adequate energy supplies and the mechanisms to regenerate them must be present for this process to occur at a sufficient rate and extent.[24-27] The rate and extent to which these cellular processes occur determine the

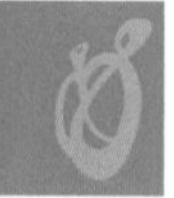

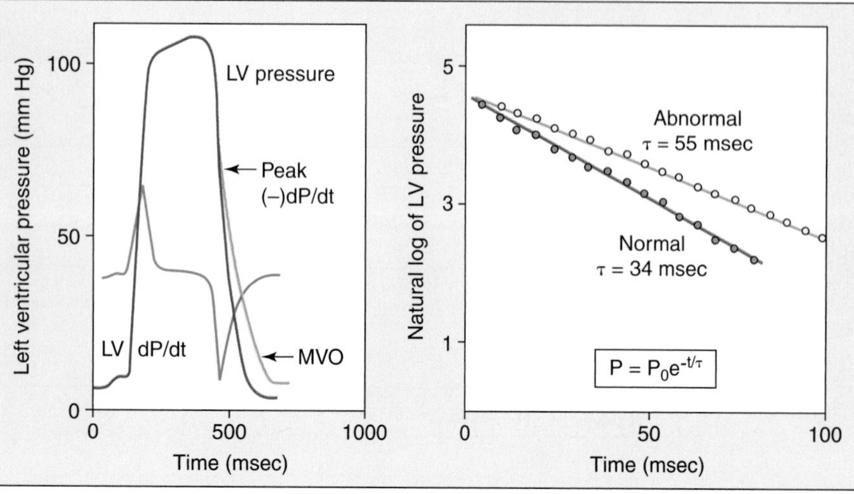

FIGURE 14–2 Schematic drawing of LV pressure and LV dP/dt showing methods used to quantitate isovolumic relaxation rate. The time constant of isovolumic pressure decline, tau (τ), is the inverse slope of the natural log of the pressure versus time relationship and can be calculated using the equation shown. Peak (−)dP/dt is the maximum rate of LV pressure decline. *MVO*, mitral valve opening. An example of a patient with normal relaxation is shown as solid lines; a patient with impaired and slowed relaxation is shown as dashed lines. Abnormal relaxation results in a decreased (−)dP/dt and an increased τ.

rate and extent of active ventricular relaxation. At the chamber level, this process results in LV pressure decline at a constant volume (isovolumic relaxation), then LV chamber filling that occurs with variable LV pressures (auxotonic relaxation). Measurements made during auxotonic relaxation are affected both by active relaxation and passive stiffness.

Isovolumic Relaxation

Isovolumic relaxation can be quantitated by measuring LV pressure using a high-fidelity micromanometer catheter and calculating the peak instantaneous rate of LV pressure decline, peak (−)dP/dt, and the time constant of isovolumic LV pressure decline, τ.[28-30] Peak (−)dP/dt is calculated as the first derivative of LV pressure with respect to time. It reflects a single instantaneous event that occurs very early during LV pressure decline. This value not only reflects changes in the isovolumic relaxation rate but also is affected by changes in mechanical factors such as preload, afterload, and heart rate. The relaxation time constant, τ, reflects the time course of LV pressure decline from peak (−)dP/dt to MVO. Tau is generally quantitated using a method which assumes that pressure declines in a monoexponential fashion. Because LV pressure is fit to monoexponential decay, the plot of the natural log of LV pressure versus time over this period forms a linear relation (Figure 14-2). τ is equal to the inverse slope of this linear relation. This relation can be expressed mathematically as $P = P_0e^{-t/\tau}$, where P is LV pressure, e is the base of the natural logarithm, t is the time in milliseconds after peak (−)dP/dt, and P_0 is the pressure at the time of peak (−)dP/dt.[28] Stated in more conceptual terms, τ is the time that it takes for LV pressure to fall by 1/e from its initial pressure (i.e., to fall by approximately two thirds of its initial value. When isovolumic pressure decline is slowed, τ is prolonged and the numeric value of τ increases. This method of calculating τ makes three assumptions: LV pressure decline is monoexponential, LV cavity pressure is equal to transmural pressure, and LV pressure will fall asymptotically to zero.[29] Alternative methods of calculating τ in which the zero pressure asymptote is not assumed to be zero include the derivative method and the use of a three-constant nonlinear regression analysis.[30] Comparison of these three methods has not demonstrated significant differences in interpretation of the effects of a pathological state on measurements of active relaxation.[30] τ, like peak (−) dP/dt is influenced by changes in loading conditions.[31] Therefore, no index of relaxation (isovolumic or auxotonic) including τ, can be considered an index of "intrinsic" relaxation rate unless loading conditions (and other modulators) are held constant or at least specified. One practical way to overcome this limitation is to examine indices of relaxation over a range of loads (Figure 14-3). Afterload can be altered acutely using mechanical or pharmacological methods. Abnormal relaxation is indicated by the shift in the position of the relaxation rate versus the afterload relationship where τ is prolonged at any equivalent systolic stress.[31] Therefore, indices of active relaxation must be measured at equivalent loading conditions or at least interpreted in light of differing loading conditions. A practical clinical application of this concept was proven in a recent clinical study in which a pharmacologically induced decrease in blood pressure resulted in an improvement in the relaxation rate.[32]

While active relaxation may, in the strictest sense, be regarded as an early "diastolic" event, the time of onset of this process depends, at least in part, upon "systolic" events such as the duration of contraction.[14] Conversely, the time of onset of relaxation can modify systolic events. Therefore the rate and extent of relaxation, in addition to being dependent on ventricular load, is also dependent on the duration of systole, the time of onset of relaxation, and the time during systole in which load is altered.[14,31,33] If the onset of relaxation is delayed, for example, by an increase in load early in systole, this may prolong the duration of systole, increase cardiac work during systole, and may prolong relaxation. Conversely, if the onset of relaxation occurs earlier, for example, because of an increase in load late in systole, this may shorten the duration of systole and may abbreviate relaxation. Thus a complex interaction between events traditionally considered to occur during "systole" can affect the measurement and interpretation of active relaxation.

Recoil/Suction

Normal LV relaxation is rapid and causes early LV diastolic pressures to fall toward and often reach zero. The resultant early transmitral pressure gradient plus the release of the potential energy created by systolic contraction create suction, or recoil that pulls blood from the left atrium toward the apex of the left ventricle. This normal recoil force can be quantitated from color m-mode echocardiography as the velocity of flow propagation (Vp). In patients with DHF, recoil is decreased because the release of the stored potential energy is apposed by the increased viscoelastic passive properties of the heart in DHF. As a consequence Vp declines, left atrial pressures rise, and blood is pushed rather than pulled into the left ventricle. While Vp is also reduced in patients with SHF, the mechanisms that underlie this abnormality are quite different. In SHF, contraction is notably reduced and therefore there are marked decreases in stored potential energy during systole and a resultant decrease in the recoil force available during diastole.

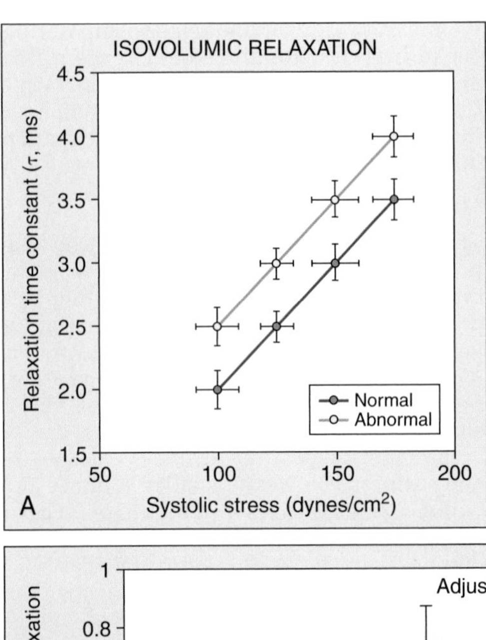

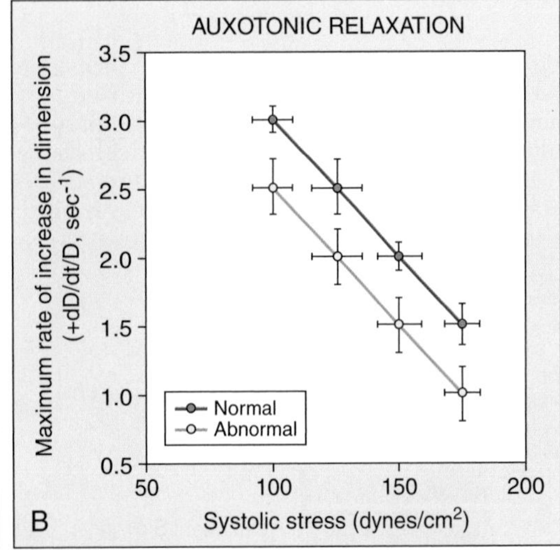

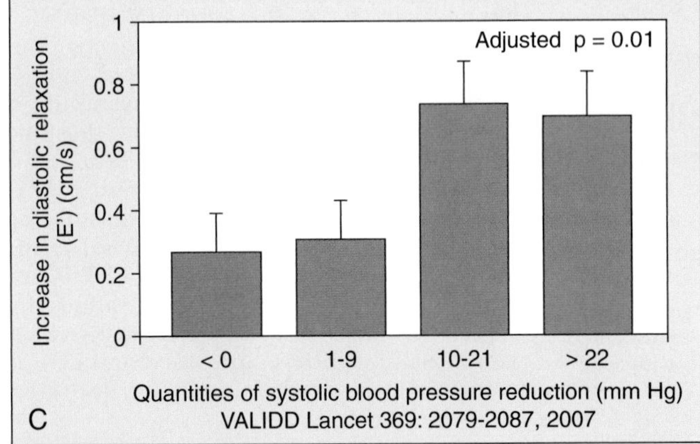

FIGURE 14–3 Examples of the relationship between indices of relaxation rate and afterload. The isovolumic time constant, τ (an index of isovolumic relaxation rate) versus LV systolic stress (an index of afterload) is plotted in **(A)**, maximum rate of increase in LV dimension, (+)dD/dt/D (an index of auxotonic diastolic filling rate) versus LV systolic stress is plotted in **(B)**. When relaxation is abnormal and slowed, both τ and (+)dD/dt/D are decreased at any equivalent systolic stress. The downward shift in these relationships indicate that relaxation is impaired. The results of the clinical study VALIDD **(C)**[32] showed that a decrease in blood pressure resulted in an increase in relaxation velocity.

Auxotonic Relaxation

The auxotonic LV filling phases of diastole can be characterized using Doppler-echocardiography, radionuclide, conductance, or MRI techniques. While each technique has advantages and disadvantages, all assess diastolic function by measuring indices of volume transients during ventricular filling. M-mode echocardiograms can be digitized to provide LV dimension versus time (dD/dt) or LV wall thickness versus time (dH/dt) data. Peak (+)dD/dt (dimension increasing) and peak (−)dH/dt (wall thinning) can be used as indices of an early auxotonic relaxation rate. In addition, LV cavity area from 2-D images can be digitized on a frame-by-frame basis with sufficient sampling frequency to examine cavity area versus time (dA/dt). If carried throughout diastolic filling, both early and late filling rates can be quantified. Transmitral LV inflow velocity during diastole can be assessed using Doppler echocardiography. This technique provides the means to assess temporal distribution of LV filling, provides indices of auxotonic filling rates, and provides indirect indices of LV chamber compliance. Early diastolic filling velocity (E wave), late diastolic filling velocity consequent to atrial contraction (A wave), the E/A ratio, E wave deceleration time, and A wave duration can be used to assess auxotonic relaxation. Radionuclide ventriculography can be used to derive time versus activity and/or time versus volume relationships from which indices of diastolic filling rate can be derived. Magnetic resonance imaging (MRI) can be used to measure transmitral flow velocities from which indices of diastolic filling rate can be derived. In addition MRI tagging can provide measurements of myocardial strain and strain rate, and twist and untwist rates. Likewise recent advances in tissue Doppler methods and strain rate imaging have provided new tools for assessment of diastolic filling and diastolic filling pressure assessment. Tissue Doppler imaging (TDI) is based on measurements of regional length and velocity, which, when normalized to initial length, can be used to derive strain and strain rate.

However, like all relaxation indices, all auxotonic indices must be interpreted in light of simultaneous changes in load, both afterload and filling load (load present during filling).[14,35,36] For example, the precise pattern of early and late diastolic transmitral flow velocities will depend on factors governing instantaneous atrial and LV pressures before and after mitral valve opening and the resultant atrial-ventricular pressure gradient (filling load). It is thus not surprising that interventions or pathological conditions that increase left atrial pressure increase early transmitral flow velocities, while interventions that reduce left atrial pressure also reduce early filling velocities. To correctly interpret changes in transmitral flow velocities, concomitant changes in filling load must be considered. These considerations can now be provided by tissue Doppler and pulmonary venous Doppler and color m-mode velocities using the scheme shown in Figure 14-6.[37]

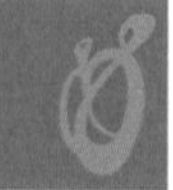

Stiffness

In addition to active relaxation, passive viscoelastic properties contribute to the process that returns the myocardium to its resting force and length. These passive viscoelastic properties are dependent both on intracellular and extracellular structures (see "Mechanisms" section). Changes in the stiffness of the ventricular chamber can be assessed by examining the pressure and volume relationship during diastole. Chamber stiffness is determined both by the stiffness of the constituent myocardium and LV mass and the LV mass/volume ratio. Changes in myocardial stiffness can be assessed by examining the myocardial stress, strain, and strain rate relationships during diastole.

FIGURE 14–4 Schematic and examples of color M-mode propagation velocity demonstrating changes in diastolic suction in patients with systolic heart failure (SHF) versus diastolic heart failure (DHF). *LV,* left ventricular; *DP,* diastolic pressure; *LAP,* left atrial pressure.

Chamber Stiffness

Chamber stiffness can be quantified by examining the relationship between diastolic LV pressure and volume. LV diastolic pressure can be changed either by a volume-dependent change in instantaneous operating stiffness or by a volume-independent change in the overall chamber stiffness (Figure 14-7). The instantaneous operating stiffness at any point along a given pressure-volume curve is equal to the slope of a tangent drawn to the curve at that point (dP/dV) (see Figure 14-7). Operating stiffness changes throughout filling, and stiffness is lower at smaller volumes and higher at larger volumes (see Figure 14-7 point a to point b, volume-dependent change in diastolic pressure and stiffness). Obtaining sufficient data to characterize the entire LV diastolic pressure versus volume curve may be difficult using currently available methods. At a minimum, an index of end-diastolic operating stiffness may be determined by examining the ratio of end-diastolic pressure (EDP) versus end-diastolic volume (EDV). Under some circumstances, end-diastolic operating stiffness may reflect overall chamber stiffness. For example, if EDP is increased with a normal EDV, end-diastolic operating stiffness (and likely overall chamber stiffness) is increased (Figures 14-7 and 14-8, as seen in DHF). If EDP is normal and EDV is increased, end-diastolic operating stiffness (and likely overall chamber stiffness) is decreased (see Figures 14-7 and 14-8, as seen in SHF). If EDP is increased and EDV is also increased, stiffness may be normal, increased, or decreased. In this later

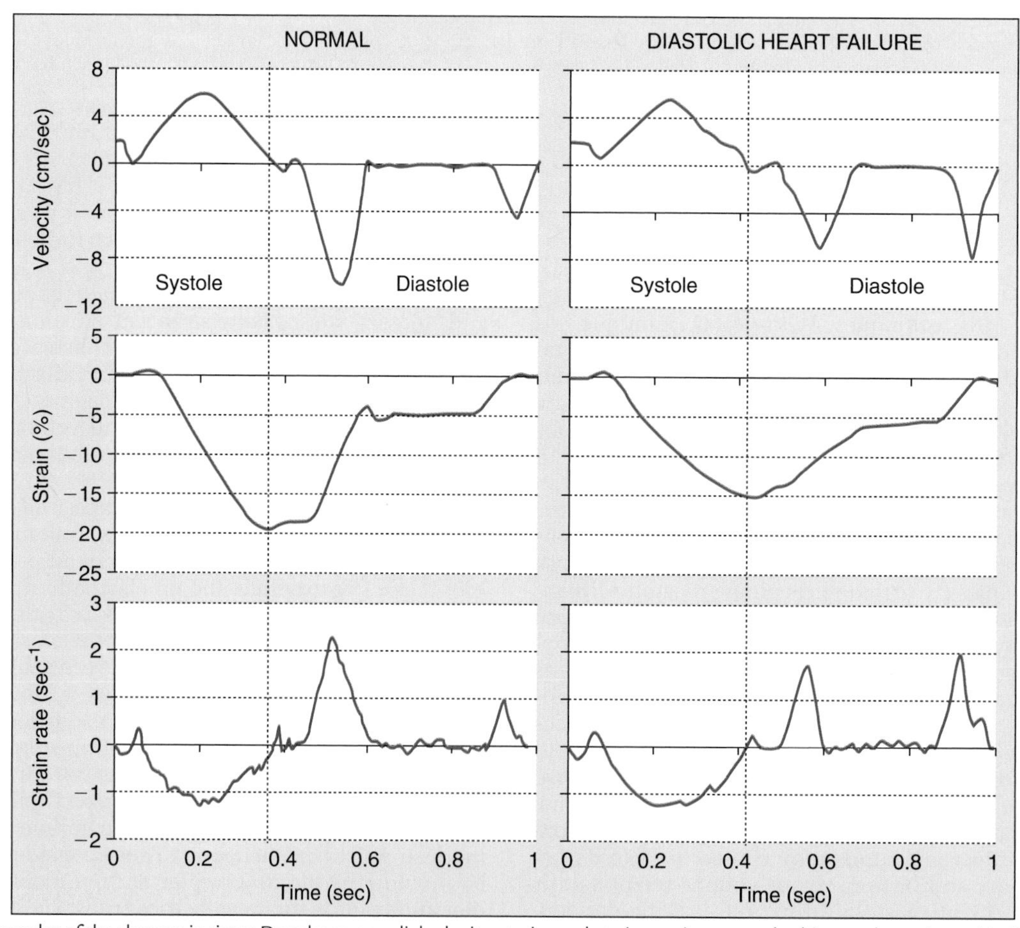

FIGURE 14–5 Examples of the changes in tissue Doppler myocardial velocity, strain, and strain rate in a normal subject and a patient with diastolic heart failure.

condition, measuring the entire pressure-volume relationship becomes essential in determining overall chamber stiffness. The shape and position of the entire pressure-volume relationship can be used to calculate an overall chamber stiffness constant (see Figure 14-7). Because the diastolic pressure-volume relationship is curvilinear and generally exponential, the relationship between dP/dV and pressure is linear, the slope (K_c) is called the "modulus of chamber stiffness" (or "chamber stiffness constant") and can be used as a single numeric value to quantitate overall chamber stiffness. K_c can be represented mathematically using a monoexponential equation: $P = P_0 e^{K_c V}$, where P is LV pressure, V is LV volume, P_0 is LV pressure at equilibrium volume, and K_c is the chamber stiffness constant. When overall chamber stiffness is increased, the pressure-volume curve shifts to the left, the slope of the dP/dV versus pressure relationship becomes steeper, and K_c is increased (volume-independent change in diastolic pressure and stiffness).[30,31] Thus diastolic pressure can be changed either by a volume-dependent change in instantaneous operating stiffness or by a volume-independent change in the overall chamber stiffness. In patients with DHF, a number of recent studies have shown that both the overall diastolic chamber stiffness and end-diastolic operative stiffness are significantly increased compared with normal control subjects.

Diastolic pressure versus volume (and stress vs. strain, described later) relationships can be derived from a single cardiac cycle or from multiple cardiac cycles. Using a single cardiac cycle, pressure versus volume coordinates during a single diastole—from mitral valve opening to mitral valve closure—must be obtained. Using multiple cardiac cycles, end-diastolic values are obtained from cardiac cycles in which end-diastolic volume or pressure are altered using pharmacological or mechanical means. To accurately compare indices of chamber stiffness between pathological states, these indices must be derived from data that share common ranges of pressure. Specifically, the range of pressure over which stiffness is calculated must be similar in each left ventricle.

A multitude of recent studies has shown definitively that LV chamber stiffness is increased in patients with DHF.[38-43] In patients with DHF, LV diastolic pressures are increased at normal LV diastolic volumes, the diastolic pressure-volume curves are shifted up and to the left, and the chamber stiffness constants are increased (Figure 14-9). By comparison, patients with SHF have been shown to have LV diastolic pressure volume curves that are shifted down and to the right with decreased chamber stiffness constants.

Myocardial Stiffness

Cardiac muscle behaves as a viscoelastic material, developing a resisting force (stress, ε) as myocardial length is increased (strain, ε) by ventricular filling. Strain is the deformation (increased length) of the muscle produced by the application of a force (increased stress). Strain (ε) is generally expressed as the percent change in length (L) from the unstressed length. Using Lagrangian strain, the unstressed length (L_0) is equal to the equilibrium length (i.e., the length of the muscle when subjected to no external forces). Myocardial stiffness can be quantitated by examining the relationship between myocardial stress and strain during diastole (see Figure 14-7). At any given strain, myocardial stiffness is equal to the slope (dσ/dε) of a tangent drawn to the stress-strain relationship at that strain. Because the stress-strain relationship is curvilinear and exponential, the relationship between dσ/dε and stress

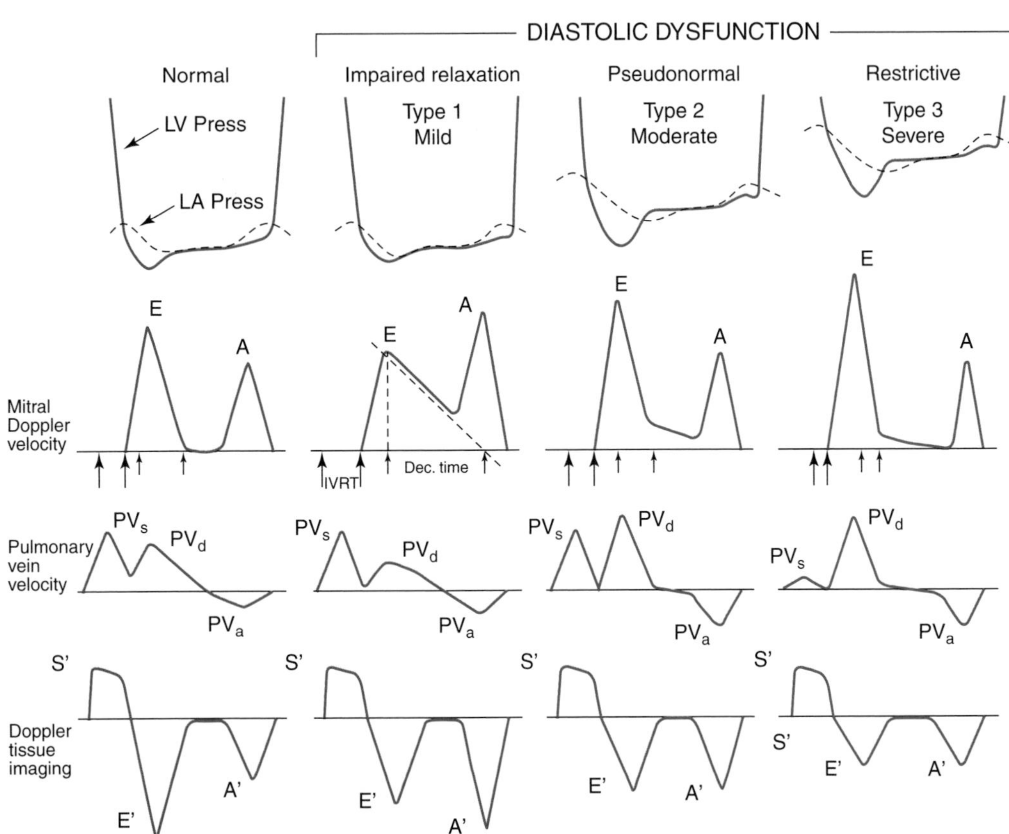

FIGURE 14–6 Schematic drawing of left ventricular (LV) and left atrial (LA) pressures during diastole, transmitral Doppler LV inflow velocity, pulmonary vein Doppler velocity, and Doppler tissue velocity. *IVRT,* isovolumic relaxation time; *dec. time,* e wave deceleration time; *E,* early LV filling velocity; *A,* velocity of LV filling contributed by atrial contraction; *PVs,* systolic pulmonary vein velocity; *PVd,* diastolic pulmonary vein velocity; *PVa,* pulmonary vein velocity resulting from atrial contraction; *S',* myocardial velocity during systole; *E',* myocardial velocity during early filling; *A',* myocardial velocity during filling produced by atrial contraction.

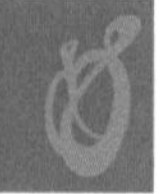

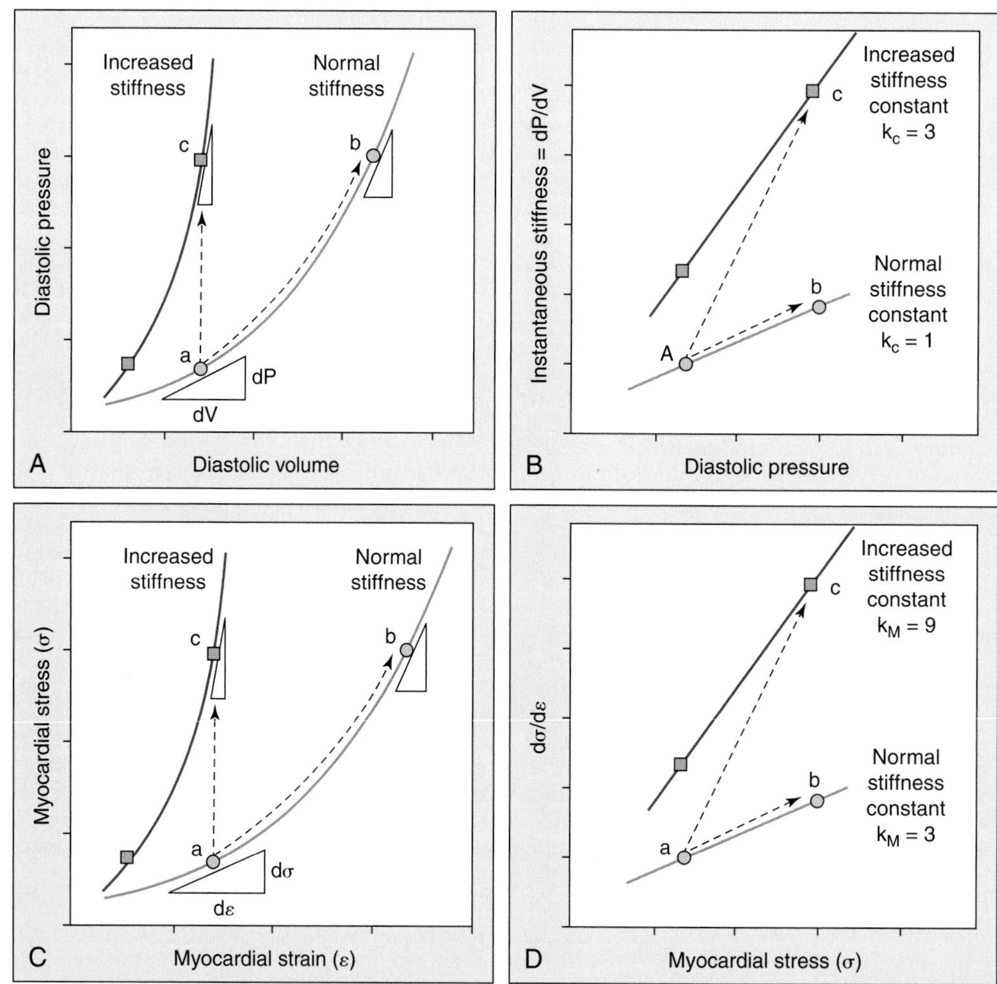

FIGURE 14–7 Schematic drawing of the LV diastolic pressure versus volume relationship showing methods used to quantitate chamber stiffness; K_c is the chamber stiffness constant **(A** and **B)**. Schematic drawing of the myocardial diastolic stress versus strain relationship showing methods used to quantitate myocardial stiffness; K_m is the myocardial stiffness constant **(C** and **D)**.

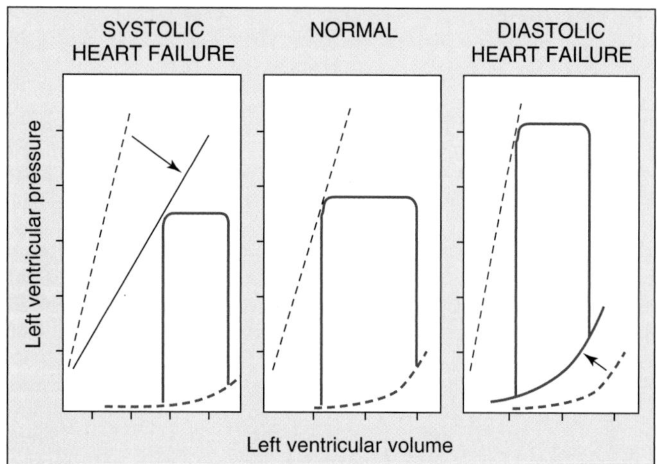

FIGURE 14–8 Schematic pressure-volume loops contrasting diastolic heart failure **(C)** with systolic heart failure **(A)** and normal **(B)**. The dashed lines represent end-systolic elastance. The dotted lines represent diastolic stiffness (or distensibility).

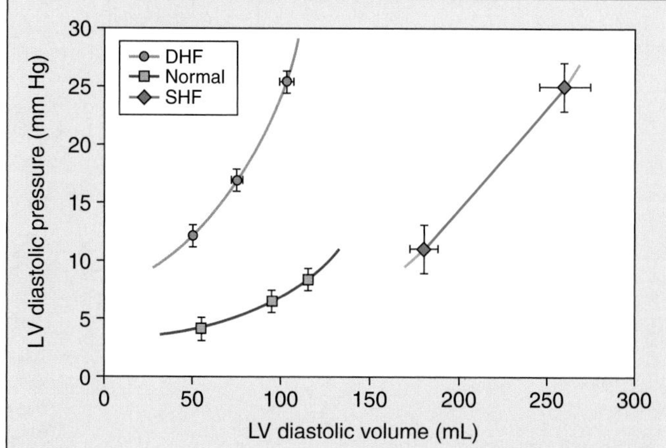

FIGURE 14–9 Diastolic pressure versus volume data from normal control subjects, patients with systolic heart failure (SHF), and diastolic heart failure (DHF). LV chamber stiffness was increased in DHF and decreased in SHF patients.

is linear and the slope of this relation, K_m, is the modulus of myocardial stiffness (or myocardial stiffness constant). When myocardial stiffness is increased, the stress-strain relationship shifts to the left, so that for any given change in myocardial length (strain), there is a greater increase in force (wall stress) that develops to resist this deformation. In addition, the slope of the dσ/dε versus stress relationship becomes steeper and K_m increases when myocardial stiffness is increased. K_m can be represented mathematically using a monoexponential equation: $\sigma = \sigma_0 (e^{K_m \varepsilon})$, σ = LV wall stress, ε = strain, σ_0 is stress at zero strain and K_m is the elastic stiffness constant.[30,31] Comparison of myocardial stiffness using

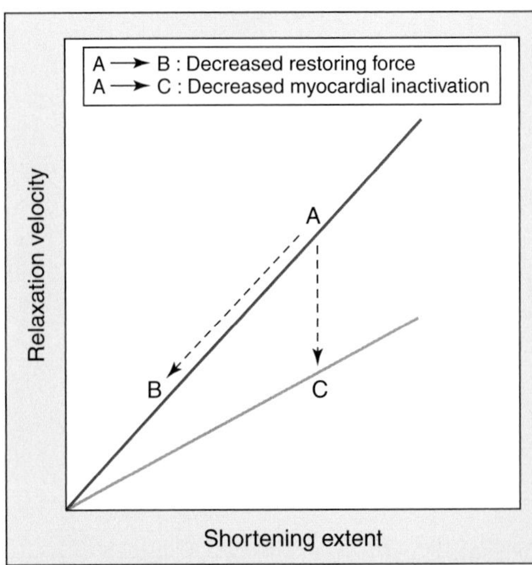

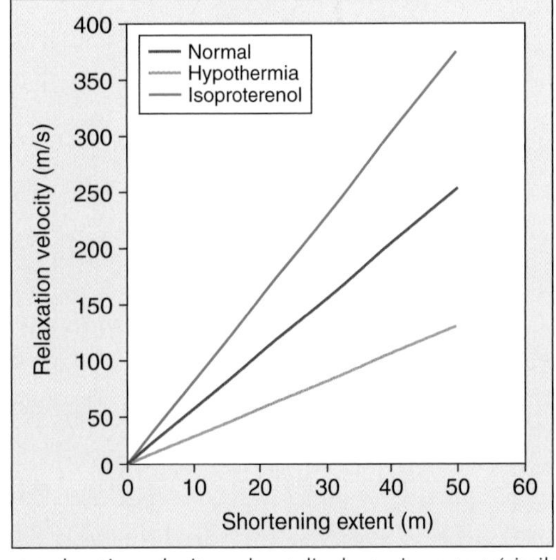

FIGURE 14–10 Example of the direct linear relationship between cardiomyocyte relaxation velocity and systolic shortening extent (similar techniques can be applied to isolated cardiac muscles). In a normal cardiomyocyte (*solid line*) relaxation, velocity decreases when shortening extent is decreased because there is a decrease in restoring force. In an abnormal cardiomyocyte (*dashed lines*), relaxation velocity is decreased to a value less than normal at any equal shortening extent because of a decrease in myocardial inactivation. Hypothermia caused a decrease in myocardial inactivation and decreased the slope of the relaxation velocity versus shortening extent relationship. Isoproterenol caused an increase in myocardial inactivation and increased the slope of the relaxation velocity versus shortening extent relationship.

these methods is only appropriate when the calculations are made over common ranges of LV wall stress.

In Vitro Quantitation of Diastolic Function

Relaxation

The process of relaxation can be measured in vitro in isolated muscle tissue or isolated cardiomyocytes. Isometric force decline and isotonic lengthening rates can be measured in an isolated muscle. In contrast, only the isotonic lengthening rate can be assessed in an isolated cardiomyocyte.[52-56] However, it should be noted that these in vitro indices of active relaxation, like the in vivo indices, must be interpreted in light of simultaneous changes in load. For example, the cardiomyocyte isotonic lengthening rate may be decreased by two possible mechanisms: (1) a decrease in restoring force or (2) abnormal myocardial inactivation (Figure 14-10). Restoring forces are created during contraction when potential energy is stored by deformation in cellular structures. This potential energy changes into kinetic energy during diastole and acts to restore the cardiomyocyte to rest or equilibrium length. Changes in myocardial inactivation alter lengthening rate independent of concomitant changes in restoring force. Studies have shown that examining the relaxation velocity versus shortening extent relationship (see Figure 14-10) provides an analytic method to distinguish between these two factors.[54-56]

If a given pathological process causes the relaxation velocity to change along a common relationship between relaxation velocity and shortening extent (see panel *A*, Figure 14-10, from point A to point B), this indicates that these changes were caused by alterations in restoring forces that occurred concomitantly with alterations in systolic function. In contrast, if a pathological process causes the relaxation velocity to change along a distinctly different relationship (see panel *A*, Figure 14-8, from point A to point C), this would indicate that there had been changes in the rate of myocardial inactivation. Two interventions (hypothermia and isoproterenol) known to produce primary alterations in myocardial inactivation were examined in normal cardiomyocytes[54-56] (see Figure 14-8, panel *B*). During hypothermia, the slope of the relaxation velocity versus shortening extent relationship decreased such that for any given shortening extent, relaxation velocity was less at 30° C than at 37° C.[54-56] During isoproterenol infusion, the slope of the relaxation velocity versus the shortening extent relationship increased significantly.[54-56] Thus the slope of the relaxation velocity versus the shortening extent relationship is sensitive to and dependent on changes in the rate of myocardial inactivation. This analytical method can be applied to isolated cardiomyocyte and muscle preparations.

Viscoelastic Stiffness

A number of mechanical and bioengineering models and experimental designs have been used to describe the constitutive material viscoelastic properties of myocardial tissue and cardiomyocytes.[57-59] One such method, applicable to both isolated cardiac muscle and cardiomyocyte consists of a two-element model composed of a nonlinear spring in parallel with a nonlinear viscous damper. Conceptually, the passive elastic spring consists of structures or processes that resist deformation in a time-independent manner (i.e., it resists deformation to the same extent irrespective of the rate of deformation). The viscous damper consists of structures or processes that resist stretch in a time-dependent manner (i.e., it resists deformation to a greater extent when the rate of deformation is increased). While this kind of analysis is difficult to perform in vivo, it can be done in vitro. There are a number of important reasons to examine elastic stiffness and viscous damping, separately and independently. This kind of analysis may provide clues to which specific cellular or extracellular mechanism is altered by a particular pathological state and which specific mechanism leads to changes in diastolic function.

To calculate elastic stiffness (β) and viscous damping (η) constants, measurements of muscle or cardiomyocyte stress, strain, and strain rate are obtained using uniaxial variable rate stretches (Figure 14-11). These data can be fit by a constitutive equation for a nonlinear viscoelastic composite biomaterial where $\sigma(\varepsilon,\varepsilon') = (Ae^{\beta\varepsilon} + B) + (C - De^{\eta\varepsilon'})$, and A, B, C, and D are curve fitting constants. The elastic stiffness constant is assessed using the slowest uniaxial stretch. Under these conditions, strain rate approximates zero, the second portion of the equation equation $(C - De^{\eta\varepsilon'})$ becomes constant, stress becomes a function of strain alone, and β can be determined. When elastic stiffness is increased, the σ versus ε relationship shifts up and left and β increases (see Figure 14-11). The

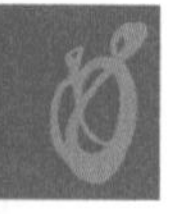

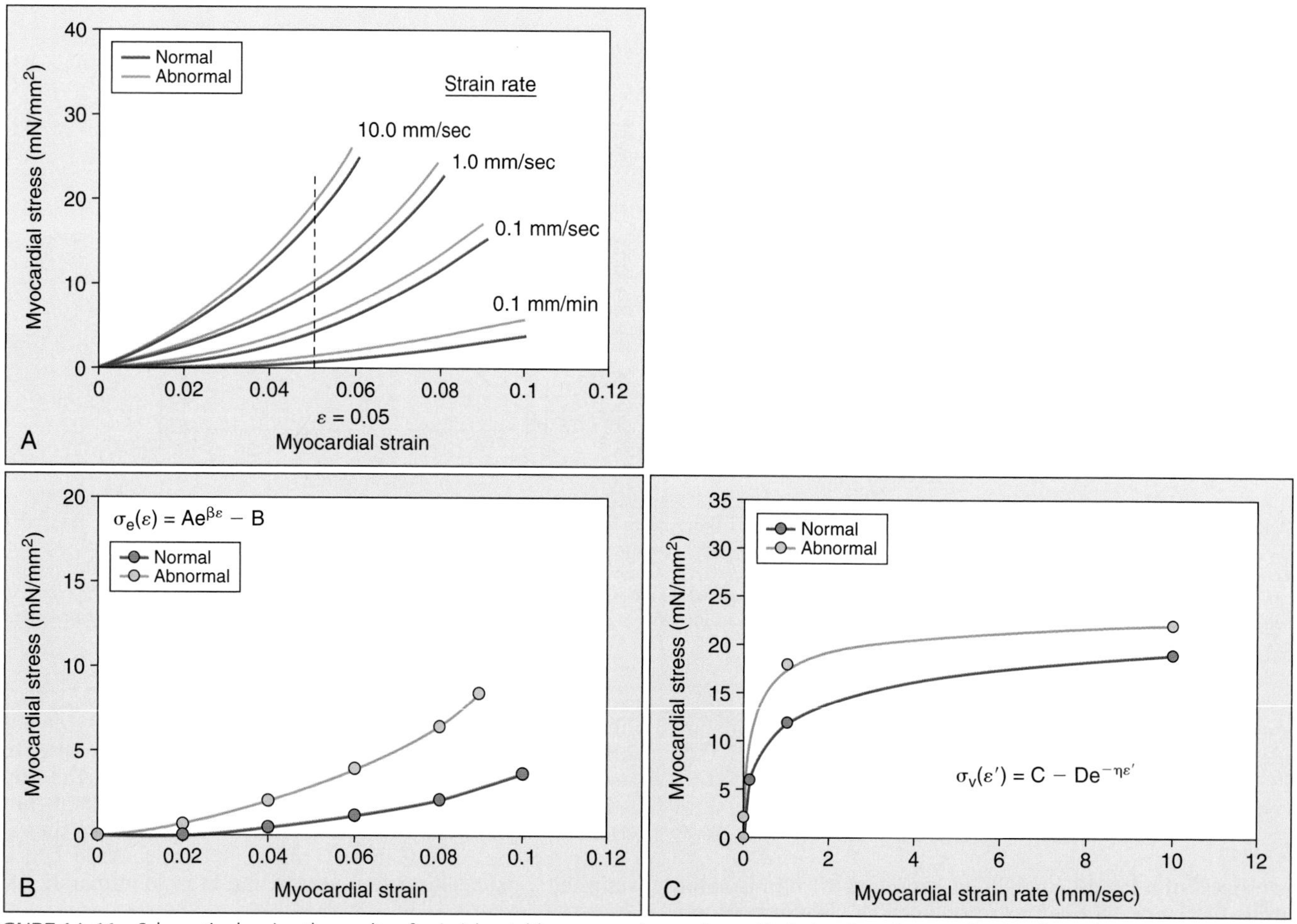

FIGURE 14–11 Schematic showing the results of uniaxial variable rate stretches performed in isolated cardiac muscles (similar techniques can be applied to isolated cardiomyocytes) **(A)**. Stress, strain, and strain rate data obtained from these methods can be used to calculate elastic stiffness and viscous damping constants. Stress versus strain data at the lowest strain rate **(B)** were fit to the equation shown to calculate the elastic stiffness constant. Stress versus strain rate data at constant strain **(C)** were fit to the equation shown to calculate the viscosity constant.

viscous damping constant is assessed using all four uniaxial variable rate stretches. From these stretches, the relationship between stress and strain rate is defined at constant strain. At any selected constant strain, the relationship between stress and strain rate is curvilinear. Under these experimental conditions, strain is constant, the first portion of the equation ($Ae^{\beta\varepsilon} + B$) becomes constant, and stress becomes a function of strain rate alone. Therefore, the stress versus strain rate data can be fit to the equation, and η determined. When viscous damping is increased, the σ versus ε' relationship shifts up and η increases (see Figure 14-9).

Recent studies were performed in patients with DHF in which cardiomyocytes were isolated from myocardial biopsies and the cardiomyocyte stiffness properties measured. These studies showed that myocardial stiffness and cardiomyocytes are increased in patients with DHF.[47-51]

MEASUREMENT OF SYSTOLIC PROPERTIES IN PATIENTS WITH DHF

There is an emerging consensus that the most important functional abnormalities in patients with DHF are the dominant abnormalities in diastolic function. However, questions have been raised about concomitant abnormalities in systolic function and arterial stiffness. To determine whether and to what extent patients with DHF have abnormalities in the systolic properties of the left ventricle, load and remodeling independent indices were examined in a study by Baicu et al. Many such indices have been proposed, but there is no single, universally applicable index of systolic properties that is independent of load and remodeling (see also Chapter 13).[60,61] It was hypothesized that if multiple indices are measured and if the results are in general agreement and viewed in aggregate, it should be possible to determine whether patients with DHF have significant abnormalities in the systolic properties of the left ventricle. Accordingly, a full assessment of the contractile behavior of the ventricle required measuring the combined indices that reflect LV systolic performance, function, and contractility, and global and regional function were examined in a group of patients with DHF.[60]

Ventricular performance is a term that is used to describe the pumping ability of the left ventricle. The performance of the ventricle as a pump may be assessed by measuring the pressure developed by the ventricle, the stroke volume ejected by the ventricle, or preferably the stroke work generated by the ventricle. Stroke work can be determined invasively in the catheterization laboratory or estimated noninvasively with the use of echocardiographically measured stroke volume multiplied by the mean arterial pressure. A limitation of the noninvasive method is that total pressure (i.e., peak systolic pressure) rather than developed pressure (i.e., LV systolic pressure minus end-diastolic pressure) is often used; this results in an overestimation of the work performed by the ventricle. Thus stroke work calculated as the product of developed pressure and stroke volume credits the ventricle for pressure and shortening work in a single integrated index. To date, studies have shown that patients with

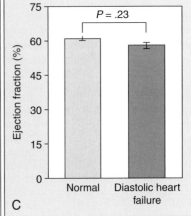

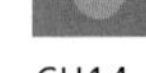
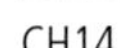

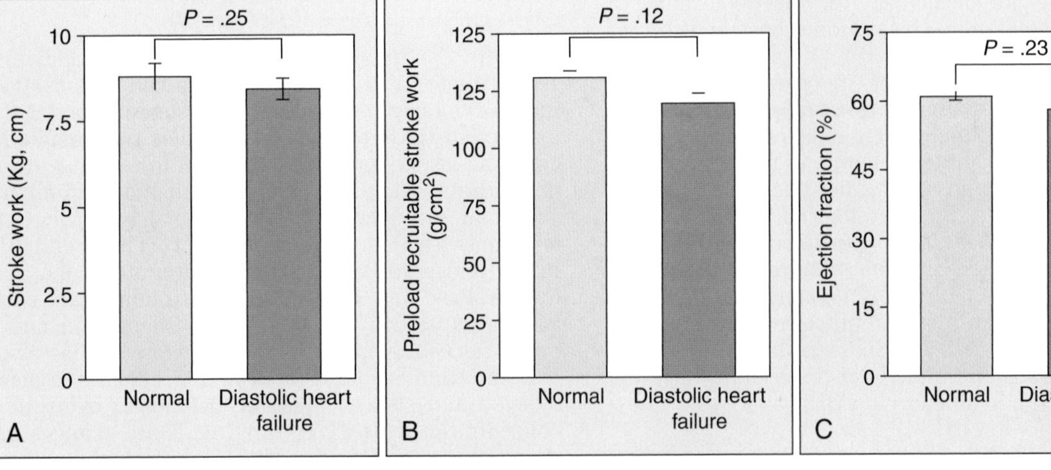

CONTRACTILITY

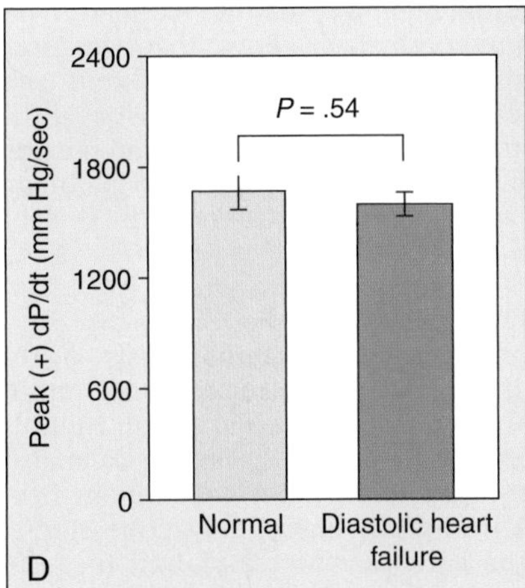

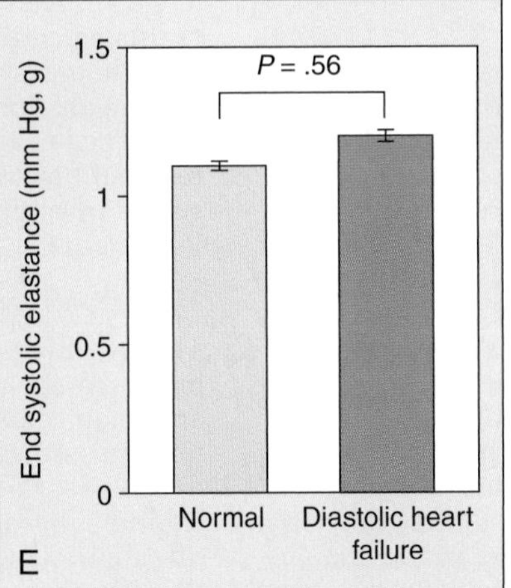

FIGURE 14–12 Systolic properties in normal control subjects and patients with diastolic heart failure (DHF). Each measurement of LV systolic chamber performance, function, and contractility was normal in the DHF patients.

DHF have normal stroke work compared with normal control subjects (Figure 14-12).[60]

A classic *ventricular function* curve can be constructed by plotting coordinates of performance (e.g., stroke work) against an index of preload (e.g., end-diastolic pressure or volume). When contractility is increased, the stroke work versus preload relationship is shifted upward, and when contractility is decreased, the relationship is shifted downward. A family of such ventricular function curves credits the ventricle for pressure development and ejection, and, importantly, it incorporates load and contractility. Thus plots of stroke work against preload allow construction of a Frank-Starling ventricular function curve or a preload recruitable stroke work relationship.[60] To date, studies have shown that patients with DHF have normal stroke work versus preload and normal preload recruitable stroke work compared with normal control subjects (see Figure 14-12).[60]

The term *ventricular contractility* refers to the contractile or inotropic state of the whole ventricle. Indices of ventricular contractility have conventionally been divided into isovolumic phase indices (e.g., peak positive dP/dt), ejection phase indices (e.g., systolic wall stress versus endocardial shortening), and indices determined at the end of ejection (e.g., end-systolic elastance). The concept of ventricular contractility is similar to that of myocardial contractility, but all indices of ventricular contractility are inextricably linked to and influenced by loading conditions and ventricular remodeling. Only if loading conditions and ventricular remodeling are considered or incorporated in the analysis can these parameters of "function" reflect changes in ventricular "contractility." For example, peak positive dP/dt can be altered by an acute change in preload, but the influence of chronic geometric changes and remodeling on dP/dt is not well defined. By contrast, systolic elastance is not affected by acute changes in preload (it is determined by altering load); however, systolic elastance is affected by chronic changes in LV volume and mass. It is for this reason that indices of end-systolic elastance should be normalized for the LV mass/volume ratio. To date, studies have shown that patients with DHF have normal dP/dt, endocardial fractional shortening versus mean systolic stress relationship, and normal mass/volume corrected end-systolic elastance compared with normal control subjects (see Figure 14-12).[60]

In summary, every index of LV systolic performance, function, and contractility examined to date was normal in DHF patients compared with normal controls.

Some studies have shown that arterial stiffness estimated as Ea is increased in DHF patients compared with controls; however, the arterial-ventricular coupling index, Ea/Ees ratio, was not different in DHF patients than in controls. In addition, when patients with hypertension-induced LVH but no DHF were compared with patients with hypertensive LVH and DHF, there were no differences in arterial stiffness.[60,42]

Patients with DHF may have some detectable abnormalities in LV systolic properties despite the presence of a normal ejection fraction.[62-68] It has been suggested that these

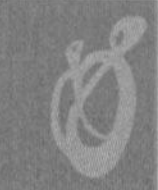

abnormalities of LV systolic properties constitute an important pathophysiological mechanism for the occurrence of heart failure in these patients. This notion is based on studies that examined the extent and velocity of LV long-axis shortening, mitral annular systolic velocity, myocardial strain, and strain rate. However, it is likely that these measurements, like all indices of LV systolic function, are affected by alterations in LV loading conditions and geometry, and changes in contractility. In addition, it is possible, if not likely, that some of these indices of LV systolic function reflect changes in ventricular remodeling independent of changes in contractility.[69-71]

Therefore, we conclude that the dominant functional abnormality in patients with DHF is abnormal diastolic function. These changes in diastolic function along with the concomitant changes in left ventricle, cardiomyocyte, and extracellular matrix structure (see later discussion) form the substrate from which patients develop DHF.

STRUCTURAL CHANGES IN PATIENTS WITH DHF

The hearts of patients with systolic heart failure differ dramatically from those of patients with diastolic heart failure in regard to both gross and microscopical anatomical features (Figures 14-13 and 14-14). These anatomical differences tend to parallel physiological and functional differences in systolic and diastolic heart failure[72-78] (see Table 14-2). Patients with diastolic heart failure generally exhibit a concentric pattern of LV remodeling and hypertrophic process that is characterized by a normal or near-normal end-diastolic volume, increased wall thickness, and high ratio of mass to volume with a high ratio of wall thickness to chamber radius. By contrast, patients with systolic heart failure exhibit a pattern of eccentric remodeling with an increase in end-diastolic volume, little increase in wall thickness, and substantial decrease in the ratio of mass to volume and thickness to radius. The aforementioned dramatic differences in organ morphology and geometry are paralleled by anatomical differences at the microscopic level. As shown in Figure 14-14, in diastolic heart failure the cardiomyocyte exhibits an increased diameter, and there is an increase in the amount of collagen with a corresponding increment in the width and continuity of the fibrillar components of the extracellular matrix.[72-78] By contrast, in systolic heart failure, the cardiomyocytes are elongated, and there are degradation and disruption of the fibrillar collagen.[72-78]

MECHANISMS CAUSING DIASTOLIC DYSFUNCTION

Conceptually the mechanisms causing abnormalities in diastolic function that lead to the development of diastolic heart failure can be divided into factors intrinsic to the myocardium itself (myocardial) and factors that are extrinsic to the myocardium (extramyocardial) (Box 14-1). Myocardial factors can be divided into structures and processes within the cardiac muscle cell (cardiomyocyte), within the extracellular matrix (ECM) that surrounds the cardiac muscle cell, and those that activate the autocrine or paracrine production of neurohormones.

Abnormalities in diastolic function can be caused by changes in extramyocardial mechanisms such as acute changes in (1) hemodynamic loading conditions including an increase in afterload caused by hypertension and (2) heterogeneity, either asynchrony or asynergy, caused by coronary artery disease. In addition, chronic changes in these extramyocardial factors can result in changes in the myocardial factors discussed next.

Cardiomyocyte

Calcium Homeostasis (see also Chapter 3)

Diastolic dysfunction can be caused by mechanisms that are intrinsic to the cardiac muscle cells themselves. These include changes in calcium homeostasis caused by (1) abnormalities in the sarcolemmal channels responsible for short- and long-term extrusion of calcium from the cytosol such as the sodium calcium exchanger and the calcium pump; (2) abnormal sarcoplasmic reticulum calcium (SR Ca^{++}) reuptake caused by a decrease in SR Ca^{++} ATPase; and (3) changes in the phosphorylation state of the proteins that modify SR Ca^{++} ATPase function such as phospholamban, calmodulin, and calsequestrin (Figure 14-15). Changes in any of these processes can result in increased cytosolic diastolic calcium concentration, prolongation in the calcium transient, and delayed and slowed diastolic decline in cytosolic calcium concentration (see Figure 14-15). These changes have been shown to occur in cardiac disease and cause abnormalities in both active relaxation and passive stiffness.[23] Studies in pathological myocardium such as pressure overload hypertrophy or dilated cardiomyopathy have shown that alterations in calcium homeostasis can slow the myocardial and cardiomyocyte relaxation rate and increase viscoelastic stiffness.[57-59] Abnormal calcium homeostasis can lead to an increase in the residual diastolic actin myosin cross-bridge cycling and persistent diastolic activation which can resist force decline and lengthening.

Myofilaments (see also Chapter 3)

The myofilament contractile proteins consist of thick filament myosin and thin filament actin proteins. Bound to actin are a complex of regulatory proteins, which include tropomyosin and troponin-T, C, and I. During relaxation, ATP hydrolysis is required for myosin detachment from actin, calcium dissociation from Tn-C, and active sequestration of calcium by the sarcoplasmic reticulum (Figure 14-16). Modification of any of these steps, the myofilament proteins involved in these steps, or the ATPase that catalyzes them can alter diastolic function.[23-27] In the relaxed state, in the absence of calcium, myosin cannot bind to actin because the binding site is occupied by troponin-I. During contraction when calcium and ATP become available, calcium is bound to Tn-C, a conformational change in this protein complex occurs, Tn-I dissociates from actin, tropomyosin shifts toward the middle of the actin filament, and myosin can bind to actin. Myosin ATPase catalyzes ATP hydrolysis, causing a conformational change in the actin myosin cross-bridge and contraction. During relaxation, additional ATP hydrolysis is required for myosin detachment from actin, calcium dissociation from Tn-C, and active sequestration of calcium by the sarcoplasmic reticulum. Modification of any of these steps or the proteins involved can alter diastolic function.

Energetics (see also Chapter 7)

Relaxation is an energy-consuming process. Energetic factors necessary to maintain normal diastolic function include the requirement that the concentration of the products of ATP hydrolysis (adenosine diphosphate, ADP and inorganic phosphate, Pi) must remain low and produce the appropriate relative ADP/ATP ratio.[24-27] Diastolic dysfunction will occur if the absolute concentration of ADP or Pi increases or if the relative ratio of ADP/ATP rises. Abnormalities in these energetics factors may be caused by a limited ability to recycle ADP to ATP because of a decrease in phosphocreatine (PCr). These kinds of abnormalities in energetics have been found in clinical pathological conditions of pressure overload and ischemia/reperfusion where diastolic function is clearly abnormal.[24-27]

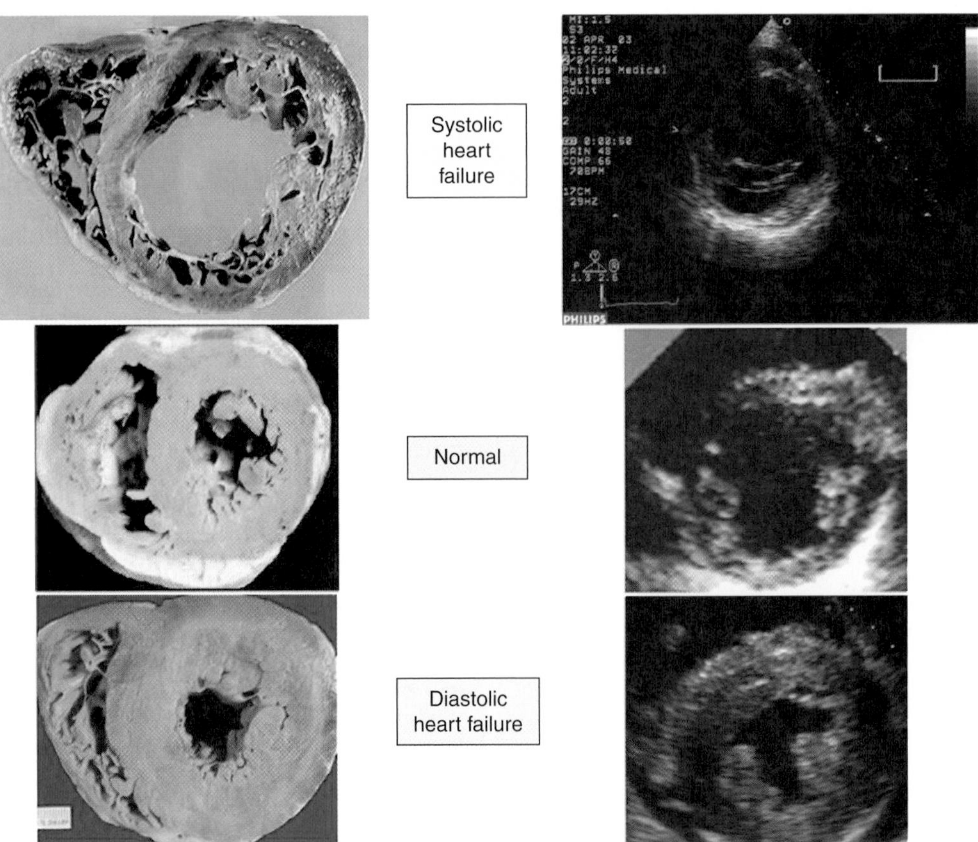

FIGURE 14–13 Examples of autopsy and echocardiographic LV short axis cross-sectional images in normal control subjects, patients with systolic heart failure (SHF), and diastolic heart failure (DHF). Patients with SHF are characterized by eccentric remodeling with increased LV volume, increased LV mass, and a decreased mass/volume ratio. Patients with DHF are characterized by concentric remodeling with increased LV mass, no change in LV volume, and an increased mass/volume ratio.

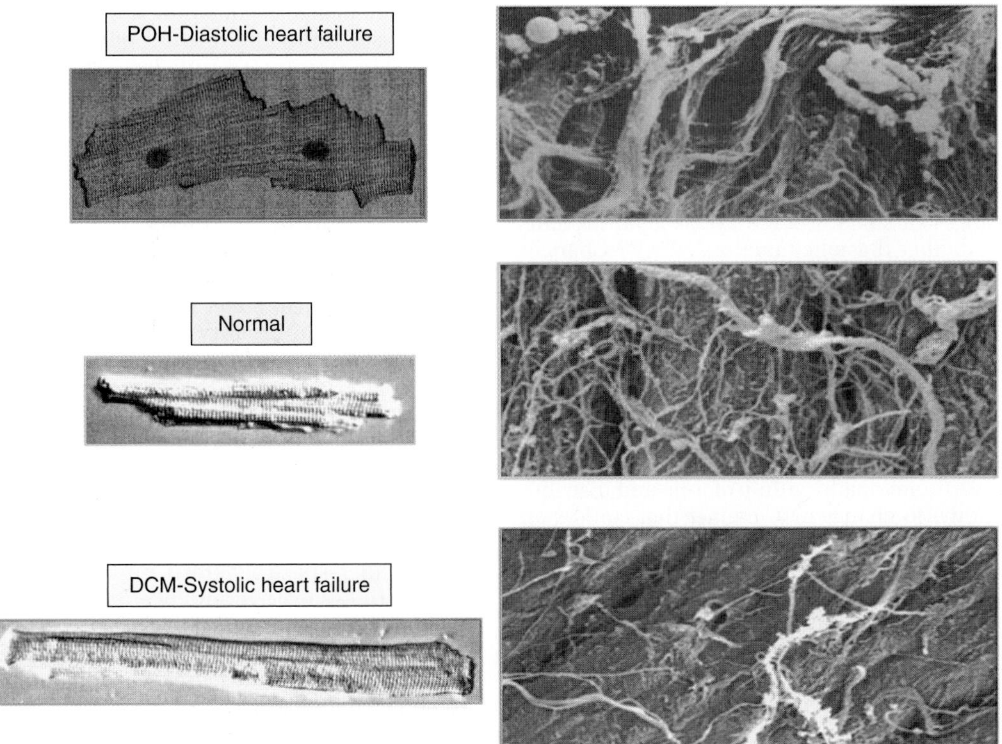

FIGURE 14–14 Examples of cardiomyocyte and extracellular matrix (ECM) changes in systolic heart failure (SHF) and diastolic heart failure (DHF) compared with normal. DHF has an increased cardiomyocyte diameter, little or no change in length, and markedly increased ECM fibrillar collagen. SHF has an increased cardiomyocyte length, little or no change in diameter, and disrupted ECM fibrillar collagen.

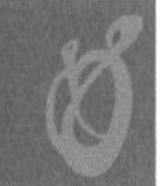

BOX 14–1 Diastolic Heart Failure: Mechanisms

A. Extramyocardial
   1. Hemodynamic load: early diastolic load, afterload
   2. Heterogeneity
   3. Pericardium
B. Myocardial
   1. Cardiomyocyte
      a. Calcium homeostasis
         1) Calcium concentration
         2) Sarcolemmal and sarcoplasmic reticulum calcium transport function
         3) Modifying proteins (phospholamban, calmodulin, calsequestrin)
      b. Myofilaments
         1) Troponin-C calcium binding
         2) Troponin-I phosphorylation
         3) Myofilament calcium sensitivity
         4) α/β-myosin heavy chain ATPase ratio
      c. Energetics
         1) ADP/ATP ratio
         2) ADP and Pi concentration
      d. Cytoskeleton
         1) Microtubules
         2) Intermediate filaments (desmin)
         3) Microfilaments (actin)
         4) Endosarcomeric skeleton (titin, nebulin)
   2. Extracellular matrix
      a. Fibrillar collagen homeostasis
      b. Basement membrane proteins
      c. Proteoglycans
      d. MMP/TIMP
   3. Neurohormonal activation
      a. Renin-angiotensin-aldosterone
      b. Sympathetic nervous system
      c. Endothelin
      d. Nitric oxide
      e. Natriuretic peptides

Abbreviations: *ATP*, adenosine triphosphate; *ADP*, adenosine diphosphate; *Pi*, inorganic phosphate; *MMP*, matrix metalloproteinase; *TIMP*, tissue inhibitor of matrix metalloproteinase.

Cytoskeleton

The cardiomyocyte cytoskeleton is composed of microtubules, intermediate filaments (desmin), microfilaments (actin), and endosarcomeric proteins (titin, nebulin, α-actinin, myomesin, M-protein).[79] Changes in some of these cytoskeletal proteins have been shown to alter diastolic function.[57-59,79-83] Changes in titin isotypes have been shown to alter relaxation and viscoelastic stiffness (Figure 14-17). During contraction, potential energy is gained when titin is compressed and during diastole, titin acts like viscoelastic springs, expends this stored potential energy, and provides a recoiling force to restore the myocardium to its resting length.[81,82] In addition, titin extension during diastole is limited and protects the myocardium from being stretched too far beyond resting length. In experimental end-stage dilated cardiomyopathy, titin isoforms and distribution have been shown to change in a manner that confers an increase in stiffness.[82] Likewise, an increase in microtubule density and distribution has been shown in some forms of pressure overload to act as a viscous load and increases myocardial and cardiomyocyte viscoelastic stiffness.[57-59,80] This change in diastolic function is reversible when microtubules are acutely depolymerized by chemical or physical agents.[57-59,80]

Extracellular Matrix (see also Chapter 5)

Changes in the structures within the extracellular matrix (ECM) can also affect diastolic function. The myocardial ECM is composed of three important constituents: (1) fibrillar protein such as collagen type I, collagen type III, and elastin; (2) proteoglycans; and (3) basement membrane proteins, such as collagen type IV, laminin, and fibronectin. It has been hypothesized that the most important component within the ECM contributing to the development of diastolic heart failure is fibrillar collagen.[84-88] Within the myocardial ECM, fibrillar collagen exists in a complex 3D, geometric distribution. This distribution is divided into three layers: (1) endomysial collagen, which surrounds and connects individual cardiomyocytes; (2) perimysial collagen, which surrounds and connects bundles of cardiomyocytes; and (3) epimysial collagen, which forms the outermost layer (Figure 14-18). Because these fibrillar proteins surround and envelope individual and groups of cardiomyocytes, it has been hypothesized that in normal myocardium they connect cardiomyocytes into fascicular structures, coordinate their mechanical activity, transmit and transduce mechanical and perhaps neurohumoral input, protect against and limit cardiomyocyte strain, and coordinate and recruit preload recruitable work. The evidence that suggests that changes in ECM fibrillar collagen play an important role in the development of diastolic dysfunction and diastolic heart failure follows three lines of evidence. First, disease processes that alter diastolic function also alter ECM fibrillar collagen particularly in terms of its amount, geometry, distribution, degree of cross-linking and ratio of collagen type I versus collagen type III. Second, treatment of these disease processes, which is successful in correcting diastolic function, is associated with normalization of fibrillar collagen. Finally, experiments in which a chronic alteration in collagen metabolism is performed results in an alteration of diastolic function.[89-94] The role played by other fibrillar proteins, the basement membrane proteins, and the proteoglycans remains largely unexplored.

The regulatory control of collagen homeostasis has a number of major determinants: transcriptional regulation of procollagen biosynthesis by physical, neurohormonal, and growth factors; postsynthetic procollagen processing influenced by matricellular and extracellular proteins and peptides; posttranslational regulation including collagen cross-linking; and fibrillar collagen degradation influenced by matrix metalloproteinases (MMPs) and their endogenous tissue inhibitors (TIMPs) (Figure 14-19). Collagen synthesis is altered by load, including preload and afterload; neurohumoral activation, including the renin-angiotensin-aldosterone system (RAAS) and sympathetic nervous system; and growth factors. Collagen degradation is under the control of proteolytic enzymes, including a family of zinc dependent enzymes—the matrix metalloproteinases (MMP).[95-97] The balance between synthesis, processing, posttranslational modification, and degradation results in the total fibrillar collagen content present in a given pathological state. Changes in each of these determinants and their regulatory processes have been shown to alter diastolic function and lead to the development of diastolic heart failure.

Fibrillar collagen biosynthesis begins within the fibroblast endoplasmic reticulum with the synthesis of procollagen α-chain monomeric proteins.[98,99] These monomers undergo hydroxylation, glycosylation, and disulfide bond formation to form the triple helical structure of a procollagen molecule. After synthesis, a procollagen molecule is secreted into the extracellular space where it must undergo a series of very ordered time-sensitive and location-sensitive sequential postsynthetic processing steps in order to become a mature cross-linked insoluble structural collagen fibril.

Once secreted into the extracellular space, postsynthetic procollagen processing can have two major outcomes: (1) ordered procollagen processing within the extracellular space that favors formation of, or incorporation into, a mature cross-linked insoluble structural collagen fibril, or (2) procollagen association with cell surface receptors, which leads to

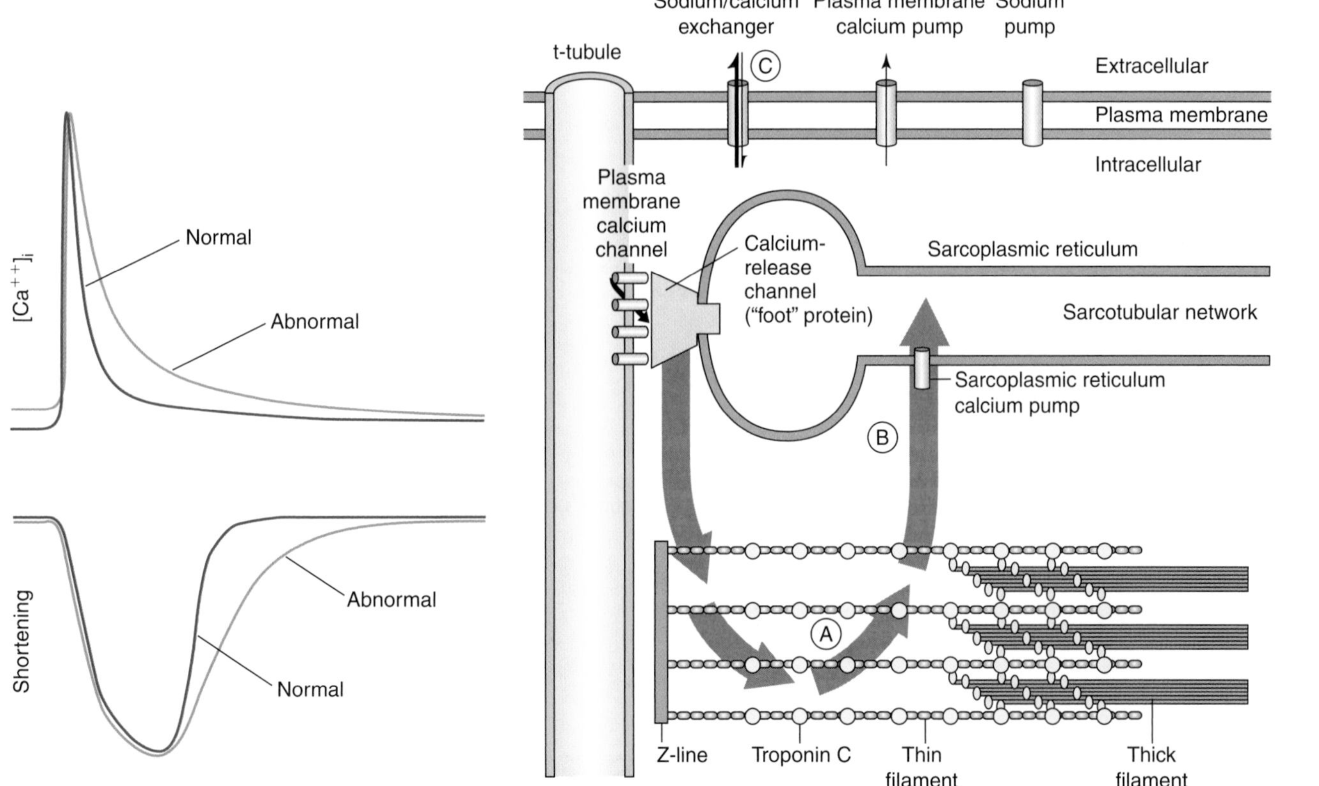

FIGURE 14–15 Left panel—Examples of normal (*solid line*) and abnormal (*dashed line*) calcium transients (*top*) and cardiomyocyte contractions (*bottom*). Calcium transient is prolonged, calcium decay is slowed, cardiomyocyte lengthening rate is slowed in a cardiomyocyte with abnormalities in calcium homeostasis. Right panel—Schematic drawing showing steps involved in calcium homeostasis during diastole. Calcium is released from myofilaments **(A)**, sequestrated into the sarcoplasmic reticulum **(B)**, and calcium is extruded into the extracellular space **(C)**. Changes in any of these steps, or the proteins that cause them, can result in the abnormalities shown in the left panel and abnormalities in relaxation and stiffness.

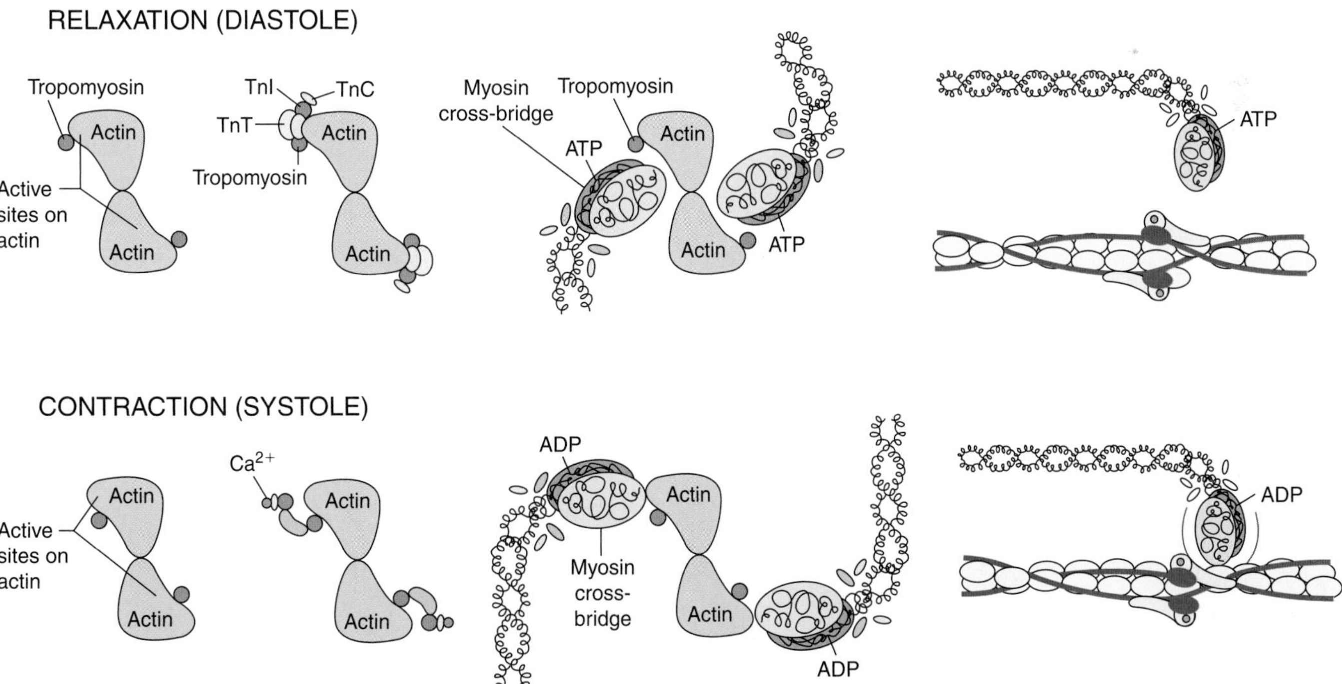

FIGURE 14–16 Schematic of myofilament proteins during contraction and relaxation. *Tn,* troponin; *ATP,* adenosine triphosphate; *ADP,* adenosine diphosphate; Ca^{2+}, calcium. Changes in the structure or function of any of these myofilament proteins may result in abnormalities in relaxation and stiffness.

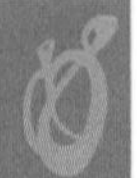

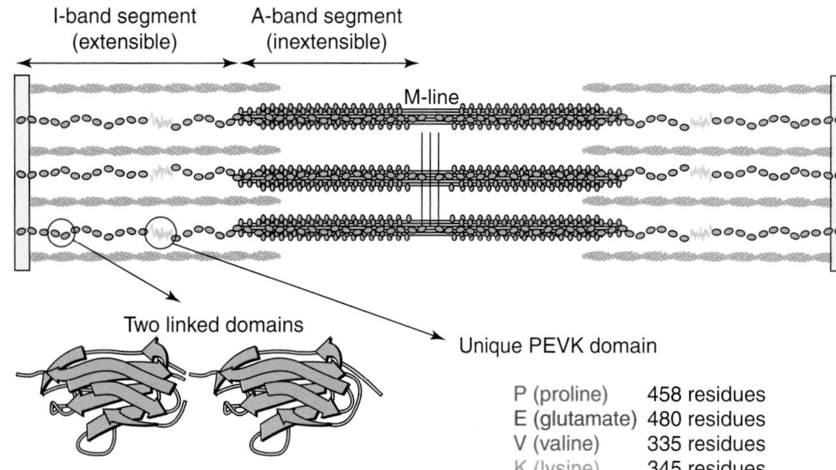

FIGURE 14–17 Schematic of titin molecule.

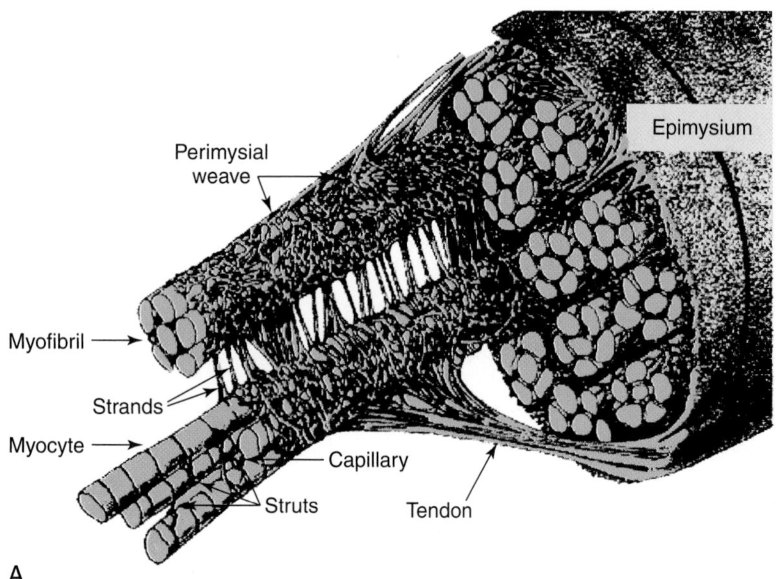

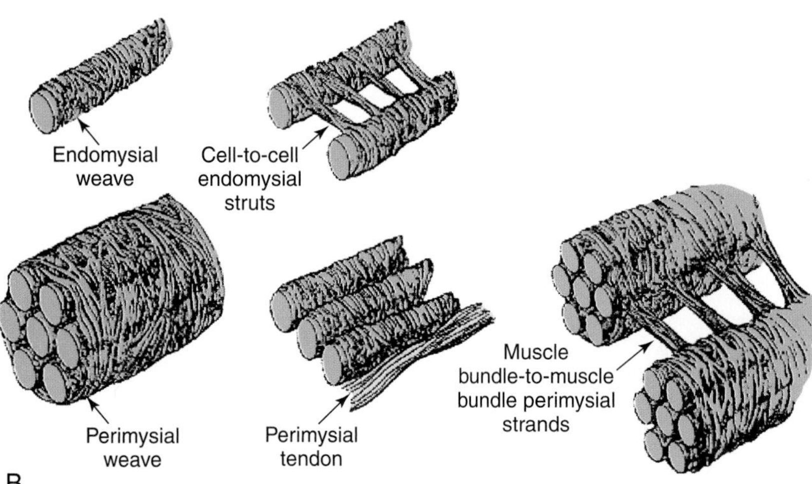

FIGURE 14–18 Schematic of fibrillar collagen distribution within the myocardial extracellular matrix.

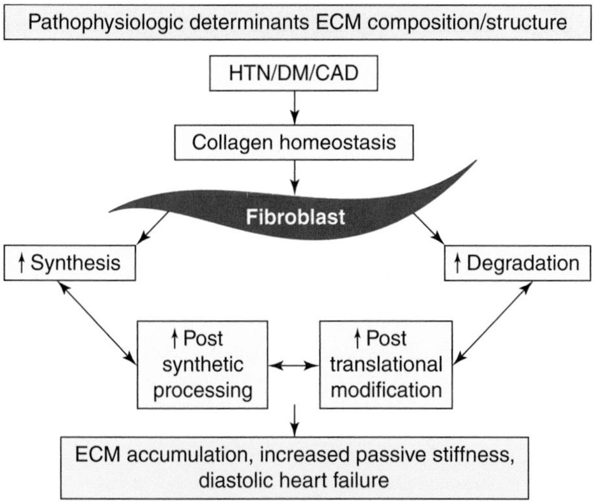

Pathophysiologic determinants ECM composition/structure
HTN/DM/CAD
Collagen homeostasis
Fibroblast
↑ Synthesis
↑ Degradation
↑ Post synthetic processing
↑ Post translational modification
ECM accumulation, increased passive stiffness, diastolic heart failure

FIGURE 14–19 Schematic of the determinants of extracellular matrix (ECM) composition and structure. Pathological processes such as hypertension (HTN), diabetes (DM), and coronary artery disease (CAD) act on the myocardial fibroblast to change rates of synthesis, processing, posttranslational modification, and degradation.

degradation of procollagen before incorporation into a mature cross-linked insoluble structural collagen fibril, and/or premature disordered procollagen processing associated with the cell surface, which does not promote formation of, or incorporation into, a mature cross-linked insoluble structural collagen fibril. To form a mature collagen fibril, procollagen is processed by extracellular determinants. The C-terminal propeptide of procollagen must be cleaved by BMP-1 (bone morphogenetic protein or related tolloid receptors). The activity of BMP-1 is enhanced by PCPE-1 (procollagen C-proteinase enhancer 1) and 2. The N-terminal propeptide of procollagen is cleaved by ADAMTS-2 (a disintegrin-like and metalloproteinase domain with a thrombospondin-type motif). The resulting collagen molecules are then cross-linked into mature collagen fibrils. The covalent intermolecular cross-linkages are catalyzed by the enzymes lysyl oxidase and hydroxylysyl oxidase. This procollagen processing is highly ordered and appears to be most efficient in leading to formation of, or incorporation into, a mature cross-linked insoluble structural collagen fibril when it occurs in the extracellular space. Factors that decrease procollagen association with the cell surface increase collagen incorporation into mature collagen fibrils. The process of procollagen processing can be influenced by "matricellular" proteins; SPARC is one example.[98,99] SPARC is a procollagen-binding protein with counteradhesive activity, which is hypothesized to coordinate procollagen processing and facilitate collagen fibril assembly and formation. Studies by Bradshaw et al have shown that when SPARC binds to newly secreted procollagen in LV myocardial tissues and fibroblasts it chaperones the procollagen molecule through processing within the extracellular space and limits binding of procollagen to cell surface receptors such as transmembrane $\alpha_1\beta_1$ integrin.[98,99] By diminishing procollagen engagement of cell surface receptors, SPARC facilitates the optimal sequence and timing of the processing steps and prevents procollagen from being prematurely degraded or improperly processed. Processing of procollagen to form a mature cross-linked insoluble structural collagen fibril does not absolutely require SPARC but SPARC enhances and facilitates this process. In studies of animal models of pressure overload, changes in matricellular and other extracellular proteins and peptides have been shown to be one mechanism that contributes to the development of diastolic dysfunction that underlies the clinical syndrome of DHF.

Myocardial collagen structure and composition can also be altered by changes in posttranslational modification (PTM).[100-105] Collagen can be cross-linked enzymatically by lysyl oxidase acting shortly after collagen fiber synthesis. In addition, and potentially more important to changes seen in DHF, collagen can also undergo nonenzymatic cross-linking that begins with formation of advanced glycation end products (AGEs). AGE-modified collagen forms nonenzymatic cross-links that change the physical properties of collagen, making collagen more resistant to degradation and increasing collagen content. Myocardial fibroblasts express cell surface receptors for AGE-modified proteins (such as RAGE, receptor for age-modified proteins). RAGE binds AGE-modified proteins and begins a signal transduction process that can result in an increase in bioactive proteins and peptides that can increase collagen synthesis, decrease degradation, and increase the number of RAGEs present.[107-113] Myocardial AGE/RAGE interaction may contribute to the development of diastolic dysfunction and DHF. Currently both clinical and animal experiments are being conducted that will test the hypothesis that in DHF there are an increased number of AGE-modified proteins and increased interaction with RAGE, which together play a causal role in the development of diastolic dysfunction and DHF.

Collagen degradation is influenced by the zinc-dependent interstitial proteases, MMPs. MMPs are generally grouped into classes according to their enzyme activity and the proteins and structures that they act upon. The activity of MMPs is regulated by TIMPs.[106] TIMPs bind to the activated MMP or proMMP in a 1:1 stoichiometric molar ratio and therefore form an important endogenous system for regulating MMP activity in vivo. Changes in MMP and TIMP levels can be measured in myocardial tissue and plasma samples. Both tissue and plasma techniques have been applied to animal models of POH and patients with clinical evidence of POH. Data suggest that changes in MMP/TIMP stoichiometry and expression play an important role in the structural and functional remodeling during the development of diastolic dysfunction and DHF. Ongoing studies are examining what ECM-regulatory mechanisms that control how MMP/TIMP dependent change LV/ECM structure/function or cause the development of diastolic dysfunction.

Neurohormonal

Both acutely and chronically, neurohumoral and cardiac endothelial activation and/or inhibition have been shown to alter diastolic function.[114-118] Chronic activation of the RAAS has been shown to increase ECM fibrillar collagen and can be associated with increased stiffness. Inhibition of RAAS prevents or reverses this increase in fibrillar collagen and generally but not consistently reduces myocardial stiffness. In addition, acute activation or inhibition of neurohumoral and cardiac endothelial systems have been shown to alter relaxation and stiffness. These acute pharmacological interventions act in a time frame too short to alter the ECM; therefore their effect on diastolic function must be caused by acting directly on the cardiomyocyte to alter one or more cellular determinants of diastolic function. For example, acutely treating patients with pressure overload with an angiotensin-converting enzyme (ACE) inhibitor, a direct NO donor, or an indirect endothelin dependent NO donor, caused LV pressure decline and LV filling to be more rapid and complete and caused the LV pressure versus volume relationship to shift to the right, decreasing stiffness. In addition, there is a cyclical release of NO in the heart, most noted subendocardially, which peaks at the time of relaxation and filling. These brief bursts of NO release provide a beat-to-beat modulation of relaxation and stiffness.[119]

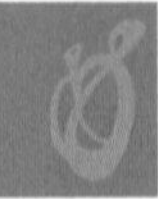

1. Ramachandran, S. V., Larson, M. G., Benjamin, E. J., et al. (1999). Congestive heart failure in subjects with normal versus reduced left ventricular ejection fraction. *J Am Coll Cardiol, 33*, 1948–1955.
2. Lenzen, M. J., Scholte op Reimer, W. J. M., Boersma, E., et al. (2004). Differences between patients with a preserved and a depressed left ventricular function: a report from the EuroHeart failure survey. *Eur Heart J, 25*, 1214–1220.
3. Hogg, K., Swedberg, K., & McMurray, J. (2004). Heart failure with preserved left ventricular systolic function. Epidemiology, clinical characteristics, and prognosis. *J Am Coll Cardiol, 43*, 317–327.
4. Bhatia, R. S., Tu, J. V., Lee, D. S., et al. (2006). Outcome of heart failure with preserved ejection fraction in a popular-based study. *N Engl J Med, 355*, 260–269.
5. Owan, T. E., Hodge, D. O., Herges, R. M., et al. (2006). Trends in prevalence and outcome of heart failure with preserved ejection fraction. *N Engl J Med, 355*, 251–259.
6. Hunt, S. A., Abraham, W. T., Chin, M. H., et al. (2009). 2009 Focused update incorporated into the ACC/AHA 2005 guidelines for the diagnosis and management of heart failure in adults. *Circulation, 119*, e391–e479.
7. Lee, D. S., Gona, P., Vasan, R. S., et al. (2009). Relation of disease pathogenesis and risk factors to heart failure with preserved or reduced ejection fraction. Insights from the Framingham Heart Study of the National Heart, Lung, and Blood Institute. *Circulation, 119*, 3070–3077.
8. Yusef, S., Pfeffer, M. A., Swedberg, K., et al. (2003). Effects of candesartan in patients with chronic heart failure and preserved left-ventricular ejection fraction: the CHARM-preserved trial. *Lancet, 362*, 777–781.
9. Ahmed, A., Rich, M. W., Fleg, J. L., et al. (2006). Effects of digoxin on morbidity and mortality in diastolic heart failure. The ancillary digitalis investigation group trial. *Circulation, 114*, 397–403.
10. Cleland, J. G. F., Tendera, M., Adamus, J., et al. (2006). The perindopril in elderly people with chronic heart failure (PEP-CHF) study. *Eur Heart J, 27*, 2338–2345.
11. Massie, B. M., Carson, P. E., McMurray, J. J., et al. (2008). Irbesartan in patients with heart failure and preserved ejection fraction. *N Engl J Med, 359*, 2456–2467.
12. van Veldhuisen, D. J., Cohen-Solal, A., Böhm, M., et al. (2009). Beta-blockade with nebivolol in elderly heart failure patients with impaired and preserved left ventricular ejection fraction: data from SENIORS (study of effects of nebivolol intervention on outcomes and rehospitalization in seniors with heart failure). *J Am Coll Cardiol, 3*(23), 2150–2158.
13. McKee, P. A., Castelli, W. P., McNamara, P. M., et al. (1971). The natural history of congestive heart failure: the Framingham study. *N Engl J Med, 285*, 1441–1446.
14. Brutsaert, D. L., & Sys, S. U. (1997). Diastolic dysfunction in heart failure. *J Card Fail, 3*(3), 225–242.
15. Paulus, W. J., Tschöpe, C., Sanderson, J. E., et al. (2007). How to diagnose diastolic heart failure: a consensus statement on the diagnosis of heart failure with normal left ventricular ejection fraction by the Heart Failure and Echocardiography Associations of the European Society of Cardiology. *Eur Heart J, 20*, 2539–2550.
16. Yturralde, R. F., & Gaasch, W. H. (2005). Diagnostic criteria for diastolic heart failure. *Prog Cardiovasc Dis, 47*(5), 314–319.
17. Lubien, E., DeMaria, A., Krishnaswamy, P., et al. (2001). Utility of B-natriuretic peptide (BNP) in detecting diastolic dysfunction: comparison with Doppler velocity recordings. *Circulation*, (in press).
18. Maeda, K., Tsutamoto, T., Wada, A., et al. (1998). Plasma brain natriuretic peptide as a biochemical marker of high left ventricular end-diastolic pressure in patients with symptomatic left ventricular dysfunction. *Am Heart J, 135*, 825–832.
19. Yamamoto, K., Burnett, J. C., Jougasaki, M., et al. (1996). Superiority of brain natriuretic peptide as a hormonal marker of ventricular systolic and diastolic dysfunction and ventricular hypertrophy. *Hypertension, 28*, 988–994.
20. Lubien, E., DeMaria, A., Krishnaswamy, P., et al. (2002). Utility of B-natriuretic peptide in detecting diastolic dysfunction. Comparison with Doppler velocity recording. *Circulation, 105*, 595–601.
21. TschÖpe, C., Kašner, M., Westermann, D., et al. (2005). The role of NT-proBNP in the diagnostics of isolated diastolic dysfunction: correlation with echocardiographic and invasive measurements. *Eur Heart J, 26*, 2277–2284.
22. Grewal, J., McKelvie, R. S., Persson, H., et al. (2008). Usefulness of N-terminal pro-brain natriuretic peptide and brain natriuretic peptide to predict cardiovascular outcomes in patients with heart failure and preserved left ventricular ejection fraction. *Am J Cardiol, 102*(6), 733–737.
23. Apstein, C. S., & Morgan, J. P. (1994). Cellular mechanisms underlying left ventricular diastolic dysfunction. In W. H. Gaasch & M. M. LeWinter (Eds.), *Left ventricular diastolic dysfunction and heart failure*. Philadelphia: Lea & Febiger.
24. Ingwall, J. S. (1998). Energetics of the normal and failing human heart: focus on the creatine kinase reaction. *Adv Org Biol, 4*, 117–141.
25. Solaro, R. J., Wolska, B. M., & Westfall, M. Regulatory proteins and diastolic relaxation. In B. H. Lorell & W. Grossman (Eds.), (1987). *Diastolic relaxation of the heart*. Boston: Kluwer Academic.
26. Alpert, N. R., LeWinter, M., Mulieri, L. A., et al. (1999). Chemomechanical energy transduction in the failing heart. *Heart Fail Rev, 4*(3), 281–295.
27. Tian, R., Nascimben, L., Ingwall, J. S., et al. (1997). Failure to maintain a low ADP concentration impairs diastolic function in hypertrophied rat hearts. *Circulation, 96*, 1313–1319.
28. Weiss, J. L., Fredericksen, J. W., & Weisfeldt, M. L. (1976). Hemodynamic determinants of the time course of fall in canine left ventricular pressure. *J Clin Invest, 58*, 83–95.
29. Smith, V. E., Zile, M. R., et al. (1992). Relaxation and diastolic properties of the heart. In H. A. Fozzard (Ed.), *The heart and cardiovascular system*. New York: Raven Press.
30. Mirsky, I., & Pasipoularides, A. (1990). Clinical assessment of diastolic function. *Prog Cardiovasc Dis, 32*, 291–318.
31. Zile, M. R., Nishimura, R. A., & Gaasch, W. H. (1994). Hemodynamic loads and left ventricular diastolic function: factors affecting the indices of isovolumetric and auxotonic relaxation. In W. H. Gaasch & N. M. LeWinter (Eds.), *LV diastolic dysfunction and heart failure*. Philadelphia: Lea & Febiger.
32. Solomon, S. D., Janardhanan, R., Verma, A., et al. (2007). Effect of angiotensin receptor blockade and antihypertensive drugs on diastolic function in patients with hypertension and diastolic dysfunction: a randomised trial. *Lancet, 369*(9579), 2079–2087.
33. Zile, M. R., & Gaasch, W. H. (1991). Load-dependent left ventricular relaxation in conscious dogs. *Am J Physiol, 261*, H669–H699.
34. Little, W. C. (2005). Diastolic dysfunction beyond distensibility: adverse effects of ventricular dilatation. *Circulation, 112*(19), 2888–2890.
35. Gaasch, W. H., Schick, E. C., & Zile, M. R. (1996). Management of left ventricular diastolic dysfunction. In T. W. Smith (Ed.), *Cardiovascular therapeutics. A companion to Braunwald's heart disease*. Philadelphia: WB Saunders.
36. Zile, M. R. (1992). Hemodynamic determinants of echocardiography derived indices of left ventricular filling. *Echocardiography, 9*, 289–300.
37. Aurigemma, G. P., Zile, M. R., & Gaasch, W. H. (2006). Contractile behavior of the left ventricle in diastolic heart failure: with emphasis on regional systolic function. *Circulation, 113*(2), 296–304.
38. Zile, M. R., Bourge, R. C., Bennett, T. D., et al. (2008). Application of implantable hemodynamic monitoring in the management of patients with diastolic heart failure: a subgroup analysis of the COMPASS-HF trial. *J Card Fail, 14*(10), 816–823.
39. Zile, M. R., Bennett, T. D., St John Sutton, M., et al. (2008). Transition from chronic compensated to acute decompensated heart failure: pathophysiological insights obtained from continuous monitoring of intracardiac pressures. *Circulation, 118*(14), 1433–1441.
40. Zile, M. R., & Lewinter, M. M. (2007). Left ventricular end-diastolic volume is normal in patients with heart failure and a normal ejection fraction: a renewed consensus in diastolic heart failure. *J Am Coll Cardiol, 49*(9), 982–985.
41. Quiñones, M. A., Zile, M. R., Massie, B. M., et al. (2006). Chronic heart failure: a report from the Dartmouth diastole discourses. *Congest Heart Fail, 12*(3), 162–165.
42. Ahmed, S. H., Clark, L. L., Pennington, W. R., et al. (2006). Matrix metalloproteinases/tissue inhibitors of metalloproteinases: relationship between changes in proteolytic determinants of matrix composition and structural, functional, and clinical manifestations of hypertensive heart disease. *Circulation, 113*(17), 2089–2096.
43. Zile, M. R., Baicu, C. F., & Gaasch, W. H. (2004). Diastolic heart failure—abnormalities in active relaxation and passive stiffness of the left ventricle. *N Engl J Med, 350*(19), 1953–1959.
44. Lam, C. S., Roger, V. L., Rodeheffer, R. J., et al. (2007). Cardiac structure and ventricular-vascular function in persons with heart failure and preserved ejection fraction from Olmsted County, Minnesota. *Circulation, 115*, 1982–1990.
45. Melenovsky, V., Borlaug, B., Rosen, B., et al. (2007). Cardiovascular features of heart failure with preserved ejection fraction versus non-failing hypertensive left ventricular hypertrophy in the urban Baltimore community. *J Am Coll Cardiol, 49*, 198–207.
46. Westermann, D., Kasner, M., Steendijk, P., et al. (2008). Role of left ventricular stiffness in heart failure with normal ejection fraction. *Circulation, 117*, 2051–2060.
47. Borbely, A., van der Velden, J., Papp, Z., et al. (2005). Cardiomyocyte stiffness in diastolic heart failure. *Circulation, 111*(6), 774–781.
48. van Heerebeek, L., Borbély, A., Niessen, H. W. M., et al. (2006). Myocardial structure and function differ in systolic and diastolic heart failure. *Circulation, 113*, 1966.
49. Borbély, A., Papp, Z., Edes, I., et al. (2009). Molecular determinants of heart failure with normal left ventricular ejection fraction. *Pharmacol Rep, 61*(1), 139–145.
50. Borbély, A., Falcao-Pires, I., van Heerebeek, L., et al. (2009). Hypophosphorylation of the stiff N2B titin isoform raises cardiomyocyte resting tension in failing human myocardium. *Circ Res, 104*(6), 780–786.
51. Borbély, A., van Heerebeek, L., & Paulus, W. J. (2009). Transcriptional and posttranslational modifications of titin: implications for diastole. *Circ Res, 104*(1), 12–14.
52. Zile, M. R., Conrad, C. H., Gaasch, W. H., et al. (1990). Preload does not affect relaxation rate in normal, hypoxic or hypertrophic myocardium. *Am J Physiol, 258*, H191–H197.
53. Zile, M. R., Gaasch, W. H., Weigner, A. W., et al. (1987). Mechanical determinants of the rate of isotonic lengthening in rat left ventricular myocardium. *Circ Res, 60*, 815–823.
54. Tsutsui, H., Urabe, Y., Mann, D., et al. (1993). Effects of chronic mitral regurgitation on diastolic function in isolated cardiocytes. *Circ Res, 72*, 1110–1123.
55. Zile, M. R., Mukherjee, R., Clayton, C., et al. (1995). Effects of chronic supraventricular pacing tachycardia on relaxation rate in isolated cardiac muscle cells. *Am J Physiol, 268*, H2104–H2113.
56. Zile, M., & Spinale, F. G. (1994). Diastolic dysfunction and tachycardia-induced heart failure: International Symposium on the Physiology of Diastole in Health and Disease. In W. Grossman & B. Lorell (Eds.), *Diastolic relaxation of the heart*. Boston: Kluwer Academic Press.
57. Zile, M. R., Cowles, M. K., Buckley, J. M., et al. (1998). Gel stretch method: a new method to measure constitutive properties of cardiac muscle cells. *Am J Physiol, 274*, H2188–H2202.
58. Zile, M. R., Richardson, K., Cowles, M. K., et al. (1998). Constitutive properties of adult mammalian cardiac muscle cells. *Circulation, 98*, 567–579.
59. Harris, T. S., Baicu, C. F., Conrad, C. H., et al. (1998). Constitutive properties of hypertrophied myocardium: cellular contributions to changes in myocardial stiffness and viscosity. *Circulation, 98*(Suppl. I), I-649.
60. Baicu, C. F., Zile, M. R., Aurigemma, G. P., et al. (2005). Left ventricular systolic performance, function, and contractility in patients with diastolic heart failure. *Circulation, 111*, 2306–2312.
61. Carabello, B. A. (2002). Evolution of the study of left ventricular function: everything old is new again. *Circulation, 105*, 2701–2703.
62. Petri, M. C., Caruana, L., Berry, C., et al. (2002). "Diastolic heart failure" or heart failure caused by subtle left ventricular systolic dysfunction. *Heart, 87*, 29–31.
63. Petrie, M., & McMurray, J. (2001). Changes in notions about heart failure. *Lancet, 358*, 432–434.
64. Yip, G., Wang, Zhang, Y., et al. (2002). Left ventricular long axis function in diastolic heart failure is reduced in both diastole and systole: time for a redefinition. *Heart, 87*, 121–125.

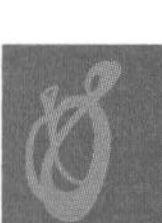

65. Nikitin, N. P., & Witte, K. K. A. (2002). Color tissue Doppler-derived long-axis left ventricular function in heart failure with preserved global systolic function. *Am J Cardiol, 90*, 1174–1177.
66. Banerjee, P., Banerjee, T., Khand, A., et al. (2002). Diastolic heart failure: neglected or misdiagnosed?. *J Am Coll Cardiol, 39*, 138–141.
67. Yu, C., Lin, H., Yang, H., et al. (2002). Progression of systolic abnormalities in patients with "isolated" diastolic heart failure and diastolic dysfunction. *Circulation, 105*, 1195–1201.
68. Steendijk, P. (2004). Heart failure with preserved ejection fraction: diastolic dysfunction, subtle systolic dysfunction, systolic-ventricular and arterial stiffening, or misdiagnosis? *Cardiovasc Res, 64*, 9–11.
69. Norton, G. R., Woodiwiss, A. J., Gaasch, W. H., et al. (2002). Heart failure in pressure overload hypertrophy: the relative roles of ventricular remodeling and myocardial dysfunction. *J Am Coll Cardiol, 39*, 664–671.
70. Anand, I. S., Daosheng, L., Chugh, S. S., et al. (1997). Isolated myocyte contractile function is normal in postinfarct remodeled rat heart with systolic dysfunction. *Circulation, 96*, 3974–3984.
71. Anand, I. S. (2002). Ventricular remodeling without cellular contractile dysfunction. *J Card Failure, 8*, S401–S408.
72. Zile, M. R., & Brutsaert, D. L. (2002). New concepts in diastolic dysfunction and diastolic heart failure, part I: diagnosis, prognosis, measurements of diastolic function. *Circulation, 105*, 1387–1393.
73. Zile, M. R., & Brutsaert, D. L. (2002). New concepts in diastolic dysfunction and diastolic heart failure, part II: causal mechanisms and treatment. *Circulation, 105*, 1503–1508.
74. Kitzman, D. W., Little, W. C., Brubaker, P. H., et al. (2002). Pathophysiological characterization of isolated diastolic heart failure in comparison to systolic heart failure. *JAMA, 288*, 2144–2150.
75. Spinale, F. G., Tomita, M., Zellner, J. L., et al. (1991). Collagen remodeling and changes in left ventricular function during development and recovery from supraventricular tachycardia. *Am J Physiol, 261*(pt 2), H308–H318.
76. Spinale, F. G., Zellner, J. L., Tomita, M., et al. (1991). Relation between ventricular and myocyte remodeling with the development and regression of supraventricular tachycardia-induced cardiomyopathy. *Circ Res, 69*, 1058–1067.
77. Hein, S., Arnon, E., Kostin, S., et al. (2003). Progression from compensated hypertrophy to failure in the pressure-overloaded human heart. *Circulation, 107*, 984–991.
78. Gaasch, W. H., Delorey, D. E., St John Sutton, M. G., et al. (2008). Patterns of structural and functional remodeling of the left ventricle in chronic heart failure. *Am J Cardiol, 102*(4), 459–462.
79. Kostin, S., Hein, S., Arnon, E., et al. (2000). The cytoskeleton and related proteins in the human failure heart. *Heart Fail Rev, 5*, 271–280.
80. Cooper, G. (2000). IV: Cardiocyte cytoskeleton in hypertrophied myocardium. *Heart Fail Rev, 5*, 187–201.
81. Bell, S. P., Nyland, L., Tischler, M. D., et al. (2000). Alterations in the determinants of diastolic suction during pacing tachycardia. *Circ Res, 87*(3), 235–240.
82. Cazolla, O., Freiburg, A., Helmes, M., et al. (2000). Differential expression of cardiac titin isoforms and modulation of cellular stiffness. *Circ Res, 86*(1), 59–67.
83. Tagawa, H., Wang, N., Narishige, T., et al. (1997). Cytoskeletal mechanics in pressure overload cardiac hypertrophy. *Circ Res, 80*, 281–289.
84. Weber, K. T., & Brilla, C. G. (1991). Pathological hypertrophy and cardiac interstitium: fibrosis and renin-angiotensin-aldosterone system. *Circulation, 83*, 1849–1865.
85. Weber, K. T., Sun, Y., & Guarda, E. (1994). Structural remodeling in hypertensive heart disease and the role of hormones. *Hypertension, 23*, 869–877.
86. Borg, T. K., & Caulfield, J. B. (1981). The collagen matrix of the heart. *Fed Proc, 40*(7), 2037–2041.
87. Weber, K. T. (1989). Cardiac interstitium in health and disease: the fibrillar collagen network. *J Am Coll Cardiol, 13*, 1637–1652.
88. Covell, J. W. (1990). Factors influencing diastolic function. Possible role of the extracellular matrix. *Circulation, 81*(Suppl. III), III-155-III-158.
89. Jalil, J. E., Doering, C. W., Janicki, J. S., et al. (1989). Fibrillar collagen and myocardial stiffness in the intact hypertrophied rat left ventricle. *Circ Res, 64*, 1041–1050.
90. Weber, K. T., Janicki, J. S., Pick, R., et al. (1990). Myocardial fibrosis and pathologic hypertrophy in the rat with renovascular hypertension. *Am J Cardiol, 65*, 1G–7G.
91. Villari, B., Campbell, S. E., Hess, O. M., et al. (1993). Influence of collagen network on left ventricular systolic and diastolic function in aortic valve disease. *J Am Coll Cardiol, 22*, 1477–1484.
92. Villari, B., Vassalli, G., Monrad, E. S., et al. (1995). Normalization of diastolic dysfunction in aortic stenosis late after valve replacement. *Circulation, 91*(9), 2353–2358.
93. Kato, S., Spinale, F. G., Tanaka, R., et al. (1995). Inhibition of collagen cross-linking: effects on fibrillar collagen and ventricular diastolic function. *Am J Physiol*, 269, H863-H868.
94. Brilla, C. G., Funck, R. C., & Rupp, H. (2000). Lisinopril-mediated regression of myocardial fibrosis in patients with hypertensive heart disease. *Circulation, 102*, 1388–1393.
95. Spinale, F. S., Coker, M. L., Bond, B. R., et al. (2000). Myocardial matrix degradation and metalloproteinase activation in the failing heart: a potential therapeutic target. *Cardiovasc Res, 46*, 225–238.
96. Nagatomo, Y., Carabello, B. A., Coker, M. L., et al. (2000). Differential effects of pressure or volume overload on myocardial MMP levels and inhibitory control. *Am J Physiol Heart Circ Physiol, 278*, H151–H161.
97. Spinale, F. G., Coker, M. L., Krombach, S. R., et al. (1999). Matrix metalloproteinase inhibition during the development of congestive heart failure. Effects on left ventricular dimensions and function. *Circ Res, 85*, 364–376.
98. Bradshaw, A. D., Baicu, C. F., Rentz, T. J., et al. (2009). Pressure overload-induced alterations in fibrillar collagen content and myocardial diastolic function: role of secreted protein acidic and rich in cysteine (SPARC) in postsynthetic procollagen processing. *Circulation, 119*(2), 269–280.
99. McCurdy, S., Baicu, C. F., Heymans, S., et al. (2010). Cardiac extracellular matrix remodeling: fibrillar collagens and secreted protein acidic and rich in cysteine (SPARC). *J Mol Cell Cardiol* 48(3), 544–549.
100. Davidson, J. M., & Berg, R. A. (1981). Posttranslational events in collagen biosynthesis. *Methods Cell Biol, 23*, 119–136.
101. Kielty, C. M., Hopkinson, I., & Grant, M. E. (1993). Collagen: structure, assembly, and organization in the ECM. In P. M. Royce & B. S. Steinmann (Eds.), *Connective tissue and its heritable disorders*. New York: Wiley-Liss.
102. Nimni, M. E. (1993). Fibrillar collagens: their biosynthesis, molecular structure, and mode of assembly. In M. A. Zern & L. M. Reid (Eds.), *Extracellular matrix*. New York: Marcel Dekker.
103. Singh, R., Barden, A., Mori, T., et al. (2001). Advanced glycation end-products: a review. *Diabetologia, 44*, 129–146.
104. Brownlee, M. (1995). The pathological implications of protein glycation. *Clin Invest Med, 18*, 275–281.
105. Cerami, A., Ulrich, P. Pharmaceutical intervention of advanced glycation endproducts. Ageing vulnerability: causes and intervention. *Novartis Found Symp* 201;235:202–216.
106. Spinale, F. (2007). Myocardial matrix remodeling and the matrix metalloproteinases: influence on cardiac form and function. *Physiol Rev, 87*(4), 1285–1342.
107. Stern, D. M., Yan, S. D., Yan, S. F., et al. (2002). Receptor for advanced glycation endproducts (RAGE) and the complications of diabetes. *Ageing Res Rev, 1*, 1–15.
108. Yan, S. D., Zhu, H., Zhu, A., et al. (2000). Receptor-dependent cell stress and amyloid accumulation in systemic amyloidosis. *Nat Med, 6*, 643–651.
109. Kislinger, T., Fu, C., Huber, B., et al. (1999). N(epsilon)-carboxymethyl)lysine adducts of proteins are ligands for receptor for advanced glycation end products that activate cell signaling pathways and modulate gene expression. *J Biol Chem, 274*, 31740–31749.
110. Sun, M., Yokoyama, M., Ishiwata, T., et al. (1998). Deposition of advanced glycation end products (AGE) and expression of the receptor for AGE in cardiovascular tissue of the diabetic rat. *Int J Exp Pathol, 79*, 207–222.
111. Schmidt, A. M., Yan, S. D., & Stern, D. (2000). The biology of RAGE and its ligands. *Biochim Biophys Acta, 1498*, 99–111.
112. Huang, J. S., Guh, J. Y., Chen, H. C., et al. (2001). Role of receptor for advanced glycation end-products and the JAK/STAT-signaling pathway in AGE-induced collagen production in NRK-49F cells. *J Cell Biochem, 81*, 102–113.
113. Yan, S. F., Ramasamy, R., Naka, Y., et al. (2003). Glycation, inflammation, and RAGE. A scaffold for the macrovascular complications of diabetes and beyond. *Circ Res, 93*, 1159–1169.
114. Haber, H. L., Powers, E. R., Gimple, L. W., et al. (1994). Intracoronary angiotensin-converting enzyme inhibition improves diastolic function in patients with hypertensive left ventricular hypertrophy. *Circulation, 89*, 2616–2625.
115. Friedrich, S. P., Lorell, B. H., Rousseau, M. F., et al. (1994). Intracardiac angiotensin-converting enzyme inhibition improves diastolic function in patients with left ventricular hypertrophy due to aortic stenosis. *Circulation, 90*, 2761–2771.
116. Paulus, W. J., & Shah, A. M. (1999). NO and cardiac diastolic function. *Cardiovasc Res, 43*, 595–606.
117. Yamamoto, K., Burnett, J. C., Jr., & Redfield, M. M. (1997). Effect of endogenous natriuretic peptide system on ventricular and coronary function in failing heart. *Am J Physiol, 273*, H2406–H2414.
118. Clarkson, P. B., Wheeldon, N. M., et al. (1996). Effects of brain natriuretic peptide on exercise hemodynamics and neurohormones in isolated diastolic heart failure. *Circulation, 93*, 2037–2042.
119. Paulus, W. J. (2000). Beneficial effects of nitric oxide on cardiac diastolic function: "the flip side of the coin." *Heart Fail Rev, 5*(4), 337–344.

CHAPTER 15

Alterations in Ventricular Structure: Role of Left Ventricular Remodeling

Inder S. Anand and Viorel G. Florea

It is now generally recognized that heart failure progresses through a process of structural remodeling (see Chapters 9 and 10) of the heart to which neurohormonal and cytokine activation make an important contribution (see Chapter 11). The term *ventricular remodeling* refers to deviation in ventricular architecture from normal, with changes in volume, wall thickness, and/or shape. The term has initially been applied to the pathological changes, related to myocardial hypertrophy and fibrosis with associated chamber dilation, that have been well described following a large myocardial infarction.[1-3] The term has also been applied to other conditions associated with ventricular dilation in a spherical configuration and eccentric myocardial hypertrophy, referred to as "dilated cardiomyopathy," and to conditions associated with concentric left ventricular (LV) hypertrophy with a normal or reduced chamber volume, as is seen in hypertensive heart disease. There is now a large body of evidence indicating that these forms of pathological ventricular remodeling are independently associated with adverse clinical outcomes, and more importantly, that interventions that attenuate or reverse these changes are usually associated with improved clinical outcomes (see Chapter 8).[4]

REMODELING CONCEPT OF HEART FAILURE

It is well known that the heart can enlarge or shrink in response to hemodynamic demands (Figure 15-1).[5] Critical to our understanding of heart failure are observations that heart failure is related to progressive alterations in structure and function of the heart. The earliest reference to the role of cardiac structure in the development of heart failure dates back to the nineteenth century.[6] In *The Principles and Practice of Medicine*, William Osler pointed to hypertrophy as a step in the development of heart failure, since it is followed by a "period of broken compensation . . . that commonly takes place slowly and results from degeneration and weakening of the heart muscle.[7]" However, in the modern era, Linzbach has been credited for being the first to recognize that alterations in cardiac structure are the primary determinants of heart failure, and that LV weight of about 200 g was critical in the natural history of the disorder.[8]

In the 1960s, a different view of LV hypertrophy and enlargement began to emerge. In accordance with Laplace's law, which dictates that afterload-induced increases in systolic wall stress are offset by increases in wall thickness, hypertrophic growth of the heart was seen as "compensatory" and hence beneficial.[9,10] Animal models of pressure overload led Meerson to suggest that cardiac growth induced by biomechanical stress plays a protective role, at least in the short term.[11] Moreover, in the 1970s and 1980s, hemodynamic measurements in patients with valvular heart disease provided support for the concept of adaptive hypertrophic growth, which when "inadequate" could lead to systolic dysfunction.[12-14]

Recent clinical studies have called into question the idea that structural changes of the ventricle are adaptive and protective. Progressive LV hypertrophy, enlargement, and cavity distortion over time have consistently been shown to be directly related to deterioration of LV performance and an increase in mortality and morbidity[15-19] irrespective of the cause of heart failure.[20]

Current concepts of ventricular remodeling have largely been derived from studies on patients and animal models of myocardial infarction.[21-24] However, the idea that changes in ventricular size and shape are a dynamic response to hemodynamic and metabolic needs imposed on the ventricle was firmly established in the early experimental work on hypertension. Studies by Chanutin and Barsdale[25] on an experimental model of arterial hypertension demonstrated that LV weight and myocyte fiber diameter increased in relation to the severity of hypertension. Later, Janice Pfeffer et al[26,27] studied the relationship between LV mass and function over time in the spontaneously hypertensive rat model. They demonstrated that despite continuous and marked LV wall thickening, the left ventricle eventually dilates and then fails. At this stage, the stimulus for LV hypertrophy is not only elevated arterial pressure, but also chamber dilation that further aggravates the hemodynamic load by increasing wall stress. This seminal finding laid the foundation for the concept that regardless of the initial insult, ventricular dilation may become a self-sustaining process of deterioration in LV structure and function. In effect, progressive chamber enlargement becomes a stimulus for further ventricular hypertrophy and dilation, without additional myocardial injury.

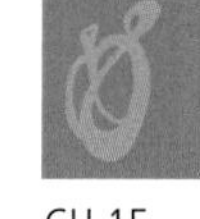

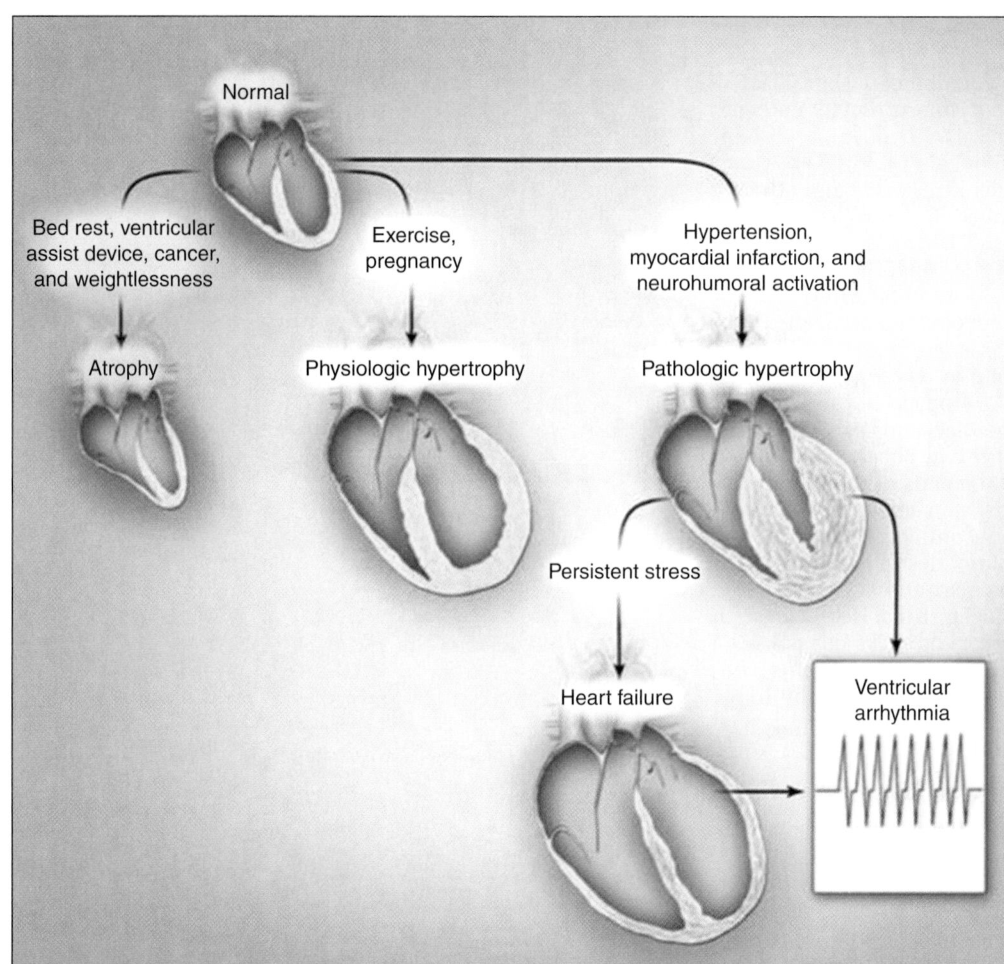

FIGURE 15–1 Conditions leading to remodeling of the heart and resulting in atrophy or hypertrophy. Depending on the circumstances, remodeling can be normal or pathological. Pathological remodeling is associated with a propensity toward decompensation, ventricular dilation, systolic dysfunction, and electrophysiological changes leading to malignant ventricular arrhythmia. (From Hill JA, Olson EN. Cardiac plasticity. *N Engl J Med* 2008;358:1370-1380.[5])

A recent consensus statement helped define remodeling as the "genomic expression resulting in molecular, cellular and interstitial changes that are manifested clinically as changes in size, shape and function of the heart after cardiac injury.[28]" The remodeling process is regulated by mechanical, genetic, and neurohormonal factors.[29] The importance of ventricular remodeling has increased with the observation that agents such as inhibitors of the sympathetic and renin-angiotensin-aldosterone systems that have beneficial effects in heart failure also generally attenuate or reverse ventricular remodeling (see Chapters 8, 45, and 46),[30-34] whereas agents that fail to improve clinical outcomes either have no effect on remodeling or have been associated with adverse remodeling.[4] Ventricular remodeling has therefore emerged as a credible surrogate endpoint and an important therapeutic target in heart failure.[35,36]

MECHANISMS OF LEFT VENTRICULAR REMODELING

Although ventricular remodeling may occur following any form of myocardial injury,[20] most of our knowledge has been acquired from the study of remodeling following myocardial infarction. Acute coronary occlusion in the clinical setting or in the experimental animal leads to loss of myocardial tissue, depression of myocardial function, and hypotension. This causes baroreceptor-mediated activation of a number of neurohormones that help stabilize the hemodynamics through an increase in heart rate, contractility, and fluid retention. However, continuous activation of these mechanisms, designed for short-term support of blood pressure,[37] may lead to progressive LV remodeling and dysfunction. Two distinct phases have been identified following myocardial infarction: early infarct expansion and late progressive LV remodeling.

Early Postinfarct Left Ventricular Remodeling

Loss of regional wall function after acute myocardial infarction results in an abrupt increase in loading conditions of the ventricle that brings on a unique pattern of remodeling involving the infarct area and border zone and the remote noninfarcted myocardium. Thinning and stretching of the acutely infarcted myocardium leads to infarct expansion, the first feature of LV remodeling.[21,22] Although later thinning of the LV wall also occurs in the noninfarcted myocardium, the cellular mechanisms are different in the two regions. In infarcted myocardium, as expected, wall thinning is pronounced and is a result of the loss of myocytes, collapse of the intercellular space, and stretching of surviving myocytes.[21-23,38,39] This may lead to bulging of the infarct zone that may result in ventricular rupture, aneurysm, mitral insufficiency, and ventricular tachyarrhythmias. In the noninfarcted regions, the myocardium thins because of a decrease in the number of myocytes across the wall.[38,39] Two mechanisms—myocyte slippage,[38] and myocyte loss from necrosis[40-42] and apoptosis[41,43]—have been proposed to explain this decrease.

It has been suggested that "myocyte slippage" plays a major role in progressive chamber dilation leading to failure,[8,38,44] though much of the literature mentioning this phenomenon is rather vague. This concept usually refers to slippage of myocytes past one another transversely or linear slippage of individual myofibrils within myocytes.[44,45] It would seem more likely that linear slippage of myocytes past one another could occur only at fascial planes because of the

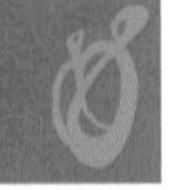

complex interdigitating connections between myocytes and the presence of intermyocyte collagen struts.[46]

It is believed that increased myocardial collagenase activity (see later discussion) disrupts intermyocyte collagen struts, leading to side-to-side slippage of myocyte (see Chapter 5).[47] Such a process could reduce wall thickness and increase the volume of the ventricle. Linzbach[44] and others[38] have noted a reduction in the number of myocytes across the wall as evidence of myocyte slippage. However, this explanation may be too simplistic. For a meaningful discussion of the slippage concept, however, we need to take into account the three-dimensional nature of myocyte-to-myocyte interconnections. Each myocyte is connected to an average of 5 to 10 neighboring myocytes via end-to-end and side-to-side intercalated disks (Figure 15-2).[48] Slippage implies disruption of intercalated disks. Once the disks are disrupted, they may be unable to reconnect, resulting in poorly coordinated contractions. If, however, disks at the ends of the main body of the cell were to be disrupted, disks on smaller side-to-side branches may remain intact, and contractile coordination between cells may be impaired but not destroyed. Thus myocyte slippage could occur if there is disruption of intercalated disks and loss of intermyocyte collagen struts. However, such widespread disruption of the intercalated disks has not been demonstrated, and this attractive hypothesis remains controversial and unproven. This issue is complicated by likely sliding and rearrangement of myocyte bundles along fascial planes, especially during contraction.

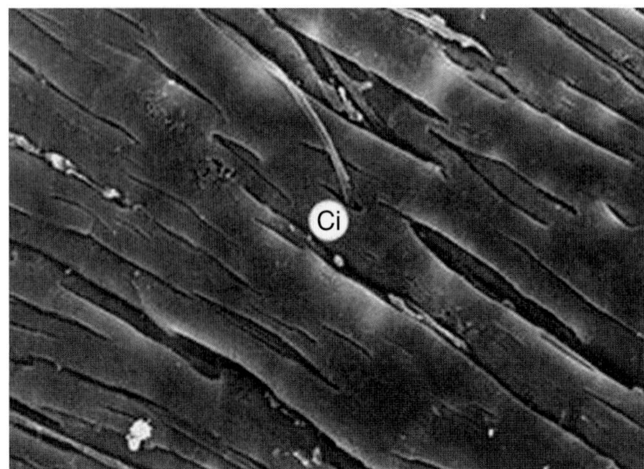

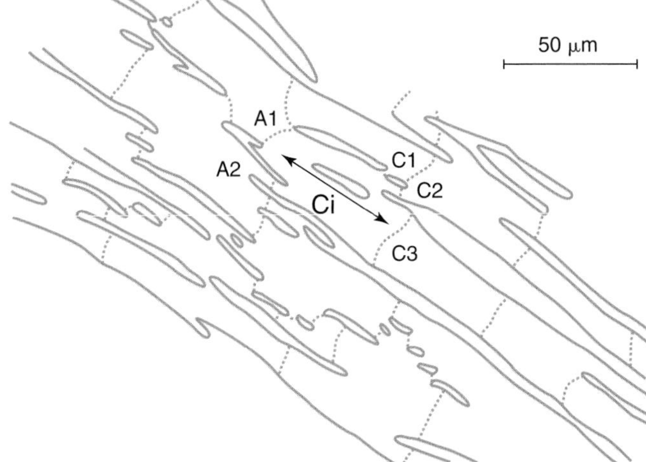

FIGURE 15–2 Scanning electron micrograph (*top*) and a drawing (*bottom*) of the cardiac myocardial fibers. The cardiocyte Ci connects with five neighboring cardiomyocytes (A_1, A_2, C_1, C_2, and C_3). (From Yamamoto S, et al. Generation of new intercellular junctions between cardiomyocytes. A possible mechanism compensating for mechanical overload in the hypertrophied human adult myocardium. *Circ Res* 1996;78:362-370.[48])

Factors Affecting the Magnitude of Remodeling after Myocardial Infarction

The magnitude of infarct expansion and development of LV remodeling depend on a number of factors. The most important determinant is the extent of myocardial damage. In the rat model, the increase in LV diastolic volume has been related to the size of the infarct and correlated with the extent of impaired systolic performance.[49,50] A critical infarct size of 17% of LV myocardium was necessary for significant infarct expansion, and the degree of expansion correlated with infarct size occurring in 66% of transmural infarcts but in none of the nontransmural infarcts.[22] Preservation of a normal LV contour was observed in only 20% of the myocardial infarction in that series.[22] Likewise, infarct expansion is observed more frequently in patients with large anterior transmural infarction compared with other regions of the left ventricle.[51-53] Distortion of the ventricular contour leading to aneurysm formation is frequent in patients with infarct expansion and is associated with increased mortality and morbidity.[1] Patients developing an aneurysm early in the course of anterior infarction have a much higher 1-year mortality than patients with anterior infarction and comparably reduced ejection fraction but without aneurysm.[54]

The loading conditions of the ventricle are also of central importance in influencing ventricular remodeling and eventual outcome. In dogs, early transient increases in afterload after an acute myocardial infarction have been shown to increase infarct expansion and thinning, and slow infarct healing.[55] In the rat, sustained increase in afterload following aortic banding also increased infarct expansion independent of infarct size.[56] Patients with hypertension and LV hypertrophy have increased morbidity and mortality after myocardial infarction.[57] Thus careful afterload reduction early in the course of myocardial infarction may have important effects on LV remodeling by reducing infarct expansion and limiting infarct size.[58]

Patency of the infarct-related coronary artery may also confer a beneficial effect on ventricular remodeling and long-term survival. In patients with acute myocardial infarction, the prompt restoration of antegrade flow in the infarct-related coronary artery, whether accomplished pharmacologically[59] or mechanically,[60] improves LV systolic function and reduces mortality. Initially, these salutary effects of reperfusion therapy were thought to be tightly linked: successful reperfusion salvaged ischemic but still viable myocardium, which led to improved LV function and, in turn, improved survival. Conversely, reperfusion of the infarct-related artery more than 12 hours after the onset of infarction was thought not to achieve these beneficial results. However, several studies suggested that the effects of reperfusion on LV function and survival might, to some extent, be independent of one another. In the Western Washington trial,[61] fibrinolytic therapy (with streptokinase) improved survival without improving LV function. In the Second International Study of Infarct Survival,[62] streptokinase reduced mortality even when given 13 to 24 hours after the onset of chest pain, at a time when myocardial salvage was unlikely. These initial studies formed the basis for the so-called open-artery hypothesis: that the restoration of antegrade flow in the infarct-related artery days, weeks, or even several months after myocardial infarction would improve survival even though LV function did not improve. The Occluded Artery Trial was a large randomized, prospective study assessing the open-artery hypothesis.[63] The study unequivocally demonstrated that the late restoration of antegrade flow did not reduce the incidence of death, reinfarction, or heart failure. In the Total Occlusion Study of Canada (TOSCA)-2 Trial,[64] opening a persistently occluded infarct-related artery beyond the acute phase of myocardial infarction effectively maintained long-term artery patency but had no effect on LV dimensions and ejection fraction.

Late Progressive Postinfarct Left Ventricular Remodeling

Early infarct expansion after myocardial infarction may be followed by progressive ventricular dilation and dysfunction over subsequent months and years, involving predominantly the noninfarcted segments. The mechanisms responsible for this inexorable deterioration of LV structure and function are not entirely clear but are related to continued activation of neurohormones and cytokines such as norepinephrine, angiotensin II, aldosterone, endothelin, and tumor necrosis factor. These factors, in combination with increased wall stress and mechanical stretch of the myocytes, upregulate a large number of signaling pathways (see later discussion), leading to structural and functional changes in the myocyte and nonmyocyte compartments that underlie a reduction in LV function and the progression of heart failure. In the discussion that follows, changes in these individual components will be described and their implications discussed.

ALTERATIONS IN THE MYOCYTE COMPARTMENT

The remodeling process results in important changes in the cardiac myocytes. These include myocyte hypertrophy, myocyte loss by necrosis[41,42,65] and apoptosis,[41,66-69] and changes in the structural proteins with downregulation of contractile and sarcomeric skeleton proteins, and upregulation of cytoskeletal and membrane-associated proteins.[70] In addition, loss of myofilaments, nuclear enlargement, development of multiple small mitochondria, and a decrease in the T-tubular system and sarcoplasmatic reticulum are common histological features of the failing myocardium.[71]

Myocyte Hypertrophy

Individual cardiac myocytes are considered terminally differentiated cells that are unable to reenter the cell cycle, and, therefore, the postnatal growth of cardiac myocytes occurs through hypertrophy of existing cells.[72-74] In nonmyocyte cells, which include both fibroblasts and endothelial cells, growth is predominantly through a hyperplastic process.[75]

Grossman and coworkers proposed that alterations in myocyte shape and size determine the type of cardiac hypertrophy.[76] In conditions with pressure overload such as aortic stenosis or hypertension, parallel addition of sarcomere causes an increase in myocyte cross-sectional area with no increase in myocyte length (Figure 15-3).[77-79] This leads to an increase in wall thickness and concentric LV hypertrophy (increase in ratio of wall thickness to chamber dimension).[76,80] In conditions with volume overload such as aortic and mitral regurgitation, ventricular volume and wall thickness increase proportionally, and this is associated with a corresponding proportional increase in both myocyte length and cross-sectional area (addition of sarcomeres both in parallel and series)[81] (see Figure 15-3). It appears that during the compensated stage of concentric LV hypertrophy, wall stress does not increase.

After a large myocardial infarction, progressive LV dilation is due to an increase in myocyte size, which occurs predominantly by laying of sarcomeres in a series, resulting in an increase in myocyte length, with only a mild increase in width and cross-sectional area[82-85] (Figure 15-4). This further increases cavity volume with no change or a decrease in wall thickness. Myocyte length is the major determinant of changes in LV size, and most of the increase in LV

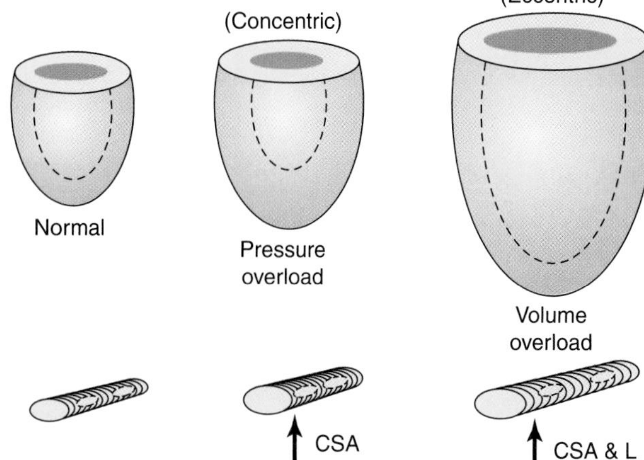

FIGURE 15–3 Schematic representation of myocyte change in left ventricular concentric and eccentric hypertension. In pressure overload hypertrophy, myocyte cross-sectional area increases and the ventricular wall becomes thicker during the compensatory phase. In volume overload hypertrophy, ventricular volume and wall thickness increase proportionally, and this is associated with a corresponding proportional increase in both myocyte length and cross-sectional area (CSA). *CSA & L*, cross-sectional area and length. (From Gerdes AM. The use of isolated myocytes to evaluate myocardial remodeling. *Trends Cardiovasc Med* 1992;2:152-155.[79])

volume can be explained by an increase in myocyte length (Figure 15-5).[82,84-86] Although LV mass increases, the increase in LV volume is proportionately greater, so that mass-to-volume ratio, an important determinant of wall stress, is reduced. Development of myocardial hypertrophy after myocardial infarction, therefore, results in eccentric hypertrophy (cavity dilation with a decrease in wall thickness to chamber dimension ratio) that increases wall stress.

In volume overload conditions such as mitral and aortic regurgitation, ventricular hypertrophy remains appropriate and helps to maintain normal wall stress for variable periods of time (see Chapter 29). Transition from a compensated to a decompensated state is associated with a further increase in chamber volume but no increase in wall thickness. This results in a decrease in mass-to-volume ratio and an increase in wall stress. The cellular mechanisms responsible for this are not entirely clear, but they could be related to an arrest in the growth of the myocytes in the transverse diameter, resulting in myocyte lengthening without further change in myocyte cross-sectional area. Studies of mitral regurgitation in the dog, and in patients at the time of mitral valve surgery also show a decrease in myocardial myosin content, proportional to degree of LV dysfunction.[81,87] Thus reduced contractility in mitral regurgitation could, in part, be due to loss of contractile elements. Although aortic and mitral regurgitation are often considered together as volume overload conditions, the two have their specific pathophysiological features.

In aortic regurgitation, the sum of the regurgitant and forward stroke volume is ejected into the aorta in systole, resulting in a wide pulse pressure and systolic hypertension. Therefore, aortic regurgitation creates both volume and pressure overload on the left ventricle. Systolic wall stress is always higher in aortic regurgitation than in mitral regurgitation,[88] and is often as high as in aortic stenosis (the classic pressure overload condition).[89] These different loading conditions in mitral and aortic regurgitation create two different types of ventricular geometry. In mitral regurgitation, there is an enlarged thin-walled left ventricle in which the mass-to-volume ratio is less than 1.0.[90] In contrast, in aortic regurgitation, the mass-to-volume ratio is normal at 1.0.[91] Whether the cellular hypertrophy, at the onset of failure, is different in these two conditions remains to be determined.

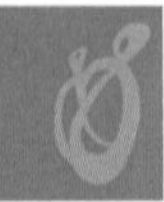

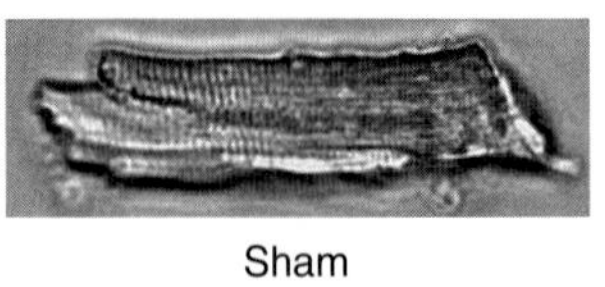

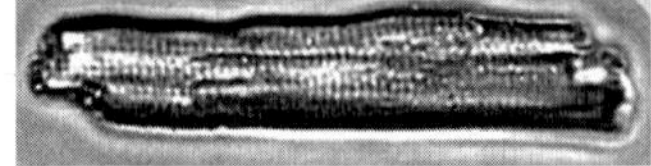

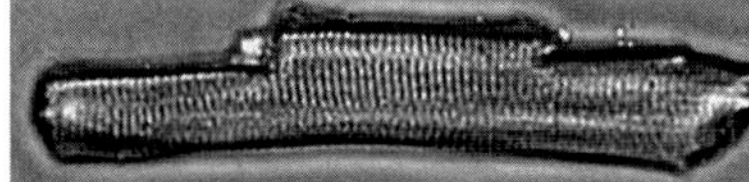

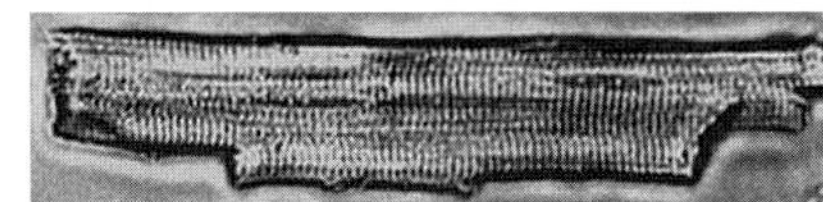

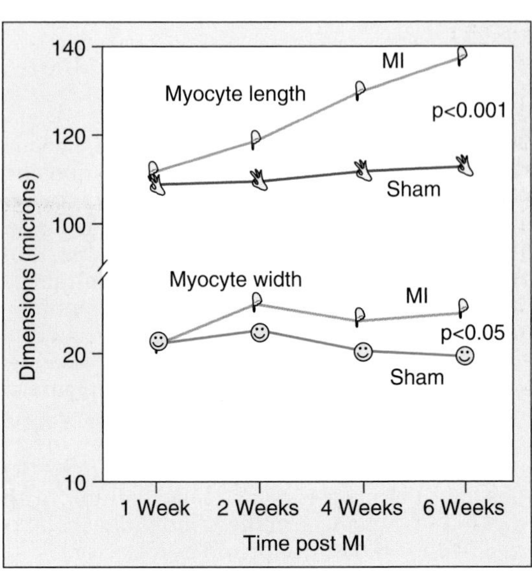

FIGURE 15–4 Cardiac myocyte remodeling in the rat infarct model. Myocyte length and width from rats 1, 2, 4, and 6 weeks after myocardial infarction are compared with those from a sham-operated animal. Note that myocyte hypertrophy after myocardial infarction is predominantly due to an increase in myocyte length. *MI,* Myocardial infarction. (From Anand IS, Liu D, Chugh SS, et al. Isolated myocyte contractile function is normal in postinfarct remodeled rat heart with systolic dysfunction. *Circulation* 1997;96(11):3974-3984.[85])

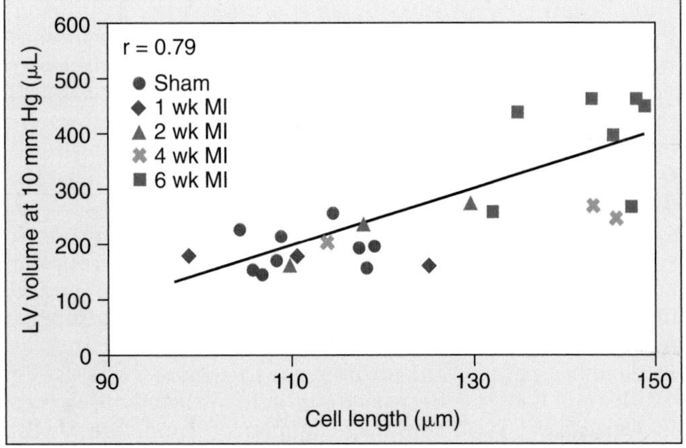

FIGURE 15–5 Scatterplot showing the relation between left ventricular volume and mean length of myocytes obtained from 1- to 6-week-old post-MI rat hearts (r = 0.79). The relationship suggests that most of the increase in LV volume after MI could be explained by an increase in myocyte length. (From Anand IS, Liu D, Chugh SS, et al. Isolated myocyte contractile function is normal in postinfarct remodeled rat heart with systolic dysfunction. *Circulation* 1997;96(11):3974-3984.[85])

In pressure-overload conditions, concentric ventricular hypertrophy (thick wall, normal chamber volume, and high mass-to-volume ratio) helps to keep wall stress normal despite high ventricular pressure. Because systolic stress (afterload) is a major determinant of ejection performance, normalization of systolic stress helps to maintain a normal stroke volume despite the need to generate high levels of systolic pressure.[12] Transition to failure is accompanied by progressive cavity enlargement and a decline in the mass-to-volume ratio, resulting in eccentric ventricular hypertrophy. In spontaneously hypertensive rats, transition to failure is preceded by myocyte lengthening without an increase in myocyte cross-sectional area.[77,78] Whether the same occurs in aortic stenosis is not known.

Data from many mammalian species suggest that the myocyte length-to-width ratio is normally regulated within a somewhat narrow range.[92,93] Although the length-to-width ratio declines slightly in concentric hypertrophy, it remains normal in volume-overload conditions such as arteriovenous fistula, mitral regurgitation, and aortic insufficiency.[81,94] There is a dramatic increase in myocyte length-to-width ratio, however, in ischemic or dilated cardiomyopathy.[84,95] Thus it appears that the onset of myocyte lengthening without transverse growth may be the critical early cellular event elevating wall stress, leading to progressive LV dilation and deterioration of LV function. In postinfarct remodeling, this process may start from the very beginning. Data are not available to confirm whether arrest of myocyte transverse growth is also responsible for the deterioration of LV function in aortic and mitral regurgitation.

Mechanisms of Myocyte Hypertrophy and Signaling Pathways

The molecular mechanisms whereby cardiac myocytes regulate the addition of new sarcomeres, in series or parallel, in response to different hemodynamic load and lead to eccentric or concentric LV hypertrophy remain unknown. A clearer understanding of these mechanisms may help develop therapeutic strategies to arrest abnormal myocardial growth.

Myocyte hypertrophy is usually accompanied by complex changes in gene reprogramming (see Chapter 3).[75] These changes include the reexpression of immature fetal cardiac genes such as those for A- and B-type natriuretic peptides (ANP and BNP) and genes that modify motor unit composition and sarcomere deposition.[96,97] However, changes in gene and protein expression may not be identical in the two forms of hypertrophy. For example, the α-adrenergic agonist phenylephrine, which acts through G protein–coupled receptors, induces a pressure-overloaded type of myocyte hypertrophy, whereas the cytokine-related agonist cardiotrophin-1 produces a volume-overloaded myocyte morphology.[98] The signaling pathways responsible for these differences are not clear.

Reversible protein phosphorylation and/or dephosphorylation play a central role in signal transduction in cardiomyocyte hypertrophy. Although multiple pathways probably mediate hypertrophy, two groups of regulatory proteins: the mitogen-activated protein kinases (MAPKs)[99,100] and Ca^{2+}/calmodulin-activated protein kinases/phosphatases[101,102] are considered to be important. The MAPK pathways consist of three major phosphorylation cascades: the extracellular signal-regulated protein kinases 1 and 2, the c-Jun N-terminal kinases, and the p38 MAPKs.[103-105] When activated, the MAPKs translocate to the nucleus, where their primary targets, the transcription factors, are located.[106] These transcription factors regulate the induction of genes that determine the ultimate biological response of the cells, including cardiac hypertrophy. Recent data suggest that differential activation of MAPKs by systolic and diastolic load may underlie difference between pressure- and volume-overload hypertrophy.[107]

The Ca^{2+}/calmodulin-activated protein kinases/phosphatases include Ca^{2+}/calmodulin-activated protein kinases (CAM kinases) and calcineurin, a Ca^{2+}/calmodulin-dependent phosphatase. Transgenic mice that overexpress components of the calcineurin signaling pathway develop a hypertrophic phenotype that can be suppressed by pharmacological inhibitors of calcineurin.[101] However, calcineurin inhibitors fail to suppress experimental hypertrophy in several animal models[108,109] and in humans with hypertension after cardiac transplantation.[110] These observations suggest that redundant signaling pathways are likely to modulate load-induced hypertrophy, with the potential for recruitment of alternate signaling cascades when a single pathway is suppressed.[111]

How is an increase in myocardial mechanical load sensed and transduced into biochemical events that lead to the addition of sarcomeres in the myocyte? Although the sensor mechanisms are unclear, they are likely to be different for the two types of hypertrophy. The role of the cytoskeleton is probably pivotal in this regard as it is not only involved in cellular stability and integrity but it also plays a significant role in transmitting signals from the cellular membrane to the nucleus.[112] Changes in different loading conditions in the heart may be sensed by the extracellular matrix and transduced by the cytoskeletal proteins, leading to phosphorylation of proteins that then translocate to the nucleus as transcription factors.[113] Integrins can act as mechanoreceptors, and transfer of force from integrins to the cytoskeleton is thought to represent a proximal step in an intracellular mechanical signaling that leads to global cytoskeletal rearrangements.[114]

Myocyte Death (see also Chapter 6)

Cell death is an important determinant of progressive cardiac remodeling and LV wall thinning. A reduction of contractile material is a prominent feature in heart failure and myocyte loss may occur either by necrosis or apoptosis.[41]

Myocyte necrosis: Necrosis generally occurs in the setting of catastrophic events, such as myocardial infarction or inflammation, and is characterized by severe membrane alterations, release of cell breakdown products, and polymorphonuclear infiltration. However, slow myocyte loss by necrosis is also a common feature of chronic heart failure.[40-42,115] During the progression of heart failure, there is activation of several neurohormones including norepinephrine, angiotensin II, and endothelin. These neurohormones are directly toxic to the myocardium, and have been shown to cause myocyte necrosis in various animal models.[116,117] Moreover, in patients with severe heart failure, circulating levels of troponin are often increased, suggesting ongoing myocyte necrosis.[118,119] Myocyte loss through necrosis probably contributes to progressive LV dilation and wall thinning. Even very low plasma concentrations of troponin are predictive of adverse outcomes in patients with chronic heart failure.[118]

Myocyte apoptosis: Apoptosis, or programmed cell death, is an evolutionarily conserved process of cell death, wherein cells die without provoking significant inflammatory response. There is convincing evidence that apoptosis contributes to the progression of heart failure. Apoptosis occurs through a cascade of subcellular events including cytochrome *c* release into the cytoplasm and activation of proteolytic caspases.[120] Activated caspases lead to fragmentation of cytoplasmic proteins, including contractile apparatus.[121] Caspase 3 (the final executioner in the apoptotic cascade) overexpression or activation has been shown to directly reduce the contractile performance of the left ventricle.[122] The degree of myosin cleavage with caspases correlates with the contractile performance of the heart.[123] It has been proposed that the release of cytochrome *c* from mitochondria and contractile protein loss in living heart muscle cells contribute to systolic dysfunction.[120] Apoptosis is involved at multiple points in the natural history of heart failure. This includes initial events such as ischemia, infarction, inflammation, and those events occurring later in established LV dysfunction. Several of the factors implicated in the pathogenesis of heart failure such as myocardial stretch,[124] norepinephrine,[125] angiotensin II,[126,127] tumor necrosis factor α (TNF-α), and oxidative stress[128,129] may provoke apoptosis.

While the presence of myocardial apoptosis has been confirmed in end-stage human heart failure[68,69] and in several animal models,[41,43,66,67] questions remain whether apoptosis is a cause or a consequence of heart failure. Myocyte apoptosis may be a factor in the transition from compensated to uncompensated heart failure.[121] This has been demonstrated in several animal models of experimentally induced LV hypertrophy and heart failure.[130-132] Several studies have demonstrated the presence of apoptosis late after myocardial infarction.[133-135] Consistent with the open artery hypothesis, patients with occluded infarct-related arteries tend to have more apoptosis as compared to the ones with patent infarct-related arteries. The presence of apoptosis, late after myocardial infarction, correlates with worsening heart failure, probably via the loss of functional myocardium and increased LV remodeling. In autopsy studies on patients dying 10 to 60 days after MI, myocyte apoptosis in the infarct zones and in areas remote from the infarct site have been found to be a major determinant of adverse LV remodeling.[133,136] This has in general translated into unfavorable hemodynamic performance and adverse clinical outcomes in heart failure.[28]

Myocyte Hyperplasia (see also Chapter 4)

Although cardiac myocytes are generally considered to be terminally differentiated cells, unable to regenerate, replicate, and replace damaged myocardium,[73,74] recent observations in human and animal models suggest that under conditions of intense and prolonged stress on the myocardium, myocytes can reenter the cell cycle and replicate.[137,138] The area of cardiac regeneration has gained considerable attention lately, especially with the finding that immature muscle cells and/or autologous stem cells can regenerate function in a previously injured heart.[138-140] Controversy exists concerning the potential for cardiovascular self-repair evidenced by chimerism in an allografted human heart. Several investigators have examined the explanted allografted female hearts transplanted into human male recipients for the presence of Y chromosome–positive cells either in the coronary vasculature or within cardiomyocytes.[141-144] Conflicting results have been obtained. Glaser et al[141] reported that regeneration is possible to a certain degree in the coronary vasculature but fails to occur within cardiomyocytes.[141] In contrast, Quaini et al[144] claimed not only that vascular regeneration occurs, but also that repair of up to 30% of the donor myocardium takes place within 1 month of transplantation. The paradigm shift, from the dogma of nonregenerating myocardium to that of a self-repairing heart, therefore requires proof and further reproduction of the data.[145]

Alterations in Myocyte Structural Proteins (see also Chapter 5)

The complexity of events involved in the pathogenesis of ventricular remodeling cannot be solely attributed to myocyte hypertrophy and cell loss. The hypertrophied myocytes in the remodeled failing heart also show alterations in most of the structural proteins (Table 15-1).[70] A brief description of the structural proteins (Figure 15-6), alterations that occur in these proteins in heart failure, and their functional consequences follows.

Contractile Proteins

The contractile apparatus includes thick filament myosin and thin filament complexes composed of α-actin, α-tropomyosin, and troponins C, I, and T. Ventricular remodeling involves transcriptional and translational downregulation of these proteins with resulting functional consequences.[70] One of the earliest changes is a decrease in α-myosin heavy chain and an increase in β-myosin heavy chain.[146] Mechanoenergetic alterations commonly accompany remodeling of the contractile machinery. The attachment and detachment of the cross-bridge cycle requires cleavage of ATP. Depression of maximal Ca^{2+}-activated myofibrillar ATPase activity (by as much as 50%) was the first biochemical abnormality described in failing human myocardium[147] and reflects a slower rate of cross-bridge cycling in the failing state. An alteration of this magnitude is likely to be an important contributor to myocyte contractile dysfunction.

Sarcomeric Skeleton Proteins

The contractile apparatus is kept in register by different proteins localized in the Z-disk, M-band of the sarcomere, and the giant filament molecule titin, which spans the entire half-sarcomere from the Z-disk to the M-line. The Z-disk is a region of overlapping tails of actin microfilaments, cross-linked by α-actinin. The M-line is the region where the myosin tails are linked and organized by the M-line proteins—myomesin, M-line protein, and myosin-binding protein C. Titin is anchored with its N-terminus at the Z-disk and reaches the M-line region with its C-terminal head portion where it interacts with the M-line protein and myomesin.[148] It spans the Z-disk of the sarcomere[149] and overlaps in the M-line region of the sarcomere,[150] thus functioning as a molecular spring and a source of elastic properties of the cardiomyocyte (see Figure 15-6). The interplay between titin and actomyosin suggests a possible role for titin in the Frank-Starling mechanism of the heart.[148] Several studies have reported that the amount of titin is reduced in the myocardium of patients with dilated cardiomyopathy and that this could be responsible for the altered ventricular compliance in this condition.[112,151] Because titin is required for sarcomere formation, lack of titin may also contribute to contractile dysfunction of failing hearts.[152]

TABLE 15–1 Myocyte Protein Families

Contractile proteins	Myosin, α-actin, α-tropomyosin, troponins C, I, and T
Sarcomeric skeleton	Titin, α-actinin, M-line proteins: M-protein, myosin-binding protein C
Cytoskeletal proteins	Tubulin, desmin, nonsarcomeric actin
Membrane-associated proteins	Vinculin, talin, dystrophin, spectrin, integrins
Proteins of the intercalated disk	Connexins, cadherins, catenins

From Kostin S, Heling A, Hein S, et al. The protein composition of the normal and diseased cardiac myocyte. *Heart Fail Rev* 1998;2:245-260.[70]

Cytoskeletal Proteins

The cytoskeleton is a complex network of microtubules (primarily tubulin), nonsarcomeric actin, and intermediate filaments (primarily desmin). Tubulin is the protein of microtubules, which are hollow tubes formed from α- and β-tubulin, with a diameter of 25 nm surrounding the nucleus and spreading, mostly in the longitudinal direction, throughout the entire cell. Microtubules undergo continuous polymerization and depolymerization, which under normal conditions results in a stable relationship between free cytosolic tubulin and structure-related tubulin (i.e., the microtubules). This dynamic process can be enhanced or arrested by the application of agents such as taxol or colchicine, which respectively promotes or prevents polymerization from the tubulin pool. Under steady-state conditions, about 70% of the total tubulin in the cell is typically in the depolymerized form. The multifunctional roles of microtubules include mitosis, intracellular transport, organization of organelles, cell motility, determination of cell shape, receptor modulation, and signaling.[153]

Desmin belongs to the family of intermediate filaments with a diameter of 12 to 15 nm ranging between microtubules (25 nm) and actin filaments (8 to 10 nm). It surrounds the Z-disks and connects the sarcomeres so that these are kept in register during contraction. Desmin filaments also link myofibrils to one another, to the sarcolemma, and to the nuclear envelope.[154] The desmin network plays a role in the underlying structural integrity of the myocyte and participates in the signaling processes necessary for integration of cellular responses to external and internal stimuli.[154]

The cytoskeleton contributes substantially to cell stability by anchoring subcellular structures, such as mitochondria, Golgi apparatus, nuclei, and myofibrils. The cytoskeleton proteins also act as a stabilizing force and as mechanotransductors through their connection with membrane-associated proteins.[155] A close cytoskeleton-integrin linkage system also exists at the level of the sarcolemma, which allows cells to respond to physical and biochemical influences exerted by the

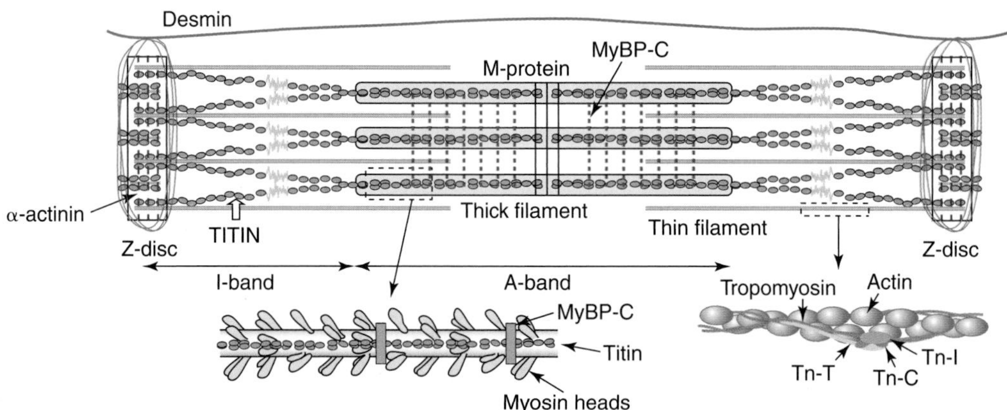

FIGURE 15–6 Diagram of the myocyte sarcomeric proteins. *MyBP-C,* myosin binding protein-C; *Tn-C,* troponin C, *Tn-I,* troponin I; *Tn-T,* troponin T. (Courtesy H. L. Granzier.)

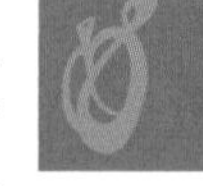

extracellular matrix. When the matrix resists movement, the linkage to the cytoskeleton is strengthened via an increased number of integrins.[156] At the intercalated disk, the cytoskeleton is anchored to sites of cadherin-mediated adhesion between adjacent plasma membranes via catenins and desmoplakins.[157]

In failing human myocardium, both tubulin and desmin are increased.[158] The increase in these proteins mainly occurs in cells that lack myofilaments and could, therefore, help maintain cellular stability. Tubulin accumulation plays a role in certain models of pressure-overload hypertrophy.[159] In feline right ventricular hypertrophy, resulting from pulmonary artery banding, isolated myocytes show contractile dysfunction and loss of compliance.[160-162] These changes are accompanied by an increase in total and polymerized tubulin. Reduction of microtubule hyperpolymerization by colchicine treatment reverses myocyte stiffness and normalizes contractile dysfunction. Taxol treatment of normal myocytes hyperpolymerizes tubulin and produces functional disturbances similar to chronic pressure overload.[160-162] The results of these studies underscore the role of the cytoskeleton in myocyte contractile dysfunction in at least one model of heart failure. Whether this is a universal finding in heart failure is debatable.

There are increasing reports of desmin-related cardiomyopathies that have, as a hallmark, abnormal deposits of desmin aggregates. A progressive increase of desmin protein and filaments was shown to accompany the transition from hypertrophy to heart failure.[163] Overexpression and altered distribution of desmin were also observed in human hearts with end-stage congestive heart failure in dilated cardiomyopathy.[158] Absence of an intact desmin filament system may also be involved in cardiomyocyte hypertrophy and cardiac dilation with compromised systolic function.[164] Whether alteration in desmin quantity is a cause or a consequence of heart failure remains to be elucidated.

Membrane-associated and Intercalated Disk Proteins

Membrane-associated proteins include dystrophin, vinculin, talin, spectrin, and integrins, which are involved in fixation of sarcomeres to the lateral sarcolemma and stabilization of the T-tubular system.[70,165,166] It was recently shown that mutations of these proteins could cause dilated cardiomyopathy.[167-169] Dystrophin connects intracellular actin and extracellular laminin independent of integrin binding[155] and plays an important role in promoting the action of the cytoskeleton as a stabilizing force and as mechanotransductor.[170]

The intercalated disk consists of three different types of specialized membranes: fasciae adherens, desmosomes, and gap junctions.[171] Fasciae adherens establish the longitudinal connections with the contractile filaments. The desmosomes are connections with intracellular desmin via the desmoplakins, and the gap junction consists of the membrane-spanning connexins. Gap junctions are responsible for the orderly spread of electrical excitation from one myocyte to the next in the heart. Gap junction channel proteins are termed "connexins." Different connexins exhibit different biophysical properties. Remodeling of gap junction and connexin expression is a conspicuous feature of human congestive heart failure and other cardiac conditions with a dysrhythmic tendency. Remodeling of gap junctions and reduced connexin[43] levels may contribute to slowing of conduction.[172,173] Evidence from studies in experimental animals strengthens the case that gap junction remodeling is a key determinant of arrhythmias in the diseased heart.[174,175]

ALTERATIONS IN THE NONMYOCYTE COMPARTMENT

While historically considered a static structure, it is now becoming recognized that the myocardial extracellular matrix (ECM) is a complex microenvironment containing a large portfolio of matrix proteins, signaling molecules, proteases, and cell types that play a fundamental role in the myocardial remodeling process.[28,176-178]

Apart from the myocyte compartment, the chronically failing heart is characterized by iterations in the extracellular matrix (ECM), particularly by fibrous tissue formation.[65] Such an adverse accumulation of ECM raises myocardial stiffness and impairs contractile behavior.[179]

Extracellular Matrix Remodeling (see Chapter 5)

The extracellular matrix of the heart is made up of a number of structural proteins including fibrillar collagen, smaller amounts of elastin, and the signaling peptides laminin and fibronectin. The complex collagen 3D weave, mainly consisting of type I collagen, interconnects individual myocytes through a collagen-integrin-cytoskeletal-myofibril arrangement. This network supports cardiac myocytes during contraction and relaxation, and also provides a mechanism for translating individual myocyte shortening and force generation into ventricular contraction; it is also responsible for much of the ventricle's passive diastolic stiffness.[180] In both human and animal studies, progressive LV remodeling and dysfunction are associated with significant changes in the ECM.[181-184]

The structural hallmark of prolonged pressure-overload hypertrophy is significantly increased collagen accumulation between individual myocytes and myocyte fascicles (Figure 15-7).[185,186] Thus the highly organized architecture of the ECM is replaced with a thickened, poorly organized ECM related to decreased capacity for ECM degradation and turnover. This "reactive" collagen deposition is characterized by both perivascular and interstitial fibrosis.[180,187,188] It is not clear whether the initiation of reactive fibrosis is triggered by myocardial ischemia or the local activation of trophic peptides such as angiotensin II, aldosterone, and catecholamines, which results in the sequential expression of transforming growth factor β_1 and fibronectin, and a relative increase in collagen I.[187-189] While the accumulation of ECM with pressure-overload hypertrophy is not exclusive to collagen, these initial structural studies gave rise to the generic term for this extracellular remodeling process as myocardial fibrosis. Autopsy and biopsy studies of patients with severe chronic hypertension or aortic stenosis frequently show changes in collagen architecture, and a severe increase in the percentage of fibrosis occupying the myocardium.[188,190] Enhanced synthesis and deposition of myocardial ECM in pressure-overload hypertrophy is directly associated with increased LV myocardial stiffness properties, which in turn cause poor filling characteristics during diastole.[186,191,192] Indeed, clinical evidence suggests that progressive ECM accumulation and diastolic dysfunction are important underlying pathophysiological mechanisms for heart failure in patients with pressure-overload hypertrophy.[193,194]

In volume-overload hypertrophy due to the persistently elevated preload, a much different pattern of ECM remodeling occurs. In large-animal models of volume-overload hypertrophy due to chronic mitral regurgitation, the LV remodeling process is accompanied by a distinctive loss of collagen fibrils surrounding individual myocytes.[87,195-198] These changes in ECM support are associated with changes in isolated LV myocyte geometry where the cardiac cells increase in length. Representative scanning electron micrographs taken from a model of canine mitral regurgitation[195] are shown in Figure 15-8 and demonstrate the profound differences in ECM structure and composition compared with normal myocardium and that of volume-overload hypertrophy. Increased ECM proteolytic activity likely contributes to the reduced ECM content and support, and thereby facilitates the overall LV remodeling process.[178]

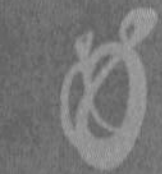

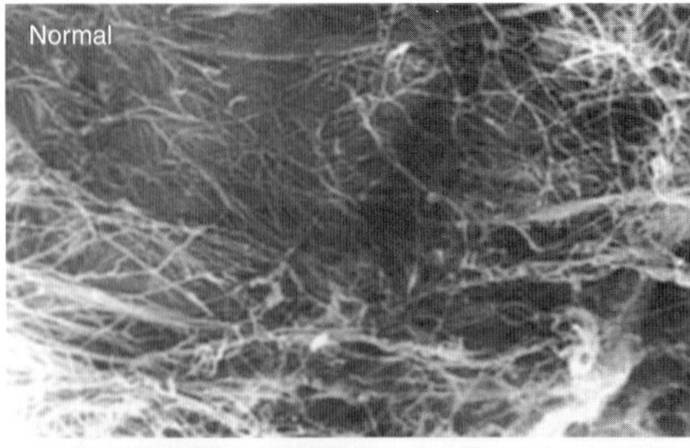

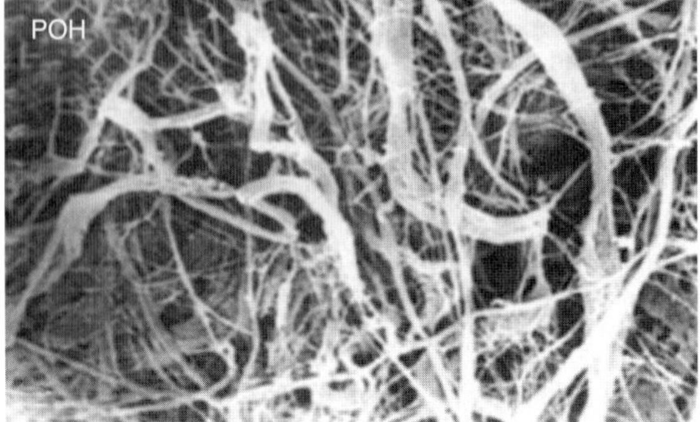

FIGURE 15–7 Scanning electron micrographs taken from normal nonhuman primate left ventricular myocardium and following the induction of pressure overload hypertrophy (POH). These microscopic studies demonstrated thickening of the collagen weave and overall increased relative content between myocytes with POH. (From Abrahams et al. Myocardial hypertrophy in *Macaca fascicularis*. Structural remodeling of the collagen matrix. *Lab Invest* 1987;56:676-683.[185])

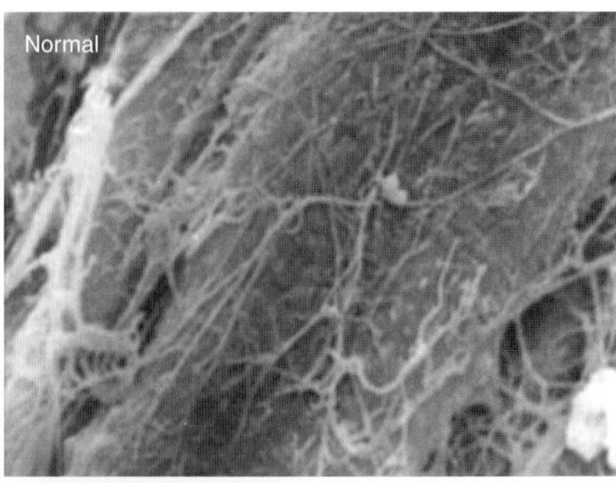

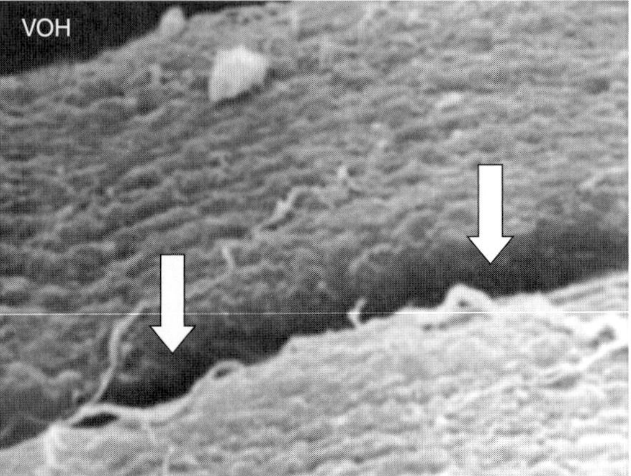

FIGURE 15–8 Scanning electron micrographs taken from normal canine left ventricular myocardium following chronic mitral regurgitation that causes a volume overload hypertrophy (VOH). In this model of VOH,[195] a loss of normal ECM architecture was demonstrated between individual myocytes (arrows), and the collagen supporting network is poorly organized. (Figure 2 from Dell'italia, L. J., Balcells, E, Meng, Q. C., et al. Volume-overload cardiac hypertrophy is unaffected by ACE inhibitor treatment in dogs. *Am J Physiol Heart Circ Physiol* 273: H961-H970, 1997.)

Although the mechanisms by which increased degradation of collagen promote LV dilation and global LV dysfunction are not entirely clear, dissolution of the collagen weave may lead to increased elasticity and contribute to muscle fiber slippage and therefore an increase in chamber size.[191] Loss of collagen struts connecting individual myocytes could, as we will see later, prevent transduction of individual myocyte contractions into myocardial force development, resulting in reduced myocardial systolic performance.

The ECM and, particularly, collagen are under dynamic control of two sets of proteins: those that favor degradation and those that tend to inhibit it. The dissolution or degradation of collagen is predominantly related to the activation of matrix metalloproteinases (MMPs), a family of zinc-containing proteins that includes collagenases, gelatinases, stromelysins, and membrane types of MMPs.[178] Active MMPs can undergo autodigestion and thereby lose proteolytic activity. However, the kinetics of this process are not fully understood and can be variable for different MMPs and conditions. A more critical control point for MMP activity is through the inhibition of the activated enzyme by the action of a group of specific MMP inhibitors termed *tissue inhibitors of metalloproteinases* (TIMP).[178] There are four known TIMP species of which TIMP-1 and TIMP-2 have been the most studied. The timps are low-molecular-weight proteins that can complex noncovalently with high efficiency to active MMPs inhibiting their activity.[199,200]

While the contributory mechanisms for the changes in plasma MMP levels remain speculative, an association between changes in plasma MMP levels to adverse LV remodeling is beginning to emerge. For example, in a Framingham Heart substudy, it was demonstrated that increased plasma MMP-9 levels were associated with LV dilation.[201] Specifically, higher plasma levels of MMP-9 were associated with an approximately twofold higher risk of adverse LV remodeling. Changes in the plasma levels of TIMP-1 have been studied in several large-scale cardiovascular studies.[201,202] Elevated TIMP-1 plasma levels have been shown to be associated with major cardiovascular risk factors and with the presence of LV hypertrophy in the Framingham Heart Study.[201] Furthermore, changes in plasma TIMP-1 levels were associated with increased mortality in another study.[202] However, it is likely that the changes in plasma MMP and TIMP levels observed in these studies will be influenced by the underlying cause of the cardiovascular disease process, and therefore, future studies will be necessary. Furthermore, these studies only measured MMP and TIMP plasma levels at one point in time, and how the temporal relation to the natural history of the LV remodeling process and progression to heart failure remains to be established. Nevertheless, these studies do provide further evidence to support the potential utility of plasma MMP and TIMP profiling in terms of prognosis.

Myocardial Fibrosis

Fibrosis in heart failure is an ongoing active process of increasing collagen concentration and not simply a response to myocyte injury.[179] There are two types of fibrosis: reparative and reactive. Reparative fibrosis occurs in response to a loss of myocardial material and is mainly interstitial. In contrast, reactive fibrosis is observed in the absence of cell loss as a reaction to changes in myocardial load or inflammation, and is primarily perivascular. During ventricular remodeling, reactive and reparative fibrosis usually coexist. After myocardial infarction, reparative fibrosis is organized as a scar and is surrounded by reactive fibrosis and myocyte hypertrophy.[203]

The mechanisms responsible for fibrosis are still controversial. Fibrosis is not directly induced by stretch or mechanical overload. Chronic volume overload due to exercise training, atrial septal defect, or aortic insufficiency is not accompanied by ventricular fibrosis.[204,205] In contrast, pressure overload is frequently associated with fibrosis. It has been proposed that ventricular fibrosis seen in arterial hypertension is caused by associated factors linked to this condition, such as ischemia[206] and neurohormones.[179] Humoral factors, particularly those of the renin-angiotensin-aldosterone system, are believed to be responsible for fibrosis. Angiotensin II and aldosterone have been implicated in the process as they stimulate collagen synthesis in cultured cardiac fibroblasts, and angiotensin II inhibits collagen degradation.[207,208]

Myocardial fibrosis has a number of deleterious effects on cardiac function. A twofold to threefold increase in myocardial collagen content alters ventricular filling properties particularly by increasing diastolic stiffness; a fourfold or greater increase in fibrosis also affects systolic function.[209] Fibrosis contributes to ventricular arrhythmias because disproportionate collagen accumulation creates myocardial electrical heterogeneity. Fibrosis is therefore one of the major biological determinants of fatal issues in cardiac remodeling, including congestive heart failure, severe arrhythmias, and sudden death.

Coronary Microvasculature

Another factor that may contribute to progressive LV remodeling and dysfunction is the inadequate growth of myocardial microvasculature accompanying myocardial hypertrophy. This results in a reduction in capillary density in the hypertrophying remote noninfarcted myocardium and increases the average diffusion distance for oxygen from the capillary wall to the mitochondria of the myocytes.[82,210] These structural abnormalities are also accompanied by a functional decrease in coronary vascular reserve.[211] Thus both structural and functional abnormalities in the microvasculature could contribute to progressive LV dilation and remodeling that occurs during development of chronic heart failure.

CHANGES IN MYOCYTE CONTRACTILE FUNCTION (see Chapter 3)

These abnormalities include changes in the contractile proteins or their regulatory elements,[146] alterations in the β-adrenergic receptor signaling pathway with downregulation of the β-adrenergic receptor,[212] an increase in β-adrenergic receptor kinase,[213] defects in energetics,[214] and alterations in cytoskeletal proteins.[158] In addition, calcium-handling proteins are altered with a decrease in sarcoplasmic reticulum Ca^{2+}-atpase (SERCA2a), and an increase in the Na^+/Ca^{2+} exchanger.[43,215,216] Such changes would be expected to cause progressive myocyte contractile dysfunction. Indeed, the contractile function of myocytes isolated from end-stage heart failure in human and various animal models is often abnormal.[81,217-219] In models of concentric hypertrophy, the earliest change is slowing of myocyte relaxation that is manifest even before the appearance of overt heart failure.[220] Later, development of depressed myocyte peak contraction and slow relaxation is accompanied by alterations in Ca^{2+} transients.[220-224] These contractile defects have been related to underlying biochemical alterations in Ca^{2+} handling proteins, a decrease in SERCA2a, and an increase in the Na^+/Ca^{2+} exchanger.[215,216] In such conditions, therefore, global LV dysfunction could be explained on the basis of myocyte contractile defects.

Thus there is a considerable weight of evidence that one or another cellular function may be abnormal in the cardiac myocyte of different models of heart failure. However, there is no indication of any single final common pathway that is universally responsible for contractile dysfunction in the isolated myocytes of the failing heart. Indeed, in certain models of heart failure, myocyte contractile function may be preserved despite depressed global LV function. In one such model, rats 6 weeks following myocardial infarction developed significant remodeling and global LV dysfunction.[85] Myocytes isolated from these hearts showed eccentric hypertrophy, and an increase in length of the myocytes that correlated well with the LV volume. Despite global LV remodeling and dysfunction, however, these hypertrophied myocytes showed normal contractile function under a variety of conditions including increasing stimulation frequency, extracellular calcium, isoproterenol, and viscous loading.[43,85,225] Similarly, volume-overload hypertrophy associated with AV fistula in cats was reported to occur without changes in myocyte contractility.[226]

How can we explain global LV dysfunction despite preserved myocyte contractile function? The first way that pump function may be depressed with normal myocyte function is related to loss of cardiac myocytes. As we have seen, myocyte loss can occur acutely (e.g., following a myocardial infarction or chronically during the remodeling process through necrotic or apoptotic cell death). Either way, myocyte loss resulting in a thin-walled and dilated LV chamber with attendant increase in wall stress could be expected to develop pump dysfunction, independent of myocyte contractile function. A second possible mechanism is related to increased collagen disruption and loss of collagen struts connecting individual myocytes (see Figure 15-8). This would have the effect of under-tethering myocytes, preventing force generated by normally contracting myocytes to be transmitted to the wall, resulting in reduced global systolic performance. A recent study designed to test this hypothesis in papillary muscles isolated from normal rats and in pressure-overload hypertrophied cats found that acute disruption of the ECM fibrillar collagen, by plasmin-activated MMP, resulted in severe reduction in force generation.[227] However, myocytes isolated from these papillary muscles showed normal contractile function.[227] These data support the hypothesis that the ECM facilitates transduction of cardiomyocyte contraction into myocardial force development, and that ECM disruption could explain depressed LV systolic performance, despite the presence of normal myocyte contractile function.

CHANGES IN GLOBAL STRUCTURE AND FUNCTION

The mechanical effects of LV remodeling set in motion several self-sustaining deleterious consequences. As the ventricle enlarges, LV geometry alters from a normal prolate ellipse to a mechanically disadvantageous spherical or globular shape (Figure 15-9). The result is an increase in meridional wall stress,[228] an abnormal distribution of fiber shortening, an increase in oxygen consumption,[228,229] and abnormal myocardial bioenergetics.[214] The spherical shape of the left ventricle leads to dilation of the atrioventricular ring and stretching of the papillary muscles, resulting in functional mitral regurgitation,[230] which contributes to a further decrease in forward cardiac output. Moreover, the high LV end-diastolic volume and pressure promote subendocardial ischemia that aggravates LV dysfunction and neurohormonal activation, decreases exercise capacity,[231] and increases the risk of ventricular arrhythmias.[232] Thus a downward spiral of worsening heart failure is initiated that ends in death of the patient.

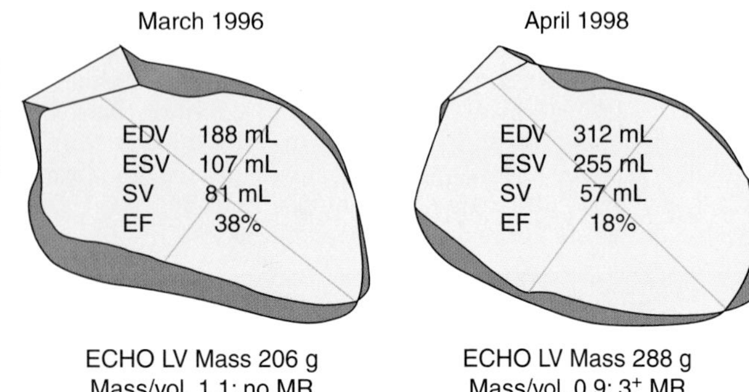

FIGURE 15-9 Left ventricular (LV) remodeling over time. Left ventricular angiogram in the right anterior oblique projection of a patient 1 month after acute myocardial infarction (March 1996) and 2 years later (April 1998). Note that 2 years after infarction, the end-diastolic volume (EDV) was three times normal, end-systolic volume (ESV) was five times normal, stroke volume (SV) was decreased, and there was a further decrease in ejection fraction (EF). There was a decrease in the ventricular mass-to-volume ratio over time, suggesting further increase in wall stress. The globular shape contributed to severe mitral regurgitation.

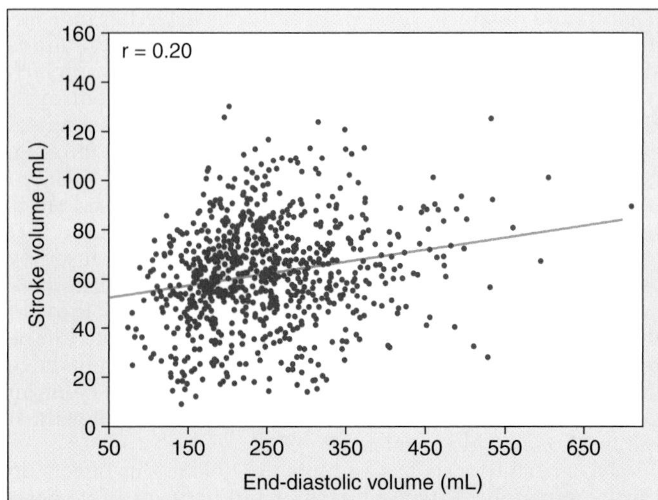

FIGURE 15-10 Lack of significant relationship between stroke volume and end-diastolic volume in 816 separate measurements of the left ventricle using magnetic resonance imaging techniques. The stroke volume is held relatively constant over a large range of end-diastolic volumes. (Unpublished data from IS Anand.)

STRUCTURAL BASES OF HEART FAILURE

In the preceding discussion we saw that the development and worsening of clinical heart failure is related to progressive ventricular dilation. It has been suggested that as the ventricle dilates, there may be an obligatory reduction of myocardial shortening or ejection fraction to maintain an optimal stroke volume.[233] An unchanged ejection fraction from a dilated left ventricle could deliver a large and potentially damaging stroke volume to the vasculature. The homeostatic mechanisms responsible for such a conceptual model are not clear but may be related to prevent a large pulse pressure from damaging the vasculature. According to this view, structural changes in LV architecture and increase in LV volume are the primary abnormalities that result in reduced wall motion mandated to generate a normal stroke volume from a large end-diastolic volume.[233] Therefore, this view challenges the traditional concept that contractile dysfunction leads to chamber dilation. The fact that the stroke volume is generally held constant, albeit at a lower than normal level, over a relatively large range of end-diastolic volumes supports this hypothesis (Figure 15-10).

COMPENSATORY VERSUS MALADAPTIVE REMODELING

A fundamental question that must be addressed before embarking on a strategy to reverse the hypertrophic and structural myocardial remodeling is whether remodeling is good or bad. Distinction is often made between a compensatory (adaptive) and a decompensatory (maladaptive) process. The organism is not endowed with any mechanism to distinguish between the effect of its response to an acute stimulus and the ultimate effects of that response when the stimulus is maintained over a prolonged period of time. An adaptive component enables the heart to maintain function in response to pressure or volume overloading in the acute phase of cardiac injury.[234] Acute distention of the viable myocardium and the operation of the Frank-Starling mechanism, through an increase in sarcomere length, are therefore entirely appropriate beneficial responses. Likewise, augmentation of chronotropic and inotropic activity through adrenergic receptor stimulation that tends to maintain pump function during the abrupt loss of contractile tissue can be considered compensatory. Progressive left ventricle dilation after myocardial infarction can also help to maintain stroke volume in the face of reduced contractile function, and has been considered an adaptive and compensatory response.[3,235] Under these circumstances, however, an increase in LV volume is not due to sarcomere stretch, but because of the addition of new sarcomeres in a series,[85] and therefore is not a mechanism of enhancing contractility on the basis of the Frank-Starling mechanism. Such a progressive remodeling and LV dilation does not normalize but increases wall stress and is associated with a poor prognosis.[19,235] Moreover, prevention of very early LV dilation with use of angiotensin-converting enzyme (ACE) inhibitors and β-blockers does not have any deleterious hemodynamic consequence.[236-238] Indeed, Sharpe et al[236] have demonstrated that attenuation of LV remodeling with early initiation of ACE inhibitors is actually associated with a greater increase in stroke volume as compared with a placebo. Furthermore, prevention of remodeling by early initiation of an ACE inhibitor or β-blocker, after myocardial infarction, in selected populations with LV dysfunction[31,34] and even in unselected populations[239] is associated with significant reduction in mortality and morbidity.[34,237,240,241] Hence, ventricular remodeling and dilation after myocardial infarction may be maladaptive from the very start, and should be a target for aggressive antiremodeling therapy.

In contrast, an increase in ventricular mass that helps to normalize wall stress in aortic stenosis and hypertension may be an appropriate compensatory response. Because systolic stress (afterload) is a major determinant of ejection performance, normalization of systolic stress helps to maintain a normal ejection fraction while generating high levels of systolic pressure.[12] However, LV hypertrophy has been shown to be an important independent risk factor for mortality and morbidity.[17] Similarly, a proportional increase in chamber volume, wall thickness, and mass in mitral and aortic regurgitation normalizes wall stress and is an obligatory response to maintain a large stroke volume that is necessitated by the regurgitant volume. Until the initial volume and pressure overload is matched by adequate hypertrophy, the process may be considered adaptive and compensatory. Eventually, with progressive dilation there is a mismatch and the process becomes maladaptive and decompensatory, and heart failure becomes clinically manifest.[242,243] There are no data to indicate when the transition from possible adaptive to maladaptive remodeling occurs; such a transition and its time course may be expected to vary greatly. However, once established beyond a certain phase, it is likely that remodeling actually contributes to progression of heart failure. Thus whether remodeling is beneficial or deleterious cannot be viewed as a stereotypical process. Today's challenge is to be able to take advantage of the adaptive features of the hypertrophic response while eliminating, or at least minimizing, the maladaptive consequences.

REVERSE REMODELING (see Chapter 8)

"Reverse remodeling" is a relatively new concept, where progressive LV dilation and deterioration in contractile function are not simply arrested, but partially reversed. Two important questions are related to the issue of reverse remodeling: "Do myocytes have the ability to remove sarcomeres?" and "Is there any time line beyond which reverse remodeling cannot be achieved?" A number of lines of evidence from surgical and pharmacological experiments have confirmed that regression of myocyte hypertrophy with removal of sarcomeres is possible. There are, however, insufficient data to address the second question. It is believed that early in the natural history of transition from hypertrophy to failure, remodeling is reversible, whereas later, with the development of extensive fibrosis, accumulation of cytoskeletal proteins, and loss of the contractile filaments, an irreversible process sets in.[112] Several therapeutic approaches for heart failure have been shown to halt or even reverse the remodeling process.

Pharmacological Approaches

Several experimental studies, aimed primarily at modulating the neurohormonal responses, have been conducted to determine whether established remodeling of a damaged left ventricle could be reversed pharmacologically. It is well known that inhibition of the renin-angiotensin system improves cardiac remodeling.[244,245] McDonald et al[246] showed that ACE inhibition and β-adrenoreceptor blockade can reverse established ventricular remodeling in a canine model of discrete myocardial damage.[246] A significant reduction of LV mass and a trend in reduction of end-diastolic volume were found in both captopril- and β-blocker-treated groups compared with the control group.[246] Tamura et al[247] have reported that administration of angiotensin II type 1 receptor blockers produced significant reverse remodeling of myocyte volume, length, and cross-sectional area in rats with spontaneously hypertensive heart failure. In this study, myocyte dimensions were reduced below pretreatment values, suggesting true reverse remodeling rather than simply arrested progression of myocyte hypertrophy.[247] Xu et al[248] studied the effect of the angiotensin II receptor blocker losartan combined with exercise training in the postinfarction rat model and demonstrated that exercise training after myocardial infarction provides a beneficial effect on cardiac function and LV remodeling by altering the gene and protein expressions that regulate myocardial fibrosis, whereas such effects were only slightly improved by the combination of exercise and losartan.[248]

Angiotensin-Converting Enzyme (ACE) Inhibitors

The first class of medications shown to beneficially affect remodeling and clinical outcomes in patients with heart failure was ACE inhibitors. In several trials performed in both asymptomatic and symptomatic patients with reduced ejection fraction, ACE inhibitors attenuated the progressive increase in end-diastolic and end-systolic volume.[32,236,249-251]

β-Blockers

In contrast to ACE inhibitors that attenuate LV remodeling, use of β-blockers is associated with significant reduction in ventricular volumes and improvement in global LV function (reverse remodeling).[30,31,33,252] β-blockers were shown to reduce myocardial apoptosis, which at least in part could explain the favorable effect on ventricular remodeling.[253]

Aldosterone Receptor Blockers

Aldosterone receptor blockers have been shown to reverse LV remodeling following myocardial infarction and in patients with heart failure.[254,255] The 4E-Left Ventricular Hypertrophy Study[256] used cardiac MRI to compare LV mass regression by the selective aldosterone blocker eplerenone to the ACE inhibitor enalapril and the combination of eplerenone/enalapril in hypertensive patients with LV hypertrophy. Eplerenone was as effective as enalapril in regression of LV hypertrophy and control of blood pressure. The combination of eplerenone and enalapril was more effective in reducing LV mass and systolic blood pressure than eplerenone alone.[256] In a single-site clinical trial, Chan et al[257] have recently demonstrated with serial cardiac magnetic resonance (CMR) that the addition of spironolactone to candesartan has significant beneficial effects on LV reverse remodeling in patients with mild to moderate chronic systolic heart failure.

Angiotensin Receptor Blockers

Several recent trials demonstrated the beneficial effect of angiotensin receptor blockers (ARBs) on LV remodeling. In the Valsartan Heart Failure Trial (Val-HeFT),[258,259] valsartan therapy attenuated LV remodeling.[260] Stratification by baseline severity of remodeling showed that patients with worse LV enlargement and systolic function are at highest risk for an event, yet appear to gain the most antiremodeling effect and clinical benefit with valsartan treatment.[261] The Losartan Intervention For Endpoint (LIFE) study[262] showed that reduction in LV mass by angiotensin II blockade was independent of blood pressure reduction, indicating that inhibition of the renin-angiotensin-aldosterone system has added benefits beyond blood pressure control.[262]

Isosorbide Dinitrate/Hydralazine Combination

In the first Vasodilator-Heart Failure Trial (V-HeFT-I),[263] isosorbide dinitrate combined with hydralazine therapy compared with placebo in patients with heart failure treated only with digoxin and diuretic resulted in a sustained increase in LV ejection fraction that was quantitatively associated with improved survival.[263] The African American Heart Failure Trial (AHeFT) confirmed these findings, even on top of ACE inhibitors and β-blockers.[264,265]

Cell Transplantation (see Chapter 4)

The past decade has seen an explosion of activity in the field of cell transplantation after myocardial injury. The first control-matched study using bone marrow stem cells was published by Strauer et al in 2002.[266] Ten patients were treated with intracoronary bone marrow mononuclear cells (BMMNCs) for 7 days after suffering a myocardial infarction. Three months later, the treated patients exhibited a decrease in infarct size when compared with controls. This study was followed by the TOPCARE-AMI (Transplantation Of Progenitor Cells And Regeneration Enhancement in Acute Myocardial Infarction) trial, which revealed improvement in ventricular function after treatment with either BMMNCs or circulating endothelial progenitor cells.[267,268] The first randomized trial, BOOST (Bone marrow transfer to enhance ST-elevation infarct regeneration), initially demonstrated improvement in ventricular function in myocardial infarction patients after treatment with BMMNCs; however, this effect was not sustained at 18 months.[269,270] The two largest randomized trials, ASTAMI[271] and Repair-AMI,[272] were published in 2006. Using similar protocols, the ASTAMI trial did not show any

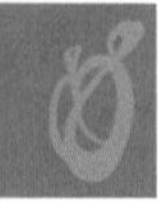

improvement in LVEF at 6 months, whereas Repair-AMI showed a 5.5% increase in mean LVEF in the treated group compared with 3% in the controls at 4 months.[271,272] The BMMNC-treated group in the Repair-AMI study also demonstrated a statistically significant decrease in the combined endpoint of death, recurrence of myocardial infarction, and hospitalization for heart failure; however, the overall event rate in both groups were low (12 events in the control group, 2 events in the treated group).[272] Thus there is no consensus whether cell therapy works. Well-designed clinical trials are needed to further define the best cell population to be used, the delivery technique, and the most appropriate timing of cell therapy after an acute myocardial infarction.

Surgical Approaches (see Chapter 55)

Several "conventional" surgical procedures have been developed to reverse the vicious cycle of ventricular remodeling that accompanies systolic heart failure with the goal to improve symptoms and survival of heart failure patients. The details of the most common surgical methods currently used to arrest or reverse cardiac remodeling are beyond the scope of this chapter and are discussed elsewhere.[273] In 2002, the National Heart, Lung, and Blood Institute funded the Surgical Treatment for Ischemic Heart Failure (STICH) trial[275] to address two pressing clinical questions regarding the management of patients with heart failure with surgically revascularizable coronary artery disease and left ventricular dysfunction. First, is contemporary coronary artery bypass graft (CABG) surgery superior to contemporary medical therapy in prolonging survival in these patients? Second, among patients with significant LV anterior wall dysfunction, does the addition of surgical ventricular reconstruction to CABG improve hospitalization-free survival? The primary outcomes of the first hypothesis are expected to be published in 2011. The results of the primary outcomes of the second hypothesis were recently published and showed that adding surgical ventricular reconstruction to CABG reduced the left ventricular volume, as compared with CABG alone. However, this anatomical change was not associated with a greater improvement in symptoms or exercise tolerance or with a reduction in the rate of death or hospitalization for cardiac causes.[275]

Removal of the hemodynamic stress in patients with either aortic stenosis or aortic insufficiency after aortic valve replacement has been shown to be associated with significant hemodynamic improvement and a decrease in LV mass.[276] Villari et al[277] analyzed serial LV hemodynamic and biopsy findings before and after valve replacement in patients with aortic valve disease. These patients initially had massive LV hypertrophy and severe collagen deposition. The results demonstrated that near-normalization of systolic load causes a rapid reduction in myocyte hypertrophy and LV mass within a few weeks after valve replacement.[277] In this early phase of regression of myocyte hypertrophy, little change in collagen and matrix was observed. However, after months and years following valve replacement, regression of interstitial fibrosis occurred, resulting in near-normalization of both muscle mass and fibrous tissue content. This initial rapid regression of hypertrophy and later regression of fibrosis was accompanied by an improvement in ventricular function and exercise capacity.[277] In an experimental model of aorto-caval fistula in rats, Gerdes et al[278] demonstrated that myocytes possess the necessary machinery to remove recently added sarcomeres in a series, returning altered pump function and dilated ventricular chamber geometry toward control values.[278]

There is now compelling evidence that prolonged, near-complete unloading of the left ventricle with the use of an LVAD is associated with reduced myocardial apoptosis[279] and structural reverse remodeling[95,280-282] that can be accompanied by functional improvement.[283-285] However, recovery that is sufficient to permit explantation of the device has been observed in only 5% to 24% of patients in various series,[286-291] with a relatively high incidence of early recurrence.[286] Birks et al[292] have recently combined mechanical and pharmacological therapy (addition of the β_2-adrenergic-receptor agonist clenbuterol to standard heart failure therapy) in 15 patients with severe heart failure due to nonischemic cardiomyopathy and found an increased frequency and a sustained reversal of LV remodeling and heart failure.[292] The reproducibility and durability of these single-center findings, and the mechanisms contributing to the findings, require further study in different groups of patients.

Cardiac Resynchronization Approach (see Chapter 47)

Beneficial effects of cardiac resynchronization therapy (CRT) on survival, New York Heart Association (NYHA) functional class, exercise capacity, and quality of life are associated with significant improvement in LV remodeling as early as 1 month after device implantation,[293-295] with further progressive reduction in LV volumes beyond 1 year in select patients.[296,297] The Cardiac Resynchronization-Heart Failure (CARE-HF) study demonstrated an early and sustained reduction in NT-pro-BNP with CRT that correlated with improvement in LV dimension and ejection fraction and mitral regurgitation.[298]

Cardiac Constraint Devices

Preclinical studies have demonstrated that passive ventricular containment with cardiac constraint devices halts progressive ventricular remodeling[299-301] and improves myocyte function and structure, as characterized by enhanced myocyte contraction and relaxation, decreased myocyte hypertrophy, and decreased interstitial fibrosis.[299,301] Ventricular restraint prevents infarct expansion, improves border zone function, and favorably modifies LV geometry and myocardial structure after myocardial infarction.[302-304] Clinical studies showed amelioration of symptoms and improvement in left ventricle chamber dimensions and ejection fraction with the Acorn CorCap Cardiac Support Device.[305,306]

Exercise Training Approach (see Chapter 57)

Although there is growing evidence that exercise training may beneficially alter the course of postmyocardial infarction remodeling and its attendant morbidity and mortality,[307-309] the question of when to start exercise training after myocardial infarction remains controversial. Experimental studies using a transmural myocardial infarction rat model showed that exercise beginning 24 hours to 7 days after myocardial infarction results in infarct thinning and expansion.[310,311] Other studies demonstrated that exercise training starting 7 days to 5 weeks after myocardial infarction causes hypertrophy of the noninfarcted wall and attenuates LV remodeling.[312,313] Wan et al[314] sought to determine whether starting exercise at 1 or 6 weeks after myocardial infarction would affect myocardial remodeling differently and found that exercise starting early or late after myocardial infarction affects myocardial remodeling and function similarly.[314]

In heart failure patients, exercise training was shown to improve peak oxygen consumption, muscle strength and mass, NYHA functional class, quality of life, and survival.[315-319] In the recently presented HF-ACTION trial (Heart failure and a controlled trial investigating outcomes of exercise training),[320] exercise training caused a nonsignificant reduction in all-cause mortality and all-cause hospitalization and was associated with a modest improvement in exercise capacity.[320] Exercise training is now recommended for patients with mild to moderate heart failure symptoms.[321,322] Haykowsky et al[323] performed a meta-analysis to determine

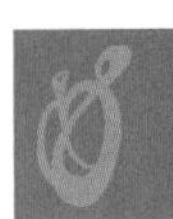

the effect of exercise training and type of exercise (aerobic vs. strength vs. combined training) on LV remodeling in heart failure and found that while aerobic training reverses patients with LV remodeling in clinically stable individuals with heart failure, this benefit was not confirmed with combined aerobic and strength training.[323]

VENTRICULAR REMODELING AS A SURROGATE ENDPOINT IN HEART FAILURE

There is now a large body of evidence indicating that ventricular remodeling is independently associated with adverse clinical outcomes, and more importantly, that agents that have beneficial effects in heart failure also generally attenuate or reverse ventricular remodeling, whereas agents that have failed to improve clinical outcomes either had no effect on remodeling or have been associated with adverse remodeling. We believe that these findings are sufficient to warrant consideration of the impact of a therapeutic intervention on ventricular remodeling, in conjunction with other findings, as credible evidence in support of a claim for improved clinical outcomes.[4,35]

A number of studies have demonstrated strong, independent correlation between ventricular dilation and subsequent mortality, particularly among patients who have suffered a myocardial infarction.[15,19,251,324] In a meta-analysis, Kramer et al[325] reviewed 25 drug/device therapy trials and 88 remodeling trials of the same therapies in patients with LV dysfunction to examine whether the magnitude of remodeling effects is associated with the odd ratios for death across all therapies are favorable, neutral, or adverse. They found that the odds ratio for death in the mortality trials was correlated with drug/device effect on LV EF ($r=-0.51$, $p<0.001$, EDV ($r=0.44$, $p=0.002$) and ESV ($r=0.48$, $p=0.002$). In logistic regressions, the odds for neutral or favorable effects in the mortality trials increased with mean increases in LVEF and with mean decreases in EDV and ESV in the remodeling trials. These data show that in patients with LV dysfunction, short-term trial-level therapeutic effects of a drug or device on LV remodeling are associated with longer-term trial-level effects on mortality. In the early Vasodilator-Heart Failure Trials (V-HeFT), hydralazine-isosorbide dinitrate combination and enalapril slowed remodeling compared with a placebo and improved survival, whereas prazosin had no effect on remodeling or outcomes.[263]

Table 15-2 compares the effect of a particular drug on ventricular remodeling and on clinical outcomes. In every case, the survival effects, unknown at the time that the volumetric data were acquired, paralleled the changes in ventricular remodeling. In the treatment and prevention arms of the Studies of Left Ventricular Dysfunction, the relative magnitude of an ACE inhibitor versus a placebo on ventricular remodeling approximated the relative magnitude of benefit on outcomes within the same population.[249,250,326,327] In the Metoprolol Randomized Interventional Trial in Heart Failure (MERIT-HF), the antiremodeling effects of metoprolol CR/XL on the left ventricle seen in the MRI substudy[33] paralleled the decrease in mortality from worsening heart failure.[328] In the Carvedilol Post-Infarction Survival Control in Left Ventricular Dysfunction (CAPRICORN) trial, carvedilol had a beneficial effect on ventricular remodeling[31] and reduced all-cause and cardiovascular mortality[237] in patients with LV dysfunction after acute myocardial infarction. In a meta-analysis, carvedilol showed greater benefits on LV remodeling compared with immediate-release metoprolol,[329] a finding which anticipated the subsequent results of the COMET trial showing improved survival for patients randomized to carvedilol, compared with those randomized to immediate-release metoprolol.[330] The Randomized Aldactone Evaluation Study (RALES) showed a 30% reduction in mortality with spironolactone in patients with advanced heart failure.[331] A later study showed improvement in the LV volume and mass with spironolactone.[255] In the AHeFTt, therapy with an isosorbide dinitrate/hydralazine combination resulted in regression in LV remodeling[264] and increased survival among black patients with advanced heart failure.[265] Ibopamine was initially observed to increase ventricular volumes,[332] and later found to be associated with excess mortality.[333] The angiotensin receptor blocker losartan was initially found to have an adverse trend on LV volumes compared with the ACE inhibitor captopril,[334] and the dual vasopeptidase inhibitor, omapatrilat had an equivalent effect on LV remodeling.[335] In each case, the remodeling data closely predicted the subsequent result of a large-scale morbidity and mortality trial.[336,337] Despite favorable early clinical findings,[338,339] endothelin receptor antagonist use has been associated with neutral to adverse effects on clinical outcomes and no benefits on LV volume or mass.[340] We have earlier shown that chronic arginine vasopressin receptor blockade does not attenuate postmyocardial infarction ventricular remodeling in the rat model.[341] In the Efficacy of Vasopressin Antagonism in Heart Failure Outcome Study With Tolvaptan (EVEREST) trial, tolvaptan initiated for acute treatment of patients hospitalized with heart failure had no effect on long-term mortality or heart failure–related morbidity.[342] Changes in LV remodeling over time also correspond to subsequent changes in mortality, independent of drug effect,[251,263] further reinforcing the role of remodeling as a surrogate marker in heart failure.

Noninvasive Assessment of Left Ventricular Remodeling (see Chapter 36)

Since the initial angiographic-based methods for assessing ventricular remodeling in humans, a variety of techniques have been developed that have been used for assessment of ventricular size, shape, and function for both clinical and research studies. Two-dimensional echocardiography has emerged as the predominant noninvasive diagnostic method for clinical use in evaluating LV function; this modality has become the most widely used technique to assess ventricular remodeling. Nevertheless, nuclear techniques that have proven both reliable and highly reproducible have also been used in a clinical and research setting and, more recently, CMR imaging has offered the potential to obtain extremely high-quality images of the heart at much higher resolution than either of the other techniques.

Echocardiography

Unlike cardiac MRI, echocardiography is not a true tomographic technique; the image obtained and the measurements made from the image are dependent on the imaging plane chosen by the sonographer. Three-dimensional measures of ventricular size—such as ventricular volume—are never derived directly from echocardiographic images but are estimated based on formulas that make assumptions about ventricular shape. Ventricular volume calculations are typically derived from 2D images and rely on some assumptions about ventricular geometry. Approaches that make the fewest assumptions about ventricular geometry—such as the modified Simpson's rule method—offer the most accurate estimations of ventricular volume.[343] Nevertheless, mistakes made on tracing a 2-D ventricular contour are amplified when volumes are calculated.

The reproducibility of echocardiography for measurement of LV dimensions, mass, and ejection fraction has been studied using a variety of study designs and statistical methods.[344,345] Although important information has been generated on interobserver and intraobserver variability, beat-by-beat variability, and interstudy (test-retest) variability in normal subjects,[344,345] similar data are not widely available in a heart failure population. Therefore the value by which

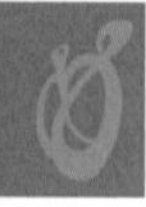

TABLE 15–2 Relationship Between Drug Effects on Left Ventricular Remodeling and on Mortality in Heart Failure

Study	Drug	LV Volumes	Mortality
SOLVD Treatment	Enalapril	Reduced[250]	Reduced[326]
SOLVD Prevention	Enalapril	Mildly reduced[249]	Mildly reduced[327]
MERIT-HF	Metoprolol CR/XL	Reduced[33]	Reduced[328]
CAPRICORN	Carvedilol	Reduced[31]	Reduced[237]
COMET	Carvedilol vs. metoprolol	Improved with carvedilol[329]	Improved with Carvedilol[330]
RALES	Spironolactone	Decreased[255]	Decreased (RALES)[331]
AHeFT	Isosorbide dinitrate/hydralazine	Decreased[264]	Decreased[265]
PRIME II	Ibopamine	Increased[332]	Increased (PRIME II)[333]
ELITE I	Losartan vs. carvedilol	NS; trend favors captopril[334]	NS; trend favors captopril (ELITE II)[337]
IMPRESS	Omapatrilat vs. lisinopril	Equivalent[335]	Equivalent (OVERTURE)[336]
RENAISSANCE	Etanercept	Equivalent*	Equivalent[373]
EARTH	Darusentan	Equivalent[340]	Equivalent for bosentan (ENABLE)[374]

AHeFT, African American Heart Failure Trial; *CAPRICORN,* Carvedilol Post-Infarction Survival Control in Left Ventricular Dysfunction; *COMET,* Carvedilol Or Metoprolol European Trial; *EARTH,* Endothelin A Receptor Antagonist Trial in Heart Failure; *ELITE,* Losartan Heart Failure Survival Study; *ENABLE,* Endothelin Antagonist Bosentan for Lowering Cardiac Events in Heart Failure; *MERIT-HF,* Metoprolol Randomized Interventional Trial in Heart Failure; *NS,* not significant; *OVERTURE,* Omapatrilat Versus Enalapril Randomized Trial of Utility in Reducing Events; *PRIME II,* Second Prospective Randomised Study of Ibopamine on Mortality and Efficacy; *RENAISSANCE,* Randomized Etanercept North American Strategy to Study Antagonism of Cytokines; *SOLVD,* Studies of Left Ventricular Dysfunction; *, Immunex (Now Amgen) RENAISSANCE Trial MRI data on file.

LV mass and volume must change to exceed methodological variability on sequential examination in heart failure patients within a multicenter study is not well established.

The noninvasive echocardiographic examination is standardized throughout the world and can be performed in virtually all medical centers. The technique is relatively inexpensive, especially compared with the more invasive angiographic or MRI-based techniques. Finally, echocardiography can offer additional information about cardiac valvular function and diastolic function that are difficult to obtain with other modalities. Nevertheless, this technique suffers from marked variation in image quality that cannot be predicted, and approximately 10% to 15% of patients cannot be adequately imaged for quantitative purposes. For these reasons, the reproducibility and overall accuracy of echocardiography may not be as high as some of the other available techniques.

Radionuclide Ventriculography

Radionuclide ventriculography is a reliable technique for measurement of LV ejection fraction.[346] Background-corrected radionuclide counts within a region of interest are used to determine ejection fraction without the need to determine absolute volumes. However, calculation of absolute LV volume has proven more complex, requiring several corrections and assumptions regarding the relation between count activity as measured in a 2D picture of the left ventricle to the absolute volume.

A strength of the radionuclide ventriculography technique is the substantial reproducibility and the low intraobserver and interobserver variability that have been reported in the literature. Several studies have assessed the reproducibility of radionuclide ventriculography in both normal subjects and patients with heart diseases. Upton et al[347] determined the intrinsic variability of radionuclide measurements of LV function at rest and during exercise in 10 normal subjects. The interobserver variabilities for ejection fraction (2.1 ± 1.0%) and for end-diastolic volume (7.5 ± 4.7 mL) at rest were considerably smaller than those reported in studies using contrast ventriculography.[348,349] The interstudy variability in ejection fraction in this study was 4.0 ± 3.8% at rest and 3.2 ± 2.5% during exercise, suggesting that at 95% confidence levels, repeat ejection fraction should not vary by more than 8% at rest and 5% during exercise. A difference in end-diastolic volume of at least 20 mL between rest and exercise studies was suggested to be required for the change to be considered meaningful.[347] A similar variability in ejection fraction of 4.4 ± 3.6% was reported by Marshall et al[350] in 20 patients with cardiac disease who had three resting radionuclide ventriculograms separated by an average of 4.3 days. Numerous studies using radionuclide techniques have documented that changes in LV volumes in heart failure patients determined by the radionuclide ventriculography technique appear to reflect long-term changes in natural history seen with this same drug therapy (see Table 15-2). Thus radionuclide ventriculography allows a relatively accurate, reproducible assessment of serial changes in LV volumetrics suitable for analysis in clinical trials of new therapies in heart failure and other cardiovascular diseases. It is less costly than Doppler echocardiography or MRI and is potentially widely available (at least in the United States), though the exact volumetric techniques are no longer widely practiced for purely clinical care purposes. A disadvantage of the radionuclide technique is that analysis of right and left ventricular volumes is not commonly undertaken in most clinical radionuclide laboratories. Moreover, the radionuclide ventriculography techniques require meticulous attention to detail and correction for attenuation.

Magnetic Resonance Imaging

In recent years, two tomographic techniques have been increasingly applied to the diagnosis of cardiovascular disease and the quantification of cardiac dimensions and function. These techniques, ultrafast computed tomography and MRI, could acquire tomographic images at multiple levels encompassing the entire heart and thereby yield a 3D data set. Computed tomography has, however, some major drawbacks in that it requires rapid infusion of intravenous contrast material and exposes patients to radiation, both of which carry an element of risk.[351,352] MRI does not have these limitations and can be performed in any imaging plane so that a data set parallel or perpendicular to the long axis of the ventricle is produced. Because a 3D data set is acquired, accurate LV volume and mass measurements can be obtained.[346]

Cardiovascular MRI has effectively become a reference standard for quantifying ventricular volumes and function and for measuring the myocardial scar burden after myocardial infarction. Imaging of late gadolinium enhancement and microvascular obstruction carries strong prognostic information for identifying patients who would benefit from antiremodeling therapy.[353] Contrast-enhanced MRI can characterize acute myocardial infarction with two well-defined contrast-enhanced patterns as follows: (1) first-pass images performed immediately after contrast injection often demonstrate areas of reduced contrast-enhanced MRI or hypoenhancement in the endocardial core of the infarct, corresponding to microvascular obstruction,[354,355] and (2) delayed images (10 to 20 minutes after contrast injection) demonstrate regional signal hyperenhancement, corresponding to myocardial necrosis.[356] A combination of contrast-enhanced perfusion MRI with functional data might be useful for the identification of myocardial viability, allowing one to distinguish permanently dysfunctional myocardium from dysfunctional segments bound to recover contractile function and contribute to LV stroke volume after myocardial infarction.[354,355,357,358] MRI enables the study of myocardial deformation and strain evolution in precise regions of the myocardium with high levels of reproducibility and accuracy.[359,360] The data combination obtained with the delayed enhancement and the tagging images allows a precise monitoring of the functional variations in the different regions.[361]

MRI is now considered the reference technique for the noninvasive assessment of LV dimensions, mass, and function. This method is accurate to about 2%[362] and, because it is highly reproducible, offers an ideal means of serial assessment of disease progression or response to treatment in an individual patient.[363] MRI has been shown to be superior to echocardiography, contrast ventriculography, and radionuclide ventriculography with regard to accuracy,[364,365] and for interobserver and interstudy reproducibility of LV cavity volumes, ejection fraction, and mass both in normal and in diseased hearts,[366-368] including patients with heart failure.[369] For research purposes, this results in a considerable reduction in the sample size required to show a given change, when compared with echocardiography. Bellenger and colleagues[370] reported that to demonstrate a 10-mL difference in end-diastolic and end-systolic volumes and a 10-g difference in mass with 90% power and p value of 0.05, only 12, 10, and 9 patients would be required using MRI as compares with a sample size of 97, 53, and 190 patients for 2D echocardiography. Similar findings have also been reported in patients with hypertension.[371] Thus because of good accuracy and superior reproducibility, MRI may be considered the gold standard for quantification of LV mass, dimensions, and ejection fraction. Even though this method may be more expensive than 2D echocardiography, its greater reproducibility may make it suitable for research studies in which the greater cost could be offset by the savings from recruiting and studying fewer patients. The combination of gadolinium enhancement, perfusion, and cine imaging should make MRI the modality of choice in the assessment of LV dysfunction and remodeling.

Several factors are limiting the routine use of MRI for the evaluation of cardiovascular disease, including limited access to MRI imagers, expense of the studies, and the duration of the procedure required to achieve images of the entire heart. Claustrophobia is a problem with some patients but may be resolved with the newer open-sided scanners. Absolute contraindications to MRI are few, but patients with implantable devices such as pacemakers and defibrillators, cochlear implants, and cerebral aneurism clips usually cannot be scanned except under very controlled and clinically urgent circumstances.[372]

CONCLUSIONS

Ventricular remodeling is a complex process that results from interactions between the initial myocardial injury or alteration in loading conditions and multiple mechanical and neurohormonal factors that are capable of modifying the cardiomyocyte phenotype and of inducing changes in the extracellular matrix. Myocyte hypertrophy, cellular necrosis and apoptosis, interstitial fibrosis, and degradation of collagen are the major features of myocardial remodeling. Each of these components of the remodeling process contributes importantly to the development and progression of heart failure. At the level of the ventricular chamber, remodeling refers to changes in ventricular geometry, volume, and mass. Although initially it may be compensatory in certain pressure and volume overload conditions, progressive ventricular remodeling is ultimately a maladaptive process, contributing to progression of symptomatic heart failure and to an adverse outcome. After acute myocardial infarction, however, progressive hypertrophy and remodeling of noninfarcted myocardium may be harmful from the start. Ventricular remodeling is emerging as an important therapeutic target and a credible surrogate endpoint in heart failure. A variety of noninvasive techniques have been used for assessment of ventricular remodeling, CMR imaging being the gold standard for quantification of LV mass, dimensions, and ejection fraction. Treatment with the goal of slowing or reversing remodeling has been shown to improve long-term outcome. Remodeling of the dilated failing ventricle can also be partially reversed when hearts are "rested" using LVAD, but it is clear that currently available therapy remains palliative. Additional research is needed to identify the molecular processes responsible for remodeling, and to improve ways to inhibit this maladaptive growth response.

FUTURE DIRECTIONS

Enormous effort has been directed toward identifying new therapeutic strategies with long-term efficacy in heart failure. The path is littered with successes and failures,[4] yet advances in myocardial biology, stem-cell research, pharmacological developments, and mechanical devices hold promise for future treatments. A comprehensive understanding of ventricular remodeling will be obligatory, since it reflects the basic mechanisms of heart failure development and progression. Although multiple studies have documented that interventions that have beneficial effects in heart failure also generally attenuate or reverse ventricular remodeling and that those that fail to improve clinical outcomes either have no effect on remodeling or have been associated with adverse remodeling, few studies have examined the mechanism by which LV reverse remodeling is mediated. Questions remain as to whether the reversal of myocyte structural remodeling is accompanied by normalization of the biology of the failing myocyte and what the mechanisms of changes are at the myocyte level. Further research should focus on the molecular and cellular mechanisms involved in adverse and reverse remodeling and on optimizing therapies to prevent remodeling and identifying appropriate patient groups to target. Major challenges remain, but patients with heart disease are likely to benefit from these efforts.

REFERENCES

1. Eaton, L. W., Weiss, J. L., Bulkley, B. H., et al. (1979). Regional cardiac dilatation after acute myocardial infarction: recognition by two-dimensional echocardiography. *N Engl J Med, 300*(2), 57–62.
2. Erlebacher, J. A., Weiss, J. L., Eaton, L. W., et al. (1982). Late effects of acute infarct dilation on heart size: a two dimensional echocardiographic study. *Am J Cardiol, 49*(5), 1120–1126.
3. McKay, R. G., Pfeffer, M. A., Pasternak, R. C., et al. (1986). Left ventricular remodeling after myocardial infarction: a corollary to infarct expansion. *Circulation, 74*(4), 693–702.
4. Anand, I. S., & Florea, V. G. (2008). Traditional and novel approaches to management of heart failure: successes and failures. *Cardiol Clin, 26*(1), 59–72.
5. Hill, J. A., & Olson, E. N. (2008). Cardiac plasticity. *N Engl J Med, 358*(13), 1370–1380.
6. Flint, A. (1870). *Diseases of the heart* (ed 2). Philadelphia: HC Lea.
7. Osler, W. (1892). *The principles and practice of medicine.* New York: Appleton.

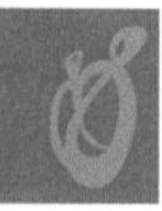

8. Linzbach, A. M. (1960). Heart failure from the point of view of quantitative anatomy. *Am J Cardiol, 5*, 370–382.
9. Hood, W. P., Jr., Rackley, C. E., & Rolett, E. L. (1968). Wall stress in the normal and hypertrophied human left ventricle. *Am J Cardiol, 22*(4), 550–558.
10. Sandler, H., & Dodge, H. T. (1963). Left ventricular tension and stress in man. *Circ Res, 13*, 91–104.
11. Meerson, F. Z. (1961). On the mechanism of compensatory hyperfunction and insufficiency of the heart. *Cor Vasa, 3*, 161–177.
12. Gunther, S., & Grossman, W. (1979). Determinants of ventricular function in pressure-overload hypertrophy in man. *Circulation, 59*(4), 679–688.
13. Huber, D., Grimm, J., Koch, R., et al. (1981). Determinants of ejection performance in aortic stenosis. *Circulation, 64*(1), 126–134.
14. Krayenbuehl, H. P., Hess, O. M., Ritter, M., et al. (1988). Left ventricular systolic function in aortic stenosis. *Eur Heart J, 9*(suppl E), 19–23.
15. Hammermeister, K. E., DeRouen, T. A., & Dodge, H. T. (1979). Variables predictive of survival in patients with coronary disease. Selection by univariate and multivariate analyses from the clinical, electrocardiographic, exercise, arteriographic, and quantitative angiographic evaluations. *Circulation, 59*(3), 421–430.
16. Koren, M. J., Devereux, R. B., Casale, P. N., et al. (1991). Relation of left ventricular mass and geometry to morbidity and mortality in uncomplicated essential hypertension. *Ann Intern Med, 114*(5), 345–352.
17. Levy, D., Garrison, R. J., Savage, D. D., et al. (1990). Prognostic implications of echocardiographically determined left ventricular mass in the Framingham Heart Study. *N Engl J Med, 322*(22), 1561–1566.
18. Vasan, R. S., Larson, M. G., Benjamin, E. J., et al. (1997). Left ventricular dilatation and the risk of congestive heart failure in people without myocardial infarction. *N Engl J Med, 336*(19), 1350–1355.
19. White, H. D., Norris, R. M., Brown, M. A., et al. (1987). Left ventricular end-systolic volume as the major determinant of survival after recovery from myocardial infarction. *Circulation, 76*(1), 44–51.
20. Florea, V. G., Mareyev, V. Y., Samko, A. N., et al. (1999). Left ventricular remodelling: common process in patients with different primary myocardial disorders. *Int J Cardiol, 68*(3), 281–287.
21. Hutchins, G. M., & Bulkley, B. H. (1978). Infarct expansion versus extension: two different complications of acute myocardial infarction. *Am J Cardiol, 41*(7), 1127–1132.
22. Hochman, J. S., & Bulkley, B. H. (1982). Expansion of acute myocardial infarction: an experimental study. *Circulation, 65*(7), 1446–1450.
23. Weisman, H. F., Bush, D. E., Mannisi, J. A., et al. (1985). Global cardiac remodeling after acute myocardial infarction: a study in the rat model. *J Am Coll Cardiol, 5*(6), 1355–1362.
24. Erlebacher, J. A. (1985). Ventricular remodeling in myocardial infarction—the rat and the human. *Am J Cardiol, 56*(13), 910.
25. Chanutin, A., & Barksdale, E. E. (1933). Experimental renal insufficiency produced by partial nephrectomy. *Arch Intern Med, 52*, 739–751.
26. Pfeffer, J. M., Pfeffer, M. A., Fishbein, M. C., et al. (1979). Cardiac function and morphology with aging in the spontaneously hypertensive rat. *Am J Physiol, 237*(4), H461–H468.
27. Pfeffer, J., Pfeffer, M., Fletcher, P., et al. (1979). Alterations of cardiac performance in rats with established spontaneous hypertension. *Am J Cardiol, 44*(5), 994–998.
28. Cohn, J. N., Ferrari, R., & Sharpe, N. (2000). Cardiac remodeling—concepts and clinical implications: a consensus paper from an international forum on cardiac remodeling. *J Am Coll Cardiol, 35*(3), 569–582.
29. Sutton, M. G., & Sharpe, N. (2000). Left ventricular remodeling after myocardial infarction: pathophysiology and therapy. *Circulation, 101*(25), 2981–2988.
30. Doughty, R. N., Whalley, G. A., Gamble, G., et al. (1997). Left ventricular remodeling with carvedilol in patients with congestive heart failure due to ischemic heart disease. Australia-New Zealand heart failure research collaborative group. *J Am Coll Cardiol, 29*(5), 1060–1066.
31. Doughty, R. N., Whalley, G. A., Walsh, H. A., et al. (2004). Effects of carvedilol on left ventricular remodeling after acute myocardial infarction: the CAPRICORN echo substudy. *Circulation, 109*(2), 201–206.
32. Greenberg, B., Quinones, M. A., Koilpillai, C., et al. (1995). Effects of long-term enalapril therapy on cardiac structure and function in patients with left ventricular dysfunction. Results of the SOLVD echocardiography substudy. *Circulation, 91*(10), 2573–2581.
33. Groenning, B. A., Nilsson, J. C., Sondergaard, L., et al. (2000). Antiremodeling effects on the left ventricle during beta-blockade with metoprolol in the treatment of chronic heart failure. *J Am Coll Cardiol, 36*(7), 2072–2080.
34. St John Sutton, M., Pfeffer, M. A., Moye, L., et al. (1997). Cardiovascular death and left ventricular remodeling two years after myocardial infarction: baseline predictors and impact of long-term use of captopril: information from the survival and ventricular enlargement (SAVE) trial. *Circulation, 96*(10), 3294–3299.
35. Konstam, M. A., Udelson, J. E., Anand, I. S., et al. (2003). Ventricular remodeling in heart failure: a credible surrogate endpoint. *J Card Fail, 9*(5), 350–353.
36. Anand, I. S., Florea, V. G., & Fisher, L. (2002). Surrogate end points in heart failure. *J Am Coll Cardiol, 39*(9), 1414–1421.
37. Harris, P. (1983). Evolution and the cardiac patient. *Cardiovasc Res, 17*(6), 313–319, 373–378, 437–445.
38. Olivetti, G., Capasso, J. M., Sonnenblick, E. H., et al. (1990). Side-to-side slippage of myocytes participates in ventricular wall remodeling acutely after myocardial infarction in rats. *Circ Res, 67*(1), 23–34.
39. Weisman, H. F., Bush, D. E., Mannisi, J. A., et al. (1988). Cellular mechanisms of myocardial infarct expansion. *Circulation, 78*(1), 186–201.
40. Beltrami, C. A., Finato, N., Rocco, M., et al. (1995). The cellular basis of dilated cardiomyopathy in humans. *J Mol Cell Cardiol, 27*(1), 291–305.
41. Anversa, P., Kajstura, J., & Olivetti, G. (1996). Myocyte death in heart failure. *Curr Opin Cardiol, 11*(3), 245–251.
42. Kajstura, J., Cheng, W., Reiss, K., et al. (1996). Apoptotic and necrotic myocyte cell deaths are independent contributing variables of infarct size in rats. *Lab Invest, 74*(1), 86–107.
43. Gupta, S., Prahash, A. J. C., & Anand, I. S. (2000). Myocyte contractile function is intact in the post-infarct remodeled rat heart despite molecular alterations. *Cardiovasc Res, 48*(1), 77–88.
44. Linzbach, A. (1976). Hypertrophy, hyperplasia and structural dilation of the human heart. *Adv Cardiol, 18*, 1–14.
45. Komamura, K., Shannon, R. P., Ihara, T., et al. (1993). Exhaustion of Frank-Starling mechanism in conscious dogs with heart failure. *Am J Physiol, 265*(4 pt 2), H1119–H1131.
46. Hoyt, R. H., Cohen, M. L., & Saffitz, J. E. (1989). Distribution and three-dimensional structure of intercellular junctions in canine myocardium. *Circ Res, 64*(3), 563–574.
47. Zhao, M. J., Zhang, H., Robinson, T. F., et al. (1987). Profound structural alterations of the extracellular collagen matrix in postischemic dysfunctional (stunned) but viable myocardium. *J Am Coll Cardiol, 10*(6), 1322–1334.
48. Yamamoto, S., James, T. N., Sawada, K., et al. (1996). Generation of new intercellular junctions between cardiocytes. A possible mechanism compensating for mechanical overload in the hypertrophied human adult myocardium. *Circ Res, 78*(3), 362–370.
49. Pfeffer, M. A., Pfeffer, J. M., Fishbein, M. C., et al. (1979). Myocardial infarct size and ventricular function in rats. *Circ Res, 44*(4), 503–512.
50. Fletcher, P. J., Pfeffer, J. M., Pfeffer, M. A., et al. (1981). Left ventricular diastolic pressure-volume relations in rats with healed myocardial infarction. Effects on systolic function. *Circ Res, 49*(3), 618–626.
51. Picard, M. H., Wilkins, G. T., Gillam, L. D., et al. (1991). Immediate regional endocardial surface expansion following coronary occlusion in the canine left ventricle: disproportionate effects of anterior versus inferior ischemia. *Am Heart J, 121*(3 pt 1), 753–762.
52. Pirolo, J. S., Hutchins, G. M., & Moore, G. W. (1986). Infarct expansion: pathologic analysis of 204 patients with a single myocardial infarct. *J Am Coll Cardiol, 7*(2), 349–354.
53. Weisman, H. F., & Healy, B. (1987). Myocardial infarct expansion, infarct extension, and reinfarction: pathophysiologic concepts. *Prog Cardiovasc Dis, 30*(2), 73–110.
54. Meizlish, J. L., Berger, H. J., Plankey, M., et al. (1984). Functional left ventricular aneurysm formation after acute anterior transmural myocardial infarction. Incidence, natural history, and prognostic implications. *N Engl J Med, 311*(16), 1001–1006.
55. Hammerman, H., Kloner, R. A., Alker, K. J., et al. (1985). Effects of transient increased afterload during experimentally induced acute myocardial infarction in dogs. *Am J Cardiol, 55*(5), 566–570.
56. Nolan, S. E., Mannisi, J. A., Bush, D. E., et al. (1988). Increased afterload aggravates infarct expansion after acute myocardial infarction. *J Am Coll Cardiol, 12*(5), 1318–1325.
57. Rabkin, S. W., Mathewson, F. A., & Tate, R. B. (1977). Prognosis after acute myocardial infarction: relation to blood pressure values before infarction in a prospective cardiovascular study. *Am J Cardiol, 40*(4), 604–610.
58. Jugdutt, B. I., & Khan, M. I. (1994). Effect of prolonged nitrate therapy on left ventricular remodeling after canine acute myocardial infarction. *Circulation, 89*(5), 2297–2307.
59. GISSI. (1986). Effectiveness of intravenous thrombolytic treatment in acute myocardial infarction. *Lancet, 1*(8478), 397–402.
60. Grines, C. L., Browne, K. F., Marco, J., et al. (1993). A comparison of immediate angioplasty with thrombolytic therapy for acute myocardial infarction. The primary angioplasty in myocardial infarction study group. *N Engl J Med, 328*(10), 673–679.
61. Kennedy, J. W., Ritchie, J. L., Davis, K. B., et al. (1983). Western Washington randomized trial of intracoronary streptokinase in acute myocardial infarction. *N Engl J Med, 309*(24), 1477–1482.
62. Randomised trial of intravenous streptokinase. (1988). oral aspirin, both, or neither among 17,187 cases of suspected acute myocardial infarction: ISIS-2. ISIS-2 (second International Study of Infarct Survival) collaborative group.. *Lancet, 2*(8607), 349–360.
63. Hochman, J. S., Lamas, G. A., Buller, C. E., et al. (2006). Coronary intervention for persistent occlusion after myocardial infarction. *N Engl J Med, 355*(23), 2395–2407.
64. Dzavik, V., Buller, C. E., Lamas, G. A., et al. (2006). Randomized trial of percutaneous coronary intervention for subacute infarct-related coronary artery occlusion to achieve long-term patency and improve ventricular function: the total occlusion study of Canada (TOSCA)-2 trial. *Circulation, 114*(23), 2449–2457.
65. Beltrami, C. A., Finato, N., Rocco, M., et al. (1994). Structural basis of end-stage failure in ischemic cardiomyopathy in humans. *Circulation, 89*(1), 151–163.
66. Sharov, V. G., Sabbah, H. N., Shimoyama, H., et al. (1996). Evidence of cardiocyte apoptosis in myocardium of dogs with chronic heart failure. *Am J Pathol, 148*(1), 141–149.
67. Teiger, E., Than, V. D., Richard, L., et al. (1996). Apoptosis in pressure overload-induced heart hypertrophy in the rat. *J Clin Invest, 97*(12), 2891–2897.
68. Olivetti, G., Abbi, R., Quaini, F., et al. (1997). Apoptosis in the failing human heart. *N Engl J Med, 336*(16), 1131–1141.
69. Narula, J., Haider, N., Virmani, R., et al. (1996). Apoptosis in myocytes in end-stage heart failure. *N Engl J Med, 335*(16), 1182–1189.
70. Kostin, S., Heling, A., Hein, S., et al. (1998). The protein composition of the normal and diseased cardiac myocyte. *Heart Fail Rev, 2*, 245–260.
71. Schaper, J., Froede, R., Hein, S., et al. (1991). Impairment of the myocardial ultrastructure and changes of the cytoskeleton in dilated cardiomyopathy. *Circulation, 83*(2), 504–514.
72. Rakusan, K. (1984). Cardiac growth, maturation and aging. In R. Zak (Ed.), *Growth of the heart in health and disease.* New York: Raven Press.
73. MacLellan, W. R., & Schneider, M. D. (2000). Genetic dissection of cardiac growth control pathways. *Annu Rev Physiol, 62*, 289–319.
74. Molkentin, J. D., & Dorn, I. G., II (2001). Cytoplasmic signaling pathways that regulate cardiac hypertrophy. *Annu Rev Physiol, 63*, 391–426.
75. Swynghedauw, B. (1999). Molecular mechanisms of myocardial remodeling. *Physiol Rev, 79*(1), 215–262.
76. Grossman, W., Jones, D., & McLaurin, L. P. (1975). Wall stress and patterns of hypertrophy in the human left ventricle. *J Clin Invest, 56*(1), 56–64.

77. Gerdes, A. M., Onodera, T., Wang, X., et al. (1996). Myocyte remodeling during the progression to failure in rats with hypertension. *Hypertension, 28*(4), 609–614.
78. Onodera, T., Tamura, T., Said, S., et al. (1998). Maladaptive remodeling of cardiac myocyte shape begins long before failure in hypertension. *Hypertension, 32*(4), 753–757.
79. Gerdes, A. M. (1992). The use of isolated myocytes to evaluate myocardial remodeling. *Trends Cardiovasc Med, 2*, 152–155.
80. Lorell, B. H., & Carabello, B. A. (2000). Left ventricular hypertrophy: pathogenesis, detection, and prognosis. *Circulation, 102*(4), 470–479.
81. Urabe, Y., Mann, D. L., Kent, R. L., et al. (1992). Cellular and ventricular contractile dysfunction in experimental canine mitral regurgitation. *Circ Res, 70*(1), 131–147.
82. Olivetti, G., Capasso, J. M., Meggs, L. G., et al. (1991). Cellular basis of chronic ventricular remodeling after myocardial infarction in rats. *Circ Res, 68*(3), 856–869.
83. Zimmer, H. G., Gerdes, A. M., Lortet, S., et al. (1990). Changes in heart function and cardiac cell size in rats with chronic myocardial infarction. *J Mol Cell Cardiol, 22*(11), 1231–1243.
84. Gerdes, A. M., Kellerman, S. E., Moore, J. A., et al. (1992). Structural remodeling of cardiac myocytes in patients with ischemic cardiomyopathy. *Circulation, 86*(2), 426–430.
85. Anand, I. S., Liu, D., Chugh, S. S., et al. (1997). Isolated myocyte contractile function is normal in postinfarct remodeled rat heart with systolic dysfunction. *Circulation, 96*(11), 3974–3984.
86. Tamura, T., Onodera, T., Said, S., et al. (1998). Correlation of myocyte lengthening to chamber dilation in the spontaneously hypertensive heart failure (SHHF) rat. *J Mol Cell Cardiol, 30*(11), 2175–2181.
87. Spinale, F. G., Ishihra, K., Zile, M., et al. (1993). Structural basis for changes in left ventricular function and geometry because of chronic mitral regurgitation and after correction of volume overload. *J Thorac Cardiovasc Surg, 106*(6), 1147–1157.
88. Wisenbaugh, T., Spann, J. F., & Carabello, B. A. (1984). Differences in myocardial performance and load between patients with similar amounts of chronic aortic versus chronic mitral regurgitation. *J Am Coll Cardiol, 3*(4), 916–923.
89. Sutton, M., Plappert, T., Spiegel, A., et al. (1987). Early postoperative changes in left ventricular chamber size, architecture, and function in aortic stenosis and aortic regurgitation and their relation to intraoperative changes in afterload: a prospective two-dimensional echocardiographic study. *Circulation, 76*(1), 77–89.
90. Carabello, B. A. (1995). The relationship of left ventricular geometry and hypertrophy to left ventricular function in valvular heart disease. *J Heart Valve Dis, 4*(suppl. 2), S132–S138, discussion S138–S139.
91. Feiring, A. J., & Rumberger, J. A. (1992). Ultrafast computed tomography analysis of regional radius-to-wall thickness ratios in normal and volume-overloaded human left ventricle. *Circulation, 85*(4), 1423–1432.
92. Gerdes, A. M., Moore, J. A., Hines, J. M., et al. (1986). Regional differences in myocyte size in normal rat heart. *Anat Rec, 215*(4), 420–426.
93. Gerdes, A. M., Kellerman, S. E., Schocken, D. D., et al. (1995). Implications of cardiomyocyte remodeling in heart dysfunction. In N. S. Dhalla, R. E. Beamish, & N. Takeda (Eds.), *The failing heart*. New York: Raven Press.
94. Gerdes, A. M., Campbell, S. E., & Hilbelink, D. R. (1988). Structural remodeling of cardiac myocytes in rats with arteriovenous fistulas. *Lab Invest, 59*(6), 857–861.
95. Zafeiridis, A., Jeevanandam, V., Houser, S. R., et al. (1998). Regression of cellular hypertrophy after left ventricular assist device support. *Circulation, 98*(7), 656–662.
96. Sugden, P. H. (1999). Signaling in myocardial hypertrophy: life after calcineurin? *Circ Res, 84*(6), 633–646.
97. Sugden, P. H. (2001). Mechanotransduction in cardiomyocyte hypertrophy. *Circulation, 103*(10), 1375–1377.
98. Wollert, K. C., Taga, T., Saito, M., et al. (1996). Cardiotrophin-1 activates a distinct form of cardiac muscle cell hypertrophy. Assembly of sarcomeric units in series VIA gp130/leukemia inhibitory factor receptor-dependent pathways. *J Biol Chem, 271*(16), 9535–9545.
99. Komuro, I., Katoh, Y., Kaida, T., et al. (1991). Mechanical loading stimulates cell hypertrophy and specific gene expression in cultured rat cardiac myocytes. Possible role of protein kinase C activation. *J Biol Chem, 266*(2), 1265–1268.
100. Yamazaki, T., Komuro, I., Kudoh, S., et al. (1995). Mechanical stress activates protein kinase cascade of phosphorylation in neonatal rat cardiac myocytes. *J Clin Invest, 96*(1), 438–446.
101. Molkentin, J. D., Lu, J. R., Antos, C. L., et al. (1998). A calcineurin-dependent transcriptional pathway for cardiac hypertrophy. *Cell, 93*(2), 215–228.
102. Passier, R., Zeng, H., Frey, N., et al. (2000). CaM kinase signaling induces cardiac hypertrophy and activates the MEF2 transcription factor in vivo. *J Clin Invest, 105*(10), 1395–1406.
103. Karin, M. (1995). The regulation of AP-1 activity by mitogen-activated protein kinases. *J Biol Chem, 270*(28), 16483–16486.
104. Hunter, T. (1997). Oncoprotein networks. *Cell, 88*(3), 333–346.
105. Force, T., Pombo, C. M., Avruch, J. A., et al. (1996). Stress-activated protein kinases in cardiovascular disease. *Circ Res, 78*(6), 947–953.
106. Lenormand, P., Sardet, C., Pages, G., et al. (1993). Growth factors induce nuclear translocation of MAP kinases (p42mapk and p44mapk) but not of their activator MAP kinase kinase (p45mapkk) in fibroblasts. *J Cell Biol, 122*(5), 1079–1088.
107. Yamamoto, K., Dang, Q. N., Maeda, Y., et al. (2001). Regulation of cardiomyocyte mechanotransduction by the cardiac cycle. *Circulation, 103*(10), 1459–1464.
108. Zhang, W., Kowal, R. C., Rusnak, F., et al. (1999). Failure of calcineurin inhibitors to prevent pressure-overload left ventricular hypertrophy in rats. *Circ Res, 84*(6), 722–728.
109. Ding, B., Price, R. L., Borg, T. K., et al. (1999). Pressure overload induces severe hypertrophy in mice treated with cyclosporine, an inhibitor of calcineurin. *Circ Res, 84*(6), 729–734.
110. Rowan, R. A., & Billingham, M. E. (1990). Pathologic changes in the long-term transplanted heart: a morphometric study of myocardial hypertrophy, vascularity, and fibrosis. *Hum Pathol, 21*(7), 767–772.
111. Homcy, C. J. (1998). Signaling hypertrophy: how many switches, how many wires. *Circulation, 97*(19), 1890–1892.
112. Hein, S., Kostin, S., Heling, A., et al. (2000). The role of the cytoskeleton in heart failure. *Cardiovasc Res, 45*(2), 273–278.
113. Juliano, R. L., & Haskill, S. (1993). Signal transduction from the extracellular matrix. *J Cell Biol, 120*(3), 577–585.
114. Wang, N., Butler, J. P., & Ingber, D. E. (1993). Mechanotransduction across the cell surface and through the cytoskeleton. *Science, 260*(5111), 1124–1127.
115. Bing, O. H., Brooks, W. W., Robinson, K. G., et al. (1995). The spontaneously hypertensive rat as a model of the transition from compensated left ventricular hypertrophy to failure. *J Mol Cell Cardiol, 27*(1), 383–396.
116. Mann, D. L., Kent, R. L., Parsons, B., et al. (1992). Adrenergic effects on the biology of the adult mammalian cardiocyte. *Circulation, 85*(2), 790–804.
117. Tan, L. B., Jalil, J. E., Pick, R., et al. (1991). Cardiac myocyte necrosis induced by angiotensin II. *Circ Res, 69*(5), 1185–1195.
118. Latini, R., Masson, S., Anand, I. S., et al. (2007). Prognostic value of very low plasma concentrations of troponin T in patients with stable chronic heart failure. *Circulation, 116*(11), 1242–1249.
119. Missov, E., Calzolari, C., & Pau, B. (1997). Circulating cardiac troponin I in severe congestive heart failure. *Circulation, 96*(9), 2953–2958.
120. Narula, J., Haider, N., Arbustini, E., et al. (2006). Mechanisms of disease: apoptosis in heart failure—seeing hope in death. *Nat Clin Pract Cardiovasc Med, 3*(12), 681–688.
121. Garg, S., Narula, J., & Chandrashekhar, Y. (2005). Apoptosis and heart failure: clinical relevance and therapeutic target. *J Mol Cell Cardiol, 38*(1), 73–79.
122. Laugwitz, K. L., Moretti, A., Weig, H. J., et al. (2001). Blocking caspase-activated apoptosis improves contractility in failing myocardium. *Hum Gene Ther 20, 12*(17), 2051–2063.
123. Moretti, A., Weig, H. J., Ott, T., et al. (2002). Essential myosin light chain as a target for caspase-3 in failing myocardium. *Proc Natl Acad Sci U S A, 99*(18), 11860–11865.
124. Cheng, W., Li, B., Kajstura, J., et al. (1995). Stretch-induced programmed myocyte cell death. *J Clin Invest, 96*(5), 2247–2259.
125. Colucci, W. S., Sawyer, D. B., Singh, K., et al. (2000). Adrenergic overload and apoptosis in heart failure: implications for therapy. *J Card Fail, 6*(2 suppl. 1), 1–7.
126. Cigola, E., Kajstura, J., Li, B., et al. (1997). Angiotensin II activates programmed myocyte cell death in vitro. *Exp Cell Res, 231*(2), 363–371.
127. Kajstura, J., Cigola, E., Malhotra, A., et al. (1997). Angiotensin II induces apoptosis of adult ventricular myocytes in vitro. *J Mol Cell Cardiol, 29*(3), 859–870.
128. Ferrari, R., Agnoletti, L., Comini, L., et al. (1998). Oxidative stress during myocardial ischaemia and heart failure. *Eur Heart J, 19*(suppl. B), B2–B11.
129. DeLong, M. J. (1998). Apoptosis: a modulator of cellular homeostasis and disease states. *Ann N Y Acad Sci, 842*, 82–90.
130. Condorelli, G., Morisco, C., Stassi, G., et al. (1999). Increased cardiomyocyte apoptosis and changes in proapoptotic and antiapoptotic genes bax and bcl-2 during left ventricular adaptations to chronic pressure overload in the rat. *Circulation, 99*(23), 3071–3078.
131. Li, Z., Bing, O. H., Long, X., et al. (1997). Increased cardiomyocyte apoptosis during the transition to heart failure in the spontaneously hypertensive rat. *Am J Physiol, 272*(5 pt 2), H2313–H2319.
132. Matturri, L., Milei, J., Grana, D. R., et al. (2002). Characterization of myocardial hypertrophy by DNA content, PCNA expression and apoptotic index. *Int J Cardiol, 82*(1), 33–39.
133. Baldi, A., Abbate, A., Bussani, R., et al. (2002). Apoptosis and post-infarction left ventricular remodeling. *J Mol Cell Cardiol, 34*(2), 165–174.
134. Palojoki, E., Saraste, A., Eriksson, A., et al. (2001). Cardiomyocyte apoptosis and ventricular remodeling after myocardial infarction in rats. *Am J Physiol Heart Circ Physiol, 280*(6), H2726–H2731.
135. Sam, F., Sawyer, D. B., Chang, D. L., et al. (2000). Progressive left ventricular remodeling and apoptosis late after myocardial infarction in mouse heart. *Am J Physiol Heart Circ Physiol, 279*(1), H422–H428.
136. Abbate, A., Biondi-Zoccai, G. G., Bussani, R., et al. (2003). Increased myocardial apoptosis in patients with unfavorable left ventricular remodeling and early symptomatic post-infarction heart failure. *J Am Coll Cardiol, 41*(5), 753–760.
137. Anversa, P., & Kajstura, J. (1998). Ventricular myocytes are not terminally differentiated in the adult mammalian heart. *Circ Res, 83*(1), 1–14.
138. Beltrami, A. P., Urbanek, K., Kajstura, J., et al. (2001). Evidence that human cardiac myocytes divide after myocardial infarction. *N Engl J Med, 344*(23), 1750–1757.
139. McMahon, J. T., & Ratliff, N. B. (1990). Regeneration of adult human myocardium after acute heart transplant rejection. *J Heart Transplant, 9*(5), 554–567.
140. Taylor, D. A., Atkins, B. Z., Hungspreugs, P., et al. (1998). Regenerating functional myocardium: improved performance after skeletal myoblast transplantation. *Nat Med, 4*(8), 929–933.
141. Glaser, R., Lu, M. M., Narula, N., et al. (2002). Smooth muscle cells, but not myocytes, of host origin in transplanted human hearts. *Circulation, 106*(1), 17–19.
142. Hruban, R. H., Long, P. P., Perlman, E. J., et al. (1993). Fluorescence in situ hybridization for the Y-chromosome can be used to detect cells of recipient origin in allografted hearts following cardiac transplantation. *Am J Pathol, 142*(4), 975–980.
143. Laflamme, M. A., Myerson, D., Saffitz, J. E., et al. (2002). Evidence for cardiomyocyte repopulation by extracardiac progenitors in transplanted human hearts. *Circ Res, 90*(6), 634–640.
144. Quaini, F., Urbanek, K., Beltrami, A. P., et al. (2002). Chimerism of the transplanted heart. *N Engl J Med, 346*(1), 5–15.
145. Taylor, D. A., Hruban, R., Rodriguez, E. R., et al. (2002). Cardiac chimerism as a mechanism for self-repair: does it happen and if so to what degree? *Circulation, 106*(1), 2–4.
146. Lowes, B. D., Minobe, W., Abraham, W. T., et al. (1997). Changes in gene expression in the intact human heart. Downregulation of alpha-myosin heavy chain in hypertrophied, failing ventricular myocardium. *J Clin Invest, 100*(9), 2315–2324.
147. Alpert, N. R., & Gordon, M. S. (1962). Myofibrillar adenosine phosphatase activity in congestive heart failure. *Am J Physiol, 202*, 940–946.
148. Labeit, S., & Kolmerer, B. (1995). Titins: giant proteins in charge of muscle ultrastructure and elasticity. *Science, 270*(5234), 293–296.

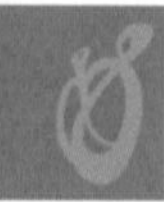

149. Gregorio, C. C., Trombitas, K., Centner, T., et al. (1998). The NH2 terminus of titin spans the Z-disc: its interaction with a novel 19-kD ligand (T-cap) is required for sarcomeric integrity. *J Cell Biol*, *143*(4), 1013–1027.
150. Obermann, W. M., Gautel, M., Weber, K., et al. (1997). Molecular structure of the sarcomeric M band: mapping of titin and myosin binding domains in myomesin and the identification of a potential regulatory phosphorylation site in myomesin. *EMBO J*, *16*(2), 211–220.
151. Hein, S., Scholz, D., Fujitani, N., et al. (1994). Altered expression of titin and contractile proteins in failing human myocardium. *J Mol Cell Cardiol*, *26*(10), 1291–1306.
152. Gregorio, C. C., Granzier, H., Sorimachi, H., et al. (1999). Muscle assembly: a titanic achievement? *Curr Opin Cell Biol*, *11*(1), 18–25.
153. Gelfand, V. I., & Bershadsky, A. D. (1991). Microtubule dynamics: mechanism, regulation, and function. *Annu Rev Cell Biol*, *7*, 93–116.
154. Lockard, V. G., & Bloom, S. (1993). Trans-cellular desmin-lamin B intermediate filament network in cardiac myocytes. *J Mol Cell Cardiol*, *25*(3), 303–309.
155. Klietsch, R., Ervasti, J. M., Arnold, W., et al. (1993). Dystrophin-glycoprotein complex and laminin colocalize to the sarcolemma and transverse tubules of cardiac muscle. *Circ Res*, *72*(2), 349–360.
156. Choquet, D., Felsenfeld, D. P., & Sheetz, M. P. (1997). Extracellular matrix rigidity causes strengthening of integrin-cytoskeleton linkages. *Cell*, *88*(1), 39–48.
157. Koch, P. J., & Franke, W. W. (1994). Desmosomal cadherins: another growing multigene family of adhesion molecules. *Curr Opin Cell Biol*, *6*(5), 682–687.
158. Heling, A., Zimmermann, R., Kostin, S., et al. (2000). Increased expression of cytoskeletal, linkage, and extracellular proteins in failing human myocardium. *Circ Res*, *86*(8), 846–853.
159. Rappaport, L., & Samuel, J. L. (1988). Microtubules in cardiac myocytes. *Int Rev Cytol*, *113*, 101–143.
160. Tsutsui, H., Ishihara, K., & Cooper, G.T. (1993). Cytoskeletal role in the contractile dysfunction of hypertrophied myocardium. *Science*, *260*(5108), 682–687.
161. Tsutsui, H., Tagawa, H., Kent, R. L., et al. (1994). Role of microtubules in contractile dysfunction of hypertrophied cardiocytes. *Circulation*, *90*(1), 533–555.
162. Tagawa, H., Wang, N., Narishige, T., et al. (1997). Cytoskeletal mechanics in pressure-overload cardiac hypertrophy. *Circ Res*, *80*(2), 281–289.
163. Wang, X., Li, F., Campbell, S. E., et al. (1999). Chronic pressure overload cardiac hypertrophy and failure in guinea pigs: II. Cytoskeletal remodeling. *J Mol Cell Cardiol*, *31*(2), 319–331.
164. Milner, D. J., Taffet, G. E., Wang, X., et al. (1999). The absence of desmin leads to cardiomyocyte hypertrophy and cardiac dilation with compromised systolic function. *J Mol Cell Cardiol*, *31*(11), 2063–2076.
165. Kostin, S., Scholz, D., Shimada, T., et al. (1998). The internal and external protein scaffold of the T-tubular system in cardiomyocytes. *Cell Tissue Res*, *294*(3), 449–460.
166. Ohlendieck, K. (1996). Towards an understanding of the dystrophin-glycoprotein complex: linkage between the extracellular matrix and the membrane cytoskeleton in muscle fibers. *Eur J Cell Biol*, *69*(1), 1–10.
167. Ortiz-Lopez, R., Li, H., Su, J., et al. (1997). Evidence for a dystrophin missense mutation as a cause of X-linked dilated cardiomyopathy. *Circulation*, *95*(10), 2434–2440.
168. Towbin, J. A. (1998). The role of cytoskeletal proteins in cardiomyopathies. *Curr Opin Cell Biol*, *10*(1), 131–139.
169. Towbin, J. A., Bowles, K. R., & Bowles, N. E. (1999). Etiologies of cardiomyopathy and heart failure. *Nat Med*, *5*(3), 266–267.
170. Kaprielian, R. R., Stevenson, S., Rothery, S. M., et al. (2000). Distinct patterns of dystrophin organization in myocyte sarcolemma and transverse tubules of normal and diseased human myocardium. *Circulation*, *101*(22), 2586–2594.
171. Severs, N. J. (1990). The cardiac gap junction and intercalated disc. *Int J Cardiol*, *26*(2), 137–173.
172. Smith, J. H., Green, C. R., Peters, N. S., et al. (1991). Altered patterns of gap junction distribution in ischemic heart disease. An immunohistochemical study of human myocardium using laser scanning confocal microscopy. *Am J Pathol*, *139*(4), 801–821.
173. Emdad, L., Uzzaman, M., Takagishi, Y., et al. (2001). Gap junction remodeling in hypertrophied left ventricles of aortic-banded rats: prevention by angiotensin II type 1 receptor blockade. *J Mol Cell Cardiol*, *33*(2), 219–231.
174. Gutstein, D. E., Morley, G. E., Tamaddon, H., et al. (2001). Conduction slowing and sudden arrhythmic death in mice with cardiac-restricted inactivation of connexin43. *Circ Res*, *88*(3), 333–339.
175. Lerner, D. L., Yamada, K. A., Schuessler, R. B., et al. (2000). Accelerated onset and increased incidence of ventricular arrhythmias induced by ischemia in Cx43-deficient mice. *Circulation*, *101*(5), 547–552.
176. Jugdutt, B. I. (2003). Ventricular remodeling after infarction and the extracellular collagen matrix: when is enough enough? *Circulation*, *108*(11), 1395–1403.
177. Miner, E. C., & Miller, W. L. (2006). A look between the cardiomyocytes: the extracellular matrix in heart failure. *Mayo Clin Proc*, *81*(1), 71–76.
178. Spinale, F. G. (2007). Myocardial matrix remodeling and the matrix metalloproteinases: influence on cardiac form and function. *Physiol Rev*, *87*(4), 1285–1342.
179. Weber, K. T., Brilla, C. G., & Janicki, J. S. (1993). Myocardial fibrosis: functional significance and regulatory factors. *Cardiovasc Res*, *27*(3), 341–348.
180. Weber, K. T., Sun, Y., Tyagi, S. C., et al. (1994). Collagen network of the myocardium: function, structural remodeling and regulatory mechanisms. *J Mol Cell Cardiol*, *26*(3), 279–292.
181. Rossi, M. A., Abreu, M. A., & Santoro, L. B. (1998). Images in cardiovascular medicine. Connective tissue skeleton of the human heart: a demonstration by cell-maceration scanning electron microscope method. *Circulation*, *97*(9), 934–935.
182. Weber, K. T., Pick, R., Janicki, J. S., et al. (1988). Inadequate collagen tethers in dilated cardiopathy. *Am Heart J*, *116*(6 pt 1), 1641–1646.
183. Gunja-Smith, Z., Morales, A. R., Romanelli, R., et al. (1996). Remodeling of human myocardial collagen in idiopathic dilated cardiomyopathy. Role of metalloproteinases and pyridinoline cross-links. *Am J Pathol*, *148*(5), 1639–1648.
184. Spinale, F. G., Tomita, M., Zellner, J. L., et al. (1991). Collagen remodeling and changes in LV function during development and recovery from supraventricular tachycardia. *Am J Physiol*, *261*(2 pt 2), H308–H318.
185. Abrahams, C., Janicki, J. S., & Weber, K. T. (1987). Myocardial hypertrophy in *Macaca fascicularis*. Structural remodeling of the collagen matrix. *Lab Invest*, *56*(6), 676–683.
186. Weber, K. T., Janicki, J. S., Shroff, S. G., et al. (1988). Collagen remodeling of the pressure-overloaded, hypertrophied nonhuman primate myocardium. *Circ Res*, *62*(4), 757–765.
187. Weber, K. T., & Brilla, C. G. (1991). Pathological hypertrophy and cardiac interstitium. Fibrosis and renin-angiotensin-aldosterone system. *Circulation*, *83*(6), 1849–1865.
188. Schaper, J., & Speiser, B. (1992). The extracellular matrix in the failing human heart. *Basic Res Cardiol*, *87*(suppl. 1), 303–309.
189. Boluyt, M. O., O'Neill, L., Meredith, A. L., et al. (1994). Alterations in cardiac gene expression during the transition from stable hypertrophy to heart failure. Marked upregulation of genes encoding extracellular matrix components. *Circ Res*, *75*(1), 23–32.
190. Villari, B., Campbell, S. E., Hess, O. M., et al. (1993). Influence of collagen network on left ventricular systolic and diastolic function in aortic valve disease. *J Am Coll Cardiol*, *22*(5), 1477–1484.
191. Kato, S., Spinale, F. G., Tanaka, R., et al. (1995). Inhibition of collagen cross-linking: effects on fibrillar collagen and ventricular diastolic function. *Am J Physiol*, *269* (3 pt 2), H863–H868.
192. Stroud, J. D., Baicu, C. F., Barnes, M. A., et al. (2002). Viscoelastic properties of pressure overload hypertrophied myocardium: effect of serine protease treatment. *Am J Physiol Heart Circ Physiol*, *282*(6), H2324–H2335.
193. Katz, A. M., & Zile, M. R. (2006). New molecular mechanism in diastolic heart failure. *Circulation*, *113*(16), 1922–1925.
194. Zile, M. R., Baicu, C. F., & Gaasch, W. H. (2004). Diastolic heart failure—abnormalities in active relaxation and passive stiffness of the left ventricle. *N Engl J Med*, *350*(19), 1953–1959.
195. Dell'italia, L. J., Balcells, E., Meng, Q. C., et al. (1997). Volume-overload cardiac hypertrophy is unaffected by ACE inhibitor treatment in dogs. *Am J Physiol*, *273*(2 pt 2), H961–H970.
196. Perry, G. J., Wei, C. C., Hankes, G. H., et al. (2002). Angiotensin II receptor blockade does not improve left ventricular function and remodeling in subacute mitral regurgitation in the dog. *J Am Coll Cardiol*, *39*(8), 1374–1379.
197. Tsutsui, H., Spinale, F. G., Nagatsu, M., et al. (1994). Effects of chronic beta-adrenergic blockade on the left ventricular and cardiocyte abnormalities of chronic canine mitral regurgitation. *J Clin Invest*, *93*(6), 2639–2648.
198. Weber, K. T., Pick, R., Silver, M. A., et al. (1990). Fibrillar collagen and remodeling of dilated canine left ventricle. *Circulation*, *82*(4), 1387–1401.
199. Brew, K., Dinakarpandian, D., & Nagase, H. (2000). Tissue inhibitors of metalloproteinases: evolution, structure and function. *Biochim Biophys Acta*, *1477*(1–2), 267–283.
200. Nagase, H., Visse, R., & Murphy, G. (2006). Structure and function of matrix metalloproteinases and TIMPs. *Cardiovasc Res*, *69*(3), 562–573.
201. Sundstrom, J., Evans, J. C., Benjamin, E. J., et al. (2004). Relations of plasma total TIMP-1 levels to cardiovascular risk factors and echocardiographic measures: the Framingham Heart Study. *Eur Heart J*, *25*(17), 1509–1516.
202. Cavusoglu, E., Ruwende, C., Chopra, V., et al. (2006). Tissue inhibitor of metalloproteinase-1 (TIMP-1) is an independent predictor of all-cause mortality, cardiac mortality, and myocardial infarction. *Am Heart J*, *151*(5), e1101–e1108.
203. Weber, K. T. (1995). *Wound healing in cardiovascular disease*. Armonk, NY: Futura.
204. Marino, T. A., Kent, R. L., Uboh, C. E., et al. (1985). Structural analysis of pressure versus volume overload hypertrophy of cat right ventricle. *Am J Physiol*, *249*(2 pt 2), H371–H379.
205. Apstein, C. S., Lecarpentier, Y., Mercadier, J. J., et al. (1987). Changes in LV papillary muscle performance and myosin composition with aortic insufficiency in rats. *Am J Physiol*, *253*(5 pt 2), H1005–H1011.
206. Silver, M. A., Pick, R., Brilla, C. G., et al. (1990). Reactive and reparative fibrillar collagen remodelling in the hypertrophied rat left ventricle: two experimental models of myocardial fibrosis. *Cardiovasc Res*, *24*(9), 741–747.
207. Brilla, C. G., & Maisch, B. (1994). Regulation of the structural remodelling of the myocardium: from hypertrophy to heart failure. *Eur Heart J*, *15*(suppl. D), 45–52.
208. Brilla, C. G., Matsubara, L. S., & Weber, K. T. (1993). Anti-aldosterone treatment and the prevention of myocardial fibrosis in primary and secondary hyperaldosteronism. *J Mol Cell Cardiol*, *25*(5), 563–575.
209. Weber, K. T., Sun, Y., & Campbell, S. E. (1995). Structural remodelling of the heart by fibrous tissue: role of circulating hormones and locally produced peptides. *Eur Heart J*, *16*(suppl. N), 12–18.
210. Anversa, P., Loud, A. V., Levicky, V., et al. (1985). Left ventricular failure induced by myocardial infarction. II. Tissue morphometry. *Am J Physiol*, *248*(6 pt 2), H883–H889.
211. Karam, R., Healy, B. P., & Wicker, P. (1990). Coronary reserve is depressed in postmyocardial infarction reactive cardiac hypertrophy. *Circulation*, *81*(1), 238–246.
212. Bristow, M. R., Ginsburg, R., Minobe, W., et al. (1982). Decreased catecholamine sensitivity and beta-adrenergic-receptor density in failing human hearts. *N Engl J Med*, *307*(4), 205–211.
213. Ungerer, M., Bohm, M., Elce, J. S., et al. (1993). Altered expression of beta-adrenergic receptor kinase and beta 1-adrenergic receptors in the failing human heart. *Circulation*, *87*(2), 454–463.
214. Saks, V. A., Belikova, Y. O., Kuznetsov, A. V., et al. (1991). Phosphocreatine pathway for energy transport: ADP diffusion and cardiomyopathy. *Am J Physiol*, *261*(suppl. 4), 30–38.
215. Reinecke, H., Studer, R., Vetter, R., et al. (1996). Cardiac Na^+/Ca^{2+} exchange activity in patients with end-stage heart failure. *Cardiovasc Res*, *31*(1), 48–54.
216. Schillinger, W., Lehnart, S. E., Prestle, J., et al. (1998). Influence of SR Ca(2+)-ATPase and Na(+)-Ca(2+)-exchanger on the force-frequency relation. *Basic Res Cardiol*, *93*(suppl. 1), 38–45.

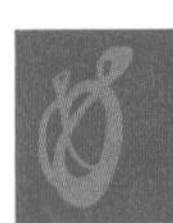

217. Davies, C. H., Davia, K., Bennett, J. G., et al. (1995). Reduced contraction and altered frequency response of isolated ventricular myocytes from patients with heart failure. *Circulation, 92*(9), 2540–2549.
218. Capasso, J. M., & Anversa, P. (1992). Mechanical performance of spared myocytes after myocardial infarction in rats: effects of captopril treatment. *Am J Physiol, 263*(3 pt 2), H841–H849.
219. Spinale, F. G., Fulbright, B. M., Mukherjee, R., et al. (1992). Relation between ventricular and myocyte function with tachycardia-induced cardiomyopathy. *Circ Res, 71*(1), 174–187.
220. Kiss, E., Ball, N. A., Kranias, E. G., et al. (1995). Differential changes in cardiac phospholamban and sarcoplasmic reticular Ca(2+)-ATPase protein levels. Effects on Ca^{2+} transport and mechanics in compensated pressure-overload hypertrophy and congestive heart failure. *Circ Res, 77*(4), 759–764.
221. Naqvi, R. U., & Macleod, K. T. (1994). Effect of hypertrophy on mechanisms of relaxation in isolated cardiac myocytes from guinea pig. *Am J Physiol, 267*(5 pt 2), H1851–H1861.
222. Hohl, C. M., Hu, B., Fertel, R. H., et al. (1993). Effects of obesity and hypertension on ventricular myocytes: comparison of cells from adult SHHF/Mcc-cp and JCR: LA-cp rats. *Cardiovasc Res, 27*(2), 238–242.
223. Naqvi, R. U., del Monte, F., O'Gara, P., et al. (1994). Characteristics of myocytes isolated from hearts of renovascular hypertensive guinea pigs. *Am J Physiol, 266*(5 Pt 2), H1886–H1895.
224. del Monte, F., O'Gara, P., Poole-Wilson, P. A., et al. (1995). Cell geometry and contractile abnormalities of myocytes from failing human left ventricle. *Cardiovasc Res, 30*(2), 281–290.
225. Prahash, A. J. C., Gupta, S., & Anand, I. S. (2000). Myocyte response to beta adrenergic stimulation is preserved in the noninfarcted myocardium of globally dysfunctional rat following myocardial infarction. *Circulation, 102*(15), 1840–1846.
226. Urabe, Y., Hamada, Y., Spinale, F. G., et al. (1993). Cardiocyte contractile performance in experimental biventricular volume-overload hypertrophy. *Am J Physiol, 264*(5 pt 2), H1615–H1623.
227. Stroud, J. D., Baicu, C. F., Isomatsu, Y., et al. (2001). Changes in extracellular collagen matrix after systolic performance in normal and pressure overloaded hypertrophied myocardium. *Circulation, 102*(18), II-627.
228. Sabbah, H. N., & Goldstein, S. (1993). Ventricular remodelling: consequences and therapy. *Eur Heart J, 14*(suppl. C), 24–29.
229. Douglas, P. S., Morrow, R., Ioli, A., et al. (1989). Left ventricular shape, afterload and survival in idiopathic dilated cardiomyopathy. *J Am Coll Cardiol, 13*(2), 311–315.
230. Kono, T., Sabbah, H. N., Rosman, H., et al. (1992). Left ventricular shape is the primary determinant of functional mitral regurgitation in heart failure. *J Am Coll Cardiol, 20*(7), 1594–1598.
231. Florea, V. G., Henein, M. Y., Anker, S. D., et al. (2000). Relation of changes over time in ventricular size and function to those in exercise capacity in patients with chronic heart failure. *Am Heart J, 139*(5), 913–917.
232. Cohn, J. N., Johnson, G. R., Shabetai, R., et al. (1993). Ejection fraction, peak exercise oxygen consumption, cardiothoracic ratio, ventricular arrhythmias, and plasma norepinephrine as determinants of prognosis in heart failure. *Circulation, 87*(suppl. 6), VI5–V16.
233. Cohn, J. N. (1995). Structural basis for heart failure. Ventricular remodeling and its pharmacological inhibition. *Circulation, 91*(10), 2504–2507.
234. Meerson, F. Z. (1962). Compensatory hyperfunction of the heart and cardiac insufficiency. *Circ Res, 10*, 250–258.
235. Gaudron, P., Eilles, C., Kugler, I., et al. (1993). Progressive left ventricular dysfunction and remodeling after myocardial infarction. Potential mechanisms and early predictors. *Circulation, 87*(3), 755–763.
236. Sharpe, N., Smith, H., Murphy, J., et al. (1991). Early prevention of left ventricular dysfunction after myocardial infarction with angiotensin-converting-enzyme inhibition. *Lancet, 337*(8746), 872–876.
237. Dargie, H. J. (2001). Effect of carvedilol on outcome after myocardial infarction in patients with left-ventricular dysfunction: the CAPRICORN randomised trial. *Lancet, 357*(9266), 1385–1390.
238. Doughty, R. N., Whalley, G. A., Walsh, H., et al. (2001). Effects of carvedilol on left ventricular remodeling in patients following acute myocardial infarction: the CAPRICORN echo substudy. *Circulation, 104*(suppl. 17), II-517 (abstract).
239. The ACE Inhibitor Myocardial Infarction Collaborative Group (1998). Indications for ACE inhibitors in the early treatment of acute myocardial infarction: systematic overview of individual data from 100,000 patients in randomized trials. *Circulation, 97*(22), 2202–2212.
240. Effect of ramipril on mortality and morbidity of survivors of acute myocardial infarction with clinical evidence of heart failure. (1993). The acute infarction ramipril efficacy (aire) study investigators. *Lancet, 342*(8875), 821–828.
241. Buch, P., Rasmussen, S., Abildstrom, S. Z., et al. (2005). The long-term impact of the angiotensin-converting enzyme inhibitor trandolapril on mortality and hospital admissions in patients with left ventricular dysfunction after a myocardial infarction: follow-up to 12 years. *Eur Heart J, 26*(2), 145–152.
242. Grossman, W. (1980). Cardiac hypertrophy: useful adaptation or pathologic process? *Am J Med, 69*(4), 576–584.
243. Katz, A. M. (1990). Cardiomyopathy of overload. A major determinant of prognosis in congestive heart failure. *N Engl J Med, 322*(2), 100–110.
244. Raya, T. E., Fonken, S. J., Lee, R. W., et al. (1991). Hemodynamic effects of direct angiotensin II blockade compared to converting enzyme inhibition in rat model of heart failure. *Am J Hypertens, 4*(4 pt 2), 334S–340S.
245. Schieffer, B., Wirger, A., Meybrunn, M., et al. (1994). Comparative effects of chronic angiotensin-converting enzyme inhibition and angiotensin II type 1 receptor blockade on cardiac remodeling after myocardial infarction in the rat. *Circulation, 89*(5), 2273–2282.
246. McDonald, K. M., Rector, T., Carlyle, P. F., et al. (1994). Angiotensin-converting enzyme inhibition and beta-adrenoceptor blockade regress established ventricular remodeling in a canine model of discrete myocardial damage. *J Am Coll Cardiol, 24*(7), 1762–1768.
247. Tamura, T., Said, S., Harris, J., et al. (2000). Reverse remodeling of cardiac myocyte hypertrophy in hypertension and failure by targeting of the renin-angiotensin system. *Circulation, 102*(2), 253–259.
248. Xu, X., Wan, W., Ji, L., et al. (2008). Exercise training combined with angiotensin II receptor blockade limits post-infarct ventricular remodelling in rats. *Cardiovasc Res, 78*(3), 523–532.
249. Konstam, M. A., Kronenberg, M. W., Rousseau, M. F., et al. (1993). Effects of the angiotensin converting enzyme inhibitor enalapril on the long-term progression of left ventricular dilatation in patients with asymptomatic systolic dysfunction. SOLVD (studies of left ventricular dysfunction) investigators. *Circulation, 88*(5 pt 1), 2277–2283.
250. Konstam, M. A., Rousseau, M. F., Kronenberg, M. W., et al. (1992). Effects of the angiotensin converting enzyme inhibitor enalapril on the long-term progression of left ventricular dysfunction in patients with heart failure. *Circulation, 86*(2), 431–438.
251. St John Sutton, M., Pfeffer, M. A., Plappert, T., et al. (1994). Quantitative two-dimensional echocardiographic measurements are major predictors of adverse cardiovascular events after acute myocardial infarction. The protective effects of captopril. *Circulation, 89*(1), 68–75.
252. Hall, S. A., Cigarroa, C. G., Marcoux, L., et al. (1995). Time course of improvement in left ventricular function, mass and geometry in patients with congestive heart failure treated with beta-adrenergic blockade. *J Am Coll Cardiol, 25*(5), 1154–1161.
253. Sabbah, H. N., Sharov, V. G., Gupta, R. C., et al. (2000). Chronic therapy with metoprolol attenuates cardiomyocyte apoptosis in dogs with heart failure. *J Am Coll Cardiol, 36*(5), 1698–1705.
254. Hayashi, M., Tsutamoto, T., Wada, A., et al. (2003). Immediate administration of mineralocorticoid receptor antagonist spironolactone prevents post-infarct left ventricular remodeling associated with suppression of a marker of myocardial collagen synthesis in patients with first anterior acute myocardial infarction. *Circulation, 107*(20), 2559–2565.
255. Tsutamoto, T., Wada, A., Maeda, K., et al. (2001). Effect of spironolactone on plasma brain natriuretic peptide and left ventricular remodeling in patients with congestive heart failure. *J Am Coll Cardiol, 37*(5), 1228–1233.
256. Pitt, B., Reichek, N., Willenbrock, R., et al. (2003). Effects of eplerenone, enalapril, and eplerenone/enalapril in patients with essential hypertension and left ventricular hypertrophy: the 4E-left ventricular hypertrophy study. *Circulation, 108*(15), 1831–1838.
257. Chan, A. K., Sanderson, J. E., Wang, T., et al. (2007). Aldosterone receptor antagonism induces reverse remodeling when added to angiotensin receptor blockade in chronic heart failure. *J Am Coll Cardiol, 50*(7), 591–596.
258. Cohn, J. N., & Tognoni, G. (2001). A randomized trial of the angiotensin-receptor blocker valsartan in chronic heart failure. *N Engl J Med, 345*(23), 1667–1675.
259. Maggioni, A. P., Anand, I., Gottlieb, S. O., et al. (2002). Effects of valsartan on morbidity and mortality in patients with heart failure not receiving angiotensin-converting enzyme inhibitors. *J Am Coll Cardiol, 40*(8), 1414–1421.
260. Wong, M., Staszewsky, L., Latini, R., et al. (2002). Valsartan benefits left ventricular structure and function in heart failure: Val-HeFT echocardiographic study. *J Am Coll Cardiol, 40*(5), 970–975.
261. Wong, M., Staszewsky, L., Latini, R., et al. (2004). Severity of left ventricular remodeling defines outcomes and response to therapy in heart failure: valsartan heart failure trial (Val-HeFT) echocardiographic data. *J Am Coll Cardiol, 43*(11), 2022–2027.
262. Lindholm, L. H., Ibsen, H., Dahlof, B., et al. (2002). Cardiovascular morbidity and mortality in patients with diabetes in the losartan intervention for endpoint reduction in hypertension study (LIFE): a randomised trial against atenolol. *Lancet, 359*(9311), 1004–1010.
263. Cintron, G., Johnson, G., Francis, G., et al. (1993). Prognostic significance of serial changes in left ventricular ejection fraction in patients with congestive heart failure. *Circulation, 87*(suppl. 6), VI17–VII23.
264. Cohn, J. N., Tam, S. W., Anand, I. S., et al. (2007). Isosorbide dinitrate and hydralazine in a fixed-dose combination produces further regression of left ventricular remodeling in a well-treated black population with heart failure: results from A-HeFT. *J Card Fail, 13*(5), 331–339.
265. Taylor, A. L., Ziesche, S., Yancy, C., et al. (2004). Combination of isosorbide dinitrate and hydralazine in blacks with heart failure. *N Engl J Med, 351*(20), 2049–2057.
266. Strauer, B. E., Brehm, M., Zeus, T., et al. (2002). Repair of infarcted myocardium by autologous intracoronary mononuclear bone marrow cell transplantation in humans. *Circulation, 106*(15), 1913–1918.
267. Assmus, B., Schachinger, V., Teupe, C., et al. (2002). Transplantation of progenitor cells and regeneration enhancement in acute myocardial infarction (TOPCARE-AMI). *Circulation, 106*(24), 3009–3017.
268. Schachinger, V., Assmus, B., Britten, M. B., et al. (2004). Transplantation of progenitor cells and regeneration enhancement in acute myocardial infarction: final one-year results of the TOPCARE-AMI trial. *J Am Coll Cardiol, 44*(8), 1690–1699.
269. Meyer, G. P., Wollert, K. C., Lotz, J., et al. (2006). Intracoronary bone marrow cell transfer after myocardial infarction: eighteen months' follow-up data from the randomized, controlled BOOST (BOne marrOw transfer to enhance ST-elevation infarct regeneration) trial. *Circulation, 113*(10), 1287–1294.
270. Wollert, K. C., Meyer, G. P., Lotz, J., et al. (2004). Intracoronary autologous bone-marrow cell transfer after myocardial infarction: the BOOST randomised controlled clinical trial. *Lancet, 364*(9429), 141–148.
271. Lunde, K., Solheim, S., Aakhus, S., et al. (2006). Intracoronary injection of mononuclear bone marrow cells in acute myocardial infarction. *N Engl J Med, 355*(12), 1199–1209.
272. Schachinger, V., Erbs, S., Elsasser, A., et al. (2006). Intracoronary bone marrow-derived progenitor cells in acute myocardial infarction. *N Engl J Med, 355*(12), 1210–1221.
273. De Bonis, M., & Alfieri, O. (2007). Surgical methods to reverse left ventricular remodeling. *Curr Heart Fail Rep, 4*(4), 214–220.

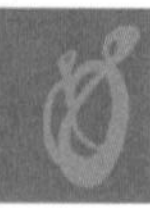

274. Velazquez, E. J., Lee, K. L., O'Connor, C. M., et al. (2007). The rationale and design of the surgical treatment for ischemic heart failure (STICH) trial. *J Thorac Cardiovasc Surg, 134*(6), 1540–1547.

275 Jones, R. H., Velazquez, E. J., Michler, R. E., et al. Coronary bypass surgery with or without surgical ventricular reconstruction. *N. Engl J Med.* 360(17), 1705–1717.

276. Monrad, E. S., Hess, O. M., Murakami, T., et al. (1988). Time course of regression of left ventricular hypertrophy after aortic valve replacement. *Circulation, 77*(6), 1345–1355.

277. Villari, B., Vassalli, G., Monrad, E. S., et al. (1995). Normalization of diastolic dysfunction in aortic stenosis late after valve replacement. *Circulation, 91*(9), 2353–2358.

278. Gerdes, A. M., Clark, L. C., & Capasso, J. M. (1995). Regression of cardiac hypertrophy after closing an aortocaval fistula in rats. *Am J Physiol, 268*(6 pt 2), H2345–H2351.

279. Francis, G. S., Anwar, F., Bank, A. J., et al. (1999). Apoptosis, Bcl-2, and proliferating cell nuclear antigen in the failing human heart: observations made after implantation of left ventricular assist device. *J Card Fail, 5*(4), 308–315.

280. Burkhoff, D., Klotz, S., & Mancini, D. M. (2006). LVAD-induced reverse remodeling: basic and clinical implications for myocardial recovery. *J Card Fail, 12*(3), 227–239.

281. Drakos, S. G., Terrovitis, J. V., Anastasiou-Nana, M. I., et al. (2007). Reverse remodeling during long-term mechanical unloading of the left ventricle. *J Mol Cell Cardiol, 43*(3), 231–242.

282. Levin, H. R., Oz, M. C., Chen, J. M., et al. (1995). Reversal of chronic ventricular dilation in patients with end-stage cardiomyopathy by prolonged mechanical unloading. *Circulation, 91*(11), 2717–2720.

283. Dipla, K., Mattiello, J. A., Jeevanandam, V., et al. (1998). Myocyte recovery after mechanical circulatory support in humans with end-stage heart failure. *Circulation, 97*(23), 2316–2322.

284. Soppa, G. K., Barton, P. J., Terracciano, C. M., et al. (2008). Left ventricular assist device-induced molecular changes in the failing myocardium. *Curr Opin Cardiol, 23*(3), 206–218.

285. Terracciano, C. M., Harding, S. E., Adamson, D., et al. (2003). Changes in sarcolemmal Ca entry and sarcoplasmic reticulum Ca content in ventricular myocytes from patients with end-stage heart failure following myocardial recovery after combined pharmacological and ventricular assist device therapy. *Eur Heart J, 24*(14), 1329–1339.

286. Dandel, M., Weng, Y., Siniawski, H., et al. (2005). Long-term results in patients with idiopathic dilated cardiomyopathy after weaning from left ventricular assist devices. *Circulation, 112*(suppl. 9), I37–I45.

287. Farrar, D. J., Holman, W. R., Mcbride, L. R., et al. (2002). Long-term follow-up of Thoratec ventricular assist device bridge-to-recovery patients successfully removed from support after recovery of ventricular function. *J Heart Lung Transplant, 21*(5), 516–521.

288. Frazier, O. H., Delgado, R. M., III, Scroggins, N., et al. (2004). Mechanical bridging to improvement in severe acute "nonischemic, nonmyocarditis" heart failure. *Congest Heart Fail, 10*(2), 109–113.

289. Frazier, O. H., & Myers, T. J. (1999). Left ventricular assist system as a bridge to myocardial recovery. *Ann Thorac Surg, 68*(2), 734–741.

290. Mancini, D. M., Beniaminovitz, A., Levin, H., et al. (1998). Low incidence of myocardial recovery after left ventricular assist device implantation in patients with chronic heart failure. *Circulation, 98*(22), 2383–2389.

291. Simon, M. A., Kormos, R. L., Murali, S., et al. (2005). Myocardial recovery using ventricular assist devices: prevalence, clinical characteristics, and outcomes. *Circulation, 112*(suppl. 9), I32–I36.

292. Birks, E. J., Tansley, P. D., Hardy, J., et al. (2006). Left ventricular assist device and drug therapy for the reversal of heart failure. *N Engl J Med, 355*(18), 1873–1884.

293. Cleland, J. G., Daubert, J. C., Erdmann, E., et al. (2005). The effect of cardiac resynchronization on morbidity and mortality in heart failure. *N Engl J Med, 352*(15), 1539–1549.

294. Linde, C., Leclercq, C., Rex, S., et al. (2002). Long-term benefits of biventricular pacing in congestive heart failure: results from the MUltisite STimulation in cardiomyopathy (MUSTIC) study. *J Am Coll Cardiol, 40*(1), 111–118.

295. Molhoek, S. G., Bax, J. J., van Erven, L., et al. (2004). Comparison of benefits from cardiac resynchronization therapy in patients with ischemic cardiomyopathy versus idiopathic dilated cardiomyopathy. *Am J Cardiol, 93*(7), 860–863.

296. Sutton, M. G., Plappert, T., Hilpisch, K. E., et al. (2006). Sustained reverse left ventricular structural remodeling with cardiac resynchronization at one year is a function of etiology: quantitative Doppler echocardiographic evidence from the multicenter in sync randomized clinical evaluation (MIRACLE). *Circulation, 113*(2), 266–272.

297. Sutton, M. S., & Keane, M. G. (2007). Reverse remodelling in heart failure with cardiac resynchronisation therapy. *Heart, 93*(2), 167–171.

298. Fruhwald, F. M., Fahrleitner-Pammer, A., Berger, R., et al. (2007). Early and sustained effects of cardiac resynchronization therapy on N-terminal pro-B-type natriuretic peptide in patients with moderate to severe heart failure and cardiac dyssynchrony. *Eur Heart J, 28*(13), 1592–1597.

299. Chaudhry, P. A., Mishima, T., Sharov, V. G., et al. (2000). Passive epicardial containment prevents ventricular remodeling in heart failure. *Ann Thorac Surg, 70*(4), 1275–1280.

300. Saavedra, W. F., Tunin, R. S., Paolocci, N., et al. (2002). Reverse remodeling and enhanced adrenergic reserve from passive external support in experimental dilated heart failure. *J Am Coll Cardiol, 39*(12), 2069–2076.

301. Sabbah, H. N., Sharov, V. G., Gupta, R. C., et al. (2003). Reversal of chronic molecular and cellular abnormalities due to heart failure by passive mechanical ventricular containment. *Circ Res, 93*(11), 1095–1101.

302. Blom, A. S., Mukherjee, R., Pilla, J. J., et al. (2005). Cardiac support device modifies left ventricular geometry and myocardial structure after myocardial infarction. *Circulation, 112*(9), 1274–1283.

303. Blom, A. S., Pilla, J. J., Arkles, J., et al. (2007). Ventricular restraint prevents infarct expansion and improves borderzone function after myocardial infarction: a study using magnetic resonance imaging, three-dimensional surface modeling, and myocardial tagging. *Ann Thorac Surg, 84*(6), 2004–2010.

304. Pilla, J. J., Blom, A. S., Gorman, J. H., III, et al. (2005). Early postinfarction ventricular restraint improves borderzone wall thickening dynamics during remodeling. *Ann Thorac Surg, 80*(6), 2257–2262.

305. Mann, D. L., Acker, M. A., Jessup, M., et al. (2007). Clinical evaluation of the CorCap Cardiac Support Device in patients with dilated cardiomyopathy. *Ann Thorac Surg, 84*(4), 1226–1235.

306. Starling, R. C., Jessup, M., Oh, J. K., et al. (2007). Sustained benefits of the CorCap Cardiac Support Device on left ventricular remodeling: three year follow-up results from the Acorn clinical trial. *Ann Thorac Surg, 84*(4), 1236–1242.

307. Giannuzzi, P., Temporelli, P. L., Corra, U., et al. (1997). Attenuation of unfavorable remodeling by exercise training in postinfarction patients with left ventricular dysfunction: results of the exercise in left ventricular dysfunction (ELVD) trial. *Circulation, 96*(6), 1790–1797.

308. Musch, T. I. (1992). Effects of sprint training on maximal stroke volume of rats with a chronic myocardial infarction. *J Appl Physiol, 72*(4), 1437–1443.

309. Shephard, R. J., & Balady, G. J. (1999). Exercise as cardiovascular therapy. *Circulation, 99*(7), 963–972.

310. Hammerman, H., Schoen, F. J., & Kloner, R. A. (1983). Short-term exercise has a prolonged effect on scar formation after experimental acute myocardial infarction. *J Am Coll Cardiol, 2*(5), 979–982.

311. Kloner, R. A., & Kloner, J. A. (1983). The effect of early exercise on myocardial infarct scar formation. *Am Heart J, 106*(5 pt 1), 1009–1013.

312. Orenstein, T. L., Parker, T. G., Butany, J. W., et al. (1995). Favorable left ventricular remodeling following large myocardial infarction by exercise training. Effect on ventricular morphology and gene expression. *J Clin Invest, 96*(2), 858–866.

313. Varin, R., Mulder, P., Richard, V., et al. (1999). Exercise improves flow-mediated vasodilatation of skeletal muscle arteries in rats with chronic heart failure. Role of nitric oxide, prostanoids, and oxidant stress. *Circulation, 99*(22), 2951–2957.

314. Wan, W., Powers, A. S., Li, J., et al. (2007). Effect of post-myocardial infarction exercise training on the renin-angiotensin-aldosterone system and cardiac function. *Am J Med Sci, 334*(4), 265–273.

315. Belardinelli, R., Georgiou, D., Cianci, G., et al. (1999). Randomized, controlled trial of long-term moderate exercise training in chronic heart failure: effects on functional capacity, quality of life, and clinical outcome. *Circulation, 99*(9), 1173–1182.

316. Coats, A. J., Adamopoulos, S., Meyer, T. E., et al. (1990). Effects of physical training in chronic heart failure. *Lancet, 335*(8681), 63–66.

317. Coats, A. J., Adamopoulos, S., Radaelli, A., et al. (1992). Controlled trial of physical training in chronic heart failure. Exercise performance, hemodynamics, ventilation, and autonomic function. *Circulation, 85*(6), 2119–2131.

318. Hambrecht, R., Gielen, S., Linke, A., et al. (2000). Effects of exercise training on left ventricular function and peripheral resistance in patients with chronic heart failure: a randomized trial. *JAMA, 283*(23), 3095–3101.

319. Piepoli, M. F., Davos, C., Francis, D. P., et al. (2004). Exercise training meta-analysis of trials in patients with chronic heart failure (EXTraMATCH). *BMJ, 328*(7433), 189.

320. O'Connor, C. M. (2008). Morbidity and mortality outcomes from aerobic exercise training in heart failure: results of the heart failure and a controlled trial investigating outcomes of exercise training (HF-ACTION) study. New Orleans: paper presented at American Heart Association's scientific sessions 2008.

321. Recommendations for exercise training in chronic heart failure patients. Working Group on Cardiac Rehabilitation and Exercise Physiology and Working Group on Heart Failure of the European Society of Cardiology. (2001). *Eur Heart J, 22*(2), 125–135.

322. Pina, I. L., Apstein, C. S., Balady, G. J., et al. (2003). Exercise and heart failure: a statement from the American Heart Association committee on exercise, rehabilitation, and prevention. *Circulation, 107*(8), 1210–1225.

323. Haykowsky, M. J., Liang, Y., Pechter, D., et al. (2007). A meta-analysis of the effect of exercise training on left ventricular remodeling in heart failure patients: the benefit depends on the type of training performed. *J Am Coll Cardiol, 49*(24), 2329–2336.

324. Pfeffer, M. A., & Pfeffer, J. M. (1987). Ventricular enlargement and reduced survival after myocardial infarction. *Circulation, 75*(5 pt, 2), IV93–IV97.

325. Kramer, D. G., Trikalinos, T. A., Kent, D. M., et al. (2010). Quantitative evaluation of drug or device effects on ventricular remodeling as predictors of therapeutic effects on mortality in patients with heart failure and reduced ejection fraction: a meta-analysis approach. *J Am Coll Cardiol.* (vol. 56), No. 5.

326. The SOLVD Investigators (1991). Effect of enalapril on survival in patients with reduced left ventricular ejection fractions and congestive heart failure. *N Engl J Med, 325*(5), 293–302.

327. The SOLVD Investigators (1992). Effect of enalapril on mortality and the development of heart failure in asymptomatic patients with reduced left ventricular ejection fractions. *N Engl J Med, 327*(10), 685–691.

328. Effect of metoprolol CR/XL in chronic heart failure (1999). Metoprolol CR/XL randomised intervention trial in congestive heart failure (MERIT-HF). *Lancet, 353*(9169), 2001–2007.

329. Packer, M., Antonopoulos, G. V., Berlin, J. A., et al. (2001). Comparative effects of carvedilol and metoprolol on left ventricular ejection fraction in heart failure: results of a meta-analysis. *Am Heart J, 141*(6), 899–907.

330. Poole-Wilson, P. A., Swedberg, K., Cleland, J. G., et al. (2003). Comparison of carvedilol and metoprolol on clinical outcomes in patients with chronic heart failure in the carvedilol or metoprolol European trial (COMET): randomised controlled trial. *Lancet, 362*(9377), 7–13.

331. Pitt, B., Zannad, F., Remme, W. J., et al. (1999). The effect of spironolactone on morbidity and mortality in patients with severe heart failure. Randomized aldactone evaluation study investigators. *N Engl J Med, 341*(10), 709–717.

332. Rousseau, M. F., Konstam, M. A., Benedict, C. R., et al. (1994). Progression of left ventricular dysfunction secondary to coronary artery disease, sustained neurohormonal activation and effects of ibopamine therapy during long-term therapy with angiotensin-converting enzyme inhibitor. *Am J Cardiol, 73*(7), 488–493.

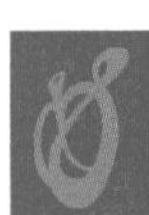

333. Hampton, J. R., van Veldhuisen, D. J., Kleber, F. X., et al. (1997). Randomised study of effect of ibopamine on survival in patients with advanced severe heart failure. Second prospective randomised study of ibopamine on mortality and efficacy (PRIME II) investigators. *Lancet, 349*(9057), 971–977.
334. Konstam, M. A., Patten, R. D., Thomas, I., et al. (2000). Effects of losartan and captopril on left ventricular volumes in elderly patients with heart failure: results of the ELITE ventricular function substudy. *Am Heart J, 139*(6), 1081–1087.
335. Udelson, J. E., Antonopoulos, G. V., Proulx, G., et al. (2000). Comparison of long-term dual vasopeptidase inhibition with omapatrilat to ACE inhibition with lisinopril on ventricular volumes in patients with heart failure. *Circulation, 102*, II-536.
336. Packer, M., Califf, R. M., Konstam, M. A., et al. (2002). Comparison of omapatrilat and enalapril in patients with chronic heart failure: the omapatrilat versus enalapril randomized trial of utility in reducing events (OVERTURE). *Circulation, 106*(8), 920–926.
337. Pitt, B., Poole-Wilson, P. A., Segal, R., et al. (2000). Effect of losartan compared with captopril on mortality in patients with symptomatic heart failure: randomised trial—the losartan heart failure survival study ELITE II. *Lancet, 355*(9215), 1582–1587.
338. Luscher, T. F., Enseleit, F., Pacher, R., et al. (2002). Hemodynamic and neurohumoral effects of selective endothelin A (ET[A]) receptor blockade in chronic heart failure: the heart failure ET(A) receptor blockade trial (HEAT). *Circulation, 106*(21), 2666–2672.
339. Spieker, L. E., Mitrovic, V., Noll, G., et al. (2000). Acute hemodynamic and neurohumoral effects of selective ET(A) receptor blockade in patients with congestive heart failure. ET 003 investigators. *J Am Coll Cardiol, 35*(7), 1745–1752.
340. Anand, I., McMurray, J., Cohn, J. N., et al. (2004). Long-term effects of darusentan on left-ventricular remodelling and clinical outcomes in the endothelina receptor antagonist trial in heart failure (EARTH): randomised, double-blind, placebo-controlled trial. *Lancet, 364*(9431), 347–354.
341. Chandrashekhar, Y., Prahash, A. J., Sen, S., et al. (2003). The role of arginine vasopressin and its receptors in the normal and failing rat heart. *J Mol Cell Cardiol, 35*(5), 495–504.
342. Konstam, M. A., Gheorghiade, M., Burnett, J. C., Jr., et al. (2007). Effects of oral tolvaptan in patients hospitalized for worsening heart failure: the EVEREST outcome trial. *JAMA, 297*(12), 1319–1331.
343. Schapira, J. N., Kohn, M. S., Beaver, W. L., et al. (1981). In vitro quantitation of canine left ventricular volume by phased-array sector scan. *Cardiology, 67*(1), 1–11.
344. Collins, H. W., Kronenberg, M. W., & Byrd, B. F., III (1989). Reproducibility of left ventricular mass measurements by two-dimensional and M-mode echocardiography. *J Am Coll Cardiol, 14*(3), 672–676.
345. Himelman, R. B., Cassidy, M. M., Landzberg, J. S., et al. (1988). Reproducibility of quantitative two-dimensional echocardiography. *Am Heart J, 115*(2), 425–431.
346. Anand, I. S., Florea, V. G., Solomon, S. D., et al. (2002). Noninvasive assessment of left ventricular remodeling: concepts, techniques, and implications for clinical trials. *J Card Fail, 8*(suppl. 6), S452–S464.
347. Upton, M. T., Rerych, S. K., Newman, G. E., et al. (1980). The reproducibility of radionuclide angiographic measurements of left ventricular function in normal subjects at rest and during exercise. *Circulation, 62*(1), 126–132.
348. Chaitman, B. R., DeMots, H., Bristow, J. D., et al. (1975). Objective and subjective analysis of left ventricular angiograms. *Circulation, 52*(3), 420–425.
349. Cohn, P. F., Levine, J. A., Bergeron, G. A., et al. (1974). Reproducibility of the angiographic left ventricular ejection fraction in patients with coronary artery disease. *Am Heart J, 88*(6), 713–720.
350. Marshall, R. C., Berger, H. J., Reduto, L. A., et al. (1978). Variability in sequential measures of left ventricular performance assessed with radionuclide angiocardiography. *Am J Cardiol, 41*(3), 531–536.
351. Katzberg, R. W. (1988). Renal effects of contrast media. *Invest Radiol, 23*(suppl. 1), S157–S160.
352. vanSonnenberg, E., Neff, C. C., & Pfister, R. C. (1987). Life-threatening hypotensive reactions to contrast media administration: comparison of pharmacologic and fluid therapy. *Radiology, 162*(1 pt 1), 15–19.
353. Jerosch-Herold, M., & Kwong, R. Y. (2008). Magnetic resonance imaging in the assessment of ventricular remodeling and viability. *Curr Heart Fail Rep, 5*(1), 5–10.
354. Lima, J. A., Judd, R. M., Bazille, A., et al. (1995). Regional heterogeneity of human myocardial infarcts demonstrated by contrast-enhanced MRI. Potential mechanisms. *Circulation, 92*(5), 1117–1125.
355. Rochitte, C. E., Lima, J. A., Bluemke, D. A., et al. (1998). Magnitude and time course of microvascular obstruction and tissue injury after acute myocardial infarction. *Circulation, 98*(10), 1006–1014.
356. Gerber, B. L., Garot, J., Bluemke, D. A., et al. (2002). Accuracy of contrast-enhanced magnetic resonance imaging in predicting improvement of regional myocardial function in patients after acute myocardial infarction. *Circulation, 106*(9), 1083–1089.
357. Kim, R. J., Fieno, D. S., Parrish, T. B., et al. (1999). Relationship of MRI delayed contrast enhancement to irreversible injury, infarct age, and contractile function. *Circulation, 100*(19), 1992–2002.
358. Ramani, K., Judd, R. M., Holly, T. A., et al. (1998). Contrast magnetic resonance imaging in the assessment of myocardial viability in patients with stable coronary artery disease and left ventricular dysfunction. *Circulation, 98*(24), 2687–2694.
359. Kramer, C. M., Lima, J. A., Reichek, N., et al. (1993). Regional differences in function within noninfarcted myocardium during left ventricular remodeling. *Circulation, 88*(3), 1279–1288.
360. Kramer, C. M., Rogers, W. J., Theobald, T. M., et al. (1997). Dissociation between changes in intramyocardial function and left ventricular volumes in the eight weeks after first anterior myocardial infarction. *J Am Coll Cardiol, 30*(7), 1625–1632.
361. Mewton, N., Croisille, P., Revel, D., et al. (2008). Left ventricular postmyocardial infarction remodeling studied by combining MR-tagging with delayed MR contrast enhancement. *Invest Radiol, 43*(4), 219–228.
362. Longmore, D. B., Klipstein, R. H., Underwood, S. R., et al. (1985). Dimensional accuracy of magnetic resonance in studies of the heart. *Lancet, 1*(8442), 1360–1362.
363. Eichstadt, H. W., Felix, R., Langer, M., et al. (1987). Use of nuclear magnetic resonance imaging to show regression of hypertrophy with ramipril treatment. *Am J Cardiol, 59*(10), 98D–103D.
364. Higgins, C. B. (1992). Which standard has the gold? *J Am Coll Cardiol, 19*(7), 1608–1609.
365. Mogelvang, J., Stokholm, K. H., Saunamaki, K., et al. (1992). Assessment of left ventricular volumes by magnetic resonance in comparison with radionuclide angiography, contrast angiography and echocardiography. *Eur Heart J, 13*(12), 1677–1683.
366. Pattynama, P. M., Lamb, H. J., van der Velde, E. A., et al. (1993). Left ventricular measurements with cine and spin-echo MR imaging: a study of reproducibility with variance component analysis. *Radiology, 187*(1), 261–268.
367. Semelka, R. C., Tomei, E., Wagner, S., et al. (1990). Interstudy reproducibility of dimensional and functional measurements between cine magnetic resonance studies in the morphologically abnormal left ventricle. *Am Heart J, 119*(6), 1367–1373.
368. Semelka, R. C., Tomei, E., Wagner, S., et al. (1990). Normal left ventricular dimensions and function: interstudy reproducibility of measurements with cine MR imaging. *Radiology, 174*(3 pt 1), 763–768.
369. Grothues, F., Smith, G. C., Moon, J. C., et al. (2002). Comparison of interstudy reproducibility of cardiovascular magnetic resonance with two-dimensional echocardiography in normal subjects and in patients with heart failure or left ventricular hypertrophy. *Am J Cardiol, 90*(1), 29–34.
370. Bellenger, N. G., Davies, L. C., Francis, J. M., et al. (2000). Reduction in sample size for studies of remodeling in heart failure by the use of cardiovascular magnetic resonance. *J Cardiovasc Magn Reson, 2*(4), 271–278.
371. Bottini, P. B., Carr, A. A., Prisant, L. M., et al. (1995). Magnetic resonance imaging compared to echocardiography to assess left ventricular mass in the hypertensive patient. *Am J Hypertens, 8*(3), 221–228.
372. Gimbel, J. R., Johnson, D., Levine, P. A., et al. (1996). Safe performance of magnetic resonance imaging on five patients with permanent cardiac pacemakers. *Pacing Clin Electrophysiol, 19*(6), 913–919.
373. Mann, D. L., Mcmurray, J. J., Packer, M., et al. (2004). Targeted anticytokine therapy in patients with chronic heart failure: results of the randomized etanercept worldwide evaluation (RENEWAL). *Circulation, 109*(13), 1594–1602.
374. Packer, M. (2002). The ENABLE (endothelin antagonist bosentan for lowering cardiac events in heart failure) study. Paper presented at 51st Annual Scientific Sessions of the American College of Cardiology.

CHAPTER 16

Alterations in the Sympathetic and Parasympathetic Nervous Systems in Heart Failure

John S. Floras

Of the several identified markers of disease progression and premature mortality in heart failure, disturbances in the adrenergic and vagal regulation of the heart and circulation have received particular attention.[1-4] Before the prescription of contemporary therapy for heart failure due to left ventricular systolic dysfunction, long-term survival was found to relate inversely to plasma norepinephrine concentrations,[3,5] and in a cohort referred for consideration of cardiac transplantation,[3] more specifically to the appearance rate of norepinephrine in the coronary sinus.[6] Diminished tonic and reflex parasympathetic heart rate modulation is also associated with adverse prognosis.[7-12] However, in many people with asymptomatic or mild to moderate symptomatic left ventricular (LV) systolic dysfunction, plasma norepinephrine concentrations and sympathetic nerve firing rates are not elevated.[13-16] These observations raise several as yet unresolved questions: (1) what mechanisms account for the presence and variable magnitude of sympathetic activation and parasympathetic withdrawal in heart failure; (2) do these adverse associations between disturbed neurogenic circulatory control and survival reflect causal relationships; and (3) will interventions that inhibit adrenergic activity or augment vagal tone improve outcome?[17-19]

This chapter will summarize evidence for disturbed autonomic neural regulation of the heart and circulation in human heart failure because of LV systolic dysfunction, and review mechanisms responsible for this derangement and their relevance to the pathophysiology and therapy of this relentlessly progressive condition. Heart failure patients with preserved systolic function (i.e., diastolic heart failure[20]) have been less well characterized, but the available data will also be reviewed. Reference to animal models will be limited to concepts that have not been tested in humans.

ASSESSMENT OF SYMPATHETIC AND PARASYMPATHETIC NERVOUS SYSTEM ACTIVITY IN HUMANS

Several distinct yet complementary methods are available for the invasive and noninvasive assessment of specific aspects of sympathetic or parasympathetic function in conscious humans (Figure 16-1). Their application has yielded important insights into mechanisms of autonomic dysregulation in heart failure, but none has entered routine clinical practice. Each has specific advantages and limitations in the setting of heart failure that should be considered when interpreting information acquired with these techniques.

Catecholamines

Sympathoadrenal activity may be determined indirectly, by quantifying plasma or urine catecholamine concentrations, or the rate of appearance of catecholamines in plasma. When obtaining basal values, blood should be withdrawn from an indwelling catheter after 30 minutes of quiet rest to minimize any excitatory effects of anxiety or antecedent activity.

Venous plasma norepinephrine concentrations relate significantly to outcome in large heart failure trials, but their predictive value for individual patients is low. This is for several reasons. Measurements obtained at rest provide little indication of the magnitude and duration of sympathetic nerve and adrenal responses to emotional and physical stimuli, such as exercise. These responses are often well differentiated and quite specific to the heart, kidney, or adrenal gland, whereas antecubital venous sampling reflects primarily neurotransmitter release from upstream forearm skeletal muscle.[21-23] Because of high neuronal and extraneuronal uptake, only a small fraction of norepinephrine released from sympathetic vesicles acts on postjunctional adrenoceptors or spills over into plasma. Under conditions of low cardiac output, plasma concentrations of norepinephrine increase due to reductions in neuronal and extraneuronal clearance. Without determining their impact on clearance, the effect of heart failure therapies on neurotransmitter release cannot be deduced with confidence from changes in the plasma concentration of catecholamines.[23-25]

The isotopic dilution method, developed by Esler's group in Melbourne,[23] overcomes several of these limitations but adds complexity and cost to the estimation of sympathoadrenal activity in a heart failure patient. Total body spillover into plasma can be determined from the dilution of tritium-labeled norepinephrine during its steady-state infusion in tracer concentrations, as follows:

$$\text{Total body NE spillover (pmol/min)} = [^3H]\ \textit{NE infusion rate (dpm/min)}$$

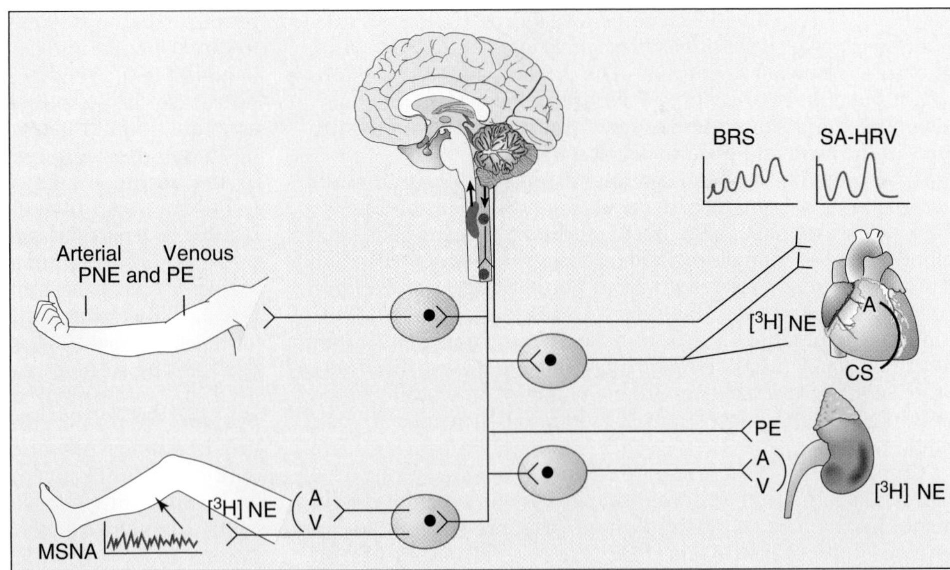

FIGURE 16–1 Assessment of sympathetic and parasympathetic function in humans. Sympathetic function: arterial (A) or venous (V) or plasma norepinephrine (PNE) and epinephrine (PE) concentrations (*upper left*); sympathetic nerve traffic to muscle (MSNA) or skin (*lower left*); total body norepinephrine ($[^3H]$ NE) spillover or regional norepinephrine spillover across the heart (*A*, aorta or arterial; *CS*, coronary sinus) (*upper right*), kidney (*lower right*) or leg (*lower left*); spectral analysis of heart rate variability (SA-HRV) (*upper right*). Parasympathetic function (*upper right*): bradycardic response to phenylephrine (*BRS*, baroreflex sensitivity); spectral analysis of heart rate variability (SA-HRV). (From Floras JS. Clinical aspects of sympathetic activation and parasympathetic withdrawal in heart failure. *J Am Coll Cardiol* 1993;22:72A-84A, with permission from the American College of Cardiology Foundation.)

plasma NE specific activity (dpm / pmol)

where NE = norepinephrine
$[^3H]$ NE = tritium - labeled NE, and
dpm = disintegrations per minute of tritium - labeled norepinephrine

If venous effluent from the heart, kidney, brain, or another vascular bed is collected simultaneously with an arterial sample, the difference in tritium-labeled norepinephrine between the vein and artery can be used to calculate its local extraction (Extr) by neuronal and extraneuronal transport mechanisms. Organ-specific norepinephrine spillover (NES) can then be determined by the equation:

$$NES = [(NE_v - NE_a) + (NE_a \times Extr)] \times PF$$

where NE_a and NE_v represent arterial and venous concentrations of unlabeled norepinephrine and PF plasma flow.

Quantification of norepinephrine metabolites provides additional insight into neuronal and extraneuronal transport. For example, spillover of tritium-labeled dihydroxyphenylglycol (DHPG), the intraneuronal metabolite, provides an index of neuronal norepinephrine reuptake and storage.[26,27] Being complex, the organ-specific isotopic dilution method has been applied to human heart failure research in only a few laboratories. Unfortunately, the catheter required for assessment of venous plasma flow rate and blood sampling is no longer available commercially.

Microneurography

Multifiber or single fiber microneurography permits direct recording from postganglionic sympathetic nerves supplying muscular or cutaneous vascular beds.[28,29] This method provides unique real-time insight into the dynamic nature of sympathetic activity and its reflex control. The peroneal and tibial nerves are the preferred sites for electrode insertion.

Muscle and skin sympathetic nerves exhibit different discharge characteristics under basal conditions and in response to a variety of physical and emotional stimuli. Sympathetic discharge directed at resistance beds in skeletal muscle (MSNA) is entrained by input from arterial and cardiopulmonary mechanoreceptors and therefore exhibits distinctive pulse-synchronicity, with bursts appearing 1.1 to 1.3 seconds after the preceding R wave of the electrocardiogram.[18,28] In healthy subjects, MSNA is activated by reductions in diastolic[30] or cardiac filling pressure,[31] exercise,[32] hypoxia,[33] hypercapnia,[33] and arousal from sleep,[34] and is inhibited by lung inflation.[17,35] Skin sympathetic nerves (SSNA) fire in response to noise, touch, or cold independently of the cardiac cycle. MSNA therefore provides greater insight than SSNA into mechanisms responsible for sympathetic activation in the setting of heart failure.

In patients with heart failure due to systolic dysfunction, MSNA is more reproducible from one week to the next than is plasma norepinephrine concentration,[36] but microneurography has its own limitations. Training and experience are required to ensure the consistent acquisition of high-quality, stable MSNA recordings devoid of skin or motor unit discharge. Burst amplitude is critically dependent upon electrode placement. The presence, in subjects with normal ventricular function, of significant positive correlations between individual values for MSNA and both renal and cardiac norepinephrine spillover,[37,38] and proportionately similar increases in both MSNA and cardiac norepinephrine spillover (CNES) in response to isometric exercise[38] are observations consistent with the concept that a common mechanism influences the strength of resting sympathetic discharge to the heart, kidney, and skeletal muscle. However, because the sympathetic nervous system is capable of targeted outflow, the possibility that in heart failure muscle sympathetic burst firing characteristics might differ from those of sympathetic nerves directed at other hemodynamically important vascular beds must be considered.

Baroreflex–Heart Rate Sequences

The arterial baroreflex regulation of heart rate by the parasympathetic and sympathetic nervous systems can be assessed in humans in several ways.[39] Because cardiac cycle length responds much more rapidly to changes in acetylcholine than to norepinephrine release, brisk sinus node responses to acute perturbations in blood pressure are mediated primarily by reflex vagal activation or withdrawal. Thus the strength, or gain, of reflex vagal heart rate regulation can be determined by quantifying the bradycardic response to a bolus of a vasoconstrictor drug such as phenylephrine or the tachycardic response to nitroprusside or nitroglycerin-induced hypotension. Responses to longer ("steady-state") infusions of these vasoactive agents are less specific because they represent the net of competing vagal and sympathetic influences.

The use of such drugs for this purpose has several limitations. Nitrate donors have direct effects on sinoatrial

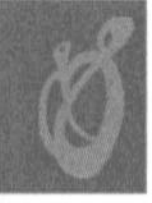

discharge.[40] By causing sustained vasoconstriction or dilation, these drugs will themselves cause mechanical distortion of baroreceptor nerve endings. The impact of these infusions is not specific to the arterial baroreceptor reflex; they may also alter the discharge frequency of mechanoreceptors situated in the atria and pulmonary vasculature.[41]

To avoid such drugs, heart rate responses to carotid sinus baroreceptor stimulation by neck suction or unloading by neck pressure have also been studied,[42] recognizing that blood pressure changes evoked by these maneuvers will elicit counterregulatory responses from aortic arch baroreceptors. Algorithms have been developed to track spontaneous fluctuations in blood pressure and heart rate from continuous noninvasive or invasive recordings and identify within these brief sequences with concordant changes in systolic blood pressure and the subsequent R-R intervals (inverse of heart rate).[39]

Common to these methods is the construction of a regression equation relating changes in pulse interval (in msec) to changes in systolic blood pressure (in mm Hg) of immediately preceding cardiac cycles. The slope of this line estimates the gain of the arterial baroreflex control of heart rate. Values obtained using the spontaneous sequence method are similar to those derived when blood pressure is altered by bolus administration of vasoactive drugs.[43,44] Importantly, the available methods do not distinguish between impairments in baroreflex sensitivity caused by altered mechanical transduction of blood pressure due to increased vascular stiffness, changes in the neural transduction of baroreceptor distortion, or altered central processing of afferent input.[45]

Baroreflex–Sympathetic Nerve Sequences

Although not specific to the arterial baroreflex, microneurographic recordings during graded infusions of pressor or vasodilator drugs have been used to evaluate the reflex regulation of central sympathetic outflow.[46] Blood pressure changes induced by such infusions are relatively slow in onset; studies in anaesthetized rabbits[47] and conscious humans[48] indicate that the arterial baroreceptors transduce high-frequency oscillations more effectively and at higher gain than low-frequency oscillations.[49]

Heart Rate Variability

Tonic vagal modulation of heart rate may also be estimated by determining its beat-to-beat variation. Time domain variables used for this purpose include the standard deviation of all normal (i.e., excluding ectopic beats) pulse intervals within a defined period,[50] the standard deviation of beat-by-beat pulse interval variations, the arithmetic mean of standard deviations derived from 5-minute intervals over a 24-hour recording period (to reflect short-term variability of heart rate), the number of differences of successive RR intervals greater than 50 msec divided by the total number of intervals, and variations on these formulas.[51]

Spectral analysis has attracted considerable interest as a noninvasive frequency domain method of estimating nonneural and neural parasympathetic and sympathetic contributions to short- and long-term oscillations in heart rate.[51-54] The North American Society of Pacing and Electrophysiology and the European Society of Cardiology have proposed a standardized approach to the acquisition and interpretation of these power spectra.[51] The algorithms most commonly employed to develop power spectra are fast Fourier transformation, autoregressive analysis, and coarse-graining spectral analysis. The latter method was developed to address the observation that harmonic contributions to heart rate variability are superimposed on a broadband nonharmonic "noise," which is most prominent from 0.00003 to 0.1 Hz (i.e., across the very low-frequency range and extending into the low-frequency spectral band [0.05–0.15 Hz])[55] and is fractal in nature.[56] Nonharmonic power can be quantified by plotting the log of spectral power as a function of the log of frequency (a $1/f_\beta$ plot).[55,57] Once the nonharmonic component is extracted, more precise estimates of the residual harmonic contributions to low- and high-frequency (0.15 to 0.50 Hz) power can be obtained.[55,57] This feature is a particular advantage in the study of heart failure patients, in whom, compared with healthy subjects, there is a greater concentration of heart rate spectral power with very low and low-frequency bands.[52,58-63]

Because vagal blockade abolishes high-frequency power, oscillations in heart rate within this band have been attributed to parasympathetic activity, with respiration as its primary rhythmic stimulus. In experimental preparations, low-frequency power increased during baroreceptor deactivation with nitroglycerin, and was prevented by prior bilateral stellectomy.[53,64] Therefore, heart rate fluctuations within these frequencies were at first considered useful representations of sympathetic neural modulation. Indeed, maneuvers known to increase central sympathetic outflow, such as standing,[54] tilt,[53,57] exercise,[65] and lower body negative pressure[57] were shown to increase low-frequency spectral power, whereas decreases were observed during sleep,[66] and after β-blockade[54] or central sympatholysis with clonidine.[66] However, below 0.15 Hz, the power spectrum is also influenced by parasympathetic oscillatory input.[53,54,65-69] To address this complexity, the ratio between low- and high-frequency power has been proposed as an estimate of the balance between these two simultaneously active neural influences.[53] Although this concept of "sympathovagal balance" has been adopted by many authors,[51] it has been rejected by others.[60,61]

Frequency domain analysis should be appreciated primarily for the insight it allows into mechanisms responsible for oscillations in regulatory systems, and for its prognostic value in populations with cardiovascular disease. At best, it provides an estimate of the extent to which parasympathetic and cardiac sympathetic nerves are capable of modulating heart rate variability within specific frequency bands. Unfortunately, because some authors do not make the important distinction between modulation of neural discharge and its intensity, and/or between sympathetic outflow directed at the heart and regional vascular beds, considerable confusion as to the research and clinical utility of this method persists, particularly within the heart failure literature.[52,58,60-62,70]

Cross-Spectral Analysis

Algorithms used to derive power spectra for heart rate can also be applied to blood pressure and respiratory signals. The mean voltage neurogram also displays fluctuations in muscle sympathetic nerve discharge, responsive to changes in blood pressure, heart rate, and respiration. The presence, in normal subjects, of synchronous and concordant changes in low- and high-frequency oscillations in both heart rate and MSNA variability elicited by interventions that raise and lower sympathetic discharge suggest that sympathetic and parasympathetic outflow can be modulated by a shared brainstem mechanism.[71]

Cross-spectral analysis between two variables of interest can be performed to determine the magnitude or gain (ratio of output/input power) of the transfer function, the coherence, and the phase delay between these signals.[72] The gain of the transfer function between systolic blood pressure (input) and pulse interval (output) oscillations within the low- or high-frequency regions (α-coefficient) has achieved widespread acceptance, for research purposes, as a noninvasive spectral index of the baroreceptor reflex control of heart rate,[39] but its agreement with the vasoactive drug method is weak.[73]

Similarly, the gain of the transfer function between blood pressure (input) and MSNA (output) can be calculated as an estimate of arterial baroreflex regulation of efferent sympathetic nerve traffic.[72]

SYMPATHETIC ACTIVATION AND PARASYMPATHETIC WITHDRAWAL IN HUMAN HEART FAILURE (see also Chapters 13, 45, and 46)

Heart Failure with Impaired Systolic Function

Sympathetic Activation

On average, plasma norepinephrine concentrations, sampled during supine rest, are elevated in patients with asymptomatic LV dysfunction and increase further with the progression to overt congestive heart failure.[1,3] Nonetheless, in a substantial proportion of patients with both symptomatic and asymptomatic LV systolic dysfunction, plasma norepinephrine concentrations are similar to those of age-matched control subjects.[13,16]

In health, approximately 25% of total body norepinephrine spillover arises from the kidney and about 2% from the heart.[23] Cardiac norepinephrine spillover is elevated in mild heart failure, before any obvious increase in total body norepinephrine spillover, renal adrenergic drive, or MSNA[15] (Figures 16-2 and 16-3). In patients with more advanced LV dysfunction, studied before the advent of contemporary heart failure therapy, norepinephrine clearance was a third lower, and total body norepinephrine spillover doubled, when compared with control subjects. Approximately 60% of the latter increase resulted from a twofold to threefold rise in renal norepinephrine spillover, and a fivefold to twentyfold elevation in cardiac norepinephrine spillover.[23,74] In the paced-ovine model of heart failure, such preferential activation of cardiac sympathetic nerve traffic results from one third lower resting cardiac than renal burst incidence in healthy sheep, affording much greater cardiac sympathoexcitatory capacity once heart failure develops.[75] Indeed, in human heart failure, mental stress and cycling exercise elicit further increases in cardiac neurotransmitter release, indicating that considerable adrenergic reserve remains.[76]

In advanced heart failure, plasma epinephrine concentrations also rise, indicating heightened adrenal sympathetic nerve activity and medullary catecholamine release.[3] Under these circumstances, epinephrine may be transported into sympathetic nerve terminals and incorporated, along with norepinephrine, into vesicles.[77] Esler et al[77] have documented cardiac epinephrine spillover, averaging 2 ng/min or 2% of the corresponding norepinephrine spillover, in untreated congestive heart failure but not healthy subjects. Neuronal release from the gut, liver, lungs, and kidneys, comprising approximately 25% of the total epinephrine plasma appearance rate, was also detected. The implication of these observations, as discussed later, is that epinephrine, a potent β_2-adrenergic receptor agonist, could come to exert both a neurotransmitter and a humoral role in heart failure.[78]

To determine whether this increased norepinephrine spillover results from greater central sympathetic outflow, or from alterations in its synthesis, release, or reuptake, Leimbach et al recorded MSNA in subjects with moderate to severe heart failure. The mean sympathetic nerve firing rate correlated with plasma norepinephrine concentrations and was significantly elevated as compared with both age-matched and younger subjects with normal ventricular function.[79] The latter observation was subsequently replicated in studies involving younger subjects with dilated cardiomyopathy.[80] Single fiber recordings in heart failure patients have demonstrated

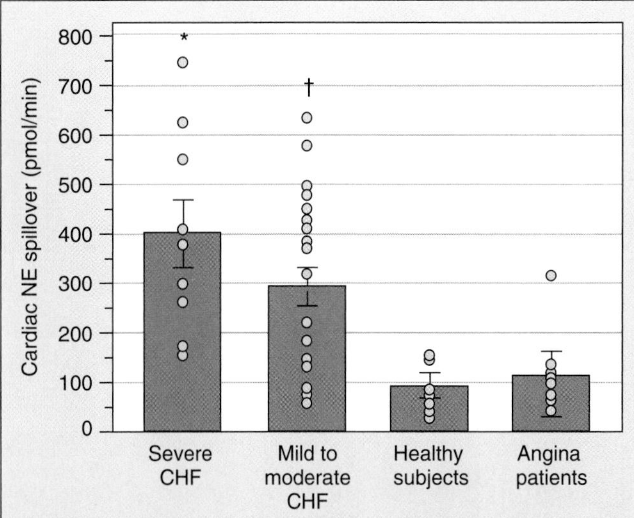

FIGURE 16–2 Individual and mean ± SEM values for cardiac NE spillover in patients with mild to moderate and severe CHF, in healthy subjects, and in patients with stable angina pectoris.
*Statistically significant difference (P <.05) between severe chronic heart failure (CHF) and both control groups. †Statistically significant difference (P <.05) between mild to moderate CHF and both healthy subjects and angina patients. (From Rundqvist B, Elam M, Bergmann-Sverrisdottir Y, et al. Increased cardiac adrenergic drive precedes generalized sympathetic activation in human heart failure. *Circulation* 1997;95:169-175.)

that these increases result not only from a higher nerve firing probability, but also multiple within-burst discharges, and the recruitment of previously silent fibers.[81] By contrast, skin sympathetic activity is not increased in patients with heart failure.[82] This dissociation indicates that systems such as the high- and low-pressure baroreceptor reflexes, which tightly regulate muscle but not skin neural discharge, elevate the set point for central sympathetic outflow in heart failure.

In subjects with mild depression of LV ejection fraction (down to 40%), group mean values for MSNA burst incidence are intermediate between those of patients with more severe heart failure and healthy control subjects.[46] There is little or no correlation with MSNA burst incidence once ejection fraction falls below 35%. Importantly, and in many patients with profound LV systolic dysfunction, muscle sympathetic nerve burst frequency or heart rate corrected burst incidence remains within the range observed in age-matched control subjects.[14,15,83-85] Notarius et al[14] recorded MSNA at rest, and during isometric and isotonic handgrip, of various intensities in age-matched subjects with normal and impaired LV systolic function (mean ejection fraction 19%). Patients with an MSNA $\dot{V}O_2$ peak less than 56% of that predicted by their age, sex, and weight and height had consistently higher MSNA at rest and during exercise than age-matched healthy subjects. In contrast, MSNA in patients whose $\dot{V}O_2$ peak was greater than 56% of their predicted value was remarkably similar to that of age-matched control subjects, despite their mean LV ejection fraction of 18% (Figure 16-4). These findings, coupled with the identification in patients with mild to moderate heart failure, by Rundqvist et al, of a selective increase in cardiac norepinephrine spillover, without any corresponding increase in mean values for muscle sympathetic nerve activity or total body norepinephrine spillover,[15] argue against generalized sympathetic activation as a cardinal characteristic of heart failure, or a consistent consequence of ventricular systolic dysfunction.

In the frequency domain, heart failure and age-matched control subjects display similar total MSNA power, harmonic power, nonharmonic power between 0 and 0.5 Hz and spectral density within the very low- (0 to 0.05 Hz) and high- (0.15 to 0.5 Hz) frequency bands.[72] However, low-frequency oscillations in the mean voltage neurogram were diminished

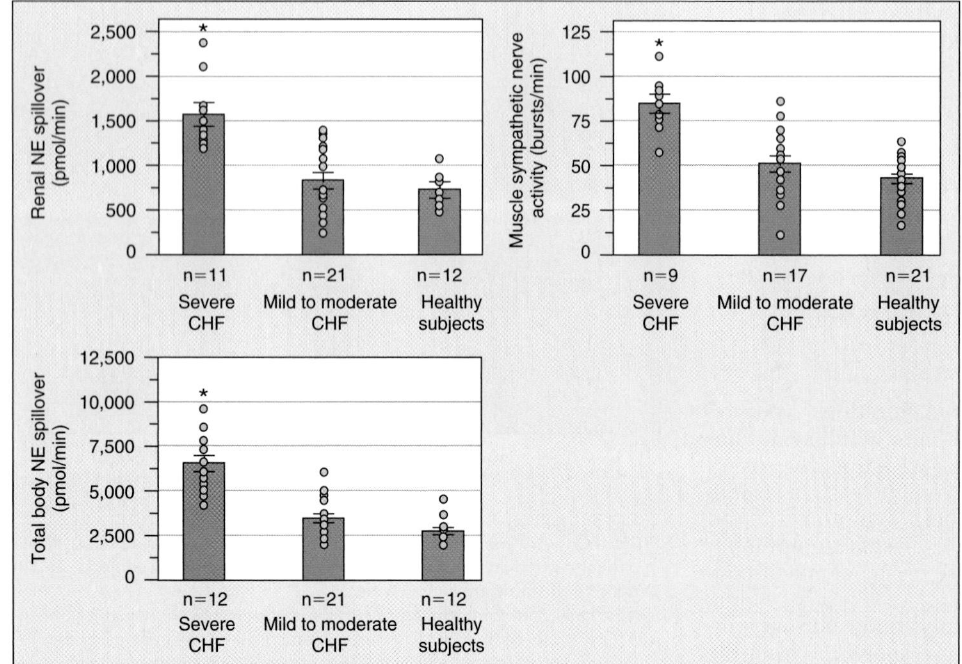

FIGURE 16–3 Individual and mean ± SEM values for renal (*top*) and total body (*middle*) NE spillover and muscle sympathetic nerve activity (*bottom*) in the groups defined in the legend to Figure 16-2. *Statistically significant difference (*P* <.05) between severe chronic heart failure (CHF) and both healthy subjects and mild to moderate CHF. (From Rundqvist B, Elam M, Bergmann-Sverrisdottir Y, et al. Increased cardiac adrenergic drive precedes generalized sympathetic activation in human heart failure. *Circulation* 1997;95:169-175.)

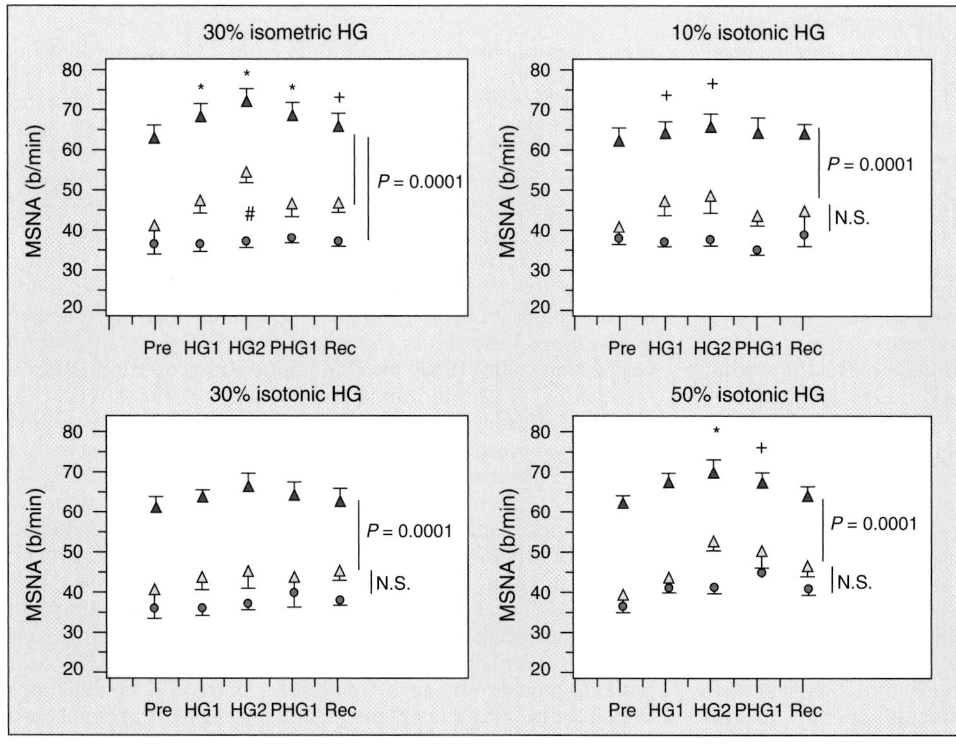

FIGURE 16–4 Muscle sympathetic nerve activity (MSNA) response to handgrip (HG) exercise for peak oxygen uptake ($\dot{V}O_2$ peak) less than 56% predicted (▲, *n* = 8), VO_2 peak greater than 56% predicted (Δ, *n* = 6) and normal subjects (•, *n* = 10). NS, not significant. Stated *P* values refer to the significance level of the main effect of group; **P* <.05 vs. pre-HG in both heart failure groups; ^+P <.05 vs. pre-HG in VO_2 peak >56% predicted only; #*P* <.05 vs. VO_2 peak >56% predicted compared with normal subjects. (From Notarius CF, Atchison DJ, Floras JS. Impact of heart failure and exercise capacity on sympathetic response to handgrip exercise. *Am J Physiol Heart Circ Physiol* 2001;280:H969-H976.)

significantly or absent, despite near-maximal sympathetic burst incidence, suggesting progressive loss of central or reflex modulation of efferent sympathetic traffic with advancing heart failure.[72,86]

Parasympathetic Alterations

A blunted heart rate response to a rise in blood pressure was first described in human heart failure by Eckberg et al.[87] Bradycardic responses to carotid sinus baroreceptor stimulation by neck suction also are attenuated.[42] Subsequently, other investigators reported that slopes for baroreflex sensitivity (expressed either as ms/mm Hg or as beats per minute/mm Hg) generated from infusions of phenylephrine and sodium nitroprusside to raise and lower systolic blood pressure, and thereby elicit reflexively increases and decreases in pulse interval, respectively, were shallower than in healthy controls, and diminished in proportion to the degree of LV systolic dysfunction,[46] New York Heart Association (NYHA) functional symptoms, the severity of mitral regurgitation, resting heart rate, and blood urea nitrogen.[46,88,89] Reflex and tonic vagal heart rate modulation, as assessed in the time domain (SDNN), correlate strongly.[89] Reductions in vagal modulation of heart rate appear to relate reciprocally to concurrent increases in sympathetic activity.[90]

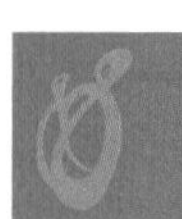

Parasympathetic and Sympathetic Contributions to Heart Rate Variability

Loss of vagal heart rate modulation can be detected in both the time and the frequency domain at the earliest stage of ischemic or dilated cardiomyopathy.[91,92-94] Soon after the onset of doxyrubicin-induced cardiomyopathy, high-frequency spectral power decreases, whereas low-frequency spectral power increases, and there is a corresponding rise in plasma norepinephrine concentrations.[95]

However, this harmonic spectral index of cardiac adrenergic modulation is in general not increased, and is often attenuated in subjects with LV systolic dysfunction. Several groups have often demonstrated an inverse, rather than a direct relationship between low-frequency spectral power and discharge frequency in muscle sympathetic nerves or cardiac norepinephrine spillover.[70,96] Moreover, and as failure advances, heart rate often becomes invariant, and consequently refractory to analysis by most frequency domain methods.[58,96,97] Guazzi et al[98] observed a "predominance" of the low-frequency component of the heart rate power spectrum in NYHA class II patients, but not in class III or IV heart failure, which they attributed to functional sympathetic denervation in the latter groups.[58,96] It should be emphasized that power spectra reflect the fidelity with which postjunctional sinoatrial receptors respond to oscillations in nerve discharge, rather than the intensity of the sympathetic stimulus.[58,99-101] Whereas values for cardiac noradrenaline spillover are not affected by postsynaptic mechanisms, saturation or downregulation of cardiac postjunctional β-adrenoceptors and impairment of postsynaptic β-adrenoreceptor signal transduction will decrease sinoatrial responsiveness to neurally released norepinephrine.[99]

Nonharmonic contributions to the heart rate power spectrum are not attenuated in heart failure, but the complexity of the heart rate signal is less than in subjects with normal ventricular function, seemingly due to less in vagal modulation.[97]

Heart Failure with Preserved Systolic Function (see Chapters 14 and 48)

Information as to sympathetic activation in heart failure with preserved ventricular systolic function is sparse. Benedict et al did not detect any increase in plasma norepinephrine concentrations of patients enrolled in the Studies of Left Ventricular Dysfunction (SOLVD) registry who had pulmonary congestion but a LV ejection fraction greater than 45%.[102] Although in a single center study of subjects 60 years or older, similar increases in mean values for plasma norepinephrine concentrations were found in cohorts with impaired and preserved systolic function[103] in general, the sympathetic nervous system would not appear to be as activated as in heart failure patients with systolic dysfunction,[104] and heart rate variability not as depressed.[105] MSNA has yet to be characterized in this specific population, but Grassi et al[106] have observed significantly higher MSNA burst incidence (but not plasma norepinephrine concentrations) in untreated men with hypertension-related LV diastolic dysfunction, as compared with hypertensive subjects with normal diastolic function or normotensive control subjects. Sudden increases in sympathoadrenal activity may be responsible for episodes of acute pulmonary edema in these individuals.[107]

CLINICAL CONSEQUENCES

Cardiac

In humans, the first manifestation of sympathetic activation is a selective increase in cardiac norepinephrine spillover.[15] Cardiac sympathetic activation and vagal withdrawal constitute adaptive mechanisms, engaged to maintain peripheral tissue perfusion in the face of compromised cardiac performance. However, once congestion becomes manifest, the heart endures the greatest proportional increase in regional norepinephrine spillover.[74] Thus the failing heart is the organ exposed to the greatest magnitude and duration of sympathetic activation.

The direct myocardial consequences of this intense cardiac adrenergic drive include myocyte necrosis and apoptosis,[108] fibrosis,[109] decreased β-adrenergic receptor number, diminished β_1-adrenoceptor responsiveness to catecholamines, and altered β-adrenergic receptor signal transduction,[110-113] altered calcium regulation by the sarcoplasmic reticulum,[114] induction of proinflammatory cytokine expression,[115] oxidative stress,[116] destruction of sympathetic nerve terminals,[117] and depletion of myocardial norepinephrine content.[26] Nonuniform topography of myocardial norepinephrine depletion and sympathetic denervation should disturb the temporal coordination of right and left ventricular contraction and relaxation and alter the dispersion of refractoriness, promoting arrhythmogenesis. In advanced heart failure, cardiac norepinephrine becomes a potent marker of premature death,[6] and if cardiac norepinephrine stores are high, sudden death.[26]

The impact in heart failure of impaired vagal tone on heart rate modulation, regulation of LV performance, and inflammatory pathways has been reviewed recently in detail.[118]

Peripheral

Excessive sympathetic drive to arteries, veins, and the kidney exacerbates the hemodynamic derangements of heart failure by increasing both preload and afterload. Stimulation of renal sympathetic nerves activates the renin-angiotensin-aldosterone axis, promotes tubular absorption of sodium and water, decreases glomerular filtration, increases renal vascular resistance, and blunts the renal responsiveness to atrial natriuretic peptide.[119,120] In young subjects with dilated cardiomyopathy, muscle sympathetic burst frequency correlates directly with resistance to blood flow in the calf, the vascular bed distal to the recording electrode.[80] This observation implicates sympathetically mediated vasoconstriction as an important mechanism for increased afterload in human heart failure. Increased sympathetic outflow may also raise ventricular afterload by decreasing conduit artery compliance.

Exercise

A reduction in exercise capacity, whether due to dyspnea or fatigue, is a common heart failure symptom.[121] Several β_2-adrenoceptor polymorphisms associated with impaired exercise performance have been identified.[122] A central factor limiting exercise capacity is chronotropic incompetence due to decreased cardiac β-adrenergic receptor density or responsiveness to endogenous catecholamines,[110] whereas augmented neurogenic vasoconstriction represents one of several peripheral limitations.[123,124] In heart failure patients (but not in healthy age-matched control subjects) maximal oxygen uptake during exercise correlates inversely to resting MSNA[83] (Figure 16-5). Cardiac norepinephrine spillover, on the other hand, bears little relation to peak $\dot{V}O_2$ in either group.[125] Reductions in blood flow below levels required to meet local metabolic demands during exercise may cause further reflexive increases in central sympathetic outflow by stimulating metaboreceptor afferents in skeletal muscle.[14]

Mortality

Before the widespread use of angiotensin-converting enzyme inhibitors and β-adrenoceptor antagonists, the life expectancy of most heart failure patients with venous plasma

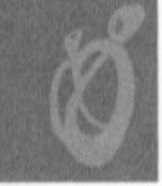

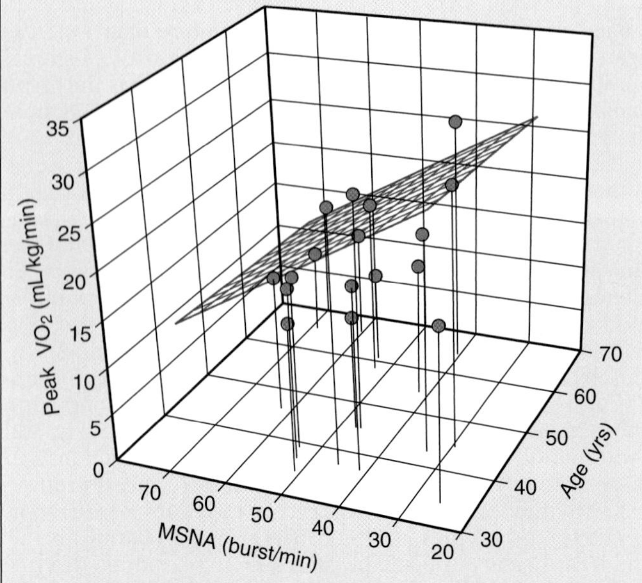

FIGURE 16–5 Relationship between peak oxygen uptake ($\dot{V}O_2$ peak) and muscle sympathetic nerve activity (MSNA) burst frequency and age in patients with heart failure. Three-dimensional graph shows individual data points and regression plane. Regression equation: $\dot{V}O_2$ peak = 40.5 − (0.347 × MSNA) − (0.0570) × age); slope of the MSNA variable is significantly different from zero (P <.02). By contrast there was no relationship between MSNA and $\dot{V}O_2$ peak in healthy controls, in whom MSNA increased significantly with age (P <.04) (not shown). (From Notarius CF, Ando SI, Rongen GA, et al. Resting muscle sympathetic nerve activity and peak oxygen uptake in heart failure and normal subjects.) *Eur Heart J* 2001;23:800-805.

norepinephrine concentrations greater than 800 pg/mL was less than 1 year.[3,5] Increased plasma norepinephrine concentrations also predict all-cause and cardiovascular mortality of asymptomatic patients with LV systolic dysfunction.[126] An inverse relationship between plasma norepinephrine concentrations and survival can still be detected in symptomatic patients receiving contemporary therapy, including β-blockade.[127] In a Brazilian study involving 122 heart failure patients, the level of MSNA was a significant independent predictor of mortality.[128]

A marked increased cardiac norepinephrine spillover rate, proportionally greater than corresponding increases in total body norepinephrine spillover, is a characteristic in the general population of survivors of sudden spontaneous ventricular arrhythmias,[129] and a particularly potent marker of 1-year mortality in advanced heart failure[6] (Figure 16-6). Estimating cardiac norepinephrine stores provides insight into the probable mode of death. In a group of 116 patients with a mean LV ejection fraction of 19%, followed on average for 18 months, those with greater than median estimated cardiac norepinephrine stores plus increased norepinephrine spillover had a twofold to threefold higher risk of sudden death, whereas patients with depleted myocardial norepinephrine stores and high cardiac norepinephrine spillover (reflecting chronically increased neurotransmitter turnover and reduced reuptake and storage) had a twofold to fourfold higher risk of death from progressive pump failure.[26,130] Noninvasive assessment of cardiac norepinephrine uptake using metaiodobenzylguanidine (MIBG) imaging has also been shown to identify heart failure patients at increased risk of death.[131,132]

Diminished baroreflex sensitivity and loss of heart rate variability are also associated with accelerated mortality from progressive myocardial failure and arrhythmias.[7-9,11,12,133] An attenuated reflex heart rate response to phenylephrine has similar prognostic implications in patients treated or not treated with β-adrenoceptor antagonists.[89] Loss of complexity in the heart rate signal, as estimated by nonharmonic

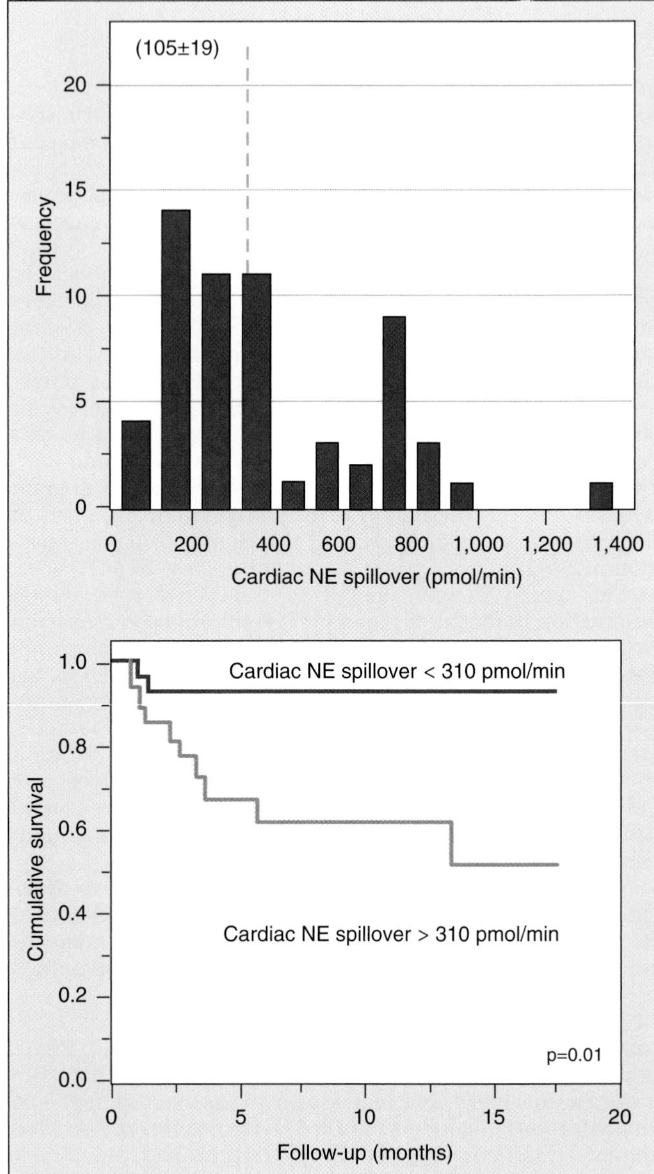

FIGURE 16–6 *Top,* Histogram depicting the frequency distribution of cardiac norepinephrine (NE) spillover rates for patients with heart failure. Dashed line indicates group median (310 pmol/min). Data above indicates mean cardiac norepinephrine spillover rate for healthy subjects, with 95% confidence limits. Cardiac norepinephrine spillover was significantly higher in patients with heart failure (402 ± 37 vs. 105 ± 19 pmol/min; P <.01). *Bottom,* Survival curves for patients dichotomized by median cardiac norepinephrine spillover rate, with reduced survival (P = .01) in patients with the highest values. (Data from Kaye DM, Lefkovitz J, Jennings GL, et al. Adverse consequences of high sympathetic nervous system activity in the failing human heart. *J Am Coll Cardiol* 1995;26:1257-1263, with permission from the American College of Cardiology Foundation.)

power-law regression parameters,[133] and low-frequency harmonic power may be the most sensitive predictors of sudden death.[11]

MECHANISMS

Alterations in the neurogenic control of the circulation with the onset and progression of heart failure can arise from one or more elements responsible for the regulation of autonomic tone, such as inhibitory and excitatory input to brainstem vasomotor neurons, cortical modulation of central nervous system integration and catecholamine turnover, and efferent

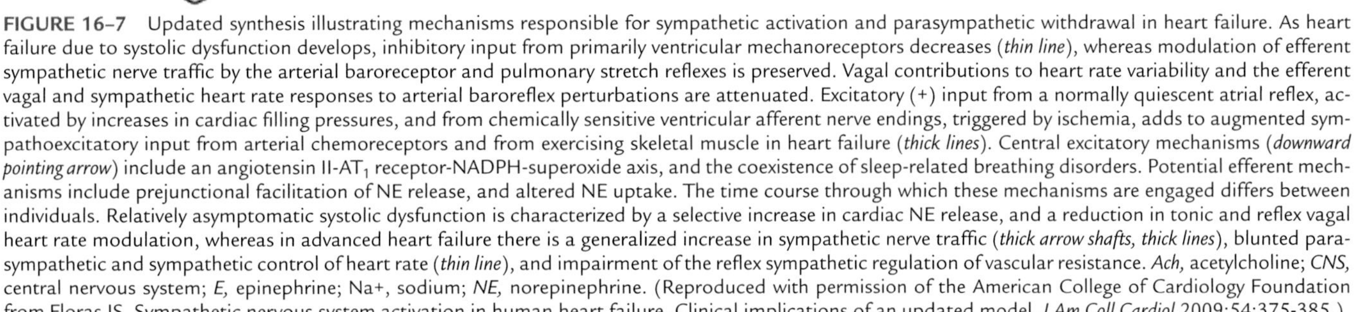

FIGURE 16–7 Updated synthesis illustrating mechanisms responsible for sympathetic activation and parasympathetic withdrawal in heart failure. As heart failure due to systolic dysfunction develops, inhibitory input from primarily ventricular mechanoreceptors decreases (*thin line*), whereas modulation of efferent sympathetic nerve traffic by the arterial baroreceptor and pulmonary stretch reflexes is preserved. Vagal contributions to heart rate variability and the efferent vagal and sympathetic heart rate responses to arterial baroreflex perturbations are attenuated. Excitatory (+) input from a normally quiescent atrial reflex, activated by increases in cardiac filling pressures, and from chemically sensitive ventricular afferent nerve endings, triggered by ischemia, adds to augmented sympathoexcitatory input from arterial chemoreceptors and from exercising skeletal muscle in heart failure (*thick lines*). Central excitatory mechanisms (*downward pointing arrow*) include an angiotensin II-AT_1 receptor-NADPH-superoxide axis, and the coexistence of sleep-related breathing disorders. Potential efferent mechanisms include prejunctional facilitation of NE release, and altered NE uptake. The time course through which these mechanisms are engaged differs between individuals. Relatively asymptomatic systolic dysfunction is characterized by a selective increase in cardiac NE release, and a reduction in tonic and reflex vagal heart rate modulation, whereas in advanced heart failure there is a generalized increase in sympathetic nerve traffic (*thick arrow shafts, thick lines*), blunted parasympathetic and sympathetic control of heart rate (*thin line*), and impairment of the reflex sympathetic regulation of vascular resistance. *Ach,* acetylcholine; *CNS,* central nervous system; *E,* epinephrine; Na+, sodium; *NE,* norepinephrine. (Reproduced with permission of the American College of Cardiology Foundation from Floras JS. Sympathetic nervous system activation in human heart failure. Clinical implications of an updated model. *J Am Coll Cardiol* 2009;54:375-385.)

mechanisms determining the release rates of and receptor responsiveness to neurotransmitters (Figure 16-7).

Afferent Influences

In healthy subjects, inputs from carotid sinus and aortic arch "arterial high pressure" and the cardiopulmonary "low pressure" mechanoreceptors provide the principal peripheral inhibitory influences on sympathetic outflow, with discharge from arterial chemoreceptors and muscle "metaboreceptors" providing excitatory information. The efferent vagal component of the baroreceptor heart rate reflex is also subject to arterial baroreceptor afferent input. At rest, healthy individuals display low sympathetic discharge and high heart rate variability. Reflex vagal and sympathoneural responses to acute perturbations in blood pressure are brisk.

Arterial Baroreceptor Reflexes

Arterial baroreceptor nerve discharge is activated by the pressure wave of systole, and diminishes or falls silent during diastole. Systolic stimulation of baroreceptor discharge will increase parasympathetic and decrease efferent sympathetic outflow reflexively. Baroreceptor silence during diastole eliminates the tonic inhibition of efferent sympathetic outflow, resulting, for example, in a burst of MSNA.[30]

Blunted arterial baroreflex control of heart rate is a characteristic feature of human heart failure.[87] Because baroreceptor afferent nerve discharge, which governs both sympathetic and vagal efferent limbs of this reflex arc, is less responsive to changes in local distending pressure in experimental models of ventricular systolic dysfunction, the prevailing view has been that arterial baroreflex regulation of vagal and sympathetic outflow in human heart failure are impaired equally.[17,134-137] However, assessment of the baroreceptor-heart rate reflex in humans relies upon the indirect estimation of sinoatrial responsiveness to two distinct and differentially regulated autonomic inputs. In heart failure, impaired efferent vagal ganglionic neurotransmission diminishes parasympathetic responsiveness to baroreceptor stimulation,[138] yet myocardial responsiveness to acetylcholine is intact in humans[139] and in experimental heart failure augmented.[140] By contrast, cardiac-specific sympathetic neural modulation is attenuated by downregulation or desensitization of β-adrenoceptors,[141] rendering the sinoatrial node less responsive to reflexively elicited changes in neurally released norepinephrine. Noncardiac sympathetic efferent responses to arterial baroreflex perturbation upstream of the effector target can be measured directly and specifically by microneurography. Heart failure, by these several mechanisms, reduces the variability and complexity of heart rate but the variability of blood pressure

TABLE 16-1 Evidence for Preserved Arterial Baroreflex Modulation of Sympathetic Activity in Human Heart Failure

Concept	Observation
MSNA pulse-synchronicity lost after sinoaortic baroreceptor denervation[18]	Pulse-synchronicity preserved, even in end-stage HF[90]
Pause with decay in DBP after pre-mature beat increases reflexively MSNA burst amplitude, duration, and area; rise in DBP after post-extrasystolic beat inhibits MSNA[18]	Extra-systolic augmentation of MSNA amplitude, duration, and area and post-extrasystolic suppression replicated in HF; duration or suppression proportional to magnitude of diastolic overshoot[147]
MSNA bursts track previous DBP with 1.2-1.3 sec lag[30]	Synchronization of sympathetic neural alternans with pulsus alternans[49]
Frequency domain estimate of arterial BR gain derived by cross-spectral analysis with BP oscillations as stimulus and MSNA oscillations as response	Transfer function gain in HF and healthy subjects similar across all frequency bands; calculated gain highest in high-frequency range[72]
Arterial BR unloading with SNP elicits reflex increase in TNES	Similar reflex increase in TNES in HF and healthy subjects[25]
LV pacing in HF increases DBP	Acute inverse DBP-MSNA relationship immediately upon conversion from to RV to LV pacing[324]
Muller maneuver increases acutely intrathoracic aortic and LV trans-mural pressure	MSNA inhibited similarly in HF and control subjects[195]

BP, Blood pressure; *BR,* baroreceptor reflex; *DBP,* diastolic blood pressure; *HF,* heart failure due to systolic dysfunction; *LV,* left ventricular; *MSNA,* muscle sympathetic nerve activity; *RV,* right ventricular; *SNP,* sodium nitroprusside; *TNES,* total body norepinephrine spillover.

is similar in patients and age-matched healthy subjects,[97] suggesting relatively preserved modulation of sympathetic outflow in this condition.

Brandle et al[142] found no differences in the time course of changes in hemodynamics and plasma norepinephrine concentrations during the development of pacing-induced heart failure in dogs with and without sinoaortic baroreceptor denervation, and concluded that impairment of the arterial baroreflex could not be responsible for sustaining the increase in sympathetic outflow in this experimental model of heart failure. Reports, in heart failure, of significant inverse relationships between stroke work index and muscle sympathetic nerve activity[143] and between cardiac output and cardiac norepinephrine spillover[144] suggest that the arterial baroreflex regulation of efferent sympathetic discharge may actually be appropriate, when hemodynamic alterations present in this condition are considered. Grassi et al, using the vasoactive drug method, described an impairment of both limbs of the reflex control of MSNA that worsened with the progression of heart failure.[46] A second study also reported diminished arterial baroflex gain, but unfortunately in this report the mean age of patients was twice that of control subjects.[88] By contrast, Dibner-Dunlap et al[145] documented similar gains in the arterial baroreflex control of MSNA in healthy and heart failure subjects, whereas reflex responses to stimuli that raised and lowered cardiac filling pressure without affecting systemic blood pressure were markedly attenuated. These investigators concluded that impairment of the cardiopulmonary (not the arterial) baroreflex was the fundamental defect in the regulation of sympathetic outflow in human heart failure[145,146] (see Figure 16-7).

Two autonomic disturbances characteristic of advanced heart failure should be considered carefully when interpreting the results of experiments involving vasoactive drugs: (1) muscle sympathetic burst firing is pulse synchronous, and its incidence (i.e., bursts/100 cardiac cycles) approaches 100%; and (2) the heart rate response to arterial baroreceptor perturbation by phenylephrine or nitroprusside is markedly attenuated. If cardiac frequency hardly changes in response to these interventions, there is little opportunity arithmetically to modify a cardiac frequency-dependent representation of sympathetic nerve firing. If the reported effect of these drug interventions on MSNA burst frequency is reexpressed in terms of cardiac frequency (or as changes in absolute units, rather than as a percentage of baseline values) the gain of the arterial baroreflex regulation of MSNA is not appreciably impaired.[18,19,46,88]

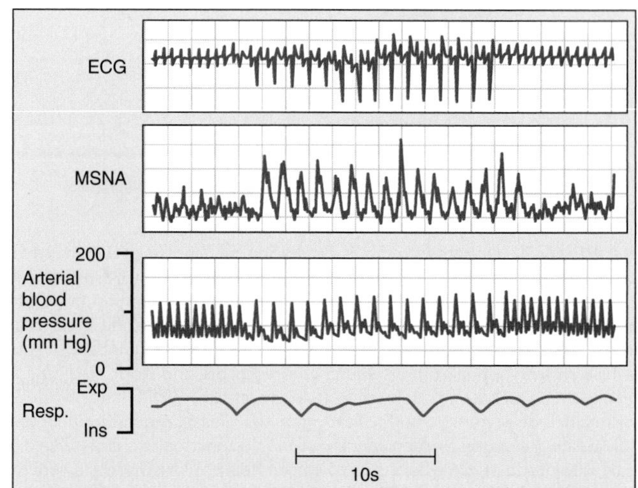

FIGURE 16–8 The electrocardiogram (ECG), mean voltage neurogram for (MSNA), blood pressure, and respiratory excursions in a young man with end-stage heart failure due to dilated cardiomyopathy. Paroxysms of ventricular bigeminy result in a doubling of the blood pressure cycle length, a longer diastolic period, and lower diastolic blood pressure. These changes are registered immediately by the arterial baroreceptors and result in a corresponding increase in the duration of the sympathetic burst and a marked increase in burst amplitude. These are reversed with restoration of sinus rhythm.

Several lines of evidence obtained using different approaches, and summarized in Table 16-1, are consistent with the concept that arterial baroreflex modulation of efferent sympathetic outflow is relatively intact in human heart failure* (Figures 16-8 and 16-9). Further evidence for preserved functionality of the arterial baroreflex arises from recent experiments involving the paced-canine and paced-ovine heart failure models. In the former, electrical stimulation of the carotid sinus nerve to increase afferent input from the unloaded arterial baroreceptor caused a significant fall in plasma norepinephrine concentration and enhanced survival.[148] In the latter, directly recorded cardiac sympathetic nerve activity (CSNA) was significantly increased, and the baroreceptor regulation of heart rate was profoundly impaired, but the arterial baroreflex control of both CSNA and renal sympathetic nerve traffic did not differ from that of normal sheep.[75,149]

In human heart failure, the renal efferent response to arterial baroreceptor unloading behaves differently. In one study, hypotension induced by nitroprusside elicited an 85%

*References 18, 19, 25, 49, 72, 147.

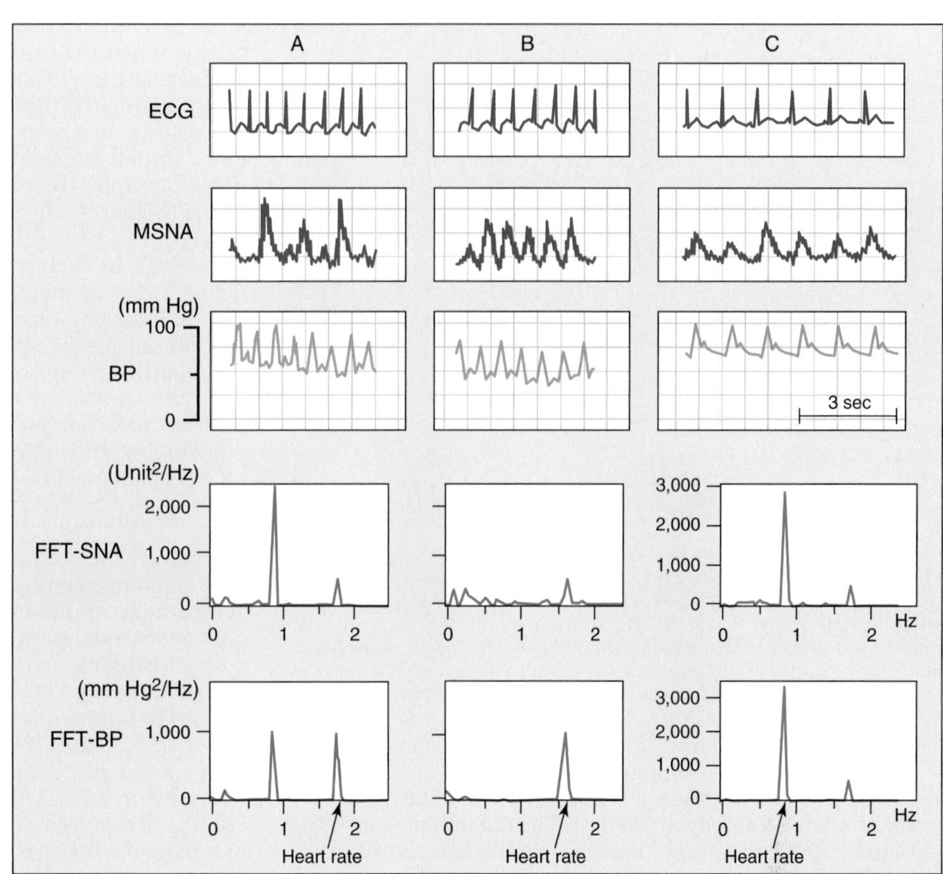

FIGURE 16–9 **A,** The ECG, muscle sympathetic nerve activity (MSNA), systemic blood pressure (BP), and power spectra of sympathetic nerve activity (FFT-SNA) and blood pressure during pulsus alternans. **B,** Recordings during intravenous nitroglycerin with disappearance of pulsus alternans. During pulsus alternans, there were relatively small changes in BP yet large oscillations in the amplitude of nerve bursts. Each sympathetic burst followed the preceding diastolic BP by 1.2 to 1.3 seconds, with a fall in amplitude as diastolic BP rose and vice versa. Power spectra were derived by use of fast Fourier transformation (FFT) from all cardiac cycles during a 7-minute period. During alternans **(A)**, there were two peaks in both the BP and the MSNA signal, one at the prevailing heart rate and a second at half this rate—that is, corresponding to the alternans frequency (0.9 Hz). MSNA power at the alternans frequency was greater than at the cardiac frequency, indicating that sympathetic alternans was present at this frequency throughout most of this 7-minute recording period. The lower frequency peak disappeared when pulsus alternans was abolished **(B)**; the residual BP and MSNA peaks are at this patient's heart rate. **C,** Similar recordings of ECG, MSNA, and BP and the power spectra for MSNA and BP in a patient with heart failure but without pulsus alternans (for purposes of comparison with A and B). A single peak of high spectral power falls on the heart rate frequency (*arrow*) in both the MSNA and BP spectra. (From Ando S, Dajani HR, Senn BL, et al. Sympathetic alternans. Evidence for arterial baroreflex control of muscle sympathetic nerve activity in congestive heart failure. *Circulation* 1997;95:316-319.)

increase in renal NE spillover in healthy control subjects, but no net change in heart failure subjects, albeit from a nearly threefold higher baseline.[150] What could not be determined from these experiments is whether the absence of sympathoexcitation represents a ceiling effect (i.e., renal NE spillover cannot be increased further from these high baseline levels, as suggested by the ovine experiments of Ramchandra et al[75]) or the integrated response to the combination of arterial and cardiopulmonary receptor unloading with a concurrent reduction in renal venous pressure. In a more recent study, low dose nitroglycerin reduced pulmonary artery pressures selectively without altering renal NE spillover in either heart failure or healthy subjects, whereas a higher, hypotensive dose was accompanied by a significant reduction only in those with systolic dysfunction.[151]

Cardiopulmonary Reflexes

In healthy subjects, cardiopulmonary reflexes elicit sympathoinhibition and forearm vasodilation, when stimulated by increasing cardiac filling pressures, volume, or inotropic state, and sympathoexcitation when unloaded by interventions such as phlebotomy, or nonhypotensive lower body negative pressure (LBNP).[41] There is substantial evidence that such responses are altered in human heart failure. When Middlekauff et al[152] performed phlebotomy, the reflex forearm vasoconstrictor response to this stimulus was attenuated in heart failure patients, whereas the renal cortical vasoconstrictor response, as assessed by positron emission tomography, was preserved. In some patients, lower body negative pressure elicits forearm vasodilation rather than vasoconstriction.[153] Activation of vagal afferents with inhibitory reflex effects on sympathetic outflow, as a result of acute increases in ventricular contractile force (possibly due to release of pericardial constraint) has been proposed as a potential mechanism for this paradoxical response.[153,154] However, sympathetic outflow was not quantified in these experiments. Subsequently, Dunlap et al reported greatly attenuated reflex MSNA responses to stimuli that raised and lowered cardiac filling pressure without affecting systemic blood pressure.[145] In our laboratory, nonhypotensive LBNP increased total body norepinephrine spillover significantly in subjects with normal ventricular systolic function, whereas there was only a trend, not significant, toward higher values in those with impaired ventricular systolic function.[155]

Such impairment would not be sufficient to account for two aspects of sympathoexcitation in heart failure: (1) a selective increase in cardiac norepinephrine spillover in mild to moderate human heart failure, without change in total body or renal norepinephrine spillover or in muscle sympathetic nerve activity,[15] and (2) the presence of direct correlations, in more advanced heart failure, between MSNA and pulmonary artery or capillary wedge pressure.[79,143] These observations suggest that a reflex that senses the degree of cardiopulmonary volume or pressure overload becomes active in heart failure. Indeed, in the pacing-induced canine model of congestion, Wang and Zucker documented sensitization of cardiac sympathetic afferents responsive to chemical stimulation, and speculated that enhancement of this reflex might contribute to increased sympathetic nerve traffic in chronic human heart failure.[156,157] This cardiac sympathetic afferent reflex was potentiated by acute volume expansion.[158]

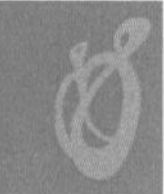

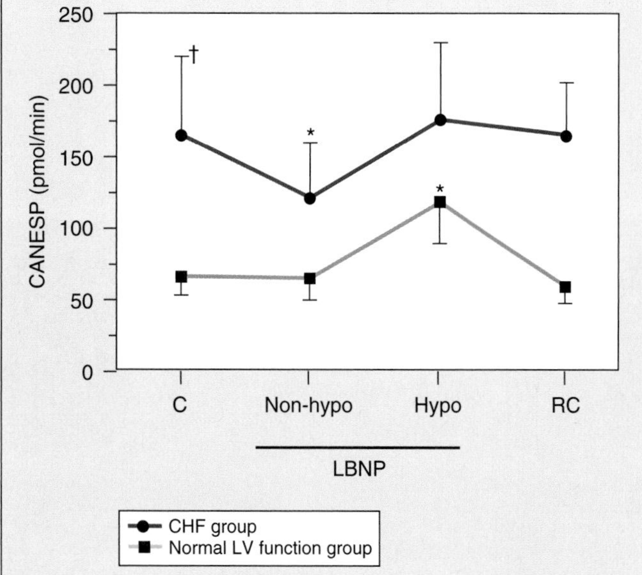

FIGURE 16–10 Cardiac norepinephrine spillover (CANESP) responses to nonhypotensive and hypotensive LBNP. ■ indicates normal LV function group; •, CHF group; *C*, control; and *RC*, recovery. *P <.05 vs. normal LV function group at control. (Data from Azevedo ER, Newton GE, Floras JS, et al. Reducing cardiac filling pressure lowers cardiac norepinephrine spillover in patients with chronic heart failure. *Circulation* 2000;101:2053-2059.)

Is there evidence in humans for activation, by increased filling pressure, of a cardiac-specific sympathoexcitatory reflex, perhaps arising from myelinated cardiac afferent nerves?[159] In patients with heart failure, there is a significant positive relationship between the pulmonary capillary wedge pressure and cardiac norepinephrine spillover.[144] Infusion of sodium nitroprusside in those with secondary pulmonary hypertension lowers cardiac norepinephrine spillover in addition to atrial and arterial pressure,[160] as does the brief application of positive airway pressure to reduce atrial and pulmonary venous transmural pressure (simultaneous reductions in intrathoracic aortic arch and LV transmural pressure should increase sympathetic outflow reflexively[161]). Nonhypotensive LBNP, applied to reduce selective cardiac filling and pulmonary pressure, decreases cardiac norepinephrine spillover in heart failure, but not in subjects with normal ventricular systolic function (Figure 16-10).[155] Because this maneuver lowers stroke volume and cardiac output, the reduction in cardiac norepinephrine spillover (but not total body norepinephrine spillover, which tends to increase) cannot be explained by activation of ventricular mechanoreceptors due to increases in systolic force.[153,154] Instead, Azevedo et al[155] attributed the sympathoinhibitory response to nonhypotensive LBNP to unloading of low-pressure mechanoreceptor afferents in the heart and lungs that reflexively and selectively excite cardiac adrenergic drive[159] (see Figure 16-7). Saline infusion causes a paradoxical increase in forearm vascular resistance in mild heart failure, an effect not seen in control subjects,[162] suggesting that in humans the efferent limb of this reflex, when stimulated acutely, might not be selective to cardiac sympathetic nerves.

Increasing the intensity of LBNP to induce systemic hypotension evoked a significant increase in cardiac norepinephrine spillover in the control group only (see Figure 16-10),[155] an observation concordant with these investigators' prior description of similar increases in total body norepinephrine spillover in heart failure and healthy subjects, yet attenuation of the reflex increase in cardiac norepinephrine spillover in response to a hypotensive infusion of sodium nitroprusside in those with impaired systolic function.[25] Together, these findings suggest that the normal arterial baroreflex-mediated increase in cardiac norepinephrine spillover, evoked reflexively by a fall in systemic blood pressure, is tempered significantly in heart failure by concurrent removal of an excitatory stimulus arising from cardiac sympathetic afferents.

To summarize, the weight of present evidence indicates that arterial baroreceptor reflex regulation of muscle and cardiac sympathetic activity is not impaired in human heart failure. Consequently, the higher sympathetic nerve firing rate characteristic of the majority of patients with systolic dysfunction can be considered an appropriate reflex response to alterations in their systemic hemodynamics. The principal defect in baroreceptor regulation of the sympathetic nervous system appears, instead, to arise from reflexes originating in mechanoreceptors situated within the heart and pulmonary vasculature.[146] In some patients with heart failure, these baroreflex-mediated responses appear sufficient to account for the prevailing level of sympathetic activity, but in many others the contribution of nonbaroreflex-mediated excitatory reflexes also must be considered.

Nonbaroreflex Mechanisms

Pulmonary Stretch Reflexes. A reflex arising from pulmonary stretch receptors distended by inspiration will inhibit sympathetic outflow.[35] In healthy subjects, breathing frequency correlates positively with MSNA burst frequency, and with reflex sympathoneural responses to hypoxia and hypercapnia.[163] The influence of breathing pattern on oscillations in adrenergic discharge is preserved in heart failure patients,[72,164] in whom decreased tidal volume, high respiratory frequency,[165] and brief periods of apnea elicit marked increases in MSNA (Figure 16-11). However, a greater tidal volume is required to inhibit completely MSNA in heart failure patients than in healthy subjects.[164] Rapidly adapting airway vagal sensory receptors, responding to inflation and deflation, are also stimulated by increases in left atrial pressure and extravascular pulmonary fluid volume.[166]

Peripheral Chemoreceptor Reflexes. The contribution of arterial chemoreceptors to sympathetic activation in experimental models of heart failure has been reviewed recently in detail by Schultz et al.[167] In healthy subjects, brief exposure to hypoxia can cause sustained increases in MSNA, persisting well after reoxygenation.[168] Augmented peripheral chemoreceptor sensitivity to hypoxia is reported to be present in approximately 40% of chronically treated heart failure patients[169,170] (see Figure 16-7). However, in two studies, inhalation of 100% O_2 to suppress peripheral chemoreceptor input had no effect on group mean values for MSNA, suggesting that chemoreceptor-mediated sympathoexcitation may not be this prevalent.[171,172] Di Vanna et al[173] described increased MSNA responses to hypoxic (peripheral) and hypercapneic (central) chemoreceptor stimulation in class II-III heart failure patients compared with control subjects. Carotid chemoreceptor reflex-induced sympathetic activation in heart failure may assume greater importance during exercise than in the resting state.[174]

Increased peripheral chemoreceptor sensitivity gives rise to several autonomic disturbances with adverse prognostic implications. These include higher plasma norepinephrine and brain natriuretic peptide concentrations, impaired arterial baroreflex control of heart rate, augmented very low-frequency heart rate and blood pressure spectral power, but loss of low-frequency heart rate variability, the development of periodic oscillations in breathing at very low frequency both during sleep and in the awake state, enhanced ventilatory responses to exercise, and a higher likelihood of developing nonsustained ventricular tachycardia.[169,170,175-178] In heart failure patients with coexisting chronic obstructive pulmonary disease, significantly higher plasma norepinephrine concentrations may reflect chronic hypoxemia.[179]

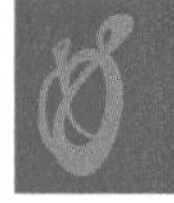

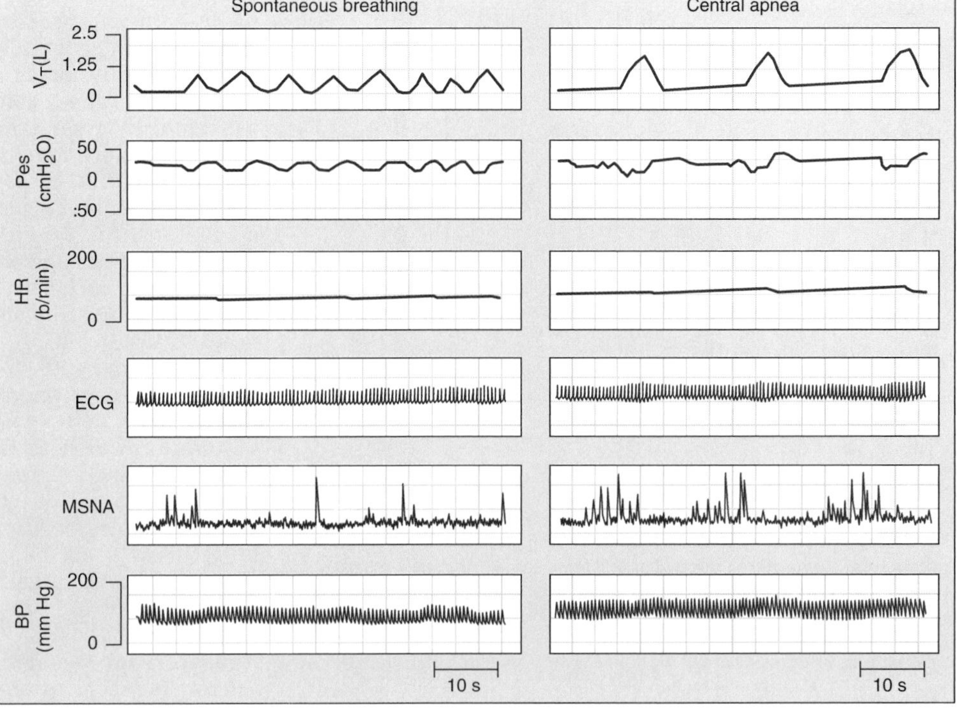

FIGURE 16–11 Tidal volume (V_T), esophageal pressure (Pes), heart rate (HR), the electrocardiogram (ECG), muscle sympathetic nerve activity (MSNA), and blood pressure (BP) in a young patient with dilated cardiomyopathy. Recordings taken during spontaneous breathing and spontaneous episodes of central apnea, while awake, only minutes apart, demonstrate marked activation of central sympathetic outflow and increased BP corresponding to periods of apnea.

Sleep-related Breathing Disorders (see also Chapter 32)

Normally, nonrapid eye movement (non-REM) sleep is characterized by reductions in central sympathetic outflow, heart rate, stroke volume, and systemic vascular resistance. Blood pressure typically falls 20% to 25% from average waking levels.[180-183] Vagal activity, and in particular the arterial baroreflex control of heart rate, is augmented.[184,185] Paroxysms of sympathetic discharge provoking surges in heart rate and blood pressure occur during rapid eye movement (REM) sleep, but in general REM comprises only 15% of sleep time.[182] Systolic dysfunction itself is associated with briefer sleep duration and interrupted sleep,[186,187] resulting in a greater integrated daily adrenergic burden. However, sleep apnea is evident in the majority of chronic symptomatic heart failure patients studied in published reports, with approximately one third exhibiting obstructive sleep apnea (OSA) and one third central sleep apnea (CSA).[188,189]

By deactivating pulmonary stretch receptors and stimulating peripheral and central chemoreceptors by hypoxia and hypercapnia, each pause in breathing during sleep elicits profound increases in MSNA.[33,190-193] This sympathetic excitation is independent of and in addition to any reflex responses to mechanoreceptor unloading resulting from pump failure or systemic hypotension in heart failure. Inspiratory efforts against a collapsed upper airway, as occurs in obstructive sleep apnea (OSA), will generate extreme negative swings in intrathoracic pressure (i.e., an abrupt increase in LV afterload). Because the failing heart is more sensitive to increases in afterload, obstruction provokes an acute fall in stroke volume and diastolic blood pressure.[194] This unloading of arterial baroreceptors elicits a reflex increase in MSNA of greater intensity in heart failure than in control subjects with normal LV function, who are better able to maintain stable systemic blood pressure in the face of this mechanical stimulus.[195] Arousal from sleep, which terminates an apneic event, is accompanied by a further surge in central sympathetic outflow, a rise in blood pressure above awake levels, and a decrease in heart rate variability due a to concurrent reduction in vagal tone.[182,195,196] In severely affected patients, these cycles of apnea and arousal recur repeatedly over the course of each night, exposing the failing heart and peripheral circulation during sleep to greater to concentration of norepinephrine than is required to maintain circulatory homeostasis. Nocturnal and daytime exposure to heightened adrenergic drive[168] could lead, over time, to chronic hypertension.[197,198]

In patients with OSA but normal LV function studied while awake, the after-effects of these nocturnal sympathoexcitatory stimuli induce sustained these nocturnal sympathoexcitatory stimuli sustained induce sustained increases in MSNA during wakefulness.[190,199,200] Coexisting obesity and hypertension[189] are important clues to the presence of obstructive sleep apnea in patients with LV systolic dysfunction. Grassi et al[201] described higher daytime MSNA in heart failure patients with obesity or hypertension, but did not report the prevalence of sleep apnea in this population. In a study involving 60 heart failure patients, of whom 43 had an apnea hypopnea index (AHI) of 15 events per hour,[85] MSNA during wakefulness was significantly higher in those with sleep apnea. In those with predominantly OSA, MSNA was increased by 11 bursts per 100 heartbeats. When OSA was abolished in a subset of such patients by 1 month of continuous positive airway pressure (CPAP), MSNA fell by 12 bursts per 100 heart beats.[85,202] In the absence of sleep apnea, MSNA of treated heart failure patients is not appreciably greater than that of aged-matched control subjects (Figure 16-12). Such data provide important evidence in human heart failure for convergence on central sympathetic neurons of input from two independent sympathoexcitatory influences (heart failure and sleep apnea) that act in concert to increase MSNA through a process of additive summation[203] (Figure 16-13). Mortality rates in patients with untreated OSA and heart failure are greater than those of heart failure patients without OSA,[204] suggesting that this additional OSA-mediated sympathoexcitation has the independent potential to accelerate the progression of systolic dysfunction.

A transition from predominantly obstructive apnea at the beginning of the night to mostly central events toward waking has been observed in some patients.[205] Also observed is a prolongation of circulation time, and a reduction in P_{CO_2} below the threshold for apnea. These observations suggest that these repetitive increases in LV afterload during airway obstructions

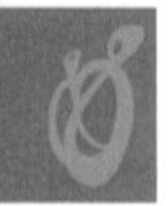

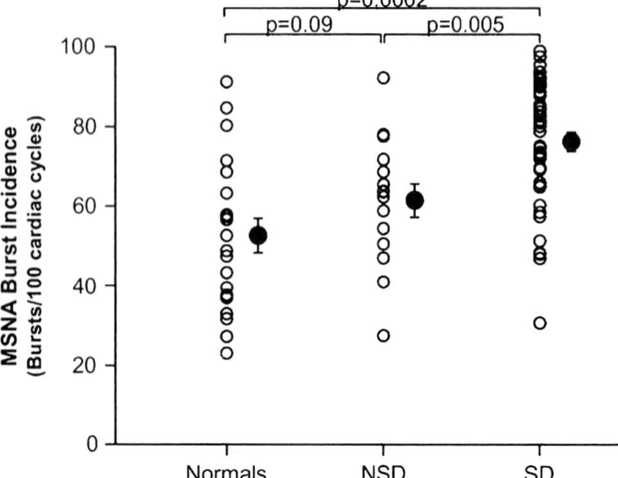

FIGURE 16–12 Scattergrams and means ± standard errors for muscle sympathetic burst incidence (bursts per 100 cardiac cycles) in treated heart failure patients with and without sleep apnea, as compared with age-matched healthy laboratory controls. Note that MSNA in treated heart failure patients without sleep apnea is not significantly greater than that of healthy subjects, whereas the coexistence of sleep apnea with heart failure is accompanied by significantly higher MSNA (P = .005). (Reproduced with permission of the American College of Cardiology Foundation from Floras JS. Sympathetic nervous system activation in human heart failure. Clinical implications of an updated model. *J Am Coll Cardiol* 2009;54:375-385.)

cause systolic function to deteriorate over the course of the night, with increased venous return and LV filling pressure stimulating hyperventilation and hypocapnia. Should this pattern progress over a period of months or years, the coexistence of obstructive apnea could predispose heart failure patients to worsening LV systolic function and central sleep apnea.

Compared with heart failure patients matched for ejection fraction and other clinical characteristics, but without sleep-related breathing disorders, those with CSA have higher nocturnal urinary norepinephrine excretion and increased plasma norepinephrine concentrations while awake. The magnitude of such activation is proportional to the frequency of arousal from sleep and the degree of apnea-related hypopnea.[206] MSNA during wakefulness is also greater in heart failure patients with, than without, CSA.[85] Mansfield et al[207] reported higher rates of cardiac and total body norepinephrine spillover in heart failure patients with CSA than in those without CSA or with OSA, and attributed these differences to greater hemodynamic decompensation in those with CSA. A direct comparison with the microneurographic literature is not possible because these investigators did not measure MSNA and used a quite low apnea-hypopnea index (>5 events per hour) to define sleep apnea.

Myocardial Ischemia and Infarction (see also Chapter 23)

Nonbaroreflex Mechanisms. Myocardial ischemia and prior infarction, very common in the heart failure population, should also exert, via several mechanisms, an additional acute or chronic effect on sympathetic outflow that is both additive and independent of the magnitude of ventricular systolic function and consequent hemodynamic derangement.[208,209]

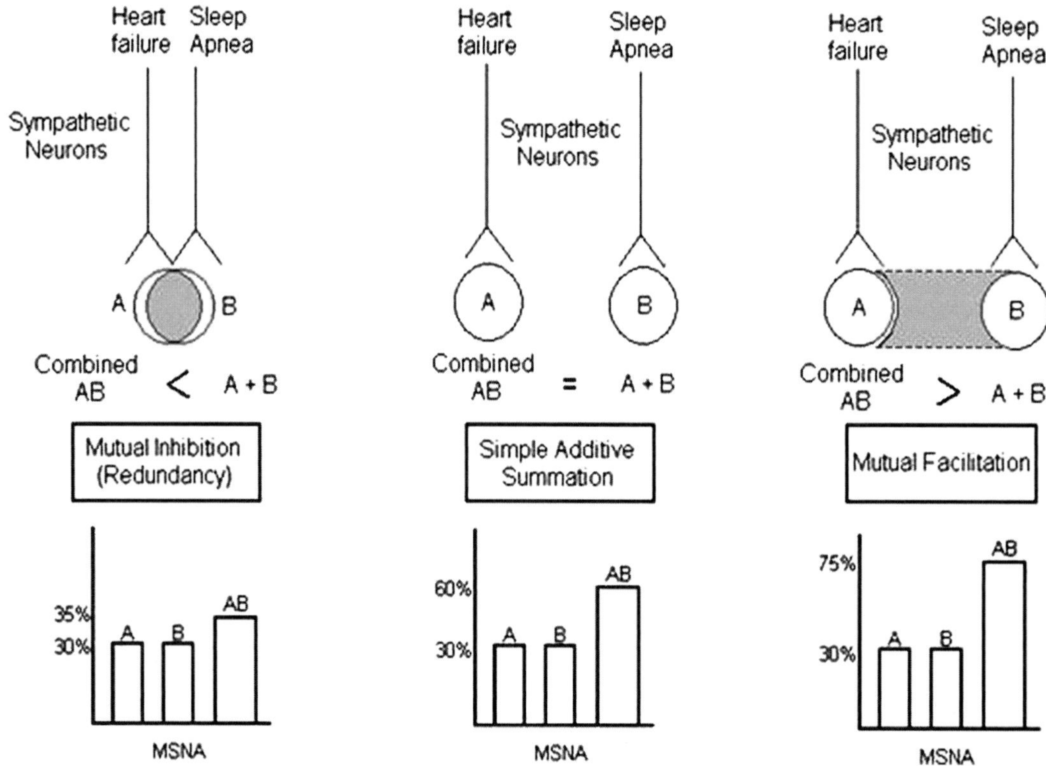

FIGURE 16–13 Convergence of afferent input from two sets of reflexes (in this example, heart failure and sleep apnea) eliciting directionally similar (in this example, excitatory) effects on muscle sympathetic nerve activity (MSNA) may summate and interact centrally through mutual inhibition (redundancy), simple additive summation, or mutual facilitation. The difference in MSNA recorded during wakefulness in heart failure patients with and without obstructive sleep apnea (OSA) [85] is eliminated when OSA is abolished.[202] This finding is consistent with the concept that these two sympathoexcitatory stimuli interact through a process of simple additive summation. (Reproduced with permission of the American College of Cardiology Foundation from Floras JS. Sympathetic nervous system activation in human heart failure. Clinical implications of an updated model. *J Am Coll Cardiol* 2009;54:375-385.)

Both anterior and inferoposterior wall ischemia elicit reflex sympathoexcitation by stimulating cardiac sympathetic afferent nerves.[210] Stimulation, by ischemia, of the vanilloid receptor-1 on cardiac spinal afferent nerves may represent one signaling pathway mediating this reflex response.[211]

Although cardiac sympathetic afferents may be stimulated by reductions in myocardial blood flow above the threshold for angina,[159] the reflex sympathoexcitatory response (which is reversed by stellectomy) is most evident during transmural ischemia.[210] If cardiac output and hence arterial blood pressure were to decrease as a consequence of ischemia, the resultant unloading of sinoaortic baroreceptors should elicit a further reflexive increase in sympathetic outflow. Vagal afferents arising from inferoposterior ventricular segments evoke a depressor response.[212-214] Prior myocardial infarction will interrupt the course of mechanoreceptor input to vagal afferents with inhibitory effects on sympathetic outflow.[209,215]

Consistent with this concept, 6 months after myocardial infarction, patients with relatively preserved ejection fraction (mean 52%) had significantly higher single fiber and multifiber MSNA burst incidences than patients with coronary artery disease or control subjects.[216] Do otherwise clinically similar patients with ischemic and nonischemic cardiomyopathy differ with respect to sympathetic activation? Higher plasma norepinephrine concentrations[217] and higher relative low-frequency heart rate spectral power[218] have been described for patients with ischemic as compared with dilated cardiomyopathy, whereas Grassi et al[219] reported virtually identical values for MSNA in these two cohorts. By contrast, in a comparative study of well-matched treated patients with ischemic and nonischemic dilated cardiomyopathy who were 5 to 10 years younger, and had much lower ejection fractions (22% vs. 33% for the Italian group), MSNA was significantly higher in those with an ischemic cardiomyopathy, and in addition, their $\dot{V}O_2$ peak was significantly less.[220]

In advanced heart failure, metabolic disturbances, such as increased free radical production, and a shift from glucose to greater fatty acid oxidation by underperfused myocytes may stimulate sympathoexcitation in nonischemic cardiomyopathy.[221,222] An increase in efferent sympathetic drive will deplete cardiac glycogen stores and stimulate fatty acid oxidation and ketogenesis; blood ketone bodies in heart failure correlate directly with plasma norepinephrine concentrations.[223]

Excitatory Reflexes Arising from Skeletal Muscle. Several neural mechanisms, arising from skeletal muscle, have the capacity to increase the set point for central sympathetic outflow in heart failure (see Figure 16-7). These include (1) a sympathoexcitatory reflex, stimulated by adenosine, with the participation of angiotensin acting via the AT_1 receptor as a neural intermediary[224,225]; (2) increases in local venous pressure[226]; (3) a muscle mechanoreflex[227] elicited by passive exercise, present in heart failure but not healthy control subjects; and (4) a muscle metaboreflex elicited by both isotonic and isometric handgrip.[14,225] The metaboreflex, which arises primarily from type IV sensory fibers, is activated at a lower workload in heart failure than in age-matched healthy control subjects. Importantly, the reflex MSNA response to exercise and postexercise skeletal muscle ischemia, elicited using a maneuver which traps ischemic metabolites in the forearm, is more prominent in heart failure patients with low peak $\dot{V}O_2$ than in patients matched for ejection fraction (<20% in both groups) with a $\dot{V}O_2$ peak greater than 56% of that predicted by their age, sex, weight, and height (see Figure 16-4).[14] This latter finding implies that comparisons between individuals of sympathetic activation obtained only under resting conditions underestimate the magnitude and adverse consequences of sympathetic activation when such heart failure patients are physically active.

Excitatory Reflexes Arising from the Kidney. An afferent signal from the uremic kidney has been shown to stimulate muscle sympathetic nerve activity of patients with chronic renal failure.[228,229] This sympathoexcitatory pathway may become active and functionally important in patients whose moderate to severe congestive heart failure is accompanied by renal insufficiency or increased venous pressure in the setting of right heart failure.

Central Integration and Interactions

Baroreceptor and chemoreceptor afferent nerves terminate in the nucleus tractus solitarius, which sends excitatory information to cell bodies situated in the caudal ventrolateral medulla (VLM). Discharge from the caudal VLM has inhibitory effects on neurons located in the rostral VLM medulla which, in turn, increase the firing rate of sympathetic preganglionic neurons in the intermediolateral cell column of the spinal cord. Input from adjacent respiratory centers, and suprabulbar subcortical regions involved in cardiovascular regulation interact with these pathways at several sites to further modulate central sympathetic outflow. A wide range of neurotransmitters, including catecholamines, nitric oxide, and peptides, mediate these interactions.[230]

By measuring norepinephrine appearance rates in the internal jugular vein, along with those of its lipophilic metabolites, 3-methoxy-4-hydroxyphenylglycol (MHPG) and 3,4-dihydroxyphenylglycol (DHPG), Esler's group has demonstrated significant increases in human heart failure in internal jugular spillover of MHPG, DHPG, epinephrine, and of the serotonin metabolite, 5-HIAA,[144,231] and a significant positive correlation between brain norepinephrine turnover and cardiac norepinephrine spillover.[231] Sampling selectively venous effluent from cortical and subcortical regions, Aggarwel et al detected fourfold higher suprabulbar subcortical turnover of norepinephrine in treated heart failure patients than in control subjects.[232] Cortical norepinephrine turnover tended to be lower. Furthermore, there was a significant positive correlation between subcortical norepinephrine turnover, and total body norepinephrine spillover in the heart failure group, an observation consistent with these authors' hypothesis that activation of noradrenergic neurons projecting rostrally from the brainstem mediates sympathetic excitation in heart failure. Because of their participation in arousal, vigilance, and circulatory control in the rat, brain norepinephrine nuclei in the locus coeruleus have received particular attention.[233] Chronic sleep disruption in heart failure (even in the absence of nocturnal breathing disorders)[187] may establish a state of heightened arousal, increasing adrenergic drive as a consequence.

With the progression of heart failure symptoms, ventilatory and sympathetic neural responses to central chemoreceptor stimulation by hypercapnia are augmented[170,173,175,234,235] and within-breath sympathoinhibition attenuated.[235] An increase in the gain of the central chemoreflex response to CO_2 could assist in establishing the cyclical breathing oscillations characteristic of central sleep apnea[236]; apneas act, in turn, to further stimulate central sympathetic outflow, with exaggerated sympathoexcitation[235] and carryover of high MSNA into the awake state.[85,206] In the most recently published series, involving of 60 consecutive patients with class I-III heart failure (mean LVEF 31%) receiving contemporary therapy, the prevalence of increased sensitivity to hypercapnia was 47%.[170]

The concept that the central nervous system simply integrates information from these several afferent inputs, and then transmits output passively has been superseded by experimental and clinical evidence demonstrating an active contribution to the autonomic disturbances of heart failure.[142] Central alterations in the gain of the arterial or cardiopulmonary baroreflex modulation of sympathetic outflow are not accessible to study in humans, but in experimental heart failure models, Zucker's group has documented central augmentation of cardiac sympathetic afferent reflex regulation of renal sympathetic nerve activity, arising from increases in central angiotensin II, decreases in local synthesis of neuronal NO, which exerts sympathoinhibitory actions at several brain sites,[237] and generation of reactive oxygen species. These actions and interactions have important sympathoexcitatory consequences.[238,239] Overexpression of inducible NO synthase in the RVLM by adenoviral vectors also increases sympathetic activity by generating reactive oxygen species.[240]

Angiotensin II inhibits vagal discharge, increases central sympathetic outflow, and interacts with the arterial baroreflex at several sites within and outside the blood-brain barrier.[241-245] In dogs without heart failure, the hypotensive response to chronic carotid baroreceptor stimulation is attenuated if angiotensin II is infused concurrently.[246] The cardiac sympathetic afferent reflex in dogs is potentiated by chronic central infusion of angiotensin II[247]; in rats with chronic heart failure this reflex can be normalized by central administration of antisense oligodeoxynucleotides to AT_1 receptor mRNA.[248] Sympathetically mediated increases in renal renin release in heart failure could therefore generate a positive feedback loop, amplifying adrenergic discharge through these central actions of angiotensin II.

In rats with congestive heart failure, an increase in renal sympathetic outflow and resetting of its regulation by the arterial baroreceptor reflex could be reversed by intracerebroventricular infusions of Fab fragments (as inhibitors of ouabain-like activity), the angiotensin II AT_1 receptor antagonist, losartan,[248-252] or an angiotensin-converting enzyme inhibitor[253] and was not observed in transgenic rats deficient in brain angiotensinogen.[254] In a rabbit heart failure model, sympathoexcitation resulted from increased rostral VLM angiotensin AT_1 receptor and NAD(P)H oxidase subunit gene expression with consequent upregulation of superoxide production.[238,255] This group has proposed that increased central angiotensin II in heart failure initiates a positive feedback loop involving a reactive oxygen species pathway that may regulate neuronal excitability by modulation of ion channel function.[256] In this model, increased central enhancement of the gain of the cardiac reflex, rather than loss of arterial baroreceptor input,[142] contributes to the increased set point for sympathetic outflow in chronic heart failure.[257-259] Central mineralocorticoid receptors also participate in the regulation of sympathetic outflow. In rats with experimental heart failure, intracerebroventricular infusion of spironolactone reduced renal sympathetic nerve firing and augmented its arterial baroreflex regulation.[260] Aldosterone of adrenal origin has also been reported to stimulate the brain renin-angiotensin system by increasing paraventricular (hypothalamic) nucleus angiotensin AT_1 receptor mRNA, protein, and NAD(P)H oxidase subunit gene expression, and concurrently plasma NE concentrations.[261] Recently described is an additional central cytokine-mediated sympathoexcitatory pathway that can be attenuated by antiinflammatory cytokines[262] or by mineralocorticoid receptor blockade.[263]

Efferent Mechanisms

Ganglionic Neurotransmission

The principal defect in the parasympathetic modulation of heart rate in experimental heart failure appears to lie at the level of vagal ganglionic neurotransmission.[138] Conversely, by stimulating sympathetic ganglionic and adrenomedullary neurotransmission, increases in angiotensin II in heart failure could augment norepinephrine and epinephrine release.[241]

Prejunctional Mechanisms and Efferent Sympathovagal Interactions

In the hamster model of dilated cardiomyopathy, early increases in cardiac norepinephrine turnover, tyrosine hydroxylase and dopamine β-hydroxylase activity, and cardiac dopamine stores are followed by depletion of myocardial norepinephrine content and destruction of sympathetic nerve terminals.[117] In a rabbit model of pacing-induced heart failure, ventricular systolic dysfunction and an increase in plasma norepinephrine were followed by a reduction in cardiac norepinephrine uptake and transporter density, and a subsequent decrease in myocardial β-receptor density, with gradual normalization after pacing ended.[264]

Radioligand-binding experiments in ventricles derived from patients with class II-IV heart failure detected a significant decrease of up to 30% in norepinephrine uptake-1 carrier density.[265] Isotopic dilution studies have identified reduced efficiency of norepinephrine uptake, such that its spillover into the coronary sinus was increased disproportionally more than its neuronal release.[130] Rundqvist et al[15] calculated the fractional extraction of norepinephrine to be 87% in healthy controls, but only 60% in heart failure patients. These abnormalities of cardiac norepinephrine uptake can be improved with chronic ß-adrenoceptor blockade[266] and, in patients with heart failure and preserved systolic function, with the angiotensin II AT_1 receptor antagonist, candesartan.[267]

The release of norepinephrine from sympathetic nerve endings and the discharge of acetylcholine from vagal nerves also can be augmented or suppressed by endogenous or exogenously administered agonists, acting on a wide variety of prejunctional receptors. Norepinephrine release from cardiac, intrathoracic, and peripheral sympathetic nerve endings, and catecholamine release from the adrenal medulla can be facilitated through stimulation of prejunctional β_2-adrenoceptors by its endogenous agonist, epinephrine.[77,78,268-272] In more advanced heart failure, circulating epinephrine may be transported into sympathetic nerve terminals, incorporated into vesicles along with norepinephrine, and released as a cotransmitter[77,273] with a potential prejunctional sympathofacilitatory action.[78]

In contrast, α_2-adrenoceptor agonists, such as clonidine, inhibit norepinephrine release. Observations concerning the functional importance of such inhibition in human heart failure suggest regional selectivity, with left ventricular[274] but not forearm α_2-adrenoceptors[275] retaining this inhibitory capacity.

Polymorphisms of prejunctional adrenergic receptors might contribute to interindividual variation in norepinephrine release. In a retrospective genetic-association study, Small et al[276] detected a sixfold increase in the risk of developing heart failure in black subjects homozygous for the hypofunctioning prejunctional α_{2C} Del322-325 polymorphism, and a tenfold increase in those who were also homozygous for the hyperfunctional postjunctional β_1Arg329 receptor, which demonstrates greater affinity, in vivo, for adenylyl cyclase, and augmented generation of contractile force in right ventricular trabeculae of nonfailing and failing hearts exposed to isoproterenol.[277] These authors proposed that this increased risk for heart failure resulted from a synergistic enhancement of polymorphisms within these two adrenergic signal-transduction pathways. However, in this initial report, no direct functional data concerning cardiac norepinephrine release, or postjunctional responsiveness, such as heart rate were provided.[276] By contrast, in healthy subjects, variability in the blood pressure and plasma norepinephrine response to the selective α_2-agonist dexmedetomidine was unaffected by this genotype,[278] and in a cohort of patients with severe heart failure, Kaye et al[279] detected no relationship between the α_{2C} Del322-325 or $ß_2$-adrenoceptor polymorphisms and the rate of cardiac norepinephrine release. Curiously, the relationship

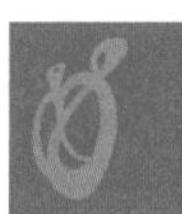

between norepinephrine release and heart rate was steeper in ß$_2$-adrenoceptor Arg 16 homozygotes, implying increased postjunctional responsiveness.

Muscarinic M_2 receptors on adrenergic nerve endings also attenuate norepinephrine release when stimulated by acetylcholine.[280-282] Intracoronary infusion of acetylcholine into subjects with LV systolic dysfunction and increased cardiac adrenergic drive decreased cardiac norepinephrine spillover, an effect not seen in control subjects with normal LV systolic function. Receptor blockade with atropine had no effect in the heart failure group, but increased cardiac norepinephrine spillover in control subjects.[283] Conversely, increased norepinephrine release from sympathetic nerve endings inhibits acetylcholine release by stimulating prejunctional α_1-adrenoceptors on vagal nerve endings.[284] More recent experiments have identified neuregulin-1 signaling as an important antiadrenergic pathway, requiring eNOS-mediated muscarinic cholinergic receptor activation.[285] Neuregulin-1 expression initially increases and then decreases with the development of congestive heart failure.[285] Other sympathetic neurotransmitters, such as NPY, that inhibit acetylcholine release[228,286,287] may also exert a vagolytic action in advanced heart failure.

In experimental preparations, prejunctional AT_1 receptors have been shown to facilitate neural and adrenal release of catecholamines when stimulated by angiotensin II[241,288-290] but it has proven difficult to replicate this action in human heart failure.[291]

Circulating activating antibodies against ß$_1$ and/or ß$_2$ adrenoceptors, present in same patients with dilated cardiomyopathy, can mimic a state of marked sympathoexcitation.[292]

THERAPEUTIC IMPLICATIONS

Parenteral catecholaminergic positive inotropic agents were among the earliest therapies for heart failure. Acutely, dobutamine infusion causes a significant reduction in cardiac norepinephrine spillover, an effect attributed to reductions in cardiac filling pressures, and activation of ventricular mechanoreceptors.[293] However, the long-term administration of sympathomimetics has been shown, consistently, to increase mortality, and the application of isotope dilution methodology to heart failure patients disproved the concept that the failing heart required inotropic support to compensate for sympathetic denervation. Use of these agents is now restricted to short-term palliation.

From the perspective of the autonomic nervous system, current pharmacological and nonpharmacological management of heart failure is predicated upon the following hypotheses: (1) in most patients, the magnitude of sympathetic activation is in excess of that required to maintain cardiovascular homeostasis; (2) as evident from the transplantation literature[294] and the device literature,[259] many of the mechanisms contributing to sympathetic activation and parasympathetic withdrawal in heart failure result from functional, reversible alterations rather than irreversible damage; and (3) interventions that counter cardiac sympathetic overactivity will improve both symptoms and prognosis. Several therapeutic strategies have been pursued, with varying degrees of success: (1) attenuation of sympathoexcitatory stimuli, (2) modulation of sympathetic nerve traffic and norepinephrine release, (3) adrenoceptor blockade, (4) central sympatholysis, and (5) augmentation of vagal tone.

By modulating sympathetic nerve traffic and NE release, opposing adrenoceptor stimulation by either neurally released or circulating catecholamines, or attenuating sympathoexcitatory stimuli such as high cardiac filling pressure and myocardial ischemia, several contemporary disease-based heart failure therapies counter, directly or indirectly, the adverse effects of excessive cardiac and systemic sympathetic activity and augment vagal tone to improve symptoms, prognosis, or both. These include relief of congestion and central sleep apnea through diuresis[295,296] (but avoiding bladder fullness[297]) prescription of angiotensin-converting enzyme inhibitors,[145,298] angiotensin receptor antagonists,[224,225,243,299,300] amiodarone,[301] antagonists of prejunctional β_2-adrenergic receptors that facilitate NE release,[302] and digitalis glycosides.[303,304] Antagonism of β_1-adrenergic-mediated stimulation of renin release, resulting in lower circulating concentrations of angiotensin II, should provide additional therapeutic benefit.[305] Although not formally tested in randomized controlled trials, chronic cardiac resynchronization therapy also appears to lower MSNA[306]; whether this adaptation represents an appropriate reflex response to atrial mechanoreceptor unloading or arterial baroreceptor stimulation has yet to be clarified. Importantly, neither these drug nor device therapies address directly nonbaroreflex stimuli to sympathetic nervous system activation, such as skeletal muscle mechanoreflexes and metaboreflexes that augment sympathoneural responses to exercise, the co-existence of sleep-related breathing disorders, or adrenoceptor polymorphisms, such as that of the hyperfunctional postjunctional β_1Arg329 receptor, which influences the response to ß-adrenoceptor blockade.[277] The identification of such conditions in individual patients affords the opportunity to add, as adjunctive treatment, new therapeutic strategies targeted at their specific sympathoexcitatory pathophysiology.

While α_1-adrenoceptor antagonists might be expected to counter the adverse effects of NE on the kidney and peripheral vasculature, this drug class has not been demonstrated to alter mortality rates in heart failure,[307] possibly due to the absence of a sustained effect on neurogenic vasoconstriction.[308]

The symptomatic, hemodynamic, and mortality benefits of long-term β_1- and nonselective β-blockade for patients with heart failure due to depressed LV systolic function have been proven in a series of landmark placebo-controlled trials involving carvedilol, bisoprolol, and metoprolol (see also Chapter 46).[156,309-312] In a randomized, double-blind comparative investigation in heart failure patients (mean LV ejection fraction of 20%), 4 months of therapy with carvedilol decreased total body and cardiac norepinephrine spillover by more than 35%. These changes did not occur in metoprolol-treated patients.[302] Because neither drug affected postganglionic MSNA, these reductions were attributed to the blockade of prejunctional neural β_2-adrenoceptors capable of facilitating norepinephrine release. Moreover, there was a significant inverse relationship between changes in CNES and reflex vagal heart rate modulation. In contrast, β-blockade had no effect on arterial baroreflex modulation of MSNA. Together, these latter findings are best explained by an efferent sympathetic-parasympathetic interaction (i.e., blockade of cardiac sympathetic prejunctional β_2-adrenoceptors), rather than by any augmentation of afferent or central components of the baroreflex arc, resulting in withdrawal of the inhibitory effects of excess cardiac norepinephrine release on vagal modulation of sinoatrial discharge.[313] Thus, in addition to protecting myocytes from the toxic effects of high local concentrations of catecholamines,[108] β-adrenoceptor antagonists such as carvedilol and metoprolol address the earliest autonomic disturbances identified in heart failure by countering the adverse effects of cardiac sympathetic overactivity and by augmenting tonic and reflex heart rate modulation while preserving normal homeostatic oscillations in MSNA.[314]

Some patients receiving the combination of angiotensin-converting enzyme inhibition, β-adrenoceptor blockade, and aldosterone antagonism continue to demonstrate persistently high sympathoadrenal activity. Moreover, β-blockade does not shield the heart, kidney, or periphery from α-adrenoceptor-mediated vasoconstriction or renal sodium retention, or from vasoconstriction caused by neurotransmitters co-released with norepinephrine such as ATP[315] or neuropeptide Y (NPY), which has a more sustained effect than NE[316] and is also a potent inhibitor of efferent vagal neurotransmission.[317] Not unexpectedly, myocardial spillover of NPY also is increased in heart failure.[318] More aggressive neuro-humoral blockade, or central abolition of sympathetic outflow, or both, have been proposed therefore as means of further reducing mortality rates. Importantly, these strategies presume that peripheral sympathetic drive is excessive in all treated heart failure patients, and its antagonism will benefit all patients. Both assumptions should be questioned critically.

Central sympathetic outflow can be attenuated directly, by stimulating α_2 and imidazoline I_1 receptors located within the rostral VLM using either clonidine, an $\alpha_2 + I_1$ receptor agonist, or I_1 agonists such as moxonidine. Acutely, the intravenous administration of 0.1 mg clonidine lowered arterial norepinephrine concentrations, cardiac norepinephrine spillover, and left ventricular +dP/dt by 47%, 58%, and 15%, respectively.[319] When administered for 2 months by transdermal patch, 0.1 mg of daily clonidine reduced muscle sympathetic burst frequency by 26% and plasma norepinephrine concentrations by 47%.[320]

Unfortunately, both in a pilot study,[321] and in a large-scale mortality trial,[322] there was an excess of deaths in patients allocated moxonidine. In retrospect, this outcome may relate more to the specific aspects of these clinical trials, than the validity of the underlying hypothesis.[19] In many of the patients recruited, plasma norepinephrine concentrations were not markedly elevated, perhaps because of prior optimization of their medical therapy for their heart failure. The dose of moxonidine selected for study may have been sympathoablative, reducing residual central sympathetic outflow to levels insufficient to support cardiac output or peripheral resistance at rest, and unlike ß-adrenoceptor antagonists, preventing appropriate increases in neurotransmitter release in response to exercise or other stimuli. An excess of mortality and sudden death might have resulted from a rebound during periods of non-adherence. In the MOXSE pilot study, there were twofold to threefold increases in plasma norepinephrine concentrations, and corresponding rebound elevations in heart rate, blood pressure, and ventricular ectopy during tapered withdrawal from active therapy.[321] The fundamental question raised by these two studies is whether the adverse effect of this therapy on outcomes should be attributed to the drug strategy itself, to excessive sympatholysis, or to intense rebound surges in central sympathetic outflow. A similar concern was raised by a trial of bucindolol in heart failure, in which a marked fall in plasma norepinephrine concentration with treatment was accompanied by an increase in mortality; although described as "sympatholysis," whether this effect was due to decreased sympathetic nerve traffic, decreased norepinephrine release, or increased clearance cannot be established.[323] This line of investigation is unlikely to advance unless these issues are resolved, and a method of identifying patients with residual sympathetic activation more reliable than venous norepinephrine concentrations or HR spectral analysis,* can be deployed routinely within the clinical setting.

Future approaches may address the central angiotensin II-AT_1 receptor–reactive oxygen species–sympathoexcitatory hypothesis of heart failure by administering centrally acting antioxidants,[325] mineralocorticoid receptor antagonists,[261,326] or statins[327-329] or by stimulating neuregulin-1/ErbB signaling to reduce cardiac sympathetic and augment vagal tone.[285] In heart failure patients, infusion of 2.5 mg of vitamin C augmented the reflex vagal heart rate modulation by approximately 30%.[330] There may be a role for nicotinic agonists[331] or vagal nerve pacing[332] to preserve parasympathetic tone as heart failure progresses, and for chronic afferent baroreceptor nerve pacing,[148] or for novel approaches to attenuate or reverse the loss of norepinephrine carrier density and augment its reuptake at cardiac sympathetic nerve endings.[333] In a rabbit model of heart failure, overexpression of the norepinephrine transporter uptake-1 protein by adenoviral gene transfer resulted in recovery of norepinephrine uptake throughout the left ventricle, greater β_1-adrenoceptor and sarcoplasmic reticulum Ca^{2+} ATPase protein expression, and improvement in cardiac structure and contractile function.[334] Direct injection of nerve growth factor into the left stellate ganglion of rats with experimental heart failure also resulted in augmented norepinephrine uptake and an increase in fractional shortening.[335]

Conversely, if directed evaluation identifies coexisting conditions that augment adrenergic outflow to the heart and periphery in excess of that needed to maintain hemodynamic stability, then therapy individualized so as to attenuate patient-specific sympathoexcitatory pathophysiology may be added to conventional disease-specific treatment. In addition to attenuating myocardial ischemia surgically, mechanically, or pharmacologically, this goal might be achieved by (1) normalizing cardiac filling pressure and relieving pulmonary congestion with natriuretic peptide infusion[155,336,337] or ultrafiltration,[338] but without inducing systemic hypotension and thereby increasing reflexively sympathetic activity and norepinephrine release[336,339,338]; (2) physical conditioning[84,340]; and (3) abolishing coexisting OSA with nocturnal continuous positive airway pressure (CPAP).[341,342] Each of these interventions has been demonstrated to both diminish sympathetic tone and augment the tonic or reflex vagal modulation of heart rate.[84,340,342-350] By contrast, if deployed prematurely (i.e., when filling pressures are not elevated diuretic therapy would have adverse consequences-activating both the sympathetic nervous and renin-angiotensin systems. However, as yet none of these interventions has been demonstrated in large clinical trials to reduce mortality rates.

Conventional pharmacological approaches to heart failure have no impact on OSA. By contrast, nocturnal nasal CPAP abolishes upper airway obstruction and four of its sympathoexcitatory consequences: apnea, hypoxia, hypercapnia, and arousal from sleep. In patients with heart failure and obstructive sleep apnea, CPAP reduces nocturnal blood pressure and heart rate (see also Chapter 32), [351] and increases the arterial baroreflex modulation of heart rate.[348] Thus the sympathoinhibitory and vagotonic effects of CPAP during sleep, alone, may be sufficient to benefit heart failure patients with co-existing OSA. Consequently, there is increasing recognition of the importance of identifying and treating OSA when present in heart failure patients.

In addition, in patients with elevated LV end-diastolic pressure, studied while awake, the acute application of CPAP augmented stroke volume,[352] increased total spectral power, nonharmonic power, low- and high-frequency power, and the ratio of high to total power[353] and diminished cardiac norepinephrine spillover.[161] In randomized trials of 1 month duration involving heart failure patients with OSA, nightly use of CPAP abolished apnea, improved LV structure and ejection fraction,[341] lowered systolic blood pressure, heart rate, and MSNA during wakefulness,[341,342] and reduced ventricular ectopy during sleep.[354] A randomized controlled trial involving patients with milder OSA (apnea-hypopnea index >5 events per hour) and an LV ejection fraction less than 55% also observed a significant increase in LV ejection fraction in conjunction with a reduction in urinary norepinephrine excretion after 3 months of CPAP treatment.[355] Data from non-randomized observational studies, involving OSA subjects without[356] and with,[204] heart failure suggest that the abolition of apneas by CPAP may also reduce mortality rates.

In a 3-month randomized trial involving heart failure patients with CSA, the nightly application of CPAP suppressed

---

*References 23, 52, 58, 60-62, 324.

the apnea-hypopnea index and reduced nocturnal urinary norepinephrine by 41%, to values similar to those obtained in clinically matched heart failure patients without CSA. CPAP also reduced plasma norepinephrine during wakefulness by 22%.[206] In a long-term trial involving 258 heart failure patients with CSA, CPAP did not improve transplant-free survival overall,[357] but this intervention reduced the apnea-hypopnea index only from 40 to 20 events per hour. However, in a post hoc efficacy analysis, CPAP improved significantly transplant-free survival of those patients in whom the apnea-hypopnea index was suppressed below 15 apneic or hypopneic events per hour. The threshold required for recruitment into the CANPAP trial.[187]

SUMMARY

In this chapter we have (1) reviewed methods for assessing sympathetic and parasympathetic function in conscious humans; (2) summarized evidence for adrenergic activation and vagal withdrawal in human heart failure, and the adverse consequences of these disturbances; and (3) discussed, in detail, mechanisms that underlie both these alterations in neurogenic circulatory control and the actions of current and emerging pharmacological and nonpharmacological interventions for this condition. Several key concepts should be reemphasized.

Patients with LV systolic dysfunction have in common impaired vagal modulation of heart rate, but differ considerably in the magnitude and mechanisms of sympathetic activation. Although the set point for central sympathetic outflow is increased in the majority of patients, in a substantial minority of those with asymptomatic or symptomatic LV systolic dysfunction values for plasma norepinephrine concentrations, muscle sympathetic nerve activity and total body norepinephrine spillover remain within the range described for control subjects. Therefore, sympathetic activation cannot be considered a defining characteristic of LV systolic dysfunction. Many current therapies for heart failure attenuate adrenergic drive and augment vagal tone. The therapeutic implication of these findings is that patients without evidence for sympathetic activation are unlikely to benefit from multiple neurohumoral antagonists or from sympatholytic interventions.[19,358]

Alterations in both inhibitory and excitatory influences on autonomic outflow contribute to these disturbances in neurogenic circulatory control. The extent to which each of these regulatory systems is impaired or activated is subject to considerable interindividual variation. Early activation of adrenergic drive to the diseased myocardium appears to be the principal mechanism linking altered neural regulation of the heart and circulation to adverse outcomes.

The currently available evidence in humans allows five conclusions with respect to mechanoreceptor reflex regulation of heart rate and sympathetic nervous system activity in human heart failure due to impaired systolic function (see Figure 16-7): (1) the arterial baroreceptor reflex regulation of heart rate by the vagus nerve is impaired; (2) in contrast, the arterial baroreflex regulation of muscle sympathetic nerve activity is rapidly responsive to changes in diastolic blood pressure; (3) pulmonary mechanoreceptor-mediated inhibition of sympathetic outflow is preserved; and (4) cardiopulmonary reflex control of muscle sympathetic nerve activity is blunted. As a consequence, efferent sympathetic outflow to the skeletal muscle is not suppressed by increased cardiac filling pressure. Rather, (5) elevated filling pressures in heart failure can increase cardiac norepinephrine spillover by stimulating a cardiac-specific sympathoexcitatory reflex.

Viewed from this perspective, the heterogeneity and time course of organ-specific sympathetic activation and parasympathetic withdrawal can be considered appropriate to individual hemodynamic profiles (Table 16-2). Patients will progress from asymptomatic to end-stage heart failure by different pathways and at different rates. In some, the initial insult may be a sudden drop in cardiac output and blood pressure, which will reflexively activate the sympathetic nervous and renin-angiotensin systems and decrease vagal tone so as to achieve a state of relative compensation.[16] If, on the other hand, relatively normal stroke volume and blood pressure can be maintained by increases in LV end-diastolic volume, rather than cardiac filling pressure, such patients would be less likely to manifest evidence, at rest, for hemodynamically mediated sympathetic activation. Indeed, by increasing the ventricular mechanoreceptor firing rate, such remodeling might even depress, reflexively, sympathetic outflow to the kidney and skeletal muscle, maintaining renal responsiveness to natriuretic influences and relatively normal peripheral resistance. Impaired cardiac reserve in such patients might only be evidenced by abnormal adrenergic or heart rate responses to exercise or mental stress.

Table 16-2 Summary and Proposed Construct Relating Time Course and Heterogeneity of Autonomic Disturbances in Human Heart Failure to Hemodynamic and Nonhemodynamic Abnormalities

Primary Abnormality	Autonomic Consequence
Acute heart failure with pulmonary congestion and hypotension	Generalized activation of sympathetic and renin-angiotensin-aldosterone systems; parasympathetic withdrawal
Chronic increase in left atrial pressure	Activation of cardiac sympathetic afferents causing reflex increase in efferent cardiac SNA
	Decrease in tonic +/− reflex vagal HR modulation
	Decreased pre-junctional muscarinic receptor-mediated inhibition of NE release
Chronic increase in left ventricular end diastolic pressure and volume	Reflex inhibition of sympathetic outflow to kidneys, skeletal muscle, and other systemic vascular beds
Chronic exposure to increased cardiac SNA	Impaired cardiac β-mediated signal transduction
	Increased pre-junctional α_1-mediated inhibition of Ach release
Chronic reduction in stroke volume and systemic blood pressure	Impaired arterial baroreflex regulation of HR
	Reflex sympathetic activation resulting from intact and responsive arterial baroreflex regulation of muscle SNA, total body NE spillover, ± cardiac NE spillover, ± renal NE spillover
Pulmonary congestion	Decreased inhibition of central sympathetic outflow by pulmonary stretch reflexes stimulated by lung inflation
	Decreased respiratory sinus arrhythmia (vagal)
Chemoreceptor and muscle metaboreceptor activation	Increased muscle SNA
	Decreased tonic and reflex vagal HR modulation
Co-existing sleep apnea	Increased muscle SNA and decreased vagal HR modulation during sleep
	Increased daytime plasma NE

Ach, Acetylcholine; *HR*, heart rate; *NE*, norepinephrine; *SNA*, sympathetic nerve activity.

From this compensated state, heart failure may progress along several pathways, with corresponding disturbances of neural regulation. If cardiac filling pressures rise initially, as required to maintain stroke volume and systemic arterial pressure, the anticipated response would be activation of the cardiac sympathetic reflex[159] and a decrease in tonic vagal heart rate modulation[359] without any corresponding changes in MSNA or total body norepinephrine spillover. Any withdrawal of muscarinic tone will release its restraining influence on cardiac norepinephrine.[283] This hypothetical scenario would account for the selective increase in cardiac norepinephrine spillover documented in mild to moderate symptomatic LV systolic dysfunction,[15] and for the positive correlation noted between cardiac norepinephrine spillover and pulmonary capillary wedge pressure.[144] Chronic exposure to increased cardiac norepinephrine release would initiate the process of sinoatrial adrenoceptor downregulation and altered β_1-adrenoceptor signal transduction. In some individuals genetic polymorphisms involving adrenergic receptors may accelerate this process.[276] Similar alterations in autonomic regulation may occur in diastolic heart failure, but this hypothesis has yet to be formally tested.

As myocardial contractile performance deteriorates, heart rate will rise through arterial baroreflex-mediated vagal withdrawal and sympathetic activation to maintain cardiac output. Over time, further unloading of arterial baroreceptors by a decline in systolic or pulse pressure will elicit further diminution of cardiac vagal modulation, generalized neurohumoral activation resulting from reflex increases in sympathetic outflow to the heart, kidney, and skeletal muscle, and loss of low-frequency MSNA spectral modulation due to impaired neuroeffector transduction. By removing the inhibitory or restraining effect of lung inflation on central sympathetic outflow—pulmonary congestion—altered lung mechanics and increased work of breathing will cause a further step-up in nerve traffic; indeed, it is those patients with short shallow breaths who display the highest values for MSNA.[165]

Arterial baroreceptor reflex-mediated increases in cardiac or peripheral sympathetic outflow (in response to decreases in stroke volume, ventricular inotropy, or blood pressure) are present in the majority of patients with LV systolic dysfunction, but the intensity of this response will differ between individuals, depending upon the magnitude of hemodynamic compromise. Other sympathoexcitatory stimuli that act to elevate the set point for central sympathetic outflow or neurotransmitter release above levels required to maintain hemodynamic stability, such as elevated atrial pressures, the coexistance of sleep-related breathing disorders, and chemoreceptor or muscle metaboreceptor activation will vary from patient to patient. The induction of inflammation may initiate an additional cascade of catecholamines.[360] Without characterizing the extent of these several sympathoexcitatory mechanisms, one cannot be certain that the magnitude of adrenergic activation in a particular patient is best can be managed solely with sympatho-modulatary therapies, such as β-adrenergic antagonism and angiotensin-converting enzyme (ACE) inhibition, or requires additional specific pharmacological and nonpharmacological interventions.

FUTURE DIRECTIONS

Therapies that modulate sympathetic and vagal outflow or antagonize the postjunctional actions of neurally released and circulating catecholamines lower mortality rate and decrease morbidity. Whether there is a direct causal relationship between these neural effects of therapy and improved outcomes and whether patients with heart failure but preserved systolic function exhibit similar alterations in sympathetic and parasympathetic function by these several baroreflex and nonbaroreflex-mediated mechanisms are two important hypotheses for future investigation.

REFERENCES

1. Francis, G. S., Goldsmith, S. R., Levine, T. B., et al. (1984). The neurohumoral axis in congestive heart failure. *Ann Intern Med*, *101*, 370–377.
2. Hirsch, A. T., Dzau, V. J., & Creager, M. A. (1987). Baroreceptor function in congestive heart failure: effect on neurohumoral activation and regional vascular resistance. *Circulation*, *75*, IV-36–IV-48.
3. Swedberg, K., Eneroth, P., Kjekshus, J., et al. (1990). Hormones regulating cardiovascular function in patients with severe congestive heart failure and their relation to mortality. CONSENSUS trial study group. *Circulation*, *82*, 1730–1736.
4. Benedict, C. R., Johnstone, D. E., Weiner, D. H., et al. (1994). Relation of neurohumoral activation to clinical variables and degree of ventricular dysfunction: a report from the registry of studies of left ventricular dysfunction. SOLVD investigators. *J Am Coll Cardiol*, *23*, 1410–1420.
5. Cohn, J. N., Levine, T. B., Olivari, M. T., et al. (1984). Plasma norepinephrine as a guide to prognosis in patients with chronic congestive heart failure. *N Engl J Med*, *311*, 819–824.
6. Kaye, D. M., Lefkovits, J., Jennings, G. L., et al. (1995). Adverse consequences of high sympathetic nervous activity in the failing human heart. *J Am Coll Cardiol*, *26*, 1257–1263.
7. Nolan, J., Batin, P. D., Andrews, R., et al. (1998). Prospective study of heart rate variability and mortality in chronic heart failure: results of the United Kingdom heart failure evaluation and assessment of risk trial (UK). *Circulation*, *98*, 1510–1516.
8. Szabo, B. M., van Veldhuisen, D. J., van der Veer, N., et al. (1997). Prognostic value of heart rate variability in chronic heart failure secondary to idiopathic or ischemic dilated cardiomyopathy. *Am J Cardiol*, *79*, 978–980.
9. La Rovere, M. T., Bigger, J. T., Marcus, F. I., et al. (1998). Baroreflex sensitivity and heart rate variability in prediction of total cardiac mortality after myocardial infarction. *Lancet*, *351*, 478–484.
10. Mortara, T. A., La Rovere, M. T., Pinna, G., et al. (1997). Arterial baroreflex modulation of heart rate in chronic heart failure. *Circulation*, *96*, 3450–3458.
11. Galinier, M., Pathak, A., Fourcade, J., et al. (2000). Depressed low frequency power of heart rate variability as an independent predictor of sudden death in chronic heart failure. *Eur Heart J*, *21*, 475–482.
12. Ponikowski, P., Anker, S. D., Chua, T. P., et al. (1997). Depressed heart rate variability as an independent predictor of death in chronic congestive heart failure is secondary to ischemia or idiopathic dilated cardiomyopathy. *Am J Cardiol*, *79*, 1645–1650.
13. Francis, G. S., Benedict, D. E., Johnstone, D. E., et al. (1990). Comparison of neuroendocrine activation in patients with left ventricular dysfunction with and without congestive heart failure. A substudy of the studies of left ventricular dysfunction (SOLVD). *Circulation*, *82*, 1724–1729.
14. Notarius, C. F., Atchison, D. J., & Floras, J. S. (2001). Impact of heart failure and exercise capacity on sympathetic response to handgrip exercise. *Am J Physiol*, *280*, H969–H976.
15. Rundqvist, B., Elam, M., Bergman-Sverrisdottir, Y., et al. (1997). Increased cardiac adrenergic drive precedes generalized sympathetic activation in human heart failure. *Circulation*, *95*, 169–175.
16. Viquerat, C. E., Daly, P., Swedberg, K., et al. (1985). Endogenous catecholamine levels in chronic heart failure. *Am J Med*, *78*, 455–460.
17. Floras, J. S. (1993). Clinical aspects of sympathetic activation and parasympathetic withdrawal in heart failure. *J Am Coll Cardiol*, *22*, 72A–84A.
18. Floras, J. S. (2001). Arterial baroreceptor and cardiopulmonary reflex control of sympathetic outflow in human heart failure. *Ann N Y Acad Sci*, *940*, 500–513.
19. Floras, J. S. (2002). The "unsympathetic" nervous system of heart failure. *Circulation*, *105*, 1753–1755.
20. Zile, M. R., Gaasch, W. H., Carroll, J. D., et al. (2001). Heart failure with a normal ejection fraction: is measurement of diastolic function necessary to make the diagnosis of diastolic heart failure? *Circulation*, *104*, 779–782.
21. Folkow, B., DiBona, G. F., Hjemdahl, P., et al. (1983). Measurements of plasma norepinephrine concentrations in human primary hypertension: a word of caution on their applicability for assessing neurogenic contributions. *Hypertension*, *5*, 399–403.
22. Floras, J. S., Jones, J. V., Hassan, M. O., et al. (1986). Failure of plasma norepinephrine to consistently reflect sympathetic activity in humans. *Hypertension*, *8*, 641–649.
23. Esler, M., Jennings, G., Korner, P., et al. (1988). Assessment of human sympathetic nervous system activity from measurements of norepinephrine turnover. *Hypertension*, *11*, 3–20.
24. Goldstein, D. S., Zimlichman, R., Stull, R., et al. (1986). Estimation of intrasynaptic norepinephrine concentrations in humans. *Hypertension*, *8*, 471–475.
25. Newton, G. E., & Parker, J. D. (1996). Cardiac sympathetic responses to acute vasodilation: normal ventricular function versus congestive heart failure. *Circulation*, *94*, 3161–3167.
26. Brunner-La Rocca, H. P., Esler, M. D., Jennings, G. L., et al. (2001). Effect of cardiac sympathetic nervous activity on mode of death in congestive heart failure. *Eur Heart J*, *22*, 1069–1071.
27. Eisenhofer, G., Esler, M. D., Meredith, I. T., et al. (1992). Sympathetic nervous function in human heart as assessed by cardiac spillovers of dihydroxyphenylglycol and norepinephrine. *Circulation*, *85*, 1775–1785.
28. Wallin, B. G., & Fagius, J. (1988). Peripheral sympathetic neural activity in conscious humans. *Ann Rev Physiol*, *50*, 565–576.
29. Macefield, V. A., Rundqvist, B., Sverrisdottir, Y. B., et al. (1999). Firing properties of single muscle vasoconstrictor neurons in the sympathoexcitation associated with congestive heart failure. *Circulation*, *100*, 1708–1713.

30. Sanders, J. S., & Ferguson, D. W. (1989). Diastolic pressure determines autonomic responses to pressure perturbations in humans. *J Appl Physiol, 66*, 800–807.
31. Floras, J. S. (1990). Sympathoinhibitory effects of atrial natriuretic factor in normal humans. *Circulation, 81*, 1860–1873.
32. Mark, A. L., Victor, R. G., Nerhed, C., et al. (1985). Microneurographic studies of the mechanisms of sympathetic nerve responses to static exercise in humans. *Circ Res, 57*, 461–469.
33. Somers, V. K., Mark, A. L., Zavala, D. C., et al. (1989). Contrasting effects of hypoxia and hypercapnia on ventilation and sympathetic activity in humans. *J Appl Physiol, 67*, 2101–2106.
34. Narkiewicz, K., & Somers, V. K. (1997). The sympathetic nervous system and obstructive sleep apnea: implications for hypertension. *J Hypertens, 15*, 1613–1619.
35. Seals, D. R., Suwarno, N. O., Joyner, M. J., et al. (1993). Respiratory modulation of muscle sympathetic nerve activity in intact and lung denervated humans. *Circ Res, 72*, 440–454.
36. Grassi, G., Bolla, G., Quart-Trevano, F., et al. (2008). Sympathetic activation in congestive heart failure: reproducibility of neuroadrenergic markers. *Eur J Heart Fail, 10*, 1186–1191.
37. Wallin, B. G., Thompson, J. M., Jennings, G. L., et al. (1996). Renal noradrenaline spillover correlates with muscle sympathetic activity in humans. *J Physiol, 491*(pt 3), 881–887.
38. Wallin, B. G., Esler, M. D., Dorward, P., et al. (1992). Simultaneous measurements of cardiac norepinephrine spillover and sympathetic outflow to skeletal muscle. *J Physiol, 453*, 59–67.
39. Parati, G., Di Rienzo, M., & Mancia, G. (2000). How to measure baroreflex sensitivity: from the cardiovascular laboratory to daily life. *J Hypertens, 19*, 157–161.
40. Casadei, B., & Paterson, D. J. (2000). Should we still use nitrovasodilators to test baroreflex sensitivity? *J Hypertens, 18*, 3–6.
41. Mark, A. L., & Mancia, G. (1983). Cardiopulmonary baroreflexes in humans. In J. T. Shepherd & F. M. Abboud (Eds.), *Handbook of physiology, section 2: the cardiovascular system, vol. III: peripheral circulation and organ blood flow, part II*. Bethesda, MD: American Physiological Society.
42. Sopher, S. M., Smith, M. L., Eckberg, D. W., et al. (1990). Autonomic pathophysiology in heart failure: carotid baroreceptor-cardiac reflexes. *Am J Physiol, 259*, H689–H696.
43. Parlow, J., Viale, J. P., Annat, G., et al. (1995). Spontaneous cardiac baroreflex in humans. Comparison with drug-induced responses. *Hypertension, 25*, 1058–1068.
44. Persson, P. B., Di Rienzo, M., Castiglioni, P., et al. (2001). Time versus frequency domain techniques for assessing baroreflex sensitivity. *J Hypertens, 19*, 1699–1705.
45. Kornet, L., Hocks, A. P., Janssen, B. J., et al. (2002). Carotid diameter variations as a non-invasive tool to examine cardiac baroreceptor sensitivity. *J Hypertens, 20*, 1165–1173.
46. Grassi, G., Seravalle, G., Cattaneo, B. M., et al. (1995). Sympathetic activation and loss of reflex sympathetic control in mild congestive heart failure. *Circulation, 92*, 3206–3211.
47. Imaizumi, T., Sugimachi, M., Harasawa, Y., et al. (1993). Contribution of wall mechanics to the dynamic properties of aortic baroreceptor. *Am J Physiol, 264*, H872–H880.
48. Bath, E., Lindblad, L. E., & Wallin, G. B. (1981). Effects of dynamic and static neck suction on muscle nerve sympathetic activity, heart rate and blood pressure in man. *J Physiol, 311*, 551–564.
49. Ando, S., Dajani, H. R., Senn, B. L., et al. (1997). Sympathetic alternans. Evidence for arterial baroreflex control of muscle sympathetic nerve activity in congestive heart failure. *Circulation, 95*, 316–319.
50. Floras, J. S., Hassan, M. O., Jones, J. V., et al. (1988). Factors influencing blood pressure and heart rate variability in hypertensive humans. *Hypertension, 11*, 273–281.
51. Task force of the European Society of Cardiology and the North American Society of Pacing and Electrophysiology. (1996). Heart rate variability: standards of measurement piacu. *Circulation, 93*, 1043–1065.
52. Malliani, A., Pagani, M., Lombardi, F., et al. (1991). Cardiovascular neural regulation explored in the frequency domain. *Circulation, 84*, 482–492.
53. Pagani, M., & Malliani, A. (1994). Power spectral analysis of heart rate variability to assess the changes in sympathovagal balance during graded orthostatic tilt. *Circulation, 90*, 1826–1831.
54. Pomeranz, B., Macaulay, R. J. B., Caudill, M. A., et al. (1985). Assessment of autonomic function in humans by heart rate spectral analysis. *Am J Physiol, 248*, H151–H153.
55. Yamamoto, Y., & Hughson, R. L. (1991). Coarse-graining spectral analysis: new method for studying heart rate variability. *J Appl Physiol, 71*, 1143–1150.
56. Goldberger, A. L. (1990). Fractal electrodynamics of the heartbeat. *Ann N Y Acad Sci, 591*, 402–409.
57. Butler, G. C., Yamamoto, Y., Xing, H. C., et al. (1993). Heart rate variability and fractal dimension during orthostatic challenges. *J Appl Physiol, 75*, 2602–2612.
58. Notarius, C. F., & Floras, J. S. (2001). Limitations of the use of spectral analysis of heart rate variability for the estimation of cardiac sympathetic activity in heart failure. *Europace, 3*, 29–38.
59. Scalvini, S., Volterrani, M., & Zanelli, E. (1998). Is heart rate variability a reliable method to assess autonomic modulation in left ventricular dysfunction and heart failure? Assessment of autonomic modulation with heart rate variability. *Int J Cardiol, 67*, 9–17.
60. Eckberg, D. L. (1997). Sympathovagal balance: a critical appraisal. *Circulation, 96*, 3224–3232.
61. Pagani, M., Lombardi, F., & Malliani, A. (1993). Heart rate variability: disagreement on the markers of sympathetic and parasympathetic activities. *J Am Coll Cardiol, 22*, 951–953.
62. Floras, J. S., Butler, G. C., Ando, S. I., et al. (2001). Differential sympathetic nerve and heart rate spectral effects of nonhypotensive lower body negative pressure. *Am J Physiol 281*, R468–R475.
63. Mortara, T. A., La Rovere, M. T., Signorini, M. G., et al. (1994). Can power spectral analysis of heart rate variability identify a high risk subgroup of congestive heart failure patients with excessive sympathetic activation? A pilot study before and after heart transplantation. *Br Heart J, 71*, 422–430.
64. Rimoldi, O., Pierini, S., Ferrari, A., et al. (1990). Analysis of short term oscillations of R-R and arterial pressure in conscious dogs. *Am J Physiol, 258*, H967–H976.
65. Nakamura, Y., Yamamoto, Y., & Muraoka, I. (1993). Autonomic control of heart rate during physical exercise and fractal dimension of heart rate variability. *J Appl Physiol, 74*, 875–881.
66. Miyajima, E., Sawada, R., Shigemasa, T., et al. (1997). LF/HF ratio as an index of sympathetic nerve activity in humans. *Hypertension, 29*, 908.
67. Butler, G. C., Yamamoto, Y., & Hughson, R. L. (1994). Heart rate variability to monitor autonomic nervous system activity during orthostatic stress. *J Clin Pharmacol, 34*, 558–562.
68. Saul, J. P., Berger, R. D., Albrecht, P., et al. (1991). Transfer function analysis of the circulation: unique insights into cardiovascular regulation. *Am J Physiol, 261*, H1231–H1245.
69. Akselrod, S., Gordon, D., Ubel, F. A., et al. (1981). Power spectrum analysis of heart rate fluctuation: a quantitative probe of beat-to-beat cardiovascular control. *Science, 213*, 220–222.
70. Kingwell, B. A., Thompson, J. M., Kaye, D. M., et al. (1994). Heart rate spectral analysis, cardiac norepinephrine spillover, and muscle sympathetic nerve activity during human sympathetic nervous activation and failure. *Circulation, 90*, 234–240.
71. Pagani, M., Montano, N., Porta, A., et al. (1997). Relationship between spectral components of cardiovascular variabilities and direct measures of muscle sympathetic nerve activity in humans. *Circulation, 95*, 1441–1448.
72. Ando, S., Dajani, H. R., & Floras, J. S. (1997). Frequency domain characteristics of muscle sympathetic nerve activity in heart failure and healthy humans. *Am J Physiol, 273*, R205–R212.
73. Pitzalis, M. V., Mastropasqua, F., Passantino, A., et al. (1998). Comparison between noninvasive indices of baroreceptor sensitivity and the phenylephrine method in post-myocardial infarction patients. *Circulation, 97*, 1362–1367.
74. Hasking, G. J., Esler, M. D., Jennings, G. L., et al. (1986). Norepinephrine spillover to plasma in patients with congestive heart failure: evidence of increased overall and cardiorenal sympathetic nervous activity. *Circulation, 73*, 615–621.
75. Ramchandra, R., Hood, S. G., Denton, D. A., et al. (2009). Basis for the preferential activation of cardiac sympathetic nerve activity in heart failure. *Proc Natl Acad Sci U S A, 106*, 924–928.
76. Kaye, D. M., Lefkovits, J., Cox, H., et al. (1995). Regional epinephrine kinetics in human heart failure: evidence for extra-adrenal, nonneural release. *Am J Physiol, 269*, H182–H188.
77. Esler, M., Eisenhofer, G., Chin, J., et al. (1991). Is adrenaline released by sympathetic nerves in man? *Clin Auton Res, 1*, 103–108.
78. Floras, J. S., Aylward, P. E., Victor, R. G., et al. (1988). Epinephrine facilitates neurogenic vasoconstriction in humans. *J Clin Invest, 81*, 1265–1274.
79. Leimbach, W. N., Wallin, B. G., Victor, R. G., et al. (1986). Direct evidence from intraneural recordings for increased central sympathetic outflow in patients with heart failure. *Circulation, 73*, 913–919.
80. Hara, K., & Floras, J. S. (1996). After-effects of exercise on haemodynamics and muscle sympathetic nerve activity in young patients with dilated cardiomyopathy. *Heart, 75*, 602–608.
81. Elam, M., & Macefield, V. (2001). Multiple firing of single muscle vasoconstrictor neurons during cardiac dysrhythmias in human heart failure. *J Appl Physiol, 91*, 717–724.
82. Middlekauff, H. R., Hamilton, M. A., Stevenson, L. W., et al. (1994). Independent control of skin and muscle sympathetic nerve activity in patients with heart failure. *Circulation, 90*, 1794–1798.
83. Notarius, C. F., Ando, S., Rongen, G. A., et al. (1999). Resting muscle sympathetic nerve activity and peak oxygen uptake in heart failure and normal subjects. *Eur Heart J, 20*, 880–887.
84. Roveda, F., Middlekauff, H. R., Rondon, M. U., et al. (2003). The effects of exercise training on sympathetic neural activation in advanced heart failure: a randomized controlled trial. *J Am Coll Cardiol, 42*, 854–860.
85. Spaak, J., Egri, Z. J., Kubo, T., et al. (2005). Muscle sympathetic nerve activity during wakefulness in heart failure patients with and without sleep apnea. *Hypertension, 46*, 1327–1332.
86. van de Borne, P., Montano, N., Pagani, M., et al. (1997). Absence of low frequency variability of sympathetic nerve activity in severe heart failure. *Circulation, 95*, 1449–1454.
87. Eckberg, D. L., Drabinsky, M., & Braunwald, E. (1971). Defective cardiac parasympathetic control in patients with heart disease. *N Engl J Med, 285*, 877–883.
88. Ferguson, D. W., Berg, W. J., Roach, P. J., et al. (1992). Effects of heart failure on baroreflex control of sympathetic neural activity. *Am J Cardiol, 69*, 523–531.
89. La Rovere, M. T., Pinna, G. D., Maestri, R., et al. (2009). Prognostic implications of baroreflex sensitivity in heart failure patients in the beta-blocking era. *J Am Coll Cardiol, 53*, 193–199.
90. Porter, T. R., Eckberg, D. L., Fritsch, J. M., et al. (1990). Autonomic pathophysiology in heart failure patients. Sympathetic-cholinergic interrelations. *J Clin Invest, 85*, 1362–1371.
91. Saul, J. P., Arai, Y., Berger, R. D., et al. (1988). Assessment of autonomic regulation in chronic congestive heart failure by heart rate spectral analysis. *Am J Cardiol, 61*, 1292–1299.
92. Binkley, P. F., Nunziata, E., Haas, G. J., et al. (1991). Parasympathetic withdrawal is an integral component of autonomic imbalance in congestive heart failure: demonstration in human subjects and verification in a paced canine model of ventricular failure. *J Am Coll Cardiol, 18*, 464–472.
93. Van Hoogenhuyze, D. V., Weinstein, N., Martin, G. J., et al. (1991). Reproducibility and relation to mean heart rate of heart rate variability in normal subjects and in patients with congestive heart failure secondary to coronary artery disease. *Am J Cardiol, 68*, 1668–1676.
94. Amorim, D. S., Dargie, H. J., Heer, K., et al. (1981). Is there autonomic impairment in congestive (dilated) heart failure? *Lancet, 1*, 525–527.
95. Nousiainen, T., Vanninen, E., Jantunen, E., et al. (2001). Neuroendocrine changes during the elevation of doxorubicin-induced left ventricular dysfunction in adult lymphoma patients. *Clin Sci, 101*, 601–607.

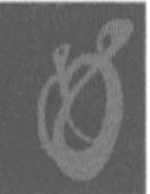

96. Notarius, C. F., Butler, G. C., Ando, S., et al. (1999). Dissociation between microneurographic and heart rate variability estimates of sympathetic tone in normal and heart failure subjects. *Clin Sci, 96*, 557–565.
97. Butler, G. C., Ando, S. I., & Floras, J. S. (1997). Fractal component of variability of heart rate and systolic blood pressure in congestive heart failure. *Clin Sci, 92*, 543–550.
98. Guzzetti, S., Cogliati, C., Turiel, M., et al. (1995). Sympathetic predominance followed by functional denervation in the progression of chronic heart failure. *Eur Heart J, 16*, 1100–1107.
99. Malik, M., & Camm, J. (1993). Components of heart rate variability — what they really mean and what we really measure. *Am J Cardiol, 72*, 821–822.
100. Casadei, B., Cochrane, S., Johnston, J., et al. (1995). Pitfalls in the interpretation of spectral analysis of the heart rate variability during exercise in humans. *Acta Physiol Scand, 153*, 125–131.
101. Piepoli, M., Adamopoulos, S., Bernardi, L., et al. (1995). Sympathetic stimulations by exercise-stress testing and by dobutamine infusion induce similar changes in heart rate variability in patients with chronic heart failure. *Clin Sci, 89*, 155–164.
102. Benedict, C. R., Weiner, D. H., Johnson, D. E., et al. (1993). Comparative neurohormonal responses in patients with preserved and impaired left ventricular function. Results of the studies of left ventricular dysfunction (SOLVD) registry. *J Am Coll Cardiol, 22*, 146A–153A.
103. Kitzman, D. W., Little, W. C., Brubaker, P. H., et al. (2002). Pathophysiological characterization of isolated diastolic heart failure in comparison to systolic heart failure. *JAMA, 288*, 2144–2150.
104. Hogg, K., & McMurray, J. (2005). Neurohumoral pathways in heart failure with preserved systolic function. *Prog Cardiovasc Dis, 47*, 357–366.
105. Arora, R., Krummerman, A., Vijayaraman, P., et al. (2004). Heart rate variability and diastolic heart failure. *Pacing Clin Electrophysiol, 27*, 299–303.
106. Grassi, G., Seravalle, G., Quarti-Trevano, F., et al. (2009). Sympathetic and baroreflex cardiovascular control in hypertension-related left ventricular dysfunction. *Hypertension, 53*, 205–209.
107. Gandhi, S. K., Powers, J. C., & Nomeir, A. M. (2001). The pathogenesis of acute pulmonary edema associated with hypertension. *N Engl J Med, 344*, 17–22.
108. Mann, D. L., Kent, R. L., Parsons, B., et al. (1992). Adrenergic effects on the biology of the adult mammalian cardiocyte. *Circulation, 85*, 790–804.
109. Akiyama-uchida, Y., Ashizawa, N., Ohtsuru, A., et al. (2002). Norepinephrine enhances fibrosis mediated by TGF-beta in cardiac fibroblasts. *Hypertension, 40*, 148–154.
110. Colucci, W. S., Ribeiro, J. P., Rocco, M. B., et al. (1989). Impaired chronotropic response to exercise in patients with congestive heart failure: role of postsynaptic beta-adrenergic desensitization. *Circulation, 80*, 314–323.
111. Dash, R., Kadambi, V. J., Schmidt, A. G., et al. (2001). Interactions between phospholamban and beta-adrenergic drive may lead to cardiomyopathy and early mortality. *Circulation, 103*, 889–896.
112. Lefkowitz, R. J., Rockman, H. A., & Koch, W. J. (2000). Catecholamines, cardiac beta-adrenergic receptors, and heart failure. *Circulation, 101*, 1634–1637.
113. Fowler, M. B., Laser, J. A., Hopkins, G. L., et al. (1986). Assessment of the beta-adrenergic receptor pathway in the intact failing human heart: progressive receptor down regulation and subsensitivity to agonist response. *Circulation, 74*, 1290–1302.
114. Marks, A. R., Reiken, S., & Marx, S. O. (2002). Progression of heart failure. Is protein kinase a hyperphosphorylation of the ryanodine receptor a contributing factor? *Circulation, 105*, 272–275.
115. Murray, D. R., Prabhu, S. D., & Chandrasekar, B. (2000). Chronic beta-adrenergic stimulation induces myocardial proinflammatory cytokine expression. *Circulation, 101*, 2338–2341.
116. Givertz, M. M., Sawyer, D. B., & Colucci, W. S. (2001). Antioxidants and myocardial contractility illuminating the "dark side" of beta-adrenergic receptor activation? *Circulation, 103*, 782–783.
117. Daly, P. A., & Sole, M. J. (1990). Myocardial catecholamines and the pathophysiology of heart failure. *Circulation, 82*, 35–43.
118. Olshansky, B., Sabbah, H. N., Hauptman, P. J., et al. (2008). Parasympathetic nervous system and heart failure: pathophysiology and potential implications for therapy. *Circulation, 118*, 863–871.
119. DiBona, G. F. (1991). Sympathetic neural control of the kidney in hypertension. *Hypertension, 19*, I-28.
120. Morali, G. A., Floras, J. S., Legault, L., et al. (1991). Muscle sympathetic nerve activity and renal responsiveness to atrial natriuretic factor during development of hepatic ascites. *Am J Med, 91*, 383–392.
121. Cohen-Solal, A., Logeart, D., Dahan, M., et al. (1999). Cardiac and peripheral responses to exercise in patients with chronic heart failure. *Eur Heart J, 20*, 931–945.
122. Wagoner, L. E., Craft, L. L., Singh, B., et al. (2000). Polymorphisms of the beta(2)-adrenergic receptor determine exercise capacity in patients with heart failure. *Circ Res, 86*, 834–840.
123. Shoemaker, J. K., Kunselman, A. R., Silber, D. H., et al. (1998). Maintained exercise pressor response in heart failure. *J Appl Physiol, 85*, 1793–1799.
124. Shoemaker, J. K., Naylor, H. L., Hogeman, C. S., et al. (1999). Blood flow dynamics in heart failure. *Circulation, 99*, 3002–3008.
125. Notarius, C. F., Azevedo, E. R., Parker, J. D., et al. (2001). Peak oxygen uptake is not determined by cardiac norepinephrine spillover in heart failure. *Eur Heart J, 23*, 800–805.
126. Benedict, C. R., Shelton, B., Johnstone, D. E., et al. (1996). Prognostic significance of plasma norepinephrine in patients with asymptomatic left ventricular dysfunction. SOLVD investigators. *Circulation, 94*, 690–697.
127. Zugck, C., Haunstetter, A., Kruger, C., et al. (2002). Impact of beta-blocker treatment on the prognostic value of currently used risk predictors in congestive heart failure. *J Am Coll Cardiol, 39*, 1615–1622.
128. Barretto, A. C., Santos, A. C., Munhoz, R., et al. (2009). Increased muscle sympathetic nerve activity predicts mortality in heart failure patients. *Int J Cardiol 135*, 302–307.
129. Meredith, I. T., Broughton, A., Jennings, G. L., et al. (1991). Evidence of a selective increase in cardiac sympathetic activity in patients with sustained ventricular arrhythmias. *N Engl J Med, 325*, 618–624.
130. Eisenhofer, G., Friberg, P., Rundqvist, B., et al. (1996). Cardiac sympathetic nerve function in congestive heart failure. *Circulation, 93*, 1667–1676.
131. Merlet, P., Benvenuti, C., Moyse, D., et al. (1999). Prognostic value of MIBG imaging in idiopathic dilated cardiomyopathy. *J Nucl Med, 40*, 917–923.
132. Tamaki, S., Yamada, T., Okuyama, Y., et al. (2009). Cardiac iodine-123 metaiodobenzylguanidine imaging predicts sudden cardiac death independently of left ventricular ejection fraction in patients with chronic heart failure and left ventricular systolic dysfunction: results from a comparative study with signal-averaged electrocardiogram, heart rate variability, and QT dispersion. *J Am Coll Cardiol, 53*, 426–435.
133. Bigger, J. T., Steinman, R. C., Rolnitzky, L. M., et al. (1996). Power law behaviour of RR-interval variability in healthy middle-aged persons, patients with recent acute myocardial infarction, and patients with heart transplants. *Circulation, 93*, 2142–2151.
134. Wang, W., Chen, J. S., & Zucker, I. H. (1990). Carotid sinus baroreceptor sensitivity in experimental heart failure. *Circulation, 81*, 1959–1966.
135. Dibner Dunlap, M. E., & Thames, M. D. (1989). Baroreflex control of renal sympathetic nerve activity is preserved in heart failure despite reduced arterial baroreceptor sensitivity. *Circ Res, 65*, 1526–1535.
136. DiBona, G. F., & Sawin, L. L. (1994). Reflex regulation of renal nerve activity in cardiac failure. *Am J Physiol, 266*, R27–R39.
137. Zucker, J. H., Wang, W., Brande, M., et al. (1995). Neural regulation of sympathetic nerve activity in heart failure. *Prog Cardiovasc Dis, 37*, 397–414.
138. Bibevski, S., & Dunlap, M. E. (1999). Ganglionic mechanisms contribute to diminished vagal control in heart failure. *Circulation, 99*, 2958–2963.
139. Newton, G. E., Parker, A. B., Landzberg, J. S., et al. (1996). Muscarinic receptor modulation of basal and beta-adrenergic stimulated function of the failing human left ventricle. *J Clin Invest, 98*, 2756–2763.
140. Dunlap, M. E., Bibevski, S., Rosenberry, T. L., et al. (2003). Mechanisms of altered vagal control in heart failure: influence of muscarinic receptors and acetylcholinesterase activity. *Am J Physiol, 285*, H1632–H1640.
141. Bristow, M. R. (1993). Changes in myocardial and vascular receptors in heart failure. *J Am Coll Cardiol, 22*, 61A–71A.
142. Brandle, M., Patel, K. P., Wang, W., et al. (1996). Hemodynamic and norepinephrine responses to pacing-induced heart failure in conscious sinoaortic-denervated dogs. *J Appl Physiol, 81*, 1855–1862.
143. Ferguson, D. W., Berg, W. J., & Sanders, J. S. (1990). Clinical and hemodynamic correlates of sympathetic nerve activity in normal humans and patients with heart failure: evidence from direct microneurographic recordings. *J Am Coll Cardiol, 16*, 1125–1134.
144. Kaye, D. M., Lambert, G. W., Lefkovits, J., et al. (1994). Neurochemical evidence of cardiac sympathetic activation and increased central nervous system norepinephrine turnover in severe congestive heart failure. *J Am Coll Cardiol, 23*, 570–578.
145. Dibner-Dunlap, M. E., Smith, M. L., Kinugawa, T., et al. (1996). Enalaprilat augments arterial and cardiopulmonary baroreflex control of sympathetic nerve activity in patients with heart failure. *J Am Coll Cardiol, 27*, 358–364.
146. Dibner-Dunlap, M. E. (1992). Arterial or cardiopulmonary baroreflex control of sympathetic nerve activity in heart failure? *Am J Cardiol, 70*, 1640–1642.
147. Grassi, G., Seravalle, G., Bertinieri, G., et al. (2002). Sympathetic response to ventricular extrasystolic beats in hypertension and heart failure. *Hypertension, 39*, 886–891.
148. Zucker, I. H., Hackley, J. F., Cornish, K. G., et al. (2007). Chronic baroreceptor activation enhances survival in dogs with pacing-induced heart failure. *Hypertension, 50*, 904–910.
149. Watson, A. M., Hood, S. G., Ramchandra, R., et al. (2007). Increased cardiac sympathetic nerve activity in heart failure is not due to desensitization of the arterial baroreflex. *Am J Physiol, 293*, H798–H804.
150. Al-Hesayen, A., & Parker, J. D. (2004). Impaired baroreceptor control of renal sympathetic activity in human chronic heart failure. *Circulation, 109*, 2862–2865.
151. Petersson, M., Friberg, P., Lambert, G., et al. (2005). Decreased renal sympathetic activity in response to cardiac unloading with nitroglycerin in patients with heart failure. *Eur J Heart Fail, 7*, 1003–1010.
152. Middlekauff, H. R., Nitzsche, E. U., Hamilton, M. A., et al. (1995). Evidence for preserved cardiopulmonary baroreflex control of renal cortical blood flow in humans with advanced heart failure. A positron emission tomography study. *Circulation, 92*, 395–401.
153. Ferguson, D. W., Thames, M. D., & Mark, A. L. (1983). Effects of propranolol on reflex vascular responses to orthostatic stress in humans: role of ventricular baroreceptors. *Circulation, 67*, 802–807.
154. Atherton, J. J., Moore, T. D., Lele, S. S., et al. (1997). Diastolic ventricular interaction in chronic heart failure. *Lancet, 349*, 1720–1724.
155. Azevedo, E. R., Newton, G. E., Floras, J. S., et al. (2000). Reducing cardiac filling pressure lowers cardiac norepinephrine spillover in patients with chronic heart failure. *Circulation, 101*, 2053–2059.
156. Wang, W., & Zucker, I. H. (1996). Cardiac sympathetic afferent reflex in dogs with congestive heart failure. *Am J Physiol, 271*, R751–R756.
157. Wang, W., Schultz, H. D., & Ma, R. (1999). Cardiac sympathetic afferent sensitivity is enhanced in heart failure. *Am J Physiol, 277*, H812–H817.
158. Wang, W., Schultz, H. D., & Ma, R. (2001). Volume expansion potentiates cardiac sympathetic afferent reflex in dogs. *Am J Physiol, 280*, H576–H581.
159. Malliani, A., & Montano, N. (2002). Emerging excitatory role of cardiovascular sympathetic afferents in pathophysiological conditions. *Hypertension, 39*, 63–68.
160. Kaye, D. M., Jennings, G. L., Dart, A. M., et al. (1998). Differential effect of acute baroreceptor unloading on cardiac and systemic sympathetic tone in congestive heart failure. *J Am Coll Cardiol, 31*, 583–587.
161. Kaye, D. M., Mansfield, D., Aggarwal, A., et al. (2001). Acute effects of continuous positive airway pressure on cardiac sympathetic tone in congestive heart failure. *Circulation, 103*, 2336–2338.

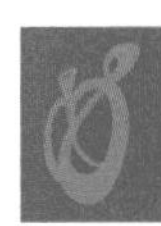

162. Volpe, M., Tritto, C., De Luca, N., et al. (1991). Failure of atrial natriuretic factor to increase with saline load in patients with dilated cardiomyopathy and mild heart failure. *J Clin Invest, 88*, 1481–1489.
163. Narkiewicz, K., van de Borne, P., Montano, N., et al. (2006). Sympathetic neural outflow and chemoreflex sensitivity are related to spontaneous breathing rate in normal men. *Hypertension, 47*, 51–55.
164. Goso, Y., Asanoi, H., Ishise, H., et al. (2001). Respiratory modulation of muscle sympathetic nerve activity in patients with chronic heart failure. *Circulation, 104*, 418–423.
165. Naughton, M. T., Floras, J. S., Rahman, M. A., et al. (1998). Respiratory correlates of muscle sympathetic nerve activity in heart failure. *Clin Sci, 95*, 277–285.
166. Kappagoda, C. T., & Ravi, K. (2006). The rapidly adapting receptors in mammalian airways and their responses to changes in extravascular fluid volume. *Exp Physiol, 91*, 647–654.
167. Schultz, H. D., Li, Y. L., & Ding, Y. (2007). Arterial chemoreceptors and sympathetic nerve activity: implications for hypertension and heart failure. *Hypertension, 50*, 6–13.
168. Xie, A., Skatrud, J. B., Puleo, D. S., et al. (2001). Exposure to hypoxia produces long-lasting sympathetic activation in humans. *J Appl Physiol, 91*, 1551–1562.
169. Ponikowski, P. P., Chua, T. P., Anker, S. D., et al. (2001). Peripheral chemoreceptor hypersensitivity: an ominous sign in patients with chronic heart failure. *Circulation, 104*, 544–549.
170. Giannoni, A., Emdin, M., Poletti, R., et al. (2008). Clinical significance of chemosensitivity in chronic heart failure: influence on neurohormonal derangement, Cheyne-Stokes respiration and arrhythmias. *Clin Sci, 114*, 489–497.
171. van de Borne, P., Oren, R., Anderson, E. A., et al. (1996). Tonic chemoreflex activation does not contribute to elevated muscle sympathetic nerve activity in heart failure. *Circulation, 94*, 1325–1328.
172. Andreas, S., Binggeli, C., Mohacsi, P., et al. (2003). Nasal oxygen and muscle sympathetic nerve activity in heart failure. *Chest, 123*, 322–325.
173. Di Vanna, A., Braga, A. M., Laterza, M. C., et al. (2007). Blunted muscle vasodilatation during chemoreceptor stimulation in patients with heart failure. *Am J Physiol, 293*, H846–H852.
174. Stickland, M. K., Miller, J. D., Smith, C. A., et al. (2007). Carotid chemoreceptor modulation of regional blood flow distribution during exercise in health and chronic heart failure. *Circ Res, 100*, 1371–1378.
175. Chua, T. P., Clark, A. L., Amadi, A. A., et al. (1996). Relation between chemosensitivity and the ventilatory response to exercise in chronic heart failure. *J Am Coll Cardiol, 27*, 650–657.
176. Chua, T. P., Ponikowski, P., Webb-Peploe, K., et al. (1997). Clinical characteristics of chronic heart failure patients with an augmented peripheral chemoreflex. *Eur Heart J, 18*, 480–486.
177. Ponikowski, P., Chua, T. P., Piepoli, M., et al. (1997). Chemoreceptor dependence of very low frequency rhythms in advanced heart failure. *Am J Physiol, 272*, H438–H447.
178. Ponikowski, P., Chua, T. P., Piepoli, M., et al. (1997). Augmented peripheral chemosensitivity as a potential input to baroreflex impairment and autonomic imbalance in chronic heart failure. *Circulation, 96*, 2586–2594.
179. Staszewsky, L., Wong, M., Masson, S., et al. (2007). Clinical, neurohormonal, and inflammatory markers and overall prognostic role of chronic obstructive pulmonary disease in patients with heart failure: data from the Val-HeFT heart failure trial. *J Card Fail, 13*, 797–804.
180. Floras, J. S., & Sleight, P. (1983). Ambulatory monitoring of blood pressure. In P. Sleight & J. V. Jones (Eds.), *Scientific foundations of cardiology.* London: Heineman n, pp. 155–164.
181. Linsell, C. R., Lightman, S. L., Mullen, P. E., et al. (1985). Circadian rhythms of epinephrine and norepinephrine in man. *J Clin Endocrinol Metab, 60*, 1210–1215.
182. Somers, V. K., Dyken, M. E., Mark, A. L., et al. (1993). Sympathetic-nerve activity during sleep in normal subjects. *N Engl J Med, 328*, 303–307.
183. Khatri, I. M., & Freis, E. D. (1967). Hemodynamic changes during sleep. *J Appl Physiol, 22*, 867–873.
184. Smyth, H. S., Sleight, P., & Pickering, G. W. (1969). Reflex regulation of arterial pressure during sleep in man. A quantitative method of assessing baroreflex sensitivity. *Circ Res, 24*, 109–121.
185. van de Borne, P., Nguyen, H., Biston, P., et al. (1994). Effects of wake and sleep stages on the 24-h autonomic control of blood pressure and heart rate in recumbent men. *Am J Physiol, 266*, H548–H554.
186. Malone, S., Liu, P. P., Holloway, R., et al. (1991). Obstructive sleep apnea in patients with dilated cardiomyopathy: effects of continuous positive airway pressure. *Lancet, 338*, 1480–1484.
187. Arzt, M., Floras, J. S., Logan, A. G., et al. (2007). Suppression of central sleep apnea by continuous positive airway pressure and transplant-free survival in heart failure: a post hoc analysis of the Canadian positive airway pressure for patients with central sleep apnea and heart failure trial (CANPAP). *Circulation, 115*, 3173–3180.
188. Javaheri, S., Parker, T. J., Liming, J. D., et al. (1998). Sleep apnea in 81 ambulatory male patients with stable heart failure: types and their prevalences, consequences, and presentations. *Circulation, 97*, 2154–2159.
189. Sin, D., Fitzgerald, F., Parker, J. D., et al. (1999). Risk factors for central and obstructive sleep apnea in 450 men and women with congestive heart failure. *Am J Respir Crit Care Med, 160*, 1101–1106.
190. Somers, V. K., Dyken, M. E., Clary, M. P., et al. (1995). Sympathetic neural mechanisms in obstructive sleep apnea. *J Clin Invest, 96*, 1897–1904.
191. Morgan, B. J., Denahan, T., & Ebert, T. J. (1993). Neurocirculatory consequences of negative intrathoracic pressure vs. asphyxia during voluntary apnea. *J Appl Physiol, 74*, 2969–2975.
192. Somers, V. K., Mark, A. L., Zavala, D. C., et al. (1989). Influence of ventilation and hypocapnia on sympathetic nerve responses to hypoxia in normal humans. *J Appl Physiol, 67*, 2095–2100.
193. Somers, V. K., Mark, A. L., & Abboud, F. M. (1988). Sympathetic activation by hypoxia and hypercapnia—implications for sleep apnea. *Clin Exp Hypertens A, A10*, 413–422.
194. Bradley, T. D., Hall, M. J., Ando, S., et al. (2001). Hemodynamic effects of simulated obstructive apneas in humans with and without heart failure. *Chest, 119*, 1827–1835.
195. Bradley, T. D., Tkacova, R., Hall, M. J., et al. (2003). Augmented sympathetic neural response to simulated obstructive sleep apnoea in human heart failure. *Clin Sci, 104*, 231–238.
196. Narkiewicz, K., Montano, N., Cogliati, C., et al. (1998). Altered cardiovascular variability in obstructive sleep apnea. *Circulation, 98*, 1071–1077.
197. Brooks, D., Horner, R. L., Kozar, L. F., et al. (1997). Obstructive sleep apnea as a cause of systemic hypertension: evidence from a canine model. *J Clin Invest, 99*, 106–109.
198. Levy, D., Larson, M. G., Vasan, R. S., et al. (1996). The progression from hypertension to congestive heart failure. *JAMA, 275*, 1557–1562.
199. Hedner, J., Ejnell, H., Sellgren, J., et al. (1988). Is high and fluctuating muscle nerve sympathetic activity in the sleep apnoea syndrome of pathogenic importance for the development of hypertension? *J Hypertens, 6*, S529–S531.
200. Carlson, J. T., Hedner, J., Elam, M., et al. (1993). Augmented resting sympathetic activity in awake patients with obstructive sleep apnea. *Chest, 103*, 1763–1768.
201. Grassi, G., Seravalle, G., Quarti-Trevano, F., et al. (2003). Effects of hypertension and obesity on the sympathetic activation of heart failure patients. *Hypertension, 42*, 873–877.
202. Usui, K., Bradley, T. D., Spaak, J., et al. (2005). Inhibition of awake sympathetic nerve activity of heart failure patients with obstructive sleep apnea by nocturnal continuous positive airway pressure. *J Am Coll Cardiol, 45*, 2008–2011.
203. Abboud, F. M., & Thames, M. D. (1983). Interaction of cardiovascular reflexes in circulatory control. In J. T. Shepherd & F. M. Abboud (Eds.), *Handbook of physiology, section 2: the cardiovascular system, vol. III: peripheral circulation and organ blood flow, part 2.* Bethesda, MD: American Physiological Society, 675-753.
204. Wang, H., Parker, J. D., Newton, G. E., et al. (2007). Influence of obstructive sleep apnea on mortality in patients with heart failure. *J Am Coll Cardiol, 49*, 1625–1631.
205. Tkacova, R., Niroumand, M., Lorenzi-Filho, G., et al. (2001). Overnight shift from obstructive to central apneas in patients with heart failure: role of PCO_2 and circulatory delay. *Circulation, 103*, 238–243.
206. Naughton, M. T., Benard, D. C., Liu, P. P., et al. (1995). Effects of nasal CPAP on sympathetic activity in patients with heart failure and central sleep apnea. *Am J Respir Crit Care Med, 152*, 473–479.
207. Mansfield, D., Kaye, D., La Rocca, H., et al. (2003). Raised sympathetic nerve activity in heart failure and central sleep apnea is due to heart failure severity. *Circulation, 107*, 1396–1400.
208. Hainsworth, R. (1991). Reflexes from the heart. *Physiol Rev, 71*, 617–658.
209. Zipes, D. P. (1990). Influence of myocardial ischemia and infarction on autonomic innervation of heart. *Circulation, 82*, 1095–1105.
210. Minisi, A. J., & Thames, M. D. (1993). Distribution of left ventricular sympathetic afferents demonstrated by reflex responses to transmural myocardial ischemia and to intracoronary and epicardial bradykinin. *Circulation, 87*, 240–246.
211. Pan, H. L., & Chen, S. R. (2004). Sensing tissue ischemia: another new function for capsaicin receptors? *Circulation, 110*, 1826–1831.
212. Wei, J. Y., Markis, J. E., Malagold, M., et al. (1983). Cardiovascular reflexes stimulated by reperfusion of ischemic myocardium in acute myocardial infarction. *Circulation, 67*, 796–801.
213. Weaver, L. C., Danos, L. M., Oehl, R. S., et al. (1981). Contrasting reflex influences of cardiac nerves during coronary occlusion. *Am J Physiol, 240*, H620–H629.
214. Felder, R. B., & Thames, M. D. (1979). Interaction between cardiac receptors and sinoaortic baroreceptors in the control of efferent cardiac sympathetic nerve activity during myocardial ischemia in dogs. *Circ Res, 45*, 728–736.
215. Minisi, A. J., & Thames, M. D. (1989). Effect of chronic myocardial infarction on vagal cardiopulmonary baroreflex. *Circ Res, 65*, 396–405.
216. Graham, L. N., Smith, P. A., Stoker, J. B., et al. (2002). Time course of sympathetic neural hyperactivity after uncomplicated acute myocardial interaction. *Circulation, 106*, 793–797.
217. Deng, M. C., Brisse, B., Erren, M., et al. (1997). Ischemic versus idiopathic cardiomyopathy: differing neurohumoral profiles despite comparable peak oxygen uptake. *Int J Cardiol, 61*, 261–268.
218. Malfatto, G., Branzi, G., Gritti, S., et al. (2001). Different baseline sympathovagal balance and cardiac autonomic responsiveness in ischemic and non-ischemic congestive heart failure. *Eur J Heart Fail, 3*, 197–202.
219. Grassi, G., Seravalle, G., Bertinieri, G., et al. (2001). Sympathetic and reflex abnormalities in heart failure secondary to ischaemic or idiopathic dilated cardiomyopathy. *Clin Sci, 101*, 141–146.
220. Notarius, C. F., Spaak, J., Morris, B. L., et al. (2007). Comparison of muscle sympathetic activity in ischemic and nonischemic heart failure. *J Card Fail, 13*, 470–475.
221. Taylor, M., Wallhaus, T. R., Degrado, T. R., et al. (2001). An evaluation of myocardial fatty acid and glucose uptake using PET with [18F] fluoro-6-thia-heptadecanoic acid and [18F] FDG in patients with congestive heart failure. *J Nucl Med, 42*, 55–62.
222. Tuunanen, H., Engblom, E., Naum, A., et al. (2006). Decreased myocardial free fatty acid uptake in patients with idiopathic dilated cardiomyopathy: evidence of relationship with insulin resistance and left ventricular dysfunction. *J Card Fail, 12*, 644–652.
223. Lommi, J., Kupari, M., Koskinen, P., et al. (1996). Blood ketone bodies in congestive heart failure. *J Am Coll Cardiol, 28*, 665–672.
224. Rongen, G. A., Brooks, S. C., Ando, S., et al. (1998). Angiotensin AT1 receptor blockade abolishes the reflex sympatho-excitatory response to adenosine. *J Clin Invest, 101*, 769–776.
225. Notarius, C. F., Atchison, D. J., Rongen, G. A., et al. (2001). Effect of adenosine receptor blockade with caffeine on sympathetic response to handgrip exercise in heart failure. *Am J Physiol, 281*, H1312–H1318.

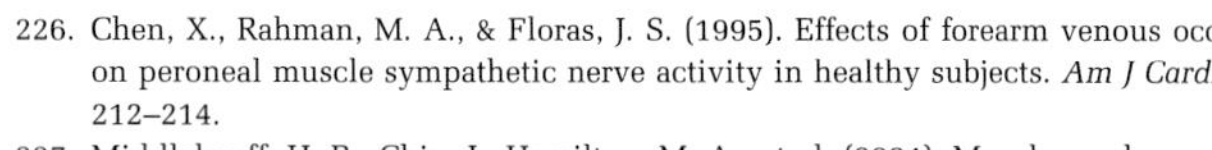

226. Chen, X., Rahman, M. A., & Floras, J. S. (1995). Effects of forearm venous occlusion on peroneal muscle sympathetic nerve activity in healthy subjects. *Am J Cardiol, 76*, 212–214.
227. Middlekauff, H. R., Chiu, J., Hamilton, M. A., et al. (2004). Muscle mechanoreceptor sensitivity in heart failure. *Am J Physiol, 287*, H1937–H1943.
228. Converse, R. L., Jr., Jacobsen, T. N., Toto, R. D., et al. (1992). Sympathetic overactivity in patients with chronic renal failure. *N Engl J Med, 327*, 1912–1918.
229. Hausberg, M., Kosch, M., Harmelink, P., et al. (2002). Sympathetic nerve activity in end-stage renal disease. *Circulation, 106*, 1974–1979.
230. Pilowsky, P. M., & Goodchild, A. K. (2002). Baroreceptor reflex pathways and neurotransmitters: 10 years on. *J Hypertens, 20*, 1675–1688.
231. Lambert, G., Kaye, D. M., Lefkovits, J., et al. (1995). Increased central nervous system monoamine neurotransmitter turnover and its association with sympathetic nervous activity in treated heart failure patients. *Circulation, 92*, 1813–1818.
232. Aggarwal, A., Esler, M., Lambert, G. W., et al. (2002). Norepinephrine turnover is increased in suprabulbar subcortical brain regions and is related to whole-body sympathetic activity in human heart failure. *Circulation, 105*, 1031–1033.
233. Elam, M., Yao, T., Svensson, T. H., et al. (1984). Regulation of locus coeruleus neurons and splanchnic, sympathetic nerves by cardiovascular afferents. *Brain Res, 290*, 281–287.
234. Narkiewicz, K., Pesek, C. A., van de Borne, P., et al. (1999). Enhanced sympathetic and ventilatory responses to central chemoreflex activation in heart failure. *Circulation, 100*, 262–267.
235. Ueno, H., Asanoi, H., Yamada, K., et al. (2004). Attenuated respiratory modulation of chemoreflex-mediated sympathoexcitation in patients with chronic heart failure. *J Card Fail, 10*, 236–243.
236. Topor, Z. L., Johannson, L., Kasprzyk, J., et al. (2001). Dynamic ventilatory response to CO(2) in congestive heart failure patients with and without central sleep apnea. *J Appl Physiol, 91*, 408–416.
237. Patel, K. P., Zhang, K., Zucker, I. H., et al. (1996). Decreased gene expression of neuronal nitric oxide synthase in hypothalamus and brainstem of rats in heart failure. *Brain Res, 734*, 109–115.
238. Gao, L., Wang, W., Li, Y. L., et al. (2004). Superoxide mediates sympathoexcitation in heart failure: roles of angiotensin II and NAD(P)H oxidase. *Circ Res, 95*, 937–944.
239. Zucker, I. H., & Liu, J. L. (2000). Angiotensin II-nitric oxide interactions in the control of sympathetic outflow in heart failure. *Heart Fail Rev, 5*, 27–43.
240. Kimura, Y., Hirooka, Y., Sagara, Y., et al. (2005). Overexpression of inducible nitric oxide synthase in rostral ventrolateral medulla causes hypertension and sympathoexcitation via an increase in oxidative stress. *Circ Res, 96*, 252–260.
241. Reid, I. A. (1992). Interactions between ANG II, sympathetic nervous system, and baroreceptor reflexes in regulation of blood pressure. *Am J Physiol, 262*, E763–E778.
242. Lumbers, E. R., McCloskey, D. I., & Potter, E. K. (1979). Inhibition by angiotensin II of baroreceptor-evoked activity in cardiac vagal efferent nerves in the dog. *J Physiol, 294*, 69–80.
243. Zucker, I. H. (2002). Brain angiotensin II: new insights into its role in sympathetic regulation. *Circ Res, 90*, 503–505.
244. Potts, P. D., Hirooka, Y., & Dampney, R. A. (1999). Activation of brain neurons by circulating angiotensin II: direct effects and baroreceptor-mediated secondary effects. *Neuroscience, 90*, 581–594.
245. Matsukawa, S., & Reid, I. A. (1990). Role of the area postrema in the modulation of the baroreflex control of heart rate by angiotensin II. *Circ Res, 67*, 1462–1473.
246. Lohmeier, T., Dwyer, T., Hildebrandt, D., et al. (2005). Influence of prolonged baroreflex activation on arterial pressure in angiotensin hypertension. *Hypertension, 46*, 1194–1200.
247. Ma, R., Schultz, H. D., & Wang, W. (1999). Chronic central infusion of ANG II potentiates cardiac sympathetic afferent reflex in dogs. *Am J Physiol, 277*, H15–H22.
248. Zhu, G. Q., Gao, L., Li, Y., et al. (2004). AT1 receptor mRNA antisense normalizes enhanced cardiac sympathetic afferent reflex in rats with chronic heart failure. *Am J Physiol, 287*, H1828–H1835.
249. DiBona, G. F., Jones, S. Y., & Brooks, V. L. (1995). ANG II receptor blockade and arterial baroreflex regulation of renal nerve activity in cardiac failure. *Am J Physiol, 269*, R1189–R1196.
250. Huang, B. S., Yuan, B., & Leenen, F. H. (2000). Chronic blockade of brain "ouabain" prevents sympathetic hyper-reactivity and impairment of acute baroreflex resetting in rats with congestive heart failure. *Can J Physiol Pharmacol, 78*, 45–53.
251. Leenen, F. H., Huang, B. S., Yu, H., et al. (1995). Brain "ouabain" mediates sympathetic hyperactivity in congestive heart failure. *Circ Res, 77*, 993–1000.
252. Zhang, W., Huang, B. S., & Leenen, F. H. (1999). Brain renin-angiotensin system and sympathetic hyperactivity in rats after myocardial infarction. *Am J Physiol, 276*, H1608–H1615.
253. Francis, J., Wei, S. G., Weiss, R. M., et al. (2004). Brain angiotensin-converting enzyme activity and autonomic regulation in heart failure. *Am J Physiol, 287*, H2138–2146.
254. Wang, H., Huang, B. S., Ganten, D., et al. (2004). Prevention of sympathetic and cardiac dysfunction after myocardial infarction in transgenic rats deficient in brain angiotensin. *Circ Res, 94*, 843.
255. Gao, L., Wang, W., Li, Y. L., et al. (2005). Sympathoexcitation by central ANG II: roles for AT1 receptor upregulation and NAD(P)H oxidase in RVLM. *Am J Physiol, 288*, H2271–H2279.
256. Zucker, I. H. (2006). Novel mechanisms of sympathetic regulation in chronic heart failure. *Hypertension, 48*, 1005–1011.
257. Liu, J. L., & Zucker, I. H. (1999). Regulation of sympathetic nerve activity in heart failure: a role for nitric oxide and angiotensin II. *Circ Res, 84*, 417–423.
258. Ma, R., Zucker, I. H., & Wang, W. (1999). Reduced NO enhances the central gain of cardiac sympathetic afferent reflex in dogs with heart failure. *Am J Physiol, 276*, H19–H26.
259. Ogletree-Hughes, M. L., Stull, L. B., Sweet, W. E., et al. (2001). Mechanical unloading restores beta-adrenergic responsiveness and reverses receptor downregulation in the failing human heart. *Circulation, 104*, 881–886.
260. Francis, J., Weiss, R. M., Wei, S. G., et al. (2001). Central mineralocorticoid receptor blockade improves volume regulation and reduces sympathetic drive in heart failure. *Am J Physiol, 281*, H2241–H2251.
261. Yu, Y., Wei, S. G., Zhang, Z. H., et al. (2008). Does aldosterone upregulate the brain renin-angiotensin system in rats with heart failure? *Hypertension, 51*, 727–733.
262. Yu, Y., Zhang, Z. H., Wei, S. G., et al. (2007). Central gene transfer of interleukin-10 reduces hypothalamic inflammation and evidence of heart failure in rats after myocardial infarction. *Circ Res, 101*, 304–312.
263. Kang, Y. M., Zhang, Z. H., Johnson, R. F., et al. (2006). Novel effect of mineralocorticoid receptor antagonism to reduce proinflammatory cytokines and hypothalamic activation in rats with ischemia-induced heart failure. *Circ Res, 99*, 758–766.
264. Kawai, H., Mohan, A., Hagen, J., et al. (2000). Alterations in cardiac adrenergic terminal function and beta-adrenoceptor density in pacing-induced heart failure. *Am J Physiol, 278*, H1708–H1716.
265. Bohm, M., La Rosee, K., Schwinger, R. H., et al. (1995). Evidence for reduction of norepinephrine uptake sites in the failing human heart. *J Am Coll Cardiol, 25*, 146–153.
266. Lotze, U., Kaepplinger, S., Kober, A., et al. (2001). Recovery of the cardiac adrenergic nervous system after long-term beta-blocker therapy in idiopathic dilated cardiomyopathy: assessment by increase in myocardial 123I-metaiodobenzylguanidine uptake. *J Nucl Med, 42*, 49–54.
267. Kasama, S., Toyama, T., Kumakura, H., et al. (2005). Effects of candesartan on cardiac sympathetic nerve activity in patients with congestive heart failure and preserved left ventricular ejection fraction. *J Am Coll Cardiol, 45*, 661–667.
268. Floras, J. S. (1992). Epinephrine and the genesis of hypertension. *Hypertension, 19*, 1–18.
269. Newton, G. E., & Parker, J. D. (1996). Acute effects of beta 1-selective and nonselective beta-adrenergic receptor blockade on cardiac sympathetic activity in congestive heart failure. *Circulation, 94*, 353–358.
270. Watson-Wright, W., Boudreau, G., Cardinal, R., et al. (1991). Beta 1- and beta 2-adrenoreceptor subtypes in canine intrathoracic efferent sympathetic nervous system regulating the heart. *Am J Physiol, 261*, R1269–R1275.
271. Huang, M. H., Smith, F. M., & Armour, J. A. (1993). Modulation of in situ canine intrinsic cardiac neuronal activity by nicotinic, muscarinic, and beta-adrenergic agonists. *Am J Physiol, 265*, R659–R669.
272. Kassis, E., Jacobsen, T. N., Mogensen, F., et al. (1986). Sympathetic reflex control of skeletal muscle blood flow in patients with congestive heart failure: evidence for beta-adrenergic circulatory control. *Circulation, 74*, 529–538.
273. Johansson, M., Rundqvist, B., Eisenhofer, G., et al. (1997). Cardiorenal epinephrine kinetics: evidence for neuronal release in the human heart. *Am J Physiol, 273*, H2178–H2185.
274. Parker, J. D., Newton, G. E., Landzberg, J. S., et al. (1995). Functional significance of presynaptic alpha-adrenergic receptors in failing and nonfailing human left ventricle. *Circulation, 92*, 1793–1800.
275. Aggarwal, A., Esler, M. D., Socratous, F., et al. (2001). Evidence for functional presynaptic alpha-2 adrenoceptors and their down-regulation in human heart failure. *J Am Coll Cardiol, 37*, 1246–1251.
276. Small, K. M., Wagoner, L. E., Levin, A. B., et al. (2002). Synergistic polymorphisms of beta1- and alpha 2c-adrenergic receptors and the risk of congestive heart failure. *N Engl J Med, 347*, 1135–1142.
277. Liggett, S. B., Mialet-Perez, J., Thaneemit-Chen, S., et al. (2006). A polymorphism within a conserved beta1-adrenergic receptor motif alters cardiac function and beta-blocker response in human heart failure. *Proc Natl Acad Sci U S A, 103*, 11288–11293.
278. Kurnik, D., Muszkat, M., Sofowora, G. G., et al. (2008). Ethnic and genetic determinants of cardiovascular response to the selective alpha-2 adrenoceptor agonist dexmedetomidine. *Hypertension, 51*, 406–411.
279. Kaye, D. M., Smirk, B., Finch, S., et al. (2004). Interaction between cardiac sympathetic drive and heart rate in heart failure: modulation by adrenergic receptor genotype. *J Am Coll Cardiol, 44*, 2008–2015.
280. Vanhoutte, P. M., & Levy, M. N. (1980). Prejunctional cholinergic modulation of adrenergic neurotransmission in the cardiovascular system. *Am J Physiol, 238*, H275–H281.
281. Matko, I., Feher, E., & Vizi, E. S. (1994). Receptor mediated presynaptic modulation of the release of noradrenaline in human papillary muscle. *Cardiovasc Res, 28*, 700–704.
282. Vanhoutte, P. M. (1974). Inhibition by acetylcholine of adrenergic neurotransmission in vascular smooth muscle. *Circ Res, 34*, 317–326.
283. Azevedo, E. R., & Parker, J. D. (1999). Parasympathetic control of cardiac sympathetic activity. Normal ventricular function versus congestive heart failure. *Circulation, 100*, 274–279.
284. McDonough, P. M., Wetzel, G. T., & Brown, J. H. (1986). Further characterization of the presynaptic alpha-1 receptor modulating (3H) ACh release from rat atria. *J Pharmacol Exp Ther, 238*, 612–617.
285. Lemmens, K., Doggen, K., & De Keulenaer, G. W. (2007). Role of neuregulin-1/ErbB signaling in cardiovascular physiology and disease: implications for therapy of heart failure. *Circulation, 116*, 954–960.
286. Smith-White, M. A., Wallace, D., & Potter, E. K. (1999). Sympathetic-parasympathetic interactions at the heart in the anaesthetised rat. *J Auton Nerv Syst, 75*, 171–175.
287. Potter, E. K. (1985). Prolonged non-adrenergic inhibition of cardiac vagal action following sympathetic stimulation: neuromodulation by neuropeptide Y? *Neurosci Lett, 54*, 117–121.
288. Clemson, B., Gaul, L., Gubin, S. S., et al. (1994). Prejunctional angiotensin II receptors. Facilitation of norepinephrine release in the human forearm. *J Clin Invest, 93*, 684–691.
289. Zimmerman, B. G. (1978). Actions of angiotensin on adrenergic nerve endings. *Fed Proc, 37*, 199–202.
290. Dendorfer, A., Raasch, W., Tempel, K., et al. (2002). Comparison of the vascular and antiadrenergic activities of four angiotensin II type I antagonists in the pithed rat. *J Hypertens, 20*, 1151–1156.
291. Goldsmith, S. R., Hasking, G. J., & Miller, E. (1993). Angiotensin II and sympathetic activity in patients with congestive heart failure. *J Am Coll Cardiol, 21*, 1107–1113.

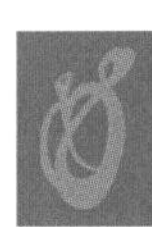

292. Magnusson, Y., Wallukat, G., Waagstein, F., et al. (1994). Autoimmunity in idiopathic dilated cardiomyopathy. Characterization of antibodies against the beta 1-adrenoceptor with positive chronotropic effect. *Circulation, 89*, 2760–2767.
293. Al-Hesayen, A., Azevedo, E. R., Newton, G. E., et al. (2002). The effects of dobutamine on cardiac sympathetic activity in patients with congestive heart failure. *J Am Coll Cardiol, 39*, 1269–1274.
294. Ellenbogen, K. A., Mohanty, P. K., Szentpetery, S., et al. (1989). Arterial baroreflex abnormalities in heart failure. Reversal after orthotopic cardiac transplantation. *Circulation, 79*, 51–58.
295. Faris, R., Flather, M. D., Purcell, H., et al. (2006). Diuretics for heart failure. *Cochrane Database Syst Rev, 1*, CD003838.
296. Solin, P., Bergin, P., Richardson, M., et al. (1999). Influence of pulmonary capillary wedge pressure on central apnea in heart failure. *Circulation, 99*, 1574–1579.
297. Fagius, J., & Karhuvaara, S. (1989). Sympathetic activity and blood pressure increases with bladder distension in humans. *Hypertension, 14*, 511–517.
298. Grassi, G., Cattaneo, B. M., Seravalle, G., et al. (1997). Effects of chronic ACE inhibition on sympathetic nerve traffic and baroreflex control of circulation in heart failure. *Circulation, 96*, 1173–1179.
299. Krum, H., Carson, P., Farsang, C., et al. (2004). Effect of valsartan added to background of ACE inhibitor therapy in patients with heart failure: results from Val-HeFT. *Eur J Heart Fail, 6*, 937–945.
300. Hikosaka, M., Yuasa, F., Mimura, J., et al. (2002). Candesartan and arterial baroreflex sensitivity and sympathetic nerve activity in patients with mild heart failure. *Cardiovasc Pharmacol, 40*, 875–880.
301. Kaye, D. M., Dart, A. M., Jennings, G. L., et al. (1999). Antiadrenergic effect of chronic amiodarone therapy in human heart failure. *J Am Coll Cardiol, 33*, 1553–1559.
302. Azevedo, E. R., Kubo, T., Mak, S., et al. (2001). Nonselective versus selective beta-adrenergic receptor blockade in congestive heart failure differential effects on sympathetic activity. *Circulation, 104*, 2194–2199.
303. Ferguson, D. W. (1989). Sympathoinhibitory responses to digitalis glycosides in heart failure patients: direct evidence from sympathetic neural recordings. *Circulation, 80*, 65–77.
304. Newton, G. E., Tong, J. H., Schofield, A. M., et al. (1996). Digoxin reduces cardiac sympathetic activity in severe congestive heart failure. *J Am Coll Cardiol, 28*, 155–161.
305. Campbell, D. J., Aggarwal, A., Esler, M., et al. (2001). Beta-blockers, angiotensin II, and ACE inhibitors in patients with heart failure. *Lancet, 358*, 1609–1610.
306. Grassi, G., Brambilla, R., Trevano, F. Q., et al. (2004). Sustained sympathoinhibitory effects of cardiac resynchronization therapy in severe heart failure. *Hypertension, 44*, 727–731.
307. Cohn, J. N., Archibald, D. G., Ziesche, S., et al. (1986). Effect of vasodilator therapy on mortality in chronic congestive heart failure. Results of a Veterans Administration cooperative study. *N Engl J Med, 314*, 1547–1552.
308. Kubo, T., Azevedo, E. R., Newton, G. E., et al. (2001). Lack of evidence for peripheral alpha(1)-adrenoceptor blockade during long-term treatment of heart failure with carvedilol. *J Am Coll Cardiol, 38*, 1463–1469.
309. MERIT-HF Study Group. (1999). Effect of metoprolol CR/XL in chronic heart failure: metoprolol CR/XL randomized intervention trial in congestive heart failure (MERIT-HF). *Lancet, 353*, 2001–2007.
310. Packer, M., Bristow, M. R., Cohn, J. N., et al. (1996). The effect of carvedilol on morbidity and mortality in patients with chronic heart failure. *N Engl J Med, 334*, 1349–1355.
311. CIBIS-II Investigators and Committees. (1999). The cardiac insufficiency bisoprolol study II (CIBIS II): a randomized trial. *Lancet, 353*, 9–13.
312. Packer, M., Coats, A. J., Fowler, M. B., et al. (2001). Effect of carvedilol on survival in severe chronic heart failure. *N Engl J Med, 344*, 1651–1657.
313. Kubo, T., Parker, J. D., Azevedo, E. R., et al. (2005). Vagal heart rate responses to chronic beta-blockade in human heart failure relate to cardiac norepinephrine spillover. *Eur J Heart Fail, 7*, 878–881.
314. Floras, J. S., Kubo, T., Azevedo, E., et al. (2006). Beta-blockade augments low frequency muscle sympathetic spectral power in human heart failure. *Circulation, 114*, II-370.
315. Rongen, G. A., Floras, J. S., Lenders, J., et al. (1997). Cardiovascular pharmacology of purines. *Clin Sci, 92*, 13–24.
316. Clarke, J., Benjamin, N., Larkin, S., et al. (1991). Interaction of neuropeptide Y and the sympathetic nervous system in vascular control in man. *Circulation, 83*, 774–777.
317. Yang, T., & Levy, M. N. (1992). Sequence of excitation as a factor in sympathetic-parasympathetic interactions in the heart. *Circ Res, 71*, 898–905.
318. Morris, M. J., Cox, H. S., Lambert, F. W., et al. (1997). Region-specific neuropeptide Y overflow at rest and during sympathetic activation in humans. *Hypertension, 29*, 137–143.
319. Azevedo, E. R., Newton, G. E., & Parker, J. D. (1999). Cardiac and systemic sympathetic activity in response to clonidine in human heart failure. *J Am Coll Cardiol, 33*, 186–191.
320. Grassi, G., Turri, C., Seravalle, G., et al. (2001). Effects of chronic clonidine administration on sympathetic nerve traffic and baroreflex function in heart failure. *Hypertension, 38*, 286–291.
321. Swedberg, K., Bristow, M., Cohn, J. N., et al. (2002). The effects of moxonidine SR, an imidazoline agonist, on plasma norepinephrine in patients with chronic heart failure. *Circulation, 105*, 1797–1803.
322. Cohn, J. N., Pfeffer, M. A., Rouleau, J., et al. (2003). Adverse mortality effect of central sympathetic inhibition with sustained-release moxonidine in patients with heart failure (MOXCON). *Eur J Heart Fail, 5*, 659–667.
323. Bristow, M. R., Krause-Steinrauf, H., Nuzzo, R., et al. (2004). Effect of baseline or changes in adrenergic activity on clinical outcomes in the beta-blocker evaluation of survival trial. *Circulation, 110*, 1437–1442.
324. Floras, J. S. (2004). Alterations in the sympathetic and parasympathetic nervous system in heart failure. In D. Mann (Ed.). *A companion to Braunwald's heart disease.* Philadelphia: Harcourt, pp. 247-277.
325. Lindley, T. E., Doobay, M. F., Sharma, R. V., et al. (2004). Superoxide is involved in the central nervous system activation and sympathoexcitation of myocardial infarction-induced heart failure. *Circ Res, 20*, 402–409.
326. Huang, B. S., & Leenen, F. H. (2005). Blockade of brain mineralocorticoid receptors or Na^+ channels prevents sympathetic hyperactivity and improves cardiac function in rats post-MI. *Am J Physiol, 288*, H2491–H2497.
327. Gao, L., Wang, W., Li, Y. L., et al. (2005). Simvastatin therapy normalizes sympathetic neural control in experimental heart failure: roles of angiotensin II type I receptors and NAD(P)H oxidase. *Circulation, 112*, 1763–1770.
328. Pliquett, R. U., Cornish, K. G., & Zucker, I. H. (2003). Statin therapy restores sympathovagal balance in experimental heart failure. *J Appl Physiol, 95*, 700–704.
329. Pliquett, R. U., Cornish, K. G., Peuler, J. D., et al. (2003). Simvastatin normalizes autonomic neural control in experimental heart failure. *Circulation, 107*, 2493–2498.
330. Piccirillo, G., Nocco, M., Moise, A., et al. (2003). Influence of vitamin C on baroreflex sensitivity in chronic heart failure. *Hypertension, 41*, 1240–1245.
331. Bibevski, S., & Dunlap, M. E. (2004). Prevention of diminished parasympathetic control of the heart in experimental heart failure. *Am J Physiol, 287*, H1780–H1785.
332. Li, M., Zheng, C., Sato, T., et al. (2004). Vagal nerve stimulation markedly improves long-term survival after chronic heart failure in rats. *Circulation, 109*, 120–124.
333. Liang, C. S. (2007). Cardiac sympathetic nerve terminal function in congestive heart failure. *Acta Pharmacol Sin, 28*, 921–927.
334. Munch, G., Rosport, K., Bultmann, A., et al. (2005). Cardiac overexpression of the norepinephrine transporter uptake-1 results in marked improvement of heart failure. *Circ Res, 97*, 928–936.
335. Kreussner, M. M., Haass, M., Buss, S. J., et al. (2006). Injection of nerve growth factor into stellate ganglia improves norepinephrine reuptake into failing hearts. *Hypertension, 47*, 209–215.
336. Johnson, W. H., Omland, T., Hall, C., et al. (2002). Neurohormonal activation rapidly decreases after intravenous therapy with diuretics and vasodilators for class IV heart failure. *J Am Coll Cardiol, 39*, 1623–1629.
337. Abramson, B. L., Ando, S., Notarius, C. F., et al. (1999). Effect of atrial natriuretic peptide on muscle sympathetic activity and its reflex control in human heart failure. *Circulation, 99*, 1810–1815.
338. Agostino, P., Marenzi, G., Lauri, G., et al. (1994). Sustained improvement in functional capacity after removal of body fluid with isolated ultrafiltration in chronic cardiac insufficiency: failure of furosemide to provide the same result. *Am J Med, 96*, 191–199.
339. Azevedo, E. R., Newton, G. E., Parker, A. B., et al. (2000). Sympathetic responses to atrial natriuretic peptide in patients with congestive heart failure. *J Cardiovasc Pharmacol, 35*, 129–135.
340. Fraga, R., Franco, F. G., Roveda, F., et al. (2007). Exercise training reduces sympathetic nerve activity in heart failure patients treated with carvedilol. *Eur J Heart Fail, 9*, 630–636.
341. Kaneko, Y., Floras, J. S., Usui, K., et al. (2003). Cardiovascular effects of continuous positive airway pressure in patients with heart failure and obstructive sleep apnea. *N Engl J Med, 348*, 1233–1241.
342. Usui, K., Parker, J. D., Newton, G. E., et al. (2006). Left ventricular structural adaptations to obstructive sleep apnea in dilated cardiomyopathy. *J Am Coll Cardiol, 173*, 1170–1175.
343. Radaelli, A., Coats, A. J., Leuzzi, S., et al. (1996). Physical training enhances sympathetic and parasympathetic control of heart rate and peripheral vessels in chronic heart failure. *Clin Sci, 92*, 92–94.
344. Toepfer, M., Meyer, K., Maier, P., et al. (1996). Influence of exercise training and restriction of activity on autonomic balance in patients with severe congestive heart failure. *Clin Sci, 91*, 116.
345. Coats, A. J. S., Adamopoulos, S., Radaelli, A., et al. (1992). Controlled trial of physical training in chronic heart failure. Exercise performance, hemodynamics, ventilation, and autonomic function. *Circulation, 85*, 2119–2131.
346. Minotti, J. R., & Massie, B. M. (1992). Exercise training in heart failure patients. Does reversing the peripheral abnormalities protect the heart? *Circulation, 85*, 2323–2325.
347. Kiilavuori, K., Toivonen, L., Naveri, H., et al. (1995). Reversal of autonomic derangements by physical training in chronic heart failure assessed by heart rate variability. *Eur Heart J, 16*, 490–495.
348. Tkacova, R., Dajani, H. R., Rankin, F., et al. (2000). Continuous positive airway pressure improves nocturnal baroreflex sensitivity in patients with obstructive sleep apnea and heart failure. *J Hypertens, 18*, 1257–1262.
349. Meredith, I. T., Friberg, P., Jennings, G. L., et al. (1991). Exercise training lowers resting renal but not cardiac sympathetic activity in humans. *Hypertension, 18*, 575–582.
350. Marin-Neto, J. A., Pintya, A. O., Gallo, L., et al. (1991). Abnormal baroreflex control of heart rate in decompensated congestive heart failure and reversal after compensation. *Am J Cardiol, 67*, 604–610.
351. Tkacova, R., Hall, M. J., Rutherford, R., et al. (1996). Effect of continuous positive airway pressure on nocturnal blood pressure in patients with heart failure and obstructive sleep apnea. *Circulation, 94*, I340.
352. Bradley, T. D., Holloway, R. M., McLaughlin, P. R., et al. (1992). Cardiac output response to continuous positive airway pressure in congestive heart failure. *Am Rev Respir Dis, 145*, 377–382.
353. Butler, G. C., Naughton, M. T., Rahman, M. A., et al. (1995). Continuous positive airway pressure increases heart rate variability in congestive heart failure. *J Am Coll Cardiol, 25*, 672–679.
354. Ryan, C. M., Usui, K., Floras, J. S., et al. (2005). Effect of continuous positive airway pressure on ventricular ectopy in heart failure patients with obstructive sleep apnoea. *Thorax, 60*, 781–785.
355. Mansfield, D., Gollogly, N. C., Kaye, D. M., et al. (2004). Controlled trial of continuous positive airway pressure in obstructive sleep apnea and heart failure. *Am J Respir Crit Care Med, 169*, 361–366.

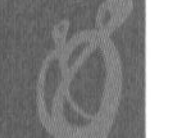

356. Marin, J. M., Carrizo, S. J., Vicente, E., et al. (2005). Long-term cardiovascular outcomes in men with obstructive sleep apnoea-hypopnoea with or without treatment with continuous positive airway pressure: an observation study. *Lancet*, *365*, 1046–1053.

357. Bradley, T. D., Logan, A. G., Kimoff, R. J., et al. (2005). Continuous positive airway pressure for central sleep apnea and heart failure. *N Engl J Med*, *353*, 2025–2033.

358. Massie, B. M. (2002). Neurohormonal blockade in chronic heart failure. How much is enough? Can there be too much? *J Am Coll Cardiol*, *39*, 79–82.

359. Horner, S. M., Murphy, C. F., Coen, B., et al. (1996). Contribution to heart rate variability by mechanoelectric feedback-stretch of the sinoatrial node reduces heart rate variability. *Circulation*, *94*, 1762–1767.

360. Flierl, M. A., Rittirsch, D., Nadeau, B. A., et al. (2007). Phagocyte-derived catecholamines enhance acute inflammatory injury. *Nature*, *449*, 721–725.

CHAPTER 17

Alterations in the Peripheral Circulation in Heart Failure

Helmut Drexler, Burkhard Hornig, and Ulf Landmesser

CARDIOVASCULAR EFFECTS OF SUSTAINED NEUROHUMORAL ACTIVATION IN HEART FAILURE

Systemic perfusion pressure is determined by cardiac output and vascular tone of peripheral arteries. When cardiac output decreases, systemic perfusion pressure is maintained mainly by peripheral vasoconstriction and sodium retention, which are both characteristic findings in patients with overt heart failure and attributable to the interaction of hemodynamic and neurohumoral factors. Several neurohumoral systems are activated in patients with chronic heart failure that cause peripheral vasoconstriction. The sympathetic nervous system is activated very early in the disease process, whereas the renin-angiotensin system is usually activated when clinical symptoms develop. Vasopressin is released mainly in very advanced stages of chronic heart failure when systemic perfusion is already threatened.[1] Furthermore, chronic severe heart failure is associated by an increased endothelial release of locally acting vasoconstricting factors such as endothelin.

These endogenous vasoconstricting factors are counterbalanced in part by endogenous vasodilators. In normal individuals, natriuretic peptides attenuate the release of norepinephrine, renin, and vasopressin and their actions on peripheral blood vessels and within the kidneys. In addition, the continuous release of endothelium-derived relaxing factor (nitric oxide) from the endothelium normally counteracts the vasoconstricting factors. In fact, the continuous basal release of nitric oxide keeps the peripheral vasculature in a dilated state. In patients with heart failure, however, the effects of circulating and locally active vasodilators are attenuated. The release of atrial natriuretic peptide is blunted in chronic heart failure and the effects of both atrial (ANP) and brain natriuretic peptide (BNP) lose their ability to suppress the release of renin or dilate peripheral blood vessels (see also Chapter 18).[2] In addition the vascular availability of nitric oxide is severely diminished in patients with chronic heart failure.[3] Thus diminished vasodilator forces leave the actions of vasoconstrictors unopposed. It is important to note that the interaction of the sympathetic and renin-angiotensin systems even amplifies their vasoconstricting effects. Increased sympathetic activity increases the release of renin and vice versa and angiotensin enhances the release of both norepinephrine and vasopressin.

BLOOD FLOW TO SKELETAL MUSCLE IN CHRONIC HEART FAILURE

Impaired cardiac contractility is not necessarily associated with clinical signs of heart failure but may be present in an asymptomatic patient. The clinical symptoms of heart failure are apparently not related to cardiac dysfunction but to activation of compensatory mechanisms such as activation of the sympathetic nerve system, renin-angiotensin system, or activation of cytokines such as tumor necrosis factor (TNF)-α or interleukin-6. In most cases of well-treated chronic heart failure, cardiac output remains close to normal during resting conditions[4] and only a minority of patients have an impaired increase of cardiac output during exercise testing that appears to be associated with a poor prognosis, particularly when peak oxygen consumption is severely reduced.[5] Muscle blood flow during exercise, however, is reduced in patients with chronic heart failure as compared with normal individuals because of diversion of blood flow away from the muscles.[6] In addition, the size and vascularization of the skeletal muscle is reduced in heart failure patients,[6] contributing to the clinical symptom of premature muscular fatigue during physical activity or exercise. Attempts to augment muscle blood flow by increasing the pumping capacity of the heart during exercise have produced only mild increases in blood flow to exercising skeletal muscle and did not result in acutely improved exercise tolerance. One explanation may be that the increased cardiac output was associated with increased skin rather than skeletal muscle perfusion; moreover, there is evidence that skeletal muscle is unable to use increased oxygen supply acutely due to impaired oxidative capacity of skeletal muscle.

In many patients with chronic heart failure, the increase in blood flow to working muscle with exercise is attenuated for each given workload compared with that in normal persons.[7] Peak oxygen consumption is also lower in patients with chronic heart failure and is accompanied

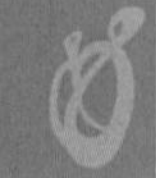

by an early increase in plasma lactate concentration.[7] The reduced maximal blood flow to working muscle occurs predominantly in oxidative working muscle[8] and is primarily caused by an abnormality of arteriolar vasodilation during exercise. Patients who exhibit improved exercise capacity after therapy with angiotensin-converting enzyme (ACE) inhibitors also exhibit improved leg blood flow.[9] The failure of muscle blood flow to increase normally during exercise in patients with chronic heart failure is primarily because of an abnormality of peripheral arteriolar vasodilation. During exercise, blood flow to working muscles increases largely due to two mechanisms: increase in cardiac output and redistribution of blood flow. Both mechanisms are altered in chronic heart failure. This increase in cardiac output with exercise is impaired. In addition, normally arterioles within the exercising muscle dilate, a mechanism that is also impaired in many patients with heart failure,[7,10,11] in part due to excessive sympathetically mediated vasoconstriction, activation of the plasma renin-angiotensin system, and possibly to increased plasma concentrations of endothelin[12] both in the pulmonary[13] and systemic circulation.[14] Although these neurohumoral factors exert potent systemic and regional vasoconstriction, they do not completely explain the impaired vasodilating capacity within skeletal muscle in patients with chronic heart failure. Impaired metabolic vasodilation during exercise cannot be restored by α-adrenoreceptor blockade with phentolamine.[1,15] Similarly, ACE inhibition does not restore impaired metabolic vasodilation during exercise after acute administration, despite a substantial reduction of plasma angiotensin II and norepinephrine concentrations.[9,16] Chronic treatment with an ACE inhibitor over several months, however, leads to a significant increase in femoral blood flow during exercise in patients with chronic heart failure and is associated with an improved oxygen consumption.[9] Chronic ACE-inhibitor therapy reversed therefore the inability of peripheral vessels to dilate.[17] These findings are in line with previous observations in large clinical trials that the full beneficial effect of ACE-inhibitor therapy emerges slowly over time.[18] Similarly, the restoration of peripheral perfusion and skeletal muscle function takes weeks to months after cardiac transplantation, suggesting that chronic heart failure leads to alterations of arterial function and structure.

STRUCTURAL ALTERATIONS OF PERIPHERAL ARTERIES IN CHRONIC HEART FAILURE

Experimental evidence indicates that angiotensin II induces hypertrophy of cultured rat aortic smooth muscle cells[19] and may be involved in the proliferative process of tissues during growth. Recent experimental observations suggest that structural vascular alterations emerge in the chronic phase of heart failure and can be reversed by high-dose ACE inhibition[20] (Figure 17-1, *A*). Unfortunately, clinical studies indicating structural alterations in peripheral resistance arteries are scarce and usually confined to skin resistance vessels that may not be representative for skeletal muscle resistance vessels. Small skeletal muscle biopsies often allow only examination of very small arterioles (<50 μm), which may not play a major role in the regulation of blood flow such as resistance vessels in the range of 80 to 200 μm. A further potential mechanism that contributes to structural alterations of peripheral arteries in chronic heart failure is a "vascular stiffness factor" owing to the increased vascular sodium content, which can be, in part, reduced with diuretic therapy in decompensated heart failure.[21] The stiffness factor represents a mechanical factor that may impair the vasodilator capacity of peripheral blood vessels either because of an increase of sodium content within the vascular wall or because edema enhances the compressive forces of perivascular tissues. A reduced density of skeletal muscle capillaries may represent another structural abnormality in experimental models[20] (Figure 17-1, *B*) and patients with chronic heart failure[22] that may contribute to the reduced vasodilator capacity in chronic heart failure, since reduction of capillary density leads to a reduction of total peripheral vascular cross-sectional area.

ALTERATION OF ENDOTHELIUM-DEPENDENT VASODILATION IN HEART FAILURE

The endothelium plays an important role in the control of vascular tone by releasing both vasodilating and vasoconstricting factors.[23] These mechanisms are important for the regulation of the microvasculature[24] and for the larger conduit arteries.[3,25] Patients with chronic heart failure are

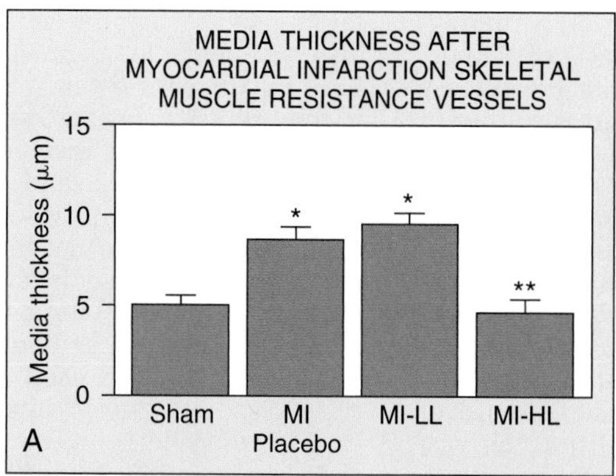

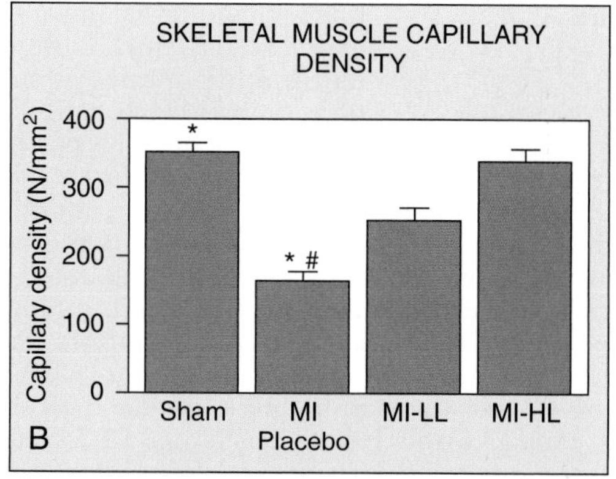

FIGURE 17–1 **A,** Media thickness of skeletal muscle resistance vessels from rat skeletal muscle 1 year after myocardial infarction. Bar graphs indicate media thickness in sham-operated animals (sham), placebo-treated animals with myocardial infarction (MI placebo), animals treated with low-dose lisinopril (MI-LL), and animals treated with high-dose lisinopril (MI-HL). Data are mean ± SEM, **P* <.01 vs. Sham; ***P* <.01 vs. MI placebo, and MI-LL; **B,** Skeletal muscle capillary density determined from quadriceps femoris muscle 1 year after myocardial infarction. Bar graphs indicate skeletal muscle capillary density in sham-operated animals (sham), placebo-treated animals with myocardial infarction (MI placebo), animals treated with low-dose lisinopril (MI-LL), and animals treated with high-dose lisinopril (MI-HL). Data are mean ± SEM, **P*<0.05 vs. MI-LL; #*P* <.01 vs. Sham, MI-LL, and MI-LH. (Modified from Schieffer B, Wollert K, Berchthold M, et al. Development and prevention of skeletal muscle structural alterations after experimental myocardial infarction. *Am J Physiol* 1995;269:H1507-H1513.)

characterized by increased systemic vasoconstriction and a reduced vasodilator response during physical exercise. While neurohumoral factors undoubtedly are involved in alterations of the peripheral vasculature, there is good evidence that abnormal function of the endothelium contributes to the abnormal vasodilator response in chronic heart failure. In this respect, the role of endothelium-derived relaxing factor (i.e., nitric oxide[26]) has received considerable attention. Nitric oxide is synthesized in the endothelial cell by the endothelial cell NO synthase from the amino acid L-arginine[27] (Figure 17-2) in the presence of cofactors such as tetrahydrobiopterin.[28]

The endothelium releases NO in response to a variety of stimuli including increased shear stress[3,25] during increased blood flow such as during physical activity, or receptor stimulation such as muscarinic or bradykinin β_2-receptors.[23,29] Following its release from the endothelial cell and uptake into the vascular smooth muscle cell, NO stimulates the guanylate cyclase to form cyclic guanosine monophosphate (cGMP), resulting in smooth muscle relaxation and vascular dilation (see Figure 17-2). With the assumption that an impaired vasodilator response to acetylcholine reflects endothelial dysfunction,[29,30] evidence for an impaired endothelium-dependent vasodilation was found in the *microcirculation* of the myocardium, leg, and forearm of patients with chronic heart failure.[31-35] These observations suggest that the impairment of endothelium-dependent, NO-mediated vasodilator function is a generalized phenomenon in patients with chronic heart failure. Yet, beyond the impaired response to endothelium-dependent stimuli, basal release of nitric oxide may be altered in chronic heart failure. In normal individuals, the arterial vasculature is kept in a somewhat dilated state by constant basal release of nitric oxide[36] as demonstrated by decreased peripheral blood flow following inhibition of NO synthesis by L-monomethyl-L-arginine (L-NMMA). However, this basal release of nitric oxide may be enhanced in patients with severe chronic heart failure. In some but not all studies, the reduction of blood flow following L-NMMA was enhanced in heart failure as compared to normal individuals. These observations raised the concept that severe heart failure is associated with increased basal release of nitric oxide to counterbalance the excessive vasoconstrictor forces jeopardizing tissue perfusion. Severe heart failure is associated with increased levels of cytokines, which may induce the expression of inducible nitric oxide within the vascular wall. This concept is supported by the observation that peripheral venous nitrate, the product of NO metabolism in blood, also has been found to increase in heart failure.[37,38] However, these observations were not made in all patient populations studied, in particular, basal release of nitric oxide may be normal in patients with more compensated states of heart failure without substantial cytokine activation.

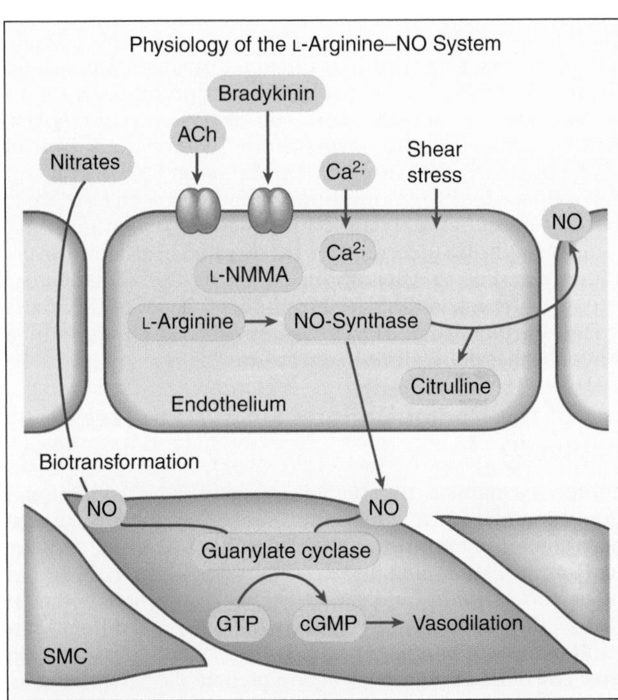

FIGURE 17–2 The physiology of the L-arginine-nitric-oxide (NO) system: Nitric oxide is synthesized in the endothelial cell from the amino-acid L-arginine by the endothelial NO-synthase. Following uptake into the vascular smooth muscle cell (SMC), NO stimulates the guanylate cyclase to form cyclic guanosine monophosphate (cGMP) resulting in vasodilation.

One consequence of impaired endothelium-mediated vasodilation of peripheral *resistance arteries* may include reduction of tissue perfusion during physical exercise, thereby contributing to impaired exercise capacity in heart failure. The disturbance of microvascular dilation within the coronary artery circulation may result in ischemia and further myocardial damage and dysfunction in patients with chronic heart failure.

Alterations in endothelial function emerge not only in peripheral resistance vessels but also in *peripheral conduit arteries*; flow-dependent vasodilation of conduit arteries in humans is to a large extent mediated by endothelial release of nitric oxide.[3,25] However, flow-dependent vasodilation is impaired in patients with chronic heart failure as compared with healthy control subjects.[3,39] Following blockade of the NO synthase by L-NMMA, flow-dependent dilation is similar in patients with heart failure and healthy subjects, suggesting that the impairment in patients is due to reduced bioavailability of nitric oxide. Importantly, the impairment of flow-dependent vasodilation is similar in patients with ischemic and dilated cardiomyopathy, suggesting that heart failure per se rather than the etiology of heart failure determines the extent of endothelial dysfunction. Because large arteries are more than just passive conduits,[40] it is possible that the impairment of flow-mediated vasodilation during exercise might lead to increased impedance to the left ventricular ejection and thereby contributes to the hemodynamic derangements characteristic of chronic heart failure.

MECHANISMS OF ENDOTHELIAL VASODILATOR DYSFUNCTION IN HEART FAILURE

Preclinical experiments suggest that endothelial dysfunction is a progressive, time-dependent process that probably plays a minor role early in heart failure. Rats in whom heart failure was induced by coronary ligation with subsequent myocardial infarction demonstrated no evidence of endothelial dysfunction 1 week after myocardial infarction. Four and 16 weeks after myocardial infarction, however, a reduced vasorelaxation was observed in aortic rings in response to acetylcholine as compared with sham-operated control animals.[41] Moreover, endothelial dysfunction in the rat infarct model appears to emerge only in rats with large myocardial infarctions, markedly impaired left ventricular function, and evidence of heart failure.[24] Several pathophysiological mechanisms appear to contribute to the impaired NO-dependent vasodilation in chronic heart failure and many of these aspects have now been studied in humans (Box 17-1).

Nitric Oxide Synthase in Heart Failure

The reduced endothelium-dependent nitric oxide–mediated vasodilator response to acetylcholine may be, in part, caused by reduced gene expression and activity of the nitric oxide

Box 17–1 Potential Mechanisms for Endothelial Dysfunction in Heart Failure

- Reduced eNOS gene expression and activity, including TNF-alpha induced shortening of eNOS mRNA half life.
- Activation of the RAAS, including increased ACE-activity and increased aldosterone concentrations
- Inactivation of NO by superoxide anions
- Endogenous inhibitors of eNOS
- Alteration of vascular signal transduction
- Impaired endothelial repair mechanisms

forming enzyme NO synthase (eNOS). Pulsatile flow[42] and the associated shear stress[40,43] are important regulators of NO production, thereby providing a potential link between impaired cardiac and vascular function as represented by impaired endothelial vasodilator function in patients with chronic heart failure. In fact, experimental and clinical studies have shown that eNOS gene expression in aortic endothelial cells and myocardial tissue is reduced in heart failure.[44,49] Moreover, nitric oxide production from cardiac microvessels from patients with end-stage heart failure is reduced as compared with normal hearts.[48] Taken together, impaired expression and activity of endothelial cell NO synthase may represent one factor contributing to impaired endothelium-dependent dilation in patients with heart failure. There is good evidence that gene expression of endothelial nitric oxide synthase is upregulated by shear stress,[43] raising the possibility that chronically reduced blood flow in chronic heart failure may be involved in the development of reduced nitric oxide synthase gene expression.

Impact of Cytokines (see also Chapter 11)

Plasma concentrations of cytokines, such as tumor necrosis factor-α (TNF-α), are increased in patients with chronic heart failure[47] and may represent a further mechanism contributing to impaired endothelium-dependent vasodilation in patients with chronic heart failure by diminishing the availability of NO.[48] Experimental evidence suggests that TNF-α can inhibit the stimulated release of nitric oxide from the endothelium[49] and that TNF-α impairs the stability of eNOS mRNA by shortening its half-life.[50] TNF-α has also been shown to increase endothelial and vascular smooth muscle cell production of superoxide anions, which decrease the half-life of nitric oxide.[51] Thus TNF-α may inhibit endothelium-dependent nitric oxide–mediated vasodilation by decreasing the bioavailability of nitric oxide through enhanced destruction and reduced synthesis of NO-synthase, although data derived from human studies are limited. It is interesting to note that TNF-α plasma concentrations were closely related with forearm blood flow responses to intrabrachial infusions of acetylcholine.[47] Moreover, the administration of etanercept, a recombinant TNF receptor that binds to and functionally inactivates TNF-α, has been shown to improve vasodilator capacity in patients with advanced heart failure, suggesting the important role of TNF-α for impaired endothelial vasoreactivity in CHF.[47a]

Inactivation of Nitric Oxide by Superoxide Anions

Another mechanism that appears to play a role in the development of endothelial dysfunction in chronic heart failure is an enhanced oxidant stress (i.e., superoxide anion production) that can rapidly inactivate nitric oxide and tetrahydrobiopterin, an important cofactor of the endothelial NO synthase.[47b,47c] There is accumulating evidence that the production of oxygen-free radicals is enhanced in chronic heart failure[52] which, in turn,

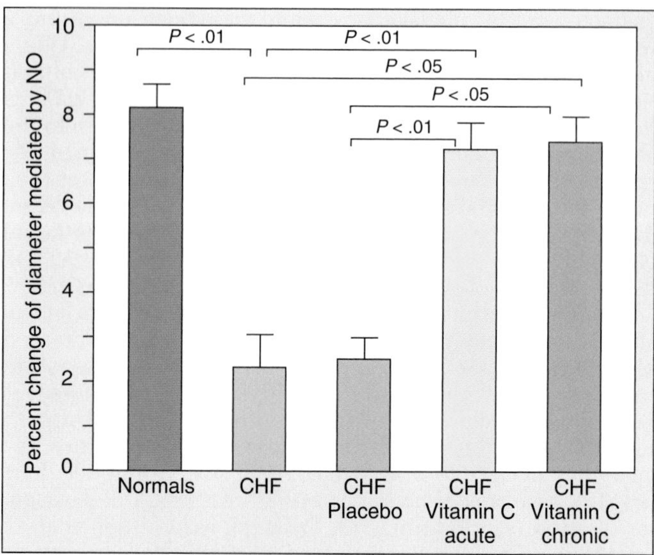

FIGURE 17–3 Reduced bioavailability of NO in heart failure. Restoration of arterial diameter by high-dose intraarterial infusion of vitamin C (acute) or 2 g vitamin C (orally) indicating inactivation of NO by radicals. Bar graphs represent the NO-mediated vasodilation of the radial artery in healthy controls (Normals), patients with chronic heart failure (CHF) and the effect of placebo (CHF-placebo), intraarterial infusion of vitamin C (CHF-vitamin C acute), and oral therapy with vitamin C over 4 weeks (CHF vitamin C chronic) in patients with chronic heart failure. (Modified from Hornig B, Arakawa N, Kohler C, et al. Vitamin C improves endothelial function of conduit arteries in patients with chronic heart failure. *Circulation* 1998;97:363-368.)

would contribute to a reduced bioavailability of nitric oxide and endothelial dysfunction in these patients. Antioxidant therapy with ascorbic acid improves endothelium-mediated vasodilation in patients with chronic heart failure by increasing the bioavailability of nitric oxide[53] (Figure 17-3), supporting the role of oxidative stress in heart failure.

The underlying mechanisms leading to increased production of oxygen-free radicals in chronic heart failure likely include increased NAD(P)H oxidase[54a] and xanthine oxidase activation.[54b] There is experimental evidence that the redox state of the vascular wall is influenced by angiotensin II and TNF by increasing the production of superoxide anions in vascular smooth muscle cells by activating the NADH/NADPH-oxidases.[54] Moreover, there is increased vascular activity of NAD(P)H oxidase[54a] and increased binding of xanthine oxidase to the endothelium in patients with CHF that is related to endothelial dysfunction.[54b] Other potential sources of increased radical formation in chronic heart failure may include the failing cardiac myocyte[55,56] and leukocytes.[57] Moreover, there is evidence that the activity of antioxidative enzyme systems, such as superoxide dismutase, are reduced within the arterial wall in heart failure.[54b]

Role of the Renin-Angiotensin System (see also Chapter 9)

Another mechanism involved in endothelial dysfunction in chronic heart failure might be an increased activity of the angiotensin-converting enzyme (ACE)[58] in the face of an activated renin-angiotensin system in chronic heart failure. ACE is identical to kininase II and degradates bradykinin. Increased activity of ACE is therefore associated with increased formation of angiotensin II and enhanced inactivation of endogenous bradykinin. The deleterious effects of angiotensin II on radical formation has been described above. The consequence of increased degradation of bradykinin results in impaired bioavailability of NO by reducing its release and synthesis from the endothelium. In addition, bradykinin exerts its vasodilating properties by endothelial release of endothelium-derived hyperpolarizing factor[59] and prostacyclin.[60] Numerous experimental studies have indicated that bradykinin tissue levels are altered in heart failure and that ACE inhibitors can improve bradykinin availability. There is also clinical evidence that ACE inhibition is associated with an increase in bradykinin plasma concentrations.[61] Moreover, there exists a specific interaction of ACE inhibitors with the bradykinin β_2-receptor.[62] Interestingly, the bradykinin β_2-receptor can act as an inverse receptor,[63] which may also play a role in interventions with ACE inhibitors. By using a specific bradykinin β_2 receptor antagonist, we recently have shown in humans that bradykinin is involved in the regulation of vascular tone in vivo.[64] In addition, the beneficial effect of ACE inhibition on endothelium-dependent vasodilation is mediated by bradykinin and/or a bradykinin β_2-receptor-mediated mechanism[65] (Figure 17-4) after acute administration. Long-term ACE inhibition improves endothelial function and the bioavailability of NO in patients with heart failure.[66] In fact, recent data would suggest that bradykinin may contribute to the vasodilation associated with chronic ACE-inhibitor therapy in patients with heart failure via the β_1-receptor.[67,67a]

Interestingly, while the antioxidant ascorbic acid improves endothelium-dependent vasodilation before starting ACE-inhibitor therapy, the beneficial effect of ascorbic acid was lost after long-term ACE inhibitor therapy[68] (Figure 17-5, *A*). Thus the beneficial effect of chronic ACE inhibition on endothelium-dependent vasodilator function may involve, indirectly, antioxidative effects (i.e., mediated by reduced formation of superoxide anions by vascular NADP/NADPH-oxidases[68]) and increased activity of extracellular superoxide dismutase (EC-SOD), a major antioxidative enzyme system within the human arterial vascular wall degrading superoxide anions. In fact, there is evidence that EC-SOD activity increases substantially after long-term therapy with an ACE inhibitor or an AT_1-receptor antagonist[68] (see Figure 17-5, *B*), including a close relationship between the increase of EC-SOD activity and the increase of the availability of nitric oxide.[68] These intervention studies in patients would suggest that increased oxidative stress in patients is related to both enhanced radical formation by NADPH oxidase, xanthine oxidase, and others, but also to impaired degradation of superoxide anions by antioxidative enzyme systems (Figure 17-6).

It should be noted that intervention studies also suggest that endothelial function of peripheral *resistance arteries* is impaired and chronic heart failure is modulated by the renin-angiotensin system: for example, ACE inhibitors affect forearm blood flow, in an endothelium-dependent matter, by mediating prostaglandins.[69] It appears that the contribution of

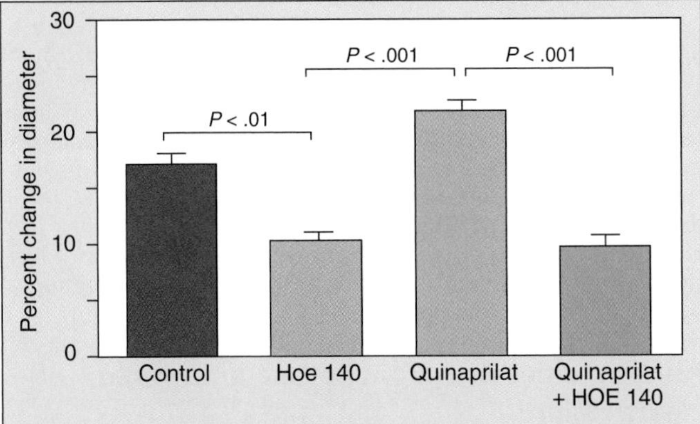

FIGURE 17–4 Contribution of bradykinin to the effect of ACE inhibition on flow-dependent dilation. Bar graphs represent the percent change of radial artery diameter during flow-dependent, endothelium-mediated vasodilation of the radial artery in healthy controls during control conditions (control), after intraarterial infusion of the bradykinin β_2-receptor antagonist HOE 140 (HOE 140), after infusion of the ACE-inhibitor quinaprilat (Quinaprilat) and after co-infusion of quinaprilat together with HOE 140 (Quinaprilat + HOE 140)

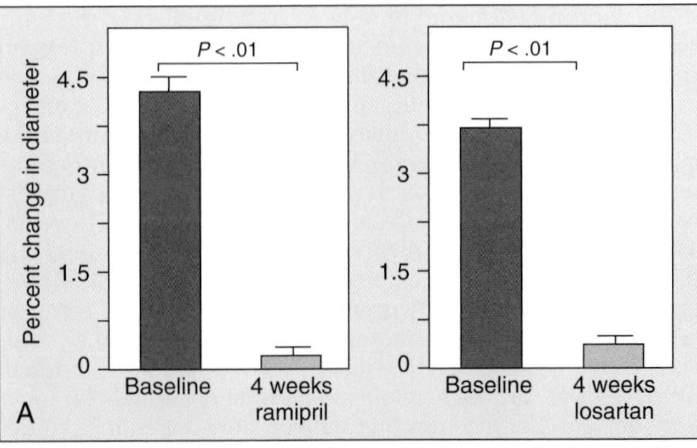

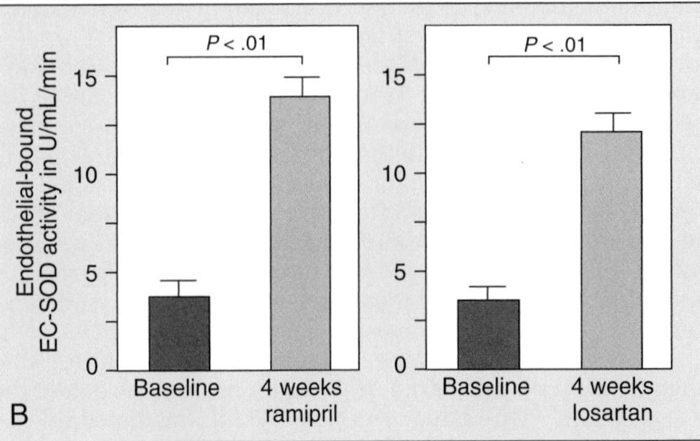

FIGURE 17–5 **A,** Antioxidative effects of pharmacological interference with the renin-angiotensin system: bar graphs indicate the effect of intraarterial infusion of vitamin C on flow-dependent, endothelium-mediated vasodilation of the radial artery of patients with coronary artery disease before and after 4 weeks of therapy with ramipril (10 mg/d) or losartan (100 mg/d). **B,** Effect of ACE inhibition and AT_1-receptor antagonism on EC-SOD activity in patients with coronary artery disease: bar graphs show the activity of endothelial-bound activity of extracellular superoxide dismutase (EC-SOD) before and after 4 weeks of therapy with ramipril (10 mg/d) or losartan (100 mg/d) in patients with coronary artery disease.

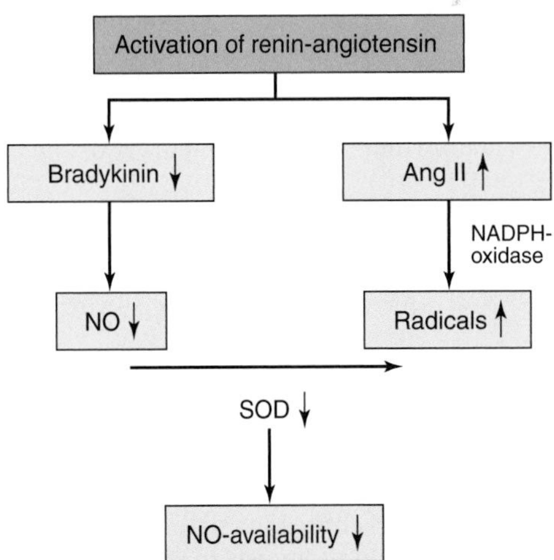

FIGURE 17–6 The activated renin-angiotensin system in heart failure leads to increased inactivation of bradykinin, resulting in impaired release of NO by endothelial cells. Since extracellular superoxide dismutase (SOD) is regulated by NO, the impaired release of NO by bradykinin is associated with reduced SOD-activity. In addition, activation of the renin-angiotensin system results in increased formation of free radicals by NADH/NADPH oxidases. The resulting increase in cellular radicals leads to enhanced inactivation of NO. Thus activation of the renin-angiotensin system results in impaired NO availability due to both reduced production and increased inactivation of NO.

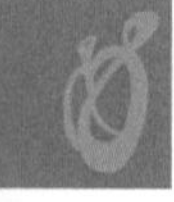

prostaglandins is operative only in individuals and patients with mild heart failure, whereas such an effect is not observed in patients with severe heart failure.

Intervention studies with angiotensin-II type 1 (AT_1-) receptor and aldosterone antagonists revealed that the renin-angiotensin system has a very complex impact on vascular functions including the endothelium. At the first glance, it may be surprising that the AT_1 receptor affects endothelial function. However, both experimental and clinical studies have shown the blockade of the AT_1 receptor is associated with improved endothelium-dependent relaxation,[64,70] suggesting a role for the AT_1 receptor in modulating endothelium-dependent mechanisms (i.e., indirectly by preventing inactivation of NO by superoxide anions). In this respect, we have demonstrated that the beneficial long-term effect of AT_1 receptor blockade on flow-dependent, endothelium-mediated vasodilation is blocked by the NO-synthase inhibitor L-NMMA, suggesting that therapy with an AT_1-receptor antagonist increases the bioavailability of NO.[68] Concomitantly, the AT_1-receptor blockade antagonist abolished the beneficial effect of antioxidant interventions. Based on experimental data, it is possible that the blockade of angiotensin II actions via the AT_1 receptor reduces NADH-oxidase activity and formation of superoxide anions.[71] The experimental observations in this respect are supported by our observation that 4 weeks of therapy with an AT_1-receptor antagonist increased the antioxidative potential of the vessel wall in patients with coronary artery disease by increasing the activity of EC-SOD[68] (see Figure 17-5, *B*). In addition, experimental data suggest that angiotensin II stimulates the AT_2 receptor during blockade of the AT_1 receptor,[72] which may cause bradykinin-mediated release of NO from endothelial cells.[72,73] In fact, long-term therapy with an AT_1 receptor has been shown to improve the vasodilation of peripheral resistance arteries in response to intraarterial infusion of bradykinin, an effect that was significantly smaller as compared with the effect of a comparable dose of an ACE inhibitor.[67]

It has recently been demonstrated by the RALES study that therapy with spironolactone on top of standard therapy, including diuretics and ACE inhibitors, improves the prognosis in patients with chronic heart failure.[74] In this respect it is interesting to note that there is evidence that spironolactone improves impaired endothelium-mediated vasodilation in patients with chronic heart failure. The beneficial effect of spironolactone was observed in patients on top of standard therapy with an ACE inhibitor and diuretics in a prospective, placebo-controlled cross-over study.[75] The improved endothelium-mediated vasomotion of forearm resistance arteries was inhibited by L-NMMA, supporting the concept that spironolactone increases bioavailability of NO consistent with experimental data that aldosterone inhibits endothelial release of NO.[76] In addition, aldosterone plasma concentrations in patients with chronic heart failure correlate inversely with arterial compliance,[77] which is in part related to endothelial release of nitric oxide.[78] Moreover, aldosterone may increase oxidative stress in the vascular wall, which, in turn, would then be attenuated by spironolactone.

Thus there is increasing evidence that the renin-angiotensin-aldosterone system can affect endothelial function in patients with chronic heart failure. Blockade of this neurohumoral activation by inhibition of ACE, aldosterone, and/or AT_1 receptors may well contribute to the beneficial long-term effects of these agents on prognosis in these patients. It is less clear to what extent blockade of the renin-angiotensin system affects other functions of the peripheral circulation, including the vascular structure of peripheral resistance vessels. However, some experimental data support that at least ACE inhibitors are capable of reversing vascular remodeling of the vasculature in heart failure,[79,80] consistent with the notion that the activated renin-angiotensin system has a profound impact on vascular function and structure in heart failure.

Alterations of Vascular Signal Transduction in Heart Failure

It has been suggested that abnormalities in vasodilator responsiveness in studies with the use of acetylcholine may be, in part, explained by a defect at the endothelial muscarinic receptor level or its signal transduction pathway. The majority of patients with heart failure have underlying ischemic heart disease and risk factors that are known to affect adversely the vascular responses to acetylcholine.[29,30,81] However, a reduced response to acetylcholine was found in chronic heart failure patients with nonischemic cardiomyopathy and without cardiovascular risk factors.[82] Because acetylcholine has direct smooth muscle contracting properties,[23] the response to this agonist represents the net effect of the release of vasodilating substances from the endothelium and direct smooth muscle contraction. Accordingly, the use of a pure endothelium-dependent vasodilator without effects on vascular smooth muscle might provide a clearer picture of endothelial vasodilator capacity. Substance P is a peptide that stimulates endothelial NO synthase through a different endothelial receptor, for example, the tachykinin receptor,[83] and has no direct effect on vascular smooth muscle cells. Substance P has been shown to dilate epicardial coronary arteries and coronary microvessels in humans[84] and forearm resistance and conduit arteries.[85] This vasodilator effect can be attenuated significantly by the NO-synthase inhibitor L-NMMA in normal subjects.[86] Interestingly, the acetylcholine-induced vasodilation of forearm resistance arteries was reduced significantly in patients with chronic heart failure, whereas the increase in blood flow in response to substance P was preserved and not impaired as compared with healthy controls. Similarly, intracoronary infusion of acetylcholine caused significantly less of an increase in coronary blood flow in heart failure patients as compared with control subjects, whereas substance P resulted in a similar increase in coronary blood flow in both groups.[87] Furthermore, the epicardial vasodilator response to substance P was also similar in both groups.[87] Thus it is possible that chronic heart failure may be associated with an abnormality of the muscarinic receptor and/or postreceptor coupling mechanisms, which could contribute to the observed reduction of the response to acetylcholine. However, it is established that endothelium-dependent dilation in response to increased flow, the most physiological test of endothelium-dependent relaxation, is markedly impaired in chronic heart failure. Moreover, vasodilation in response to stimulation of vasopressin type II (V2) receptors[88] is dependent on endothelial nitric oxide release and can be blocked by L-NMMA but not by indomethacin.[89,90] When the V2 receptor agonist desmopressin was infused into the brachial artery of heart failure patients and control subjects, the ensuing vasodilation was attenuated significantly in patients.[91] Moreover, inhibition of nitric oxide synthesis by L-NMMA reduced desmopressin responses to a significantly greater extent in control subjects as compared with patients.[91] Accordingly, these data clearly indicate that impaired endothelium-dependent vasodilation in patients with chronic heart failure is not limited to a specific defect of the muscarinic receptor or its signal transduction pathway.

Abnormalities of L-arginine Use in Chronic Heart Failure

L-arginine is the amino acid from which the endothelial NO-synthase synthesizes NO. Therefore, it has been supposed that an L-arginine deficit contributes to impaired NO-dependent vasodilation. Some experimental and clinical studies suggest that L-arginine has a beneficial effect on peripheral endothelial function, blood flow, and even exercise capacity. However, L-arginine improved endothelium-mediated vasodilation only in some, but not in all, studies performed in patients with chronic heart failure.[92-94] The effect of L-arginine may not be limited to improvements in endothelium-dependent relaxation; in fact, there is some evidence that L-arginine supplementation inhibits monocyte adhesion and platelet aggregation.[95,96] Yet, the potential beneficial effect of L-arginine is difficult to explain, since L-arginine plasma concentrations are sufficiently high for a maximal saturation of endothelial NO synthase.[97] This phenomenon is called the "L-arginine paradox." There are, however, experimental[98] and clinical data suggesting that endogenous competitive L-arginine antagonists such as asymmetrical dimethyl-L-arginine (ADMA) inhibit NO-synthesis from L-arginine as demonstrated in hypercholesterolemia and chronic heart failure.[99,100] Furthermore, data from our group suggest that ADMA plasma concentrations are inversely related to endothelium-mediated vasodilation and exercise capacity in patients with chronic heart failure.[101] In this respect, the bioavailability of NO may be determined by the ratio between L-arginine and ADMA. ADMA is inactivated by DDAH, an enzyme that is redox-sensitive.[102] Oxidative stress contributes to increased ADMA plasma concentrations and L-arginine supplementation might develop antioxidative effects. In hypercholesterolemia, intracellular ADMA levels are increased and L-arginine availability is impaired, despite normal L-arginine plasma concentrations.[103] However, little is known about the expression and activity of DAHH in heart failure, nor do we have data on intracellular L-arginine and ADMA levels in endothelial cells in this condition. However, the markedly increased ADMA levels show a profound alteration of the L-arginine-NO system in heart failure, which may have additional implications beyond endothelium-dependent mechanisms (i.e., impact on the bioavailability of NO in skeletal muscle, which could affect muscle contraction and oxygen consumption [see later discussion]). In addition, oxidant stress-sensitive arginase activity may explain a limited L-arginine availability.[101a] In the clinical setting, the supplementation of high dosages of L-arginine (5 to 20 g/day) during long-term therapy are necessary to achieve an effect and may be associated with altered taste and gastrointestinal side effects. Thus L-arginine supplementation may represent a "proof of the principle" rather than a practical therapeutic option.

Role of Physical Activity for Endothelial Function in Chronic Heart Failure (see also Chapter 57)

One functional consequence of an impaired endothelial function is that the vessels lose their ability to release NO in response to increased blood flow such as during physical activity[104] (i.e., impairment of flow-dependent, endothelium-mediated vasodilation).[39] Experimental work showed that chronically reduced blood flow is associated with reduced endothelial release of NO while increased flow is translated into increased release of NO[105,106] due to upregulation of eNOS and EC-SOD gene expression related to enhanced shear stress.[107] Consistent with these experimental observations, physical training improves endothelial function by increasing the bioavailability of NO (Figure 17-7). The positive effect of physical training appears to be restricted to the extremity exposed to physical training. The beneficial effect of training is quickly lost within weeks after the end of training.[3] These observations suggest that endothelial function is regulated locally and modulated by the extent of daily physical activity. These beneficial effects of physical training have now been demonstrated by different groups in healthy controls,[108] patients with chronic heart failure,[109,110] coronary artery disease,[111] hypercholesterolemia,[112] and arterial hypertension[113] in peripheral resistance[109,110] along with conduit arteries[3] and in the coronary circulation.[111] The positive effects of physical training on endothelial function are multifactorial, including increased expression of eNOS, EC-SOD, and potentially mobilization of endothelial progenitor cells.[111a] The effect of physical training on EC-SOD appears to be dependent on the upregulation of eNOS, since EC-SOD activity is reduced in eNOS knockout mice, but can be increased by physical training associated with increased eNOS gene expression.[114] ACE-activity is increased in patients with chronic heart failure and/or arteriosclerosis,[58,115] leading to increased formation of angiotensin II and increased inactivation of endogenous bradykinin, resulting in decreased NO levels. In contrast, increased sheer stress reduces ACE-gene expression and results in increased NO activity.[116] Since NO has profound effects on vascular structure and remodeling, exercise induced changes in blood flow may affect NO levels through changes in ACE-activity, with resultant favorable changes in vascular structure. While there is some experimental evidence that mechanism is important in animal models of arteriosclerosis (i.e., normalization of vascular structure and increased inner arterial lumen diameter)[117], there are no data that support this mechanism is in experimental or clinical heart failure.

Abnormalities of Vascular Smooth Muscle Responsiveness in Chronic Heart Failure

Beyond impaired endothelium-dependent vascular responses, it is possible that the responses of the underlying vascular smooth muscle to vasodilators, such as nitric oxide or

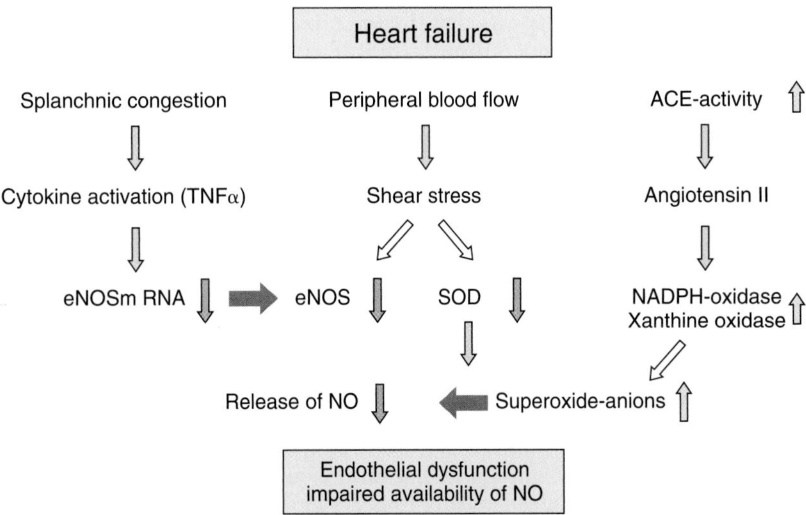

FIGURE 17–7 Shows the effect of 4 weeks of physical training on flow-dependent, endothelium-dependent vasodilation (FDD) in patients with chronic heart failure. Bar graphs indicate percent change of radial artery diameter during FDD before (baseline) and after training (training) and 6 weeks after end of the training. (Modified from Hornig B, Maier V, Drexler H. Physical training improves endothelial function in patients with chronic heart failure. *Circulation* 1996;93:210-214.)

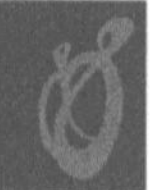

adenosine, is altered in severe chronic heart failure. Nitric oxide stimulates the guanylyl cyclase in vascular smooth muscle cells and the resultant increase in cGMP leads to muscular relaxation, causing vasodilation. It is conceivable that a reduced responsiveness of this system to nitric oxide stimulation also could contribute to vasodilator dysfunction in chronic heart failure. A reduced response to nitroglycerin was first observed by Zelis et al[15] in their landmark study of the peripheral circulation in 1968. Some more recent studies did not find significant differences in the vascular responses to direct-acting donors of nitric oxide or endothelium-independent vasodilators; however, the clinical characteristics of these patients were different (i.e., less edematous and in a more compensated state). The initial observations were confirmed in patients with severe heart failure (i.e., nitroglycerin resulted in a significantly smaller increase in mean blood flow velocity of the superficial artery after intraarterial infusion in patients with chronic heart failure as compared with control subjects). Therefore a reduced responsiveness of vascular smooth muscle to nitric oxide–dependent cGMP-mediated or nonspecific vasodilation appears to represent a contributing factor in severe chronic heart failure.

Beyond impaired vasodilator capacity in heart failure, enhanced synthesis and release of vascular vasoconstricting factor may emerge in heart failure (i.e., originating from the cyclooxygenase metabolic pathway).[59,118,119] In this respect, patients with chronic heart failure showed a blunted response to acetylcholine as compared with control subjects.[34] When these experiments were repeated after cyclooxygenase inhibition with indomethacin, the vasodilator responses to acetylcholine were unchanged in normal subjects, but significantly increased in patients. Despite this improvement, the response still was significantly attenuated compared with normal subjects.[34] In addition, intraarterial infusion of sodium-nitroprusside in chronic heart failure patients treated with aspirin resulted in significantly greater vasodilation as compared with patients not pretreated with aspirin.[17] Both findings are compatible with the view that an abnormal production of cyclooxygenase-dependent vasoconstricting factor(s) seems to be present in the peripheral circulation of patients with chronic heart failure. Such an effect may blunt the vasodilatory effects of both endogenous nitric oxide liberated by endothelial agonists such as acetylcholine and exogenous nitric oxide derived from nitric oxide donors such as sodium nitroprusside or nitroglycerin.

Thus there is abundant evidence that chronic heart failure is associated with impaired endothelium-dependent vasodilator function of peripheral resistance and conduit arteries. This impaired endothelium-dependent vasodilation is to a large extent secondary to a reduced bioavailability of nitric oxide. Nevertheless, it appears that the impaired endothelial function in chronic heart failure is multifactorial, including reduced expression of endothelial nitric oxide synthase, L-arginine substrate limitations, activation of the renin-angiotensin system, and enhanced oxidant stress, further reducing nitric oxide availability.

POTENTIAL FUNCTIONAL IMPLICATIONS FOR PATIENTS WITH CHRONIC HEART FAILURE

Because endothelial vasodilator function is involved in the control of tissue perfusion, the question arises whether impaired exercise-induced release of nitric oxide contributes to reduced aerobic exercise capacity and worsening LV remodeling in patients with chronic heart failure. Moreover, it would be important to know whether improved endothelial function increases exercise capacity in chronic heart failure.

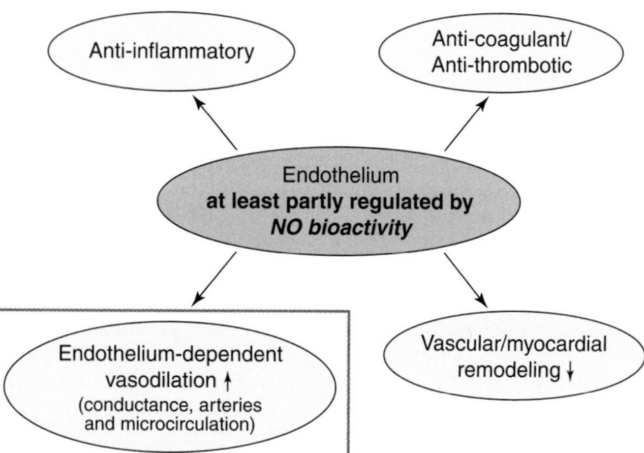

FIGURE 17–8 Role of endothelial function in heart failure.

If so, the endothelium would represent an attractive therapeutic target in these patients (Figure 17-8).

The beneficial effects of physical training in patients with chronic heart failure are established and are associated with improved endothelial vasodilator function. Several mechanisms have been proposed to account for the clinical benefit of physical training, including improvement of left ventricular diastolic function, autonomic balance, and ventilatory and/or skeletal muscle function. In particular, skeletal muscle atrophy, impaired metabolism, and reduced skeletal muscle oxidative capacity appear to contribute to the reduced exercise capacity in chronic heart failure. Exercise training improves force of contraction, metabolism, and oxidative capacity of skeletal muscle. Force of contraction in skeletal muscle is modulated by nitric oxide through reduced Ca^{2+} activation of actin filaments, resulting in decreased myofibrillar calcium sensitivity.[120] Skeletal muscle fibers express two isoforms of the nitric oxide synthase: neuronal and endothelial. In chronic heart failure, expression of the inducible nitric oxide synthase has been shown to emerge in skeletal muscle of patients.[121] Therefore, increased nitric oxide availability within the skeletal muscle may reduce the contractile force in these patients. In addition, endogenous nitric oxide released from microvascular endothelium plays an important role in the modulation of cellular respiration in skeletal muscle.[122] The suppression of tissue oxygen consumption in response to bradykinin (presumably stimulating endothelial release of nitric oxide) is blunted in the skeletal muscle of dogs with heart failure,[123] indicating a defective endogenous nitric oxide–mediated modulation of tissue oxygen consumption in skeletal muscle after development of heart failure. It is conceivable that defective biosynthesis of nitric oxide in skeletal muscle can be improved by physical training. Interestingly, the preservation of endothelial vasodilator function by physical training is associated by preserved resting hemodynamics and alleviation of clinical manifestations of heart failure,[124] consistent with the ideas that the beneficial effects of physical training are mediated in part by endothelial mechanisms.

The significant relationship between improvement of endothelial function and exercise capacity supports the notion that improved endothelial function contributes to increased exercise capacity, particularly since there is experimental evidence suggesting that limb blood flow during exercise is dependent on nitric oxide.[125] However, improved endothelial function can probably account only for a small incremental increase in exercise capacity. A complex physiology exists for hyperemia, exercise, and nitric oxide. The role of nitric oxide in exercise-induced increase in blood flow still remains controversial and the effects of inhibition of nitric oxide synthesis in this respect are modest at best. Increases in blood flow during exercise or following arterial occlusions are mediated by several mediators and blockade of several systems is necessary to attenuate reactive hyperemia. In normal individuals, peak vasodilatory capacity can be increased by physical training without influencing basal or stimulated activity of the nitric oxide vasodilator system,[126] although exercise training undoubtedly augments endothelial nitric oxide synthesis and flow-dependent dilation of skeletal muscle arterioles through nitric oxide and prostaglandins.[127] Following physical training, an increase in flow reserve or reactive hyperemia has been observed both in animals and in humans. In fact, physical training in patients has been associated with increases in skeletal muscle blood flow during exercise, reactive hyperemia, and peak oxygen consumption possibly by enhancing vascular conduction and growth.[128] However, increased metabolic vasodilation in response to arterial occlusion may not be associated necessarily with increased training-induced endothelium-dependent vasodilation during exercise in chronic heart failure. Indeed, a recent study observed that the increased vasodilatory responses following arterial occlusion and endothelium-dependent stimuli following physical training in patients with chronic heart failure do not correlate, suggesting that the determinants of peak reactive hyperemic blood flow and endothelium-dependent vasodilation are not linked.[109] However, increased availability of nitric oxide during exercise provided by regular physical training may contribute to exercise capacity without affecting total increases in skeletal muscle blood flow by affecting the distribution of blood flow within the skeletal muscle. Interestingly, a recent pilot study has suggested that intense aerobic interval exercise training is substantially more effective as compared with continuous moderate exercise in restoring endothelium-dependent vasodilation in patients with CHF[109a]; however, this has to be confirmed in a larger study. Intense exercise training was also associated with a more pronounced beneficial effect on cardiac remodeling.[109a]

In chronic heart failure, skeletal muscle underperfusion emerges predominately in oxidative working muscle.[8] Inhibition of nitric oxide synthesis by L-nitro-arginine methyl ester (L-NAME) is most effective in limiting blood flow to oxidative working muscles, but the inhibitory effect of L-NAME on blood flow in these muscle fibers appears to be attenuated in chronic heart failure.[129] Thus redistribution of blood flow within skeletal muscle appears to emerge in heart failure caused by endothelial dysfunction possibly secondary to chronic deconditioning. It may be speculated that improved oxygen delivery with physical training is related partially to the reversal of impaired endothelium-dependent relaxation within oxidative muscle fibers. In this respect, it is noteworthy that activity of the neuronal NO synthase can be upregulated by endurance training.

Nitric oxide also is involved in the central regulation of sympathetic outflow, raising the possibility that both neuronal and endothelial nitric oxide synthesis may contribute to the regulation of vasomotor tone.[130] It is possible that the sympathoinhibitory effects of nitric oxide may be reduced in chronic heart failure and thus contribute to sustained sympathetic activation.

Several other interventions targeting the endothelium have been studied in chronic heart failure. ACE inhibition has been shown to improve endothelium-dependent vasodilation.[69,131] Accordingly, it is conceivable that the related beneficial effects of ACE inhibitors on exercised-induced blood flow and exercise capacity in heart failure[9] is, in part, caused by improved endothelium-dependent vasodilation. Antioxidants such as vitamin C are effective in restoring endothelium-dependent vasodilation[53]; however, their potential to improve exercise capacity is limited.[132]

In conclusion, endothelial dysfunction may play a role in the redistribution of blood flow during exercise and adversely affect exercise capacity. Conditions such as chronic heart failure that reduce the availability of endothelium-derived nitric oxide also impair the normal exercise-induced blood flow response. This in turn may lead to diminished exercise capacity.

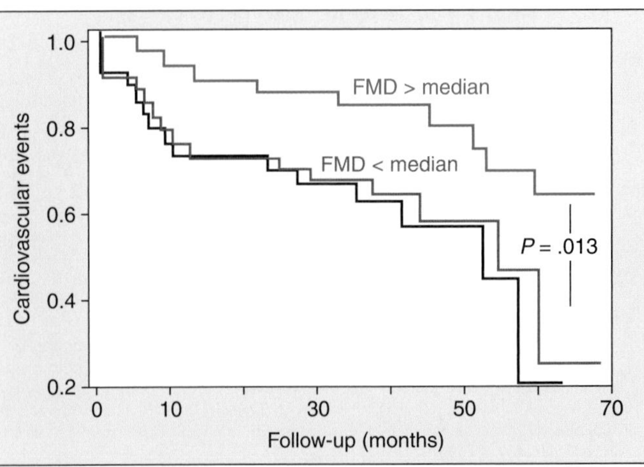

FIGURE 17–9 Effect of endothelial function on prognosis in heart failure. Endothelial dysfunction (i.e., impaired endothelium-dependent vasodilation) has been associated with a markedly adverse outcome in patients with CHF in several studies. The figure shows the relationship between endothelium-dependent vasodilation (measured at the radial artery) and cardiovascular events (cardiac death, hospitalization due to worsening of heart failure—NYHA class IV/pulmonary edema, or necessity for heart transplantation) in the follow-up of patients with CHF. The study cohort was divided into those with flow-dependent vasodilation (FDD), greater median (6.2%) and lesser median. (Modified from Fischer D, Rossa S, Landmesser U, et al. Endothelial dysfunction in patients with chronic heart failure is independently associated with increased incidence of hospitalization, cardiac transplantation, or death. *Eur Heart J* 2005;26(1):65-69.)

PROGNOSTIC IMPLICATIONS OF ENDOTHELIAL DYSFUNCTION

There is now accumulating evidence suggesting that an impaired nitric oxide–mediated vasodilation may have prognostic implications in patients with CHF. Indeed, impaired endothelium-dependent vasodilation was associated with an increased risk of hospitalization for heart failure and death in patients with CHF (Figure 17-9).[133-135] Thus in a limited number of patients with chronic heart failure and endothelium-mediated vasomotion studies, a correlation of endothelial dysfunction with future cardiovascular outcome has been shown by several authors using different techniques to characterize endothelial function. It should be noted, however, that the number of cardiovascular events was rather small in all of these studies.

Experimental data, however, suggest that endothelial NO synthase (and consequently endothelial function) is important for outcome in postmyocardial infarction. In this respect, a recent experimental study showed that mice lacking endothelial NO synthase have a substantially reduced survival rate after a myocardial infarction.[136] Moreover, we have observed that statin-induced beneficial effects on outcome after myocardial infarction were dependent on endothelial NO synthase, since they were not observed in eNOS-deficient animals.[137]

REFERENCES

1. Francis, G. S., Benedict, C., Johnstone, D. E., et al. (1990). for the SOLVD investigators. Comparison of neuro-endocrine activation in patients with left ventricular dysfunction with and without congestive heart failure. *Circulation, 82*, 1724–1729.
2. Cody, R. J., Atlas, S. A., Laragh, J. H., et al. (1986). Atrial natriuretic factor in normal subjects and heart failure patients: plasma levels and renal, hormonal and hemodynamic responses to peptide infusion. *J Clin Invest, 78*, 1362–1374.
3. Hornig, B., Maier, V., & Drexler, H. (1996). Physical training improves endothelial function in patients with chronic heart failure. *Circulation, 93*, 210–214.

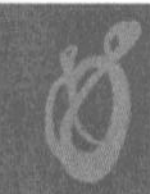

4. Wilson, J. R., Rayos, G., Yeoh, T. K., et al. (1995). Dissociation between peak exercise oxygen consumption and hemodynamic dysfunction in potential heart transplantation candidates. *J Am Coll Cardiol, 26*, 429–435.
5. Chomsky, D. B., Lang, C. C., Rayos, G. H., et al. (1996). Hemodynamics of exercise testing. A valuable tool in the selection of cardiac transplantation candidates. *Circulation, 94*, 3176–3183.
6. Wilson, J. R., Martin, J. L., Schwartz, D., et al. (1984). Exercise intolerance in patients with chronic heart failure: role of impaired nutritive flow to skeletal muscle. *Circulation, 69*, 1079–1087.
7. Zelis, R., Longhurst, J., Capone, R. J., et al. (1974). A comparison of regional blood flow and oxygen utilization during dynamic forearm exercise in normal subjects and patients with chronic heart failure. *Circulation, 50*, 137–143.
8. Drexler, H., Faude, F., Höing, S., et al. (1987). Blood flow distribution within skeletal muscle during exercise in the presence of chronic heart failure: effect of milrinone. *Circulation, 76*, 1344–1352.
9. Drexler, H., Banhardt, U., Meinertz, T., et al. (1989). Contrasting peripheral short-term and long-term effects of converting enzyme inhibition in patients with chronic heart failure. A double-blind, placebo-controlled trial. *Circulation, 79*, 491–502.
10. Sullivan, M. J., Knight, J. D., Higginbotham, M. B., et al. (1989). Relation between central and peripheral hemodynamics during exercise in patients with chronic heart failure. *Circulation, 80*, 769–781.
11. LeJemtel, T. H., Maskin, C. S., Lucido, D., et al. (1986). Failure to augment maximal limb blood flow in response to one-leg versus two-leg exercise in patients with severe heart failure. *Circulation, 74*, 245–251.
12. McMurray, J. J., Ray, S. G., Abdulla, I., et al. (1992). Plasma endothelin in chronic heart failure. *Circulation, 85*, 1374–1379.
13. Giaid, A., Yanagisawa, M., Langleben, D., et al. (1993). Expression of endothelin-1 in the lungs of patients with pulmonary hypertension. *N Engl J Med, 328*, 1732–1739.
14. Kiowski, W., Bertel, O., Sütsch, G., et al. (1995). Vasodilator effects of the endothelin-1 receptor antagonist bosentan in patients with severe chronic heart failure. *J Am Coll Cardiol, 25*, 296A (abstract).
15. Zelis, R., Mason, D. T., & Braunwald, E. (1968). A comparison of the effects of vasodilator stimuli on peripheral resistance vessels in normal subjects and patients with congestive heart failure. *J Clin Invest, 47*, 960–970.
16. Wilson, J. R., & Ferraro, N. (1985). Effect of renin-angiotensin system on limb circulation and metabolism during exercise in patients with heart failure. *J Am Coll Cardiol, 6*, 556–563.
17. Jeserich, M., Pape, L., Just, H., et al. (1995). Effect of long-term ACE-inhibition on vascular function in patients with chronic heart failure. *Am J Cardiol, 76*, 1079–1082.
18. Captopril Multicenter Research Group. (1983). A placebo-controlled trial of captopril in refractory chronic heart failure. *J Am Coll Cardiol, 2*, 755–763.
19. Geisterfer, A. A. T., Peach, M. J., & Owens, G. K. (1988). Angiotensin II induces hypertrophy not hyperplasia of cultured rat aortic smooth muscle cells. *Circ Res, 62*, 749–756.
20. Schieffer, B., Wollert, K., Berchthold, M., et al. (1995). Development and prevention of skeletal muscle structural alterations after experimental myocardial infarction. *Am J Physiol, 269*, H1507–H1513.
21. Sinoway, L. I., Minotti, J., Musch, T., et al. (1987). Enhanced metabolic vasodilation secondary to diuretic therapy in decompensated congestive heart failure secondary to coronary artery disease. *Am J Cardiol, 60*, 107–111.
22. Drexler, H., Riede, U., Münzel, T., et al. (1992). Alterations of skeletal muscle in chronic heart failure. *Circulation, 85*, 1751–1759.
23. Vane, J. R., Anggard, E. E., & Botting, R. M. (1990). Regulatory functions of the endothelium. *N Engl J Med, 323*, 27–36.
24. Drexler, H., & Lu, W. (1992). Endothelial dysfunction of hindquarter resistance vessels in experimental heart failure. *Am J Physiol, 262*, H1640–H1645.
25. Joannides, R., Haefeli, W. E., Linder, L., et al. (1995). Nitric oxide is responsible for flow-dependent dilatation of human peripheral conduit arteries in vivo. *Circulation, 91*, 1314–1319.
26. Palmer, R. M. J., Ferrige, A. G., & Moncada, S. (1987). Nitric oxide accounts for the biological activity of endothelium-derived relaxing factor. *Nature, 327*, 524–526.
27. Palmer, R. M. J., Ashton, D. S., & Moncada, S. (1988). Vascular endothelial cells synthesize nitric oxide from L-arginine. *Nature, 333*, 664–666.
28. Nathan, C. (1992). Nitric oxide as a secretory product of mammalian cells. *FASEB J, 6*, 3051–3064.
29. Linder, L., Kiowski, W., Buhler, F. R., et al. (1990). Indirect evidence for release of endothelium-derived relaxing factor in human forearm circulation in vivo. Blunted response in essential hypertension. *Circulation, 81*, 1762–1767.
30. Panza, J. A., Casino, P. R., Kilcoyne, C. M., et al. (1993). Role of endothelium-derived nitric oxide in the abnormal endothelium-dependent vascular relaxation of patients with essential hypertension. *Circulation, 87*, 1468–1474.
31. Treasure, C. B., Vita, J. A., Cox, D. A., et al. (1990). Endothelium-dependent dilation of the coronary microvasculature is impaired in dilated cardiomyopathy. *Circulation, 81*, 772–779.
32. Katz, S. D., Biasucci, L., Sabba, C., et al. (1992). Impaired endothelium-mediated vasodilation in the peripheral vasculature of patients with congestive heart failure. *J Am Coll Cardiol, 19*, 918–925.
33. Kubo, S. H., Rector, T. S., Bank, A. J., et al. (1991). Endothelium-dependent vasodilation is attenuated in patients with heart failure. *Circulation, 84*, 1589–1596.
34. Katz, S. D., Schwarz, M., Yuen, J., et al. (1993). Impaired acetylcholine-mediated vasodilation in patients with congestive heart failure. Role of endothelium-derived vasodilating and vasoconstricting factors. *Circulation, 88*, 55–61.
35. Drexler, H., Hayoz, D., Münzel, T., et al. (1992). Endothelial function in chronic congestive heart failure. *Am J Cardiol, 69*, 1596–1601.
36. Vallance, P., Collier, J., & Moncada, S. (1989). Effects of endothelium-derived nitric oxide on peripheral arteriolar tone in man. *Lancet, 2*, 997–1000.
37. Winlaw, D. S., Smythe, G. A., Keogh, A. M., et al. (1994). Increased nitric oxide production in heart failure. *Lancet, 344*, 373–374.
38. Habib, F., Dutka, D., Crossman, D., et al. (1994). Enhanced basal nitric oxide production in heart failure: another failed counter-regulatory vasodilator mechanism? *Lancet, 344*, 371–373.
39. Hayoz, D., Drexler, H., Münzel, T., et al. (1993). Flow-mediated arteriolar dilation is abnormal in congestive heart failure. *Circulation, 87*(suppl. VII), VII-92–VII-96.
40. Ramsey, M. W., & Jones, C. J. H. (1994). Large arteries are more than passive conduits. *Br Heart J, 72*, 3–4.
41. Teerlink, J. R., Clozel, M., Fischli, W., et al. (1993). Temporal evolution of endothelial dysfunction in a rat model of chronic heart failure. *J Am Coll Cardiol, 22*, 615–620.
42. Rubanyi, G., Romero, C. J., & Vanhoutte, P. M. (1986). Flow-induced release of endothelium-derived relaxing factor. *Am J Physiol, 250*, H1145–H1149.
43. Uematsu, M., Ohara, Y., Navas, J. P., et al. (1995). Regulation of endothelial cell nitric oxide synthase mRNA expression by shear stress. *Am J Physiol, 269*, C1371–C1378.
44. Smith, C. J., Sun, D., Hoegler, C., et al. (1996). Reduced gene expression of vascular endothelial NO synthase and cyclooxygenase-1 in heart failure. *Circ Res, 78*, 58–64.
45. Drexler, H., Kästner, A., Strobel, A., et al. (1998). Expression, activity, and functional significance of inducible nitric oxide synthase in the failing human heart. *J Am Coll Cardiol, 32*, 955–963.
46. Kichuk, M. R., Seyedi, N., Zhang, X., et al. (1996). Regulation of nitric oxide production in human coronary microvessels and the contribution of local kinin formation. *Circulation, 94*, 44–51.
47. Katz, S. D., Ramanath, R., Berman, J. W., et al. (1994). Pathophysiological correlation of increased serum tumor necrosis factor in patients with chronic heart failure. Relation to nitric oxide dependent vasodilation in the forearm circulation. *Circulation, 90*, 12–16.

47a. Fichtlscherer, S., Rossig, L., Breuer, S., et al. (2001). Tumor necrosis factor antagonism with etanercept improves systemic endothelial vasoreactivity in patients with advanced heart failure. *Circulation, 104*, 3023–3025.

47b. Landmesser, U., Dikalov, S., Price, S. R., et al. (2003). Oxidation of tetrahydrobiopterin leads to uncoupling of endothelial cell nitric oxide synthase in hypertension. *J Clin Invest, 111*(8), 1201–1209.

47c. Moens, A. L., Takimoto, E., Tocchetti, C. G., et al. (2008). Reversal of cardiac hypertrophy and fibrosis from pressure overload by tetrahydrobiopterin: efficacy of recoupling nitric oxide synthase as a therapeutic strategy. *Circulation, 117*(20), 2626–2636.

48. Aoki, N., Siegfried, M., & Lefer, A. M. (1989). Anti-EDRF effect of tumor necrosis factor in isolated, perfused cat carotid arteries. *Am J Physiol, 256*(suppl. II), H1509–H1512.
49. Yoshimuzi, M., Perella, M. A., Burnett, J. C., et al. (1993). Tumor necrosis factor down regulates an endothelial nitric oxide synthase mRNA by shortening its half-life. *Circ Res, 73*, 205–209.
50. Levine, B., Kalman, J., Mayer, L., et al. (1990). Elevated circulation levels of tumor necrosis factor in severe chronic heart failure. *N Engl J Med, 323*, 236–241.
51. Matsabura, T., & Ziff, M. (1986). Increased superoxide anion release from human endothelial cells in response to cytokines. *J Immunol, 137*, 3295–3298.
52. Belch, J. J. F., Bridges, A. B., Scott, N., et al. (1991). Oxygen free radicals and congestive heart failure. *Br Heart J, 65*, 245–248.
53. Hornig, B., Arakawa, N., Kohler, C., et al. (1998). Vitamin C improves endothelial function of conduit arteries in patients with chronic heart failure. *Circulation, 97*, 363–368.
54. Griendling, K. K., Minieri, C. A., Ollerenshaw, J. D., et al. (1994). Angiotensin II stimulates NADH and NADPH oxidase activity in cultured vascular smooth muscle cells. *Circ Res, 74*, 1141–1148.

54a. Dworakowski, R., Walker, S., Momin, A., et al. (2008). Reduced nicotinamide adenine dinucleotide phosphate oxidase-derived superoxide and vascular endothelial dysfunction in human heart failure. *J Am Coll Cardiol, 51*(14), 1349–1356.

54b. Landmesser, U., Spiekermann, S., Dikalov, S., et al. (2002). Vascular oxidative stress and endothelial dysfunction in patients with chronic heart failure: role of xanthine-oxidase and extracellular superoxide dismutase. *Circulation, 106*(24), 3073–3078.

55. Mohazzab, H. K. M., Zhang, X., Kichuk, M. R., et al. (1995). Potential sites and changes of superoxide anion production in failing and non-failing explanted human cardiac myocytes. *Circulation, 92*(suppl. I), 32 (abstract).
56. Sole, M., Schimmer, J., Golstein, D., et al. (1995). Oxidative stress contributes to decompensation of the failing heart. *Circulation, 92*(suppl. I), 31 (abstract).
57. Prasad, K., Kalra, J., & Bharadwaj, B. (1987). Phagocytic activity in blood of dogs with chronic heart failure. *Clin Invest Med, 10*, 1354–1357.
58. Studer, R., Reinecke, H., Müller, B., et al. (1994). Increased angiotensin-I-converting enzyme gene expression in the failing human heart. *J Clin Invest, 94*, 301–310.
59. Mombouli, J. V., Illiano, S., Nagao, T., et al. (1992). Potentiation of endothelium-dependent relaxations to bradykinin by angiotensin I converting enzyme inhibitors in canine coronary arteries involves both endothelium-derived relaxing and hyperpolarizing factors. *Circ Res, 71*, 137–144.
60. Barrow, S. E., Dollerey, C. T., Heavey, D. J., et al. (1986). Effect of vasoactive peptides on prostacyclin synthesis in man. *Br J Pharmacol, 87*, 243–247.
61. Pellacani, A., Brunner, H. R., & Nussberger, J. (1994). Plasma kinins increase after angiotensin-converting enzyme inhibition in human subjects. *Clin Sci, 87*, 567–574.
62. Benzing, T., Fleming, I., Blaukat, A., et al. (1999). Angiotensin-converting enzyme inhibitor ramiprilat interferes with the sequestration of the B2 kinin receptor within the plasma membrane of native endothelial cells. *Circulation, 99*, 2034–2040.
63. Leeb-Lundberg, L. M., Mathis, S. A., & Herzig, M. C. S. (1994). Antagonists of bradykinin that stabilize a G-protein uncoupled state of the B2 receptor act as inverse agonists in rat myometrial cells. *J Biol Chem, 269*, 25970–25973.
64. Groves, P., Kurz, S., Just, H., et al. (1995). Role of endogenous bradykinin in human coronary artery vasomotor control. *Circulation, 92*, 3424–3430.
65. Hornig, B., Kohler, C., & Drexler, H. (1997). Role of bradykinin in mediating vascular effects of ACE-inhibitors in humans. *Circulation, 95*, 1115–1118.
66. Varin, R., et al. (2000). Improvement of endothelial function by chronic angiotensin-converting enzyme inhibition in heart failure. *Circulation, 102*, 351–356.

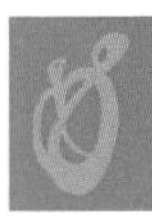

67. Davie, A. P., Dargie, H. J., & McMurray, J. J. V. (1999). Role of bradykinin in the vasodilator effects of losartan and enalapril in patients with heart failure. *Circulation, 100*, 268–273.

67a. Witherow, F. N., Helmy, A., Webb, D. J., et al. (2001). Bradykinin contributes to the vasodilator effects of chronic angiotensin-converting enzyme inhibition in patients with heart failure. *Circulation, 104*, 2177–2181.

68. Hornig, B., Landmesser, U., Kohler, C., et al. (2001). Comparative effect of ACE inhibition and angiotensin II type 1 receptor antagonism on bioavailability of nitric oxide in patients with coronary artery disease. Role of superoxide dismutase. *Circulation, 103*, 799–805.

69. Hirsch, H., Bijou, R., Yuen, J., et al. (1993). Enalapril-induced vasodilation is attenuated by indomethacin in congestive heart failure and completely abolished in normal subjects. *Circulation, 88*, I293.

70. Prasad, A., Tupas-Habib, T., Schenke, W. H., et al. (2000). Acute and chronic angiotensin-1 receptor antagonism reverses endothelial dysfunction in atherosclerosis. *Circulation, 101*, 2349.

71. Warnholtz, A., Nickenig, G., Schulz, E., et al. (1999). Increased NADH-oxidase-mediated superoxide production in the early stages of atherosclerosis: evidence for the involvement of the renin-angiotensin system. *Circulation, 99*, 2027–2033.

72. Tsutsumi, Y., Matsubara, H., Masaki, H., et al. (1999). Angiotensin I type 2 receptor overexpression activates the vascular kinin system and causes vasodilation. *J Clin Invest, 104*, 925–935.

73. Gohlke, P., Pees, C., & Unger, T. (1998). AT2 receptor stimulation increases aortic cyclic cGMP in SHRSP by a kinin-dependent mechanism. *Hypertension, 31*, 349–355.

74. Pitt, B., Zannad, F., Remme, W. J., et al. (1999). The effect of spironolactone on morbidity and mortality in patients with severe heart failure. *N Engl J Med, 341*, 709–717.

75. Farquharson, C. A. J., & Struthers, A. D. (2000). Spironolactone increases nitric oxide bioactivity, improves endothelial vasodilator dysfunction and suppresses vascular angiotensin I/angiotensin II conversion in patients with chronic heart failure. *Circulation, 101*, 594–597.

76. Ikeda, U., Kanbe, T., Nakayama, I., et al. (1995). Aldosterone inhibits nitric oxide synthesis in rat vascular smooth muscle cells induced by interleukin-1ß. *Eur J Pharmacol, 290*, 69–73.

77. Duprez, D. A., DeBuyerze, M. L., Rietzschel, E. R., et al. (1998). Inverse relationship between aldosterone and large artery compliance in chronically treated heart failure patients. *Eur Heart J, 19*, 1371–1376.

78. Ramsey, M. W., Goodfellow, J., Jones, C. J. H., et al. (1995). Endothelial control of arterial distensibility is impaired in chronic heart failure. *Circulation, 92*, 3212–3219.

79. Schieffer, B., Wollert, K. C., Berchthold, M., et al. (1995). Development and prevention of skeletal muscle structural alterations after experimental myocardial infarction. *Am J Physiol, 269*, H1507–H1513.

80. Mulder, P., et al. (1996). Peripheral artery structure and endothelial function in heart failure: effect of ACE inhibition. *Am J Physiol, 271*, H469–H477.

81. Creager, M. A., Cooke, J. P., Mendelsohn, M. E., et al. (1990). Impaired vasodilation of forearm resistance vessels in hypercholesterolemic humans. *J Clin Invest, 86*, 228–234.

82. Nakamura, M., Yoshida, H., Arakawa, N., et al. (1996). Endothelium-dependent vasodilatation is not selectively impaired in patients with chronic heart failure secondary to valvular heart disease and congenital heart disease. *Eur Heart J, 17*, 1875–1881.

83. Saito, R., Nonaka, S., Konishi, H., et al. (1991). Pharmacological properties of the tachykinin receptor subtype in the endothelial cell and vasodilation. *Ann N Y Acad Sci, 632*, 457–459.

84. Crossman, D. C., Larkin, S. W., Fuller, R. W., et al. (1989). Substance P dilates epicardial coronary arteries and increases coronary blood flow in humans. *Circulation, 80*, 475–484.

85. McEvan, J. R., Benjamin, N., Larkin, S., et al. (1988). Vasodilatation by calcitonin gene-related peptide and by substance P: a comparison of their effects on resistance and capacitance vessels of human forearms. *Circulation, 77*, 1072–1080.

86. Panza, J. A., Casino, P. R., Kilcoyne, C. M., et al. (1994). Impaired endothelium-dependent vasodilation in patients with essential hypertension: evidence that the abnormality is not at the muscarinic receptor level. *J Am Coll Cardiol, 23*, 1610–1616.

87. Holdright, D. R., Clarke, D., Fox, K., et al. (1994). The effects of intracoronary substance P and acetylcholine on coronary blood flow in patients with idiopathic dilated cardiomyopathy. *Eur Heart J, 15*, 1537–1544.

88. Hirsch, A. T., Dzau, V. J., Majzoub, J. A., et al. (1989). Vasopressin-mediated forearm vasodilation in normal humans. Evidence for a vascular vasopressin V2 receptor. *J Clin Invest, 84*, 418–426.

89. Liard, J. F. (1994). L-NAME antagonizes vasopressin V2-induced vasodilatation in dogs. *Am J Physiol, 266*, H99–H106.

90. Tagawa, T., Imaizumi, T., Shiramoto, M., et al. (1995). V2 receptor-mediated vasodilation in healthy humans. *J Cardiovasc Pharmacol, 25*, 387–392.

91. Rector, T. S., Bank, A. J., Tschumperlin, L. K., et al. (1996). Abnormal desmopressin induced forearm vasodilatation in patients with heart failure: dependence on nitric oxide synthase activity. *Clin Pharmacol Ther, 60*, 667–674.

92. Hirooka, Y., Egashira, K., Imaizumi, T., et al. (1994). Effects of L-arginine on impaired acetylcholine-induced and ischemic vasodilation of the forearm in patients with chronic heart failure. *Circulation, 90*, 658–668.

93. Rector, T. S., Bank, A. J., Mullen, K. A., et al. (1996). Randomized, double-blind, placebo-controlled study of supplemental oral L-arginine in patients with heart failure. *Circulation, 93*, 2135–2141.

94. Chin-Dusting, J. P. H., Kaye, D. M., Lefkovits, J., et al. (1996). Dietary supplementation with L-arginine fails to restore endothelial function in the forearm resistance arteries of patients with severe heart failure. *J Am Coll Cardiol, 27*, 1207–1213.

95. Adams, M. R., Forsyth, C., Jessup, W., et al. (1995). Oral L-arginine inhibits platelet aggregation but does not enhance endothelium-dependent dilation in healthy young men. *J Am Coll Cardiol, 26*, 1054–1061.

96. Wolf, A., Zalpour, C., Thielmeier, G., et al. (1997). Dietary L-arginine supplementation normalizes platelet aggregation in hypercholesterolemic humans. *J Am Coll Cardiol, 29*, 479–485.

97. Harrison, D. G. (1997). Cellular and molecular mechanisms of endothelial cell dysfunction. *J Clin Invest, 100*, 2153–2157.

98. Bode-Böger, S. M., Böger, R. H., Kienke, S., et al. (1996). Elevated L-arginine/dimethylarginine ratio contributes to enhanced systemic NO production by dietary L-arginine in hypercholesterolemic rabbits. *Biochem Biophys Res Commun, 219*, 598–603.

99. Böger, R. H., Bode-Böger, S. M., Szuba, A., et al. (1998). Asymmetric dimethylarginine (ADMA): a novel risk factor for endothelial dysfunction. *Circulation, 98*, 1842–1847.

100. Feng, Q., Lu, X., Fortin, A. J., et al. (1998). Elevation of an endogenous inhibitor of nitric oxide synthesis in experimental congestive heart failure. *Cardiovasc Res, 37*, 667–675.

101. Hornig, B., Arakawa, N., Boeger, R., et al. (1998). Plasma levels of ADMA are increased and inversely related to endothelium-mediated vasodilation in patients with chronic heart failure; a new predictor of endothelial function. *Circulation, 17*, I-318.

101a. Steppan, J., Ryoo, S., Schuleri, K. H., et al. (2006). Arginase modulates myocardial contractility by a nitric oxide synthase 1-dependent mechanism. *Proc Natl Acad Sci U S A, 103*(12), 4759–4764.

102. Mac Allister, R. J. (1996). Regulation of nitric oxide synthesis by dimethylarginine dimethylaminohydrolase. *Br J Pharmacol, 119*, 1533–1540.

103. Ito, A., Tsao, P. S., Adimoolam, S., et al. (1999). Novel mechanism for endothelial dysfunction: dysregulation of dimethylarginine dimethylaminohydrolase. *Circulation, 99*, 3092–3095.

104. Drexler, H., Zeiher, A. M., Wollschläger, H., et al. (1989). Flow-dependent coronary artery vasodilation in humans. *Circulation, 80*, 466–474.

105. Miller, V. M., & Vanhoutte, P. M. (1988). Enhanced release of endothelium-derived factor(s) by chronic increases in blood flow. *Am J Physiol, 2455*, H446–H451.

106. Miller, V. M., & Burnett, J. C., Jr. (1992). Modulation of NO and endothelin by chronic increases in blood flow in canine femoral arteries. *Am J Physiol, 261*, H103–H108.

107. Nishida, K., Harrison, D. G., Navas, J. P., et al. (1992). Molecular cloning and characterization of the consecutive bovine endothelial cell nitric oxide synthase. *J Clin Invest, 90*, 2092–2096.

108. Jungersten, L., Ambring, A., Wall, B., et al. (1997). Both physical fitness and acute exercise regulate nitric oxide formation in healthy humans. *J Appl Physiol, 82*, 760–764.

109. Katz, S. D., Yuen, J., Bijou, R., et al. (1997). Training improves endothelium-dependent vasodilation in resistance vessels of patients with chronic heart failure. *J Appl Physiol, 82*, 1488–1492.

109a. Tjønna, A. E., Lee, S. J., Rognmo Ø, et al. (2008). Aerobic interval training versus continuous moderate exercise as a treatment for the metabolic syndrome: a pilot study. *Circulation, 118*(4), 346–354.

110. Hambrecht, R., Fiehn, E., Weigl, C., et al. (1998). Regular physical exercise corrects endothelial dysfunction and improves exercise capacity in patients with chronic heart failure. *Circulation, 98*, 2709–2715.

111. Hambrecht, R., Wolf, A., Gielen, S., et al. (2000). Effect of exercise on coronary endothelial function in patients with coronary artery disease. *N Engl J Med, 342*, 454–460.

111a. Sandri, M., Adams, V., Gielen, S., Linke, A., et al. (2005). Effects of exercise and ischemia on mobilization and functional activation of blood-derived progenitor cells in patients with ischemic syndromes: results of 3 randomized studies. *Circulation, 111*(25), 3391–3399.

112. Lewis, T. V., Dart, A. M., Chin-Dusting, J. P., et al. (1999). Exercise training increases basal nitric oxide production from the forearm of hypercholesterolemic patients. *Artioscler Thromb Vasc Biol, 19*, 2782–2787.

113. Higashi, Y., Sasdaki, S., Kurisu, S., et al. (1999). Regular aerobic exercise augments endothelium-dependent vascular relaxations in normotensive as well as in hypertensive subjects: role of endothelium-derived nitric oxide. *Circulation, 100*, 1194–1202.

114. Fukai, T., Siegried, M. R., Ushio-Fukai, M., et al. (2000). Regulation of extracellular superoxide dismutase by nitric oxide in vascular smooth muscle. *J Clin Invest, 105*, 1631–1639.

115. Diet, F., Pratt, R. E., Berry, G. J., et al. (1996). Increased accumulation of tissue ACE in human atherosclerotic coronary disease. *Circulation, 94*, 2756–2767.

116. Rieder, M. J., Carmona, R., Krieger, J. E., et al. (1997). Suppression of angiotensin-converting enzyme expression by shear stress. *Circ Res, 80*, 312–319.

117. Kramsch, D. M., Aspen, A. J., et al. (1981). Reduction of coronary atherosclerosis by moderate conditioning exercise in monkeys on an atherogenic diet. *N Engl J Med, 305*, 1483–1489.

118. Katusic, Z. S., Shepherd, J. T., & Vanhoutte, P. M. (1988). Endothelium-dependent contractions to calcium ionophore A23187, arachidonic acid, and acetylcholine in canine basilar arteries. *Stroke, 19*, 476–479.

119. Kaiser, L., Spickard, R. C., & Olivier, N. B. (1989). Heart failure depresses endothelium-dependent responses in canine femoral artery. *Am J Physiol, 256*, H962–H967.

120. Andrade, F. H., Reid, M. B., Allen, D. G., et al. (1998). Effect of nitric oxide on single skeletal muscle fibres from the mouse. *J Physiol, 509*, 577–586.

121. Riede, U. N., Förstermann, U., Drexler, H., et al. (1998). Inducible nitric oxide synthase in skeletal muscle of patients with chronic heart failure. *J Am Coll Cardiol, 32*, 964–969.

122. Shen, W., Hintze, T. H., & Wollin, M. S. (1995). Nitric oxide: an important signaling mechanism between vascular endothelium and parenchymal cells in the regulation of oxygen consumption. *Circulation, 92*, 1086–1095.

123. Shen, W., Wollin, M. S., & Hintze, T. H. (1997). Defective endogenous nitric oxide-mediated modulation of cellular respiration in canine skeletal muscle after the development of heart failure. *J Heart Lung Transplant, 16*, 1026–1034.

124. Wang, J., Yi, G. H., Knecht, M., et al. (1997). Physical training alters the pathogenesis of pacing-induced heart failure through endothelium-mediated mechanisms in awake dogs. *Circulation, 96*, 2683–2692.

125. Maxwell, A. J., Schauble, E., Bernstein, D., et al. (1998). Limb blood flow during exercise is dependent on nitric oxide. *Circulation, 98*, 369–374.

126. Green, D. J., Fowler, D. T., O'Driscoll, J. G., et al. (1996). Endothelium-derived nitric oxide activity in forearm vessels of tennis players. *J Appl Physiol, 81*, 943–948.

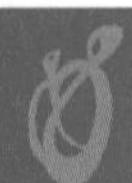

127. Koller, A., Huang, A., Sun, D., et al. (1995). Exercise training augments flow-dependent dilation in rat skeletal muscle arterioles. Role of endothelial nitric oxide and prostaglandins. *Circ Res*, *76*, 544–550.
128. Demopoulos, L., Testa, M., Zulio, M., et al. (1996). Low level physical training improves peak oxygen consumption in patients with congestive heart failure despite long-term beta adrenergic blockade by enhancing vascular conductance and growth. *J Am Coll Cardiol*, *27*, 754-751.
129. Hirai, T., Zelis, R., & Musch, T. I. (1995). Effects of nitric oxide synthase inhibition on the muscle blood flow response to exercise in rats with heart failure. *Cardiovasc Res*, *30*, 469–476.
130. Balon, T. W., & Nadler, J. L. (1994). Nitric oxide release is present from incubated skeletal muscle preparations. *J Appl Physiol*, *77*, 2519–2521.
131. Hornig, B., Arakawa, N., Haussmann, D., et al. (1998). Differential effects of quinaprilat and enalaprilat on endothelial function of conduit arteries in patients with chronic heart failure. *Circulation*, *98*, 2842–2848.
132. Nightingale, A. K., Crilley, J. G., Pegge, N. C., et al. (2007). Chronic oral ascorbic acid therapy worsens skeletal muscle metabolism in patients with chronic heart failure. *Eur J Heart Fail*, *9*, 287–291 .
133. Fischer, D., Rossa, S., Landmesser, U., et al. (2005). Endothelial dysfunction in patients with chronic heart failure is independently associated with increased incidence of hospitalization, cardiac transplantation, or death. *Eur Heart J*, *26*(1), 65–69.
134. Heitzer, T., Baldus, S., von Kodolitsch, Y., et al. (2005). Systemic endothelial dysfunction as an early predictor of adverse outcome in heart failure. *Arterioscler Thromb Vasc Biol*, *25*(6), 1174–1179.
135. Katz, S. D., Hryniewicz, K., Hriljac, I., et al. (2005). Vascular endothelial dysfunction and mortality risk in patients with chronic heart failure. *Circulation*, *111*(3), 310–314.
136. Scherrer-Crosbie, M., et al. (2001). Endothelial nitric oxide synthase limits left ventricular remodeling after myocardial infarction in mice. *Circulation*, *104*, 1286–1291.
137. Landmesser, U., Engberding, N., Bahlmann, F. H., et al. (2004). Statin-induced improvement of endothelial progenitor cell mobilization, myocardial neovascularization, left ventricular function, and survival after experimental myocardial infarction requires endothelial nitric oxide synthase. *Circulation*, *110*(14), 1933–1999.

CHAPTER 18

Alterations in Renal Function in Heart Failure

Guido Boerrigter, Lisa Costello-Boerrigter, and John C. Burnett, Jr.

The kidney is the major organ responsible for the excretion of waste products and toxins and also plays a crucial role in the control of fluid, electrolyte, and acid-base homeostasis. In addition, it is the source of renin and erythropoietin and involved in the formation of vitamin D. Consequently, renal impairment can affect the function of the body in fundamental ways by altering the internal milieu. While the heart appears to be the main culprit in "heart" failure, the contributing and disease-modifying role of the kidney has recently become highlighted. Renal dysfunction can be due to both hemodynamic impairment and preexisting intrinsic renal disease, which can adversely affect cardiac function and contribute to the pathogenesis of cardiovascular disease. Importantly, decreased glomerular filtration rate (GFR), usually estimated with creatinine-based equations, has emerged as a powerful independent predictor of outcomes in patients with heart failure (HF) (Figure 18-1).[1-4] In addition, deteriorating renal function and diuretic resistance during HF therapy are prominent therapeutic challenges (see also Chapter 44).[5-7] Indeed, the requirement to maintain a sufficient renal perfusion pressure is an important limitation to the dosing of vasodilating drugs that are commonly used for the treatment of congestive heart failure (CHF).

Here we will review the basic physiology and pathophysiology of the kidney in heart failure, discuss the emerging concept of the "cardiorenal syndrome," and finally focus on novel therapeutic strategies that enhance pathways based on the second messenger cyclic guanosine monophosphate (cGMP).

THE RENAL REGULATION OF SALT AND WATER

The kidneys control intravascular volume through the regulation of salt and water excretion and receive about 25% of the cardiac output. A kidney can be divided anatomically and physiologically into the cortex, outer medulla, and inner medulla.The single renal nephron (Figure 18-2), one of several hundred thousands that make up a kidney, is the basic functional unit of the kidney and includes the glomerulus, which filters the blood delivering plasma ultrafiltrate to the renal tubule.[8] The normal glomerulus is impermeable to macromolecules, and only in disease states becomes permeable to molecules such as albumin, which when lost in the urine impairs the ability to regulate intravascular volume through reductions in plasma oncotic pressure. The loss of plasma oncotic pressure favors edema formation as occurs in disease states such as in the nephrotic syndrome and has been reported in severe CHF with increases in renal venous pressure. Indeed, the high prevalence of CHF in chronic kidney disease may in part be mediated by increased glomerular permeability with microalbuminuria, the latter of which is a robust signature of increased cardiovascular risk.[9]

Glomerular function is also regulated by glomerular hydrostatic pressure, which is controlled by arterial blood pressure and segmental vascular resistances at the level of preglomerular and postglomerular vessels (i.e., afferent and efferent arterioles). Renal perfusion pressure can be reduced by systemic arterial hypotension as in HF or by renovascular disease (i.e., renal artery stenosis). Importantly, the role of increased renal venous pressure has recently been highlighted. Damman et al and Mullens et al reported that central venous pressure was a more important factor in determining reduced GFR and worsening renal function than renal blood flow or cardiac index (Figure 18-3).[10-12] Indeed, prior physiological studies had indicated that increasing renal venous pressure in volume-expanded healthy canines increased renal interstitial pressure and decreased fractional excretion of sodium, glomerular filtration rate, and renal blood flow (Figure 18-4).[13] While increasing renal venous pressure would be expected to increase hydrostatic pressure in the glomerulus and thus promote filtration, given the tight renal capsule it can also compress the tubules, which would reduce the hydrostatic pressure gradient across the glomerular membrane.[14] Prospective studies are needed to assess whether tailoring therapies according to renal venous pressure (via central venous pressure) improves outcomes. Neurohumoral factors also regulate glomerular function either by altering glomerular pressure via hemodynamic actions or by direct action on the glomerular membrane. Glomerular filtration rate can also be reduced if the number of nephrons is reduced due to intrinsic renal disease, even though remaining nephrons can compensate somewhat.

From the glomerulus, the filtrate flows successively through the proximal tubule, the loop of Henle, the distal tubule, and finally the collecting duct to reach the renal pelvis as urine. The sections of the tubule vary in permeabilities for water and solutes due to the differential expression of transporters and channels, the activity of which can be affected by hormones and drugs (see Figure 18-2). The proximal tubule is regulated by hormonal and physical factors in the control of sodium reabsorption.[15] It is a key site also associated with enhanced reabsorption of sodium in overt CHF, thus contributing to sodium retention and edema formation. The juxtaglomerular apparatus is the location of renin-secreting cells and the macula densa and lies at the junction between the loop of Henle and the distal nephron at which the tubule comes in close proximity to the afferent arteriole.[16] The juxtaglomerular apparatus and macula densa sense alterations in intratubular sodium concentration, which depends on GFR and proximal reabsorption. Increased delivery of sodium to the macula densa and juxtaglomerular apparatus decreases renin secretion, whereas decreased sodium delivery as a result of decreased GFR or increased proximal reabsorption as would occur in CHF, increases renin releases and activate the renin-angiotensin-aldosterone (RAAS) cascade.[17] The loop of Henle is therefore an important segment of the renal nephron and is responsible for reabsorption of sodium through direct alterations in sodium transport, and through changes in renal medullary blood flow. The final mediator of renal sodium regulation is the collecting duct, which is under the influence of both natriuretic and antinatriuretic factors.[18] These include aldosterone, which promotes active sodium reabsorption, and arginine vasopressin, which regulates the reabsorption of water. Natriuretic factors, such as the cardiac peptides ANP and BNP (see later discussion), also act primarily in the distal nephron. In overt CHF, this segment is overwhelmed by sodium-retaining factors to overcome the natriuretic effects of ANP and BNP, resulting in profound reabsorption of sodium and further edema formation and congestion. Understanding the single nephron in both structure and function provides insights into therapeutic approaches to enhance GFR, decrease sodium and water reabsorption, and therefore restore proper sodium and water homeostasis. With regard to therapy, it should be noted that loop diuretics act in the loop of Henle but not in the distal tubule or collecting duct, so that some of the sodium delivered to the distal nephron will be reabsorbed there. Indeed, chronic loop diuretic therapy can lead to hypertrophy and hyperplasia of distal nephron segments.[71] Furthermore, addition of thiazide-like diuretics, which act in the distal nephron, to loop diuretics can induce a powerful diuresis ("sequential nephron blockade").

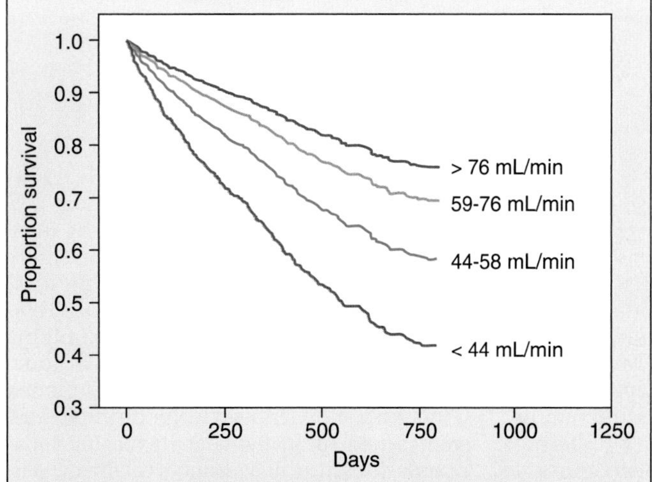

FIGURE 18–1 Proportional relationship of calculated glomerular filtration rate (using the Cockcroft-Gault equation) with mortality in Cox-adjusted survival analysis. Patients had heart failure (New York Heart Association class III or IV, left ventricular ejection fraction <35%) and were enrolled in the Second Perspective Randomized study of Ibopamine on Mortality and Efficacy (PRIME-II) trial, which investigated the oral dopamine agonist ibopamine. (With permission from Hillege HL, Girbes AR, de Kam PJ, et al. Renal function, neurohormonal activation, and survival in patients with chronic heart failure. *Circulation* 2000;102(2):203-210.[1])

THE "CARDIORENAL SYNDROME"

Given the interdependence of the heart and kidney and the apparent worse outcome of HF patients with coexisting renal dysfunction, the concept of a "cardiorenal syndrome" (CRS)

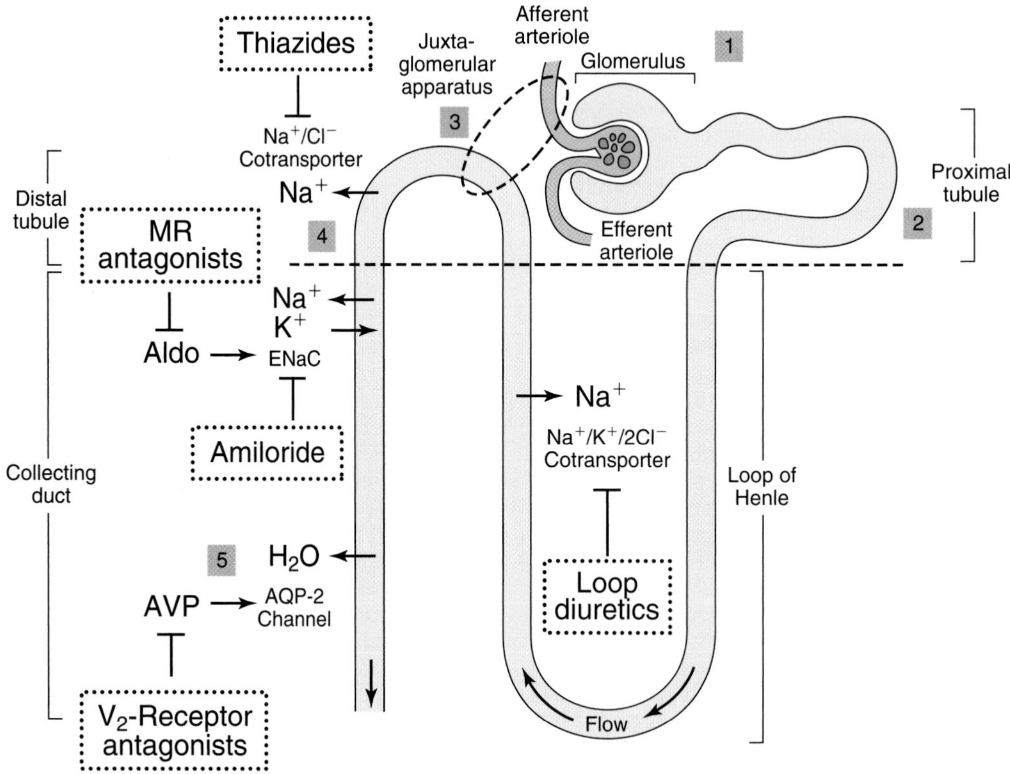

FIGURE 18–2 Schematic of a single nephron with major sites of action of some conventional diuretics and the natriuretic peptides. The juxtaglomerular apparatus, located at the junction of the afferent arteriole and the distal tubule, contains renin-secreting cells. Natriuretic peptides have diverse renal actions: they can (1) increase glomerular filtration, (2) oppose proximal reabsorption of sodium by opposing angiotensin II and the sympathetic nervous system, (3) inhibit tubuloglomerular feedback and the secretion of renin, (4) inhibit sodium reabsorption in the distal tubule, and (5) promote free water excretion by opposing arginine vasopressin. *Aldo,* aldosterone; *AQP-2,* aquaporin 2 water channel; *AVP,* arginine vasopressin; *ENaC,* epithelial sodium channel; *MR,* mineralocorticoid; *V_2-Receptor,* vasopressin 2 receptor.

was proposed.[19] In a broader sense it could be defined as a syndrome in which either the heart or the kidney fails to compensate for the functional impairment of the other organ, resulting in a vicious cycle that will ultimately lead to decompensation of the entire circulatory system. In a narrower sense, CRS could be defined as worsening renal function or diuretic resistance in patients treated for HF. Given that the term is somewhat vague and not consistently defined, Ronco et al recently suggested the following classification:[20]

Type 1 CRS: abrupt worsening of cardiac function (e.g., acute cardiogenic shock or decompensated CHF) leading to acute kidney injury

Type 2 CRS: chronic abnormalities in cardiac function (e.g., chronic CHF) causing progressive chronic kidney disease

Type 3 CRS: abrupt worsening of renal function (e.g., heart failure, arrhythmia, ischemia)

Type 4 CRS: state of chronic kidney disease (e.g., chronic glomerular disease) contributing to decreased cardiac function, cardiac hypertrophy, and/or increased risk of adverse cardiovascular events

Type 5 CRS: systemic condition (e.g., sepsis) causing both cardiac and renal dysfunction

Of course, CRS types could overlap. While the usefulness of this classification for patient treatment or clinical trial

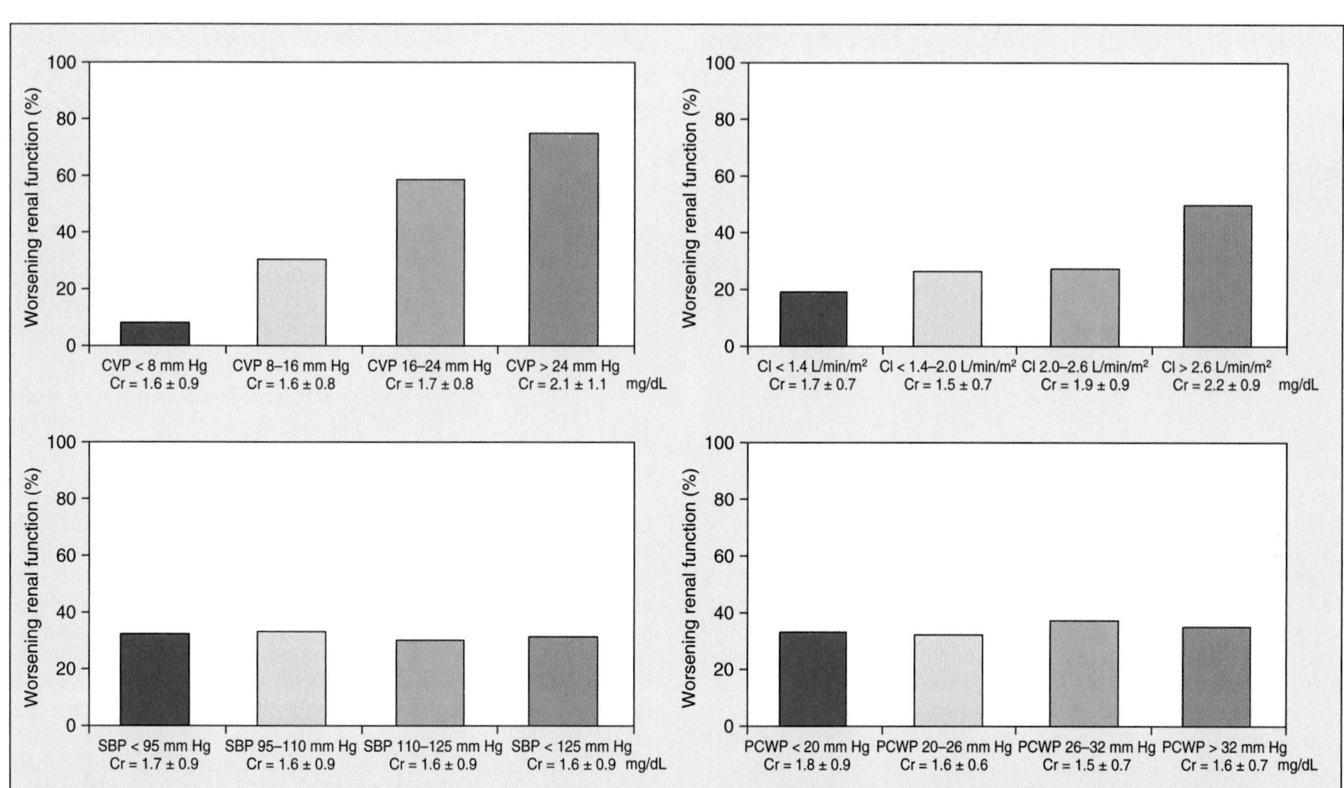

FIGURE 18–3 Prevalence of worsening renal function (defined as an increase of serum creatinine of 0.3 mg/dL) during hospitalization according to categories of admission central venous pressure (CVP), cardiac index (CI), systolic blood pressure (SBP), and pulmonary capillary wedge pressure (PCWP). (With permission from Mullens W, Abrahams Z, Francis GS, et al. Importance of venous congestion for worsening of renal function in advanced decompensated heart failure. *J Am Coll Cardiol* 2009;53(7):589-596.[12])

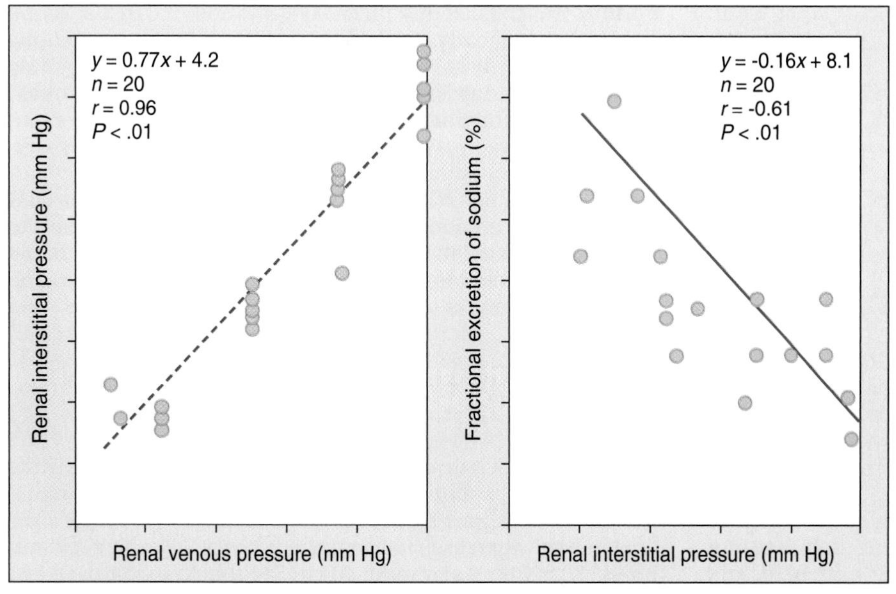

FIGURE 18–4 Relationship of renal venous pressure and renal interstitial pressure (*left panel*) and renal interstitial pressure and fractional excretion of sodium (*right panel*) in volume-expanded healthy canines. (With permission from Burnett JC Jr, Knox FG. Renal interstitial pressure and sodium excretion during renal vein constriction. *Am J Physiol* 1980;238(4):F279-F282.[13])

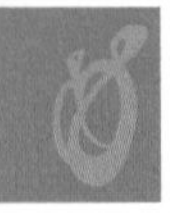

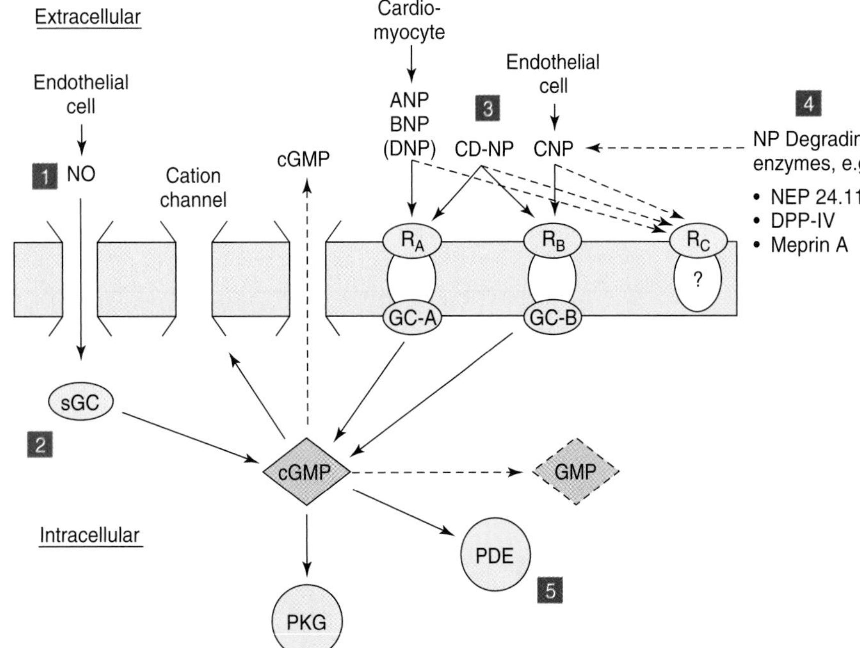

FIGURE 18–5 Simplified schematic of guanylyl cyclase (GC) pathways, which have cyclic guanosine monophosphate (cGMP) as their second messenger. Nitric oxide is produced by endothelial cells and activates soluble GC in the target cell. ANP and BNP stimulate GC-A (also called NP receptor A), while CNP stimulates GC-B (also called NP receptor B). DNP is a GC-agonist first discovered in snake venom. CD-NP is a chimeric peptide composed of the ring structure and amino terminus of CNP and the carboxyterminus of DNP; it activates both GC-A and GC-B. Natriuretic peptides also bind to the non-GC-linked natriuretic peptide C receptor, the biological significance of which beyond NP clearance is currently unclear. Cyclic GMP modulates cGMP-dependent protein kinase G, cGMP-regulated PDEs, and cGMP-regulated cation channels. The cGMP signal is terminated by PDEs that hydrolyze cGMP to GMP, or by extrusion into the extracellular space. The NPs are degraded by a variety of peptidases. Cyclic GMP signaling can be enhanced by (1) the use of NO mimetics such as nitrovasodilators, (2) direct sGC stimulators, (3) exogenous NPs, (4) inhibiting NP degrading enzymes, and (5) inhibiting the activity of cGMP-hydrolyzing PDEs. *ANP,* atrial natriuretic peptide; *BNP,* B-type natriuretic peptide; *cGMP,* cyclic guanosine monophosphate; *GMP,* guanosine monophosphate; *GC,* guanylyl cyclase; *DNP, Dendroaspis* natriuretic peptide; *DPP4,* dipeptidyl peptidase IV; *NEP,* neutral endopeptidase; *NO,* nitric oxide; *PDE,* phosphodiesterase; *PKG,* protein kinase G; R_A*,* natriuretic peptide receptor A; *sGC,* soluble guanylate cyclase.

design remains to be established, it illustrates the scope of the problem of cardiorenal disease.

Recognizing that hemodynamic interaction between kidney and heart are not sufficient to explain the poor prognosis of coexisting renal and cardiac dysfunction, Bongartz et al highlighted "cardiorenal connectors" (i.e., factors that adversely affect both the kidney and the heart):[21]

- The renin-angiotensin-aldosterone system (RAAS).
- Relative deficiency of nitric oxide (NO) compared with reactive oxygen species (ROS)
- Inflammation
- The sympathetic nervous system

There is substantial overlap and mutual reinforcement among these factors, contributing to accelerated cardiorenal deterioration on many different levels, such as sodium retention, inflammation, fibrosis, and left ventricular hypertrophy. One therapeutic strategy would be to block some or all of these factors. An alternative strategy would be to enhance endogenous pathways that oppose these factors. Increasing evidence points to the renal cGMP system as fundamental in the regulation of sodium excretion and GFR. Later we will discuss what is known about cGMP and therapeutic strategies to improve renal function and the cardiorenal axis in CHF by targeting cGMP pathways especially in the kidney.

THE CARDIORENAL AXIS AND CYCLIC GMP

3′, 5′-cyclic guanosine monophosphate (cGMP) is the second messenger of signaling systems that use distinct guanylyl cyclases (GCs; E.C. 4.6.1.2), which convert guanosine 5′-triphosphate (GTP) to cGMP.[22] Currently, one cytosolic (soluble) and seven membrane-bound (particulate) GCs have been identified. As illustrated in Figure 18-5, they are soluble GC (nitric oxide (NO)-sensitive GC) with its endogenous ligand NO, GC-A (also called natriuretic peptide A receptor [NPR-A]) with its endogenous ligands ANP and BNP, and GC-B (also called NPR-B) with its endogenous ligand CNP. Other GCs are GC-C (ligands: guanylin and uroguanylin, heat-stable enterotoxins) and GC-D, -E, -F, and -G for which the endogenous ligands remain unknown. Cyclic GMP affects the activity of effector molecules, specifically cGMP-dependent protein kinases (PKG), cGMP-regulated phosphodiesterases (PDEs), and cGMP-regulated cation channels. Further, cGMP itself is also a substrate of several PDEs, which hydrolyze cGMP to GMP and thus terminate the cGMP signal.[23]

It is important to recognize that despite having a common second messenger, activating different cGMP-dependent pathways will not necessarily result in similar actions. Specifically, receptors can differ both in their tissue and their intracellular distribution. Within the cell GC-A activation as compared to sGC stimulation increases distinct cGMP pools that are compartmentalized by the activity of PDEs.[24] These findings are consistent with the observation of distinct action profiles. Specifically, ANP, BNP, and NO have vasodilating actions, but only ANP and BNP are natriuretic. Regarding renal function, intrarenal administration of the NO synthase inhibitor N^G-monomethyl-L-arginine (L-NMMA) in experimental acute CHF reduces renal blood flow without affecting GFR and sodium excretion, whereas natriuretic peptide receptor blockade does not affect renal blood flow but decreases GFR and sodium excretion.[25] It should also be noted that there can be reciprocal regulation of different cGMP pathways such that in vascular smooth muscle cells activation of GC-A leads to an attenuated response to sGC and vice versa.[26]

THE NO-sGC-cGMP PATHWAY: A POTENT RENOVASODILATING MECHANISM

Soluble GC (sGG) is a heterodimeric heme enzyme consisting of an α- and β-subunit and a prosthetic heme group with a ferrous iron.[27] Binding of NO to the heme iron modifies the enzyme and increases its catalytic activity. The bioavailability of NO is frequently reduced in CHF due to oxidative stress

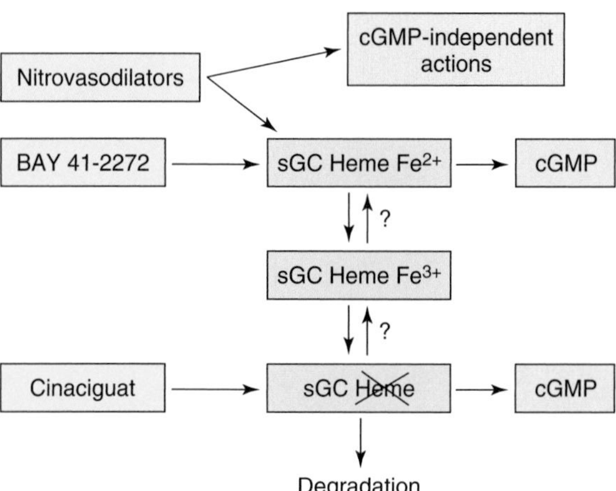

FIGURE 18–6 Schematic illustrating three different forms of soluble guanylate cyclase and their respective responsiveness to nitrovasodilators, heme-dependent sGC stimulators (e.g., BAY 41-2272), and heme-independent sGC activators (e.g., cinaciguat [also known as BAY 58-2667]). Nitric oxide (NO) and nitrovasodilators only stimulate sGC when it, contains the heme moiety with a ferrous iron (Fe^{2+}); furthermore, NO and nitrovasodilators have cGMP-independent actions. BAY 41-2272 also activates only the NO-sensitive sGC but without the cGMP-independent actions of NO and nitrovasodilators. Cinaciguat activates heme-free sGC, which is insensitive to NO, and also inhibits its degradation. The question marks indicate that little is known about the transition between the different forms, their prevalence in health and disease, and their potential restoration to the reduced, NO-sensitive form. *cGMP,* cyclic guanosine monophosphate; *Fe,* iron; *sGC,* soluble guanylate cyclase. (From Boerrigter G, Burnett JC Jr. Soluble guanylate cyclase: not a dull enzyme. *Circulation* 2009;119(21):2752-2754.[70])

leading to attenuated NO/sGC/cGMP signaling in vascular and renal tissues contributing to endothelial dysfunction. Furthermore, recent studies showed that the heme of sGC can be oxidized or removed, rendering the enzyme insensitive to endogenous NO or conventional nitrovasodilators (Figure 18-6). This endothelial or vascular dysfunction provides a rationale for the therapeutic enhancement of the NO/sGC/cGMP pathway, which is discussed later with conventional and novel sGC activators.

Soluble GC stimulation with nitrovasodilators has been used for over a century.[28] Importantly, long-term administration of nitrovasodilators is associated with the development of tolerance and cGMP-independent actions, which may have beneficial but also detrimental actions. The detrimental actions of nitrovasodilators include oxidative stress, mitochondrial toxicity, endothelial dysfunction, and protein nitrosation.[29-31] These adverse effects can partially be prevented by hydralazine, which possesses antioxidant properties. This may explain the results of clinical trials in which patients who received a combination of a nitrate (isosorbide dinitrate) and hydralazine had improved outcomes compared with a placebo before the introduction of ACE inhibitors and more recently in African Americans even on top of therapy with ACE inhibitors and β-blockers.[32,72]

In a key study Ko et al reported in 1994 that the molecule YC-1 activates sGC directly (i.e., independently of NO), prompting studies to develop such agents for cardiovascular therapeutic purposes such as CHF.[33] Two new classes of direct sGC stimulators, one NO-independent but heme-dependent, the other both NO- and heme-independent, have been developed and are potent renal and systemic vasodilating compounds. The former class only stimulates sGC if the heme iron is in the ferrous state (Fe^{2+}), whereas the latter class stimulates the enzyme preferentially when the heme is absent.[34]

The first orally available NO-independent but heme-dependent sGC stimulator to be described is BAY 41-2272.[35] This novel agent binds to a regulatory site on sGC and activates it synergistically with NO and can thus be considered an "NO sensitizer." In experimental CHF induced by rapid right ventricular pacing, BAY 41-2272 decreased mean arterial pressure, pulmonary capillary wedge pressure and systemic and renal vascular resistances and increased cardiac output and renal blood flow.[36] The hemodynamic actions were similar to nitroglycerin with the important exception of right atrial pressure, which decreased with nitroglycerin but was unchanged with BAY 41-2272. This difference could be explained by recognizing that BAY 41-2272 acts synergistically with NO, which may be more abundant in arteries than veins. In contrast, nitroglycerin is bioactivated preferentially in the veins. Further drug optimization led to the development of riociguat, which is currently in clinical trials for pulmonary hypertension.[37]

The first reported NO- and heme-independent sGC activator is cinaciguat (also referred to as BAY 58-2667), which activates sGC as it competes with and replaces the heme moiety, which in the non-nitrosylated state inhibits enzyme activity.[38] Interestingly, heme-oxidized sGC is usually ubiquitinated and destined for proteosomal degradation; however, cinaciguat stabilizes the heme-free enzyme and prevents its degradation.[39] Stasch et al reported that in various experimental cardiovascular disease conditions the potency of nitrovasodilators was reduced, whereas it was increased for cinaciguat, strongly suggesting an increased prevalence of oxidized or heme-free sGC.[40] These findings provide evidence for a potential additional pathophysiological mechanism contributing to renal and systemic endothelial and vascular smooth muscle cell dysfunction in CHF.

Cinaciguat also has an additive effect with NO and lowers blood pressure in rats and healthy canines. In experimental pacing-induced CHF, cinaciguat was a potent renovasodilator and had hemodynamic actions similar to nitroglycerin with reductions in mean arterial and pulmonary capillary wedge pressure, systemic and renal vascular resistance, and increases in cardiac output and renal blood flow (Figure 18-7).[41] Unlike BAY 41-2272, cinaciguat decreased right atrial pressure. GFR and urinary sodium excretion were preserved despite the hypotensive actions. There was also no activation of renin or aldosterone, whereas ANP and BNP decreased, consistent with cardiac unloading.

Cinaciguat therefore displays promising cardiorenal properties in experimental CHF and preserves renal function. Most recently, an unblinded, uncontrolled proof-of-concept study was reported. Specifically, Lapp et al assessed the effect of cinaciguat on hemodynamic and symptomatic status in patients admitted to the hospital with acute decompensated CHF, NYHA class III/IV symptoms, PCWP of 18 mm Hg or more, parenteral pharmacotherapy, and invasive hemodynamic monitoring.[42] Cinaciguat significantly reduced PCWP, right atrial pressure, and systemic and pulmonary vascular resistances, while cardiac output increased. A PCWP reduction of 4 mm Hg was achieved in 53%, 83%, and 90% after 2, 4, and 6 hours, respectively, which was associated with an improvement in symptomatic status as assessed by a dyspnea score. This study shows that also in human CHF there exists a pool of oxidized or heme-free sGC that can be activated by cinaciguat with favorable cardiac preload and afterload reduction, warranting further studies especially looking at the kidney.

THE NATRIURETIC PEPTIDE PATHWAYS: ACTIVATORS OF RENAL PARTICULATE GUANYLYL CYCLASES

The natriuretic peptides ANP and BNP are secreted by the heart in response to cardiac overload such as CHF and via the GC-A stimulate the production of cGMP. They have natriuretic, diuretic, vasodilating, and renin- and aldosterone-suppressing actions that help to unload the heart. Moreover, ANP and BNP have antihypertrophic, antifibrotic,

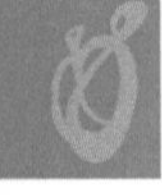

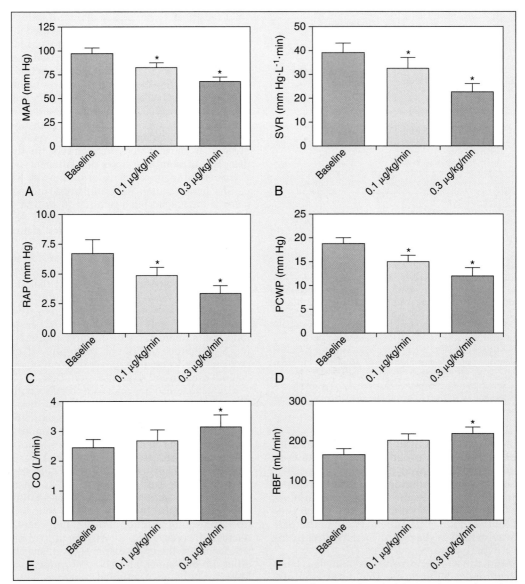

FIGURE 18–7 Effect of cinaciguat (BAY 58-2667) administration on (A) mean arterial pressure (MAP), (B) systemic vascular resistance, (C) right atrial pressure (RAP), (D) pulmonary capillary wedge pressure (PCWP), (E) cardiac output (CO), and (F) renal blood flow (RBF). * Indicates $P < .05$ compared with baseline. (From Boerrigter G, Costello-Boerrigter LC, Cataliotti A, et al. Targeting heme-oxidized soluble guanylate cyclase in experimental heart failure. *Hypertension* 2007;49(5):1128-1133.[41])

and positive lusitropic properties.[43-45] CNP of endothelial origin functions via activation of NPR-B and is a more autocrine/paracrine peptide in endothelial cell/vascular smooth muscle cell control, with vasodilating actions, especially in the venous circulation.[46] CNP, however, is not natriuretic. Importantly, in more advanced CHF stages, the response to endogenous and exogenous NPs is blunted, which can at least partially be overcome by administration of exogenous NPs, providing a rationale for pharmacologically augmenting the NP system. This is possible in various ways (e.g., administration of exogenous NPs or prolonging the bioactivity of endogenous NPs by inhibiting their degradation [see Figure 18-2]).

B-TYPE NATRIURETIC PEPTIDE

Supporting the use of BNP as a therapy in human CHF were studies in experimental CHF, one of which reported that BNP augmented the diuretic and natriuretic response to furosemide, increased GFR, and prevented an increase in aldosterone induced by furosemide alone.[47] Nesiritide is a recombinant form of human BNP and was approved for the treatment of acute decompensated CHF in the United States in 2001 (see also Chapters 43 and 44). In the VMAC trial, which led to BNP approval by the FDA, nesiritide resulted a larger decrease in pulmonary capillary wedge pressure at 3 and 24 hours as compared with a placebo and nitroglycerin, although symptomatic status was not improved compared with nitroglycerin.[48] It should be noted that subsequent meta-analyses of publicly available studies suggested that nesiritide was associated with an increase in serum creatinine and mortality.[49,50] The mechanism for these findings is unclear but possibly the nesiritide dose administered, particularly the bolus, may have contributed to hypotension, which due to BNP's half-life would be more prolonged as compared with, for example, nitroglycerin. Subsequent small studies reported no indication for detrimental or beneficial renal effects of nesiritide in acute decompensated CHF.[51-54]

Supporting the use of BNP as a therapy in human CHF were studies in experimental CHF, one of which reported importantly, in the NAPA trial, nesiritide or placebo (n = 138) was given to patients with a left ventricular ejection fraction of 40% or less undergoing bypass surgery with anticipated cardiopulmonary bypass (Figure 18-8).[55] Patients

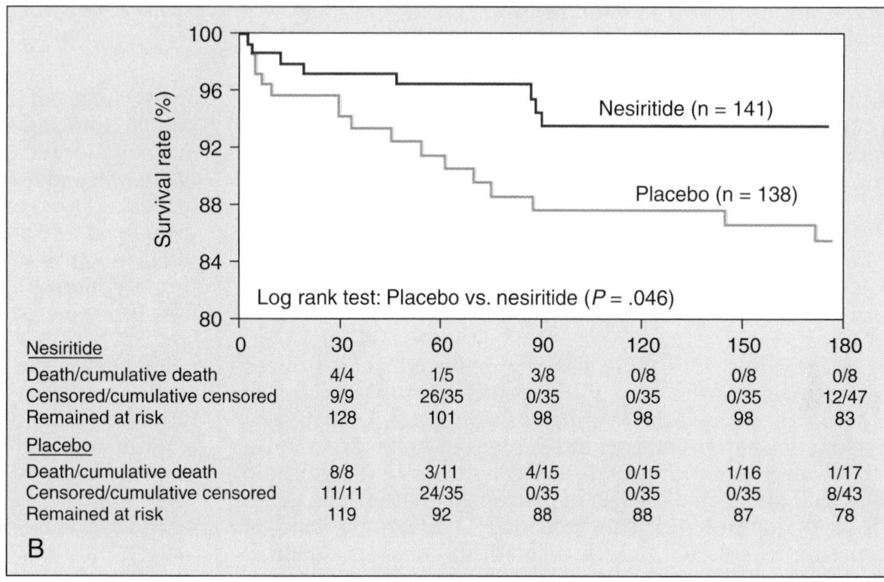

Nesiritide	0	30	60	90	120	150	180
Death/cumulative death		4/4	1/5	3/8	0/8	0/8	0/8
Censored/cumulative censored		9/9	26/35	0/35	0/35	0/35	12/47
Remained at risk		128	101	98	98	98	83
Placebo							
Death/cumulative death		8/8	3/11	4/15	0/15	1/16	1/17
Censored/cumulative censored		11/11	24/35	0/35	0/35	0/35	8/43
Remained at risk		119	92	88	88	87	78

FIGURE 18–8 Adjusted mean maximum decrease in glomerular filtration rate (GFR) from baseline through hospital discharge or by study day 14, whichever came first, using an analysis of covariance model. Error bars indicate standard error of the mean **(A)**. Kaplan-Meier survival curve to day 180 by treatment group in the "safety population," which is a subset of the total study population added during the study to assess long-term safety **(B)**. *BL*, Baseline; *GFR*, glomerular filtration rate; *sCr*, serum creatinine. (From Mentzer RM Jr, Oz MC, Sladen RN, et al. Effects of perioperative nesiritide in patients with left ventricular dysfunction undergoing cardiac surgery: the NAPA trial. *J Am Coll Cardiol* 2007;49(6):716-726.[55])

randomized to nesiritide had a smaller rise in serum creatinine, larger urine output, shorter hospital stay, and a lower 180-day mortality. Similarly, in a study of patients with reduced renal function undergoing cardiac bypass surgery, randomization to nesiritide as compared with control improved postoperative renal function.[56] Another possible indication where studies are pursued is nesiritide as a treatment to ameliorate remodeling after a myocardial infarction in an effort to reduce CHF, which is supported by a recent report demonstrating cardioprotective properties of BNP in human MI.[57] Importantly, a 7000-patient acute CHF trial (ASCEND) is nearing completion addressing the safety and efficacy of BNP.[58]

CHIMERIC NATRIURETIC PEPTIDES: CD-NP

Snake venom has been the source of several peptides that have been useful in the development of cardiovascular drugs and include agents such as the ACE inhibitor captopril and the glycoprotein IIb/IIIa antagonist eptifibatide. Schweitz et al reported the in vitro biological actions of a newly discovered peptide, *Dendroaspis* natriuretic peptide (DNP), which was isolated from the venom of the green mamba. DNP, like ANP and BNP, activates GC-A and binds to the natriuretic peptide clearance receptor, but it does not activate GC-B. GC-A and the natriuretic peptide clearance receptor, but not GC-B.[59] We reported that DNP in vivo was potently natriuretic and diuretic and possessed cardiac unloading actions but with significant hypotensive properties.[60,61] These in vivo actions of DNP are consistent with GC-A activation as such effects mimic ANP and BNP but not CNP.

A structural feature of DNP is that it possesses the longest C-terminus of the known natriuretic peptides consisting of 15 amino acids (AA) as compared with 5 AA for ANP, 6 AA for BNP, and none for CNP. This long C-terminus of DNP may make DNP highly resistant to degradation by neutral endopeptidase, which is highly expressed in the kidney, contributing to potent natriuretic and diuretic actions.[62] Further, the lack of a C-terminus for CNP may explain the observation that of the three known endogenous natriuretic peptides CNP is the most susceptible to degradation by NEP, which could limit its renal actions.[63]

We recently reported that fusion of the 15 AA C-terminus of DNP onto the C-terminus position resulted in a synthetic chimeric NP that in vivo possessed the cardiac unloading actions of CNP with minimal hypotensive properties compared with BNP together with the additional renal effects of natriuresis and diuresis (Figure 18-9).[64] We also observed that this designer peptide called CD-NP retained properties of CNP in vitro in activating cGMP in cardiac fibroblasts and inhibiting cell proliferation. Further, in vitro studies also reported that CD-NP activates both GC-A and GC-B (B>A).[65] Thus this chimeric NP possesses potentially beneficial efficacy and safety for the treatment of cardiorenal disease states such as CHF. A first- in-human study was recently completed in normal human subjects and demonstrated activation of plasma and

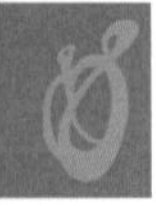

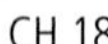

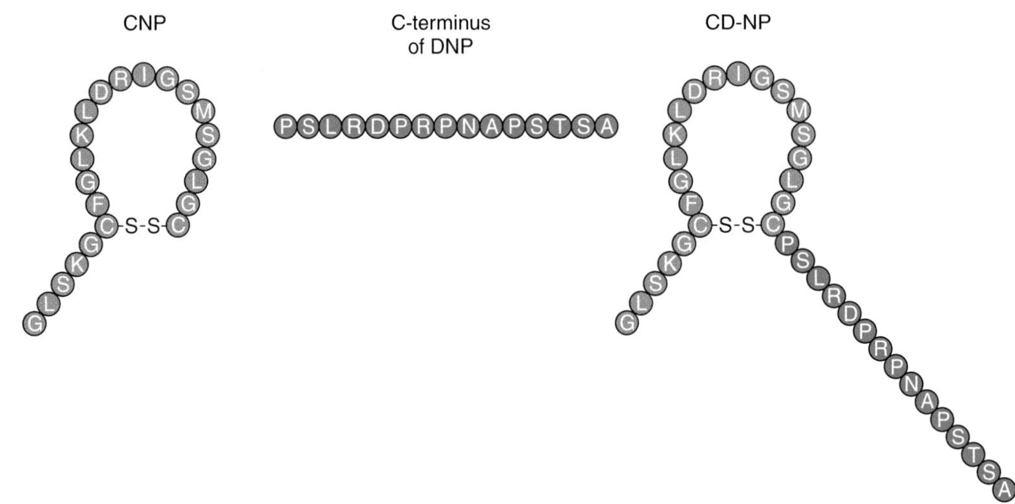

FIGURE 18–9 CD-NP is a chimeric peptide consisting of the amino terminus and ring structure of C-type natriuretic peptide and the carboxy terminus of *Dendroaspis* natriuretic peptide.

urinary cGMP, natriuresis, and aldosterone suppression with minimal actions on arterial pressure.[66] Human trials in CHF are currently under way.

PHOSPHODIESTERASE INHIBITION

It is now well established that the cGMP signal is effectively terminated by the action of specific phosphodiesterases (PDEs) that hydrolyze cGMP to GMP. Inhibition of the isoenzyme PDE5 (e.g., with sildenafil, vardenafil, tadalafil) reduces vascular tone particularly in the corpus cavernosum and the pulmonary vasculature, leading to its application in erectile dysfunction and pulmonary arterial hypertension. In a mouse model of pressure overload due to aortic banding, chronic sildenafil attenuated cardiac hypertrophy, dilation, and fibrosis, and improved cardiac function.[67] Importantly, cardiac hypertrophy was not only prevented but, once established, could be reversed with sildenafil. This was associated with decreased activation of hypertrophic factors such as calcineurin, the mitogen-activated kinase ERK1/2, Akt, and PI3Kα.

In experimental CHF, chronic PDE5 inhibition with sildenafil reduced systemic vascular resistance and increased cardiac output but did not affect cardiac filling pressures or renal function.[68] In addition, chronic PDE5 inhibition augmented the renal response to acutely administered BNP. This combined therapy augmented GFR, further reduced tubular reabsorption of sodium, and increased sodium and water excretion. An emerging strategy for optimizing renal function in CHF is to activate GC receptors linked to the NPs and to inhibit the degradation of cGMP by PDE5. Indeed, we have reported the increase in renal PDE5 activity in experimental CHF underscoring the rationale for combined NP and PDE5 inhibition in CHF to enhance renal function.[69]

OPTIMIZING sGC-pCG SIGNALING IN THE KIDNEY IN CHF

As illustrated in Figure 18-5, cGMP is generated by activation of pGC receptors to which the NPs bind or by stimulation of sGC by NO. We recently investigated the contribution of the renal NP/pGC/cGMP and NO/sGC/cGMP pathways in preserving renal function in acute CHF in which there are acute increases in the circulating NPs together with an intact renal NO system.[25] We used a large animal model of acute CHF. Renal hemodynamic and tubular function were assessed in the presence and absence of antagonism of the endogenous GC receptors or inhibition of NO release. Particulate GC antagonism reduced GFR and sodium excretion but did not alter renal blood flow. In contrast, NO inhibition only decreased renal blood flow and did not alter either GFR or urinary sodium excretion. These studies demonstrate distinct roles for cGMP pathways (pGC vs. sGC) in the preservation of renal function in CHF in which GFR and sodium reabsorption are more linked to the NPs and pGC while renal blood flow is more linked to NO and sGC. These studies support the concept of "physiological compartmentalization" of cGMP in the kidney. Thus optimization of the cGMP pathways in the kidney would involve targeting GC-A/-B and sGC with inhibition of PDE5. Such a strategy is currently being defined in experimental CHF with severe renal dysfunction.

SUMMARY

Renal dysfunction is an important independent predictor of adverse outcomes in CHF and frequently poses a therapeutic challenge, underscoring the need for new treatment strategies. Cyclic GMP in the kidney is a second messenger vital in the optimal regulation of renal function. Novel drugs are now available to enhance this signaling pathway with novel NO-independent and dependent sGC stimulators, GC-A and GC-B agonists, and PDE inhibitors. Given promising preclinical and clinical data, it is likely that the cGMP system will remain an attractive area of research and drug development. Indeed, in strategies targeting cardiorenal function in CHF, the focus has been on antagonizing endogenous neurohumoral systems. Cyclic GMP research has now opened a new direction in CHF therapeutics with an innovative way to enhance signaling pathways that possess properties of cardiorenal protection warranting further basic and clinical research.

REFERENCES

1. Hillege, H. L., Girbes, A. R., de Kam, P. J., et al. (2000). Renal function, neurohormonal activation, and survival in patients with chronic heart failure. *Circulation, 102*(2), 203–210.
2. Dries, D. L., Exner, D. V., Domanski, M. J., et al. (2000). The prognostic implications of renal insufficiency in asymptomatic and symptomatic patients with left ventricular systolic dysfunction. *J Am Coll Cardiol, 35*(3), 681–689.
3. Hillege, H. L., Nitsch, D., Pfeffer, M. A., et al. (2006). Renal function as a predictor of outcome in a broad spectrum of patients with heart failure. *Circulation, 113*(5), 671–678.
4. Smilde, T. D., van Veldhuisen, D. J., Navis, G., et al. (2006). Drawbacks and prognostic value of formulas estimating renal function in patients with chronic heart failure and systolic dysfunction. *Circulation, 114*(15), 1572–1580.
5. Gottlieb, S. S., Abraham, W., Butler, J., et al. (2002). The prognostic importance of different definitions of worsening renal function in congestive heart failure. *J Card Fail, 8*(3), 136–141.
6. Forman, D. E., Butler, J., Wang, Y., et al. (2004). Incidence, predictors at admission, and impact of worsening renal function among patients hospitalized with heart failure. *J Am Coll Cardiol, 43*(1), 61–67.

7. Damman, K., Jaarsma, T., Voors, A. A., et al. (2009). Both in- and out-hospital worsening of renal function predict outcome in patients with heart failure: results from the coordinating study evaluating outcome of advising and counseling in heart failure (COACH). *Eur J Heart Fail, 11*(9), 847–854.
8. Brenner, B. M., Baylis, C., & Deen, W. M. (1976). Transport of molecules across renal glomerular capillaries. *Physiol Rev, 56*(3), 502–534.
9. Sarafidis, P. A., & Bakris, G. L. (2006). Microalbuminuria and chronic kidney disease as risk factors for cardiovascular disease. *Nephrol Dial Transplant, 21*(9), 2366–2374.
10. Damman, K., Navis, G., Smilde, T. D., et al. (2007). Decreased cardiac output, venous congestion and the association with renal impairment in patients with cardiac dysfunction. *Eur J Heart Fail, 9*(9), 872–878.
11. Damman, K., van Deursen, V. M., Navis, G., et al. (2009). Increased central venous pressure is associated with impaired renal function and mortality in a broad spectrum of patients with cardiovascular disease. *J Am Coll Cardiol, 53*(7), 582–588.
12. Mullens, W., Abrahams, Z., Francis, G. S., et al. (2009). Importance of venous congestion for worsening of renal function in advanced decompensated heart failure. *J Am Coll Cardiol, 53*(7), 589–596.
13. Burnett, J. C., Jr., & Knox, F. G. (1980). Renal interstitial pressure and sodium excretion during renal vein constriction. *Am J Physiol, 238*(4), F279–F282.
14. Winton, F. (1931). The influence of venous pressure on the isolated mammalian kidney. *J Physiol, 72*, 49–61.
15. Chan, Y. L., Malnic, G., & Giebisch, G. (1983). Passive driving forces of proximal tubular fluid and bicarbonate transport: gradient dependence of H^+ secretion. *Am J Physiol, 245*(5 pt 1), F622–F633.
16. Schnermann, J. (1998). Juxtaglomerular cell complex in the regulation of renal salt excretion. *Am J Physiol, 274*(2 pt 2), R263–R279.
17. Knox, F. G., Mertz, J. I., Burnett, J. C., Jr., et al. (1983). Role of hydrostatic and oncotic pressures in renal sodium reabsorption. *Circ Res, 52*(5), 491–500.
18. Bengele, H. H., Lechene, C., & Alexander, E. A. (1980). Sodium and chloride transport along the inner medullary collecting duct: effect of saline expansion. *Am J Physiol, 238*(6), F504–F508.
19. Shlipak, M. G., & Massie, B. M. (2004). The clinical challenge of cardiorenal syndrome. *Circulation, 110*(12), 1514–1517.
20. Ronco, C., Haapio, M., House, A. A., et al. (2008). Cardiorenal syndrome. *J Am Coll Cardiol, 52*(19), 1527–1539.
21. Bongartz, L. G., Cramer, M. J., Doevendans, P. A., et al. (2005). The severe cardiorenal syndrome: "Guyton revisited." *Eur Heart J, 26*(1), 11–17.
22. Boerrigter, G., Lapp, H., & Burnett, J. C. (2009). Modulation of cGMP in heart failure: a new therapeutic paradigm. *Handb Exp Pharmacol, 191*(191), 485–506.
23. Conti, M., & Beavo, J. (2007). Biochemistry and physiology of cyclic nucleotide phosphodiesterases: essential components in cyclic nucleotide signaling. *Annu Rev Biochem, 76*, 481–511.
24. Castro, L. R., Verde, I., Cooper, D. M., et al. (2006). Cyclic guanosine monophosphate compartmentation in rat cardiac myocytes. *Circulation, 113*(18), 2221–2228.
25. Martin, F. L., Supaporn, T., Chen, H. H., et al. (2007). Distinct roles for renal particulate and soluble guanylyl cyclases in preserving renal function in experimental acute heart failure. *Am J Physiol Regul Integr Comp Physiol, 293*(4), R1580–R1585.
26. Madhani, M., Okorie, M., Hobbs, A. J., et al. (2006). Reciprocal regulation of human soluble and particulate guanylate cyclases in vivo. *Br J Pharmacol, 149*(6), 797–801.
27. Schmidt, P. M., Schramm, M., Schroder, H., et al. (2004). Identification of residues crucially involved in the binding of the heme moiety of soluble guanylate cyclase. *J Biol Chem, 279*(4), 3025–3032.
28. Brunton, T. (1867). Use of nitrite of amyl in angina pectoris. *Lancet, 2*, 97–98.
29. Caramori, P. R., Adelman, A. G., Azevedo, E. R., et al. (1998). Therapy with nitroglycerin increases coronary vasoconstriction in response to acetylcholine. *J Am Coll Cardiol, 32*(7), 1969–1974.
30. Hess, D. T., Matsumoto, A., Kim, S. O., et al. (2005). Protein S-nitrosylation: purview and parameters. *Nat Rev Mol Cell Biol, 6*(2), 150–166.
31. Munzel, T., Sayegh, H., Freeman, B. A., et al. (1995). Evidence for enhanced vascular superoxide anion production in nitrate tolerance. A novel mechanism underlying tolerance and cross-tolerance. *J Clin Invest, 95*(1), 187–194.
32. Taylor, A. L., Ziesche, S., Yancy, C., et al. (2004). Combination of isosorbide dinitrate and hydralazine in blacks with heart failure. *N Engl J Med, 351*(20), 2049–2057.
33. Ko, F. N., Wu, C. C., Kuo, S. C., et al. (1994). YC-1, a novel activator of platelet guanylate cyclase. *Blood, 84*(12), 4226–4233.
34. Evgenov, O. V., Pacher, P., Schmidt, P. M., et al. (2006). NO-independent stimulators and activators of soluble guanylate cyclase: discovery and therapeutic potential. *Nat Rev Drug Discov, 5*(9), 755–768.
35. Stasch, J. P., Becker, E. M., Alonso-Alija, C., et al. (2001). NO-independent regulatory site on soluble guanylate cyclase. *Nature, 410*(6825), 212–215.
36. Boerrigter, G., Costello-Boerrigter, L. C., Cataliotti, A., et al. (2003). Cardiorenal and humoral properties of a novel direct soluble guanylate cyclase stimulator BAY 41-2272 in experimental congestive heart failure. *Circulation, 107*(5), 686–689.
37. Grimminger, F., Weimann, G., Frey, R., et al. (2009). First acute haemodynamic study of soluble guanylate cyclase stimulator riociguat in pulmonary hypertension. *Eur Respir J, 33*(4), 785–792.
38. Schmidt, P., Schramm, M., Schroder, H., et al. (2003). Mechanisms of nitric oxide independent activation of soluble guanylyl cyclase. *Eur J Pharmacol, 468*(3), 167–174.
39. Meurer, S., Pioch, S., Pabst, T., et al. (2009). Nitric oxide-independent vasodilator rescues heme-oxidized soluble guanylate cyclase from proteasomal degradation. *Circ Res, 105*(1), 33–41.
40. Stasch, J. P., Schmidt, P. M., Nedvetsky, P. I., et al. (2006). Targeting the heme-oxidized nitric oxide receptor for selective vasodilatation of diseased blood vessels. *J Clin Invest, 116*(9), 2552–2561.
41. Boerrigter, G., Costello-Boerrigter, L. C., Cataliotti, A., et al. (2007). Targeting heme-oxidized soluble guanylate cyclase in experimental heart failure. *Hypertension, 49*(5), 1128–1133.
42. Lapp, H., Mitrovic, V., Franz, N., et al. (2009). Cinaciguat (BAY 58-2667) improves cardiopulmonary hemodynamics and has a favorable safety profile in patients with acute decompensated heart failure. *Circulation, 119*(21), 2781–2788.
43. Tsuruda, T., Boerrigter, G., Huntley, B. K., et al. (2002). Brain natriuretic peptide is produced in cardiac fibroblasts and induces matrix metalloproteinases. *Circ Res, 91*(12), 1127–1134.
44. Holtwick, R., van Eickels, M., Skryabin, B. V., et al. (2003). Pressure-independent cardiac hypertrophy in mice with cardiomyocyte-restricted inactivation of the atrial natriuretic peptide receptor guanylyl cyclase-A. *J Clin Invest, 111*(9), 1399–1407.
45. Lainchbury, J. G., Burnett, J. C., Jr., Meyer, D., et al. (2000). Effects of natriuretic peptides on load and myocardial function in normal and heart failure dogs. *Am J Physiol Heart Circ Physiol, 278*(1), H33–H40.
46. Stingo, A. J., Clavell, A. L., Heublein, D. M., et al. (1992). Presence of C-type natriuretic peptide in cultured human endothelial cells and plasma. *Am J Physiol, 263*(4 pt 2), H1318–H1321.
47. Cataliotti, A., Boerrigter, G., Costello-Boerrigter, L. C., et al. (2004). Brain natriuretic peptide enhances renal actions of furosemide and suppresses furosemide-induced aldosterone activation in experimental heart failure. *Circulation, 109*(13), 1680–1685.
48. VMAC-Investigators. (2002). Intravenous nesiritide vs nitroglycerin for treatment of decompensated congestive heart failure: a randomized controlled trial. *JAMA, 287*(12), 1531–1540.
49. Sackner-Bernstein, J. D., Skopicki, H. A., & Aaronson, K. D. (2005). Risk of worsening renal function with nesiritide in patients with acutely decompensated heart failure. *Circulation, 111*(12), 1487–1491.
50. Sackner-Bernstein, J. D., Kowalski, M., Fox, M., et al. (2005). Short-term risk of death after treatment with nesiritide for decompensated heart failure: a pooled analysis of randomized controlled trials. *JAMA, 293*(15), 1900–1905.
51. Witteles, R. M., Kao, D., Christopherson, D., et al. (2007). Impact of nesiritide on renal function in patients with acute decompensated heart failure and pre-existing renal dysfunction: a randomized, double-blind, placebo-controlled clinical trial. *J Am Coll Cardiol, 50*(19), 1835–1840.
52. Burnett, J. C., Jr., & Korinek, J. (2008). The tumultuous journey of nesiritide: past, present, and future. *Circ Heart Fail, 1*, 6–8.
53. Arora, S., Clarke, K., Srinivasan, V., et al. (2007). Effect of nesiritide on renal function in patients admitted for decompensated heart failure. *QJM, 100*(11), 699–706.
54. Costanzo, M. R., Johannes, R. S., Pine, M., et al. (2007). The safety of intravenous diuretics alone versus diuretics plus parenteral vasoactive therapies in hospitalized patients with acutely decompensated heart failure: a propensity score and instrumental variable analysis using the Acutely Decompensated Heart Failure National Registry (ADHERE) database. *Am Heart J, 154*(2), 267–277.
55. Mentzer, R. M., Jr., Oz, M. C., Sladen, R. N., et al. (2007). Effects of perioperative nesiritide in patients with left ventricular dysfunction undergoing cardiac surgery: the NAPA trial. *J Am Coll Cardiol, 49*(6), 716–726.
56. Chen, H. H., Sundt, T. M., Cook, D. J., et al. (2007). Low dose nesiritide and the preservation of renal function in patients with renal dysfunction undergoing cardiopulmonary-bypass surgery: a double-blind placebo-controlled pilot study. *Circulation, 116*(suppl. 11), I134–I138.
57. Chen, H. H., Martin, F. L., Gibbons, R. J., et al. (2009). Low-dose nesiritide in human anterior myocardial infarction suppresses aldosterone and preserves ventricular function and structure: a proof of concept study. *Heart, 95*(16), 1315–1319.
58. Newton, P. J., Betihavas, V., & Macdonald, P. (2009). The role of b-type natriuretic peptide in heart failure management. *Aust Crit Care, 22*(3), 117–123.
59. Schweitz, H., Vigne, P., Moinier, D., et al. (1992). A new member of the natriuretic peptide family is present in the venom of the green mamba (*Dendroaspis angusticeps*). *J Biol Chem, 267*(20), 13928–13932.
60. Lisy, O., Jougasaki, M., Heublein, D. M., et al. (1999). Renal actions of synthetic *Dendroaspis* natriuretic peptide. *Kidney Int, 56*(2), 502–508.
61. Lisy, O., Lainchbury, J. G., Leskinen, H., et al. (2001). Therapeutic actions of a new synthetic vasoactive and natriuretic peptide, *Dendroaspis* natriuretic peptide, in experimental severe congestive heart failure. *Hypertension, 37*(4), 1089–1094.
62. Chen, H. H., Lainchbury, J. G., & Burnett, J. C., Jr. (2002). Natriuretic peptide receptors and neutral endopeptidase in mediating the renal actions of a new therapeutic synthetic natriuretic peptide *Dendroaspis* natriuretic peptide. *J Am Coll Cardiol, 40*(6), 1186–1191.
63. Kenny, A. J., Bourne, A., & Ingram, J. (1993). Hydrolysis of human and pig brain natriuretic peptides, urodilatin, C-type natriuretic peptide and some C-receptor ligands by endopeptidase-24.11. *Biochem J, 291*(pt 1), 83–88.
64. Lisy, O., Huntley, B. K., McCormick, D. J., et al. (2008). Design, synthesis, and actions of a novel chimeric natriuretic peptide: CD-NP. *J Am Coll Cardiol, 52*(1), 60–68.
65. Dickey, D. M., Burnett, J. C., Jr., & Potter, L. R. (2008). Novel bifunctional natriuretic peptides as potential therapeutics. *J Biol Chem, 283*(50), 35003–35009.
66. Lee, C. Y., Chen, H. H., Lisy, O., et al. (2009). Pharmacodynamics of a novel designer natriuretic peptide, CD-NP, in a first-in-human clinical trial in healthy subjects. *J Clin Pharmacol, 49*(6), 668–673.
67. Takimoto, E., Champion, H. C., Li, M., et al. (2005). Chronic inhibition of cyclic GMP phosphodiesterase 5A prevents and reverses cardiac hypertrophy. *Nat Med, 11*(2), 214–222.
68. Chen, H. H., Huntley, B. K., Schirger, J. A., et al. (2006). Maximizing the renal cyclic 3'-5'-guanosine monophosphate system with type V phosphodiesterase inhibition and exogenous natriuretic peptide: a novel strategy to improve renal function in experimental overt heart failure. *J Am Soc Nephrol, 17*(10), 2742–2747.
69. Supaporn, T., Sandberg, S. M., Borgeson, D. D., et al. (1996). Blunted cGMP response to agonists and enhanced glomerular cyclic 3',5'-nucleotide phosphodiesterase activities in experimental congestive heart failure. *Kidney Int, 50*(5), 1718–1725.
70. Boerrigter, G., & Burnett, J. C., Jr. (2009). Soluble guanylate cyclase: not a dull enzyme. *Circulation, 119*(21), 2752–2754.
71. Reilly, R. F., Ellison, D. H. (2000). Mammalian distal tubule: physiology, pathophysiology, and molecular anatomy. *Physiol Rev, 80*, 277–313.
72. Cohn, J. N., Archibald, D. G., Ziesche, S., et al. (1986). Effect of vasodilator therapy on mortality in chronic congestive heart failure. Results of a Veterans Administration Cooperative Study. *N Engl J Med*, 314, 1547–1552.

CHAPTER 19

Alterations in Diaphragmatic and Skeletal Muscle in Heart Failure

Thierry H. Le Jemtel and Donna M. Mancini

Skeletal and diaphragmatic muscle alterations have been extensively reviewed in patients and experimental models of heart failure (HF) due to left ventricular (LV) systolic dysfunction.[1-7] Accordingly, the first aim of this chapter is to provide a concise summary of the vascular atrophic and metabolic skeletal muscle (SM) alterations that have been reported in patients with HF. The second aim is to review recent human and experimental investigations that have focused on the underlying mechanisms of SM alterations and possible novel therapeutic strategies. The third aim of the chapter is to provide an update on diaphragmatic muscle alterations in HF and the impact of diaphragmatic muscle alterations on the symptomatic progression of HF syndrome.

SKELETAL MUSCLE IN HEART FAILURE

The view that alterations of skeletal muscle (SM) vasculature metabolism and mass play an important role in limiting peak functional capacity in patients with heart failure (HF) is now well accepted.[8,9] Vascular metabolic and atrophic alterations have been thoroughly documented in skeletal and diaphragmatic muscle of patients with HF.[10-14] However, the cascade of events and mechanisms that are responsible for SM alterations remain somewhat controversial in HF. Most investigators agree that reduced physical activity (disuse) plays an important role in the pathogenesis of SM alterations in HF and that HF-related SM alterations do not substantially differ from those observed in other chronic conditions, such as chronic obstructive pulmonary disease (COPD) or chronic kidney disease (CKD).[15] Paradoxically, while disuse was becoming increasingly recognized as an important determinant of HF-related SM alterations, alleviating disuse by exercise training was recently reported to have a modest impact on SM alterations as assessed by the change peak functional capacity in the HF-ACTION trial (see also Chapter 57).[16] Confronted with exercise training's limited benefits, investigators are seeking novel approaches to reverse or better prevent the development of SM alterations in patients with HF. Investigative efforts focusing on molecular pathways that mediate SM alterations in patients with CHF are presently under way with the aim of developing innovative therapeutic strategies.

Besides disuse, HF is associated with low-level systemic inflammation (see also Chapter 11) that fosters development of SM alterations. (see also Chapter 57)[17,18] As SM alterations become more severe, inflammatory mediators are released into the circulation, thereby deepening systemic inflammation that in turn promote SM atrophy. Accentuation of the muscle mechanoreflex in HF heightens sympathetic nervous activation (SNA) during exercise, resulting in vasoconstriction and metabolic derangements that may exacerbate SM alterations.[19] Progression of SM alterations in HF appears to be largely dependent on local factors and is not directly related to deterioration of LV systolic or diastolic function.

Skeletal Muscle Alterations and Stages of Heart Failure

Skeletal muscle alterations develop and worsen concomitantly to the occurrence and deterioration of symptoms in patients with HF. Progression of HF due to LV systolic dysfunction is currently being summarized in four stages: Stage A attests to a high risk of developing HF; Stage B includes LV remodeling in the absence of symptoms[20]; Stage C is defined by the occurrence and progression of symptoms; Stage D denotes the presence of a low cardiac output. From a clinical standpoint, SM alterations are most relevant at stage C where both enhancement of LV systolic function and reversal of SM alterations are required for sustained functional improvement while at stage D enhancement of LV systolic function alone results in immediate functional improvement. In summary, partial or complete reversal of SM alterations is required at stage C to restore the functional capacity of HF patients to that of age-and gender-matched controls.[21]

Vascular Alterations

While lower limb blood flow may increase up to 20 times from rest to peak exercise in healthy subjects, lower limb flow can increase only 2 to 3 times in patients with advanced HF due to LV systolic dysfunction.[11,22] Thus the vasodilatory response of the lower limb SM beds to exercise is relatively much more impaired than that of the cardiac output in severe HF. Some investigators have failed to observe a limited vasodilatory response of SM beds to exercise in patients with severe HF.[23-25] Cause of HF (primarily due to valvular disease rather than end-stage cardiomyopathy), and technical issues in the measurement of skeletal muscle blood flow (use of single thermistor for the thermodilution technique and measurement of blood flow draining other tissues than skeletal muscles) may in part explain the disparate findings. At stage C of HF, SM perfusion during exercise is primarily limited by an impaired vasodilatory response of lower limb SM beds and not by the cardiac output response to exercise. At stage D of CHF, SM perfusion during exercise is limited by the cardiac output response as it is in normal subjects.[22] The findings regarding SM microcirculation are controversial in severe HF.[4] Capillary density has been reported to be normal or decreased depending on normalization to the muscle fibers' number and size. Duscha et al measured vascular density in the skeletal muscle of patients with HF.[26] Using cell-specific antibodies to measure vascular density, these investigators found decreased numbers of endothelial cells per fiber, which indicates a reduced capillary density. However, since capillary density varies with fiber type, and fiber-type switching is a dynamic process in patients with HF, studies on capillary density ratio should be interpreted with caution. Other investigators have reported a normal skeletal muscle capillary density in patients with HF.[27] Thickness of the capillary basement membrane is increased in the pronator teres muscle of patients with HF.[28] Finally, the resistance of the microvasculature is only minimally increased in the cutaneous tissue in patients with HF.[29] Of note, although vascular endothelial dysfunction (an important determinant of capillary behavior during exercise) is impaired in HF, oxygen extraction by exercising SM is nearly complete in severely symptomatic patients.[30] Similarly, reduced SM oxidative capacity does not limit oxygen extraction by exercising muscles in HF.[31] The oxygen content of the deep femoral vein that exclusively drains skeletal muscle is less than 1 to 2 mL/100 mL in patients with severe HF.[30] In summary, while skeletal muscle capillary density is likely to be altered in HF and oxidative capacity is reduced, they do not limit oxygen extraction by exercising muscles.

The mechanisms of vascular SM alterations are incompletely understood in HF. Few studies have dealt with vascular smooth muscle function while vascular endothelial function and particularly nitric oxide (NO)-mediated control of vasomotor tone has been extensively studied in HF.[32-35] Endothelial function was first evaluated in the upper limb vasculature by measuring forearm blood flow in response to methacholine, an endothelium-dependent dilator, and nitroprusside, an endothelium-independent dilator.[35] Blood flow was measured by venous plethysmography. The response to methacholine was significantly lower in patients with HF, when compared with age-matched controls, while the response to nitroprusside tended to be lower, although it did not reach statistical significance. The blunted response to methacholine implies that patients with HF have an impaired reserve of vascular endothelium. Endothelial function was studied in the lower limb vasculature of patients with HF using Doppler ultrasonography of the superficial femoral artery.[34] Patients did not have comorbid vascular disease that could have contributed to endothelial dysfunction. The maximal velocity of blood using a volume sampler positioned in the center of the vessel was evaluated during intraarterial administration of acetylcholine, an endothelial-dependent dilator, and nitroglycerin, an endothelial-independent dilator. Maximal blood flow velocity did not increase in response to acetylcholine at concentrations of 10-5M, while it increased by fivefold in healthy subjects. Maximal blood flow velocity in response to nitroglycerin at 10-7M was substantially reduced in patients when compared with the response elicited in healthy subjects. Following administration of a dose of nitroglycerin at 5 to 10 M, patients with HF experienced an increase in maximal blood flow velocity similar to that produced by nitroglycerin at 7 to 10 M in healthy subjects. The lack of response to acetylcholine clearly demonstrates the absence of functional reserve of the vascular endothelium in patients with HF. However, reduced vascular endothelial function in patients with HF may in part be due to reduced functional integrity of the cyclic GMP pathway that is evidenced by the depressed response to nitroglycerin. The mechanisms that are responsible and mediate the progression of vascular endothelial function in patients with HF are still poorly understood. Furthermore, the state of vascular function under basal conditions in patients with CHF is still debated. Administration of L-NMMA (N-monomethyl-L-arginine), a selective inhibitor of the production of NO from arginine, yielded similar forearm blood flow decreases in patients with CHF and in healthy subjects.[36,37] However, others observed the expected decrease in blood flow following administration of L-NMMA in healthy subjects, but did not observe a decrease in patients with CHF.[38] Experimental data indicate that increases in oxidative stress associated with heart failure may accelerate NO degradation, and thus may impact on NO availability.[39]

In the rat model, heart failure induced by ligation of the left anterior descending artery causes progressive peripheral vascular endothelial dysfunction.[40] The systemic vascular response to acetylcholine was not decreased until 4 weeks after coronary ligation and progressively worsened through week 16. Similar data are not available in human subjects. The mechanisms that mediate vascular endothelial dysfunction early in the course of heart failure are likely to be different from those responsible at later stages. In patients with symptomatic HF, the improvement induced by vitamin C administration and subsequent decreased extracellular SOD (superoxide dismutase) activity implies that increased oxidative stress may accelerate NO degradation, and may be partially responsible for vascular endothelial dysfunction.[41] Our data suggest that there is increased expression of endothelial NO synthase (eNOS) when normalized to Von Willebrand factor in the vastus lateralis muscle of patients with CHF.[42] Increased eNOS endothelial expression implies the development of an adaptive mechanism to compensate for accelerated NO degradation.

Skeletal Muscle Mass

Calf muscle mass was reported to be significantly lower in patients with severe HF as evidenced by a peak $\dot{V}O_2$ of 13 mL/min/kg when compared with age- and gender-matched controls. Approximately two thirds of these patients have a reduced calf mass that correlates only weakly ($r = 0.48$) with peak oxygen uptake.[10] Overall the data regarding SM mass are disparate in patients with HF with some investigators reporting a normal muscle mass in patients with average peak oxygen uptake of 13.4 mL/kg/min while others are reporting a reduced muscle mass in patients with average peak oxygen uptake of 18.0 mL/kg/min.[43] In contrast to the controversial data on muscle mass, most investigators report decreased muscle strength when normalized to fiber cross-sectional areas in patients with HF.[4] Slowing of relaxation and steady decline in strength have been reported during low-frequency stimulation of slow-twitch muscles in rats with congestive HF.[44] Reduced isometric force and calcium-activated actomyosin (AM) ATPase activity in patients with HF may be due to a decline in density of contractile proteins, in the rate of cross-bridge attachment, or in both.[45] A reduction in contractile protein content appears to be the most likely explanation of reduced muscle strength since SM contractile protein function has been reported to be unaltered in patients with HF.[46]

Exertional shortness of breath and fatigue are the cornerstones of the clinical syndrome of HF. Exertional symptoms induce physical inactivity that results in disuse. The syndrome of HF is a low level inflammatory state. Both disuse and systemic inflammation are initially responsible for loss of SM mass and atrophy in patients with HF (Figure 19-1). Thereafter, SM atrophy steadily progresses in the absence of intervention. The progression of SM atrophy appears to be more closely related to an ongoing interaction between atrophy and local inflammation than to deterioration of LV dysfunction and HF (see Figure19-1). The lack of correlation between progression of SM alterations and deterioration of LV function accounts in part for the discordant reports of SM alterations in HF due to LV systolic dysfunction. Furthermore, SM alterations are not easily quantifiable in patients and many SM parameters have no direct clinical correlates.

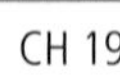

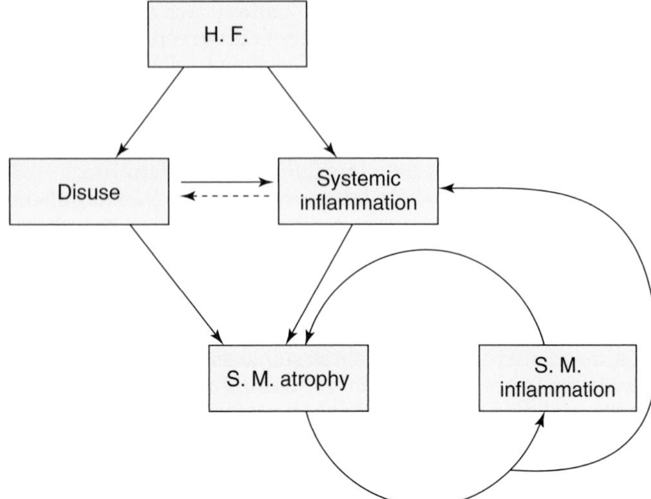

FIGURE 19–1 Heart failure (HF) results in reduced physical activity (disuse) as shortness of breath and fatigue during exercise tend to limit physical activity. Patients with HF exhibit a low-level inflammatory state as evidenced by mildly elevated levels of circulating inflammatory mediators. Both disuse and systemic inflammation promote skeletal muscle (SM) atrophy that leads to SM inflammation and further loss of SM mass. In addition, SM inflammation fosters systemic inflammation that combined with disuse exacerbates SM atrophy. Disuse is associated with systemic inflammation that may negatively impact on functional capacity. Once loss of SM mass occurs, it tends to progress independently from the initiating cause.

Skeletal muscle atrophy promotes local inflammation that in turn exacerbates SM atrophy via multiple mechanisms. In addition, SM inflammation exacerbates systemic inflammation that results in further muscle atrophy. Akin to LV remodeling, which may progress independently from the initial cardiac event and is influenced by the presence of comorbid conditions such as diabetes or hypertension, SM alterations develop and progress in HF independently from LV dysfunction. As previously mentioned, magnitude of SM alterations and severity of LV dysfunction are not closely related.

Although intuitively plausible, experimental data do not support disuse as a cause of SM atrophy in HF. In a rat coronary ligation model of HF, changes in SM morphology and gene expression could not be explained by reduced activity.[47] However, limited activity of animals housed in cages and sham thoracotomy in control animals may have substantially reduced the likelihood of recording different activity levels between failing and control animals. A strong argument for the role of disuse in the pathogenesis of SM alterations comes from the observation that conditions which share disuse as a common trait but are as different as COPD, CKD, and chronic HF result in comparable SM alterations.[48] Physical inactivity in patients with CHF affect primarily the lower limb SM because patients—due to exertional shortness of breath and fatigue—curtail walking and climbing stairs long before they curtail physical activities involving the upper limbs when they experience symptoms at rest.[49] Thus studies of forearm SM in HF need to include a precise staging of symptoms and possibly the occupation of patients before they develop HF. Since these parameters are quite subjective and often poorly reported, the findings of forearm muscle studies in HF are commonly difficult to interpret.

The modest effect of exercise training on peak functional capacity in the HF-ACTION trial appears to argue against disuse playing an important role in the pathogenesis of SM alterations in HF. However, several carefully conducted single - center studies have thoroughly demonstrated the beneficial effects of exercise training on SM in patients with HF.[50,51] The unimpressive findings of the HF-ACTION trial underline how difficult it is to enforce strict adherence to exercise training in a large study population. The findings of the HF-ACTION trial do not invalidate the previously well-documented beneficial effects of exercise training on functional capacity and SM mass in smaller populations of HF patients.

Skeletal Muscle Fiber Composition

Adult human SM is composed of four fiber types: type I, IIa, IIb, and IIx. The fiber types are defined by their myosin heavy chain isoforms and are identified based on differential immunocytochemistry staining for myosin ATPase.[52] Type I fibers are slow-twitch fibers, so-called because they have a slowly propagated action potential. They develop low tension and primarily use aerobic or oxidative metabolism to generate ATP. They typically contain an abundance of mitochondria and use ATP very slowly, and are therefore fatigue-resistant fibers. Type I fibers are necessary for endurance activity; this includes posture, repetitive movements, and also long-distance exercise. In contrast, type IIb/x fibers are fasttwitch fibers that develop large tensions and rely on anaerobic metabolism to generate ATP. They have fewer mitochondria and use ATP very quickly. They are responsible for muscle power, in short bursts, but fatigue easily because anaerobic or glycolytic energy pathways are much less efficient in generating ATP. Type IIa fibers are a hybrid of fast and slow-twitch; they have the capacity to achieve great tension, but also have some measure of endurance. As expected, they rely on both aerobic and anaerobic metabolism to generate energy.[52] It may be that type IIa fibers are in the process of fiber type switching.

Patients with HF have an increased number of type IIb/x fibers (anaerobic, glycolytic) as compared with type I (aerobic, oxidative).[12,14,54] When compared with deconditioning-related SM atrophy, HF-related SM atrophy is more selective for type II. Mancini[10] et al reported an increased percentage of type IIb fibers and trends toward a decreased percentage of type I in the gastrocnemius muscle of patients with CHF. However, due to reduced areas of type IIb fibers, the relative contribution of each fiber type in a given cross-sectional area of muscle was not different between CHF patients and normal subjects. Interestingly, the percentage of type IIb fibers correlated inversely with peak oxygen uptake. Drexler[14] et al also found that fiber distribution was shifted toward type II fibers in the vastus lateralis of patients with HF. There was also decreased volume density of the mitochondria and surface density of the mitochondrial cristae, implying that oxidative transport coupling was compromised. Decreased mitochondrial density and surface density of mitochondrial cristae occurred mostly in patients with peak $\dot{V}O_2$ averaging 12 mL/kg/min. Patients whose peak $\dot{V}O_2$ was normal (more than 25 mL/kg/min) had normal mitochondrial parameters compared with controls. The decreased mitochondrial volume correlated with peak aerobic capacity, suggesting a major contribution of altered skeletal muscle metabolism to exercise intolerance. Recently, Mettauer[55] et al compared intrinsic mitochondrial function in the vastus lateralis muscle of patients with CHF to that of sedentary and active controls. The basal and stimulated oxidative parameters of the entire mitochondrial population were similar in CHF patients and sedentary controls, but were reduced when compared with the active controls. In agreement with previous reports,[12,56] the content of intramitochondrial Krebs cycle citrate synthase was lowest in HF patients. The level in sedentary subjects was also reduced, as compared with active subjects, but not as low as that found in patients with CHF. Total cytosolic creatine kinase (CK), skeletal muscle–specific CK (MM-CK), and lactate dehydrogenase (LDH) were lower in CHF patients. In experimental preparations, including myocardial infarction and moderate heart failure, angiotensin-converting enzyme inhibition completely prevents the fiber switch from type I to II in the skeletal muscle.[57,58] Similar observations were made in the gastrocnemius muscle of patients with CHF following angiotensin-converting enzyme (ACE) inhibition or angiotensin receptor blockade for 6 months.[59]

Skeletal Muscle Metabolism

Skeletal muscle metabolism has been studied by radioactive phosphorus nuclear magnetic resonance (31P-NMR) spectroscopy in patients with HF. Concomitant use of 31P-NMR to study SM metabolism and venous plethysmography to measure limb blood flow demonstrated that early SM acidosis during exercise occurs in the absence of an associated decrease in flow in patients with HF.[60,61] 31P-NMR spectroscopy consistently demonstrates the following abnormalities in the SM of patients with HF: accelerated rate of use of phosphocreatine (PCr, a high-energy phosphate), accumulation of inorganic phosphate (Pi, a by-product of ATP use), early intracellular acidification (low pH), and delayed PCr recovery after exercise. These abnormalities of SM metabolism were first reported in the forearm. Immediately after exercise, patients exhibited a greater than normal increase in the Pi/PCr ratio and a decrease in pH.[62-64] The lack of correlation between forearm blood flow assessed immediately after exercise by plethysmography and the previously mentioned metabolic abnormalities was offered as evidence that reduced SM perfusion is not responsible for the metabolic abnormalities.[60,61,63] Taking into account that forearm blood flow was most likely normal in the patients studied by 31P-NMR spectroscopy, a lack of correlation between flow and metabolism was expected. Thus the anticipated lack of correlation between SM blood flow and metabolism has no bearing on the pathophysiology of SM alterations in HF. It is likely that forearm SM metabolic alterations were related to some degree of deconditioning among the patients studied by 31P-NMR spectroscopy. Chati[65] et al have clearly demonstrated that the rate of use of PCr, accumulation of Pi, and intracellular acidification are not different in the SM of patients with HF and sedentary normal subjects. Adamopoulos[66] et al showed that physical conditioning substantially corrects SM metabolic alterations in patients with HF. After undergoing 8 weeks of home-based bicycle exercise training in a randomized-crossover trial, patients exhibited less PCr depletion and faster PCr recovery. Acidification was unaffected by physical conditioning. Metabolic abnormalities similar to those documented in the forearm were subsequently demonstrated in the thigh and leg of patients with CHF.[64,67] On the basis of a significant correlation between the slope of PCr decrease when related to workload and peak oxygen uptake, Okita[67] et al concluded that the metabolic abnormalities in the thigh muscles limit exercise capacity in patients with HF. Studying the calf, Mancini[64] et al failed to observe a correlation between the slope of the Pi/PCr over $\dot{V}O_2$ ratio and muscle enzyme activities. In summary, SM metabolic alterations have been thoroughly documented by 31P-NMR spectroscopy in patients with HF. Overall, patients with HF experience SM metabolic alterations that are similar to those reported after deconditioning. Extent of SM atrophy and severity of SM fibrosis and inflammation rather than impairment in SM metabolism are likely to underlie 31P-NMR spectroscopy SM metabolic alterations. In patients with HF, 31P-NMR spectroscopy findings need to be normalized to the amount of underlying intact SM and extent of SM fibrosis and fat deposits.

Excitation Contraction Coupling

Excitation contraction (EC) coupling of the basic SM contractile unit of the sarcomere is abnormal in HF. Skeletal muscles from animals with HF exhibit Ca^{2+} spark frequency, decreased Ca^{2+} spark amplitude, and increased Ca^{2+} spark duration consistent with leaky sarcoplasmic reticulum (SR) Ca^{2+} release and with decreased SR Ca^{2+} content.[68] Heart failure is associated with elevated levels of circulating catecholamines and widespread activation of adrenergic signaling pathways. The type 1 ryanodine receptor (RyR1) becomes leaky in HF as chronic adrenergic stimulation results in cAMP-dependent protein kinase (PKA) hyperphosphorylation of the channel, which in turn dissociates calstabin-1, the stabilizing protein that keeps the RyR1 channel in a closed state from the channel.[68] Whether Ca^{2+} leak has any clinical correlates remains to be demonstrated in patients with HF. Data regarding SR Ca^{2+} pumping in HF differ in fast- and slow-twitch muscles and according the level of fatigue.[44] In agreement with data in aging, SRCa^{2+} pumping appears to be most impaired in slow-twitch muscles of animals with HF. Data regarding SM protein and mRNA expression of sarcoplasmic reticulum calcium (SERCA) ATPase are divergent in HF.[1,69] Predominant muscle fiber composition and nature of the HF model may in part account for the disparate findings that have been occasionally correlated with early muscle fatigue.

Mechanisms of Skeletal Muscle Atrophy

The mechanisms that mediate SM wasting and atrophy have not been extensively investigated in patients with HF. Loss of SM mass can result from decreased protein synthesis, increased protein degradation, or both. Several key signaling pathways involved in protein degradation and synthesis are illustrated in Figure 19-2.[70] These pathways will be discussed in the following sections.

Protein Degradation. Recent experimental data in a mouse model of chronic HF due to ligation of the left coronary artery indicate that the ubiquitin-proteasome pathway plays an important role in HF-induced SM atrophy.[71] Ubiquitin protein ligases target specific proteins for ubiquitination. Proteins are marked by ubiquitin and subsequently rapidly degraded through the 26S proteasome, an ATP-dependent pathway that yields peptides and intact ubiquitin.[4] In experimental preparations, the ubiquitin-proteasome pathway was found to be activated as evidenced by selective induction of muscle-specific ubiquitin ligase atrogin-1 muscle atrophy Fbox (MAFbx), resulting in critical (FoxO) transcriptional factor activation.[71] Transgenic overexpression of MLC/mLgf-1 that encodes for a locally active isoform of IGF-1 prevents proteasome activation breakdown of SM structural proteins and atrophy.[71] Thus at least experimentally ubiquitin-mediated proteolytic degradation appears to be partly responsible for LV systolic dysfunction-related SM wasting. However, preliminary data from our laboratory did not support activation of the ubiquitin-proteasome pathway in patients with severe HF and overt SM atrophy. Whether the ubiquitin-proteasome pathway is activated at an earlier stage of HF when patients have not yet developed full-blown SM atrophy is currently unknown.

Experimental data regarding the seminal role of IGF-1 in the development of SM atrophy have been provided in a model of SM wasting induced by chronic administration of angiotensin II (AII).[72] The chronic AII administration model of SM wasting results in systemic AII levels that are similar to that measured in patients with decompensated HF who are not receiving ACE inhibitors. Chronic administration of AII downregulates IGF-1 signaling via the Akt/mTOR/p7056k pathway that is critical for caspase-3 activation, actin cleavage, ubiquitination, and apoptosis.[72] Caspase 3 activation is an essential step in muscle protein degradation. It cleaves actomyosin in proteins that are degraded by the ubiquitin-proteasome pathway.[73] Caspase 3 activation is blocked by muscle-specific expression of IGF-1 via the Akt/mTOR/p7056k pathway.[72]

In summary, experimental data support that AII-mediated downregulation of IGF-1 in SM is causally related to AII-induced muscle wasting,[72] Whether the beneficial effects of

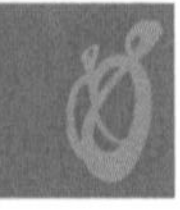

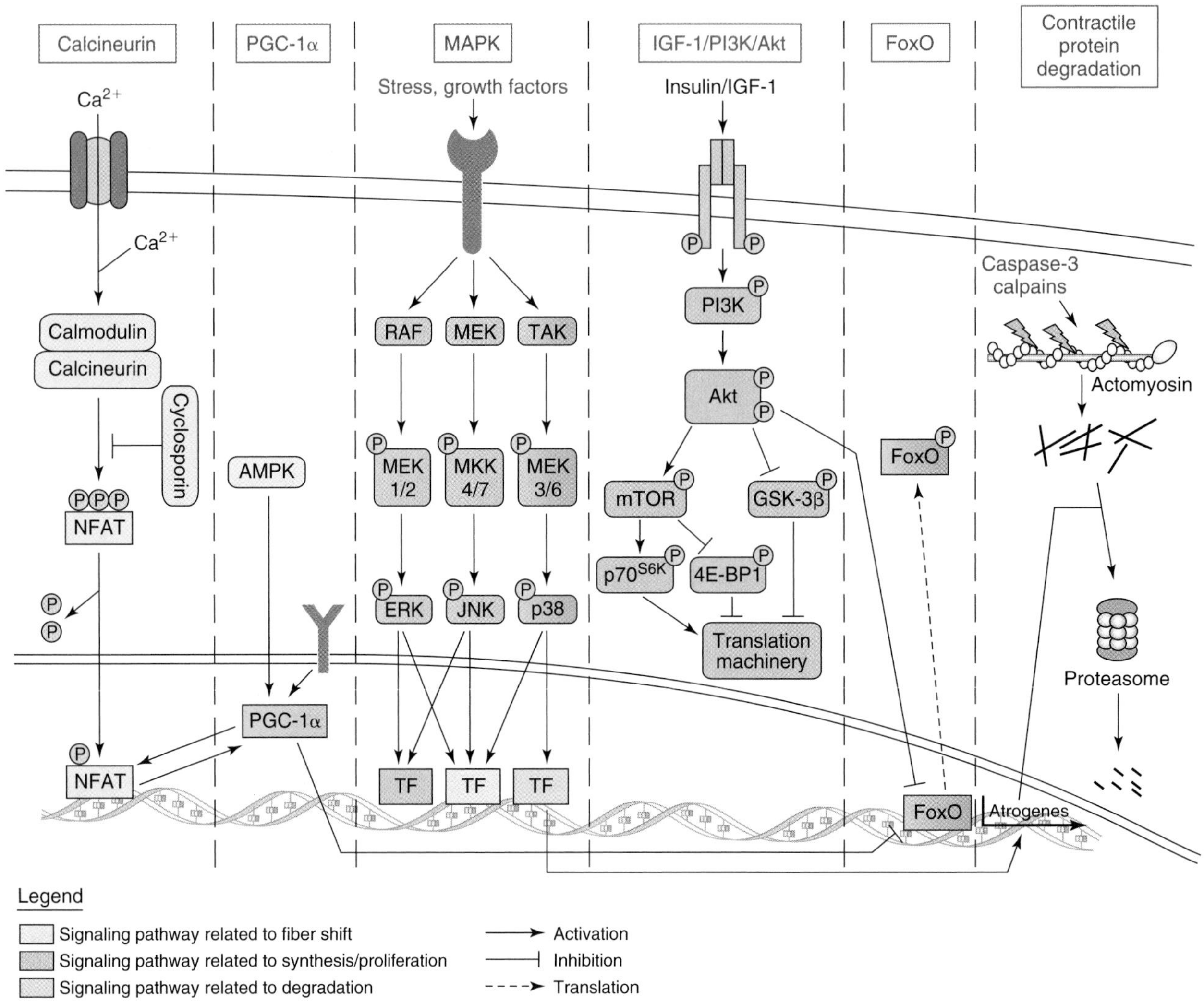

Calcineurin | PGC-1α | MAPK | IGF-1/PI3K/Akt | FoxO | Contractile protein degradation

Ca^{2+}
Stress, growth factors
Insulin/IGF-1
Ca^{2+}
Caspase-3 calpains
Calmodulin
Calcineurin
Cyclosporin
RAF MEK TAK
PI3K
Akt
Actomyosin
MEK 1/2 MKK 4/7 MEK 3/6
AMPK
mTOR
GSK-3β
FoxO
NFAT
p70S6K
4E-BP1
ERK JNK p38
Translation machinery
Proteasome
PGC-1α
NFAT
TF TF TF
FoxO
Atrogenes

Legend
Signaling pathway related to fiber shift
Signaling pathway related to synthesis/proliferation
Signaling pathway related to degradation
Activation
Inhibition
Translation

FIGURE 19–2 Signaling pathways underlying fiber type of switching and protein synthesis and degradation in skeletal muscle.
Six potential signaling pathways are illustrated. The interaction between the pathways is not depicted.

1. Calcineurin, a calcium-activated phosphatase, modulates fiber shift by activating the nuclear factor of activated T-cells (NFAT) transcription factor.
2. Peroxisome proliferator-activated receptor-γ (PPAR) coactivator 1α (PGC-1a) is highly expressed in type I fibers and participates in the biogenesis of mitochondria to promote oxidative metabolism. It can be activated by cAMP and nuclear receptors such as PPAR.
3. The MAPK pathway can be divided into three distinct pathways (i.e., ERK, JNK, and p38), which activate common and distinct transcription factors. ERK and JNK pathways stimulate proliferation and a shift toward type I fibers. The p38 pathway decreases proliferation and promotes protein degradation.
4. The IGF-1/phosphatidylinositol 3-kinase (PI3K)/Akt pathway is a key regulator of protein homeostasis. When activated by IGF-1, Akt induces synthesis and survival signals through many targets, including mammalian target of rapamycin (mTOR), and glycogen synthase kinase-3β (GSK-3β). Akt can phosphorylate and inactivate Forkhead box-containing protein O (FoxOs), thus contributing to reduced protein degradation.
5. FoxOs are a family of transcription factors that regulate the transcription of atrophying genes, such as Atrogin-1 and MuRF1. FoxOs also contribute to fiber shift.
6. The proteasome ensures degradation of intracellular protein using a two-step process. First, actomyosin is fragmented into polypeptides by caspase 3 or calpains, which are then ubiquitinated and degraded by the 26S proteasome enzymes. (From Caron M. Comparative assessment of the quadriceps and diaphragm in patients with COPD. *Appl Physiol* 2009;107:954.)

ACE inhibition on SM in HF patients are mediated through the IGF-1 pathway or result from a direct effect on SM vasculature via improvement of vascular endothelial function remains to be determined. In addition to AII elevated cytokines, SM levels can directly activate the ubiquitin-proteasome pathway and thereby result in SM protein degradation.[74]

Protein Synthesis. The syndrome of HF is associated with deficiencies in several anabolic hormones.[75,76] In male patients with HF deficiencies in circulating total testosterone, dehydroepiandrosterone (DHA) and IIGF-1 are common and correlate with a poor prognosis.[76] Testosterone produces SM hypertrophy by increasing fractional muscle protein synthesis.[77] The exact molecular pathways that mediate testosterone hypertrophic effects are incompletely understood. Testosterone appears to stimulate IGF-expression and downregulates IGF-binding protein-4 in the muscle.[78] At supraphysiological doses, testosterone appears to act through androgen receptors' independent mechanisms. In most tissues, androgen receptors are either saturated or downregulated at the lower end of normal concentrations.[78] In patients with HF serum levels of free testosterone and dehydroepiandrosterone are decreased in proportion to HF severity[76] in a placebo-controlled trial of 70 elderly patients with moderately severe HF testosterone was recently shown to improve exercise capacity muscle strength glucose metabolisms and baroreflex sensitivity.[79] Despite beneficial effects on insulin resistance, testosterone had no apparent effects on myocardial performance and LV function. The increase in exercise capacity was related to serum levels of testosterone and not to changes in LV function. Independently of its possible effects on muscle metaboreflex that may contribute to improved peak functional capacity, testosterone improved insulin sensitivity with an increase in total body mass and a decrease in fat mass.[79] Long-acting therapy seems to be well tolerated by elderly patients with moderately severe HF.

Besides their effects on SM protein degradation and cell death, growth hormone (GH) resistance and reduction in SM IGF-1 concentration contribute to SM atrophy in HF by directly reducing protein synthesis and by lessening muscle satellite cell recruitment and differentiation.[80] Cell-based therapy is presently under investigation for the treatment of muscular dystrophy.[81] Cell-based therapy is an attractive approach for SM regeneration in patients with disuse-induced atrophy.[82,83] Ghrelin, a novel GH-releasing peptide, stimulates physiological release of IGF-1 through a mechanism that is independent from hypothalamic GH-releasing hormone.[84] Administration of ghrelin for 3 weeks improves functional capacity and alleviates SM atrophy in patients with chronic HF and COPD.[85] Lastly the role of peroxisome proliferator-activated receptor γ coactivator 1α (PGC1α) in the pathogenesis of disuse-induced SM atrophy remains to be investigated in patients with chronic HF or COPD.[86]

Mechanisms of Skeletal Muscle Inflammation

Chronic HF is a low-level inflammatory state as evidenced by modest elevation of circulating IL-1 and IL-6 and TNF-α(see Chapter 11).[17] The initiating factors of SM inflammation are incompletely understood in HF. Disuse-induced atrophy promotes SM inflammation through activation of several signaling pathways (see Figure 19-2). Increased SNA promotes vasoconstriction and thereby reduces oxygen delivery to exercising SM. Concomitant activation of the renin-angiotensin system results in elevated A II SM concentration that increases local oxidative stress and lowers SM concentration of IGF-1. Reduced oxygen delivery and IGF-1 SM concentration combined with increased oxidative stress may accelerate protein degradation while decreasing protein synthesis. The increase in muscle SNA is mostly due to accentuation of muscle mechanoreceptors in HF while accentuation and desensitization of muscle metaboreceptors have been reported in HF depending on the severity of metabolic derangements, the degree of metaboreceptor desensitization, and the mode of exercise: static versus rhythmic.[87-90] Loss of SM mass, reduction in SM blood flow and blood flow distribution within SM, and fiber type composition contribute to muscle reflex alterations in HF.[19] In normal subjects, muscle reflex activation helps raise blood pressure and thereby maintain muscle perfusion during muscle acidosis. In HF, muscle reflex activation occurs at the onset of exercise, resulting in vasoconstriction and limited SM perfusion. Increased SM SNA and AII concentration promote local inflammation by reducing O_2 delivery and local IGF-1 concentration and increasing oxidative stress. In turn SM inflammation upregulates expression of cytokines, especially IL-6 and TNF-α and expression of inducible nitric oxide synthase (iNOS).[91] Elevated IL-6 and TNF-α concentrations activates the NF κB signaling pathway that modulates immune and inflammatory SM responses, thereby exacerbating SM wasting.[92] Increased SM IL-6 concentration has been associated with SM and diaphragmatic atrophy in rats and the Janus activated kinase (JAK)-I, activator of transcription (STAT) and cAMP-activated protein kinase (AMPK) signaling pathways.[93] Increased Akt activation increases activity of (FoxO) transcription factors, which control SM cell proliferation growth atrophy and metabolism.[72] As previously mentioned, increased FoxO activity precipitates SM protein degradation through the ubiquitin-proteasome pathway in rats with HF. SM inflammation exacerbates SM atrophy through stimulation of multiple cytokine-activated signaling pathways.

In summary, chronic conditions and particularly chronic HF are associated with reduced physical activity, resulting in disuse and low-level systemic inflammation (Figure 19-3). Both disuse and systemic inflammation promote loss of SM mass and ultimately SM atrophy. Continuous loss of SM mass activates multiple signaling pathways that mediate SM inflammation. In turn SM inflammation activates signaling pathways that promote further loss of SM mass and exacerbates local inflammation. The negative interaction between atrophy and inflammation within the SM appears to progress independently from the initial event and may be related to the presence of comorbid conditions, including hormonal deficiencies, diabetes mellitus, and obesity/sleep disorder breathing. An important goal of therapy in HF patients is to reverse or optimally prevent the development of SM alterations to restore a normal functional capacity.

Diaphragm and Respiratory Muscle in Heart Failure

Skeletal muscles are not simply a mechanical system, but sensory organs that sense effort, tension, displacement, and fatigue via tendon organs, muscle spindles, joint receptors,

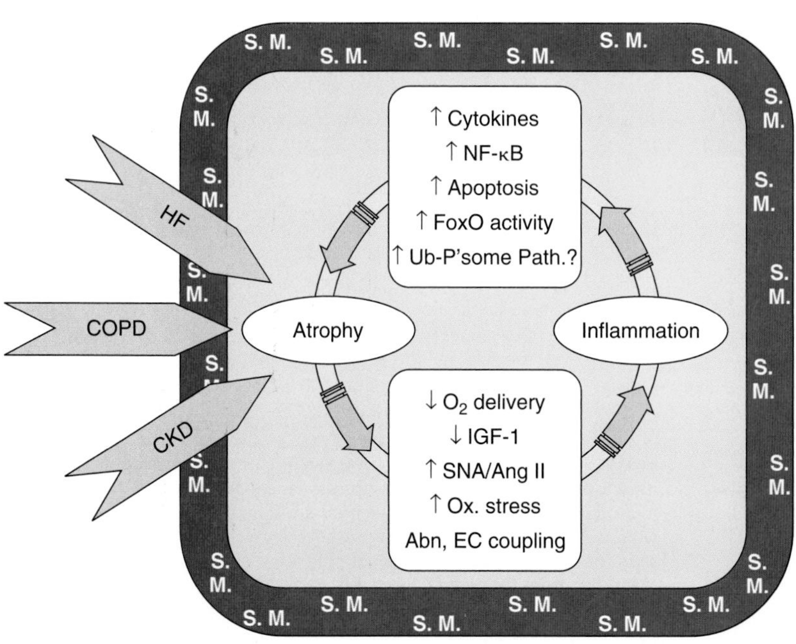

FIGURE 19–3 Chronic conditions such as heart failure (HF), chronic obstructive pulmonary disease (COPD), and chronic kidney disease (CKD) have a substantial impact on skeletal muscles (SM). Patients with HF, COPD, or CKD experience SM wasting and ultimately atrophy. Besides abnormal excitation contraction (EC) coupling, atrophy is associated with increased sympathetic nervous activation (SNA), angiotensin II (Ang II), and oxidative (Ox) stress, reduced O_2 delivery, and IGF-1 concentration that mediate SM inflammation. In turn, SM inflammation is associated with increased cytokine levels, nuclear factor κB (NF κB) signaling, rate of apoptosis, and FoxO transcription factors. Whether the ubiquitin-proteasome pathway (Ub-P'some Path) is activated in patients with HF is unclear. Inflammation-related SM alterations foster SM atrophy and thereby a negative atrophy-inflammation interaction with SM. Whereas chronic conditions are initially responsible for SM atrophy, its progression appears to be largely dependent on local SM factors, including a negative atrophy-inflammation interaction and to a lesser extent on the deterioration of the initiating chronic condition.

and small nerve endings. It is the sensory aspect of skeletal muscles that mediates the symptoms of exercise intolerance in both healthy and disease states.[7,94,95] The first portion of this chapter focused on the limb skeletal muscle and we will now shift our attention to the respiratory muscles. Both groups of muscles are exposed to the same generalized heightened neurohormonal activation, cytokine release, and oxidative stress that is associated with the heart failure state, but unlike the limb musculature, which is underused with disease progression, the diaphragm and respiratory muscles encounter an ever-increasing workload as lung compliance decreases. Table 19-1 contrasts the skeletal muscle characteristics of the locomotor and respiratory muscles in heart failure.

Mechanism of Dyspnea

A unified mechanism for dyspnea based on respiratory muscle function is that breathlessness occurs when the activity of the respiratory muscles is increased and/or the respiratory muscles are weak.[7,94] Varying respiratory muscle strength and workload will result in differences in perception of load and dyspnea.[96-99] Dyspnea is a conscious sensation that results from an unusual perception of discomfort during breathing.[4-7] As it is a sensation, it has a significant affective component that can be modified by cognitive and contextual influences. Dyspnea occurs in both normal and diseased states, and originates from the stimulation of mechanoreceptors, chemoreceptors, or proprioreceptors. The magnitude of a stimulus to the receptor is transduced by the firing frequency in an afferent nerve to the central nervous system. The central impression constructed is interpreted based on past experience to generate a conscious sensation.[7]

Respiratory muscle fatigue may also contribute to dyspnea via biochemical changes in the muscles.[100,101] Dempsey et al have shown that fatiguing contractions of the inspiratory muscles result in an accumulation of metabolites that activate type IV phrenic afferents, resulting in an increase in sympathetic vasoconstrictor activity via a supraspinal reflex (i.e., inspiratory muscle metaboreflex).[100] This reflex is important during heavy sustained exercise and modulates the competition for blood flow between the respiratory and locomotor muscles. Activation of this reflex redirects blood flow from the periphery to the ventilatory muscles.

Additionally, increased respiratory drive during exercise may be due to metabolic stimuli arising from limb skeletal muscle.[102,103] Previous studies have demonstrated how changes in metabolism in skeletal muscle stimulate respiration. Oelberg et al[104] used magnetic resonance spectroscopy to demonstrate that skeletal muscle pH correlates with minute ventilation (Figure 19-4). It is not clear whether such stimulation occurs through central or peripheral pathways.[105]

TABLE 19–1 Comparison of Locomotor and Respiratory Muscles

	Locomotor Muscles	Respiratory Muscles
Reduced fiber CSA	Yes	Yes
Fiber type	Type IIb >> Type I	Type I >>> Type II
Oxidative enzyme activity	Decreased	Increased
Glycolytic enzyme activity	Increased	Decreased
Oxidative stress	Increased	Increased
Workload	Decreased	Increased
Atrophy	Yes	Yes
Mitochondrial changes	Decreased	Increased
Contractility	Decreased	Decreased

Diaphragmatic Histochemical Changes in Heart Failure

Histochemical and metabolic changes that occur in respiratory muscles may serve to accentuate the sensation of dyspnea in heart failure patients. A diaphragmatic myopathy has been demonstrated in an animal model of chronic heart failure[106] with decreased contractile and relaxation parameters.[107] Impaired diaphragmatic performance was correlated to a total cross-bridge number and altered calcium regulation.[108] Elevated tumor necrosis factor has been suggested to explain the diaphragmatic dysfunction.[109] Malnutrition has been shown to affect diaphragmatic weight and histochemistry.[110,111]

Various histologic abnormalities in the diaphragm of patients undergoing cardiac transplantation have been described.[111-113] In one study, costal diaphragmatic biopsies were obtained from 7 normal subjects and 10 patients at the time of transplant or LV assist placement.[112] The distribution of myosin heavy chain isoforms I, IIa, and IIb (MHC) by SDS gel electrophoresis was measured along with the activities of the oxidative (citrate synthase), lipolytic (β-hydroxyacyl CoA dehydrogenase), and glycolytic (lactate dehydrogenase) enzymes. In normal subjects, the distribution of MHC isoforms I, IIa, and IIb was 35%, 49%, and 17%, respectively, versus 54%, 40%, and 6% in the HF subjects. Therefore, in the patients with HF, slow myosin heavy chains were significantly increased ($P < .01$) and glycolytic fast-twitch fibers significantly reduced compared with normal subjects ($P < .01$). Additionally, oxidative and lipolytic enzymatic activities were greater and glycolytic enzyme activity was significantly less in HF than normal subjects (Figure 19-5) (all $P < .01$). Thus in the diaphragm in HF, there is a shift from fast to slow myosin isoforms with an increase in oxidative capacity and a decrease in glycolytic capacity. These changes are consistent with those elicited by endurance training. The endurance changes described in the diaphragm probably were the consequence of the increased work of breathing that occurs in this patient population. These findings were subsequently found in animal models.[106,107]

However, despite the shift to more oxidative metabolism, evidence of decreased contractility and strength was

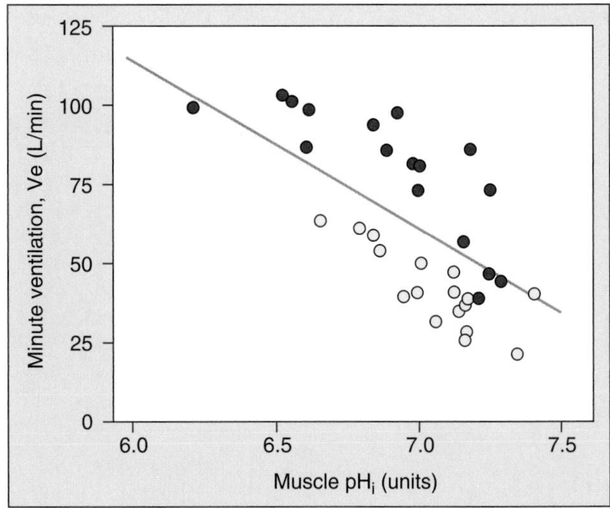

FIGURE 19–4 The correlation between minute ventilation and quadriceps muscle pH (determined by magnetic resonance spectroscopy) during exercise in patients with heart failure. The data are from three exercise bouts in one subject. Bilateral lower extremity positive pressure of 45 Torr was used to separate out the effects of arterial pH, pain, or central motor command. (Modified from Oelberg D, Evans AB, Hrovat MI, et al. Skeletal muscle chemoreflex and pHi in exercise ventilatory control. *J Appl Physiol* 1998;84:676-682 with permission.)

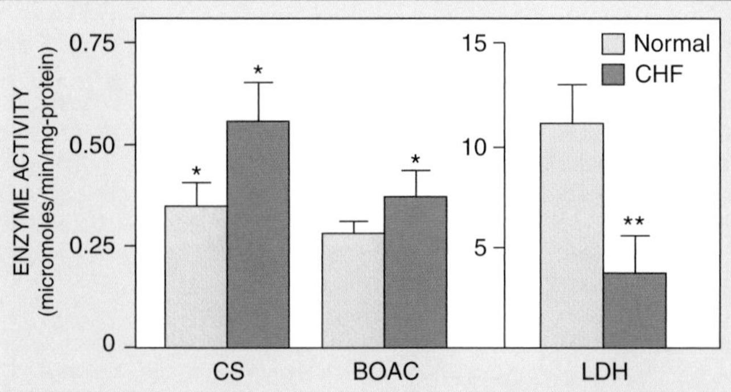

FIGURE 19–5 Abnormal costal muscle enzyme activity in patients with heart failure. Costal diaphragmatic biopsy samples were obtained from 7 normal subjects and 10 patients. Activity of citrate synthase (CS, a marker of oxidative metabolism) and B-hydroxyacyl-CoA dehydrogenase (BOAC, a marker of lipolytic enzymatic activity) were greater and glycolytic enzyme activity as assessed by the activity of lactate dehydrogenase (LDH) was significantly less in heart failure than normal subjects. (Modified from Tikunov B, Levine B, Mancini DM. Chronic congestive heart failure elicits adaptations of endurance exercise in diaphragmatic muscle. *Circulation* 1997;95:910-916 with permission.)

described in animal models. A rat HF model demonstrated similar histochemical changes as described in HF patients.[114] However, the mitochondrial function of the rat costal diaphragmatic muscle was reduced as measured in skinned muscle fibers using an oxygen electrode. ADP sensitivity of the mitochondria was increased but returned to normal in the presence of creatine. Decreased concentration of the mitochondrial isoform of creatine kinase has been previously demonstrated. Thus though the diaphragmatic muscle had an appropriate training response to the heightened work of breathing, the performance of the muscle was still attenuated due to the altered mitochondrial function.[115]

Myogenic regulatory factors regulate the expression of myosin heavy chains. In a rat model of heart failure, the expression of Myo D, myogenin, and MRF4 was examined in the diaphragm of heart failure and control rats. Myogenin is expressed at higher concentrations in slow-twitch muscle, whereas Myo D expression is increased in fast-twitch fibers. In the heart failure rats there was a selective downregulation of Myo D, leading to a lower percentage of fast-twitch fibers. The trigger for the downregulation of the Myo D is unknown but thought to be due to neurohormonal and cytokine activation.[116]

Respiratory Muscle Function

Respiratory muscle function is commonly quantitated by measurement of respiratory muscle strength.[117] Maximal inspiratory pressure is measured with the subject inhaling against at a resistance at functional residual volume to maximize the force–length relationship of the muscles. This measurement is volitional and as such may overestimate the degree of muscle weakness but this measurement has been shown to be reproducible. Inspiratory muscle weakness is arbitrarily defined as a maximum inspiratory pressure (PImax) less than 70% of predicted value. A reduction in inspiratory and expiratory respiratory muscle strength in patients with HF from both systolic and diastolic dysfunction has been shown in many studies.[118-121] Studies measuring diaphragmatic strength using esophageal and transdiaphragmatic pressure during maximal sniffs and phrenic nerve stimulation have also demonstrated reduction in diaphragmatic strength in HF patients.

When both respiratory muscle and limb muscle strength are measured in HF patients, a more marked reduction in respiratory rather than peripheral muscle strength has been observed. Chua et al failed to find a correlation between PImax and quadriceps strength.[122] Ambrosino[121] reported reductions in maximal inspiratory and expiratory pressures that paralleled the severity of heart failure. HF patients with relatively preserved exercise capacity had reduced PImax.

PImax has been shown to have prognostic value independent of peak $\dot{V}O_2$. Meyer et al[123] measured PImax in 244 consecutive HF patients and found this measurement to be a strong univariate and multivariate predictor of survival. Improvement in PImax has been found in patients with heart failure following initiation of angiotensin-converting enzyme inhibitor therapy, CPAP, and respiratory muscle training. However, serial changes in inspiratory strength were not predictive of prognosis.[124]

Respiratory Muscle Perfusion

Limb skeletal muscle underperfusion has been described in patients with heart failure.[125] Animal and human studies suggest that with HF, respiratory muscle underperfusion may also occur. The diaphragm, the major respiratory muscle, has a complex and generous blood supply provided by the internal mammary, intercostal, and phrenic arteries and the costophrenic arcades. Because of its rich perfusion, the diaphragm is relatively resistant to ischemia, even during exercise, when large increases in perfusion of the diaphragm are needed. Examination of regional muscle perfusion in the dog during exercise has demonstrated that the muscle group with the largest increase in perfusion is the diaphragm.[126] In animal models of HF, the increase in diaphragmatic blood flow during submaximal exercise[127] was greatest in those animals with the most severe HF. Presumably the increased blood flow was required for increased work of breathing. During exercise, dramatic increases in blood flow occur in the diaphragm. This response is accentuated in HF.

Diaphragmatic ischemia and fatigue have been demonstrated in a canine model of cardiogenic shock produced by tamponade.[128] In spontaneously breathing dogs with tamponade, respiratory muscle failure preceded cardiac arrest. Preterminal increased neural excitation to the respiratory muscles was observed, implying an impairment of the contractile process. Diaphragmatic blood lactate was increased. Thus in this canine model of HF, respiratory muscle fatigue was probably due to respiratory muscle underperfusion.

Near-infrared spectroscopy is a technique that can be used to noninvasively assess skeletal muscle oxygenation.[129] This technique primarily relies on the optical properties of hemoglobin. Both oxygenated and deoxygenated forms absorb light at 800 nm, whereas at 760 nm absorption is primarily by the deoxygenated forms. By monitoring the difference between these two wavelengths, venous hemoglobin deoxygenation can be assessed.[130] Application of near-infrared spectroscopy during maximal exercise has demonstrated accessory respiratory muscle deoxygenation in HF but not normal subjects.[131]

Whether this respiratory muscle deoxygenation represents underperfusion, ischemia, and/or fatigue was investigated by measuring the development of low-frequency muscle fatigue following exercise in HF patients. Davies et al[132] demonstrated a decrease in maximum inspiratory and expiratory pressure following bicycle exercise in HF patients. This suggested respiratory muscle fatigue. However, measurements of maximal inspiratory and expiratory pressures are motivation dependent, and the observed reduction may have occurred from central mechanisms. To investigate objectively whether low-frequency diaphragmatic fatigue occurs in HF patients, supramaximal bilateral transcutaneous phrenic nerve stimulation before and after maximal bicycle exercise was performed.[133] Maximal transdiaphragmatic pressure was derived before and after exercise using the twitch interpolation technique. In both normal and HF subjects, maximal inspiratory and expiratory pressures decreased significantly with peak exercise. However, the maximal transdiaphragmatic pressure derived from the twitch interpolation technique

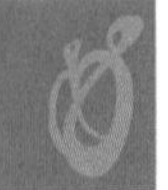

was unchanged in both normal and HF subjects. Thus low-frequency diaphragmatic muscle fatigue did not occur in patients with heart failure despite accessory respiratory muscle deoxygenation during exercise.

Increased activity of the respiratory muscles and/or respiratory muscle weakness rather than fatigue may be sufficient to evoke the sensation of dyspnea. Measurement of the tension-time index and thus the work of the diaphragm per breath demonstrated dramatic increases in patients with heart failure at rest and during exercise (Figure 19-6).[133] The tension-time index is calculated for each breath. It is the product of the ratio of the time in inspiration divided by the time per breath (Ti/Ttot), and the ratio of the mean transdiaphragmatic pressure to maximal transdiaphragmatic pressure. It approximates the oxygen consumption of the diaphragm. Fatigue of the diaphragm is thought to occur when the tension-time index reaches a ratio of 0.15 or greater.[134] However, this fatiguing ratio may be lower in ischemic muscle, or with high tidal volumes, breathing frequency and minute ventilation. In the majority of the patients studied, the tension time index at end exercise was 0.1 and thus approached fatiguing levels.

The relationship between parameters of respiratory muscle function and ratings of perceived dyspnea during submaximal exercise was also examined.[133] Significant linear correlations were observed between a rating of perceived dyspnea (i.e., the Borg scale) at a fixed exercise workload (25 watts) and parameters of respiratory muscle strength (maximal inspiratory and expiratory pressures), and work (tension-time index), but not with lung volumes (tidal volume, minute ventilation). McParland also demonstrated a strong correlation between inspiratory muscle weakness and dyspnea during daily activities in stable ambulatory HF patients, as quantitated by the Dyspnea Index.[118]

The endurance of the respiratory muscles in HF patients is also diminished. Respiratory muscle endurance can be assessed by progressive isocapnic hyperpnea using a rebreathing circuit to measure maximal sustainable ventilatory capacity.[135] Both maximal voluntary ventilation and maximal sustainable ventilatory capacity are significantly reduced in HF patients compared with normal subjects consistent with lowered respiratory muscle endurance.

Respiratory Muscle Training

Modification of respiratory muscle function with an appropriate shift in perceived dyspnea could demonstrate the importance of respiratory muscle function in the development of dyspnea. If respiratory muscles were a key modulator of the sensation of dyspnea, then selective respiratory muscle training should attenuate exertional dyspnea and may also improve exercise performance particularly in patients limited by dyspnea. Accordingly, the effect of selective respiratory muscle training on exertional dyspnea and exercise capacity has been examined in heart failure subjects. In our original series, we examined the effect of respiratory muscle training in 14 HF patients.[136] Supervised respiratory muscle training was performed for 3 months. Maximal sustainable ventilatory capacity, maximal mouth pressures, pulmonary function tests, and submaximal and maximal exercise capacity were measured before and after training.

As with aerobic training there are many different training regimens that can be employed involving either endurance or isometric type of exercise. The training protocol we devised included a variety of elements including isocapnic hyperpnea at a predetermined maximal sustainable ventilatory level, strength training with repetitive maximal inspiratory and expiratory mouth pressures, pulmonary rehabilitation exercises, and resistive breathing using a commercial available device (THRESHOLD Health Scan, Cedar Grove, NJ). Thus the impact of both strength and endurance training of

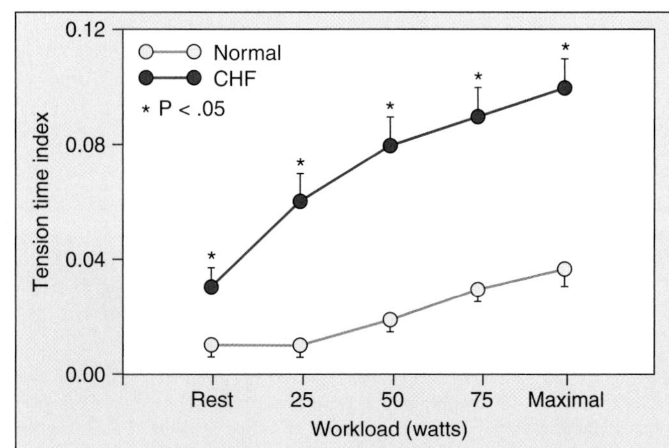

FIGURE 19-6 Plot of tension-time index at rest and at submaximal and maximal exercise in normal subjects and heart failure (CHF) patients. The tension-time index is a measure of the work of the diaphragm per breath. (Modified from Mancini DM, Henson D, LaManca J, et al. Respiratory muscle function and dyspnea in patients with chronic congestive heart failure. *Circulation* 1992;86:909-918.)

the respiratory muscles in HF patients was investigated. Of the 14 patients enrolled in the study, only 8 completed the training protocol. The six dropouts were followed and comprised a comparison group by which to assess the reproducibility of the measurements. Respiratory muscle endurance was significantly improved with training as evidenced by increases in maximal sustainable ventilatory capacity of 57%. Respiratory muscle strength, and submaximal and maximal exercise capacity were also significantly improved with selective respiratory muscle training. Dyspnea was subjectively improved in the majority of trained patients. In contrast, no significant improvements in maximal sustainable ventilatory capacity, maximal mouth pressures, 6-minute walk, or peak $\dot{V}O_2$ were observed in the six patients who did not complete the training program.

Since our initial study several other investigators[137-142] (Table 19-2) have studied respiratory muscle training in these patients using predominantly resistive pressure threshold load devices or computer-controlled biofeedback trainers. Training has been performed at a wide range of inspiratory pressure loads ranging from 15 to 60% of PImax. Though the training regimens have varied the overall results have been consistent with demonstration of improvement in respiratory muscle strength, peak $\dot{V}O_2$, and 6-minute walk tests. The consistency of the improvement in overall peak $\dot{V}O_2$ has led to studies to identify the mechanism for the enhanced exercise capacity.

Chiappa et al hypothesized that the improvement in peak $\dot{V}O_2$ may result from a redistribution of blood from the lungs to the locomotor muscles.[143] Inspiratory muscle loading results in a reduction of blood flow to resting and exercising muscle, which following respiratory muscle training is alleviated in patients with HF and respiratory muscle weakness. Borghi Silva et al[144] also have demonstrated that unloaded ventilation improves submaximal exercise and skeletal muscle perfusion in nine patients with HF.

Conversely, if skeletal muscle metaboreceptors modulate the sensation of dyspnea, then selectively improving leg muscles may similarly alleviate dyspnea. As aerobic training results in training of both the leg and respiratory muscles, selective low-level leg training was performed in 17 HF patients. Low-level bicycle and treadmill exercise, where minute ventilation was below 25 L/min, was performed along with leg callisthenic exercises. Perceived dyspnea during submaximal exercise was reduced in patients with low-level training, suggesting that skeletal muscle function impacts this sensation.[145]

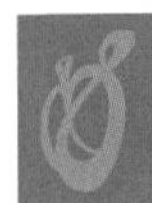

TABLE 19–2 Clinical Trials of Respiratory Muscle Training in Heart Failure

	n	NYHA	LVEF (%)	Training Protocol	Outcome
Mancini[136]	14	I-IV	22 ± 9	Isocapnic hyperpnea Resistive Breathing @ 30% PImax Strength Training	Increase PImax Increase MVV Increase 6 min walk Increase $\dot{V}O_2$
Weiner[138]	20	II-III	<30	Resistive Breathing 15-60% PImax	Increase PImax Increase resp muscle endurance Increase 12 min walk test No change peak $\dot{V}O_2$
Laoutaris[139]	37	II-III	24 ± 1	60% PImax	Increase PImax Increase $\dot{V}O_2$ Increase 6 min walk
Dall'ago[137]	32		<45	30% PImax	Increase PImax Increase $\dot{V}O_2$ Increase 6 min walk
Laoutaris[141]	38	II-III	28 ± 1	60% PImax vs 15% PImax (control)	Increase PImax Increase Peak $\dot{V}O_2$ Increase 6 min walk
Laoutaris[142]	23	II-III	29 ± 1	60% PImax 15% PImax	Increase PImax Increase Peak $\dot{V}O_2$ Increase 6 min walk

CONCLUSION

Dyspnea is an extremely common symptom in patients with heart failure. In these patients, the increased work of breathing results from a combination of factors, including excessive ventilatory response during exercise, from increased dead space ventilation, and from ventilation perfusion mismatching; an increased impedance to breathing from bronchial hyperreactivity due to venous engorgement; and decreased lung compliance from elevated filling pressures and subsequent chronic fibrotic changes. This increased work of breathing is transduced into the sensation of dyspnea by stimulation of receptors in weak, atrophic, underperfused, and probably metabolically abnormal respiratory muscles. Additionally the atrophic and metabolically abnormal limb skeletal muscles may also exacerbate this sensation through an excessive muscle reflex activity.

In conclusion, the symptoms of fatigue and dyspnea both largely originate in skeletal muscle. The size, histology, metabolism, and vasculature of the skeletal muscle are all impacted by the neurohormonal, cytokine, and inflammatory activation that characterize heart failure and results in the classic symptoms of this disease.

REFERENCES

1. Lunde, P. K., Sjaastad, I., Schiotz Thorud, H. M., et al. (2001). Skeletal muscle disorders in heart failure. *Acta Physiol Scand*, *171*, 277–294.
2. Clark, A. L., Poole-Wilson, A., & Coats, A. J. S. (1996). Exercise limitation in chronic heart failure: central of the periphery. *J Am Coll Cardiol*, *28*, 1092–1102.
3. Gosker, H. R., Wouters, E. F. M., van der Vusse, G. J., et al. (2000). Skeletal muscle dysfunction in chronic obstructive pulmonary disease and chronic heart failure: underlying mechanisms and therapy perspectives. *Am J Clin Nutr*, *71*, 1033–1047.
4. Duscha, B. D., Schulze, C., Robbins, J. L., et al. (2008). Implications of chronic heart failure on peripheral vasculature and skeletal muscle before and after exercise training. *Heart Fail Rev*, *13*, 21–37.
5. Fishman, A., & Ledlie, J. (1979) *Dyspnea. Bull Eur Physiopathol Respir*, *15*, 789.
6. Wasserman, K., & Casaburi, R. (1988). Dyspnea. Physiological and pathological mechanisms. *Annu Rev Med*, *39*, 503–515.
7. Killian, K., & Jones, N. (1988). Respiratory muscle and dyspnea. *Clin Chest Med*, *9*, 237–248.
8. Joyner, M. J. (2004). Congestive heart failure. more bad news from exercising muscle? *Circulation*, *110*, 2978–2979.
9. Mann, D. L., & Reid, M. B. (2003). Exercise training and skeletal muscle inflammation in chronic heart failure: feeling better about fatigue. *J Am Coll Cardiol*, *42*, 869–872.
10. Mancini, D. M., Walter, G., Reichek, N., et al. (1992). Contribution of skeletal muscle atrophy to exercise intolerance and altered muscle metabolism in heart failure. *Circulation*, *85*, 1364–1373.
11. Le Jemtel, T. H., Maskin, C. S., Lucido, D., et al. (1986). Failure to augment maximal limb blood flow in response to one-leg versus two-leg exercise in patients with severe heart failure. *Circulation*, *74*, 245–251.
12. Sullivan, M. J., Green, H. J., & Cobb, F. R. (1990). Skeletal muscle biochemistry in ambulatory patients with long-term heart failure. *Circulation*, *81*, 518–527.
13. Minotti, J. R., Christoph, I., Oka, M., et al. (1991). Impaired skeletal muscle function in patients with congestive heart failure: relationship to systemic exercise performance. *J Clin Invest*, *88*, 2077–2082.
14. Drexler, H., Riede, U., Munzel, T., et al. (1992). Alterations of skeletal muscle in chronic heart failure. *Circulation*, *85*, 1751–1759.
15. Troosters, T., Gosselink, R., & Decramer, M. (2004). Chronic obstructive pulmonary disease and chronic heart failure. Two muscle diseases? *J Cardiopulm Rehabil*, *24*, 137–145.
16. O'Connor, C. M., Whellan, D. J., Lee, K. L., et al. (2009). Efficacy and safety of exercise training in patients with chronic heart failure. HF-action randomized controlled trial. *JAMA*, *301*, 1439–1450.
17. Testa, M., Yeh, M., Lee, P., et al. (1996). Circulating levels of cytokines and their endogenous modulators in patients with mild to severe congestive heart failure due to coronary artery disease and hypertension. *J Am Coll Cardiol*, *28*, 964–971.
18. Mann, D. L. (2002). Inflammatory mediators and the failing heart: past, present, and the foreseeable future. *Circ Res*, *91*, 988–998.
19. Sinoway, L. I., & Jianhua, L. (2005). A perspective on the muscle reflex: implications for congestive heart failure. *J Appl Physiol*, *99*, 5–22.
20. Golberg, L. R., & Jessup, M. (2006). Stage B heart failure management of asymptomatic left ventricular systolic dysfunction. *Circulation*, *113*, 2851–2860.
21. Mancini, D., Goldsmith, R., Levin, H., et al. (1998). Comparison of exercise performance in patients with chronic severe heart failure versus left ventricular assist devices. *Circulation*, *98*, 1178–1183.
22. Gonzalez-Alonso, J., & Colbert, J. A. L. (2003). Reductions in systemic and skeletal muscle blood flow and oxygen delivery limit maximal aerobic capacity in humans. *Circulation*, *107*, 824–830.
23. Wilson, J. R., Martin, J. L., & Ferraro, N. (1984). Impaired skeletal muscle nutritive flow during exercise in patients with congestive heart failure: role of cardiac pump dysfunction as determined by the effect of dobutamine. *Am J Cardiol*, *53*, 1308–1315.
24. Arnold, J. M. O., Ribeiro, J. P., & Colucci, W. S. (1990). Muscle blood flow during forearm exercise in patients with severe heart failure. *Circulation*, *82*, 465–472.
25. Isnard, R., Lechat, P., Kalotka, H., et al. (1996). Muscular blood flow response to submaximal leg exercise in normal subjects and in patients with heart failure. *J Appl Physiol*, *81*, 2571–2579.
26. Duscha, B. D., Kraus, W. E., Keteyian, S. J., et al. (1999). Capillary density of skeletal muscle. *J Am Coll Cardiol*, *33*, 1956–1963.
27. Lipkin, D. P., Jones, D. A., Round, J. M., et al. (1988). Abnormalities of skeletal muscle in patients with chronic heart failure. *Int J Cardiol*, *18*, 187–195.
28. Longhurst, J., Capone, R. J., & Zelis, R. (1975). Evaluation of skeletal muscle capillary basement membrane thickness in congestive heart failure. *Chest*, *67*, 195–198.
29. Mahy, I. R., & Tooke, J. E. (1995). Peripheral microvascular function in human heart failure. *Clin Sci*, *88*, 501–508.
30. Katz, S. D., Maskin, C., Jondeau, G., et al. (2000). Near-maximal fractional oxygen extraction by active skeletal muscle in patients with chronic heart failure. *J Appl Physiol*, *88*, 2138–2142.
31. Ventura-Clapier, R. (2009). Exercise training, energy metabolism, and heart failure. *Appl Physiol Nutr Metab*, *34*, 336–339.
32. Teerlink, J. R., Clozel, M., Fischli, W., et al. (1993). Temporal evolution of endothelial dysfunction in a rat model of chronic heart failure. *J Am Coll Cardiol*, *22*, 615–620.
33. Kaiser, L., Spickard, R. C., & Olivier, N. B. (1989). Heart failure depresses endothelium-dependent responses in canine femoral artery. *Am J Physiol*, *256*, H962–H967.
34. Katz, S. D., Biasucci, L., Sabba, C., et al. (1992). Impaired endothelium-mediated vasodilation in the peripheral vasculature of patients with congestive heart failure. *J Am Coll Cardiol*, *19*, 918–925.

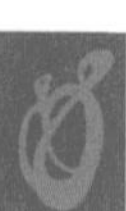

35. Kubo, S. H., Rector, T. S., Bank, A. J., et al. (1991). Endothelium-dependent vasodilation is attenuated in patients with heart failure. *Circulation, 84,* 1589–1596.
36. Drexler, H., Hayoz, D., Munzel, T., et al. (1992). Endothelial function in chronic heart failure. *Am J Cardiol, 69,* 1596–1601.
37. Kubo, S. H., Rector, T. S., & Bank, A. J. (1994). Lack of contribution of nitric oxide to basal vasomotor tone in heart failure. *Am J Cardiol, 74,* 1133–1136.
38. Hambrecht, R., Fiehn, E., Weigl, C., et al. (1998). Regular physical exercise corrects endothelial dysfunction and improves exercise capacity in patients with chronic heart disease. *Circulation, 98,* 2709–2715.
39. Bauersachs, J., Bouloumie, A., Fraccarrollo, D., et al. (1999). Endothelial dysfunction in chronic myocardial infarction despite increased vascular endothelial nitric oxide synthase and soluble guanylate cyclase expression: role of enhanced vascular superoxide production. *Circulation, 100,* 292–298.
40. Thomas, G. D., Zhang, W., & Victor, R. G. (2001). Impaired modulation of sympathetic vasoconstriction in contracting skeletal muscle of rats with chronic myocardial infarctions: role of oxidative stress. *Circ Res, 88,* 816–823.
41. Hornig, B., Maier, V., & Drexler, H. (1996). Physical training improves endothelial function in patients with chronic heart failure. *Circulation, 93,* 210–214.
42. Ennezat, P. V., Van Belle, E., Asseman, P., et al. (2007). Steady nitric oxide synthase expression in heart failure. *Acta Cardiol, 62,* 265–268.
43. Lang, C. C., Chomsky, D. B., Rayos, G., et al. (1997). Skeletal muscle mass and exercise performance in stable ambulatory patients with heart failure. *J Appl Physiol, 82,* 257–261.
44. Lunde, P. K., Dahlstedt, A. J., Bruton, J. D., et al. (2001). Contraction and intracellular Ca^{2+} handling in isolated skeletal muscle of rats with congestive heart failure. *Circ Res, 88,* 1299–1305.
45. Szentesi, P., Bekedam, M. A., van Beek-Harmsen, B. J., et al. (2005). Depression of force production and ATPase activity in different types of human skeletal muscle fibers from patients with chronic heart failure. *J Appl Physiol, 99,* 2189–2195.
46. Okada, Y., Toth, M. J., & Vanburen, P. (2008). Skeletal muscle contractile protein function is preserved in human heart failure. *J Appl Physiol, 104,* 952–957.
47. Simonini, A., Long, C. S., Dudley, G. A., et al. (1996). Heart failure in rats causes changes in skeletal muscle morphology and gene expression that are not explained by reduced activity. *Circ Res, 79,* 128–136.
48. Le Jemtel, T. H., Padeletti, M., & Jelic, S. (2007). Diagnostic and therapeutic challenges in patients with coexistent chronic obstructive pulmonary disease and chronic heart failure. *J Am Coll Cardiol, 49,* 171–180.
49. Jondeau, G., Katz, S. D., Toussaint, J. F., et al. (1993). Regional specificity of peak hyperemic response in patients with congestive heart failure: correlation with peak aerobic capacity. *J Am Coll Cardiol, 22,* 1399–1402.
50. Linke, A., Adams, V., Schulze, P. C., et al. (2005). Antioxidative effects of exercise training in patients with chronic heart failure. Increase in radical scavenger enzyme activity in skeletal muscle. *Circulation, 111,* 1763–1770.
51. Wisloff, U., Stoylen, A., & Loennechen, J. P. (2007). Superior cardiovascular effect of aerobic interval training versus moderate continuous training in heart failure patients. A randomized study. *Circulation, 115,* 3086–3094.
52. Schiaffino, S., & Reggiani, C. (1996). Molecular diversity of myofibrillar proteins: gene regulation and functional significance. *Physiol Rev, 76,* 371–423.
53. Armstrong, R. B. (1988). Muscle fiber recruitment patterns and their metabolic correlates. In H. S. Horton & R. L. Terjung (Eds.), *Exercise, nutrition, and energy metabolism.* New York: Macmillan.
54. Schaufelberger, M., Eriksson, B. O., Grimby, G., et al. (1995). Skeletal muscle fiber composition and capillarization in patients with chronic heart failure: relation to exercise capacity and central hemodynamics. *J Card Fail, 1,* 267–272.
55. Mettauer, B., Zoll, J., Sanchez, H., et al. (2001). Oxidative capacity of skeletal muscle in heart failure patients versus sedentary or active control subjects. *J Am Coll Cardiol, 38,* 947–954.
56. Opasich, C., Aquilani, R., Dossena, M., et al. (1996). Biochemical analysis of muscle biopsy in overnight fasting patients with severe heart failure. *Eur Heart J, 17,* 1686–1693.
57. Sabbah, H. N., Shimoyama, H., Sharov, V. G., et al. (1996). Effects of ACE inhibition and β-blockade on skeletal muscle fiber types in dogs with moderate heart failure. *Am J Physiol, 270,* H115–H120.
58. Schieffer, B., Wollert, K. C., Berchtold, M., et al. (1995). Development and prevention of skeletal muscle structural alterations after experimental myocardial infarction. *Am J Physiol, 269,* H1507–H1513.
59. Vescovo, G., Dalla Libera, L., Serafini, F., et al. (1998). Improved exercise tolerance after losartan and enalapril in heart failure. *Circulation, 98,* 1742–1749.
60. Massie, B. M., Conway, M., Yonge, R., et al. (1987). Skeletal muscle metabolism in patients with congestive heart failure: relation to clinical severity and blood flow. *Circulation, 76,* 1009–1119.
61. Weiner, D. H., Fink, L. I., Maris, J., et al. (1986). Abnormal skeletal muscle bioenergetics during exercise in patients with heart failure: role of reduced muscle blood flow. *Circulation, 73,* 1127–1136.
62. Chati, Z., Zannad, F., Jeandel, C., et al. (1996). Physical deconditioning may be a mechanism for the skeletal muscle energy phosphate metabolism abnormalities in chronic heart failure. *Am Heart J, 131,* 560–566.
63. Massie, B. M., Conway, M., Rajagopalan, B., et al. (1988). Skeletal muscle metabolism during exercise under ischemic conditions in congestive heart failure: evidence for abnormalities unrelated to blood flow. *Circulation, 78,* 320–326.
64. Mancini, D. M., Coyle, E., Coggan, A., et al. (1989). Contribution of intrinsic skeletal muscle changes to 31P-NMR skeletal muscle metabolic abnormalities in patients with chronic heart failure. *Circulation, 80,* 1338–1346.
65. Chati, Z., Zannad, F., Robin-Lherbier, B., et al. (1994). Contribution of specific skeletal muscle metabolic abnormalities to limitation of exercise capacity in patients with chronic heart failure: a phosphorus 31 nuclear magnetic resonance study. *Am Heart J, 128,* 781–792.
66. Adamopoulos, S., Coats, A. J. S., Brunotte, F., et al. (1993). Physical training improves skeletal muscle metabolism in patients with chronic heart failure. *J Am Coll Cardiol, 21,* 1101–1106.
67. Okita, K., Yonezawa, K., & Nishijima, H. (1998). Skeletal muscle metabolism limits exercise capacity in patients with chronic heart failure. *Circulation, 98,* 1886–1891.
68. Bellinger, A. M., Mongillo, M., & Marks, A. R. (2008). Stressed out: the skeletal muscle ryanodine receptor as a target of stress. *J Clin Invest, 118,* 445–453.
69. Peters, D. G., Mitchell, H. L., McCune, S. A., et al. (1997). Skeletal muscle sarcoplasmic reticulum Ca^{2+}-ATPase gene expression in congestive heart failure. *Circ Res, 81,* 703–710.
70. Caron, M. A., Debigare, R., Dekhuijzen, P., et al. (2009). The respiratory muscles in chronic obstructive pulmonary disease: comparative assessment of the quadriceps and the diaphragm in patients with COPD. *J Appl Physiol, 107,* 952–961.
71. Schulze, P. C., Fang, J., Kassik, K. A., et al. (2005). Transgenic overexpression of locally acting insulin-like growth factor-1 inhibits ubiquitin-mediated muscle atrophy in chronic left-ventricular dysfunction. *Circ Res, 97,* 418–426.
72. Song, H. Y., Li, Y., Du, J., et al. (2005). Muscle-specific expression of IGF-1 blocks angiotensin II-induced skeletal muscle wasting. *J Clin Invest, 115,* 451–458.
73. Du, J., Wang, X., Miereles, C., et al. (2004). Activation of caspase-3 is an initial step triggering accelerated muscle proteolysis in catabolic conditions. *J Clin Invest, 113,* 115–123.
74. Pedersen, B. K., & Febbraio, M. A. (2006). Muscle as an endocrine organ: focus on muscle-derived interleukin-6. *Physiol Rev, 88,* 1370–1406.
75. Sacca, L. (2009). Heart failure as a multiple hormonal deficiency syndrome. *Circ Heart Fail, 2,* 151–156.
76. Jankowska, E. A., Bartosz, B. B., Majda, J., et al. (2006). Anabolic deficiency in men with chronic heart failure prevalence and detrimental impact on survival. *Circulation, 114,* 1829–1837.
77. Ankrust, P., Ueland Gullestad, L., et al. (2009). Testosterone: a novel therapeutic approach in chronic heart failure? *J Am Coll Cardiol, 54,* 928–929.
78. Bhasin, S., Woodhouse, L., & Storer, T. W. (2001). Proof of the effect of testosterone on skeletal muscle. *J Endocrinol, 170,* 27–38.
79. Caminiti, G., Volterrani, M., Iellamo, F., et al. (2009). Effect of long-acting testosterone treatment on functional exercise capacity, skeletal muscle performance, insulin resistance and baroreflex in elderly patients with chronic heart failure. *J Am Coll Cardiol, 54,* 919–927.
80. Velloso, C. P. (2008). Regulation of muscle mass by growth hormone and IGF-1. *Br J Pharmacol, 154,* 557–568.
81. Blau, H. M. (2008). Cell therapies for muscular dystrophy. *N Engl J Med, 359,* 1403–1405.
82. Scime, A., & Rudnicki, M. A. (2006). Anabolic potential and regulation of skeletal muscle satellite cell populations. *Curr Opin Clin Nutr Metab Care, 9,* 214–219.
83. Sun, D., Martinez, C. O., Ochoa, O., et al. (2009). Bone marrow-derived cell regulation of skeletal muscle regeneration. *FASEB J, 23,* 382–395.
84. Nagaya, N., Moriya, J., Yasumura, Y., et al. (2004). Effects of ghrelin administration on left ventricular function, exercise capacity and muscle wasting in patients with chronic heart failure. *Circulation, 110,* 3674–3679.
85. Nagaya, N., Itoh, T., Murakami, S., et al. (2005). Treatment of cachexia with ghrelin in patients with COPD. *Chest, 28,* 1187–1193.
86. Handschin, C., & Spiegelman, B. M. (2008). The role of exercise and PGC1α in inflammation and chronic disease. *Nature, 454,* 463–469.
87. Smith, S. A., Williams, M. A., Mitchell, J. H., et al. (2005). The capsaicin-sensitive afferent neuron in skeletal muscle is abnormal in heart failure. *Circulation, 111,* 2056–2065.
88. Piepoli, M. F., Kaczmarek, A., & Francis, D. P. (2006). Reduced peripheral skeletal muscle and abnormal reflex physiology in chronic heart failure. *Circulation, 114,* 126–134.
89. Li, J., Sinoway, A. N., Gao, Z., et al. (2004). Muscle mechanoreflex and metaboreflex responses after myocardial infarction in rats. *Circulation, 110,* 3049–3054.
90. Middlekauff, H. R., Nitzsche, E. U., Hamilton, M. A., et al. (2001). Exaggerated muscle mechanoreceptor control of reflex renal vasoconstriction. *J Appl Physiol, 90,* 1714–1719.
91. Gielen, S., Adams, V., Mobius-Winkle, S., et al. (2003). Anti-inflammatory effects of exercise training in the skeletal muscle of patients with chronic heart failure. *J Am Coll Cardiol, 42,* 861–868.
92. Mourkioti, F., & Rosenthal, N. (2008). NF-κB signaling in skeletal muscle: prospects for intervention in muscle diseases. *J Mol Med, 86,* 747–759.
93. Sofie, P. M., Gayan-Ramirez, G., Van Den Bergh, A., et al. (2005). Interleukin-6 causes myocardial failure and skeletal muscle atrophy in rats. *Circulation, 111,* 996–1005.
94. Killian, K., & Jones, N. (1988). Respiratory muscle and dyspnea. *Clin Chest Med, 9,* 237–248.
95. Jones, G., Killian, K., Summers, E., et al. (1985). Inspiratory muscle forces and endurance in maximum resistive loading. *J Appl Physiol, 58,* 1608–1615.
96. Campbell, E., Gandevia, S., Killian, K., et al. (1980). Changes in the perception of inspiratory resistive loads during partial curarization. *J Physiol, 309,* 93–100.
97. Stubbing, D., Ramsdale, E., Killian, K., et al. (1983). Psychophysics of inspiratory muscle force. *J Appl Physiol, 54,* 1216–1221.
98. Campbell, E., & Howell, J. (1976). The sensation of breathlessness. *Br Med Bull, 19,* 36.
99. Roussos, C., & Macklem, P. (1982). The respiratory muscles. *N Engl J Med, 307,* 786–797.
100. Johnson, B., Babcock, M., Suman, Q., et al. (1993). Exercise-induced diaphragmatic fatigue in healthy humans. *J Physiol, 460,* 385–405.
101. Hagberg, J., Coyle, E., Carroll, J., et al. (1982). Exercise hyperventilation in patients with McArdle's disease. *J Appl Physiol, 52,* 991.
102. Fregosi, R. F., & Seals, D. R. (1993). Hypoxic potentiation of the ventilatory response to dynamic forearm exercise. *J Appl Physiol, 74,* 2365–2372.
103. McCully, K., Mancini, D., & Levine, S. (1999). Nuclear magnetic resonance spectroscopy: its role in providing valuable insight into diverse clinical problems. *Chest, 116,* 1434–1441.

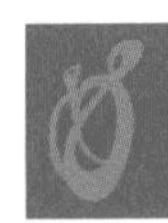

104. Oelberg, D., Evans, A. B., Hrovat, M. I., et al. (1998). Skeletal muscle chemoreflex and pHi in exercise ventilatory control. *J Appl Physiol, 84*, 676–682.
105. Levine, M., Weinstein, J., Diver, D., et al. (1989). Progressive improvement in pulmonary vascular resistance after percutaneous mitral valvuloplasty. *Circulation, 79*, 1061–1067.
106. Lecarpentier, Y., Coirault, C., Langeron, O., et al. (1999). Impaired load dependence of diaphragm relaxation during congestive heart failure in the rabbit. *J Appl Physiol, 87*(4), 1339–1345.
107. Lecarpentier, Y., Pery, N., Coirault, C., et al. (1993). Intrinsic alterations of diaphragm muscle in experimental cardiomyopathy. *Am Heart J, 126*(3 pt 2), 770–776.
108. Lecarpentier, Y., Chemla, D., Blanc, F. X., et al. (1998). Mechanics, energetics, and crossbridge kinetics of rabbit diaphragm during congestive heart failure. *FASEB J, 12*(11), 981–989.
109. Ferrari, R., Bachetti, T., Confortini, R., et al. (1995). Tumour necrosis factor soluble receptors in patients with various degrees of congestive heart failure. *Circulation, 92*, 1479–1486.
110. Arora, N., & Rocheter, D. (1982). Effect of body weight and muscularity on human diaphragm muscle mass, thickness, and area. *J Appl Physiol, 52*, 64–70.
111. Thurlbeck, W. (1978). Diaphragm and body weight in emphysema. *Thorax, 33*, 483–487.
112. Lindsay, D., Lovegrove, C., Dunn, M., et al. (1992). Histological abnormalities of diaphragmatic muscle may contribute to dyspnoea in heart failure. *Circulation, 86*, 515A.
113. Tikunov, B., Levine, B., & Mancini, D. M. (1997). Chronic congestive heart failure elicits adaptations of endurance exercise in diaphragmatic muscle. *Circulation, 95*, 910–916.
114. DeSousa, E., Veksler, V., Bigard, X., et al. (2001). Dual influence of disease and increased load and diaphragmatic muscle in heart failure. *J Mol Cell Cardiol, 33*, 699–701.
115. Van Hees, H., vander Heijden, H., Hafmans, T., et al. (2008). Impaired contractility and structural abnormalities in the diaphragm of congestive heart failure rats. *Int J Cardiol, 128*, 326–335.
116. DaSilva-Lopes, S., Carvalho, F., Campos, G., et al. (2008). Down regulation of Myo-D gene expression in rat diaphragm muscle with heart failure. *Int J Exp Pathol, 89*, 216–222.
117. Robeiro, J., Chiappa, G., Neder, J., et al. (2009). Respiratory muscle function and exercise intolerance in heart failure. *Curr Heart Fail Rep, 6*, 95–101.
118. McParland, C., Krishnan, B., Wang, Y., et al. (1992). Inspiratory muscle weakness and dyspnea in chronic heart failure. *Am Rev Respir Dis, 146*, 467–472.
119. Hammond, M., Bauer, K., Sharp, J., et al. (1990). Respiratory muscle strength in congestive heart failure. *Chest, 98*, 1091–1094.
120. Nishimura, Y., Maeda, H., Tanaka, K., et al. (1994). Respiratory muscle strength and hemodynamics in chronic heart failure. *Chest, 105*, 355–359.
121. Ambrosino, N., Opasich, C., Crotti, P., et al. (1994). Breathing pattern, ventilatory drive and respiratory muscle strength in patients with chronic heart failure. *Eur Respir J, 7*, 17–22.
122. Chua, T., Anker, S., Harrington, D., et al. (1995). Inspiratory muscle strength is a determinant of maximum oxygen consumption in chronic heart failure. *Brit Heart J, 74*, 381–385.
123. Meyer, F. J., Borst, M. M., Zugck, C., et al. (2001). Respiratory muscle dysfunction in congestive heart failure: clinical correlation and prognostic significance. *Circulation, 103*, 2153–2158.
124. Frankenstein, L., Meyer, F. J., Sigg, C., et al. (2008). Is serial determination of inspiratory muscle strength a useful prognostic marker in chronic heart failure? *Eur J Cardiovasc Prev Rehabil, 15*, 156–161.
125. Zelis, R., Nellis, S. H., Longhurst, J., et al. (1975). Abnormalities in the regional circulations accompanying congestive heart failure. *Prog Cardiovasc Dis, 18*, 181–199.
126. Fixler, D., Atkins, J., Mitchell, J., et al. (1976). Blood flow to respiratory, cardiac, and limb muscles in dogs during graded exercise. *Am J Physiol, 231*, 1515–1519.
127. Musch, T., & Terrell, J. (1990). Elevated diaphragmatic blood flow during submaximal exercise in rats with CHF. *Circulation, 82*(suppl III), III-156.
128. Aubier, M., Trippenbach, T., & Roussous, C. (1981). Respiratory muscle fatigue during cardiogenic shock. *J Appl Physiol, 51*, 499–508.
129. Wilson, J. R., Mancini, D. M., McCully, K., et al. (1989). Noninvasive detection of skeletal muscle underperfusion with near-infrared spectroscopy in patients with heart failure. *Circulation, 80*, 1668–1674.
130. Mancini, D. M., Farrell, L., & Wilson, J. R. (1992). Validation of near-infrared spectroscopy in man. *Circulation, 86*(suppl I), I-401A (abstract).
131. Mancini, D., Nazzaro, D., Ferraro, N., et al. (1991). Demonstration of respiratory muscle deoxygenation during exercise in patients with heart failure. *J Am Coll Cardiol, 18*, 492–498.
132. Davies, S., Jordan, S., Pride, N., et al. (1990). Respiratory muscle failure on exercise in chronic heart failure. *Circulation, 82*(suppl III), III-24.
133. Mancini, D. M., Henson, D., LaManca, J., et al. (1992). Respiratory muscle function and dyspnea in patients with chronic congestive heart failure. *Circulation, 86*, 909–918.
134. Aubier, M., Farkas, G., DeTroyer, A., et al. (1981). Detection of diaphragmatic fatigue in man by phrenic stimulation. *J Appl Physiol, 50*, 538–544.
135. Mancini, D. M., LaManca, J., Levine, S., et al. (1992). Respiratory muscle endurance is decreased in patients with heart failure. *Circulation, 86*(suppl I), I-515A.
136. Mancini, D. M., Henson, D., LaManca, J., et al. (1995). Benefit of selective respiratory muscle training on exercise capacity in patients with chronic congestive heart failure. *Circulation, 91*, 320–329.
137. Dall'Ago, P., Chiappa, G. R., Guths, H., et al. (2006). Inspiratory muscle training in patients with heart failure and inspiratory muscle weakness: a randomized trial. *J Am Coll Cardiol, 47*, 757–763.
138. Weiner, P., Waizman, J., Magadle, R., et al. (1999). The effect of specific inspiratory muscle training on the sensation of dyspnea and exercise tolerance in patients with congestive heart failure. *Clin Cardiol, 22*, 727–732.
139. Laoutaris, I., Dritsas, A., Brown, M. D., et al. (2004). Inspiratory muscle training using incremental endurance test alleviates dyspnea and improves functional status in patients with chronic heart failure. *Eur J Cardiovasc Prev Rehabil, 11*, 480–496.
141. Laoutaris, I. D., Dritsas, A., Brown, M. D., et al. (2007). Immune response to inspiratory muscle training in patients with chronic heart failure. *Eur J Cardiovasc Prev Rehabil, 14*, 679–685.
142. Laoutaris, I. D., Dritsas, A., Brown, M. D., et al. (2008). Effects of inspiratory muscle training on autonomic activity, endothelial vasodilator function, and N-terminal pro-brain natriuretic peptide levels in chronic heart failure. *J Cardiopulm Rehabil Prev, 28*, 99–106.
143. Chiappa, G. R., Roseguini, B. T., Vieira, P. J., et al. (2008). Inspiratory muscle training improves blood flow to resting and exercising limbs in patients with chronic heart failure. *J Am Coll Cardiol, 51*, 1663–1671.
144. Borghii-Silva, A., Carrascosa, C., Oliveira, C. C., et al. (2008). Effects of respiratory muscle unloading on leg muscle oxygenation and blood volume during high-intensity exercise in chronic heart failure. *Am J Physiol Heart Circ Physiol, 294*, H2465–H2472.
145. Beniaminovitz, A., Lang, C., LaManca, J., et al. (2002). Selective low level leg muscle training alleviates dyspnea in patients with heart failure. *J Am Coll Cardiol, 40*, 1602–1608.

CHAPTER 20

Alterations in Cardiac Metabolism

Linda R. Peterson, Joel Schilling, and Heinrich Taegtmeyer

This chapter is based on two broad concepts. The *first concept* considers the heart as an efficient converter of energy.[1] It addresses the hypothesis that defective energy metabolism is a cause for contractile dysfunction of the heart (see Chapter 7). The *second concept* considers heart failure as a systemic disease that begins with adaptation and ends with maladaptation of the heart in response to different stimuli. This chapter covers the entire spectrum, from altered energy metabolism to cardiac hypertrophy and failure. It also addresses the hypothesis that metabolism not only provides energy for contraction, but also generates signals that regulate cardiac-specific gene programs, including programs of adaptation and maladaptation of the heart to environmental stimuli (Figure 20-1).

By definition, energy is the capacity for doing work. The transfer of energy includes ATP and phosphocreatine, but it is not limited to energy-rich phosphate compounds. A discussion of myocardial energy metabolism in heart failure should therefore include a brief review of normal energy transfer in the heart, a review of methods used to detect abnormal energy transfer in the heart, and of evolving paradigms on metabolic adaptation and maladaptation of the failing heart. An inevitable question is whether metabolic derangements are causes or consequences of heart failure. The answer is clear in cases of myocardial ischemia and in the relatively rare cases of genetically determined cardiomyopathies. The answer is less clear in the majority of patients suffering from dilated cardiomyopathies.

Over the years, it has been speculated that the failing heart is "energy starved (see Chapter 7)."[2] Although ^{31}P-NMR spectroscopy can detect metabolic abnormalities already in asymptomatic patients with cardiomyopathy, the concept of energy starvation has rested primarily on a reductionist approach focusing on some of the final reactions (e.g., the creatine kinase reaction). In this chapter, we use a more inclusive perspective that encompasses consideration of all energy-metabolizing pathways. Such an approach seems justified in light of (1) emerging pharmacological and surgical strategies directed at shifting substrate flux through specific metabolic pathways, (2) the rapidly emerging concepts of peroxisome proliferator activated receptor signaling in the control of cardiac energy metabolism,[3] and (3) metabolically inducible forms of heart failure.

The complex and highly regulated systems of energy transfer have been the subject of biochemistry studies for most of the past century[4] and provide many likely sites for defective metabolism. In the heart, defective energy metabolism has been characterized best in the case of myocardial ischemia, where the lack of oxygen results in severe impairment of the efficient system of oxidative phosphorylation. Drugs that target specific "bottleneck" reactions in intermediary metabolism of the heart hold the promise of improving cardiac function in ischemic heart disease and in dilated cardiomyopathies (see Chapter 50). Although conceptually attractive, this concept may be an oversimplification. In the following section, we will see why.

PERSPECTIVES

Metabolism and Function Are Tightly Coupled

Catabolic energy substrate metabolism transfers energy from chemical bonds to ATP, the immediate precursor for conversion to mechanical energy. Heart muscle derives its energy for contraction from the oxidation of a variety of fuels, including glucose, lactate, and especially long-chain fatty acids.[5] When fatty acids are abundant, the myocardium increases fatty acid metabolism, which suppresses glucose metabolism. Conversely, myocardial fatty acid oxidation is suppressed when higher fuel efficiency (from glucose metabolism) is required.[6,7]

Metabolism is an integral part of the heart's physiological function (Figure 20-2). A decrease in energy demand and contractile function (e.g., during sleep or with β-adrenergic receptor blockade) results in a decrease in energy turnover. Vice versa, as first shown by Langendorff's classic studies in the isolated perfused cat heart, a decrease in energy supply (e.g., during ischemia) results in a decrease in contractile function.[8] Because the heart can store only a small amount of energy (and because energy is the capacity for doing work), it follows that supply of, and demand for, energy-providing substrates in the heart are finely regulated and need to be in balance. The tight coupling of contractile function and myocardial oxygen consumption in the mammalian heart has been known for nearly a century.[9] The evidence of this relationship between function and metabolism

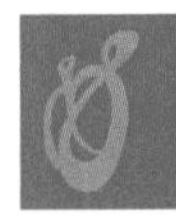

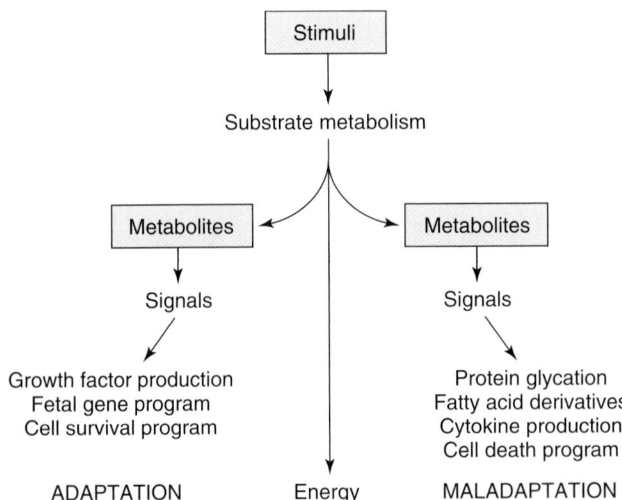

FIGURE 20–1 The pleiotropic role of metabolites in energy metabolism, substrate storage, cell structure, cell signaling, gene expression, and apoptosis (programmed cell death). See text for discussion. (Adapted from Young ME, McNulty P, Taegtmeyer H. Adaptation and maladaptation of the heart in diabetes: Part II. Potential mechanisms. *Circulation* 2002; 105:1861-1870).

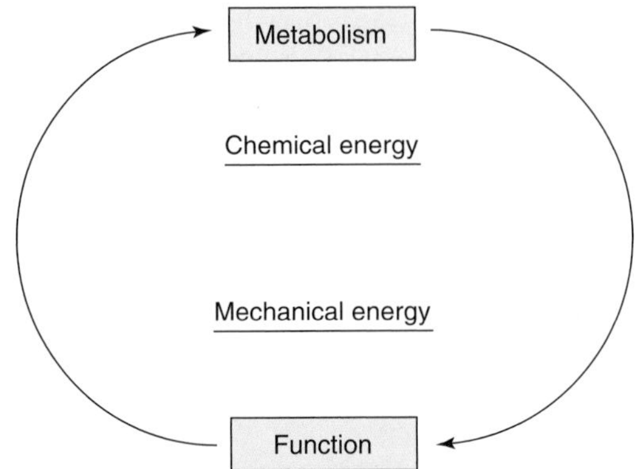

FIGURE 20-2 The metabolic machinery in the heart converts chemical energy into mechanical energy. The tight coupling of energy substrate metabolism and contractile function of the heart underlies a system of high adaptability and efficiency. (Adapted from Taegtmeyer H. Cardiac metabolism as a target for the treatment of heart failure. *Circulation* 2004; 110(8): 894-896.)

and function is seen routinely in the clinical practice of cardiology (e.g., the hearts of patients with a decreased supply of oxygen [ischemia] exhibit decreased contractile function). In simple terms: The prerequisite for normal contractile function is the normal flux of energy, a concept already known to the ancient Greeks: παντα ρει, meaning "all is in flux" (Heraclitus, 540-475 BC).

Heart muscle derives its energy from the oxidative metabolism of fuels (for review, see Taegtmeyer).[1] Because the heart is capable of oxidizing a variety of biological fuels, we have termed it a "metabolic omnivore". The essence of energy substrate metabolism in the heart is to maintain a dynamic state of equilibrium. Heart muscle burns chemical energy (fuels) and converts it into physical energy (pump function). In doing so, the heart distributes energy in the form of substrates and oxygen to the rest of the body. Hence the concept that heart failure is a disease of impaired energy transfer, beginning and ending with the heart.

It goes without saying that when the heart's ability to convert chemical into mechanical energy is impaired for any reason, the consequences affect every organ of the body. The general concept that the failing heart is in an energy-deprived state helps us to understand why in a number of clinical trials inotropic agents failed to produce a beneficial long-term effect. These drugs improve symptoms of heart failure, but do so at the expense of cardiac energy expenditure, which can only be expected to worsen cardiac performance.

The Plasticity of Cardiac Metabolism

As mentioned, the heart is able to use multiple different fuels for generation of ATP. Fatty acids (either from free fatty acids or hydrolyzed triglycerides) are the main substrate used and glucose is typically a secondary substrate, but the heart can also use ketones, lactate, and amino acids.[1,10] One of the main determinants of the heart's substrate choice is substrate availability. Under resting conditions in the fed and immediate postprandial state, the fuel for respiration is influenced by the composition of the diet, which affects both blood hormone and substrate levels. For example, increases in postprandial plasma glucose and insulin levels increase the heart's glucose uptake and use. During fasting, the main fuel of the heart is fatty acids.[10] During exercise, with increased lactate production, the heart increases lactate and glucose use.[11] Thus there is "plasticity" of the heart's substrate metabolism (i.e., it can readily and rapidly switch substrate preference based on substrate availability under physiologic conditions). Special physiological conditions also influence substrate choice and a return to the fetal gene program and aging. In the fetal state, the heart uses predominantly glucose rather than fatty acids.[12] Interestingly, the aging heart is also associated with predominantly glucose use rather than fatty acid metabolism.[13] As discussed later, the failing heart (due to idiopathic cardiomyopathy) also predominantly uses glucose, like the fetal and aging heart.

Energy Transfer in the Heart

The heart transforms chemical energy from its substrates into ATP and then uses ATP for cellular function. The main source of ATP is oxidative phosphorylation (see Chapter 2). The high rate of ATP turnover of the heart is reflected in the heart's high rates of oxygen consumption, the high cellular density of mitochondria, and the high capillary density in heart muscle (2500 capillaries/mm^3 in the heart vs. 400 capillaries/mm^3 in red skeletal muscle). Mitochondria in heart muscle are not only more abundant but they also contain a far greater number of cristae (the location of respiratory chain enzymes) than mitochondria of other organs. Classic studies on the ultrastructure of the normal rat myocardium have shown that mitochondria account for 35.8% of myocyte cell volume with a mitochondria/myofibril ratio of 0.75. This ratio increases in the early phase of hypertrophy induced by aortic constriction[14] and decreases below normal values with prolongation of pressure overload.[15] The latter decrease is due to a decrease in the volume fraction of mitochondria, in combination with an increase in the volume fraction of myofibrils.[16] Mitochondria isolated from hypertrophied, nonfailing rabbit hearts exhibit significantly increased respiratory activity compared with controls,[17] whereas mitochondria from failing hearts exhibit respiratory rates near or below normal values and decreased respiratory control.[18]

Although all of the mechanisms by which respiration is coupled to energy expenditure in vivo are not known, the efficacy of oxidative phosphorylation is well established. For example, one mole of glucose yields 36 moles of ATP when oxidized, whereas the same amount of glucose yields only 2 moles of ATP when metabolized to lactate under anaerobic conditions. In addition, this less productive anaerobic glycolysis is suppressed by oxygen.[19] In the context of oxidative metabolism, it is also well established that efficient energy transfer occurs through a series of moiety-conserved cycles (Figure 20-3).[1] In the heart, these moiety-conserved cycles begin with the circulation itself, continue with the cyclic

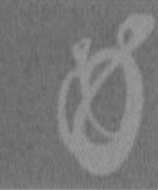

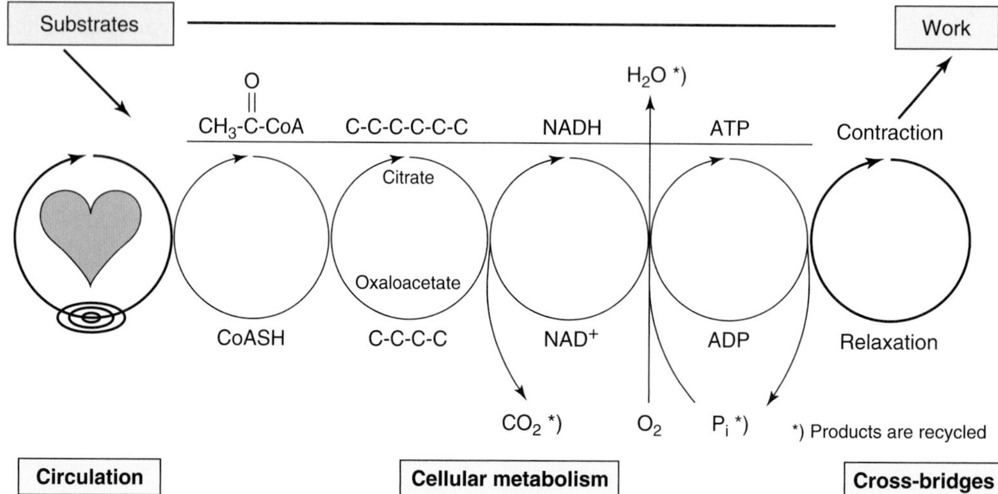

FIGURE 20-3 A series of moiety-conserved cycles underlies the efficient energy transfer from substrates to work. The moiety-conserved cycles can be likened to the wheels of a bicycle and provide a mechanism for immediate response to changes in energy demand. The higher the flux of energy, the greater the rate of turnover of the cycles. The concentration of cycle intermediates (moieties) remains stable over a wide range of energy fluxes. (Adapted from Sherma S, Androgue JV, Goldman L et al: Energy metabolism of the heart: from basic concepts to clinical applications. *Curr Prob Cardiol* 1994; 19:57-111.)

metabolic processes in the cell, and end with the cycling of the actin and myosin cross-bridges. Moiety-conserved cycles can be likened to the wheels of a bicycle because these cycles of energy are much more efficient than linear pathways (e.g., anaerobic glycolysis), just as the wheels of a bicycle area more efficient mechanism for locomotion than the more linear mechanism of walking.[20]

In addition to the concept of interconnected cycles, it is a convenient practice to divide energy transfer into three stages (Figure 20-4). Stage 1 involves the uptake of substrates into the cell, their conversion into acetyl-CoA, and oxidation in the Krebs cycle. Stage 2 consists of the final acceptance of electrons from reducing equivalents to molecular oxygen in the respiratory chain, which is coupled to the rephosphorylation of ADP to ATP in the proton motive force. Stage 3 is the transfer of energy from the mitochondria to the rest of the cell for contractile and other work. This division of substrate metabolism into stages helps to define sites at which energy transfer may become impaired and to identify potential sites for pharmacological intervention. In short, each stage can be the site of a metabolic block causing impaired energy transfer and contractile dysfunction. For example, impaired uptake of glucose is a feature of the heart, in type 1 diabetes,[20] impaired oxidation of long-chain fatty acids is a feature of lipotoxic heart failure,[21] impaired Krebs cycle flux is a feature of limited cofactor availability for certain dehydrogenases,[22] and impaired respiratory chain flux is a feature of ischemia with a redirection of metabolic fluxes from aerobic to anaerobic metabolism.[23,24] These concepts will be expanded upon in the section on metabolic adaptation and maladaptation.

Lastly, for practical purposes it is also useful to distinguish between *control* and *regulation* of metabolism. *Metabolic control* is the power to change the state of metabolism in response to an external signal, whereas *metabolic regulation* is geared toward maintaining a constant internal state.[25] In such a system, large changes in flux through metabolic pathways correspond to small changes in myocardial metabolite concentrations.[26] It follows that regulatory sites of metabolism, or "pacemaker" enzymes,[27] are not only targets for the change of metabolic fluxes by physiological effectors, but also emerging targets for pharmacological agents. Examples include the "fuel gauge" 5′-AMP-dependent protein kinase (AMPK) and the evolving class of partial fatty acid oxidation inhibitors (and other metabolically active drugs) in the management of ischemic heart disease. In the former case, AMPK is the primary sensor of energy charge in the mammalian cell.[28] Most effectors of intracellular ATP depletion are probably mediated through this kinase pathway rather than through direct effects of adenine nucleotides. AMPK promotes glucose uptake and long-chain fatty acid oxidation by different mechanisms,[29] and the activity of this kinase can be altered both acutely (e.g., increased workload) and chronically (e.g., ischemia and pressure-overload-induced hypertrophy).[30] In the latter case, partial inhibition of fatty acid oxidation shifts the fuel balance to the energetically more efficient oxidation of glucose.

METHODS FOR DETECTING DEFECTIVE SUBSTRATE METABOLISM IN THE FAILING HEART

Substrate Uptake by Arteriovenous (AV) Differences

At the beginning of the past century, the oxygen requirement of the mammalian heart was established by the German physiologist Hans Winterstein.[31] The British physiologist C. Lovatt Evans studied the effect of various mechanical conditions on the gaseous metabolism and efficiency of the mammalian heart.[32] However, it was not until the advent of cardiac catheterization and cannulation of the coronary sinus that the hypothesis of defective energy metabolism in the failing heart could be tested in earnest. The results firmly established that heart muscle derives its energy for contraction from the oxidation of energy-providing substrates[33] and suggested that oxygen consumption is an index of energy production. Despite decreased efficiency of the failing human heart, the results were disappointing because no qualitative change in substrate metabolism was observed through measurement of AV differences.[34] These early studies found that like the normal human heart, the failing heart under fasting conditions derived about 30% of its energy requirements from carbohydrates, 5% from amino acids, 7% from ketone bodies, and the remaining 58% from fatty acids.[34] Thus, these early measurements of AV differences of substrates failed to provide insight into mechanisms of impaired cardiac function. However, it should be noted that these early studies were limited in that they did not use nonradiolabeled tracer infusions, such as C-13 palmitate, which facilitate the discrimination of exogenous substrate use from endogenous substrate

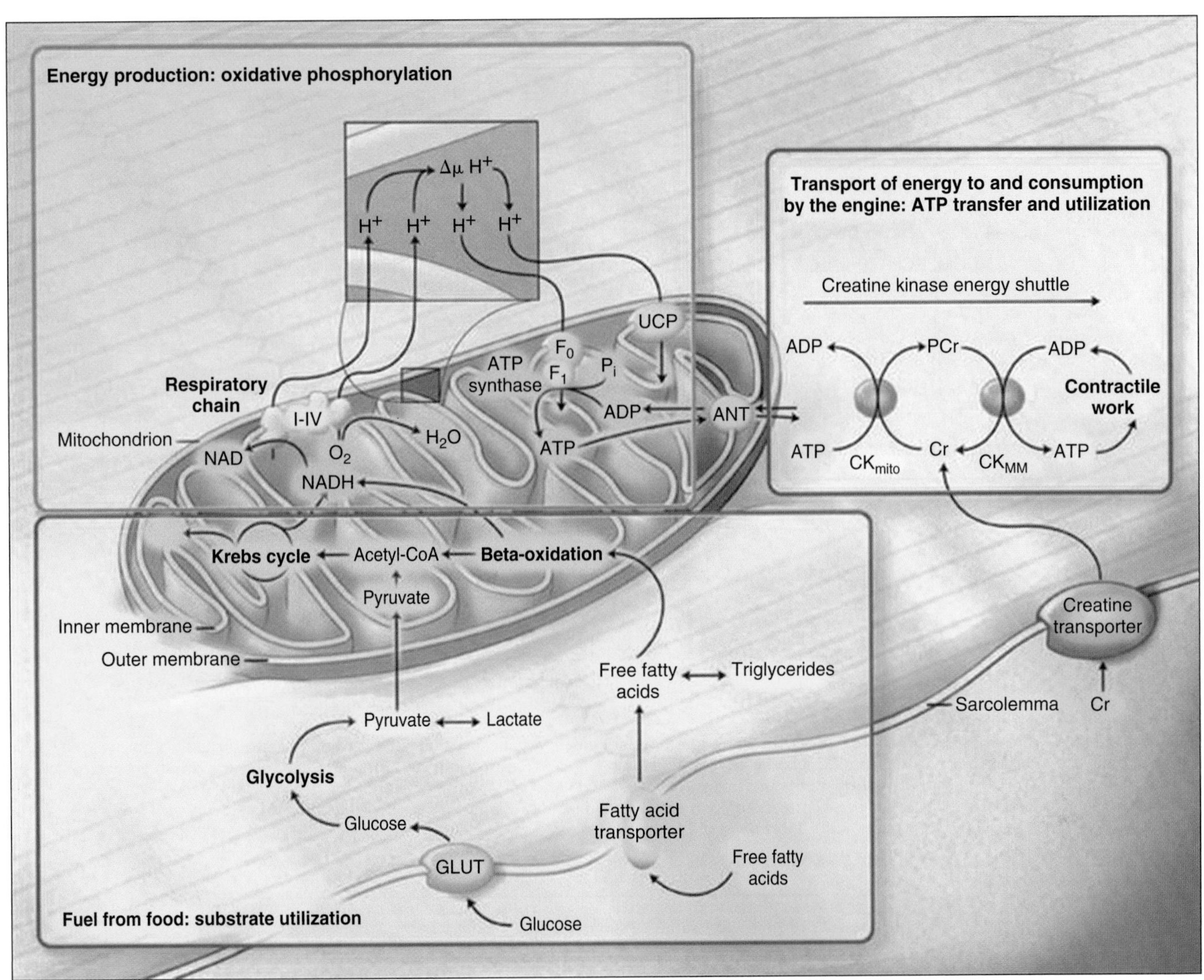

FIGURE 20-4 Energy transfer in the cardiac myocyte occurs in three stages. Each stage may be the site of metabolic derangements causing or accompanying contractile dysfunction of the heart. The first stage is substrate uptake and metabolism (outlined in red). In this stage substrates are broken down by β-oxidation and glycolysis to form acetyl coenzyme A (CoA), from which the Krebs cycle produces NADH and CO_2. The second stage is energy production through oxidative phosphorylation (outlined in blue). Respiratory chain complexes in the mitochondria transfer electrons from NAHD to oxygen. This creates a proton electrochemical gradient (Δμ H⁺) across the inner mitochondrial membrane in addition to water and NAD. This gradient drives ATP synthase. Uncoupling proteins (UCPs) use this electrochemical gradient to create heat instead of ATP. The third stage is energy transfer via the creatine kinase shuttle (outlined in green). ATP is transferred to and consumed by myofibrillar ATPase and other reactions. *GLUT*, glucose transporter; P_i, inorganic phosphate; *ANT*, adenine nucleotide translocase; *PCr*, phosphocreatine; *Cr*, free creatine; CK_{mito}, mitochondrial creatine kinase isoenzyme; and CK_{MM}, myofibrillar creatine kinase isoenzyme. (Reproduced with permission from Neubauer S. The failing heart—an engine out of fuel. *N Engl J Med* 2007;356:1140-1151.)

production. More recent A-V balance studies have taken advantage of this technique to evaluate myocardial uptake and use of exogenous versus endogenous substrates.[12] In addition, some of the early AV balance studies of heart failure did not evaluate substrate metabolism in patients with concomitant diabetes or obesity, which would be expected to affect substrate delivery and thus myocardial substrate use.

NMR Spectroscopy (see Chapter 7)

NMR spectroscopy of energy-rich phosphates and other biological compounds detects the magnetic spin of atomic nuclei and is used to monitor changes in metabolic content and enrichment in the intact heart. Commonly used nuclei include ^{1}H, ^{2}H, ^{13}C, ^{15}N, ^{17}O, ^{31}P, ^{23}N, and ^{39}K. ^{31}P NMR spectroscopy is one of the most commonly used types of NMR spectroscopy, which yields distinct quantitative resonance peaks for monophosphate esters, inorganic phosphates, phosphocreatine, and the three phosphorus atoms of ATP (γ-ATP, α-ATP, and β-ATP). The sizes of these peaks are related to the concentration of these metabolites. A decrease in the myocardial PCr/ATP ratio occurs relatively early in heart failure and results from a decrease in creatine transporter function, which leads to lower [Cr] and [PCr] levels. A decreased PCr/ATP ratio (<1.6) is a predictor of mortality in patients with dilated cardiomyopathy (Figure 20-5).[35] Decreased PCr/ATP ratio is also an early finding in inherited hypertrophic cardiomyopathy, even without frank left ventricular (LV) hypertrophy.[36] Heart failure impairs the creatine kinase energy-transfer mechanism, reducing ATP flux rates by approximately 50% in mild to moderate heart failure. ADP concentrations increase in heart failure.[2] A decrease in myocardial ATP level generally only occurs in advanced heart failure. An overview of the evolution of changes in high-energy phosphate metabolism created by heart failure (along with the changes in myocardial metabolism and oxidative phosphorylation) is shown in Figure 20-6. Although most clinical ^{31}P NMR studies of heart failure have measured the PCr/ATP ratio, it is possible to quantify concentrations of myocardial metabolites by normalizing their NMR signal to that of a standard of known concentration.

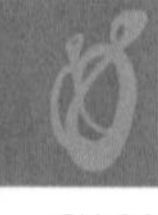

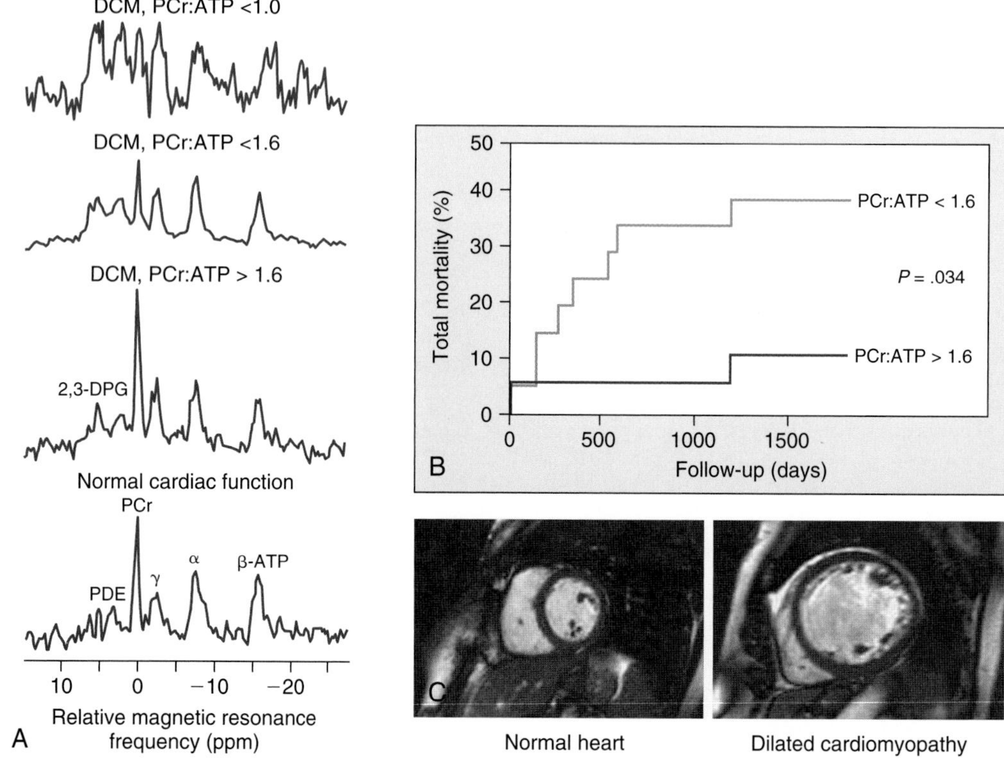

FIGURE 20-5 **A,** Illustrates top to bottom: a ^{31}P-NMR spectra in a normal human, a patient with dilated cardiomyopathy but a favorable PCr/ATP ratio of greater than 1.6, a patient with dilated cardiomyopathy and an unfavorable PCr/ATP ratio less than 1.6, and a cardiomyopathy patient with a severely decreased PCr/ATP (<1.0), who died within 7 days after this image was taken. **B,** A Kaplan-Meier analysis showing prognosis differences based on PCr/ATP. **C,** Shows magnetic resonance imaging (MRI) of a normal heart compared with a dilated cardiomyopathy. (Reproduced with permission from Neubauer S. The failing heart–an engine out of fuel. *N Engl J Med* 2007;356:1140-1151.)

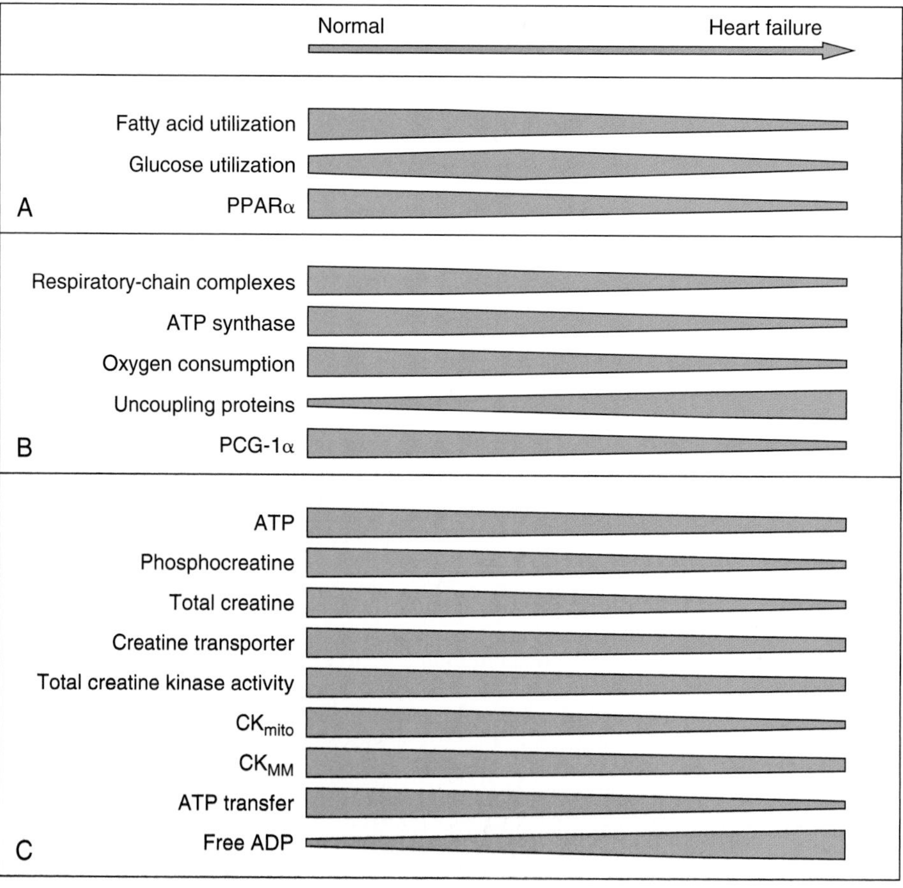

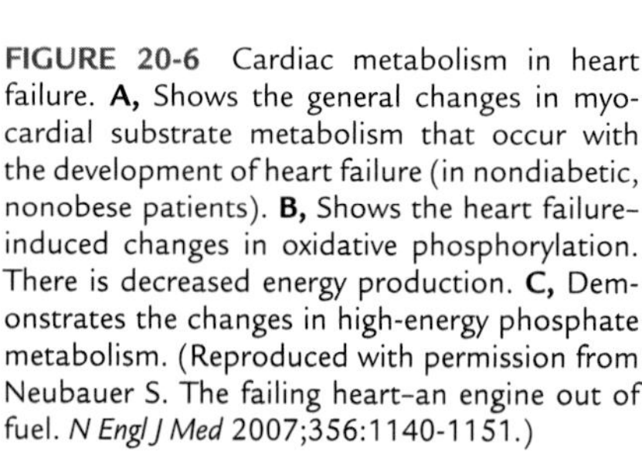

FIGURE 20-6 Cardiac metabolism in heart failure. **A,** Shows the general changes in myocardial substrate metabolism that occur with the development of heart failure (in nondiabetic, nonobese patients). **B,** Shows the heart failure–induced changes in oxidative phosphorylation. There is decreased energy production. **C,** Demonstrates the changes in high-energy phosphate metabolism. (Reproduced with permission from Neubauer S. The failing heart–an engine out of fuel. *N Engl J Med* 2007;356:1140-1151.)

^{1}H-NMR spectroscopy is useful for assessing myocardial fatty acid metabolism both in animal models and in humans with heart failure.[37] The spectra generated from ^{1}H-NMR are used to determine intramyocellular triglyceride *deposition* (as opposed to flux). The spectra are acquired from a region of interest in the interventricular septum to avoid contamination from epicardial fat. As shown in Figure 20-7, the spectral peak due to water is very large in comparison with the peaks due to myocardial triglycerides. However, the agreement between ^{1}H-NMR spectroscopy measurement of myocardial triglycerides and traditional biochemical methods is very good, and ^{1}H-NMR spectroscopy is reproducible. The amount of myocardial triglyceride deposition correlates with increased ventricular mass, concentric remodeling, and decreased regional systolic function (Figure 20-8).[37] This noninvasive technique is particularly valuable for the robust myocardial phenotyping of patients with heart failure due to different causes and for monitoring responses to metabolic modulation therapies.

Radionuclear Imaging: A Focus on Positron Emission Tomography

Tracing metabolic pathways with short-lived radionuclear tracers has found more widespread clinical applications than NMR spectroscopy, mainly in the diagnosis and management of ischemic heart disease. Although single-photon emission computed tomography (SPECT) imaging can be used to evaluate myocardial glucose or fatty acid metabolism, SPECT cannot quantify myocardial metabolism rates, so its utility for measuring metabolism has been limited. In contrast, positron emission tomography (PET) can be used to quantify myocardial oxygen and substrate metabolism (see also Chapter 36). In general, two types of positron-emitting tracers are used in PET imaging: generator-derived substrate analogs, such as [^{18}F]2-deoxy-2-fluoro-D-glucose (FDG), and cyclotron-derived [^{11}C]-labeled tracers, such as [1-^{11}C]-glucose. The main advantages of generator-produced tracers are that an onsite cyclotron is not needed and the cost is often cheaper than cyclotron-produced tracers. The main advantage of cyclotron-produced tracers is that (in conjunction with compartmental modeling) they can provide more comprehensive information about intracellular myocardial metabolism. While complete detail on all metabolic tracers ever used or being developed for myocardial metabolic measurements is beyond the scope of this chapter, it is important to note that clinically the most commonly used metabolic tracer is FDG. The method for calculation of myocardial glucose metabolism rates using FDG requires use of a "lumped constant" that represents the ratio of the use of 2-deoxyglucose relative to glucose. The uptake and retention of FDG is linear with time and follows zero-order kinetics.[38] For research purposes, more detailed measurements of metabolism and intracellular fate of substrates is now possible using [1-^{11}C]-labeled glucose, fatty acids, and lactate due to the development of new compartmental models that are used in conjunction with the PET-derived time-activity curves from the myocardium and the blood.[39] For example, clearance of labeled long-chain fatty acids is biexponential, suggesting both rapid and slow turnover pools.[40] The size and slope of the exponential components of the ^{11}C time-activity curve reflect immediate and delayed oxidation of labeled fatty acids. Most recently, a methodology designed to measure endogenous triglyceride oxidation in animals using [1-^{11}C] palmitate and 3-dimensional PET has shown promise for the potential use of PET for the noninvasive measurement of endogenous triglyceride oxidation.[41]

Still, the most important clinical use for metabolic PET imaging is the assessment of myocardial viability (see Chapter 36).[42] Regional responses in substrate metabolism to myocardial ischemia can be visualized entirely noninvasively. The basis of viability studies is the finding that ischemic, noncontractile, *but viable* myocardium has markedly impaired blood flow but normal or enhanced glucose metabolism due to a return to the fetal gene program.[43] Thus demonstration of enhanced FDG uptake and normal or decreased coronary

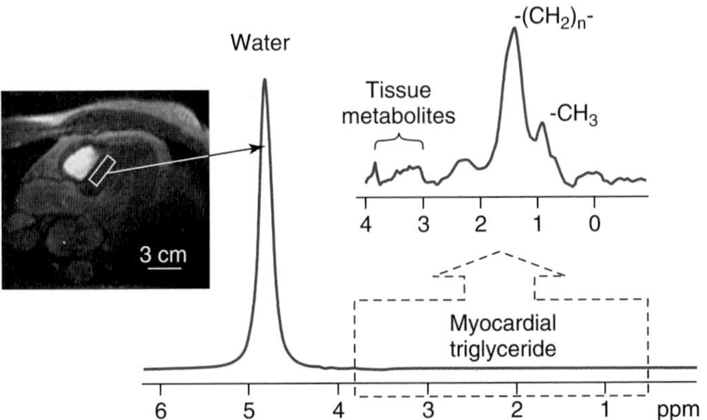

FIGURE 20-7 *Far left:* Magnetic resonance image of the heart showing a region of interest in the ventricular septum. The ^{1}H-NMR spectra generated from the region of interest are next to the MRI image. The largest peak is from water. The myocardial triglyceride peaks have been enlarged. (Reproduced with permission from Szczepaniak LS, Dobbins RL, Metzger GJ, et al. Myocardial triglycerides and systolic function in humans: in vivo evaluation by localized proton spectroscopy and cardiac imaging. *Magn Res Med* 2003;49:417-423.)

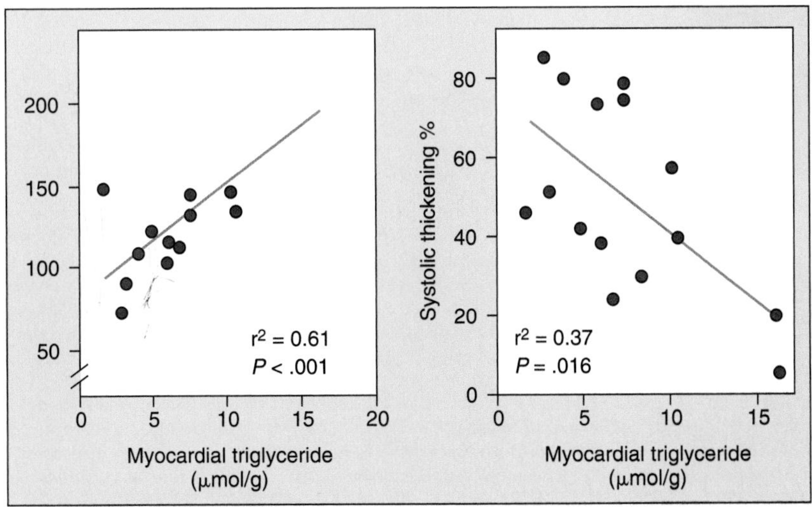

FIGURE 20-8 Demonstrates that as myocardial triglyceride deposition increases, left ventricular (LV) mass increases and systolic function decreases. (Reproduced with permission from Szczepaniak LS, Dobbins RL, Metzger GJ, et al. Myocardial triglycerides and systolic function in humans: in vivo evaluation by localized proton spectroscopy and cardiac imaging. *Magn Res Med* 2003;49:417-423.)

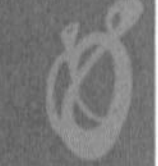

flow (metabolism/perfusion mismatch) is the current gold standard for identification of potentially reversible contractile dysfunction with revascularization (Figure 20-9).

Results from PET studies of myocardial metabolism in nonischemic heart failure in nonobese, nondiabetic patients are somewhat mixed but generally demonstrate a shift toward glucose and away from fatty acid metabolism.[44] For example, in a PET study of human idiopathic cardiomyopathy using [^{11}C] palmitate, the mean LV myocardial use of fatty acids was significantly less than that of control subjects.[45] In heart failure from a different cause (i.e., due to genetic defects in fatty acid oxidation), it is not the total fatty acid use that is altered as much as the rates of β-oxidation of fatty acids are decreased.[46] In contrast, in one study of hypertrophic cardiomyopathy due to a particular mutation (Asp175Asn in the α-tropomyosin gene), myocardial oxygen consumption and fatty acid metabolism were increased.[47] Taken together, these studies demonstrate that all heart failure is not created equally in terms of myocardial metabolism. Different causes lead to different patterns of myocardial metabolic substrate preference even if decreased function is common to all. This suggests that myocardial metabolic changes observed in heart failure are not solely in response to functional changes. Moreover, it suggests that new treatment strategies aimed at improving myocardial metabolism will have to be *individualized* to the metabolic pattern peculiar to a particular cause of heart failure.

Treatment of heart failure patients with standard heart failure medications aimed at the neurohormonal axis may also have effects on myocardial metabolism and energetics. For example, the β-blocker carvedilol leads to a readily detectable decrease of fatty acid uptake by the heart and an increase in glucose uptake, suggesting increased reliance on glucose an energy-providing substrate. ACE inhibitor therapy also appeared to improve myocardial energetics in heart failure. The findings are consistent with the concept of a change in the biological properties of the failing human heart with β-blockade that includes substrate preference[48] and substrate-induced improvement in cardiac efficiency.[49]

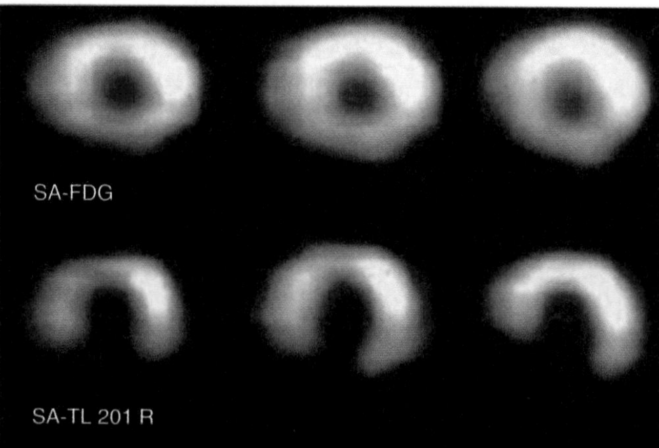

FIGURE 20-9 Assessment of myocardial viability. The top short axis positron emission tomography (PET) images show uptake of FDG in all myocardial segments, consistent with intact glucose metabolism. The bottom images show markedly decreased perfusion in the inferior wall *(white arrows)* assessed by thallium-201 uptake. Demonstration of enhanced FDG uptake and normal or decreased coronary flow (metabolism/perfusion mismatch) is the current gold standard for identification of potentially reversible contractile dysfunction with revascularization. (Reproduced with permission from Cornel JH, Bax JJ, Fioretti PM, et al. Prediction of improvement of ventricular function after revascularization. 18F-fluorodeoxyglucose single-photon emission computed tomography versus low-dose dobutamine echocardiography. *Eur Heart J* 1997;18(6):941-948.)

Transcript Analyses

Another dimension in the evaluation of metabolic disturbances underlying heart failure is the assessment of gene expression in myocardial biopsy samples. With the exception of rare disorders such as glycogen storage disease and lipotoxic heart disease (see later discussion), histology and immunocytochemistry have limited usefulness as tools for diagnosing metabolic disturbances of the failing heart. As outlined previously, the use of AV differences, ^{31}P-NMR, and PET have brought to light a number of defects in energy substrate metabolism. These findings and the concept of energy starvation of the failing heart are now the basis for further studies examining cardiac gene expression of key regulators in energy substrate metabolism. Moreover, the advent of quantitative RT-PCR and targeted gene expression arrays have facilitated a more complete assessment of metabolic gene expression changes in the failing heart.

Consistent with the observed reduction in fatty acid oxidation capacity in heart failure from dilated cardiomoypathy, the mRNA expression of enzymes that mediate long-chain fatty acid metabolism is downregulated[50,51] (Figure 20-10). Similar downregulation in the expression of genes encoding fatty acid oxidation enzymes is observed in animal models of hypertrophy and heart failure.[52]

Many of the genes for proteins of fatty acid uptake and oxidation are regulated by the nuclear receptor peroxisome proliferator activated receptor α (PPARα).[53] This transcription factor forms a heterodimer with the retinoic X receptor α (RXRα) and complexes with coactivators, most prominently PGC1α.[54] One of the natural ligands for PPARα was recently determined to be 16:0;18:1 glycerol-3-phosphocholine; however, other fatty acid moieties may also be able to activate this nuclear receptor. In animal models of cardiac hypertrophy, gene expression and DNA binding activity of PPARα

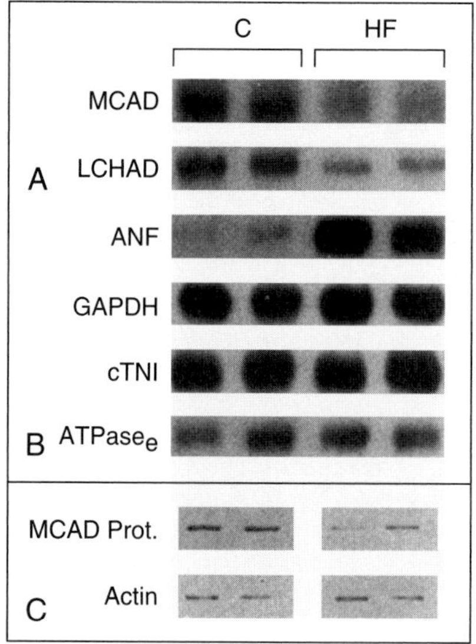

FIGURE 20-10 Downregulation of enzymes of long-chain fatty acid metabolism in patients with dilated cardiomyopathy. FAO enzyme mRNA and protein levels in left ventricle from failing human hearts. **A,** Representative autoradiographs of Northern *(top)* and Western *(bottom two rows)* blot analysis from left ventricle of two controls **(C)** and two subjects with heart failure. **B,** Bars represent mean steady-state mRNA or protein levels shown as arbitrary units (AU), normalized (= 100) to control *(solid bars)* and standardized to the signal obtained with an 18S rRNA probe or to the total protein (MCAD protein). Hatched bars indicate heart failure; cTNI, cardiac troponin I. *Significant difference (P <.5) compared with control values. (Reproduced with permission from Sack MN, Rader TA, Park S, et al. Fatty acid oxidation enzyme gene expression is downregulated in the failing heart. *Circulation* 1996;94:2837-2842.)

decrease as does the expression of various enzymes involved in β-oxidation,[53] suggesting a possible transcriptional mechanism for diminished rates of fatty acid oxidation. These observations are consistent with data demonstrating that PPARα is downregulated in the failing human heart.[55] In addition to PPARα, the heart also expresses high levels of the nuclear receptors PPARβ/δ and ERRα. Although the regulation of these transcription factors in heart failure is less clear, both PPARβ/δ and ERRα upregulate many of the same fatty acid oxidation genes as PPARα.[56] In addition, PPARβ/δ and ERRα are distinct from PPARα in that they induce genes involved in glucose uptake and mitochondrial oxidative phosphorylation, respectively. Mice overexpressing PPARβ/δ in the myocardium are resistant to high-fat diet-induced cardiomyopathy and show increased protection from ischemia reperfusion injury.[56] In contrast, animals with a cardiac-specific deletion of PPARβ/δ develop cardiomyopathy.[57] These data are consistent with the concept that PPARβ/δ-induced transcriptional programs are cardioprotective. ERRα also plays a protective role when the heart is exposed to stresses such as pressure overload, as evidenced by the rapid development of heart failure in ERRα knockout mice subjected to aortic banding.[58] Recent evidence also suggests that ERRα-regulated pathways are downregulated in humans with heart failure.[59]

In contrast to long-chain fatty acids, the transcriptional regulation of glucose metabolism in heart failure is less well understood. Cardiac hypertrophy is associated with increased reliance on glucose oxidation,[60] whereas late-stage cardiomyopathy is associated with decreased glucose uptake.[61] Recent studies suggest that glucose transporters 1 and 4 are both downregulated in patients with end-stage heart failure at the transcriptional level.[51] In addition, pacing-induced heart failure in a canine model caused decreased mRNA levels of lactate dehydrogenase. In the same model, the activities of 3-phosphoglycerate kinase and pyruvate kinase were also downregulated,[62] consistent with an impairment of glucose use in the later stages of heart failure. Thus not only do different causes of heart failure affect the heart's substrate metabolism profile, but severity of heart failure also affects it.

In addition to changes in transcript levels of enzymes regulating energy substrate metabolism, genes controlling the transfer of high-energy phosphates across the inner mitochondrial membrane also show alterations in the failing heart. For instance, a recent report showed a downregulation of adenine nucleotide translocator 1 (ANT1) in a rodent model of chronic heart failure.[63] In contrast, others have found that hearts from patients with dilated cardiomyopathy have decreased transcript levels of adenine nucleotide translocator 2, whereas adenine nucleotide translocator 1 protein content increased.[64] Overall, these findings suggest that in the failing heart, changes in expression of regulators of energy transfer pathways are likely contributors to the progression of contractile dysfunction.

Transcripts for mitochondrial proteins are also decreased in the failing heart. For instance, in a mouse model of heart failure, mitochondrial DNA-encoded gene transcripts, including the subunits of complex I (ND1, 2, 3, 4, 4L, and 5), complex III (cytochrome b), complex IV (cytochrome oxidase), and rRNA (12S and 16S) are all decreased. These transcriptional changes were accompanied by changes in the enzymatic activity of complexes I, III, and IV.[65] These findings are consistent with other observations of decreased mitochondrial respiration in the failing human heart, and defective mitochondrial structure and function in animal models of heart failure.[66] However, with the exception of certain inherited cardiomyopathies exhibiting mutations for mitochondrial enzymes of long-chain fatty acid metabolism,[50] it cannot be determined with certainty whether mitochondria play a primary or a secondary role in contributing to heart failure.

The regulation of genes involved in both fatty acid oxidation and mitochondrial oxidative capacity/biogenesis are controlled by the nuclear receptor coactivators PGC-1α and-β.[67] These proteins are highly expressed in the heart where they direct gene expression through interactions with nuclear receptor (PPARα, PPARβ/δ, ERRα) and nonnuclear receptor transcription factors (NRF-1/2, MEF2). The highly inducible nature of these proteins allows them to rapidly reprogram metabolism in response to a variety of stressors. In both humans and animal models of hypertrophy and heart failure from dilated cardiomyopathy PGC-1 coactivators are downregulated. This is further supported by the observation that mice lacking both PGC-1 isoforms die of heart failure early in life.[68] Thus although a metabolic shift toward glucose metabolism and away from fatty acid metabolism may in some ways be adaptive (e.g., glucose metabolism is more oxygen efficient than fat metabolism), a marked decrease fatty acid metabolism appears to be maladaptive. The decrease in fatty acid metabolism may be detrimental because the heart can produce more ATP from each long-chain fatty acid compared with each glucose molecule. So, a marked downregulation of myocardial fatty acid enzymes and fatty acid metabolism would result in less energy production for the failing heart.

Genomic Analysis

Genomic analysis of enzymes of lipid metabolism has the potential to contribute to both diagnosis and prognosis in heart failure. At least a dozen separate inherited disorders of mitochondrial fatty acid β-oxidation have been described in humans (Table 20-1).[69] The severe clinical manifestations of these inborn errors in human fatty acid oxidizing enzymes include dilated cardiomyopathy and sudden death, underlining the importance of *normal* fatty acid metabolism for *normal* function of the *normal* heart.[70] The most commonly recognized defect is medium-chain acyl-CoA dehydrogenase (MCAD) deficiency. In addition, polymorphisms of the PPARα gene have been shown to influence human LV growth

TABLE 20-1 Defects of Mitochondrial Fatty Acid Oxidation

Fatty acid oxidation defect
Muscular CPT (adult-onset CPT II) deficiency
Hepatic CPT (CPT I) deficiency
MCAD deficiency
LCAD deficiency
ETF deficiency
ETF: QO deficiency
SCAD deficiency
LCHAD deficiency
Carnitine transport defect
2,4-Dienoyl-CoA reductase deficiency
Hepatomuscular CPT (infantile CPT II) deficiency
Carnitine/acylcarnitine translocase deficiency
SCHAD deficiency

Adapted from Coates PM, Tanaka K. Molecular basis of mitochondrial fatty acid oxidation defects. *J Lipid Res* 1992;33:1099-1110.

Abbreviations: *CPT,* carnitine palmitoyltransferase; *CPT II,* carnitine palmitoyltransferase II; *CPT I,* carnitine palmitoyltransferase I; *MCAD,* medium-chain acyl-CoA dehydrogenase; *LCAD,* long-chain acyl-CoA dehydrogenase; *ETF,* electron transfer flavoprotein; *QO,* ubiquinone oxidoreductase; *SCAD,* short-chain acyl-CoA dehydrogenase; *LCHAD,* long-chain 3-hydroxyacyl-CoA dehydrogenase; *SCHAD,* short-chain 3-hydroxyacyl-CoA dehydrogenase.

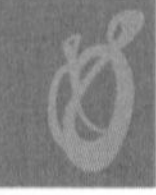

in response to exercise and hypertension[71] and to modify the response to β-blockers in patients with recent myocardial infarction.[72] Further characterization of the phenotypic impact of polymorphisms within metabolic regulatory proteins has prognostic and therapeutic potential for patients with heart failure.

METABOLIC ADAPTATION AND MALADAPTATION OF THE HEART

Perhaps one of the most exciting developments in the field of cardiac metabolism is the recognition that the heart possesses defined mechanisms to adapt to external stimuli. Sustained and/or multiple stimuli may also lead to metabolic remodeling and maladaptation of the heart.

Steps Leading to Metabolic Remodeling

Studies carried out in isolated perfused heart preparations have shown that the heart responds to changes in its environment by redirecting substrate fluxes through those pathways that are energetically most efficient in a given metabolic or physiological environment. Examples are the suppression of glucose oxidation when there is an oversupply of fatty acids, and conversely, the suppression of long-chain fatty acid oxidation in the presence of high concentrations of glucose and insulin.[5] An acute increase in the workload of the heart results in instantaneous mobilization and oxidation of glycogen and a shift from fat to carbohydrates (glucose and lactate) as the main fuel for respiration.[73] In the heart, in vivo, this shift is tied to greater efficiency of energy conversion.[74]

Sustained changes in the heart's environment, caused by altering substrate supply or by changing LV pressure, induce isoform-specific switches in sarcomeric and metabolic proteins.[75] Qualitative and quantitative changes in metabolic gene expression result in a shift from fat to glucose in the hypertrophied and atrophied heart.[76] In contrast, the heart in obesity and diabetes further increases its reliance on fatty acids as fuel for respiration,[77] changes that are orchestrated at least in part through altered expression of metabolic genes.

The dynamic nature of this oscillation between uses of different substrates is not always appreciated. As outlined previously, this adaptation can either be acute (alterations in preexisting proteins) or chronic (alterations in gene expression, remodeling), depending upon the intensity and duration of the stimulus.[60] It is reasonable to propose that metabolic adaptation often precedes or parallels functional adaptation of the heart. While this metabolic change may initially be generally adaptive to a stimulus in the short-term, it may also have detrimental effects over the long-term and lead to contractile dysfunction and failure (maladaptation).

Hypertrophy from Pressure Overload

The impact of workload on cardiac metabolism, gene expression, and function has been intensely studied. Alterations in workload on the heart have both acute and chronic effects on myocardial metabolism. When the workload is increased, the heart rapidly responds by increasing the flux of carbon through metabolic pathways. In doing so, the heart balances the rates of energy-generating reactions (e.g., oxidative phosphorylation) with that of energy-consuming reactions (e.g., cross-bridge cycling). More specifically, increased workload on the heart rapidly results in increased glucose uptake, glycogenolysis, glycolytic flux, and pyruvate oxidation (whether derived from extracellular glucose, extracellular lactate, or intracellular glycogen), with little effect on fatty acid oxidation.[78]

If the increased workload on the heart is sustained, the heart responds with characteristic alterations in morphology, increased cell size, and gene expression (e.g., reexpression of fetal genes), paralleled by a process of metabolic remodeling. In general terms, the hypertrophied heart increases its reliance on glucose as a fuel, while decreasing fatty acid oxidation.[79] This upregulation of glucose metabolism occurs even before there is an increase in LV mass.[80] Somewhat unexpectedly, with a sustained *decrease* in workload, the heart also responds with an upregulation of glucose metabolism.[76] It appears that any sustained changes in workload results in similar patterns of metabolic remodeling and in a switch from an energetically less efficient (fatty acids) to an energetically more efficient (glucose) fuel for respiration.

Two important questions arise when considering metabolic adaptation of the hypertrophied heart. (1) What is the mechanism for substrate switching and (2) why does substrate switching occur? In the past, mechanistic studies of substrate switching have focused on the regulation of the pyruvate dehydrogenase complex (PDC). Recent evidence suggests, however, that the nuclear receptor PPARα plays a key regulatory role in substrate switching,[81] whereas PDC activity remains relatively unaffected in response to sustained pressure overload. PPARα binds to the promoter of, and subsequently induces the transcription of, multiple genes encoding for proteins involved in fatty acid metabolism. These include fatty acid translocase (FAT/CD36), heart-specific fatty acid binding protein (hFABP), acyl-CoA synthetase I (ACSI), malonyl-CoA decarboxylase (MCD), muscle-specific carnitine palmitoyltransferase I (mCPTI), medium-chain acyl-CoA dehydrogenase (MCAD), and long-chain acyl-CoA dehydrogenase (LCAD). PPARα is itself activated by fatty acids, thereby forming a positive feed-forward mechanism for fatty acid–induced fatty acid oxidation. Pressure overload represses this mechanism by decreasing the expression of PPARα itself, and its coactivator, PGC1. PPARα-DNA binding activity is also reduced through covalent modification (phosphorylation) in response to pressure overload. The result is decreased expression of fatty acid metabolizing genes in the hypertrophied heart, and therefore decreased fatty acid oxidation capacity. In addition, several other transcription factors (e.g., Sp1, Coup-TF) known to be activated in the response to pressure overload have been implicated in the repression of fatty acid oxidation genes.[82] What is less clear is the mechanism by which reliance on glucose as a metabolic fuel increases in the hypertrophied heart. One possibility is that the increased glucose oxidation is the result of decreased fatty acid oxidation through a mechanism complementing the one described nearly 40 years ago by Randle and his group.[7] In the normal heart, fatty acids suppress glucose oxidation to a greater extent than glycolysis, and glycolysis to a greater extent than glucose uptake. Conversely, glucose also suppresses fatty acid oxidation[5] through a mechanism that involves malonyl-CoA-induced inhibition of the fatty acid transporter protein CPTI.[83] Although increased glycolytic rates in the hypertrophied heart are consistent with the Randle hypothesis, rates of pyruvate oxidation are not increased to the same extent,[84] and insulin's effects on glucose oxidation are attenuated.[85] Therefore, a loss of coordination between glucose oxidation and glycolysis exists. Other potential factors involved in increased glucose use in response to pressure overload include decreased expression of PDK4 (a PPARα target gene), chronic activation of AMPK, and elevated cytosolic levels of Ca^{2+}.[86]

Why does substrate switching occur in the hypertrophied heart? A classic explanation for this phenomenon is at the energetic level. Glucose is a more efficient energy source compared with fatty acids (i.e., more ATP generated per O_2 consumed). This is particularly important when oxygen demand outstrips oxygen supply, as may be the case in the hypertrophied heart. Furthermore, evidence exists suggesting that glycolytically derived ATP is preferentially used by ion channels, the activities of which are increased in the hypertrophied heart. However, substrate switching may have roles beyond its stereotypical function as a provider of ATP, potentially creating essential signals within the cardiomyocyte required for adaptation and remodeling. For example, as mentioned previously, fatty acids affect the expression of several target genes through transcription factor activation. Work performed in the liver as a model system for metabolically controlled gene transcription has shown that glucose metabolites alter the expression of specific genes, such as pyruvate kinase, acetyl CoA-carboxylase α, and fatty acid synthase.[87] Specific glucose-sensing transcription factors (e.g., SP1, USF) become activated through reversible covalent modification (phosphorylation and/or glycosylation) when glucose metabolites accumulate within the cell.[88] These transcription factors are present in the heart, and both are activated in response to pressure overload.[75] Evidence is accumulating for their involvement in the induction of several fetal genes.[89] Glucose has also been suggested to be involved in the induction of growth factors and the activation of translation factors, and may therefore be involved in the trophic response to pressure overload. Indeed, heart-specific overexpression of GLUT1 or the knockout of hFABP in the heart results in substrate switching and cardiac hypertrophy, suggesting increased glucose use is sufficient to trigger the hypertrophic response.[90]

As outlined previously, it appears that metabolic adaptation, including a switch to glucose use, may be important for the heart not only as a means of efficient ATP generation, but also for the generation of intracellular signals involved in the hypertrophic response to pressure overload. PPARα plays a key role in this substrate switching, since activation of PPARα in the hypertrophied heart prevents downregulation of fatty acid oxidation and blocks the increased reliance on glucose in response to pressure overload in rats.[91] Such PPARα activation results in contractile dysfunction in the hypertrophied heart, supporting the idea that switching to glucose use is essential for the heart to maintain contractile function in response to pressure overload. Furthermore, the induction of the fetal gene skeletal α-actin was abolished by PPARα activation. The activation of this contractile protein in response to pressure overload has previously been shown to be dependent upon the activation of the glucose-sensing transcription factor, Sp1. Despite the block of metabolic and gene expression adaptation, the trophic response to pressure overload was unaffected by PPARα activation.[91] Increased reliance on myocardial glucose metabolism therefore appears essential for the maintenance of contractile function and the initially adaptive trophic response to pressure overload.

METABOLIC REMODELING OF THE HEART IN OBESITY, INSULIN RESISTANCE, AND DIABETES

Adaptation and Maladaptation of the Heart in Obesity

There is increasing awareness of the link between obesity and cardiovascular disease (see Chapter 22), and cardiac remodeling in obesity.[92] Obesity is a growing public health concern, and affects approximately one third of the U.S. population and a growing percentage worldwide. Obesity is also a major risk factor for the development of heart failure. It is estimated that between 11% and 14% of all heart failure is due to obesity alone, and that a much greater percentage of all heart failure is due to obesity and its frequent comorbidities, diabetes, hypertension, and coronary disease.[93] In morbidly obese patients, overfeeding the heart with energy-providing substrates results in the accumulation of triglycerides in cardiac myocytes and impaired contractile function. This is not a new concept. "Fat in all the wrong places"[94] was already described by Virchow who observed in his *Cellular Pathology* that "genuine fatty degeneration (metamorphosis) of the heart is a real transformation of its substance, going on in the interior of the fibers."[95] Although extreme cardiac fatty metamorphosis (adipositas cordis), manifested by a heart so stuffed with lipids that it floats in water, is relatively rare, impairment of myocardial triglyceride and fatty acid metabolism on a more modest scale also appears to have deleterious effects on the function of the heart.[96]

"Lipotoxicity" in a general sense describes the effects of excessive uptake of fatty acids by the heart. When first described in animal models, however, lipotoxicity referred to a specific pathway in which increased fatty acid uptake exceeded β-oxidation and led to fatty acid *deposition*, ceramide production, increased iNOS activity, and apoptosis.[75] Since this initial description, it has been discovered that fatty acid *deposition*-induced apoptosis may also result from reactive oxygen species generation[97] (Figure 20-11). Excessive fatty acid *oxidation* may also play a role in the development of obesity-related cardiac dysfunction through pathways that do not result in apoptosis. For example, a study of *db/db* mice showed that increased myocardial fatty acid oxidation precedes contractile dysfunction, suggesting that excessive fatty acid oxidation may contribute to dysfunction. A mouse model with transgenic overexpression of a fatty acid transport protein in the heart also demonstrated increased cardiac fatty acid oxidation, leading to diastolic cardiac dysfunction.[98] Excessive free radical generation from oxidative processes in general may contribute to dysfunctional calcium handling and dysfunction rather than apoptosis-induced dysfunction.[99]

In humans, there is growing evidence that alterations in myocardial fatty acid metabolism accompany decreased cardiac function. Fat deposition has been demonstrated in pathological examination of failing human hearts from obese and diabetic patients.[100] This fat deposition can now be measured in vivo noninvasively, using ^{1}H-NMR as described previously.[37] Fat deposition may be reversible, as shown in one study of obese, diabetic patients placed on a very low-calorie diet, in whom a decrease in myocardial lipid accumulation was accompanied by an improvement in diastolic function.[101] Nonetheless, it remains unclear whether the lipid deposition per se results in human cardiac dysfunction, or if it is a marker of an altered metabolic milieu and myocardial metabolic metabolism that leads to dysfunction. Obesity and its frequent comorbidity, insulin resistance, also are associated with increased myocardial fatty acid uptake, use, and oxidation in asymptomatic young women without frank cardiac systolic dysfunction compared with age-matched controls.[102] Weight loss can decrease the high rates of myocardial fatty acid metabolism associated with obesity.[103] Weight loss (from bariatric surgery or diet therapy) also improves whole body metabolic abnormalities, cardiac diastolic dysfunction, and occasionally systolic function.[104] The fact that weight loss results in an improvement in diastolic and sometimes systolic dysfunction suggests that in humans, apoptosis is not likely the predominant mechanism by which obesity causes heart failure.[105]

Adaptation and Maladaptation of the Heart in Diabetes

Although the question whether there is a diabetes-specific cardiomyopathy has been debated for decades (see Chapter 26), there is increasing evidence that diabetes has detrimental

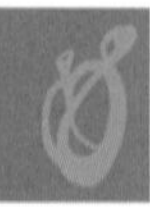

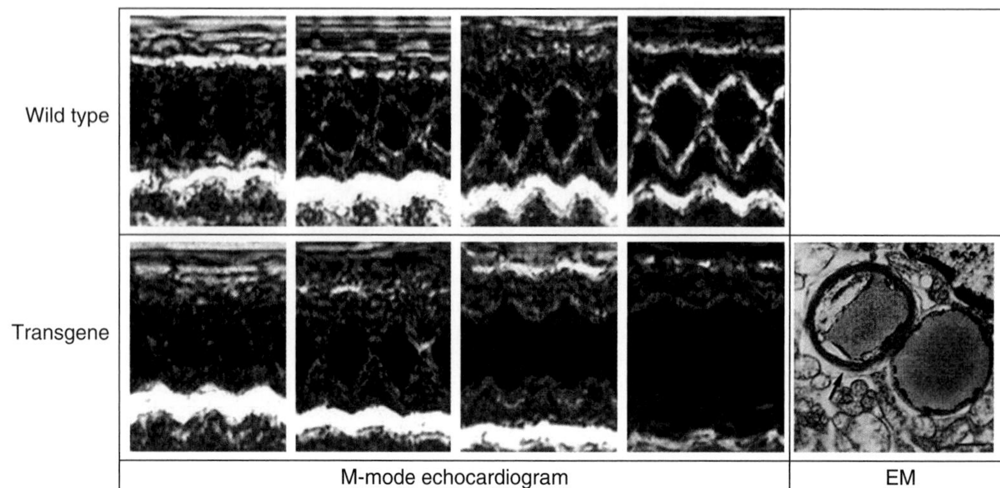

FIGURE 20-11 Cardiac hypertrophy and failure in a mouse heart model of lipotoxicity. The panels are (from left to right) serial 2-dimensional guided M-mode echocardiographic images obtained from wild-type *(upper panel)* and MHC-ACS1 07 *(lower panel)* mice at 2, 3, 4, and 6 weeks of age. Images shown are from a representative pair of age- and sex-matched wild-type transgenic animals. The last panel on the right is a transmission electronmicrograph of cardiac tissue from 18-day-old MHC-ACS mice shown at 15,000× magnification. Numerous lipid droplets are observed in ventricular myocytes. Some droplets at this stage are surrounded by multiple concentric layers of membrane *(arrow)*. (Modified with permission from Chiu HC, Kovacs A, Ford DA, et al. A novel mouse model of lipotoxic cardiomyopathy. *J Clin Invest* 2001;107:813-822.)

effects on cardiac function not accounted for by coronary or other cardiac disease. Patients with diabetes mellitus have an increased lifetime risk of congestive heart failure[106] and are overrepresented in large heart failure databases.[107] Other evidence for a "diabetic cardiomyopathy" in humans includes a number of morphological, functional, energetic, and biochemical observations. Moreover, heart disease in general is the leading cause of death among patients with diabetes mellitus. This excess heart disease is observed both in patients with type 1, characterized by severe impairment or absence of insulin secretion, and in patients with type 2, characterized by a combination of peripheral tissue insulin resistance and inadequate compensatory insulin secretion. Insulin resistance is a feature of both types of diabetes.

The prevalence of type 2 diabetes has increased dramatically in parallel with the obesity epidemic.[75,108] Thus the adaptation of the heart in diabetes warrants further discussion. There is a depression of glucose oxidation in the diabetic heart. This is likely due to inhibition of PDC. The activity of PDC is affected by both allosteric modulation and covalent modification. In the diabetic state, increased fatty acid and ketone body use results in increased intramitochondrial acetyl-CoA levels, which allosterically inhibit PDC. Furthermore, activation of PPARα by fatty acids induces pyruvate dehydrogenase kinase 4 (PDK4), which phosphorylates and inhibits PDC.[91] Despite the apparent opposite metabolic adaptation, the heart in diabetes shows gene expression of myosin isoforms that is similar to that of the pressure-overloaded heart.[109] In pressure overload, the reexpression of these particular fetal genes is proposed to be due to increased glucose metabolites within the cardiomyocytes involved in the induction of fetal genes. At first sight this does not seem to be consistent with the diabetic heart's metabolic profile. However, if there is hyperglycemia, the rate of glucose transport in the hearts of diabetic animals is often similar to that of normal animals because substrate use is very dependent on plasma substrate concentration. Due to the severe attenuation of pyruvate oxidation, glucose oxidation rates are lower than rates of glucose uptake, resulting in the accumulation of glycolytic intermediates in the heart during diabetes. Thus in diabetes, myocardial glucose uptake and oxidation are not as tightly coupled as in the normal heart, which has consequences on cardiac gene expression.

It is also very evident that diabetes is as much a disorder of fatty acid metabolism as it is a disorder of glucose metabolism.[110] Just like in the fasted state, the normal heart oxidizes predominantly fatty acids.[111] In the diabetic milieu, the increased fatty acid availability is accompanied by even greater rates of fatty acid oxidation.[112] Current concepts support the view that the greater reliance on fat oxidation in the diabetic heart is due to activation of PPARα and subsequent induction of PPARα-regulated fatty acid oxidation enzymes.[113] For example, induction of MCD in the heart of streptozotocin-induced diabetic rats (a model of type I diabetes) likely plays a role in the decreased malonyl-CoA levels (an inhibitor of fatty acyl-CoA entry into the mitochondrion) and increased fatty acid oxidation.[114] Models of type 2 diabetes also demonstrate an increase in myocardial fatty acid oxidation at a young age and lipid accumulation at older ages.[115] As mentioned in the section previously discussed on obesity, this increase in fatty acid oxidation and/or lipid accumulation may have direct, lipotoxic effects on cardiac function. However, β-oxidation of fatty acids may not always match excessive fatty acid delivery to the heart, resulting in subsequent elevation of intracellular fatty acids and lipids, which have been associated with diabetic cardiomyopathy in rodent models.[116] In this respect, the diabetic heart appears similar to the obese heart, although some studies suggest that the former has even greater fat accumulation (Figure 20-12).[100] There appear to be multiple mechanisms that contribute to this type of lipid accumulation-driven lipotoxicity, including chronically activated PKCs, generation of reactive oxygen species (ROS), and ceramide-induced apoptosis. In addition, it is not surprising that dysregulation of myocardial fatty acid metabolism may decrease cardiac function in the diabetic heart, since fatty acids and fatty acid metabolites have multiple cellular functions (Figure 20-13). They are mediators of signal transduction (e.g., activation of various protein kinase C (PKC) isoforms, initiation of apoptosis), ligands for nuclear transcription factors (e.g., PPARα), and essential components of biological membranes.

Some of the more recent studies of the human heart in diabetes demonstrate similar metabolic features as seen in animal models. In patients with type I diabetes, there is an increase in myocardial oxygen consumption and fatty acid metabolism, and a lower glucose use/level of plasma insulin,

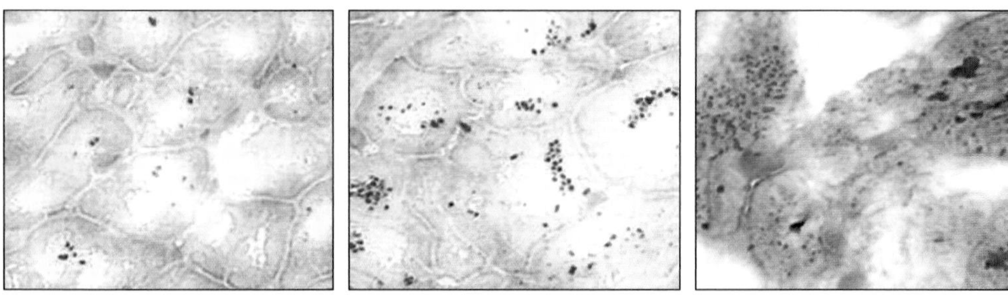

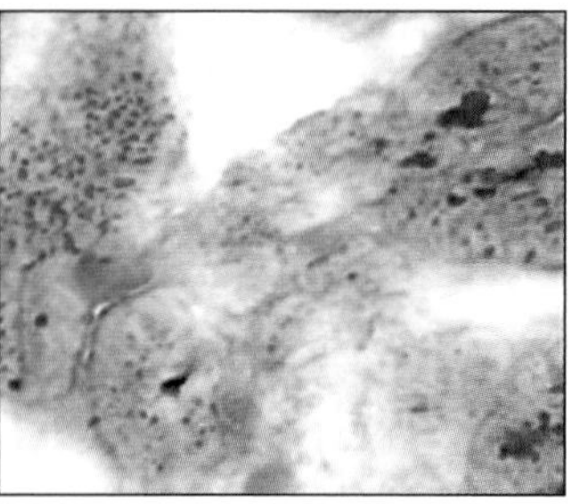

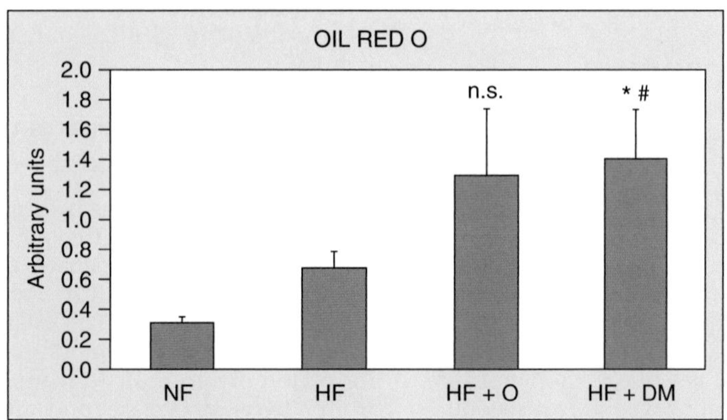

FIGURE 20-12 Cardiac lipotoxicity. *Top:* Photomicrographs of low, intermediate, and high lipid accumulation in the myocardium, as stained by Oil red O. *Bottom:* The amount of intramyocardial triglyceride in explanted hearts from nonfailing donors (NF) not suitable for transplant, nonobese heart failure patients(HF), obese heart failure patients (HF + O), and diabetic heart failure patients (HF + DM). The patients with diabetes and heart failure had higher intramyocardial fat levels (* $P < .05$). (Adapted from Sharma S, Androgue JV, Golfman L, et al: Intramyocardial lipid accumulation in the failing human heart resembles the lipotoxic rat heart. *FASEBJ*. 2004; 18:1692-1700.)

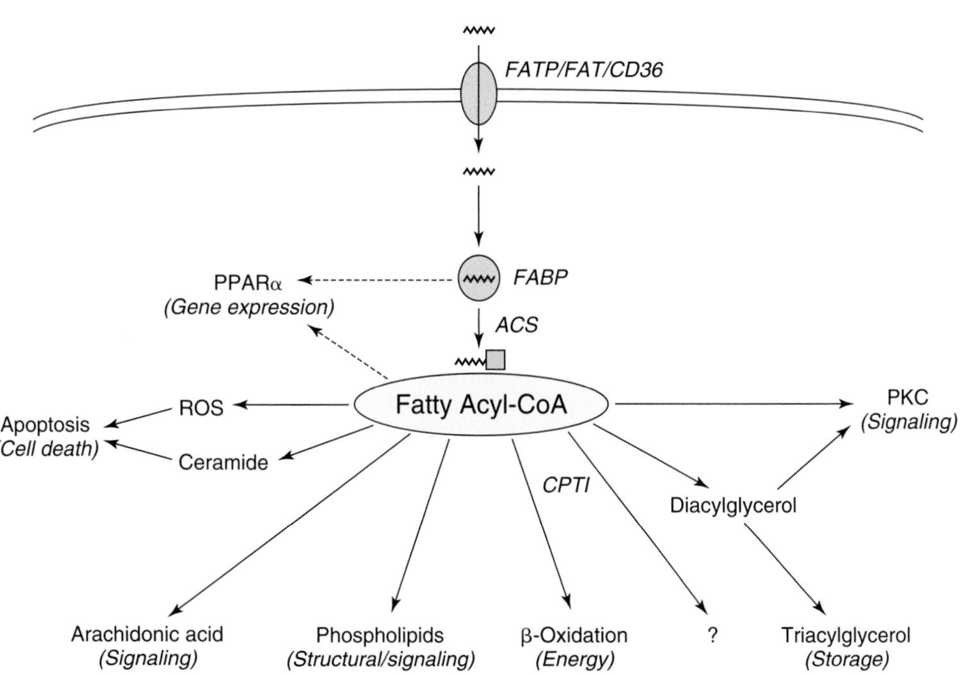

FIGURE 20-13 The multiple fates of activated fatty acids in the cardiac myocytes. See text for further discussion.

suggesting insulin resistance.[117,118] However, the myocardium can still respond to changes in insulin and free fatty acid levels by changing its substrate preference. This suggests that the metabolic regulatory phenomena such as the Randle cycle or "Randle phenomenon" still are germane to the diabetic heart. In patients with type 2 diabetes without heart failure, there is increased myocardial fatty acid use. In type 2 diabetics, there is also evidence of increased myocardial fatty acid accumulation.[100] As noted previously, lipid accumulation in diabetics without heart failure may be decreased with weight loss. Myocardial energetics in diabetes are also altered, with decreased PCr/ATP compared with controls. Moreover, this detrimentally altered energetic state *is directly related to impaired diastolic function.*[119] At least one study has also related hyperglycemia with diastolic dysfunction as well.[120] Whether therapies aimed at manipulating diabetes-induced alterations in myocardial metabolism and/or energetics improves cardiac function is as yet unknown.

To make matters more complicated, diabetes is often associated with hypertension, obesity, and the metabolic syndrome.[108] The addition of other pathophysiological conditions (particularly hypertension) on top of diabetes complicates and exacerbates its myocardial metabolic abnormalities. For example, induction of diabetes in rats with pressure-overload-induced hypertrophy results in rapid cardiac failure.[121] This phenomenon is similar to the observation that reactivation of PPARα in the hypertrophied heart results in contractile dysfunction.[91] The attenuation of fatty acid oxidation due to pressure overload and increased fatty acid availability because of concomitant diabetes theoretically should accelerate lipid deposition within the cardiomyocyte, thereby accelerating lipotoxicity. Thus forcing a hypertrophied heart to use fatty acids in the diabetic milieu results in a maladapted heart, exhibiting contractile dysfunction.

CROSSTALK BETWEEN CYTOKINE SIGNALING PATHWAYS, INNATE IMMUNITY, AND METABOLISM

Nitric Oxide: Effects on Metabolism

Since the identification of nitric oxide (NO) as an endothelial-derived relaxation factor (EDRF), which is a mediator of various vasodilatory agents, including bradykinin, the role of NO has been implicated in various cellular systems.[122] NO is a simple free radical gas with a relatively short half-life in biological systems (estimated at approximately 4 seconds) due to its high reactivity.[122] The ability of NO to diffuse freely through membranes enables it to have paracrine and autocrine functions (see Chapter 17).

Nitric oxide is a modulator of cardiac metabolism, both oxidative and nonoxidative. In the former case, NO inhibits mitochondrial oxygen consumption through its effects on aconitase, complexes I and II of the electron transport chain, and cytochrome *c* oxidase, most likely due to a direct interaction of NO with these iron-containing proteins.[123] Exposure of the heart to NO donors has been shown to inhibit oxygen consumption.[124] Conversely, inhibition of NOS with L-arginine analogues increases mitochondrial oxygen consumption.[124] Selective NOS isoform knockout mice suggest that NO derived from eNOS, the most highly expressed NOS isoform in the heart, acts as a physiological inhibitor of mitochondrial oxygen consumption.[125]

NO also affects glucose uptake and glycolytic flux. In contrast to skeletal muscle, NO appears to inhibit cardiac glucose metabolism.[126,127] Exposure of the heart to NO donors decreases glucose uptake, while glucose uptake is stimulated by NOS inhibitors.[126] In addition, eNOS knockout mouse hearts have elevated rates of glucose uptake when perfused *ex vivo,* compared with wild-type hearts. It has been postulated that these effects of NO are mediated by cGMP. Inhibition of the glycolytic enzyme, phosphofructokinase, by NO is also due to elevated intracellular cGMP levels and subsequent activation of cGMP-dependent protein kinase (PKG).

Results of studies regarding the effects of NO on fatty acid metabolism are mixed. Indirect observations suggest that the NO may decrease fatty acid oxidation. For example, activation of acetyl-CoA carboxylase by NO results in increased intracellular levels of malonyl-CoA, an inhibitor of long-chain fatty acyl-CoA transport into the mitochondrion.[126] As mitochondrial fatty acid metabolism is an aerobic process, the inhibition of the mitochondrial electron transport chain components by NO would presumably contribute to inhibition of β-oxidation. However, studies in the dog heart show both an increase in free fatty acid uptake and a decrease in the respiratory quotient (RQ) in response to NO donors, indicative of increased reliance on fatty acid oxidation.[124] This increased reliance on fatty acid oxidation with NO would fit well with the known decrease in glucose metabolism with NO stimulation.

The physiological relevance of nitric oxide signaling in the myocardium has been underscored by the observation that β-3 adrenergic signaling in the heart activates NO-generating pathways. The activation of β-3 receptors on cardiac myocytes reduces contractility through an NO-dependent mechanism,[128] consistent with the described effects of NO on metabolism. Nebivolol is a third-generation β-blocker that is a highly selective β-1 antagonist, but also a β-3 receptor agonist. This drug produces NO-dependent vasodilation and cardiodepression,[128] which in some circumstances is thought to improve the balance between energy delivery and use. The SENIORs trial investigated this drug in elderly patients with clinical heart failure and demonstrated a significant improvement in clinical outcomes related to therapy with nebivolol.[129]

Modulation of Myocardial Metabolism by Inflammatory Cytokines

In the past decade, it has been suggested that numerous cytokines are involved in the pathogenesis of heart failure.[130] Among these, tumor necrosis factor α (TNF-α) has received special attention (see Chapter 11). Although the precise mechanisms by which TNF-α and other cytokines elicit their effects on contractile function are still not fully understood, induction of apoptosis, uncoupling of β-adrenergic receptors from adenylate cyclase, and modulation of the extracellular matrix have emerged as possible candidates. In addition, cytokines have dramatic effects on cardiac energy metabolism.[131] Studies in cardiomyocytes have shown that both TNF-α and interleukin-1α inhibit mitochondrial respiration and decrease PDC activity.[132] In addition, interleukin-1β increases nonoxidative glucose metabolism and decreases mitochondrial enzyme activity (complex I and complex II).[133] The exact mechanisms by which these cytokines modulate energy substrate metabolism are not known, but may depend on the production of NO, the effects of which were discussed previously.

The effects of inflammatory signaling on myocardial metabolism and function are readily apparent in the syndrome of septic shock. It is now recognized that more than 50% of patients with bacterial sepsis will develop inflammatory-induced transient myocardial dysfunction.[129] The inflammatory cascade responsible for the syndrome of gram-negative sepsis is triggered by the host receptor TLR4, which recognizes bacterial lipopolysaccharide (LPS).[134] In animal models of sepsis, the injection of LPS produces LV dysfunction that is dependent on TLR4 activation.[146] The cardiometabolic effects of LPS include decreased fatty acid oxidation capacity and myocardial triglyceride accumulation.[147] Consistent with these observations, LPS downregulates the expression of genes involved in fatty acid oxidation including PPARα, ERRα, MCAD, and MCP-1.[148] In addition, the nuclear receptor coactivators PGC-1α and PGC-1β, which regulate fatty acid oxidation and mitochondrial function pathways, are profoundly downregulated during TLR4-induced inflammatory stress. Recent data suggest that LPS-mediated modulation of myocardial metabolism occurs through a PGC-1-dependent mechanism.

The suppression of myocardial fatty acid oxidation pathways by inflammation has been further illustrated in a transgenic mouse with cardiac-specific overexpression of TNF-α.[135] Similar to the acute model of LPS stimulation, TNF-α transgenic mice have reduced fatty acid oxidation capacity and downregulation of the genes encoding PGC-1α, PPARα, and many FAO enzymes. In this system, TNF induction of TGF-β was shown to mediate the observed downregulation of PPARα-mediated gene transcription through a Smad3-dependent mechanism. Taken together, it is clear that inflammatory signaling reprograms myocardial metabolism, leading

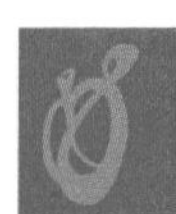

to reduced rates of fatty acid oxidation. In addition to direct relevance to sepsis-induced myocardial dysfunction, the crosstalk between inflammatory and metabolic pathways illustrated by LPS and TNF stimulation models may also be salient to the metabolic reprogramming observed in chronic heart failure, which is often associated with increased inflammation, particularly in end-stage heart failure.

Modulation of Programmed Cell Death and Cell Survival by Glucose and Fatty Acid Metabolites

Recent studies have shown that energy metabolism interacts with various pathways regulating programmed cell death and cell survival.[136] There is evidence to suggest that in the heart metabolites serve as signals for programs of adaptation and maladaptation (see Figure 20-1).[137-139] For example, the pleiotropic functions of glucose in the heart include a strong cardioprotective component. Provision of glucose during hypoxic stress,[140] overexpression of the glucose transporter GLUT1, and chronic hyperglycemia all reduce cardiac apoptosis.[153,154] With respect to the protective effects of glucose and insulin on cell function of the heart, three observations are of importance. First, in the reperfused heart, insulin itself increases postischemic cardiac power without increasing rates of glucose oxidation during early reperfusion.[141] This suggests that insulin itself improves the efficiency of the heart without a concomitant increase in rates of glucose oxidation and may be tied to the insulin signal transduction in cascade. Key regulators of this pathway are the insulin receptor, insulin receptor substrate (IRS), PI3 kinase, and Akt/protein kinase B.[142] PI3 kinase regulates cardiac growth,[143] while Akt activation reduces cardiomyocyte death and induces cardiac hypertrophy.[144] Downstream from the activation of mTOR and its targets is dependent on hexose 6-phosphate.[145] Akt is antiapoptotic and promotes both glucose uptake and glycogen synthesis.[146] Activation of Akt by insulin affords myocardial protection through the insulin signaling cascade,[147] and it appears that the inhibition of early apoptotic events by Akt is dependent upon the first committed step of glycolysis, and, more specifically, by the action of hexokinase II, which is bound to the mitochondria.[148] Increased hexokinase activity also protects against acute oxidant-induced cell death.[149]

Deletion of GLUT4 or glucose deprivation, on the other hand, enhances cardiac injury during ischemia.[30,150] Possible mechanisms by which glucose protects the cell from apoptosis include the prevention of intracellular Ca^{2+} accumulation, the activation of Akt,[144] and/or the upregulation of the antiapoptotic protein Bcl-2.[151] Three different pathways have been implicated in this response, including glucose deprivation-induced ATP depletion and stimulation of the mitochondrial death pathway cascade, hypoglycemia-induced oxidative stress and activation of the JNK/MAPK signaling pathways,[152] and glucose deprivation–induced stabilization of p53 leading to an increase in p53-associated apoptosis.[152]

In contrast to glucose, fatty acids are implicated in the induction of programmed cell death.[21] A study in Zucker diabetic fatty rats found that high levels of myocardial triacylglycerol were associated with increased DNA laddering (a marker of apoptosis).[153] Both myocardial triacylglycerol accumulation and DNA were attenuated by treating the animals with a lipid-lowering drug.[154] One proposed mechanism of lipoapoptosis is the increased synthesis of ceramide from palmitoyl acyl-CoA.[153] Ceramide is a potent inhibitor of complex III of the electron transport chain, and promotes the accumulation of reactive oxygen species (ROS).[155] Ceramide also upregulates iNOS expression, NO production, and peroxynitrite generation. The latter is an inducer of apoptosis.[153] Studies in cell culture have shown that fatty acid–induced apoptosis can also be regulated by ceramide-independent pathways. One such pathway appears to be mediated by the generation of ROS.[97]

Metabolism as a Target for Pharmacological Intervention in Heart Failure (see Chapter 50)

The complex and highly regulated network of metabolic pathways provides many potential targets for drug intervention. Prominent among those are drugs directed at shifting the heart's energy supply from oxidation of fatty acids to the more energy efficient oxidation of glucose. This shift can be brought about by either lowering fatty acid availability in the plasma, by inhibiting fatty acid oxidation, or by direct targeting of mitochondrial metabolism. Lastly, drugs may be aimed at the restoration of moiety-conserved cycles.

Trimetazidine

Trimetazidine, a piperazine compound, is an antianginal drug widely used in France, and belongs to the group of partial fatty acid oxidation inhibitors (so-called PFox inhibitors). Trimetazidine has cardioprotective effects in animal models of ischemia.[156] In clinical trials of chronic stable angina pectoris, trimetazidine was as effective as nifedipine and propranolol for the treatment of stable angina.[157] In contrast to nifedipine and propranolol, trimetazidine elicited beneficial effects independent of any hemodynamic changes.

Trimetazidine is cardioprotective because it modulates energy substrate metabolism, and it may also have antioxidative properties. Trimetazidine decreases long-chain fatty acid oxidation by inhibition of 3 ketoacyl-CoA thiolase.[158] This decrease in fatty acid oxidation leads to an increase in carbohydrate oxidation. This switch in energy substrate preference results in improved coupling between glycolysis and glucose oxidation, thereby decreasing proton and Na^+ accumulation. There are a few small clinical trials showing that trimetazidine improves heart failure.[159] In one randomized study, those heart failure patients receiving trimetazidine realized improvements in their functional class and LV function. In a PET study, trimetazidine modestly decreased myocardial fatty acid oxidation without changing overall oxygen consumption, implying but not proving an increase in glucose oxidation.[160] However, trimetazidine has limited availability and is not FDA approved for use in the United States.

Ranolazine

Like trimetazidine, ranolazine belongs to the family of piperazine derivatives, which partially inhibit fatty acid oxidation and hence enhance glucose oxidation.[161] There is also some evidence that ranolazine may reduce calcium overload in ischemic myocardium. Activity of PDC, a key regulator of glucose oxidation, increases after ranolazine treatment, most likely due to decreased inhibitory effects of end products of β-oxidation (NADH, acetyl-CoA)[162] or due to changes in the phosphorylation state. There are also data showing that ranolazine improves myocardial efficiency and LV systolic function in animal models of chronic heart failure.[163] To date there are no data on ranolazine's effects on myocardial metabolism in humans with heart failure, so it has no indication for heart failure treatment at present.

Lipid-Lowering Agents

Drugs and other therapies, such as weight loss, that decrease fatty acid and/or triglyceride delivery to the heart are attractive targets for decreasing excessive myocardial fatty acid uptake and accumulation. Weight loss decreases myocardial fatty acid use in obese humans.[103] Thiazolidinediones (predominantly PPARγ agonists) reduce plasma lipid levels and (in one study) increase myocardial glucose use. However, results regarding their effect on steatosis are mixed, with some studies demonstrating decreased and others showing increased lipid accumulation in nonadipose tissues.[164,165] Another drug, acipimox, known to markedly and acutely decrease plasma free fatty acid levels, *impaired* cardiac efficiency and cardiac work in dilated cardiomyopathy patients.[166] However, the patients in this study would not have been expected to have excessive cardiac fatty acid metabolism before treatment since they were not diabetic. Thus it is perhaps not surprising that they did not benefit. It may be that patients with heart failure related to underlying diabetes and obesity, who have marked myocardial lipid abnormalities at the outset, may have the most to gain from lipid-lowering therapies.

Propionyl-L-Carnitine

Propionyl-L-carnitine (PLC) has been shown to improve postischemic contractile performance in the heart, presumably through redistribution of long-chain acyl-CoA esters to less toxic intermediates.[167,168] In the failing heart, PLC may improve energy metabolism by three possible mechanisms. First, PLC provides propionate. As a precursor of succinyl-CoA, propionate may replenish citric acid cycle intermediates.[169] Secondly, PLC may raise the levels of free CoASH and improves flux through α-ketoglutarate dehydrogenase. Third, PLC may redistribute carnitine levels between cytosol and mitochondria and improve fatty acid oxidation in the stressed heart.[170] Collectively, it appears that PLC (and possibly also carnitine[171]) improves substrate flux, and possibly also contractile function of the heart. Indeed, alterations in substrate metabolism produced by carnitine deficiency result in inadequate ATP production under high workload conditions that cause impaired cardiac contractile performance, and carnitine deficiency may also induce a number of changes in gene expression of key enzymes required for normal cardiac function and metabolism.[172,173] Chronic cardiomyopathy has been described in children with a defect in carnitine uptake,[174] and systemic carnitine deficiency has been identified as a treatable cardiomyopathy.[175]

SUMMARY AND OUTLOOK

The human heart is an efficient energy converter and consumes several kilograms of ATP each day.[1] ATP production is linked to a highly regulated system of energy substrate metabolism and is tightly coupled to both oxygen consumption and contractile function of the heart. Intermediary metabolites provide essential signals for pathways of adaptation and maladaptation of the heart to external stimuli (Figure 20-14).

Because heart failure is a systemic disease that begins and ends with the heart, an appreciation of the principles of myocardial energy metabolism seems critical for the understanding of heart failure. At the present time we possess a wealth of information on the biochemistry of the heart. To a large extent it still has to be determined how this information can be integrated into the diagnosis and management of heart failure. Defective energy metabolism of the heart is both cause and consequence of heart failure and can be detected in the whole heart by noninvasive methods, or in myocardial biopsy samples by gene or protein expression assays or by biochemical analyses. Pharmacological and nutritional interventions targeted at the specific myocardial metabolic alterations of particular causes of heart failure hold promise for reversing defective energy metabolism and improving contractile function of the heart. An appreciation of the pivotal role of metabolism in the process of adaptation and maladaptation of the heart to external stimuli provides essential clues for the pathophysiology and treatment of heart failure.

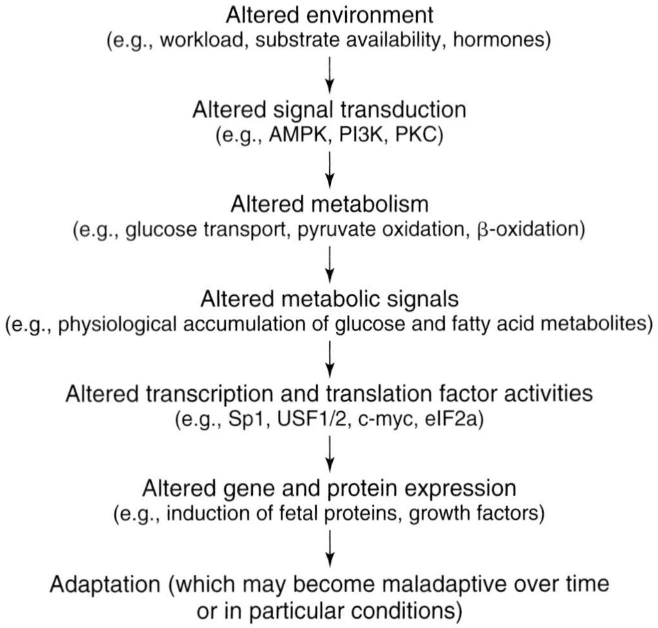

Altered environment
(e.g., workload, substrate availability, hormones)
↓
Altered signal transduction
(e.g., AMPK, PI3K, PKC)
↓
Altered metabolism
(e.g., glucose transport, pyruvate oxidation, β-oxidation)
↓
Altered metabolic signals
(e.g., physiological accumulation of glucose and fatty acid metabolites)
↓
Altered transcription and translation factor activities
(e.g., Sp1, USF1/2, c-myc, eIF2a)
↓
Altered gene and protein expression
(e.g., induction of fetal proteins, growth factors)
↓
Adaptation (which may become maladaptive over time or in particular conditions)

FIGURE 20-14 The sequence of steps leading from altered environment to altered gene and protein expression. See text for details.

REFERENCES

1. Taegtmeyer, H. (1994). Energy metabolism of the heart: from basic concepts to clinical applications. *Curr Prob Cardiol*, *19*, 57–116.
2. Neubauer, S. (2007). The failing heart–an engine out of fuel. *N Engl J Med*, *356*, 1140–1151.
3. Barger, P. M., Browning, A. C., Garner, A. N., et al. (2001). p38 Mitogen-activated protein kinase activates peroxisome proliferator-activated receptor alpha: a potential role in the cardiac metabolic stress response. *J Biol Chem*, *276*, 44495–44501.
4. Holmes, F. L. (1992). *Between biology and medicine: the formation of intermediary metabolism*. Berkeley, Calif: University of California at Berkeley.
5. Taegtmeyer, H., Hems, R., & Krebs, H. A. (1980). Utilization of energy-providing substrates in the isolated working rat heart. *Biochem J*, *186*, 701–711.
6. Taegtmeyer, H., & Lesch, M. (1980). Altered protein and amino acid metabolism in myocardial hypoxia and ischemia. In K. Wildenthal (Ed.). *Degradative processes in heart and skeletal muscle*. New York: Elsevier/North Holland Biomedical Press.
7. Hue, L., & Taegtmeyer, H. (2009). The Randle cycle revisited: a new head for an old hat. *Am J Physiol Endocrinol Metab*, *297*, E578–E591.
8. Langendorff, O. (1895). Untersuchungen am uberlebenden Saugethierherzen. *Pflugers Arch Gesamte Physiol Menschen Tiere*, *61*, 291–332.
9. Rohde, E. (1912). Über den Einfluss der mechanischen Bedingungen auf die Tätigkeit und den Sauerstoffverbrauch des Warmblüterherzens. *Naunyn Schmiedeberg's Arch Exp Pathol Pharmakol*, *68*, 401–410.
10. Bing, R. J., Siegel, A., Ungar, I., et al. (1954). Metabolism of the human heart. II. Studies on fat, ketone and amino acid metabolism. *Am J Med*, *16*, 504–515.
11. Gertz, E. W., Wisneski, J. A., Stanley, W. C., et al. (1988). Myocardial substrate utilization during exercise in humans. *J Clin Invest*, *82*, 2017–2025.
12. Lopaschuk, G. D., Collins-Nakai, R. L., & Itoi, T. (1992). Developmental changes in energy substrate use by the heart. *Cardiovasc Res*, *26*, 1172–1180.
13. Kates, A. M., Herrero, P., Dence, C., et al. (2003). Impact of aging on substrate metabolism by the human heart. *J Am Coll Cardiol*, *41*, 293–299.
14. Meerson, F. Z. (1974). Development of modern components of the mechanism of cardiac hypertrophy. *Circ Res*, *35*, 58–63.
15. Wollenberger, A., & Schulze, W. (1961). Mitochondrial alterations in the myocardium of dogs with aortic stenosis. *J Biophys Biochem Cytol*, *10*, 285.
16. Page, E., & McCallister, L. P. (1973). Quantitative electron microscopic description of heart muscle cells. *Am J Cardiol*, *31*, 172.
17. Zak, R., & Rabinowitz, M. (1979). Molecular aspects of cardiac hypertrophy. *Annu Rev Physiol*, *41*, 539–552.
18. Sordahl, L. A., Liddicoat, J. E., Diethrich, E. B., et al. (1970). Respiratory activity of mitochondria from isolated human and dog hearts maintained in a portable preservation chamber. *J Mol Cell Cardiol*, *1*, 379–388.
19. Krebs, H. A., Williamson, D. H., Bates, M. W., et al. (1971). The role of ketone bodies in caloric homeostasis. In G. Weber (Ed.), *Advances in enzyme regulations*. New York: Pergamon Press.
20. Doria, A., Nosadini, R., Avogaro, A., et al. (1991). Myocardial metabolism in type 1 diabetic patients without coronary artery disease. *Diabet Med*, *8*, Spec No: S104–S107.
21. Unger, R. H., & Orci, L. (2001). Diseases of liporegulation: new perspective on obesity and related disorders. *FASEB J*, *15*, 312–321.
22. Cooney, G. J., Taegtmeyer, H., & Newsholme, E. A. (1981). Tricarboxylic acid cycle flux and enzyme activities in the isolated working rat heart. *Biochem J*, *200*, 701–703.
23. Taegtmeyer, H. (1978). Metabolic responses to cardiac hypoxia: increased production of succinate by rabbit papillary muscles. *Circ Res*, *43*, 808–815.

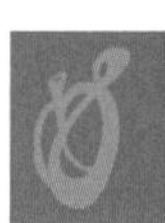

24. Bolukoglu, H., Goodwin, G. W., Guthrie, P. H., et al. (1996). Metabolic fate of glucose in reversible low-flow ischemia of the isolated working rat heart. *Am J Physiol, 270*, H817–H826.
25. Fell, D. (1997). *Understanding the control of metabolism*. Miami: Portland Press.
26. Brown, G. C. (1992). Control of respiration and ATP synthesis in mammalian mitochondria and cells. *Biochem J, 284*, 1–13.
27. Newsholme, E. A., & Start, C. (1973). *Regulation in metabolism*. London: J Wiley & Sons.
28. Hardie, D. G., & Carling, D. (1997). The AMP-activated protein kinase–fuel gauge of the mammalian cell?. *Eur J Biochem, 246*, 259–273.
29. Russell, R. R., Bergeron, R., Shulman, G. I., et al. (1999). Translocation of myocardial GLUT-4 and increased glucose uptake through activation of AMPK by AICAR. *Am J Physiol, 277*, H643–H649.
30. Tian, R., Musi, N., D'Agostino, J., et al. (2001). Increased adenosine monophosphate-activated protein kinase activity in rat hearts with pressure-overload hypertrophy. *Circulation, 104*, 1664–1669.
31. Winterstein, H. (1904). Ueber die Sauerstoffatmung des isolierten Saeugetierherzens. *Z Allg Physiol, 4*, 339–359.
32. Evans, C. L., & Matsuoka, Y. (1915). The effect of various mechanical conditions on the gaseous metabolism and efficiency of the mammalian heart. *J Physiol (Lond), 49*, 378–405.
33. Bing, R. J., Siegel, A., Vitale, A. G., et al. (1953). Metabolism of the human heart in vivo. *Am J Med, 15*, 284.
34. Blain, J. M. (1956). Studies in myocardial metabolism. VI. Myocardial metabolism in congestive heart failure. *Am J Med, 20*, 820–833.
35. Neubauer, S., Horn, M., Cramer, M., et al. (1997). Myocardial phosphocreatine-to-ATP ratio is a predictor of mortality in patients with dilated cardiomyopathy. *Circulation, 96*, 2190–2196.
36. Ashrafian, H., Redwood, C., Blair, E., et al. (2003). Hypertrophic cardiomyopathy: a paradigm for myocardial energy depletion. *Trends Genet, 19*, 263–268.
37. Szczepaniak, L. S., Dobbins, R. L., Metzger, G. J., et al. (2003). Myocardial triglycerides and systolic function in humans: in vivo evaluation by localized proton spectroscopy and cardiac imaging. *Magn Reson Med, 49*, 417–423.
38. Nguyen, V. T., Mossberg, K. A., Tewson, T. J., et al. (1990). Temporal analysis of myocardial glucose metabolism by 2-[18F]fluoro-2-deoxy-D-glucose. *Am J Physiol, 259*, H1022–H1031.
39. Herrero, P., Dence, C. S., Coggan, A. R., et al. (2007). L-3-^{11}C-lactate as a PET tracer of myocardial lactate metabolism: a feasibility study. *J Nucl Med, 48*, 2046–2055.
40. Schelbert, H., Henze, E., & Sochor, H. (1986). Effects of substrate availability on myocardial 11C palmitate kinetics by positron emission tomography in normal subjects and patients with ventricular dysfunction. *Am Heart J, 111*, 1055–1065.
41. Kisrieva-Ware, Z., Coggan, A. R., Sharp, T. L., et al. (2009). Assessment of myocardial triglyceride oxidation with PET and 11C-palmitate. *J Nucl Cardiol, 16*, 411–421.
42. Schelbert, H. R. (2002). 18F-deoxyglucose and the assessment of myocardial viability. *Semin Nucl Med, 32*, 60–69.
43. Rajabi, M., Kassiotis, C., Razeghi, P., et al. (2007). Return to the fetal gene program protects the stressed heart: a strong hypothesis. *Heart Fail Rev, 12*, 331–343.
44. Davila-Roman, V. G., Vedala, G., Herrero, P., et al. (2002). Altered myocardial fatty acid and glucose metabolism in idiopathic dilated cardiomyopathy. *J Am Coll Cardiol, 40*, 271–277.
45. Geltman, E. M., Smith, J. L., Beecher, D., et al. (1983). Altered regional myocardial metabolism in congestive cardiomyopathy detected by positron tomography. *Am J Med, 74*, 773–785.
46. Bergmann, S. R., Herrero, P., Sciacca, R., et al. (2001). Characterization of altered myocardial fatty acid metabolism in patients with inherited cardiomyopathy. *J Inherit Metab Dis, 24*, 657–674.
47. Tuunanen, H., Kuusisto, J., Toikka, J., et al. (2007). Myocardial perfusion, oxidative metabolism, and free fatty acid uptake in patients with hypertrophic cardiomyopathy attributable to the Asp175Asn mutation in the alpha-tropomyosin gene: a positron emission tomography study. *J Nucl Cardiol, 14*, 354–365.
48. Eichhorn, E. J., & Bristow, M. R. (1996). Medical therapy can improve the biological properties of the chronically failing heart. A new era in the treatment of heart failure. *Circulation, 94*, 2285–2296.
49. Beanlands, R. S., Nahmias, C., Gordon, E., et al. (2000). The effects of beta(1)-blockade on oxidative metabolism and the metabolic cost of ventricular work in patients with left ventricular dysfunction: a double-blind placebo-controlled, positron-emission tomography study. *Circulation, 102*, 2070–2075.
50. Sack, M. N., Rader, T. A., Park, S., et al. (1996). Fatty acid oxidation enzyme gene expression is downregulated in the failing heart. *Circulation, 94*, 2837–2842.
51. Razeghi, P., Young, M. E., Alcorn, J. L., et al. (2001). Metabolic gene expression in fetal and failing human heart. *Circulation, 104*, 2923–2931.
52. Finck, B. N., & Kelly, D. P. (2007). Peroxisome proliferator-activated receptor gamma coactivator-1 (PGC-1) regulatory cascade in cardiac physiology and disease. *Circulation, 115*, 2540–2548.
53. Young, M. E., Patil, S., Ying, J., et al. (2001). Uncoupling protein 3 transcription is regulated by peroxisome proliferator-activated receptor (alpha) in the adult rodent heart. *FASEB J, 15*, 833–845.
54. Qi, C., Zhu, Y., & Reddy, J. K. (2000). Peroxisome proliferator-activated receptors, coactivators, and downstream targets. *Cell Biochem Biophys, 32*, 187–204.
55. Razeghi, P., Young, M. E., Cockrill, T. C., et al. (2002). Downregulation of myocardial myocyte enhancer factor 2C and myocyte enhancer factor 2C-regulated gene expression in diabetic patients with nonischemic heart failure. *Circulation, 106*, 407–411.
56. Burkart, E. M., Sambandam, N., Han, X., et al. (2007). Nuclear receptors PPARbeta/delta and PPARalpha direct distinct metabolic regulatory programs in the mouse heart. *J Clin Invest, 117*, 3930–3939.
57. Cheng, L., Ding, G., Qin, Q., et al. (2004). Cardiomyocyte-restricted peroxisome proliferator-activated receptor-delta deletion perturbs myocardial fatty acid oxidation and leads to cardiomyopathy. *Nat Med, 10*, 1245–1250.
58. Huss, J. M., Imahashi, K., Dufour, C. R., et al. (2007). The nuclear receptor ERRalpha is required for the bioenergetic and functional adaptation to cardiac pressure overload. *Cell Metab, 6*, 25–37.
59. Sihag, S., Cresci, S., Li, A. Y., et al. (2009). PGC-1alpha and ERRalpha target gene downregulation is a signature of the failing human heart. *J Mol Cell Cardiol, 46*, 201–212.
60. Taegtmeyer, H. (2000). Genetics of energetics: transcriptional responses in cardiac metabolism. *Ann Biomed Eng, 28*, 871–876.
61. Taylor, M., Wallhaus, T., DeGrado, T., et al. (2001). An evaluation of myocardial fatty acid and glucose uptake using PET with [18F]fluoro-6-thia-heptadecanoic acid. *J Nucl Med, 42*, 55–62.
62. Dzeja, P. P., Pucar, D., Redfield, M. M., et al. (1999). Reduced activity of enzymes coupling ATP-generating with ATP-consuming processes in the failing myocardium. *Mol Cell Biochem, 201*, 33–40.
63. Ning, X. H., Zhang, J., Liu, J., et al. (2000). Signaling and expression for mitochondrial membrane proteins during left ventricular remodeling and contractile failure after myocardial infarction. *J Am Coll Cardiol, 36*, 282–287.
64. Dorner, A., Schulze, K., Rauch, U., et al. (1997). Adenine nucleotide translocator in dilated cardiomyopathy: pathophysiological alterations in expression and function. *Mol Cell Biochem, 174*, 261–269.
65. Ide, T., Tsutsui, H., Hayashidani, S., et al. (2001). Mitochondrial DNA damage and dysfunction associated with oxidative stress in failing hearts after myocardial infarction. *Circ Res, 88*, 529–535.
66. Scheuer, J. (1993). Metabolic factors in myocardial failure. *Circulation, 87*, 54–57.
67. Finck, B. N., & Kelly, D. P. (2006). PGC-1 coactivators: inducible regulators of energy metabolism in health and disease. *J Clin Invest, 116*, 615–622.
68. Lai, L., Leone, T. C., Zechner, C., et al. (2008). Transcriptional coactivators PGC-1alpha and PGC-lbeta control overlapping programs required for perinatal maturation of the heart. *Genes Dev, 22*, 1948–1961.
69. Coates, P. M., & Tanaka, K. (1992). Molecular basis of mitochondrial fatty acid oxidation defects. *J Lipid Res, 33*, 1099–1110.
70. Kelly, D. P., & Strauss, A. W. (1994). Inherited cardiomyopathies. *N Engl J Med, 330*, 913–919.
71. Jamshidi, Y., Montgomery, H., Hense, H., et al. (2002). Peroxisome proliferator–activated receptor alpha gene regulates left ventricular growth in response to exercise and hypertension. *Circulation, 105*, 950–955.
72. Cresci, S., Jones, P. G., Sucharov, C. C., et al. (2009). Interaction between PPARA genotype and beta-blocker treatment influences clinical outcomes following acute coronary syndromes. *Pharmacogenomics, 9*, 1403–1417.
73. Goodwin, G. W., Cohen, D. M., & Taegtmeyer, H. (2001). [5-3H]glucose overestimates glycolytic flux in isolated working rat heart: role of the pentose phosphate pathway. *Am J Physiol Endocrinol Metab, 280*, E502–E508.
74. Korvald, C., Elvenes, O. P., & Myrmel, T. (2000). Myocardial substrate metabolism influences left ventricular energetics in vivo. *Am J Physiol Heart Circ Physiol, 278*, H1345–H1351.
75. Young, M. E., McNulty, P., & Taegtmeyer, H. (2002). Adaptation and maladaptation of the heart in diabetes: part II: potential mechanisms. *Circulation, 105*, 1861–1870.
76. Doenst, T., Goodwin, G. W., Cedars, A. M., et al. (2001). Load-induced changes in vivo alter substrate fluxes and insulin responsiveness of rat heart in vitro. *Metabolism, 50*, 1083–1090.
77. Stanley, W. C., Lopaschuk, G. D., & McCormack, J. G. (1997). Regulation of energy substrate metabolism in the diabetic heart. *Cardiovasc Res, 34*, 25–33.
78. Goodwin, G. W., Taylor, C. S., & Taegtmeyer, H. (1998). Regulation of energy metabolism of the heart during acute increase in heart work. *J Biol Chem, 273*, 29530–29539.
79. Allard, M. F., & Lopaschuk, G. D. (1996). Ischemia and reperfusion injury in the hypertrophied heart. *EXS, 76*, 423–441.
80. Taegtmeyer, H., & Overturf, M. L. (1988). Effects of moderate hypertension on cardiac function and metabolism in the rabbit. *Hypertension, 11*, 416–426.
81. Barger, P. M., Browning, A. C., Garner, A. N., et al. (2001). p38 MAP kinase activates PPAR(alpha): a potential role in the cardiac metabolic stress response. *J Biol Chem, 276*, 44495–44501.
82. van Bilsen, M., Van der Vusse, G. J., & Reneman, R. S. (1998). Transcriptional regulation of metabolic processes: implications for cardiac metabolism. *Pflugers Arch, 437*, 2–14.
83. McGarry, J. D., Mills, S. E., Long, C. S., et al. (1983). Observations on the affinity for carnitine and malonyl-CoA sensitivity of carnitine palmitoyl transferase I in animal and human tissues. Demonstration of the presence of malonyl-CoA in non-hepatic tissues of the rat. *Biochem J, 214*, 21–28.
84. Lydell, C. P., Chan, A., Wambolt, R. B., et al. (2002). Pyruvate dehydrogenase and the regulation of glucose oxidation in hypertrophied rat hearts. *Cardiovasc Res, 53*, 841–851.
85. Allard, M. F., Wambolt, R. B., Longnus, S. L., et al. (2000). Hypertrophied rat hearts are less responsive to the metabolic and functional effects of insulin. *Am J Physiol Endocrinol Metab, 279*, E487–E493.
86. Hayashi, T., Hirshman, M. F., Kurth, E. J., et al. (1998). Evidence for 5'AMP-activated protein kinase mediation of the effect of muscle contraction on glucose transport. *Diabetes, 47*, 1369–1373.
87. Girard, J., Ferre, P., & Foufelle, F. (1997). Mechanisms by which carbohydrates regulate expression of genes for glycolytic and lipogenic enzymes. *Annu Rev Nutr, 17*, 325–352.
88. Vaulont, S., Vasseur-Cognet, M., & Kahn, A. (2000). Glucose regulation of gene transcription. *J Biol Chem, 275*, 31555–31558.
89. Karns, L., Kariya, K., & Simpson, P. (1995). M-CAT, CArG, and Sp1 elements are required for alpha 1-adrenergic induction of the skeletal alpha-actin promoter during cardiac myocyte hypertrophy. Transcriptional enhancer factor-1 and protein kinase C as conserved transducers of the fetal program in cardiac growth. *J Biol Chem, 270*, 410–417.
90. Tian, R., D'Agostino, J., Jain, M., et al. (2000). Increasing basal glucose entry by cardiac-specific overexpression of GLUT1 causes hypertrophy and insulin resistance in mouse hearts. *Circulation, 102*(8) (abstract).

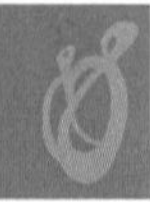

91. Young, M. E., Laws, F. A., Goodwin, G. W., et al. (2001). Reactivation of peroxisome proliferator-activated receptor alpha is associated with contractile dysfunction in hypertrophied rat heart. *J Biol Chem*, *276*, 44390–44395.
92. Abel, E. D., Litwin, S. E., & Sweeney, G. (2008). Cardiac remodeling in obesity. *Physiol Rev*, *88*, 389–419.
93. Kenchaiah, S., Evans, J. C., Levy, D., et al. (2002). Obesity and the risk of heart failure. *N Engl J Med*, *347*, 305–313.
94. Friedman, J. J. (2002). Fat in all the wrong places. *Nature*, *415*, 268–269.
95. Virchow, R. (1858). *Die Zellularpathologie und ihre Begründung auf physiologische und pathologische Gewebelehre*. Berlin: A Hirschwald.
96. Harmancey, R., Wilson, C. R., & Taegtmeyer, H. (2008). Adaptation and maladaptation of the heart in obesity. *Hypertension*, *52*, 181–187.
97. Listenberger, L. L., Ory, D. S., & Schaffer, J. E. (2001). Palmitate-induced apoptosis can occur through a ceramide-independent pathway. *J Biol Chem*, *276*, 14890–14895.
98. Chiu, H. C., Kovacs, A., Blanton, R. M., et al. (2005). Transgenic expression of fatty acid transport protein 1 in the heart causes lipotoxic cardiomyopathy. *Circ Res*, *96*, 225–233.
99. Andrade, F. H., Reid, M. B., & Westerblad, H. (2001). Contractile response of skeletal muscle to low peroxide concentrations: myofibrillar calcium sensitivity as a likely target for redox-modulation. *FASEB J*, *15*, 309–311.
100. Sharma, S., Adrogue, J. V., Golfman, L., et al. (2004). Intramyocardial lipid accumulation in the failing human heart resembles the lipotoxic rat heart. *FASEB J*, *18*, 1692–1700.
101. Hammer, S., Snel, M., Lamb, H. J., et al. (2008). Prolonged caloric restriction in obese patients with type 2 diabetes mellitus decreases myocardial triglyceride content and improves myocardial function. *J Am Coll Cardiol*, *52*, 1006–1012.
102. Peterson, L. R., Herrero, P., Schechtman, K. B., et al. (2004). Effect of obesity and insulin resistance on myocardial substrate metabolism and efficiency in young women. *Circulation*, *109*, 2191–2196.
103. Viljanen, A. P. M., Karmi, A., Borra, R., et al. (2009). Effect of calorie restriction on myocardial fatty acid uptake, left ventricular mass, and cardiac work in obese adults. *Am J Cardiol*, *103*, 1721–1726.
104. Leichman, J. G., Wilson, E. B., Scarborough, T., et al. (2008). Dramatic reversal of derangements in muscle metabolism and left ventricular function after bariatric surgery. *Am J Med*, *121*, 966–973.
105. Ramani, G. V., McCloskey, C., Ramanathan, R. C., et al. (2008). Safety and efficacy of bariatric surgery in morbidly obese patients with severe systolic heart failure. *Clin Cardiol*, *31*, 516–520.
106. Garcia, M. J., McNamara, P. M., Gordon, T., et al. (1974). Morbidity and mortality in diabetics in the Framingham population. Sixteen year follow-up study. *Diabetes*, *23*, 105–111.
107. Solang, L., Malmberg, K., & Ryden, L. (1999). Diabetes mellitus and congestive heart failure. Further knowledge needed. *Eur Heart J*, *20*, 789–795.
108. Taegtmeyer, H., McNulty, P., & Young, M. E. (2002). Adaptation and maladaptation of the heart in diabetes: part I: general concepts. *Circulation*, *105*, 1727–1733.
109. Depre, C., Young, M. E., Ying, J., et al. (2000). Streptozotocin-induced changes in cardiac gene expression in the absence of severe contractile dysfunction. *J Mol Cell Cardiol*, *32*, 985–996.
110. McGarry, J. D. (1992). What if Minkowski had been ageusic? An alternative angle on diabetes. *Science*, *258*, 766–770.
111. Bing, R. J. (1955). The metabolism of the heart. *Harvey Lect*, *50*, 27–70.
112. Ungar, I., Gilbert, M., Siegel, A., et al. (1955). Studies on myocardial metabolism: IV. Myocardial metabolism in diabetes. *Am J Med*, *18*, 385–396.
113. Finck, B. N., Lehman, J. J., Leone, T. C., et al. (2002). The cardiac phenotype induced by PPARα overexpression mimics that caused by diabetes mellitus. *J Clin Invest*, *109*, 121–130.
114. Sakamoto, J., Barr, R. L., Kavanagh, K. M., et al. (2000). Contribution of malonyl-CoA decarboxylase to the high fatty acid oxidation rates seen in the diabetic heart. *Am J Physiol Heart Circ Physiol*, *278*, H1196–H1204.
115. Aasum, E., Hafstad, A. D., Severson, D. L., et al. (2003). Age-dependent changes in metabolism, contractile function, and ischemic sensitivity in hearts from db/db mice. *Diabetes*, *52*, 434–441.
116. Young, M. E., Guthrie, P. H., Razeghi, P., et al. (2002). Impaired long-chain fatty acid oxidation and contractile dysfunction in the obese Zucker rat heart. *Diabetes*, *51*, 2587–2595.
117. Peterson, L. R., Herrero, P., McGill, J., et al. (2008). Fatty acids and insulin modulate myocardial substrate metabolism in humans with type 1 diabetes. *Diabetes*, *57*, 32–40.
118. Herrero, P., Peterson, L. R., McGill, J. B., et al. (2006). Increased myocardial fatty acid metabolism in patients with type 1 diabetes mellitus. *J Am Coll Cardiol*, *47*, 598–604.
119. Diamant, M., Lamb, H. J., Groeneveld, Y., et al. (2003). Diastolic dysfunction is associated with altered myocardial metabolism in asymptomatic normotensive patients with well-controlled type 2 diabetes mellitus. *J Am Coll Cardiol*, *42*, 328–335.
120. Sánchez-Barriga, J. J., Rangel, A., Castañeda, R., et al. (2000). Left ventricular diastolic dysfunction secondary to hyperglycemia in patients with type II diabetes. *Arch Med Res*, *32*, 44–47.
121. Factor, S. M., Bhan, R., Minase, T., et al. (1981). Hypertensive-diabetic cardiomyopathy in the rat: an experimental model of human disease. *Am J Pathol*, *102*, 19–28.
122. Moncada, S., Palmer, R. M., & Higgs, E. A. (1991). Nitric oxide: physiology, pathophysiology, and pharmacology. *Pharmacol Rev*, *43*, 109–142.
123. Stumpe, T., Decking, U. K., & Schrader, J. (2001). Nitric oxide reduces energy supply by direct action on the respiratory chain in isolated cardiomyocytes. *Am J Physiol Heart Circ Physiol*, *280*, H2350–H2356.
124. Recchia, F. A., McConnell, P. I., Loke, K. E., et al. (1999). Nitric oxide controls cardiac substrate utilization in the conscious dog. *Cardiovasc Res*, *44*, 325–332.
125. Loke, K. E., McConnell, P. I., Tuzman, J. M., et al. (1999). Endogenous endothelial nitric oxide synthase-derived nitric oxide is a physiological regulator of myocardial oxygen consumption. *Circ Res*, *84*, 840–845.
126. Depre, C., Gaussin, V., Ponchaut, S., et al. (1998). Inhibition of myocardial glucose uptake by cGMP. *Am J Physiol*, *274*, H1443–H1449.
127. Young, M. E., Radda, G. K., & Leighton, B. (1997). Nitric oxide stimulates glucose transport and metabolism in rat skeletal muscle in vitro. *Biochem J*, *322*, 223–228.
128. Rozec, B., Erfanian, M., Laurent, K., et al. (2009). Nebivolol, a vasodilating selective beta(1)-blocker, is a beta(3)-adrenoceptor agonist in the nonfailing transplanted human heart. *J Am Coll Cardiol*, *53*, 1532–1538.
129. Rudiger, A., & Singer, M. (2007). Mechanisms of sepsis-induced cardiac dysfunction. *Crit Care Med*, *35*, 1599–1608.
130. Kapadia, S., Dibbs, Z., Kurrelmeyer, K., et al. (1998). The role of cytokines in the failing human heart. *Cardiol Clin*, *16*, 645–656.
131. Mann, D. L., Knueferman, P., & Baumgarten, G. (2000). Cytokines in ischemic heart disease and heart failure. *Dialog Cardiovasc Med*, *5*, 135–146.
132. Zell, R., Geck, P., Werdan, K., et al. (1997). TNF-alpha and IL-1 alpha inhibit both pyruvate dehydrogenase activity and mitochondrial function in cardiomyocytes: evidence for primary impairment of mitochondrial function. *Mol Cell Biochem*, *177*, 61–67.
133. Tatsumi, T., Matoba, S., Kawahara, A., et al. (2000). Cytokine-induced nitric oxide production inhibits mitochondrial energy production and impairs contractile function in rat cardiac myocytes. *J Am Coll Cardiol*, *35*, 1338–1346.
134. Lin, W. J., & Yeh, W. C. (2005). Implication of Toll-like receptor and tumor necrosis factor alpha signaling in septic shock. *Shock*, *24*, 206–209.
135. Sekiguchi, K., Tian, Q., Ishiyama, M., et al. (2007). Inhibition of PPAR-alpha activity in mice with cardiac-restricted expression of tumor necrosis factor: potential role of TGF-beta/Smad3. *Am J Physiol Heart Circ Physiol*, *292*, H1443–H1451.
136. Depre, C., & Taegtmeyer, H. (2000). Metabolic aspects of programmed cell survival and cell death in the heart. *Cardiovasc Res*, *45*, 538–548.
137. Jackson, S. P., & Tjian, R. (1988). O-glycosylation of eukaryotic transcription factors: implications for mechanisms of transcriptional regulation. *Cell*, *55*, 125–133.
138. Clark, R. J., McDonough, P. M., Swanson, E., et al. (2003). Diabetes and the accompanying hyperglycemia impairs cardiomyocyte calcium cycling through increased nuclear O-GlcNAcylation. *J Biol Chem*, *278*, 44230–44237.
139. Young, M. E., Yan, J., Razeghi, P., et al. (2007). Proposed regulation of gene expression by glucose in rodent heart. *Gene Regul Syst Bio*, *1*, 251–262.
140. Malhotra, R., & Brosius, F. C. (1999). Glucose uptake and glycolysis reduce hypoxia-induced apoptosis in cultured neonatal rat cardiac myocytes. *J Biol Chem*, *274*, 12567–12575.
141. Doenst, T., Richwine, R. T., Bray, M. S., et al. (1999). Insulin improves functional and metabolic recovery of reperfused working rat heart. *Ann Thorac Surg*, *67*, 1682–1688.
142. Saltiel, A. R., & Kahn, C. R. (2001). Insulin signalling and the regulation of glucose and lipid metabolism. *Nature*, *414*, 799–806.
143. Shioi, T., Kang, P. M., Douglas, P. S., et al. (2000). The conserved phosphoinositide 3-kinase pathway determines heart size in mice. *EMBO J*, *19*, 2537–2548.
144. Matsui, T., Tao, J., del Monte, F., et al. (2001). Akt activation preserves cardiac function and prevents injury after transient cardiac ischemia in vivo. *Circulation*, *104*, 330–335.
145. Sharma, S., Guthrie, P. H., Chan, S. S., et al. (2007). Glucose phosphorylation is required for insulin-dependent mTOR signalling in the heart. *Cardiovasc Res*, *76*, 71–80.
146. Cook, S. A., Matsui, T., Li, L., et al. (2002). Transcriptional effects of chronic Akt activation in the heart. *J Biol Chem*, *277*, 22528–22533.
147. Jonassen, A. K., Sack, M. N., Mjos, O. D., et al. (2001). Myocardial protection by insulin at reperfusion requires early administration and is mediated via Akt and p70s6 kinase cell-survival signaling. *Circ Res*, *89*, 1191–1198.
148. Gottlob, K., Majewski, N., Kennedy, S., et al. (2001). Inhibition of early apoptotic events by Akt/PKB is dependent on the first committed step of glycolysis and mitochondrial hexokinase. *Genes Dev*, *15*, 1406–1418.
149. Robey, R. B., Ma, J., Santos, A. V., et al. (2002). Regulation of mesangial cell hexokinase activity and expression by heparin-binding epidermal growth factor-like growth factor. *J Biol Chem*, *277*, 14370–14378.
150. Bialik, S., Cryns, V. L., Drincic, A., et al. (1999). The mitochondrial apoptotic pathway is activated by serum and glucose deprivation in cardiac myocytes. *Circ Res*, *85*, 403–414.
151. Schaffer, S. W., Croft, C. B., & Solodushko, V. (2000). Cardioprotective effect of chronic hyperglycemia: effect on hypoxia-induced apoptosis and necrosis. *Am J Physiol Heart Circ Physiol*, *278*, 1948–1954.
152. Moley, K. H. (2000). Mueckler MM. Glucose transport and apoptosis. *Apoptosis*, *5*, 99–105.
153. Zhou, Y. T., Grayburn, P., Karim, A., et al. (2000). Lipotoxic heart disease in obese rats: implications for human obesity. *Proc Natl Acad Sci U S A*, *97*, 1784–1789.
154. Zhu, P., Lu, L., Xu, Y., et al. (2000). Troglitazone improves recovery of left ventricular function after regional ischemia in pigs. *Circulation*, *101*, 1165–1171.
155. Gudz, T. I., Tserng, K. Y., & Hoppel, C. L. (1997). Direct inhibition of mitochondrial respiratory chain complex III by cell-permeable ceramide. *J Biol Chem*, *272*, 24154–24158.
156 d'Alche, P., Clauser, P., Morel, M., et al. (1991). Assessment with potential mapping of the cardiac protective effect of a drug. Example of trimetazidine. *J Pharmacol Methods*, *26*, 43–51.
157. Detry, J. M., Sellier, P., Pennaforte, S., et al. (1994). Trimetazidine: a new concept in the treatment of angina. Comparison with propranolol in patients with stable angina. Trimetazidine European multicenter study group. *Br J Clin Pharmacol*, *37*, 279–288.
158. Kantor, P. F., Lucien, A., Kozak, R., et al. (2000). The antianginal drug trimetazidine shifts cardiac energy metabolism from fatty acid oxidation to glucose oxidation by inhibiting mitochondrial long-chain 3-ketoacyl coenzyme A thiolase. *Circ Res*, *86*, 580–588.
159. Vitale, C., Wajngaten, M., Sposato, B., et al. (2004). Trimetazidine improves left ventricular function and quality of life in elderly patients with coronary artery disease. *Eur Heart J*, *25*, 1814–1821.

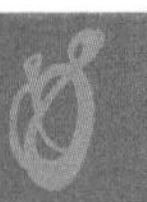

160. Tuunanen, H., Engblom, E., Naum, A., et al. (2008). Trimetazidine, a metabolic modulator, has cardiac and extracardiac benefits in idiopathic dilated cardiomyopathy. *Circulation, 118*, 1250–1258.
161. Zacharowski, K., Blackburn, B., & Thiemermann, C. (2001). Ranolazine, a partial fatty acid oxidation inhibitor, reduces myocardial infarct size and cardiac troponin T release in the rat. *Eur J Pharmacol, 418*, 105–110.
162. Clarke, B., Wyatt, K. M., & McCormack, J. G. (1996). Ranolazine increases active pyruvate dehydrogenase in perfused normoxic rat hearts: evidence for an indirect mechanism. *J Mol Cell Cardiol, 28*, 341–350.
163. Chandler, M. P., Stanley, W. C., Morita, H., et al. (2002). Short-term treatment with ranolazine improves mechanical efficiency in dogs with chronic heart failure. *Circ Res, 91*, 278–280.
164. Lautamaki, R., Airaksinen, K. E., Seppanen, M., et al. (2005). Rosiglitazone improves myocardial glucose uptake in patients with type 2 diabetes and coronary artery disease: a 16-week randomized, double-blind, placebo-controlled study. *Diabetes, 54*, 2787–2794.
165. Wilmsen, H. M., Ciaraldi, T. P., Carter, L., et al. (2003). Thiazolidinediones upregulate impaired fatty acid uptake in skeletal muscle of type 2 diabetic subjects. *Am J Physiol Endocrinol Metab, 285*, E354–E362.
166. Tuunanen, H., Engblom, E., Naum, A., et al. (2006). Free fatty acid depletion acutely decreases cardiac work and efficiency in cardiomyopathic heart failure. *Circulation, 114*, 2130–2137.
167. Di Lisa, F., Menabò, R., & Siliprandi, N. (1989). L-propionyl-carnitine protection of mitochondria in ischemic rat hearts. *Mol Cell Biochem, 88*, 169–173.
168. Liedtke, A. J., DeMaison, L., & Nellis, S. H. (1988). Effects of L-propionylcarnitine on mechanical recovery during reflow in intact hearts. *Am J Physiol, 255*, 169–176.
169. Russell, R. R., Mommessin, J. I., & Taegtmeyer, H. (1995). Propionyl-L-carnitine-mediated improvement in contractile function of rat hearts oxidizing acetoacetate. *Am J Physiol, 268*, H441–H447.
170. Paulson, D. J., Traxler, J., Schmidt, M., et al. (1986). Protection of the ischaemic myocardium by L-propionyl-carnitine: effects on the recovery of cardiac output after ischemia and reperfusion, carnitine transport and fatty acid oxidation. *Cardiovasc Res, 20*, 536–541.
171. Opie, L. H. (1979). Role of carnitine in fatty acid metabolism of normal and ischemic myocardium. *Am Heart J, 97*, 375–388.
172. Kaido, M., Fujimura, H., Ono, A., et al. (1997). Mitochondrial abnormalities in a murine model of primary carnitine deficiency. *Eur Neurol, 38*, 302–309.
173. Paulson, D. J. (1998). Carnitine deficiency-induced cardiomyopathy. *Mol Cell Biochem, 180*, 33–41.
174. Stanley, C. A., DeLeeuw, S., Coates, P. M., et al. (1991). Chronic cardiomyopathy and weakness or acute coma in children with a defect in carnitine uptake. *Ann Neurol, 30*, 709–716.
175. Tripp, M. E., Katcher, M. L., Peters, H. A., et al. (1981). Systemic carnitine deficiency presenting as familial endomyocardial fibroelastosis. *N Engl J Med, 305*, 385–390.

CHAPTER 21

Alterations in Nutrition and Body Mass in Heart Failure

Wolfram Doehner, Stephan von Haehling, and Stefan D. Anker

The treatment of chronic heart failure (CHF) has made significant advances over the past 2 decades. Even more so, our understanding of the disease has developed from a hemodynamic model of mere pumping failure to a complex approach, including multiple body systems and peripheral organs and tissues. Improved acute and chronic therapy and a steadily older growing population have resulted in an increasing prevalence and incidence of CHF.

The prevalence of CHF has been estimated at around 0.3% to 2.4%, which implies that 5 million people in the United States are affected.[1] Heart failure accounts for 970,000 hospitalizations and 12 to 15 million outpatient office visits in this country per year. Overall, the incidence of CHF is steadily increasing in most European countries and in the United States. Heart failure is primarily a diagnosis among the elderly and with the aging of the population a further increase in prevalence with epidemic proportion is anticipated. Current estimates amount to an overall incidence of 0.1% to 0.5% per year, with doubling of the numbers with each decade reaching 3% in those over the age of 75.

More patients survive acute cardiac events and live for a prolonged period of time in a state of compensated cardiac failure. Consequently, complications of long-term disease progression are increasingly coming to the fore in the clinical presentation of patients. Systemic metabolic impairment emerged as characteristic feature inherent to chronic heart failure. Imbalanced hormonal signaling leads to adaptive and eventually maladaptive changes in metabolic flux and hence in maintenance of structural tissue and energy storage. Weight loss and the development of cachexia in the course of disease have been recognized as a severe complication of CHF with further deterioration of clinical symptoms and a particular grave prognosis.

Despite improved medical and interventional therapy of cardiac disease, CHF mortality remains high and, in fact, is even increasing due to the factors indicated previously. About half of the patients with CHF die within 4 years of diagnosis.[2] This truly devastating prognosis is comparable to that of some types of cancer.[3]

The situation worsens considerably once cardiac cachexia has been diagnosed. Although a uniform definition of cardiac cachexia has been subject to debate over years (see later discussion), most researchers have unanimously agreed on the particular poor prognosis of the cachectic patient. In unselected patients with CHF, mortality rates were as high as 50% in the cachectic subset compared with 17% in the noncachectic subset at 18 months of follow-up.[4] Already a comparatively small amount of documented tissue loss is associated with a significant increase in mortality. Considerations of a certain cutoff for weight loss to identify patients at higher risk are of particular relevance for clinical evaluation and identification of patients with cachexia and are discussed in further detail later.

Cachexia is not only associated with poor outcome, but also with advanced symptomatic status, poor quality of life, and an unfavorable response to drug treatment. Although anorexia is certainly a common characteristic in HF and a contributing factor of weight loss, this feature alone cannot explain the metabolic changes observed during this perturbation. It is among the most common misconceptions that feeding and enhanced nutritional and caloric supplementation may be sufficient to adequately reverse the process of losing weight in patients with cachexia. Weight loss in the cachectic patient predominantly affects muscle protein; however, bone and fat tissue are likewise affected later in the course of the disease. The timelines differ widely between patients. We are only beginning to understand the factors that trigger the progression from clinically and weight-stable ambulatory CHF to cardiac cachexia. Cachexia is not a unique feature of CHF, but is also seen in advanced stages of a range of chronic illnesses, including cancer, chronic kidney and liver disease, rheumatoid arthritis, acquired immunodeficiency syndrome (AIDS), and others. Based on observed similarities in the signaling and regulatory processes in cachectic patients of varying origin, a common final pathway of weight loss in chronic disease has been hypothesized.[5]

In this chapter an overview of the current knowledge of metabolic imbalance, nutritional aspects, and the significance of cardiac cachexia in CHF is presented.

BODY COMPOSITION AND HEART FAILURE FROM THE HISTORIC AND PUBLIC PERSPECTIVE: THE OBESITY PARADOX

Weight loss and the development of cachexia in association with cardiac illness have been known to physicians for centuries as a "signum mali ominis," indicating end-stage disease and poor quality of life. Cachexia (Greek: *kakós'* "bad"; *hexis'* "condition") constitutes its terminal phase and develops in advanced stages of various chronic illnesses (e.g., CHF, chronic obstructive pulmonary disease, or cancer). Already in ancient Greece, a picturesque clinical description of cachexia was provided by Hippocrates: "The flesh is consumed and becomes water,... the abdomen fills with water, the feet and legs swell, the shoulders, clavicles, chest, and thighs melt away.... The illness is fatal.[6]" Despite the manifest change in the patient's shape and appearance, a systematic investigation into this aspect was not extended beyond the state of mere observation until recently. Weakness and a reduced urge to eat were easily accepted as underlying mechanism of weight loss.[7] Increasing investigation of the significance and underlying mechanisms of weight loss and body composition changes in CHF revealed the significant impact of metabolic failure as a characteristic feature of CHF pathophysiology that contributes to both the morbidity and mortality of the patients.

Body weight is a dynamic parameter and has a certain rhythm over the life span.[8] Currently, public awareness of body weight and body composition is more concerned with overweight and weight gain than weight loss, and therefore most of the programs in adults are aimed at the reduction of body size.[9] In fact the aim to be slim and to lose weight has been thoroughly implemented in the public consciousness as surrogates for physical and mental well-being. This makes it hard to establish a more differential view on the association between body composition and morbidity and mortality. It should be noted, however, that the principles that have been proven for healthy populations may not be applicable in full in the setting of chronic diseased patients. In fact, convincing evidence has been accumulated that the WHO criteria of normal body mass index (BMI, Figure 21-1) may not be applicable to patients with CHF with regard to optimum survival.

More recent data from a collaborative analysis of 57 prospective studies with more than 890,000 participants, mostly in western Europe and North America, revealed also on an epidemiological level that BMI less than 22.5 kg/m^2 is associated inversely with overall mortality, mainly because of strong inverse associations with respiratory disease and lung cancer.[10]

In a number of CHF populations from large multicenter controlled studies, it emerged that patients with overweight and mild obesity have better survival rates than patients with the a BMI less than 25kg/m^2, the upper limit of normal according to WHO criteria. From the Digitalis Investigation Group (DIG) trial, 7767 patients were analyzed, showing a linear rather than a U-shaped association between BMI and survival.[11] Even after multivariable adjustment, overweight and obese patients were at lower risk for death (HR 0.88, 95% CI 0.80 to 0.96, and HR 0.81, 95% CI 0.72 to 0.92, respectively) compared with normal BMI. In the study population of the Candesartan in Heart Failure: Assessment of Reduction in Mortality and Morbidity (CHARM) program, 7599 patients with CHF (NYHA II-IV) with a broad spectrum of left ventricular ejection fraction (mean 39%) were analyzed for BMI and survival; 1831 patients died during follow-up (mean 37.7 months). Optimum survival was observed in the subgroup of patients with a BMI of 30 to 34.9 kg/m^2, with a graded increase in mortality risk in the groups with lower BMI (see Figure 21-1).[12] Moreover, the increased risk of death in patients with BMI greater than 35 was not statistically significant. These associations were not altered by age, smoking, or LVEF.

In a post hoc analysis of 5010 patients from the Valsartan Heart Failure Trial (Val-HeFT), again, a stepwise linear association between BMI and mortality rate was observed (Table 21-1).[13] In a meta-analysis of nine observational trials in CHF populations, the affect of body weight on all-cause mortality was evaluated in a total of 28,209 patients with a mean follow-up period of 2.7 years.[14] The investigators reported the uniform finding that in all studies included in the analysis, overweight and obesity were associated with lower all-cause mortality and cardiovascular mortality rates.

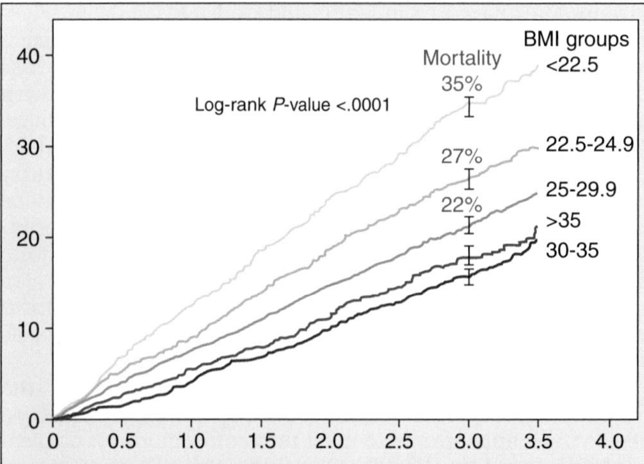

FIGURE 21–1 Mortality in the CHARM trial program in patient subgroups according to BMI. Lowest mortality was observed in the BMI subgroup 30 to 34.9, with a stepwise increase in risk in the lower BMI groups. (Adapted from Kenchaiah S, Pocock SJ, Wang D, et al. Body mass index and prognosis in patients with chronic heart failure: insights from the candesartan in heart failure: assessment of reduction in mortality and morbidity (CHARM) program. *Circulation* 2007;116:627-636.)

TABLE 21–1 Mortality Rate on Patients with CHF in the Valsartan Heart Failure Trial (Val-HeFT) *P* <.0001

BMI Subgroup	BMI (kg/m^2)	Mortality Rate (%)
Underweight	<22	27.2
Normal weight	22-24.9	21.7
Overweight	25-29.9	17.9
Obese	>30	16.5

The constant finding that higher BMI is not associated with increased mortality in CHF is opposite to the U-shaped curve of the association between BMI and survival that is known from populational analyses. This finding led the researchers to coin the term "obesity paradox."[11] Interestingly, the "paradox" aspect may be viewed as a reflection of the expectation that is fueled from the epidemiological studies in healthy subjects. An important conclusion from these findings is that metabolic balance and body composition need to be viewed from a different perspective in patients with a chronic disease such as CHF as compared with healthy subjects. Insights and "common knowledge" on weight and body composition from a normal healthy population may not be uncritically translated to such patient populations as significant differences may exist in the metabolic homeostasis in chronic patients.

Definition of Cardiac Cachexia

Clinical decisions in modern medicine rely to a large degree on quantifiable variables as the basis for clear-cut definitions and guidelines for identification and management of medical conditions. Unfortunately, there is no universal definition available for appropriate identification of cachectic patients or patients at risk.[15] It remains hitherto at the discretion of the individual physician to observe this important aspect in the progression of the diseases. Additional confusion is caused by the inconsistent nomenclature used when describing body wasting. Indeed, descriptive terms such as "cachexia," "anorexia," "sarcopenia," "malnutrition," and even "hypercatabolism" are often used as synonyms. While

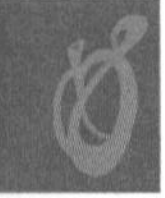

sarcopenia refers to age-associated "normal" muscle wasting,[16] weight may largely remain balanced because muscle is replaced by fat tissue. Opposite to cachexia, weight loss due to malnutrition and anorexia is fully reversible with adequate food intake. Loss of appetite or anorexia causes primarily loss of fat mass rather than muscle tissue. Malnutrition is also associated with body wasting, predominantly of fat tissue. Lastly, the term "hypercatabolism" cannot be evaluated during clinical examination and does not appreciate anabolic processes as the other side of the metabolic balance.[17]

Several definitions of cardiac cachexia have been put forward in different studies using a range of clinical tests such as skinfold thickness, fat tissue content, BMI, and others.

The recently proposed definition derived from the SOLVD (Studies of Left Ventricular Dysfunction) database seems most appropriate to meet the requirements of clinical usefulness and applicability.[18] In the SOLVD study population of 1929 patients with CHF, a nonedematous weight loss of greater than 6% of total body weight over a period of 6 or more months has been identified to be the strongest predictor of mortality among cutoffs from 5% to 15%. This finding had been validated in the study population of the V-HeFT II trial, confirming the strong and independent prognostic power of this cutoff to predict mortality in patients with CHF.

Several aspects are of importance to underscore applicability of this definition. First, the dynamic process of tissue loss rather than a single time BMI assessment is appreciated as the underlying principle of cachexia, avoiding bias from constitutional asthenic body composition. The observed weight loss carries the significant information of an ongoing detrimental spiral of tissue degradation (Figure 21-2).[19]

Second, a weight loss of greater than 6% of body weight is in comparison, a small difference that is in contrast to the rather traditional perception of cachectic patients. Further, the simple method to obtain a weight history ensures practicality and applicability of the definition in any clinical condition at no cost. Notably, the severity of cardiac cachexia may not always correlate with classic criteria of disease severity as a New York Heart Association (NYHA) functional class, left ventricular ejection fraction, or exercise duration.[20] Cardiac cachexia even may not be associated with morphological cardiac changes as seen by magnetic resonance imaging or echocardiography.[21,22]

A series of conferences was held in recent years aiming to achieve a consensus for a common definition of cachexia in chronic illness. According to the recently published consensus document resulting from these conferences,[5] cachexia has to be considered in adult patients with chronic illness, who experience weight loss of 5% or more in upto 12 months (or have a body mass index <20), and comply with at least three out of five clinical or laboratory criteria (Table 21-2). With this definition of cachexia, the interventional trial results will be more applicable to cachexia of different causes, and the quest for an effective treatment may be reaching some landmarks in the near future.

Mechanisms of Altered Body Composition in Chronic Heart Failure

Cardiac cachexia as a clinical entity is acknowledged as a complex syndrome with multiple factors mutually interrelated. Patients usually experience progressive weight loss with body composition alterations and disturbed homeostasis of several body systems. There is evidence for activation of neuroendocrine and inflammatory systems, increased lipolysis, muscle wasting, lack of appetite, and malabsorption.[23,24] The importance of individual pathways and their exact interplay are still incompletely understood.

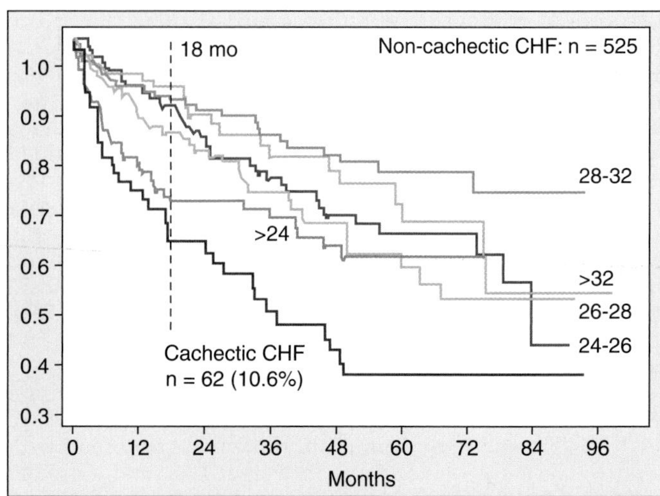

FIGURE 21-2 Mortality of patients with CHF in subgroups according to BMI and with stable body weight (numbers show range of BMI per group) in comparison to patients with observed weight loss 7.5% of body weight (*black curve*). Best survival was seen in patients with mild obesity (BMI 28 to 32). However, highest mortality occurred in patients with documented weight loss. (Adapted from Davos CH, Doehner W, Rauchhaus M, et al. Body mass and survival in patients with chronic heart failure without cachexia: the importance of obesity. *J Card Fail* 2003;9:29-35.)

TABLE 21-2 Consensus Definition of Cachexia in an Adult Patient: Diagnostic Criteria

Presence of an underlying disease
AND
Weight loss of ≥ 5% in 12 months or less (or body mass index <20)
PLUS
≥3 out of 5 criteria • Decreased muscle strength • Fatigue • Anorexia • Low fat-free mass index • Abnormal biochemistry • Inflammation • Anemia • Low serum albumin

Adapted from Evans WJ, Morley JE, Argilés J, et al. Cachexia: a new definition. *Clin Nutr* 2008;27:793-9.

Nutrition and Regulation of Feeding

Loss of appetite and inadequate food intake are important components contributing to the development of weight loss and cachexia in CHF. This anorexia may occur as a consequence of symptomatic disablement of the patients from weakness, dyspnea, fatigue, or lethargy.[25] Also intestinal edema leading to nausea, diminished absorption, and protein-losing enteropathy have been described in this context.[26] Notably, iatrogenic factors may unfavorably contribute to the decreased appetite and food intake of patients as a consequence of multiple daily drug regimens. Also imposed dietary restrictions may have a role, which, in view of those previously mentioned, needs to be viewed with great care on an individual basis.

Regulation of feeding is a complex regulated balance within a satiety-hunger homeostatic model (Figure 21-3), with a multitude of factors involved. The fine-tuned regulation of appetite is characterized by pleiotropism and redundancy—two key principles in balanced physiology. Many of the factors involved are increasingly investigated and will briefly be discussed with reference to specific observations

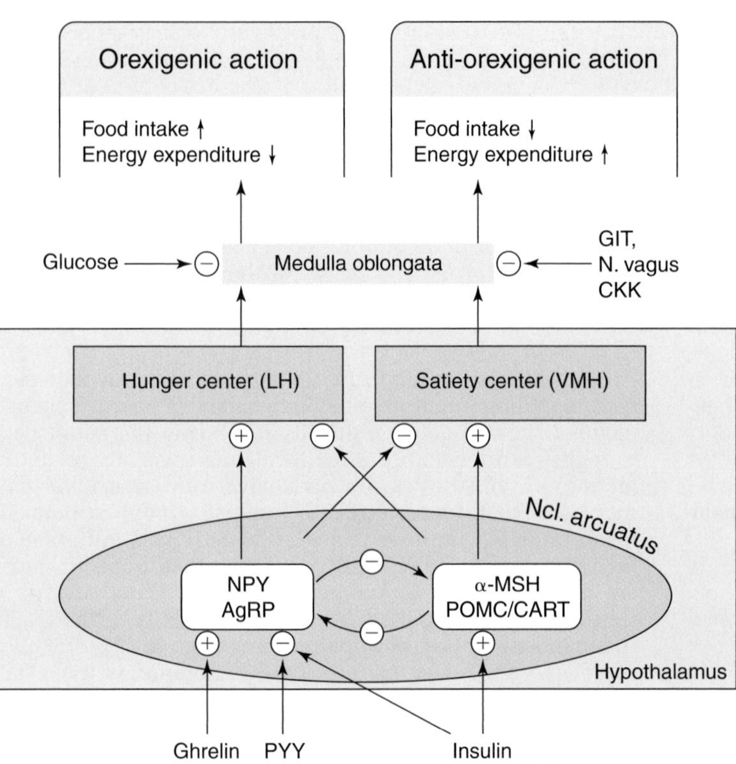

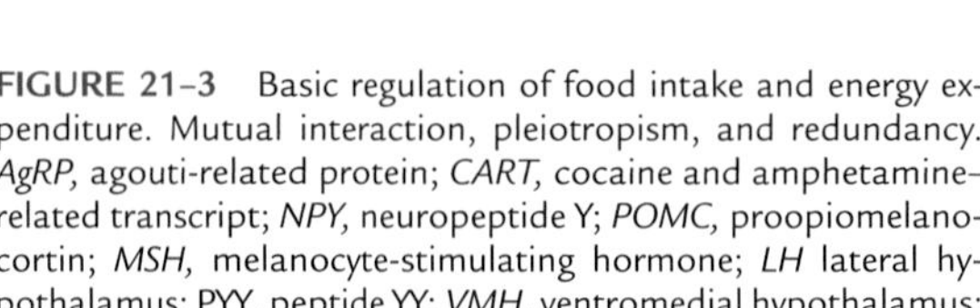
FIGURE 21–3 Basic regulation of food intake and energy expenditure. Mutual interaction, pleiotropism, and redundancy. *AgRP,* agouti-related protein; *CART,* cocaine and amphetamine-related transcript; *NPY,* neuropeptide Y; *POMC,* proopiomelanocortin; *MSH,* melanocyte-stimulating hormone; *LH* lateral hypothalamus; PYY, peptide YY; *VMH,* ventromedial hypothalamus; CCK, cholecystokinin.

in CHF. The hypothalamus has been identified as the central regulating site of appetite with a lateral "feeding area" and a medial "satiety center."[27] Stimulation of the first increased the urge for food intake; the latter triggers cessation of eating. Numerous mediators take part in controlling these centers in the hypothalamus. For a given person under normal conditions, a balanced equilibrium between both pathways results in an individually defined set point of fairly stable body weight and composition. Excessive fluctuations on either side, however, cause weight and body composition changes, which may develop into medical conditions or disease.

Neuropeptide Y

Neuropeptide Y (NPY) is a neurotransmitter in the central and peripheral nervous system, which is stored mainly in the hypothalamus as the central site of appetite regulation.[28] NPY is a central player in appetite regulation with a potent orexigenic capacity (i.e., stimulating food intake). NPY excretion from the hypothalamus increases during fasting and exercise. Besides increased appetite, a range of pathways is modulated that starts a cascade of hormonal signaling. Parasympathetic activity and induction of corticotropin-releasing factor are stimulated, the latter yielding release of adrenocorticotropic hormone and cortisol. Sympathetic activity and energy expenditure, on the other hand, are being suppressed. The NPY pathway in turn is suppressed by insulin and the adipocyte-derived polypeptide leptin (see later discussion).[29]

A study in 30 patients with CHF and 16 healthy controls demonstrated elevated plasma levels of NPY in the patients with CHF ($P < .01$).[30] Although vasoconstriction is an effect of endogenous NPY, intravenous infusion of the peptide had no hemodynamic effect.[31]

Leptin

Leptin (Greek: *leptos,* "thin") was the first adipocyte-derived hormone to be discovered.[32,33] Leptin is produced exclusively by adipocytes and its identification surmounted the paradigm that fat tissue merely serves as a passive energy depot. Accordingly a close correlation exists between size of adipose tissue and serum leptin levels with higher levels in women compared with men.[34] It circulates in the bloodstream either free or protein bound and can cross the blood-brain barrier. A large number of OBRb, one of five isoforms of the leptin receptor, the is expressed in the choroid plexus and hypothalamus, and hence leptin is viewed as the link between adipose tissue and central nervous system mediating the central regulation of satiety and energy metabolism. Beyond its central effects, leptin may have pleiotropic peripheral actions. Leptin receptors are also expressed in several peripheral tissues such as pancreatic islets, liver, kidney, lung, adrenal glands, heart, and skeletal muscle.[35,36,37] These would include interaction with several metabolic and hormonal pathways (e.g., lipogenesis in adipose tissue, growth hormone signaling, and insulin sensitivity).[38,39] In turn, leptin is under multihormonal control (such as insulin, glucocorticoids, catecholamines).

It is a key regulator of food intake and energy homeostasis. Leptin levels increase with accumulating fat tissue and decline during body fat deprivation. Indeed, it has been shown that a 10% reduction in body weight led to a 53% reduction in serum leptin, whereas a 10% body weight increase caused a 300% increase in serum leptin.[40] Leptin's effects on body metabolism are mediated by multifactorial pathways including insulin, glucocorticoids, catecholamines, and in particular the melanocortin system. The activation of this system via pro-opiomelanocortin (POMC) cells, α-melanocyte stimulating hormone (MSH), and the type 4 melanocortin receptor (MC4R) eventually leads to the suppression of food intake (antiorexigenic effect) and increases in energy expenditure. On the other hand, leptin suppresses the antagonistic (i.e., orexigenic) pathway of NPY/agouti-related protein (AgRP).[41,42] Additionally, both systems are targeted by several peripheral metabolic signals, including insulin, glucose, ghrelin, and peptide YY.[43,44]

In CHF, preserved[45] and even elevated leptin levels have been observed.[46] In cachectic patients serum leptin levels are significantly lower than in noncachectic patients, rather in the range of normal values.[47] Notably, the significantly reduced fat tissue amount in cachectic patients[48] may explain

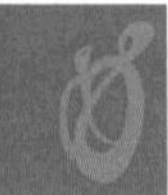

the pseudonormal leptin levels. Indeed, adjustment for fat tissue amount reveals that both cachectic and noncachectic CHF patients are relatively hyperleptinemic.[46] These findings argue against a predominant role of leptin-regulated reduced appetite in the development of cardiac cachexia. Indirect effects of hyperleptinemia may nevertheless have a contributing role such as via insulin resistance and acquired growth hormone resistance, which are both observed to relate to hyperleptinemia in CHF.[46,49]

Melanocortins

Melanocortins primarily stimulate the melanogenesis and/or steroidogenesis in melanocytes and adrenal cortical cells, respectively. Melanocortins can bind and activate five different melanocortin receptors.[50] Food intake and energy expenditure are mainly regulated through MC4R, which are widely distributed within the central nervous system, including the hypothalamus, the thalamus, and the spinal cord.[51]

Melanocortins are antiorexigenic and loss of normal melanocortin signaling leads to hyperphagia and obesity.[52,53,54] The overactivity of this system, on the other hand, would lead to suppression of food intake and upregulation of energy expenditure.[55] Evidence is mounting that increased melanocortin activity plays a role in the pathogenesis of cachexia.[56,57] This appears to be mainly due to an increased production of systemic proinflammatory cytokines.[58] In experimental settings in cancer or renal failure, melanocortin antagonists were shown to improve food intake and lean body mass. This approach seems feasible for cachexia therapy in chronic disease; however, studies are warranted to test applicability to humans.[59]

Ghrelin

Ghrelin is mainly produced in the fundus region of the stomach,[60,61] but it is also expressed in other organs, including the duodenum, jejunum, ileum, and colon (with gradually decreasing expression), where it promotes gastric motility.[60] It is also found in the pancreas,[62] in the arcuate nucleus of the hypothalamus, in the kidneys,[63] and the placenta.[64] Active ghrelin binds to the growth hormone secretagogue receptor (GHS-R), a G protein–coupled receptor.[65,66] Physiologically, ghrelin induces the release of growth hormone and has appetite-regulating and antiinflammatory properties. Growth hormone is released in a dose-dependent manner from the pituitary gland upon binding of ghrelin to the GHS-R.[60] In humans, high doses of ghrelin also increase the levels of adrenocorticotropic hormone—prolactin and cortisol.[67]

Ghrelin expressing neurons in the hypothalamus have direct contact with neurons containing NPY, agouti-related protein (AgRP), and proopiomelanocortin (POMC; see Figure 21-3).[68] Hence, ghrelin is likely to exert its effect on feeding by stimulating the release of NPY and AgRP,[69] while reducing the release of POMC.[68] Although peptides generally do not pass the blood-brain barrier, ghrelin injected into the periphery is able to stimulate the hypothalamus[70] and food intake.[71] The signaling of ghrelin via afferent nerve fibers of the vagus[72] has been observed, which among other target areas project to the stomach and bowel.

The ghrelin-induced inhibition of the expression of proinflammatory cytokines has been reported in a time- and dose-dependent fashion,[73] and downregulated proliferation of murine anti-CD3 activated T cells has been described.[74] Moreover, ghrelin accounted for downregulated circulating proinflammatory cytokines in a rat model of endotoxemia[75] and attenuated proinflammatory response in human endothelial cells.[76]

Elevated plasma ghrelin levels have been shown in cachectic heart failure patients compared with noncachectic CHF patients in association with elevated levels of growth hormone and TNF-α.[77] In an uncontrolled pilot study in predominantly cachectic CHF patients, infusion of ghrelin showed promising cardiovascular results.[78] Intravenous gherelin administration of 4 μg/kg body weight resulted in increased food intake and lean body mass. LVEF increased and plasma levels of B-type natriuretic peptide decreased over the 3-week treatment period. Similar results regarding heart function, body weight, and body composition have been described in animal models of heart failure.[79] Currently, several trials aim to reproduce these data in a double-blind, placebo-controlled fashion but results are inconsistent[80,81] and further research is needed to establish the therapeutic potential of ghrelin.

Adiponectin

Adiponectin is another fat tissue–derived hormone with feedback signaling function to regulate balanced energy substrate metabolism and body composition. Playing the counterpart to leptin, adiponectin plasma levels are inversely related to fat stores[82] and low adiponectin levels are associated with increased insulin resistance,[83] whereas high adiponectin levels indicate improved insulin sensitivity.[84] Adiponectin levels are increased in CHF.[85,86] Elevated adiponectin levels are directly related to symptomatic status[87] and severity of LV dysfunction,[88] and adiponectin has been identified as an independent marker of impaired prognosis in CHF.[89] This is somewhat surprising because CHF is commonly associated with impaired insulin sensitivity (see later discussion). More research is needed to uncover the pathophysiological relevance of adiponectin in CHF.

Chronic Immune Activation (see Chapter 11)

The hormonal regulation of body composition, feeding, and metabolic flux as outlined previously has tight and multiple interconnections with chronic inflammatory activation, a commonly observed characteristic in CHF. Since the initial description of elevated TNF α levels in CHF,[90] a number of different hypotheses have been suggested to explain the origin of immune activation in this disease. The production of proinflammatory cytokines has been attributed to secretion by mononuclear cells, although the myocardium seems to be another important source. However, it appears that only the *failing* myocardium is capable of TNF α production.[91] Some evidence suggests that catecholamines augment myocardial cytokine release. Other concepts suggest a response to myocardial injury[92] and underperfusion of peripheral tissues[93] as underlying mechanisms. It has also been proposed that increased bowel wall edema may cause impairment of bowel wall barrier function. This leads to increased translocation of bacterial components, such as lipopolysaccharide (LPS), a cell wall component from gram-negative bacteria and one of the strongest inducers of proinflammatory cytokines and especially TNF α.[94] Indeed, it has been shown that very small (pathophysiological) amounts of this substance are capable of inducing TNF α secretion.[95] Notably, LPS levels are particularly elevated in the bloodstream of patients with CHF during edematous decompensation (i.e., when clinical signs of severe tissue congestion are present.[96] It is well possible that the aforementioned hypotheses rather complement than exclude one another, but it is certainly true that inflammatory activation is much more than an epiphenomenon in CHF.

Anabolic Failure

Growth Hormone (GH)

The peptide hormone from the anterior pituitary gland has a central role in the regulation of energy stores and exerts strong anabolic effects. The pleiotropic effects of GH are mediated by activation of insulin-like growth factor-1 (IGF-1) and somatomedins.[97] The main site of IGF-1 synthesis is the liver but peripheral tissues are also capable of its production.[98]

Direct actions of GH include an increase in muscle protein synthesis[99] but also effects on glucose, lipid, and sodium metabolism. Lipolytic effects account for enhanced fat use. Thus GH plays a significant role in the regulation of substrate metabolism and body composition in man.

Despite the plausible and intriguing therapeutic concept to prevent tissue wasting and cachexia by administration of recombinant GH, results from a series of studies were disappointing.[100,101,102] An explanation of the failing approach may come from an observation of an acquired GH resistance in CHF[103] characterized by a threefold increase in GH levels in cachectic patients compared with noncachectic patients with CHF and healthy subjects paralleled by lower than normal IGF-1 levels.

Insulin Resistance (see also Chapters 20 and 26)

Besides the central function as a regulator of glucose homeostasis, energy flux and substrate use in general, insulin is the strongest anabolic hormone in human physiology. In the setting of CHF, impaired insulin signaling function (i.e., insulin resistance) was reported more than a decade ago.[104] Overt diabetes mellitus is a common co-morbidity in CHF, and the Euro Heart Failure Survey reported an incidence as high as 27%.[105] As insulin resistance occurs years if not decades before the clinical criteria of diabetes mellitus are met, the incidence may be much higher. Indeed, subclinical impairment of glucose metabolism has been reported for 43% of patients with CHF.[106] It is also well established that diabetes mellitus is an important risk factor for the development of CHF.[107]

Importantly, insulin resistance occurs as a consequence of CHF and independently and on top of the metabolic syndrome, a clear risk factor for ischemic-type heart failure. Insulin resistance in CHF correlates directly with the severity of the symptomatic status.[108] In a study of 41 patients and 21 healthy control subjects, insulin sensitivity (assessed by intravenous glucose tolerance testing) was reduced by 31% in patients with CHF compared with controls ($P < .01$), and fasting insulin levels were higher in patients than in controls ($P < .01$).[38] Serum leptin levels remained the only independent predictor of insulin resistance. Moreover, a recent study identified insulin resistance as a prognosticator in patients with CHF independent of previously established prognostic factors.[109] It has been shown that skeletal muscle GLUT 4 transport protein—the rate-limiting step of glucose uptake and subsequent use as energy substrate—is reduced in CHF well in parallel to CHF severity (Figure 21-4).[110] Mechanisms that cause insulin resistance in patients with CHF are not entirely understood but are likely a complex cluster of mechanisms including hormonal interaction, immune activation, oxidative stress, hemodynamic impairment, and tissue hypoperfusion, skeletal muscle adaptation to disabled lifestyle, and others (Figure 21-5).[111]

Pathophysiological mechanisms and clinical and prognostic implications suggest insulin resistance as a potential treatment target, in particular when body wasting and cachexia are involved. The novel class of insulin sensitizers or glitazones would be a plausible option. The use of TZD in CHF is, however, limited by their characteristic to increase fluid retention and edema, suggesting progression of heart failure[112] disease and increased hospitalization.[113] There are recent studies reporting promising data in favor of this concept with regard to prognostic benefit[114,115] and myocardial functional assessment.[116] However, given the ongoing controversy on increased cardiovascular risk following TZD therapy, their use in CHF patients is currently not recommended.[117]

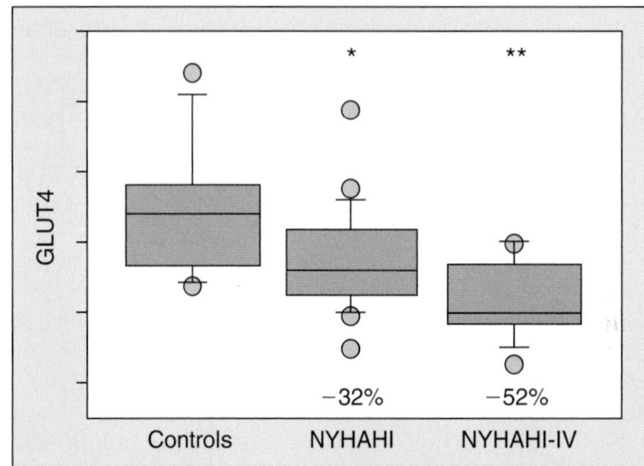

FIGURE 21-4 Reduced GLUT 4 transport protein in skeletal muscle in patients with CHF according to CHF severity (NYHA I/II n = 18, NYHA III/IV n = 11). +$P < .05$, ++$P < .01$ vs. controls (n = 7). (Adapted from Doehner W, Gathercole D, Cicoira M, et al. Reduced glucose transporter GLUT4 in skeletal muscle predicts insulin resistance in nondiabetic chronic heart failure patients independently of body composition. *Int J Cardiol* 2010; 138:19-24.)

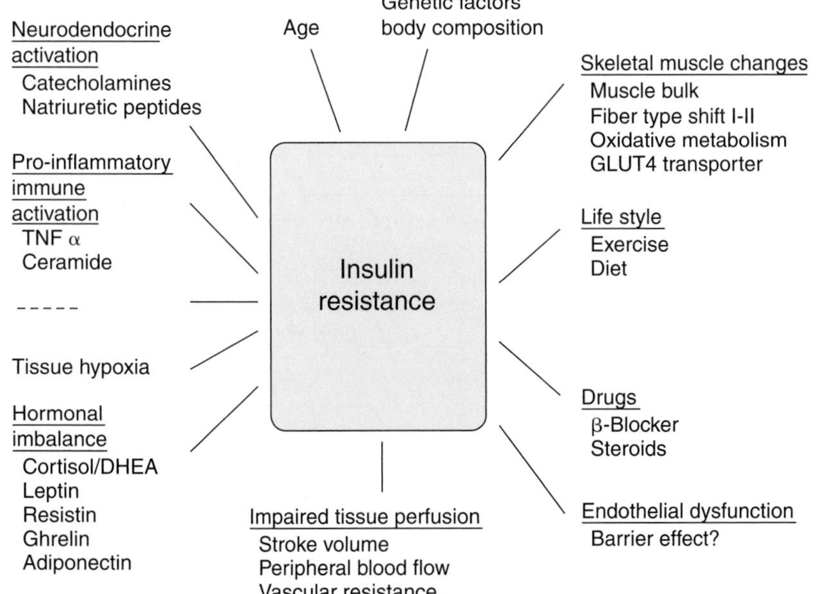

FIGURE 21-5 Factors contributing to impaired insulin sensitivity in CHF. (Adapted from Doehner W., von Haehling S., Anker SD. (2005). Chronische Herzinsuffizienz: eine metabolische Erkrankung, Von der Pathophysiologie zu neuen Therapieansatzen. Kardiologie up2date, 1, 45–58.)

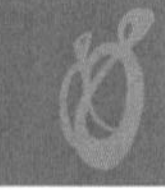

MECHANISMS OF WASTING IN DIFFERENT BODY COMPARTMENTS

Investigations of specific tissue compartments reveal detailed characteristics of body wasting, beyond the clinically overt loss of total body weight. Lean body mass depletion is a dominant feature of cardiac cachexia. Muscle atrophy is observed in up to 68% of patients with CHF.[118] Reduction in muscle tissue is of utmost importance in association to progressing symptomatic status of the patients. It has been shown, however, that bone and fat mass also are decreasing later in the course of the disease, all adding to the observed net weight loss of the patients.

Muscle (see also Chapter 19)

The major site of protein loss has been observed in skeletal muscle. Time course studies revealed that the process of tissue degradation in skeletal muscle starts early in the course of the disease, before overt weight loss even becomes apparent. In a study of noncachectic and cachectic patients with stable CHF and, healthy controls of similar age were assessed using dual energy absorption (DEXA) technology.[119] Noncachectic CHF patients displayed reduced lean tissue in the legs as compared with healthy subjects (−9%, $P<.01$). Interestingly, no weight difference was observed, suggesting replacement of muscle with nonfunctional tissue. Cachectic patients had further reduced lean (−20% vs. noncachectic CHF, −21% vs. control), fat (−37% vs. noncachectic CHF, −33% vs. control), and bone tissue (−16% vs. noncachectic CHF, −18% vs. control) (all $P<.0001$; Figure 21-6). The ubiquitin-proteasome pathway has been identified as the pathway for accelerated proteolysis in various catabolic conditions. IGF-1 and insulin have been shown to suppress the expression of atrogin-1, a muscle-specific ubiquitin ligase that induces atrophy.[120] This ability of IGF-1 and insulin constitute important new actions of these hormones that must contribute in a major way to their capacity to stimulate muscle growth.

A number of metabolic derangements have been described in the skeletal muscle of CHF patients (Table 21-3). Biopsy studies have shown defects in oxidative and lipolytic enzymes, succinate dehydrogenase, citrate synthetase, and β-hydroxyacyl dehydrogenase.[121] The reduced exercise capacity in CHF patients results largely from muscle wasting.[122] In fact, skeletal muscle quantitative and qualitative changes might explain some of the major symptoms, such as early fatigue, exercise limitation, and exertional dyspnea, better than abnormalities of central hemodynamic parameters.[123,124]

These peripheral abnormalities may even account for the progression of the disease by maintaining a vicious cycle of deterioration of CHF, coined the "muscle hypothesis" (Figure 21-7).[125]

However, after onset of tissue wasting and the observation of cachexia, peripheral blood flow becomes a stronger predictor of exercise capacity than muscle mass.[126] This suggests impaired nutritional flow to the skeletal muscle as a major reason for reduced maximal exercise capacity of CHF patients. Impaired skeletal muscle metabolism, seen in the lower and upper limbs during exercise in patients with CHF, was related to systemic exercise tolerance.[127] In MRI studies, it has been shown that also myocardium tissue is lost in patients who develop cachexia, although the amount may not significantly contribute to the weight change observed.[21,22]

Fat Tissue (see also Chapter 20)

Lipolysis is controlled mainly by the enzyme *hormone-sensitive lipase.* It is chiefly activated by catecholamines via β-adrenoceptors. The natriuretic peptides (atrial, B-type, and C-type natriuretic peptides) were recently identified to be involved in fat-cell metabolism.[128] The natriuretic peptides control lipid mobilization and lipid oxidation by increasing intracellular cGMP and lipolysis.[129] They also reduce leptin production, increase circulating free fatty acids, and increase insulin resistance.[130]

Insulin is the main antilipolytic substance. Loss of adipose tissue in patients with cachexia could be mediated by increased lipolysis or reduced lipogenesis.[131] Study data from patients with cancer cachexia point to the fact that the predominant mechanism is increased lipolysis. Indeed, fasting plasma glycerol levels, which reflect triglyceride breakdown, are higher in cancer patients with weight loss than in those without.[132,133] This has not been demonstrated in patients with cardiac cachexia or patients with CHF; however, it is tempting to speculate that increased levels in catecholamines and possibly natriuretic peptides may be responsible for the loss of adipose tissue that has been observed in such patients.[119]

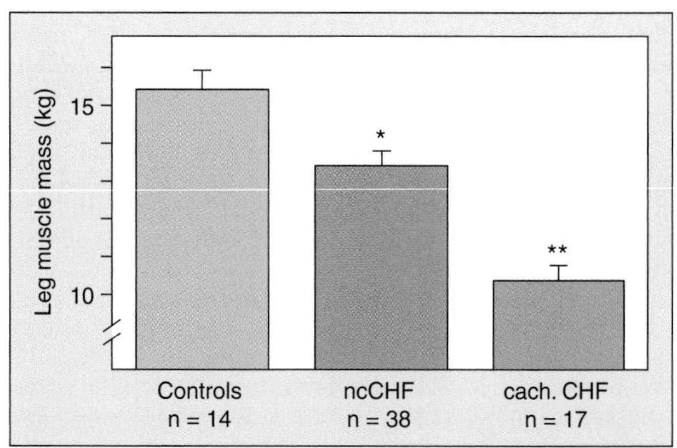

FIGURE 21-6 Leg muscle tissue mass of body composition in noncachectic (ncCHF), cachectic (cach) CHF patients and controls. Body composition measurements determined by dual x-ray absorptiometry. $*P<.05$; $***P<.001$ vs. controls, nc CHF vs. cCHF $P<.001$. (Adapted from Anker SD, Ponikowski PP, Clark AL, et al. Cytokines and neurohormones relating to body composition alterations in the wasting syndrome of chronic heart failure. *Eur Heart J* 1999;20:683-693.)

TABLE 21-3	Skeletal Muscle Changes in Heart Failure
Functional deficit	Weakness Fatigability
Structural change	Loss of muscle mass Atrophy, fibrosis, no apoptosis Fiber type switch type I-type Iib reduced GLUT4 transport protein
Loss of mitochondria	Endothelial damage
Blood flow	Reduced capillary density Impaired vasodilation Reduced peak leg blood flow
Metabolism	Proteolysis Impaired oxidative metabolism
Abnormal lipolytic activity Insulin resistance Glycolysis, acidosis	
Inflammation	Increased cytokine and oxygen radical load
Neuroendocrine factors	GH resistance, epinephrine, norepinephrine
Genetic factors	Myostatin, IGF

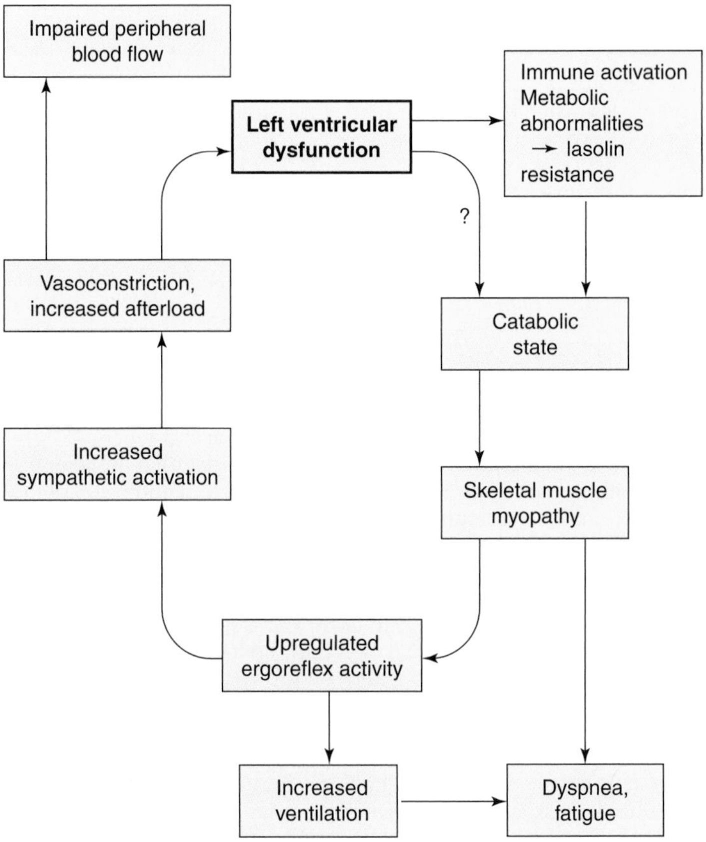

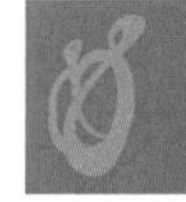

Impaired peripheral blood flow

Left ventricular dysfunction

Immune activation
Metabolic abnormalities
→ lasolin resistance

?

Vasoconstriction, increased afterload

Catabolic state

Increased sympathetic activation

Skeletal muscle myopathy

Upregulated ergoreflex activity

Increased ventilation

Dyspnea, fatigue

FIGURE 21–7 The muscle hypothesis of chronic heart failure. An initial reduction in left ventricular function activates a self-enhancing cycle of skeletal muscle abnormalities and central feedback signaling. This contributes to exercise intolerance and further sympathetic activation that in turn worsens the left ventricular function, maintaining a vicious cycle of deterioration. (Adapted from Coats AJ, Clark AL, Piepoli M, et al. Symptoms and quality of life in heart failure: the muscle hypothesis. *Br Heart J* 1994;72(suppl 2):S36-S39.)

TNF-α, which is also overexpressed in both CHF[134] and cardiac cachexia,[90] plays a major role in fat cell lipolysis and inhibiting insulin signaling. The latter is an important aspect in the development of insulin resistance.

Bone

Bone undergoes constant remodeling (i.e., a process of coordinated resorption and formation of skeletal tissue). Few studies have investigated alterations in bone mass in patients with CHF. Genuine osteoporosis has also been observed in advanced stages of the disease.[135] In their study of 31 adult male cardiac transplant recipients and 14 adult men with CHF awaiting cardiac transplantation, Lee et al found that bone mineral density in the proximal femur was below normal in both groups compared with age-matched control subjects. CHF patients had a trend toward elevations of parathyroid hormone, 1,25-dihydroxyvitamin D, and urinary calcium excretion compared with transplant patients. Eight of 31 transplant patients and 2 of 14 CHF patients presented with vertebral compression fractures (P <.001). In fact, reduced 1,25(OH)(2)D levels (Vit D39) in inverse relation to increased osteoporosis and frailty score were reported in CHF patients.[136]

Lower serum levels of calcium in CHF patients have been observed compared with controls with bone mineral content and bone mineral density being lower in cachectic, but not noncachectic patients than controls (P <.01).[137] An earlier study investigated markers of bone turnover in 101 patients with advanced CHF (NYHA class III-IV).[138] For this purpose, patients had parathyroid hormone, 1,25-dihydroxyvitamin D, serum osteocalcin, urinary hydroxyproline, and pyridinium analyzed. Osteoporosis was present in 7% to 19% (depending on the site of assessment), osteopenia in 42% to 47% of patients with a gender difference toward higher numbers in women (P = .007). Notable, low serum vitamin D metabolites were associated with biochemical evidence of increased bone turnover.[138] Many of the details of the underlying mechanisms of bone wasting in cardiac cachexia still need to be elucidated in future studies.

THERAPEUTIC APPROACHES TO METABOLIC IMBALANCE, WEIGHT LOSS, AND CACHEXIA IN CHF

The significant contribution of metabolic abnormality to CHF pathophysiology with implications for both morbidity and mortality is increasingly recognized. Despite the emerging evidence there is currently no approved therapeutic option to specifically target metabolic failure, weight loss, or cachexia in CHF.

In the following section an overview is provided on three different aspects of metabolically targeted therapeutic approaches: impact of current state of the art medical therapy in CHF, specific nutritional considerations in CHF, and potential novel medical treatment strategies. For some of these, benefit has been shown from retrospective analyses; some have even shown their efficacy in clinical pilot studies. Others have yet to prove their therapeutic benefit based on intriguing theoretical concepts.

Impact of Current CHF Therapy on Body Composition and Metabolic Balance

Angiotensin-converting Enzyme Inhibitors and Angiotensin Receptor Antagonists (see also Chapter 45)

A substantial body of evidence has been accumulated to demonstrate the benefit of inhibition of the renin-angiotensin system for morbidity and mortality in CHF. Besides neurohormonal inhibition as the main effect of angiotensin-converting enzyme (ACE) inhibitors and angiotensin receptor blockers (ARB), a range of additional effects of these compounds have been identified that add to the favorable properties.

Retrospective analyses have shown that ACE inhibitors may prevent or delay the risk of weight loss in patients with CHF. A substudy from the SOLVD database showed that 817 of 1929 patients had a weight loss of 5% during follow-up.[18] Enalapril at a dose of ≥20 mg once daily significantly reduced the risk of weight loss 6% body weight by 19% as compared with placebo (P = .0054). Data from the Cardiovascular Health Study (CHS), a community-based prospective cohort study of 5888 older adults, showed that ACE inhibitor use was associated with less annual weight loss when used as an antihypertensive treatment and in CHF treatment.[139]

Additionally, ACE inhibitors have been implicated in the improvement of insulin resistance.[140] A substudy of the HOPE trial (Heart Outcomes Prevention Evaluation) demonstrated a delay of new onset of diabetes among high-risk patients with established vascular disease following ramipril therapy.[141] Indeed, among those who received the placebo (n = 2883), a total of 155 patients (5.4%) developed new-onset diabetes during 4.5 years of follow-up as compared with 102 patients (3.6%, P <.001) who received ramipril (n = 2837). In a meta-analysis from 22 clinical trials, including 143,153 patients who did not have diabetes at randomization, a significant risk reduction for development of diabetes with ARB (OR 0.57, 95% CI 0.46 to 0.72) or ACE inhibitor (OR 0.67, 95% CI 5.56 to 0.80, both P <.0001).[142]

β-*Blockers (see also Chapter 46)*

A range of β-blockers, such as metoprolol, bisoprolol, carvedilol, and nebivolol, have proven their beneficial effect in CHF therapy. In addition to their effect on survival, β-blockers may exert beneficial effects on weight development. This effect might be explained by the inhibition of catecholamine-induced lipolysis[143] and decreased resting energy expenditure.[144]

A subanalysis of the COPERNICUS (Carvedilol Prospective Randomized Cumulative Survival) database showed that carvedilol-treated patients showed a significant increase in weight compared with placebo-treated patients.[145] At 12 months of follow-up, mean changes in weight in the carvedilol versus the placebo group were +1.1 kg versus +0.2 kg (P <.001). A similar finding has been reported from the CIBIS II-study (Cardiac Insufficiency Bisoprolol Study). Bisoprolol at a target dose of 10 mg once daily prevented or delayed the risk of weight loss in patients with CHF[146] with a 0.84-kg weight gain at 12 months and 1.2 kg at 24 months compared with a placebo.

This effect appears to be mainly due to an increase in body fat mass as data from a small prospective study found increases in body fat content with β-blocker therapy.[147] Hryniewicz et al studied patients with CHF before and after 6 months of β-blocker therapy.[148] Interestingly, 6 months of β-blocker therapy yielded a significantly greater weight gain in patients classified as cachectic than in the noncachectic patients (+5.2 ± 9.6 vs. +0.8 ± 5.0 kg, P = .027).

Metabolic effects in CHF patients may also be translated from findings in patients with severe burns in whom β-blockers have been shown to reverse excess protein catabolism.[149] In this study by Herndon et al with severely burned children, propranolol treatment yielded a decrease in resting energy expenditure and increased muscle-protein balance by 82% over baseline. The fat-free mass did not change substantially. In addition to these effects, it has been observed in an animal model that β-blockers may mediate an increase in skeletal muscle mass.[150]

With regard to insulin sensitivity, the heterogeneity between β-blockers may not allow a common conclusion as the negative and positive impact of β-blockers has been reported. In contrast to nonselective β-blockers, β_1-selective blockers appear to be without significant negative influences on glucose metabolism.[151,152] It has been shown that β_1-selective blockers have no important adverse effect on glucose metabolism and do not prolong hypoglycemia or mask hypoglycemic symptoms.[153] In fact, beneficial effects of metoprolol and atenolol on insulin sensitivity in subjects with hypertension and impaired glucose tolerance have been reported,[154] but the controversy continues and conflicting results have also been reported.[155] Further analyses are needed to show if there is a specific effect of β-blockers on glucose metabolism in CHF patients.

BOX 21–1 Pleiotropic Effects of Statins

Effects on endothelial function
- Induction of eNOS
- Increased NO release
- Reduced oxidative stress

Mobilization of endothelial progenitor cells
Antiinflammatory properties
Reduced proteasome activity
Antitumor activities
Induction of apoptosis

Statins (see also Chapter 24)

Statins are well established to significantly reduce plasma cholesterol and hence cardiovascular risk.[156,157] However, a reduction in recurrent coronary events can be observed as early as 16 weeks after therapy initiation,[158] by far too short to ascribe the risk reduction to cholesterol reduction alone.[159] Moreover, statins seem to be able to ameliorate morbidity and mortality in patients with coronary artery disease irrespective of plasma cholesterol values. Thus effects beyond mere cholesterol reduction, so-called pleiotropic effects of statins, are intensely discussed and have been subject to vigorous research over the past several years (Box 21-1). Some of them might be particularly helpful in the treatment of CHF and possibly cardiac or other forms of cachexia.

Statins have been found to improve endothelial function by a number of different mechanisms, including induction of endothelial nitric oxide synthase (eNOS),[160] increase in nitric oxide release,[161] and reduced oxidative stress.[162] Statins are also able to mobilize endothelial progenitor cells from the bone marrow,[163,164] and possess antiinflammatory properties.[165,166,167] The antiinflammatory properties of statins may be particularly useful in cachectic patients. Additionally, it has been shown that lovastatin can inhibit proteasome activity in cell lysates of a human breast cancer cell line.[168] Statins have also been shown to possess antitumor activities. Indeed, lovastatin was demonstrated to inhibit the cell cycle of a murine fibroblast cell line[169] and a human bladder carcinoma cell line[170] in the G1 phase. In addition to this effect, the induction of apoptosis might be another important antitumor activity.[171]

The use of statins in CHF has recently suffered a significant setback. Based on favorable findings in retrospective observations and meta-analyses, the prospective CORONA (Controlled Rosuvastatin Multinational Trial in Heart Failure) study enrolled 5011 patients with ischemic CHF and an impaired LVEF to test the effect of rosuvastatin 10 mg daily versus placebo in a double-blind fashion.[172] After a median follow-up of 32.8 months, no significant difference between the two groups could be detected for the primary outcome (composite of death from cardiovascular causes, nonfatal myocardial infarction, or nonfatal stroke). The primary endpoint was observed in 692 patients in the rosuvastatin and

732 patients in the placebo group (hazard ratio 0.92, 95% CI 0.83 to 1.02, $P = .12$). The only beneficial effect that was noted in the rosuvastatin group was a reduction in the total number of hospitalizations for worsening heart failure ($P = .01$). It has been discussed that the pleiotropic effect is not a class effect of statins, and that rosuvastatin may not possess effects that are beneficial in CHF. Interestingly, rosuvastatin did reduce levels of C-reactive protein during follow-up ($P < .0001$), which, however, failed to translate into beneficial effects.

A second large-scale randomized controlled study, the GISSI-HF trial (Gruppo Italiano per lo Studio della Sopravvivenza nell'Insufficienza Cardiaca) tested the impact of n-3 polyunsaturated fatty acids (PUFA) and rosuvastatin in patients with CHF.[173] Patients with CHF (NYHA class II-IV), irrespective of cause, and left ventricular ejection fraction were included and randomly assigned to rosuvastatin 10 mg daily (n = 2285) or placebo (n = 2289). Median follow-up was 3.9 years (IQR 3.0 to 4.4). Death from any cause occurred in 657 (29%) versus 644 (28%) patients in the rosuvastatin versus the placebo group (adjusted HR 1.00; 95.5% CI 0.898 to 1.122, $P = .943$). Also the other primary endpoint, death or admission to hospital for cardiovascular reasons, was stunningly similar between groups (adjusted HR 1.01; 99% CI 0.908 to 1.112, $P = .903$). These findings were despite a 27% decreased LDL cholesterol in the rosuvastatin group at 3 years. Based on these two large trials, treatment of CHF patients in general with statins seems unlikely to translate into clinical benefit. Whether particular patients with cachexia may benefit from statin therapy needs to be clarified.

Nutrition

Energy and substrate input are naturally major determinants of the body's metabolic balance. Accordingly, nutritional supply contributes significantly to the development of prevention of tissue wasting. Patients with CHF are prone to reduced appetite and reduced food intake.[174] Besides changes in the fine-tuned balance in the regulation of hunger and satiety (see previous discussion), dietary advice on salt and calorie intake, social isolation, derangements in bowel perfusion, and an altered intestinal barrier[175] may all contribute to reduced food intake in CHF patients. These alterations are likely to cause both deficiencies in micronutrients and macronutrients that may fuel the wasting process.

Large-scale studies on appetite and food intake in CHF are not available. Since both the intake of micronutrients and macronutrients may be affected in patients with CHF and those with cardiac cachexia, it may be necessary to optimize food intake of all components that are affected. This, however, is not always possible, and clinical guidelines on this issue for patients with CHF are missing. Some general rules, however, appear to apply for patients with CHF as for those with cardiac cachexia.

A diet high in sodium is generally viewed as potentially harmful in CHF because it may cause fluid overload and consequently acute hemodynamic decompensation. Rare cases of micronutrient deficiency as a cause of CHF have been reported for selenium and thiamine (vitamin B_1).[176] One study suggests that thiamine supplementation per se may improve cardiac function.[177] Low levels of selenium have been reported in patients with CHF. In a study in 21 patients with CHF (NYHA class II-III, mean LVEF 29±6%), baseline selenium levels were approximately 20% lower than those in healthy control subjects ($P = .0004$).[178] Lower levels of copper and zinc were also reported in this study (both $P < .05$).[178]

Patients with CHF are usually receiving loop diuretics, which increase urinary excretion of micronutrients. This affects, for example, magnesium and calcium.[176] Witte et al performed a placebo-controlled, randomized, double-blind study of multiple micronutrient supplementation in 30 patients with CHF.[179] Patients received capsules containing thiamine (daily dose: 200 mg), vitamin C (500μ mg) and E (400 mg), magnesium (150 mg), selenium (50 μg), zinc (15 mg), coenzyme Q10 (150 mg), and various other substances. Interestingly, 9 months of treatment yielded an improvement in LVEF by 5.3 ± 1.4% in the micronutrient group ($P < .05$ vs. placebo). It is not clear how this effect had been mediated but it may be that a reduction in oxidative stress took place. Indeed, many micronutrients can scavenge free radicals.[180] This may ensue through direct action as with vitamins C and E or through indirect action. In agreement with this, vitamin C has also been shown to improve endothelial dysfunction.

As discussed previously, wasting takes place not only in muscle tissue but also in fat and bone tissue. The constituent amino acids are capable of being transformed into all three macronutrients (i.e., protein, carbohydrate, and fat[181]). Therefore, amino acid supplementation has been studied in some clinical settings, and some models indicate that patients with CHF require a greater amount of protein than healthy adults of the same age.[181] Thus the current dietary reference of 0.8 g protein per kg of body weight may be too low for patients with CHF and those with cardiac cachexia.[181]

Low plasma levels of glutamine were found in critically ill patients and patients with chronic illness associated with muscle wasting.[182,183] After 4 weeks of treatment with glutamine, a nonessential amino acid that is involved in cellular integrity and immune function, patients with cancer cachexia gained 0.95 ± 0.66 kg compared with control subjects who lost 0.26 ± 0.78 kg.[184] This change was due to a significant increase in fat-free mass in the active treatment group (+1.12 ± 0.68 kg vs. −1.34 ± 0.78 kg, $P = .02$). Patients in the active treatment group received not only glutamine, but a mixture of β-hydroxy-β-methylbutyrate (3 g/day), L-arginine (14 g/day), and L-glutamine (14 g/day). Patients in the control group received a mixture of nonessential amino acids in double-blind fashion.

Branched-chain amino acids, namely, leucine, isoleucine, and valine, have been suggested as a useful supplementation in the treatment of cachexia[185] because they may exert anabolic effects by promoting protein synthesis and by inhibiting proteolysis. This effect appears to be most potently exerted by leucine.[186] Supplementation of any amino acid is certainly not beneficial. Homocysteine, for example, is known to possess negative inotropic properties.[187] In patients with CHF, high levels of homocysteine were found in association with low levels of vitamins B_6, B_9 (folate), B_{12}, and magnesium. Indeed, a correlation has been shown between circulating homocysteine levels and certain vitamins because homocysteine degradation is dependent on the presence of vitamins B_6, B_9, and B_{12}.[188] Gorelik et al have shown that the intake of vitamin B_9 did not reach the recommended daily amount (400 μg) in 57 patients with CHF who were hospitalized and 40 healthy controls.[189]

The use of n-3 polyunsaturated fatty acids derived from fish oil has been studied in a canine model of heart failure.[190] A total of 28 dogs, 15 of which were cachectic, were fed fish oil supplement or placebo for 8 weeks. Interestingly, active treatment decreased plasma levels of IL-1 ($P = .02$) and improved cachexia ($P = .01$) compared with the placebo group.

As an alternative to the supplementation of single substances, Rozentryt et al studied the effects of high caloric enteral support in a small, randomized, placebo-controlled study in 29 patients with cardiac cachexia.[191] Patients were randomized in a 3:1 fashion to either high caloric enteral support (600 kcal daily in addition to their normal diet) or a placebo for 6 weeks. Weight increased by 2.6 kg after 12 weeks' follow-up. Moreover, 6-minute walking distance improved from 366 ± 108 m to 433 ± 106 m; $P = .02$.

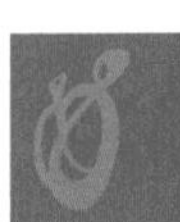

It is important to understand, however, that increased food intake and high caloric or specific substrate supplementation alone may not be sufficient to prevent or reverse the overall catabolic process underlying the development of weight loss and cachexia. As noted earlier, the complex pathophysiology of tissue wasting includes impairment of resorption, assimilation, storage, and metabolic use of substrates. Increased nutritional supply to the system needs to be accompanied by improved energy and substrate metabolic efficiency of the body's tissues and increased anabolic drive and attenuated catabolic stimulation to prevent or reverse a continued catabolic spiral toward cachexia.

Nutritional Considerations

The daily sodium intake should be restricted to 2 g in all patients with advanced CHF or cardiac cachexia.[174] Thus all food rich in salt should be avoided. This is particularly true for cheese, sausages, crisps, canned soup and vegetables, ham, bacon, canned meat, and canned or smoked fish.[174] Prolonged periods of fasting are potentially harmful, and cachectic patients should be advised to eat small, frequent meals.[192] Fluid intake should be restricted to 1.5 to 2.0 liters per day, especially in patients with severe symptoms or those requiring high doses of diuretics.[174] At least one study suggests that multiple micronutrient supplementation is potentially beneficial.[179] Such supplements should contain antioxidant supplements and B-group vitamins. Statin therapy should be initiated with caution, because retrospective data indicate that low levels of total cholesterol, LDL, and triglycerides are associated with poor outcomes in CHF patients.[193,194] However, statin therapy is still associated with survival benefits in patients with CHF. Thus statins may be beneficial in CHF patients not because but despite of their cholesterol lowering effects (see later discussion).[195]

It is also recommended to avoid food and lifestyle factors that trigger the acute phase response such as an excess of carbohydrates or saturated fats, alcohol, and smoking.[196] Food that counteracts inflammatory responses, on the other hand, can be recommended. This includes fish oil supplements, olives, walnuts, flaxseed oil, any fruits or vegetables, garlic, ginger, turmeric, sunflower seeds, eggs, herring, or nuts.[196] Enteral nutrition should always be given preference over parenteral nutrition; however, if the latter cannot be avoided, the general guidelines can be followed: 35 kcal per kg of body weight per day, 1.2 g of protein per kg per day, and a 70:30 glucose:lipid ratio for the nonprotein energy.[8]

Pharmacotherapy of Cardiac Cachexia

Despite the emerging data of weight loss and cachexia as a significant impact on morbidity and mortality on CHF, there is currently no approved therapy available to prevent, reduce, or reverse the tissue wasting in these patients. A range of compounds are available and in use for other conditions. Their value for the setting in CHF, however, is unclear if not controversial. The following section provides an overview on therapeutic strategies currently under evaluation or in use in other settings of wasting and cachexia, such as, above others, in cancer and HIV (Box 21-2).

BOX 21–2 Potential Therapeutic Options to Improve Metabolic Status

Appetite Stimulants
- Megestrol acetate
- Medroxyprogesterone acetate
- Cyproheptadine
- Dronabinol

Anabolic Steroids (Selection)
- Danazol
- Fluoxymesterone
- Methandrostenolone
- Methyltestosterone
- Nandrolone decanoate
- Nandrolone phenpropionate
- Oxandrolone
- Oxymetholone
- Stanozolol

Antiinflammatory Substances
- TNF-α inhibitory potential
- Adenosine
- Amiodarone
- Etanercept
- IC14 (LPS receptor blocker, not approved)
- Infliximab
- Pentoxifylline
- Thalidomide

Proteasome Inhibitors

Appetite Stimulants

Appetite stimulating compounds are naturally of great interest in the context of anticachectic therapy. Synthetic derivates from the steroid hormone progesterone, such as medroxyprogesterone acetate and megestrol acetate, have shown their efficacy in stimulating appetite in cachectic patients in a number of randomized controlled trials.[197,198] The precise mechanism by which the resulting weight gain is mediated is presently unknown but a range of effects, including stimulation of neuropeptide Y,[199] inhibition of proinflammatory cytokines,[200] and modulation of calcium channels in the ventromedial hypothalamus,[201] are discussed. Clinical studies focused on cancer- and AIDS-associated wasting and no studies in patients with cardiac cachexia are available.

Cannabinoids

Cannabinoids are known to stimulate appetite. Two indications are currently approved for delta-9-tetrahydrocannabinol: chemotherapy-associated nausea and vomiting and AIDS-associated anorexia and wasting. The active ingredient of cannabis is delta-9-tetrahydrocannabinol. Dronabinol, nabilone, and levonantradol are synthetic cannabinoids for oral application. Patients in AIDS-[202] and cancer-related[203,204] weight loss studies, however, have not shown a significant weight gain.

Cardiac side effects of cannabinoids such as tachycardia, hypotension, and decreased cardiac function[205] seem to contraindicate the use in patients with cardiac cachexia.

Anabolic Steroids

Anabolic steroids are chemically related to testosterone, yielding an increase in protein synthesis and hence an increase in muscle mass. Due to an extensive first-pass metabolism in the liver, the oral bioavailability of testosterone is poor. Intramuscular injections, implantable pellets, buccal, and transdermal systems are available for delivery. Other anabolic steroids such as methyltestosterone, danazol, oxandrolone, and others are available for oral administration.

While testosterone replacement was shown to improve functional capacity and symptoms in general heart failure patients,[206,207] no study has been performed in patients with cardiac cachexia. Observations in patients with cachexia due to COPD and in HIV patients[208] showed significant increase in body weight, particularly in lean tissue.[209]

Antiinflammatory Substances (see also Chapter 11)

A vast array of substances from different drug classes has been shown to suppress inflammation, especially the production or the action of proinflammatory cytokines.[210] Despite the intriguing pathophysiological concept, however (see previous discussion), results so far were disappointing.

One approach used etanercept, which is a TNF-α receptor 2 fusion protein that binds and thus inactivates the cytokine. A large trial program using etanercept included the RENAISSANCE trial (Randomized Etanercept North AmerIcan Strategy to Study ANtagonism of CytokinEs) and the RECOVER trial (Research into Etanercept: CytOkine Antagonism in VEntriculaR Dysfunction) plus the combined analysis (RENEWAL). The program was terminated early following a recommendation of its Independent Data Safety Monitoring Board (DSMB)[211] when interim analyses revealed a lack of efficacy of the treatment.

Infliximab is a chimeric (mouse/human) IgG_1 monoclonal antibody that binds both soluble and membrane-bound TNF-α□. It is clinically used with good effect in the treatment of Crohn disease. The ATTACH (Anti-TNF-α Therapy Against Chronic Heart failure) trial, a multicenter, randomized, double-blind, placebo-controlled study in CHF, was stopped prematurely because of an increased risk of death (RR 2.84, 95% CI 1.01 to 7.97, $P<.05$) with the higher dose of infliximab (i.e., 10 mg/kg body weight).[212] Like with etanercept, it is not easy to explain the disappointing results. Infliximab was shown to be directly cytotoxic to cells expressing TNF-α on their membranes. This effect is beneficial in eliminating activated T cells in Crohn's disease, but it is deleterious in CHF, in which failing myocytes express TNF-α on their surfaces.[213]

Inhibition of Lipopolysaccharide Bioactivity

Since LPS is discussed as a trigger of inflammatory activation in CHF (see previous discussion), this pathway, including the Toll-like receptor 4, may serve as a therapeutic target.[214] IC14, an antibody that blocks CD14-mediated LPS binding to Toll-like receptor 4, has been shown to downregulate LPS-induced TNF-α production in whole blood samples from patients with CHF.[215]

A rather unexpected finding was that patients with CHF and higher plasma cholesterol levels have better (not worse) survival rates than those with lower levels.[193,194] Additional in vitro data showed a linear relationship between plasma cholesterol levels and LPS-stimulated TNF-α production.[216] This suggests that LPS is inactivated by cholesterol, which lends support to the endotoxin-lipoprotein hypothesis.[217] This hypothesis suggests that micelle formation by cholesterol around LPS could be beneficial in CHF.

Immune Modulation by Thalidomide (see also Chapter 11)

Thalidomide was part of one of the largest drug tragedies in the history of medicine because of the initially unrecognized induction of congenital abnormalities, most frequently phocomelia.[218] The drug was later found to inhibit angiogenesis,[219] resulting in limb malformation, after only a single dose taken within a specific period during pregnancy.

The potent TNF-α selective antiinflammatory capacity of thalidomide[220] and amino-substituted analogues may yield positive immune modulatory effects.[221] This led to the suggestion of using thalidomide in the treatment of CHF[222] and cachexia.[223] Results from early small studies suggest increased LVEF[223] and improved the 6-minute walking distance.[224,225] Others, however, were unable to find effects on LVEF or any other echocardiographic parameters after treatment with thalidomide.[226] The potential role in cardiac cachexia warrants further investigation.

Proteasome Inhibitors

To date, four different classes of proteasome inhibitors have been described that are either reversible or irreversible inhibitors of specific activities of the proteasome.[227] Bortezomib was given approval by the U.S. Food and Drug Administration for the treatment of multiple myeloma and mantle cell lymphoma in patients who had received at least one prior therapy. No studies are available that have specifically evaluated whether bortezomib or possibly other proteasome inhibitors are able to reverse weight loss in cachectic patients.

Pentoxifylline (see also Chapter 11)

It was initially characterized as a hemorheologic agent; however, recent studies suggested that pentoxifylline may inhibit TNF-α formation.[228] A number of clinical studies have been performed in patients with CHF. Increased LVEF in parallel to reduced TNF-α plasma levels were observed.[229,230] In other randomized, double-blind, placebo-controlled studies, a significant increase in NYHA class and improved LVEF[231] were observed. Other studies were, however, unable to confirm the former findings in CHF.[232] Beneficial effects in the treatment of cancer cachexia have been reported to prevent muscle atrophy and suppress protein breakdown by inhibition of the ubiquitin-proteasome pathway.[233,234] Future studies need to define the role of pentoxifylline in the setting of cachexia.

CONCLUSION AND OUTLOOK

The pathophysiology of cardiac cachexia is exceedingly complex, and we still do not understand when and how CHF progresses into this syndrome. Metabolic imbalance, hormonal dysregulation, and proinflammatory cytokines play important parts in the interrelated system (Figure 21-8). Despite convincing concepts on pathophysiological grounds, a range of approaches failed when tested in clinical studies. We are currently not able to interfere with appetite regulation in a promising way, although initial steps have been undertaken and may prove beneficial in future studies.

No studies are currently available that have specifically targeted cardiac cachexia using a pharmacological approach. Nutritional recommendations to prevent of reverse cardiac cachexia remain speculative, and no large-scale, randomized, controlled trials have been performed.

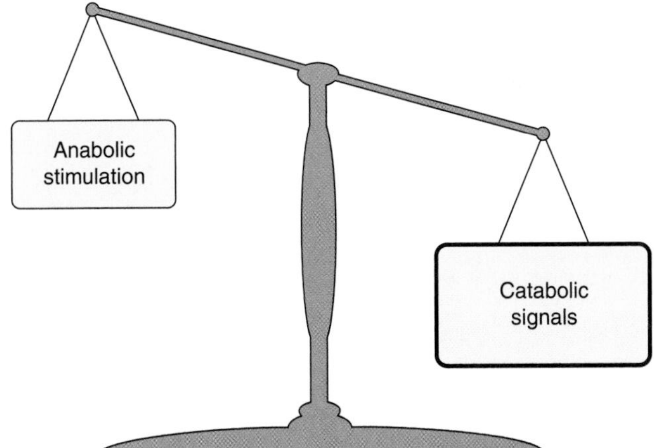

FIGURE 21–8 Pathophysiology of cachexia in chronic illness: An overall catabolic dominance results from a combined effect of impaired regulatory systems, such as neuroendocrine activation, metabolic hormonal signaling failure, inflammatory activation, impaired central regulation of appetite, and others.

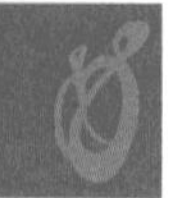

With better understanding of the complex interaction of metabolic abnormalities within the pathophysiology of CHF we may advance the pharmacological therapeutic options in CHF beyond the neuroendocrine activation. Targeting immune activation, feeding, and metabolic balance are promising areas for future therapeutic concepts. Novel compounds constantly coming along the pharmaceutical development pipelines and future research will show whether those may translate into clinical improvement of patients with CHF.

REFERENCES

1. American Heart Association. Heart disease and stroke statistics. (2005). *Update.* Dallas: American Heart Association.
2. Remme, W. J., & Swedberg, K. (2001). Guidelines for the diagnosis and treatment of chronic heart failure. *Eur Heart J, 22,* 1527–1560.
3. Stewart, S., MacIntyre, K., Hole, D. J., et al. (2001). More "malignant" than cancer? Five-year survival following a first admission for heart failure. *Eur J Heart Fail, 3,* 315–312.
4. Anker, S. D., Ponikowski, P., Varney, S., et al. (1997). Wasting as independent risk factor for mortality in chronic heart failure. *Lancet, 349,* 1050–1053.
5. Evans, W. J., Morley, J. E., Argilés, J., et al. (2008). Cachexia: a new definition. *Clin Nutr, 27,* 793–799.
6. Katz, A. M., & Katz, P. B. (1962). Diseases of the heart in the works of Hippokrates. *Br Heart J, 24,* 257–264.
7. Doehner, W., & Anker, S. D. (2002). Cardiac cachexia in early literature: a review of research prior to Medline. *Int J Cardiol, 85,* 7–14.
8. Wallace, J. I., & Schwartz, R. S. (2002). Epidemiology of weight loss in humans with special reference to wasting in the elderly. *Int J Cardiol, 85,* 15–21.
9. Dansinger, M. L., Tatsioni, A., Wong, J. B., et al. (2007). Meta-analysis: the effect of dietary counseling for weight loss. *Ann Intern Med, 147,* 41–50.
10. Whitlock, G., Lewington, S., Prospective Studies Collaboration, et al. (2009). Body-mass index and cause-specific mortality in 900,000 adults: collaborative analyses of 57 prospective studies. *Lancet, 373*(9669), 1083–1096.
11. Curtis, J. P., Selter, J. G., Wang, Y., et al. (2005). The obesity paradox: body mass index and outcomes in patients with heart failure. *Arch Intern Med, 165,* 55–61.
12. Kenchaiah, S., Pocock, S. J., Wang, D., et al. (2007). Body mass index and prognosis in patients with chronic heart failure: insights from the candesartan in heart failure: assessment of reduction in mortality and morbidity (CHARM) program. *Circulation, 116,* 627–636.
13. Cicoira, M., Maggioni, A. P., Latini, R., et al. (2007). Body mass index, prognosis and mode of death in chronic heart failure: results from the valsartan heart failure trial. *Eur J Heart Fail, 9,* 397–402.
14. Oreopoulos, A., Padwal, R., Kalantar-Zadeh, K., et al. (2008). Body mass index and mortality in heart failure: a meta-analysis. *Am Heart J, 156,* 13–22.
15. Lainscak, M., Filippatos, G., Gheorghiade, M., et al. (2007). Cachexia: common, deadly, with an urgent need for precise definition and new therapies. *Am J Cardiol 2008, 101,*8E-10E.
16. Evans, W. J. (1995). What is sarcopenia? *J Gerontol A Biol Sci Med Sci, 50*(spec no), 5–8.
17. Springer, J., Filippatos, G., Akashi, Y. J., et al. (2006). Prognosis and therapy approaches of cardiac cachexia. *Curr Opin Cardiol, 21,* 229–233.
18. Anker, S. D., Negassa, A., Coats, A. J., et al. (2003). Prognostic importance of weight loss in chronic heart failure and the effect of treatment with angiotensin-converting-enzyme inhibitors: an observational study. *Lancet, 361,* 1077–1083.
19. Davos, C. H., Doehner, W., Rauchhaus, M., et al. (2003). Body mass and survival in patients with chronic heart failure without cachexia: the importance of obesity. *J Card Fail, 9,* 29–35.
20. Anker, S. D., Chua, T. P., Ponikowski, P., et al. (1997). Hormonal changes and catabolic/anabolic imbalance in chronic heart failure and their importance for cardiac cachexia. *Circulation, 96,* 526–534.
21. Florea, V. G., Henein, M. Y., Rauchhaus, M., et al. (2002). The cardiac component of cardiac cachexia. *Am Heart J, 144,* 45–50.
22. Florea, V. G., Moon, J., Pennell, D. J., et al. (2004). Wasting of the left ventricle in patients with cardiac cachexia: a cardiovascular magnetic resonance study. *Int J Cardiol, 97,* 15–20.
23. von Haehling, S., Doehner, W., & Anker, S. D. (2007). Nutrition, metabolism and the complex pathophysiology of cachexia in chronic heart failure. *Cardiovasc Res, 73,* 298–309.
24. Strassburg, S., Springer, J., & Anker, S. D. (2005). Muscle wasting in cardiac cachexia. *Int J Biochem Cell Biol, 37,* 1938–1947.
25. Akashi, Y. J., Springer, J., & Anker, S. D. (2005). Cachexia in chronic heart failure: prognostic implications and novel therapeutic approaches. *Curr Heart Fail Rep, 2,* 198–203.
26. Schwengel, R. H., Gottlieb, S. S., & Fisher, M. L. (1994). Protein-energy malnutrition in patients with ischemic and nonischemic dilated cardiomyopathy and congestive heart failure. *Am J Cardiol, 73,* 908–910.
27. Ganong, W. F. (1999). Central regulation of visceral function. In *Review of medical physiology.* Stamford, Conn: Appleton & Lange.
28. Williams, G., Cai, X. J., Elliott, J. C., et al. (2004). Anabolic neuropeptides. *Physiol Behav, 81,* 211–222.
29. Kokot, F., & Ficek, R. (1999). Effects of neuropeptide Y on appetite. *Miner Electrolyte Metab, 25,* 303–305.
30. Feng, Q., Lambert, M. L., Callow, I. D., et al. (2000). Venous neuropeptide Y receptor responsiveness in patients with chronic heart failure. *Clin Pharmacol Ther, 67,* 292–298.
31. Ullman, B., Pernow, J., Lundberg, J. M., et al. (2002). Cardiovascular effects and cardiopulmonary plasma gradients following intravenous infusion of neuropeptide Y in humans: negative dromotropic effect on atrioventricular node conduction. *Clin Sci, 103,* 535–542.
32. Zhang, Y., Proenca, R., Maffei, M., et al. (1994). Positional cloning of the mouse obese gene and its human homologue. *Nature, 372,* 425–432.
33. Houseknecht, K. L., Baile, C. A., Matteri, R. L., et al. (1998). The biology of leptin: a review. *J Anim Sci, 76,* 1405–1420.
34. Kennedy, A., Gettys, T. W., Watson, P., et al. (1997). The metabolic significance of leptin in humans: gender-based differences in relationship to adiposity, insulin sensitivity, and energy expenditure. *J Clin Endocrinol Metab, 82,* 1293–1300.
35. Tartaglia, L. A., Dembski, M., Weng, X., et al. (1995). Identification and expression cloning of a leptin receptor, OB-R. *Cell, 83,* 1263–1271.
36. Lee, G. H., Proenca, R., Montez, J. M., et al. (1996). Abnormal splicing of the leptin receptor in diabetic mice. *Nature, 379,* 632–635.
37. Emilsson, V., Liu, Y. L., Cawthorne, M. A., et al. (1997). Expression of the functional leptin receptor mRNA in pancreatic islets and direct inhibitory action of leptin on insulin secretion. *Diabetes, 46,* 313–316.
38. Doehner, W., Rauchhaus, M., Godsland, I. F., et al. (2002). Insulin resistance in moderate chronic heart failure is related to hyperleptinaemia, but not to norepinephrine or TNF-alpha. *Int J Cardiol, 83,* 73–81.
39. Ronti, T., Lupattelli, G., & Mannarino, E. (2006). The endocrine function of adipose tissue: an update. *Clin Endocrinol, 64,* 355–365.
40. Considine, R. V., Sinha, M. K., Heiman, M. L., et al. (1996). Serum immunoreactive-leptin concentrations in normal-weight and obese humans. *N Engl J Med, 334,* 292–295.
41. Horvath, T. L. (2005). The hardship of obesity: a soft-wired hypothalamus. *Nat Neurosci, 8,* 561–565.
42. Cone, R. D. (2005). Anatomy and regulation of the central melanocortin system. *Nat Neurosci, 8,* 571–578.
43. Schwartz, M. W., & Morton, G. J. (2002). Keeping hunger at bay. *Nature, 418,* 595–597.
44. Cowley, M. A., Smart, J. L., Rubinstein, M., et al. (2001). Leptin activates anorexigenic POMC neurons through a neural network in the arcuate nucleus. *Nature, 411,* 480–484.
45. Toth, M. J., Gottlieb, S. S., Fisher, M. L., et al. (1997). Plasma leptin concentrations and energy expenditure in heart failure patients. *Metabolism, 46,* 450–453.
46. Doehner, W., Pflaum, C. D., Rauchhaus, M., et al. (2001). Leptin, insulin sensitivity and growth hormone binding protein in chronic heart failure with and without cardiac cachexia. *Eur J Endocrinol, 145,* 727–735.
47. Murdoch, D. R., Rooney, E., Dargie, H. J., et al. (1999). Inappropriately low plasma leptin concentration in the cachexia associated with chronic heart failure. *Heart, 82,* 352–356.
48. Doehner, W., & Anker, S. D. (2000). The significance of leptin in humans—do we know it yet? *Int J Cardiol, 76,* 122–124.
49. Leyva, F., Anker, S. D., Egerer, K., et al. (1998). Hyperleptinaemia in chronic heart failure. Relationships with insulin. *Eur Heart J, 19,* 1547–1551.
50. Coll, A. P. (2007). Effects of pro-opiomelanocortin (POMC) on food intake and body weight: mechanisms and therapeutic potential? *Clin Sci, 113,* 171–182.
51. Mountjoy, K. G., Mortrud, M. T., Low, M. J., et al. (1994). Localization of the melanocortin-4 receptor (MC4-R) in neuroendocrine and autonomic circuits in the brain. *Mol Endocrinol, 8,* 1298–1308.
52. Krude, H., Biebermann, H., Luck, W., et al. (1998). Severe early-onset obesity, adrenal insufficiency and red hair pigmentation caused by POMC mutations in humans. *Nat Genet, 19,* 155–157.
53. Yeo, G. S., Farooqi, I. S., Aminian, S., et al. (1998). A frameshift mutation in MC4R associated with dominantly inherited human obesity. *Nat Genet, 20,* 111–112.
54. Vaisse, C., Clement, K., Guy-Grand, B., et al. (1998). A frameshift mutation in human MC4R is associated with a dominant form of obesity. *Nat Genet, 20,* 113–114.
55. Shimizu, H., Inoue, K., & Mori, M. (2007). The leptin-dependent and -independent melanocortin signaling system: regulation of feeding and energy expenditure. *J Endocrinol, 193,* 1–9.
56. Laviano, A., Inui, A., Marks, D. L., et al. (2008). Neural control of the anorexia-cachexia syndrome. *Am J Physiol Endocrinol Metab, 295,* E1000–E1008.
57. DeBoer, M. D., & Marks, D. L. (2006). Therapy insight: use of melanocortin antagonists in the treatment of cachexia in chronic disease. *Nat Clin Pract Endocrinol Metab, 2,* 459–466.
58. Mak, R. H., & Cheung, W. (2007). Cachexia in chronic kidney disease: role of inflammation and neuropeptide signaling. *Curr Opin Nephrol Hypertens, 16,* 27–31.
59. DeBoer, M. D. (2007). Melanocortin interventions in cachexia: how soon from bench to bedside? *Curr Opin Clin Nutr Metab Care, 10,* 457–462.
60. Kojima, M., Hosoda, H., Date, Y., et al. (1999). Ghrelin is a growth-hormone-releasing acylated peptide from stomach. *Nature, 402,* 656–660.
61. Date, Y., Kojima, M., Hosoda, H., et al. (2000). Ghrelin, a novel growth hormone-releasing acylated peptide, is synthesized in a distinct endocrine cell type in the gastrointestinal tracts of rats and humans. *Endocrinology, 141,* 4255–4261.
62. Date, Y., Nakazato, M., Hashiguchi, S., et al. (2002). Ghrelin is present in pancreatic alpha-cells of humans and rats and stimulates insulin secretion. *Diabetes, 51,* 124–129.
63. Mori, K., Yoshimoto, A., Takaya, K., et al. (2000). Kidney produces a novel acylated peptide, ghrelin. *FEBS Lett, 486,* 213–216.
64. Gualillo, O., Caminos, J., Blanco, M., et al. (2001). Ghrelin, a novel placental-derived hormone. *Endocrinology, 142,* 788–794.
65. Howard, A. D., Feighner, S. D., Cully, D. F., et al. (1996). A receptor in pituitary and hypothalamus that functions in growth hormone release. *Science, 273,* 974–977.
66. McKee, K. K., Palyha, O. C., Feighner, S. D., et al. (1997). Molecular analysis of rat pituitary and hypothalamic growth hormone secretagogue receptors. *Mol Endocrinol, 11,* 415–423.
67. Arvat, E., Maccario, M., Di Vito, L., et al. (2001). Endocrine activities of ghrelin, a natural growth hormone secretagogue (GHS), in humans: comparison and interactions with hexarelin, a nonnatural peptidyl GHS, and GH-releasing hormone. *J Clin Endocrinol Metab, 86,* 1169–1174.
68. Cowley, M. A., Smith, R. G., Diano, S., et al. (2003). The distribution and mechanism of action of ghrelin in the CNS demonstrates a novel hypothalamic circuit regulating energy homeostasis. *Neuron, 37,* 649–661.

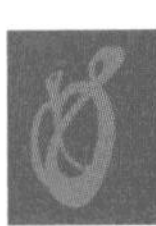

69. Chen, H. Y., Trumbauer, M. E., Chen, A. S., et al. (2004). Orexigenic action of peripheral ghrelin is mediated by neuropeptide Y and agouti-related protein. *Endocrinology, 145*, 2607–2612.
70. Hewson, A. K., & Dickson, S. L. (2000). Systemic administration of ghrelin induces Fos and Egr-1 proteins in the hypothalamic arcuate nucleus of fasted and fed rats. *J Neuroendocrinol, 12*, 1047–1049.
71. Wren, A. M., Small, C. J., Abbott, C. R., et al. (2001). Ghrelin causes hyperphagia and obesity in rats. *Diabetes, 50*, 2540–2547.
72. Sakata, I., Yamazaki, M., Inoue, K., et al. (2003). Growth hormone secretagogue receptor expression in the cells of the stomach-projected afferent nerve in the rat nodose ganglion. *Neurosci Lett, 342*, 183–186.
73. Gnanapavan, S., Kola, B., Bustin, S. A., et al. (2002). The tissue distribution of the mRNA of ghrelin and subtypes of its receptor, GHS-R, in humans. *J Clin Endocrinol Metab, 87*, 2988.
74. Xia, Q., Pang, W., Pan, H., et al. (2004). Effects of ghrelin on the proliferation and secretion of splenic T lymphocytes in mice. *Regul Pept, 122*, 173–178.
75. Chang, L., Zhao, J., Yang, J., et al. (2003). Therapeutic effects of ghrelin on endotoxic shock in rats. *Eur J Pharmacol, 473*, 171–176.
76. Li, W. G., Gavrila, D., Liu, X., et al. (2004). Ghrelin inhibits proinflammatory responses and nuclear factor-kappaB activation in human endothelial cells. *Circulation, 109*, 2221–2226.
77. Nagaya, N., Uematsu, M., Kojima, M., et al. (2001). Elevated circulating level of ghrelin in cachexia associated with chronic heart failure: relationships between ghrelin and anabolic/catabolic factors. *Circulation, 104*, 2034–2038.
78. Nagaya, N., Moriya, J., Yasumura, Y., et al. (2004). Effects of ghrelin administration on left ventricular function, exercise capacity, and muscle wasting in patients with chronic heart failure. *Circulation, 110*, 3674–3679.
79. Nagaya, N., Uematsu, M., Kojima, M., et al. (2001). Chronic administration of ghrelin improves left ventricular dysfunction and attenuates development of cardiac cachexia in rats with heart failure. *Circulation, 104*, 1430–1435.
80. Akashi, Y. J., Palus, S., Datta, R., et al. (2008). No effects of human ghrelin on cardiac function despite profound effects on body composition in a rat model of heart failure. *Int J Cardiol* (Pubmed ahead of print).
81. Akamizu, T., Iwakura, H., Ariyasu, H., et al. (2008). Effects of ghrelin treatment on patients undergoing total hip replacement for osteoarthritis: different outcomes from studies in patients with cardiac and pulmonary cachexia. *J Am Geriatr Soc, 56*, 2363–2365.
82. Ukkola, O., & Santaniemi, M. (2002). Adiponectin: a link between excess adiposity and associated comorbidities? *J Mol Med, 80*, 696–702.
83. Santaniemi, M., Kesäniemi, Y. A., & Ukkola, O. (2006). Low plasma adiponectin concentration is an indicator of the metabolic syndrome. *Eur J Endocrinol, 155*, 745–750.
84. Díez, J. J., & Iglesias, P. (2003). The role of the novel adipocyte-derived hormone adiponectin in human disease. *Eur J Endocrinol, 148*, 293–300.
85. Nørrelund, H., Wiggers, H., Halbirk, M., et al. (2006). Abnormalities of whole body protein turnover, muscle metabolism and levels of metabolic hormones in patients with chronic heart failure. *J Intern Med, 26*, 11–21.
86. McEntegart, M. B., Awede, B., Petrie, M. C., et al. (2007). Increase in serum adiponectin concentration in patients with heart failure and cachexia: relationship with leptin, other cytokines, and B-type natriuretic peptide. *Eur Heart J, 28*, 829–835.
87. George, J., Patal, S., Wexler, D., et al. (2006). Circulating adiponectin concentrations in patients with congestive heart failure. *Heart, 92*, 1420–1424.
88. Nakamura, T., Funayama, H., Kubo, N., et al. (2006). Association of hyperadiponectinemia with severity of ventricular dysfunction in congestive heart failure. *Circ J, 70*, 1557–1562.
89. Kistorp, C., Faber, J., Galatius, S., et al. (2005). Plasma adiponectin, body mass index, and mortality in patients with chronic heart failure. *Circulation, 112*, 1756–1762.
90. Levine, B., Kalman, J., Mayer, L., et al. (1990). Elevated circulating levels of tumor necrosis factor in severe chronic heart failure. *N Engl J Med, 323*, 236–241.
91. Mann, D. L. (2001). Recent insights into the role of tumor necrosis factor in the failing heart. *Heart Fail Rev, 6*, 71–80.
92. Matsumori, A., Yamada, T., Suzuki, H., et al. (1994). Increased circulating cytokines in patients with myocarditis and cardiomyopathy. *Br Heart J, 72*, 561–566.
93. Tsutamoto, T., Hisanaga, T., Wada, A., et al. (1998). Interleukin-6 spillover in the peripheral circulation increases with the severity of heart failure, and the high plasma level of interleukin-6 is an important prognostic predictor in patients with congestive heart failure. *J Am Coll Cardiol, 31*, 391–398.
94. Anker, S. D., Egerer, K. R., Volk, H. D., et al. (1997). Elevated soluble CD14 receptors and altered cytokines in chronic heart failure. *Am J Cardiol, 79*, 1426–1430.
95. Genth-Zotz, S., von Haehling, S., Bolger, A. P., et al. (2002). Pathophysiologic quantities of endotoxin-induced tumor necrosis factor-alpha release in whole blood from patients with chronic heart failure. *Am J Cardiol, 90*, 1226–1230.
96. Niebauer, J., Volk, H. D., Kemp, M., et al. (1999). Endotoxin and immune activation in chronic heart failure: a prospective cohort study. *Lancet, 353*, 1838–1842.
97. Ho, K. K., O'Sullivan, A. J., & Hoffman, D. M. (1996). Metabolic actions of growth hormone in man. *Endocr J, 43*(suppl), S57–S63.
98. Underwood, L. E., & Van Wyk, J. J. (1992). Normal and aberrant growth. In J. D. Wilson & D. D. Foster (Eds.). *Williams textbook of endocrinology.* Philadelphia: WB Saunders.
99. Tirapegui, J. (1999). Effect of insulin-like growth factor-1 (IGF-1) on muscle and bone growth in experimental models. *Int J Food Sci Nutr, 50*, 231–236.
100. Osterziel, K. J., Strohm, O., Schuler, J., et al. (1998). Randomised, double blind, placebo-controlled trial of human recombinant growth hormone in patients with chronic heart failure due to dilated cardiomyopathy. *Lancet, 351*, 1233–1237.
101. Frustaci, A., Gentiloni, N., & Russo, M. A. (1996). Growth hormone in the treatment of dilated cardiomyopathy. *N Engl J Med, 335*, 672–673.
102. Isgaard, J., Bergh, C. H., Caidahl, K., et al. (1998). A placebo-controlled study of growth hormone in patients with congestive heart failure. *Eur Heart J, 19*, 1704–1711.
103. Anker, S. D., Volterrani, M., Pflaum, C. D., et al. (2001). Acquired growth hormone resistance in patients with chronic heart failure: implications for therapy with growth hormone. *J Am Coll Cardiol, 38*, 443–452.
104. Swan, J. W., Walton, C., Godsland, I. F., et al. (1994). Insulin resistance in chronic heart failure. *Eur Heart J, 15*, 1528–1532.
105. Cleland, J. G., Swedberg, K., Follath, F., et al. (2003). The Euroheart failure survey programme—a survey on the quality of care among patients with heart failure in Europe. Part 1: patient characteristics and diagnosis. *Eur Heart J, 24*, 442–463.
106. Suskin, N., McKelvie, R. S., Burns, R. J., et al. (2000). Glucose and insulin abnormalities relate to functional capacity in patients with congestive heart failure. *Eur Heart J, 21*, 1368–1375.
107. Iribarren, C., Karter, A. J., Go, A. S., et al. (2001). Glycemic control and heart failure among adult patients with diabetes. *Circulation, 103*, 2668–2673.
108. Swan, J. W., Anker, S. D., Walton, C., et al. (1997). Insulin resistance in chronic heart failure: relation to severity and etiology of heart failure. *J Am Coll Cardiol, 30*, 527–532.
109. Doehner, W., Rauchhaus, M., Ponikowski, P., et al. (2005). Impaired insulin sensitivity as an independent risk factor for mortality in patients with stable chronic heart failure. *J Am Coll Cardiol, 46*, 1019–1026.
110. Doehner, W., Gathercole, D., Cicoira, M., et al. (2010). Reduced glucose transporter GLUT4 in skeletal muscle predicts insulin resistance in non-diabetic chronic heart failure patients independently of body composition. *Int J Cardiol.*
111. Doehner, W. (2006). Xanthine oxidase inhibitors and insulin sensitizers. In K. G. Hofbauer, S. D. Anker, & A. Inui (Eds.). *Pharmacotherapy of cachexia.* Boca Raton, Fla: CRC Press.
112. Lipscombe, L. L., Gomes, T., Lévesque, L. E., et al. (2007). Thiazolidinediones and cardiovascular outcomes in older patients with diabetes. *JAMA, 298*(22), 2634–2643.
113. Giles, T. D., Miller, A. B., Elkayam, U., et al. (2008). Pioglitazone and heart failure: results from a controlled study in patients with type 2 diabetes mellitus and systolic dysfunction. *J Card Fail, 14*(6), 445–452.
114. Masoudi, F. A., Inzucchi, S. E., Wang, Y., et al. (2005). Thiazolidinediones, metformin, and outcomes in older patients with diabetes and heart failure: an observational study. *Circulation, 111*, 583–590.
115. Rajagopalan, R., Rosenson, R. S., Fernandes, A. W., et al. (2004). Association between congestive heart failure and hospitalization in patients with type 2 diabetes mellitus receiving treatment with insulin or pioglitazone: a retrospective data analysis. *Clin Ther, 26*, 1400–1410.
116. Dargie, H. J., Hildebrandt, P. R., Riegger, G. A., et al. (2007). A randomized, placebo-controlled trial assessing the effects of rosiglitazone on echocardiographic function and cardiac status in type 2 diabetic patients with New York Heart Association Functional Class I or II heart failure. *J Am Coll Cardiol, 49*, 1696–1704.
117. Nissen, S. E., & Wolski, K. (2007). Effect of rosiglitazone on the risk of myocardial infarction and death from cardiovascular causes. *N Engl J Med, 356*, 2457–2471.
118. Mancini, D. M., Walter, G., Reichek, N., et al. (1992). Contribution of skeletal muscle atrophy to exercise intolerance and altered muscle metabolism in heart failure. *Circulation, 85*, 1364–1373.
119. Anker, S. D., Ponikowski, P. P., Clark, A. L., et al. (1999). Cytokines and neurohormones relating to body composition alterations in the wasting syndrome of chronic heart failure. *Eur Heart J, 20*, 683–693.
120. Sandri, M., Sandri, C., Gilbert, A., et al. (2004). Foxo transcription factors induce the atrophy related ubiquitin ligase atrogin-1 and cause skeletal muscle atrophy. *Cell, 117*(3), 399–412.
121. Coats, A. J. (2002). Origin of symptoms in patients with cachexia with special reference to weakness and shortness of breath. *Int J Cardiol, 85*(1), 133–139.
122. Anker, S. D., Swan, J. W., Volterrani, M., et al. (1997). The influence of muscle mass, strength, fatigability and blood flow on exercise capacity in cachectic and non-cachectic patients with chronic heart failure. *Eur Heart J, 18*(2), 259–269.
123. Franciosa, J. A., Park, M., & Levine, T. B. (1981). Lack of correlation between exercise capacity and indexes of resting left ventricular performance in heart failure. *Am J Cardiol, 47*, 33–39.
124. Harrington, D., Anker, S. D., Chua, T. P., et al. (1997). Skeletal muscle function and its relation to exercise tolerance in chronic heart failure. *J Am Coll Cardiol, 30*, 1758–1764.
125. Coats, A. J., Clark, A. L., Piepoli, M., et al. (1994). Symptoms and quality of life in heart failure: the muscle hypothesis. *Br Heart J, 72*(suppl 2), S36–S39.
126. Wilson, J. R., Martin, J. L., Schwartz, D., et al. (1984). Exercise intolerance in patients with chronic heart failure: role of impaired nutritive flow to skeletal muscle. *Circulation, 69*(6), 1079–1087.
127. Nagai, T., Okita, K., Yonezawa, K., Yamada, Y., et al. (2004). Comparisons of the skeletal muscle metabolic abnormalities in the arm and leg muscles of patients with chronic heart failure. *Circ J, 68*(6), 573–579.
128. Birkenfeld, A. L., Boschmann, M., Moro, C., et al. (2005). Lipid mobilization with physiological atrial natriuretic peptide concentrations in humans. *J Clin Endocrinol Metab, 90*, 3622–3628.
129. Lafontan, M., Moro, C., Berlan, M., et al. (2008). Control of lipolysis by natriuretic peptides and cyclic GMP. *Trends Endocrinol Metab, 19*, 130–137.
130. Moro, C., Klimcakova, E., Lolmède, K., et al. (2007). Atrial natriuretic peptide inhibits the production of adipokines and cytokines linked to inflammation and insulin resistance in human subcutaneous adipose tissue. *Diabetologia, 50*, 1038–1047.
131. Ryden, M., & Arner, P. (2007). Fat loss in cachexia—is there a role for adipocyte lipolysis? *Clin Nutr, 26*, 1–6.
132. Drott, C., Persson, H., & Lundholm, K. (1989). Cardiovascular and metabolic response to adrenaline infusion in weight-losing patients with and without cancer. *Clin Physiol, 9*, 427–439.
133. Zuijdgeest-van Leeuwen, S. D., van den Berg, J. W., Wattimena, J. L., et al. (2000). Lipolysis and lipid oxidation in weight-losing cancer patients and healthy subjects. *Metabolism, 49*, 931–936.

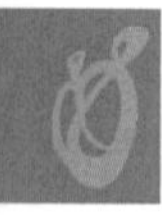

134. von Haehling, S., Jankowska, E. A., & Anker, S. D. (2004). Tumour necrosis factor-alpha and the failing heart—pathophysiology and therapeutic implications. *Basic Res Cardiol, 99*, 18–28.
135. Lee, A. H., Mull, R. L., Keenan, G. F., et al. (1994). Osteoporosis and bone morbidity in cardiac transplant recipients. *Am J Med, 96*, 35–41.
136. Abou-Raya, S., & Abou-Raya, A. (2008). Osteoporosis and congestive heart failure (CHF) in the elderly patient: double disease burden. *Arch Gerontol Geriatr, 49*, 250–254.
137. Anker, S. D., Clark, A. L., Teixeira, M. M., et al. (1999). Loss of bone mineral in patients with cachexia due to chronic heart failure. *Am J Cardiol, 83*, 612–615.
138. Shane, E., Mancini, D., Aaronson, K., et al. (1997). Bone mass, vitamin D deficiency, and hyperparathyroidism in congestive heart failure. *Am J Med, 103*, 197–207.
139. Schellenbaum, G. D., Smith, N. L., Heckbert, S. R., et al. (2005). Weight loss, muscle strength, and angiotensin-converting enzyme inhibitors in older adults with congestive heart failure or hypertension. *J Am Geriatr Soc, 53*, 2030–2031.
140. Paolisso, G., Balbi, V., Gambardella, A., et al. (1995). Lisinopril administration improves insulin action in aged patients with hypertension. *J Hum Hypertens, 9*, 541–546.
141. Yusuf, S., Gerstein, H., Hoogwerf, B., et al. (2001). Ramipril and the development of diabetes. *JAMA, 286*, 1882–1885.
142. Elliott, W. J., & Meyer, P. M. (2007). Incident diabetes in clinical trials of antihypertensive drugs: a network meta-analysis. *Lancet, 369*, 201–207.
143. Langin, D. (2006). Adipose tissue lipolysis as a metabolic pathway to define pharmacological strategies against obesity and the metabolic syndrome. *Pharmacol Res, 53*, 482–491.
144. Lamont, L. S., Brown, T., Riebe, D., et al. (2000). The major components of human energy balance during chronic beta-adrenergic blockade. *J Cardiopulm Rehabil, 20*, 247–250.
145. Anker, S. D., Coats, A. J., Roecker, E. B., et al. (2002). Does carvedilol prevent and reverse cardiac cachexia in patients with severe heart failure? Results of the COPERNICUS study. *Eur Heart J, 23*, 394 (abstract).
146. Anker, S. D., Lechat, P., & Dargie, H. J. (2003). Prevention and reversal of cachexia in patients with chronic heart failure by bisoprolol: results from the CIBIS II-study. *J Am Coll Cardiol, 41*, 156A–157A (abstract).
147. Lainscak, M., Keber, I., & Anker, S. D. (2006). Body composition changes in patients with systolic heart failure treated with beta blockers: a pilot study. *Int J Cardiol, 106*, 319–322.
148. Hryniewicz, K., Androne, A. S., Hudaihed, A., et al. (2003). Partial reversal of cachexia by beta-adrenergic receptor blocker therapy in patients with chronic heart failure. *J Card Fail, 9*, 464–468.
149. Herndon, D. N., Hart, D. W., Wolf, S. E., et al. (2001). Reversal of catabolism by beta-blockade after severe burns. *N Engl J Med, 345*, 1223–1229.
150. Rehfeldt, C., Weikard, R., & Reichel, K. (1994). The effect of the beta-adrenergic agonist clenbuterol on the growth of skeletal muscles of rats. *Arch Tierernahr, 45*, 333–344.
151. Ekberg, G., & Hansson, B. G. (1977). Glucose tolerance and insulin release in hypertensive patients treated with the cardioselective beta-receptor blocking agent metoprolol. *Acta Med Scand, 202*, 393–397.
152. William-Olsson, T., Fellenius, E., Bjorntorp, P., et al. (1979). Differences in metabolic responses to beta-adrenergic stimulation after propranolol or metoprolol administration. *Acta Med Scand, 205*, 201–206.
153. Sawicki, P. T., & Siebenhofer, A. (2001). Beta blocker treatment in diabetes mellitus. *J Intern Med, 250*, 11–17.
154. Fagerberg, B., Berglund, A., Holme, E., et al. (1990). Metabolic effects of controlled-release metoprolol in hypertensive men with impaired or diabetic glucose tolerance: a comparison with atenolol. *J Intern Med, 227*, 37–43.
155. Pollare, T., Lithell, H., Selinus, I., et al. (1989). Sensitivity to insulin during treatment with atenolol and metoprolol: a randomised, double blind study of effects on carbohydrate and lipoprotein metabolism in hypertensive patients. *BMJ, 298*, 1152–1157.
156. Shepherd, J., Cobbe, S. M., Ford, I., et al. (1995). Prevention of coronary heart disease with pravastatin in men with hypercholesterolemia. West of Scotland coronary prevention study group. *N Engl J Med, 333*, 1301–1307.
157. The Long-Term Intervention with Pravastatin in Ischaemic Disease (LIPID) Study Group. (1998). Prevention of cardiovascular events and death with pravastatin in patients with coronary heart disease and a broad range of initial cholesterol levels. *N Engl J Med, 339*, 1349–1357.
158. Schwartz, G. G., Olsson, A. G., Ezekowitz, M. D., et al. (2001). Effects of atorvastatin on early recurrent ischemic events in acute coronary syndromes: the MIRACL study: a randomized controlled trial. *JAMA, 285*, 1711–1718.
159. Vaughan, C. J., Gotto, A. M., Jr., & Basson, C. T. (2000). The evolving role of statins in the management of atherosclerosis. *J Am Coll Cardiol, 35*, 1–10.
160. Laufs, U., La Fata, V., Plutzky, J., et al. (1998). Upregulation of endothelial nitric oxide synthase by HMG CoA reductase inhibitors. *Circulation, 97*, 1129–1135.
161. Feron, O., Dessy, C., Desager, J. P., et al. (2001). Hydroxy-methylglutaryl-coenzyme A reductase inhibition promotes endothelial nitric oxide synthase activation through a decrease in caveolin abundance. *Circulation, 103*, 113–118.
162. Wassmann, S., Laufs, U., Baumer, A. T., et al. (2001). HMG-CoA reductase inhibitors improve endothelial dysfunction in normocholesterolemic hypertension via reduced production of reactive oxygen species. *Hypertension, 37*, 1450–1457.
163. Condorelli, G., Borello, U., De Angelis, L., et al. (2001). Cardiomyocytes induce endothelial cells to trans-differentiate into cardiac muscle: implications for myocardium regeneration. *Proc Natl Acad Sci U S A, 98*, 10733–10738.
164. Vasa, M., Fichtlscherer, S., Adler, K., et al. (2001). Increase in circulating endothelial progenitor cells by statin therapy in patients with stable coronary artery disease. *Circulation, 103*, 2885–2890.
165. Solheim, S., Seljeflot, I., Arnesen, H., et al. (2001). Reduced levels of TNF alpha in hypercholesterolemic individuals after treatment with pravastatin for 8 weeks. *Atherosclerosis, 157*, 411–415.
166. Albert, M. A., Danielson, E., Rifai, N., et al. (2001). Effect of statin therapy on C-reactive protein levels: the pravastatin inflammation/CRP evaluation (PRINCE): a randomized trial and cohort study. *JAMA, 286*, 64–70.
167. Ridker, P. M., Cannon, C. P., Morrow, D., et al. (2005). C-reactive protein levels and outcomes after statin therapy. *N Engl J Med, 352*, 20–28.
168. Rao, S., Porter, D. C., Chen, X., et al. (1999). Lovastatin-mediated G1 arrest is through inhibition of the proteasome, independent of hydroxymethyl glutaryl-CoA reductase. *Proc Natl Acad Sci U S A, 96*, 7797–7802.
169. Vogt, A., Qian, Y., McGuire, T. F., et al. (1996). Protein geranylgeranylation, not farnesylation, is required for the G1 to S phase transition in mouse fibroblasts. *Oncogene, 13*, 1991–1999.
170. Jakóbisiak, M., Bruno, S., Skierski, J. S., et al. (1991). Cell cycle-specific effects of lovastatin. *Proc Natl Acad Sci U S A, 88*, 3628–3632.
171. Rubins, J. B., Greatens, T., Kratzke, R. A., et al. (1998). Lovastatin induces apoptosis in malignant mesothelioma cells. *Am J Respir Crit Care Med, 157*, 1616–1622.
172. Kjekshus, J., Apetrei, E., Barrios, V., et al. (2007). Rosuvastatin in older patients with systolic heart failure. *N Engl J Med* (Epub ahead of print).
173. Investigators, GISSI-HF, Tavazzi, L., Maggioni, A. P., et al. (2008). Effect of rosuvastatin in patients with chronic heart failure (the GISSI-HF trial): a randomised, double-blind, placebo-controlled trial. *Lancet, 372*, 1231–1239.
174. Gibbs, C. R., Jackson, G., & Lip, G. Y. (2000). ABC of heart failure. Non-drug management. *BMJ, 320*, 366–369.
175. Sandek, A., Bauditz, J., Swidsinski, A., et al. (2007). Altered intestinal function in patients with chronic heart failure. *J Am Coll Cardiol, 50*, 1561–1569.
176. Witte, K. K., Clark, A. L., & Cleland, J. G. (2001). Chronic heart failure and micronutrients. *J Am Coll Cardiol, 37*, 1765–1774.
177. Shimon, I., Almog, S., Vered, Z., et al. (1995). Improved left ventricular function after thiamine supplementation in patients with congestive heart failure receiving long-term furosemide therapy. *Am J Med, 98*, 485–490.
178. de Lorgeril, M., Salen, P., Accominotti, M., et al. (2001). Dietary and blood antioxidants in patients with chronic heart failure. Insights into the potential importance of selenium in heart failure. *Eur J Heart Fail, 3*, 661–669.
179. Witte, K. K., Nikitin, N. P., Parker, A. C., et al. (2005). The effect of micronutrient supplementation on quality-of-life and left ventricular function in elderly patients with chronic heart failure. *Eur Heart J, 26*, 2238–2244.
180. Witte, K. K., & Clark, A. L. (2002). Nutritional abnormalities contributing to cachexia in chronic illness. *Int J Cardiol, 85*, 23–31.
181. Lennie, T. A. (2006). Nutritional recommendations for patients with heart failure. *J Cardiovasc Nurs, 21*, 261–268.
182. Oudemans-van Straaten, H. M., Bosman, R. J., Treskes, M., et al. (2001). Plasma glutamine depletion and patient outcome in acute ICU admissions. *Intensive Care Med, 27*, 84–90.
183. Schols, A. M., Deutz, N. E., Mostert, R., et al. (1993). Plasma amino acid levels in patients with chronic obstructive pulmonary disease. *Monaldi Arch Chest Dis, 48*, 546–548.
184. May, P. E., Barber, A., D'Olimpio, J. T., et al. (2002). Reversal of cancer-related wasting using oral supplementation with a combination of beta-hydroxy-beta-methylbutyrate, arginine, and glutamine. *Am J Surg, 183*, 471–479.
185. Laviano, A., Muscaritoli, M., Cascino, A., et al. (2005). Branched-chain amino acids: the best compromise to achieve anabolism? *Curr Opin Clin Nutr Metab Care, 8*, 408–414.
186. Buse, M. G., & Reid, S. S. (1975). Leucine. A possible regulator of protein turnover in muscle. *J Clin Invest, 56*, 1250–1261.
187. Kennedy, R. H., Owings, R., Shekhawat, N., et al. (2004). Acute negative inotropic effects of homocysteine are mediated via the endothelium. *Am J Physiol Heart Circ Physiol, 287*, H812–H817.
188. Herrmann, M., Taban-Shomal, O., Hubner, U., et al. (2006). A review of homocysteine and heart failure. *Eur J Heart Fail, 8*, 571–576.
189. Gorelik, O., Almoznino-Sarafian, D., Feder, I., et al. (2003). Dietary intake of various nutrients in older patients with congestive heart failure. *Cardiology, 99*, 177–181.
190. Freeman, L. M., Rush, J. E., Kehayias, J. J., et al. (1998). Nutritional alterations and the effect of fish oil supplementation in dogs with heart failure. *J Vet Intern Med, 12*, 440–448.
191. Rozentryt, P., Michalak, A., Nowak, J. U., et al. (2005). *The effects of enteral supplementation in patients with cardiac cachexia—a prospective, randomised, double-blind, placebo controlled trial.* Rome: 3rd Cachexia Conference Abstract Book.
192. Mustafa, I., & Leverve, X. (2001). Metabolic and nutritional disorders in cardiac cachexia. *Nutrition, 17*, 756–760.
193. Rauchhaus, M., Clark, A. L., Doehner, W., et al. (2003). The relationship between cholesterol and survival in patients with chronic heart failure. *J Am Coll Cardiol, 42*, 1933–1940.
194. Horwich, T. B., Hamilton, M. A., Maclellan, W. R., et al. (2002). Low serum total cholesterol is associated with marked increase in mortality in advanced heart failure. *J Card Fail, 8*, 216–224.
195. von Haehling, S., & Anker, S. D. (2005). Statins for heart failure: at the crossroads between cholesterol reduction and pleiotropism? *Heart, 91*, 1–2.
196. Azhar, G., & Wei, J. Y. (2006). Nutrition and cardiac cachexia. *Curr Opin Nutr Metab Care, 9*, 18–23.
197. Yavuzsen, T., Davis, M. P., Walsh, D., et al. (2005). Systematic review of the treatment of cancer-associated anorexia and weight loss. *J Clin Oncol, 23*, 8500–8511.
198. Neri, B., Garosi, V. L., & Intini, C. (1997). Effect of medroxyprogesterone acetate on the quality of life of the oncologic patient: a multicentric cooperative study. *Anticancer Drugs, 8*, 459–465.
199. McCarthy, H. D., Crowder, R. E., Dryden, S., et al. (1994). Megestrol acetate stimulates food and water intake in the rat: effects on regional hypothalamic neuropeptide Y concentrations. *Eur J Pharmacol, 265*, 99–102.
200. Mantovani, G., Macciò, A., Massa, E., et al. (2001). Managing cancer-related anorexia/cachexia. *Drugs, 61*, 499–514.

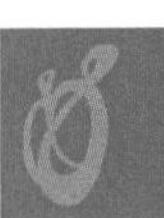

201. Costa, A. M., Spence, K. T., Plata-Salamán, C. R., et al. (1995). Residual Ca^{2+} channel current modulation by megestrol acetate via a G-protein alpha s-subunit in rat hypothalamic neurones. *J Physiol, 487*, 291–303.
202. Beal, J. E., Olson, R., Laubenstein, L., et al. (1995). Dronabinol as a treatment for anorexia associated with weight loss in patients with AIDS. *J Pain Symptom Manage, 10*, 89–97.
203. Nelson, K., Walsh, D., Deeter, P., et al. (1994). A phase II study of delta-9-tetrahydrocannabinol for appetite stimulation in cancer-associated anorexia. *J Palliat Care, 10*, 14–18.
204. Strasser, F., Luftner, D., Possinger, K., et al. (2006). Comparison of orally administered cannabis extract and delta-9-tetrahydrocannabinol in treating patients with cancer-related anorexia-cachexia syndrome: a multicenter, phase III, randomized, double-blind, placebo-controlled clinical trial from the cannabis-in-cachexia-study-group. *J Clin Oncol, 24*, 3394–3400.
205. John, M. (2006). Appetite stimulants. In K. G. Hofbauer, S. D. Anker, & A. Inui (Eds.). *Pharmacotherapy of cachexia*. Boca Raton, Fla: Taylor & Francis.
206. Malkin, C. J., Pugh, P. J., West, J. N., et al. (2006). Testosterone therapy in men with moderate severity heart failure: a double-blind randomized placebo controlled trial. *Eur Heart J, 27*, 57–64.
207. Pugh, P. J., Jones, T. H., & Channer, K. S. (2003). Acute haemodynamic effects of testosterone in men with chronic heart failure. *Eur Heart J, 24*, 909–915.
208. Cuerda, C., Zugasti, A., Bretón, I., et al. (2005). Treatment with nandrolone decanoate and megestrol acetate in HIV-infected men. *Nutr Clin Pract, 20*, 93–97.
209. Yeh, S. S., DeGuzman, B., & Kramer, T. (2002). Reversal of COPD-associated weight loss using the anabolic agent oxandrolone. *Chest, 122*, 421–428.
210. von Haehling, S., & Anker, S. D. (2005). Future prospects of anticytokine therapy in chronic heart failure. *Expert Opin Investig Drugs, 14*, 163–176.
211. Mann, D. L., McMurray, J. J., Packer, M., et al. (2004). Targeted anticytokine therapy in patients with chronic heart failure: results of the randomized etanercept worldwide evaluation (RENEWAL). *Circulation, 109*, 1594–1602.
212. Chung, E. S., Packer, M., Lo, K. H., et al. (2003). Randomized, double-blind, placebo-controlled, pilot trial of infliximab, a chimeric monoclonal antibody to tumor necrosis factor-alpha, in patients with moderate-to-severe heart failure: results of the anti-TNF therapy against congestive heart failure (ATTACH) trial. *Circulation, 107*, 3133–3140.
213. Torre-Amione, G., Kapadia, S., Lee, J., et al. (1996). Tumor necrosis factor-alpha and tumor necrosis factor receptors in the failing human heart. *Circulation, 93*, 704–711.
214. Foldes, G., von Haehling, S., & Anker, S. D. (2006). Toll-like receptor modulation in cardiovascular disease: a target for intervention? *Expert Opin Investig Drugs, 15*, 857–871.
215. Genth-Zotz, S., von Haehling, S., Bolger, A. P., et al. (2006). The anti-CD14 antibody IC14 suppresses ex vivo endotoxin stimulated tumor necrosis factor-alpha in patients with chronic heart failure. *Eur J Heart Fail, 8*, 366–372.
216. Sharma, R., von Haehling, S., Rauchhaus, M., et al. (2005). Whole blood endotoxin responsiveness in patients with chronic heart failure: the importance of serum lipoproteins. *Eur J Heart Fail, 7*, 479–484.
217. Rauchhaus, M., Coats, A. J., & Anker, S. D. (2000). The endotoxin-lipoprotein hypothesis. *Lancet, 356*, 930–933.
218. Calabrese, L., & Resztak, K. (1998). Thalidomide revisited: pharmacology and clinical applications. *Expert Opin Investig Drugs, 7*, 2043–2060.
219. D'Amato, R. J., Loughnan, M. S., Flynn, E., et al. (1994). Thalidomide is an inhibitor of angiogenesis. *Proc Natl Acad Sci U S A, 91*, 4082–4085.
220. Sampaio, E. P., Sarno, E. N., Galilly, R., et al. (1991). Thalidomide selectively inhibits tumor necrosis factor production by stimulated human monocytes. *J Exp Med, 173*, 699–703.
221. Muller, G. W., Chen, R., Huang, S. Y., et al. (1999). Amino-substituted thalidomide analogs: potent inhibitors of TNF-alpha production. *Bioorg Med Chem Lett, 9*, 1625–1630.
222. Davey, P. P., & Ashrafian, H. (2000). New therapies for heart failure: is thalidomide the answer? *QJM, 93*, 305–311.
223. Gullestad, L., Semb, A. G., Holt, E., et al. (2002). Effect of thalidomide in patients with chronic heart failure. *Am Heart J, 144*, 847–850.
224. Agoston, I., Dibbs, Z. I., Wang, F., et al. (2002). Preclinical and clinical assessment of the safety and potential efficacy of thalidomide in heart failure. *J Card Fail, 8*, 306–314.
225. Gullestad, L., Ueland, T., Fjeld, J. G., et al. (2005). Effect of thalidomide on cardiac remodeling in chronic heart failure: results of a double-blind, placebo-controlled study. *Circulation, 112*, 3408–3414.
226. Orea-Tejeda, A., Arrieta-Rodriguez, O., Castillo-Martinez, L., et al. (2006). Effects of thalidomide treatment in heart failure patients. *Cardiology, 108*, 237–242.
227. von Haehling, S., Genth-Zotz, S., Anker, S. D., et al. (2002). Cachexia: a therapeutic approach beyond cytokine antagonism. *Int J Cardiol, 85*, 173–183.
228. Zabel, P., Schonharting, M. M., Schade, U. F., et al. (1991). Effects of pentoxifylline in endotoxinemia in human volunteers. *Prog Clin Biol Res, 367*, 207–213.
229. Sliwa, K., Skudicky, D., Candy, G., et al. (1998). Randomised investigation of effects of pentoxifylline on left-ventricular performance in idiopathic dilated cardiomyopathy. *Lancet, 351*, 1091–1093.
230. Sliwa, K., Woodiwiss, A., Kone, V. N., et al. (2004). Therapy of ischemic cardiomyopathy with the immunomodulating agent pentoxifylline: results of a randomized study. *Circulation, 109*, 750–755.
231. Skudicky, D., Bergemann, A., Sliwa, K., et al. (2001). Beneficial effects of pentoxifylline in patients with idiopathic dilated cardiomyopathy treated with angiotensin-converting enzyme inhibitors and carvedilol: results of a randomized study. *Circulation, 103*, 1083–1088.
232. Bahrmann, P., Hengst, U. M., Richartz, B. M., et al. (2004). Pentoxifylline in ischemic, hypertensive and idiopathic-dilated cardiomyopathy: effects on left-ventricular function, inflammatory cytokines and symptoms. *Eur J Heart Fail, 6*, 195–201.
233. Bossola, M., Pacelli, F., & Doglietto, G. B. (2007). Novel treatments for cancer cachexia. *Expert Opin Investig Drugs, 16*, 1241–1253.
234. Goldberg, R. M., Loprinzi, C. L., Mailliard, J. A., et al. (1995). Pentoxifylline for treatment of cancer anorexia and cachexia? A randomized, double-blind, placebo-controlled trial. *J Clin Oncol, 13*, 2856–2859.

CHAPTER 22

Epidemiology of Heart Failure

Raghava S. Velagaleti and Ramachandran S. Vasan

Heart failure (HF) is a syndrome associated with high morbidity and mortality and considerable economic burden.[1] It is the third most prevalent cardiovascular disease and the third leading cause of cardiovascular death in the United States.[2] Once diagnosed, HF continues to portend a grim prognosis despite advances in treatment. Recognizing the importance of the preclinical phases of HF and the possibility of prevention, the American Heart Association and American College of Cardiology classify HF into four stages (Figure 22-1): presence of risk factors, but with normal cardiac structure and function (Stage A), subclinical changes in left ventricular structure and/or function (Stage B), clinical HF (Stage C), and advanced HF (Stage D).[3] Understanding the epidemiology of the preclinical and clinical stages of HF may facilitate preventative strategies. In this chapter, we provide (1) an overview of HF stages A and B, and (2) detail the epidemiology of clinical HF.

EPIDEMIOLOGY OF HF RISK FACTORS

Several etiological factors have been described for HF (Table 22-1).[4] Of these, coronary heart disease (CHD) and hypertension account for approximately three fourths of all HF, although their relative importance differs according to age, sex, and race.[5] Also, the relative contribution of the various risk factors to HF occurrence in the community may be changing over time. Data from the Framingham Heart Study demonstrate that from the 1950s onward there has been a steady decline in the contribution of valvular disease to HF burden, whereas that of CHD has increased substantially.[6] When not initially apparent, the diagnosis of the specific cause of HF is often difficult; in one study of 1230 individuals with initially unexplained cardiomyopathy, 50% were ultimately classified as idiopathic after a comprehensive workup, including endomyocardial biopsy.[7]

EPIDEMIOLOGY OF CHD IN RELATION TO HF RISK

Angiographic coronary artery disease is present in approximately half of all patients with new-onset HF.[8] In various investigations, CHD has been reported to account for 23% to 73% of HF in the patients evaluated. In the HF series that focused on patients with a reduced LV ejection fraction, CHD is usually the most common cause.[9] Data from the National Health and Nutrition Examination Survey (NHANES-I) show that presence of CHD confers an eightfold higher HF risk.[10] Framingham data indicate a differential contribution of CHD to HF burden in men versus women; the population attributable risk (PAR) for HF associated with CHD was 39% in men and 18% in women.[11] These observations highlight the importance of CHD as a determinant of HF occurrence both from individual risk and population burden perspectives.

A separate issue of concern is the trend in the incidence of HF after myocardial infarction (MI). Data from Framingham demonstrate a rise in post-MI HF between 1971 and 2000, mostly due to an increase in HF incidence in the very early post-MI period.[12] This is likely due to improved survival of people with MI[13] leading to an increase in population "at risk" for HF and thereby contributing to an increase in HF prevalence.

EPIDEMIOLOGY OF HYPERTENSION IN RELATION TO HF RISK

In the United States, approximately 74 million people have hypertension (see also Chapter 28), with millions more having blood pressures in the "high normal" range.[3] Data from the Framingham study show that hypertension is an antecedent of the vast majority of individuals with HF in the community.[11] The relative risk of HF in people with hypertension is twofold and threefold higher in men and women, respectively, compared with those without hypertension.[11] Both systolic blood pressure and pulse pressure independently carry a 55% increased risk of HF per standard deviation increment after accounting for standard risk factors[14] and a 30% increased risk of HF per standard deviation increment after additionally accounting for prevalent and incident MI.[15] The effect of increased blood pressure on HF risk persists for many years, as evidenced by the independent contributions of recent and remote blood pressure elevations to HF risk, after adjustment for current measurements.[15,16]

The population burden of hypertension-associated HF is substantial, as evidenced by a PAR of 39% in men and 59% in women in a Framingham study investigation.[11] Although the prevalence of hypertension is high and may be increasing over time,[17] the PAR for hypertension (for HF risk) is decreasing, likely due to improving blood pressure control in the community, and attendant attenuation of blood pressure-CVD risk relations.[18,19] Despite these improvements, a substantial number

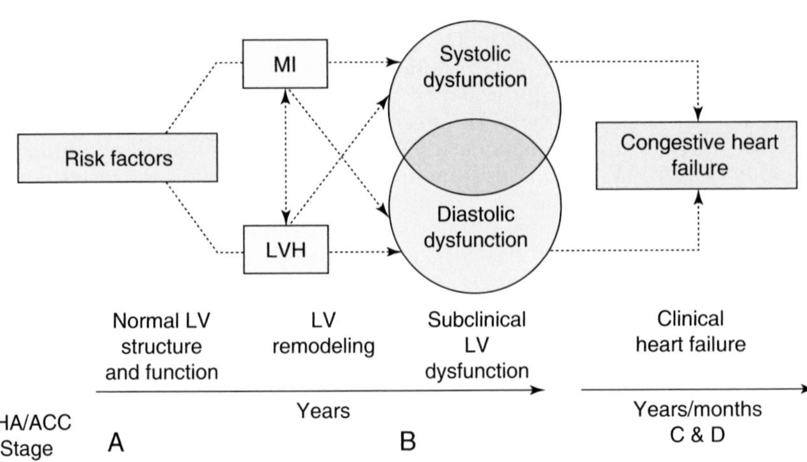

FIGURE 22-1 Progression to HF. HF develops over several years starting with the onset of risk factors, progressing to alterations in LV structure and function, and culminating in clinical HF. (Adapted from Vasan, et al. The role of hypertension in the pathogenesis of heart failure. A clinical mechanistic overview, *Arch Intern Med* 1996;156:1789-1796; and Parikh N, Vasan RS. Epidemiology of heart failure. In Colucci WS, editor. *Atlas of heart failure*, ed 5, Philadelphia, 2008, Springer.)

TABLE 22-1 Risk Factors for HF

	MAJOR	MINOR
Clinical Risk Factors	* Age * Male sex * Hypertension * Electrocardiograhic left ventricular (LV) hypertrophy * Myocardial infarction * Diabetes mellitus * Valve disease * Overweight/obesity	* Excessive alcohol consumption * Cigarette smoking * Dyslipidemia * Renal insufficiency * Sleep-disordered breathing * Low physical activity * Low socioeconomic status * Coffee consumption * Dietary sodium intake * Increased heart rate * Impaired pulmonary function * Mental stress and depression
Toxic Risk Precipitants	* Chemotherapeutic agents (doxorubicin, daunorubicin, cyclophosphamide, 5-fluorouracil)	* Cocaine * Nonsteroidal antiinflammatory agents * Thiazolidinediones * Doxazosin
Biochemical Risk Predictors	* Albuminuria * Natriuretic peptides	* Homocysteine * Insulin-like growth factor I * Tumor necrosis factor α * Interleukin-6 * C-reactive protein
Morphologic Risk Predictors	* LV dilatation * Increased LV mass * Asymptomatic LV systolic dysfunction * LV diastolic filling impairment	
Genetic Risk Predictors	* Family history of cardiomyopathy	* Genetic polymorphisms

"Major" risk factors—established firmly by multiple investigations.
"Minor" risk factors—less consistently related to HF risk.

of people have poorly controlled or refractory hypertension,[20] offering the possibility of further reductions in hypertension-associated HF by targeting these individuals.

EPIDEMIOLOGY OF OBESITY IN RELATION TO HF RISK (see Chapter 20)

Approximately a third of U.S. adults are obese[21] (defined as body mass index [BMI] of 30 kg/m^2), and an additional third are overweight (BMI between 25.0 and 29.9 kg/m^2). Observations from the Framingham Heart Study show that the risk for incident HF increases by 5% and 7% in men and women, respectively, per unit increase in BMI.[22] There is a graded increase in HF risk across categories of BMI in both men and women (Figure 22-2), and compared with people with normal BMI, those with obesity carry approximately twice the HF risk after accounting for established HF risk factors.[22] The HF risk portended by obesity seems to be partially ameliorated by concomitant physical activity; participants of the Physicians Health Study who were overweight or obese but had regular physical activity had HF risk that was intermediate to those who were lean and active and those who were obese but not active.[23] Potential explanations for the association between overweight/obesity and HF occurrence include greater prevalence of other HF risk factors and higher prevalence and incidence of MI in this group, and obesity-associated LV remodeling.[24] A recent investigation from Framingham also reported the increased risk for incident HF portended by elevated resistin (an adipokine) levels, providing clues to a potential direct mechanistic link between increased adiposity and HF risk.[25]

There has been a substantial increase in both the prevalence and incidence of overweight and obesity over the past few decades,[26,27] including an increased prevalence of extreme obesity (BMI ≥40 kg/m^2).[28] However, there has been a parallel decline in prevalence of other HF risk factors (notably hypertension, smoking, and hyperlipidemia) among those overweight and obese in the same timespan,[29] suggesting that people with these conditions are being increasingly targeted for cardiovascular risk factor modification, and raising the possibility that the obesity epidemic may not translate into an HF epidemic.

STRUCTURAL AND/OR FUNCTIONAL ALTERATIONS THAT PREDISPOSE TO HEART FAILURE

A variety of cardiac structural and functional abnormalities detected either indirectly (e.g., with electrocardiography or chest roentgenography) or directly (e.g., with echocardiography or cardiac magnetic resonance imaging [CMR]) have been shown to antedate clinical HF. Electrocardiographic LV hypertrophy, QRS prolongation, QT prolongation, and evidence of a prior MI predict incident HF.[30,31] Similarly, a cardiothoracic ratio greater than 0.5 on a chest x-ray is associated with twofold higher odds of HF.[32]

LV Structural Alterations (see Chapter 15)

The advent of echocardiography and CMR has enhanced our ability to directly visualize changes in cardiac structure and in global and regional cardiac function. Left ventricular mass

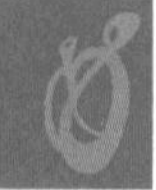

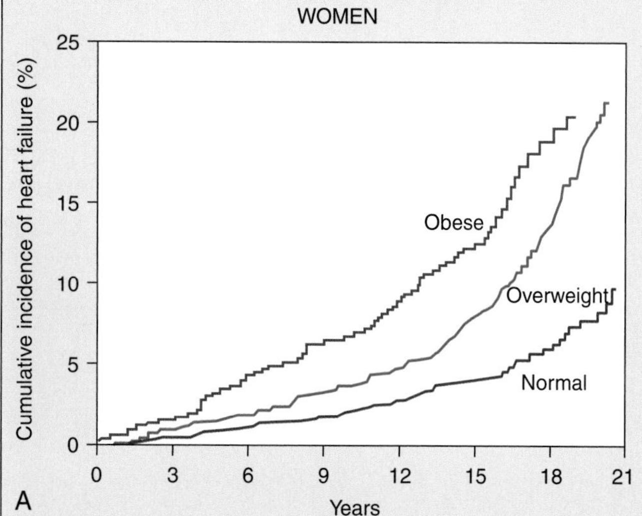

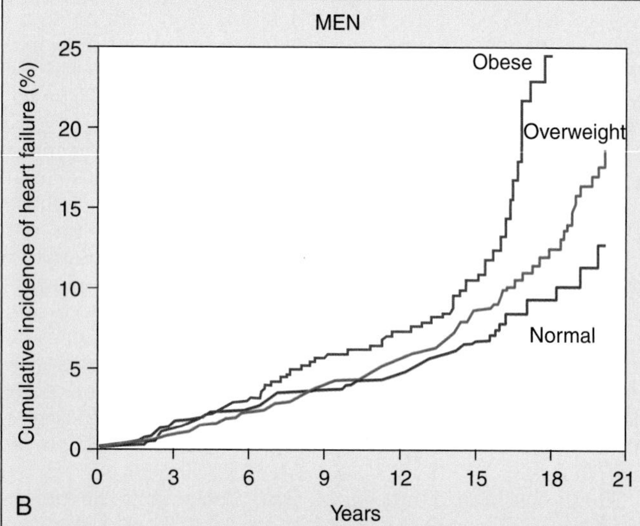

FIGURE 22-2 Cumulative incidence of heart failure according to category of body-mass index at the baseline examination. The body-mass index was 18.5 to 24.9 in normal subjects, 25.0 to 29.9 in overweight subjects, and 30.0 or more in obese subjects. (Modified from Kenchaiah S, Evans JC, Levy D, et al. Obesity and the risk of heart failure. *N Engl J Med* 2002;347:305-313; and Mann DL. Management of heart failure with a depressed ejection fraction. In Libby PL, Bonow RO, Mann DL, et al, editors. *Braunwald's heart disease*, ed 8, Philadelphia, 2004, Elsevier.)

(calculated using validated formulas from measurements of LV dimensions) has been consistently identified as a predictor of HF risk.[33-35] LV mass also predicts future occurrence of depressed LV systolic function in participants with an initial normal ejection fraction.[36] Estimates of the magnitude of increment in HF risk with an increase in LV mass vary according to the quantitative denominator (i.e., per standard deviation or gram increment, etc.), method of indexation, modality of assessment (echocardiography or CMR, etc.), and the covariates adjusted for.

Increased LV end-systolic and end-diastolic internal dimensions are powerful risk factors for HF. Observations from the Framingham Heart Study show that in people without a prior MI, each standard deviation increment in height-indexed LV end-systolic and end-diastolic dimensions is associated with a 43% and 47% increased risk of HF, respectively.[37] LV dilation in the immediate postinfarction period and dilation 6 months post-MI also predict incident HF.[38,39]

Asymptomatic LV Dysfunction

Asymptomatic LV dysfunction (comprising either systolic dysfunction, diastolic dysfunction, or both) has been conventionally accepted as an antecedent of HF. However, the proportion of HF preceded by either systolic or diastolic dysfunction is unclear. Estimates of prevalence of asymptomatic LV systolic dysfunction vary depending on the criteria used (Table 22-2).[40] The prevalence of mild and moderate to severe asymptomatic LV diastolic dysfunction is approximately 20% and 7%, respectively, in the general adult population, and 48% and 17%, respectively, in those at high risk for HF (Table 22-3).[41] Prospectively, the rates of HF incidence among HF-free people with ejection fraction (EF) ≤50% and those with EF greater than 50% have been estimated to be 5.8 and 0.7, respectively, per 100 person-years.[42] Individuals with EF ≤50% carry an HF risk that is approximately five times greater than those with EF greater than 50%, after adjusting for standard cardiovascular risk factors.[42] Several other measures of systolic and diastolic function, notably endocardial fractional shortening, transmitral Doppler peak E, and Doppler E/A ratio, also predict incident HF.[43]

The natural history of asymptomatic LV diastolic dysfunction has not been well described. Of note, the prevalence of diastolic dysfunction in the community is either the same or higher in men compared with women, in contrast to the relative prevalences of diastolic HF (that has a female preponderance).[44,45] The reason for this paradox is unclear.

Screening for Ventricular Remodeling

There has been considerable interest in screening for LV remodeling as a way of identifying people at high risk for developing HF.[46] However, although people with the aforementioned structural and functional alterations are at higher risk for HF compared with those without, the prevalence of HF in groups identified by using these traits individually is low, suggesting that widespread echocardiographic screening may not be cost-effective.[40] The performance of natriuretic peptides for the detection of LV systolic dysfunction or elevated LV mass in the community is suboptimal, implying limited usefulness for identifying those who could potentially benefit from cardiac imaging.[47] An alternate approach may be to use clinical factors as an initial screen to identify a subset of individuals who would be most likely to benefit from additional imaging tests. A recent report identified clinical measures that predict LV dilation and/or dysfunction; such "clinical rules" may help identify people who may benefit from screening with imaging.[48] In addition, combining several imaging indices in the form of a composite score may further help identify those at very high risk for HF. One investigation used a score based on five echocardiographic measures that demonstrated good stratification; the incidence of HF ranged from 4% to 48% across strata of risk index.[49] Such "staged" screening strategies (a serial testing strategy using a clinical score to identify candidates for imaging; an imaging score to identify those at high risk for HF, who could then be targeted for preventive intervention) may offer greater utility at a lower cost. However, the cost-effectiveness of these approaches has not been evaluated.

EPIDEMIOLOGY OF CHRONIC HF

Prevalence

There are approximately 5 million people with HF in the United States.[2] There has been a doubling of HF prevalence in the past 25 years,[50] and by the year 2040, it is estimated to further increase to 10 million. The prevalence of heart failure

TABLE 22–2 Prevalence of Asymptomatic LV Systolic Dysfunction

Study	Country	Participants	Mean Age/ Age Range	% Men	LSVD Criteria	Prevalence of Asymptomatic LVSD
EF >40 or Equivalent						
Strong Heart Study	United States	3184	58	37	EF ≤0.54	12.5
HyperGEN	United States	2086	55	38	EF ≤0.54	12.9
Davies et al	England	3960	61	50	EF ≤0.50	3.3
MONICA project	Germany	1566	50	48	EF ≤0.48	1.1
Hedberg et al	Sweden	412	75	50	WMI <1.7	3.2
Nielsen et al	Denmark	126	70	55	WMI ≤1.5 or FS <0	1.0
Rotterdam Study	Netherlands	2267	66	45	FS ≤0.25	2.9
Helsinki Ageing Study	Finland	501	76-86	27	FS ≤0.25	8.6
EF ≤40 or Equivalent						
Strong Heart Study	United States	3184	58	37	EF <0.40	2.1
HyperGEN	United States	2086	55	38	EF <0.40	3.4
Davies et al	England	3960	61	50	EF <0.40	0.9
MONICA project	Germany	1467	50	48	EF <0.35	5.9
MONICA project	Germany	1467	50	48	EF <0.30	1.4
Qualitatively "Reduced" EF						
Cardiovascular Health Study	United States	5532	73	42	Qualitative	2.5
Morgan et al	England	817	76	46	Qualitative	3.9

increases with age: from less than 1% in the 20-to-39-year age group to more than 20% in people age 80 years or older.[51] There is an increasing trend in HF prevalence; in the decade 1989-1999, HF prevalence increased by 1 per 1000 and 0.9 per 1000 in women and men, respectively.[52] The aging of the U.S. population, and an improved survival and "salvage" of patients with MI (with subsequent progression to pump failure) will likely contribute to increasing prevalence over the next few decades.

The relative prevalence of HF with normal EF versus reduced EF varies with characteristics of the study sample and of the threshold used to define a "normal" EF (Figure 22-3 displays the relative prevalence of HF with normal EF and reduced EF reported in various epidemiological studies; Table 22-4 lists the sample age and HF definition characteristics of studies from which Figure 22-3 data are drawn).[41] Overall each group (reduced and preserved EF) accounts for approximately one half of HF cases.[53,54] The prevalence of HF with normal EF increases substantially with age.[55] There has been an increasing trend in the incidence of HF with a normal EF,[56] likely reflecting increasing awareness of the condition and willingness of clinicians to make the diagnosis. HF with normal EF is more commonly associated with female gender, hypertension, and atrial fibrillation, and less commonly with MI and electrocardiographic left bundle branch block.[57]

TABLE 22–3 Prevalence of Asymptomatic LV Diastolic Dysfunction

Variables	No. of Participants	Diastolic Dysfunction: Mild	Diastolic Dysfunction: Moderate to Severe
General Adult Population			
All	1991	20.6 (18.7-22.6)	6.8 (5.6-8.0)
Men	952	22.3 (19.5-25.3)	6.2 (4.7-8.1)
Women	1039	19.1 (16.7-21.8)	7.3 (5.7-9.1)
High-risk Population (Aged >65 yr and with Hypertension or Coronary Artery Disease)			
All	396	47.6 (42.1-53.1)	16.5 (12.6-20.9)
Men	196	48.7 (40.7-56.8)	14.6 (9.5-21.0)
Women	200	46.5 (38.8-54.3)	18.2 (12.7-24.9)

Prevalence of asymptomatic diastolic dysfunction as assessed by Doppler echocardiographic analysis of 2042 men and women greater than 45 years of age.

Incidence

More than half a million new cases of heart failure are diagnosed each year in the United States, and this incidence is expected to rise to 772,000 new cases per year by 2040 (Figure 22-4).[41] This increase in incidence is mainly due to the aging of the population, as HF incidence doubles with each successive decade above age 45 for both men and women.[58] An analysis from Framingham showed that when adjusted for age, there has been no increasing trend in HF incidence for men, and may be slightly decreasing in women,[59] whereas data from Olmsted County show no change in HF incidence for either gender.[60]

Lifetime Risk

The lifetime risk of developing heart failure is estimated at 20% in both men and women (Figure 22-5).[61] An age-related increase in HF risk is counterbalanced by a decreasing life

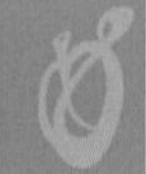

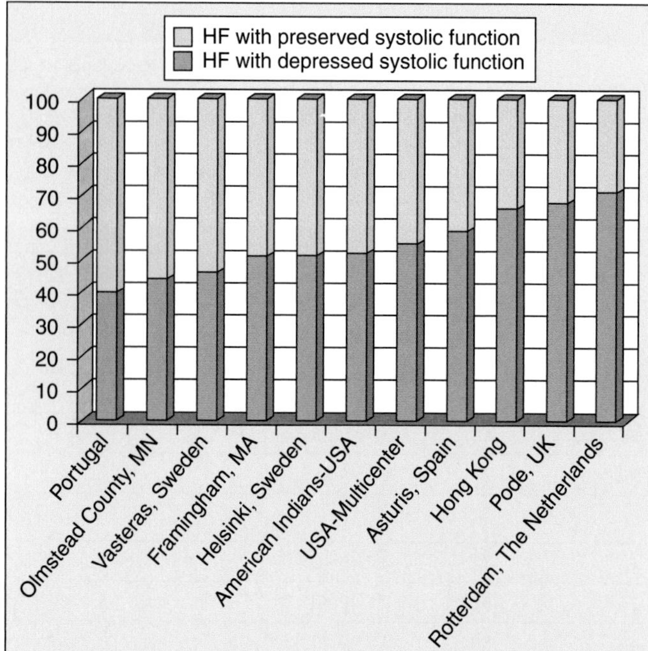

FIGURE 22–3 Prevalence of HF with normal systolic function in community based studies. Prevalence of HF with preserved systolic function varied across studies, ranging from 40% (in Portugal) to 71% (in Rotterdam). (Adapted from Owan TE, Redfield MM. Epidemiology of diastolic heart failure. *Prog Cardiovasc Dis* 2005;47:320-332 and Parikh N, Vasan RS. Epidemiology of heart failure. In Colucci WS, editor. *Atlas of heart failure*, ed 5, Philadelphia 2008, Springer.)

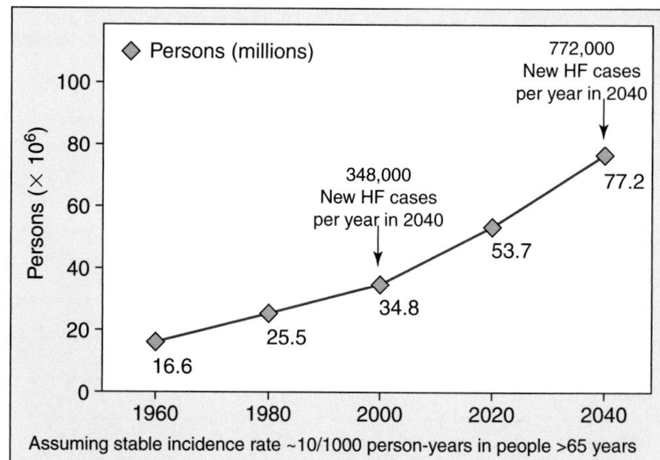

FIGURE 22–4 Projected increase in HF incidence. Projections are based on current HF incidence rates. (Adapted from Owan TE, Redfield MM. Epidemiology of diastolic heart failure. *Prog Cardiovasc Dis* 2005;47:320-332; and Parikh N, Vasan RS. Epidemiology of heart failure. In Colucci WS, editor. *Atlas of heart failure*, ed 5, Philadelphia, 2008, Springer.)

TABLE 22–4 Characteristics of Epidemiological Studies Reporting Prevalence of HF with Normal Systolic Function (also see Figure 22-3)

Study Location	Population	Age	Definition of Preserved Systolic Function
Portugal	5434	>25	EF ≥0.45
Olmstead County, MN	2042	≥45	EF ≥0.50
Framingham, MA	73	Mean = 73	EF ≥0.50
Helsinki, Sweden	501	75-86	FS ≥0.25
American Indians-USA	3638	45-74	EF >0.54
USA-Multicenter	4242	≥65	Qualitative normal function
Asturias, Spain	391	>40	EF ≥0.50
Hong Kong	Not reported	All ages	EF >0.45
Poole, UK	817	70-84	Qualitative normal function
Rotterdam, The Netherlands	5540	≥55	FS >0.25

expectancy with advancing age, so that the lifetime risk of HF remains relatively stable at 20% at all ages above 40 years. Even without antecedent CHD, the lifetime risk of developing heart failure at age 40 years is estimated at 11.4% for men, and 15.4% for women.[61] A significant proportion of lifetime risk of HF is accounted for by lifestyle factors; in a recent report, those with four or more of six healthy lifestyle habits (consumption of breakfast cereals, fruits and vegetables, maintenance of normal body weight, regular exercise, refraining from smoking, and moderate alcohol intake) had half the lifetime risk for HF compared with those who adhered to none.[62]

Morbidity and Mortality

HF accounts for 12 to 15 million office visits and 6.5 million days of hospital stay each year in the United States.[63] The number of HF hospitalizations has risen to more than a million per year over the past decade,[2] and they now account for at least 20% of all admissions for persons older than 65 years.[64] The estimated annual cost of caring for HF patients is $37 billion.[2] In one prospective study, the 1-year costs for prevalent (at the time of study entry) and incident (during study period) HF with normal EF were $32,000 and $45,000, respectively, and corresponding estimated costs for HF with reduced EF were approximately $33,000 and $49,000, respectively.[65] In addition, HF patients usually have multiple comorbid conditions,[66] which influence the risk for both hospitalization and death,[67] especially in those with HF with normal EF.[68]

There are approximately 50,000 HF deaths in the United States annually. An earlier report from the Framingham Heart Study revealed 1-year and 5-year survival rates of 57% and 24% in men, and 64% and 38% in women, respectively.[69] Mortality increased with increasing age at 27% per decade.[69] Median survival after the onset of HF was 1.7 years and 3.2 years in men and women, respectively.[70] An examination of the temporal trends in survival after HF onset demonstrated a modest improving trend between the years 1950 and 1999 (Figure 22-6). However, in a more recent Framingham evaluation, the median survival was 2.1 years and a 5-year mortality rate 74%, with equally dismal prognosis in both men and women, and in both those with HF with preserved EF and normal EF.[57]

Of note is a striking geographic heterogeneity in HF mortality rates (Figure 22-7).[71] The highlighted areas indicate an "HF belt" across the United States that consists of states with the highest HF death rates. Higher prevalence of hypertension and CHD, varying access to early diagnosis compounded by regional differences in HF management, and differences in death certificate coding practices may explain this occurrence.

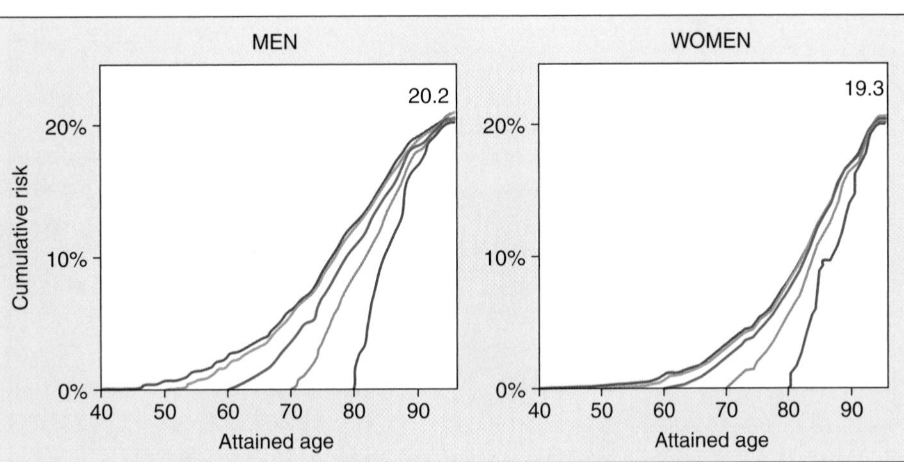

FIGURE 22–5 Lifetime HF incidence. Lifetime risk of developing HF was estimated at various ages (between 40 years and 80 years of age) among 3757 men and 4472 women in the Framingham Heart Study from 1971 to 1996. (Adapted from Lloyd-Jones DM, Larson MG, Leip EP, et al. Lifetime risk for developing congestive heart failure: the Framingham Heart Study. *Circulation* 2002;106:3068-3072; and Parikh N, Vasan RS. Epidemiology of heart failure. In Colucci WS, editor. *Atlas of heart failure*, ed 5, Philadelphia, 2008, Springer.)

EPIDEMIOLOGY OF STAGE D HF

Few investigations have addressed the epidemiology of Stage D HF. In a study of a population-based cross-sectional random sample of people aged 45 years from Olmsted County, 0.2% had Stage D HF, and the prevalence increased with advancing age. Stage D HF accounted for 0.4% of all stages of HF, and 2% of clinical HF.[72] Stage D was associated with markedly reduced survival (20% in 5 years).[72] An analysis of the Acute Decompensated Heart Failure Registry (ADHERE) compared those with Stage D HF to people with acute decompensated HF (ADHF) and noted that people with Stage D were younger, more likely male, had a higher prevalence of dyslipidemia and CHD, and were more likely to receive intravenous vasoactive therapy compared with those with ADHF.[73] The 1-year survival rate free of death or hospitalization was only 33%.[73] The pathophysiological significance or clinical implications of these differences between Stage D HF and ADHF are unclear.

EPIDEMIOLOGY OF ACUTE HF (see Chapter 43)

Acute HF (also referred to as ADHF or "acute HF syndromes") is the rapid occurrence of symptoms and signs of HF, or the deterioration of stable chronic HF, leading to the requirement of hospitalization and/or intensive therapy (see also Chapters 43 and 44).[74] It may occur in the presence or absence of preexisting cardiac disease, and may be new-onset HF or worsening of previously stable HF.[75] Thus acute HF has a broad spectrum of clinical presentations and an evolving clinical definition.[76]

Approximately 65% to 87% of acute HF episodes are worsening of chronic HF.[77] Factors precipitating hospitalizations include pneumonia or other respiratory infections, myocardial ischemia, arrhythmias, or worsening renal function.[78] The in-hospital mortality rates are 3% to 4%; older age, lower systolic blood pressure, lower serum sodium, and elevated serum creatinine are independently associated with a greater mortality risk.[79] The 60- to 90-day postdischarge mortality rate and readmission rate are 8.6% and 29.6%, respectively; the most important predictors for these complications include older age, lower weight and systolic blood pressure, lower serum sodium, elevated serum creatinine, and associated pulmonary disease.[80] The relative prevalence of normal and reduced EF in people with acute HF is similar to those with chronic HF.[81] The 60- to 90-day postdischarge mortality risk and rehospitalization rates are similar in the two types of HF.[81] A heartening recent trend is the improvement in conformity to quality of care measures in people hospitalized with acute HF, with attendant improvement in in-hospital mortality and morbidity.[82]

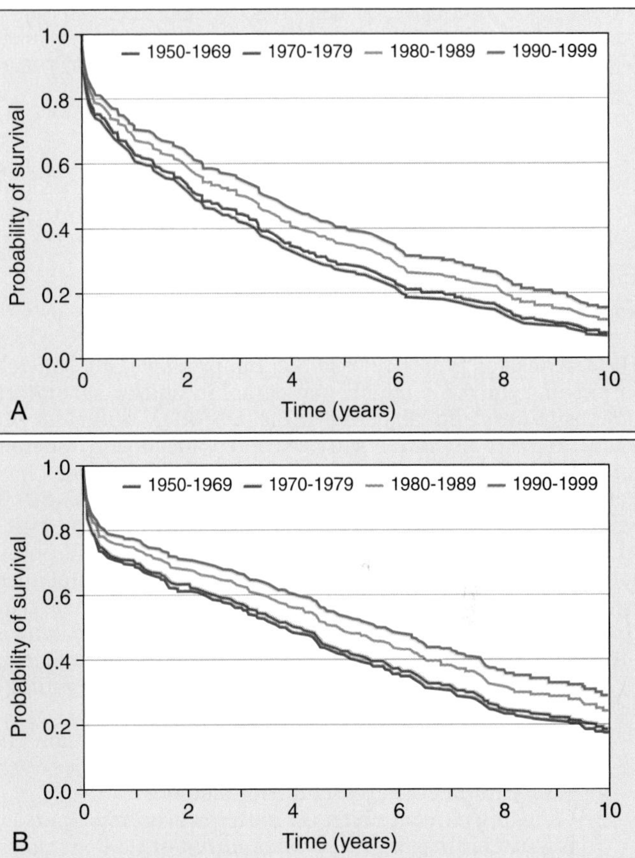

FIGURE 22-6 Age-adjusted survival after the onset of heart failure (ages 65-74 years) **A,** Temporal trends in age-adjusted survival after the onset of heart failure in men. **B,** Temporal trends in age-adjusted survival after the onset of heart failure in woman. (Adapted from Levy D, Kenchaiah S, Larson MG, et al. Long-term trends in the incidence of and survival with heart failure. *N Engl J Med* 2002;347:1397-1402; and Parikh N, Vasan RS. Epidemiology of heart failure. In Colucci WS, editor. *Atlas of heart failure*, ed 5, Philadelphia, 2008, Springer.)

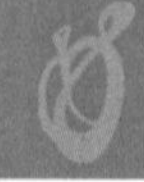

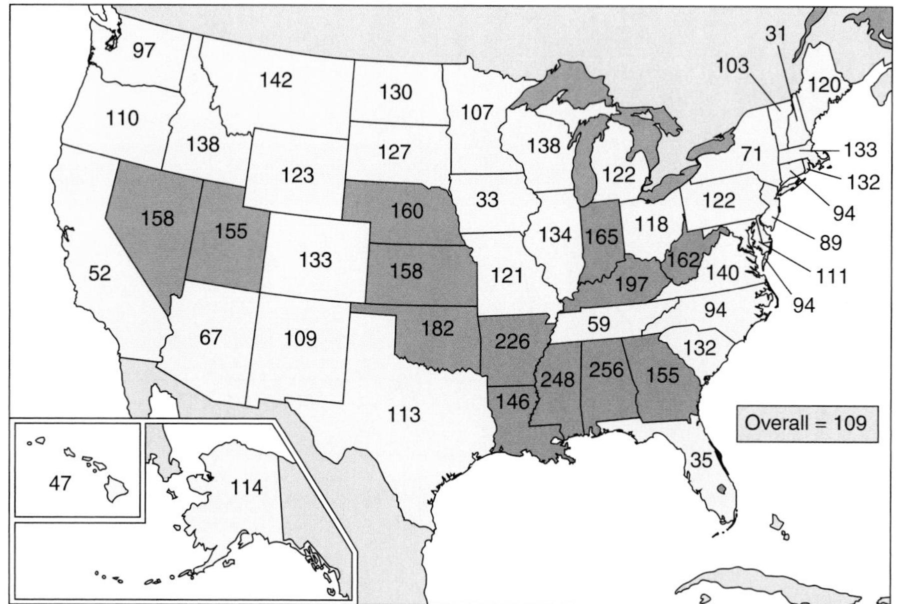

FIGURE 22–7 Geographic variation in U.S. HF death rates. Displayed numbers indicate state-specific, age-adjusted death rates per 100,000 persons in the time period 1990-1996, for men and women 65 years of age. (From Changes in mortality from heart failure—United States, 1980-1995. *MMWR Morb Mortal Wkly Rep* 1998;47:633-637; and Parikh N, Vasan RS. Epidemiology of heart failure. In Colucci WS, editor. *Atlas of heart failure*, ed 5, Philadelphia, 2008, Springer.)

DIFFICULTIES IN INTERPRETING EVALUATIONS ADDRESSING HF EPIDEMIOLOGY

HF diagnosis is typically based on the presence of a constellation of symptoms, signs, radiographic and/or laboratory abnormalities, and objective measures of LV function. As such, there is no universally accepted diagnostic schema, and several sets of criteria (with varying performance characteristics) have been used in epidemiological studies.[83,84] Published differences in the epidemiological characteristics of HF between different geographical regions, different populations, and across time periods may therefore be influenced by varying diagnostic methodologies as opposed to true differences; the magnitude of epidemiological differences attributable to differences in criteria used to diagnose HF is unknown. The major issues in evaluating the epidemiology of HF are:

1. Differences between studies in criteria used for HF diagnosis[84]
2. Nonuniform case ascertainment methods[85]
3. Changing clinical diagnosis patterns over time: increasing use of imaging[86] and laboratory testing (e.g., natriuretic peptide measurements) over time
4. Difficulties in reconciling findings between studies addressing overall trends versus cause-specific trends (e.g., post-MI HF vs. hypertensive HF) or type-specific trends (HF with normal vs. reduced EF)
5. Differences in morbidity statistics due to clinical practice patterns related to hospitalizations, changes in reimbursement, and differences in coding of diagnosis-related groups
6. Differences due to sources of information regarding the epidemiology of HF: longitudinal studies versus registries versus clinic databases

Data regarding the trends and epidemiological pattern of HF should therefore be interpreted with caution in light of these caveats.

FUTURE DIRECTIONS

HF is the only cardiovascular disease increasing in prevalence, and as noted previously, it continues to be associated with a very high morbidity and mortality burden. Improved characterization of (1) those at risk for HF, (2) determinants of poor prognosis in people with established HF, and (3) elucidation of factors associated with varying responses to therapy may aid in the prevention of and reduction in mortality associated with HF.

BIOMARKERS FOR HF RISK PREDICTION

There has been considerable interest recently in the use of circulating biomarkers for prediction and stratification of HF risk.[87,88] Circulating biomarkers of inflammation, renin-angiotensin-aldosterone axis, neurohormonal activation, fibrinolytic potential, and oxidative stress have all been reported as associated with cardiovascular remodeling and/or HF risk.[89-94] Similarly, cardiac troponins T and I, BNP, and interleukin receptors have been shown to predict outcomes in patients with HF.[95-97] However, the incremental utility of these markers in improving risk prediction is unclear at present. Experiences from coronary event risk prediction efforts suggest that contribution of biomarkers to overall risk prediction may be more modest than anticipated.[98] However, biomarkers may be useful in improving the stratification of individuals deemed to be at "intermediate risk" of developing HF based on clinical factors alone.[99]

INVESTIGATION OF HF GENOMICS

The sequencing of the human genome[100] and publication of the HapMap template[101] allow us to elucidate genetic attributes that may help in predicting both HF risk and its prognosis. The most common type of genetic variation is the single nucleotide polymorphism (SNP) and the recently developed

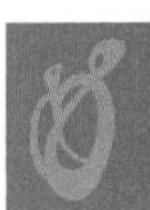

technique of genomewide association study (GWAS) may allow us to identify genetic predictors in the near future. GWAS may also help identify molecular targets for therapy and predictors of pharmacological response, thus offering the possibility of "personalized medicine." However, no GWAS targeting HF has been published to date.

OTHER MOLECULAR APPROACHES TO HF EVALUATION

Another avenue for improving the clinical and epidemiological description of HF is the use of transcriptomics.[102] The "transcriptome" is a complete qualitative and quantitative description of the messenger RNA in a cell. By elucidating the specific gene programs expressed under a given set of conditions, transcriptomic analyses allow us to identify the determinants of disease manifestations and the interplay between genetic and environmental factors. As an example, one recent investigation identified a profile of 46 overexpressed genes that delineated HF patients into those with good versus poor prognosis with 74% sensitivity and 90% specificity.[103]

CONCLUSION

HF is a complex syndrome with numerous risk factors and determinants of outcome. Significant progress has been made in identifying the major risk factors and the population patterns of HF and associated trends. Newer technologies offer further promise of clarifying the clinical and epidemiological course of this condition.[104] The development of universally accepted definitions for diagnosis and classification of HF will simplify and aid epidemiological research, and help in instituting initiatives for prevention.

REFERENCES

1. Heart Failure Society of America. (2006). HFSA 2006 comprehensive heart failure practice guideline. *J Card Fail, 12*, e1–e2.
2. Lloyd-Jones, D., Adams, R., Carnethon, M., et al. (2009). Heart disease and stroke statistics–2009 update: a report from the American Heart Association statistics committee and stroke statistics subcommittee. *Circulation, 119*, e21–e181.
3. Hunt, S. A., Abraham, W. T., Chin, M. H., et al. (2009). 2009 focused update incorporated into the ACC/AHA 2005 guidelines for the diagnosis and management of heart failure in adults: a report of the American College of Cardiology Foundation/American Heart Association task force on practice guidelines: developed in collaboration with the International Society for Heart and Lung Transplantation. *Circulation, 119*, e391–e479.
4. Kenchaiah, S., Narula, J., & Vasan, R. S. (2004). Risk factors for heart failure. *Med Clin North Am, 88*, 1145–1172.
5. Velagaleti, R. S., & Vasan, R. S. (2007). Heart failure in the twenty-first century: is it a coronary artery disease or hypertension problem? *Cardiol Clin, 25*, 487–495.
6. Kannel, W. B., Ho, K., & Thom, T. (1994). Changing epidemiological features of cardiac failure. *Br Heart J, 72*, S3–S9.
7. Felker, G. M., Thompson, R. E., Hare, J. M., et al. (2000). Underlying causes and long-term survival in patients with initially unexplained cardiomyopathy. *N Engl J Med, 342*, 1077–1084.
8. Fox, K. F., Cowie, M. R., Wood, D. A., et al. (2001). Coronary artery disease as the cause of incident heart failure in the population. *Eur Heart J, 22*, 228–236.
9. Cowie, M. R., Wood, D. A., Coats, A. J., et al. (1999). Incidence and aetiology of heart failure: a population-based study. *Eur Heart J, 20*, 421–428.
10. He, J., Ogden, L. G., Bazzano, L. A., et al. (2001). Risk factors for congestive heart failure in US men and women: NHANES I epidemiologic follow-up study. *Arch Intern Med, 161*, 996–1002.
11. Levy, D., Larson, M. G., Vasan, R. S., et al. (1996). The progression from hypertension to congestive heart failure. *JAMA, 275*, 1557–1562.
12. Velagaleti, R. S., Pencina, M. J., Murabito, J. M., et al. (2008). Long-term trends in the incidence of heart failure after myocardial infarction. *Circulation, 118*, 2057–2062.
13. Parikh, N. I., Gona, P., Larson, M. G., et al. (2009). Long-term trends in myocardial infarction incidence and case fatality in the National Heart, Lung, and Blood Institute's Framingham heart study. *Circulation, 119*, 1203–1210.
14. Haider, A. W., Larson, M. G., Franklin, S. S., et al. (2003). Systolic blood pressure, diastolic blood pressure, and pulse pressure as predictors of risk for congestive heart failure in the Framingham heart study. *Ann Intern Med, 138*, 10–16.
15. Lee, D. S., Massaro, J. M., Wang, T. J., et al. (2007). Antecedent blood pressure, body mass index, and the risk of incident heart failure in later life. *Hypertension, 50*, 869–876.
16. Vasan, R. S., Massaro, J. M., Wilson, P. W., et al. (2002). Antecedent blood pressure and risk of cardiovascular disease: the Framingham heart study. *Circulation, 105*, 48–53.
17. Hajjar, I., & Kotchen, T. A. (2003). Trends in prevalence, awareness, treatment, and control of hypertension in the United States, 1988-2000. *JAMA, 290*, 199–206.
18. Ingelsson, E., Gona, P., Larson, M. G., et al. (2008). Altered blood pressure progression in the community and its relation to clinical events. *Arch Intern Med, 168*, 1450–1457.
19. Mosterd, A., D'Agostino, R. B., Silbershatz, H., et al. (1999). Trends in the prevalence of hypertension, antihypertensive therapy, and left ventricular hypertrophy from 1950 to 1989. *N Engl J Med, 340*, 1221–1227.
20. Wang, T. J., & Vasan, R. S. (2005). Epidemiology of uncontrolled hypertension in the United States. *Circulation, 112*, 1651–1662.
21. Ogden, C. L., Carroll, M. D., Curtin, L. R., et al. (2006). Prevalence of overweight and obesity in the United States, 1999-2004. *JAMA, 295*, 1549–1555.
22. Kenchaiah, S., Evans, J. C., Levy, D., et al. (2002). Obesity and the risk of heart failure. *N Engl J Med, 347*, 305–313.
23. Kenchaiah, S., Sesso, H. D., & Gaziano, J. M. (2009). Body mass index and vigorous physical activity and the risk of heart failure among men. *Circulation, 119*, 44–52.
24. Lauer, M. S., Anderson, K. M., Kannel, W. B., et al. (1991). The impact of obesity on left ventricular mass and geometry. The Framingham heart study. *JAMA, 266*, 231–236.
25. Frankel, D. S., Vasan, R. S., D'Agostino, R. B., Sr, et al. (2009). Resistin, adiponectin, and risk of heart failure the Framingham offspring study. *J Am Coll Cardiol, 53*, 754–762.
26. Parikh, N. I., Pencina, M. J., Wang, T. J., et al. (2007). Increasing trends in incidence of overweight and obesity over 5 decades. *Am J Med, 120*, 242–250.
27. Li, C., Ford, E. S., McGuire, L. C., et al. (2007). Increasing trends in waist circumference and abdominal obesity among US adults. *Obesity (Silver Spring), 15*, 216–224.
28. Freedman, D. S., Khan, L. K., Serdula, M. K., et al. (2002). Trends and correlates of class 3 obesity in the United States from 1990 through 2000. *JAMA, 288*, 1758–1761.
29. Gregg, E. W., Cheng, Y. J., Cadwell, B. L., et al. (2005). Secular trends in cardiovascular disease risk factors according to body mass index in US adults. *JAMA, 293*, 1868–1874.
30. Rautaharju, P. M., Prineas, R. J., Wood, J., et al. (2007). Electrocardiographic predictors of new-onset heart failure in men and in women free of coronary heart disease (from the atherosclerosis in communities [ARIC] study). *Am J Cardiol, 100*, 1437–1441.
31. Dhingra, R., Pencina, M. J., Wang, T. J., et al. (2006). Electrocardiographic QRS duration and the risk of congestive heart failure: the Framingham heart study. *Hypertension, 47*, 861–867.
32. Kannel, W. B., D'Agostino, R. B., Silbershatz, H., et al. (1999). Profile for estimating risk of heart failure. *Arch Intern Med, 159*, 1197–1204.
33. Bluemke, D. A., Kronmal, R. A., Lima, J. A., et al. (2008). The relationship of left ventricular mass and geometry to incident cardiovascular events: the MESA (multi-ethnic study of atherosclerosis) study. *J Am Coll Cardiol, 52*, 2148–2155.
34. De Simone, G., Gottdiener, J. S., Chinali, M., et al. (2008). Left ventricular mass predicts heart failure not related to previous myocardial infarction: the cardiovascular health study. *Eur Heart J, 29*, 741–747.
35. Gardin, J. M., McClelland, R., Kitzman, D., et al. (2001). M-mode echocardiographic predictors of six- to seven-year incidence of coronary heart disease, stroke, congestive heart failure, and mortality in an elderly cohort (the cardiovascular health study). *Am J Cardiol, 87*, 1051–1057.
36. Drazner, M. H., Rame, J. E., Marino, E. K., et al. (2004). Increased left ventricular mass is a risk factor for the development of a depressed left ventricular ejection fraction within five years: the cardiovascular health study. *J Am Coll Cardiol, 43*, 2207–2215.
37. Vasan, R. S., Larson, M. G., Benjamin, E. J., et al. (1997). Left ventricular dilatation and the risk of congestive heart failure in people without myocardial infarction. *N Engl J Med, 336*, 1350–1355.
38. de Kam, P. J., Nicolosi, G. L., Voors, A. A., et al. (2002). Prediction of 6 months left ventricular dilatation after myocardial infarction in relation to cardiac morbidity and mortality. Application of a new dilatation model to GISSI-3 data. *Eur Heart J, 23*, 536–542.
39. Migrino, R. Q., Young, J. B., Ellis, S. G., et al. (1997). End-systolic volume index at 90 to 180 minutes into reperfusion therapy for acute myocardial infarction is a strong predictor of early and late mortality. The global utilization of streptokinase and t-pa for occluded coronary arteries (gusto)-i angiographic investigators. *Circulation, 96*, 116–121.
40. Wang, T. J., Levy, D., Benjamin, E. J., et al. (2003). The epidemiology of "asymptomatic" left ventricular systolic dysfunction: implications for screening. *Ann Intern Med, 138*, 907–916.
41. Owan, T. E., & Redfield, M. M. (2005). Epidemiology of diastolic heart failure. *Prog Cardiovasc Dis, 47*, 320–332.
42. Wang, T. J., Evans, J. C., Benjamin, E. J., et al. (2003). Natural history of asymptomatic left ventricular systolic dysfunction in the community. *Circulation, 108*, 977–982.
43. Aurigemma, G. P., Gottdiener, J. S., Shemanski, L., et al. (2001). Predictive value of systolic and diastolic function for incident congestive heart failure in the elderly: the cardiovascular health study. *J Am Coll Cardiol, 37*, 1042–1048.
44. Fischer, M., Baessler, A., Hense, H. W., et al. (2003). Prevalence of left ventricular diastolic dysfunction in the community. Results from a Doppler echocardiographic-based survey of a population sample. *Eur Heart J, 24*, 320–328.
45. Redfield, M. M., Jacobsen, S. J., Burnett, J. C., Jr., et al. (2003). Burden of systolic and diastolic ventricular dysfunction in the community: appreciating the scope of the heart failure epidemic. *JAMA, 289*, 194–202.
46. Lee, D. S., Wang, T. J., & Vasan, R. S. (2006). Screening for ventricular remodeling. *Curr Heart Fail Rep, 3*, 5–13.
47. Vasan, R. S., Benjamin, E. J., Larson, M. G., et al. (2002). Plasma natriuretic peptides for community screening for left ventricular hypertrophy and systolic dysfunction: the Framingham heart study. *JAMA, 288*, 1252–1259.
48. Rovai, D., Morales, M. A., Di Bella, G., et al. (2007). Clinical diagnosis of left ventricular dilatation and dysfunction in the age of technology. *Eur J Heart Fail, 9*, 723–729.
49. Stevens, S. M., Farzaneh-Far, R., Na, B., et al. (2009). Development of an echocardiographic risk-stratification index to predict heart failure in patients with stable coronary artery disease: the heart and soul study. *JACC Cardiovasc Imaging, 2*, 11–20.

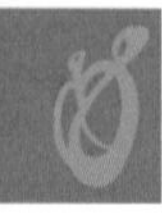

50. Smith, W. M. (1985). Epidemiology of congestive heart failure. *Am J Cardiol, 55*, 3A–8A.
51. Lloyd-Jones, D. M., Larson, M. G., Leip, E. P., et al. (2002). Lifetime risk for developing congestive heart failure: the Framingham heart study. *Circulation, 106*, 3068–3072.
52. McCullough, P. A., Philbin, E. F., Spertus, J. A., et al. (2002). Confirmation of a heart failure epidemic: findings from the resource utilization among congestive heart failure (REACH) study. *J Am Coll Cardiol, 39*, 60–69.
53. Bursi, F., Weston, S. A., Redfield, M. M., et al. (2006). Systolic and diastolic heart failure in the community. *JAMA, 296*, 2209–2216.
54. Hogg, K., Swedberg, K., & McMurray, J. (2004). Heart failure with preserved left ventricular systolic function; epidemiology, clinical characteristics, and prognosis. *J Am Coll Cardiol, 43*, 317–327.
55. Zile, M. R., & Brutsaert, D. L. (2002). New concepts in diastolic dysfunction and diastolic heart failure: part I: diagnosis, prognosis, and measurements of diastolic function. *Circulation, 105*, 1387–1393.
56. Owan, T. E., Hodge, D. O., Herges, R. M., et al. (2006). Trends in prevalence and outcome of heart failure with preserved ejection fraction. *N Engl J Med, 355*, 251–259.
57. Lee, D. S., Gona, P., Vasan, R. S., et al. (2009). Relation of disease pathogenesis and risk factors to heart failure with preserved or reduced ejection fraction: insights from the Framingham heart study of the National Heart, Lung, and Blood Institute. *Circulation, 119*, 3070–3077.
58. Kannel, W. B. (2000). Incidence and epidemiology of heart failure. *Heart Fail Rev, 5*, 167–173.
59. Levy, D., Kenchaiah, S., Larson, M. G., et al. (2002). Long-term trends in the incidence of and survival with heart failure. *N Engl J Med, 347*, 1397–1402.
60. Roger, V. L., Weston, S. A., Redfield, M. M., et al. (2004). Trends in heart failure incidence and survival in a community-based population. *JAMA, 292*, 344–350.
61. Lloyd-Jones, D. M., Larson, M. G., Leip, E. P., et al. (2002). Lifetime risk for developing congestive heart failure: the Framingham heart study. *Circulation, 106*, 3068–3072.
62. Djousse, L., Driver, J. A., & Gaziano, J. M. (2009). Relation between modifiable lifestyle factors and lifetime risk of heart failure. *JAMA, 302*, 394–400.
63. O'Connell, J. B., & Bristow, M. R. (1994). Economic impact of heart failure in the United States: time for a different approach. *J Heart Lung Transplant, 13*, S107–S112.
64. Jessup, M., & Brozena, S. (2003). Heart failure. *N Engl J Med, 348*, 2007–2018.
65. Liao, L., Jollis, J. G., Anstrom, K. J., et al. (2006). Costs for heart failure with normal vs reduced ejection fraction. *Arch Intern Med, 166*, 112–118.
66. Krum, H., & Gilbert, R. E. (2003). Demographics and concomitant disorders in heart failure. *Lancet, 362*, 147–158.
67. Brown, A. M., & Cleland, J. G. (1998). Influence of concomitant disease on patterns of hospitalization in patients with heart failure discharged from Scottish hospitals in 1995. *Eur Heart J, 19*, 1063–1069.
68. Shah, S. J., & Gheorghiade, M. (2008). Heart failure with preserved ejection fraction: treat now by treating comorbidities. *JAMA, 300*, 431–433.
69. Ho, K. K., Anderson, K. M., Kannel, W. B., et al. (1993). Survival after the onset of congestive heart failure in Framingham heart study subjects. *Circulation, 88*, 107–115.
70. Ho, K. K., Pinsky, J. L., Kannel, W. B., et al. (1993). The epidemiology of heart failure: the Framingham study. *J Am Coll Cardiol, 22*, 6A–13A.
71. Changes in mortality from heart failure–United States, 1980-1995. (1998). *MMWR Morb Mortal Wkly Rep, 47*, 633–637.
72. Ammar, K. A., Jacobsen, S. J., Mahoney, D. W., et al. (2007). Prevalence and prognostic significance of heart failure stages: application of the American College of Cardiology/American Heart Association heart failure staging criteria in the community. *Circulation, 115*, 1563–1570.
73. Costanzo, M. R., Mills, R. M., & Wynne, J. (2008). Characteristics of "Stage D" heart failure: insights from the Acute Decompensated Heart Failure National Registry longitudinal module (ADHERE LM). *Am Heart J, 155*, 339–347.
74. Nieminen, M. S., Bohm, M., Cowie, M. R., et al. (2005). Executive summary of the guidelines on the diagnosis and treatment of acute heart failure: the task force on acute heart failure of the European Society of Cardiology. *Eur Heart J, 26*, 384–416.
75. Fonarow, G. C., Adams, K. F., Jr., Abraham, W. T., et al. (2005). Risk stratification for in-hospital mortality in acutely decompensated heart failure: classification and regression tree analysis. *JAMA, 293*, 572–580.
76. Gheorghiade, M., Zannad, F., Sopko, G., et al. (2005). Acute heart failure syndromes: current state and framework for future research. *Circulation, 112*, 3958–3968.
77. Fonarow, G. C. (2008). Epidemiology and risk stratification in acute heart failure. *Am Heart J, 155*, 200–207.
78. Fonarow, G. C., Abraham, W. T., Albert, N. M., et al. (2008). Factors identified as precipitating hospital admissions for heart failure and clinical outcomes: findings from OPTIMIZE-HF. *Arch Intern Med, 168*, 847–854.
79. Abraham, W. T., Fonarow, G. C., Albert, N. M., et al. (2008). Predictors of in-hospital mortality in patients hospitalized for heart failure: insights from the organized program to initiate lifesaving treatment in hospitalized patients with heart failure (OPTIMIZE-HF). *J Am Coll Cardiol, 52*, 347–356.
80. O'Connor, C. M., Abraham, W. T., Albert, N. M., et al. (2008). Predictors of mortality after discharge in patients hospitalized with heart failure: an analysis from the organized program to initiate lifesaving treatment in hospitalized patients with heart failure (OPTIMIZE-HF). *Am Heart J, 156*, 662–673.
81. Fonarow, G. C., Stough, W. G., Abraham, W. T., et al. (2007). Characteristics, treatments, and outcomes of patients with preserved systolic function hospitalized for heart failure: a report from the OPTIMIZE-HF registry. *J Am Coll Cardiol, 50*, 768–777.
82. Fonarow, G. C., Heywood, J. T., Heidenreich, P. A., et al. (2007). Temporal trends in clinical characteristics, treatments, and outcomes for heart failure hospitalizations, 2002 to 2004: findings from Acute Decompensated Heart Failure National Registry (ADHERE). *Am Heart J, 153*, 1021–1028.
83. Di Bari, M., Pozzi, C., Cavallini, M. C., et al. (2004). The diagnosis of heart failure in the community. Comparative validation of four sets of criteria in unselected older adults: the ICARe Dicomano study. *J Am Coll Cardiol, 44*, 1601–1608.
84. Mosterd, A., Deckers, J. W., Hoes, A. W., et al. (1997). Classification of heart failure in population based research: an assessment of six heart failure scores. *Eur J Epidemiol, 13*, 491–502.
85. Vasan, R. S., Benjamin, E. J., & Levy, D. (1995). Prevalence, clinical features and prognosis of diastolic heart failure: an epidemiologic perspective. *J Am Coll Cardiol, 26*, 1565–1574.
86. Lopez-Jimenez, F., Goraya, T. Y., Hellermann, J. P., et al. (2004). Measurement of ejection fraction after myocardial infarction in the population. *Chest, 125*, 397–403.
87. Braunwald, E. (2008). Biomarkers in heart failure. *N Engl J Med, 358*, 2148–2159.
88. Lee, D. S., & Vasan, R. S. (2005). Novel markers for heart failure diagnosis and prognosis. *Curr Opin Cardiol, 20*, 201–210.
89. Collet, J. P., Montalescot, G., Vicaut, E., et al. (2003). Acute release of plasminogen activator inhibitor-1 in ST-segment elevation myocardial infarction predicts mortality. *Circulation, 108*, 391–394.
90. Lieb, W., Larson, M. G., Benjamin, E. J., et al. (2009). Multimarker approach to evaluate correlates of vascular stiffness: the Framingham heart study. *Circulation, 119*, 37–43.
91. Vasan, R. S., Sullivan, L. M., Roubenoff, R., et al. (2003). Inflammatory markers and risk of heart failure in elderly subjects without prior myocardial infarction: the Framingham heart study. *Circulation, 107*, 1486–1491.
92. Vasan, R. S., Beiser, A., D'Agostino, R. B., et al. (2003). Plasma homocysteine and risk for congestive heart failure in adults without prior myocardial infarction. *JAMA, 289*, 1251–1257.
93. Velagaleti, R. S., Gona, P., Levy, D., et al. (2008). Relations of biomarkers representing distinct biological pathways to left ventricular geometry. *Circulation, 118*, 2252–2258.
94. Wang, T. J., Larson, M. G., Levy, D., et al. (2004). Plasma natriuretic peptide levels and the risk of cardiovascular events and death. *N Engl J Med, 350*, 655–663.
95. Latini, R., Masson, S., Anand, I. S., et al. (2007). Prognostic value of very low plasma concentrations of troponin T in patients with stable chronic heart failure. *Circulation, 116*, 1242–1249.
96. Januzzi, J. L., Jr., Peacock, W. F., Maisel, A. S., et al. (2007). Measurement of the interleukin family member ST2 in patients with acute dyspnea: results from the PRIDE (pro-brain natriuretic peptide investigation of dyspnea in the emergency department) study. *J Am Coll Cardiol, 50*, 607–613.
97. Horwich, T. B., Patel, J., MacLellan, W. R., et al. (2003). Cardiac troponin I is associated with impaired hemodynamics, progressive left ventricular dysfunction, and increased mortality rates in advanced heart failure. *Circulation, 108*, 833–838.
98. Wang, T. J., Gona, P., Larson, M. G., et al. (2006). Multiple biomarkers for the prediction of first major cardiovascular events and death. *N Engl J Med, 355*, 2631–2639.
99. Pencina, M. J., D'Agostino, R. B., Sr, D'Agostino, R. B., Jr., et al. (2008). Evaluating the added predictive ability of a new marker: from area under the ROC curve to reclassification and beyond. *Stat Med, 27*, 157–172.
100. International Human Genome Sequencing Consortium (2004). Finishing the euchromatic sequence of the human genome. *Nature, 431*, 931–945.
101. The International HapMap Consortium (2003). The international HapMap project. *Nature, 426*, 789–796.
102. Heidecker, B., & Hare, J. M. (2007). The use of transcriptomic biomarkers for personalized medicine. *Heart Fail Rev, 12*, 1–11.
103. Heidecker, B., Kasper, E. K., Wittstein, I. S., et al. (2008). Transcriptomic biomarkers for individual risk assessment in new-onset heart failure. *Circulation, 118*, 238–246.
104. Vasan, R. S. (2006). Biomarkers of cardiovascular disease: molecular basis and practical considerations. *Circulation, 113*, 2335–2362.

CHAPTER 23

Heart Failure as a Consequence of Ischemic Heart Disease

James D. Flaherty, Robert O. Bonow, and Mihai Gheorghiade

Despite significant progress in the prevention and treatment of cardiovascular disease over the past 30 years, national statistics indicate that the incidence and prevalence of heart failure (HF) continue to rise.[1] This has occurred during a time period in which death rates from coronary artery disease (CAD) and stroke have declined. HF and CAD are age-related conditions (the prevalence of HF is 1% between the ages of 50 and 59 years, but 10% above the age of 75 years).[2] The increased survival after myocardial infarction (MI) and advances in medical and device therapies (e.g., β-blockers and implantable cardioverter-defibrillators [ICDs]) for the prevention of sudden cardiac death (SCD) have increased the pool of patients with the potential to develop chronic HF.[3-5]

PREVALENCE OF CORONARY ARTERY DISEASE IN HEART FAILURE

CAD has emerged as the dominant causal factor in HF (see Chapter 22). Survivors of acute MI, even when not complicated by HF, have a relatively high incidence of subsequent HF hospitalization.[6] This is due not only to the initial ventricular insult caused by the MI, but also the progressive nature of CAD (Figure 23-1). The Framingham Heart Study suggests that the factors contributing to HF are changing, as evidenced by a decrease in valvular heart disease and left ventricular (LV) hypertrophy, but an increase in MI as a risk factor from 1950 to 1998.[3] In this analysis, the odds of a prior MI as a cause of HF increased by 26% per decade in men and 48% per decade in women. In contrast, hypertension as a cause of HF decreased by 13% per decade in men and 25% in women, and valvular heart disease as a cause of HF decreased by 24% per decade in men and 17% in women.

In the Studies of Left Ventricular Dysfunction (SOLVD) registry, which enrolled 6273 patients, CAD was determined as the underlying cause of chronic HF in approximately 70% of patients, whereas hypertension was invoked as the primary cause in only 7% of cases.[7] Of note, there was a history of hypertension in 43% of patients. There were striking racial differences observed in this registry. HF was considered due to CAD in 73% of Caucasian patients, but only 36% of African American patients.

Pooling data from 26 multicenter trials of chronic HF since 1986 with greater than 43,000 patients revealed that 62% carried a diagnosis of CAD[8-33] (Table 23-1). This number may actually underestimate the true prevalence of CAD in this population as in clinical practice and in most studies there is no systemic assessment of coronary artery anatomy. In addition, most of these trials excluded patients with a recent MI, angina, or objective evidence of active ischemia. In a study of 136 patients (<75 years old) hospitalized with de novo HF, a review of the clinical, angiographic, and myocardial perfusion imaging data was used to determine that CAD was the primary cause in greater than 50% of cases.[34] In this study alone, two thirds of all patients who underwent angiography had obstructive CAD (defined as >50% luminal stenosis), although CAD was not considered the primary causal factor in all cases. In a recent analysis of a large U.S. acute HF registry, myocardial ischemia was found to be a leading precipitating factor for hospitalization.[35]

PROGNOSTIC SIGNIFICANCE OF CORONARY ARTERY DISEASE IN HEART FAILURE

The presence of CAD in patients with HF has been shown to be independently associated with a worsened long-term outcome in numerous studies.[36] Atherosclerosis is an important contributing cause of death in HF patients through a variety of mechanisms, including SCD, progressive ventricular failure, MI, renal failure, and stroke. In patients with HF, the long-term prognosis is directly related to the angiographic extent and severity of CAD.[37,38] This has been demonstrated both in HF patients with LV systolic dysfunction (LVSD) and in those with preserved systolic function.[39]

Recent data suggest that the mechanism of SCD may differ between ischemic and nonischemic HF, with acute coronary events representing the major cause of SCD in patients with CAD.[40,41] In the Assessment of Treatment with Lisinopril and Survival (ATLAS) study, 54% of patients with chronic HF and CAD who died suddenly had autopsy evidence of acute MI.[40] In another autopsy study of 180 patients with known ischemic cardiomyopathy, acute MI was responsible for 57% of the deaths.[41] This study revealed that, before autopsy data were available, many deaths due to acute MI in patients with HF were misclassified as due to progressive HF or arrhythmias. In another study of patients with HF and LVSD, 25% of repeat hospitalizations were attributed to ACS.[42] However, approximately 10% of patients with a history of HF who were subsequently hospitalized for ACS were originally classified as having a nonischemic cause. These findings further emphasize the importance of accurately assessing for the presence of CAD in patients with HF.

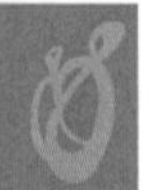

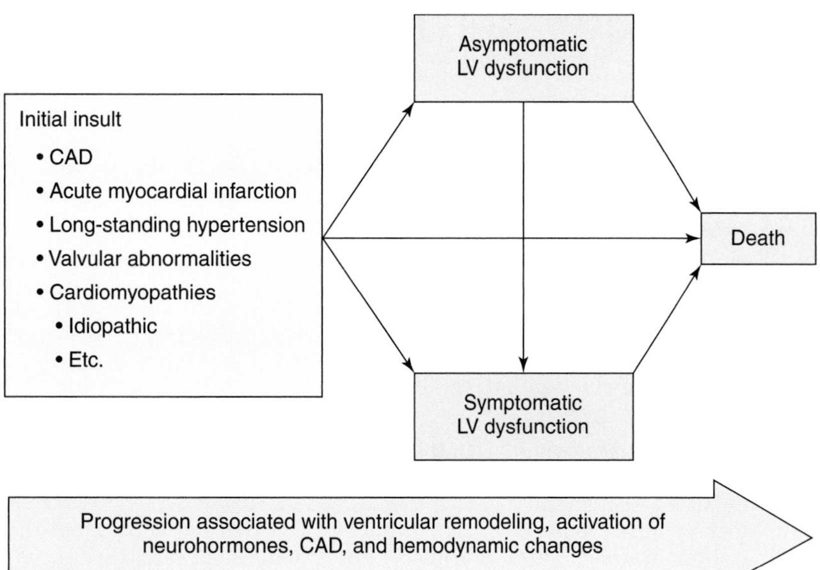

FIGURE 23–1 Coronary artery disease (CAD) contributes to left ventricular (LV) dysfunction not only during an initial insult (e.g., myocardial infarction) but throughout its progression. In addition, progression of chronic heart failure is associated with ventricular remodeling, activation of neurohormones, and hemodynamic changes.

PATHOPHYSIOLOGY OF ACUTE HEART FAILURE IN PATIENTS WITH CAD

Underlying Coronary Artery Disease

Patients hospitalized with acute HF differ from patients with chronic ambulatory HF with respect to prognosis and early management.[43] Patients with CAD who develop acute HF do so with either an ACS or a non-ACS presentation. Although the majority of such patients do not have ACS, there is considerable overlap in these two presentations with respect to clinical characteristics (Table 23-2, *A*) and potential therapies (Table 23-2, *B*). However, the approach to the patient with ACS has become more standardized in clinical practice guidelines compared with the acute HF patient with a non-ACS presentation. Myocardial injury is common in both, but in ACS patients it is usually the principal cause of HF, whereas in non-ACS patients myocardial injury may be the result of worsening HF. In these latter patients, cardiac troponin levels are frequently elevated in patients with acute HF, representing myocardial injury. These values typically do not reach the established threshold values for ACS, but are still associated with worse outcomes.[44-49]

Low-level myocardial injury in patients with acute HF and underlying CAD may be the result of the marked hemodynamic and neurohormonal abnormalities that are frequently present in acute HF, but less likely to be present in chronic ambulatory HF. In acute HF, a high LV diastolic pressure can result in subendocardial ischemia. The excessive neurohormal activation can exacerbate ischemia via increased cardiac contractility and reduced coronary perfusion because of endothelial dysfunction. In addition, patients with acute HF and CAD often have hibernating or stunned myocardium.[50] Together, all of these factors may result in myocardial injury.[52]

Patients with acute HF and a low blood pressure have a much higher mortality compared to patients who are normotensive or hypertensive at the time of admission.[51 and 52] Low systemic blood pressure combined with elevated LV diastolic pressure reduces coronary perfusion, and in this setting, the autoregulation between coronary artery perfusion pressure and coronary vasoactive tone may be lost or impaired in patients with obstructive epicardial CAD. This may contribute to myocardial injury (as reflected by cardiac enzyme elevation) and worse outcomes. This may help to explain why patients with acute HF and underlying CAD have a worse outcome than those without CAD and have improved outcomes if they have a history of myocardial revascularization.[48,53]

Acute Coronary Syndromes

Approximately 10% to 20% of patients with ACS have concomitant acute HF and roughly 10% of ACS patients develop HF in-hospital.[54-59] In the EuroHeart Survey II on HF, 42% of all de novo HF cases were due to ACS.[60] Patients with ACS and ST-segment elevation typically have a high degree of myocardial injury. ACS patients with HF but without ST-segment elevation also have significant cardiac enzyme elevation, but a smaller degree of injury.[47] The short-term risk of adverse outcomes in ACS patients with HF is directly proportional to the level of troponin elevation.[61] Most of these patients do not have a history of HF or LVSD.[54,56]

Patients with ACS complicated by HF have markedly increased short- and long-term mortality rates compared with ACS patients without HF.[54-56,61-69] ACS patients who develop HF after the initial presentation have even higher mortality rates.[55,59] The prognosis of ACS complicated by HF is directly related to the Killip class.[55,57,59] Compared with Killip class I patients, patients with an ACS in Killip class II or III HF are four times more likely to die in-hospital.[56,59] The risk goes up to tenfold for patients with cardiogenic shock (Killip class IV). Among ACS patients who recover from transient HF, the majority develop recurrent HF.[6]

PATHOPHYSIOLOGY OF CHRONIC HEART FAILURE IN PATIENTS WITH CAD AND REDUCED EJECTION FRACTION

HF in the setting of CAD is a heterogeneous condition with several possible factors contributing to clinical manifestations of HF and LVSD and/or diastolic dysfunction. First and foremost, the sequelae of MI, with loss of functioning myocytes, development of myocardial fibrosis, and subsequent LV remodeling, result in chamber dilation and neurohormonal activation that lead to progressive deterioration of the remaining viable myocardium.[70] This is a well-recognized clinical process that can be ameliorated after acute MI by the use of angiotensin-converting enzyme (ACE) inhibitor therapy, β-blocking agents, and myocardial revascularization.[71-74] Second, the majority of patients surviving MI have significant

TABLE 23–1	Prevalence of Coronary Artery Disease (CAD) in 26 Multicenter Chronic Heart Failure Trials Reported by the *New England Journal of Medicine* Since 1986		
Trial	**Year**	***N***	**CAD**
VHEFT-1	1986	642	282
CONSENSUS	1987	253	146
Milrinone	1989	230	115
PROMISE	1991	1088	590
SOLVD-T	1991	2569	1828
VHEFT-2	1991	804	427
SOVLD-P	1992	4228	3518
RADIANCE	1993	178	107
Vesnarinone	1993	477	249
STAT-CHF	1995	674	481
Carvedilol	1996	1094	521
PRAISE	1996	1153	732
DIG	1997	6800	4793
VEST	1998	3833	2236
RALES	1999	1663	907
DIAMOND	1999	1518	1017
Nesiritide	2000	127	58
COPERNICUS	2001	2289	1534
BEST	2001	2708	1587
Val-HeFT	2001	5010	2880
MIRACLE	2002	453	108
COMPANION	2004	1520	842
SCD-HeFT	2005	2521	1310
CARE-HF	2005	813	309
RethinQ	2007	172	90
Dronedarone	2008	627	407
Total		**43,444**	**27,074**

Coronary artery disease was documented to be present in nearly 65% of patients.

atherosclerotic disease in coronary arteries other than the infarct-related artery.[75] Thus superimposed on the left ventricle with irreversibly damaged myocardium, there is often a considerable degree of jeopardized myocardium served by a stenotic coronary artery either within the infarct zone or remote from the infarcted tissue. This may result in myocardial ischemia/hibernation, contributing to LV dysfunction and the risk of recurrent MI producing further deterioration in LV function or SCD. Finally, endothelial dysfunction, a characteristic feature of atherosclerotic CAD, may also contribute importantly and independently to the progression of LV dysfunction (Figure 23-2).[76]

Left Ventricular Remodeling (see also Chapter 15)

According to St. John Sutton and Sharpe, LV remodeling is the process by which the left ventricle's size, shape, and function are altered in response to acute and chronic injury or overload, a process that is regulated by mechanical, neurohormonal, and genetic factors (Figure 23-3).[70] The severe loss of myocardial cells after acute MI results in an abrupt increase in loading conditions that induces a unique pattern of remodeling involving the infarct zone, the infarct border zone, and the remote noninfarcted myocardium.[70] Myocyte necrosis initiates a process of reparative changes, which

TABLE 23–2A	Characteristics of Patients with AHFS and CAD Versus Patients with ACS Complicated by HF	
	AHFS and CAD	**ACS Complicated by HF**
Dyspnea	Common	Common
Chest discomfort	Uncommon	Common
Prior HF	Common	Uncommon
BNP/N-terminal pro-BNP	Elevated	Elevated
Troponin	Normal or elevated*	Usually elevated
Left ventricular systolic function	Normal or depressed	Normal or depressed
Diagnostic testing for CAD† (ischemia/viability/angiography)	Uncommon	Standard (per guidelines)
Myocardial revascularization	Uncommon†	Standard (per guidelines)
Secondary prevention for CAD	Underused	Standard (per guidelines)
In-hospital mortality	Relatively low	Relatively high
Early after-discharge death or rehospitalization	High	High

*Typically low-level elevation.
†During index hospitalization.
ACS, Acute coronary syndrome; *AHFS,* acute heart failure syndrome; *BNP,* B-type natriuretic peptide; *CAD,* coronary artery disease; *HF,* heart failure

TABLE 23–2B	Therapies for AHFS and CAD Versus ACS Complicated by HF	
	AHFS and CAD	**ACS Complicated by HF**
Immediate Therapies		
Nitrates	Yes	Yes
Antiplatelet agents	Yes	Yes
Anticoagulation	No	Yes
Inotropes	Avoid if possible	Avoid if possible
Statins	Yes	Yes
Renin-Angiotensin System Modulation		
ACE-I or ARB	Yes	Yes
Aldosterone blockade (if LVSD)	Yes	Yes
β-blockers	Yes	Yes
Early angiography/revascularization	Yes*	Yes*

*If jeopardized myocardium present (ischemia or viability).
(From Flaherty JD, Bax JJ, De Luca L, et al. Acute heart failure syndromes in patients with coronary artery disease: early assessment and treatment. *J Am Coll Cardiol* 2009;53:254-263.)
ACE-I, Angiotensin-converting enzyme inhibitor; *ARB,* angiotensin receptor blocker; *LVSD,* left ventricular systolic dysfunction.

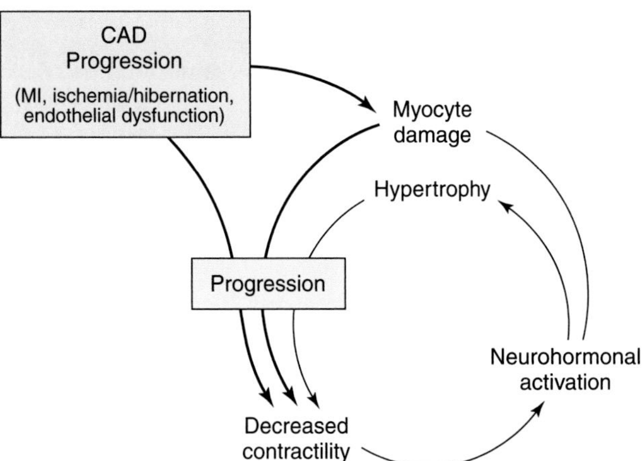

FIGURE 23–2 Progression of coronary artery disease (CAD) leads to decreased contractility, which stimulates neurohormonal activation of chamber remodeling, hypertrophy, and myocyte damage. *CAD,* Coronary artery disease; *MI,* myocardial ischemia. (Adapted from Gheorghiade M, Bonow RO. Chronic heart failure in the United States: a manifestation of coronary artery disease. *Circulation* 1998;97:282-289.)

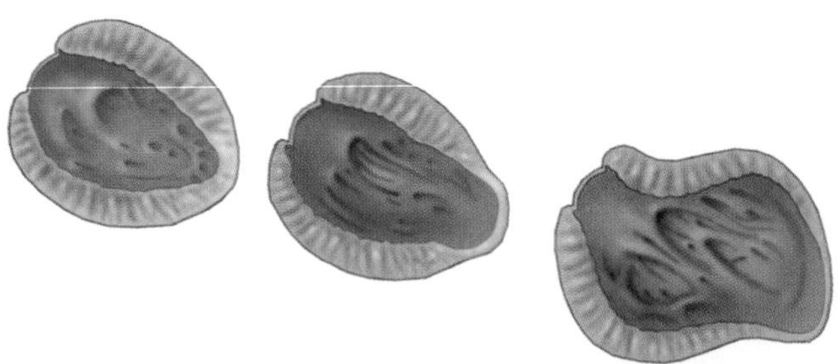

FIGURE 23–3 Remodeling of left ventricle after ST-elevation myocardial infarction (STEMI). *Left,* Apical STEMI (white zone of left ventricle). Over time, the infarct zone elongates and thins. Progressive remodeling of the left ventricle occurs (*center* and *right*), ultimately converting the left ventricle from an oval shape to a spherical shape. Pharmacological and catheter-based reperfusion strategies for STEMI have a favorable impact on this process by minimizing the extent of myocardial necrosis (*left*) through prompt restoration of flow in the epicardial infarct vessel. (Modified from McMurray JJV, Pfeffer MA, editors. *Heart failure updates*, London, 2003, Martin Dunitz.)

consist of dilation, hypertrophy, and the formation of collagen scar. This process usually continues into the chronic phase until the heart, strengthened by collagen scarring, offsets the dilating forces. Other factors may influence this process, including the location and transmurality of the infarct, the extent of myocardial stunning beyond the initial infarction, infarct-related artery patency, and local trophic factors.[70] Three components participate in this process: the myocytes, the extracellular matrix, and the microcirculation. Postinfarction remodeling has been arbitrarily divided into an early phase (within 72 hours) and a late phase (beyond 72 hours). In patients with transmural MI, the early phase involves expansion of the infarct, with thinning and bulging that may result in ventricular rupture, aneurysm, mitral insufficiency, and ventricular tachyarrhythmias. Late remodeling involves the left ventricle globally and is associated morphologically with dilation, hypertrophy, and myocyte hypertrophy (see Figure 23-3).[70] These processes all may contribute to deterioration in contractile function. In summary, LV remodeling consists of ventricular thinning and dilation in the infarct zone, myocyte hypertrophy in the noninfarct zones, fibrosis, and activation of neurohormones. These processes impact the biology of the cardiac myocyte and nonmyocyte components of the myocardium and contribute independently to the progression of HF.[77]

Myocardial Ischemia

Under basal conditions, episodes of reversible myocardial ischemia caused by a severe coronary artery stenosis superimposed on the left ventricle with depressed systolic function may produce transient worsening of LV function. This exacerbates dyspnea on exertion and fatigue. In many patients, these HF symptoms, stimulated by exercise, represent an anginal equivalent that may occur in the absence of chest pain.

Transient LV dysfunction can aggravate symptoms during stress or spontaneous ischemia in patients with CAD and HF. Ischemia can also produce a rapid and massive increase in the concentration of all three endogenous catecholamines (norepinephrine, epinephrine, dopamine) in the myocardial interstitial fluid, which is mediated by inhibition of neuronal reuptake mechanisms.[78] High myocardial catecholamine concentration may have a deleterious effect on cardiac myocytes.[79-81]

Ischemia may also lead to myocyte apoptosis, which may result in progression of LV dysfunction without a clear ischemic event.[82] This situation also indicates that ischemia from a chronic stenosis can produce substantial myocyte loss in the absence of significant necrosis or fibrosis. Ischemia may also cause an increase in endothelin production that may have a negative effect on LV function.[83] Aggressive medical and surgical interventions designed to ameliorate ischemia appear to have a substantial impact on limiting apoptosis.

Hibernation/Stunning (see also Chapter 36)

Episodes of transient myocardial ischemia may cause prolonged LVSD that persists after the ischemic insult itself has resolved. This process is termed *stunning,* which is similar to more severe and protracted myocardial stunning that results from coronary occlusion and reperfusion (Figure 23-4, *A*).[84] Recurrent episodes of myocardial ischemia that produce repetitive myocardial stunning may contribute to overall LV dysfunction and HF symptoms.

Another important mechanism for systolic dysfunction with additive effects on LV performance is myocardial hibernation. Once considered a process in which myocardial contraction is downregulated in response to chronic reduction in myocardial blood supply,[85-87] the current evidence supports the hypothesis that persistent contractile dysfunction in patients with chronic CAD represents a process of programmed disassembly of contractile elements following repeated episodes of reversible ischemia (Figure 23-4, *B*).[88-92] Thus rather than a "protective" mechanism, hibernation represents a disadvantageous process that, left uncorrected, may lead to apoptosis and myocyte loss, replacement fibrosis, graded and reciprocal changes in α- and β-adrenergic receptor density, progressive LVSD, and the risk of ventricular arrhythmias (Figure 23-5). This process may affect a substantial number of HF patients. Among patients with HF, CAD, and LVSD, approximately 50% have evidence of viable but dysfunctional myocardium.[93-95]

Diagnosis

Hibernating myocardium should be suspected in all patients with CAD and chronic LV dysfunction of any degree, regional and global.[95] Up to 50% of patients with CAD and chronic LV dysfunction have significant areas of dysfunctional but viable myocardium.[96] Hibernating myocardium can be determined with the use of imaging techniques that detect myocardial contractile reserve, preserved metabolic activity, or cell membrane integrity within the region of dysfunctional myocardium.[74,97-100] Intact perfusion, cell membrane integrity, and intact mitochondria can be evaluated with single photon emission tomography using thallium-201 and/or technetium-99m labeled traces. Preserved glucose metabolism can be

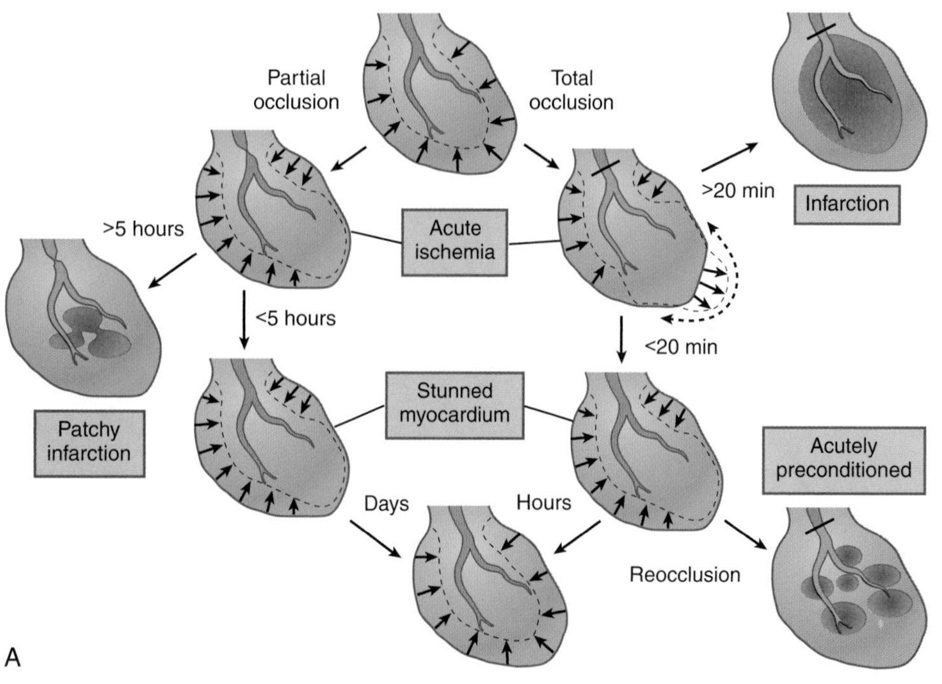

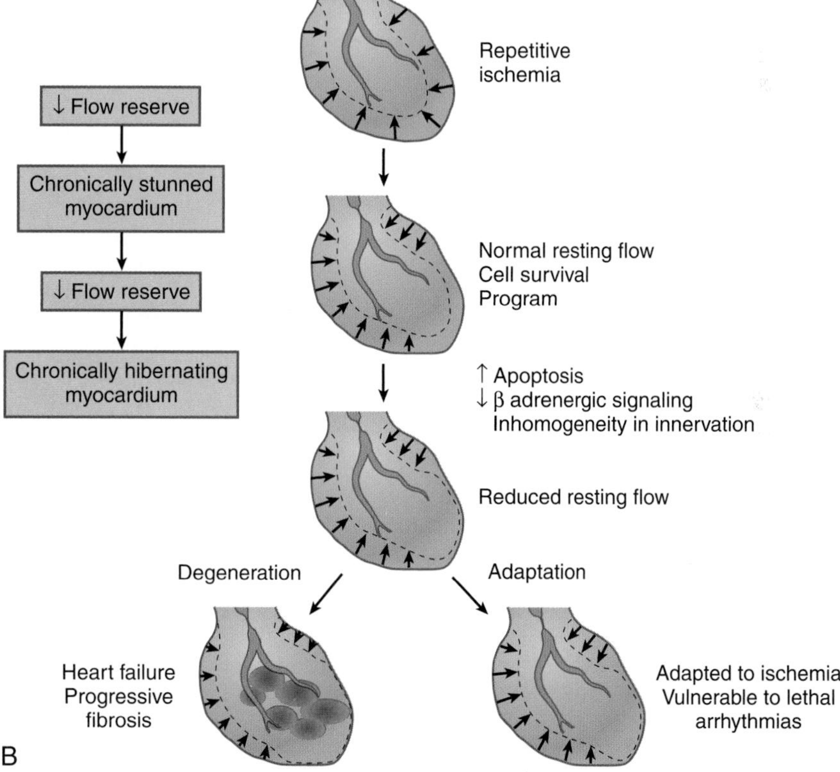

FIGURE 23–4 Effects of ischemia on left ventricular (LV) function and irreversible injury. The ventriculograms illustrate contractile dysfunction (*dashed lines* and *arrows*). **A,** Consequences of acute ischemia. A brief total occlusion (*right*) or a prolonged partial occlusion (caused by an acute high-grade stenosis, *left*) leads to acute contractile dysfunction proportional to the reduction in blood flow. Irreversible injury begins after 20 minutes following a total occlusion but is delayed for up to 5 hours following a partial occlusion (or with significant collaterals) caused by short-term hibernation. When reperfusion is established before the onset of irreversible injury, stunned myocardium develops and the time required for recovery of function is proportional to the duration and severity of ischemia. With prolonged ischemia, stunning in viable myocardium coexists with subendocardial infarction and accounts for reversible dysfunction. Brief episodes of ischemia preceding prolonged ischemia elicits protection against infarction (acute preconditioning). **B,** Effects of chronic repetitive ischemia on function distal to a stenosis. As stenosis severity increased, coronary flow reserve decreases and the frequency of reversible ischemia increases. Reversible repetitive ischemia initially leads to chronic preconditioning against infarction and stunning (not shown). Subsequently, there is a gradual progression from contractile dysfunction with normal resting flow (chronically stunned myocardium) to contractile dysfunction with depressed resting flow (hibernating myocardium). This transition is related to the physiological significance of a coronary stenosis and can occur in a time period as short as 1 week or develop chronically in the absence of severe angina. The cellular response during the progression to chronic hibernating myocardium is variable, with some patients exhibiting successful adaptation with little cell death and fibrosis and others developing degenerative changes difficult to distinguish from subendocardial infarction. (From Canty JM. Coronary blood flow and myocardial ischemia. In Libby P, Bonow RO, Mann DL, et al, editors. *Braunwald's heart disease*, Philadelphia, 2008, Elsevier.)

assessed by positron emission tomography using F18-fluorodeoxyglucose. Contractile reserve can be unmasked by infusion of low-dose dobutamine during echocardiography. The use of these techniques has been associated with improved survival in patients with chronic HF and significant viability who underwent myocardial revascularization.[97-101]

Cardiac magnetic resonance imaging is also an established technique to assess myocardial viability and the potential for recovery of LV function.[102-104] Resting cine MRI can be used to assess LV end-diastolic wall thickness. An end-diastolic wall thickness less than 5 to 6 mm is a marker of transmural MI and virtually excludes the presence of viable myocardium. In dysfunctional myocardium with preserved end-diastolic wall thickness (6 mm), detection of contractile reserve during low-dose dobutamine infusion confirms the presence of viable myocardium. Gadolinium-based contrast agents have been

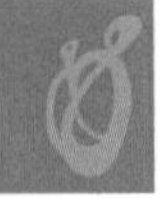

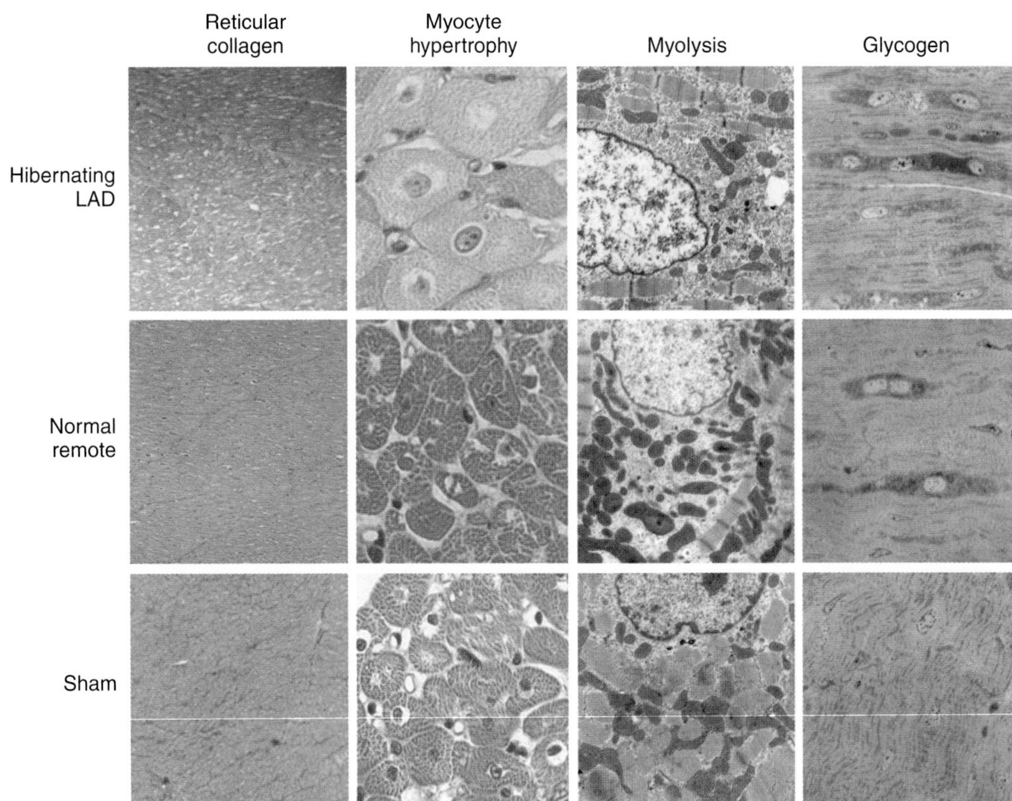

FIGURE 23–5 Myocyte cellular changes in hibernating myocardium. The increased myocyte loss results in compensatory myocyte cellular hypertrophy in hibernating myocardium. Whereas reticular collagen is regionally increased (about 2%), there is no evidence of infarction. The electron microscopic characteristics of hibernating myocardium demonstrate myofibrillar loss, an increased number of small mitochondria, and increased glycogen content. Although these are markedly different from normal myocardium (sham), biopsies of normal remote, nonischemic segments show similar morphological changes, indicating that these structural abnormalities are not directly related to ischemia nor are they the cause of regional contractile dysfunction.
LAD, left anterior descending artery. (From Canty JM, Fallavollita JA. Hibernating myocardium. *J Nucl Cardiol* 2005;12:104.)

used to detect nonviable myocardium because these agents accumulate selectively in areas of scar tissue.[102,103] It should be noted that this technique is extremely sensitive to detect scar tissue (with very high spatial resolution), but the absence of scar tissue does not permit discrimination between normal tissue and hibernating or stunned myocardium.

Clinical Implications

The presence of viable but dysfunctional myocardium can be used to predict a favorable response to myocardial revascularization and pharmacological therapy.[101,105,106] The restoration of blood flow with revascularization or treatment with agents that improve endothelial function and blood flow, such as statins and β-blockers, may improve contractility in a hibernating area.[105-108] In contrast, agents like dobutamine and milrinone, especially at high doses, may precipitate myocardial necrosis and are associated with worse long-term outcomes in patients with CAD and HF.[109-112] Hibernating myocardium is associated with global alterations in LV volume and shape, not just impairment of underperfused segments.[99] This explains why myocardial revascularization of hibernating territories can promote reverse remodeling globally.[113]

Endothelial Dysfunction (see Chapter 17)

Available data suggest that the coronary endothelium plays an important role not only in the control of blood flow and vascular patency but also in the physiological modulation of myocardial structure and function.[114] Thus endothelial dysfunction, an inherent component of the pathophysiology of atherosclerotic CAD, may directly affect ventricular function.[115]

According to Bell and associates,[116] the coronary endothelium has numerous physiological roles including:

- Regulation of vascular tone through the release of mediators such as nitric oxide (NO), prostacyclin, and endothelin
- Maintenance of a permeable barrier to provide for exchange and active transport of substances into the artery wall
- Synthesis and secretion of cytokines and growth factors
- Alterations of lipoproteins in the arterial wall
- Provision of a nonthrombogenic surface and a nonadherence surface for leukocytes
- Maintenance of basement membrane collagen proteoglycans[117]

Endothelial Vasodilators

The endothelial release of NO relaxes vascular smooth muscle cells in association with activation of guanyl cyclase and increased levels of cyclic glucose monophosphate. NO is the most potent endogenous vasodilator and is responsible for the maintenance of vasovascular tone. NO also inhibits smooth muscle cell proliferation and migration, leukocyte adhesion, and platelet aggregation.[118,119]

Endothelial Vasoconstrictors

The major endothelin-derived vasoconstrictive substances include angiotensin-II and endothelin. Angiotensin-II is a potent vasoconstrictor that also exerts a variety of effects on vascular structure and function.[120] Studies of angiotensin II indicate the involvement of the renin-angiotensin system in many aspects of vascular homeostasis. Angiotensin II increases the production of plasminogen activator inhibitor type 1, the primary endogenous inhibitor of tissue plasminogen activator, and promotes vascular growth in addition to stimulating the production of other growth factors.[121] Angiotensin II also enhances platelet aggregation, sensitizes the platelets to the effects of direct platelet agonists, and stimulates the production of endothelin.[122] Endothelin is the most potent endogenous vasoconstrictor yet identified and promotes proliferation of smooth muscle cells and secretion of extracellular matrix, which contribute to the formation of atherosclerotic plaque.[123]

Disordered endothelial function in patients with CAD stimulates vasoconstriction, smooth muscle migration and proliferation, increased lipid deposition in the vessel wall, and possibly coronary thrombosis. This promotes myocardial ischemia, which may further contribute directly or indirectly to progression of LV dysfunction.[115,124-126] The release of endothelin is also increased in failing myocardium.[127] Angiotensin II contributes to the release of endothelin and the excessive degradation of nitric oxide.[125] Taken together, these observations make a case for an interplay between the failing myocardium and the coronary endothelium that potentiates the progression of both CAD and LV dysfunction.

Properties of the normal endothelium serve to relax vascular tone, and inhibit smooth muscle growth, platelet aggregation, and leukocyte adhesion. Many drugs that reduce mortality and reinfarction in patients with CAD have the potential to improve endothelial function, including lipid lowering agents, ACE inhibitors, nonselective β-blockers, and aspirin.[128-131] For example, marked reduction of serum cholesterol is associated with a rapid recovery of endothelial function, improvement of myocardial perfusion, and reduction of myocardial ischemia.[132-138] An improvement in tissue perfusion is an important goal in patients with HF in terms of both the peripheral and the coronary circulation.

In summary, endothelial dysfunction may further reduce blood flow, promote progression of coronary atherosclerosis, and have direct negative effects on the myocardial cells and the interstitium.[139,140]

Clinical Manifestations

Reinfarction. Patients with HF and CAD are at increased risk for reinfarction. An analysis of the SOLVD trial found that patients who experienced MI had an approximately two-fold higher rate of hospitalization for HF and about a four-fold increase in death compared with patients who did not experience MI.[141] Similarly, an analysis of the Survival and Ventricular Enlargement (SAVE) trial found that patients with evidence of a previous MI before enrollment were at significantly greater risk for cardiovascular death, LV enlargement, or both.[142] In clinical trials, the rate of infarction or reinfarction is relatively low, with a fatal MI rate of 3%.[143] However, in one study, more than half of patients with HF and CAD who died suddenly had autopsy evidence of an acute ischemic event (e.g., coronary clot, recent infarct),[40] suggesting that the number of patients with plaque rupture is not accounted for in clinical trials.

Sudden Cardiac Death. The risk of SCD after MI has significantly declined in recent years.[144] However, the occurrence of HF post-MI is associated with a markedly increased risk of SCD.[144] In several clinical HF trials, SCD accounted for 20% to 60% of deaths, depending on the severity of HF.[145] In the Metoprolol CR/XL Randomised Intervention Trial in Congestive Heart Failure (MERIT-HF), 64% of patients in NYHA class II who subsequently died had SCD compared with 59% of patients in class III and 33% of patients in class IV.[146] Several factors have been implicated in the high rate of SCD in patients with HF. These include subendocardial ischemia, ventricular hypertrophy, stretching of myocytes, a high sympathetic tone, abnormal baroreceptor responsiveness

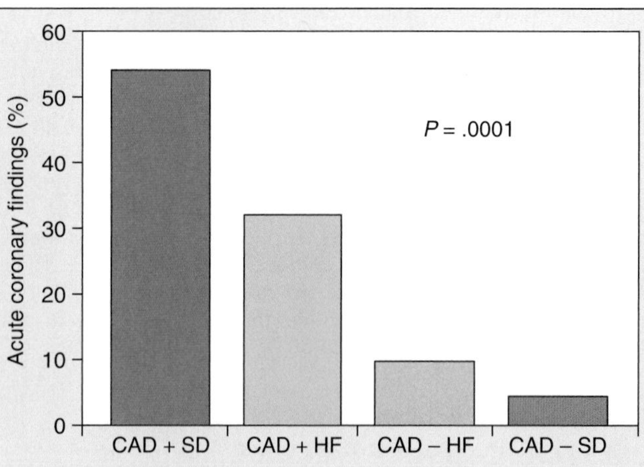

FIGURE 23–6 Relation of acute coronary findings to mode of death and presence of coronary artery disease in the ATLAS trial. Patients with SCD had the highest prevalence of acute coronary findings. (Key: + Indicates presence of CAD; –, absence of). (From Uretsky BF, Thygesen K, Armstrong PW, et al. Acute coronary findings at autopsy in heart failure patients with sudden death: results from the assessment of treatment with lisinopril and survival (ATLAS) trial. *Circulation* 2000;102:611-616.)

lowering the threshold for a malignant arrhythmia, potassium and magnesium depletion, and coronary artery emboli from atrial or LV thrombi.[145] However, CAD probably contributes directly to SCD.[145] Patients with CAD and systolic HF have dilated hearts, large regions of myocardial scar, and obstructive epicardial coronary stenoses. CAD and its major structural consequences (i.e., plaque rupture, thrombosis, and infarction) constitute the most common structural basis of SCD.[147,148]

Uretsky et al reported the relative importance of an acute coronary event as a trigger for SCD in patients with HF who were studied in the Assessment of Treatment with Lisinopril and Survival (ATLAS) trial, which included 3164 patients with moderate to severe systolic HF.[40] There were 1383 deaths (43.7%) during the follow-up period of 3 to 5 years. An autopsy was performed in only 188 patients, and the postmortem data were available in only 171 patients (12.4% of the total patients who died). Patients who died in this study were older and had both more symptoms and a higher prevalence of CAD than the surviving patients. The patients who died and did not undergo autopsy were similar to those who died and were subjected to autopsy. Acute coronary findings were observed in 54% of the patients with significant CAD who died suddenly (Figure 23-6). The ATLAS study was the first to demonstrate that recent coronary events are frequently unrecognized in patients with moderate to advanced HF symptoms who die suddenly, especially in patients with CAD.

Other studies have documented a high frequency of plaque rupture or coronary thrombosis in patients with CAD who suffered SCD.[147,149] However, it should be noted that these studies reported a much higher incidence of ruptured plaque, ranging from 57% to 81%, than the ATLAS autopsy study.[40,147,149] However, the prevalence of clinical acute coronary findings in the same series ranged from 21% to 41%, which was similar to the ATLAS study.[40] Because the autopsy findings reported in ATLAS were based on routine clinical examinations, it is unlikely that the examinations involved the degree of detail necessary to observe ruptured plaque and small thrombi. Therefore, it is possible that the rate of acute coronary events may have been even higher than reported. This study underlines the importance of strategies to prevent and treat acute coronary events to successfully prevent SCD in patients with HF. For example, in the ATLAS trial, two thirds of patients had CAD but only 40% of this group was taking aspirin.[40]

Among patients with HF who receive an ICD for the primary prevention of SCD, those who receive shocks have a markedly increased short-term risk of death compared with those who do not receive shocks. This risk may be much higher in patients with CAD.[150,151] A recent analysis of the Sudden Cardiac Death in Heart Failure Trial (SCD-HeFT) revealed that patients with HF due to CAD who received an appropriate ICD shock had a threefold increased risk of mortality compared with patients with HF and a nonischemic cause who received an appropriate ICD shock. This suggests that among patients with HF, those with CAD can develop fundamental alterations in the underlying arrhythmic substrate that predisposes them to SCD.

CORONARY ARTERY DISEASE AND DIASTOLIC HEART FAILURE

The vast majority of HF trials conducted over the past 30 years have studied patients with LVSD. However, HF with relatively preserved systolic function is present in approximately half of all patients hospitalized with HF.[152-159] Among patients with HF and preserved systolic function, approximately 60% have documented CAD.[156] Over the past two decades, the relative proportion of patients with HF and preserved systolic function has risen steadily relative to those with LVSD.[153] Patients with HF and preserved systolic function tend to be older than those with HF and LVSD. Thus the relative rise in this category of HF is reflective of an aging population. This rise has also corresponded to increased rates of CAD, hypertension, diabetes, and atrial fibrillation in this population. Among patients hospitalized with HF, the early and long-term risk of death is similar for patients with preserved systolic function and LVSD.[154,157-159] However, patients with HF and preserved systolic function are more likely to die from other cardiac comorbidities, including CAD, rather than progressive HF when compared with patients with HF and LVSD.[160,161]

When systolic function is preserved, it is assumed that the majority of these patients have HF signs and symptoms on the basis of abnormal LV diastolic function.[162] A variety of factors predispose to abnormalities in diastolic functional behavior of the left ventricle and lead to elevating filling pressures, impaired forward output, or both, despite normal systolic function.[163] Myocardial ischemia is one of the leading factors. Pulmonary congestion can be caused by reversible episodes of ischemia, which impair LV relaxation and impair LV filling pressure.[164]

The prognosis in patients with HF and preserved systolic function in the presence of CAD may be directly related to the angiographic burden of CAD. O'Connor et al demonstrated that patients with HF and preserved systolic function have a worse 5-year survival if they have left main or 3-vessel CAD versus those with 1- to 2-vessel CAD.[42] Similarly, according to the Coronary Artery Surgery Study (CASS) registry, the 6-year survival rate of patients with normal ejection fraction and HF symptoms was 92% in patients with no CAD, 83% in patients with 1- or 2-vessel CAD, and 68% in patients with 3-vessel disease.[165]

There is a need for reappraisal on whether systolic function is truly normal at the time when HF symptoms are present in patients diagnosed with HF and "normal" systolic function. The majority of studies of this syndrome did not report the timing of the evaluation demonstrating normal systolic function relative to the episodes of HF itself.[166] In other studies, the evaluation was performed days to weeks after the episode.[167] Transient ischemia may cause regional systolic dysfunction, which in many patients was severe and extensive enough to cause a brief but profound reduction in global LV function.[167] The pathophysiological changes in regional and global systolic function form the basis for exercise radionuclide ventriculography and exercise echocardiography as diagnostic tests for myocardial ischemia due to CAD. It may be that many patients with apparently normal systolic function and HF caused by CAD do not have isolated diastolic dysfunction but instead have transient systolic and diastolic dysfunction at the time when myocardial ischemia induces HF symptoms.

DIABETES, HEART FAILURE, AND CAD (see also Chapter 24)

In terms of cardiovascular risk, a diagnosis of diabetes is comparable to a diagnosis of CAD.[168,169] The prevalence of documented CAD in diabetic patients has been shown to be as high as 55%, compared with 2% to 4% for the general population.[170] Diabetic patients with a history of MI have a markedly worse prognosis than individuals with only one of these conditions.[168,169] A significant number of patients with HF have diabetes: 23% in the CONSENSUS trial, 25% in SOLVD, 20% in V-HeFT, 20% in ATLAS, 27% in RESOLVD, 42% in the OPTIMIZE-HF registry, and 44% in the ADHERE registry.[9,11,40,171,172-174] Diabetes is an independent risk factor for the development of HF.[175-177] In the Framingham Heart Study, the relative risk for developing HF in diabetic patients was 3.8 for men and 5.5 for women, respectively, compared with nondiabetic patients.[177] The risk of developing HF in diabetic patients has been directly related to glycemic control.[178,179] In the United Kingdom Prospective Diabetic Study (UKPDS), for each 1% increase in glycosylated hemoglobin level, the risk of HF rose by 12%.[179]

The presence of diabetes in patients with HF is associated with substantially higher mortality rates.[180-189] Several studies suggest that the increased risk in diabetic patients with HF compared with nondiabetic patients with HF is limited to individuals with concomitant CAD.[186-189] Diabetic patients with CAD also have worse outcomes following myocardial revascularization.[190] Derangements associated with diabetes, including hyperglycemia, insulin resistance, dyslipidemia, inflammation, and thrombosis, contribute to the development of hypertension, endothelial cell dysfunction, accelerated atherogenesis, and coronary thrombosis.[190,191] In addition, diabetic patients exhibit more complex and diffuse anatomical patterns of CAD, including more lipid-rich plaques and intracoronary thrombi but less compensatory vascular remodeling.[190,192-194]

Diabetes directly contributes to HF in patients with LVSD, diastolic dysfunction, or both.[195,196] The increased mortality in patients with HF in the presence of diabetes has been observed in patients with either LVSD or preserved systolic function.[182] Ventricular dysfunction in patients with HF and diabetes has been termed "diabetic cardiomyopathy" and is the result of the complex interplay between the sympathetic nervous system and the renin-angiotensin-aldosterone system (RAAS), increased levels of circulation cytokines, alterations in heart rate variability, and increased oxidative stress.[197] Chronic hyperglycemia leads to the glycation of collagen and elevated serum levels of advanced glycation end products, which results in increased myocardial stiffness.[198] Pathologically this cardiomyopathy is characterized by myocyte atrophy, interstitial fibrosis, increased periodic acid–Schiff (PAS) positive material, intramyocardial microangiopathy, and depletion of myocardial catecholamines.[199] In diabetic patients with HF and LVSD, myocardial fibrosis and the deposition advanced glycation end products predominate, while in those with HF and preserved systolic function, increased cardiomyocyte resting tension is a more important mechanism.[196]

Therapeutic Options

Recognition that progression of CAD may contribute importantly to progression of HF, in at least a subset of patients, shifts the focus from medical management designed solely to reduce neurohormonal activation and alleviate congestive symptoms to a strategy designed to employ aggressive secondary prevention measures. Those efforts to slow the progression of CAD include attention to reducing the risk of acute coronary events by plaque stabilization, reducing ischemia, and enhancing endothelial function. It is noteworthy that the classes of drugs that have shown conclusively to improve survival in HF-ACE inhibitors, angiotensin receptor blockers (ARBs), β-blockers, and aldosterone antagonists, address those factors. The beneficial effects of these drugs may relate as much to their vascular protective effects as to their neurohormonal blocking effects. Patients hospitalized with HF are frequently undertreated for CAD. For example, ACS patients with acute HF are less likely to receive antiplatelet agents, β-blockers, ACE inhibitors, or statins than ACS patients without HF.[42,45,46,51,158] In addition to pharmacological therapy, myocardial revascularization, surgical therapy, and cardiac device therapy may play an important role in the treatment of patients with HF in the setting of CAD.

Immediate Management of the Hospitalized Patient

The immediate management of acute HF usually occurs in the emergency department.[200] There is considerable overlap in the presentation and management of acute HF patients with CAD and ACS versus CAD and non-ACS (Tables 23-2, *A*, and 23-2, *B*). In patients with underlying CAD who are not hypotensive, nitrates may provide a rapid reduction of myocardial ischemia and improve coronary perfusion. In patients with severe pulmonary edema, the combination of high-dose nitrates and low-dose diuretics (vs. low-dose nitrates and high-dose diuretics) led to significantly decreased rates of mechanical ventilation and MI.[201] A regimen for acute HF consisting of lower doses of diuretics has been proposed as a method of preserving renal function. In a large acute HF registry, the use of intravenous nitroglycerin or nesiritide was associated with lower in-hospital mortality compared with treatment with dobutamine or milrinone.[202] However, compared with intravenous nesiritide in acute HF patients, of whom greater than 60% had documented CAD, intravenous nitroglycerin has been associated with less deterioration of renal function and a trend toward less mortality at 30 days.[203-204]

Inotropes may be particularly harmful when used in HF patients with CAD. Experimentally, the use of dobutamine in a model of HF with hibernating myocardium led to increased myocardial necrosis.[205] Hospitalized HF patients with troponin elevation have significantly higher in-hospital mortality when inotropes are used.[49] In the Outcomes of a Prospective Trial of Intravenous Milrinone for Exacerbations of Chronic Heart Failure (OPTIME-CHF) trial, use of the phosphodiesterase inhibitor milrinone in patients with CAD was associated with increased postdischarge mortality compared with a placebo.[111] In general, a decrease in coronary perfusion as a result of a decrease in blood pressure and/or an increase in heart rate resulting from inotropes with vasodilator properties, or inotropes used in conjunction with vasodilators, may be particularly deleterious in HF patients with CAD.[112,206]

Long-term Therapies for the Heart Failure Patient with CAD

Renin-Angiotensin-Aldosterone System Modulators. The RAAS regulates sodium balance, fluid volume, and blood pressure, which has a profound impact on HF and CAD (see also Chapter 45).[207] The use of ACE inhibitors or ARBs is strongly indicated in HF patients with LVSD and is also indicated for the secondary prevention of cardiovascular events in all patients with CAD.[208-210]

Endothelial dysfunction plays a fundamental role in many forms of cardiovascular disease and is the final common pathway through which most cardiovascular risk factors contribute to inflammation and atherosclerosis. Angiotensin II is a powerful vasoconstrictor, and also stimulates smooth muscle cells (hyperplasia), fibroblast proliferation, collagen deposition, inflammation, and thrombosis. All these maladaptations can be mitigated by the use of ACE inhibitors or ARBs.[129,207,211] In the SOLVD and the SAVE trials, the ACE inhibitors enalapril and captopril not only reduced overall mortality in patients with CAD, but also reduced the rate of nonfatal MI and unstable angina.[141,212] In the SAVE trial, a 25% decrease in MI with captopril occurred despite the selection criteria, which excluded patients with residual ischemia who were considered at great risk of reinfarction.[212] The reduction of acute ischemic events would not have been anticipated only on the basis of the hemodynamic or neurohormonal effects of ACE inhibitors. Moreover, in the SOLVD trial, the reduction of unstable angina and MI with enalapril was not evident until more than 6 months after randomization.[141] This suggests that the beneficial effects of enalapril on ischemic events was not due to an immediate effect related to a primary or secondary reduction in LV afterload.

The addition of eplerenone, an aldosterone antagonist, to optimal medical therapy in ACS patients with acute HF and LVSD significantly reduced death and rehospitalization in the Eplerenone Post-Acute Myocardial Infarction Heart Failure Efficacy and Survival Study (EPHESUS) trial (Figure 23-7).[104] The reduction in death corresponded with a decrease in SCD, which may be due to the inhibition of myocardial fibrosis.[213] Recently, direct renin inhibitors have been added to the armamentarium of RAAS inhibition. These agents effectively suppress angiotensin II and aldosterone levels without the rebound increase in plasma renin activity seen with ACE inhibitors and ARB therapy.[214] Aliskiren, the first commercially available direct renin inhibitor for the treatment of hypertension, is being investigated for use in patients with HF and LVSD in the Aliskiren Trial on Acute Heart Failure Outcomes (ASTRONAUT).

β-Blockers. β-blockers are effective for the reduction of death and rehospitalization in patients with HF and CAD.[98] The continuation or predischarge initiation of β-blockers in patients hospitalized with HF is associated with improved medication adherence and an early survival advantage (see also Chapter 46).[215-217] Patients with viable but dysfunctional myocardium derive greater improvement in LV function and remodeling from β-blocker therapy than those without viability.[96,113]

The improvement in survival with β-blockers in the MERIT-HF and CIBIS II trials was more pronounced in patients with HF and documented CAD than in patients with a presumed nonischemic cause.[145,218] However, improvement in survival was slightly more pronounced in patients with presumed nonischemic HF and mild to moderate HF studied in the U.S. Carvedilol Trials and in patients with severe HF patients studied in the Carvedilol Prospective Randomized Cumulative Survival (COPERNICUS) Trial.[18,19] These differential effects were minor since the reduction in mortality in each of these four trials was less than 30% and there was a nonsignificant difference in mortality benefit between ischemic and nonischemic patients.[219] In MERIT-HF, mortality was slightly higher in diabetic patients with HF who were treated with metoprolol succinate than in nondiabetic patients with HF, while carvedilol showed similar reductions for diabetic and nondiabetic patients in both the U.S. Carvedilol Trials and COPERNICUS. The benefit of carvedilol in CAD patients was later confirmed in post-MI patients in the CAPRICORN study (Carvedilol Post-Infarct Survival Control in LV Dysfunction).[220] In 1959 patients with a LV ejection fraction of 40% or less (with or without HF symptoms) carvedilol, in addition to ACE inhibition and antiplatelet therapy, reduced the mortality and reinfarction rate by 29%; the risk reduction was similar for diabetic patients (Figure 23-8).[220] The differences observed with β-blockers in outcomes based on the presence

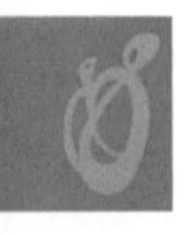

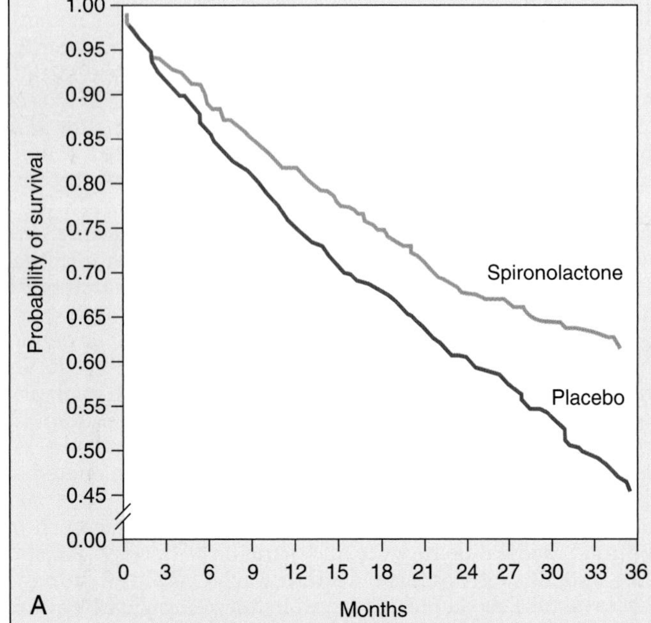

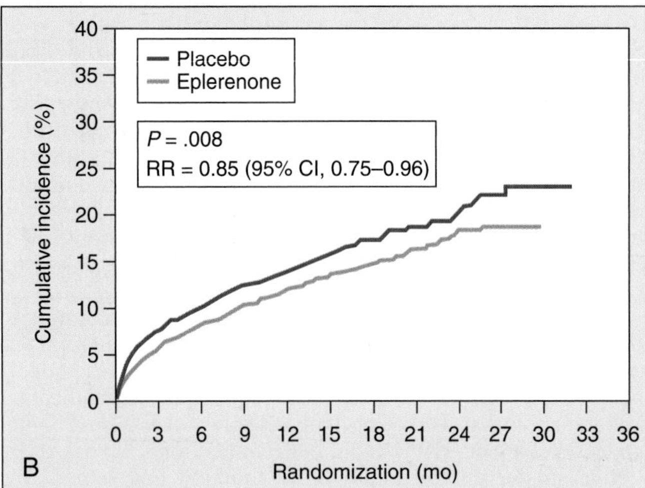

FIGURE 23–7 Trial using aldosterone antagonists. *EPHESUS,* Eplerenone Post-Acute Myocardial Infarction Heart Failure Efficacy and Survival Study; *RALES,* Randomized Aldactone Evaluation Study; *RR,* relative risk. (Modified from Pitt B, Zannad F, Remme WJ, et al. The effect of spironolactone on morbidity and mortality in patients with severe heart failure. Randomized aldactone evaluation study investigators. *N Engl J Med* 1999;341:709; and Pitt B, Remme W, Zannad F, et al. Eplerenone, a selective aldosterone blocker, in patients with left ventricular dysfunction after myocardial infarction. *N Engl J Med* 2003;348:1309.)

of CAD in HF patients may be due to cause-related differences in pathophysiological derangements on the β-adrenergic signal transduction pathway.[221] This may also relate to the more severe symptoms of patients enrolled in COPERNICUS, differences in β_1-selectivity versus β_1-nonselectivity, or other pharmacological differences between β-blocking agents, such as α-blockade, antioxidant effect, and lipophilicity.[222]

Lipid-lowering Agents. Statin therapy is strongly recommended in patients with CAD.[223] The benefits of statins may be due to plaque stabilization and improvements in endothelial function. The Cholesterol and Recurrent Events (CARE) trial, which demonstrated beneficial effects of pravastatin in patients with mild elevation of serum cholesterol after MI, prospectively randomized a subset of patients with an ejection fraction between 25% and 40%[224]; these patients had similar characteristics to those entered into post-MI ACE inhibitor trials, such as SAVE.[142] Pravastatin significantly

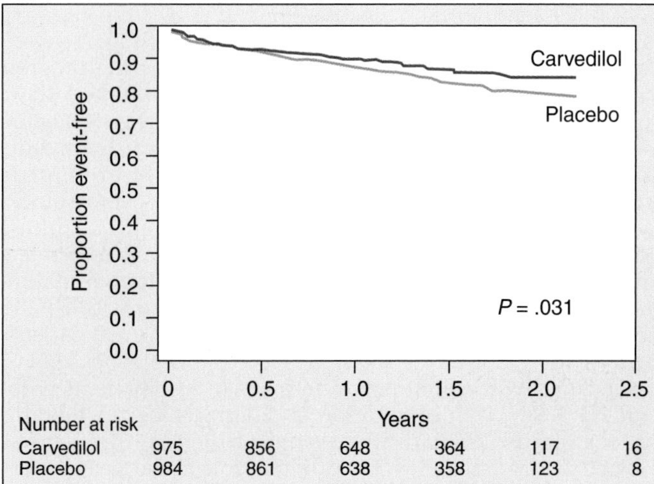

FIGURE 23–8 Effect of carvedilol on morbidity and mortality in patient with left ventricular dysfunction after acute myocardial infarction in the CAPRICORN study. (From Dargie HJ. Effect of carvedilol on outcome after myocardial infarction in patients with left-ventricular dysfunction: the CAPRICORN randomised trial. *Lancet* 2001;357:1385-1390).

decreased cardiac events in this subgroup. Similarly, in the Scandinavian Simvastatin Survival Study (4S), simvastatin decreased the development of HF symptoms after MI; among patients who experienced HF, simvastatin decreased mortality from 32% to 25%.[225] Furthermore, in patients with either stable CAD or ACS, the use of high-dose statin therapy is associated with a decreased risk for HF hospitalization compared with low-dose statin therapy.[226, 227]

In unselected HF patients, the use of statins is associated with lower mortality, including the elderly and patients with preserved systolic function.[228-230] However, the Controlled Rosuvastatin Multinational Trial in Heart Failure (CORONA) showed that rosuvastatin therapy in older patients (60 years or older of age) with chronic HF and LVSD did not lead to a decrease in all-cause death (Figure 23-9, *A*), although there was a reduction in HF hospitalizations.[231] There was also a trend toward fewer coronary events in the patients treated with rosuvastatin. In the Gruppo Italiano per lo Studio della Sopravvievenza nell'Insufficienza Cardiaca Heart Failure (GISSI-HF) trial, the use of rosuvastatin in patients with chronic HF (mean age 68 years, 90% with LVSD, 40% ischemic cause) did not decrease mortality or cardiovascular hospitalization at 4 years (Figure 23-9, *B*).[232] These data suggest that statin therapy may be important for the prevention of HF and ischemic events in patients with CAD, but may be unable to impact mortality in patients with chronic HF and LVSD.

Fish consumption and dietary supplementation with n-3 polyunsaturated fatty acids (PUFA), in individuals with and without established CAD, is associated with reduced cardiovascular mortality.[176,233,234] In a separate GISSI-HF trial, the use of n-3 PUFA in patients with chronic HF (mean age 67 years, 90% with LVSD, 50% ischemic cause) led to a 2% absolute risk reduction in mortality (27% vs. 29% at 4 years, $P = .041$) and a similar reduction in cardiovascular hospitalization.[235] It is suspected that n-3 PUFA may exert their beneficial effect via the reduction of arrhythmic events and not ischemic events. As the use of ICD therapy in this trial was low (7%), the impact of this therapy on patients with chronic HF and LVSD with appropriate indications for ICD therapy is unclear.

Antiplatelet and Anticoagulation Therapy. The use of antiplatelet therapy (i.e., aspirin or clopidogrel) is strongly indicated in the presence of CAD for the secondary prevention of cardiovascular events.[236] Dual antiplatelet therapy, clopidogrel added to aspirin, has been shown to be beneficial

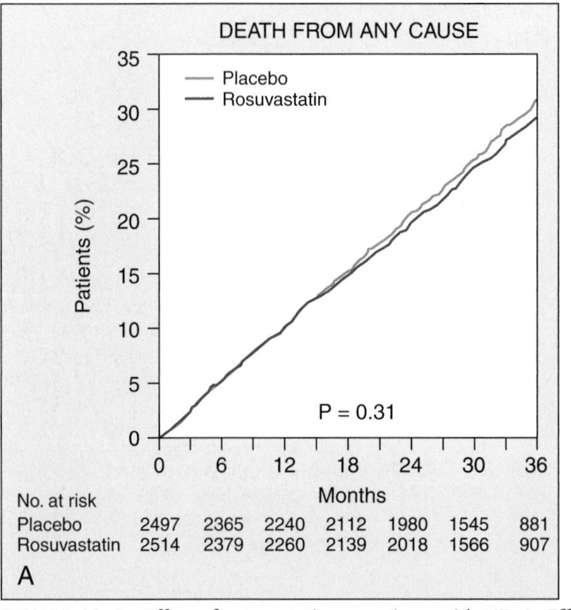

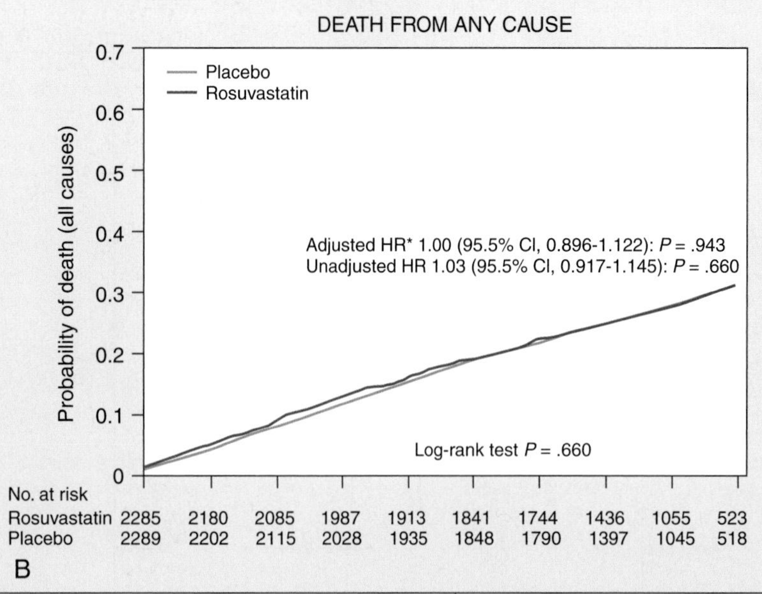

FIGURE 23–9 Effect of rosuvastatin on patients with HF. **A,** Effects of rosuvastatin on all-cause death in older patients (60 years of age) with chronic HF and LVSD in the CORONA study. **B,** Effects of rosuvastatin on all-cause death in patients with chronic HF with depressed and preserved systolic function in the GISSI-HF trial. (Modified from Kjekshus J, Apetrei E, Barrios V, et al. Rosuvastatin in older patients with systolic heart failure. *N Engl J Med* 2007;357:2248-2261; and GISSI-HF Investigators. Effect of rosuvastatin in patients with chronic heart failure. *Lancet* 2008;372:1231-1239.)

in ACS patients for the prevention of recurrent ischemic events and was associated with an 18% reduction in subsequent HF.[237] There is experimental evidence that aspirin inhibits the acute arterial and venous vasodilator response to ACE inhibitors in patients with chronic HF.[238] However, there is no prospective evidence that this potential interaction is clinically relevant. Nevertheless, it may be prudent to limit the combination of aspirin and ACE inhibitor therapy in HF patients to those with established CAD.

LVSD is independently associated with an increased risk of ischemic stroke.[239] The use of oral anticoagulation is strongly indicated in HF patients with atrial fibrillation and patients with confirmed or suspected LV thrombus. However, to date, there is a lack of evidence that the use oral anticoagulation in HF patients without atrial fibrillation has a beneficial effect on cardiovascular events, including embolic stroke.[240, 241]

Myocardial Revascularization. The role of surgical management of HF patients with stable coronary artery disease is not certain (see also Chapter 55). To date no randomized clinical trials have evaluated the outcomes of revascularization in patients with advanced ischemic cardiomyopathy. The three major randomized clinical trials that have compared coronary artery bypass graft surgery with medical management, the Veterans Administration Cooperative Study, the European Coronary Surgery Study, and the Coronary Artery Surgery Study, all excluded patients with heart failure or severe LVSD. In the absence of clinical trial data, registries and databases have been used to guide decision making for patients with ischemic cardiomyopathy. For example, a recent report from the Duke database compared coronary artery bypass graft (CABG) surgery versus medical therapy over a 25-year period. Medical therapy was used in 1052 patients and CABG in 339.[72] Unadjusted and adjusted survival (Cox proportional hazards model) strongly favored CABG after 30 days and at 10 years. This analysis included all groups by extent of coronary artery disease, and by different subgroups (Figure 23-10). Adjusted overall survival at 1 year, 5 years, and 10 years was 83% versus 74%; 61% versus 37%; 42% versus 13% for CABG versus medical therapy (all P <.0001).

Because the results of registries and databases have generally favored myocardial revascularization over medical therapy, no formal prospective randomized clinical trials of this therapy were initiated until 2002 when the National Institutes of Health initiated funding for the STICH (Surgical Treatment for Ischemic Heart Failure) trial. Patients who have suffered a large anterior MI often develop HF that may not improve with revascularization alone if this territory has a large transmural scar with LV aneurysm formation. In these patients, surgical LV restoration (with or without concomitant CABG) has been shown to improve LV systolic function and NYHA functional class. The STICH trial is a prospective randomized study that includes 2800 patients randomized from 100 centers. Patients with CAD and LVSD amenable to CABG were randomized to combinations of three different treatment strategies: CABG, surgical ventricular reconstruction (SVR), and intensive medical therapy. The trial is powered to address two primary hypotheses: (1) CABG combined with medical therapy improves long-term survival when compared with medical therapy alone; and (2) SVR provides an additional long-term survival benefit when combined with CABG and medical therapy. The results of the second arm of the study have been reported recently. SVR reduced the end-systolic volume index by 19%, as compared with a reduction of 6% with CABG alone. Cardiac symptoms and exercise tolerance improved from baseline to a similar degree in the two study groups. However, there was no significant difference in a composite of death from any cause and hospitalization for cardiac causes, which was the primary outcome of the trial (Figure 23-11). The results of the STICH trial may indicate that a stricter definition of what constitutes an LV aneurysm may need to be applied in future studies of SVR.[242]

Revascularization may improve outcomes in patients with HF and dysfunctional but viable myocardium. In a meta-analysis of greater than 3000 patients with LVSD, revascularization was associated with markedly decreased yearly mortality (3.2% vs. 16.0%, P <.0001) if viability was present.[101] In patients without hibernating myocardium, revascularization did not improve survival. A different retrospective observational study examined the role of myocardial revascularization in approximately 4000 patients with chronic HF.[243] At 1 year, patients who underwent revascularization had substantially reduced mortality (11.8% vs. 21.6%; HR 0.52; 95% CI, 0.47 to 0.58). The survival curves continued to diverge through 7 years of follow-up. Moreover, studies have

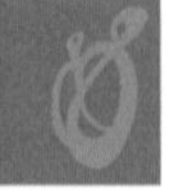

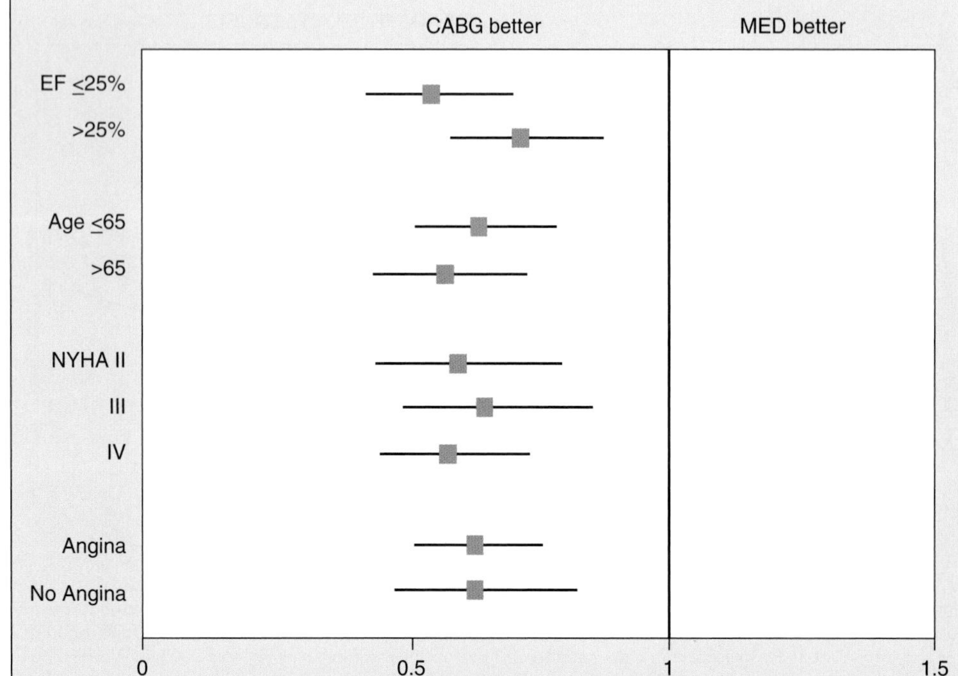

FIGURE 23–10 Subgroup analysis of coronary artery revascularization versus medical therapy in patients with heart failure. Hazard rations (95% confidence interval) for mortality for a number of baseline characteristics all favored CABG. *CABG,* coronary artery bypass grafting; *EF,* ejection fraction; *MED,* medical therapy; *NYHA,* New York Heart Association. (Modified from O'Connor CM, Velazquez EJ, Gardner LH, et al. Comparison of coronary artery bypass grafting versus medical therapy on long-term outcome in patients with ischemic cardiomyopathy: a 25-year experience from the Duke cardiovascular disease databank. *Am J Cardiol* 2002;90:101.)

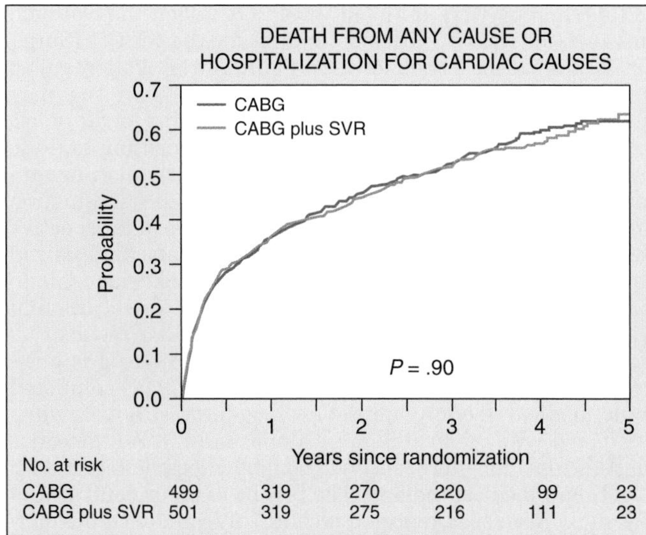

FIGURE 23–11 Effect of coronary artery bypass surgery with or without surgical ventricular reconstruction on all-cause death and hospitalization for cardiac causes in the STICH trial. (Modified from Jones RH, Velazquez EJ, Michler RE, et al. Coronary bypass surgery with or without surgical ventricular reconstruction. *N Engl J Med* 2009;360:1705-1717.)

shown that outcomes in patients with HF in the setting of an ACS are improved by a strategy of early myocardial revascularization.[244] This includes patients with and without ST-segment elevation and those in cardiogenic shock.[245] Despite this, patients with ACS complicated by HF are less likely to undergo revascularization than ACS patients without HF. [6,244] Non-ACS patients hospitalized with acute HF have improved early survival if they have a history of myocardial revascularization, although this a retrospective finding.[47,53] This relationship has been observed in acute HF patients with LVSD or preserved systolic function (see Figure 23-11). These data generate the hypothesis that early revascularization will be beneficial in acute HF patients with ischemia due to CAD. A management strategy for the acute HF failure based on the presence, extent, and severity of CAD could help identify appropriate candidates for optimal medical therapy for CAD and, when indicated, myocardial revascularization (Figure 23-12). The performance of in-hospital angiography in patients with acute HF and CAD is associated with an increased use of aspirin, statins, β-blockers, ACE inhibitors, and myocardial revascularization and improved postdischarge outcomes.[246]

Cardiac Device and Mitral Valve Therapy

Patients with HF and an LV ejection fraction of ≤35% should be strongly considered for ICD implantation.[247] In addition, the presence of electrical dyssynchrony (QRS complex >120 ms) and/or mechanical LV dyssynchrony (as assessed by echocardiographic techniques) is another important therapeutic target in a select group of HF patients with LVSD. The use of cardiac resynchronization therapy in these patients can improve symptoms and prolong survival.[248]

HF accompanied by mitral regurgitation is associated with worse outcomes, particularly among patients with moderate to severe regurgitation.[249] Advancements in surgical mitral valve repair techniques and the emergence of percutaneous mitral valve procedures to reduce mitral regurgitation are promising to play a role in the future management of HF patients.[250-255]

CONCLUSIONS

The progression of LV dysfunction, worsening of HF, and death in many patients with CAD may be related to the progressive nature of CAD, in addition to the neurohormonal mechanisms that exacerbates myocardial dysfunction. This progression does not require a discrete coronary event such as an acute MI. Myocardial ischemia or hibernation (or both) may contribute to symptoms of HF. In addition, myocardial hibernation appears to be an unstable process that may progress with time to myocyte loss, apoptosis, and replacement fibrosis, leading to more LV dysfunction. As previously noted, endothelial dysfunction may also lead to progression of myocardial dysfunction. Measures specifically targeting reduction in the risk of subacute ischemic events and improvement in

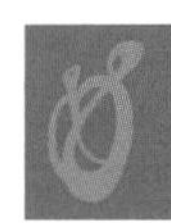

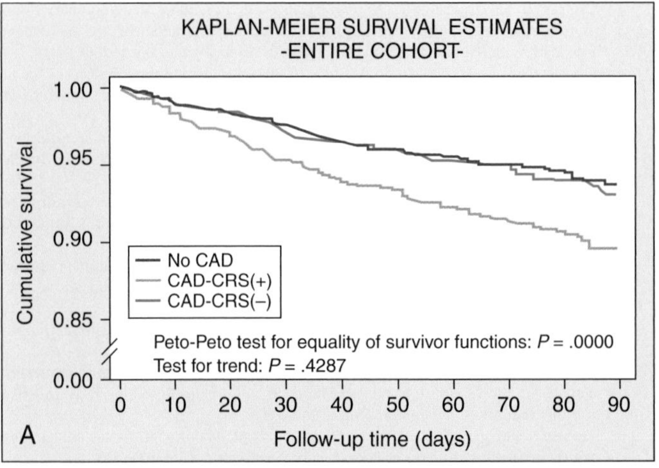

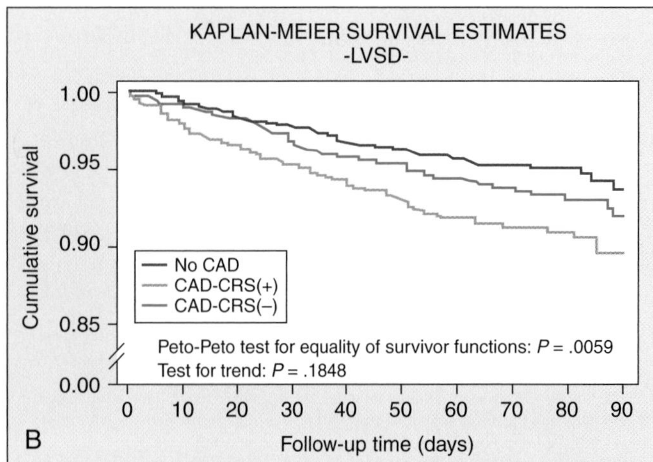

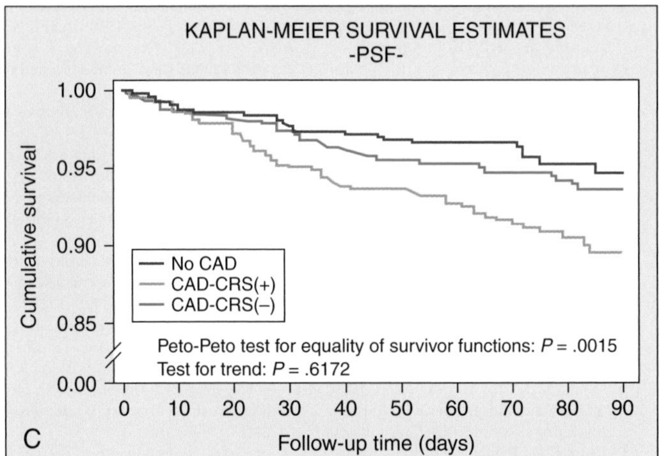

FIGURE 23–12 Impact of a history of myocardial revascularization on early postdischarge survival (60 to 90 days) in the Organized Program to Initiate Lifesaving Treatment in Hospitalized Patients with Heart Failure (OPTIMIZE-HF). Kaplan-Meier survival curves according to revascularization. **A,** Entire cohort. **B,** Patients with left ventricular systolic dysfunction (LVSD). *CRS,* Coronary Revascularization Status. **C,** Patients with preserved systolic function (PSF). (From Rossi JS, Flaherty JD, Fonarow GC, et al. Influence of coronary artery disease and coronary revascularization status on outcomes in patients with acute heart failure syndromes: a report from OPTIMIZE-HF. *Euro J Heart Fail* 2008;10:1215-1223.)

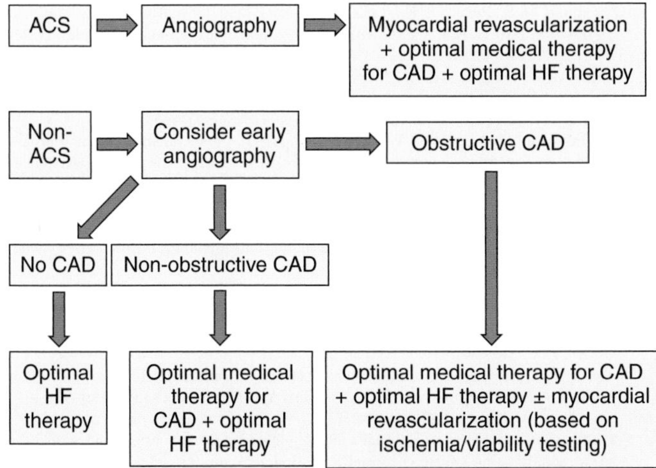

FIGURE 23–13 A proposed algorithm for the management of acute heart failure patients on the basis of presence, extent, and severity of CAD. *For those patients with remote or no history of coronary angiography. *ACS,* acute coronary syndrome; *CAD,* coronary artery disease; *HF,* heart failure. (From Flaherty JD, Bax JJ, De Luca L, et al. Acute heart failure syndromes in patients with coronary artery disease: early assessment and treatment. *J Am Coll Cardiol* 2009;53:254-263.)

endothelial function may be important in blunting the progression of HF and in improving prognosis. If mortality from HF is to be reduced, CAD must be recognized as a leading cause of HF in the United States. Although some patients may be candidates for myocardial revascularization or surgical and device therapy to improve LV function, all patients are candidates for aggressive secondary prevention strategies designed to reduce progression of CAD.

REFERENCES

1. Jessup, M., Abraham, W. T., Casey, D. E., et al. (2009). 2009 focused update: ACC/AHF guidelines for the diagnosis and management of heart failure in adults: a report of the American College of Cardiology/American Heart Association task force on practice guidelines. *Circulation, 119*, 1977–2016.
2. Ho, K. K., Pinsky, J. L., Kannel, W. B., et al. (1993). The epidemiology of heart failure: the Framingham study. *J Am Coll Cardiol, 22*, 6A–13A.
3. Levy, D., Vasan, R. S., Benjamin, E. J., et al. (2000). Temporal trends in heart failure risk factors from 1950-1998. *Circulation, 102*(suppl 2), II-780 (abstract).
4. Moss, A. J., Zareba, W., Hall, W. J., et al. (2002). Prophylactic implantation of a defibrillator in patients with myocardial infarction and reduced ejection fraction. *N Engl J Med, 346*, 877–883.
5. Exner, D. V., Klein, G. J., & Prystowsky, E. N. (2001). Primary prevention of sudden death with implantable defibrillator therapy in patients with cardiac disease: can we afford to do it? (Can we afford not to?). *Circulation, 104*, 1564–1570.
6. Torabi, A., Cleland, J. G. F., Khan, N. K., et al. (2008). The timing of development and subsequent clinical course of heart failure after a myocardial infarction. *Eur Heart J, 29*, 859–870.
7. Bourassa, M. G., Gurne, O., Bangdiwala, S. I., et al. (1993). Natural history and patterns of current practice in heart failure. The studies of left ventricular dysfunction (SOLVD) investigators. *J Am Coll Cardiol, 22*, 14A–19A.

8. Cohn, J. N., Archibald, D. G., Ziesche, S., et al. (1986). Effect of vasodilator therapy on mortality in chronic congestive heart failure. Results of a Veterans Administration cooperative study. *N Engl J Med*, *314*, 1547–1552.
9. The CONSENSUS Trial Study Group. (1987). Effects of enalapril on mortality in severe congestive heart failure. Results of the cooperative North Scandinavian enalapril survival study (CONSENSUS). *N Engl J Med*, *316*, 1429–1435.
10. DiBianco, R., Shabetai, R., Kostuk, W., et al. (1989). A comparison of oral milrinone, digoxin, and their combination in the treatment of patients with chronic heart failure. *N Engl J Med*, *320*, 677–683.
11. The SOLVD Investigators. (1991). Effect of enalapril on survival in patients with reduced left ventricular ejection fractions and congestive heart failure. *N Engl J Med*, *325*, 293–302.
12. Cohn, J. N., Johnson, G., Ziesche, S., et al. (1991). A comparison of enalapril with hydralazine-isosorbide dinitrate in the treatment of chronic congestive heart failure. *N Engl J Med*, *325*, 303–310.
13. Packer, M., Carver, J. R., Rodeheffer, R. J., et al. (1991). Effect of oral milrinone on mortality in severe chronic heart failure. The PROMISE study research group. *N Engl J Med*, *325*, 1468–1475.
14. The Studies of Left Ventricular Dysfunction Investigators. (1992). Effect of enalapril on mortality and the development of heart failure in asymptomatic patients with reduced left ventricular ejection fractions. *N Engl J Med*, *327*, 685–691.
15. Packer, M., Gheorghiade, M., Young, J. B., et al. (1993). Withdrawal of digoxin from patients with chronic heart failure treated with angiotensin-converting-enzyme inhibitors. RADIANCE study. *N Engl J Med*, *329*, 1–7.
16. Feldman, A. M., Bristow, M. R., Parmley, W. W., et al. (1993). Effects of vesnarinone on morbidity and mortality in patients with heart failure. Vesnarinone study group. *N Engl J Med*, *329*, 149–155.
17. Singh, S. N., Fletcher, R. D., Fisher, S. G., et al. (1995). Amiodarone in patients with congestive heart failure and asymptomatic ventricular arrhythmia. Survival trial of antiarrhythmic therapy in congestive heart failure. *N Engl J Med*, *333*, 77–82.
18. Packer, M., Bristow, M. R., Cohn, J. N., et al. (1996). The effect of carvedilol on morbidity and mortality in patients with chronic heart failure. U.S. carvedilol heart failure study group. *N Engl J Med*, *334*, 1349–1355.
19. Packer, M., O'Connor, C. M., Ghali, J. K., et al. (1996). Effect of amlodipine on morbidity and mortality in severe chronic heart failure. Prospective randomized amlodipine survival evaluation study group. *N Engl J Med*, *335*, 1107–1114.
20. The Digitalis Investigation Group. (1997). The effect of digoxin on mortality and morbidity in patients with heart failure. *N Engl J Med*, *336*, 525–533.
21. Cohn, J. N., Goldstein, S. O., Greenberg, B. H., et al. (1998). A dose-dependent increase in mortality with vesnarinone among patients with severe heart failure. Vesnarinone trial investigators. *N Engl J Med*, *339*, 1810–1816.
22. Pitt, B., Zannad, F., Remme, W. J., et al. (1999). The effect of spironolactone on morbidity and mortality in patients with severe heart failure. Randomized aldactone evaluation study investigators. *N Engl J Med*, *341*, 709–717.
23. Torp-Pedersen, C., Moller, M., Bloch-Thomsen, P. E., et al. (1999). Dofetilide in patients with congestive heart failure and left ventricular dysfunction. Danish investigations of arrhythmia and mortality on dofetilide study group. *N Engl J Med*, *341*, 857–865.
24. Colucci, W. S., Elkayam, U., Horton, D. P., et al. (2000). Intravenous nesiritide, a natriuretic peptide, in the treatment of decompensated congestive heart failure. Nesiritide study group. *N Engl J Med*, *343*, 246–253.
25. Packer, M., Coats, A. J., Fowler, M. B., et al. (2001). Effect of carvedilol on survival in severe chronic heart failure. *N Engl J Med*, *344*, 1651–1658.
26. The Beta-Blocker Evaluation of Survival Trial Investigators. (2001). A trial of the beta-blocker bucindolol in patients with advanced chronic heart failure. *N Engl J Med*, *344*, 1659–1667.
27. Cohn, J. N., & Gianni, Tognoni (2001). A randomized trial of the angiotensin-receptor blocker valsartan in chronic heart failure. *N Engl J Med*, *345*, 1667–1675.
28. Abraham, W. T., Fisher, W. G., Smith, A. L., et al. (2002). Cardiac resynchronization in chronic heart failure. *N Engl J Med*, *346*, 1845–1853.
29. Bristow, M. R., Saxon, L. A., Boehmer, J., et al. (2004). Cardiac resynchronization therapy with or without an implantable defibrillator in advanced chronic heart failure. *N Engl J Med*, *350*, 2140–2150.
30. Bardy, G. H., Lee, K. L., Mark, D. B., et al. (2005). Amiodarone or an implantable cardioverter-defibrillator for congestive heart failure. *N Engl J Med*, *352*, 225–237.
31. Cleland, J. G. F., Daubert, J. C., Erdmann, E., et al. (2005). The effect of cardiac resynchronization on morbidity and mortality in heart failure. *N Engl J Med*, *352*, 1539–1549.
32. Beshai, J. F., Grimm, R. A., Nagueh, S. F., et al. (2007). Cardiac-resynchronization therapy in heart failure with narrow QRS complexes. *N Engl J Med*, *357*, 2461–2471.
33. Køber, L., Torp-Petersen, C., McMurray, J. J. V., et al. (2008). Increased mortality after dronedarone therapy for severe heart failure. *N Engl J Med*, *358*, 2678–2687.
34. Fox, K. F., Cowie, M. R., Wood, D. A., et al. (2001). Coronary artery disease as the cause of incident heart failure in the population. *Eur Heart J*, *22*, 228–236.
35. Fonarow, G. C., Abraham, W. T., Albert, N. M., et al. (2008). Factors identified as precipitating hospital admissions for heart failure and clinical outcomes: findings from OPTIMIZE-HF. *Arch Intern Med*, *168*, 847–854.
36. Follath, F., Cleland, J. G., Klein, W., et al. (1998). Etiology and response to drug treatment in heart failure. *J Am Coll Cardiol*, *32*, 1167–1172.
37. Felker, G. M., Shaw, L. K., & O'Connor, C. M. (2002). A standardized definition of ischemic cardiomyopathy for use in clinical research. *Circulation*, *39*, 210–208.
38. Bart, B. A., Shaw, L. K., McCants, B. S. C. B., Jr., et al. (1997). Clinical determinants of mortality in patients with angiographically diagnosed ischemic or nonischemic cardiomyopathy. *J Am Coll Cardiol*, *30*, 1002–1008.
39. O'Connor, C. M., Gatis, W. A., Shaw, L., et al. (2000). Clinical characteristics and long-term outcomes of patients with heart failure and preserved systolic function. *Am J Cardiol*, *86*, 863–867.
40. Uretsky, B. F., Thygesen, K., Armstrong, P. W., et al. (2000). Acute coronary findings at autopsy in heart failure patients with sudden death: results from the assessment of treatment with lisinopril and survival (ATLAS) trial. *Circulation*, *102*, 611–616.
41. Orn, S., Cleland, J. G. F., Romo, M., et al. (2005). Recurrent infarction causes the most deaths following myocardial infarction with left ventricular dysfunction. *Am J Med*, *118*, 752–758.
42. Cleland, J. G. F., Thygesen, K., Uretsky, B. F., et al. (2001). Cardiovascular critical event pathways for the progression of heart failure; a report from the ATLAS study. *Eur Heart J*, *22*, 1601–1612.
43. Flaherty, J. D., Bax, J. J., De Luca, L., et al. (2009). Acute heart failure syndromes in patients with coronary artery disease: early assessment and treatment. *J Am Coll Cardiol*, *53*, 254–263.
44. Horwich, T. B., Patel, J., MacLellan, W. R., et al. (2003). Cardiac troponin I is associated with impaired hemodynamics, progressive left ventricular dysfunction, and increased mortality rates in advanced heart failure. *Circulation*, *108*, 833–838.
45. You, J. J., Austin, P. C., Alter, D. A., et al. (2007). Relation between cardiac troponin I and mortality in acute decompensated heart failure. *Am Heart J*, *153*, 462–470.
46. Metra, M., Nodari, S., Parrinello, G., et al. (2007). The role of plasma biomarkers in acute heart failure: serial changes and independent prognostic value of NT-proBNP and cardiac troponin-T. *Eur J Heart Fail*, *9*, 776–786.
47. Tavazzi, L., Maggioni, A. P., Lucci, D., et al. (2006). Nationwide survey on acute heart failure in cardiology ward services in Italy. *Eur Heart J*, *27*, 1207–1215.
48. Gheorghiade, M., Gattis Stough, W., Adams, K. F., Jr., et al. (2005). The Pilot Randomized Study of nesiritide versus dobutamine in heart failure (PRESERVD-HF). *Am J Cardiol*, *96*, 18G–25G.
49. Peacock, W. F., De Marco, T., Fonarow, G. C., et al. (2008). Cardiac troponin and outcome in acute heart failure. *N Engl J Med*, *358*, 2117–2126.
50. Beohar, N., Erdogan, A. K., Lee, D. C., et al. (2008). Acute heart failure syndromes and coronary perfusion. *J Am Coll Cardiol*, *52*, 13–16.
51. Gheorghiade, M., Zannad, F., Sopko, G., et al. (2005). Acute heart failure syndromes: current state and framework for future research. *Circulation*, *112*, 3958–3968.
52. Gheorghiade, M., Abraham, W. T., Albert, N. M., et al. (2006). Systolic blood pressure at admission, clinical characteristics, and outcomes in patients hospitalized with acute heart failure. *JAMA*, *296*, 2217–2226.
53. Rossi, J. S., Flaherty, J. D., Fonarow, G. C., et al. (2008). Influence of coronary artery disease and coronary revascularization status on outcomes in patients with acute heart failure syndromes: a report from OPTIMIZE-HF. *Eur J Heart Fail*, *10*, 1215–1223.
54. Roe, M. T., Chen, A. Y., Riba, A. L., et al. (2006). Impact of congestive heart failure in patients with non-ST-segment elevation acute coronary syndromes. *Am J Cardiol*, *97*, 1707–1712.
55. Khot, U. N., Jia, G., Moliterno, D. J., et al. (2003). Prognostic importance of physical examination for heart failure in non-ST-elevation acute coronary syndromes: the enduring value of Killip classification. *JAMA*, *290*, 2174–2181.
56. Steg, P. G., Dabbous, O. H., Feldman, L. J., et al. (2004). Determinants and prognostic impact of heart failure complicating acute coronary syndromes: observations from the Global Registry of Acute Coronary Events (GRACE). *Circulation*, *109*, 494–499.
57. Di Chiara, A., Fresco, C., Savonitto, S., et al. (2006). Epidemiology of non-ST elevation acute coronary syndromes in the Italian cardiology network: the BLITZ-2 study. *Eur Heart J*, *27*, 393–405.
58. Shibata, M. C., Collinson, J., Taneja, A. K., et al. (2006). Long term prognosis of heart failure after acute coronary syndromes without ST elevation. *Postgrad Med J*, *82*, 55–59.
59. Spencer, F. A., Meyer, T. E., Gore, J. M., et al. (2002). Heterogeneity in the management and outcomes of patients with acute myocardial infarction complicated by heart failure: the National Registry of Myocardial Infarction. *Circulation*, *105*, 2605–2610.
60. Nieminen, M. S., Brutsaert, K., Dickstein, K., et al. (2006). EuroHeart failure survey II: a survey on hospitalized acute heart failure patients: description of population. *Eur Heart J*, *27*, 2725–2736.
61. Gattis, W. A., O'Connor, C. M., Hasselblad, V., et al. (2004). Usefulness of an elevated troponin-I in predicting clinical events in patients for acute heart failure and acute coronary syndrome (from the RITZ-4 trial). *Am J Cardiol*, *93*, 1436–1437.
62. Emanuelsson, H., Karlson, B. W., & Herlitz, J. (1994). Characteristics and prognosis of patients with acute myocardial infarction in relation to occurrence of congestive heart failure. *Eur Heart J*, *15*, 761–768.
63. O'Connor, C. M., Hathaway, W. R., Bates, E. R., et al. (1997). Clinical characteristics and long-term outcome of patients in whom congestive heart failure develops after thrombolytic therapy for acute myocardial infarction: development of a predictive model. *Am Heart J*, *133*, 663–673.
64. Hasdai, D., Topol, E. J., Kilaru, R., et al. (2003). Frequency, patient characteristics, and outcomes of mild-to-moderate heart failure complicating ST-segment elevation acute myocardial infarction: lessons from 4 international fibrinolytic therapy trials. *Am Heart J*, *145*, 73–79.
65. Ali, A. S., Rybicki, B. A., Alam, M., et al. (1999). Clinical predictors of heart failure in patients with first acute myocardial infarction. *Am Heart J*, *138*, 1133–1139.
66. Spencer, F. A., Meyer, T. E., Goldberg, R. J., et al. (1999). Twenty year trends (1975-1995) in the incidence, in-hospital and long-term death rates associated with heart failure complicating acute myocardial infarction: a community-wide perspective. *J Am Coll Cardiol*, *34*, 1378–1387.
67. Wu, A. H., Parsons, L., Every, N. R., et al. (2002). Hospital outcomes in patients presenting with congestive heart failure complicating acute myocardial infarction: a report from the Second National Registry of Myocardial Infarction (NRMI-2). *J Am Coll Cardiol*, *40*, 1389–1394.
68. Segev, A., Strauss, B. H., Tan, M., et al. (2006). Prognostic significance of admission heart failure in patients with non-ST-elevation acute coronary syndromes. *Am J Cardiol*, *98*, 470–473.
69. Haim, M., Battler, A., Behar, S., et al. (2004). Acute coronary syndromes complicated by symptomatic and asymptomatic heart failure: does current treatment comply with guidelines? *Am Heart J*, *147*, 859–864.

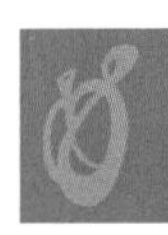

70. St. John Sutton, M. G., & Sharpe, N. (2000). Left ventricular remodeling after myocardial infarction: pathophysiology and therapy. *Circulation, 101*, 2981–2988.
71. Sanchez, J. A., & Mentzer, R. M., Jr. (1998). Coronary revascularization in patients with chronic heart failure. *Coron Artery Dis, 9*, 685–689.
72. O'Connor, C. M., Velazquez, E. J., Gardner, L. H., et al. (2002). Comparison of coronary artery bypass grafting versus medical therapy on long-term outcome in patients with ischemic cardiomyopathy (a 25-year experience from the Duke cardiovascular disease databank). *Am J Cardiol, 90*, 101–107.
73. Challapalli, S., Bonow, R. O., & Gheorghiade, M. (1998). Medical management of heart failure secondary to coronary artery disease. *Coron Artery Dis, 9*, 659–674.
74. Ragosta, M., & Beller, G. A. (1998). The assessment of patients with congestive heart failure as a manifestation of coronary artery disease. *Coron Artery Dis, 9*, 645–651.
75. Goldstein, J. A., Demetriou, D., Grines, C. L., et al. (2000). Multiple complex coronary plaques in patients with acute myocardial infarction. *N Engl J Med, 343*, 915–922.
76. Gheorghiade, M., & Bonow, R. O. (1998). Chronic heart failure in the United States: a manifestation of coronary artery disease. *Circulation, 97*, 282–289.
77. Mann, D. L. (1999). Mechanisms and models in heart failure: a combinatorial approach. *Circulation, 100*, 999–1008.
78. Lameris, T. W., de Zeeuw, S., Alberts, G., et al. (2000). Time course and mechanism of myocardial catecholamine release during transient ischemia in vivo. *Circulation, 101*, 2645–2650.
79. Tomai, F., Crea, F., Chiariello, L., et al. (1999). Ischemic preconditioning in humans: models, mediators, and clinical relevance. *Circulation, 100*, 559–563.
80. Rona, G. (1985). Catecholamine cardiotoxicity. *J Mol Cell Cardiol, 17*, 291–306.
81. Cruickshank, J. M., Neil-Dwyer, G., Degaute, J. P., et al. (1987). Reduction of stress/catecholamine-induced cardiac necrosis by beta 1-selective blockade. *Lancet, 2*, 585–589.
82. Scarabelli, T., Stephanou, A., Rayment, N., et al. (2001). Apoptosis of endothelial cells precedes myocyte cell apoptosis in ischemia/reperfusion injury. *Circulation, 104*, 253–256.
83. Hiramatsu, T., Forbess, J., Miura, T., et al. (1995). Effects of endothelin-1 and endothelin-A receptor antagonist on recovery after hypothermic cardioplegic ischemia in neonatal lamb hearts. *Circulation, 92*, II400–II404.
84. Bolli, R. (1992). Myocardial "stunning" in man. *Circulation, 86*, 1671–1691.
85. Wijns, W., Vatner, S. F., & Camici, P. G. (1998). Hibernating myocardium. *N Engl J Med, 339*, 173–181.
86. Lim, H., Fallavollita, J. A., Hard, R., et al. (1999). Profound apoptosis-mediated regional myocyte loss and compensatory hypertrophy in pigs with hibernating myocardium. *Circulation, 100*, 2380–2386.
87. Shan, K., Bick, R. J., Poindexter, B. J., et al. (2000). Altered adrenergic receptor density in myocardial hibernation in humans: a possible mechanism of depressed myocardial function. *Circulation, 102*, 2599–2606.
88. Luisi, A. J., Fallavollita, J. A., Suzuki, G., et al. (2002). Spacial inhomogeneity of sympathetic nerve function in hibernating myocardium. *Circulation, 106*, 779–781.
89. Fallavollita, J. A., Malm, B. J., & Canty, J. M. (2003). Hibernating myocardium retains metabolic and contractile reserve despite regional reductions in flow, function, and oxygen consumption at rest. *Circ Res, 92*, 48–55.
90. Canty, J. M., Suzuki, G., Banas, M. K., et al. (2004). Hibernating myocardium: chronically adapted to ischemia but vulnerable to sudden death. *Circ Res, 94*, 1142–1149.
91. Thijssen, V. L. J. L., Borgers, M., Lenders, M. H., et al. (2004). Temporal and spatial variations in structural protein expression during the progression from stunned to hibernating myocardium. *Circulation, 110*, 3313–3321.
92. Iyer, V. S., & Canty, J. M. (2005). Regional desensitization of β-adrenergic receptor signaling in swine with chronic hibernating myocardium. *Circ Res, 97*, 789–795.
93. Auerbach, M. A., Schoder, H., Hoh, C., et al. (1999). Prevalence of myocardial viability as detected by positron emission tomography in patients with ischemic cardiomyopathy. *Circulation, 99*, 2921–2926.
94. Cleland, J. G., Pennel, D., Ray, S., et al. (1999). The carvedilol hibernation reversible ischaemia trial: marker of success (CHRISTMAS). The CHRISTMAS study steering committee and investigators. *Eur J Heart Fail, 1*, 191–196.
95. Challapalli, S., Hendel, R. C., & Bonow, R. O. (1998). Clinical profile of patients with congestive heart failure due to coronary artery disease: stunned/hibernating myocardium, ischemia, scar. *Coron Artery Dis, 9*, 629–644.
96. Al-Mohammad, A., Mahy, I. R., Norton, M. Y., et al. (1998). Prevalence of hibernating myocardium in patients with severely impaired ischemic left ventricles. *Heart, 80*, 559–564.
97. Dilsizian, V., & Bonow, R. O. (1993). Current diagnostic techniques of assessing myocardial viability in patients with hibernating and stunned myocardium. *Circulation, 87*, 1–20.
98. Bonow, R. O. (1996). Identification of viable myocardium. *Circulation, 94*, 2674–2680.
99. Schinkel, A. F., Bax, J. J., Poldermans, D., et al. (2007). Hibernating myocardium: diagnosis and patient outcomes. *Curr Probl Cardiol, 32*, 375–410.
100. Camici, P. G., Prasad, S. K., & Rimoldi, O. E. (2008). Stunning, hibernation, and assessment of myocardial viability. *Circulation, 117*, 103–114.
101. Allman, K. C., Shaw, L. J., Hachamovitch, R., et al. (2002). Myocardial viability testing and the impact of revascularization on prognosis in patients with coronary artery disease and left ventricular dysfunction: a meta-analysis. *J Am Coll Cardiol, 39*, 1151–1158.
102. Kim, R. J., Wu, E., Rafael, A., et al. (2000). The use of contrast-enhanced magnetic resonance imaging to identify reversible myocardial dysfunction. *N Engl J Med, 343*, 1445–1453.
103. Bucciarelli-Ducci, C., Wu, E., Lee, D. C., et al. (2006). Contrast-enhanced cardiac magnetic resonance in the evaluation of myocardial infarction and myocardial viability in patients with ischemic heart disease. *Curr Probl Cardiol, 31*, 125–168.
104. Soriano, C. J., Ridocci, F., Estornell, J., et al. (2005). Noninvasive diagnosis of coronary artery disease in patients with heart failure and systolic dysfunction of uncertain etiology using late gadolinium-enhanced cardiovascular magnetic resonance. *J Am Coll Cardiol, 45*, 743–748.
105. Bello, D., Shah, D. J., & Farah, G. M. (2003). Gadolinium cardiovascular magnetic resonance predicts reversible myocardial dysfunction and remodeling in patients with heart failure undergoing beta-blocker therapy. *Circulation, 108*, 1945–1953.
106. Seghatol, F. F., Shah, D. J., Deluzio, S., et al. (2004). Relation between contractile reserve and improvement in left ventricular function with beta-blocker therapy in patients with heart failure secondary to ischemic or idiopathic dilated cardiomyopathy. *Am J Cardiol, 93*, 854–859.
107. McFarlane, S. I., Muniyappa, R., Francisco, R., et al. (2002). Clinical review 145: pleiotropic effects of statins: lipid reduction and beyond. *J Clin Endocrinol Metab, 87*, 1451–1458.
108. Gould, K. L. (1998). New concepts and paradigms in cardiovascular medicine: the noninvasive management of coronary artery disease. *Am J Med, 104*, 2S–17S.
109. Schulz, R., Guth, B. D., Pieper, K., et al. (1992). Recruitment of an inotropic reserve in moderately ischemic myocardium at the expense of metabolic recovery. A model of short-term hibernation. *Circ Res, 70*, 1282–1295.
110. Chen, C., Li, L., Chen, L. L., et al. (1995). Incremental doses of dobutamine induce a biphasic response in dysfunctional left ventricular regions subtending coronary stenoses. *Circulation, 92*, 756–766.
111. Felker, G. M., Benza, R. L., Chandler, A. B., et al. (2003). Heart failure etiology and response to milrinone in decompensated heart failure: results from the OPTIME-CHF study. *J Am Coll Cardiol, 41*, 997–1003.
112. Elkayam, U., Tasissa, G., Binanay, C., et al. (2007). Use and impact of inotropes and vasodilator therapy in hospitalized patients with severe heart failure. *Am Heart J, 153*, 98–104.
113. Carluccio, E., Biagioli, P., Alumni, G., et al. (2006). Patients with hibernating myocardium show altered left ventricular volumes and shape, which revert after revascularization. *J Am Coll Cardiol, 47*, 969–977.
114. Azevedo, E. R., Stewart, D. J., & Parker, J. D. (2001). Increased extraction of endothelin-1 across the failing human heart. *Am J Cardiol, 88*, 180–182, A6.
115. Harrison, D. G. (1994). Endothelial dysfunction in atherosclerosis. *Basic Res Cardiol, 89*(suppl 1), 87–102.
116. Bell, D. M., Johns, T. E., & Lopez, L. M. (1998). Endothelial dysfunction: implications for therapy of cardiovascular diseases. *Ann Pharmacother, 32*, 459–470.
117. Moncada, S., & Higgs, A. (1993). The L-arginine-nitric oxide pathway. *N Engl J Med, 329*, 2002–2012.
118. Zeiher, A. M., Drexler, H., Saurbier, B., et al. (1993). Endothelium-mediated coronary blood flow modulation in humans. Effects of age, atherosclerosis, hypercholesterolemia, and hypertension. *J Clin Invest, 92*, 652–662.
119. Rubanyi, G. M. (1993). The role of endothelium in cardiovascular homeostasis and diseases. *J Cardiovasc Pharmacol, 22*(suppl 4), S1–S14.
120. Cody, R. J. (1997). The integrated effects of angiotensin II. *Am J Cardiol, 79*, 9–11.
121. Mehta, J. L., Li, D. Y., Yang, H., et al. (2002). Angiotensin II and IV stimulate expression and release of plasminogen activator inhibitor-1 in cultured human coronary artery endothelial cells. *J Cardiovasc Pharmacol, 39*, 789–794.
122. Brown, N. J., & Vaughan, D. E. (2000). Prothrombotic effects of angiotensin. *Adv Intern Med, 45*, 419–429.
123. Neylon, C. B. (1999). Vascular biology of endothelin signal transduction. *Clin Exp Pharmacol Physiol, 26*, 149–153.
124. Loscalzo, J., & Vita, J. A. (1994). Ischemia, hyperemia, exercise, and nitric oxide: complex physiology and complex molecular adaptations. *Circulation, 90*, 2556–2559.
125. Levin, E. R. (1995). Endothelins. *N Engl J Med, 333*, 356–363.
126. Luskutoff, D. J., Sawdey, M., & Mimuro, J. (1989). Type 1 plasminogen activator inhibitor. *Prog Hemost Thromb, 9*, 87–115.
127. Sakai, S., Miyauchi, T., Sakurai, T., et al. (1996). Endogenous endothelin-1 participates in the maintenance of cardiac function in rats with congestive heart failure: marked increase in endothelin-1 production in the failing heart. *Circulation, 93*, 1214–1222.
128. Kario, K., Matsuo, T., Hoshide, S., et al. (1999). Lipid-lowering therapy corrects endothelial cell dysfunction in a short time but does not affect hypercoagulable state even after long-term use in hyperlipidemic patients. *Blood Coagul Fibrinolysis, 10*, 269–276.
129. Adams, K. F., Jr. (1998). Angiotensin-converting enzyme inhibition and vascular remodeling in coronary artery disease. *Coron Artery Dis, 9*, 675–684.
130. Intengan, H. D., & Schiffrin, E. L. (2000). Disparate effects of carvedilol versus metoprolol treatment of stroke-prone spontaneously hypertensive rats on endothelial function of resistance arteries. *J Cardiovasc Pharmacol, 35*, 763–768.
131. Quyyumi, A. A. (1998). Effects of aspirin on endothelial dysfunction in atherosclerosis. *Am J Cardiol, 82*, 31S–33S.
132. Gould, K. L., Martucci, J. P., Goldberg, D. I., et al. (1994). Short-term cholesterol lowering decreases size and severity of perfusion abnormalities by positron emission tomography after dipyridamole in patients with coronary artery disease. A potential noninvasive marker of healing coronary endothelium. *Circulation, 89*, 1530–1538.
133. Eichstadt, H. W., Eskotter, H., Hoffman, I., et al. (1995). Improvement of myocardial perfusion by short-term fluvastatin therapy in coronary artery disease. *Am J Cardiol, 76*, 122A–125A.
134. Van Boven, A. J., Jukema, J. W., Zwinderman, A. H., et al. (1996). Reduction of transient myocardial ischemia with pravastatin in addition to the conventional treatment in patients with angina pectoris. REGRESS study group. *Circulation, 94*, 1503–1505.
135. Andrews, T. C., Raby, K., Barry, J., et al. (1997). Effect of cholesterol reduction on myocardial ischemia in patients with coronary disease. *Circulation, 95*, 324–328.
136. Mostaza, J. M., Gomez, M. V., Gallardo, F., et al. (2000). Cholesterol reduction improves myocardial perfusion abnormalities in patients with coronary artery disease and average cholesterol levels. *J Am Coll Cardiol, 35*, 76–82.
137. Baller, D., Notohamiprodjo, G., Gleichmann, U., et al. (1999). Improvement in coronary flow reserve determined by positron emission tomography after 6 months of cholesterol-lowering therapy in patients with early stages of coronary atherosclerosis. *Circulation, 99*, 2871–2875.
138. Segal, R., Pitt, B., Poole Wilson, P., et al. (2000). Effects of HMG-CoA reductase inhibitors (statins) in patients with heart failure. *Eur J Heart Fail, 2*(suppl 2), 96.

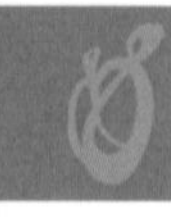

139. Drexler, H. (1999). Nitric oxide synthases in the failing human heart: a doubled-edged sword? *Circulation, 99*, 2972–2975.
140. Cannon, R. O., III (2000). Cardiovascular benefit of cholesterol-lowering therapy: does improved endothelial vasodilator function matter? *Circulation, 102*, 820–822.
141. Yusuf, S., Pepine, C. J., Garces, C., et al. (1992). Effect of enalapril on myocardial infarction and unstable angina in patients with low ejection fractions. *Lancet, 340*, 1173–1178.
142. St John, S. M., Pfeffer, M. A., Moye, L., et al. (1997). Cardiovascular death and left ventricular remodeling two years after myocardial infarction: baseline predictors and impact of long-term use of captopril: information from the survival and ventricular enlargement (SAVE) trial. *Circulation, 96*, 3294–3299.
143. O'Connor, C. M., Carson, P. E., Miller, A. B., et al. (1998). Effect of amlodipine on mode of death among patients with advanced heart failure in the PRAISE trial. Prospective randomized amlodipine survival evaluation. *Am J Cardiol, 82*, 881–887.
144. Adabag, A. S., Therneau, T. M., Gersh, B. J., et al. (2008). Sudden death after myocardial infarction. *JAMA, 300*, 2022–2029.
145. Stevenson, W. G., Stevenson, L. W., Middlekauff, H. R., et al. (1993). Sudden death prevention in patients with advanced ventricular dysfunction. *Circulation, 88*, 2953–2961.
146. MERIT-HF Study Group. (1999). Effect of metoprolol CR/XL in chronic heart failure: metoprolol CR/XL randomised intervention trial in congestive heart failure (MERIT-HF). *Lancet, 353*, 2001–2007.
147. Davies, M. J. (1992). Anatomic features in victims of sudden coronary death. Coronary artery pathology. *Circulation, 85*, I19–I24.
148. Zipes, D. P., & Wellens, H. J. (1998). Sudden cardiac death. *Circulation, 98*, 2334–2351.
149. Farb, A., Tang, A. L., Burke, A. P., et al. (1995). Sudden coronary death. Frequency of active coronary lesions, inactive coronary lesions, and myocardial infarction. *Circulation, 92*, 1701–1709.
150. Poole, J. E., Johnson, G. W., Hellkamp, A. S., et al. (2008). Prognostic importance of defibrillator shocks in patients with heart failure. *N Engl J Med, 359*, 1009–1017.
151. Moss, A. J., Greenberg, H., Case, R. B., et al. (2004). Long-term clinical course of patients after termination of ventricular tachyarrhythmia by an implanted defibrillator. *Circulation, 110*, 3760–3765.
152. Cleland, J. G. F., Swedberg, K., Follath, F., et al. (2003). The EuroHeart failure survey programme—a survey on the quality of care among patients with heart failure in Europe: part 1: patient characteristics and diagnosis. *Eur Heart J, 24*, 442–463.
153. Owan, T. E., Hodge, D. O., Herges, R. M., et al. (2006). Trends in prevalence and outcome of heart failure with preserved ejection fraction. *N Engl J Med, 355*, 251–259.
154. Fonarow, G. C., Gattis Stough, W., Abraham, W. T., et al. (2007). Characteristics, treatments and outcomes of patients with preserved systolic function hospitalized with heart failure: a report from OPTIMIZE-HF. *J Am Coll Cardiol, 50*, 768–777.
155. Judge, K. W., Pawitan, Y., Caldwell, J., et al. (1991). Congestive heart failure symptoms in patients with preserved left ventricular systolic function: analysis of the CASS registry. *J Am Coll Cardiol, 18*, 377–382.
156. Bhatia, R. S., Tu, J. V., Lee, D. S., et al. (2007). Outcome of heart failure with preserved ejection fraction in a population based study. *N Engl J Med, 355*, 260–269.
157. Lenzen, M. J., Scholte op Reimer, W. J. M., Boersma, E., et al. (2004). Differences between patients with preserved and a depressed left ventricular function: a report from the EuroHeart failure survey. *Eur Heart J, 25*, 1214–1220.
158. Tribouilloy, C., Rusinaru, D., Mahjoub, H., et al. (2008). Prognosis of heart failure with preserved ejection fraction: a 5 year prospective population-based study. *Eur Heart J, 29*, 339–347.
159. Siirilä-Waris, K., Lassus, J., Melin, et al. (2006). Characteristics, outcomes, and predictors of 1-year mortality in patients hospitalized for acute heart failure. *Eur Heart J, 27*, 3011–3017.
160. Shah, S. J., & Gheorghiade, M. (2008). Heart failure with preserved ejection fraction. *JAMA, 300*, 431–433.
161. Ahmed, A., Rich, M. W., Fleg, J. L., et al. (2006). Effects of digoxin on morbidity and mortality in diastolic heart failure. *Circulation, 114*, 397–403.
162. Gandhi, S. K., Powers, J. C., Nomeir, A. M., et al. (2001). The pathogenesis of acute pulmonary edema associated with hypertension. *N Engl J Med, 344*, 17–22.
163. Grossman, W. (1991). Diastolic dysfunction in congestive heart failure. *N Engl J Med, 325*, 1557–1564.
164. Aroesty, J. M., McKay, R. G., Heller, G. V., et al. (1985). Simultaneous assessment of left ventricular systolic and diastolic dysfunction during pacing-induced ischemia. *Circulation, 71*, 889–900.
165. Judge, K. W., Pawitan, Y., Caldwell, J., et al. (1991). Congestive heart failure symptoms in patients with preserved left ventricular systolic function: analysis of the CASS registry. *J Am Coll Cardiol, 18*, 377–382.
166. Vasan, R. S., Benjamin, E. J., & Levy, D. (1995). Prevalence, clinical features and prognosis of diastolic heart failure: an epidemiologic perspective. *J Am Coll Cardiol, 26*, 1565–1574.
167. Choudhury, L., Gheorghiade, M., & Bonow, R. O. (2002). Coronary artery disease in patients with heart failure and preserved systolic function. *Am J Cardiol, 89*, 719–722.
168. Haffner, S. M., Lehto, S., Ronnemaa, T., et al. (1998). Mortality from coronary heart disease in subjects with type 2 diabetes and in nondiabetic subjects with and without prior myocardial infarction. *N Engl J Med, 339*, 229–234.
169. Sowers, J. R., Epstein, M., & Frohlich, E. D. (2001). Diabetes, hypertension, and cardiovascular disease: an update. *Hypertension, 37*, 1053–1059.
170. Hammond, T., Tanguay, J. F., & Bourassa, M. G. (2000). Management of coronary artery disease: therapeutic options in patients with diabetes. *J Am Coll Cardiol, 36*, 355–365.
171. Carson, P., Johnson, G., Fletcher, R., et al. (1996). Mild systolic dysfunction in heart failure (left ventricular ejection fraction >35%): baseline characteristics, prognosis and response to therapy in the vasodilator in heart failure trials (V-HeFT). *J Am Coll Cardiol, 27*, 642–649.
172. McKelvie, R. S., Yusuf, S., Pericak, D., et al. (1999). Comparison of candesartan, enalapril, and their combination in congestive heart failure: randomized evaluation of strategies for left ventricular dysfunction (RESOLVD) pilot study. The RESOLVD pilot study investigators. *Circulation, 100*, 1056–1064.
173. Greenberg, B. H., Abraham, W. T., Albert, N. M., et al. (2007). Influence of diabetes on characteristics and outcomes in patients hospitalized with heart failure. *Am Heart J, 154*, 647–654.
174. Adams, K. F., Fonarow, G. C., Emerman, C. L., et al. (2005). Characteristics and outcomes of patients hospitalized for heart failure in the United States. *Am Heart J, 149*, 209–216.
175. Gottdiener, J. S., Arnold, A. M., Aurigemma, G. P., et al. (2000). Predictors of congestive heart failure in the elderly. *J Am Coll Cardiol, 35*, 1628–1637.
176. He, J., Ogden, L. G., Bazzano, L. A., et al. (2001). Risk factors for congestive heart failure in U.S. men and woman. *Arch Intern Med, 161*, 996–1002.
177. Kannel, W. B., Hjortland, M., & Castelli, W. P. (1974). Role of diabetes in congestive heart failure: the Framingham study. *Am J Cardiol, 34*, 29–34.
178. Iribarren, C., Karter, A. J., Go, A. S., et al. (2001). Glycemic control and heart failure among adult patients with diabetes. *Circulation, 103*, 2668–2673.
179. Stratton, I. M., Adler, A. I., Neil, A. W., et al. (2000). Association of glycaemia with macrovascular complications of type 2 diabetes. *BMJ, 321*, 405–412.
180. Lee, D. L., Austin, P. C., Rouleau, J. L., et al. (2003). Predicting mortality among patients hospitalized for heart failure. *JAMA, 290*, 2581–2587.
181. Pocock, S. J., Wang, D., Pfeffer, M. A., et al. (2006). Predictors of mortality and morbidity in patients with chronic heart failure. *Eur Heart J, 27*, 65–75.
182. Gustafsson, I., Brendorp, B., Seibæk, M., et al. (2004). Influence of diabetes and diabetes-gender interaction on the risk of death in patients hospitalized with congestive heart failure. *J Am Coll Cardiol, 43*, 771–777.
183. Bertoni, A. G., Hundley, W. G., Massing, M. W., et al. (2004). Heart failure prevalence, incidence, and mortality in the elderly with diabetes. *Diabetes Care, 27*, 699–703.
184. Vaur, L., Gueret, P., Lievre, M., et al. (2003). Development of congestive heart failure in type 2 diabetes patients with microalbuminuria or proteinuria. *Diabetes Care, 26*, 855–860.
185. From, A. M., Leibson, C. L., Bursi, F., et al. (2006). Diabetes in heart failure: prevalence and impact on outcome in the population. *Am J Med, 119*, 591–599.
186. Domanski, M., Krause-Steinrauf, H., Deedwania, P., et al. (2003). The effect of diabetes on outcomes of patients with advanced heart failure in the BEST trial. *J Am Coll Cardiol, 42*, 914–922.
187. Brophy, J. M., Dagenais, G. R., McSherry, F., et al. (2004). A multivariate model for predicting mortality in patients with heart failure and systolic dysfunction. *Am J Med, 116*, 300–304.
188. de Groote, P., Lamblin, N., Mouquet, F., et al. (2004). Impact of diabetes mellitus on long-term survival in patients with congestive heart failure. *Eur Heart J, 25*, 656–662.
189. Dries, D. L., Sweitzer, N. K., Drazner, M. H., et al. (2001). Prognostic impact of diabetes mellitus in patients with heart failure according to etiology of left ventricular systolic dysfunction. *J Am Coll Cardiol, 38*, 421–428.
190. Flaherty, J. D., & Davidson, C. J. (2005). Diabetes and coronary revascularization. *JAMA, 293*, 1501–1508.
191. Nesto, R. W. (2004). Correlation between cardiovascular disease and diabetes mellitus. *Am J Med, 116*(suppl 5A), 11S–22S.
192. Waller, B. F., Palumbo, P. J., Lie, J. T., et al. (1980). Status of the coronary arteries at necropsy in diabetes mellitus with onset after 30 years. *Am J Med, 69*, 498–506.
193. Moreno, P. R., Murcia, A. M., Palacios, I. F., et al. (2000). Coronary composition and macrophage infiltration in atherectomy specimens from patient with diabetes mellitus. *Circulation, 102*, 2180–2184.
194. Nicholls, S. J., Tuzcu, E. M., Kalidindi, S., et al. (2008). Effect of diabetes on progression of coronary atherosclerosis and arterial remodeling. *J Am Coll Cardiol, 52*, 255–262.
195. MacDonald, M. R., Petrie, M. C., Hawkins, N. M., et al. (2008). Diabetes, left ventricular systolic dysfunction and chronic heart failure. *Eur Heart J, 29*, 1224–1240.
196. van Heerebeek, L., Hamdani, N., Handoko, L., et al. (2008). Diastolic stiffness of the failing diabetic heart. *Circulation, 117*, 43–51.
197. Lee, T. S., Satlsman, K. A., Ohashi, H., et al. (1989). Activation of protein kinase C by elevation of glucose concentration: proposal of a mechanism in the development of diabetic vascular complications. *Proc Natl Acad Sci U S A, 86*, 5141–5145.
198. Berg, T. J., Snorgaard, O., Faber, J., et al. (1999). Serum levels of advanced glycation end products are associated with left ventricular diastolic function in patients with type 1 diabetes. *Diabetes Care, 22*, 1186–1190.
199. Grundy, S. M., Benjamin, I. J., Burke, G. L., et al. (1999). Diabetes and cardiovascular disease: a statement for healthcare professionals from the American Heart Association. *Circulation, 100*, 1134–1146.
200. Gheorghiade, M., & Pang, P. S. (2009). Acute heart failure syndromes. *J Am Coll Cardiol, 53*, 557–573.
201. Cotter, G., Metzkor, E., Kaluski, E., et al. (1998). Randomised trial of high-dose isosorbide dinitrate plus low-dose furosemide versus high-dose furosemide plus low-dose isosorbide dinitrate in severe pulmonary oedema. *Lancet, 351*, 389–393.
202. Abraham, W. T., Adams, K. F., Fonarow, G. C., et al. (2005). In-hospital mortality in patients with acute compensated heart failure requiring intravenous vasoactive medications: an analysis from the Acute Decompensated Heart Failure Registry (ADHERE). *J Am Coll Cardiol, 46*, 57–64.
203. Investigators, V. M. A. C. (2002). Intravenous nesiritide vs. nitroglycerin for treatment of decompensated congestive heart failure. *JAMA, 287*, 1531–1540.
204. Sackner-Bernstein, J. D., Skopicki, H. A., & Aaronson, K. D. (2005). Risk of worsening renal function with nesiritide in patients with acutely decompensated heart failure. *Circulation, 111*, 1487–1491.
205. Schultz, R., Rose, J., Martin, C., et al. (1993). Development of short-term myocardial hibernation. *Circulation, 88*, 684–695.
206. Felker, G. M., Benza, R. L., Chandler, A. B., et al. (2003). Heart failure etiology and response to milrinone in decompensated heart failure: results from the OPTIME-CHF study. *J Am Coll Cardiol, 41*, 997–1003.
207. Schmieder, R. E. (2005). Mechanisms for the clinical benefits of angiotensin II receptor blockers. *Am J Hypertension, 18*, 720–730.

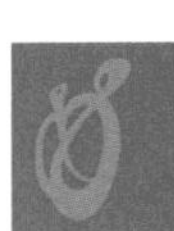

208. The Heart Outcomes Prevention Evaluation (HOPE) Study Investigators. (2000). Effects of an angiotensin-converting-enzyme inhibitor, ramipril, on cardiovascular events in high-risk patients. *N Engl J Med, 342*, 145–153.
209. The EUROPA Investigators. (2003). Efficacy of perindopril in reduction of cardiovascular events among patients with stable coronary artery disease: randomised, double-blind, placebo-controlled, multicentre trial. *Lancet, 362*, 782–788.
210. The ONTARGET Investigators. (2008). Telmisartan, ramipril, or both in patients at high risk for vascular events. *N Engl J Med, 358*, 1547–1559.
211. O'Keefe, J. H., Wetzel, M., Moe, R. R., et al. (2001). Should an angiotensin-converting enzyme inhibitor be standard therapy for patients with atherosclerotic disease?. *J Am Coll Cardiol, 37*, 1–8.
212. Rutherford, J. D., Pfeffer, M. A., Moye, L. A., et al. (1994). Effects of captopril on ischemic events after myocardial infarction. Results of the survival and ventricular enlargement trial. SAVE investigators. *Circulation, 90*, 1731–1738.
213. Nishioka., et al. (2007). Eplerenone attenuates myocardial fibrosis in the angiotensin II-induced hypertensive mouse. *J Cardiovasc Pharmacol, 49*, 261–268.
214. Seed, A., et al. (2007). Neurohumoral effects of the new orally active rennin inhibitor, aliskiren, in chronic heart failure. *Euro J Heart Fail, 9*, 1120–1127.
215. Gattis, W. A., O'Connor, C. M., Gallup, D. S., et al. (2004). Predischarge initiation of carvedilol in patients hospitalized for decompensated heart failure. *J Am Coll Cardiol, 43*, 1534–1541.
216. Fonarow, G. C., Abraham, W. T., Albert, N. M., et al. (2007). Carvedilol use at discharge in patients hospitalized for heart failure is associated with improved survival. *Am Heart J, 153*, 82e1M–82e11.
217. Fonarow, G. C., Abraham, W. T., Albert, N. M., et al. (2008). Influence of beta-blocker continuation or withdrawal on outcomes in patients hospitalized with heart failure. *J Am Coll Cardiol, 52*, 190–199.
218. The CIBIS-II Investigators. (1999). The cardiac insufficiency bisoprolol study II (CIBIS-II): a randomised trial. *Lancet, 353*, 9–13.
219. Cleland, J. G., Alamgir, F., Nikitin, N. P., et al. (2001). What is the optimal medical management of ischemic heart failure? *Prog Cardiovasc Dis, 43*, 433–455.
220. The Capricorn Investigators. (2001). Effect of carvedilol on outcome after myocardial infarction in patients with left-ventricular dysfunction: the CAPRICORN randomised trial. *Lancet, 357*, 1385–1390.
221. Bristow, M. R., Anderson, F. L., Port, J. D., et al. (1991). Differences in beta-adrenergic neuroeffector mechanisms in ischemic versus idiopathic dilated cardiomyopathy. *Circulation, 84*, 1024–1039.
222. Bristow, M. R. (2000). Beta-adrenergic receptor blockade in chronic heart failure. *Circulation, 101*, 558–569.
223. NCEP Expert Panel. (2001). Executive summary of the third report of the national cholesterol education panel (NCEP) expert panel on detection, evaluation, and treatment of high blood cholesterol in adults (adult treatment panel III). *JAMA, 285*, 2486–2497.
224. Sacks, F. M., Pfeffer, M. A., Moye, L. A., et al. (1996). The effect of pravastatin on coronary events after myocardial infarction in patients with average cholesterol levels. *N Engl J Med, 335*, 1001–1009.
225. Kjekshus, J., Pedersen, T. R., Olsson, A. G., et al. (1997). The effects of simvastatin on the incidence of heart failure in patients with coronary heart disease. *J Card Fail, 3*, 249–254.
226. Khush, K. K., Waters, D. D., Bittner, V., et al. (2007). Effect of high-dose atorvastatin on hospitalizations for heart failure. *Circulation, 115*, 576–583.
227. Scirica, B. M., Morow, D. A., Cannon, C. P., et al. (2006). Intensive statin therapy and the risk of hospitalization for heart failure after an acute coronary syndrome in the PROVE IT-TIMI 22 study. *J Am Coll Cardiol, 47*, 2326–2331.
228. Go, A. S., Lee, W. Y., Yang, J., et al. (2006). Statin therapy and risks for death and hospitalization in chronic heart failure. *JAMA, 296*, 2105–2111.
229. Foody, J. M., Shah, R., Galusha, D., et al. (2006). Statins and mortality among elderly patients hospitalized with heart failure. *Circulation, 113*, 1086–1092.
230. Fukuta, H., Sane, D. C., Brucks, S., et al. (2005). Statin therapy may be associated with lower mortality in patients with diastolic heart failure. *Circulation, 112*, 357–363.
231. Kjekshus, J., Apetrei, E., Barrios, V., et al. (2007). Rosuvastatin in older patients with systolic heart failure. *N Engl J Med, 357*, 2248–2261.
232. GISSI-HF Investigators. (2008). Effect of rosuvastatin in patients with chronic heart failure. *Lancet, 372*, 1231–1239.
233. GISSI-Prevenzione Investigators. (1999). Dietary supplementation with n-3 polyunsaturated fatty acids and vitamin E after myocardial infarction. *Lancet, 354*, 447–455.
234. Yamagishi, K., Iso, H., Date, C., et al. (2008). Fish, n-3 polyunsaturated fatty acids, and mortality from cardiovascular disease in a nationwide community-based cohort of Japanese men and women. *J Am Coll Cardiol, 52*, 988–996.
235. GISSI-HF Investigators. (2008). Effect of n-3 polyunsaturated fatty acids in patients with chronic heart failure. *Lancet, 372*, 1223–1230.
236. Smith, S. C., Allen, J., Blair, S. N., et al. (2006). AHA/ACC guidelines for secondary prevention for patients with coronary and other atherosclerotic vascular disease. *J Am Coll Cardiol, 47*, 2130–2139.
237. Yusuf, S., Zhao, F., Mehta, S. R., et al. (2001). Effects of clopidogrel in addition to aspirin in patients with acute coronary syndromes without ST-segment elevation. *N Engl J Med, 345*, 494–502.
238. MacIntrye, I. M., Jhund, P. S., & McMurray, J. V. (2005). Aspirin inhibits the acute arterial and venous vasodilator response to captopril in patients with chronic heart failure. *Cardiovasc Drugs Ther, 19*, 261–265.
239. Hays, A. G., Sacco, R. L., Rundek, T., et al. (2006). Left ventricular systolic dysfunction and the risk of ischemic stroke in a multiethnic population. *Stroke, 37*, 1715–1719.
240. Cleland, J. G. F., Findlay, I., Jafri, S., et al. (2004). The warfarin/aspirin study in heart failure. *Am Heart J, 148*, 157–164.
241. Cokkinos, D. V., Haralabopoulos, G. C., Kostis, J. B., et al. (2006). Efficacy of antithrombotic therapy in chronic heart failure. *Eur J Heart Fail, 8*, 428–432.
242. Jones, R. H., Velazquez, E. J., Michler, R. E., et al. (2009). Coronary bypass surgery with or without surgical ventricular reconstruction. *N Engl J Med, 360*, 1705–1717.
243. Tsuyuki, R. T., Shrive, F. M., Galbraith, D., et al. (2006). Revascularization in patients with heart failure. *Can Med Assoc J, 175*, 361–373.
244. Steg, P. G., Kerner, A., Van de Werf, F., et al. (2008). Impact of in-hospital revascularization with non-ST-elevation acute coronary syndrome and congestive heart failure. *Circulation, 118*, 1163–1171.
245. Hochman, J. S., Sleeper, L. A., Webb, J. S., et al. (2006). Early revascularization and long-term survival in cardiogenic shock complicating acute myocardial infarction. *JAMA, 295*, 2511–2515.
246. Add Flaherty, J. D., Rossi, J. S., Fonarow, G. C., et al. (2009). Influence of coronary angiography on the utilization of therapies in patients with acute heart failure syndromes: findings from OPTIMIZE-HF. *Am Heart J, 157*, 1018–1025.
247. Zipes, D. P., Camm, A. J., Borggrefe, M., et al. (2006). ACC/AHA/ESC 2006 guidelines for management of patients with ventricular arrhythmias and the prevention of sudden cardiac death: a report of the American College of Cardiology/American Heart Association task force and the European Society of Cardiology committee for practice guidelines. *J Am Coll Cardiol, 48*, e247–e346.
248. McAlister, F. A., Ezekowitz, J., Hooton, N., et al. (2007). Cardiac resynchronization therapy for patients with left ventricular systolic dysfunction: a systematic review. *JAMA, 297*, 2502–2514.
249. Trichon, B. H., Felker, G. M., Shaw, L. K., et al. (2003). Relation of frequency and severity of mitral regurgitation to survival among patients with left ventricular systolic dysfunction and heart failure. *Am J Cardiol, 91*, 538–543.
250. Acker, M. A., Bolling, S., Shemin, R. J., et al. (2006). Mitral valve surgery in heart failure: insights from the Acorn clinical trial. *J Thorac Cardiovasc Surg, 132*, 568–577.
251. Bishay, E. S., McCarthy, P. M., Cosgrove, D. M., et al. (2000). Mitral valve surgery in patients with severe left ventricular dysfunction. *Eur J Cardiothorac Surg, 17*, 213–221.
252. Webb, J. G., Harnek, J., Munt, B. I., et al. (2006). Percutaneous transvenous mitral annuloplasty. *Circulation, 113*, 851–855.
253. Fedak, P. W. M., McCarthy, P. M., & Bonow, R. O. (2008). Evolving concepts and technologies in mitral valve repair. *Circulation, 117*, 963–974.
254. Athanasuleas, C. L., Buckberg, G. D., Stanley, A. W. H., et al. (2004). Surgical ventricular restoration in the treatment of congestive heart failure due to post-infarction ventricular dilation. *J Am Coll Cardiol, 44*, 1439–1445.
255. Velazquez, E. J., Lee, K. L., O'Connor, C. M., et al. (2007). The rationale and design of the surgical treatment for ischemic heart failure (STICH) trial. *J Thorac Cardiovasc Surg, 134*, 1540–1547.

CHAPTER 24

Heart Failure as a Consequence of Dilated Cardiomyopathy

Biykem Bozkurt

DEFINITION

The term "dilated cardiomyopathy" (DCM) refers to a spectrum of heterogeneous myocardial disorders (Table 24-1) that are characterized by ventricular dilation and depressed myocardial contractility in the absence of abnormal loading conditions (such as hypertension or valvular disease) or ischemic heart disease sufficient to cause global systolic impairment.[1] The dilated cardiomyopathies constitute the largest group of myopathic disorders that are responsible for systolic heart failure. Indeed, more than 75 specific diseases can produce a dilated cardiomyopathic phenotype. Thus DCM can be envisioned as the final common pathway for a myriad of cardiac disorders that either damage the heart muscle or, alternatively, disrupt the ability of the myocardium to generate force and subsequently cause chamber dilation.

In clinical practice and recent multicenter trials in heart failure, the cause of heart failure has often been categorized into two categories: ischemic and nonischemic cardiomyopathy and the term "DCM" has been interchangeably used with "nonischemic cardiomyopathy." Though this approach may be practical, it has certain drawbacks. It fails to recognize that the term "nonischemic cardiomyopathy" may include cardiomyopathies due to volume or pressure overload—such as hypertension or valvular heart disease—which are not conventionally accepted under the definition of DCM.[1]

EPIDEMIOLOGY OF DILATED CARDIOMYOPATHY

The reported incidence of DCM varies annually about 5 to 8 cases per 100,000 of the population. The true incidence may be underestimated due to underreporting or underdetection of asymptomatic cases of DCM, which may occur in as many as 50% to 60% of heart failure patients. In most multicenter, randomized trials in heart failure, approximately 30% to 40% of the enrolled patients have nonischemic dilated cardiomyopathy.[2,3] According to the Acute Decompensated Heart Failure National Registry (ADHERE), one of the largest databases on acute heart failure, 47% of the patients admitted to the hospital with heart failure have nonischemic cardiomyopathy.[4] The age-adjusted prevalence of DCM in the United States averages 36 cases per 100,000 population and DCM accounts for 10,000 deaths annually.[5]

Compared with whites, African Americans have almost a threefold increase in risk for developing DCM. This increased risk for developing DCM in African Americans is not explained by differences in hypertension, cigarette smoking, alcohol use, or socioeconomic factors.[6] Moreover, African Americans have approximately a 1.5- to 2.0-fold higher risk of dying from DCM when compared with age-matched whites with DCM. While the reason(s) for these differences are not known, there are several potential explanations, including differences in the genetic predisposition, the cause of heart failure, the number of risk factors for development of heart failure, the rate of progression of heart failure, access to medical care and/or differences in response to therapy. Recent data from the second Vasodilator-Heart Failure Trial (V-HeFT II),[7] Beta-Blocker Evaluation of Survival Trial,[8] and Studies of Left Ventricular Dysfunction (SOLVD)[9] suggest that African American patients with heart failure may not benefit from commonly used doses of currently recommended therapies to the same extent as White patients, although unanimity of opinion does not exist with regard to this issue.[10]

In general, heart failure is more common in men than women (see also Chapters 22 and 49). Epidemiological data suggesting sex-related differences in the occurrence and prognosis of heart failure are conflicting and may be confounded by differing causes of heart failure. The overall effect of female gender on the prognosis of heart failure is not clear at this time, in large measure because many of the early clinical trials in heart failure have been comprised predominantly of male subjects. Women with heart failure in the Framingham Heart Study (even after controlling for age and cause of heart failure)[11] and women in the National Health and Nutrition Examination Survey-I (NHANES-I)[12] had improved survival compared with men. Studies of Left Ventricular Dysfunction (SOLVD), in which only 15% of the patients were women, reported no difference in gender-related survival.[13] However, the SOLVD registry, which included approximately 20% female patients, suggested that women had significantly higher annual risk of heart failure–related mortality and higher rates of hospitalization than age-matched male subjects.[14] Analyses from MERIT-HF[15] and CIBIS-II[16] β-blocker treatment trials in heart failure suggest that female sex may be a significant independent predictor of survival in patients with heart failure, independent of ischemic or nonischemic cause. One of the challenges in defining gender-specific causes and prognostic factors in dilated cardiomyopathy is that hypertension, which represents the major and strongest risk factor for development of heart failure in women, has been categorized under "nonischemic cardiomyopathy" in most large-scale clinical trials. In the Framingham Heart Study, hypertension was the cause of heart failure in 59% of women.[17] There aren't many trials reporting specific causes of nonischemic cardiomyopathy in women; therefore, the "true" incidence of dilated cardiomyopathy in women, independent of hypertension is not well known. One of these few studies was the EuroHeart Failure Survey II (EHFS), in which women had less incidence of dilated cardiomyopathy compared with men.[18]

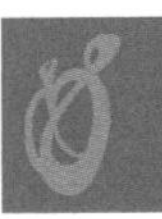

TABLE 24–1 Causes of Dilated Cardiomyopathy
Idiopathic
Idiopathic dilated cardiomyopathy Idiopathic arrhythmogenic right ventricular dysplasia
Familial (hereditary)
Autosomal dominant X-chromosomal Polymorphism
Toxic
Ethanol Cocaine Adriamycin Catecholamine excess Phenothiazines, antidepressants Cobalt Carbon monoxide Lead Lithium Cyclophosphamide Methysergide
Inflammatory: Infectious Cause
Viral (coxsackie virus, parvovirus, adenovirus, echovirus, influenza virus, HIV) Spirochete (leptospirosis, syphilis) Protozoal (Chagas disease, toxoplasmosis, trichinosis)
Inflammatory: Noninfectious Cause
Collagen vascular disease (scleroderma, lupus erythematosus, dermatomyositis, rheumatoid arthritis) Kawasaki Hypersensitivity myocarditis
Miscellaneous Acquired Cardiomyopathy
Postpartum cardiomyopathy Obesity
Metabolic/Nutritional
Thiamine Kwashiorkor pellagra Scurvy Hypervitaminosis D Selenium deficiency Carnitine deficiency
Endocrine
Diabetes mellitus Acromegaly Thyrotoxicosis Myxedema Uremia Cushing disease Pheochromocytoma
Electrolyte Imbalance
Hypophosphatemia Hypocalcemia
Physiological Agents
Tachycardia Heat stroke Hypothermia Radiation
Autoimmune Disorders

Further studies will be helpful to define the role of gender on the development and prognosis of DCM.

Advancing age is a risk factor for mortality in heart failure. As reported in the SOLVD registry, the risk of death at 1 year for a person over the age of 64 years with heart failure was 1.5 times greater than for subjects who were less than 64 years of age.[14] Advancing age has been reported as an independent risk factor for mortality in DCM in several studies.[19] Indeed, Sugrie et al reported the relative risk of dying from DCM increases by 0.59 with every 10 years of increase in age.[20] Interestingly, though the number of hospitalizations for heart failure continues to increase among the elderly, with advances in the pharmacological and device treatment, the prognosis of heart failure and DCM has significantly improved over the past 20 years.[21]

The prevalence, cause, and prognosis of dilated cardiomyopathy can differ according to the geographical location and sociodemographics of the affected populations. For example, in Western developed countries, dilated nonischemic cardiomyopathy accounts for approximately 30% to 40% of the heart failure population, of which idiopathic cardiomyopathy is the most frequent cause. The prevalence of DCM in Japan appears to be about half, and in Africa and Latin America approximately double that of the Western populations.[22] As populations go through epidemiological, socioeconomic transitions, and health care modifications, the features of DCM will continue to change. Failure of treatment and eradication of AIDS globally and especially in Africa, rising prevalence of ethanol or substance abuse in Western countries, the development of obesity, new metabolic and dietary trends in North America, and the success in treatment of protozoal diseases in Latin America will continue to play a dynamic role in the epidemiology of DCM.

NATURAL HISTORY OF DILATED CARDIOMYOPATHY

The natural history of DCM is not well established for two reasons: first, as noted at the outset, DCM represents a heterogeneous spectrum of myocardial disorders that may each progress at different rates,[23] and second, the onset of the disease may be insidious, particularly in the case of familial and/or idiopathic dilated cardiomyopathies. Indeed, approximately 4% to 13% of the patients with DCM will have asymptomatic left ventricular (LV) dysfunction and LV dilation. For these patients the overall prognosis is unclear. However, once DCM patients become symptomatic, the available evidence suggests that the prognosis is relatively poor, with 25% mortality at 1 year and 50% mortality at 5 years (Figure 24-1).[19] The cause of death appears to be primarily pump failure in approximately 70% of patients with DCM, whereas sudden cardiac death accounts for approximately 30% of all deaths in patients with DCM. However, it should be recognized that many of the natural history studies of DCM were performed before angiotensin-converting enzyme (ACE) inhibitors and β-blockers were routinely used. More recent studies suggest that the prognosis for patients with DCM and mild LV dilation may be more favorable, perhaps reflecting earlier diagnosis and better treatment.[20] Furthermore, it should be recognized that approximately 25% of DCM patients with the recent onset of symptoms of heart failure will improve spontaneously, including patients who have been referred for cardiac transplantation.[24] This statement notwithstanding, patients with symptoms lasting more than 3 months who have severe clinical decompensation generally have less chance of recovery.[24]

As shown in Box 24-1, there are a number of other parameters that predict a poor prognosis in patients with DCM, including left and right ventricular enlargement, left and right ventricular ejection fraction, persistent S_3 gallop, right-sided heart failure, elevated LV filling pressures, moderate to severe mitral regurgitation, pulmonary hypertension, ECG findings of first- or second-degree atrioventricular block, left bundle branch block or marked intraventricular conduction delay, recurrent ventricular tachycardia, reduced heart rate variability, late potentials of QRS in signal average EKG, myocytolysis

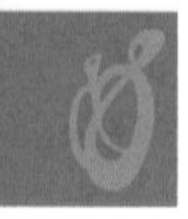

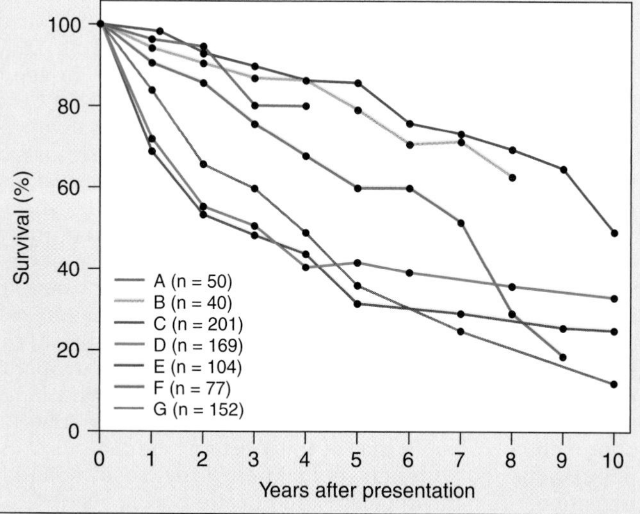

FIGURE 24–1 Survival of patients with idiopathic dilated cardiomyopathy in seven published series (A to G). n = number of patients enrolled. To identify each specific series, please refer to the article by Dec and Fuster.[26] (Dec GW, Fuster V. Idiopathic dilated cardiomyopathy. *N Engl J Med* 1994;331:1564-1575, reproduced with permission from the *New England Journal of Medicine*.)

BOX 24–1 Factors Predicting a Poor Prognosis in Patients with Dilated Cardiomyopathy

Left ventricular enlargement
Right ventricular enlargement
Left and right ventricular ejection fraction
Elevated LV filling pressures
Persistent S_3 gallop
Right-sided heart failure
Pulmonary hypertension
Moderate to severe mitral regurgitation
ECG findings: first- or second-degree atrioventricular block or LBBB
Recurrent ventricular tachycardia
Reduced heart rate variability
Late potentials of QRS in signal average EKG
Myocytolysis on endomyocardial biopsy
Elevated levels of neurohormones (BNP, NE, PRA, and ET-1)
Elevated levels of cytokines (TNF-α and IL-6)
Elevation of serum CK/MB, troponin T, troponin I levels
Peak oxygen consumption <10-12 mL/kg/min
Reduced contractile response with dobutamine
Serum sodium <137 mmol/L
Advanced New York Heart Association class
Advanced age (>64 years)

on endomyocardial biopsy, elevated levels of neurohormones (norepinephrine, plasma renin activity, atrial natriuretic peptide, brain natriuretic peptide, and endothelin-1), elevated levels of cytokines (tumor necrosis factor α and interleukin-6), persistently elevated markers of myocardial cell death (elevation of serum troponin T levels, an increased ratio of creatine kinase MB_2/MB_1 peak oxygen consumption less than 10 to 12 mL/kg/min, serum sodium less than 137 mmol/L, New York Heart Association class rating, age older than 64 years, and reduced contractile response with dobutamine. Concomitant renal or hepatic dysfunction may limit the use of optimal diuretics or ACE inhibitors and therefore may have an impact on prognosis that is not easily appreciated. Finally, it should be emphasized that comorbid conditions, such as diabetes and hypertension, increase the risk of developing heart failure approximately fivefold.

Ischemic Versus Dilated Cardiomyopathy

In general practice and clinical research trials, the term "ischemic cardiomyopathy" is defined as cardiomyopathy due to ischemic heart disease. The classification of cardiomyopathies proposed by the WHO/ISFC Task Force in 1995,[1] however, defines ischemic cardiomyopathy as "a dilated cardiomyopathy with impaired contractile performance not explained by the extent of coronary disease or ischemic damage" reserved for the remodeling process of the noninfarcted myocardium. In this chapter, we will use the term "ischemic cardiomyopathy" defined as cardiomyopathy due to ischemic heart disease rather than the WHO/ISFC Task Force definition.

The existing clinical studies suggest that patients with idiopathic dilated cardiomyopathy have a lower total mortality.[25] The risk of sudden cardiac death, however, appears to be relatively higher in patients with DCM in some studies.[25] The differential treatment benefit seen in DCM patients compared with patients with ischemic cardiomyopathy that has been observed in several randomized clinical trials such as with digoxin[26] or amiodarone[27] suggest that there may be therapeutic differences between ischemic and nonischemic heart failure. Similar earlier reports of survival difference with β-blockers[28] or amlodipine[29] in patients with dilated but not ischemic cardiomyopathy, have not been reproduced in subsequent large-scale randomized trials,[2,28] in which the benefit was similar in both the ischemic and nonischemic heart failure patients. This has raised the question whether there truly is a difference in response to treatment according to the cause of heart failure. On the other hand, the absence of a rigorous definition of "nonischemic heart failure" in many studies may account for this discrepancy and make interpretation of the results difficult. Further studies to clarify the effects of the cause of heart failure could be particularly important to achieve further treatment benefit over and above the conventional treatment strategies that target heart failure as a single disease entity.

PATHOPHYSIOLOGY

Dilated cardiomyopathy may be viewed as a progressive disorder initiated after an "index event" that either damages the heart muscle, with a resultant loss of functioning cardiac myocytes, or alternatively disrupts the ability of the myocardium to generate force, thereby preventing the heart from contracting normally. This index event may have an abrupt onset, as in the case of acute exposure to toxins, or it may have a gradual or insidious onset, as in the case hemodynamic pressure or volume overloading, or it may be hereditary, as in the case of many of the familial cardiomyopathies. Regardless of the nature of the inciting event, the feature that is common to each of these index events is that they all, in some manner, produce a decline in pumping capacity of the heart. The anatomic and pathophysiological abnormalities that occur in LV remodeling are discussed in Chapter 15. Patients with dilated cardiomyopathy generally have dilation of all four chambers of the heart (Figure 24-2). Despite the fact that there is thinning of the LV wall in patients with DCM, there is massive hypertrophy at the level of the intact heart, and at the level of the cardiac myocyte, which has a characteristic elongated appearance that is observed in myocytes obtained from hearts subjected to chronic volume overload (Figure 24-3). The coronary arteries are usually normal in DCM, although it should be emphasized the end-stage "ischemic cardiomyopathies" may also have a dilated phenotype. The cardiac valves are anatomically normal; however, there is usually tricuspid and mitral annular dilation due to cavity enlargement,

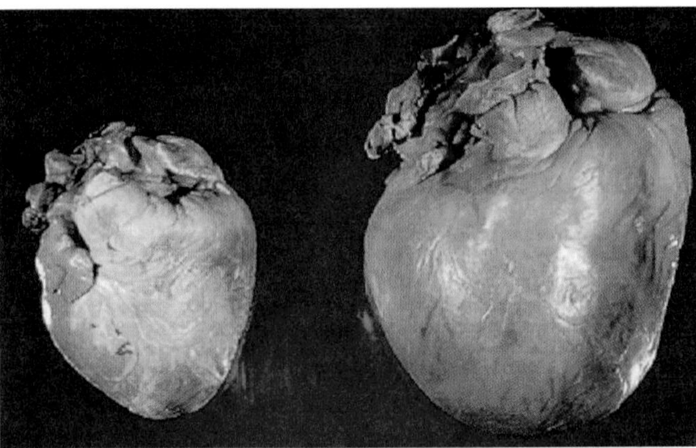

FIGURE 24–2 Pathology of normal heart (*left*) and a dilated cardiomyopathic ventricle (*right*). The dilated cardiomyopathic ventricle is characterized by enlargement of all four cardiac chambers, and a more spherical shape, in comparison to the normal ventricle. (From Kasper EK, Hruban RH, Baughman KL. Idiopathic dilated cardiomyopathy. In Abelman WH, editor. *Atlas of heart diseases: cardiomyopathies, myocarditis and pericardial disease*, Philadelphia, 1995, Current Medicine, reproduced with permission from Current Medicine.)

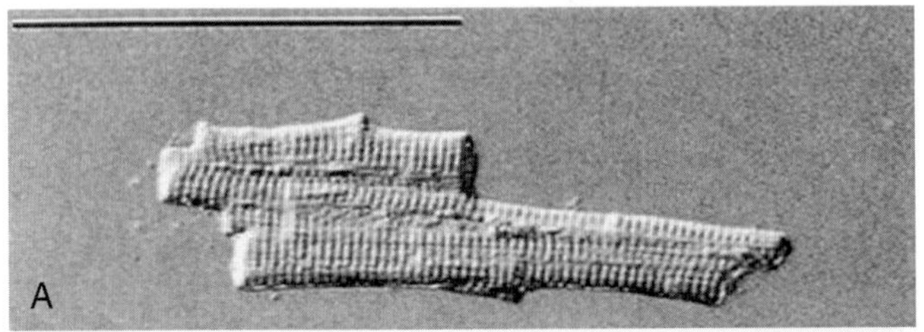

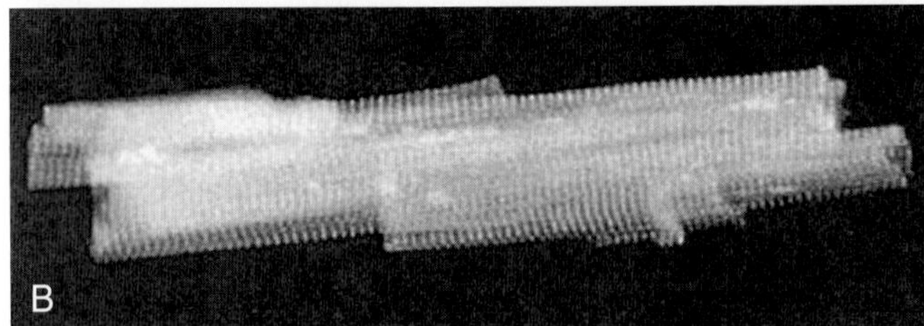

FIGURE 24–3 Cardiac myocyte structure (*top*) in normal myocardium and in dilated cardiomyopathy (*bottom*). Cardiac myocytes isolated from myocardium from patients with DCM have an elongated shape as the result of the sarcomeres being formed in series. (From Gerdes AM, Kellerman SE, Moore JA, et al. Structural remodeling of cardiac myocytes in patients with ischemic cardiomyopathy. *Circulation* 1992;86:426-430, reproduced with permission from Lippincott Williams & Wilkins.)

distortion of subvalvular apparatus, and stretching of the papillary muscles giving rise to valvular regurgitation. Intracavitary thrombi are common usually in the ventricular apex.

Myocardial Diseases Presenting as Dilated Cardiomyopathy

As shown in Figure 24-4, the most common causes of DCM are idiopathic, alcoholic/toxic, inflammatory, familial, and miscellaneous other (inflammatory noninfectious, acquired, metabolic, and nutritional causes). However, it should be recognized that the exact prevalence of the various forms of dilated cardiomyopathy will vary based on the demographics of the patient population. In the section that follows, we will review the various specific causes that lead to the development of DCM.

Idiopathic Dilated Cardiomyopathy

Although the term "idiopathic dilated cardiomyopathy" has become synonymous with that of dilated cardiomyopathy in some heart failure parlance, the term "idiopathic" was originally intended to characterize the subset of DCM patients in whom no known etiological cause for ventricular dilation and depressed myocardial contractility was apparent. However, with increasing sophistication in diagnostic testing, clinicians have become aware that many cases of so-called idiopathic dilated cardiomyopathy may occur as the result of inherited and/or spontaneous mutations of genes that regulate cardiac structure and/or function, such as the genes for cytoskeletal proteins, or as a consequence of undiagnosed hypertension, autoimmune diseases, viral illness, or toxin exposure. Nonetheless, in the context of the present chapter we use the terminology of idiopathic dilated cardiomyopathy to refer to those patients with DCM whose etiological cause remains unknown. As shown in Figure 24-4, idiopathic dilated cardiomyopathy represents the largest subset of patients with DCM; however, as alluded to previously, it is likely that the proportion of patients with idiopathic dilated cardiomyopathy will diminish with increased sophistication in diagnostic testing.

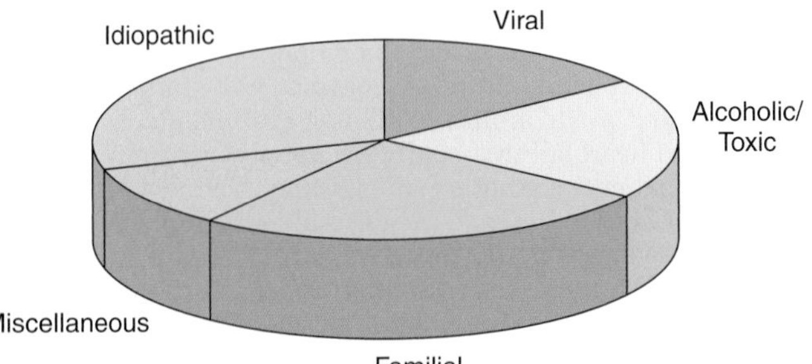

FIGURE 24–4 Causes of dilated cardiomyopathy. As shown, the most frequent causes of DCM are: idiopathic dilated cardiomyopathy; familial cardiomyopathy; alcoholic/toxic cardiomyopathy; viral cardiomyopathy; and miscellaneous other (inflammatory noninfections, acquired, metabolic, and nutritional causes).

Familial Cardiomyopathy

There is growing evidence that many cases of previously diagnosed "idiopathic" dilated cardiomyopathies have a genetic basis. It is estimated that at least 20% to 30% of dilated cardiomyopathy cases are familial. This topic is discussed in detail in Chapter 27.

Alcoholic/Toxic Cardiomyopathy

Alcoholic Cardiomyopathy. Chronic alcoholism is one of the most important causes of dilated cardiomyopathy in the Western world.[30] It is estimated that two thirds of the adult population use alcohol to some extent and more than 10% are heavy users. In the United States, in both sexes and all races, long-term heavy alcohol consumption (of any beverage type) has been quoted as the leading cause of a nonischemic, dilated cardiomyopathy by some investigators.[30] A large proportion of chronic alcoholics demonstrate impairment of cardiac function. The clinical diagnosis of alcoholic cardiomyopathy can be made when biventricular dysfunction and dilation are persistently observed in a heavy drinker, in the absence of other known causes for myocardial disease. Thus the diagnosis of alcoholic cardiomyopathy remains a diagnosis of exclusion. The prevalence of alcoholic cardiomyopathy is variable and ranges from 23% to 40%. Alcoholic cardiomyopathy most commonly occurs in men 30 to 55 years of age who have been heavy consumers of alcohol for more than 10 years. Women represent approximately 14% of the alcoholic cardiomyopathy cases but women may be more vulnerable to the development of alcohol-related cardiomyopathy, since it has been reported that alcoholic cardiomyopathy develops in women with a less total lifetime exposure to alcohol compared with men.[30] In all races, death rates due to alcoholic heart muscle disease are greater in men compared with women, and are greater in

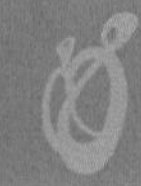

African American men and women compared with white men and women with alcoholic cardiomyopathy.[30] Even before the clinically overt heart failure, LV contractile dysfunction can be demonstrated in alcoholics. Although chronic alcoholic liver disease and heart failure usually are not observed clinically in the same patient, cirrhotic patients may have asymptomatic LV dysfunction, in which case atrial fibrillation is usually the initial presenting manifestation of cardiac dysfunction. The point at which these abnormalities appear during the course of an individual's lifetime of drinking, such that the abnormalities can be called a dilated cardiomyopathy, is not well established and is highly individualized.

The risk of developing alcoholic cardiomyopathy appears to be related to both the mean daily alcohol intake and the duration of drinking. In general, alcoholic patients consuming greater than 90 g of alcohol a day (approximately seven to eight standard drinks per day) for more than 5 years are at risk for the development of asymptomatic alcoholic cardiomyopathy. On the other hand, mild to moderate alcohol consumption has recently been reported to be protective against development of heart failure in the general population. According to the Framingham Heart Study, moderate alcohol consumption is not associated with increased risk for congestive heart failure, and in fact appears to be protective against development of congestive heart failure.[31] Similarly, in a prospective cohort study of elderly persons, moderate alcohol consumption was associated with a decreasing risk of heart failure.[32] These paradoxical findings (i.e., alcohol may be protective against development of heart failure in certain populations when used in moderation, but detrimental in others, especially when used in excess over longer periods of time) suggest that duration of exposure and individual genetic susceptibility play an important role in pathogenesis. Persistent DCM develops in only 1% to 2% of chronic drinkers, and the role of genetic predisposition, or the presence of synergistic cardiovascular factors such as hypertension or arrhythmias in the development of alcohol-related cardiomyopathy are not clear at the present time.

Studies in experimental animals have demonstrated that both acute and chronic ethanol administration impairs cardiac contractility. Alcohol results in acute and chronic depression of myocardial contractility even when ingested by normal individuals in quantities consumed during social drinking.[33] Compensatory mechanisms such as vasodilation or sympathetic stimulation may mask the direct acute myocardial depressant effects of alcohol. Despite the known deleterious effects of alcohol, it has been difficult to produce heart failure in animal models in which ethanol has been administered. Thus the direct causal relationship between alcohol consumption and the development of cardiomyopathy has not been rigorously demonstrated in experimental models, despite the long-recognized clinical relationship between alcohol consumption and the development of DCM. The pathophysiology and progression of alcoholic cardiomyopathy are complex and involve changes in many aspects of myocyte function. The potential mechanisms that have been invoked to explain the depressed myocardial function include the direct toxic effects of alcohol on striated muscle, since most alcoholics have manifestations of skeletal myopathy and cardiomyopathy. Shifts in the relative expression of the contractile proteins α-myosin heavy chain to β-MHC have been reported in animal models after exposure to ethanol.[30] Alcohol and its metabolite acetaldehyde can also cause alterations in cellular calcium, magnesium, or phosphate homeostasis. The toxic effects of acetaldehyde or the formation of fatty acid ethyl esters may also impair mitochondrial oxidative phosphorylation. In acute ethanol toxicity free radical damage and/or ischemia may occur, possibly due to increased xanthine oxidase activity or β-adrenergic stimulation, respectively. In addition, ethanol and its metabolites interfere with numerous membrane and cellular functions such as transport and binding of calcium, mitochondrial respiration, lipid metabolism, myocardial protein synthesis, signal transduction, and excitation contraction coupling.[34] Both autopsy and endomyocardial biopsy specimens from alcoholic cardiomyopathy patients reveal marked mitochondrial swelling, with fragmentation of cristae, swelling of endoplasmic reticulum, entrance of mitochondria into the nucleus potentially promoting attack of mitochondria by nuclear proteins and the attack of nuclear DNA by proteins of the mitochondrial intermembrane space,[35] cytoskeletal disorganization, and destruction of myofibrils (Figure 24-5). Several studies suggest that heavy drinking alters both lymphocyte and granulocyte production and function, raising the possibility that myocardial damage secondary to prolonged alcohol consumption might initiate autoreactive mechanisms comparable to those observed in viral or idiopathic myocarditis. The point at which the changes in mitochondrial, sarcoplasmic reticulum, contractile protein, and calcium homeostasis culminate in intrinsic cell dysfunction is incompletely understood. There are several early reports that support the role for myocyte loss as a final mechanism underlying alcohol-induced cardiac dysfunction. Application of insulin-like growth factor (IGF)-1 has been reported to attenuate the apoptotic effects of ethanol in primary neonatal myocyte cell cultures.[30]

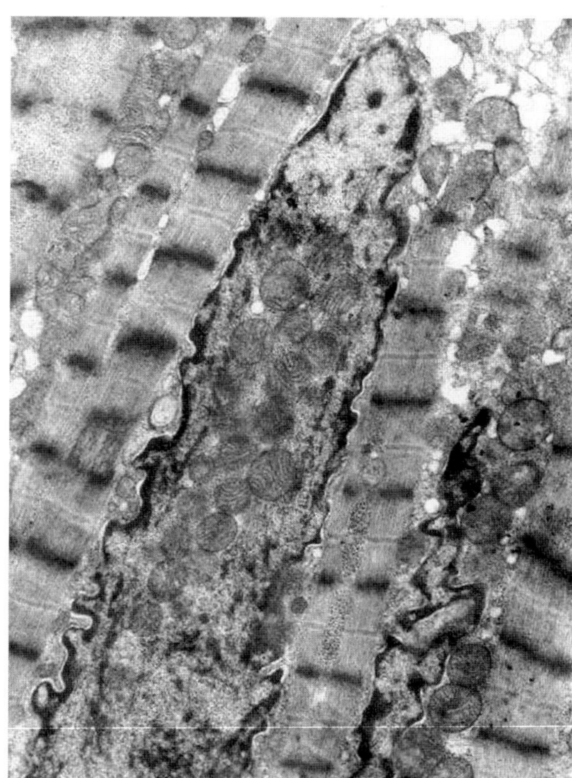

FIGURE 24–5 Electron microscopy of cardiomyocytes of patients with alcoholic cardiomyopathy revealing the presence of nuclei with mitochondria accumulated in their core, associated with chromatin displacement to periphery of the nucleus. (From Bakeeva LE, Skulachev VP, Sudarikova YV, et al. Mitochondria enter the nucleus [one further problem in chronic alcoholism]. *Biochemistry (Mosc)* 2001;66(12):1335-1341, reproduced with permission from *Biochemistry*.)

Recent reports suggest that certain genetic traits influence the occurrence, pathogenesis, and progression of alcoholic cardiomyopathy, which may explain interindividual variations in the sensitivity of the myocardium to alcohol-induced myocardial damage. In addition, nutritional deficiencies, commonly thiamine deficiency, may play an additive role to the direct myocardial damage of ethanol. Thus the cardiomyopathy that develops following chronic alcohol consumption may be multifactorial in origin.

The management of patients with alcohol cardiomyopathy begins with total abstinence from alcohol, in addition to the conventional management of heart failure, as described later. There are currently no studies of specific pharmacotherapies in patients with alcoholic cardiomyopathy other than the standard therapy of heart failure; however, there are numerous reports that detail the reversibility of depressed LV dysfunction after the cessation of drinking.[36] Many heart failure programs limit alcoholic beverage consumption to no more than alcoholic beverage serving daily for all patients with LV dysfunction, regardless of the cause being alcohol related or not.[37] Even if the depressed LV function does not normalize completely, the symptoms and signs of congestive heart failure improve after abstinence.[36] However, the overall prognosis remains poor, with a mortality of 40% to 50% within 3 to 6 years, if the patient is not abstinent.[30] Survival is significantly lower for patients who continue to drink compared with patients with idiopathic DCM or alcoholic cardiomyopathy patients who abstain.[30]

Cocaine Cardiomyopathy. Long-term abuse of cocaine, a drug which causes postsynaptic nervous system norepinephrine reuptake blockade and possible presynaptic release of dopamine and norepinephrine, may eventuate in dilated cardiomyopathy even without presence of coronary artery disease, vasculitis, or regional myocardial injury. This has been termed as "cocaine-related cardiomyopathy" and perhaps reflects the direct toxicity of the cocaine on the myocardium. Depressed LV function has been reported in 4% to 9% of asymptomatic cocaine abusers.[38] Similarly, Om et al reported 18% of cocaine abusers who underwent cardiac catheterization had normal coronary arteries with low ejection fraction and global hypokinesia.[39]

The cardiovascular evaluation of a patient with cocaine abuse usually reflect the following: The electrocardiogram may reveal increased QRS voltage, early repolarization, ischemic or nonspecific ST-T changes, or pathological Q waves. Episodes of ST elevation may be seen during Holter monitoring. An echocardiogram usually reveals LV hypertrophy. Segmental wall motion abnormalities usually suggest myocardial injury; however, as mentioned previously, approximately 18% of patients with cocaine abuse manifest global hypokinesia and depressed myocardial function. Cardiac catheterization in these patients may reveal normal coronaries or mild coronary artery disease not significant enough to explain the extent of myocardial dysfunction. However, accelerated coronary atherosclerosis, coronary vasculitis, coronary spasm, or coronary thrombosis are perhaps more common findings in cocaine-related heart disease.

Cocaine may produce LV dysfunction through its direct toxic effects on the myocardium by provoking coronary arterial spasm (and hence myocardial ischemia), and by causing increased release of catecholamines, which may be directly toxic to cardiac myocytes. These effects will decrease myocardial oxygen supply and may increase demand if heart rate and blood pressure rise. The vasoactive effects of cocaine are further complicated with enhanced platelet aggregation, anticardiolipin antibody formation, and endothelial release of potent vasoconstrictors such as endothelin-1. Upregulation of tissue plasminogen activator inhibitors, increased platelet aggregation, and decreased fibrinolysis by cocaine predispose to coronary thrombosis and or microvascular disease.[38] Myocarditis with inflammatory lymphocytes and eosinophils has also been reported in 20% of patients dying of natural or homicidal causes in whom cocaine was detected, raising the possibility of hypersensitivity myocarditis due to cocaine or associated contaminants.[40] Alternatively, the myocarditis may occur directly in response to the necrosis that is caused by cocaine. Scattered foci of myocyte necrosis, contraction band necrosis, and foci of myocyte fibrosis have been reported in patients with cocaine abuse. Additionally, experimental studies and clinical case reports suggest that cocaine may also cause lethal arrhythmias. Cocaine prolongs repolarization by a depressant effect on potassium current and may generate early after depolarizations.[38]

Other than abstinence, very little is known about the treatment of cocaine-induced cardiac dysfunction. Indeed, there are case reports of reversibility of cardiac function after cessation of drug use. In patients who develop cardiomyopathy, the traditional therapy for LV dysfunction is appropriate. Given that some of the toxicity of cocaine is caused by catecholamine excess and/or myocardial ischemia, the use of β-adrenergic blocking agents appeared to be a logical treatment, both in terms of preventing further disease progression, and for treating the ventricular arrhythmias that are prone to develop in this setting. Two decades ago, the treatment of cocaine-induced cardiovascular effects favored the use of β-blockers, especially propranolol. As the clinical use of propranolol increased, reports of accentuation of cocaine-induced hypertension and myocardial ischemia began to surface, blaming the unopposed α effects of the β-blockers. Although these reports were isolated, the routine use of propranolol and subsequently all β-adrenergic blockers decreased to the point that β-blockers were considered relatively contraindicated in treating cocaine-induced cardiovascular emergencies. The end result is that an entire generation of potent and selective β-adrenergic blocking agents have been overlooked, both for acute and chronic treatment of cocaine-related cardiac disease, due to the possibility of "unopposed α effects." The focus of treatment shifted from the cardiovascular effects to combating central nervous stimulation. As a result, benzodiazepines have been the drug of choice in treating the cerebrovascular and subsequent systemic hyperadrenergic complications of cocaine, and nitroprusside or phentolamine being advocated for peripheral vasodilatory effects. It is now becoming apparent that treatment of cardiovascular effects of cocaine should involve a multifactorial approach to combat both central nervous system and peripheral vasospastic effects of cocaine. In this regard β-adrenergic blocking agents, especially β-blocking agents with both α- and β-blocking properties such as labetalol or carvedilol, may play an important role in treating cocaine-related cardiomyopathy or chronic heart failure. It should also be noted that β-blockers are not recommended to be used in the acute setting of cocaine-related acute coronary syndrome.

Anthracycline. Cardiotoxicity is a well-known side effect of several cytotoxic drugs, especially of the anthracyclines and can lead to long-term morbidity (see also Chapter 58). Anthracyclines, such as doxorubicin (Adriamycin) and daunorubicin, produce cardiac toxicity, possibly by increasing oxygen-free radical generation, platelet activating factor, prostaglandins, histamine, calcium, and C-13 hydroxy metabolites, or by interfering with sarcolemmal sodium potassium pump and mitochondrial electron transport chain. The formation of oxygen-free radicals that are generated by iron-catalyzed pathways appears to be the most important pathway in the pathogenesis of anthracycline-induced cardiomyopathy because it has been noted that iron-chelating agents that prevent generation of oxygen-free radicals, such as dexrazoxane, are cardioprotective. The prognosis of anthracycline-induced cardiomyopathy relates to the time course of treatment and preexisting additional risk factors for myocardial injury such as radiation, coexisting coronary artery disease, and preexisting cardiac dysfunction. In general, patients with anthracycline-induced cardiomyopathy have a worse survival than that seen with idiopathic DCM (Figure 24-6). Prevention of anthracycline-induced myocardial damage by use of free radical "scavengers" and antioxidants may reduce cardiotoxicity in some patients. Other chemotherapeutic agents in cancer associated with cardiac toxicity complications are the monoclonal antibody trastuzumab (Herceptin), high-dose cyclophosphamide,

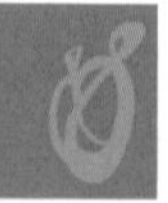

taxoids, mitomycin-C, 5-fluorouracil, and the interferons. In contrast to anthracycline-induced cardiac toxicity, trastuzumab-related cardiac dysfunction does not appear to increase with cumulative dose or to be associated with ultrastructural changes in the myocardium and is generally reversible. This topic is discussed in further detail in Chapter 58.

Other Myocardial Toxins. In addition to the classic toxins described previously, as shown in Table 24-1, there are a number of other toxic agents that may lead to LV dysfunction and heart failure, including cobalt and catecholamines. One such agent, ephedra, which has been used for the purposes of athletic performance enhancement and weight loss, has been linked to a high rate of serious adverse outcomes including LV systolic dysfunction, development of heart failure, and cardiac deaths ultimately resulting in the ban of this agent by the U.S. Food and Drug Administration.

Inflammation-induced Cardiomyopathy

Over the past 10 to 15 years there has been increasing evidence, which suggests that inflammation and/or inflammatory processes may contribute to the overall pathogenesis of dilated cardiomyopathy. Moreover, there is increasing evidence that biological properties of inflammatory mediators, such as proinflammatory cytokines, are also sufficient to produce a dilated cardiac phenotype.[41] As will be discussed later and in Chapter 11, both infectious and noninfectious inflammatory processes may lead to the development of DCM. Although a great many infections and noninfectious processes may impact the myocardium, and may transiently lead to systolic dysfunction and congestive symptomatology, the great majority of these infections and noninfectious processes do not lead to the development of DCM. Therefore, in the section that follows, we will focus primarily on those disease states that are considered to lead to DCM.

Inflammation-induced Cardiomyopathy: Infectious Causes

Viral Cardiomyopathy. The subject of viral myocarditis and is covered in detail in Chapter 31.

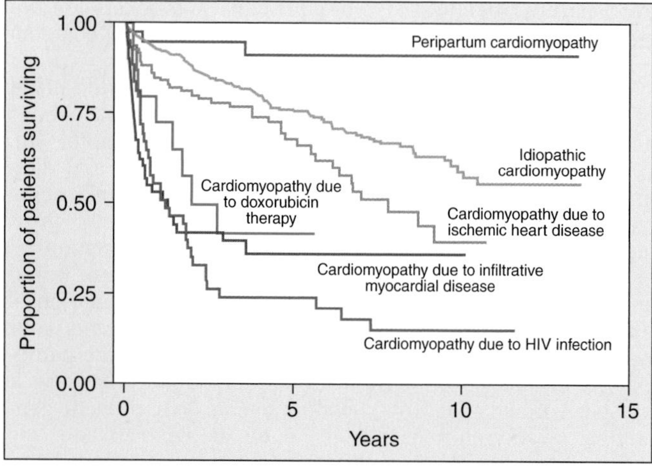

FIGURE 24–6 Survival according to different causes of dilated cardiomyopathy. In a cohort of patients who underwent endomyocardial biopsy as part of an evaluation for heart failure due to unexplained cardiomyopathy, when compared with the patients with idiopathic cardiomyopathy, survival significantly better in patients with peripartum cardiomyopathy and significantly worse among the patients with cardiomyopathy due to infiltrative myocardial disease, HIV infection, therapy with doxorubicin, and ischemic heart disease. (Felker GM, Thompson RE, Hare JM, et al. Underlying causes and long-term survival in patients with initially unexplained cardiomyopathy. *N Engl J Med* 2000;342:1077-1084, reproduced with permission from the *New England Journal of Medicine.*)

Acquired Immunodeficiency Syndrome (AIDS). Several investigators have reported that there is an association between AIDS and dilated cardiomyopathy. Reviews and studies published before the introduction of highly active antiretroviral therapy regimens have correlated the incidence and course of human immunodeficiency virus (HIV) infection in relation to dilated cardiomyopathy in both children and adults. In a long-term echocardiographic follow-up by Barbaro et al,[42] 8% of initially asymptomatic HIV-positive patients were diagnosed with dilated cardiomyopathy during the 60-month follow-up. All patients with dilated cardiomyopathy were in NYHA functional class III or IV. The mean annual incidence rate was 15.9 cases per 1000 patients. The extent of immunodeficiency of the patients, as assessed by the CD4 count, influenced the incidence of dilated cardiomyopathy; specifically, there was a higher incidence among patients with a CD4 count of less than 400 cells per cubic millimeter.

Current hypotheses concerning the pathogenesis of cardiomyopathy associated with infection with the human immunodeficiency virus include infection of myocardial cells with HIV type 1 or coinfection with other cardiotropic viruses, postviral cardiac autoimmunity, autonomic dysfunction, cardiotoxicity from illicit drugs, and pharmacological agents (such as nucleoside analogues and pentamidine), nutritional deficiencies, and prolonged immunosuppression. Recently it has been demonstrated that targeted myocardial expression of HIV transactivator in transgenic mice results in cardiomyopathy and mitochondrial damage,[43] emphasizing the role of the HIV infection itself in AIDS cardiomyopathy. The role of HIV type 1 infection of cardiac myocytes in the development of dilated cardiomyopathy in HIV has not been fully characterized. Even though human myocardial cells are not known to express CD4 cells, autopsy series of persons dying from AIDS-related illnesses demonstrate histological evidence of myocarditis in approximately 50% of the patients.[44] By in situ hybridization techniques in cardiac tissue sections, HIV nucleic acid sequences were detected in 27% of the patients who died of AIDS (Figure 24-7).[45] Symptomatic heart failure is seen in approximately half of these patients with myocardial involvement. Whether early treatment with angiotensin-converting enzyme inhibitors and/or β-blockers will prevent and/or retard disease progression in these patients is unknown at this time. The treatment of patients with symptomatic HIV

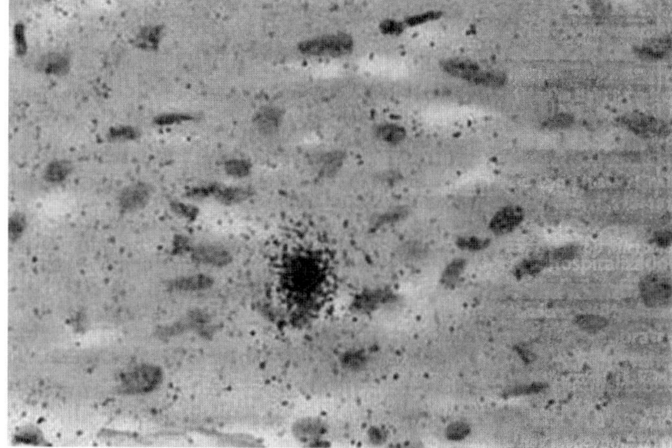

FIGURE 24–7 In situ hybridization of HIV RNA probe in a section of myocardial tissue obtained at autopsy from AIDS patients. There is intense staining within and around one myocyte. Using sulfur-35-labeled ribonucleic acid probes, HIV nucleic acid sequences were detected in cardiac tissue sections (hematoxylin and eosin, 400×). (From Grody WW, Cheng L, Lewis W. Infection of the heart by the human immunodeficiency virus. *Am J Cardiol* 1990;66:203-206, reproduced with permission from the *American Journal of Cardiology.*)

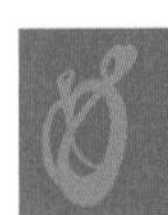

cardiomyopathy is the same as the conventional treatment for patients with DCM. The prognosis of HIV cardiomyopathy remains poor, with more than a 50% mortality rate in 2 to 3 years (see Figure 24-6).

Chagas Disease (see also Chapter 33). Although Chagas disease is a relatively uncommon cause of DCM in North America, Chagas disease remains a leading cause of death in many areas of Central and South America (see Chapter 33). Indeed, 50,000 people die of Chagas disease each year.[46] *Trypanosoma cruzi*, the causative organism for Chagas disease is found only in the Western hemisphere, where it primarily infects wild and domestic mammals and insects. Humans become involved when infected vectors infest the simple houses that are common in Latin America. It is estimated that 16 to 18 million people have chronic *T. cruzi* infection. Chagas control programs in certain South American countries have demonstrated significant decline in the seropositive subjects from 47.8% to 17.1%, most marked among children and teenagers from 29.9% to 1.9%, suggesting reduction in transmission of the disease.[46] There are three different clinical and pathophysiological phases of disease: the acute, indeterminate, and chronic phases. Sudden cardiac death can occur during each phase; however, DCM is a late manifestation of the disease and is generally seen during the chronic phase. Acute Chagas disease is usually a mild illness with a case fatality rate of less than 5%. The systemic spread of the parasites from the site of entry and their initial multiplication may be accompanied by fever, malaise, and edema of the face and lower extremities, and generalized lymphadenopathy and hepatosplenomegaly. Muscles, including the heart, are often heavily parasitized, and severe myocarditis develops in a small proportion of patients. The acute illness resolves spontaneously over a period of 4 to 6 weeks in most patients, who then enter the indeterminate phase of *T. cruzi* infection. In this phase there are no symptoms, but there are lifelong, low-grade parasitemias in association with antibodies to many *T. cruzi* antigens. Many people in this phase have subtle signs of cardiac or gastrointestinal involvement long before the disease becomes symptomatic. Most infected people remain in the indeterminate phase for life. However, this carrier state can be a major cause of transfusion-associated transmission of the parasite. Symptomatic chronic Chagas disease develops in an estimated 10% to 30% of infected persons, years or even decades after the *T. cruzi* infection is acquired. The heart is most commonly affected, and the pathological changes may include biventricular enlargement, thinning of ventricular walls, apical aneurysms, and mural thrombi. Widespread lymphocytic infiltration is often seen in stained specimens of cardiac tissue and diffuse interstitial fibrosis and atrophy of myocardial cells. The conduction system is often affected, typically resulting in right bundle branch block, left anterior fascicular block, or complete atrioventricular block. The symptoms reflect the dysrhythmias, cardiomyopathy, and thromboembolism that develop over time. Death usually results from rhythm disturbances or progressive heart failure. The overall prognosis for patients with Chagas cardiomyopathy and heart failure is poor, with 50% of patients dying within a period of 47 months. The presence of complete heart block, atrial fibrillation, left bundle branch block, and complex ventricular ectopy auger a poor prognosis.

The leading hypothesis with respect to the pathogenesis of Chagas cardiomyopathy is that patients develop progressive myocardial damage due to parasite persistence and autoimmune responses. [46] The neurogenic hypothesis of Chagas cardiomyopathy suggests that the cardiac parasympathetic neurones are irreversibly damaged by the parasite during the acute phase of the disease. As a consequence, the cardiac sympathetic nervous system is unopposed and the cardiotoxic effects of a permanent and excessive sympathetic activation are responsible for the relentless progression of myocardial damage. However, activation of the sympathetic nervous system and of the renin-angiotensin-aldosterone system, is a late event in the natural history of Chagas disease and patients with parasite persistence but no segmental myocardial damage do not have neurohormonal activation.[46] Myocardial ischemia and coronary microcirculation abnormalities have also been demonstrated in animal models and in humans with Chagas disease.

The pharmacological treatment for *T. cruzi* infection remains unsatisfactory. Extensive clinical experience has been accumulated with two drugs: benznidazole and nifurtimox. Both shorten the acute phase of *T. cruzi* infection and decrease mortality, but they achieve parasitological cures in only about 50% of treated patients; moreover, these drugs cause substantial toxicity.[46] Other than treatment of the infection, treatment of cardiomyopathy is the same as the conventional treatment of patients with DCM.

Inflammation-induced Cardiomyopathy: Noninfectious Causes

Hypersensitivity Myocarditis. Hypersensitivity to a variety of agents may result in allergic reactions that involve the myocardium, characterized by peripheral eosinophilia, and a perivascular infiltration of the myocardium by eosinophils, lymphocytes, and histiocytes. These infiltrates may be occasionally associated with necrosis. A variety of drugs, most commonly the sulfonamides, penicillins, methyldopa, and other agents such as amphotericin B, streptomycin, phenytoin, isoniazid, tetanus toxoid, hydrochlorothiazide, and chlorthalidone have been reported to cause allergic hypersensitivity myocarditis. Most patients are not clinically ill, but may die suddenly, presumably secondary to an arrhythmia. Hypersensitivity myocarditis is recognized only rarely clinically, but may be sufficient to produce global and/or regional myocardial dysfunction detected by noninvasive methods. This entity is often first diagnosed on postmortem examination, and occasionally on endomyocardial biopsy.[47]

Systemic Lupus Erythematosus (SLE). Although a number of cardiac abnormalities have been reported in patients with SLE, the development of DCM is not a prominent manifestation of this disease process. Global LV dysfunction has been reported in 5%, segmental LV wall motion abnormalities in 4%, and right ventricular enlargement in 4% of patients with SLE. In general the abnormalities in cardiac function usually correlate with disease activity. The myocardial involvement is frequently found at autopsy or at endomyocardial biopsy and is less easily detected clinically. The myocardial lesions are characterized by an increase in interstitial connective tissue and myocardial scarring. Recent studies suggest that depolarization abnormalities on signal average ECG accompanied with echocardiographic evidence of abnormal LV filling may reflect the presence of myocardial fibrosis and could be a marker of subclinical myocardial involvement in SLE patients.[48] Cardiac involvement may manifest itself by conduction system abnormalities such as complete atrioventricular heart block. Neonatal lupus especially is characterized by congenital heart block, and cardiomyopathy, cutaneous lupus lesions, hepatobiliary disease, and thrombocytopenia.

Scleroderma. The development of DCM is rare in patients with scleroderma. A recent echocardiographic study showed that although there was no difference in LV dimensions or fractional shortening in patients with scleroderma, there was indication of systolic impairment in the majority of patients.[49] A distinctive focal myocardial lesion ranging from contraction band necrosis to replacement fibrosis without morphological abnormalities of the coronary arteries is noted in approximately half of the patients with scleroderma. This is postulated to be due to intermittent vascular spasm with intramyocardial Raynaud phenomenon. Thus progressive systemic sclerosis can lead to conduction abnormalities, arrhythmias, heart failure, angina pectoris with normal

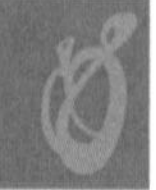

coronary arteries, myocardial fibrosis, pericarditis, and sudden death. Late contrast enhancement with gadolinium may be used to characterize patchy fibrosis and myocardial edema interspersed with normal myocardium in scleroderma. Cardiac involvement in systemic sclerosis portends an ominous prognosis, and is probably most directly related to the extent of myocardial fibrosis.

Rheumatoid Arthritis. Cardiac involvement in rheumatoid arthritis generally results from the development of myocarditis and/or pericarditis. However, the development of DCM is rare in these patients. In a retrospective study of 172 patients with juvenile rheumatoid arthritis, symptomatic cardiac involvement occurred in 7.6% of patients, including pericarditis, perimyocarditis, and myocarditis. Both myocarditis and pericarditis are regarded as poor prognostic factors in rheumatoid arthritis.[50] Myocardial involvement in rheumatoid arthritis is thought to be secondary to disturbances in the microcirculation secondary to microvasculitis, and occurs in the absence of any clinical symptoms of ECG changes.

Kawasaki Disease. Kawasaki disease is an acute febrile illness associated with mucosal inflammation, skin rash, and cervical lymphadenopathy. This disease is recognized most often in children less than 4 years of age. Kawasaki disease represents an acute vasculitic syndrome of unknown cause that primarily affects small- and medium-sized arteries, including coronary arteries. Coronary arterial aneurysms are seen in 25% to 55% of the acute Kawasaki cases. Of these, 4.7% progress to premature atherosclerotic ischemic heart disease. Myocardial infarction is noted in approximately 2% of patients, and cardiovascular death is reported in 0.8%. Although the development of DCM is not typical for Kawasaki disease, repetitive infarctions secondary to coronary arterial aneurysms may lead to a dilated cardiomyopathic phenotype.

Peripartum Cardiomyopathy. Peripartum cardiomyopathy is a disease of unknown cause in which severe LV dysfunction occurs during the last trimester of pregnancy or the early puerperium. It is reported in 1 in 1300 to 1 in 4000 live births. In the past, the diagnosis of this entity was made on clinical grounds; however, modern echocardiographic techniques have allowed more accurate diagnoses by excluding cases of diseases that mimic the clinical symptoms and signs of heart failure. Risk factors for peripartum cardiomyopathy include advanced maternal age, multiparity, African descent, twinning, and long-term tocolysis. Anticoagulation is strongly recommended, especially if ventricular dysfunction is persistent. Although its cause remains unknown, most theories have focused on the hemodynamic and immunological stresses of pregnancy. An immune pathogenesis is supported by the frequent finding of lymphocytic myocarditis on myocardial biopsy and the fact that multiparity or previous exposure to fetal antigens is a significant risk factor.[51]

The prognosis of peripartum cardiomyopathy is related to the recovery of ventricular function. In contrast to patients with idiopathic dilated cardiomyopathy, significant improvement in myocardial function is seen in 30% to 50% of patients in the first 6 months after presentation (see Figure 24-6).[51] However, for those patients who do not recover to normal or near-normal function, the prognosis is similar to other forms of dilated cardiomyopathy.[52] Cardiomegaly that persists for more than 4 months after diagnosis indicates a poor prognosis, with a 50% mortality at 6 years.

Diagnosis is based upon the clinical presentation of congestive heart failure and objective evidence of LV systolic dysfunction. Conventional pharmacological therapy for congestive heart failure, such as diuretics, digoxin, angiotensin-converting enzyme inhibitors, angiotensin receptor blockers, and β-adrenergic blockers, are routinely used and are quite effective. Aggressive use of implantable defibrillators and advances in medical therapy have significantly reduced the risk of sudden death and all-cause mortality rates. More recently, the use of bromocriptine, a dopamine D2 receptor agonist, has been investigated in the treatment of PPM. Oxidative stress in the setting of pregnancy or in the postpartum period leads to the cleavage of the conventional prolactin molecule into a form which appears to have a detrimental effect on the myocardium by promoting apoptosis, vasoconstriction, and inflammation. In several human case reports of postpartum cardiomyopathy, treatment with bromocriptine resulted in improvement in clinical status and LV function. For those patients who remain refractory to conventional pharmacological therapy, cardiac transplantation and mechanical circulatory support are viable options. For greater than 50% of peripartum cardiomyopathy patients, LV function normalizes with pharmacological therapy. However, subsequent pregnancies almost always are associated with recurrence of LV systolic dysfunction. Caution is advised against subsequent pregnancy, especially if LV dysfunction is persistent.

Endocrine and Metabolic Causes of Cardiomyopathy

Obesity. Obesity cardiomyopathy is defined as congestive heart failure due entirely or predominantly to obesity. Heart failure in the markedly obese usually develops over a long period of time, and can be directly related to the duration of obesity (see chapter 20). Initially the dyspnea and edema in these patients are simply related to alterations in LV compliance, diastolic heart failure with resultant elevated filling pressures. However, with chronicity, some of these patients will develop significant LV hypertrophy, increased LV mass, and some subsequently develop DCM. Although the precise reasons for obesity-related heart failure are not known, it is thought that the excessive adipose accumulation results in an increase in circulating blood volume; subsequently, it results in a persistent increase in cardiac output, cardiac work, and systemic blood pressure, which ultimately lead to myocardial failure.[53] Furthermore, there is increased prevalence of hypertension and coronary artery disease in obese patients, which may also contribute to the development of DCM in these patients. Recently, cardiac myocyte injury by lipotoxicity has been implicated as a potential mechanism, especially in individuals with metabolic syndrome and insulin resistance. Cardiac lipotoxicity is hypothesized to arise from an imbalance between fatty acid uptake and use, leading to the inappropriate accumulation of free fatty acids and neutral lipids within cardiomyocytes. This lipid overload causes cellular dysfunction, cell death, and eventual organ dysfunction.[54] Obesity-related hypoventilation and sleep apnea may also contribute to the pathophysiology. A recent study examining the relation between obesity and heart failure in participants in the Framingham Heart Study[55] reported that after adjustment for established risk factors, there was an increase in the risk of heart failure of 5% for men and 7% for women for each increment of 1 in the body mass index. When compared with subjects with a normal body mass index, obese subjects had a doubling of the risk of heart failure. Obesity alone was estimated to account for 11% of cases of heart failure in men and 14% of those in women.[55] Given the high prevalence of obesity in Western countries in the past decade, strategies to promote optimal body weight may reduce the population burden of heart failure. In addition to its recognized risk for development of heart failure, intuitively, one would anticipate that obesity would adversely affect the outcome of patients with established heart failure. Interestingly however, there is a recognized paradox with obesity and heart failure, and that is, in patients with established heart failure, obesity is associated with better clinical outcomes.[56] (Figure 24-8). This paradox, though not clearly understood, may partly be due to comparison of individuals in a noncatabolic state with the ability to gain weight to individuals who are lean or cachectic due to advanced heart failure;

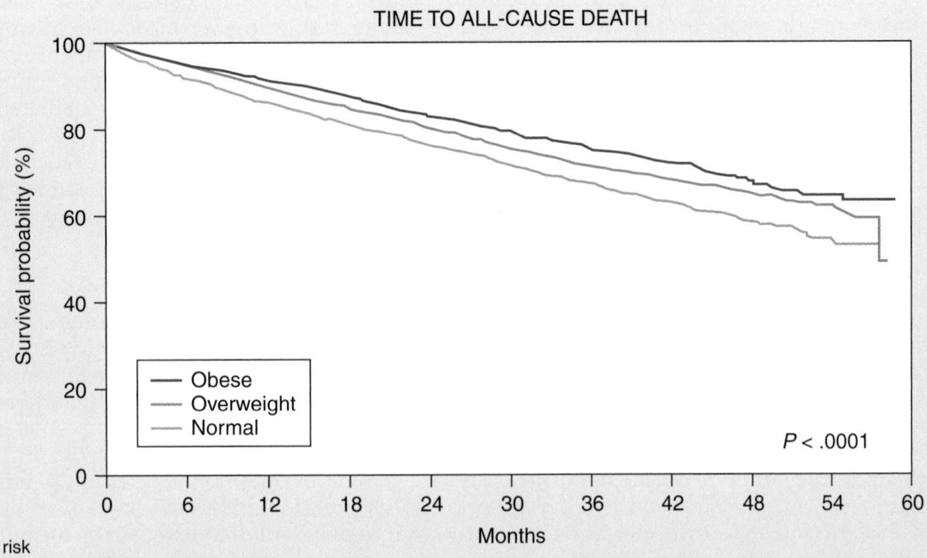

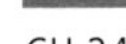

TIME TO ALL-CAUSE DEATH

Survival probability (%): 0, 20, 40, 60, 80, 100

Obese / Overweight / Normal

$P < .0001$

Months: 0, 6, 12, 18, 24, 30, 36, 42, 48, 54, 60

No. at risk	0	6	12	18	24	30	36	42	48	54	60
Normal weight	2583	2374	2227	2089	1958	1746	1352	973	527	100	12
Overweight	3084	2936	2776	2612	2469	2199	1748	1276	730	172	20
Obese	1960	1868	1789	1712	1616	1466	1124	785	406	97	10

FIGURE 24–8 Kaplan-Meier survival curves by body mass index in the obese, overweight, and normal-weight groups in patients with heart failure. The number of patients at risk for death at each 6-month interval is shown below the figure. (From Bozkurt B, Deswal A. Obesity as a prognostic factor in chronic symptomatic heart failure. *Am Heart J* 2005;150:1233-1239, reproduced with permission from *American Heart Journal*.)

selective survival of different subtypes of obese individuals; earlier detection or misdiagnosis of heart failure in obese patients due to increased prevalence of dyspnea and edema; differences in cause of heart failure in obese (hypertension, diabetes) versus nonobese (coronary artery disease); the endocrine/paracrine role of the adipose tissue, which may also participate in metabolic turnover or rapid degradation of certain chemokines; and neurohormones including natriuretic peptides. Ongoing studies will provide more insight into the obesity paradox in heart failure. Although there are anecdotal reports regarding symptomatic improvement following weight reduction in obesity-induced heart failure, large-scale clinical trials on the role of weight loss in heart failure patients with obesity have not yet been performed.[57,58] The safety and efficacy of weight loss drugs, such as orlistat or sibutramine, have not been tested in large-scale trials in cardiac patients. There has been concern against use of sibutramine in heart failure due to reports of development of cardiomyopathy, and this medication is contraindicated in heart failure.[59] In small-scale pilot studies, orlistat appeared to be tolerated and effective in weight loss in heart failure patients with obesity, but ongoing investigations are under way regarding its hepatic safety profile.[60] Similarly, there are no large-scale studies on safety or efficacy of weight loss with lifestyle modification with diet or exercise in obese heart failure patients. Since the prevalence of obesity is increasing in the general and in the heart failure population, examination of obesity and prevention and treatment options will be critical in heart failure patients.

Diabetic Cardiomyopathy (see chapter 24). Since its first description in 1972, a considerable amount of experimental, pathological, epidemiological, and clinical data have accumulated to support the existence of "diabetic cardiomyopathy." So far, a large body of literature suggests that the occurrence of diabetic cardiomyopathy is an independent phenomenon from macroangiographic changes in coronary arteries and hypertension. Diabetes is now well recognized as an independent risk factor for the development of heart failure despite correcting for age, hypertension, obesity, hypercholesterolemia, and coronary artery disease. This subject is covered in further detail in Chapter 20 of this textbook.

Hyperthyroidism. Hyperthyroidism has been implicated in causing dilated cardiomyopathy; however, in view of the increased cardiac contractile function of patients with hyperthyroidism, the development of heart failure is unexpected and raises the question whether there truly is a direct causal association between hyperthyroidism and cardiomyopathy. Patients with hyperthyroidism may occasionally have exertional dyspnea or other symptoms and signs of heart failure. Many of these clinical manifestations may be attributed to the direct effects of thyroid hormone on cardiovascular hemodynamics. In most patients with hyperthyroidism, cardiac output is high, and the subnormal response to exercise may be the result of an inability to increase heart rate maximally or to lower vascular resistance further, as normally occurs with exercise. The term "high-output failure" is not appropriate for all cases of cardiomyopathy related to hyperthyroidism because the ability of the heart to maintain increased cardiac output at rest and with exercise is usually preserved.[61] Occasional patients with severe, long-standing hyperthyroidism have poor cardiac contractility, low cardiac output, and symptoms and signs of heart failure, including a third heart sound and pulmonary congestion. This complex of findings most commonly occurs with persistent sinus tachycardia or atrial fibrillation and is the result of so-called tachycardia-related heart failure. In older patients with heart disease, the increased workload that results from hyperthyroidism may further impair cardiac function and thus result in dilated cardiomyopathy. The presence of ischemic or hypertensive heart disease may compromise the ability of the myocardium to respond to the metabolic demands of hyperthyroidism. Histological examination usually reveals a nonspecific pattern, including foci of lymphocytic and eosinophilic infiltration, fibrosis, fatty infiltration, and myofibril hypertrophy. Although enhanced adrenergic activity contributes to the hyperdynamic state in hyperthyroidism, β-adrenergic blockade does not fully return the heart rate or contractility to normal, which may suggest a primary cardiac effect of thyroid hormone with contributory effects of catecholamines.[61]

Hypothyroidism. Abnormalities in cardiac systolic and diastolic performance have been reported both in experimental and clinical studies of hypothyroidism; however, the

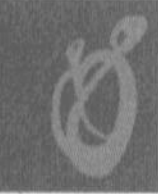

classic findings of myxedema do not usually indicate cardiomyopathy. The most common signs are bradycardia, mild hypertension, a narrowed pulse pressure, and attenuated activity on the precordial examination. Pericardial effusions and nonpitting edema (myxedema) can occur in patients with severe, long-standing hypothyroidism. The low cardiac output is caused by bradycardia, a decrease in ventricular filling, and a decrease in cardiac contractility. Systemic vascular resistance may increase by as much as 50%, and diastolic relaxation and filling are slowed.[61] However, heart failure is rare, because the cardiac output is usually sufficient to meet the lowered demand for peripheral oxygen delivery. Positron-emission tomographic studies of oxygen consumption in patients with hypothyroidism have revealed that myocardial work efficiency is lower than in normal subjects. From 10% to 25% of patients have diastolic hypertension, which combined with the increase in vascular resistance, raises cardiac afterload and cardiac work.[61] Abnormal systolic force may improve with thyroid hormone replacement but does not return to normal levels, suggesting the possibility of persistent myocardial dysfunction.[62] Thyroid hormone replacement should be initiated at low doses and titrated slowly as LV failure may be precipitated. Interestingly, patients with heart failure also have low serum triiodothyronine concentrations, and the decrease is proportional to the degree of heart failure. Whether such changes in thyroid hormone metabolism contribute to further impairment of cardiovascular function in patients with heart failure is not known.[61]

Acromegaly and Growth Hormone Deficiency. Impaired cardiovascular function has recently been demonstrated to potentially reduce life expectancy both in growth hormone deficiency and excess. Experimental and clinical studies have supported the evidence that growth hormone and insulin-like growth factor-1 (IGF-1) are implicated in cardiac development.[63] In most patients with acromegaly, a specific cardiomyopathy, characterized by myocardial hypertrophy with interstitial fibrosis, lymphomononuclear infiltration, and areas of monocyte necrosis, results in biventricular concentric hypertrophy.[63] Myocardial dysfunction is a major cause of morbidity and mortality in acromegaly, and appears to be related to both the severity and duration of growth hormone excess. In contrast, patients with childhood or adult-onset growth hormone deficiency may suffer both from structural cardiac abnormalities, such as narrowing of cardiac walls, and functional impairment that combine to reduce diastolic filling and impair LV response to peak exercise. In addition, growth hormone deficiency patients may have an increase in vascular intima-media thickness and a higher occurrence of atheromatous plaques, which can further aggravate the hemodynamic conditions and contribute to increased cardiovascular and cerebrovascular risk. Several studies have suggested that the cardiovascular abnormalities can be partially reversed by suppressing growth hormone and IGF-1 levels in acromegaly or after growth hormone replacement therapy in growth hormone deficiency patients.[63] Receptors for both growth hormone and IGF-1 are expressed by cardiac myocytes; therefore, growth hormone may act directly on the heart or via the induction of local or systemic IGF-1, while IGF-1 may act by endocrine, paracrine, or autocrine mechanisms. Animal models of pressure and volume overload have demonstrated upregulation of cardiac IGF-1 production and expression of growth hormone and IGF-1 receptors, implying that the local regulation of these factors is influenced by hemodynamic changes.[63] Moreover, experimental studies suggest that growth hormone and IGF-1 have stimulatory effects on myocardial contractility, possibly mediated by changes in intracellular calcium handling. Thus recently, much attention has been focused on the ability of growth hormone to increase cardiac mass, suggesting its possible use in the treatment of chronic heart failure. Initial studies demonstrated that treatment with growth hormone may result in improvement in the hemodynamic and clinical status of patients with heart failure; however, two randomized, placebo-controlled studies did not show any significant growth hormone–mediated improvement in cardiac performance in patients with dilated cardiomyopathy despite significant increases in IGF-1.[64] Although these data need to be confirmed in more extensive studies, such promising results seem to open new perspectives for growth hormone treatment in humans.

Nutritional Causes of Cardiomyopathy

Thiamine Deficiency. Thiamine serves as a cofactor for several enzymes involved primarily in the carbohydrate catabolism and is found in high concentrations in the heart, skeletal muscle, liver, kidneys, and brain. The most common cause of thiamine deficiency in Western countries is chronic alcoholism and anorexia nervosa. AIDS and pregnancy can account for other rare causes of thiamine deficiency.[65] A state of severe depletion can develop in patients on a strict thiamine-deficient diet in approximately 18 to 21 days. The major manifestations of thiamine deficiency in humans involve the cardiovascular (wet beriberi) and nervous (dry beriberi, or neuropathy and/or Wernicke-Korsakoff syndrome) systems. The cardiovascular signs and symptoms include dyspnea, fatigue, leg edema, and palpitations. Tachycardia is common and there are usually increased jugular venous pressure and warm extremities. Biventricular heart failure is present and the circulation is usually hyperkinetic. Ultimately circulatory collapse, metabolic acidosis, or shock can develop, at which time the disease has advanced from chronic beriberi to fulminating beriberi heart failure (Shoshin beriberi). Severe lactic acidemia in the presence of a high cardiac output and extremely low oxygen consumption are the classic features of acute fulminant cardiovascular beriberi, which, if unrecognized and untreated, can lead to high cardiac output failure and death. Treatment for beriberi should consist of administration of thiamine along with other conventional treatment of circulatory support and heart failure.

Carnitine Deficiency. L-carnitine and its derivative, propionyl-L-carnitine, are organic amines necessary for oxidation of fatty acids, the deficiency of which may be associated with a syndrome of progressive skeletal myopathy and lipid vacuoles on muscle biopsy.[66] They have also been shown to reduce intracellular accumulation of toxic metabolites during ischemia, demonstrate protective effects on muscle metabolism injuries, inhibit caspases, and decrease the levels of TNF-α and sphingosine, and reduce apoptosis of skeletal muscle cells and thus have been implied in the treatment of congestive heart failure. Several metabolic genes, including the muscle carnitine palmitoyl transferase-1, the key enzyme for the transport of long-chain acyl-coenzyme A (acyl-CoA) compounds into mitochondria, are downregulated in the failing human heart.[67] Inhibitors of carnitine palmitoyl-transferase I (CPT I), such as etomoxir, have been developed as agents for treating diabetes mellitus. Despite initial promising preclinical and phase II clinical results, a double-blind randomized multicenter clinical trial with etomoxir in heart failure was stopped prematurely, because unacceptably high liver transaminase levels were detected in four patients taking etomoxir.[68]

Selenium Deficiency. Selenium deficiency is associated with cardiomyopathy and congestive heart failure in geographic areas where dietary selenium intake is low.[69] This has been named as the Keshan disease due to the geographical prevalence of a specific form of dilated cardiomyopathy in northeast China, in which the soil has a low selenium content. Chronic selenium deficiency may also occur in individuals with malabsorption and long-term selenium-deficient parenteral nutrition. Selenium deficiency is implicated in causing

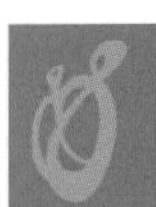

cardiomyopathy as a result of the depletion of selenium-associated antioxidant enzymes; selenoenzymes, which protect cell membranes from damage by free radicals. The cardiomyopathy is manifested by insidious onset of congestive heart failure or a complication of sudden death or thromboembolic phenomena. The heart shows biventricular enlargement and histologically exhibits edema, mitochondrial swelling, hypercontraction bands, widespread myocytolysis, and extensive fibrosis.[69]

Hematological Causes of Cardiomyopathy

Cardiomyopathy Due to Iron Overload: Hemochromatosis and Thalassemia. Iron-overload cardiomyopathy manifests itself as systolic or diastolic dysfunction secondary to increased deposition of iron in the heart and occurs with common genetic disorders such as primary hemochromatosis and β-thalassemia major.

Hereditary hemochromatosis is an inherited disorder of iron metabolism and is the most common hereditary disease of northern Europeans with a prevalence of approximately 5 per 1000. It is an autosomal recessive disorder of iron metabolism characterized by increased iron absorption and deposition in the liver, pancreas, heart, joints, and pituitary gland. Without treatment, death may occur from cirrhosis, primary liver cancer, diabetes, or cardiomyopathy. In 1996, HFE, the gene for hereditary hemochromatosis, was mapped on the short arm of chromosome 6.[70] Two mutations have been implicated in hereditary hemochromatosis: C282Y and H63D, resulting in excessive iron absorption. The former occurs in a homozygous state seen in 75% to 100% of the patients. The frequency of the latter mutation, the H63D mutation, is significantly increased in patients with idiopathic dilated cardiomyopathy.[70] The high correlation of the HFE to hemochromatosis has caused it to be considered as a candidate gene for population-based genetic testing for diagnosis and detection of predisposition to hemochromatosis. In addition, mechanisms of iron transport and metabolism are unfolding and are providing clues to the enigma of iron homeostasis and the pathophysiology of iron overload.

The complications of hemochromatosis can be devastating, but its clinical management is simple and effective if the disease is identified early in its progression.

Although the exact mechanism of iron-induced heart failure remains to be elucidated, the toxicity of iron in biological systems is attributed to its ability to catalyze the generation of oxygen-free radicals. It has been shown that chronic iron overload results in dose-dependent increases in myocardial iron burden, decreases in the protective antioxidant enzyme activity, increased free-radical production, and increased mortality.[71] These findings suggest that the mechanism of iron-induced heart dysfunction involves, at least in part, free radical-mediated processes. Myocardial iron deposition is most prominent in and around contractile elements and less common in the conduction system, in contrast to sarcoidosis and amyloidosis in which the pathological process commonly involves the conduction system.[71] The mechanism by which iron produces cellular dysfunction is not yet clear, as fibrosis may not be prominent. This also implies that the disease process is reversible if the tissue iron concentration can be controlled. Myocardial iron deposits do not occur until other organs such as liver, pancreas, and connective tissues are saturated with iron. Thus the extracardiac manifestations are present before the cardiomyopathy develops.[71]

Iron overload can occur either as a result of inappropriate excess iron absorption, as in the case of hemochromatosis or thalassemia major, or due to multiple transfusions. The most important manifestations of heart disease in hemochromatosis are congestive heart failure and cardiac arrhythmia. During the initial phases of the cardiomyopathy, the hemodynamic profile represents a restrictive pattern. As the severity of cardiomyopathy advances, dilated cardiomyopathy with biventricular enlargement and heart failure ensues. The spectrum of arrhythmia ranges from minor abnormalities on the electrocardiogram to supraventricular arrhythmia, atrioventricular conduction block, and ventricular tachyarrhythmia presumably due to myocardial dysfunction and iron deposition in the conduction system and AV node. The ECG most commonly shows decreased voltage and nonspecific ST- and T-wave changes; Q waves are uncommon. Among patients with β-thalassemia major, biventricular, dilated cardiomyopathy remains the leading cause of mortality. In some patients, a restrictive type of LV cardiomyopathy or pulmonary hypertension is noted. The clinical course, although variable and occasionally fulminant, is more benign in recent than in older series.

The diagnosis of hemochromatosis is suggested by elevated serum ferritin and increased ratio of iron to total iron binding capacity (TIBC). The most sensitive screening test for hemochromatosis is saturation of the transferrin with iron; a fasting value greater than 50% is strongly suggestive of the disease. The most definitive test for calculation of iron stores in the body is by measurement of iron concentration by liver biopsy. Magnetic resonance imaging can also be very useful to identify the iron-laden organs and cardiac involvement. Though not required to demonstrate cardiac involvement in every case, endomyocardial biopsy can be useful in assessment of cardiac iron deposition. The echocardiogram usually reveals increased systolic and diastolic ventricular dimensions and reduced LV ejection fraction.

Before phlebotomy and chelation therapy, survival among patients with hemochromatosis and heart failure was less than 20% in 5 years. The actuarial survival rates of the individuals who are homozygous for the C282Y mutation of the hemochromatosis gene C282Y have been reported to be 95%, 93%, and 66%, respectively at 5, 10, and 20 years.[72] Similarly, in patients with thalassemia major, cardiac failure is one of the most frequent causes of death. Chelation therapy, including newer forms of oral chelators, such as deferoxamine, and phlebotomy have dramatically improved the outcome of hemochromatosis. Similarly, chelation therapy has improved prognosis in β-thalassemia major both by reducing the incidence of heart failure and by reversing cardiomyopathy. It is important to start therapy early because treatment may prevent or reverse cardiac involvement. Early diagnosis and treatment by phlebotomy before tissue damage has occurred are essential because life span seems to be normal in treated patients but markedly shortened in those who are not. Additionally, genetic counseling with evaluation of first-degree relatives is mandatory.[71] New imaging modalities, especially magnetic resonance imaging, are expected to improve early diagnosis and risk stratification for treatment. By increasing the proportion of patients on optimal chelation, survival in patients with hemachromatosis or β-thalassemia may further improve.

Physical Agents

Tachycardia-induced Dilated Cardiomyopathy. The concept that incessant or chronic tachycardia can lead to reversible LV dysfunction is supported both by animal models of chronic pacing and human studies documenting improvement in ventricular function with tachycardia rate or rhythm control. Sustained rapid pacing in experimental animal models can produce severe biventricular systolic dysfunction. In humans, descriptions of reversal of cardiomyopathy with rate or rhythm control of incessant or chronic tachycardias have been reported with atrial tachycardias, accessory pathway reciprocating tachycardias, atrioventricular node reentry, and atrial fibrillation with rapid ventricular responses.[73] Control of the rapid ventricular responses in atrial fibrillation has been shown to improve ventricular function. It should also

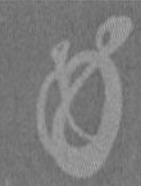

be noted that in patients with atrial fibrillation and congestive heart failure, a routine strategy of rhythm control does not reduce cardiovascular mortality, but may improve quality of life and LV function when compared with a strategy of rate control alone.[74] The diagnosis of tachycardia-induced cardiomyopathy is usually made following observation of a marked improvement in systolic function after normalization of heart rate. Clinicians should be aware that patients with unexplained systolic dysfunction may have tachycardia-induced cardiomyopathy, and that controlling the arrhythmia may result in improvement and even complete normalization of systolic function.[73] Tachycardia-induced cardiomyopathy may be a more common mechanism of LV dysfunction than recognized and aggressive treatment of the arrhythmia should be considered.

Autoimmune Mechanisms

There has been increasing evidence suggesting that abnormalities in cellular and humoral immunity may contribute to the overall pathogenesis of dilated cardiomyopathy. Circulating autoantibodies to a variety of cardiac antigens including G protein–linked receptors (such as those to β_1-adrenoreceptors and muscarinic receptors), mitochondrial antigens, adenosine diphosphate, adenosine triphosphate carrier proteins, and cardiac myosin heavy chain have been identified in patients with dilated cardiomyopathy.[75] In this regard it is interesting to note that immunization with certain cardiac muscle (but not skeletal) antigens such as α-myosin heavy chain can result in the development of a dilated cardiac phenotype in certain susceptible strains of mice. Moreover, a recent meta-analysis has shown that there is increased expression of the antigens of genes located at the major histocompatibility complex (MHC) on chromosome 6, which is the locus that is responsible for regulating immune responses. This study showed that HLA class II antigens such as DR4 or DQw4 were present in 63% of the patients with cardiomyopathy as compared with 26% in the control subjects.[76] Features that support an autoimmune cause in patients who have myocarditis and DCM include familial aggregation, a weak association with HLA-DR4 haplotype, abnormal expression of HLA class II antigens in cardiac tissue, and detection of organ- and disease-specific cardiac autoantibodies by immunofluorescence and immunoabsorption techniques. Nonetheless, a precise interpretation of the previous findings has been complicated by the knowledge that low titers of autoantibodies, which can be part of the normal immunological repertoire, are not always pathogenic. For example, tissue injury secondary to ischemia or infection may lead to autoantibody production because of alterations of self-antigens or exposure of antigens that are normally sequestered from the immune system. In such situations, the generation of autoantibodies is the result, and not the cause, of the tissue injury. Furthermore, observations about autoimmune responses are generally made in patients with established disease; accordingly, any inferences regarding cause and effect are, invariably, indirect and circumstantial.

CLINICAL RECOGNITION

The most common initial presenting manifestations of DCM are related to the presence of left heart failure, and include progressive exertional dyspnea, fatigue, weakness, diminished exercise capacity, orthopnea, paroxysmal nocturnal dyspnea, nocturnal cough, fluid retention, and edema. With the development of right heart failure, abdominal distention, right upper quadrant pain, early satiety, postprandial fullness, and nausea appear and edema worsens. Some cases will eventually develop cardiac cachexia and wasting from advanced heart failure. In systemic embolization, pulmonary emboli can be seen in 1% to 4% of cases and are more commonly seen with cardiomegaly. Palpitations can occur with atrial fibrillation and ventricular arrhythmias. Ventricular arrhythmias are common toward advanced stages of cardiomyopathy; however, syncope and sudden cardiac death are rare initial presentations.

Diagnostic Evaluation

The diagnostic evaluation of patients with dilated cardiomyopathy is, in general, similar to that for patients with ischemic heart disease and is further discussed in Chapter 35.

Laboratory Testing

Initial Laboratory Tests. Initial laboratory evaluation of patients having heart failure should include complete blood count, urinalysis, serum electrolytes (including calcium and magnesium), blood urea nitrogen, serum creatinine, fasting blood glucose (glycohemoglobin), lipid profile, liver function tests, and thyroid-stimulating hormone.[37] Furthermore, screening for hemochromatosis and human immunodeficiency virus is reasonable in suspected patients who have cardiomyopathy. Diagnostic tests for rheumatological diseases, amyloidosis, or pheochromocytoma are reasonable in patients with clinical suspicion.[37] Beyond these routine tests, the positive predictive value and/or utility of additional laboratory studies remains low unless supported by specific elements of the history and physical. One possible exception to this statement is the use of the natriuretic peptides: brain natriuretic peptide (BNP) or N-terminal pro BNP (NT-proBNP), as biochemical markers for both diagnostic and prognostic strategies in heart failure patients (see Chapter 34).

BNP. B-type natriuretic peptide (BNP) is a neurohormone secreted mainly in the cardiac ventricles in response to volume expansion and pressure overload. BNP or NT-proBNP can be used for identifying patients with asymptomatic LV systolic dysfunction for diagnosis of heart failure in patients with dyspnea,[77] and for prognosis and risk stratification of patients with heart failure.[78] Despite recognition that falling BNP levels during hospitalization correlate with clinical improvement and lower readmission rates,[79] so far it cannot be assumed that BNP levels can be used effectively as targets for adjustment of therapy in individual patients. Many patients taking optimal doses of medications continue to show markedly elevated levels of BNP,[80] and some patients demonstrate BNP levels within the normal range despite advanced heart failure. The value of serial measurements of BNP to guide therapy for patients with HF is also not well established.[80] Furthermore, the use of BNP measurements to guide the titration of drug doses has not been shown conclusively to improve outcomes more effectively than achievement of the target doses of drugs shown in clinical trials.[79] BNP is elevated probably in all forms of cardiomyopathy including DCM. There have been reports of higher BNP levels in patients with hypertrophic cardiomyopathy than patients with idiopathic DCM.[81] This may be related to the difference in proportional production of BNP by markedly hypertrophied and pressure-loaded ventricles.

Chest Radiography. In the early phases of DCM, cardiac enlargement may be minimal and may not be detected by chest radiography. However, in general the chest x-ray usually reveals LV enlargement or generalized cardiomegaly that involves all four cardiac chambers. Depending upon the patient's volume status there may or may not be findings of pulmonary congestion. Cephalization of blood flow or pulmonary vascular redistribution are early signs of volume overload, followed by the development of interstitial edema with appearance of Kerley B lines and fluid in the interlobar fissures, followed by frank alveolar edema in advanced volume

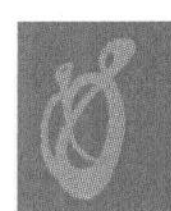

overload. Pleural effusions may be present and the azygous vein and superior vena cava may be dilated, especially with right ventricular failure. Current heart failure guidelines recommend that a chest radiograph (PA and lateral) should be performed initially in all patients having heart failure.[37]

Electrocardiography (ECG). If the patient with DCM has signs or symptoms referable to heart failure, the ECG usually reveals sinus tachycardia. However, it is important to note that sinus bradycardia may also be present in many patients with end-stage DCM. The ECG morphology is seldom normal, and often shows nonspecific repolarization or ST-segment abnormalities. Conduction abnormalities, especially left bundle branch block, left anterior hemiblock, nonspecific intraventricular conduction delays, and occasionally first-degree atrioventricular block are common in patients with long-standing symptoms, and they may be markers of increasing interstitial fibrosis or myocyte hypertrophy. Left atrial or biatrial enlargement may be present. Pathological anterior, anterolateral, or diffuse Q waves mimicking myocardial infarction, or poor R wave progression may be seen with viral myocarditis or when there is extensive LV fibrosis even without a discrete myocardial scar. A variety of atrial and ventricular tachyarrhythmias and atrioventricular conduction disturbances may also be seen. Atrial fibrillation develops in approximately 20% of the patients. Premature ventricular contractions are not an uncommon finding on routine ECGs in patients with DCM. Current heart failure guidelines recommend that a twelve-lead electrocardiogram should be performed initially in all patients having heart failure.[37]

Ambulatory Electrocardiographic (Holter) Monitoring. There is an inverse relationship between the severity of ventricular arrhythmia and LV ejection fraction. Thus it is perhaps not surprising that the majority of DCM patients will have PVCs when monitored over a 24-hour period; moreover, approximately half of the patients with DCM will have nonsustained ventricular tachycardia on routine ambulatory 24-hour Holter monitoring. However, the predictive value of ambulatory Holter monitoring as a routine screening tool in asymptomatic patients for identification of risk for sudden cardiac death has not been validated. There are conflicting data from studies involving small groups of patients regarding the role of routine ambulatory ECG monitoring as a significant independent risk factor for sudden cardiac death. Thus at the present time routine screening with Holter monitoring in asymptomatic heart failure patients is not recommended as a reliable means to predict those patients who will develop sudden cardiac death.[37]

Signal Average ECG. In patients with syncope or coronary artery disease, the presence of late potentials on a signal average ECG identifies those patients at high risk for developing ventricular tachycardia and sudden death. Although late potentials are less frequent in patients with DCM, the current evidence suggests that an abnormal signal average ECG also can predict ventricular arrhythmias and sudden cardiac death in patients with DCM. However, studies evaluating the utility of a positive signal-averaged electrocardiogram to identify a subgroup of dilated heart failure patients at risk for sudden death have yielded disparate results. Indeed, the sensitivity of the signal average ECG varies between 22% and 100% and the specificity ranges from 45% to 96% in various studies.[82] Therefore, although the signal average ECG may be useful for predicting future events in some patients with DCM, the inherent problems with the sensitivity, specificity, and predictive value suggest that the signal average ECG may not be a reliable tool for screening asymptomatic patients who are at a high risk for sudden cardiac death. Current heart failure guidelines do not recommend routine use of signal-averaged electrocardiography for the evaluation of patients having heart failure.[37]

Echocardiography. Two-dimensional and Doppler echocardiography are extremely useful techniques for assessing LV function, LV dimensions, and valvular structures in DCM patients (see also Chapter 36). Generally, patients will have global LV dilation, LV wall thinning, global hypokinesis, and an LV ejection fraction less than 35% to 40%. Segmental wall motion abnormalities may be seen with altered regional wall stress due to elevated filling pressures and depressed contractility, or with acute myocarditis due to segmental myocardial injury. Interestingly, the presence of segmental wall motion abnormalities suggests a more favorable outcome than if global hypokinesis is present.[83] Left ventricular apical thrombi can be identified in as many as 40% of the patients with DCM. Small pericardial effusion can sometimes be demonstrated, especially if an infectious or noninfectious inflammatory cause is responsible for producing the DCM.

Doppler echocardiography usually reveals mild degrees of mitral and tricuspid regurgitation and sometimes trace pulmonary insufficiency. The mechanisms of mitral and tricuspid regurgitation have been attributed to ventricular enlargement, annular dilation, lengthening of chordae tendinea, abnormalities in contractility of the papillary muscles, and displacement of the coaptation point of the mitral leaflets. The Doppler mitral inflow patterns can also provide useful information on elevated LV filling pressures, which are suggested by the appearance of high E/A ratio ("pseudonormalization") and short isovolumic relaxation time and deceleration time. The elevated early filling wave results from an elevated left atrial pressure, whereas the rapid deceleration time reflects a further decrease in LV compliance. These Doppler findings have been associated with a poor prognosis in DCM.

Newer modalities of echocardiography have been instrumental in diagnosis and risk stratification of heart failure and selection of appropriate therapies in heart failure patients. Doppler tissue imaging is widely used in documentation of dyssynchrony, diastolic dysfunction, evaluation of filling pressures, wall motion abnormalities, demonstration of myocardial structural abnormalities, and characterization of infiltrative or hypertrophic cardiomyopathy. Speckled strain imaging has been useful in assessment of load independent contractile performance of the left ventricle. Three-dimensional imaging has been useful in better delineation of valvular abnormalities and structural abnormalities of the heart. At present time, according to the ACCF/AHA Guidelines for the Diagnosis and Management of Heart Failure in Adults, two-dimensional echocardiography with Doppler should be performed during initial evaluation of all patients having heart failure to assess LVEF, LV size, wall thickness, and valve function.[37]

Radionuclide Techniques (see Chapter 36). Multigated radionuclide angiocardiography (MUGA) is a very useful test for the initial assessment of LV ejection fraction in patients with DCM. Both the right and LV ejection fractions can be quantified reliably with this technique; moreover, the interobserver and intertest variability appear to be less than with echocardiography. Electrocardiographically gated myocardial perfusion single-photon emission computed tomography SPECT imaging is also a state-of-the-art technique for the combined evaluation of myocardial perfusion and LV function with LVEF quantification within a single study. Due to shorter half life, ^{99m}Tc-sestamibi or ^{99m}Tc-tetrofosmin are the preferred agents for a gated SPECT study. Though frequently used to determine presence of ischemia as a potential cause of cardiomyopathy, stress testing with thallium 201 myocardial scintigraphy may not be a highly specific technique for differentiating patients with ischemic heart disease from those with DCM because patients with DCM may have both reversible and fixed perfusion abnormalities that are related to the presence of myocardial fibrosis.[84] Nevertheless, noninvasive

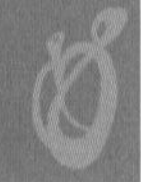

imaging with nuclear perfusion scanning may be considered to determine presence of ischemia and coronary artery disease in patients with heart failure and LV dysfunction (see also Chapter 36).[37] In addition to the previous methodologies, radionuclide techniques have also been used to detect the presence of myocardial inflammation. Both gallium-67 (a marker for inflammation) and indium-III labeled antimyosin antibodies (a marker for myocyte necrosis) have been used to detect myocarditis in small uncontrolled studies.[85] These techniques are supportive of the diagnosis of myocarditis when clinically suspected (Figure 24-9), but do not have the specificity or the sensitivity to be used reliably as screening tools for patients with myocarditis.[85]

Cardiovascular Magnetic Resonance (CMR) (see Chapter 36). Cardiovascular magnetic resonance is very helpful in assessing myocardial anatomy, regional and global function, and viability in one setting in heart failure patients (see also Chapter 36). It allows assessment of perfusion and acute tissue injury (edema and necrosis), detection of fibrosis, infiltration, and iron overload, which can help diagnose the underlying cause of DCM. It is a reliable technique for monitoring of disease progression, especially for infiltrative disease such as cardiomyopathy due to iron overload. It also has a prognostic role as evidence on the predictive value of CMR-derived parameters in heart failure is rapidly emerging. In the setting of ischemic cardiomyopathy, there is usually delayed hyperenhancement in segmental areas of subendocardium, whereas in nonischemic CMP, there is usually patchy midwall, epicardial, or global endocardial hyperenhancement (Figure 24-10). In DCM, midwall fibrosis determined by CMR is a predictor of the combined endpoint of all-cause mortality and cardiovascular hospitalization and sudden cardiac death. This suggests a potential role for CMR in the risk stratification of patients with DCM, which may have value in determining the need for device therapy.[86]

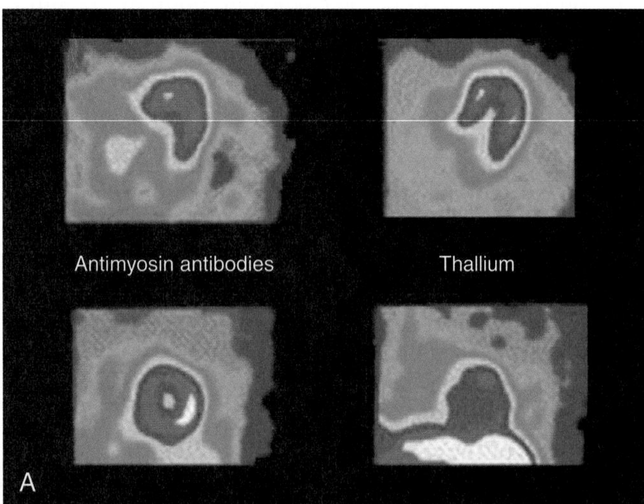

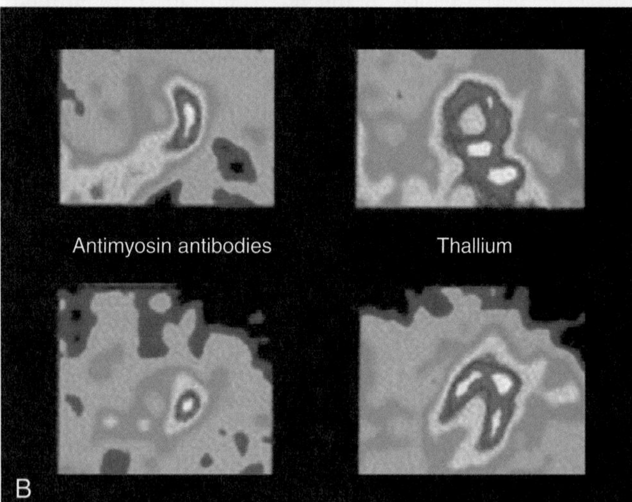

FIGURE 24-9 Dual-isotope rest imaging with ^{111}In-antimyosin antibody and ^{201}Thallium SPECT in patients with myocarditis. **A,** Scintigraphic pattern of diffuse myocarditis showing diffuse antimyosin antibody uptake throughout the whole LV myocardium and normal ^{201}Thallium uptake. **B,** Scintigraphic pattern of focal myocarditis showing antimyosin antibody uptake on the apex and the lateral LV wall, and a normal ^{201}Thallium scan. (From Sarda L, Colin P, Boccara F, et al. Myocarditis in patients with clinical presentation of myocardial infarction and normal coronary angiograms. *J Am Coll Cardiol* 2001;37(3):786-792, reproduced with permission from *Journal of American College of Cardiology*.)

Cardiac Catheterization. Coronary arteriography is primarily used as a basis for planning further treatment options in patients who have ischemic heart disease. Current heart failure guidelines state that coronary arteriography is reasonable for patients having heart failure who have known or suspected coronary artery disease.[37] In the majority of patients with DCM, the coronary arteries are normal with no atherosclerotic lesions; however, in a small portion there may be evidence of mild, nonobstructive, isolated atherosclerotic lesions that may not be sufficient to explain the extent of cardiomyopathy. Therefore, in these cases, other causes for the cardiomyopathy should be sought. The ventriculogram generally reveals a dilated ventricle with depressed contractility. The LV end-diastolic pressures are usually elevated. Right heart catheterization may be considered a useful means for adjusting medical therapy in patients with advanced symptoms, with hemodynamic instability, or impaired perfusion in whom the adequacy of filling pressures cannot be determined from clinical assessment, especially when they are considered for vasodilator and/or inotropic and/or mechanical support, or for assessing the suitability of certain patients for cardiac transplantation.[37]

Endomyocardial Biopsy. The routine use of right ventricular endomyocardial biopsy as a diagnostic tool for evaluating patients with newly diagnosed DCM is not recommended.[37] However, endomyocardial biopsy can be useful in patients having heart failure when a specific diagnosis is suspected that would influence therapy. It may yield a new diagnosis in up to 20% of patients, and may provide a potentially new and/or beneficial form of therapy in 5% of the patients.[87] Therefore, it may be considered in patients with suspected treatable systemic or infiltrative myocardial diseases, such as sarcoidosis, hypereosinophilic syndrome, hypersensitivity myocarditis, amyloidosis, hemochromatosis, doxorubicin-induced cardiomyopathy, or fulminant myocarditis. Moreover, as noted previously, in certain types of fulminant myocarditis, especially giant cell myocarditis, there is the suggestion that aggressive immunosuppression may attenuate disease progression. Therefore, endomyocardial biopsy may be especially useful in diagnosing patients who have a fulminant course, and/or who progressively decompensate despite optimal medical therapy. In experienced laboratories, the risk of perforation of the heart from the biopsy is approximately 1/200 (0.5%) and the risk of death from the procedure is 3 in 10,000 (0.03%).[87] Therefore, in electing to perform a myocardial biopsy, the clinician must weigh the potential benefits of rendering a new diagnosis for which a specific form of therapy exists against the risks associated with performing myocardial biopsy in his or her institution.[87]

Treatment Strategies for Dilated Cardiomyopathy

The first priority in implementing treatment strategies for patients with DCM is to determine if the condition has a cause for which there is a specific form of treatment. Table 24-2 lists a number of "cause-specific" treatment strategies designed to treat the underlying disease process that is responsible for

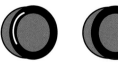

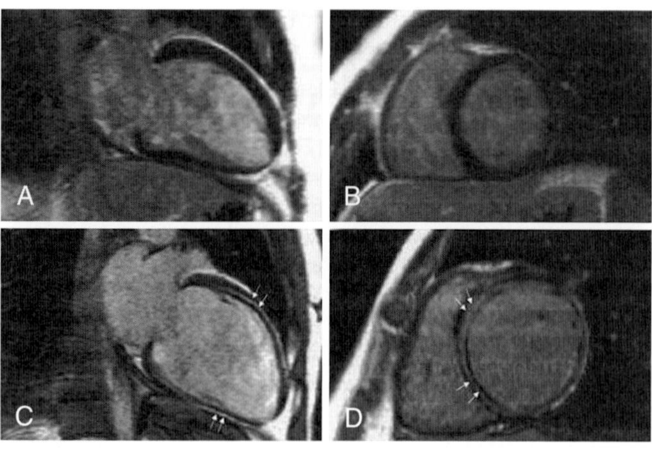

Midwall hyperenhancement

• Idiopathic dilated cardiomyopathy
• Myocarditis

• Myocarditis
• Chagas disease

Epicardial hyperenhancement

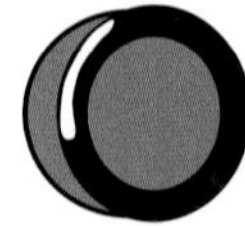

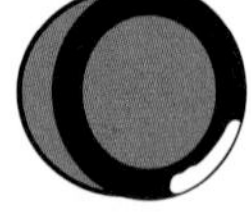

• Myocarditis
• Chagas disease
• Sarcoidosis

Global endocardial hyperenhancement

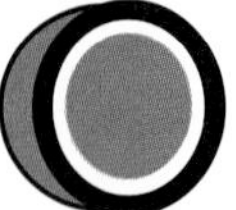

• Systemic sclerosis
• Amyloidosis

E

FIGURE 24–10 Late gadolinium enhancement patterns in dilated cardiomyopathy in vertical long axis (**A** and **C**) and short axis (**B** and **D**). A patient without late enhancement is shown in **A** and **B**, and a patient with marked midwall enhancement is shown in **C** and **D**. The enhancement pattern (*arrows*) is distinct from that associated with coronary artery disease because of endocardial sparing and noncoronary territory distribution. **E,** A schematic representation of hyperenhancement patterns that are characteristic for nonischemic cardiomyopathy. Note that midwall or epicardial hyperenhancement strongly suggests a nonischemic cause. (A-D, From Assomull RG, Prasad SK, Lyne J, et al. Cardiovascular magnetic resonance, fibrosis, and prognosis in dilated cardiomyopathy. *J Am Coll Cardiol* 2006;48(10):1977-1985. E, Reprinted with permission from Shah DJ, Judd RM, Kim RJ. Myocardial viability. In Edelman RR, Hesselink JR, Zlatkin MB, et al, editors. *Clinical magnetic resonance imaging*, ed 3, New York, 2006, Elsevier.)

TABLE 24–2 Primary Treatment Approaches to Dilated Cardiomyopathies

Cause for DCM	Primary Treatment
Alcoholic	Abstinence
Cocaine	Abstinence
Anthracycline	Cessation of anthracycline therapy
Systemic lupus erythematosus	Steroids, cytotoxic agents
Viral myocarditis	Prednisone and immunosuppressant therapy for fulminant course
Chagas disease	Benzonidazole, nifurtimox
Scleroderma	Steroids, Ca channel blockers for Raynaud
Kawasaki disease	IV immunoglobulin replacement
Thiamine, selenium, or carnitine deficiency	
Hyperthyroidism/hypothyroidism	Achieve euthyroid state
AIDS	Increase CD4 count
Uremia	Dialysis
Pheochromocytoma	Removal of tumor
Tachycardia induced	AV nodal ablation, β-blockers

causing the dilated cardiomyopathy. The second priority in implementing treatment strategies for DCM is to initiate supportive "heart failure" therapy, the goals of which should be to (1) prolong life; (2) avoid the need for future hospitalizations; (3) improve functional capacity and the quality of life; and (4) to prevent heart failure progression. In the section that follows, we will only discuss those treatment strategies that appear (at the time of this writing) to be unique to the treatment of heart failure for patients with DCM.

Standard Medical Therapy. Current ACCF/AHA Guidelines for the Diagnosis and Management of Heart Failure recommend use of standard medical therapy for patients with chronic heart failure regardless of ischemic or nonischemic cause, or DCM diagnosis.[37] Existing studies suggest that both patients with ischemic cardiomyopathy and DCM have significant survival benefit from the use of angiotensin-converting enzyme (ACE) inhibitors and β-blockers (see Chapters 45 and 46),[2,13,88] and they are indicated for all patients with current or prior symptoms of heart failure and reduced LVEF.[37] In patients who are ACE inhibitor-intolerant, angiotensin II receptor blockers are recommended as alternatives. Currently, the recommended β-blockers for treatment of heart failure include metoprolol succinate, carvedilol, and bisoprolol both for ischemic or nonischemic cardiomyopathy patients. Additionally, diuretics and salt restriction are recommended in patients with current or prior symptoms of heart failure who have evidence of fluid retention.[37] There is no information on potential differential effects of diuretics on morbidity or mortality in ischemic versus nonischemic heart failure.

Aldosterone antagonism with spironolactone has been reported to reduce mortality in patients with advanced heart failure, both in dilated or ischemic cardiomyopathy.[89]

According to the results of the RALES trial,[89] spironolactone (25 to 50 mg/day) is recommended for patients with recent or current symptoms of heart failure at rest despite the use of ACE inhibitors, diuretics, digoxin, and a β-blocker, regardless of the cause of heart failure, in patients with NYHA class III-IV heart failure and LVEF less than 35%, with adjustment of potassium supplements and close laboratory follow-up. Current ACCF/AHA Guidelines for the Diagnosis and Management of Heart Failure recommend the addition of an aldosterone antagonist in selected patients with moderately severe to severe symptoms of heart failure and reduced LVEF who can be carefully monitored for preserved renal function and normal potassium concentration.[37] Under circumstances where monitoring for hyperkalemia or renal dysfunction is not anticipated to be feasible, the risks may outweigh the benefits of aldosterone antagonists.[90,91] Routine combined use of an ACE inhibitor, ARB, and aldosterone antagonist is not recommended.[37]

In the past decade, several studies have shown that angiotensin receptor blockers (ARBs), when added to background therapy with ACE inhibitors, can result in improvement in combined morbidity and mortality in patients with chronic heart failure,[3,92] both in ischemic or nonischemic dilated cardiomyopathy patients. According to current guidelines, in persistently symptomatic patients with reduced LVEF who are already being treated with conventional therapy, the addition of angiotensin II receptor blockers may be considered.[37] It is important to recognize that in chronic heart failure, the angiotensin receptor blocker trials[3,92] were conducted predominantly in patients with mild to moderate heart failure (NYHA class II to III), whereas the RALES trial[89] (the only aldosterone receptor antagonist trial in chronic heart failure including patients with nonischemic cause) was conducted in patients with severe heart failure (NYHA class III-IV). At the present time, there are no large-scale, prospective, randomized clinical trials with aldosterone receptor blockers in mild to moderate chronic heart failure patients, and there are no head-to-head trials comparing ARBs and aldosterone receptor blockers in the treatment of heart failure, either for ischemic or nonischemic patients.

Digitalis can be beneficial in patients with current or prior symptoms of heart failure and reduced LVEF to decrease hospitalizations for heart failure.[37] Pooled results from the Prospective Randomized Study of Ventricular Function and Efficacy of Digoxin (PROVED) and the Randomized Assessment of Digoxin and Inhibitors of Angiotensin-Converting Enzyme (RADIANCE) trials indicate that digoxin increases LV ejection fraction more in patients with DCM than in patients with ischemic heart disease, and that withdrawal of digoxin leads to a significantly greater likelihood of clinical deterioration in the DCM patients.[93] In the Digitalis Investigators' Group trial,[26] digoxin was associated with a significant reduction in a combined endpoint of death or hospitalization as a result of worsening heart failure in patients in sinus rhythm. This benefit was somewhat greater in patients with nonischemic cause than in those with ischemic cause.[26] That is, patients with DCM were noted to have a 33% risk reduction in the combined endpoint of death and heart failure hospitalization compared with a 21% risk reduction in patients with ischemic cardiomyopathy. The cause of this therapeutic difference is unclear at this point. In a recent retrospective cohort of hospitalized patients with heart failure with LV systolic dysfunction on contemporary background, heart failure treatment including angiotensin-converting enzyme inhibitors and β-blockers, digoxin use was not associated with improvement in survival either in DCM or ischemic cardiomyopathy patients.[94]

Recently, the addition of a fixed dose of isosorbide dinitrate plus hydralazine to standard therapy for heart failure including ACE inhibitors and β-blockers has been shown to be efficacious in increasing survival among black patients with advanced (NYHA class III-IV) heart failure and LV systolic dysfunction.[95] Interestingly, in 77% to 78% of the patients in this trial, the cause of heart failure was categorized as nonischemic (40% due to hypertension), but the subgroup analysis of outcomes according to the cause of heart failure has not been reported.[95] At the present time, the combination of hydralazine and nitrates is recommended to improve outcomes in African Americans, with moderate to severe symptoms of heart failure on optimal therapy with ACE inhibitors, β-blockers, and diuretics.[95] A combination of hydralazine and a nitrate might be reasonable in patients with current or prior symptoms of heart failure and reduced LVEF who cannot be given an ACE inhibitor or ARB because of drug intolerance, hypotension, or renal insufficiency.[37]

The use of the first generation of calcium antagonists (diltiazem, verapamil, or nifedipine) with negative inotropic effects is considered potentially harmful in patients with heart failure.[37] Recent studies with the second generation of calcium channel blockers, such as amlodipine and felodipine, suggest that these agents may be safer, but do not confer survival benefit in patients with heart failure. Initial reports of survival benefit with amlodipine (PRAISE-I)[29] in patients with dilated but not ischemic cardiomyopathy have failed to be reproduced by the subsequent large-scale randomized trial (PRAISE-II), in which the survival was similar in both the ischemic and nonischemic HF patients. Studies with felodipine showed similar results. In the V-HeFT III trial, felodipine when used as supplementary vasodilator therapy in patients with chronic heart failure was safe but had no additional benefit.[96] At the present time, regardless of the cause of heart failure, calcium channel blockers with negative inotropic effects are not recommended in patients with heart failure and reduced LVEF. Similarly, other drugs known to adversely affect the clinical status of patients with heart failure and reduced LVEF should be avoided or withdrawn whenever possible, including nonsteroidal antiinflammatory drugs and most antiarrhythmic drugs.[37]

Antiarrhythmic Therapy Implantable Devices. The role of implantable defibrillators for secondary prevention of sudden cardiac death is clearly established both for the ischemic and nonischemic cardiomyopathy patients (see Chapter 47). Implantable defibrillators decrease sudden death risk in patients with LV dysfunction who have survived sudden cardiac death or sustained ventricular tachycardia or fibrillation.[37,97] For primary prevention, there is a large body of literature supporting the prophylactic use of implantable defibrillators to prevent sudden cardiac death in ischemic cardiomyopathy patients with reduced LVEF postmyocardial infarction,[37,98] and there is recent evidence supporting use in patients with nonischemic dilated cardiomyopathy.[99] Two earlier studies, the Amiodarone versus Implantable Cardioverter-Defibrillator Trial (AMIOVIRT)[100] and the DEFINITE trial,[101] failed to show a significant survival benefit with implantable cardioverter-defibrillator (ICD) therapy in patients with nonischemic cardiomyopathy and heart failure, whereas the Sudden Cardiac Death in Heart Failure Trial (SCD-HeFT) trial[99] provided the first large-scale evidence of survival benefit with ICDs for primary prevention of sudden cardiac death in patients with DCM. In this trial, in patients with NYHA class II or III heart failure and an LV ejection fraction of 35%, the single-lead, shock-only ICD therapy reduced overall mortality by 23%, whereas amiodarone had no favorable effect on survival. The cause of heart failure was nonischemic in 48%, and the results did not vary according to either ischemic or nonischemic cause. A recent meta-analysis of trials enrolling 1854 heart failure patients with nonischemic cardiomyopathy suggested a 31% significant reduction in total mortality among patients with an ICD or cardiac resynchronization therapy defibrillator (CRT-D) therapy (Figure 24-11).[102]

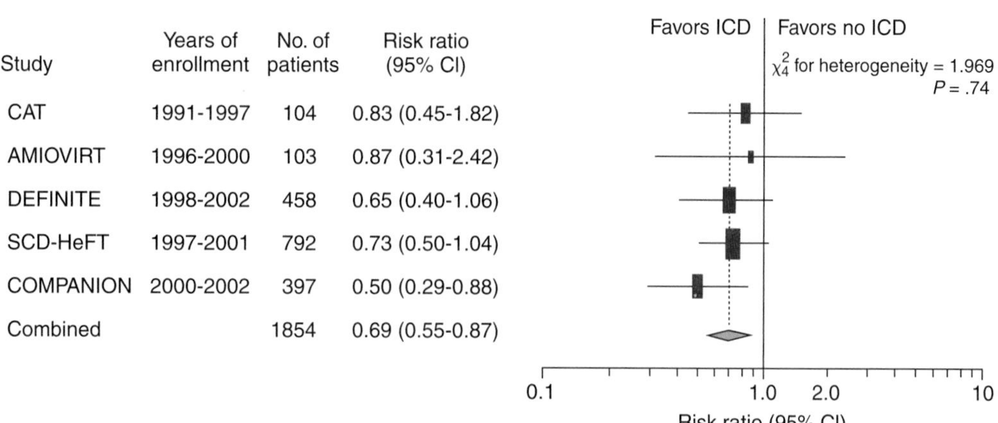

FIGURE 24–11 All-cause mortality among patients with nonischemic cardiomyopathy randomized to ICD or CRT-D versus medical therapy in primary prevention revealing significant survival benefit with device therapy in nonischemic cardiomyopathy patients. Number of patients with nonischemic cardiomyopathy enrolled is reported. Size of the data marker corresponds to the relative weight assigned in the pooled analysis using fixed-effects models. ICD indicates implantable cardioverter-defibrillator; *CRT-D,* cardiac resynchronization plus defibrillator; *CI,* confidence interval. (From Desai AS, Fang JC, Maisel WH, et al. Implantable defibrillators for the prevention of mortality in patients with nonischemic cardiomyopathy: a meta-analysis of randomized controlled trials. *JAMA* 2004;292:2874-2879, reproduced with permission from *JAMA*. Copyright © (2011) American Medical Association. All rights reserved.)

It should be noted that for patients with standard indications for ICD therapy, but without indication for cardiac pacing, dual-chamber pacing offers no clinical advantage over ventricular backup pacing and may be detrimental by increasing the combined endpoint of death or hospitalization for heart failure.[103] Current ACCF/AHA Guidelines for the Diagnosis and Management of Heart Failure recommend implantable cardioverter-defibrillator therapy for primary prevention of sudden cardiac death to reduce total mortality in patients with nonischemic dilated cardiomyopathy or ischemic heart disease with an LVEF less than or equal to 35%, and NYHA functional class II or III symptoms while receiving chronic optimal medical therapy, and who have reasonable expectation of survival with a good functional status for more than 1 year. [37]

Medical Antiarrhythmic Therapy. Studies addressing the role of antiarrhythmic therapy in prolonging survival or preventing sudden death in heart failure have yielded disparate results. The Survival Trial of Antiarrhythmic Therapy in Congestive Heart Failure with Amiodarone (CHF-STAT)[27] revealed that amiodarone treatment was effective in suppressing ventricular arrhythmias and improving ventricular function; however, it did not reduce the incidence of sudden death or prolong survival among patients with heart failure, except for a trend toward reduced mortality among those with nonischemic cardiomyopathy. In the trial by Grupo de Estudio de la Sobrevida en la Insuficiencia Cardiaca en Argentina (GESICA),[104] low-dose amiodarone resulted in reduction in total mortality, sudden cardiac death, and heart failure death in both the dilated nonischemic and ischemic patients. As mentioned previously, in the SCD-HeFT trial,[99] amiodarone failed to have any beneficial effect on survival when compared against a placebo in heart failure patients regardless of cause. Presently, antiarrhythmic medical therapy is reserved for individualized treatment of symptomatic arrhythmias, especially for suppression of ventricular arrhythmias after ICD implantation or supraventricular arrhythmias such as atrial fibrillation.

It is important to emphasize that β-blockers have also been shown to reduce sudden cardiac death risk by approximately 30% in patients with ischemic or nonischemic heart failure in addition to their overall benefit in reducing mortality and heart failure hospitalizations.[2,28,88]

Cardiac Resynchronization Therapy. Many patients with dilated cardiomyopathy have cardiac conduction abnormalities, such as left bundle branch block or intraventricular conduction delays, which can lead to ventricular dyssynchrony and reduction in stroke volume as a consequence. In patients with heart failure, the presence of left bundle branch block (LBBB) or IVCD further degrades ventricular function, contributing directly to the severity of their heart failure symptoms. Biventricular pacing with transvenous leads in the right atrium, right ventricle, and left ventricle via the coronary sinus can restore cardiac resynchronization (see Chapter 47). Several recent studies: the Multicenter InSync Randomized Clinical Evaluation (MIRACLE)[105]; Multisite Stimulation in Cardiomyopathy (MUSTIC)[106]; Comparison of Medical Therapy, Pacing, and Defibrillation in Heart Failure (COMPANION)[107]; and Cardiac Resynchronization-Heart Failure (CARE-HF)[108] trials validated the safety and efficacy of cardiac resynchronization therapy in advanced heart failure. Data from these studies have shown statistically significant improvements in LV ejection fraction, New York Heart Association class, exercise tolerance, and quality of life. Furthermore, the COMPANION trial demonstrated that in patients with advanced heart failure and a prolonged QRS interval, cardiac-resynchronization therapy decreased the combined risk of death from any cause or first hospitalization, and when combined with an implantable defibrillator, significantly reduced mortality.[107] However, in the COMPANION trial, the decrease in the risk of death was not significant with cardiac resynchronization therapy alone. The more recent CARE-HF trial[108] demonstrated that in patients with heart failure, class III or IV heart failure due to LV systolic dysfunction (LVEF <35%) and cardiac dyssynchrony (QRS >120 msec and or other evidence of dyssynchrony), cardiac resynchronization improved symptoms and the quality of life, and reduced the risk of death. In these trials the benefit was present both in ischemic or nonischemic heart failure patients. The proposed mechanisms involved in improving ventricular function with biventricular pacing include improved septal contribution to ventricular ejection, increased diastolic filling times, reduced mitral regurgitation, and prevention of progressive remodeling. Resynchronization therapy may also reduce arrhythmias by stabilization of the arrhythmia substrate and by improving the heart failure status. The current ACCF/AHA Guidelines for the Diagnosis and Management of Heart Failure recommend that patients with LVEF of less than or equal to 35%, sinus rhythm, and NYHA functional class III or ambulatory class IV symptoms, on optimal medical therapy, and a QRS duration greater than or equal to 0.12 seconds, should receive cardiac resynchronization therapy, with or without an ICD.[37] It should be noted that the most recent MADIT-CRT trial demonstrated that in heart failure patients with mild cardiac symptoms (NYHA class I or II), with an ejection fraction of 30% or less and a QRS duration of 130 msec or more, cardiac resynchronization with defibrillator therapy using biventricular pacing did not reduce all-cause mortality, but reduced the combined endpoint of heart failure free survival.[109] The benefit did not differ between ischemic or nonischemic cause. The superiority of cardiac resynchronization therapy was driven by a 41% reduction in the risk of heart failure events, a finding that was evident primarily in a prespecified subgroup of patients with a QRS duration of 150 msec or more. Cardiac resynchronization therapy was associated with a significant reduction in LV volumes and improvement in the ejection fraction. There was no significant difference between the two groups in the overall risk of death, with a 3% annual mortality rate in each treatment group. The result of this, and other future trials, may expand the indication for cardiac resynchronization therapy to relatively asymptomatic patients (NYHA class I or II) with a low ejection fraction and wide QRS complex. It should also be noted that cardiac resynchronization therapy does not confer benefit in heart failure patients with narrow QRS.[110] In a recent trial conducted in patients with heart failure with LVEF less than 35%, QRS of 130 msec, and NYHA class III heart failure, approximately 47% of the patients had heart failure due to nonischemic cause. There was a significant improvement in NYHA class and the 6-minute walking test in the nonischemic stratum but no difference in peak oxygen consumption or quality of life scores with cardiac resynchronization therapy.[110]

Anticoagulants (see also Chapter 52). Patients with dilated cardiomyopathy have multiple factors that predispose to thromboembolic events. However, the appropriateness of chronic anticoagulant therapy in DCM has been controversial. The Warfarin and Antiplatelet Therapy in Chronic Heart failure (WATCH) trial, a multicenter, randomized, international trial comparing the efficacy of aspirin, clopidogrel, and warfarin in heart failure patients, was the largest trial of antithrombotic therapies conducted in chronic heart failure patients. It reportedly failed to show any major differences among the three medications to prevent the combined endpoint of nonfatal myocardial infarction, stroke, and mortality.[111] Currently, the Warfarin versus Aspirin in Patients with Reduced Cardiac Ejection Fraction (WARCEF) study, a National Institutes of Health–funded, randomized, double-blind clinical trial, is continuing enrollment to determine whether aspirin or warfarin would improve event-free survival (death or stroke) among patients with LVEF at 35%, who do not have atrial fibrillation or mechanical prosthetic heart valves, and will provide valuable information regarding the role of anticoagulation in heart failure patients. In the absence of controlled trials, the available data do not support the use of anticoagulants in heart failure patients other than those with a history of atrial fibrillation, previous stroke, or other thromboembolic events, or with visible protruding or mobile thrombus on echocardiography.

Lipid Modifying Agents

Statins. The non–lipid-lowering or pleiotropic effects of 3-hydroxy-3-methylglutaryl coenzyme A reductase inhibitors (statins) have been hypothesized to beneficially alter mechanisms involved in heart failure. In the past, evidence from experimental studies, retrospective analyses, and limited clinical investigations have suggested that statin therapy may improve ventricular function, heart failure status, and clinical outcomes independent of heart failure cause, and through mechanisms other than statin effects on dyslipidemia. However, two recently published, large, prospective randomized trials did not demonstrate any significant clinical benefit of statins in heart failure patients.[112,113] Despite significant reduction in low-density lipoprotein and high sensitivity C-reactive protein, data from Gruppo Italiano per lo Studio della Sopravvivenza nell'Infarto miocardico—Heart Failure (GISSI-HF) trial suggested that rosuvastatin at a 10-mg daily dose did not have any effect on clinical outcomes in chronic heart failure patients of any cause.[112] In the Controlled Rosuvastatin in Multinational Trial in Heart Failure (CORONA), again rosuvastatin treatment did not show any benefit in cardiovascular mortality in older patients with systolic heart failure.[113] At the present time, there is no evidence to support initiating statin therapy in patients with DCM or nonischemic heart failure. This is concept was covered in detail in Chapter 50.

Polyunsaturated Fatty Acids (PUFA). Interestingly, in the GISSI-HF trial, long-term administration of 1 g per day of omega n-3 polyunsaturated fatty acids was very effective in reducing both all-cause mortality and cardiovascular admissions, both in ischemic or nonischemic chronic heart failure patients (Figure 24-12). In this trial, 30% of the patients enrolled were with dilated cardiomyopathy, and the benefit of n-3 PUFA was demonstrated in all predefined subgroups, including nonischemic causes.[114] This trial suggests that omega n-3 polyunsaturated fatty acids are helpful in improving clinical outcomes in patients with heart failure.

Immunosuppression and Immunomodulation in DCM. Although an autoimmune pathogenesis has been postulated for dilated cardiomyopathy, immunosuppressive therapy has not been shown to be effective in clinical trials. The failure of the Myocarditis Treatment Trial[115] to show a significant benefit for immunosuppressive therapy is discussed in Chapter 31.

Based on its possible immunomodulatory effects, intravenous immunoglobulin has been studied as a potential beneficial agent in patients with dilated cardiomyopathy. Although the exact mechanism of action of intravenous immunoglobulin is not known, a number of different mechanisms have been proposed, including Fc receptor blockade, neutralization of autoantibodies, modulation of cytokine activity, and activation of an inhibitory Fc receptor. It is an effective therapy for Kawasaki disease in children, and it has been reported to improve ventricular function in children with new-onset dilated cardiomyopathy, and in women with postpartum cardiomyopathy.[116] The initial promising results observed in the adult population were not confirmed by the randomized, placebo-controlled, multicenter Intervention in Myocarditis and Acute Cardiomyopathy (IMAC) trial. This topic was further covered in Chapter 11.

The technique of immunoadsorption, removal of autoantibodies with immunoadsorption by passing a patient's plasma over columns that contain immobilized antibodies against immunoglobulin (IgG) kappa and lambda light chains and IgG heavy chains has been reported to be beneficial in DCM. Wallukat et al were the first to show that this technique efficiently removed circulating antibodies directed against the β_1-adrenoreceptor and were associated with an improvement in NYHA functional class in patients with dilated cardiomyopathy.[117] This study was soon followed by other small studies that reported improvement in short-term hemodynamic effects, significant lowering of anti-β_1-adrenoreceptor antibodies, significant improvement in LV ejection fraction, and a decrease in LV end-diastolic dimension.[118,119] Therapy with immunoadsorption and subsequent immunoglobulin G substitution has been demonstrated to result in a marked decrease in myocardial HLA-class II antigen expression (Figure 24-13), reduction in CD4 and CD8 lymphocyte cell

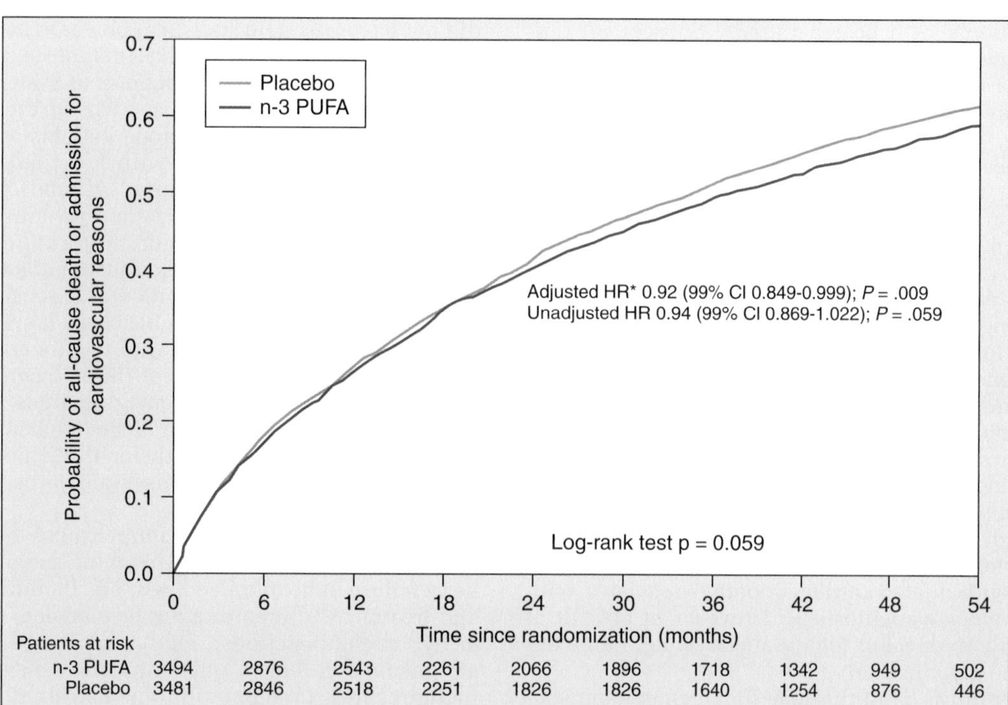

FIGURE 24–12 Kaplan-Meier curves for time to all-cause death or admission to hospital for cardiovascular reasons with n-3 polyunsaturated fatty acids (n-3 PUFA) versus placebo. Estimates were calculated with a Cox proportional hazards model, with adjustment for admission to hospital for heart failure in the previous year, previous pacemaker, and aortic stenosis. (From Tavazzi L, Maggioni AP, Marchioli R, et al. Effect of n-3 polyunsaturated fatty acids in patients with chronic heart failure (the GISSI-HF trial): a randomised, double-blind, placebo-controlled trial. *Lancet* 2008;372:1223-1230, reproduced with permission from *Lancet*.)

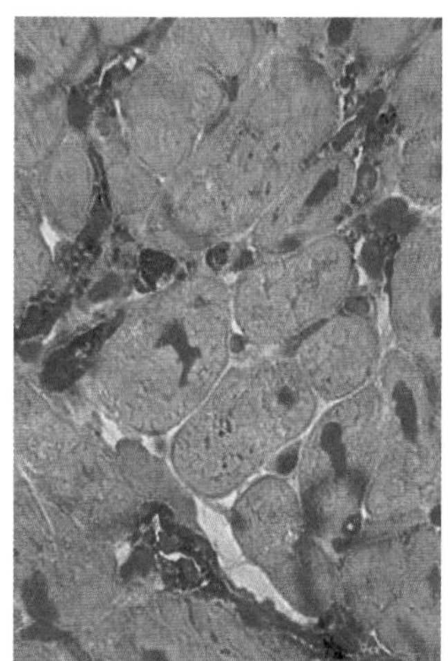

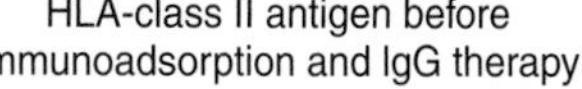

HLA-class II antigen before immunoadsorption and IgG therapy

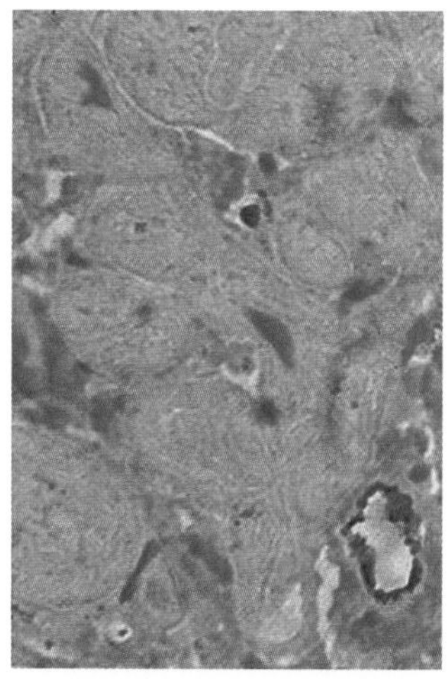

HLA-class II antigen after immunoadsorption and IgG therapy

FIGURE 24–13 Changes in HLA class II antigen expression of same patient before and after 3-month therapy with IA and subsequent IgG substitution (magnification 400×). (From Staudt A, Schäper F, Stangl V, et al. Immunohistological changes in dilated cardiomyopathy induced by immunoadsorption therapy and subsequent immunoglobulin substitution. *Circulation* 2001;103:2681-2686.)

counts after 3 months, and improvements in LV function and functional status in selected patients with dilated cardiomyopathy.[120] Despite the evidence of mitigation of certain features of myocardial inflammation in select patients, it is important to emphasize the existing gaps in our knowledge with respect to immunoadsorption in patients with dilated cardiomyopathy. At the present time it is unclear whether all patients with dilated cardiomyopathy will benefit from immunoadsorption therapy, or whether patients with elevated levels of circulating autoantibodies should be treated. Second, the mechanism(s) of action of immunoadsorption is not known. Although studies have demonstrated decreases in circulating autoantibodies, it is not at all clear that a cause-and-effect relationship has been established. Immunoadsorption can lead to a decline in systemic vascular resistance independent of the removal of circulating autoantibodies. Thus part of the hemodynamic benefit that has been observed may be related to vasodilation and not an improvement in LV function. Third, the optimal strategy for immunoadsorption has yet to be determined. Different investigators use different protocols and different immunoadsorbent devices. It is not clear from existing studies whether immunoadsorption alone, which would be expected to modulate humoral immunity, will be sufficient in the long term, or whether it may be necessary to incorporate strategies that lead to suppression of cellular-mediated immunity as well.

One recent strategy of device-based nonspecific immunomodulation therapy, involving reinjection of patients' blood that has been exposed to ex vivo oxidative stress by ozone and ultraviolet light, failed to show any reduction in mortality and cardiovascular hospitalizations in chronic heart failure patients with NYHA functional class II-IV and LV systolic dysfunction. Interestingly, by subgroup analysis, patients with nonischemic cause and NYHA class II heart failure appeared to benefit from immunomodulation therapy (see also Chapter 11). Immunomodulation or immunosuppressive therapies await further validation and identification of specific patients these treatment strategies may benefit.

Growth Hormone (see chapter 21). There has been growing enthusiasm for the use of growth hormone in patients with DCM, based on the rationale that there may be inadequate compensatory cardiac hypertrophy in this disorder. Growth hormone and insulin-like growth factor 1 are involved in several physiological processes such as the control of muscle mass and function, body composition, and regulation of nutrient metabolism. Earlier reports suggested that growth hormone therapy could increase myocardial mass and reduce the size of the LV chamber, resulting in improvement in hemodynamics, myocardial energy metabolism, and the clinical

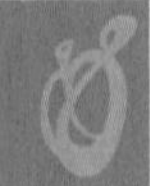

status of the patients with heart failure.[121] Subsequent randomized, placebo-controlled studies of recombinant human growth hormone did not show significant improvement in cardiac performance or clinical status of patients with dilated cardiomyopathy, despite significant increases in LV mass related to changes in serum IGF-1 concentrations.[64] Whether longer treatment with recombinant growth hormone would result in an improved clinical outcome in the patients with DCM is unknown.

Gene Therapy (see also Chapter 50). After a decade of preclinical and early phase 1 clinical investigations, gene therapy is proving likely to be a viable alternative to conventional therapies for heart failure. So far in preclinical studies, three types of gene transfer studies have been investigated to enhance myocardial contractility. These include modulating calcium homeostasis (overexpression of SERCa2 by rat or transgenic mice DCM models), manipulating β-adrenergic receptor signaling (transfection or overexpression of the β-adrenergic receptor gene in rat or rabbit DCM models), and augmenting cardiomyocyte resistance to apoptosis (adenoviral gene transfer of antiapoptotic Bcl-2 and Akt in gp130 knockout mice with dilated cardiomyopathy associated with massive cardiomyocyte apoptosis).[122] However, at present, it has been difficult to develop highly effective gene delivery techniques in the myocardium.

Since the identification of the gene for Duchenne muscular dystrophy in 1987, many groups have reported successful approaches for the adenoviral vector delivery of dystrophin, the Duchenne muscular dystrophy gene product, resulting in restoration of dystrophin-associated glycoprotein complex proteins to the sarcolemma and amelioration of muscular dystrophy symptoms in animal models.[123] Although dystrophin is the most extensively studied gene that is implicated in DCM, correction of the dystrophin defects, associated with X-linked cardiomyopathy, has not been fully studied in humans yet.[122]

Angiogenesis and cell therapy are discussed in Chapter 51.

Treatment of Anemia. Anemia is very common in heart failure both in nonischemic and ischemic cardiomyopathy patients, and is associated with very poor outcomes. Preliminary data have suggested that treatment of anemia with erythropoietin-stimulating agents is associated with improvement in cardiac function, functional class, and reduction in hospitalizations.[124] However, in a recent randomized placebo-controlled trial of 319 patients, treatment with darbepoetin alfa did not significantly improve exercise duration, NYHA class, or quality of life score in heart failure patients, regardless of ischemic or nonischemic cause.[125] A more definitive, randomized, multicenter clinical trial (Reduction of Events With Darbepoetin Alfa in Heart Failure—RED-HF) is being conducted to determine the efficacy of treatment of anemia with darbepoetin alfa on mortality or heart failure hospitalizations in subjects with symptomatic LV systolic dysfunction and anemia. Until more data are available, the safety or efficacy of these agents or other strategies of treatment of anemia remains unclear in heart failure patients.

Vitamins, Nutritional Supplements. Except for omega n-3 polyunsaturated fatty acids, which have been proven to be beneficial in improving clinical outcomes in heart failure patients (see Lipid Modifying Agents section), other dietary or nutritional supplements such as vitamin E or coenzyme Q-10 failed to consistently or significantly improve LV systolic function, quality of life, or other clinical outcomes in patients with heart failure and LV systolic dysfunction in Western populations.[126] At the present time, use of nutritional supplements as treatment for heart failure is not indicated in patients with current or prior symptoms of heart failure or DCM.[37]

Exercise Training (see also chapter 57). Many observational or small studies have advocated exercise training to improve clinical outcomes in heart failure patients, but most did not have adequate statistical power to measure the effects of exercise training on clinical outcomes. The recent Controlled Trial Investigating Outcomes of Exercise Training (HF-ACTION), the largest randomized trial on the role efficacy and safety of exercise training among patients with heart failure, enrolled over 2000 patients with heart failure and reduced ejection fraction, 48% of whom had nonischemic causes. In this trial, exercise training resulted in nonsignificant trends for reductions in all-cause mortality, cardiovascular mortality, and hospitalizations. After adjustment for highly prognostic predictors, exercise training was associated with modest but significant reductions for all-cause mortality or hospitalization and cardiovascular mortality or heart failure hospitalizations.[127] The results did not differ according to ischemic or nonischemic cause. Current guidelines recommend that exercise training be considered for medically stable outpatients with heart failure, both for ischemic or nonischemic cardiomyopathy patients. This topic is discussed further in detail in Chapter 57.

Treatment of Acute Decompensated Heart Failure in DCM. The standard management of acute decompensated heart failure in hospitalized patients, including identification and treatment of precipitating factors such as hypertension, arrhythmias, infections, pulmonary emboli, renal failure, and medical or dietary noncompliance; diagnostic strategies, including measurement of B-type natriuretic peptide; assessment of adequacy of systemic perfusion, monitoring of volume status; treatment with diuretics, oxygen, salt restriction, vasodilators, inotropic agents, or vasopressors when indicated; invasive hemodynamic monitoring in certain patients with instability and uncertainty of filling pressures; continuation of standard oral heart failure therapies; close monitoring of renal function and electrolytes; and coordination of prehospital and posthospital care are very similar in ischemic or nonischemic DCM patients.[37] Recent trials with vasopressin receptor antagonists, nesiritide, or adenosine receptor antagonists initiated for acute treatment of patients hospitalized with heart failure failed to demonstrate any benefit in long-term mortality or heart failure–related morbidity, regardless of ischemic or nonischemic cause. This topic is further discussed in detail in Chapter 43.

Mechanical Circulatory Support Devices. Over the past 2 decades, mechanical circulatory support devices have steadily evolved in the clinical management of end-stage heart failure and have emerged as a standard of care for the treatment of acute and chronic heart failure refractory to conventional medical therapy for both ischemic or nonischemic dilated cardiomyopathy patients. Possible indications for using mechanical circulatory support are acute cardiogenic shock as a bridge to transplantation, a bridge to recovery, and more recently, as destination therapy. Because of potential of tissue recovery, DCM patients have been of special interest for studying the reversal of remodeling and improvement in contractile function with cardiac support devices. These modalities are further discussed in Chapter 56.

Surgical Treatment of Dilated Cardiomyopathy. For decades, there have been numerous surgical interventions to improve LV performance, reverse or attenuate LV remodeling, lessen contribution from valvular regurgitation in patients with DCM. These interventions ranged from ventricular reconstruction surgery, LV support with dynamic cardiomyoplasty (with use of latissimus dorsi muscle), passive containment devices or Mysplint devices, and mitral valve surgery to partial left ventriculectomy. Despite initial enthusiasm, most long-term studies with partial left ventriculectomy have not demonstrated sustained improvement in clinical outcomes; thus partial left ventriculectomy is not recommended in patients with nonischemic CMP.[37] Left ventricular support with passive containment devices has been associated with sustained beneficial impact on LV size and shape in patients

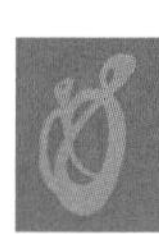

with DCM, but long-term survival benefit has not been demonstrated. Further studies are being conducted and may provide insight into which patients may benefit from these procedures. This topic is discussed in detail in Chapter 55.

ACKNOWLEDGMENTS

The research reviewed herein was supported, in part, by research funds from the Department of Veterans Affairs and the NIH (R01HL073017, R01HL089543, K30RR022295). Dr. Bozkurt is a recipient of the Veterans Affairs MERIT Review Entry Program award.

REFERENCES

1. Richardson, P., McKenna, W., Bristow, M., et al. (1996). Report of the 1995 World Health Organization/International Society and Federation of Cardiology task force on the definition and classification of cardiomyopathies. *Circulation, 93*, 841–842.
2. MERIT-HF Study Group. (1999). Effect of metoprolol CR/XL in chronic heart failure: metoprolol CR/XL randomised intervention trial in congestive heart failure (MERIT-HF). *Lancet, 353*, 2001–2007.
3. Cohn, J. N., & Tognoni, G. (2001). A randomized trial of the angiotensin-receptor blocker valsartan in chronic heart failure. *N Engl J Med, 345*, 1667–1675.
4. Adams, K. F., Jr., Fonarow, G. C., Emerman, C. L., et al. (2005). Characteristics and outcomes of patients hospitalized for heart failure in the United States: rationale, design, and preliminary observations from the first 100,000 cases in the Acute Decompensated Heart Failure National Registry (ADHERE). *Am Heart J, 149*, 209–216.
5. Manolio, T. A., Baughman, K. L., Rodeheffer, R., et al. (1992). Prevalence and etiology of idiopathic dilated cardiomyopathy (summary of a National Heart, Lung, and Blood Institute workshop. *J Cardiol, 69*, 1458–1466.
6. Dries, D. L., Exner, D. V., Gersh, B. J., et al. (1999). Racial differences in the outcome of left ventricular dysfunction. *N Engl J Med, 340*, 609–616.
7. Carson, P., Ziesche, S., Johnson, G., et al. (1999). Racial differences in response to therapy for heart failure: analysis of the vasodilator-heart failure trials. Vasodilator-Heart failure trial study group. *J Card Fail, 5*, 178–187.
8. BEST Investigators. (2001). A trial of the beta-blocker bucindolol in patients with advanced chronic heart failure. *N Engl J Med, 344*, 1659–1667.
9. Exner, D. V., Dries, D. L., Domanski, M. J., et al. (2001). Lesser response to angiotensin-converting-enzyme inhibitor therapy in black as compared with white patients with left ventricular dysfunction. *N Engl J Med, 344*, 1351–1357.
10. Dries, D. L., Strong, M. H., Cooper, R. S., et al. (2002). Efficacy of angiotensin-converting enzyme inhibition in reducing progression from asymptomatic left ventricular dysfunction to symptomatic heart failure in black and white patients. *J Am Coll Cardiol, 40*, 311–317.
11. Ho, K. K., Anderson, K. M., Kannel, W. B., et al. (1993). Survival after the onset of congestive heart failure in Framingham heart study subjects. *Circulation, 88*, 107–115.
12. Schocken, D. D., Arrieta, M. I., Leaverton, P. E., et al. (1992). Prevalence and mortality rate of congestive heart failure in the United States. *J Am Coll Cardiol, 20*, 301–306.
13. The SOLVD Investigators. (1991). Effect of enalapril on survival in patients with reduced left ventricular ejection fractions and congestive heart failure. *N Engl J Med, 325*, 293–302.
14. Bourassa, M. G., Gurne, O., Bangdiwala, S. I., et al. (1993). Natural history and patterns of current practice in heart failure. The studies of left ventricular dysfunction (SOLVD) investigators. *J Am Coll Cardiol, 22*, 14A–19A.
15. Ghali, J. K., Pina, I. L., Gottlieb, S. S., et al. (2002). Metoprolol CR/XL in female patients with heart failure: analysis of the experience in metoprolol extended-release randomized intervention trial in heart failure (MERIT-HF). *Circulation, 105*, 1585–1591.
16. Simon, T., Mary-Krause, M., Funck-Brentano, C., et al. (2001). Sex differences in the prognosis of congestive heart failure: results from the cardiac insufficiency bisoprolol study (CIBIS II). *Circulation, 103*, 375–380.
17. Levy, D., Larson, M. G., Vasan, R. S., et al. (1996). The progression from hypertension to congestive heart failure. *JAMA, 275*, 1557–1562.
18. Nieminen, M. S., Harjola, V. P., Hochadel, M., et al. (2008). Gender related differences in patients presenting with acute heart failure. *Results from EuroHeart failure survey II. Eur J Heart Fail, 10*, 140–148.
19. Dec, G. W., & Fuster, V. (1994). Idiopathic dilated cardiomyopathy. *N Engl J Med, 331*, 1564–1575.
20. Sugrue, D. D., Rodeheffer, R. J., Codd, M. B., et al. (1992). The clinical course of idiopathic dilated cardiomyopathy. A population-based study. *Ann Intern Med, 117*, 117–123.
21. Kubo, T., Matsumura, Y., Kitaoka, H., et al. (2008). Improvement in prognosis of dilated cardiomyopathy in the elderly over the past 20 years. *J Cardiol, 52*, 111–117.
22. Amoah, A. G., & Kallen, C. (2000). Aetiology of heart failure as seen from a national cardiac referral centre in Africa. *Cardiology, 93*, 11–18.
23. Felker, G. M., Thompson, R. E., Hare, J. M., et al. (2000). Underlying causes and long-term survival in patients with initially unexplained cardiomyopathy. *N Engl J Med, 342*, 1077–1084.
24. Steimle, A. E., Stevenson, L. W., Fonarow, G. C., et al. (1994). Prediction of improvement in recent onset cardiomyopathy after referral for heart transplantation. *J Am Coll Cardiol, 23*, 553–559.
25. Ehlert, F. A., Cannom, D. S., Renfroe, E. G., et al. (2001). Comparison of dilated cardiomyopathy and coronary artery disease in patients with life-threatening ventricular arrhythmias: differences in presentation and outcome in the AVID registry. *Am Heart J, 142*, 816–822.
26. The Digitalis Investigation Group. (1997). The effect of digoxin on mortality and morbidity in patients with heart failure. *N Engl J Med, 336*, 525–533.
27. Singh, S. N., Fletcher, R. D., Fisher, S. G., et al. (1995). Amiodarone in patients with congestive heart failure and asymptomatic ventricular arrhythmia. Survival trial of antiarrhythmic therapy in congestive heart failure. *N Engl J Med, 333*, 77–82.
28. CIBIS-II Investigators and Committees. (1999). The cardiac insufficiency bisoprolol study II (CIBIS-II): a randomised trial. *Lancet, 353*, 9–13.
29. Packer, M., O'Connor, C. M., Ghali, J. K., et al. (1996). Effect of amlodipine on morbidity and mortality in severe chronic heart failure. Prospective randomized amlodipine survival evaluation study group. *N Engl J Med, 335*, 1107–1114.
30. Piano, M. R. (2002). Alcoholic cardiomyopathy: incidence, clinical characteristics, and pathophysiology. *Chest, 121*, 1638–1650.
31. Walsh, C. R., Larson, M. G., Evans, J. C., et al. (2002). Alcohol consumption and risk for congestive heart failure in the Framingham heart study. *Ann Intern Med, 136*, 181–191.
32. Abramson, J. L., Williams, S. A., Krumholz, H. M., et al. (2001). Moderate alcohol consumption and risk of heart failure among older persons. *JAMA, 285*, 1971–1977.
33. Lang, R. M., Borow, K. M., Neumann, A., et al. (1985). Adverse cardiac effects of acute alcohol ingestion in young adults. *Ann Intern Med, 102*, 742–747.
34. Preedy, V. R., Atkinson, L. M., Richardson, P. J., et al. (1993). Mechanisms of ethanol-induced cardiac damage. *Br Heart J, 69*, 197–200.
35. Bakeeva, L. E., Skulachev, V. P., Sudarikova, Y. V., et al. (2001). Mitochondria enter the nucleus (one further problem in chronic alcoholism). *Biochemistry (Mosc), 66*, 1335–1341.
36. Pavan, D., Nicolosi, G. L., Lestuzzi, C., et al. (1987). Normalization of variables of left ventricular function in patients with alcoholic cardiomyopathy after cessation of excessive alcohol intake: an echocardiographic study. *Eur Heart J, 85*, 535–540.
37. Jessup, M., Abraham, W. T., Casey, D. E., et al. (2009). 2009 focused update: ACCF/AHA guidelines for the diagnosis and management of heart failure in adults: a report of the American College of Cardiology Foundation/American Heart Association task force on practice guidelines: developed in collaboration with the International Society for Heart and Lung Transplantation. *Circulation, 119*, 1977–2016.
38. Chakko, S., & Myerburg, R. J. (1995). Cardiac complications of cocaine abuse. *Clin Cardiol, 18*, 67–72.
39. Om, A., Warner, M., Sabri, N., et al. (1992). Frequency of coronary artery disease and left ventricle dysfunction in cocaine users. *Am J Cardiol, 69*, 1549–1552.
40. Virmani, R., Robinowitz, M., Smialek, J. E., et al. (1988). Cardiovascular effects of cocaine: an autopsy study of 40 patients. *Am Heart J, 115*, 1068–1076.
41. Bozkurt, B., Kribbs, S., Clubb, F. J., Jr., et al. (1998). Pathophysiologically relevant concentrations of tumor necrosis factor-α promote progressive left ventricular dysfunction and remodeling in rats. *Circulation, 97*, 1382–1391.
42. Barbaro, G., Di Lorenzo, G., Grisorio, B., et al. (1998). Incidence of dilated cardiomyopathy and detection of HIV in myocardial cells of HIV-positive patients. Gruppo Italiano per lo Studio Cardiologico dei Pazienti Affetti da AIDS. *N Engl J Med, 339*, 1093–1099.
43. Raidel, S. M., Haase, C., Jansen, N. R., et al. (2002). Targeted myocardial transgenic expression of HIV Tat causes cardiomyopathy and mitochondrial damage. *Am J Physiol Heart Circ Physiol, 282*, H1672–H1678.
44. Kaul, S., Fishbein, M. C., & Siegel, R. J. (1991). Cardiac manifestations of acquired immune deficiency syndrome: a 1991 update. *Am Heart J, 122*, 535–544.
45. Grody, W. W., Cheng, L., & Lewis, W. (1990). Infection of the heart by the human immunodeficiency virus. *Am J Cardiol, 66*, 203–206.
46. Rossi, M. A., & Bestetti, R. B. (1995). The challenge of chagasic cardiomyopathy. The pathologic roles of autonomic abnormalities, autoimmune mechanisms and microvascular changes, and therapeutic implications. *Cardiology, 86*, 1–7.
47. Burke, A. P., Saenger, J., Mullick, F., et al. (1991). Hypersensitivity myocarditis. *Arch Pathol Lab Med, 115*, 764–769.
48. Paradiso, M., Gabrielli, F., Masala, C., et al. (2001). Evaluation of myocardial involvement in systemic lupus erythematosus by signal-averaged electrocardiography and echocardiography. *Acta Cardiol, 56*, 381–386.
49. Kazzam, E., Caidahl, K., Hallgren, R., et al. (1991). Non-invasive assessment of systolic left ventricular function in systemic sclerosis. *Eur Heart J, 12*, 151–156.
50. Goldenberg, J., Ferraz, M. B., Pessoa, A. P., et al. (1992). Symptomatic cardiac involvement in juvenile rheumatoid arthritis. *Int J Cardiol, 34*, 57–62.
51. Elkayam, U., Tummala, P. P., Rao, K., et al. (2001). Maternal and fetal outcomes of subsequent pregnancies in women with peripartum cardiomyopathy. *N Engl J Med, 344*, 1567–1571.
52. O'Connell, J. B., Costanzo-Nordin, M. R., Subramanian, R., et al. (1986). Peripartum cardiomyopathy: clinical, hemodynamic, histologic and prognostic characteristics. *J Am Coll Cardiol, 8*, 52–56.
53. Alpert, M. A. (2001). Obesity cardiomyopathy: pathophysiology and evolution of the clinical syndrome. *Am J Med Sci, 321*, 225–236.
54. Schulze, P. C. (2009). Myocardial lipid accumulation and lipotoxicity in heart failure. *J Lipid Res, 50*(11), 2137–2138.
55. Kenchaiah, S., Evans, J. C., Levy, D., et al. (2002). Obesity and the risk of heart failure. *N Engl J Med, 347*, 305–313.
56. Bozkurt, B., & Deswal, A. (2005). Obesity as a prognostic factor in chronic symptomatic heart failure. *Am Heart J, 150*, 1233–1239.
57. Alpert, M. A., Lambert, C. R., Panayiotou, H., et al. (1995). Relation of duration of morbid obesity to left ventricular mass, systolic function, and diastolic filling, and effect of weight loss. *Am J Cardiol, 76*, 1194–1197.
58. Ristow, B., Rabkin, J., & Haeusslein, E. (2008). Improvement in dilated cardiomyopathy after bariatric surgery. *J Card Fail, 14*, 198–202.
59. Sayin, T., & Guldal, M. (2005). Sibutramine: possible cause of a reversible cardiomyopathy. *Int J Cardiol, 99*, 481–482.
60. Beck-da-Silva, L., Higginson, L., Fraser, M., et al. (2005). Effect of orlistat in obese patients with heart failure: a pilot study. *Congest Heart Fail, 11*, 118–123.
61. Klein, I., & Ojamaa, K. (2001). Thyroid hormone and the cardiovascular system. *N Engl J Med, 344*, 501–509.

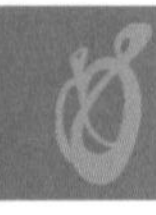

62. Lee, R. T., Plappert, M., & Sutton, M. G. (1990). Depressed left ventricular systolic ejection force in hypothyroidism. *Am J Cardiol, 65*, 526–527.
63. Colao, A., Marzullo, P., Di Somma, C., et al. (2001). Growth hormone and the heart. *Clin Endocrinol (Oxf), 54*, 137–154.
64. Osterziel, K. J., Strohm, O., Schuler, J., et al. (1998). Randomised, double-blind, placebo-controlled trial of human recombinant growth hormone in patients with chronic heart failure due to dilated cardiomyopathy. *Lancet, 351*, 1233–1237.
65. Djoenaidi, W., Notermans, S. L., & Dunda, G. (1992). Beriberi cardiomyopathy. *Eur J Clin Nutr, 46*, 227–234.
66. Retter, A. S. (1999). Carnitine and its role in cardiovascular disease. *Heart Dis, 1*, 108–113.
67. Razeghi, P., Young, M. E., Ying, J., et al. (2002). Downregulation of metabolic gene expression in failing human heart before and after mechanical unloading. *Cardiology, 97*, 203–209.
68. Holubarsch, C. J., Rohrbach, M., Karrasch, M., et al. (2007). A double-blind randomized multicentre clinical trial to evaluate the efficacy and safety of two doses of etomoxir in comparison with placebo in patients with moderate congestive heart failure: the ERGO (etomoxir for the recovery of glucose oxidation) study. *Clin Sci (Lond), 113*, 205–212.
69. Cheng, T. O. (2002). Selenium deficiency and cardiomyopathy. *J R Soc Med, 95*, 219–220.
70. Mahon, N. G., Coonar, A. S., Jeffery, S., et al. (2000). Haemochromatosis gene mutations in idiopathic dilated cardiomyopathy. *Heart, 84*, 541–547.
71. Gochee, P. A., & Powell, L. W. (2001). What's new in hemochromatosis. *Curr Opin Hematol, 8*, 98–104.
72. Wojcik, J. P., Speechley, M. R., Kertesz, A. E., et al. (2002). Natural history of C282Y homozygotes for hemochromatosis. *Can J Gastroenterol, 16*, 297–302.
73. Umana, E., Solares, C. A., & Alpert, M. A. (2003). Tachycardia-induced cardiomyopathy. *Am J Med, 114*, 51–55.
74. Shelton, R. J., Clark, A. L., Goode, K., et al. (2009). A randomised, controlled study of rate versus rhythm control in patients with chronic atrial fibrillation and heart failure: (CAFE-II study). *Heart, 95*, 924–930.
75. Limas, C. J., Goldenberg, I. F., & Limas, C. (1989). Autoantibodies against β-adrenoceptors in human idiopathic dilated cardiomyopathy. *Circ Res, 64*, 97–103.
76. Carlquist, J. F., Menlove, R. L., Murray, M. B., et al. (1991). HLA class II (DR and DQ) antigen associations in idiopathic dilated cardiomyopathy. *Circulation, 83*, 515–522.
77. Maisel, A. S., Krishnaswamy, P., Nowak, R. M., et al. (2002). Rapid measurement of B-type natriuretic peptide in the emergency diagnosis of heart failure. *N Engl J Med, 347*, 161–167.
78. Koglin, J., Pehlivanli, S., Schwaiblmair, M., et al. (2001). Role of brain natriuretic peptide in risk stratification of patients with congestive heart failure. *J Am Coll Cardiol, 38*, 1934–1941.
79. Troughton, R. W., Frampton, C. M., Yandle, T. G., et al. (2000). Treatment of heart failure guided by plasma aminoterminal brain natriuretic peptide (N-BNP) concentrations. *Lancet, 355*, 1126–1130.
80. Dhaliwal, A. S., Deswal, A., Pritchett, A., et al. (2009). Reduction in BNP levels with treatment of decompensated heart failure and future clinical events. *J Card Fail, 15*, 293–299.
81. Mizuno, Y., Yoshimura, M., Harada, E., et al. (2000). Plasma levels of A- and B-type natriuretic peptides in patients with hypertrophic cardiomyopathy or idiopathic dilated cardiomyopathy. *Am J Cardiol, 86*, 1036–1040, A11.
82. Mancini, D. M., Wong, K. L., & Simson, M. B. (1993). Prognostic value of an abnormal signal-averaged electrocardiogram in patients with nonischemic congestive cardiomyopathy. *Circulation, 87*, 1083–1092.
83. Wallis, D. E., O'Connell, J. B., Henkin, R. E., et al. (1989). Segmental wall motion abnormalities in dilated cardiomyopathy. *J Am Coll Cardiol, 13*, 311–315.
84. Glamann, D. B., Lange, R. A., Corbett, J. R., et al. (1992). Utility of various radionuclide techniques for distinguishing ischemic from nonischemic dilated cardiomyopathy. *Arch Intern Med, 152*, 769–772.
85. Dec, G. W., Palacios, I., Yasuda, T., et al. (1990). Antimyosin antibody cardiac imaging: its role in the diagnosis of myocarditis. *J Am Coll Cardiol, 16*, 97–104.
86. Assomull, R. G., Prasad, S. K., Lyne, J., et al. (2006). Cardiovascular magnetic resonance, fibrosis, and prognosis in dilated cardiomyopathy. *J Am Coll Cardiol, 48*, 1977–1985.
87. Mason, J. W. (1989). Clinical merit of endomyocardial biopsy. *Circulation, 79*, 971–979.
88. Packer, M., Bristow, M. R., Cohn, J. N., et al. (1996). The effect of carvedilol on morbidity and mortality in patients with chronic heart failure. U.S. carvedilol heart failure study group. *N Engl J Med, 334*, 1349–1355.
89. Pitt, B., Zannad, F., Remme, W. J., et al. (1999). The effect of spironolactone on morbidity and mortality in patients with severe heart failure. Randomized aldactone evaluation study investigators. *N Engl J Med, 341*, 709–717.
90. Bozkurt, B., Agoston, I., & Knowlton, A. A. (2003). Complications of inappropriate use of spironolactone in heart failure: when an old medicine spirals out of new guidelines. *J Am Coll Cardiol, 41*, 211–214.
91. Juurlink, D. N., Mamdani, M. M., Lee, D. S., et al. (2004). Rates of hyperkalemia after publication of the randomized aldactone evaluation study. *N Engl J Med, 351*, 543–551.
92. McMurray, J. J., Ostergren, J., Swedberg, K., et al. (2003). Effects of candesartan in patients with chronic heart failure and reduced left-ventricular systolic function taking angiotensin-converting-enzyme inhibitors: the CHARM-Added trial. *Lancet, 362*, 767–771.
93. Adams, K. F., Jr., Gheorghiade, M., Uretsky, B. F., et al. (1997). Patients with mild heart failure worsen during withdrawal from digoxin therapy. *J Am Coll Cardiol, 30*, 42–48.
94. Dhaliwal, A. S., Bredikis, A., Habib, G., et al. (2008). Digoxin and clinical outcomes in systolic heart failure patients on contemporary background heart failure therapy. *Am J Cardiol, 102*, 1356–1360.
95. Taylor, A. L., Ziesche, S., Yancy, C., et al. (2004). Combination of isosorbide dinitrate and hydralazine in blacks with heart failure. *N Engl J Med, 351*, 2049–2057.
96. Cohn, J. N., Ziesche, S., Smith, R., et al. (1997). Effect of the calcium antagonist felodipine as supplementary vasodilator therapy in patients with chronic heart failure treated with enalapril: V-HeFT III. Vasodilator-Heart failure trial (V-HeFT) study group. *Circulation, 96*, 856–863.
97. AVID Investigators. (1997). A comparison of antiarrhythmic-drug therapy with implantable defibrillators in patients resuscitated from near-fatal ventricular arrhythmias. *N Engl J Med, 337*, 1576–1583.
98. Moss, A. J., Zareba, W., Hall, W. J., et al. (2002). Prophylactic implantation of a defibrillator in patients with myocardial infarction and reduced ejection fraction. *N Engl J Med, 346*, 877–883.
99. Bardy, G. H., Lee, K. L., Mark, D. B., et al. (2005). Amiodarone or an implantable cardioverter-defibrillator for congestive heart failure. *N Engl J Med, 352*, 225–237.
100. Strickberger, S. A., Hummel, J. D., Bartlett, T. G., et al. (2003). Amiodarone versus implantable cardioverter-defibrillator: randomized trial in patients with nonischemic dilated cardiomyopathy and asymptomatic nonsustained ventricular tachycardia-AMIOVIRT. *J Am Coll Cardiol, 41*, 1707–1712.
101. Kadish, A., Dyer, A., Daubert, J. P., et al. (2004). Prophylactic defibrillator implantation in patients with nonischemic dilated cardiomyopathy. *N Engl J Med, 350*, 2151–2158.
102. Desai, A. S., Fang, J. C., Maisel, W. H., et al. (2004). Implantable defibrillators for the prevention of mortality in patients with nonischemic cardiomyopathy: a meta-analysis of randomized controlled trials. *JAMA, 292*, 2874–2879.
103. Wilkoff, B. L., Cook, J. R., Epstein, A. E., et al. (2002). Dual-chamber pacing or ventricular backup pacing in patients with an implantable defibrillator: the dual chamber and VVI implantable defibrillator (DAVID) trial. *JAMA, 288*, 3115–3123.
104. Doval, H. C., Nul, D. R., Grancelli, H. O., et al. (1994). Randomised trial of low-dose amiodarone in severe congestive heart failure. Grupo de Estudio de la Sobrevida en la Insuficiencia Cardiaca en Argentina (GESICA). *Lancet, 344*, 493–498.
105. Abraham, W. T., Fisher, W. G., Smith, A. L., et al. (2002). Cardiac resynchronization in chronic heart failure. *N Engl J Med, 346*, 1845–1853.
106. Linde, C., Leclercq, C., Rex, S., et al. (2002). Long-term benefits of biventricular pacing in congestive heart failure: results from the multisite stimulation in cardiomyopathy (MUSTIC) study. *J Am Coll Cardiol, 40*, 111–118.
107. Bristow, M. R., Saxon, L. A., Boehmer, J., et al. (2004). Cardiac-resynchronization therapy with or without an implantable defibrillator in advanced chronic heart failure. *N Engl J Med, 350*, 2140–2150.
108. Cleland, J. G., Daubert, J. C., Erdmann, E., et al. (2005). The effect of cardiac resynchronization on morbidity and mortality in heart failure. *N Engl J Med, 352*, 1539–1549.
109. Moss, A. J., Hall, W. J., Cannom, D. S., et al. (2009). Cardiac-resynchronization therapy for the prevention of heart-failure events. *N Engl J Med, 361*, 1329–1338.
110. Beshai, J. F., Grimm, R. A., Nagueh, S. F., et al. (2007). Cardiac-resynchronization therapy in heart failure with narrow QRS complexes. *N Engl J Med, 357*, 2461–2471.
111. Massie, B. M., Krol, W. F., Ammon, S. E., et al. (2004). The warfarin and antiplatelet therapy in heart failure trial (WATCH): rationale, design, and baseline patient characteristics. *J Card Fail, 10*, 101–112.
112. Tavazzi, L., Maggioni, A. P., Marchioli, R., et al. (2008). Effect of rosuvastatin in patients with chronic heart failure (the GISSI-HF trial): a randomised, double-blind, placebo-controlled trial. *Lancet, 372*, 1231–1239.
113. Kjekshus, J., Apetrei, E., Barrios, V., et al. (2007). Rosuvastatin in older patients with systolic heart failure. *N Engl J Med, 357*, 2248–2261.
114. Tavazzi, L., Maggioni, A. P., Marchioli, R., et al. (2008). Effect of n-3 polyunsaturated fatty acids in patients with chronic heart failure (the GISSI-HF trial): a randomised, double-blind, placebo-controlled trial. *Lancet, 372*, 1223–1230.
115. Mason, J. W., O'Connel, J. B., Herskowitz, A., et al. (1995). A clinical trial of immunosuppressive therapy for myocarditis. *N Engl J Med, 333*, 269–275.
116. Bozkurt, B., Villaneuva, F. S., Holubkov, R., et al. (1999). Intravenous immune globulin in the therapy of peripartum cardiomyopathy. *J Am Coll Cardiol, 34*, 177–180.
117. Wallukat, G., Reinke, P., Dorffel, W. V., et al. (1996). Removal of autoantibodies in dilated cardiomyopathy by immunoadsorption. *Int J Cardiol, 54*, 191–195.
118. Felix, S. B., Staudt, A., Dorffel, W. V., et al. (2000). Hemodynamic effects of immunoadsorption and subsequent immunoglobulin substitution in dilated cardiomyopathy: three-month results from a randomized study. *J Am Coll Cardiol, 35*, 1590–1598.
119. Muller, J., Wallukat, G., Dandel, M., et al. (2000). Immunoglobulin adsorption in patients with idiopathic dilated cardiomyopathy. *Circulation, 101*, 385–391.
120. Staudt, A., Schaper, F., Stangl, V., et al. (2001). Immunohistological changes in dilated cardiomyopathy induced by immunoadsorption therapy and subsequent immunoglobulin substitution. *Circulation, 103*, 2681–2686.
121. Fazio, S., Sabatini, D., Capaldo, B., et al. (1996). A preliminary study of growth hormone in the treatment of dilated cardiomyopathy. *N Engl J Med, 334*, 809–814.
122. Isner, J. M. (2002). Myocardial gene therapy. *Nature, 415*, 234–239.
123. Dubowitz, V. (2002). Special centennial workshop-101st ENMC international workshop: therapeutic possibilities in Duchenne muscular dystrophy, 30th November-2nd December 2001, *Neuromuscul Disord* (12). The Netherlands: Naarden.
124. Silverberg, D. S., Wexler, D., Blum, M., et al. (2000). The use of subcutaneous erythropoietin and intravenous iron for the treatment of the anemia of severe, resistant congestive heart failure improves cardiac and renal function and functional cardiac class, and markedly reduces hospitalizations. *J Am Coll Cardiol, 35*, 1737–1744.
125. Ghali, J. K., Anand, I. S., Abraham, W. T., et al. (2008). Randomized double-blind trial of darbepoetin alfa in patients with symptomatic heart failure and anemia. *Circulation, 117*, 526–535.
126. Watson, P. S., Scalia, G. M., Galbraith, A., et al. (1999). Lack of effect of coenzyme Q on left ventricular function in patients with congestive heart failure. *J Am Coll Cardiol, 33*, 1549–1552.
127. O'Connor, C. M., Whellan, D. J., Lee, K. L., et al. (2009). Efficacy and safety of exercise training in patients with chronic heart failure: HF-ACTION randomized controlled trial. *JAMA, 301*, 1439–1450.

CHAPTER 25

Heart Failure as a Consequence of Restrictive Cardiomyopathy

Ali J. Marian

Hypertrophic cardiomyopathy (HCM) is a fascinating disease. Since its first description by French pathologist Liouville in the nineteenth century, HCM has continued to intrigue various experts from pathologists to clinicians and more recently geneticists. The continued interest in HCM has largely paralleled technological advances in medicine. Accordingly, HCM was primarily a pathological entity for the first half of the twentieth century[1,2] and was largely unrecognized as a clinical entity until the second half of the twentieth century.[3-5] During the latter era, phenotypic description of HCM was based on the development of modern diagnostic tools, such as cardiac catheterization and echocardiography. In the 1960s, Braunwald et al coined the term "idiopathic hypertrophic subaortic stenosis," or "IHSS," and provided the first comprehensive hemodynamic characteristics of left ventricular (LV) outflow tract obstruction in patients with HCM.[6-8] Hence, HCM was mainly recognized as a disease characterized by outflow tract obstruction. The recognition of outflow tract obstruction as a major phenotypic feature of HCM soon led to the description of surgical septal myectomy through a transaortic approach as an effective technique to reduce the outflow tract obstruction, a procedure that is widely known as the Morrow procedure.[9] More recently, Sigwart introduced catheter-based septal ablation typically performed through injection of alcohol into the septal branches of the left anterior descending coronary artery.[10] The latter technique is also effective in reducing the LV outflow tract gradient and for symptomatic relief.

The widespread use of M mode and 2-dimensional echocardiography in the 1970s expanded the phenotypic spectrum of HCM beyond the obstructive form to include concentric LV hypertrophy and asymmetric septal hypertrophy (ASH).[11] Soon Doppler echocardiography emerged as a robust noninvasive method to demonstrate and quantify the LV flow tract obstruction and to characterize cardiac diastolic dysfunction in HCM.[12-14] More recently, tissue Doppler imaging has been applied to delineate myocardial dysfunction, despite preserved global systolic function, and to demonstrate its potential utility to diagnose the disease early and independent of expression of cardiac hypertrophy.[15]

Seidman et al discovered the first causal gene for HCM in 1990 and ushered in the era of molecular genetics.[16] The discovery was a watershed event and it was soon followed by identification of over a dozen causal genes and several hundred mutations and modifier loci.[17] These advances in the molecular genetic basis of HCM have raised interest in genetic-based screening, diagnosis, and risk stratification. However, it has also become clear that the phenotype in HCM is determined not only by the causal mutations but also by the modifier genes and various other genetic and nongenetic factors.

Sudden cardiac death (SCD) has always been the main concern of the patients and physicians alike. The concern is highlighted by the fact that HCM is a major cause of SCD in the young and that SCD often occurs in apparently healthy and asymptomatic individuals.[18] The difficult challenge is in appropriate risk stratification and identification of the subgroup of individuals who are at high risk for SCD considering that HCM overall is a relatively benign disease.[19] SCD in the young is always tragic, particularly when it occurs in apparently healthy and athletic individuals without any noticeable warnings. In those with warning signs, however, conventional pharmacological interventions, while effective for symptomatic relief, are not known to reduce the risk of SCD. Thus the choice is primarily limited to the effective use of implantable defibrillators in those at high risk for SCD.[20] Recent experimental data in animal models of HCM have raised the potential utility of new pharmacological interventions in the prevention and regression of cardiac phenotype and possibly reducing the risk of cardiac arrhythmias.[21-23] Clinical studies are needed to test the potential utility of new pharmacological interventions in reversing or preventing cardiac phenotype and reducing the risk of SCD in humans with HCM.

DEFINITION

HCM is a genetic disease of cardiac myocytes. Thus it is primarily a disease of the myocardium. Clinically HCM is diagnosed by the presence of primary cardiac hypertrophy (i.e., cardiac hypertrophy that cannot be fully explained by the loading conditions, valvular diseases, or other external factors).[17] Typically the LV cavity is normal or even small in size because of concentric hypertrophy and global LV systolic function is normal or even hyperdynamic.[17]

Diagnostic Challenges

Clinical diagnosis, typically based on the echocardiographic findings of cardiac hypertrophy, is usually straightforward. However, there are many diagnostic challenges. The most common is the presence of systemic hypertension, which affects approximately one third of the adult population in the United States and hence may exist concomitantly in patients with HCM. In the presence of systemic hypertension, it is difficult to diagnose HCM with a high level of certainty and yet a significant number of patients with systemic hypertension exhibit a disproportionate hypertrophic response. Such patients

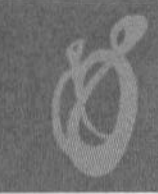

may have an underlying causal mutation for HCM or may have a genetic background that renders them prone to an enhanced hypertrophic response to systemic hypertension. In the former scenario, systemic hypertension could serve as a contributing factor to phenotypic expression of cardiac hypertrophy in HCM. Nevertheless, while conventional, the presence of systemic hypertension or even valvular abnormalities alone is not sufficient to exclude HCM definitively. This dilemma is often encountered in competitive professional athletes who exhibit significant cardiac hypertrophy, necessitating the distinction between pathological hypertrophy of HCM and the physiological hypertrophy of exercise. The distinction is crucial because HCM is the most common discernible cause of SCD in professional athletes and its diagnosis bars them from competitive sports. Clinical clues such as the extent, severity, and the type of cardiac hypertrophy, hyperdynamic left ventricle, small LV cavity size, the presence of outflow tract obstruction, and tissue Doppler or magnetic resonance abnormalities of the myocardium could help to differentiate true HCM from other hypertrophic conditions.

The clinical diagnosis of HCM based on the presence of primary cardiac hypertrophy is also compounded by phenocopy conditions, which are diseases that cause gross cardiac hypertrophy and mimic HCM. Phenocopy conditions include various storage diseases, mitochondrial diseases, triplet repeat syndromes, and others.[24,25] The distinction between true HCM and phenocopy conditions is important as their pathogenesis and treatment differ significantly. The clinical distinction, however, is often difficult because the gross phenotype, namely cardiac hypertrophy, is very similar between true HCM and its phenocopy conditions. Phenotypic features such as the presence of a hyperdynamic left ventricle and outflow tract obstruction would favor the diagnosis of true HCM. In contrast, the presence of depressed global cardiac systolic function, cardiac dilation, conduction defects, or involvement of other organs—such as deafness, neurological abnormalities, and skeletal myopathy—suggest the possibility of a phenocopy condition. Often it is necessary to perform an endomyocardial biopsy for histological examination, including detection of myocyte disarray, which is considered the pathological hallmark of true HCM. Likewise, specific histological staining of myocardial sections could help to diagnose storage diseases. As an example, the phenocopy condition caused by mutations in the $\gamma 2$ subunit of adenosine monophosphate kinase (AMPK) is due to storage of glycogen in the heart.[25-27] The phenotype is characterized by cardiac hypertrophy, conduction defect, and the preexcitation pattern on the electrocardiogram. Finally, genetic-based diagnosis is expected to provide a clear distinction between true HCM and phenocopy conditions. With advances in the molecular genetic basis of HCM and the phenocopy conditions, one would expect genetic-based screening to provide for a robust distinction between true HCM and its phenocopy. The genetic-based distinction is likely to gain clinical significance as new specific treatments for HCM and phenocopy conditions are developed.

The shortcomings of the current clinical diagnosis of HCM, which is primarily based on an echocardiographic finding of "unexplained" cardiac hypertrophy, have raised the interest in genetic-based diagnosis. Genetic-based diagnosis is expected to provide the opportunity for the preclinical diagnosis of those with causal mutations. Genetic-based diagnosis not only provides the opportunity for an early diagnosis but could have considerable implications for early interventions to prevent the evolution of the phenotype and the risk of SCD. However, for the genetic-based diagnosis to supplant the clinical diagnosis of HCM and become routine, further advances in our understanding of the genetic causes of HCM and in genetic screening techniques would be necessary. Despite the apparent advantages of genetic-based diagnosis and intervention, phenotypic variability of HCM, even in those with an identical causal mutation, and the complexity of factors that determine the clinical outcome somewhat limit the clinical utility of genetic-based risk stratification. Thus clinical decision making in the management of the patients with HCM should comprise all constituents of the determinants of the phenotype, whether genetic or environmental.

PREVALENCE

HCM is a relatively common disease with an estimated prevalence of approximately 1 in 500 in the general population.[28] The estimate was based on the presence of LV wall thickness of 15 mm or greater on an echocardiogram in a relatively young population between the ages of 23 and 35 years. This estimate may underestimate the true prevalence of HCM because of the stringent diagnostic criteria used to define HCM because many patients with the causal mutation may express a milder degree of cardiac hypertrophy. Likewise, the estimate was determined in a relatively young population and many young individuals with causal mutations may not exhibit the phenotype yet because of age-dependent expression of the phenotype. Thus a higher prevalence in an older population would be expected. Another caveat is the potential presence of concomitant systemic hypertension, which by definition in most situations excludes the diagnosis of HCM. The prevalence estimate, however, potentially includes those with the phenocopy conditions, defined as conditions that grossly are similar to HCM but are not true HCM as their pathogenesis differs significantly. The prevalence of phenocopy conditions in those with the clinical diagnosis of HCM is unknown but may comprise a significant number of all cases diagnosed clinically as HCM. Thus to determine the precise prevalence of true HCM, large-scale genetic studies in conjunction with clinical studies will be needed.

PHENOTYPIC MANIFESTATIONS

Clinical Presentation

Patients with HCM exhibit a diverse array of clinical phenotypes, ranging from a benign asymptomatic course to that of severe diastolic heart failure and SCD. Most patients with HCM are asymptomatic or mildly symptomatic. The most common symptoms are dyspnea, which typically occurs upon exertion; chest pain, which is atypical for being of coronary origin; palpitations, lightheadedness and less frequently syncope. Syncope is usually due to cardiac arrhythmias and less frequently due to hypotension. Recurrent syncope often is a major predictor of SCD and merits full evaluation and treatment.[29,30] Supraventricular arrhythmias including atrial fibrillation and ventricular arrhythmias are the most common cardiac arrhythmias and are important determinants of clinical outcomes.[31,32] Likewise, a small subgroup of patients with HCM exhibits electrocardiographic findings of Wolff-Parkinson-White (WPW) syndrome and therefore may develop AV nodal reciprocating arrhythmias. In the presence of an electrocardiographic pattern of preexcitation, the possibility of phenocopy conditions should be considered.[26,27]

SCD in HCM

Despite the heterogeneity of the clinical phenotype, the most pressing issue for patients, whether symptomatic or not, and physicians is the risk of SCD. The risk is of particular concern in young competitive athletes because HCM is the most common cause of SCD in this group in the United States.[18,33] Indeed HCM is responsible for approximately half of the cases of SCD in athletes younger than 35 years of age in the U.S. population.[18] This is in contrast to Italy where arrhythmogenic right ventricular cardiomyopathy appears to be the

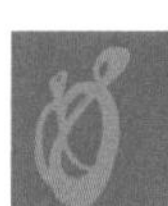

most common cause of SCD in professional athletes.[34] In both conditions the death is tragic, as SCD often occurs as the first manifestation of the disease in apparently young healthy individuals.[18] SCD typically occurs during or immediately after exercise and often on the sports field.

There is no reliable predictor of SCD in HCM. However, several clinical, pathological, and genetic factors have been identified as major risk factors for SCD in patients with HCM, including a previous episode of cardiac arrest, recurrent syncope, severe cardiac hypertrophy, presence of multiple runs of nonsustained ventricular tachycardia or sustained ventricular tachycardia, and a strong family history of SCD.[35-38] The putative risk factors for SCD in patients with HCM are listed in Box 25-1.

SCD also may occur in the absence of discernible risk factors but the overall risk is low. In the risk stratification and counseling of patients with HCM for SCD, it is important to consider the global risk because the positive predictive value of each putative risk marker is relatively low.[37,38] In general, HCM is a relatively benign disease with an estimated annual mortality of about 1% in the adult population but higher, ranging from 2% to 3%, in children.[19,39-41]

Morphological and functional features

Cardiac hypertrophy is the quintessential morphological phenotype of HCM, though the degree of cardiac hypertrophy may be mild and gross hypertrophy may be absent in a small fraction of the patients. Likewise, a typical feature of HCM is the asymmetric nature of cardiac hypertrophy with the predominant involvement of the interventricular septum. Indeed, an interventricular septal to posterior wall thickness ratio of 1:3 is considered a major feature. However, cardiac hypertrophy involves the septum and the posterior wall in approximately one third of cases and in a small group of patients hypertrophy is localized to the apex, lateral wall, or posterior wall. Patients with apical HCM may exhibit the unique phenotype of giant T wave inversion in the precordial leads on an electrocardiogram. Patients with apical HCM may experience significant cardiovascular morbidity but have a relatively benign prognosis with a 15-year survival rate of approximately 95%.[42]

The LV cavity size is usually small or at least not dilated. The LV outflow tract is often narrow and could be obstructed to blood flow further because of systolic anterior motion (SAM) of the anterior leaflet of the mitral valve. In a small fraction of patients, the mitral valve may have anatomic malposition and/or an elongated anterior leaflet. The left ventricle is hyperdynamic and LV ejection fraction, a global index of systolic function, is usually increased or preserved. However, more sensitive indices of LV regional function such as tissue Doppler imaging show impaired myocardial systolic and diastolic function.[43] The typical feature of HCM is impaired cardiac diastolic function and elevated LV end-diastolic pressure, which is the primary reason for symptoms of heart failure in HCM. Occasionally the phenotype of HCM (i.e., concentric cardiac hypertrophy with hyperdynamic left ventricle) evolves into the phenotype of dilated cardiomyopathy (DCM),

BOX 25–1 Potential Risk Factors for SCD in Patients with HCM

Established Risk Factors
- Prior episode of cardiac arrest (aborted SCD)
- Family history of SCD (more than 1 premature SCD)
  - Causal mutations, including double mutations
  - Modifier genes
- History of syncope
- Sustained and repetitive nonsustained ventricular tachycardia
- Severe cardiac hypertrophy

Probable Risk Factors
- Left ventricular outflow tract obstruction
- Abnormal blood pressure response to exercise
- Severe interstitial fibrosis and myocyte disarray
- Early onset of clinical manifestations (young age)
- Presence of myocardial ischemia

Left ventricular outflow tract obstruction (LVOT) at rest is present in approximately 25% of patients with HCM (Figure 25-1). The obstruction is in part caused by anatomical narrowing of the LVOT because of septal and subaortic hypertrophy and in part by dynamic obstruction due to a hyperdynamic left ventricle with a small cavity and SAM of the mitral valve leaflet. LVOT gradient could be provoked using amyl nitrate, exercise, or dobutamine in the majority of patients with HCM. The presence of LVOT obstruction is associated with significant mortality and morbidity in patients with HCM.[44] The LVOT obstruction has characteristic LV systolic pressure peripheral pulse waveforms with two components of early and late systolic waves, the latter referred to as a "bifid pulse."

Histopathological features

Cardiac myocyte hypertrophy with pleiotropic nuclei is a common feature. However, the histopathological hallmark of HCM is cardiac myocyte disarray, which is defined as malaligned, distorted, and often short and hypertrophic myocytes oriented in different directions (Figure 25-2). Disarray may comprise 20% to 30% of the myocardium as opposed to less than 5% of the myocardium in the normal heart.[45] Myocyte disarray is commonly found throughout the myocardium but considered more remarkable in the interventricular septum. Myocyte disarray is associated with the risk of SCD in young patients with HCM.[46] Likewise, interstitial fibrosis is a common feature of HCM and is associated with cardiac arrhythmias.[46] Other histopathological phenotypes include a subaortic thickening of the endocardium further compromising the outflow tract, thickening of media of intramural coronary arteries, malpositioned mitral valve, and elongated leaflets. Histopathological phenotypes such as myocyte disarray, hypertrophy, and interstitial fibrosis are associated with the risk of SCD, mortality, and morbidity in patients with HCM.

MOLECULAR GENETICS

HCM is a genetic disease. It is familial in approximately two thirds of cases and sporadic in the remainder. The mode of inheritance in familial HCM is autosomal dominant.[47] Therefore, 50% of the offspring, males and females equally, will inherit the mutation and will develop the disease sometime in life. An autosomal recessive mode of inheritance has also been described.[48] Sporadic cases are caused by inheritance of germ line de novo mutations from the parents.[49] The causal mutation in a sporadic case will be passed on to the offspring in an autosomal dominant fashion.

The pioneering work of Dr. Christine Seidman et al led to identification of the first causal mutation, namely the R403Q mutation in *MYH7* encoding the β-myosin heavy chain (MyHC) protein in families with HCM.[16] The discovery was soon followed by identification of mutations in *TNNT2* and *TPM1*, coding for cardiac troponin T and α-tropomyosin proteins, respectively, in families with HCM. Since then more than a dozen causal genes and several hundred mutations in families with HCM have been identified (Table 25-1). Thus HCM is a genetically heterogeneous disease. Nevertheless, all known causal genes, with the exception of those that cause phenocopy states, encode sarcomeric proteins (Figure 25-3).

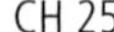

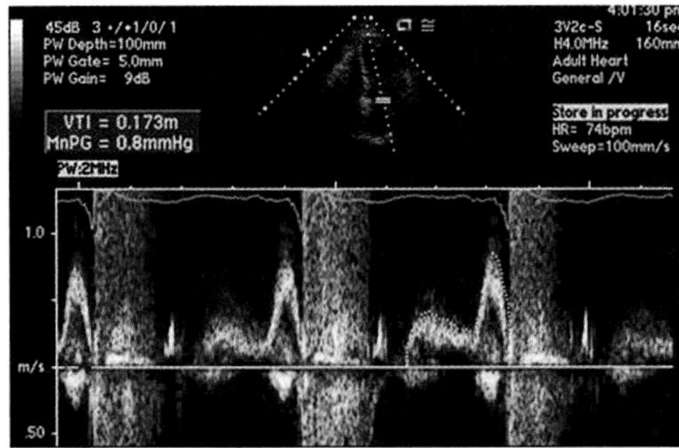

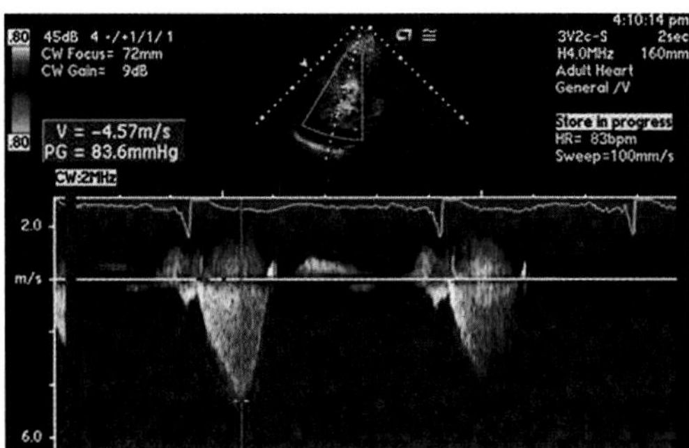

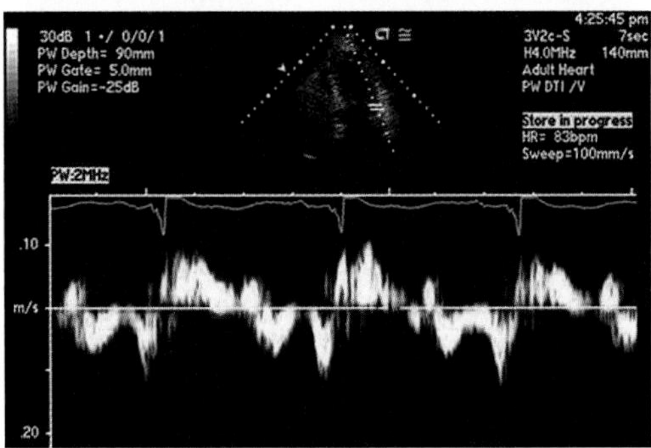

FIGURE 25–1 Echo/Doppler evaluation of cardiac function in a patient with HCM and severe outflow tract obstruction. **A,** Mitral inflow velocities showing diastolic dysfunction evidenced by decreased E and increased A velocities. **B,** Doppler measurement of left ventricular outflow tract gradient, which is about 40 mm Hg. **C,** Reduced systolic and early diastolic velocities, which are early markers for HCM.

Therefore, HCM is considered a disease of sarcomeric proteins.[50] Perhaps clinically diagnosed HCM could be differentiated into those caused by sarcomeric protein mutations and true HCM, and those caused by mutations in nonsarcomeric proteins and phenocopy conditions, such as glycogen storage disorders.

Causal Genes

Causal genes by definition are those that, whenever mutated, cause HCM, albeit with variable penetrance and expressivity. During the past 2 decades about two thirds of all causal genes for HCM have been identified. The most common causal genes for HCM are *MYH7* and *MYBPC3*, encoding β-MyHC and myosin binding protein C (MyBP-C). Each is responsible for approximately 25% of the HCM cases.[51-54] Several hundred different mutations in *MYH7* and *MYBPC3* in families and individuals with HCM have been identified. Most *MYH7* mutations are located within the globular head of the β-MyHC, which is the site of ATPase activity and binding to cardiac α-actin. A few mutations in the hinge arm and the rod tail of the β-MyHC also have been described.[55,56] Otherwise, there is no obvious predilection toward concentration of the mutations in a specific domain. A noteworthy difference in the *MYH7* and *MYBPC3* mutations is the prevalence of insertion/deletion mutations in *MYBPC3* as opposed to *MYH7* wherein the vast majority of the mutations are missense mutations. The next most common causal genes are *TNNT2* and *TNNI3*, which encode cardiac troponin T and cardiac troponin I, respectively, each accounting for approximately 3% to 5% of HCM families.[51,57,58]

There are a large number of uncommon causal genes for HCM, including *TPM1* encoding α-tropomyosin, *ACTC* encoding cardiac α-actin, *TTN* encoding titin, *MYL3* encoding essential myosin light chain, and *MYL2*, which codes for the regulatory myosin light chain.[59-61,62-64] The spectrum of the causal gene expands beyond the thin and thick filaments of the sarcomere to include genes encoding the Z-disk proteins, such as *TCAP* encoding telethonin, *MYOZ2* coding for myozenin 2 or calsarcin 1 and muscle LIM protein (*CSRP3*).[65-67] Finally, mutations in *TNNC1*, *MYH6*, *MYLK2*, *PLN*, and *CAV3* coding for cardiac troponin C, α-MyHC, myosin light chain kinase, phospholamban, and caveolin 3 have been reported in patients with HCM.[65,68-71] However, their causal role in HCM is less certain.

TABLE 25–1 Causal Genes for HCM

Established Causal Gene	Protein	Prevalence
MYH7	β-Myosin heavy chain	~25%
MYBPC	Myosin binding protein-C	~25%
TNNT2	Cardiac troponin T	~2%-5%
TNNI3	Cardiac troponin I	~2%-5%
TPM1	α-tropomyosin	~2%-5%
MYOZ2	Myozenin 2 (calsarcin 1)	1:250
ACTA1	Cardiac α-actin	<1%
TTN	Titin	<1%
MYL3	Essential myosin light chain	<1%
MYL2	Regulatory myosin light chain	<1%
TCAP	Tcap (Telethonin or titin-cap)	Rare
Possible Causal Genes		
PLN	Phospholamban	Rare
CAV3	Caveolin 3	Rare
MYH6	α-Myosin heavy chain	Rare
MYLK2	Cardiac myosin light peptide kinase	Rare
TNNCI	Cardiac troponin C	Rare

Most HCM mutations are missense mutations that typically affect a highly conserved amino acid. However, frame-shift

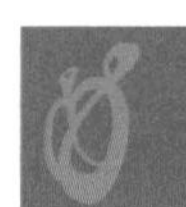

mutations resulting from an insertion or a nucleotide and splice junction mutations are also found more commonly in *MYBPC3* than the other causal genes.[51,53,72] The frameshift mutations typically lead to premature truncation of the protein, which may not be stably expressed.[73] An important point with implications for genetic testing is the low frequency of each causal HCM mutation and that most mutations are "private." Another noteworthy point is the presence of double mutations, which have been reported in a small fraction of patients with HCM but are recognized more often because systemic screening of many genes are included in genetic analysis.[74,75]

An important point in genetic studies of HCM is the issue of causality, which is often difficult to establish particularly in sporadic cases or small families whereby the cosegregation of the phenotype with inheritance of the disease cannot be established. Likewise, "there is no perfect protein" because any protein may have a polymorphic variant, including nonsynonymous variants. Thus identification of a nonsynonymous variant in an individual with the phenotype should not be interpreted as a causal mutation. One should consider the frequency of the variant in the general population, conservation of the involved amino acid across species, and the biological and functional effects of variants when considering causality. In general, the analogous element of the Koch postulates of causality needs to be fulfilled as much as possible.[76]

Modifier Genes

Genes that have variants that affect the expression and severity of the phenotype of a single gene disorder are referred to as "modifier genes." The variants are referred to as the "modifier alleles." Modifier alleles, unlike causal mutations, are neither necessary nor sufficient to cause HCM. However, when present, they influence phenotypic expression of the disease. In the case of HCM, variants of the modifier genes could influence the severity of cardiac hypertrophy, risk of SCD, and susceptibility to cardiac arrhythmias or heart failure. Modifier genes are partially responsible for the phenotypic variability of HCM.[77] Phenotypic variability of HCM is notable among individuals with different causal mutations and among individuals who have identical causal mutations[77] (Figure 25-4). The influence of the modifier genes on phenotypic expression of HCM is best illustrated in familial HCM, wherein members of the family share an identical causal mutation and yet exhibit significant variation in phenotypic expression.

The interindividual variability in the phenotypic expression of HCM is partially due to the presence of single-nucleotide polymorphisms (SNPs) and structural variants often referred to as copy number variants (CNVs) in the genome. There are several million SNPs and several thousands CNVs in the genome.[78,79] The CNVs, although less frequent than the SNPs, affect about three fourths of all variant nucleotides in the genome.[78] Accordingly, patients with HCM are expected to have considerable SNPs and SVs in their genome, which could affect phenotypic expression of HCM.

We recently performed a genomewide scan in members of a very large family with HCM caused by an insertion mutation in *MYBPC3* and mapped five modifier loci that influence expression of cardiac hypertrophy.[80] The loci, located on 3q26.2 (two separate loci), 10p13, 17q24, and 16q12.2 impart considerable effect on the magnitude of cardiac hypertrophy. The effect sizes range from an approximately 8-to approximately 90-g shift in the LV mass, depending on the heterozygosity or homozygosity of the modifier alleles. The mapped modifier loci encompass several biologically plausible candidate genes including Grb2 and ITGA8, which have been implicated in modulating cardiac hypertrophy and fibrosis in mice.[81,82]

Through candidate gene analysis, several genes have been implicated as the modifiers for cardiac hypertrophy in HCM. Among them is the *ACE*, which encodes the angiotensin-1–converting enzyme 1.[83,84] The insertion/deletion polymorphism in the *ACE*, which is associated with plasma and tissue levels of ACE1,[85] is associated with the severity of cardiac hypertrophy and the risk of SCD in HCM.[83,84,86] Several other genes have been implicated but not established as potential modifiers in HCM.[17,77] Overall, given the complexity of the molecular biology of cardiac hypertrophy, a large number of genes are expected to influence phenotypic expression of HCM, each imparting a modest effect on the severity of cardiac hypertrophy or the risk of SCD.

PATHOGENESIS

Identification of the causal genes for HCM has provided the impetus for molecular mechanistic studies that have led to partial elucidation of the molecular pathogenesis of HCM. Nonetheless, the precise molecular events that link the causal mutations to the clinical or morphological phenotypes are largely unknown but appear to involve a diverse array of signaling pathways.[87] One may simplify the link between the genetic mutations and the clinical phenotype into three major stages: initial structural and functional defects (Figure 25-5) in the protein encoded by the causal mutation, which affect not only the protein itself but also its interactions with the other proteins. This is then followed by activation of the signaling molecules, which in turn leads to transcriptional activation of gene expression. The latter leads to molecular, histological, and morphological phenotypes of HCM.[87] The initial functional defects are diverse, which is partly reflective of the diversity of the causal genes and mutations and partly reflective of the diversity of the function of each protein. Among the initial functional defects are altered Ca^{+2} sensitivity of myofibrillar ATPase activity,[88-90] actomyosin cross-bridge kinetics,[91] and Ca^{+2} sensitivity of myofibrillar force generation.[92-94] The initial functional abnormalities could impart mechanical, biochemical, and bioenergetic stress on cardiac myocytes and activate a series of stress-responsive signaling molecules that induce gene expression. It appears that diverse arrays of genes are expressed and signaling molecules are activated in response to the causal mutations.[95,96] Myocardial bioenergetic deficit as evidenced by changes in the ratio of cardiac phosphocreatine (PCr) to adenosine triphosphate (ATP) has been implicated as a common intermediary phenotype in HCM.[97-99] Metabolic abnormalities including altered myocardial bioenergetics, however, are common to various forms of cardiac hypertrophy and may be a consequence of cardiac stress.[100,101] Other mechanisms may include a direct role for the sarcomeric or Z-disk proteins in instigating the hypertrophic signaling pathways, such as potential activation of the protein phosphatase 2B calcineurin pathway by mutations in myozenin 2.[13,67] Likewise, preferential degradation of the truncated mutant proteins by the ubiquitin-proteasome pathway has been implicated in the pathogenesis of HCM.[102] The initial functional defect is reflected in the whole heart by impaired myocardial contraction and relaxation, which is present before and in the absence of cardiac hypertrophy.[103,104] Thus cardiac hypertrophy and interstitial fibrosis are considered secondary to activation of a diverse array of hypertrophic and profibrotic molecules in response of the initial functional defects imparted by the causal mutation. Accordingly, cardiac hypertrophy, the clinical diagnostic phenotype of HCM, and interstitial fibrosis are potentially reversible through blockade of the intermediary signaling molecules.

In patients with an autosomal-dominant HCM, only one copy of the causal gene and only half of the sarcomeric protein is mutated. Therefore, in HCM caused by missense mutations, which encompasses the majority of the cases, the mutant protein exerts a dominant-negative effect to express the phenotype (poison-peptide hypothesis). A small number of the causal mutations in HCM are splice-junction or frame-shift mutations. They lead to expression of truncated proteins that could be degraded by the ubiquitin-proteasome pathway and hence lead to a null allele status. The effect of such mutations, therefore, is "haplo-insufficiency."[73,102] The molecular event that leads to HCM in haplo-insufficiency states remains unclear.

The pathogenesis of myocyte disarray, the pathological hallmark of HCM, appears to be independent of the pathogenesis of cardiac hypertrophy and fibrosis. We have implicated impaired myocyte alignment through the ß-catenin-cadherins at the adherens junctions as a potential mechanism for myocyte disarray.[23] Alternative mechanisms include activation of the signaling pathways involved in myocyte axis formation and altered myocardial architecture by excess extracellular matrix proteins.

Determinants of Cardiac Phenotype in Hypertrophic Cardiomyopathy

The clinical phenotype is the outcome of complex and intertwined interactions between the constituents that contribute to the phenotype. In monogenic diseases such as HCM, the causal mutation is the prerequisite and a major determinant of the phenotype. The phenotype, however, ensues from interactions of the causal mutation with a variety of genetic and nongenetic factors (Figure 25-6). In a sense, the clinical phenotype of single gene disorders is a complex phenotype, determined not only by the causal mutation but also by the modifier genes, noncoding RNAs including microRNAs, posttranslational modification of proteins, and environmental factors. While there is considerable information on the significance of each component in influencing cardiac structure and function in general, their roles in affecting expression of the phenotype in HCM are poorly understood. Nevertheless, the complexity of the factors that determine the clinical phenotype points to the limitation of the genotype-phenotype correlation studies in humans with HCM. Thus in risk stratification of patients with HCM, it is important that all components that contribute to the phenotype are included in the analysis. Likewise, the findings in a small subset of patients with HCM could be restricted to the particular study population and not applicable to the general population of HCM.

Despite the recognized limitations of the genotype-phenotype correlation studies performed in relatively small populations, the causal mutations impart significant impact on the clinical phenotype, including the severity of cardiac hypertrophy and the risk of SCD.[72,105,106] The data suggests that, despite the presence of considerable variability, mutations in *MYH7*, as opposed to those in *MYBPC3*, are associated with a relatively high penetrance with the expression of significant cardiac hypertrophy relatively early in life.[105] Conversely, mutations in *MYBPC3* generally appear to be associated with a mild phenotype that typically occurs late in life.[72] The relatively low penetrance of certain mutations raises an important clinical point in the management of the relatives of patients with HCM because the normal phenotype in those at risk may reflect the low penetrance. Such individuals may develop the disease later in life.[107] Thus unless the inheritance of the causal mutation is excluded through genetic screening, those at risk should be evaluated periodically. The prognostic impact of the mutations on the risk of SCD is associated with the influence on the severity of cardiac hypertrophy.[108] It also appears that individuals with mutations leading to premature truncation of the protein are associated with more severe phenotypes than the missense mutations.[53] Mutations in *TNNT2* and *TNNI3* are associated with a relatively milder degree of cardiac hypertrophy but more prominent cardiac myocyte disarray and increased risk of SCD.[109] Nonetheless, no phenotype is specific to a specific gene or mutations, and benign and malignant phenotypes have been associated with the common causal genes.[110]

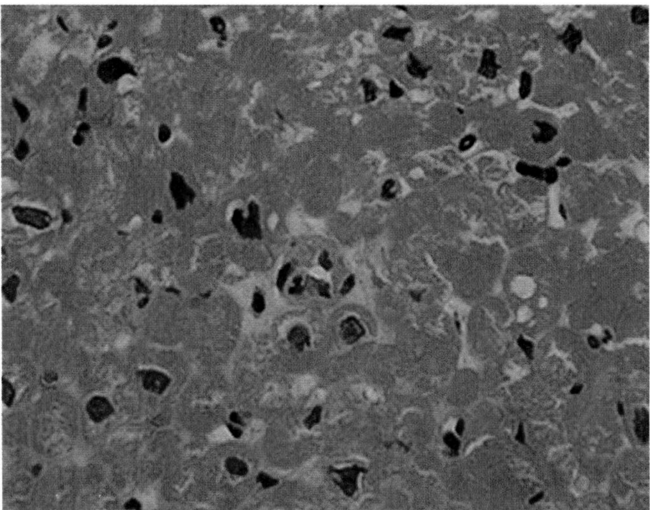

FIGURE 25–2 H&E stained thin myocardial section from a patient with hypertrophic cardiomyopathy who died suddenly. There is altered myocardial architecture with evidence of myocyte hypertrophy and disarray.

A noteworthy determinant of the clinical phenotype in HCM is the presence of double mutations, whether in *cis* or in *trans*.[51,74,75] Likewise, the presence of concomitant diseases such as hypertension could increase the penetrance and accelerate expression and severity of cardiac hypertrophy. The impact of hypertension on the phenotypic expression of HCM mutations could be illustrated in "hypertensive hypertrophic cardiomyopathy of the elderly," which may prove to be a form of HCM in conjunction with concomitant hypertension.[111] The impacts of heavy physical exercise, particularly isometric exercises on expression of cardiac hypertrophy and the risk of SCD are yet to be clarified. One may surmise that since hypertrophy is the secondary response of the heart to the causal mutations, heavy exercise could promote cardiac growth and enhance expression of cardiac hypertrophy, and consequently the risk of SCD HCM. Experimental data in a mouse model suggest otherwise.[112] Regardless, because HCM is the most common cause of SCD in young competitive athletes, patients with HCM are advised not to participate in competitive or contact sports.[113]

A fascinating feature of mutations in the sarcomeric protein is phenotypic plasticity. Accordingly, patients with HCM caused by mutations in *MYH7*, *TNNT2*, or *TNNI3* can develop the phenotypes of dilated cardiomyopathy (DCM) or restrictive cardiomyopathy (RCM) during the course of the disease.[114-116] Moreover, mutations in sarcomeric proteins could present from the outset with HCM, DCM, RCM, or LV noncompaction syndrome.[117-119] The molecular basis of such phenotypic plasticity is largely unknown but may reflect the topography of the causal mutations imparting different structural and functional effects on the mutant proteins and/or the effects of modifier genes and noncoding RNAs. The data suggest mutations that cause HCM are associated with enhanced Ca^{+2} sensitivity of the myofibrillar force generation and ATPase activity.[93,120-126] In contrast, mutations leading to DCM are associated with reduced Ca^{+2} sensitivity of the myofibrillar force generation and ATPase activity.[93,120-126] Likewise, we have shown that mutations in *TNNT2* that cause the contrasting phenotypes of HCM and DCM in humans impart differential effects on protein-protein interactions among the constituents of the sarcomeric filaments.[89]

Hypertrophic Cardiomyopathy Phenocopy

A phenocopy is a phenotype that falsely mimics the true phenotype. In the case of HCM, a phenocopy condition will express a phenotype that grossly resembles HCM, mainly "unexplained cardiac hypertrophy." Phenocopy conditions typically have a different cause and their pathogenesis differs from the disease that they imitate. Accordingly, the phenotype of cardiac hypertrophy in the absence of increased loading conditions could occur in a variety of other conditions, such as storage diseases, mitochondrial disorders, and triplet repeat syndromes (Table 25-2). The prevalence of phenocopy in patients with the clinical diagnosis of HCM is unclear but is estimated to be around 5% to 10%. The prevalence of phenocopy conditions may be higher in children, probably because of early manifestations of the phenocopy conditions.

The most common HCM phenocopy in children is Noonan syndrome, an uncommon autosomal dominant disorder characterized by dysmorphic facial features, pulmonic stenosis, mental retardation, bleeding disorders, and cardiac hypertrophy. In one report approximately one third of children with the clinical diagnosis of HCM had Noonan syndrome.[127] The known causal genes are protein-tyrosine phosphatase, nonreceptor type 11 (*PTPN11*), *SOS*, *KRAS*, and *RAF1* genes that collectively account for approximately two thirds of the cases.[128-131] Leopard syndrome (*l*entigines, *e*lectrocardiographic conduction abnormalities, *o*cular hypertelorism, *p*ulmonic stenosis, *a*bnormal genitalia, *r*etardation of growth, and *d*eafness) is an allelic variant of Noonan syndrome. It is caused primarily by mutations in *RAF1*.[129]

Glycogen storage diseases are relatively common causes of HCM phenocopy. Danon disease is a storage disease caused by mutations in *LAMP2* that codes for lysosome-associated membrane protein 2.[25] Likewise, mutations in *PRKAG2*, which encode the γ2 regulatory subunit of AMP-activated protein kinase (AMPK), lead to glycogen storage in the heart and cardiac hypertrophy, AV conduction defects, and a pattern of preexcitation on the electrocardiogram.[26,27,132,133] Another example of storage diseases mimicking HCM is the Fabry disease, which is an autosomal recessive lysosomal storage disease.[134,135] The estimated prevalence of Fabry disease in the adult population with a clinical diagnosis of HCM is approximately 3%.[135] Cardiac phenotype results from the deposits of glycosphingolipids in the heart. Other features of Fabry disease are angiokeratoma, renal insufficiency, proteinuria, neuropathy, transient ischemic attack, stroke, anemia, and corneal deposits.[136,137] The cardiac phenotype includes hypertrophy, which is often indistinguishable from true HCM, high QRS voltage, conduction defects, cardiac arrhythmias, valvular regurgitation, coronary artery disease, myocardial infarction, and aortic annular dilation. Fabry disease is caused by mutations in the *GLA* gene on chromosome Xq22, which encodes the lysosomal hydrolase α-Gal A protein.[136] Mutations lead to deficient activity of α-galactosidase A (α-Gal A), also known as "ceramide trihexosidase." Because the causal gene is located on the X chromosome, the disease predominantly affects males and to a lesser extent, female carriers. Fabry disease is diagnosed by the measuring α-Gal A levels and activity in leukocytes. The distinction between true HCM and Fabry disease is important because enzyme replacement therapy using human α-Gal A (agalsidase α) or recombinant human α-Gal A (agalsidase β), is somewhat effective in slowing progression of Fabry disease.[138-140]

Cardiac involvement in triplet repeat syndromes, a group of disorders caused by the expansion of naturally occurring trinucleotide repeats in the genes, includes cardiac hypertrophy that is usually diagnosed as HCM. HCM phenocopy is found frequently in patients with Friedreich ataxia, an autosomal recessive neurodegenerative disease caused by expansion of *GAA* repeat sequences in the intron of *FRDA*.[141] HCM phenocopy in patients with Friedreich ataxia could evolve into DCM. Likewise, cardiac involvement may present as DCM from the outset.

Another important cause of HCM phenocopy is defective mitochondrial oxidative phosphorylation pathways. A prototypic example is Kearns-Sayre syndrome (KSS), which is characterized by a triad of progressive external

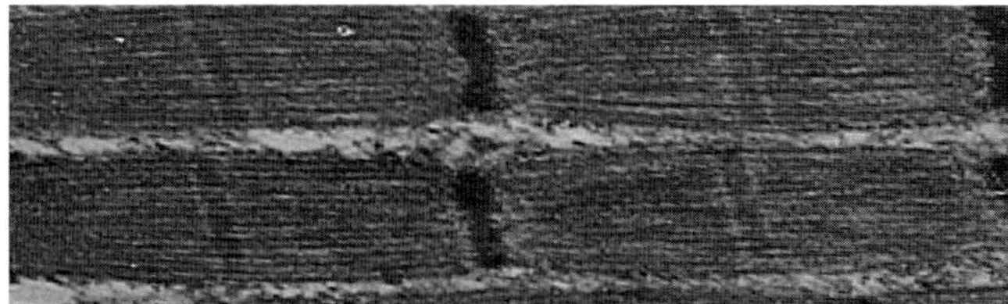

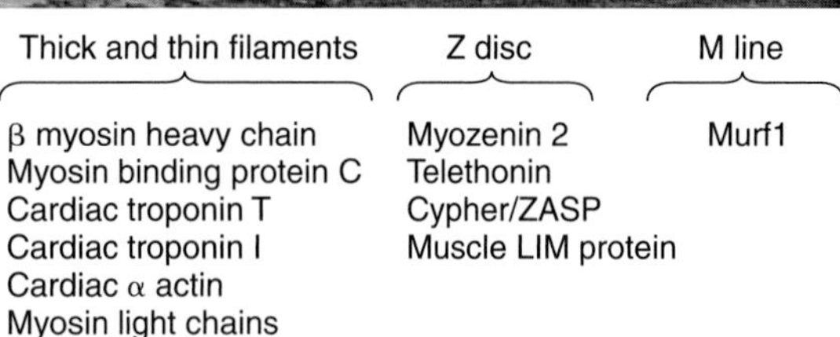

FIGURE 25–3 The vast majority of clinically diagnosed HCM is caused by mutations in sarcomeric proteins. Sarcomeres are comprised of thick and thin filaments and the S disk.

TABLE 25–2 HCM Phenocopy Conditions

Disease	Causal Gene	Protein
AMPK-mediated glycogen storage	*PRKAG2*	Protein kinase A, γ subunit
Pompe disease	*GAA*	α-1,4-glucosidase (acid maltase)
Fabry disease	*GLA*	α-galactosidase A
Danon disease	*LAMP2*	Lysosome-associated membrane protein 2
Myosin VI	*MYO6*	Unconventional myosin 6
Kearns-Sayre syndrome	*MtDNA*	Mitochondrial DNA
Friedreich ataxia	*FRDA*	Frataxin
Myotonic dystrophy	*DMPK*	Myotonin protein kinase
	DMWD	
Noonan syndrome	*PTPN11*	Protein tyrosine phosphatase, nonreceptor type 11
	SOS	Son of Sevenless
	RAF1	Murine leukemia viral oncogene homolog 1
	KRAS	Kirsten rat sarcoma virus homolog
Neimann-Pick disease	*NPC*	Neimann-Pick
Refsum disease	*PAHX (PHYH)*	Phytanoyl-CoA hydroxylase

ophthalmoplegia, pigmentary retinopathy, and cardiac conduction defects.[142] Patients with KSS frequently exhibit cardiac hypertrophy diagnosed as HCM. The list of conditions that cause HCM phenocopy is extensive and involves metabolic diseases, such as Refsum disease, glycogen storage disease type II (Pompe disease), Niemann-Pick disease, Gaucher disease, hereditary hemochromatosis, and CD36 deficiency.

MANAGEMENT OF PATIENTS WITH HYPERTROPHIC CARDIOMYOPATHY

Genetic Screening

There is considerable interest in genetic testing for HCM by patients and physicians. The interest stems from the potential clinical utility of genetic testing for an accurate diagnosis

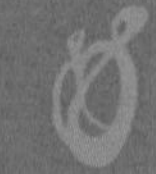

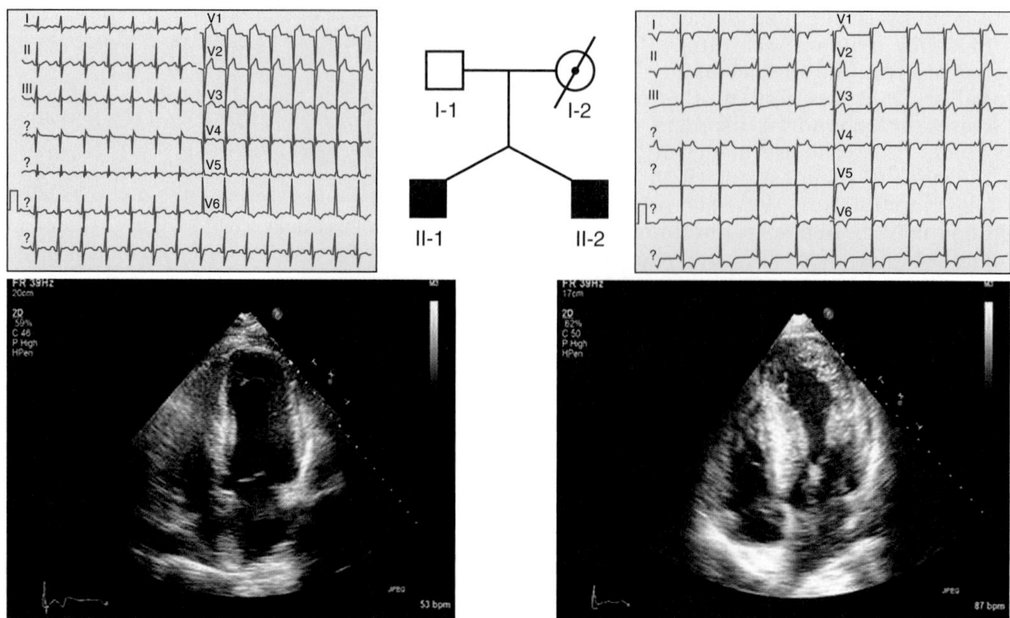

FIGURE 25–4 Phenotypic variability. A truncated pedigree shows twin brothers with HCM caused by S48P mutation in *MYOZ2*. There is significant variability in the degree of cardiac hypertrophy on 12-lead ECGs and echocardiograms between the two brothers.

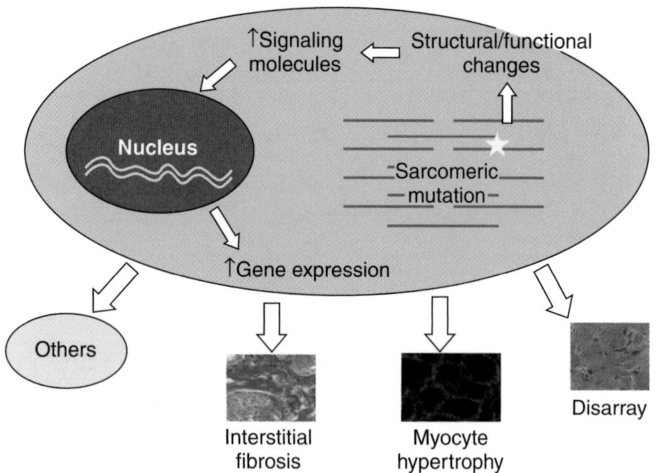

FIGURE 25–5 Pathogenesis of HCM, simplified into three stages of initial structural and functional defects followed by activation of signaling molecules, which lead to secondary gene expression and to HCM phenotype.

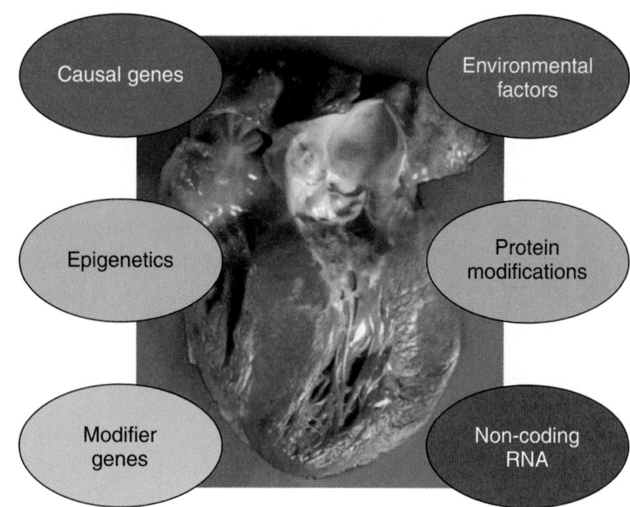

FIGURE 25–6 Major expected determinants of clinical phenotype in patients with hypertrophic cardiomyopathy.

of HCM, preclinical diagnosis of mutation carriers independent of and before clinical manifestations of the disease, and possibly prognostication, particularly as it regards the risk of SCD. The demand for genetic testing has led to the development of academic and commercial centers for genetic testing of HCM. Clinicians and patients, therefore, need to familiarize themselves with the strengths and limitations of genetic testing and the implications of the findings. Perhaps the best case scenario for genetic testing is in familial HCM wherein the causal mutation has already been identified and all members of the family could be tested for inheritance of the causal mutation. Genetic testing in such a scenario could lead to accurate distinction of those who have or have not inherited the causal mutation. The implications are twofold: First, with an early and accurate identification of the mutation carriers, the physician could closely monitor such individuals and intervene early. Early pharmacological interventions in animal models of HCM show the potential to prevent evolution of cardiac phenotype in HCM.[22] Inheritance of the causal mutations indicates that the individual will develop HCM, but the severity of HCM cannot be predicted accurately based on the inheritance of the causal mutation. The second implication is the accurate identification of those who have not inherited the causal mutation and, for practical purposes, are not at risk of developing HCM except for very rare circumstances.

In the most common scenario for genetic testing, neither the causal gene nor the mutation is known. In large families, one may perform linkage analysis and map the causal gene and identify the mutation. The approach, however, is possible in research laboratories only and is expensive. In smaller size families, linkage analysis does not offer sufficient power to map and identify the causal mutation. In small size families and in sporadic cases, therefore, one is restricted to the candidate gene approach. The screening is complicated by the allelic and nonallelic heterogeneity of HCM and the relatively low prevalence of each causal mutation. Therefore the approach currently focuses on the screening of each individual for the most common causal genes, namely, *MYH7, MYBPC3, TNNI3, TNNT2, TPM1,* and *ACTC1*. Typically, the coding regions and the exon-intron boundaries are sequenced to identify the causal mutation. The approach is successful in approximately half of cases. Inclusion of less common causal genes and genes coding for the relatively common phenocopy conditions are expected to increase the chance of finding the

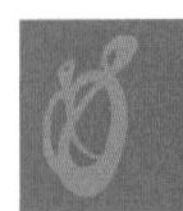

causal mutation slightly. The overall yield of genetic screening at the present time is at best about 60%.

One major clinical implication of genetic testing is the distinction between the phenocopy conditions and sarcomeric HCM. The distinction is important because the treatment of the two conditions differs significantly and enzyme replacement therapy for many phenocopy conditions has shown beneficial effects, as discussed previously. The utility of genetic testing for prognostication is hindered by the presence of considerable phenotypic variability and influence of many other factors on the phenotype, as discussed earlier. Accordingly, information garnered through identification of the causal mutation alone in the assessment of the risk of SCD is inadequate but could supplement the clinical data for risk stratification and management of patients with HCM. In this aspect, a comprehensive approach that uses not only the information content of the causal genes and mutations but also encompasses the potential impacts of the double causal mutations and the modifier alleles and the clinical predictors is necessary to improve risk stratification in patients with HCM.

Management of Risk of Sudden Cardiac Death

The risk of SCD is the primary concern of patients and physicians alike. The risk factors for SCD were discussed previously and listed in Box 25-1. Pharmacological treatment has not been shown to reduce the risk of SCD in HCM. In contrast, implantation of AICD is effective in secondary and primary prevention of SCD in patients with HCM.[143] However, the specific indication of AICD implantation in various clinical scenarios is less settled. Those with a prior episode of cardiac arrest should undergo complete cardiovascular evaluation and AICD implantation, which has been shown to be effective in secondary prevention of SCD.[143] Coronary angiography to detect atherosclerosis should be performed in a subgroup considered susceptible to atherosclerosis followed by appropriate intervention. A family history of premature SCD is an important risk factor for SCD, particularly whenever it occurs in two or more individuals. Whether a family history of premature SCD alone is sufficient for AICD implantation is debatable. Given the presence of extensive phenotypic variability, additional risk stratification and an individual-based approach is preferable. Recurrent syncope is a major risk factor and necessitates extensive evaluation to determine the cause. In addition to detailed history taking, physical examination, 12-lead ECG, and comprehensive echocardiography, the evaluation should include extended Holter monitoring and event recording, tilt-table testing whenever autonomic dysfunction and orthostatic hypotension are suspected, and electrophysiological studies in specific circumstances. Those with sustained or repetitive episodes of nonsustained ventricular tachycardia on Holter or rhythm monitoring are candidates for AICD implantation. AICD is effective in reducing the risk of SCD in those at high risk of SCD.[143]

Severe LV hypertrophy, while a risk factor for SCD, and LV outflow tract obstruction, probably are not sufficient indications for routine implantation of an AICD. Those with risk factors for SCD undergoing surgical septal myectomy should be reevaluated postoperatively, as surgical septal myectomy appears to impart a favorable outcome on the risk of SCD.[144] In contrast, patients with risk factors for SCD undergoing catheter-based alcohol septal ablation probably should also undergo an AICD implantation because there have been occasional reports of ventricular tachycardia postcatheter-based alcohol septal ablation.[145,146]

Pharmacological Treatment

Current pharmacological treatment of patients with HCM is largely empirical and unchanged over the past two decades. A large number of patients with HCM are asymptomatic or minimally symptomatic. Therefore, only periodic clinical and laboratory evaluations that also include assessment of the risk of SCD are recommended. Routine periodic evaluation of such patients should include obtaining 12-lead ECG, 2-dimensional and Doppler echocardiography, and Holter monitoring, the latter particularly in those who have risk factors for SCD. The main focus is on the risk of SCD and early interventions, as AICD appears to be effective even in primary prevention of SCD in high-risk patients with HCM.[143] In asymptomatic individuals at low risk of SCD, no intervention is necessary because none of the existing therapies has been shown to slow or reverse evolution of the cardiac phenotype in HCM.

The cornerstone of pharmacological treatment of symptomatic patients is β-blockers. β-blockers with intrinsic sympathetic activity should be avoided as they could worsen the symptoms. Calcium channel blockers, namely, verapamil and diltiazem but not nifedipine, are the agents of choice in those who do not tolerate β-blockers or are added to β-blockers, whenever symptoms persist. However, in patients with LV outflow tract obstruction, the vasodilatory effects of Ca^{2+} channel blockers could precipitate or worsen LV outflow tract obstruction. Disopyramide, which possesses a negative inotropic effect, is effective in reducing LV outflow tract obstruction and ameliorating symptoms.[147] However, it does not affect the overall survival or the risk of SCD.[147] Diuretics are used in those with symptoms of diastolic heart failure, albeit cautiously to avoid volume depletion and precipitation of hypotension. Amiodarone is used primarily for treatment of atrial and ventricular arrhythmias. Patients with new-onset atrial fibrillation should be treated with electrical cardioversion to restore normal sinus rhythm. In general, patients with severe cardiac hypertrophy or outflow tract obstruction who develop atrial fibrillation develop severe symptoms. Every attempt should be made to convert to and maintain such patients in normal sinus rhythm. However, this may prove difficult because of the underlying pathology in HCM. Those with chronic or intermittent atrial fibrillation should be anticoagulated to reduce risk of systemic embolization and stroke. Pharmacological treatment of such patients includes β-blockers, verapamil, and amiodarone, and possibly d-l, sotalol, and dofetilide. Catheter-based ablation should be considered in HCM patients with atrial fibrillation refractory to medical therapy.

Surgical Myectomy (Morrow Technique) and Catheter-based Septal Ablation (Alcohol Septal Ablation)

A subset of patients with HCM remain symptomatic and refractory to medical therapy, some because of severe diastolic heart failure and others because of severe outflow tract obstruction. Those with a significant LV outflow tract obstruction at rest or provoked and an interventricular septal thickness of 15 mm or greater are candidates for surgical myectomy or catheter-based alcohol septal ablation. Both approaches are effective in relieving the outflow tract obstruction and improving symptoms. Therefore, the choice is largely determined by the presence of concomitant diseases, such as significant valvular lesions and coronary artery disease, which necessitates concomitant surgery and preference for surgical myectomy. Likewise, surgical myectomy is more desirable in those at high risk for SCD. In contrast, the presence of comorbidities that increase the surgical risk significantly favors percutaneous interventions. The advantages and disadvantages of these two techniques are summarized in Table 25-3.

Surgical myectomy (myomectomy), which is referred to as the "Morrow procedure," involves partial resection of the base of the septum through a transaortic approach. It is the procedure of choice in HCM patients who have concomitant

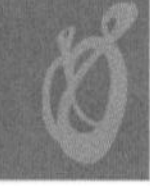

TABLE 25–3 Comparison of Surgical Myectomy and Ethanol Septal Ablation

	Surgical Myectomy	Ethanol Septal Ablation
Approach	Cardiopulmonary bypass	Cardiac catheterization
Hospital stay	5-7 days	1-2 days
Perioperative mortality	1%-5%	1%-5%
Procedural success	>95%	>85%
Short-term symptomatic relief	Excellent	Excellent
Long-term symptomatic relief	Excellent	Excellent
Long-term safety	Established	Risk of ventricular arrhythmias
Impact on survival	Favorable	Unknown
Septal infarction/ fibrosis	None	Present
Recurrence of LVOT gradient	Rare	Uncommon
Repeat procedure	Rare	Uncommon
Atrioventricular block requiring permanent pacemaker	~2%	10%-20%
Late ventricular arrhythmias	Rare	Uncommon
Postoperative atrial fibrillation	Common	Rare
Significant aortic regurgitation	Infrequent	None
Ventricular septal defect	Rare	None
Correction of concomitant problems	Amenable	NA

coronary artery disease or valvular disorders or have an anatomy that is not amenable to catheter-based septal ablation. It is also preferable in patients at high risk for SCD because the risk of SCD appears to be low after a surgical myectomy.[144] The overall surgical mortality is 1% to 5% but higher in the elderly and those requiring concomitant surgeries, such as coronary artery bypass surgery or valvular repair/replacement.[148,149] The long-term beneficial effects of surgical myectomy in relieving the outflow tract gradient and improving symptoms are well established.[148,149] The recurrence rate and the need for permanent pacemaker implantation are relatively low.

Transcatheter alcohol septal ablation is performed by infusing 1 to 3 mL of pure ethanol into the main septal perforators of the left anterior descending artery. It is also very effective in reducing the outflow tract gradient and improving symptoms.[146,150] Infusion of ethanol into the septal branches induces local myocardial necrosis, which is associated with LV remodeling and partial regression of cardiac hypertrophy.[150,151] The periprocedure mortality rate is low. A major complication is the development of advanced conduction defect requiring permanent pacemaker implantation in 10% to 20% of the patients.[152,153] An uncommon and sometimes late complication of alcohol septal ablation is ventricular arrhythmias, mandating implantation of AICD.[145,146] Overall, transcoronary septal ablation is a very effective procedure for reduction of LV outflow tract obstruction and improvement of symptoms. Its effects on long-term survival and risk of SCD remain to be established.

Experimental Therapies

The ultimate goal of pharmacological interventions in human patients with HCM is not only to improve symptoms and reduce the risk of SCD but also to prevent the clinical manifestation of the disease in total. However, current pharmacological agents have not been shown to reduce mortality, regress cardiac hypertrophy, or prevent the development of the phenotype. Experimental data in animal models of human HCM have raised the potential utility of 3-hydroxy-3-methylglutaryl-coenzyme A (HMG-CoA) reductase inhibitors (statins), inhibitors of the renin-angiotensin-aldosterone system, and antioxidant *N*-acetylcysteine in prevention, attenuation, and regression of evolving phenotypes in HCM.[21-23,154,155] However, whether the results obtained in animal models caused by specific mutations in a more homogeneous genetic background and under controlled environmental conditions could be extended to humans who have heterogeneous genetic and environmental factors remains to be determined. Two pilot studies have shown the potential beneficial effects of the angiotensin II receptor blocker losartan in human patients with HCM.[156,157] A pilot study with atorvastatin, however, showed no beneficial effect on cardiac mass or function in patients with HCM.[158] Large-scale clinical studies in HCM patients genotyped for the causal mutations would be necessary to establish the potential beneficial effects of experimental therapies.

REFERENCES

1. Liouville, H. (1869). Retrecissement cardiaque sous aortique. *Gaz Med (Paris), 24*, 161–165.
2. Schmincke, A. (1907). Ueber linkseitige muskulose conusstenosen. *Dtsch Med Wochenschr, 33*, 2082.
3. Davies, L. G. (1952). A familial heart disease. *Br Heart J, 14*(2), 206–212.
4. Teare, D. (1958). Asymmetrical hypertrophy of the heart in young adults. *Br Heart J, 20*(1), 1–8.
5. Brock, R., & Fleming, P. R. (1956). Aortic subvalvar stenosis: a report of 5 cases diagnosed during life. *Guys Hosp Rep, 105*(4), 391–408.
6. Braunwald, E., & Ebert, P. A. (1962). Hemodynamic alterations in idiopathic hypertrophic subaortic stenosis induced by sympathomimetic drugs. *Am J Cardiol, 10*, 489–495.
7. Braunwald, E., Lambrew, C. T., Rockoff, S. D., et al. (1964). Idiopathic hypertrophic subaortic stenosis. I. A description of the disease based upon an analysis of 64 patients. *Circulation, 30*(suppl. 4), 3–119.
8. Pierce, G. E., Morrow, A. G., & Braunwald, E. (1964). Idiopathic hypertrophic subaortic stenosis. 3. Intraoperative studies of the mechanism of obstruction and its hemodynamic consequences. *Circulation, 30*(suppl. 4), 152–213.
9. Morrow, A. G., Lambrew, C. T., & Braunwald, E. (1964). Idiopathic hypertrophic subaortic stenosis. II. Operative treatment and the results of pre- and postoperative hemodynamic evaluations. *Circulation, 30*(suppl. 4), 120–151.
10. Sigwart, U. (1995). Non-surgical myocardial reduction for hypertrophic obstructive cardiomyopathy. *Lancet, 346*(8969), 211–214.
11. Henry, W. L., Clark, C. E., & Epstein, S. E. (1973). Asymmetric septal hypertrophy. Echocardiographic identification of the pathognomonic anatomic abnormality of IHSS. *Circulation, 47*(2), 225–233.
12. Boughner, D. R., Schuld, R. L., & Persaud, J. A. (1975). Hypertrophic obstructive cardiomyopathy. Assessment by echocardiographic and Doppler ultrasound techniques. *Br Heart J, 37*(9), 917–923.
13. Joyner, C. R., Harrison, F. S., Jr., & Gruber, J. W. (1971). Diagnosis of hypertrophic subaortic stenosis with a Doppler velocity flow detector. *Ann Intern Med, 74*(5), 692–696.
14. Takenaka, K., Dabestani, A., Gardin, J. M., et al. (1986). Left ventricular filling in hypertrophic cardiomyopathy: a pulsed Doppler echocardiographic study. *J Am Coll Cardiol, 7*(6), 1263–1271.
15. Nagueh, S. F., Bachinski, L., Meyer, D., et al. (2001). Tissue Doppler imaging consistently detects myocardial abnormalities in patients with familial hypertrophic cardiomyopathy and provides a novel means for an early diagnosis prior to and independent of hypertrophy. *Circulation, 104*, 128–130.
16. Geisterfer-Lowrance, A. A., Kass, S., Tanigawa, G., et al. (1990). A molecular basis for familial hypertrophic cardiomyopathy: a beta cardiac myosin heavy chain gene missense mutation. *Cell, 62*(5), 999–1006.
17. Marian, A. J. (2008). Genetic determinants of cardiac hypertrophy. *Curr Opin Cardiol, 23*(3), 199–205.
18. Maron, B. J., Shirani, J., Poliac, L. C., et al. (1996). Sudden death in young competitive athletes. Clinical, demographic, and pathological profiles. *JAMA, 276*(3), 199–204.
19. Cannan, C. R., Reeder, G. S., Bailey, K. R., et al. (1995). Natural history of hypertrophic cardiomyopathy. A population-based study, 1976 through 1990. *Circulation, 92*(9), 2488–2495.
20. Maron, B. J., Shen, W. K., Link, M. S., et al. (2000). Efficacy of implantable cardioverter-defibrillators for the prevention of sudden death in patients with hypertrophic cardiomyopathy. *N Engl J Med, 342*(6), 365–373.

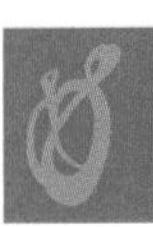

21. Patel, R., Nagueh, S. F., Tsybouleva, N., et al. (2001). Simvastatin induces regression of cardiac hypertrophy and fibrosis and improves cardiac function in a transgenic rabbit model of human hypertrophic cardiomyopathy. *Circulation, 104*(3), 317–324.
22. Senthil, V., Chen, S. N., Tsybouleva, N., et al. (2005). Prevention of cardiac hypertrophy by atorvastatin in a transgenic rabbit model of human hypertrophic cardiomyopathy. *Circ Res, 97*(3), 285–292.
23. Tsybouleva, N., Zhang, L., Chen, S., et al. (2004). Aldosterone, through novel signaling proteins, is a fundamental molecular bridge between the genetic defect and the cardiac phenotype of hypertrophic cardiomyopathy. *Circulation, 109*(10), 1284–1291.
24. Elliott, P., & McKenna, W. J. (2004). Hypertrophic cardiomyopathy. *Lancet, 363*(9424), 1881–1891.
25. Arad, M., Maron, B. J., Gorham, J. M., et al. (2005). Glycogen storage diseases presenting as hypertrophic cardiomyopathy. *N Engl J Med, 352*(4), 362–372.
26. Gollob, M. H., Green, M. S., Tang, A. S., et al. (2001). Identification of a gene responsible for familial Wolff-Parkinson-White syndrome. *N Engl J Med, 344*(24), 1823–1831.
27. Blair, E., Redwood, C., Ashrafian, H., et al. (2001). Mutations in the gamma(2) subunit of AMP-activated protein kinase cause familial hypertrophic cardiomyopathy: evidence for the central role of energy compromise in disease pathogenesis. *Hum Mol Genet, 10*(11), 1215–1220.
28. Maron, B. J., Gardin, J. M., Flack, J. M., et al. (1995). Prevalence of hypertrophic cardiomyopathy in a general population of young adults. Echocardiographic analysis of 4111 subjects in the CARDIA study. Coronary artery risk development in (young) adults. *Circulation, 92*(4), 785–789.
29. Elliott, P. M., Poloniecki, J., Dickie, S., et al. (2000). Sudden death in hypertrophic cardiomyopathy: identification of high risk patients. *J Am Coll Cardiol, 36*(7), 2212–2218.
30. Nienaber, C. A., Hiller, S., Spielmann, R. P., et al. (1990). Syncope in hypertrophic cardiomyopathy: multivariate analysis of prognostic determinants. *J Am Coll Cardiol, 15*(5), 948–955.
31. Olivotto, I., Cecchi, F., Casey, S. A., et al. (2001). Impact of atrial fibrillation on the clinical course of hypertrophic cardiomyopathy. *Circulation, 104*(21), 2517–2524.
32. Monserrat, L., Elliott, P. M., Gimeno, J. R., et al. (2003). Non-sustained ventricular tachycardia in hypertrophic cardiomyopathy: an independent marker of sudden death risk in young patients. *J Am Coll Cardiol, 42*(5), 873–879.
33. Basavarajaiah, S., Shah, A., & Sharma, S. (2007). Sudden cardiac death in young athletes. *Heart, 93*(3), 287–289.
34. Corrado, D., Basso, C., Schiavon, M., et al. (1998). Screening for hypertrophic cardiomyopathy in young athletes. *N Engl J Med, 339*(6), 364–369.
35. Miller, M. A., Gomes, J. A., & Fuster, V. (2007). Risk stratification of sudden cardiac death in hypertrophic cardiomyopathy. *Nat Clin Pract Cardiovasc Med, 4*(12), 667–676.
36. Marian, A. J. (2003). On predictors of sudden cardiac death in hypertrophic cardiomyopathy. *J Am Coll Cardiol, 41*(6), 994–996.
37. Frenneaux, M. P. (2004). Assessing the risk of sudden cardiac death in a patient with hypertrophic cardiomyopathy. *Heart, 90*(5), 570–575.
38. Elliott, P. M., Gimeno, B., Jr., Mahon, N. G., et al. (2001). Relation between severity of left-ventricular hypertrophy and prognosis in patients with hypertrophic cardiomyopathy. *Lancet, 357*(9254), 420–424.
39. Kofflard, M. J., Waldstein, D. J., Vos, J., et al. (1993). Prognosis in hypertrophic cardiomyopathy observed in a large clinic population. *Am J Cardiol, 72*(12), 939–943.
40. Kofflard, M. J. M., ten Cate, F. J., van der Lee, C., et al. (2003). Hypertrophic cardiomyopathy in a large community-based population: clinical outcome and identification of risk factors for sudden cardiac death and clinical deterioration. *J Am Coll Cardiol, 41*(6), 987–993.
41. Yetman, A. T., Hamilton, R. M., Benson, L. N., et al. (1998). Long-term outcome and prognostic determinants in children with hypertrophic cardiomyopathy. *J Am Coll Cardiol, 32*(7), 1943–1950.
42. Eriksson, M. J., Sonnenberg, B., Woo, A., et al. (2002). Long-term outcome in patients with apical hypertrophic cardiomyopathy. *J Am Coll Cardiol, 39*(4), 638–645.
43. Nagueh, S. F., McFalls, J., Meyer, D., et al. (2003). Tissue Doppler imaging predicts the development of hypertrophic cardiomyopathy in subjects with subclinical disease. *Circulation, 108*(4), 395–398.
44. Maron, M. S., Olivotto, I., Betocchi, S., et al. (2003). Effect of left ventricular outflow tract obstruction on clinical outcome in hypertrophic cardiomyopathy. *N Engl J Med, 348*(4), 295–303.
45. Davies, M. J., & McKenna, W. J. (1995). Hypertrophic cardiomyopathy—pathology and pathogenesis. *Histopathology, 26*(6), 493–500.
46. Varnava, A. M., Elliott, P. M., Mahon, N., et al. (2001). Relation between myocyte disarray and outcome in hypertrophic cardiomyopathy. *Am J Cardiol, 88*(3), 275–279.
47. Greaves, S. C., Roche, A. H., Neutze, J. M., et al. (1987). Inheritance of hypertrophic cardiomyopathy: a cross sectional and M mode echocardiographic study of 50 families. *Br Heart J, 58*(3), 259–266.
48. Olson, T. M., Karst, M. L., Whitby, F. G., et al. (2002). Myosin light chain mutation causes autosomal recessive cardiomyopathy with mid-cavitary hypertrophy and restrictive physiology. *Circulation, 105*, 2337–2340.
49. Greve, G., Bachinski, L., Friedman, D. L., et al. (1994). Isolation of a de novo mutant myocardial beta MHC protein in a pedigree with hypertrophic cardiomyopathy. *Hum Mol Genet, 3*(11), 2073–2075.
50. Thierfelder, L., Watkins, H., MacRae, C., et al. (1994). Alpha-tropomyosin and cardiac troponin T mutations cause familial hypertrophic cardiomyopathy: a disease of the sarcomere. *Cell, 77*(5), 701–712.
51. Richard, P., Charron, P., Carrier, L., et al. (2003). Hypertrophic cardiomyopathy: distribution of disease genes, spectrum of mutations, and implications for a molecular diagnosis strategy. *Circulation, 107*(17), 2227–2232.
52. Van Driest, S. L., Jaeger, M. A., Ommen, S. R., et al. (2004). Comprehensive analysis of the beta-myosin heavy chain gene in 389 unrelated patients with hypertrophic cardiomyopathy. *J Am Coll Cardiol, 44*(3), 602–610.
53. Erdmann, J., Raible, J., Maki-Abadi, J., et al. (2001). Spectrum of clinical phenotypes and gene variants in cardiac myosin-binding protein C mutation carriers with hypertrophic cardiomyopathy. *J Am Coll Cardiol, 38*(2), 322–330.
54. Andersen, P. S., Havndrup, O., Bundgaard, H., et al. (2004). Genetic and phenotypic characterization of mutations in myosin-binding protein C (MYBPC3) in 81 families with familial hypertrophic cardiomyopathy: total or partial haploinsufficiency. *Eur J Hum Genet, 12*(8), 673–677.
55. Marian, A. J., Yu, Q. T., Mares, A., Jr., et al. (1992). Detection of a new mutation in the beta-myosin heavy chain gene in an individual with hypertrophic cardiomyopathy. *J Clin Invest, 90*(6), 2156–2165.
56. Blair, E., Redwood, C., de Jesus, O. M., et al. (2002). Mutations of the light meromyosin domain of the beta-myosin heavy chain rod in hypertrophic cardiomyopathy. *Circ Res, 90*(3), 263–269.
57. Torricelli, F., Girolami, F., Olivotto, I., et al. (2003). Prevalence and clinical profile of troponin T mutations among patients with hypertrophic cardiomyopathy in Tuscany. *Am J Cardiol, 92*(11), 1358–1362.
58. Mogensen, J., Murphy, R. T., Kubo, T., et al. (2004). Frequency and clinical expression of cardiac troponin I mutations in 748 consecutive families with hypertrophic cardiomyopathy. *J Am Coll Cardiol, 44*(12), 2315–2325.
59. Watkins, H., McKenna, W. J., Thierfelder, L., et al. (1995). Mutations in the genes for cardiac troponin T and alpha-tropomyosin in hypertrophic cardiomyopathy. *N Engl J Med, 332*(16), 1058–1064.
60. Olson, T. M., Doan, T. P., Kishimoto, N. Y., et al. (2000). Inherited and de novo mutations in the cardiac actin gene cause hypertrophic cardiomyopathy. *J Mol Cell Cardiol, 32*(9), 1687–1694.
61. Mogensen, J., Klausen, I. C., Pedersen, A. K., et al. (1999). Alpha-cardiac actin is a novel disease gene in familial hypertrophic cardiomyopathy. *J Clin Invest, 103*(10), R39–R43.
62. Hayashi, T., Arimura, T., Itoh-Satoh, M., et al. (2004). Tcap gene mutations in hypertrophic cardiomyopathy and dilated cardiomyopathy. *J Am Coll Cardiol, 44*(11), 2192–2201.
63. Andersen, P. S., Havndrup, O., Bundgaard, H., et al. (2001). Myosin light chain mutations in familial hypertrophic cardiomyopathy: phenotypic presentation and frequency in Danish and South African populations. *J Med Genet, 38*(12), E43.
64. Van Driest, S. L., Ellsworth, E. G., Ommen, S. R., et al. (2003). Prevalence and spectrum of thin filament mutations in an outpatient referral population with hypertrophic cardiomyopathy. *Circulation, 108*(4), 445–451.
65. Hayashi, T., Arimura, T., Ueda, K., et al. (2004). Identification and functional analysis of a caveolin-3 mutation associated with familial hypertrophic cardiomyopathy. *Biochem Biophys Res Commun, 313*(1), 178–184.
66. Geier, C., Perrot, A., Ozcelik, C., et al. (2003). Mutations in the human muscle LIM protein gene in families with hypertrophic cardiomyopathy. *Circulation, 107*(10), 1390–1395.
67. Osio, A., Tan, L., Chen, S. N., et al. (2007). Myozenin 2 is a novel gene for human hypertrophic cardiomyopathy. *Circ Res, 100*(6), 766–768.
68. Davis, J. S., Hassanzadeh, S., Winitsky, S., et al. (2002). A gradient of myosin regulatory light-chain phosphorylation across the ventricular wall supports cardiac torsion. *Cold Spring Harb Symp Quant Biol, 67*, 345–352.
69. Hoffmann, B., Schmidt-Traub, H., Perrot, A., et al. (2001). First mutation in cardiac troponin C, L29Q, in a patient with hypertrophic cardiomyopathy. *Hum Mutat, 17*(6), 524.
70. Carniel, E., Taylor, M. R., Sinagra, G., et al. (2005). Alpha-myosin heavy chain: a sarcomeric gene associated with dilated and hypertrophic phenotypes of cardiomyopathy. *Circulation, 112*(1), 54–59.
71. Minamisawa, S., Sato, Y., Tatsuguchi, Y., et al. (2003). Mutation of the phospholamban promoter associated with hypertrophic cardiomyopathy. *Biochem Biophys Res Commun, 304*(1), 1–4.
72. Charron, P., Dubourg, O., Desnos, M., et al. (1998). Clinical features and prognostic implications of familial hypertrophic cardiomyopathy related to the cardiac myosin-binding protein C gene. *Circulation, 97*(22), 2230–2236.
73. Rottbauer, W., Gautel, M., Zehelein, J., et al. (1997). Novel splice donor site mutation in the cardiac myosin-binding protein-C gene in familial hypertrophic cardiomyopathy. Characterization of cardiac transcript and protein. *J Clin Invest, 100*(2), 475–482.
74. Blair, E., Price, S. J., Baty, C. J., et al. (2001). Mutations in cis can confound genotype-phenotype correlations in hypertrophic cardiomyopathy. *J Med Genet, 38*(6), 385–388.
75. Richard, P., Isnard, R., Carrier, L., et al. (1999). Double heterozygosity for mutations in the beta-myosin heavy chain and in the cardiac myosin binding protein C genes in a family with hypertrophic cardiomyopathy. *J Med Genet, 36*(7), 542–545.
76. Marian, A. J., & Roberts, R. (2002). On Koch's postulates, causality and genetics of cardiomyopathies. *J Mol Cell Cardiol, 34*(8), 971–974.
77. Marian, A. J. (2002). Modifier genes for hypertrophic cardiomyopathy. *Curr Opin Cardiol, 17*(3), 242–252.
78. Levy, S., Sutton, G., Ng, P. C., et al. (2007). The diploid genome sequence of an individual human. *PLoS Biol, 5*(10), e254.
79. Korbel, J. O., Urban, A. E., Affourtit, J. P., et al. (2007). Paired-end mapping reveals extensive structural variation in the human genome. *Science, 318*(5849), 420–426.
80. Daw, E. W., Chen, S. N., Czernuszewicz, G., et al. (2007). Genome-wide mapping of modifier chromosomal loci for human hypertrophic cardiomyopathy. *Hum Mol Genet, 16*(20), 2463–2471.
81. Zhang, S., Weinheimer, C., Courtois, M., et al. (2003). The role of the Grb2-p38 MAPK signaling pathway in cardiac hypertrophy and fibrosis. *J Clin Invest, 111*(6), 833–841.
82. Bouzeghrane, F., Mercure, C., Reudelhuber, T. L., et al. (2004). [Alpha]8[beta]1 integrin is upregulated in myofibroblasts of fibrotic and scarring myocardium. *J Mol Cell Cardiol, 36*(3), 343–353.
83. Lechin, M., Quinones, M. A., Omran, A., et al. (1995). Angiotensin-I converting enzyme genotypes and left ventricular hypertrophy in patients with hypertrophic cardiomyopathy. *Circulation, 92*(7), 1808–1812.

84. Marian, A. J., Yu, Q. T., Workman, R., et al. (1993). Angiotensin-converting enzyme polymorphism in hypertrophic cardiomyopathy and sudden cardiac death. *Lancet, 342*(8879), 1085–1086.
85. Rigat, B., Hubert, C., Alhenc-Gelas, F., et al. (1990). An insertion/deletion polymorphism in the angiotensin I-converting enzyme gene accounting for half the variance of serum enzyme levels. *J Clin Invest, 86*(4), 1343–1346.
86. Tesson, F., Dufour, C., Moolman, J. C., et al. (1997). The influence of the angiotensin I converting enzyme genotype in familial hypertrophic cardiomyopathy varies with the disease gene mutation. *J Mol Cell Cardiol, 29*(2), 831–838.
87. Marian, A. J. (2000). Pathogenesis of diverse clinical and pathological phenotypes in hypertrophic cardiomyopathy. *Lancet, 355*(9197), 58–60.
88. Nagueh, S. F., Chen, S., Patel, R., et al. (2004). Evolution of expression of cardiac phenotypes over a 4-year period in the beta-myosin heavy chain-Q403 transgenic rabbit model of human hypertrophic cardiomyopathy. *J Mol Cell Cardiol, 36*(5), 663–673.
89. Lombardi, R., Bell, A., Senthil, V., et al. (2008). Differential interactions of thin filament proteins in two cardiac troponin T mouse models of hypertrophic and dilated cardiomyopathies. *Cardiovasc Res, 79*(1), 109–117.
90. Lowey, S., Lesko, L. M., Rovner, A. S., et al. (2008). Functional effects of the hypertrophic cardiomyopathy R403Q mutation are different in an alpha- or beta-myosin heavy chain backbone. *J Biol Chem, 283*(29), 20579–20589.
91. Palmer, B. M., Fishbaugher, D. E., Schmitt, J. P., et al. (2004). Differential cross-bridge kinetics of FHC myosin mutations R403Q and R453C in heterozygous mouse myocardium. *Am J Physiol Heart Circ Physiol, 287*(1), H91–H99.
92. Heller, M. J., Nili, M., Homsher, E., et al. (2003). Cardiomyopathic tropomyosin mutations that increase thin filament Ca^{2+}-sensitivity and tropomyosin N-domain flexibility. *J Biol Chem, 278*, 41742–41748.
93. Szczesna-Cordary, D., Guzman, G., Zhao, J., et al. (2005). The E22K mutation of myosin RLC that causes familial hypertrophic cardiomyopathy increases calcium sensitivity of force and ATPase in transgenic mice. *J Cell Sci, 118*(16), 3675–3683.
94. Lang, R., Gomes, A. V., Zhao, J., et al. (2002). Functional analysis of a troponin I (R145G) mutation associated with familial hypertrophic cardiomyopathy. *J Biol Chem, 277*(14), 11670–11678.
95. Hwang, J. J., Allen, P. D., Tseng, G. C., et al. (2002). Microarray gene expression profiles in dilated and hypertrophic cardiomyopathic end-stage heart failure. *Physiol Genomics, 10*(1), 31–44.
96. Lim, D. S., Roberts, R., & Marian, A. J. (2001). Expression profiling of cardiac genes in human hypertrophic cardiomyopathy: insight into the pathogenesis of phenotypes. *J Am Coll Cardiol, 38*(4), 1175–1180.
97. Sieverding, L., Jung, W. I., Breuer, J., et al. (1997). Proton-decoupled myocardial 31P NMR spectroscopy reveals decreased PCr/Pi in patients with severe hypertrophic cardiomyopathy. *Am J Cardiol, 80*(3A), 34A–40A.
98. Jung, W. I., & Dietze, G. J. (1999). 31P nuclear magnetic resonance spectroscopy: a noninvasive tool to monitor metabolic abnormalities in left ventricular hypertrophy in human. *Am J Cardiol, 83*(12A), 19H–24H.
99. Crilley, J. G., Boehm, E. A., Blair, E., et al. (2003). Hypertrophic cardiomyopathy due to sarcomeric gene mutations is characterized by impaired energy metabolism irrespective of the degree of hypertrophy. *J Am Coll Cardiol, 41*(10), 1776–1782.
100. Jung, W. I., Sieverding, L., Breuer, J., et al. (1998). 31P NMR spectroscopy detects metabolic abnormalities in asymptomatic patients with hypertrophic cardiomyopathy. *Circulation, 97*(25), 2536–2542.
101. Roberts, R., & Marian, A. J. (2003). Can an energy-deficient heart grow bigger and stronger? *J Am Coll Cardiol, 41*(10), 1783–1785.
102. Sarikas, A., Carrier, L., Schenke, C., et al. (2005). Impairment of the ubiquitin-proteasome system by truncated cardiac myosin binding protein C mutants. *Cardiovasc Res, 66*(1), 33–44.
103. Nagueh, S. F., Bachinski, L. L., Meyer, D., et al. (2001). Tissue Doppler imaging consistently detects myocardial abnormalities in patients with hypertrophic cardiomyopathy and provides a novel means for an early diagnosis before and independently of hypertrophy. *Circulation, 104*(2), 128–130.
104. Nagueh, S. F., Kopelen, H. A., Lim, D. S., et al. (2000). Tissue Doppler imaging consistently detects myocardial contraction and relaxation abnormalities, irrespective of cardiac hypertrophy, in a transgenic rabbit model of human hypertrophic cardiomyopathy. *Circulation, 102*(12), 1346–1350.
105. Charron, P., Dubourg, O., Desnos, M., et al. (1998). Genotype-phenotype correlations in familial hypertrophic cardiomyopathy. A comparison between mutations in the cardiac protein-C and the beta-myosin heavy chain genes. *Eur Heart J, 19*(1), 139–145.
106. Anan, R., Greve, G., Thierfelder, L., et al. (1994). Prognostic implications of novel beta cardiac myosin heavy chain gene mutations that cause familial hypertrophic cardiomyopathy. *J Clin Invest, 93*(1), 280–285.
107. Maron, B. J., Niimura, H., Casey, S. A., et al. (2001). Development of left ventricular hypertrophy in adults in hypertrophic cardiomyopathy caused by cardiac myosin-binding protein C gene mutations. *J Am Coll Cardiol, 38*(2), 315–321.
108. Abchee, A., & Marian, A. J. (1997). Prognostic significance of beta-myosin heavy chain mutations is reflective of their hypertrophic expressivity in patients with hypertrophic cardiomyopathy. *J Investig Med, 45*(4), 191–196.
109. Varnava, A. M., Elliott, P. M., Baboonian, C., et al. (2001). Hypertrophic cardiomyopathy: histopathological features of sudden death in cardiac troponin T disease. *Circulation, 104*(12), 1380–1384.
110. Van Driest, S. L., Ackerman, M. J., Ommen, S. R., et al. (2002). Prevalence and severity of "benign" mutations in the beta-myosin heavy chain, cardiac troponin T, and alpha-tropomyosin genes in hypertrophic cardiomyopathy. *Circulation, 106*(24), 3085–3090.
111. Niimura, H., Patton, K. K., McKenna, W. J., et al. (2002). Sarcomere protein gene mutations in hypertrophic cardiomyopathy of the elderly. *Circulation, 105*(4), 446–451.
112. Konhilas, J. P., Watson, P. A., Maass, A., et al. (2006). Exercise can prevent and reverse the severity of hypertrophic cardiomyopathy. *Circ Res, 98*(4), 540–548.
113. Maron, B. J., & Fananapazir, L. (1992). Sudden cardiac death in hypertrophic cardiomyopathy. *Circulation, 85*(suppl. 1), I57–I63.
114. Fujino, N., Shimizu, M., Ino, H., et al. (2002). A novel mutation Lys273Glu in the cardiac troponin T gene shows high degree of penetrance and transition from hypertrophic to dilated cardiomyopathy. *Am J Cardiol, 89*(1), 29–33.
115. Mogensen, J., Kubo, T., Duque, M., et al. (2003). Idiopathic restrictive cardiomyopathy is part of the clinical expression of cardiac troponin I mutations. *J Clin Invest, 111*(2), 209–216.
116. Fujino, N., Shimizu, M., Ino, H., et al. (2001). Cardiac troponin T Arg92Trp mutation and progression from hypertrophic to dilated cardiomyopathy. *Clin Cardiol, 24*(5), 397–402.
117. Li, D., Czernuszewicz, G. Z., Gonzalez, O., et al. (2001). Novel cardiac troponin T mutation as a cause of familial dilated cardiomyopathy. *Circulation, 104*(18), 2188–2193.
118. Klaassen, S., Probst, S., Oechslin, E., et al. (2008). Mutations in sarcomere protein genes in left ventricular noncompaction. *Circulation, 117*(22), 2893–2901.
119. Kamisago, M., Sharma, S. D., DePalma, S. R., et al. (2000). Mutations in sarcomere protein genes as a cause of dilated cardiomyopathy. *N Engl J Med, 343*(23), 1688–1696.
120. Yanaga, F., Morimoto, S., & Ohtsuki, I. (1999). Ca^{2+} sensitization and potentiation of the maximum level of myofibrillar ATPase activity caused by mutations of troponin T found in familial hypertrophic cardiomyopathy. *J Biol Chem, 274*(13), 8806–8812.
121. Morimoto, S., Lu, Q. W., Harada, K., et al. (2002). Ca(2+)-desensitizing effect of a deletion mutation Delta K210 in cardiac troponin T that causes familial dilated cardiomyopathy. *Proc Natl Acad Sci U S A, 99*(2), 913–918.
122. Davis, J., Wen, H., Edwards, T., et al. (2008). Allele and species dependent contractile defects by restrictive and hypertrophic cardiomyopathy-linked troponin I mutants. *J Mol Cell Cardiol, 44*(5), 891–904.
123. Chang, A. N., Harada, K., Ackerman, M. J., et al. (2005). Functional consequences of hypertrophic and dilated cardiomyopathy causing mutations in alpha-tropomyosin. *J Biol Chem, 280*, 34343–34349.
124. Burton, D., Abdulrazzak, H., Knott, A., et al. (2002). Two mutations in troponin I that cause hypertrophic cardiomyopathy have contrasting effects on cardiac muscle contractility. *Biochem J, 362*(pt 2), 443–451.
125. Bottinelli, R., Coviello, D. A., Redwood, C. S., et al. (1998). A mutant tropomyosin that causes hypertrophic cardiomyopathy is expressed in vivo and associated with an increased calcium sensitivity. *Circ Res, 82*(1), 106–115.
126. Bing, W., Knott, A., Redwood, C., et al. (2000). Effect of hypertrophic cardiomyopathy mutations in human cardiac muscle alpha-tropomyosin (Asp175Asn and Glu180Gly) on the regulatory properties of human cardiac troponin determined by in vitro motility assay. *J Mol Cell Cardiol, 32*(8), 1489–1498.
127. Nugent, A. W., Daubeney, P. E. F., Chondros, P., et al. (2005). Clinical features and outcomes of childhood hypertrophic cardiomyopathy: results from a national population-based study. *Circulation, 112*(9), 1332–1338.
128. Tartaglia, M., Mehler, E. L., Goldberg, R., et al. (2001). Mutations in *PTPN11*, encoding the protein tyrosine phosphatase SHP-2, cause Noonan syndrome. *Nat Genet, 29*(4), 465–468.
129. Pandit, B., Sarkozy, A., Pennacchio, L. A., et al. (2007). Gain-of-function RAF1 mutations cause Noonan and LEOPARD syndromes with hypertrophic cardiomyopathy. *Nat Genet, 39*(8), 1007–1012.
130. Tartaglia, M., Pennacchio, L. A., Zhao, C., et al. (2007). Gain-of-function *SOS1* mutations cause a distinctive form of Noonan syndrome. *Nat Genet, 39*(1), 75–79.
131. Carta, C., Pantaleoni, F., Bocchinfuso, G., et al. (2006). Germline missense mutations affecting *KRAS* isoform B are associated with a severe Noonan syndrome phenotype. *Am J Hum Genet, 79*(1), 129–135.
132. Gollob, M. H., Seger, J. J., Gollob, T. N., et al. (2001). Novel *PRKAG2* mutation responsible for the genetic syndrome of ventricular preexcitation and conduction system disease with childhood onset and absence of cardiac hypertrophy. *Circulation, 104*(25), 3030–3033.
133. Arad, M., Benson, D. W., Perez-Atayde, A. R., et al. (2002). Constitutively active AMP kinase mutations cause glycogen storage disease mimicking hypertrophic cardiomyopathy. *J Clin Invest, 109*(3), 357–362.
134. Chimenti, C., Pieroni, M., Morgante, E., et al. (2004). Prevalence of Fabry disease in female patients with late-onset hypertrophic cardiomyopathy. *Circulation, 110*(9), 1047–1053.
135. Sachdev, B., Takenaka, T., Teraguchi, H., et al. (2002). Prevalence of Andersen-Fabry disease in male patients with late onset hypertrophic cardiomyopathy. *Circulation, 105*(12), 1407–1411.
136. Brady, R. O., & Schiffmann, R. (2000). Clinical features of and recent advances in therapy for Fabry disease. *JAMA, 284*(21), 2771–2775.
137. Desnick, R. J., Brady, R., Barranger, J., et al. (2003). Fabry disease, an under-recognized multisystemic disorder: expert recommendations for diagnosis, management, and enzyme replacement therapy. *Ann Intern Med, 138*(4), 338–346.
138. Eng, C. M., Guffon, N., Wilcox, W. R., et al. (2001). Safety and efficacy of recombinant human alpha-galactosidase A—replacement therapy in Fabry's disease. *N Engl J Med, 345*(1), 9–16.
139. Schiffmann, R., Murray, G. J., Treco, D., et al. (2000). Infusion of alpha-galactosidase A reduces tissue globotriaosylceramide storage in patients with Fabry disease. *Proc Natl Acad Sci U S A, 97*(1), 365–370.
140. Wilcox, W. R., Banikazemi, M., Guffon, N., et al. (2004). Long-term safety and efficacy of enzyme replacement therapy for Fabry disease. *Am J Hum Genet, 75*(1), 65–74.
141. Meyer, C., Schmid, G., Gorlitz, S., et al. (2007). Cardiomyopathy in Friedreich's ataxia—assessment by cardiac MRI. *Mov Disord, 22*(11), 1615–1622.
142. Karpati, G., Carpenter, S., Larbrisseau, A., et al. (1973). The Kearns-Shy syndrome. A multisystem disease with mitochondrial abnormality demonstrated in skeletal muscle and skin. *J Neurol Sci, 19*(2), 133–151.
143. Maron, B. J., Spirito, P., Shen, W. K., et al. (2007). Implantable cardioverter-defibrillators and prevention of sudden cardiac death in hypertrophic cardiomyopathy. *JAMA, 298*(4), 405–412.
144. McLeod, C. J., Ommen, S. R., Ackerman, M. J., et al. (2007). Surgical septal myectomy decreases the risk for appropriate implantable cardioverter defibrillator discharge in obstructive hypertrophic cardiomyopathy. *Eur Heart J, 28*(21), 2583–2588.

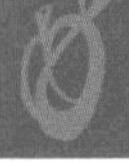

145. McGregor, J. B., Rahman, A., Rosanio, S., et al. (2004). Monomorphic ventricular tachycardia: a late complication of percutaneous alcohol septal ablation for hypertrophic cardiomyopathy. *Am J Med Sci, 328*(3), 185–188.
146. Sorajja, P., Valeti, U., Nishimura, R. A., et al. (2008). Outcome of alcohol septal ablation for obstructive hypertrophic cardiomyopathy. *Circulation, 118*(2), 131–139.
147. Sherrid, M. V., Barac, I., McKenna, W. J., et al. (2005). Multicenter study of the efficacy and safety of disopyramide in obstructive hypertrophic cardiomyopathy. *J Am Coll Cardiol, 45*(8), 1251–1258.
148. Schonbeck, M. H., Brunner-La Rocca, H., Vogt, P. R., et al. (1998). Long-term follow-up in hypertrophic obstructive cardiomyopathy after septal myectomy. *Ann Thorac Surg, 65*(5), 1207–1214.
149. Schulte, H. D., Bircks, W. H., Loesse, B., et al. (1993). Prognosis of patients with hypertrophic obstructive cardiomyopathy after transaortic myectomy. Late results up to twenty-five years. *J Thorac Cardiovasc Surg, 106*(4), 709–717.
150. van Dockum, W. G., ten Cate, F. J., ten Berg, J. M., et al. (2004). Myocardial infarction after percutaneous transluminal septal myocardial ablation in hypertrophic obstructive cardiomyopathy: evaluation by contrast-enhanced magnetic resonance imaging. *J Am Coll Cardiol, 43*(1), 27–34.
151. Nagueh, S. F., Lakkis, N. M., Middleton, K. J., et al. (1999). Changes in left ventricular diastolic function 6 months after nonsurgical septal reduction therapy for hypertrophic obstructive cardiomyopathy. *Circulation, 99*(3), 344–347.
152. Chang, S. M., Nagueh, S. F., Spencer, W. H., III, et al. (2003). Complete heart block: determinants and clinical impact in patients with hypertrophic obstructive cardiomyopathy undergoing nonsurgical septal reduction therapy. *J Am Coll Cardiol, 42*(2), 296–300.
153. Talreja, D. R., Nishimura, R. A., Edwards, W. D., et al. (2004). Alcohol septal ablation versus surgical septal myectomy: comparison of effects on atrioventricular conduction tissue. *J Am Coll Cardiol, 44*(12), 2329–2332.
154. Lim, D. S., Lutucuta, S., Bachireddy, P., et al. (2001). Angiotensin II blockade reverses myocardial fibrosis in a transgenic mouse model of human hypertrophic cardiomyopathy. *Circulation, 103*(6), 789–791.
155. Marian, A. J., Senthil, V., Chen, S. N., et al. (2006). Antifibrotic effects of antioxidant *N*-acetylcysteine in a mouse model of human hypertrophic cardiomyopathy mutation. *J Am Coll Cardiol, 47*(4), 827–834.
156. Araujo, A. Q., Arteaga, E., Ianni, B. M., et al. (2005). Effect of losartan on left ventricular diastolic function in patients with nonobstructive hypertrophic cardiomyopathy. *Am J Cardiol, 96*(11), 1563–1567.
157. Yamazaki, T., Suzuki, J., Shimamoto, R., et al. (2007). A new therapeutic strategy for hypertrophic nonobstructive cardiomyopathy in humans. A randomized and prospective study with an angiotensin II receptor blocker. *Int Heart J, 48*(6), 715–724.
158. Bauersachs, J., Stork, S., Kung, M., et al. (2007). HMG CoA reductase inhibition and left ventricular mass in hypertrophic cardiomyopathy: a randomized placebo-controlled pilot study. *Eur J Clin Invest, 37*(11), 852–859.

CHAPTER 26

Heart Failure as a Consequence of Diabetic Cardiomyopathy

Peter Van Buren and Martin M. LeWinter

THE EPIDEMIOLOGY OF DIABETES AND HEART FAILURE

Diabetes mellitus (DM) is a burgeoning public health problem. In the United States, its incidence increased by 61% between 1990 and 2001.[1] It is estimated that more than 20 million Americans now have DM with an additional 50 million categorized as prediabetic based on elevated fasting blood glucose levels.[2] Thus in view of its magnitude as a public health problem and, as is discussed later, its prominent importance as a risk factor for heart failure (HF), DM can be viewed as an epidemic that is directly contributing to the prevalence of another epidemic, that being heart failure.

The Framingham investigators were the first to quantify and call attention to the markedly increased risk of HF in patients with DM (see Chapter 22). In their seminal study,[3] the presence of DM increased the risk of HF by about twofold in men and fivefold in women. This effect, which is *independent of the presence of coexistent coronary artery disease* (CAD) *and/or hypertension*, has been confirmed in numerous subsequent studies (see references 4-9 for examples) and holds true for both type 1 and type 2 DM. Most studies report an overall independent relative risk for development of HF in patients with DM on the order of 1.5 to 2.0. In a more recent Framingham report,[4] the percentage of HF cases accounted for *solely by DM* was 6% in men and 12% in women. Conversely, among Medicare recipients with a primary hospital discharge diagnosis of HF, a striking 38% had concomitant DM.[10] Both the risk of development of HF[11] and the chance of hospitalization for HF[12] are positively correlated with hemoglobin A1c levels.

As will be seen, the most common clinically recognized effect of DM on the myocardium is diastolic dysfunction (see also Chapter 14). However, the population of patients with nonischemic, dilated cardiomyopathy has an overrepresentation of DM patients,[13] indicating a direct association of DM with both systolic and diastolic HF. Although the increased risk of HF associated with DM is unequivocal, the true magnitude of risk may be somewhat confounded by the fact that HF itself induces insulin resistance.[14]

In addition to its role as a major HF risk factor per se, DM also contributes independently to the risk of developing HF as a complication of acute myocardial infarction (MI), which is independent of infarct size,[15] and to the progression and mortality of established HF[16-18] (Figure 26-1). As noted earlier,[1] DM is a stronger risk factor for development of HF in women than men. It also appears that women with DM and HF have worse outcomes than their male counterparts.[19-21]

For a more detailed reading on this topic the reader is referred to the review by Masoudi and Inzucchi.[22]

Diabetic Cardiomyopathy: Mechanisms of Myocardial Damage

The powerful epidemiologic evidence linking DM to HF led to consideration of the possibility that DM is directly causal in the development of cardiac dysfunction. The earliest suggestion of this is credited to Rubler et al,[23] who described four patients with diabetic nephropathy and cardiomyopathy in the absence of angiographically detectable CAD. Subsequently, the existence of a diabetic cardiomyopathy has become well accepted.[22,24-26] Although diabetic cardiomyopathy can cause HF and/or evidence of myocardial dysfunction on its own, it is much more common for it to act in concert with the comorbidities of CAD, hypertension, and obesity. The contribution of diabetic cardiomyopathy to HF is inevitably difficult to sort out when these other common accompaniments of DM are present.

Diabetes is a complex disorder and multiple interconnected features of the disease mechanistically contribute to the development of diabetic cardiomyopathy.[22,24-26] Each of these features can cause multiple functional consequences and generally more than one is operative in an individual patient. Moreover, the relative importance of one or another underlying mechanism is dependent on whether the patient has type 1 or type 2 DM, the duration of disease, and very likely its management. In addition, much of the mechanistic information about diabetic cardiomyopathy has been derived from various animal models, all of which exhibit various differences when compared with the human disease. As shown in Figure 26-2, despite this complexity three key metabolic derangements—hyperglycemia, increased nonesterified fatty acid (FA) concentration, and hyperinsulinemia—appear to play central roles in this disease process (see also Chapter 20).[24-26]

Hyperglycemia

Reactive Oxygen Species (see Chapter 12). In type 2 DM, where hyperinsulinemia is present, hyperglycemia may result in increased glucose oxidation and generation of superoxide, peroxynitrate, and other reactive oxygen species (ROS) in tissues such as the myocardium that are not strongly insulin resistant[26-29] (see Figure 26-2). ROS react with cellular proteins and nucleic acids, leading to various deleterious effects. These include oxidation and nitration of proteins directly involved in contraction and relaxation; uncoupling of mitochondrial oxidative phosphorylation, leading to impaired energetics; and DNA damage and cell death.[24,26-33] ROS can directly affect both calcium cycling and contractile protein function. DM-induced oxidative changes in both the sarcoplasmic reticulum ATPase

(SERCA-2) and myosin can directly inhibit the function of these proteins.[33,35] ROS also appear to play a central role in the pathogenesis of diabetic cardiomyopathy by directly contributing to hyperglycemia-mediated activation of protein kinase C[33] and protein glycation and the subsequent formation of advanced glycation end products (AGEs) (discussed in more detail later).

The importance of ROS is highlighted by the fact that increased expression of the antioxidants metallothionein or superoxide dismutase (SOD) in mouse models of DM prevented the development of cardiomyopathy.[29,35,36]

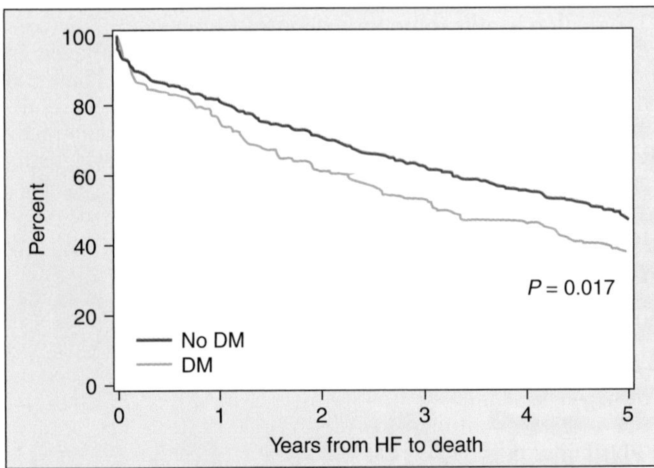

FIGURE 26–1 The effect of diabetes on survival in patients with established heart failure (HF). (Reproduced from AM, Leibson CL, Bursi F, et al. Diabetes in heart failure: prevalence and impact on outcome in the population. *Am J Med* 2006;119:591-599 [reprinted with permission of the *American Journal of Medicine*.]). DM, Diabetes mellitus

Inhibition of ROS production through overexpression of SOD in hyperglycemic endothelial cells has been shown to prevent increased glucose flux through the aldose reductase pathway, increased intracellular AGE formation, and the increase in PKC activation associated with hyperglycemia and DM.[37] Peroxynitrite ($ONOO^-$), which causes protein nitration, has been specifically linked to mitochondrial dysfunction in a mouse model.[38]

Protein Glycation and AGE Formation. Protein glycation and the production of AGEs are important components of hyperglycemia-mediated myocardial damage.[39-42] Protein glycation results from enhanced production of dicarbonyl species (glyoxal, methylglyoxal, and 3-deoxyglucosone) that nonenzymatically react with protein amino groups under conditions of hyperglycemia and oxidative stress. The initial process of protein glycation involves the reaction of a carbonyl group of glucose with the amino group of a protein to form a Schiff base (Figure 26-3). This process differs from glycosylation because the reaction is not driven by an enzymatic catalyst. This initial reaction is reversible but the carbonyl-protein adduct is eventually converted to a more stable Amadori product. Amadori products are gradually modified to form AGEs, which are very long-lasting and retard the degradation of proteins, most notably collagen. This series of chemical reactions is known collectively as the Maillard reaction (see Figure 26-3). AGEs can also form protein cross-links.[39,40,43-46] Largely through the work of Cerami et al, protein glycation and AGE formation have been recognized for many years as important mechanisms of the complications of DM.[47]

The effects of protein glycation are twofold. Glycation can directly affect protein function[34,35,39,40,45] and AGEs interact with the cell membrane receptor for advanced glycation end products (RAGE),[39,48-52] which are present in a number of cells including fibroblasts. As shown in Figure 26-4, activation of

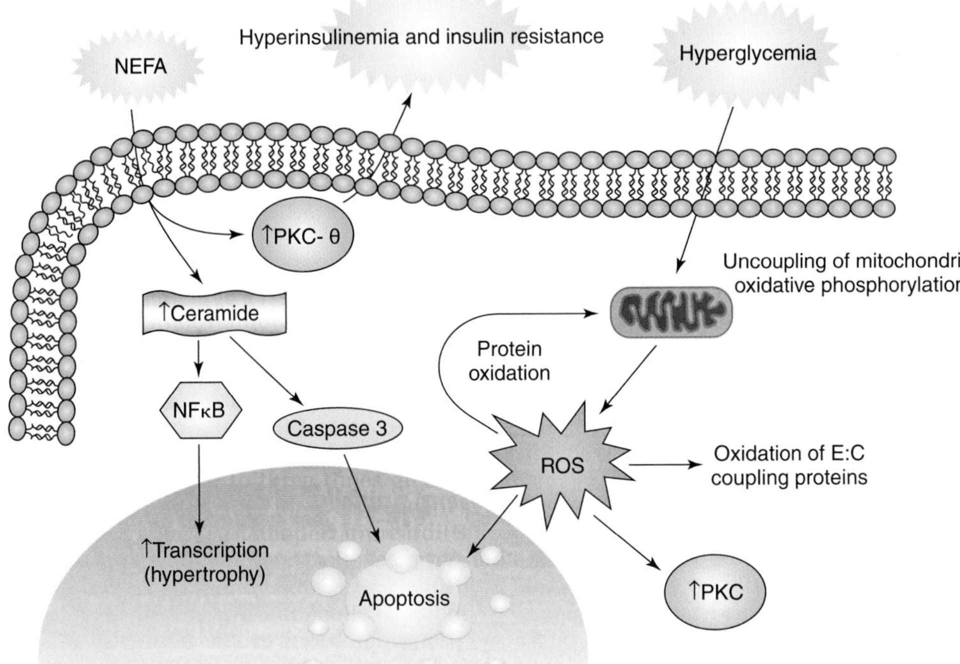

FIGURE 26–2 An overview of the effects of hyperglycemia, increased nonesterified fatty acids, and insulin resistance as mechanisms of myocardial damage in diabetes (see text for details). *NEFA,* nonesterified fatty acids; *ROS,* reactive oxygen species; *PKC,* protein kinase C.

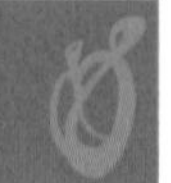

RAGE by AGEs increases the activity of several signaling proteins and inflammatory cytokines, most notably nuclear factor κB (NF κB), tissue growth factor-β (TGF-β), interleukin-2 (IL-2), and tumor necrosis factor α (TNF-α). In addition RAGE activation promotes ROS production. RAGE expression increases with increased abundance of its ligands, thus creating a vicious cycle. RAGE blockade slows the progression of experimental atherosclerosis,[49-51] whereas overexpression of RAGE in murine cardiocytes resulted in slowing of calcium dynamics leading to depressed myocyte contraction.[52]

Both contractile and calcium cycling proteins are modified by glycation and/or AGEs. In vitro, the function of myosin[35,53] and myofilament assembly are adversely affected by glycation.[54] In addition, SERCA-2 and the ryanodine receptor have been shown to be subject to glycation and AGE formation in the streptozotocin (STZ) rat model of DM.[55,56] SERCA-2 glycation was reversed by insulin treatment. Intracellular AGE formation is likely closely related to the aforementioned excess superoxide production.

As shown in Figure 26-4, AGEs can also form in the extracellular matrix of the myocardium as adducts to collagen.[39,40,42,44-46,57] Here, AGEs can form cross-links between adjacent fibrils, which increases the stiffness of collagen. Moreover, the presence of crosslinks renders collagen more resistant to degradation by matrix metalloproteinases (MMPs). The aforementioned AGE-RAGE interaction results in a proinflammatory, profibrotic signaling cascade that ultimately results in changes in MMPs and tissue inhibitors of MMPs (TIMPs) that favor collagen accumulation.[34,35,39,40,45] Thus the net result of AGEs is an increase in the content of collagen, which itself is abnormally crosslinked. These processes make AGEs a prime candidate mechanism in the development of DM-associated diastolic dysfunction in humans.[58] This concept is supported by the fact that AGEs stiffen collagen in nonmyocardial tissue in humans and in the hearts of animal diabetic models.[59,60] Although scant information is available in human myocardium, AGEs have been detected by light microscopy using antibody labeling.[61,62] Recently, using

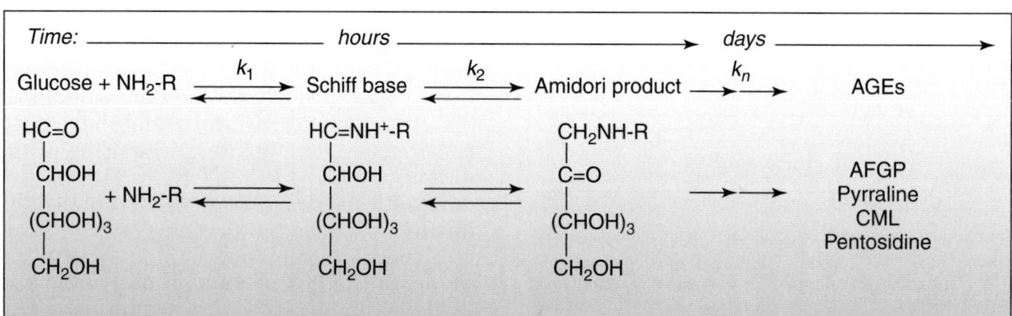

FIGURE 26–3 The Maillard reaction sequence, in which protein glycation gradually leads to the formation of AGEs. *AFGP,* antifreeze glycoprotein; *CML,* carboxymethyl lysine. (From Fraser D.A., Hanssen K.F.(2005). Making sense of advanced glycation endproducts and their relevance to diabetic complications. International Diabetes monitor. 17(3):1-7.)

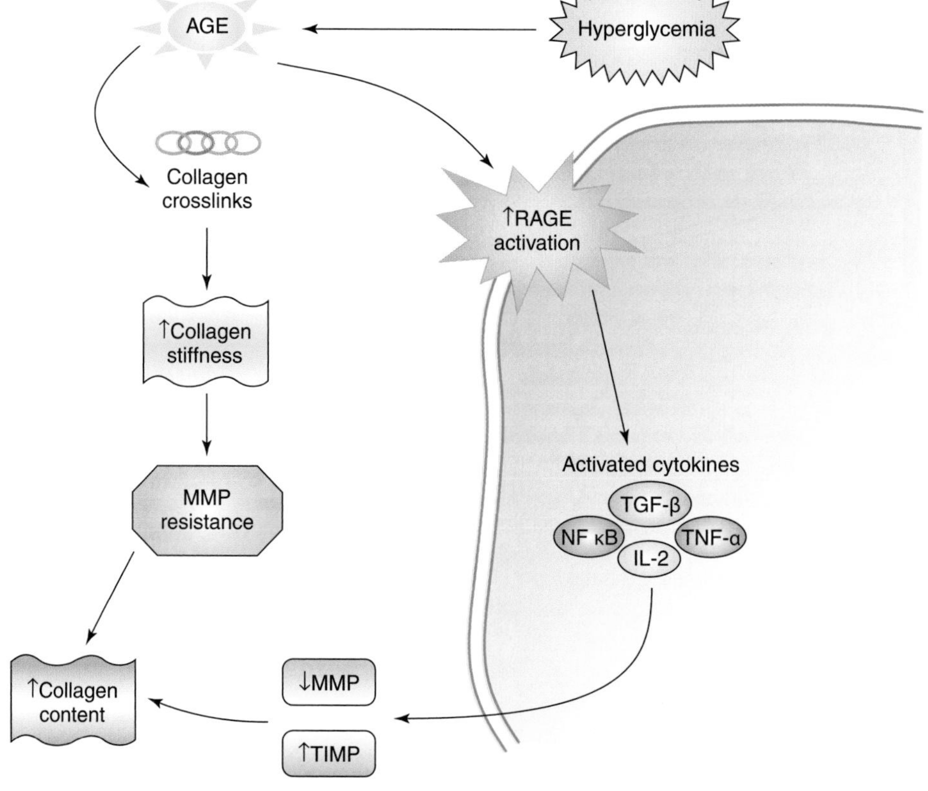

FIGURE 26-4 Schema of the effects of AGE formation on collagen cross-linking and content (see text).

immunoelectron microscopic techniques, we detected AGEs associated with collagen fibrils in human myocardial biopsies obtained from patients with DM at the time of coronary artery bypass grafting (Figure 26-5, *left panel*). Finally, in diabetic animal models the AGE crosslink breaker alagebrium has been shown to decrease myocardial fibrosis and improve ventricular function.[59]

Protein Kinase C Signaling (see also Chapter 2). A number of circulating neurohormones, most importantly angiotensin II, are increased in DM.[63] Angiotensin II can directly affect intracellular signaling by binding to one of a family of seven transmembrane receptors. β_1- and β_2-adrenergic, α-adrenergic, and endothelin signaling occurs through this same receptor family[64] (Figure 26-6). Common to all of these receptors is the close intracellular association with specific GTP binding proteins (or G proteins, consisting of α, β, and γ subunits and an effector enzyme). When an agonist binds to the receptor, GDP is released from the a subunit allowing GTP to bind and leading to disassociation of the a subunit-effector enzyme and the ß, γ subunit from the agonist-receptor. G protein subunit isoform variation allows for association with specific effector enzymes. Upon activation of the receptor, Ga coupled phospholipase-Cβ is activated, hydrolyzing the membrane bound phospholipid, phosphatidylinositol 4,5 bisphosphate, to yield diacylglycerol (DAG) and inositol 1,4,5- triphosphate. DAG is the primary activator of most protein kinase C (PKC) isoforms. In DM, DAG synthesis is increased, in part via ROS-mediated activation of the DNA repair enzyme poly (ADP ribose) polymerase (PARP).[28] Thus both enhanced 7 transmembrane receptor activation and increased DAG synthesis contribute to PKC activation in DM.[30] In animal models of DM, increases in the myocardial activity of PKC isoforms α, β, ε, and δ have been observed.[65]

A number of PKC isoforms are known to directly affect both myofilament function and calcium cycling.[66,67] At the myofilament level, PKC can phosphorylate troponin I, troponin

IMMUNOELECTRON MICROGRAPHS OF HUMAN MYOCARDIUM

Collagen fibrils

Myofilaments

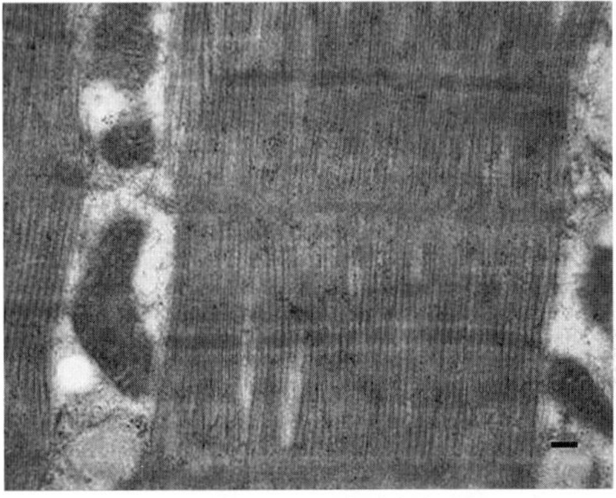

FIGURE 26–5 Immunoelectron micrographic sections of myocardial collagen fibrils (*left*) and myofilaments (*right*) labeled for carboxymethyl lysine advanced glycation end-products with colloidal gold in myocardial biopsy tissue from a patient with diabetes undergoing coronary bypass grafting. Small black dots are colloidal gold particles indicating antigen-antibody complexes.

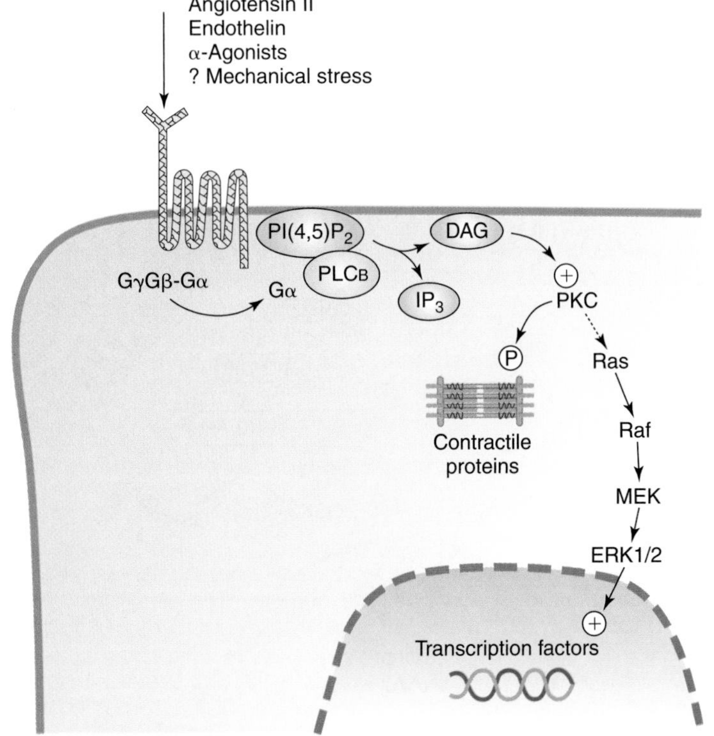

FIGURE 26–6 Schema of G protein signaling pathways (see text).

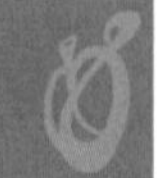

T, myosin binding protein C, myosin regulatory light chain, and titin. In animal models of HF and in human end-stage HF phosphorylation of troponins I and T directly modulates thin filament function leading to a depression in maximal contractile force, a process that is likely mediated by PKC.[66,67] In addition PKC activates protein phosphatase 1, which dephosphorylates phospholamban and inhibits SERCA-2 activity.[68] Sodium-calcium exchanger function may also be impaired by PKC.[69]

PKC also activates extracellular signal-related kinases 1 and 2 (ERK 1/2) of the mitogen-activated protein kinase (MAPK) family.[64,70] Activation of the ERK 1/2 pathway has been demonstrated to be an important mediator of the hypertrophic response in heart failure.[71] Current evidence suggests that the cascade is triggered by PKC-mediated activation of the "small" GTP binding protein, Ras. Ras activates Raf (a MAPK), which phosphorylates ERK 1/2, resulting in the activation of several transcription factors and inducing a hypertrophy gene program (see Figure 26-3). The ERK 1/2 pathway is also activated by several growth factors and mechanical stress-mediated signaling mechanisms.[70] Thus PKC signaling likely contributes to cardiac hypertrophy in DM (see later discussion).

Nonesterified Fatty Acids

As shown in Figure 26-2, nonesterified FA concentration and oxidation are characteristically increased in DM.[22,24-26] Triglycerides are also elevated and may be observed as lipid droplets in cardiac myocytes in animal models of type 2 DM.[72] The high concentration of FAs is itself a mechanism of the insulin resistance characteristic of type 2 DM.[25,26] This may be related to activation of PKC-θ, which interferes with the binding of insulin to insulin receptor-1 [25]. Excessive FA oxidation in the cardiac myocyte results in accumulation of toxic, long chain FAs in the cytoplasm as the capacity of the mitochondria to process FAs is exceeded.[24-26,72] Lipotoxicity caused by increased cardiac myocyte FA and long chain FAs may directly impair cardiac contractility due to alterations in membrane-associated ion channel and pump function.[73] For example, excess FAs induce opening of the K_{ATP} channel resulting in shortening of the action potential duration.[74]

Accumulation of FAs also leads to increased use of alternative metabolic pathways that increase ceramide generation.[24-26] This may in part be mediated by peroxisome-proliferator–activated receptor-α induction.[75] Ceramide is an important activator of NF κB and caspase 3, which in turn activate proapoptotic and proinflammatory signaling pathways. Increased ROS may also contribute to apoptotic signaling. Increased myocardial apoptosis has been demonstrated in animal DM models[76] and in patients with DM.[77] A recent study reported a markedly increased proportion of apoptotic cells in biopsy specimens from nonischemic cardiomyopathy patients with DM versus those without DM.[78]

Hyperinsulinemia

Hyperinsulinemia is present only in type 2 DM, and therefore does not contribute to cardiomyopathy in type 1 DM. Cardiac hypertrophy is perhaps the most important consequence of hyperinsulinemia.[24,79,80] Patients with DM have been shown to have increased cardiac mass independent of co-existent hypertension.[79,80] Multiple mechanisms are probably responsible for hypertrophy in DM.[24] PKC signaling is enhanced by hyperinsulinemia and, as mentioned earlier, can directly contribute to the hypertrophic response.[70,71] Insulin acutely augments glucose uptake via activation of a tyrosine kinase receptor–mediated Akt-1 pathway[81] (Figure 26-7). Akt-1 inactivates glycogen synthase kinase-3β, an inhibitor of nuclear factor in activated lymphocytes (NFAT-3), a key hypertrophy mediator. Hyperinsulinemia-mediated increased sympathetic activation may also function to augment Akt-1 activity.[81] The tyrosine kinase pathway also contributes to PKC activation (see Figure 26-7). Finally, insulin is an activator of the MAPK hypertrophic pathway.[82]

Diabetic Microvasculopathy

When the concept of diabetic cardiomyopathy was first proposed, "small vessel" disease (i.e., diabetic microvasculopathy) was offered as the likely mechanism. Subsequently, correlations between manifestations of microvascular disease (e.g., nephropathy, retinopathy) and the presence of HF or subclinical diastolic dysfunction have been reported.[83-86] However, a clear mechanistic link between diabetic

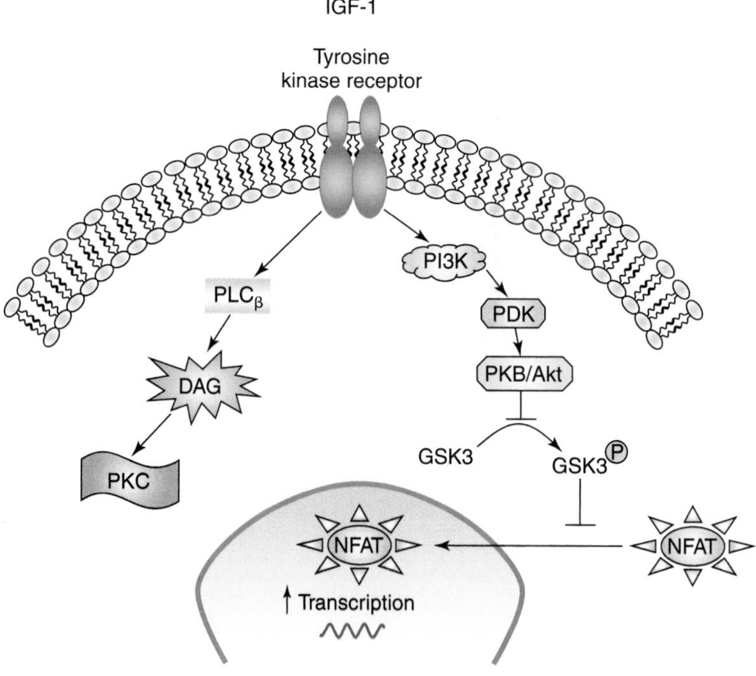

FIGURE 26-7 Schema of insulin activation of a tyrosine kinase-mediated signaling pathway that contributes to cardiac hypertrophy and PKC activation (see text).

cardiomyopathy and microvasculopathy has not as yet been established.[86]

Functional and Morphological Manifestations of Diabetic Cardiomyopathy

Animal Models

Much of our understanding of the mechanisms and functional consequences of diabetic cardiomyopathy is derived from animal models. STZ, a direct pancreatic islet cell toxin, has been the most widely employed means to induce DM, most commonly in rats.[24,26] STZ mimics human type I DM with hyperglycemia and hypoinsulinemia. Alloxan[87] has been used mainly in larger animals to produce relatively mild type 1 DM. Type 2 insulin resistance models have also been widely employed, for example, leptin deficient db/db mice[88] and the Zucker fatty rat.[89] Depressed systolic function has been observed in virtually all of these models but tends to be more prominent in type 1 DM. In type 2 models, changes in diastolic function are generally more prominent, resembling human type 2 DM.[90] By echocardiography, these changes include increased isovolumic relaxation time and alterations in mitral inflow and pulmonary venous flow patterns.[84,90-92] Changes in systolic function are also common in type 2 models but typically include decreases in fiber shortening and ejection rates, with fractional shortening unchanged. Correspondingly, isolated heart preparations reveal slowed rates of pressure development and decline. Similar changes are observed in isolated cardiac myocytes.[93]

Alterations in Calcium Cycling

In animal models of both type I and type II DM, alterations in calcium cycling are well documented.* These include reductions in the rate of calcium release from the sarcoplasmic reticulum (SR), peak cytosolic systolic calcium concentration, the rate of SR calcium sequestration, and SERCA-2 activity. As noted earlier, ROS and AGEs may play a role via posttranslational modification of the proteins involved in calcium cycling. Thus in STZ rats, SERCA-2 and the ryanodine receptor have been shown to be glycated with both non-crosslinked and crosslinked AGEs.[55,56] As noted earlier, overexpression of the AGE receptor results in slowing of calcium dynamics,[52] further supporting a role for AGEs in the pathophysiology of diabetic cardiomyopathy in STZ rats.

These changes in calcium cycling proteins contribute to changes in cardiac function by reducing calcium available for activation of the myofilaments and decreasing late systolic calcium clearance, resulting in continued cross-bridge formation in early diastole and impaired and/or incomplete relaxation. Transgenic overexpression of SERCA-2 in an STZ mouse reversed the contractile and relaxation deficits, consistent with an important functional role for altered calcium cycling in this model.[96] Reduced calcium extrusion by the sarcolemmal sodium calcium exchanger may also contribute to abnormalities in relaxation, as may the increased expression of phospholamban, which binds to SERCA-2 and inhibits its function.[26,34]

In excitable strips dissected from human epicardial biopsies from patients at the time of coronary artery bypass grafting, the force frequency relation was found to be moderately depressed in patients with DM.[97] The force frequency relation is a key mechanism of adaptation to increased functional demands on the myocardium. It is profoundly depressed in end-stage, failing myocardium, and has been related to altered calcium cycling.[98] Thus force frequency relation depression in DM patients could reflect the same underlying abnormality.

Alterations in the Myofilament (see also Chapter 3)

Sarcomere shortening is the result of cyclic cross-bridge formation between the myosin "head" formed by the myosin heavy chain (MHC) and active sites on actin. The process is regulated by the thin filament associated proteins, troponin (Tn) C, I, and T, and tropomyosin. Ventricular myocardium is composed of two MHC isoforms, α and β. Normal rodent myocardium is composed predominantly of α-MHC while normal human myocardium is predominantly β-MHC.[99] Major increases in the proportion of the β-MHC isoform are observed in rodent models of HF and STZ DM.[100,101] Compared with α-MHC, β-MHC exhibits slower kinetics as it interacts with actin. This myosin isoform shift likely contributes to the depressed contractile parameters observed in STZ DM. Since nonfailing human myocardium is composed of predominantly β-MHC, any myosin isoform shift toward the β isoform in *patients* with DM would be small and thus not likely to be functionally important.[99] In STZ rats, an increase in TnI phosphorylation has been reported, which may affect contractile protein function.[102] In humans, maximal myofilament contractile force and calcium sensitivity is decreased in detergent-treated (skinned) myocardial strips obtained from patients with DM.[103] These preparations are used to assess myofilament function independent of changes in calcium cycling. The changes in myofilament function in this human study were associated with an increase in TnI and TnT phosphorylation. TnI and TnT phosphorylation have complex effects on myofilament contractile function[67] and could also contribute to impaired ventricular contraction and relaxation. Finally, depressed optimal frequency of work production and power generation in skinned strips from female but not male coronary artery bypass patients with DM has been reported.[104] This could possibly help explain poorer outcomes in women with HF and DM.

As with calcium cycling proteins, posttranslational modification of myofilament proteins by ROS and AGEs may also contribute to myofilament dysfunction. In this regard, in addition to detecting AGEs in association with collagen fibrils, we have also identified AGEs in myofilament sections in biopsy specimens from patients with DM (see Figure 26-5, *right panel*).

Ultrastructural Changes and Passive Myocardial Stiffness in Diabetes Mellitus (see also Chapter 5)

Myocardial collagen content is determined by the balance between synthetic pathways and degradation by matrix metalloproteinases (MMPs).[105] MMP activity is modulated by tissue inhibitors of MMPs (TIMPs). AGEs, renin-angiotensin-aldosterone system activation, and other elements of neurohormonal and proinflammatory signaling are key profibrotic modulators of this balance and play important roles in DM.[106]

Animal models of DM often demonstrate increased collagen content, but this is more consistent and prominent in human myocardium.[106] Factor et al quantified fibrosis in postmortem specimens from patients with DM, hypertension, and their combination.[107,108] In addition to increased collagen in DM patients, they noted a striking synergistic effect of the combination of DM and hypertension on collagen content. The apparent differences between animal models and patients may simply reflect differing duration of disease. van Heerebeek et al[62] recently published a report in which left ventricular (LV) endomyocardial biopsies from patients with DM and HF and either normal or reduced ejection fraction (EF) were compared. LV chamber stiffness was increased in both DM patient groups. Collagen volume fraction was greater in DM patients with reduced EF, but this study did not contain a group without DM for comparison. Despite evidence that myocardial collagen

*References 26, 34, 52, 55, 56, 94, 95.

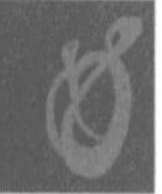

content is increased as well as abnormal noninvasively derived indexes of diastolic function in patients (see later discussion), there are no reports of direct measurements of myocardial passive stiffness in animal models or patients with DM.

Cardiac myocyte hypertrophy is the other main ultrastructural feature of diabetic cardiomyopathy, and has been discussed earlier.

Clinical Features of Diabetic Cardiomyopathy

Role of Diabetic Cardiomyopathy as a Mechanism of Heart Failure Symptoms

Although the increased risk of developing HF in patients with DM has been amply documented, in individual patients its precise contribution to the clinical presentation is rarely known. Thus in the case of a common disease such as nonischemic dilated cardiomyopathy (defined by the absence of significant coronary stenoses on angiography) it is impossible to know with confidence whether DM or some other cause is responsible. Patients with HF and normal or preserved EF (diastolic HF) typically have some other co-existing substrate for HF such as hypertension or CAD. The high incidence of HF following acute or chronic MI in patients with DM is likely accounted for to a significant extent by preexisting diabetic cardiomyopathy, but here again additional factors are usually present in individual patients. Recently, the association between obesity and other features of the metabolic syndrome and diastolic heart failure (often with a restrictive hemodynamic pattern) has been emphasized and related to the amount of epicardial fat.[109] Interestingly, on myocardial biopsy these patients have lipid droplets evident in cardiac myocytes, as has been reported previously in DM. In metabolic syndrome patients, once again, it is impossible to know how much underlying type 2 DM and/or insulin resistance contributes to HF versus other features of the metabolic syndrome.

Diabetic Cardiomyopathy and Diastolic Dysfunction

Although the precise contribution of DM to the syndrome of HF is usually uncertain in individual cases, a large proportion, possibly in excess 30% to 40%, of patients with DM without hypertension, known CAD, or other overt evidence of cardiac disease, have evidence of diastolic dysfunction based on noninvasive assessments.[85,110,111] This has been documented in a number of echocardiographic-Doppler reports of abnormal mitral inflow profiles[83,85,112] and, more recently, abnormal tissue Doppler velocity patterns[113,114] indicative of diastolic dysfunction in DM patients with normal EF. These abnormalities have been correlated with $HgbA_{1c}$ levels, measures of insulin resistance, presence of microvascular complications of DM, and, most interestingly, plasma AGE levels.[58] Thus asymptomatic diastolic dysfunction appears to be the most common and earliest detectable manifestation of diabetic cardiomyopathy in patients. Once again, however, when symptoms of HF appear in patients other comorbidities are often present.

Increased Left Ventricular Mass

As discussed earlier, LV mass is on average increased in DM patients. In the Multi-Ethnic Study of Atherosclerosis (MESA) cohort of subjects without clinical cardiovascular disease, in whom cardiac magnetic resonance imaging is being used to quantify cardiac structure and function, African Americans and Hispanics with DM had more prominent increases in LV mass than whites or Asians.[115]

Management of Heart Failure in Patients with Diabetes

There is no current evidence that HF should be managed differently in patients with DM compared with nondiabetic patients, although few studies have addressed this topic. Thus published American College of Cardiology/American Heart Association (ACC/AHA) guidelines[116] for medical management of ischemic and nonischemic systolic HF should be followed, with the usual cornerstones of β-adrenergic and renin-angiotensin-aldosterone system blockade. Until more definitive, evidence-based data are available, the management of diastolic HF remains empirical, but generally targeted at optimal management of contributing comorbid factors.

What little information that is available in regard to responses to medical therapy in HF patients with DM has been carefully reviewed by Masoudi and Inzucchi.[22] Thus a meta-analysis by Shekelle et al[117] revealed essentially identical outcome responses to angiotensin-converting enzyme (ACE) inhibitors in diabetic and nondiabetic patients with systolic HF. A community-based observational study by Masoudi et al[118] came to a similar conclusion. As pointed out by Masoudi and Inzucchi,[22] ACE inhibitors should be used especially cautiously in DM patients with type IV renal tubular acidosis and/or other aspects of diabetic nephropathy. There is virtually no information available about the use of angiotensin receptor blockers specific to patients with DM and systolic HF, although the same caution in regard to type IV renal tubular acidosis applies.

β-blockers also appear to be equally efficacious and safe in diabetic and nondiabetic patients with dilated cardiomyopathy.[119] With respect to aldosterone antagonists, patients with DM were not reported separately in the Randomized Aldactone Evaluation Study (RALES) of spironolactone in systolic HF,[120] but in the Eplerenone Post–Acute Myocardial Infarction Heart Failure Efficacy and Survival Study (EPHESUS) of eplerenone in patients with HF post-MI[121] improvement in outcomes were indistinguishable in patients with and without DM.

Management of Diabetes in Patients with Heart Failure

The Question of Tight Glycemic Control

In all patients the management of DM begins with diet, weight loss, and regular exercise. Blood glucose and $HgbA_{1c}$ levels should be monitored to ensure satisfactory glycemic control. The question of whether tight control of blood glucose is advantageous in the general management of DM has been a topic of debate for many years. The UK Prospective Diabetes Study (UKPDS)[122] provided strong evidence that tight control results in better microvascular outcomes. The evidence with respect to macrovascular complications such as MI and stroke is mixed, however. Nathan et al[123] reported marked improvement in macrovascular outcomes with tight control in patients with *type 1* DM. However, in the Action in Diabetes and Vascular disease: PreterAx and DiamicroN-MR Controlled Evaluation (ADVANCE) trial[124] of intensive control ($HgbA_{1c}$ of 6.5% or less) versus standard treatment ($HgbA_{1c}$ 7.0% to 7.9%) in *type 2* DM, intensive control resulted in significant reduction in nephropathy but no significant effects on macrovascular outcomes. Similarly, the recent Action to Control Cardiovascular Risk in Diabetes (ACCORD) study[125] concluded that tight control does not significantly reduce nonfatal MI or stroke. Moreover, tight control resulted in significantly *higher* mortality than standard treatment. Importantly, UKPDS, ADVANCE, and ACCORD did not demonstrate a reduction in incidence rates of HF. However, there are no prospective data about the effects of tight control in patients with established HF. An observational study by Eshagian et al[126] reported that patients with advanced systolic HF with $HgbA_{1c}$ greater than 7% actually had reduced mortality compared with patients with $HgbA_{1c}$ less than 7%. Although firm recommendations cannot be made at this time as to the role of tight control in patients with DM and HF, the available evidence suggests that it need not be a specific therapeutic goal. However, in individual patients this must be tempered by the beneficial microvascular effects of tight control.

Pharmacological Therapy

Many patients will of course require insulin to achieve satisfactory control. The effects of insulin on the course of HF and ventricular remodeling are controversial. The antiinflammatory effects of insulin and its salutary effects on cardiac myocyte energy metabolism would be expected to be useful in patients with HF. On the other hand, as discussed earlier, hyperinsulinemia may contribute to cardiac hypertrophy. Nichols et al[127] reviewed the Kaiser Permanente database and found that patients with DM receiving insulin had a greater chance of developing HF than those receiving oral hypoglycemics. Moreover, Smooke et al[128] retrospectively analyzed a cohort of patients with advanced systolic HF and found that insulin use was associated with increased mortality. While observational studies cannot distinguish between adverse effects of insulin versus the likelihood that insulin use simply identifies patients with both more severe DM and more severe underlying myocardial disease, these results point out the considerable uncertainties in this area. At present, one cannot argue strongly for or against insulin in situations where its use is optional.

For patients with DM receiving oral drugs for glycemic control, options have markedly increased over the last decade.[22,129,130] Currently available classes of drugs are summarized in Table 26-1. None of these drugs has been prospectively tested in sufficiently powered, long-term outcome trials in patients with established HF.

The sulfonylureas (glyburide, glipizide, glimepiride) have fallen somewhat out of favor in recent years because, at least in older studies, there was a suggestion of increased cardiovascular risk and their side effect profile is not as favorable as a number of other agents.[22]

The biguanide metformin, which continues to be widely used, had previously been considered contraindicated in HF because of early reports of lactic acidosis possibly caused by the drug. The latter resulted in an FDA-mandated package insert warning. Over the years, it became apparent that lactic acidosis is exceedingly rare and occurs only in the sickest HF patients.[22] Moreover, prospective studies[22] indicate that metformin reduces cardiovascular risk and a retrospective analysis suggests improved survival in HF patients receiving metformin.[131] Accordingly, in 2006 the package insert warning was removed. Metformin is thus a very reasonable choice for many patients with DM and HF.

TABLE 26-1 Classes and Mechanisms of Action of Drugs Used to Treat Diabetes

Class	Examples	Mechanism
Sulfonylureas	Glyburide	Increase insulin secretion by binding to sulfonylurea receptor
Meglitinides	Repaglinide	Same as sulfonylureas, shorter duration of action
Biguanides	Metformin	Decrease hepatic glucose production
α-Glucosidase	Acarbose	Reduces GI carbohydrate absorption inhibitors
Thiazolidinediones	Rosiglitazone Pioglitazone	PPARγ agonists that increase insulin sensitivity
Incretins	Exenatide	Increase glucose-dependent insulin production; decrease glucagon production by activating GLP-1 receptor
Dipeptidyl peptidase IV inhibitors	Sitagliptin	Inhibit degradation of GLP-1 receptors, potentiating incretin effects

The peroxisome-proliferator–activated receptor γ agonist thiazolidinediones (TZDs) (pioglitazone, rosiglitazone) are highly effective for long-term glycemic control and exert a number of effects, including improvements in lipids, antiinflammatory properties, vasodilation, and blood pressure lowering that are attractive in patients with HF.[132,133] They are in general well tolerated,[130] do not have adverse effects on cardiac remodeling,[134,135] and, at least in animal models, may improve diastolic function.[136] There is also some evidence of improved long-term outcomes in patients with HF.[131] However, a large prospective study evaluating overall, long-term cardiovascular risk in patients receiving pioglitazone[137] had a negative result for its primary endpoint, although there was a significant but modest improvement in a secondary combined endpoint of mortality, MI, and stroke. More recently, a meta-analysis[138] revealed an increase in coronary events for rosiglitazone, but not pioglitazone. While the evidence for such an effect is at present inconclusive, this report has caused considerable concern.

Even though TZDs have properties that may be beneficial in patients with HF, it became apparent early on that they routinely cause weight gain and peripheral edema.[129,132,133] The mechanism is salt and water retention in the distal tubule of the kidney and possibly local effects on vascular permeability. Use of these drugs can precipitate HF in a small number of patients (<1%) without a prior HF history. In patients with known HF or those who are at high risk for HF, the incidence of exacerbation or precipitation is clearly further increased, although the precise magnitude of increased risk is difficult to quantify. Accordingly, current guidelines[139] recommend that TZDs not be used in patients with class III or IV HF and that they be used very cautiously in patients with less severe HF. Because of the current uncertainty with respect to the coronary event risk of rosiglitazone, it is prudent to avoid initiating therapy with this drug in patients with concomitant coronary artery disease until this issue is resolved. In patients already receiving the drug with excellent glycemic control, this decision should be individualized.

Certain of the newer oral agents may be particularly useful in HF patients. As indicated, however, little objective information is available as yet. The incretin mimetics include both injectable preparations (glucagon-like peptide-1 [GLP-1] analogues and mimetics) and the orally administered dipeptidyl peptidase IV inhibitors (sitagliptin, vildagliptin). In animal experiments, GLP-1 administration had salutary effects in HF.[140] In small clinical studies improvement in EF recovery after acute MI[141] and in EF and functional measures in chronic HF patients[142] were observed. The α-glucosidase inhibitors (e.g., acarbose) act exclusively in the GI tract to block carbohydrate absorption. They have significant GI side effects but no systemic side effects such as salt and water retention. In the Study to Prevent Non-Insulin-Dependent Diabetes Mellitus (STOP-NIDDM)[143] in patients with insulin resistance without overt DM, acarbose markedly reduced the risk of MI.

The increased pharmacological options available for glycemic control allow considerable individualization in patients with co-existing HF. There are modest reasons to avoid sulfonylureas, and TZDs must be used with appropriate caution in patients with HF. Of the more commonly used agents, metformin appears to be an excellent choice in many patients.

Selected Future Directions

Prevention of insulin resistance and type 2 diabetes and their complications, including cardiomyopathy, can be accomplished with straightforward measures such as weight loss

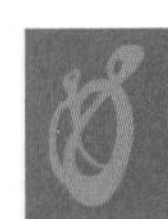

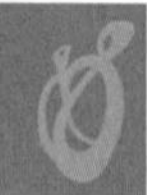

and exercise. This is especially important in young people[144] and will certainly be a major focus going forward. With respect to treatment, one of the most promising future directions is development of anti-AGE agents. One crosslink breaker, alagebrium, has undergone limited clinical trials and other agents designed to reduce formation of AGEs and/or reduce RAGE signaling are in development.[39,46,49] Reduction of ROS formation and interference with PKC signaling are other promising therapeutic targets. Last, additional studies directed toward optimization of the management of DM in patients with HF are badly needed.

REFERENCES

1. Mokdad, A. H., Ford, E. S., Bowman, B. A., et al. (2003). Prevalence of obesity, diabetes, and obesity-related health risk factors, 2001. *JAMA* (289), 76.
2. Rosamond, W., Flegal, K., Friday, G., et al. (2007). Heart disease and stroke statistics - 2007 update: a report from the American Heart Association committee and stroke statistics subcommittee. *Circulation, 115*, e69.
3. Kannel, W. B., Hjortland, M., & Castelli, W. P. (1974). Role of diabetes in congestive heart failure: the Framingham study. *Am J Cardiol, 34*, 29–34.
4. Levy, D., Larson, M. G., Vasan, R. S., et al. (1996). The progression from hypertension to congestive heart failure. *JAMA, 275*, 1557.
5. Gottdiener, J. S., Arnold, A. M., Aurigemma, G. P., et al. (2000). Predictors of congestive heart failure in the elderly: the cardiovascular health study. *J Am Coll Cardiol, 35*, 1628.
6. Nichols, G. A., Hillier, T. A., Erbey, J. R., et al. (2001). Congestive heart failure in type 2 diabetes: prevalence, incidence, and risk factors. *Diabetes Care, 24*, 1614.
7. Parker, A. B., Yusuf, S., & Naylor, C. D. (2002). The relevance of subgroup-specific treatment effects: the studies of left ventricular dysfunction (SOLVD) revisited. *Am Heart J, 144*, 941.
8. Arnold, J. M., Yusuf, S., Young, J., et al. (2003). Prevention of heart failure in patients in the heart outcomes prevention evaluation (HOPE) study. *Circulation, 107*, 1284.
9. Davis, B. R., Piller, L. B., Cutler, J. A., et al. (2006). Role of diuretics in the prevention of heart failure: the antihypertensive and lipid-lowering treatment to prevent heart attack trial. *Circulation, 113*, 2201.
10. Havranek, E. P., Masoudi, F. A., Westfall, K. A., et al. (2002). Spectrum of heart failure in older patients: results from the national heart failure project. *Am Heart J, 143*, 412–417.
11. Iribarren, C., Karter, A. J., Go, A. S., et al. (2001). Glycemic control and heart failure among adult patients with diabetes. *Circulation, 103*, 2668.
12. Held, C., Gerstein, H. C., Yusuf, S., et al. (2007). Glucose levels predict hospitalization for congestive heart failure in patients at high cardiovascular risk. *Circulation, 115*, 1371.
13. Bertoni, A. G., Tsai, A., Kasper, E. K., et al. (2003). Diabetes and idiopathic cardiomyopathy: a nationwide case-control study. *Diabetes Care, 26*, 2791.
14. Ashrafian, H., Frenneaux, M. P., & Opie, L. H. (2007). Metabolic mechanisms in heart failure. *Circulation, 116*, 434.
15. Jaffe, A. S., Spadaro, J. J., Schechtman, K., et al. (1984). Increased congestive heart failure after myocardial infarction of modest extent in patients with diabetes mellitus. *Am Heart J, 108*, 31.
16. Das, S. R., Drazner, M. H., Yancy, C. W., et al. (2004). Effects of diabetes mellitus and ischemic heart disease on the progression from asymptomatic left ventricular dysfunction to symptomatic heart failure: a retrospective analysis from the studies of left ventricular dysfunction (SOLVD) prevention trial. *Am Heart J, 148*, 883.
17. Domanski, M., Krause-Steinrauf, H., Deedwania, P., et al. (2003). The effect of diabetes on outcomes of patients with advanced heart failure in the BEST trial. *J Am Coll Cardiol, 42*, 914.
18. From, A. M., Leibson, C. L., Bursi, F., et al. (2006). Diabetes in heart failure: prevalence and impact on outcome in the population. *Am J Med, 119*, 591.
19. Hellerman, J. P., Jacobsen, S. J., Gersh, B. J., et al. (2002). Heart failure after myocardial infarction: a review. *Am J Med, 113*, 341.
20. Gustaffson, I., Brendorp, B., Seibaek, M., et al. (2004). Influence of diabetes and diabetes-gender interaction on the risk of death in patients hospitalized with congestive heart failure. *J Am Coll Cardiol, 43*, 771.
21. Pijna, I. L., & Buchter, C. (2003). Heart failure in women. *Cardiol Rev, 11*, 337.
22. Masoudi, F. A., & Inzucchi, S. E. (2006). Diabetes mellitus and heart failure: epidemiology, mechanisms, and pharmacotherapy. *Am J Cardiol, 99*(suppl 1), 113.
23. Rubler, S., Dlugash, J., Yuceoglu, Y. Z., et al. (1972). A new type of cardiomyopathy associated with diabetic glomerulosclerosis. *Am J Cardiol, 30*, 595.
24. Poormina, I. G., Parikh, P., & Shannon, R. P. (2006). Diabetic cardiomyopathy: the search for a unifying hypothesis. *Circulation, 98*, 596.
25. An, D., & Rodrigues, B. (2006). Role of changes in cardiac metabolism in development of diabetic cardiomyopathy. *Am J Physiol Heart Circ Physiol, 291*, H1489.
26. Boudina, S., & Abel, E. D. (2007). Diabetic cardiomyopathy revisited. *Circulation, 115*, 3213.
27. Nishikawa, T., Edelstein, D., Du, X. L., et al. (2000). Normalizing mitochondrial superoxide production blocks three pathways of hyperglycaemic damage. *Nature, 404*, 787.
28. Du, X., Matsumura, T., Edelstein, D., et al. (2003). Inhibition of GAPDH activity by poly(ADP-ribose)polymerase activates three major pathways of hyperglycemic damage in endothelial cells. *J Clin Invest, 112*, 1049.
29. Cai, L., Wang, Y., Zhou, G., et al. (2006). Attenuation by metallothionein of early cardiac cell death via suppression of mitochondrial oxidative stress results in a prevention of diabetic cardiomyopathy. *J Am Coll Cardiol, 48*, 1688.
30. Koya, D., & King, G. L. (1998). Protein kinase C activation and the development of diabetic complications. *Diabetes, 47*, 859.
31. Nishikawa, T., Edelstein, D., & Brownlee, M. (2000). The missing link: a single unifying mechanism for diabetic complications. *Kidney Int Suppl, 77*, S26.
32. Cai, L., & Kang, Y. J. (2001). Oxidative stress and diabetic cardiomyopathy: a brief review. *Cardiovasc Toxicol, 1*, 181.
33. Guo, M., Wu, M. H., Korompai, F., et al. (2003). Upregulation of PKC genes and isozymes in cardiovascular tissues during early stages of experimental diabetes. *Physiol Genomics, 12*, 139.
34. Cesario, D. A., Brar, R., & Shivkumar, K. (2006). Alterations in ion channel physiology in diabetic cardiomyopathy. *Endocrinol Metab Clin North Am, 35*, 601.
35. Ramamurthy, B., Höök, P., Jones, A. D., et al. (2001). Changes in myosin structure and function in response to glycation. *FASEB J, 15*, 2415.
36. Wang, J., Song, Y., Elsherif, L., et al. (2006). Cardiac metallothionein induction plays the major role in the prevention of diabetic cardiomyopathy by zinc supplementation. *Circulation, 113*, 544.
37. Shen, X., Zheng, S., Metreveli, N. S., et al. (2006). Protection of cardiac mitochondria by overexpression of MnSOD reduces diabetic cardiomyopathy. *Diabetes, 55*, 798.
38. Turko, I. V., Li, L., Akulak, K. S., et al. (2003). Protein tyrosine nitration in the mitochondria from diabetic mouse heart. Implications to dysfunctional mitochondria in diabetes. *J Biol Chem, 278*, 33972.
39. Kass, D. A. (2003). Getting better without AGE: new insights into the diabetic heart. *Circ Res, 92*, 704.
40. Aronson, D. (2003). Cross-linking of glycated collagen in the pathogenesis of arterial and myocardial stiffening of aging and diabetes. *J Hypertens, 21*, 3.
41. Thormally, P. J. (2005). Dicarbonyl intermediates in the Maillard reaction. *Ann N Y Acad Sci, 1043*, 111.
42. Li, S. Y., Du, M., Dolence, E. K., et al. (2005). Aging induces cardiac diastolic dysfunction, oxidative stress, accumulation of advanced glycation endproducts and protein modification. *Aging Cell, 4*, 57.
43. Wolffenbuttel, B. H., Boulanger, C. M., Crijns, F. R., et al. (1998). Breakers of advanced glycation end products restore large artery properties in experimental diabetes. *Proc Natl Acad Sci U S A, 95*, 4630.
44. Vaitkevicius, P. V., Lane, M., Spurgeon, H., et al. (2001). A cross-link breaker has sustained effects on arterial and ventricular properties in older rhesus monkeys. *Proc Natl Acad Sci U S A, 98*, 1171.
45. Herrmann, K. L., McCulloch, A. D., & Omens, J. H. (2002). Glycated collagen cross-linking alters cardiac mechanics in volume-overload hypertrophy. *Am J Physiol, 284*, H1277.
46. Liu, J., Masurekar, M. R., Vatner, D. E., et al. (2003). Glycation end-product cross-link breaker reduces collagen and improves cardiac function in aging diabetic heart. *Am J Physiol Heart Circ Physiol, 285*, H2587.
47. Cerami, A., Vlassara, H., & Brownlee, M. (1988). Role of advanced glycosylation products in complications of diabetes. *Diabetes Care, 11*(suppl 1), 73.
48. Huang, J. S., Guh, J. Y., Chen, H. C., et al. (2001). Role of receptor for advanced glycation end-product (RAGE) and the JAK/STAT-signaling pathway in AGE-induced collagen production in NRK-49F cells. *J Cell Biochem, 81*, 102.
49. Yan, S. F., Ramasamy, R., Naka, Y., et al. (2003). Glycation, inflammation, and RAGE: a scaffold for the macrovascular complications of diabetes and beyond. *Circ Res, 93*, 1159.
50. Naka, Y., Bucciarelli, L. G., Wendt, T., et al. (2004). RAGE axis: animal models and novel insights into the vascular complications of diabetes. *Arterioscler Thromb Vasc Biol, 24*, 1342.
51. Kim, W., Hudson, B. I., Moser, B., et al. (2005). Receptor for advanced glycation end products and its ligands: a journey from the complications of diabetes to its pathogenesis. *Ann N Y Acad Sci, 1043*, 553.
52. Petrova, R., Yamamoto, Y., Muraki, K., et al. (2002). Advanced glycation end product-induced calcium handling impairment in mouse cardiac myocytes. *J Mol Cell Cardiol, 34*, 1425.
53. Coirault, C., Guellich, A., Barbry, T., et al. (2007). Oxidative stress of myosin contributes to skeletal muscle dysfunction in rats with chronic heart failure. *Am J Physiol Heart Circ Physiol, 292*, H1009.
54. Katayama, S., Haga, Y., & Saeki, H. (2004). Loss of filament-forming ability of myosin by non-enzymatic glycosylation and its molecular mechanism. *FEBS Lett, 575*, 9.
55. Bidasee, K. R., Nallani, K., Yu, Y., et al. (2003). Chronic diabetes increases advanced glycation end products on cardiac ryanodine receptors/calcium-release channels. *Diabetes, 52*, 1825.
56. Bidasee, K. R., Zhang, Y., Shao, C. H., et al. (2004). Diabetes increases formation of advanced glycation end products on sarco(endo)plasmic reticulum Ca^{2+}-ATPase. *Diabetes, 53*, 463.
57. Monnier, V. M., Mustata, G. T., Biemel, K. L., et al. (2005). Cross-linking of the extracellular matrix by the Maillard reaction in aging and diabetes: an update on "a puzzle nearing resolution. " *Ann N Y Acad Sci, 1043*, 533.
58. Berg, T. J., Snorgaard, O., Faber, J., et al. (1999). Serum levels of advanced glycation end products are associated with left ventricular diastolic function in patients with type 1 diabetes. *Diabetes Care, 22*, 1186.
59. Candido, R., Forbes, J. M., Thomas, M. C., et al. (2003). A breaker of advanced glycation end products attenuates diabetes-induced myocardial structural changes. *Circ Res, 92*, 785.
60. Schafer, S., Huber, J., Wihler, X. C., et al. (2006). Impaired left ventricular relaxation in type 2 diabetic rats is related to myocardial accumulation of N(epsilon)-(carboxymethyl) lysine. *Eur J Heart Fail, 8*, 206.
61. Nakamura, Y., Horii, Y., Nishino, T., et al. (1993). Immunohistochemical localization of advanced glycosylation end products in coronary atheroma and cardiac tissue in diabetes mellitus. *Am J Pathol, 143*, 1649.
62. van Heerebeek, L., Hamdani, N., Handoko, M. L., et al. (2008). Diastolic stiffness of the failing diabetic heart: importance of fibrosis, advanced glycation end products, and myocyte resting tension. *Circulation, 117*, 43.
63. Lim, S. H., MacFayden, R. J., & Lip, G. Y. H. (2004). Diabetes mellitus, the renin-angiotensin-aldosterone system, and the heart. *Arch Intern Med, 164*, 1737.
64. Wieland, T., Lutz, S., & Chidiac, P. (2007). Regulators of G protein signalling: a spotlight on emerging functions in the cardiovascular system. *Curr Opin Pharmacol, 7*, 201.

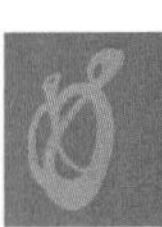

65. Liu, X., Wang, J., Takeda, N., et al. (1999). Changes in cardiac protein kinase C activities and isozymes in streptozotocin-induced diabetes. *Am J Physiol, 277*, E798.
66. Noguchi, T., Kihara, Y., Begin, K. J., et al. (2003). Altered myocardial thin-filament function in the failing Dahl salt-sensitive rat heart: amelioration by endothelin blockade. *Circulation, 107*, 630.
67. Noguchi, T., Hunlich, M., Camp, P. C., et al. (2004). Thin filament-based modulation of contractile performance in human heart failure. *Circulation, 110*, 982.
68. Braz, J. C., Gregory, K., Pathak, A., et al. (2004). PKC-alpha regulates cardiac contractility and propensity toward heart failure. *Nat Med, 10*, 248.
69. Shigekawa, M., Katanosaka, Y., & Wakabayashi, S. (2007). Regulation of the cardiac Na^+/Ca^{2+} exchanger by calcineurin and protein kinase C. *Ann N Y Acad Sci, 1099*, 53.
70. Pan, J., Singh, U. S., Takahashi, T., et al. (2005). PKC mediates cyclic stretch-induced cardiac hypertrophy through Rho family GTPases and mitogen-activated protein kinases in cardiomyocytes. *J Cell Physiol, 202*, 536.
71. Flesch, M., Margulies, K. B., Mochmann, H. C., et al. (2001). Differential regulation of mitogen-activated protein kinases in the failing human heart in response to mechanical unloading. *Circulation, 104*, 2273.
72. Young, M. E., Guthrie, P. H., Razeghi, P., et al. (2002). Impaired long-chain fatty acid oxidation and contractile dysfunction in the obese Zucker rat heart. *Diabetes, 51*, 2587.
73. Zhou, Y. T., Grayburn, P., Karim, A., et al. (2000). Lipotoxic heart disease in obese rats: implications for human obesity. *Proc Natl Acad Sci U S A, 97*, 1784.
74. Liu, G. X., Hanley, P. J., Ray, J., & Daut, J. (2001). Long-chain acyl-coenzyme A esters and fatty acids directly link metabolism to K(ATP) channels in the heart. *Circ Res, 88*, 918.
75. Finck, B. N., Han, X., Courtois, M., et al. (2003). A critical role for PPAR alpha-mediated lipotoxicity in the pathogenesis of diabetic cardiomyopathy: modulation by dietary fat content. *Proc Natl Acad Sci U S A, 100*, 1226.
76. Barouch, L. A., Berkowitz, D. E., Harrison, R. W., et al. (2003). Disruption of leptin signaling contributes to cardiac hypertrophy independently of body weight in mice. *Circulation, 108*, 754.
77. Frustaci, A., Kajstura, J., Chimenti, C., et al. (2000). Myocardial cell death in human diabetes. *Circ Res, 87*, 1123.
78. Kuethe, F., Sigusch, H. H., Bornstein, S. R., et al. (2007). Apoptosis in patients with dilated cardiomyopathy and diabetes: a feature of diabetic cardiomyopathy?*Horm Metab Res, 39*, 672.
79. Ilercil, A., Devereux, R. B., Roman, M. J., et al. (2002). Associations of insulin levels with left ventricular structure and function in American Indians: the strong heart study. *Diabetes, 51*, 1543.
80. Iacobellis, G., Ribaudo, M. C., Zappaterreno, A., et al. (2003). Relationship of insulin sensitivity and left ventricular mass in uncomplicated obesity. *Obes Res, 11*, 518.
81. Morisco, C., Condorelli, G., Trimarco, V., et al. (2005). Akt mediates the cross-talk between beta-adrenergic and insulin receptors in neonatal cardiomyocytes. *Circ Res, 96*, 180.
82. Wang, C. C., Goalstone, M. L., & Draznin, B. (2004). Molecular mechanisms of insulin resistance that impact cardiovascular biology. *Diabetes, 53*, 2735.
83. Poirier, P., Bogaty, P., Philippon, F., et al. (2003). Preclinical diabetic cardiomyopathy: relation of left ventricular diastolic dysfunction to cardiac autonomic neuropathy in men with uncomplicated well-controlled type 2 diabetes. *Metabolism, 52*, 1056.
84. Cheung, N., Wang, J. J., Rogers, S. L., et al. (2008). Diabetic retinopathy and risk of heart failure. *J Am Coll Cardiol, 51*, 1573.
85. Galderisi, M. (2006). Diastolic dysfunction and diabetic cardiomyopathy: evaluation by Doppler echocardiography. *J Am Coll Cardiol, 48*, 1548.
86. Brooks, B. A., Franjic, B., Ban, C. R., et al. (2008). Diastolic dysfunction and abnormalities of the microcirculation in type 2 diabetes. *Diabetes Obes Metab*, 10, 739–46.
87. Hansen, P. S., Clarke, R. J., Buhagiar, K. A., et al. (2007). Alloxan-induced diabetes reduces sarcolemmal Na^+-K^+ pump function in rabbit ventricular myocytes. *Am J Physiol Cell Physiol, 292*, C1070.
88. Aasum, E., Hafstad, A. D., Severson, D. L., et al. (2003). Age-dependent changes in metabolism, contractile function, and ischemic sensitivity in hearts from db/db mice. *Diabetes, 52*, 434.
89. Conti, M., Renaud, I. M., Poirier, B., et al. (2004). High levels of myocardial antioxidant defense in aging nondiabetic normotensive Zucker obese rats. *Am J Physiol Regul Integr Comp Physiol, 286*, R793.
90. Lacombe, V. A., Viatchenko-Karpinski, S., Terentyev, D., et al. (2007). Mechanisms of impaired calcium handling underlying subclinical diastolic dysfunction in diabetes. *Am J Physiol Regul Integr Comp Physiol, 293*, R1787.
91. Hattori, Y., Matsuda, N., Kimura, J., et al. (2000). Diminished function and expression of the cardiac Na+-Ca2+ exchanger in diabetic rats: implication in Ca2+ overload. *J Physiol, 527*(pt 1), 85.
92. Joffe, II, Travers, K. E., Perreault-Micale, C. L., et al. (1999). Abnormal cardiac function in the streptozotocin-induced non-insulin-dependent diabetic rat: noninvasive assessment with Doppler echocardiography and contribution of the nitric oxide pathway. *J Am Coll Cardiol, 34*, 2111.
93. Kralik, P. M., Ye, G., Metreveli, N. S., et al. (2005). Cardiomyocyte dysfunction in models of type 1 and type 2 diabetes. *Cardiovasc Toxicol, 5*, 285.
94. Belke, D. D., Swanson, E. A., & Dillmann, W. H. (2004). Decreased sarcoplasmic reticulum activity and contractility in diabetic db/db mouse heart. *Diabetes, 53*, 3201.
95. Vasanji, Z., Cantor, E. J. F., Juric, D., et al. (2006). Alterations in cardiac contractile performance and sarcoplasmic reticulum function in sucrose-fed rats is associated with insulin resistance. *Am J Physiol Cell Physiol, 291*, C772.
96. Trost, SU, Belke, DD, Bluhm, WF, et al. (2002). Overexpression of the sarcoplasmic reticulum Ca(2+)-ATPase improves myocardial contractility in diabetic cardiomyopathy. *Diabetes, 51*, 1166.
97. Mulieri, L. A., Leavitt, B. J., Hasenfuss, G., et al. (1992). Contraction frequency dependence of twitch and diastolic tension in human dilated cardiomyopathy (tension-frequency relation in cardiomyopathy). *Basic Res Cardiol, 87*(suppl 1), 199.
98. Mulieri, L. A., Hasenfuss, G., Leavitt, B., et al. (1992). Altered myocardial force-frequency relation in human heart failure. *Circulation, 85*, 1743.
99. Noguchi, T., Camp, P., Jr., Alix, S. L., et al. (2003). Myosin from failing and non-failing human ventricles exhibit similar contractile properties. *J Mol Cell Cardiol, 35*, 91.
100. LeWinter, M. M., & VanBuren, P. (2005). Sarcomeric proteins in hypertrophied and failing myocardium: an overview. *Heart Fail Rev, 10*, 173.
101. Rundell, V. L. M., Geenen, D. L., Buttrick, P. M., et al. (2004). Depressed cardiac tension cost in experimental diabetes is due to altered myosin heavy chain isoform expression. *Am J Physiol Heart Circ Physiol, 287*, H408.
102. Malhotra, A., Reich, D., Reich, D., et al. (1997). Experimental diabetes is associated with functional activation of protein kinase C epsilon and phosphorylation of troponin I in the heart, which are prevented by angiotensin II receptor blockade. *Circ Res, 81*, 1027.
103. Jweied, E. E., McKinney, R. D., Walker, L. A., et al. (2005). Depressed cardiac myofilament function in human diabetes mellitus. *Am J Physiol Heart Circ Physiol, 289*, H2478.
104. Fukagawa, N. K., Palmer, B. M., Barnes, W. D., et al. (2005). Acto-myosin crossbridge kinetics in humans with coronary artery disease: influence of sex and diabetes mellitus. *J Mol Cell Cardiol, 39*, 743.
105. Rao, V. U., & Spinale, F. G. (1999). Controlling myocardial matrix remodeling: implications for heart failure. *Cardiol Rev, 7*, 136.
106. Asbun, J., & Villareal, F. J. (2006). The pathogenesis of myocardial fibrosis in the setting of diabetic cardiomyopathy. *J Am Coll Cardiol, 47*, 693.
107. Factor, S. M., Minase, T., & Sonnenblick, E. H. (1980). Clinical and morphological features of human hypertensive-diabetic cardiomyopathy. *Am Heart J, 99*, 446.
108. van Hoeven, K. H., & Factor, S. M. (1990). A comparison of the pathological spectrum of hypertensive, diabetic, and hypertensive-diabetic heart disease. *Circulation, 82*, 848.
109. Szczepaniak, L. S., Victor, R. G., Orci, L., et al. (2007). Forgotten but not gone: the rediscovery of fatty heart, the most common unrecognized disease in America. *Circ Res, 101*, 759.
110. Piccini, J. P., Klein, L., Gheorghiade, M., et al. (2004). New insights into diastolic heart failure: role of diabetes mellitus. *Am J Med, 116*(suppl 5A), 64S.
111. Owan, T. E., Hodge, D. O., Herges, R. M., et al. (2006). Trends in prevalence and outcome of heart failure with preserved ejection fraction. *N Engl J Med, 355*, 251.
112. Diamant, M., Lamb, H. J., Groeneveld, Y., et al. (2003). Diastolic dysfunction is associated with altered myocardial metabolism in asymptomatic normotensive patients with well-controlled type 2 diabetes mellitus. *J Am Coll Cardiol, 42*, 328.
113. Kosmala, W., Kucharski, W., Przewlocka-Kosmala, M., et al. (2004). Comparison of left ventricular function by tissue Doppler imaging in patients with diabetes mellitus without systemic hypertension versus diabetes mellitus with systemic hypertension. *Am J Cardiol, 94*, 395.
114. Di Bonito, P., Moio, N., Cavuto, L., et al. (2005). Early detection of diabetic cardiomyopathy: usefulness of tissue Doppler imaging. *Diabet Med, 22*, 1720.
115. Bertoni, A. G., Goff, D. C., Jr., D'Agostino, R. B., Jr., et al. (2006). Diabetic cardiomyopathy and subclinical cardiovascular disease: the multi-ethnic study of atherosclerosis (MESA). *Diabetes Care, 29*, 588.
116. American College of Cardiology/American Heart Association Task Force on Practice Guidelines (2005). ACC/AHA 2005 guideline update for the diagnosis and management of chronic heart failure in the adult. *Circulation, 112*, e154.
117. Shekelle, P. G., Rich, M. W., Morton, S. C., et al. (2003). Efficacy of angiotensin-converting enzyme inhibitors and beta-blockers in the management of left ventricular systolic dysfunction according to race, gender, and diabetic status: a meta-analysis of major clinical trials. *J Am Coll Cardiol, 41*, 1529.
118. Masoudi, F. A., Rathore, S. S., Wang, Y., et al. (2004). National patterns of use and effectiveness of angiotensin-converting enzyme inhibitors in older patients with heart failure and left ventricular systolic dysfunction. *Circulation, 110*, 724.
119. Packer, M., Coats, A. J., Fowler, M. B., et al. (2001). Effect of carvedilol on survival in severe chronic heart failure. *N Engl J Med, 344*, 1651.
120. Pitt, B., Zannad, F., Remme, W. J., Cody, R., et al. (1999). The effect of spironolactone on morbidity and mortality in patients with severe heart failure. *N Engl J Med, 341*, 709.
121. Pitt, B., Remme, W., Zannad, F., et al. (2003). Eplerenone, a selective aldosterone blocker, in patients with left ventricular dysfunction after myocardial infarction. *N Engl J Med, 348*, 1309.
122. UK Prospective Diabetes Study Group. (1998). Effect of intensive blood-glucose control with metformin on complications in overweight patients with type 2 diabetes (UKPDS 34). *Lancet, 352*, 854.
123. Nathan, D. M., Cleary, P. A., Backlund, J. Y., et al. (2005). Intensive diabetes treatment and cardiovascular disease in patients with type 1 diabetes. *N Engl J Med, 353*, 2643.
124. The ADVANCE Collaborative Group. (2008). Intensive blood glucose control and vascular outcomes in patients with Type 2 diabetes. *N Engl J Med, 358*, 2560.
125. The Action to Control Cardiovascular Risk in Diabetes Study Group. (2008). Effects of intensive glucose lowering in Type 2 diabetes. *N Engl J Med, 358*, 2545.
126. Eshaghian, S., Horwich, T. B., & Fonarow, G. C. (2006). An unexpected inverse relationship between HbA1c levels and mortality in patients with diabetes and advanced systolic heart failure. *Am Heart J, 151*, 91.
127. Nichols, G. A., Koro, C. E., Gullion, C. M., et al. (2005). The incidence of congestive heart failure associated with antidiabetic therapies. *Diabetes Metab Res Rev, 21*, 51.
128. Smooke, S., Horwich, T. B., & Fonarow, G. C. (2005). Insulin-treated diabetes is associated with a marked increase in mortality in patients with advanced heart failure. *Am Heart J, 149*, 168.
129. McGuire, D. K., & Inzucchi, S. E. (2008). New drugs for the treatment of diabetes mellitus. Part I. Thiazolidinediones and their evolving cardiovascular implications. *Circulation, 117*, 440.
130. Inzucchi, S. E., & McGuire, D. K. (2008). New drugs for the treatment of diabetes. Part II. Incretin-based therapy and beyond. *Circulation, 117*, 574.
131. Masoudi, F. A., Inzucchi, S. E., Wang, Y., et al. (2005). Thiazolidinediones, metformin, and outcomes in older patients with diabetes and heart failure. *Circulation, 111*, 583.

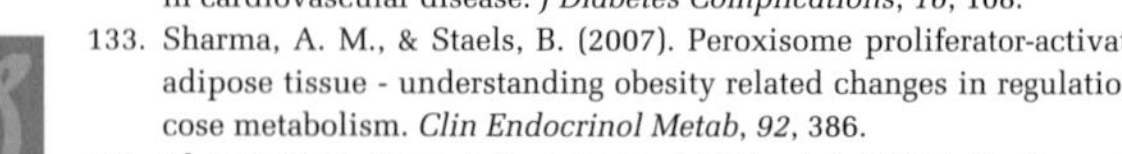

132. Takano, H., & Komuro, I. (2002). Roles of peroxisome proliferator-activated receptor γ in cardiovascular disease. *J Diabetes Complications, 16*, 108.
133. Sharma, A. M., & Staels, B. (2007). Peroxisome proliferator-activated receptor γ and adipose tissue - understanding obesity related changes in regulation of lipid and glucose metabolism. *Clin Endocrinol Metab, 92*, 386.
134. Ghazzi, M. N., Perez, J. E., Antonucci, T. K., et al. (1997). Cardiac and glycemic benefits of troglitazone treatment in NIDDM. The troglitazone study group. *Diabetes, 46*, 433.
135. St John Sutton, M., Rendell, M., et al. (2002). A comparison of the effects of rosiglitazone and glyburide on cardiovascular function and glycemic control in patients with type 2 diabetes. *Diabetes Care, 25*, 2058.
136. Tsuji, T., Mizushige, K., Noma, T., et al. (2001). Pioglitazone improves left ventricular diastolic function and decreases collagen accumulation in prediabetic stage of a type II diabetic rat. *J Cardiovasc Pharmacol, 38*, 868.
137. Dormandy, J. A., Charbonnel, B., Eckland, D. J., et al. (2005). Secondary prevention of macrovascular events in patients with type 2 diabetes in the proactive study (prospective pioglitazone clinical trial in macrovascular events): a randomised controlled trial. *Lancet, 366*, 1279.
138. Nissen, S. E., & Wolski, K. (2007). Effect of rosiglitazone on the risk of myocardial infarction and death from cardiovascular causes. *N Engl J Med, 356*, 2457.
139. Nesto, R. W., Bell, D., Bonow, R. O., et al. (2003). Thiazolidinedione use, fluid retention, and congestive heart failure: a consensus statement from the American Heart Association and American Diabetes Association. *Circulation, 108*, 2941.
140. Nikolaidis, L. A., Elahi, D., Hentosz, T., et al. (2004). Recombinant glucagon-like peptide-1 increases myocardial glucose uptake and improves left ventricular performance in conscious dogs with pacing-induced dilated cardiomyopathy. *Circulation, 110*, 955.
141. Nikolaidis, L. A., Mankad, S., Sokos, G. G., et al. (2004). Effects of glucagon-like peptide-1 in patients with acute myocardial infarction and left ventricular dysfunction after successful reperfusion. *Circulation, 109*, 962.
142. Sokos, G. G., Nikolaidis, L. A., Mankad, S., et al. (2006). Glucagon-like peptide-1 infusion improves left ventricular ejection fraction and functional status in patients with chronic heart failure. *J Card Fail, 12*, 694.
143. Chiasson, J. L., Josse, R. G., Gomis, R., et al. (2002). Acarbose for prevention of type 2 diabetes mellitus: the STOP-NIDDM randomised trial. *Lancet, 359*, 2072.
144. Mayer-Davis, E. J. (2008). Type 2 diabetes in youth: epidemiology and current research toward prevention and treatment. *J Am Diet Assoc, 108*(4 suppl. 1), S45.

CHAPTER 27

Heart Failure as a Consequence of Genetic Cardiomyopathy

Jeffrey A. Towbin and John Lynn Jefferies

Cardiomyopathies are major causes of morbidity and mortality, and over the past 20 years, limited improvements in outcome have been reported.[1] However, improvement in the understanding of the major forms of cardiomyopathy has occurred over that time, in large part due to advances in genetics and genomics.[2,3] In addition, new forms of cardiomyopathy have been described and classified over that time frame, in large part due to our improved genetic-based understanding of heart muscle disease. Further, the improved understanding gained in heart muscle disease has led to understanding of similarities and differences in heart and skeletal muscle and their often overlapping clinical presentations.

A new classification scheme was recently developed for the cardiomyopathies in which five forms of disease were formally classified as distinct forms of cardiomyopathy.[4] These forms include dilated cardiomyopathy (DCM), hypertrophic cardiomyopathy (HCM) (see Chapter 25), restrictive cardiomyopathy (RCM), arrhythmogenic right ventricular cardiomyopathy (ARVC), and left ventricular noncompaction (LVNC). These were further classified into genetic/inherited forms and acquired/noninherited forms.[4] All of these forms of disease occur in childhood and adulthood, although ARVC is almost always identified in young adults. In all forms, heart failure may be conspicuous at the time of presentation or, in many cases, late in the course of the disease.

To understand the mechanisms responsible for the development of the clinical phenotypes of cardiomyopathies and resulting heart failure, an understanding of normal cardiac structure is necessary.

NORMAL CARDIAC STRUCTURE

Cardiac muscle fibers consist of separate cellular units (myocytes) connected in series.[5] In contrast to skeletal muscle fibers, cardiac fibers do not assemble in parallel arrays but bifurcate and recombine to form a complex 3-dimensional network. Cardiac myocytes are joined at each end to adjacent myocytes at the intercalated disk, the specialized area of interdigitating cell membrane (Figure 27-1). The intercalated disk contains gap junctions (containing connexins), and mechanical junctions, consisting of adherens junctions (containing N-cadherin, catenins, and vinculin) and desmosomes (containing desmin, desmoplakin, desmocollin, desmoglein). Cardiac myocytes are surrounded by a thin membrane (sarcolemma) and the interior of each myocyte contains bundles of longitudinally arranged myofibrils. The myofibrils are formed by repeating sarcomeres, the basic contractile units of cardiac muscle consisting of interdigitating thin (actin) and thick (myosin) filaments (see Figure 27-1) that give the muscle its characteristic striated appearance.[6,7] The thick filaments are composed primarily of myosin but additionally contain myosin binding proteins C, H, and cardiac X. The thin filaments are composed of cardiac actin, α-tropomyosin (α-TM), and cardiac troponins T, I, and C (cTnT, cTnI, cTnC). In addition, myofibrils contain a third filament formed by the giant filamentous protein, titin, which extends from the Z-disk to the M-line and acts as a molecular template for the layout of the sarcomere. The Z-disk at the borders of the sarcomere is formed by a lattice of interdigitating proteins that maintain myofilament organization by crosslinking antiparallel titin and thin filaments from adjacent sarcomeres (Figure 27-2). Other proteins in the Z-disk include α-actinin, nebulette, telethonin/T-cap, capZ, MLP, myopalladin, myotilin, Cypher/Z-band alternatively spliced PDZ-motif protein (ZASP), filamin, and FATZ.[6-8]

Finally, the extrasarcomeric cytoskeleton, a complex network of proteins linking the sarcomere with the sarcolemma and the extracellular matrix (ECM), provides structural support for subcellular structures and transmits mechanical and chemical signals within and between cells. The extrasarcomeric cytoskeleton has intermyofibrillar and subsarcolemmal components, with the intermyofibrillar cytoskeleton composed of intermediate filaments (IFs), microfilaments, and microtubules.[9,10] Desmin IFs form a three-dimensional scaffold throughout the extrasarcomeric cytoskeleton with desmin filaments surrounding the Z-disk, allowing for longitudinal connections to adjacent Z-disks and lateral connections to subsarcolemmal costameres.[10] Microfilaments composed of nonsarcomeric actin (mainly γ-actin) also form complex networks linking the sarcomere (via α-actinin) to various components of the costameres. Costameres are subsarcolemmal domains located in a periodic, gridlike pattern, flanking the Z-disks and overlying the I bands along the cytoplasmic side of the sarcolemma. These costameres are sites of interconnection between various cytoskeletal networks linking sarcomere and sarcolemma and are thought to function as anchor sites for stabilization of the sarcolemma and for integration of pathways involved in mechanical force transduction. Costameres contain three principal components: the focal adhesion-type complex, the spectrin-based complex, and the dystrophin/dystrophin-associated protein complex (DAPC).[11,12] The focal adhesion-type complex, consisting of cytoplasmic

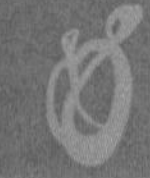

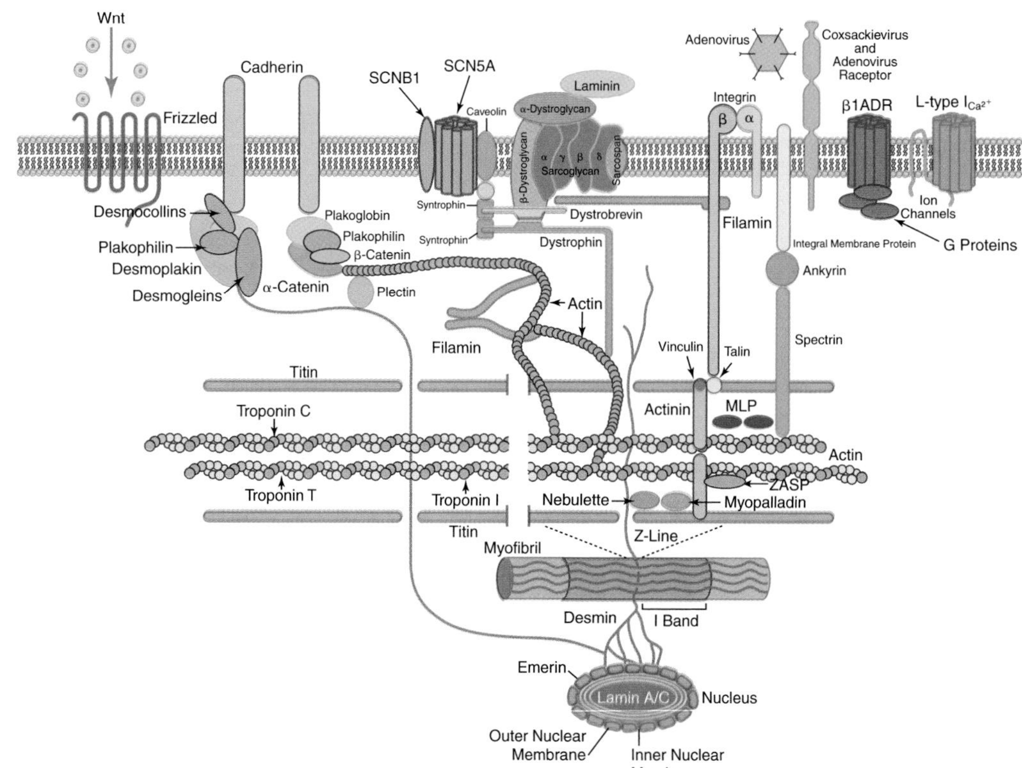

FIGURE 27–1 Cardiac myocyte cytoarchitecture. Schematic of the interactions between dystrophin and the dystrophin-associated proteins in the sarcolemma and intracellular cytoplasm (dystroglycans, sarcoglycans, syntrophins, dystrobrevin, sarcospan) at the carboxy-terminal end of the dystrophin. The integral membrane proteins interact with the extracellular matrix via α-dystroglycan-laminin α_2 connections. The amino-terminus of dystrophin binds actin and connects dystrophin with the sarcomere intracellularly, the sarcolemma, and extracellular matrix. Additional sarcolemmal proteins include ion channels, adrenergic receptors, integrins, and the Coxsackie and adenoviral receptor. Cell-cell junctions, including cadherins, the plakin, and other desmosomal family proteins are also notable. Also shown is the interaction between intermediate filament proteins (i.e., desmin) with the nucleus. *MLP,* muscle LIM protein; *β_1ADR, β*-1 adrenergic receptor; *ZASP,* Z-band alternatively spliced PDZ-motif protein.

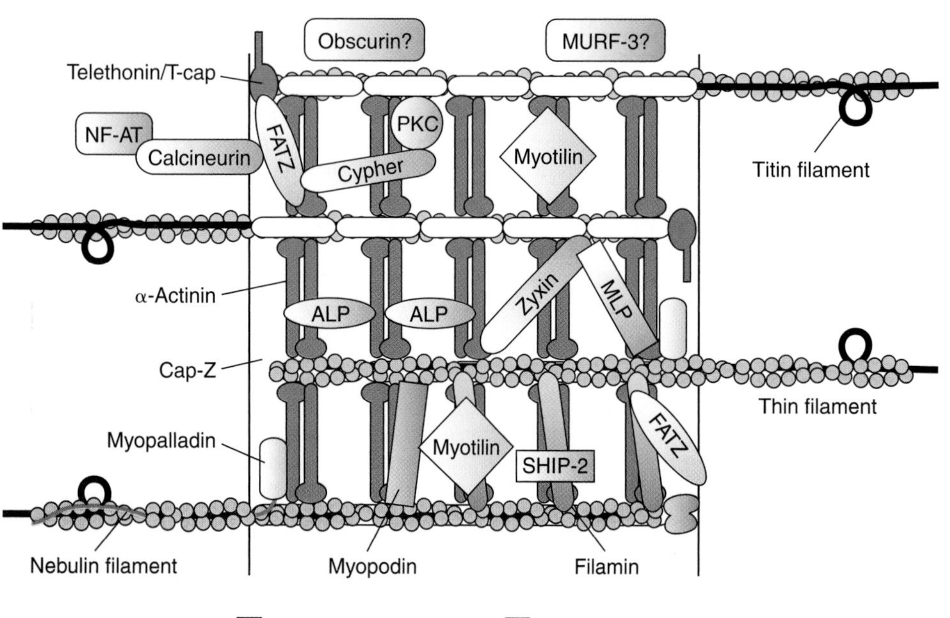

FIGURE 27–2 Z-disk architecture. The Z-disk of the sarcomere consists of multiple interacting proteins that anchor the sarcomere. (Reported with permission from Clark KA, McElhinny AS, Beckerle MC, et al. Striated muscle cytoarchitecture: an intricate web of form and function. *Annu Rev Cell Dev Biol* 2002;18:637-706.)

proteins (i.e., vinculin, talin, tensin, paxillin, zyxin), connect with cytoskeletal actin filaments and with the transmembrane proteins α-, β-dystroglycan; α-, β-, γ-, δ-sarcoglycans; dystrobrevin; and syntrophin. Several actin-associated proteins are located at sites of attachment of cytoskeletal actin filaments with costameric complexes, including α-actinin and the muscle LIM protein, MLP. The C-terminus of dystrophin binds β-dystroglycan (see Figure 27-1), which in turn interacts with α-dystroglycan to link to the ECM (via α-2-laminin). The N-terminus of dystrophin interacts with actin. Also notable, voltage gated sodium channels colocalize with dystrophin, β-spectrin, ankyrin, and syntrophins while potassium channels interact with the sarcomeric Z-disk and intercalated disks.[13,14] Since arrhythmias and conduction system diseases are common in children and adults with DCM, this could play an important role. Hence, disruption of the links from the sarcolemma to ECM at the dystrophin C-terminus and of those to the sarcomere and nucleus via N-terminal dystrophin interactions could lead to a "domino effect" disruption of systolic function and development of arrhythmias.

DILATED CARDIOMYOPATHY

Dilated cardiomyopathy (DCM) is the most common form of cardiomyopathy (see also Chapter 24). It is characterized primarily by left ventricular (LV) dilation and systolic dysfunction (Figure 27-3) with associated right ventricular (RV) dysfunction and diastolic abnormalities. In children, the annual incidence of DCM is 0.57 cases per 100,000 per year overall, but is higher in boys than in girls (0.66 vs. 0.47 cases per 100,000; $P < .001$), in blacks than in whites (0.98 vs. 0.46 cases per 100,000; $P < .001$), and in infants (<1 year) than in children (4.40 vs. 0.34 cases per 100,000; $P < .001$). The majority of children (66%) are thought to have idiopathic disease.[15] The mortality rate in the United States due to cardiomyopathy is greater than 10,000 deaths per annum, with DCM being the major contributor.[1] The total cost of health care in the United States focused on cardiomyopathies is in the billions of dollars and only limited success has been achieved. To achieve improved care and outcomes in children and adults, understanding of the causes of these disorders has been sought.

Dilated cardiomyopathy has become a popular target of research over the past 10 to 15 years, with multiple genes identified during that time period. These genes appear to encode two major subgroups of proteins, cytoskeletal and sarcomeric proteins.[2] The cytoskeletal proteins identified to date include dystrophin, desmin, lamin A/C, δ-sarcoglycan, β-sarcoglycan, and metavinculin. In the case of sarcomere-encoding genes, the same genes identified for HCM appear to be culprits, and include β-myosin heavy chain, myosin binding protein C, actin, α-tropomyosin, and cardiac troponin T. A new group of sarcomeric genes, those encoding Z-disk proteins, have also been identified and include cypher/ZASP, muscle LIM protein, and α-actinin-2.[2,3] In addition, phospholamban and G4.5/Tafazzin have also been reported. Another form of DCM, the acquired disorder viral myocarditis, has the same clinical features as DCM including heart failure, arrhythmias, and conduction block.[3] The most common causes of myocarditis are viral, including the enteroviruses (coxsackieviruses and echovirus), adenoviruses, and parvovirus B19, among other cardiotropic viruses. Evidence exists that suggests that viral myocarditis and DCM (genetic) have similar mechanisms of disease based on the proteins targeted.

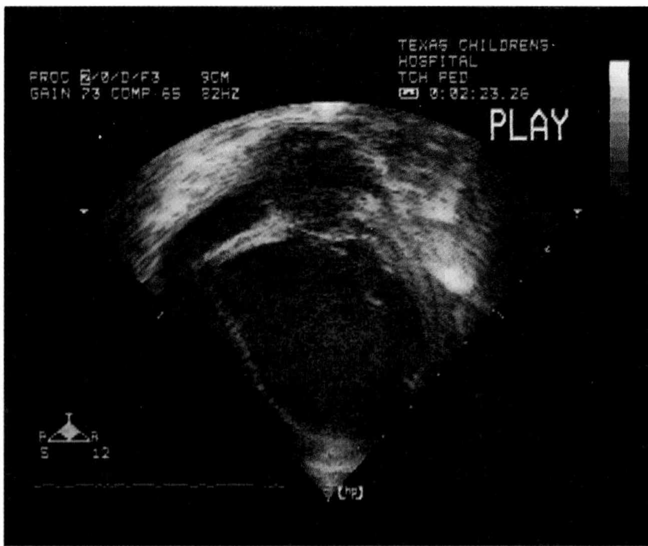

FIGURE 27–3 Echocardiography in dilated cardiomyopathy. Apical four-chamber view demonstrating a dilated left ventricle. In real-time, the systolic function is depressed.

TABLE 27–1 Dilated Cardiomyopathy (DCM) Genetics

CHR Locus	Gene	Protein
Xp21.2	*DYS*	Dystrophin
Xq28	*G4.5*	Tafazzin
1q21	*LMNA*	Lamin A/C
1q32	*TNNT2*	Cardiac troponin T
1q42-43	*ACTN*	α-Actinin-2
2q31	*TTN*	Titin
2q35	*DES*	Desmin
5q33	*SGCD*	δ-Sarcoglycan
6q22.1	*PLN*	Phospholamban
10q22.3-23.2	*ZASP/Cypher*	ZASP
10q22-q23	*VCL*	Metavinculin
11p11	*MYBPC3*	Myosin-binding protein-C
11p15.1	*MLP*	Muscle LIM protein
14q12	*MYH7*	β-Myosin heavy chain
15q14	*ACTC*	Cardiac actin
15q22	*TPM1*	α-Tropomyosin

Clinical Genetics of Dilated Cardiomyopathy

Dilated cardiomyopathy was initially believed to be inherited in a small percentage of cases until Michels et al showed that approximately 20% of probands had family members with echocardiographic evidence of DCM when family screening was performed.[16] More recently, inherited, familial DCM (FDCM) has been shown to occur in 30% to 40% of cases with autosomal dominant inheritance being the predominant pattern of transmission; X-linked, autosomal recessive, and mitochondrial inheritance is less common.[2]

Molecular Genetics of Dilated Cardiomyopathy

Over the past decade, progress has been made in the understanding of the genetic cause of FDCM (Table 27-1). Initial progress was made studying families with X-linked forms of DCM, with the autosomal dominant forms of DCM beginning to unravel over the past few years. In the case of X-linked forms of DCM, two disorders have been well characterized, X-linked cardiomyopathy (XLCM), which presents in adolescence and young adults, and Barth syndrome, which is most frequently identified in infancy.[17,18]

X-LINKED CARDIOMYOPATHIES

X-Linked Dilated Cardiomyopathy (XLCM)

First described in 1987 by Berko and Swift as DCM occurring in males in the teen years and early 20s with rapid progression from CHF to death due to ventricular tachycardia/

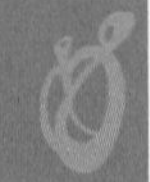

ventricular fibrillation (VT/VF) or transplantation, these patients are distinguished by elevated serum creatine kinase muscle isoforms (CK-MM).[17] Female carriers tend to develop mild to moderate DCM in the fifth decade and the disease is slowly progressive. Towbin et al were the first to identify the disease-causing gene and characterize the functional defect.[19] In this report, the dystrophin gene was shown to be responsible for the clinical abnormalities and protein analysis by immuno-blotting demonstrated severe reduction or absence of dystrophin protein in the heart of these patients. These findings were later confirmed by Muntoni et al when a mutation in the muscle promoter and exon 1 of dystrophin was identified in another family with XLCM.[20] Subsequently, multiple mutations have been identified in dystrophin in patients with XLCM.

Dystrophin is a cytoskeletal protein that provides structural support to the myocyte by creating a latticelike network to the sarcolemma. In addition, dystrophin plays a major role in linking the sarcomeric contractile apparatus to the sarcolemma and extracellular matrix.[21,22] Furthermore, dystrophin is involved in cell signaling, particularly through its interactions with nitric oxide synthase. The dystrophin gene is responsible for Duchenne and Becker muscular dystrophy (DMD/BMD) when mutated as well.[23] These skeletal myopathies present early in life (DMD is diagnosed before age 12 years while BMD is seen in teenage males older than 16 years of age) and the vast majority of patients develop DCM before their twenty-fifth birthday. In most patients, CK-MM is elevated similar to that seen in XLCM; in addition, manifesting female carriers develop disease late in life, similar to XLCM. Furthermore, immunohistochemical analysis demonstrates reduced levels (or absence) of dystrophin, similar to that seen in the hearts of patients with XLCM.

Murine models of dystrophin deficiency demonstrate abnormalities of muscle physiology based on membrane structural support abnormalities.[24] In addition to the dysfunction of dystrophin, mutations in dystrophin secondarily affect proteins that interact with dystrophin. At the amino-terminus (N-terminus), dystrophin binds to the sarcomeric protein actin, a member of the thin filament of the contractile apparatus. At the carboxy-terminus (C-terminus), dystrophin interacts with α-dystroglycan, a dystrophin-associated membrane-bound protein, which is involved in the function of the dystrophin-associated protein complex (DAPC), which includes β-dystroglycan, the sarcoglycan subcomplex (α-, β-, γ-, δ-, and ε-sarcoglycan), syntrophins, and dystrobrevins (see Figure 27-1).[25] In turn, this complex interacts with α_2-laminin and the extracellular matrix.[26] Like dystrophin, mutations in these genes lead to muscular dystrophies with or without cardiomyopathy, supporting the contention that this group of proteins are important to the normal function of the myocytes of the heart and skeletal muscles.[26] In both cases, mechanical stress appears to play a significant role in the age-onset dependent dysfunction of these muscles.[24] The information gained from the studies on XLCM, DMD, and BMD, led us to hypothesize that DCM is a disease of the cytoskeleton/sarcolemma, which affects the sarcomere, a "final common pathway" of DCM.[27,28] We also have suggested that dystrophin mutations play a role in idiopathic DCM in males. This is supported when we showed that 3 of 22 boys with DCM had dystrophin mutations and all were later found to have elevated CK-MM as well.[29] In addition, eight families with DCM and possible X-linked inheritance were also screened, and in three of eight families, dystrophin mutations were noted. Again, CK-MM was elevated in all subjects carrying mutations.[30]

Barth Syndrome

Initially described as X-linked cardioskeletal myopathy with abnormal mitochondria and neutropenia by Neustein et al and Barth et al, this disorder typically presents in male infants as CHF associated with neutropenia (cyclic) and 3-methylglutaconic aciduria.[31,32] Mitochondrial dysfunction is noted on EM and electron transport chain biochemical analysis. Recently, abnormalities in cardiolipin have been noted.[33] Echocardiographically these infants typically have LV dysfunction with LV dilation, endocardial fibroelastosis, or a dilated hypertrophic left ventricle. In some cases these infants succumb due to CHF/sudden death VT/VF, or sepsis due to leukocyte dysfunction. The majority of these children survive infancy and do well clinically, although DCM usually persists. In some cases, cardiac transplantation has been performed. Histopathological evaluation typically demonstrates the features of DCM, although endocardial fibroelastosis may be prominent and the mitochondria are abnormal in shape and abundance.

The genetic basis of Barth syndrome was first described by Bione et al who cloned the disease-causing gene, *G4.5*.[34] This gene encodes a novel protein called tafazzin, whose gene product is an acyltransferase and results in cardiolipin abnormalities.[33] Mutations in *G4.5* result in a wide clinical spectrum, which includes apparent classic DCM, hypertrophic DCM, endocardial fibroelastosis (EFE), or LVNC.[2,35]

Autosomal Dominant Dilated Cardiomyopathy

The most common form of inherited DCM is the autosomal dominant form of disease.[3] These patients present as classic "pure" DCM or DCM associated with conduction system disease (CDDC). In the latter case, patients usually present in the third decade of life with mild conduction system disease, which can progress to complete heart block over decades. DCM usually presents late in the course but is out-of-proportion to the degree of conduction system disease.[36] The echocardiographic and histological findings in both subgroups are classic for DCM, although the conduction system may be fibrotic in patients with CDDC. In both groups of DCM patients, VT, VF, and TdP occur and may result in sudden death.

Genetic heterogeneity exists for autosomal dominant DCM with more than 15 loci mapped for pure DCM and five loci for CDDC. In the case of pure DCM, 10 genes have been identified to date, including three by our group (δ-sarcoglycan, α-actinin-2, ZASP), and actin, desmin, troponin T, β-myosin heavy chain, titin, metavinculin, myosin binding protein C, α-tropomyosin, muscle LIM protein (MLP), β-sarcoglycan, and phospholamban (see Table 27-1).[2,37-39]

The majority of genes identified to date encode either cytoskeletal or sarcomeric proteins. In the case of cytoskeletal proteins (desmin, δ-sarcoglycan, metavinculin, MLP), defects of force transmission are considered to result in the DCM phenotype, while defects of force generation have been speculated to cause sarcomeric protein-induced DCM.[27]

Cardiac actin is a sarcomeric protein that is a member of the sarcomeric thin filament interacting with tropomyosin and the troponin complex. As previously noted, actin plays a significant role in linking the sarcomere to the sarcolemma via its binding to the N-terminus of dystrophin and the mutations in actin, which resulted in DCM as described by Olson et al appear to be directly involved in the binding of dystrophin.[40] The DCM-causing mutations are believed to result by causing force transmission abnormalities. Further, actin interacts in the sarcomere with TnT and β-MHc, two other genes resulting in either DCM or HCM depending on the position of the mutation.[41] In the case of TnT and β-MHC, force generation abnormalities have been speculated as the responsible mechanism.

Desmin is a cytoskeletal protein that forms intermediate filaments specific for muscle.[10] This muscle-specific 53 kDa subunit of class III intermediate filaments forms connections between the nuclear and plasma membranes of cardiac, skeletal, and smooth muscle. Desmin is found at the Z lines and the intercalated disks of muscle and its role in muscle

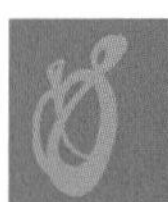

function appears to involve attachment or stabilization of the sarcomere. Mutations in this gene appear to cause abnormalities of force and signal transmission similar to that believed to occur with actin mutations.[42]

Another DCM-causing gene, δ-sarcoglycan, is a member of the sarcoglycan subcomplex of the DAPC.[37] This gene encodes for a protein involved in stabilization of the myocyte sarcolemma and signal transduction. Mutations identified in familial and sporadic cases resulted in reduction of the protein within the myocardium. In the absence of δ-sarcoglycan, the remaining sarcoglycans (δ, β, γ, Σ) cannot assemble properly in the endoplasmic reticulum.[43] Mouse models of δ-sarcoglycan deficiency demonstrate dilated, hypertrophic cardiomyopathy, sarcolemmal fragility, and disrupted vasculin smooth muscle, which leads to vascular spasm, including coronary spasm.[44] Other human mutations in δ-sarcoglycan cause a form of autosomal recessive limb girdle muscular dystrophy (LGMD2F), which rarely is associated with heart disease.

The final cytoskeletal protein-encoding gene, metavinculin, encodes vinculin and its splice variant metavinculin. Vinculin is ubiquitously expressed and metavinculin is coexpressed with vinculin in heart, skeletal, and smooth muscle, with this protein complex localized to subsarcolemmal costameres in the heart where they are localized to subsarcolemmal costameres in the heart where they interact with α-actinin, talin, and γ-actin to form a microfilamentous network linking the cytoskeleton and the sarcolemma. In addition, these proteins are present in adherens junctions in intercalated disks and participate in cell-cell adhesion. Mutations in metavinculin has been shown to disrupt the intercalated disks and alter actin filament cross-linking.[45,46]

Mutations in the sarcomere may produce hypertrophic cardiomyopathy or dilated cardiomyopathy. In the latter case, abnormalities in force generation or transmission are thought to contribute to the development of this phenotype.[41] In addition to mutations in the thin filament protein actin, mutations in the thick filament protein-encoding gene β-myosin heavy chain has been shown to cause DCM with associated sudden death in at least one infant, and DCM in older children and adults.[41,47] Mutations in this gene are thought to perturb the actin-myosin interaction and force generation or alter cross-bridge movement during contraction. Mutations in cardiac troponin T, a thin filament protein, have been speculated to disrupt calcium-sensitive troponin C binding.[47] Mutations in phospholamban have also been identified, which further support calcium handling as a potentially important mechanism in the development of DCM.[48,49] Interestingly, Haghihi et al identified homozygous mutations causing dilated cardiomyopathy and heart failure, while heterozygotes had cardiac hypertrophy.[49] Recessive mutation in troponin I is thought to impair the interaction with troponin T, while α-tropomyosin mutations have also been identified and were predicted to alter the surface charge of the protein leading to impaired interaction with actin.[50]

A recent area of interest for evaluation at the molecular level is the Z disk.[51] Knoll et al identified mutations in muscle LIM protein (MLP) and demonstrated that this results in defects in the interaction with telethonin.[52] Using mouse models, they also demonstrated that MLP acts as a stretch sensor and that mutant MLP causes defects in this activity. More recently, mutations in MLP in families and sporadic cases were described and, in addition, abnormalities in the T-tubule system and Z disk architecture by electron microscopy was identified, which correlates with the histopathology seen in MLP-knockout mice.[53] This was further supported by the finding of reduced expression of MLP in chronic human heart failure.[54] In addition, mutations in α-actinin-2, which is involved in cross-linking actin filaments and shares a common actin binding domain with dystrophin, were also identified in familial DCM, which disrupts its binding to MLP.[3] Vatta et al identified mutations in the Z-band alternatively spliced PDZ-motif protein ZASP, the human homolog of the mouse cypher gene, which when disrupted leads to DCM.[55] Multiple mutations in this gene were identified in families and sporadic cases of DCM and with LV noncompaction. This protein, which interacts with α-actinin-2, disrupts the actin cytoskeleton when mutated. Another gene, titin, which encodes the giant sarcomeric cytoskeletal protein titin that contributes to the maintenance of the sarcomere organization and myofibrillar elasticity, interacts with these proteins at the Z disk/I band transition zone.[56] Mutations have been identified in familial DCM as well.[57]

As seen in pure autosomal dominant DCM, genetic heterogeneity also exists for CDDC. To date, CDDC genes have been mapped to chromosomes 1p1-1q1, 2q14-21, 3p25-22, and 6q23. The only gene thus far identified was reported to be lamin A/C on chromosome 1q21, which encodes a nuclear envelope intermediate filament protein.[58,59]

Lamin A/C

The lamins are located in the nuclear lamina at the nucleoplasmic side of the inner nuclear membrane, and lamin A and C are expressed in heart and skeletal muscle.[60] Mutations in this gene were initially reported to cause the autosomal dominant form of Emery-Dreifuss muscular dystrophy, which has skeletal myopathy associated with DCM and conduction system disease.[61,62] It has also been found to cause a form of autosomal dominant limb girdle muscular dystrophy (LGMD1B), which is also associated with conduction system disease.[63] Multiple mutations have been identified in patients with DCM and conduction system disease which, in some cases, had mildly elevated CK. This gene defect appears to be relatively common in patients with CDDC. The mechanism(s) responsible for the development of DCM and conduction system abnormalities and skeletal myopathy are being determined.[64] Comprehending may be aided by understanding how other genes that encode interacting proteins result in disease, such as thymopoietin.[65]

Muscle Is Muscle: Cardiomyopathy and Skeletal Myopathy Genes Overlap

Interestingly, nearly all of the genes identified for inherited DCM are also known to cause skeletal myopathy in humans and/or mouse models. In the case of dystrophin, mutations cause Duchenne and Becker muscular dystrophy while δ-sarcoglycan mutations cause limb girdle muscular dystrophy (LGMD2F). Lamin A/C has been shown to cause autosomal dominant Emery-Dreifuss muscular dystrophy (EDMD) and LGMD1B, whereas actin mutations are associated with nemaline myopathy. Desmin, G4.5, α-dystrobrevin, Cypher/ZASP, MLP, α-actinin-2, titin, β-sarcoglycan mutations also have associated skeletal myopathy suggesting that cardiac and skeletal muscle function is interrelated and that possibly the skeletal muscle fatigue seen in patients with DCM with and without CHF may be due to primary skeletal muscle disease and not only related to the cardiac dysfunction. It also suggests that the function of these muscles has a "final common pathway" and that both cardiologists and neurologists should consider evaluation of both sets of muscles.

Further support for this concept comes from studies of animal models. Mutations in δ-sarcoglycan in hamsters results in cardiomyopathy while mutations in all sarcoglycan subcomplex genes in mice cause skeletal and cardiac muscle disease. Mutations in other DAPC genes and dystrophin in murine models also consistently demonstrate abnormalities of skeletal and cardiac muscle function. Arber et al also produced a mouse deficient in muscle LIM protein (MLP), a structural protein that links the actin cytoskeleton to the contractile apparatus.[53] The resultant mice develop severe DCM, CHF, and disruption of cardiac myocyte cytoskeletal architecture. Murine mutations in titin, cypher, α-dystrobrevin, desmin,

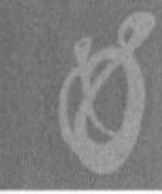

and other all demonstrate cardiac and skeletal muscle disease. Finally, Badorff et al has shown that the DCM that develops after viral myocarditis has a mechanism similar to the inherited forms.[66] Using coxsackievirus B3 (CVB3) infection of mice, the authors showed that the CVB3 genome encodes for a protease (enteroviral protease 2A), which cleaves dystrophin at the third hinge region of dystrophin, resulting in force transmission abnormalities and DCM. In addition, Xiong et al showed that abnormal dystrophin increases susceptibility to viral infection and resultant myocarditis.[67] Interestingly, a similar dystrophin mutation, which affects the first hinge region of dystrophin in patients with XLCM, was previously reported by our laboratory, demonstrating a consistent mechanism of DCM development, abnormalities of the cytoskeleton/sarcolemma, and sarcomere. In addition, we have shown that N-terminal dystrophin is reduced or absent in hearts of patients with all forms of DCM (ischemic, acquired, genetic, idiopathic) and that reduction of mechanical stress by use of left ventricular assist devices (LVADs) results in reverse remodeling of dystrophin and of the heart itself.[68]

HYPERTROPHIC CARDIOMYOPATHY

Hypertrophic cardiomyopathy (HCM) is characterized by ventricular hypertrophy predominantly affecting the left ventricle. Most commonly, the clinical phenotype includes asymmetrical septal hypertrophy and hypercontractile systolic function in the face of diastolic dysfunction. This "stiff" appearing heart occasionally develops dilated atria due to restrictive physiology. In some patients, the left ventricle has concentric hypertrophy. Left ventricular outflow tract obstruction (LVOTO) and arrhythmias are variable findings. While heart failure due to diastolic dysfunction or to a "burned out" form in which systolic dysfunction develops, the most well-known clinical feature of HCM is its propensity for sudden cardiac death.

The genetics of HCM is most commonly associated with autosomal dominant inheritance and approximately 70% of subjects can be found to have mutations in sarcomere-encoding genes. This is covered in detail in Chapter 25. Other forms of inheritance, such as X-linked, mitochondrial, or autosomal recessive are also seen, most commonly in childhood and the causes differ from the classic form of sarcomeric disease. Some of these other forms of "inappropriate" LV hypertrophy are described later.

Infiltrative Forms of Hypertrophic Cardiomyopathy

A variety of disorders that have apparent LV hypertrophy and features of hypertrophic cardiomyopathy occur due to infiltrative disorders. The classic form of infiltrative disease in this category is Pompe disease, a disorder typically presenting in the first weeks of life.[69] More recently, other forms of infiltrative disease have been identified with later onset disease, such as Fabry disease, Danon disease, and LV hypertrophy due to mutations in AMP-activated protein kinase (AMP-K) encoded by the PRKAG2 gene.[70-73] These disorders, along with those caused by mitochondrial abnormalities and genetic dysmorphism syndromes, such as Noonan syndrome and LEOPARD syndrome, are caused by abnormalities not primarily affecting the sarcomere.[93] Therapy is similar to the sarcomeric form of the disease, unless systolic dysfunction occurs. In this case, heart failure therapy should be instituted.

Pompe Disease (Type II Glycogen Storage Disease)

Genetic deficiency of acid α-1,4 glucosidase, an enzyme involved in the breakdown of glycogen to glucose, results in a wide clinical spectrum ranging from the rapidly fatal infantile onset of type II glycogen storage disease (GSD) to a slowly progressive adult-onset myopathy. The infantile-onset form (Pompe disease) typically manifests during the first 5 months of life, and patients usually die before their second year.[69] This rare inborn error of glycogen metabolism occurs in less than 1 per 100,000 births. Massive glycogen accumulation occurs, leading to the clinical findings of enlarged tongue, striking hepatomegaly, hypotonia with decreased deep tendon reflexes, and cardiomyopathy (usually HCM) with congestive heart failure. The glycogen accumulation can be noted histologically in the skeletal muscles, liver, and heart. Children usually succumb in the first 2 years of life. The diagnosis may be predicted from the pathognomonic electrocardiogram (ECG).[19] The disease has autosomal recessive inheritance; the gene coding for the lysosomal enzyme was originally mapped to chromosome 17 at subband 17q23-q25.[74]

Allelic variation at the acid α-glucosidase locus is presumed to be the most important factor in diversity of type II GSD.[75] It has been shown that various combinations of homoallelic and heteroallelic mutant genotypes are the basis for this clinical heterogeneity. Zhong et al identified a missense mutation in one allele of a patient with Pompe disease.[76] This base pair substitution resulted in a loss of restriction endonuclease sites, which allowed them to demonstrate mRNA expression deficiency from the second allele using polymerase chain reaction (PCR)-amplified RNA. This was the first evidence of single base pair missense mutations in patients with this disease. In addition to molecular analysis, the diagnosis can be made biochemically by analysis of α-glucosidase in blood lymphocytes or skin fibroblasts. Prenatal diagnosis is possible by amniocentesis or chorionic villus sampling by assay of α-glucosidase. Enzyme therapy is now possible and appears to reverse the cardiac phenotype.[77]

Fabry Disease

An X-linked recessive disorder with mild expression occasionally seen in carrier females, this entity is caused by deficiency of the enzyme α-galactosidase (α-Gal) and is found in 1 of 40,000 people. Young adults may be prone to renal failure and myocardial infarctions. Fabry disease usually has its onset in adolescence and usually manifests with sensations of burning pain in the hands and feet.[78] These sensations tend to be associated with fever, heart, cold, and exercise. With increasing age, multiple angiokeratoma become noticeable, especially around the umbilicus and genitalia. Corneal opacities are often noted. Progressive renal failure develops with age. CNS manifestations include seizures and headaches, and hemiplegia associated with an increased risk of stroke. Primary cardiac manifestations in affected males are hypertrophic cardiomyopathy and mitral insufficiency and the diagnosis depends on echocardiography.[79] The LV myocardium and mitral valve tend to be areas of greatest storage of lipid material. On electrocardiogram, the PR interval is usually short. Deposition of sphingolipids in the coronary arteries leads to myocardial ischemia and infarction.[80]

The disease-causing gene was originally localized to the long arm of the X chromosome in the Xq22 region, and the full-length cDNA was isolated and sequenced, demonstrating a 1393-bp cDNA with a 60-nucleotide 5′ untranslated region, and encoding a precursor peptide of 429 amino acids.[81] The gene was found to contain seven exons; mutations and phenotypic correlation have been described.[82]

Nakao et al studied 1603 men by echocardiography and demonstrated significant LVH in 230 subjects (14%) of which 7 (3%) had proven α-Gal deficiency.[83] These patients had concentric LVH. More recently, Sachdev et al identified five patients with HCM diagnosed after age 40 years and one with earlier-onset (younger than 40 years) HCM, all with low α-Gal activity.[84] In five of the six patients, the hypertrophy was concentric, while one had asymmetrical hypertrophy. In one case, LV outflow tract obstruction was noted. Nonsustained ventricular tachycardia occurred in two patients and another patient had 2-degree AV block initially and then atrial fibrillation. Therefore, it appears that these abnormalities in α-Gal activity result in some cases of HCM or "unexplained" LVH. Enzyme replacement therapy may have a role in the treatment of Fabry disease with optimal results being seen with institution of therapy before evidence of myocardial fibrosis.[85]

Danon Disease

Danon disease is an X-linked dominant disorder characterized by intracytoplasmic vacuoles containing autophagic material and glycogen in cardiac and skeletal muscle cells, cardiomyopathy, and skeletal myopathy, with or without conduction defect, Wolff-Parkinson-White syndrome, or mental retardation.[86] The underlying abnormality affects lysosomal function and is due to mutations in the lysosomal associated membrane protein 2 (LAMP2) and the biopsy demonstrates vacuolization (Figure 27-4).[87] The clinical phenotypic expression of Danon disease is variable. Charron et al screened 50 cases of HCM for LAMP2 mutations and identified mutations in two patients with HCM and skeletal myopathy.[88] Both of these individuals presented during their teenage years and other younger affected individuals in the family were also identified as young as 7 years of age. Wolff-Parkinson-White syndrome and high voltage QRS complexes on electrocardiogram were notable along with high creatine kinase plasma levels. In addition, late LV dilation and dysfunction occurred with symptoms of heart failure. Atrial and ventricular arrhythmias and conduction disease was notable along with death during their 20s. Visual acuity abnormality was also common because of choriocapillary ocular atrophy. This disease appears to be underrecognized and may play a significant role in pediatric heart failure.

AMP-Activated Protein Kinase (AMP-K)

AMP-activated protein kinase (AMP-K), encoded by the γ-2 regulatory subunit of the *PRKAG2* gene on chromosome 7q31, is an enzyme that modulates glucose uptake and glycolysis.[89] Dominant mutations in this gene were first identified by Gollob et al and Blair et al in 2001 in subjects with hypertrophic cardiomyopathy, Wolff-Parkinson-White (WPW) preexcitation, and atrioventricular block.[90,91] The genetic locus on chromosome 7q3 was first described by MacRae et al in 1995 in families with HCM and WPW and was felt to be clinically different than the patients with other forms of adult HCM.[101] Blair et al[113] made the case that mutations in AMP-K resulted in HCM due to compromise of energy production and use, but Arad et al provided evidence that this disorder is a form of glycogen-storage disease.[73] Cardiac pathology differed from other forms of HCM, with no myocyte and myofibrillar disarray seen but instead pronounced formation of vacuoles, which were filled with glycogen-associated granules. The myocytes were enlarged and interstitial fibrosis was minimal. Using a yeast system in which a similar enzyme is functional, Arad et al introduced the same mutations found in the patients and showed that the enzyme activity is persistent (i.e., does not turn off), leading to glycogen accumulation. The authors confirmed these findings by developing a murine model that mimics the human disorder.[92]

ENERGY-DEPENDENT FORMS OF HYPERTROPHIC CARDIOMYOPATHY

Mitochondrial Cardiomyopathies

The human mitochondrial genome is a small, circular DNA molecule that is maternally inherited.[93] Mitochondrial DNA (mtDNA) encodes 13 of the 69 proteins required for oxidative metabolism, 22 transfer RNAs (tRNAs) and 2 ribosomal RNAs (rRNAs) required for their translation (Figure 27-5). Because mtDNA has much less redundancy than the nuclear genome (in which essentially identical information is received from both parents), and tRNAs and rRNAs are present in multiple copies, the mitochondrial genome is an excellent target for mutations giving rise to human disease.[94] Mitochondria enjoy a symbiotic relationship with the cell. These subcellular organelles are dependent on nucleocytoplasmic mechanisms for most structural components, but do contribute vital peptides that are central to cellular respiration. Mitochondria contain a permeable outer membrane and a highly restrictive inner membrane that guards the chemical microenvironment of the matrix compartment. Adaptive mechanisms exist for the passage of large and small molecules across the inner membrane. Translocases shuttle monocarboxylic acids, amino acids, acylcarnitine conjugates, small ions, and other metabolites in and out of the mitochondrial matrix. Energy is required for importation of proteins into the mitochondria because the nuclear gene–synthesized mitochondrial proteins are precursor molecules that require presequence cleavage. The 13 mtDNA genes

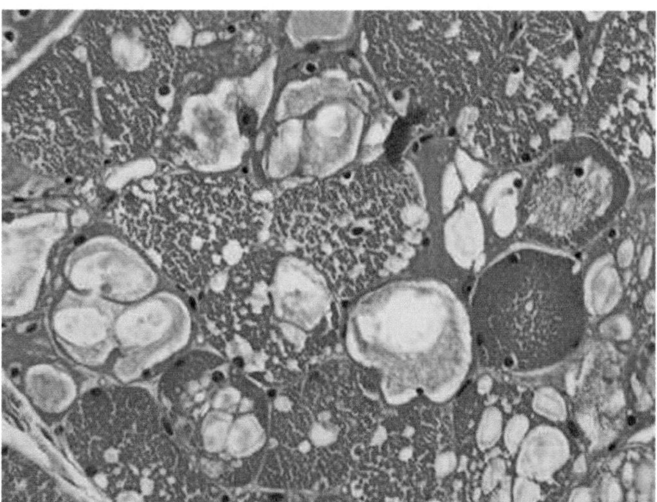

FIGURE 27–4 LAMP-2 deficiency cardiomyopathy. LAMP-2 deficiency is an X-linked lysosomal storage disorder causing cardiomyopathy and skeletal myopathy. Biopsies commonly demonstrate the vacuoles notable in this specimen.

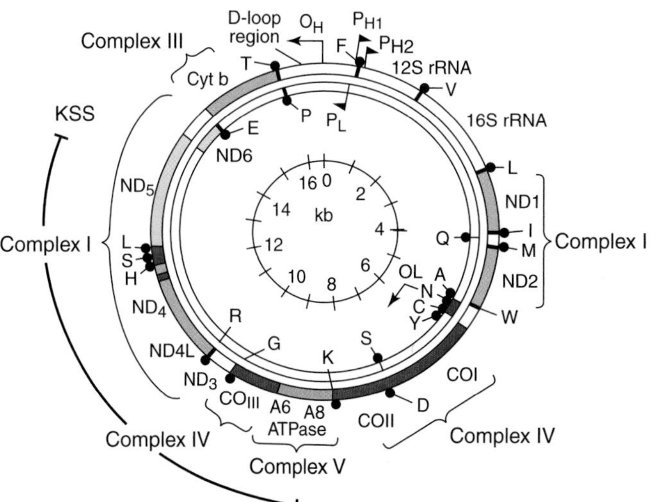

FIGURE 27–5 Mitochondrial (mtDNA) genome. Circular mtDNA encoding proteins of the mitochondria, including a portion of the proteins of the electron transport chain.

are located in the respiratory chain (Figure 27-6) and include seven complex I subunits (ND1, 2, 3, 4L, 4, 5, and 6); one complex III subunit (cytochrome b); three complex IV subunits (COI, II, III); and two complex V subunits (ATPase 6 and 8).[95] Coordination must exist between nuclear and mitochondrial genomes to permit assembly of the complex holoenzymes. Each cell contains numerous mitochondria and each mitochondrion contains multiple copies of mtDNA. This genetic material derives exclusively from the female gamete and any mutation must be passed from female parent to all progeny, male and female. The replicative segregation of mutant mtDNA copies within the cell determines whether this biological disadvantage is expressed. In most mitochondrial disorders, patients carry a mix of mutant and normal mitochondria, a condition known as heteroplasmy, with the proportions varying from tissue-to-tissue and individual-to-individual within a pedigree in a manner correlating with severity of phenotype.[94]

Mitochondrial diseases often produce disturbances of brain and muscle function, presumably because these two organs are so metabolically active, and therefore the metabolic demand is high during growth and development.[96] Cardiac disease is most commonly seen with respiratory chain defects.[97] Ragged red fibers are present in muscle biopsy specimens almost invariably when the molecular defect involves mtDNA (except in infants).[98] These defects represent the genetics of ATP production. The diverse clinical syndromes associated with various respiratory chain complexes are thought to result from involvement of tissue-nonspecific (generalized) subunits in other cases and the residual enzyme activity in affected tissues.[99] The cardiac diseases associated with mitochondrial defects include both hypertrophic cardiomyopathy and dilated cardiomyopathy, and LV noncompaction.[182,183] No theory has thus far been advanced to explain the cause of these phenotypically different cardiac abnormalities. It is possible, however, that the dilated form occurs after an initial hypertrophic response (i.e., it is a "burned-out" dilated form of HCM).

Kearns-Sayre Syndrome

This mitochondrial myopathy is characterized by ptosis, chronic progressive external ophthalmoplegia, abnormal retinal pigmentation, cardiac conduction defects, and DCM. Channer et al reported a case of rapidly developing progressive congestive heart failure and DCM requiring transplantation in a patient with Kearns-Sayre syndrome.[100] Approximately 20% of Kearns-Sayre syndrome patients have cardiac involvement and the majority usually have conduction defects causing progressive heart block. These patients generally have large, heterogeneous deletions in the mitochondrial chromosome. Poulton et al showed germ line deletions of mtDNA in a family with Kearns-Sayre syndrome using polymerase chain reaction (PCR) to amplify across the deletion, with primers flanking these deletions.[101] The patient was shown to have a deletion in muscle mtDNA and at low levels in blood that was identical to that found in the mother and sister. The probands, however, had more deleted DNA, correlating with more severe symptomatology. Other mutations have also been described.[102]

MERRF Syndrome

This syndrome is characterized by myoclonic epilepsy with ragged red muscle fibers (MERRF) and is caused by a single nucleotide substitution in tRNA LYS that apparently interferes with mitochondrial translation.[103] Shoffner et al showed an A to G transition mutation as the cause of the disease associated with defects in complexes I and IV.[104] This abnormality causes decline in ATP-generating capacity, with onset of disease that includes cardiomyopathy. Other reports outline various disease-causing mutations.[105]

OVERLAP DISORDERS

Left Ventricular Noncompaction

This disorder has previously been considered to be a rare disease and has been identified by a variety of names including spongy myocardium, fetal myocardium, and noncompaction of the LV myocardium.[106,107] The abnormality is believed to represent an arrest in the normal process of myocardial compaction, the final stage of myocardial morphogenesis, resulting in persistence of multiple prominent ventricular trabeculations and deep intertrabecular recesses (Figure 27-7).

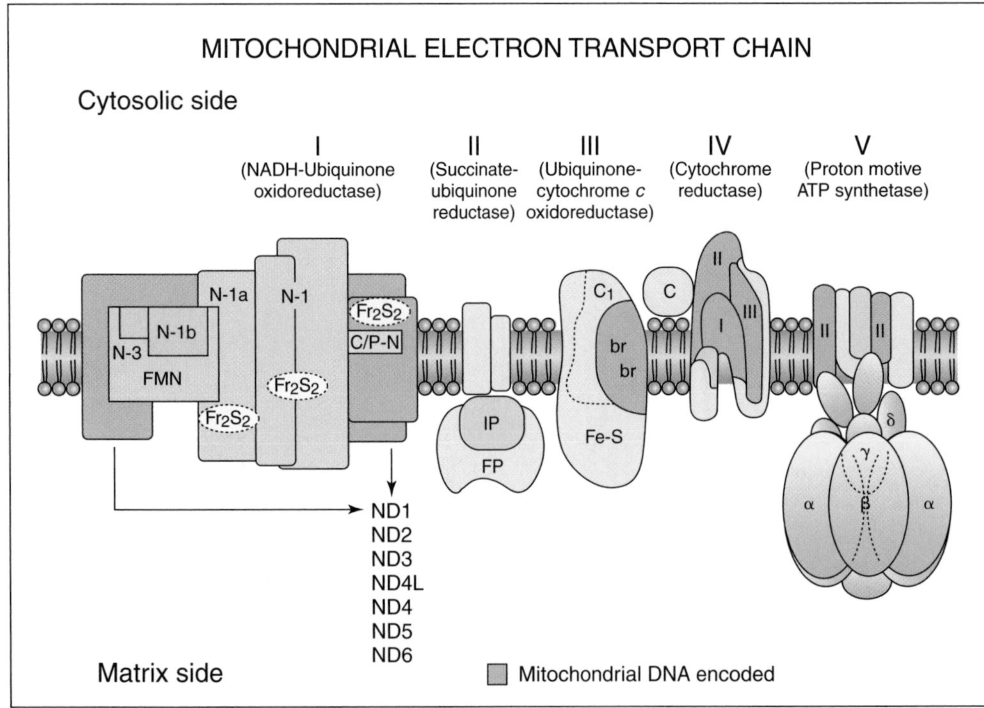

FIGURE 27-6 Electron transport chain. The machinery of mitochondrial ATP production. The electron transport chain consist of 5 critical complexes. Disturbed function of any complex leads to energy production-utilization mismatch.

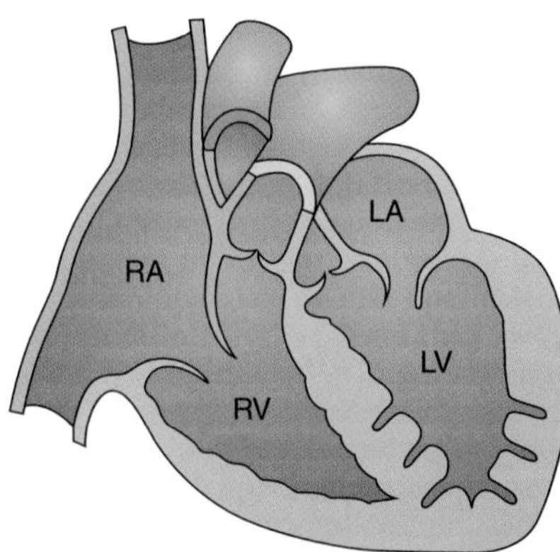

FIGURE 27–7 Illustration of LV noncompaction. Note the spongy appearance of the ventricular myocardium and the relative wall thickness. (Modified from Towbin JA, Bowles NE. The failing heart. *Nature* 2002;415:227-233.)

The myocardium typically demonstrates trabeculations and deep intertrabecular recesses at the apex (Figure 27-8) and the echocardiographic findings include trabeculations and deep intertrabecular recesses (Figure 27-9) and color Doppler suggestion of blood traversing the recesses (Figure 27-10). This cardiomyopathy is somewhat difficult to diagnose unless the physician has a high level of suspicion during echocardiographic evaluation. In fact, on careful review of echocardiograms and other clinical data, it appears that LV noncompaction is relatively common in children and is also seen in adults.[107,108] In the most recent American Heart Association/American College of Cardiology (AHA/ACC) Cardiomyopathy Classification, LVNC for the first time was recognized as a formal form of classified cardiomyopathy.

Two forms of LV noncompaction occur: (1) isolated noncompaction and (2) noncompaction associated with congenital heart disease such as septal defects (ventricular and/or atrial septal defect), pulmonic stenosis, and hypoplastic left heart syndrome, among others.[109,110] In the isolated form and the form associated with congenital heart disease, metabolic derangements may be notable.[111]

Clinical Features

Left ventricular noncompaction most commonly presents in infancy with signs and symptoms of heart failure but some patients are identified during later childhood, adolescence, or adulthood. Pignatelli et al recently reported the findings on 36 children identified over a 5-year period, with the median age at presentation being 90 days (range 1 day to 17 years).[108] In this study, 40% of the children had low cardiac output or congestive heart failure and only one child (3%) had syncope. The most common presenting symptom other than heart failure was asymptomatic electrocardiographic or radiographic abnormalities, with 42% being asymptomatic. In addition, 14% of children had associated dysmorphic features while 19% of affected children had first-degree relatives with cardiomyopathy. The children with dysmorphic features were diagnosed with DiGeorge syndrome in one child and one child had congenital adrenal hyperplasia.

Genetics

When LV noncompaction is inherited, it can be transmitted as an X-linked, mitochondrial, autosomal recessive or autosomal dominant trait.[112] In approximately 20% to 30% of cases, familial inheritance has been identified. The X-linked form usually is associated with isolated noncompaction and a mutation in the *G4.5* (tafazzin) gene located on chromosome Xq28.[110] This gene has also been identified in patients with Barth syndrome.

In autosomal dominant inherited cases, mutations in the Z-line protein encoding ZASP, located on chromosome 10q22, have been identified in isolated noncompaction, while

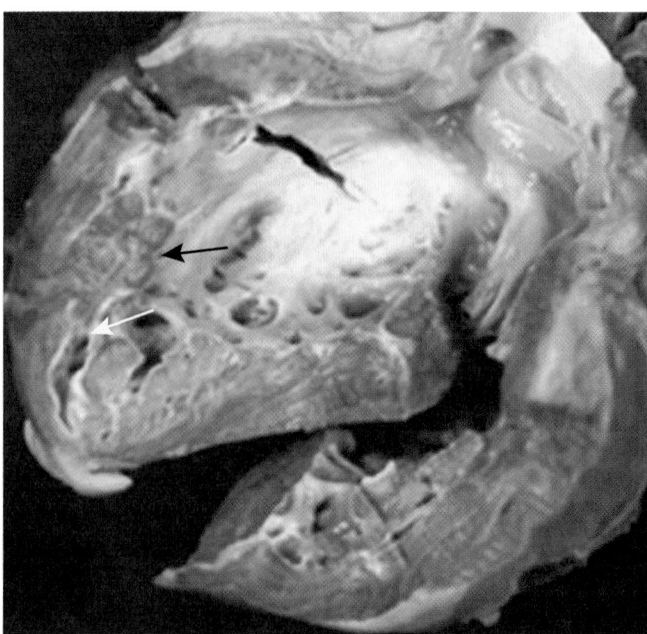

FIGURE 27–8 Anatomical specimen with LV noncompaction. LV trabeculations (*black arrow*) and intertrabecular recesses (*white arrow*) are notable at the apex of this heart of a child with LVNC.

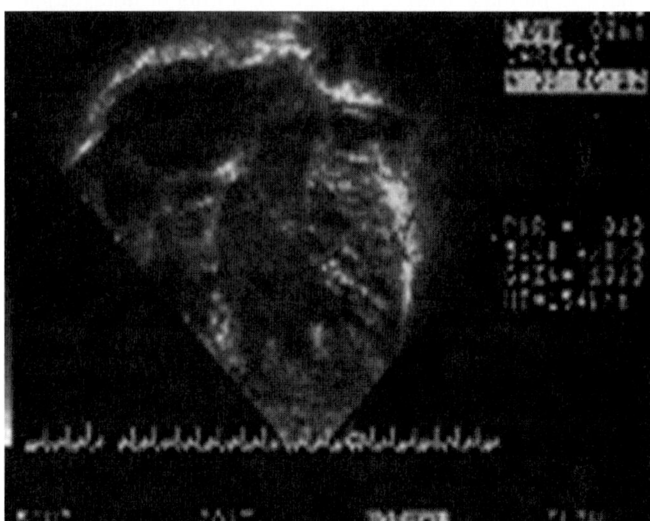

FIGURE 27–9 Echocardiographic features of LV noncompaction. Apical four-chamber view of LVNC with apical and free wall trabeculations and ventricular hypertrophy.

mutations in the gene encoding α-dystrobrevin, a cytoskeletal protein located on chromosome, have been identified in patients with noncompaction associated with congenital heart disease.[55,110] No genes have been identified thus far for autosomal recessive-inherited noncompaction while mutations in mitochondrial DNA have been seen in patients with noncompaction.[109,111]

Therapy and Outcome

The specific therapy depends on the clinical and echocardiographic findings. In patients with systolic dysfunction and heart failure, anticongestive therapy identical to those used in patients with dilated cardiomyopathy is appropriate. In particular, angiotensin-converting enzyme (ACE) inhibitors such as captopril and enalapril, and β-adrenergic blocking agents such as metoprolol or carvedilol are useful. Diuretics may also be needed. However, in those patients exhibiting findings more consistent with a hypertrophic cardiomyopathy or

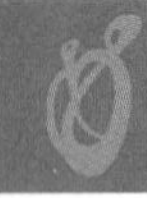

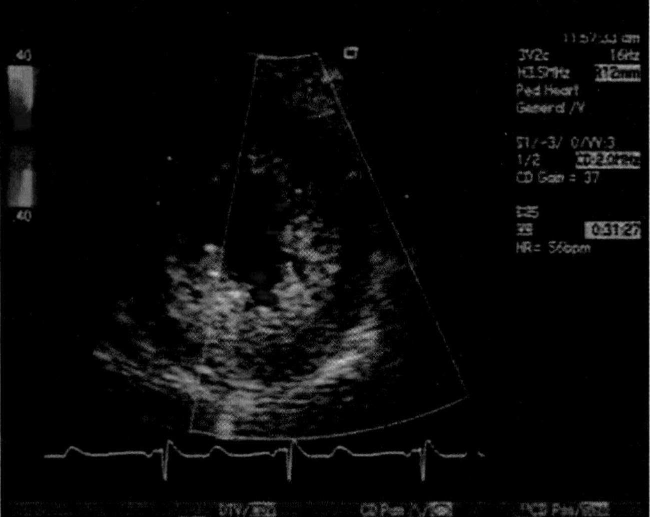

FIGURE 27–10 Echocardiographic features of LV noncompaction. A parasternal short-axis view with color Doppler demonstrates hypertrophy of the LV apex with deep trabeculations filled with blood (red flow).

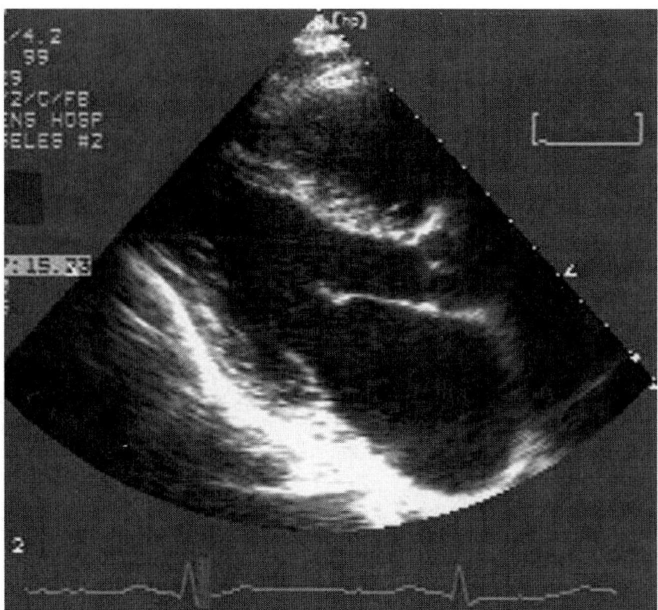

FIGURE 27–11 Restrictive cardiomyopathy. A parasternal long-axis view demonstrates a moderately dilated left atrium with normal LV size, thickness, and systolic function and no mitral regurgitation or shunt lesions.

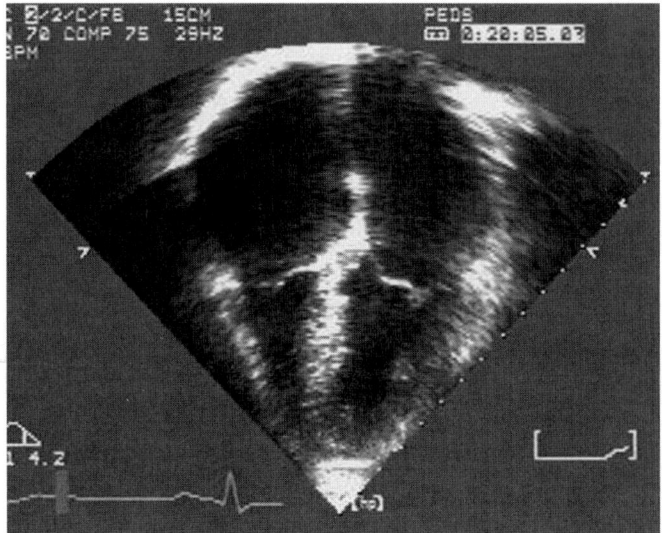

FIGURE 27–12 Restrictive cardiomyopathy. Apical four-chamber view with biatrial enlargement and mild interventricular septal hypertrophy.

a diastolic dysfunction physiological phenotype, β-blocker therapy alone with propranolol or atenolol is more appropriate. In patients with either of these forms of noncompaction with associated mitochondrial or metabolic dysfunction, some investigators add a "vitamin cocktail" to the cardiac therapy with coenzyme Q10, carnitine, riboflavin, and thiamine commonly used alone or in combination.

In patients having associated congenital heart disease, appropriate therapeutic approaches may include simple pharmacological therapy with diuretics for volume overload associated with left to right shunts, more complex pharmacological therapy for patients with restrictive physiology and pulmonary hypertension, or invasive therapy with catheter intervention or surgical repairs, depending on the lesions. Intimate understanding of the cardiac function abnormalities, evidence of thrombi (which should be treated with anticoagulation), and the metabolic status of the patient must be attended to by the interventional cardiologist, cardiac anesthesiologist, and surgeon in approaching these patients invasively. In addition, cardiac rhythm disturbances need to be identified and therapies such as pacemakers, implantable defibrillators, and intracardiac ablations considered.

The clinical outcome of patients with noncompaction has been reported to be poor with death occurring due to heart failure or sudden death presumably arrhythmia-related or stroke-related due to embolization of LV thrombi.[106,110] However, Pignatelli et al demonstrated a 5-year survival rate of 86%; when transplanted patients were added, the 5-year survival rate (free at transplantation) was 75%.[108]

Restrictive Cardiomyopathy

Restrictive cardiomyopathy (RCM), the rarest of the cardiomyopathies, is a diastolic disorder in which the atria are dilated in the face of normal ventricular size, thickness, and systolic function (Figure 27-11). In some cases, ventricular hypertrophy may coexist and, in this case, is commonly described as HCM with restrictive physiology instead of RCM function (Figure 27-12).[113] Sudden death is common although diastolic heart failure occurs in some cases. RCM may be associated with skeletal myopathy, conduction system disease, or can occur as an isolated disorder. In childhood, this disorder has a rapidly progressive course with sudden death occurring within 2 years of clinical presentation. These patients most typically have syncope without prior symptoms. In some patients, chest pain, atrial or ventricular arrhythmias, or a family history of RCM or sudden death leads to the diagnosis.

Genetic Basis of Restrictive Cardiomyopathy

The disease, when inherited, is most commonly an autosomal dominant trait.[112] In the past, complex forms of RCM were studied and genes identified as causative. For instance, patients with RCM associated with conduction system disease and/or skeletal myopathy were found to result from mutations in desmin. Further, infiltrative forms of disease caused by amyloid or sarcoid, were also identified. More recently, studies of families and sporadic cases have been successful in defining RCM as a result of mutations in sarcomere-encoding genes. The most common of these genes appears to be troponin I, although mutations in the β-myosin heavy chain gene (β-MyHC) have also been reported.[113] More studies are required to further pinpoint the causes of RCM and to determine the mechanism(s) differentiating the severity of diastolic dysfunction that separates RCM and HCM as clinical disorders.

Arrhythmogenic Right Ventricular Cardiomyopathy

Arrhythmogenic right ventricular cardiomyopathy (ARVC) is characterized by replacement of RV myocardium with adipose or fibrofatty tissue that occasionally extends to the left ventricle.[114] Clinically the disease manifests as rhythm disturbances of RV origin, ranging from innocuous ventricular ectopy to potentially life-threatening ventricular tachycardia and fibrillation resulting in syncope or sudden death. In fact, ARVC represents a significant cause of sudden death, particularly in young athletes. ARVC exhibits wide phenotypic variability with onset of symptoms typically in the second to fourth decades of life, although some patients present in their early teen years. In some affected patients, heart failure occurs. The lack of standardized diagnostic criteria led to the formulation of major and minor criteria by the European Society of Cardiology/International Federation of Cardiology task force in 1994. An updated "Task Force" set of diagnostic criteria for ARVC are currently being devised. Unfortunately, limitations persist in disease identification due in part to the constellation of structural and functional abnormalities and the reliance on multiple diagnostic modalities that have potentially low sensitivity and/or specificity.[114] Echocardiographic findings typically include RV dilation, focal aneurysms, and wall motion abnormalities. Electrocardiograms (ECGs) may reveal T wave inversions in the right precordial leads, premature ventricular contractions, ventricular tachycardia with left bundle branch pattern, or ε waves that correspond to late potentials seen on signal-averaged electrocardiogram (SAECG).[115] Endomyocardial biopsy will often identify the histopathological changes characteristic of ARVC, including replacement of the myocardium with fibrous tissue and fat (Figure 27-13). A recent study by Asimaki et al suggests that a high sensitivity and specificity for diagnosis may be possible with immunohistochemical analysis.[116] Cardiac magnetic resonance (CMR) imaging has provided another adjunctive test in recent years but it too has similar limitations.[117] Molecular genetics perhaps offers the greatest promise for future inroads into improved diagnostic accuracy and guiding future treatment strategies.[114] Recent genetic studies have helped to define the underlying "final common pathway" involved in the development of the clinical disorder.

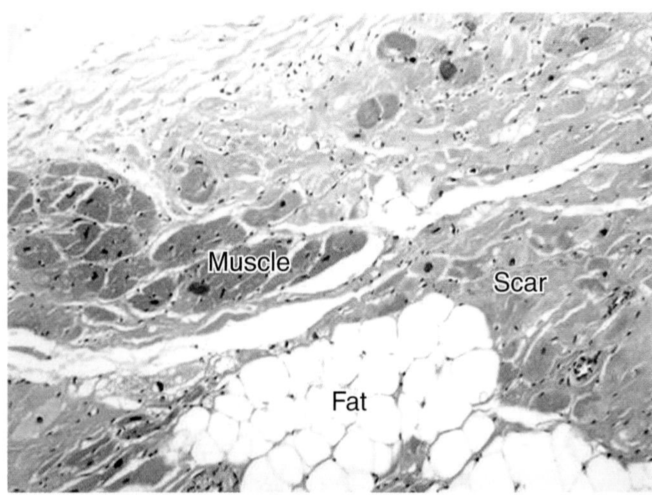

FIGURE 27–13 Histopathology of arrhythmogenic RV cardiomyopathy. Myocardial histopathology demonstrating myocardium (muscle) surrounded by fibrous tissue (scar) and fat (adipose tissue).

Clinical Genetics of Arrhythmogenic Right Ventricular Cardiomyopathy

The exact prevalence of the disease is unknown; however, limited studies suggest there are roughly 6 in 10,000 affected individuals in the general population with significantly higher rates observed in geographic regions such as northeast Italy. Approximately 30% of ARVC is familial, most often exhibiting autosomal dominant inheritance. Less common autosomal recessive forms, Naxos disease and Carvajal syndrome, have been associated with palmoplantar keratoderma and woolly hair. In many affected individuals, particularly those with Carval syndrome, a primary LV form of the disease occurs. ARVC displays incomplete penetrance with variable phenotypic expression.

Genetic Basis of Arrhythmogenic Right Ventricular Cardiomyopathy

As with the other forms of cardiomyopathy and arrhythmia disorders, the genes responsible for ARVC encode proteins of a "final common pathway," in this case cell-cell junctions.[118] To date, eight genes for autosomal dominant inherited ARVC and two genes for autosomal recessive ARVC have been identified. In all cases to date, the causative gene encodes a desmosomal protein or a protein that interacts with and modulates or modifies the function of a desmosomal protein. The genes responsible for the dominant form of ARVC include desmoplakin (*DSP*), plakophillin-2 (*PKP2*), desmoglein-2 (*DSG2*), desmocollin-2 (*DSC2*), plakoglobin (*JUP*), transforming growth factor β-3 (TGFβ3), and, most recently, transmembrane protein 43 (TMEM43). The ryanodine receptor (RyR2) has also been reported but doubt regarding its authenticity as an ARVC-causing gene has been raised. Gerull et al have suggested that PKP2 mutations are the most common cause of this form of disease, responsible for approximately 25% of all cases (Table 27-2). However, we have found that a high percentage of subjects and families with ARVC and PKP2 mutations have reduced penetrance and, in fact, the disease is caused by either second mutations in PKP2 (compound heterozygosity) or mutations in a second desmosome-encoding gene (digenic heterozygosity).

In the case of the autosomal recessive forms of ARVC, Naxos disease is caused by homozygous mutations in JUP, while Carvajal syndrome occurs due to homozygous mutations in DSP.[119]

Animal Models of Arrhythmogenic Right Ventricular Cardiomyopathy

Animal models have demonstrated that the intercalated disks of cardiomyocytes are "pulled apart" and, in many cases, total loss of the desmosomes of the intercalated disk occurs. In addition, in the case of DSP mutants, lipid infiltration appears to be caused by disturbance of the *wnt* signaling pathway. To date, animal models for desmoplakin, RyR2, and plakophilin-2 (PKP2) have been reported.

Ryanodine Receptor Mutant Murine Models. Based on the original report by Tiso et al outlining mutations in RyR2 (located on chromosome 1q42-q43) in subjects reported to have ARVC type 2 (ARVC2), animal modeling studies were initated.[120] Using homologous recombination in embryonic stem cells, a point mutation in exon 8 of the RyR2 gene (*R176Q*) was engineered in C57Black/6 (C57BL/6) mice using a knock-in strategy by Kannankeril et al.[121] This mutation, which was previously shown to cosegregate with ARVD in humans leading to the effort-induced polymorphic VT and mild ARVD histologically characteristic of the ARVD2 form of disease, demonstrated germ line transmission in these mice and once grown were studied clinically and by use of pathological analysis. Histological analysis of hearts from mutant ($RyR2^{R176Q/+}$) and wild-type (WT) mice revealed no evidence of structural abnormalities or fibrofatty infiltration. Noninvasive imaging demonstrated mild systolic dysfunction, and electrocardiographic evaluation identified no spontaneous

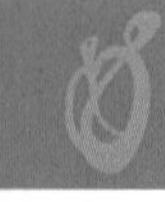

TABLE 27–2 Arrhythmogenic RV Cardiomyopathy (ARVC) Genetics

Locus Name	Inheritance	Map Position	Gene
ARVD1	AD	14q23	*TGFB3*
ARVD2	AD	1q42-q43	*RyR2*
ARVD3	AD	14q12	?
ARVD4	AD	2q32	?
ARVD5	AD	3p23	*TMEM43*
ARVD6	AD	10p12	?
ARVD7	AD	10p22	?
ARVD8	AD	6p24	*Desmoplakin*
ARVD9	AD	12p11	*Plakophilin 2*
Naxos	AR	17q21	*Plakoglobin*
Carvajal	AR	6p24	*Desmoplakin*

arrhythmias in telemetered animals. However, intracardiac electrophysiological studies using programmed stimulation elicited differences in inducibility of VT in the mutant mice versus the WT animals. The aggressive stimulation protocol induced multiple short episodes of VT <0.5 seconds in length in both groups. Using isoproterenol infusion, however, the authors demonstrated an increased number and duration of VT episodes in the mutant mice. In addition, spontaneous ventricular ectopy was induced in the mutant animals but not in the WT mice. This model was inconclusive regarding the phenotype but appeared more consistent with a CPVT phenotype than that of a classic form of ARVC.

Plakophilin-2 Mutant Murine Models. Plakophilins are proteins of the armadillo family of proteins that function in embryonic development and in the adult. Proteins of the armadillo family are characterized by domains composed of variable numbers of repeats of the *arm* motif, 42 amino acids in length, and this family includes β-catenin, plakoglobin (γ-catenin), and plakophilins. Arm repeat proteins bind to the cytoplasmic end of glycoproteins of the cadherin family of cell adhesion molecules, thus forming plaques to which bundles of cytoskeletal filaments are tethered. The plakophilin subfamily of *arm* repeat proteins include four members (PKP1-4), juxtamembranous components of plaques of desmosomes that tightly associate with other arm proteins, cadherins, and desmoplakin, and participate in intermediate filament anchorage. In addition, plakophilins translocate to the nucleus.

Grossmann et al created a null mutation of the plakophilin-2 (*PKP2*) gene by homologous recombination in embryonic stem cells whereby an early stop of *PKP2* translation after exon 1 (43 amino acids) was engineered.[122] Generation of homozygous mutants led to no live offspring, consistent with embryonic lethality. Normal development occurred until embryonic day 10.75 (E10.75), at which time blood accumulation in the pericardial and peritoneal cavities was noted. At E11.5, the number of viable embryos declined significantly. In addition, reduced trabeculations within the ventricles and atrial wall thinning was observed. Confocal microscopy demonstrated lack of the normal colocalization of desmoplakin to the junctions and intercalated disks, instead being dispersed over the cytoplasm, mostly distant from the intercalated disks. In addition, PKP2 was absent and desmoglein-2, another desmosomal cadherin protein, could not be localized in significant levels in these mutant hearts. Electron microscopy confirmed these findings and abnormalities of cytoskeletal organization. In the latter case, intermediate filament arrays appearing as extensive swirls of disordered filaments around dense desmoplakin aggregates were seen. Hence, these findings were consistent with the concept that abnormalities of PKP2 lead to cardiac abnormalities with an unusual form of cardiomyopathy due to desmosomal destabilization. These findings are supportive of the human mutations in PKP2 that are believed to cause ARVC.

Junctional Plakoglobin Mutant Murine Models. Junctional plakoglobin (JUP), also known as Gamma-catenin, was the first member of the armadillo family of proteins discovered. It is a constituent of the cytoplasmic plaque of desmosomes and other cell adherens junctions and is involved in anchorage of cytoskeletal filaments to specific cadherins and consists of 13 arm repeats flanked by unique N-terminal and C-terminal sequences. JUP associates with the desmosomal cadherin proteins desmoglein 1-3 and desmocollin 1-3 to form plaques, which also contain desmoplakin and PKP2.

Using homologous recombination in which mutation in the junction between exons 3 and 4 of the plakoglobin gene was engineered in embryonic stem cells and injected into C57Black/6 (C57BL/6) mice, Ruiz et al generated null JUP mice.[123] Homozygous mutants ($JUP^{-/-}$) were found to be embryonic lethal between days 12 to 16 of embryogenesis (E12-E16) while heterozygous mutants ($JUP^{+/-}$) and WT animals were born with normal development. Evaluation of homozygous embryos between days E10-E16 of gestation demonstrated mild growth retardation at E12 and reduced blood supply, especially to the liver and placenta. The pericardial cavity was swollen and filled with blood and the hearts of these embryos was frequently ruptured within the ventricular walls. Heart rates were increased in these mutants and ventricular contraction was reduced in E11.5 embryos, consistent with systolic dysfunction. Immunofluorescence microscopy showed extensive expression of JUP at E10.5 in WT animals but expression was absent in homozygous mutants. The morphology of the intercalated disks was grossly altered as well. Desmoplakin was found to colocalize in many places with β-catenin but desmoglein was absent in these junctions. Hence, the homozygous mutant animals lack desmosomes, which are replaced by extended adherens, junctions that contain desmosomal proteins such as desmoplakin but have impaired architectural stability and function. Interestingly, the skin of these animals was unaffected.

The findings in this animal model support the concept that mutant JUP results in a form of cardiomyopathy. In humans, homozygous mutations in JUP, located on human chromosome 17q21, result in the cardiocutaneous disorder called Naxos disease in which ARVC is a major component.[124] Although the animal model described here is not a perfect re-creation of the human condition, it serves to be a proof of concept.

Desmoplakin Mutant Murine Models. Desmoplakin (*DSP*), localized to chromosome 6p24, was initially identified as the mutant gene causing autosomal recessive Carvajal syndrome. It was later shown to cause autosomal dominant ARVC8 and is a major component of desmosomes, complex intercellular junctions assembled through cooperative interactions between multiple proteins.[125] The majority of patients with DSP have the classic form of ARVC, although a substantial number of affected individuals have associated LV disease.

Using the Cre-LoxP system, a cardiac-restricted exon 2 deletion in DSP was created in mice. These animals were engineered by crossing mice in which the second exon of the murine desmoplakin gene (*Dsp*) is flanked by LoxP sequence (floxed DP mice; 129/SvJ strain) with mice expressing Cre recombinase under the control of the α-MHC promoter (α-MHC-Cre mice; FVB/N strain). Homozygous ($DP^{-/-}$) mutant mice had a high rate of embryonic lethality. These homozygous mutant mouse embryos exhibited growth arrest at embryonic stage E10-E12, appeared pale, had no circulating red blood cells in their organs, and were growth retarded. Histopathological evaluation revealed poorly formed hearts with no chamber specification and unorganized cardiac myocytes. In addition, red blood cells were localized to the pericardial sac instead of within the cardiac chambers. Furthermore, an excess number of cells resembling adipocytes, dispersed between myocytes and localized to adjacent areas, were also detected. In comparison, their cardiac phenotype was normal in $DP^{+/+}$ and $DP^{+/-}$ embryos, with and without the α-MHC-Cre transgene. Those $DP^{-/-}$ mice surviving the embryonic period (approximately 5% of the litter) died typically within the first 2 weeks postnatally. On the other hand, $DP^{+/-}$ mice were born with normal development but had age-dependent penetrance of heart involvement, including a 20% incidence of SCD by 6 months of life. Gross pathological analysis of both $DP^{+/-}$ and $DP^{-/-}$ animals demonstrated grossly enlarged cardiac chambers and increased heart weight with an increased heart weight-to-body ratio being highest in the homozygous mutants and lowest in the WT animals. Both right ventricle and left ventricle were enlarged equally and this enlargement occurred at approximately the same age. The gross anatomical findings were further supported by echocardiographic measurements, which revealed thin ventricular walls, increased LV end-diastolic and end-systolic dimensions, and depressed systolic function with reduced ejection fraction. Furthermore, baseline resting electrocardiographic evaluation identified spontaneous ventricular ectopy, including premature ventricular contractions, ventricular couplets, and short runs of VT in heterozygous mutants but no ventricular arrhythmias in WT mice. Histological examination revealed poorly organized myocytes with large areas of patchy fibrosis; in the $DP^{-/-}$ animals, fibrosis was seen in up to 30% to 40% of the myocardium. Excess accumulation of fat droplets was notable in both $DP^{-/-}$ and $DP^{+/-}$ mutant mice using oil red O staining, and was seen predominantly at the site of fibrosis.

In addition to these pathological abnormalities, the authors showed that junctional plakoglobin, a member of the armadillo repeat protein family that plays a role in regulation of gene expression, interacts and competes with β-catenin, the effector of the canonical Wnt signaling, having a negative effect on this pathway. They were able to show that plakoglobin was translocated to the nucleus in cardiac-restricted DP-deficient mice and that expression levels of gene targets of the canonical Wnt/β-catenin pathway (*c-myc* and cyclin D1) were reduced. Expression of adipogenic genes were increased, as was TUNEL-positive cells, but in the absence of DNA laddering consistent with low levels of apoptosis.

Another animal model of mutant desmoplakin was recently described by our group. This model, a transgenic mouse with cardiac-restricted overexpression of a C-terminal DSP mutant (R2834H), demonstrated histological evidence of increased cardiomyocyte apoptosis, cardiac fibrosis, and neutral lipid accumulation (Figure 27-14). Echocardiography and CMR imaging revealed ventricular enlargement and cardiac dysfunction of both ventricles (see Figure 27-14), which was confirmed on necropsy. RV wall thickness was also reduced. The mutant mice also displayed interruption of the DSP-desmin interaction at intercalated disks and marked ultrastructural abnormalities of the intercalated disks. The intercalated disks were irregularly shaped with markedly widened gaps between adjacent anchoring sarcomeres, affecting both the adherens junctions and desmosomes. In addition, changes in other desmosomal and junctional components were notable, including increased expression and redistribution of JUP, PKP2, and β-catenin, and changes in gap junction components including redistribution of connexin 43.

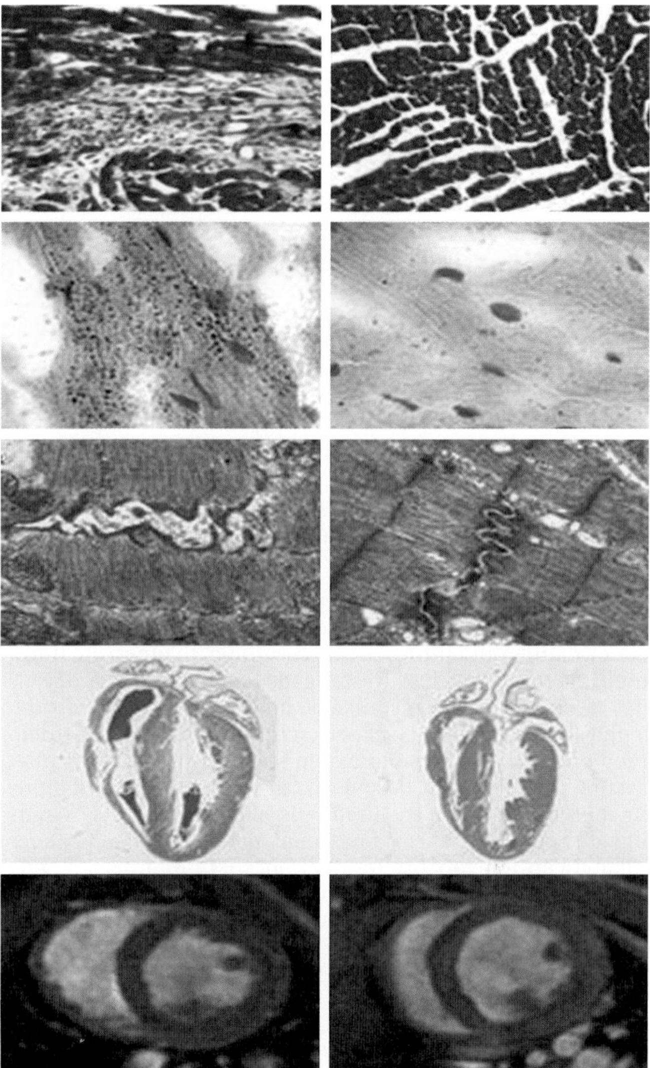

FIGURE 27–14 Desmoplakin transgenic mouse model (DSP) of arrhythmogenic RV cardiomyopathy. The leftward panels demonstrate findings in the DSP mutant mouse while the rightward panels demonstrate findings in the nontransgenic (NTG) mice. From top to bottom, the DSP mutants show fibrosis (blue stain), lipid infiltration (oil red O stain), disrupted intercalated disk appearing to be "pulled apart," dilated thin-walled right ventricle on gross anatomy, and biventricular dilation by cardiac magnetic resonance imaging compared with the NTG counterparts.

Mechanisms of Arrhythmogenic Right Ventricular Cardiomyopathy

ARVC is a disease of desmosomal dysfunction as demonstrated by the human genetics and animal models. In addition to dysfunction of the key desmosomal proteins (Figure 27-15) and disruption of protein-protein interactions of the desmosomal proteins, mechanical stress forces complete the phenotypic presentation with disruption of the intercalated disks, leading to dilation and dysfunction of the ventricles. Arrhythmias occur and sudden death is thought to result from ventricular tachyarrhythmias. Signaling pathway function, particularly the wnt pathway, also appears to play a key role.

CONCLUSIONS AND FUTURE DIRECTIONS

Heart failure, when caused by cardiomyopathies, appears to occur due to disruption of "final common pathways" and the resultant physiological disturbances that ensue. These disruptions may be due to purely genetic causes, such as mutations

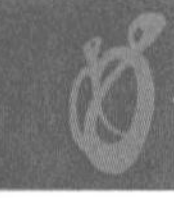

FIGURE 27–15 Desmosome proteins and structure. Illustration of the desmosome, the proteins comprising the desmosome, and the cell-cell contacts between myocytes. Key proteins, including plakoglobin, plakophillin, and desmoplakin are shown, with the link of desmoplakin to the intermediate filaments (desmin) also seen. Disruption of protein structure plus mechanical stress leads to disrupted protein-protein binding and the "pulling apart" of cell-cell contacts seen in these patients and animal models.

in a single gene that results in a dysfunctional protein, which leads to a domino effect of downstream protein interaction abnormalities and ultimately a phenotype. In other situations, multiple mutations in the same gene (compound heterozygosity) or in different genes (digenic heterozygosity) may lead to a phenotype that may be classic, more severe, or even overlapping with other disease forms. In some cases, different intersecting pathways may become disturbed, resulting in complex phenotypes. Further, acquired causes may play a role by causing disruption of these functional pathways. For instance, dilated cardiomyopathy results from disruption in the "final common pathway" linking the sarcomere and sarcolemma and mutations in the affected genes are responsible for cardiac and skeletal muscle dysfunction. The mechanisms of disease, which include disruption of the linkage due to protein-protein interaction abnormalities that occur from dysfunctional proteins, and the interplay of other factors such as mechanical stress and stretch, are being elucidated in detail with the development of animal models of the human disease. Many of the genes identified are now clinically available in fee-for-service laboratories. Novel therapies have resulted from the improved understanding of this clinical phenotype, as noted previously. Similarly, the genetic basis and mechanistic understanding of HCM as a disturbance of sarcomeric function has occurred over the past 2 decades and genetic tests are clinically available. The development of novel targeted therapies has been somewhat slow in coming but is expected to develop in the near future. In the case of LVNC, the "new kid on the block," genetic understanding is in the early phases. The future of cardiomyopathy care is poised to shift in the next decade due to these new developments, and the growing science of stem cell therapy. Since children have "pure" disease states, unfettered by comorbidities, the dream of "cures" of muscle disease (cardiac, skeletal muscle) will likely be realized more fully in this population. We must move toward that goal.

REFERENCES

1. Jessup, M., & Brozena, S. C. (2007). Guidelines for the management of heart failure: differences in guideline perspectives. *Cardiol Clin, 25*, 497–506.
2. Towbin, J. A., & Bowles, N. E. (2002). The failing heart. *Nature, 415*, 227–233.
3. Morita, H., Seidman, J., & Seidman, C. E. (2005). Genetic causes of human heart failure. *J Clin Invest, 115*, 518–526.
4. Maron, B. J., Towbin, J. A., Thiene, G., et al. (2006). Contemporary definitions and classification of the cardiomyopathies: an American Heart Association scientific statement from the council on clinical cardiology, heart failure and transplantation committee; quality of care and outcomes research and functional genomics and translational biology interdisciplinary working groups; and council on epidemiology and prevention. *Circulation, 113*, 1807–1816.
5. Schwartz, S. M., Duffy, J. Y., Pearl, J. M., et al. (2001). Cellular and molecular aspects of myocardial dysfunction. *Crit Care Med, 29*, S214–S219.
6. Gregorio, C. C., & Antin, P. B. (2000). To the heart of myofibril assembly. *Trends Cell Biol, 10*, 355–362.
7. Clark, K. A., McElhinny, A. S., Beckerle, M. C., et al. (2002). Striated muscle cytoarchitecture: an intricate web of form and function. *Annu Rev Cell Dev Biol, 18*, 637–706.
8. Vigoreaux, J. O. (1994). The muscle Z band: lessons in stress management. *J Muscle Res Cell Motil, 15*, 237–255.
9. Barth, A. I., Nathke, I. S., & Nelson, W. J. (1997). Cadherins, catenins and APC protein: interplay between cytoskeletal complexes and signaling pathways. *Curr Opin Cell Biol, 9*, 683–690.
10. Capetanaki, Y. (2002). Desmin cytoskeleton: a potential regulator of muscle mitochondrial behavior and function. *Trends Cardiovasc Med, 12*, 339–348.
11. Sharp, W. W., Simpson, D. G., Borg, T. K., et al. (1997). Mechanical forces regulate focal adhesion and costamere assembly in cardiac myocytes. *Am J Physiol, 273*, H546–H556.
12. Straub, V., Rafael, J. A., Chamberlain, J. S., et al. (1997). Animal models for muscular dystrophy show different patterns of sarcolemmal disruption. *J Cell Biol, 139*, 375–385.
13. Furukawa, T., Ono, Y., Tsuchiya, H., et al. (2001). Specific interaction of the potassium channel beta-subunit minK with the sarcomeric protein T-cap suggests a T-tubule-myofibril linking system. *J Mol Biol, 313*, 775–784.
14. Kucera, J. P., Rohr, S., & Rudy, Y. (2002). Localization of sodium channels in intercalated disks modulates cardiac conduction. *Circ Res, 91*, 1176–1182.
15. Towbin, J. A., Lowe, A. M., Colan, S. D., et al. (2006). Incidence, causes, and outcomes of dilated cardiomyopathy in children. *JAMA, 296*, 1867–1876.
16. Michels, V. V., Moll, P. P., Miller, F. A., et al. (1992). The frequency of familial dilated cardiomyopathy in a series of patients with idiopathic dilated cardiomyopathy. *N Engl J Med, 326*, 77–82.
17. Berko, B. A., & Swift, M. (1987). X-linked dilated cardiomyopathy. *N Engl J Med, 316*, 1186–1191.
18. Towbin, J. A., Bowles, K. R., & Bowles, N. E. (1999). Etiologies of cardiomyopathy and heart failure. *Nat Med, 5*, 266–267.
19. Towbin, J. A. (1993). Molecular genetic aspects of cardiomyopathy. *Biochem Med Metab Biol, 49*, 285–320.
20. Muntoni, F., Cau, M., Ganau, A., et al. (1993). Brief report: deletion of the dystrophin muscle-promoter region associated with X-linked dilated cardiomyopathy. *N Engl J Med, 329*, 921–925.
21. Cox, G. F., & Kunkel, L. M. (1997). Dystrophies and heart disease. *Curr Opin Cardiol, 12*, 329–343.
22. Kaprielian, R. R., Stevenson, S., Rothery, S. M., et al. (2000). Distinct patterns of dystrophin organization in myocyte sarcolemma and transverse tubules of normal and diseased human myocardium. *Circulation, 101*, 2586–2594.
23. Koenig, M., Hoffman, E. P., Bertelson, C. J., et al. (1987). Complete cloning of the Duchenne muscular dystrophy (DMD) cDNA and preliminary genomic organization of the DMD gene in normal and affected individuals. *Cell, 50*, 509–517.
24. Petrof, B. J., Shrager, J. B., Stedman, H. H., et al. (1993). Dystrophin protects the sarcolemma from stresses developed during muscle contraction. *Proc Natl Acad Sci U S A, 90*, 3710–3714.
25. Ozawa, E., Yoshida, M., Suzuki, A., et al. (1995). Dystrophin-associated proteins in muscular dystrophy. *Hum Mol Genet, 4*(spec No), 1711–1716.
26. Emery, A. E. (2002). The muscular dystrophies. *Lancet, 359*, 687–695.
27. Towbin, J. A. (1998). The role of cytoskeletal proteins in cardiomyopathies. *Curr Opin Cell Biol, 10*, 131–139.
28. Bowles, N. E., Bowles, K. R., & Towbin, J. A. (2000). The "final common pathway" hypothesis and inherited cardiovascular disease. The role of cytoskeletal proteins in dilated cardiomyopathy. *Herz, 25*, 168–175.
29. Feng, J., Yan, J., Buzin, C. H., et al. (2002). Mutations in the dystrophin gene are associated with sporadic dilated cardiomyopathy. *Mol Genet Metab, 77*, 119–126.
30. Feng, J., Yan, J. Y., Buzin, C. H., et al. (2002). Comprehensive mutation scanning of the dystrophin gene in patients with nonsyndromic X-linked dilated cardiomyopathy. *J Am Coll Cardiol, 40*, 1120–1124.
31. Neustein, H. B., Lurie, P. R., Dahms, B., et al. (1979). An X-linked recessive cardiomyopathy with abnormal mitochondria. *Pediatrics, 64*, 24–29.
32. Barth, P. G., Scholte, H. R., Berden, J. A., et al. (1983). An X-linked mitochondrial disease affecting cardiac muscle, skeletal muscle and neutrophil leucocytes. *J Neurol Sci, 62*, 327–355.
33. Schlame, M., Towbin, J. A., Heerdt, P. M., et al. (2002). Deficiency of tetralinoleoyl-cardiolipin in Barth syndrome. *Ann Neurol, 51*, 634–637.
34. Bione, S., D'Adamo, P., Maestrini, E., et al. (1996). A novel X-linked gene, G4.5, is responsible for Barth syndrome. *Nat Genet, 12*, 385–389.
35. Bleyl, S. B., Mumford, B. R., Thompson, V., et al. (1997). Neonatal, lethal noncompaction of the left ventricular myocardium is allelic with Barth syndrome. *Am J Hum Genet, 61*, 868–872.
36. Graber, H. L., Unverferth, D. V., Baker, P. B., et al. (1986). Evolution of a hereditary cardiac conduction and muscle disorder: a study involving a family with six generations affected. *Circulation, 74*, 21–35.
37. Tsubata, S., Bowles, K. R., Vatta, M., et al. (2000). Mutations in the human delta-sarcoglycan gene in familial and sporadic dilated cardiomyopathy. *J Clin Invest, 106*, 655–662.
38. Karkkainen, S., & Peuhkurinen, K. (2007). Genetics of dilated cardiomyopathy. *Ann Med, 39*, 91–107.
39. Towbin, J. A., & Bowles, N. E. (2006). Dilated cardiomyopathy: a tale of cytoskeletal proteins and beyond. *J Cardiovasc Electrophysiol, 17*, 919–926.
40. Olson, T. M., Michels, V. V., Thibodeau, S. N., et al. (1998). Actin mutations in dilated cardiomyopathy, a heritable form of heart failure. *Science, 280*, 750–752.
41. Kamisago, M., Sharma, S. D., DePalma, S. R., et al. (2000). Mutations in sarcomere protein genes as a cause of dilated cardiomyopathy. *N Engl J Med, 343*, 1688–1696.
42. Li, D., Tapscoft, T., Gonzalez, O., et al. (1999). Desmin mutation responsible for idiopathic dilated cardiomyopathy. *Circulation, 100*, 461–464.

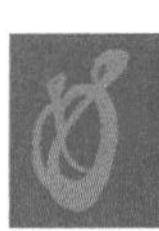

43. Ozawa, E., Mizuno, Y., Hagiwara, Y., et al. (2005). Molecular and cell biology of the sarcoglycan complex. *Muscle Nerve, 32*, 563–576.
44. Wheeler, M. T., Allikian, M. J., Heydemann, A., et al. (2004). Smooth muscle cell-extrinsic vascular spasm arises from cardiomyocyte degeneration in sarcoglycan-deficient cardiomyopathy. *J Clin Invest, 113*, 668–675.
45. Olson, T. M., Illenberger, S., Kishimoto, N. Y., et al. (2002). Metavinculin mutations alter actin interaction in dilated cardiomyopathy. *Circulation, 105*, 431–437.
46. Maeda, M., Holder, E., Lowes, B., et al. (1997). Dilated cardiomyopathy associated with deficiency of the cytoskeletal protein metavinculin. *Circulation, 95*, 17–20.
47. Chang, A. N., & Potter, J. D. (2005). Sarcomeric protein mutations in dilated cardiomyopathy. *Heart Fail Rev, 10*, 225–235.
48. Schmitt, J. P., Semsarian, C., Arad, M., et al. (2003). Consequences of pressure overload on sarcomere protein mutation-induced hypertrophic cardiomyopathy. *Circulation, 108*, 1133–1138.
49. Haghighi, K., Kolokathis, F., Pater, L., et al. (2003). Human phospholamban null results in lethal dilated cardiomyopathy revealing a critical difference between mouse and human. *J Clin Invest, 111*, 869–876.
50. Olson, T. M., Kishimoto, N. Y., Whitby, F. G., et al. (2001). Mutations that alter the surface charge of alpha-tropomyosin are associated with dilated cardiomyopathy. *J Mol Cell Cardiol, 33*, 723–732.
51. Pyle, W. G., & Solaro, R. J. (2004). At the crossroads of myocardial signaling: the role of Z-discs in intracellular signaling and cardiac function. *Circ Res, 94*, 296–305.
52. Knoll, R., Hoshijima, M., Hoffman, H. M., et al. (2002). The cardiac mechanical stretch sensor machinery involves a Z disc complex that is defective in a subset of human dilated cardiomyopathy. *Cell, 111*, 943–955.
53. Arber, S., Hunter, J. J., Ross, J., Jr., et al. (1997). MLP-deficient mice exhibit a disruption of cardiac cytoarchitectural organization, dilated cardiomyopathy, and heart failure. *Cell, 88*, 393–403.
54. Zolk, O., Caroni, P., & Bohm, M. (2000). Decreased expression of the cardiac LIM domain protein MLP in chronic human heart failure. *Circulation, 101*, 2674–2677.
55. Vatta, M., Mohapatra, B., Jimenez, S., et al. (2003). Mutations in Cypher/ZASP in patients with dilated cardiomyopathy and left ventricular non-compaction. *J Am Coll Cardiol, 42*, 2014–2027.
56. Granzier, H. L., & Labeit, S. (2004). The giant protein titin: a major player in myocardial mechanics, signaling, and disease. *Circ Res, 94*, 284–295.
57. Gerull, B., Gramlich, M., Atherton, J., et al. (2002). Mutations of TTN, encoding the giant muscle filament titin, cause familial dilated cardiomyopathy. *Nat Genet, 30*, 201–204.
58. Fatkin, D., MacRae, C., Sasaki, T., et al. (1999). Missense mutations in the rod domain of the lamin A/C gene as causes of dilated cardiomyopathy and conduction-system disease. *N Engl J Med, 341*, 1715–1724.
59. Brodsky, G. L., Muntoni, F., Miocic, S., et al. (2000). Lamin A/C gene mutation associated with dilated cardiomyopathy with variable skeletal muscle involvement. *Circulation, 101*, 473–476.
60. Stuurman, N., Heins, S., & Aebi, U. (1998). Nuclear lamins: their structure, assembly, and interactions. *J Struct Biol, 122*, 42–66.
61. Bonne, G., Di Barletta, M. R., Varnous, S., et al. (1999). Mutations in the gene encoding lamin A/C cause autosomal dominant Emery-Dreifuss muscular dystrophy. *Nat Genet, 21*, 285–288.
62. Raffaele Di Barletta, M., Ricci, E., Galluzzi, G., et al. (2000). Different mutations in the LMNA gene cause autosomal dominant and autosomal recessive Emery-Dreifuss muscular dystrophy. *Am J Hum Genet, 66*, 1407–1412.
63. Muchir, A., Bonne, G., van der Kooi, A. J., et al. (2000). Identification of mutations in the gene encoding lamins A/C in autosomal dominant limb girdle muscular dystrophy with atrioventricular conduction disturbances (LGMD1B). *Hum Mol Genet, 9*, 1453–1459.
64. Decostre, V., Ben Yaou, R., & Bonne, G. (2005). Laminopathies affecting skeletal and cardiac muscles: clinical and pathophysiological aspects. *Acta Myol, 24*, 104–109.
65. Taylor, M. R., Slavov, D., Gajewski, A., et al. (2005). Thymopoietin (lamina-associated polypeptide 2) gene mutation associated with dilated cardiomyopathy. *Hum Mutat, 26*, 566–574.
66. Badorff, C., Lee, G. H., Lamphear, B. J., et al. (1999). Enteroviral protease 2A cleaves dystrophin: evidence of cytoskeletal disruption in an acquired cardiomyopathy. *Nat Med, 5*, 320–326.
67. Xiong, D., Lee, G. H., Badorff, C., et al. (2002). Dystrophin deficiency markedly increases enterovirus-induced cardiomyopathy: a genetic predisposition to viral heart disease. *Nat Med, 8*, 872–877.
68. Vatta, M., Stetson, S. J., Jimenez, S., et al. (2004). Molecular normalization of dystrophin in the failing left and right ventricle of patients treated with either pulsatile or continuous flow-type ventricular assist devices. *J Am Coll Cardiol, 43*, 811–817.
69. Winchester, B., Bali, D., Bodamer, O. A., et al. (2008). Methods for a prompt and reliable laboratory diagnosis of Pompe disease: report from an international consensus meeting. *Mol Genet Metab, 93*, 275–281.
70. Cable, W. J., Kolodny, E. H., & Adams, R. D. (1982). Fabry disease: impaired autonomic function. *Neurology, 32*, 498–502.
71. Sugie, K., Yamamoto, A., Murayama, K., et al. (2002). Clinicopathological features of genetically confirmed Danon disease. *Neurology, 58*, 1773–1778.
72. Yang, Z., McMahon, C. J., Smith, L. R., et al. (2005). Danon disease as an underrecognized cause of hypertrophic cardiomyopathy in children. *Circulation, 112*, 1612–1617.
73. Arad, M., Benson, D. W., Perez-Atayde, A. R., et al. (2002). Constitutively active AMP kinase mutations cause glycogen storage disease mimicking hypertrophic cardiomyopathy. *J Clin Invest, 109*, 357–362.
74. D'Ancona, G. G., Wurm, J., & Croce, C. M. (1979). Genetics of type II glycogenosis: assignment of the human gene for acid alpha-glucosidase to chromosome 17. *Proc Natl Acad Sci U S A, 76*, 4526–4529.
75. Beratis, N. G., LaBadie, G. U., & Hirschhorn, K. (1983). Genetic heterogeneity in acid alpha-glucosidase deficiency. *Am J Hum Genet, 35*, 21–33.
76. Zhong, N., Martiniuk, F., Tzall, S., et al. (1991). Identification of a missense mutation in one allele of a patient with Pompe disease, and use of endonuclease digestion of PCR-amplified RNA to demonstrate lack of mRNA expression from the second allele. *Am J Hum Genet, 49*, 635–645.
77. Kishnani, P. S., Steiner, R. D., Bali, D., et al. (2006). Pompe disease diagnosis and management guideline. *Genet Med, 8*, 267–288.
78. Masson, C., Cisse, I., Simon, V., et al. (2004). Fabry disease: a review. *Joint Bone Spine, 71*, 381–383.
79. Colucci, W. S., Lorell, B. H., Schoen, F. J., et al. (1982). Hypertrophic obstructive cardiomyopathy due to Fabry's disease. *N Engl J Med, 307*, 926–928.
80. Broadbent, J. C., Edwards, W. D., Gordon, H., et al. (1981). Fabry cardiomyopathy in the female confirmed by endomyocardial biopsy. *Mayo Clin Proc, 56*, 623–628.
81. Bishop, T. R., Frelin, L. P., & Boyer, S. H. (1986). Nucleotide sequence of rat liver delta-aminolevulinic acid dehydratase cDNA. *Nucleic Acids Res, 14*, 10115.
82. Eng, C. M., Niehaus, D. J., Enriquez, A. L., et al. (1994). Fabry disease: twenty-three mutations including sense and antisense CpG alterations and identification of a deletional hot-spot in the alpha-galactosidase A gene. *Hum Mol Genet, 3*, 1795–1799.
83. Nakao, S., Takenaka, T., Maeda, M., et al. (1995). An atypical variant of Fabry's disease in men with left ventricular hypertrophy. *N Engl J Med, 333*, 288–293.
84. Sachdev, B., Takenaka, T., Teraguchi, H., et al. (2002). Prevalence of Andersen-Fabry disease in male patients with late onset hypertrophic cardiomyopathy. *Circulation, 105*, 1407–1411.
85. Weidemann, F., Niemann, M., Breunig, F., et al. (2009). Long-term effects of enzyme replacement therapy on Fabry cardiomyopathy: evidence for a better outcome with early treatment. *Circulation, 119*, 524–529.
86. Danon, M. J., Oh, S. J., DiMauro, S., et al. (1981). Lysosomal glycogen storage disease with normal acid maltase. *Neurology, 31*, 51–57.
87. Nishino, I., Fu, J., Tanji, K., et al. (2000). Primary LAMP-2 deficiency causes X-linked vacuolar cardiomyopathy and myopathy (Danon disease). *Nature, 406*, 906–910.
88. Charron, P., Villard, E., Sebillon, P., et al. (2004). Danon's disease as a cause of hypertrophic cardiomyopathy: a systematic survey. *Heart, 90*, 842–846.
89. Cheung, A. T., Wang, J., Ree, D., et al. (2000). Tumor necrosis factor-alpha induces hepatic insulin resistance in obese Zucker (fa/fa) rats via interaction of leukocyte antigen-related tyrosine phosphatase with focal adhesion kinase. *Diabetes, 49*, 810–819.
90. Gollob, M. H., Green, M. S., Tang, A. S., et al. (2001). Identification of a gene responsible for familial Wolff-Parkinson-White syndrome. *N Engl J Med, 344*, 1823–1831.
91. Blair, E., Redwood, C., Ashrafian, H., et al. (2001). Mutations in the gamma(2) subunit of AMP-activated protein kinase cause familial hypertrophic cardiomyopathy: evidence for the central role of energy compromise in disease pathogenesis. *Hum Mol Genet, 10*, 1215–1220.
92. Arad, M., Moskowitz, I. P., Patel, V. V., et al. (2003). Transgenic mice overexpressing mutant PRKAG2 define the cause of Wolff-Parkinson-White syndrome in glycogen storage cardiomyopathy. *Circulation, 107*, 2850–2856.
93. Attardi, G. (1986). The elucidation of the human mitochondrial genome: a historical perspective. *BioEssays, 5*, 34–39.
94. Clarke, A. (1990). Mitochondrial genome: defects, disease, and evolution. *J Med Genet, 27*, 451–456.
95. Anderson, S., Bankier, A. T., Barrell, B. G., et al. (1981). Sequence and organization of the human mitochondrial genome. *Nature, 290*, 457–465.
96. Petty, R. K., Harding, A. E., & Morgan-Hughes, J. A. (1986). The clinical features of mitochondrial myopathy. *Brain, 109*(pt 5), 915–938.
97. Vogel, H. (2001). Mitochondrial myopathies and the role of the pathologist in the molecular era. *J Neuropathol Exp Neurol, 60*, 217–227.
98. Wallace, D. C., Zheng, X. X., Lott, M. T., et al. (1988). Familial mitochondrial encephalomyopathy (MERRF): genetic, pathophysiological, and biochemical characterization of a mitochondrial DNA disease. *Cell, 55*, 601–610.
99. Capaldi, R. A., Halphen, D. G., Zhang, Y. Z., et al. (1988). Complexity and tissue specificity of the mitochondrial respiratory chain. *J Bioenerg Biomembr, 20*, 291–311.
100. Channer, K. S., Channer, J. L., Campbell, M. J., et al. (1988). Cardiomyopathy in the Kearns-Sayre syndrome. *Br Heart J, 59*, 486–490.
101. Poulton, J., Deadman, M. E., Ramacharan, S., et al. (1991). Germ-line deletions of mtDNA in mitochondrial myopathy. *Am J Hum Genet, 48*, 649–653.
102. Moraes, C. T., Schon, E. A., DiMauro, S., et al. (1989). Heteroplasmy of mitochondrial genomes in clonal cultures from patients with Kearns-Sayre syndrome. *Biochem Biophys Res Commun, 160*, 765–771.
103. Suomalainen, A., Kollmann, P., Octave, J. N., et al. (1993). Quantification of mitochondrial DNA carrying the tRNA(8344Lys) point mutation in myoclonus epilepsy and ragged-red-fiber disease. *Eur J Hum Genet, 1*, 88–95.
104. Shoffner, J. M., Lott, M. T., Lezza, A. M., et al. (1990). Myoclonic epilepsy and ragged-red fiber disease (MERRF) is associated with a mitochondrial DNA tRNA(Lys) mutation. *Cell, 61*, 931–937.
105. Fukuhara, N. (1995). Clinicopathological features of MERRF. *Muscle Nerve, 3*, S90–S94.
106. Chin, T. K., Perloff, J. K., Williams, R. G., et al. (1990). Isolated noncompaction of left ventricular myocardium. A study of eight cases. *Circulation, 82*, 507–513.
107. Stollberger, C., & Finsterer, J. (2004). Left ventricular hypertrabeculation/noncompaction. *J Am Soc Echocardiogr, 17*, 91–100.
108. Pignatelli, R. H., McMahon, C. J., Dreyer, W. J., et al. (2003). Clinical characterization of left ventricular noncompaction in children: a relatively common form of cardiomyopathy. *Circulation, 108*, 2672–2678.
109. Stollberger, C., Finsterer, J., & Blazek, G. (2002). Left ventricular hypertrabeculation/noncompaction and association with additional cardiac abnormalities and neuromuscular disorders. *Am J Cardiol, 90*, 899–902.
110. Ichida, F., Hamamichi, Y., Miyawaki, T., et al. (1999). Clinical features of isolated noncompaction of the ventricular myocardium: long-term clinical course, hemodynamic properties, and genetic background. *J Am Coll Cardiol, 34*, 233–240.

111. Scaglia, F., Towbin, J. A., Craigen, W. J., et al. (2004). Clinical spectrum, morbidity, and mortality in 113 pediatric patients with mitochondrial disease. *Pediatrics, 114*, 925–931.
112. Hershberger, R. E., Lindenfeld, J., Mestroni, L., et al. (2009). Genetic evaluation of cardiomyopathy–a Heart Failure Society of America practice guideline. *J Card Fail, 15*, 83–97.
113. Mogensen, J., & Arbustini, E. (2009). Restrictive cardiomyopathy. *Curr Opin Cardiol, 24*, 214–220.
114. Marcus, F. I., Zareba, W., Calkins, H., et al. (2009). Arrhythmogenic right ventricular cardiomyopathy/dysplasia clinical presentation and diagnostic evaluation: results from the North American multidisciplinary study. *Heart Rhythm, 6*, 984–992.
115. Steriotis, A. K., Bauce, B., Daliento, L., et al. (2009). Electrocardiographic pattern in arrhythmogenic right ventricular cardiomyopathy. *Am J Cardiol, 103*, 1302–1308.
116. Asimaki, A., Tandri, H., Huang, H., et al. (2009). A new diagnostic test for arrhythmogenic right ventricular cardiomyopathy. *N Engl J Med, 360*, 1075–1084.
117. Casolo, G., Di Cesare, E., Molinari, G., et al. (2004). Diagnostic work up of arrhythmogenic right ventricular cardiomyopathy by cardiovascular magnetic resonance (CMR). Consensus statement. *Radiol Med, 108*, 39–55.
118. Saffitz, J. E. (2009). Arrhythmogenic cardiomyopathy and abnormalities of cell-to-cell coupling. *Heart Rhythm, 6*, S62–S65.
119. Uzumcu, A., Norgett, E. E., Dindar, A., et al. (2006). Loss of desmoplakin isoform I causes early onset cardiomyopathy and heart failure in a Naxos-like syndrome. *J Med Genet, 43*, e5.
120. Tiso, N., Salamon, M., Bagattin, A., et al. (2002). The binding of the RyR2 calcium channel to its gating protein FKBP12.6 is oppositely affected by ARVD2 and VTSIP mutations. *Biochem Biophys Res Commun, 299*, 594–598.
121. Kannankeril, P. J., Mitchell, B. M., Goonasekera, S. A., et al. (2006). Mice with the R176Q cardiac ryanodine receptor mutation exhibit catecholamine-induced ventricular tachycardia and cardiomyopathy. *Proc Natl Acad Sci U S A, 103*, 12179–12184.
122. Grossmann, K. S., Grund, C., Huelsken, J., et al. (2004). Requirement of plakophilin 2 for heart morphogenesis and cardiac junction formation. *J Cell Biol, 167*, 149–160.
123. Ruiz, P., Brinkmann, V., Ledermann, B., et al. (1996). Targeted mutation of plakoglobin in mice reveals essential functions of desmosomes in the embryonic heart. *J Cell Biol, 135*, 215–225.
124. Whittock, N. V., Eady, R. A., & McGrath, J. A. (2000). Genomic organization and amplification of the human plakoglobin gene (JUP). *Exp Dermatol, 9*, 323–326.
125. Kaplan, S. R., Gard, J. J., Carvajal-Huerta, L., et al. (2004). Structural and molecular pathology of the heart in Carvajal syndrome. *Cardiovasc Pathol, 13*, 26–32.

CHAPTER 28

Heart Failure as a Consequence of Hypertension

Thomas D. Giles and Gary E. Sander

Hypertension, if defined simply by JNC (Joint National Committee) criteria as a systemic arterial blood pressure (BP) greater than 140/90 mm Hg, is present in at least one third of the U.S. population. Ninety-one percent of cases of heart failure are preceded by hypertension when a BP level of 140/90 mm Hg is used as the sole diagnostic criterion. Hypertension is thus the most important modifiable risk factor for heart failure.[1,2,3] However, it is now evident that the optimal BP of adults over 40 years of age is less than 115/75 mm Hg and furthermore that the increase in cardiovascular risk rises sharply above that number.[4] Simply stated, there is no threshold BP pressure that identifies those with hypertension from those without the disease; hence BP is best understood as a biomarker of hypertension as a disease. In fact, a definition of hypertension independent of BP thresholds was proposed by a Writing Group of the American Society of Hypertension.[5] Throughout this review, unless otherwise specified, the term hypertension will be used to refer to the disease state rather than as simply an elevation of BP greater than 140/90 mm Hg.

Hypertension is a disease of the cardiovascular system that primarily manifests itself as an increase in systemic arterial blood pressure and may be associated with the development of myocardial disease (i.e., cardiomyopathy). There are numerous causes of increased blood pressure involving genetic and environmental factors. *Heart failure* is not a disease, but rather a clinical syndrome that manifests itself late in the course of a cardiomyopathy. Hypertensive cardiomyopathy is a pathophysiological process that may lead to the development of heart failure. The importance of heart failure as a complication of hypertension is seen when viewing the untreated natural history.[6]

The presence of a resting arterial blood pressure chronically greater than 140/90 mm Hg has been defined as hypertension by the JNC VI report.[7] However, it has become increasingly apparent that sustained BP that exceeds the optimal level for an individual does damage target organs, including the heart. The threshold for departure from optimal BP has not yet been identified, but cardiovascular abnormalities, including increased left ventricular mass and reduced vasodilator capacity, have been demonstrated in the normotensive offspring of subjects with hypertension, with more prominent abnormalities in those with two hypertensive parents.[8] Hypertensive heart disease, perhaps better identified as hypertensive cardiomyopathy—the ultimate cause of heart failure associated with hypertension—in its simplest form results from the increased workload of the heart, a true *hyperergopathic cardiomyopathy*.[9]

Hypertension seldom exists for a prolonged time without association with other factors that modify the response of the myocardium. These factors include genotype, gender and body size, and comorbid conditions such as coronary artery disease, diabetes mellitus, obesity, excessive alcohol intake, neurohumoral factor [renin-angiotensin-aldosterone system (RAAS), sympathetic nervous system (SNS)] activation, and many others. Hypertension thus becomes an important factor in the production of a *pluricausal* cardiomyopathy (cardiomyopathy resulting from more than one cause) and resultant heart failure; in fact, most heart failure is the result of *pluricausal* cardiomyopathy. Therefore, hypertension alone may produce cardiomyopathy and heart failure, but may also interact with other factors that are important in increasing the risk of developing myocardial disease and dysfunction.

EPIDEMIOLOGY

Much of what is known concerning the epidemiology of hypertension and heart failure has come from the Framingham study (see Chapter 22). As early as 1972, elevated BP (>140/90 mm Hg) was identified as the most frequent cause of heart failure, especially in the 30- to 62-year age group, occurring six times more frequently relative to individuals identified as normotensive.[2] In 1996, the progression from elevated BP alone to hypertension with congestive heart failure was reported in participants in the Original Framingham Heart Study and Framingham Offspring Study, which had been initiated on January 1, 1970.[10] During this interval a total of 5,143 subjects were observed with a mean follow-up 14.1 years. Elevated BP preceded the development of heart failure in 91% of the 392 new cases (Figure 28-1). The hazard for developing heart failure in hypertensive, compared with normotensive, subjects was approximately twofold in men and threefold in women after adjustment for age and heart failure risk factors in proportional hazards regression models. The 5-year survival rate for hypertensive heart failure was 24% for men and 31% for women.

Although much attention has been devoted to diastolic BP, the role of an elevated systolic BP is perhaps more important in the development of hypertensive heart disease. Heart failure is often preceded by isolated systolic hypertension as defined by a systolic BP greater than 160 mm Hg with a diastolic BP less than 90 mm Hg.[11] The importance of systolic BP in the production of hypertensive cardiomyopathy is supported by the finding that systolic pressure is a stronger determinant on left ventricular geometry and function than is diastolic pressure.[12]

The role of hypertension in the development of heart failure is of particular importance in the older patient population (see Chapter 49). More than 75% of heart failure patients in the United States are older than 65 years of age; heart failure is the leading cause of hospitalization in older adults.[13] Elevated BP is prevalent in older patients; heart failure in this group is often associated with preserved left ventricular systolic function and is perhaps due to diastolic dysfunction. Heart failure with preserved systolic function accounts for up to 50% of all cases of congestive heart failure in adults more than 65 years of age. In the Helsinki Aging Study, 8.2% of the cohort of subjects born in 1904, 1909, and 1914 developed heart failure; of these, 72% had normal left

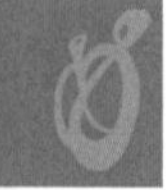

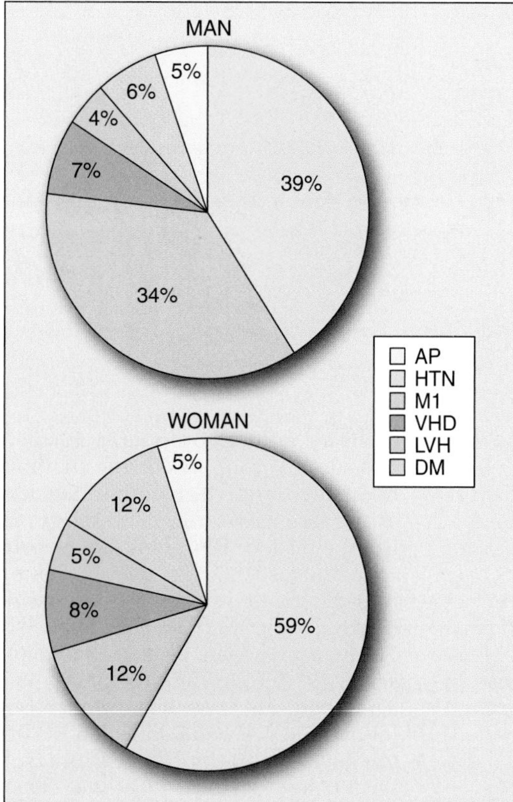

FIGURE 28–1 The epidemiology of heart failure. The prominent role played by hypertension in the development of heart failure is shown by data from the Framingham study. (From Levy D, Larson MG, Vasan RS, et al. The progression from hypertension to congestive heart failure. *JAMA* 1996;275:1557-1562.)

ventricular function determined by echocardiography.[14] Diastolic heart failure was found in 51% of patients and hypertension was the underlying cause in 54% of these subjects. Black patients with elevated BP are at increased risk for the development of heart failure (see Chapter 49). In a study of 301 black patients with congestive heart failure, systemic hypertension was the most common cause and was the primary cause in 61%.[15]

Some common comorbid conditions that contribute, along with hypertension, to the development of pluricausal cardiomyopathy and heart failure are coronary atherosclerosis, diabetes mellitus, and alcohol consumption. Among hypertensive subjects in the Framingham study, myocardial infarction, diabetes, left ventricular hypertrophy, and valvular heart disease were further predictive of increased risk for heart failure in both men and women.[10] Cardiovascular morbidity and mortality are increased 4.4 fold in type 2 diabetic patients in comparison with nondiabetic subjects even in the absence of classical risk factors including hypertension.[16] The coexistence of diabetes with elevated BP results in cardiomyopathy and heart failure in excess of that which would be expected from either one alone.[17-19] Increased alcohol consumption may also play a role in the development of heart failure in hypertensive individuals.[20]

Pathophysiology of Hypertensive Cardiomyopathy

The characteristic change that occurs in the heart secondary to a chronic increase in systemic arterial BP is left ventricular hypertrophy (LVH). At some point the hypertrophy ceases to be "physiological" in nature and becomes "pathological."[21] Although the characteristics of LVH are dependent on numerous factors that include age, sex, genotype, endocrine, autocrine, and paracrine influences, what is central to the development of ventricular hypertrophy is the reaction of the myocardium to increased wall stress secondary to increased pressures.

Mechanical Effects of Hypertension on the Left Ventricle. In individuals with normal blood pressure, factors that have been shown to influence left ventricular mass are genotype, gender, and body size.[22] The genetic influence on LV mass has been demonstrated in studies of monozygotic and dizygotic twins and population studies. Left ventricular mass index is increased in the offspring of parents with hypertension before increased systemic arterial pressure was present either at rest, or with exercise.[8] The influence of gender on LV mass becomes apparent at puberty and then persists throughout adulthood. Body size is important in determining LV mass, particularly lean body mass (75% of the variance). All of the previous determinants of LV mass influence the loading conditions of the ventricle and are, therefore, hemodynamic stimuli to the production of LVH. Thus in the normal individual, cardiac work (i.e., stroke volume times mean systolic pressure) is closely related to LV mass. Since stroke work is determined by the force required to overcome vascular impedance, it is interesting that the development of heart failure is related more to pulse pressure (an indirect assessment of vascular compliance) than to mean arterial pressure or previous myocardial infarction.[23] This reflects a loss of proximal arterial elastance associated with a decrease in elastin and an increase in type 4 collagen. Also important is the influence of heart rate, which determines the amount of work performed over time.

It has been suggested that a gender-specific LV mass can be determined and that theoretically, every value of observed LV mass that exceeds 100% of the predicted value may be considered as abnormally elevated. Thus by extension, a BP that is greater than "optimal" may, by increasing cardiac work, be associated with an abnormal increase in LV mass that may not, by current criteria, reach the threshold of "clinical hypertrophy."

The adaptive response of the left ventricle to an increased workload is primarily aimed at maintaining normal wall tension (see Chapter 15). Assuming the ventricle to be a sphere or ellipsoid, the average meridional wall stress is defined as force per unit area acting at the midplane of the heart in the direction of apex to base. Meridional or longitudinal wall stress (σ_m) is a function of the intracavitary pressure (P), the internal radius of the ventricle (R), and wall thickness (h): ($\sigma_m = PR/2h$). During normal ventricular systole, increases in LV pressure are matched by increases in wall thickness resulting from the thickening of the normal ventricular wall, thereby maintaining normal wall tension. However, when there is exposure to a chronic increase in ventricular pressure, as with elevated BP, the increase in wall thickness and muscle mass represents a structural change. The increase in thickness of the LV wall tends to maintain systolic wall stress (σ_m) within a narrow range despite variations in ventricular size or systolic pressure. There is an inverse relationship between LV systolic pressure and the radius/thickness (R/2h) or end-diastolic volume/mass ratio.

The concept of wall stress provides a means of interpretation for the patterns of hypertrophy apparent at the gross anatomical level. These patterns are concentric remodeling, concentric hypertrophy, and eccentric hypertrophy (see Chapter 15). Concentric remodeling is the first step in the restructuring of the heart and consists of an increase in wall thickness relative to LV end-diastolic dimensions without an increase in myocardial mass; this pattern is particularly apparent in the left ventricle. Remodeling is accomplished by a rearrangement of the cells of the myocardium so that the left ventricular cavity is reduced in its internal dimension. This concentric remodeling, by increasing LV wall thickness and reducing LV chamber diameter, maintains normal wall tension despite the increased systemic arterial pressure.

Concentric hypertrophy occurs when there is an increased myocardial mass with normal or reduced ventricular internal dimensions. Eccentric hypertrophy occurs when the ventricle becomes dilated; calculated myocardial mass is increased. When this occurs, the ventricle loses its mechanical advantage[24,25] and LV dilation increases the risk of heart failure.[26]

Cellular Biochemical and Molecular Aspects of Hypertensive Cardiomyopathy. All components of the myocardium—myocytes, interstitial cells, and the microcirculation—are involved in the myocardial remodeling process of hypertensive cardiomyopathy; formed elements of the blood, including monocytes and macrophages, may also play a role in the development of cardiomyopathy (see Chapter 11). Myocytes account for approximately 25% of all of the cells in the myocardium, but represent 70% of the myocardial mass. The number of cardiac myocytes is genetically determined and reaches a final amount within the first year after birth, when mitotic activity ceases.[26] Hypertrophy of myocytes occurs in response to the chronic increase in systolic wall tension produced by increased systemic arterial blood pressure. Thus the mechanical forces imposed by increased myocardial work provides a basis for the progression of myocardial disease in hypertension from progressive cardiomyopathy to the appearance of heart failure.[21,27-29] Initially, myocyte hypertrophy is accomplished by the addition of myofibrils in parallel, thus increasing the cross-sectional area of the individual myocytes.[21] This response to increased wall tension appears to involve expression of immediate early genes (IEGs), such as those encoding transcription factors, e.g., *c-fos, c-myc, c-jun,* and *egr-1*.[30-33] The IEG response is followed by an expression of a fetal genetic pattern, which may be characterized by the reexpression of ventricular mRNA for atrial natriuretic peptide (ANP), β-myosin heavy chain (β-MHC), and skeletal muscle α-actin. There is subsequently upregulation of several constitutively expressed genes, including vMLC-2 and cardiac muscle (CM) α-actin. Downregulation of certain genes such as sarcoplasmic reticulum (SR) Ca^{2+}-release channel (the ryanodine receptor) and SR Ca^{2+}-ATPase-2 (SERCA-2), which are responsible for cycling Ca^{2+} into and out of the SR, also occurs in this stage of myocyte hypertrophy.

The interstitium of the myocardium is pivotal to the remodeling of the heart that takes place during the process of the development of hypertensive heart disease. Fibrillar connective tissue, which constitutes the interstitium of the myocardium, contains mainly types I and III collagen. This fibrillar collagen network maintains the architecture of the myocardium and provides a means of tethering and orienting the myocytes, and is responsible for distributing diastolic filling stress throughout the ventricle. An abnormal increase of collagen (e.g., fibrosis) may be responsible for increased myocardial stiffness (i.e., loss of compliance). Hypertension may also be associated with increased perivascular interstitial fibrosis. After a prolonged period of hypertension, parenchymal cell injury and loss of myocytes develop, leading to replacement or reparative fibrosis in response to microscopic scarring resulting from myocyte necrosis. In contrast to the apparently benign myocyte hypertrophy without fibrosis that is seen in athletes who develop physiological LVH, biopsies from patients with hypertension *and* LVH demonstrate increased collagen content and extensive fibrosis; the degree of this fibrosis is a critical determinant of the severity of diastolic dysfunction. An inverse correlation between diastolic filling volume and percent of myocardial fibrosis as assessed by endomyocardial biopsy has been reported.[34]

A study exploring the fibrotic changes in diastolic heart failure (DHF) divided 86 hypertensive patients into groups according to the presence of DHF (32 with, 54 without) and the extent of diastolic dysfunction (20 with normal function, 38 with impaired relaxation, 10 with pseudonormalization, and 16 with restrictive filling). Serum carboxy-terminal telopeptide of procollagen type I, carboxy-terminal telopeptide of procollagen type I, amino-terminal propeptide of procollagen type III, MMP-2, and MMP-9 levels ($P < .001$ for all, controlled for age and gender) were greater in patients with DHF than in those without (see Chapters 5 and 14). When the results were controlled for age and gender, levels of serum carboxy-terminal telopeptide of procollagen type I, tissue inhibitor of MMP-1, amino-terminal propeptide of procollagen type III (all $P < .001$), carboxy-terminal telopeptide of procollagen type I ($P = .008$), and MMP-2 ($P = .03$) were greater in more severe phases of diastolic dysfunction. Within phases of diastolic dysfunction, serum carboxy-terminal telopeptide of procollagen type I, amino-terminal propeptide of procollagen type III, MMP-2, and MMP-9 were elevated in those with DHF compared with those without DHF (all $P < .001$), thus demonstrating active fibrosis.[35] The process governing this fibrosis is not well understood. Fibroblast stimulation is essential for reactive and reparative fibrosis. Recently data have suggested that the mineralocorticoid aldosterone may be important for the fibroblast activation.[36] Treatment with the aldosterone-antagonist spironolactone (25 mg/day) improved echocardiographic evidence of diastolic dysfunction in patients with hypertensive heart disease.[37]

Coronary vessels with a luminal diameter less than 100 μm constitute the resistance vessels of the myocardium and mainly control coronary blood flow. Since these vessels comprise more than 70% of the intramural arterial tree, rarefaction or inadequate growth in relation to hypertrophy of myocytes might diminish oxygen and substrate delivery despite the increased requirement due to hypertrophy. The actual demonstration of alterations of microvessels in hypertension has been somewhat controversial; however, the majority of evidence points to remodeling of the vessels, including hyperplasia of smooth muscle cells, edema, and increased content of collagen and other matrix components.[38] Hormonal stimulation and growth factors are involved (e.g., RAAS). Changes in the coronary circulation contribute to myocardial ischemia, both with and without the presence of epicardial coronary artery disease.

Clinical Presentations of Hypertensive Cardiomyopathy

The pathway from elevated BP to hypertension to heart failure involves LVH, interactions with comorbidities, and cardiac remodeling. The clinical presentation may be one of several intermediate phenotypes.

Left Ventricular Hypertrophy. The earliest clinical indication of hypertensive cardiomyopathy is the detection of asymptomatic LVH. LVH is, as discussed previously, initially adaptive because it permits the maintenance of normal systolic wall stress, fiber shortening, and stroke volume. In a large group of patients with ECG defined LVH enrolled in the LIFE (Losartan Intervention for Endpoint Reduction in Hypertension) study, 19% had normal geometry, 11% had concentric remodeling, 47% had eccentric hypertrophy, and 23% had concentric hypertrophy.[39] The ECG criteria used in LIFE (Cornell voltage-duration product >2440 and/or SV1 +/− RV5-6 >38 mm) identify hypertensive patients with a greater than 70% prevalence of anatomical LVH as documented by echocardiography, allowing accurate identification of high-risk status by this commonly used technique.[40,41]

LVH is more closely related to 24-hour BP than to casual (office) BP[40]; even transient increases in pressure may cause LVH.[42] However, the presence of "white coat hypertension" does not necessarily lead to major structural or functional cardiac abnormalities,[43] but may do so.[44] The presence of LVH by ECG predicts the development of heart failure in subsequent years. In the echocardiographic substudy of the LIFE study, inappropriate LVH (observed/predicted LV mass >128%) had a greater incidence of decreased LV systolic function.[45]

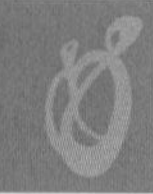

Heart Failure in Hypertensive Cardiomyopathy. The clinical presentation of hypertensive cardiomyopathy follows the morphological and functional changes associated with ventricular hypertrophy and remodeling. Even though hypertension is associated with alterations in right ventricular function, the clinical presentations involve changes primarily in the left ventricle.

Heart Failure with Preserved Systolic Function (Diastolic Dysfunction). Heart failure may be present clinically in patients with hypertension when measured systolic function is normal (see Chapters 14 and 48). Such presentations may be due to diastolic dysfunction that result in impaired filling of the left ventricle due to decreased lusitropy (inability of the ventricle to relax properly). In patients having acute pulmonary edema associated with hypertension and a normal LVEF (>0.50), the edema is due to the exacerbation of diastolic dysfunction by increases in systemic arterial pressure and intravascular volume and not to transient systolic dysfunction or mitral regurgitation.[46] Diastolic dysfunction is usually apparent early in hypertension after the development of pathological hypertrophy associated with concentric remodeling or concentric hypertrophy. Patients usually are initially aware of symptoms with exertion but increasing symptoms become apparent at rest.[47] The symptoms of diastolic dysfunction are associated with abnormal diastolic filling pressures required to fill the left ventricle, which result in interstitial lung edema or which limit ventricular filling and thus compromise cardiac output. These symptoms are those of dyspnea and fatigue. Furthermore, pathologically hypertrophied myocardium is a substrate for cardiac arrhythmias. Thus palpitations may be a symptom of hypertensive cardiomyopathy. Physical examination may show jugular venous distention, pulmonary rales, an abnormal cardiac apical impulse (occasionally bifid) and an abnormal early (protodiastolic, S_3) or late (atrial, S_4) gallop sounds. A more laterally displaced cardiac apical impulse, more systemic venous hypertension, and peripheral edema usually characterize advanced hypertensive cardiomyopathy associated with eccentric ventricular remodeling.

Systolic dysfunction and heart failure associated with hypertensive cardiomyopathy may eventually develop late as a complication of the hypertensive process. Although resting systolic function remains normal in hypertensives for a considerable period of time even when LVH is present, systolic dysfunction may become more apparent with exercise.[48] Thus while diastolic dysfunction may be present, it is the same myocardium in systole and diastole—abnormal in both instances.

Hypertension and Pluricausal Cardiomyopathy

Myocardial Ischemia, Coronary Heart Disease, and Hypertension. Myocardial ischemia may be present in patients with hypertension in the face of normal coronary arteries by angiography due to small vessel disease as elaborated earlier.[49] Therefore, patients with hypertension often have symptoms of chest discomfort not due to epicardial coronary artery obstruction. However, hypertension is a risk factor for the development of coronary atherosclerosis. The contribution of hypertension to the progression of ventricular dysfunction in the face of coronary atherosclerosis and subsequent complications, including transient myocardial ischemia and myocardial infarction, is considerable (see Chapter 23).

Myocardial ischemia produced by atherosclerotic epicardial obstruction of coronary arteries is worsened by the presence of hypertensive cardiomyopathy. Hypertrophic cardiomyopathy increases the resistance to blood flow across the myocardial wall; since there is increased wall tension, subendocardial perfusion is impaired, and this may contribute to transient myocardial ischemia and myocardial stunning. Increases in ventricular impedance to ejection by infusion of methoxamine over a 4-hour period has been demonstrated to produce relative infarct expansion and thinning in the early phase of infarct healing in dogs.[50] Similarly, aortic banding in the rat has been shown to increase infarct expansion independent of infarct size.[51]

Myocardial infarction results in the segmental loss of myocardium that results in increased physical burden for the remaining myocardium.[52-54] The ventricular remodeling that follows myocardial infarction occurring in a heart with hypertensive cardiomyopathy must contend with increased wall tension, now secondary to both ventricular dilation and increased arterial pressure that are consequences of pathological hypertrophy already present in the remaining, noninfarcted myocardium. Hypertensive hypertrophic cardiomyopathy is associated with increased morbidity and mortality after myocardial infarction. Moreover, necropsy studies have shown a positive correlation between a history of systemic hypertension and ventricular expansion and rupture. Thus both experimental and clinical data demonstrate the powerful effects of the mechanical aspects of hypertension in complications of coronary atherosclerosis.

Interactions of Diabetes Mellitus with Hypertension in Heart Failure. Diabetes mellitus is associated with the development of cardiomyopathy independent of the increased atherosclerosis often seen in these patients. The risk of heart failure is greatly increased in diabetic patients (see Chapter 26) as evidenced by data from the Framingham Heart Study.[55] In this study, diabetic male patients had more than twice the incidence rate of heart failure compared with nondiabetic cohorts, while diabetic women showed a fivefold increased risk. The cardiomyopathy of diabetes is markedly increased in the presence of increased systemic arterial pressure.[18,19] Mechanisms for the production of diabetic cardiomyopathy include increased oxidative stress, nonenzymatic glycosylation of proteins, alterations in intracellular signaling, and abnormalities in myocardial metabolism.[18,19] Abnormalities in diastolic function assessed by echocardiography occur in 27% to 69% of asymptomatic diabetic patients and may be followed by the development of clinical heart failure.[56]

Prevention and Treatment of Hypertensive Cardiomyopathy and Heart Failure

Prevention of Heart Failure in Hypertension. Increased emphasis is being placed on preventive strategies to decrease the incidence and prevalence of heart failure. The American College of Cardiology/American Heart Association (ACC/AHA) Guidelines for the Evaluation and Management of Heart Failure describe criteria for four stages of heart failure (i.e., A-D).[57] Stages A and B are not really heart failure but rather early stages of cardiomyopathy. Notably, hypertension (stage A) and left ventricular hypertrophy (stage B) are important antecedents for the development of heart failure (Table 28-1).

It has been suggested that treatment of hypertension *alone* may result in a reduction in relative risk of developing heart failure by approximately 50%[58,59] (Figure 28-2). The effect of the treatment of hypertension on the development of heart failure in patients with isolated systolic hypertension is striking. Risk was reduced by 51% in the Swedish Trial of Old Persons Hypertension (STOP) Trial (Figure 28-3, A),[60] and by 55% in the Systolic Hypertension in Elderly Program (SHEP) trial (see Figure 28-3, B).[61] Other analyses show that whereas HF accounted for more than half of the deaths in hypertensive patients before the advent of adequate antihypertensive drugs, its contribution to mortality has fallen considerably.[62,63] The risk reduction for heart failure by treating hypertension is strikingly illustrated in a meta-analysis of the efficacy of various antihypertensive therapies used as first-line agents.[64]

In patients with hypertension, a reduction in LV mass during treatment is a favorable prognostic marker that predicts a lesser risk for subsequent cardiovascular morbid events. Such

TABLE 28–1 The Early Stages of Heart Failure

Stage	Description	Examples
A	Patients at high risk of developing heart failure (HF) because of the presence of conditions that are strongly associated with the development of HF. Such patients have no identified structural or functional abnormalities of the pericardium, myocardium, or cardiac valves and have never shown signs or symptoms of HF.	*Systemic hypertension*; coronary artery disease; diabetes mellitus; history of cardiotoxic drug therapy or alcohol abuse; personal history of rheumatic fever; family history of cardiomyopathy
B	Patients who have developed structural heart disease that is strongly associated with the development of HF but who have never shown signs or symptoms of HF.	*Left ventricular hypertrophy* or fibrosis; left ventricular dilation or hypocontractility; asymptomatic valvular heart disease; previous myocardial infarction.

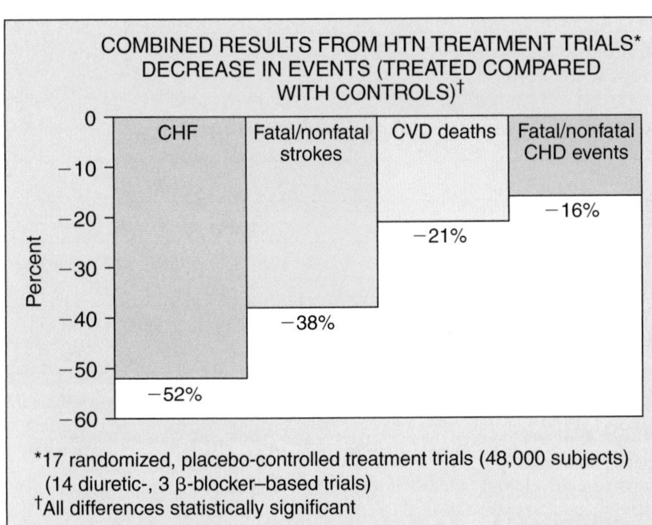

FIGURE 28–2 Effect of antihypertensive treatment on the incidence of heart failure, strokes, cardiovascular deaths, and coronary heart disease events (48,000 subjects). (Modified from Hebert PR, Moser M, Mayer, et al. Recent evidence on drug therapy of mild to moderate hypertension and decreased risk of coronary heart disease. *Arch Intern Med* 1993;153[5]:578-581 and Moser M, Herbert PR. Prevention of disease progression, left ventricular hypertrophy and congestive heart failure in hypertension treatment trials. *J Am Coll Cardiol* 1996;27:1214-1218.)

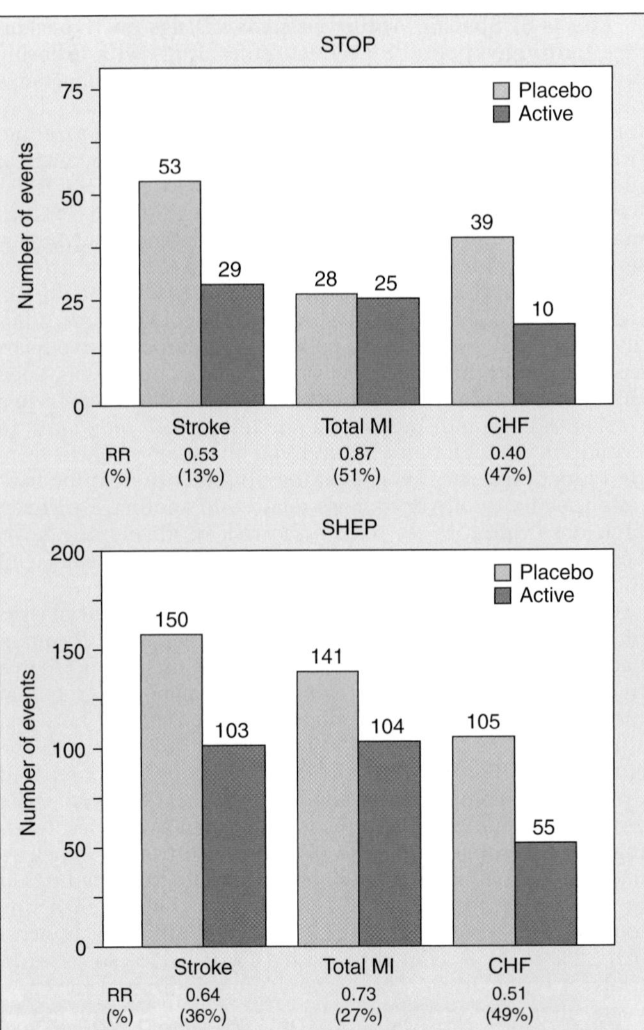

FIGURE 28–3 Reduction of cardiovascular events by treating hypertension in the elderly. **A,** Results of the Swedish Trial of Old Persons Hypertension trial (STOP). **B,** Results of the Systolic Hypertension in the Elderly Program (SHEP) trial. (From Dahlöf B, Lindholm LH, Hannson L, et al. Morbidity and mortality in the Swedish trial in old patients with hypertension [STOP hypertension]. *Lancet* 1991;338:1281-1285 and SHEP Cooperative Research Group. Prevention of stroke by antihypertensive drug treatment in older persons with isolated systolic hypertension. Final results of the systolic hypertension in the elderly program [SHEP]. *JAMA* 1991;266:3255-3264.)

an association is independent of baseline LV mass, baseline clinic and ambulatory BP, and degree of BP reduction.[65]

An attempt to gain insight into the importance of regression of LVH on cardiovascular outcomes was made with the Losartan Intervention For Endpoint reduction in hypertension study (LIFE). The trial was conducted in 9193 participants older than 55 years of age who had hypertension and ECG LVH. Patients were randomized to treatment with either losartan-based or atenolol-based therapy and followed for 4 years. Blood pressure reduction was equal for both treatment groups. Losartan-based therapy was associated with greater prevention of cardiovascular morbidity and mortality and fewer instances of new-onset diabetes than atenolol-based therapy. An analysis with the ECG indices of LVH as time-varying covariates showed a partial (less than one third) relation with the effect of losartan-based treatment on the primary outcome. There was no difference in the losartan-based and atenolol-based treatment groups for admission to the hospital for heart failure.[66]

Yet further evidence supporting the critical importance of BP reduction comes from the CARDIO-SIS trial,[67] in which 1111 nondiabetic and thus lower risk patients with systolic BP of 150 mm Hg or greater were randomly assigned to a target systolic pressure of 140 mm Hg or to a lower target of less than 130 mm Hg. Antihypertensive medications were not specified and were tailored by the treating physician to individually bring the patient to target. After randomization, patients were followed for 2 years. Over 2 years of observation, systolic and diastolic BP decreased by 23.5 mm Hg and 8.9 mm Hg, respectively, in the usual-control arm and 27.3 mm Hg and 10.4 mm Hg in the tight-control arm. The primary endpoint of electrocardiographic LVH occurred in 17% of patients treated to the usual systolic BP target and in 11.4% of patients treated to less than 130 mm Hg. This translated into a significant 37% reduction in risk. A prespecified secondary endpoint, a composite of death from any cause, MI, stroke, transient ischemic attack, atrial fibrillation, admission for heart failure, angina, or coronary revascularization, occurred in 9.4% of individuals treated to the usual target and 4.8% of those treated to a lower systolic pressure goal.

Effects of Specific Antihypertensive Drugs on Hypertensive Cardiomyopathy. BP reduction by drugs with differing mechanisms of action may provide clues to the importance of nonhemodynamic mechanisms in reducing LV mass. Confounding such an analysis is the observation that a reduction in BP and LV mass may result from nonpharmacological means alone, and the resulting reduction in LV mass is similar to that achieved with antihypertensive drugs.[68] Such findings make it difficult to determine if different classes of antihypertensive drugs vary in ability to reduce LVH.

Several meta-analyses have suggested that RAAS blocking drugs are more effective in reducing LVH than other classes.[69-71] BP reduction in patients with hypertensive heart disease results in a decrease in LV mass. Thus it has been difficult to determine whether there is additional benefit to a further reduction of LV mass at any level of BP reduction. In principle, the higher the BP, and thus the greater benefit from BP reduction alone, the greater the difficulty in defining benefits specific to one drug class relative to another. However, high dose diuretics do reduce the risk of developing heart failure compared with low dose diuretics or β-blockers, but increase the risk of sudden death.

The issues of the quantitative efficacy of different classes of blood pressure lowering drugs in preventing coronary heart disease (CHD) and stroke, and of who should receive treatment, has been addressed in a meta-analysis that included 108 trials that studied differences in BP between study drug and placebo (or control group not receiving the study drug) (BP difference trials), and 46 trials that compared drugs (drug comparison trials)[72] (Table 28-2). Seven trials with three randomized groups fell into both categories, totaling 958,000 subjects.[4] In the BP difference trials, β-blockers had a special effect over and above that due to BP reduction in preventing recurrent CHD events in people with a history of CHD: risk reduction 29% (95% confidence interval [CI] 22% to 34%) compared with 15% (CI, 11% to 19%) in trials of other drugs. The extra effect was limited to a few years after myocardial infarction, with a risk reduction of 31% compared with 13% in people with CHD with no recent infarct (P = .04). In the other BP difference trials (excluding CHD events in trials of β-blockers in people with CHD), there was a 22% reduction in CHD events (17% to 27%) and a 41% (33% to 48%) reduction in stroke for a BP reduction of 10 mm Hg systolic or 5 mm Hg diastolic, similar to the reductions of 25% (CHD) and 36% (stroke) expected for the same difference in BP from the cohort study meta-analysis, indicating that the benefit is explained by pressure reduction in itself. The five main classes of drugs (thiazides, β-blockers, angiotensin-converting enzyme inhibitors (ACEI), angiotensin receptor blockers (ARB), and calcium channel blockers) were similarly effective (within a few percentage points) in preventing CHD events and strokes, with the exception that calcium channel blockers had a greater preventive effect on stroke (relative risk, 0.92; 95% CI, 0.85 to 0.98). The percentage reductions in CHD and stroke were similar in people with and without cardiovascular disease and regardless of blood pressure before treatment (down to 110 mm Hg systolic and 70 mm Hg diastolic). When these results were combined with those from other studies, analysis showed that in people aged 60 to 69 with a diastolic pressure before treatment of 90 mm Hg, three drugs at half standard dose in combination reduced the risk of CHD by an estimated 46% and of stroke by 62%; one drug at standard dose had about half this effect. Drugs other than calcium channel blockers and noncardioselective β-blockers reduced the incidence of heart failure by 24% (19% to 28%), and calcium channel blockers by 19% (6% to 31%). With the exception of the extra protective effect of β-blockers given shortly after a myocardial infarction and the minor additional effect of calcium channel blockers in preventing stroke, all classes of antihypertensive drugs have a similar effect in reducing CHD events and stroke for a given reduction in pressure, thus apparently excluding effects other than BP itself. The proportional reduction in cardiovascular disease events was the same or similar regardless of pretreatment BP and the presence or absence of existing cardiovascular disease. Lowering systolic pressure by 10 mm Hg or diastolic pressure by 5 mm Hg using any of the main classes of drugs reduced CHD events (fatal and nonfatal) by about a quarter and stroke by about a third, regardless of the presence or absence of vascular disease and of pretreatment BP. Heart failure is also reduced by about 25%.

However, in these trials BP was measured as brachial cuff pressure; only recently has there been recognition of differential effects of antihypertensive drugs upon central aortic pressure, and of the potential impact of these differences in central pressure reductions on target organs. Data from the Anglo-Cardiff Collaborative Trial II demonstrated that cardiovascular risk factors affect the pulse pressure ratio and that central pressure cannot be reliably inferred from peripheral pressure. These observations suggested that assessment of central pressure may improve the identification and management of patients with elevated cardiovascular risk.[73]

TABLE 28–2 Risk Reduction in Heart Failure by Type of Drug Treatment

Class of Drug	No. of Trials	No. of Episodes	Relative Risk* (95% CI)
Blood Pressure Difference Trials			
Single drug therapy			
Calcium channel blockers	13	1519	0.81 (0.69-0.94)
Thiazides	5	222	0.59 (0.45-0.78)
β-Blockers	13	2846	0.77 (0.69-0.87)
Angiotensin-converting enzyme inhibitors	16	3834	0.74 (0.68-0.81)
Angiotensin receptor blockers	3	1675	0.82 (0.73-0.92)
All drug classes except calcium channel blockers	36†	8553†	0.76 (0.72-0.81)
Combination drug therapy	7	144	0.57 (0.36-0.92)
Drug Comparison Trials			
Calcium channel blockers vs. any other drug class	21	4572	1.22 (1.10-1.35)
Drug comparisons not involving calcium channel blockers:			
Thiazides	2	2335	0.91 (0.64-1.30)
β-Blockers	2	335	1.04 (0.84-1.29)
Angiotensin-converting enzyme inhibitors	9	5063	0.98 (0.91-1.06)
Angiotensin receptor blockers	7	2436	1.00 (0.93-1.08)

*Relative risk <1.0 indicates specified drug class reduces risk of heart failure; >1.0 increases risk.

†All trial totals are less than column totals because one trial had two treated groups sharing same placebo group.

Results are shown from 64 blood pressure difference trials and 31 drug comparison trials of blood pressure lowering drugs.

(Reprinted with permission Law MR, Morris JK, Wald NJ. Use of blood pressure lowering drugs in the prevention of cardiovascular disease: meta-analysis of 147 randomised trials in the context of expectations from prospective epidemiological studies. *BMJ* 2009;338:1245-1253.)

In a separate trial,[74] central pulse pressure was reduced significantly by perindopril, the dihydropyridine lercanidipine, and bendrofluazide, whereas atenolol had no effect. Lercanidipine reduced the augmentation index, whereas atenolol increased it. However, aortic pulse wave velocity was not changed by any of the drugs. The vasodilating β-blocker nebivolol has also been demonstrated to reduce both forearm vascular resistance, central aortic pressure, and augmentation index to a greater extent than nonvasodilating β-blockers[75,76] (Figure 28-4). An analysis from the Strong Heart Study suggests that noninvasive measurements of central aortic pressure more closely identify the presence of vascular disease, as detected by carotid ultrasound, than do standard brachial pressure readings and are also more predictive of outcomes.[77] That central aortic pressure and augmentation indexes are differentially reduced by different drug classes despite the presence of similar effects on brachial artery blood pressure was shown in the CAFE (Conduit Artery Function Evaluation) substudy of the ASCOT (Anglo-Scandinavian Cardiac Outcomes Trial); importantly, central pulse pressure was significantly associated with a post hoc-defined composite outcome of total cardiovascular events/procedures and development of renal impairment.[78] Furthermore, in end-stage renal disease patients, the insensitivity of central aortic pressure to decreased blood pressure is an independent predictor of mortality.[79]

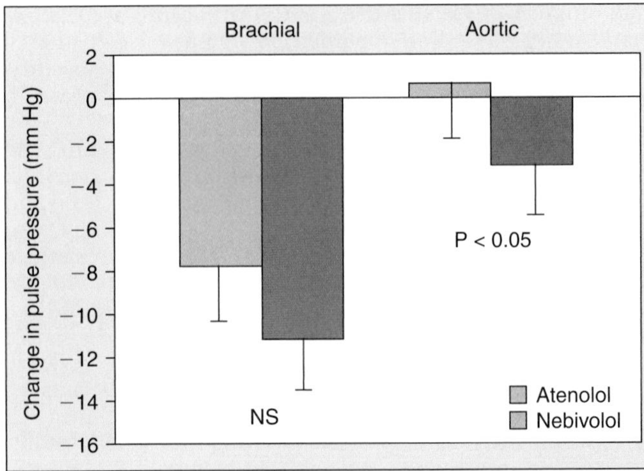

FIGURE 28-4 Differential effects of brachial versus central aortic pressure of atenolol compared with nebivolol. (Modified from Pederson ME, Cockcroft JR. The vasodilatory beta-blockers. *Curr Hypertens Rep* 2007;9[4]: 269-277.)

Hypertension, Diabetes Mellitus, and Heart Failure. Understanding of BP management in diabetes began to change with the publications of the United Kingdom Prospective Diabetes Study beginning in 1998[80,81] in which 1148 hypertensive diabetics were randomized to "tight" (<150/85 mm Hg) versus "less tight" (<180/105 mm Hg) BP control. Within the "tight" control group, 400 diabetics were assigned to ACE inhibitors and 358 patients to β-blockers. The "less tight" control group (n = 390) could not receive either of these classes of drugs. Diabetic-related deaths were significantly reduced equally well with β-blockers as with ACEI. However, the less tightly controlled group had significantly more diabetic-related deaths (P = .019). There was no reduction in all cause mortality (P = .17) or myocardial infarction (P = .13); however, there was a significant reduction in heart failure (P = .0043), strokes (P = .013), and microvascular disease (P = .0092) in the tightly controlled diabetic group. Furthermore, microvascular endpoints (renal failure, death, vitreous hemorrhage or photocoagulation) were reduced equally well with β-blockers as with ACEI in the tightly controlled group and less well in the less tightly controlled group. It is now known that the benefits seen in the UKPDS extend to blood pressures of less than 110 mm Hg systolic BP. These findings have been further reinforced in the SANDS using the surrogate marker of intimal/medial thickness in American Indians with type 2 diabetes.[82]

Studies Treating Isolated Systolic Hypertension: SHEP and Syst-Eur. Systolic BP is recognized as an important marker for cardiovascular disease. The overall cardiovascular mortality is two to three times greater in diabetics compared with nondiabetics for every level of systolic pressure.[16] This observation led to expectations for BP interventions in diabetics with isolated systolic hypertension. The Systolic Hypertension in the Elderly Program (SHEP) showed that a diuretic-based therapy in diabetics was effective in heart failure by heart failure by 49% (see Figure 28-3, *B*), and by reducing major cardiovascular events by 34%, strokes by 22% (not significant), nonfatal myocardial infarctions and fatal coronary heart disease events by 54%, CHD events by 56% and all cause mortality by 26% (not significant).[8] Post hoc analysis of the Systolic Hypertension in Europe (SYS-EUR) Trial showed that overall cardiovascular mortality was reduced in diabetics.[83] The dihydropyridine nitrendipine given with or without an ACEI and/or a diuretic reduced stroke risk in 492 diabetics by 69% compared with placebo (P = .02) and reduced cardiac events by 57% (not significantly different compared with placebo). With an adjusted analysis for baseline differences, overall mortality, cardiovascular mortality, cardiovascular events and stroke events and cardiac events were all significantly reduced in the 492 diabetic patients, but not in the 4203 non diabetic patients.

Hypertension Optimal Treatment Trial. The Hypertension Optimal Treatment (HOT) Trial, a prospective, open-labeled, blinded endpoint (PROBE) design trial, enrolled subjects with a diastolic pressure of 100 to 115 mm Hg.[84] Participants received antihypertensive medicines according to an algorithm in which felodipine, either an ACEI or a β-blocker, and a diuretic were given to achieve one of three levels of blood pressure goals (<90 mm Hg, <85 mm Hg, or <80 mm Hg). Compared with the treatment goal of less than 90 mm Hg versus *less than* 80 mm Hg, major cardiovascular events among the 1501 diabetics were reduced by 51% (P = .005 for trend), an observation not explained by the trend in the reduction in myocardial infarction (P = .11) and stroke (P = .34). Furthermore, there was no significant reduction in overall mortality (P = .068). However, in the subset of patients with diabetes, there was a significant reduction with lower diastolic pressure targets.

Heart Outcomes Prevention Evaluation Study. The Heart Outcomes Prevention Evaluation (HOPE) study was a randomized, double blind two by two factorial design study involving 9541 subjects, who had to be at least 55 years of age and have a high risk for vascular disease, which could include coronary artery disease, stroke, peripheral vascular disease, or diabetes mellitus with one other risk factor (hypertension, elevated total cholesterol, low HDL cholesterol, cigarette smoking, or documented microalbuminuria).[85] The risk of cardiovascular disease was significantly reduced when 10 mg of ramipril was given once daily. There was a 22% reduction in myocardial infarction, stroke, and cardiovascular death and all cause mortality. The diabetic subgroup (n = 3577) and the patients with microalbuminuria (n = 1956) treated with ramipril significantly benefited relative to the placebo group.

Candesartan in Heart Failure-Assessment of Reduction in Mortality and Morbidity (CHARM)-Preserved Study. A total of 3023 patients with heart failure symptoms and LVEF of 40% received candesartan (32 mg/day) or placebo for 36.6 months.[86] Candesartan reduced BP by a mean of 7/3 mm Hg, and, when adjusted for covariates, reduced the primary endpoint (cardiovascular death and heart failure hospitalization) by 14%, a finding of borderline significance ($P = .051$). Although there was no effect on cardiovascular mortality, candesartan treatment resulted in a significant decrease in hospitalizations for heart failure.

I-PRESERVE. In the I-PRESERVE trial, 4128 patients who were 60 years old with heart failure and LVEF greater than 45% were randomized to irbesartan (300 mg) or placebo and followed for 49.5 months[87] (see Figure 28-4). The patient population was typical for diastolic heart failure; the mean age was 72 years, 60% were women, 88% had a history of hypertension, and 63% had a hypertensive cause for heart failure. Irbesartan reduced BP by a mean of 3.8/2.1 mm Hg. There was, however, no difference in the occurrence of the primary endpoint (death or hospitalization for cardiovascular causes), mortality, heart failure hospitalization, or quality of life.

Together with CHARM-Preserved, this trial RAAS inhibition again reinforces the concept that extent of BP control, rather than any specific pharmacological mechanism of drug action in the absence of significant blood pressure reduction, is the determinant of clinical outcome.

Valsartan in Diastolic Dysfunction (VALIDD) Trial. VALIDD was designed to address the role of diastolic dysfunction as an important pathophysiological intermediate between hypertension and heart failure, testing the possibility that inhibitors of the RAAS, which can reduce ventricular hypertrophy and myocardial fibrosis, can improve diastolic function to a greater extent than can other antihypertensive agents (Figure 28-5).[88] Patients with hypertension and evidence of diastolic dysfunction were randomly assigned to receive either valsartan (titrated to 320 mg once daily) or matched placebo. Patients in both groups also received concomitant antihypertensive agents that did not inhibit RAAS to reach targets less than 135 mm Hg systolic pressure and less than 80 mm Hg diastolic pressure. The primary endpoint was the change in diastolic relaxation velocity between baseline and 38 weeks as determined by tissue Doppler imaging. Analyses were done with the intention to treat 186 patients who were randomly assigned to receive valsartan and 198 who received a placebo. Over 38 weeks, there was a 12.8/7.1 mm Hg reduction in pressure in the valsartan group and a 9.7 mm Hg reduction in the placebo group that was not significant between the two groups. Diastolic relaxation velocity increased in both groups, with no significant difference between the groups ($P = .29$). Thus this carefully conducted trial, together with the two other angiotensin receptor blocker trials described earlier, have demonstrated that lowering BP improves diastolic function irrespective of the type of antihypertensive agent used.

Antihypertensive and Lipid-Lowering Treatment to Prevent Heart Attack Trial (ALLHAT). ALLHAT was designed to determine whether newer antihypertensive agents (lisinopril or amlodipine) reduce the incidence of cardiovascular disease when compared with diuretics (chlorthalidone or doxazosin). ALLHAT randomized a total of 33,357 patients (aged ≥ 55 years) with hypertension and at least one other coronary heart disease (CHD) risk factor to receive chlorthalidone (12.5 to 25 mg/day) amlodipine (2.5 to 10 mg/day); or lisinopril (10 to 40 mg/day). The primary outcome was combined fatal coronary heart disease or nonfatal myocardial infarction, analyzed by intention-to-treat. Secondary outcomes were all-cause mortality, stroke, combined CHD (primary outcome, coronary revascularization, or angina with hospitalization), and combined cardiovascular death (combined CHD, stroke, treated angina without hospitalization, heart failure or hospitalized/fatal heart failure). As shown in Figure 28-6, there was a significant 38% decreased risk of heart failure and a 35% decreased risk of hospitalization/fatal heart failure in the chlorthalidone treated group when compared with the amlodipine treated group, consistent with prior reports with calcium channel blockers in hypertension. There was also a significant 19% decreased risk of heart failure and a nonsignificant 10% decreased risk of hospitalization/fatal heart failure in the chlorthalidone treated group when compared with the lisinopril treated group. The treatment effects were consistent among subgroups by gender,

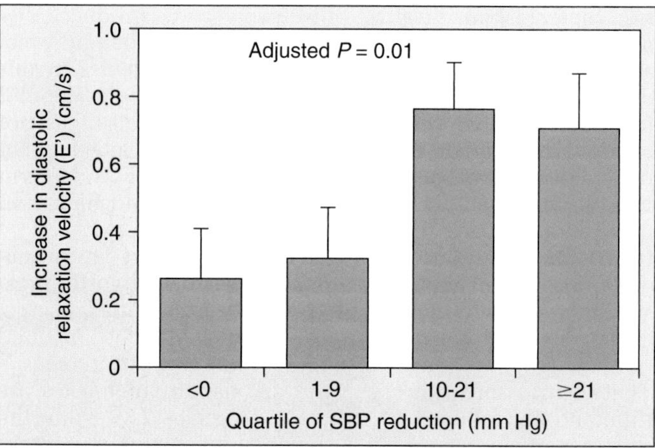

FIGURE 28–5 Change in diastolic function by quartile reduction in systolic blood pressure (SBP). (Modified from Solomon SD, Janardhanan R, Verma A, et al. Effect of angiotensin receptor blockade and antihypertensive drugs on diastolic function in patients with hypertension and diastolic dysfunction: a randomised trial. *Lancet* 2007;369[9579]:2079-2087.)

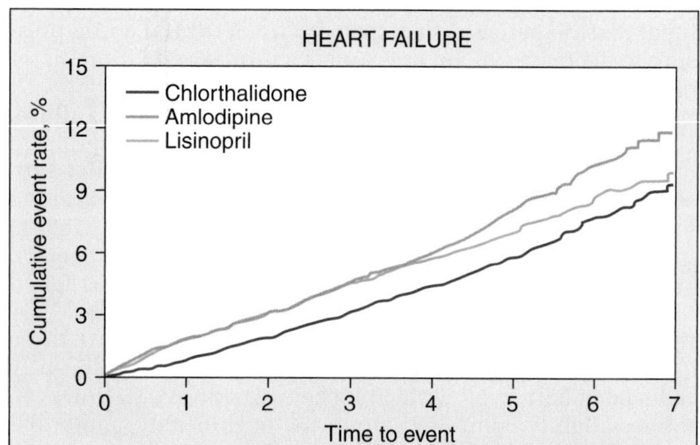

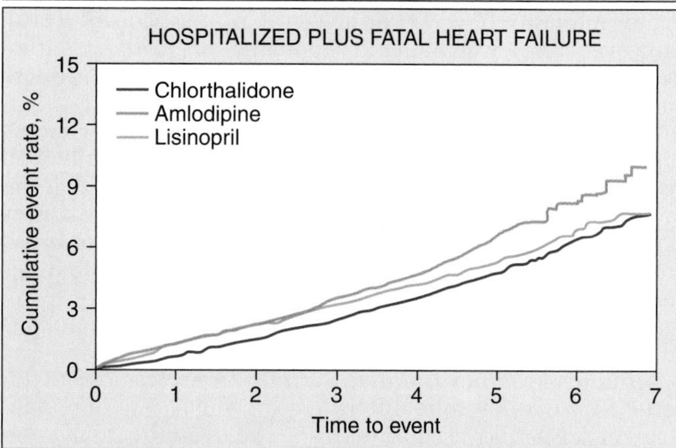

FIGURE 28–6 Cumulative event rates for heart failure and hospitalization with fatal heart failure in the ALLHAT trial. **Top,** Event rates for heart failure. **Bottom,** Event rates for hospitalization plus fatal heart failure. (Modified from The ALLHAT Officers and Coordinators for the ALLHAT Collaborative Research Group. Major outcomes in high-risk hypertensive patients randomized to angiotensin-converting enzyme inhibitor or calcium channel blocker vs. diuretic: the antihypertensive and lipid-lowering treatment to prevent heart attack trial [ALLHAT] *JAMA* 2002;288:2981-2997.) Copyright (2011) American Medical Association. All rights reserved.

diabetic status, and underlying CHD status. Whether the salutary effects of chlorthalidone in ALLHAT represent better control of blood pressure, superior control of "congestion" with a diuretic, or an unknown effect on the development and progression of heart failure are not known.[89] Data from a separate arm of the ALLHAT showed that there was a twofold increase in the incidence of heart failure (8.1% vs. 4.4%) for doxazosin when compared with chlorthalidone.[90]

CONCLUSION

Hypertension is the number one modifiable risk factor for the development of heart failure associated both with reduced and preserved left ventricular systolic function. Data from multiple clinical trials have demonstrated convincingly that reducing elevated systemic arterial pressures produces marked decreases in the incidence of heart failure. Yet, only one third of patients with known hypertension have BP controlled to the minimum of 140/80 mm Hg. Only 35.8% of participants in the Third National Health and Nutrition Examination Survey (NHANES III, conducted 1988-1994) and NHANES 1999-2000 achieved the target of systolic blood pressure (SBP) less than 130 mm Hg and diastolic blood pressure (DBP) less than 80 mm Hg, and 40.4% had hypertensive blood pressure levels (SBP ≥ 140 or DBP ≥ 90 mm Hg). NHANES 1999-2000 percentages did not change significantly from NHANES III ($P = .10$ and $P = .56$, respectively).

Although hypertension alone may result in heart failure, heart failure usually results when hypertension coexists with other diseases that affect the myocardium (e.g., coronary atherosclerosis, diabetes mellitus). In particular, aggressive treatment of increased blood pressure in patients with diabetes mellitus is warranted to reduce cardiovascular morbidity in general, and heart failure in particular.

Thus the choice of drugs for the treatment of hypertension should be based upon their efficacy in preventing heart failure rather than their ability to induce LVH regression. However, the direct acting vasodilators hydralazine and minoxidil should probably not be first line therapy because they do not cause LV regression either in experimental animals or in humans and better drugs are available. American and European guidelines suggest that the most effective agents in reducing heart failure are diuretics, ACEI, ARB, and β-blockers.[91,92] The Antihypertensive and Lipid-Lowering treatment to prevent Heart Attack Arial (ALLHAT) trial demonstrated that the α_1-blocking agent doxazosin was less effective in preventing heart failure than were diuretic, calcium channel blocker, or ACE inhibitor[90]; this class is also no longer recommended as first-line therapy.

It is, however, critically important to recognize that the selection of antihypertensive agents may be driven by the need to treat comorbidities. It is very interesting to note that there is evidence that RAAS inhibition in type 2 diabetic patients with nephropathy may have renoprotective effects beyond that of blood pressure reduction alone, thus necessitating early use of RAAS inhibition in patients in this category.[93]

Based on recent trials, the JNC VII has slightly modified its recommendations for the treatment of hypertension in diabetics.[94] The treatment goal remained less than 130/85 mm Hg; ACE inhibitors remained initial therapy in the presence of albuminuria or proteinuria. However, from the initial drug selection α_1-blockers were eliminated and β-blockers were added.

Much of the role of hypertension on the heart may be attributed to the increased mechanical effects of an increased BP, which does not preclude the influence of other neurohormonal and local cellular mechanisms in the production of pathological left ventricular hypertrophy. Nevertheless, it is apparent that the major step in preventing hypertension-associated heart failure is to control BP.[95] This is supported by the 2009 ACC/AHA guidelines in which control of systolic and diastolic hypertension is a class I recommendation (level of evidence A) for the treatment of diastolic heart failure.[96]

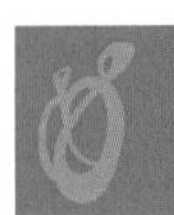

REFERENCES

1. He, J., & Whelton, P. K. (1997). Epidemiology and prevention of hypertension. *Med Clin North Am, 81*, 1077–1097.
2. Kannel, W. B., Castelli, W. P., McNamara, P. M., et al. (1972). Role of blood pressure in the development of congestive heart failure. *N Engl J Med, 287*, 781–787.
3. He, J., Ogden, L. G., Bazzano, L. A., et al. (2001). Risk factors for congestive heart failure in US men and women: NHANES I epidemiologic follow-up study. *Arch Intern Med, 161*, 996–1002.
4. Lewington, S., Clarke, R., Qizilbash, N., et al. (2002). Prospective studies collaboration age-specific relevance of usual blood pressure to vascular mortality: a meta-analysis of individual data for one million adults in 61 prospective studies. *Lancet, 360*(9349), 1903–1913.
5. Giles, T. D., Berk, B. C., Black, H. R., et al. (2005). Expanding the definition and classification of hypertension. *J Clin Hypertens (Greenwich), 7*(9), 505–512.
6. Perera, G. A. (1955). Hypertensive vascular disease: description and natural history. *J Chronic Dis, 1*, 33–42.
7. Joint National Committee on Prevention. (1997). Detection, Evaluation, and Treatment of High Blood Pressure. The sixth report of the joint national committee on prevention, detection, evaluation, and treatment of high blood pressure. *Arch Intern Med, 157*, 2413–2446.
8. Celentano, A., Galderisi, M., Garofalo, M., et al. (1988). Blood pressure and cardiac morphology in young children of hypertensive subjects. *J Hypertens, 6*(suppl. 4), S107–S109.
9. Thomas, M. G., Sander, G. E., & Giles, T. D. (1988). Hyperergopathic cardiomyopathy. In T. D. Giles, & G. E. Sander (Eds.), Cardiomyopathy. Littleton, Colo: PSG.
10. Levy, D., Larson, M. G., Vasan, R. S., et al. (1996). The progression from hypertension to congestive heart failure. *JAMA, 275*, 1557–1562.
11. Kostis, J. B., Davis, B. R., Cutler, J., et al. (1997). Prevention of heart failure by antihypertensive drug treatment in older persons with isolated systolic hypertension. SHEP cooperative research group. *JAMA, 278*, 212–216.
12. Papaemetriou, V., Devereux, R. B., Narayan, P., et al. (2001). Similar effects of isolated systolic and combined hypertension on left ventricular geometry and function: the LIFE study. *Am J Hypertens, 14*, 768–774.
13. Hunt, S. A., Abraham, W. T., Casey Jr., D. E., et al. (2005). ACC/AHA 2005 guideline update for the diagnosis and management of chronic heart failure in the adult: a report of the American College of Cardiology/American Heart Association Task Force on practice guidelines (writing committe to update the 2001 guidelines for the evaluation and management of heart failure). *J Am Coll Cardiol, 46*, e1–e82.
14. Kupari, M., Lindroos, M., Iivanainen, A. M., et al. (1997). Congestive heart failure in old age: prevalence, mechanisms and 4-year prognosis in the Helsinki ageing study. *J Intern Med, 241*, 387–394.
15. Mathew, J., Davidson, S., Narra, L., et al. (1996). Etiology and characteristics of congestive heart failure in blacks. *Am J Cardiol, 78*, 1447–1450.
16. Schernthaner, G. (1996). Cardiovascular mortality and morbidity in type-2 diabetes mellitus. *Diabetes Res Clin Pract, 31*, S3–S13.
17. Factor, S. M., Broczuk, A., Charron, M. J., et al. (1996). Myocardial alterations in diabetes and hypertension. *Diabetes Res Clin Pract, 31*, S133–S142.
18. Factor, A. M., Minase, T., & Sonnenblick, E. H. (1980). Clinical and morphological features of human hypertensive-diabetic cardiomyopathy. *Am Heart J, 99*, 446–448.
19. Giles, T. D., & Sander, G. E. (1989). Myocardial disease in the hypertensive diabetic. *Am J Med, 87*(suppl. A), 23S–28S.
20. Olubodun, J. O., & Lawal, S. O. (1996). Alcohol consumption and heart failure in hypertensives. *Int J Cardiol, 53*, 81–85.
21. Grossman, W., Jones, D., & McLaurin, L. P. (1975). Wall stress and patterns of hypertrophy in the human left ventricle. *J Clin Invest, 56*, 56–64.
22. de Simone, G., Pasanisi, F., & Contaldo, F. (2001). Link of nonhemodynamic factors to hemodynamic determinants of left ventricular hypertrophy. *Hypertension, 38*, 13–18.
23. Kostis, J. B., Lawrence-Nelson, J., Ranjan, R., et al. (2001). Association of increased pulse pressure with the development of heart failure in SHEP. Systolic Hypertension in the Elderly (SHEP) Cooperative Research Group. *Am J Hypertens, 14*, 798–803.
24. Burch, G. E., Ray, C. T., & Cronvich, J. S. (1952). Certain mechanical peculiarities of the human pump in normal and diseased states. *Circulation, 5*, 504–513.
25. Vasan, R. S., Larson, M. G., Benjamin, E. F., et al. (1997). Left ventricular dilatation and the risk of congestive heart failure in people without myocardial infarction. *N Engl J Med, 336*, 1350–1355.
26. Zak, R. (1974). Development and proliferative capacity of cardiac muscle cells. *Circ Res, 35*, 17–26.
27. Vasan, R. S., & Levy, D. (1996). The role of hypertension in the pathogenesis of heart failure. A clinical mechanistic overview. *Arch Intern Med, 156*, 1789–1796.
28. Echeverria, H. H., Bilsker, M. S., Myerburg, R. J., et al. (1983). Congestive heart failure: echocardiographic insights. *Am J Med, 75*, 750–755.
29. Kitzman, D. W., Higginbotham, M. B., Cobb, F. R., et al. (1991). Exercise intolerance in patients with heart failure and preserved left ventricular systolic function: failure of the Frank-Starling mechanism. *J Am Coll Cardiol, 17*, 1065–1072.
30. Izumo, S., Nadal-Ginard, B., & Mahdavi, V. (1988). Protooncogene induction and reprogramming of cardiac gene expression produced by pressure overload. *Proc Natl Acad Sci U S A, 85*, 339–343.
31. Schwartz, K., de la Bastie, D., Bouvert, P., et al. (1986). Alpha-skeletal muscle actin mRNAs accumulate in hypertrophied adult rat hearts. *Circ Res, 59*, 551–555.
32. Gardner, D. G., Deschepper, C. F., Ganong, W. F., et al. (1986). Extra-atrial expression of the gene for atrial natriuretic factor. *Proc Natl Acad Sci U S A, 83*, 6697–6701.
33. Sugden, P. H., Fuller, S. J., et al. (1997). Cellular and molecular biology of the myocardium: growth and hypertrophy. In P. A. Poole-Wilson, W. S. Colucci, & B. M. Massie (Eds.), *Heart failure: scientific principles and clinical* practice. New York: Churchill Livingstone.
34. Sugihara, N., Genda, A., Shimizu, M., et al. (1988). Diastolic dysfunction and its relation to myocardial fibrosis in essential hypertension. *J Cardiol, 18*, 353–361.

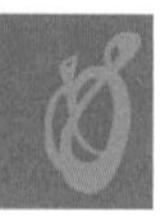

35. Martos, R., Baugh, J., Ledwidge, M., et al. (2007). Diastolic heart failure: evidence of increased myocardial collagen turnover linked to diastolic dysfunction. *Circulation, 115*(7), 888–895.
36. Weber, K. T., Sun, Y., & Guarda, E. (1994). Structural remodeling in hypertensive heart disease and the role of hormones. *Hypertension, 23*, 869–877.
37. Mottram, P. M., Haluska, B., Leano, R., et al. (2004). Effect of aldosterone antagonism on myocardial dysfunction in hypertensive patients with diastolic heart failure. *Circulation, 110*, 558–565.
38. Linzbach, A. J. (1960). Heart failure from the point of view of quantitative anatomy. *Am J Cardiol, 5*, 370–382.
39. Wachtell, K., Rokkedal, J., Bella, J. N., et al. (2001). Effect of electrocardiographic left ventricular hypertrophy on left ventricular systolic function in systemic hypertension (the LIFE study). Losartan intervention for endpoint. *Am J Cardiol, 87*, 54–60.
40. Devereux, R. B., Pickering, T. G., & Harshfield, G. A. (1983). Left ventricular hypertrophy in patients with hypertension: importance of blood pressure response to regular recurring stress. *Circulation, 68*, 470–476.
41. Devereux, R. B., Bella, J., Boman, K., et al. (2001). Echocardiographic left ventricular geometry in hypertensive patients with electrocardiographic left ventricular hypertrophy: the LIFE study. *Blood Press, 10*, 74–82.
42. Julius, S., Li, Y., Brant, D., et al. (1989). Neurogenic pressor episodes fail to cause hypertension but do induce cardiac hypertrophy. *Hypertension, 13*, 422–429.
43. Cavallini, M. C., Roman, M. J., Pickering, T. G., et al. (1995). Is white coat hypertension associated with arterial disease or left ventricular hypertrophy? *Hypertension, 26*, 413–419.
44. Kuwajima, I., Suzuki, Y., Jujisawa, A., et al. (1993). Is white coat hypertension innocent? Structure and function of the heart in the elderly. *Hypertension, 21*, 836–844.
45. Palmieri, V., Wachtell, K., Gerdts, E., et al. (2001). Left ventricular function and hemodynamic features of inappropriate left ventricular hypertrophy in patients with systemic hypertension: the LIFE study. *Am Heart J, 141*, 784–791.
46. Gandhi, S. K., Powers, J. C., Momeir, A. M., et al. (2001). The pathogenesis of acute pulmonary edema associated with hypertension. *N Engl J Med, 344*, 56–59.
47. Fouad-Tarazi, F. M. (1994). Left ventricular diastolic dysfunction in hypertension. *Curr Opin Cardiol, 9*, 551–560.
48. Devereux, R. B., & Roman, M. J. (1995). Hypertensive cardiac hypertrophy: pathophysiologic and clinical characteristics. In J. H. Laragh, & B. M. Brenner (Eds.), *Hypertension: pathophysiology, diagnosis, and* management. New York: Raven Press.
49. Houghton, J. L., Frank, M. F., Carr, A. A., et al. (1990). Relations among impaired coronary flow reserve, left ventricular hypertrophy and thallium perfusion defects in hypertensive patients without obstructive coronary artery disease. *J Am Coll Cardiol, 15*, 43–51.
50. Pfeffer, M. A., & Braunwald, E. (1990). Ventricular remodeling after myocardial infarction: experimental observations and clinical implications. *Circulation, 81*, 1161–1172.
51. Nolan, S. E., Mannisi, J. A., Bush, D. E., et al. (1988). Increased afterload aggravates infarct expansion after acute myocardial infarction. *J Am Coll Cardiol, 12*, 1318–1325.
52. Rabkin, S. W., Mathewson, F. A. L., & Tate, R. B. (1977). Prognosis after acute myocardial infarction: relation to blood pressure values before infarction in a prospective cardiovascular study. *Am J Cardiol, 40*(4), 604–610.
53. Christensen, D. J., Ford, M., & Reading, J. (1977). Effect of hypertension on myocardial rupture after acute myocardial infarction. *Chest, 72*, 618–622.
54. Schuster, E. H., & Bulkley, B. H. (1979). Expansion of transmural myocardial infarction: a pathophysiologic factor in cardiac rupture. *Circulation, 60*, 1532–1538.
55. Kannel, W. B., Hjortland, M., & Castelli, W. P. (1974). Role of diabetes in congestive heart failure: the Framingham study. *Am J Cardiol, 34*, 29–34.
56. Zarich, S. W., Arbuckle, B. E., Cohen, L. R., et al. (1988). Diastolic abnormalities in young asymptomatic diabetic patients assessed by pulsed Doppler echocardiography. *J Am Coll Cardiol, 12*, 114–120.
57. Hunt, S. A., Abraham, W. T., Casey, Jr., D. E., et al. (2005). ACC/AHA2005 guideline update for the diagnosis and management of chronic heart failure in the adult: a report of the American College of Cardiology/American Heart Association Task Force on practice Guidelines(Writing Committee to update the 2001 Guidelines for the Evaluation and management of Heart Failure). *J Am Coll Cardiol 46*, e1–e82.
58. Hebert, P. R., & Moser, M. (1993). Mayer, el al. Recent evidence on drug therapy of mild to moderate hypertension and decreased risk of coronary heart disease. *Arch Intern Med, 153*(5), 578–581.
59. Moser, M., & Herbert, P. R. (1996). Prevention of disease progression, left ventricular hypertrophy and congestive heart failure in hypertension treatment trials. *J Am Coll Cardiol, 27*, 1214–1218.
60. Dahlöf, B., Lindholm, L. H., Hansson, L., et al. (1991). Morbidity and mortality in the Swedish trial in old patients with hypertension (STOP-hypertension). *Lancet, 338*, 1281–1285.
61. SHEP Cooperative Research Group. (1991). Prevention of stroke by antihypertensive drug treatment in older persons with isolated systolic hypertension. Final results of the systolic hypertension in the elderly program (SHEP). *JAMA, 266*, 3255–3264.
62. Doyle, A. E. (1988). Does hypertension predispose to coronary disease? Conflicting epidemiological and experimental evidence. *Am J Hypertens, 1*, 319–324.
63. Yusuf, S., Thom, T., & Abbott, R. D. (1989). Changes in hypertension treatment and in congestive heart failure mortality in the United States. *Hypertension, 13*(suppl. I), I74–I79.
64. Psaty, B. M., Smith, N. L., Siscovick, D. S., et al. (1997). Health outcomes associated with antihypertensive therapies used as first-line agents. A systematic review and meta-analysis. *JAMA, 277*, 739–745.
65. Verdecchia, P., Schillaci, G., Borgioni, C., et al. (1998). Prognostic significance of serial changes in left ventricular mass in essential hypertension. *Circulation, 97*, 48–54.
66. Dahlöf, B., Devereux, R. B., Kjeldson, S. E., et al. (2002). Cardiovascular morbidity and mortality in the losartan intervention for endpoint reduction in hypertension study (LIFE): a randomised trial against atenolol. *Lancet, 359*, 995–1003.
67. Verdecchia, P., Staessen, J. A., Angeli, F., et al. (2009). Usual versus tight control of systolic blood pressure in nondiabetic patients with hypertension (CARDIO-SIS): an open-label randomised trial. *Lancet, 374*, 525–533.
68. Liebson, P. R., Grandits, G. A., Dianzumba, S., et al. (1995). Comparison of five antihypertensive monotherapies and placebo for change in left ventricular mass in patients receiving nutritional-hygienic therapy in the treatment of mild hypertension study (TOMHS). *Circulation, 91*, 698–706.
69. Dahlöf, B., Pennert, K., & Hansson, L. (1992). Reversal of left ventricular hypertrophy in hypertensive patients. A meta-analysis of 109 treatment studies. *Am J Hypertens, 5*, 95–110.
70. Cruickshank, J. M., Lewis, J., Moore, V., et al. (1992). Reversibility of left ventricular hypertrophy by differing types of antihypertensive therapy. *J Hum Hypertens, 6*, 85–90.
71. Schmieder, R. E., Martus, P., & Klingbeil, A. (1996). Reversal of left ventricular hypertrophy in essential hypertension. A meta-analysis of randomized double studies. *JAMA, 275*, 1507–1513.
72. Law, M. R., Morris, J. K., & Wald, N. J. (2009). Use of blood pressure lowering drugs in the prevention of cardiovascular disease: meta-analysis of 147 randomised trials in the context of expectations from prospective epidemiological studies. *BMJ, 338*, 1245–1253.
73. McEniery, C. M., Yasmin, McDonnell B, et al. (2008). Central pressure: variability and impact of cardiovascular risk factors: the Anglo-Cardiff collaborative trial II. Hypertension, *51*(6), 1476–1482.
74. Mackenzie, I. S., McEniery, C. M., Dhakam, Z., et al. (2009). Comparison of the effects of antihypertensive agents on central blood pressure and arterial stiffness in isolated systolic hypertension. *Hypertension, 54*(2), 409–413.
75. Cockcroft, J. R., Chowienczyk, P. J., Brett, S. E., et al. (1995). Nebivolol vasodilates human forearm vasculature: evidence for an L-arginine/NO-dependent mechanism. *J Pharmacol Exp Ther, 274*, 1067–1071.
76. Pederson, M. E., & Cockcroft, J. R. (2007). The vasodilatory beta-blockers. *Curr Hypertens Rep, 9*(4), 269–277.
77. Roman, M. J., Devereux, R. B., Kizer, J. R., et al. (2007). Central pressure more strongly relates to vascular disease and outcome than does brachial pressure: the strong heart study. *Hypertension, 50*(1), 197–203.
78. Williams, B., Lacy, P. S., Thom, S. M., et al. (2006). Differential impact of blood pressure-lowering drugs on central aortic pressure and clinical outcomes: principal results of the conduit artery function evaluation (CAFE) study. *Circulation, 113*(9), 1213–1225.
79. Guerin, A. P., Blacher, J., Pannier, B., et al. (2001). Impact of aortic stiffness attenuation on survival of patients in end-stage renal failure. *Circulation, 103*(7), 987–992.
80. UK Prospective Diabetes Study Group. (1998). Tight blood pressure control and risk of macrovascular and microvascular complications in type 2 diabetes: UKPDS 38. *BMJ, 317*(7160), 703–713.
81. UK Prospective Diabetes Study Group. (1998). Efficacy of atenolol and captopril in reducing risk of macrovascular and microvascular complications in type 2 diabetes: UKPDS 39. *BMJ, 317*(7160), 713–720.
82. Howard, B. V., Roman, M. J., Devereux, R. B., et al. (2008). Effect of lower targets for blood pressure and LDL cholesterol on atherosclerosis in diabetes: the SANDS randomized trial. *JAMA, 299*(14), 1678–1689.
83. Staessen, J. A., Fagard, R., Thijs, L., et al. (1997). Randomised double-blind comparison of placebo and active treatment for older patients with isolated systolic hypertension. *Lancet, 350*, 757–764.
84. Hansson, L., Zanchetti, A., Carruthers, S. G., et al. (1998). Effects of intensive blood-pressure lowering and low-dose aspirin in patients with hypertension: principal results of the hypertension optimal treatment (HOT) randomised trial. *Lancet, 351*, 1755–1762.
85. The Heart Outcomes Prevention Evaluation Study Investigators. (2000). Effects of an angiotensin-converting-enzyme inhibitor, ramipril, on cardiovascular events in high-risk patients. *N Engl J Med, 342*, 145–153.
86. Yusuf, S., Pfeffer, M. A., Swedberg, K., et al. (2003). Effects of candesartan in patients with chronic heart failure and preserved left-ventricular ejection fraction: the CHARM-Preserved trial. *Lancet, 362*, 777–781.
87. Massie, B. M., Carson, P. E., McMurray, J. J., et al. (2008). Irbesartan in patients with heart failure and preserved ejection fraction. *N Engl J Med, 359*, 2456–2467.
88. Solomon, S. D., Janardhanan, R., Verma, A., et al. (2007). Effect of angiotensin receptor blockade and antihypertensive drugs on diastolic function in patients with hypertension and diastolic dysfunction: a randomised trial. *Lancet, 369*(9579), 2079–2087.
89. The ALLHAT Officers and Coordinators for the ALLHAT Collaborative Research Group (2002). Major outcomes in high-risk hypertensive patients randomized to angiotensin-converting enzyme inhibitor or calcium channel blocker vs diuretic: the antihypertensive and lipid-lowering treatment to prevent heart attack trial (ALLHAT). *JAMA, 288*, 2981–2997.
90. The ALLHAT Officers and Coordinators for the ALLHAT Collaborative Research Group (2002). Major outcomes in high-risk hypertensive patients randomized to angiotensin-converting enzyme inhibitor or calcium channel blocker vs diuretic: the antihypertensive and lipid-lowering treatment to prevent heart attack trial (ALLHAT). *JAMA, 288*, 2981–2997.
91. The Task Force for the Diagnosis and Treatment of Chronic Heart Failure of the European Society of Cardiology. (2005). Guidelines for the diagnosis and treatment of chronic heart failure: executive summary (update 2005). *Eur Heart J, 26*, 1115–1140.
92. Jessup, M., Abraham, W. T., Casey, D. E., et al. (2009). 2009 Focused update: ACCF/AHA guidelines for the diagnosis and management of heart failure in adults: a report of the American College of Cardiology Foundation/American Heart Association task force on practice management of heart failure developed in collaboration with the International Society for Heart and Lung Transplantation. *J Am Coll Cardiol, 53*, 1343–1382.
93. Parving, H. H., Lehnert, H., Bröchner-Mortensen, J., et al. (2001). The effect of irbesartan on the development of diabetic nephropathy in patients with type 2 diabetes. *N Engl J Med, 345*(12), 870–878.
94. Chobanian, A. V., Bakris, G. L., Black, H. R., et al. (2003). The seventh report of the joint national committee on prevention, detection, evaluation, and treatment of high blood pressure: the JNC 7 report. *JAMA, 289*(19), 2560–2572.
95. Moser, M., & Hebert, P. R. (1996). Prevention of disease progression, left ventricular hypertrophy and congestive heart failure in hypertension treatment trials. *J Am Coll Cardiol, 27*, 1214–1218.
96. Hunt, S. A., Abraham, W. T., Chin, M. H., et al. (2009). 2009 Focused update: ACCF/AHA guidelines for the diagnosis and management of heart failure in adults: a report of the American College of Cardiology Foundation/American Heart Association task force on practice guidelines (2009 writing group to review new evidence and update the 2005 guidelines for the management of patients with chronic heart failure writing on behalf of the 2005 heart failure writing committee). *Circulation, 119*, 1977–2057.

CHAPTER 29

Heart Failure as a Consequence of Valvular Heart Disease

Blase A. Carabello

Valvular heart disease is emerging as a progressively more common cause of congestive heart failure. Recent demographic data from New York City demonstrate that while admissions due to coronary artery disease have fallen over the last decade, admissions for the treatment of valvular heart disease have progressively increased.[1] This has occurred primarily because valvular heart disease in western culture today is often a consequence of aging and our population is getting older. While the incidence of valve disease due to rheumatic fever has fallen dramatically, both aortic stenosis and mitral regurgitation have increased with the aging population. A persistent background incidence of infective endocarditis adds additional cases of both aortic and mitral insufficiency.

All valvular heart diseases impart a hemodynamic load on the left and/or right ventricles. If this load is severe and acute, or severe and prolonged, it causes heart failure and death. The importance of valvular disease is further heightened because proper recognition and management of these diseases removes the hemodynamic overload and can either prevent or reverse the heart failure syndrome, a situation rare in the realm of heart failure where most diseases that cause it confer persistent systolic and/or diastolic dysfunction.

On the following pages, each valvular heart disease will be addressed regarding mechanisms by which acute and chronic hemodynamic overload leads to heart failure, the medical and surgical options for treating heart failure, and proper timing of intervention so as to prevent heart failure from occurring or at least from becoming permanent.

Aortic Insufficiency

Acute Aortic Insufficiency

Acute aortic insufficiency such as might occur due to perforation of an aortic leaflet by infective endocarditis is usually a surgical emergency. The hemodynamics of acute aortic insufficiency is demonstrated in Figure 29-1.[2] While the clinician is accustomed to finding a myriad of hyperdynamic signs produced by chronic aortic insufficiency, these are usually absent in acute disease. In chronic aortic insufficiency, eccentric hypertrophy allows the ventricle to generate increased total stroke volume to help compensate for that which is regurgitated. This large total stroke volume is ejected into the aorta where it produces a widened pulse pressure and a hyperdynamic circulation responsible for Corrigan pulse, de Musset sign, Quincke pulse, etc. However, in acute disease, left ventricular (LV) dilation has not developed and thus, acute aortic insufficiency causes little increase in total stroke volume, a sudden fall in forward output, and a fall in systemic blood pressure. At the same time, backward flow into the left ventricle stretches sarcomeres toward their maximum. This volume overload does allow the ventricle to generate increased force by the Frank Starling mechanism, but also exposes the unprepared small ventricle to a large increase in diastolic pressure. While the lungs are partially protected by this increased pressure by preclosure of the mitral valve, the ventricle is not. The driving gradient for generating coronary blood flow is the aortic diastolic pressure minus the LV filling pressure (which compresses the endocardium preventing coronary inflow.) As can be seen in Figure 29-2, these pressures may become equal midway through diastole, reducing coronary blood flow, in turn, leading to myocardial ischemia and worsening muscle function.[3] While unproven, it is likely that it is this sequence of events that often generates a rapid downhill course so that a patient with acute aortic insufficiency can go from mild decompensation to death within hours. Medical therapy is often to no avail. Vasodilators, which might help to increase forward flow, further decrease blood pressure leading to worsening myocardial perfusion. Pressor agents, some of which increase blood pressure by causing vasoconstriction, are also likely to worsen the amount of regurgitation severely limiting the usefulness of these agents. Agents, which increase heart rate, can help by decreasing the time for aortic runoff but these drugs also increase myocardial oxygen consumption, potentially worsening ischemia. Intraaortic balloon pumping is obviously contraindicated and ineffective since diastolic inflation of the balloon dramatically worsens the amount of aortic insufficiency. Thus, in acute aortic insufficiency, acute severe volume overload forces the operation of the left ventricle to the high right-hand side of the pressure volume relationship leading to pulmonary congestion. The sharp reduction in forward output further compounds the heart failure syndrome. Reduced output diminishes systemic blood pressure, leading to reflex vasoconstriction in turn worsening regurgitation.

The therapy for this syndrome requires aggressive action. As indicated previously, while it is often hoped that medical therapy may stabilize the patient and give more time for antibiotics (in infective endocarditis), to become effective, continued hemodynamic deterioration usually occurs despite medical therapy. Even the mildest symptoms and signs of heart failure, such as slight orthopnea or tachycardia unexplained by the patient's fever, should be taken as an early warning that aortic valve replacement should be imminent.[4] It should be recognized that despite the worry that replacement valve may become infected, this worry is usually not justified even in mechanical valves where the reinfection rate is less than 10%.[5] The reinfection rate with homographs appears to be even lower and this valve has become the preferred prosthesis in patients with active infection.[6]

Chronic Aortic Insufficiency

Common causes of chronic aortic insufficiency include annuloaortic ectasia, Marfan syndrome, rheumatic heart disease, and endocarditis that was not severe enough to require immediate valve replacement. In chronic aortic insufficiency, volume overload

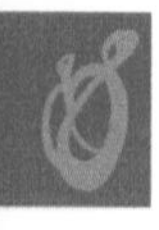

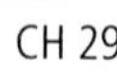

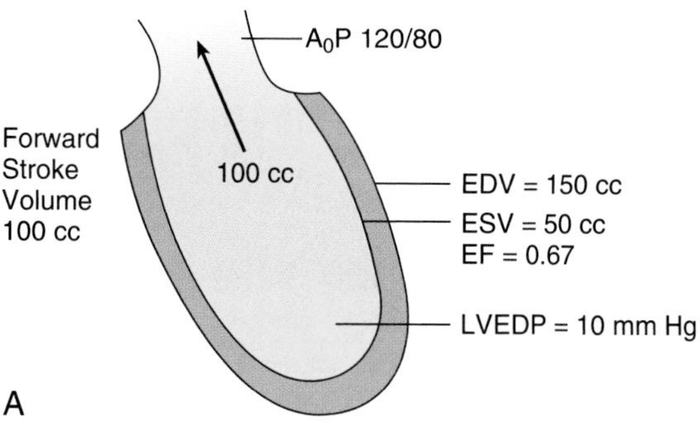

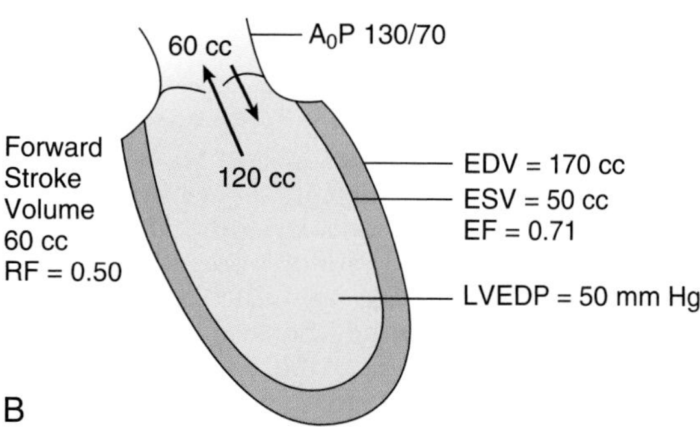

FIGURE 29–1 **A,** Normal physiology. **B,** Pathophysiology of acute aortic regurgitation. In response to acute volume overload, end-diastolic volume (EDV) increases modestly, allowing for a modest increase in total stroke volume. This small increase widens pulse pressure only slightly. The regurgitant volume is summed with that returning from the pulmonary veins, causing LV volume overload. This overload on the unprepared left ventricle causes a large increase in LV end-diastolic pressure (LVEDP). At the same time, forward stroke volume is reduced. Thus all the manifestations of heart failure are present even though myocardial function is normal. *EF,* ejection fraction; *ESV,* end-systolic volume; *RF,* regurgitant fraction. (Reprinted from Carabello BA. Hemodynamic determinants of prognosis. In Cohn LH, DiSesa VJ, editors. *Aortic regurgitation: medical and surgical management*, New York, 1986, Marcel Dekker.)

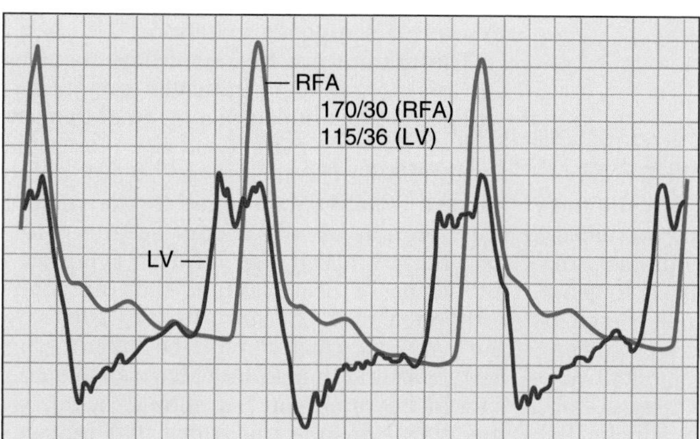

FIGURE 29–2 Hemodynamic effects of aortic regurgitation. End-diastolic aortic and ventricular pressure become equal in middiastole, a point at which there can be no significant coronary blood flow. *RFA,* right femoral artery; *LV,* left ventricle. (Reprinted with permission from Carabello BA, Gazes PC. *Cardiology pearls*, ed 2, Philadelphia, 2001, Hanley & Belfus.)

leads to the development of eccentric hypertrophy where sarcomeres laid down in series increase the length of individual myocytes. Increased myocyte length leads to increased LV volume, allowing total stroke volume to increase. This mechanism may be quite effective, allowing the patient with even severe chronic aortic insufficiency to be totally asymptomatic. Indeed young patients who have developed the disease from endocarditis can often engage in sports activities (although

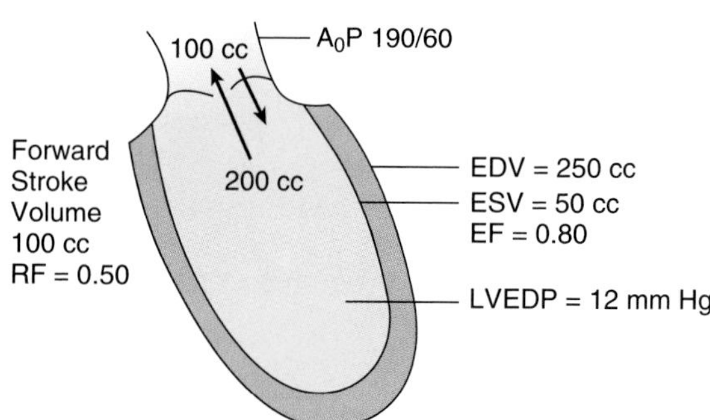

FIGURE 29–3 Pathophysiology of chronic compensated aortic regurgitation. Compared with Figure 29-1*B*, eccentric hypertrophy has developed, allowing a large increase in end-diastolic volume (EDV), increasing total stroke volume and in turn returning forward stroke volume toward normal. The larger ventricle can now accommodate the volume overload at much lower LV end-diastolic pressure (LVEDP). The large total stroke volume results in a widened pulse pressure, which is responsible for many of the signs of chronic aortic regurgitation. *EF,* ejection fraction; *ESV,* end-systolic volume; *RF,* regurgitant fraction. (Reprinted from Carabello BA. Hemodynamic determinants of prognosis. In Cohn LH, DiSesa VJ, editors. *Aortic regurgitation: medical and surgical management*, New York, 1986, Marcel Dekker.)

this is contraindicated if there is substantial left ventricle dilation) without symptoms. At the same time, increased ventricular size allows the regurgitant volume to be accommodated at a lower filling pressure, in turn relieving or preventing the symptoms of congestion that are seen in acute aortic insufficiency when the ventricle is small (Figure 29-3).[2] Accordingly, severe aortic insufficiency may be extremely well compensated with a normal forward output and normal filling pressure. As noted previously, the large stroke volume produced in aortic insufficiency causes a wide pulse pressure and systolic hypertension. Thus there is an element of increased afterload seen in aortic insufficiency that is not present in mitral insufficiency.[7] This increased afterload leads to an element of concentric hypertrophy in addition to the eccentric hypertrophy generated by the volume overload.[8] Concentric hypertrophy helps to normalize systolic wall stress, allowing ejection fraction (EF) to be normal. However, as the disease progresses, this mechanism may become inadequate to normalize stress, wall stress increases, and ejection fraction is reduced.[9] At this time, symptoms may develop because the systolic dysfunction engendered by increased systolic wall stress places the ventricle on a higher portion of its operating pressure volume relationship. In addition, the concentric hypertrophy that develops diminishes diastolic function, further contributing to the syndrome of heart failure. Apart from the abnormal loading, which helps generate the heart failure syndrome, muscle dysfunction may also intervene. The mechanisms of myocardial dysfunction are not yet well worked out for aortic insufficiency. However, it is known that coronary blood flow, especially to the endocardium, is reduced in these patients. Thus ischemia especially during exercise may contribute to the syndrome.[10] In an important rabbit model of aortic insufficiency, increased extracellular matrix deposition leads to increased myocardial stiffness and to myocyte destruction, thus contributing both to diastolic and systolic dysfunction.[11] In patients with aortic insufficiency, increased fibrosis and decreased myosin content in the myocardium has also been detected and both obviously could lead respectfully to diastolic and systolic dysfunction.[12]

Management of Congestive Heart Failure in Aortic Insufficiency

Avoidance of CHF

Aortic insufficiency is a mechanical problem, which places an overload on the myocardium. This mechanical problem can be corrected by valve replacement or occasionally by valve

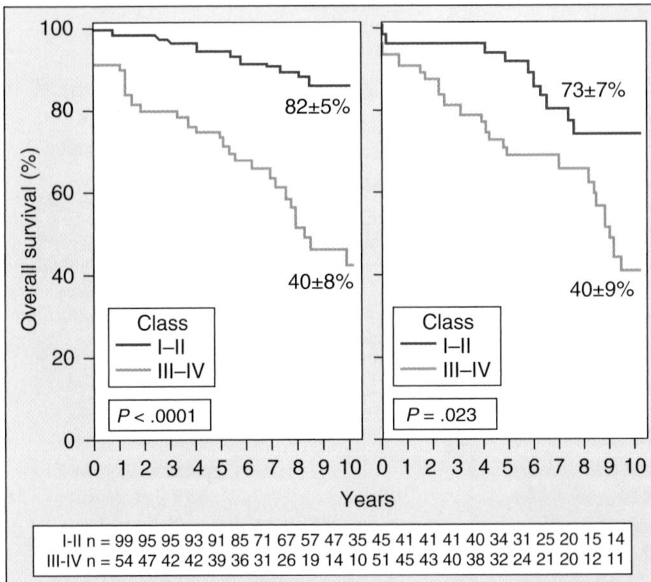

FIGURE 29–4 The importance of symptoms. Whether ejection fraction was normal (*left panel*) or reduced (*right panel*), survival in patients with aortic regurgitation was most influenced by symptom severity. (From Klodas E, Enriquez-Sarano M, Tajik AJ, et al. Surgery for aortic regurgitation in women: contrasting indications and outcomes compared with men. *Circulation* 1996;94:2472-2478.)

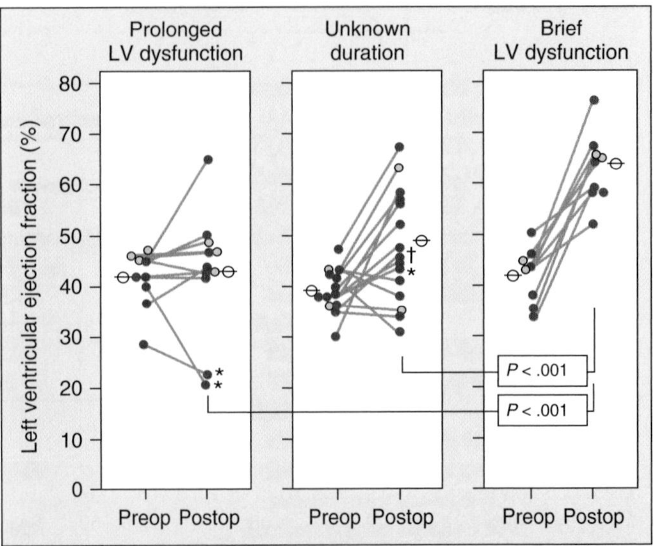

FIGURE 29–5 The effects of the duration of left ventricular (LV) dysfunction on recovery of function after valve replacement. If ejection fraction was reduced for 15 months or less before surgery (*right panel*), ejection fraction improved; improvement was less likely (*left panel*) if ejection fraction had been depressed for longer periods. (From Bonow RO, Rosing DR, Maron BJ, et al. Reversal of LV dysfunction after aortic valve replacement for chronic aortic regurgitation: influence of duration of preoperative LV dysfunction. *Circulation* 1984;70:570-579.)

repair. Close surveillance of the patient with aortic insufficiency allows for the timing of this correction to occur before irreversible muscle damage has developed and also in time to allow for a normal life expectancy following valve replacement. Further, as surgical techniques and prosthetic valves have improved, their risk has diminished—making earlier timing of surgery progressively more attractive because as risk diminishes, benefit increases.

Symptoms. Once even mild symptoms of congestive heart failure develop in chronic aortic insufficiency, prognosis worsens as shown in Figure 29-4.[13] Although it seems intuitive that the symptoms from valvular heart disease would have the same implications as those from other types of heart disease, the higher risk of prosthetic valves and surgery decades ago, generated a strategy of withholding surgery until it was inevitable. Typically, patients were not operated upon until their symptoms were far advanced. However, once the detrimental cascade of congestive heart failure has been initiated, a downhill course can be expected until that cascade is halted. Fortunately, in valvular heart disease, the cascade can be reversed and prognosis restored to normal. Thus, even mild symptoms are an indication for mechanical intervention in this disease especially in light of improved modern surgical techniques.

Asymptomatic Left Ventricular Dysfunction

While many patients develop symptoms when LV dysfunction develops or may become symptomatic even before there are objective signs of LV dysfunction, other patients remain asymptomatic despite LV dysfunction. Lack of symptoms may result from denial or unknown factors limiting perception by the patient. Nonetheless, it is generally accepted that some patients may remain asymptomatic despite relatively far advanced contractile dysfunction. To prevent dysfunction from becoming irreversible, it must be detected and corrected in a timely fashion. Figure 29-5 demonstrates that even if fairly advanced LV dysfunction has developed, it returns to normal if correction occurs within 15 months of onset.[14] Because by definition the patient under consideration is asymptomatic, the clinician needs a tool other than patient complaint to alert him or her that dysfunction is developing. Currently, echocardiographic surveillance is the standard technique for early detection of LV dysfunction, although it may be that in the future brain natriuretic peptide (BNP) or other serological examinations will be determined to be useful. Several studies have examined echocardiographic markers associated with poor versus good outcome following surgery. These can be summarized most simply as stating that when ejection fraction falls below 0.50 or when end systolic dimension exceeds 50 to 55 mm, postsurgical outcome is reduced.[15] Presumably, these markers of poor outcome indicate that LV dysfunction is becoming irreversible and therefore, are an indication for mechanical relief from the volume and pressure overload.

Following surgery, ejection fraction usually improves if it was reduced preoperatively. As noted, this is especially true if correction of the mechanical lesion is provided within 15 months of the onset of LV dysfunction. Improvement in function is predicated upon a fall in afterload as both the pressure and radius terms of the La Place equation (stress = pressure × radius/2x thickness) are reduced following surgery and also due to improved myocardial function.[9] Improved function following surgery is predicated upon a reduction in collagen content and an improvement in myosin content.[16]

Medical Therapy

Because aortic insufficiency increases LV afterload, afterload reducing agents have been used in an attempt to forestall the onset of LV dysfunction. In a controlled study, nifedipine compared to digoxin forestalled the need for surgery as indicated by the development of symptoms or LV dysfunction by 2 to 3 years.[17] However, a more recent study of randomized patients receiving nifedipine versus a true placebo (instead of digoxin), employed a third arm, enalapril.[18] It found no benefit to vasodilator use. Thus the AHA/ACC Guidelines for the management of valvular heart disease reduced the indication for vasodilator use in aortic insufficiency from a class 1 indication (beneficial) to a class 2b indication (uncertain benefit).[15] However, in the patient with heart failure due to aortic insufficiency in whom surgery cannot be performed, standard heart failure therapy should be initiated.

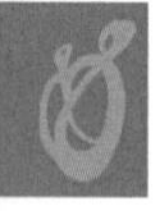

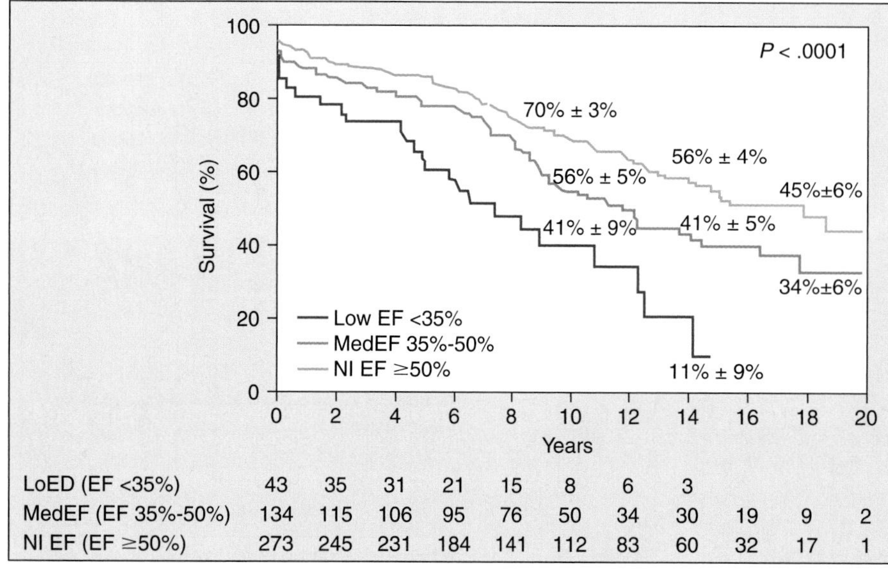

	0	2	4	6	8	10	12	14	16	18	20
LoED (EF <35%)	43	35	31	21	15	8	6	3			
MedEF (EF 35%-50%)	134	115	106	95	76	50	34	30	19	9	2
Nl EF (EF ≥50%)	273	245	231	184	141	112	83	60	32	17	1

FIGURE 29-6 Postoperative survival for patients with aortic insufficiency is plotted according to preoperative ejection fraction. (From Chaliki HP, Mohty D, Avierinos JF, et al. Outcomes after aortic valve replacement in patients with severe aortic regurgitation and markedly reduced LV function are impaired. *Circulation* 2002;106[21]:2687-2693).

It has generally been held that β-blockers should be contraindicated in aortic insufficiency. It was thought that slowing of the heart rate would increase the period during which regurgitation could occur, worsening the volume overload. However, a recent report suggests that some patients with severe aortic insufficiency actually benefitted from β-blockade.[19] In a retrospective study, aortic insufficiency patients taking β-blockers had improved survival compared with those who were not receiving them. Most had heart failure and the presence of coronary disease and hypertension did not account for β-blockade benefit. While this finding goes against current wisdom and must be confirmed, it may be that the beneficial effects of β-blockade in heart failure in general outweigh the potential negative potential of increasing the diastolic leak in aortic insufficiency. It should also be noted that paradoxically, the β-blockade group actually had slightly faster heart rates than the unblocked group and it was the group with the fastest heart rates that benefitted most from β-blockade.

Far Advanced Left Ventricular Dysfunction

The question often arises, "Has left ventricular dysfunction ever become so far advanced that surgery is impossible?" As indicated in Figure 29-5, even patients with very low ejection fractions may benefit from aortic valve replacement especially if LV dysfunction has been of short duration. Thus, no specific ejection fraction provides a cutoff that prohibits surgery, although as demonstrated in Figure 29-6 low ejection fraction negatively impacts prognosis.[20] It does seem logical that since one of the major mechanisms of improvement following surgery is reduction in afterload, that the absence of afterload excess preoperatively is a bad prognostic sign and thus in the patient with severe aortic insufficiency and a reduced ejection fraction, who also has low, rather than elevated systolic blood pressure, outcome may be reduced. The exact prognosis in such patients awaits further study.

Mitral Regurgitation

Acute Mitral Regurgitation

In acute mitral regurgitation such as might occur with rupture of a chordae tendineae, there is the sudden opening of a new pathway for ejection from the left ventricle. This pathway produces two unwanted consequences leading to congestive heart failure. First, there is volume overload of the unprepared left atrium and left ventricle as the regurgitant flow is summed with flow returning from the pulmonary veins. This volume overload acutely raises left atrial and LV diastolic pressures, in turn leading to pulmonary congestion and dyspnea. At the same time, forward cardiac output is reduced by the amount of flow lost to regurgitation. As shown in Figure 29-7, there is partial compensation for this insult as the volume overload stretches existing sarcomeres in the left ventricle to their maximum, increasing end-diastolic volume and the pumping capacity of the left ventricle.[21] Also, the reduced afterload created by the new ejection pathway into the relatively low pressure of the left atrium enhances ejection and reduces end-systolic volume. Increased end-diastolic volume and decreased end-systolic volume increase total stroke volume in part compensating for that which is lost to regurgitation. However, this increase is inadequate to normalize forward stroke volume. In this instance, LV contractile function is normal; ejection fraction is markedly increased due to the favorable loading conditions on the left ventricle, yet, all of the hemodynamic and clinical facets of congestive heart failure are present. If the regurgitant lesion is severe, reduced forward stroke volume leads to lower blood pressure while at the same time, the patient develops pulmonary edema. In such patients, arterial vasodilators may allow for a preferential increase in forward flow while diminishing regurgitant flow, in turn improving the hemodynamic situation.[22] However, if hypotension is already present, the use of vasodilators may further lower blood pressure and cannot be used. In such cases, intraaortic balloon pumping is used to maintain mean arterial pressure while reducing afterload and increasing forward stroke volume until surgical correction of the defect can be performed.

If the acute regurgitation is less severe, it may be attended by only mild symptoms, which can be treated successfully with diuretics. Currently, at issue is what constitutes the best management in patients who have been rendered asymptomatic by relatively minimal medical therapy. As shown in Figure 29-7, eccentric cardiac hypertrophy may develop over time, allowing for normalization of forward stroke volume. At the same time, atrial and ventricular chamber enlargement can accommodate the regurgitant volume, resulting in normal filling pressure and thus the symptoms of pulmonary congestion are relieved. Such patients may remain asymptomatic for months or years thereby avoiding cardiac surgery. However, one study has found that a few such patients rendered asymptomatic by medical therapy may have been at risk for sudden death although asymptomatic.[23,24] Thus whether successful medical therapy is in fact beneficial or whether it simply masks the potential risk for sudden death awaits further study.

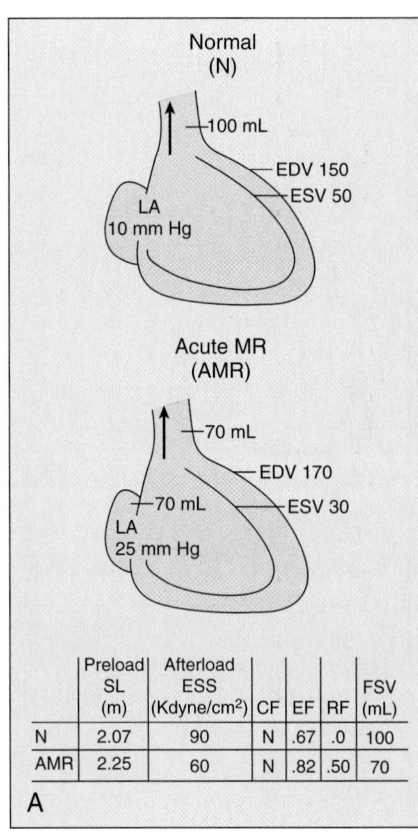

	Preload SL (m)	Afterload ESS (Kdyne/cm²)	CF	EF	RF	FSV (mL)
N	2.07	90	N	.67	.0	100
AMR	2.25	60	N	.82	.50	70

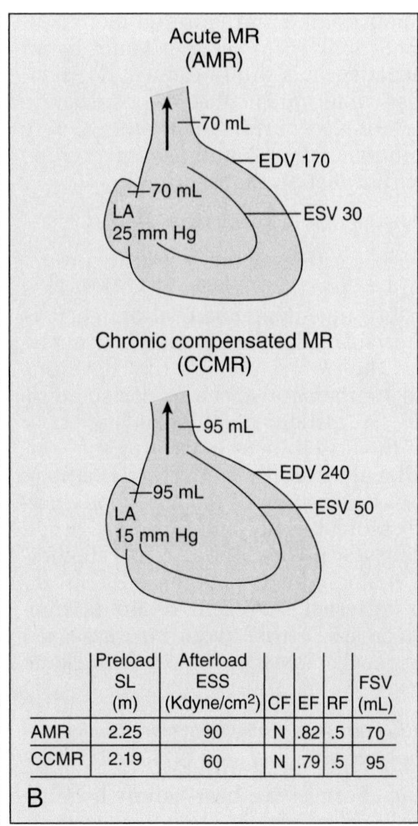

	Preload SL (m)	Afterload ESS (Kdyne/cm²)	CF	EF	RF	FSV (mL)
AMR	2.25	90	N	.82	.5	70
CCMR	2.19	60	N	.79	.5	95

FIGURE 29–7 Normal physiology (*left panel*) is compared with that of acute mitral regurgitation (MR) and chronic compensated mitral regurgitation (*right panel*). In acute MR, volume overload increases end-diastolic volume (EDV), whereas the new pathway for ejection into the left atrium (LA) reduces afterload, in turn reducing end-systolic volume. These factors increase total stroke volume but not enough to compensate for that which is lost to regurgitation; thus, forward stroke volume is reduced. The volume overload on the small left atrium and left ventricle increase left atrial pressure, leading to pulmonary congestion. In chronic compensated MR (right panel), eccentric hypertrophy develops, allowing an increase in both total and forward stroke volumes; the now-enlarged left-sided chambers accommodate the volume overload at lower filling pressure. *CF,* contractile function; *EF,* ejection fraction; *ESS,* end-systolic stress; *ESV,* end-systolic volume; *FSV,* forward stroke volume; *RF,* regurgitant fraction; *SL,* sarcomere length. (From Carabello B. Mitral regurgitation: basic pathophysiologic principles. *Mod Concepts Cardiovasc Dis* 1988;57:53-58.)

Chronic Mitral Regurgitation

It appears that moderate mitral regurgitation can be tolerated for years or perhaps, indefinitely. In studies of patients undergoing mitral valve replacement for mitral regurgitation, regurgitant fraction almost always exceeds 50%.

In a dog model of mitral regurgitation that causes myocardial dysfunction, there is almost complete recovery of function if mitral valve repair reduces regurgitant fraction to less than 35%.[25] Thus it seems that it requires a regurgitant fraction of between 40% and 50% to create and maintain LV dysfunction. Figure 29-7 demonstrates that the major compensatory mechanism for mitral regurgitation is the development of eccentric cardiac hypertrophy. Here individual myocytes add sarcomeres in series so that the individual cell becomes longer, increasing ventricular volume. In addition, the volume overload causes sarcomere stretch, increasing preload. Thus increased preload together with normal contractile function of an enlarged left ventricle allows for increased total stroke volume, increasing forward stroke volume toward normal. At the same time, enlargement of the left atrium and left ventricle allows for accommodation of the regurgitant volume at fairly normal filling pressure. In this compensated phase of mitral regurgitation, patients might be entirely asymptomatic even during vigorous activities. It should be noted, however, that such patients may have activation of the adrenergic nervous system, which can maintain both contractile and pump function at normal levels despite concealed intrinsic muscle dysfunction.[26,27]

If mitral regurgitation is severe, eventually muscle dysfunction does occur. While once believed that mitral regurgitation was well tolerated for prolonged periods of time, it is now evident that most patients with severe mitral regurgitation develop adverse clinical events within 5 years of recognition of severe disease.[28,29] The mechanisms of this dysfunction are now being worked out. In both an experimental model of mitral regurgitation and in man, at the papillary muscle level there is a loss of contractile proteins and contractile elements, obviously reducing muscle function.[30] The second cause of the muscle dysfunction that develops is a shift in the force-frequency relationship such that the muscle develops less force with peak force developed at a slower heart rate than normal. These changes imply that abnormalities in calcium handling are at the source of the dysfunction.[31]

In addition, the hypertrophy that occurs in mitral regurgitation is both adaptive and maladaptive. It is adaptive because it allows the chamber to pump an increase in total volume. It is maladaptive because as volume increases, the radius term in the La Place equation also increases, thereby increasing both systolic and diastolic stress. While mitral regurgitation is usually viewed as a lesion that reduces LV afterload (and it does in acute mitral regurgitation), as the radius increases, afterload returns first to normal and then even to higher than normal levels when LV dysfunction has developed. This abnormality of chamber geometry further contributes to LV dysfunction in chronic mitral regurgitation.[32]

Besides the changes in chamber geometry noted previously, the hypertrophy that develops in mitral regurgitation, seems to be qualitatively different than that which occurs in pressure overload. In LV pressure overload, hypertrophy accrues primarily by an increase in synthesis of contractile

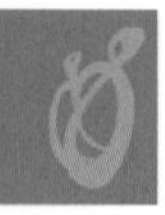

proteins.[33] However, in both canine and lapinine models of mitral regurgitation, hypertrophy seems to accrue not by an increase in synthesis but rather by a diminution in degradation rate.[34] These changes would mean that the contractile proteins in mitral regurgitation are turning over more slowly and thus are older than normal, which could in some way be implicated in the muscle dysfunction that accrues.

Reversal of Left Ventricular Dysfunction in Mitral Regurgitation

Both in man and in dog, correction of the mitral regurgitation can lead to an improvement in contractility.[35,36] This improvement is presumably time-dependent, although it is not clear at what point the ventricular dysfunction is irreversible. Of interest, much of the LV dysfunction that develops in experimental mitral regurgitation also can be corrected by initiation of β-blockade.[37] The benefits of β-blockade are now not surprising in view of their usefulness in treating the contractile dysfunction of dilated cardiomyopathy (see Chapters 24 and 46). Presumably, overactivation of the adrenergic nervous system leads to myocardial damage and this damage can be corrected by protecting the myocardium from catecholamines. The efficacy of β-blockade in patients with mitral regurgitation has yet to be tested. A recent report in man shows that β-blockade decreased stroke work but increased stroke volume, potential mechanisms by which β-blockade could be beneficial.[38]

Strategies for Detection and Correction of Congestive Heart Failure in Chronic Primary Mitral Regurgitation

Once even mild symptoms of congestive heart failure develop in the patient with chronic mitral regurgitation, prognosis is reduced.[39] Thus it seems clear that mitral valve repair or replacement should be performed at the onset of symptoms. There is no evidence that medical therapy at this point in the disease is beneficial, although no human trials of either β-blockers or ace inhibitors have been performed in a scale large enough to know whether these therapies might be of benefit.

As with aortic regurgitation, patients with mitral regurgitation may develop LV dysfunction without developing symptoms. Once ejection fraction declines below 60%[39] or once the left ventricle is unable to contract to an end-systolic dimension of 45 mm,[40] prognosis worsens (Figure 29-8). In fact recent data suggest that for EF to return to normal postoperatively, end-systolic dimension should not exceed 40 mm.[41] It is likely, therefore, that these markers indicate the presence of enough muscle dysfunction to impact prognosis. Thus mitral valve surgery should be performed when ejection fraction falls toward 60% or when end-systolic dimension increases toward 40 mm.[15]

In protecting the patient with mitral valve regurgitation from congestive heart failure, it is crucial that during surgery all, or at least part, of the mitral valve apparatus and its natural connections be preserved.[42-45] It is clear that the mitral valve apparatus contributes substantially to LV contraction and to maintaining the shape of the left ventricle. If the apparatus is destroyed, there is a substantial and irreversible decline in the ejection performance following surgery.[42] Even if a prosthetic valve is inserted, the posterior connections between the papillary muscles, the chordae, and the posterior leaflet can be maintained and this amount of preservation is beneficial to the outcome.[45] However, it should be noted that despite the wealth of evidence that preservation of the mitral apparatus during surgery is crucial, only approximately 60% of mitral valves are being repaired in the United States today. Indeed, there is substantial variation in repair rate from institution to institution with some institutions reporting a 95% repair rate.

Strategies to control mitral regurgitation less invasively using transcatheter mitral repair are currently undergoing testing in clinical trials. The MitraClip (Evalve, Inc.) uses a triaxial catheter-based system to create a double-orifice mitral

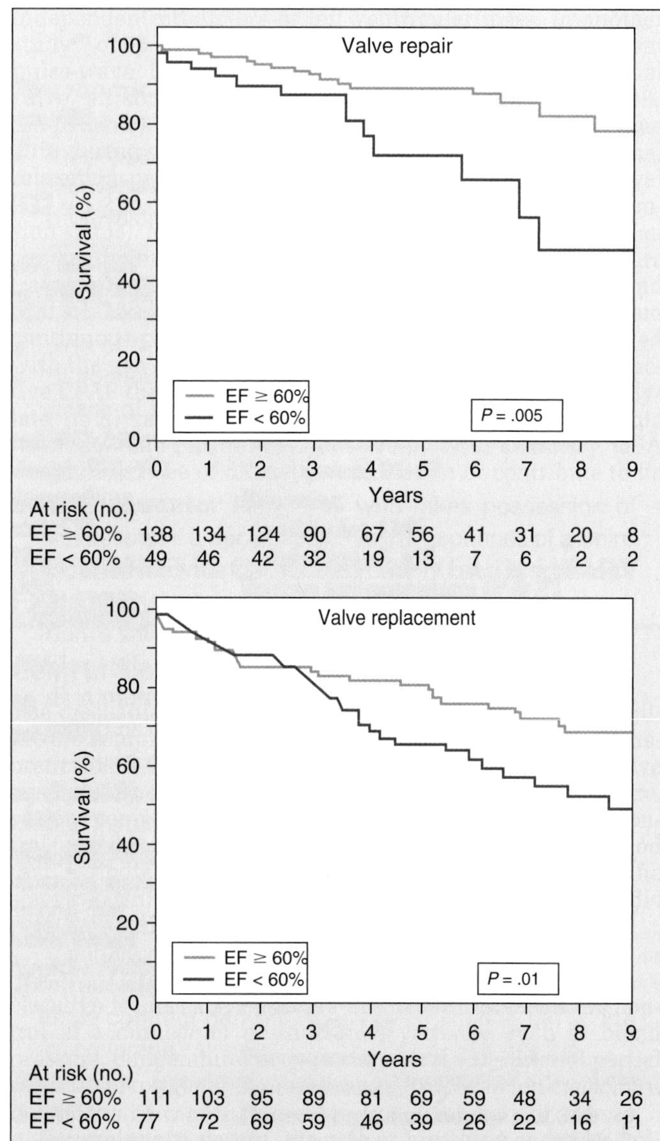

FIGURE 29-8 Survival following mitral valve surgery for mitral regurgitation. Whether repair or replacement is done, survival is excellent as long as the preoperative ejection fraction (EF) exceeds 0.60. (From Enriquez-Sarano M, Tajik AJ, Schaff HV, et al. Echocardiographic prediction of survival after surgical correction of organic mitral regurgitation. *Circulation* 1994;90: 830-837.)

valve similar to the Alfieri surgical technique. The ongoing Endovascular Valve Edge-to-Edge REpair STudy (EVEREST II) and Real World ExpAnded MuLtIcenter Study of the MitraClip System (REALISM) trials are prospective, multicenter, randomized studies to evaluate the safety and effectiveness of an endovascular approach to the treatment of mitral valve regurgitation using the MitraClip edge-to-edge implant (ClinicalTrials.gov Identifier: NCT00209274). Patients are randomized 2:1 to the study and control arms, respectively. The primary endpoints of the trial are freedom from surgery for valve dysfunction, death, and moderate to severe (3+) or severe (4+) mitral regurgitation at 12 months and freedom from major adverse events at 30 days or hospital discharge, whichever is longer. The study is powered to show noninferiority of effectiveness of the MitraClip compared with a treatment strategy of mitral valve repair or replacement surgery. The study is also powered to show superiority of safety at 30 days of an endovascular treatment strategy with the MitraClip compared with a treatment strategy of mitral valve repair or replacement surgery. Although this trial is not recruiting heart

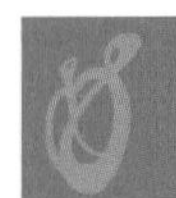

failure patients per se, the patients must be symptomatic from their mitral regurgitation or have evidence of LV dysfunction.

The MOBIUS leaflet repair system (Edwards, Inc.) is another edge-to-edge technique that uses a percutaneous stitch to create a double-orifice mitral valve.[50] There are also several direct annuloplasty techniques that imitate a surgical annuloplasty procedure, including the Mitralign System (Mitralign, Inc.), the AccuCinch (Guided Delivery Systems), and the QuantumCor device (QuantumCor). In addition, there are transcatheter coronary sinus techniques that reduce the septal-lateral dimensions of the mitral annulus using a reshaping device that is implanted in the coronary sinus. Several systems, including the MONARC device (Edwards, Inc.), the Percutaneous Mitral Annuloplasty device (PTMA, Viacor), and the CARILLON Mitral Contour System (Cardiac Dimensions) are in early phase testing. Whether these systems can be used in patients with heart failure and dilated ventricles remains to be determined.

Secondary Mitral Regurgitation

As systolic function worsens in patients with ischemic or dilated cardiomyopathy, ventricular dilation and wall motion abnormalities frequently lead to mitral incompetence. In this case the burden of volume overload caused by regurgitation is added to the already serious problem of the primary disease. The presence of functional MR worsens the prognosis of heart failure.[46] But what is not certain is whether the MR is the cause of the worsened prognosis or simply a marker of poorer LV function. The exact implications of secondary mitral regurgitation and its management are currently undergoing intense scrutiny (see also Chapter 55). In a seminal study, surgical correction of mitral regurgitation using a simple ring angioplasty substantially decreased the amount of mitral regurgitation, had a 70% one year survival rate and significantly reduced cardiac volumes while improving ejection fraction.[47] However, follow-up of these patients found no survival benefit compared with medical therapy.[48] Other studies have found little or no benefit to correcting MR in the face of severe heart failure.[49]

Aortic Stenosis

Acute Aortic Stenosis

The occurrence of acute aortic stenosis is limited to the sudden malfunction of a prosthetic aortic valve in which thrombus or other material prevents the valve leaflets from opening properly. Unlike chronic aortic stenosis where the obstruction to outflow develops gradually, allowing the left ventricle time for hypertrophic compensation, in acute aortic stenosis sudden obstruction increases afterload and impairs left ventricle ejection. Depending on the severity of the obstruction, the amount of impairment may range from mild to catastrophic. The only satisfactory therapy is immediate release of the obstruction by replacing the prosthesis, or, if a clot is the cause of the obstruction, thrombolytic agents have been used safely for dissolution of thrombus on the aortic valve.[51]

Chronic Aortic Stenosis

Little hemodynamic consequence develops as the aortic valve becomes narrowed from its normal aperture to one half its normal orifice area. However, further narrowing creates progressive obstruction to LV outflow resulting in a pressure gradient between the left ventricle and aorta. This gradient represents the additional pressure work that the left ventricle must perform to drive blood past the stenotic valve. It is generally agreed that an adaptive response to this pressure overload is the development of concentric LV hypertrophy.[52,53] Examining the Laplace equation, when pressure in the numerator is increased, it can be offset by increased wall thickness in the denominator. Thus even though there is an increase in LV pressure, wall stress can remain normal and afterload on an individual muscle fiber can be maintained in the normal range despite the presence of aortic stenosis.

However, while the LV hypertrophy is adaptive in some cases of aortic stenosis, it is maladaptive in others. Even if the amount of hypertrophy that develops is just enough to offset the increased LV pressure, the increased wall thickness requires a higher filling pressure to distend the ventricle to a given volume than if thickness were normal. Although the characteristics of the muscle in concentric hypertrophy can be normal, increased thickness mandates diastolic dysfunction. In addition as the pressure overload becomes more severe and more prolonged, collagen content of the myocardium increases, further increasing ventricular stiffness and decreasing diastolic function.[54,55]

With regards to systole, as noted previously, the amount of hypertrophy that develops may exactly offset the pressure overload to maintain normal stress. However, in some patients, especially men, the amount of hypertrophy is not adequate to normalize wall stress, wall stress rises, and ejection fraction is depressed.[56,57] In other patients, especially older women, the amount of hypertrophy that develops appears to be in excess of that which is needed to normalize stress. Stress becomes subnormal and ventricular function becomes supernormal at the chamber level. However, although systolic function is normal, or even supernormal, diastolic function is compromised. Recently attention has been called to another pattern of muscle distribution in aortic stenosis, that of concentric remodeling.[58,59] In such patients there is an increase in wall thickness with a decrease in LV radius so that stress normalization occurs without an increase in LV mass. Patients with this pattern demonstrate better LV function than those with LV hypertrophy. However such patients also have reduced stroke volume because LV end-diastolic volume is reduced. This may cause the symptoms of low output heart failure with a normal ejection fraction.

Irrespective of the effects of hypertrophy in normalizing or failing to normalize wall stress, LV muscle function eventually declines. The cellular mechanisms leading to the transition from compensated to decompensated LV hypertrophy remains a topic of intense investigation.[60] Several mechanisms have been delineated but none entirely explain the LV dysfunction which is present. In concentric hypertrophy, especially that which has been acquired in adults, coronary blood flow to the subendocardium is reduced especially during activity.[61] Thus it is likely that subendocardial ischemia plays a role in the LV dysfunction of aortic stenosis, although there is little evidence that ischemia is present at rest. In the case of aortic stenosis where persistently high wall stress has been created by inadequate hypertrophy, there is a densification of the microtubules compromising a portion of the cytoskeleton of the heart.[62] These tubules act as internal stents increasing internal load on the myocytes, inhibiting LV contraction. In other circumstances, abnormalities in calcium handling appear to be part of the mechanism causing contractile dysfunction. Finally, while many believe in a gradual transition from normal to compensated hypertrophy to hypertrophy with failure, this concept has recently been challenged.[63] Buermans et al found genetic expression differed in animals with hypertrophy destined to develop failure from those that remained compensated very early in the course of hypertrophy, well before failure developed. These data suggest diverging pathways to decompensated versus compensated hypertrophy rather than one transitioning to the other.

Treatment of Heart Failure from Aortic Stenosis

Heart failure from aortic stenosis responds well only to aortic valve replacement. In almost all cases of aortic stenosis complicated by heart failure, afterload mismatch plays at least

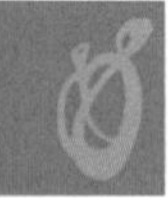

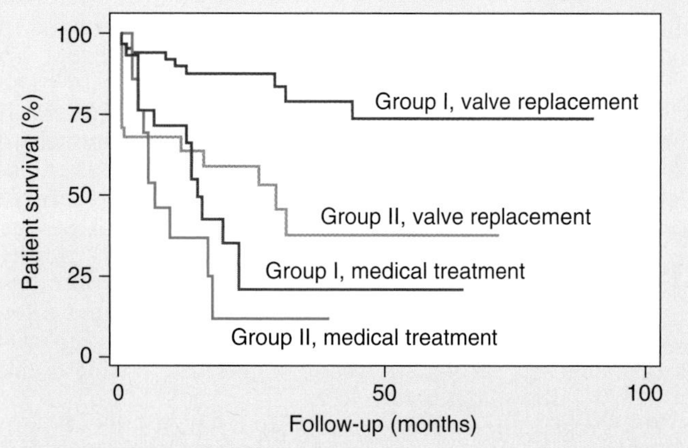

FIGURE 29–9 Postoperative outcome for aortic stenosis patients with low preoperative ejection fraction and low transvalvular gradient is demonstrated. Group I patients demonstrated preoperative inotropic reserve during dobutamine infusion while group II patients did not. An obvious advantage to surgical intervention in group I patients is demonstrated. (From Monin JL, Quere JP, Monchi M, et al. Low-gradient aortic stenosis: operative risk stratification and predictors for long-term outcome: a multicenter study using dobutamine stress hemodynamics. *Circulation* 2003;108:319-324.)

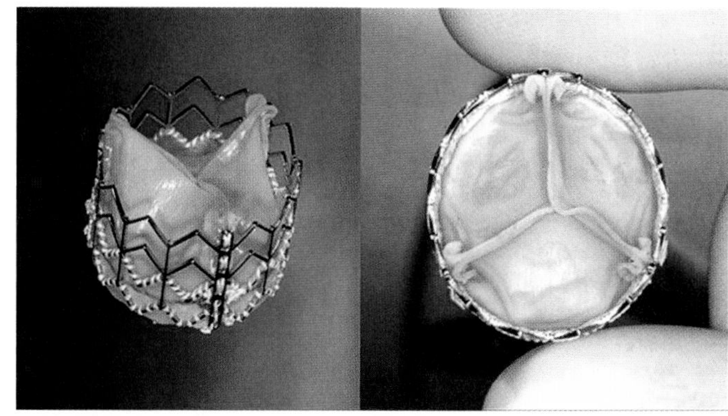

FIGURE 29–10 The SAPIEN transcatheter aortic prosthesis is mounted on a balloon-expandable stainless steel stent that is placed in the subcoronary position. The trileaflet bovine pericardial prosthesis is attached to the stent and treated with an anticalcification treatment. The stent has a polyethylene terephthalate fabric skirt that decreases perivalvular leaks. (From Zajarias A, Cribier AG. Outcomes and safety of percutaneous aortic valve replacement. *J Am Coll Cardiol* 2009;53:1829-1836.)

a partial role in causing LV dysfunction.[57] By replacing the valve, LV pressure overload is reduced, afterload is reduced, and ejection fraction improves. Even patients with severely reduced preoperative ejection fraction can have the ejection fraction return to normal following aortic valve replacement. This is especially true if the mean transvalvular gradient exceeds 40 mm Hg. In patients with reduced ejection fraction and transvalvular gradient of less than 30 mm Hg, output and gradient are reduced because of severe muscle dysfunction.[64] While in many cases this dysfunction is irreversible and prognosis is poor,[64-67] recent studies have demonstrated an advantage to aortic valve replacement even in this group of patients, especially if they demonstrate inotropic reserve preoperatively.[68] However, while operative risk is high in patients lacking inotropic reserve, even those patients who survive surgery may have a dramatic improvement in LV function.[69] Additionally, it appears that those patients with the most severely stenotic valves are the ones who benefit the most from valve replacement. The conundrum has been that at rest, two different groups appear to exist even though each has a similar valve area.[70,71] In one group, there is mild stenosis but a myopathic ventricle from another cause is unable to open the valve completely. In this case, the cardiomyopathy is primary and the mild stenosis does not constitute the major pathophysiological problem. In such cases, it is unlikely that aortic valve replacement will be helpful although this hypothesis is virtually untested. In other cases where severe stenosis has led to LV dysfunction, valve replacement appears warranted.[67] The two groups can be divorced by increasing cardiac output either with exercise or pharmacologically. If output increases and gradient fails to increase proportionally, valve area increases substantially and it is these patients who are likely to do better with medical than surgical therapy. In other cases where gradient increases proportionally with the output, there is likely severe aortic stenosis and it is this group with low ejection fraction and low gradient most likely to benefit from the aortic valve replacement (Figure 29-9).

While aortic valve replacement is the only effective therapy for aortic stenosis, many patients with the disease have acquired so many comorbidities as they have aged that aortic valve replacement is too risky to perform. However development of percutaneous valve replacement may expand the availability of aortic valve replacement for patients too infirm to undergo surgery. The ongoing PARTNERS trial (Placement of AoRTic TraNscathetER Valve Trial; [ClinicalTrials.gov Identifier NCT00530894] is a randomized open label clinical trial that is intended to determine the safety and effectiveness of a SAPIEN® Transcatheter Heart Valve (Edwards) (Figure 29-10) in high-risk, symptomatic patients with severe aortic stenosis. There are two cohorts: Cohort A will compare the percutaneous transcatheter heart valve (transfemoral or transapical) against surgery, whereas Cohort B will compare the percutaneous transcatheter heart valve (transfemoral) against medical therapy in patients who cannot tolerate aortic valve surgery. The endpoint for both cohorts is freedom from death. Although patients with severe LV dysfunction (EF < 0.20) are excluded from this study, patients with heart failure and aortic stenosis will be studied. This trial will likely provide important new information regarding the treatment of patients with aortic stenosis who have developed heart failure.

Mitral Stenosis

Mitral stenosis inhibits LV filling by preventing decompression of the left atrium during diastole. In turn, left atrial pressure and pulmonary venous pressure are elevated leading to pulmonary congestion. These changes in LV and left atrial loading cause heart failure (diminished cardiac output and increased pulmonary venous pressure), yet, in most cases LV muscle function in mitral stenosis is normal.[72] However, in some cases of aggressive rheumatic fever (the usual cause of mitral stenosis), myocarditis and depressed LV function may ensue.[73]

Interestingly, about a third of patients with mitral stenosis have reduced LV ejection performance. In most cases, this accrues from abnormal loading of the left ventricle.[72] Reduced forward output initiates reflex vasoconstriction, increasing LV afterload— cause for reduced ejection performance. At the same time, inhibition of LV inflow prevents the use of preload reserve to overcome the afterload access and ejection fraction remains depressed. However, after mitral valve commissurotomy, ejection fraction often returns to normal indicating that it was these abnormalities in loading that were primarily responsible for the preprocedure LV dysfunction.

LV filling is primarily driven by an early transmitral gradient in diastole. This gradient accrues (1) from ventricular suction as the restoring forces created by systolic compression of the ventricle are released in diastole and, (2) from increased left atrial pressure as the atrium fills following mitral valve closure in systole. In mitral stenosis, however, obstruction to inflow into the left ventricle reduces LV filling. The obstruction

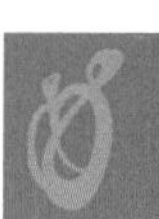

is compensated in part by an increased pressure head delivered by the right ventricle. Thus mitral stenosis leads to pulmonary hypertension. In addition to the mitral gradient, pulmonary vasoconstriction develops, further increasing pulmonary artery pressure.[74] Eventually pulmonary hypertension leads to right ventricular dysfunction, which clearly worsens outcome in mitral stenosis; thus surgery should be timed before the onset of severe pulmonary hypertension.

The issue of right ventricular contractile function in mitral stenosis has not been resolved. Pulmonary hypertension in experimental animals induces right ventricular muscle dysfunction. However, studies of right ventricular function in mitral stenosis in man have not confirmed muscle dysfunction,[75] but it must be pointed out that ventricular loading on the right ventricle has been extremely difficult to study. The shape of the right ventricle has defied easy expression of wall stress used to calculate afterload. Thus stress-strain relations used to analyze LV function have been difficult to use in estimating right ventricular function.

Therapy

Ultimately the only satisfactory therapy for the treatment of mitral stenosis is relief of the obstruction at the mitral valve. In cases of mild disease with mild symptoms, diuretics alone may be sufficient to lower left atrial pressure and render the patient asymptomatic. There is no evidence that this kind of therapy results in either sudden death or increased mortality. However, once the symptoms of mitral stenosis advances beyond NVHA class II or if asymptomatic pulmonary hypertension develops, surgical outcome is worsened. Thus mechanical correction of the lesion should take place before symptoms become far advanced or before pulmonary hypertension has been well established. In most cases, balloon valvulotomy produces a durable improvement in the orifice area with enhanced postoperative diastolic function and a rapid decline in pulmonary artery pressure toward normal. In cases where valvulotomy is impossible, mitral valve replacement produces a similar benefit.

Tricuspid Regurgitation

Most cases of tricuspid regurgitation are secondary to right ventricular pressure overload induced either from LV disease or from pulmonary parenchymal or pulmonary artery disease. However, occasionally tricuspid regurgitation is primary due to either tricuspid valve endocarditis or other abnormalities in the tricuspid valve. Recent animal studies indicate that tricuspid regurgitation, unlike mitral regurgitation, even when severe and prolonged does not cause intrinsic muscle dysfunction.[76] Rather, tricuspid regurgitation increases systemic venous pressure leading to the symptoms of right ventricular failure. Presumably, in some way, differences in loading between the right ventricle in tricuspid regurgitation and the left ventricle in mitral regurgitation are responsible for the differences in myocyte adaptation to the volume overload of each chamber.

The usual therapy for tricuspid regurgitation is to improve the primary disease responsible for it. Thus if left-sided failure has resulted in pulmonary hypertension and secondary tricuspid regurgitation, improvement in left-sided failure will result in reduced pulmonary pressure, reducing the tricuspid regurgitation.

Conclusion

Valvular heart disease accounts for only about 5% of all cases of heart failure. However, because this group of diseases is easily recognized and reversed it should be a focus of the clinician's attention. Proper timing of surgical intervention is crucial in managing this group of illnesses and the burgeoning improvement in surgical practice has pushed this timing earlier and earlier in the course of these diseases. The advent of percutaneous devices may advance the timing of mechanical intervention yet further or may make such intervention available to patients considered too risky for a standard surgical approach.[77]

REFERENCES

1. Supino, Phyllis G.,Borer, Jeffrey S., Preibisz, Jacek and Bornstein, Abraham. (2002). The epidemiology of valvular heart disease: a growing public health problem. In J. S. Borer, & O. W. Isom (Eds.), *Pathophysiology, evaluation and management of valvular heart diseases*. Basel, Switzerland: Karger.
2. Carabello, B. A., (1986). Aortic regurgitation: hemodynamic determinants of prognosis. In L. H. Cohn, & V. J. DiSesa (Eds.), *Aortic regurgitation: medical and surgical management* New York: Marcel Dekker.
3. Carabello, B. A., & Gazes, P. C. (2001). *Cardiology pearls* (2nd ed). Philadelphia: Hanley & Belfus.
4. Larbalestier, R. I., Kinchia, N. M., Aranki, S. F., et al. (1992). Acute bacterial endocarditis-optimizing surgical results. *Circulation, 86*(Suppl. 2), II-68–II-74, 2.
5. al Jubair, K., al Fagih, M. R., Ashmeg A, et al. (1992). Cardiac operations during active endocarditis. *J Thorac Cardiovasc Surg, 104*, 487–490.
6. Musci, M., Weng, Y., Hubler, M., et al. (2009). Homograft aortic root replacement in native or prosthetic active infective endocarditis: Twenty-year single-center experience. *J Thorac Cardiovasc Surg*, Epub ahead of print.
7. Wisenbaugh, T., Spann, J. F., & Carabello, B. A. (1984). Differences in myocardial performance and load between patients with similar amounts of chronic aortic versus chronic mitral regurgitation. *J Am Coll Cardiol, 3*, 916–923.
8. Feiring, A. J., & Rumberger, J. A. (1992). Ultrafast computed tomography analysis of regional radius-to-wall thickness ratios in normal and volume-overloaded human left ventricle. *Circulation, 85*, 1423–1432.
9. Taniguchi, K., Nakano, S., Kawashima, Y., et al. (1990). Left ventricular ejection performance, wall stress, and contractile state in aortic regurgitation before and after aortic valve replacement. *Circulation, 82*, 798–807.
10. Gascho, J. A., Mueller, T. M., Eastham, C., et al. (1982). Effect of volume-overload hypertrophy on the coronary circulation in awake dogs. *Cardiovasc Res, 16*(5), 288–292.
11. Borer, J. S., Truter, S. L., Herrold, E. M., et al. (2002). The cellular and molecular basis of heart failure in regurgitant valvular diseases: the myocardial extracellular matrix as a building block for future therapy. *Adv Cardiol, 39*, 7–14.
12. Schwarz, F., Flameng, W., Schaper, J., et al. (1978). Myocardial structure and function in patients with aortic valve disease and their relation to postoperative results. *Am J Cardiol, 41*, 661–669.
13. Klodas, E., Enriquez-Sarano, M., Tajik, A. J., et al. (1996). Surgery for aortic regurgitation in women: contrasting indications and outcomes compared with men. *Circulation, 94*, 2472–2478.
14. Bonow, R. O., Rosing, D. R., Maron, B. J., et al. (1984). Reversal of left ventricular dysfunction after aortic valve replacement for chronic aortic regurgitation: influence of duration of preoperative left ventricular dysfunction. *Circulation, 70*, 570–579.
15. American College of Cardiology/American Heart Association Task Force on Practice Guidelines, Society of Cardiovascular Anesthesiologists, & Society for Cardiovascular Angiography and Interventions. (2006). 2006 guidelines for the management of patients with valvular heart disease: a report of the American College of Cardiology/American Heart Association task force on practice guidelines (writing committee to revise the 1998 guidelines for the management of patients with valvular heart disease): developed in collaboration with the Society of Cardiovascular Anesthesiologists: endorsed by the Society of Cardiovascular Angiography and Interventions and the Society of Thoracic Surgeons. *Circulation, 114*(5), e84-231.
16. Krayenbuehl, H. P., Hess, O. M., Monrad, E. S., et al. (1989). Left ventricular myocardial structure in aortic valve disease before, intermediate, and late after aortic valve replacement. *Circulation, 79*(4), 744–755.
17. Scognamiglio, R., Rahimtoola, S. H., Fasoli, G., et al. (1994). Nifedipine in asymptomatic patients with severe aortic regurgitation and normal left ventricular function. *N Engl J Med, 331*, 689–694.
18. Evangelista, A., Tornos, P., Sambola, A., et al. (2005). Long-term vasodilator therapy in patients with severe aortic regurgitation. *N Engl J Med, 353*(13), 1342–1349.
19. Sampat, U., Varadarajan, P., Turk, R., et al. (2009). Effect of beta-blocker therapy on survival in patients with severe aortic regurgitation. *J Am Coll Cardiol, 54*(5), 452–457.
20. Chaliki, H. P., Mohty, D., Avierinos, J. F., et al. (2002). Outcomes after aortic valve replacement in patients with severe aortic regurgitation and markedly reduced left ventricular function. *Circulation, 106*(21), 2687–2693.
21. Carabello, B. A. (1988). Mitral regurgitation: basic pathophysiologic principles. *Mod Concepts Cardiovasc Dis, 57*, 53–58.
22. Yoran, C., Yellin, E. L., Becker, R. M., et al. (1979). Mechanism of reduction of mitral regurgitation with vasodilator therapy. *Am J Cardiol, 43*, 773–777.
23. Grigioni, F., Enriquez-Sarano, M., Ling, L. H., et al. (1999). Sudden death in mitral regurgitation due to flail leaflet. *J Am Coll Cardiol, 34*, 2078–2085.
24. Carabello, B. A. (1999). Sudden death in mitral regurgitation: why was I so surprised? *J Am Coll Cardiol, 34*(7), 2078–2085.
25. Nagatsu, M., Ishihara, K., Zile, M. R., et al. (1994). The effects of complete versus incomplete mitral valve repair in experimental mitral regurgitation. *J Thorac Cardiovasc Surg, 107*(2), 416–423.
26. Nagatsu, M., Zile, M. R., Tsutsui, H., et al. (1994). Native beta-adrenergic support for left ventricular dysfunction in experimental mitral regurgitation normalizes indexes of pump and contractile function. *Circulation, 89*(2), 818–826.
27. Mehta, R. H., Supiano, M. A., Oral, H., et al. (2000). Relation of systemic sympathetic nervous system activation to echocardiographic left ventricular size and performance and its implications in patients with mitral regurgitation. *Am J Cardiol, 85*(11), 1193–1197.

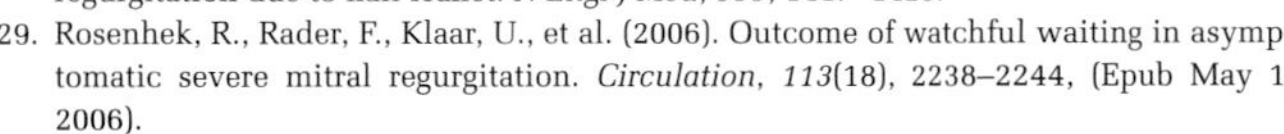

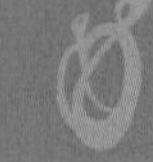

28. Ling, L. H., Enrique-Sarano, M., Seward, J. B., et al. (1996). Clinical outcome of mitral regurgitation due to flail leaflet. *N Engl J Med, 335*, 1417–1423.
29. Rosenhek, R., Rader, F., Klaar, U., et al. (2006). Outcome of watchful waiting in asymptomatic severe mitral regurgitation. *Circulation, 113*(18), 2238–2244, (Epub May 1, 2006).
30. Urabe, Y., Mann, D. L., Kent, R. L., et al. (1992). Cellular and ventricular contractile dysfunction in experimental canine mitral regurgitation. *Circ Res, 70*(1), 131–147.
31. Mulieri, L. A., Leavitt, B. J., Kent, R. L., et al. (1993). Myocardial force-frequency defect in mitral regurgitation heart failure is reversed for forskolin. *Circulation, 88*(6), 2700–2704.
32. Carabello, B. A. (2000). The pathophysiology of mitral regurgitation. *J Heart Valve Dis, 9*(5), 600–608, (review).
33. Nagatamo, Y., Carabello, B. A., Hamawaki, M., et al. (1999). Translational mechanisms accelerate the rate of protein synthesis during canine pressure-overload hypertrophy. *Am J Physiol, 277*(6 pt 2), H2176–H2184.
34. Matsuo, T., Carabello, B. A., Nagatamo, Y., et al. (1998). Mechanisms of cardiac hypertrophy in canine volume overload. *Am J Physiol, 275*(1 pt 2), H65–H74.
35. Nakano, K., Swindle, M. M., Spinale, F., et al. (1991). Depressed contractile function due to canine mitral regurgitation improves after correction of the volume overload. *J Clin Invest, 87*(6), 2077–2086.
36. Starling, M. R. (1995). Effects of valve surgery on left ventricular contractile function in patients with long-term mitral regurgitation. *Circulation, 92*, 811–818.
37. Tsutsui, H., Spinale, F. G., Nagatsu, M., et al. (1994). Effects of chronic β-adrenergic blockade on the left ventricular and cardiocyte abnormalities of chronic canine mitral regurgitation. *J Clin Invest, 93*, 2639–2648.
38. Stewart, R. A., Raffel, O. C., Kerr, A. J., et al. (2008). Pilot study to assess the influence of beta-blockade on mitral regurgitant volume and left ventricular work in degenerative mitral valve disease. *Circulation, 118*(10), 1041–1046.
39. Enriquez-Sarano, M., Tajik, A. J., Schaff, H. V., et al. (1994). Echocardiographic prediction of survival after surgical correction of organic mitral regurgitation. *Circulation, 90*, 830–837.
40. Wisenbaugh, T., Dkudicky, D., & Sareli, P. (1994). Prediction of outcome after valve replacement for rheumatic mitral regurgitation in the era of chordal preservation. *Circulation, 89*, 191–197.
41. Matsumura, T., Ohtaki, F., Tanaka, K., et al. (2003). Echocardiographic prediction of left ventricular dysfunction after mitral valve repair for mitral regurgitation as an indicator to decide the optimal timing of repair. *J Am Coll Cardiol, 42*(3), 458–463.
42. Enriquez-Sarano, M., Schaff, H. V., Orszulak, T. A., et al. (1995). Valve repair improves the outcome of surgery for mitral regurgitation: a multivariate analysis. *Circulation, 91*, 1022–1028.
43. Rozich, J. D., Carabello, B. A., Usher, B. W., et al. (1992). Mitral valve replacement with and without chordal preservation in patients with chronic mitral regurgitation: mechanisms for differences in postoperative ejection performance. *Circulation, 86*, 1718–1726.
44. Horskotte, D., Schultz, H. D., Bircks, W., et al. (1993). The effect of chordal preservation on late outcome after mitral valve replacement: a randomized study. *J Heart Valve Dis, 2*, 150–158.
45. David, T. E., Uden, D. E., & Strauss, H. D. (1983). The importance of the mitral apparatus in left ventricular function after correction of mitral regurgitation. *Circulation, 68*, II76–II82.
46. Trichon, B. H., Fleker, G. M., Shaw, L. K., et al. (2003). Relation of frequency and severity of mitral regurgitation to survival among patients with left ventricular systolic dysfunction and heart failure. *Am J Cardiol, 91*(5), 538–543.
47. Bach, D. S., & Bolling, S. F. (1996). Improvement following correction of secondary mitral regurgitation in end-stage cardiomyopathy with mitral annuloplasty. *Am J Cardiol, 78*(8), 966–969.
48. Wu, A. H., Aaronson, K. D., Bolling, S. F., et al. (2005). Impact of mitral valve annuloplasty on mortality risk in patients with mitral regurgitation and left ventricular systolic dysfunction. *J Am Coll Cardiol, 45*(3), 381–387.
49. Mihaljevic, T., Lam, B. K., Rajeswaran, J., et al. (2007). Impact of mitral valve annuloplasty combined with revascularization in patients with functional ischemic mitral regurgitation. *J Am Coll Cardiol, 49*(22), 2191–2201.
50. Piazza, N., Asgar, A., Ibrahim, R., et al. (2009). Transcatheter mitral and pulmonary valve therapy. *J Am Coll Cardiol, 53*(20), 1837–1851.
51. Roudaut, R., Lafitte, S., Roudaut, M. F, et al. (2009). Management of prosthetic heart valve obstruction: fibrinolysis versus surgery. Early results and long-term follow-up in a single-centre study of 263 cases. *Arch Cardiovasc Dis, 102*(4), 269–277.
52. Sasayama, S., Ross, J., Jr., Franklin, D., et al. (1976). Adaptations of the left ventricle to chronic pressure overload. *Circ Res, 38*, 172–178.
53. Gunther, S., & Grossman, W. (1979). Determinants of ventricular function in pressure-overload hypertrophy in man. *Circulation, 59*(4), 679–688.
54. Murakami, T., Hess, O. M., Gage, J. E., et al. (1986). Diastolic filling dynamics in patients with aortic stenosis. *Circulation, 73*, 1162–1174.
55. Villari, B., Campbell, S. E., Hess, O. M., et al. (1993). Influence of collagen network on left ventricular systolic and diastolic function in aortic valve disease. *J Am Coll Cardiol, 22*, 1477–1484.
56. Carabello, B. A., Green, L. H., Grossman, W., et al. (1980). Hemodynamic determinants of prognosis of aortic valve replacement in critical aortic stenosis and advanced congestive heart failure. *Circulation, 62*, 42–48.
57. Huber, D., Grimm, J., Koch, R., et al. (1981). Determinants of ejection performance in aortic stenosis. *Circulation, 64*, 126–134.
58. Kupari, M., Turto, H., & Lommi, J. (2005). Left ventricular hypertrophy in aortic valve stenosis: preventive or promotive of systolic dysfunction and heart failure? *Eur Heart J, 26*, 1790–1796.
59. Dumesnil, J. G., Pibarot, P., & Carabello, B. (Sep 8, 2009). Paradoxical low flow and/or low gradient severe aortic stenosis despite preserved left ventricular ejection fraction: implications for diagnosis and treatment. *Eur Heart J*, (Epub ahead of print).
60. Lorell, B. H., & Carabello, B. A. (2000). Left ventricular hypertrophy: pathogenesis, detection, and prognosis. *Circulation, 102*(4), 470–479 (review).
61. Marcus, M. L., Doty, D. B., Hiratzka, L. F., et al. (1982). Decreased coronary reserve: a mechanism for angina pectoris in patients with aortic stenosis and normal coronary arteries. *N Engl J Med, 307*, 1362–1367.
62. Zile, M. R., Green, G. R., Schuyler, G. T., et al. (2001). Cardiocyte cytoskeleton in patients with left ventricular pressure overload hypertrophy. *J Am Coll Cardiol, 37*(4), 1080–1084.
63. Buermans, H. P. J., Redout, E. M., Schiel, A. E., et al. (2005). Micro-array analysis reveals pivotal divergent mRNA expression profiles early in the development of either compensated ventricular hypertrophy or heart failure. *Physiol Genomics, 21*, 314–323.
64. Connolly, H. M., Oh, J. K., Orszulak, T. A., et al. (1997). Aortic valve replacement for aortic stenosis with severe left ventricular dysfunction: prognostic indicators. *Circulation, 95*, 2395–2400.
65. Brogan, W. C., III, Grayburn, P. A., Lange, R. A., et al. (1993). Prognosis after valve replacement in patients with severe aortic stenosis and a low transvalvular pressure gradient. *J Am Coll Cardiol, 21*, 1657–1660.
66. Connolly, H. M., Oh, J. K., Schaff, H. V., et al. (2000). Severe aortic stenosis with low transvalvular gradient and severe left ventricular dysfunction: result of aortic valve replacement in 52 patients. *Circulation, 101*, 1940–1946.
67. Pereira, J. J., Lauer, M. S., Bashier, M., et al. (2002). Survival after aortic valve replacement for severe aortic stenosis with low transvalvular gradients and severe left ventricular dysfunction. *J Am Coll Cardiol, 39*(8), 1364–1365.
68. From Monin, J. L., Quere, J. P., Monchi, M., et al. (2003). Low-gradient aortic stenosis: operative risk stratification and predictors for long-term outcome: a multicenter study using dobutamine stress hemodynamics. *Circulation, 108*, 319–324.
69. Quere, J. P., Monin, J. L., Levy, F., et al. (2006). Influence of preoperative left ventricular contractile reserve on postoperative ejection fraction in low-gradient aortic stenosis. *Circulation, 113*(14), 1738–1744, (Epub April 3, 2006).
70. Cannon, J. D., Zile, M. R., Crawfor, F. A., et al. (1992). Aortic valve resistance as an adjunct to the Gorlin formula in assessing the severity of aortic stenosis in symptomatic patients. *J Am Coll Cardiol, 20*, 1517–1523.
71. DeFilippi, C. R., Willett, D. L., Brickner, M. E., et al. (1995). Usefulness of dobutamine echocardiography in distinguishing severe from nonsevere valvular aortic stenosis in patients with depressed left ventricular function and low transvalvular gradients. *Am J Cardiol, 75*, 191–194.
72. Gash, A. K., Carabello, B. A., Cepin, D., et al. (1983). Left ventricular ejection performance and systolic muscle function in patients with mitral stenosis. *Circulation, 67*(1), 148–154.
73. Mohan, J. C., Khalilullah, M., & Arora, R. (1989). Left ventricular intrinsic contractility in pure rheumatic mitral stenosis. *Am J Cardiol, 64*, 240.
74. Mahoney, P. D., Loh, E., Blitz, L. R., et al. (2001). Hemodynamic effects of inhaled nitric oxide in women with mitral stenosis and pulmonary hypertension. *Am J Cardiol, 87*(2), 188–192.
75. Wroblewski, E., James, F., Spann, J. F., et al. (1981). Right ventricular performance in mitral stenosis. *Am J Cardiol, 47*(1), 51–55.
76. Ishibashi, Y., Rembert, J. C., Carabello, B. A., et al. (2001). Normal myocardial function in severe right ventricular volume overload hypertrophy. *Am J Physiol Heart Circ Physiol, 28*(1), H11–H16.
77. Berry, D. (2009). Percutaneous aortic valve replacement: an important advance in cardiology. *Eur Heart J, 30*(18), 2167–2169.

CHAPTER 30

Heart Failure as a Consequence of Congenital Heart Disease

Julian Booker and Wayne Franklin

In Western societies, the most common cause of heart failure in adults is "acquired" and generally arises secondary to coronary artery disease and/or hypertension (see Chapters 22, 23, and 28).[1,6] The lifetime risk of developing acquired heart failure in North America and Europe is approximately one in five for a 40-year-old. However, the true incidence of heart failure in adults with congenital heart disease is not known, particularly in the United States where universal health care data bases are not available. Moreover, as will be discussed later, the cause of heart failure in adults with congenital heart disease is exceedingly complex, and manifests either as systolic and/or diastolic dysfunction of the left, right, or a single ventricle, which makes it difficult to obtain epidemiological data regarding the true incidence of heart failure in this population. In the following chapter we will address what types of patients with adult congenital heart disease develop heart failure, and discuss what treatment options are available.

ROLE OF CONGENITAL HEART DISEASE

The term congenital heart disease refers to structural abnormalities of the heart, pericardium, and/or great vessels that are present from birth.[7] Some defects can be functionally significant at birth or may become so throughout life into adulthood. The rate of congenital heart disease is about six to eight per 1000 live births. However, many of these, such as small atrial septal defects, will never become clinically significant.[8-10] Extrapolation of these data indicate that there may be as many as 1.3 million persons with congenital heart disease in the United States alone[10] with 800,000 or more being adults.[11-13]

Approximately 15% of the children born with CHD will have potentially life-threatening defects.[10] Many of these patients will have complex or cyanotic lesions. These defects include various combinations of shunts, obstructive lesions, chamber malformation and discordance between the cardiac chambers including the great vessels. The abnormal anatomy leads to derangements in intracardiac pressure and volumes with nonphysiological flow.[14] If no other form of cardiac injury supervenes, adults with congenital heart disease may live chronically for years with an indolent disease process that is slowly progressive until the individual presents with overt symptoms of heart failure. In contrast to the majority of HF in the adult where the culprit abnormality is acquired (e.g., coronary artery disease or viral myocarditis), some congenital defects that predispose to eventual cardiomyopathy and HF are present at birth. Because of this, it has been referred to as the "original heart failure syndrome.[14]"

Surgical intervention is the cornerstone of the therapy for complex congenital heart disease. In the presurgical era, only 20% of children with complex congenital heart disease could be expected to reach adulthood. Today, nearly 90% of all patients with congenital heart disease will live to adulthood.[15] The higher prevalence is primarily related to improved survival, which coincides with the development and subsequent improvement in surgical techniques and postoperative medical care. The goal of surgery is to approximate normal anatomical and hemodynamic function as closely as possible. A minority of patients are able to undergo a truly corrective procedure and thus surgical repairs are typically palliative. The chronic abnormalities in hemodynamics frequently result in HF years to decades later. Even when corrective procedures lead to a seemingly structurally normal heart, there is evidence that subtle physiological derangements may persist. Most varieties of complex congenital heart disease ultimately lead to some form of heart failure. The timing and the type of cardiac failure will depend upon the extent of the congenital defect in conjunction with the success of surgical and medical intervention. As a result, a portion of the burden of adult HF can be directly attributed to congenital heart disease.

Heart failure in adults with congenital heart disease is characterized using the bimodal classification system focusing on systolic dysfunction and diastolic dysfunction of the left, right, or single ventricle. The clinical severity of disease is most frequently graded using the New York Heart Association (NYHA) classification of heart failure symptoms, which focuses on functional status. NYHA classification is a prime determinant of outcomes in persons with acquired heart disease, and this trend continues to hold true for the subcategory of heart failure secondary to congenital heart disease.

Piran et al looked at a cohort of 188 patients with either a system right ventricle or single ventricle physiology and evaluated the prevalence of heart failure. Ventricular function was assessed by echocardiography or radionuclide angiography. In Mustard patients, congenitally corrected transposition of the great vessels and Fontan patients the prevalence of heart failure by Framingham criteria was 22%, 32%, and 40% respectively. Within this subgroup, 82.4% were classified as either NYHA class I or II, 13.3% were NYHA class III, and 4.3% were NYHA class IV (Figure 30-1).[16] Long-term follow-up revealed a substantial difference in mortality between symptomatic and asymptomatic patients (47.1% vs. 5% at 15 years). The most powerful predictors of mortality were similar to what would be expected in a typical heart failure population: (1) NYHA classification, (2) ejection fraction of the systemic ventricle, and (3) age at onset.[16] When the cause of death of a large cohort of patients with adults with congenital heart disease was reviewed, the second most common cause of death was

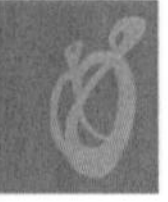

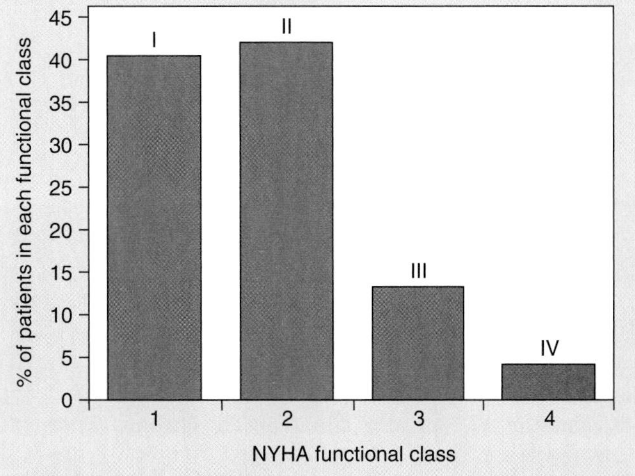

FIGURE 30–1 New York Heart Association (NYHA) functional classification of patients with systemic right ventricle or single ventricles (percentage of patients in each functional class). For deceased patients, this information was also obtained from last follow-up. (From Piran S, Veldtman G, et al. Heart failure and ventricular dysfunction in patients with single or systemic right ventricles. *Circulation* 2002;105:1189-1194.)

reported as heart failure. Heart failure accounted for 21% of the total number of deaths. "Sudden death" which constituted 26% of the total mortality was the leading cause of death and most likely consisted of some patients with heart failure.[17] These findings were corroborated by Nieminen et al who found that over a 45-year period of follow-up, 40% of patients died as a direct result of heart failure.[18]

Systemic Right Ventricle

There is a widely held misconception that the right ventricle plays a limited role in the overall hemodynamic requirements of the circulatory system. Compared with the left ventricle, it has a very complex and poorly understood physiology and anatomy. Because of these differences, the role of the right ventricle in the cardiac cycle and cardiac output is often understated and likely underestimated. In contrast to the left ventricle, the right ventricle is well suited to tolerate the dramatic changes in volume and preload that may occur with changes in intrathoracic pressure and venous return, whereas its ability to meet acute increases in afterload is limited.[19]

In the normal heart, the right ventricle supports the pulmonary circulation. However, in congenital heart disease, the morphological right ventricle may be forced to meet the higher resistance of the systemic circulation such as in patients with transposition of the great arteries or in the single ventricle physiology with a right ventricle. Mechanically, the morphological right ventricle is not equipped to withstand systemic resistance indefinitely. The right ventricle undergoes adaptive changes like hypertrophy to help sustain systemic pressures though maladaptive changes like ventricular dilation invariably follow. As a result, a large portion of heart failure in complex congenital heart disease results from dysfunction of the morphological right ventricle.

It is unclear as to whether the pressure overload alone is responsible for the failure of the right ventricle. Impaired flow reserve and myocardial perfusion defects have been noted, which suggest insufficient blood flow.[20,21] The insufficient blood flow does not appear to be a result of coronary artery disease, but rather supply-demand mismatch from elevated wall tension and inadequate coronary distribution to the right ventricle to accommodate the increased demand.[22] Evaluation by gadolinium-enhanced cardiac magnetic resonance (CMR) imaging reveals islands of myocardium consistent with regional fibrosis

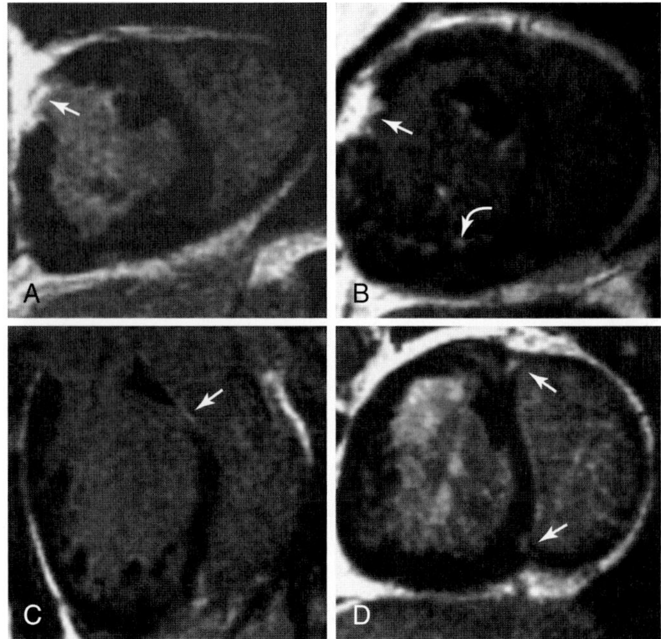

FIGURE 30–2 Magnetic resonance imaging in systemic right ventricle. **A,** Full-thickness late gadolinium enhancement of anterior wall of right ventricle. **B,** RV anterior wall enhancement (*arrow*) and multiple foci of late gadolinium enhancement, suggesting fibrosis of RV trabeculae (*curved arrow*). **C,** Late gadolinium enhancement of a spontaneously closed perimembranous VSD (*arrow*). **D,** Superior and inferior left ventricle and RV insertion point enhancement (*arrows*). (From Babu-Narayan SV, Goktekin O, Moon JC, et al. Late gadolinium enhancement cardiovascular magnetic resonance of the systemic right ventricle in adults with previous atrial redirection surgery for transposition of the great arteries. *Circulation* 2005;111:2091-2098.)

(Figure 30-2).[23,24] As a result, failure of the systemic right ventricle ultimately leads to heart failure that is clinically similar to classical heart failure that arises secondary to left ventricular (LV) failure.

L-TGA (Levo-Transposition of the Great Arteries)

The nomenclature for congenitally corrected transposition of the great arteries varies from cc-TGA ro L-TGA to atrioventricular, ventriculo-arterial discordance, to more simply ventricular inversion. Anatomically, this results in the aorta arising from the right ventricle and the pulmonary artery originating from the left ventricle. Congenitally corrected TGA, either alone or in combination with other congenial cardiac defects, is a relatively rare entity occurring in less than 1% of all congenital heart lesions. Isolated cc-TGA (i.e., with no additional congenital cardiac defects) is exceedingly rare, occurring in less than 2% of cases.[28] Associated cardiac lesions in the setting of cc-TGA are to be expected, with pulmonic or subpulmonic valvular stenosis occurring in 74%, ventricular septal defect in 74%, and systemic atrioventricular (tricuspid) valve abnormalities in 38% of patients. Also, complete heart block occurs in upto 2% of patients per year. The population of patients with cc-TGA is largely heterogeneous and there are relatively small numbers of patients with this primary lesion, which makes epidemiological studies difficult.

Unlike cyanotic congenital heart disease where childhood palliative or corrective surgery is frequently necessary for long-term survival, this is not always the case with cc-TGA. Many of these patients survive through adolescence and their first presentation of clinical ventricular failure is in adulthood. Historically, if an operation was performed, it involved repair of associated hemodynamically significant lesions. If subpulmonic outflow tract obstruction was present, then a valved conduit bypassed the obstruction, leaving the morphological left ventricle as the subpulmonic ventricle and the

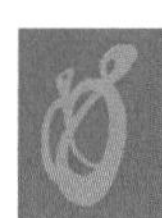

morphological right ventricle supporting the systemic circulation. In some surgical studies, long-term survival after surgical intervention has been disappointing, with approximately 50% to 60% post-operative survival at 10 years. Seventy percent to 100% of the deaths could be directly attributable to progressive morphological right ventricular (RV) failure.[25-27]

A study by Presbitero et al found that 24% of patients in their fifth decade of life had heart failure. By the sixth decade of life, 77% were diagnosed with heart failure. Failure of the systemic right ventricle is part of the natural history of the disease but the heterogeneous nature of the population makes prediction of its occurrence difficult. Twelve percent had developed significant AV valve regurgitation in their fourth decade of life. However, this number rose to approximately 70% by the sixth decade.[28] It is unclear whether AV valve regurgitation was a result of worsening ventricular failure or if the resulting volume overload precipitated the failure. Nonetheless, systemic AV valve regurgitation may be a marker for imminent systemic RV failure.

Over the last 2 decades, more cc-TGA patients have undergone the "double-switch" operation. In these patients, the morphological left ventricle has become conditioned to meet the workload of the pulmonary circulation. The majority of these patients have some degree of pulmonic LVOT obstruction, usually subpulmonic stenosis. In these patients, the afterload that the subpulmonic left ventricle has to overcome is higher than what would be seen by a normal subpulmonic right ventricle. However, a significant minority of cc-TGA patients will have insufficient (or absent) subpulmonic stenosis to adequately prepare the morphological left ventricle. These untrained left ventricles will not be adequately conditioned to contend with the systemic pressures after the double switch has taken place. In these patients, as the first stage of their "double-switch operation," this subgroup may undergo pulmonary artery banding, which increases the afterload that the subpulmonic left ventricle must face and serves to retrain the left ventricle. The left ventricle can be converted to the systemic position, and the right ventricle is switched to subpulmonic position.

D-TGA (Dextro-Transposition of the Great Arteries)

Dextroposition-transposition of the great arteries (d-TGA, ventriculo-arterial discordance, or complete transposition) is incompatible with long-term life, since most unrepaired babies died within their first year of life. The result of the congenital defect is two separate circulations, without mixing. Like other cyanotic congenital heart disease, surgical intervention is usually required to reach adulthood. Long-term survival requires a redirection of the circulation to create two circulatory paths via two inter-atrial baffles that are in series.

The atrial switch operations as described by Senning in 1959[29] and Mustard in 1964[30] revolutionized treatment of patients with d-TGA. Before the development of the atrial switch procedure, there was an approximate 90% mortality within the first year of life. With the advent of the procedure, greater than 90% long-term survival has been possible. Physiologically, the result of the atrial switch is similar to that of cc-TGA, where the morphological right ventricle becomes the systemic ventricle. As with cc-TGA, dysfunction of the systemic right ventricle plays a significant role in heart failure in d-TGA though the reported incidence of RV dysfunction is highly variable ranging up to 66%.[31] The time of onset of right ventricular dysfunction has been shown to be equally variable.[32-34] Reich et al found that concomitant LV diastolic function may play as important a role in heart failure in d-TGA.

After many years with a systemic right ventricle after the Mustard or Senning procedure, surgical options for long-term survival are limited, leaving only a heart transplantation/ventricular assist device or the "switch conversion" procedure. The arterial switch conversion is a two step process designed to "retrain" the left ventricle take over as the systemic pump chamber, similar in theory to the "double-switch" operation for cc-TGA. This is achieved by placing a pulmonary artery band in position to increase the afterload against the left ventricle. This surgically implemented increase in afterload causes the left ventricle to hypertrophy in the presence of systemic vascular resistance. It is unclear as to how long to leave the pulmonary artery band in place, and sometimes several rounds of band-tightening need to be done to "mimic" the systemic resistance. At least 18 months is often the usual time for retraining. Then, when the left ventricle is deemed sufficiently "retrained," the atrial baffles are taken down, an atrial septum is created, and an arterial switch operation is performed, in which the great arteries are transected above the valve leaflets, and switched so the pulmonary artery arises from the former aortic valve (now called the "neopulmonic valve") and the aorta arises from the former pulmonic valve (now called the "neoaortic valve"). The procedure has shown promise in pediatric population but has had decidedly mixed reviews in adults. Two large case series have shown that the procedure is feasible in the adult population but a relatively low long-term survival has not met expectations.[35,36] In a study by Poirier and Mee, age greater than 12 years old was associated with a higher chance of LV failure and mortality.[36] A second study by Cochrane et al demonstrated an 80% one year actuarial survival.[37] These findings have been corroborated by a number of smaller case series, which taken together may suggest that at present cardiac transplantation or mechanical support may be the preferred option over the arterial switch conversion.[38-41] However, once past the immediate postoperative period, some studies report that 89% of patients will normalize RV function and up to 91% will normalize LV function.[36]

Jatene et al first reported in 1976 an attempt at a true anatomic correction for d-TGA in which they describe the "arterial switch operation.[42]" Reported long-term results have been very good with reports of approximately 90% survival at 10 years.[43,44] Quality of life following the arterial switch is superior to that of patients who undergo the atrial switch operation.[45] Ninety-six percent of patients report no subjective limitations in their daily activity.[44] There is a small but distinct percentage of patients who have problems with coronary perfusion related to coronary ischemia, either from an abnormal coronary course or from the long-term sequelae of coronary reimplantation at the time of operation, which can lead to ostial disease.[46] The long-term outcomes of these arterial switch patients have yet to be determined since most are now in their late teens and early 20s.

Fontan and Single Ventricle Physiology

A sizable number of the individuals with complex congenital heart defects have a functionally single ventricle. By definition, a single ventricle is defined anatomically by the lack of nontrabeculated portion of a ventricle, which is the ventricular inlet of either ventricle. Clinically this can present itself as a double inlet or common inlet ventricle with a primary larger functioning ventricle and a smaller rudimentary ventricle. In patients with single ventricle physiology, there is mixing of arterial and venous blood. This mixing can result in cyanosis if there is inadequate pulmonary blood flow, or in pulmonary overcirculation (with possible development of subsequent pulmonary hypertension later) if there is significantly too much pulmonary blood flow from a left-to-right shunt.

The Fontan procedure serves as definitive palliation for single ventricle patients.[47] The Fontan procedure has evolved since its inception in 1971, although the basic premise remains the same. The original operation performed by Fontan et al was a direct atriopulmonary connection, creating a direct anastomotic connection between the right atrium and main pulmonary artery.[48] In recent years, this technique has been supplanted by the "modified Fontan" variation, incorporating a lateral tunnel through the right atrium or, in more recent

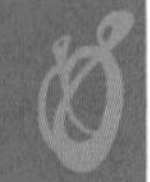

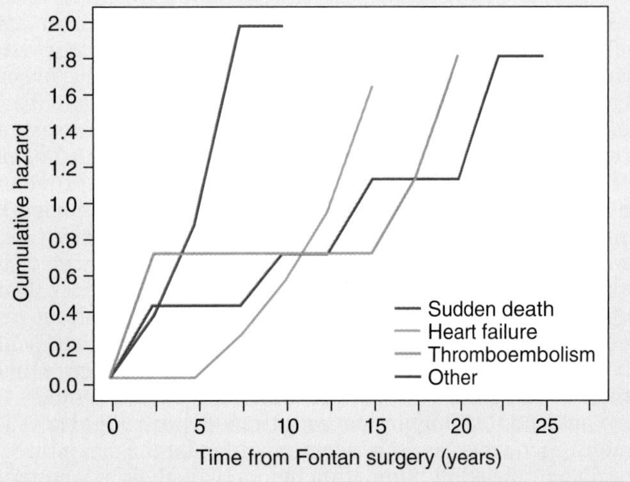

FIGURE 30–3 Cumulative hazard by mode of death following the Fontan procedure. Cumulative hazard values over time are depicted for sudden, heart failure-related, thromboembolic, and other deaths. (From Khairy P, Fernandes SM, Mayer JE Jr, et al. Long-term survival, modes of death, and predictors of mortality in patients with Fontan surgery. *Circulation* 2008;117:85-92.)

years, an extra cardiac conduit, in which a Gore-Tex tube from the IVC to the right pulmonary artery is used to bypass the hypoplastic right heart. The Fontan circulation, also known as the total cavopulmonary connection (TCPC), results in direct diversion of systemic venous blood with passive flow through the pulmonary circuit since there is no RV pump. The Fontan operation is now the most common surgery performed for congenital hearts defects after the age of 2 years. An entire generation of patients with single ventricles, who underwent the palliative Fontan operation, has now reached adulthood.

We now know the tendency of the Fontan circulation to do well for 20 years but then have progressive clinical decline with the end-stage of this process often referred to as the "failed Fontan." The "failed Fontan" term refers to a several clinical events that contribute to low cardiac output. The failed Fontan circuit can exist in isolation but can also be seen in combination with ventricular systolic dysfunction. More specifically, the failing Fontan state deals with inefficiency of the atriopulmonary circulation, complicated by the lack of a true RV pump to assist with pulmonary blood flow. Other complications that contribute to this state are recurrent atrial tachycardias (often intra-atrial reentrant tachycardia) and elevated right-atrial-Fontan circuit pressure.

Normal Fontan physiology relies upon a normal, low pulmonary vascular resistance.[49] Deterioration of the atriopulmonary circuit can be caused by inadequate flow at two levels: (1) inadequate systemic venous return, or (2) inadequate pulmonary venous return. Restriction of systemic venous return may be iatrogenic, related to thrombus formation or some other obstructive process. Also, any increase in the pulmonary vascular resistance (such as from respiratory infections, sleep apnea, or pulmonary emboli) can lead to decreased pulmonary circulation and may ultimately result in hemodynamic compromise, which can present as ascites and lower extremity edema. The role that thrombi play in the deterioration of the Fontan circuit cannot be overstated. The classic Fontan predisposes to massive atrial dilation, which may have less laminar flow and potential areas of stasis blood. This altered homodynamic milieu predisposes to a "slow flow state" and thrombus formation. Thrombus at any level of the systemic venous return, but particularly those involving the right atrium or pulmonary artery emboli are frequently responsible for failure of the circuit. However, compression of the pulmonary veins by a severely dilated atrium is significantly less common but a recognized entity nonetheless.

Clinically, it can be difficult to differentiate symptoms related to the failed Fontan circuit from those related to ventricular failure as there may be significant overlap. The failed Fontan state may lead to cardiopulmonary compromise and a clinical syndrome analogous to "right-sided" heart failure in the biventricular heart, including lower extremity edema, protein losing enteropathy, easy fatigability, and exercise intolerance. Additionally, these patients are at risk for macroreentrant atrial arrhythmias (such as intraatrial reentrant tachycardia) from severe right atrial dilation and/or atrial surgical scars. Also, cyanosis can develop from small leaks in the Fontan circuit (that cause a right-to-left shunt into the left atrium) or venovenous collaterals (such as from the subclavian vein to the pulmonary veins). Tachycardia or cyanosis are two conditions that warrant further investigation immediately. Concomitant left ventricular failure results in pulmonary congestion and an overall clinical scenario similar to that of biventricular failure.

Vigilant surveillance is necessary because failure of the Fontan circuit is common, especially in patients who are 20 years status-post initial Fontan palliation. There are a number of risk factors that have been shown to place a patient at an increased risk of Fontan circuit failure. The presence of the atriopulmonary connection (known as the "classic Fontan"), younger age at the time of operation, absence of a baffle fenestration, distorted pulmonary artery anatomy, the presence of a right-sided tricuspid valve as only atrioventricular valve, a mean pulmonary artery pressure greater than or equal to 19 mm Hg, worse NYHA classification,[50] and the presence of a permanent pacemaker. In contrast, a morphological left ventricle with normal arterial concordance or single right ventricle tends to be protective. However, in patients with the Fontan repair, independent predictors of *heart failure*-related death are the presence of a single morphological right ventricle, elevated right atrial pressure, and protein-losing enteropathy.[51]

Careful observation for the development of heart failure is critical to care of these patients. The primary treatment option for failure of the Fontan circuit is surgical. The Fontan revision procedure, a corrective surgical procedure performed when a Fontan circuit has failed, has become relatively commonplace at our institution over the past several years. The Fontan revision involves debulking the enlarged right atrium, converting the classic Fontan or one of its earlier iterations to a lateral tunnel or extracardiac conduit, performing a modified Maze operation, and placement of an epicardial pacemaker.[52] Some indications for revision include supraventricular tachycardia, persistent cyanosis, protein-losing enteropathy, or simply "failing Fontan physiology." Careful patient selection and close clinical follow-up postoperatively is mandatory.

Volume Overload Lesions

RV failure may also develop in response to RV volume overload as a consequence of increased flow to the right ventricle. The most common congenitally related causes are atrial septal defects or a regurgitant atrioventricular valve, which frequently is seen in the setting of the Ebstein abnormality. Patients with repaired tetralogy of Fallot may have cardiac failure from volume *and* pressure overload as a consequence of chronic pulmonary insufficiency.[53-55] The increased volume leads to compensatory dilation of the right ventricle, which initially helps to augment cardiac output by improving contractility via the Starling mechanism. Over time, the dilation becomes maladaptive and RV contractility declines once dilation exceeds an optimum size.

Hemodynamically significant volume overload lesions should be corrected surgically. Most atrial septal defects have the option of being closed percutaneously or surgically. The option of percutaneous closure means that once

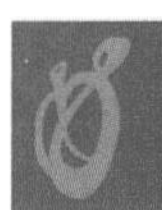

a hemodynamically significant lesion is identified, it may be electively repaired as soon as possible to prevent or reverse the complications of the chronic volume overload state. Heart failure related to surgical repair of the tetralogy of Fallot and chronic pulmonary valve regurgitation generally should be addressed either with surgical pulmonary valve replacement or percutaneous pulmonary valve implantation. These patients have undergone at least one operation and in many cases multiple operations by the time they reach adulthood. Surgical repair of the pulmonary insufficiency may not be durable and the prospect of additional repairs via repeat sternotomies is challenging. Therefore the goal is often to defer as long as possible before pulmonary valve replacement in an attempt to limit the total number of cardiac operations but prevent permanent negative cardiac remodeling. There are recent data that advocates routine noninvasive surveillance with cardiac magentic resonance (CMR) imaging and surgical repair before the right ventricle volume index reaches 170 cc/m^2.[56]

MEDICAL TREATMENT OF HEART FAILURE IN ADULTS WITH CONGENITAL HEART DISEASE

The hemodynamic model has been traditionally used to describe the heart failure that arises in adults with congenital heart disease. This model states that the heart consists of two positive displacement pumps in series and that heart failure is caused by dysfunction of one or both of the pumps. Treatment dictated by this model has focused primarily on improving pump contractility and/or decreasing the resistance that the pump must work against. The pharmacological focus of this therapy involves inotropes, diuretics, and vasodilators.

In recent years, there has been a paradigm shift in the understanding of adult heart failure. The neurohormonal model now forms the basis for understanding and treating heart failure. Along with the increased activation of several neurohormonal systems (see Chapters 9 and 10), there is a commensurate increase in cytokine release (see Chapter 11).[57-60] The altered neurohormonal milieu is associated with the clinical signs and symptoms of heart failure and resultant cardiac remodeling.[61,62] The degree of neurohormonal imbalance is directly related to heart failure related mortality,[63] LV dysfunction,[64,65] and poor functional capacity.[61,62] Subsequent studies examining the effects of neuroendocrine inhibitors, such as β-blockers,[66-70] angiotensin-converting enzyme (ACE) inhibitors,[71-73] angiotensin receptor blockers,[74-77] and aldosterone inhibitors,[78,79] have led to the formulation of the neurohormonal hypothesis for heart failure. There is a small but growing body of evidence that the maladaptive neurohormonal response plays a large role in heart failure related to congenital defects, much in the same way that it does in heart failure from acquired heart disease. As in heart failure of acquired heart disease, there is activation of multiple tiers of the neuroendocrine system. There is concomitant activation of the sympathoadrenergic (Figure 30-4), renin-angiotensin-aldosterone (RAAS) (Figure 30-5), and the endothelin systems (see Figure 30-4)[14,80-85] and release of inflammatory cytokines.[86,87] Similarly, the degree of elevation of these neurohormones corresponds with the clinical severity of heart failure (see Figure 30-5).[14]

Outpatient Medical Management

There are very limited data available regarding medical therapy for treating heart failure that develops patients with adult congenital heart disease. Accordingly, at the time of this writing there are insufficient clinical data to develop "evidence-based" treatment algorithms. Indeed, data are primarily limited to retrospective analysis, case series, and case reports for treating these patients. Indeed, virtually no prospective trials exist in the adult congenital heart disease literature. Thus far most of the therapies that are used in clinical practice with adult congenital heart disease patients has been extrapolated from heart failure studies in the adult with acquired heart disease that affects the left ventricle.

The foundation of pharmacotherapy for symptomatic heart failure in patients with adult congenital heart disease includes diuretic therapy to control vascular congestion and pulmonary edema. Caution should be exercised when using diuretics in those patients who have undergone Fontan repair. Fontan physiology leads to passive, nonpulsatile filling of the pulmonary vascular bed, which is therefore entirely preload dependent. Accordingly preload reduction with or without volume depletion can be detrimental to overall cardiac output. Similarly, patients with Eisenmenger syndrome or pulmonary outflow tract obstruction with RV hypertrophy and subsequent diastolic dysfunction are similarly dependent upon preload.

The renin-angiotensin aldosterone system (RAAS) is activated by decreased renal perfusion caused by intravascular volume depletion or low cardiac output, sodium restriction, or increased adrenergic drive, and is activated in patients with adult congenital heart disease (see Figure 30-4). Although a number of studies in adults with advanced heart failure have demonstrated the benefits of ACE inhibitors on LV function and LV remodeling in NYHA class I-IV heart failure patients (see Chapter 45),[72,88-90] treatment with ramipril for 1 year had no effect on RV ejection fraction, nor right ventricle size in a small prospective randomized study of patients with systemic right ventricles after a Mustard or Senning procedure (Figure 30-7).[91]

Angiotensin receptor blockers (ARB) act to inhibit the renin-angiotensin axis at its final common pathway by directly blocking angiotensin-II from binding to its receptor (see Chapters 9 and 45). Data from the CHARM-Alternative,[75] ELITE, ELITE II, and STRETCH trials among others demonstrate the effect that ARBs have on LV dysfunction and heart failure. Data from the CHARM-Added trial[74] suggests that concomitant therapy with an ACE inhibitor has added benefit. In heart failure, activation of the RAAS leads to increased expression of aldosterone. Increased expression of aldosterone may lead to a number of pathological states, including endothelial damage, myocardial fibrosis, and hypertrophy (see Chapter 45).[92-97] Based on the wealth of data on ARBs and aldosterone antagonists in acquired heart failure, these agents may also be considered early in the course of treatment for heart failure that arises in the setting of adult congenital heart disease.

One of the most powerful drug classes in the armamentarium for the treatment of heart failure treatment is that of the β-blockers (see Chapter 46). Chronically elevated levels of catecholamines can be cardiotoxic and cause apoptosis of myocytes.[98-100] Catecholamines are also potent activators of the RAAS.[101,102] Moreover, β-blockade helps to prevent and/or reverse negative cardiac remodeling. Clinical trials such as the U.S. Carvedilol,[103] MERIT-HF,[69] and CIBIS-II[66] have repeatedly demonstrated the importance of β-blockade not only for suppression of arrhythmias, but also for progressive pump failure in acquired forms of heart failure. Based on current data in acquired heart disease, β-blockers may also be considered for the treatment for heart failure that arises in the setting of adult congenital heart disease. The dosing and precautions about starting these agents in patients with adult congenital heart disease are identical to those with acquired forms of heart disease (see Chapter 46).

Inpatient Medical Management

Intravenous administration remains the primary mode of delivery for medications used to treat decompensated heart failure requiring hospitalization. As with the outpatient

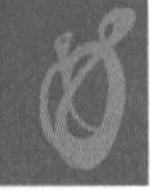

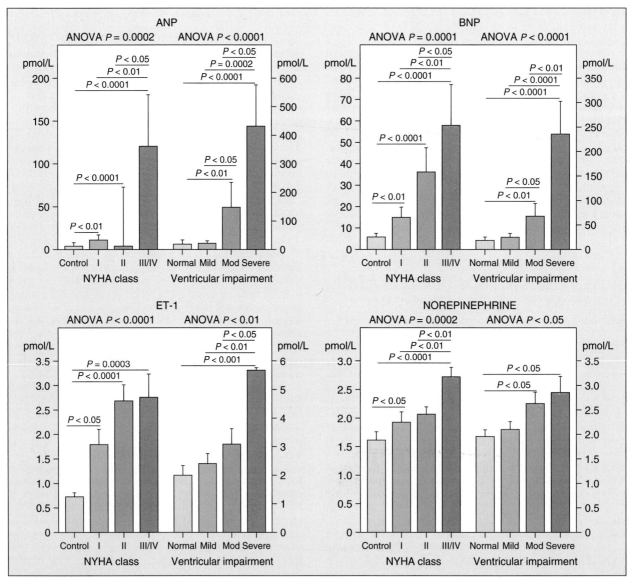

FIGURE 30–4 Neurohormone levels in all subjects according to NYHA functional class and in adults with congenital heart disease according to systemic ventricular function. Note differing *y*-scales for each measure. As shown, there was a highly significant stepwise increase in the concentrations of all four neurohormones with increasing disease severity. Neurohormonal activation was evident even in patients with asymptomatic disease when compared with control subjects. (From Bolger AP, Sharma R, Li W, et al. Neurohormonal activation and the chronic heart failure syndrome in adults with congenital heart disease. *Circulation* 2002;106:92-99 and modified from Franklin WJ, Webb GD. Heart failure in adults with congenital heart disease. In Chang AC, Towbin JA, editors. *Heart failure in children and young adults*, ed 1, Philadelphia, 2006, Elsevier.)

population, the diuretics remain a cornerstone of the treatment of symptomatic heart failure. They can be used frequently in the treatment of heart failure associated with congenital heart defects. However, as with outpatient therapy, extreme caution should be taken when using diuretics in patients post-Fontan repair.

In hypotension with or without low cardiac output, vasopressors, inotropes, or a combination of the two should be used (see Chapter 43). There is very limited data on the use of inotropes to treat decompensated heart failure in congenital heart failure. At our institution, dopamine and dobutamine are considered first-line therapy if inotropic support is required. Vasopressin, epinephrine, and norepinephrine may be added in various combinations if either more α-agonism or β-agonism is required. There appears to be a growing role for the phosphodiesterase inhibitor milrinone in the treatment of congenital heart disease. In the pediatric population, phosphodiesterase inhibition has been successful at not only prevention but also the treatment of a postoperative low cardiac output state following cardiac surgery[104-106] and specifically following Fontan palliation.[107] The hemodynamic impact of milrinone, specifically, inotropy, lusitropy, and vasodilation appears to be favorable for the treatment of certain congenital heart failure syndromes. There are no trials published on using vasopressin antagonists in patients with adult congenital heart disease.

Surveillance

The clinical history and physical examination are still the most important components of successful follow-up of heart failure patients with congenital heart disease. Close follow-up of symptoms and volume status are paramount. The cardiopulmonary stress test or the exercise tolerance test may provide objective data, which can help determine the functional status of the patient and the extent of heart failure.

Ventricular dysfunction, either left or right,[108-110] portends a poorer prognosis in the setting of heart failure than does normal ventricular function. Elevated pulmonary artery pressure is also a predictor of worse outcomes. These variables are important not only for prognostic information but they are critical in the decision-making process for proper medical and surgical management. Two-dimensional echocardiography can provide anatomical information and functional information. The addition of the Doppler examination allows for assessment of cardiac hemodynamics including pulmonary artery pressure. As a result of multiple cardiac operations, many adults with complex congenital heart disease frequently have poor acoustic windows, which may yield suboptimal visualization by echocardiography. Many patients with complex congenital heart disease will have a systemic morphological right ventricle or a single common ventricle. A potential obstacle to examining the function of the morphological RV function or single common ventricle has related to difficulties in accurate, noninvasive assessment of their function. Unlike the left ventricle, the complex anatomy of the right ventricle precludes traditional echocardiographic estimation of RV ejection fraction. Echocardiographic techniques used to assess RV function rely heavily on surrogates of ejection fraction, like annular excursion measured by tissue Doppler or require complex geometric assumptions to calculate the ejection fraction.[111-113]

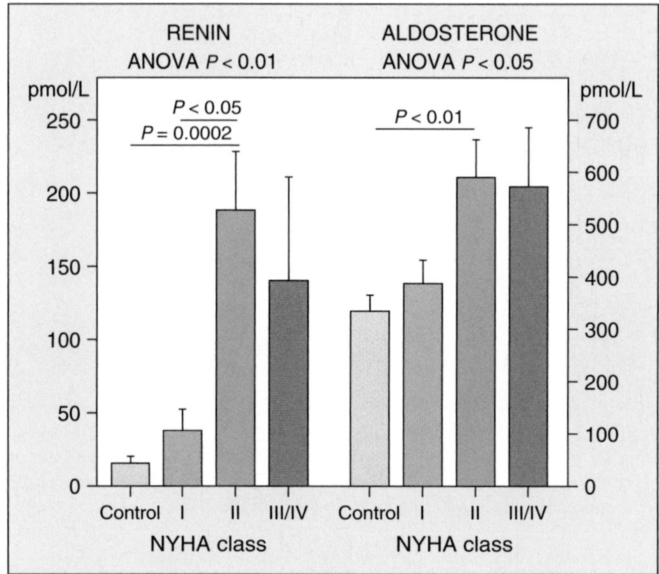

FIGURE 30–5 Renin and aldosterone levels in adult congenital heart disease patients according to NYHA functional class. As shown, activation of the renin-aldosterone axis was apparent in symptomatic adult congenital heart disease patients versus control subjects or versus those without symptoms. (From Bolger AP, Sharma R, Li W, et al. Neurohormonal activation and the chronic heart failure syndrome in adults with congenital heart disease. *Circulation* 2002;106:92-99.)

CMR imaging is a newer imaging modality, which is not limited by some of the shortcomings of echocardiography but has a set of its own that prevents it from being all inclusive. CMR has excellent spatial resolution. This allows for accurate structural information and shunt quantification. One of the most important aspects of CMR, it provides the practitioner the tools for accurate volumetric analysis including reproducible calculation of both the left and right ventricular ejection fractions.[114-116] Unfortunately, patients with defibrillators and pacemakers are generally not able to undergo CMR evaluation because of the strong magnetic field. If either of the aforementioned modalities is unavailable, then radionuclide angiography or a gated SPECT study, both nuclear imaging techniques, can be used to provide reasonable assessment of ventricular ejection fraction without geometric assumptions. However, these tests require radiation and give limited structural and functional information.[117] Serial evaluation of cardiac function should be performed routinely since results will guide therapy. If more detailed hemodynamic data are required, cardiac catheterization can be performed by clinicians trained in congenital heart disease.

Mechanical Support (see also Chapter 56)

Over the past 2 decades, the use of mechanical circulatory support has become more prevalent. For many patients with acute, severe decompensation, temporary mechanical

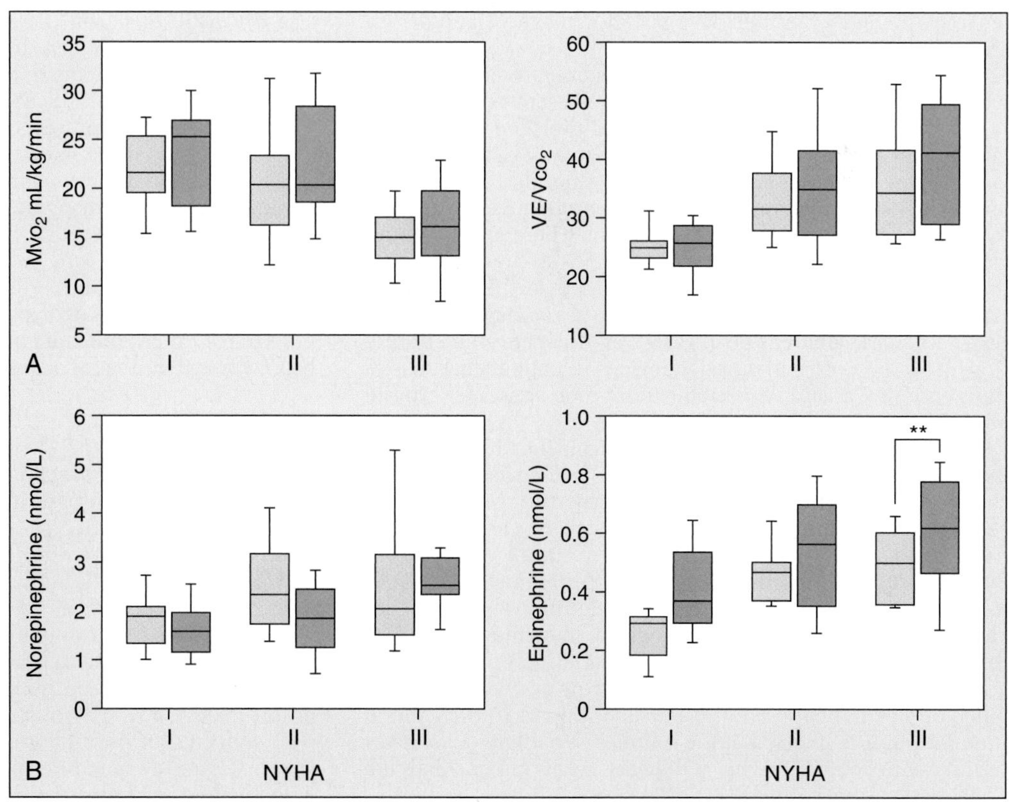

FIGURE 30–6 Exercise limitation and neurohormonal activation in adults with congenital heart disease and patients with heart failure due to other causes. **A,** The relationship between peak oxygen consumption ($M\dot{V}O_2$) and the ventilatory response to exercise (VE/VCO_2) with NYHA functional class in 47 patients with noncachectic chronic heart failure due to ischaemic or dilated cardiomyopathy no white bars in figure and in 28 adult patients with congenital heart disease of varying type no gray bars in figure. There are no statistical differences between the two groups at each level of functional impairment. **B,** The relationship between plasma norepinephrine and epinephrine levels with NYHA functional class in the same 47 patients with chronic heart failure and in 52 adult patients with congenital heart disease of varying type. There are no statistical differences between the two groups in respect to norepinephrine. Epinephrine levels tend to be higher at all levels of functional impairment in adults with congenital heart disease and are significantly so with respect to NYHA class III (key ** $P < .01$). (From Bolger AP, Gatzoulis MA. Towards defining heart failure in adults with congenital heart disease. *Int J Cardiol* 2004;97([suppl 1]15-23.)

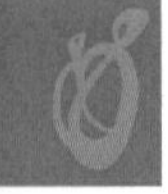

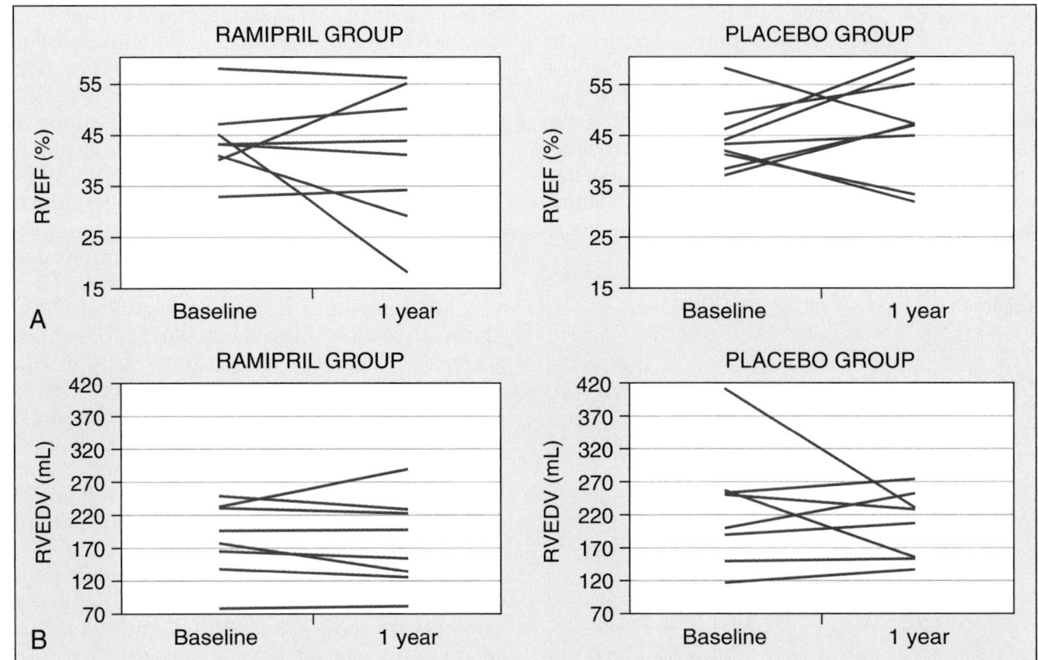

FIGURE 30–7 Effect of ramipril on RV structure and function in patients with systemic right ventricles. **A,** Right ventricular ejection fraction at baseline and after 1 year of therapy with ramipril or a placebo. (*RVEF,* right ventricular ejection fraction). **B,** Right ventricular end-diastolic volume at baseline and after 1 year of therapy with ramipril or a placebo. (*RVEDD,* right ventricular end-diastolic volume). **C,** Right ventricular end-systolic volume at baseline and after 1 year of therapy with ramipril or a placebo. (*RVESD,* Right ventricular end-systolic volume). (From Therrien J, Provost Y, Harrison J, et al. Effect of angiotensin receptor blockade on systemic right ventricular function and size: a small, randomized, placebo-controlled study. *Int J Cardiol* 2008;129:187-192.)

support is often required. Intraaortic balloon counterpulsation is widely used as a temporizing therapy in the treatment of adult heart failure. In the failing Fontan circuit, intraaortic balloon counterpulsation (IABP) has been shown to improve pulmonary circulation by lowering LV end-diastolic pressure resulting in reduction in left atrial pressure.[118] The additional hemodynamic support helps to reestablish the Fontan circulation.[118,119] However, anecdotal experience and further studies of IABP use in Fontans have not shown benefit and do not support its widespread use.

The ventricular assist device is a semipermanent device used to augment cardiac output in the setting of severe cardiomyopathy and decompensated heart failure. The devices can either be primarily extracorporeal or primarily intracorporeal. Use of the ventricular assist device as either destination therapy, bridge to transplantation, or bridge to recovery has been well established in the adult population. There is a small but growing body of evidence supporting VAD use in some capacity for congenital heart disease–related heart failure.[120-123] And, devices such as the Berlin heart have been implanted into patients as small as 4 kg. However, there are some limitations to using ventricular assist devices in patients because of their complex anatomy, which can include abnormal arterial and venous connections.

Extracorporeal membrane oxygenation (ECMO) has been used for many years for critically ill pediatric patients. It serves as a means to temporarily oxygenate patients with refractory hypoxemia due to respiratory or cardiovascular causes. Survival in both children and adults who receive ECMO support for cardiac reasons is approximately 40%.[124] Although there is evidence that heart failure related to congenital heart disease may have worse outcomes on ECMO than does cardiomyopathy.[125] The population of adults with congenital heart disease continues to grow as does the prevalence of mechanical cardiopulmonary support in the general population. It is likely that the number of patients with heart failure and congenital heart defects receiving mechanical assist devices will grow in parallel.

Surgical Therapy

A variety of surgical options may be available as salvage therapy as these patients develop heart failure. The most common surgical options for each abnormality have been discussed earlier in their respective sections. The final surgical option for some patients is cardiac transplantation. According to UNOS, nearly 7% of the cardiac transplants performed in 2007 were as a direct result of cardiac failure secondary to congenital heart disease. This is an increase from the 5% of heart transplants in 2002, but is still inadequate for the amount of congenital heart patients with advanced heart failure. In addition, patients with a history of congenital heart disease often pose many problems surgically. They often have abnormal or distorted anatomy as a result of their defects. Many will have undergone multiple cardiac operations during their lifetime, which places them at high risk for adhesions and bleeding. There is often an extensive history of exposure to blood products. In light of high levels of circulating antibodies, finding a suitable blood donor may be problematic. At experienced centers, the 1-year mortality rates for cardiac transplant for congenital anomalies has been worse than that of acquired cardiomyopathies.[126-128]

Future Challenges

Since patients with heart failure are one of the fastest growing subsections of cardiology, and since the majority of children with congenital heart disease are now surviving into adulthood, the number of adults with congenital heart disease and heart failure will undoubtedly to continue to expand. This necessitates preparation for this new population, which should include better evidence-based therapies and more clinicians with expertise in this field. In addition, as mechanical circulatory support continues to improve, cardiac transplantation for these heart defects may be needed less often. This will continue to provide great challenges and opportunities in cardiovascular medicine as we strive to provide the best care for these complex patients.

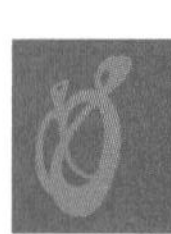

REFERENCES

1. McMurray, J. J., & Stewart, S. (2000). Epidemiology, aetiology, and prognosis of heart failure. *Heart, 83*, 596–602.
2. Kannel, W. B. (2000). Incidence and epidemiology of heart failure. *Heart Fail Rev, 5*, 167–173.
3. Swedberg, K., Cleland, J., Dargie, H., et al. (2005). Guidelines for the diagnosis and treatment of chronic heart failure: executive summary (update 2005): the task force for the diagnosis and treatment of chronic heart failure of the European Society of Cardiology. *Eur Heart J, 26*, 1115–1140.
4. Levy, D., Kenchaiah, S., Larson, M. G., et al. (2002). Long-term trends in the incidence of and survival with heart failure. *N Engl J Med, 347*, 1397–1402.
5. Mendez, G. F., & Cowie, M. R. (2001). The epidemiological features of heart failure in developing countries: a review of the literature. *Int J Cardiol, 80*, 213–219.
6. McKee, P. A., Castelli, W. P., McNamara, P. M., et al. (1971). The natural history of congestive heart failure: the Framingham study. *N Engl J Med, 285*, 1441–1446.
7. Mitchell, S. C., Korones, S. B., & Berendes, H. W. (1971). Congenital heart disease in 56,109 births. Incidence and natural history. *Circulation, 43*, 323–332.
8. Hoffman, J. I., & Christianson, R. (1978). Congenital heart disease in a cohort of 19,502 births with long-term follow-up. *Am J Cardiol, 42*, 641–647.
9. Hoffman, J. I., & Kaplan, S. (2002). The incidence of congenital heart disease. *J Am Coll Cardiol, 39*, 1890–1900.
10. Wren, C., Reinhardt, Z., & Khawaja, K. (2008). Twenty-year trends in diagnosis of life-threatening neonatal cardiovascular malformations. *Arch Dis Child Fetal Neonatal Ed, 93*, F33–F35.
11. Hoffman, J. I., Kaplan, S., & Liberthson, R. R. (2004). Prevalence of congenital heart disease. *Am Heart J, 147*, 425–439.
12. Marelli, A. J., Mackie, A. S., Ionescu-Ittu, R., et al. (2007). Congenital heart disease in the general population: changing prevalence and age distribution. *Circulation, 115*, 163–172.
13. Warnes, C. A., Liberthson, R., Danielson, G. K., et al. (2001). Task force 1: the changing profile of congenital heart disease in adult life. *J Am Coll Cardiol, 37*, 1170–1175.
14. Bolger, A. P., Sharma, R., Li, W., et al. (2002). Neurohormonal activation and the chronic heart failure syndrome in adults with congenital heart disease. *Circulation, 106*, 92–99.
15. Garson, A., Jr., Allen, H. D., Gersony, W. M., et al. (1994). The cost of congenital heart disease in children and adults. A model for multicenter assessment of price and practice variation. *Arch Pediatr Adolesc Med, 148*, 1039–1045.
16. Piran, S., Veldtman, G., Siu, S., et al. (2002). Heart failure and ventricular dysfunction in patients with single or systemic right ventricles. *Circulation, 105*, 1189–1194.
17. Oechslin, E. N., Harrison, D. A., Connelly, M. S., et al. (2000). Mode of death in adults with congenital heart disease. *Am J Cardiol, 86*, 1111–1116.
18. Nieminen, H. P., Jokinen, E. V., & Sairanen, H. I. (2007). Causes of late deaths after pediatric cardiac surgery: a population-based study. *J Am Coll Cardiol, 50*, 1263–1271.
19. Yacoub, M. H. (1979). The case for anatomic correction of transposition of the great arteries. *J Thorac Cardiovasc Surg, 78*, 3–6.
20. Singh, T. P., Humes, R. A., Muzik, O., et al. (2001). Myocardial flow reserve in patients with a systemic right ventricle after atrial switch repair. *J Am Coll Cardiol, 37*, 2120–2125.
21. Hauser, M., Bengel, F. M., Hager, A., et al. (2003). Impaired myocardial blood flow and coronary flow reserve of the anatomical right systemic ventricle in patients with congenitally corrected transposition of the great arteries. *Heart, 89*, 1231–1235.
22. Hornung, T. S., Kilner, P. J., Davlouros, P. A., et al. (2002). Excessive right ventricular hypertrophic response in adults with the mustard procedure for transposition of the great arteries. *Am J Cardiol, 90*, 800–803.
23. Babu-Narayan, S. V., Goktekin, O., Moon, J. C., et al. (2005). Late gadolinium enhancement cardiovascular magnetic resonance of the systemic right ventricle in adults with previous atrial redirection surgery for transposition of the great arteries. *Circulation, 111*, 2091–2098.
24. Hartke, L. P., Gilkeson, R. C., O'Riordan, M. A., et al. (2006). Evaluation of right ventricular fibrosis in adult congenital heart disease using gadolinium-enhanced magnetic resonance imaging: initial experience in patients with right ventricular loading conditions. *Congenit Heart Dis, 1*, 192–201.
25. McGrath, L. B., Kirklin, J. W., Blackstone, E. H., et al. (1985). Death and other events after cardiac repair in discordant atrioventricular connection. *J Thorac Cardiovasc Surg, 90*, 711–728.
26. Termignon, J. L., Leca, F., Vouhe, P. R., et al. (1996). "Classic" repair of congenitally corrected transposition and ventricular septal defect. *Ann Thorac Surg, 62*, 199–206.
27. van Son, J. A., Danielson, G. K., Huhta, J. C., et al. (1995). Late results of systemic atrioventricular valve replacement in corrected transposition. *J Thorac Cardiovasc Surg, 109*, 642–652, discussion 652–653.
28. Presbitero, P., Somerville, J., Rabajoli, F., et al. (1995). Corrected transposition of the great arteries without associated defects in adult patients: clinical profile and follow up. *Br Heart J, 74*, 57–59.
29. Senning, A. (1959). Surgical correction of transposition of the great vessels. *Surgery, 45*, 966–980.
30. Mustard, W. T. (1964). Successful two-stage correction of transposition of the great vessels. *Surgery, 55*, 469–472.
31. Reich, O., Voriskova, M., Ruth, C., et al. (1997). Long-term ventricular performance after intra-atrial correction of transposition: left ventricular filling is the major limitation. *Heart, 78*, 376–381.
32. Graham, T. P., Jr. (1982). Hemodynamic residua and sequelae following intra-atrial repair of transposition of the great arteries: a review. *Pediatr Cardiol, 2*, 203–213.
33. Graham, T. P., Jr., Burger, J., Bender, H. W., et al. (1985). Improved right ventricular function after intra-atrial repair of transposition of the great arteries. *Circulation, 72*, II45–II51.
34. Wong, K. Y., Venables, A. W., Kelly, M. J., et al. (1988). Longitudinal study of ventricular function after the Mustard operation for transposition of the great arteries: a long term follow up. *Br Heart J, 60*, 316–323.
35. Poirier, N. C., & Mee, R. B. (2000). Left ventricular reconditioning and anatomical correction for systemic right ventricular dysfunction. *Semin Thorac Cardiovasc Surg Pediatr Card Surg Annu, 3*, 198–215.
36. Poirier, N. C., Yu, J. H., Brizard, C. P., et al. (2004). Long-term results of left ventricular reconditioning and anatomic correction for systemic right ventricular dysfunction after atrial switch procedures. *J Thorac Cardiovasc Surg, 127*, 975–981.
37. Cochrane, A. D., Karl, T. R., & Mee, R. B. (1993). Staged conversion to arterial switch for late failure of the systemic right ventricle. *Ann Thorac Surg, 56*, 854–861, discussion 861–862.
38. Benzaquen, B. S., Webb, G. D., Colman, J. M., et al. (2004). Arterial switch operation after Mustard procedures in adult patients with transposition of the great arteries: is it time to revise our strategy? *Am Heart J, 147*, E8.
39. Burkhart, H. M., Dearani, J. A., Williams, W. G., et al. (2004). Late results of palliative atrial switch for transposition, ventricular septal defect, and pulmonary vascular obstructive disease. *Ann Thorac Surg, 77*, 464–468, discussion 468-469.
40. Cetta, F., Bonilla, J. J., Lichtenberg, R. C., et al. (1997). Anatomic correction of dextrotransposition of the great arteries in a 36-year-old patient. *Mayo Clin Proc, 72*, 245–247.
41. Padalino, M. A., Stellin, G., Brawn, W. J., et al. (2000). Arterial switch operation after left ventricular retraining in the adult. *Ann Thorac Surg, 70*, 1753–1757.
42. Lincoln, C., Hasse, J., Anderson, R. H., et al. (1976). Surgical correction in complete levotransposition of the great arteries with an unusual subaortic ventricular septal defect. *Am J Cardiol, 38*, 344–351.
43. de Koning, W. B., van Osch-Gevers, M., Harkel, A. D., et al. (2008). Follow-up outcomes 10 years after arterial switch operation for transposition of the great arteries: comparison of cardiological health status and health-related quality of life to those of a normal reference population. *Eur J Pediatr*,167(9), 995–1004.
44. von Bernuth, G. (2000). 25 years after the first arterial switch procedure: mid-term results. *Thorac Cardiovasc Surg, 48*, 228–232.
45. Culbert, E. L., Ashburn, D. A., Cullen-Dean, G., et al. (2003). Quality of life of children after repair of transposition of the great arteries. *Circulation, 108*, 857–862.
46. Raisky, O., Bergoend, E., Agnoletti, G., et al. (2007). Late coronary artery lesions after neonatal arterial switch operation: results of surgical coronary revascularization. *Eur J Cardiothorac Surg, 31*, 894–898.
47. Jahangiri, M., Ross, D. B., Redington, A. N., et al. (1994). Thromboembolism after the Fontan procedure and its modifications. *Ann Thorac Surg, 58*, 1409–1413, discussion 1413–1414.
48. Fontan, F., Mounicot, F. B., Baudet, E., et al. (1971). "Correction" of tricuspid atresia. 2 cases "corrected" using a new surgical technic. *Ann Chir Thorac Cardiovasc, 10*, 39–47.
49. Gewillig, M., & Kalis, N. (2000). Pathophysiological aspects after cavopulmonary anastomosis. *Thorac Cardiovasc Surg, 48*, 336–341.
50. Driscoll, D. J., Offord, K. P., Feldt, R. H., et al. (1992). Five- to fifteen-year follow-up after Fontan operation. *Circulation, 85*, 469–496.
51. Khairy, P., Fernandes, S. M., Mayer, J. E., Jr., et al. (2008). Long-term survival, modes of death, and predictors of mortality in patients with Fontan surgery. *Circulation, 117*, 85–92.
52. Morales, D. L., Dibardino, D. J., Braud, B. E., et al. (2005). Salvaging the failing Fontan: lateral tunnel versus extracardiac conduit. *Ann Thorac Surg, 80*, 1445–1451, discussion 1451–1452.
53. Davlouros, P. A., Kilner, P. J., Hornung, T. S., et al. (2002). Right ventricular function in adults with repaired tetralogy of Fallot assessed with cardiovascular magnetic resonance imaging: detrimental role of right ventricular outflow aneurysms or akinesia and adverse right-to-left ventricular interaction. *J Am Coll Cardiol, 40*, 2044–2052.
54. Geva, T., Sandweiss, B. M., Gauvreau, K., et al. (2004). Factors associated with impaired clinical status in long-term survivors of tetralogy of Fallot repair evaluated by magnetic resonance imaging. *J Am Coll Cardiol, 43*, 1068–1074.
55. Helbing, W. A., Niezen, R. A., Le Cessie, S., et al. (1996). Right ventricular diastolic function in children with pulmonary regurgitation after repair of tetralogy of Fallot: volumetric evaluation by magnetic resonance velocity mapping. *J Am Coll Cardiol, 28*, 1827–1835.
56. Therrien, J., Provost, Y., Merchant, N., et al. (2005). Optimal timing for pulmonary valve replacement in adults after tetralogy of Fallot repair. *Am J Cardiol, 95*, 779–782.
57. Sigurdsson, A., & Swedberg, K. (1996). The role of neurohormonal activation in chronic heart failure and postmyocardial infarction. *Am Heart J, 132*, 229–234.
58. Benedict, C. R., Johnstone, D. E., Weiner, D. H., et al. (1994). Relation of neurohumoral activation to clinical variables and degree of ventricular dysfunction: a report from the registry of studies of left ventricular dysfunction. SOLVD investigators. *J Am Coll Cardiol, 23*, 1410–1420.
59. Packer, M. (1988). Neurohormonal interactions and adaptations in congestive heart failure. *Circulation, 77*, 721–730.
60. Packer, M., Lee, W. H., Kessler, P. D., et al. (1987). Role of neurohormonal mechanisms in determining survival in patients with severe chronic heart failure. *Circulation, 75*, IV80–IV92.
61. Sigurdsson, A., Amtorp, O., Gundersen, T., et al. (1994). Neurohormonal activation in patients with mild or moderately severe congestive heart failure and effects of ramipril. The ramipril trial study group. *Br Heart J, 72*, 422–427.
62. Wei, C. M., Lerman, A., Rodeheffer, R. J., et al. (1994). Endothelin in human congestive heart failure. *Circulation, 89*, 1580–1586.
63. Cohn, J. N., Levine, T. B., Olivari, M. T., et al. (1984). Plasma norepinephrine as a guide to prognosis in patients with chronic congestive heart failure. *N Engl J Med, 311*, 819–823.
64. Thomas, J. A., & Marks, B. H. (1978). Plasma norepinephrine in congestive heart failure. *Am J Cardiol, 41*, 233–243.
65. Eriksson, S. V., Eneroth, P., Kjekshus, J., et al. (1994). Neuroendocrine activation in relation to left ventricular function in chronic severe congestive heart failure: a subgroup analysis from the cooperative North Scandinavian enalapril survival study (CONSENSUS). *Clin Cardiol, 17*, 603–606.
66. CIBIS-II Investigators and Committees. (1999). The cardiac insufficiency bisoprolol study II (CIBIS-II): a randomised trial. *Lancet, 353*, 9–13.

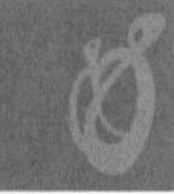

67. Packer, M., O'Connor, C. M., Ghali, J. K., et al. (1996). Effect of amlodipine on morbidity and mortality in severe chronic heart failure. Prospective randomized amlodipine survival evaluation study group. *N Engl J Med, 335*, 1107–1114.
68. Waagstein, F., Bristow, M. R., Swedberg, K., et al. (1993). Beneficial effects of metoprolol in idiopathic dilated cardiomyopathy. Metoprolol in dilated cardiomyopathy (MDC) trial study group. *Lancet, 342*, 1441–1446.
69. MERIT-HF Study Group. (1999). Effect of metoprolol CR/XL in chronic heart failure: metoprolol CR/XL randomised intervention trial in congestive heart failure (MERIT-HF). *Lancet, 353*, 2001–2007.
70. Poole-Wilson, P. A., Swedberg, K., Cleland, J. G., et al. (2003). Comparison of carvedilol and metoprolol on clinical outcomes in patients with chronic heart failure in the carvedilol or metoprolol European trial (COMET): randomised controlled trial. *Lancet, 362*, 7–13.
71. The, C. O. N. S. E. N. S. U. S. (1987). Trial Study Group. Effects of enalapril on mortality in severe congestive heart failure. Results of the cooperative North Scandinavian enalapril survival study (CONSENSUS). *N Engl J Med, 316*, 1429–1435.
72. The SOLVD Investigators. (1991). Effect of enalapril on survival in patients with reduced left ventricular ejection fractions and congestive heart failure. *N Engl J Med, 325*, 293–302.
73. Yusuf, S., Sleight, P., Pogue, J., et al. (2000). Effects of an angiotensin-converting-enzyme inhibitor, ramipril, on cardiovascular events in high-risk patients. The heart outcomes prevention evaluation study investigators. *N Engl J Med, 342*, 145–153.
74. McMurray, J. J., Ostergren, J., Swedberg, K., et al. (2003). Effects of candesartan in patients with chronic heart failure and reduced left-ventricular systolic function taking angiotensin-converting-enzyme inhibitors: the CHARM-Added trial. *Lancet, 362*, 767–771.
75. Granger, C. B., McMurray, J. J., Yusuf, S., et al. (2003). Effects of candesartan in patients with chronic heart failure and reduced left-ventricular systolic function intolerant to angiotensin-converting-enzyme inhibitors: the CHARM-Alternative trial. *Lancet, 362*, 772–776.
76. Pitt, B., Poole-Wilson, P. A., Segal, R., et al. (2000). Effect of losartan compared with captopril on mortality in patients with symptomatic heart failure: randomised trial–the losartan heart failure survival study ELITE II. *Lancet, 355*, 1582–1587.
77. Pitt, B., Segal, R., Martinez, F. A., et al. (1997). Randomised trial of losartan versus captopril in patients over 65 with heart failure (evaluation of losartan in the elderly study, ELITE). *Lancet, 349*, 747–752.
78. Pitt, B., Remme, W., Zannad, F., et al. (2003). Eplerenone, a selective aldosterone blocker, in patients with left ventricular dysfunction after myocardial infarction. *N Engl J Med, 348*, 1309–1321.
79. Pitt, B., Zannad, F., Remme, W. J., et al. (1999). The effect of spironolactone on morbidity and mortality in patients with severe heart failure. Randomized aldactone evaluation study investigators. *N Engl J Med, 341*, 709–717.
80. Lang, R. E., Unger, T., Ganten, D., et al. (1985). Alpha atrial natriuretic peptide concentrations in plasma of children with congenital heart and pulmonary diseases. *Br Med J (Clin Res Ed), 291*, 1241.
81. Lees, M. H. (1966). Catecholamine metabolite excretion of infants with heart failure. *J Pediatr, 69*, 259–265.
82. Scammell, A. M., & Diver, M. J. (1987). Plasma renin activity in infants with congenital heart disease. *Arch Dis Child, 62*, 1136–1138.
83. Yoshibayashi, M., Nishioka, K., Nakao, K., et al. (1991). Plasma endothelin levels in healthy children: high values in early infancy. *J Cardiovasc Pharmacol, 17*(suppl 7), S404–S405.
84. Iivainen, T. E., Groundstroem, K. W., Lahtela, J. T., et al. (2000). Serum N-terminal atrial natriuretic peptide in adult patients late after surgical repair of atrial septal defect. *Eur J Heart Fail, 2*, 161–165.
85. Tulevski, I. I., Groenink, M., van Der Wall, E. E., et al. (2001). Increased brain and atrial natriuretic peptides in patients with chronic right ventricular pressure overload: correlation between plasma neurohormones and right ventricular dysfunction. *Heart, 86*, 27–30.
86. Sharma, R., Bolger, A. P., Li, W., et al. (2003). Elevated circulating levels of inflammatory cytokines and bacterial endotoxin in adults with congenital heart disease. *Am J Cardiol, 92*, 188–193.
87. Yilmaz, E., Ustundag, B., Sen, Y., et al. (2007). The levels of Ghrelin, TNF-alpha, and IL-6 in children with cyanotic and acyanotic congenital heart disease. *Mediators Inflamm*, 2007:32403.
88. Packer, M., Poole-Wilson, P. A., Armstrong, P. W., et al. (1999). Comparative effects of low and high doses of the angiotensin-converting enzyme inhibitor, lisinopril, on morbidity and mortality in chronic heart failure. ATLAS study group. *Circulation, 100*, 2312–2318.
89. Swedberg, K., Held, P., Kjekshus, J., et al. (1992). Effects of the early administration of enalapril on mortality in patients with acute myocardial infarction. Results of the cooperative new Scandinavian enalapril survival study II (CONSENSUS II). *N Engl J Med, 327*, 678–684.
90. Swedberg, K., Held, P., Kjekshus, J., et al. (1992). Effects of the early administration of enalapril on mortality in patients with acute myocardial infarction. Results of the cooperative new Scandinavian enalapril survival study II (CONSENSUS II). *N Engl J Med, 327*, 678–684.
91. Therrien, J., Provost, Y., Harrison, J., et al. (2008). Effect of angiotensin receptor blockade on systemic right ventricular function and size: a small, randomized, placebo-controlled study. *Int J Cardiol, 129*, 187–192.
92. Brilla, C. G., & Weber, K. T. (1992). Mineralocorticoid excess, dietary sodium, and myocardial fibrosis. *J Lab Clin Med, 120*, 893–901.
93. Robert, V., Heymes, C., Silvestre, J. S., et al. (1999). Angiotensin AT1 receptor subtype as a cardiac target of aldosterone: role in aldosterone-salt-induced fibrosis. *Hypertension, 33*, 981–986.
94. Rocha, R., Stier, C. T., Jr., Kifor, I., et al. (2000). Aldosterone: a mediator of myocardial necrosis and renal arteriopathy. *Endocrinology, 141*, 3871–3878.
95. Silvestre, J. S., Heymes, C., Oubenaissa, A., et al. (1999). Role of cardiac aldosterone in post-infarction ventricular remodeling in rats. *Arch Mal Coeur Vaiss, 92*, 991–996.
96. Weber, K. T., & Brilla, C. G. (1992). Factors associated with reactive and reparative fibrosis of the myocardium. *Basic Res Cardiol, 87*(suppl 1), 291–301.
97. Young, M., Head, G., & Funder, J. (1995). Determinants of cardiac fibrosis in experimental hypermineralocorticoid states. *Am J Physiol, 269*, E657–E662.
98. Mann, D. L., & Bristow, M. R. (2000). Mechanisms and models in heart failure: the biomechanical model and beyond. *Circulation, 111*, 2837–2849.
99. Communal, C., Singh, K., Pimentel, D. R., et al. (1998). Norepinephrine stimulates apoptosis in adult rat ventricular myocytes by activation of the beta-adrenergic pathway. *Circulation, 98*, 1329–1334.
100. Mann, D. L., Kent, R. L., Parsons, B., et al. (1992). Adrenergic effects on the biology of the adult mammalian cardiocyte. *Circulation, 85*, 790–804.
101. Hirsch, A. T., Pinto, Y. M., Schunkert, H., et al. (1990). Potential role of the tissue renin-angiotensin system in the pathophysiology of congestive heart failure. *Am J Cardiol, 66*, 22D–30D,, discussion 30D-32D.
102. Johnson, J. A., Davis, J. O., & Witty, R. T. (1971). Effects of catecholamines and renal nerve stimulation on renin release in the nonfiltering kidney. *Circ Res, 29*, 646–653.
103. Willerson, J. T. (ed.). (1996). Effect of carvedilol on mortality and morbidity in patients with chronic heart failure. *Circulation, 94*, 592.
104. Hoffman, T. M., Wernovsky, G., Atz, A. M., et al. (2002). Prophylactic intravenous use of milrinone after cardiac operation in pediatrics (PRIMACORP) study. Prophylactic intravenous use of milrinone after cardiac operation in pediatrics. *Am Heart J, 143*, 15–21.
105. Hoffman, T. M., Wernovsky, G., Atz, A. M., et al. (2003). Efficacy and safety of milrinone in preventing low cardiac output syndrome in infants and children after corrective surgery for congenital heart disease. *Circulation, 107*, 996–1002.
106. Khazin, V., Kaufman, Y., Zabeeda, D., et al. (2004). Milrinone and nitric oxide: combined effect on pulmonary artery pressures after cardiopulmonary bypass in children. *J Cardiothorac Vasc Anesth, 18*, 156–159.
107. Sorensen, G. K., Ramamoorthy, C., Lynn, A. M., et al. (1996). Hemodynamic effects of amrinone in children after Fontan surgery. *Anesth Analg, 82*, 241–246.
107. Konstam, M. A., Gheorghiade, M., Burnett, J. C., Jr., et al. (2007). Effects of oral tolvaptan in patients hospitalized for worsening heart failure: the EVEREST outcome trial. *JAMA, 297*(12), 1319–1331.
108. Field, M. E., Solomon, S. D., Lewis, E. F., et al. (2006). Right ventricular dysfunction and adverse outcome in patients with advanced heart failure. *J Card Fail, 12*, 616–620.
109. Kjaergaard, J., Akkan, D., Iversen, K. K., et al. (2007). Right ventricular dysfunction as an independent predictor of short- and long-term mortality in patients with heart failure. *Eur J Heart Fail, 9*, 610–616.
110. La Vecchia, L., Varotto, L., Zanolla, L., et al. (2006). Right ventricular function predicts transplant-free survival in idiopathic dilated cardiomyopathy. *J Cardiovasc Med (Hagerstown), 7*, 706–710.
111. De Simone, R., Wolf, I., Mottl-Link, S., et al. (2005). Intraoperative assessment of right ventricular volume and function. *Eur J Cardiothorac Surg, 27*, 988–993.
112. Kaul, S., Tei, C., Hopkins, J. M., et al. (1984). Assessment of right ventricular function using two-dimensional echocardiography. *Am Heart J, 107*, 526–531.
113. Ochiai, Y., Morita, S., Tanoue, Y., et al. (1999). Use of transesophageal echocardiography for postoperative evaluation of right ventricular function. *Ann Thorac Surg, 67*, 146–152, discussion 153.
114. Helbing, W. A., Rebergen, S. A., Maliepaard, C., et al. (1995). Quantification of right ventricular function with magnetic resonance imaging in children with normal hearts and with congenital heart disease. *Am Heart J, 130*, 828–837.
115. Jauhiainen, T., Jarvinen, V. M., Hekali, P. E., et al. (1998). MR gradient echo volumetric analysis of human cardiac casts: focus on the right ventricle. *J Comput Assist Tomogr, 22*, 899–903.
116. Markiewicz, W., Sechtem, U., & Higgins, C. B. (1987). Evaluation of the right ventricle by magnetic resonance imaging. *Am Heart J, 113*, 8–15.
117. Wackers, F. J., Berger, H. J., Johnstone, D. E., et al. (1979). Multiple gated cardiac blood pool imaging for left ventricular ejection fraction: validation of the technique and assessment of variability. *Am J Cardiol, 43*, 1159–1166.
118. Nawa, S., Sugawara, E., Murakami, T., et al. (1988). Efficacy of intra-aortic balloon pumping for failing Fontan circulation. *Chest, 93*, 599–603.
119. Chowdhury, U. K., Kothari, S. S., & Subramaniam, G. K. (2007). Intra-aortic balloon counterpulsation in a patient with the failing Fontan circulation. *Cardiol Young, 17*, 102–104.
120. Merkle, F., Boettcher, W., Stiller, B., et al. (2003). Pulsatile mechanical cardiac assistance in pediatric patients with the Berlin heart ventricular assist device. *J Extra Corpor Technol, 35*, 115–120.
121. Petrofski, J. A., Hoopes, C. W., Bashore, T. M., et al. (2003). Mechanical ventricular support lowers pulmonary vascular resistance in a patient with congenital heart disease. *Ann Thorac Surg, 75*, 1005–1007.
122. Blume, E. D., Naftel, D. C., Bastardi, H. J., et al. (2006). Outcomes of children bridged to hearttransplantationwithventricularassistdevices:amulti-institutionalstudy. *Circulation, 113*, 2313–2319.
123. Undar, A., McKenzie, E. D., McGarry, M. C., et al. (2004). Outcomes of congenital heart surgery patients after extracorporeal life support at Texas Children's Hospital. *Artif Organs, 28*, 963–966.
124. Dalton, H. J., Rycus, P. T., & Conrad, S. A. (2005). Update on extracorporeal life support 2004. *Semin Perinatol, 29*, 24–33.
125. Fiser, W. P., Yetman, A. T., Gunselman, R. J., et al. (2003). Pediatric arteriovenous extracorporeal membrane oxygenation (ECMO) as a bridge to cardiac transplantation. *J Heart Lung Transplant, 22*, 770–777.
126. Pigula, F. A., Gandhi, S. K., Ristich, J., et al. (2001). Cardiopulmonary transplantation for congenital heart disease in the adult. *J Heart Lung Transplant, 20*, 297–303.
127. Simmonds, J., Burch, M., Dawkins, H., et al. (2008). Heart transplantation after congenital heart surgery: improving results and future goals. *Eur J Cardiothorac Surg, 34*(2), 313–317.
128. Speziali, G., Driscoll, D. J., Danielson, G. K., et al. (1998). Cardiac transplantation for end-stage congenital heart defects: the Mayo Clinic experience. Mayo cardiothoracic transplant team. *Mayo Clin Proc, 73*, 923–928.

CHAPTER 31

Heart Failure as a Consequence of Viral and Nonviral Myocarditis

Naveen Pereira and Leslie T. Cooper Jr.

The focus of this chapter is the special case of heart failure due to viral infection and postviral autoimmunity. Although a wide variety of toxic, metabolic, and infectious injuries can lead to myocarditis, viruses are a major cause of myocarditis in North America and Europe. The spectrum of viruses detected in patients with cardiomyopathy is changing from enteroviruses, in particular Coxsackie B (CVB), in the late twentieth century, to parvovirus B19, several herpes viruses, and a host of less prevalent viruses today. The clinical syndromes and histopathology associated with newer viruses differ somewhat from typical enterovirus myocarditis. Yet almost all of the knowledge regarding the cellular and molecular pathogenesis of viral cardiomyopathy derive from studies of virulent CVB or encephalomyocarditis virus strains in genetically predisposed rodents and cell culture systems. In these models, direct viral injury and innate and subsequently adaptive, lymphocyte-mediated, tissue specific immunity leads to acute myocarditis and often dilated cardiomyopathy (DCM) (see Chapter 24). In contrast, the pathogenesis of DCM due to newer viruses such as parvovirus B19 is not well understood. For most viruses, the diagnosis requires molecular analysis of endomyocardial biopsy tissue. Studies differ on the prognostic importance of viral genomes in the heart. The role of antiviral and immunomodulatory treatments for patients with cardiomyopathy associated with viral genomes or features of postviral autoimmunity are now being evaluated in randomized clinical trials.

Cause

Myocarditis, defined histologically as inflammation of the myocardium, can be considered in two broad categories: viral, which includes the immune-mediated damage following the initial injury, and nonviral. Viral myocarditis is a significant cause of fulminant and acute DCM.[1] Viral persistence in the absence of typical inflammation is seen in up to 67% of patients with chronic DCM.[2] Some viruses, particularly parvovirus B19, can cause diastolic dysfunction and chest pain and DCM possibly through endothelial cell dysfunction and microvascular ischemia.[3] Virus associated myocardial damage may be mediated through direct toxicity or through an innate and acquired immune response.[4] Thus viral cardiomyopathy may occur without cellular inflammation. In contrast, nonviral myocarditis may be caused by a variety of toxic, metabolic, allergic, and infectious disorders. These uncommon forms of myocarditis, including giant cell myocarditis (GCM), eosinophilic myocarditis, and granulomatous myocarditis, will be discussed in the latter sections of this chapter.

Bowles et al demonstrated enteroviral genome in the heart tissue of myocarditis patients in 1986.[5] Through the 1990s enteroviruses, typically detected by polymerase chain reaction (PCR), were commonly associated with acute and chronic dilated cardiomyopathy. Beginning in the mid-1990s, adenovirus genomes were identified in patients undergoing heart transplantation and those with acute myocarditis.[6] In contrast to enterovirus, adenovirus infection was associated with little cellular inflammation. The importance of viral infection has been documented in multiple case series in which viral infection is linked to poor clinical outcomes. For example, Shirali et al demonstrated that children with viral genomes detected on endomyocardial biopsy (EMB) samples had a 5-year survival rate of 66% compared with PCR-negative patients who had a 95% 5-year survival rate following heart transplantation.[7]

The frequency of enteroviral and adenoviral genome identification has decreased in the past decade. Newer viruses associated with DCM and myocarditis include the hepatitis C virus, particularly in Asia; cytomegalovirus (CMV); and Epstein-Barr virus (EBV).[8,9] Recently, parvovirus B19 has been frequently linked to dilated cardiomyopathy (DCM) anginal chest pain, and isolated diastolic dysfunction.[10] human herpesvirus 6 (HHV6) and multiple viral coinfections have been associated with chest pain and progressive cardiomyopathy, respectively.[11,12]

Pathogenesis of Postviral Cardiomyopathy

The pathogenesis of postviral DCM is complex and involves the interaction of viral and host genetic susceptibility and environmental variables, including trace elements (Figure 31-1). Since the original description of CVB myocarditis,[13,14] the molecular pathogenesis of viral and postviral autoimmune myocarditis has been elucidated from studies of inbred rodent strains and cultured cells that are susceptible to virulent CVB strains.[15,16] The severity of CVB infection is modified by variations in the 5' untranslated region of the viral genome.[17] However, primary cell culture studies have also revealed that most wild-type CVB strains are not cardiovirulent[18] and that the host cell plays a major role in CVB phenotype. Briefly, CVB virus first enters cells by binding with decay accelerating factor for primary attachment and the coxsackie adenovirus receptor (CAR), a junctional molecule, for internalization.[19-21] CAR expression increases in experimental autoimmune myocarditis and in human DCM, which may partly explain the affinity for the heart. However, other organs with high CAR expression, such as the liver, do not display much CVB-damage, demonstrating that host organ factors besides receptor expression are important in viral pathogenesis.[22]

Following entry into cells, CVB shuts down host RNA synthesis by inhibition of

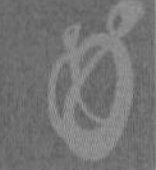

FIGURE 31–1 Pathogenesis of myocarditis. The current understanding of the cellular and molecular pathogenesis of postviral and autoimmune myocarditis is based solely on animal models. In these models, the progression from acute injury to chronic dilated cardiomyopathy may be simplified into a three-stage process. Acute injury leads to cardiac damage, exposure of intracellular antigens such as cardiac myosin, and activation of the innate immune system. Over weeks, specific immunity that is mediated by T lymphocytes and antibodies directed against pathogens and similar endogenous heart epitopes cause robust inflammation. In most patients, the pathogen is cleared and the immune reaction is downregulated with few sequelae. However, in other patients, the virus is not cleared and causes persistent myocyte damage, and heart-specific inflammation may persist because of mistaken recognition of endogenous heart antigens as pathogenic entities. APC denotes antigen-presenting cell. (Cooper LT Jr. Myocarditis. *N Engl J Med* 2009;360:1526-1538.)

eukaryotic initiation factor 4γ and other host proteins.[23] CVB causes cell cycle arrest by ubiquitin-dependent proteolysis of cyclin D1.[24] Necrosis and apoptosis cause myocyte death within hours of infection.[4]

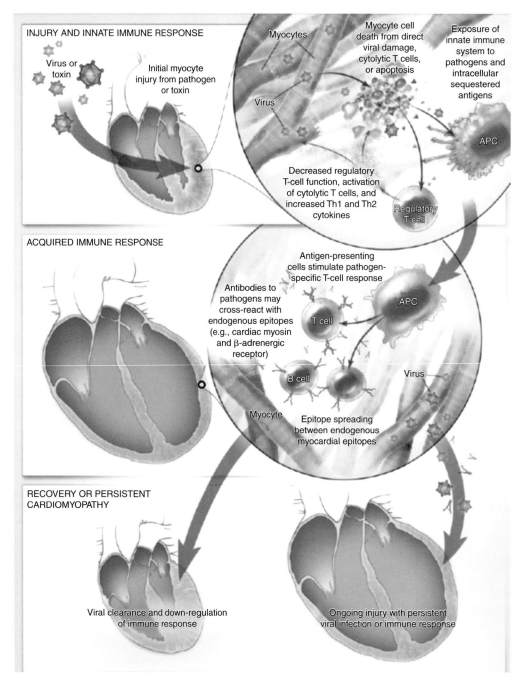

The innate immune response is essential for host defense. Early in the course of an infection (see also Chapter 11), CVB upregulates toll-like receptor (TLR) 4 on macrophages, stimulates antigen presenting cell maturation, leads to proinflammatory cytokine release,[25] and decreases regulatory T-cell function.[26] Human cardiac myosin, which is released in the course of acute viral myocarditis, can stimulate TLR 2 and 8 as an endogenous ligand. TLR 2 and 8 activation on monocytes releases proinflammatory cytokines.[27] In the first few days after infection, dendritic cells and other resident myocardial cells produce cytokines, including interferon-γ, tumor necrosis factor-β, interleukin-1, and interleukin-6 by a myeloid differentiation factor (MyD)-88 dependent pathway.[28] The character of the initial immune response, in particular higher levels of a Th1 and Th2 cytokines, are associated with the development of cardiomyopathy.[29] One effort to translate these insights from animal models into prognostically useful information is the recently completed IMAC-2 study, which seeks to correlate circulating cytokine levels and gene polymorphisms with left ventricular (LV) recovery in patients with acute DCM.

Inflammatory lesions develop from natural killer, CD4 and CD8 positive lymphocytes. T lymphocytes are key mediators of experimental autoimmune myocarditis.[30,31] Experimental studies in mice suggest that low-avidity, circulating T cells that evade central and peripheral tolerance can cause immune-mediated heart disease if stimulated with large amounts of self-antigens.[32] A T helper subset, TH17 cells, that produce IL-17[33] have recently been implicated in myocarditis as well.[34]

In contrast to effector T-cell subsets, regulatory T-cell populations, such as CD4(+)CD25(+)FOXp3(+) T cells are important negative regulators of inflammation in CVB myocarditis.[35,36] Regulatory T-cell subsets have not yet been studied in human myocarditis, but offer an exciting opportunity for mechanistic studies with the potential for significant diagnostic and therapeutic impact.

Autoantibodies to a variety of cardiac antigens are present in up to 80% of patients with myocarditis and DCM.[37] Epitopes on CVB and streptococcal M protein are shared with cardiac myosin, which can lead to anti–self-immunity through antigenic mimicry.[38] After the initial injury and viral clearance, cardiac myosin may provide an endogenous source of antigen in chronic myocarditis. Antibodies to cardiac myosin can cause myocyte damage by binding to the β-adrenergic receptor and stimulating protein kinase A.[39]

A major challenge is to distinguish immune autoreactivity, which occurs commonly in the course of normal viral clearance, from autoimmune disease, in which anticardiac antibodies and T cells are actually contributing to cardiomyopathy. Therefore a major theme of ongoing research includes a search for biomarkers that reflect inflammation and infection and that impact prognosis in clinically suspected myocarditis.[40]

Host factors that impact viral virulence include trace element deficiency. In murine models of CVB myocarditis, copper and selenium deficiency are associated with increased viral virulence.[41] Mercury exposure exacerbates infection with virulent strains of encephalomyocarditis virus,[42] herpes simplex virus type 2,[43] and a myocarditic strain of coxsackie B3 virus,[44,45]possibly through sequestration of selenopeptides.[46] In a case series from Italy, mercury concentration in the myocardium was reportedly higher in DCM patients (178.5 μg/g) than it was in control subjects (0.008 μg/g).[47]

Myocardial damage in enteroviral infections may also occur independently of any immune reaction. Protein products of the enteroviral genome, including viral protease 2a and 3a can cleave host proteins, including dystrophin, and lead to cardiomyopathy.[48] Dystrophin deficiency markedly increases enterovirus-induced cardiomyopathy.[49] Active CVB infection is associated with disruption of dystrophin in patients who die of myocardial infarction, suggesting that CVB can contribute to the pathogenesis of myocardial infarction and DCM.[50]

In contrast to the relatively abundant data on viral myocarditis, the pathogenesis of nonviral myocarditis is poorly understood, largely because of the rarity of the diseases and fewer model systems. In the case of giant cell myocarditis, CD4 positive T lymphocytes are the main effectors of inflammation,[51] although anticardiac myosin antibodies are also elevated in a minority of patients.[39] In the case of cardiac sarcoidosis or idiopathic granulomatous myocarditis, T lymphocytes are also thought to be the main effector cells involved in disease pathogenesis.[52] In contrast, myocarditis following smallpox vaccination seems to be an allergic type of reaction characterized by an eosinophil rich infiltrate, interleukin-4 and interleukin-5.[53]

DIAGNOSIS OF CARDIOMYOPATHY DUE TO MYOCARDITIS

Typical Presentations in Heart Failure

The question of whether myocarditis is a cause of heart failure arises typically in a patient who has acute decompensated heart failure and less often in patients who have been found to have asymptomatic dilated cardiomyopathy. Factors associated with heart failure suggestive of myocarditis are listed in Box 31-1. Less commonly patients with myocarditis can present as hypertrophic cardiomyopathy due to the presence of myocardial edema or as restrictive cardiomyopathy in older patients.[54] Recently, there have been reports of patients with myocarditis presenting as arrhythmogenic right ventricular dysplasia.[55] Patients with infiltrative cardiomyopathy such as in amyloidosis can also develop concomitant myocarditis.[56] Patients with chronic heart failure can also decompensate due to development of interval myocarditis and the diagnosis of this phenomenon has been made retrospectively, either during autopsy or examination of the explanted heart.[57] Occasionally patients who have sudden cardiac death or chest pain and preserved ejection fraction can have myocarditis.[58]

BOX 31–1 Factors Associated with Heart Failure Suggestive of Myocarditis

1. Viral prodrome
2. Elevated troponins in the absence of acute coronary syndrome
3. Ischemic ECG changes in the absence of obstructive coronary artery disease
4. Acute, new onset heart failure with hemodynamic perturbations
5. Elevated ESR
6. Peripheral eosinophilia
7. Failure to respond to standard medical therapy
8. Declining left ventricular ejection fraction despite standard medical therapy
9. Refractory ventricular arrhythmias
10. Second- or third-degree AV block

Clinical Features

The various heart failure syndromes that patients with myocarditis can have are outlined in Box 31-2. In patients with heart failure due to myocarditis there appears to be a male preponderance as seen in the Myocarditis Treatment Trial in which 62% of the patients were male.[59] A prodrome of fever, myalgias, and gastrointestinal or respiratory symptoms is variably reported and may reflect systemic effects of acute viral infection in patients with viral myocarditis and commonly precedes acute fulminant myocarditis usually within 2 weeks before hospitalization. There appears to be a short duration of heart failure symptoms in patients with acute fulminant myocarditis, typically lasting less than 1 to 2 weeks.[60] These clinical features are important to recognize since these patients decompensate rapidly and usually require inotrope or mechanical circulatory support. Acute fulminant myocarditis is usually due to acute lymphocytic myocarditis but rarely can be caused by acute giant cell myocarditis. The differentiation of the two conditions is important and requires endomyocardial biopsy.[61] Patients with heart failure due to myocarditis could have symptoms of chest pain due to accompanying pericarditis or ischemia from underlying vasculitis or coronary vasospasm.[62] The presence of significant ventricular arrhythmias should alert the clinician to the possibility of nonviral causes of myocarditis, such as cardiac sarcoidosis and giant cell myocarditis.[63]

A variety of specific disorders should be considered in the patient with suspected myocarditis. Patients with Lyme myocarditis can have accompanying atrioventricular conduction abnormalities and often have traveled or live in endemic regions or give a history of a tick bite.[64] Patients with drug-induced hypersensitivity myocarditis are typically older, on multiple medications, and have systemic complaints of rash, fever, and possibly

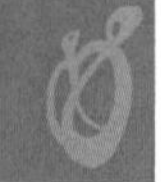

BOX 31–2 Heart Failure Syndromes as a Consequence of Viral and Nonviral Myocarditis

1. Acute coronary syndrome with "normal coronaries"
   a. Acute lymphocytic myocarditis
   b. Giant cell myocarditis
2. Acute heart failure with hemodynamic compromise
   a. Acute fulminant lymphocytic myocarditis
   b. Giant cell myocarditis
   c. Eosinophilic myocarditis
3. Heart failure with ventricular arrhythmias and high degree AV block
   a. Giant cell myocarditis
   b. Cardiac sarcoidosis
   c. Lyme myocarditis (consider coinfection with Babesia and Ehrlichia)
   d. Chagas myocarditis
4. Heart failure with eosinophilia
   a. Eosinophilic myocarditis
   b. Hypersensitivity myocarditis

Drugs: azithromycin, benzodiazepines, clozapine, cephalosporins, dapsone, dobutamine, gefitinib, lithium, loop diuretics, methyldopa, mexiletine, nonsteroidal antiinflammatories, penicillins, phenobarbital, smallpox vaccination, streptomycin, sulfonamides, tetanus toxoid, tetracycline, thiazide diuretics, tricyclic antidepressants

Other: bee venom, wasp venom, black widow spider venom, scorpion venom, snake venom

5. Heart failure associated with systemic diseases
   a. Churg-Strauss
   b. Systemic lupus erythematosus
   c. Inflammatory bowel disease
   d. Thyrotoxicosis
   e. Takayasu arteritis
   f. Wegener granulomatosis
   g. Celiac disease
   h. Kawasaki disease
   i. Sarcoidosis (idiopathic granulomatous myocarditis)

eosinophilia on peripheral blood.[65] Eosinophilia with a concomitant pulmonary infiltrate should alert the treating physician to possible Churg-Strauss syndrome. Eosinophilic myocarditis may also occur in the setting of malignancy, parasitic infection, after vaccination, and early in the course of Loeffler endomyocardial fibrosis.[66] Hypereosinophilic syndrome, a diagnosis of exclusion is rare and affects predominantly males, resulting sometimes in endomyocarditis and intracardiac thrombi. Chagas cardiomyopathy should be suspected in patients from endemic areas of rural Central and or South America, who can have accompanying arrhythmias including AV block but who can also be asymptomatic (see Chapter 33).[67] Patients with HIV who have cardiomyopathy are usually asymptomatic and the incidence appears to be decreasing with the advent of effective antiretroviral therapy. The causes of cardiomyopathy in HIV are multifactorial including toxicity of antiretroviral agents, nutritional deficiencies, and autoimmune factors such as development of antimyosin antibodies. Presentation with myocarditis due to the virus itself is unusual, but the gp120 protein can directly cause myocyte dysfunction.[68, 69] Rarer causes of myocarditis in these patients are concomitant opportunistic infections such as toxoplasmosis and aspergillosis.

Biochemical Markers (see also Chapter 37)

There are no available biomarkers at present that clearly differentiate myocarditis from other causes of acute heart failure since acute decompensated heart failure in itself can cause elevations of cardiac enzymes that indicate cardiomyocyte death. Cardiac troponin T and I elevations are seen in a minority of patients with acute myocarditis but suggest the diagnosis, especially in the absence of obstructive coronary artery disease. Standard markers of myocardial damage including troponin I have a high specificity (89%) but limited sensitivity (34%) in the diagnosis of myocarditis especially with a shorter duration (less than 4 weeks) of symptoms when analyzed in the Myocarditis Treatment Trial population.[70] With the advent of CMR, myocarditis is being increasingly recognized as a cause of chest pain in patients with raised troponin levels and normal epicardial coronary arteries. Clinical and experimental data suggest that cardiac troponin I is increased much more frequently than creatinine kinase MB subunits (CK-MB) in patients with myocarditis.[71] Natriuretic peptides such as NT-proBNP may be elevated in patients with myocarditis and cardiac dysfunction, and with troponin levels could be used to monitor patients on immunomodulatory therapy and is a marker of persistent cardiac dysfunction.[72] Patients with myocarditis who have increased serum levels of soluble Fas and soluble Fas ligand at initial presentation have an increased short-term risk of death.[73] High interleukin-10 levels are also a marker of poor prognosis and predict patients who will develop cardiogenic shock in acute fulminant myocarditis.[74] Erythrocyte sedimentation rate although commonly used has a low sensitivity and specificity for acute myocarditis.

Noninvasive Cardiac Testing (see also Chapter 36)

The ECG in acute myocarditis may show sinus tachycardia with nonspecific ST-segment and T-wave abnormalities. Occasionally, the ECG changes are suggestive of an acute myocardial infarction; and may include ST-segment elevation in two or more contiguous leads (54%), widespread ST-segment depressions (18%), and pathological Q waves (18% to 27%).[75] Global T-wave inversions may also be present. In a small proportion of patients, various degrees of heart block may occur. Ventricular arrhythmias may also be present, but occur more commonly in cardiac sarcoidosis and giant cell myocarditis.[76]

An echocardiogram should be performed in all patients with suspected acute myocarditis; however, echocardiographic findings while useful in confirming the presence of reduced LV ejection fraction are not specific for myocarditis. Nondiagnostic findings such as regional wall motion abnormalities, increased LV wall thickness, and absence of LV cavity dilation in the presence of LV systolic dysfunction, diastolic dysfunction, and changes in echocardiographic texture have been reported.[77] Echocardiographic patterns of dilated, hypertrophic, restrictive, and ischemic cardiomyopathies have also been described in histologically proven myocarditis. In the Myocarditis Treatment Trial, increased sphericity and LV volume occurred in acute, active myocarditis. Left ventricular cavity size may initially be normal primarily due to increased LV wall thickness in very early myocarditis and subsequent increase over time may occur due to resolution of inflammation and edema, and adverse remodeling. Echocardiography may be useful in distinguishing acute fulminant myocarditis from acute myocarditis by echocardiographic criteria as suggested by Felker et al.[78] Patients with fulminant myocarditis had near normal left ventricular diastolic dimensions with increased septal thickness at presentation likely due to a greater inflammatory component and edema, while those with acute myocarditis had increased diastolic dimensions but normal septal thickness. The increased wall thickness has been shown to be spontaneously reversible in acute fulminant myocarditis over time or after treatment with corticosteroids in acute eosinophilic myocarditis.[79]

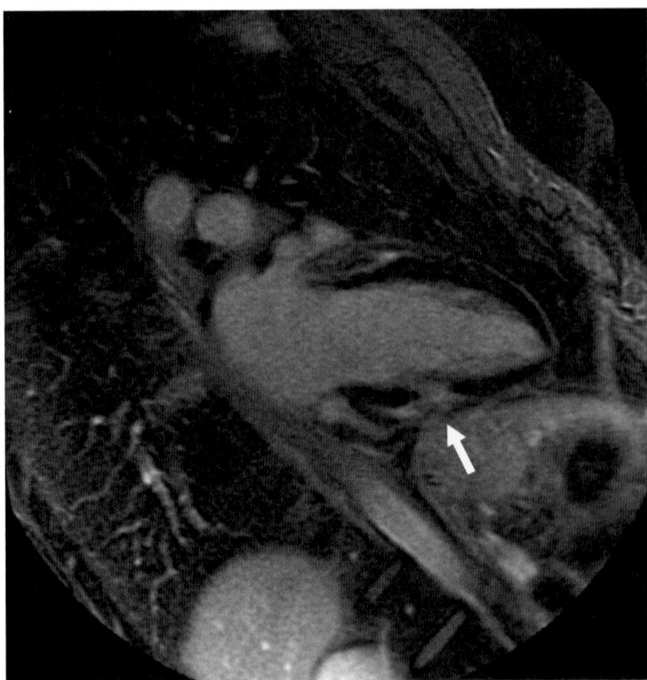

FIGURE 31–2 Contrast-enhanced cardiac magnetic resonance image of the heart showing focal late enhancement (*arrow*) of gadolinium in a patient with myocarditis.

Cardiac magnetic resonance (CMR) imaging is being increasingly used as a diagnostic test in acute dilated cardiomyopathy and suspected acute myocarditis due to the noninvasive nature of the test and its ability to detect inflammation in myocardial tissue (see Chapter 36).[80,81] CMR is able to provide information similar to echocardiography that may serve as corroborative evidence for the presence of myocarditis such as the presence of ventricular systolic dysfunction, pericardial effusion, and increased LV mass. Techniques used for tissue characterization include T2-weighted imaging for myocardial edema, contrast enhanced fast spin echo T1-weighted images for hyperemia, and delayed gadolinium enhancement for necrosis or fibrosis (Figure 31-2 and Box 31-3). The combination of these markers enhances the diagnostic capability of CMR and when compared with histopathology the sensitivity is 63% with a specificity of 89% for a diagnosis of myocarditis.[82] Although CMR has great potential for noninvasive diagnosis and prognosis, motion artifacts and arrhythmias can affect image accuracy and quality. The main limitations of the published CMR studies are that most have used clinical parameters to define myocarditis, and all have used patients with acute myocardial infarction on normal controls for comparison. As of March 2009, only 289 patients had been reported in eight controlled trials of CMR for the diagnosis of myocarditis.

Endomyocardial Biopsy

The gold standard in diagnosing myocarditis is histopathology. Therefore endomyocardial biopsy has played an important role in the evaluation of a patient with suspected myocarditis. In patients with unexplained cardiomyopathy, endomyocardial biopsy identified approximately 9% of patients with myocarditis.[83] In the Myocarditis Treatment Trial, the average incidence of positive endomyocardial biopsy was 10% in patients with heart failure of less than 2 years of duration using traditional Dallas criteria, which are outlined in Table 31-1[59] (Figure 31-3*A*). The sensitivity of EMB for myocarditis increased if immunoperoxidase staining for specific cells and/or MHC antigen expression is used. Such stains are commonly

BOX 31–3 Select Diagnostic Tests in Myocarditis

1. Endomyocardial biopsy
   a. Dallas criteria for myocarditis require an inflammatory infiltrate with necrosis and/or degeneration of adjacent myocytes without evidence of Chagas' disease or features of ischemic heart disease
   b. Immunoperoxidase-based stains are used to identify more sensitive markers for myocardial inflammation such as MHC antigens HLA-A, B, C, and HLA-DR, and surface antigens such as anti-CD3, anti-CD4, anti-CD20, and anti-CD68.
   c. Viral genomes can be detected using molecular methods such as the polymerase chain reaction (PCR)
2. Cardiac magnetic resonance imaging
   a. T1-weighted spin-echo images with gadolinium enhancement using appropriate absolute or normalized to skeletal muscle quantitative measurements
   b. T2-weighted spin-echo images showing gadolinium enhancement with a high signal intensity ratio normalized to skeletal muscle or the presence of myocardial edema

TABLE 31–1 Dallas Criteria for the Diagnosis of Myocarditis*
First Biopsy
Active myocarditis (with or without fibrosis)
Borderline myocarditis (not diagnostic and requiring no further biopsy)
No evidence of myocarditis
Subsequent Biopsies
Ongoing (persistent) myocarditis
Resolving (healing) myocarditis
Resolved (healed) myocarditis

*The histological diagnosis of active myocarditis requires an inflammatory infiltrate with necrosis and/or degeneration of adjacent myocytes without evidence of Chagas disease or features of ischemic heart disease.

used in recent reports, including the European Study of Epidemiology and Treatment of Cardiac Inflammatory Diseases Study, and large case series from Padua and Tubigen[84,85-87] (see Figure 31-3, *B*). Viral genomes can be identified in heart tissue using polymerase chain reaction (PCR) techniques. Endomyocardial biopsy for histopathological or molecular analysis is limited by sampling error and procedural risks.

The overall complication rate in experienced centers is approximately 6%; 2.7% occurring during sheath insertion and 3.3% occurring as a result of the biopsy procedure itself. The most common complications being arterial puncture, arrhythmias, pneumothorax, and damage to the tricuspid valve and the most grievous being cardiac perforation, which occurs in 0.5% of cases.[88] These complications can be minimized by use of ultrasound guidance to access the vein and the use of echocardiography during tissue procurement. The relative insensitivity of the endomyocardial biopsy in diagnosing myocarditis has been demonstrated in autopsy and explanted hearts and more recently by CMR studies. The risks are likely lower if a smaller tip bioptome is used.[89] The accepted indications and recommendations for endomyocardial biopsy have been driven primarily by prognostic and therapeutic considerations. In a consensus statement endorsed by the American Heart Association, American College of Cardiology, and European Society of Cardiology, the indications for endomyocardial biopsy in various heart failure scenarios were outlined and shown in Table 31-2.[61] The

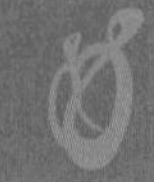

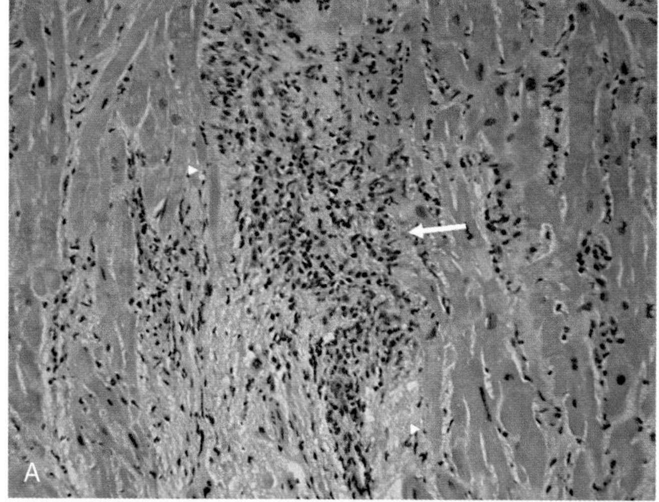

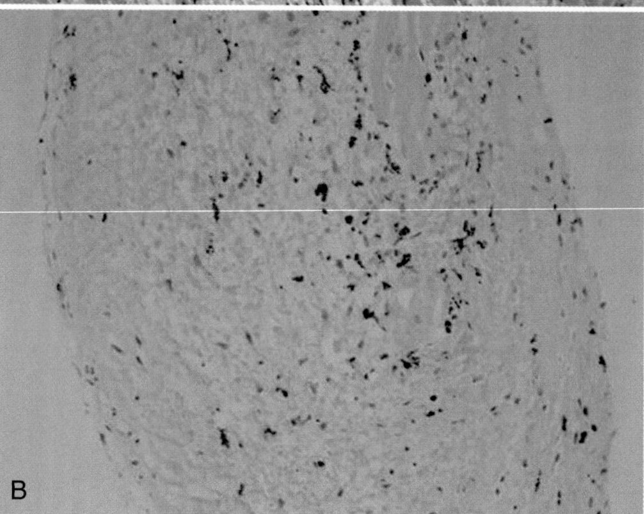

FIGURE 31–3 **A,** Acute myocarditis on hematoxylin and eosin stained section. A lymphocytic and histiocytic infiltrate (*arrow*) is associated with myocyte damage (*arrowhead*). **B,** CD68 immunostain for macrophages in a patient with peripartum cardiomyopathy.

class 1 indications for endomyocardial biopsy are primarily for clinical scenarios that are suggestive of fulminant or GCM, conditions with unique prognoses and treatments.

Clinical Aspects of Nonviral Myocarditis

Although most cases of acute DCM are relatively mild and resolve with few short-term sequelae, certain signs and symptoms predict GCM, a disorder with a mean transplant-free survival time of only 5.5 months.[90] GCM is associated with a variety of autoimmune disorders, thymoma,[91] and drug hypersensitivity.[92] At presentation ventricular tachycardia is present in 15%, complete heart block in 5%, and an acute coronary syndrome in 6%, rates higher than are typically seen in noninflammatory DCM. In follow-up, 29% of GCM patients developed ventricular tachycardia and 15% developed AV block (8% complete).[93] The sensitivity of EMB for GCM in patients who subsequently had definitive pathology evaluation from ventricular tissue cores, explanted or autopsied hearts is 80% to 85%.[94] Thus clinical clues to suggest GCM and prompt an EMB include association with other autoimmune disorders or thymoma, failure to respond to usual care, and the presence of complete heart block or ventricular tachycardia.

Patients with acute heart failure due to GCM respond well to heart transplantation. Alternatively, treatment with combination immunosuppression may improve transplant-free survival time compared with patients with GCM not receiving immunosuppressive treatment. In a multicenter registry, patients treated without immunosuppressive therapy had a median transplant-free survival time of 3.0 months, compared with a 12.3-month (P = .003) median transplant-free survival time for patients treated with cyclosporine-based immunosuppression. In a prospective series of 11 patients with GCM treated with cyclosporine-based immunosuppression, there was one death and two heart transplants in the first year of therapy.[63] Therefore a diagnosis of GCM on endomyocardial biopsy will likely impact prognosis and treatment.

Cardiac sarcoidosis is present in approximately 25% of patients with systemic sarcoidosis.[95] However, symptoms referable to cardiac sarcoidosis occur in only 5% of sarcoid patients.[95, 96] Up to 50% of patients with sarcoid granulomas in the heart have no evidence of extracardiac disease. Patients with cardiac sarcoidosis may sometimes be distinguished from those with DCM by a high rate of heart block (8% to 67%) and ventricular arrhythmias (29%).[97-100] The rates of ventricular tachycardia and heart block are therefore similar in cardiac sarcoidosis and GCM, but cardiac sarcoidosis generally has a more chronic course. Because the sensitivity of EMB is low in patients with suspected cardiac sarcoidosis, CMR has been used to infer cardiac involvement and follow disease activity.[101,102]

Hypersensitivity myocarditis (HSM) is an uncommon disorder with a wide range of presentations, including sudden death, rapidly progressive heart failure, or more chronic DCM. Drug-associated, toxin-associated, and infectious causes of myocarditis are listed in Box 31-4. Clinical clues that are reported in a minority of cases include rash, fever, and peripheral eosinophilia.[103] A temporal relation with recently initiated medications or the use of multiple medications is usually present.[104] The ECG is often abnormal with nonspecific ST-segment changes or infarct patterns similar to other forms of acute myocarditis. The prevalence of clinically undetected HSM in explanted hearts ranges from 2.4% to 7%[105] and has been associated with dobutamine.[106]

Early suspicion and recognition of HSM may lead to withdrawal of offending medications and administration of high-dose corticosteroids.

Eosinophilic myocarditis associated with the hypereosinophilic syndrome is a form of eosinophilic myocarditis that typically evolves over weeks to months. The presentation is usually biventricular heart failure, although arrhythmias may lead to sudden death. Usually there is a hypereosinophilia that precedes or coincides with the onset of cardiac symptoms; however, the eosinophilia may be delayed.[107] Eosinophilic myocarditis may also occur in the setting of malignancy, parasite infection, and early in the course of endocardial fibrosis.

TREATMENT

Physical Activity (see also Chapter 57)

In murine models, exercise early in the course of CVB myocarditis has been shown to enhance viral replication, myocardial inflammation, and necrosis.[108] Myocarditis was also identified as a common cause of sudden death in young Swedish male military recruits between 1979 and 1992[109] and in other case series. Although adequate clinical data are unavailable, it is not unreasonable to recommend that patients refrain from competitive sports and athletic activity until up to 6 months after the onset of the disease and/or myocardial dysfunction and inflammation is felt to have resolved by ECG, echocardiographic, and biochemical data.

Antiinflammatory Agents

Nonsteroidal antiinflammatory drugs (NSAIDS) have not shown any efficacy in the treatment of myocarditis, despite histological evidence of inflammatory infiltrates in myocarditis.

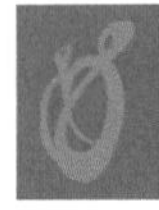

TABLE 31–2 The Role of Endomyocardial Biopsy in Various Heart Failure Clinical Scenarios

Scenario Number	Clinical Scenario	Class of Recommendation (I, IIa, IIb, III)	Level of Evidence (A,B,C)
1	New onset heart failure of less than 2 weeks' duration associated with a normal size or dilated left ventricle and hemodynamic compromise	I	B
2	New onset heart failure of 2 weeks to 3 months' duration associated with a dilated left ventricle, and new ventricular arrhythmias, second- or third-degree heart block, or failure to respond to usual care within 1 to 2 weeks	I	B
3	Heart failure of greater than 3 months' duration associated with a dilated left ventricle and new ventricular arrhythmias, second- or third-degree heart block, or failure to respond to usual care within 1 to 2 weeks	IIa	C
4	Heart failure associated with a dilated cardiomyopathy of any duration associated with suspected allergic reaction and/or eosinophilia	IIa	C
5	Heart failure associated with suspected anthracycline cardiomyopathy	IIa	C
6	Heart failure associated with unexplained restrictive cardiomyopathy	IIa	C
7	Unexplained cardiomyopathy in children	IIa	C
8	New onset heart failure of 2 weeks to 3 months duration associated with a dilated left ventricle, without new ventricular arrhythmias, or second- or third-degree heart block, and that responds to usual care within 1 to 2 weeks	IIb	B
9	Heart failure of greater than 3 months duration associated with a dilated left ventricle, without new ventricular arrhythmias, or second or third degree heart block, and that responds to usual care within 1 to 2 weeks	IIb	C
10	Heart failure associated with unexplained hypertrophic cardiomyopathy	IIb	C

Modified from Cooper LT, Baughman KL, Feldman AM, et al. The role of endomyocardial biopsy in the management of cardiovascular disease: a scientific statement from the American Heart Association, the American College of Cardiology, and the European Society of Cardiology. *Circulation* 2007;116(19):2216-2233. Source: American Heart Association.

BOX 31–4 Infectious and Toxin- or Drug-Associated Causes of Myocarditis

Infectious Causes

Viral: adenovirus, arborvirus, Chikungunya virus, cytomegalovirus, echovirus, enterovirus (Coxsackie B), Epstein-Barr virus, flavivirus (*dengue fever* and *yellow fever*), hepatitis B virus, hepatitis C virus, herpes viruses (human herpesvirus-6), human immunodeficiency virus (*HIV/AIDS*), influenza A and B viruses, parvovirus (parvovirus B-19), mumps virus, poliovirus, rabies virus, respiratory syncytial virus, rubeola virus, rubella virus, varicella virus, variola virus (*smallpox*)

Bacterial: Burkholderia pseudomallei (melioidosis), *Brucella, Chlamydia* (especially *Chlamydia pneumonia* and *Chlamydia psittacosis, Corynebacterium diphtheriae* (*diphtheria*), *Francisella tularensis* (tularemia), *Haemophilus influenzae,* Gonococcus, Clostridium, *Legionella pneumophila* (Legionnaire's disease), Mycobacterium (tuberculosis), *Neisseria meningitidis, Salmonella, Staphylococcus,* Streptococcus A (rheumatic fever), *Streptococcus pneumoniae,* syphilis, tetanus, tularemia, *Vibrio cholerae*

Spirochetal: Borrelia burgdorferi (Lyme disease), *Borrelia recurrentis* (relapsing fever), leptospira, *Treponema pallidum* (syphilis)

Rickettsial: Coxiella burnetii (Q fever), *Orientia tsutsugamushi* (scrub typhus), *Rickettsia prowazekii* (typhus), *Rickettsia rickettsii* (Rocky Mountain spotted fever)

Fungal: Actinomyces, Aspergillus, Blastomyces, Candida, Coccidioides, Cryptococcus, Histoplasma, Mucor species, *Nocardia, Sporothrix schenckii, Strongyloides stercoralis*

Protozoal: Balantidium, Entamoeba histolytica (amebiasis), *Leishmania, Plasmodium falciparum* (malaria), *Sarcocystis, Trypanosoma cruzi* (Chagas' disease), *Trypanosoma brucei* (African sleeping sickness),*Toxoplasma gondii* (toxoplasmosis)

Helminthic: Ascaris, Echinococcus granulosus, Heterophyes, Paragonimus westermani, Schistosoma, Strongyloides stercoralis, Taenia solium (cysticercosis), *Toxocara canis* (visceral larva migrans), *Trichinella spiralis, Wuchereria bancrofti* (filariasis)

Toxin- or Drug-associated Causes

Aminophylline, amphetamines, anthracyclines, catecholamines, chloramphenicol, cocaine, cyclophosphamide, doxorubicin, ethanol, 5-fluorouracil, imatinib mesylate, interleukin-2, methysergide, phenytoin, trastuzumab, zidovudine, arsenic, carbon monoxide, copper, iron, lead

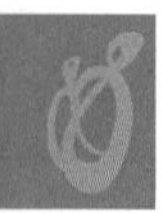

In fact, they may lead to increased mortality by exacerbating the inflammatory process in the myocardium and increasing the virulence of the infectious agent.[110-112] Tea catechins in experimental autoimmune myocarditis have been shown to reduce inflammation and improve myocardial function, especially when administered early in the course of disease.

Antiarrhythmic Therapy

The arrhythmic risk may subside after the acute phase of myocarditis; however, determining when this has occurred is often difficult. Arrhythmias may resolve with therapy, for example, atrioventricular nodal block in sarcoidosis or Lyme carditis, and may not warrant placement of a permanent pacemaker.[113] Patients with acute myocarditis should be hospitalized for electrocardiographic monitoring. The 2006 ACC/AHA/ESC guidelines for the management of arrhythmias recommended that acute arrhythmia emergencies be managed conventionally in the setting of myocarditis.[114] For patients with life-threatening ventricular arrhythmias, ICD therapy may be appropriate if they are not in the acute phase of myocarditis and are on optimal medical therapy with reasonable prognosis for recovery of functional status. Amiodarone or dofetilide have been used as antiarrhythmic therapy when indicated in these patients. In the absence of clinical data, there is a low threshold in clinical practice to implant an ICD in patients with heart failure due to giant cell myocarditis and sarcoidosis.

Specific Therapy

Patients with Lyme myocarditis are treated with a combination of antibiotics including intravenous ceftriaxone or cefotaxime or penicillin G, followed by amoxicillin and doxycycline for at least 4 weeks.[115,116] Myocarditis in systemic lupus erythematosus may be treated with augmentation of immunosuppression such as high dose steroids and cyclophosphamide.[117] Hypersensitivity and eosinophilic myocarditis generally responds well to high dose corticosteroids and withdrawal of the offending agent.

TREATMENT OF ACUTE HEART FAILURE

Acute heart failure syndromes should be managed as per the current AHA/ACCF, ESC, and HFSA guidelines (see also Chapter 43).[118-120] Diuretics should be given to manage volume status, appropriate use of vasodilator therapy and close observation under a monitored setting for functional decline and arrhythmias should be undertaken. Low-dose inotropes can be used in patients with poor end-organ perfusion; however, patients with acute fulminant myocarditis can decline rapidly and intervention in the form of mechanical circulatory support may need to be instituted.

Intraaortic balloon pumps, ventricular assist devices, or extracorporeal membrane oxygenation (ECMO) as a bridge to transplantation or recovery has been used successfully.[121,122] ECMO support may be especially beneficial for patients with fulminant myocarditis with profound shock, where short-term recovery is expected.[123,124] For patients with cardiogenic shock due to acute (nonfulminant) myocarditis, recovery is more likely to be less rapid and implantation of a ventricular assist device as a bridge to transplantation or recovery may be a more effective strategy.[125, 126]

Neurohormonal Blockade in Myocarditis

Patients with heart failure and myocarditis in general respond well to supportive measures and pharmaceutical intervention including neurohormonal blockade, an approach used in the traditional patient with chronic heart failure.

The use of angiotensin-converting enzyme inhibitors/angiotensin receptor blockers (ACEI/ARBs) has not been prospectively tested in patients with myocarditis and data supporting its use is extrapolated from the heart failure trials and animal studies (see Chapter 45). Captopril has been found to reduce inflammatory infiltrates, myocardial necrosis,[127] LV mass, and liver congestion.[128] Candesartan has been shown in a murine model of viral myocarditis to significantly improve survival as compared with controls. Therefore it is not unreasonable to use ACEI or ARB in patients with myocarditis and LVEF less than 40%.

The use of nonspecific β-blockers in animal studies of myocarditis have promising results. The first study of carteolol, a nonselective β-blocker, demonstrated improvement of inflammation and reduction in wall thickness.[129] Carvedilol demonstrated a similar beneficial effect in a model of encephalomyocarditis virus. Viral replication and myocardial necrosis were reduced and survival time increased.[130,131] In human studies, lack of β-blocker therapy in patients with clinically suspected myocarditis was a marker of poor prognosis.[132] β-blockers, preferably nonselective, should therefore be used in patients with heart failure and myocarditis in accordance with current guidelines.

A selective aldosterone antagonist, eplerenone, when used in a mouse model of myocarditis, was found to result in significantly decreased fibrosis in affected hearts probably by its antiinflammatory effect on metalloproteinases and collagen formation.[133] Aldosterone inhibitors improve mortality and heart failure symptoms and should be used in that subset of heart failure patients with myocarditis in accordance with current heart failure guidelines.

Antiviral Therapy

Key trials of antiviral and immunomodulatory treatments for myocarditis are listed in Table 31-3. Antiviral therapy has limited applicability in patients with *acute* cardiomyopathy due to viral myocarditis for several reasons. First, detecting the presence of a viral genome in myocardium is challenging due to various technical factors and routine use of endomyocardial biopsy for this purpose is not recommended due to attendant risks.[61] Secondly, antiviral therapy for acute cardiomyopathy would be most effective when administered at the time of inoculation with the virus or soon thereafter, a timeline that is not practical to follow in human cases of acute myocarditis except in immunosuppressed patients who are being closely monitored. Thirdly, data regarding the use of antiviral agents for the treatment of acute myocarditis is limited to animal models and small case series. In one small case series, three of four patients with life-threatening myocarditis treated with pleconaril improved.[134] Antiviral therapy with ribavarin when administered at the time of virus inoculation was shown to improve survival in treated mice and interferon-α A/D in a similar murine model of viral myocarditis, was found to reduce the severity of myocardial inflammation and necrosis, and viral titers.[135,136] Only certain specific interferon subtypes like IFN A6, A9, and B administered by DNA inoculation in murine models of cytomegalovirus myocarditis have been found to inhibit myocarditis and inflammation.

In contrast, in the setting of chronic, dilated cardiomyopathy with enteroviral or adenoviral persistence detected by PCR, treatment with interferon-β was associated with viral clearance/eradication in all patients, a significant increase in LV ejection fraction and a significant decrease in LV dimensions in approximately 70% of the treatment group.[137] Similar results have been seen in an open labeled randomized trial in patients with dilated cardiomyopathy treated with interferon-α. Although antiviral therapy cannot be recommended for the routine treatment of acute myocarditis at this

TABLE 31–3 Important Clinical Trials of Immunomodulatory and Antiviral Therapies in Cardiomyopathy Due to Myocarditis

Trial	Heart Failure Syndrome	Diagnostic Criteria Used (% patients)	Number of Patients*	Therapy Including Duration	Heart Failure Therapy	Primary Endpoint	Secondary Endpoint	Period of Follow-up
Mason, 1995	Heart failure <2 years, EF ≤ 45%	Active or borderline myocarditis = 64%	N = 111 P = 47 T = 64	Prednisone plus cyclosporine or azathioprine; 6 months	Digitalis ACEI	Improvement in LVEF; no treatment benefit seen	Survival, immune activation markers; no significant difference	28 weeks
McNamara, 1999	Acute heart failure, EF ≤ 40%	Active myocarditis = 7% Borderline myocarditis = 5% Inflammatory markers = 5%	N = 62 P = 29 T = 33	Intravenous immunoglobulin, one time dose	ACEI β-blockers	Improvement in LVEF; no difference between placebo and treatment group	Survival and peak $\dot{V}O_2$; no difference seen between 2 groups	6 and 12 months
Wojnicz, 2001	Chronic heart failure, EF ≤ 40%	Active myocarditis = 8% Borderline myocarditis = 19% Upregulation of HLA Class I = 100%	N = 84 P = 43 T = 41	Prednisone plus azathioprine; 3 months	ACEI β-blockers Digitalis Nitrates Spironolactone Amiodarone	Composite of death, heart transplantation, and hospital readmission; no treatment benefit	Improvement in LVEF, NYHA class, LV chamber size	2 years
Kuhl, 2003	Fatigue, chest pain, arrhythmias	Active or borderline myocarditis = 0% Viral genome = 100% Inflammatory markers = 30%	N = 22 EF >50% =10 EF <50% = 12	Interferon-β; 6 months	ACEI β-blockers Digitalis	Viral clearance, improvement in LV size, LVEF; 100% viral clearance, 70% improvement in LV function	NA	6 months
Frustaci, 2003	Chronic heart failure, EF ≤ 40%	Active myocarditis = 100% Viral genome = 50%	N = 41	Prednisone and azathioprine; 6 months	ACEI β-blockers Digitalis	Improvement in LVEF, NYHA class; treatment benefit for patients with no viral genome in the myocardium	NA	1 year
Cooper, 2008	Acute heart failure, arrhythmias	Giant cell myocarditis by histology = 100%	N = 11	Prednisone, cyclosporine; 1 year ± OKT3 10 days	ACEI or ARB β-blockers Digitalis Hydralazine Amiodarone	Survival or transplant; treatment benefit observed in 90% of patients	Histological parameters; improvement was observed at 4 weeks	1 year
Frustaci, 2009	Chronic heart failure, EF <45%	Active myocarditis = 100% Viral genome = 0%	N = 85 P = 42 T = 43	Prednisone, 5 months; and azathioprine, 6 months	ACEI β-blockers Digitalis	Improvement in LV function; 88% improved in treatment group, none in placebo	NA	6 months

*N = total number of patients; P = placebo; and T = treatment arm.

time, there may be a role in patients with chronic dilated cardiomyopathy who fail to respond to usual care.

Immunosuppression and Immunomodulatory Therapy

Myocardial injury sustained in myocarditis appears to be due to a predominantly immune response involving T lymphocytes and production of auto-antibodies. Hence it would seem that immunosuppression would be a useful treatment modality. However, despite earlier anecdotal reports of the promise of immunosuppression, the Myocarditis Treatment Trial failed to show a survival or functional (change in LV ejection fraction) benefit with the use of azathioprine or cyclosporine with prednisone in patients with histologic myocarditis and LV ejection fraction less than 45%.[59] The study did have many limitations, including different treatment arms with small patient numbers in each arm, discrepancy in biopsy interpretation in up to 36% of patients, use of traditional histologic criteria for patient inclusion, and short duration of symptoms (less than a month) in up to 50% of patients. The duration of symptoms appears to be important as suggested by a recent meta-analysis of immunosuppression and immunomodulation trials wherein trials performed in DCM of less than 6 months duration were negative, and the trials in DCM of greater than 6 months duration were generally positive due to the large improvement in the placebo groups in subjects with acute myocarditis.[138] The utility of using Dallas criteria to identify patients with chronic DCM who will respond to immunomodulatory therapy has been questioned. Up to 40% of patients with chronic DCM will have immunohistochemical evidence of myocardial inflammation, defined by HLA or cell-specific antigen expression on endomyocardial biopsy. In two randomized trials, immunosuppression with azathioprine and prednisone resulted in an improvement in LVEF, NYHA functional class, LV volume, and LV end diastolic diameter.[139] The improvement in one trial was sustained over a period of 2 years in approximately 70% of patients in the immunosuppression arm compared with 30%

of patients in the placebo arm. However, there was no difference in the primary endpoint of death, hospitalization, or readmission rates.

In a case controlled series of patients with active myocarditis and chronic heart failure, unresponsive to conventional therapy, the presence of cardiac autoantibodies and absence of viral genome seem to predict response to treatment with prednisone and azathioprine.[140] Similar results were recently reported in patients with chronic heart failure and active myocarditis and lack of viral genome in myocardial tissue when treated with immunosuppression with an improvement in LVEF from mean of 26% to 46% at 6 months.[141] As is the case for antiviral therapy, the role for immunosuppression may be limited to carefully selected patients with chronic myocarditis (identified by immunoperoxidase based criteria) and those with specific causes such as systemic lupus erythematosus, sarcoidosis, or giant cell myocarditis.

Intravenous immunoglobulin (IVIG) has been shown to be effective in case series of acute myocarditis due to Kawasaki disease and in murine viral myocarditis.[142] In a pediatric population with clinically suspected acute myocarditis, the use of IVIG was associated with improved LV ejection fraction. However, there was no clear survival benefit and β-blockers were not routinely used.[143,144] In the Intervention for Myocarditis and Acute Cardiomyopathy (IMAC-1) trial, adult patients with recent onset myocarditis (less than 5% had active myocarditis) or dilated cardiomyopathy of less than 6 months in duration received IVIG or a placebo. The treatment and placebo groups showed no significant differences.[145] The lack of benefit in this trial is possibly explained by the absence of significant histological myocarditis in treated patients but more importantly could be due to the beneficial effect of IVIG being most pronounced in the acute viremic phase by supplying exogenous neutralizing antibody. A recent systematic review that included IMAC and other smaller studies concluded that there is insufficient evidence to recommend its use in acute myocarditis in adults at this time.[146]

Animal studies have suggested a role for immunomodulatory agents such as interleukin-10 and pimobendan, a phosphodiesterase III inhibitor, in acute viral myocarditis, but these agents remain untested in human studies. Immunoadsorption and other immunomodulatory therapy are currently being tested in human populations.

Prognosis

The outcome of patients with heart failure due to myocarditis depends largely on the presenting clinical scenario. Prognosis is excellent for adult acute lymphocytic myocarditis patients with mild symptoms and preserved LV ejection fraction. The patient with acute fulminant myocarditis appears to have a similar good prognosis if appropriately supported through the acute illness.[60] Patients who have an acute myocardial infarction pattern similarly do well usually with complete recovery of LV ejection fraction. Patients with giant cell myocarditis have a poor prognosis with a 5-year survival rate of approximately 20%; however, immunosuppression may attenuate the course of this disease extending median transplant-free survival time from 3 to 12 months.[63] In patients with acute dilated cardiomyopathy, 67% of who were confirmed to have myocarditis by biopsy, 40% demonstrate improvement in LV function with supportive therapy before the modern era of heart failure treatment.[147] Current prognosis in such patients with acute dilated cardiomyopathy and the routine use of ACE-I and β-blockers seems to be good with transplant-free survival rate being 95% at 1 year. In a large single center, case series, patients with acute lymphocytic myocarditis had a 5-year transplant-free survival rate of approximately 50% compared with patients who were diagnosed with borderline myocarditis who seem to have a better prognosis, with the 5-year survival rate being greater than 80%.[148] In the era of contemporary heart failure therapy, the composite endpoint of death, transplant, and hospital readmission in patients with chronic heart failure, LVEF less than 40% who have increased HLA expression does not seem to be any different as compared with other patients with chronic heart failure being approximately 20% with or without immunosuppression at 2 years. When patients with myocarditis undergo heart transplantation overall survival is similar to survival for other causes of cardiac transplantation,[149] although in the case of giant cell myocarditis and rarely sarcoidosis there is a risk of recurrence of the disease in the transplanted heart.

REFERENCES

1. Cooper, L. T., Jr. (2009). Myocarditis. *N Engl J Med*, *360*(15), 1526–1538.
2. Kuhl, U., Pauschinger, M., Noutsias, M., et al. (2005). High prevalence of viral genomes and multiple viral infections in the myocardium of adults with "idiopathic" left ventricular dysfunction. *Circulation*, *111*, 887–893.
3. Vallbracht, K., Schwimmbeck, P., Kuhl, U., et al. (2005). Differential aspects of endothelial function of the coronary microcirculation considering myocardial virus persistence, endothelial activation, and myocardial leukocyte infiltrates. *Circulation*, *111*(14), 1784–1791.
4. Esfandiarei, M., & McManus, B. M. (2008). Molecular biology and pathogenesis of viral myocarditis. *Ann Rev Pathol Mech Dis*, *3*, 127–155.
5. Bowles, N. E., Richardson, P. J., Olsen, E. G., et al. (1986). Detection of Coxsackie-B-virus-specific RNA sequences in myocardial biopsy samples from patients with myocarditis and dilated cardiomyopathy. *Lancet*, *1*(8490), 1120–1123.
6. Pauschinger, M., Bowles, N. E., Fuentes-Garcia, F. J., et al. (1999). Detection of adenoviral genome in the myocardium of adult patients with idiopathic left ventricular dysfunction. *Circulation*, *99*(10), 1348–1354.
7. Shirali, G., Ni, J., Chinnock, R., et al. (2001). Association of viral genome with graft loss in children after cardiac transplantation. *N Engl J Med*, *344*(20), 1545–1547.
8. Matsumori, A. (2005). Hepatitis C virus infection and cardiomyopathies. *Circ Res*, *96*(2), 144–147, (comment).
9. Pankuweit, S., Portig, I., Eckhardt, H., et al. (2000). Prevalence of viral genome in endomyocardial biopsies from patients with inflammatory heart muscle disease. *Herz*, *25*(3), 221–226.
10. Tschope, C., Bock, C. T., Kasner, M., et al. (2005). High prevalence of cardiac parvovirus B19 infection in patients with isolated left ventricular diastolic dysfunction. *Circulation*, *111*(7), 879–886.
11. Kühl, U., Pauschinger, M., Seeberg, B., et al. (2005). Viral persistence in the myocardium is associated with progressive cardiac dysfunction. *Circulation*, *112*, 1965–1970.
12. Mahrholdt, H., Wagner, A., Deluigi, C., et al. (2006). Presentation, patterns of myocardial damage, and clinical course of viral myocarditis. *Circulation*, *114*(15), 1581–1590.
13. Dalldorf, G., & Sickles, G. (1948). Unidentified filterable agent isolated from feces of children with paralysis. *Science*, *108*, 61–62.
14. Gifford, R., & Dalldorf, G. (1951). Morbid anatomy of experimental Coxsackie virus infection. *Am J Pathol*, *27*, 1047–1063.
15. Wolfgram, L. J., Beisel, K. W., Herskowitz, A., et al. (1986). Variations in the susceptibility to coxsackievirus B3-induced myocarditis among different strains of mice. *J Immunol*, *136*(5), 1846–1852.
16. Tam, P. (2006). Coxsackievirus myocarditis: interplay between virus and host in the pathogenesis of heart disease. *Viral Immunol*, *19*(2), 133–146.
17. Kim, K., Tracy, S., Tapprich, W., et al. (2005). 5'-Terminal deletions occur in coxsackievirus B3 during replication in murine hearts and cardiac myocyte cultures and correlate with encapsidation of negative-strand viral RNA. *J Virol*, *79*(11), 7024–7041.
18. Tracy, S., Hofling, K., Pirruccello, S., et al. (2000). Group B coxsackievirus myocarditis and pancreatitis: connection between viral virulence phenotypes in mice. *J Med Virol*, *62*, 70–81.
19. Coyne, C. B., & Bergelson, J. M. (2005). CAR: a virus receptor within the tight junction. *Adv Drug Deliv Rev*, *57*(6), 869–882.
20. Kuhn, R. (1997). Identification and biology of receptors for the Coxsackie B virus group. *Curr Top Microbiol Immunol*, *223*, 209–226.
21. Coyne, C. B., & Bergelson, J. M. (2006). Virus-induced Abl and Fyn kinase signals permit coxsackievirus entry through epithelial tight junctions. *Cell*, *124*(1), 119–131, (see comment).
22. Tracy, S., & Gauntt, C. (2008). Group B coxsackievirus virulence. *Curr Top Microbiol Immunol*, *323*, 49–63.
23. Yalamanchili, P., Datta, U., & Dasgupta, A. (1997). Inhibition of host cell transcription by poliovirus: cleavage of transcription factor CREB by poliovirus-encoded protease 3Cpro. *J Virol*, *71*(2), 1220–1226.
24. Luo, H., Zhang, J., Dastvan, F., et al. (2003). Ubiquitin-dependent proteolysis of cyclin D1 is associated with coxsackievirus-induced cell growth arrest. *J Virol*, *77*(1), 1–9.
25. Fairweather, D., Frisancho-Kiss, S., & Rose, N. (2005). Viruses as adjuvants for autoimmunity: evidence from coxsackievirus-induced myocarditis. *Rev Med Virol*, *15*(1), 17–27.
26. Frisancho-Kiss, S., Davis, S., Nyland, J., et al. (2007). Cutting edge: cross-regulation by TLR4 and T cell Ig mucin-3 determines sex differences in inflammatory heart disease. *J Immunol*, *178*(11), 6710–6714.
27. Zhang, P., Cox, C. J., Alvarez, K. M., et al. (2009). Cutting edge: cardiac myosin activates innate immune responses through TLRs. *J Immunol*, *183*(1), 27–31.
28. Fuse, K., Chan, G., Liu, Y., et al. (2005). Myeloid differentiation factor-88 plays a crucial role in the pathogenesis of coxsackievirus B3-induced myocarditis and influences type I interferon production. *Circulation*, *112*(15), 2276–2285.

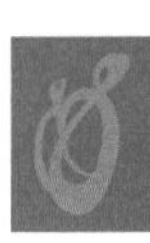

29. Fairweather, D., Frisancho-Kiss, S., Gatewood, S., et al. (2004). Mast cells and innate cytokines are associated with susceptibility to autoimmune heart disease following coxsackievirus B3 infection. *Autoimmunity, 37*(2), 131–145.
30. Eriksson, U., Ricci, R., Hunziker, L., et al. (2003). Dendritic cell-induced autoimmune heart failure requires cooperation between adaptive and innate immunity. *Nat Med, 9*(12), 1484–1490.
31. Kodama, M., Hanawa, H., Saeki, M., et al. (1994). Rat dilated cardiomyopathy after autoimmune giant cell myocarditis. *Circ Res, 75*(2), 278–284.
32. Zehn, D., & Bevan, M. (2006). T cells with a low avidity for a tissue-restricted antigen routinely evade central and peripheral tolerance and cause autoimmunity. *Immunity, 25*, 261–270.
33. Wilson, N., Boniface, K., Chan, J., et al. (2007). Development, cytokine profile and function of human interleukin 17-producing helper T cells. *Nat Immunol, 8*(9), 950–957.
34. Rangachari, M., Mauermann, N., Marty, R., et al. (2006). T-bet negatively regulates autoimmune myocarditis by suppressing local production of interleukin 17. *J Exp Med, 203*(8), 2009–2019.
35. Huber, S., Feldman, A., & Sartini, D. (2006). Coxsackievirus B3 induces T regulatory cells, which inhibit cardiomyopathy in tumor necrosis factor-alpha transgenic mice. *Circ Res, 99*(10), 1109–1116.
36. Ono, M., Shimizu, J., Miyachi, Y., et al. (2006). Control of autoimmune myocarditis and multiorgan inflammation by glucocorticoid-induced TNF receptor family-related protein(high), Foxp3-expressing CD25+ and CD25– regulatory T cells. *J Immunol, 176*(8), 4748–4756.
37. Caforio, A. L., Tona, F., Bottaro, S., et al. (2008). Clinical implications of anti-heart autoantibodies in myocarditis and dilated cardiomyopathy. *Autoimmunity, 41*(1), 35–45.
38. Li, Y., Heuser, J., Cunningham, L., et al. (2006). Mimicry and antibody-mediated cell signaling in autoimmune myocarditis. *J Immunol, 177*(11), 8234–8240.
39. Mascaro-Blanco, A., Alvarez, K., Yu, X., et al. (2008). Consequences of unlocking the cardiac myosin molecule in human myocarditis and cardiomyopathies. *Autoimmunity, 41*(6), 442–453.
40. Heidecker, B., Kasper, E. K., Wittstein, I. S., et al. (2008). Transcriptomic biomarkers for individual risk assessment in new-onset heart failure. *Circulation, 118*(3), 238–246, (see comment).
41. Beck, M. A., Shi, Q., Morris, V. C., et al. (1995). Rapid genomic evolution of a non-virulent coxsackievirus B3 in selenium-deficient mice results in selection of identical virulent isolates. *Nat Med, 1*(5), 433–436.
42. Koller, L. (1975). Methylmercury: effect on oncogenic and nononcogenic viruses in mice. *Am J Vet Res, 36*(10), 1501–1504.
43. Christensen, M., Ellermann-Eriksen, S., Rungby, J., et al. (1996). Influence of mercuric chloride on resistance to generalized infection with herpes simplex virus type 2 in mice. *Toxicology, 114*(1), 57–66.
44. South, P., Morris, V., Levander, O., et al. (2001). Mortality in mice infected with an amyocarditic coxsackievirus and given a subacute dose of mercuric chloride. *J Toxicol Environ Health A, 63*(7), 511–523.
45. Ilback, N., Lindh, U., Wesslen, L., et al. (2000). Trace element distribution in heart tissue sections studied by nuclear microscopy is changed in Coxsackie virus B3 myocarditis in methyl mercury-exposed mice. *Biol Trace Elem Res, 78*(1-3), 131–147.
46. Cooper, L. T., Rader, V., & Ralston, N. V. (2007). The roles of selenium and mercury in the pathogenesis of viral cardiomyopathy. *Congest Heart Fail, 13*(4), 193–199.
47. Frustaci, A., Magnavita, N., Chimenti, C., et al. (1999). Marked elevation of myocardial trace elements in idiopathic dilated cardiomyopathy compared with secondary cardiac dysfunction. *J Am Coll Cardiol, 33*(6), 1578–1583.
48. Badorff, C., Lee, G., Lamphear, B., et al. (1999). Enteroviral protease 2A cleaves dystrophin: evidence of cytoskeletal disruption in an acquired cardiomyopathy. *Nat Med, 5*, 320–326.
49. Badorff, C., & Knowlton, K. U. (2004). Dystrophin disruption in enterovirus-induced myocarditis and dilated cardiomyopathy: from bench to bedside. *Med Microbiol Immunol, 193*(2-3), 121–126.
50. Andreoletti, L., Venteo, L., Douche-Aourik, F., et al. (2007). Active coxsackieviral B infection is associated with disruption of dystrophin in endomyocardial tissue of patients who died suddenly of acute myocardial infarction. *J Am Coll Cardiol, 50*(23), 2207–2214, (see comment).
51. Kodama, M., Hanawa, H., Saeki, M., et al. (1994). Rat dilated cardiomyopathy after autoimmune giant cell myocarditis. *Circ Res, 75*(2), 278–284.
52. Kim, J. S., Judson, M. A., Donnino, R., et al. (2009). Cardiac sarcoidosis. *Am Heart J, 157*(1), 9–21.
53. Murphy, J., Wright, R., Bruce, G., et al. (2003). Eosinophilic-Lymphocytic myocarditis after smallpox vaccination. *Lancet, 362*, 1378–1380.
54. Takata, Y., Teraoka, K., Abe, M., et al. (1993). Sudden cardiac death from hypertrophic cardiomyopathy and acute idiopathic (Fiedler) myocarditis: autopsy report. *Intern Med, 32*(10), 815–819.
55. Pieroni, M., Dello Russo, A., Marzo, F., et al. (2009). High prevalence of myocarditis mimicking arrhythmogenic right ventricular cardiomyopathy differential diagnosis by electroanatomic mapping-guided endomyocardial biopsy. *J Am Coll Cardiol, 53*(8), 681–689, (see comment).
56. Rahman, J., Helou, E., Gelzer-Bell, R., et al. (2004). Noninvasive diagnosis of biopsy-proven cardiac amyloidosis. *J Am Coll Cardiol, 43*(3), 410–415.
57. Frustaci, A., Verardo, R., Caldarulo, M., et al. (2007). Myocarditis in hypertrophic cardiomyopathy patients presenting acute clinical deterioration. *Eur Heart J, 28*(6), 733–740.
58. Maron, B. J., Doerer, J. J., Haas, T. S., et al. (2009). Sudden deaths in young competitive athletes: analysis of 1866 deaths in the United States, 1980-2006. *Circulation, 119*(8), 1085–1092.
59. Mason, J. W., O'Connell, J. B., Herskowitz, A., et al. (1995). A clinical trial of immunosuppressive therapy for myocarditis. *N Engl J Med, 333*(5), 269–275.
60. Hare, J. M., & Baughman, K. L. (2001). Fulminant and acute lymphocytic myocarditis: the prognostic value of clinicopathological classification. *Eur Heart J, 22*(4), 269–270.
61. Cooper, L. T., Baughman, K. L., Feldman, A. M., et al. (2007). The role of endomyocardial biopsy in the management of cardiovascular disease: a scientific statement from the American Heart Association, the American College of Cardiology, and the European Society of Cardiology. *Circulation, 116*(19), 2216–2233.
62. McCully, R. B., Cooper, L. T., & Schreiter, S. (2005). Coronary artery spasm in lymphocytic myocarditis: a rare cause of acute myocardial infarction. *Heart, 91*(2), 202.
63. Cooper, L. T., Jr., Hare, J. M., Tazelaar, H. D., et al. (2008). Usefulness of immunosuppression for giant cell myocarditis. *Am J Cardiol, 102*(11), 1535–1539.
64. Silver, E., Pass, R. H., Kaufman, S., et al. (2007). Complete heart block due to Lyme carditis in two pediatric patients and a review of the literature. *Congenit Heart Dis, 2*(5), 338–341.
65. Ben m'rad, M., Leclerc-Mercier, S., Blanche, P., et al. (2009). Drug-induced hypersensitivity syndrome: clinical and biologic disease patterns in 24 patients. *Medicine, 88*(3), 131–140.
66. Cooper, L. T., & Zehr, K. J. (2005). Biventricular assist device placement and immunosuppression as therapy for necrotizing eosinophilic myocarditis. *Nat Clin Pract Cardiovasc Med, 2*(10), 544–548.
67. Bilate, A. M. B., & Cunha-Neto, E. (2008). Chagas disease cardiomyopathy: current concepts of an old disease. *Rev Inst Med Trop Sao Paulo, 50*(2), 67–74.
68. Brucato, A., Colombo, T., Bonacina, E., et al. (2004). Fulminant myocarditis during HIV seroconversion: recovery with temporary left ventricular mechanical assistance. *Ital Heart J, 5*(3), 228–231.
69. Chen, F., Shannon, K., Ding, S., et al. (2002). HIV type 1 glycoprotein 120 inhibits cardiac myocyte contraction. *AIDS Res Hum Retroviruses, 18*(11), 777–784.
70. Smith, S. C., Ladenson, J. H., Mason, J. W., et al. (1997). Elevations of cardiac troponin I associated with myocarditis. Experimental and clinical correlates. *Circulation, 95*(1), 163–168.
71. Lauer, B., Niederau, C., Kuhl, U., et al. (1997). Cardiac troponin T in patients with clinically suspected myocarditis. *J Am Coll Cardiol, 30*(5), 1354–1359.
72. Nasser, N., Perles, Z., Rein, A. J., et al. (2006). NT-proBNP as a marker for persistent cardiac disease in children with history of dilated cardiomyopathy and myocarditis. *Pediatr Cardiol, 27*(1), 87–90.
73. Fuse, K., Kodama, M., Okura, Y., et al. (2000). Predictors of disease course in patients with acute myocarditis. *Circulation, 102*(23), 2829–2835.
74. Fuse, K., Kodama, M., Okura, Y., et al. (2005). Short-term prognostic value of initial serum levels of interleukin-10 in patients with acute myocarditis. *Eur J Heart Fail, 7*(1), 109–112.
75. Angelini, A., Calzolari, V., Calabrese, F., et al. (2000). Myocarditis mimicking acute myocardial infarction: role of. *Heart, 84*(3), 245–250.
76. Cooper, L. T. (2005). Giant cell and granulomatous myocarditis. *Heart Fail Clin, 1*(3), 431–437.
77. Skouri, H. N., Dec, G. W., Friedrich, M. G., et al. (2006). Noninvasive imaging in myocarditis. *J Am Coll Cardiol, 48*(10), 2085–2093.
78. Felker, G. M., Boehmer, J. P., Hruban, R. H., et al. (2000). Echocardiographic findings in fulminant and acute myocarditis. *J Am Coll Cardiol, 36*(1), 227–232.
79. Hiramitsu, S., Morimoto, S., Kato, S., et al. (2001). Transient ventricular wall thickening in acute myocarditis: a serial echocardiographic and histopathologic study. *Jpn Circ J, 65*(10), 863–866.
80. Laissy, J. P., Messin, B., Varenne, O., et al. (2002). MRI of acute myocarditis: a comprehensive approach based on various imaging sequences. *Chest, 122*(5), 1638–1648.
81. Friedrich, M. G., Strohm, O., Schulz-Menger, J., et al. (1998). Contrast media-enhanced magnetic resonance imaging visualizes myocardial changes in the course of viral myocarditis. *Circulation, 97*(18), 1802–1809.
82. Friedrich, M. G., Sechtem, U., Schulz-Menger, J., et al. (2009). Cardiovascular magnetic resonance in myocarditis: a JACC white paper. *J Am Coll Cardiol, 53*(17), 1475–1487.
83. Felker, G., Thompson, R., Hare, J., et al. (2000). Underlying causes and long-term survival in patients with initially unexplained cardiomyopathy. *N Engl J Med, 342*(15), 1077–1084.
84. Caforio, A. L., Calabrese, F., Angelini, A., et al. (2007). A prospective study of biopsy-proven myocarditis: prognostic relevance of clinical and aetiopathogenetic features at diagnosis. *Eur Heart J, 28*(11), 1326–1333, (see comment).
85. Kindermann, I., Kindermann, M., Kandolf, R., et al. (2008). Predictors of outcome in patients with suspected myocarditis. *Circulation, 118*(6), 639–648.
86. Kuhl, U., Noutsias, M., Seeberg, B., et al. (1996). Immunohistological evidence for a chronic intramyocardial inflammatory process in dilated cardiomyopathy. *Heart, 75*(3), 295–300.
87. Hufnagel, G., Pankuweit, S., Richter, A., et al. (2000). The European study of epidemiology and treatment of cardiac inflammatory. *Herz, 25*(3), 279–285.
88. Deckers, J., Hare, J., & Baughman, K. (1992). Complications of transvenous right ventricular endomyocardial biopsy in adult patients with cardiomyopathy: a seven-year survey of 546 consecutive diagnostic procedures in a tertiary referral center. *J Am Coll Cardiol, 19*, 43–47.
89. Holzmann, M., Nicko, A., Kuhl, U., et al. (2008). Complication rate of right ventricular endomyocardial biopsy via the femoral approach: a retrospective and prospective study analyzing 3048 diagnostic procedures over an 11-year period. *Circulation, 118*(17), 1722–1728.
90. Cooper, L. T., Berry, G. J., & Shabetai, R. (1997). Giant cell myocarditis: natural history and treatment. *N Engl J Med, 336*, 1860–1866.
91. Kilgallen, C., Jackson, E., Bankoff, M., et al. (1998). A case of giant cell myocarditis and malignant thymoma: a postmortem diagnosis by needle biopsy. *Clin Cardiol, 21*(1), 48–51.

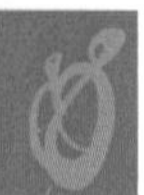

92. Daniels, P., Tazelaar, H., Edwards, W., et al. (2000). Hypersensitivity myocarditis presenting histologically with fulminant giant cell myocarditis. *Cardiovasc Pathol, 9*(5), 287–291.
93. Okura, Y., Dec, G., Hare, J., et al. (2000). A multicenter registry comparison of cardiac sarcoidosis and giant cell myocarditis. *Circulation, 102*(18 suppl. II), 3897.
94. Shields, R. C., Tazelaar, H. D., Berry, G. J., et al. (2002). The role of right ventricular endomyocardial biopsy for idiopathic giant cell myocarditis. *J Card Fail, 8*(2), 74–78.
95. Silverman, K. J., Hutchins, G. M., & Bulkley, B. H. (1978). Cardiac sarcoid: a clinicopathologic study of 84 unselected patients with systemic sarcoidosis. *Circulation, 58*(6), 1204–1211.
96. Sekiguchi, M., Yazaki, Y., Isobe, M., et al. (1996). Cardiac sarcoidosis: diagnostic, prognostic, and therapeutic considerations. *Cardiovasc Drugs Ther, 10*(5), 495–510.
97. Yazaki, Y., Isobe, M., Hiramitsu, S., et al. (1998). Comparison of clinical features and prognosis of cardiac sarcoidosis and idiopathic dilated cardiomyopathy. *Am J Cardiol, 82*, 537–540.
98. Fleming, H. A., & Bailey, S. M. (1981). Sarcoid heart disease. *J R Coll Physicians Lond, 15*(4), 245–246.
99. Cooper, L., Okura, Y., Hare, J., et al. (2001). Survival in biopsy-proven cardiac sarcoidosis is similar to survival in lymphocytic myocarditis and dilated cardiomyopathy. In A. Kimchi (Ed.). *Heart Disease: New Trends in Research, Diagnosis, and Treatment*. Englewood, NJ: Medimond.
100. Okura, Y., Dec, G. W., Hare, J. M., et al. (2003). A clinical and histopathologic comparison of cardiac sarcoidosis and idiopathic giant cell myocarditis. *J Am Coll Cardiol, 42*(2), 322–328.
101. Smedema, J. P., Snoep, G., van Kroonenburgh, M. P. G., et al. (2005). Cardiac involvement in patients with pulmonary sarcoidosis assessed at two university medical centers in the Netherlands. *Chest, 128*(1), 30–35, (see comment).
102. Schulz-Menger, J., Wassmuth, R., Abdel-Aty, H., et al. (2006). Patterns of myocardial inflammation and scarring in sarcoidosis as assessed by cardiovascular magnetic resonance. *Heart, 92*(3), 399–400.
103. Fineschi, V., Neri, M., Riezzo, I., et al. (2004). Sudden cardiac death due to hypersensitivity myocarditis during clozapine treatment. *Int J Legal Med, 118*(5), 307–309.
104. Taliercio, C., Olney, B., & Lie, J. (1985). Myocarditis related to drug hypersensitivity. *Mayo Clin Proc, 60*, 463–468.
105. Hawkins, E., Levine, T., Goss, S., et al. (1995). Hypersensitivity myocarditis in the explanted hearts of transplant recipients: reappraisal of pathologic criteria and their clinical implications. *Pathol Annu, 30*, 287–305.
106. Spear, G. (1995). Eosinophilic explant carditis with eosinophilia: hypersensitivity to dobutamine infusion. *J Heart Lung Transplant, 14*(4), 755–760.
107. Morimoto, S., Kato, S., Hiramitsu, S., et al. (2003). Narrowing of the left ventricular cavity associated with transient ventricular wall thickening reduces stroke volume in patients with acute myocarditis. *Circ J, 67*(6), 490–494.
108. Kiel, R. J., Smith, F. E., Chason, J., et al. (1989). Coxsackievirus B3 myocarditis in C3H/HeJ mice: description of an inbred model and the effect of exercise on virulence. *Eur J Epidemiol, 5*(3), 348–350.
109. Friman, G., Larsson, E., & Rolf, C. (1997). Interaction between infection and exercise with special reference to myocarditis and the increased frequency of sudden deaths among young Swedish orienteers 1979-92. *Scand J Infect Dis Suppl, 104*, 41–49.
110. Khatib, R., Reyes, M. P., Smith, F., et al. (1990). Enhancement of coxsackievirus B4 virulence by indomethacin. *J Lab Clin Med, 116*(1), 116–120.
111. Costanzo-Nordin, M. R., Reap, E. A., O'Connell, J. B., et al. (1985). A nonsteroid anti-inflammatory drug exacerbates Coxsackie B3 murine myocarditis. *J Am Coll Cardiol, 6*(5), 1078–1082.
112. Rezkalla, S., Khatib, R., Khatib, G., et al. (1988). Effect of indomethacin in the late phase of coxsackievirus myocarditis in a murine model. *J Lab Clin Med, 112*(1), 118–121.
113. Hanawa, H., Izumi, T., Saito, Y., et al. (1998). Recovery from complete atrioventricular block caused by idiopathic giant cell myocarditis after corticosteroid therapy. *Jpn Circ J, 62*(3), 211–214.
114. Zipes, D., Camm, A., Borggrefe, M., et al. (2006). ACC/AHA/ESC 2006 guideline for management of patients with ventricular arrhythmias and the prevention of sudden cardiac death. *Circulation, 114*(10), e385–e484.
115. Fish, A. E., Pride, Y. B., & Pinto, D. S. (2008). Lyme carditis. *Infect Dis Clin North Am, 22*(2), 275–288.
116. Costello, J. M., Alexander, M. E., Greco, K. M., et al. (2009). Lyme carditis in children: presentation, predictive factors, and clinical course. *Pediatrics, 123*(5), e835–e841, (see comment).
117. Apte, M., McGwin, G., Jr., Vila, L. M., et al. (2008). Associated factors and impact of myocarditis in patients with SLE from LUMINA, a multiethnic US cohort. *Rheumatology, 47*(3), 362–367.
118. Jessup, M., Abraham, W. T., Casey, D. E., et al. (2009). 2009 Focused update: ACCF/AHA guidelines for the diagnosis and management of heart failure in adults: a report of the American College of Cardiology Foundation/American Heart Association task force on practice guidelines: developed in collaboration with the International Society for Heart and Lung Transplantation. *Circulation, 119*(14), 1977–2016.
119. Swedberg, K., Cleland, J., Dargie, H. J., et al. (2005). Guidelines for the diagnosis and treatment of chronic heart failure (update 2005). *Eur Heart J, 26*, 1115–1140.
120. HFSA guidelines for management of patients with heart failure caused by left ventricular systolic dysfunction–pharmacological approaches. Heart Failure Society of America. (2000). *Pharmacotherapy, 20*(5), 495–522.
121. Farrar, D. J., Holman, W. R., McBride, L. R., et al. (2002). Long-term follow-up of Thoratec ventricular assist device bridge-to-recovery patients successfully removed from support after recovery of ventricular function. *J Heart Lung Transplant, 21*(5), 516–521.
122. Chen, Y. S., & Yu, H. Y. (2005). Choice of mechanical support for fulminant myocarditis: ECMO vs. VAD. *Eur J Cardiothorac Surg, 27*(5), 931–932, author reply 932 (comment)..
123. Pages, O., Aubert, S., Combes, A., et al. (2009). Paracorporeal pulsatile biventricular assist device versus extracorporal membrane oxygenation-extracorporal life support in adult fulminant myocarditis. *J Thorac Cardiovasc Surg, 137*(1), 194–197.
124. Duncan, B., Bohn, D., Atz, A., et al. (2001). Mechanical circulatory support for the treatment of children with acute fulminant myocarditis. *J Thorac Cardiovasc Surg, 122*(3), 440–448.
125. Reinhartz, O., Hill, J., Al-Khaldi, A., et al. (2005). Thoratec ventricular assist devices in pediatric patients: update on clinical results. *ASAIO J, 51*(5), 501–503.
126. Topkara, V., Dang, N. C., Barili, F., et al. (2006). Ventricular assist device use for the treatment of acute viral myocarditis. *J Thorac Cardiovasc Surg, 131*(5), 1190–1191.
127. Rezkalla, S. H., Raikar, S., & Kloner, R. A. (1996). Treatment of viral myocarditis with focus on captopril. *Am J Cardiol, 77*(8), 634–637.
128. Rezkalla, S., Kloner, R. A., Khatib, G., et al. (1990). Effect of delayed captopril therapy on left ventricular mass and myonecrosis during acute coxsackievirus murine myocarditis. *Am Heart J, 120*(6 pt 1), 1377–1381.
129. Tominaga, M., Matsumori, A., Okada, I., et al. (1991). Beta-blocker treatment of dilated cardiomyopathy. Beneficial effect of carteolol in mice. *Circulation, 83*, 2021–2028.
130. Yue-Chun, L., Li-Sha, G., Jiang-Hua, R., et al. (2008). Protective effects of carvedilol in murine model with the coxsackievirus B3-induced viral myocarditis. *J Cardiovasc Pharmacol, 51*(1), 92–98.
131. Pauschinger, M., Rutschow, S., Chandrasekharan, K., et al. (2005). Carvedilol improves left ventricular function in murine coxsackievirus-induced acute myocarditis association with reduced myocardial interleukin-1beta and MMP-8 expression and a modulated immune response. *Eur J Heart Fail, 7*(4), 444–452.
132. Kindermann, I., Kindermann, M., Kandolf, R., et al. (2008). Predictors of outcome in patients with suspected myocarditis. *Circulation, 118*(6), 639–648, (erratum appears in *Circulation*, 2008;118(12): e493.)
133. Xiao, J., Shimada, M., Liu, W., et al. (2009). Anti-inflammatory effects of eplerenone on viral myocarditis. *Eur J Heart Fail, 11*(4), 349–353.
134. Rotbart, H. A., & Webster, A. D. (2001). Pleconaril Treatment Registry Group. Treatment of potentially life-threatening enterovirus infections with pleconaril. *Clin Infect Dis, 32*(2), 228–235.
135. Matsumori, A., Crumpacker, C. S., & Abelmann, W. H. (1987). Prevention of viral myocarditis with recombinant human leukocyte interferon alpha A/D in a murine model. *J Am Coll Cardiol, 9*(6), 1320–1325.
136. Okada, I., Matsumori, A., Matoba, Y., et al. (1992). Combination treatment with ribavirin and interferon for Coxsackie B3 replication. *J Lab Clin Med, 120*, 569–573.
137. Kuhl, U., Pauschinger, M., Schwimmbeck, P., et al. (2003). Interferon-beta treatment eliminates cardiotropic viruses and improves left ventricular function in patients with myocardial persistence of viral genomes and left ventricular dysfunction. *Circulation, 107*, 2703–2708.
138. Stanton, C., Mookadam, F., Cha, S., et al. (2007). Greater symptom duration predicts response to immunomodulatory therapy in dilated cardiomyopathy. *Int J Cardiol*, Epub ahead of print.
139. Wojnicz, R., Nowalany-Kozielska, E., Wojciechowska, C., et al. (2001). Randomized, placebo-controlled study for immunosuppressive treatment of inflammatory dilated cardiomyopathy: two-year follow-up results. *Circulation, 104*(1), 39–45.
140. Frustaci, A., Chimenti, C., Calabrese, F., et al. (2003). Immunosuppressive therapy for active lymphocytic myocarditis: virological and immunologic profile of responders versus nonresponders. *Circulation, 107*, 857–863.
141. Frustaci, A., Russo, M. A., & Chimenti, C. (2009). Randomized study of the efficacy of immunosuppressive therapy in patients with virus-negative inflammatory cardiomyopathy: the TIMIC study. *Eur Heart J, 30*(16), 1995–2002.
142. Takada, H., Kishimoto, C., & Hiraoka, Y. (1995). Therapy with immunoglobulin suppresses myocarditis in a murine coxsackievirus B3 model: antiviral and anti-inflammatory effects. *Circulation, 92*(6), 1604–1611.
143. Drucker, N. A., Colan, S. D., Lewis, A. B., et al. (1994). Gamma-globulin treatment of acute myocarditis in the pediatric population. *Circulation, 89*(1), 252–257.
144. Tedeschi, A., Airaghi, L., Giannini, S., et al. (2002). High-dose intravenous immunoglobulin in the treatment of acute myocarditis. A case report and review of the literature. *J Intern Med, 251*(2), 169–173.
145. McNamara, D. M., Holubkov, R., Starling, R. C., et al. (2001). Controlled trial of intravenous immune globulin in recent-onset dilated cardiomyopathy. *Circulation, 103*(18), 2254–2259.
146. Hia, C. P., Yip, W. C., Tai, B. C., et al. (2004). Immunosuppressive therapy in acute myocarditis: an 18 year systematic review. *Arch Dis Child, 89*(6), 580–584.
147. Dec, G. W., Jr., Palacios, I. F., Fallon, J. T., et al. (1985). Active myocarditis in the spectrum of acute dilated cardiomyopathies. Clinical features, histologic correlates, and clinical outcome. *N Engl J Med, 312*(14), 885–890.
148. Magnani, J. W., Danik, H. J., Dec, G. W., Jr., et al. (2006). Survival in biopsy-proven myocarditis: a long-term retrospective analysis of the histopathologic, clinical, and hemodynamic predictors. *Am Heart J, 151*(2), 463–470.
149. Moloney, E. D., Egan, J. J., Kelly, P., et al. (2005). Transplantation for myocarditis: a controversy revisited. *J Heart Lung Transplant, 24*(8), 1103–1110.

CHAPTER 32

Heart Failure as a Consequence of Sleep-Disordered Breathing

Shahrokh Javaheri

Chronic congestive heart failure is a highly prevalent and progressive disorder, has a huge economic impact, and is a cause of excess morbidity and mortality worldwide. One factor that may contribute to progression of left ventricular remodeling, and consequently to morbidity and mortality of left-sided heart failure, is sleep-related breathing disorders. Sleep apnea is highly prevalent among patients with left-sided heart failure and, when untreated, contributes to excess mortality. In contrast, effective treatment of sleep apnea improves survival of patients with heart failure. Physicians caring for patients with heart failure need to be aware of sleep-related breathing disorders and various therapeutic options, which are distinct from the standard treatment of heart failure.

HISTORY AND REDISCOVERY OF CHEYNE-STOKES BREATHING

In 1818, John Cheyne[1] observed an unusual pattern of breathing in a patient whose autopsy later revealed a fatty heart. Thirty-six years later, William Stokes[2] also observed the gradual crescendo-decrescendo changes in breathing with intervening apnea. Figure 32-1 is a polysomnographic depiction of Cheyne-Stokes breathing in a sleeping patient with heart failure.[3]

George Cheyne, another Scottish physician who practiced in the early 1700s, might actually have been the first person to observe Cheyne-Stokes breathing as a pathological entity.[4,5] However, the best description of Cheyne-Stokes breathing is by a British physician, John Hunter,[6,7] about 37 years before John Cheyne's report.[1] The eponym, therefore, does not credit the main discoverer of the breathing pattern. For this reason, this breathing disorder is referred to as Hunter-Cheyne-Stokes breathing.

Hunter-Cheyne-Stokes breathing has been considered a rare entity associated with severe heart failure and potentially an indicator of terminal prognosis. The reason for its seeming rarity is that the disorder is only occasionally obvious during wakefulness.[8] The reason for heralding a poor prognosis stems from clinical observation that when Hunter-Cheyne-Stokes breathing is observed during wakefulness, it is associated with impending mortality.

Since 1990, however, Hunter-Cheyne-Stokes breathing has been reanalyzed. Many researchers have reported a high prevalence of this disorder in heart failure.[8-19] The reanalysis is largely related to the availability of polysomnography to diagnose breathing disorders during sleep, the state in which the disorder commonly manifests. In addition to frequent co-occurrence of Hunter-Cheyne-Stokes breathing and central sleep apnea (CSA), polysomnography has also revealed presence of obstructive sleep apnea (OSA) in patients with heart failure.

Other important factors that have contributed to further research and increased recognition of sleep apnea is the high rates of morbidity and mortality among patients with heart failure.[20] As discussed later in this chapter, study findings have strongly suggested that sleep apnea contributes to mortality in patients with heart failure and that effective treatment improves survival rates.

POLYSOMNOGRAPHY, SLEEP STAGES, AND DEFINITIONS OF SLEEP APNEA AND HYPOPNEA

Polysomnography (from the Latin *Somnus*, god of sleep in Roman mythology) is electrophysiological recording of brain waves (usually two channels) and eye movements, along with chin electromyography. These recordings allow the state of wakefulness to be differentiated from the state of sleep and enable recognition of different stages of sleep.[21] To recognize sleep-related breathing disorders, naso-oral airflow (measured by a thermocouple and a pressure sensor), thoracoabdominal excursions (measured by strain gauges, inductive plethysmography, or impedance pneumography), and arterial oxyhemoglobin saturation (measured by pulse oximetry) are also recorded.[22] Monitoring of the electrocardiogram and of the electromyogram of the anterior tibialis muscles allows, respectively, detection of nocturnal arrhythmias and a sleep disorder called *periodic limb movements*, which are common in patients with congestive heart failure.[23]

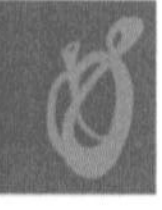

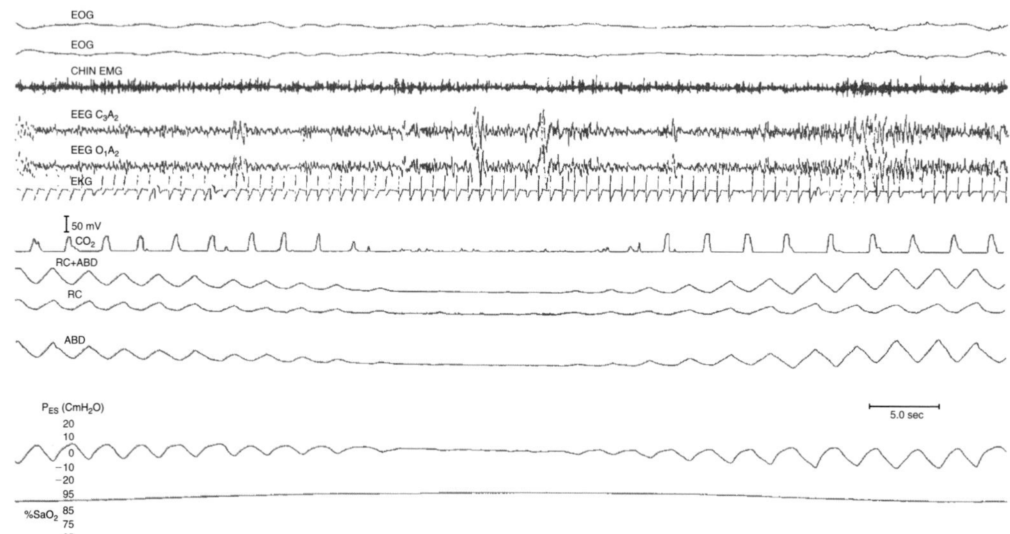

FIGURE 32–1 Polysomnographic example of classic Cheyne-Stokes respiration in stage 2 sleep. *Top to bottom,* Two electro-oculograms (1st and 2nd tracings), chin electromyogram (3rd tracings), two electroencephalograms (4th and 5th tracings), electrocardiogram (6th tracing), abdominal excursion (7th tracing), esophageal pressure excursions (8th tracing), and arterial oxyhemoglobin saturation (9th tracing). Note the smooth and gradual changes in the thoracoabdominal excursions and esophageal pressure of the crescendo and decrescendo arms of the cycle. There is intervening central apnea. Central apnea is characterized by absence of effort to breathe. This is reflected in the absence of naso-oral airflow and excursions in the thoracoabdominal and pleural pressure (as measured by esophageal pressure) tracings. An arousal, characterized by an increase in chin electromyographic and electroencephalographic speeding (alpha waves), occurs at the peak of hyperventilation. Desaturation in somewhat delayed because of long circulation time in heart failure. A 5-second time scale is shown on right bottom corner.

Sleep is not a homogeneous state. According to electroencephalographic criteria, eye movements, and chin electromyography, sleep is divided into periods of rapid-eye-movement (REM) and non–rapid-eye-movement (non-REM) states.[21] Non-REM sleep consists of stages 1 to 4 and accounts for about 80% of total sleep time in adults. REM sleep, which accounts for 20% of total sleep time in adults, is characterized by rapid eye movements (hence the name) that occur intermittently (phasic REM, in contrast to tonic REM), skeletal muscle atonia (characterized by a decrease in the amplitude of the chin electromyogram), and dreaming. REM sleep is therefore a state of brain activity in a paralyzed body. Because of the paralysis, the dream is not enacted.

An adult normally enters sleep in stage 1 (currently referred to as *N1* instead of *S1; N* stands for "non–rapid-eye-movement sleep"), which in few minutes progresses to deeper sleep stages of N2 (formerly S2) and N3 (formerly S3 and S4). In N3, brain waves are tall (≥75 μV) and wide (≥0.5 seconds). These are *delta waves,* for which reason N3 may be referred to as *delta sleep.*

After about 90 minutes of non-REM sleep, the first episode of REM sleep occurs, and then the first cycle of sleep is completed.[21] Several sleep cycles occur each night. In a total dark time of 8 hours and a total sleep time of 7.5 hours (sleep efficiency of 94%), there are five cycles, in which non-REM sleep accounts for about 6 hours and REM sleep for 1.5 hours of total sleep time.

For sleep to be refreshing, it should be quantitatively adequate and should also progress normally along its various stages without much interruption. However, in the presence of breathing disorders, sleep becomes fragmented. Sleep fragmentation is characterized by excessive electroencephalographic arousals, awakenings, and a shift toward lighter sleep stages. Consequences of sleep fragmentation are lack of refreshing sleep, excessive daytime sleepiness, fatigue, memory lapses, and difficulty concentrating.

Various sleep-related breathing disorders exist. *Apnea* is defined as the absence of inspiratory airflow for 10 seconds or more, recorded by a naso-oral pressure probe and a thermocouple. Apnea has three forms: central (see Figure 32-1), obstructive (Figure 32-2), and mixed. In central apnea, the absence of airflow results from the absence of activation of inspiratory pump muscles, including the diaphragm. It is therefore characterized by simultaneous absence of naso-oral airflow and of thoracoabdominal excursions (see Figure 32-1). In obstructive apnea, in contrast, the inspiratory thoracic pump muscles, such as the diaphragm, are active. The absence of airflow is a result of upper airway occlusion. This is secondary to inward collapse of the relaxed dilator muscles of the oropharynx, which cannot resist the negative intra-airway pressure during inspiration.

On polysomnograms, obstructive apnea is characterized by the absence of naso-oral airflow in spite of continual thoracoabdominal excursions (see Figure 32-2). Mixed apnea has an initial central component followed by an obstructive component.

Hypopnea is a reduction in breathing. It may be defined as reduced naso-oral airflow or thoracoabdominal excursions of 10 seconds or more in duration, resulting in either a drop in arterial oxyhemoglobin saturation of at least 4% or an electroencephalographic arousal (Figure 32-3). Like apnea, hypopnea may be either obstructive or central; however, this distinction is very difficult because these two kinds of hypopnea are frequently not reported separately.

To determine the severity of sleep-related breathing disorders, the apnea-hypopnea index (AHI) is calculated as the number of apneic and hypopneic episodes per hour of sleep. An AHI of 5 or more is considered abnormal and has been used as the criterion for polysomnographic diagnosis.[24] When an obstructive AHI of 5 or more is associated with excessive daytime sleepiness, the combination is referred to as *obstructive sleep apnea (hypopnea) syndrome.*

The number of electroencephalographic arousals per hour of sleep, referred to as an *arousal index,* is used as an indication of sleep fragmentation. The severity of hypoxemia during sleep is usually assessed by the lowest oxyhemoglobin saturation and the time spent below saturation of 90%.

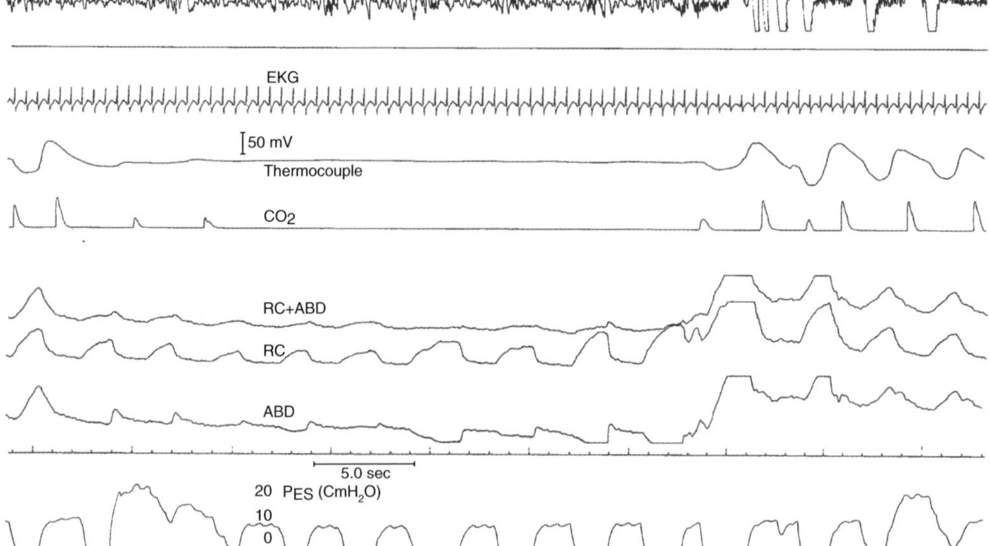

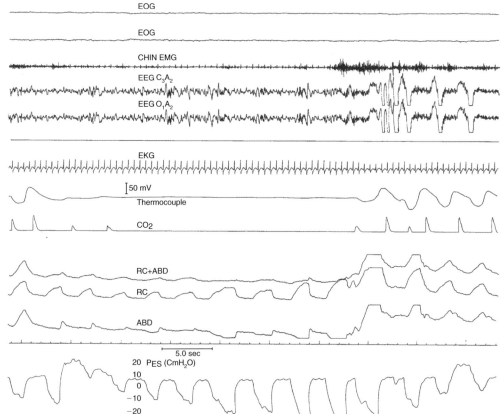

FIGURE 32–2 Polysomnographic example of obstructive sleep apnea in stage 2 sleep. *Top to bottom,* Two electro-oculograms (1st and 2nd tracings), chin electromyogram (3rd tracing), two electroencephalograms (4th and 5th tracings), electrocardiogram (7th tracing), naso-oral airflow measured by thermocouple (8th tracing) and by CO_2 signal (9th tracing), combined rib cage and abdominal excursions (10th tracing), rib cage excursion (11th tracing), abdominal excursion (12th tracing), time in seconds (13th tracing), and esophageal pressure (14th tracing). Note absence of airflow in the presence of effort observed on rib cage, abdominal, and esophageal pressure tracings. Breathing resumes with the onset of arousal (increase in chin electromyographic and electroencephalographic alpha waves) and consequent relief of upper airway occlusion. Also note the paradoxical thoracoabdominal excursions (rib cage and abdominal tracings), which commonly occur with upper airway occlusion. These excursions can be observed visually at the bedside.

Periodic breathing is a pattern of breathing characterized by cyclic fluctuations in the amplitude of tidal volume.[25] It consists of periodically recurring cycles of apnea or hypopnea, or both, followed by hyperpnea. The apnea and hypopnea may be obstructive (i.e., resulting from upper airway occlusion) or central in nature, and both forms may occur in patients with heart failure.[6,9] Hunter-Cheyne-Stokes breathing (see Figure 32-1) is a form of periodic breathing that occurs primarily in systolic heart failure. In contrast to apnea and hypopnea, however, Hunter-Cheyne-Stokes breathing is a subjective description and is not readily quantifiable. For these reasons, the term *central sleep apnea* is preferable, and it also avoids misrepresentation, inasmuch as the credit for the discovery of Hunter-Cheyne-Stokes breathing has not been given to the original discoverers.

EFFECTS OF SLEEP ON CARDIOPULMONARY SYSTEMS

In wakefulness, in comparison with sleep, the balance of autonomic nervous system reverses.[26-28] Normally, during non-REM sleep, as the depth of sleep increases from N1 to N3, sympathetic activity decreases progressively. During phasic REM sleep, however, surges in sympathetic activity occur. These changes in sympathetic nervous system have been best shown by the use of peroneal nerve microneurography to monitor muscle sympathetic nerve activity.[29-31] Intermittent sampling of blood and of lumbar and brain ventricular cerebrospinal fluid have also revealed significant reduction in norepinephrine level during sleep, particularly in delta sleep.[32,33] In addition, and in contrast to a reduction in sympathetic activity, parasympathetic activity increases during sleep.[27,34]

As a result of such changes in autonomic nervous system activity in non-REM sleep, systemic blood pressure, heart rate, and cardiac output decrease.[35-37] In phasic REM sleep, however, blood pressure and pulse rate increase.[29] Because non-REM sleep accounts for about 80% of total sleep time in adults overall, sleep should be a restful period for the cardiovascular system.

With onset of sleep and withdrawal of the nonchemical respiratory drive of wakefulness, minute ventilation decreases and arterial partial pressure of carbon dioxide (P_{CO_2}) rises.[37-40] Furthermore, in the absence of respiratory influences of wakefulness drive, breathing during sleep is primarily under metabolic control, exhibiting extreme sensitivity to small changes in P_{CO_2}.[38-40]

Sleep-induced cardiovascular and respiratory quiescence, however, could become punctuated by periodic breathing. Among the consequences of periodic breathing are arousals. Electroencephalographically, cortical arousals are characterized by return of alpha waves (see Figures 32-1 to 32-3), which are normally observed during relaxed wakefulness. Arousals are associated with transient reinstitution of wakefulness drive, increased sympathetic activity, and decreased

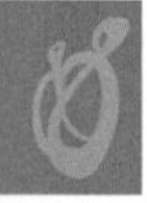

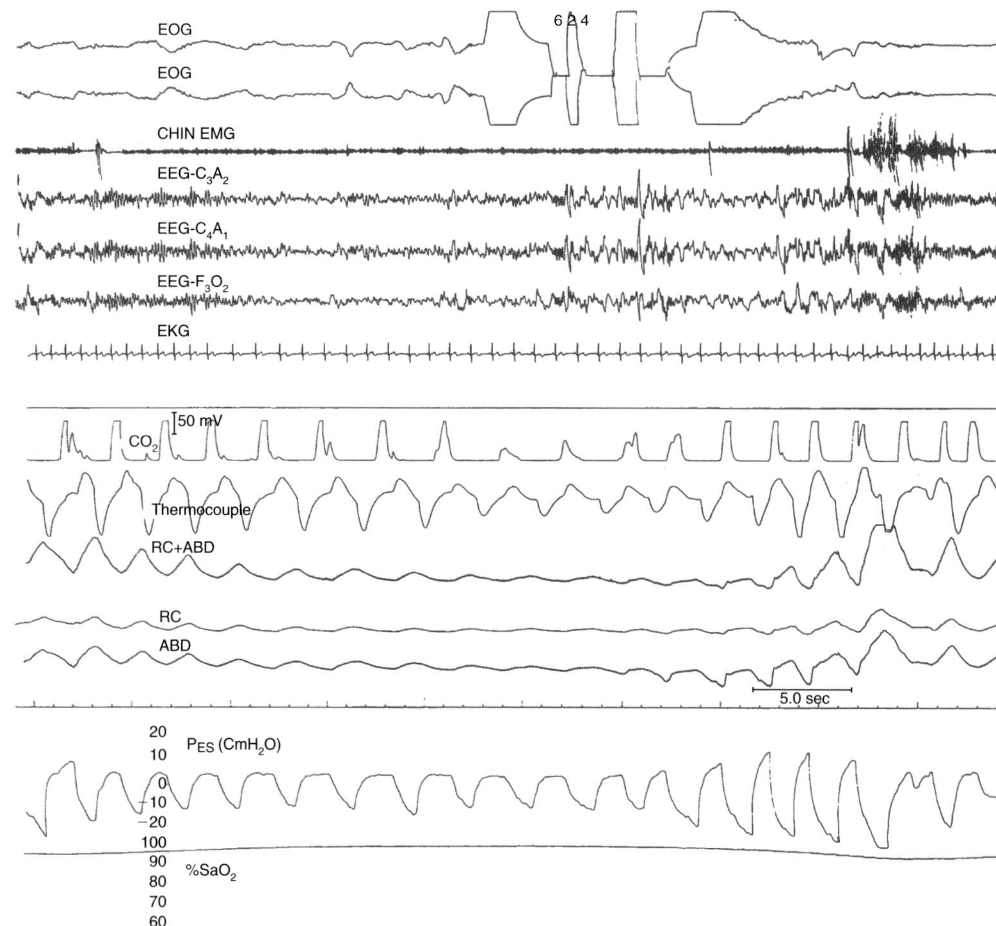

FIGURE 32–3 Polysomnographic example of hypopnea occurring in rapid-eye-movement sleep. *Top to bottom,* Two electro-oculograms (1st and 2nd tracings), chin electromyogram (3rd tracing), three electroencephalogram (4th, 5th, and 6th tracings), electrocardiogram (7th tracing), naso-oral airflow measured by CO_2 signal (9th tracing) and by thermocouple (10th tracing), combined rib cage and abdominal excursions (11th tracing), rib cage excursion (12th tracing), and abdominal excursion (13th tracing), time in seconds (14th tracing), esophageal pressure (15th tracing), and saturation (15th tracing). Note reduction in airflow and in rib cage and abdominal excursions, all of which increase with the arousal (increase in chin electromyographic amplitude, and electroencephalographic speeding with alpha waves).

parasympathetic activity.[41-43] Consequently, heart rate, blood pressure, and ventilation increase, and P_{CO_2} decreases. Therefore, arousals, in addition to disrupting sleep and causing sleep fragmentation, also result in adverse cardiovascular and respiratory consequences.

SLEEP APNEA IN SYSTOLIC HEART FAILURE

Prevalence of sleep-related breathing disorders has been studied in patients with heart failure arising from a variety of causes, although most systematically in heart failure caused by left ventricular systolic dysfunction (see also Chapter 13).

Studies of patients with stable heart failure and left ventricular systolic dysfunction have revealed that half of consecutive patients suffer from sleep apnea defined as an AHI of 15 or more per hour. Table 32-1 depicts prevalence of sleep apnea, both central and obstructive, in a few studies in which full nighttime polysomnography, or at least four respiratory channels, were used.[44-51]

The most detailed systematic prospective study in systolic heart failure[44] involved 100 ambulatory male subjects with stable, treated heart failure. Several aspects of this study must be emphasized. Of 114 consecutive patients who were eligible to take part in the study, 100 accepted. Exclusion criteria were unstable cardiovascular status and presence of comorbid disorders (e.g., chronic obstructive pulmonary disease). Patients were recruited from a cardiology unit and a primary care clinic, and no questions regarding the risk factors for sleep apnea (e.g., snoring, witnessed apnea, waking up tired) were asked. Each patient spent 2 nights in the sleep laboratory, the first night for habituation. Polysomnography with simultaneous Holter monitoring was performed during the second night. According to an AHI of a minimum of 5 or 15 per hour as the threshold 68% and 49%, respectively, of the 100 patients had the sleep disorder. At the time of this study, 10% of the patients were taking β-blockers. However, widespread use of β-blockers has had no effect on prevalence of sleep apnea among patients with heart failure[13-16,19,20] (see Table 32-1). According to studies of 1250 patients from around the world, 52% have an AHI of 15 or more per hour; 31% have CSA and 21% have OSA (Figure 32-4). In most of these studies, 80% to 90% of the patients were taking a β-blocker.

In comparison, in a large population study of subjects aged 30 to 60 years without clinically recognized heart failure,[24] only 9% had an AHI of 15 or more per hour. As noted earlier, an AHI of 5 or more per hour has been used to define presence of significant number of disordered breathing events in obstructive sleep apnea (hypopnea) syndrome.[24] Therefore, because sleep apnea (see Table 32-1) is much more prevalent among patients with heart failure than in the general population, systolic heart failure is a leading risk factor for sleep apnea.

TABLE 32–1 Worldwide Prevalence of Sleep Apnea in Systolic Heart Failure

Country (Year)	No. of Subjects	% of Patients with AHI ≥ 15/Hour	% of Patients Taking β-Blockers
United States (2006)[44]	100	49	10
United States* (2008)[50]	108	61	82
Canada (2007)[45]	287	47	80
United Kingdom (2007)[46]	55	53	78
Germany* (2007)[49]	700	52	85

*Electroencephalography was not recorded.

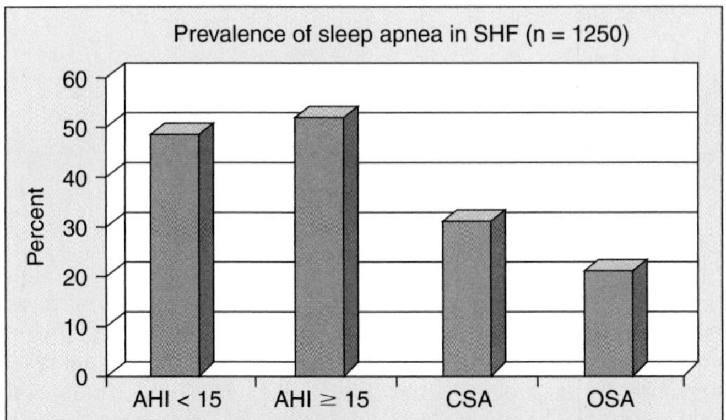

FIGURE 32–4 Prevalence of sleep apnea in systolic heart failure (SHF). The data represent a series of world sleep studies (referenced in Table 13-2). AHI, apnea-hypopnea index; CSA, central sleep apnea; OSA, obstructive sleep apnea. (Adapted from Javahari S. Cardiovascular disorders. In Kryger MH, editor. *Atlas of clinical sleep medicine,* Philadelphia, 2010, Elsevier.)

Phenotype of Heart Failure Patients with Obstructive and Central Sleep Apnea

As noted earlier, both forms of sleep apnea, central and obstructive, commonly occur in the same patient. Depending on the predominant form of sleep apnea, the phenotype of patients varies, and if these specific characteristics are recognized, they should help the clinician to suspect the presence of either OSA or CSA (Figures 32-5 and 32-6).

Obesity and habitual snoring are important risk factors for OSA in patients with heart failure[10,12,44] (see Figure 32-5), as they are in the general population.[24] However, there is no significant difference in subjective excessive daytime sleepiness between patients with heart failure who do and those who do not have either OSA and CSA (see Figure 32-5).[10,44] We believe that this is related partly to the overlapping nocturnal and diurnal symptoms of chronic heart failure with sleep apnea.

Because patients with heart failure and sleep apnea do not report subjective excessive daytime sleepiness, clinical suspicion for its presence remains low. This is particularly the case for patients with heart failure and CSA because such patients are commonly not obese and do not snore much and CSA remains occult.[8] However, the presence of some important risk factors should increase suspicion for CSA: atrial fibrillation, high New York Heart Association class, very low left ventricular ejection fraction, frequent nocturnal arrhythmias, and low arterial P_{CO_2} (see Figure 32-6).[44] There are also some important gender issues, which are addressed in the following section.

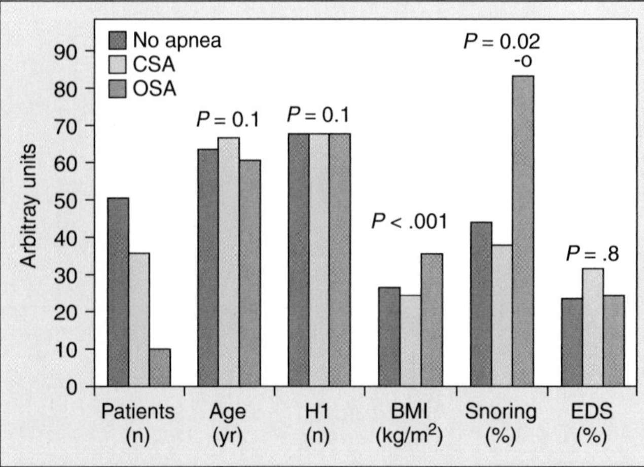

FIGURE 32–5 Demographics, historical data, and physical examination findings in patients who had heart failure without sleep apnea, with central sleep apnea (CSA), and with obstructive sleep apnea (OSA). Patients with obstructive sleep apnea were heavier and had a higher prevalence of habitual snoring than did patients with CSA. There was no difference in prevalence of excessive daytime sleepiness (EDS) between the patients with sleep apnea and the patients without sleep apnea. BMI, body mass index; Ht, height. (Modified from Javaheri S. Sleep disorders in systolic heart failure: A prospective study of 100 male patients. The final report. *Int J Cardiol* 2006;106:21-28; adapted from Javahari S. Cardiovascular disorders. In Kryger MH, editor. *Atlas of clinical sleep medicine,* Philadelphia, 2010, Elsevier.)

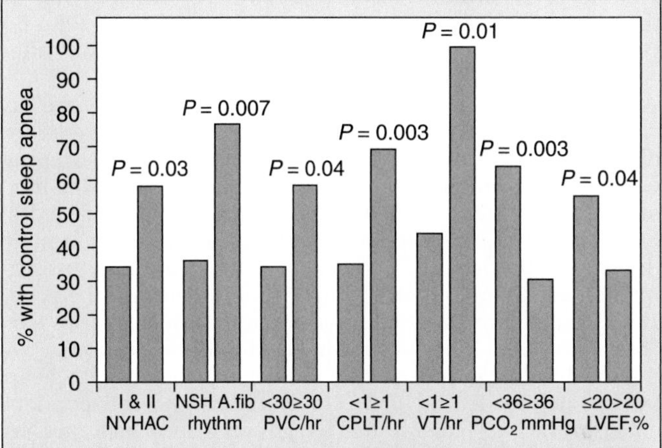

FIGURE 32–6 Clinical and laboratory characteristics that are more likely to be associated with central sleep apnea. A.fib, Atrial fibrillation; CPLT, couplets; LVEF, left ventricular ejection fraction; NSR, normal sinus rhythm; NYHAC, New York Heart Association Class; PVC, premature ventricular contractions; VT, ventricular tachycardia. (Modified from Javaheri S. Sleep disorders in systolic heart failure: A prospective study of 100 male patients. The final report. *Int J Cardiol* 2006;106:21-28; adapted from Javahari S. Cardiovascular disorders. In Kryger MH, editor. *Atlas of clinical sleep medicine,* Philadelphia, 2010, Elsevier.)

Gender and Sleep Apnea in Systolic Heart Failure

In general population, the prevalence of OSA is significantly higher among men than among women.[24] This is probably the case in heart failure as well and for CSA in particular. According to the results of several studies in systolic heart failure,[11-15] 40% of the male subjects have CSA, which is significantly higher than the 18% prevalence of CSA among female subjects (Figure 32-7).

The reasons for a low prevalence of OSA and CSA in women are not well understood, but female hormones may play an important role. The results of population studies of subjects without heart failure[52,53] suggest that menopause may be a risk factor for OSA and that the risk is probably

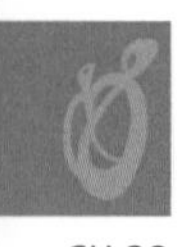

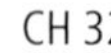

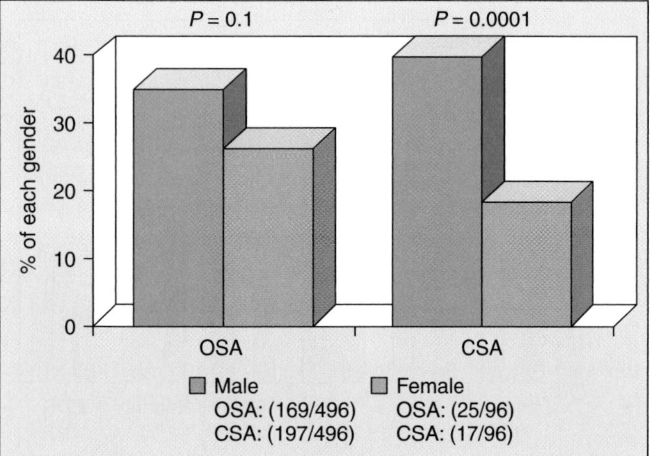

FIGURE 32–7 Prevalence of obstructive sleep apnea (OSA) and central sleep apnea (CSA) in men and women with systolic heart failure. The prevalence of CSA is much lower among women than among men. A similar trend is found in OSA, although it is not statistically significant. (Data from Allen E, Turk JL, Murley R, editors. *The case books of John Hunter FRS*, New York, 1993, Parthenon, pp 29-30; and from Javaheri S, Shukla R, Zeigler H, Wexler L: Central sleep apnea, right ventricular dysfunction, and low diastolic blood pressure are predictors of mortality in systolic heart failure. *J Am Coll Cardiol*, 49:2028-2034, 2007.)

reduced by hormone replacement therapy.[53] In women with systolic heart failure, risk for CSA was six times higher in those aged 60 years or older than in those younger than 60 years.[12] A similar difference exists for OSA before and after age 60 years.[12]

Progesterone is a known respiratory stimulant, and its various effects on respiratory system may in part explain the lower prevalence of CSA and OSA among menstruating women. Progesterone increases ventilation[54] and the tone of the dilator muscles of the upper airway.[55] Furthermore, premenopausal women have a significantly lower apneic threshold—the level of P_{CO_2} below which rhythmic breathing ceases—than do men,[56] which should decrease the probability that a woman would develop apnea during sleep (see "Mechanisms of Sleep Apnea in Heart Failure" section).

However, large prospective studies of women with heart failure are needed in order to elucidate the independent effects of various factors, such as age and menopause, on CSA and OSA. A similar view has been expressed for studies of women without heart failure.[57]

SLEEP APNEA IN ISOLATED DIASTOLIC HEART FAILURE

Depending on age, a considerable number of patients with symptoms of congestive heart failure may suffer from isolated diastolic heart failure with preserved left ventricular ejection fraction (see Chapter 14).

Little is known about prevalence of sleep-related breathing disorders and their effect on isolated diastolic heart failure. Both sleep apnea and diastolic heart failure are prevalent in older populations and the consequences of sleep apnea (such as sympathetic activation, nocturnal and diurnal hypertension, and hypoxemia[58]) impair left ventricular diastolic function and eventually result in remodeling of cardiac chamber. In this regard, the largest study,[59] consisting of 2058 participants in the Sleep Heart Health Study revealed—after accounting for age, gender, ethnicity, smoking, alcohol consumption, body mass index, systolic blood pressure, antihypertensive medication use, diabetes, and prevalent myocardial infarction—that apnea, hypopnea, and hypoxemia indices were independent predictors of left ventricular mass. In another study[60] of 66 consecutive patients with OSA who underwent pulse-wave Doppler echocardiography of the transmitral valve, an abnormal relaxation pattern was present in 38% (25 patients). In multivariate analysis, saturation of less than 70% during sleep was an independent predictor of abnormal relaxation pattern (odds ratio = 4, 95% confidence interval [CI] = 1.2 to 15.3, P = .02, irrespective of age and hypertension status). Meanwhile, effective treatment of OSA has been shown to improve left ventricular function and structure (reverse remodeling).[61,62] In one randomized, double-blind trial of 12 weeks' duration, the placebo condition (sham continuous positive airway pressure [CPAP]) was compared with the use of a CPAP device with minimal pressure; effective CPAP therapy resulted in a significant increase in early/late (E/A) ratio and a significant decrease in isovolumic relaxation and mitral deceleration time.[62] In summary, OSA could be a cause of diastolic dysfunction or contribute to its progression.

MECHANISMS OF SLEEP APNEA IN HEART FAILURE

Central Sleep Apnea

The mechanisms of periodic breathing and CSA in heart failure are complex and multifactorial. Numerous articles on theoretical and experimental aspects of periodic breathing have been published[63-68] and reviewed elsewhere.[69] In heart failure, various components of the negative feedback system that controls breathing undergo alterations that increase the likelihood that periodic breathing will develop. In addition, specific sleep-related mechanisms underlie augmentation of periodic breathing and the genesis of central apnea during sleep.

Negative Feedback Control System and Periodic Breathing

Negative feedback systems are involved in homeostatic control of a number of physiological variables such as blood pressure, temperature, and arterial blood P_{CO_2}, arterial partial pressure of oxygen (P_{O_2}), and arterial hydrogen ion concentration [H^+].

In respiratory system, the rate of breathing and tidal volume are normally regulated so that arterial blood gases are precisely controlled. For example, when a breathing disturbance, such as a short pause in breathing, occurs, the P_{CO_2} increases and the P_{O_2} decreases, and ventilation normally increases appropriately to minimize the effects of the disturbance. However, in the presence of certain conditions such as systolic heart failure, ventilatory overshoot may occur, resulting in ventilatory instability.

The three major components of the negative feedback system involved in homeostatic control of breathing are (1) the chemoreceptors (the controller), (2) the lungs (the plant), and (3) the communication channels between the chemoreceptors and the lungs (the circulating arterial blood from the lungs to the chemoreceptors, and the nerves from the brain to the respiratory muscles).

In systolic heart failure, the structure and function of the various components of this negative feedback system become altered in a way that favors instability in control of breathing, which results in periodic breathing. These alterations include increased arterial circulation time (which delays the transfer of information regarding changes in P_{O_2} and P_{CO_2} from pulmonary capillary blood to the chemoreceptors), enhanced gain of the chemoreceptors (enhanced CO_2/O_2 chemosensitivity, the high responders), and enhanced plant gain (decreased functional residual capacity); collectively, these alterations result in increased loop gain and increase the likelihood of periodic breathing in systolic heart failure.[59-68] Because these alterations are not state (sleep or wake)–specific, periodic breathing may occur both during wakefulness and sleep (although most frequently during sleep).

In systolic heart failure, arterial circulation time is lengthened as a result of increased blood volume in the pulmonary venous system and the left heart chambers; this lengthening is augmented by a low stroke volume.

A breathing pause results in hypoxemia and hypercapnia in pulmonary capillary blood. With a normal circulation time, these reactions are quickly aborted. In the presence of prolonged circulation time, however, it takes a long time for the chemoreceptors to detect the onset of the breathing pause–induced hypoxemia and hypercapnia; consequently, the pause persists without any compensatory ventilatory effort to abort the reactions. In addition, because the pause is prolonged, the chemoreceptors continue to be stimulated by the abnormal blood gas tensions for some time before they receive any feedback information regarding compensatory changes in PO_2 and PCO_2 in the pulmonary capillary blood. Prolonged circulation time, therefore, converts a negative feedback system to a positive one.

The second factor that increases the likelihood that periodic breathing and central apnea will occur is the increased gain of the chemoreceptors.[68] In patients with heart failure who have increased sensitivity to changes in carbon dioxide (or PO_2), the chemoreceptors elicit a large ventilatory response whenever the PCO_2 rises (or PO_2 decreases). The consequent intense hyperventilation, by driving the PCO_2 below the apneic threshold, results in central apnea. As a result of central apnea, PCO_2 rises, and the cycles of hyperventilation and hypoventilation persist.[68]

The third factor that may contribute to the development of periodic breathing in heart failure is decreased functional residual capacity, which causes underdamping. For a given change in ventilation (e.g., a 10-second cessation of breathing), underdamping results in augmented changes in the controlled variables—that is, PO_2 and PCO_2—which in turn elicit pronounced compensatory ventilatory responses. Overcompensation tends to destabilize breathing. In systolic heart failure, functional residual capacity decreases because of pulmonary congestion or edema, pleural effusion, and reduced compliance of the respiratory system.

Specific Sleep Mechanisms and Genesis of Central Sleep Apnea

The Concept of Apneic Threshold. The mechanisms involved in the genesis of CSA relate specifically to the state of sleep and removal of nonchemical drive of wakefulness on breathing. As a result, sleep unmasks the apneic threshold and, in addition, breathing becomes extremely PCO_2-sensitive.[69-71]

As mentioned previously, apneic threshold is defined as the level of PCO_2 below which rhythmic breathing ceases. The difference between two PCO_2 setpoints—the prevailing PCO_2 minus the PCO_2 at the apneic threshold—is a critical factor for occurrence of central apnea. The smaller this difference is, the greater is the likelihood that apnea will occur,[69-71] because it takes only a small rise in ventilation to lower the prevailing PCO_2 toward and below the apneic threshold.

Normally, with onset of sleep, ventilation decreases and PCO_2 increases. As long as the prevailing PCO_2 is above the apneic threshold, rhythmic breathing continues. However, in some patients with heart failure, prevailing PCO_2 does not rise at sleep onset, and CSA occurs because of the proximity of the prevailing PCO_2 to the apneic threshold.[71,72] This could happen because of the lack of normally observed decrease in ventilation at sleep onset; then pulmonary capillary pressure rises, possibly as a result of increased venous return in the supine position. The stiffer the left ventricle is, the higher is the increase in pulmonary capillary pressure. The latter results in increases in respiratory rate and ventilation, which prevent the normally observed rise in PCO_2 at sleep onset.

In summary, during sleep, the unmasking of the apneic threshold, the proximity of the apneic threshold to the prevailing PCO_2, and the extreme sensitivity of breathing to small changes in PCO_2 are critical for the occurrence of CSA.

Obstructive Sleep Apnea

Another profound effect of sleep on breathing relates to the neuromuscular control of upper airway dilator muscles.[73] During wakefulness, these muscles receive adequate stimulation; for example, the genioglossus muscle maintains upper airway patency in the presence of negative inspiratory airway pressure generated by contraction of the diaphragm. However, during sleep, these dilator muscles relax. Consequently, subjects with a narrow upper airway become particularly prone to develop complete occlusion (OSA) or narrowing (obstructive sleep hypopnea) of the airway. The mechanisms underlying OSA and obstructive hypopnea during sleep therefore relate to the neuromuscular control of the upper airway muscles and altered upper airway anatomy. These mechanisms are the same in patients who have OSA without heart failure.

Obesity, which causes narrowing of the upper airway, in part as a result of fat deposition in the throat, is a major risk factor for OSA in general population[24] and in patients with heart failure.[10,12,44] The author and colleagues[8,10,44] conducted studies in which polysomnograms were scored blindly and independently of demographics of the patients with systolic heart failure; obesity was found to be the important risk factor for OSA (see Figure 32-6). Snoring, another manifestation of upper airway narrowing, is also very common among such patients (see Figure 32-6).

Sleep Apnea in Isolated Diastolic Heart Failure. Both CSA and OSA have been observed in patients with diastolic heart failure,[74] although the latter is the most prevalent form of sleep apnea. The pathophysiological processes in diastolic heart failure are related to a stiff, noncompliant left ventricle that cannot fill adequately at normal diastolic pressure. As left ventricular end-diastolic pressure increases, symptoms of pulmonary congestion and edema develop. Pulmonary congestion is associated with narrowing of the PCO_2 reserve (the difference between the prevailing PCO_2 and the PCO_2 at the apneic threshold), which increases the likelihood that sleep apnea will develop.[75] Meanwhile, OSA is common in obesity, systemic hypertension, and aging, which are conditions also associated with left ventricular dysfunction.

PATHOLOGICAL CONSEQUENCES OF SLEEP APNEA IN HEART FAILURE

There are three immediate adverse consequences of sleep apnea (see Figures 32-1 and 32-2): (1) arterial blood gas abnormalities, (2) arousals, and (3) large negative swings in intrathoracic pressure. These conditions adversely affect various cardiovascular functions and structure[76-81] (Figure 32-8) and are most detrimental in the presence of established left ventricular systolic and diastolic dysfunction and coronary artery disease.

Arterial Blood Gas Abnormalities and Their Consequences

Periodic breathing is characterized by episodes of apnea and hypopnea, which cause hypoxemia and hypercapnia, and episodes of hyperpnea, which results in reoxygenation and hypocapnia.

Hypoxemia may decrease myocardial oxygen delivery, increase sympathetic nervous system activity, and causes pulmonary arteriolar vasoconstriction. In addition, hypoxia and reoxygenation promote endothelial cell dysfunction.

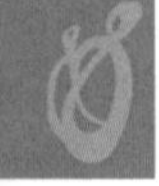

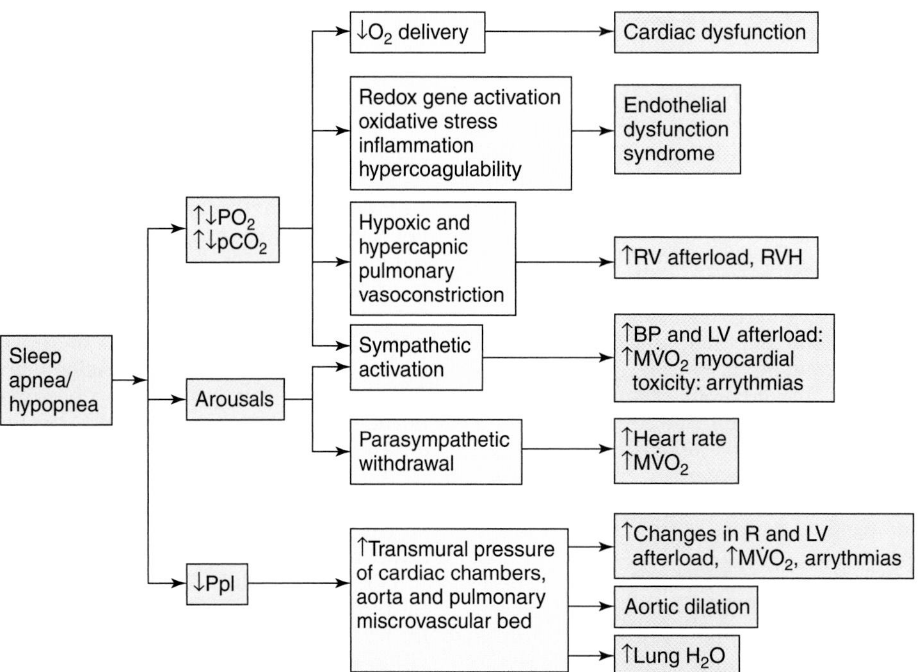

FIGURE 32–8 The consequences of recurrent sleep apnea and hypopnea include hypoxemia and reoxygenation in association with hypercapnia and hypocapnia, respectively, during apnea, followed by hyperpnea. The other consequences are arousals and negative swings in intrathoracic pressure. These consequences, in conjunction, could eventually result in significant cardiovascular dysfunction. Hypoxemia may result in diminished oxygen delivery to the myocardium, which in turn could result in arrhythmias and systolic and diastolic dysfunction. Hypoxemia and reoxygenation could result in activation of redox-sensitive genes, oxidative stress inflammation, and hypercoagulability, leading to endothelial dysfunction syndrome. Both alveolar hypoxia and hypercapnia (as a result of sleep apnea or hypopnea) result in hypoxic and hypercapnic pulmonary vasoconstriction that increases right ventricular (RV) afterload and its myocardial oxygen consumption. This eventually could result in right ventricular hypertrophy (RVH) and cor pulmonale. Hypoxemia and hypercapnia, along with arousals, could also lead to sympathetic activation that would increase blood pressure (BP). This would result in increased left ventricular (LV) afterload, increased myocardial oxygen consumption ($M\dot{V}O_2$), and arrhythmias. In addition, this increase in sympathetic activation and release of myocardial norepinephrine could result in myocardial toxicity and apoptosis. Arousals also result in parasympathetic withdrawal, which increases the heart rate and myocardial oxygen consumption. Negative swings in intrathoracic pressure increase the transmural pressure of the left and right ventricles, both of which increase the wall tension of the ventricles, leading to an increase in myocardial oxygen consumption. In addition, increasing the transmural pressure also affects the aorta and predisposes to aortic dilation and potentially dissection. Furthermore, increased pleural pressure of the atria predisposes to development of atrial fibrillation. Finally, negative interstitial pressure increases transcapillary fluid flow, facilitating the development of pulmonary edema. Overall, therefore, the consequences of sleep apnea and hypopnea in conjunction could result in cardiovascular dysfunction. Ppl, pleural (intrathoracic) pressure. (Adapted from Javahari S. Cardiovascular disorders. In Kryger MH, editor. *Atlas of clinical sleep medicine,* Philadelphia, 2010, Elsevier.)

Direct Effects of Hypoxia on Myocardium

Decreased myocardial oxygen delivery may result in an imbalance between myocardial oxygen consumption and demand and hence in myocardial hypoxia, particularly if coronary artery disease is already present. Potential clinical consequences include nocturnal angina, myocardial infarction, arrhythmias, and sudden cardiac death during sleep. Hypoxia may also impair myocardial contractility[82-86] and diastolic function.[58]

Hypoxia and Reoxygenation, Reactive Oxygen Species, Oxidative Stress, Inflammation, and Endothelial Dysfunction

A number of human and animal studies, coupled with laboratory studies of cell culture, have demonstrated the pivotal role of hypoxia-reoxygenation, which, through production of reactive oxygen species, results in oxidative stress, diminished availability of nitric oxide, and increased expression of number of redox-sensitive genes; this last result occurs through activation of certain transcription factors such as hypoxia-inducible factor-1α (HIF-1α) and nuclear factor κB (NF κB).[80,87-92] HIF-1α encodes production of endothelin-1 (the most potent vasoconstrictor with proinflammatory properties), vascular endothelial growth factor, and platelet-derived growth factor. Activation of NF κB which plays a pivotal role in production of inflammatory cytokines (such as tumor necrosis factor α and interleukin-6), enhancing expression of adhesion molecules, promoting leukocyte rolling, and endothelial adherence,[93-95] all of which lead to atherosclerosis.[96] Hypoxia and reoxygenation impairs endothelial function and induces endothelial and myocyte apoptosis.[97-100]

Hypoxia and Pulmonary Arteriolar Vasoconstriction

Alveolar hypoxia (partly through release of endothelin[101]) and hypercapnia cause pulmonary arteriolar vasoconstriction and hypertension, which could adversely affect right ventricular function. In particular, OSA is a known cause of pulmonary hypertension[102] and cor pulmonale (pickwickian syndrome).

Hypocapnia

Episodes of hyperpnea after apnea and hypopnea result in hypocapnia. Hypocapnia (arterial $P_{CO_2} \leq 35$ mm Hg) may impair myocardial oxygen delivery and uptake by causing coronary artery vasoconstriction[103] and shifting the oxygen-hemoglobin dissociation curve to the left. Hypocapnia may also be a cause of arrhythmias. Among hypocapnic subjects with systolic heart failure, the prevalence of CSA and arrhythmias is high.[104]

Arousals

Disordered breathing events are frequently followed by arousals, which are associated with increased sympathetic activity and decreased parasympathetic activity.[41-43] Consequently, there is a transient rise in blood pressure and heart rate with associated adverse cardiovascular consequences.

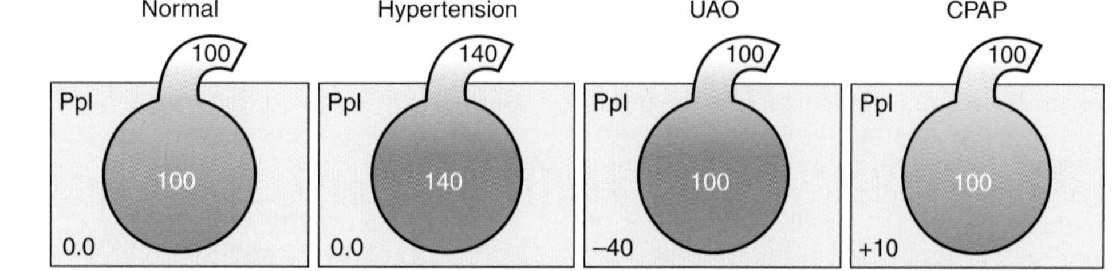

FIGURE 32–9 Transmural (Tm) pressure (Pr) of left ventricle (LV) during systole. As a result of obstructive apnea caused by upper airway occlusion (UAO), a negative pleural pressure (Ppl) of −40 mm Hg is generated. This increases left ventricular transmural pressure from 100 to 140 mm Hg, which is equivalent to an increase in systolic aortic blood pressure from 100 to 140 mm Hg. Note the reduction in left ventricular transmural pressure with application of nasal continuous positive airway pressure (CPAP).

In addition, arousals result in sleep fragmentation, lack of refreshing sleep, daytime fatigue, lack of concentration, and sleepiness.

Exaggerated Negative Intrathoracic Pressure and Its Consequences

Negative intrathoracic pressures as high as 60 to 80 cm H_2O may be generated during episodes of obstructive apnea. After central apnea, hyperpnea occurs, and relatively large negative pressure deflections, particularly in the presence of stiff lungs and chest wall, may also be observed. However, pleural pressure changes are generally more pronounced in OSA than in CSA (see Figures 32-1 and 32-2). The increased negative pressure increases the transmural pressure (pressure inside minus pressure outside) of the intrathoracic vascular structures, including the aorta, pulmonary vascular bed, atria, and ventricles (Figure 32-9).

Numerous studies have addressed the cardiovascular consequences of both negative and positive pressure deflections affecting right and left ventricular function.[105-108] According to the Laplace law, increased transmural myocardial pressure increases wall tension and myocardial oxygen consumption. Atria, because they are more compliant than ventricles, are subject to stretch, which could result in atrial arrhythmias, such as atrial fibrillation observed with sleep apnea. Negative intrathoracic pressure surrounding intrathoracic aorta could contribute to aortic dilation. Negative intrathoracic pressure is also reflected in the perivascular space, decreasing the perivascular pressure. This increases extravascular lung water by favoring fluid transudation across pulmonary microvascular bed and by diminishing lymph outflow from the lungs.[109] Sleep apnea may therefore contribute to excess lung water and pulmonary edema in congestive heart failure (see Figure 32-5).

SLEEP APNEA AUGMENTS THE HYPERADRENERGIC STATE OF HEART FAILURE

During normal sleep, in comparison with wakefulness, the balance of activity of the sympathetic and parasympathetic nervous systems reverses. However, CSA and OSA increase sympathetic activity, as measured by microneurography blood and urinary norepinephrine levels.[110-116] Effective treatment of OSA and CSA with positive airway pressure devices decreases sympathetic activity.[112,114-117] Similarly, treatment of CSA with nasal oxygen decreases sympathetic activity, as measured by urinary norepinephrine level.[118] These findings have important implications because in heart failure, increased sympathetic activity is associated with poor survival rate.

Sleep apnea causes sympathetic activity to increase for several reasons. These include hypoxemia and hypercapnia, arousals, and apnea itself.

In heart failure with left ventricular systolic dysfunction, sympathetic activity is increased as a result of blunting of baroreceptor activity. Blood gas abnormalities associated with sleep apnea augment sympathetic activity through stimulation of chemosensitive carotid bodies,[119-121] which are upregulated in heart failure. In contrast to the inhibitory function of the baroreceptors, increased carotid body activity augments sympathetic outflow by the central nervous system.

Lack of lung inflation (apnea) and arousals are also associated with increased central sympathetic outflow and, along with altered blood gases, collectively contribute and augment the hyperadrenergic state of heart failure.

Sympathetic activation has multiple adverse cardiac consequences, particularly in the setting of left ventricular dysfunction and coronary artery disease. These include increased systemic vascular resistance and left ventricular afterload, venoconstriction with increased right ventricular load, increased myocardial contractility, tachycardia, and arrhythmias (see also Chapter 10). Furthermore, increased myocardial norepinephrine levels cause myocyte toxicity through calcium overload mediated by cyclic adenosine monophosphate[122] and myocyte apoptosis mediated by protein kinase A.[123] These two toxic effects of norepinephrine are prevented by β-adrenergic blockade.[122,123]

β-Blockers have been used successfully to minimize long-term sympathetic activation in systolic heart failure. The improvement by β-blockers in survival among patients with heart failure may result in part from counterbalancing the sympathetic activity caused by sleep-related breathing disorders. Furthermore, by improving cardiac function, β-blockers may further improve sleep-related breathing disorders; however, any residual breathing disorders result in failure of maximal sympathetic deactivation, particularly during sleep.

In summary, pathophysiological consequences of sleep apnea in heart failure result in a hyperadrenergic state superimposed on an already overactive sympathetic nervous system. Sleep apnea is also associated with oxidative stress, increased levels of inflammatory cytokines, and endothelial dysfunction. The interaction between sleep apnea and heart failure could result in a vicious cycle, increasing mortality among patients with heart failure, which is discussed next.

PROGNOSTIC SIGNIFICANCE OF SLEEP APNEA IN HEART FAILURE

Systolic heart failure is a complex disorder in which multiple pathophysiological processes are involved in and contribute to its progression. In the contemporary management of systolic heart failure, the identification and treatment of neurohormones and the use of angiotensin-converting enzyme inhibitors and β-blockers have improved patients' quality of life and survival. In spite of the many therapeutic triumphs, however, heart failure remains a major public health problem with considerable morbidity and mortality. Of utmost importance are the identification and treatment of residual comorbid factors that contribute to the progression of heart failure. One comorbid condition is sleep apnea; results of studies, reviewed in the following discussion, strongly suggest that both OSA and CSA are associated with excess mortality in patients with heart failure and that effective treatment improves survival.

Many observational studies of subjects who have OSA with or without known heart disease strongly suggest that this disorder is associated with increased mortality. In studies of OSA without known heart failure,[124-143] the most systematic is the Wisconsin Sleep Cohort population study,[130] in which 1522 subjects (not patients or individuals referred to a sleep laboratory) were monitored for up to 18 years. Severe OSA (defined as AHI ≥ 30 per hour of sleep) was associated with increased risk of all-cause mortality independently of age, gender, body mass index, and other potential confounders ($P < .0008$). After excluding the 120 persons who reported using CPAP, the researchers found that the hazard ratios were 3.8 (95% CI = 1.6 to 9.0) for all-cause mortality and 5.2 (95% CI = 1.4 to 19.2) for cardiovascular mortality. Similarly, in the Busselton Health Study,[131] the adjusted hazard ratio for all cause mortality was 6.2 (95% CI = 2 to 19) in moderate to severe OSA.

Yaggi and associates[137] monitored 1022 patients for a median of about 3 years. Subjects were referred for evaluation of OSA. They were aged 50 years or older (mean = 61 years), and 68% had an AHI of 5 or more per hour (mean = 35). After adjustment for age, gender, smoking, body mass index, and a number of cardiovascular risk factors(hypertension, diabetes, and hyperlipidemia), OSA was associated with a significantly increased risk for a composite endpoint of death and stroke (hazard ratio = 1.97, 95% CI = 1.12 to 3.38, $P = .01$). In patients with severe OSA (AHI ≥ 36/hour), the hazard ratio was increased to 3.3 for the composite endpoint. Similar results were reported in a study from Israel[135]; according to a Cox proportional analysis in which only AHI and body mass index were used, severe sleep apnea (AHI > 30/hour) was associated with a significantly increased risk for all-cause mortality (hazard ratio = 2.13, 95% CI = 1.36 to 2.34).

The prospective Sleep Heart Health Study,[139] in which 6441 men and women were monitored for an average of 8.2 years, revealed that severe OSA was associated with a statistically significant increased risk of death primarily in men aged 40 to 70 years (adjusted hazard ratio = 2.1, 95% CI = 1.3 to 3.30). It should be emphasized that in this cohort, 52% had hypertension and 18% had another cardiovascular disease at the time of baseline measurement. Marin and associates[136] monitored 1651 Spanish patients (mean follow-up period, 10.1 years) and reported that severe OSA (AHI ≥ 30/hour) was associated with a statistically significant increased risk of cardiovascular death (odds ratio = 2.87, 95% CI = 1.17 to 7.51). Meanwhile, the circadian pattern of death differs between patients with OSA and those without OSA: OSA patients die mostly at night.[139]

The studies just described were all correlational. However, the notion that OSA is a cause of mortality is supported by several observational studies in which researchers reported improved survival in CPAP-adherent patients with OSA, in comparison with those who were nonadherent.[136,138,142] In Marin and associates' study,[136] the odds ratio of cardiovascular mortality for severe OSA in CPAP-treated patients was 1.05 (95% CI = 0.39 to 2.21), in comparison with 2.87 in patients with similarly severe but untreated OSA. In Campos-Rodriguez and colleagues' study,[143] the 5-year cumulative survival rates were significantly lower (85.5%) in patients who did not use CPAP (adherence < 1 hour) than in those who were adherent (>6 hours; 96.4%). Another study, from Germany,[138] revealed that treatment of mild to moderate OSA with CPAP was associated with a cardiovascular risk reduction of 64%.

With regard to heart failure, several studies[18,45,144-156] focused on mortality associated with sleep apnea, both OSA and CSA. With regard to OSA,[45,144] a prospective study[45] revealed that the death rate among 37 patients who had untreated heart failure with OSA was significantly higher than among the 113 patients without (or with mild) OSA. The death rate was significant after confounding factors were controlled. Furthermore, the authors reported no deaths among the 14 patients with heart failure and OSA who were treated with CPAP devices. However, the number of subjects was small, and this difference was significant at $P = .07$. In a larger study in Japan[144] of 65 patients with moderate to severe OSA, use of a CPAP device was associated with significant reduction in the rate of hospitalization and mortality in comparison with 23 untreated OSA patients with systolic heart failure. The rate of survival was improved only in CPAP-adherent patients (Figure 32-10). The finding in patients with OSA and heart failure that CPAP adherence improves survival is similar to that in patients with OSA but without heart failure cited earlier (see "Obstructive Sleep Apnea" section under "Mechanisms of Sleep Apnea in Heart Failure" section). A similar observation was reported in patients with systemic hypertension; improvement was noted primarily in those who were CPAP adherent[157] (for reviews, see Becker and Javaheri[158]).

Multiple investigators have studied CSA and mortality; most[145-154] showed that CSA is associated with excess mortality among patients with systolic heart failure. Two studies[156,157] yielded different results; one[156] revealed a tendency for excess mortality among patients with heart failure and CSA, but this finding was not significant, probably because

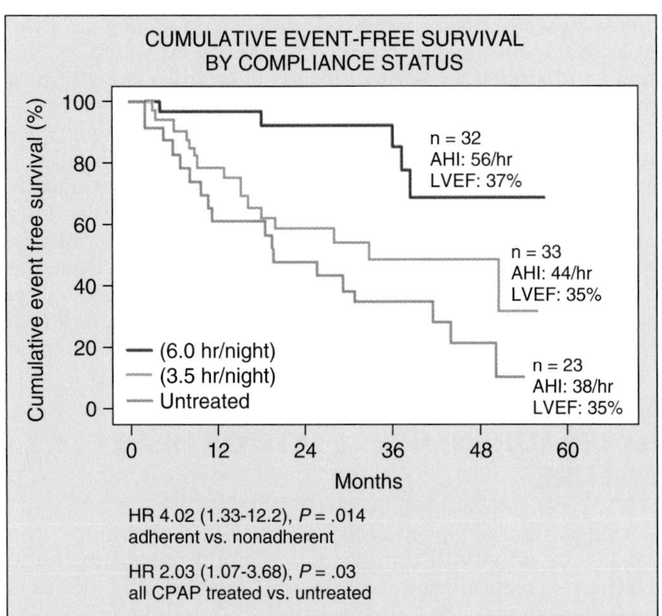

FIGURE 32-10 Probability of hospitalization and mortality in patients with heart failure and obstructive sleep apnea. This probability decreases if patients are treated with continuous positive airway pressure (CPAP) and adhere to therapy. AHI, apnea-hypopnea index; HR, hazard ratio; LVEF, left ventricular ejection fraction. (Modified from Oldenburg O, Lamp B, Faber L, et al. Sleep-disordered breathing in patients with symptomatic heart failure: a contemporary study of prevalence in and characteristics of 700 patients. *Eur J Heart Fail* 2007;9:251; and from Javahari S. Cardiovascular disorders. In Kryger MH, editor. *Atlas of clinical sleep medicine,* Philadelphia, 2010, Elsevier.)

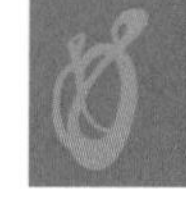

of the small number of patients. In addition, patients with heart failure who exhibited periodic breathing while awake suffered excess mortality.

The author and colleagues[153] monitored 88 patients with heart failure, of whom 56 had CSA (mean AHI = 35/hour) and 32 did not (mean AHI = 2/hour). The median follow-up time was 51 months. After controlling for 24 confounding variables, the investigators found that CSA was associated with excess mortality (hazard ratio = 2.14, $P = .02$). The average length of survival among patients who had heart failure but not CSA was 90 months, in comparison with 45 months among those with CSA (Figure 32-11). The hypothesis that CSA contributes to excess mortality among patients with systolic heart failure is supported by the observation that effective treatment of CSA with CPAP devices improves survival.[152]

INDICATIONS FOR POLYSOMNOGRAPHY IN HEART FAILURE

The following sections discuss a number of clinical and laboratory findings that, when present in patients with heart failure, should increase clinical suspicion for sleep apnea and prompt the physician to perform a diagnostic sleep study.

Risk Factors for Obstructive Sleep Apnea

Indications to perform a sleep study for evaluation of OSA in patients without heart failure are equally applicable to patients with heart failure. The protean manifestations and risk factors of OSA in general population include obesity, habitual snoring, witnessed apnea, waking up unrested, excessive daytime sleepiness, and hypertension. However, subjective excessive daytime sleepiness may be absent in patients with heart failure and OSA (see Figure 32-5).

Nocturnal Angina

Both in general population and in patients with heart failure, with or without known coronary artery disease, nocturnal angina should increase suspicion of sleep apnea.

Paroxysmal Nocturnal Dyspnea

This symptom may actually be perception of shortness of breath that occurs during the hyperpneic phase of periodic breathing.

Restless Sleep

This complaint may reflect periodic arousals and movements following episodes of apnea and hypopnea.

Low Arterial Partial Pressure of Carbon Dioxide

Several studies[10,13,44,159,160] have shown that among patients with heart failure and low arterial P_{CO_2}, the prevalence of CSA is high. The predictive value of low P_{CO_2} (≤35 mm Hg) is about 80%.[103] However, many patients with heart failure have CSA without daytime hypocapnia.[161]

Atrioventricular Arrhythmias

Several studies have shown that among patients with heart failure and sleep apnea, the prevalence of atrial fibrillation[10,12,44,162] and ventricular arrhythmias[10,33,163,164] is higher. Presence of these arrhythmias should increase suspicion of the presence of CSA.

Progressive Left Ventricular Systolic or Diastolic Dysfunction

Patients with heart failure and progressive ventricular dysfunction or those whose status remains New York Heart Association class III or IV in spite of intensive medical therapy should undergo a diagnostic sleep study.

Pacemaker and Cardioverter Defibrillator

In a European multicenter study[165] of a large number of patients who had received a pacemaker (for sinus node dysfunction, atrioventricular block, or congestive heart failure), 50% were found to have sleep apnea. The results of this study confirmed those of an earlier study[19] showing that 40% of patients with heart failure who received a cardioverter

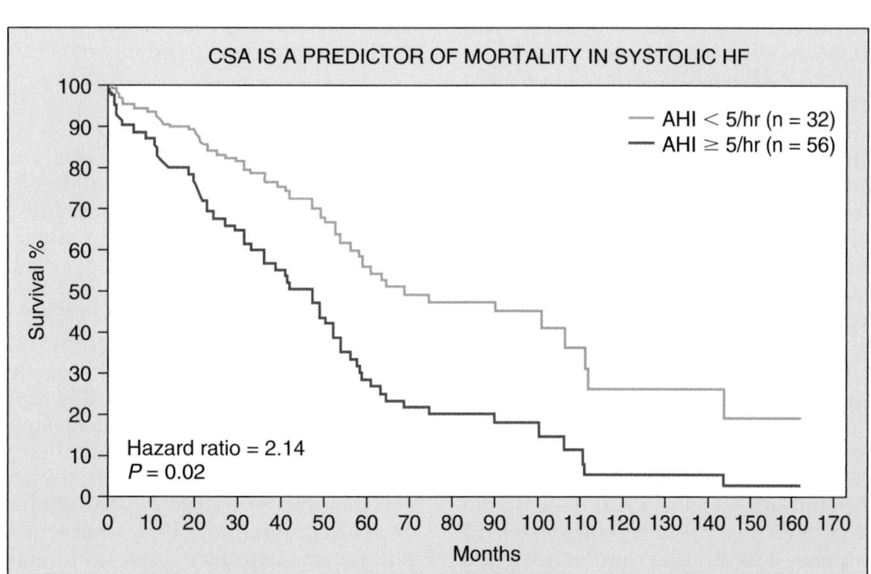

FIGURE 32–11 Probability of survival in patients with systolic heart failure (HF) according to the presence or absence of central sleep apnea (CSA). AHI, apnea-hypopnea index. (Modified from Javaheri S, Shukla R, Zeigler H, et al. Central sleep apnea, right ventricular dysfunction, and low diastolic blood pressure are predictors of mortality in systolic heart failure. *J Am Coll Cardiol* 2007;49:2028; and from Javahari S. Cardiovascular disorders. In Kryger MH, editor. *Atlas of clinical sleep medicine,* Philadelphia, 2010, Elsevier.)

defibrillator had sleep apnea and that the rate of mortality was highest in those with CSA. The author and colleagues suggest that patients with implanted pacemakers undergo polysomnography for diagnosis of sleep-related breathing disorders and appropriate therapy.

Awaiting Cardiac Transplantation

Prevalence of sleep apnea is high among patients awaiting cardiac transplantation, inasmuch as they suffer from severe left ventricular dysfunction.[15] The waiting period for transplantation is long, and a large number of patients die from consequences of heart failure while waiting. Appropriate therapy for sleep apnea could improve survival of these patients and thereby increase their chance of living long enough to undergo cardiac transplantation.

TABLE 32–2	Treatment of Obstructive Sleep Apnea in Heart Failure
Improvement in cardiac function	
Promotion of sleep hygiene	
Cessation of smoking	
Weight reduction when applicable	
Avoidance of alcoholic beverages, narcotics, benzodiazepines, and sildenafil at bedtime	
Treatment of nasal congestion	
Positive airway pressure devices (CPAP, bilevel, PSSV)	
Mandibular advancement devices	
Upper airway procedures	
Nocturnal use of supplemental oxygen	

CPAP, continuous positive airway pressure; PSSV, pressure support servo-ventilation.

TREATMENT OF SLEEP APNEA IN HEART FAILURE

Obstructive Sleep Apnea

Treatment options for OSA in heart failure (Table 32-2) are similar to those in the absence of heart failure. The treatment of choice is CPAP, which has been shown to improve cardiovascular function and survival. Meanwhile, improvement in sleep hygiene and avoidance of both alcoholic beverages and benzodiazepines (both of which may result in relaxation of the muscles of the upper airway) are also recommended. Single-dose administration of sildenafil has also been shown to worsen OSA, and associated desaturation,[166] presumably by vasodilation of the vascular bed in the upper airway, compromising the surface area. We also recommend avoiding use of this and related medications before sleep.

Weight Loss

Obesity is the major risk factor for OSA, and both obesity and OSA are associated with heart failure. Both obesity[167] and OSA are also associated with increased mortality, primarily from cardiovascular causes. The author and colleagues therefore recommend weight loss for obese patients with heart failure.

Noninvasive Positive Airway Pressure Devices

These devices consist of a nasal (or naso-oral) mask that, through a piece of tubing, is connected to an electrically driven blower that provides an adjustable amount of positive pressure to the airway. Application of the device increases the transmural pressure of the upper airway, preventing closure (pneumatic splint). Online heated humidification is added to prevent upper airway dryness.

There are several forms of these devices. Nasal CPAP devices are programmed to deliver a constant inspiratory and expiratory pressure. For subjects who feel expiratory pressure is excessive, bilevel pressure devices, in which expiratory pressure is set at a lower level than the inspiratory pressure, may be used. There are also devices that provide an expiratory pressure that is lower than inspiratory pressure and variable inspiratory pressure (pressure support servo-ventilation).

The level of pressure necessary to maintain upper airway patency may vary from 5 to 20 cm H_2O and is determined in a sleep titration study. With the subject asleep and wearing the mask, the pressure of the device is gradually increased till obstructive apnea, hypopnea, desaturation, and snoring are eliminated. The device is set at that pressure, and it is recommended for use any time the subject sleeps, including naps.

These devices have been successfully used to treat OSA both in general population and in patients with heart failure.[168-171] Overnight application of nasal CPAP resulted in significant improvement in disordered breathing and arterial oxyhemoglobin desaturation.[168] In four randomized trials,[169-172] all of which included a control group, patients with heart failure and OSA were studied; in three trials,[169-171] long-term use of CPAP improved left ventricular ejection fraction. In the fourth study,[172] ejection fraction did not increase, but compliance with CPAP was less than in the other studies. As noted previously, long-term use of CPAP has been shown to improve survival of patients with heart failure and OSA who use it adequately (see Figure 32-10). For patients who do not comply with CPAP use because of complaints of high expiratory pressure, bilevel mechanical devices are recommended.

Other Therapeutic Modalities

Many other modalities, including oral appliances (which advance the mandible to prevent upper airway closure), upper airway surgery (to remove excess pharyngeal soft tissue such as tonsils and the uvula), and nocturnal nasal oxygen (to prevent or minimize desaturation during sleep), are available. However, no long-term systematic studies have been performed. In patients with heart failure, every attempt should be made to treat OSA with positive airway pressure devices, which are invariably effective.

Central Sleep Apnea

In contrast to OSA, which is easily treated with CPAP, CSA is generally difficult to treat, and response to any given therapy (CPAP, medications) is variable: Some patients respond and some do not. Figure 32-7 depicts the author's current approach to treatment of this disorder in heart failure.

Optimization of Cardiopulmonary Function

Optimal therapy for heart failure with diuretics, angiotensin-converting enzyme inhibitors, β-blockers, and cardiac resynchronization therapy (CRT) may improve or eliminate periodic breathing by several mechanisms (for reviews, see Javaheri[173,174] and De Backer and Javaheri[175]). These mechanisms include improved arterial circulation time (as stroke volume increases and cardiopulmonary blood volume decreases), increased P_{CO_2} reserve (resulting from decreased pulmonary capillary pressure), and increased functional residual capacity (caused by decrease in cardiac size, pleural effusion, and intravascular and extravascular lung water). β-Blockers, by increasing stroke volume and decreasing pulmonary capillary pressure, should be particularly helpful

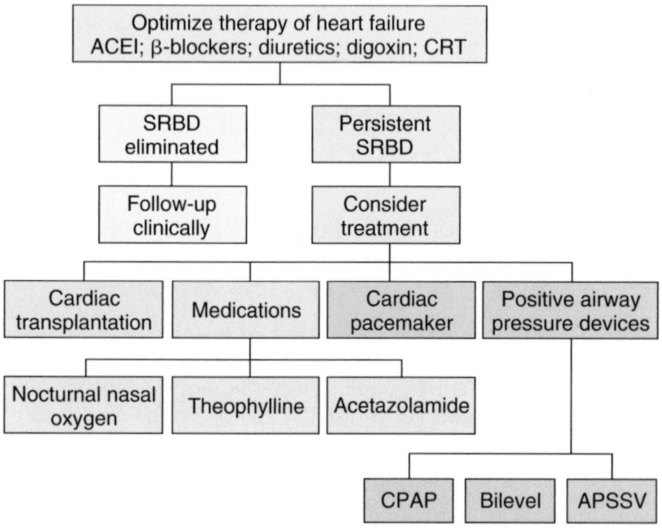

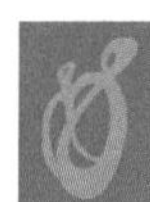

Optimize therapy of heart failure
ACEI; β-blockers; diuretics; digoxin; CRT
SRBD eliminated
Persistent SRBD
Follow-up clinically
Consider treatment
Cardiac transplantation
Medications
Cardiac pacemaker
Positive airway pressure devices
Nocturnal nasal oxygen
Theophylline
Acetazolamide
CPAP
Bilevel
APSSV

FIGURE 32–12 Treatment of central sleep apnea in heart failure. ACEI, angiotensin-converting enzyme inhibitor; APSSV, adaptive pressure support servo-ventilation; CPAP, continuous positive airway pressure; CRT, cardiac resynchronization therapy; SRBD, sleep-related breathing disorder. (Adapted from De Backer W, Javaheri S. Treatment of sleep apnea in heart failure. *Sleep Med Clin* 2007;2:63-638.)

in improving periodic breathing in systolic heart failure. An additional beneficial effect of β-blockers may relate to their counterbalancing of nocturnal sympathetic hyperactivity by decreasing repetitive arousals and desaturation. One particular side effect of β-blockers, however, relates to their effect on melatonin. Melatonin, a sleep-promoting chemical, is secreted through the cyclic adenosine monophosphate–mediated β-receptor signal transduction system, and most β-blockers have been shown to decrease melatonin secretion.[176,177] One of the exceptions is carvedilol.

Several studies have shown that CRT, by improving hemodynamics, improves CSA.[178-181] In one study 77 patients with heart failure who were eligible for CRT were studied before CRT and, on average, 5 months after CRT.[180] In patients with CSA, AHI decreased from 31/hour to 17/hour ($P < .001$). Improvement in CSA occurred only in patients whose hemodynamics improved with CRT. CRT is generally ineffective in OSA.

Atrial overdrive pacing may improve sleep apnea by the same mechanism as CRT but to a lesser extent.

After optimization of cardiopulmonary function, if periodic breathing persists, several approaches are possible (Figure 32-12).

Cardiac Transplantation (see also Chapter 54)

After cardiac transplantation,[182-186] CSA is generally eliminated. This observation, along with human studies (reviewed previously) and animal studies,[66] indicate that heart failure is the cause of CSA. Unfortunately, however, OSA may develop a few months after transplantation.[182-186] In the largest study,[186] in which 45 patients underwent polysomnography a few months after cardiac transplantation, 36% had developed moderate to severe OSA, with an AHI of 15 or more per hour. This group of patients, in comparison with those who had no or mild OSA, had gained the most weight after transplantation. OSA was associated with systemic hypertension and poor quality of life. Because of steroid use and improved quality of life, weight gain is common in transplant recipients, and obesity is the major risk factor for OSA. It is therefore important that cardiac transplant recipients be monitored for weight gain and development of OSA.

Oxygen

As early as 1908, Pembrey[186] demonstrated that administration of oxygen resulted in improvement in periodic breathing in a few patients with congestive heart failure. Several systematic studies of subjects with systolic heart failure[187-194] have shown that supplemental nasal oxygen administered during sleep ameliorates CSA. Oxygen administration may also decrease arousals and light sleep. In addition, randomized, placebo-controlled, double-blind studies have revealed that short-term (1- to 4-week) administration of supplemental nocturnal oxygen improved maximum exercise capacity[191] and decreased overnight excretion of urinary norepinephrine.[192] The latter finding may be a better indicator of the overall sympathetic activity than serum norepinephrine spot sampling. In addition, investigators in three randomized clinical trials[193-195] (9, 12, and 52 weeks in duration) reported that nocturnal oxygen therapy significantly improved CSA, desaturation, left ventricular ejection fraction, and quality of life in patients with systolic heart failure. In the two longest studies, left ventricular ejection fraction increased by 5% to 6% in oxygen-treated subjects but did not change significantly in the control subjects.

Mechanisms of therapeutic effect of nasal oxygen on CSA are complex[196] and may include increasing the difference between the prevailing P_{CO_2} and the P_{CO_2} at the apneic threshold and decreasing ventilatory response to carbon dioxide and increasing body stores (e.g., lung contents) of oxygen, which increases damping. Consequently, breathing during sleep should stabilize (see "Mechanisms of Sleep Apnea in Heart Failure" section).

Although many years of experience and studies have demonstrated beneficial effects of nocturnal oxygen therapy in patients with CSA and heart failure, prospective placebo-controlled, long-term studies have not been performed to determine the potential to decrease mortality among patients with systolic heart failure.

Noninvasive Positive Airway Pressure Devices

As noted previously, these devices have been successfully used to treat OSA in patients with heart failure. They have also been used to treat CSA, but efficacy has been variable.

Continuous Positive Airway Pressure and Bilevel Pressure Devices. Both these types of devices have been used to treat CSA in patients with heart failure.[152,168,197-204] However, most studies have focused on CPAP.

One-night use of CPAP has been shown to eliminate CSA in 43% of the subjects with systolic heart failure.[168] OSA, in contrast, is invariably eliminated with overnight CPAP titration.

In patients with CSA who have responded to CPAP, the AHI decreased from 36 per hour to 4 per hour, and desaturation was virtually eliminated. CPAP level varied from 5 to 12 cm H_2O. In these patients, the number of premature ventricular contractions, couplets, and episodes of ventricular tachycardia decreased.[168] This effect was presumed to result from decreased sympathetic activity and improved oxygenation. CPAP had no significant effect on ventricular irritability in patients whose disordered breathing did not improve.

In one study,[168] 53% of CSA patients did not respond to CPAP. Others investigators have also reported negative results.[198-200,202] This observation may explain why CPAP therapy did not improve survival of patients with heart failure and CSA in the Canadian Continuous Positive Airway Pressure for Patients with Central Sleep Apnea and Heart Failure (CANPAP) trial.[202] In the CANPAP trial, patients with heart failure and CSA were randomly assigned to receive CPAP or no CPAP for a mean duration of 2 years. There was no difference between these groups in the primary endpoint of death or transplantation ($P = .54$), nor was there a significant difference in the frequency of hospitalization between groups

(0.56 vs. 0.61 hospitalizations per patient year, $P = .45$). The trial was terminated prematurely in part because of excess early mortality in the CPAP recipients in comparison with the control group ($P = .02$). In their analysis, the authors did not categorize patients with heart failure as CPAP responders and nonresponders. In a pro and con discussion[205] about these observations, we suggested that excess mortality occurred primarily in nonresponders. Consequently, the post hoc analysis of the data[152] revealed significant improvement in survival of CPAP responders (Figure 32-13). The reasons why CPAP may have increased mortality are multiple,[205] including adverse hemodynamic effects of increased intrathoracic pressure (decreasing venous return and cardiac output), which is quite deleterious in patients who continue to have persistent CSA while receiving CPAP.

Caution should therefore be exercised with use of nasal CPAP. If CSA persists during an overnight CPAP titration, we recommend a trial with pressure support servo-ventilation devices.

Pressure Support Servo-Ventilation Devices. These devices are distinctively different from CPAP and bilevel pressure devices. First, they provide variable (not constant) and proportional amounts of ventilatory support during different phases of periodic breathing. The support is minimal during the hyperpneic phase of periodic breathing and maximal during periods of diminished breathing and central apnea. Like a buffer that keeps the pH of a solution relatively stable, these devices keep ventilation relatively stable (buffer positive airway pressure).

In addition, these devices are equipped with a backup rate that initiates a breath after a short preset time (a few seconds) of no spontaneous breathing.

Several short-term studies provide evidence of the efficacy of these devices in the treatment of heart failure[206-214] and also in the treatment of idiopathic CSA[215] and CSA associated with the use of opioids.[216]

These devices should be used in patients with heart failure who are not responsive to or are noncompliant with CPAP treatment. Randomized clinical trials are in progress to determine long-term efficacy.

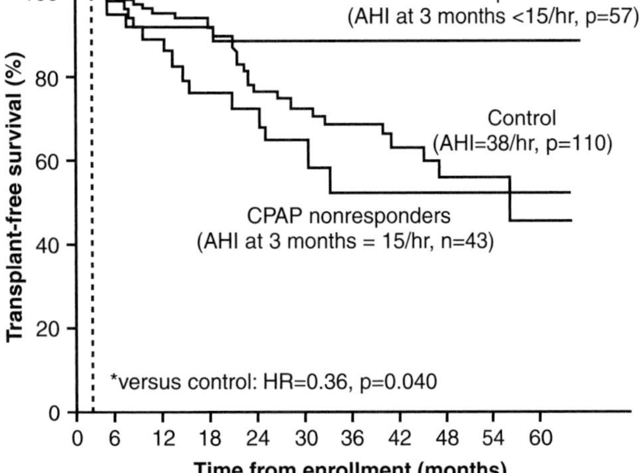

FIGURE 32–13 Probability of survival in patients with systolic heart failure (HF) comparing continuous positive airway pressure (CPAP) responders to a control group (patients with systolic heart failure and similar apnea-hypopnea index [AHI]) and to CPAP nonresponders. CPAP responders had a significantly increased probability of survival compared to the control group. CPAP nonresponders tended to have a poor survival when compared to the control group, although this was not significant. CSA, central sleep apnea; HR, hazard ratio. (Modified from Artzm. Floras, J. S., Logan, A. G., et al. (2007). Supression of central sleep apnea by continuous positive airway pressure and transplant free survival in heart failure, *Circulation* 115; 3173-3180 and adapted from Javaheri S, cardiovascular disorders Atlas of clinical Sleep Medicine.)

Acetazolamide. Acetazolamide acts as a respiratory stimulant and a mild diuretic. It has been used for prevention and treatment of periodic breathing at high altitude and idiopathic CSA.[217,218] In a double-blind, placebo-controlled crossover study[219] in 12 patients with systolic heart failure and severe CSA, patients who received acetazolamide exhibited significantly lower central AHI (34 per hour) than did placebo recipients (57 per hour) after 5 nights. Arterial oxyhemoglobin desaturation also improved significantly in the experimental group. Acetazolamide was administered as a single dose at about 3 mg/kg one half hour before bedtime, in order to minimize the side effects associated with multiple doses, particularly with long-term use. Patients reported improved subjective perception of overall sleep quality, feeling rested on awakening, falling asleep unintentionally, and fatigue. Acetazolamide could have two other advantageous effects when used in patients with heart failure and CSA: acting as a mild diuretic and minimizing alkalemia (caused by loop diuretics), which is commonly present in patients with heart failure. At this dose, the effect on pH is mild. In this study,[219] arterial blood pH decreased from 7.43 before bedtime to 7.37 in the morning.

The mechanism of action of acetazolamide is related to an increase in P_{CO_2} reserve, noted previously.[70]

Theophylline. Aminophylline and theophylline have long been known to alleviate CSA in premature infants and adults. Open-label studies have demonstrated the efficacy of this drug in the treatment of CSA in patients with heart failure.[3,220] In a double-blind, randomized, placebo-controlled, crossover study of 15 patients with treated, stable systolic heart failure, similar results were reported.[221] Administration of theophylline, twice daily by mouth, at therapeutic plasma concentrations (11 µg/mL; range, 7 to 15/µg/mL) decreased the AHI by about 50% and improved arterial oxyhemoglobin saturation.[221]

The mechanisms of action of theophylline in improving central apnea remain unclear.[221] At therapeutic serum concentrations, theophylline competes with adenosine at some of its receptor sites. In the central nervous system, adenosine is a respiratory depressant, and theophylline stimulates respiration[222,223] by competing with adenosine. It is therefore conceivable that an increase in ventilation by theophylline could decrease central apnea during sleep. Theophylline does not increase ventilatory response to carbon dioxide.[223]

Potential arrhythmogenic effects and phosphodiesterase inhibition are common concerns with long-term use of theophylline in patients with heart failure. Therefore, further controlled studies are necessary to establish its safety. If theophylline is used to treat CSA, frequent and careful follow-up is necessary.

Benzodiazepines. It has been hypothesized that by decreasing arousals, benzodiazepines may decrease CSA. However, two studies,[198,224] including a placebo-controlled, double-blind study,[224] failed to show any improvement in CSA in patients with systolic heart failure. Therefore, their use for this purpose is not recommended.

Inhaled Carbon Dioxide. Several studies have demonstrated that low-level inhalation of carbon dioxide virtually eliminates CSA.[225-229] However, some of these studies also have also shown that carbon dioxide inhalation increases arousals, which are associated with increased sympathetic and decreased parasympathetic activity. Because of the adverse cardiovascular effects of sympathetic overactivity in heart failure, the use of carbon dioxide to treat CSA is not recommended.

CONCLUSIONS

Heart failure is a widespread problem with significant economic effects. Because of the increase in average life span and improvements in therapy for ischemic coronary artery

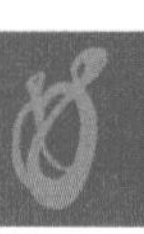

disease and hypertension, the number of people living with heart failure will remain high.

Heart failure is associated with excess morbidity and mortality, despite recent advances in its treatment. Multiple factors may contribute to the progressively declining course of heart failure. One such cause could be the occurrence of repetitive episodes of apnea, hypopnea, and hyperpnea, which are common in patients with heart failure. Episodes of apnea, hypopnea, and hyperpnea cause sleep disruption, arousals, intermittent hypoxemia, hypercapnia, hypocapnia, and changes in intrathoracic pressure. These pathophysiological consequences of sleep-related breathing disorders have deleterious effects on the cardiovascular system and may be most pronounced in the setting of established heart failure and coronary artery disease. Several studies have revealed that patients with systolic heart failure and sleep apnea, both OSA and CSA, have significantly shorter survival than do patients without sleep apnea. Furthermore, several observational studies have demonstrated that appropriate treatment of sleep-related breathing disorders, both OSA and CSA, improves survival of patients with heart failure.

REFERENCES

1. Cheyne, J. (1818). A case of apoplexy, in which the fleshy part of the heart was converted into fat. *Dublin Hosp Rep Commun, 2*, 216–223.
2. Stokes, W. (1846). Observations on some cases of permanently slow pulse. *Dublin Q J Med Sci, 2*, 73–85.
3. Dowdell, W. T., Javaheri, S., & McGinnis, W. (1990). Cheyne-Stokes respiration presenting as sleep apnea syndrome. Clinical and polysomnographic features. *Am Rev Respir Dis, 141*, 871–879.
4. Cheyne, G. (1976). *The English Malady Scholars.* New York: Facsimilies and Reprints, Inc. (pp 208–213).
5. Tenney, S. M. (1994). Cheyne, Cheyne and Stokes. *News Physiol Sci, 9*, 96–97.
6. Ward, M. (1973). Periodic respiration. A short historical note. *Ann R Coll Surg Engl, 52*, 330–334.
7. Allen, E., Turk, J. L., & Murley, R. (1993). *The Case Books of John Hunter FRS.* New York: Parthenon.
8. Javaheri, S., Parker, T. J., Wexler, L., et al. (1995). Occult sleep-disordered breathing in stable congestive heart failure. *Ann Intern Med, 122*, 442, 487, [Erratum, Ann Intern Med 1995;123:77].
9. Hanly, P. J., Millar, T. W., Steljes, D. G., et al. (1989). Respiration and abnormal sleep in patients with congestive heart failure. *Chest, 96*, 480–488.
10. Javaheri, S., Parker, T. J., Liming, J. D., et al. (1998). Sleep apnea in 81 ambulatory male patients with stable heart failure: types and their prevalences, consequences, and presentations. *Circulation, 97*, 2154–2159.
11. Tremel, F., Pépin, J. -L., Veale, D., et al. (1999). High prevalence and persistence of sleep apnoea in patients referred for acute left ventricular failure and medically treated over 2 months. *Eur Heart J, 20*, 1201–1209.
12. Sin, D. D., Fitzgerald, F., Parker, J. D., et al. (1999). Risk factors for central and obstructive sleep apnea in 450 men and women with congestive heart failure. *Am J Respir Crit Care Med, 160*, 1101–1106.
13. Solin, P., Bergin, P., Richardson, M., et al. (1999). Influence of pulmonary capillary wedge pressure on central apnea in heart failure. *Circulation, 99*, 1574–1579.
14. Yasuma, F., Nomura, H., Hayashi, H., et al. (1989). Breathing abnormalities during sleep in patients with chronic heart failure. *Circ J, 53*, 1506–1510.
15. Lofaso, F., Verschueren, P., Rande, J. L. D., et al. (1994). Prevalence of sleep-disordered breathing in patients on a heart transplant waiting list. *Chest, 106*, 1689–1694.
16. Traversi, E., Callegari, G., Pozzoli, M., et al. (1997). Sleep disorders and breathing alterations in patients with chronic heart failure. *G Ital Cardiol, 27*, 423.
17. Staniforth, A. D., Kinnear, W. J. M., Starling, R., et al. (1998). Nocturnal desaturation in patients with stable heart failure. *Heart, 79*, 394–399.
18. Lanfranchi, P. A., Braghiroli, A., Bosimini, E., et al. (1999). Prognostic value of nocturnal Cheyne-Stokes respiration in chronic heart failure. *Circulation, 99*, 1435–1440.
19. Fries, R., Bauer, D., Heisel, A., et al. (1999). Clinical significance of sleep-related breathing disorders in patients with implantable cardioverter defibrillators. *Pace, 22*, 223–227.
20. American Heart Association. (2009). Heart disease and stroke statistics—2009 update. *Circulation, 119*, e1–e161.
21. Carskadon, M. A., & Dement, W. C. (2000). Normal human sleep; an overview. In M. G. Kryger, T. Roth, & M. C. Dement (Eds.). *Principles and practice of sleep medicine* (ed 3, pp. 5–25). Philadelphia: WB Saunders.
22. Kryger, M. H. (2000). Monitoring respiratory and cardiac function. In M. G. Kryger, T. Roth, & M. C. Dement (Eds.), *Principles and practice of sleep medicine* (ed 3, pp. 1217–1230). Philadelphia: WB Saunders.
23. Hanly, P. J., & Zuberi-Khokhar, N. (1996). Periodic limb movements during sleep in patients with congestive heart failure. *Chest, 109*, 1497, 1502.
24. Young, T., Palta, M., Dempsey, J., et al. (1993). The occurrence of sleep-disordered breathing among middle-aged adults. *N Engl J Med, 328*, 1230–1235.
25. Cherniack, N. S. (1999). Apnea and periodic breathing during sleep. *N Engl J Med, 341*, 985–987.
26. Mancia, G. (1993). Autonomic modulation of the cardiovascular system during sleep. *N Engl J Med, 238*, 347–349.
27. Mancia, G., & Zanchetti, A. (1980). Cardiovascular regulation during sleep. In J. Orem, & C. D. Barnes (Eds.). *Physiology in sleep* (pp. 1–55). New York: Academic Press.
28. Baust, W., Weidinger, H., & Kirchner, F. (1968). Sympathetic activity during natural sleep and arousal. *Arch Ital Biol, 106*, 379–390.
29. Somers, V. K., Dyken, M. E., Mark, A. L., et al. (1993). Sympathetic-nerve activity during sleep in normal subjects. *N Engl J Med, 328*, 303–307.
30. Hornyak, M., Cejnar, M., Elam, M., et al. (1991). Sympathetic muscle nerve activity during sleep in man. *Brain, 114*, 1281–1295.
31. Okada, H., Iwase, S., Mano, T., et al. (1991). Changes in muscle sympathetic nerve activity during sleep in humans. *Neurology, 41*, 1961–1966.
32. Ziegler, M. G., Lake, C. R., Wood, J. H., et al. (1976). Circadian rhythm in cerebrospinal fluid noradrenaline of man and monkey. *Nature, 264*, 656–658.
33. Linsell, C. R., Lightman, S. L., Mullen, P. E., et al. (1985). Circadian rhythms of epinephrine and norepinephrine in man. *J Clin Endocrinol Metab, 160*, 1210–1215.
34. Vaughn, B. V., Quint, S. R., Messenheimer, J. A., et al. (1995). Heart period variability in sleep. *Electroenceph Clin Neurophysiol, 94*, 155–162.
35. Khatri, I. M., & Freis, E. D. (1967). Hemodynamic changes during sleep. *J Appl Physiol, 22*, 867–873.
36. Coote, J. H. (1982). Respiratory and circulatory control during sleep. *J Exp Biol, 100*, 223–244.
37. Shepard, J. W., Jr. (1985). Gas exchange and hemodynamics during sleep. *Med Clin North Am, 69*, 1243–1264.
38. Phillipson, E. A. (1978). Control of breathing during sleep. *Am Rev Respir Dis, 118*, 909.
39. Dempsey, J. A., & Skatrud, J. B. (1988). Fundamental effects of sleep state on breathing. *Curr Pulmonol, 9*, 267–304.
40. Skatrud, J. B., & Dempsey, J. A. (1983). Interaction of sleep state and chemical stimuli in sustaining rhythmic ventilation. *J Appl Physiol, 55*, 813–822.
41. Morgan, B.J., Crabtree, D.C., Puleo. D.S., et al. (1996). Neurocirculatory consequences of abrupt change in sleep state in humans. *J Appl Physiol* 80:1627.
42. Davies, R. J. O., Belt, P. J., Roberts, S. J., et al. (1993). Arterial blood pressure responses to graded transient arousal from sleep in normal humans. *J Appl Physiol, 74*, 1123–1130.
43. Horner, R. L., Brooks, D., Kozar, L. F., et al. (1995). Immediate effects of arousal from sleep on cardiac autonomic outflow in the absence of breathing in dogs. *J Appl Physiol, 79*, 151–162.
44. Javaheri, S. (2006). Sleep disorders in systolic heart failure: A prospective study of 100 male patients. The final report. *Int J Cardiol, 106*, 21–28.
45. Wang, H., Parker, J. D., Newton, G. E., et al. (2007). Influence of obstructive sleep apnea on mortality in patients with heart failure. *J Am Coll Cardiol, 49*, 1625–1631.
46. Vazir, A., Hastings, P. C., Dayer, M., et al. (2007). A high prevalence of sleep disorder breathing in men with mild symptomatic chronic heart failure due to left ventricular systolic dysfunction. *Eur J Heart Fail, 9*, 243–250.
47. Zhao, Z., Sullivan, C., Liu, Z., et al. (2007). Prevalence and clinical characteristics of sleep apnea in Chinese patients with heart failure. *Int J Cardiol, 118*, 122–132.
48. Christ, M., Sharkova, Y., Fenske, H., et al. (2007). Brain natriuretic peptide for prediction of Cheyne-Stokes respiration in heart failure patients. *Int J Cardiol, 116*, 62–69.
49. Oldenburg, O., Lamp, B., Faber, L., et al. (2007). Sleep disordered breathing in patients with symptomatic heart failure: a contemporary study of prevalence in and characteristics of 700 patients. *Eur J Heart Fail, 9*, 251–257.
50. MacDonald, M., Fang, J., Pittman, S. D., et al. (2008). The current prevalence of sleep disordered breathing in congestive heart failure patients treated with beta-blockers. *J Clin Sleep Med, 4*, 38–42.
51. Schulz, R., Blau, A., Borgel, J., et al. (2007). Sleep apnoea in heart failure. *Eur Respir J, 29*, 1201–1205.
52. Young, T., Peppard, P. E., & Gottlieb, D. J. (2002). Epidemiology of obstructive sleep apnea. *Am J Respir Crit Care Med, 165*, 1217–1239.
53. Bixler, E. O., Vgontzas, A. N., Lin, H. M., et al. (2001). Prevalence of sleep-disordered breathing in women: effects of gender. *Am J Respir Crit Care Med, 163*, 608–613.
54. Javaheri, S., & Guerra, L. F. (1990). Effects of domperidone and medroxyprogesterone acetate on ventilation in man. *Respir Physiol, 81*, 359–370.
55. St. John, W. M., Bartlett, D., Jr., Knuth, K. V., et al. (1986). Differential depression of hypoglossal nerve activity by alcohol. Protection by pretreatment with medroxyprogesterone acetate. *Am Rev Respir Dis, 133*, 46–48.
56. Zhou, X. S., Shahabuddin, S., Zahn, B. R., et al. (2000). Effect of gender on the development of hypocapnic apnea/hypopnea during NREM sleep. *J Appl Physiol, 89*, 192–199.
57. Young, T. (2001). Menopause, hormone replacement therapy, and sleep-disordered breathing. *Am J Respir Crit Care Med, 163*, 597.
58. Cargill, J. I., Kiely, D. G., & Lipworth, B. J. (1995). Adverse effects of hypoxaemia on diastolic filling in humans. *Clin Sci (Lond), 89*, 165–169.
59. Chami, H. A., Devereux, R. B., Gottdiener, J. S., et al. (2008). Left ventricular morphology and systolic function in sleep-disordered breathing. *Circulation, 117*, 2599–2607.
60. Fung, J. W. H., Li, T. S. T., Choy, D. K. L., et al. (2002). Severe obstructive sleep apnea is associated with left ventricular diastolic dysfunction. *Chest, 121*, 422–429.
61. Shivalkar, B., Van De Heyning, C., Kerremans, M., et al. (2006). Obstructive sleep apnea syndrome. More insights on structural and functional cardiac alterations, and the effects of treatment with continuous positive pressure. *J Am Coll Cardiol, 47*, 1433–1439.
62. Arias, M. A., Garcia-Rio, F., Alonso-Fernandez, A., et al. (2005). Obstructive sleep apnea syndrome affects left ventricular diastolic function. *Circulation, 112*, 375–383.
63. Cherniack, N. S. (1981). Respiratory dysrhythmias during sleep. *N Engl J Med, 305*, 325–330.
64. Cherniack, N. S., & Longobardo, G. S. (1973). Cheyne-Stokes breathing: an instability in physiologic control. *N Engl J Med, 288*, 952–957.
65. Khoo, M. C. K., Gottschalk, A., & Pack, A. I. (1991). Sleep-induced periodic breathing and apnea: a theoretical study. *J Appl Physiol, 70*, 2014.
66. Guyton, A. C., Crowell, J. W., & Moore, J. W. (1956). Basic oscillating mechanisms of Cheyne-Stokes breathing. *Am J Physiol, 187*, 395–398.
67. Hall, M. J., Xie, A., Rutherford, R., et al. (1996). Cycle length of periodic breathing in patients with and without heart failure. *Am J Respir Crit Care Med, 154*, 376–381.

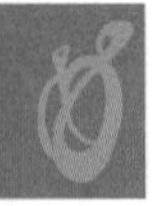

68. Javaheri, S. (1999). A mechanism of central sleep apnea in patients with heart failure. *N Engl J Med, 341*, 949–954.
69. Javaheri, S., & Dempsey, J. (2007). Mechanisms of sleep apnea and periodic breathing in systolic heart failure. *Sleep Med Clin, 2*, 623–630.
70. Nakayama, H., Smith, C. A., Rodman, J. R., et al. (2002). Effect of ventilatory drive on CO_2 sensitivity below eupnea during sleep. *Am J Crit Care Med, 165*, 1251–1258.
71. Xie, A., Skatrud, J. B., Puleo, D. S., et al. (2002). Apnea-hypopnea threshold for CO_2 in patients with congestive heart failure. *Am J Respir Crit Care Med, 165*, 1245–1250.
72. Tkacova, R., Hall, M. L., Luie, P. P., et al. (1997). Left ventricular volume in patients with heart failure and Cheyne-Stokes respiration during sleep. *Am J Respir Crit Care Med, 156*, 1549–1555.
73. Schwab, R. J., Kuna, S., & Remmers, J. E. (2005). Anatomy and physiology of upper airway obstruction. In M. G. Kryger, T. Roth, & M. C. Dement (Eds.), *Principles and practice of sleep medicine* (ed 4, pp. 984–1000). Philadelphia: WB Saunders.
74. Chan, J., Sanderson, J., Chan, W., et al. (1997). Prevalence of sleep-disordered breathing in diastolic heart failure. *Chest, 111*, 1488–1493.
75. Chenuel, B., Smith, C., Skatrud, J., et al. (2006). Increased propensity of apnea in response to acute elevations in left atrial pressure during sleep in the dog. *J Appl Physiol, 101*, 76–83.
76. Somers, V., & Javaheri, S. (2005). Cardiovascular effects of sleep-related breathing disorders. In M. G. Kryger, T. Roth, & M. C. Dement (Eds.), *Principles and practice of sleep medicine* (ed 4, pp. 1180–1191). Philadelphia: WB Saunders.
77. Mc Nicholas, W. T., & Javaheri, S. (2007). Pathophysiological mechanisms of cardiovascular disease in obstructive sleep apnea. *Sleep Med Clin, 2*, 539–547.
78. Lévy, P., Pepin, J. L., Tamisier, R., et al. (2007). Prevalence and impact of central sleep apnea in heart failure. *Sleep Med Clin, 2*, 615–621.
79. Lavie, L., & Lavie, P. (2009). Molecular mechanisms of cardiovascular disease in OSAHS: the oxidative stress link. *Eur Respir J, 33*, 1467–1484.
80. Somers, V. K., White, D. P., Amin, R., et al. (2008). Sleep apnea and cardiovascular disease. *J Am Coll Cardiol, 52*, 686–717.
81. Allen, D. G., Morris, P. G., Orchard, C. H., et al. (1985). A nuclear magnetic resonance study of metabolism in the ferret heart during hypoxia and inhibition of glycolysis. *J Physiol, 361*, 185–204.
82. Wyman, R. M., Farhi, E. R., Bing, O. H. L., et al. (1989). Comparative effects of hypoxia and ischemia in the isolated, blood-perfused dog heart: Evaluation of left ventricular diastolic chamber distensibility and wall thickness. *Circ Res, 64*, 121–128.
83. Nayler, W. G., Yepez, C. E., & Poole-Wilson, P. A. (1978). The effect of β-adrenoceptor and Ca^{2+} antagonist drugs on the hypoxia-induced increase in resting tension. *Cardiovasc Res, 12*, 666–674.
84. Nakamura, Y., Wiegner, A. W., & Bing, O. H. L. (1986). Measurement of relaxation in isolated rat ventricular myocardium during hypoxia and reoxygenation. *Cardiovasc Res, 20*, 690.
85. Kusuoka, H., Weisfeildt, M. L., Zweier, J. L., et al. (1986). Mechanism of early contractile failure during hypoxia in intact ferret heart: evidence for modulation of maximal Ca^{2+}-activated force by inorganic phosphate. *Circ Res, 59*, 270–282.
86. Yu, A. Y., Shimoda, L. A., Iyer, N. V., et al. (1999). Impaired physiological responses to chronic hypoxia in mice partially deficient for hypoxia-inducible factor 1α. *J Clin Invest, 103*, 691–696.
87. Koong, A. C., Chen, E. Y., & Giaccia, A. J. (1994). Hypoxia causes the activation of nuclear factor ϰB through the phosphorylation of IϰBα on tyrosine residues. *Cancer Res, 54*, 1425–1430.
88. Royds, J. A., Dower, S. K., Qwarnstrom, E. E., et al. (1998). Response of tumor cells to hypoxia: role of p53 and NFϰB. *J Clin Pathol Mol Pathol, 51*, 55.
89. Ryan, S., McNicholas, W.T., & Taylor, C. T. (2005). Selective activation of inflammatory pathways by intermittent hypoxia in obstructive sleep apnea syndrome. *Circulation, 112*, 2660–2667.
90. Adhikary, G., Kline, D., Yuan, G., et al. (2001). Gene regulation during intermittent hypoxia: evidence for the involvement of reactive oxygen species. *Adv Exp Med Biol, 499*, 297–302.
91. Samarasinghe, D. A., Tapner, M., & Farrell, G. C. (2000). Role of oxidative stress in hypoxia-reoxygenation injury to cultured rat hepatic sinusoidal endothelial cells. *Hepatology, 31*, 1600–1605.
92. Prabhakar, N. R. (2001). Physiological and genomic consequences of intermittent hypoxia. Invited review: oxygen sensing during intermittent hypoxia: cellular and molecular mechanisms. *J Appl Physiol, 90*, 1986–1994.
93. Ichikawa, H., Flores, S., Kvietys, P. R., et al. (1997). Molecular mechanisms of anoxia/reoxygenation-induced neutrophil adherence to cultured endothelial cells. *Circ Res, 81*, 922–931.
94. Gonzalez, N. C., & Wood, J. G. (2001). Leukocyte-endothelial interactions in environmental hypoxia. *Adv Exp Med Biol, 502*, 39–60.
95. Biegelsen, E. S., & Loscalzo, J. (1999). Endothelial function and atherosclerosis. *Coron Artery Dis, 10*, 241.
96. Britten, M. B., Zeiher, A. M., & Schächinger, V. (1999). Clinical importance of coronary endothelial vasodilator dysfunction and therapeutic options. *J Intern Med, 245*, 315–327.
97. Mombouli, J. V., & Vanhoutte, P. M. (1999). Endothelial dysfunction: from physiology to therapy. *J Mol Cell Cardiol, 31*, 61–74.
98. Faller, D. V. (1999). Endothelial cell responses to hypoxic stress. *Clin Exp Pharmacol Physiol, 26*, 74–84.
99. Aoki, M., Nata, T., Morishita, R., et al. (2001). Endothelial apoptosis induced by oxidative stress through activation of NF-ϰB. Antiapoptotic effect of antioxidant agents on endothelial cells. *Hypertension, 38*, 48–55.
100. Shirakami, G., Nakao, K., Saito, Y., et al. (1991). Acute pulmonary alveolar hypoxia increases lung and plasma endothelin-1 levels in conscious rats. *Life Sci, 48*, 969–976.
101. Young, T., Nieto, J., Javaheri, S. Systemic and pulmonary hypertension in obstructive sleep apnea. In MG, Kryger T, Roth MC, Dement (Eds.), *Principles and practice of sleep medicine*, ed 5, Philadelphia, in press, WB Saunders.
102. Nakao, K., Ohgushi, M., Yoshimura, M., et al. (1997). Hyperventilation as a specific test for diagnosis of coronary artery spasm. *Am J Cardiol, 80*, 545–549.
103. Javaheri, S., & Corbett, W. S. (1998). Association of low $PaCO_2$ with central sleep apnea and ventricular arrhythmias in ambulatory patients with stable heart failure. *Ann Intern Med, 128*, 204–207.
104. Buda, A. J., Pinsky, M. R., Ingels, N. B., Jr., et al. (1979). Effect of intrathoracic pressure on left ventricular performance. *N Engl J Med, 301*, 453–459.
105. Fessler, H. E., Brower, R. G., Wise, R. A., et al. (1988). Mechanism of reduced LV afterload by systolic and diastolic positive pleural pressure. *J Appl Physiol, 65*, 1244–1250.
106. Virolainen, J., Ventilä, M., Turto, H., et al. (1995). Effect of negative intrathoracic pressure on left ventricular pressure dynamics and relaxation. *J Appl Physiol, 79*, 455–460.
107. Brinker, J. A., Weiss, J. L., Lappe, D. L., et al. (1980). Leftward septal displacement during right ventricular loading in man. *Circulation, 61*, 626–632.
108. Fletcher, E. C., Proctor, M., Yu, J., et al. (1999). Pulmonary edema develops after recurrent obstructive apneas. *Am J Respir Crit Care Med, 160*, 1688–1696.
109. Van de Borne, P., Oren, R., Abouassaly, C., et al. (1998). Effect of Cheyne-Stokes respiration on muscle sympathetic nerve activity in severe congestive heart failure secondary to ischemic or idiopathic dilated cardiomyopathy. *Am J Cardiol, 81*, 432–436.
110. Shimizu, T., Takahashi, Y., Kogawa, S., et al. (1997). Muscle sympathetic nerve activity during central, mixed and obstructive apnea: are there any differences? *Psychiatry Clin Neurosci, 51*, 397–404.
111. Naughton, M. T., Benard, D. C., Liu, P. P., et al. (1995). Effects of nasal CPAP on sympathetic activity in patients with heart failure and central sleep apnea. *Am J Respir Crit Care Med, 152*, 473–479.
112. Somers, V. K., Dyken, M. E., Clary, M. P., et al. (1995). Sympathetic neural mechanisms in obstructive sleep apnea. *J Clin Invest, 96*, 1897–1904.
113. Fletcher, E. C., Miller, J., Schaaf, J. W., et al. (1987). Urinary catecholamines before and after tracheostomy in patients with obstructive sleep apnea and hypertension. *Sleep, 10*, 35–44.
114. Waravdekar, N. V., Sinoway, L. I., Zwillich, C. W., et al. (1996). Influence of treatment on muscle sympathetic nerve activity in sleep apnea. *Am J Respir Crit Care Med, 153*, 1333–1338.
115. Narkiewicz, K., Kato, M., Phillips, B. G., et al. (1999). Nocturnal continuous positive airway pressure decreases daytime sympathetic traffic in obstructive sleep apnea. *Circulation, 100*, 2332–2335.
116. Pepperell, J., Maskell, N. A., Jones, D. R., et al. (2003). A randomized controlled trial of adaptive ventilation for Cheyne-Stokes breathing in heart failure. *Am J Respir Crit Care Med, 168*, 1109–1114.
117. Staniforth, A. D., Kinneart, W. J. M., Hetmanski, D. J., et al. (1998). Effect of oxygen on sleep quality, cognitive function and sympathetic activity in patients with chronic heart failure and Cheyne-Stokes respiration. *Eur Heart J, 19*, 922–928.
118. Fletcher, E. C., Lesske, J., Behm, R., et al. (1992). Carotid chemoreceptors, systemic blood pressure, and chronic episodic hypoxia mimicking sleep apnea. *J Appl Physiol, 72*, 1978–1984.
119. Morgan, B. J., Crabtree, D. C., Palta, M., et al. (1995). Combined hypoxia and hypercapnia evokes long-lasting sympathetic activation in humans. *J Appl Physiol, 79*, 205–213.
120. Rose, C. E., Jr., Althaus, J. A., Kaiser, D. L., et al. (1983). Acute hypoxemia and hypercapnia: increase in plasma catecholamines in conscious dogs. *Am J Physiol, 245*, H924–H929.
121. Hardy, J. C., GrayWhisler, K. S., et al. (1994). Sympathetic and blood pressure responses to voluntary apnea are augmented by hypoxemia. *J Appl Physiol, 77*, 2360–2365.
122. Mann, D. L., Kent, R. L., Parsons, B., et al. (1992). Adrenergic effects on the biology of the adult mammalian cardiocyte. *Circulation, 85*, 790–804.
123. Communal, C., Singh, K., Pimental, D. R., et al. (1998). Norepinephrine stimulates apoptosis in adult rat ventricular myocytes by activation of the β-adrenergic pathway. *Circulation, 98*, 1329–1334.
124. He, J., Kryger, M. H., Zorick, F. J., et al. (1988). Mortality and apnea index in obstructive sleep apnea: experience in 385 male patients. *Chest, 94*, 531–538.
125. Partinen, M., Jamieson, A., & Guilleminault, C. (1988). Long-term outcome for obstructive sleep apnea syndrome patients: mortality. *Chest, 94*, 1200–1204.
126. Partinen, M., & Guilleminault, C. (1990). Daytime sleepiness and vascular morbidity at seven-year follow-up in obstructive sleep apnea patients. *Chest, 97*, 27–32.
127. Peker, Y., Hedner, J., Norum, J., et al. (2002). Increased incidence of cardiovascular disease in middle-aged men with obstructive sleep apnea. *Am J Respir Crit Care Med, 166*, 159–165.
128. Peker, Y., Hedner, J., Kraiczi, H., et al. (2000). Respiratory disturbance index: an independent predictor of mortality in coronary artery disease. *Am J Respir Crit Care Med, 162*, 81–86.
129. Mooe, T., Franklin, K. A., Holmström, K., et al. (2001). Sleep-disordered breathing and coronary artery disease: long-term prognosis. *Am J Respir Crit Care Med, 164*, 1910–1913.
130. Young, T., Finn, L., Peppard, P., et al. (2008). Sleep disordered breathing and mortality: eighteen-year follow-up of the Wisconsin Sleep Cohort. *Sleep, 31*, 1071–1078.
131. Marshall, N. S., Wong, K. K., Liu, P. Y., et al. (2008). Sleep apnea as an independent risk factor for all-cause mortality: The Busselton Health Study. *Sleep, 31*, 1079–1085.
131a. Bliwise, D. L., Bliwise, N. G., Partinen, M., et al. (1988). Sleep apnea and mortality in an aged cohort. *Am J Public Health, 78*, 544–547.
132. Ancoli-Israel, S., Klauber, M. R., Kripke, D. F., et al. (1989). Sleep apnea in female patients in a nursing home. Increased risk of mortality. *Chest, 96*, 1054–1058.
133. Mant, A., King, M., Saunders, N. A., et al. (1995). Four-year follow-up of mortality and sleep-related respiratory disturbance in non-demented seniors. *Sleep, 18*, 433–438.
134. Ancoli-Israel, S., Kripke, D. F., Klauber, M. R., et al. (1996). Morbidity, mortality and sleep-disordered breathing in community swelling elderly. *Sleep, 19*, 277–282.
135. Lavie, P., Lavie, L., & Herer, P. (2005). All-cause mortality in males with sleep apnoea syndrome; declining mortality rates with age. *Eur Respir J, 25*, 514.
136. Marin, J. M., Carrizo, S. J., Vicente, E., & Agusti, A. G. (2005). Long-term cardiovascular outcomes in men with obstructive sleep apnoea-hypopnoea with or without treatment with continuous positive airway pressure: an observational study. *Lancet, 365*, 1046.
137. YaggiConcato, H. K., Kernan, W. N., et al. (2005). Obstructive sleep apnea as a risk factor for stroke and death. *N Engl J Med, 353*, 2034–2041.

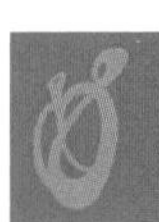

138. Buchner, N. J., Sanner, B. M., Borgel, J., et al. (2007). Continuous positive airway pressure treatment of mild to moderate obstructive sleep apnea reduces cardiovascular risk. *Am J Respir Crit Care Med, 176*, 1274–1280.
139. Gami, A. S., Howard, D. E., Olson, E. J., et al. (2005). Day-night pattern of sudden death in obstructive sleep apnea. *N Engl J Med, 352*, 1206–1214.
140. Punjabi, M. N., Caffo, B. S., Goodwin, J. L., et al. (2009). Sleep-disordered breathing and mortality: a prospective cohort study. *PLoS Med, 8*, 1–9.
141. Sahlin, C., Sandberg, O., Gustafson, Y., et al. (2008). Obstructive sleep apnea is a risk factor for death in patients with stroke. *Arch Intern Med, 168*, 297–301.
142. Doherty, L. S., Kiely, J. L., Swan, V., et al. (2005). Long-term effects of nasal continuous positive pressure therapy cardiovascular outcomes in sleep apnea syndrome. *Chest, 127*, 2076–2084.
143. Campos-Rodriguez, F., Pena-Gritnan, N., Reyes-Nunez, N., et al. (2005). Mortality in obstructive sleep apnea-hypopnea patients treated with positive airway pressure. *Chest, 128*, 624–633.
144. Kasai, T., Narui, K., Dohi, T., et al. (2008). Prognosis of patients with heart failure and obstructive sleep apnea treated with continuous positive airway pressure. *Chest, 133*, 690–696.
145. Findley, L. J., Zwillich, C. W., Ancoli-Israel, S., et al. (1985). Cheyne-Stokes breathing during sleep in patients with left ventricular heart failure. *South Med J, 78*, 11–15.
146. Hanly, P., & Zuberi-Khkhar, N. (1996). Increased mortality associated with Cheyne-Stokes respiration in patients with congestive heart failure. *Am J Respir Crit Care Med, 153*, 272–276.
147. Sin, D. D., Logan, A. G., Fitzgerald, F. S., et al. (2000). Effects of continuous positive airway pressure on cardiovascular outcomes in heart failure patients with and without Cheyne-Stokes respiration. *Circulation, 102*, 61–66.
148. Leite, J. J., Mansur, A. J., de Freitas, H. F. G., et al. (2003). Periodic breathing during incremental exercise predicts mortality in patients with chronic heart failure evaluated for cardiac transplantation. *J Am Coll Cardiol, 41*, 2175–2181.
149. Brack, T., Thuer, I., Clarenbach, C. F., et al. (2007). Daytime Cheyne-Stokes respiration in ambulatory patients with severe congestive heart failure is associated with increased mortality. *Chest, 132*, 1463–1471.
150. Corra, U., Pistono, M., Mezzani, A., et al. (2006). Sleep and exertional periodic breathing. *Circulation, 113*, 44–50.
151. La Rovere, M. T., Pinna, G. D., Maestri, R., et al. (2007). Clinical relevance of short-term day-time breathing disorders in chronic heart failure patients. *Eur J Heart Fail, 9*, 949–954.
152. Arzt, M., Floras, J. S., Logan, A. G., et al. (2007). Suppression of central sleep apnea by continuous positive airway pressure and transplant-free survival in heart failure. A post-hoc analysis of the Canadian Continuous Positive Airway Pressure for Patients with Central Sleep Apnea and Heart Failure Trial (CANPAP). *Circulation, 115*, 3173–3180.
153. Javaheri, S., Shukla, R., Zeigler, H., et al. (2007). Central sleep apnea, right ventricular dysfunction and low diastolic blood pressure are predictors of mortality in systolic heart failure. *J Am Coll Cardiol, 49*, 2028–2034.
154. Ancoli-Israel, S., DuHamel, E. R., Stepnnowsky, C., et al. (2003). The relationship between congestive heart failure, sleep apnea and mortality in older men. *Chest, 124*, 1400–1405.
155. Andreas, S., Hagenah, G., Möller, C., et al. (1996). Cheyne-Stokes respiration and prognosis in congestive heart failure. *Am J Cardiol, 78*, 1260–1264.
156. Roebuck, T., Solin, P., Kaye, D. M., et al. (2004). Increased long term mortality in heart failure due to sleep apnoea in not yet proven. *Eur Respir J, 23*, 735–740.
157. Pepperell, J. C., Ramdassingh-Dow, S., Crosthwaite, N., et al. (2002). Ambulatory blood pressure after therapeutic and subtherapeutic nasal continuous positive airway pressure for obstructive sleep apnea: a randomized parallel trial. *Lancet, 359*, 204.
158. Becker, H., & Javaheri, S. (2007). Systemic and pulmonary arterial hypertension in obstructive sleep apnea. *Sleep Med Clin, 2*, 549–557.
159. Hanly, P., Zuberi, N., & Gray, R. (1993). Pathogenesis of Cheyne-Stokes respiration in patients with congestive heart failure. Relationship to arterial Pco_2. *Chest, 104*, 1079–1084.
160. Naughton, M., Bernard, D., Tam, A., et al. (1993). Role of hyperventilation in the pathogenesis of central sleep apneas in patients with congestive heart failure. *Am Rev Respir Dis, 148*, 330–338.
161. Javaheri, S. (2000). Central sleep apnea and heart failure. *Circulation, 342*, 293.
162. Blackshear, J. L., Kaplan, J., Thompson, R. C., et al. (1995). Nocturnal dyspnea and atrial fibrillation predict Cheyne-Stokes respirations in patients with congestive heart failure. *Arch Intern Med, 155*, 1297.
163. Davis, S. W., John, L. M., Wedzicha, J. A., et al. (1991). Overnight studies in severe chronic left heart failure: arrhythmias and oxygen desaturation. *Br Heart J, 65*, 77.
164. Cripps, T., Rocker, G., & Strading, J. (1992). Nocturnal hypoxia and arrhythmias in patients with impaired left ventricular function. *Br Heart J, 68*, 382.
165. Garrigue, S., Pepin, J. L., Defaye, P., et al. (2007). High prevalence of sleep apnea syndrome in patients with long-term pacing: the European Multicenter Polysomnographic Study. *Circulation, 115*, 1703–1709.
166. Roizenblatt, S., Guilleminault, C., Poyares, D., et al. (2006). A double-blind, placebo-controlled, crossover study of sildenafil in obstructive sleep apnea. *Arch Intern Med, 166*, 1763–1767.
167. Calle, E. E., Thun, M. J., Petrelli, J. M., et al. (1999). Body-mass index and mortality in a prospective cohort of U.S. adults. *N Engl J Med, 341*, 1097.
168. Javaheri, S. (2000). Effects of continuous positive airway pressure on sleep apnea and ventricular irritability in patients with heart failure. *Circulation, 101*, 392–397.
169. Kaneko, Y., Floras, J. S., Usui, K., et al. (2003). Cardiovascular effects of continuous positive airway pressure in patients with heart failure and obstructive sleep apnea. *N Engl J Med, 248*, 1233–1241.
170. Mansfield, D. R., Gollogly, C., & Kaye, D. M. (2004). Controlled trail of continuous positive airway pressure in obstructive sleep apnea and heart failure. *Am J Respir Crit Care Med, 169*, 361–366.
171. Egea, C. J., Aizpuru, F., Pinto, J. A., et al. (2008). Cardiac function after CPAP therapy in patients with chronic heart failure and sleep apnea: a multicenter study. *Sleep Med*, 660–666.
172. Smith, L. A., Vennelle, M., Gardner, R. S., et al. (2007). Auto-titrating continuous positive airway pressure therapy in patients with chronic heart failure and obstructive sleep apnoea: a randomized placebo-controlled trial. *Eur Heart J, 28*, 1221–1227.
173. Javaheri, S. (2007). Treatment of obstructive and central sleep apnoea in heart failure: practical options. *Eur Respir Rev, 16*, 183–188.
174. Javaheri, S. Heart failure. In M. G, Kryger, T. Roth & M. C. Dement (Eds.), *Principles and practice of sleep medicine*, ed 5, Philadelphia, in press, WB Saunders.
175. De Backer, W., & Javaheri, S. (2007). Treatment of sleep apnea in heart failure. *Sleep Med Clin, 2*, 631–638.
176. Arendt, J., Bojkowsxki, C., Franey, C., et al. (1985). Immunoassay of 6-hydroxymelatonin sulfate in human plasma and urine: abolition of the urinary 24-hour rhythm with atenolol. *J Clin Endocrinol Metab, 60*, 1166–1173.
177. Stoschitzky, K., Sakotnik, A., Lercher, P., et al. (1999). Influence of beta-blockers on melatonin release. *Eur J Clin Pharmacol, 55*, 111–115.
178. Sinha, A. M., Skobel, E. C., Breithardt, O. A., et al. (2004). Cardiac resynchronization therapy improves central sleep apnea and Cheyne-Stokes respiration in patients with chronic heart failure. *J Am Coll Cardiol, 44*, 68–71.
179. Gabor, J. Y., Newman, D. A., Barnard-Roberts, V., et al. (2005). Improvement in Cheyne-Stokes respiration following cardiac resynchronization therapy. *Eur Respir J, 26*, 95–100.
180. Oldenburg, O., Faber, L., Vogt, J., et al. (2007). Influence of cardiac resynchronization therapy on different types of sleep disordered breathing. *Eur J Heart Fail, 9*, 820–826.
181. Kara, T., Novak, M., Nykodym, J., et al. (2008). Short-term effects of cardiac resynchronization therapy on sleep-disordered breathing in patients with systolic heart failure. *Chest, 134*, 87–93.
182. Collop, N. A. (1993). Cheyne-Stokes ventilation converting to obstructive sleep apnea following heart transplantation. *Chest, 104*, 1288–1289.
183. Klink, M. E., Sethi, G. K., Copeland, J. G., et al. (1993). Obstructive sleep apnea in heart transplant patients. A report of five cases. *Chest, 104*, 1090–1092.
184. Madden, B. P., Shenoy, V., Dalrymple-Hay, M., et al. (1997). Absence of bradycardic response to apnea and hypoxia in heart transplant recipients with obstructive sleep apnea. *J Heart Lung Transplant, 16*, 394–397.
185. Javaheri, S., Abraham, W., Brown, C., et al. (2004). Prevalence of obstructive sleep apnea and periodic limb movement in 45 subjects with heart transplantation. *Eur Heart J, 25*, 260–266.
186. Pembrey, M. S. (1908). Observations on Cheyne-Stokes respiration. *J Pathol Bacteriol, 12*, 259–266.
187. Hanly, P. F., Millar, T. W., Steljes, D. G., et al. (1989). The effect of oxygen on respiration and sleep in patients with congestive heart failure. *Ann Intern Med, 111*, 777–782.
188. Javaheri, S., Ahmed, M., Parker, T. J., et al. (1999). Effects of nasal O_2 on sleep-related disordered breathing in ambulatory patients with stable heart failure. *Sleep, 22*, 1101 –1106.
189. Franklin, K. A., Eriksson, P., Sahlin, et al. (1997). Reversal of central sleep apnea with oxygen. *Chest, 111*, 163–169.
190. Andreas, S., Clemens, C., Sandholzer, H., et al. (1996). Improvement of exercise capacity with treatment of Cheyne-Stokes respiration in patients with congestive heart failure. *J Am Coll Cardiol, 27*, 1486–1490.
191. Staniforth, A. D., Kinnear, W. J., Starling, R., et al. (1998). Effect of oxygen on sleep quality, cognitive function and sympathetic activity in patients with chronic heart failure and Cheyne-Stokes respiration. *Eur Heart J, 19*, 922–928.
192. Sasayama, S., Izumi, T., Seino, Y., et al. (2006). Effects of nocturnal oxygen therapy on outcome measures in patients with chronic heart failure and Cheyne-Stokes respiration. *Circ J, 70*, 1–7.
193. Sasayama, S., Izumi, T., Matsuzaki, M., et al. (2009). Improvement of quality of life with nocturnal oxygen therapy in heart failure patients with central sleep apnea. *Circ J, 73*, 1255–1262.
194. Toyama, T., Seki, R., Kasama, S., et al. (2009). Effectiveness of nocturnal home oxygen therapy to improve exercise capacity, cardiac function and cardiac sympathetic nerve activity in patients with chronic heart failure and central sleep apnea. *Circ J, 73*, 299–304.
195. Sasayama, S., Izumi, T., Matsuzaki, M. (2009). Improvement of quality of life with nocturnal oxygen therapy in heart failure patients with central sleep apnea. *Circ J, 73*: 1255–1262.
196. Javaheri, S. (2003). Pembrey's dream: the time has come for a long-term trial of nocturnal supplemental nasal oxygen to treat central sleep apnea in congestive heart failure. *Chest, 123*, 322–325.
197. Naughton, M. T., Liu, P. P., Benard, D. C., et al. (1995). Treatment of congestive heart failure and Cheyne-Stokes respiration during sleep by continuous positive airway pressure. *Am J Respir Crit Care Med, 151*, 92–97.
198. Guilleminault, C., Clerk, A., Labanowski, M., et al. (1993). Cardiac failure and benzodiazepines. *Sleep, 16*, 524–528.
199. Buckle, P., Millar, T., & Kryger, M. (1992). The effects of short-term nasal CPAP on Cheyne-Stokes respiration in congestive heart failure. *Chest, 102*, 31–35.
200. Davies, R. J. O., Harrington, K. J., Omerod, J. M., et al. (1993). Nasal continuous positive airway pressure in chronic heart failure with sleep-disordered breathing. *Am Rev Respir Dis, 147*, 630–634.
201. Keily, J. L., Deegan, P., Buckley, A., et al. (1998). Efficacy of nasal continuous positive airway pressure therapy in chronic heart failure. Importance of underlying cardiac rhythm. *Thorax, 53*, 956–962.
202. Bradley, T., Logan, A., Kimoff, J., et al. (2006). Continuous positive airway pressure for central sleep apnea and heart failure. *N Engl J Med, 353*, 2025–2033.
203. Kohnlein, T., Welte, T., Tan, L. B., et al. (2002). Assisted ventilation for heart failure patients with Cheyne-Stokes respiration. *Eur Respir J, 20*, 934–941.
204. Kasai, T., Narui, K., Dohi, T., et al. (2008). Efficacy of nasal bi-level positive airway pressure in congestive heart failure patients with Cheyne-Stokes respiration and central apnea. *Circ J, 72*, 1100–1105.

205. Javaheri, S. (2006). CPAP should not be used for central sleep apnea in congestive heart failure patients. *J Clin Sleep Med, 2*, 399–402.
206. Teschler, H., Döhring, J., Wang, Y. M., et al. (2001). Adaptive pressure support servo-ventilation. *Am J Respir Crit Care Med, 164*, 614–619.
207. Pepperell, J., Maskell, N. A., Jones, D. R., et al. (2003). a randomized controlled trial of adaptive ventilation for Cheyne-Stokes breathing in heart failure. *Am J Respir Crit Care Med, 168*, 1109–1114.
208. Philippe, C., Stoica-Herman, M., Drouot, X., et al. (2006). Compliance with and effectiveness of adaptive servoventilation versus continuous positive airway pressure in the treatment of Cheyne-Stokes respiration in heart failure over a six month period. *Heart, 92*, 337–342.
209. Szollosi, I., O'Driscoll, D. M., Dayer, M. J., et al. (2006). Adaptive servo-ventilation and deadspace: effects on central sleep apnoea. *J Sleep Res, 15*, 199–205.
210. Kasai, T., Narui, K., Dohi, T., et al. (2006). First experience of using new adaptive servo-ventilation device for Cheyne-Stokes respiration with central sleep apnea among Japanese patients with congestive heart failure. *Circ J, 70*, 1148–1154.
211. Fietze, I., Blau, A., Glos, M., et al. (2008). Bi-level positive pressure ventilation and adaptive servo ventilation in patients with heart failure and Cheyne-Stokes respiration. *Sleep Med, 9*, 652–659.
212. Oldenburg, O., Schmidt, A., Lamp, B., et al. (2008). Adaptive servoventilation improved cardiac function in patients with chronic heart failure and Cheyne-Stokes respiration. *Eur J Heart Fail, 10*, 581–586.
213. Arzt, M., Wensel, R., Montalvan, S., et al. (2008). Effects of dynamic bilevel positive airway pressure support on central sleep apnea in men with heart failure. *Chest, 134*, 61–66.
214. Randerath, W., Galetke, W., Stieglitz, S., et al. (2008). Adaptive servo-ventilation in patients with coexisting obstructive sleep apnoea/hypopnoea and Cheyne-Stokes respiration. *Sleep Med, 9*, 823–830.
215. Banno, K., Okamura, K., & Kryger, M. (2006). Adaptive servo-ventilation in patients with idiopathic Cheyne-Stokes breathing. *J Clin Sleep Med, 2*, 181–186.
216. Javaheri, S., Malik, A., Smith, J., et al. (2008). Adaptive pressure support servoventilation: a novel treatment for sleep apnea associated with use of opioids. *J Clin Sleep Med, 4*, 305–310.
217. White, D. P., Zwillich, C. W., Pickett, C. K., et al. (1982). Central sleep apnea. *Arch Intern Med, 142*, 1816–1819.
218. DeBacker, W. A., Verbraecken, J., Willeman, M., et al. (1995). Central apnea index decreases after prolonged treatment with acetazolamide. *Am J Respir Crit Care Med, 151*, 87–91.
219. Javaheri, S. (2006). Acetazolamide improves central sleep apnea in heart failure: a double-blind prospective study. *Am J Respir Crit Care Med, 173*, 234–237.
220. Dowell, A. R., Heyman, A., Sicker, H. O., et al. (1965). Effect of aminophylline on respiratory-center sensitivity in Cheyne-Stokes respiration and in pulmonary emphysema. *N Engl J Med, 273*, 1447–1453.
221. Javaheri, S., Parker, T. J., Wexler, L., et al. (1996). Effect of theophylline on sleep-disordered breathing in heart failure. *N Engl J Med, 335*, 562.
222. Javaheri, S., Evers, J. A. M., & Teppama, L. J. (1989). Increase in ventilation caused by aminophylline in the absence of changes in ventral medullary extracellular fluid pH and carbon dioxide tension. *Thorax, 44*, 121–125.
223. Javaheri, S., & Guerra, L. (1990). Lung function, hypoxic and hypercapnic ventilatory responses, and respiratory muscle strength in normal subjects taking oral theophylline. *Thorax, 45*, 743–747.
224. Biberdorf, D. J., Steens, R., Millar, T. W., et al. (1993). Benzodiazepines in congestive heart failure: effects of temazepam on arousability and Cheyne-Stokes respiration. *Sleep, 16*, 529–538.
225. Steens, R. D., Millar, T. W., Xiaoling, S., et al. (1994). Effect of 3% CO_2 on Cheyne-Stokes respiration in congestive heart failure. *Sleep, 17*, 61–68.
226. Andreas, S., Weidel, K., Hagenah, G., et al. (1998). Treatment of Cheyne-Stokes respiration with nasal oxygen and carbon dioxide. *Eur Respir J, 12*, 414–419.
227. Khayat, R. N., Xie, A., Patel, A. K., et al. (2003). Cardiorespiratory effects of added dead space in patients with heart failure and central sleep apnea. *Chest, 123*, 1551–1560.
228. Lorenzo-Filho, G., Rankin, F., Bies, I., et al. (1999). Effects of inhaled carbon dioxide and oxygen on Cheyne-Stokes respiration in patients with heart failure. *Am J Respir Crit Care Med, 159*, 1490–1498.
229. SzollosiI, Jones M, Morrel, M. J., et al. (2004). Effect of CO_2 inhalation on central sleep apnea and arousals from sleep. *Respiration, 71*, 493–498.

CHAPTER 33

Heart Failure in Developing Countries

Gustavo F. Méndez Machado

In the *epidemiological transition,* the basic human needs for water, food, shelter, and medical care are met with a consequent reduction in the burden of infectious, parasitic, nutritional, and perinatal diseases, to the point that life expectancy rises above 50 to 55 years.[1] At this point, the number of deaths from cardiovascular disease (CVD) exceed those from infectious and parasitic diseases, and the population disease pattern has changed to one dominated by chronic diseases.[2]

Currently, CVD accounts for about 25% of all deaths worldwide; as a health burden in developed countries, it accounts for almost 50% of all deaths (see also Chapter 22).[3] The CVD epidemic in developed countries has declined since 1980: CVD-related mortality fell by nearly 50% in Australia, Canada, France, England, Japan, and the United States.[4-6] However, awareness of the possibility that CVD has become an epidemic in developing countries has grown enormously, as a result of (1) the epidemiological transition, (2) the rapid onset of traditional cardiovascular risk factors (smoking and obesity), (3) the rapid rates of population aging, and (4) the process of migration from rural areas.[7,8] This information has encouraged to several researchers to study the health effects of CVD in these countries.

Indeed, in 1998, 86% of disability-adjusted life years (DALYs, which is a combination of years of life lost through premature death and years lived with disability) related to CVD occurred in developing countries, and in 1999 alone, CVDs contributed to a third of global deaths, 78% in low- and middle-income countries.[9] According to a report from Columbia University,[10] heart disease and stroke are far more urgent threats to global health in developing countries; CVD in younger people (aged 35 to 64) accounts for almost 40% of all deaths from heart disease. These analyses have encouraged several institutions and organizations worldwide to establish health policy strategies to tackle the problem of CVD in developing countries: assessment of cost-effectiveness interventions, risk assessment of the population, population-based strategies, and tobacco control. The focus is always on primary prevention.[10-12]

Since 1990, heart failure has emerged as a major health problem in developed countries, imposing an escalating burden on their health care systems.[13-15] This burden is reflected by an increase in the number of hospitalizations in nearly all developed countries in Europe and North America.[16] Nowadays, heart failure is the leading cause of admission to hospital with a medical problem in the United States. In the United States alone, approximately 5 million patients have heart failure, and more than 550,000 patients receive diagnoses of heart failure for the first time each year. Heart failure is the main reason for 12 to 15 million office visits and 6.5 million days of hospitalization each year. The number of deaths from heart failure has increased steadily despite advances in treatment, partly because the numbers of patients with heart failure have increased as a result of better treatment of ischemic heart disease and myocardial infarction.[17]Of all patients receiving Medicare, those with heart failure constitute the largest group and more Medicare dollars are spent for the diagnosis and treatment of heart failure than for any other diagnosis. Estimates of the crude incidence of heart failure in the general population in developed countries range from 1 to 5 cases per 1000 per year, with a crude prevalence ranging from 3 to 20 per 1000.[14] Coronary artery disease is the most common cause of heart failure, follow by hypertension, which frequently coexists with coronary artery disease.[18]

Most of the published data on the population features of heart failure is based on work in white populations within developed nations, but some data are available from developing countries. It is possible that heart failure would have a greater effect on the health care systems in those countries, in view of the enhanced awareness about CVD. This chapter draws this information together to provide a better sense of the epidemiology of heart failure in developing countries.

Méndez and Cowie[19] were unable to find population-based studies of heart failure in developing countries. All the published studies were case series, hospital-based studies, or national surveys of hospitalized patients with the diagnosis of heart failure. The lack of truly population-based studies is presumably related to the difficulty of conducting community epidemiological studies of heart failure. However, the information published does enable very interesting comparisons between different areas within developing countries and between those countries and developed nations.

AFRICA

CVD is increasingly recognized as a significant cause of morbidity and mortality in most African countries, including sub-Saharan Africa, where it accounts for almost 10% of all medical admissions.[20,21] Sub-Saharan Africa is the only world region where CVD is not the leading cause of death; high mortality rates there are secondary to infectious and nutritional diseases.[2,11]

Cardiomyopathy in Africa has been endemic since the 1940s, primarily in the forms of dilated cardiomyopathy and endomyocardial fibrosis. Dilated cardiomyopathy accounts for 10% to 17% of the diagnoses made in autopsy studies were of patients with heart failure and for 17% to 48% of diagnoses in all patients hospitalized for heart failure.[22] Dilated cardiomyopathy is found in all ages groups and in all regions of Africa; endomyocardial fibrosis, in contrast, is a disease of children and young adults that is confined to tropical and equatorial regions of Africa.[22]

Most cases of dilated cardiomyopathy have been classified as idiopathic; however, the role of infection and myocarditis in the pathogenesis of dilated cardiomyopathy in Africans has revealed striking regional variation. In Nigeria, infection with *Toxoplasma gondii* and coxsackievirus B is thought to play a major role in the pathogenesis of dilated cardiomyopathy. In Kenya,

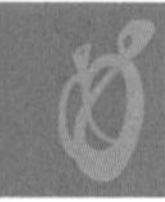

in contrast, where up to 50% of the cases reported manifest histological signs of myocarditis, no serological evidence of a previous or recent coxsackievirus B infection or other viral infection has been found.[23] In general, it seems that in the African population, the main combination of genetic and environmental factors is present to produce the development of dilated cardiomyopathy and endomyocardial fibrosis.

In 1966, Parry,[23a] in Addis Ababa, Ethiopia, described the main causes of heart failure in young Africans on the basis of clinical symptoms and autopsy studies. He stated that the two most common causes of heart failure in the young adult African were "African cardiomyopathy" (dilated cardiomyopathy) or mitral stenosis resulting from rheumatic heart disease. Other causes of cardiomyopathy have been described in different geographical regions in Africa: for example, left ventricular endomyocardial fibrosis was common in Uganda (especially in a Rwandan-Burundian ethnic group), Zaire, Ghana, and the West Coast Africa but uncommon in Kenya and Tanzania.[24,25] The presence of hypertensive heart failure, peripartum cardiomyopathy, and annular subvalvular aneurysm of the left ventricle were also mentioned, but no exact frequencies were specified.

In a hospital series of 315 patients admitted to the Katsina Hospital in the northern part of Nigeria with the diagnosis of heart failure, 7% of all admissions were medical and pediatric.[26] The cause was determined by clinical assessment and without echocardiography or coronary angiography. In almost half of the patients, the diagnosis was cardiomyopathy, with a congestive pattern in 60% of the cases. Peripartum cardiomyopathy was the main diagnosis in women, which accounted for 29% of all cases of heart failure in women and 16% of all cases in all patients. All of the cases occurred in Hausa women who lived in the Northern part of Nigeria. In contrast, in the southern part of Nigeria, heart failure resulting from peripartum cardiomyopathy was rare (2% of cases); hypertension represented 35% of cases and endomyocardial fibrosis, 17% of cases.

Recently, Stewart and associates published their findings in the Heart of Soweto Study,[27] in which all of the 1960 patients admitted to the Chris Hani Baragwanath Hospital in the township of Soweto with the diagnosis of heart failure underwent diagnostic echocardiography. The probable cause was established by two independent cardiologists. Patients with heart failure had a mean age of 55 years and were predominantly women (57%) and black Africans (88%). The most common diagnoses were hypertensive heart failure (33%), idiopathic dilated cardiomyopathy (28%), and right-sided heart failure (27%); ischemic cardiomyopathy was diagnosed far less often (12%). In another study from Uniben Hospital in Benin City, hypertensive heart failure also was the main cause in 55 patients hospitalized with the diagnosis of heart failure.[28]

In developing areas of the world, acute rheumatic fever and rheumatic heart disease are estimated to affect nearly 20 million people and are the leading causes of cardiovascular death during the first five decades of life.[29] Rheumatic heart disease accounts for 10% of all patients hospitalized with heart failure in Nigeria.[26] Oyoo and Ogola[21] published a hospital-based study of heart failure in 91 patients admitted to the Kenyatta National Hospital in Nairobi, Kenya. Congestive heart failure accounted for 3% of all medical admissions. The main cause of heart failure was rheumatic heart disease (32%); this, dilated cardiomyopathy (25%), and hypertensive heart disease (17%) constituted the majority of causes of admissions for heart failure. The incidence of rheumatic heart disease is known to be very high in Africa; estimates range from fewer than 1 to more than 15 per 1000 per year, representing 30% of all hospital admissions for CVD in Africa.[20,30]

In 2008, Kengne and associates[31] established that even in sub-Saharan Africa, heart failure accounts for more than 30% of all hospital admissions in specialized cardiac units and that in this population, approximately 11% of all patients with heart failure had type 2 diabetes. As a result of the increase in the prevalence of diabetes, this disease has emerged as a major comorbid condition or cause.

CENTRAL AND SOUTH AMERICA

Since 1970, Central and South American countries have undergone profound changes in demographic, sociocultural, and epidemiological profiles. Therefore, it is likely that deaths secondary to noncommunicable diseases exceed deaths from communicable diseases for the first time. The change has been swift: The proportion of annual deaths from CVDs has increased from 20% to 27% since 1980.[32] CVD is now the leading cause of death in 31 of the 35 countries in Central and South America that report mortality statistics.[32]

The National Register of Heart Failure in Chile[33] reported 372 patients admitted with the diagnosis of heart failure to 14 hospitals across all nation. The mean age was 69 years, and 59% were men. The major causes were hypertension (35%), ischemic heart disease (32%), valvular heart disease (15%), and idiopathic dilated cardiomyopathy (7%). Patients' medical histories included hypertension (69%), type 2 diabetes (35%), myocardial infarction (22%), and atrial fibrillation (28%). Ejection fraction was less than 40% in 69% of the patients. The mean hospital stay was 11 days, and the in-hospital mortality rate was 5%. In the analysis of patients admitted to the hospital with the diagnosis of heart failure, the same register reported that preserved ejection fraction was defined as exceeding 50%. In these patients, the mean age was 66 years, and 73% were women. The major comorbid conditions were hypertension (76%) and atrial fibrillation (62%). The main limitation of this register is that it did not provide information about the procedure used to identify the main causes, and length of hospital stay varied widely, with no report of mortality from heart failure.

In Argentina in 1999, Amarilla and associates[34] reported a survey of 751 patients admitted with the diagnosis of heart failure to 31 hospitals nationwide. The main causes were ischemic heart disease (30%), hypertension (21%), valvular heart disease (17%), dilated cardiomyopathy (14%), and Chagas' disease (3%). In 2004, Macin and colleagues[35] reported the analysis of 192 patients admitted to the Institute of Cardiology of Corrientes, Argentina, with the diagnosis of heart failure. Of these patients, 73% were male, and the mean age was 65 years. The main causes were ischemic heart disease (45%), hypertension (26%), and valvular heart disease (10%). The mortality rate over 10 months was 39%.

In Mexico, the author and colleagues published the efficacy of a heart failure clinic in the improvement of quality of life of patients with heart failure in a tertiary hospital in Veracruz, Mexico.[36] The main causes were ischemic heart disease (47%) and idiopathic dilated cardiomyopathy (44%). The cause was evaluated by two cardiologists, and in all patients, coronary angiography was performed. The mortality rate at 6 months was 12% (95% confidence interval, 2% to 22%).

In Brazil in 2002, there were 372,604 hospital admissions with a mortality rate of 7%, which represented 3% of all hospital admissions.[37] In 2008, Mangini and associates[38] published an analysis of 212 patients with a diagnosis of decompensated heart failure who were admitted to an emergency department of the Heart Institute (InCor) in Sao Paulo, Brazil. Of these patients, 56% were male, and the mean age was 60 years. The main causes were ischemic heart disease (29%), hypertension (21%), valvular heart disease (15%), and Chagas' disease–related cardiomyopathy (15%). The in-hospital mortality rate was 10%. In 2006, Braga and colleagues[39] reported on a series of 356 patients referred for management of heart failure to the Clinic of the Federal University of Bahia,

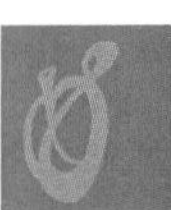

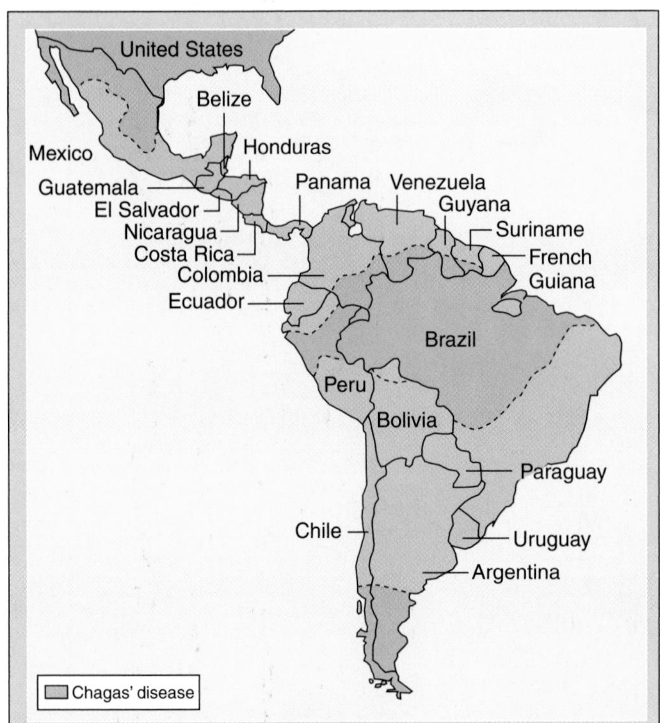

FIGURE 33-1 Distribution of Chagas' disease in Central and South America. (Modified from Acquatella H: Chagas' disease. In Abelmann WH, Braunwald E, editors. *Atlas of heart disease. Cardiomyopathies, myocarditis, and pericardial disease,* Philadelphia, 1995, Current Medicine, pp 8.1-8.18; and Liu PP, Schultheiss HP. Myocarditis. In Libby P, Bonow RO, Mann DL, et al, editors. *Braunwald's heart disease,* Philadelphia, 2008, Elsevier, pp 1779.)

Brazil. Of these patients, 53% were male, and the mean age was 54 years. The main causes were Chagas' disease–related cardiomyopathy (48%), hypertension (19%), idiopathic dilated cardiomyopathy (11%), ischemic cardiomyopathy (9%), and valvular heart disease (3%). In previous studies in Brazil,[40] investigators reported causes such as ischemic heart disease (33%), dilated cardiomyopathy (26%), valvular heart disease (22%), and Chagas' disease–related cardiomyopathy (6%). All these investigators acknowledged a high prevalence of Chagas' disease in that it is an endemic cause of dilated cardiomyopathy in this part of the world, with geographical variation within the same country (Figure 33-1).

Chagas' disease[41] is caused by a single-celled flagellate (*Trypanosoma cruzi*) that is transmitted by arthropods. The disease occurs mainly in Latin America, and the resulting cardiac problems are the main cause of morbidity and mortality (Figure 33-2). Accordingly to estimates, the prevalence of *T. cruzi* infestation in Latin American immigrants is 16 per 1000 in Australia, 9 per 1000 in Canada, 25 per 1000 in Spain, and 8 to 50 per 1000 in the United States. The transmission of Chagas' disease is no longer confined to the Americas because it can be transmitted through blood transfusions and organ transplantation. The rate of mortality is higher among patients with Chagas' disease–related cardiomyopathy than among patients with other types of cardiomyopathy; the most common causes of death are fatal arrhythmias, progressive heart failure, and brain embolism. Cases of Chagas' disease have been reported from all over Latin America (Argentina to Mexico).[42,43]

ASIA

Since 2000, CVD has become the leading cause of death in many Asian countries, such as China,[44] India,[45] Singapore,[46] and Turkey.[47]

Hung and co-authors[48] described a 1997 retrospective study, with a 1-year follow-up period, about the epidemiology of heart failure from 11 hospitals of the Hospital Authority, Hong Kong. All patients admitted with a primary diagnosis of heart failure were identified. Of the cases of heart failure, 4589 (74%) were new and 1614 (26%) were old cases. Of the patients, 56% were female, and the mean age was 77 years. This is the first study in Asia in which incidence and prevalence of heart failure were reported. The incidence of heart failure was 0.7 per 1000 population. The incidences were 20 per 1000 women and 14 per 1000 men older than 85 years; the prevalences among patients older than 85 years was 30 per 1000 women and 20 per 1000 men, and the 1-year mortality rate was 32%. The main limitation of this study was that it provided no information about cause or whether heart failure was systolic or diastolic.

In an early (1999) study from the Prince of Wales Hospital, Hong Kong, Yip and associates[49] showed that the main causes of heart failure were hypertension (50%), coronary artery disease (35%), dilated cardiomyopathy (10%), type 2 diabetes (30%), and rheumatic heart disease (12%); in many patients, more than one factor was implicated. Of patients with coronary artery disease, 69% had hypertension, and of hypertensive patients, 48% had coronary artery disease.

Joshi and coworkers[50] published an analysis of 125 consecutive patients admitted to the Government Medical College in Nagpur, India, with the clinical diagnosis of heart failure. The main causes were rheumatic heart disease (52%) and ischemia or hypertensive heart disease or both (27%). A similar statistic could be found in neighborhood countries; for example, in Pakistan, the current situation regarding rheumatic fever and rheumatic heart disease was almost the same as in India.[51]

In Singapore,[46] congestive heart failure accounted for 4.5% of all hospital admissions and 2.5% of overall mortality in the population aged 65 years and older. A total of 15,774 hospital admissions were identified between 1991 to 1998; cardiovascular deaths occurred in 5.6%. Although analysis of cause was not conducted in all cases, it seems that as a result of the increasing survival of patients with myocardial infarction, ischemic heart disease could be the main cause of heart failure in this country.

Because of their unique geographical situation, Israel and Turkey have showed specific patterns of heart failure. In 2003,[52] the National Heart Failure Survey in Israel reported on 4102 consecutive patients admitted to the 25 public hospital nationwide. Of these patients, 57% were male, and the mean age was 73 years. The most frequent comorbid conditions were coronary artery disease (82%), hypertension (75%), type 2 diabetes (50%), and atrial fibrillation (33%). The in-hospital and 30 day mortality were 5% and 8% respectively. At one year, the mortality rate was 28%. In Turkey,[47] a survey of 16 academic hospitals included 661 consecutive cases of patients admitted with the diagnosis of heart failure. Of these patients, 63% were male, and the mean age was 61 years. Ischemic heart disease was the main cause, followed by hypertension and rheumatic heart disease.

CONCLUSIONS AND FUTURE DIRECTIONS

Heart failure has imposed a high burden on the health care systems in developed countries since 1980. It is becoming increasingly apparent that the same burden will be reproduced in developing nations as a result of their epidemiological transition. As shown in Figure 33-3, the causes of heart failure in developing countries vary by continent. Unfortunately, there is a dearth of information about how the epidemiological patterns of heart failure are changing in such nations. Moreover, no proper population epidemiological

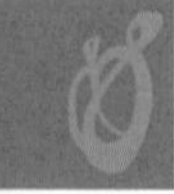

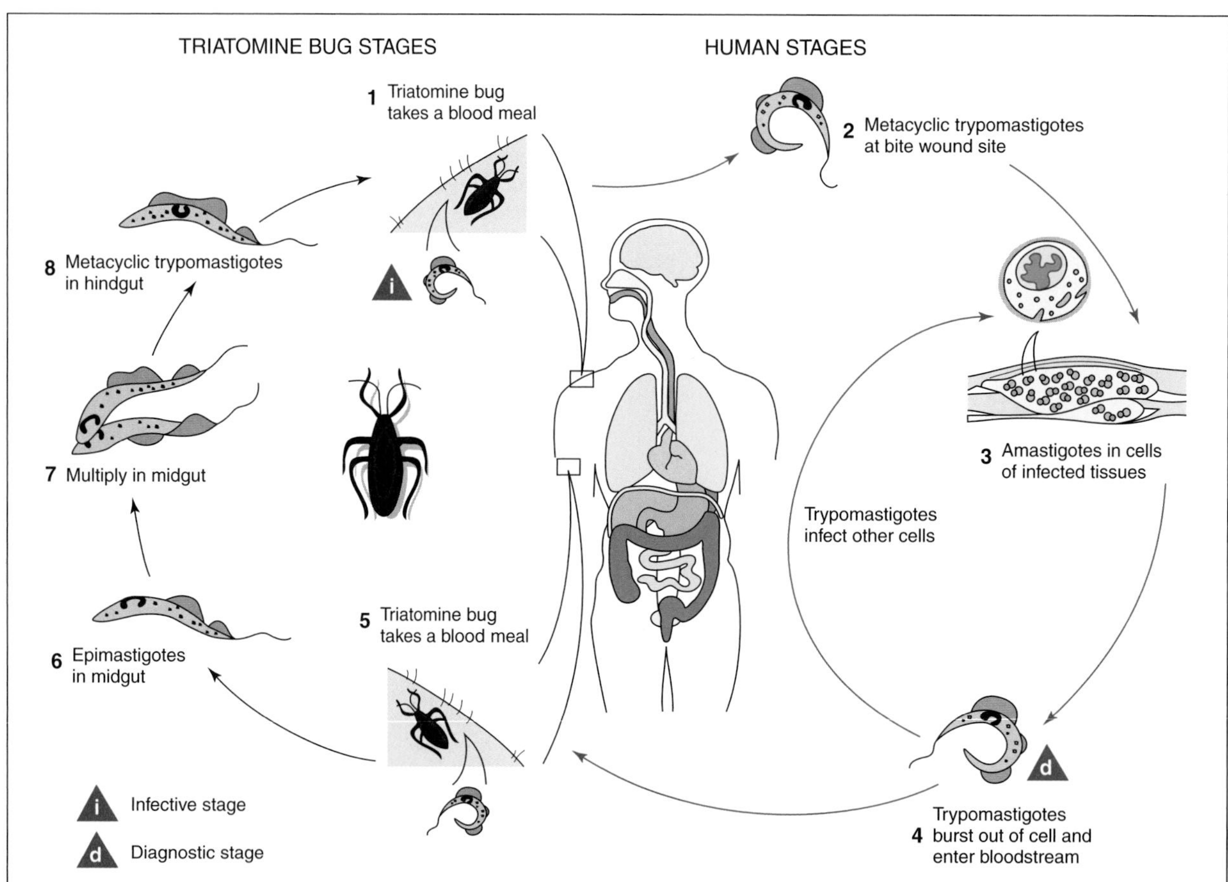

FIGURE 33–2 Life cycle of American trypanosome, which causes Chagas' disease. The trypomastigote stage of American trypanosomes is an invasive but nonreplicative form that enters several different cell types; in those cells, the parasite develops into a replicative amastigote form, some of which develop further into invasive trypomastigotes in dying host cells. (1) In taking a blood meal, the triatomine bug passes metacyclic trypomastigotes in its feces; trypomastigotes enter the bite wound or mucosal membranes, such as the conjunctiva. (2) Metacyclic trypomastigotes penetrate various cells at the bite wound site. Inside cells, they transform into amastigotes. (3) Amastigotes multiply by binary fission in cells of infected tissues. Trypomastigotes can infect other cells and transform into intracellular amastigotes in new infection sites. Clinical manifestations can result during this infective stage. (4) Intracellular amastigotes transform into trypomastigotes and then burst out of the cell and enter the bloodstream. (5) The triatomine bug takes a blood meal from the human host, and trypomastigotes are ingested. (6) Epimastigotes develop in the midgut of the triatomine bug. (7) Epimastigotes multiply in the midgut and are transformed into metacyclic trypomastigotes. (8) Metacyclic trypomastigotes move to the bug's hindgut and are passed in feces. (From Blum JA, Zellweger MJ, Burri C, et al. Cardiac involvement in African and American trypanosomiasis. *Lancet Infect Dis* 2008;8:631-641.)

studies have been performed to clarify the changing patterns. Such studies are important from more than only the academic point of view; they would be of value for health policy makers. Up to now, published data are chiefly from hospital-based series and national registers that are subject to selection bias (which may be substantial). Objective confirmation of the clinical diagnosis of heart failure is often lacking; the use of echocardiography and coronary angiography is confined to reports dating only as recently as 2000 from relatively wealthy countries. The determination of cause is another limitation in such studies and is also open to criticism, and any conclusion must be tempered with a considerable degree of caution. Table 33-1 summarizes the available data on the relative importance of the different causes of heart failure. Properly conducted population-based studies in these countries are urgently needed to establish the true size of the problem and the relative importance of the different causes. Preventive and public health strategies must rely on the specific information obtained from such studies.

In terms of future directions, proper population-based studies on the epidemiological patterns of heart failure must be conducted in developing countries to understand the effects of heart failure in those populations, with special emphasis in the incidence, prevalence, and etiological determinants. The medical community and general population must acknowledge public information about the principal risk factors for the development of heart failure; the main purpose is to tackle the future increase of heart failure in these countries. Finally, developed countries should collaborate with their expertise and economic resources to obtain adequate information about the epidemiological patterns of heart failure in developing economies. Such information will be useful for establishing preventive and public health strategies to diminish the effects of heart failure in those countries.

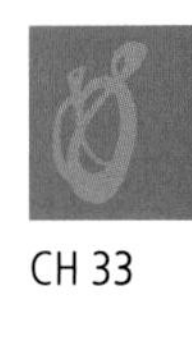

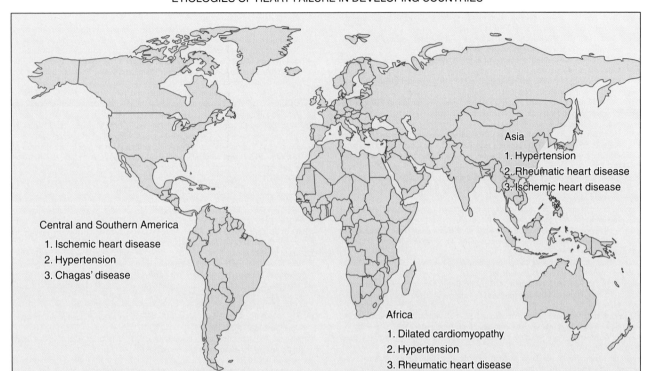

FIGURE 33–3 Causes of heart failure in developing countries.

TABLE 33–1 The Relative Importance of the Different Causes of Heart Failure in the Published Literature

	Cause (%)						
Africa	**DCM**	**HT**	**IHD**	**RHD**	**EMF**	**PPCM**	**Chagas' Disease**
Soweto[27]	28	33	9	8	NR	4	NR
Northern Nigeria[26]	31	11	0	13	0	16	NR
Southern Nigeria[26]	9	35	3	10	17	2	NR
Kenya[21]	25	17	2	32	NR	NR	NR
Central and South America	**DCM**	**HT**	**IHD**	**VHD**	**EMF**	**PPCM**	**Chagas' Disease**
Chile[33]	7	35	32	15	NR	NR	NR
Argentina[34]	14	21	30	17	1	NR	3
Argentina[35]	NR	36	45	10	NR	NR	NR
Mexico[36]	44	NR	47	NR	NR	NR	NR
Brazil[38]	8	21	29	15	NR	NR	15
Brazil[39]	11	19	9	3	NR	NR	48
Brazil[40]	26	7	33	22	NR	NR	6
Asia	**DCM**	**HT**	**IHD**	**RHD**	**DM**	**PPCM**	**Chagas' Disease**
Hong Kong[48]	10	50	35	12	30	NR	NR
India[50]	NR	**27 combined**		52	NR	NR	NR

Please see text for interpretation of data.

DCM, dilated cardiomyopathy; DM, diabetes mellitus; EMF, endomyocardial fibrosis; HT, hypertension; IHD, ischemic heart disease; PPCM, peripartum cardiomyopathy; NR, not reported; RHD, rheumatic heart disease; VHD, valvular heart disease.

REFERENCES

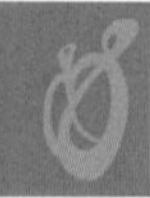

1. Omram, A. R. (1971). The epidemiologic transition: a theory of epidemiology of population change. *Milbank Memorial Fund Q, 49*, 509–538.
2. Pearson, T. A. (1999). Cardiovascular disease in developing countries: myths, realities, and opportunities. *Cardiovasc Drugs Ther, 13*, 95–104.
3. Lopez, A. D. (1993). Assessing the burden of mortality from cardiovascular diseases. *World Health Stat Q, 46*, 91–96.
4. Reddy, K. S., & Yusuf, S. (1998). Emerging epidemic of cardiovascular disease in developing countries. *Circulation, 97*, 596–601.
5. Howson, C. P., Reddy, K. S., Ryan, T. J., et al. (1998). *Control of cardiovascular diseases in developing countries. Research, development and institutional strengthening* (ed 1). Washington, DC: National Academy Press.
6. Unal, B., Critchley, J. A., & Capewell, S. (2004). Explaining the decline in coronary heart disease mortality in England and Wales between 1981 and 2000. *Circulation, 109*, 1101–1107.
7. Beaglehole, R. (1992). Cardiovascular disease in developing countries. *BMJ, 305*, 1170–1171.
8. Miranda, J. J., Kinra, S., Casas, J. P., et al. (2008). Non-communicable diseases in low- and middle-income countries: context, determinants and health policy. *Trop Med Int Health, 13*, 1225–1234.
9. Boutayeb, A., & Boutayeb, S. (2005). The burden of non communicable diseases in developing countries. *Int J Equity Health, 4*, 2.
10. Leeder, S., Raymond, S., Greenberg, H., et al. (2004). *A race against time. The challenge of cardiovascular disease in developing economies* (ed 1). New York: Trustees of Columbia University.
11. Gaziano, T. A. (2007). Reducing the growing burden of cardiovascular disease in the developing world. *Health Aff (Millwood), 26*, 13–24.
12. Gaziano, T. A., Opie, L. H., & Weinstein, M. C. (2006). Cardiovascular disease prevention with a multidrug regimen in the developing world: a cost-effectiveness analysis. *Lancet, 368*, 679–686.
13. McMurray, J. J. V., McDonagh, T. A., Morrison, C. E., et al. (1993). Trends in hospitalisation for heart failure in Scotland 1980-1990. *Eur Heart J, 14*, 1158–1162.
14. Cowie, M. R., Mosterd, A., Wood, D. A., et al. (1997). The epidemiology of heart failure. *Eur Heart J, 18*, 208–225.
15. Stewart, S., MacIntyre, K., MacLeod, M. M. C., et al. (2001). Trends in hospitalization for heart failure in Scotland 1990-1996. An epidemic that has reached its peak?. *Eur Heart J, 22*, 209–217.
16. McMurray, J. J. V., & Stewart, S. (2000). Epidemiology, aetiology, and prognosis of heart failure. *Heart, 83*, 596–602.
17. Hunt, S. A., Abraham, W. T., Chin, M. H., et al. (2005). ACC/AHA 2005 guideline update for the diagnosis and management of chronic heart failure in the adult: a report of the American College of Cardiology/American Heart Association Task Force on Practice Guidelines (Writing Committee to Update the 2001 Guidelines for the Evaluation and Management of Heart Failure): developed in collaboration with the American College of Chest Physicians and the International Society for Heart and Lung Transplantation: endorsed by the Heart Rhythm Society. *Circulation, 112*, 154–235.
18. Cowie, M. R. (1999). Annotated references in epidemiology. *Eur J Heart Fail, 1*, 101–107.
19. Méndez, G. F., & Cowie, M. R. (2001). The epidemiological features of heart failure in developing countries: a review of the literature. *Int J Cardiol, 80*, 213–219.
20. Muna, W. F. T. (1993). Cardiovascular disorders in Africa. *World Health Stat Q, 46*, 125–133.
21. Oyoo, G. O., & Ogola, E. N. (1999). Clinical and socio demographic aspects of congestive heart failure patients at Kenyatta National Hospital, Nairobi. *East Afr Med J, 76*, 23–27.
22. Mayosi, B. M., & Somers, K. (2007). Cardiomyopathy in Africa: heredity versus environment. *Cardiovasc J Afr, 18*, 175–179.
23. Sliwa, K., Damasceno, A., & Mayosi, B. M. (2005). Epidemiology and etiology of cardiomyopathy in Africa. *Circulation, 112*, 3577–3583.

23a. Parry, E. H. O. (1996). Diagnosis and management of heart failure in the young adult African. *B M J*, 1966; 2:1119–1122.

24. Hutt, M. S. R. (1983). Epidemiology aspects of endomyocardial fibrosis. *Postgrad Med J, 59*, 142–144.
25. Davies, J. N. P., & Coles, R. M. (1960). Some considerations regarding obscure diseases affecting the mural endocardium. *Am Heart J, 59*, 600–631.
26. Antony, K. K. (1980). Pattern of cardiac failure in Northern Savanna Nigeria. *Trop Geogr Med, 32*, 118–125.
27. Stewart, S., Wilkinson, D., Hansen, C., et al. (2008). Predominance of heart failure in the Heart of Soweto Study cohort. Emerging challenges for Urban African Communities. *Circulation, 118*, 2360–2367.
28. Obasohan, A. O., & Ajuyah, C. O. (1996). How common is heart failure due to systemic hypertension alone in hospitalised Nigerians?. *J Hum Hypertens, 10*, 801–804.
29. Gerber, M. A., Baltimore, R. S., Eaton, C. B., et al. (2009). Prevention of rheumatic fever and diagnosis and treatment of acute streptococcal pharyngitis: a scientific statement from the American Heart Association Rheumatic Fever, Endocarditis, and Kawasaki Disease Committee of the Council on Cardiovascular Disease in the Young, the Interdisciplinary Council on Functional Genomics and Translational Biology, and the Interdisciplinary Council on Quality of Care and Outcomes Research: endorsed by the American Academy of Pediatrics. *Circulation, 119*, 1541–1551.
30. World Health Organization. (2000). *The world health report 2000—health systems: improving performance*. Geneva, Switzerland: World Health Organization.
31. Kengne, A. P., Dzudie, A., & Sobngwi, E. (2008). Heart failure in sub-Saharan Africa: a literature review with emphasis on individuals with diabetes. *Vasc Health Risk Manag, 4*, 123–130.
32. Nicholls, E. S., Peruga, A. P., & Restrepo, H. E. (1993). Cardiovascular disease mortality in the Americas. *World Health Stat Q, 46*, 134–150.
33. Castro, P., Vukasovic, J. L., Garces, S. E., et al. (2004). Cardiac failure in Chilean hospitals: results of the National Registry of Heart Failure, ICARO. *Rev Med Chile, 132*, 655–662.
34. Amarilla, G. A., Carballido, R., Tacchi, C. D., et al. (1999). National Survey of Chronic Heart Failure in Argentina. Variables in related to in-hospital mortality rate (preliminary results CONAREC VI). *Rev Argent Cardiol, 67*, 53–62.
35. Macin, S. M., Perna, E. R., Canella, J. P. C., et al. (2004). Differences in clinical profile and outcome in patients with decompensated heart failure and systolic dysfunction or preserved systolic function. *Rev Esp Cardiol, 57*, 45–52.
36. Méndez, G. F., Betancourt, L., & Galicia-Mora, G. (2007). The impact of heart failure clinic in the improvement on the quality of life of heart failure patients in Mexico. *Int J Cardiol, 115*, 242–243.
37. Albanesi-Filho, F. M. (2005). What is the current scenario for heart failure in Brazil?. *Arq Bras Cardiol, 85*, 155–156.
38. Mangini, S., Sierra Silveira, F., Pereira Silva, C., et al. (2008). Decompensated heart failure in the emergency department of a cardiology hospital. *Arq Bras Cardiol, 90*, 400–406.
39. Braga, J. C., Reis, F., Aras, R., et al. (2006). [Clinical and therapeutic aspects of heart failure due to Chagas disease.]. *Arq Bras Cardiol, 86*, 297–302.
40. Pereira, A. C., Cuce, M. R., Wajngarten, M., et al. (1998). Heart failure in a large tertiary hospital of São Paulo. *Arq Bras Cardiol, 71*, 15–20.
41. Blum, J. A., Zellweger, M., Burri, C., et al. (2008). Cardiac involvement in African and American trypanosomiasis. *Lancet Infect Dis, 8*, 631–641.
42. Marin-Nieto, J. A., Cunha-Neto, E., Maciel, B. C., et al. (2007). Pathogenesis of chronic Chagas heart disease. *Circulation, 115*, 1109–1123.
43. Sierra-Johnson, J., Olivera-Mar, A., Monteon-Padilla, V. M., et al. (2005). Epidemiological and clinical outlook of chronic Chagas' heart disease in Mexico. *Rev Saude Publica, 39*, 754–760.
44. Chonghua, Y., Zhaosu, W., & Yingkai, W. (1993). The changing pattern of cardiovascular diseases in China. *World Health Stat Q, 46*, 113–118.
45. Reddy, K. S. (1993). Cardiovascular diseases in India. *World Health Stat Q, 46*, 101–107.
46. Ng, T. P., & Niti, M. (2003). Trends and ethnic differences in hospital admissions and mortality for congestive heart failure in the elderly on Singapore, 1991 to 1998. *Heart, 89*, 865–870.
47. Ergin, A., Eryol, N. K., Unal, S., et al. (2004). Epidemiological and pharmacological profile of congestive heart failure at Turkish academic hospitals. *Anadolu Kardiyol Derg, 4*, 32–38.
48. Hung, Y. T., Cheung, N. T., Ip, S., et al. (2000). Epidemiology of heart failure in Hong Kong, 1997. *Hong Kong Med J, 6*, 159–162.
49. Yip, G. W. K., Ho, P. P. Y., Woo, K. S., et al. (1999). Comparison of frequencies of left ventricular systolic and diastolic heart failure in Chinese living in Hong Kong. *Am J Cardiol, 84*, 563–567.
50. Joshi, P. P., Mohanan, C. J., Sengupta, S. P., et al. (1999). Factors precipitating congestive heart failure—role of patient non-compliance. *J Assoc Physicians India, 47*, 294–295.
51. Kaplan, E. L. (2004). Rheumatic heart disease in rural Pakistan. *Heart, 90*, 361–362.
52. Garty, M., Shotan, A., Gottlieb, S., et al. (2007). The management, early and one year outcome in hospitalized patients with heart failure: a national Heart Failure Survey in Israel—HFSIS 2003. *Isr Med Assoc J, 9*, 227–233.

CHAPTER 34

The Prognosis of Heart Failure

James B. Young

In a heart failure clinic, a response to the leading question "What brings you in to see us today?" is often "My doctor told me I have only 6 months to live and I must get a heart transplant." Most patients come with family, loved ones, or concerned friends and companions. All are anxious and frightened, sometimes to the point of being terrified. This type of encounter is not solely relegated to the heart failure clinic, of course, and the challenge of determining prognosis in any patient is extraordinary and a grave responsibility. The manner in which a clinician determines likelihood of outcomes, particularly major morbid events, and communicates this information to patients and their attendants, is crucial in long-term management. After all, this information might be life-altering in many patients with serious disease. An accurate prognosis of favorable outcomes that dispels misinformation that suggests imminent bad events is, of course, invaluable therapy for many patients who had been incorrectly informed that they were to die soon. Caregivers' tasks are to make patients feel better, cure disease when possible, and prevent or attenuate progression to more substantive difficulties. An accurate prognosis is, therefore, essential in designing treatment protocols and judging therapeutic risks and benefits of any intervention to achieve these goals.

The results of the Framingham Heart Study suggested that, over a lifetime, the average resident of Framingham, Massachusetts, had a 20% risk of developing congestive heart failure (see Chapter 22).[1] As a result, innumerable patients have come for evaluation and asked clinicians to determine their prognosis. Box 34-1 lists several issues important to pursue in prognosticating for the patient with heart failure. This turns out to be a difficult task because no single factor seems the best and most powerful prognosticator.[2-4] It is clearly important to determine whether a patient's symptoms or clinical findings are indeed related to heart failure. Prognosis is dependent on the clinician's having made a correct diagnosis. The cause of the difficulty and identification of events precipitating the patient's presentation affect prognosis and must be enumerated. The nuances of cardiac pump performance, such as presence of diastolic or systolic left ventricular dysfunction, are also critical in predicting outcomes. Obviously, acute and chronic therapeutic interventions, such as treatment with β-blockers or defibrillators, can alter prognosis and must be considered. Guidelines for the evaluation and management of chronic heart failure in the adult are now in use and endorsed by many professional societies.[5-7] All emphasize the importance of treating patients with evidence-based strategies that are based on the severity of disease at presentation and long-term prognosis. End-of-life considerations are an important focus of these guidelines as well, and prognosis is a prime driver in the identification of patients who should be guided toward the hospice and palliative care environment.[8]

Box 34-2 is a compendium of clinical variables that influence outcomes in patients with heart failure who have participated in clinical trials and registries.[2,3] Once symptomatic heart failure develops, the outlook for patients can be poor, with an average 5-year mortality rate as high as 75% among men and 60% among women; this prognosis is worse than those for many cancers. However, there is a high degree of variability among individual patients. The Rochester Epidemiology Project supervised by the Mayo Clinic group emphasized the adverse prognostic effect of heart failure in the study of all patients who received an initial diagnosis of congestive heart failure in Olmsted County, Minnesota, in 1991.[9,10] That year, of a population of 106,470 citizens, 216 demonstrated "new-onset congestive heart failure." Among patients with newly diagnosed heart failure, the 5-year survival rate was 35%. Of the patients in whom ejection fraction was known, 43% had preserved systolic function; in this particular cohort, the survival rate was no different than that among patients with depressed left ventricular systolic function. Further analyses of the incidence of congestive heart failure and prognosis in patients who received diagnoses in 1981, in comparison with those who received diagnoses a decade later, suggested that survival rates of both groups of patients were similar. Levy and colleagues[11] from the Framingham Heart Study demonstrated that since about 1960, the incidence of heart failure has seemingly declined among women but not among men; however, survival after the syndrome onset has improved slightly but is still relatively poor among women. The 5-year mortality rate for newly diagnosed congestive heart failure in the Framingham Cohort was 70% among men who received diagnoses between 1950 and 1969 and almost 60% among men who received diagnoses between 1990 and 1999. The prognosis of heart failure can, in fact be dismal.

According to results of more recent clinical studies of patients hospitalized for all forms of decompensated heart failure, the rate of in-patient hospital mortality is about 4%, the rate of 90-day mortality after discharge is close to 9%, and about 30% of patients require rehospitalization within 90 days.[12,13] Rates of in-hospital mortality for acutely decompensated heart failure can be compared with the rate of mortality among patients with acute myocardial infarction, Killip class I without heart failure or left ventricular dysfunction. Among such patients, the current mortality rate is approximately 3%.[14]

Another contemporary analysis of outcomes was the Heart Failure—A Controlled Trial Investigating Outcomes of Exercise Training (HF-ACTION), in which, for about 30 months, researchers monitored almost 2500 patients with a mean age of 59 years, who had a median left ventricular ejection fraction of 25%, and of whom one third had New York Heart Association (NYHA) functional class III or IV symptoms; 56% were hospitalized for or died of cardiovascular problems.[14,15] Collectively, these observations emphasize the high variability in prognosis of patients with heart failure when different populations are analyzed.

BOX 34–1 Determining the Prognosis of a Patient with Heart Failure: Important Questions to Ask

- Does the patient actually have heart failure?
- What is the cause of the heart failure syndrome?
- What events precipitated presentation or clinical deterioration?
- What comorbid conditions are present?
- What are the characteristics of cardiac pump and circulatory (including pulmonary) performance?
- How compensated, decompensated, or congested is the patient?
- What acute and chronic therapeutic strategies are in place?
- What changes in therapeutic strategies can be made to alter prognosis beneficially?

The clinical variables in Box 34-2 that are related to outcome in patients with heart failure have been verified, at the least, in univariant analysis; many of them are independently significant when multifactorial analysis techniques are employed. Nonetheless, it is difficult to determine which prognostic variable is most important in predicting an individual patient's outcome either in clinical trials or during day-to-day management. This has been a persistent dilemma for decades, and it is particularly problematic when researchers try to design clinical trials in which event rates determine statistical power and size calculations.[16]

Cowburn and coworkers[17] and Lee and Packer[18] summarized peer-reviewed publications of studies containing more than 200 subjects with chronic, usually congestive, heart failure in which a multivariate analysis of prognostic factors was reported. The original report was subsequently expanded with more observations included.[2,3] The variables listed in Box 34-2 could be ranked with regard to importance and power of predicting outcomes in cohorts of patients with heart failure. In general, the highest ranking variables associated with adverse clinical outcome included hyponatremia,[18,19] The

BOX 34–2 Clinical Variables Relevant to Prognosis of Patients with Heart Failure

Demographics
Age
Gender
Race

Cause of Heart Failure
Alcohol use
Amyloidosis
Anthracycline
Coronary artery disease
Genetic factors
Hemachromatosis
Idiopathic dilated cardiomyopathy
Myocarditis
Valvular heart disease
Ventricular hypertrophy

Comorbid Conditions
Anemia
Chronic lung disease
Diabetes mellitus
Hepatic abnormalities
Hyperthyroidism or hypothyroidism
Obesity/cachexia (body mass)
Pulmonary hypertension
Renal insufficiency
Sleep apnea

Symptoms
Angina pectoris
Depression
Dyspnea syndromes
Edematous states
NYHA class
Syncope

Hemodynamics
Cardiac index
Exercise PuAP
Left ventricular ejection fraction
PCWP
PuAP
PuAP-PCWP
Right ventricular ejection fraction

Findings in Exercise Testing
Anaerobic threshold
Blood pressure response
Development of arrhythmias
Heart rate response (including recovery)
Ischemic electrocardiographic response
O_2 uptake slope
Peak/maximal V_{O_2}
Six-minute walk time
V_E/V_{CO_2}

Metabolic Findings
Acidosis or alkalosis
Azotemia
Hepatic dysfunction
Serum sodium level

Chest Radiographic Findings
Congestion
Cardiac-thoracic ratio

Electrocardiographic Findings
Heart rate variability
Width of QRS interval
QT interval
Rhythm
T-wave alternans
Voltage

Cytokines
Pro-inflammatory/antiinflammatory ratio
Sedimentation rate
TNF-α; IL-1, IL-6, IL-10

Hormones
Aldosterone
B-natriuretic peptide
Epinephrine
Norepinephrine

Endomyocardial Biopsy Findings
Degree of cellular disarray
Degree of fibrosis
Infiltrative processes
Inflammation

presence of coronary artery disease,[20-22] severely depressed left ventricular ejection fraction,[23] and elevated levels of neuro-hormones such as epinephrine, norepinephrine, plasma renin, and natriuretic peptides.[24,25] NYHA functional classification,[26] left ventricular end-systolic volume,[27,28] stroke work index,[29] persistent atrial fibrillation, left ventricular internal dimension,[28] peak oxygen consumption on metabolic exercise treadmill testing,[29,30] pulmonary capillary wedge pressure,[29] hepatic dysfunction,[31] evidence of diastolic filling abnormalities on Doppler echocardiography, hypertension, hypotension, age, and chest radiographic cardiothoracic ratio were also frequent, but less consistently present, as independent markers of adverse outcome in the population with heart failure.[2,3,18] The number of variables associated with poor outcome is dizzying. In general, patients who have the greatest perturbation of cardiac and circulatory systems had the poorest outcomes. This is not surprising. Fairly consistent was the fact that patients with coronary artery disease seemed to have worse prognoses; another trend, although not as consistent, was that patients with systolic left ventricular dysfunction had adverse outcomes more often than did patients with congestive heart failure but reasonably normal ejection fraction. Gender is a controversial issue with regard to prognosis; some reports have suggested that women have worse outcomes, whereas others have indicated that being male is predictive of greater morbidity.[32,33]

The observation that few variables are consistently predictive of adverse outcome is disturbing, and this makes clinicians' conversations with patients more difficult. Indeed, clinicians must realize that heart failure is an extraordinarily complicated and heterogeneous syndrome. Box 34-3 summarizes the variability that exists in identifying specific parameters that are consistently predictive of morbid events. The power of any population-based multivariable analysis to identify factors depends on sample size: Larger clinical cohorts with diverse representation are more likely to reveal factors predictive of adverse outcomes. Heterogeneity of observations also results from the fact that demographics (age, gender, race, and heart failure cause) are highly variable. For example, when attempting to identify adverse prognostic factors in the setting of heart failure with coronary artery disease, researchers must not contaminate the population with individuals who do not have this diagnosis. However, this happens in many clinical trials. An adverse prognostic variable for an individual with idiopathic dilated cardiomyopathy is quite different from that for patients with hypertension and heart failure caused primarily by diastolic dysfunction.[12]

The varying stages of presentation of heart failure also probably affect the ability to identify adverse outcomes. For example, an individual presenting with new-onset and untreated heart failure probably has adverse prognostic variables that are different from those in a stable patient who does not have congestion and has been taking a β-blocker and an angiotensin-converting enzyme (ACE) inhibitor for many years.[12,13] The presence of a defibrillator or cardiac resynchronization device can have an even more extraordinary effect and improve outcomes when used according to guidelines in specific populations.[5] The time at which information is obtained is highly variable in reports. For example, some studies have relied on initial hemodynamic characterization of patients, which usually occurs at a time when congestive states are at their worst; pulmonary capillary wedge pressure may be more or less important at hospital admission than at discharge. Similarly, determination of exercise tolerance and, in particular, measurement of peak oxygen consumption are complicated by this issue. Many patients can improve their exercise capacity and hemodynamics with aggressive therapeutics. The time the measurement is made in the course of the illness should, therefore, be critical, but little information is available about the prognostic effect of changing observations over time and during short- and long-term follow-up.[4] Furthermore, does an increase in myocardial oxygen consumption at peak exercise after treatment mean that a patient has a better prognosis? Should researchers instead determine how ill the patient is at his or her best?

BOX 34–3 Difficulties with Identification of Specific Prognostic Factors in Heart Failure Trials, Registries, and Populations

Small cohort sizes
Heterogeneity of population studied
Narrow entry criteria (bias of ascertainment)
Selective data acquisition
Variable duration of follow-up
Measurements with high variability
Variables that are often interrelated and compete in mathematical model
Flawed techniques from mathematical and statistical point of view

Particularly contentious, and noted in Box 34-3, is the fact that, for variables studied in large clinical trials, there is great ascertainment bias in the study population; in many heart failure studies, cohorts do not represent patients in community-based clinics.[1,9,10] Some trials, for example, have focused solely on male veterans, who, for the most part, are younger than cohorts identified in community settings and may represent an entirely different socioeconomic group.[34] Selective inclusion of clinical information also creates difficulties. Only when hemodynamics or exercise capacity is measured, for example, are these variables included in any multivariable analysis and have a chance of demonstrating predictive value. Many variables are interrelated and therefore, from a mathematical standpoint, compete in prognostic models, so that one or more variables are eliminated as an independent predictor of outcome. Peak oxygen consumption and treadmill exercise time or exercise hemodynamics are examples of this problem. The astuteness of clinicians and the skill of technicians determine the quality of certain testing procedures, particularly echocardiography, radionuclide ventriculography, hemodynamic measurement, and determination of peak myocardial oxygen uptake. The variables identified in compulsively performed clinical trials to determine prognosis might not have the same power when studied in a rudimentary manner during clinical practice. Introduction of therapies during patient follow-up can be variable and might also account for why different prognostic tests yield significant results in one patient but not in another. If the entry criteria for a study are narrow, bias of ascertainment can limit the power of any specific observation. For example, congestive heart failure is defined as a clinical syndrome in patients with both normal and low ejection fraction. This measure is usually an independent predictor of mortality. However, if the cohort includes only patients with ejection fractions of less than 20%, and a narrow standard deviation for this measure exists in the cohort, ejection fraction, per se, is usually not identified as an adverse prognostic factor.[16]

PROGNOSTIC VARIABLES

Demographic Variables

Race, sex, and age are frequently implicated as important variables in the determination of a patient's prognosis in the setting of heart failure. The Framingham database suggested that

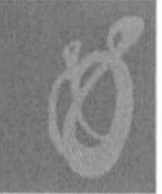

female patients have a better prognosis than do male patients and that women might have higher ejection fraction than do male counterparts with comparable symptoms, but the latter suggestion is a matter of contention (see Chapter 22).[11,26,32-35] The Studies Of Left Ventricular Dysfunction (SOLVD) demonstrated an interesting disparity when its registry database was compared with the two SOLVD clinical trials with regard to gender-related outcomes. SOLVD clinical trials excluded patients with an ejection fraction greater than 35% with the "treatment" and "prevention" programs, and the results suggested that women actually had worse outcomes than did men.[34,36,37] The SOLVD registry, however, did not require depressed left ventricular ejection fraction for entry and did not suggest that women did any worse than did their male counterparts. Also important is the fact that when heart failure is due to coronary artery disease, little difference in outcomes was noted when men were compared to women. Perhaps outcomes are more adversely affected by the cause of heart failure and other factors than by the gender of the patient.

Controversy has also arisen with regard to the effect of race on heart failure outcome. African Americans have been observed to have a worse prognosis than do white Americans. Differences in causes of heart failure, however, might once again explain some of these observations, as might socioeconomic status and access to health care. According to the SOLVD registry, coronary artery disease was a cause of heart failure syndrome in 73% of white Americans but in only 36% of African American participants.[37] Conversely, hypertension was a primary cause of chronic heart failure in 32% of African Americans in the SOLVD registry but in only 4% of the white patients. As with gender in the SOLVD registry, rates of cardiovascular-related mortality and total rates of mortality were no different when African American and white cohorts were compared, but the African American cohort was younger and had a higher proportion of women than the white cohort.

One of the more consistent and forceful predictors of adverse outcome in heart failure is age.[38,39] This seems intuitive. As has been repeatedly demonstrated, the incidence and prevalence of chronic heart failure increase with age. When studies exclude patients older than 75 years, age may not be an independent predictor of mortality, as was the case in the Vasodilator and Heart Failure Trial (V-HeFT).[40] In the older cohort of V-HeFT patients, however, the risk of death or hospital readmission for worsening congestive heart failure over a 12-month period approached 50%.

Causes of Heart Failure

Patients in whom coronary artery disease is the cause of chronic heart failure generally fare worse than do patients with dilated cardiomyopathy.[20-22] A few exceptions have been noted. In the treatment trial of SOLVD, a difference in prognosis could not be demonstrated when patients with ischemic and nonischemic heart disease were compared.[41] However, many patients who did not enter the SOLVD trial with the diagnosis of ischemic heart disease suffered subsequent myocardial infarction; therefore, just because coronary artery disease is not diagnosed at trial onset does not indicate that coronary anatomy is normal.

Valvular heart disease carries unique implications with regard to prognosis once heart failure is diagnosed (see Chapter 29).[42] For example, in a cohort of patients undergoing percutaneous coronary interventions for atherosclerotic obstructions, the presence of residual mitral regurgitation was linked to a higher rate of long-term mortality. This was particularly pronounced when left ventricular ejection fraction was less than 40%; among patients with grade 3 or 4+ mitral regurgitation, the 36-month survival rate was less than 50%.[43] When significant aortic stenosis was present and if the valve was not repaired or replaced, length of survival was only 1 or 2 years.[44] In the past, there has been reluctance to operate on patients with aortic stenosis when left ventricular systolic dysfunction was present because of the added risk of adverse surgical outcome. In patients with substantial mitral stenosis, symptoms of congestive heart failure appear frequently despite preservation of left ventricular systolic function. In aortic regurgitation, earlier and more aggressive intervention with vasodilator drugs appears to alter the clinical course.

Despite the fact that viral infections probably cause a significant number of "idiopathic" cardiomyopathies, it is difficult to demonstrate lymphocyte myocarditis on endomyocardial biopsy (see Chapter 31).[45-47] However, no survival difference was noted between patients in whom myocarditis was diagnosed by Dallas criteria at the time of endomyocardial biopsy and patients with idiopathic dilated cardiomyopathy but without this biopsy finding.[45] Anecdotal reports do suggest that patients with acute, fulminant lymphocytic myocarditis have higher mortality rates. Also, giant cell myocarditis, a difficulty of unknown origin, appears to be particularly problematic, with extremely high acute fatality rates.[47] In autopsy series of patients who died with acquired immunodeficiency syndrome (AIDS), lymphocytic myocarditis was noted frequently. In the patients with myocarditis, approximately half had had symptoms of heart failure before death. Nonetheless, endomyocardial biopsy is not routinely indicated to determine prognosis in most patients with heart failure.[5-7]

Although the assumption is under contention, peripartum cardiomyopathy (see Chapter 24) has been thought to be an autoimmune or inflammatory type of myocarditis and has several prognostic subsets. Many patients with peripartum cardiomyopathy improve within several months of diagnosis, and biopsies in those patients usually yield negative findings (myocardial tissue does not demonstrate lymphocytic infiltration).[48]

Patients with hypertrophic cardiomyopathy (see Chapter 25) have historically been particularly plagued by sudden cardiac death. Patients with nonsustained ventricular tachycardia have a higher risk of lethal events in this setting. In patients with a family history of the combination of hypertrophic cardiomyopathy and sudden cardiac death, the degree of left ventricular hypertrophy seems important with regard to predicting adverse outcome in this syndrome.[49]

Alcoholic cardiomyopathy has been suggested to be a powerful predictor of mortality in some cases (see Chapter 24). There may be a genetic predisposition to the development of cardiomyopathy with heavy alcohol use, and women, who rarely develop hepatic cirrhosis, seem less susceptible than men.[50] Of interest is that varying degrees of alcohol consumption have been noted to have a relationship to left ventricular dysfunction. In some people, even modest levels of alcohol consumption causes difficulties. Arrhythmias associated with ethanol consumption (particularly atrial fibrillation) can worsen prognosis as well.

Cardiomyopathy caused by chemotherapy for malignancy is most often related to anthracycline administration (see Chapter 58).[51] Anthracycline-related cardiomyopathy is linked to dosage and, depending on the aggressiveness of cancer treatment, can arise in 5% to 20% of patients who receive these agents. Individuals who develop acute anthracycline-related cardiomyopathy usually have very malignant courses with poor responses to general medical therapies for heart failure. This manifestation can result in death within a few months. Mild to moderate heart failure after anthracycline exposure is more heterogeneous with regard to prognosis. In these cases, it is more difficult to predict adverse outcomes, and the course of illness may be related as much to the presence of additional risk factors for cardiomyopathy, such as concomitant radiation therapy, preexisting cardiac dysfunction from hypertension or coronary artery disease, and valvular abnormalities. All things considered, patients with

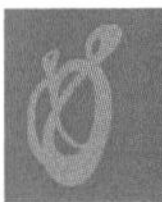

anthracycline-related cardiomyopathy appear to have worse rates of survival than do comparatively managed patients with idiopathic dilated cardiomyopathy.

Infiltrative processes that cause cardiomyopathy in heart failure, such as amyloidosis and hemachromatosis, can be diagnosed through endomyocardial biopsy. Among patients with these conditions, the actuarial survival rate is poor; response to standard therapies is generally unsatisfactory. Among patients in whom these diagnoses are made in a setting of frank congestive heart failure, it is rare to live beyond 2 years.[52]

Some forms of idiopathic dilated cardiomyopathy appear to have worse prognosis when all other factors are considered equal. Familial dilated cardiomyopathy, for example, appears to be associated with increased risk of mortality in comparison with sporadically appearing forms of idiopathic dilated cardiomyopathy. The reasons of this are unknown.[53]

Comorbid Conditions that Affect Outcome of Heart Failure

Comorbid conditions that affect the outcomes of heart failure include hypertension, diabetes mellitus, pulmonary hypertension, and renal insufficiency. Although hypertension increases the risk of developing heart failure significantly, only minimal evidence suggests that hypertension is an independent outcome risk predictor once heart failure is present. In fact, patients with lower blood pressures seem to have worse outcomes and prognosis.[23] Hypertension is certainly related to symptomatic deterioration in acutely decompensated congestive heart failure, and it prompts many visits to emergency departments and many hospital admissions.[54] Diabetes is another prominent risk factor for the development of heart failure and, interestingly, is a stronger risk factor in women than in men.[55] The combination of hypertension and diabetes seems particularly problematic; the risk of developing heart failure is quintupled. Pulmonary hypertension, whether secondary to left ventricular dysfunction or other primary pulmonary vascular problems, affects survival by causing right ventricular dysfunction with failure and precipitating malignant arrhythmias.[56] Attention has been focused on sleep apnea in heart failure because nocturnal desaturation associated with periodic respirations promotes pulmonary hypertension, right ventricular dysfunction, and worsening heart failure with increased neurohormonal levels.[57]

Renal insufficiency might result from low cardiac output and medication administration, as well as from underlying diseases such as diabetes and hypertension. Renal dysfunction can therefore be associated with worse outcomes in patients with heart failure.[58] Hepatic dysfunction can present because of worsening passive congestion of the liver. Sometimes this difficulty can be severe enough to cause cirrhosis of the liver, hence the term *cardiac cirrhosis*.[31]

Diseases that already shorten life expectancy, such as chronic obstructive pulmonary disease or metastatic malignancy, are, when combined with heart failure, associated with increased rates of mortality. However, most clinical trials and registries of patients with heart failure have excluded individuals with significant lung disease or other chronic illnesses, and so the precise effect of these diseases on ventricular dysfunction and its complications is largely unknown.

Clinical Manifestation (see Chapter 35)

Severe congestive states in the heart failure syndrome have been consistent predictors of adverse outcomes in most clinical trials. Even when extremely gross assessments of symptomatic severity (such as NYHA functional classification) are used, mortality rates appear higher in more symptomatic patients. Quality-of-life score, classification of daily activities, and motion meters have all provided some degree of prognostic information. Patients in whom depression or mood-altering disorders are diagnosed are at increased risk of death and decompensation. The presence of peripheral or pulmonary edema is associated with worse outcomes. Longer duration of symptoms is predictive of high mortality and a lower likelihood that depressed ejection fraction will improve. Syncope, whether associated with an arrhythmia or not, portends adverse outcomes, as does angina pectoris or recent myocardial infarction.

As noted, although this issue is under contention, the relationship of congestive symptoms to systolic and diastolic dysfunction may be important with regard to predicting morbid events. Congestive heart failure in individuals who have normal and near-normal ejection fraction is being observed more frequently. Sudden decompensated heart failure with acute symptoms caused by predominantly diastolic dysfunction can be seen in the setting of acute myocardial infarction or severe hypertension.

Prognosis in patients with primarily left ventricular diastolic dysfunction and a congestive state may be different than in patients with left ventricular systolic dysfunction. When clinicians try to determine outcomes in patients with diastolic dysfunction and congestive heart failure, it is more important to determine the cause of the diastolic dysfunction. Infiltrative processes such as amyloidosis and hemachromatosis cause much worse outcomes. When diastolic dysfunction complicates systolic dysfunction, chances of survival may also be worse.

Ventricular Performance and Hemodynamics

Systolic left ventricular function has been repeatedly one of the most powerful independent predictors of morbidity in patients with heart failure who enter clinical trials (see Chapter 13). In general, an ejection fraction less than 25% is predictive of major adverse outcomes in comparison with ejection fractions greater than 35%. However, left ventricular ejection fraction should be used alone only with caution to determine prognosis. Many other variables play a role. A noncongested, active, mesomorphic individual with well-controlled blood pressure and an ejection fraction of 20% can do quite well for many years by taking β-blockers and ACE inhibitors or vasodilators. Nonetheless, most practitioners rely on left ventricular ejection fraction, by one method or another, to differentiate between systolic and diastolic dysfunction and to get some idea about severity of disease and likelihood of an adverse outcome. Some information suggests that a serial yearly decrease in ejection fraction is associated with increased risk of mortality, but guidelines do not recommend regular measurement of ejection fraction in patients with heart failure. Of most importance is that clinicians not use ejection fraction exclusively to determine a patient's prognosis.

Right ventricular ejection fraction is much more difficult to determine accurately than is left ventricular ejection fraction. Nonetheless, right ventricular ejection fraction of more than 35% at rest or during exercise was associated with higher survival in patients with heart failure than was oxygen consumption at peak exercise in one study.[59]

Hemodynamics has been used to assess the severity of heart failure when heart transplantation is considered.[60] Particularly important is the presence of the degree of congestion, manifesting as high right atrial pressures and pulmonary hypertension; "irreversible" pulmonary hypertension is predictive of adverse outcome in general and after cardiac transplantation. However, resting hemodynamics have turned out not to correspond directly with symptoms, physical findings, or exercise capacity more generally. Assessing risk by resting hemodynamic profile has therefore yielded disappointing results. This seems particularly true when patients are admitted to the hospital with decompensated heart failure.[61]

The routine referral of a patient for right-sided heart hemodynamic measurement did not improve outcomes in one large multicenter clinical trial.[61] Right ventricular hemodynamics should be measured only in complicated cases in which specific details of management need to be addressed. When hemodynamic measurements have been used, however, cardiac index of less than 2 L/min/m^2 and pulmonary resistance higher than 2.5 Wood units were predictive of substantially higher mortality rates.

Exercise Testing (see also Chapter 57)

Functional status and cardiac reserve of patients with chronic heart failure can be objectively characterized by determining exercise tolerance.[29,30] Particularly important is the precise measurement of peak oxygen consumption. It has become probably the most important test to determine whether ambulatory patients are ill enough to list for cardiac transplantation.[60] Patients who have a peak oxygen uptake of less than 10 mL/kg/min at a respiratory exchange rate greater than 1.10—which suggest that the patient has reached anaerobic threshold and peak exercise capability—is associated with a 1-year mortality risk that can be as high as 77%, in comparison with 21% when the peak oxygen uptake is in the range of 10 to 18 mL/kg/min. Mancini and colleagues used this particular finding to determine optimal timing for cardiac transplantation; they suggested that patients with a peak oxygen uptake below 14 mL/kg/min were mostly likely to benefit from cardiac transplantation, and this number has become an important guideline for transplantation programs.[29,30]

Peak oxygen uptake can, however, be affected by age, gender, muscle mass, aerobic conditioning, and medication therapy. Thus, some individuals with peak oxygen uptake of less than 14 mL/kg/min do well despite the presence of significant left ventricular dysfunction. Some authors have used percentage of predictive peak oxygen uptake rather than the absolute value to stratify risk. In multivariate analysis, 50% or 55% of predicted peak oxygen uptake (when the respiratory exchange ratio is greater than 1.10) has generally been selected as the most significant predictor of cardiac death.[60] Adjustments have to be made if the patient is taking a β-blocker.[62]

Attempts have been made to enhance the predictive power of peak oxygen uptake during exercise by coupling this measure to other data such as central hemodynamics, presence or absence of T-wave alternans, abnormal heart rate recovery, and ratio of ventilation to ventilatory carbon dioxide uptake (V_E/V_{CO_2}). Additional findings that may help classify patients into more serious heart failure categories include peak exercise heart rate, systolic blood pressure, minute ventilation, and anaerobic threshold. These observations have played a role in creating outcome prediction formulas or algorithms, discussed subsequently.

Although metabolic exercise testing to determine ventilatory responses in heart failure is quite important, specialized equipment and highly trained personnel are needed to accurately perform. Conversely, a simple 6-minute walking test also provides valuable prognostic information.[63] Many clinical trials have now used the 6-minute walk test to classify patients with heart failure into syndrome severity categories. A significant correlation between distance walked during 6 minutes and survival is noted. A total distance walked of less than about 300 meters in the SOLVD study carried an annual mortality risk of 11%, in contrast to 4% among patients who could walk more than about 450 meters.[63]

Metabolic Parameters

Many metabolic perturbations occur as heart failure alters flow to the central nervous system and mesentery. In patients with severe congestive heart failure, the serum sodium measurement probably reflects the degree of neurohormonal perturbation and intensity of diuretic therapy. Low serum sodium is associated with high morbidity rates. Elevated uric acid level is probably a result of renal perfusion abnormalities and also is associated with adverse outcomes. Liver enzyme levels can be elevated as a result of hepatic congestion. Hypothyroidism and hyperthyroidism frequently coexist with heart failure, can worsen symptoms, and may affect survival.

Chest Radiography

Routine chest radiography has been criticized as a tool to establish prognosis in heart failure; however, critical review of this simple, relatively inexpensive, and easy test has revealed pertinent findings that might be helpful.[28] Cardiothoracic ratio has been noted to be an independent predictor of survival. There is, however, a poor correlation between cardiothoracic ratio and left ventricular ejection fraction. Nonetheless, volume overload, manifesting as either pleural effusions or pulmonary parenchymal congestion, has been noted to be an independent predictor of mortality in some multivariate analyses.

Electrocardiography

In view of studies demonstrating the beneficial effects of cardiac resynchronization in patients with QRS intervals longer than 120 msec and with depressed ejection fraction, electrocardiography has had a resurgence in use during evaluation of patients with heart failure.[64] The combination of first-degree atrial ventricular block with intraventricular conduction delay can be particularly problematic, and now that cardiac resynchronization devices are available, clinicians must quite carefully evaluate a routine 12-lead surface electrocardiogram, particularly for QRS prolongation. Of course, the presence of arrhythmias such as atrial fibrillation, nonsustained ventricular tachycardia, and simply frequent premature ventricular contractions is important.

Support for signal average electrocardiography has waxed and waned with regard to stratifying risk for patients with dilated and ischemic cardiomyopathies.[65,66] Some investigators have noted that this technique is predictive of adverse outcome, but the sensitivity of signal average electrocardiographic parameters appears low overall, and the use of this technique remains controversial. QT dispersion has been used to stratify risk for patients with heart failure as well.[67,68] Patients who have atrial fibrillation and demonstrate complete left bundle branch block, however, present challenges to analysis of QT dispersion. In contrast, heart rate variability, a surrogate index of cardiac autonomic balance, appears to be, in some studies, a more powerful predictor of mortality and morbidity.[69,70] Electrocardiographic measurement of baroreflex sensitivity, an indirect measure of cardiac autonomic disruption, has also been used to stratify risk for patients with heart failure, but this technique has not been often used in the author's experience. Routine electrophysiological studies in patients with congestive heart failure have demonstrated that the inducing of ventricular tachycardia by programmed ventricular stimulation does not appear to be predictive of adverse outcome in nonselected patient populations.[71] However, in patients with heart failure who have a history of sudden cardiac death, syncope, or coronary artery disease, inducible ventricular tachycardia does seem to be associated with high morbidity rates. Of interesting is that electrophysiological study data do not often drive decision making regarding insertion of defibrillator devices in large practices. Rather, the general clinical characteristics of a patient with heart failure drive decisions to insert a defibrillator according to practice guidelines.

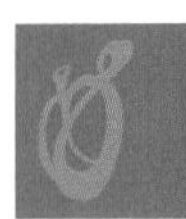

Inflammatory Markers of Heart Failure (see also Chapter 11)

Cytokines are small protein molecules that are produced not by specialized glands, as are hormones, but rather by many different tissues and individual cells. Unlike hormones, cytokines are not liberated continuously but are upregulated and downregulated in response to specific stimuli. Cytokines exert their effect in a paracrine manner on adjacent cells or in an autocrine manner on the producing cell itself. Major systemic effects may not be obvious with cytokine upregulation. Interest has emerged in cytokine analysis in the setting of heart failure because of the link between heart failure pathogenesis and inflammation more generally.[72-74] However, the routine measurement of cytokines has not proved useful for individual patients.[74] Nonetheless, cytokines can produce left ventricular dysfunction, precipitate pulmonary edema, cause cardiomyopathy, and induce ventricular remodeling (causing hypertrophy). Cytokines are also linked to anorexia and cachexia in patients with very severe heart failure (tumor necrosis factor, for example, is also called *cachectin*). In general, proinflammatory cytokines have been the ones associated with adverse outcome (tumor necrosis factor and interleukins-1 and -6, for example).

The erythrocyte sedimentation rate, a nonspecific index of inflammation, can be correlated with severity of illness of patients with heart failure.[75,76] Indeed, Paul Wood observed in 1936 that sedimentation rates were low in patients with pulmonary congestion and peripheral edema.[75] More recently, the erythrocyte sedimentation rate has been shown to vary in these patients, depending on individual patients' presentation. Patients with low or normal sedimentation rates in the setting of heart failure generally had more severe hemodynamic abnormalities than have patients with elevated sedimentation rates.

Neuroendocrine Activation

One of the most important insights into heart failure pathophysiology is that neuroendocrine activation appears early in the syndrome and can be subtle; several classic studies documented that renin-angiotensin-aldosterone abnormalities was associated with poor prognosis in the absence of treatment with neurohormonal modulating agents (ACE inhibitors, angiotensin receptor–blocking drugs, aldosterone antagonists, and β-blockers).[77] More recently, elevated levels of C- and N-terminal atrial and brain natriuretic peptide indicate worse outcomes in patients with heart failure.[78] These natriuretic peptide measurements can be used to both diagnose heart failure and guide clinicians during prognostication and treatment. It is not clear whether routine measurements of neurohormones other than natriuretic peptides will add further prognostic information in individuals.

Plasma endothelin been recognized as an independent, significant prognostic marker in congestive heart failure as well.[79] Endothelin is an extremely potent vasoconstricting, endogenous hormone that causes pulmonary hypertension. Big endothelin-I is the biologically inactive precursor of endothelin-1 and has been shown to be associated with short-term mortality from heart failure.

Endomyocardial Biopsy

The routine performance of endomyocardial biopsy in patients with heart failure, as previously mentioned, is not now endorsed as a routinely applied method to help with prognostication.[5] In some cases, however, the procedure can be useful. Adverse outcomes are associated with certain biopsy findings, including the presence of inflammation, particularly giant cell myocarditis, as discussed. Morphometric analysis of biopsy specimens that focuses on the degree of fibrosis and hypertrophy has been considered, but, again, it is not routinely used. Because endomyocardial biopsy is important for diagnosing doxorubicin (Adriamycin)–induced cardiomyopathy and for differentiating this difficulty from other infiltrative disease processes such as amyloidosis and hemochromatosis, endomyocardial biopsy cannot be completely dismissed, even though it should not be routinely performed.

PREDICTING OUTCOMES IN HEART FAILURE

In prognosticating during day-to-day management of individuals with heart failure, the clinician should focus attention on readily available clinical information that includes symptom severity (usually NYHA functional classification), left ventricular ejection fraction, cause of the difficulty, routine biochemical markers (particularly serum sodium, creatinine, blood urea nitrogen, and uric acid levels; liver function tests), and select hormones such as natriuretic peptides.[80-90]

Several algorithms have been tested to assist clinicians in determining which patients might benefit from cardiac transplantation, pharmacotherapeutic prescriptions, and device interventions.[81,85] Aaronson and colleagues[81] proposed a noninvasive risk-stratification model that was based on clinical findings during determination of peak oxygen uptake. This particular model contains seven variables: whether ischemia is present, resting heart rate, left ventricular ejection fraction, presence of a QRS duration longer than 200 msec, mean resting blood pressure, peak oxygen uptake, and serum sodium level. A heart failure score can be developed and related to subsequent morbidity and mortality. Adding invasively obtained data to this formula, including mean pulmonary capillary wedge pressure, improved predictive power of this approach somewhat. This model defines low-, medium-, and high-risk groups: 1-year event-free survival rates are 93%, 72%, and 43%, respectively.

Campana and coworkers[88] also tested a prognosticating model with similar but not the same factors. This model included cause of heart failure, functional class, presence of an S3 gallop, cardiac output, mean arterial pressure, and either pulmonary artery diastolic pressure or pulmonary capillary wedge pressure. This model obviously requires invasive measurements of hemodynamics. According to the risk score generated, patients were stratified into low-, intermediate-, and high-risk groups, whose 1-year event-free survival rates were 95%, 75%, and 40%, respectively, which were quite similar to those of the Aaronson model.

The model that is perhaps most elegant and easy to use and that has been a subject of great interest is the Seattle Heart Failure Prognostication Model.[86,88] Previous heart failure risk models, such as the ones described previously, stratify patients into group ranges without a specific and individualized risk assignment. The Seattle Heart Failure risk prediction tool produces an individualized estimate of survival and is based on readily available clinical characteristics and not invasive measurements of hemodynamics. Levy and colleagues[86] at the University of Washington Health Sciences Center derived the model by retrospectively investigating predictors of outcome among 1125 patients with heart failure who had been entered into randomized clinical trials whose entry criteria required symptomatic NYHA class III or IV, an ejection fraction of less than 30%, and medication with an ACE inhibitor and diuretics. A stepwise Cox proportional hazard model was used to create a multivariate risk model that identified age, gender, ischemic cause, functional classification, ejection fraction, systolic blood pressure, potassium-sparing diuretic use, statin use, allopurinol use, hemoglobin, percent lymphocyte count, uric acid level, serum sodium level, total

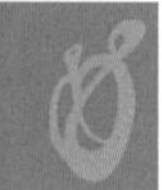

cholesterol level, and diuretic dose as significant predictors of death. The model was then prospectively validated in five additional cohorts totaling almost 10,000 patients and 17,000 person-years of follow-up. The model provided an accurate estimate of 1-, 2-, and 3-year survival with the use of easily obtained clinical characteristics. Particularly attractive is the fact that the model can be freely accessed at http://depts.washington.edu/shfm (accessed February 6, 2010) and individual patient characteristics entered to determine the effects of various interventions. Figure 34-1 demonstrates that for a 65-year-old man with class III symptoms and an ejection fraction of 30% with a normal blood pressure, no anemia, and preserved serum sodium level, starting "guideline-driven, evidence-based" drug therapy will improve the chance of 5-year survival from 33% to 74%. Another advantage is that the likelihood of improving outcomes with interventions in appropriate patients with defibrillators and resynchronization pacing can be assessed.

Of course, these prediction models have limitations. Nonetheless, the use of mathematical models to help predict outcome in heart failure cohorts helps physicians determine which patients might be appropriate candidates for particular therapies.

THE CONVERSATION

Prognostication in a patient with heart failure is critical in patient management, and patients deserve careful, thoughtful, and compassionate analysis of the data and then information that will guide them through the important challenges of self-care. Fortunately, most patients with heart failure have a reasonable prognosis. Nonetheless, bad news is often given, and cardiologists do not have adequate training in the delivery of this information. It is stressful to the clinician and, unlike physicians in the fields of oncology and neurology, cardiologists have paid less attention to this challenge. One strategy used by some authorities is summarized by the mnemonic SPIKES.[91] "S" stands for "setting up the conversation"; the clinician has a strategy regarding the discussion before entering the room with the patient and family or attendants. The clinician should anticipate that the patient and the family are experiencing anxiety, and although the clinician might wish to avoid the conversation entirely, the conversation must take place. "P" represents "perception": What does the patient know about the disease and multiple issues that might be complicating the clinical situation? Does the patient know the facts, or does the patient have misperceptions that have been conveyed by less educated caregivers? The clinician must educate the patient. If the prognosis is not that bad, that point should be highlighted, but the clinician should not be excessively optimistic. "I" represents "invitation," which means that the clinician must determine how much information the patient desires. "K" is for "knowledge": The clinician should educate the patient by using a discussion format that the patient can understand. "E" means "empathy": The clinician should give the patient a few minutes to let the information and discussion resonate and then use empathetic statements to react to the patient's emotions. The clinician should not be patronizing or paternalistic. The clinician should be sensitive to the wishes of the patient. Forceful persuasion should not be used in discussing therapeutic options. The final "S" stands for "summarize and strategize": Make sure that the patient understands what has been discussed and, in particular, what the next steps are. A few common barriers to these discussions include the clinician's feeling responsible for buoying a patient's hope, ignoring the clinician's own feelings, making assumptions (that are often quite wrong) about the knowledge level and sophistication of the patient, assuming that all patients want "everything possible" done and that cure is the goal, and talking more than listening.[92] These insights could be helpful during difficult conversations with some patients with heart failure.

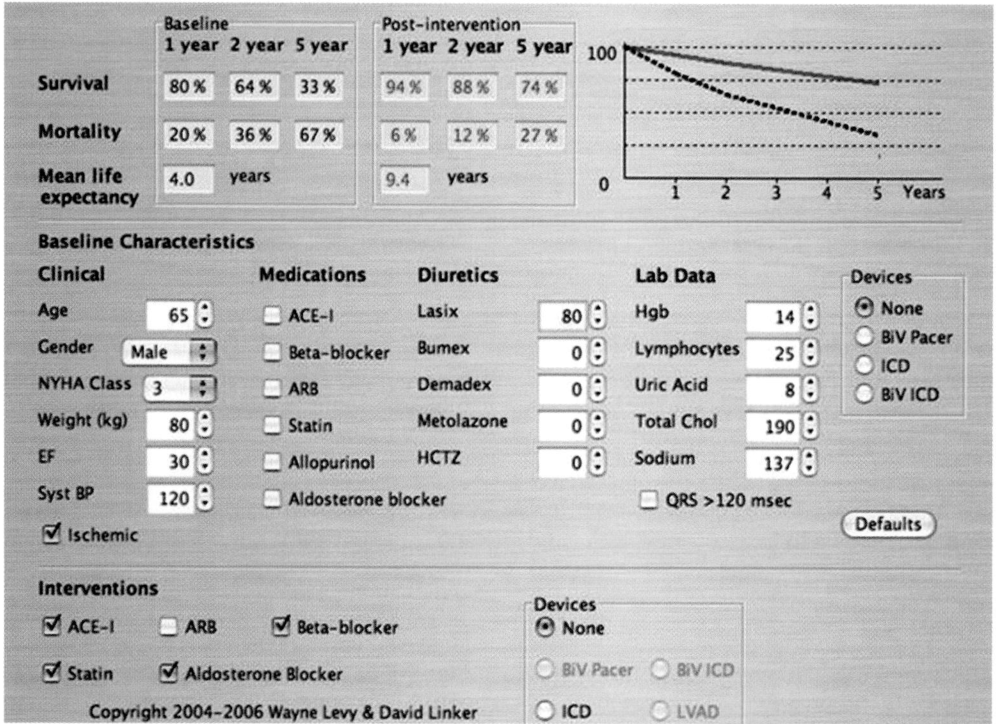

FIGURE 34–1 Seattle Heart Failure Prognostication Model. This online model for predicting risk in heart failure is easily accessed (http://depts.washington.edu/shfm; accessed November 1, 2009) and can help with determining mathematical survival likelihood with a variety of interventions. In this example, the predicted 1-year survival rate increased from 80% to 94% when an angiotensin-converting enzyme inhibitor, a β-blocker, an aldosterone antagonist, and a "statin" were added to the medication treatment protocol of a 65-year-old man with normal blood pressure, narrow QRS interval, coronary artery disease, and an ejection fraction of 30%. (Courtesy Dr. Wayne Levy and Dr. David Linker.)

REFERENCES

1. Lloyd-Jones, D. M., Larson, M. G., Leip, E. P., et al. (2002). Lifetime risk for developing congestive heart failure. The Framingham Heart Study. *Circulation, 106*, 3068–3072.
2. Young, J. B. (2000). Prognosis of heart failure. In J. D. Hosenpud, & B. H. Greenberg (Eds.). *Congestive heart failure* (ed 2, pp. 655–671). Philadelphia: Lippincott, Williams & Wilkins.
3. Young, J. B. (2004). The prognosis of heart failure. In D. L. Mann (Ed.). *Heart failure. A companion to Braunwald's Heart Disease* (pp. 389–505). Philadelphia: WB Saunders.
4. Cohn, J. N. (1989). Prognostic factors in heart failure: Poverty amidst a wealth of variables. *J Am Coll Cardiol, 14*, 571–572.
5. Jessup, M., Abraham, W. T., Chen, M. H., et al. (2009). 2009 Focused update:ACC/AHA guidelines for the diagnosis and management of heart failure in adults. *Circulation, 119*, 1977–2016.
6. Dickstein, K., Cohen-Solal, A., Fillippatos, G., et al. (2008). European Society of Cardiology Guidelines for the diagnosis and treatment of acute and chronic heart failure 2008. *Eur Heart J, 29*, 2388–2442.
7. Heart Failure Society of America. (2006). 2006 Comprehensive heart failure practice guideline. *J Card Fail, 12*, e1–e122.
8. Goodlin, S. J., Hauptman, P. J., Arnold, R., et al. (2004). Consensus statement: palliative and supportive care in advanced heart failure. *J Card Fail, 10*, 200–2009.
9. Senni, M., Triboulloy, C. M., Rodeheffer, R. J., et al. (1998). Congestive heart failure in the community: a study of all incident cases in Olmstead County, Minnesota, in 1991. *Circulation, 98*, 2282–2289.
10. Senni, M., Triboulloy, C. M., Rodeheffer, R. J., et al. (1999). Congestive heart failure in the community: trends and incidence and survival in a 10 year period. *Arch Intern Med, 159*, 29–34.
11. Levy, D., Kenchaiah, S., Larson, M. G., et al. (2002). Long-term trends in the incidence of and survival with heart failure. *N Engl J Med, 347*, 1397–1402.
12. O'Connor, C. M., Abraham, W. T., Albert, N. M., et al. (2008). Predictors of mortality after discharge in patients hospitalized with heart failure: an analysis from the Organized Program To Initiate lifesaving treatMent In hospitaliZEd patients with Heart Failure (OPTIMIZE-HF). *Am Heart J, 156*, 662–673.
13. Abraham, W. T., Fonarow, G. C., Albert, N. M., et al. (2008). Predictors of in-hospital mortality in patients hospitalized for heart failure: insights from the Organized Program To Initiate lifesaving treatMent In hospitaliZEd patients with Heart Failure (OPTIMIZE-HF). *J Am Coll Cardiol, 52*, 347–356.
14. Sutton, G. C., & Chatterjee, K. (2008). *Heart failure: current clinical understanding.* London: Remidica Publishing.
15. Flynn, K. E., Pina, I. L., Whellan, D. J., et al. (2009). Effects of exercise training on health status in patients with chronic heart failure: HF-ACTION randomized clinical trial. *JAMA, 301*, 1451–1459.
16. Dickstein, K. (2009). Diagnosing heart failure: the mathematician and the clinician. *J Am Coll Cardiol, 54*, 1522–1523.
17. Cowburn, P. J., Cleland, J. G. F., Coats, A. J. S., et al. (1998). Risk stratification in heart failure. *Eur Heart J, 19*, 696–712.
18. Lee, W. H., & Packer, M. (1986). Prognostic importance of serum sodium concentration and its modification by converting enzyme inhibition in patients with severe chronic heart failure. *Circulation, 73*, 257–267.
19. Leier, C. V., DeiCas, L., & Metra, M. (1994). Clinical relevance and management of the major electrolyte abnormalities in congestive heart failure: hyponatremia; hypokalemia, and hypomagnesemia. *Am Heart J, 128*, 564–572.
20. Chandler, S. L., & Kay, H. R. (1987). Clinical determinants of mortality and chronic congestive heart failure secondary to idiopathic dilated or to ischemic cardiomyopathy. *Am J Cardiol, 59*, 634–638.
21. Rockman, H. A., Juneau, C., Chatterjee, K., et al. (1989). Long-term predictors of sudden and low cardiac output death in chronic congestive heart failure secondary to coronary artery disease. *Am J Cardiol, 64*, 1544–1548.
22. Saxon, L. A., Stevenson, W. G., Middlekauf, H. R., et al. (1993). Predicting death from progressive heart failure secondary to ischemic or idiopathic dilated cardiomyopathy. *Am J Cardiol, 72*, 62–65.
23. Fonarow, G. C., Adams, K. F., Jr., Abraham, W. T., et al. (2005). Risk stratification for in-hospital mortality in acutely decompensated heart failure: classification and regression tree analysis. *JAMA, 293*, 572–580.
24. Cohn, J. N., Johnson, G. R., Shabetai, R., et al. (1983). Ejection fraction, peak exercise oxygen consumption, cardiothoracic ratio, ventricular arrhythmias in plasma norepinephrine as determinants of prognosis in heart failure. *Circulation, 87*, V15–V116.
25. DeLemos, J. A., Morrow, D. A., Bentley, J. H., et al. (2001). The prognostic value of B-type natriuretic peptide in patients with acute coronary syndromes. *N Engl J Med, 345*, 1014–1021.
26. Ho, K. K. L., Anderson, K. M., Grossman, W., et al. (1993). Survival after the onset of congestive heart failure. The Framingham Heart Study subjects. *Circulation, 88*, 107–115.
27. Migrino, R. Q., Young, J. B., Ellis, S. J., et al. (1997). The relationship of early left ventricular volume to subsequent mortality after myocardial infarction: a substudy of GUSTO. *Circulation, 96*, 116–121.
28. Ostojic, M., Young, J. B., & Hess, K. R. (1989). Prediction of left ventricular ejection fraction using a unique method of chest x-ray and ECG analysis. A noninvasive index of cardiac performance based on the concept of heart volume and mass inter-relationship. *Am Heart J, 117*, 590–598.
29. Mancini, D., Katz, S., Donchez, L., et al. (1996). Coupling of hemodynamic measurements with oxygen consumption during exercise did not improve risk stratification in patients with heart failure. *Circulation, 94*, 2492–2496.
30. Mancini, D. M., Eisen, H., Kussmaul, W., et al. (1991). Value of peak exercise oxygen consumption for optimal timing of cardiac transplantation in ambulatory patients with heart failure. *Circulation, 83*, 778–786.
31. Batin, P. D., Wickens, M., McEntegard, D., et al. (1995). The importance of abnormalities of liver function test and predicting mortality in chronic heart failure. *Eur Heart J, 16*, 1613–1618.
32. Adams, K. F., Dunlap, S. H., Sueta, C. A., et al. (1996). Relation between gender, etiology, and survival in patients with symptomatic heart failure. *J Am Coll Cardiol, 28*, 1781–1788.
33. Ghali, J. K., Weiner, D. H., Greenberg, B., et al. (1997). Does gender have an impact on survival in patients with heart failure? Findings from the SOLVD registry. *J Am Coll Cardiol, 29*, 246A.
34. Mendes, L. A., Davidoff, R., Coupples, L. A., et al. (1997). Congestive heart failure in patients with coronary artery disease: the gender paradox. *Am Heart J, 134*, 207–212.
35. Simon, T., Mary-Krause, M., Funck-Brentano, C., et al. (2001). Sex differences in the prognosis of congestive heart failure; results from the Cardiac Insufficiency Bisoprolol Study (CIBIS II). *Circulation, 103*, 375–380.
36. Young, J. B., Weiner, D. H., Yusuf, S., et al. (1995). Patterns of medication use in patients with heart failure: a report from the registry of Studies of Left Ventricular Dysfunction (SOLVD). *South Med J, 88*, 514–523.
37. Bangdivala, S. I., Weiner, D. H., Bourassa, M. G., et al. (1992). Studies of Left Ventricular Dysfunction registry. *Am J Cardiol, 70*, 347–353.
38. Rich, M. W., Becikhman, V., Wittenberg, C., et al. (1995). A multidisciplinary intervention to prevent the readmission of elderly patients with congestive heart failure. *N Engl J Med, 333*, 1190–1195.
39. Hughes, C. V., Wong, M., Johnson, G., et al. (1993). Influence of age on mechanisms and prognosis of heart failure. *Circulation, 87*, v5–v15.
40. Cohn, J. N., Archibald, D. G., Ziesch, S., et al. (1986). Effect of vasodilator therapy on mortality of chronic congestive heart failure. *N Engl J Med, 314*, 1547–1554.
41. The SOLVD Investigators. (1991). Effect of enalapril on survival in patients with reduced left ventricular ejection fractions and symptomatic congestive heart failure. *N Engl J Med, 325*, 293–302.
42. Bonow, R. O., Carabello, B. A., Chatterjee, K., et al. (2008). 2008 Focused update incorporated into the ACC/AHA guidelines for the management of patients with valvular heart disease: a report of the American College of Cardiology/American Heart Association Task Force on Practice Guidelines (Writing Committee to Revise the 1998 Guidelines for the Management of Patients With Valvular Heart Disease): endorsed by the Society of Cardiovascular Anesthesiologists, Society for Cardiovascular Angiography and Interventions, and Society of Thoracic Surgeons. *Circulation, 118*(15), e523–e661.
43. Ellis, S. G., Whitlow, P. I., Raymond, R. E., et al. (2002). Impact of mitral regurgitation on long term survival after percutaneous coronary intervention. *Am J Cardiol, 89*, 315–318.
44. Ross, J., Jr. (1981). Left ventricular function in the timing and surgical treatment of valvular heart disease. *Ann Intern Med, 94*, 498–510.
45. Mason, J. W., O'Connell, J. B., Herskowitz, A., et al. (1995). Clinical trial of immunosuppressive therapy of myocarditis. The Myocarditis Treatment Trial Investigators. *N Engl J Med, 333*, 269–275.
46. Grogan, M., Redfield, M. M., Bailey, K. R., et al. (1995). Long-term outcome of patients with biopsy proved myocarditis. Comparison with idiopathic dilated cardiomyopathy. *J Am Coll Cardiol, 26*, 804–815.
47. Cooper, L. T., Jr., Berry, G. J., & Shabetai, R. (1997). Idiopathic giant cell myocarditis: natural history and treatment. Multicenter Giant Cell Myocarditis Study Group Investigators. *N Engl J Med, 336*, 1860–1866.
48. Sliwa, K., Fett, J., & Elkayam, U. (2006). Peripartum cardiomyopathy. *Lancet, 368*, 687–693.
49. Maron, B. J., McKenna, W. J., Danielson, G. K., et al. (2003). ACC/ESC clinical expert consensus document on hypertrophic cardiomyopathy. *J Am Coll Cardiol, 42*, 1687–1713.
50. Piano, M. R. (2002). Alcoholic cardiomyopathy. Incidence, clinical characteristics and pathophysiology. *Chest, 121*, 1238–1250.
51. Shan, K., Lincoff, A. M., & Young, J. B. (1996). Anthracycline induced cardiotoxicity. *Ann Intern Med, 125*, 47–58.
52. Desai, A., & Fang, J. C. (2008). Heart failure with preserved ejection fraction: hypertension, diabetes, sleep apnea/obesity, hypertrophic and infiltrative cardiomyopathies. *Heart Fail Clin, 4*, 87–97.
53. Canady, M., Hogye, M., Kallai, A., et al. (1995). Familial cardiomyopathy: a worse prognosis compared with sporadic forms. *Br Heart J, 74*, 171–173.
54. Lip, G. Y., Felmeden, D. C., Li-Saw-Hee, F. L., et al. (2000). Hypertensive heart disease. A complex syndrome or a hypertensive "cardiomyopathy"? *Eur Heart J, 21*, 1653–1665.
55. Vaughn, T., & Bell, D. S. H. (2006). Diabetic cardiomyopathy. *Heart Fail Clin, 2*, 71–80.
56. Rubin, L. J., & Badesch, D. B. (2005). Evaluation and management of the patient with pulmonary arterial hypertension. *Ann Intern Med, 143*, 282–292.
57. Wang, H., Parker, J. D., Newton, G. E., et al. (2007). Influence of sleep apnea on mortality in patients with heart failure. *J Am Coll Cardiol, 49*, 1625–1631.
58. McAlister, F. A., Exekowiz, J., Tonelli, M., et al. (2004). Renal insufficiency and heart failure. Prognostic and therapeutic implications from a prospective cohort study. *Circulation, 109*, 1004–1009.
59. Disalvo, T. G., Mathier, M., Semigran, M. J., et al. (1995). Preserved right ventricular ejection fraction predicts exercise capacity and survival in advanced heart failure. *J Am Coll Cardiol, 25*, 1143–1151.
60. Mehra, M. R., Kobashigawa, J., Starling, R., et al. (2006). Listing criteria for heart transplantation. International Society for Heart and Lung Transplantation guidelines for the care of cardiac transplant candidates. *J Heart Lung Transplant, 25*, 1024–1124.
61. ESCAPE Trial Investigators. (2005). Evaluation Study of Congestive Heart Failure and Pulmonary artery catheterization Effectiveness. The ESCAPE Trial. *JAMA, 294*, 1625–1633.
62. O'Neil, J. O., Young, J. B., Pothier, C. E., et al. (2005). Peak oxygen consumption as a predictor of death in patients with heart failure receiving beta blockers. *Circulation, 111*, 2313–2318.

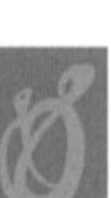

63. Bittner, V., Weiner, D. H., Yusuf, S., et al. (1993). Prediction of mortality and morbidity with a six minute walk test in the patient with left ventricular dysfunction. *JAMA, 270*, 1702–1707.
64. Strickberger, S. A., Conti, J., Daud, E. G., et al. (2005). Patient selection for cardiac resynchronization therapy. AHA Scientific Advisory. *Circulation, 111*, 2146–2150.
65. Brembilla-Perrot, B., Terrier de la Chasse, A., Jacquemin, L., et al. (1997). The signal averaged electrocardiogram is of limited value in patients with bundle branch block and cardiomyopathy in predicting inducible ventricular tachycardia or death. *Am J Cardiol, 79*, 154–159.
66. Silverman, M. E., Pressel, M. D., Brackett, J. C., et al. (1995). Prognostic value of the signal averaged electrocardiogram and prolonged QRS in ischemic and nonischemic cardiomyopathy. *Am J Cardiol, 75*, 460–464.
67. Pinski, D. J., Sciacca, R. R., & Steinberg, J. S. (1997). QT dispersion is a marker of risk in patients awaiting heart transplantation. *J Am Coll Cardiol, 29*, 1576–1584.
68. Fei, L., Goldman, J. H., Prasad, K., et al. (1996). QT dispersion and RR variations on 12 lead ECG's in patients with congestive heart failure secondary to idiopathic dilated cardiomyopathy. *Eur Heart J, 17*, 258–263.
69. Brouwer, J., van Veldhuisen, D., Manin, T., et al. (1996). Prognostic value of heart rate variability during long-term follow-up in patients with mild to moderate heart failure. *J Am Coll Cardiol, 28*, 1183–1189.
70. Nolan, J. P., Batin, P. D., Lindsey, S. J., et al. (1996). Reduced heart rate variability and mortality in chronic heart failure. *Circulation, 94*, 1498.
71. Zipes, D. P., Camm, A. J., Borggrefe, M., et al. (2006). ACC/AHA/ESC Guideline for management of patients with ventricular arrhythmias and the prevention of sudden cardiac death—executive summary. *J Am Coll Cardiol*, 8(5):e247–346.
72. Levine, B., Kalmen, J., Mayer, L., et al. (1990). Elevated circulating levels of tumor necrosis factor in severe chronic heart failure. *N Engl J Med, 323*, 236–241.
73. Torre-Amione, G., Kapadia, S., Benedict, C., et al. (1996). Pro-inflammatory cytokine levels in patients with depressed left ventricular ejection fraction: a report from the Studies of Left Ventricular Dysfunction (SOLVD). *J Am Coll Cardiol, 27*, 1201–1206.
74. Mann, D. L., McMurray, J. J., Packer, M., et al. (2004). Targeted anticytokine therapy in patients with chronic heart failure: results of the randomized etanercept worldwide evaluation. *Circulation, 109*, 1594–1602.
75. Wood, P. (1936). The erythrocyte sedimentation rate in heart disease. *Q J Med, 36*(5), 1–19.
76. Haber, H. L., Leavy, J. A., Kessler, P. D., et al. (1991). The erythrocyte sedimentation rate in congestive heart failure. *N Engl J Med, 324*, 353–358.
77. Givertz, M. M., & Braunwald, E. (2004). Neurohormones in heart failure: predicting outcomes, optimizing care. *Eur Heart J, 25*, 281–282.
78. Sa, D. D., & Chen, H. H. (2008). The role of natriuretic peptides in heart failure. *Curr Heart Fail Rep, 5*, 177–184.
79. De Luca, L., Mebazaa, A., Filippatos, G., et al. (2008). Overview of emerging pharmacology agents for acute heart failure syndromes. *Eur J Heart Fail, 10*, 201–213.
80. Lee, D. S., Austin, P. C., Rouleau, J. L., et al. (2003). Predicting mortality among patients hospitalized with heart failure: derivation and validation of a clinical model. *JAMA, 290*, 2581–2587.
81. Aaronson, K. D., Schwartz, J. S., Chen, T. M., et al. (1997). Development and prospective validation of a clinical index to predict survival in ambulatory patients referred for cardiac transplant evaluation. *Circulation, 95*, 2660–2667.
82. Brophy, J. M., Dagenias, G. R., McSherry, F., et al. (2004). Multivariate model for predicting mortality in patients with heart failure and systolic dysfunction. *Am J Med, 116*, 300–304.
83. Lund, L. H., Aaronson, K. D., & Mancini, D. M. (2003). Predicting survival in ambulatory patients with severe heart failure on beta blocker therapy. *Am J Cardiol, 92*, 1350–1354.
84. Klelling, T. M., Joseph, S., & Aaronson, K. D. (2004). Heart failure survival score continues to predict clinical outcomes in patients with heart failure receiving beta blockers. *J Heart Lung Transplant, 23*, 1414–1422.
85. Keogh, A. M., Baron, D. W., & Hickie, J. B. (1990). Prognostic guides in patients with idiopathic or chronic dilated cardiomyopathy assessed for cardiac transplantation. *Am J Cardiol, 65*, 903–908.
86. Levy, W. C., Mozaffarian, D., Linker, D. T., et al. (2006). The Seattle Heart Failure Model: prediction of survival in heart failure. *Circulation, 113*, 1424–1433.
87. Mozaffarian, D., Anker, S. D., Anand, I., et al. (2007). Prediction of mode of death in heart failure: the Seattle Heart Failure Model. *Circulation, 116*, 392–398.
88. Campana, C., Gavazzi, A., Beruni, C., et al. (1993). Predictors of prognosis in patients awaiting heart transplantation. *J Heart Lung Transplant, 12*, 756–765.
89. Steinhart, B., Thorpe, K. E., Bayoumi, A. M., et al. (2009). Improving the diagnosis of heart failure using a validated prediction model. *J Am Coll Cardiol, 54*, 1515–1521.
90. Poses, R. M., Smith, W. R., McClish, D. K., et al. (1997). Physicians survival predictions for patients with acute congestive heart failure. *Arch Intern Med, 157*, 1001–1007.
91. Baile, W. F., Buckman, R., Lenzi, R., et al. (2000). SPIKES"—a six step protocol for delivering bad news: applications to the patient with cancer. *Oncologist, 5*, 302–311.
92. Giving bad news. *Medical Oncology Communication Skills Training Learning Modules*, Learning Module 2. 2002, pgs 7-9 (online publication): http://depts.washington.edu/oncotalk. Accessed February 4, 2010.

CHAPTER 35

Clinical Evaluation of Heart Failure

W. H. Wilson Tang and Gary S. Francis

Heart failure is a clinical syndrome that manifests in different stages with a wide spectrum of bedside observations. Hence, the evaluation of the patient with heart failure may vary, but it is a critically important task. The physician must use clinical acumen and laboratory resources properly and skillfully. Heart failure is much like fever or anemia, in that it should not be considered as a "stand-alone" diagnosis but should be described with its associated cause (or causes), such as coronary artery disease, hypertension, valvular heart disease, or arrhythmia. This evaluation is clearly not to be a "one-time" occurrence but rather an ongoing process, and it may evolve according to how the clinical course unfolds. Additional diagnostic information may be necessary to support the diagnosis and to determine the precise mechanism of the symptoms, the severity of the problem, the natural history of the disorder, and the prognosis for an individual patient.

Historically, the clinical concept of heart failure has been descriptive of volume overload (which may explain the common use of the term "congestive heart failure"). Today the availability of hemodynamic and imaging measures, ability to quantify the degree of cardiac insufficiency, and description of morphological abnormalities are increasingly becoming part of the process of bedside clinical evaluation. With the adaptation of the staging system that extends beyond the presentation of signs and symptoms of heart failure, the evaluation process requires the implementation of a combination of complex clinical and laboratory skills. In particular, patients with "preclinical" heart failure can be identified only by careful imaging or other techniques that reveal underlying structural abnormalities. Thus, the departure from a purely symptomatic evaluation and management in favor of a notion of a process of disease progression allows for the opportunity to explore how to best evaluate patients afflicted by this condition.

This chapter provides a broad framework of clinical evaluation across the spectrum of heart failure to gain an appreciation of how the heart failure began, how the signs and symptoms develop over time, and the pace at which the signs and symptoms appear. Such information is critical for determining prognosis and devising precise management strategies, specific therapies, and interventions, including pharmacological treatment, percutaneous coronary intervention, surgery, and use of mechanical devices.

CLINICAL EVALUATION OF PRESENTING SYMPTOMS: THE MEDICAL HISTORY

One of the first principles of the clinical evaluation of heart failure is to determine whether the patient is indeed presenting with heart failure. Although this may sound obvious and self-fulfilling, presenting signs and symptoms of heart failure are often nonspecific. Despite these ambiguities, a series of questions should be addressed to every patient in order to understand the contributors and trajectory of disease progression: When did the symptoms start? Are the symptoms stable or are they getting worse? Are symptoms provoked, or do they occur at rest? Are there accompanying symptoms (such as chest pain or calf claudication, palpitations, and dizziness)? How do the symptoms affect everyday activities? Illness narratives are particularly important, and sometimes patients may provide some clues as to how their conditions evolved, even though many of these questions may not yield immediate answers (and sometimes the answers may be elicited from significant others or family members). Sometimes, several rounds of interviewing are necessary. It can be a time-consuming process, and the person taking the history must be patient.

It is important to determine the stage in which the patient might be in the natural history of the disorder. Risk factors for the development of heart failure must be identified in order to anticipate heart failure (so-called stage A heart failure, according to the heart failure guidelines of Hunt and associates[1]) (Figure 35-1). Such risk factors include hypertension, coronary artery disease, diabetes mellitus, valvular heart disease, history of myocardial infarction, family history of cardiomyopathy, or exposure to cardiotoxins (such as excessive use of alcohol, use of anthracycline, occupational exposure, use of ephedra-containing supplements, or use of illicit drugs). Table 35-1 lists the prevalence and population attributable risk of some of these risk factors. Figure 35-2 illustrates a risk scoring system that may be used to predict the risk of developing heart failure, on the basis of common clinical variables.[2] Some of these risk factors may not be apparent, and it is commonly necessary for patients to trace back their past exposures or their family histories in order to provide clues to possible underlying causes, particularly in those with nonischemic causes.

Even in the absence of symptoms, some patients may have structural and functional abnormalities of the heart and circulation that antedate the onset of symptoms (so-called stage B heart failure[1]). These structural abnormalities include left ventricular

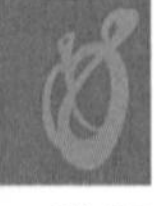

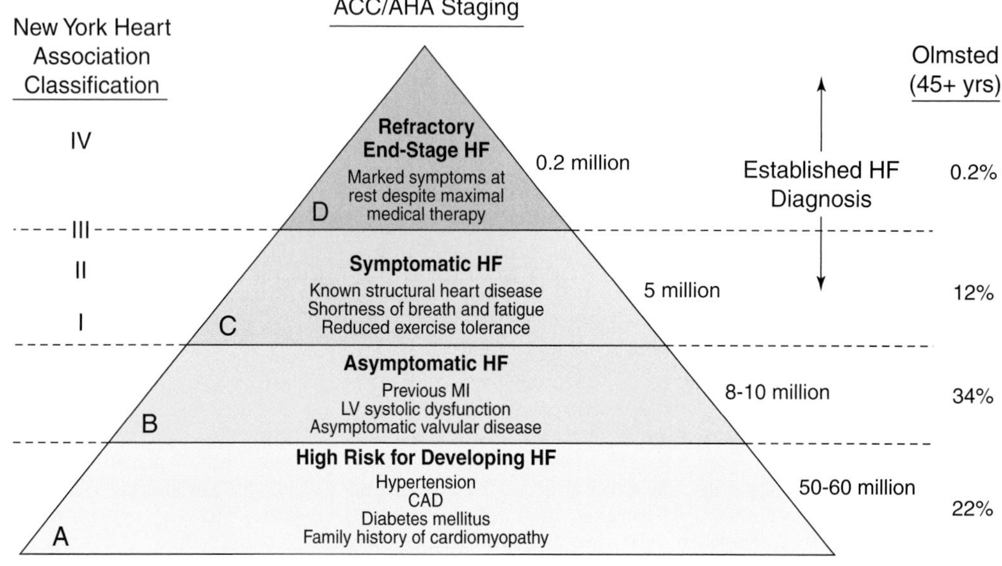

FIGURE 35–1 Heart failure (HF) staging and prevalence of stages in the Olmstead County Epidemiology Study. ACC, American College of Cardiology; *AHA,* American Heart Association; *CAD,* coronary artery disease; *LV,* left ventricular; *MI,* myocardial infarction. (Data on the right side of the figure is from Ammar KA, Jacobsen SJ, Mahoney DW, et al. Prevalence and prognostic significance of heart failure stages: application of the American College of Cardiology/American Heart Association heart failure staging criteria in the community. *Circulation* 2007;115:1563-1570.)

hypertrophy, asymptomatic left ventricular dysfunction, asymptomatic valvular dysfunction, or wall-motion abnormalities from prior myocardial infarction. Because heart failure will probably develop in these early stages in some patients, preventive therapy or risk factor modification should be instituted, as well as early use of neurohormonal antagonists, including angiotensin-converting enzyme (ACE) inhibitors and, in selected cases, β-blockers and statin therapy.

Symptoms of heart failure may be well controlled with outpatient medical therapy (stage C^1) or may become refractory to conventional therapy (stage D^1). After the physician establishes that symptoms may be caused by the syndrome of heart failure, ongoing review of the patient's clinical status is crucial for the appropriate selection and monitoring of therapy. It is traditional to classify patients by extent of disability according to the New York Heart Association (NYHA) functional classification (see Figure 35-1).[3] Although this classification system is notoriously subjective, it has stood the test of time and continues to be widely applied to patients with heart failure. Several other clinical scoring systems have been developed to define heart failure in population-based studies (Table 35-2).[4] There is an important distinction between staging and functional classification assessment: The NYHA functional classification applies only to patients with overt heart failure (stages C and D), and whereas a patient's NYHA class can improve or worsen, heart failure staging can only advance forward. In other words, once a patient's condition reaches stage C, even if the patient becomes asymptomatic with treatment, the condition would not be restaged B because symptoms have already manifested themselves.

The pace at which heart failure develops and progresses can be highly variable, and sometimes it is difficult to distinguish stage C from stage D. The timing and need for various diagnostic assessments therefore depend on decisions regarding the appropriateness and timing of specialized interventions (such as revascularization and heart transplantation). For example, a young woman with decompensated heart failure resulting from acute inflammatory myocarditis may require full diagnostic workup and mechanical circulatory support to maximize the chances of recovery. In contrast, an elderly patient who has long-standing rheumatic valve disease with stable symptoms of heart failure and has not undergone surgical therapy may benefit from routine clinical follow-up if there are no interim changes in signs and symptoms. Often neglected is the preference of the patient with regard to undergoing diagnostic testing and various medical and

TABLE 35–1 Prevalence and Population Attributable Risk Factors for Developing Heart Failure

Risk Factor	Age- and Risk Factor -Adjusted Hazard Ratio	% Prevalence	Population Attributable Risk
Hypertension (BP ≥ 140/90 mm Hg)			
Men	2.1	60	39
Women	3.4	62	59
Myocardial infarction			
Men	6.3	10	34
Women	6.0	3	13
Angina			
Men	1.4	11	5
Women	1.7	9	5
Diabetes			
Men	1.8	8	6
Women	3.7	5	12
Left ventricular hypertrophy (electrocardiography)			
Men	2.2	4	4
Women	2.9	3	5
Valvular heart disease			
Men	2.5	5	7
Women	2.1	8	8

Age	
Years	Points
≤71	−1
72-75	0
76-78	1
≥79	2

Coronary artery disease	
Status	Points
No	0
Possible	2
Definite	5

LV Hypertrophy	
Status	Points
No	0
Yes	2

Systolic blood pressure	
mm Hg	Points
≤90	−4
95-100	−3
105-115	−2
120-125	−1
130-140	0
145-150	1
155-165	2
170-175	3
180-190	4
195-200	5
>200	6

Heart rate	
bpm	Points
≤50	−2
55-60	−1
65-70	0
75-80	1
85-90	2
≥95	3

Smoking	
Status	Points
Never	0
Past	1
Current	4

Creatinine	
g/dL	Points
≤4.8	−3
4.5-4.7	−2
4.2-4.4	−1
3.9-4.1	0
3.6-3.8	1
3.3-3.5	2
≥3.2	3

Fasting glucose	
mg/dL	Points
≤80	−1
85-125	0
130-170	1
175-220	2
225-265	3
≥270	5

Creatinine	
mg/dL	Points
≤0.7	−2
0.8-0.9	−1
1.0-1.1	0
1.2-1.4	1
1.5-1.8	2
1.9-2.3	3
≥2.3	6

Key:
Systolic BP to nearest 5 mm Hg
Heart rate to nearest 5 bpm
Albumin to nearest 0.1 g/dL
Glucose to nearest 5 mg/dL
Creatinin to nearest 0.1 mg/dL

HF = Heart failure

Health ABC HF risk score	HF Risk group	5-yr HF risk
≤2 points	Low	<5%
3-5 points	Average	5-10%
6-9 points	High	10-20%
≥10 points	Very high	>20%

FIGURE 35-2 Risk scoring system for predicting the development of heart failure. *BP,* blood pressure; *bpm,* beats per minute; LV, left ventricular. (From Butler J, Kalogeropoulos A, Georgiopoulou V, et al. Incident heart failure prediction in the elderly: the Health ABC Heart Failure score. *Circ Heart Fail* 2008;1:125-133.)

surgical interventions, as well as their clinical consequences. This is particularly important in patients with advanced heart failure, whose choices may be limited to improving the quality versus length of life.[5]

When a patient first presents with new heart failure or decompensated heart failure, identification and correction of a *precipitating cause* is very important (Box 35-1). In some cases, this is obvious (such as dietary indiscretion), but in other cases, it may be far more subtle. A prospective substudy of a large clinical trial demonstrated that the most common acute precipitants of heart failure exacerbations were noncompliance with salt restriction (22%), pulmonary infections (15%), and arrhythmias (13%). More alarming is the prevalence of iatrogenic causes of decompensation, such as use of antiarrhythmic agents (15%) or calcium channel blockers (13%), or inappropriate reductions in medications for heart failure (10%).[6] Furthermore, different precipitating factors may also have different implications. For example, 60- to 90-day outcomes are poorer for heart failure decompensation caused by ischemia or worsening renal function than for that caused by poor blood pressure control or arrhythmia (because the latter are more likely to be reversible with appropriate treatment).[7]

Much effort has been made to develop objective assessment of health-related quality of life in heart failure, such as the Minnesota Living with Heart Failure questionnaire[8] (Box 35-2) or the Kansas City Cardiomyopathy Questionnaire[9] (Table 35-3). These disease-specific instruments have been developed to improve the measurement of health status and quality of life; the findings would help physicians gain insight into disease severity or to quantify changes over time. Many of these have been used in substudies of clinical trials and are now beginning to be incorporated into standardized registries as part of patient assessment tools and performance measures.

The cardinal symptoms of heart failure are dyspnea (shortness of breath) and fatigue that occur either at rest or with exertion, or in both situations. Some patients may attribute their dyspnea to being "out of shape" or even to "old age." Many patients may have lived with it for so long that they do not even notice the degree of slow but steady deterioration. Conversely, some patients present initially with severe acute pulmonary edema that can be rarely mistaken for any other condition. Most patients manifest heart failure somewhere between these two extremes, and the most recent guideline updates have emphasized that the clinical manifestation can be congestion, lack of congestion, or lack of symptoms.[1] As in the eliciting of any medical history, many of the answers may be apparent only to experts, and most arise in casual conversations regarding activities of daily living. A good example is when patients are asked about their fluid status and dietary salt intake. Most patients insist that they have

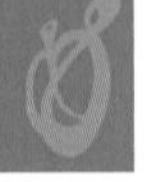

TABLE 35–2 Diagnostic Criteria for Heart Failure in Population-Based Studies

Framingham Criteria*

Major Criteria	Minor Criteria	Major or Minor Criteria
Paroxysmal nocturnal dyspnea or orthopnea	Ankle edema, night cough, dyspnea on exertion	Weight loss >4.5 kg in 5 days in response to treatment
Neck-vein distention	Hepatomegaly	
Rales	Pleural effusion	
Cardiomegaly	Vital capacity decreased 50% from maximal capacity	
Acute pulmonary edema	Tachycardia (heart rate >120/min)	
S3 gallop		
Increased venous pressure > 6 cm H_2O		
Circulation time > 25 sec		
Hepatojugular reflux		

Boston Criteria and NHANES Clinical Score†

Categories	Criteria	NHANES	Boston
History	Dyspnea		
	• At rest	—	4
	• On level ground	1	2
	• On climbing	1	1
	• Stop when walking at own pace or on level ground after 100 yards (91.44 m)	2	—
	Orthopnea	—	4
	Paroxysmal nocturnal dyspnea	—	3
Physical examination	Heart rate		
	• 91–110 beats/min	1	1
	• 110 beats/min	2	2
	Jugular venous pressure (>6 cm H_2O)		
	• Alone	1	2
	• Plus hepatomegaly or edema	2	3
	Rales/crackles		
	• Basilar crackles	1	1
	• More than basilar crackles	2	2
	Wheezing	—	3
	S3 gallop	—	3
Chest radiography	Alveolar pulmonary edema	—	4
	Alveolar fluid plus pleural fluid	3	—
	Interstitial pulmonary edema	2	3
	Interstitial edema plus pleural fluid	3	—
	Bilateral pleural effusion	—	3
	Cardiothoracic ratio >0.5 (posteroanterior projection)	—	3
	Upper zone flow redistribution	1	2

*Diagnosis of heart failure: two major criteria, or one major and two minor criteria, are required.

†Boston criteria for diagnosis of heart failure: "definite" (score 8–12 points), "possible" (score 5–7 points), or "unlikely" (score ≤ 4 points). NHANES-1 criteria for diagnosis of heart failure: score ≥ 3 points.

From Rector, T.S., Cohn, J.N. Assessment of patient outcome with the Minnesota Living with Heart Failure questionnaire: reliability and validity during a randomized, double-blind, placebo-controlled trial of pimobendan. Pimobendan Multicenter Research Group. *Am Heart J*, 1992;124(4):1017-25.

NHANES, National Health and Nutrition Examination Survey.

made every effort to reduce sodium intake. However, careful review of their dietary habits may reveal otherwise or simply clear ignorance of salt-laden food intake. Probing into specifics often helps physicians better understand patients' conditions and their immediate environment. Patients may also be focused on any abnormal signs and symptoms that may be attributable to heart failure or its treatment side effects. Good rapport with patients and their families is vital in eliciting information regarding adherence to medical advice and reviewing abilities to provide appropriate self-care.

Dyspnea

Dyspnea is the uncomfortable awareness of breathing. When it occurs at rest or at a level of physical activity at which it is not expected, it is abnormal. Dyspnea is a nonspecific symptom that occurs with a wide variety of cardiac, pulmonary, and chest wall disorders. For example, it can also result from acute anxiety, acute coronary insufficiency, and anemia. Patients with heart failure may manifest various types of dyspnea, including exertional dyspnea, orthopnea, paroxysmal nocturnal dyspnea, dyspnea at rest, and, with acute pulmonary edema, respiratory distress. An increase in respiratory rate (usually > 16 breaths/minute) usually accompanies dyspnea and may signal the onset of acute decompensation of stable heart failure.

The mechanisms of dyspnea, fatigue, and exercise intolerance in patients with heart failure are still not well understood, inasmuch as they are not simply a result of increased pulmonary capillary wedge pressure and decreased cardiac output.[10-14] There is little correlation between pulmonary capillary wedge pressure and exertional dyspnea in individual patients with heart failure, unless frank pulmonary is present.[15] It is well known that in auscultation, the lungs may sound clear in a substantial proportion of patients with shortness of breath and heart failure.[16]

All patients with heart failure should be carefully queried regarding the threshold of dyspnea onset during exercise.

BOX 35–1 Factors That May Precipitate the Worsening of Heart Failure

Myocardial ischemia or infarction
Excess dietary sodium or excess fluid intake
Medication noncompliance
Iatrogenic volume overload
Uncontrolled hypertension
Arrhythmia
- Atrial fibrillation or flutter
- Ventricular tachyarrhythmias
- Bradyarrhythmias

Comorbid conditions
- Fever, infections, or sepsis
- Thyroid dysfunction
- Anemia
- Renal insufficiency
- Nutritional deficiencies (such as thiamine deficiency)
- Pulmonary diseases (chronic obstructive pulmonary disease, pulmonary embolism, hypoxemia)

Inappropriate reduction of medications for heart failure
Adverse drug effects
- Alcohol
- Overzealous administration of negative inotropic agents (such as β-blockers, calcium channel blockers, antiarrhythmic agents)
- Nonsteroidal antiinflammatory drugs
- Thiazolidinediones and other medications that can cause fluid retention
- Corticosteroids

BOX 35–2 Minnesota Living With Heart Failure Questionnaire

Did your heart failure prevent you from living as you wanted during the last month by:
1. causing swelling in your ankles, legs, etc.?
2. making you sit or lie down to rest during the day?
3. making your walking about or climbing stairs difficult?
4. making your working around the house or yard difficult?
5. making your going places away from home difficult?
6. making your sleep at night difficult?
7. making your relating to or doing things with your friends and family difficult?
8. making your working to earn a living difficult?
9. making your recreational pastimes, sports, or hobbies difficult?
10. making your sexual activities difficult?
11. making you eat less of the foods you like?
12. making you short of breath?
13. making you tired, fatigued, or low on energy?
14. making you stay in a hospital?
15. costing you money for medical care?
16. giving you side effects from medicine?
17. making you feel you are a burden to your family or friends?
18. making you feel a loss of self-control in your life?
19. making you worry?
20. making it difficult for you to concentrate or remember things?
21. making you feel depressed?

TABLE 35–3 Kansas City Cardiomyopathy Questionnaire

1. Please indicate how much you are limited by *heart failure* (shortness of breath or fatigue) in your ability to do the following activities *over the past 2 weeks?* (extremely limited, quite a bit limited, moderately limited, slightly limited, not at all limited, or limited for other reasons or did not do the activity)
   - Dress yourself
   - Showering/bathing
   - Walking 1 block on level ground
   - Doing yard work, housework, or carrying groceries
   - Climbing a flight of stairs without stopping
   - Hurrying or jogging (as if to catch a bus)
2. *Compared with 2 weeks ago,* have your symptoms of *heart failure* (shortness of breath, fatigue, or ankle swelling) changed? (much worse, slightly worse, not changed, slightly better, much better, I've had no symptoms over the last 2 weeks)
3. Over the *past 2 weeks,* how much have the following signs/symptoms bothered you? (extremely, quite a bit, moderately, slightly, not at all bothersome; no such signs/symptoms)
   - Swelling in your feet, ankles, or legs
   - Fatigue
   - Shortness of breath
4. Over the *past 2 weeks,* how many times did you have *swelling* in your feet, ankles, or legs when you woke up in the morning? (every morning, 3 or more times a week but not every day, 1–2 times a week, less than once a week, never over the past 2 weeks)
5. Over the *past 2 weeks,* on average, how many times has *fatigue* limited your ability to do what you want? (all the time, several times/day, at least once/day, 3 or more times/week but not every day, 1–2 times/week, less than once/week, never over the past 2 weeks)
6. Over the *past 2 weeks,* on average, how many times have you been forced to sleep sitting up in a chair or with at least 3 pillows to prop you up because of *shortness of breath?* (every night, 3 or more times/week but not every day, 1–2 times/week, less than once/week, never over the past 2 weeks)
7. *Heart failure* symptoms can worsen for a number of reasons. How sure are you that you know what to do, or whom to call, if your *heart failure* gets worse? (not at all sure, not very sure, somewhat sure, mostly sure, completely sure)
8. How well do you understand what things you are able to do to keep your *heart failure* symptoms from getting worse (for example, weighing yourself, eating a low salt diet, etc.)? (Do not understand at all, do not understand very well, somewhat understand, mostly understand, completely understand)
9. Over the *past 2 weeks,* how much has your *heart failure* limited your enjoyment of life? (extremely, quite a bit, moderately, slightly, not limited)
10. If you had to spend the rest of your life with your *heart failure* the way it is *right now,* how would you feel about this? (not at all satisfied, mostly dissatisfied, somewhat satisfied, mostly satisfied, completely satisfied)
11. Over the *past 2 weeks,* how often have you felt discouraged or down in the dumps because of your *heart failure?* (all the time, most of the time, occasionally, rarely, never)
12. How much does your *heart failure* affect your lifestyle? Please indicate how your *heart failure* may have limited your participation in the following activities *over the past 2 weeks.* (severe limited, limited quite a bit, moderately limited, slightly limited, did not limit at all, does not apply or did not do for other reasons)
   - Hobbies, recreational activities
   - Working or doing household chores
   - Visiting family or friends out of your home
   - Intimate relationships with loved ones

From Green, C.P., Porter, C.B., Bresnahan, D.R., et al. Development and evaluation of the Kansas City Cardiomyopathy Questionnaire: a new health status measure for heart failure. *J Am Coll Cardiol* 2000; 35:1245-1255.

Specific examples of how and when the dyspnea occurs should be sought. The mechanism of dyspnea should be considered. Shortness of breath may be caused by concomitant pulmonary disease or respiratory muscle dysfunction.[17] Increased ventilatory drive or exercise hyperventilation is believed to be a common cause of dyspnea in patients with heart failure,[18-21] but the precise mechanism of dyspnea has not been pinpointed. The mechanism of increased ventilatory drive in patients with heart failure is multifactorial and incompletely understood, but it may be related to increased peripheral chemosensitivity in the skeletal muscles and accumulation of lactic acid. Both of these may lead to exercise hyperpnea,[22,23] which tires the patient out at increasingly earlier points in exercise. This concept is consistent with the "muscle hypothesis," according to which dyspnea in patients with heart failure actually begins in the skeletal muscles.[22,23] Exertional dyspnea can also occur when there is markedly elevated left ventricular filling pressure.

Multiple, complex mechanisms are operative in the production of exertional dyspnea in patients with heart failure, and probably no single mechanism is dominant. Nevertheless, the augmented ventilatory response to exercise in heart failure (such as increased breathing rate in relation to the amount of exercise) is correlated with hemodynamic alterations,[24] whereas peak ventilatory oxygen uptake (Vo_2) is not. According to the dominant theory of increased exercise ventilatory response of heart failure, increases in carbon dioxide output in relation to peak oxygen consumption lead to bicarbonate buffering and accumulation of lactic acid.[23] Lactic acid builds up at relative low levels in patients with heart failure and acts as an additional stimulus to breathing. This buildup may also contribute to the sensation of dyspnea. In some patients, there is also an increase in airway dead space because of reduced perfusion of ventilated lung tissue, which leads to inefficient gas exchange. Despite this, arterial carbon dioxide concentration is driven to low levels during peak exercise in most patients with heart failure. According to the "muscle hypothesis" of exertional dyspnea, peripheral (i.e., skeletal muscle) chemoreceptors are stimulated by higher levels of arterial oxygen and carbon dioxide concentrations in heart failure, which leads to overactivation of ergoreflexes.[25] This overactivation increases both ventilatory drive and sympathetic nervous system activity through the activation of a central mechanism. Physical training in patients with heart failure may reduce exaggerated ergoreflex activity and thereby improve the response to exercise.[26] Clearly, exertional dyspnea in patients with heart failure is complex, multifactorial, and not simply a result of increased filling pressures. Reflex control mechanisms involving the heart, lungs, brain, and skeletal muscles and a buildup of lactic acid in the working muscles are probably involved; they would lead to an increased ventilatory response to exercise.

Fatigue

As with dyspnea, the mechanism of fatigue in patients with heart failure is uncertain. Cardiac fatigue was widely assumed to be simply a result of low cardiac output, but since 2000, it has become clear that abnormalities of skeletal muscles and other noncardiac comorbid conditions such as anemia may contribute to fatigue. Abnormalities of high-energy phosphates in the skeletal muscles of patients with heart failure are well documented (see also Chapter 19),[27-31] even in the presence of normal regional blood flow.[29] Muscle fatigue is related to abnormal phosphocreatinine depletion, acidosis, or both in the working muscle. The anaerobic regeneration of adenosine triphosphate (ATP) is impaired in the skeletal muscles of patients with heart failure. There is also a shift in fiber distribution: The percentage of the fast-twitch, glycolytic, easily fatigable type IIb fibers is increased.[27] Patients with heart failure have major histological alterations in skeletal muscle and biochemical alterations,[32] including the development of skeletal muscle atrophy.[33] Significant ultrastructural abnormalities[34] lead to diminished oxidative capacity of working muscle.[35,36] Chronic fatigue begets further inactivity, which leads to further deconditioning and a greater extent of disability. In the late stages of heart failure, low cardiac output and anemia related to chronic disease probably also contribute to fatigue. Patients who are ambulatory with heart failure should be encouraged to stay physically active,[37,38] and participation in a structured exercise training program can improve exercise tolerance.[39-41]

Other Symptoms of Heart Failure

An occasional patient with heart failure presents with palpitations, lightheadedness, or even frank syncope. In the authors' experience, this is unusual. However, heart block, arrhythmias with circulatory collapse, or even atrial fibrillation or premature beats may be a presenting feature of heart failure, which is especially common in specific conditions such as acute myocarditis, sarcoid cardiomyopathy, or Chagas' disease. Right upper quadrant pain caused by acute liver congestion or early satiety may be another presenting symptom. Additional presenting symptoms might include nocturnal angina, weight loss (weight gain is more common), and cough. Other signs and symptoms of heart failure are usually present. Sometimes symptoms of heart failure are more subtle and are often mistakenly misdiagnosed as "bronchitis" (dry productive cough), "asthma" (wheezing due to cardiac asthma), or "insomnia" (Hunter-Cheyne-Stokes respiration). Many endocrine abnormalities can be associated with heart failure and may be treatable. In asymptomatic people it is not uncommon for cardiomegaly to be diagnosed on a routine chest radiograph or for left bundle branch block or arrhythmia to be detected on an electrocardiogram; both situations are forerunners to the development of heart failure and cardiac dysfunction.

CLINICAL EVALUATION OF PRESENTING SIGNS: PHYSICAL EXAMINATION

A careful physical examination is always warranted in the evaluation of patients with heart failure. The purpose of the examination is to help determine the cause and severity of the heart failure. Obtaining additional information about the hemodynamic profile, documenting the response to therapy, and determining the prognosis are important additional goals of the physical examination.

General Inspection of the Patient

The diagnosis of heart failure is relatively straightforward by simple medical history and physical examination. It is not unusual for an experienced physician to sense the severity of the heart failure syndrome within the first few minutes of walking into the examination room, meeting the patient, and observing the patient carefully. Hospitalized patients often have labored or uncomfortable breathing. They may not be able to finish a sentence because of shortness of breath. Lying down may be difficult because of orthopnea. Altered respiratory signs such as coughing, Hunter-Cheyne-Stokes respiration, and cyanosis are sometimes observed. Peripheral cyanosis, which is limited to exposed skin, usually indicates inadequate perfusion or low cardiac output. In contrast, central cyanosis is uncommon, but when it occurs, it is found predominantly in the tongue, uvula, and buccal mucosa; its presence indicates intracardiac or intrapulmonary shunting. Some patients demonstrate cachexia, a particularly poor prognostic sign. The presence of severe peripheral edema and ascites are obvious in visual inspection.

Examination of the arterial pulse is very important. The absence of pulses should be noted, as should the character of the pulse detected. Pulsus alternans (a strong beat alternating with a weak beat), although unusual, is virtually diagnostic for severe advanced heart failure. Pulsus paradoxus (a substantial diminishment in the amplitude of the arterial pulse during inspiration) is found in pericardial tamponade. It is usually confirmed by measuring blood pressure carefully during the phases of inspiration and expiration. Pulsus paradoxus is also seen in an occasional patient with severe asthma, pulmonary embolism, pregnancy, or marked obesity and in patients with superior vena cava syndrome. Patients with aortic stenosis may have diminished upstroke of the carotid pulse, whereas patients with severe, chronic aortic regurgitation manifest accentuated pulses and a series of findings related to a large stroke volume. Peripheral pulses may be absent in patients with coarctation of the aorta. Therefore, a thorough assessment of the pulses is always warranted.

Assessment of the Volume Status of the Patient

Pertinent features of the cardiac physical examination, such as jugular venous distention and tissue congestion, are especially important in the accurate assessment of the patient with heart failure. It can be useful to dichotomize the signs of heart failure as those of volume overload and those of low cardiac output (see Figure 35-3).[42] Signs of volume overload include increased jugular venous distention, prominent V waves, gallop heart rhythm (or third heart sound [S3]), rales and pleural effusion, anasarca, ascites, and peripheral edema. On occasion, specific organomegaly is present; examples include enlarged and sometimes tender liver, enlarged spleen (rare), and cardiomegaly. According to the Evaluation Study of Congestive Heart Failure and Pulmonary Artery Catheterization Effectiveness (ESCAPE) trial,[43] the presence of orthopnea and increased jugular venous distention may be useful for detecting increased intracardiac filling pressures, whereas a global assessment of inadequate perfusion ("cold profile") may be useful for detecting reduced cardiac index.

Despite the historical use of the term *congestive heart failure,* it is not unusual for patients with advanced heart failure to consistently demonstrate no evidence of volume overload.[16] For reasons that are unclear, such patients do not seem to retain significant amounts of salt and water; hence, they are subject to overdiuresis, which leads in some cases to *prerenal azotemia.* Patients should be examined while they are lying down, with the head tilted at 45 degrees. The physician should examine a patient from the patient's right side (oslerian tradition). The most important assessment of volume status is careful examination of the jugular venous pressure; unfortunately, this is somewhat of a lost art.[16,44,45] It is important to understand that jugular venous pressure often reflects left- and right-sided filling pressures but that a substantial number of patients with heart failure have relatively normal intracardiac filling pressures and no distended neck veins. In patients with mild heart failure, the jugular venous pressure may be normal when the patient is lying with the head tilted at 45 degrees, but it rises to abnormal levels with compression to the right upper quadrant. This is referred to as *hepatojugular reflux.* To elicit this sign, the right upper quadrant should be compressed firmly, gradually, and continuously for 1 minute while the neck veins are observed. The presence of hepatojugular reflux that very slowly dissipates on release of hand pressure is a sign that intracardiac filling pressures are abnormally increased.[46]

Despite the common lack of abdominal complaints, some patients do accumulate fluid in the form of ascites or visceral edema. Examination of the abdomen should be performed to determine the presence of ascites, hepatosplenomegaly, or pulsatile, tender liver. Splenomegaly is rare in heart failure. However, hepatomegaly is common, and acute congestion can lead to rather severe right upper quadrant tenderness that mimics cholecystitis. On occasion, patients with acute decompensation and severe right upper quadrant pain may even go to the operating room for cholecystectomy with the suspicion of acute cholecystitis, where the actual problem is found to be acute hepatic congestion. Liver transaminase levels are often elevated during acute passive congestion, and in severe right-sided heart failure, levels of clotting factors and total bilirubin may be increased. Raised intra-abdominal pressures have been recognized in patients with congestion and decompensated heart failure, which further illustrates the evidence and hemodynamic impact of abdominal congestion.[47]

Normal, hyperdynamic, or sustained precordial pulsations may be present. Cardiomegaly tends to displace the point of maximal impulse, which is also sustained in cases of severe left ventricular hypertrophy. Physical examination of the precordial pulsation, however, is inadequate for assessing

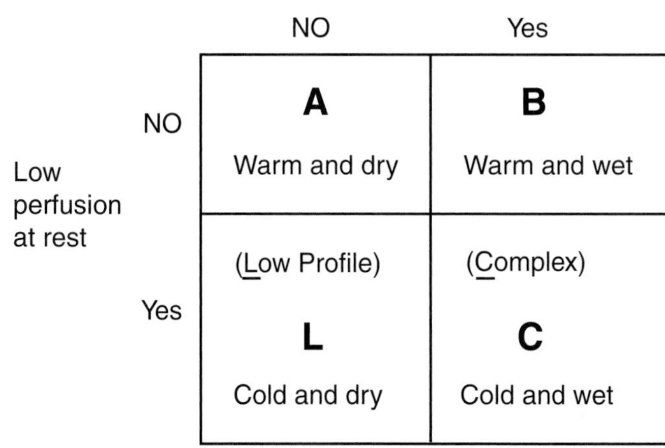

NO
Yes
NO
Yes
Low perfusion at rest
A
Warm and dry
B
Warm and wet
(Low Profile)
(Complex)
L
Cold and dry
C
Cold and wet
Signs/Symptoms of Congestion:
Orthopnea/PND
Jugular venous distension
Hepatomegaly
Edema
Rales (rare in chronic heart failure)
Elevated est. PAsys
Valsalva square wave
Abdominal-jugular reflux
Possible Evidence of Low Perfusion:
Narrow pulse pressure
Sleepy/obtunded
Low serum sodium
Cool extremities
Hypotension with ACE inhibitor
Renal dysfunction

FIGURE 35–3 Clinical presentation of acute heart failure syndrome based on congestion and perfusion. (From Nohria, A., Lewis E., Stevenson, L. W. (2002). Medical management of advanced heart failure. JAMA, *287*, 628-640.)

the degree of left ventricular dysfunction. In some patients, a third heart sound is audible and palpable at the apex. Patients with enlarged or hypertrophied right ventricles may have a sustained and prolonged left parasternal impulse that extends throughout systole.

A third heart sound (or gallop rhythm) is most commonly present in patients with volume overload who have tachycardia and tachypnea. It may be absent in many patients with advanced heart failure, but the presence of a third heart sound can signify severe hemodynamic compromise.[48] The murmurs of mitral and tricuspid regurgitation are frequently present in patients with advanced heart failure, although severe regurgitation is frequently present in the absence of an audible murmur. The presence of jugular venous distention and a third heart sound imply a poor prognosis[49] and disease progression[50] and should always be sought and recorded in the notes.

Of interest is that signs of pulmonary congestion (such as rales, pulmonary edema, and elevated jugular venous pressure) are frequently absent even in patients with raised pulmonary capillary wedge pressure.[16] Similar to patients with long-standing mitral stenosis, patients with chronic, severe heart failure tend to have robust lymphatic drainage of the pulmonary interstitial spaces. The absence of rales does not preclude impending pulmonary edema, and direct hemodynamic measurements may sometimes be necessary. Instead, tachypnea (and in some extreme cases, hypoxia) is often associated with significant pulmonary congestion.

An increase in circulating volume is often associated with evidence of excessive adrenergic activity. This evidence includes diaphoresis, tachycardia, pallor, and coldness of the extremities. The adrenergic nervous system is similarly activated during low cardiac output. Relief of congestion is always an important primary goal in the management of patients with chronic heart failure; thus, the identification of the volume overload state is a critical step in the physical examination.[51]

Signs of Low Cardiac Output

Patients in a low-output state may exhibit a wide variety of clinical signs (from cool, dry skin, pallor, or peripheral cyanosis to normal color, warmth, and appearance). In some cases, pulses may be diminished and blood pressure may be low with a narrow pulse pressure. Some patients demonstrate virtually no signs of inadequate blood flow despite a low cardiac output. They may be alert and cognitively responsive despite extreme diminishment in cardiac index (i.e., <1.5 L/min/m^2). This finding is probably related to the body's remarkable ability to redistribute flow to vital organs (including the brain) in the presence of very diminished cardiac output. In contrast, with acute cardiogenic shock (e.g., acute myocardial infarction), patients may develop cool skin, pallor, changes in mental status or cognitive deficits, oliguria, peripheral cyanosis, and hypothermia. Pulsus alternans, if present, is virtually pathognomonic of a low-output state[52] but is more often seen in terminally ill patients. Compensatory tachycardia (especially in young patients) and low blood pressures are more common in the setting of profound signs and symptoms of heart failure, and they are of concern in low-output states. Clinical assessment of inadequate perfusion can yield reasonably accurate findings.[43]

Signs of Cachexia (see also Chapter 21)

The importance of cachexia in patients with severe end-stage heart failure is currently the subject of intense research.[53,54] It is believed that unintentional weight loss and cachexia portend a very poor prognosis. Although the mechanism of cachexia is not entirely understood, it may be related to various cytokines, including tumor necrosis factor α, whose levels are known to be increased in patients with heart failure with poor prognosis.[55]

LABORATORY EVALUATION OF THE PATIENT WITH HEART FAILURE

As shown in Tables 35-4 and 35-5, the diagnostic sensitivity and specificity of the clinical history and physical examination for diagnosing patients with heart failure are relatively poor. For this reason, laboratory testing has assumed a progressively greater role in establishing the diagnosis of heart failure.

Biochemical Evaluation: Biomarker Testing (see also Chapter 37)

It is recommended that patients with new-onset heart failure undergo a battery of routine laboratory tests when the condition is first diagnosed. This is also recommended for patients with chronic heart failure and acute decompensation, when there is a change in therapeutic intervention, or in periodic monitoring for clinical stability. Very often, a basic metabolic panel that includes measurement of electrolytes and renal markers is useful, sometimes with additional thyroid or liver function tests or measurement of markers of glycemic or lipid control.[56,57] The recognition of anemia in patients with heart failure who have a poor prognosis has also prompted periodic evaluation of hemoglobin levels and iron profiles, but some patients may have reversible abnormalities.[58]

Several cardiac biomarkers may provide incremental diagnostic and prognostic information, such as B-type (brain) natriuretic peptide (BNP) and cardiac troponin.[59] BNP and its amino-terminal fragment (NT-proBNP) in particular have provided important diagnostic utility for heart failure in the acute clinical setting (Figure 35-4). There are still ongoing clinical studies to determine the appropriateness of their uses in guiding therapy, because clinical trials supporting the drugs and devices received their approval *before* broad adoption of biomarker testing. Testing for markers for inflammation (such as erythrocyte sedimentation rate, C-reactive protein, or other specific rheumatological disease markers) can sometimes be helpful in unmasking myocarditis or other inflammatory causes, but routine measurements are yet to be adopted.[59] Viral antibody titers have also found to yield little information and are rarely indicated, inasmuch as the appropriate treatment with positive viral antibody titers remains unclear at this point. Other commonly measured biomarkers indicate renal function (blood urea nitrogen and serum creatinine levels), electrolyte balance (sodium and potassium levels), oxidative process (uric acid level), liver function (total bilirubin level, aminotransferase levels, prothrombin time), and hematological status (hemoglobin, red blood cell distribution width); the majority of them are important prognostic indicators of disease severity. The use of cardiac biomarker evaluation in heart failure is discussed further in Chapter 37.

Electrocardiographic Evaluation: Electrocardiography

Electrocardiographic evaluation remains a valuable and broadly available laboratory test for patients with heart failure. An electrocardiogram should be routinely obtained and studied for evidence of underlying structural alterations (e.g., left ventricular hypertrophy, prior myocardial infarctions), for rhythm abnormalities as a cause or consequence of heart failure decompensation (e.g., atrial fibrillation, frequent ectopic beats, or other sustained arrhythmias), and for the presence of conduction abnormalities (such as bundle branch block or intraventricular conduction delays) that may lead to electrical dyssynchrony. Frequently, Holter monitoring or event monitoring can assist with the detection of such abnormalities.

The QT interval should be noted because many types of therapy can further prolong the QT interval and provoke lethal arrhythmias. In patients who have undergone cardiac resynchronization therapy (CRT), acute changes in the QRS complex or structure may also signify underlying pacing or programming alterations (although such changes may or may not result in reversal of cardiac remodeling, and they are not a prerequisite for symptomatic improvement). The presence of ectopic beats, although benign in most cases, may also lead to cardiac insufficiency when the burden is high.

Morphological Evaluation: Chest Radiography, Echocardiography, and Magnetic Resonance Imaging (see also Chapter 36)

The authors believe that chest radiography remains important in the assessment of patients with heart failure. Radiographic evidence of pulmonary congestion may precede the presence of rales. Careful examination of the cardiac size and shape, as well as the pulmonary vasculature, remains part of routine evaluation of all patients with heart failure. In recipients of CRT implantation, posteroanterior and lateral views of chest radiographs may help determine inappropriate left ventricular lead positioning that may contribute to persistent symptoms (Figure 35-5).

Echocardiographic evaluation remains an essential diagnostic tool for assessing cardiac structure and function. The focus has traditionally been on left ventricular ejection fraction, and the degree of underlying chamber dilation (or hypertrophy) can be overlooked. In fact, it is seldom recognized that the estimation of effective stroke volume (i.e., the ejection fraction relative to the left ventricular end-diastolic volume) is more appropriate in determining whether the signs and symptoms can be explained by cardiac causes. Therefore, chamber size is an important indicator of compensatory progression of disease, and the propensity for long-term recovery. Other aspects of chamber dilation can lead to valvular regurgitation (from annular dilation) or mechanical dyssynchrony from prolonged interventricular and intraventricular conduction delays. Doppler study estimates of right ventricular or pulmonary artery systolic pressure are helpful surrogates for measurements of pulmonary hypertension. Doppler patterns of mitral, tricuspid, and pulmonary vein flow can provide estimates of intracardiac pressures and diastolic staging, and tissue Doppler indices can characterize the myocardial abnormalities related to diastolic dysfunction and restrictive physiology.

The clinical utility of mechanical dyssynchrony assessment remains debated. Left atrial enlargement and left ventricular hypertrophy are common findings in diastolic heart failure, whereas left ventricular outflow track obstruction (at rest or provoked by amyl nitrite), caused by asymmetrical septal hypertrophy or systolic anterior motion of the mitral leaflet, may occur in the setting of hypertrophic cardiomyopathy. The presence of thrombus in the left ventricular appendage or the left atrium or left atrial appendage can be a surrogate indicator of low cardiac output status, and should warrant aggressive evaluation. The presence of wall motion abnormalities or abnormalities of cardiac structure and performance are obvious hallmarks of stage B heart failure. This topic is further discussed in Chapter 36.

Magnetic resonance imaging (MRI) has been considerably useful in the morphological and functional assessment of the heart. At present, however, this technology is used mainly to gain additional information. Cardiac MRI, like echocardiography, requires viewing in multiple oblique planes of the heart. The imaging techniques are designed to render blood dark or bright and to depict various aspects of motion, flow, and perfusion (Figure 35-6). Different techniques have been used for assessing cardiac function with MRI. New magnetic

TABLE 35–4 Sensitivity, Specificity, and Predictive Accuracy of Symptoms and Signs for Diagnosing Heart Failure

Symptoms or Signs	Sensitivity (%)	Specificity (%)	Predictive Accuracy (%)
Exertional dyspnea	66	52	23
Orthopnea	21	81	2
Paroxysmal	33	76	26
History of edema	23	80	22
Resting heart rate	7	99	6
Rales	13	91	21
Third heart sound	31	95	61
Jugular	10	97	2
Edema (on examination)	10	93	3

From Harlan WR, Oberman A, Grimm R, et al. Chronic congestive heart failure in coronary artery disease: clinical criteria. *Ann Intern Med* 1977;86:133-138.

TABLE 35–5 Utility of Components of History and Physical Examination in Detecting Pulmonary Capillary Wedge Pressure Exceeding 22 mm Hg

			Predictive Value		Likelihood Ratio	
Finding	Sensitivity	Specificity	Positive	Negative	Positive	Negative
Rales (≥1/3 lung field)	15	89	69	38	1.32	1.04
S3	62	32	61	33	0.92	0.85
Ascites (≥moderate)	21	92	81	40	2.44	1.15
Edema (≥2+)	41	66	67	40	1.20	1.11
Orthopnea (≥2 pillow)	86	25	66	51	1.15	1.80
Hepatomegaly (>4 fb)	15	93	78	39	2.13	1.09
Hepatojugular reflux	83	27	65	49	1.13	1.54
JVP ≥ 12 mm Hg	65	64	75	52	1.79	1.82
JVP < 8 mm Hg	4.3	81	28	33	0.23	0.85

From Drazner MH, Hellkamp AS, Leier CV, et al. Value of clinician assessment of hemodynamics in advanced heart failure: the ESCAPE trial. *Circ Heart Fail* 2008;1:170-177.
fb, fingerbreadths; JVP, jugular venous pressure.

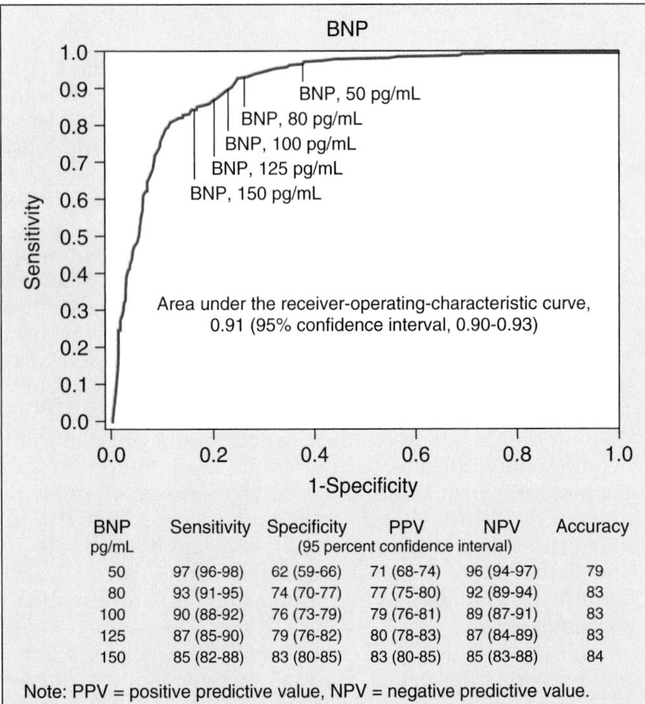

BNP pg/mL	Sensitivity	Specificity	PPV	NPV	Accuracy
	(95 percent confidence interval)				
50	97 (96-98)	62 (59-66)	71 (68-74)	96 (94-97)	79
80	93 (91-95)	74 (70-77)	77 (75-80)	92 (89-94)	83
100	90 (88-92)	76 (73-79)	79 (76-81)	89 (87-91)	83
125	87 (85-90)	79 (76-82)	80 (78-83)	87 (84-89)	83
150	85 (82-88)	83 (80-85)	83 (80-85)	85 (83-88)	84

Note: PPV = positive predictive value, NPV = negative predictive value.

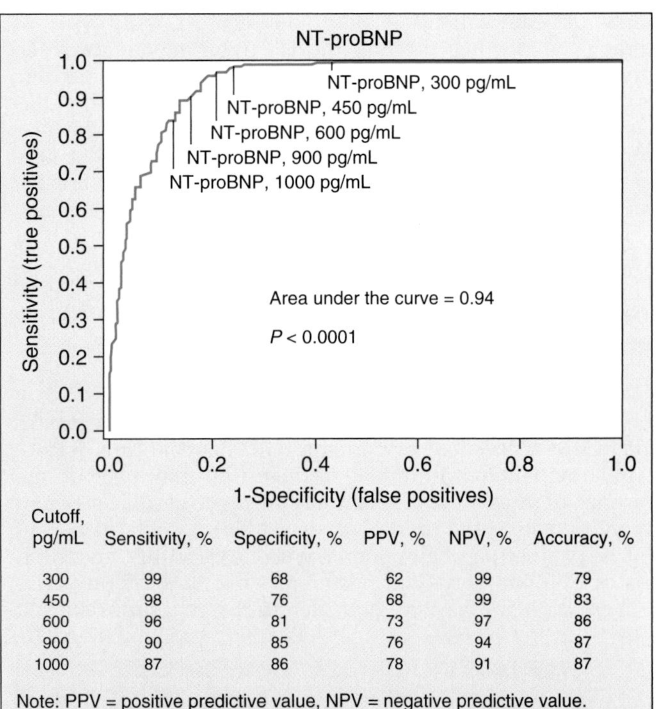

Cutoff, pg/mL	Sensitivity, %	Specificity, %	PPV, %	NPV, %	Accuracy, %
300	99	68	62	99	79
450	98	76	68	99	83
600	96	81	73	97	86
900	90	85	76	94	87
1000	87	86	78	91	87

Note: PPV = positive predictive value, NPV = negative predictive value.

FIGURE 35–4 Receiver operator characteristic curves for diagnostic accuracies for B-type natriuretic peptide (BNP) (*left*) and amino-terminal pro-B-type natriuretic peptide (NT-proBNP) (*right*). *CHF,* congestive heart failure; V_E, ventilation; V_{CO_2}, carbon dioxide production. (*Left,* From Maisel AS, Krishnaswamy P, Nowak RM, et al. Rapid measurement of B-type natriuretic peptide in the emergency diagnosis of heart failure. *N Engl J Med* 2002;347:161-167. *Right,* From Januzzi JL Jr, Camargo CA, Anwaruddin S, et al. The N-terminal Pro-BNP Investigation of Dyspnea in the Emergency Department (PRIDE) study. *Am J Cardiol* 2005;95:948-954.)

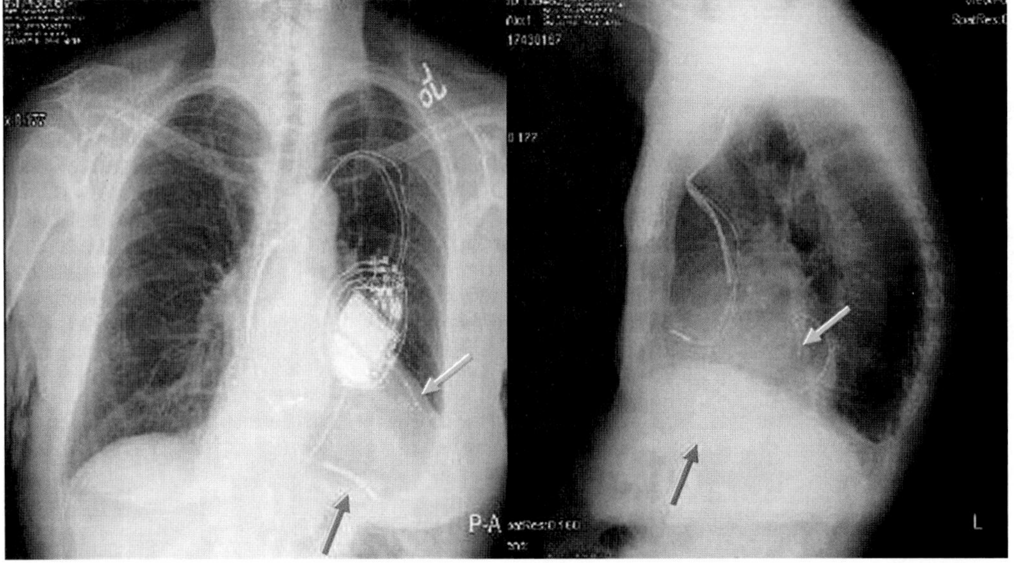

FIGURE 35–5 Appropriate lead placement (*arrows*) for cardiac resynchronization therapy in chest radiography.

resonance sequences enable the study of cardiac motion (myocardial tagging, blood flow velocity (phase contrast method), and myocardial scarring (late enhancement technique), and specific patterns may indicate the presence of infiltrative diseases (such as amyloidosis, sarcoidosis, hemachromatosis) or myocarditis (see also Chapter 36).

Ischemic Evaluation: Myocardial Viability and Coronary Anatomy (see Chapters 23 and 36)

Coronary artery disease is the cause of heart failure in about two thirds of patients with left ventricular systolic dysfunction, and up to one third of patients with nonischemic cardiomyopathy experience chest pain that mimics angina (see also Chapter 23).[56,60] Researchers have also pointed out that underdiagnosis or misdiagnosis of ischemic heart disease among patients with heart failure is common if angiographic evaluation was not undertaken as part of the heart failure workup.[61,62]

Patients with systolic heart failure and severe coronary artery disease have, by definition, ischemic cardiomyopathy, and in some cases this reduction in myocardial function may be improved with percutaneous coronary intervention (PCI) or surgical revascularization. Most patients with heart failure should be considered candidates for diagnostic coronary angiography to determine whether significant coronary artery disease is present, especially in patients for

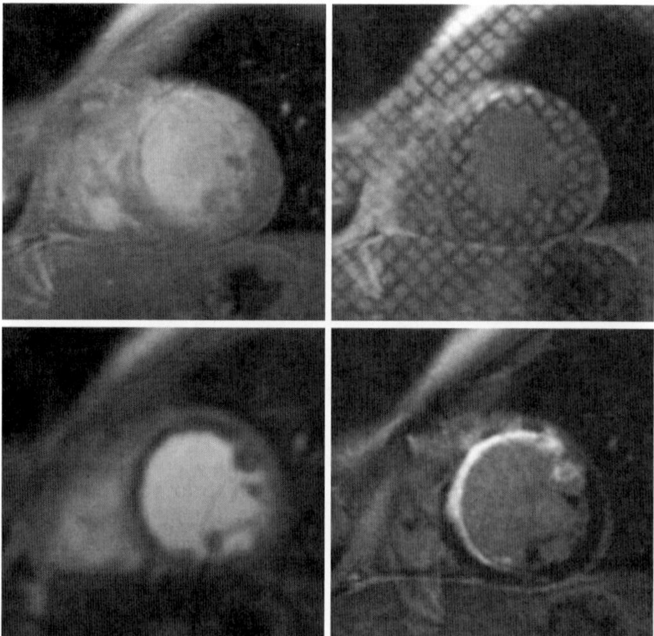

FIGURE 35-6 Cardiac magnetic resonance imaging (MRI) assessment of myocardial viability with cine-imaging (*top left*), myocardial tagging imaging (*top right*), TurboFlash perfusion imaging with gadolinium (*bottom left*), and delay-enhanced imaging with gadolinium (*bottom right*).

whom revascularization is often very beneficial. This clearly remains highly controversial because such an invasive procedure may not be needed in most patients with a good clinical history and in whom clinical suspicion of heart failure is low because of the lack of cardiovascular risk factors. However, coronary artery disease may not be easily predicted from the medical history, physical examination findings, and echocardiogram.[63] For a patient who has angina pectoris and heart failure, an even more compelling argument can be made for performing diagnostic coronary angiography. On the other hand, severe coronary artery disease and reduced left ventricular function are present but anginal symptoms are minimal, demonstration of myocardial viability is of paramount importance (and is discussed in Chapter 37). Also, diagnostic evaluation for coronary artery disease provides only a "snapshot" at the time of evaluation, and atherosclerotic diseases may progress over time, leading to progressive ischemia.

In the case of cardiac MRI, assessment of myocardial viability is of utmost importance to detect ischemic but viable myocardium for potential therapeutic interventions. In patients with heart failure, of whom 60% to 70% suffer from coronary artery disease, these techniques are helpful for therapeutic and prognostic stratification. Late-enhancement MRI has become a tool for determining lesion size in patients with myocardial infarction. The spatial and temporal relationship measured through differential uptake and release of contrast material in the viable tissue versus scar tissue can provide the location as well as extent of the scar.

Functional Evaluation: Cardiopulmonary Exercise Testing (see Chapter 57)

For many activities of daily living, a fundamental requirement is the ability to perform aerobic work. Functional capacity is usually measured in metabolic equivalents (METs) where 1 MET represents 3.5 mL of O_2/kg/min. Exercise testing is a valuable tool in the diagnosis and assessment of patients with heart failure[38] (Table 35-6). It has long been recognized that the simple history and physical examination, as well as various subjective functional classification systems, can be too nonspecific and relatively insensitive. Therefore, exercise testing can add substantial precision in the initial evaluation of the patient with heart failure. This is particularly true when heart transplantation is a consideration or when quantitative information on assessing an individual patient's disability is necessary.

The primary goal of metabolic exercise testing is to determine the functional status and prognosis of the patient objectively (see also Chapter 57). Exercise testing in patients with heart failure was first widely applied in the late 1970s to test the response of patients to various drug therapies.[13] Although it has become apparent that response of exercise to short-term drug therapy is not predictive of long-term drug efficacy,[64] useful information regarding how to gauge the degree of disability more precisely has emerged from these studies. More recently, exercise testing has been used to assess the severity of heart failure and to help determine the prognosis for individual patients. In retrospect, it has become clear that measurements of the peak V_{O_2} and the slope of the ratio of ventilation (V_E) to carbon dioxide production (V_{CO_2}) (V_E/V_{CO_2}) are powerful predictors of prognosis. Serial improvement in peak V_{O_2}, either in response to therapy or occurring spontaneously, has also been demonstrated to have prognostic value.[65] However, the V_E/V_{CO_2} slope remains the strongest predictor of prognosis, better even than peak V_{O_2}.[66] The usefulness of cardiac output estimation during standard metabolic exercise testing is under intense investigation.[67]

Metabolic exercise testing is of value in determining whether the heart or lungs are causing the dyspnea. Increased ventilation (V_E) with regard to carbon dioxide production is a hallmark finding of patients with heart failure[66,68] (Figure 35-7). The slope of the V_E/V_{CO_2} ratio offers important prognostic information, perhaps even more than V_{O_2}.[68,69] However, the increase in V_E/V_{CO_2} slope observed in patients with heart failure is nonspecific[70]; it can also be abnormally steep in patients with primary lung disease.[71]

Assessment of functional capacity is typically performed on a motorized treadmill or a stationary bicycle ergometer. The functional capacity can be estimated or measured directly by gas exchange methods (V_{O_2}) from the highest work level achieved. Estimates of functional capacity such as exercise duration are less reliable than direct measurements of gas exchange. Peak V_{O_2} and anaerobic ventilatory threshold are

TABLE 35–6 Weber Classification of Functional Impairment in Aerobic Capacity and Anaerobic Threshold as Measured during Incremental Exercise Testing

Class	Degree of Impairment	V_{O_2} Max (mL/min/kg)	Anaerobic Threshold (mL/min/kg)
A	None to mild	>20	> 14
B	Mild to moderate	16–20	11–14
C	Moderate to severe	10–16	8–11
D	Severe	6–10	5–8
E	Very severe	<6	≤4

V_{O_2}, ventilatory oxygen uptake.

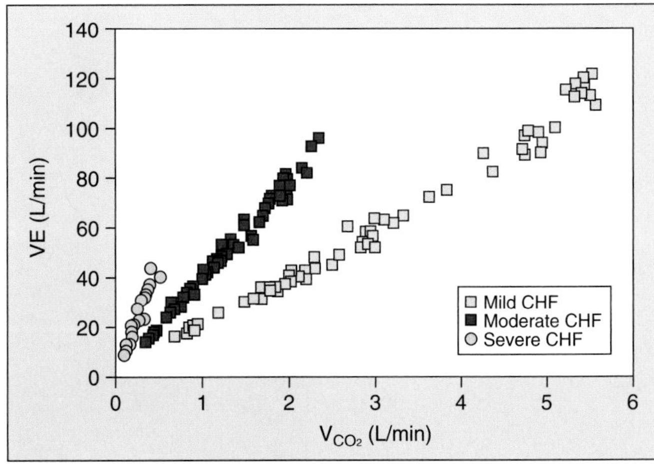

FIGURE 35–7 Plot of minute ventilation (VE) versus the rate of carbon dioxide production (V_{CO_2}) in patients with different degrees of severity of chronic heart failure (CHF). (From Coats AJ. Heart failure: What causes the symptoms of heart failure? *Heart* 2001;86:574-578.)

highly reproducible and therefore recommended for evaluation of patients with heart failure.[38] The peak V_{O_2} is currently the standard used by most laboratories. However, maximal exercise testing has well-known limitations in the setting of heart failure.[72] Because patients generally have a reduced level of physical activity, peak V_{O_2} may not be a relevant indicator of everyday exercise capacity. The 6-minute walk or shuttle-walk tests, on the other hand, are simpler and do not require special equipment.[73,74] Simply assessing exercise duration can also provide important prognostic information. However, it is controversial whether these submaximal exercise tests are accurate predictors of prognosis,[75,76] inasmuch as the results may depend on the patient's motivation and the operator's enthusiasm. The point of aerobic threshold is, however, insensitive to patient motivation. In this regard, submaximal exercise testing may be an ideal test of everyday activity capacity, but there is no uniform agreement on how to best perform it. A prime use of metabolic exercise testing is in the evaluation of patients for heart transplantation. A peak V_{O_2} of more than 14 mL/kg/min is considered "too well" for transplantation in many centers.[77] Because this information was derived from a relatively aged population before the widespread use of β-adrenergic blockers, this criterion has posed some problems with younger individuals, in whom extremely poor functional capacity is not below this cutoff range. In the most recent guidelines about advanced heart failure,[78] the criteria have therefore been refined to include an age- and gender-predicted comparison, and a peak V_{O_2} of more than 50% of predicted normal is now often considered as being impaired to the point at which heart transplantation might be considered.

Additional information from the exercise test includes the chronotropic response to exercise, which is indicative of abnormal parasympathetic activation, a well-described feature of heart failure.[79] Abnormal return of parasympathetic activity after exercise (that is, reduction in heart rate to 12 beats or less 1 minute after cessation of exercise) is also abnormal in many patients with heart failure.

Hemodynamic Evaluation: Cardiac Catheterization

In certain individual circumstances, it may be prudent to consider invasive hemodynamic evaluation and monitoring as part of the clinical evaluation of patients with heart failure. This was the predominant mode of quantifying disease during the development of neurohormonal antagonists. The main shift in practice occurred as a result of both fading interest in using intravenous vasoactive therapies and increasing concerns regarding the lack of incremental long-term benefit (or even harm) in using such strategies.

The results of the ESCAPE trial have clarified the usefulness of invasive monitoring to some degree.[80] Currently, patients who are doing poorly with severe congestion, ascites, anasarca, or obvious signs and symptoms of low cardiac output might be considered for hospitalization with hemodynamic monitoring. When constrictive physiology or restrictive cardiomyopathy is suspected, right-sided heart catheterization should also be considered. With improved imaging techniques, the role of right-sided heart catheterization is diminishing, although it is still useful as a confirmatory test in patients with complex or unusual forms of heart failure. Most right-sided heart catheterizations performed in patients with heart failure today are used to help guide therapy rather than to make a specific diagnosis. Clearly, it is no longer a routine diagnostic component of the evaluation algorithm.

Histological Evaluation: Endomyocardial Biopsy

The role of diagnostic endomyocardial biopsy in patients with heart failure has diminished,[81] because of the results from the Myocarditis Treatment Trial, which implied a sense of futility regarding various treatment strategies for acute myocarditis.[82] It is unclear whether certain forms of cardiomyopathy and myocarditis can be managed better with the aid of diagnostic endomyocardial biopsy,[82] especially with some recent support for immunosuppression and immunoabsorption in the setting of chronic persistent myocarditis without viral persistence. If acute inflammatory myocarditis is suspected, endomyocardial biopsy should still be considered, especially with the current availability of newer molecular markers.[83] Selected patients may in fact respond to various immunosuppressant therapies, but success cannot be predicted reliably.[84]

Although the role of endomyocardial biopsy is diminishing in the evaluation of patients with heart failure, it is important that clinicians keep in mind that specific entities can be diagnosed through only this technique. Endomyocardial biopsy is a requirement for the diagnosis of acute myocarditis, inasmuch as the clinical diagnosis of this entity is notoriously insensitive. Some types of heart failure, including fulminant myocarditis, giant-cell myocarditis, sarcoidosis, and amyloid heart disease, are quite distinct and are variably responsive to different management strategies. For example, amyloid heart disease is usually refractory to both conventional therapy and heart transplantation. Patients with fulminant myocarditis may recover spontaneously after aggressive hemodynamic support.[85] Patients with giant-cell myocarditis often have a rapid downhill course and may be eligible for immunosuppressive protocols or heart transplantation.[86] Therefore, although its use is now more limited, endomyocardial biopsy clearly has a role when specific types of cardiomyopathy are suggested on clinical grounds, and the biopsy information may be quite helpful in planning therapy. Table 35-7 outlines the 14 clinical scenarios in which endomyocardial biopsy should be considered, as recommended by a published consensus statement.[84]

Genetic Evaluation (see Chapter 27)

Clinical genetic testing for monogenetic mutations of sarcomeric and metabolic genes in inherited cardiomyopathies has become available in commercial testing laboratories. Many of the inherited cardiomyopathies have been extensively reviewed in Chapter 27. Several important hurdles facing routine genetic testing remain. First, mapping specific gene mutations can be highly complex, and some of the affected genes are large, which can translate into labor-intensive and expensive ventures. Second, despite the association between a family history of heart failure and underlying genetic predispositions, only a small proportion of mutations are known to lead to inherited cardiomyopathies. This means that a negative result of a test for unexplained cardiomyopathies cannot provide the confidence to rule out any underlying genetic mutations. Third, treatment options have yet to catch up with the availability of genetic information to help clinicians to tailor their management strategies. For now, the most efficient use of genetic testing remains identification of at risk individuals for inherited cardiomyopathies who then require careful evaluation and close monitoring, particularly in the case of hypertrophic cardiomyopathy and arrhythmogenic right ventricular dysplasia.[87] For specific diseases such as Fabry's disease or transthyretin amyloidosis, genetic tests are available for confirmatory purposes also. Nevertheless, pharmacogenomic-guided therapy is still under intensive clinical investigations. Some of the challenges of pharmacogenetics are discussed in Chapter 42.

FUTURE DIRECTIONS

The current approach to clinical evaluation of heart failure is still confined to the traditional patient-doctor encounter, including the elicitation of the medical history for suspect symptoms, bedside examinations to detect clinical signs of congestion and perfusion, and the decision to conduct confirmatory or monitored testing in search for therapeutic interventions. These require the patient's physical presence and may capture only a "snapshot" of the clinical picture. Simple longitudinal information such as daily weighings, self-reports of health status, and vital sign measurements have been widely used but are often plagued with nonadherence, subjectivity, and selectivity in self-reporting. The next step in clinical evaluation relies on the ability of technological advances to quantify disease severity both at the time of clinical encounter and at home. Some of these advances are already available as implantable devices that yield adjunctive parameters; others have linked disease management with home care programs. Examples of information yielded by this technology include arrhythmia detection and management, intracardiac impedance monitoring, and even detection of intracardiac filling pressures. External devices, both standalone and portable versions, are also becoming increasingly available to measure physiological and electrocardiographic information. When the appropriate configurations and methods are established, such "ambulatory" insight can provide insight and clarity into the clinical profile, which could transform the way physicians evaluate (and ultimately manage) patients with heart failure.

TABLE 35–7 Indications for Endomyocardial Biopsy: 14 Clinical Scenarios

Scenario	Recommendation (Strength/Level)
1. New-onset heart failure of <2 weeks' duration associated with a normal-sized or dilated left ventricle and hemodynamic compromise	I/B
2. New-onset heart failure of 2 weeks' to 3 months' duration associated with a dilated left ventricle and new ventricular arrhythmias, second- or third-degree heart block, or failure to respond to usual care within 1-2 weeks	I/B
3. Heart failure of ≥3 months' duration associated with a dilated left ventricle and new ventricular arrhythmias, second- or third-degree heart block, or failure to respond to usual care within 1-2 weeks	IIa/C
4. Heart failure associated with a dilated cardiomyopathy of any duration associated with suspected allergic reaction and/or eosinophilia	IIa/C
5. Heart failure associated with suspected anthracycline cardiomyopathy	IIa/C
6. Heart failure associated with unexplained restrictive cardiomyopathy	IIa/C
7. Suspected cardiac tumors	IIa/C
8. Unexplained cardiomyopathy in children	IIa/C
9. New-onset heart failure of 2 weeks' to 3 months' duration associated with a dilated left ventricle, without new ventricular arrhythmias or second- or third-degree heart block, that responds to usual care within 1-2 weeks	IIb/B
10. Heart failure of >3 months' duration associated with a dilated left ventricle, without new ventricular arrhythmias or second- or third-degree heart block, that responds to usual care within 1-2 weeks	IIb/C
11. Heart failure associated with unexplained hypertrophic cardiomyopathy	IIb/C
12. Suspected arrhythmogenic right ventricular dysplasia	IIb/C
13. Unexplained ventricular arrhythmias	IIb/C
14. Unexplained atrial fibrillation	III/C

From Cooper LT, Baughman KL, Feldman AM, et al. The role of endomyocardial biopsy in the management of cardiovascular disease: a scientific statement from the American Heart Association, the American College of Cardiology, and the European Society of Cardiology. *Circulation* 2007;116:2216-2233.

REFERENCES

1. Hunt, S. A., Abraham, W. T., Chin, M. H., et al. (2009). Focused update incorporated into the ACC/AHA 2005 Guidelines for the Diagnosis and Management of Heart Failure in Adults: a report of the American College of Cardiology Foundation/American Heart Association Task Force on Practice Guidelines: developed in collaboration with the International Society for Heart and Lung Transplantation. *Circulation, 119*(14), e391–e479.
2. Butler, J., Kalogeropoulos, A., Georgiopoulou, V., et al. (2008). Incident heart failure prediction in the elderly: the Health ABC Heart Failure score. *Circ Heart Fail, 1*, 125–133.
3. Criteria Committee of the New York Heart Association. (1994). *Nomenclature and criteria for diagnosis of diseases of the heart and great vessels* (ed 9). Boston: Little, Brown.
4. Mosterd, A., Deckers, J. W., Hoes, A. W., et al. (1997). Classification of heart failure in population based research: an assessment of six heart failure scores. *Eur J Epidemiol, 13*, 491–502.
5. Lewis, E. F., Johnson, P. A., Johnson, W., et al. (2001). Preferences for quality of life or survival expressed by patients with heart failure. *J Heart Lung Transplant, 20*, 1016–1024.
6. Tsuyuki, R. T., McKelvie, R. S., Arnold, M. O., et al. (2001). Acute precipitants of congestive heart failure exacerbations. *Arch Intern Med, 161*, 2337–2342.

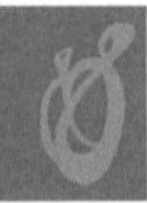

7. Fonarow, G. C., Abraham, W. T., Albert, N. M., et al. (2008). Factors identified as precipitating hospital admissions for heart failure and clinical outcomes: findings from OPTIMIZE-HF. *Arch Intern Med, 168*, 847–854.
8. Rector, T. S., & Cohn, J. N. (1992). Assessment of patient outcome with the Minnesota Living with Heart Failure questionnaire: reliability and validity during a randomized, double-blind, placebo controlled trial of pimobendan. *Am Heart J, 124*, 1017.
9. Green, C. P., Porter, C. B., Bresnahan, D. R., et al. (2000). Development and evaluation of the Kansas City Cardiomyopathy Questionnaire: a new health status measure for heart failure. *J Am Coll Cardiol, 35*, 1245–1255.
10. ACC/AHA guidelines for the management of patients with valvular heart disease. (1998). A report of the American College of Cardiology/American Heart Association. Task Force on Practice Guidelines (Committee on Management of Patients with Valvular Heart Disease). *J Am Coll Cardiol, 32*, 1486–1588.
11. Benge, W., Litchfield, R. L., & Marcus, M. L. (1980). Exercise capacity in patients with severe left ventricular dysfunction. *Circulation, 61*, 955–959.
12. Franciosa, J. A., Park, M., & Levine, T. B. (1981). Lack of correlation between exercise capacity and indexes of resting left ventricular performance in heart failure. *Am J Cardiol, 47*, 33–39.
13. Franciosa, J. A., Ziesche, S., & Wilen, M. (1979). Functional capacity of patients with chronic left ventricular failure. Relationship of bicycle exercise performance to clinical and hemodynamic characterization. *Am J Med, 67*, 460–466.
14. Francis, G. S., Goldsmith, S. R., & Cohn, J. N. (1982). Relationship of exercise capacity to resting left ventricular performance and basal plasma norepinephrine levels in patients with congestive heart failure. *Am Heart J, 104*(4 Pt 1), 725–731.
15. Fink, L. I., Wilson, J. R., & Ferraro, N. (1986). Exercise ventilation and pulmonary artery wedge pressure in chronic stable congestive heart failure. *Am J Cardiol, 57*, 249–253.
16. Stevenson, L. W., & Perloff, J. K. (1989). The limited reliability of physical signs for estimating hemodynamics in chronic heart failure. *JAMA, 261*, 884–888.
17. Mancini, D. M., Henson, D., LaManca, J., et al. (1992). Respiratory muscle function and dyspnea in patients with chronic congestive heart failure. *Circulation, 86*, 909–918.
18. Clark, A. L., Poole-Wilson, P. A., & Coats, A. J. (1996). Exercise limitation in chronic heart failure: central role of the periphery. *J Am Coll Cardiol, 28*, 1092–1102.
19. MacGowan, G. A., Cecchetti, A., & Murali, S. (1997). Ventilatory drive during exercise in congestive heart failure. *J Card Fail, 3*, 257–262.
20. Wasserman, K. (1982). Dyspnea on exertion. Is it the heart or the lungs? *JAMA, 248*, 2039–2043.
21. Wilson, J. R., & Mancini, D. M. (1993). Factors contributing to the exercise limitation of heart failure. *J Am Coll Cardiol, 22*(4 Suppl A), 93A–98A.
22. Chua, T. P., Clark, A. L., Amadi, A. A., et al. (1996). Relation between chemosensitivity and the ventilatory response to exercise in chronic heart failure. *J Am Coll Cardiol, 27*, 650–657.
23. Ponikowski, P., Francis, D. P., Piepoli, M. F., et al. (2001). Enhanced ventilatory response to exercise in patients with chronic heart failure and preserved exercise tolerance: marker of abnormal cardiorespiratory reflex control and predictor of poor prognosis. *Circulation, 103*, 967–972.
24. Johnson, R. L., Jr. (2001). Gas exchange efficiency in congestive heart failure II. *Circulation, 103*, 916–918.
25. Wasserman, K. (1989). The peripheral circulation and lactic acid metabolism in heart, or cardiovascular, failure. *Circulation, 80*, 1084–1086.
26. Piepoli, M., Clark, A. L., Volterrani, M., et al. (1996). Contribution of muscle afferents to the hemodynamic, autonomic, and ventilatory responses to exercise in patients with chronic heart failure: effects of physical training. *Circulation, 93*, 940–952.
27. Mancini, D. M., Coyle, E., Coggan, A., et al. (1989). Contribution of intrinsic skeletal muscle changes to 31P NMR skeletal muscle metabolic abnormalities in patients with chronic heart failure. *Circulation, 80*, 1338–1346.
28. Mancini, D. M., Ferraro, N., Tuchler, M., et al. (1988). Detection of abnormal calf muscle metabolism in patients with heart failure using phosphorus-31 nuclear magnetic resonance. *Am J Cardiol, 62*, 1234–1240.
29. Massie, B., Conway, M., Yonge, R., et al. (1987). Skeletal muscle metabolism in patients with congestive heart failure: relation to clinical severity and blood flow. *Circulation, 76*, 1009–1019.
30. Massie, B. M., Conway, M., Yonge, R., et al. (1987). 31P Nuclear magnetic resonance evidence of abnormal skeletal muscle metabolism in patients with congestive heart failure. *Am J Cardiol, 60*, 309–315.
31. Wilson, J. R., Fink, L., Maris, J., et al. (1985). Evaluation of energy metabolism in skeletal muscle of patients with heart failure with gated phosphorus-31 nuclear magnetic resonance. *Circulation, 71*, 57–62.
32. Sullivan, M. J., Green, H. J., & Cobb, F. R. (1990). Skeletal muscle biochemistry and histology in ambulatory patients with long-term heart failure. *Circulation, 81*, 518–527.
33. Mancini, D. M., Walter, G., Reichek, N., et al. (1992). Contribution of skeletal muscle atrophy to exercise intolerance and altered muscle metabolism in heart failure. *Circulation, 85*, 1364–1373.
34. Drexler, H., Riede, U., Munzel, T., et al. (1992). Alterations of skeletal muscle in chronic heart failure. *Circulation, 85*, 1751–1759.
35. Schaefer, S., Gober, J. R., Schwartz, G. G., et al. (1990). In vivo phosphorus-31 spectroscopic imaging in patients with global myocardial disease. *Am J Cardiol, 65*, 1154–1161.
36. Sullivan, M. J., Green, H. J., & Cobb, F. R. (1991). Altered skeletal muscle metabolic response to exercise in chronic heart failure. Relation to skeletal muscle aerobic enzyme activity. *Circulation, 84*, 1597–1607.
37. Working Group on Cardiac Rehabilitation & Exercice Physiology and Working Group on Heart Failure of the European Society of Cardiology. Recommendations for exercise training in chronic heart failure patients. (2001). *Eur Heart J, 22*, 125–135.
38. Fleg, J. L., Pina, I. L., Balady, G. J., et al. (2000). Assessment of functional capacity in clinical and research applications: an advisory from the Committee on Exercise, Rehabilitation, and Prevention, Council on Clinical Cardiology, American Heart Association. *Circulation, 102*, 1591–1597.
39. Minotti, J. R., & Massie, B. M. (1992). Exercise training in heart failure patients. Does reversing the peripheral abnormalities protect the heart? *Circulation, 85*, 2323–2325.
40. Sullivan, M. J., Higginbotham, M. B., & Cobb, F. R. (1989). Exercise training in patients with chronic heart failure delays ventilatory anaerobic threshold and improves submaximal exercise performance. *Circulation, 79*, 324–329.
41. Sullivan, M. J., Higginbotham, M. B., & Cobb, F. R. (1988). Exercise training in patients with severe left ventricular dysfunction. Hemodynamic and metabolic effects. *Circulation, 78*, 506–515.
42. Nohria, A., Lewis, E., & Stevenson, L. W. (2002). Medical management of advanced heart failure. *JAMA, 287*, 628–640.
43. Drazner, M. H., Hellkamp, A. S., Leier, C. V., et al. (2008). Value of clinician assessment of hemodynamics in advanced heart failure: the ESCAPE trial. *Circ Heart Fail, 1*, 170–177.
44. Economides, E., & Stevenson, L. W. (1998). The jugular veins: knowing enough to look. *Am Heart J, 136*, 6–9.
45. Perloff, J. K. (2001). The jugular venous pulse and third heart sound in patients with heart failure. *N Engl J Med, 345*, 612–614.
46. Wiese, J. (2000). The abdominojugular reflux sign. *Am J Med, 109*, 59–61.
47. Mullens, W., Abrahams, Z., Skouri, H. N., et al. (2008). Elevated intra-abdominal pressure in acute decompensated heart failure: a potential contributor to worsening renal function? *J Am Coll Cardiol, 51*, 300–306.
48. Tribouilloy, C. M., Enriquez-Sarano, M., Mohty, D., et al. (2001). Pathophysiologic determinants of third heart sounds: a prospective clinical and Doppler echocardiographic study. *Am J Med, 111*, 96–102.
49. Drazner, M. H., Rame, J. E., Stevenson, L. W., et al. (2001). Prognostic importance of elevated jugular venous pressure and a third heart sound in patients with heart failure. *N Engl J Med, 345*, 574–581.
50. Drazner, M. H., Rame, J. E., & Dries, D. L. (2003). Third heart sound and elevated jugular venous pressure as markers of the subsequent development of heart failure in patients with asymptomatic left ventricular dysfunction. *Am J Med, 114*, 431–437.
51. Lucas, C., Johnson, W., Hamilton, M. A., et al. (2000). Freedom from congestion predicts good survival despite previous class IV symptoms of heart failure. *Am Heart J, 140*, 840–847.
52. Lee, Y. C., & Sutton, F. J. (1982). Pulsus alternans in patients with congestive cardiomyopathy. *Circulation, 65*, 1533–1534.
53. Anker, S. D., Ponikowski, P., Varney, S., et al. (1997). Wasting as independent risk factor for mortality in chronic heart failure. *Lancet, 349*, 1050–1053.
54. Anker, S. D., & Rauchhaus, M. (1999). Insights into the pathogenesis of chronic heart failure: immune activation and cachexia. *Curr Opin Cardiol, 14*, 211–216.
55. Dunlay, S. M., Weston, S. A., Redfield, M. M., et al. (2008). Tumor necrosis factor–alpha and mortality in heart failure: a community study. *Circulation, 118*, 625–631.
56. Hunt, S. A., Abraham, W. T., Chin, M. H., et al. (2005). ACC/AHA 2005 Guideline Update for the Diagnosis and Management of Chronic Heart Failure in the Adult: a report of the American College of Cardiology/American Heart Association Task Force on Practice Guidelines (Writing Committee to Update the 2001 Guidelines for the Evaluation and Management of Heart Failure): developed in collaboration with the American College of Chest Physicians and the International Society for Heart and Lung Transplantation: endorsed by the Heart Rhythm Society. *Circulation, 112*(12), e154–e235.
57. Heart Failure Society of America. (2006). Executive summary: HFSA 2006 Comprehensive Heart Failure Practice Guideline. *J Card Fail, 12*, 10–38.
58. Tang, W. H., Tong, W., Jain, A., et al. (2008). Evaluation and long-term prognosis of new-onset, transient, and persistent anemia in ambulatory patients with chronic heart failure. *J Am Coll Cardiol, 51*, 569–576.
59. Tang, W. H., Francis, G. S., Morrow, D. A., et al. (2007). National Academy of Clinical Biochemistry Laboratory Medicine practice guidelines: clinical utilization of cardiac biomarker testing in heart failure. *Circulation, 116*(5), e99–e109.
60. Gheorghiade, M., & Bonow, R. O. (1998). Chronic heart failure in the United States: a manifestation of coronary artery disease. *Circulation, 97*, 282–289.
61. Baba, R., Tsuyuki, K., Kimura, Y., et al. (1999). Oxygen uptake efficiency slope as a useful measure of cardiorespiratory functional reserve in adult cardiac patients. *Eur J Appl Physiol Occup Physiol, 80*, 397–401.
62. Brookes, C. I., Hart, P., Keogh, B. E., et al. (1995). Angiography and the aetiology of heart failure. *Postgrad Med J, 71*, 480–482.
63. Bortman, G., Sellanes, M., Odell, D. S., et al. (1994). Discrepancy between pre- and post-transplant diagnosis of end-stage dilated cardiomyopathy. *Am J Cardiol, 74*, 921–924.
64. Smith, R. F., Johnson, G., Ziesche, S., et al. (1993). Functional capacity in heart failure. Comparison of methods for assessment and their relation to other indexes of heart failure. The V-HeFT VA Cooperative Studies Group. *Circulation, 87*(6 Suppl), VI88–VI93.
65. Florea, V. G., Henein, M. Y., Anker, S. D., et al. (2000). Prognostic value of changes over time in exercise capacity and echocardiographic measurements in patients with chronic heart failure. *Eur Heart J, 21*, 146–153.
66. Chua, T. P., Ponikowski, P., Harrington, D., et al. (1997). Clinical correlates and prognostic significance of the ventilatory response to exercise in chronic heart failure. *J Am Coll Cardiol, 29*, 1585–1590.
67. Lang, C. C., Agostoni, P., & Mancini, D. M. (2007). Prognostic significance and measurement of exercise-derived hemodynamic variables in patients with heart failure. *J Card Fail, 13*, 672–679.
68. Robbins, M., Francis, G., Pashkow, F. J., et al. (1999). Ventilatory and heart rate responses to exercise: better predictors of heart failure mortality than peak oxygen consumption. *Circulation, 100*, 2411–2417.
69. Weber, K. T., Kinasewitz, G. T., Janicki, J. S., et al. (1982). Oxygen utilization and ventilation during exercise in patients with chronic cardiac failure. *Circulation, 65*, 1213–1223.
70. Russell, S. D., McNeer, F. R., & Higginbotham, M. B. (1998). Exertional dyspnea in heart failure: a symptom unrelated to pulmonary function at rest or during exercise. Duke University Clinical Cardiology Studies (DUCCS) Exercise Group. *Am Heart J, 135*, 398–405.
71. Johnson, R. L., Jr. (2000). Gas exchange efficiency in congestive heart failure. *Circulation, 101*, 2774–2776.
72. Francis, G. S., & Rector, T. S. (1994). Maximal exercise tolerance as a therapeutic end point in heart failure—are we relying on the right measure? *Am J Cardiol, 73*, 304–306.

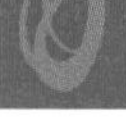

73. Guyatt, G. H., Sullivan, M. J., Thompson, P. J., et al. (1985). The 6-minute walk: a new measure of exercise capacity in patients with chronic heart failure. *Can Med Assoc J, 132*, 919–923.
74. Morales, F. J., Martinez, A., Mendez, M., et al. (1999). A shuttle walk test for assessment of functional capacity in chronic heart failure. *Am Heart J, 138*(2 Pt 1), 291–298.
75. Opasich, C., Pinna, G. D., Mazza, A., et al. (2001). Six-minute walking performance in patients with moderate-to-severe heart failure; is it a useful indicator in clinical practice? *Eur Heart J, 22*, 488–496.
76. Sharma, R., & Anker, S. D. (2001). The 6-minute walk test and prognosis in chronic heart failure—the available evidence. *Eur Heart J, 22*, 445–448.
77. Mancini, D. M., Eisen, H., Kussmaul, W., et al. (1991). Value of peak exercise oxygen consumption for optimal timing of cardiac transplantation in ambulatory patients with heart failure. *Circulation, 83*, 778–786.
78. Mehra, M. R., Kobashigawa, J., Starling, R., et al. (2006). Listing criteria for heart transplantation: International Society for Heart and Lung Transplantation guidelines for the care of cardiac transplant candidates—2006. *J Heart Lung Transplant, 25*, 1024–1042.
79. Lauer, M. S., Francis, G. S., Okin, P. M., et al. (1999). Impaired chronotropic response to exercise stress testing as a predictor of mortality. *JAMA, 281*, 524–529.
80. Binanay, C., Califf, R. M., Hasselblad, V., et al. (2005). Evaluation study of congestive heart failure and pulmonary artery catheterization effectiveness: the ESCAPE trial. *JAMA, 294*, 1625–1633.
81. Hrobon, P., Kuntz, K. M., & Hare, J. M. (1998). Should endomyocardial biopsy be performed for detection of myocarditis? A decision analytic approach. *J Heart Lung Transplant, 17*, 479–486.
82. Mason, J. W., O'Connell, J. B., Herskowitz, A., et al. (1995). A clinical trial of immunosuppressive therapy for myocarditis. The Myocarditis Treatment Trial Investigators. *N Engl J Med, 333*, 269–275.
83. Kawai, C. (1999). From myocarditis to cardiomyopathy: mechanisms of inflammation and cell death: learning from the past for the future. *Circulation, 99*, 1091–1100.
84. Cooper, L. T., Baughman, K. L., Feldman, A. M., et al. (2007). The role of endomyocardial biopsy in the management of cardiovascular disease: a scientific statement from the American Heart Association, the American College of Cardiology, and the European Society of Cardiology. *Circulation, 116*, 2216–2233.
85. McCarthy, R. E., 3rd, Boehmer, J. P., Hruban, R. H., et al. (2000). Long-term outcome of fulminant myocarditis as compared with acute (nonfulminant) myocarditis. *N Engl J Med, 342*, 690–695.
86. Cooper, L. T., Jr., Berry, G. J., & Shabetai, R. (1997). Idiopathic giant-cell myocarditis—natural history and treatment. Multicenter Giant Cell Myocarditis Study Group Investigators. *N Engl J Med, 336*, 1860–1866.
87. Hershberger, R. E., Lindenfeld, J., Mestroni, L., et al. (2009). Genetic evaluation of cardiomyopathy—a Heart Failure Society of America practice guideline. *J Card Fail, 15*, 83–97.

CHAPTER 36

Use of Cardiac Imaging in the Evaluation of Heart Failure

Hisham Dokainish, Matthias Friedrich, Maria C. Ziadi, and Rob S. Beanlands

Noninvasive cardiac imaging plays a critical initial role in the diagnosis and subsequent management of patients with heart failure. Echocardiography, cardiac magnetic resonance (CMR) imaging, and nuclear cardiac imaging are all noninvasive tests commonly used in patients with heart failure. This chapter describes the utility of these noninvasive cardiac imaging techniques in the diagnosis and management of patients with both systolic and diastolic heart failure, including sections on assessing heart failure with a depressed and preserved ejection fraction, assessment of right ventricular (RV) function, the role of imaging with regard to implanting cardiac devices, and future directions for cardiac imaging in heart failure.

ASSESSMENT OF THE LEFT VENTRICLE: VOLUMES, EJECTION FRACTION

Echocardiography

In the clinical setting, 2-dimensional echocardiography is the noninvasive imaging test most commonly used to assess left ventricular (LV) volume, as well as calculating LV ejection fraction (LVEF); these measurements are necessary for determining the proper management of patients with heart failure.[1-4] Although M-mode measurements can be used, more accurate measurements of LV systolic and diastolic volumes are obtained by biplane Simpson's method or the area-length method used in the apical two- and four-chamber views (Figure 36-1).[5] The use of harmonic imaging has greatly improved endocardial–blood border differentiation in technically difficult studies, and the use of intravenous contrast material further increases the accuracy of assessing LV echocardiographic volumes.[6] Although 2-dimensional echocardiography is relatively well correlated with LV volumes that are obtained by CMR imaging, the correlation with CMR imaging is better in 3-dimensional echocardiography.[7-9] Once LV systolic and diastolic volumes are measured, LV stroke volume can be readily calculated as LV end-diastolic volume − LV end-systolic volume.[5] The LVEF is calculated as the ratio of stroke volume to LV end-diastolic volume.[5]

Spectral Doppler imaging can also be used to determine cardiac output in patients with heart failure, and pulsed-wave Doppler imaging is used in the left ventricular outflow tract to determine stroke volume (Figure 36-2).

Cardiac Magnetic Resonance Imaging

CMR imaging has emerged as an important imaging technique with regard to the morphological and functional assessment of patients with heart failure. CMR imaging requires acquisition of multiple oblique planes in relation to the heart (Figure 36-3). The imaging techniques are designed to render blood dark or bright and to depict various aspects of cardiac motion, blood flow, and myocardial perfusion. CMR imaging is considered the reference standard for the quantitative assessment of systolic function.[10] If CMR imaging is used strictly for the assessment of LV function, the acquisition time of a scan usually does not exceed 10 minutes. The accurate quantification of volumes can be used to calculate LVEF, stroke volume, and cardiac index. This is of particular importance in patients with heart failure and a normal ejection fraction (e.g., in restrictive cardiomyopathy or cardiac amyloidosis), in whom low-output states can be determined even if the ejection fraction is normal. Different techniques have been used for assessing cardiac function with magnetic resonance imaging (MRI). New magnetic resonance sequences allow for the assessment of 3-dimensional cardiac motion by labeling ("tagging") specific myocardial regions (Figure 36-4). The rotational and translational motion of the left ventricle can be determined by following the motion of the tags, which has been likened to the wringing of a wet towel. During systole, there is clockwise twisting motion at the base and a counterclockwise rotation at the apex (Figure 36-5). The untwisting motion occurs very early in diastole and is directly related to myocardial relaxation. The rate of untwisting may be used as a measure of the rate and completeness of relaxation and may serve as an estimate of early diastolic filling. Despite the strengths of CMR imaging for assessing cardiac structure and function in patients with heart failure, the applicability of this technique is currently limited, insofar as patients with implantable cardioverter-defibrillators or biventricular pacemakers, or both, cannot be placed within the electromagnetic waves of the magnet, which may interfere with function of the intracardiac defibrillators or biventricular pacemakers. However, CMR imaging–compatible pacemakers are now available in Europe (Advisa MRI SureScan pacemaker), which suggests that this problem may be ameliorated in the future.

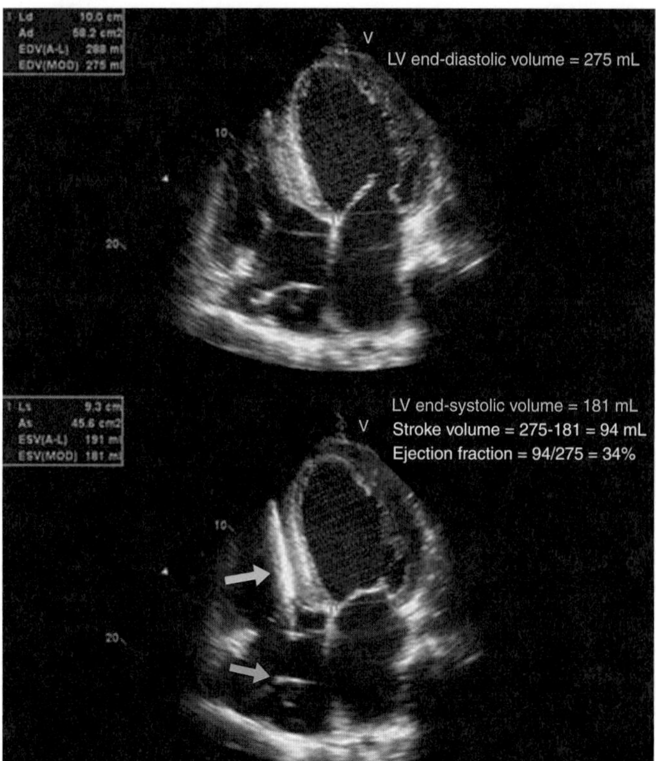

FIGURE 36–1 Calculation of left ventricular (LV) stroke volume and ejection fraction by method of discs in a patient with ischemic cardiomyopathy. The LV end-diastolic volume was 275 mL (*top*), and the LV end-systolic volume was 181 mL (*bottom*). Therefore, LV stroke volume was 94 mL, and the LV ejection fraction was 34%. Note the implantable cardiac defibrillator wire in the right ventricle (*yellow arrow*) with a pacemaker lead visualized in the right atrium (*blue arrow*).

Nuclear Imaging

Radionuclide Angiography

Radionuclide angiography is a highly reproducible for measuring LV function when performed either by *first-pass* or by *multiple-gated acquisition techniques.*[11,12] Technetium-99m (^{99m}Tc)–labeled red blood cells are used to define the blood pool. First-pass techniques yield a high target-to-background ratio, more distinct visualization of the separate cardiac chambers, and rapid imaging. In contrast, the multiple-gated technique enables repeated assessment of cardiac function, high count density, and acquisition of images in multiple projections, and it is therefore best for the assessment of LVEF.

Echocardiography–Gated SPECT with Myocardial Perfusion Imaging

Although gated single photon emission computed tomography (SPECT) with ^{99m}Tc or thallium-201 (^{201}Tl) has been validated against other techniques for assessing LV function,[13,14] SPECT is generally viewed as less accurate than radionuclide angiography because of its greater variability. The best use for this technique has been the determination of wall motion to determine whether a perfusion defect represents scar or attenuation artefact.[15]

Echocardiography–Gated PET with Myocardial Perfusion Imaging

This method enables better tissue characterization of perfusion, metabolism, and function.[16] Because the timing of image acquisition is immediately after stress, rubidium-82 (^{82}Rb)–labeled positron emission tomography (PET) is better able to estimate LVEF and volumes at peak stress than is SPECT, and it also yields additional diagnostic information about disease severity.[16,17]

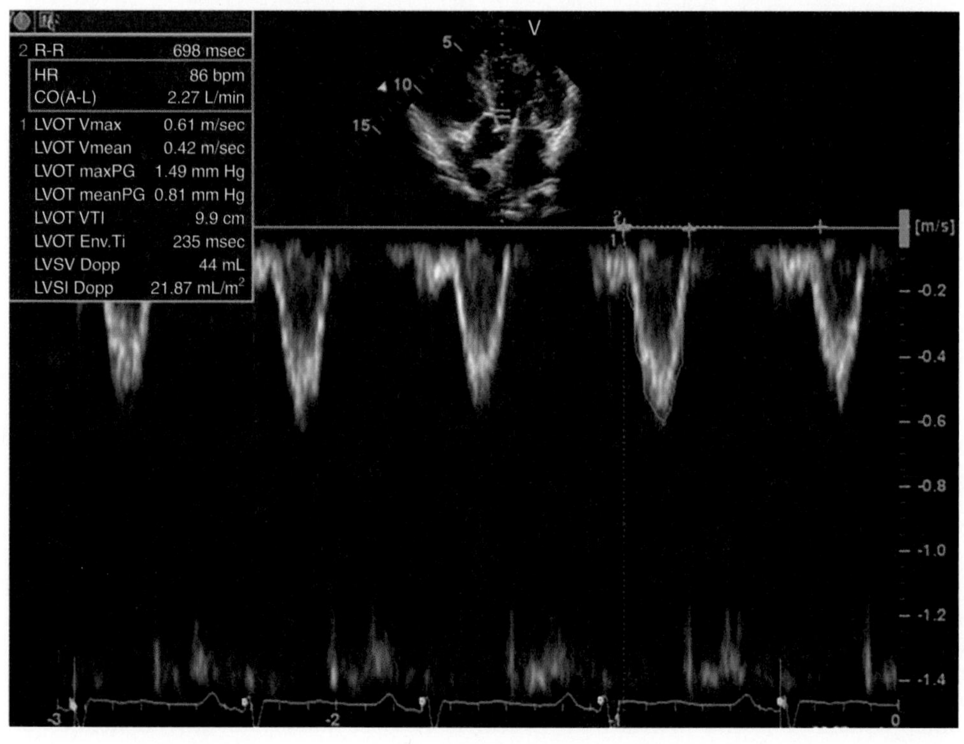

FIGURE 36–2 Use of spectral Doppler imaging for the calculation of cardiac output in a patient with advanced nonischemic cardiomyopathy. With the use of pulsed-wave Doppler imaging in the apical five-chamber view, the sample volume is placed in the left ventricular outflow tract (LVOT). Integrating the LVOT spectral tracing (*blue lines*) yields a velocity time integral (VTI). After the LVOT area is calculated as the square of the diameter of the LVOT × 0.785, the stroke volume can be determined as LVOT area × LVOT VTI. The cardiac output (L/minute) can then be calculated as the heart rate × stroke volume. In the example in this figure, the calculated cardiac output was 2.2 L/min, which is depressed.

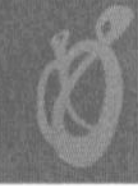

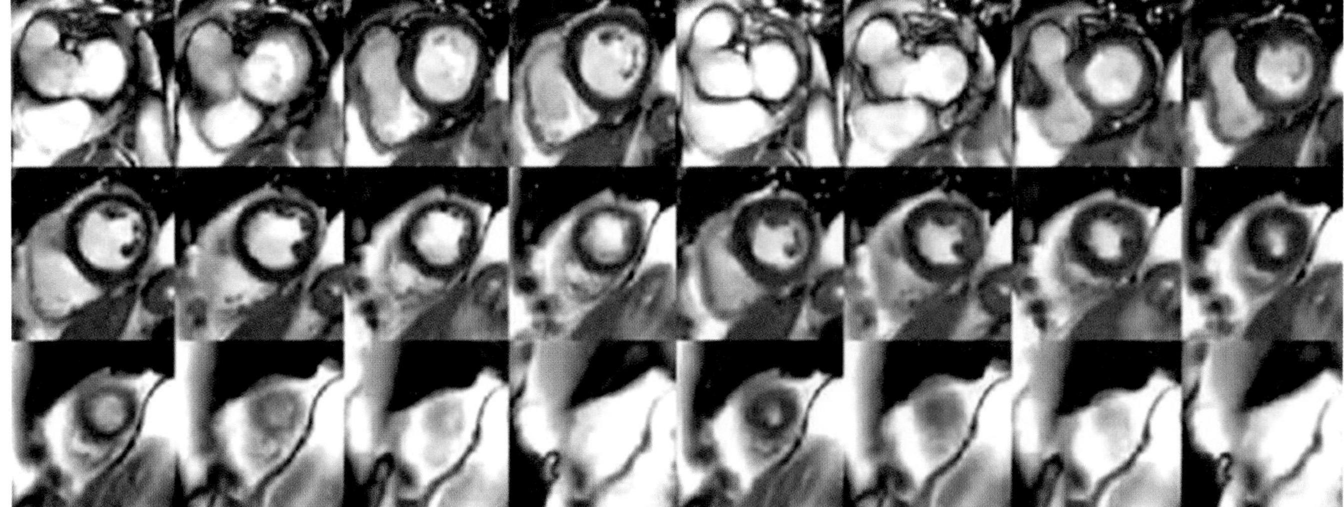

FIGURE 36–3 Example of short-axis stack in cardiac magnetic resonance imaging in a patient with heart failure and depressed left ventricular ejection fraction.

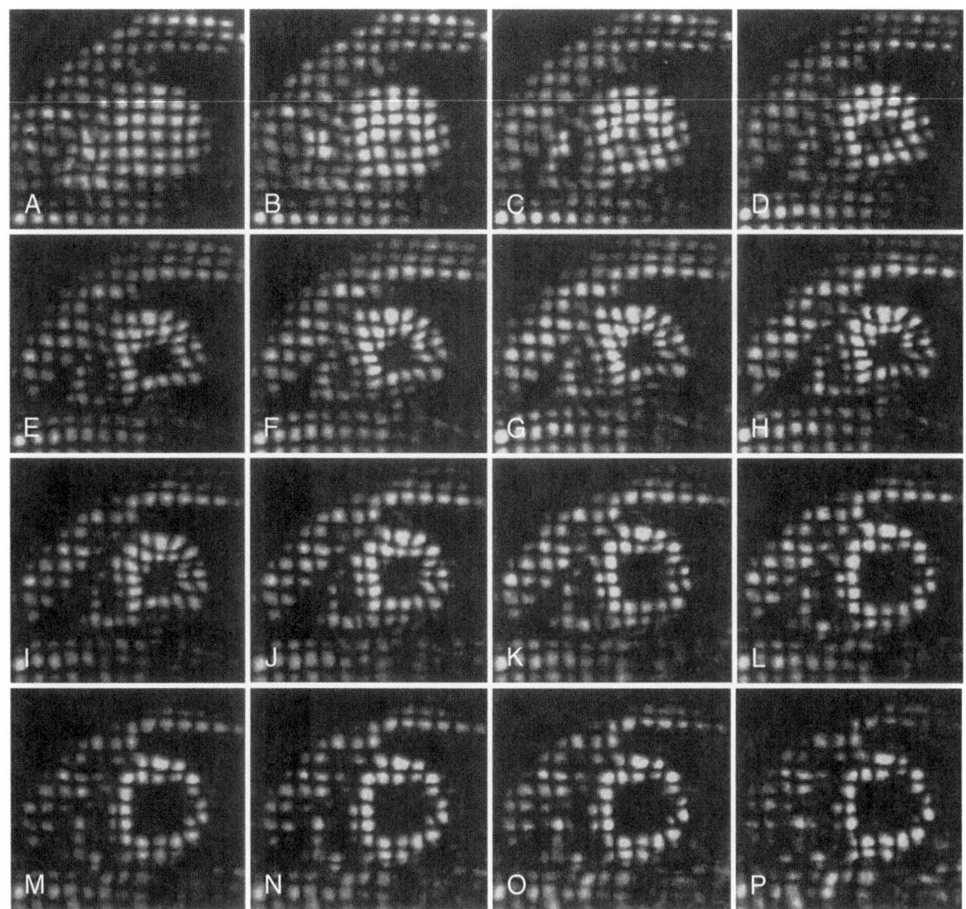

FIGURE 36–4 Series of magnetic resonance images in a control patient with normal left ventricular function (temporal resolution 35 msec). The horizontal and vertical lines (myocardial tags) are superimposed on the conventional magnetic resonance image. From the movement of the grid crossing points, the contraction and relaxation behavior of the left ventricle can be determined. During isovolumic contraction, there is a counterclockwise rotation at the apex, followed by systolic shortening. During isovolumic relaxation, there is a clockwise rotation ("untwisting"), followed by diastolic lengthening. This systolic-diastolic contraction-relaxation behavior is altered in patients with diastolic dysfunction, with prolongation of diastolic back-rotation. (From Mandinov L, Eberli F, Seiler C, et al: Diastolic heart failure. *Cardiovasc Res* 2000;45:813-825.)

DETECTION OF MYOCARDIAL ISCHEMIA AND MYOCARDIAL INFARCTION

Echocardiography

Identification of ischemia as the cause of heart failure is of great importance in patients with systolic dysfunction, insofar as revascularization can improve LV function and the patient's functional status. Echocardiography can demonstrate the presence of previous ischemic injury, most typically myocardial infarction, which can be visualized as thin (<6 mm in diameter), echo-dense ("bright") LV walls that contract poorly in relation to other normal LV myocardial segments. The absence of segmental wall motion abnormalities (e.g., global hypokinesis) does not necessarily preclude an ischemic cause of heart failure. Similarly, segmental abnormalities do not necessarily preclude a nonischemic cause. For example, patients with dilated cardiomyopathy from sarcoidosis may have regional myocardial disease.[4,18,19]

Stress echocardiography, conducted either with exercise treadmill or bicycle or pharmacologically (with dobutamine), has been shown to help accurately identify ischemic and

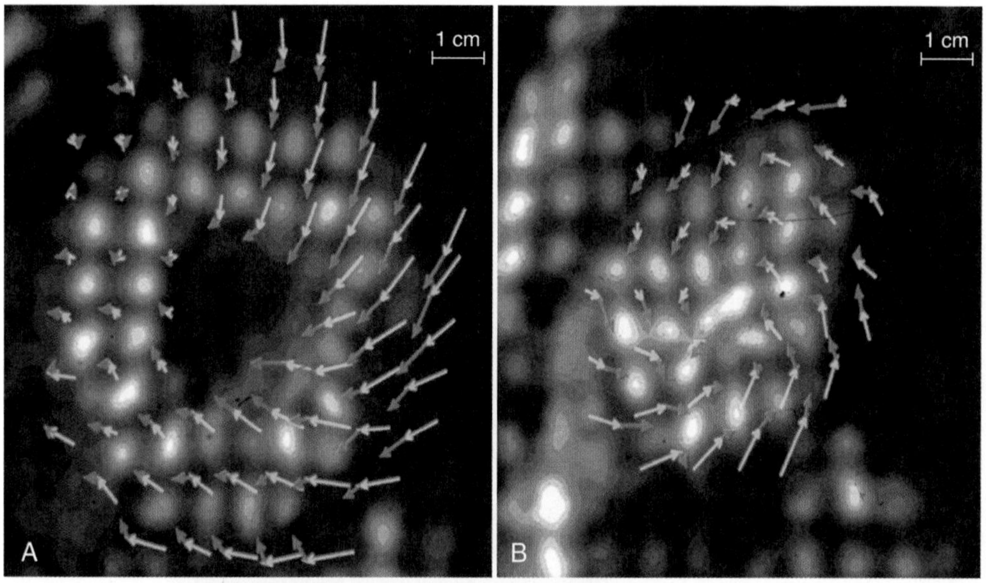

FIGURE 36–5 Ejection phase of the left ventricle at the base (**A**) and at the apex (**B**) of a healthy subject. End-systolic acquisitions are overlaid with corresponding local trajectories. There is a clockwise rotation at the base and a counterclockwise rotation at the apex. This motion pattern has been described as a systolic wringing motion, and its analysis provides a more sophisticated approach to quantifying regional left ventricular systolic function than do the traditional methods of analyzing endocardial shortening and simple wall thickening. (From Stuber M, Scheidegger MB, Fischer SE, et al: Alterations in the local myocardial motion pattern in patients suffering from pressure overload due to aortic stenosis. *Circulation* 1999;100:361-368.)

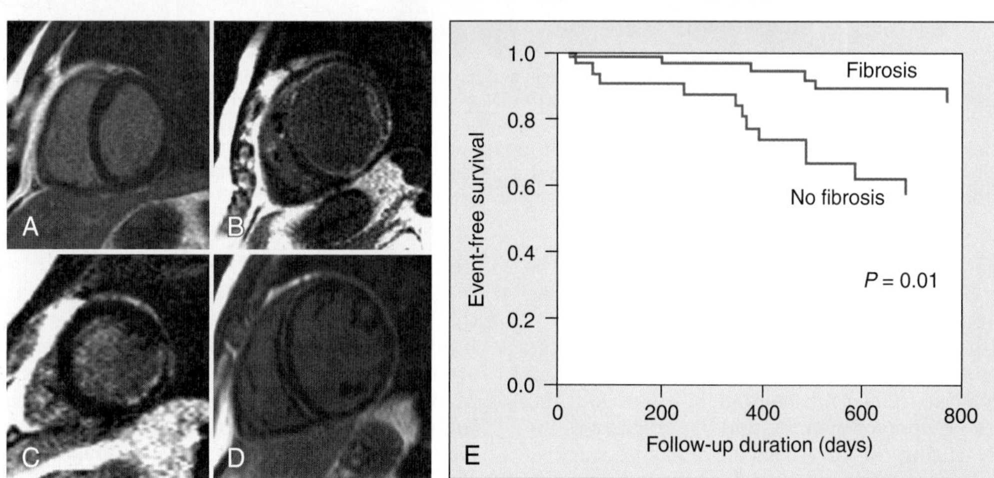

FIGURE 36–6 **A-D,** Cardiac MRIs in patients with dilated cardiomyopathy (DCM). **A,** DCM is evident without gadolinium enhancement. **B,** In a patient with known previous myocardial infarction that resulted in heart failure, late gadolinium enhancement is seen throughout the subendocardium, causing thinning particularly in the septum and inferolateral wall. **C,** In a patient with the presumed clinical diagnosis of coronary angiography, late gadolinium-enhanced CMR imaging clearly shows an inferolateral infarction despite the normal coronary arteries; the patient's heart failure is probably related to coronary disease and not to DCM. **D,** In a patient with DCM, the midwall of the septum in the ventricular circumferential fibers is enhanced by late gadolinium. This pattern of fibrosis is recognized by pathologists but had not been previously visualized in vivo. **E,** Kaplan-Meier survival curves of the occurrence of major cardiac events in patients with proven DCM according to the presence of intramural fibrosis. Fibrosis was a powerful predictor of outcome, which was poorer in relation to worsening cardiac volumes and ejection fraction. (**A** to **D,** From McCrohon JA, Moon JC, Prasad SK, et al: Differentiation of heart failure related to dilated cardiomyopathy and coronary artery disease using gadolinium-enhanced cardiovascular magnetic resonance. *Circulation* 2003;108:54. **E,** From Assomull RG, Prasad SK, Lyne J, et al: Cardiovascular magnetic resonance, fibrosis, and prognosis in dilated cardiomyopathy. *J Am Coll Cardiol* 2006;48:1977.)

infarcted myocardial segments, and the findings are correlated with patient's prognosis.[20-22] For evaluating suspected ischemic heart disease, the advantages of stress echocardiography include relatively low cost, rapid performance and availability of results, relative ease of performing the study (because of low technological requirements), and lack of radiation exposure.[20,21] Disadvantages include the need for expert readers to minimize erroneous interpretation and technical difficulties in scanning certain patients, particularly those with significant lung disease or morbid obesity.[20,21]

Cardiac Magnetic Resonance Imaging

Late gadolinium enhancement can be used to reliably differentiate patients with ischemic cardiomyopathy from patients with nonischemic cardiomyopathy[23] without the need for stress perfusion imaging (Figure 36-6). Gadolinium, an agent used for extracellular imaging, normally does not enter the myocardium because cardiac muscle is packed tightly. After myocardial infarction, however, the extracellular space is expanded because of cellular rupture, which allows for a distribution of the gadolinium within the myocardial scar. The optimal time for gadolinium imaging for late enhancement is after 10 to 15 minutes. The myocardial scar secondary to myocardial ischemia invariably involves the subendocardial layer because of the transmyocardial perfusion pressure gradient, whereas myocardial scars that are secondary to nonischemic injury typically demonstrate a regional distribution that is fairly distinct from that seen with myocardial ischemia or infarction.[24] Specific patterns have been associated with several myocardial diseases such as myocarditis (see Chapter 31),[25] dilated cardiomyopathy (see Chapter 24),[23] and hypertrophic cardiomyopathy (see Chapter 25).[26] With cardiac sarcoidosis,[27] there is evidence of a transmural myocardial scar; however, the distribution of this myocardial scarring does not necessarily reflect coronary artery anatomy. Gadolinium should be used cautiously in some patients with heart failure and reduced renal function, insofar as gadolinium-induced

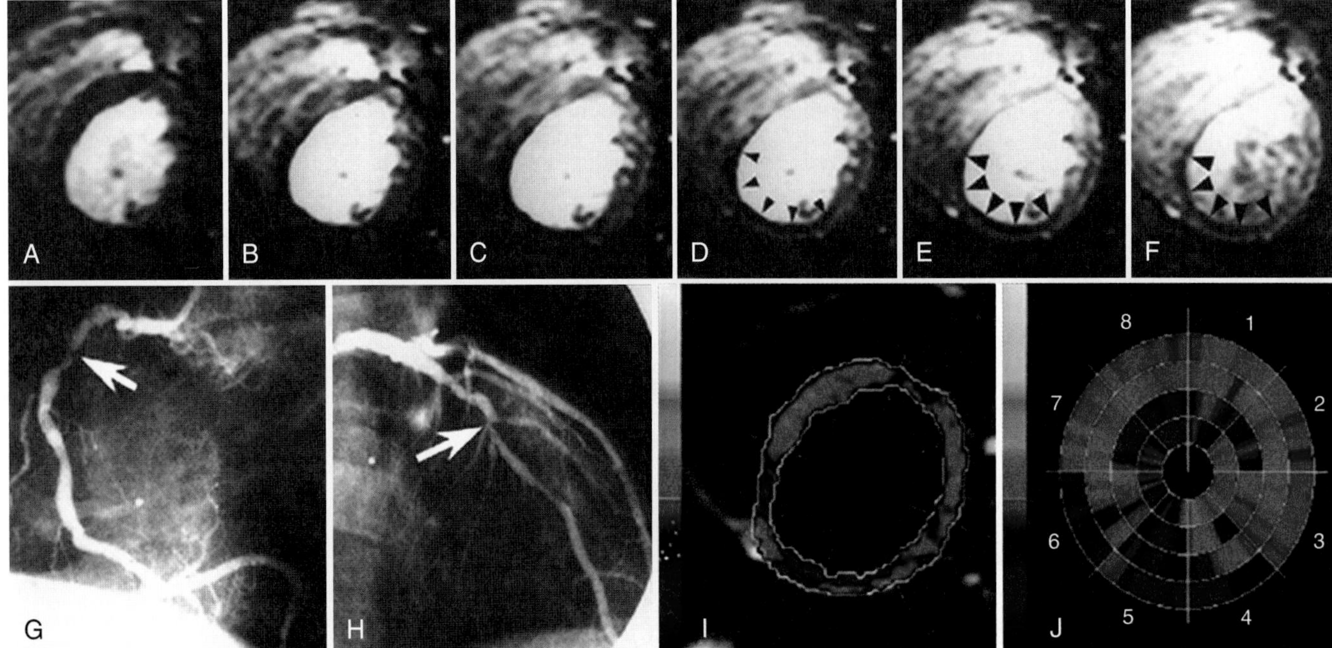

FIGURE 36–7 Perfusion cardiovascular magnetic resonance (CMR) images and parametric maps in a patient with stenosis of the right coronary and left anterior descending arteries (*arrows* in **G** and **H**). A single slice (**A** through **F**) shows delayed wash of gadolinium in the inferior wall during the first pass (*arrowheads*). In the parametric map (**I**), this abnormality is shown in *blue.* Image **J** is a segmental display of perfusion in a bull's eye plot (32-segment model). In the polar map (**K**), areas of abnormal perfusion are shown in *blue,* and both the inferoseptal and anteroseptal abnormal areas, corresponding to right coronary and left anterior descending artery stenoses, respectively, are apparent. (From Schwitter J, Nanz D, Kneifel S, et al: Assessment of myocardial perfusion in coronary artery disease by magnetic resonance: a comparison with positron emission tomography and coronary angiography. *Circulation* 2001;103:2230-2235.)

nephrotoxicity has been reported. However, it should be emphasized that the deleterious effects of gadolinium on renal function remain controversial.

Both dobutamine and adenosine stress testing can be used with CMR imaging in order to detect clinically significant coronary artery disease. A fast intravenous bolus of gadolinium is administered by power injector, and the changes in the myocardial signal during the first pass are measured at rest and during stress. Low-signal areas of perfusion can be readily detected during stress (Figure 36-7*A* to *F*). Dobutamine infusions in conjunction with CMR imaging have been shown to yield very reproducible results,[28,29] and these studies are especially useful in patients with suboptimal echocardiographic image quality.[30] CMR imaging with stress perfusion has the potential for significant widespread use because of the combination of enhanced resolution with no ionizing radiation. The sensitivity may be increased by the use of myocardial tagging (see Figure 36-4).[31] Adenosine can be used with CMR imaging for assessing myocardial perfusion. Studies have shown that the prognostic utility of CMR imaging with adenosine stress is similar to that of CMR imaging with dobutamine stress.[32] The clinical evaluation of myocardial blood flow is often qualitative; however, with experience, the degree of diagnostic accuracy may exceed that obtained with SPECT.[33] Practical and accurate algorithms for a quantitative analysis of CMR imaging with myocardial perfusion have been developed (see Figure 36-7*K*) and offer high degrees of diagnostic accuracy[34-36] and reproducibility.[37] Furthermore, imaging of myocardial perfusion under stress can be combined with late gadolinium enhancement to delineate areas of nonviability.

Nuclear Imaging

Myocardial perfusion imaging (MPI) is used to identify and predict the functional consequences of coronary artery disease.[17] Moreover, MPI can be used to differentiate between myocardial scar and ischemia (Figure 36-8), as well as distinguish at-risk individuals who are the most likely to benefit from interventional therapies in comparison with medical therapy alone (Figure 36-9).[38,39] Myocardial perfusion defects that appear reversible on at-rest images are indicative of stress-induced ischemia, whereas myocardial perfusion defects that are irreversible, or "fixed," on at-rest images are indicative of myocardial scarring. Findings on SPECT that imply high risk include a large myocardial perfusion defect, multiple myocardial perfusion defects in more than one coronary territory, abnormal at-rest LVEF, transient RV visualization, transient ischemic LV dilation, increased lung uptake, and post-stress LV dysfunction with a normal at-rest LVEF.[40] In the setting of chronic stable coronary artery disease, basing intervention decisions on coronary anatomy alone is often problematic and does not necessarily lead to improved outcomes.[38,39,41] Hachamovitch and colleagues[39] demonstrated that the magnitude of inducible myocardial ischemia[38] is predictive of a survival benefit with revascularization. Thus, the clinical decision to perform coronary artery revascularization in patients with heart failure hinges on the severity of symptoms and the magnitude of inducible myocardial ischemia (see Figure 23-13).[38]

ASSESSMENT OF VIABILITY IN PATIENTS WITH ISCHEMIC CARDIOMYOPATHY

The myocardium has several acute and chronic ways of adapting to temporary or sustained reductions in myocardial blood flow (Figure 36-10), known as stunning, hibernation, and ischemic preconditioning (see also Chapter 23) is understood as an increased tolerance toward ischemia, caused by brief, preceding episode of ischemia. *Myocardial stunning* has been defined as reversible myocardial contractile dysfunction in the presence of normal resting myocardial blood flow.[42] Recovery of function occurs spontaneously. *Myocardial hibernation* is defined as reversible myocardial contractile dysfunction in the presence of myocardial hypoperfusion. *Ischemic preconditioning* is understood as an increased tolerance toward ischemia, caused by

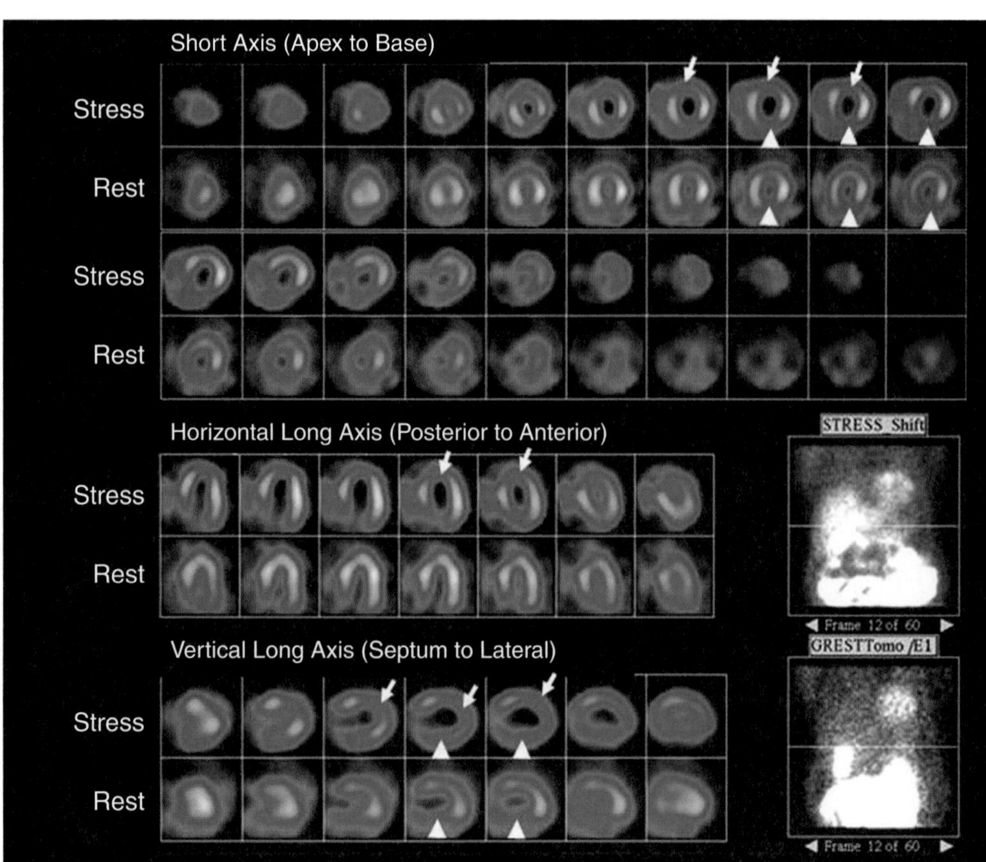

FIGURE 36–8 Myocardial perfusion images. Single photon emission computed tomography (SPECT) images at rest (*lower panels*) and during stress (*upper panels*), revealing a mixture of nontransmural scar and moderate ischemia involving the apex and middle to distal anterior wall (*arrows*), which are consistent with coronary artery disease in the left anterior artery distribution. The images also reveal a moderate to severe fixed perfusion defect in the inferior and inferolateral walls, which is suggestive of nontransmural scar of the right coronary artery and left circumflex arterial distribution (*arrowhead*). Transient ischemic dilation (1.88) was identified with the stress images. Gated images demonstrated a moderately dilated left ventricle (end-diastolic volume = 209 mL; end-systolic volume = 137 mL) with a drop in left ventricular ejection fraction (LVEF) on the post-stress images (at rest, LVEF = 50%; after stress, LVEF = 35%).

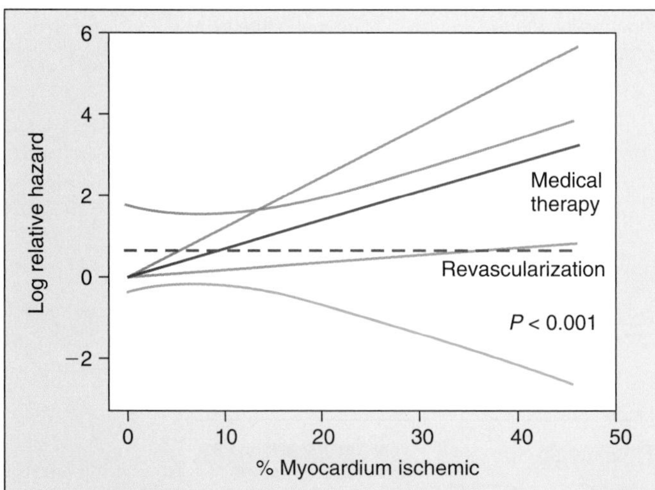

FIGURE 36–9 Role of myocardial perfusion imaging in risk stratifying patients with coronary artery disease. As shown, Cox proportional hazards modeling suggests that hazard ratios for both medical therapy and for revascularization increase as a function of increasing area of ischemic myocardium; however, the relative risk is significantly lower for patients who underwent revascularization. (From Hachamovitch R, Rozanski A, Hayes SW, et al. Predicting therapeutic benefit from myocardial revascularization procedures: are measurements of both resting left ventricular ejection fraction and stress-induced myocardial ischemia necessary? *J Nucl Cardiol* 2006;13:768-778.)

brief, preceding episodes of ischemia. Recovery of function occurs only with restoration of myocardial blood flow. The goal of assessing viability is to optimize selection of patients with heart failure whose symptoms may improve after revascularization. Echocardiography, CMR imaging, and nuclear imaging can be used to demonstrate myocardial viability.

Echocardiography

In patients with heart failure and a depressed ejection fraction secondary to myocardial ischemia, the identification of myocardial viability is important, insofar as such patients may have hibernating myocardium and may benefit from myocardial revascularization.[43,44] Three typical patterns are seen during dobutamine stress echocardiography. Patients with ischemic cardiomyopathy and viable myocardium commonly manifest a typical "biphasic response" to dobutamine stress: that is, segmental function in viable segments improves with low-dose dobutamine (typically 5 to 10 μg/kg/min) and deteriorates with higher doses (20 to 40 μg/kg/min), as the viable segments become ischemic.[20-22] A second possible response is one of continuing improvement in segmental function and global LVEF with increasing doses of dobutamine ("contractile reserve"), wherein viable segments do not become ischemic at high doses of dobutamine. This response can occur in patients with nonischemic cardiomyopathy, with or without concomitant mild coronary artery disease. A third common finding is no change in global LVEF or segmental function (i.e, a "flat response"), or a worsening of LV function with dobutamine. In general, patients with a

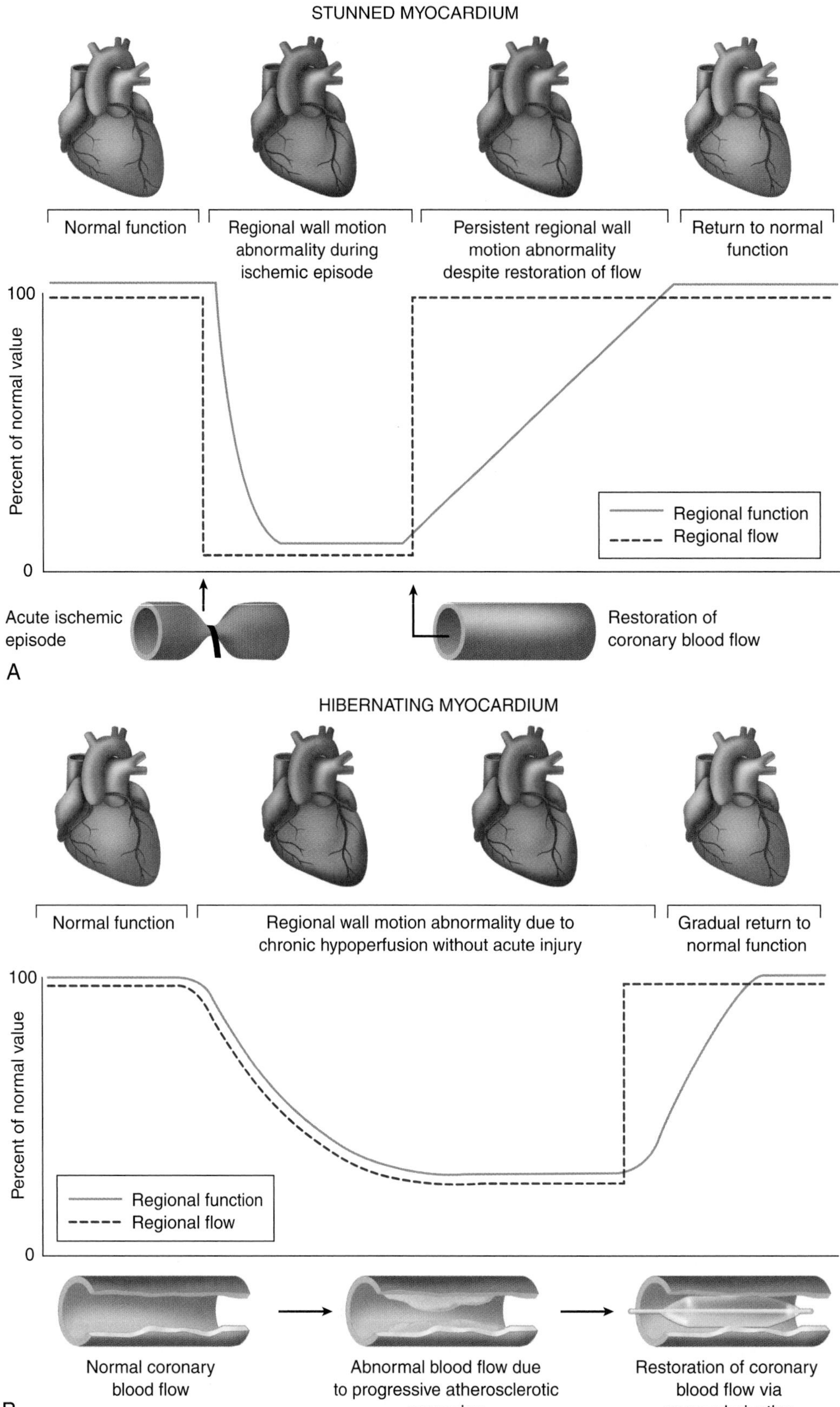

FIGURE 36–10 Pathophysiological processes of stunning and hibernation, representing different mechanisms of acute and chronic reversible left ventricular dysfunction. (Adapted from Dilsizian V. Myocardial viability: reversible left ventricular dysfunction. In Dilsizian V, Narula J, Braunwald E, editors. *Atlas of nuclear cardiology,* Philadelphia, 2006, Current Medicine. With kind permission of Springer Science +Business Media.)

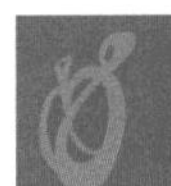

TABLE 36–1 Advantages and Disadvantages of Different Cardiac Imaging Modalities for Detecting Myocardial Viability

Imaging Technique	Advantages	Disadvantages
Cardiac SPECT	• Well-established • Widely available • Lower cost • High sensitivity • Observational outcome literature • Commonly first choice	• Depth-dependent attenuation correction • Moderate specificity • Lower spatial resolution (in comparison with PET and CMR imaging)
Cardiac PET with CT	• Acceptable spatial resolution • Best molecular sensitivity • Use of natural occurring elements • Quantitative capabilities • Rapid patient throughput • Depiction of flow, metabolism, function, and coronary anatomy in the same session	• High radiation dose • High cost • Poorer availability • Dependence of FDG uptake on the patient's metabolic state
CMR imaging	• Increasingly available • Best noninvasive definition of myocardial structure • Moderate sensitivity and specificity • Depiction of structure, function, perfusion, and scar in the same session • No radiation	• Contraindicated or used with caution in patients with renal failure • Limited outcome literature (in patients with viability imaging and severe left ventricular dysfunction) • Contraindicated in patients with metallic objects and devices • Heart rate and rhythm not visualized
Stress echocardiography with dobutamine	• Availability • No radiation • High specificity	• Lower sensitivity • High interobserver and intercenter variation • Accuracy reduced by severity of resting dysfunction • Moderate observational literature (no randomized trials)

Comparison of noninvasive imaging techniques for assessment of myocardial viability in patients with heart failure. Although stress echocardiography with dobutamine, cardiac magnetic resonance (CMR) imaging, cardiac single photon emission computed tomography (SPECT), and cardiac positron emission tomography (PET) with computed tomography (CT) all are helpful and validated techniques for assessment of myocardial viability, each has its particular advantages and disadvantages.

FDG, fluorodeoxyglucose.

(From Camici PG, Prasad SK, Rimoldi OE. Stunning, hibernation, and assessment of myocardial viability. *Circulation* 2008:117:103-114.)

biphasic response demonstrate the best response to revascularization, followed by those with evidence of contractile reserve.[43,44] Patients with a flat or worsening response to dobutamine typically do not benefit from or fare poorly with revascularization and are often advised to continue medical management. When LV recovery after revascularization is assessed segmentally, SPECT and PET demonstrate excellent sensitivity, whereas echocardiography and CMR imaging with dobutamine stress have superior specificity and positive predictive value (Table 36-1).[45]

Cardiac Magnetic Resonance Imaging

CMR imaging is an established technique for assessing myocardial viability, as well as predicting the potential for recovery of LV function after myocardial revascularization (see also Chapter 23). Prior studies have shown that an LV end-diastolic wall thickness of less than 5 to 6 mm depicted on a resting cine MRI is a marker of transmural myocardial infarction and virtually precludes the presence of viable myocardium. In the event of poorly contracting LV myocardium with preserved end-diastolic wall thickness (≥6 mm), detection of contractile reserve during low-dose dobutamine infusion confirms the presence of viable myocardium.[46,47] This approach is considered very specific and is thus very helpful for therapeutic decision making for patients with suspected ischemia-induced chronic contractile dysfunction. Because CMR imaging can visualize both viable and nonviable tissue, side by side with cine loops of ventricular contraction, late gadolinium enhancement (discussed previously; see Figure 36-6) is useful in assessing myocardial viability. Gadolinium accumulation accurately reflects irreversible myocardial injury,[48] and late enhancement imaging accurately visualizes scars in acute and in chronic infarction[49,50] and is predictive of the functional recovery of dysfunctional segments after myocardial revascularization.[51] In some patients, the late enhancement series can be combined with a low-dose dobutamine infusion in the same session.[29]

Nuclear Imaging

MPI is the imaging method most widely used for assessing myocardial viability in patients with heart failure. After injection of a selected radiotracer (e.g., ^{201}Tl), the isotope is extracted from the blood by viable myocytes and is retained within the myocytes for some time. For a dysfunctional segment or territory, the probability of functional recovery after revascularization is directly related to the magnitude of tracer uptake. The magnitude of global LV functional recovery after revascularization is dependent on the extent of viable myocardial tissue. In a clinical trial of patients with heart failure, of whom only a minority had angina, hibernation, stress-induced ischemia, or both (angina and hibernation or ischemia), were demonstrated in approximately 70% of the patients by SPECT; this finding suggests a significant population of patients with heart failure may benefit from viability testing.

SPECT Imaging with Thallium-201

After intravenous injection of ^{201}Tl, the extent of its initial myocardial uptake is proportional to regional blood flow. The peak myocardial concentration of ^{201}Tl within the myocardium occurs within 5 minutes after injection, with rapid clearance from the intravenous compartment. Although the initial uptake and distribution of ^{201}Tl are primarily a function of myocardial blood flow, the subsequent distribution of ^{201}Tl is a function of the concentration gradient between the level of ^{201}Tl in the blood and the level in cardiac myocytes. The presence of ^{201}Tl after redistribution is indicative of myocyte cellular viability. However, because the absence of ^{201}Tl uptake on the redistribution images does not necessarily preclude myocyte viability, a number of imaging protocols

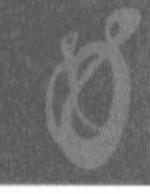

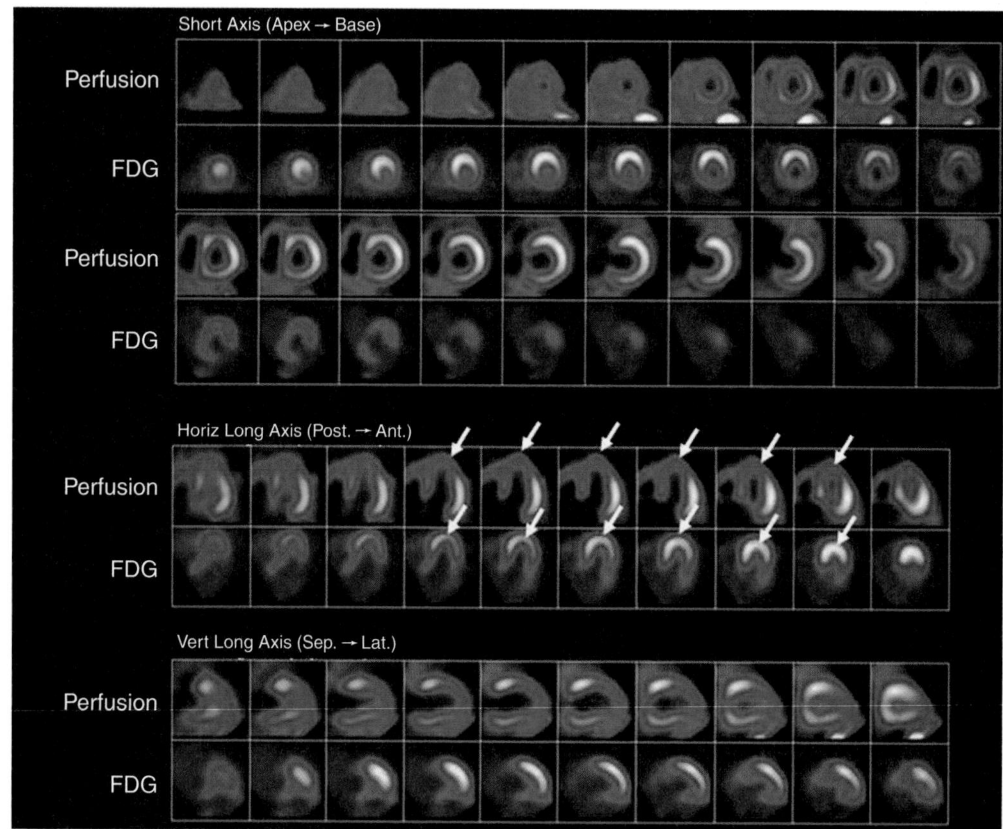

FIGURE 36–11 Use of positron emission tomography (PET) to determine myocardial viability. Myocardial uptake of perfusion with rubidium-82 (^{82}Rb) is depicted in the upper panels, whereas myocardial uptake of perfusion with 2-[fluorine-18]-fluoro-2-deoxy-D-glucose (^{18}FDG) is depicted in the lower panels. There is large area of decreased perfusion with preserved FDG metabolism (perfusion-metabolic mismatch) involving the apex (*arrows*), the septum, and the entire anterior and anteroseptal walls, which is consistent with hibernating myocardium in the distribution of the left anterior descending artery.

have been developed to increase the sensitivity and specificity of this technique for detecting viability. At present, stress-redistribution-reinjection imaging and late rest-redistribution imaging are the two protocols most commonly applied for viability assessment.[52] With rest-redistribution ^{201}Tl imaging, images are obtained after tracer reinjection at rest, and images are obtained 3 to 4 hours after redistribution. With late redistribution ^{201}Tl imaging, ^{201}Tl injection 24 to 48 hours after the initial stress allows for more time for redistribution to occur. However, image quality may be suboptimal with this technique. For defining viable tissue, tracer uptake on redistribution-reinjection images or on late rest-redistribution imaging must exceed 50% to determine viability.[52]

SPECT Imaging with Technetium 99m–Labeled Agents

As with ^{201}Tl imaging, stress-induced perfusion abnormalities and resting isotope uptake of 50% to 60% are predictive of functional recovery.[53] Sestamibi SPECT has been performed after the administration of nitrates, which improves specificity and sensitivity.[52,54] In comparison with PET, SPECT underestimates viability.[55,56]

PET with 2-[Fluorine-18]-Fluoro-2-Deoxy-D-Glucose

2-[Fluorine-18]-fluoro-2-deoxy-D-glucose (^{18}FDG) can be used for the assessment of glucose metabolism in the heart, and this method is very sensitive in detecting myocardial viability.[45,54,57,58] When at-rest perfusion is integrated with measurement of myocardial glucose metabolism and LV function, the pattern of reduced perfusion with preserved metabolism (*perfusion-metabolism mismatch)* is considered essential for myocardial hibernation[59] and is predictive of improved functional outcomes and survival outcomes (Figure 36-11).[57,60] Although patients with severe ventricular dysfunction and coronary disease may benefit from revascularization,[61,62] perioperative morbidity and mortality rates are significant. The prospective PET and Recovery Following Revascularization (PARR-2) trial showed that among patients with severe LV dysfunction, those who underwent ^{18}FDG PET to detect viable myocardium and guide therapy tended to have better 1-year outcomes than did those who received standard care.[63]

Figure 36-12 depicts the outcome of medical management in comparison with revascularization in patients with or without myocardial viability, as determined by dobutamine echocardiography or FDG PET. As shown, the outcomes with revascularization were superior to those with medical treatment in this observational study.

ASSESSMENT OF VALVE FUNCTION IN PATIENTS WITH HEART FAILURE

Echocardiography

Doppler echocardiography plays a pivotal role in determining the primary or secondary relation of valve function or dysfunction to cardiac performance and hemodynamics. Mitral valve disease can be a primary cause of cardiac dysfunction in settings such as myxomatous mitral valve disease, rheumatic mitral valve disease, endocarditis, congenital mitral valve disease, or ischemic mitral valve dysfunction.[64] In general, a mitral valve regurgitation lesion that is more than "moderate" in severity (regurgitant volume > 50 mL) can result in LV remodeling and lead to heart failure ("primary mitral regurgitation").[65,66] Mitral valve regurgitation can also be secondary to the LV dilation that occurs with advancing heart failure. Two-dimensional echocardiography can readily distinguish the cause of mitral valve dysfunction—whether

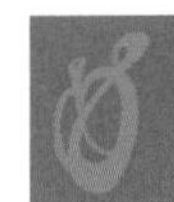

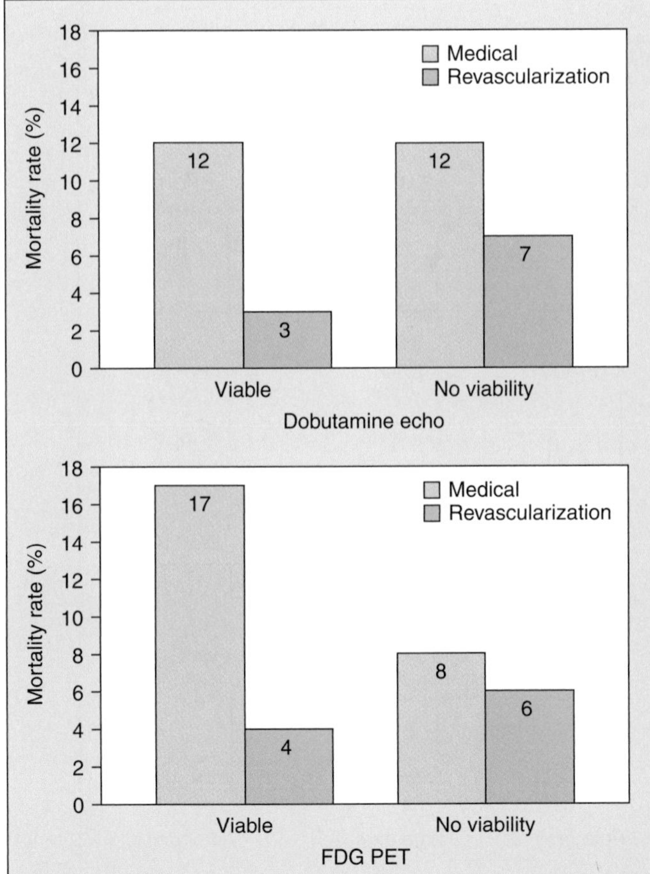

FIGURE 36–12 Role of myocardial viability testing using dobutamine echocardiography and positron emission tomography (PET). Mortality rates were lower among patients who underwent revascularization than among those who received medical therapy when myocardial viability was present, determined either by dobutamine echocardiography (1645 patients) or 2-[fluorine-18] fluoro-2-deoxy-D-glucose (^{18}FDG) PET (1002 patients). (Adapted from Schnikel AFL, Bax JJ, Poldermans D, et al. Hibernating myocardium: diagnosis and patient outcomes. *Curr Prob Cardiol* 2007;32:375-410.)

primary or secondary, myxomatous or ischemic—and Doppler analysis, including spectral and color imaging, can accurately calculate regurgitant volumes.[65,66] For significant primary mitral valve regurgitation, surgical correction is appropriate if the patient is symptomatic, if LV dilation (LV end-systolic dimension > 4.0 cm) is present, or if the LVEF exceeds 60%.[65] However, if the LV is severely dysfunctional (LVEF < 30%) or if the mitral valve regurgitation is secondary to LV dilation, the results of surgical mitral valve correction are often suboptimal, and medical management may be more appropriate.[65]

Severe and chronic aortic valve disease (stenosis or regurgitation) can result in significant LV systolic dysfunction. Two-dimensional echocardiography can readily reveal the cause of aortic valve disease (degenerative, rheumatic, congenital or bicuspid, or secondary to aortic root disease), and Doppler imaging can accurately reflect the severity of aortic valve disease.[65-67] In general, in the setting of significant aortic valve stenosis or regurgitation (more than moderately severe), if a patient is symptomatic or has signs of LV dilation or systolic dysfunction, surgery is warranted.[65] In asymptomatic severe aortic valve stenosis or regurgitation, echocardiography can be helpful for determining surgical timing.[65-67] For patients with low-gradient aortic stenosis (moderate stenosis with LVEF < 35%), low-dose dobutamine stress echocardiography can be helpful for distinguishing true, severe aortic stenosis from "pseudo"–aortic stenosis and for demonstrating the presence of LV contractile reserve.[65,68,69] In general, patients with true stenosis or contractile reserve respond favorably to aortic valve replacement.[65,68,69]

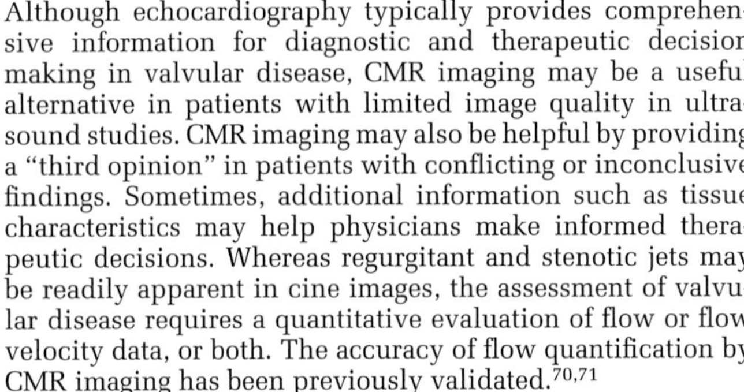

Cardiac Magnetic Resonance Imaging

Although echocardiography typically provides comprehensive information for diagnostic and therapeutic decision making in valvular disease, CMR imaging may be a useful alternative in patients with limited image quality in ultrasound studies. CMR imaging may also be helpful by providing a "third opinion" in patients with conflicting or inconclusive findings. Sometimes, additional information such as tissue characteristics may help physicians make informed therapeutic decisions. Whereas regurgitant and stenotic jets may be readily apparent in cine images, the assessment of valvular disease requires a quantitative evaluation of flow or flow velocity data, or both. The accuracy of flow quantification by CMR imaging has been previously validated.[70,71]

In regurgitant valvular heart disease, regurgitant volume and fraction can be measured by comparing left ventricular stroke volume with systolic aortic flow. CMR imaging allows for measuring effective cardiac output and can therefore provide an important objective parameter of heart failure related to low output. In stenotic valvular disease, flow quantification can be used to identify increased transvalvular flow velocity and calculate pressure gradients.[72] A planimetric quantification of the aortic valve area provides reliable results and avoids the limitations introduced by irregularly turbulent jets and varying pressure gradients.[73-75] This may be of special importance in patients with associated heart failure, inasmuch as the pressure gradient is often unreliable in low-output states.

HEART FAILURE WITH A DEPRESSED EJECTION FRACTION (see Chapters 14 and 48)

Echocardiography

Assessment of Left Ventricular Mass and Left Atrial Size

In diastolic heart failure, also referred to as heart failure with a preserved ejection fraction (LV > 46% to 50%), elevated left atrial pressures (which reflect LV filling pressures in the absence of obstructive mitral valve disease) lead to increased pulmonary venous pressures and dyspnea at rest or during exertion.[76-80] In order for left atrial (LA) pressures to be elevated in the absence of significantly depressed LVEF, LV relaxation and compliance generally are impaired (see Chapter 14).[76,77,80] Therefore, increased LV mass (≥90 g/m^2 for women and ≥115 g/m^2 for men; i.e., LV hypertrophy) is common in patients with diastolic heart failure.[5,76,80] Because LA pressures are elevated in this scenario, LA enlargement (≥30 mL/m^2) is usually observed.[76-81] In previous studies, increasing degrees of LV mass have been correlated with increasing LV diastolic dysfunction and filling pressures.[82] Similarly, increasing LA size is correlated with increasing LV filling pressures and worse outcome in patients with diastolic heart failure.[81,83] In cases of ischemic or infiltrative heart disease, significant LV hypertrophy may be absent, and yet LA volumes are often enlarged.[77,84]

Identification of Diastolic Dysfunction and Elevated Left Ventricular Filling Pressures

Clinically, diastolic dysfunction secondary to impaired LV relaxation and increased LV stiffness is usually demonstrated by Doppler echocardiography.[76-81] The best correlate of symptoms and survival in diastolic heart failure is elevation of left atrial (or left ventricular filling) pressure, readily estimated through comprehensive echocardiography with Doppler measurement.[76,77] Pulsed Doppler interrogation of transmitral and

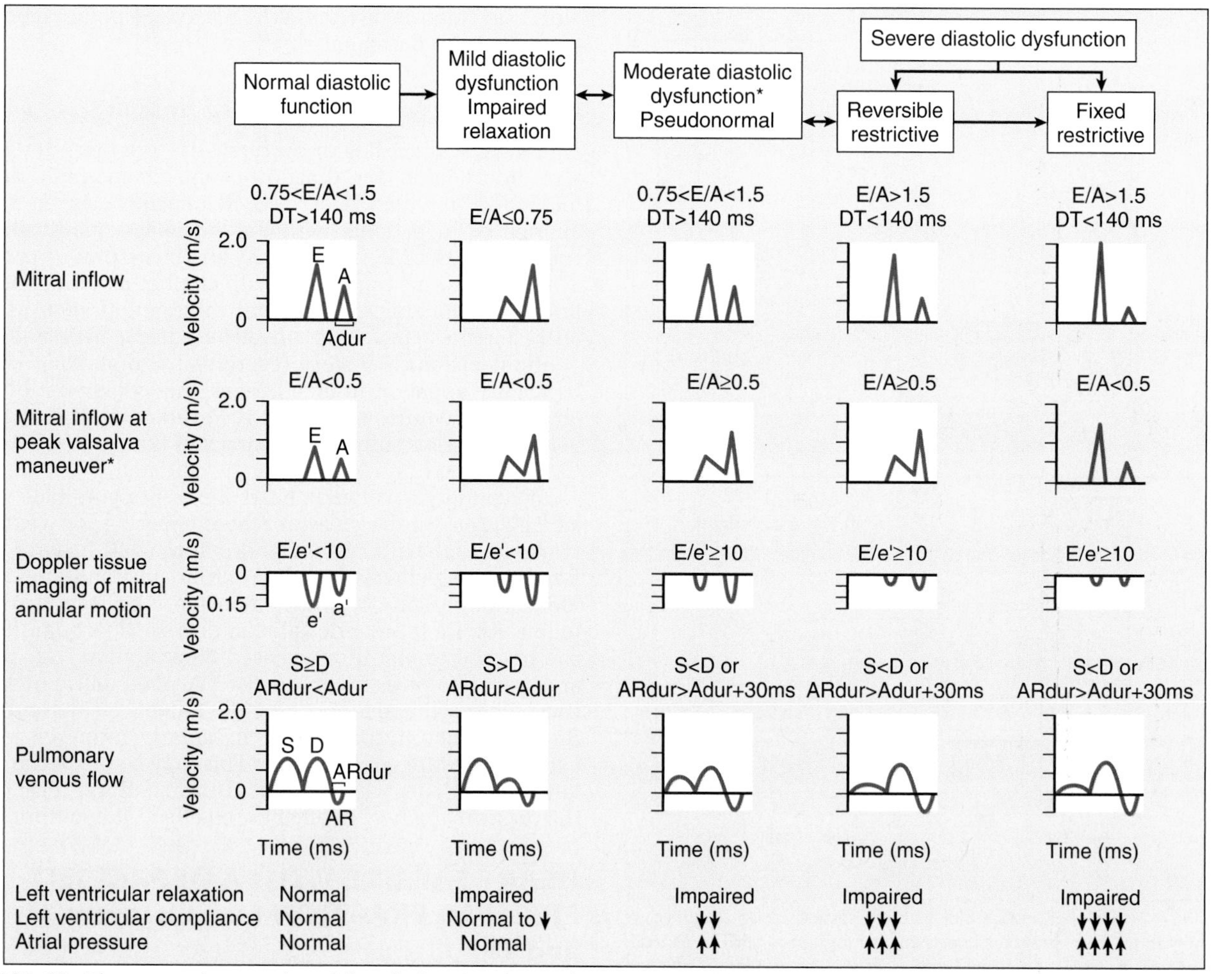

	Normal diastolic function	Mild diastolic dysfunction Impaired relaxation	Moderate diastolic dysfunction* Pseudonormal	Severe diastolic dysfunction: Reversible restrictive	Severe diastolic dysfunction: Fixed restrictive
Mitral inflow	0.75<E/A<1.5 DT>140 ms	E/A≤0.75	0.75<E/A<1.5 DT>140 ms	E/A>1.5 DT<140 ms	E/A>1.5 DT<140 ms
Mitral inflow at peak valsalva maneuver*	E/A<0.5	E/A<0.5	E/A≥0.5	E/A≥0.5	E/A<0.5
Doppler tissue imaging of mitral annular motion	E/e'<10	E/e'<10	E/e'≥10	E/e'≥10	E/e'≥10
Pulmonary venous flow	S≥D ARdur<Adur	S>D ARdur<Adur	S<D or ARdur>Adur+30ms	S<D or ARdur>Adur+30ms	S<D or ARdur>Adur+30ms
Left ventricular relaxation	Normal	Impaired	Impaired	Impaired	Impaired
Left ventricular compliance	Normal	Normal to ↓	↓↓	↓↓↓	↓↓↓↓
Atrial pressure	Normal	Normal	↑↑	↑↑↑	↑↑↑↑

FIGURE 36–13 The proposed progression of diastolic function abnormalities, as assessed through comprehensive Doppler echocardiography with correlation of invasively measured diastolic properties. A comprehensive Doppler assessment, as illustrated in this figure, can yield important information regarding relaxation, filling pressures, and (indirectly) diastolic stiffness in most patients, but careful data acquisition and informed interpretation are required. (From Redfield MM. Heart failure with a normal ejection fraction. In Libby P, Bonow RO, Mann DL, et al, editors. *Braunwald's heart disease,* Philadelphia, 2008, Elsevier, pp 641-656.)

pulmonary venous flows is crucial for the assessment of LV filling pressures. Figure 36-13 depicts the grades of diastolic dysfunction that have clinical and prognostic utility. Markedly elevated LV filling pressure are represented by "restrictive filling" in echocardiography (Figure 36-14).[78-80] The Doppler ratio of early transmitral velocity to early mitral diastolic tissue velocity (E/Ea) has been validated as a reasonably reliable noninvasive indicator of LV filling pressure in patients with preserved or depressed LVEF.[85-88] When obtained from the septal annulus, an E/Ea ratio exceeding 15 indicates a pulmonary capillary wedge pressure of 20 mm Hg or more. When the E/Ea ratio is less than 8, the pulmonary capillary wedge pressure is usually normal. An E/Ea ratio between 8 and 15 is usually inconclusive, and other information is needed in order to estimate pulmonary capillary wedge pressure. One useful formula that has been suggested is LV end-diastolic pressure (in millimeters of mercury) = 1.3 (E/Ea) + 2. Secondary echocardiographic markers of significant diastolic dysfunction include an enlarged LA volume (>30 mL/m^2) and evidence of elevated pulmonary artery pressures (>30 mm Hg).[78-81]

Cardiac Magnetic Resonance Imaging

Assessment of LV Mass and LA Size

CMR calculation of LV mass is highly accurate[89,90] and reproducible,[91] even in irregularly shaped ventricles.[92] Atrial volumes may have prognostic significance[93] and can be monitored in clinical scenarios such as atrial fibrillation.[94] Volumes can be calculated on the basis of geometrical assumptions and multislice volumetric methods.[95]

Identification of Diastolic Dysfunction and Demonstration of Elevated LV Filling Pressures

Parameters of diastolic function that are assessed in CMR imaging include transmitral and pulmonary venous flow and myocardial annular motion.[96,97] Rates of time to peak filling,[98] peak left atrial filling,[99] and left ventricular filling[100] can also be assessed; the latter can be combined with measurements of early diastolic tissue velocity on the basis of concepts developed in echocardiography.[101] Like echocardiography, phase-contrast CMR flow sequences can be used to assess filling pressures by quantification of the E/Ea ratio as part of a comprehensive protocol in a patient with heart failure.[101]

In myocardial tagging, prepulses are used to selectively saturate spins within the field of view to produce a grid or set of stripes with transiently nullified tissue. The deformation of these patterns during the cardiac cycle allows for analyzing contraction, relaxation, or both patterns of the myocardium (see Figures 36-4 and 36-5). This has been used for 2-dimensional[102] and 3-dimensional[103] strain analysis, including strain analysis of diastolic dysfunction in LV hypertrophy.[104] A large population-based study demonstrated adequate reproducibility of strain analysis.[105] Markers for early diastolic

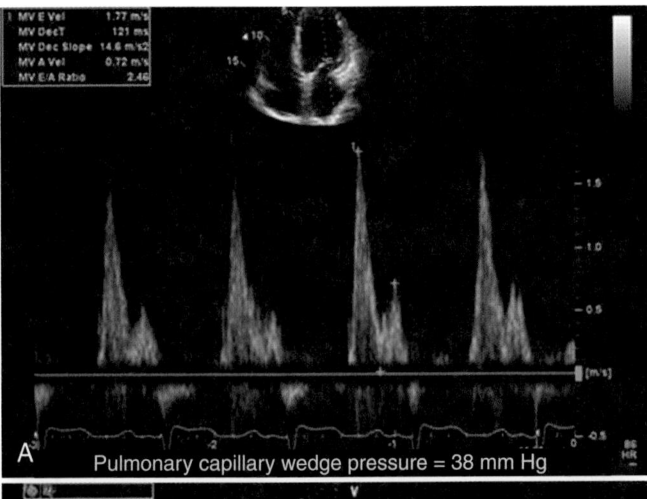

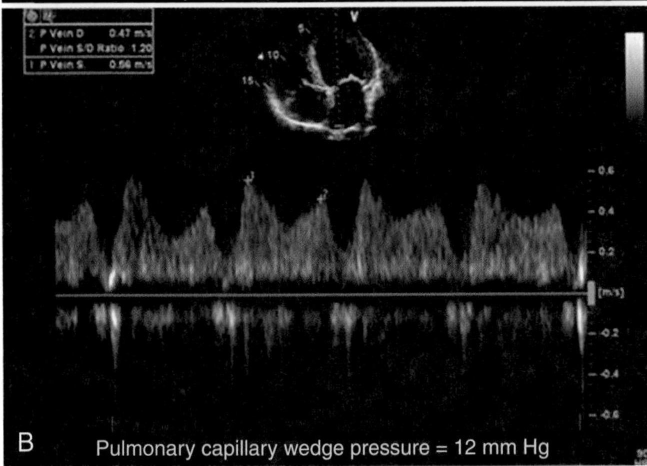

FIGURE 36–14 Utility of Doppler estimates of left ventricular (LV) filling pressures, derived from examinations of mitral valve (*MV*) inflow velocities (**A**) and pulmonary (*P*) vein flow velocities (**B**). **A,** A patient with known depressed LV ejection fraction presented with acute dyspnea. Transmitral Doppler imaging revealed an early (*E*) mitral valve velocity of 1.77 m/sec, a late (*A*) mitral valve velocity of 0.72 m/sec, with an E/A ratio of 2.46. The mitral deceleration time (*DecT*) was 121 msec. Together, these parameters are indicators of a restrictive filling pattern, which is predictive of a pulmonary capillary wedge pressure of 25 mm Hg or higher. In this patient, the right-sided heart catheterization study revealed a pulmonary capillary wedge pressure of 38 mm Hg. **B,** A patient with dilated cardiomyopathy and a depressed ejection fraction presented with dyspnea. Pulmonary venous Doppler imaging revealed a systolic (*S*) wave velocity of 0.56 m/sec, a diastolic (*D*) wave velocity of 0.47 m/sec, and an S/D ratio of 1.2, all consistent with normal LV filling pressure. Subsequent right-sided heart catheterization study revealed a pulmonary capillary wedge pressure of 12 mm Hg. A pulmonary embolus was subsequently diagnosed as the cause of dyspnea.

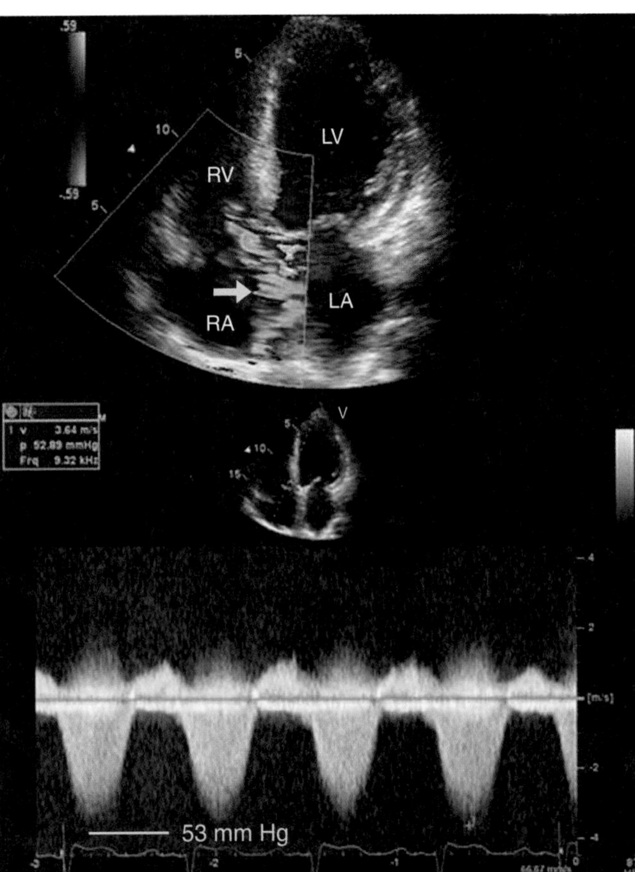

FIGURE 36–15 Use of Doppler velocity of tricuspid valve regurgitation in the estimation of pulmonary artery systolic pressure. In a patient with ischemic cardiomyopathy and marked dyspnea, color Doppler echocardiography (*top*) revealed moderately severe, eccentric tricuspid valve regurgitation (*yellow arrow*). Continuous wave Doppler echocardiography (*bottom*) revealed a peak tricuspid valve regurgitation velocity of 3.64 m/sec, or 53 mm Hg by modified Bernoulli equation. When this was added to a right atrial pressure estimate of 10 mm Hg, the estimated pulmonary artery systolic pressure was 63 mm Hg, which was consistent with moderate pulmonary hypertension secondary to left-sided heart failure. *Frq*, frequency; *LA*, left atrium; *LV*, left ventricle; *P*, pressure; *RA*, right atrium; *RV*, right ventricle; *V*, velocity.

untwisting motion of the basal and apical segments have been used to assess diastolic function[106,107] and were shown to be independent of preload.[108]

Nuclear Imaging

Although 2-dimensional echocardiography is most commonly used, radionuclide angiography or gated SPECT and PET can provide information as well. Equilibrium radionuclide angiography techniques[109] can be used to assess LV diastolic filling properties; such assessment relies on analysis of the LV time-activity curve, which represents relative volume changes throughout the cardiac cycle. This method yields results that are well correlated with those of Doppler echocardiography.[110]

ASSESSMENT OF RIGHT VENTRICULAR FUNCTION

Echocardiography

Echocardiography is a noninvasive method commonly used for assessing RV function and dysfunction. Variables for assessment of the right ventricle include RV transverse diameter (normal value < 3.8 cm in the apical four-chamber view),[5] assessment of RV fractional area change (normal ≥ 40%), tricuspid annular longitudinal displacement by M-mode echocardiography (normal > 1.5 cm),[111] Doppler systolic annular velocity of tricuspid tissue (normal > 9 cm/sec),[112,113] and RV systolic strain and strain rate (normal > 16% and > 1.1 m/sec, respectively).[114] In the setting of RV failure, several secondary echocardiographic phenomena can be observed: right atrial dilation (>30 mL/m^2), evidence of elevated RA pressure by dilated hepatic veins and a dilated inferior vena cava, the presence of pulmonary artery hypertension, tricuspid valve regurgitation (Figure 36-15), dilation of the pulmonary artery, and pulmonary valve insufficiency.[111,115] Doppler echocardiography has proven invaluable for estimating pulmonary artery pressures. The velocity of tricuspid valve regurgitation reflects the difference in systolic pressure between the right

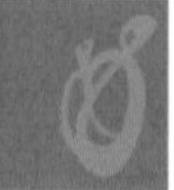

ventricle and the right atrium. As shown in Figure 36-15, the peak velocity of the tricuspid valve regurgitant jet can be obtained and converted to an estimated pressure by means of the modified Bernoulli equation (4 × [tricuspid valve regurgitation peak velocity]^2). When the calculated pressure is added to an estimated right atrial pressure of 10 mm Hg, it is possible to obtain reliable estimates of pulmonary artery systolic pressures.

Echocardiography is particularly useful for differentiation between secondary RV failure (caused by left-sided heart dysfunction, in which LA pressures are elevated), cor pulmonale (in which pulmonary artery pressure is elevated but the left heart chambers are normal), and primary RV failure (in which case there is no evidence of left-sided heart disease or significant parenchymal pulmonary disease).[115] Both in secondary RV failure and in cor pulmonale, pulmonary artery hypertension results in increased RV diameter, and depressed Doppler systolic annular velocity of tissue and RV strain have been shown to be adverse prognosticators.[111-115]

Cardiac Magnetic Resonance Imaging

Because it is often difficult to obtain echocardiographic imaging of the right ventricle, CMR imaging has become a pivotal imaging tool for determining RV structure and function.[116] With regard to heart failure, this is often of critical importance for planning surgical repair[117] in congenital heart disease, as well as follow-up after surgery.[118,119] Because of the irregular shape of the right ventricle, the assessment of RV mass is more difficult than the assessment of LV mass, which has ellipsoidal geometry.[120] However, reasonable estimates of RV structure have been obtained with CMR imaging in axial views.[121] Reference values obtained with state-of-the-art CMR sequences are available,[100,122,123] including data for various ethnic backgrounds.[124] In RV heart failure (e.g., chronic pulmonary hypertension), ventricular interaction is an important contributor to the impairment of cardiac output. The underlying mechanism entails a leftward shift of the interventricular septum that leads to underfilling of the left ventricle, which can easily be identified by CMR studies[125,126] and whose detection is often helpful for diagnosing pulmonary hypertension. As in echocardiography, retrograde flow velocity of a tricuspid valve regurgitant jet can be measured in CMR flow studies and can be used to estimate systolic RV pressure. This measurement, however, not widely performed.

Nuclear Imaging

Equilibrium gated radionuclide angiography is used with ^{99m}Tc-labeled red blood cells. Right ventricular ejection fraction (RVEF) can be abnormally decreased in patients with pulmonary hypertension. Patients with lesions in the proximal right coronary artery may exhibit decreases in RVEF during exercise.[11] With SPECT, RV uptake may be qualitatively assessed with the raw projection data and with the reconstructed data. The intensity of the RV uptake is 50% of peak intensity of LV uptake.[15] RV uptake increases in the presence of RV hypertrophy.[11] As on radionuclide angiography, reduced RV uptake evident on SPECT may be a sign of coronary artery disease in the distribution of the right coronary artery.[15] In the setting of chronic obstructive pulmonary disease, smoking, and severe LVEF impairment, sequestration of nitrogen-13–labeled ammonia ($^{13}NH_3$) in the lungs can be increased on PET, for which it would be necessary to delay the time between radiotracer injection and image acquisition to enhance image quality. This is an indirect marker of RV and LV performance that may provide additional data.[16]

ROLE OF CARDIAC IMAGING IN IMPLANTABLE CARDIAC DEVICES (see also Chapter 47)

Echocardiography

The role of echocardiography in the selection of patients for, and the optimization of, cardiac resynchronization therapy (CRT) has been extensively investigated.[127] LV septal-posterior wall systolic delay, demonstrated in M-mode echocardiography, was one of the first echocardiographic parameters shown to indicate significant LV dyssynchrony.[128] Doppler tissue imaging has been of value in demonstrating different time to peak systolic velocity in opposing walls (>65 msec being evidence of significant dyssynchrony) or in the maximum delay of any of six walls in the apical views (>100 msec being significant).[129,130] The standard deviation of time to opposing wall delay of more than 33 msec, on the 12 segments visible in the three apical views, has also been shown to denote significant intraventricular dyssynchrony and to be predictive of response to therapy.[131] Newer modalities involving speckle-based LV strain in systole, as well as 3-dimensional echocardiography, have also been employed to identify significant dyssynchrony.[132] The PROSPECT trial has highlighted reproducibility challenges in the measurement of these echocardiographic indicators of LV dyssynchrony.[133] For implantable cardioverter-defibrillator therapy, echocardiography is commonly used for demonstrating depressed LVEF (<30%), which is an indication for implantation of the defibrillator for the primary prevention of sudden cardiac death in patients with ischemic cardiomyopathy.[134]

Cardiac Magnetic Resonance Imaging

Data derived from CMR studies may provide important information for planning interventional therapy. Among several parameters,[135] strain analysis with tagged images may be particularly useful in mapping conduction abnormalities in three dimensions, which would significantly increase the success rate of CRT.[136] Furthermore, CMR imaging has been successfully used to predict outcome of CRT by assessing scar patterns with late enhancement CMR imaging.[137] Currently, the selection of patients for implantation of cardioverters-defibrillators is largely based on LVEF. However, markers for increased susceptibility of myocardial tissue to arrhythmic events may prove to be of critical value in decision making. The presence of nonischemic, intramural scars, as defined by midwall layers of late enhancement, is predictive of inducible ventricular tachycardia[138] in dilated cardiomyopathy. This finding was associated with increased susceptibility to arrhythmia in hypertrophic cardiomyopathy.[139,140] There is also a strong association between heterogeneous signal intensity of peri-infarct regions and inducible arrhythmia, which probably reflects the pathological substrate for arrhythmic foci after myocardial infarction.[141]

Nuclear Imaging

Radionuclide angiography has been used to quantify LV dyssynchrony by analysis of phase histograms and their standard deviation,[142] as well as to assess the effects of CRT. Gated SPECT and MPI with phase analysis could also be used to predict response to CRT.[143] PET has provided insight into the changes in myocardial perfusion, metabolism, and myocardial efficiency after CRT. Thus far, the effect of CRT on myocardial blood flow and metabolism has been investigated in several studies.[144-147] In ongoing studies, researchers are evaluating the role of phase analysis and FDG PET in directing CRT. Development of novel strategies to identify substrates associated with a high risk of sudden cardiac death could improve selection of patients for device-based primary prevention of arrhythmia-related death.

FUTURE DIRECTIONS IN CARDIAC IMAGING

Echocardiography

3-Dimensional Echocardiography

Many contemporary echocardiographic machines perform full 3-dimensional volume analysis of the heart with use of a hand-held ultrasonographic probe. LV systolic and diastolic volumes can be measured from the full volume data set, and they compare favorably with those obtained by MRI (Figure 36-16).[148] LV ejection fraction has also shown to be better estimated with 3-dimensional echocardiography than with 2-dimensional echocardiography and is more closely related to those obtained with MRI.[149] Furthermore, 3-dimensional echocardiographic LV and LA volumes have been predictive of prognosis in patients with heart failure.[150] Future advances in transthoracic and transesophageal echocardiography will probably be influenced or determined by 3-dimensional echocardiography.[151]

Speckle-Based Tracking Echocardiography

Speckle-based tracking is a method of non-Doppler 2-dimensional imaging ("speckle echocardiography") to track myocardial motion in various planes. Reflection scattering and interference of the ultrasound beam in the myocardial tissue produces on the images the formation of speckles, which can be tracked from frame to frame throughout the cardiac cycle; this provides information on displacement, velocity, deformation, and deformation rate (strain and strain rate, respectively) that is independent of angulation and cardiac translational motion.[152] Speckle-based tracking allows for the assessment of LV rotational movement, which is referred to as *torsion* or *twist* (Figure 36-17). Speckle-based echocardiography has provided detailed information on myocardial mechanics in hypertensive heart disease, hypertrophic cardiomyopathy, and diastolic and systolic LV failure and in cases of pulmonary hypertension.[152-155] Currently, such speckle-based measurements are being studied to assess their role in predicting patient outcomes in heart failure. State-of-the-art and future applications are combining speckle-based imaging with 3-dimensional echocardiography to obtain a 3-dimensional velocity and strain map of the left ventricle.[156]

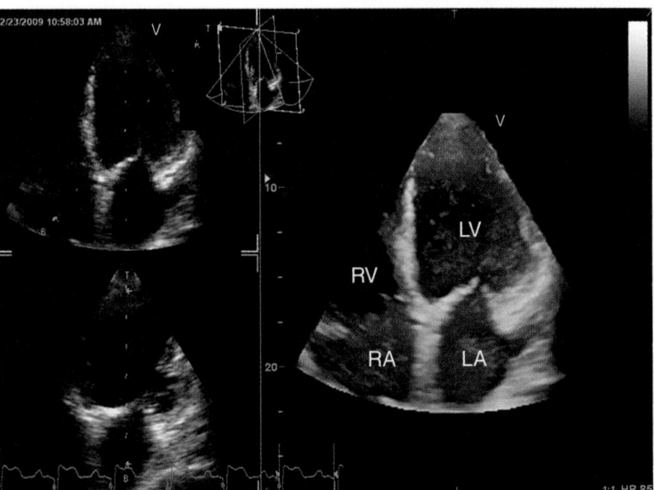

FIGURE 36–16 In a patient with ischemic cardiomyopathy, 3-dimensional echocardiography was used for assessment of increasing dyspnea on exertion. It revealed significantly dilated left and right ventricles and a calculated left ventricular ejection fraction of 28%. Left-sided heart catheterization study revealed severe three-vessel coronary artery disease. *LA*, left atrium; *LV*, left ventricle; *RA*, right atrium; *RV*, right ventricle; *V*, velocity.

Cardiac Magnetic Resonance Imaging

Role of Strain and Strain Rate Imaging in Patients with Heart Failure

As discussed previously, myocardial strain and strain rate can also be assessed with CMR imaging. Sequences with tagging pulses imprint a grid, or set of parallel stripes, onto the images of myocardial tissue (see Figures 36-4 and 36-5). The deformation of the visible patterns over the cardiac cycle allows for analyzing regional ventricular function,[157] as well as myocardial strain and strain rate. Among various parameters, systolic circumferential strain appears to be the most promising. Patients at risk for heart failure show distinct patterns of abnormal strain,[104] and standardized CMR protocols have been proposed and validated with a normal population.[105]

Nuclear Imaging

Assessment of Cardiac Sympathetic Innervation

Neurotransmitter assessment and cardiac receptor imaging represent promising advances in molecular imaging that could facilitate the understanding of the pathophysiological processes involved in progression of heart failure.[158,159] The normal heart usually extracts norepinephrine from arterial blood, whereas in patients with moderate heart failure, the coronary sinus norepinephrine concentration exceeds the arterial concentration, which indicates that there is increased adrenergic stimulation of the heart. However, as heart failure progresses, there is a significant decrease in the myocardial concentration of norepinephrine. The mechanism responsible for cardiac norepinephrine depletion in severe heart failure is not clear; it may be related to an "exhaustion" phenomenon resulting from the prolonged adrenergic activation of the cardiac adrenergic nerves in heart failure. Iodine-123–labeled metaiodobenzylguanidine (^{123}I-MIBG), a radiopharmaceutical that is normally taken up by adrenergic nerve endings, is not taken up normally in patients with cardiomyopathy, which suggests that norepinephrine reuptake is also impaired in heart failure. ^{123}I-MIBG imaging of cardiac sympathetic innervation has been predictive of outcomes in heart failure.[160,161] Researchers in the Prognostic Significance of ^{123}I-MIBG Myocardial Scintigraphy in Heart Failure (ADMIRE-HF) study examined the prognostic usefulness of the assessment of myocardial sympathetic innervation, as determined by the heart-to-mediastinum ratio on planar ^{123}I-MIBG imaging as either normal (>1.6) or abnormal (<1.6), for identifying patients with New York Heart Association (NYHA) class II or III heart failure with an ejection fraction of less than 35% who were at increased risk of experiencing an adverse cardiac event. Patients were monitored for a maximum of 2 years. Results showed that the composite endpoint—the first occurrence of NYHA heart failure class progression, potentially life-threatening arrhythmic event, or cardiac death—occurred significantly ($P < .0001$) more frequently in patients who had low uptake of the tracer.[162] Interestingly, ^{123}I-MIBG imaging had independent prognostic capability complementary to B-type natriuretic peptide (BNP) and helped distinguish between patients who were likely to die from heart failure progression and those who would have an arrhythmic event. Patients with the lowest

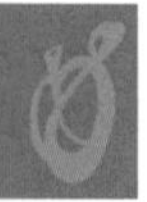

uptakes (heart-to-mediastinum ratio < 1.2) tended to die from heart failure progression, whereas arrhythmic events tended to occur in patients with heart-to-mediastinum ratios in the range of 1.2 to 1.6; this finding suggests that molecular imaging may be used to guide defibrillator therapy in the future.[162]

Molecular Imaging with PET

Carbon-11 (^{11}C)–labeled meta-hydroxyephedrine (HED, *N*-methyl-metaraminol) is a catecholamine analogue, developed for PET, of sympathetic nerve terminals of the heart and is used as an index of norepinephrine reuptake transporter density and synaptic norepinephrine levels. In conjunction with FDG viability imaging, ^{11}C-labeled HED imaging may prove useful in identifying patients with ischemic cardiomyopathy who are at risk for sudden cardiac death.[163] The branched-chain fatty acid β-methyl-*p*-[^{123}I]-iodophenyl-pentadecanoic acid (^{123}BMIPP) undergoes limited beta-oxidation after myocardial ischemia, despite restoration of myocardial blood flow.[164] These findings support the concept that ^{123}BMIPP imaging can be used to

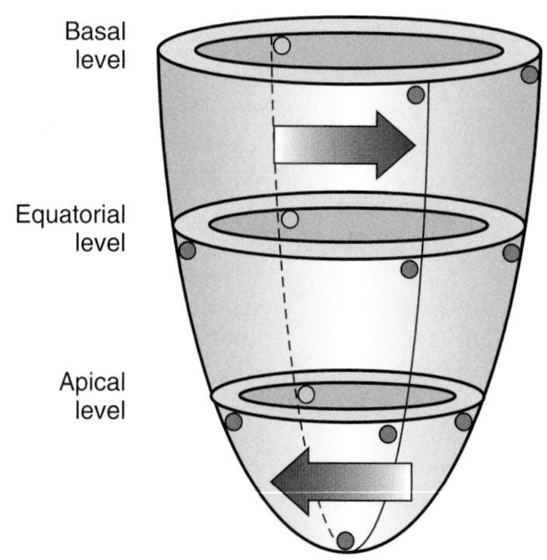

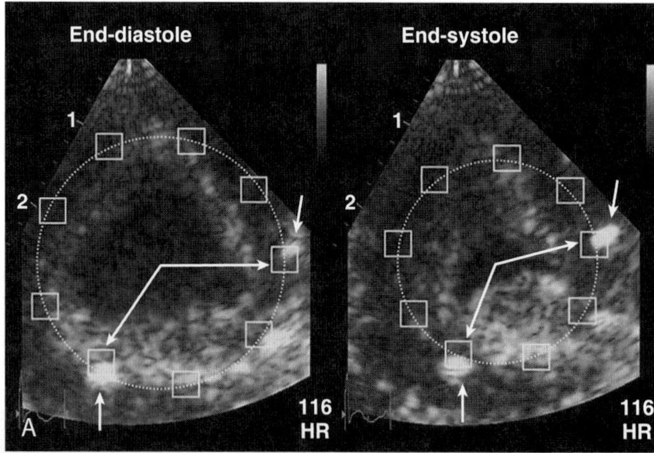

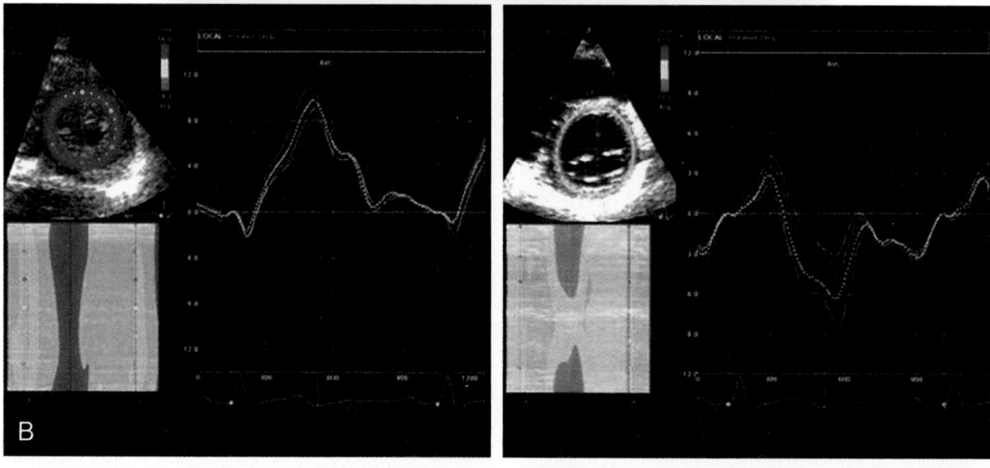

FIGURE 36–17 **A, Top,** Viewed from the apex, the apical rotation is counterclockwise (*top thick arrow*) and basal rotation is clockwise (*bottom thick arrow*). **A, Bottom,** Speckled tracking regions of interest are denoted by *white boxes* in the echocardiographic image of the animal model. Rotational changes are noted by the *dotted white arrows* during end-diastole and end-systole frames. **B,** Cardiac rotation in a normal person. The extent of rotation is colorized in these speckle-based tracking images. **B, Left,** Apical short-axis view with counterclockwise rotation (*blue*). Maximal rotation occurred at end-systole, shown as the graph above the baseline. The extent of rotation of multiple segments is shown in different colors. The rectangle below the speckle-based image shows colorized rotation of different segments during one cardiac cycle, which is a color M-mode of left ventricular apical rotation. **B, Right,** The basal segment of the left ventricle, with clockwise rotation by color and graph. Because rotation is clockwise, the graph is recorded below the baseline.

Continued

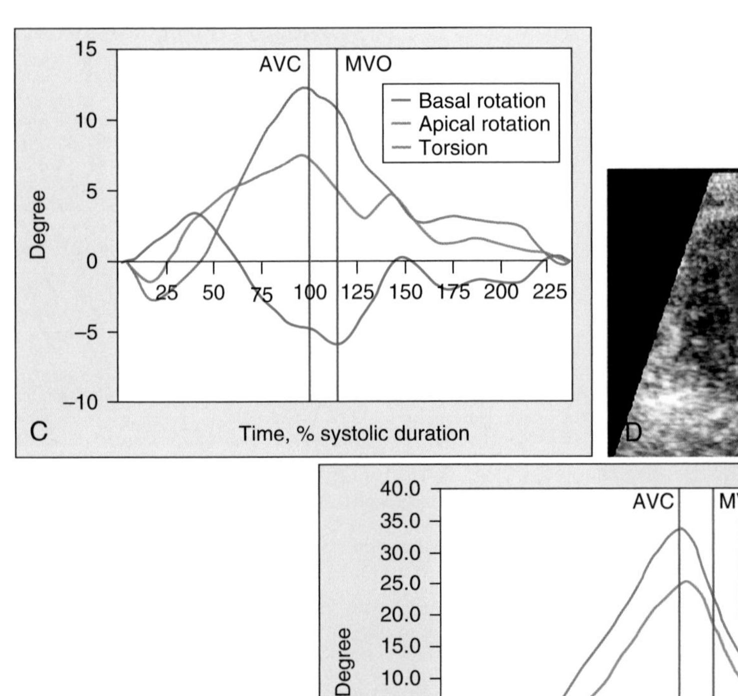

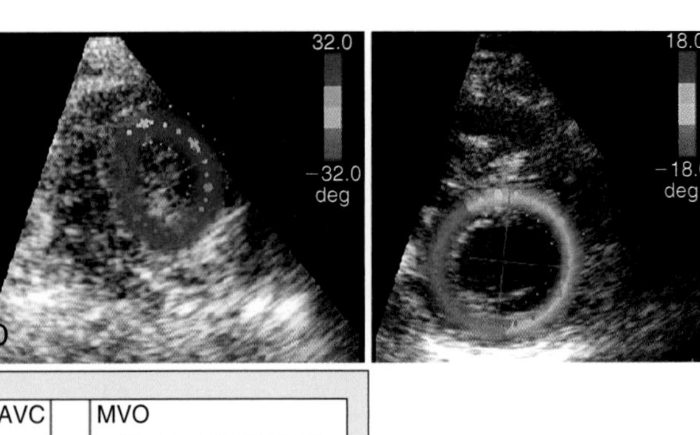

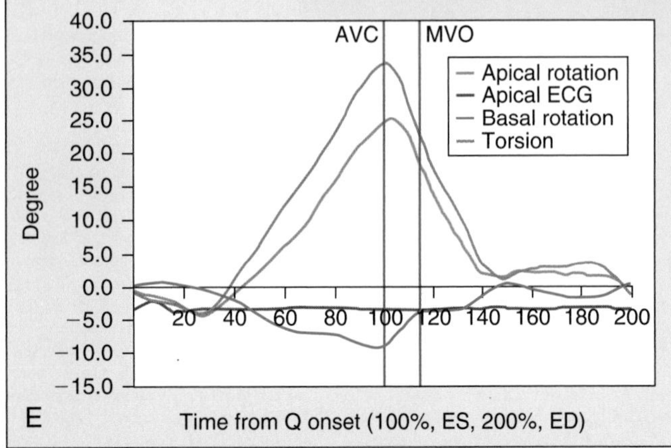

FIGURE 36–17, Cont'd **C,** The mean apical rotation (7-degree counterclockwise) and basal rotation (5-degree clockwise rotation) at the time of aortic valve closing (AVC) are shown. They resulted in a net torsion of 12 degrees. Untwisting of the torsion starts the myocardial relaxation process. **D, Left,** Apical short-axis view with speckle-based imaging, showing exaggerated counterclockwise rotation in a patient with abnormal myocardial relaxation. **D, Right,** Basal short-axis view, showing clockwise rotation. **E,** Quantification of the extent of the rotation and resulting torsion is shown in this graph from the same patient as in **D.** Apical counterclockwise rotation is 25 degrees (above the baseline), and the peak basal clockwise rotation (below the baseline) is 9 degrees. Both apical rotation and basal rotation are greater than those of a normal person. Therefore, torsion is higher than in a normal person at 34 degrees. *ED*, end-diastole; *ES*, end-systole; *MVD*, mitral valve opening. (From Connolly HM, Oh JK. Echocardiography. In Libby P, Bonow RO, Mann DL, et al, editors. *Braunwald's heart disease,* Philadelphia, 2008, Elsevier, pp 227-325.)

provide a metabolic imprint of a stress-induced ischemic episode, which has been referred to as *ischemic memory.* Another potentially useful tracer is ^{11}C acetate, which has been used for studying myocardial oxidative metabolism and regional myocardial blood flow, and hence determining myocardial efficiency, in patients with dilated cardiomyopathy.[165]

PET is also able to quantify absolute myocardial blood flow.[17] This facilitates the detection of hemodynamically significant stenotic lesions in the coronary arteries and may facilitate detection of multivessel disease as well.[166] Absolute flow quantification by PET has been used extensively to determine the effects of drugs and devices on myocardial blood flow.[167] Whether this approach adds benefit in terms of diagnosis or prognosis in patients with heart failure remains to be determined.

Use of Dual Imaging Techniques in Patients with Heart Failure

Multimodal imaging PET and computed tomography (CT) systems have become established in clinical practice.[168] There is also a trend toward increasing use of hybrid SPECT and CT systems for conventional nuclear imaging. Moreover, the combination of PET with MRI may afford further advantages.[169] However, several technical issues need to be resolved before the true added value of these hybrid imaging systems can be assessed. These hybrid technologies are expected to expand the role of cardiac imaging in patients with heart failure.

REFERENCES

1. Hunt, S. A., Abraham, W. T., Chin, M. H., et al. (2005). ACC/AHA 2005 guideline update for the diagnosis and management of chronic heart failure in the adult: a report of the American College of Cardiology/American Heart Association Task Force on Practice Guidelines (Writing Committee to Update the 2001 Guidelines for the Evaluation and Management of Heart Failure): developed in collaboration with the American College of Chest Physicians and the International Society for Heart and Lung Transplantation: endorsed by the Heart Rhythm Society. *Circulation, 112,* e154–e235.
2. Dickstein, K., Cohen-Solal, A., Filippatos, G., et al. (2008). ESC guidelines for the diagnosis and treatment of acute and chronic heart failure 2008: the Task Force for the Diagnosis and Treatment of Acute and Chronic Heart Failure 2008 of the European Society of Cardiology. Developed in collaboration with the Heart Failure Association of the ESC (HFA) and endorsed by the European Society of Intensive Care Medicine (ESICM). *Eur Heart J, 29,* 2388–2442.
3. Senni, M., Rodeheffer, R. J., Tribouilloy, C. M., et al. (1999). Use of echocardiography in the management of congestive heart failure in the community. *J Am Coll Cardiol, 33,* 164–170.
4. Kirkpatrick, J. N., Vannan, M. A., Narula, J., et al. (2007). Echocardiography in heart failure: applications, utility, and new horizons. *J Am Coll Cardiol, 50,* 381–396.
5. Lang, R. M., Bierig, M., Devereux, R. B., et al. (2005). Recommendations for chamber quantification: a report from the American Society of Echocardiography's Guidelines and Standards Committee and the Chamber Quantification Writing Group, developed in conjunction with the European Association of Echocardiography, a branch of the European Society of Cardiology. *J Am Soc Echocardiogr, 18,* 1440–1463.
6. Mulvagh, S. L., Rakowski, H., Vannan, M. A., et al. (2008). American Society of Echocardiography consensus statement on the clinical applications of ultrasonic contrast agents in echocardiography. *J Am Soc Echocardiogr, 21,* 1179–1201.
7. Gopal, A. S., Shen, Z., Sapin, P. M., et al. (1995). Assessment of cardiac function by three-dimensional echocardiography compared with conventional noninvasive methods. *Circulation, 92,* 842–853.
8. Pouleur, A. C., le Polain de Waroux, J. B., Pasquet, A., et al. (2008). Assessment of left ventricular mass and volumes by three-dimensional echocardiography in patients with or without wall motion abnormalities: comparison against cine magnetic resonance imaging. *Heart, 94,* 1050–1057.

9. Jenkins, C., Bricknell, K., Chan, J., et al. (2007). Comparison of two- and three-dimensional echocardiography with sequential magnetic resonance imaging for evaluating left ventricular volume and ejection fraction over time in patients with healed myocardial infarction. *Am J Cardiol, 99*, 300–306.
10. Hendel, R. C., Patel, M. R., Kramer, C. M., et al. (2006). ACCF/ACR/SCCT/SCMR/ASNC/NASCI/SCAI/SIR 2006 appropriateness criteria for cardiac computed tomography and cardiac magnetic resonance imaging: a report of the American College of Cardiology Foundation Quality Strategic Directions Committee Appropriateness Criteria Working Group, American College of Radiology, Society of Cardiovascular Computed Tomography, Society for Cardiovascular Magnetic Resonance, American Society of Nuclear Cardiology, North American Society for Cardiac Imaging, Society for Cardiovascular Angiography and Interventions, and Society of Interventional Radiology. *J Am Coll Cardiol, 48*, 1475–1497.
11. Klocke, F. J., Baird, M. G., Lorell, B. H., et al. (2003). ACC/AHA/ASNC guidelines for the clinical use of cardiac radionuclide imaging—executive summary: a report of the American College of Cardiology/American Heart Association Task Force on Practice Guidelines (ACC/AHA/ASNC Committee to Revise the 1995 Guidelines for the Clinical Use of Cardiac Radionuclide Imaging). *J Am Coll Cardiol, 42*, 1318–1333.
12. Zaret, B. L. (2008). Cardiac performance. In B. L. Zaret, & G. A. Beller (Eds.), *Clinical nuclear cardiology. State of the art and future directions* (pp. 175–187). St. Louis: Mosby.
13. Chua, T., Yin, L. C., Thiang, T. H., et al. (2000). Accuracy of the automated assessment of left ventricular function with gated perfusion SPECT in the presence of perfusion defects and left ventricular dysfunction: correlation with equilibrium radionuclide ventriculography and echocardiography. *J Nucl Cardiol, 7*, 301–311.
14. Faber, T. L., Vansant, J. P., Pettigrew, R. I., et al. (2001). Evaluation of left ventricular endocardial volumes and ejection fractions computed from gated perfusion SPECT with magnetic resonance imaging: comparison of two methods. *J Nucl Cardiol, 8*, 645–651.
15. Hansen, C. L., Goldstein, R. A., Akinboboye, O. O., et al. (2007). Myocardial perfusion and function: single photon emission computed tomography. *J Nucl Cardiol, 14*, e39–e60.
16. Machac, J., Bacharach, S. L., Bateman, T. M., et al. (2006). Positron emission tomography myocardial perfusion and glucose metabolism imaging. *J Nucl Cardiol, 13*, e121–e151.
17. Ziadi, M. C., Beanlands, R. S. B., deKemp, R., et al. Diagnosis and prognosis in cardiac disease using cardiac PET perfusion imaging. In Zaret BL, Beller GA, editors. *Clinical nuclear cardiology. State of the art and future directions.* St. Louis, Mosby, in press.
18. Diaz, R. A., Nihoyannopoulos, P., Athanassopoulos, G., et al. (1991). Usefulness of echocardiography to differentiate dilated cardiomyopathy from coronary-induced congestive heart failure. *Am J Cardiol, 68*, 1224–1227.
19. Cheesman, M. G., Leech, G., Chambers, J., et al. (1998). Central role of echocardiography in the diagnosis and assessment of heart failure. British Society of Echocardiography. *Heart, 80* (Suppl. 1), S1–S5.
20. Armstrong, W. F., & Zoghbi, W. A. (2005). Stress echocardiography: current methodology and clinical applications. *J Am Coll Cardiol, 45*, 1739–1747.
21. Douglas, P. S., Khandheria, B., Stainback, R. F., et al. (2008). ACCF/ASE/ACEP/AHA/ASNC/SCAI/SCCT/SCMR 2008 appropriateness criteria for stress echocardiography: a report of the American College of Cardiology Foundation Appropriateness Criteria Task Force, American Society of Echocardiography, American College of Emergency Physicians, American Heart Association, American Society of Nuclear Cardiology, Society for Cardiovascular Angiography and Interventions, Society of Cardiovascular Computed Tomography, and Society for Cardiovascular Magnetic Resonance: endorsed by the Heart Rhythm Society and the Society of Critical Care Medicine. *Circulation, 117*, 1478–1497.
22. Elhendy, A., Sozzi, F., van Domburg, R. T., et al. (2005). Effect of myocardial ischemia during dobutamine stress echocardiography on cardiac mortality in patients with heart failure secondary to ischemic cardiomyopathy. *Am J Cardiol, 96*, 469–473.
23. McCrohon, J. A., Moon, J. C., Prasad, S. K., et al. (2003). Differentiation of heart failure related to dilated cardiomyopathy and coronary artery disease using gadolinium-enhanced cardiovascular magnetic resonance. *Circulation, 108*, 54–59.
24. Mahrholdt, H., Wagner, A., Deluigi, C. C., et al. (2006). Presentation, patterns of myocardial damage, and clinical course of viral myocarditis. *Circulation, 114*, 1581–1590.
25. Mahrholdt, H., Goedecke, C., Wagner, A., et al. (2004). Cardiovascular magnetic resonance assessment of human myocarditis: a comparison to histology and molecular pathology. *Circulation, 109*, 1250–1258.
26. Wilson, J. M., Villareal, R. P., Hariharan, R., et al. (2002). Magnetic resonance imaging of myocardial fibrosis in hypertrophic cardiomyopathy. *Tex Heart Inst J, 29*, 176–180.
27. Smedema, J. P., Snoep, G., van Kroonenburgh, M. P., et al. (2005). Evaluation of the accuracy of gadolinium-enhanced cardiovascular magnetic resonance in the diagnosis of cardiac sarcoidosis. *J Am Coll Cardiol, 45*, 1683–1690.
28. Nagel, E., Lehmkuhl, H. B., Bocksch, W., et al. (1999). Noninvasive diagnosis of ischemia-induced wall motion abnormalities with the use of high-dose dobutamine stress MRI: comparison with dobutamine stress echocardiography. *Circulation, 99*, 763–770.
29. Kramer, C. M., Barkhausen, J., Flamm, S. D., et al. (2008). Standardized cardiovascular magnetic resonance imaging (CMR) protocols, society for cardiovascular magnetic resonance: Board of Trustees Task Force on Standardized Protocols. *J Cardiovasc Magn Reson, 10*, 35.
30. Nagel, E., Lehmkuhl, H. B., Klein, C., et al. (1999). Influence of image quality on the diagnostic accuracy of dobutamine stress magnetic resonance imaging in comparison with dobutamine stress echocardiography for the noninvasive detection of myocardial ischemia. *Z Kardiol, 88*, 622–630.
31. Kuijpers, D., Ho, K. Y., van Dijkman, P. R., et al. (2003). Dobutamine cardiovascular magnetic resonance for the detection of myocardial ischemia with the use of myocardial tagging. *Circulation, 107*, 1592–1597.
32. Jahnke, C., Nagel, E., Gebker, R., et al. (2007). Prognostic value of cardiac magnetic resonance stress tests: adenosine stress perfusion and dobutamine stress wall motion imaging. *Circulation, 115*, 1769–1776.
33. Schwitter, J., Wacker, C. M., van Rossum, A. C., et al. (2008). MR-IMPACT: comparison of perfusion–cardiac magnetic resonance with single-photon emission computed tomography for the detection of coronary artery disease in a multicentre, multivendor, randomized trial. *Eur Heart J, 4*, 480–489.
34. Schwitter, J., Nanz, D., Kneifel, S., et al. (2001). Assessment of myocardial perfusion in coronary artery disease by magnetic resonance: a comparison with positron emission tomography and coronary angiography. *Circulation, 103*, 2230–2235.
35. Ibrahim, T., Nekolla, S. G., Schreiber, K., et al. (2002). Assessment of coronary flow reserve: comparison between contrast-enhanced magnetic resonance imaging and positron emission tomography. *J Am Coll Cardiol, 39*, 864–870.
36. Nagel, E., Klein, C., Paetsch, I., et al. (2003). Magnetic resonance perfusion measurements for the noninvasive detection of coronary artery disease. *Circulation, 108*, 432–437.
37. Elkington, A. G., Gatehouse, P. D., Ablitt, N. A., et al. (2005). Interstudy reproducibility of quantitative perfusion cardiovascular magnetic resonance. *J Cardiovasc Magn Reson, 7*, 815–822.
38. Hachamovitch, R., Hayes, S. W., Friedman, J. D., et al. (2003). Comparison of the short-term survival benefit associated with revascularization compared with medical therapy in patients with no prior coronary artery disease undergoing stress myocardial perfusion single photon emission computed tomography. *Circulation, 107*, 2900–2907.
39. Hachamovitch, R., Rozanski, A., Hayes, S. W., et al. (2006). Predicting therapeutic benefit from myocardial revascularization procedures: are measurements of both resting left ventricular ejection fraction and stress-induced myocardial ischemia necessary? *J Nucl Cardiol, 13*, 768–778.
40. Wackers, F. J., Coronary artery disease: exercise stress. In B. L. Zaret, G. A. Beller, editors. *Clinical nuclear cardiology. State of the art and future directions.* St. Louis, in press, Mosby, pp 215–232.
41. Shaw, L. J., Berman, D. S., Maron, D. J., et al. (2008). Optimal medical therapy with or without percutaneous coronary intervention to reduce ischemic burden: results from the Clinical Outcomes Utilizing Revascularization and Aggressive Drug Evaluation (COURAGE) trial nuclear substudy. *Circulation, 117*, 1283–1291.
42. Di Carli, M. F., Prcevski, P., Singh, T. P., et al. (2000). Myocardial blood flow, function, and metabolism in repetitive stunning. *J Nucl Med, 41*, 1227–1234.
43. Bax, J. J., Poldermans, D., Elhendy, A., et al. (1999). Improvement of left ventricular ejection fraction, heart failure symptoms and prognosis after revascularization in patients with chronic coronary artery disease and viable myocardium detected by dobutamine stress echocardiography. *J Am Coll Cardiol, 34*, 163–169.
44. Sawada, S., Bapat, A., Vaz, D., et al. (2003). Incremental value of myocardial viability for prediction of long-term prognosis in surgically revascularized patients with left ventricular dysfunction. *J Am Coll Cardiol, 42*, 2099–2105.
45. Camici, P. G., Prasad, S. K., & Rimoldi, O. E. (2008). Stunning, hibernation, and assessment of myocardial viability. *Circulation, 117*, 103–114.
46. Baer, F. M., Voth, E., Schneider, C. A., et al. (1995). Comparison of low-dose dobutamine-gradient-echo magnetic resonance imaging and positron emission tomography with [18F]fluorodeoxyglucose in patients with chronic coronary artery disease. A functional and morphological approach to the detection of residual myocardial viability. *Circulation, 91*, 1006–1015.
47. Baer, F. M., Theissen, P., Crnac, J., et al. (2000). Head to head comparison of dobutamine-transoesophageal echocardiography and dobutamine-magnetic resonance imaging for the prediction of left ventricular functional recovery in patients with chronic coronary artery disease. *Eur Heart J, 21*, 981–991.
48. Rehwald, W. G., Fieno, D. S., Chen, E. L., et al. (2002). Myocardial magnetic resonance imaging contrast agent concentrations after reversible and irreversible ischemic injury. *Circulation, 105*, 224–229.
49. Kim, R. J., Fieno, D. S., ParrishTB, et al. (1999). Relationship of MRI delayed contrast enhancement to irreversible injury, infarct age, and contractile function. *Circulation, 100*, 1992–2002.
50. Wagner, A., Mahrholdt, H., Holly, T. A., et al. (2003). Contrast-enhanced MRI and routine single photon emission computed tomography (SPECT) perfusion imaging for detection of subendocardial myocardial infarcts: an imaging study. *Lancet, 361*, 374–379.
51. Kim, R. J., Wu, E., Rafael, A., et al. (2000). The use of contrast-enhanced magnetic resonance imaging to identify reversible myocardial dysfunction. *N Engl J Med, 343*, 1445–1453.
52. Schinkel, A. F., Poldermans, D., Elhendy, A., et al. (2007). Assessment of myocardial viability in patients with heart failure. *J Nucl Med, 48*, 1135–1146.
53. Bax, J. J., van der Wall, E. E., & Harbinson, M. (2004). Radionuclide techniques for the assessment of myocardial viability and hibernation. *Heart, 90*(Suppl. 5), v26–v33.
54. Schinkel, A. F., Bax, J. J., Poldermans, D., et al. (2007). Hibernating myocardium: diagnosis and patient outcomes. *Curr Probl Cardiol, 32*, 375–410.
55. Chareonthaitawee, P., Gersh, B. J., Araoz, P. A., et al. (2005). Revascularization in severe left ventricular dysfunction: the role of viability testing. *J Am Coll Cardiol, 46*, 567–574.
56. Sawada, S. G., Allman, K. C., Muzik, O., et al. (1994). Positron emission tomography detects evidence of viability in rest technetium-99m sestamibi defects. *J Am Coll Cardiol, 23*, 92–98.
57. Bax, J. J., Poldermans, D., Elhendy, A., et al. (2001). Sensitivity, specificity, and predictive accuracies of various noninvasive techniques for detecting hibernating myocardium. *Curr Probl Cardiol, 26*, 147–186.
58. Schelbert, H. R., Beanlands, R., Bengel, F., et al. (2003). PET myocardial perfusion and glucose metabolism imaging: part 2—guidelines for interpretation and reporting. *J Nucl Cardiol, 10*, 557–571.
59. Beanlands, R. S., deKemp, R. A., Smith, S., et al. (1997). F-18-fluorodeoxyglucose PET imaging alters clinical decision making in patients with impaired ventricular function. *Am J Cardiol, 79*, 1092–1095.

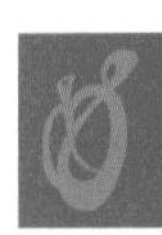

60. Haas, F., Augustin, N., Holper, K., et al. (2000). Time course and extent of improvement of dysfunctioning myocardium in patients with coronary artery disease and severely depressed left ventricular function after revascularization: correlation with positron emission tomographic findings. *J Am Coll Cardiol, 36*, 1927–1934.
61. Beanlands, R. S., Hendry, P. J., Masters, R. G., et al. (1998). Delay in revascularization is associated with increased mortality rate in patients with severe left ventricular dysfunction and viable myocardium on fluorine 18-fluorodeoxyglucose positron emission tomography imaging. *Circulation, 98*, II51–II56.
62. Tarakji, K. G., Brunken, R., McCarthy, P. M., et al. (2006). Myocardial viability testing and the effect of early intervention in patients with advanced left ventricular systolic dysfunction. *Circulation, 113*, 230–237.
63. Beanlands, R. S., Nichol, G., Huszti, E., et al. (2007). F-18-fluorodeoxyglucose positron emission tomography imaging–assisted management of patients with severe left ventricular dysfunction and suspected coronary disease: a randomized, controlled trial (PARR-2). *J Am Coll Cardiol, 50*, 2002–2012.
64. Gaasch, W. H., & Meyer, T. E. (2008). Left ventricular response to mitral regurgitation: implications for management. *Circulation, 118*, 2298–2303.
65. Bonow, R. O., Carabello, B. A., Chatterjee, K., et al. (2008). 2008 Focused update incorporated into the ACC/AHA 2006 guidelines for the management of patients with valvular heart disease: a report of the American College of Cardiology/American Heart Association Task Force on Practice Guidelines (Writing Committee to Revise the 1998 Guidelines for the Management of Patients With Valvular Heart Disease): endorsed by the Society of Cardiovascular Anesthesiologists, Society for Cardiovascular Angiography and Interventions, and Society of Thoracic Surgeons. *Circulation, 118*, e523–e661.
66. Zoghbi, W. A., Enriquez-Sarano, M., Foster, E., et al. (2003). Recommendations for evaluation of the severity of native valvular regurgitation with two-dimensional and Doppler echocardiography. *J Am Soc Echocardiogr, 16*, 777–802.
67. Baumgartner, H., Hung, J., Bermejo, J., et al. (2009). Echocardiographic assessment of valve stenosis: EAE/ASE recommendations for clinical practice. *J Am Soc Echocardiogr, 22*, 1–23.
68. Monin, J. L., Monchi, M., Gest, V., et al. (2001). Aortic stenosis with severe left ventricular dysfunction and low transvalvular pressure gradients: risk stratification by low-dose dobutamine echocardiography. *J Am Coll Cardiol, 37*, 2101–2107.
69. Monin, J. L., Quere, J. P., Monchi, M., et al. (2003). Low-gradient aortic stenosis: operative risk stratification and predictors for long-term outcome: a multicenter study using dobutamine stress hemodynamics. *Circulation, 108*, 319–324.
70. Higgins, C. B., Wagner, S., Kondo, C., et al. (1991). Evaluation of valvular heart disease with cine gradient echo magnetic resonance imaging. *Circulation, 84*, 198–207.
71. Globits, S., & Higgins, C. B. (1995). Assessment of valvular heart disease by magnetic resonance imaging. *Am Heart J, 129*, 369–381.
72. Caruther, S. D., Lin, S. J., Brown, P., et al. (2003). Practical value of cardiac magnetic resonance imaging for clinical quantification of aortic valve stenosis: comparison with echocardiography. *Circulation, 108*, 2236–2243.
73. Friedrich, M. G., Schulz-Menger, J., Poetsch, T., et al. (2002). Quantification of valvular aortic stenosis by magnetic resonance imaging. *Am Heart J, 144*, 329–334.
74. John, A. S., Dill, T., Brandt, R. R., et al. (2003). Magnetic resonance to assess the aortic valve area in aortic stenosis: how does it compare to current diagnostic standards? *J Am Coll Cardiol, 42*, 519–526.
75. Kupfahl, C., Honold, M., Meinhardt, G., et al. (2004). Evaluation of aortic stenosis by cardiovascular magnetic resonance imaging: comparison with established routine clinical techniques. *Heart, 90*, 893–901.
76. Zile, M. R., Baicu, C. F., & Gaasch, W. H. (2004). Diastolic heart failure—abnormalities in active relaxation and passive stiffness of the left ventricle. *N Engl J Med, 350*, 1953–1959.
77. Paulus, W. J., Tschope, C., Sanderson, J. E., et al. (2007). How to diagnose diastolic heart failure: a consensus statement on the diagnosis of heart failure with normal left ventricular ejection fraction by the Heart Failure and Echocardiography Associations of the European Society of Cardiology. *Eur Heart J, 28*, 2539–2550.
78. Oh, J. K., Hatle, L., Tajik, A. J., et al. (2006). Diastolic heart failure can be diagnosed by comprehensive two-dimensional and Doppler echocardiography. *J Am Coll Cardiol, 47*, 500–506.
79. Lester, S. J., Tajik, A. J., Nishimura, R. A., et al. (2008). Unlocking the mysteries of diastolic function: deciphering the Rosetta Stone 10 years later. *J Am Coll Cardiol, 51*, 679–689.
80. Nagueh, S. F., Appleton, C. P., Gillebert, T. C., et al. (2009). Recommendations for the evaluation of left ventricular diastolic function by echocardiography. *J Am Soc Echocardiogr, 22*, 107–133.
81. Abhayaratna, W. P., Seward, J. B., Appleton, C. P., et al. (2006). Left atrial size: physiologic determinants and clinical applications. *J Am Coll Cardiol, 47*, 2357–2363.
82. Dokainish, H., Sengupta, R., Pillai, M., et al. (2008). Assessment of left ventricular systolic function using echocardiography in patients with preserved ejection fraction and elevated diastolic pressures. *Am J Cardiol, 101*, 1766–1771.
83. Dokainish, H., Zoghbi, W. A., Lakkis, N. M., et al. (2005). Incremental predictive power of B-type natriuretic peptide and tissue Doppler echocardiography in the prognosis of patients with congestive heart failure. *J Am Coll Cardiol, 45*, 1223–1226.
84. Koyama, J., Ray-Sequin, P. A., & Falk, R. H. (2003). Longitudinal myocardial function assessed by tissue velocity, strain, and strain rate tissue Doppler echocardiography in patients with AL (primary) cardiac amyloidosis. *Circulation, 107*, 2446–2452.
85. Nagueh, S. F., Middleton, K. J., Kopelen, H. A., et al. (1997). Doppler tissue imaging: a noninvasive technique for evaluation of left ventricular relaxation and estimation of filling pressures. *J Am Coll Cardiol, 30*, 1527–1533.
86. Kasner, M., Westermann, D., Steendijk, P., et al. (2007). Utility of Doppler echocardiography and tissue Doppler imaging in the estimation of diastolic function in heart failure with normal ejection fraction: a comparative Doppler-conductance catheterization study. *Circulation, 116*, 637–647.
87. Dokainish, H., Zoghbi, W. A., Lakkis, N. M., et al. (2004). Optimal noninvasive assessment of left ventricular filling pressures: a comparison of tissue Doppler echocardiography and B-type natriuretic peptide in patients with pulmonary artery catheters. *Circulation, 109*, 2432–2439.
88. Rivas-Gotz, C., Manolios, M., Thohan, V., et al. (2003). Impact of left ventricular ejection fraction on estimation of left ventricular filling pressures using tissue Doppler and flow propagation velocity. *Am J Cardiol, 91*, 780–784.
89. Fieno, D. S., Jaffe, W. C., Simonetti, O. P., et al. (2002). TrueFISP: assessment of accuracy for measurement of left ventricular mass in an animal mode. *J Magn Reson Imaging, 15*, 526–531.
90. Plein, S., Bloomer, T. N., Ridgway, J. P., et al. (2001). Steady-state free precession magnetic resonance imaging of the heart: comparison with segmented k-space gradient-echo imaging. *J Magn Reson Imaging, 14*, 230–236.
91. Alfakih, K., Bloomer, T., Bainbridge, S., et al. (2004). A comparison of left ventricular mass between two-dimensional echocardiography, using fundamental and tissue harmonic imaging, and cardiac MRI in patients with hypertension. *Eur J Radiol, 52*, 103–109.
92. Semelka, R. C., Tomei, E., Wagner, S., et al. (1990). Interstudy reproducibility of dimensional and functional measurements between cine magnetic resonance studies in the morphologically abnormal left ventricle. *Am Heart J, 119*, 1367–1373.
93. Sachdev, V., Shizukuda, Y., Brenneman, C. L., et al. (2005). Left atrial volumetric remodeling is predictive of functional capacity in nonobstructive hypertrophic cardiomyopathy. *Am Heart J, 149*, 730–736.
94. Therkelsen, S. K., Groenning, B. A., Svendsen, J. H., et al. (2005). Atrial and ventricular volume and function in persistent and permanent atrial fibrillation, a magnetic resonance imaging study. *J Cardiovasc Magn Reson, 7*, 465–473.
95. Hudsmith, L. E., Cheng, A. S., Tyler, D. J., et al. (2007). Assessment of left atrial volumes at 1.5 tesla and 3 tesla using FLASH and SSFP cine imaging. *J Cardiovasc Magn Reson, 9*, 673–679.
96. Paelinck, B. P., Lamb, H. J., Bax, J. J., et al. (2004). MR flow mapping of dobutamine-induced changes in diastolic heart function. *J Magn Reson Imaging, 19*, 176–181.
97. Rathi, V. K., Doyle, M., Yamrozik, J., et al. (2008). Routine evaluation of left ventricular diastolic function by cardiovascular magnetic resonance: a practical approach. *J Cardiovasc Magn Reson, 10*, 36.
98. Tseng, W. Y., Liao, T. Y., & Wang, J. L. (2002). Normal systolic and diastolic functions of the left ventricle and left atrium by cine magnetic resonance imaging. *J Cardiovasc Magn Reson, 4*, 443–457.
99. Westwood, M. A., Wonke, B., Maceira, A. M., et al. (2005). Left ventricular diastolic function compared with T2* cardiovascular magnetic resonance for early detection of myocardial iron overload in thalassemia major. *J Magn Reson Imaging, 22*, 229–233.
100. Maceira, A. M., Prasad, S. K., Khan, M., et al. (2006). Reference right ventricular systolic and diastolic function normalized to age, gender and body surface area from steady-state free precession cardiovascular magnetic resonance. *Eur Heart J, 27*, 2879–2888.
101. Paelinck, B. P., de Roos, A., Bax, J. J., et al. (2005). Feasibility of tissue magnetic resonance imaging: a pilot study in comparison with tissue Doppler imaging and invasive measurement. *J Am Coll Cardiol, 45*, 1109–1116.
102. Marcus, J. T., Götte, M. J., van Rossum, A. C., et al. (1997). Myocardial function in infarcted and remote regions early after infarction in man: assessment by magnetic resonance tagging and strain analysis. *Magn Reson Med, 38*, 803–810.
103. Kuijer, J. P., Marcus, J. T., Götte, M. J., et al. (2002). Three-dimensional myocardial strains at end-systole and during diastole in the left ventricle of normal humans. *J Cardiovasc Magn Reson, 4*, 341–351.
104. Edvardsen, T., Rosen, B. D., Pan, L., et al. (2006). Regional diastolic dysfunction in individuals with left ventricular hypertrophy measured by tagged magnetic resonance imaging—the Multi-Ethnic Study of Atherosclerosis (MESA). *Am Heart J, 151*, 109–114.
105. Castillo, E., Osman, N. F., Rosen, B. D., et al. (2005). Quantitative assessment of regional myocardial function with MR-tagging in a multi-center study: interobserver and intraobserver agreement of fast strain analysis with harmonic phase (HARP) MRI. *J Cardiovasc Magn Reson, 7*, 783–791.
106. Rademakers, F. E., Buchalter, M. B., Rogers, W. J., et al. (1992). Dissociation between left ventricular untwisting and filling. Accentuation by catecholamines. *Circulation, 85*, 1572–1581.
107. Stuber, M., Scheidegger, M. B., Fischer, S. E., et al. (1999). Alterations in the local myocardial motion pattern in patients suffering from pressure overload due to aortic stenosis. *Circulation, 100*, 361–368.
108. Dong, S. J., Hees, P. S., Siu, C. O., et al. (2001). MRI assessment of LV relaxation by untwisting rate: a new isovolumic phase measure of tau. *Am J Physiol Heart Circ Physiol, 281*, H2002–H2009.
109. Eguchi, M., Tsuchihashi, K., Hotta, D., et al. (2000). Technetium-99m sestamibi/tetrofosmin myocardial perfusion scanning in cardiac and noncardiac sarcoidosis. *Cardiology, 94*, 193–199.
110. Spirito, P., Maron, B. J., & Bonow, R. O. (1986). Noninvasive assessment of left ventricular diastolic function: comparative analysis of Doppler echocardiographic and radionuclide angiographic techniques. *J Am Coll Cardiol, 7*, 518–526.
111. Lindqvist, P., Calcutteea, A., & Henein, M. (2008). Echocardiography in the assessment of right heart function. *Eur J Echocardiogr, 9*, 225–234.
112. Meluzin, J., Spinarova, L., Bakala, J., et al. (2001). Pulsed Doppler tissue imaging of the velocity of tricuspid annular systolic motion; a new, rapid, and non-invasive method of evaluating right ventricular systolic function. *Eur Heart J, 22*, 340–348.
113. Dokainish, H., Sengupta, R., Patel, R., et al. (2007). Usefulness of right ventricular tissue Doppler imaging to predict outcome in left ventricular heart failure independent of left ventricular diastolic function. *Am J Cardiol, 99*, 961–965.
114. Gondi, S., & Dokainish, H. (2007). Right ventricular tissue Doppler and strain imaging: ready for clinical use?. *Echocardiography, 24*, 522–532.
115. Lee, K. S., Abbas, A. E., Khandheria, B. K., et al. (2007). Echocardiographic assessment of right heart hemodynamic parameters. *J Am Soc Echocardiogr, 20*, 773–782.

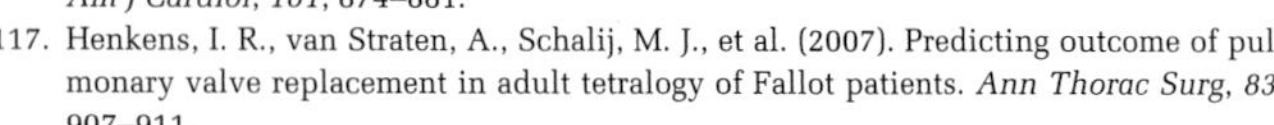

116. Chow, P. C., Liang, X. C., Lam, W. W., et al. (2008). Mechanical right ventricular dyssynchrony in patients after atrial switch operation for transposition of the great arteries. *Am J Cardiol, 101*, 874–881.
117. Henkens, I. R., van Straten, A., Schalij, M. J., et al. (2007). Predicting outcome of pulmonary valve replacement in adult tetralogy of Fallot patients. *Ann Thorac Surg, 83*, 907–911.
118. Schoen, S. P., Kittner, T., Bohl, S., et al. (2006). Transcatheter closure of atrial septal defects improves right ventricular volume, mass, function, pulmonary pressure, and functional class: a magnetic resonance imaging study. *Heart, 92*, 821–826.
119. Coats, L., Khambadkone, S., Derrick, G., et al. (2006). Physiological and clinical consequences of relief of right ventricular outflow tract obstruction late after repair of congenital heart defects. *Circulation, 113*, 2037–2044.
120. Grothues, F., Moon, J. C., Bellenger, N. G., et al. (2004). Interstudy reproducibility of right ventricular volumes, function, and mass with cardiovascular magnetic resonance. *Am Heart J, 147*, 218–223.
121. Alfakih, K., Plein, S., Bloomer, T., et al. (2003). Comparison of right ventricular volume measurements between axial and short axis orientation using steady-state free precession magnetic resonance imaging. *J Magn Reson Imaging, 18*, 25–32.
122. Alfakih, K., Plein, S., Thiele, H., et al. (2003). Normal human left and right ventricular dimensions for MRI as assessed by turbo gradient echo and steady-state free precession imaging sequences. *J Magn Reson Imaging, 17*, 323–329.
123. Hudsmith, L. E., Petersen, S. E., Francis, J. M., et al. (2005). Normal human left and right ventricular and left atrial dimensions using steady state free precession magnetic resonance imaging. *J Cardiovasc Magn Reson, 7*, 775–782.
124. Tandri, H., Daya, S. K., Nasir, K., et al. (2006). Normal reference values for the adult right ventricle by magnetic resonance imaging. *Am J Cardiol, 98*, 1660–1664.
125. Marcus, J. T., Vonk-Noordegraff, A., Roeleveld, R. J., et al. (2001). Impaired left ventricular filling due to right ventricular pressure overload in primary pulmonary hypertension: noninvasive monitoring using MRI. *Chest, 119*, 1761–1765.
126. Gan, C. T., Lankhaar, J. W., Marcus, J. T., et al. (2006). Impaired left ventricular filling due to right-to-left ventricular interaction in patients with pulmonary arterial hypertension. *Am J Physiol Heart Circ Physiol, 290*, H1528–H1533.
127. Gorcsan, J., III, Abraham, T., Agler, D. A., et al. (2008). Echocardiography for cardiac resynchronization therapy: recommendations for performance and reporting—a report from the American Society of Echocardiography Dyssynchrony Writing Group endorsed by the Heart Rhythm Society. *J Am Soc Echocardiogr, 21*, 191–213.
128. Gorcsan, J., III (2008). Role of echocardiography to determine candidacy for cardiac resynchronization therapy. *Curr Opin Cardiol, 23*, 16–22.
129. Van de Veire, N. R., Bleeker, G. B., de Sutter, J., et al. (2007). Tissue synchronisation imaging accurately measures left ventricular dyssynchrony and predicts response to cardiac resynchronisation therapy. *Heart, 93*, 1034–1039.
130. Penicka, M., Bartunek, J., De Bruyne, B., et al. (2004). Improvement of left ventricular function after cardiac resynchronization therapy is predicted by tissue Doppler imaging echocardiography. *Circulation, 109*, 978–983.
131. Yu, C. M., Zhang, Q., Fung, J. W., et al. (2005). A novel tool to assess systolic asynchrony and identify responders of cardiac resynchronization therapy by tissue synchronization imaging. *J Am Coll Cardiol, 45*, 677–684.
132. Lim, P., Buakhamsri, A., Popovic, Z. B., et al. (2008). Longitudinal strain delay index by speckle tracking imaging: a new marker of response to cardiac resynchronization therapy. *Circulation, 118*, 1130–1137.
133. Chung, E. S., Leon, A. R., Tavazzi, L., et al. (2008). Results of the Predictors of Response to CRT (PROSPECT) trial. *Circulation, 117*, 2608–2616.
134. Moss, A. J., Zareba, W., Hall, W. J., et al. (2002). Prophylactic implantation of a defibrillator in patients with myocardial infarction and reduced ejection fraction. *N Engl J Med, 346*, 877–883.
135. England, B., Lee, A., Tran, T., et al. (2005). Magnetic resonance criteria for future trials of cardiac resynchronization therapy. *J Cardiovasc Magn Reson, 7*, 827–834.
136. Helm, R. H., Byrne, M., Helm, P. A., et al. (2007). Three-dimensional mapping of optimal left ventricular pacing site for cardiac resynchronization. *Circulation, 115*, 953–961.
137. White, J. A., Yee, R., Yuan, X., et al. (2006). Delayed enhancement magnetic resonance imaging predicts response to cardiac resynchronization therapy in patients with intraventricular dyssynchrony. *J Am Coll Cardiol, 48*, 1953–1960.
138. Nazarian, S., Bluemke, D. A., Lardo, A. C., et al. (2005). Magnetic resonance assessment of the substrate for inducible ventricular tachycardia in nonischemic cardiomyopathy. *Circulation, 112*, 2821–2825.
139. Adabag, M. S., Maron, B. J., Appelbaum, E., et al. (2008). Occurrence and frequency of arrhythmias in hypertrophic cardiomyopathy in relation to delayed enhancement on cardiovascular magnetic resonance. *J Am Coll Cardiol, 51*, 1369–1374.
140. Kwon, D. H., Setser, R. M., Popovic, Z. B., et al. (2008). Association of myocardial fibrosis, electrocardiography and ventricular tachyarrhythmia in hypertrophic cardiomyopathy: a delayed contrast enhanced MRI study. *Int J Cardiovasc Imaging, 6*, 617–625.
141. Schmidt, A., Azevedo, C. F., Cheng, A., et al. (2007). Infarct tissue heterogeneity by magnetic resonance imaging identifies enhanced cardiac arrhythmia susceptibility in patients with left ventricular dysfunction. *Circulation, 115*, 2006–2014.
142. Siegrist, P. T., Comte, N., Holzmeister, J., et al. (2008). Effects of AV delay programming on ventricular resynchronisation: role of radionuclide ventriculography. *Eur J Nucl Med Mol Imaging, 35*, 1516–1522.
143. Henneman, M. M., Chen, J., Dibbets-Schneider, P., et al. (2007). Can LV dyssynchrony as assessed with phase analysis on gated myocardial perfusion SPECT predict response to CRT? *J Nucl Med, 48*, 1104–1111.
144. Thompson, K., Saab, G., Birnie, D., et al. (2006). Is septal glucose metabolism altered in patients with left bundle branch block and ischemic cardiomyopathy? *J Nucl Med, 47*, 1763–1768.
145. Nowak, B., Stellbrink, C., Sinha, A. M., et al. (2004). Effects of cardiac resynchronization therapy on myocardial blood flow measured by oxygen-15 water positron emission tomography in idiopathic-dilated cardiomyopathy and left bundle branch block. *Am J Cardiol, 93*, 496–499.
146. Lindner, O., Sorensen, J., Vogt, J., et al. (2006). Cardiac efficiency and oxygen consumption measured with ^{11}C-acetate PET after long-term cardiac resynchronization therapy. *J Nucl Med, 47*, 378–383.
147. Ypenburg, C., Schalij, M. J., Bleeker, G. B., et al. (2006). Extent of viability to predict response to cardiac resynchronization therapy in ischemic heart failure patients. *J Nucl Med, 47*, 1565–1570.
148. Sugeng, L., Mor-Avi, V., & Lang, R. M. (2008). Three-dimensional echocardiography: coming of age. *Heart, 94*, 1123–1125.
149. Nikitin, N. P., Constantin, C., Loh, P. H., et al. (2006). New generation 3-dimensional echocardiography for left ventricular volumetric and functional measurements: comparison with cardiac magnetic resonance. *Eur J Echocardiogr, 7*, 365–372.
150. Tamborini, G., Brusoni, D., Torres Molina, J. E., et al. (2008). Feasibility of a new generation three-dimensional echocardiography for right ventricular volumetric and functional measurements. *Am J Cardiol, 102*, 499–505.
151. Suh, I. W., Song, J. M., Lee, E. Y., et al. (2008). Left atrial volume measured by real-time 3-dimensional echocardiography predicts clinical outcomes in patients with severe left ventricular dysfunction and in sinus rhythm. *J Am Soc Echocardiogr, 21*, 439–445.
152. Perk, G., Tunick, P. A., & Kronzon, I. (2007). Non-Doppler two-dimensional strain imaging by echocardiography—from technical considerations to clinical applications. *J Am Soc Echocardiogr, 20*, 234–243.
153. Wang, J., Khoury, D. S., Yue, Y., et al. (2008). Preserved left ventricular twist and circumferential deformation, but depressed longitudinal and radial deformation in patients with diastolic heart failure. *Eur Heart J, 29*, 1283–1289.
154. Wang, J., Khoury, D. S., Yue, Y., et al. (2007). Left ventricular untwisting rate by speckle tracking echocardiography. *Circulation, 116*, 2580–2586.
155. Dokainish, H., Sengupta, R., Pillai, M., et al. (2008). Usefulness of new diastolic strain and strain rate indexes for the estimation of left ventricular filling pressure. *Am J Cardiol, 101*, 1504–1509.
156. De Boeck, B. W., Kirn, B., Teske, A. J., et al. (2008). Three-dimensional mapping of mechanical activation patterns, contractile dyssynchrony and dyscoordination by two-dimensional strain echocardiography: rationale and design of a novel software toolbox. *Cardiovasc Ultrasound, 6*, 22.
157. Osman, N. F., Kerwin, W. S., McVeigh, E. R., et al. (1999). Cardiac motion tracking using cine harmonic phase (HARP) magnetic resonance imaging. *Magn Reson Med, 42*, 1048–1060.
158. Valette, H., Syrota, A., & Merlet, P. (1996). Use of PET radiopharmaceuticals to probe cardiac receptors. In M. Schwaiger (Ed.), *Cardiac positron emission tomography* (pp. 331–351). Boston: Kluwer.
159. Bengel, F. M., & Schwaiger, M. (2004). Assessment of cardiac sympathetic neuronal function using PET imaging. *J Nucl Cardiol, 11*, 603–616.
160. Matsui, T., Tsutamoto, T., Maeda, K., et al. (2002). Prognostic value of repeated 123I-metaiodobenzylguanidine imaging in patients with dilated cardiomyopathy with congestive heart failure before and after optimized treatments—comparison with neurohumoral factors. *Circ J, 66*, 537–543.
161. Gerson, M. C., Craft, L. L., McGuire, N., et al. (2002). Carvedilol improves left ventricular function in heart failure patients with idiopathic dilated cardiomyopathy and a wide range of sympathetic nervous system function as measured by iodine 123 metaiodobenzylguanidine. *J Nucl Cardiol, 9*, 608–615.
162. Hughes S. *ADMIRE-HF: New imaging test helps better define risk in heart failure* (online article): http://www.theheart.org/article/956053.do. Accessed January 13, 2010.
163. Fallavollita, J. A., Luisi, A. J., Jr., Michalek, S. M., et al. (2006). Prediction of arrhythmic events with positron emission tomography: PAREPET study design and methods. *Contemp Clin Trials, 27*, 374–388.
164. Messina, S. A., Aras, O., & Dilsizian, V. (2007). Delayed recovery of fatty acid metabolism after transient myocardial ischemia: a potential imaging target for "ischemic memory." *Curr Cardiol Rep, 9*, 159–165.
165. Beanlands, R. S., & Schwaiger, M. (1995). Changes in myocardial oxygen consumption and efficiency with heart failure therapy measured by ^{11}C acetate PET. *Can J Cardiol, 11*, 293–300.
166. Yoshinaga, K., Katoh, C., Noriyasu, K., et al. (2003). Reduction of coronary flow reserve in areas with and without ischemia on stress perfusion imaging in patients with coronary artery disease: a study using oxygen 15–labeled water PET. *J Nucl Cardiol, 10*, 275–283.
167. Kaufmann, P. A., & Camici, P. G. (2005). Myocardial blood flow measurement by PET: technical aspects and clinical applications. *J Nucl Med, 46*, 75–88.
168. Di Carli, M. F., & Hachamovitch, R. (2007). New technology for noninvasive evaluation of coronary artery disease. *Circulation, 115*, 1464–1480.
169. Pichler, B. J., Wehrl, H. F., Kolb, A., et al. (2008). Positron emission tomography/magnetic resonance imaging: the next generation of multimodality imaging? *Semin Nucl Med, 38*, 199–208.

CHAPTER 37

The Use of Biomarkers in the Evaluation of Heart Failure

Leo Slavin, Lori B. Daniels, and Alan S. Maisel

The approach to the diagnosis of acute heart failure is complex and challenging because it has heterogeneous manifestations and nonspecific signs and symptoms.[1] Classically, students are taught that a careful history in patients presenting with congestive heart failure (CHF) elicits symptoms of dyspnea, orthopnea, and paroxysmal nocturnal dyspnea, whereas the physical examination reveals elevated jugular venous pressure, rales, an S3 gallop, and pitting peripheral edema (see also Chapter 35). However, it is well documented that in practice, the clinical manifestation of heart failure, even in combination with chest radiographs, electrocardiograms, and standard laboratory assessments, frequently does not clinch the diagnosis. Often clinicians must consider other causes of dyspnea, such as chronic obstructive pulmonary disease or pneumonia, which can delay necessary treatment. The growth and development of various classes of biomarkers are improving the understanding of the pathogenesis, diagnosis, and prognosis in heart failure.

BIOMARKERS IN HEART FAILURE

Morrow and de Lemos[2] proposed three criteria required for a biomarker to be clinically useful. First, the assay should be precise, accurate, and rapidly available to the clinician at relatively low cost. Second, the biomarker should provide additional information that is not surmised from findings of the clinical evaluation. Third, the absolute measured value should help in clinical decision making.[2] Currently, few biomarkers can fulfill all these requirements. Biomarkers that do meet these criteria reflect the different mechanisms (such as biomechanical stretch, inflammation, and myocyte injury) that are involved in the pathophysiology and natural history of heart failure. These markers individually and jointly provide important information for assessing the progression of disease, diagnosing acute exacerbations, and establishing prognosis.

Markers of Myocardial Stretch

Natriuretic Peptides

Biology. Three major natriuretic peptides—atrial natriuretic peptide (ANP), B-type natriuretic peptide (BNP), and C-type natriuretic peptide—counter the effects of volume overload or adrenergic activation of the cardiovascular system. ANP is synthesized primarily in the atria, stored in granules, and, under minor triggers such as exercise, released into the circulation.[3] BNP has minimal storage in granules and is synthesized and secreted in bursts primarily by the ventricles.[3] C-type natriuretic peptide is a product of endothelial cells and may be protective in post–myocardial infarction remodeling.[4] Upon release into the circulation, ANP and BNP bind to various tissues and induce vasodilation, natriuresis, and diuresis.[5]

Left ventricular pressure or volume overload results in myocardial wall stress that initiates the synthesis of precursor pro–B-type natriuretic peptide (pre-proBNP). Pre-proBNP is initially cleaved to proBNP and then to BNP, the biologically active form, and the inactive N-terminal fragment, NT-proBNP (Figure 37-1). The mechanism of action of natriuretic peptides is mediated through membrane-bound natriuretic peptide receptors (NPRs). NPR-A preferentially binds ANP and BNP, and NPR-B primarily binds C-type natriuretic peptide. The natriuretic peptide–receptor interaction activates the enzyme guanylyl cyclase, which leads to the production of cyclic guanosine monophosphate. Clearance of natriuretic peptides is mediated through NPR-C, degradation by neutral endopeptidase, and by direct renal clearance (Table 37-1).

Patients with heart failure are in a state of BNP insufficiency that results from a deficiency of the active BNP form plus molecular resistance to its effects.[6] Studies have demonstrated that the BNP detected in acute heart failure is primarily the high–molecular-weight proBNP rather than the biologically active form.[7] Some authors have suggested that abnormal cellular processing of BNP is a factor in the relative BNP-deficiency state in heart failure.[8] In addition, upregulation of phosphodiesterases leads to rapid clearance of the secondary messenger, cyclic guanosine monophosphate, despite high activation of the NPRs by natriuretic peptides.[9]

What constitutes a normal natriuretic peptide level depends on the specific clinical setting. Two studies revealed that BNP levels in normal adults without cardiovascular disease increase with age and appear to be higher in women; NT-proBNP levels show greater age dependence than do BNP levels.[10,11] According to general guidelines, 90% of young, healthy adults have a BNP level of less than 25 pg/mL and an NT-proBNP level of 70 pg/mL or lower.[12] In patients presenting with acute dyspnea, a BNP cutoff level of less than 100 pg/mL and an NT-proBNP cutoff level of less than 300 pg/mL should be used to rule out heart failure.[13,14]

Natriuretic Peptides in Acute Heart Failure. BNP and NT-proBNP levels have become powerful diagnostic tools in the evaluation of patients presenting with dyspnea in a variety of clinical settings. In the Breathing Not Properly Multinational Study, BNP levels were measured in 1586 patients with shortness of breath upon arrival in the emergency department (ED). Use of this information resulted in a higher diagnostic accuracy, with an area under the receiver-operating characteristic curve (AUC) of 0.91.[13] A BNP cutoff level of 100 pg/mL was 90% sensitive and 76% specific for the diagnosis of heart failure as the cause of dyspnea (Figure 37-2). The data were similar for NT-proBNP levels in the ProBNP Investigation of Dyspnea in the Emergency Department (PRIDE) study, in which NT-proBNP level was measured in 600 emergency department

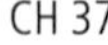

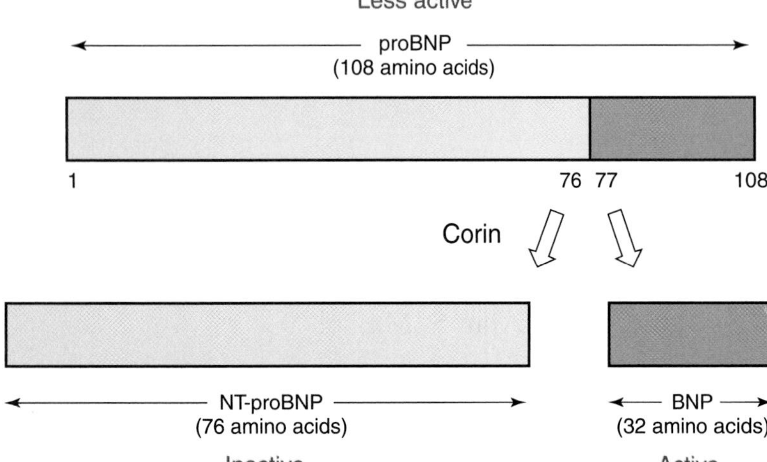

FIGURE 37–1 Synthesis of B-type natriuretic peptide (BNP) and amino terminal B-type natriuretic peptide (NT-proBNP).

TABLE 37–1 Biochemical Properties of BNP versus NT-proBNP

Property	BNP	NT-proBNP
Amino acids	32	76
Molecular weight (kDa)	3.5	8.5
Half-life (min)	22	60-120
Clearance		
• Primary	Neutral endopeptidase	Renal
• C-R	NPR-C	Renal
• Hemodialysis	No	No
Point-of-care	Yes	Pending
Correlation with GFR	Moderate	Strong
Biologically active	Yes	No
Clinical range (pg/mL)	0–5,000	0–35,000

Adapted from Daniels LB, Maisel AS. Natriuretic peptides. *J Am Coll Cardiol* 2007;50:2357-2368.

BNP, B-type natriuretic peptide; *C-R*, clearance receptor; *GFR*, glomerular filtration rate; *NPR*, natriuretic peptide receptor; *NT-proBNP*, *N*-terminal pro-*B*-type natriuretic peptide.

patients with dyspnea; its sensitivity and specificity were demonstrated in the diagnosis of CHF (AUC = 0.94).[14] A NT-proBNP cutoff level of less than 300 pg/mL was proposed to rule out heart failure as the cause of dyspnea.

The use of natriuretic peptides has also proved to be significantly cost effective. In the BNP for Acute Shortness of breath EvaLuation (BASEL) study, 452 patients in the emergency department with dyspnea were randomly assigned to conditions involving a single measurement of BNP level versus no such measurement. The researchers reported a 10% reduction in the rate of admissions and a 3-day decrease in the median length of stay with the use of BNP level, which amounted to a total cost savings of $1800 per patient without an increase in mortality or repeated hospitalization.[15] These results were also obtained with NT-proBNP level in the Improved Management of Patients with Congestive Heart Failure (IMPROVE-CHF) study.[16]

Elevated Natriuretic Peptide Levels in Other Clinical Settings. For optimal use of natriuretic peptides, it is important to be aware of clinical scenarios other than acute heart failure that can cause natriuretic peptide levels to rise. Patients with a history of heart failure but without an acute exacerbation can have intermediate BNP levels, as shown in the Breathing Not Properly trial.[13] Acute coronary syndrome is also associated with elevated levels of natriuretic peptides: Acute ischemia causes transient diastolic dysfunction, which results in increased left ventricular end-diastolic pressure, a rise in wall stress, and increased synthesis of BNP.[17] The role of BNP is perhaps most useful in differentiating between cardiac and pulmonary causes of shortness of breath. Although natriuretic peptide values can be elevated to intermediate levels in patients with underlying lung disease, they tend to remain significantly lower than in patients presenting with CHF.[18] The Breathing Not Properly trial demonstrated that natriuretic peptide levels were useful in diagnosing heart failure, which was present in 87 of the 417 patients with a history of chronic obstructive pulmonary disease or asthma (BNP levels, 587 vs. 109 pg/mL, $P < .0001$).[13] In addition, right-sided heart dysfunction from hemodynamically significant pulmonary embolism, severe lung disease, and pulmonary hypertension can lead to elevated levels of natriuretic peptides.[19-22] Therefore, when levels of natriuretic peptide levels are intermediate in an acutely dyspneic patient, it is important to consider other life-threatening causes of dyspnea.

Hyperdynamic states of sepsis, cirrhosis, and hyperthyroidism can also be associated with elevated levels of natriuretic peptides.[23-25] These levels are also increased in the setting of atrial fibrillation.[26] The Breathing Not Properly trial demonstrated that BNP still performed well in patients with atrial fibrillation; the AUC was 0.84, in comparison with 0.91 for the entire cohort. Increasing the cutoff to 200 pg/mL for these patients improved specificity and the positive predictive value for diagnosing heart failure.[27]

Caveats. In addition to wall stress, other factors have been associated with elevated natriuretic peptide levels. Aging appears to be associated with elevated levels of BNP, independent of the degree of diastolic dysfunction.[10,11] Possible mechanisms may include altered renal function, changes in the biosynthesis and processing of natriuretic peptides on a cellular level, or a reduction in the clearance receptor NPR-C.[28] Women appear to have higher natriuretic peptide levels than do men the same age.[10,11] Although the reasons for this sex difference are unclear, some authors have proposed that differences in estrogen or testosterone may be responsible.[10,29]

The association between natriuretic peptide levels and renal function is complex. In the setting of renal dysfunction, increased concentrations of natriuretic peptides may stem from elevation in atrial pressure, systemic pressure, or ventricular mass. Many patients with renal disease have hypertension that results in significant left ventricular hypertrophy, and comorbid cardiac conditions are also common.

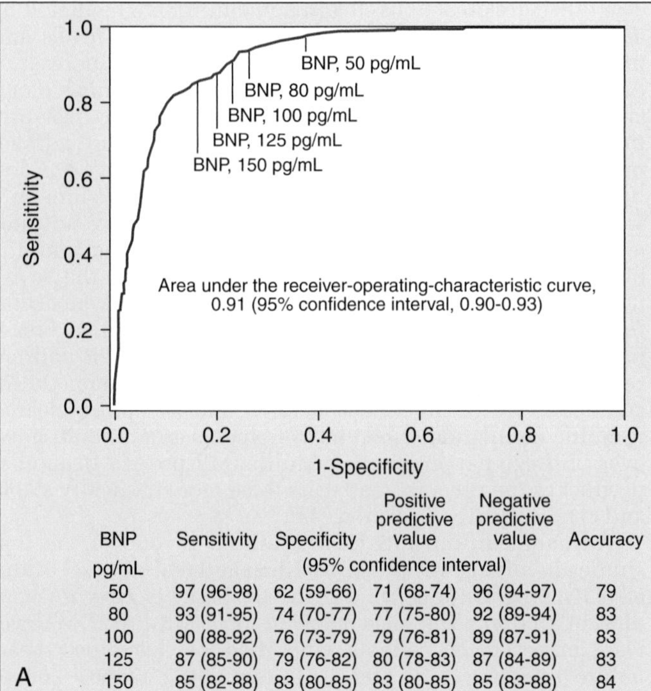

BNP pg/mL	Sensitivity	Specificity	Positive predictive value	Negative predictive value	Accuracy
	(95% confidence interval)				
50	97 (96-98)	62 (59-66)	71 (68-74)	96 (94-97)	79
80	93 (91-95)	74 (70-77)	77 (75-80)	92 (89-94)	83
100	90 (88-92)	76 (73-79)	79 (76-81)	89 (87-91)	83
125	87 (85-90)	79 (76-82)	80 (78-83)	87 (84-89)	83
150	85 (82-88)	83 (80-85)	83 (80-85)	85 (83-88)	84

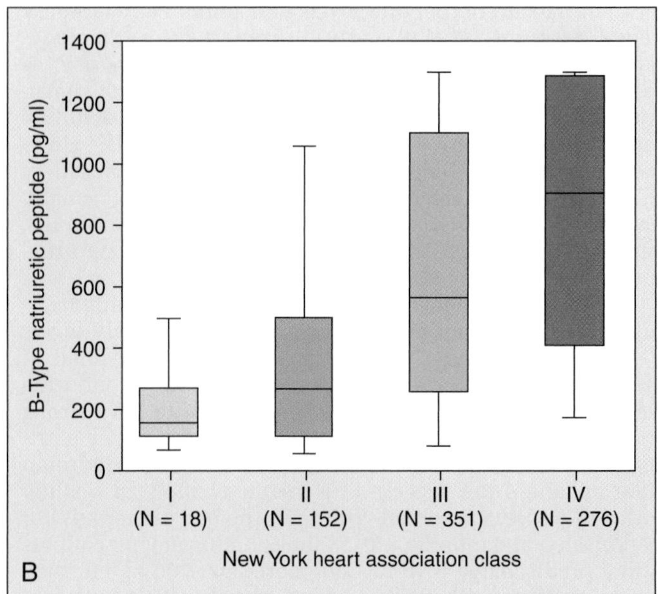

FIGURE 37–2 **A,** Receiver-operating-characteristic curve from the Breathing Not Properly Multinational Study for various cutoff levels of B-type natriuretic peptides in differentiating dyspnea caused by heart failure from dyspnea with other causes. **B,** Box plots showing the median levels of B-type natriuretic peptide among patients in different New York Heart Association classifications. (From Maisel AS, Krishnaswamy P, Nowak RM, et al. Rapid measurement of B-type natriuretic peptide in the emergency diagnosis of heart failure. *N Engl J Med* 2002;347:161-167.)

This interplay between the heart and kidneys in patients with reduced renal function accounts for one component of the increase in natriuretic peptide levels, reflecting elevated "true" physiological natriuretic peptide levels.[30] The Breathing Not Properly study revealed a weak but significant correlation between glomerular filtration rate (GFR) and BNP level, and the researchers suggested higher cutoff levels for patients with a GFR of less than 60 mL/min/1.7 m^2.[31]

Interpretation of NT-proBNP levels in the setting of renal dysfunction is more challenging because clearance is not mediated by NPR-C or neutral endopeptidase and is more dependent on renal function. GFR seems to be more strongly correlated with NT-proBNP (r = −0.55) than with BNP, although the discrepancy may be somewhat less prominent in patients with acute CHF (r = −0.33 for NT-proBNP level, and r = −0.18 for BNP level).[32,33] An analysis from the PRIDE study demonstrated that NT-proBNP levels in patients with GFR of less than 60 mL/min/1.7 m^2 were still the strongest predictors of outcome, and the researchers suggested a higher cutoff level, of more than 1200 pg/mL, for the diagnosis of heart failure.[33] In contrast, there is no significant relationship between NT-proBNP levels and GFR in relatively healthy patients with mild renal insufficiency.[34] Despite the relationship between natriuretic peptide levels and GFR, both BNP and NT-proBNP levels still provide important diagnostic and prognostic information in patients with renal dysfunction.

Several studies have demonstrated an inverse relationship between body mass index and BNP levels.[11,35-37] The reasons for this are not fully elucidated, although some authors have postulated a theory of increased clearance mediated though elevated levels of NPR-C in adipocytes[38]; data for this are conflicting.[34,39] A study of patients who had undergone bariatric surgery showed an increase in both BNP and NT-proBNP levels after the surgery, which suggests that downregulation of natriuretic peptide production in obesity, rather than increased clearance, may be responsible for the lower levels of natriuretic peptides in the obese population.[40] Despite lower circulating levels, natriuretic peptide values retain their diagnostic capability in obese patients, albeit at lower cutoff levels.[37]

Flash pulmonary edema, CHF with causes upstream from the left ventricle (i.e., acute mitral regurgitation and mitral stenosis), and pericardial disease do not lead to substantial elevations in natriuretic peptides.[30] In flash pulmonary edema, because of the small amounts of natriuretic peptides that are preformed and residing in secretory granules, and because of the delay between wall stress and upregulation of gene expression, the levels of natriuretic peptides are disproportionately low in comparison to symptoms.[30] Patients with constrictive pericardial disease can present with symptoms of right-sided heart failure; however, because the stiff pericardium limits the myocardium's stretching, natriuretic peptide levels are typically normal or minimally elevated.[30,41]

Prognosis. There has been a tremendous increase in data demonstrating the prognostic power of natriuretic peptides in a variety of clinical settings. Several researchers reported that natriuretic peptide levels in patients presenting to the emergency department with heart failure are predictive of future cardiovascular events. Every 100-pg/mL increase is associated with a 35% increase in the risk of death in heart failure.[42] The prospective, multicenter Rapid ED Heart Failure Outpatient Trial (REDHOT), involving 464 patients presenting to the emergency department with heart failure, showed that BNP level was predictive of future heart failure–related events and of mortality and was superior to the emergency department physician's assessment of severity of illness. In patients with chronic heart failure, BNP level provides powerful prognostic information regarding survival and deterioration of functional status.[43] In more than 4300 outpatients with chronic heart failure in the Valsartan Heart Failure Trial (Val-HeFT), patients with the greatest rise in BNP level despite therapy had the highest rates of morbidity and mortality.[44]

In addition to heart failure, both BNP and NT-proBNP levels have strong prognostic value in patients with coronary artery disease, acute coronary syndrome, and valvular heart disease and in the prediction of sudden cardiac death.[45-50]

Monitoring Therapy

Inpatient. Several investigators evaluated the relationship between natriuretic peptide levels and pulmonary capillary wedge pressure (PCWP) derived from invasive hemodynamic catheters.[51] Because in various clinical scenarios, as described above, there can be discordance between natriuretic peptide levels and clinical manifestation, natriuretic peptide levels are not always correlated with PCWP.[52] However, in patients with decompensated heart failure caused by volume overload, a treatment-induced drop in PCWP usually leads to a rapid decrease in BNP levels (35 to 50 pg/mL/hour), especially in the first 24 hours of therapy, if adequate urine output is maintained.[53]

In the management of hospitalized patients with heart failure, it is probably not necessary to measure daily levels of natriuretic peptides. Instead, measurements obtained at admission and before discharge can be useful in tailoring the intensity of therapy and has been shown to have strong prognostic implications.[54,55] A third measurement of natriuretic peptide level in the first 24 to 48 hours after admission often enhances the success of a treatment plan. In a study with 114 patients admitted with CHF, the rate of mortality or readmission at 6 months was 15 times higher among patients with a predischarge BNP level of more than 700 pg/mL than among patients with BNP levels of less than 350 pg/mL at discharge.[56]

Outpatient. Monitoring natriuretic peptide levels in the outpatient setting might help improve patient care. Changes in natriuretic peptide levels could potentially, help physicians titrate neurohormonal blockade agents and diuretics more aggressively and safely. Prospective studies in this area have yielded somewhat conflicting results. In the Systolic Heart Failure Treatment Supported by BNP (STARS-BNP) study, 220 patients with heart failure and left ventricular dysfunction were randomly assigned to receive therapy guided by natriuretic peptide levels versus standard of care; natriuretic peptide–guided treatment that targeted a BNP level of less than 100 pg/mL significantly reduced death and hospital stay for heart failure.[57] The smaller (130-patient) Strategies for Tailoring Advanced Heart Failure Regimens in the Outpatient Settings: Brain NatrIuretic Peptides Versus the Clinical CongesTion ScorE (STARBRITE) study failed to show significant improvement in the primary outcome of nonhospital days alive in patients whose treatment was guided by BNP levels. However, STARBRITE enrolled patients with more severe disease and used a higher BNP cutoff level.[58] In both studies, clinicians who adjusted medical therapy on the basis of natriuretic peptide levels prescribed higher doses of angiotensin converting enzyme (ACE) inhibitors and β-blockers.

In patients monitored in clinics, it is important to establish the "steady state" level of natriuretic peptide that corresponds to a patient's optimized fluid status. Significant deviations from this baseline level allows for rapid diagnosis and institution of therapy, with more aggressive diuresis and follow-up when levels rise substantially.[59] Values that are considerably reduced from baseline can signal overdiuresis and impending prerenal azotemia. In view of significant intraindividual variability in natriuretic peptide levels, a change of at least 50% in the steady-state natriuretic peptide level might be a reasonable impetus for a more aggressive evaluation and modification of treatment.[30]

Adrenomedullin

Biology. Adrenomedullin level, like natriuretic peptide levels, is elevated in the setting of myocardial stress. Adrenomedullin is a vasoactive peptide consisting of 52 amino acids that shares homology with calcitonin gene–related peptide.[60] The downstream actions of adrenomedullin are mediated by an increase in cyclic adenosine monophosphate levels and nitric oxide, which lead to potent vasodilation, an increase in cardiac output, and diuresis and natriuresis.[61-65] This biologically active modulator is produced from the precursor preproadrenomedullin, which is produced by the heart, adrenal medulla, lungs, kidneys, and vascular endothelium.[66,67] Adrenomedullin levels are increased in endothelial dysfunction, which is common in patients with heart failure and indicates a poor prognosis. In patients with heart failure, the magnitude of increase in adrenomedullin corresponds with the severity of heart failure and is inversely related to left ventricular function.[66,68] Adrenomedullin levels increase with worsening symptoms of heart failure and elevated PCWP and are reduced with appropriate therapy.[66] Because adrenomedullin combines with complement factor H and is rapidly cleared from the circulation, direct measurements are difficult; however, midregional proadrenomedullin (MR-proADM), another product of the precursor, appears to be more clinically stable and can be readily measured.[69,70]

Adrenomedullin and Heart Failure. In one of the first studies involving MR-proADM, Khan and colleagues[71] evaluated its prognostic capability in 983 patients after myocardial infarction. The data showed that MR-proADM level was increased in patients who died or developed heart failure (median, 1.19 nmol/L [interquartile range, 0.09 to 5.39 nmol/L]), in comparison with survivors (median, 0.71 nmol/L [interquartile range, 0.25 to 6.66 nmol/L], $P < .0001$). The AUCs for MR-proADM, NT-proBNP, and the combination of both markers for prediction of death or heart failure were 0.77, 0.79, and 0.84, respectively,[71] which demonstrate that MR-proADM level is a powerful predictor of adverse outcome in patients after myocardial infarction and provides additive information with natriuretic peptides.

The prognostic implications of elevated MR-proADM levels in outpatients with both ischemic and nonischemic causes of CHF were evaluated by Adlbrecht and associates.[72] In 786 patients admitted with CHF, they demonstrated that MR-proADM level was a significant predictor of death (hazard ratio = 1.77, $P < .001$) at 24 months.[72] Adrenomedullin also has predictive capability in asymptomatic patients with risk factors for coronary artery disease. In a study of 121 patients, Nishida and colleagues[73] reported that patients with elevated adrenomedullin levels had a higher risk of future cardiovascular events.

MR-proADM has also been evaluated in patients with acute decompensated heart failure. Gegenhuber and associates[74] evaluated the utility of natriuretic peptides, MR-proADM, and other biomarkers in predicting mortality in 137 patients with acute decompensated heart failure. The AUCs for the prediction of 1-year mortality were similar for BNP level (0.716; 95% confidence interval [CI], 0.633 to 0.790), midregional pro–A-type natriuretic peptide (MR-proANP) (0.725; 95% CI, 0.642 to 0.798), MR-proADM (0.708; 95% CI, 0.624 to 0.782), and copeptin (0.688; 95% CI, 0.603 to 0.764).[74] In the Biomarkers in the Assessment of Congestive Heart failure (BACH) study, MR-proADM level was compared with BNP and NT-proBNP levels in predicting mortality at 90 days in patients hospitalized for decompensated heart failure.[75] Of 1641 patients recruited, 568 (approximately one third) ultimately received a diagnosis of heart failure. The data showed that MR-proADM level was more accurate than BNP or NT-proBNP level at predicting outcome at 90 days.[75]

Summary of MR-proADM. Adrenomedullin is a relatively new biomarker that reflects biomechanical stretch and increases with pressure or volume overload. Although experience with adrenomedullin is limited, available data indicate that its levels are correlated with natriuretic peptide levels and may provide superior prognostic information in patients with acute and chronic heart failure.

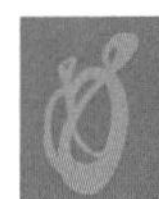

ST2 Receptor

Biology. ST2 is a member of the interleukin (IL)–1 receptor family and has two primary isoforms: a transmembrane receptor form (ST2L) and a soluble receptor form (soluble ST2), each regulated by different promoters.[76-78] Microarray analysis demonstrates marked upregulation of the transcript for both forms of ST2; the soluble form displays more robust expression in mechanically stimulated cardiomyocytes.[78,79] In response to mechanical strain, there is also an increase in the transcription and translation of the ligand, IL-33.[80] The IL-33/ST2 signaling cascade is thought to play a critical role in the regulation of myocardial response to pressure overload, which inhibits development of fibrosis.[81-83] Genetic knockouts of ST2 in mouse models demonstrated significant cardiac hypertrophy, interstitial fibrosis, and cavity dilation in response to transverse aortic constriction.[78,84] A similar phenotype is generated by infusion of soluble ST2, which is believed to serve as a decoy receptor, thereby decreasing the beneficial IL-33 interaction with ST2L. In this way, the ratio of soluble ST2 to IL-33 may regulate the IL-33/ST2L system.[78]

ST2 and Acute Coronary Syndrome. Clinically, ST2 levels increase early in the course of acute myocardial infarction and are inversely correlated with systolic function.[79] When ST2 levels were analyzed in more than 800 patients presenting to the hospital with an acute ST wave–elevation myocardial infarction (STEMI), the concentration of ST2 at the time of presentation was independently associated with in-hospital and 30-day mortality, after adjustments for age, hemodynamics, infarct territory, Killip class, and time from symptom onset to treatment.[85] Sabatine and colleagues[86] confirmed the utility of ST2 as a prognostic biomarker in 1239 patients presenting with STEMI in the Clopidogrel as Adjunctive Reperfusion Therapy—Thrombolysis in Myocardial Infarction (CLARITY-TIMI 28) trial. After adjusting for baseline characteristics and NT-proBNP level, the researchers showed that a concentration of ST2 above the median was a powerful predictor of cardiovascular death and heart failure, independent of baseline characteristics. The combination of ST2 and NT-proBNP levels significantly improved risk stratification in this patient population.[86]

ST2 and Heart Failure. In 161 patients with severe chronic New York Heart Association (NYHA) class III or IV heart failure, Weinberg and associates[87] demonstrated that change in ST2 levels over a 2-week period was an independent predictor of subsequent mortality or need for transplantation. ST2 has also proved to be an important biomarker in patients presenting with acute decompensated heart failure. In the PRIDE study,[88] ST2 concentrations were measured in 593 dyspneic patients in the emergency department and were found to be higher among patients with acute heart failure than in patients with other causes of dyspnea (0.50 vs. 0.15 ng/mL; $P < .001$). An ST2 level of 0.20 ng/mL or higher was strongly predictive of death at 1 year in the entire cohort (hazard ratio = 5.6; 95% CI, 2.2 to 14.2; $P < .001$). The 1-year mortality rate was less than 4.5% among patients in the lowest decile of ST2 levels but 45% among those in the highest decile (Figure 37-3).[88] In another study, researchers investigated change in ST2 concentrations during the course of a hospitalization in 150 patients with acute heart failure.[89] Multiple biomarkers were measured, including ST2, BNP, NT-proBNP, and blood urea nitrogen levels six times between admission and discharge. Among patients whose ST2 values decreased by 15.5% or more during the study period, the incidence of death was 7%, whereas those whose ST2 levels failed to decrease by 15.5% had a 33% chance of dying within 90 days.[89] Rehman and coworkers further examined the patient-specific characteristics of ST2 in 346 patients hospitalized with acute heart failure, demonstrating that, even after they controlled for established and clinical characteristics, ST2 remained a predictor of mortality (hazard ratio = 2.04; 95% CI, 1.3 to 3.24; $P = .003$)[90] (see Figure 37-3). The highest mortality rate was observed in the subgroup that had elevated concentrations of both natriuretic peptides and ST2 (see Figure 37-3).[90]

Summary of ST2. ST2, induced by myocardial response to pressure or volume overload, has important clinical implications for patients with acute and chronic heart failure and acute coronary syndrome. ST2 level is a powerful prognosticator of future cardiovascular morbidity and mortality, providing incremental information to natriuretic peptides.[91]

Markers of Inflammation

An abnormal inflammatory response in patients with heart failure is a mechanism for disease progression and deterioration (see also Chapter 11).[92] Ischemia and other biological insults to the heart trigger an innate immune response that leads to the upregulation of proinflammatory cytokines.[91] The activation of these mediators results in apoptosis, hypertrophy, and dilation, which in turn accelerate disease progression (Figure 37-4).[91] Many features of heart failure, including hemodynamic compromise and vascular abnormalities, can be explained through the effects of proinflammatory cytokines, including C-reactive protein (CRP), tumor necrosis factor–α (TNF-α), IL-6, and IL-18.[93-96]

C-Reactive Protein

Biology. CRP is synthesized by hepatocytes in response mainly to IL-6.[97] CRP is an acute-phase reactant, its levels becoming significantly elevated shortly within the onset of an inflammatory process. It is, however, a nonspecific marker; its levels are commonly increased in the settings of infection, inflammatory diseases, acute coronary syndrome, smoking, and neoplastic processes.[98] CRP reduces the release of nitric oxide and increases expression of endothelin-1 and of endothelial adhesion molecules.[99] These features are suggestive of mechanisms by which CRP plays an important role in vascular diseases.

hsCRP and Future Development of Heart Failure. In four major population-based investigations (the Cardiovascular Health Study; the Framingham Heart Study; the Health, Aging and Body Composition [Health ABC] Study; and the Rotterdam Study), researchers have studied the development of heart failure in asymptomatic populations. In a total of 15,282 elderly patients with a follow-up period of 3.6 to 6.2 years, there was a significant association between elevated levels of high-sensitivity C-reactive protein (hsCRP) and development of heart failure (Table 37-2).[98,100-103] Subsets of patients with the highest levels of hsCRP had double the risk of developing heart failure. In the Health ABC study, high levels of other inflammatory cytokines such as TNF-α and IL-6 were also predictive of the development of heart failure.[102] The Rotterdam Study demonstrated that the association between hsCRP and heart failure was weaker in women and did not persist after the adjustment for traditional cardiovascular risk factors.[103]

hsCRP and Patients at High Risk. Large volumes of data have been collected to examine the relationship between hsCRP and the development of heart failure in high-risk patients, particularly those admitted with acute coronary syndrome (Table 37-3).[98,104-112] The initial study, in which Pietilä and colleagues[104] monitored 188 patients with acute myocardial infarction for 2 years, revealed that patients with higher peak CRP levels within the period immediately after myocardial infarction had increased risk of death and of development of heart failure. Subsequent analysis of more than 10,000 patients confirmed that elevated levels of CRP or hsCRP within 24 hours of acute myocardial infarction were predictive of short- and long-term development of heart failure. One of the largest studies of this association was a substudy from the Thrombolysis in Myocardial Infarction

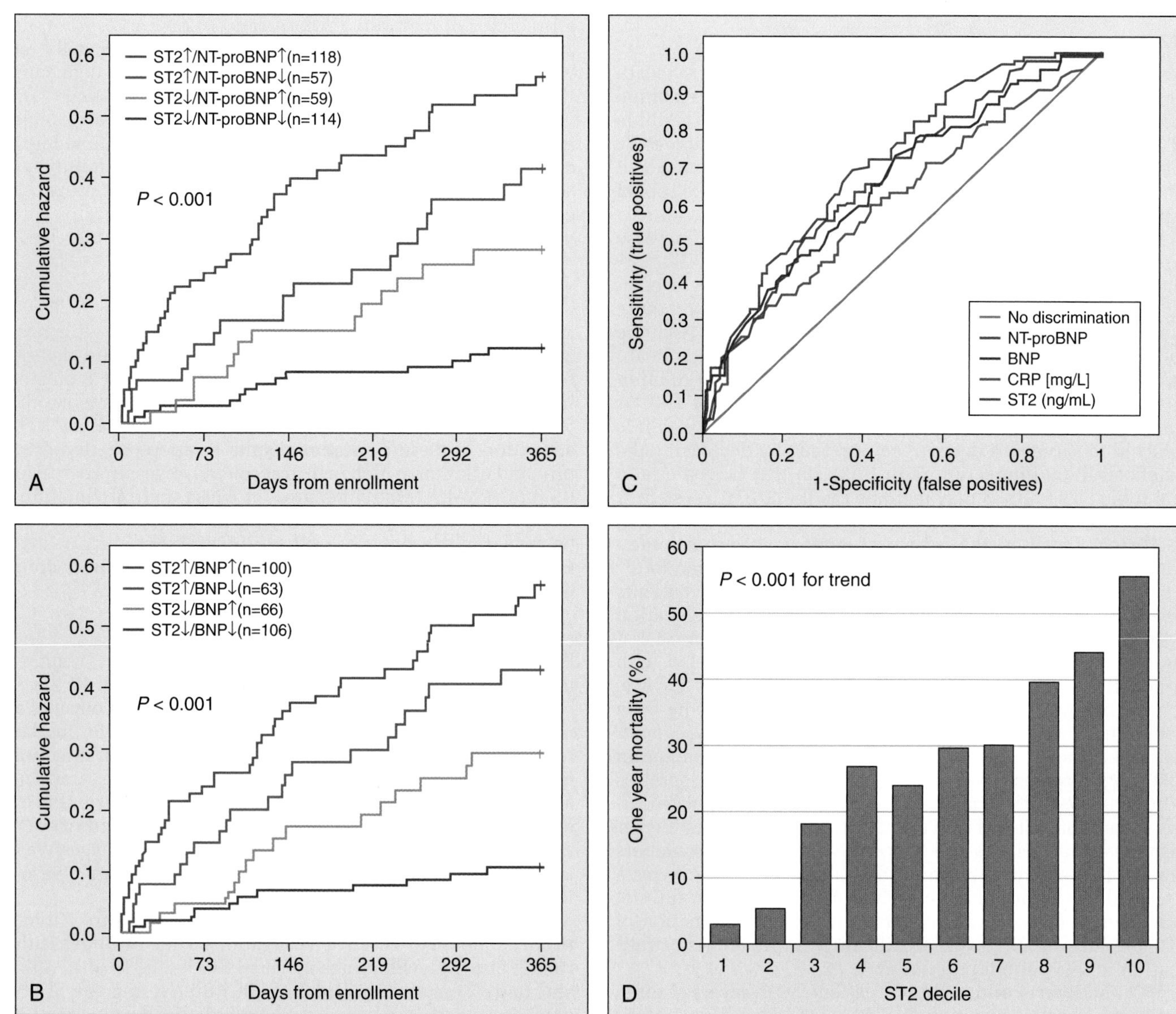

FIGURE 37–3 Mortality rates among patients hospitalized with acute heart failure as a function of ST2 and amino-terminal B-type natriuretic peptide (NT-proBNP) concentration **(A)** or B-type natriuretic peptide (BNP) concentration **(B)**. **C,** Receiver-operator characteristic curve analysis, in which ST2 level was compared with BNP, NT-proBNP and C-reactive protein levels for predicting death at 1 year after hospitalization for acute heart failure. **D,** Frequency of mortality at 1 year as a function of ST2 decile. (From Rehman SU, Mueller T, Januzzi JL Jr. Characteristics of the novel interleukin family biomarker ST2 in patients with acute heart failure. *J Am Coll Cardiol* 2008;52:1458-1465.)

(TIMI) trials, in which increased concentrations of hsCRP within 48 hours of symptoms were strongly associated with development of heart failure.[105] More recently, analysis of data from more than 4000 patients with STEMI and non-STEMI revealed higher event rates for cardiovascular endpoints (cardiovascular death, recurrent myocardial infarction, stroke, and heart failure) with increasing quartile of hsCRP.[106] Patients with chronic stable angina have a similar association between hsCRP levels and the development of heart failure.[113,114]

hsCRP and Prognosis in Heart Failure. The prognostic implications of hsCRP on patients with chronic heart failure has been evaluated in multiple studies with a combined total of more than 6600 patients (Table 37-4).[98,115-123] There is a significant association between increasing level of hsCRP and worse cardiovascular outcome, including mortality, poorer left ventricular systolic function, higher prevalence of NYHA class III or IV symptoms, and poorer quality of life. This association appears to translate to both ischemic and nonischemic causes of heart failure.[98,115-123]

In contrast, there is a paucity of data regarding the prognostic significance of hsCRP in acute heart failure. Alonso-Martínez and associates[124] prospectively studied the role of hsCRP in 76 patients admitted with acute heart failure. The data showed that elevated hsCRP levels were associated with increased rates of readmission at 18 months. Subsequently, Mueller and colleagues[125] evaluated 214 patients with acute heart failure to determine the impact of CRP on rates of all-cause mortality at 24 months. Patients in the highest tertile of CRP had significantly higher in-hospital and all-cause mortality rates at 24 months. In a study in Finland, researchers evaluated clinical and biochemical predictors of 1-year mortality in patients hospitalized for acute heart failure. The data showed that elevated CRP was independently predictive of mortality at 1 year.[126] Villacorta and coworkers[127] confirmed that finding in 119 patients hospitalized in Brazil for acute heart failure: CRP proved to be the most important prognosticator of mortality at 1 year. Although the role of CRP as a prognostic biomarker in patients hospitalized with heart failure is yet to be firmly established, limited data suggest that it may complement other biomarkers in predicting mortality in this clinical setting.

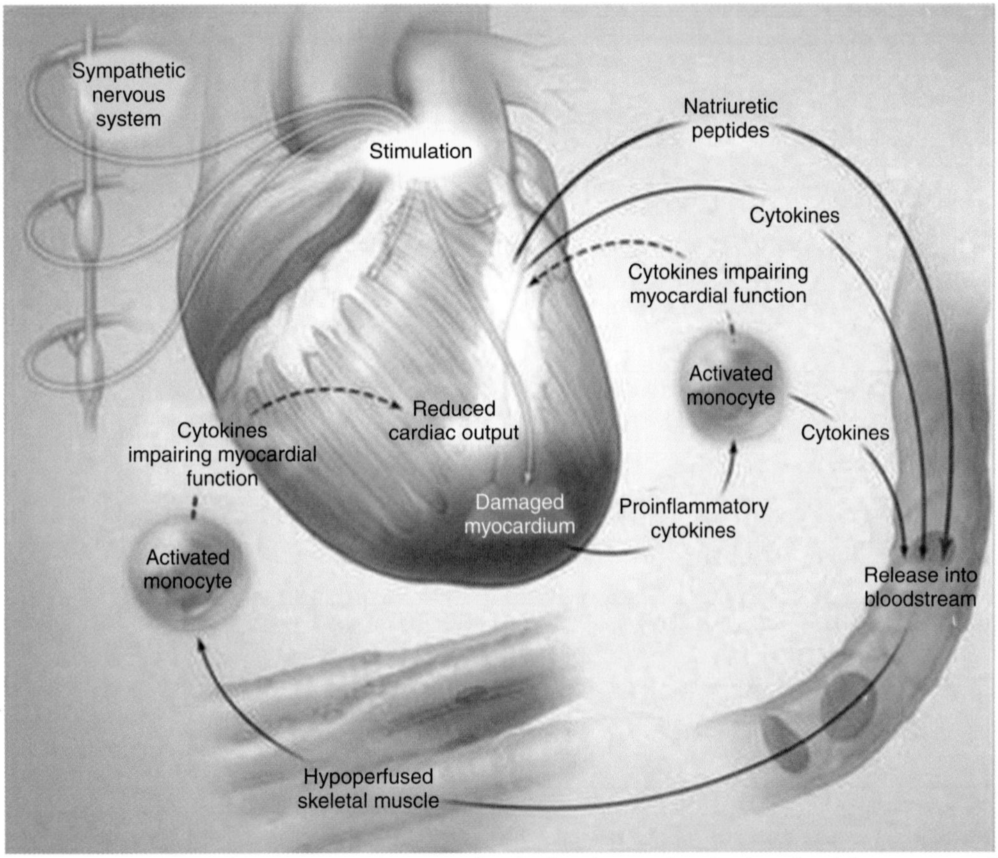

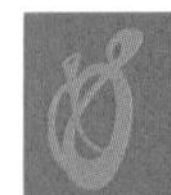

FIGURE 37–4 Cytokine hypothesis of heart failure. Injury to the myocardium leads to increased production of proinflammatory cytokines (tumor necrosis factor α, interleukin-6, and interleukin-18), leading to depressed cardiac function. Decreased cardiac output causes hypoperfusion of the skeletal muscle, which activates monocytes to produce proinflammatory cytokines, further impairing cardiac function. (From Braunwald E. Biomarkers in heart failure. *N Engl J Med* 2008;358:2148-2159.)

Summary of CRP. CRP is perhaps the most important marker of inflammation and is analyzed routinely in clinical practice. It has validated utility in predicting the development of heart failure in populations at low and high risk, as well as prognostic value in patients with chronic heart failure. In practice, interpretation of CRP levels is somewhat hampered by the fact that different cutoff levels were used in different studies, which makes it difficult to interpret individual CRP levels. Determining the real-world clinical utility of hsCRP necessitates further investigation with uniform studies that use similar assays and cutoff levels.

Markers of Myocardial Cell Death

Troponin

Biology. Myocardial cell death occurs in heart failure and may represent the common final pathway to refractory failure. Although cardiac troponin levels are well-validated markers of myocyte injury during myocardial infarction, the pathophysiological mechanisms underlying troponin elevations in heart failure are probably distinct from those underlying acute coronary syndrome.[128] Multiple mechanisms, including inflammation, interstitial fibrosis, increased wall stress, oxidative stress, and neurohormonal activation, are responsible for adverse cardiac remodeling that leads to progressive heart failure.[129-132] Troponin is a cardiac structural protein that is part of the troponin-tropomyosin complex, with a small amount present in the cytosol.[128] Mild elevations in troponin levels have been documented in a number of cardiovascular diseases, including heart failure. Hypotheses for why troponin levels may be elevated in the setting of heart failure, even in the absence of overt ischemia, include myocardial injury, loss of cell membrane integrity, excessive wall tension that leads to subendocardial ischemia, apoptosis, or some combination.[91,133,134]

Troponin and Acute Heart Failure. Several small studies have reported elevated cardiac troponin levels in patients with decompensated heart failure, in the absence of acute coronary syndrome, and found associations between elevated levels of troponin and poor prognosis.[135-138] La Vecchia and associates evaluated the clinical associations and prognostic implications of detectable cardiac troponin I (cTnI) in 34 patients with severe heart failure.[139] Modest elevations of cTnI (0.7 ± 0.3 ng/mL) were associated with lower left ventricular ejection fraction, and there was a trend toward higher pulmonary artery pressures. In patients who evinced clinical improvement after admission, cTnI levels became undetectable after a few days.[139] However, in patients with refractory heart failure who ultimately died in the hospital, detectable levels of cTnI persisted throughout the observation period.[139] In a larger subsequent study, cTnI's role in predicting adverse outcomes was evaluated in 238 patients with advanced heart failure who were referred for cardiac transplantation.[128] Patients with detectable cTnI levels of 0.04 ng/mL or higher had higher levels of BNP, impaired hemodynamics (indicated by lower cardiac index and higher PCWP), progression of left ventricular dysfunction, and increased mortality (relative risk, 2.05; 95% CI, 1.22 to 3.43).[128]

Researchers for the Acute Decompensated Heart Failure National Registry (ADHERE) evaluated the association between cardiac troponin level and adverse events in 84,872 patients with acute decompensated heart failure.[140] Patients with positive troponin levels (6.2%) had lower systolic blood pressure on admission, a lower ejection fraction, and higher rates of in-hospital mortality (8.0% vs. 2.7%; $P < .001$) than did those with undetectable troponin levels (odds ratio for

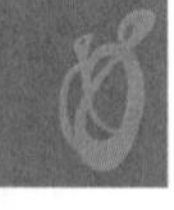

TABLE 37–2 Association Between hsCRP and Future Development of Heart Failure in Population-Based Studies

Reference	Study Title (country)	*N*	Age (% Male)	Mean Follow-up Period (Years)	Incidence of Heart Failure	hsCRP Comparisons*	Hazard Ratio (95% CI)	Adjusted for
Gottdiener et al[100]	Predictors of congestive heart failure in the elderly. The Cardiovascular Health Study (United States)	5888	73 ± 5 years (42%)	5.5	597 (19.3%)	≥7.40 mg/L vs. ≤0.95 mg/L (5th vs. 1st quintile)	1.91 (1.43–2.57)	Age, sex, CHD or stroke at baseline, diabetes, SBP, LVEF ankle-arm index, internal carotid thickness, FEV_1, creatinine
Vasan et al[101]	Inflammatory markers and risk of HF in elderly subjects without prior myocardial infarction. The Framingham Heart Study (United States)	732	78 ± 4 years (33%)	5.2	56 (7.6%)	≥5 mg/L vs. <5 mg/L (optimal cutoff)	2.81 (1.22–6.50)	Age, sex, smoking, diabetes, valve disease, AF, previous cardiovascular disease, LV hypertrophy, total cholesterol/HDL
Cesari et al[102]	Inflammatory markers and onset of cardiovascular events. Results from the Health ABC Study (United States)	2225	70–79 years (45%)	3.6	92 (4.1%)	≥2.51 mg/L vs. ≤1.15 mg/L (3rd vs. 1st tertile)	2.60 (1.45–4.67)	Age, sex, race, smoking, diabetes, hypertension, BMI, HDL cholesterol, triglycerides, albumin
Kardys et al[103]	CRP and risk of heart failure. The Rotterdam Study (The Netherlands)	6437	≥55 years; 69 ± 9 years (40%)	6.5	551 (8.6%)	≥3.5 mg/L vs. ≤0.9 mg/L (4th vs. 1st quartile)	2.08 (1.58–2.74)	Age, sex, smoking, hypertension, diabetes, BMI, HDL cholesterol

*hsCRP method in all studies except the Framingham Heart Study (standard method).

AF, atrial fibrillation; *BMI*, body mass index; *CI*, confidence interval; FEV_1, forced expiratory volume in 1 second; *HDL*, high-density lipoprotein; *HF*, heart failure; *hsCRP*, high-sensitivity C-reactive protein; *LV*, left ventricular; *LVEF*, left ventricular ejection fraction; *SBP*, systolic blood pressure.

Modified from Araújo JP, Lourenço P, Azevedo A, et al. Prognostic value of high-sensitivity C-reactive protein in heart failure: a systematic review. *J Card Fail* 2009;15:256-266.

death, 2.55; 95% CI, 2.24 to 2.89; $P < .001$). The study confirmed the powerful prognostic utility of elevated troponin levels in predicting mortality in patients hospitalized with decompensated heart failure (Figure 37-5).[140]

Troponin and Chronic Heart Failure. The role of myocyte injury in prognosis of stable outpatients with heart failure was evaluated by Hudson and colleagues.[141] The authors assessed the association of elevated cardiac troponin T (cTnT) levels with the severity, cause, and prognosis of heart failure in 136 stable, ambulatory patients. Patients with elevated cTnT levels had an increased risk of death from or hospitalization for heart failure (relative risk, 2.7; 95% CI, 1.7 to 4.3; $P = .001$) and of death alone (relative risk, 4.2; 95% CI, 1.8 to 9.5, $P = .001$) at 14 months.[141] In a larger outpatient data set from the Val-HeFT study, Latini and associates[142] measured levels of cTnT and high-sensitive troponin T (hsTnT) in 4053 patients with chronic stable heart failure. Levels of cTnT were detectable in 10.4% of the population with the cTnT assay (lower limit of detection, 0.01 ng/mL), in comparison with levels of htTNT in 92.0% with the new hsTnT assay (lower limit of detection, 0.001 ng/mL). Patients in whom cTnT level was elevated or in whom hsTnT level was above the median (0.012 ng/mL) had more severe heart failure and worse prognoses.[142] Increased concentration of cTnT (cTnT level > 0.01 ng/mL) was associated with an increased risk of death (hazard ratio, 2.08; 95% CI, 1.72 to 2.52; $P < .0001$) and increased risk of first hospitalization for heart failure (hazard ratio, 1.55; 95% CI, 1.25 to 1.93; $P < .0001$) in multivariable models. For each 0.01-ng/mL increase in hsTnT level, risk of death increased 5% (95% CI, 4% to 7%).[142]

Troponin Summary. Cardiac troponin level, an indicator of myocardial necrosis, is an established biomarker in the evaluation and management of acute coronary syndrome. There is clear evidence that even low levels of detectable troponin in patients with heart failure have significant prognostic implications in terms of morbidity and mortality. Such data hold true for patients with both acute decompensated and chronic heart failure.

Markers of Renal Function (see also Chapter 18)

Neutrophil Gelatinase–Associated Lipocalin

In patients with heart failure who develop concurrent renal dysfunction, management is challenging, requiring a careful balance between diuretic and vasodilator therapy. The cardiorenal syndrome is a well-documented phenomenon and is common among patients with acute heart failure; approximately 60% of these patients manifest at least a 0.1-mg/dL rise in creatinine level during hospitalization.[143] However, nephrotoxic insult, as manifested by an increase in serum creatinine level, usually takes at least 24 hours to become evident. A biomarker that rapidly increases with acute kidney injury could prove to be very powerful in guiding therapy in these complex clinical scenarios.

Biology. Neutrophil gelatinase–associated lipocalin (NGAL) is a small (25-kDa) molecule that belongs to a superfamily of lipocalins and is normally secreted in low amounts in the lungs, kidneys, trachea, stomach, and colon.[144,145] Levels of NGAL are elevated in various pathological states, including acute or chronic kidney injury, neoplasia, chronic

TABLE 37–3 Association Between hsCRP and Future Development of Heart Failure in High-Risk Population

Reference	Study (Country)	*N*	Age (% Male)	Follow-up Period	Incidence of Heart Failure	hsCRP Comparisons	Hazard Ratio (95% CI)	Adjusted for
Berton et al[107]	C-reactive protein in acute myocardial infarction: association with heart failure (Italy)	220	66.7 years (mean) (74%)	1 year	86 (39.1%)	≥15 mg/L vs. <15 mg/L (optimal cutoff)	4.3 (-)	Age, gender, hypertension, diabetes, BMI, CK, previous MI or angor, thrombolytic therapy, LVEF
Suleiman et al[108]	Admission C-reactive protein levels and 30-day mortality in acute myocardial infarction (Israel)	448	60 ± 12 years (78%)	30 days	121 (27.0%)	>23.3 mg/L vs. <6.9 mg/L (3rd vs. 1st tertile)	2.60 (1.50–4.60)	Age, gender, smoking, diabetes, hypertension, Killip class, BP, creatinine, aspirin, statin, anterior and ST-elevation MI, thrombolysis vs. primary angioplasty, wall motion score index
Suleiman et al[109]	Early inflammation and risk of long-term development of heart failure and mortality in survivors of acute myocardial infarction: predictive role of C-reactive protein (Israel)	1044	60 ± 13 years (89%)	23 months (median)	112 (10.7%)	≥37.9 mg/L vs. ≤5.0 mg/L (4th vs. 1st quartile)	2.80 (1.40–5.90)	Age, gender, smoking, hypertension, diabetes, BB, previous HF, Killip class, anterior MI, BP, heart rate, peak CK, LVEF
Scirica et al[105]	Clinical application of C-reactive protein across the spectrum of acute coronary syndromes (United States)	1992	61.1 years (mean) (70%)	30 days and 10 months	—	>25.4 mg/L vs. <3.4 mg/L (4th vs. 1st quartile)	30 days: 8.20 (-)10 months: 2.60 (-)	Age, gender, smoking, diabetes, prior MI, peripheral arterial or cerebrovascular disease, hypercholesterolemia BMI, Killip class, statin, aspirin, treatment with orbofiban
Bursi et al[110]	C-reactive protein and heart failure after myocardial infarction in the community (United States)	329	69 ± 16 years (52%)	1 year	92 (28.0%)	> 15 mg/L vs. < 3 mg/L (3rd vs. 1st tertile)	2.83 (1.27–4.82)	Age, sex, comorbid conditions, previous MI, Killip class, troponin T
Kavsak et al[111]	Elevated C-reactive protein in acute coronary syndrome presentation is an independent predictor of long-term mortality and heart failure (United States)	446	62 ± 14 years (59%)	2 and 8 years	—	>7.44 mg/L vs. <3 mg/L (arbitrary cutoff)	2 years: 4.14 (-) 8 years: 3.69 (-)	Age, sex, presentation, and peak troponin I
Hartford et al[112]	C-reactive protein, interleukin-6, secretory phospholipase A2 group IIA and intercellular adhesion molecule–1 in the prediction of late outcome events after acute coronary syndromes (Sweden)	757	65 years (73%)	2 years for morbidity (median)	76 (10.0%)	>16 mg/L vs. <2 mg/L (4th vs. 1st quartile)	1.40 (1.10–1.90)	Age, sex, smoking, diabetes, hypertension, hypercholesterolemia, obesity, previous MI, Killip class, creatinine, aspirin, statin, BB, ACE inhibitor

(Continued)

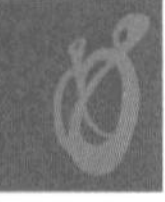

TABLE 37–3 Association Between hsCRP and Future Development of Heart Failure in High-Risk Population—cont'd

Reference	Study (Country)	*N*	Age (% Male)	Follow-up Period	Incidence of Heart Failure	hsCRP Comparisons	Hazard Ratio (95% CI)	Adjusted for
Mielniczuk et al[106]	Estimated glomerular filtration rate, inflammation, and cardiovascular events after an acute coronary syndrome (Canada)	4178	60.4 years (75%)	2 years	166 (4.0%)	> 45.2 mg/L vs. < 8.0 mg/L (4th vs. 1st quartile)	2.89 (1.70-4.80)	Age, sex, race, smoking diabetes, hypertension, prior MI, cholesterol, triglycerides, LVEF, GFR
Sabatine et al[113]	Prognostic significance of the Centers for Disease Control/ American Heart Association high-sensitivity C-reactive protein cut points for cardiovascular and other outcomes in patients with stable coronary artery disease (Multicentric)	3771	63.7 years (mean) (81.1%)	4.8 years (median)	106 (2.8%)	>3 mg/L vs. <1 mg/L (arbitrary cutoff)	2.83 (1.54-5.22)	Age, sex, smoking, diabetes, hypertension, previous MI, SBP, DBP, BMI, cholesterol, GFR, BB, statin
Williams et al[114]	C-reactive protein, diastolic dysfunction, and risk of heart failure in patients with coronary heart disease: Heart and Soul Study (United States)	985	67 ± 11 years (81.4%)	3 years	99 (10.0%)	>3 mg/L vs. ≤3 mg/L (arbitrary cutoff)	2.10 (1.20-3.60)	Sex, smoking, physical activity, BMI, statin, aspirin, LDL and HDL cholesterol, creatinine clearance, MI events, LVEF

ACE, angiotensin-converting enzyme; *BB*, β-blocker; *BMI*, body mass index; *BP*, blood pressure; *CI*, confidence interval; *CK*, creatine kinase; *DBP*, diastolic blood pressure; *GFR*, glomerular filtration rate; *HDL*, high-density lipoprotein; *HF*, heart failure; *hsCRP*, high-sensitivity C-reactive protein; *LDL*, low-density lipoprotein; *LVEF*, left ventricular ejection fraction; *MI*, myocardial infarction; *SBP*, systolic blood pressure.

From Araújo JP, Lourenço P, Azevedo A, et al. Prognostic value of high-sensitivity C-reactive protein in heart failure: a systematic review. *J Card Fail* 2009;15:256-266.

inflammatory processes, and atherosclerosis.[144] Cellular action of NGAL is mediated by binding to two types of cellular receptors: 24p3R (a brain-type organic cation transporter) and the megalin multiscavenger complex (found on the brush-boarder surface of renal tubular cells).[146,147] NGAL interacts with these receptors and forms a complex with its ligand, iron siderophores; this leads to receptor-mediated endocytosis and to intercellular and intracellular iron trafficking.[144] By depleting iron and iron-binding molecules critical for bacterial survival, NGAL exerts bacteriostatic effects.[145] In addition to its antimicrobial properties, in vitro experiments have demonstrated that NGAL is a stress-induced renal biomarker. In renal tubules, NGAL messenger RNA is upregulated within a few hours of exposure to harmful stimuli.[144] NGAL production is rapidly induced and expressed in mice upon intraperitoneal injection of cisplatin, and the subsequent rise in levels of NGAL precedes the rise in serum creatinine or urine *N*-acetyl glucosaminidase levels.[148]

NGAL and Acute Kidney Injury. The promise of NGAL as an early marker of acute kidney injury has been demonstrated in small clinical studies.[149-152] In 71 children undergoing cardiopulmonary bypass, Mishra and associates[149] evaluated NGAL levels in both serum and urine at baseline and 2 hours after the procedure. Multivariate analysis confirmed that the level of urinary NGAL was the most powerful independent predictor of severe kidney injury; a cutoff level of 50 μg/L was strongly predictive of acute kidney injury onset (AUC = 0.99; sensitivity, 100%; specificity, 98%).[149] Hirsch and colleagues[150] evaluated the utility of NGAL in predicting contrast material–induced nephropathy (CIN) in 91 children with congenital heart disease who underwent cardiac catheterization. In patients who subsequently developed contrast material–induced nephropathy, there was a significant increase in urinary NGAL and serum NGAL 2 hours after the procedure, according to a cutoff level of 100 ng/mL (urine NGAL, 0.92; serum NGAL, 0.91; sensitivity, 73%; specificity, 100% for both).[150] Other studies have confirmed these observations, which suggests that NGAL measurement may be a very powerful predictor of acute kidney injury, regardless of the mode of injury.[151,152]

NGAL and Heart Failure. Data on the utility of NGAL in heart failure are limited. A small study of 90 patients showed that, in comparison with age- and sex-matched healthy control subjects, patients with left ventricular dysfunction, as expected, had a lower GFR and higher NT-proBNP levels and urinary albumin excretion.[153] The median urinary NGAL levels were significantly higher in the group with left ventricular dysfunction (175 vs. 37 μg/gCr, P = .0001). Both serum creatinine level and estimated GFR were significantly correlated with urinary NGAL levels.[153] In another study involving 46 elderly patients with CHF, higher levels of NGAL were found in patients with heart failure than in healthy age-matched control subjects (458 vs. 37.8 ng/mL, P = .0001).[154] Moreover, NGAL level was found to increase in parallel with severity of heart failure and proved to be prognostic, inasmuch as among patients with a baseline NGAL level exceeding 783 ng/mL, the mortality rate was significantly higher (hazard ratio = 4.08, P = .001).[154] In CHF, reduction in GFR arises in large part from reduced renal perfusion, which serves as a hypoxic trigger for acute tubular necrosis.[155]

NGAL Summary. NGAL level represents a first in its class: a renal stress biomarker that signifies acute kidney injury. Its

TABLE 37–4 Prognostic Value of hsCRP in Heart Failure

Reference	Study (Country)	*N*	Age (% Male)	Follow-up Period	Readmission for Worsening Heart Failure or Death	hsCRP Comparisons	Hazard Ratio (95% CI)	Adjusted for
Anand et al[159]	C-reactive protein in heart failure. Prognostic value and the effect of valsartan (Val-HeFT: Multicentric)	4202	63 ± 11 years (80%)	36 months	1255 (29.9%)	≥7.3 mg/L vs. <1.4 mg/L (4th vs. 1st quartile)	1.53 (1.28–1.84)	Age, sex, CHD, NHYA class, LVEF, hemoglobin, GFR, uric acid, BNP, aldosterone, renin, norepinephrine, statin, aspirin, BB, valsartan vs. placebo
Yin et al[115]	Independent prognostic value of elevated high-sensitivity C-reactive protein in chronic heart failure (Taiwan)	108	62 ± 16 years (66%)	403 days (median)	35 (32.4%)	>2.97 mg/L vs. <2.97 mg/L (optimal cutoff)	3.05 (1.15–8.05)	Age, sex, CHD, LVEF, left ventricular filling pressure, TNF-α, statin
Xue et al[116]	Prognostic value of high-sensitivity C-reactive protein in patients with chronic heart failure (China)	128	62 ± 15 years (79%)	378 days (mean)	42 (32.8%)	>3.2 mg/L vs. <3.2 mg/L (optimal cutoff)	3.81 (2.14–9.35)	Age, sex, CHD, LVEF, troponin T, statin
Windram et al[117]	Relationship of high-sensitivity C-reactive protein to prognosis and other prognostic markers in outpatients with heart failure (United Kingdom)	957	71 ± 10 years (71%)	36 months	163 (17.0%; only death)	>11 mg/L vs. <2.8 mg/L (4th vs. 1st quartile)	3.00 (2.1–4.1)	Age, sex, smoking diabetes, white blood cell count, BB, statin, NSAID
Yin et al[118]	Multimarker approach to risk stratification among patients with advanced chronic heart failure (Taiwan)	152	56 ± 14 years (77%)	186 days (median)	63 (41.4%)	>4.92 mg/L vs. <4.92 mg/L (median)	2.16 (1.17–3.99)	Age, sex, etiology, SBP, LVEF, sodium, creatinine clearance, troponin I, NT-proBNP
Tang et al[119]	Usefulness of C-reactive protein and left ventricular diastolic performance for prognosis in patients with left ventricular systolic heart failure (United States)	136	57 ± 14 years (76%)	33 months (mean)	36 (26.5%)	>5.96 mg/L vs. <5.96 mg/L (optimal cutoff)	2.26 (1.11–4.63)	LVEF, echocardiographic indexes of diastolic dysfunction, BNP
Lamblin et al[120]	High-sensitivity C-reactive protein: potential adjunct for risk stratification in patients with stable heart failure (France)	546	56 ± 12 years (82%)	972 days (median)	113 (20.7%)	>3 mg/L vs. <3 mg/L (optimal cutoff)	1.78 (1.17–2.72)	Age, sex, cause, hypertension, diabetes, BMI, NYHA class, LVEF, BNP
Chirinos et al[121]	Usefulness of C-reactive protein as an independent predictor of death in patients with ischemic cardiomyopathy (United States)	123	64 ± 10 years (100%)	3 years	—	For each 10-mg/L increase	1.26 (1.02–1.55)	Age, number of vessels involved with coronary disease, LVEF, sodium, creatinine, hematocrit, ACE inhibitor, BB

(Continued)

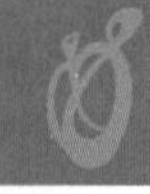

TABLE 37–4 Prognostic Value of hsCRP in Heart Failure—cont'd

Reference	Study (Country)	*N*	Age (% Male)	Follow-up Period	Readmission for Worsening Heart Failure or Death	hsCRP Comparisons	Hazard Ratio (95% CI)	Adjusted for
Ronnow et al[122]	C-reactive protein predicts death in patients with non-ischemic cardio-myopathy (United States)	203	62 ± 13 years (59%)	2.4 years (mean)	40 (19.7%)	>23.3 mg/L vs. <23.3 mg/L (3rd tertile vs. 1st and 2nd tertiles)	20.0 0 (1.04–3.80)	Age, sex, smoking, family history, hypertension, hyperlipidemia, diabetes, renal failure, BMI, LVEF
Ishikawa et al[123]	Prediction of mortality by high-sensitivity C-reactive protein and brain natriuretic peptide in patients with dilated cardio-myopathy (Japan)	84	56 ± 2 years (81%)	42 months (mean)	—	>1 mg/L vs. <1 mg/L (arbitrary cutoff)	3.30 (1.2–9.0)	Age, sex, NYHA class, LVEF, cardiac index, hemoglobin, creatinine, BNP, IL-6, endothelin, norepinephrine

ACE, angiotensin-converting enzyme; *BB,* β-blocker; *BMI,* body mass index; *BNP,* B-type natriuretic peptide; *CHD,* coronary heart disease; *CI,* confidence interval; *CRP,* C-reactive protein; *GFR,* glomerular filtration rate; *HF,* heart failure; *hsCRP,* high-sensitivity C-reactive protein; *IL-6,* interleukin-6; *LVEF,* left ventricular ejection fraction; *NSAID,* nonsteroidal antiinflammatory drug; *NT-*proBNP, *N*-terminal pro-B-type natriuretic peptide; *NYHA,* New York Heart Association; *SBP,* systolic blood pressure; *TNF-α,* tumor necrosis factor-α.
From Araújo JP, Lourenço P, Azevedo A, et al. Prognostic value of high-sensitivity C-reactive protein in heart failure: a systematic review. *J Card Fail* 2009;15:256-266.

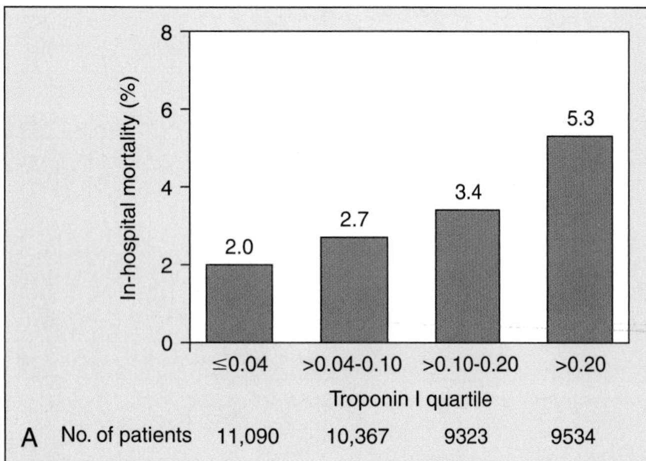

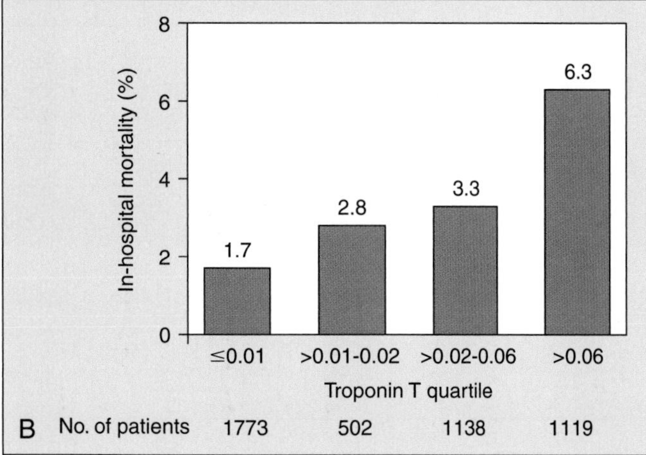

FIGURE 37–5 In-hospital mortality rates in comparison with troponin I (**A**) or troponin T (**B**) quartiles in patients admitted with decompensated heart failure. (From Peacock WF 4th, De Marco T, Fonarow GC, et al. Cardiac troponin and outcome in acute heart failure. *N Engl J Med* 2008;358: 2117-2126.)

utility in predicting the development of renal insufficiency with good sensitivity and specificity has been shown in small studies involving cardiopulmonary bypass and angiography. Future studies may further define the role of NGAL level in assisting clinicians to achieve a proper balance between diuretics, vasodilators, and inotropes when treating patients with acute heart failure.

MULTIMARKER APPROACH AND FUTURE DIRECTION

The evolution of numerous biomarkers has created valuable assets for the classification and management of heart failure. There is growing interest in the use of multimarker strategies to stratify patients with heart failure, similar to acute coronary syndromes. The interaction in heart failure between biomechanical strain, inflammation, and cellular injury allows a variety of biomarkers to jointly lead to better understanding of the pathogenesis, clinical diagnosis, and prognosis of heart failure.[91] These markers are complementary to the clinical data and enhance prediction of morbidity and mortality.

In evaluating the association between cTnI and mortality in advanced heart failure, Horwich and coworkers[128] demonstrated that using both cTnI and BNP levels further improves prognostic value.[128] Patients with both detectable cTnI level and a BNP level exceeding 485 pg/mL had a twelve-fold higher risk of death than did those with both undetectable cTnI level and a BNP level of less than 485 pg/mL. The prognostic value of this combination was confirmed with the hsTnT assay.[142] Prediction was also enhanced with measurements of natriuretic peptides and MR-proADM, ST2, or CRP.[71,88,156] In 983 consecutive patients who had suffered myocardial infarction, Khan and associates showed that the combination of MR-proADM provided further risk stratification for patients with NT-proBNP levels above the median ($P < .001$).[71] The PRIDE study verified the prognostic capability of the multimarker approach. Of the 184 patients with NT-proBNP level of 986 pg/mL or higher, 56 (30.4%) died. All but 1 of the decedents within this group had an ST2 level of 0.2 ng/mL or higher.[88] In contrast, of the 28 patients with NT-proBNP levels of

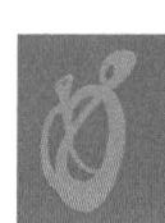

986 pg/mL or higher and ST2 levels of *less* than 0.2 pg/mL, only 1 (3.5%) died at 1 year.[88]

Dunlay and colleagues[157] used CRP, BNP, and cTnT levels in 593 patients with heart failure to evaluate the prognostic utility of a multimarker approach. Among patients with CRP (<11.8 mg/L), BNP (<350 pg/mL), and cTnT (≤0.01 ng/mL) levels all lower than the median, the 1-year mortality rate was low (3.3%), whereas among those with two or three biomarkers higher than the median, the mortality rate was markedly increased (30.8% and 35.5%, respectively). A strategy involving two biomarkers offered greater improvement in predicting 1-year mortality risk than did use of a single biomarker. In this study, however, the addition of a third biomarker conferred no added benefit over a two-biomarker approach.[157]

Short-term prognosis with a multimarker strategy was also evaluated in a study of 577 consecutive patients admitted with severe decompensated NYHA class III or IV low-output heart failure, to determine the combined prognostic value of admission BNP, cTnI, and hsCRP levels at 31 days.[158] The total mortality rate in the group was 17.7%. Multivariate Cox analysis revealed that elevated levels of BNP, cTnI, and hsCRP were independent predictors of mortality.[158] There was a significant, gradually increased risk of 31-day cardiac death with increased numbers of elevated biomarkers ($P < .001$).[158]

The multimarker approach provides powerful prognostic information in both compensated and decompensated heart failure. Combinations of biomarkers allow clinicians to better stratify risk for patients and perhaps tailor more aggressive therapy for those with a higher predicted risk. As new biomarkers are developed and implemented, more powerful multimarker approaches are likely to follow.

CONCLUSION

Biomarker use has skyrocketed since 2000. Natriuretic peptide levels, because of their low cost and rapid and accurate ability to provide additional information not surmised from clinical evaluation, are the standard biomarkers. But work with natriuretic peptide levels has also shown that they are not to be used as stand-alone tests; rather they are best used as adjuncts to other tests used by health care providers. There are many caveats to using natriuretic peptide levels, as there will be with all future biomarkers; thus, there is always much to learn about them. Finally, because complex pathological conditions are widespread, panels of multiple biomarkers will be needed in evaluation, risk stratification, and, ultimately, treatment initiation and follow-up.

REFERENCES

1. Stevenson, L. W., & Perloff, J. K. (1989). The limited reliability of physical signs for establishing hemodynamics in chronic heart failure. *JAMA, 261*, 884–888.
2. Morrow, D. A., & de Lemos, J. A. (2007). Benchmarks for the assessment of novel cardiovascular biomarkers. *Circulation, 115*, 949–952.
3. Yasue, H., Yoshimura, M., Sumida, H., et al. (1994). Localization and mechanism of secretion of B-type natriuretic peptide in comparison with those A-type natriuretic peptide in normal subjects and patients with heart failure. *Circulation, 90*, 195–203.
4. Yoshimura, M., Yasue, H., Okumura, K., et al. (1993). Different secretion patterns of atrial natriuretic peptide and brain natriuretic peptide in patients with congestive heart failure. *Circulation, 87*, 464–469.
5. Nakao, K., Ogawa, Y., Suga, S., et al. (1992). Molecular biology and biochemistry of the natriuretic peptide system. II: natriuretic peptide receptors. *J Hypertens, 10*, 1111–1114.
6. Chen, H. H. (2007). Heart failure: a state of brain natriuretic peptide deficiency or resistance or both!. *J Am Coll Cardiol, 49*, 1089–1091.
7. Shimizu, H., Masuta, K., Aono, K., et al. (2002). Molecular forms of human brain natriuretic peptide in plasma. *Clin Chim Acta, 316*, 129–135.
8. Lam, C. S., Burnett, J. C., Jr., Costello-Boerrigter, L., et al. (2007). Alternate circulating pro–B-type natriuretic peptide and B-type natriuretic peptide forms in the general population. *J Am Coll Cardiol, 49*, 1193–1202.
9. Forfia, P. R., Lee, M., Tunin, R. S., et al. (2007). Acute phosphodiesterase 5 inhibition mimics hemodynamic effects of B-type natriuretic peptide effects in failing but not normal canine heart. *J Am Coll Cardiol, 49*, 1079–1088.
10. Redfield, M. M., Rodeheffer, R. J., Jacobsen, S. J., et al. (2002). Plasma brain natriuretic peptide concentration: impact of age and gender. *J Am Coll Cardiol, 40*, 976–982.
11. Wang, T. J., Larson, M. G., Levy, D., et al. (2002). Impact of age and sex on plasma natriuretic peptide levels in healthy adults. *Am J Cardiol, 90*, 254–258.
12. Daniels, L. B., Allison, M. A., Clopton, P., et al. (2008). Use of natriuretic peptides in pre-participation screening of college athletes. *Int J Cardiol, 124*, 411–414.
13. Maisel, A. S., Krishnaswamy, P., Nowak, R. M., et al. (2002). Rapid measurement of B-type natriuretic peptide in the emergency diagnosis of heart failure. *N Engl J Med, 347*, 161–167.
14. Januzzi, J. L., Jr., CamargoAnwaruddin, C. A. S., et al. (2005). The N-terminal Pro-BNP Investigation of Dyspnea in the Emergency Department (PRIDE) study. *Am J Cardiol, 95*, 948–954.
15. Mueller, C., Scholer, A., Laule-Kilian, K., et al. (2004). Use of B-type natriuretic peptide in the evaluation and management of acute dyspnea. *N Engl J Med, 350*, 647–654.
16. Moe, G. W., Howlett, J., Januzzi, J. L., et al. (2007). N-terminal pro–B-type natriuretic peptide testing improves the management of patients with suspected acute heart failure: primary results of the Canadian prospective randomized multicenter IMPROVE-CHF study. *Circulation, 115*, 3103–3110.
17. Morita, E., Yasue, H., Yoshimura, M., et al. (1992). Increasing plasma levels of brain natriuretic peptide in patients with acute myocardial infarction. *Circulation, 88*, 82–91.
18. Morrison, L. K., Harrison, A., Krishnaswamy, P., et al. (2002). Utility of a rapid B-natriuretic peptide assay in differentiating congestive heart failure from lung disease in patients presenting with dyspnea. *J Am Coll Cardiol, 39*, 202–209.
19. Kucher, N., Printzen, G., & Goldhaber, S. Z. (2003). Prognostic role of brain natriuretic peptide in acute pulmonary embolism. *Circulation, 107*, 2545–2547.
20. Nagaya, N., Nishikimi, T., Okano, Y., et al. (1998). Plasma brain natriuretic peptide levels increase in proportion to the extent of right ventricular dysfunction in pulmonary hypertension. *J Am Coll Cardiol, 31*, 202–208.
21. Bando, M., Ishhi, Y., Sugiyama, Y., et al. (1999). Elevated plasma brain natriuretic peptide levels in chronic respiratory failure with cor pulmonale. *Respir Med, 93*, 507–514.
22. Nagaya, N., Nishikimi, T., Uematsu, M., et al. (2000). Plasma brain natriuretic peptide as a prognostic indicator in patients with primary pulmonary hypertension. *Circulation, 102*, 865–870.
23. Rudiger, A., Gasser, S., Fischler, M., et al. (2006). Comparable increase of B-type natriuretic peptide and amino-terminal pro–B-type natriuretic peptide levels in patients with severe sepsis, septic shock, and acute heart failure. *Crit Care Med, 34*, 2140–2144.
24. Schultz, M., Faber, J., Kistorp, C., et al. (2004). N-terminal-pro–B-type natriuretic peptide (NT-pro-BNP) in different thyroid function states. *Clin Endocrinol (Oxf), 60*, 54–59.
25. Yildiz, R., Yildirim, B., Karincaoglu, M., et al. (2005). Brain natriuretic peptide and severity of disease in non-alcoholic cirrhotic patients. *J Gastroenterol Hepatol, 20*, 1115–1120.
26. Ellinor, P. T., Low, A. F., Patton, K., et al. (2005). Discordant atrial natriuretic peptide and brain natriuretic peptide levels in lone atrial fibrillation. *J Am Coll Cardiol, 45*, 82–86.
27. Knudsen, C. W., Omland, T., Clopton, P., et al. (2005). Impact of atrial fibrillation on the diagnostic performance of B-type natriuretic peptide concentration in dyspneic patients: an analysis from the Breathing Not Properly Multinational Study. *J Am Coll Cardiol, 46*, 838–844.
28. Kawai, K., Hata, K., Tanaka, K., et al. (2004). Attenuation of biologic compensatory action of cardiac natriuretic peptide system with aging. *Am J Cardiol, 93*, 719–723.
29. Chang, A. Y., Abdullah, S. M., Jain, T., et al. (2007). Association among androgens, estrogens, and natriuretic peptides in young women: observations from the Dallas Heart Study. *J Am Coll Cardiol, 49*, 109–116.
30. Daniels, L. B., & Maisel, A. S. (2007). Natriuretic peptides. *J Am Coll Cardiol, 50*, 2357–2368.
31. McCullough P. A., Duc, P., Omland, T., et al. (2003). B-type natriuretic peptide and renal function in the diagnosis of heart failure: an analysis from the Breathing Not Properly Multinational Study. *Am J Kidney Dis, 41*, 571–579.
32. Lamb, E. J., Vickery, S., & Price, C. P. (2006). Amino-terminal pro-brain natriuretic peptide to diagnose congestive heart failure in patients with impaired kidney function. *J Am Coll Cardiol, 48*, 1060–1061.
33. Anwaruddin, S., Lloyd-Jones, D. M., Baggish, A., et al. (2006). Renal function, congestive heart failure, and amino-terminal pro-brain natriuretic peptide measurement: results from the ProBNP Investigation of Dyspnea in the Emergency Department (PRIDE) study. *J Am Coll Cardiol, 47*, 91–97.
34. Costello-Boerrigter, L. C., Boerrigter, G., Redfield, M. M., et al. (2006). Amino-terminal pro–B-type natriuretic peptide and B-type natriuretic peptide in the general community: determinants and detection of left ventricular dysfunction. *J Am Coll Cardiol, 47*, 345–353.
35. Mehra, M. R., Uber, P. A., Park, M. H., et al. (2004). Obesity and suppressed B-type natriuretic peptide levels in heart failure. *J Am Coll Cardiol, 43*, 1590–1595.
36. Wang, T. J., Larson, M. G., Levy, D., et al. (2004). Impact of obesity on plasma natriuretic peptide levels. *Circulation, 109*, 594–600.
37. Daniels, L. B., Clopton, P., Bhalla, V., et al. (2006). How obesity affects the cut-points for B-type natriuretic peptide in the diagnosis of acute heart failure. Results from the Breathing Not Properly Multinational Study. *Am Heart J, 151*, 999–1005.
38. Sarzani, R., Dessi-Fulgheri, P., Paci, V. M., et al. (1996). Expression of natriuretic peptide receptors in human adipose and other tissues. *J Endocrinol Invest, 19*, 581–585.
39. Krauser, D. G., Lloyd-Jones, D. M., Chae, C. U., et al. (2005). Effect of body mass index on natriuretic peptide levels in patients with acute congestive heart failure: a ProBNP Investigation of Dyspnea in the Emergency Department (PRIDE) substudy. *Am Heart J, 149*, 744–750.
40. van Kimmenade, R., van Dielen, F., Bakker, J., et al. (2006). Is brain natriuretic peptide production decreased in obese subjects?. *J Am Coll Cardiol, 47*, 886–887.
41. Leya, F. S., Arab, D., Joyal, D., et al. (2005). The efficacy of brain natriuretic peptide levels in differentiating constrictive pericarditis from restrictive cardiomyopathy. *J Am Coll Cardiol, 45*, 1900–1902.

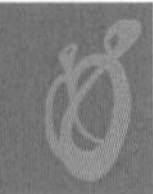

42. Doust, J. A., Pietrzak, E., Dobson, A., et al. (2005). How well does B-type natriuretic peptide predict death and cardiac events in patients with heart failure: systematic review. *BMJ, 330*, 625.
43. Maisel, A., Hollander, J. E., Guss, D., et al. (2004). Primary results of the Rapid Emergency Department Heart Failure Outpatient Trial (REDHOT). A multicenter study of B-type natriuretic peptide levels, emergency department decision making, and outcomes in patients presenting with shortness of breath. *J Am Coll Cardiol, 44*, 1328–1333.
44. Anand, I. S., Fisher, L. D., Chiang, Y. T., et al. (2003). Changes in brain natriuretic peptide and norepinephrine over time and mortality and morbidity in the Valsartan Heart Failure Trial (Val-FeFT). *Circulation, 107*, 1278–1283.
45. Schnabel, R., Lubos, E., Rupprecht, H. J., et al. (2006). B-type natriuretic peptide and the risk of cardiovascular events and death in patients with stable angina: results from the AtheroGene study. *J Am Coll Cardiol, 47*, 552–558.
46. Kragelund, C., Gronning, B., Kobel, L., et al. (2005). N-terminal pro–B-type natriuretic peptide and long-term mortality in stable coronary heart disease. *N Engl J Med, 352*, 666–675.
47. Bibbins-Domingo, K., Gupta, R., Na, B., et al. (2007). N-terminal fragment of the prohormone brain-type natriuretic peptide (NT-proBNP), cardiovascular events, and mortality in patients with stable coronary heart disease. *JAMA, 297*, 169–176.
48. Lindahl, B., Lindback, J., Jernberg, T., et al. (2005). Serial analyses of N-terminal pro–B-type natriuretic peptide in patients with non–ST-segment elevation acute coronary syndromes: a Fragmin and fast Revascularisation during In Stability in Coronary artery disease (FRISC)–II substudy. *J Am Coll Cardiol, 45*, 533–541.
49. Berger, R., Huelsman, M., Strecker, K., et al. (2002). B-type natriuretic peptide predicts sudden death in patients with chronic heart failure. *Circulation, 105*, 2392–2397.
50. Tapanainen, J. M., Lindgren, K. S., Makikallio, T. H., et al. (2004). Natriuretic peptides as predictors of non-sudden and sudden cardiac death after acute myocardial infarction in the beta-blocking era. *J Am Coll Cardiol, 43*, 757–763.
51. Taub, P. R., Daniels, L. B., & Maisel, A. S. (2009). Usefulness of B-type natriuretic peptide levels in predicting hemodynamic and clinical decompensation. *Heart Fail Clin, 5*, 169–175.
52. Forfia, P. R., Watkins, S. P., Rame, J. E., et al. (2005). Relationship between B-type natriuretic peptides and pulmonary capillary wedge pressure in the intensive care unit. *J Am Coll Cardiol, 45*, 1667–1671.
53. Kazanegra, R., Cheng, V., Garcia, A., et al. (2001). A rapid test for B-type natriuretic peptide correlates with falling wedge pressures in patients treated for decompensated heart failure: a pilot study. *J Card Fail, 7*, 21–29.
54. Cheng, V., Kazanagra, R., Garcia, A., et al. (2001). A rapid bedside test for B-type peptide predicts treatment outcomes in patients admitted for decompensated heart failure: a pilot study. *J Am Coll Cardiol, 37*, 386–391.
55. Bettencourt, P., Ferreira, S., Azevedo, A., et al. (2002). Preliminary data on the potential usefulness of B-type natriuretic peptide levels in predicting outcome after hospital discharge in patients with heart failure. *Am J Med, 113*, 215–219.
56. Logeart, D., Thabut, G., Jourdain, P., et al. (2004). Predischarge B-type natriuretic peptide assay for identifying patients at high risk of re-admission after decompensated heart failure. *J Am Coll Cardiol, 43*, 625–641.
57. Jourdain, P., Jondeau, G., Funck, F., et al. (2007). Plasma brain natriuretic peptide–guided therapy to improve outcome in heart failure: the STARS-BNP multicenter study. *J Am Coll Cardiol, 49*, 1733–1739.
58. Shah, M. R., Claise, K. A., Bowers, M. T., et al. (2005). Testing new targets of therapy in advanced heart failure: the design and rationale of the Strategies for Tailoring Advanced Heart Failure Regimens in the Outpatient Setting: BRain NatrIuretic Peptide Versus the Clinical CongesTion ScorE (STARBRITE) trial. *Am Heart J, 150*, 893–898.
59. Lee, S. C., Stevens, T. L., Sandberg, S. M., et al. (2002). The potential of brain natriuretic peptide as a biomarker for New York Heart Association class during the outpatient treatment of heart failure. *J Card Fail, 8*, 149–154.
60. Kitamura, K., Kangawa, K., Kawamoto, M., et al. (1993). Adrenomedullin: a novel hypotensive peptide isolated from human pheochromocytoma. *Biochem Biophys Res Commun, 192*, 553–560.
61. Takahashi, K., Satoh, F., Hara, E., et al. (1997). Production and secretion of adrenomedullin from glial cell tumors and its effects on cAMP production. *Peptides, 18*, 1117–1124.
62. Nakamura, M., Yoshida, H., Makita, S., et al. (1997). Potent and long-lasting vasodilatory effects of adrenomedullin in humans. Comparisons between normal subjects and patients with chronic heart failure. *Circulation, 95*, 1214–1221.
63. Parkes, D. G., & May, C. N. (1995). ACTH-suppressive and vasodilator actions of adrenomedullin in conscious sheep. *J Neuroendocrinol, 7*, 923–929.
64. Parkes, D. G., & May, C. N. (1997). Direct cardiac and vascular actions of adrenomedullin in conscious sheep. *Br J Pharmacol, 120*, 1179–1185.
65. Vari, R. C., Adkins, S. D., & Samson, W. K. (1996). Renal effects of adrenomedullin in the rat. *Proc Soc Exp Biol Med, 211*, 178–183.
66. Kato, J., Kobayashi, K., Etoh, T., et al. (1996). Plasma adrenomedullin concentration in patients with heart failure. *J Clin Endocrinol Metab, 81*, 180–183.
67. Kitamura, K., Sakata, J., Kangawa, K., et al. (1993). Cloning and characterization of cDNA encoding a precursor for human adrenomedullin. *Biochem Biophys Res Commun, 194*, 720–725.
68. Jougasaki, M., Rodeheffer, R. J., Redfield, M. M., et al. (1996). Cardiac secretion of adrenomedullin in human heart failure. *J Clin Invest, 97*, 2370–2376.
69. Hinson, J. P., Kapas, S., & Smith, D. M. (2000). Adrenomedullin, a multifunctional regulatory peptide. *Endocr Rev, 21*, 138–167.
70. Struck, J., Tao, C., Morgenthaler, N. G., et al. (2004). Identification of an adrenomedullin precursor fragment in plasma of sepsis patients. *Peptides, 25*, 1369–1372.
71. Khan, S. Q., O'Brien, R. J., Struck, J., et al. (2007). Prognostic value of midregional pro-adrenomedullin in patients with acute myocardial infarction. The LAMP (Leicester Acute Myocardial Infarction Peptide) study. *J Am Coll Cardiol, 49*, 1525–1532.
72. Adlbrecht, C., Hülsmann, M., Strunk, G., et al. (2009). Prognostic value of plasma midregional pro-adrenomedullin and C-terminal–pro–endothelin-1 in chronic heart failure outpatients. *Eur J Heart Fail, 11*, 361–366.
73. Nishida, H., Horio, T., Suzuki, Y., et al. (2008). Plasma adrenomedullin as an independent predictor of future cardiovascular events in high-risk patients: comparison with C-reactive protein and adiponectin. *Peptides, 29*, 599–605.
74. Gegenhuber, A., Struck, J., Dieplinger, B., et al. (2007). Comparative evaluation of B-type natriuretic peptide, mid-regional pro–A-type natriuretic peptide, mid-regional pro-adrenomedullin, and Copeptin to predict 1-year mortality in patients with acute destabilized heart failure. *J Card Fail, 13*, 42–49.
75. Coletta, A. P., Clark, A. L., & Cleland, J. G. (2009). Clinical trials update from the Heart Failure Society of America and the American Heart Association meetings in 2008: SADHART-CHF, COMPARE, MOMENTUM, thyroid hormone analogue study, HF-ACTION, I-PRESERVE, beta-interferon study, BACH, and ATHENA. *Eur J Heart Fail, 11*, 214–219.
76. Tominaga, S. (1989). A putative protein of a growth specific cDNA from BALB/c-3T3 cells is highly similar to the extracellular portion of mouse interleukin 1 receptor. *FEBS Lett, 258*, 301–304.
77. Townsend, M. J., Fallon, P. G., Matthews, D. J., et al. (2000). T1/ST2-deficient mice demonstrate the importance of T1/ST2 in developing primary T helper cell type 2 responses. *J Exp Med, 191*, 1069–1076.
78. Kakkar, R., & Lee, R. T. (2008). The IL-33/ST2 pathway: therapeutic target and novel biomarker. *Nat Rev Drug Discov, 7*, 827–840.
79. Weinberg, E. O., Shimpo, M., De Keulenaer, G. W., et al. (2002). Expression and regulation of ST2, an interleukin-1 receptor family member, in cardiomyocytes and myocardial infarction. *Circulation, 106*, 2961–2966.
80. Schmitz, J., Owyang, A., Oldham, E., et al. (2005). IL-33, an interleukin-1–like cytokine that signals via the IL-1 receptor–related protein ST2 and induces T helper type 2–associated cytokines. *Immunity, 23*, 479–490.
81. Diez, J., Gonzalez, A., Lopez, B., et al. (2005). Mechanisms of disease: pathologic structural remodeling is more than adaptive hypertrophy in hypertensive heart disease. *Nat Clin Pract Cardiovasc Med, 2*, 209–216.
82. Sadoshima, J., & Izumo, S. (1997). The cellular and molecular response of cardiac myocytes to mechanical stress. *Annu Rev Physiol, 59*, 551–571.
83. Manabe, I., Shindo, T., & Nagai, R. (2002). Gene expression in fibroblasts and fibrosis: involvement in cardiac hypertrophy. *Circ Res, 91*, 1103–1113.
84. Sanada, S., Hakuno, D., Higgins, L. J., et al. (2007). IL-33 and ST2 comprise a critical biomechanically induced and cardioprotective signaling system. *J Clin Invest, 117*, 1538–1549.
85. Shimpo, M., Morrow, D. A., Weinberg, E. O., et al. (2004). Serum levels of the interleukin-1 receptor family member ST2 predict mortality and clinical outcome in acute myocardial infarction. *Circulation, 109*, 2186–2190.
86. Sabatine, M. S., Morrow, D. A., Higgins, L. J., et al. (2008). Complementary roles for biomarkers of biomechanical strain ST2 and N-terminal prohormone B-type natriuretic peptide in patients with ST-elevation myocardial infarction. *Circulation, 117*, 1936–1944.
87. Weinberg, E. O., Shimpo, M., Hurwitz, S., et al. (2003). Identification of serum soluble ST2 receptor as a novel heart failure biomarker. *Circulation, 107*, 721–726.
88. Januzzi, J. L., Jr., Peacock, W. F., Maisel, A. S., et al. (2007). Measurement of the interleukin family member ST2 in patients with acute dyspnea: results from the PRIDE (Pro-Brain Natriuretic Peptide Investigation of Dyspnea in the Emergency Department) study. *J Am Coll Cardiol, 50*, 607–613.
89. Boisot, S., Beede, J., Isakson, S., et al. (2008). Serial sampling of ST2 predicts 90-day mortality following destabilized heart failure. *J Card Fail, 14*, 732–738.
90. Rehman, S. U., Mueller, T., & Januzzi, J. L., Jr. (2008). Characteristics of the novel interleukin family biomarker ST2 in patients with acute heart failure. *J Am Coll Cardiol, 52*, 1458–1465.
91. Braunwald, E. (2008). Biomarkers in heart failure. *N Engl J Med, 358*, 2148–2159.
92. Levine, B., Kalman, J., Mayer, L., et al. (1990). Elevated circulating levels of tumor necrosis factor in severe chronic heart failure. *N Engl J Med, 323*, 236–241.
93. Seta, Y., Shan, K., Bozkurt, B., et al. (1996). Basic mechanisms in heart failure: the cytokine hypothesis. *J Card Fail, 2*, 243–249.
94. Bozkurt, B., Kribbs, S. B., Clubb, F. J., Jr., et al. (1998). Pathophysiologically relevant concentrations of tumor necrosis factor–alpha promote progressive left ventricular dysfunction and remodeling in rats. *Circulation, 97*, 1382–1391.
95. Steele, I. C., Nugent, A. M., Maguire, S., et al. (1996). Cytokine profile in chronic cardiac failure. *Eur J Clin Invest, 26*, 1018–1022.
96. Kubota, T., McTiernan, C. F., Frye, C. S., et al. (1997). Dilated cardiomyopathy in transgenic mice with cardiac-specific overexpression of tumor necrosis factor-alpha. *Circ Res, 81*, 627–635.
97. Yamauchi-Takihara, K., Ihara, Y., & Ogata, A. (1995). Hypoxic stress induces cardiac myocyte–derived interleukin-6. *Circulation, 91*, 1520–1524.
98. Araújo, J. P., Lourenço, P., Azevedo, A., et al. (2009). Prognostic value of high-sensitivity C-reactive protein in heart failure: a systematic review. *J Card Fail, 15*, 256–266.
99. Venugopal, S. K., Devaraj, S., & Jialal, I. (2005). Effect of C-reactive protein on vascular cells: evidence for a proinflammatory, proatherogenic role. *Curr Opin Nephrol Hypertens, 14*, 33–37.
100. Gottdiener, J. S., Arnold, A. M., Aurigemma, G. P., et al. (2000). Predictors of congestive heart failure in the elderly: the Cardiovascular Health Study. *J Am Coll Cardiol, 35*, 1628–1637.
101. Vasan, R. S., Sullivan, L. M., Roubenoff, R., et al. (2003). Inflammatory markers and risk of heart failure in elderly subjects without prior myocardial infarction: the Framingham Heart Study. *Circulation, 107*, 1486–1491.
102. Cesari, M., Penninx, B. W., Newman, A. B., et al. (2003). Inflammatory markers and cardiovascular disease (The Health, Aging and Body Composition [Health ABC] Study). *Am J Cardiol, 92*, 522–528.
103. Kardys, I., Knetsch, A. M., Bleumink, G. S., et al. (2006). C-reactive protein and risk of heart failure. The Rotterdam Study. *Am Heart J, 152*, 514–520.
104. Pietilä, K. O., Harmoinen, A. P., Jokiniitty, J., et al. (1996). Serum C-reactive protein concentration in acute myocardial infarction and its relationship to mortality during 24 months of follow-up in patients under thrombolytic treatment. *Eur Heart J, 17*, 1345–1349.

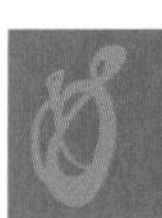

105. Scirica, B. M., Morrow, D. A., Cannon, C. P., et al. (2007). Clinical application of C-reactive protein across the spectrum of acute coronary syndromes. *Clin Chem, 53*, 1800–1807.
106. Mielniczuk, L. M., Pfeffer, M. A., & Lewis, E. F. (2008). Estimated glomerular filtration rate, inflammation, and cardiovascular events after an acute coronary syndrome. *Am Heart J, 155*, 725–731.
107. Berton, G., Cordiano, R., Palmieri, R., et al. (2003). C-reactive protein in acute myocardial infarction: association with heart failure. *Am Heart J, 145*, 1094–1101.
108. Suleiman, M., Aronson, D., Reisner, S. A., et al. (2003). Admission C-reactive protein levels and 30-day mortality in patients with acute myocardial infarction. *Am J Med, 115*, 695–701.
109. Suleiman, M., Khatib, R., Agmon, Y., et al. (2006). Early inflammation and risk of long-term development of heart failure and mortality in survivors of acute myocardial infarction: predictive role of C-reactive protein. *J Am Coll Cardiol, 47*, 962–968.
110. Bursi, F., Weston, S. A., Killian, J. M., et al. (2007). C-reactive protein and heart failure after myocardial infarction in the community. *Am J Med, 120*, 616–622.
111. Kavsak, P. A., MacRae, A. R., Newman, A. M., et al. (2007). Elevated C-reactive protein in acute coronary syndrome presentation is an independent predictor of long-term mortality and heart failure. *Clin Biochem, 40*, 326–329.
112. Hartford, M., Wiklund, O., Mattsson Hultén, L., et al. (2007). C-reactive protein, interleukin-6, secretory phospholipase A2 group IIA and intercellular adhesion molecule–1 in the prediction of late outcome events after acute coronary syndromes. *J Intern Med, 262*, 526–536.
113. Sabatine, M. S., Morrow, D. A., Jablonski, K. A., et al. (2007). Prognostic significance of the Centers for Disease Control/American Heart Association high-sensitivity C-reactive protein cut points for cardiovascular and other outcomes in patients with stable coronary artery disease. *Circulation, 115*, 1528–1536.
114. Williams, E. S., Shah, S. J., Ali, S., et al. (2008). C-reactive protein, diastolic dysfunction, and risk of heart failure in patients with coronary disease: Heart and Soul Study. *Eur J Heart Fail, 10*, 63–69.
115. Yin, W. H., Chen, J. W., Jen, H. L., et al. (2004). Independent prognostic value of elevated high-sensitivity C-reactive protein in chronic heart failure. *Am Heart J, 147*, 931–938.
116. Xue, C., Feng, Y., Wo, J., et al. (2006). Prognostic value of high-sensitivity C-reactive protein in patients with chronic heart failure. *N Z Med J, 119*, U2314.
117. Windram, J. D., Loh, P. H., Rigby, A. S., et al. (2007). Relationship of high-sensitivity C-reactive protein to prognosis and other prognostic markers in outpatients with heart failure. *Am Heart J, 153*, 1048–1055.
118. Yin, W. H., Chen, J. W., Feng, A. N., et al. (2007). Multimarker approach to risk stratification among patients with advanced chronic heart failure. *Clin Cardiol, 30*, 397–402.
119. Tang, W. H., Shrestha, K., Van Lente, F., et al. (2008). Usefulness of C-reactive protein and left ventricular diastolic performance for prognosis in patients with left ventricular systolic heart failure. *Am J Cardiol, 101*, 370–373.
120. Lamblin, N., Mouquet, F., Hennache, B., et al. (2005). High-sensitivity C-reactive protein: potential adjunct for risk stratification in patients with stable congestive heart failure. *Eur Heart J, 26*, 2245–2250.
121. Chirinos, J. A., Zambrano, J. P., Chakko, S., et al. (2005). Usefulness of C-reactive protein as an independent predictor of death in patients with ischemic cardiomyopathy. *Am J Cardiol, 95*, 88–90.
122. Ronnow, B. S., Reyna, S. P., Muhlestein, J. B., et al. (2005). C-reactive protein predicts death in patients with non-ischemic cardiomyopathy. *Cardiology, 104*, 196–201.
123. Ishikawa, C., Tsutamoto, T., Fujii, M., et al. (2006). Prediction of mortality by high-sensitivity C-reactive protein and brain natriuretic peptide in patients with dilated cardiomyopathy. *Circ J, 70*, 857–863.
124. Alonso-Martínez, J. L., Llorente-Diez, B., Echegaray-Agara, M., et al. (2002). C-reactive protein as a predictor of improvement and readmission in heart failure. *Eur J Heart Fail, 4*, 331–336.
125. Mueller, C., Laule-Kilian, K., Christ, A., et al. (2006). Inflammation and long-term mortality in acute congestive heart failure. *Am Heart J, 151*, 845–850.
126. Siirilä-Waris, K., Lassus, J., Melin, J., et al. (2006). Characteristics, outcomes, and predictors of 1-year mortality in patients hospitalized for acute heart failure. *Eur Heart J, 27*, 3011–3017.
127. Villacorta, H., Masetto, A. C., & Mesquita, E. T. (2007). C-reactive protein: an inflammatory marker with prognostic value in patients with decompensated heart failure. *Arq Bras Cardiol, 88*, 585–589.
128. Horwich, T. B., Patel, J., MacLellan, W. C., et al. (2003). Cardiac troponin I is associated with impaired hemodynamics, progressive left ventricular dysfunction, and increased mortality rates in advanced heart failure. *Circulation, 108*, 833–838.
129. Mann, D. L. (1999). Mechanisms and models in heart failure. *Circulation, 100*, 999–1008.
130. Olivetti, G., Abbi, R., Quaini, F., et al. (1997). Apoptosis in the failing human heart. *N Engl J Med, 336*, 1131–1141.
131. Logeart, D., Beyne, P., Cusson, C., et al. (2001). Evidence of cardiac myolysis in severe nonischemic heart failure and the potential role of increased wall strain. *Am Heart J, 141*, 247–253.
132. Anversa, P., & Kajstura, J. (1998). Myocyte cell death in the diseased heart. *Circ Res, 82*, 1231–1233.
133. Wu, A. H. B., & Ford, L. (1999). Release of cardiac troponin in acute coronary syndromes: ischemia or necrosis? *Clin Chim Acta, 284*, 161–174.
134. Ilva, T., Lassus, J., Siirilä-Waris, K., et al. (2008). Clinical significance of cardiac troponins I and T in acute heart failure. *Eur J Heart Fail, 10*, 772–779.
135. Sato, Y., Yamada, T., Taniguchi, R., et al. (2001). Persistently increased serum concentrations of cardiac troponin T in patients with idiopathic dilated cardiomyopathy are predictive of adverse outcomes. *Circulation, 103*, 369–374.
136. Missov, M., Calzolari, C., & Pau, B. (1997). Circulating cardiac troponin I in severe congestive heart failure. *Circulation, 96*, 2953–2958.
137. Setsuta, K., Seino, Y., Takahashi, N., et al. (1999). Clinical significance of elevated levels of cardiac troponin T in patients with chronic heart failure. *Am J Cardiol, 84*, 608–611.
138. Del Carlo, C. H., & O'Connor, C. M. (1999). Cardiac troponins in congestive heart failure. *Am Heart J, 138*, 646–653.
139. La Vecchia, L. L., Mezzena, G., Zanolla, L., et al. (2000). Cardiac troponin I as a diagnostic and prognostic marker in severe heart failure. *J Heart Lung Transplant, 19*, 644–652.
140. Peacock, W. F., 4th, De Marco, T., Fonarow, G. C., et al. (2008). Cardiac troponin and outcome in acute heart failure. *N Engl J Med, 358*, 2117–2126.
141. Hudson, M. P., O'Connor, C. M., Gattis, W. A., et al. (2004). Implications of elevated cardiac troponin T in ambulatory patients with heart failure: a prospective analysis. *Am Heart J, 147*, 546–552.
142. Latini, R., Masson, S., Anand, I. S., et al. (2007). Prognostic value of very low plasma concentrations of troponin T in patients with stable chronic heart failure. *Circulation, 116*, 1242–1249.
143. Ronco, C., Haapio, M., House, A. A., et al. (2008). Cardiorenal syndrome. *J Am Coll Cardiol, 52*, 1527–1539.
144. Bolignano, D., Donato, V., Coppolino, G., et al. (2008). Neutrophil gelatinase–associated lipocalin (NGAL) as a marker of kidney damage. *Am J Kidney Dis, 52*, 595–605.
145. Schmidt-Ott, K. M., Mori, K., Li, J. Y., et al. (2007). Dual action of neutrophil gelatinase–associated lipocalin. *J Am Soc Nephrol, 18*, 407–413.
146. Devireddy, L. R., Gazin, C., Zhu, X., et al. (2005). A cell-surface receptor for lipocalin 24p3 selectively mediates apoptosis and iron uptake. *Cell, 123*, 1293–1305.
147. Hvidberg, V., Jacobsen, C., Strong, R. K., et al. (2005). The endocytic receptor megalin binds the iron transporting neutrophil-gelatinase–associated lipocalin with high affinity and mediates its cellular uptake. *FEBS Lett, 579*, 773–777.
148. Mishra, J., Mori, K., Ma, Q., et al. (2004). Neutrophil gelatinase–associated lipocalin: a novel early urinary biomarker for cisplatin nephrotoxicity. *Am J Nephrol, 24*, 307–315.
149. Mishra, J., Dent, C., Tarabishi, R., et al. (2005). Neutrophil gelatinase–associated lipocalin (NGAL) as a biomarker for acute renal injury after cardiac surgery. *Lancet, 365*, 1231–1238.
150. Hirsch, R., Dent, C., Pfriem, H., et al. (2007). NGAL is an early predictive biomarker of contrast-induced nephropathy in children. *Pediatr Nephrol, 22*, 2089–2095.
151. Wagener, G., Jan, M., Kim, M., et al. (2006). Association between increases in urinary neutrophil gelatinase–associated lipocalin and acute renal dysfunction after adult cardiac surgery. *Anesthesiology, 105*, 485–491.
152. Bachorzewska-Gajewska, H., Malyszko, J., Sitniewska, E., et al. (2006). Neutrophil-gelatinase–associated lipocalin and renal function after percutaneous coronary interventions. *Am J Nephrol, 26*, 287–292.
153. Damman, K., van Veldhuisen, D. J., Navis, G., et al. (2008). Urinary neutrophil gelatinase associated lipocalin (NGAL), a marker of tubular damage, is increased in patients with chronic heart failure. *Eur J Heart Fail, 10*, 997–1000.
154. Bolignano, D., Basile, G., Parisi, P., et al. (2009). Increased plasma neutrophil gelatinase–associated lipocalin levels predict mortality in elderly patients with chronic heart failure. *Rejuvenation Res, 12*, 7–14.
155. Ljungman, S., Laragh, J. H., & Cody, R. J. (1990). Role of the kidney in congestive heart failure. Relationship of cardiac index to kidney function. *Drugs, 39*(Suppl 4), 10–21.
156. Ng, L. L., Pathik, B., Loke, I. W., et al. (2006). Myeloperoxidase and C-reactive protein augment the specificity of B-type natriuretic peptide in community screening for systolic heart failure. *Am Heart J, 152*, 94–101.
157. Dunlay, S. M., Gerber, Y., Weston, S. A., et al. (2009). Prognostic value of biomarkers in heart failure: application of novel methods in the community. *Circ Heart Fail, 2*, 393–400.
158. Zairis, M. N., Tsiaousis, G. Z., Georgilas, A. T., et al. (2009 Jan 19). Multimarker strategy for the prediction of 31 days cardiac death in patients with acutely decompensated chronic heart failure. *Int J Cardiol*, [Epub ahead of print].
159. Anand, I. S., Latini, R., Florea, V. G., et al. (2005). In C-reactive protein in heart failure: prognostic value and the effect of valsartan. *Circulation*, 112, 428–434.

CHAPTER 38

Measuring Quality Outcomes in Heart Failure

Edward P. Havranek

Systematic efforts to measure and improve the quality of medical care date back to the early 1900s[1] but have gained momentum only since about 2000. The pursuit of higher quality care is best viewed as an extension of clinical care in the movement toward increasing scientific rigor that has characterized the explosive growth in medical science since World War II. The forces behind the movement toward improved quality of care are both internal, coming from within medicine, and external, from society at large.[2] Thus, measures of the quality of care must be useful within health care organizations for the purpose of guiding internal quality improvement efforts and across health care organizations for the purpose of motivating organizations to improve care. Within organizations, quality measurement became important as quality improvement methods developed in manufacturing by W. Edwards Deming[3,4] began to be transferred to service organizations such as health care (Figure 38-1). Across organizations, measurement of quality of care has assumed increasing importance as quality measures have become publicly reported and comparisons have been made to determine reimbursement in "pay-for-performance" schemas.

Heart failure has occupied a prominent position in efforts to improve quality of care. Along with acute myocardial infarction, atrial fibrillation, and pneumonia, it was a condition targeted by Medicare for quality improvement efforts in 1998.[5] The reasons for this focus on heart failure are several: Mortality is high, heart failure is a common condition, and because of its chronicity and frequently severe morbidity, hospitalization is often needed. In combination, these factors result in exceptionally high cost to the health care system. Heart failure is thought to be the diagnosis entailing the highest cost among Medicare patients.[6] Finally, basic care for heart failure is strongly evidence-based, which has facilitated the development of consensus on quality measures.

GENERAL PRINCIPLES OF QUALITY MEASUREMENT

Defining Quality

Quality is an elusive concept that, particularly when applied to health care, defies definition. As detailed in a report from the Institute of Medicine,[2] high-quality health care is agreed to be described along six dimensions (Table 38-1).

A Measurement Framework

Although quality should be described by measurement of the *outcomes* of care, this may not always be possible. Circumstances may dictate that, under the framework first proposed by Donabedian[7,8] (Table 38-2), quality be measured by *processes* or *structures* of care.

Outcomes. Measuring outcomes such as mortality, hospital admission, and functional capacity have the obvious advantage of being recognized as relevant and important. Most outcomes are measured precisely, and those measurements may be readily available from administrative records.

However, measuring outcomes is generally not sufficient for guiding quality improvement efforts within organizations, since outcomes cannot be acted on directly. Although the ultimate goal might be reduction in operative mortality at a hospital, the goal cannot be accomplished unless the preoperative, intraoperative, and postoperative processes that potentially contribute to mortality can be identified, measured, and changed. Outcome events may not be suitable for comparing quality of care across organizations because numbers of cases are so small that differences in event rates may not be statistically significant; rather, the events may occur by chance.[9] Organizations using continuous quality improvement techniques need to remeasure quality at relatively frequent intervals; when numbers of outcomes are small, it can be difficult to judge whether differences over time are random or are the result of the organization's quality improvement effort. Finally, fair comparison of outcomes requires that the risk of the outcome intrinsic to the patient be equalized across the organizations being compared; this process is known as "risk adjustment."[10,11] The development of statistical models for risk adjustment is a laborious process, and retrospective statistical adjustment for risk is always subject to error from unmeasured confounding.

In addition to statistical concerns regarding the use of outcomes to measure quality of care, there are philosophical concerns regarding the selection of which outcome or outcomes to measure. Care for heart failure is an excellent example, in which mortality seems to be the obvious outcome to measure, as it has been in clinical trials (see also Chapter 34). If, however, mortality is being used to assess the quality of a hospital's care, problems arise in specifying the time frame used to define mortality. Mortality over long terms, such as 1 year, is affected by care related to the index hospitalization, but it also may be affected by care during subsequent hospitalizations, perhaps at other institutions, and to outpatient care outside the control of the index hospital. Shorter observational time frames such as 30 days may better reflect care during the index hospitalization, but it may be too short to detect

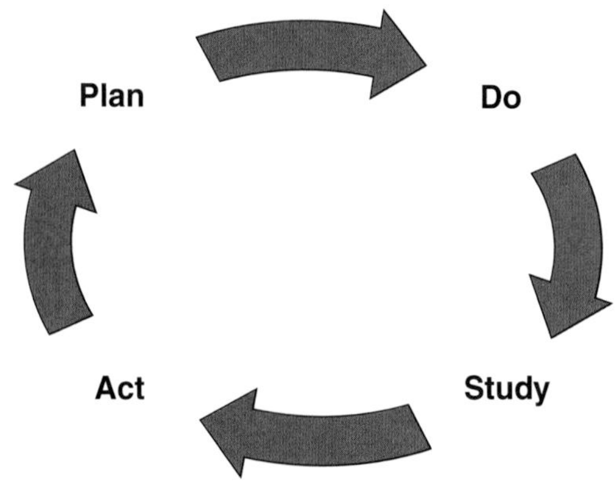

FIGURE 38–1 The role of quality measurement in continuous quality improvement. Quality measurement occurs during the study phase of the "plan-do-study-act" (PDSA), or Shewhart, cycle (attributed to W. Edwards Deming).

TABLE 38–1 Institute of Medicine Scheme for Describing Quality of Care[2]

Health care should be...	
Safe	Avoids injuries to patients from the care that is intended to help them
Effective	Provides services on the basis of scientific knowledge to all who could benefit and refrains from providing services to those not likely to benefit (avoiding underuse and overuse, respectively)
Patient-centered	Provides care that is respectful of and responsive to individual patient preferences, needs, and values and ensures that patient values guide all clinical decisions
Timely	Reduces waits and sometimes harmful delays for both those who receive and those who give care
Efficient	Avoids waste, including waste of equipment, supplies, ideas, and energy
Equitable	Provides care that does not vary in quality because of personal characteristics such as gender, ethnicity, geographical location, and socioeconomic status

differences related to high-quality care, such as initiation of β-blocker therapy (see also Chapter 46).

In addition to problems defining time frame, care that reduces mortality may not always satisfy the imperative that care be patient-centered. Again, heart failure provides an excellent example. It is well known to clinicians who specialize in heart failure that elderly patients and patients with advanced disease may value functional capacity and quality of life over duration of survival.[12,13] High-quality care for such individuals would generally not involve life-prolonging therapy such as defibrillator implantation as it might for other patients, and a lower mortality rate among such individuals would not necessarily reflect higher quality care.

Processes. Because of these difficulties in using outcomes to measure quality of care, investigators often rely on measurement of processes of care.[14] In order for a process to serve as a measure of quality, there must be consensus that there is a strong link between the process and a desirable outcome. It must also be actionable; that is, it must describe an aspect of care that is within the health care provider's control. Process measures are expressed as the percentage of eligible patients receiving a given aspect of care, and both numerator (the parameters specifying that the treatment was delivered) and denominator (the population eligible for the treatment) must be carefully and explicitly defined. Specifications for process measures necessarily involve a trade-off between specificity and sensitivity. For example, there is undeniable evidence from multiple clinical trials that angiotensin-converting enzyme (ACE) inhibitors decrease mortality and improve functional capacity in patients with heart failure caused by systolic dysfunction (see also Chapter 45). The strength of this evidence base is reflected in recommendations for ACE inhibitor use in guidelines of care for heart failure promulgated by several cardiology professional societies, and this evidence has served as the basis for measures of quality of care. Specification of these measures must strike a balance between being sensitive (designed to apply to the largest number of patients possible) and specific (designed to apply only to the subset of patients who are unequivocally eligible). In a sensitive measure, the numerator might include only patients receiving a dose consistent with benefit in clinical trials, and the denominator might include all patients who have an ejection fraction of less than 40% and have no absolute contraindication to an ACE inhibitor, such as prior angioedema or known bilateral renal artery stenosis. In a specific measure, the numerator might include patients receiving any dose, and the denominator might include all patients who have an ejection fraction of less than 40% and have no absolute or relative contraindications (such as renal insufficiency). Although specific measures have the advantage of greater validity for clinicians, they may be less useful because they do not address care for larger segments of the population of patients with heart failure than do more sensitive measures. More specific measures also tend to yield higher rates, which are less useful for guiding quality improvement because they are subject to "ceiling effects"; it is more difficult to improve rates from 90% to 100% than it is to effect an improvement from 50% to 60%.

Once numerator and denominator have been specified, process measures are typically subjected to pilot testing to determine feasibility and reliability. *Feasibility* implies that the data needed to calculate the measure can be obtained at reasonable cost within a reasonable time frame. The cost of collecting data to determine process measures is a hidden disadvantage of such measures. Because computerized medical records are not used in many hospitals and practices, data collection may require chart review, which is expensive. Tests of *reliability* typically involve assessment of reproducibility across providers and across data collectors.

TABLE 38–2 A Classification of Quality Measures

Measure	Advantages	Disadvantages
Outcomes	Validity is usually obvious Measurement is usually more precise	Numbers of events may be too small to judge whether observed differences are random or significant Statistical risk adjustment is required Time frame for observation may be difficult to specify Not directly actionable
Processes	Greater numbers of events are available for analysis	Validity may be less obvious when links with outcomes are less well established Greater effort is necessary to specify May be more costly to measure
Structures	May be most actionable	Validity is frequently questioned because of weakest links with outcomes

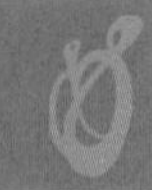

Structures. Finally, quality of care can be judged by assessing structures used to deliver care. Structures may include equipment and facilities, training and numbers of staff, administrative processes, and other materials. The links between structures and outcomes are generally not as strong as those demonstrable between processes and outcomes, and structures are less amenable to standardized evaluation across organizations. This approach has not been widely applied and has not been applied in heart failure. One example of a structural measure of quality is the use of procedural volumes to assess high-quality care.[15-17] Although in general there is a positive association between higher procedural volume and better outcomes, the associations are not strong, and variability in outcome at a given volume can be large. Computerized entry of physicians' orders and "closed" intensive care units, in which only critical care subspecialists serve as attending physicians, have also been used as measures of quality.[18]

The Role of the Organization of the Health Care System

The quality of health care must be viewed in the context in which it is delivered. Although many examples of integrated delivery systems exist, the current U.S. health care system is best characterized as being made up of a rather large number of independent components. Outpatient care is delivered jointly by primary care and specialist physicians who do have common medical records or administrative relationships. Hospital care may be provided by the same physicians who provide outpatient care, but it is increasingly delivered by hospital-based physicians. Physicians and hospitals are loosely affiliated and do not have administrative relationships. Additional independent components of the health care system include pharmacies, home health agencies, and long-term care facilities. Under these circumstances, responsibility for care of a patient with a chronic condition who requires frequent hospitalization is diffuse. When responsibility cannot be assigned, actionable quality measures are very difficult to formulate, and quality improvement efforts are fragmentary at best.

In addition to barriers created by fragmentation in the delivery system, financial incentives are often misaligned with efforts to measure and improve quality.[19] One of the best examples is the fate of hospital-based programs that manage the transition from inpatient to outpatient care for patients with heart failure. Such programs have been shown to produce beneficial outcomes, including reduced rates of readmission. Because hospital revenue may decline with decreased readmission rates under most reimbursement patterns currently in place, however, many transition management programs have been discontinued. Health care organizations that make investments in measuring and improving care are unlikely to see returns on those investments.

The Role of Health Information Technology

As discussed, measurement of process indicators is always necessary for purposes of internal quality improvement and sometimes necessary for comparing performance across organizations. Collection of data for calculating these measures is typically labor intensive. This can make data collection prohibitively expensive; furthermore, by the time data have been collected and measures calculated, conditions within organizations may have changed so that relevance of the data is questioned. Automated and ongoing query of properly structured electronic medical records can dramatically reduce the time and expense associated with data collection. Automated electronic record review often fails to identify contraindications to therapy. As a result, process measures derived from automated review often falsely identify failure to adhere to quality measures. They are thus more suitable for serial measurement within organizations rather than comparisons across organizations. In one study of over 1000 patients with diabetes at 21 Veterans Affairs facilities,[20] rates of best-practice diagnostic testing and medication use were lower with automated than manual chart review. In a more recent study, Baker and colleagues[21] focused on heart failure and obtained similar results. They reviewed patients' charts when an automated algorithm identified quality problems in 517 outpatients with heart failure. They found that performance was better, ranging from a 1.9% absolute increase on a β-blocker measure to a 23.2% absolute increase on a measure of warfarin in atrial fibrillation when additional chart review was performed.

Ongoing debate concerns whether use of an electronic record by itself improves quality. The subject was reviewed by Chaudhry and associates,[22] who focused on 76 studies conducted in the United States on multifunctional information systems; a comprehensive database of all studies they reviewed is available.[23] Although only one small early study they reported focused on heart failure,[24] studies of care that adhered to guidelines for preventive services (such as influenza vaccination) and for chronic illnesses (such as hypertension) revealed improvement, whereby decision support was linked with electronic records. There seemed to be consistent reduction in medication errors associated with computerized entry of physicians' orders.

THE CURRENT STATE OF QUALITY OF CARE FOR HEART FAILURE IN THE UNITED STATES

Of the six dimensions of quality measurement as defined by the Institute of Medicine[2] (see Table 38-1), three are relevant to the assessment of the quality of care for heart failure.

Effectiveness

Using the dimension of effectiveness to measure the quality of care implies that structures or processes of care known to be efficacious and effective are applied to the population of patients known to benefit, and the net result of this application is the achievement of desired outcomes. The key elements of this scheme are that (1) measured structures or processes are known to be *efficacious* to the highest level of certainty possible, (2) the measures are applied to a *defined population* rather than to individuals, and (3) the *net effects* on outcomes are considered.

A process for developing measures of effectiveness has been defined explicitly by the American College of Cardiology and the American Heart Association (ACC/AHA).[14] Once a target for the quality effort has been defined, the relevant literature is reviewed and synthesized. In practice, this review and synthesis are usually provided by guidelines, ideally developed independently of influence from commercial entities that might benefit materially from implementation of the process measure. In general, ACC/AHA class I and class III indications for therapy identify potential performance measures; class I indications are the "procedures/treatments that *should* be performed," and class III indications are the "procedures/treatments that *should not* be performed since they are not helpful and may be harmful."[14] Potential process measures are developed by specifying a numerator and a denominator for the measure and a period of time to which the measure will be applied. Not all class I and class III recommendations survive this process; in many cases, a sufficiently explicit specification may not be feasible. For instance, addition of an aldosterone antagonist is a class I recommendation for patients with severe symptoms except "under circumstances where monitoring for hyperkalemia or renal dysfunction is not anticipated to be feasible" because "the risks may outweigh the benefits."[14]

Although the specification of the guideline recommendation accurately reflects the known efficacy of these agents from randomized trials and the limits on their effectiveness from outcomes research, something that is "not anticipated to be feasible"[14] cannot be reliably turned into something measurable. Finally, measures are subjected to assessment of how interpretable, actionable, and feasible they are (Table 38-3). Measures not passing these three tests may still be useful to individual organizations as quality metrics[25] rather than performance measures in order to achieve self-directed quality goals.

Independent practice guidelines have been available for heart failure since 1994,[26] have been updated regularly, and are contemporary through 2009.[27,28] Few class I recommendations have been turned into process measures (Table 38-4). Currently, only assessment of left ventricular ejection fraction, prescription of an ACE inhibitor or angiotensin receptor blocker (ARB) to patients with reduced systolic function, provision of discharge instructions, and delivery of advice to quit smoking are addressed for hospitalized patients with heart failure.

TABLE 38–3 Criteria for Designating Possible Process Measures for Clinical Use

Interpretable	The degree to which a practitioner is likely to understand what the results mean and can take action if necessary
Actionable	The degree to which the performance measure is under the control of the entity being assessed
Feasible	The ease with which the required data can be collected and the measure can be assessed reproducibly; pilot testing is generally needed

Imperfect adherence to these measures has been documented extensively, with a general trend toward improvement over time; trends toward improved performance on the measures, however, have leveled off (Figure 38-2*A*). Rates of ejection fraction determination were 66% to 70% and rates of ACE inhibitor prescription were 68% to 72% at the beginning of Centers for Medicare and Medicaid Services' (CMS's) scrutiny of care for heart failure in the period 1998 to 2001.[5] According to the available data from the Medicare program for the period October 2007 through September 2008, national average rates of adherence to the discharge instruction measure were 17%; to the ejection fraction determination measure, 89%; and to the ACE inhibitor/ARB prescription measure, 88%.[28a] Certain patients' characteristics (including older age, presence of chronic kidney disease, and nonblack race) and providers' characteristics (smaller hospital size, nonteaching status, absence of advanced cardiac facilities, for-profit or public structure) have been associated with lower rates of guideline adherence.[29,30]

Whether adherence to the widely reported measures of the quality of care for heart failure has a net effect on outcomes remains somewhat controversial; thus, some authors have questioned whether the currently reported measures are sufficient.[31,32] Werner and Bradlow[33] examined the relationship between performance on the process measures for heart failure and risk-adjusted mortality rate during the inpatient stay and at 30 days and 1 year for 3657 hospitals with data available in the Hospital Compare database.[28a] They compared mortality rates in hospitals with performance above the 75th percentile with those in hospitals whose performance was below the 25th percentile. Absolute mortality reductions were small and of borderline statistical significance: 0.1% for inpatient mortality (P = .03), 0.2% for 30-day mortality

TABLE 38–4 Relationship between Guideline Recommendations and Performance Measures

Elements of Care for ACC/AHA 2009 Guideline Class I Recommendations for Patients with Heart Failure	ACC/AHA Performance Measure*	JCAHO/CMS Performance Measure*
Recommended elements of clinical assessment (history and physical examination: weight, blood pressure, activity level, volume status)	√	
Initial and follow-up laboratory testing, chest radiography, and electrocardiography	√	
Assessment of left ventricular systolic function	√	√
Assessment for coronary heart disease		
Diuretics for volume overload		
Use of ACE inhibitors and ARBs	√	√
Use of β-blockers	√	
Use of warfarin with concomitant atrial fibrillation	√	
Avoidance of potentially harmful medications		
Use of implantable defibrillators as primary prevention		
Use of implantable defibrillators as secondary prevention		
Use of cardiac resynchronization therapy		
Use of aldosterone antagonists		
Use of hydralazine/nitrates in African Americans		
Provision of written discharge instructions/patient education	√	√
Arrangement for posthospitalization follow-up		
Provision of end-of-life care when appropriate		
Multidisciplinary disease management for patients at high risk		

ACC/AHA, American College of Cardiology/American Heart Association; ACE, angiotensin-converting enzyme; ARB, angiotensin receptor blocker; JCAHO/CMS, Joint Commission on Accreditation of Healthcare Organizations/Centers for Medicare and Medicaid Services.

*Counseling for smoking cessation is an inpatient performance measure but is not an explicit guideline recommendation.

($P = .01$), and 0.2% for 1-year mortality ($P = .08$). Fonarow et al[34] reported associations between mortality at 60 to 90 days and performance on the CMS inpatient quality measures in a sub-sample consisting of 10% of patients enrolled in a multicenter heart failure registry. There was a significant reduction in likelihood of death or rehospitalization (odds ratio, 0.51; $P = .002$) for patients who were prescribed ACE inhibitors or ARBs at discharge, but no differences were found for the other measures. Mehta and coworkers,[35] reviewing the literature on process-outcome links for myocardial infarction and heart failure, cited four regional studies that demonstrated a reduction in heart failure–related mortality associated with use of ACE inhibitors. For elderly heart failure patients hospitalized between 2002 and 2006, there was no overall change in mortality despite significant improvement in performance on quality indicators. (see Figure 38-2*B*).

Patient-Centeredness

Patient-centeredness was further defined in the Institute of Medicine report[2] as

- Respect for patients, values, preferences, and expressed needs
- Coordination and integration of care

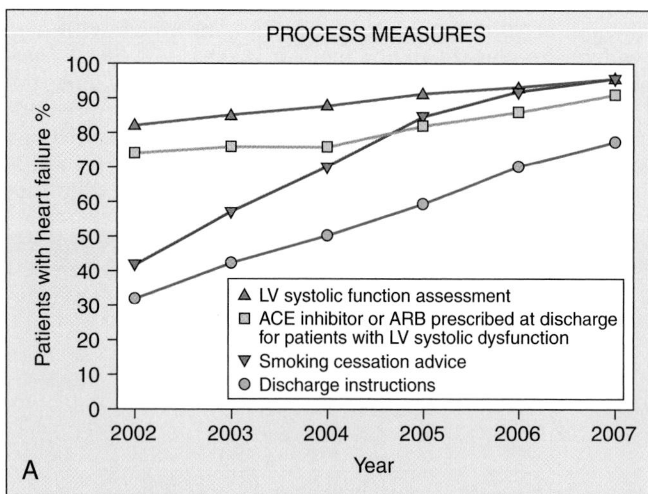

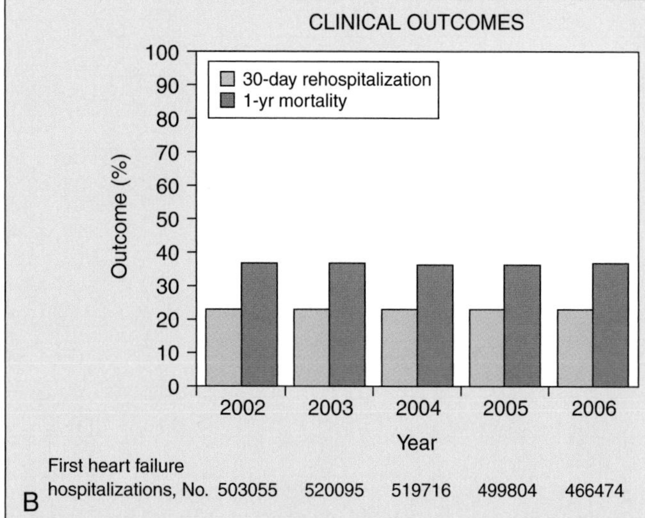

FIGURE 38-2 Temporal trends in process measures and clinical outcomes for Medicare patients hospitalized with heart failure. ACE, angiotensin-converting enzyme; ARB, angiotensin receptor blocker; LV, left ventricular. (From Fonarow GC, Peterson ED. Heart failure performance measures and outcomes: real or illusory gains. *JAMA* 2009;302 (7):792-794.) copyright © American Medical Association. All rights reserved (2011).

- Information, communication, and education
- Physical comfort
- Emotional support
- Involvement of family and friends

Each of these aspects has relevance for heart failure. Measurement of patient-centeredness in heart failure quality measures, however, has been rudimentary at best. One of the quality indicators adopted jointly by the Joint Commission on Accreditation of Healthcare Organizations (JCAHO) and CMS was the proportion of patients who received instruction at discharge regarding their medications, follow-up, and other care, which thus addresses the issue of information, communication, and education.

Provision of care in which patients' preferences are respected could be evaluated by assessing whether processes that provide end-of-life care when appropriate are in place. The degree to which physical comfort and emotional support are addressed could be evaluated with use of appropriate survey instruments. Coordination and integration of care should be an important goal of care for heart failure, but because of the barriers created by the organization and financing of care in the United States, the use of this dimension to evaluate quality across organizations seems premature. Evaluation of this dimension within some organizations, such as closed-panel health maintenance organizations, or globally budgeted systems, such as the U.S. Department of Veterans Affairs, may be of value. Improvement of transitions from hospital to outpatient care is currently under investigation as part of the Department of Veterans Affairs' Chronic Heart Failure Quality Enhancement Research Initiative (CHF QUERI).[37] A number of well-validated questionnaires have been used to measure health status in heart failure, a concept that encompasses physical capacity, emotional health, and quality of life. These questionnaires have not been used to compare the quality of care for heart failure across organizations. Emotional support is a common need among patients with heart failure; estimates of the prevalence of depression in patients with chronic heart failure have ranged from 23% to 47%.[38,39] There is as yet no consensus regarding routine screening for and management of depression in patients with heart failure.

Equity

Variation (by age, gender, race/ethnicity, and geography) in the quality of care for heart failure has been investigated. When issues of equity in medical care are studied, it must be kept in mind that differences in care do not necessarily constitute disparities in care.[40] For a difference to be considered a disparity, possible contraindications, patient preferences, clinical characteristics, and differences in eligibility must be accounted for. Differences in structures or processes of care should also be associated with differences in outcomes, Because it may not be clear whether a difference results from overtreatment in one group or undertreatment in the other.

Age

In general, advanced age is independently associated with lower rates of guideline-concurrent care.

Yancy and associates[41] reported that with increase in age, by tertile, the less likely patients would be to receive ACE inhibitors, β-blockers, aldosterone antagonists, and devices. Fonarow and colleagues[42] reported that in a large national registry of hospitalized patients with heart failure, patients older than 75 were less likely to receive guideline-based care than were younger patients. Forman and colleagues,[43] reporting results from a national quality improvement registry, found that older age was associated with lower rates of medical therapy. For instance, β-blockers were prescribed to 90.9% of eligible patients younger than 65 years but to only 82.7% of patients older than 85 years. In an analysis restricted to patients older than 65, another study did not reveal significant gradients with regard to age in the prescription of ACE inhibitors.[44]

Whether these age-related differences represent unacceptable variation in care remains somewhat open to interpretation. Eligibility may not be equivalent for older and younger patients. The studies that demonstrated the efficacy of drugs that reduce mortality in heart failure may not have enrolled sufficient numbers of elderly subjects.[45] Presence of contraindications may vary with age in ways that are difficult to measure. Enrollment criteria for studies of ACE inhibitors and aldosterone antagonists included serum creatinine level to exclude patients with significant kidney disease; however, this measure reflects renal function relatively poorly in older individuals. Preferences for life-prolonging therapy, a factor difficult to infer from chart review, may be lesser in the elderly. Nonetheless, there is adequate documentation in the literature that age bias affects medical decision making, and clinicians specializing in heart failure should make efforts to ensure that guideline-based therapy is not withheld from older patients without good reason.

Gender

In general, investigators have failed to demonstrate consistent patterns of differences by gender in the quality of care for heart failure after accounting for a lower incidence of ischemic heart disease and older age in women.

Within the context of a nationwide quality assessment of hospitalized patients with heart failure, Fonarow and colleagues[42] found no differences between men and women in the likelihood of receiving guideline-based medical therapy. Similar data sources[41,46] have revealed similar results; most, but not all, measures have shown no gender differences. A review of studies comparing treatment for heart failure and acute myocardial infarction by gender in Medicare patients[47] concluded that "within multivariate models, gender differences in treatment were small and in many cases insignificant. These national datasets fail to reveal a strong sex bias in treatment among patients aged ≥65 years." Readmission rates and mortality did not differ appreciably by gender after other demographic and clinical characteristics were controlled.

In contrast to findings of no significant gender differences in medication use in heart failure, there may be significant differences in device use. Use of implantable defibrillators and biventricular resynchronization pacing is not a formal quality indicator, and indications have changed considerably as a result of studies and changes in Medicare payment rules. Nonetheless, data from registries[48,49] and from a national sample of Medicare data[50] indicate that women are less likely to receive implantable defibrillators than are men with comparable indications.

This pattern is consistent with prior findings that women are less likely to undergo other cardiac procedures such as catheterization.[51] Whether gender bias is playing a role in differential procedure use remains somewhat uncertain, but quality measurement in heart failure, when expanded to device use, should include efforts to ensure equity, both in process and in outcome,[52,53] across gender.

Race and Ethnicity

Investigation into possible inequities in care by race and ethnicity is inevitably complicated by the confounding effects of socioeconomic status; minority individuals in the United States are more likely to be poor and to lack health insurance. Race and ethnicity are so tightly linked to socioeconomic status that, for the purposes of identifying disparities, separating them is not useful. Also complicating the investigation is the fact that robust adjustment is needed because the epidemiological profile of heart failure differs between white people and African Americans. African Americans are more likely to have a hypertensive cause, and less likely to have an ischemic cause, of heart failure[54-56] (Table 38-5). They also have similar or better survival rates, despite higher readmission rates.[57,58] In general, African American and white patients have similar rates of guideline-based care for heart failure. Care for Latino, Asian descent, and Native American patients has not been well characterized.

In a national quality-of-care registry,[54] African Americans were slightly more likely to be treated with ACE inhibitors. Similar findings have been noted in nationwide surveys by Medicare[57] and the Department of Veterans Affairs.[58-60] In a study of the same Medicare cohort,[61] lower socioeconomic status (determined from the average for the patients' area of residence) was not associated with likelihood of receiving guideline-based therapy, but it was associated with higher 1-year mortality rates. These studies, conducted in settings in which access to care based on insurance status is not an issue (Medicare and the Veterans Affairs system), suggest that when access to care is similar across racial lines, medical treatment for heart failure is equitable.

The situation with regard to use of implanted defibrillators is somewhat different: The available data have consistently demonstrated that African American patients are less likely than white patients to receive implanted defibrillators.[48,49,62,63] These studies are hampered by the fact that registries of patients receiving defibrillators and registries of patients hospitalized with heart failure may not accurately reflect the population of patients eligible for defibrillator implantation. Access may be different according to geography.[64,65] It is tempting to ascribe remaining disparities to bias and prejudice, but direct measurements of bias and prejudice have not been made.

Geography

Relatively little attention has been paid to potential differences in the quality of care for heart failure by location. Researchers have looked for small area variation[66] and for rural-urban differences.

Using chart review data from a sample of over 30,000 Medicare heart failure discharges, Havranek and coworkers[29] assessed variation across 306 hospital referral regions in the United States. A smoothing technique was used to account

TABLE 38–5 Differences in Causes of Heart Failure, by Race*

	OPTIMIZE-HF[54]		U.S. Carvedilol Heart Failure Study[55]		SOLVD[56]	
Cause	**African American**	**White**	**Black**	**Nonblack**	**African American**	**White**
Hypertension	39%	19%	66%	48%	62%	35%
Ischemia	30%	49%	32%	52%	54%	78%

OPTIMIZE-HF, Organized Program to Initiate Lifesaving Treatment in Hospitalized Patients with Heart Failure; *SOLVD*, Studies of Left Ventricular Dysfunction.

*A higher likelihood of hypertensive cardiomyopathy in African Americans may explain the higher likelihood that evidence-based medical treatment will be initiated for African American patients.

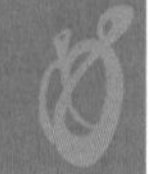

for random variation. Rates of left ventricular ejection fraction documentation ranged from 30.1% to 67.2%, and rates of ACE inhibitor prescription varied from 55.8% to 87.1% (Figure 38-3). Small, rural, nonteaching hospitals without advanced cardiac facilities tended to have lower rates on quality indicators. Nawal Lutfiyya and associates[67] examined differences in care for several conditions, including heart failure, provided in rural critical access hospitals in comparison with urban acute care hospitals. Critical access hospitals are designated for differential reimbursement by the CMS on the basis of rural location at least 35 miles from another hospital, provision of 24-hour emergency services, short average length of stay, and a size of no more than 25 beds. Rural hospitals were less likely than urban hospitals to document left ventricular function in patients with a diagnosis of heart failure (85.8% vs. 63.3%), but for patients with documented systolic dysfunction, they were equally likely to prescribe ACE inhibitors. Despite these process differences, Ross and colleagues[68] reported no differences in risk-adjusted 30-day mortality rates for heart failure across the continuum from rural to urban hospitals in a nationwide sample of Medicare records.

These studies suggest that regional differences in quality of care for heart failure may be related to limited availability of cardiac services in rural areas and that overall variation is lower than has been documented for other medical care. Data, however, are limited to the Medicare population and to a narrow range of quality indicators.

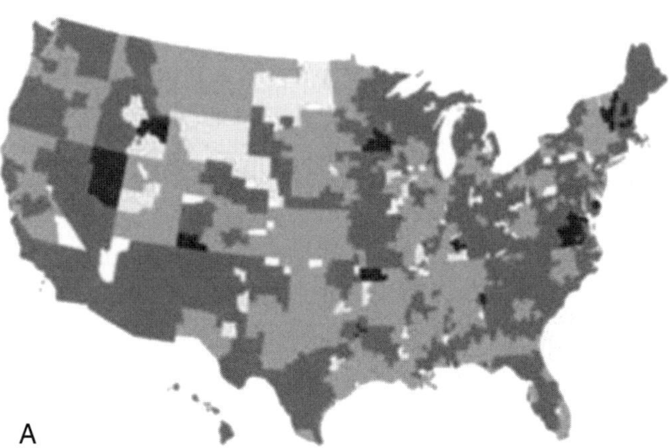

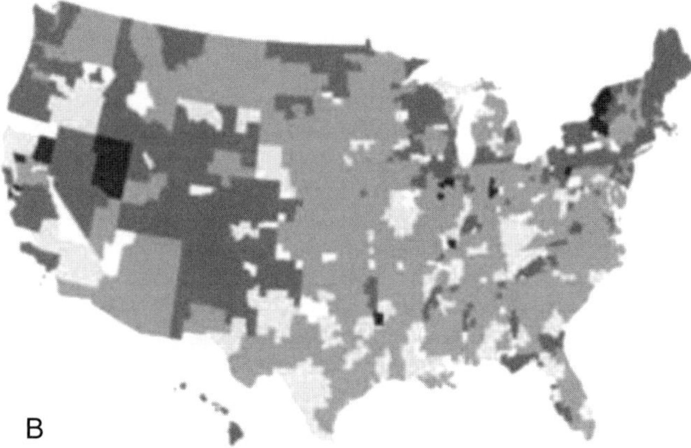

FIGURE 38-3 **A**, Variation in rates of documentation of ejection fraction by hospital referral region. *Darker shading* indicates higher rates. **B,** Variation in rates of angiotensin-converting enzyme (ACE) inhibitor prescription by hospital referral region. *Darker shading* indicates higher rates. (From Havranek EP, Wolfe P, Masoudi FA, et al. Provider and hospital characteristics associated with geographic variation in the evaluation and management of elderly patients with heart failure. *Arch Intern Med* 2004;164:1186-1191.)

Uses of Quality Measures

Continuous Quality Improvement

Measurement of quality, typically in the form of process measures, is a necessary component of continuous quality improvement within organizations (see Figure 38-1). Although internal efforts are typically directed at the measures used to compare effectiveness across organizations, high-performing organizations may be replacing these measures with quality metrics[69] not used for cross-organizational comparison. An example might be a quality improvement initiative to ensure that all patients with heart failure who are eligible for an implantable cardioverter-defibrillator, according to the most recent guidelines, have received a referral.

Public Reporting

Data on provider performance have been made public by government organizations since at least 1986, when the predecessor of CMS, the Health Care Financing Organization (HCFA), published a list of 269 hospitals whose risk-adjusted in-hospital mortality rates were high enough to be considered outliers.[70] A review published in 2000 found that rigorous evaluations of the impact of public reporting of performance data had been published for seven organizations that had released data[71]. These data covered a wide range of services and conditions, including obstetrics, cardiac surgery, myocardial infarction, and hip fracture. Since then, the type and volume of provider performance data reported by government agencies to the public has continued to grow. Despite the technical difficulties in producing valid measurements, outcomes of care are increasingly being reported. In this regard, an ACC/AHA task force[72] proposed standards for outcome measures intended for public reporting, in view of the high potential for the publication of misleading information (Box 38-1). Such measures must be explicitly defined, be constructed according to reliable data, and account for preexisting differences in patients' risk of the outcome in question. Reporting of the measures must account for the inherent uncertainty of statistical models.

CMS began reporting process measures for heart failure in 2004, 30-day mortality rates in 2007,[73] and 30-day readmission rates in 2009 on its Hospital Compare website.[28a] The outcome measures employ risk adjustment models[10,11] that generally conform to the ACC/AHA recommendations cited previously.

BOX 38–1 Preferred Attributes of Models Used for Publicly Reported Outcomes

Clear and explicit definition of an appropriate patient sample
Clinical coherence of model variables
Sufficiently high-quality and timely data
Designation of an appropriate reference time before which covariates are derived and after which outcomes are measured
Use of an appropriate outcome and a standardized period of outcome assessment
Application of an analytical approach that takes into account the multilevel organization of data
Disclosure of the methods used to compare outcomes, including disclosure of performance of risk-adjustment methodology in derivation and validation samples

From Krumholz HM, Brindis RG, Brush JE, Cohen DJ, et al. Standards for statistical models used for public reporting of health outcomes: an American Heart Association Scientific Statement from the Quality of Care and Outcomes Research Interdisciplinary Writing Group. *Circulation*. 2006; (24)113:456-462.

Similar data are reported by JCAHO.[73a] The process measures cover the four inpatient measures discussed previously: left ventricular function assessment, use of ACE inhibitors or ARBs, smoking cessation advice, and discharge instructions. The mortality and readmission measures are reported as relative to the national averages with appropriate error estimates and are further characterized as being above, below, or no different from the average. In practice, the number of hospitals characterized as have rates below the average has been quite small.

The effect of public reporting is difficult to gauge. Its purpose is presumably to enable health care to more closely resemble an efficient market, with consumers and purchasers gravitating toward providers with the best performance and away from underperforming providers. There is some evidence that this is taking place with regard to consumer's choice of health plan,[74,75] although most of the information available to them is about quality of service rather than quality of care. There is essentially no evidence that choice of hospitals is affected by the availability of quality-of-care information, even when that information is about potentially actionable choices such as coronary artery surgery.[71,74] Public reporting does, however, appear to motivate hospitals to initiate quality improvement efforts.[74] It has been suggested that public reporting may have unintended adverse consequences[76]: It may increase the likelihood that providers will avoid caring for patients at high risk or the likelihood that socioeconomically disadvantaged patients, with less access to information, will have no choice except underperforming providers. No reported data have demonstrated that this is the case. In the end, therefore, it is difficult to argue that measures of quality should *not* be made available to the public. The most important effect of public reporting, although not quantifiable, may be changing providers' fundamental attitudes about their responsibilities for transparency and accountability.

Pay for Performance

There have been efforts in the United States and in the United Kingdom to improve quality by providing financial incentives to providers that score well on performance measures. In the United States, data are available from the Premier Hospital Quality Incentive Demonstration Project and the Physician Group Practice Demonstration Project, conducted by CMS. Although pay for performance is being used by commercial insurers[77] and Medicaid,[78] results from these programs have not been reported. In the United Kingdom, the National Health Service has reported results from the Quality and Outcomes Framework. Care for heart failure was featured in all these projects.

The Premier Hospital Quality Incentive Demonstration Project was initiated by CMS in October 2003. Participants were part of the Premier nationwide network of not-for-profit hospitals; as of July 2009, 227 hospitals were participating. Hospitals scoring in the top decile on composite quality measures for acute myocardial infarction, heart failure, coronary artery bypass grafting, pneumonia, and total hip or knee replacement were given a bonus of an additional 2% of their diagnostic group–related payment; those in the second decile received a 1% bonus. In the third year, comparable decreases in payment were instituted for the bottom two deciles. A report of the initial result of the project[79] demonstrated overall improvement in composite measures of quality in participating hospitals, in comparison with a similar group of nonparticipating hospitals. For heart failure, care on a composite appropriate care measure encompassing left ventricular function assessment, use of ACE inhibitors, provision of discharge instructions, and smoking cessation assessment improved from 76.1% to 84.0% in the control hospitals and from 76.1% to 88.3% in the hospitals receiving financial incentives. The initial 3-year project was extended for 3 more years, through the end of September 2009. During the extension phase, risk-adjusted mortality and readmission rates were added to the roster of quality measures. Results for the extension period are not yet available, although trends from the first 3 years have been reported to have continued through the end of the fourth year.[80] Evaluations of the program independent of CMS, however, have yielded contrasting results. Ryan[81] used econometric modeling of 30-day risk-adjusted rates of mortality from heart failure, as well as from pneumonia, acute myocardial infarction, and coronary artery surgery, and could find no benefit associated with the program. Another study of acute myocardial infarction alone also demonstrated no effect on mortality.[82]

The Physician Group Practice Demonstration Project had a slightly different structure and was based not only on quality measures but also on cost savings.[83] Ten large geographically diverse group practices were chosen for the project. If a group demonstrated savings for Medicare in the targeted patient populations, it became eligible for an annual performance bonus funded by those cost savings. The amount of the bonus was based on performance on quality measures for heart failure, diabetes, coronary heart disease, hypertension, and cancer screening. Because this was an outpatient-based project, the heart failure measures were significantly more comprehensive than those previously used for cross-organizational comparison, addressing use of ACE inhibitors, β-blockers, warfarin in the presence of atrial fibrillation, ejection fraction assessment, patient education, and monitoring of weight at the time of writing and blood pressure. The 3-year program began in 2005, and final results are not yet available. It has been reported that of the 10 groups, 5 earned bonuses for the first year of the program.[83,84]

The Quality and Outcomes Framework program in the United Kingdom was not a demonstration project but rather a full-faith wholesale change in the reimbursement structure for physicians in England to one that includes incentives for performance in clinical care, practice organization, and patients' experience.[85] Care for heart failure was not assessed under this framework; the current discussion is limited to its use in the general assessment of pay-for-performance schema. A study of the performance of 42 primary care practices before and after introduction of the program revealed modest improvements in quality.[86] The authors concluded that "once targets were reached, the improvement in the quality of care...slowed, and the quality of care declined for two conditions that had not been linked to incentives."

The bulk of the evidence suggests that providing financial incentives to organizations produces modest gains in quality that are limited to the care being scrutinized. Incentive structures different from those employed thus far may produce better results.[87,88] There are also remaining questions about whether such programs will exacerbate inequities in care by giving incentives to providers that do not care for the underserved.[89-91]

FUTURE DIRECTIONS

Aligning financial incentives with quality, adopting information technology wisely, and widening the range of care processes measured are all necessary if the quality of care for heart failure is to improve in the future. Such changes, however, should be viewed as enabling and will not be sufficient to achieve the optimal level of care.

This chapter began by noting that much of the approach to quality measurement and improvement currently practiced in health care comes from thinking developed in manufacturing by Deming. One of the consistent themes in Deming's

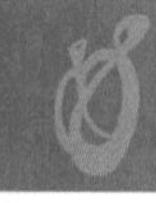

BOX 38–2 Deming's 14 Points for Transformation[3]

1. Create constancy of purpose toward improvement of product and service.
2. Adopt the new philosophy.
3. Cease dependence on inspection to achieve quality.
4. End the practice of awarding business on the basis of price tag.
5. Improve constantly and forever the system of production and service.
6. Institute training on the job.
7. Institute leadership. The aim of supervision should be to help people to do a better job.
8. Drive out fear.
9. Break down barriers between departments.
10. Eliminate slogans, exhortations, and targets for the workforce.
11. Eliminate work standards, objectives, numbers, and numeric goals. Substitute leadership.
12. Remove barriers that rob people of their right to pride of workmanship.
13. Institute a program of education and self-improvement.
14. Transformation is everybody's job.

work is that improving the quality of the products of a system must result from fundamental change in the attitudes and behaviors of the participants in the system. In his 14 points[3] (Box 38-2), he urged managers to cease dependence on inspection and to eliminate exhortations and targets. In a sense, current national efforts to improve quality through the reporting of and payment for quality measures are inspection, exhortation, and targets. Progress toward improving the quality of health care requires fundamental change in the attitudes and behaviors of participants in the system rather than more intensive scrutiny.[92] Lessons from such fields as education, organizational psychology, and behavioral economics are probably helpful in effecting the needed cultural change.[93] The motivation for making these changes must begin to come from within organizations rather than be imposed from the outside.

Providing care of the highest possible quality is the most important basic value of health care professionals. Professionals deserve to work in a system that grows directly from this value, and patients deserve to be treated in such a system.

REFERENCES

1. Codman, EA (1990). The product of a hospital. 1914. *Arch Pathol Lab Med, 114*, 1106–1111.
2. *Institute of Medicine Committee on Quality of Health Care in America. Crossing the quality chasm: a new health system for the 21st century.* (2001). Washington, DC: National Academy Press.
3. Deming WE. *Out of the crisis*, Cambridge, MA, 1982, Massachusetts Institute of Technology Center for Advanced Educational Services
4. Deming, W. E. (1994). *The New Economics for Industry, Government, Education* (ed 2). Cambridge MA: Massachusetts Institute of Technology Center for Advanced Educational Services.
5. Jencks, S. F., Huff, E. D., & Cuerdon, T. (2003). Change in the quality of care delivered to Medicare beneficiaries, 1998-1999 to 2000-2001. *JAMA, 289*, 305–312.
6. Masoudi, F. A., Havranek, E. P., & Krumholz, H. M. (2002). The burden of chronic congestive heart failure in older persons: magnitude and implications for policy and research. *Heart Failure Reviews, 7*, 9–16.
7. Donabedian, A. (1966). Evaluating the quality of medical care. *Millbank Mem Fund Q, 44*, 166–206.
8. Donabedian, A. (1978). The quality of medical care. *Science, 200*, 856–864.
9. Normand, S. T., & Zou, K. H. (2002). Sample size considerations in observational health care quality studies. *Stat Med, 21*, 331–345.
10. Krumholz, H. M., Wang, Y., Mattera, J. A., et al. (2006). An administrative claims model suitable for profiling hospital performance based on 30-day mortality rates among patients with heart failure. *Circulation, 113*, 1693–1701.
11. Keenan, P. S., Normand, S. T., Lin, Z., et al. (2008). An administrative claims measure suitable for profiling hospital performance on the basis of 30-day all-cause readmission rates among patients with heart failure. *Circ Cardiovasc Qual Outcomes, 1*, 29–37.
12. Havranek, E. P., Lowes, B. L., Abraham, W. T., et al. (1999). Utilities are valid measures of health related quality of life in patients with heart failure. *J Card Fail, 5*, 85–91.
13. Stevenson, L. W., Hellkamp, A. S., Leier, C. V., et al. (2008). Changing preferences for survival after hospitalization with advanced heart failure. *J Am Coll Cardiol, 52*, 1702–1708.
14. Spertus, J. A., Eagle, K. A., Krumholz, H. M., et al. (2005). ACC/AHA methodology for the selection and creation of performance measures for quantifying the quality of cardiovascular care: a report of the ACC/AHA Task Force on Performance Measures. *J Am Coll Cardiol, 45*, 1147–1156.
15. Hannan, E. L., Siu, A. L., Kumar, D., et al. (1995). The decline in coronary artery bypass graft surgery mortality in New York state: the role of surgeon volume. *JAMA, 273*, 209–213.
16. Tu, J. V., Austin, P., & Chan, B. (2001). Relationship between annual volume of patients treated by admitting physician and mortality after acute myocardial infarction. *JAMA, 285*, 3116–3122.
17. O'Neill, W. W. (2009). A case against low-volume percutaneous coronary intervention centers [Comment]. *Circulation, 120*, 546–548.
18. Jha, A. K., Orav, E. J., Ridgway, A. B., et al. (2008). Does the Leapfrog program help identify high-quality hospitals? *Jt Comm J Qual Patient Saf, 34*, 318–325.
19. Havranek, E. P., Krumholz, H. M., Dudley, R. A., et al. (2003). Aligning quality and payment for heart failure care: defining the challenges. *J Card Fail, 9*, 251–254.
20. Kerr, E. A., Smith, D. M., Hogan, M. M., et al. (2002). Comparing clinical automated, medical record, and hybrid data sources for diabetes quality measures. *Jt Comm J Qual Improv, 28*, 555–565.
21. Baker, D. W., Persell, S. D., Thompson, J. A., et al. (2007). Automated review of electronic health records to assess quality of care for outpatients with heart failure. *Ann Intern Med, 146*, 270–277.
22. Chaudhry, B., Wang, J., Wu, S., et al. (2006). Systematic review: impact of health information technology on quality, efficiency, and costs of medical care. *Ann Intern Med, 144*, 742–752.
23. Agency for Healthcare Research and Quality. *Health Information Technology Costs & Benefits Database Project* (online database): http://healthit.ahrq.gov/portal/server.pt?open=514&objID=5562&mode=2&holderDisplayURL=http://prodportallb.ahrq.gov:7087/publishedcontent/publish/communities/a_e/ahrq_funded_projects/healthit_cost__benefits/home.html. Accessed January 22, 2010.
24. Perlini, S., Piepoli, M., Marti, G., et al. (1990). Treatment of chronic heart failure: an expert system advisor for general practitioners. *Acta Cardiol, 45*, 365–378.
25. Bonow, R. O., Masoudi, F. A., Rumsfeld, J. S., et al. (2008). ACC/AHA classification of care metrics: performance measures and quality metrics: a report of the American College of Cardiology/American Heart Association Task Force on Performance Measures. *J Am Coll Cardiol, 52*, 2113–2117.
26. Konstam, M., Dracup, K., Baker, D., et al. (June 1994). *Heart failure: evaluation and care of patients with left-ventricular systolic dysfunction. Clinical Practice Guideline no. 11 (AHCPR Publication No. 94-0612).* Rockville MD: Agency for Health Care Policy and Research, Public Health Service, U.S. Department of Health and Human Services.
27. Jessup, M., Abraham, W. T., Casey, D. E., et al. (2009) writing on behalf of the 2005 Guideline Update for the Diagnosis and Management of Chronic Heart Failure in the Adult Writing Committee. 2009 focused update: ACCF/AHA guidelines for the diagnosis and management of heart failure in adults: a report of the American College of Cardiology/American Heart Association Task Force on Practice Guidelines. *J Am Coll Cardiol, 53*, 1343–1382.
28. Hunt, S. A., Abraham, W. T., Chin, M. H., et al. (2009). 2009 focused update incorporated into the ACC/AHA 2005 guidelines for the diagnosis and management of heart failure in adults: a report of the American College of Cardiology Foundation/American Heart Association Task Force on Practice Guidelines. *J Am Coll Cardiol, 53*, e1–e90.

28a. U.S. Department of Health and Human Services: *Find and compare hospitals* (government webpage): http://www.hospitalcompare.hhs.gov. Accessed January 24, 2010.

29. Havranek, E. P., Wolfe, P., Masoudi, F. A., et al. (2004). Provider and hospital characteristics associated with geographic variation in the evaluation and management of elderly patients with heart failure. *Arch Intern Med, 164*, 1186–1191.
30. Vogeli, C., Kang, R., Landrum, M. B., et al. (2009). Quality of care provided to individual patients in US hospitals: results from an analysis of national Hospital Quality Alliance data. *Med Care, 47*, 591–599.
31. Bonow, R. O. (2008). Measuring quality in heart failure: do we have the metrics? *Circ Cardiovasc Qual Outcomes, 1*, 9–11.
32. Fonarow, G. C., & Peterson, E. D. (2009). Heart failure performance measures and outcomes: real or illusory gains. *JAMA, 302*, 792–794.
33. Werner, R. M., & Bradlow, E. T. (2006). Relationship between Medicare's hospital compare performance measures and mortality rates. *JAMA, 296*, 2694–2702.
34. Fonarow, G. C., Abraham, W. T., & Albert, N. M. (2007) for the OPTIMIZE-HF Investigators and Hospitals. Association between performance measures and clinical outcomes for patients hospitalized with heart failure. *JAMA, 297*, 61–70.
35. Mehta, R. H., Peterson, E. D., & Califf, R. M. (2007). Performance measures have a major effect on cardiovascular outcomes: a review. *Am J Med, 120*, 398–402.
36. Curtis, L. H., Greiner, M. A., Hammill, B. G., et al. (2008). Early and long-term outcomes of heart failure in elderly persons, 2001-2005. *Arch Intern Med, 168*, 2481–2488.
37. U.S. Department of Veterans Affairs. *Chronic heart failure (CHF) Quality Enhancement Research Initiative* (website): http://www.queri.research.va.gov/chf/default.cfm. Accessed January 22, 2010.
38. Havranek, E. P., Ware, M. G., & Lowes, B. L. (1999). The prevalence of depression in patients with heart failure. *Am J Cardiol, 84*, 348–350.
39. Gottlieb, S. S., Khatta, M., Friedman, E., et al. (2004). The influence of age, gender, and race on the prevalence of depression in heart failure patients. *J Am Coll Cardiol, 43*, 1542–1549.
40. Rathore, S. S., & Krumholz, H. M. (2004). Differences, disparities, and biases: clarifying racial variations in health care use. *Ann Intern Med, 141*, 635–638.
41. Yancy, C. W., Fonarow, G. C., Albert, N. M., et al. (2009). Influence of patient age and sex on delivery of guideline-recommended heart failure care in the outpatient cardiology practice setting: findings from IMPROVE HF. *Am Heart J, 157*, 754–762.

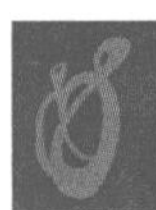

42. Fonarow, G. C., Abraham, W. T., Albert, N. M., et al. (2009) for the OPTIMIZE-HF Investigators and Hospitalset al. Age- and gender-related differences in quality of care and outcomes of patients hospitalized with heart failure (from OPTIMIZE-HF). *Am J Cardiol, 104*, 107–115.
43. Forman, D. E., Cannon, C. P., Hernandez, A. F., et al. (2009). for the Get With the Guidelines Steering Committee and Hospitals. Influence of age on the management of heart failure: findings from Get With the Guidelines-Heart Failure (GWTG-HF). *Am Heart J, 157*, 1010–1017.
44. Masoudi, F. A., Rathore, S. R., Wang, Y. F., et al. (2004). National patterns of use and effectiveness of angiotensin-converting enzyme inhibitors in older patients with heart failure and left ventricular systolic dysfunction. *Circulation, 110*, 724–731.
45. Masoudi, F. A., Havranek, E. P., Wolfe, P., et al. (2003). Most hospitalized older persons do not meet the enrollment criteria for clinical trials in heart failure. *Am Heart J, 146*, 250–257.
46. Rathore, S. S., Foody, J. M., Wang, Y., et al. (2005). Sex, quality of care, and outcomes of elderly patients hospitalized with heart failure: findings from the National Heart Failure Project. *Am Heart J, 149*, 121–128.
47. Gold, L. D., & Krumholz, H. M. (2006). Gender differences in treatment of heart failure and acute myocardial infarction: a question of quality or epidemiology? *Cardiol Rev, 14*, 180–186.
48. Hernandez, A. F., Fonarow, G. C., Liang, L., et al. (2007). Sex and racial differences in the use of implantable cardioverter-defibrillators among patients hospitalized with heart failure. *JAMA, 298*, 1525–1532.
49. El-Chami, M. F., Hanna, I. R., Bush, H., et al. (2007). Impact of race and gender on cardiac device implantations. *Heart Rhythm, 4*, 1420–1426.
50. Curtis, L. H., Al-Khatib, S. M., Shea, A. M., et al. (2007). Sex differences in the use of implantable cardioverter-defibrillators for primary and secondary prevention of sudden cardiac death. *JAMA, 298*, 1517–1524.
51. Redberg, R. F. (2005). Gender, race, and cardiac care: why the differences? *J Am Coll Cardiol, 46*, 1852–1854.
52. Redberg, R. F. (2007). Disparities in use of implantable cardioverter-defibrillators: moving beyond process measures to outcomes data. *JAMA, 298*, 1564–1566.
53. Peterson, P. N., Daugherty, S. L., Wang, Y., et al. (2009). Gender differences in procedure-related adverse events in patients receiving implantable cardioverter-defibrillator therapy. *Circulation, 119*, 1078–1084.
54. Yancy, C. W., Abraham, W. T., Albert, N. M., et al. (2008). Quality of care of and outcomes for African Americans hospitalized with heart failure: findings from the OPTIMIZE-HF (Organized Program to Initiate Lifesaving Treatment in Hospitalized Patients With Heart Failure) registry. *J Am Coll Cardiol, 51*, 1675–1684.
55. Yancy, C. W., Fowler, M. B., Colucci, W. S., et al. (2001). for the U.S. Carvedilol Heart Failure Study Group. Race and the response to adrenergic blockade with carvedilol in patients with chronic heart failure. *N Engl J Med, 344*, 1358–1365.
56. Exner, D. V., Dries, D. L., Domanski, M. J., et al. (2001). Lesser response to angiotensin-converting–enzyme inhibitor therapy in black as compared with white patients with left ventricular dysfunction. *N Engl J Med, 344*, 1351–1357.
57. Rathore, S. S., Foody, J. M., Wang, Y., et al. (2003). Race, quality of care, and outcomes of elderly patients hospitalized with heart failure. *JAMA, 289*, 2517–2524.
58. Deswal, A., Petersen, N. J., Souchek, J., et al. (2004). Impact of race on health care utilization and outcomes in veterans with congestive heart failure. *J Am Coll Cardiol, 43*, 778–784.
59. Deswal, A., Petersen, N. J., Urbauer, D. L., et al. (2006). Racial variations in quality of care and outcomes in an ambulatory heart failure cohort. *Am Heart J, 152*, 348–354.
60. Gordon, H. S., Johnson, M. L., & Ashton, C. M. (2002). Process of care in Hispanic, black, and white VA beneficiaries. *Med Care, 40*, 824–833.
61. Rathore, S. S., Masoudi, F. A., Wang, Y., et al. (2006). Socioeconomic status, treatment, and outcomes among elderly patients hospitalized with heart failure: findings from the National Heart Failure Project. *Am Heart J, 152*, 371–378.
62. Thomas, K. L., Al-Khatib, S. M., Kelsey, R. C., 2nd, et al. (2007). Racial disparity in the utilization of implantable-cardioverter defibrillators among patients with prior myocardial infarction and an ejection fraction of ≤35%. *Am J Cardiol, 100*, 924–929.
63. Farmer, S. A., Kirkpatrick, J. N., Heidenreich, P. A., et al. (2009). Ethnic and racial disparities in cardiac resynchronization therapy. *Heart Rhythm, 6*, 325–331.
64. Hasnain-Wynia, R., Baker, D. W., Nerenz, D., et al. (2007). Disparities in health care are driven by where minority patients seek care: examination of the hospital quality alliance measures. *Arch Intern Med, 167*, 1233–1239.
65. Jha, A. K., Orav, E. J., Li, Z., et al. (2007). Concentration and quality of hospitals that care for elderly black patients. *Arch Intern Med, 167*, 1177–1182.
66. Wennberg, J. E., & Cooper, M. M. (Eds.). (1999). *The quality of medical care in the United States: a report on the Medicare Program, The Dartmouth Atlas of Health Care 1999*. Chicago: American Health Association Press.
67. Nawal Lutfiyya, M., Bhat, D. K., Gandhi, S. R., et al. (2007). A comparison of quality of care indicators in urban acute care hospitals and rural critical access hospitals in the United States. *Int J Qual Health Care, 19*, 141–149.
68. Ross, J. S., Normand, S. L., Wang, Y., et al. (2008). Hospital remoteness and thirty-day mortality from three serious conditions. *Health Aff (Millwood), 27*, 1707–1717.
69. Bonow, R. O., Bennett, S., Casey, D. E., et al. (2005). ACC/AHA clinical performance measures for adults with chronic heart failure: a report of the American College of Cardiology/American Heart Association Task Force on Performance Measures. *J Am Coll Cardiol, 46*, 1144–1178.
70. Vladeck, B. C., Goodwin, E. J., Myers, L. P., et al. (1988). Consumers and hospital use: the HCFA "death list." *Health Aff (Millwood), 7*, 122–125.
71. Marshall, M. N., Shekelle, P. G., Leatherman, S., et al. (2000). The public release of performance data: what do we expect to gain? A review of the evidence. *JAMA, 283*, 1866–1874.
72. Krumholz, H. M., Brindis, R. G., Brush, J. E., et al. (2006). Standards for statistical models used for public reporting of health outcomes: an American Heart Association Scientific Statement from the Quality of Care and Outcomes Research Interdisciplinary Writing Group: cosponsored by the Council on Epidemiology and Prevention and the Stroke Council. Endorsed by the American College of Cardiology Foundation. *Circulation, 113*, 456–462.
73. Krumholz, H. M., & Normand, S. T. (2008). Public reporting of 30-day mortality for patients hospitalized with acute myocardial infarction and heart failure. *Circulation, 118*, 1394–1397.
73a. The Joint Commission. *Find a health care organization* (website): http://www.qualitycheck.org. Accessed January 25, 2010.
74. Fung, C. H., Lim, Y. W., Mattke, S., et al. (2008). Systematic review: the evidence that publishing patient care performance data improves quality of care. *Ann Intern Med, 148*, 111–123.
75. Faber, M., Bosch, M., Wollersheim, H., et al. (2009). Public reporting in health care: how do consumers use quality-of-care information? A systematic review. *Med Care, 47*, 1–8.
76. Werner, R. M., & Asch, D. A. (2005). The unintended consequences of publicly reporting quality information. *JAMA, 293*, 1239–1244.
77. Rosenthal, M. B., Landon, B. E., Normand, S. T., et al. (2006). Pay for performance in commercial HMOs. *N Engl J Med, 355*, 18951902.
78. Kuhmerker, K., & Hartman, T. (2007). *Pay-for-performance in state Medicaid programs: a survey of state Medicaid directors and programs*. New York: The Commonwealth Fund.
79. Lindenauer, P. K., Remus, D., Roman, S., et al. (2007). Public reporting and pay for performance in hospital quality improvement. *N Engl J Med, 356*, 486–496.
80. U.S. Department of Health and Human Services, Centers for Medicare and Medicaid Services. *Premier Hospital Quality Incentive Demonstration* (website): http://www.cms.hhs.gov/HospitalQualityInits/35_hospitalpremier.asp. Accessed January 22, 2010.
81. Ryan, A. M. (2009). Effects of the Premier Hospital Quality Incentive Demonstration on Medicare patient mortality and cost. *Health Serv Res, 44*, 821–842.
82. Glickman, S. W., Ou, F. S., DeLong, E. R., et al. (2007). Pay for performance, quality of care, and outcomes in acute myocardial infarction. *JAMA, 297*, 2373–2380.
83. Leavitt MO. *Report to Congress: Physician Group Practice Demonstration Project first evaluation report* (online report): http://www.cms.hhs.gov/DemoProjectsEvalRpts/downloads/PGP_Final_Congress.pdf. Accessed January 22, 2010
84. U.S. Government Accountability Office. *Report to Congressional Committees: Medicare physician payment care coordination programs used in demonstration show promise, but wider use of payment approach may be limited* (Report no. GAO-08–65, February 2008): http://www.gao.gov/new.items/d0865.pdf. Accessed January 22, 2010.
85. Roland, M. (2004). Linking physicians' pay to quality of care—a major experiment in the United Kingdom. *N Engl J Med, 351*, 1448–1454.
86. Campbell, S. M., Reeves, D., Kontopantelis, E., et al. (2009). Effects of pay for performance on the quality of primary care in England. *N Engl J Med, 361*, 368–378.
87. Fisher, E. S. (2006). Paying for performance—risks and recommendations. *N Engl J Med, 355*, 1845–1847.
88. Glickman, S. W., Boulding, W., Roos, J. M., et al. (2009). Alternative pay-for-performance scoring methods: implications for quality improvement and patient outcomes. *Med Care, 47*, 1062–1068.
89. Werner, R. M., Goldman, L. E., & Dudley, R. A. (2008). Comparison of change in quality of care between safety-net and non–safety-net hospitals. *JAMA, 299*, 2180–2187.
90. Karve, A. M., Ou, F. S., Lytle, B. L., et al. (2008). Potential unintended financial consequences of pay-for-performance on the quality of care for minority patients. *Am Heart J, 155*, 571–576.
91. Casalino, L. P., Elster, A., Eisenberg, A., et al. (2007). Will pay-for-performance and quality reporting affect health care disparities? *Health Aff (Millwood), 26*, w405–w414.
92. Werner, R. M., & McNutt, R. (2009). A new strategy to improve quality: rewarding actions rather than measures. *JAMA, 301*, 1375–1377.
93. Frølich, A., Talavera, J. A., Broadhead, P., et al. (2007). A behavioral model of clinician responses to incentives to improve quality. *Health Policy, 80*, 179–193.

CHAPTER 39

Clinical Trial Design in Heart Failure

G. Michael Felker and John R. Teerlink

Since 1980, there has been a dramatic and remarkable shift in the nature and use of scientific evidence for the clinical practice of medicine. What has occurred is a transition from a paradigm in which clinical practice was guided primarily by individual clinical experience or inference from physiological data to a paradigm focused on the rigorous evaluation of therapies on the basis of randomized, controlled clinical trials (RCTs). This era of evidence-based medicine, although now the dominant paradigm in medical education and practice, is a relatively recent phenomenon; the phrase "evidence-based medicine" first appeared in the literature in 1992.[1] Central to the development of evidence-based medicine is a broad consensus that RCTs represent the most robust form of evidence on which to base clinical practice.[2] The widespread use of RCTs in assessing new therapies for cardiovascular disease has coincided with marked progress in cardiovascular therapeutics in general and for heart failure in particular. Despite these advances, most clinical practice guidelines remain based on less robust levels of evidence (such as expert opinion).[3] A comprehensive discussion of all of the issues involved in the design and conduct of RCTs is beyond the scope of a single book chapter, and this chapter is not an attempt to replicate widely available clinical trial textbooks.[4,5] Instead, this chapter provides a perspective on the current state of clinical trial design in heart failure, so that clinicians can better understand and interpret the results of these fundamental building blocks of clinical evidence. Particular attention is devoted to new developments in trial design and conduct, as well as the unique aspects of clinical trials in specific clinical settings, including acute heart failure (AHF), surgical and device-based interventions, and trials of monitoring devices in heart failure.

FUNDAMENTAL COMPONENTS OF RANDOMIZED CONTROLLED TRIALS

The field of cardiovascular medicine has led the way in the development of high-quality clinical evidence, primarily on the basis of robustly designed multicenter RCTs. This rigor in clinical research in the cardiovascular field has been facilitated by the high prevalence of disease, which allows for enrollment of large numbers of patients, and the high event rates in these populations, which increases the feasibility of conducting adequately powered trials. The large multicenter trials are based on a foundation of basic science investigations, observational studies, and clinical experience. Those other types of investigation are different from RCTs in that RCTs entail randomization (the random assignment of study subjects to a given treatment or exposure), the use of a parallel control group (subjects who are treated and evaluated identically except not given the intervention to be studied), the uniform ascertainment of prespecified endpoints, and the robust statistical estimation of both the magnitude and validity of the observed treatment effect. Each of these fundamental "building blocks" of the modern RCT is described as follows, with a focus on the large, multicenter, phase III studies that provide definite evidence of efficacy and drive the approval of new therapies. Challenges related to trial design for earlier phase studies are discussed in a later section.

Hypothesis and Study Design

As with any experiment, the generation of the hypothesis to be tested is the first step in the design of a clinical trial, and a properly developed hypothesis provides significant guidance in the other aspects of the trial design. Although large, multicenter RCTs may contain multiple planned subgroups, secondary endpoints, and ancillary studies, the primary hypothesis of an RCT should be stated clearly and succinctly. The hypotheses for RCTs are in two broad categories: *superiority designs* and *noninferiority designs*. In superiority trials, the primary hypothesis is the assertion that the outcome of interest in patients randomly assigned to the study intervention will be superior to the outcome in the control group. In technical statistical terms, "proving" the study hypothesis actually involves rejecting the contrary assertion (i.e., the null hypothesis) that there is no difference in the outcome of interest between the intervention recipients and the control group, within a prespecified statistical certainty (typically 95%, or $P < .05$). Of importance is that failure to demonstrate a statistically significant difference between the intervention and control groups is not the same as demonstrating that there is no difference between the two treatments: "lack of evidence of a difference" is not the same as "evidence of a lack of difference."[6]

New therapies may be easier to administer, may be better tolerated, may have a better safety profile, or may be less expensive, but not all these aspects may be accounted for in the primary efficacy endpoint of a traditional superiority design. Whether a new treatment yields outcomes equivalent to those of standard therapy is therefore often an important clinical question and has important implications for both the hypothesis and the overall study. In the design of noninferiority, or equivalence, trials, the hypothesis and statistical techniques must be framed in specific ways that are often underappreciated.[7,8] Because there would be little rationale for establishing equivalence with placebo, the purpose of noninferiority trials is to compare a new intervention with established therapy; thus, they are sometimes termed *active-control trials.* An essential prerequisite of an active-control trial is that the control therapy has already been sufficiently demonstrated to yield better results than does placebo. This issue is particularly relevant to regulatory agencies that evaluate trials for potential drug approval, and specific guidelines have been developed for the selection of the active comparator.[9] Noninferiority trial designs are fundamentally based on the hypothesis that the new intervention does not yield results different from those of the control treatment to a clinically important degree, often termed the *noninferiority margin* and frequently expressed as Δ. In other words, the null hypothesis to be rejected in equivalence studies is that the control is superior to the investigational therapy by a clinical important margin (Δ). If that null hypothesis is rejected, then the two therapies can be claimed to be at least equivalent. The use of confidence intervals in assessing treatment effect can be a significant aid in the interpretation of equivalence studies, as shown in Figure 39-1.[10] Both the noninferiority design and Δ must be prespecified and justified on clinical and statistical grounds. Although the necessity of prespecified statistical approaches for noninferiority designs has been increasingly recognized, accurate reporting and interpretation of noninferiority designs continue to be problematic.[11,12] Formal guidelines that may serve to improve standardization of reporting for noninferiority designs have been published .[10]

In conjunction with the general design of the trial (superiority vs. noninferiority), the therapeutic intervention being tested must be carefully defined. In the simplest form of RCT, a single intervention is compared with a placebo control condition in a traditional parallel group design. However, as trials have become larger and more expensive and as therapeutic regimens have become increasingly complex, designs in which multiple hypotheses can be tested have become more common. In factorial designs, subjects are randomly assigned to multiple, balanced combinatorial groups. One attractive aspect of factorial designs is the ability to address two clinical questions simultaneously in the same patient population without sacrificing statistical power for either question. In reality, the preservation of statistical power in factorial study designs depends on whether there is an interaction between the two treatments, which may be independent (i.e., no interaction), additive, or subadditive. Although factorial designs may substantially increase efficiency in clinical trials, they must be interpreted carefully, particularly with regard to interactions between the two treatments.[13] Because of the increasing size, complexity, and expense of international multicenter RCTs, factorial designs have become increasingly common in cardiovascular studies.[14]

Another study design that is often considered is a crossover design, in which each patient serves as his or her own control. In its simplest form, a crossover design involves assigning patients randomly to the intervention or control group and then changing treatments (intervention changes to control and vice versa) after a designated period. Crossover designs may allow for smaller sample sizes because of limiting variability (because each patient is his or her own control, by definition the intervention group and control group are identical except for the intervention). In order for crossover designs to be valid, there must be no carryover effect: that is, the effect of the intervention must be the same whether patients receive it first or second. For these reasons, crossover designs are typically more appropriate for early-phase trials focused on surrogate endpoints[15] than for curable conditions

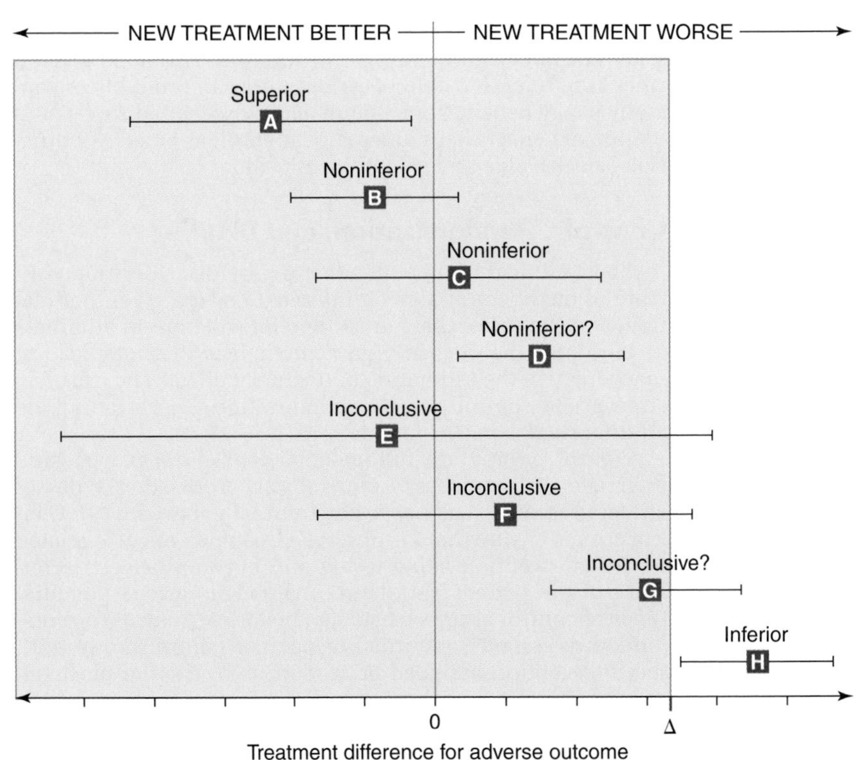

FIGURE 39-1 Possible scenarios of observed treatment differences for adverse outcomes (harms) in noninferiority trials. *Error bars* indicate two-sided 95% confidence intervals (CIs). The *tinted area* is the zone of inferiority. If the CI lies wholly to the left of zero (A), the new treatment is superior. If the CI lies to the left of Δ and includes zero (B and C), the new treatment is noninferior but not shown to be superior. If the CI lies wholly to the left of Δ and wholly to the right of zero (D), the new treatment is noninferior in the sense already defined, but it is also inferior in the sense that a null treatment difference is excluded. This puzzling case is rare; detecting it requires a very large sample size. This finding can also result from too wide a noninferiority margin. If the CI includes Δ and zero (E and F), the difference is nonsignificant, but the result regarding noninferiority is inconclusive. If the CI includes Δ and is wholly to the right of zero (G), the difference is statistically significant, but the result is inconclusive with regard to possible inferiority of magnitude Δ or worse. If the CI is wholly to the right of Δ (H), the new treatment is inferior. (Adapted from Piaggio G, Elbourne DR, Altman DG, et al, for the CONSORT Group. Reporting of noninferiority and equivalence randomized trials: an extension of the CONSORT statement. *JAMA* 2006;295:1152-1160.)

(once a disease is cured, the subject cannot revert to the disease state) or outcome trials (once an event occurs, the patient cannot revert to an event-free state.)

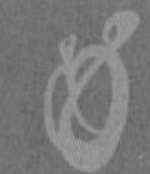

Patient Population

The patients selected for an RCT must be thought to have a reasonable possibility of benefiting from therapy according to preclinical data, observational studies, earlier phase studies, or a combination of these. In order to ethically justify the random assignment of human subjects between two therapies, there should be genuine clinical uncertainty about which treatment is preferable in a given patient population. In selecting the patient population in whom to test the study hypothesis, the researchers balance a variety of potentially conflicting considerations, including anticipated therapeutic effect, event rates, safety profiles, enrollment rates, and generalizability. The patient population for a given study is defined by the inclusion and exclusion criteria, which define what types of patients can and cannot be enrolled in a given study. Inclusion criteria are frequently designed to select patients with specific pathophysiological markers that suggest the potential to benefit from the putative mechanism of action of the therapy to be tested. In heart failure trials, such markers of potential response may be based on ventricular structure and function (e.g., ejection fraction, ventricular dimensions), symptom severity (e.g., New York Heart Association [NYHA] class), specific symptoms (e.g., edema), or other disease markers (e.g., elevated levels of B-type natriuretic peptide [BNP]). If an intervention is not expected to be efficacious or could lead to unacceptable risks in certain subjects, exclusion criteria would ensure that it is not studied in these patients.

In addition to subjects' possibility of responding to the given therapy, the patient population should be at some meaningful risk for the primary endpoint, particularly when the primary endpoint is an event such as death or hospitalization for heart failure. Selecting patients with high event rates allows for relatively smaller sample sizes (and more economical studies for the same treatment effect). In heart failure trials, such inclusion criteria are usually designed to select populations with high event rates and typically include ejection fraction, functional capacity, NYHA class, prior hospitalizations, or elevated neurohormone levels. However, not only is it desirable to select a population with a high event rate, but also these patients should have a high *disease-specific* event rate. For example, patients with advanced cancers have a high mortality rate, but it is unlikely that a heart failure therapy in such patients would have a significant effect on the rates of death. Consequently, exclusion criteria are usually chosen to exclude patients with comorbid conditions or characteristics that would place them at significant risk of an event caused by reasons other than heart failure or that would confound the interpretation of the endpoint.

A major issue in the selection of inclusion and exclusion criteria for RCTs is the balance between limiting variability (by studying a more homogeneous population) and maximizing generalizability (by studying as heterogeneous a population as possible). Studying more homogeneous populations limits background variance, which allows for a trial to be more sensitive to smaller effect sizes (i.e., an increased "signal-to-noise" ratio). Exclusion criteria are often designed to limit this variance. For example, patients with relatively rare causes of heart failure, such as myocarditis, are routinely excluded from most heart failure studies because the different natural history of such disorders increases variance in possible treatment response. Conversely, defining the population too narrowly may have important implications for study enrollment, generalizability, and labeling of approved therapies.

Implications of Patient Selection: Enrollment, Generalizability, and Labeling Considerations

Expeditious completion of RCTs is of significant concern for patients, investigators, and sponsors. Rapid enrollment of patients in the study will result in answering the study question as quickly as possible, which will either support approval of the therapy, for the greater benefit of other patients, or lead to the discontinuation of a potentially harmful or useless intervention. In addition, rapid enrollment reduces costs to the investigators and the sponsor and frees up resources for other lines of investigation. Stringent inclusion and exclusion criteria can be a significant impediment to patient recruitment, resulting in a tension between enrolling the "perfect" patients for a trial and rapid recruitment rates.

A basic principle of evidence-based medicine is that results from clinical trials should be applied to patients who are generally similar to those enrolled in the trial. In general, even when study populations are broadly defined, there is a tendency for patients enrolled in RCTs not to be representative of the broader population. In particular, women, minorities, elderly patients, and patients with significant comorbid conditions are often underrepresented in clinical trials.[16] As a result, the patients at highest risk tend to be excluded from clinical trials, and event rates for a given disease in clinical trials are typically lower than in population-based samples. This issue may be exacerbated by defining the study population too narrowly. Because it is important to be able to apply the results of a clinical trial to clinical practice, there has been considerable discussion of ways in which to make trials more generalizable by recruiting the most representative group of patients. Many approaches have been used to address this issue, including consecutive screening and enrollment, greater emphasis on enrollment in community hospitals or the primary care setting, and developing a registry of all the patients who were candidates for enrollment in the study. Comparisons between the candidates and the patients actually enrolled in the trial could provide insight into differences between the groups. The problems engendered by patient selection are important; however, the primary purpose of the clinical trial is to test a hypothesis in a scientifically valid manner, and any approaches to broaden the study population must not undermine the rigor of the trial. Although general rules are difficult to define, earlier phases in proof-of-concept studies may benefit from a more narrowly defined study population, whereas later phases should enroll as broad a population as is feasible and scientifically valid.

Controls, Randomization, and Blinding

A robust clinical trial is intended to provide an accurate estimate of the effect of a given intervention in a given population, and the researchers must therefore attempt to eliminate or minimize the chance of systematic bias that may lead to inaccuracy in the estimation of treatment effect. The use of an appropriate control group, randomization, and blinding are all important aspects of modern RCTs.

Control groups are fundamental in a clinical trial, and their use distinguishes a clinical trial from other types of clinical research (such as a longitudinal cohort study). Control groups ensure that the observed treatment effect is related to the intervention being tested and not to other characteristics of the patient population. Although various potential types of control groups exist (e.g., historical controls or non–randomly assigned controls), a parallel control group with the intervention assigned at random is by far the most rigorous method for evaluating new therapies. Randomization serves to ensure that the baseline characteristics of patients in both the treatment and control groups are similar and that any differences in the baseline characteristics between the treatment recipients and the control group arise by random chance rather than through systematic bias. Although methods for adjusting for known confounding factors are powerful tools (e.g., multivariable analyses), these approaches cannot account for all the potential differences between groups and are not a substitute for randomization. The ability to control for both known and unknown confounding factors provided by randomization imparts tremendous power to properly designed trials; thus, these types of trials have become the standard for investigations of new therapeutic interventions.

In this simplest case, study subjects are randomly assigned to one treatment condition or another as they are enrolled, in a 1:1 ratio (simple randomization). Other variations on the traditional random assignment of patients may be helpful in the conduct of RCTs. In block randomization, patients are assigned on the basis of prespecified "blocks," so that the numbers of patients assigned to the control group and the intervention group remain relatively balanced throughout the study. The sizes of the blocks may be varied at random throughout the trial to prevent investigators from preferentially trying to assign patients to a specific study condition. If particular patient characteristics are a priori thought to be likely to affect the response to therapy, stratified randomization may be used to ensure that these characteristics are balanced between the intervention and control groups. For example, if the effect of a therapy on patients with an ischemic cause of heart failure is of particular interest, stratified randomization can be used to ensure a balance of treatment assignment among those patients.

The process of keeping patients, investigators, and other study personnel unaware of the assigned treatment group is often termed *blinding* or *masking*. Masking the conditions for patients limits the placebo effect, inasmuch as patients are unaware whether they are receiving the investigational therapy. Masking the conditions for investigators limits bias that could be introduced by the knowledge of treatment assignment. For example, investigators may monitor patients more closely or use concomitant therapies differently according to whether patients are assigned to intervention or control groups. Although double-blind trials are the standard, blinding may be challenging or impossible with some types of trials, such as those with surgical or device-based interventions (described later in this chapter). In other sorts of trials, blinding may be compromised by investigators' inferences based on accessory clinical information (e.g., reduced heart rate may suggest random assignment to a condition with a β-blocker vs. placebo).[17] Although no procedures can completely eliminate unanticipated unmasking of conditions to investigators, careful attention to this issue in the design and conduct of RCTs is critical. In studies in which blinding is not possible, the use of objectively measured endpoints and endpoint committees who are unaware of conditions to adjudicate events can significantly limit potential bias. Although breaking of a blinding code is occasionally required for issues of patient safety, it should be done rarely and only with careful consideration.

Follow-up and Adherence

Adherence to the study protocol both by investigators and by study subjects is crucial for the validity of a clinical trial but often gets relatively little attention. Lack of adherence to the study protocol can complicate analysis and interpretation of trial data substantially and can undermine the validity of the results. Investigators must select sites carefully and use appropriate regulatory monitoring. To maximize patient adherence, inclusion and exclusion criteria must explicitly or implicitly result in selection patients who are more likely to adhere to follow-up and study procedures. As with many other aspects of trial design, there is a need to balance between optimizing the study conduct (by enrolling a population likely to complete follow-up procedures and adhere to treatment) and ensuring generalizability of the results (by enrolling a broadly representative population). Patients who adhere to treatment are likely to be very different in a variety of ways from those who do not, and data have confirmed that greater adherence (even to placebo procedures) is associated with improved outcomes; this suggests that adherence is a marker of other favorable health behaviors.[18]

One somewhat controversial method for maximizing adherence to the protocol is the use of run-in periods, in which potential study subjects demonstrate adherence to study protocol for some period before randomization. These run-in periods may be either placebo conditions (in which compliance is assessed) or "active" conditions (in which patients' tolerance of the study intervention is assessed). Although such active run-in periods can enhance the statistical power of trials by tending to exclude subjects who would not tolerate the study drug, they can also substantially complicate analysis. For example, the U.S. Carvedilol Heart Failure Study Group used a 3-week active run-in period to ensure tolerability of carvedilol before randomization to carvedilol or placebo condition.[19] During the run-in period, 17 patients experienced worsening heart failure and 7 died; none of them were described in the report on morbidity and mortality. This early clinical worsening led to significant controversy over the interpretation of the carvedilol trials, and researchers remain divided on how to handle events that occur during a run-in period. In general, run-in periods may be more acceptable in earlier phases of proof-of-concept studies in which tolerability of the drug is a major unanswered concern (as in the U.S. Carvedilol Heart Failure Studies[19]) but may not provide sufficiently generalizable results for definitive-phase outcome studies (such as Metoprolol CR/XL Randomised Intervention Trial in congestive Heart Failure [MERIT-HF][20] and CarvedilOl ProspEctive RaNdomIzed CUmulative Survival [COPERNICUS][21]).

Adherence to the study protocol is substantially influenced by duration of the study and type of intervention: Subjects are much more likely to be adherent in short-term studies of acute interventions, than in interventions that are complicated, time-consuming, painful, or inconvenient. In studies in which interventions are long term and challenging, specific attention to promoting adherence is critical. In the National Institutes of Health (NIH)–sponsored Heart Failure and A Controlled Trial Investigating Outcomes of Exercise TraiNing (HF-ACTION) study, the intervention group's adherence to exercise training was specifically maximized and carefully quantified.[22] To the extent possible, follow-up procedures should be frequent enough, long enough, and temporally convenient to affirm the worth of the patient's participation and demonstrate respect for their time and schedule. Adherence may also be enhanced by reminders of follow-up visits or tests and by adequate and flexible time windows. Reimbursement for travel or for time-consuming procedures affirms respect for the patient's autonomy, although the amount cannot be viewed as coercive.

Endpoints

The selection of the endpoints is crucial in the design of the clinical trial, with broad implications for the analysis and interpretation of the study. The *primary endpoint* reflects the central hypothesis of the trial. It should pertain to the desired benefit of the treatment strategy, and its reliable assessment should be feasible. Endpoint selection must also take into account the context of the overall stage of development of the therapy. In early-phase trials, *surrogate endpoints* (discussed in detail later) are often selected in order to identify a signal for moving forward with larger trials or

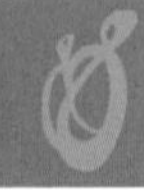

selecting a dosing regimen. In more definitive studies, *clinical endpoints* are typically designed to determine whether a patient feels better or lives longer, as demonstrated by improvement in survival, decrease in morbidity, or improvement in symptoms and quality of life. Endpoints that are considered important to evaluate rigorously are termed *secondary endpoints;* these must be viewed in the context of the primary results, particularly when there are many secondary endpoints. The advantages and disadvantages of various types of endpoints in heart failure studies are discussed as follows.

Mortality Endpoints

The best outcome of a therapy is improvement in the survival rate, and in common diseases with high mortality rates (such as heart failure), even modest reductions can have an important effect on public health. The clinical relevance of mortality as an endpoint is undisputed, but the question of whether to study all-cause mortality or disease-specific mortality is salient. All-cause mortality as an endpoint has many advantages: such mortality is self-evidently relevant, easy to assess, and not subject to bias in interpretation. However, many authorities have argued that evaluating all-cause mortality can dilute the significance of beneficial effects of therapies that target one specific cause of death (e.g., an implantable defibrillator device's effect on sudden cardiac death) and that in these cases, disease-specific mortality is a more useful endpoint.[23] The advantages of this approach include a higher sensitivity to the treatment effect, a resistance to the influence of random variations in other outcomes unlikely to be affected by treatment, and a relative absence of confounding. The major disadvantage of disease-specific mortality as an endpoint relates to the challenges in accurately assigning a cause of death in an unbiased manner. The specific mode of death is often difficult to classify, and interobserver agreement is often poor.[24,25] Clinical events committees (reviewed later), which review events in a blinded manner by using prespecified rules, may improve event adjudication. Regardless of the endpoint selected, total mortality rates must always be evaluated, so as to ensure that unforeseen adverse effects of the therapy are appropriately detected.

Despite the obvious advantages of mortality endpoints, they may not be feasible in many clinical situations. Some therapies may not target mechanisms that are anticipated to play a major role in mortality, or their projected effect size may be minimal, necessitating prohibitively large trials. In addition, as life-saving therapies are serially incorporated into the "standard of care," it becomes increasingly difficult to demonstrate improvements in mortality rate.[26] These trends have led to the increasing use of primary endpoints that focus on other aspects of the patient experience beyond mortality alone.

Morbidity Endpoints

Morbidity endpoints typically focus on nonfatal events. In heart failure trials, the most commonly used such event by far is hospitalization. As with mortality endpoints, the issue of all-cause versus disease-specific endpoints must be considered, and hospitalizations for all causes, for cardiovascular events, or for heart failure have been used in various trials. Heart failure accounts for about half of all hospitalizations in most heart failure trials—in all trials, fewer events are related to heart failure in comparison to total number of hospitalizations (a lower event rate would necessitate a larger sample size)—but, as expected, there is a compensatory greater reduction in the heart failure–specific hospitalizations in most trials, in comparison to total admissions (an increased effect size would necessitate a smaller sample size).[27] On balance, these considerations have generally favored the use of the more specific endpoint, and "hospitalization for heart failure" is the most common morbidity endpoint in contemporary studies of chronic heart failure.

Of importance is that there are limitations associated with the use of morbidity endpoints such as hospitalization. Morbidity endpoints should generally not be used in isolation from mortality, because a treatment that improves survival may lead to more hospitalizations (patients are living long enough to experience nonfatal events: the "survivor effect"). For this reason, hospitalizations are generally combined with mortality in composite endpoints (death or hospitalization). In addition, hospitalizations may be influenced by economic and cultural considerations, as well as regional differences, which may cloud interpretation of hospitalization data. Finally, rigorous definitions and adjudication are required for hospitalizations, which adds a level of complexity and expense to the trial. For example, how hospitalizations for cardiac procedures (such as an elective surgery for implantable cardioverter-defibrillators [ICDs] or heart transplantation) are handled must be defined in a prespecified manner in the study protocol. Furthermore, definitions of what counts as a hospitalization must be prespecified. For example, in the Omapatrilat Versus Enalapril Randomized Trial of Utility in Reducing Events (OVERTURE), differences in the definitions of hospitalizations for heart failure had a significant effect on the results of the trial.[28] The protocol-specified primary endpoint—the combined risk of death or hospitalization for heart failure requiring intravenous treatment—resulted in a nonsignificant decrease in events ($P = .187$), a result that fulfilled prespecified criteria for noninferiority but not for superiority. However, post hoc analysis of the primary endpoint with the definition used in the Studies of Left Ventricular Dysfunction (SOLVD) treatment trial, the combined risk of death or all hospitalizations for heart failure, revealed an 11% lower risk in patients treated with omapatrilat (nominal $P = .012$).

Symptom-Based Endpoints

Endpoints for evaluating the symptomatic status of patients are a logical approach to the "feel better or live longer" goal of major clinical trials. A therapy that markedly improves symptom status, quality of life, or other measures of a patient's sense of well-being is beneficial, as long as it does not have an adverse effect on morbidity and mortality. The objective, quantitative assessment of inherently subjective phenomena, however, presents a substantial challenge. Assessments of symptom severity by physicians (most commonly according to NYHA class) have been widely used in clinical trials, but such assessments are highly subjective, lack granularity, and are very vulnerable to investigator bias. A large body of literature concerning quality of life (QOL) has developed, and two QOL instruments specifically for use in chronic heart failure have been validated: the Minnesota Living with Heart Failure Questionnaire[29] and the Kansas City Cardiomyopathy Questionnaire.[30] Although somewhat time consuming to fill out, both these instruments have proved useful in a variety of research settings, including clinical trials. Other measures of specific symptoms, especially dyspnea, have been studied, through the use of visual analog scales or Likert scales, in several trials for acute decompensated heart failure, but such methods have not been extensively validated.[31] Investigators have begun to compare various methods for assessing symptoms in heart failure, but more research in this area is clearly needed.[32]

Composite Measures as Heart Failure Endpoints

Because heart failure is a disease characterized by high mortality rates, frequent hospitalizations, and impaired quality of life, there has been substantial interest in ways in which these various components can be integrated into a single

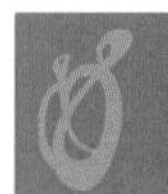

comprehensive endpoint. In addition, there has been increasing interest in using endpoints that reflect the entire clinical course of the patient. Although Cox proportional hazards analysis—clearly been a useful (and almost universally employed) analysis strategy in chronic heart failure studies—has been used to study time to first event, this technique may lead to "overweighting" less morbid events that occur earlier in the course of follow-up. This potentially introduces major problems in interpretation, in that less severe events happening earlier in the study (such as a brief hospitalization for heart failure) are counted, whereas more severe events (such as death) that happen after an initial event would be ignored in the primary analysis of the trial outcomes. An example of this potential discrepancy is the use of a composite endpoint of time to death or first hospitalization for heart failure, which is standard for chronic heart failure: A patient who is hospitalized for heart failure 2 weeks after randomization but then survives and feels well for 5 years would be viewed as having a worse outcome than one who dies 2 months after randomization. In this sense, the combined endpoint weighs the clinical course in a way that is incongruous with the way it would be viewed by patients and providers.

To deal with this aspect of time to event analysis, various alternative strategies to creating composite endpoints that incorporate the entire follow-up experience have been proposed. One such method is the use of a clinical composite score initially proposed by Packer,[33] in which a patient's overall status is classified as worsened, unchanged, or improved over the course of follow-up, according to prespecified rules. As it was initially proposed for chronic heart failure, patients are classified as worse if they have experienced any major adverse clinical event (e.g., death, hospitalization for heart failure) or if there was evidence of worsening on the final visit (according to either the patient's global assessment or the NYHA class determined by the physician). Patients are classified as improved if they have evidence of significant improvement on the final visit (according to either the patient's global assessment or the physician-determined NYHA class) and did not have any event that would have classified them as worse. If a patient is neither worse nor improved, they are classified as unchanged.

A similar framework has been adopted for acute decompensated heart failure.[34] A more granular method based on similar principles is the global rank method, wherein all patients participating in a trial are ranked on the basis of a prespecified hierarchy of events.[35] For example, in a study of chronic heart failure, all patients who died would be ranked lowest (based on the time to death), patients who did not die but were hospitalized would be ranked second lowest, and patients who did not experience an event would be ranked according to symptomatic status (as measured by a QOL instrument). Another method is to measure "total days alive and out of the hospital" over the course of follow-up. This type of endpoint, which is particularly suited to trials with shorter follow-up periods, incorporates the possibility of frequent hospitalizations and prolonged length of stay into the assessment of efficacy, while also appropriately weighting mortality. This endpoint was used in both the Outcomes of a Prospective Trial of Intravenous Milrinone for Exacerbations of Chronic Heart Failure (OPTIME-CHF) study[36] and the Evaluation Study of Congestive Heart Failure and Pulmonary Artery Catheterization Effectiveness (ESCAPE).[37] Researchers have further refined this approach by adjusting days out of the hospital by using serial measures of health status, creating a global assessment termed the *patient journey score*.[38,39] Although all these approaches have theoretical advantages, they are somewhat more complex to describe and interpret than are traditional endpoints and have thus far not supplanted the traditional endpoint (time to death or hospitalization for heart failure) in studies of chronic heart failure.

Surrogate Endpoints

A surrogate endpoint is defined by the U.S. Food and Drug Administration (FDA) as "a laboratory measurement or physical sign that is used in therapeutic trials as a substitute for a clinically meaningful end point that is a direct measure of how a patient feels, functions, or survives and is expected to predict the effect of the therapy."[40] In order to be valid, the surrogate endpoint must have been demonstrated to reliably predict the outcome that it is replacing in terms of four criteria: (1) The biological relevance of the surrogate endpoint must be clearly established through a consistent relationship between it and outcomes in multiple studies; (2) changes in the surrogate endpoint should be predictive of changes in the outcome, independent of treatment; (3) direct proportionality between changes in the surrogate endpoint and in the relevant outcome must be established; and (4) this relationship needs to be replicated in many different patient populations under different conditions.[40] Many physiological variables have been posited as possible surrogate endpoints for heart failure studies, including measures of functional capacity (such as 6-minute walk or peak ventilatory oxygen uptake), ventricular function and volumes, ventricular arrhythmias, hemodynamic changes, and levels of neurohormones or other biomarkers.[41] As currently defined and studied, none of these candidates fulfills the requirements of a true surrogate endpoint, and thus none of these variables is sufficient for the definitive evaluation of the efficacy of a new therapy for heart failure.

In practice, surrogates do serve a useful role in earlier phases of therapeutic development in order to look for signals of efficacy and safety and in selecting the best dose to use in more definitive trials. Whether researchers can identify valid surrogate endpoints that can be used in more definitive trials is a subject of substantial controversy and ongoing interest.[42] Advocates of greater use of surrogate endpoints argue that their establishment would allow for smaller more focused clinical trials and therefore speed the development of new therapies.[43] However, in view of the numerous examples of therapies for which surrogate endpoints proved to be misleading (including inotropic agents,[44] antiarrhythmic drugs,[45] tumor necrosis factor blockers[46]), efficacy studies focused on clinical endpoints such as mortality, morbidity, and symptoms will appropriately remain the definitive approach to establishing efficacy and safety for the foreseeable future.

Multiple Primary Endpoints

Clinical trials occasionally have two (or, rarely, more) primary endpoints. There are many reasons that investigators might wish to test multiple hypotheses in one trial; multiple questions may be pertinent to the treatment, which endpoint best captures the treatment effect may be uncertainty, or special considerations are needed for regulatory submissions. Multiple hypotheses may be tested with a variety of trial designs, often with active input from regulatory agencies. However, a statistical cost must be paid for these multiple hypotheses, often in some form of "α allocation," in which a fraction of the available type I, or α, error (usually 0.05) is allocated between the multiple endpoints and an adjustment is made for the fact that multiple statistical comparisons are being performed.[47] In addition, allocation of α to multiple endpoints often necessitates an increase in the trial sample size to maintain the power to detect meaningful differences.

Two trials illustrate methods to deal with multiple primary endpoints and the complexities that they may introduce. The Multicenter InSync Randomized Clinical Evaluation (MIRACLE) had three primary efficacy endpoints (Minnesota Living with Heart Failure score, NYHA class, and

6-minute walk test).[48,49] For the trial to be considered supportive of efficacy, all three endpoints had to be significant at $P < .05$, two at $P < .025$, or one at $P < .0167$. All three endpoints were significantly different at $P \le .005$, and thus the trial met the prespecified criteria for efficacy.[49] In the Carvedilol Post-Infarct Survival Control in Left Ventricular Dysfunction (CAPRICORN) trial, the original all-cause mortality endpoint ($\alpha = 0.05$) was changed to a coprimary endpoint of all-cause mortality ($\alpha = 0.005$) and a combined endpoint of hospitalizations for cardiovascular events and all-cause mortality ($\alpha = 0.045$). If either of these endpoints had been positive, the CAPRICORN results would have been interpreted as positive. Unfortunately, there was no significant difference in the combined endpoint of mortality and hospitalizations for cardiovascular events ($P = .297$), and although the mortality rate was decreased in the carvedilol recipients ($P = .031$), it did not reach the new, specified level of significance.[50]

Secondary Endpoints

The multicenter RCT represents a substantial investment of time, energy, and money on the part of subjects, investigators, and sponsors. It is therefore appropriate to gain as much knowledge as possible from the collected database. As a consequence, in addition to the primary endpoint, a variety of other endpoints called *secondary endpoints* are often analyzed. Although the evaluation of secondary endpoints can serve as an important resource for understanding the full impact of a given therapy, their interpretation must be tempered by statistical reality. Specifically, if $P = .05$ for statistical significance, there is a 5% chance that a "positive" result is actually falsely positive (type I error), which suggests a difference in outcome where none actually exists. Some protocols address this issue by prespecifying only a few secondary endpoints or even a single "primary" secondary endpoint. In the case of trials that yielded negative or neutral results with regard to the primary endpoint, researchers must strenuously avoid the tendency to analyze secondary endpoints (or post hoc subgroups with regard to the primary endpoint) and base claims of efficacy on them.

Safety Endpoints

The collection and interpretation of adverse effects is essential in determining the safety profile and in assessing the overall value of an intervention, and trials must therefore also be designed with outcome measures that will detect these events. Anticipated adverse events may be related either to the disease process studied or to the known effects of a drug. There is extensive regulatory guidance with regard to the investigator's and sponsor's responsibilities in reporting adverse events, but the basic processes are encompassed by the principle of actively protecting patients' safety and optimizing the information available for the evaluation of possible patterns of adverse events. These data also inform the writing of the package insert for the use of the therapy in clinical practice.

Sample Size and Statistical Power

The need for clinical trials arises from the practical limitation that not every patient with a given condition can be studied. Consequently, the investigator must use statistical methods to *estimate the probability* that the findings of the study are representative of the whole population of interest. Sample size and statistical power are interrelated concepts that are critical for the interpretation and validity of RCTs. *Sample size* calculations determine how many patients are "enough" to reliably detect the treatment effect under investigation, whereas the *statistical power* is a measure of the ability with a given sample size to detect a real treatment effect if one exists. Detailed discussions of issue and methods of sample size calculations and methods can be found in statistical textbooks and have been reviewed in detail elsewhere.[51]

The hypothesis of the study influences the sample size in two important ways. First, the type of hypothesis selected affects the power of the study. In general, sample sizes for a noninferiority trial are larger than those for a superiority trial. In addition, hypotheses can be defined as one-sided or two-sided, which affects the sample size. One-sided hypotheses test only one direction of the effect of the therapy (e.g., only improvement); two-sided hypotheses test both directions. Although most investigators may be interested in demonstrating only that an intervention is better than control conditions, they must always recall that therapies can also be harmful. An important example is the Cardiac Arrhythmia Suppression Trial (CAST), which was initially designed with a one-sided hypothesis ($\alpha = 0.025$) for improvement in survival; because these drugs were already marketed and widely assumed to be safe, no harm was expected. In what has become a case study for many issues in RCT design in heart failure, CAST was terminated early because of excess mortality.[45] Consequently, most contemporary trials now use a two-sided hypothesis for sample size determination.

A clinical trial is an approximation of the "truth" in the entire population of interest, and investigators must decide how precise an approximation the clinical trial should be. Two major types of errors can limit the validity of a trial. *Systematic errors* are inherent in the design of the study and usually arise from some type of bias, which can be addressed by randomization, blinding, and appropriate control groups, as described previously. *Random errors* are the result of chance and are classified as type I or type II errors.

Type I error represents the probability that the null hypothesis is incorrectly rejected, so that the alternative hypothesis is accepted (false-positive result). The probability that this will occur is referred to as the *statistical significance level,* or α. Typically, $\alpha = 0.05$, which means that there is a maximum of a 5% chance of incorrectly rejecting the null hypothesis, but other α levels may be considered more appropriate in a specific clinical circumstances. For example, if the investigators wished to be very confident that a therapy was better than a control condition, perhaps with regard to dangerous side effects, then a more stringent α might be selected (e.g., $\alpha = 0.01$), whereas in a study of a disease for which there is no therapy, investigators might be willing to accept an α of 0.10. Although it has become standard for the great majority of RCTs, there is nothing "magical" about an α of 0.05; it simple represents a broad consensus of the chance of a false-positive result that is "acceptable" in the conduct of clinical research.

The type II error represents the probability of failing to reject the null hypothesis when it is actually false (false-negative result). The type II error is called β, and it is typically set by investigators to be between 0.05 and 0.20. The type II error is more commonly expressed as the *statistical power,* which represents the probability of correctly rejecting the null hypothesis and is represented mathematically by the relation $[1\text{-}\beta]$. Type II error is generally associated with "underpowered" clinical trials, in which "no difference" is claimed between two conditions of a study on the basis of $P > .05$, even though the study had insufficient power for the investigators to make such a conclusion. Such underpowered clinical trials remain unfortunately common in the literature, and they present a variety of problems in clinical research. Patients in underpowered studies experience the risks of being in the study but may not contribute to the generalizable knowledge and care of future patients. Underpowered trials have been deemed unethical by many investigators.[52]

Sample size and statistical power are profoundly affected by factors that can be estimated only before the conduct of the trial: the *effect size* (how much better the intervention will be than control conditions with regard to the primary endpoint) and the *event rate* (how frequent events will be in the control group). With regard to effect size, the investigators cannot know what the magnitude of the real difference is, if any, before performing the study, and therefore must select the effect size in which the study should be able to reveal differences. Determining the effect size of a study is a daunting task: What reduction in an endpoint is important enough to detect? For mortality, the answer would be "as small a difference as possible," but for other endpoints, such as hospitalizations or symptom scores, the decision can be much less clear. Evidence from previous similar studies tends to be very limited, with large uncertainty in the point estimates (especially in pilot studies); published studies are highly selected, and investigators may themselves be overly optimistic. Because extremely large effect sizes (50% or greater) are exceedingly unlikely for new therapies for heart failure, a reasonably conservative estimate of effect size is required in planning the trial in order to avoid an underpowered trial that leaves the underlying hypothesis unaddressed. For example, the Defibrillators in Non-Ischemic Cardiomyopathy Treatment Evaluation (DEFINITE) trial of ICD therapy enrolled 229 patients on the basis of an optimistic anticipated treatment effect of 50%.[53] The results of the trial showed a 35% reduction in events with ICD therapy, but this did not reach statistical significance ($P = .08$) because the study was not powered to detect this degree of effect.

For typical studies in which clinical events (such as death or hospitalization) serve as endpoints, the primary determinant of statistical power is not the total number of subjects enrolled but the total number of events experienced. For this reason, estimation of both the anticipated treatment effect and the event rates in the control group is critical for the planning of clinical trials. Because baseline event rates are typically lower in clinical trials than in the community samples, such estimates of event rates are often derived from previous clinical trials in which a similar population was enrolled. One alternative approach to ensure a desired statistical power is to predetermine the number of events necessary to demonstrate the effect size and to enroll and monitor patients until this predetermined number of events is reached; thus, estimates of the control event rate would be eliminated as a major determinant of sample size (although they would be a major determinant of the study timeline). Alternatively, the sample size could be reestimated during the course of the trial, when interim evaluations of the event rate (with treatment assignment masked) are performed and the study sample size adjusted accordingly.[54] Ultimately, investigators may be forced to work backward from the number of available patients, which may be constrained by demographics, accessibility, or finances, to the effect size that the study can detect.

The statistical tests used to determine whether one group is significantly different from another are sensitive to the variability within the groups. The smaller the variation within the groups, the smaller the groups can be to detect a difference between them. This facet of statistical analysis has three main implications. First, because measurement error contributes to the variability in the groups, investigators are constantly searching for more precise instruments to capture the full treatment effect reliably. Second, study protocols are usually designed to enroll more homogeneous patient populations to limit another source of variation in the samples. Third, an estimate of the anticipated variability in the groups needs to be established before the study begins, so as to determine the sample size. For many endpoints, the degree of uncertainty in the group estimate can be approximated by analysis of previous heart failure trials, but for novel endpoints or nonvalidated instruments, the variability must also be determined by an informed guess.

Many other factors are important to consider once the inputs just described are determined. The effect size must be adjusted for the possibility of crossovers in therapy, including patients who discontinue therapy, thereby switching from active therapy to a "control" condition ("dropouts") and patients who switch from the control group to active therapy during the conduct of the trial ("drop-ins"). Drop-ins are particularly problematic if the therapy being tested (or a similar therapy) becomes clinically available during the follow-up period. In the COmparison of Medical Therapy, Pacing, ANd DefibrillatION in Heart Failure (COMPANION) trial of cardiac resynchronization therapy (CRT) and CRT defibrillator (CRT-D) devices, more than 20% of patients assigned to receive the pharmacotherapy devices had ICDs or CRT-D devices implanted clinically over the course of follow-up; this substantially complicated the interpretation of the final study results.[55] In general, both drop-ins and drop-outs tend to decrease the statistical power of a study, and this development must be adjusted for appropriately in the planning of clinical trials (especially trials with very long follow-up periods or in which problems with compliance can be reasonably anticipated). For example, in the HF-ACTION study of chronic exercise training in heart failure, sample size estimates included adjustment for anticipated numbers of drop-outs (attrition resulting from nonadherence to exercise training) and drop-ins (control patients undertaking an exercise training regimen).[22]

Data Analysis and Reporting

To protect the integrity of the trial, an analysis plan should be prospectively written; it defines the primary and secondary endpoints, the statistical procedures that will be used to analyze them, and the significance level to be tested. Such a plan protects against the temptation to change the way the data is analyzed once the results are known, and it greatly enhances the validity of the findings. Several important concepts in data interpretation are discussed in the following sections, including the intention-to-treat principle, the interpretation of the significance testing, and subgroup and post-hoc analyses.

Intention-to-Treat Analysis

Intention-to-treat analyses are counterintuitive. In an *analysis by treatment received* (*as-treated analysis*), the effect of a therapy is judged only in patients who actually receive the therapy; in an *intention-to-treat analysis,* patients are evaluated on the basis of the group to which they were randomly assigned, regardless of whether they actually received the therapy. Although as-treated analyses may seem more intuitive, they have the potential to introduce significant biases. Patients who do not adhere to a given therapy may differ significantly from those who do and often have higher event rates than do adherent patients. In addition, compliance may not be balanced between groups, particularly for therapies with significant side effects. Thus, the exclusion of subjects who do not continue the assigned therapy for whatever reason tends to bias the interpretation toward a conclusion of greater efficacy of the therapy being evaluated because only compliant patients are studied. Such an approach may confirm biological efficacy but does not establish real-world effectiveness; in clinical practice, the overall performance of a given therapy must take into account patients who cannot or will not adhere.[56] Intention-to-treat analysis provides an estimate of treatment effect that tends to be more conservative, and it remains the "gold standard" for the interpretation of RCTs. In studies with high rates of noncompliance, as-treated analyses may be performed as a secondary analysis in order to investigate biological efficacy, but such analyses should be seen as supplementary to the intention-to-treat analysis.

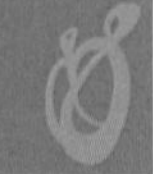

Interpretation of Endpoints

The statistical analysis of the primary and secondary endpoints should be described in detail in the analysis plan, and these analyses should be performed per protocol on the cleaned data in an unblinded manner. The interpretation of the results is often a complicated process; the power of the study must be assessed first, and the results must be interpreted in that context. The interpretation of study results should incorporate an analysis of the point estimate of the effect size, the confidence intervals around that point estimate, and the degree of statistical certainty (as reflected in the probability [*P* value]) of that result. Often, the clinical trial results are inappropriately interpreted in relation to a single value (the *P* value), and the trials are dichotomized as "negative" or "positive" on the basis of the *P* value. Data should be interpreted in the context of overall study power, as well as in comparison with other studies in similar populations. For example, in the DEFINITE study,[53] ICD therapy was associated with a 35% reduction in mortality (hazard ratio = 0.65; 95% confidence interval, 0.40 to 1.06; $P = .08$), which did not meet the prespecified criteria for statistical significance ($P = .05$). Technically, this was a "negative" study in that it did not meet its prespecified criteria to establish efficacy. However, a more nuanced interpretation would be that the results suggested the possibility of a 35% reduction in mortality with ICD therapy (on the basis of the point estimate), but the study was not powered enough to conclusively prove this effect with 95% probability (it was "proved" with a 92% probability). In the context of other studies in which ICD therapy was proved efficacious for primary prevention in patients with left ventricular dysfunction, DEFINITE can be seen as a highly supportive but ultimately underpowered study, rather than simply a "negative" one.

For studies that are used to conclusively demonstrate efficacy and support regulatory approval, the focus is typically on only the prespecified primary endpoint; if the primary endpoint is not met at the level prespecified, the study results cannot support the assertion of efficacy. This discipline in endpoint interpretation has many advantages: it interprets the trial in the manner in which the investigators felt was optimal, it is the tenet around which the trial was designed, and it is independent of any post-hoc data-driven bias, thus protecting the type I error of the trial. For example, in the CAPRICORN trial,[50] the primary endpoint was originally all-cause mortality ($\alpha = 0.05$). During the study, the data and safety monitoring committee (DSMC) noted a low overall mortality rate in an early masked analysis and believed that power might have been insufficient to detect a difference with the mortality endpoint. The steering committee then decided to adopt two coprimary endpoints. Both—combined morbidity and mortality ($P = .30$) and all-cause mortality ($P = .03$)—were "negative" according to the revised definitions and α allocation, and so CAPRICORN, a study in which mortality was reduced 23%, was technically a negative trial. However, the challenge to clinicians and regulatory agencies is to interpret this trial for application in clinical practice. Despite some debate, carvedilol had beneficial effects in patients with NYHA classes II to IV heart failure (U.S. Carvedilol Program and COPERNICUS) and β-blockers had a recognized benefit in other postmyocardial settings; thus, the reduction in all-cause mortality was thought to be sufficient to warrant the FDA's approval of carvedilol for heart failure.

Subgroup Analysis and Other Post Hoc Testing

Subgroups may be defined in a number of ways, ranging from protocol-specified to purely post hoc analyses. Protocol-specified subgroups are the least susceptible to bias but must be interpreted cautiously because of their low statistical power and the increased chance of type I error (false-positive results) inherent in multiple comparisons. The MERIT-HF trial[20] prospectively defined subgroup analyses to be performed in the data analysis plan, including prespecifying the subgroups, stating that they were to be performed only for safety concerns, specifying the endpoints that were to be studied, and mandating that each had at least 180 events. These subgroup analyses demonstrated broad and consistent safety of metoprolol in all of the prespecified subgroups. Other subgroup analysis may not be prespecified but may be highly relevant to the biological properties of the disease or treatment. The OPTIME-CHF study[57] of the inotropic drug milrinone, which is known to increase myocardial oxygen demand, revealed that the drug was particularly harmful in patients with ischemic causes of heart failure, in comparison with patients with nonischemic causes. Although such analyses should be interpreted with caution, their validity is supported by a high degree of biological plausibility. In evaluating the validity of such subgroups analyses, researchers should assess the statistical interaction between the treatment and the subgroup (e.g., subjects with ischemic vs. nonischemic causes) in the total population, and analysis should proceed only if there is evidence of a statistically significant differential response between subgroups (as reflected in the *P* value for the interaction term). Other alternative and more robust statistical methods have also been proposed for improving the statistical validity of subgroup analyses.[58] Unfortunately, many subgroup analyses are data-driven post hoc tests that are extraordinarily biased and susceptible to substantial type I error. These analyses are often performed after the data have been perused for "interesting" trends and these trends are then selected for "statistical" testing. Such data-driven subgroup analysis and other post hoc analyses should be limited as much as possible and, when performed, interpreted with the utmost caution.

Publication Issues

Clinical trials in heart failure often involve thousands of patients and hundreds of investigators and study personnel. The results of these studies have important effect on the care and management of patients with heart failure, and there is therefore an ethical mandate that these results are published fully and in a timely manner. Unfortunately, a number of major heart failure studies that did not meet their primary endpoint to some extent either have never been published or were presented only as brief papers without supporting details.[59] Part of this publication bias is inherent in all negative reports (it is much more difficult to publish a negative finding than a positive one), but many trials do not even make it to the manuscript peer-review stage. However, intellectual honesty and a responsibility to the participating patients necessitates that negative findings be clearly and objectively presented. In order to facilitate transparency and increase the publication of negative trial results, the Food and Drug Modernization Act (passed in 1997) requires all clinical trials of "experimental treatments for serious or life-threatening diseases" to be registered on an appropriate public registry (such as http://www.clinicaltrials.gov).

Publication of RCTs should include detailed descriptions of the patient population, study intervention, procedures for control and blinding, follow-up, study endpoints, and calculations of sample size and power. Standardized criteria for reporting of RCTs have been created in order to improve the consistency of reporting the results of RCTs. Flow diagrams showing the number of patients screened, enrolled, randomly assigned, and analyzed in a standardized manner (Figure 39-2) are useful.[60]

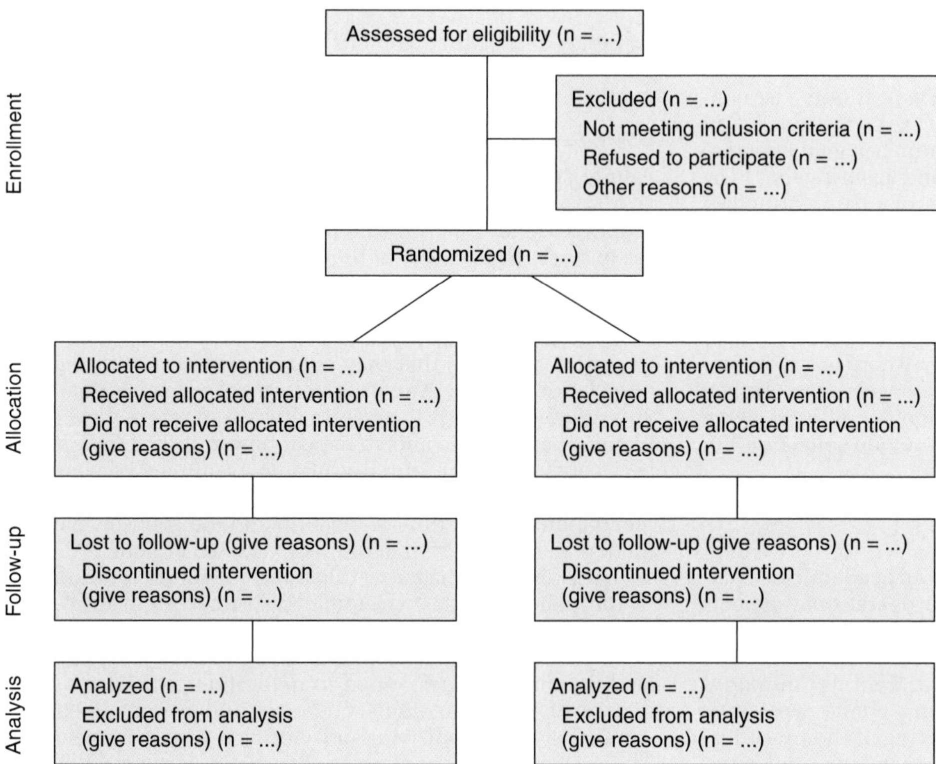

FIGURE 39-2 Example of flow diagram for reporting the results of randomized controlled trials in accordance with the Consolidated Standards of Reporting Trials (CONSORT) statement. (Adapted from Moher D, Schulz KF, Altman D, for the CONSORT Group. et al. The CONSORT statement: revised recommendations for improving the quality of reports of parallel-group randomized trials. *JAMA* 2001;285:1987-1991.) Copyright © (2011) American Medical Association. All rights reserved.

OPERATIONAL ASPECTS OF RANDOMIZED CONTROLLED TRIALS

A large multicenter RCT is a monumental endeavor, the success of which requires the combined efforts of investigators, study coordinators, project leaders, statisticians, data managers, study monitors, study sponsors, and (of most importance) research subjects. The organizational structure of a clinical trial serves to "operationalize" the scientific principles outlined in the previous section, and it is a critical aspect of a successful clinical trial. As clinical trials have grown in size and complexity and as regulatory requirements have become more complex, the operational structure necessary to perform large clinical trials has expanded as well. Although the organizational structure for a clinical trial must be tailored to the specific needs of that study, many general operational components are relevant to almost all large trials: the presence of a sponsor, a coordinating center, a leadership body, and a DSMC. Figure 39-3 is a generalized representation of the operational components of a typical large RCT in heart failure, which are discussed in detail in the following sections.

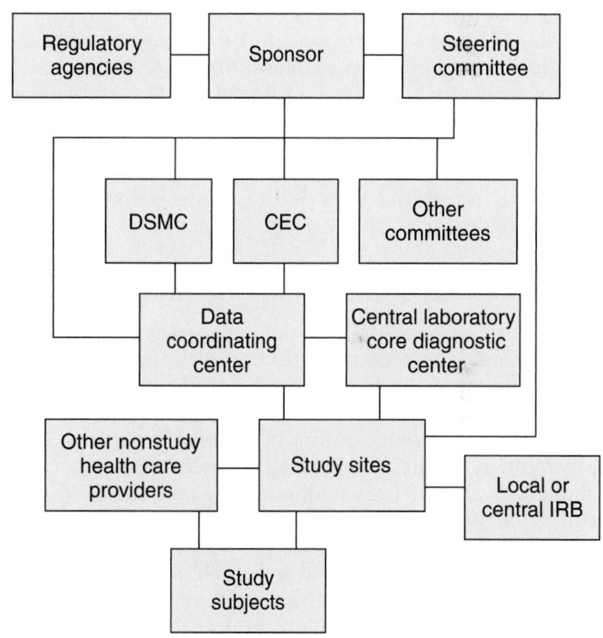

FIGURE 39-3 Generalized organizational scheme of a clinical trial. *CEC,* clinical event committee; *DSMC,* data and safety monitoring committee; *IRB,* institutional review board.

Study Leadership

Multicenter clinical trials are typically led by a steering committee of investigators who provide guidance on the scientific and operational aspects of the trial. For large or complicated studies, study leadership may be divided between a smaller executive committee (charged with making day-to-day operational decisions) that meets frequently (often weekly or biweekly) and a larger steering committee (charged with making larger decisions about the overall trial conduct) that meets less often (e.g., quarterly). Ideally, study committees ensure the scientific validity of the trial. Study committees are typically involved in all phases of study conduct, from protocol development to making decisions during the course of the study to preserve the trial's integrity and the patient's safety and to analyzing and presenting study results. The independence of the study committees is essential, and conflicts of interest should be minimized.

Study Sponsor

The study sponsor is the entity that funds the clinical trial; it may be governmental, a foundation, a commercial entity, or some combination of the three. The responsibilities of the sponsor are clearly delineated for studies involving investigational drugs and devices by the Food and Drug Administration. The sponsor of an Investigational New Drug (IND) application

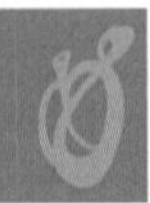

is responsible for "selecting qualified investigators, providing them with the information they need to conduct an investigation properly, ensuring proper monitoring of the investigation(s), ensuring that the investigation(s) is conducted in accordance with the general investigational plan and protocols contained in the IND, maintaining an effective IND with respect to the investigations, and ensuring that FDA and all participating investigators are promptly informed of significant new adverse effects or risks with respect to the drug". These important responsibilities require multiple areas of expertise and an intimate role in the daily activities of the trial. For many sponsors, this intimate involvement can give the appearance of a conflict of interest for the sponsor, and some sponsors do not have the time, expertise, or personnel to perform such functions. Therefore, for large clinical trials, study sponsors typically engage another entity to serve as the coordinating center and thereby provide some or all of these functions.

Coordinating Center

The coordinating center, which may be an academic or commercial organization, is crucial in the operational aspects of the clinical trial. As the name implies, the coordinating center serves as the operational hub of activities related to the clinical trial, including the selection, training, and monitoring of sites; collection and monitoring of adverse events; randomization of study subjects; supplying of the investigational drug; and collecting, cleaning, analyzing, and summarizing study data. Coordinating Center staff typically include project leaders, clinical research associates, data managers, medical monitors, regulatory personnel, and biostatisticians. Because of its central role in the clinical trial, the coordinating center must maintain the utmost integrity and must prevent conflicts of interest. In very large trials, the roles of the clinical coordinating center and the data coordinating center may be split between different entities, or regional coordinating centers may serve to coordinate activities in individual regions or countries in a "hub and spoke" model.

Data and Safety Monitoring Committee

The DSMC is an essential component of any large RCT of a new treatment. These committees comprise individuals who are independent of the investigators and the sponsor—and in view of the power of DSMCs in clinical trials, a complete lack of any real or apparent conflict of interest is critical. DSMC membership typically includes individuals with expertise in biostatistics, clinical trial methodology, and the field under investigation (e.g., heart failure). DSMCs usually have charters that very specifically delineate their relationship to the sponsor, their operating procedures, their meeting schedules, and either the guiding principles for their duties or explicit statements of the tasks and the procedures that they will use to complete them. DSMC meetings are scheduled at regular intervals either chronologically or on the basis of numbers of events or enrollment. These meetings often have an open session portion, in which the principal investigator, steering committee, or sponsor can address any questions that DSMC members might have, but the data are reviewed in closed sessions with only DSMC members present. As discussed in the next section, the DSMC is often responsible for developing, implementing, and interpreting statistical "stopping rules" for the trial, which may terminate a trial before completion because of undue harm, efficacy, or futility. DSMCs may also be responsible for reviewing unmasked data and making recommendations on altering sample size of the study or changing entry criteria for safety issues. Unless extraordinary reasons can be presented, a DSMC is an ethical necessity for any significant RCT of a new therapy. In very early phase trials or confirmatory studies of approved therapies, alternative methods may be used, as opposed to a formal DSMC, but ongoing attention to patient safety is critical in all clinical trials.[61]

DSMC Responsibilities: Administrative Analyses and Safety Analyses

Administrative analyses are the evaluations of the data by the DSMC that are related to the integrity and conduct of the trial. The DSMC may be given the responsibility to perform analyses to assess the validity of the design assumptions or to make recommendations regarding recruitment and thereby possibly make changes in the entry criteria. The DSMC can analyze the baseline data and check for any randomization imbalances in important variables that may suggest problems with the randomization scheme. An important role of administrative analyses and the DSMC is in assessing the event rate in view of the planned sample size and statistical power. If the DSMC members believe that the initially planned sample size would be inadequate to address the hypothesis, they may make recommendations to the study leadership and the sponsor to enroll more patients, extend the follow-up period, or both.

The DSMC has primary ethical responsibility for the safety of the patients and, consequently, has access to unmasked data on all adverse events. If there is evidence of an increased rate of adverse events among the treatment recipients, further analysis might be performed to determine correlates or predictors of the unfavorable outcome, and recommendations can be made to modify the entry criteria or trial procedures. These forms of safety analyses can be performed with minimal impact on the overall power of the trial, but repeated testing of the primary efficacy endpoint can have significant implications, as discussed in the next section.

One of the most important potential activities of the DSMC is to make recommendations to study leadership regarding the premature discontinuation of a clinical trial. Trials may be stopped early because of evidence of harm, conclusively established efficacy, or futility. Definitive evidence that the new therapy being tested is unsafe is a self-evident reason for stopping a trial prematurely. Conversely, if there is clear evidence of a beneficial effect of the treatment, it is in the best interest of the general population that the therapy be made available to all qualified patients. Finally, if a trial has minimal chance of producing any meaningful result, it is important to be able to inform the subjects of this futility and stop the trial. The recommendations of the DSMC are therefore complex decisions that integrate a multitude of inputs; consequently, strict stopping rules are not practical. However, predefined statistical procedures for assessing negative and positive trends, as well as futility in continuing a trial, are essential for providing the basis for these decisions. The statistical tests used in interim analyses have a number of challenges: First, they must address the issue of the statistical cost of repeated testing. Second, they must be designed to address the specific question; tests that may be applicable to the decision to stop a study may not be the most appropriate for assessing the futility of continuing a trial. Third, there must be a method for extrapolating from an incomplete data set.

Repeated testing of a hypothesis increases the probability of a false-positive result.[62] This fundamental principle of statistics has important ramifications for interim analyses in trials. For example, if five interim analyses are conducted with $\alpha = 0.05$, then the false-positive error is almost 15%, or three times greater than the standard acceptable α error. Thus, to account for these repeated tests of the study hypothesis, multiple methods have been developed. The general procedure in these interim analyses is to create, either arbitrarily or by statistical modeling, a critical boundary against which to compare the study's test statistic value at the interim analysis (Z_i). If the study's Z_i has crossed the boundary, then the null hypothesis may be rejected (Figure 39-4).[63] The most commonly used statistical methods for DSMCs in RCTs are group-sequential procedures and conditional power (or stochastic curtailment) methods, which are discussed briefly as follows.

A number of group-sequential procedures have been used, ranging from the ad hoc selection of a high critical value arbitrarily selected so that when final adjustments are made for repeated testing, the final α level is protected (Haybittle-Peto method[64]), to more precise methods of guaranteeing a precise type I error (see Figure 39-4). The O'Brien-Fleming group-sequential method has a very low likelihood of accepting the null hypothesis early in the trial, but the α at the interim test point (α_i) increases with subsequent analyses to be nearly equal to the overall α at the last analysis.[65,66] For example, if the overall α is selected to be 0.05 and there are five interim analyses, the first interim α (α_1) is 0.00001, and the α_5 is 0.046. This method has the advantage of protecting against premature discontinuation of the study at early interim analyses, for which there are relatively few events, and yet allowing the possibility of termination for decidedly negative results. Other approaches have been developed to allow for greater flexibility in the timing and frequency of the interim analyses and still limit the overall type I error.[67]

Conditional power analysis, or stochastic curtailment, is an attempt to predict the probability that the null hypothesis will ultimately be rejected if the desired sample size is attained, according to the accumulated data up to that point.[68] If the probability that the trial will be either positive or negative is very low, the decision may be made to stop the study before completion. In practice, however, such futility stopping rules apply most frequently to the ability of the trial to demonstrate a significant benefit.

These approaches often employ symmetrical stopping boundaries (i.e., the same boundaries are applied for both a negative result and a positive result), but clinical decisions may be asymmetrical. Many investigators and DSMC members are willing to enroll more patients to clearly establish the effectiveness of a new therapy (a relatively high upper boundary) but are less comfortable allowing a trial to continue if there is a strong suggestion of harm (a lower threshold for discontinuation). Asymmetrical stopping boundaries are an attempt to take into account the investigators' level of concern about the safety of the new therapy.[69] For example, in the MERIT-HF study of metoprolol XL—which was performed at a time when there were significant concerns about the safety of giving β-blockers to patients with heart failure—the researchers used asymmetrical boundary procedures from the onset of the study.[70]

The statistical methods just described provide a foundation upon which a DSMC can build their decision as to whether to recommend continuation or termination of a trial, but they are only one contribution to a very complicated structure. Other elements important to consider include evaluating the comparability of the groups for baseline variables; ensuring that evaluation of the endpoint was unbiased; verifying patient adherence; searching for internal consistency by looking for concordance with other outcomes and among subgroups; checking for external consistency in comparison to known mechanisms of action and results from other similar trials or agents in the same class; ensuring that the length of follow-up has been adequate for making a decision; and considering the potential public effect of either terminating or continuing the trial. Once all of these factors are integrated, the DSMC attempts to make a decision on the basis of protecting patient safety and respecting the scientific integrity of the clinical trial.

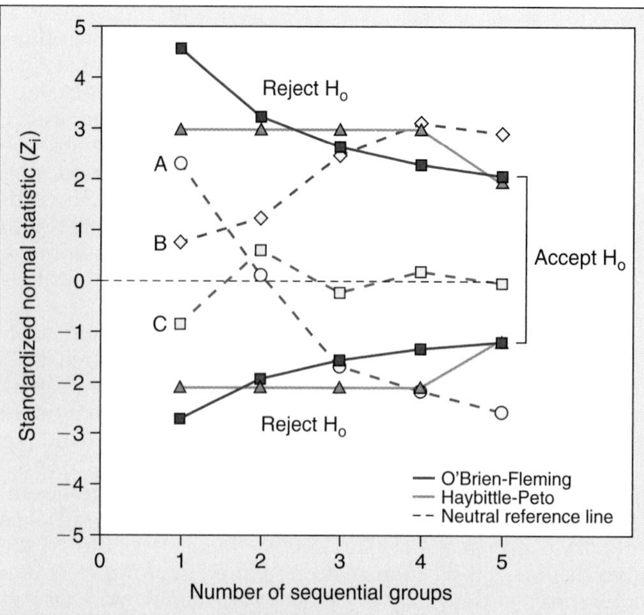

FIGURE 39-4 Asymmetrical stopping boundaries (*solid symbols*) for the standardized normal statistic with five interim analyses in which two group sequential methods were used [O'Brien-Fleming (solid purple squares) and Haybittle-Peto (solid orange triangles)]. The fifth analysis is the final analysis of the study, and in this example, the boundary for rejecting the null hypothesis (H_0) for benefit (a positive Z_i value) is more stringent than the boundary for demonstrating harm. Dashed lines A, B, and C (*open symbols*) represent hypothetical trials. In trial A (open circles, blue line), the early suggestion of benefit rapidly disappears, so that at the third or fourth interim analysis, a data and safety monitoring committee (DSMC) might consider terminating the study early to avoid harm. In trial B (open diamonds, red line), outcome also nears a boundary at the third interim analysis, but this time for benefit. The study might be continued after the third analysis, but it is discontinued for benefit after the fourth analysis. Results of trial C (open squares,green line) remain neutral during the course of the entire study; it is possible that a conditional power analysis would suggest at the fourth interim analysis that there was little chance for the trial to produce a meaningful result and the trial could be stopped for futility, depending on the prespecified definitions. (Adapted from Friedman LM, Furberg CD, DeMets DL. *Fundamentals of clinical trials,* ed 3, New York, 1998, Springer-Verlag. With kind permission of Springer Science+Business Media.)

Endpoint or Clinical Events Committee

The endpoint committee, or clinical events committee, is meant to address the considerable variability that exists between the treating physicians, hospitals, regions, countries, and continents with regard to clinical practice and event definitions. The major advantage of a clinical events committee is that it can standardize the definitions for and interpretation of clinical events, which increases the validity and comparability of the trial results. The ability to validate endpoints in a blinded manner is very important in assessing endpoints that are difficult to adjudicate (e.g., mode of death) or "softer" endpoints (e.g., myocardial infarction or hospitalization for heart failure).[24,25] Of course, the definitions that the clinical events committee uses for an event may not effectively encompass the variability of clinical practice in different regions. For example, the endpoint of the OVERTURE study[28] included only hospitalizations for heart failure in which the patients required intravenous medications, as a means of mandating higher severity of illness for the disease-specific hospitalization event. Unfortunately for the trial, aggressive oral diuretic therapy is the standard of care in some regions, and consequently, some admissions for heart failure did not count toward the endpoint. Although some study sponsors prefer not to have blinded event adjudication by a clinical events committee because of the extra expense involved, there is clear evidence of the positive effects of clinical events committees on overall trial validity.[71]

Site Investigators

The site investigators and nurse coordinators are the people who make the study work, by enrolling patients, caring for and following them, completing case report forms, and observing for important adverse or other effects. As with the sponsor of a trial, the site investigators also have specific responsibilities defined by the FDA, which include ensuring that an investigation is conducted according to the signed investigator statement, the investigational plan, and applicable regulations; protecting the rights, safety, and welfare of subjects under the investigator's care; control of drugs under investigation; and obtaining informed consent from study participants. Investigators must also have a high degree of integrity, especially in the face of financial incentives and continual pressure from the study leadership, coordinating center and sponsor to enroll as many patients as rapidly as possible.

Maximizing study enrollment is a substantial and ever-increasing challenge. To yield useful results, a large RCT in heart failure must enroll a large number of patients who have a chronic and often debilitating disease in a human experiment that may results in significant inconvenience or discomfort, with no guarantee of individual benefit. Almost invariably, initial projections about the rate of enrollment are overly optimistic, in comparison with when the trial is actually conducted. For the study to finish successfully, the investigators', study coordinators', and other clinical personnel's efforts at the study site must be sustained and ongoing. Increasingly complex regulatory requirements and diminished reimbursement for clinical research have exacerbated the difficulty in enrolling patients in heart failure trials in the United States and Western Europe. The proportion of patients in large international trials enrolled in other parts of the world, especially Eastern Europe, South America, India, and China, has accordingly increased dramatically. Although this increasing globalization of clinical trials potentially enhances the generalizability of results, it also introduces substantial concerns. For regulatory agencies such as the FDA, there is uncertainty in how to interpret clinical trial data that were collected primarily from patients with different genetic backgrounds, different comorbid conditions, different health behaviors, and different medical care. In addition, ethical considerations mandate that the developing world not be used to provide research subjects to investigate therapies that are then marketed primarily in the United States at prices that would make them difficult to obtain in the developing countries. This issue has received substantial attention in both the media and the scientific community.[72,73]

Study Subjects

Patients who consent to participate in RCTs agree to undergo possible inconvenience, discomfort, and often poorly defined risks for the purpose of obtaining generalizable knowledge. The motivations for patients to participate in clinical research have been studied extensively.[74] Many patients who participate in clinical trials do so with the expectation that participation will be of benefit to them, either through the study intervention itself or through the greater medical attention associated with being a study participant; others do so primarily because of a sense of altruism.[75,76] Whatever their motivation for participation, clinical trial participants should be treated with the utmost respect and gratitude. Their willingness to participate in the human experiment of a clinical trial helps provide the evidence for advancing scientific knowledge and improving the practice of medicine for all patients.

RANDOMIZED CONTROLLED TRIALS IN THE CONTEXT OF DRUG DEVELOPMENT: TRANSITIONAL STUDIES

Although many of the issues discussed are generalizable to all types of clinical trials, much of the preceding discussion has focused on large, multicenter RCTs with clinical endpoints, which are the types of pivotal trials that provide evidence in support of the regulatory approval and clinical use of drugs. Of importance, however, is that these definitive trials are the end of a long development process. Development programs of new therapies have traditionally been divided into three phases, each with distinct objectives and potential issues in trial design for each. The purpose of phase I studies is to assess the safety of a new therapy in humans, with the specific objectives to characterize the metabolism, pharmacokinetics, pharmacodynamics, dose-response ratio, tolerability, and possible dose-limiting side effects of the therapy before further investigation. The size of these studies varies greatly but generally ranges from 20 to 80 patients. In phase II studies, the dose and effectiveness of the therapy are evaluated for one or more specific indications in patients who have the condition of interest, and the common short-term side effects and risks associated with the drug are determined. In pragmatic terms, phase II studies are critical in defining the dose to be used in the larger phase III studies and to confirm the proof of concept of the therapy being tested, as well as providing information on the magnitude of effect to be studied. Because of the limited time and financial resources generally available at this phase of investigation, these studies may evaluate a limited number and range of doses and employ surrogate endpoints for clinical outcomes. Phase III trials are large studies designed to convincingly demonstrate the efficacy of the therapy, to provide safety information for a more complete evaluation of its benefit-to-risk ratio, and to ultimately define how the therapy should be used. These trials often include from several hundred to thousands of patients.

Although these phases of investigation are useful for discussing trial design and goals, some points regarding this paradigm must be remembered. These phases do not represent a plan that guarantees regulatory approval of the therapy; rather, they serve as a guideline about the types of information that the regulatory agencies require to assess a new therapy. A therapy may already be known to be effective for a different, often related indication (e.g., hypertension, myocardial infarction), and in this case, its evaluation in heart failure may involve a single phase III trial. Consequently, most pharmaceutical and device manufacturers enter into discussions with the FDA and other regulatory agencies early in the course of development and again before conducting phase III studies, both to ensure that their approaches are likely to be acceptable for approval, if positive, and to minimize risk to the participating subjects. The distinction between phase II and phase III trials has become progressively blurred and new study designs have been developed to transition rapidly from phase II and phase III studies and yet retain much of the study architecture.

The initial steps in the clinical development process are meant to provide a bridge between the basic scientific tenets that suggested such therapies could be useful and the definitive studies that convince investigators that the therapy can beneficially influence outcomes in a patient population. This "bench-to-bedside" transition is complicated by numerous factors, but it ultimately requires the confirmation that the therapy performs in humans in its intended manner (i.e., proof of concept) and the determination of appropriate dosages to allow more widespread testing of hypotheses (i.e., dose selection). These studies have often been considered phase II studies, but for the purposes of this discussion, they are referred to as *transitional studies,* to emphasize their role in serving as a transition from basic discovery to large-scale evaluation of efficacy. Various approaches to these critical steps in the evaluation of new therapies are summarized in Table 39-1.[77]

The selection of patients for these transitional studies is greatly influenced by the endpoints, so as to optimize the possibility of demonstrating meaningful differences between

TABLE 39–1 Approaches to the Design of Transitional (Phase II) Trials

Approach	Method	Advantages	Disadvantages
Intuitive	Drug administered by a select group of investigators who observe effects in open-label, unblinded studies and make recommendations	• Rapid, cheap, and ease to conduct	• Investigators cannot reliably discern clinical benefit • Purely subjective
Mechanistic	Administer drug in multiple dosages and select dosage that has optimal biological effect thought to best reflect drug's mechanism of action	• Often quantitative • Testable hypothesis • Rational	• Limited ability of preclinical research to reliably identify relationship of importance of mechanism in animals to that in humans • Biological effect of drug may be impossible to measure in patients • Drug may have multiple effects that may supersede its intended actions • Difficult to determine the degree of the biological effect necessary to demonstrate efficacy • Short-term biological effects may not be maintained over long term • No clear relation between mechanistic efficacy and effect on clinical outcomes
Efficacy-pilot	Administer drug in multiple dosages and select dosage that has optimal effect on an array of clinical endpoints	• Clinical relevance	• Usually no single endpoint is selected, so not clear whether results are informative • Differences are typically small, and trends are often conflicting • Does not yield benefit-to-risk information
Safety-pilot	Administer drug in multiple dosages and select dosage that has optimal safety profile	• Clinical relevance	• Mechanism of action and clinical efficacy are assumed to be established • Difficult to determine the correct dose of a new drug on basis of its safety profile • Unlikely that safety can effectively be assessed in intermediate-sized trial (<500 patients) • Does not yield benefit-to-risk information

Adapted from Packer M. Current perspectives on the design of phase II trials of new drugs for the treatment of heart failure. *Am Heart J* 2000;139:S202-S206.

the therapy and the control group (either placebo or active-control condition). The inclusion and exclusion criteria for these studies are typically much more restrictive than in later, larger trials. Selection is based on the presence of a particularly relevant aspect of the pathophysiological features or mechanism of heart failure (e.g., elevated neurohormonal concentrations), more severe manifestation of a particular symptom or greater probability for an improvement (e.g., limited exercise tolerance), or higher risk for a specific adverse effect or safety-related issue (e.g., ventricular arrhythmias). Many protocols focus on defining the "ideal" patient for the therapy, under the assumption that if the therapy is not effective in this ideal patient, it would not be effective or safe in other patient populations. The advantage of these enriched populations is that the higher event rates may overcome the relatively small sample size of these transitional studies. The disadvantage of these narrowly defined groups is that they are often not representative of the broader population in which the subsequent trial will be performed and thus have limited predictive value for that setting. In addition, selecting the "ideal" patient requires a degree of understanding of the underlying mechanisms of both the drug and the pathophysiological features of heart failure, an understanding that may be unavailable. Despite these limitations, the approach of patient selection directed at including an enriched population is the most favorable for these transitional studies.

Selection of Dose Range and Endpoints in Transitional Studies

A key goal of transitional studies of new therapies is to identify the most appropriate dosage to use in larger trials. The selection of the appropriate dose range is confined by two limits. The upper limit is typically defined by the safety profile of the drug (the maximally tolerated dosage), and the lower limit is usually defined by efficacy (the minimally effective dosage). A common approach, particularly if little is known about the dose range, is an ascending-dose design. Alternatively, a parallel design may be invoked in which many dose groups are studied in order to determine the optimal dosage. However, the more numerous the dosage groups are, the more difficult it is to demonstrate meaningful differences in efficacy or safety, unless the sample size is substantial. For many reasons, primarily economic, it is rare that study researchers will investigate a truly broad range of doses. Because of these challenges, newer approaches to study design (discussed in the next section) have evolved to include a wide range of dosages that are based on the best informed extrapolations from both animal data and human pharmacological data (preferably in patients with heart failure) but make provisions for dropping dosage conditions as the study proceeds.

Transitional studies are typically smaller than phase III definitive studies and, as such, rarely have sufficient power to use clinical endpoints. Selection of appropriate surrogate endpoints, as defined previously, is therefore a key aspect of designing transitional studies. The search for useful surrogate endpoints in heart failure has been fraught with difficulty, and at present there are no universally accepted surrogate endpoints for this condition. In general, potential surrogates used in transitional studies may be focused on physiological variables, clinical composites, or safety, each of which is discussed as follows.

In many transitional studies, physiological variables, such as hemodynamic measurements, ejection fraction, or levels of a biomarker (e.g., natriuretic peptides), are used as endpoints. Such endpoints are theoretically attractive because they appear to reflect the underlying mechanism of drug effect; for example, inotropic drugs work by increasing cardiac output, and therefore hemodynamic changes seem to be an appropriate surrogate endpoint. However, this approach presupposes a level of understanding of both the mechanism of drug action and heart failure physiology; this understanding is often lacking. In addition, drug efficacy and drug safety may involve very different mechanisms, and therefore drugs that maximize a physiological effect related to efficacy (e.g., cardiac output) may have an unacceptable rate of adverse effects (e.g., arrhythmias). The history of drug development in heart failure contains numerous examples of drugs that were developed on the basis of maximizing physiological surrogates but failed in larger studies because of unanticipated adverse effects. For example, blockade of the effects of tumor necrosis factor α with etanercept had clear biological plausibility and had been shown to increase the physiological surrogate of ejection fraction in transitional studies.[78-80] Despite these very promising early results, this therapy was not shown to be beneficial when tested in larger efficacy trials.[46] It is important to recognize that the failure of these drugs was not necessarily a failure of the concept that these drugs addressed; rather, it was attributable to unrecognized potential adverse effects. Mechanistic endpoints remain attractive in as much as they provide a rationale for the application of the therapy to patients with heart failure. If specific mechanisms are well enough defined in humans and the results are interpreted with appropriate caution, mechanistic transitional studies may still provide a basis on which to select a dose range for subsequent study.

A second category of endpoints in transitional studies are clinical efficacy measures. To the extent to which such measures often reflect patient symptoms and functional status, these are not true surrogate endpoints, but they often serve this purpose in transitional studies. When used in transitional studies, multiple clinical endpoints are often combined in a single composite in order to clarify the overall clinical effect of a given therapy. Such endpoints may include measures of clinical events (especially worsening of heart failure, hospitalizations, and death), supplemented by assessments of exercise tolerance, symptoms, or quality of life. The advantage of these endpoints is that they are clinically relevant. However, the size of such studies, the brief duration of follow-up, and the relatively low event rates usually preclude selection of one of these measures as the primary endpoint for transitional studies, and rarely do they reach statistical significance. In the absence of this statistical rigor, the small differences between groups and nonsignificant trends of these assessments must be carefully interpreted. This subjective interpretation is often complicated by results that demonstrate conflicting trends, which further limits the usefulness of any conclusions regarding dosage and design of the subsequent larger trials. In addition, these studies rely on the assumption that the clinical efficacy measures are predictive of the more important clinical outcome measures, such as morbidity and mortality. Unfortunately, this assumption has been incorrect in numerous instances. For instance, inotropic drugs such as milrinone appear to improve symptoms but have an adverse effect on mortality rate. In contrast, many angiotensin-converting enzyme inhibitors and β-blockers did not improve exercise tolerance but did improve prognosis. Finally, these types of endpoints do not yield any information regarding the ultimate benefit-to-risk ratio of the therapy, which is necessary for truly assessing efficacy.

The third category of endpoints in transitional studies focuses on safety issues. In these studies, either one or many of the potential pertinent safety concerns are selected as the endpoint, with the goal of determining the dosage with the best profile for adverse events. Examples of these endpoints include arrhythmias, hypotension, renal dysfunction, electrolyte abnormalities, and other dose-limiting side effects specific to the therapy. This approach is an attempt to directly address the concern raised by previous drug development programs, in which the failure to recognize serious adverse effects resulted in exposure of thousands of patients to increased risk and in the ultimate termination of the development program. These studies may be able to assist with dosage selection, if there are marked safety issues, and the investigators and sponsor are willing to accept a significant degree of uncertainty about these safety estimates. Unfortunately, these studies also fall prey to the limitations noted previously: The studies are generally too small with brief follow-up durations to provide definitive evidence of either safety or harm. In addition, the clinically effective dose is presumed to be known already, and no important difference in efficacy is presumed among the dosages selected for the safety study. As discussed previously, these safety studies also do not provide information about the overall balance of the safety and efficacy of the therapy. Regardless of the endpoint selected, however, any reasonably sized study should have independent unblinded monitoring to protect the safety of the subjects, such as an independent DSMC.

NOVEL APPROACHES TO DESIGN OF CLINICAL TRIALS IN HEART FAILURE

A fundamental problem for drug development in heart failure is that, of the drugs that have successfully progressed through phase II studies, few have actually proved effective in larger, more definitive studies. The imperative to develop newer, more effective, and economical development strategies is clear, but the potential solutions are constrained by the nature of heart failure. The pathophysiological processes of heart failure are multifactorial and highly integrated, which results both in considerable difficulty in predicting the response to a therapy and in a high likelihood of unintended effects. This variability increases the difficulty in drawing valid conclusions from small pilot studies. Many patients with heart failure are elderly and have other comorbid conditions; thus, competing risks that may not exist for other disease states are present in heart failure. Furthermore, in view of the proven efficacy of currently available therapies such as β-blockers and angiotensin-converting enzyme inhibitors, overall rate of events in patients with heart failure is declining, which necessitates progressively larger numbers of subjects in order to demonstrate meaningful differences. As with any experimental science in which multiple dynamic factors are present, clinical trials adapt to these changes. Previously, this adaptation was achieved in a less formal manner, which often undermined the ability of a trial to provide valid statistical inference. In contemporary clinical science, there are new approaches to modify trials so that they may be responsive to dynamic information, which may be broadly categorized as adaptive designs.[81]

Adaptive design of a clinical trial is "a design that allows adaptations or modifications to some aspects of the trial after its initiation without undermining the validity and integrity of the trial."[82] Three general types of adaptation may be described. In *prospectively designed adaptation,* there is a protocol-specified plan for using adaptive techniques to modify the study. Examples of prospective adaptation include sequential trial designs, interim analyses to apply predefined stopping rules for benefit, harm, or futility or for sample size re-estimation. Application of contemporary statistical techniques, such as conditional probabilities, allows for the prospective construction of boundaries as the basis for stopping rules, which may not only protect patient welfare but also spare the sponsor and patients further burdens when a trial is futile. *Ongoing* or *ad hoc adaptation* includes adjustment in the inclusion and exclusion criteria, dose or dosing regimen, and treatment or follow-up duration. These changes may introduce bias, inasmuch as the target population, the intervention itself, or both are altered by these modifications. Although statistical methods to account for these changes may help to preserve scientific validity, substantial changes in midstudy almost always introduce complications into the analysis and interpretation of study results. *Retrospective adaptive design* is the most flexible but also most vulnerable to bias and to undermining the validity of a trial. Examples of retrospective (but before unmasking) adaptation include changing the primary or other endpoints and changing the hypothesis from superiority to noninferiority, or vice versa.

Adaptive methods have been widely applied in the study of oncology but rarely in the study of heart failure. Because of the potential efficiency of these methods, however, they will probably be implemented in heart failure trials more frequently in the future. Some examples include adaptive randomization, adaptive hypotheses, and treatment switching, as well as some specific adaptive trial designs. In *adaptive randomization*, various methods can be used to adjust the probability that a subject will be randomly assigned to a specific condition of the trial according to some characteristic of the patients previously enrolled. This technique can balance variance within the enrolled population with regard to such things as investigational site or covariates such as comorbid conditions, age, and gender. For trials in which there are ethical concerns about the treatment conditions, adaptive randomization techniques can allocate patients to the most appropriate treatment groups on the basis of the response of prior patients.[83] These techniques have implications for subsequent hypothesis testing and sample size determination, but methods exist to adjust for these adaptations in randomization. *Adaptive hypotheses,* in which the hypothesis of the study is adapted to the evolving clinical picture, include the incorporation of data from other studies to guide the study under consideration, to include new dosages of the study treatment, or to make changes according to the recommendations of the DSMC.[84] Finally, adaptive techniques for evaluating *treatment switching* may also prove useful in future heart failure trials. This technique is particularly helpful in parallel-group active control studies, in which the patients are randomly assigned to either the active control condition or the study medication condition and are allowed to switch from one treatment to another for lack of response or evidence of disease progression.[85,86] Potential applications include AHF studies, in which the acuity and severity of symptoms preclude a true no-therapy control and many patients may switch conditions.

Various adaptive approaches to designing transitional studies of new heart failure therapies have also been used.[87,88] One design that is receiving increased consideration is the "drop-the-loser," or select-drop, design for dose selection or multicondition phase III trials.[89,90] These designs were initially described in the context of cancer therapy studies and addressed the problem of how to select among multiple different treatment regimens varying in dosages and agents.[91-93] In this design, patients are randomly assigned to one of a few different treatment regimens or to a placebo/standard therapy control condition, and, often with the use of a combined endpoint, each group in which treatment fails in comparison with the control group is dropped sequentially until one regimen is selected. This endpoint can incorporate both efficacy measures and safety or adverse events as stopping rules for the groups. Multiple methods of adaptive allocation of patients in dose-escalation studies can also be used to minimize patients' exposure to adverse effects while maximizing treatment with potentially efficacious doses. Two of these methods include the continued reassessment method[94] and a hybrid frequentist-bayesian approach.[95] Statistical methods for these sequential group designs have been developed,[96] and statistical research has incorporated bayesian analyses and decision theory.[97-99]

A significant potential limitation of applying this approach to dosage-finding studies is that relevant information about the agent being studied may be unavailable, inasmuch as each group is analyzed independently and so information on the overall pattern of dose-response may be lost. Some investigators have suggested using a prospectively planned combination of active groups for comparisons in transitional studies; others have sought to leverage the data from multiple-dosage groups by developing dose-response curves with regard to outcomes of interest in order to select appropriate doses. However, the select-drop designs have the advantage of comparing many dosages through the use of clinical endpoints with the potential of producing more clinically relevant information while enrolling fewer patients. These advantages are most evident in trials that are designed to combine phases II and III studies. An example of the combined phase II/III design is the Platelet Glycoprotein IIb/IIIa in Unstable Angina: Receptor Suppression Using Integrilin Therapy (PURSUIT) trial,[100,101] in which a prespecified interim analysis revealed no significant evidence of an unacceptable safety profile in the high-dose condition, and so the low-dose condition was dropped. The PURSUIT trial had positive efficacy results with the high-dose condition that ultimately led to FDA approval of the drug. A more recent example includes the Placebo-controlled Randomized study of the selective A1 adenosine receptor antagonist KW-3902 for patients hospitalized with acute HF and volume Overload to assess Treatment Effect on Congestion and renal function Trial (PROTECT) phase II/III program, consisting of two sequential studies of the effect of rolofylline in patients with AHF. The PROTECT pilot study[34] demonstrated improved clinical outcomes and provided crucial information for dosage selection and allowed for a relatively seamless transition to the phase III PROTECT trial.

The combined phase II/III trial design has a number of advantages, including continuous enrollment during both phases of the study with the consequent potential time efficiency and the ability to apply outcome data from the patients who were in the phase II stage of the trial to the phase III primary endpoint. In this combined design, however, it may be difficult to perform the study with more than three or four groups, which limits the ability to explore a full dose-response range. In addition, there is less flexibility in the assessment of secondary endpoints, the inclusion and exclusion criteria need to be broad enough for a large-scale phase III trial, and the procedures used to select the appropriate dosage may complicate the assessment of the primary endpoint. If safety assessments are used to guide the selection of the dosage, then the most effective dose may not be selected, whereas if the criteria for dose-selection in the transitional study stage include efficacy assessments, then the sample size of the whole trial needs to be increased, or an adjustment to the overall α error must be made, or both. It is hoped that these and other newer approaches to the design of transitional clinical trials will help address the specific challenges in establishing proof of concept and selecting the dose for new therapeutic agents in heart failure.

Underlying many of these advances in adaptive design is the application of bayesian analysis.[102] Bayesian approaches differ fundamentally from traditional, frequentist methods. In the frequentist model, parameters must be viewed as fixed so that probabilities of experimental observations can be calculated. This model explains why changing trial design (or parameters of a study) poses such difficulties for frequentist analysis. As soon as parameters are changed, the basis for the statistical inference is undermined. However, in the bayesian approach, all components of the trial, all uncertainty, are measured by probabilities, calculated from the known factors in the trial. Thus, there is more flexibility in these approaches to adapt to changes in clinical trial design. The bayesian approach incorporates continuous updating of the models as information becomes available, but it can require significant computer power and complex mathematical models. The full potential of this statistical approach has not been realized in a clinical development program to date, but there is growing enthusiasm in the both the research community[103] and in regulatory agencies[104,105] for this model. Figure 39-5 provides an example of how a program might be designed to incorporate some of the novel approaches just described.[106]

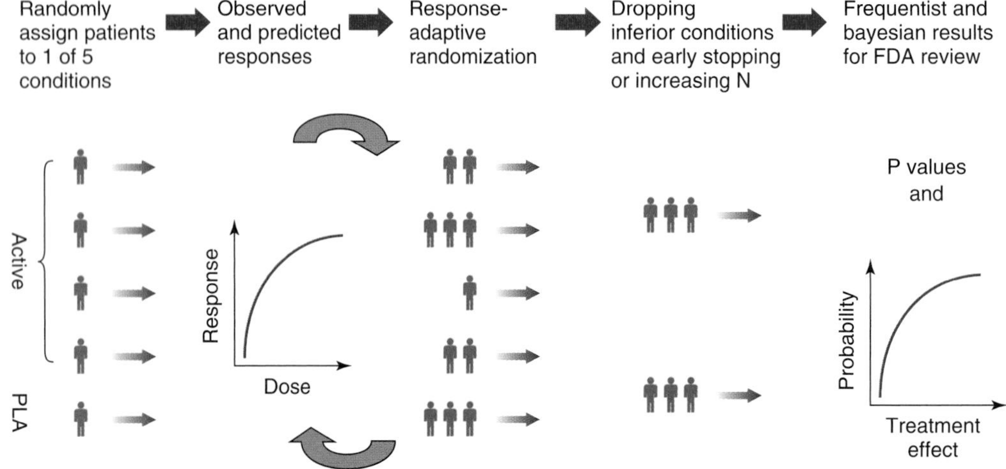

FIGURE 39–5 Example of an adaptive trial design involving the use of bayesian statistics. The trial starts as a dose-ranging study, in which four dose levels are compared with placebo; patients are enrolled on the basis of a response-adaptive randomization with an iterative interaction between the responses of those previously enrolled and the random assignment of new patients. As probability thresholds are crossed for selecting groups of different dose recipients, inferior doses are sequentially dropped, leaving the one dose for the phase III trial. The patients continue to be enrolled under the same protocol with whatever amendments are necessitated, and an interim analysis is performed to assess for early stopping or adjustment of sample size. After completion of the trial, frequentist analyses may be performed, but the evaluation by The European Agency for the Evaluation of Medicinal Products (EMEA) or the U.S. Food and Drug Administration (FDA) will be based on a bayesian assessment of the totality of the clinical package. *PLA,* placebo. (Adapted from Chow SC, Chang M. Adaptive design methods in clinical trials—a review. *Orphanet J Rare Dis* 2008;3:11. Permission granted from BioMed central.)

RANDOMIZED CONTROLLED TRIALS IN SPECIFIC CLINICAL SETTINGS

Acute Decompensated Heart Failure

Although many of the factors just described are applicable to studies of AHF, AHF trials have specific challenges that are only becoming completely recognized and that have been the subject of extensive discussion in conferences since 2005.[107,108]

The population of patients with AHF is extraordinarily heterogeneous, and entry criteria for a trial must be defined by the mechanism of action of the study medication or device. First, the patient population must actually have AHF, as opposed to other conditions that may imitate AHF, such as an exacerbation of chronic obstructive pulmonary disease or acute coronary syndromes. Because heart failure has traditionally been a clinical diagnosis without clear objective diagnostic criteria, enrollment of "pure" AHF populations in clinical trials has been a major challenge. The use of biomarkers such as natriuretic peptides and troponins to identify patients with AHF and exclude patients with acute coronary syndromes has been a major advance in clinical trials of AHF.[34]

A second important issue in study design is the targeting of appropriate subgroups within the heterogeneous AHF population as a whole. Ideally, studies should target the patients most likely to benefit from a particular intervention and exclude those more likely to be harmed by it. Renal function and blood pressure are very important factors to consider in the selection of patients for given clinical trials. Patients with low blood pressures and those who experience hypotension during hospitalization have poor outcomes,[109] and so interventions with vasodilating properties should be restricted to patients with higher baseline blood pressures. Although researchers in many studies of vasodilating drugs may wish to avoid patients with renal dysfunction, therapies with putative renoprotective properties should target patients at high risk for worsening renal failure, typically patients who already have poor baseline renal function.[34] Enrolling all patients with acute heart failure rather than targeting therapy to a specific group on the basis of the mechanism of action of the new therapy may be partially responsible for the failure of some AHF trials.

Study procedures in clinical trials of AHF therapies also have some unique aspects. First, because of the dynamic nature of an AHF clinical course, there are multiple distinct times and corresponding clinical conditions at which a patient may be enrolled.[108] During the initial or early-intervention phase, patients are more symptomatic and have received less potentially confounding therapy, which allows for optimal opportunity to demonstrate a symptomatic or other clinical benefit, but there is also greater diagnostic uncertainty. The advent of BNP assays has assisted in considerably limiting this uncertainty, and an emphasis on the early involvement of emergency department personnel has enabled early enrollment in some contemporary trials, with encouraging results.[34] Some agents may be more suitable for treating the patient during the in-hospital phase, in which the goals of therapy are to promote further improvement in the signs and symptoms of AHF, whereas other agents may be more useful in the predischarge phase. One study of tolvaptan included patients from all phases of the hospitalization, leveraging the availability of an oral formulation.[110,111] A second issue is the challenge of background therapy in AHF trials. Because no therapy for AHF is currently evidence based, background therapy may vary widely between patients, thereby complicating interpretation of the efficacy and safety of new therapies. Finally, defining the proper follow-up period for acutely administered therapies is also a challenge. Most AHF therapies are given for short durations, often 24 to 72 hours, and so the best time interval over which to assess safety is unknown. In most studies, researchers examine events up to 180 days after randomization, although both investigators and regulators acknowledge that most therapies would probably not continue to have safety effects this remotely. Fortunately, most AHF studies do not have to face difficulties of adherence.

Endpoint selection for AHF studies remains a major challenge in clinical trial design and has been reviewed in detail.[111a] Traditionally, many drug development programs have used demonstration of a hemodynamic benefit as support for efficacy of the therapy; such drugs include nesiritide,[112] levosimendan,[113] and tezosentan.[114] However, there is considerable regulatory skepticism about the ability of improvements in hemodynamics to translate into improved clinical outcomes, and hemodynamics alone are no longer considered a valid endpoint in AHF studies. Although mortality is of unequivocal importance, many investigators have questioned the likelihood that a 24-hour infusion of an intravenous therapy could have a significant effect after discharge. This has led to a focus on morbidity (e.g., rehospitalization) or symptomatic endpoints (e.g., dyspnea) and has resulted in a disparate array of endpoints and composites that have been used in published phase III clinical trials in AHF (Table 39-2).[34,36,37,110-112,115-118] These can be classified as short-term symptomatic endpoints (e.g., dyspnea improvement), endpoints reflecting events during the index hospitalization (e.g., worsening heart failure that necessitates rescue therapy), or postdischarge endpoints (e.g., death or rehospitalization).

One of the most prominent symptoms that patients report is dyspnea, and dyspnea has been evaluated in many studies as a secondary endpoint; in the pivotal Vasodilatation in the Management of Acute CHF (VMAC) trial, dyspnea was assessed as a coprimary endpoint with change in pulmonary capillary wedge pressure.[112] However, dyspnea is very difficult to evaluate as an endpoint, especially when confounded by the presence of invasive hemodynamics, as in those trials.[119] The Randomized Interventions with TeZosentan (RITZ-1)[120] and Value of Endothelin Receptor Inhibition with Tezosentan in Acute Heart Failure Study (VERITAS)[115] were the first AHF trials in which a symptom (dyspnea) was used as endpoint without the confounding effects of invasive hemodynamics. There are two main instruments for assessing changes in dyspnea. A Likert scale, on which the patient reports a relative change from baseline symptoms with categorical statements ranging from "markedly improved" to "markedly worsened," is very useful for assessing rapid changes in dyspnea, but the patient must compare current symptoms with those at a previous time, such as when study therapy was initiated. On the Visual Analog Scale (VAS), the patient rates the absolute current level of dyspnea on a scale from 0 to 100 at specific times, which allows comparative assessments over longer time scales. Other approaches to the assessment of dyspnea have also been proposed in an effort to provide more objective evaluations of this important subjective symptom.[31]

Recognizing the subjective nature of the dyspnea assessments and their inability to capture the entirety of a patient's response to a therapy, other investigators have developed composite endpoints. In the Second Randomized Multicenter Evaluation of Intravenous Levosimendan Efficacy (REVIVE-II),[117] the patient-reported global assessment had to be moderately or markedly improved at 6 hours, at 24 hours, and at 5 days without evidence of clinical deterioration, for the patient's condition to be considered "improved," whereas evidence of worsening of heart failure or death categorized the patient's condition as "worsened"; those meeting none of these criteria were considered "unchanged." This categorical variable was based on an endpoint developed for chronic heart failure studies.[33] To evaluate the efficacy and safety of newer agents, other clinical development programs are extending this approach to include such effects as worsening of renal function in phase II and phase III trials. As discussed previously, the advantages of using composite endpoints are that the totality of the patient experience can be evaluated and the event rate is increased, but the disadvantage is that they limit differentiation of the severity of events, so that death is weighted similarly to worsening of heart failure. Other approaches, such as a global ranking method, may address some of these challenges in future AHF trials.[35] In general, it seems unlikely that any single endpoint will effectively capture all aspects of the AHF clinical course, and thus it is unlikely that one endpoint will fit all types of RCTs for AHF. This area of clinical trial design for AHF is a topic of very active debate, and many currently ongoing trials will inform the next generation of studies.

Clinical Trials with Devices and Surgery

Device-based and surgical therapies for heart failure have proliferated since 2000. Indeed, the majority of advances in heart failure therapeutics have been driven by devices (e.g., ICDs, CRT, and left ventricular assist devices [LVADs]) rather than by new pharmacological therapies. In comparison with traditional RCTs of new drug therapies, the appropriate evaluation of new devices and surgical techniques presents substantial challenges. In particular, issues related to the technical aspects of the procedure, the more pronounced placebo effect, masking and endpoint selection may be uniquely difficult.

One unique challenge of device and surgical trials that is absent from trials of drugs is the extent to which variations in operator technical skill may affect the efficacy and safety of the therapy. Unlike studies of pharmacological therapies, clinical trials of surgical interventions or devices must account for operator skill level and incorporate an assessment of technical success into study design. "Technical success" itself may be quantified, depending on the intervention. For example, in a study of CRT, successful placement of the lead for the coronary sinus can be reasonably assumed to lead to successful delivery of therapy, and this success can be reliably judged at the time of the procedure. More complicated surgical procedures, such as mitral valve repair or surgical ventricular restoration, are likely to have many more gradations of "technical success," and efficacy may be influenced by small differences in technique that are not readily quantifiable and may not be apparent at the time of the intervention. Various strategies exist for dealing with issues of operator skill level and procedural success. One option, which was used in the MIRACLE study of CRT, is a pilot phase in which operators demonstrate a basic level of technical expertise before being permitted to enroll patients in main trial.[48] Once a procedure is more clinically established (e.g., coronary artery bypass grafting), formal testing of operator skills may be unnecessary, but procedural success rates should be carefully tracked during the course of the trial to the extent possible. For trials of interventions that require a high degree of technical skill, investigators frequently select sites with extensive prior experience and skill ("expert sites"). Although such a strategy may provide the most rigorous evaluation of the efficacy of the procedure or device to be tested, it does raise the issue of generalizability of the results in clinical practice with less experienced operators. This contrast between "efficacy" (the ability of a therapy to improve outcomes in a carefully controlled clinical trial context) and effectiveness (the ability of a therapy to improve outcomes when implemented into broader clinical practice) has been demonstrated for several procedures, most recently with surgical ventricular restoration procedures, in which excellent results demonstrated by expert operators have not been replicated in broader clinical practice.[121,122]

Another issue closely related to the issue of technical success is applying the principle of intention-to-treat analysis in trials of device or surgical interventions. Although it may be appropriate in the initial development of new devices or procedures (i.e., proof of concept) to randomly assign only patients in whom the device implantation is successful (as was done in the MIRACLE study and the Chronicle Offers Management to Patients with Advanced Signs and Symptoms of Heart Failure [COMPASS] study[48,123]), it is important to recognize that such a design does not fully account for the risks of a given intervention in comparison with usual care. Outside of research trials, patients who undergo a procedure that is not technically successful are exposed to the procedural risks

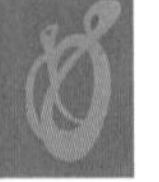

TABLE 39–2 Selected Large Phase II and III Acute Heart Failure Trials and Their Endpoints

Study	Year of Publication	Intervention	Primary Endpoint(s)	Key Secondary Endpoints	Long-Term Clinical Outcomes
Vasodilation in the Management of Acute CHF (VMAC)[112]	2002	48-Hour nesiritide infusion vs. nitroglycerine infusion vs. placebo	Coprimary: • Δ PCWP at 3 hours • Δ Dyspnea (Likert) at 3 hours	• PCWP at 24 hours • Dyspnea at 24 and 48 hours • Global clinical status	Tertiary endpoints: • 48-hour hypotension, headaches • 30-day mortality, myocardial infarction, readmission, and renal dysfunction • 6-month mortality (not powered for definitive analysis)
Outcomes of a Prospective Trial of Intravenous Milrinone for Exacerbations of Chronic Heart Failure (OPTIME-CHF)[36]	2002	48-Hour milrinone infusion vs. placebo	Cumulative days of hospitalization for cardiovascular cause or number of days at death within 60 days after random assignment	• Proportion of cases failing therapy because of adverse events or worsening heart failure (sustained SBP < 80 mm Hg, myocardial ischemia, arrhythmias, persistent CHF, inadequate diuresis, organ hypoperfusion) • Heart failure score • Global health (VAS)	Primary endpoint
Evaluation Study of Congestive Heart Failure and Pulmonary Artery Catheterization Effectiveness (ESCAPE)[37]	2005	Therapy guided by pulmonary artery catheter plus clinical assessment vs. clinical assessment alone	Days alive and out of hospital during the first 6 months	• Adverse events related to catheter use • 6-Minute walk duration • Quality of life vs. time trade-off • MLHF	Primary endpoint
Value of Endothelin Receptor Inhibition with Tezosentan in Acute Heart Failure Study (VERITAS)[115]	2007	24- to 72-hour tezosentan infusion vs. placebo	Coprimary: • Change in dyspnea (at 3, 6, and 24 hours rated on VAS scale of 0–100) over 24 hours (area under the curve) • Death or worsening heart failure (pulmonary edema, shock, new or increased IV therapy, mechanical cardiac or pulmonary support, renal replacement therapy) at 7 days	• Death or major cardiovascular events at 30 days • Improved hemodynamic measures over 24 hours • Length of stay • Days hospitalized within 30 days • 6-Month mortality	Secondary endpoints
Survival of Patients with Acute Heart Failure in Need of Intravenous Inotropic Support (SURVIVE)[116]	2007	Levosimendan infusion vs. dobutamine infusion as long as clinically indicated in patients with AHFS who require inotropic support	All-cause mortality at 180 days	• All-cause mortality at 31 days • Days alive or out of hospital at 180 days • Cardiovascular mortality at 180 days • Change in BNP level at 24 hours • Dyspnea at 24 hours • Patient-assessed global status at 24 hours	Primary and secondary endpoints
Second Randomized Multicenter Evaluation of Intravenous Levosimendan Efficacy (REVIVE II)[117]	Not yet published (presented 2005)	Levosimendan infusion vs. placebo in hemodynamically stable patients with AHFS	Composite of clinical signs and symptoms of heart failure over 5 days expressed as three-stage endpoint: • Better (moderately or markedly improved global assessment at 6 hours, 24 hours, and 5 days with no worsening) • Same • Worse (death from any cause; persistent or worsening heart failure necessitating intravenous diuretics, vasodilators, or inotropic agents at any time; or moderately or markedly worse patient-assessed global status at 6 hours, 24 hours, or 5 days)	Change in BNP; mortality at 90 days	Secondary endpoint

(Continued)

TABLE 39–2 Selected Large Phase II and III Acute Heart Failure Trials and Their Endpoints—cont'd

Study	Year of Publication	Intervention	Primary Endpoint(s)	Key Secondary Endpoints	Long-Term Clinical Outcomes
Efficacy of Vasopressin Antagonism in Heart Failure Outcome Study with Tolvaptan (EVEREST)[110,111]	2007	Tolvaptan vs. placebo up to 112 weeks	Short-term composite: • Changes in global clinical status (VAS) and body weight at day 7 or discharge Long-term dual endpoints: • All-cause mortality (superiority and noninferiority) • Cardiovascular death or hospitalization for heart failure (superiority only)	Composite components: • In isolation at days 1 and 7 or discharge • Dyspnea at day 1 • Peripheral edema at day 7 or discharge • Kansas City Cardiomyopathy Questionnaire responses at 1 week and 6 months • Body weight • Changes in serum sodium	Main safety endpoint
Acute Study of Clinical Effectiveness of Nesiritide in Decompensated Heart Failure (ASCEND-HF)[118]	Enrolling	Nesiritide infusion vs. placebo	Coprimary: • Composite of all-cause mortality and heart failure rehospitalization through 30 days • Dyspnea at 6 and 24 hours	• Overall well-being (Likert) 6 and 24 hours • Days alive and outside of hospital within 30 days	Primary endpoint
Placebo-controlled Randomized study of the selective A1 adenosine receptor antagonist KW-3902 for patients hospitalized with acute HF and volume Overload to assess Treatment Effect on Congestion and renal function Trial (PROTECT)[34]	Enrolling	Rolofylline infusion vs. placebo	Composite of clinical signs and symptoms of heart failure over 7 days, expressed as three-stage endpoint: • Better (moderately or markedly improved global assessment at 24 and 48 hours with no worsening) • Same • Worse (death from any cause, persistent or worsening heart failure through day 7, or creatinine increase ≥ 0.3 mg/dL at 7 and 14 days)	• Safety • Within trial costs	Secondary endpoint

AHFS, acute heart failure syndrome; BNP, B-type natriuretic peptide; CHF, congestive heart failure; IV, intravenous; MLHF, Minnesota Living with Heart Failure questionnaire; PCWP, postcapillary wedge pressure; SBP, systolic blood pressure; VAS, Visual Analog Scale.
Adapted from Allen LA. End points for clinical trials in acute heart failure syndromes. *J Am Coll Cardiol* 2009;53:2248-2258.

with none of the putative benefits. It is important, therefore, that more definitive trials of new devices or surgical procedures include in the analysis all patients randomly assigned to receive the intervention (intention-to-treat analysis), even if the procedure could not be completed.[55]

Two other major challenges for device and surgical trials are controlling for the placebo effect and masking. There is a significant literature on the increasing magnitude of a placebo effect as it relates to the invasiveness of the therapy (e.g., placebo injections have a much greater treatment effect than do placebo pills).[124] The presence of a strong placebo effect has led to the use of sham procedures for controls, in which control patients undergo some aspects of the procedure to be tested (such as general anesthesia) but do not undergo the actual therapeutic intervention. In studies of implanted devices such as CRT devices, a common strategy is to implant the device in all patients but activate it only in the intervention recipients. For example, in the MIRACLE study, all patients received a CRT device but were randomly assigned to have the device activated or in backup pacing mode.[48] As noted previously for the intention-to-treat principle, such a strategy is useful for proof-of-concept studies but may be less valid in definitive outcome trials, inasmuch as it does not provide complete information about the relative risks and benefits in comparison to usual care (because all patients would be exposed to the risks of the device but only half the patients would be exposed to the benefits). For studies of interventions associated with substantial risk (such as cardiac surgery), random assignment to sham procedures has generally been considered unethical.

Masking of conditions for both patients and providers is considered a hallmark of robust clinical trial design and a solution to the issue of the placebo effect, but it may be impossible with some device or surgical interventions. In some device studies, such as MIRACLE, the researchers have attempted to maintain a double-blind situation by having a separate group of physicians manage the device without masking, whereas the overall care for the patient and assessment endpoints was provided in a blinded manner by the heart failure specialist. As a practical matter, some therapies, such as ventricular assist device therapy, are impossible to mask, a limitation which may be addressed in part by careful selection of the study endpoints and the use of endpoint committees that are unaware of patients' conditions to adjudicate events.[125]

In view of these challenges, careful selection of the primary study endpoint is crucial for the success of trials of surgical and device-based therapy. Use of the most objective possible endpoint (e.g., mortality or mortality plus hospitalizations) is obviously preferable in order to minimize the biases introduced by incomplete masking and the placebo effect. For example, in the COMPANION study, a primary endpoint was the composite of all-cause mortality and all-cause hospitalizations, which was considered robust and less likely to be influenced by the device placebo effect and the lack of masking.[55] The absence of a sham-operated control group and the lack of masking were unavoidable in the Randomized Evaluation of Mechanical Assistance for the Treatment of Congestive Heart Failure (REMATCH) and were addressed by selecting the most objective endpoint possible: all-cause mortality.[125]

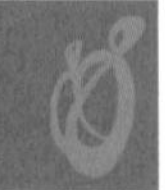

Because the very poor prognosis in end-stage heart failure, the REMATCH study was able to demonstrate a substantial treatment effect on all-cause mortality despite a small sample size. When design considerations make such "hard" clinical endpoints impractical, more objectively measured endpoints (e.g., peak ventilatory oxygen uptake [V_{O_2}], left ventricular dimensions) should generally be preferred over more subjective ones (NYHA class, quality of life) in order to minimize the extent of the placebo effect and the effect of the lack of masking.

A specific challenge of device-based therapies, such as therapy with mechanical cardiac support devices, concerns how to best assess incremental changes in technology (e.g., improvements in pump design). In contrast to drugs, improvements in device technology tend to be small and incremental, and it is often impractical to perform a new RCT to compare each new improvement to standard therapy. This creates a tension between the desire to introduce new device improvements into clinical use and the need to rigorously evaluate their efficacy and safety. In the case of mechanical cardiac support devices such as LVADs, a variety of alternative approaches to a traditional RCT have been proposed for dealing with this problem, including the use of concurrent non–randomly assigned controls and hybrid designs incorporating both randomly assigned and historical controls (Figure 39-6).[126] The advent of the Interagency Registry for Mechanically Assisted Circulatory Support (INTERMACS), an ongoing registry of patients who have received destination LVAD therapy in the United States, may help establish appropriate benchmarks that may help to serve as concurrent controls for new devices.

Clinical Trials of Monitoring Tools and Strategies

In addition to the ongoing development of new therapies, developments in both genomics and device technology have resulted in an increasing array of monitoring tools (both molecular and device based) with potential to improve the diagnosis and treatment of heart failure. Although such diagnostic tools have traditionally been held to a lower regulatory standard of evidence (e.g., simply establishing that they can accurately measure what they claim to measure) than have therapeutic interventions, such tools should ideally undergo the same rigorous evaluation for safety and efficacy before being adopted into clinical practice. There has been an increasing trend toward using RCTs to carefully evaluate monitoring strategies. Trials of such diagnostic tools present specific challenges in terms of trial design that are discussed in detail as follows.

For a diagnostic or monitoring device to be clinically useful, it must meet all of several criteria. Fundamentally, a device must be able to make measurements that are accurate, are reproducible, and can be delivered to clinicians in a timely and understandable manner. Although necessary, this criterion is not sufficient; for a diagnostic device to be of proven clinical use, that information must be actionable in a way that can be demonstrated to improve patient outcomes. In clinical trials of monitoring strategies, researchers should therefore evaluate not only whether a monitoring tool can accurately measure something but also whether the knowledge of such data by clinicians leads to therapeutic decisions that improve patient outcomes. In this sense, monitoring trials help evaluate both the tool itself and the therapeutic strategy tied to this information.

Numerous important clinical trials have been designed to rigorously evaluate a variety of monitoring devices and strategies, pulmonary artery catheters,[37] chronically implanted hemodynamic monitors,[123] serial measurements of biomarkers (such as natriuretic peptides),[127] or intensified disease management algorithms based on vital signs and weight.[128] In general, study protocols have varied in the degree to which they have predetermined how investigators would change therapy according to the information provided. In ESCAPE, specific hemodynamic goals and guidelines for achieving them were defined by protocol for the intervention group.[129] In other trials, such as the Systolic Heart Failure Treatment Supported by BNP (STARS-BNP) study of BNP-guided therapy, interventions based on the provided diagnostic information were left to the discretion of individual physicians.[127] Both approaches have obvious advantages and disadvantages. Providing specific guidance limits variability (all investigators respond to the diagnostic information in a similar way) but also ties the efficacy of the monitoring device to a specific treatment paradigm, which creates the possibility that the monitoring device could be useful but the treatment algorithm could be incorrect. Conversely, by leaving clinical decisions solely to the individual investigator, the study is a more direct evaluation of the utility of the diagnostic information per se, but it also introduces substantial heterogeneity that may complicate analysis, particularly in smaller trials.

Particularly challenging in this type of trial are issues of appropriate control groups and masking. Ideally, the experience of control subjects in RCTs is identical to that of the intervention recipients, with the exception of the intervention itself. Monitoring trials present a significant challenge to this paradigm. For some interventions, such as pulmonary artery catheterization or an implanted diagnostic device such as the Medtronic Chronicle, the invasive nature of the monitoring tool itself is associated with specific risks that must be weighed in assessing the balance of risks and benefits. One method for dealing with this potential bias is to have both groups undergo placement of the monitoring device but provide the diagnostics information only to physicians of the intervention recipients. This approach allows for single-blind conditions (i.e., the patients do not know whether they are in the "guided" condition or not). As noted in the "Clinical Trials with Devices and Surgery" section, this approach addresses some problems but creates others. Although such a design provides a more rigorous evaluation of the utility of the diagnostic information provided, it does not address the overall balance of risks and benefits of the device, in particular if the device is invasive or if hospitalization is required for implantation. As an example, in the COMPASS trial, the Chronicle device was implanted in all study patients, but only patients in whom implantation was successful were randomly assigned to have the information from the device available to their physician (intervention group) or not (control group). Although such a design provides a rigorous evaluation of the utility of *information* from a diagnostic device, it does not elucidate the overall risks and benefits of a strategy based on implanting such a device and on using data generated from the device to guide therapy. To clarify this distinction, in COMPASS there were three patients who could not undergo the implantation and therefore were not randomly assigned, 277 elective hospitalizations for device implantation, and 15 hospitalizations for complications related to the device. A true evaluation of the overall safety and efficacy of a monitoring strategy based on an implanted device would have to "count" all adverse events related to the intervention.[130]

A related issue in all monitoring studies is the frequency of interaction with patients in the intervention group versus those in the control group. More frequent interaction with health care providers alone appears to decrease event rates in chronic heart failure,[131] which potentially confounds the extent to which any observed benefit is related to a greater frequency of health care interactions or to the monitoring tool itself. To improve the rigor of monitoring strategy studies, the intensity of follow-up between the intervention and control groups should generally be as identical as possible;

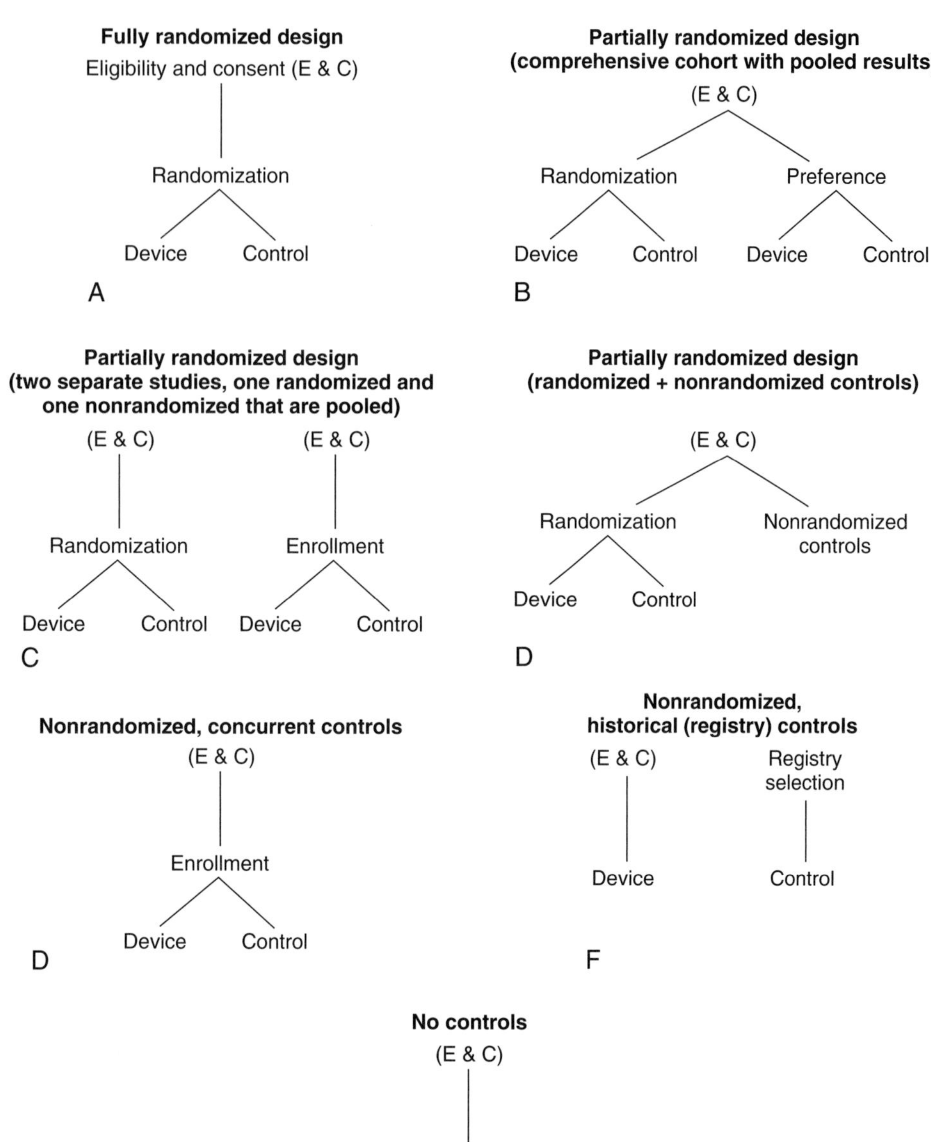

FIGURE 39–6 Possible modifications of traditional design for randomized controlled trials of mechanical cardiac support devices. (Adapted from Neaton JD, Normand SL, Gelijns A, et al. Designs for mechanical circulatory support device studies. *J Card Failure* 2007;13:63-74.)

this may involve "sham" contacts. For example, in the COMPASS trial, it was recognized that more frequent contact with intervention recipients might risk unmasking the condition to patients and might also have a more direct effect on outcomes; therefore, control patients received calls in a random schedule designed to match the frequency of contacts with the intervention recipients.[123]

NEW DIRECTIONS

Best practices for RCTs in general continues to evolve, and improvement in clinical trial methodology and education is an important part of the National Institutes of Health Roadmap Initiative.[132] Interestingly, this has resulted in an increase in "meta-research": that is, research into the methodology of research. In view of the extent to which cardiovascular medicine has been at the forefront of evidence-based medicine research, it is not surprising that cardiovascular trials will continue to drive innovation in the field of clinical trials. As described in this chapter, a variety of novel developments—including greater use of adaptive designs, bayesian statistical methods, novel endpoints, and new operational structures such as clinical trials networks—will continue to alter the landscape of clinical trials in heart failure. Developments in pharmacogenomics will also have substantial effects on clinical trial methodology. The next steps in expanding the concepts of "personalized medicine" will be prospectively incorporating such genomic or phenotypic markers into inclusion and exclusion criteria rather than confining them to ancillary studies or retrospective analyses. The use of genetic polymorphisms to better target anticoagulation therapy with warfarin has also come into mainstream clinical practice and is now part of the FDA labeling for warfarin.[133] These types of "pharmacogenomic" indications for drugs will become more numerous and will create both substantial opportunities, as well as significant challenges, for both researchers and regulatory bodies. Clinical trial methodology will need to continue adapting to new scientific and regulatory developments, in order to continue providing a robust foundation of evidence to guide clinical practice and improve the care of patients with heart failure.

1. Evidence Based Medicine Working Group. (1992). Evidence-based medicine. A new approach to teaching the practice of medicine. *JAMA, 268*, 2420–2425.
2. Gibbons, R. J., Smith, S., & Antman, E. (2003). American College of Cardiology/ American Heart Association Clinical Practice Guidelines: Part I: where do they come from? *Circulation, 107*, 2979–2986.
3. Tricoci, P., Allen, J. M., Kramer, J. M., et al. (2009). Scientific evidence underlying the ACC/AHA Clinical Practice Guidelines. *JAMA, 301*, 831–841.
4. Hennekens, C. H. (Ed.), (1999). *Clinical trials in cardiovascular disease. A companion to Braunwald's Heart Disease.* Philadelphia: WB Saunders.
5. Friedman, L. M., Furberg, C. D., & DeMets, D. L. (1999). *Fundamentals of clinical trials.* New York: Springer-Verlag.
6. White, H. D. (1998). Thrombolytic therapy and equivalence trials. *J Am Coll Cardiol, 31*, 494–496.
7. Fleming, T. R. (2000). Design and interpretation of equivalence trials. *Am Heart J, 139*, S171–S176.
8. Siegel, J. P. (2000). Equivalence and noninferiority trials. *Am Heart J, 139*, S166–S170.
9. International Conference on Harmonization. (1999). Choice of control group in clinical trials. *Fed Regist, 64*, 51767–51780.
10. Piaggio, G., Elbourne, D. R., Altman, D. G., et al. (2006). for the CONSORT Group. Reporting of noninferiority and equivalence randomized trials: an extension of the CONSORT statement. *JAMA, 295*, 1152–1160.
11. Gotzsche, P. C. (2006). Lessons from and cautions about noninferiority and equivalence randomized trials. *JAMA, 295*, 1172–1174.
12. Le Henanff, A., Giraudeau, B., Baron, G., et al. (2006). Quality of reporting of noninferiority and equivalence randomized trials. *JAMA, 295*, 1147–1151.
13. McAlister, F. A., Straus, S. E., Sackett, D. L., et al. (2003). Analysis and reporting of factorial trials: a systematic review. *JAMA, 289*, 2545–2553.
14. The Heart Outcomes Prevention Evaluation Study I. (2000). Vitamin E supplementation and cardiovascular events in high-risk patients. *N Engl J Med, 342*, 154–160.
15. Dittrich, H. C., Gupta, D. K., Hack, T. C., et al. (2007). The effect of KW-3902, an adenosine A1 receptor antagonist, on renal function and renal plasma flow in ambulatory patients with heart failure and renal impairment. *J Card Fail, 13*, 609–617.
16. Heiat, A., Gross, C. P., & Krumholz, H. M. (2002). Representation of the elderly, women, and minorities in heart failure clinical trials. *Arch Intern Med, 162*, 1682–1688.
17. Byington, R. P., Curb, J. D., & Mattson, M. E. (1985). Assessment of double-blindness at the conclusion of the Beta-Blocker Heart Attack Trial. *JAMA, 253*, 1733–1736.
18. Granger, B. B., Swedberg, K., Ekman, I., et al. (2005). Adherence to candesartan and placebo and outcomes in chronic heart failure in the CHARM programme: double-blind, randomised, controlled clinical trial. *Lancet, 366*, 2005–2011.
19. Packer, M., Bristow, M. R., Cohn, J. N., et al. (1996). The effect of carvedilol on morbidity and mortality in patients with chronic heart failure. *N Engl J Med, 334*, 1349–1355.
20. MERIT-HF Study Group. (1999). Effect of metoprolol CR/XL in chronic heart failure: Metoprolol CR/XL Randomised Intervention Trial in Congestive Heart Failure (MERIT-HF). *Lancet, 353*, 2001–2007.
21. Packer, M., Coats, A. J. S., Fowler, M. B., et al. (2001). Effect of carvedilol on survival in severe chronic heart failure. *N Engl J Med, 344*, 1651–1658.
22. Whellan, D. J., O'Connor, C. M., Lee, K. L., et al. (2007). Heart Failure and A Controlled Trial Investigating Outcomes of Exercise TraiNing (HF-ACTION): design and rationale. *Am Heart J, 153*, 201–211.
23. Yusuf, S., & Negassa, A. (2002). Choice of clinical outcomes in randomized trials of heart failure therapies: disease-specific or overall outcomes?. *Am Heart J, 143*, 22–28.
24. Petersen, J. L., Haque, G., Hellkarnp, A. S., et al. (2006). Comparing classifications of death in the Mode Selection Trial: agreement and disagreement among site investigators and a clinical events committee. *Contemp Clin Trials, 27*, 260–268.
25. Mahaffey, K. W., Harrington, R. A., Akkerhuis, M., et al. (2001). Disagreements between central clinical events committee and site investigator assessments of myocardial infarction endpoints in an international clinical trial: review of the PURSUIT study. *Curr Controlled Trials Cardiovasc Med, 2*, 187–194.
26. Teerlink, J. R. (2002). Recent heart failure trials of neurohormonal modulation (OVERTURE and ENABLE): approaching the asymptote of efficacy?. *J Card Fail, 8*, 124–127.
27. O'Connor, C. M., Gattis, W. A., & Ryan, T. J. (2000). The role of clinical nonfatal end points in cardiovascular phase II/III clinical trials. *Am Heart J, 139*, S143–S154.
28. Packer, M., Califf, R. M., Konstam, M. A., et al. (2002). Comparison of omapatrilat chronic and enalapril in patients with heart failure—the Omapatrilat Versus Enalapril Randomized Trial of Utility in Reducing Events (OVERTURE). *Circulation, 106*, 920–926.
29. Rector, T. S., & Cohn, J. N. (1992). Assessment of patient outcome with the Minnesota Living with Heart Failure questionnaire: reliability and validity during a randomized, double-blind, placebo-controlled trial of pimobendan. Pimobendan Multicenter Research Group. *Am Heart J, 124*, 1017–1025.
30. Heidenreich, P. A., Spertus, J. A., Jones, P. G., et al. (2006). Health status identifies heart failure outpatients at risk for hospitalization or death. *J Am Coll Cardiol, 47*, 752–756.
31. Pang, P. S., Cleland, J. G., Teerlink, J. R., et al. (2008). A proposal to standardize dyspnoea measurement in clinical trials of acute heart failure syndromes: the need for a uniform approach. *Eur Heart J, 29*, 816–824.
32. Allen, L. A., Metra, M., Milo-Cotter, O., et al. (2008). Improvements in signs and symptoms during hospitalization for acute heart failure follow different patterns and depend on the measurement scales used: an international, prospective registry to evaluate the evolution of Measures of Disease Severity in Acute Heart Failure (MEASURE-AHF). *J Card Fail, 14*, 777–784.
33. Packer, M. (2001). Proposal for a new clinical end point to evaluate the efficacy of drugs and devices in the treatment of chronic heart failure. *J Card Fail, 7*, 176–182.
34. Cotter, G., Dittrich, H. C., Weatherley, B. D., et al. (2008). The PROTECT pilot study: a randomized, placebo-controlled, dose-finding study of the adenosine A1 receptor antagonist rolofylline in patients with acute heart failure and renal impairment. *J Card Fail, 14*, 631–640.
35. Felker, G. M., Anstrom, K. J., & Rogers, J. G. (2008). A global ranking approach to end points in trials of mechanical circulatory support devices. *J Card Fail, 14*, 368–372.
36. Cuffe, M. S., Califf, R. M., Adams, K. F., Jr., et al. (2002). Short-term intravenous milrinone for acute exacerbation of chronic heart failure: a randomized controlled trial. *JAMA, 287*, 1541–1547.
37. Binanay, C., Califf, R. M., Hasselblad, V., et al. (2005). Evaluation Study of Congestive Heart Failure and Pulmonary Artery Catheterization Effectiveness: the ESCAPE trial. *JAMA, 294*, 1625–1633.
38. Stevenson, L. W., & Lewis, E. (2006). Mapping the journey. *J Am Coll Cardiol, 47*, 1612–1614.
39. Cleland, J. G. F., Charlesworth, A., Lubsen, J., et al. (2006). A comparison of the effects of carvedilol and metoprolol on well-being, morbidity, and mortality (the "patient journey") in patients with heart failure: a report from the Carvedilol Or Metoprolol European Trial (COMET). *J Am Coll Cardiol, 47*, 1603–1611.
40. Prentice, R. L. (1989). Surrogate endpoints in clinical trials—definition and operational criteria. *Stat Med, 8*, 431–440.
41. Anand, I. S., Florea, V. G., & Fisher, L. (2002). Surrogate end points in heart failure. *J Am Coll Cardiol, 39*, 1414–1421.
42. De Gruttola, V. G., Clax, P., DeMets, D. L., et al. (2001). Considerations in the evaluation of surrogate endpoints in clinical trials: summary of a National Institutes of Health Workshop. *Controlled Clin Trials, 22*, 485–502.
43. Cohn, J. N. (2004). New therapeutic strategies for heart failure: left ventricular remodeling as a target. *J Card Fail, 10*, S200–S201.
44. Packer, M., Carver, J. R., Rodeheffer, R. J., et al. (1991). Effect of oral milrinone on mortality in severe chronic heart failure. The PROMISE Study Research Group. *N Engl J Med, 325*, 1468–1475.
45. Echt, D. S., Liebson, P. R., Mitchell, L. B., et al. (1991). Mortality and morbidity in patients receiving encainide, flecainide, or placebo. The Cardiac Arrhythmia Suppression Trial. *N Engl J Med, 324*, 781–788.
46. Mann, D. L., McMurray, J. J. V., Packer, M., et al. (2004). Targeted anticytokine therapy in patients with chronic heart failure: results of the Randomized Etanercept Worldwide Evaluation (RENEWAL). *Circulation, 109*, 1594–1602.
47. Pocock, S. J., Geller, N. L., & Tsiatis, A. A. (1987). The analysis of multiple end-points in clinical trials. *Biometrics, 43*, 487–498.
48. Abraham, W. T. (2000). Rationale and design of a randomized clinical trial to assess the safety and efficacy of cardiac resynchronization therapy in patients with advanced heart failure: the Multicenter InSync Randomized Clinical Evaluation (MIRACLE). *J Card Fail, 6*, 369–380.
49. Abraham, W. T., Fisher, W. G., Smith, A. L., et al. (2002). Cardiac resynchronization in chronic heart failure. *New Engl J Med, 346*, 1845–1853.
50. Dargie, H. J. (2001). Effect of carvedilol on outcome after myocardial infarction in patients with left-ventricular dysfunction: the CAPRICORN randomised trial. *Lancet, 357*, 1385–1390.
51. Donner, A. (1984). Approaches to sample-size estimation in the design of clinical trials—a review. *Stat Med, 3*, 199–214.
52. Halpern, S. D., Karlawish, J. H., & Berlin, J. A. (2002). The continuing unethical conduct of underpowered clinical trials. *JAMA, 288*, 358–362.
53. Kadish, A., Dyer, A., Daubert, J. P., et al. (2004). Prophylactic defibrillator implantation in patients with nonischemic dilated cardiomyopathy. *N Engl J Med, 350*, 2151–2158.
54. Gould, A. L. (2001). Sample size re-estimation: recent developments and practical considerations. *Stat Med, 20*, 2625–2643.
55. Bristow, M. R., Saxon, L. A., Boehmer, J., et al. (2004). Cardiac-resynchronization therapy with or without an implantable defibrillator in advanced chronic heart failure. *N Engl J Med, 350*, 2140–2150.
56. Sommer, A., & Zeger, S. L. (1991). On estimating efficacy from clinical trials. *Stat Med, 10*, 45–52.
57. Felker, G. M., Benza, R. L., Chandler, A. B., et al. (2003). Heart failure etiology and response to milrinone in decompensated heart failure: results from the OPTIME-CHF study. *J Am Coll Cardiol, 41*, 997–1003.
58. Moye, L. A., & Deswal, A. (2001). Trials within trials: confirmatory subgroup analyses in controlled clinical experiments. *Controlled Clin Trials, 22*, 605–619.
59. van Veldhuisen, D. J., & Poole-Wilson, P. A. (2001). The underreporting of results and possible mechanisms of negative drug trials in patients with chronic heart failure. *Int J Cardiol, 80*, 19–27.
60. Moher, D., Schulz, K. F., & Altman, D. (2001). for the CONSORT Group.The CONSORT statement: revised recommendations for improving the quality of reports of parallel-group randomized trials. *JAMA, 285*, 1987–1991.
61. Monitoring SCT Working Group, Dixon, D. O., Freedman, R. S., et al. (2006). Guidelines for data and safety monitoring for clinical trials not requiring traditional data monitoring committees. *Clin Trials, 3*, 314–319.
62. Armitage, P. (1991). Interim analysis in clinical trials. *Stat Med, 10*, 925–937.
63. Friedman, L. M., Furberg, C. D., & DeMets, D. L. (1998). Monitoring response variables. In *Fundamentals of clinical trials* (3rd ed). New York: Springer-Verlag, pp 246–275.
64. Peto, R. F., Pike, M. C., Armitage, P. F., et al. (1976). Design and analysis of randomized clinical trials requiring prolonged observation of each patient. I. Introduction and design. *Br J Cancer, 34*, 585–612.
65. Pocock, S. J. (1982). Interim analyses for randomized clinical trials—the Group Sequential Approach. *Biometrics, 38*, 153–162.
66. O'Brien, P. C., & Fleming, T. R. (1979). A multiple testing procedure for clinical trials. *Biometrics, 35*, 549–556.
67. DeMets, D. L., & Lan, K. K. G. (1994). Interim analysis—the alpha spending function approach. *Stat Med, 13*, 1341–1352.
68. Davis, B. R., & Hardy, R. J. (1994). Data monitoring in clinical trials—the case for stochastic curtailment. *J Clin Epidemiol, 47*, 1033–1042.
69. DeMets, D. L., & Ware, J. H. (1982). Asymmetric group sequential boundaries for monitoring clinical trials. *Biometrika, 69*, 661–663.

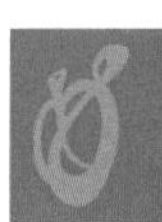

70. Fagerberg, B. (2000). Screening, endpoint classification, and safety monitoring in the Metoprolol CR/XL Randomised Intervention Trial in Congestive Heart Failure (MERIT-HF). *Eur J Heart Fail, 2*, 315–324.
71. Naslund, U., Grip, L., Fischer-Hansen, J., et al. (1999). The impact of an end-point committee in a large multicentre, randomized, placebo-controlled clinical trial—results with and without the end-point committee's final decision on end-points. *Eur Heart J, 20*, 771–777.
72. Participants in the 2001 Conference on Ethical Aspects of Research in Developing Countries. Ethics. Fair benefits for research in developing countries. (2002). *Science, 298*, 2133–2134.
73. Glickman, S. W., McHutchison, J. G., Peterson, E. D., et al. (2009). Ethical and scientific implications of the globalization of clinical research. *N Engl J Med, 360*, 816–823.
74. Yuval, R., Halon, D. A., Merdler, A., et al. (2000). Patient comprehension and reaction to participating in a double-blind randomized clinical trial (ISIS-4) in acute myocardial infarction. *Arch Intern Med, 160*, 1142–1146.
75. Yuval, R., Uziel, K., Gordon, N., et al. (2001). Perceived benefit after participating in positive or negative/neutral heart failure trials: the patients' perspective. *Eur J Heart Fail, 3*, 217–223.
76. Yuval, R., Halon, D. A., & Lewis, B. S. (2001). Patients' point of view in heart failure trials. *JAMA, 285*, 883–884.
77. Packer, M. (2000). Current perspectives on the design of phase II trials of new drugs for the treatment of heart failure. *Am Heart J, 139*, S202–S206.
78. Deswal, A., Bozkurt, B., Seta, Y., et al. (1999). Safety and efficacy of a soluble P75 tumor necrosis factor receptor (Enbrel, etanercept) in patients with advanced heart failure. *Circulation, 99*, 3224–3226.
79. Bozkurt, B., Torre-Amione, G., Warren, M. S., et al. (2001). Results of targeted anti-tumor necrosis factor therapy with etanercept (Enbrel) in patients with advanced heart failure. *Circulation, 103*, 1044–1047.
80. Bozkurt, B., Kribbs, S. B., Clubb, F. J., Jr., et al. (1998). Pathophysiologically relevant concentrations of tumor necrosis factor-alpha promote progressive left ventricular dysfunction and remodeling in rats. *Circulation, 97*, 1382–1391.
81. Chow, S. -C., & Chang, M. (2007). *Adaptive design methods in clinical trails.* Boca Raton, FL: Chapman & Hall/CRC.
82. Chow, S. C., Chang, M., & Pong, A. (2005). Statistical consideration of adaptive methods in clinical development. *J Biopharm Stat, 15*, 575–591.
83. Coad, D. S., & Ivanova, A. (2005). The use of the triangular test with response-adaptive treatment allocation. *Stat Med, 24*, 1483–1493.
84. Hommel, G. (2001). Adaptive modifications of hypotheses after an interim analysis. *Biom J, 43*, 581–589.
85. Nagelkerke, N., Fidler, V., Bernsen, R., et al. (2000). Estimating treatment effects in randomized clinical trials in the presence of non-compliance. *Stat Med, 19*, 1849–1864.
86. Branson, M., & Whitehead, J. (2002). Estimating a treatment effect in survival studies in which patients switch treatment. *Stat Med, 21*, 2449–2463.
87. Simon, R., Thall, P. F., & Ellenberg, S. S. (1994). New designs for the selection of treatments to be tested in randomized clinical trials. *Stat Med, 13*, 417–429.
88. DeMets, D. L. (2000). Design of phase II trials in congestive heart failure. *Am Heart J, 139*, S207–S210.
89. Ellenberg, S. S. (2000). Select-drop designs in clinical trials. *Am Heart J, 139*, S158–S160.
90. Sampson, A. R., & Sill, M. W. (2005). Drop-the-losers design: normal case. *Biom J, 47*, 257–268.
91. Ellenberg, S. S., & Eisenberger, M. A. (1985). An efficient design for phase III studies of combination chemotherapies. *Cancer Treat Rep, 69*, 1147–1154.
92. Thall, P. F., Simon, R., & Ellenberg, S. S. (1989). A two-stage design for choosing among several experimental treatments and a control in clinical trials. *Biometrics, 45*, 537–547.
93. Coad, D. S., & Ivanova, A. (2005). Sequential urn designs with elimination for comparing $K \geq 3$ treatments. *Stat Med, 24*, 1995–2009.
94. O'Quigley, J., Pepe, M., & Fisher, L. (1990). Continual reassessment method: a practical design for phase 1 clinical trials in cancer. *Biometrics, 46*, 33–48.
95. Chang, M., & Chow, S. C. (2005). A hybrid bayesian adaptive design for dose response trials. *J Biopharm Stat, 15*, 677–691.
96. Hughes, M. D. (1993). Stopping guidelines for clinical trials with multiple treatments. *Stat Med, 12*, 901–915.
97. Stallard, N., Thall, P. F., & Whitehead, J. (1999). Decision theoretic designs for phase II clinical trials with multiple outcomes. *Biometrics, 55*, 971–977.
98. Thall, P. F., & Cheng, S. C. (2001). Optimal two-stage designs for clinical trials based on safety and efficacy. *Stat Med, 20*, 1023–1032.
99. Zohar, S., & Chevret, S. (2001). The continual reassessment method: comparison of bayesian stopping rules for dose-ranging studies. *Stat Med, 20*, 2827–2843.
100. Inhibition of platelet glycoprotein IIb/IIIa with eptifibatide in patients with acute coronary syndromes. (1998). The PURSUIT Trial Investigators. Platelet Glycoprotein IIb/IIIa in Unstable Angina: Receptor Suppression Using Integrilin Therapy. *N Engl J Med, 339*, 436–443.
101. Lee, K. L. (2000). Sample size and interim analysis issues for dose selection. *Am Heart J, 139*, S161–S165.
102. Berry, D. A. (2006). Bayesian clinical trials. *Nat Rev Drug Discov, 5*, 27–36.
103. Berry, D. A. (2005). Introduction to bayesian methods III: use and interpretation of bayesian tools in design and analysis. *Clin Trials, 2*, 295–300.
104. Lipscomb, B., Ma, G., & Berry, D. A. (2005). Bayesian predictions of final outcomes: regulatory approval of a spinal implant. *Clin Trials, 2*, 325–333.
105. Temple, R. (2005). How FDA currently makes decisions on clinical studies. *Clin Trials, 2*, 276–281.
106. Chow, S. C., & Chang, M. (2008). Adaptive design methods in clinical trials—a review. *Orphanet J Rare Dis, 3*, 11.
107. Gheorghiade, M., & Pang, P. S. (2009). Acute heart failure syndromes. *J Am Coll Cardiol, 53*, 557–573.
108. Gheorghiade, M., Zannad, F., Sopko, G., et al. (2005). Acute heart failure syndromes: current state and framework for future research. *Circulation, 112*, 3958–3968.
109. Gheorghiade, M., Abraham, W. T., Albert, N. M., et al. (2006). Systolic blood pressure at admission, clinical characteristics, and outcomes in patients hospitalized with acute heart failure. *JAMA, 296*, 2217–2226.
110. Gheorghiade, M., Konstam, M. A., Burnett, J. C., Jr., et al. (2007). Short-term clinical effects of tolvaptan, an oral vasopressin antagonist, in patients hospitalized for heart failure: The EVEREST Clinical Status Trials. *JAMA, 297*, 1332–1343.
111. Konstam, M. A., Gheorghiade, M., Burnett, J. C., Jr., et al. (2007). Effects of oral tolvaptan in patients hospitalized for worsening heart failure: the EVEREST Outcome Trial. *JAMA, 297*, 1319–1331.
111a. Allen, L. A., Hernandez, A. F., O'Conner, C. M., et al. (2009). End points for clinical trials in acute heart failure syndromes. *J Am Coll Cardiol, 53*, 2248–2258.
112. Publication Committee for the VMAC Investigators (Vasodilatation in the Management of Acute CHF). (2002). Intravenous nesiritide vs nitroglycerin for treatment of decompensated congestive heart failure: a randomized controlled trial. *JAMA, 287*, 1531–1540.
113. Follath, F., Cleland, J. G., Just, H., et al. (2002). Efficacy and safety of intravenous levosimendan compared with dobutamine in severe low-output heart failure (the LIDO study): a randomised double-blind trial. *Lancet, 360*, 196–202.
114. Louis, A., Cleland, J. G., Crabbe, S., et al. (2001). Clinical Trials Update: CAPRICORN, COPERNICUS, MIRACLE, STAF, RITZ-2, RECOVER and RENAISSANCE and cachexia and cholesterol in heart failure. Highlights of the Scientific Sessions of the American College of Cardiology, 2001. *Eur J Heart Fail, 3*, 381–387.
115. McMurray, J. J., Teerlink, J. R., Cotter, G., et al. (2007). Effects of tezosentan on symptoms and clinical outcomes in patients with acute heart failure: the VERITAS randomized controlled trials. *JAMA, 298*, 2009–2019.
116. Mebazaa, A., Nieminen, M. S., Packer, M., et al. (2007). Levosimendan vs dobutamine for patients with acute decompensated heart failure: The SURVIVE Randomized Trial. *JAMA, 297*, 1883–1891.
117. Cleland, J. G., Freemantle, N., Coletta, A. P., & Clark, A. L. (2006). Clinical trials update from the American Heart Association: REPAIR-AMI, ASTAMI, JELIS, MEGA, REVIVE-II, SURVIVE, and PROACTIVE. *Eur J Heart Fail, 8*, 105–110.
118. Hernandez, A. F., O'Connor, C. M., Starling, R. C., et al. (2009). Rationale and design of the Acute Study of Clinical Effectiveness of Nesiritide in Decompensated Heart Failure Trial (ASCEND-HF). *Am Heart J, 157*, 271–277.
119. Teerlink, J. R. (2003). Dyspnea as an end point in clinical trials of therapies for acute decompensated heart failure. *Am Heart J, 145*, S26–S33.
120. Coletta, A. P., & Cleland, J. G. (2001). Clinical trials update: highlights of the scientific sessions of the XXIII Congress of the European Society of Cardiology—WARIS II, ESCAMI, PAFAC, RITZ-1 and TIME. *Eur J Heart Fail, 3*, 747–750.
121. Hernandez, A. F., Velazquez, E. J., Dullum, M. K., et al. (2006). Contemporary performance of surgical ventricular restoration procedures: data from the Society of Thoracic Surgeons' National Cardiac Database. *Am Heart J, 152*, 494–499.
122. Athanasuleas, C. L., Buckberg, G. D., Stanley, A. W. H., et al. (2004). Surgical ventricular restoration in the treatment of congestive heart failure due to post-infarction ventricular dilation. *J Am Coll Cardiol, 44*, 1439–1445.
123. Bourge, R. C., Abraham, W. T., Adamson, P. B., et al. (2008). Randomized controlled trial of an implantable continuous hemodynamic monitor in patients with advanced heart failure: the COMPASS-HF Study. *J Am Coll Cardiol, 51*, 1073–1079.
124. Kaptchuk, T. J., Goldman, P., Stone, D. A., et al. (2000). Do medical devices have enhanced placebo effects? *J Clin Epidemiol, 53*, 786–792.
125. Rose, E. A., Moskowitz, A. J., Packer, M., et al. (1999). The REMATCH trial: rationale, design, and end points. Randomized Evaluation of Mechanical Assistance for the Treatment of Congestive Heart Failure. *Ann Thorac Surg, 67*, 723–730.
126. Neaton, J. D., Normand, S. L., Gelijns, A., et al. (2007). Designs for mechanical circulatory support device studies. *J Card Fail, 13*, 63–74.
127. Jourdain, P., Jondeau, G., Funck, F., et al. (2007). Plasma brain natriuretic peptide–guided therapy to improve outcome in heart failure: The STARS-BNP Multicenter Study. *J Am Coll Cardiol, 49*, 1733–1739.
128. Cleland, J. G. F., Louis, A. A., Rigby, A. S., et al. (2005). Noninvasive home telemonitoring for patients with heart failure at high risk of recurrent admission and death: the Trans-European Network-Home-Care Management System (TEN-HMS) study. *J Am Coll Cardiol, 45*, 1654–1664.
129. Shah, M. R., O'Connor, C. M., Sopko, G., et al. (2001). Evaluation Study of Congestive Heart Failure and Pulmonary Artery Catheterization Effectiveness (ESCAPE): design and rationale. *Am Heart J, 141*, 528–535.
130. Teerlink, J. R. (2008). Learning the points of COMPASS-HF: assessing implantable hemodynamic monitoring in heart failure patients. *J Am Coll Cardiol, 51*, 1080–1082.
131. Kasper, E. K., Gerstenblith, G., Hefter, G., et al. (2002). A randomized trial of the efficacy of multidisciplinary care in heart failure outpatients at high risk of hospital readmission. *J Am Coll Cardiol, 39*, 471–480.
132. Zerhouni, E. A. (2005). US biomedical research: basic, translational, and clinical sciences. *JAMA, 294*, 1352–1358.
133. Anderson, J. L., Horne, B. D., Stevens, S. M., et al. (2007). Randomized trial of genotype-guided versus standard warfarin dosing in patients initiating oral anticoagulation. *Circulation, 116*, 2563–2570.

CHAPTER 40

Development and Implementation of Practice Guidelines in Heart Failure

Kirkwood F. Adams Jr.

The rapid growth of medical knowledge since the 1970s has created many advances in the treatment of chronic illness, and the treatment of cardiovascular disease has been at the center of this advancement. Unfortunately, timely translation of this progress into everyday care of patients with cardiovascular disorders remains problematic. Development of practice guidelines has emerged as a major strategy for optimizing the use of new and existing therapeutic modalities of proven benefit. To be effective, these guidelines must not only clearly delineate which therapies are efficacious but also account for the many practical aspects necessary to fully implement specific treatments in the care of patients. When professional groups address these two issues, both the art and science of medicine can be employed to obtain better patient outcomes in cardiovascular diseases long associated with high mortality rates, severe morbidity, and poor quality of life.

This chapter describes in detail the theoretical aspects of guideline development and discusses how they have evolved since 1990. The principles and methods of guideline development, which are closely linked to the evidence-based medicine movement, continue to change as the discipline matures. In addition, the process by which these abstract principles and methods are applied to generate practice guidelines for a specific clinical problem, heart failure, is examined.[1-10] Review of key guidelines for heart failure illustrates the difficulties inherent in formulating a clinically useful document to translate new advances into standard care. The condition of heart failure—a complex syndrome with many clinical manifestations and therapeutic alternatives that vary from very well established to uncertain—is well suited for the guideline approach.

RATIONALE FOR GUIDELINE DEVELOPMENT

Justification

Many rationales can be presented to justify the development of clinical practice guidelines. Three particularly cogent arguments are as follows: (1) Medical knowledge continues to accumulate at such a rapid pace that individual clinicians cannot readily and adequately synthesize the new information and adapt more effective strategies of care for the many diseases they confront in practice; (2) accepted standards for care are needed for even the simplest monitoring of practice to occur; and (3) translation of clinical trials into day-to-day practice is often difficult because of gaps in knowledge of how to apply therapies in actual practice. These three specific justifications for development of practice guidelines are discussed in detail as follows.

The rapid growth in medical knowledge, both physiological and therapeutic, is commonly acknowledged, but the effects of the this growth remain underappreciated. The constant appearance of new advances in medical knowledge has created the expectation that disease outcomes will improve not only in a commensurate way but also rapidly after research developments. Novel methods of care are developing simultaneously in many different fields, and so the burden of processing new medical knowledge has become immense. Individual practitioners cannot rapidly synthesize these developments into their daily practice unaided.

Frequently, guidelines are used as standards for quality or process control; this application has remained controversial for many health care providers. A more universally accepted rationale is that a practice guideline will accelerate and make more uniform the application of advances in medical care and thus improve health care delivery and outcomes. Substantial variation in medical practice for the same disease process in various geographic areas has long been recognized.[11] This variation may be somewhat justified on the basis of true regional differences in expression of a clinical condition. However, careful review of utilization data versus clinical profile suggests that much of the existing variation cannot be accounted for on this basis. Well-prepared guidelines offer an excellent basis for standards of care in the monitoring process.

Many clinicians believe that clinical trial results alone are sufficient to dictate practice standards and to provide adequate rationale

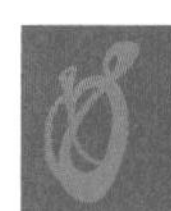

BOX 40–1 Inherent Assumptions Underlying Practice Guidelines

Clinical decisions must be made.

- Lack of action is not an option
- Correct course of action is not readily apparent

There exists a reasonably valid method to address knowledge base and evaluate medical evidence.

There exist data beyond randomized clinical trials that enhance medical decision making.

Uncertainties remain with regard to approaches to treatment after review of totality of medical evidence. Expert opinion has a role in management decisions.

Experts with interest and commitment to the clinical problem and guideline process must be available.

and direction for implementing new therapies (see Chapter 39). However, as outlined in detail in this review, translating advances in medical knowledge into changes in clinical practice is quite complex for many conditions. Many considerations beyond interpretation of a particular clinical trial as positive or negative come into play. Practice guidelines offer one strategy to bridge the gap between clinical trial results and implementation of new therapeutic modalities in community practice.

Inherent Assumptions

The creation of these position documents can be justified cogently; however, the feasibility of developing a valid and useful practice guideline depends on certain inherent assumptions that are often as much a belief system as verifiable facts (Box 40-1). Whether these assumptions are met or not depends on the clinical condition under consideration. Guidelines are most justified (1) when certain decisions clearly must be made about the specifics in the care of the patient and (2) when potential approaches to care are either certain (need widespread adoption) or uncertain (need clarification). Practice guidelines offer particular utility for disease processes that have serious consequences for individual and public health, in which failure to act has obvious consequences. There must be an acceptable method for evaluation of medical evidence related to the disease state. Data on therapeutic options should be more complex than rigorous clinical trials that are easy to interpret. Experts who focus on the study and care of the clinical problem and who can act with independent integrity must be available to execute the guideline process. These underlying assumptions appear to be valid for the syndrome of heart failure.

ROLE OF EVIDENCE-BASED MEDICINE

Since 1990, evidence-based medicine has evolved as a significant alternative to traditional approaches to medical decision making and has become a critical underpinning of the methods for guideline development.[12] Traditional medical decision making certainly involves use of scientific principles, including the pathophysiological basis of disease, and integrates clinical experience with the results of clinical studies, especially randomized trials. Despite elements in common with evidence-based medicine, traditional approaches reach therapeutic decisions in a fundamentally different way, on the basis of evaluation of advantages and disadvantages in individual encounters with patients. Such ad hoc decision making does not arise from a plan considered in advance and is not a consequence of a predefined approach; instead, it occurs on spontaneously. In contrast, evidence-based medicine stresses the need for medical decisions to be based on the best scientific data, particularly results from randomized controlled trials and systematic observational studies, which are typically beyond the individual physician's experience.[13] But where do clinical experience and the individual patient fit into the evidence-based medicine decision making? Interestingly, even cursory examination of key papers prepared during development of this discipline reveals the importance of applying the "best evidence" with regard to the peculiarities and particulars of the individual case.[14,15] Perhaps the best way to resolve this apparent fusion of two contradictory approaches is to recognize that medicine is an applied science rather than a natural science.[16,17] The understanding of medical heuristics remains incomplete and must advance only if decisions about care are to be optimized.[18]

Evidence-based medicine has been linked to guideline development from the beginning of this discipline, inasmuch as the principles of this approach apply not only to the actions of individual physicians but also to the creation of practice policies or codified documents to define patient management.[19] Archie Cochrane, among many other authors, recognized that formal methods were needed to evaluate multiple studies of the same medical problem.[20] Systematic reviews complement practice guidelines and represent another important aspect of evidence-based medicine.[21] As expected, the emphasis of evidence-based medicine on objective analysis of randomized clinical trial results and on general adherence to formalized methods has created conflict concerning the quality of practice guidelines that have been developed.[22,23] A detailed discussion of the nature of medical evidence is presented later in this chapter; debate rages concerning the relative value and, even for some clinicians, the usefulness of certain forms of medical evidence. Traditional approaches depend heavily on observational data that have tainted this form of evidence for many clinicians. A major conceptual point concerns specifying the nature of observational or nonrandomized data that are evaluated. Traditionally, decision making depends heavily on personal observational data that are rarely collected systematically or by a prospective method, are not subject to rigorous statistical analysis guided by prespecified goals, and are not replicated in any formal way. If rigorous methods are applied in the collection of observational data, however, substantial information can be obtained about drug efficacy, and the results of randomized and nonrandomized approaches are often complementary and additive to use of therapies in real patients.[24-29] The concepts of a practical clinical trial and restricted cohort design provide novel examples of bridging design methods that can advance the discipline of evidence-based medicine.[30-33] Guideline-creating bodies continue to address potential methodological issues and effectively voice counterarguments in seeking to balance the inherent tensions and conflicts described previously.[34,35]

PROCESS OF GUIDELINE DEVELOPMENT

The Role of Experts

Guidelines are developed by groups of committed individuals judged to be experts on a particular clinical problem; that is, they have special skill and knowledge gained from training and experience related to the clinical focus of guideline development. Experts are identified on the basis of visible accomplishments, such as publication of clinical and research activities linked to broad clinical experience.

Experts on a panel influence every aspect of guideline development. Some of their key roles include defining the clinical focus of the guideline, delineating the specific evidence to be considered, providing access to key data that may not be published or fully reported, creating a synthesis of the available evidence, developing a hierarchy of and weighing the evidence gathered, and determining the strength of recommendations made in the guideline.

Experts must define the scope of the clinical problem to be studied according to their clinical experience and their sense of the important aspects of the problem. Experts guarantee access to the broadest possible knowledge base. Medical evidence published from a variety of sources is frequently incomplete. Negative results of clinical trials might not be written in manuscript form or accepted, especially in a timely manner, even if they are prepared for publication. Details concerning important negative findings may be available only through experts. In some instances, critical aspects of important clinical trials are not adequately represented in trial publications. Access to this information may be limited to opinion leaders.

Experts synthesize the available evidence in a way that cannot be done by nonexperts. They evaluate the biological plausibility of a particular therapy. Biological plausibility is an important determinant of the ultimate weight of evidence or strength of conclusion for a particular therapeutic strategy. Although drug efficacy for cardiovascular disease is commonly not understood precisely, a therapy grounded in well-established basic pathophysiological theory is accorded more support. Expert opinion must particularly address gaps in therapeutic evidence, because for many important aspects of patient care, even cohort data are unavailable. Evidence from properly constructed expert opinion is indispensable in translating scientific evidence into actual clinical practice. Experts are responsible for the tone and effect of the final guideline document. Their ability to create a cogent, literate, user-friendly publication with practicality based on a sound science foundation is crucial.

Overview of Guideline Development

Numerous steps are involved in the development and implementation of a practice guideline (Box 40-2). Key points in this process are discussed as follows both as abstract concepts and through concrete examples from experience gained in the development of the Heart Failure Society of America (HFSA) practice guideline[7].

The initial step is to define the scope of the specific clinical problem. This first part of the process is typically problematic, and its successful completion should be the initial goal of the guideline group. For example, heart failure is a syndrome with a number of distinct clinical manifestations and pathophysiological processes that necessitate many different treatment strategies that are established in varying degrees. The resources at hand, adequacy of evidence for specific aspects of the disease process, and likelihood of developing a consensus may determine the scope of the guideline. The initial HFSA guideline, published in 1999, had a narrow focus concentrating on the pharmacological treatment of chronic, symptomatic left ventricular dysfunction. Other distinct subsets of the clinical syndrome of heart failure (i.e. acute, decompensated heart failure and "diastolic dysfunction") were not considered. After this first effort, the HFSA completed development of a second, comprehensive practice guideline that included most aspects of heart failure and was published in 2006. Guideline content evolves when the commissioning body is a society, and this continuity and progression are strengths of practice guidelines developed by such groups.

The second essential step in guideline development is to identify the key evidence to be considered in formulating the document. In the case of the HSFA guideline, this process was heavily dependent on the committee members involved. Other guideline groups have been more complex, consisting of committee members teamed with a research staff to ensure that a more formal and systematic review of all available evidence is produced.[36] Systematic efforts help ensure the completeness and adequacy of the review process. Systematic reviews can be a costly process and are probably best targeted at specific areas with particularly rich or complex data. Dedicated research staff associated with the committee or contract research organizations are generally essential to the systematic review process. However, the responsibility for interpreting the results of any systematic review rests ultimately on the clinical experts commissioned to develop the guideline.

The third step involves establishing a strategy for evaluating the medical knowledge concerning treatments and care plans that may be applied to a particular condition. Substantial effort has been expended to define the role that particular types of evidence should play and to establish rules to assess the quality of available evidence.

The fourth step of guideline development concerns the process of writing and reviewing the guideline before its acceptance by the commissioning body. The development of a written document is the essential part of this phase. It provides a mechanism for precision of thought and a means to elicit careful review, criticism, and refinement of controversial and problematic issues. Ideally, during this important phase, exchanges among reviewers in a point and counterpoint process can be applied to specific aspects of the guideline to further clarify and enhance the final document. Style and language concerning specific recommendations must be consistent. This aspect of the guideline process is labor intensive, inasmuch as the writing process is difficult and should be done by the health care experts on the guideline committee or writing group.

Robust internal and external reviews during finalization of the practice guideline are crucial as well. Reviewers can be external to the committee or organization, and their comments can be assimilated to a variable extent. These reviewers offer fresh perspectives and added expertise to the developmental process. Different perspectives usually provide balance and focus to the effort. In the HFSA guideline process, the organization's executive council served as the primary reviewers (Figure 40-1). This allowed integration of a substantial amount of additional expertise and experience into the final guideline. However, reviews confined within the organization commissioning the guideline may have certain limitations related to biases of the group. Both internal organizational review and the different medical perspectives of outside experts constitute the best approach.

The fifth step in guideline development and implementation is dissemination of the document. Many avenues are available, and media exposure should be diverse. Comprehensive guidelines are typically lengthy in full format but can be condensed to a series of pocket cards and made available online by hypertext links from recommendations to background sections in order to furnish more detail and reference materials. Web-based documents that can be downloaded to portable computing devices have become popular; they

BOX 40–2 Steps in the Development of a Practice Guideline

Determining the scope of the practice guideline
Identification of the medical evidence relevant to the guideline
Specifying type of evidence and relative weight of evidence
Formulating strength of evidence in recommendations
Establishing therapeutic justification for recommended therapies
Formulating strength of recommendations for specific therapies
Creation of document, including establishment of structure
Developing a review process for the document
Dissemination of the practice guideline
Determining the life cycle of the document

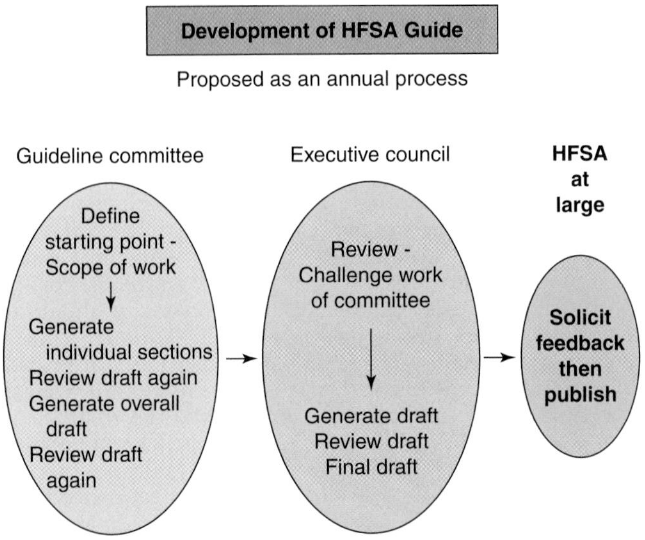

Development of HFSA Guide

Proposed as an annual process

Guideline committee	Executive council	HFSA at large
Define starting point - Scope of work → Generate individual sections; Review draft again; Generate overall draft; Review draft again	Review - Challenge work of committee → Generate draft; Review draft; Final draft	Solicit feedback then publish

FIGURE 40–1 The series of steps involved in the development and review of the practice guideline produced by the Heart Failure Society of America (HFSA). Two unique features of this guideline process were the active involvement of the executive council of the society and the relative lack of external review.

present the opportunity for point-of-care use, and they ease the search for specific information.

Another important aspect of the guideline development process focuses on minimizing the impact that conflicts of interest may have on the formation of the guideline document. Although conflicts of interest rightly focused on financial issues, they may arise for many reasons and should include any type of individual bias that will render unobjective the evaluation of medical evidence or declaration of recommendations. Information concerning sources of support, whether personal or for research purposes, should be collected periodically during the development process and available for scrutiny after publication of the document. The individual members of the guideline group should be the most aware of potential conflicts and should recuse themselves from aspects of the guideline development in which they believe they may be biased. Presence of some degree of conflict of interest is inevitable because of the necessary composition of guideline groups. Prospective recognition and awareness of the potential for conflicts of interest is critical.

The final step of guideline development concerns the life cycle of the document produced. In most instances, it is advantageous to have the guideline evolve as a "living" document, of which subsequent revisions are based on new advances in knowledge and on responses from practitioners who attempt to use the guideline in everyday practice. For example, because of new knowledge about heart failure from ongoing randomized clinical trials and other research, information about new advances must be incorporated into guideline documents. Even a yearly review of critical aspects of the heart failure guideline is not unrealistic, in view of the pace of new advances. Development of a "living" document has clearly become a major goal for the societies formulating heart failure guidelines, but substantial commitment by society members is necessary to sustain it.

APPROACHES TO MEDICAL EVIDENCE

Review of medical evidence is naturally the most essential process in guideline development; it ensures that accurate and useful recommendations concerning the efficacy and use of particular treatment strategies are formulated[37,38] (Box 40-3). Ongoing efforts aim to improve this process by iterative experience with guideline formulation and better definition of key aspects.[39-41] This complex process can be subdivided into a series of critical elements: (1) the method for identifying key evidence and determining types and strengths of evidence of interest, (2) evaluation of the scientific validity of each piece of evidence reviewed, and (3) construction of a strategy for weighing the different types of evidence to reach a conclusion or recommendation in favor of or against a particular therapeutic intervention. These three major milestones are discussed in detail as follows so that the nuances inherent in this part of the guideline process can be better understood.

BOX 40–3 Process for Evaluating Medical Evidence to Establish a Practice Guideline

Review of medical evidence for efficacy of treatments
- Types of evidence available
- Critical review of clinical trial data
- Integration of expert opinion

Beyond positivity or negativity of evidence
- Degree of positivity or negativity
- Replication
- Biological plausibility
- Totality of evidence

Determining degree of therapeutic justification
- Efficacy
- Safety
- Tolerability
- Practicality
- Justifiability

Evidence-based approach to practical use of therapy
- Dosing
- Monitoring for side effects and efficacy
- Duration of therapy
- Adjustment of concomitant prescriptions

Identification of Evidence

A variety of techniques are used to identify the key medical evidence to be reviewed in the guideline process. The widespread availability of computerized databases of medical literature (e.g., PubMed) that can be searched in an organized manner has facilitated this process. Literature searches are designed to identify key articles or reports through the use of appropriate search terms. Other methods to identify evidence, however, are essential to complement this process. Reviews of references compiled for key articles or reports of trials and other clinical research may be additional sources of evidence. Members of the guideline writing group should review results of searches performed and provide input, because they may be aware of additional important references.

Types of Evidence

Some details concerning the specific types of evidence applicable to the development of practice guidelines and the assignment of relative merit for this evidence are of interest (Table 40-1). Evidence derived from cohort studies is increasingly consulted in guideline development, because the accumulation of clinical trial data enables guideline committees to address issues important in practice, rather than the primary focus of the trial work. Cohort studies consist of both prospective and retrospective subgroup analyses of clinical trials, case-control or propensity analyses in which matched subsets of trial populations are used, and analyses of dose-response studies that may involve all or a portion of the clinical trial population. This type of evidence has well-recognized

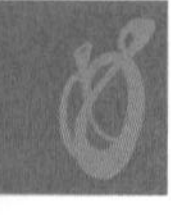

TABLE 40–1 Relative Weight of Evidence Used to Develop Practice Guidelines

Category	Types of Evidence (Highest to Lowest)
Category A	Randomized controlled clinical trials
Category B	Cohort and case-control studies Post hoc analysis, subgroup analysis, and meta-analysis
Category C	Expert opinion: • Observational studies and epidemiological findings • Registry studies • Safety reporting from large-scale use in practice

inherent limitations. Studies of this type are usually post hoc in nature and involve subgroups of the study population that were not created by a random process. Whenever possible, these analyses should be based on pre hoc hypotheses. Prospective stratification of the randomization process may be included to help provide balance for anticipated subgroup comparisons or to avoid bias in the comparison of therapy. Often a series of subgroup analyses are performed; this raises the potential for a chance finding that results from errors that arise from multiple hypothesis testing. In addition, there are often issues related to the power of such studies to detect treatment differences and to the generalizability of any positive or negative results. Despite these limitations, studies in this category often have a significant influence on guideline development because they address issues of great clinical importance that frequently cannot be resolved on the basis of classical randomized clinical trial data. Rather than relying solely on expert opinion, guideline developers can use cohort analyses as a formalized way to address some of these issues.

Observational evidence may take the form of epidemiological studies or expert opinion. Epidemiological studies by definition cannot establish the relationship between a particular treatment and any beneficial or detrimental effects. However, these studies can suggest the strength of association between a specific treatment and important clinical outcomes (see also Chapter 22). Expert opinion, discussed later in this chapter, is another form of observational data that makes up the body of evidence considered in the guideline process. It is typically a critical part of any guideline that has merit in clinical practice. The guideline document should clearly identify the nature of the evidence for specific recommendations, so that those areas covered by expert opinion can be clearly identified.

Strength of Evidence

The practice guideline document should indicate the strength of evidence for each specific recommendation through the use of a grading system similar to that shown in Table 40-1. This allows practitioners to better understand the nature of the evidence that underlies particular recommendations. Precise characterization of strength of evidence is classified by expert analysis and varies to some extent between guidelines. Some practice guidelines are more conservative with regard to criteria to qualify evidence most highly (strength of evidence level A in Table 40-1); at least two positive clinical trials are necessary to achieve this level of evidence. As experience with the application of guidelines accumulates, it will be clearer whether the current system is accurate in predicting long-term trends in accepted therapy and new knowledge about treatments.

Interpretation of Randomized Clinical Trials

Much effort has been expended in the development of specific criteria by which randomized trials should be evaluated. How trials are reported must be reviewed in detail. Was the design of the trial reported prospectively? Are the statistical methods fully detailed, and were they followed in the analysis of the trial data? Were the key data revealed in the primary or pivotal report of the trial results?

Issues Specific to Statistical Analysis

A full description of issues related to statistical analysis of clinical trial data is beyond the scope of this chapter. However, several points seem to arise frequently when data from specific trials are used for guideline development. A key question is whether a trial met its primary endpoint. Positivity, as defined in the analytical plan for the study, should be determined clearly from the study report. Although controversy may arise over the mathematical definition of statistical significance, the clinical trial design should allow ready determination of the primary endpoint and the significance level specified for achievement of the primary endpoint. Some heart failure trials have featured multiple primary endpoints, identified either prospectively or retrospectively. Multiple primary endpoints require some decision about the distribution of the probability values necessary to minimize type I or α error at the level of $P < .05$.

Another important concern is the interpretation of results concerning secondary endpoints, such as hospitalization for worsening heart failure. These are often of significant interest, as in the case of the prevention condition of the Studies of Left Ventricular Dysfunction (SOLVD) trial, and are translated into guideline recommendations even though the primary endpoint of the trial was not met. Consistency of favorable results for secondary endpoints is important as well. For instance, the total number of hospitalizations may be unaffected or increased, whereas heart failure–related hospitalizations are reduced.

Limitations of Positive Randomized Clinical Trials

Aspects other than the dichotomous outcome of a study must be considered when results from a particular clinical trial are used in everyday practice. Two important aspects to consider are the sample size and the generalizability of the study findings.

Large-scale clinical trials with many events generally provide the most accurate evidence for guideline development, especially for evaluating the effect of therapies on endpoints such as mortality and morbidity. Studies whose designs require a specified number of events, rather than achievement of a prespecified sample size that is based on estimates of event rates, are more likely to achieve this aim. Numerous small to moderate-sized heart failure trials have yielded findings that have not been replicated by additional larger studies. Various explanations have been offered for this failure to replicate initial studies. These explanations, however, have essentially reinforced the concept that a large number of events in patients with heart failure are necessary to ensure that a positive finding on mortality and morbidity endpoints is not spurious.

Clinical trials always involve selected patients from within a population with the diagnosis of a particular disease or syndrome. Selection bias takes many forms and may significantly restrict the implications of positive trial results. Inclusion and exclusion criteria may result in too narrow a study population to have wide clinical applicability. Although the screening process is generally not well reported, it is important to review what was used to obtain the population studied, as well as the inclusion and exclusion criteria. Requirements for a certain degree of illness or the absence of specific comorbid factors are typical and may restrict application of the trial results. The monitoring process necessary to ensure safety is another aspect that may influence generalizability of the study results. Because of concerns about generalizability despite positivity of specific trial results, restrictions may be placed on the recommendations given in the practice guideline.

Weighing the Evidence: Hierarchy of Relative Value

Traditionally, the process of weighing the evidence begins with the development of a hierarchy concerning the scientific validity and value of different types of medical evidence. This allows the objective assessment of the relative weight of arguments for and against a particular treatment.[42] Results of randomized clinical trials continue to be accorded the highest rating among the types of evidence available. However, the known limitations of results from clinical trials and the value of other types of evidence have caused guideline development to engage in a much more complex process concerning the evaluation of medical evidence. This process is probably best described as an integration of many types of evidence, including expert opinion that results in formulation of a consensus in support of or against particular therapies or management strategies.

Expert Opinion as Evidence

The value of expert opinion of evidence useful in guideline development remains a point of controversy. For critics, expert opinion is simply another form of observational evidence derived from clinical work in day-to-day patient care. This experience is subject to the known biases and limitations of experience of individual practitioners caring for a small number of patients in a specific practice setting. For proponents of expert opinion, this type of evidence represents the expert's complex synthesis of disease pathophysiology, direct study of patients, and interchange of experience and ideas with colleagues. Ideally, the nature of the patient care experience for most experts should be fundamentally different from that of individual practitioners in most care settings. Clinical experts should have substantial experience, derived from direct care for many patients, that is the focus of the practice guideline under development. In addition, as thought or opinion leaders, they should also be exposed to the experiences of many practitioners in a variety of practice settings. Through contact with numerous health care providers who may refer or discuss patients' cases with them, experts can encounter rare safety issues and assess efficacy of particular treatments across a very wide spectrum of cases.

The guideline process requires a team of experts acting in concert, not a series of isolated individuals. At best, expert opinion is built up from the experience of many experts involved in development of the guideline. When committee members work together, their collective experience is stronger than that of an individual practitioner. When the composite experience of experts consistently either does or does not favor a particular therapy, the evidence is heavily weighted.

Inclusion of evidence based on expert opinion sets the stage for potential conflicts between the subjective assessments of experts and the objective evidence from trials and other data. These conflicts appear to take two forms. One concerns the assessment of clinical trial results by the experts. In particular cases, flaws may be evident to one expert and not another. Reservations regarding the generalizability of trial results and the gaps in knowledge left by trial data may differ between panel members. The second area of potential conflict concerns the expert's experience with particular therapies from his or her own practice. In ideal circumstances, the assessment of clinical value by the panel experts is congruent with the highest quality of objective evidence available, typically results of randomized clinical trials. Thus, the expert's view of the value of a therapy in daily practice outside the confines of a clinical trial and the potential implications of the trial results for patient care is contrasted to the evidence-based approach.

When subjective expert opinion is not congruent with more objective scientific evidence, either for or against a therapy, how is the discrepancy resolved? Subjective opinion should focus on cogent arguments based on known potential issues with objective evidence. Unfortunately, there are no absolute rules for discarding trial results or deciding that the limitations of the trial are sufficient to countermand a traditionally positive statistical result. Most guidelines are intended to resolve these very difficult issues through a consensus opinion of the panel members involved. Strategies for reaching consensus on recommendations based on expert opinion are not well defined. However, an open, dynamic discussion seems crucial in order to prevent consensus from being driven by one or more experts with strong opinions. Working from written documents facilitates this process and provides the opportunity for feedback to the group. When expert opinion reaches a strong consensus, it may override positive or negative results from pieces of evidence of any type (including data from individual clinical trials). In contrast, the evidence in a few instances may be so controversial that it prevents the attainment of consensus. When a clear consensus cannot be reached, one action is to present more than one possible approach concerning application of a particular therapy. This may take the form of a majority-minority report or the form of two alternatives valued equally by the panel. Addressing controversial issues is critical for the practical success of a guideline, because the struggles encountered by the panel will be like those faced by clinicians in their everyday practice. A belief inherent to the guideline process is that considered judgment by credible experts in these controversial areas is more likely to be correct than ad hoc decisions made "on the spot" by physicians in practice.

EFFICACY IN BROADER CONTEXT

The press that reports novel medical findings, as well as individual practitioners, often focus solely on whether a trial's results were interpreted as positive or negative. Evaluation of trial data in the development of practice guidelines should go beyond whether the results meet a particular statistical definition of significance for the trial's primary endpoint. The additional elements analyzed from clinical trial data tend to refine and clarify study results.[43] The major elements in this evaluation process typically include (1) the endpoints studied, (2) degree of positivity or negativity of trial results, (3) whether key findings have been replicated by other work or whether the trial was conducted on the basis of results of a series of studies, and (4) how the trial results fit into the totality of evidence supporting or contraindicating a particular therapy.

Endpoints Studied

For heart failure, the strength of recommendation has tended to be influenced significantly by the effect that therapies have on morbidity and mortality. Drugs or procedures that reduce the risk of these outcomes are strongly recommended, whereas therapies that only reduce symptoms and improve quality of life receive less support. This orientation can be attributed to the profound effect that heart failure has on these clinical events of major interest. In addition, some clinicians perceive that these endpoints, particularly mortality, have the advantage of objectivity needed to clearly establish efficacy even in the setting of controlled clinical trials. Other endpoints, such as symptom scores or quality of life, are sufficiently subjective to make measurement difficult. The tools used to quantitate these endpoints are often hard to apply to

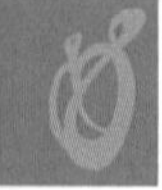

how patients seem in clinical experience. Because these factors generate a degree of uncertainty about the endpoints, the recommendations are more conservative.

Degree of Positivity or Negativity

Randomized studies may have sufficient power to be statistically positive, but therapy may produce only mild clinical benefit that hardly mandates a change in standard practice. In contrast, therapeutic trials may, in rare cases, demonstrate a profound clinical benefit that merits particular focus in a practice guideline. β-Blockade for heart failure (see Chapter 46), in which the magnitude of clinical benefit is great, is one example.

Replication and Modification

Replication is the key to advancement in basic science. The results of many well-conceived single experiments are confirmed in this manner, and "failed experiments" with unusual results may be substantiated and may lead to new insights and discoveries. Fortunately, for many favorable therapies, data from a series of clinical trials are available to strengthen evidence for efficacy. Strict replication is, of course, much more difficult to achieve in clinical trials, even with the best of intent; for example, in trials performed sequentially in time, both the patient populations studied and the concomitant therapies given may be different. Despite these limitations, it is important that clinical studies with similar populations and comparable background therapy yield concurrent results. Unfortunately, because medical science involves human subjects, replication is often difficult, and evaluation of a treatment may depend on the result of a single randomized trial. Failure to consistently replicate a finding is less problematic if there are a sufficient number of clearly positive trials.

Experience in the basic laboratory suggests that another strategy—conducting serial studies with the results of previous work to optimize future study designs—should be applied more frequently in clinical research. Unfortunately, because of the time typically necessary to organize and complete human studies, this helpful strategy is less frequently used in clinical science than is replication. Because of current limitations in funding, it is very difficult to continue investigation when initial results regarding therapy are negative, even if the dose selected or the patient population is eventually understood to be incorrect.

BEYOND EFFICACY: IS TREATMENT JUSTIFIED?

Practice guidelines must, from the available evidence, determine more than whether a treatment is efficacious or not. Treatment may have salutary effects on certain aspects of a clinical problem but still be difficult to justify as part of standard care. Therapeutic justification is one way to conceptualize how net clinical benefit and practicality are evaluated against a practice guideline. Several characteristics of therapy significantly affect how widespread the application of new treatments can and should be. Increasingly, committees carefully consider not only the risk-benefit ratio but also the cost effectiveness of novel therapies. Safety considerations may not be completely straightforward. In the case of certain desperately ill patients, greater risk for adverse reactions may be acceptable, and the quality of evidence for efficacy may be less rigorous.

Cost and cost-benefit analysis have not been major considerations during most guideline development, whether for heart failure or in other areas. However, because of the increasing recognition of the financial burden of new therapies and the crisis looming in Medicare as the number of recipients increases dramatically, financial issues have become a major focus in cardiovascular medicine. In practice guideline development, committees cannot generally ignore this aspect of care much longer.

Safety is evidently a priority, but tolerability and practicality are also important considerations when advances in care are applied in actual practice. A therapy may be safe but still associated with bothersome minor side effects. These side effects may not produce significant medical problems, but they may be sufficient to cause patients to stop being compliant with therapy. Practicality is of particular concern for pharmacological therapy that often must be taken over a prolonged period on an outpatient basis. Convenience of administration becomes a critical test in this setting; once-a-day therapy is a common goal.

DETERMINING STRENGTH OF RECOMMENDATION

The analytical process used to determine the strength of recommendations in a practice guideline is difficult to present in clear-cut way.[44] Determining value on the basis of the totality of available evidence seems to be critical when the strength of recommendations is formulated. *Totality of evidence,* as discussed in detail in the next section, refers to the impression gained about a treatment on the basis of a synthesis of all types of scientific data, favorable and unfavorable, concerning a therapy. The goal of therapeutic development is to achieve the best solution to problems of cost, convenience, and safety while ensuring that the treatment is efficacious. Formulating strength of recommendations takes all these aspects of therapy into account.

Totality of Therapeutic Evidence

The full body of scientific evidence for a therapy includes not only results of human experimentation but also expert opinion and findings from epidemiological and basic science studies. It is accepted that agreement between various types of evidence, especially from studies with different methods, adds weight to the likelihood that a particular therapy is of value. Evidence-based medicine is often equated with the summary evaluation of a few clinical trials. However, best judgment seems to result from integration of available trial data with information from the basic laboratory and the findings of observational and epidemiological studies. Therapies supported by multiple lines of evidence are perceived as necessary components of disease management. In contrast, treatments shown to be effective only by limited clinical trial data and lacking other supporting evidence are often recommended more weakly. Similar situations arise when therapies are supported by studies with small sample sizes or by trials in which subjects were selected in such a way that it is difficult to extrapolate results to everyday clinical practice. Clinical trial results concerning treatment may be conflicting in different studies for the same or related endpoints. Issues of whether a drug class effect is present may be problematic as well because even drugs with similar mechanisms can produce different side effects, or dose requirements may differ in a way that may reduce or prevent positivity in randomized clinical trials.

Scale of Strength

There is no uniform system for specifying strength of recommendations, but guidelines usually have three levels of favorable recommendation: for example, "is recommended," "should be considered," or "may be considered." The rating system is usually asymmetrical, with several degrees of favorable recommendation but only a single category for therapies not thought to be effective. The phrase "is recommended" is generally taken to mean that the therapy specified should be used in as many patients as possible with the disease process in question. Exceptions to use should be carefully delineated in the guideline document. Less positive recommendations can take the form of "should be considered" or "may be considered"; these indicate that the therapy can be applied in the majority of patients or on an individual basis, respectively. Language and the review of evidence related to strength of recommendation should be as consistent as possible within the guideline document.

GUIDELINE DEVELOPMENT: PRACTICAL ASPECTS OF DRUG THERAPY

As noted previously, despite the intent to rely on data derived from clinical trials in the creation of a practice guideline, the findings from these studies have important limitations. Many elements required for the actual implementation of a therapeutic strategy are often not addressed (Figure 40-2). For example, key factors for practicing physicians include ideas about dosing and duration of therapy, familiarity with the class and with a particular drug within the class, convenience of drug administration, side effect profile (as distinct from safety), and cost.

Practical Aspects of Drug Administration

Optimal dosing is not generally defined for cardiovascular pharmaceutical agents by clinical trial data. Trial designs usually have specific target dosages, but invariably many patients fail to reach these dosages during the course of the trial. Dose-response studies are very rare for important clinical endpoints such as morbidity and mortality. The duration of therapy necessary may not be evaluated, and the methods for upward titration and therapeutic monitoring may not be established easily from available clinical trial data. In heart failure in particular, information on how the new therapy fits with previously established treatment may be uncertain. These issues become less abstract when the fundamental aspects of pharmacological treatment are considered. When administering pharmaceutical therapy, practitioners must write a specific prescription for a defined dose, taken at a specific frequency, and taken for a designated period of time. Practitioners must also carefully consider how the new medication will interact with other drugs the patient may be taking. In many instances, clinical trial data does not provide any of this information.

A number of other factors affect ease of use of pharmacological therapy. In some cases, physicians may be familiar with a drug for one use and will more readily accept the agent for another application. Convenience of administration is an important determinant of whether an agent is adopted. The complexity of dosing, the route of administration, and the nature of the monitoring process all affect individual therapeutic decisions in clinical practice. Cost continues to be an important factor in many practice settings, especially in managed care organizations.

IMPLICATIONS OF PRACTICE GUIDELINES FOR CARDIOVASCULAR PRACTICE

Crafting a guideline is difficult enough; achieving adherence is even more problematic. Individualized treatment based on personal observation has been a touchstone of medical practice for several millennia. According to this concept, individual variation in disease expression and in

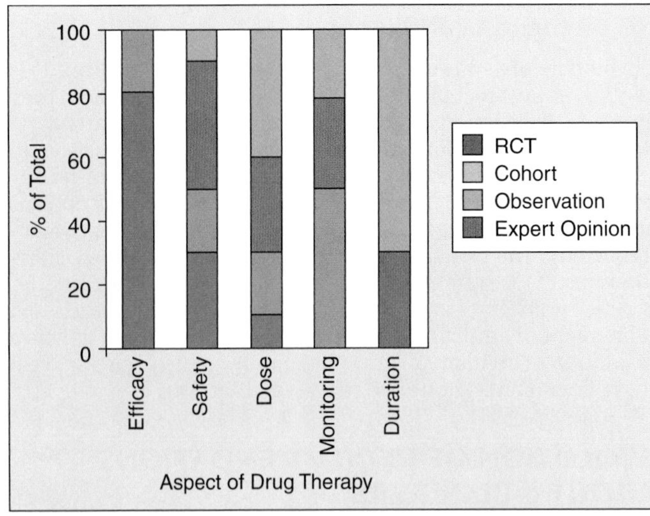

FIGURE 40–2 Estimated frequency of types of evidence available to guide specific aspects of pharmacological therapy for heart failure. Many issues that face practitioners who prescribe medication must be resolved with observational data and expert opinion. *RCT*, randomized controlled trial.

response to therapy is of more therapeutic importance than basic pathophysiological processes and mechanisms of drug action. Patients with a given disease are seen as being more different from than similar to one another. Arising with the origin of medical practice, the philosophy of individualizing therapy on the basis of personal physician experience may have been easier to accept when knowledge was scant; diseases that could be diagnosed often had a significant spontaneous recovery rate, and there was little understanding of how to identify favorable treatments. After a long period of profound uncertainty, the circumstances of medical practice that promoted extreme individualization of care have been substantially altered since the 1970s, certainly in the field of cardiovascular medicine. Application of the scientific method to clinical medicine has provided objective evidence and reproducible understanding of the effects of therapies, particularly pharmacological treatments. In addition, individualization of therapy on the basis of personal observation is especially likely to be incorrect because of several characteristics of cardiovascular disease, including heart failure: (1) Drug effects may be modest and yet important in a condition with high mortality and morbidity rates, (2) the medical problem is chronic, and the outcomes of treated patients vary widely and are difficult to quantitate from experience in practice, and (3) the drug may effect a complex array of favorable outcomes, wherein the pattern of benefit varies from one patient to the next. Because using observations from an individual's practice is a problematic way to assess therapeutic value in cardiovascular medicine, standards of care and practice guidelines are needed.

A number of treatment strategies are now sufficiently well established that it is simply not up to an individual practitioner to deviate from their use. This conclusion does not detract from the art of medicine. In some clinical situations, certain nuances in disease manifestation and response to therapy should influence the application of treatment in particular patients. Optimizing care in these situations may well stress individual practitioner experience over clinical science derived from experimentation. The main challenge facing practitioners today is to be able to distinguish these situations: when knowledge is insufficient to set exact standards versus when practice guidelines are not recommendations but requirements. Resolution of this dilemma will be difficult, but it is imperative because of the continuous advance of medical knowledge and the proper expectation on the part of patients that their care will be optimized.

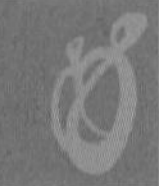

Recommend or Require?

Developers of a clinical practice guideline must confront this central issue—recommending versus requiring—when they envision translation of their recommendations into everyday practice. The definition of the word *guideline* serves to illustrate this controversy: an indication or outline of policy or conduct, in which *indication* means that certain actions are advisable (suggested or recommended) or necessary (required). The critical word *or* represents the nature of this dilemma. Most clinicians, of course, prefer not to consider practice guidelines as absolute standards. With the continued refinement of clinical trial methods and the ability to develop a totality of evidence, however, many are suggesting that these documents should be perceived that way.

EVOLUTION OF RECOMMENDATIONS ABOUT β-BLOCKERS

In the treatment of heart failure caused by left ventricular systolic dysfunction, the evolution of β-adrenergic blockade as a major therapeutic modality provides an excellent case study of therapeutic concepts developed over time during guideline development.[45,46] A review of the recommendations concerning these agents illustrates how the guideline process has resolved some difficult dilemmas even for a very efficacious therapy.

β-Blockade for Symptomatic Left Ventricular Systolic Dysfunction (see Chapter 46)

The HFSA guideline in 1999 was limited to pharmacological therapy and was the first heart failure guideline to recommend β-blockade as routine therapy for patients with symptomatic heart failure caused by left ventricular systolic dysfunction. This recommendation was accompanied by a level A strength of evidence (see Table 40-2), but the decision to provide this strength of recommendation was based on the profound overall body of knowledge supporting the role of β-blockers in treating heart failure. Use of these agents exemplifies how guideline care is closer to required rather than merely recommended. Both the totality of evidence and the quality of the clinical trial data available to support this therapy are striking. There is ample evidence from basic laboratory studies that β-adrenergic receptors are downregulated in response to sympathetic activation and that chronic sympathetic activation is harmful to cardiac structure and function.[45-47] Epidemiological data also link excess adrenergic activity to poor prognosis in patients with left ventricular systolic dysfunction.[48] Many small mechanistic trials have demonstrated convincing evidence that β-blockade enhances ventricular function in patients with heart failure.[49,50] These small-scale trials were eventually followed by several large-scale mortality trials, which documented the striking ability of β-blockade to lower risk of death and hospitalization in patients with symptomatic left ventricular systolic dysfunction.[51-53] Available clinical trial data contain excellent information concerning safety and tolerability and illustrate the justification for this therapy, in part by showing that the rates of mortality and morbidity remained high despite conventional therapy with angiotensin-converting enzyme (ACE) inhibitors and other agents as given to the "placebo" recipients. This total weight of medical evidence and knowledge concerning cost versus benefit, convenience, and safety provides very strong support for routine use of these agents in as many patients as possible who have heart failure and left ventricular systolic dysfunction.

However, gaps are present even in the rich body of evidence supporting β-blockade. Studies to help understand dose, initiation of therapy, and method of titration in clinical practice settings are limited.[54] Dose titration is reasonably well defined from trial data for surrogate endpoints, but no definitive results concerning the dosages needed for optimal outcomes are available. Information is available about target dosages, and moderate-size prospective trials with surrogate endpoints suggest some benefit at low dosages and greater benefit at target dosages.[55] Retrospective studies have suggested that heart rate response may help guide therapy with β_1 selective agents.[56] Withdrawal trials, designed to study the response of patients after discontinuation of ongoing therapy, provide a few data, but their results strongly suggest that therapy should be indefinite as long as ventricular dysfunction persists.[57,58] Data from available trials and expert experience were sufficient to outline approaches to titration and the course that should be taken if patients' conditions worsen while they receive therapy.

A major clinical issue concerning β-blockade is when to initiate therapy in patients with known systolic dysfunction. Hospitalization for cardiovascular disease provides an excellent opportunity for the initiation of life-saving therapy, and strategies based on this approach have been developed for lipid-lowering agents and other drugs. Fortunately, data are available concerning the potential effectiveness of this approach with β-blockade for heart failure. The Initiation Management Predischarge process for Assessment of Carvedilol Therapy for Heart Failure (IMPACT-HF) trial demonstrated convincingly that this approach resulted in higher likelihood of β-blocker use at 60 days after discharge, and patients treated this way were more likely to achieve target dosages.[59] This moderate-sized randomized clinical trial (n = 382) could not provide reliable outcomes data, but it did provide solid information about the safety of this approach. On the basis of these results, the 2006 HFSA guideline recommended institution of β-blockade at discharge after successful treatment of an episode of acute heart failure. Results of a subsequent large-scale observational study strongly suggest that institution of β-blockade in hospital results in better short-term outcomes.[60]

Another important clinical issue not fully addressed by trial results concerns the use of β-blockers in elderly patients. Investigators in the Cooperative Cardiovascular Project used proportional-hazards modeling to examine the likelihood of 2-year survival in patient subgroups when β-blockers were prescribed at the time of hospital discharge after an acute myocardial infarction.[61] Results of adjusted analysis indicated a substantial reduction in mortality at 2 years among patients aged 80 years or older who were treated with β-blockade. Analysis of subgroup data from the Metoprolol CR/XL Randomized Intervention Trial in congestive Heart Failure (MERIT-HF) also yielded support for the efficacy of β-blockade in older patients.[62]

β-Blockade in Patients with Severe Heart Failure

When the initial HFSA guideline was formulated, information concerning β-blockade in patients with severe heart failure caused by left ventricular systolic dysfunction was very limited. It was known that decompensation of heart failure during initiation of β-blockade was more common in these patients and that some patients had to be permanently withdrawn from therapy. Because of these difficulties and the limited amount of available data, even in view of observational experience, the recommendation was for such patients to avoid β-blocker use.

After publication of the original HFSA guideline, results from the large-scale CarvedilOl ProspEctive RaNdomIzed CUmulative Survival (COPERNICUS) study, which enrolled patients with severe heart failure, were reported.[63] Patients in this trial had severe left ventricular dysfunction (ejection fraction < 25%) and symptoms of heart failure at rest or on minimal exertion despite attempts at diuresis and optimization of medical therapy. Interestingly, New York Heart Association

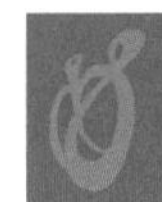

TABLE 40–2 Structure of Recommendations and Grading of Evidence Among Major Heart Failure Guidelines

HFSA 2006	ACC/AHA 2009	ESC 2008	CCS 2006
Strength of Recommendation (Highest to Lowest)			
Is recommended	Class I: Procedure or treatment should be performed or administered	Class I: Evidence or general agreement that a given treatment or procedure is beneficial, useful, or effective	Class I: Evidence or general agreement that a given procedure or treatment is beneficial, useful, and effective
Should be considered	Class IIa: It is reasonable to perform procedure or administer treatment; additional studies with focused objectives are needed	Class II: Conflicting evidence or a divergence of opinion about the usefulness or efficacy of the given treatment or procedure Class IIa: Weight of evidence or opinion is in favor of usefulness or efficacy	Class II: Conflicting evidence or a divergence of opinion about the usefulness or efficacy of the procedure or treatment Class IIa: Weight of evidence is in favor of usefulness or efficacy
May be considered	Class IIb: Procedure or treatment may be considered; additional studies with broad objectives are needed; additional registry data would be helpful	Class IIb: Usefulness or efficacy is less well established by evidence or opinion	Class IIb: Usefulness or efficacy is less well established by evidence or opinion
Not recommended	Class III: Procedure or treatment should not be performed or administered because it is not helpful and may be harmful	Class III: There is evidence or general agreement that the given treatment or procedure is not useful or effective and in some cases may be harmful	Class III: There is evidence or general agreement that the procedure or treatment is not useful or effective and in some cases may be harmful
Strength of Evidence (Highest to Lowest)			
A: At least one RCT	A: Multiple populations evaluated; data derived from multiple RCTs or meta-analyses	A: Data derived from multiple RCTs or meta-analyses	A: Data derived from multiple RCTs or meta-analyses
B: Cohort and case control studies; post hoc analysis, subgroup analysis, and meta-analysis; prospective observational studies or registries	B: Limited populations evaluated; data derived from a single RCT or nonrandomized studies	B: Data derived from a single RCT or large nonrandomized studies	B: Data derived from a single RCT or nonrandomized studies
C: Expert opinion; observational studies and epidemiological findings; safety reporting from large-scale use in practice	C: Very limited populations evaluated; only consensus opinion of experts, case studies, or standard of care	C: Consensus of opinion of the experts or small studies, retrospective studies, registries	C: Consensus of opinion of experts or small studies

ACC/AHA, American College of Cardiology Foundation/American Heart Association; *CCS*, Canadian Cardiovascular Society; *ESC*, European Society of Cardiology; *HFSA*, Heart Failure Society of America; *RCT*, randomized controlled trial.

The guidelines all have the same number of categories for grading recommendations which correlate well overall. The second category (labeled should be considered in the HFSA 2006 guideline) is the most difficult to describe and is the most dissimilar among the guidelines. Hopefully the reader can use the examples given in future tables to understand the nuances among the guideline for this strength of recommendation.

functional class was not assigned to these patients, but the mortality rate among the placebo recipients was close to 20% at 1 year, which confirmed the severity of the heart failure in the study population. Despite this degree of heart failure, β-blockade with carvedilol was well tolerated by the study patients and was associated with a marked reduction in all-cause mortality, a reduction comparable with that achieved in studies of patients with less severe symptoms. The study was stopped early by the data and safety monitoring board because of the highly significant benefit of β-blockade. Of note, this study did not include patients with severe heart failure and persistent congestion. Patients were treated to relieve congestive symptoms before randomization. A retrospective analysis of the MERIT-HF data in patients with a comparable degree of ventricular dysfunction and 1-year mortality rate also revealed a similar mortality benefit from extended-release metoprolol.[64] These favorable results led to a revision in the HFSA guideline in 2006 to include use of β-blockade in patients with severe heart failure who were thought to be adequately decongested.

β-Blockade for Asymptomatic Left Ventricular Dysfunction

In contrast to the strong recommendation for use of β-blockade in patients with symptoms, the initial HFSA guideline in 1999 gave a much more subdued recommendation for patients with no symptoms. The difficulty for guidelines in this area arose from the lack of data from randomized clinical trials to support the use of β-blockade. This illustrates a common problem for the guideline process: How accurately can the findings from one part of the disease spectrum be extrapolated to another? In contrast, in the ensuing 2001 guidelines from the American College of Cardiology Foundation/American Heart Association (ACC/AHA)[4] and the 2006 HFSA heart failure guidelines, a recommendation, about as strong that for patients with symptoms, was given in regard to β-blocker therapy in patients with asymptomatic left ventricular dysfunction.[4] Interestingly, no data from new randomized, controlled trials were available to support this strength of recommendation. This illustrates a case in which a very strong recommendation was given despite a low level of evidence. More recently, a prospective, randomized controlled trial demonstrated a favorable effect of β-blockade on left ventricular remodeling in this patient population, at least providing surrogate endpoint data in favor of this approach.[65]

Summary

These specific issues regarding the practical aspects of β-blocker therapy amply illustrate the beneficial effect that consideration of all forms of scientific data can have on guideline development. This approach makes it possible to provide the comprehensive set of guideline recommendations necessary for use of this therapy in clinical practice.

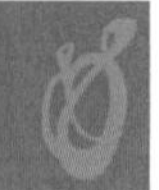

INTEGRATION OF AVAILABLE GUIDELINES

Increasing enthusiasm for practice guidelines in heart failure has led to the creation of several detailed documents by major cardiovascular societies, including the HFSA, the European Society of Cardiology (ESC), the ACC/AHA, and the Canadian Cardiovascular Society (CCS) (Table 4-2). Many authorities worry that this development adds unnecessary complexity and confusion by producing sets of guidelines that may differ meaningfully and even contradict one other. Another perspective considers multiple guidelines as an advantage, because many recommendations rest on less-than-ideal evidence (observational studies or expert opinion). In this setting, multiple guidelines by groups substantially independent of one another help address other important concerns about the role of experts. Similarities and differences among the individual guidelines help health care providers more effectively individualize management decisions. Finally, when the guidelines are concordant on key therapy, their consistency provides a much more convincing foundation for quality-of-care indicators and assurance programs.

To illustrate these points, positions taken by the individual guidelines on several common clinical scenarios in heart failure are presented in tabular form and reviewed in detail in the following sections. These guidelines share a sufficiently similar approach to formulating position statements (providing a strength of recommendation and a strength of evidence), and so comparison is possible. There as some differences in how evidence is graded and assessed in the various guidelines, but results of randomized clinical trials are considered best, whereas expert opinion is assigned the lowest value.

Left Ventricular Systolic Dysfunction

One area that illustrates substantial agreement among the guidelines concerns the medical treatment of left ventricular systolic dysfunction (Table 40-3). ACE inhibitor and β-blocker therapy are recommended on the basis of high-grade evidence for all patients with reduced ejection fraction, whether symptoms are present or not. Aldosterone antagonists are uniformly considered a standard of care in patients with severe heart failure, and digoxin is recommended for patients who remain symptomatic despite ACE inhibitor and β-blocker therapy as tolerated. Loop diuretics are recommended even though the evidence less than desirable. Exercise training represents an evolving area of care and is likely to be more uniformly recommended on the basis of clinical trial results. In contrast, the recommendations for hydralazine-nitrate therapy are more variable, but both U.S. guidelines now recommend this therapy as a standard of care in African-American patients with symptomatic systolic dysfunction.

Cardiac Resynchronization

Clinical improvement after cardiac resynchronization pacing is variable and provides a good illustration of how guidelines may include specific criteria for therapy to increase the likelihood of a favorable response (Table 40-4). The guidelines are in agreement about key characteristics of candidates for this device, with emphasis on QRS duration, presence of significant symptoms, and severe left ventricular systolic dysfunction in the setting of aggressive pharmacological treatment. The guidelines also indicate that strength of evidence is high for appropriate candidates according to data from randomized clinical trials that focused on outcomes. Contrasting strengths of recommendation among the guidelines also may be of benefit when this treatment is considered in broad patient populations. The HFSA guideline is the most conservative, with a "should be considered" strength of recommendation, similar to class IIa in the other guidelines. The HFSA device section begins with caveats concerning comorbid conditions and the likelihood of rapid death from severe underlying heart failure. This approach allows for more flexibility in decision making for individual patients than "is recommended" or a class I indication.

Inotropic Therapy in Acute Heart Failure (see Chapter 43)

The value of inotropic therapy (defined as dobutamine or milrinone) in patients with decompensated heart failure has long been hotly debated as appropriate attention has focused on the potentially harmful aspects of this drug class. A combination of results from the basic laboratory and prospective observational studies enabled the guideline committees to make a strong recommendation concerning this treatment, even though data from randomized trials are limited (Table 40-5). Their recommendations identify the potential for harm from this therapy and highlight the lack of convincing clinical benefit in broad populations of patients with acute heart failure.[66] Nevertheless, heart failure specialists who care for critically ill patients with acute heart failure, including those in cardiogenic shock, rely on these drugs. These agents may provide a bridge to recovery or surgical intervention (left ventricular assist device or cardiac transplantation). Committees agreed that the key to making a recommendation was to define the appropriate patient population in which this treatment may be considered, which is done in a very similar way in all the guidelines. Lack of enthusiasm even in the patient population identified is evident from the low strength of recommendation given by three of the four guidelines. This sends a strong message for careful consideration before this therapy is applied even in the recommended patient population, a conclusion that remains unchanged by results with newer agents in this class.[67] This element of the acute heart failure guideline illustrates the significant role that observational data can play, especially when combined with evidence from the basic laboratory and clinical trials.[68-70]

Polypharmacy

The use of multiple medications is recognized as critical in the treatment of systolic heart failure and is part of management in essentially all patients. However, this approach is problematic because of the relative lack of evidence from randomized controlled trials in which the benefits of specific combinations of therapy are tested (Table 40-6). Background therapy differs in various placebo-controlled trials; this leads to subgroup analysis and extrapolation, which weaken strength of evidence. In contrast, pathophysiological considerations and the available data on certain combinations of medication prompt interest in combination treatment. To add to the controversy, the major heart failure guidelines demonstrate both consensus and disagreement about the relative values of specific combinations of life-saving drugs. Careful review of the various guidelines reveals differences in regard to strength of evidence and target patient populations for specific combinations.

Recommendations concerning aldosterone antagonists illustrate how some of these significant issues play out among the key guidelines (see Table 40-6). These agents have been shown to be life-saving in patients with severe heart failure treated with ACE inhibitors, but essentially not in such patients treated with β-blockers, and convincing data about less symptomatic patients are not available. This creates dilemmas regarding strength of recommendation and evidence when clinicians consider prescribing these drugs in

TABLE 40–3 Recommendations Concerning Key Therapeutic Areas for Heart Failure Caused by Left Ventricular Systolic Dysfunction

	HFSA 2006		ACC/AHA 2009		ESC 2008		CCS 2006	
Clinical Scenario	**SoR**	**SoE***	**SoR**	**SoE***	**SoR**	**SoE***	**SoR**	**SoE***
ACE inhibitors, all NYHA classes with or without history of myocardial infarction	Is recommended	A	Class I	A	Class I	A	Class I	A
β-Blockers, NYHA class I post myocardial infarction	Is recommended	B	Class I	A	Class I	A	Class I	A
β-Blockers, NYHA classes II to III	Is recommended	A	Class I	A	Class I	A	Class I	A
Aldosterone antagonists, NYHA classes III to IV	Is recommended	A	Class I	B	Class I	B	Class I	B
Digoxin, symptoms despite ACE inhibitor and β-blocker as tolerated	Is recommended: classes II to III Is recommended: class IV	A B	NYHA class ≥ II	B	Class IIa NYHA class ≥ II	B	Class IIa NYHA class ≥ II	B
Loop diuretics, all NYHA classes	Is recommended	B	Class I	C	Class I	B	Class I	C
Anticoagulants in CHF with atrial fibrillation	Is recommended	A	Class I	A	Class I	A	Class I	A
Anticoagulants in CHF without atrial fibrillation	May be considered	C	Class IIb	B	Insufficient evidence		Class IIb	C
Exercise training	Not mentioned		Class I	B	Insufficient evidence		Class IIa	B
Hydralazine nitrate	Is recommended for African American patients Should consider in other patients	A C	Class I, African American patients Class IIa, in other patients	B B	Class IIa, all patients	B	Class IIb, all patients	B

*For definition of A, B, and C, see Table 40-2.

ACC/AHA, American College of Cardiology Foundation/American Heart Association; *ACE,* angiotensin-converting enzyme; *CHF,* congestive heart failure; *CCS,* Canadian Cardiovascular Society; *ESC,* European Society of Cardiology; *HFSA,* Heart Failure Society of America; *SoE,* strength of evidence; *SoR,* strength of recommendation.

combination with β-blockade and in combination with other drugs in patients who do not have severe heart failure. Recommendations concerning aldosterone antagonists as part of combination therapy are restricted because of persistent concern about their adverse effects on serum potassium level and renal function in this setting.[71] Risk of serious hyperkalemia has led all the guidelines to specifically not recommend the triple combination of angiotensin receptor blocker, ACE inhibitor, and aldosterone blocker. This reaction could be excessively conservative inasmuch as some patients have low potassium levels despite oral replacement and may need aldosterone blockade to achieve adequate serum concentrations.

TRANSLATING CLINICAL TRIAL DATA INTO PRACTICE

Problem of Perspective

The application of new therapies in practice is generally a slow process. Many practitioners ascribe to the tenet "First, do no harm." Most respond to and evaluate medical advances from the traditional perspective of medical decision making rather than the perspective of evidence-based medicine (Table 40-7). It is clear that practitioners in direct daily contact with patients, many of whom have symptoms not related to organic disease or self-limited acute conditions, often rely on a hierarchy of medical evidence different from that used in guideline development. This perspective continues to limit the rapid application of new treatments that might be expected from favorable clinical trial results alone.

Specific Issues

Three other translational problems also contribute to the fact that clinical gains are often less than expected in accordance with favorable clinical trial results. First, knowledge gained concerning disease states and results from clinical trials often do not as easily improve outcomes in general populations of patients. Selection bias for trial enrollment may avoid issues of safety and side effects that may be more common in general medical populations. Second, medical practitioners are inherently resistant to change. Unexpected problems related to new therapeutic approaches may arise, and so many practitioners adopt a conservative approach to novel treatment. Third, therapeutic advances often necessitate new methods of care for a particular disease state; these methods may or may not be easy to adapt to outpatient or inpatient practice and are frequently expensive to implement. Some new therapeutic advances require fundamental changes in physicians' perception of disease processes that are simply hard to accept.

Strategies for implementing changes in practice processes and implementing new standards of care have not been well studied or understood. Unfortunately, the changes necessitated by many therapeutic advances are significant in terms of practice organization, facilities, and personnel. Funding to support the necessary adaptations often does not accompany the change in expectations regarding treatment, particularly

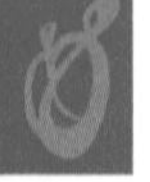

TABLE 40–4 Similarity and Contrast Among Guidelines in Recommendations for Cardiac Resynchronization Therapy

General Considerations	HFSA 2006		ACC/AHA 2009		ESC 2008		CCS 2006	
Specific recommendations	Intervention made in view of functional status and prognosis on the basis of severity of underlying heart failure and comorbid conditions (recommended, C)		Not mentioned		Not mentioned		The decision to implant a device in a patient with heart failure should be made with assessment and discussion between the heart failure and arrhythmia specialists (class I, level C)	
Criteria for use								
QRS duration	≥120 msec		≥120 msec		≥120 msec		≥120 msec	
LVEF criteria	≤35%		≤35%		≤35%		≤35%	
Optimize medications	Required 3-6 months		Required		Required		Required	
Clinical Scenarios	**SoR**	**SoE***	**SoR**	**SoE***	**SoR**	**SoE***	**SoR**	**SoE***
Class III	Should be considered	A	Class I	A	Class I	A	Class I	A
Class IV	May be considered Selected ambulatory patients	B	Class I Ambulatory patients	A	Class I Any class IV	A	Class I	A
Classes I to II	Not recommended	C	Insufficient evidence		Insufficient evidence		Insufficient evidence	

*For definition of A, B, and C, see Table 40-2.

ACC/AHA, American College of Cardiology Foundation/American Heart Association; *CCS,* Canadian Cardiovascular Society; *ESC,* European Society of Cardiology; *HFSA,* Heart Failure Society of America; *LVEF,* left ventricular ejection fraction; *SoE,* strength of evidence; *SoR,* strength of recommendation.

TABLE 40–5 Recommendations for Inotropic Therapy (Dobutamine or Milrinone) for Acute Heart Failure

Aspect	HFSA 2006	ACC/AHA 2009	ESC 2008	CCS 2006
Indications for use	Intravenous inotropic agents (milrinone or dobutamine) may be considered to relieve symptoms and improve end-organ function in patients with advanced heart failure characterized by LV dilation, reduced LVEF, and diminished peripheral perfusion or end-organ dysfunction (low-output syndrome), particularly if these patients have marginal systolic blood pressure (<90 mm Hg), have symptomatic hypotension despite adequate filling pressure, or are unresponsive to or intolerant of intravenous vasodilators. These agents may be considered in similar patients with evidence of fluid overload if they respond poorly to intravenous diuretics or manifest diminished or worsening renal function.	Patients with either predominantly low-output syndrome (e.g., symptomatic hypotension) or combined congestion and low output may be considered for intravenous inotropic agents such as dopamine, dobutamine, and milrinone. Inotropic agents are of greatest value in patients with relative hypotension and intolerance of or no response to vasodilators and diuretics.	Inotropic agents should be considered in patients with low-output states, in the presence of signs of hypoperfusion or congestion despite the use of vasodilators or diuretics, or both, to improve symptoms. Inotropic agents should be administered only in patients with low SBP or a low measured cardiac index in the presence of signs of hypoperfusion or congestion. Therapy should be reserved for patients with dilated, hypokinetic ventricles.	Patients with low cardiac output and SBP less than 90 mm Hg should be given a positive inotrope (e.g., dobutamine, 2-5 μg/kg/min, or milrinone, 0.275 μg/kg/min). Depending on the hemodynamic profile, treatment should include combined intravenous diuretics and inotropic agents. Once SBP is improved by inotropic agents, vasodilator therapy can be added to lower filling pressures further.
Strength of recommendation	May be considered	Class III	Class IIa	Class I
Strength of evidence*	C	C	B	B

*For definition of B and C, see Table 40-2.

ACC/AHA, American College of Cardiology Foundation/American Heart Association; *CCS,* Canadian Cardiovascular Society; *ESC,* European Society of Cardiology (2008); *HFSA,* Heart Failure Society of America (2006); *LV,* left ventricular; *LVEF,* left ventricular ejection fraction; *SBP,* systolic blood pressure.

TABLE 40–6 Strategy for Addition of Medical Therapy to ACE Inhibitor and β-Blocker*

In Addition to ACE Inhibitor and β-Blocker	HFSA 2006		ACC/AHA 2009		ESC 2008		CCS 2006	
	SoR	SoE†	SoR	SoE†	SoR	SoE†	SoR	SoE†
Clinical Scenario: NYHA Class II								
ARB	Should be considered	A	Class IIb	B	Class I	A	Class I	A
Aldosterone antagonist	Should be considered	C	Class IIb	B	Insufficient evidence		Insufficient evidence	
Hydralazine nitrate: African American patients	Should be considered	B	Class IIa	A	Class IIa	B	Class IIa	A
Hydralazine nitrate: non-African American patients	Should be considered	C	Class IIa	A	Class IIa	B	Insufficient evidence	
Clinical Scenario: NYHA Class III								
ARB	Should be considered	A	Class IIb	B	Class I	A*	Class I	A
Aldosterone antagonist	Should be considered	A	Class I	B	Class I	B	Class I	B
Hydralazine nitrate: African American patients	Is recommended	A	Class IIa	A	Class IIa	B	Class IIa	A
Hydralazine nitrate: non-African American patients	Should be considered	C	Class IIa	A	Class IIa	B	Insufficient evidence	

*Order in which agents are added is not well delineated by the guidelines. The triple combination of ACE inhibitors, ARB, and aldosterone antagonist is not recommended by each of the guidelines because it heightens risk of hyperkalemia and worsening renal function.

†For definition of A, B, and C, see Table 40-2.

ACC/AHA, American College of Cardiology Foundation/American Heart Association (2009); *ACE*, angiotensin-converting enzyme; *ARB*, angiotensin receptor blocker; *CCS*, Canadian Cardiovascular Society; *ESC*, European Society of Cardiology; *HFSA*, Heart Failure Society of America (2006); *NYHA*, New York Heart Association; *SoE*, strength of evidence; *SoR*, strength of recommendation.

TABLE 40–7 Factors That Affect Concerns About Therapy Among Various Groups in the Medical Care System

Group	Concerns
Clinical trialists	Results of randomized trials
Guideline makers	Randomized trials, cohort results Observational data, expert opinion
Process reviewers	Absolute consensus on therapy Clear-cut criteria to identify patients to be treated
Practicing physicians	Absence of side effects, cost, convenience Familiarly, safety Efficacy

TABLE 40–8 Unique Barriers to the Use of β-Blockade for Heart Failure

Traditional Approach	Treatment Approach with β-Blockade
Treat for immediate improvement in symptoms	Give β-blocker for long-term benefit, not for immediate symptom relief
Use new approaches in sickest patients first	Do not use in sickest patients (those with active class IV heart failure with fluid or in hospital)
Do not add drugs to regimen when patients experience improvement in symptoms	Add β-blockade as a part of a multiple-drug regimen for heart failure

when advances are related to pharmacological therapy. The practicality of making process changes is often ignored by guideline makers and by professionals who monitor compliance with guidelines.

Clinical Example: β-Blockade

β-Blockade for heart failure is a striking example of a therapy once contraindicated that is now indicated. A number of barriers have prevented the use of β-blockade for heart failure from becoming widespread. In addition to barriers that characterize many new therapies, such as necessary changes in practice processes and the need for education concerning the therapy, a number of unique challenges have been associated with the use of β-blockade (Table 40-8). Many strategies have been used to overcome these latter barriers to the translation of new advances into clinical practice. Creation of practice guidelines has emerged as one of the principal strategies and is a seemingly effective approach.

CONCLUSION

Development and promulgation of practice guidelines seem to be fixtures of modern medical care.[72] Considerable consensus supports the idea that a systematic process is necessary to evaluate new approaches to management, especially when patients suffer from debilitating, expensive, and fatal diseases such as heart failure. Despite many landmark studies that promote reliance on evidence-based medicine, significant gaps in knowledge persist, especially from the point of view of the health care provider, who, for example, must write a highly specific prescription for pharmacological therapy that details dose, frequency, and duration of a specific medication, with or without adjustment of other therapies. Many specific decisions were traditionally made on an ad hoc basis by physicians and other health care providers. In most cases, there was observational experience, but given that individual physicians were making these decisions, the nature of the observational experience was biased and often of limited value for many diseases.

BOX 40–4 Humanistic Principles Critical for Guideline Development

Achieve consensus
Avoid a single dominant voice
Maintain independence
Remain humble
Show up for work consistently

Development of specific practice guidelines is emerging as a critical part of translational strategy. The understanding of the strengths and limitations of clinical trial data as agents of change in clinical practice has deepened, and the importance of the thought process inherent in guideline development has become more evident. Effective long-term guidelines are living documents with short life cycles that accelerate along with the understanding of the steps necessary to translate advances in heart failure into clinical care. Properly conceived, these standards should significantly enhance the applications of advances in medical science to the actual day-to-day care of patients. As the economic reality increasingly clashes with rising patient and provider expectations for quality and success, novel approaches to care delivery will be paramount to avoid loss of morale and the practice of inferior medicine on a large scale.[73,74]

Although in this setting the justification for guidelines is apparent, the developmental process for these standards of care needs continued investigation and refinement. External pressures and emphasis on timeliness will increasingly complicate an already very difficult academic challenge. To quote Sackett, "Truth is not often best determined by scheduling a press conference."[75] A number of humanistic principles have become as critical to guideline development as scientific acuity and discipline (Box 40-4). Dedication to the art and science of medicine and the spirit of cooperative endeavor is more necessary than ever for success in guideline development.

REFERENCES

1. Guideline Committee for the Heart Failure Society of America. (1999). HFSA guidelines for the management of patients with heart failure caused by left ventricular systolic dysfunction—pharmacological approaches. *J Card Fail, 5*, 357–382.
2. Konstam, M. A., Dracup, K., Baker, D., et al. (1994). *Heart failure: evaluation and care of patients with left ventricular systolic dysfunction.* Rockville, MD: Agency for Health Care Policy and Research, U.S. Dept. of Health and Human Services.
3. Guidelines for the evaluation and management of heart failure. (1995). Report of the American College of Cardiology/American Heart Association Task Force on Practice Guidelines (Committee on Evaluation and Management of Heart Failure). *Circulation, 92*, 2764–2784.
4. Hunt, S. A., Baker, D. W., Chin, M. H., et al. (2001). ACC/AHA Guidelines for the evaluation and management of chronic heart failure in the adult: executive summary. A Report of the American College of Cardiology/American Heart Association Task Force on Practice Guidelines (Committee to Revise the 1995 Guidelines for the Evaluation and Management of Heart Failure): Developed in Collaboration With the International Society for Heart and Lung Transplantation; Endorsed by the Heart Failure Society of America. *Circulation, 104*, 2996–3007.
5. The treatment of heart failure. (1997). Task Force of the Working Group for Heart Failure of the European Society of Cardiology. *Eur Heart J, 18*, 736–753.
6. Liu, P., Arnold, M., Belenkie, J., et al. (2001). for the Canadian Cardiovascular Society The 2001 Canadian Cardiovascular Society consensus guideline update for the management and prevention of heart failure. *Can J Cardiol, 17*(Suppl E), 5E–25E.
7. Adams, K. F., Lindenfeld, J., Arnold, J. M. O., et al. (2006). Executive summary: HFSA 2006 comprehensive heart failure practice guideline. *J Card Fail, 12*, 10–38.
8. Arnold, J. M., Liu, P., Demers, C., et al. (2006). Canadian Cardiovascular Society consensus conference recommendations on heart failure 2006: diagnosis and management. *Can J Cardiol, 22*, 23–45.
9. Task Force for Diagnosis and Treatment of Acute and Chronic Heart Failure 2008 of European Society of Cardiology, Dickstein, K., Cohen-Solal, A., et al. (2008). ESC Guidelines for the diagnosis and treatment of acute and chronic heart failure 2008: the Task Force for the Diagnosis and Treatment of Acute and Chronic Heart Failure 2008 of the European Society of Cardiology. Developed in collaboration with the Heart Failure Association of the ESC (HFA) and endorsed by the European Society of Intensive Care Medicine (ESICM). *Eur Heart J, 29*, 2388–2442.
10. Hunt, S. A., Abraham, W. T., Chin, M. H., et al. (2009). 2009 Focused update incorporated into the ACC/AHA 2005 Guidelines for the Diagnosis and Management of Heart Failure in Adults. A report of the American College of Cardiology Foundation/American Heart Association Task Force on Practice Guidelines. Developed in collaboration with the International Society for Heart and Lung Transplantation. *J Am Coll Cardiol, 53*, e1–e90.
11. Wenneberg, J., & Gittelsohn, A. (1973). Small area variations in health care delivery. *Science, 182*, 1102–1108.
12. Eddy, D. M. (1990). Practice policies: where do they come from? *JAMA, 263*, 1265–1275.
13. Evidence-Based Medicine Working Group. (1992). Evidence-based medicine. A new approach to teaching the practice of medicine. *JAMA, 268*, 2420–2425.
14. Sackett, D. L., Rosenberg, W. M., Gray, J. A., et al. (1996). Evidence based medicine: what it is and what it isn't. *Clin Orthop Relat Res, 2007*(455), 3–5.
15. Straus, S. E., & Sackett, D. L. (1999). Applying evidence to the individual patient. *Ann Oncol, 10*, 29–32.
16. Saunders, J. (2000). The practice of clinical medicine as an art and as a science. *Med Humanit, 26*, 18–22.
17. Montgomery, K. (2009). Thinking about thinking: implications for patient safety. *Healthc Q, 12*(Spec No Patient), e191–e194.
18. McDonald, C. J. (1996). Medical heuristics: the silent adjudicators of clinical practice. *Ann Intern Med, 124*, 56–62.
19. Eddy, D. M. (2005). Evidence-based medicine: a unified approach. *Health Aff (Millwood), 24*, 9–17.
20. Cochrane's legacy [Comment]. (1992). *Lancet, 340*, 1131–1132.
21. Manchikanti, L. (2008). Evidence-based medicine, systematic reviews, and guidelines in interventional pain management, part I: introduction and general considerations. *Pain Physician, 11*, 161–186.
22. Tricoci, P., Allen, J. M., Kramer, J. M., et al. (2009). Scientific evidence underlying the ACC/AHA clinical practice guidelines. *JAMA, 301*, 831–841.
23. Shaneyfelt, T. M., & Centor, R. M. (2009). Reassessment of clinical practice guidelines: go gently into that good night. *JAMA, 301*, 868–869.
24. Concato, J., Shah, N., & Horwitz, R. I. (2000). Randomized, controlled trials, observational studies, and the hierarchy of research designs. *N Engl J Med, 342*, 1887–1892.
25. Benson, K., & Hartz, A. J. (2000). A comparison of observational studies and randomized, controlled trials. *N Engl J Med, 342*, 1878–1886.
26. Avorn, J. (2007). In defense of pharmacoepidemiology—embracing the yin and yang of drug research. *N Engl J Med, 357*, 2219–2221.
27. Black, N. (1996). Why we need observational studies to evaluate the effectiveness of health care. *BMJ, 312*, 1215–1218.
28. Black, N. (2008). Complementarity comes of age. *Transplantation, 86*, 28–29.
29. Takemoto, S. K., Arns, W., Bunnapradist, S., et al. (2008). Expanding the evidence base in transplantation: the complementary roles of randomized controlled trials and outcomes research. *Transplantation, 86*, 18–25.
30. Tunis, S. R., Stryer, D. B., & Clancy, C. M. (2003). Practical clinical trials: increasing the value of clinical research for decision making in clinical and health policy. *JAMA, 290*, 1624–1632.
31. Horwitz, R. I., & Feinstein, A. R. (1979). Methodologic standards and contradictory results in case-control research. *Am J Med, 66*, 556–564.
32. Kopec, J. A., & Esdaile, J. M. (1990). Bias in case-control studies. A review. *J Epidemiol Community Health, 44*, 179–186.
33. Schneeweiss, S., Patrick, A. R., Stürmer, T., et al. (2007). Increasing levels of restriction in pharmacoepidemiologic database studies of elderly and comparison with randomized trial results. *Med Care, 45*(Suppl 2), S131–S142.
34. Antman, E. M., & Peterson, E. D. (2009). Tools for guiding clinical practice from the American Heart Association and the American College of Cardiology: what are they and how should clinicians use them? *Circulation, 119*, 1180–1185.
35. Antman, E. M., & Gibbons, R. J. (2009). Clinical practice guidelines and scientific evidence. *JAMA, 302*, 143–144.
36. Shaneyfelt, T. M., Mayo-Smith, M. F., & Rothwangl, J. (1999). Are guideline following guidelines: the methodological quality of clinical practice guidelines in the peer-reviewed medical literature. *JAMA, 281*, 1900–1905.
37. Montori, V. M., & Guyatt, G. H. (2008). Progress in evidence-based medicine. *JAMA, 300*, 1814–1816.
38. Atkins, D., Eccles, M., Flottorp, S., et al. (2004). Systems for grading the quality of evidence and the strength of recommendations I: critical appraisal of existing approaches The GRADE Working Group. *BMC Health Serv Res, 4*, 38.
39. Guyatt, G. H., Oxman, A. D., Vist, G. E., et al. (2008). GRADE: an emerging consensus on rating quality of evidence and strength of recommendations. *BMJ, 336*, 924–926.
40. Atkins, D., Briss, P. A., Eccles, M., et al. (2005). Systems for grading the quality of evidence and the strength of recommendations II: pilot study of a new system. *BMC Health Serv Res, 5*, 25.
41. Atkins, D., Best, D., Briss, P. A., et al. (2004). Grading quality of evidence and strength of recommendations. *BMJ, 328*, 1490–1494.
42. Yusuf, S., Cairns, J. A., Camm, A. J., et al. (1998). Grading of recommendations and levels of evidence used in evidence based cardiology. In S. Yusuf, J. A. Cairns, & A. J. Camm (Eds.). *Evidence based cardiology.* London: BMJ Books, p xxvi.
43. Califf, R. M. (1998). Considerations in the design, conduct, and interpretation of quantitative clinical evidence. In E. J. Topol (Ed.). *Comprehensive cardiovascular medicine* (pp. 1203–1221). Philadelphia: Lippincott-Raven.
44. Guyatt, G. H., Oxman, A. D., Kunz, R., et al. (2008). GRADE: going from evidence to recommendations. *BMJ, 336*, 1049–1051.
45. Bristow, M. R., Ginsburg, R., Fowler, M., et al. (1986). β_1- and β_2-adrenergic receptor subpopulations in normal and failing human ventricular myocardium: coupling of both receptor subtypes to muscle contraction and selection β_1-receptor downregulation in heart failure. *Circ Res, 59*, 297–309.
46. Mann, D. L., Kent, R. L., Parsons, B., et al. (1992). Adrenergic effects on the biology of the adult mammalian cardiocyte. *Circulation, 85*, 790–804.
47. Engelhardt, S., Hein, L., Wiesman, F., et al. (1999). Progressive hypertrophy and heart failure in beta$_1$-adrenergic receptor transgenic mice. *Proc Natl Acad Sci, 96*, 7059–8064.
48. Cohn, J., Levine, T., Olivari, M., et al. (1984). Plasma norepinephrine as a guide to prognosis in patients with chronic congestive heart failure. *N Engl J Med, 311*, 819–823.
49. Swedberg, K., Hjalmarson, A., Waagstein, F., et al. (1979). Prolongation of survival in congestive cardiomyopathy by beta-receptor blockade. Beneficial effects of metoprolol in idiopathic dilated cardiomyopathy. *Lancet, 1*, 374–376.

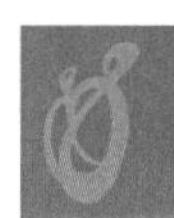

50. Bristow, M. R. (2000). Beta adrenergic blockade in chronic heart failure. *Circulation, 101*, 558–569.
51. Packer, M., Bristow, M. R., Cohn, J. N., et al. (1996). The effect of carvedilol on morbidity and mortality in patients with chronic heart failure. *N Engl J Med, 334*, 1349–1355.
52. The Cardiac Insufficiency Bisoprolol Study II (CIBIS-II). (1999). A randomised trial. *Lancet, 353*, 9–13.
53. Effect of metoprolol CR/XL in chronic heart failure. (1999). Metoprolol CR/XL Randomized Intervention Trial in congestive Heart Failure (MERIT-HF). *Lancet, 353*, 2001–2007.
54. Tandon, P., McAlister, F. A., Tsuyuki, R. T., et al. (2004). The use of beta-blockers in a tertiary care heart failure clinic: dosing, tolerance, and outcomes. *Arch Intern Med, 164*, 769–774.
55. Bristow, M. R., Gilbert, E. M., Abraham, W. T., et al. (1996). Carvedilol produces dose-related improvements in left ventricular function and survival in subjects with chronic heart failure. *Circulation, 94*, 2807–2816.
56. Wikstand, J., Hjalmarson, A., Waagstein, F., et al. (2002). for the MERIT-HF Study Group. Dose of metoprolol CR/XL and clinical outcomes in patients with heart failure. *J Am Coll Cardiol, 40*, 491–498.
57. Waagstein, F., Caidahl, K., Wallentin, I., et al. (1989). Long-term beta-blockade in dilated cardiomyopathy: effects of short-term and long-term metoprolol followed by withdrawal and readministration of metoprolol. *Circulation, 80*, 551–563.
58. Morimoto, S., Shimizu, K., Yamada, K., et al. (1999). Can beta-blocker therapy be withdrawn from patients with dilated cardiomyopathy? *Am Heart J, 137*, 456–459.
59. Gattis, W. A., O'Connor, C. M., Gallup, D. S., et al. (2004). on behalf of the IMPACT-HF Investigators. Predischarge initiation of carvedilol in patients hospitalized for decompensated heart failure. *J Am Coll Cardiol, 43*, 1534–1541.
60. Fonarow, G. C., Abraham, W. T., Albert, N. M., et al. (2007). Association between performance measures and clinical outcomes for patients hospitalized with heart failure. *JAMA, 297*, 61–70.
61. Gottlieb, S. S., McCarter, R. J., & Vogel, R. A. (1998). Effect of beta-blockade on mortality among high-risk and low-risk patients after myocardial infarction. *N Engl J Med, 339*, 489–497.
62. Deedwania, P. C., Gottlieb, S., Ghali, J. K., et al. (2004). Efficacy, safety and tolerability of beta-adrenergic blockade with metoprolol CR/XL in elderly patients with heart failure. *Eur Heart J, 25*, 1300–1309.
63. Packer, M., Coats, A. J. S., Fowler, M. B., et al. (2001). Effect of carvedilol on survival in severe chronic heart failure. *N Engl J Med, 344*, 1651–1658.
64. Goldstein, S., Fagerberg, B., Hjalmarson, A., et al. (2001). for the MERIT-HF Study Group. Metoprolol controlled release/extended release in patients with severe heart failure. *J Am Coll Cardiol, 38*, 932–938.
65. Colucci, W. S., Kolias, T. J., Adams, K. F., et al. (2007). Metoprolol reverses left ventricular remodeling in patients with asymptomatic systolic dysfunction: the REversal of VEntricular Remodeling with Toprol-XL (REVERT) trial. *Circulation, 116*, 49–56.
66. Cuffe, M. S., Califf, R. M., Adams, K. F., Jr., et al. (2002). Short-term intravenous milrinone for acute exacerbation of chronic heart failure: a randomized controlled trial. *JAMA, 287*, 1541–1547.
67. Mebazaa, A., Nieminen, M. S., Packer, M., et al. (2007). Levosimendan vs dobutamine for patients with acute decompensated heart failure: the SURVIVE Randomized Trial. *JAMA, 297*, 1883–1891.
68. Adams, K. F., Fonarow, G. C., Emerman, C. L., et al. (2005). Characteristics and outcomes of patients hospitalized for heart failure in the United States: rationale, design, and preliminary observations from the first 100,000 cases in the Acute Decompensated Heart Failure National Registry (ADHERE). *Am Heart J, 149*, 209–216.
69. Fonarow, G. C., Adams, K. F., Abraham, W. T., et al. (2005). Risk stratification for in-hospital mortality in acutely decompensated heart failure: Classification and regression tree analysis. *JAMA, 293*, 572–580.
70. Abraham, W. T., Adams, K. F., Fonarow, G. C., et al. (2005). In-hospital mortality in patients with acute decompensated heart failure treated with intravenous inotropes versus vasodilators: an analysis from the Acute Decompensated Heart Failure National Registry(ADHERE). *J Am Coll Cardiol, 46*, 57–64.
71. Juurlink, D. N., Mamdani, M. M., Lee, D. S., et al. (2004). Rates of hyperkalemia after publication of the Randomized Aldactone Evaluation Study. *N Engl J Med, 351*, 543–551.
72. Woolf, S. H. (1990). Practice guidelines: a new reality in medicine. *Arch Intern Med, 150*, 1811–1818.
73. Haburchak, D. R., Mitchell, B. C., & Boomer, C. J. (2008). Quixotic medicine: physical and economic laws perilously disregarded in health care and medical education. *Acad Med, 83*, 1140–1145.
74. Wachter, R. M. (2006). Expected and unanticipated consequences of the quality and information technology revolutions. *JAMA, 295*, 2780–2783.
75. Sackett, D. L. (1997). A science for the art of consensus. *J Natl Cancer Inst, 89*, 1003–1005.

CHAPTER 41

Disease Prevention in Heart Failure

Viorel G. Florea and Jay N. Cohn

Despite advances in the therapy of cardiovascular disorders, heart failure remains a challenging disease process with a high prevalence (Figure 41-1) and a dismal long-term prognosis (see Chapter 22).[1] Although the rate of fatal events in patients with heart failure has been declining,[2] the crude number of deaths attributed to the condition has been increasing,[1] primarily because the incidence of the condition has increased (Figure 41-2). The aging of the population and improved length of survival of patients with acute myocardial infarction are believed to be some factors contributing to the growing burden of chronic heart failure. More than 500,000 new cases of heart failure are diagnosed each year, and this incidence is expected to rise to 772,000 new cases per year by 2040.[3] The burden of heart failure will obviously not be eliminated by an improvement in the survival of patients who are already affected with the disease; instead, a drastic reduction in the incidence of heart failure is necessary to prevent an increase in the burden. It is therefore important that a population-level strategy be developed to prevent the lifetime risk of heart failure that applies to the large number of individuals at risk. Such a strategy would complement the current approaches that are aimed at intensive management of patients with manifest heart failure (Figure 41-3).

Because of the sizable public health burden posed by heart failure and the limitations in health care resources, it is crucial that the primary drivers of this problem be identified. In 2001, a new approach to the classification of heart failure was adopted by the American College of Cardiology/American Heart Association; this approach included stage A, characterized by no structural disorder of the heart or heart failure symptoms but risk factors that clearly predispose carriers toward the development of heart failure.[4] It is estimated that 74 million people in the United States are living with risk factors for heart failure (i.e., are in stage A of heart failure).[5] The new classification scheme adds a useful dimension to the understanding of heart failure: the recognition that there are established risk factors and structural prerequisites for the development of heart failure and that therapeutic interventions performed even before the appearance of left ventricular dysfunction or symptoms can prevent the development of heart failure. In 2008, the American Heart Association published a scientific statement on heart failure prevention.[6] The progression of heart failure mandates that an all-out effort be made to prevent its development in the first place, and the best time to intervene would be before or at stage A.

A number of risk factors have been identified that may lead to heart failure. These exert their adverse effects through functional and structural influence on the left ventricle, characterized as ventricular remodeling and defined as progressive ventricular hypertrophy, enlargement, and cavity distortion over time.[7,8] These risk factors include hypertension, diabetes mellitus, atherosclerotic disease, metabolic syndrome, obesity, chronic obstructive pulmonary disease (COPD), and the use of many therapeutic and recreational agents that can exert important cardiotoxic effects. Hypertension and myocardial infarction together account for approximately 75% of the population-attributable risk of heart failure,[9] and both are generally preventable with currently known and available strategies. The burden of heart failure risk factors, and comorbid conditions and their treatment on incident heart failure are examined in this chapter. As the primary mechanisms of the development of heart failure may be cardiac (structural remodeling, decreased compliance, impaired contractility) or peripheral (fluid retention, vascular remodeling), this discussion is an attempt to characterize the specific mechanisms of the effect of the comorbid conditions and their treatment on the development of heart failure.

DIASTOLIC AND SYSTOLIC HEART FAILURE

Although the existence of diastolic heart failure, as distinguished from systolic heart failure, was recognized before 1940,[10] the mechanisms that ultimately produce these two phenotypes of chronic heart failure remain, at present, largely unknown.[11] Furthermore, whereas diastolic dysfunction is common in systolic heart failure,[12] left ventricular systolic performance, function, and contractility in general remain normal in diastolic heart failure.[13] The myocardium and left ventricle of most patients with heart failure have, in fact, many similarities and are abnormal during both systole and diastole, regardless of ejection fraction. The myocardium in patients with ischemic cardiomyopathy or hypertensive heart disease is similarly characterized by increased left ventricular mass, myocyte hypertrophy, and increased interstitial collagen.[14,15] Hypertrophic myocardium in these and other conditions exhibits similar abnormalities of calcium handling and similar functional abnormalities of contraction and relaxation,[16] regardless of ejection fraction. Myocardium from patients with dilated cardiomyopathy and from those with hypertrophic cardiomyopathy demonstrates similar delay in diastolic cytosolic calcium reuptake, in association with delayed relaxation.[16]

Although classifying systolic and diastolic heart failure has been challenging,[17] the key element differentiating the two types of heart failure is the presence or absence of ventricular dilation and remodeling.[7] The presence of conditions that are considered risk factors, such as hypertension or diabetes, leads to myocyte apoptosis and necrosis.[18] The resultant fibrosis forms the basis of impaired ventricular relaxation and reduced ventricular compliance.[19] When this process is slow and chronic, the ventricle may maintain its size and shape (does not remodel) and therefore preserves its ejection fraction.[20] In acute insults to the ventricle, as in myocardial infarction, alterations in the topography of

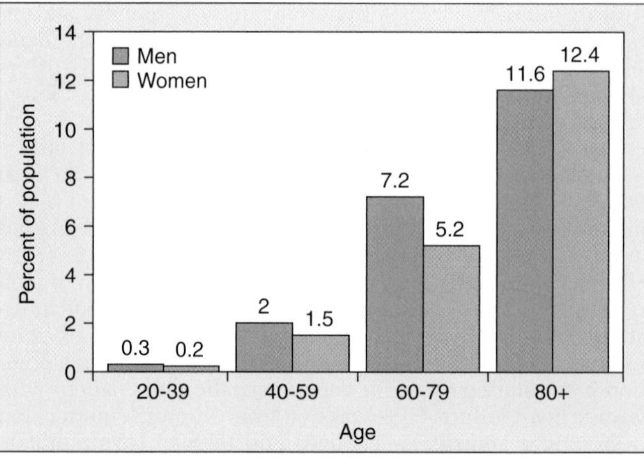

FIGURE 41–1 Prevalence of heart failure by age and gender (National Health and Nutrition Examination Survey: 1999-2004). (From Rosamond W, Flegal K, Furie K, et al. Heart disease and stroke statistics 2008 update. A report from the American Heart Association Statistics Committee and Stroke Statistics Subcommittee. *Circulation* 2007;117[4]:e25-e146.)

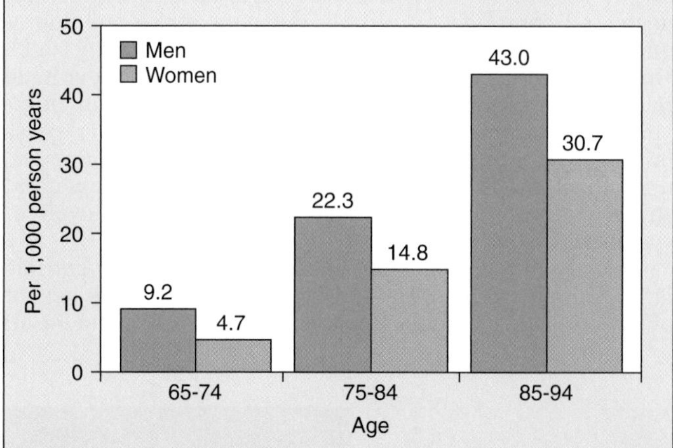

FIGURE 41–2 Incidence of heart failure by age and gender. (From Rosamond W, Flegal K, Furie K, et al. Heart disease and stroke statistics 2008 update. A report from the American Heart Association Statistics Committee and Stroke Statistics Subcommittee. *Circulation* 2007;117[4]:e25-e146.)

both the infarcted and noninfarcted regions of the ventricle may lead to progressive ventricular enlargement.[21] The decrease in global left ventricular ejection fraction results largely from ventricular dilation and remodeling (Figure 41-4).[22]

The distinctive features of remodeling in diastolic heart failure and systolic heart failure are illustrated in Figure 41-5 (see also Chapter 14).[23,24] In systolic heart failure, the left ventricular cavity size is increased, the ventricular shape and geometry are altered with a greater increase in transverse than in long axis, the wall stress is increased, and the ejection fraction is reduced. The mass is increased, but the mass-to-cavity ratio remains unchanged or is decreased. In diastolic heart failure, the cavity size remains unchanged or may even decrease, and there is usually an increase in wall thickness and mass; however, mass-to-cavity ratio is substantially increased, the end-diastolic wall stress is increased, systolic wall stress remains normal, and the ejection fraction remains normal or may even be higher than normal.[13,23]

Ejection fraction provides no information regarding functional capacity.[25] Rather, in patients with normal ejection fraction[26] and in those with low ejection fraction,[27] functional status is linked partly to the ventricular capacity for diastolic distention and preload recruitment during exertion. Konstam and associates[27] observed that among patients with low ejection fraction, diastolic distention during exercise, accompanied by associated stroke volume augmentation, distinguishes asymptomatic patients from those with symptoms of heart failure. Therefore, in both patients with heart failure and low ejection fraction and those with heart failure and more normal ejection fraction, the myocardium and left ventricle function abnormally during both systole and diastole. Ejection fraction in patients with chronic heart failure, rather than signifying distinct pathophysiological processes, principally distinguishes the pattern of hypertrophic left ventricular remodeling: hypertrophic cavity dilation versus hypertrophic concentric thickening without cavity dilation.

DISTINGUISHING FLUID RETENTION FROM ABNORMALITIES IN VENTRICULAR PERFORMANCE

The clinical syndrome of heart failure usually results from both impaired left ventricular performance and circulatory congestion (see Chapter 18). This congestion is aggravated

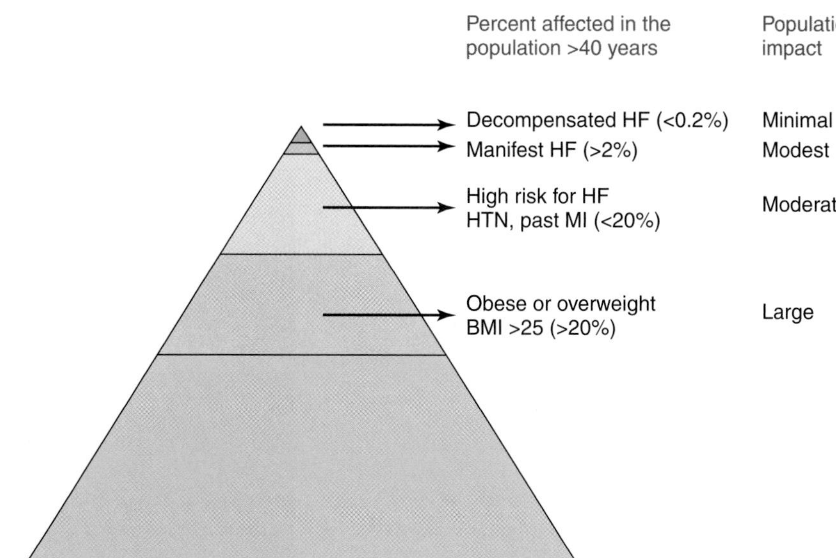

FIGURE 41–3 The pyramid of heart failure (HF) in the population and the potential effect of a range of preventive and treatment strategies in lowering age-specific mortality rates. BMI, body mass index; HTN, hypertension; MI, myocardial infarction. (From Young J, Narula J. Preface prevention should take center stage. *Cardiol Clin* 2007;25[4]:xi-xiii; data from Yusuf S, Pitt B. A lifetime of prevention: the case of heart failure. *Circulation* 2002;106:2997-2998.)

by renal sodium retention. Consequently, heart failure may develop as a result of the effects of disease or drugs either on left ventricular function or structure or on renal sodium excretion.

Hypertension and Heart Failure

Considerable evidence from experimental and clinical studies and epidemiological investigations indicates the critical role of hypertension in the pathogenesis of heart failure (see Chapter 28). Elevated levels of diastolic and especially systolic blood pressure are major risk factors for the development of heart failure.[28,29] Also, hypertension is frequently accompanied by metabolic risk factors and obesity, which themselves increase the risk of heart failure. On the basis of the 44-year follow-up data of the Framingham Heart Study, 75% of patients with heart failure have antecedent hypertension.[1,9] The population attributable risk for heart failure associated with hypertension is 39% in men and 59% in women.[28] Because nearly 33% of adults in the United States have hypertension,[30] strategies to control blood pressure are an integral part of any effort to prevent heart failure.

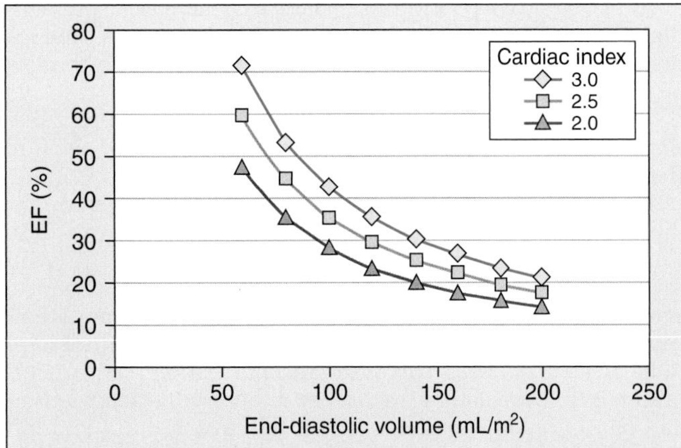

FIGURE 41-4 Relationship between left ventricular end-diastolic volume and ejection fraction (EF) at three levels of cardiac index and at a constant heart rate of 70 beats/minute. In chronic heart failure, a low EF indicates little about contractility or left ventricular load; it mostly identifies a left ventricle that has remodeled with dilation. (From Konstam MA. "Systolic and diastolic dysfunction" in heart failure? Time for a new paradigm. *J Card Fail* 2003;9:1-3.)

Both acute and chronic hypertension have been linked to the risk of heart failure. Sudden elevation of blood pressure (such as in hypertensive emergencies) can lead to acute left ventricular strain and acute heart failure[31] and is a common precipitating cause for decompensation in a patient with chronic heart failure.[32] Progression from chronic hypertension to structural ventricular changes and then to asymptomatic diastolic and systolic ventricular dysfunction is well established by natural history investigations in longitudinal epidemiological cohort studies, such as the Framingham Heart Study.[28]

Elevated blood pressure places greater hemodynamic burden on the myocardium and leads to left ventricular hypertrophy[33,34] (Figure 41-6). Left ventricular hypertrophy is associated with increased myocardial stiffness and decreased compliance, initially during exercise and subsequently at rest.[35-37] The initial concentric hypertrophy (thick wall, normal chamber volume, and high mass-to-volume ratio) helps keep wall tension normal despite high intraventricular pressure (Figure 41-7). Because systolic stress (afterload) is a major determinant of ejection performance, normalization of systolic stress helps maintain a normal stroke volume despite the need to generate high levels of systolic pressure.[38]

Because the impedance load facing the left ventricle is dependent on pressure at all pressure levels, the benefit of lowering this vascular load may be demonstrated in all

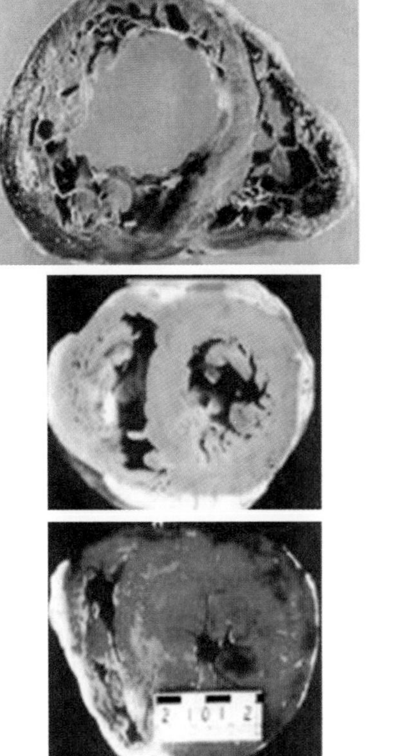

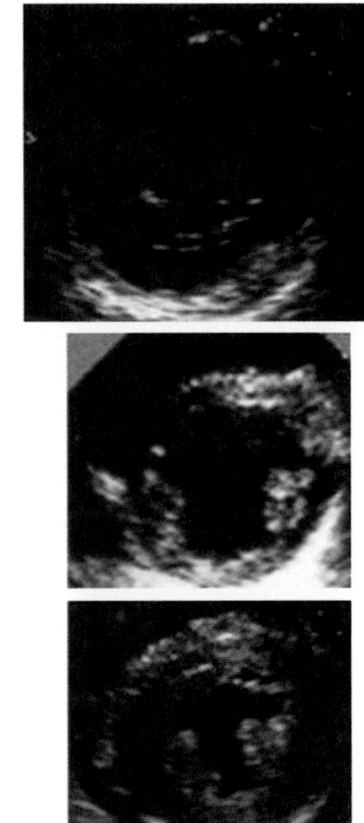

FIGURE 41-5 Ventricular remodeling in systolic and diastolic heart failure. *Left,* Autopsy samples; *right,* cross-sectional 2-dimensional echocardiographic views of systolic (*top*) and diastolic (*bottom*) heart failure, in comparison with normal heart function (*middle*). In systolic heart failure, the left ventricular cavity is markedly dilated, and wall thickness is not increased. In diastolic heart failure, the cavity size is normal or decreased, and wall thickness is markedly increased. (From Chatterjee K, Massie B. Systolic and diastolic heart failure: differences and similarities. *J Card Fail* 2007;13:569-576.)

patients with left ventricular dysfunction, regardless of the absolute pressure level. Furthermore, changes in brachial artery pressure may not serve as an adequate guide to reductions in impedance load on the left ventricle. Constriction and stiffening of small arteries at branch points and in the microcirculation augment reflected waves that may impose a late systolic aortic pressure load on left ventricular emptying that is not detectable in the arm. Therapy that relaxes these small arteries may therefore exert a greater benefit than is apparent from standard blood pressure measurement. In addition, however, some of the benefits of antihypertensive therapy on the development of heart failure may be mediated by nonpressure mechanisms. Improved endothelial function may favorably affect coronary perfusion, and some drugs may inhibit structural changes in the left ventricle independent of pressure reduction.

Aggressive control of blood pressure is the most effective approach to reduce the incidence of heart failure in a hypertensive population.[39] A number of clinical trials have demonstrated the benefit of treating hypertension in the prevention of heart failure (see also Chapter 28).[40-44] Primary prevention trials have demonstrated up to a 50% reduction in the incidence of heart failure in patients with hypertension who are treated with blood pressure–lowering agents.[45,46] The Hypertension in the Very Elderly trial achieved a 64% relative risk reduction in heart failure with the diuretic indapamide, with or without the angiotensin-converting enzyme (ACE) inhibitor perindopril (Figure 41-8).[47]

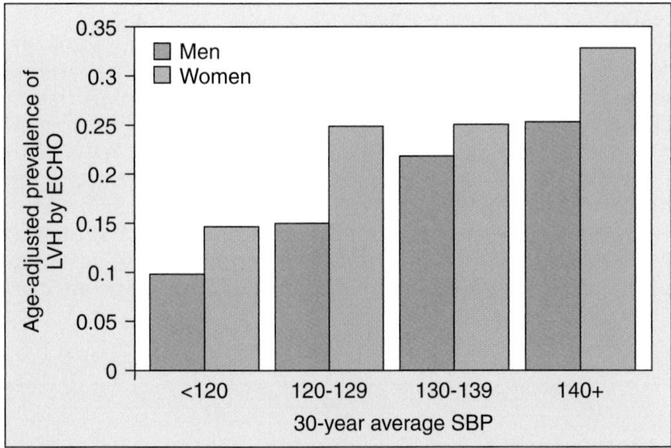

FIGURE 41–6 Prevalence of left ventricular hypertrophy (LVH), demonstrated by echocardiography (ECHO), as a function of 30-year average systolic blood pressure (SBP). (From Lauer MS, Anderson KM, Levy D. Influence of contemporary versus 30-year blood pressure levels on left ventricular mass and geometry: the Framingham Heart Study. *J Am Coll Cardiol* 1991;18:1287-1294.)

Inhibition of the renin-angiotensin system with ACE inhibitors or angiotensin receptor blockers (ARBs) appears to exert a greater benefit on left ventricular hypertrophy and remodeling than would be predicted from their pressure-lowering effect. Their effectiveness in reducing morbid events in nonhypertensive patients with atherosclerotic disease may involve pressure-independent as well as pressure-dependent mechanisms.[48,49]

β-Blockers are also effective in preventing heart failure in hypertensive patients, partly through pressure reduction and partly through inhibition of structural remodeling of the left ventricle. Diuretic therapy also is effective in preventing heart failure, not only through blood pressure reduction but also by intravascular volume contraction, which reduces the risk of congestion. Diuretics are not known to affect remodeling directly. Calcium channel antagonists, especially amlodipine, contribute to prevention of heart failure by their powerful vascular effects that reduce blood pressure and diminish reflected waves. These drugs probably do not directly inhibit left ventricular remodeling. The failure of α-blockers to prevent heart failure or to slow its progression is consistent with the lack of effectiveness of these drugs in inhibiting structural cardiac remodeling.

Diabetes Mellitus and Heart Failure (see Chapter 26)

The number of patients with diabetes mellitus continues to rise in industrial societies, mainly because of changes in lifestyle (excessive calorie and fat intake and decreased physical activity). Among Americans 20 years of age or older, 9.6% have diabetes, and among those 60 years of age or older, 21% have diabetes mellitus.[1] Since 1990, the prevalence of patients with a diagnosis of diabetes increased 61%.[50] Data from the Framingham Heart Study indicate a doubling in the incidence of diabetes since 1980, most dramatically during the 1990s. Most of the increase in absolute incidence of diabetes occurred in individuals with a body mass index (BMI) of 30 kg/m^2 or higher.[51] Researchers at the Mayo Clinic found that the prevalence of diabetes increased 3.8% per year since 1990. Among patients in whom heart failure was first diagnosed in 1999, the odds of having diabetes were nearly four times higher than for those with heart failure diagnosed 20 years earlier.[52] Worldwide, the prevalence of diabetes for all age groups was estimated to be 2.8% in 2000 and is projected to be 4.4% in 2030.[53] The total number of people with diabetes mellitus is projected to rise from 171 million in 2000 to 366 million in 2030.[53] In developing nations, the prevalence of diabetes is expected to increase between 2000 and 2010; rates in African and Asian countries are projected to rise by two to three times their current levels.[54,55]

Diabetes and insulin resistance are important risk factors for the development of heart failure.[56] The presence of

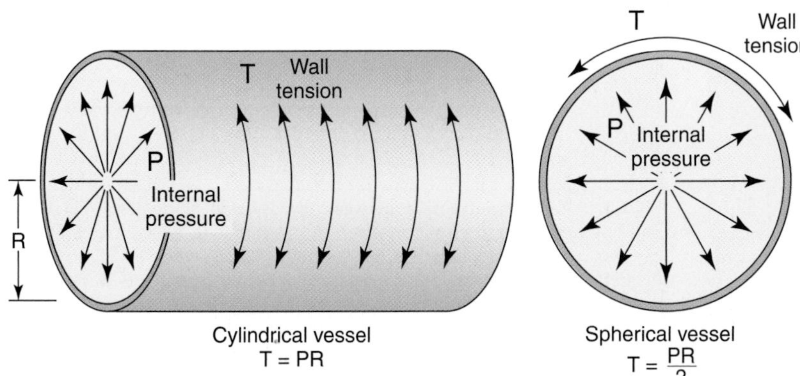

FIGURE 41–7 LaPlace's law. The larger the vessel radius (R) is, the higher the wall tension (T) must be to withstand a given internal fluid pressure (P). For a given vessel radius and internal pressure, a spherical vessel has half the wall tension of a cylindrical vessel.

clinical diabetes mellitus markedly increases the likelihood of heart failure in patients without structural heart disease[57] and adversely affects the outcomes of patients with established heart failure.[58,59] In a study of patients with type 2 diabetes mellitus, older than 50 years, and whose urinary albumin was greater than 20 mg/L, 4% of patients developed heart failure over the study period, of whom 36% died.[60] The Framingham Heart Study showed that the prevalence of heart failure was twice as high among diabetic men and five times as high among diabetic women aged between 45 and 74 years as in age-matched nondiabetic controls.[61] After the age of 65 years, the association became even stronger, with a fourfold higher prevalence in diabetic men and an eightfold higher prevalence in diabetic women.[61] A study of the predictors of heart failure among women with coronary disease revealed that diabetes was the strongest risk factor.[62] Diabetic women with elevated BMI or depressed creatinine clearance were at highest risk. Diabetic patients with fasting blood glucose levels higher than 300 mg/dL had an adjusted risk of developing heart failure three times higher than that of diabetic patients with controlled fasting blood glucose levels.[62]

The occurrence of heart failure represents a major and adverse prognostic turn in a diabetic patient's life. Heart failure is the most common admission diagnosis for diabetic patients, and more than one third of patients with type 2 diabetes die of heart failure.[61,63-65] Of patients requiring hospitalization for heart failure in the United States, 44% have diabetes; this percentage seems to be increasing with time.[66] In a community-based cohort of 665 subjects with heart failure in Olmsted County, Minnesota, the 5-year survival rate was 46% among patients with heart failure alone but only 37% among those with heart failure and diabetes mellitus.[52]

The basic reason for the increased prevalence of heart failure among diabetic patients is the presence of a distinct diabetic cardiomyopathy that is structurally characterized by cardiomyocyte hypertrophy, microangiopathy, endothelial dysfunction, and myocardial fibrosis.[18,67] At the cellular level, diabetic cardiomyopathy is associated with defects in subcellular organelles and downregulation of catecholamine receptors as a result of chronically elevated catecholamine levels.[68,69] Also, in animal models with the onset of hyperglycemia, changes in myocardial calcium transportation and alterations in contractile proteins occur, both of which lead to systolic and diastolic dysfunction that worsens as the collagen content of the myocardium increases.[68,70,71] Doppler imaging studies have been used to provide load-independent assessments of cardiac relaxation. These studies not only have confirmed evidence of diastolic dysfunction in asymptomatic patients with diabetes but also have demonstrated a direct relationship between the extent of diastolic dysfunction and glycemic control (Figure 41-9).[72] Although diastolic dysfunction is the hallmark of diabetic cardiomyopathy, concomitant subtle systolic dysfunction is present even at earlier stages of the disease.[63]

Although neither the Diabetes Control and Complications Trial in type 1 diabetes nor the U.K. Prospective Database Study (UKPDS) in type 2 diabetes showed a reduction in cardiovascular events with intensive glycemic control,[73,74] a prospective, observational component of UKPDS revealed a continuous relationship between glycemic exposure and the development of heart failure with no threshold of risk, so that for each 1% absolute reduction in glycosylated hemoglobin (HbA_{1c}), there was an associated 16% decrease in hospitalization for heart failure (Figure 41-10).[75] Similar findings were also reported in a large cohort study in the United States.[76] Another study revealed that fasting glucose levels are predictive of hospitalizations for congestive heart failure, with a 10% increase in the risk of heart failure–related hospitalization for each 18-mg/dL (1-mmol) increase in fasting glucose level.[77]

Attaining optimal glycemic control should be a goal in both the prevention and treatment of heart failure in patients with diabetes. The Action to Control Cardiovascular Risk in Diabetes (ACCORD) study indicated a previously unrecognized harm of intensive glucose lowering in patients with type 2 diabetes at high risk[78]; however, these results were not confirmed in the Action in Diabetes and Vascular disease: PreterAx and DiamicroN-MR Controlled Evaluation (ADVANCE) trial[79] and should not necessarily be interpreted as diminishing the importance of glycemic control.[80]

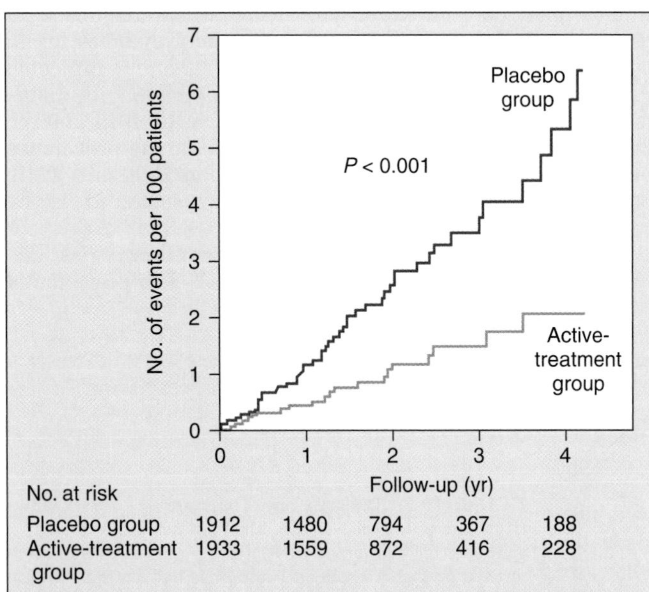

FIGURE 41-8 Kaplan-Meier estimates of the rate of heart failure according to study group in the Hypertension in the Very Elderly trial. For subjects receiving active treatment, in comparison with those receiving placebo, the unadjusted hazard ratio was 0.36 (95% confidence interval, 0.22 to 0.58). (From Beckett NS, Peters R, Fletcher AE, et al. Treatment of hypertension in patients 80 years of age or older. *N Engl J Med* 2008;358:1887-1898.

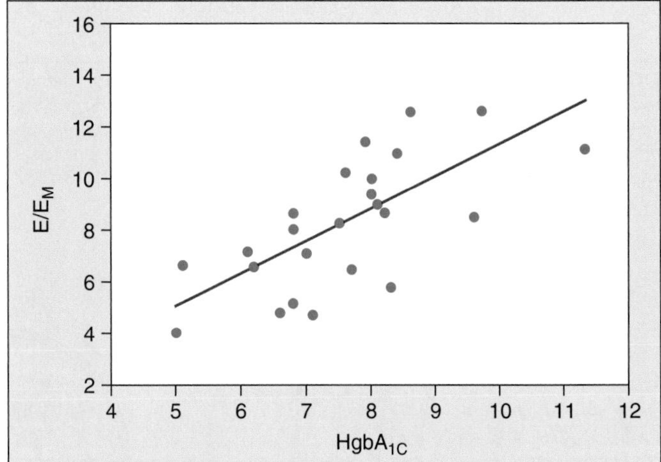

FIGURE 41-9 Relationship between glycosylated hemoglobin ($HgbA_{1c}$) and left ventricular diastolic function in patients with type 1 diabetes and without overt heart failure (r = .68, P <.0002). E/E_M = relation of peak early diastolic transmitral flow (E) to myocardial relaxation velocity during early diastole (E_M). (From Shishehbor MH, Hoogwerf BJ, Schoenhagen P, et al. Relation of hemoglobin A_{1c} to left ventricular relaxation in patients with type 1 diabetes mellitus and without overt heart disease. *Am J Cardiol* 2003;91:1514-1517, 1519.)

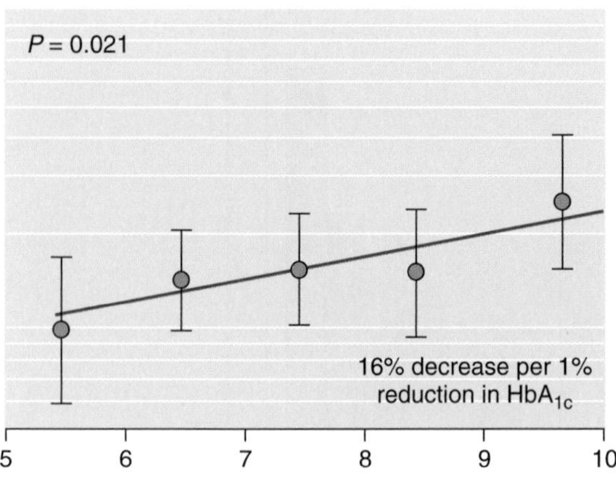

FIGURE 41–10 Relative risk of heart failure in relation to glycosylated hemoglobin ($HgbA_{1c}$) in the U.K. Prospective Diabetes Study. (From Stratton IM, Adler AI, Neil HA, et al. Association of glycaemia with macrovascular and microvascular complications of type 2 diabetes (UKPDS 35): prospective observational study. *BMJ* 2000;321:405-412.)

The choice of oral hypoglycemic agent that may be used is restricted. For instance, metformin is contraindicated in the presence of either heart failure or renal impairment, and precautions also apply to the use of the thiazolidinediones.[81,82] In addition to treating hyperglycemia, it is crucial to control all other cardiovascular and metabolic risks and to prevent complications in patients with diabetes. ACE inhibitors or ARBs can prevent the development of end-organ disease and the occurrence of clinical events in diabetic patients, even in those who do not have hypertension.[48,83] Long-term treatment with several ACE inhibitors or ARBs has been shown to decrease the risk of renal disease in diabetic patients,[84,85] and prolonged therapy with the ACE inhibitor ramipril has been shown to lower the likelihood of heart failure, myocardial infarction, and cardiovascular death.[48] Likewise, the use of ARBs in patients with diabetes mellitus and hypertension or left ventricular hypertrophy has been shown to reduce the incidence of first hospitalization for heart failure, in addition to having other beneficial effects on renal function.[86-88]

Atherosclerotic Disease and Heart Failure (see Chapter 23)

Patients with known atherosclerotic disease (e.g., of the coronary, cerebral, or peripheral blood vessels) are at increased risk of developing heart failure. The role of coronary artery disease and myocardial infarction as a major antecedent of heart failure has been well established.[89,90] Both in Europe and in the United States, coronary artery disease has been reported to be the most common cause of heart failure.[91,92] Autopsy series indicate that 33% of patients with heart failure have prevalent but undetected major coronary artery disease.[93] Even in patients with heart failure classified clinically as "nonischemic cardiomyopathy," up to 25% may have evidence of coronary artery disease at autopsy.[94] Indeed, patients with "nonischemic cardiomyopathy" may develop clinical ischemic events, which suggests that coronary artery disease may not be just an "innocent bystander" in these patients.[95] The presence of underlying coronary artery disease contributes to the morbidity and mortality of patients with heart failure.[96] In addition to epicardial disease, microvascular coronary disease is also both widespread and often underrecognized.[97] Clinically silent coronary atherosclerosis is highly prevalent in the general population, including children and young adults.[98,99] These data suggest that coronary atherosclerotic disease (epicardial or microvascular, clinically overt or silent) can lead to acute or chronic ischemia, thereby predisposing to left ventricular dysfunction and symptomatic heart failure. According to the 2008 update of heart disease and stroke statistics,[1] the proportions of persons with a first myocardial infarction who develop heart failure in 5 years are 7% of men and 12% of women at 40 to 69 years of age and 22% of men and 25% of women at 70 years of age or older.

The risk of coronary artery disease and myocardial infarction can be reduced by modification of classic risk factors (e.g., controlling hypertension).[45,46] The risk factors can be modified favorably through lifestyle changes, including reduction of weight and cessation of tobacco use. Several large trials of patients with myocardial infarction have shown a reduction in the incidence of heart failure with several treatment strategies.[100-104] ACE inhibitors reduce incidence of heart failure by 23% among patients who have coronary artery disease and normal systolic function and by 37% among patients who have reduced left ventricular systolic function.[45] In one large-scale trial, long-term treatment with an ACE inhibitor decreased the risk of the primary endpoint of cardiovascular death, myocardial infarction, and stroke among patients with high-risk established vascular disease who had no evidence of heart failure or of reduced left ventricular ejection fraction at the time of randomization, but the incidence of new heart failure was not a primary or secondary endpoint.[48] Among patients with stable coronary artery disease and no heart failure, another ACE inhibitor significantly reduced the incidence of death, myocardial infarction, or cardiac arrest.[105] A more recent large trial of ACE inhibition versus placebo failed to show a reduction in the primary composite endpoint, although a post hoc analysis did show some reduction in hospitalization for heart failure.[106]

Observational studies and small clinical investigations have suggested that hydroxymethylglutaryl–coenzyme A reductase inhibitors (statins) may be beneficial in patients with ischemic and nonischemic heart failure.[107-110] The first prospective randomized clinical outcome trial with statins that focused specifically on heart failure, Controlled Rosuvastatin in Multinational Trial in Heart Failure (CORONA), demonstrated no significant differences in the primary composite endpoint of death from cardiovascular causes, nonfatal myocardial infarction, or nonfatal stroke.[111] The role of statins in heart failure thus remains uncertain, and additional trials may be needed to resolve this uncertainty.

Metabolic Syndrome and Heart Failure (see Chapter 20)

The term "metabolic syndrome" refers to a cluster of risk factors for cardiovascular disease and type 2 diabetes mellitus. According to the National Cholesterol Education Program Adult Treatment Panel III, metabolic syndrome is diagnosed when three or more of the following five risk factors are present[112]: (1) fasting plasma glucose of 100 mg/dL or higher; (2) high-density lipoprotein (HDL) cholesterol level lower than 40 mg/dL in men or lower than 50 mg/dL in women; (3) triglyceride levels of 150 mg/dL or higher; (4) waist circumference of 102 cm or more in men or 88 cm or more in women; and (5) systolic blood pressure of 130 mm Hg or higher or diastolic blood pressure of 85 mm Hg or higher, or the presence of drug treatment for hypertension. The prevalence of metabolic syndrome reaches epidemic levels and ranges from 6.7% among people 20 to 29 years of age to 43.5% for people 60 to 69 years of age and 42.0% for those 70 years of age or older.[113,114] The age-adjusted prevalence of metabolic syndrome is similar for men (24.0%) and women (23.4%).[113]

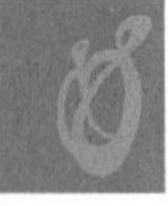

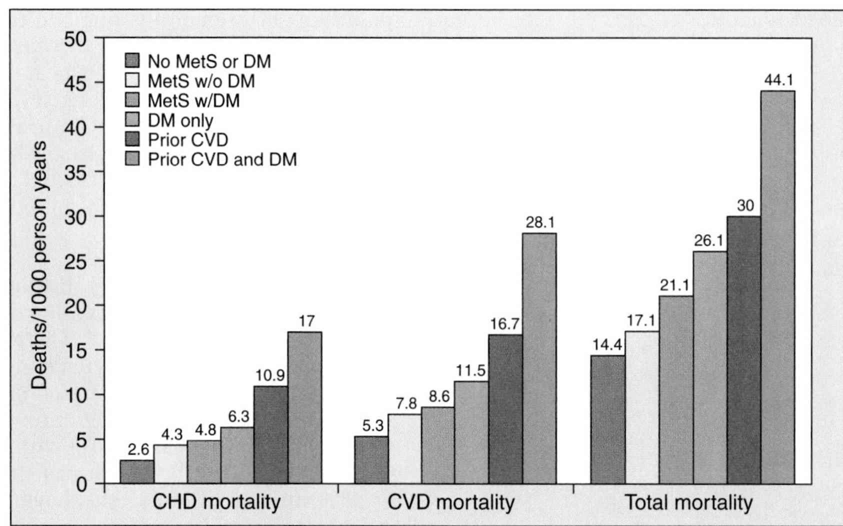

FIGURE 41–11 Mortality rates among adults in the United States, 30 to 75 years of age, with metabolic syndrome (MetS), with and without diabetes mellitus (DM) and preexisting cardiovascular disease (CVD). CHD, coronary heart disease; w/, with; w/o, without. (From Malik S, Wong ND, Franklin SS, et al. Impact of the metabolic syndrome on mortality from coronary heart disease, cardiovascular disease, and all causes in United States adults. *Circulation* 2004;110:1245-1250.)

Although the designation of metabolic syndrome as a unique pathophysiological condition and as a predictor of disease has been questioned,[115] most clinicians and researchers have long maintained that certain metabolic risk factors are prone to occur in clusters and that this clustering increases the risk of diabetes,[116] heart failure,[117] and overall cardiovascular morbidity and mortality.[118] According to the National Health and Nutrition Examination Survey (NHANES) data, people who did not have metabolic syndrome had the lowest risk for cardiovascular events, those with metabolic syndrome had an intermediate level of risk, and those with diabetes mellitus had the highest risk (Figure 41-11).[119]

Mechanisms underlying elevated cardiovascular risk associated with metabolic syndrome appear to involve subclinical organ damage.[120] Among patients with hypertension but without diabetes, those with metabolic syndrome seem more likely to have microalbuminuria, left ventricular hypertrophy, and increased carotid intima thickness than did those without metabolic syndrome.[120] In addition, the greater the number of metabolic syndrome components present, the more severe were the microalbuminuria and left ventricular hypertrophy.[120] Alterations in metabolic pathways, inflammatory reactions, and other cellular processes may increase the risk of atherosclerosis in the insulin-resistant state. For example, there is growing evidence for cellular interactions between signaling pathways involved in actions of insulin and the renin-angiotensin system.[121,122] Nuclear peroxisome proliferator-activated receptors (PPARs) also appear to play a role in the atherogenic mechanisms underlying metabolic syndrome. The PPARs regulate the expression of a variety of genes, and they modulate lipid metabolism, glycemic control, and vascular inflammation and tone.[123] Modulation of PPAR-related actions by cardiovascular risk factors, such as obesity and overweight, can lead to promotion of atherosclerotic disease.[123]

Treatment of metabolic syndrome consists of aggressive management of each of its individual components, including impaired fasting glucose concentration, dyslipidemia, and hypertension. The Diabetes Prevention Program Research Group evaluated the benefits of lifestyle intervention (weight loss and increased physical activity) in comparison with the antihyperglycemic agent metformin for prevention of diabetes in persons with elevated fasting and postload glucose concentrations.[124] Both treatments decreased the incidence of new-onset diabetes, but lifestyle intervention led to a 39% lower incidence of diabetes than did metformin treatment ($P < .001$).[124] Despite public education programs urging adults and children to modify lifestyles by including healthy food choices and more physical activity, most Americans do not follow recommended dietary or exercise guidelines for maintaining health.[125] An analysis of data from more than 153,000 U.S. adults included in the Behavioral Risk Factor Surveillance System revealed that only 3% of adults followed a healthy lifestyle.[125] Moreover, almost 10% followed no weight, dietary, or smoking recommendations.[125]

Drugs targeting PPAR-α (e.g., fenofibrate and gemfibrozil) are used in the treatment of metabolic syndrome. Fibrates decrease triglyceride level, increase HDL cholesterol, and may have some anti-inflammatory effects; however, their effect on cardiovascular disease outcomes continues to be evaluated.[126] Among patients with impaired glucose tolerance and cardiovascular disease or risk factors, the use of the angiotensin-receptor blocker valsartan along with lifestyle modification led to a relative reduction of 14% in the incidence of diabetes but did not reduce the rate of cardiovascular events.[127] A number of other trials are currently in progress to determine the most effective intervention for patients with the metabolic syndrome.[128]

Obesity and Heart Failure (see Chapter 20)

Obesity continues to be a leading public health concern in the United States.[129,130] The trend toward increasing obesity in this country is alarming.[131] Between 1980 and 2002, the prevalence of obesity doubled among adults aged 20 years or older, and the prevalence of overweight tripled in children and adolescents aged 6 to 19 years.[132,133] The age-adjusted prevalence of overweight and obesity (BMI ≥ 25 kg/m^2) increased from 64.5% in the period 1999 to 2000 to 66.3% in the period 2003 to 2004. The prevalence of obesity (BMI $\geq$ 30 kg/m^2) increased during this period from 30.5% to 32.2%. Extreme obesity (BMI ≥ 40.0 kg/m^2) increased from 4.7% to 4.8%.[133] The World Health Organization estimates that by 2015, the number of overweight people globally will increase to 2.3 billion, and more than 700 million will be obese.[1] Once considered problems only in high-income countries, overweight and obesity are now dramatically on the rise in low- and middle-income countries, particularly in urban settings.[1]

In several studies, BMI has been evaluated as a risk factor for left ventricular remodeling and overt heart failure. In these investigations, obesity has been associated consistently with left ventricular hypertrophy and dilation,[134-137] which are known precursors of heart failure.[138,139] In the Framingham Heart Study population, overweight and lesser degrees of obesity were associated with an increased risk of heart failure (Figure 41-12).[140] Extreme obesity has also been associated with heart failure.[141] Excess body weight is a strong predictor of mortality[142-144] and is associated with a significant increase in the risk of stroke.[145] Some investigators claim, and rightly so, that if the prevalence of obesity remains unchecked in the United States, the favorable trends in cardiovascular disease morbidity and mortality will probably be reversed.[146]

There are several plausible mechanisms for the association between obesity and heart failure. Increased BMI is a risk factor for hypertension,[147] diabetes mellitus,[147,148] and dyslipidemia,[131] all of which augment the risk of myocardial infarction,[149,150] an important antecedent of heart failure.[29,57,151,152] In addition, hypertension and diabetes mellitus independently increase the risk of heart failure.[28,29,57,151,152] Elevated BMI is associated with altered left ventricular remodeling,[134-138] possibly as a result of increased hemodynamic load,[153,154] neurohormonal activation,[155] and increased oxidative stress.[155,156] Adipose tissue acts as an endocrine organ, secreting hormones and other substances that create a proinflammatory state and promote formation of atherosclerotic plaques.[157] Recently, Zhou and colleagues[158] raised the possibility of a direct effect of obesity on the myocardium by demonstrating cardiac steatosis and lipoapoptosis in an animal model of obesity.

Efforts to promote optimal body weight are likely to have an effect on a number of manifestations of cardiovascular disease, including heart failure. A number of strategies have been used to treat obesity, including diet, exercise, behavior therapy, medications, and surgery. To select among these treatments, clinicians must evaluate the obesity-related risks to the individual patient and balance those risks against any

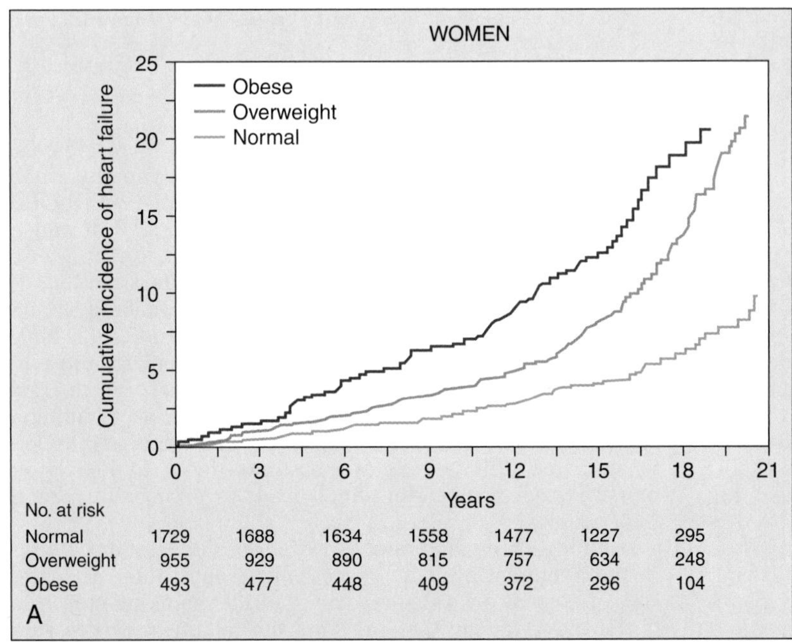

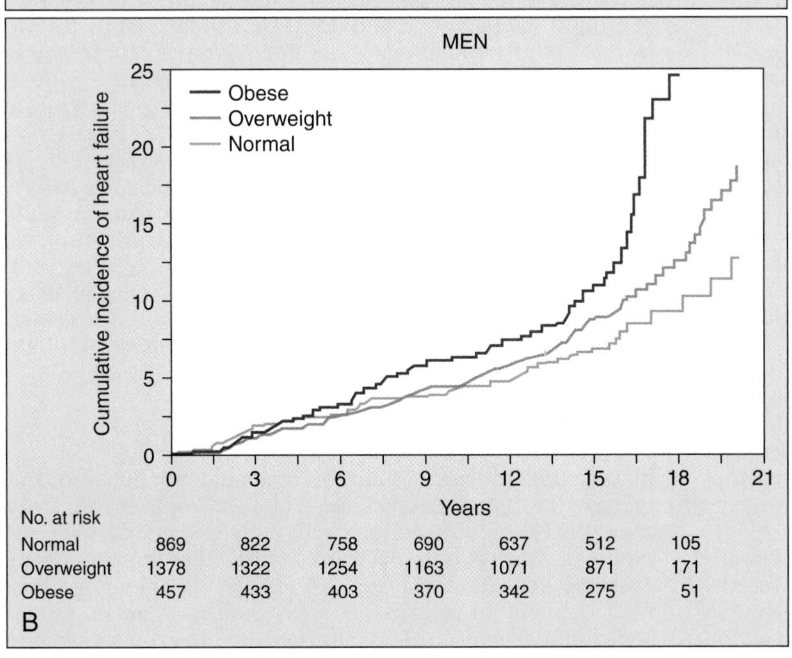

FIGURE 41–12 Cumulative incidence of heart failure according to category of body mass index at the baseline examination. The body mass index was 18.5 to 24.9 in normal subjects, 25.0 to 29.9 in overweight subjects, and 30.0 or more in obese subjects. (From Kenchaiah S, Evans JC, Levy D, et al. Obesity and the risk of heart failure. *N Engl J Med* 2002;347:305-313.)

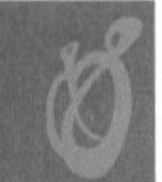

possible problems with the treatment. Because all medications inherently carry more risks than do diet and exercise, medications should be chosen only for people in whom the benefit justifies the risk.[159] This process of evaluation is particularly important because drug treatment for obesity has been tarnished by a number of problems over the years. Since the introduction of thyroid hormone to treat obesity in 1893, almost every drug that has been tried in obese patients has caused such undesirable outcomes that it had to be terminated. Thus, any new drug for the treatment of obesity must be used cautiously unless the safety profile would make it acceptable for almost everyone. If an individual is to lose weight, he or she must enter a state of negative energy balance, in which the energy taken in as food is less on average than the energy needed for daily activities. Comparatively few drugs are currently available for the treatment of overweight patients.[159-162] Medications for promoting weight loss are indicated primarily as an adjunct in patients who are unresponsive to nonpharmacological methods and who are at substantial medical risk because of their obesity.[163] Gastric bypass surgery is an option in cases of obesity that is highly refractory to therapeutic intervention and in which BMIs are above 40 kg/m^2. One study attested to the benefits of bypass in selected patients, demonstrating a significant reduction in cardiovascular, cancer, diabetes, and all causes of death.[164]

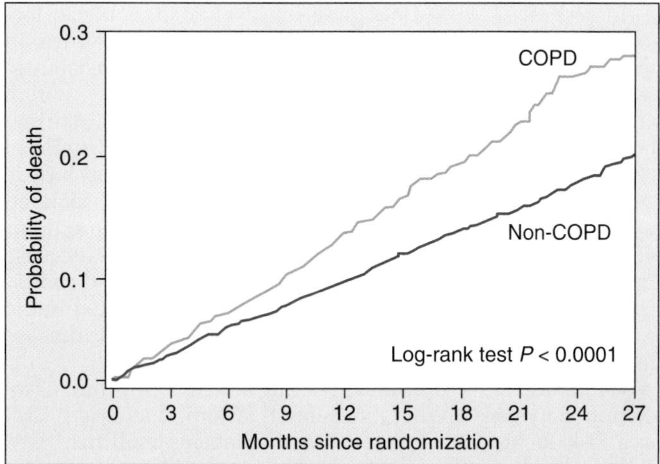

FIGURE 41–13 Kaplan-Meier curves of death among the 5010 patients enrolled in the Valsartan Heart Failure Trial according to the presence or absence of chronic obstructive pulmonary disease (COPD). (From Staszewsky L, Wong M, Masson S, et al. Clinical, neurohormonal, and inflammatory markers and overall prognostic role of chronic obstructive pulmonary disease in patients with heart failure: data from the Val-HeFT heart failure trial. *J Card Fail* 2007;13:797-804.)

Chronic Obstructive Pulmonary Disease and Heart Failure

Although precise statistics on the prevalence of COPD are surprisingly scanty, it is estimated that approximately 14 million people in the United States have this condition.[165] COPD is now the fourth leading cause of death in the United States, and it is the only common cause of death whose incidence is increasing.[165] The importance of COPD as a cause of death is probably underestimated, inasmuch as COPD is probably a contributor to other common causes of death. The prevalence of and rates of mortality from COPD are also increasing.[166] The World Health Organization predicts that by 2020, COPD will be the fifth most prevalent disease worldwide and the third most common cause of death.[167] Reasons for the dramatic increase in COPD include reductions in mortality from other causes, such as cardiovascular diseases in industrialized countries and infectious diseases in developing countries, along with a marked increase in cigarette smoking and environmental pollution in developing countries.[165]

The risk ratio of developing heart failure in patients with COPD is 4.5, in comparison with age-matched controls without COPD, after adjustments for cardiovascular risk factors.[168] Among the comorbid conditions commonly associated with heart failure, COPD is the one that most delays the diagnosis of heart failure and is most often blamed for nonadherence to therapeutic guidelines, especially β-blockade.[169] The rate-adjusted hospital prevalence of heart failure is three times greater among patients discharged with a diagnosis of COPD than among patients discharged without mention of COPD.[170] The Kaiser Permanente Medical Program reported that the age-adjusted relative rate of hospitalization for heart failure was 5.55 and the odds ratio of heart failure as a comorbid condition was 8.48 in COPD patients, in comparison with persons without COPD.[171] The prevalence of COPD ranges from 20% to 32% among patients with heart failure.[172-176] Patients with heart failure and concomitant COPD have more symptoms and worse outcomes that are not explained by poorer left ventricular function (Figure 41-13).[177]

The relationship between COPD and heart failure remains to be elucidated. A working hypothesis to account for the high prevalence of left ventricular systolic dysfunction in patients with COPD is that low-grade systemic inflammation in COPD accelerates progression of coronary atherosclerosis, which ultimately results in ischemic cardiomyopathy. Such a hypothesis is based on the fact that patients with COPD have higher elevation of inflammatory markers,[177,178] and it fits the clinical observation of a higher incidence of troponin elevation[177] and left ventricular wall motion abnormalities[179] noted in patients with COPD and left ventricular dysfunction. Patients with heart failure and concomitant COPD have higher activation of neurohormones, particularly norepinephrine and plasma renin.[177] COPD may also lead to right ventricular failure from pulmonary hypertension, a common complication of COPD.[180] The cause of pulmonary hypertension in COPD is generally assumed to be hypoxic pulmonary vasoconstriction, which leads to permanent medial hypertrophy.[180]

Although bronchodilators, corticosteroids, and antibiotics in the treatment of acute exacerbations constitute the mainstay of current drug therapy for COPD,[165] smoking cessation is the only strategy that prevents the relentless progression of airflow obstruction[181] and improves the long-term survival in the COPD population.[182] Long-term oxygen therapy was also shown to reduce mortality and improve quality of life in patients with severe COPD and chronic hypoxemia (partial pressure of arterial oxygen <55 mm Hg).[183] The presence of COPD affects the treatment of heart failure, inasmuch as COPD is still viewed as a contraindication to β-blockade. Therefore, patients with heart failure caused by left ventricular systolic dysfunction who also have COPD are often deprived of the most beneficial pharmacological intervention. A large body of data indicates that patients with COPD may tolerate selective β-blockade, and these medications should not necessarily be denied to patients with heart failure and concomitant COPD.[173]

Rheumatoid Arthritis and Heart Failure

Rheumatoid arthritis is a chronic systemic inflammatory and progressive disease characterized by persistent inflammatory synovitis, joint destruction, and increased mortality.[184,185] Cardiovascular disease has been identified as the underlying cause of a substantial proportion of deaths among patients with rheumatoid arthritis.[186] Heart failure is an important contributory cause of cardiovascular disease–associated death in patients with rheumatoid arthritis.[187] This excess mortality results primarily from the increased incidence of heart failure among patients with rheumatoid arthritis in comparison with subjects without rheumatoid arthritis.[187] Nicola and associates[188] studied 575 patients with no history of heart failure at the time rheumatoid arthritis was diagnosed and 583 controls with no rheumatoid arthritis; the relative risk of new-onset heart failure during the subsequent 30 years was 1.9-fold higher among the patients with rheumatoid arthritis after adjustment for age, gender, standard cardiovascular risk factors, and the presence of ischemic heart disease.

The most plausible explanation for the increased risk of heart failure in rheumatoid arthritis is the persistent inflammatory state that characterizes the rheumatic state.[189,190] A distinguishing feature of heart failure in rheumatoid arthritis is that it is far more likely to involve diastolic dysfunction than systolic function.[188] Patients with rheumatoid arthritis have a significantly higher risk of coronary artery disease than do subjects without rheumatoid arthritis.[191] Coronary artery disease in patients with rheumatoid arthritis is characterized by less extensive atherosclerotic plaque and greater evidence of inflammation and plaque instability than in subjects without rheumatoid arthritis.[189] Patients with rheumatoid arthritis are less likely than patients without this condition to report symptoms of angina and more likely to experience unrecognized myocardial infarction and sudden cardiac death.[191]

The issues related to inhibition of tumor necrosis factor α (TNF-α) are particularly complex. TNF-α, an inflammatory cytokine released by activated monocytes, macrophages, and T lymphocytes, promotes inflammatory responses that are central to the pathogenesis and progression of rheumatoid arthritis.[192] TNF-α is also known to mediate cardiac injury through a variety of biological mechanisms, thus contributing to the progression of heart failure.[193] These observations led to several large randomized controlled trials designed to assess the efficacy of TNF-α inhibitor therapy in the treatment of heart failure. Unfortunately, these efforts were unsuccessful; the trials were stopped prematurely because of lack of efficacy and a suggestion of worsening heart failure in the patients treated with TNF-α inhibitor.[194,195] These data suggested that TNF-α inhibitors may promote or worsen heart failure in patients with rheumatoid arthritis. However, high disease activity and systemic inflammation (typically associated with high levels of circulating cytokines) have consistently been shown to increase cardiovascular risk in rheumatoid arthritis[186,196,197]; therefore, inhibition of TNF-α should reduce heart failure risk in patients with rheumatoid arthritis. Therein lies the dilemma: it is biologically plausible that by dramatically reducing systemic inflammation, treatment with TNF-α inhibitors would result in an overall reduction of heart failure risk; however, it is also possible that these agents increase heart failure risk in persons with rheumatoid arthritis, as they have been suggested to do in the general population.[193] Listing and colleagues, addressing this question,[198] found that TNF-α inhibitor treatment that effectively reduces the inflammatory activity of rheumatoid arthritis is more likely to be beneficial than harmful with regard to the risk of heart failure, especially if patients receive no concomitant therapy with glucocorticoids or cyclooxygenase-2 (COX-2) inhibitors. Furthermore, their data suggested that TNF-α inhibition does not increase the risk of worsening of prevalent heart failure.[198] Unfortunately, although this study offered some useful insights, the results fell short of providing clinically useful guidance and left many questions unanswered.[199] Thus, although TNF-α inhibitors represent a major advance in the treatment of rheumatic disease, their effects on heart failure in rheumatoid arthritis are unknown.

BOX 41–1 Drugs Associated with Left Ventricular Systolic Dysfunction or Worsening Heart Failure

Drugs Causing Left Ventricular Systolic Dysfunction
Cytotoxic agents
- Anthracycline
- Trastuzumab

Antipsychotics
- Clozapine
- Atypical antipsychotic agents

Carbamazepine
Tricyclic antidepressants
Chloroquine
Hydroxychloroquine
Interferon-α
Interleukin-2
TNF-α antagonists

Drugs Exacerbating Heart Failure
NSAIDs
COX-2 inhibitors
Corticosteroids
Thiazolidinediones
Calcium channel antagonists
- Non-dihydropyridine agents

β-Adrenoreceptor antagonists

Unproven Associations
Doxazosin
β_2-Adrenoreceptor agonists

COX-2, cyclooxygenase-2; NSAIDs, nonsteroidal anti-inflammatory drugs; TNF-α, tumor necrosis factor α.
From Murphy CA, Dargie HJ. Drug-induced cardiovascular disorders. *Drug Saf* 2007;30:783-804.

Drug-induced Heart Failure

Although heart failure is caused predominantly by cardiovascular conditions such as hypertension, coronary heart disease, and valvular heart disease, it can also be an adverse reaction induced by drug therapy (Box 41-1). Many therapeutic and recreational agents can exert important cardiotoxic effects that lead to left ventricular systolic dysfunction or overt heart failure. Two drug groups are of particular concern: cytotoxic drugs and nonsteroidal anti-inflammatory drugs (NSAIDs). Some drugs may predispose to heart failure by causing hypertension and other cardiovascular risk factors (Box 41-2). In addition, some drugs have the propensity to adversely affect hemodynamic mechanisms in patients with an already existing heart condition. Drugs may cause heart failure by various mechanisms, including direct myocyte injury, alteration of biochemical processes, or stimulation of allergic reactions. The outcome can vary in severity from benign to fatal. Because numerous drugs in various drug classes may precipitate or worsen heart failure, a detailed history of drug exposure in patients with signs or symptoms of heart failure is mandatory.

Cytotoxic Drugs (see Chapter 58)

The introduction of doxorubicin in the mid-1900s improved cancer therapy immeasurably. However, it soon became apparent that doxorubicin was associated with significant cardiotoxicity, and this has proved a consistent problem with all subsequent anthracycline preparations. Although rapid-onset left ventricular systolic dysfunction has been reported to follow anthracycline administration,[200] these drugs are

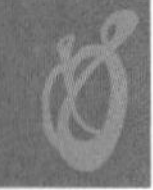

BOX 41–2 Drugs Associated with Cardiovascular Risk Factors

Drug	Effect
Corticosteroids	Hypertension, dyslipidemia, diabetes mellitus)
Ciclosporin and tacrolimus	Hypertension, dyslipidemia
NSAIDs and COX-2 inhibitors	Hypertension (minimal)
Erythropoietin	Hypertension
Combined oral contraceptives	Hypertension
Venlafaxine	Hypertension
HAART	Hypertension, dyslipidemia

COX-2, cyclooxygenase-2; *HAART,* highly active antiretroviral therapy; *NSAIDs,* nonsteroidal anti-inflammatory drugs. (Modified from Murphy CA, Dargie HJ. Drug-induced cardiovascular disorders. *Drug Saf* 2007;30:783-804.)

usually associated with the development of chronic cardiomyopathy many years after their use.

The mechanism of doxorubicin-induced cardiotoxicity involves increased oxidative and nitrosative stress,[201-204] matrix metalloproteinase activation,[205] and alteration of cardiac energetics,[206] which eventually lead to cell death by apoptosis or cell necrosis.[207-209] However, the exact mechanisms have not been fully established. Cardiotoxicity with doxorubicin is dose dependent. the risk is minimized by restricting the cumulative doxorubicin dosage to less than 400 mg/m^2. Dosages exceeding 550 mg/m^2 have significantly increased rates of cardiomyopathy: the incidence of heart failure has been reported as 18% at dosages between 551 and 600 mg/m^2, increasing further to 36% at higher doses.[210,211] The expression of COX-2 limits doxorubicin-induced injury in rat cardiomyocytes; this observation may suggest that concomitant use of NSAIDs could constitute a risk for the development of cardiac injury during anthracycline therapy.[212]

Largely because of the antineoplastic efficacy of anthracyclines, cardiotoxicity has not led to withdrawal of these agents from general use. Instead, attempts have been made to identify methods of reducing the cardiac risk. Optimal therapeutic approaches for cardioprotection with the use of anthracyclines remain undefined.[213] Minimizing anthracycline dosage is practiced, as is its co-administration with other cytotoxic drugs tailored to specific tumors.[214] A slower rate of drug infusion seems to result in reduced cardiotoxicity,[215] but the antitumor effect may be compromised. Concomitant administration of antioxidant agents such as dexrazoxane, coenzyme Q10 (ubidecarenone),[216] probucol,[207] and statins may be cardioprotective.[214] Results of one study suggested that CB_1 cannabinoid receptor antagonists may represent a new cardioprotective strategy against doxorubicin-induced cardiotoxicity.[217]

All patients exposed to anthracyclines should be considered at risk of cardiomyopathy, but older age, prior irradiation, concomitant administration of other chemotherapeutic agents, and underlying heart disease heighten this risk.[213,218,219] Cardiac biomarkers, such as troponins and natriuretic peptides, may facilitate risk stratification, but their role is not yet defined.[211] Although some reports of cardiomyopathy regression exist,[220] anthracycline-induced cardiomyopathy should be considered as an irreversible process. There is specific evidence of symptomatic benefit with β-blockers,[221,222] but management is similar to that for any cause of left ventricular systolic dysfunction.

Trastuzumab (see Chapter 58)

The human epidermal growth factor receptor 2 (HER-2) is a transmembrane tyrosine kinase receptor involved in growth regulation. HER-2 is overexpressed in approximately 20% of breast cancers, and its presence is associated with a poor prognosis. Trastuzumab is a humanized monoclonal antibody that targets the HER-2 receptor and has proven to be very effective in treating these tumors. Unfortunately, there is an independent risk of cardiomyopathy in association with trastuzumab.[223,224] The incidence of heart failure was shown to be 2.6% when trastuzumab was used as first-line monotherapy, rising to 8.5% in second- or third-line monotherapy, which included previous treatment with anthracyclines in a majority of patients.[224] In the protocol in which patients were randomly assigned to receive either trastuzumab or placebo in combination with paclitaxel or an anthracycline, the incidences of heart failure were 4.2% with paclitaxel alone, 8.8% with paclitaxel and trastuzumab, 9.6% with anthracycline alone, and 28.0% with anthracycline and trastuzumab.[224]

The mechanism underlying trastuzumab-induced cardiotoxicity is unknown but has been suggested to represent an exacerbation of anthracycline-induced cardiac effects.[224] Despite cardiotoxic effects, the beneficial therapeutic ratio for trastuzumab in treating HER-2–positive breast cancer is considered a strong rationale for the continuing use of HER-2 antibodies with other treatment modalities in breast cancer.[225] Encouragingly, there is evidence that trastuzumab-induced cardiomyopathy, unlike that induced by anthracyclines, may be reversible on drug cessation,[226,227] although this evidence remains unverified.

Nonsteroidal Anti-inflammatory Drugs

Renal perfusion is reduced in heart failure, and prostaglandins become increasingly important in controlling renal plasma flow and fluid homeostasis. NSAIDs, however, reduce prostaglandin synthesis, thus decreasing glomerular filtration and resulting in salt and water retention.[214,228] NSAIDs act by inhibiting both COX-1 and COX-2. It was long thought that the analgesic aspect was generated by COX-2 inhibition and that the adverse gastrointestinal effects were mediated by COX-1. This led to the development of selective COX-2 inhibitors, such as celecoxib and valdecoxib. COX-2 inhibitors still have some of the adverse effects observed with NSAIDs: namely, the ability to increase blood pressure and to exacerbate heart failure through salt and water retention.[214,228] Gastrointestinal complications are less common with COX-2 inhibitors,[229] and these drugs were initially thought to be successful. However, soon after their release on the market, it became evident that some COX-2 inhibitors increase the risk of myocardial infarction and stroke.[229-231] A comparison of celecoxib and placebo in adenoma prevention did reveal higher rates of a composite endpoint of myocardial infarction, stroke, and heart failure in patients treated with celecoxib.[232]

Through a number of mechanisms, COX-2 inhibition may increase the risk of cardiovascular events. COX-2 inhibitors can increase systemic blood pressure slightly[233] but may accelerate atherosclerosis through effects on mitochondrial oxidative phosphorylation or monocyte chemotaxis.[234] There is probably also a prothrombotic effect of COX-2 inhibition.[235] Thromboxane is a prothrombotic prostanoid that depends on COX-1 for its production, whereas the production of prostacyclin (epoprostenol), an antithrombotic agent, depends on COX-2. Preferential COX-2 inhibition leads to reduced levels of prostacyclin, with a lesser effect on thromboxane, thereby potentially leading to a prothrombotic state.

Thus, it appears that both NSAIDs and COX-2 inhibitors are associated with a higher risk of cardiovascular events, including heart failure, myocardial infarction, and stroke. Although some COX-2 inhibitors have been withdrawn from the market, NSAIDs have been available for many years, both by prescription and over the counter. A large number of patients depend on these analgesics to control pain; in the absence of alternative effective treatments, the removal of these drugs from circulation is not a feasible option. In clinical practice, physicians must be aware of the adverse effects of all the medicines they prescribe and, in investigating ill health, must always consider drugs as a cause, particularly when no alternative cause is apparent. On the other hand, a drug with a strong association with a particular cardiovascular adverse effect could be entirely blameless, and alternative causes should not be discounted.

Thiazolidinediones

The thiazolidinediones rosiglitazone and pioglitazone are oral hypoglycemic agents that have been shown to improve glycemic control and may act to slow the progression of β cell failure.[236] Although improved glycemic control has been linked to better clinical outcomes in diabetes[74,237,238] and thiazolidinediones have been suggested to have potential cardiovascular benefits,[239-242] concerns have arisen with regard to the adverse cardiac effects of these drugs. Use of thiazolidinediones is associated with weight gain and edema,[243] and there is evidence that both rosiglitazone and pioglitazone increase the risk of congestive heart failure.[239,241,244-246] In a population-based study of older patients with diabetes, thiazolidinedione treatment was associated with an increased risk of congestive heart failure, acute myocardial infarction, and mortality in comparison with other combinations of oral hypoglycemic agent treatments.[82] A box warning for congestive heart failure was added for these agents, recommending against the use of thiazolidinediones in persons with preexisting congestive heart failure.[247] Two meta-analyses have also suggested that rosiglitazone may be associated with an increased risk of acute myocardial infarction and death.[245,248]

Cardiotoxic Effects of Recreational Agents (see Also Chapter 24)

Many recreational agents can exert important cardiotoxic effects predisposing to heart failure. These include tobacco, as well as alcohol, cocaine, amphetamines, and other illicit drugs.[250] Patients should be strongly advised about the cardiovascular hazards of recreational agents.[117] Several epidemiological studies have revealed no correlation between the amount of alcohol ingested and the subsequent development of heart failure; nevertheless, it is strongly believed that any patient with a history of alcohol abuse or with current substantial routine alcohol consumption and new-onset heart failure without other obvious cause should be counseled to become abstinent.[117] Many heart failure programs limit alcoholic beverage consumption to no more than one alcoholic beverage serving daily for all patients with left ventricular dysfunction, regardless of cause.[251,252]

FUTURE DIRECTIONS

Thus far, research aimed at preventing heart failure in individuals at high risk has been modest in comparison with the extensive efforts at discovering new treatments for patients after heart failure has developed. Because preventive efforts are likely to be applicable to much larger numbers of individuals, such efforts could lead to greater population-level benefits. It is therefore important that strategies of prevention of heart failure be developed that apply to the large number of at-risk individuals. Such a strategy would complement the current approaches that are aimed at intensive management of patients with manifest heart failure. The current knowledge of both prevention and treatment of hypertension, obesity, and atherosclerotic vascular disease has the potential to greatly reduce the incidence and mortality from heart failure. Future endeavors to reduce heart failure burden must include the prevention of risk factors themselves, not just management of existing risk factors or established disease.

REFERENCES

1. Rosamond, W., Flegal, K., Furie, K., et al. (2007). Heart disease and stroke statistics 2008 update. A report from the American Heart Association Statistics Committee and Stroke Statistics Subcommittee. *Circulation, 117*(4), e25–e146.
2. Levy, D., Kenchaiah, S., Larson, M. G., et al. (2002). Long-term trends in the incidence of and survival with heart failure. *N Engl J Med, 347*, 1397–1402.
3. Owan, T. E., & Redfield, M. M. (2005). Epidemiology of diastolic heart failure. *Prog Cardiovasc Dis, 47*, 320–332.
4. Hunt, S. A., Baker, D. W., Chin, M. H., et al. (2001). ACC/AHA guidelines for the evaluation and management of chronic heart failure in the adult: executive summary. A report of the American College of Cardiology/American Heart Association Task Force on practice guidelines (Committee to Revise the 1995 Guidelines for the Evaluation and Management of Heart Failure): developed in collaboration with the International Society for Heart and Lung Transplantation; endorsed by the Heart Failure Society of America. *Circulation, 104*, 2996–3007.
5. Velagaleti, R. S., & Vasan, R. S. (2007). Heart failure in the twenty-first century: is it a coronary artery disease or hypertension problem? *Cardiol Clin, 25*, 487–495.
6. Schocken, D. D., Benjamin, E. J., Fonarow, G. C., et al. (2008). Prevention of heart failure: a scientific statement from the American Heart Association Councils on Epidemiology and Prevention, Clinical Cardiology, Cardiovascular Nursing, and High Blood Pressure Research; Quality of Care and Outcomes Research Interdisciplinary Working Group; and Functional Genomics and Translational Biology Interdisciplinary Working Group. *Circulation, 117*, 2544–2565.
7. Cohn, J. N., Ferrari, R., & Sharpe, N. (2000). Cardiac remodeling—concepts and clinical implications: a consensus paper from an international forum on cardiac remodeling. Behalf of an International Forum on Cardiac Remodeling. *J Am Coll Cardiol, 35*, 569–582.
8. Florea, V. G., Mareyev, V. Y., Samko, A. N., et al. (1999). Left ventricular remodelling: common process in patients with different primary myocardial disorders. *Int J Cardiol, 68*, 281–287.
9. Lloyd-Jones, D. M., Larson, M. G., Leip, E. P., et al. (2002). Lifetime risk for developing congestive heart failure: the Framingham Heart Study. *Circulation, 106*, 3068–3072.
10. Fishberg, A. M. (1937). *Heart failure*. Philadelphia: Lea & Febiger.
11. Chatterjee, K., & Massie, B. (2007). Systolic and diastolic heart failure: differences and similarities. *J Card Fail, 13*, 569–576.
12. Bursi, F., Weston, S. A., Redfield, M. M., et al. (2006). Systolic and diastolic heart failure in the community. *JAMA, 296*, 2209–2216.*
13. Baicu, C. F., Zile, M. R., Aurigemma, G. P., et al. (2005). Left ventricular systolic performance, function, and contractility in patients with diastolic heart failure. *Circulation, 111*, 2306–2312.
14. Huysman, J. A., Vliegen, H. W., Van der Laarse, A., et al. (1989). Changes in nonmyocyte tissue composition associated with pressure overload of hypertrophic human hearts. *Pathol Res Pract, 184*, 577–581.
15. Pearlman, E. S., Weber, K. T., Janicki, J. S., et al. (1982). Muscle fiber orientation and connective tissue content in the hypertrophied human heart. *Lab Invest, 46*, 158–164.
16. Gwathmey, J. K., Copelas, L., MacKinnon, R., et al. (1987). Abnormal intracellular calcium handling in myocardium from patients with end-stage heart failure. *Circ Res, 61*, 70–76.
17. Florea, V. G. (2007). Classifying systolic and diastolic heart failure. *JAMA, 297*, 1058–1059 [author reply *JAMA* 2007;297:1059].
18. Factor, S. M., Minase, T., & Sonnenblick, E. H. (1980). Clinical and morphological features of human hypertensive-diabetic cardiomyopathy. *Am Heart J, 99*, 446–458.
19. Weber, K. T., Brilla, C. G., & Janicki, J. S. (1993). Myocardial fibrosis: functional significance and regulatory factors. *Cardiovasc Res, 27*, 341–348.
20. Lauer, M. S., Anderson, K. M., & Levy, D. (1991). Influence of contemporary versus 30-year blood pressure levels on left ventricular mass and geometry: the Framingham Heart Study. *J Am Coll Cardiol, 18*, 1287–1294.
21. Pfeffer, M. A., & Braunwald, E. (1990). Ventricular remodeling after myocardial infarction. Experimental observations and clinical implications. *Circulation, 81*, 1161–1172.
22. Cohn, J. N. (1995). Critical review of heart failure: the role of left ventricular remodeling in the therapeutic response. *Clin Cardiol, 18*(9) (Suppl. 4), IV4–IV12.†
23. Aurigemma, G. P., Zile, M. R., & Gaasch, W. H. (2006). Contractile behavior of the left ventricle in diastolic heart failure: with emphasis on regional systolic function. *Circulation, 113*, 296–304.
24. Konstam, M. A. (2003). "Systolic and diastolic dysfunction" in heart failure? Time for a new paradigm. *J Card Fail, 9*, 1–3.
25. Baker, B. J., Wilen, M. M., Boyd, C. M., et al. (1984). Relation of right ventricular ejection fraction to exercise capacity in chronic left ventricular failure. *Am J Cardiol, 54*, 596–599.
26. Kitzman, D. W., Higginbotham, M. B., Cobb, F. R., et al. (1991). Exercise intolerance in patients with heart failure and preserved left ventricular systolic function: failure of the Frank-Starling mechanism. *J Am Coll Cardiol, 17*, 1065–1072.
27. Konstam, M. A., Kronenberg, M. W., Udelson, J. E., et al. (1992). Effectiveness of preload reserve as a determinant of clinical status in patients with left ventricular systolic dysfunction. The SOLVD Investigators. *Am J Cardiol, 69*, 1591–1595.

---

*Reference 12 is an important study showing that patients with reduced ejection fraction have more severe diastolic dysfunction.

†Reference 22 is a critical review of the mechanisms of heart failure that support the remodeling concept of heart failure.

28. Levy, D., Larson, M. G., Vasan, R. S., et al. (1996). The progression from hypertension to congestive heart failure. *JAMA, 275*, 1557–1562.[‡]
29. Wilhelmsen, L., Rosengren, A., Eriksson, H., et al. (2001). Heart failure in the general population of men—morbidity, risk factors and prognosis. *J Intern Med, 249*, 253–261.
30. Fields, L. E., Burt, V. L., Cutler, J. A., et al. (2004). The burden of adult hypertension in the United States 1999 to 2000: a rising tide. *Hypertension, 44*, 398–404.
31. Gandhi, S. K., Powers, J. C., Nomeir, A. M., et al. (2001). The pathogenesis of acute pulmonary edema associated with hypertension. *N Engl J Med, 344*, 17–22.
32. Gheorghiade, M., Zannad, F., Sopko, G., et al. (2005). Acute heart failure syndromes: current state and framework for future research. *Circulation, 112*, 3958–3968.
33. Kannel, W. B., Gordon, T., & Offutt, D. (1969). Left ventricular hypertrophy by electrocardiogram. Prevalence, incidence, and mortality in the Framingham study. *Ann Intern Med, 71*, 89–105.
34. Urbina, E. M., Gidding, S. S., Bao, W., et al. (1995). Effect of body size, ponderosity, and blood pressure on left ventricular growth in children and young adults in the Bogalusa Heart Study. *Circulation, 91*, 2400–2406.
35. Devereux, R. B. (1989). Left ventricular diastolic dysfunction: early diastolic relaxation and late diastolic compliance. *J Am Coll Cardiol, 13*, 337–339.
36. Inouye, I., Massie, B., Loge, D., et al. (1984). Abnormal left ventricular filling: an early finding in mild to moderate systemic hypertension. *Am J Cardiol, 53*, 120–126.
37. Smith, V. E., Schulman, P., Karimeddini, M. K., et al. (1985). Rapid ventricular filling in left ventricular hypertrophy: II. Pathologic hypertrophy. *J Am Coll Cardiol, 5*, 869–874.
38. Gunther, S., & Grossman, W. (1979). Determinants of ventricular function in pressure-overload hypertrophy in man. *Circulation, 59*, 679–688.
39. Chobanian, A. V., Bakris, G. L., Black, H. R., et al. (2003). Seventh report of the Joint National Committee on Prevention, Detection, Evaluation, and Treatment of High Blood Pressure. *Hypertension, 42*, 1206–1252.
40. Effects of treatment on morbidity in hypertension. II. Results in patients with diastolic blood pressure averaging 90 through 114 mm Hg. (1970). *JAMA, 213*, 1143–1152.
41. Izzo, J. L., Jr., & Gradman, A. H. (2004). Mechanisms and management of hypertensive heart disease: from left ventricular hypertrophy to heart failure. *Med Clin North Am, 88*, 1257–1271.
42. Kostis, J. B., Davis, B. R., Cutler, J., et al. (1997). Prevention of heart failure by antihypertensive drug treatment in older persons with isolated systolic hypertension. SHEP Cooperative Research Group. *JAMA, 278*, 212–216.
43. Dahlof, B., Lindholm, L. H., Hansson, L., et al. (1991). Morbidity and mortality in the Swedish Trial in Old Patients with Hypertension (STOP-Hypertension). *Lancet, 338*, 1281–1285.
44. Moser, M., & Hebert, P. R. (1996). Prevention of disease progression, left ventricular hypertrophy and congestive heart failure in hypertension treatment trials. *J Am Coll Cardiol, 27*, 1214–1218.
45. Baker, D. W. (2002). Prevention of heart failure. *J Card Fail, 8*, 333–346.
46. Vasan, R. S., & Levy, D. (1996). The role of hypertension in the pathogenesis of heart failure. A clinical mechanistic overview. *Arch Intern Med, 156*, 1789–1796.
47. Beckett, N. S., Peters, R., Fletcher, A. E., et al. (2008). Treatment of hypertension in patients 80 years of age or older. *N Engl J Med, 358*, 1887–1898.
48. Yusuf, S., Sleight, P., Pogue, J., et al. (2000). Effects of an angiotensin-converting-enzyme inhibitor, ramipril, on cardiovascular events in high-risk patients. The Heart Outcomes Prevention Evaluation Study Investigators. *N Engl J Med, 342*, 145–153.
49. Yusuf, S., Teo, K. K., Pogue, J., et al. (2008). Telmisartan, ramipril, or both in patients at high risk for vascular events. *N Engl J Med, 358*, 1547–1559.
50. Mokdad, A. H., Ford, E. S., Bowman, B. A., et al. (2001). Prevalence of obesity, diabetes, and obesity-related health risk factors. *JAMA, 2003*(289), 76–79.
51. Fox, C. S., Pencina, M. J., Meigs, J. B., et al. (2006). Trends in the incidence of type 2 diabetes mellitus from the 1970s to the 1990s: the Framingham Heart Study. *Circulation, 113*, 2914–2918.
52. From, A. M., Leibson, C. L., Bursi, F., et al. (2006). Diabetes in heart failure: prevalence and impact on outcome in the population. *Am J Med, 119*, 591–599.[§]
53. Wild, S., Roglic, G., Green, A., et al. (2004). Global prevalence of diabetes: estimates for the year 2000 and projections for 2030. *Diabetes Care, 27*, 1047–1053.
54. Amos, A. F., McCarty, D. J., & Zimmet, P. (1997). The rising global burden of diabetes and its complications: estimates and projections to the year 2010. *Diabet Med, 14*(Suppl. 5), S1–S85.
55. Zimmet, P., Alberti, K. G., & Shaw, J. (2001). Global and societal implications of the diabetes epidemic. *Nature, 414*, 782–787.
56. Taegtmeyer, H., McNulty, P., & Young, M. E. (2002). Adaptation and maladaptation of the heart in diabetes: part I: general concepts. *Circulation, 105*, 1727–1733.
57. He, J., Ogden, L. G., Bazzano, L. A., et al. (2001). Risk factors for congestive heart failure in US men and women: NHANES I epidemiologic follow-up study. *Arch Intern Med, 161*, 996–1002.
58. Krumholz, H. M., Chen, Y. T., Wang, Y., et al. (2000). Predictors of readmission among elderly survivors of admission with heart failure. *Am Heart J, 139*(1) (Pt 1), 72–77.
59. Shindler, D. M., Kostis, J. B., Yusuf, S., et al. (1996). Diabetes mellitus, a predictor of morbidity and mortality in the Studies of Left Ventricular Dysfunction (SOLVD) trials and registry. *Am J Cardiol, 77*, 1017–1020.
60. Vaur, L., Gueret, P., Lievre, M., et al. (2003). Development of congestive heart failure in type 2 diabetic patients with microalbuminuria or proteinuria: observations from the DIABHYCAR (type 2 DIABetes, HYpertension, CArdiovascular Events and Ramipril) study. *Diabetes Care, 26*, 855–860.
61. Kannel, W. B., & McGee, D. L. (1979). Diabetes and cardiovascular disease. The Framingham study. *JAMA, 241*, 2035–2038.

‡Reference 28 describes an important population-based study showing that hypertension is the most common risk factor for heart failure.

§Reference 52 is an update from the Rochester Epidemiology Project that details the increasing prevalence of diabetes-related heart failure.

62. Bibbins-Domingo, K., Lin, F., Vittinghoff, E., et al. (2004). Predictors of heart failure among women with coronary disease. *Circulation, 110*, 1424–1430.
63. Bell, D. S. (2007). Heart failure in the diabetic patient. *Cardiol Clin, 25*, 523–538.
64. Cook, C. B., Tsui, C., Ziemer, D. C., et al. (2006). Common reasons for hospitalization among adult patients with diabetes. *Endocr Pract, 12*, 363–370.
65. Reis, S. E., Holubkov, R., Edmundowicz, D., et al. (1997). Treatment of patients admitted to the hospital with congestive heart failure: specialty-related disparities in practice patterns and outcomes. *J Am Coll Cardiol, 30*, 733–738.
66. Adams, K. F., Jr., Fonarow, G. C., Emerman, C. L., et al. (2005). Characteristics and outcomes of patients hospitalized for heart failure in the United States: rationale, design, and preliminary observations from the first 100,000 cases in the Acute Decompensated Heart Failure National Registry (ADHERE). *Am Heart J, 149*, 209–216.
67. Fang, Z. Y., Prins, J. B., & Marwick, T. H. (2004). Diabetic cardiomyopathy: evidence, mechanisms, and therapeutic implications. *Endocr Rev, 25*, 543–567.[¶]
68. Ganguly, P. K., Pierce, G. N., Dhalla, K. S., et al. (1983). Defective sarcoplasmic reticular calcium transport in diabetic cardiomyopathy. *Am J Physiol, 244*(6), E528–E535.
69. Huggett, R. J., Scott, E. M., Gilbey, S. G., et al. (2003). Impact of type 2 diabetes mellitus on sympathetic neural mechanisms in hypertension. *Circulation, 108*, 3097–3101.
70. Giacomelli, F., & Wiener, J. (1979). Primary myocardial disease in the diabetic mouse. An ultrastructural study. *Lab Invest, 40*, 460–473.
71. Poirier, P., Bogaty, P., Garneau, C., et al. (2001). Diastolic dysfunction in normotensive men with well-controlled type 2 diabetes: importance of maneuvers in echocardiographic screening for preclinical diabetic cardiomyopathy. *Diabetes Care, 24*, 5–10.
72. Shishehbor, M. H., Hoogwerf, B. J., Schoenhagen, P., et al. (2003). Relation of hemoglobin A_{1c} to left ventricular relaxation in patients with type 1 diabetes mellitus and without overt heart disease. *Am J Cardiol, 91*, 1514–1517.
73. The effect of intensive treatment of diabetes on the development and progression of long-term complications in insulin-dependent diabetes mellitus. The Diabetes Control and Complications Trial Research Group. (1993). *N Engl J Med, 329*, 977–986.
74. Intensive blood-glucose control with sulphonylureas or insulin compared with conventional treatment and risk of complications in patients with type 2 diabetes (UKPDS 33). UK Prospective Diabetes Study (UKPDS) Group. (1998). *Lancet, 352*, 837–853.
75. Stratton, I. M., Adler, A. I., Neil, H. A., et al. (2000). Association of glycaemia with macrovascular and microvascular complications of type 2 diabetes (UKPDS 35): prospective observational study. *BMJ, 321*, 405–412.
76. Iribarren, C., Karter, A. J., Go, A. S., et al. (2001). Glycemic control and heart failure among adult patients with diabetes. *Circulation, 103*, 2668–2673.
77. Held, C., Gerstein, H. C., Yusuf, S., et al. (2007). Glucose levels predict hospitalization for congestive heart failure in patients at high cardiovascular risk. *Circulation, 115*, 1371–1375.
78. Gerstein, H. C., Miller, M. E., Byington, R. P., et al. (2008). Effects of intensive glucose lowering in type 2 diabetes. *N Engl J Med, 358*, 2545–2559.
79. Patel, A., MacMahon, S., Chalmers, J., et al. (2008). Intensive blood glucose control and vascular outcomes in patients with type 2 diabetes. *N Engl J Med, 358*, 2560–2572.
80. Dluhy, R. G., & McMahon, G. T. (2008). Intensive glycemic control in the ACCORD and ADVANCE trials. *N Engl J Med, 358*, 2630–2633.
81. Gilbert, R. E., Connelly, K., Kelly, D. J., et al. (2006). Heart failure and nephropathy: catastrophic and interrelated complications of diabetes. *Clin J Am Soc Nephrol, 1*, 193–208.
82. Lipscombe, L. L., Gomes, T., Levesque, L. E., et al. (2007). Thiazolidinediones and cardiovascular outcomes in older patients with diabetes. *JAMA, 298*, 2634–2643.
83. Effects of ramipril on cardiovascular and microvascular outcomes in people with diabetes mellitus: results of the HOPE study and MICRO-HOPE substudy. Heart Outcomes Prevention Evaluation Study Investigators. (2000). *Lancet, 355*, 253–259.
84. Kasiske, B. L., Kalil, R. S., Ma, J. Z., et al. (1993). Effect of antihypertensive therapy on the kidney in patients with diabetes: a meta-regression analysis. *Ann Intern Med, 118*, 129–138.
85. Lewis, E. J., Hunsicker, L. G., Bain, R. P., et al. (1993). The effect of angiotensin-converting-enzyme inhibition on diabetic nephropathy. The Collaborative Study Group. *N Engl J Med, 329*, 1456–1462.
86. Berl, T., Hunsicker, L. G., Lewis, J. B., et al. (2003). Cardiovascular outcomes in the Irbesartan Diabetic Nephropathy Trial of patients with type 2 diabetes and overt nephropathy. *Ann Intern Med, 138*, 542–549.
87. Brenner, B. M., Cooper, M. E., de Zeeuw, D., et al. (2001). Effects of losartan on renal and cardiovascular outcomes in patients with type 2 diabetes and nephropathy. *N Engl J Med, 345*, 861–869.
88. Zanella, M. T., & Ribeiro, A. B. (2002). The role of angiotensin II antagonism in type 2 diabetes mellitus: a review of renoprotection studies. *Clin Ther, 24*, 1019–1034.
89. Bourassa, M. G., Gurne, O., Bangdiwala, S. I., et al. (1993). Natural history and patterns of current practice in heart failure. The Studies of Left Ventricular Dysfunction (SOLVD) Investigators. *J Am Coll Cardiol, 22*(4) (Suppl. A), 14A–19A.
90. Kenchaiah, S., Narula, J., & Vasan, R. S. (2004). Risk factors for heart failure. *Med Clin North Am, 88*, 1145–1172.
91. Cowie, M. R., Wood, D. A., Coats, A. J., et al. (1999). Incidence and aetiology of heart failure: a population-based study. *Eur Heart J, 20*, 421–428.
92. Gheorghiade, M., & Bonow, R. O. (1998). Chronic heart failure in the United States: a manifestation of coronary artery disease. *Circulation, 97*, 282–289.
93. Uretsky, B. F., Thygesen, K., Armstrong, P. W., et al. (2000). Acute coronary findings at autopsy in heart failure patients with sudden death: results from the Assessment of Treatment with Lisinopril And Survival (ATLAS) trial. *Circulation, 102*, 611–616.
94. Repetto, A., Dal Bello, B., Pasotti, M., et al. (2005). Coronary atherosclerosis in end-stage idiopathic dilated cardiomyopathy: an innocent bystander? *Eur Heart J, 26*, 1519–1527.
95. Hedrich, O., Jacob, M., & Hauptman, P. J. (2004). Progression of coronary artery disease in non-ischemic dilated cardiomyopathy. *Coron Artery Dis, 15*, 291–297.

¶Reference 67 is an extensive review article on the natural history of diabetic cardiomyopathy.

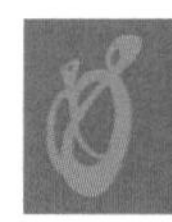

96. Bart, B. A., Shaw, L. K., McCants, C. B., Jr., et al. (1997). Clinical determinants of mortality in patients with angiographically diagnosed ischemic or nonischemic cardiomyopathy. *J Am Coll Cardiol, 30*, 1002–1008.
97. Mohri, M., & Takeshita, A. (1999). Coronary microvascular disease in humans. *Jpn Heart J, 40*, 97–108.
98. Kavey, R. E., Daniels, S. R., Lauer, R. M., et al. (2003). American Heart Association guidelines for primary prevention of atherosclerotic cardiovascular disease beginning in childhood. *Circulation, 107*, 1562–1566.
99. Tuzcu, E. M., Kapadia, S. R., Tutar, E., et al. (2001). High prevalence of coronary atherosclerosis in asymptomatic teenagers and young adults: evidence from intravascular ultrasound. *Circulation, 103*, 2705–2710.
100. Effect of ramipril on mortality and morbidity of survivors of acute myocardial infarction with clinical evidence of heart failure. The Acute Infarction Ramipril Efficacy (AIRE) Study Investigators. (1993). *Lancet, 342*, 821–828.
101. Janosi, A., Ghali, J. K., Herlitz, J., et al. (2003). Metoprolol CR/XL in postmyocardial infarction patients with chronic heart failure: experiences from MERIT-HF. *Am Heart J, 146*, 721–728.
102. Pfeffer, M. A., Braunwald, E., Moye, L. A., et al. (1992). Effect of captopril on mortality and morbidity in patients with left ventricular dysfunction after myocardial infarction. Results of the Survival And Ventricular Enlargement trial. The SAVE Investigators. *N Engl J Med, 327*, 669–677.¶
103. Pitt, B., White, H., Nicolau, J., et al. (2005). Eplerenone reduces mortality 30 days after randomization following acute myocardial infarction in patients with left ventricular systolic dysfunction and heart failure. *J Am Coll Cardiol, 46*, 425–431.
104. Yusuf, S., Zhao, F., Mehta, S. R., et al. (2001). Effects of clopidogrel in addition to aspirin in patients with acute coronary syndromes without ST-segment elevation. *N Engl J Med, 345*, 494–502.
105. Fox, K. M. (2003). Efficacy of perindopril in reduction of cardiovascular events among patients with stable coronary artery disease: randomised, double-blind, placebo-controlled, multicentre trial (the EUROPA study). *Lancet, 362*, 782–788.
106. Braunwald, E., Domanski, M. J., Fowler, S. E., et al. (2004). Angiotensin-converting-enzyme inhibition in stable coronary artery disease. *N Engl J Med, 351*, 2058–2068.
107. Go, A. S., Lee, W. Y., Yang, J., et al. (2006). Statin therapy and risks for death and hospitalization in chronic heart failure. *JAMA, 296*, 2105–2111.
108. Horwich, T. B., MacLellan, W. R., & Fonarow, G. C. (2004). Statin therapy is associated with improved survival in ischemic and non-ischemic heart failure. *J Am Coll Cardiol, 43*, 642–648.
109. Ramasubbu, K., Estep, J., White, D. L., et al. (2008). Experimental and clinical basis for the use of statins in patients with ischemic and nonischemic cardiomyopathy. *J Am Coll Cardiol, 51*, 415–426.
110. Sola, S., Mir, M. Q., Lerakis, S., et al. (2006). Atorvastatin improves left ventricular systolic function and serum markers of inflammation in nonischemic heart failure. *J Am Coll Cardiol, 47*, 332–337.
111. Kjekshus, J., Apetrei, E., Barrios, V., et al. (2007). Rosuvastatin in older patients with systolic heart failure. *N Engl J Med, 357*, 2248–2261.
112. Grundy, S. M., Cleeman, J. I., Daniels, S. R., et al. (2005). Diagnosis and management of the metabolic syndrome: an American Heart Association/National Heart, Lung, and Blood Institute Scientific Statement. *Circulation, 112*, 2735–2752.
113. Ford, E. S., Giles, W. H., & Dietz, W. H. (2002). Prevalence of the metabolic syndrome among US adults: findings from the third National Health and Nutrition Examination Survey. *JAMA, 287*, 356–359.
114. Kereiakes, D. J., & Willerson, J. T. (2003). Metabolic syndrome epidemic. *Circulation, 108*, 1552–1553.
115. Kahn, R., Buse, J., Ferrannini, E., et al. (2005). The metabolic syndrome: time for a critical appraisal: joint statement from the American Diabetes Association and the European Association for the Study of Diabetes. *Diabetes Care, 28*, 2289–2304.
116. Grundy, S. M., Brewer, H. B., Jr., Cleeman, J. I., et al. (2004). Definition of metabolic syndrome: report of the National Heart, Lung, and Blood Institute/American Heart Association conference on scientific issues related to definition. *Circulation, 109*, 433–438.
117. Hunt, S. A., Abraham, W. T., Chin, M. H., et al. (2005). ACC/AHA 2005 guideline update for the diagnosis and management of chronic heart failure in the adult: a report of the American College of Cardiology/American Heart Association Task Force on Practice Guidelines (Writing Committee to Update the 2001 Guidelines for the Evaluation and Management of Heart Failure): developed in collaboration with the American College of Chest Physicians and the International Society for Heart and Lung Transplantation: endorsed by the Heart Rhythm Society. *Circulation, 112*(12), e154–e235.
118. Lakka, H. M., Laaksonen, D. E., Lakka, T. A., et al. (2002). The metabolic syndrome and total and cardiovascular disease mortality in middle-aged men. *JAMA, 288*, 2709–2716.
119. Malik, S., Wong, N. D., Franklin, S. S., et al. (2004). Impact of the metabolic syndrome on mortality from coronary heart disease, cardiovascular disease, and all causes in United States adults. *Circulation, 110*, 1245–1250.
120. Leoncini, G., Ratto, E., Viazzi, F., et al. (2005). Metabolic syndrome is associated with early signs of organ damage in nondiabetic, hypertensive patients. *J Intern Med, 257*, 454–460.
121. Miranda, P. J., DeFronzo, R. A., Califf, R. M., et al. (2005). Metabolic syndrome: definition, pathophysiology, and mechanisms. *Am Heart J, 149*, 33–45.**
122. Prasad, A., & Quyyumi, A. A. (2004). Renin-angiotensin system and angiotensin receptor blockers in the metabolic syndrome. *Circulation, 110*, 1507–1512.
123. Tenenbaum, A., Motro, M., Schwammenthal, E., et al. (2004). Macrovascular complications of metabolic syndrome: an early intervention is imperative. *Int J Cardiol, 97*, 167–172.

¶Reference 102 describes one of the first trials assessing the effect of angiotensin-converting enzyme inhibition on mortality and morbidity in patients with left ventricular dysfunction after myocardial infarction.
**Reference 121 is an important description of metabolic syndrome.

124. Knowler, W. C., Barrett-Connor, E., Fowler, S. E., et al. (2002). Reduction in the incidence of type 2 diabetes with lifestyle intervention or metformin. *N Engl J Med, 346*, 393–403.
125. Reeves, M. J., & Rafferty, A. P. (2000). Healthy lifestyle characteristics among adults in the United States. *Arch Intern Med, 2005*(165), 854–857.
126. Miranda, P. J., DeFronzo, R. A., Califf, R. M., et al. (2005). Metabolic syndrome: evaluation of pathological and therapeutic outcomes. *Am Heart J, 149*, 20–32.
127. The NAVIGATOR Study Group. (2010). Effect of valsartan on the incidence of diabetes and cardiovascular events. *N Engl J Med*, 362, 1477-1490.
128. Gerstein, H., Yusuf, S., et al. (2008). Origin Trial Investigators, Rationale, design, and baseline characteristics for a large international trial of cardiovascular disease prevention in people with dysglycemia: the ORIGIN Trial (Outcome Reduction with an Initial Glargine Intervention). *Am Heart J, 155*, 26–32, e132-e632.
129. National Task Force on the Prevention and Treatment of Obesity. (2000). Overweight, obesity, and health risk.*Arch Intern Med, 160*, 898–904.
130. Flegal, K. M., Graubard, B. I., Williamson, D. F., et al. (2005). Excess deaths associated with underweight, overweight, and obesity. *JAMA, 293*, 1861–1867.
131. Clinical Guidelines on the Identification. (1998). Evaluation, and Treatment of Overweight and Obesity in Adults—The Evidence Report. National Institutes of Health. *Obes Res, 6*(Suppl. 2), S51–S209.
132. Hedley, A. A., Ogden, C. L., Johnson, C. L., et al. (2004). Prevalence of overweight and obesity among US children, adolescents, and adults, 1999-2002. *JAMA, 291*, 2847–2850.
133. Ogden, C. L., Carroll, M. D., Curtin, L. R., et al. (2006). Prevalence of overweight and obesity in the United States, 1999-2004. *JAMA, 295*, 1549–1555.
134. Alpert, M. A., Lambert, C. R., Terry, B. E., et al. (1995). Influence of left ventricular mass on left ventricular diastolic filling in normotensive morbid obesity. *Am Heart J, 130*, 1068–1073.
135. Hammond, I. W., Devereux, R. B., Alderman, M. H., et al. (1988). Relation of blood pressure and body build to left ventricular mass in normotensive and hypertensive employed adults. *J Am Coll Cardiol, 12*, 996–1004.
136. Lauer, M. S., Anderson, K. M., Kannel, W. B., et al. (1991). The impact of obesity on left ventricular mass and geometry. The Framingham Heart Study. *JAMA, 266*, 231–236.
137. Messerli, F. H., Sundgaard-Riise, K., Reisin, E. D., et al. (1983). Dimorphic cardiac adaptation to obesity and arterial hypertension. *Ann Intern Med, 99*, 757–761.
138. Gardin, J. M., McClelland, R., Kitzman, D., et al. (2001). M-mode echocardiographic predictors of six- to seven-year incidence of coronary heart disease, stroke, congestive heart failure, and mortality in an elderly cohort (the Cardiovascular Health Study). *Am J Cardiol, 87*, 1051–1057.
139. Vasan, R. S., Larson, M. G., Benjamin, E. J., et al. (1997). Left ventricular dilatation and the risk of congestive heart failure in people without myocardial infarction. *N Engl J Med, 336*, 1350–1355.
140. Kenchaiah, S., Evans, J. C., Levy, D., et al. (2002). Obesity and the risk of heart failure. *N Engl J Med, 347*, 305–313.
141. Alpert, M. A. (2001). Obesity cardiomyopathy: pathophysiology and evolution of the clinical syndrome. *Am J Med Sci, 321*, 225–236.††
142. Adams, K. F., Schatzkin, A., Harris, T. B., et al. (2006). Overweight, obesity, and mortality in a large prospective cohort of persons 50 to 71 years old. *N Engl J Med, 355*, 763–778.
143. Hu, F. B., Willett, W. C., Li, T., et al. (2004). Adiposity as compared with physical activity in predicting mortality among women. *N Engl J Med, 351*, 2694–2703.
144. McGee, D. L. (2005). Body mass index and mortality: a meta-analysis based on person-level data from twenty-six observational studies. *Ann Epidemiol, 15*, 87–97.
145. Hu, G., Tuomilehto, J., Silventoinen, K., et al. (2007). Body mass index, waist circumference, and waist-hip ratio on the risk of total and type-specific stroke. *Arch Intern Med, 167*, 1420–1427.
146. Balkau, B., Deanfield, J. E., Despres, J. P., et al. (2007). International Day for the Evaluation of Abdominal Obesity (IDEA): a study of waist circumference, cardiovascular disease, and diabetes mellitus in 168,000 primary care patients in 63 countries. *Circulation, 116*, 1942–1951.
147. Stamler, J. (1991). Epidemiologic findings on body mass and blood pressure in adults. *Ann Epidemiol, 1*, 347–362.
148. Chan, J. M., Rimm, E. B., Colditz, G. A., et al. (1994). Obesity, fat distribution, and weight gain as risk factors for clinical diabetes in men. *Diabetes Care, 17*, 961–969.
149. Kannel, W. B., & McGee, D. L. (1979). Diabetes and glucose tolerance as risk factors for cardiovascular disease: the Framingham study. *Diabetes Care, 2*, 120–126.
150. Manson, J. E., Colditz, G. A., Stampfer, M. J., et al. (1990). A prospective study of obesity and risk of coronary heart disease in women. *N Engl J Med, 322*, 882–889.
151. Chen, Y. T., Vaccarino, V., Williams, C. S., et al. (1999). Risk factors for heart failure in the elderly: a prospective community-based study. *Am J Med, 106*, 605–612.
152. Kannel, W. B., D'Agostino, R. B., Silbershatz, H., et al. (1999). Profile for estimating risk of heart failure. *Arch Intern Med, 159*, 1197–1204.
153. Alexander, J. K., Dennis, E. W., Smith, W. G., et al. (1962). Blood volume, cardiac output, and distribution of systemic blood flow in extreme obesity. *Cardiovasc Res Cent Bull, 1*(Winter), 39–44.
154. Messerli, F. H., Sundgaard-Riise, K., Reisin, E., et al. (1983). Disparate cardiovascular effects of obesity and arterial hypertension. *Am J Med, 74*, 808–812.
155. Engeli, S., & Sharma, A. M. (2001). The renin-angiotensin system and natriuretic peptides in obesity-associated hypertension. *J Mol Med, 79*, 21–29.
156. Vincent, H. K., Powers, S. K., Stewart, D. J., et al. (1999). Obesity is associated with increased myocardial oxidative stress. *Int J Obes Relat Metab Disord, 23*, 67–74.
157. Lau, D. C., Dhillon, B., Yan, H., et al. (2005). Adipokines: molecular links between obesity and atherosclerosis. *Am J Physiol Heart Circ Physiol, 288*(5), H2031–H2041.
158. Zhou, Y. T., Grayburn, P., Karim, A., et al. (2000). Lipotoxic heart disease in obese rats: implications for human obesity. *Proc Natl Acad Sci U S A, 97*, 1784–1789.

††Reference 141 is an important discussion of the pathophysiology and evolution of obesity-related cardiomyopathy.

159. Bray, G. A. (2007). Medical therapy for obesity—current status and future hopes. *Med Clin North Am, 91*, 1225–1253, xi.
160. Bray, G. A., & Greenway, F. L. (2007). Pharmacological treatment of the overweight patient. *Pharmacol Rev, 59*, 151–184.
161. Li, Z., Maglione, M., Tu, W., et al. (2005). Meta-analysis: pharmacologic treatment of obesity. *Ann Intern Med, 142*, 532–546.
162. Padwal, R., Li, S. K., & Lau, D. C. (2003). Long-term pharmacotherapy for overweight and obesity: a systematic review and meta-analysis of randomized controlled trials. *Int J Obes Relat Metab Disord, 27*, 1437–1446.
163. Yanovski, S. Z., & Yanovski, J. A. (2002). Obesity. *N Engl J Med, 346*, 591–602.
164. Adams, T. D., Gress, R. E., Smith, S. C., et al. (2007). Long-term mortality after gastric bypass surgery. *N Engl J Med, 357*, 753–761.
165. Barnes, P. J. (2000). Chronic obstructive pulmonary disease. *N Engl J Med, 343*, 269–280.
166. American Thoracic Society. (1995). Standards for the diagnosis and care of patients with chronic obstructive pulmonary disease. *Am J Respir Crit Care Med, 152*(5) (Pt 2), S77–S121.
167. Lopez, A. D., & Murray, C. C. (1998). The global burden of disease, 1990-2020. *Nat Med, 4*, 1241–1243.
168. Curkendall, S. M., DeLuise, C., Jones, J. K., et al. (2006). Cardiovascular disease in patients with chronic obstructive pulmonary disease, Saskatchewan Canada cardiovascular disease in COPD patients. *Ann Epidemiol, 16*, 63–70.
169. Egred, M., Shaw, S., Mohammad, B., et al. (2005). Under-use of beta-blockers in patients with ischaemic heart disease and concomitant chronic obstructive pulmonary disease. *Q J Med, 98*, 493–497.
170. Holguin, F., Folch, E., Redd, S. C., et al. (2005). Comorbidity and mortality in COPD-related hospitalizations in the United States, 1979 to 2001. *Chest, 128*, 2005–2011.
171. Sidney, S., Sorel, M., Quesenberry, C. P., Jr., et al. (2005). COPD and incident cardiovascular disease hospitalizations and mortality: Kaiser Permanente Medical Care Program. *Chest, 128*, 2068–2075.
172. Havranek, E. P., Masoudi, F. A., Westfall, K. A., et al. (2002). Spectrum of heart failure in older patients: results from the National Heart Failure project. *Am Heart J, 143*, 412–417.
173. Le Jemtel, T. H., Padeletti, M., & Jelic, S. (2007). Diagnostic and therapeutic challenges in patients with coexistent chronic obstructive pulmonary disease and chronic heart failure. *J Am Coll Cardiol, 49*, 171–180.[‡‡]
174. O'Connor, C. M., Stough, W. G., Gallup, D. S., et al. (2005). Demographics, clinical characteristics, and outcomes of patients hospitalized for decompensated heart failure: observations from the IMPACT-HF registry. *J Card Fail, 11*, 200–205.
175. Render, M. L., Weinstein, A. S., & Blaustein, A. S. (1995). Left ventricular dysfunction in deteriorating patients with chronic obstructive pulmonary disease. *Chest, 107*, 162–168.
176. Rutten, F. H., Cramer, M. J., Grobbee, D. E., et al. (2005). Unrecognized heart failure in elderly patients with stable chronic obstructive pulmonary disease. *Eur Heart J, 26*, 1887–1894.
177. Staszewsky, L., Wong, M., Masson, S., et al. (2007). Clinical, neurohormonal, and inflammatory markers and overall prognostic role of chronic obstructive pulmonary disease in patients with heart failure: data from the Val-HeFT heart failure trial. *J Card Fail, 13*, 797–804.
178. Sin, D. D., & Man, S. F. (2003). Why are patients with chronic obstructive pulmonary disease at increased risk of cardiovascular diseases? The potential role of systemic inflammation in chronic obstructive pulmonary disease. *Circulation, 107*, 1514–1519.
179. Steele, P., Ellis, J. H., Van Dyke, D., et al. (1975). Left ventricular ejection fraction in severe chronic obstructive airways disease. *Am J Med, 59*, 21–28.
180. Naeije, R. (2005). Pulmonary hypertension and right heart failure in chronic obstructive pulmonary disease. *Proc Am Thorac Soc, 2*, 20–22.
181. Anthonisen, N. R., Connett, J. E., Kiley, J. P., et al. (1994). Effects of smoking intervention and the use of an inhaled anticholinergic bronchodilator on the rate of decline of FEV_1. The Lung Health Study. *JAMA, 272*, 1497–1505.
182. Anthonisen, N. R., Skeans, M. A., Wise, R. A., et al. (2005). The effects of a smoking cessation intervention on 14.5-year mortality: a randomized clinical trial. *Ann Intern Med, 142*, 233–239.
183. Tarpy, S. P., & Celli, B. R. (1995). Long-term oxygen therapy. *N Engl J Med, 333*, 710–714.
184. Boers, M., Dijkmans, B., Gabriel, S., et al. (2004). Making an impact on mortality in rheumatoid arthritis: targeting cardiovascular comorbidity. *Arthritis Rheum, 50*, 1734–1739.
185. Gabriel, S. E., Crowson, C. S., Kremers, H. M., et al. (2003). Survival in rheumatoid arthritis: a population-based analysis of trends over 40 years. *Arthritis Rheum, 48*, 54–58.
186. Maradit-Kremers, H., Nicola, P. J., Crowson, C. S., et al. (2005). Cardiovascular death in rheumatoid arthritis: a population-based study. *Arthritis Rheum, 52*, 722–732.
187. Nicola, P. J., Crowson, C. S., Maradit-Kremers, H., et al. (2006). Contribution of congestive heart failure and ischemic heart disease to excess mortality in rheumatoid arthritis. *Arthritis Rheum, 54*, 60–67.
188. Nicola, P. J., Maradit-Kremers, H., Roger, V. L., et al. (2005). The risk of congestive heart failure in rheumatoid arthritis: a population-based study over 46 years. *Arthritis Rheum, 52*, 412–420.
189. Aubry, M. C., Maradit-Kremers, H., Reinalda, M. S., et al. (2007). Differences in atherosclerotic coronary heart disease between subjects with and without rheumatoid arthritis. *J Rheumatol, 34*, 937–942.
190. Maradit-Kremers, H., Nicola, P. J., Crowson, C. S., et al. (2007). Raised erythrocyte sedimentation rate signals heart failure in patients with rheumatoid arthritis. *Ann Rheum Dis, 66*, 76–80.
191. Maradit-Kremers, H., Crowson, C. S., Nicola, P. J., et al. (2005). Increased unrecognized coronary heart disease and sudden deaths in rheumatoid arthritis: a population-based cohort study. *Arthritis Rheum, 52*, 402–411.

‡‡Reference 173 is a state-of-the-art discussion of the diagnostic and therapeutic challenges in patients with coexistent chronic obstructive pulmonary disease and chronic heart failure.

192. Choy, E. H., & Panayi, G. S. (2001). Cytokine pathways and joint inflammation in rheumatoid arthritis. *N Engl J Med, 344*, 907–916.
193. Mann, D. L. (2002). Inflammatory mediators and the failing heart: past, present, and the foreseeable future. *Circ Res, 91*, 988–998.
194. Chung, E. S., Packer, M., Lo, K. H., et al. (2003). Randomized, double-blind, placebo-controlled, pilot trial of infliximab, a chimeric monoclonal antibody to tumor necrosis factor-alpha, in patients with moderate-to-severe heart failure: results of the anti-TNF Therapy Against Congestive Heart Failure (ATTACH) trial. *Circulation, 107*, 3133–3140.
195. Mann, D. L., McMurray, J. J., Packer, M., et al. (2004). Targeted anticytokine therapy in patients with chronic heart failure: results of the Randomized Etanercept Worldwide Evaluation (RENEWAL). *Circulation, 109*, 1594–1602.
196. Gonzalez-Gay, M. A., Gonzalez-Juanatey, C., Pineiro, A., et al. (2005). High-grade C-reactive protein elevation correlates with accelerated atherogenesis in patients with rheumatoid arthritis. *J Rheumatol, 32*, 1219–1223.
197. Sattar, N., McCarey, D. W., Capell, H., et al. (2003). Explaining how "high-grade" systemic inflammation accelerates vascular risk in rheumatoid arthritis. *Circulation, 108*, 2957–2963.
198. Listing, J., Strangfeld, A., Kekow, J., et al. (2008). Does tumor necrosis factor alpha inhibition promote or prevent heart failure in patients with rheumatoid arthritis? *Arthritis Rheum, 58*, 667–677.
199. Gabriel, S. E. (2008). Tumor necrosis factor inhibition: a part of the solution or a part of the problem of heart failure in rheumatoid arthritis? *Arthritis Rheum, 58*, 637–640.
200. Dazzi, H., Kaufmann, K., & Follath, F. (2001). Anthracycline-induced acute cardiotoxicity in adults treated for leukaemia. Analysis of the clinico-pathological aspects of documented acute anthracycline-induced cardiotoxicity in patients treated for acute leukaemia at the University Hospital of Zurich, Switzerland, between 1990 and 1996. *Ann Oncol, 12*, 963–966.
201. Doroshow, J. H., & Davies, K. J. (1986). Redox cycling of anthracyclines by cardiac mitochondria. II. Formation of superoxide anion, hydrogen peroxide, and hydroxyl radical. *J Biol Chem, 261*, 3068–3074.
202. Myers, C. E., McGuire, W. P., Liss, R. H., et al. (1977). Adriamycin: the role of lipid peroxidation in cardiac toxicity and tumor response. *Science, 197*, 165–167.
203. Pacher, P., Beckman, J. S., & Liaudet, L. (2007). Nitric oxide and peroxynitrite in health and disease. *Physiol Rev, 87*, 315–424.
204. Pacher, P., Liaudet, L., Bai, P., et al. (2003). Potent metalloporphyrin peroxynitrite decomposition catalyst protects against the development of doxorubicin-induced cardiac dysfunction. *Circulation, 107*, 896–904.
205. Bai, P., Mabley, J. G., Liaudet, L., et al. (2004). Matrix metalloproteinase activation is an early event in doxorubicin-induced cardiotoxicity. *Oncol Rep, 11*, 505–508.
206. Tokarska-Schlattner, M., Zaugg, M., Zuppinger, C., et al. (2006). New insights into doxorubicin-induced cardiotoxicity: the critical role of cellular energetics. *J Mol Cell Cardiol, 41*, 389–405.
207. Kumar, D., Kirshenbaum, L. A., Li, T., et al. (2001). Apoptosis in Adriamycin cardiomyopathy and its modulation by probucol. *Antioxid Redox Signal, 3*, 135–145.
208. Ueno, M., Kakinuma, Y., Yuhki, K., et al. (2006). Doxorubicin induces apoptosis by activation of caspase-3 in cultured cardiomyocytes in vitro and rat cardiac ventricles in vivo. *J Pharmacol Sci, 101*, 151–158.
209. Wu, S., Ko, Y. S., Teng, M. S., et al. (2002). Adriamycin-induced cardiomyocyte and endothelial cell apoptosis: in vitro and in vivo studies. *J Mol Cell Cardiol, 34*, 1595–1607.
210. Lefrak, E. A., Pitha, J., Rosenheim, S., et al. (1973). A clinicopathologic analysis of Adriamycin cardiotoxicity. *Cancer, 32*, 302–314.
211. Sparano, J. A., Brown, D. L., & Wolff, A. C. (2002). Predicting cancer therapy-induced cardiotoxicity: the role of troponins and other markers. *Drug Saf, 25*, 301–311.
212. Dowd, N. P., Scully, M., Adderley, S. R., et al. (2001). Inhibition of cyclooxygenase-2 aggravates doxorubicin-mediated cardiac injury in vivo. *J Clin Invest, 108*, 585–590.
213. Singal, P. K., & Iliskovic, N. (1998). Doxorubicin-induced cardiomyopathy. *N Engl J Med, 339*, 900–905.
214. Murphy, C. A., & Dargie, H. J. (2007). Drug-induced cardiovascular disorders. *Drug Saf, 30*, 783–804.[§§]
215. Shapira, J., Gotfried, M., Lishner, M., et al. (1990). Reduced cardiotoxicity of doxorubicin by a 6-hour infusion regimen. A prospective randomized evaluation. *Cancer, 65*, 870–873.
216. Conklin, K. A. (2005). Coenzyme q10 for prevention of anthracycline-induced cardiotoxicity. *Integr Cancer Ther, 4*, 110–130.
217. Mukhopadhyay, P., Batkai, S., Rajesh, M., et al. (2007). Pharmacological inhibition of CB1 cannabinoid receptor protects against doxorubicin-induced cardiotoxicity. *J Am Coll Cardiol, 50*, 528–536.
218. Slordal, L., & Spigset, O. (2006). Heart failure induced by non-cardiac drugs. *Drug Saf, 29*, 567–586.
219. Von Hoff, D. D., Layard, M. W., Basa, P., et al. (1979). Risk factors for doxorubicin-induced congestive heart failure. *Ann Intern Med, 91*, 710–717.
220. Saini, J., Rich, M. W., & Lyss, A. P. (1987). Reversibility of severe left ventricular dysfunction due to doxorubicin cardiotoxicity. Report of three cases. *Ann Intern Med, 106*, 814–816.
221. Hjalmarson, A., & Waagstein, F. (1994). The role of beta-blockers in the treatment of cardiomyopathy and ischaemic heart failure. *Drugs, 47*(Suppl. 4), 31–39 (discussion, *Drugs* 1994;*47*[Suppl. 4]:39–40).
222. Shaddy, R. E., Olsen, S. L., Bristow, M. R., et al. (1995). Efficacy and safety of metoprolol in the treatment of doxorubicin-induced cardiomyopathy in pediatric patients. *Am Heart J, 129*, 197–199.
223. Cobleigh, M. A., Vogel, C. L., Tripathy, D., et al. (1999). Multinational study of the efficacy and safety of humanized anti-HER2 monoclonal antibody in women who have HER2-overexpressing metastatic breast cancer that has progressed after chemotherapy for metastatic disease. *J Clin Oncol, 17*, 2639–2648.

§§Reference 214 is an excellent review of specific forms of drug-induced cardiovascular disease.

224. Suter, T. M., Cook-Bruns, N., & Barton, C. (2004). Cardiotoxicity associated with trastuzumab (Herceptin) therapy in the treatment of metastatic breast cancer. *Breast, 13*, 173–183.
225. Perez, E. A. (2004). Cardiac issues related to trastuzumab. *Breast, 13*, 171–172.
226. Ewer, M. S., Vooletich, M. T., Durand, J. B., et al. (2005). Reversibility of trastuzumab-related cardiotoxicity: new insights based on clinical course and response to medical treatment. *J Clin Oncol, 23*, 7820–7826.
227. Guarneri, V., Lenihan, D. J., Valero, V., et al. (2006). Long-term cardiac tolerability of trastuzumab in metastatic breast cancer: the M.D. Anderson Cancer Center experience. *J Clin Oncol, 24*, 4107–4115.
228. Bleumink, G. S., Feenstra, J., Sturkenboom, M. C., et al. (2003). Nonsteroidal anti-inflammatory drugs and heart failure. *Drugs, 63*, 525–534.
229. Bombardier, C., Laine, L., Reicin, A., et al. (2000). Comparison of upper gastrointestinal toxicity of rofecoxib and naproxen in patients with rheumatoid arthritis. VIGOR Study Group. *N Engl J Med, 343*, 1520–1528, 2 pp following 1528.
230. Bresalier, R. S., Sandler, R. S., Quan, H., et al. (2005). Cardiovascular events associated with rofecoxib in a colorectal adenoma chemoprevention trial. *N Engl J Med, 352*, 1092–1102.
231. Nussmeier, N. A., Whelton, A. A., Brown, M. T., et al. (2005). Complications of the COX-2 inhibitors parecoxib and valdecoxib after cardiac surgery. *N Engl J Med, 352*, 1081–1091.
232. Solomon, S. D., McMurray, J. J., Pfeffer, M. A., et al. (2005). Cardiovascular risk associated with celecoxib in a clinical trial for colorectal adenoma prevention. *N Engl J Med, 352*, 1071–1080.
233. Pope, J. E., Anderson, J. J., & Felson, D. T. (1993). A meta-analysis of the effects of nonsteroidal anti-inflammatory drugs on blood pressure. *Arch Intern Med, 153*, 477–484.
234. Fosslien, E. (2005). Cardiovascular complications of non-steroidal anti-inflammatory drugs. *Ann Clin Lab Sci, 35*, 347–385.
235. Krotz, F., Schiele, T. M., Klauss, V., et al. (2005). Selective COX-2 inhibitors and risk of myocardial infarction. *J Vasc Res, 42*, 312–324.
236. Kahn, S. E., Haffner, S. M., Heise, M. A., et al. (2006). Glycemic durability of rosiglitazone, metformin, or glyburide monotherapy. *N Engl J Med, 355*, 2427–2443.
237. Effect of intensive blood-glucose control with metformin on complications in overweight patients with type 2 diabetes (UKPDS 34). UK Prospective Diabetes Study (UKPDS) Group. (1998). *Lancet, 352*, 854–865.
238. Stettler, C., Allemann, S., Juni, P., et al. (2006). Glycemic control and macrovascular disease in types 1 and 2 diabetes mellitus: meta-analysis of randomized trials. *Am Heart J, 152*, 27–38.
239. Dormandy, J. A., Charbonnel, B., Eckland, D. J., et al. (2005). Secondary prevention of macrovascular events in patients with type 2 diabetes in the PROactive Study (PROspective pioglitAzone Clinical Trial In macroVascular Events): a randomised controlled trial. *Lancet, 366*, 1279–1289.
240. Haffner, S. M., Greenberg, A. S., Weston, W. M., et al. (2002). Effect of rosiglitazone treatment on nontraditional markers of cardiovascular disease in patients with type 2 diabetes mellitus. *Circulation, 106*, 679–684.
241. Lincoff, A. M., Wolski, K., Nicholls, S. J., et al. (2007). Pioglitazone and risk of cardiovascular events in patients with type 2 diabetes mellitus: a meta-analysis of randomized trials. *JAMA, 298*, 1180–1188.
242. Mazzone, T., Meyer, P. M., Feinstein, S. B., et al. (2006). Effect of pioglitazone compared with glimepiride on carotid intima-media thickness in type 2 diabetes: a randomized trial. *JAMA, 296*, 2572–2581.
243. Berlie, H. D., Kalus, J. S., & Jaber, L. A. (2007). Thiazolidinediones and the risk of edema: a meta-analysis. *Diabetes Res Clin Pract, 76*, 279–289.
244. Lago, R. M., Singh, P. P., & Nesto, R. W. (2007). Congestive heart failure and cardiovascular death in patients with prediabetes and type 2 diabetes given thiazolidinediones: a meta-analysis of randomised clinical trials. *Lancet, 370*, 1129–1136.
245. Singh, S., Loke, Y. K., & Furberg, C. D. (2007). Long-term risk of cardiovascular events with rosiglitazone: a meta-analysis. *JAMA, 298*, 1189–1195.
246. Singh, S., Loke, Y. K., & Furberg, C. D. (2007). Thiazolidinediones and heart failure: a teleo-analysis. *Diabetes Care, 30*, 2148–2153.
247. *Safety labeling changes approved by FDA Center for Drug Evaluation and Research (CDER).* August 14, (2007). Washington, DC: U.S. Food and Drug Administration.
248. Nissen, S. E., & Wolski, K. (2007). Effect of rosiglitazone on the risk of myocardial infarction and death from cardiovascular causes. *N Engl J Med, 356*, 2457–2471.
249. Ghuran, A., & Nolan, J. (2000). Recreational drug misuse: issues for the cardiologist. *Heart, 83*, 627–633.
250. Abramson, J. L., Williams, S. A., Krumholz, H. M., et al. (2001). Moderate alcohol consumption and risk of heart failure among older persons. *JAMA, 285*, 1971–1977.
251. Walsh, C. R., Larson, M. G., Evans, J. C., et al. (2002). Alcohol consumption and risk for congestive heart failure in the Framingham Heart Study. *Ann Intern Med, 136*, 181–191

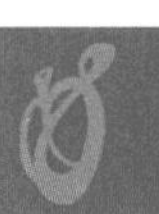

CHAPTER 42

Pharmacogenomics and Pharmacogenetics in Heart Failure

Dennis M. McNamara and Arthur M. Feldman

Medical therapy for systolic heart failure has evolved significantly since the nineteen eighties. Large randomized and placebo-controlled clinical trials have identified families of pharmacological agents and devices that can improve survival and decrease the frequency of hospitalizations for heart failure among patients in whom systolic dysfunction is diagnosed. As each new study has met the strict requirements of peer review and the new agents have been added to the pharmacopeia, the clinical management of patients has become complex because new drugs have been added to the standard regimen, rather than replacing older agents. For an African American patient with ischemic cardiomyopathy and class III heart failure, heart failure guidelines recommmend treatment with an angiotensin-converting enzyme (ACE) inhibitor, a β-blocker, an aldosterone receptor antagonist, isosorbide dinitrate, hydralazine, aspirin, and a statin. All seven of these therapies are recommended because they have improved survival in similar cohorts with systolic heart failure.

A common finding in all clinical trials has been that each new agent developed for the treatment of heart failure improves outcomes in some but not all patients with heart failure. Attempts to identify which patients will respond to a specific drug or device (or which patients might have an adverse response to a drug or device) initially focused evaluating whether subgroup analysis of predefined phenotypic identifiers—for example, age, gender, ejection fraction, or cause of heart failure—could enable this prediction. These efforts proved fruitless. However, early subgroup analysis of large randomized and multinational studies suggested that an individual's genotype could be used to predict drug response. For example, several studies demonstrated marked differences in drug response among patients from various continents, and another study suggested that patients who self-identified as African American might have had a different response to drug therapy than did patients who self-identified as being non–African American. Thus, investigators began to assess whether an individual's genotype could be used to predict drug response; this evolving area of investigation is referred to as "pharmacogenetics" or "pharmacogenomics." By identifying the genomic factors that are predictive of drug efficacy, this new field of science provides the opportunity to "personalize" care for an individual patient, lower the risk of an adverse response to an unnecessary agent, and decrease overall health care costs.

Studies of pharmacogenomics initially focused on genetic variants in single genes that encoded for drug targets, including receptors, enzymes, and signaling pathways that regulated the action of specific agents that were known to alter the pathobiological processes of heart failure. For example, variants were identified in the ACE gene (see Chapter 9). Mutation of the ACE gene resulted in the transcription of a protein with enhanced enzyme activity, which caused elevations in the levels of angiotensin II, a neurohormone known to contribute to the maladaptive remodeling that characterizes the progression of heart failure. Similarly, variants were also identified in the β-adrenergic receptors, a family of receptors that link the neurohormonal ligands epinephrine and norepinephrine with downstream activation of the neurohormone signaling cascade (see Chapter 10). These variants resulted in the transcription of an adrenergic receptor whose physiological characteristics differed from those of receptors that were transcribed from the wild-type gene. In some cases, the genetic variant increased ligand-receptor coupling and could increase the risk of heart failure, whereas in other cases, the genetic variant was associated with attenuated signaling. These genetic variants include deletions or insertions; the inclusion or exclusion of the coding region of a gene; single-nucleotide polymorphisms that alter the nucleotide sequence within a single nucleotide triplet, which may result in the transcription of a protein with a different amino acid sequence; or mutations that alter a larger segment of the coding region of the gene, resulting in a dysfunctional protein. Variants such as deletions, insertions, single-nucleotide polymorphisms, and larger mutations can also occur in either the 5′ regulatory region of the gene or in the region that encodes the 3′ untranslated tail. In the former region, the genetic variant can alter the ability of regulatory proteins to bind to the promoter region of the gene, thereby either increasing or decreasing transcription. In contrast, mutations in the 3′ untranslated region can alter RNA stability. Thus, a wide array of genotypic abnormalities can influence the amount, the structure, or the function of cardiac proteins that are important in the pathophysiological processes of heart failure.

The analysis of genetic variants in DNA samples was once labor intensive, time consuming, and expensive. However, the burgeoning in genomic technology, particularly silicon chip technology, has enabled scientists to simultaneously identify a large number of genetic variants in a single sample or multiple samples of DNA. This analysis can be performed rapidly, can be automated, and is now relatively inexpensive. However, it requires an a priori knowledge of the nucleotide sequence and gene of interest. In addition, because of the complexity and redundancy of critical pathways, it is unlikely that any single locus will determine therapeutic response, and the key to genomic targeting may be in polygenic analysis involving several loci for any given clinical or therapeutic paradigm.

More recently, investigators have begun to pursue genome-wide association studies (GWASs). This powerful technology enables investigators to identify characteristic markers that can help predict outcomes or response to drugs in a large population; however, these studies do not enable the investigator to identify the specific genes that participate in the individual's response to a drug or device. However, these two types of identification are not mutually exclusive, and when used together, they will help increase the understanding of the role of genetics in predicting how drugs work in individual patients.

This chapter reviews the major genomic polymorphisms affecting the pathogenesis of heart failure and therapeutics, and it explores how advances in GWASs may accelerate the advance toward the current goal of "personalized" genomic therapy for the treatment of heart failure.

RENIN-ANGIOTENSIN-ALDOSTERONE PATHWAY: THERAPEUTICS AND GENOMICS

The majority of medical therapies for heart failure that improve survival inhibit the renin-angiotensin-aldosterone systemic (RAAS) pathway (Figure 42-1) (see Chapter 45). Myocardial injury and diminished cardiac function result in sympathetic activation and in the release of the protease renin, which initiates the pathway. β-Blockers, ACE inhibitors, angiotensin receptor antagonists, and aldosterone receptor antagonists all inhibit steps in the RAAS pathway. Functional genomic polymorphisms appear to influence therapy targeted at the RAAS pathway, including β_1-receptor variant 389 Gly/Arg, the ACE allelic deletion/insertion (D/I) polymorphism, the aldosterone synthase promoter polymorphism, and the G protein β_3 subunit (GNB3) 894T haplotype (Table 42-1). A review of the functional nature of these polymorphisms, their effect on the pathogenesis of heart failure, and their effects on therapy demonstrates the potential utility of pharmacogenetic analysis.

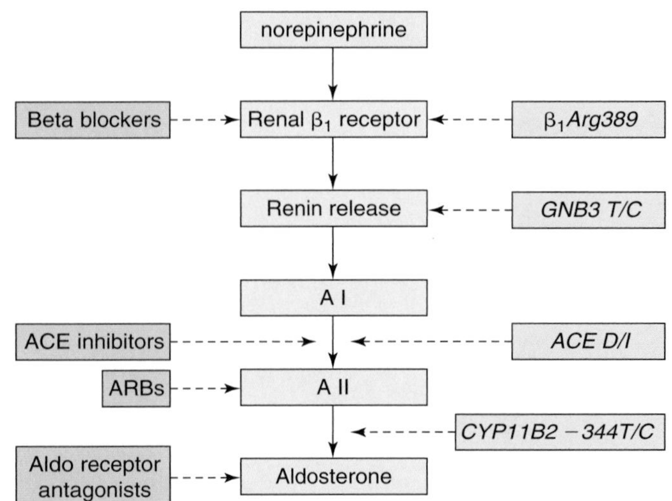

FIGURE 42–1 Renin-angiotensin-aldosterone systemic (RAAS) pathway and site of action of drug therapies and functional polymorphisms. Major pharmacological therapies that improve survival in heart failure (in *white boxes:* β-blockers, angiotensin-converting enzyme [ACE] inhibitors, angiotensin receptor blockers [ARBs], and aldosterone [Aldo] receptor antagonists) all act on RAAS. Major genetic polymorphisms (in *gray boxes:* β_1-receptor Arg389 variant, G protein β 3 subunit [GNB3 T haplotype linked to low plasma renin], ACE D/I [deletion/insertion], and aldosterone synthase [CYP11B2] promoter) influence outcomes and the effects of therapy. A I, angiotensin I; A II, angiotensin II.

THE ANGIOTENSIN-CONVERTING ENZYME DELETION/INSERTION POLYMORPHISM

The ACE deletion/insertion (D/I) biallelic polymorphism of intron 16[1,2] is the polymorphism most extensively studied in cardiovascular disease, and its potential implications for the progression of heart failure have long been recognized.[3] The D allele has been linked to increased activity of ACE, and higher levels of the peptide mediator angiotensin II in multiple clinical situations, including hypertension and post–myocardial infarction status.[4-7] In view of the importance of ACE in the pathogenesis of heart failure, it was predicted that the ACE D allele would be associated with accelerated disease progression and would act as a disease modifier. Indeed, this has been demonstrated in multiple investigations of heart failure.[3,8,9]

Pharmacogenetics of the ACE D Allele: β-Blockers and Angiotensin-Converting Enzyme Inhibitors

The adverse influence of the ACE D allele on survival with heart failure is predicted from the increase in the activity of ACE, which is associated with the deletion. As a result, therapies that directly target and limit angiotensin activation would potentially have more effect in subjects with the ACE D allele. Indeed, the effect of both β-blockers[10] and ACE inhibitors[11] is greatest in patients with heart failure who have the homozygous ACE DD genotype. This was demonstrated in the Genetic Risk Assessment of Cardiac Events (GRACE) study, a prospective investigation of pharmacogenetics and clinical outcomes in systolic heart failure, conducted at the University of Pittsburgh. The effect of the ACE D allele on survival was evident exclusively in subjects not treated with β-blockers[10,11] (Figure 42-2). This pharmacogenetic interaction of β-blockers and the ACE D allele is mediated through the β_1-receptor[12] and probably reflects the suppression of renin release by β-receptor antagonists.

Although the effect of the ACE D allele was most evident for subjects not taking β-blockers, it could still be eliminated in this subset by treatment with high-dose ACE inhibitors[11] (Figure 42-3). The genetic risk of accelerated progression of heart failure conferred by inheritance of the ACE D allele can therefore be effectively eliminated by pharmacotherapies designed to limit the effects of ACE activity: ACE inhibitors and β-receptor antagonists. The potential for "pharmacogenetic targeting" with this single locus is apparent when the effects of these two therapies is investigated within ACE genotype subsets. The effect of therapy consisting of both ACE inhibitor and β-blocker is predicted according to ACE genotype; the effects are strongest in patients with the ACE DD genotype, intermediate in patients with the heterozygous ACE DI genotype, and minimal in patients with the homozygous ACE II genotype (Figure 42-4).

The adverse influence of the ACE D allele on progression of heart failure and on survival has been consistently demonstrated. In an examination of more than 3000 subjects with hypertension, investigators found poorer survival rates among subjects with the ACE DD genotype.[13] Results of investigation of subjects after myocardial infarction suggested that the D allele is also associated with increased left ventricular remodeling.[14] The mechanism remains linked to angiotensin activation, inasmuch as in subjects with advanced heart failure, the D allele is associated with high serum levels of ACE, angiotensin II, and aldosterone.[15] Not surprisingly, the ACE D/I genotype also appears to be predictive of the time course of blood pressure response to ACE inhibitors but not other to antihypertensives.[16]

Genetic variability in the ACE pathway is not limited to the ACE D/I polymorphisms, and additional RAAS polymorphisms also influence blood pressure response to ACE inhibitors. In a study of more than 1400 hypertensive patients, the effects of ACE inhibitor therapy on blood pressure were linked to polygenetic variation in both the angiotensinogen and angiotensin II receptor genes.[17] In a second study of 450 patients with heart failure, haplotypes of the angiotensinogen gene were associated with poorer outcomes.[18]

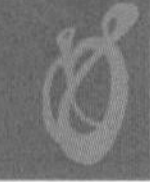

TABLE 42–1 Genetic Polymorphisms and Heart Failure Therapeutics

Signaling Pathway	Gene (References)	Polymorphism	Functional Significance	Potential Therapeutic Influence
Renin-angiotensin-aldosterone systemic (RAAS) pathway	ACE[8-12]	D/I	ACE D: higher ACE activity and A II levels	ACE inhibitors β-blockers
	Aldosterone synthase (CYP11B2)[49-51]	Promoter-344 T/C	-344 C: increased transcriptional activity and aldosterone production	ACE inhibitors Aldosterone receptor antagonistsI/H
β-Adrenergic receptors	β_1AR[23-26]	Arg389Gly	Arg: increased adrenergic signal	β-Blockers ACE inhibitors
	β_1AR[32,33]	Gly49Ser	Gly: enhanced downregulation	β-Blockers
	β_2AR[34,35]	Gly16Arg, Gln27Gly	Receptor downregulation	β-Blockers
α-Adrenergic signaling	α_{2c} Receptor[36,37,39-41]	α_{2c} Deletion	Deletion: decreased uptake of norepinephrine	β-Blockers
	G protein β_3 subunit (GNB3)[62,63]	C825T	825T: increased α-adrenergic signaling, lower plasma renin	ACE inhibitorsI/H
Nitric oxide	Endothelial nitric oxide synthase (NOS3)[60,61]	Asp298Glu	Asp: associated with lower NOS3 activity	ACE inhibitorsI/H

ACE, angiotensin-converting enzyme; β_1AR, β_1-adrenergic receptor; β_2AR, β_2-adrenergic receptor; D/I, deletion/insertion; I/H, isosorbide dinitrate and hydralazine; NOS3, endothelial nitric oxide synthase.

β-Receptor Polymorphisms and β-Receptor Antagonists

The therapeutic efficacy of β-blockers in heart failure reflects not only the inhibition of renin release but also the direct effect of the receptor antagonist on myocardial β_1- and β_2-receptors (see Chapter 10). Two β_1- and three β_2-receptor polymorphisms influence receptor function or downregulation in vitro. The pharmacogenetic interactions of these polymorphisms with β-receptor agonists and antagonists have been investigated in subjects with asthma and hypertension. The β_1-receptor variants have been explored most extensively in subjects with heart failure.[19-22] The Gly389Arg polymorphism is located in the intracellular region of the receptor. The Arg389 allele is more responsive to agonist stimulation and is the dominant allele. In the genetic substudy of the Beta-Blocker Evaluation of Survival Trial (BEST) of bucindolol in heart failure, subjects with the Arg389Arg genotype (approximately half the study group) had a much greater benefit from β-blockade than did subjects heterozygous or homozygous for the Gly389 allele, which was less responsive to the agonist.[23] In BEST, treatment with bucindolol was much less effective in African American patients, and it has been hypothesized that this may reflect lower frequency of the Arg389 allele among African Americans.[24]

The finding that subjects homozygous for the more active β_1-receptor variant receive more benefit from the β antagonist bucindolol conforms to an attractive hypothesis; however, attempts to replicate this finding with metoprolol and carvedilol have not been successful.[25] For subjects randomly assigned to receive either metoprolol succinate or placebo in the Metoprolol CR/XL Randomised Intervention Trial in Congestive Heart Failure (MERIT-HF), a genetic substudy demonstrated no effect of the Arg389 allele on either heart failure survival or the effect of therapy.[26] These results may reflect differences in the receptor sensitivities of the two agents, as well as the partial agonist properties of bucindolol. In addition, of relevance is that in contrast to BEST, the MERIT-HF genetic substudy was completed in a more homogeneous European cohort. In a large prospective cohort of more than 2000 subjects, the effect of the Gly389 allele on β-blocker therapy was modified by the coinheritance of the Gln41Gln genotype of G protein receptor kinase (GRK5), a downstream mediator of adrenergic signaling.[27]

Further evidence for the influence of β-receptor genotype on β-blocker therapy was obtained in studies of left ventricular remodeling. A study of carvedilol therapy in nonischemic cardiomyopathy demonstrated a marked increase in left ventricular ejection fraction (LVEF) in subjects with improvements of 19 ejection fraction (EF) units among subjects with Arg389Arg, 9 EF units among subjects with Gly389Gly, and 6 EF units among subjects with Gly389Gly. These results were consistent with the observed survival effect in the BEST trial.[28] Meta-analysis of three additional studies demonstrated improvements in LVEF, which were 5 EF units greater in subjects with Arg389Arg than in subjects with Gly389Arg or Gly389Gly.[29]

Although the Arg389Gly polymorphism is the most extensively studied, clinical investigations suggest that the Ser49Gly polymorphism also influences outcomes in heart failure.[30] This polymorphism is a variant that alters protein function secondary to a change in the amino acid sequence of the extracellular region. Receptors with the less common allele, Gly49, have an increased rate of receptor downregulation in vitro in response to agonist stimulation,[31] and the Gly49 receptor is linked more with an enhanced response to β-blocker therapy.[32] According to investigations in hypertension, haplotype analysis, which incorporates data from both polymorphisms, best predicts the effect of β-blockade treatment.[33] Common polymorphisms also exist in the extracellular region of the β_2-adrenergic receptors (Gly16Arg and Gln27Gly) and also influence receptor downregulation in vitro. One report suggested that the subjects with heart failure who are homozygous for the Arg16Gln27 haplotype have an increased risk of death or transplantation.[34] A separate study of left ventricular remodeling revealed no influence of the β_2-receptor polymorphisms on left ventricular size and ejection fraction.[35] In contrast to the findings with β_1-receptor polymorphisms, those with β_2-receptor polymorphisms appear less consistent in subjects with heart failure, and there is less evidence of their influence on the effectiveness of β-blockade.

α_{2c}-Adrenergic Receptor Deletion

It is increasingly recognized that most if not all pharmacogenetic influences on specific therapies (e.g., β-blockers in heart failure) are polygenic and involve multiple loci. Variations in α-adrenergic receptors are important genomic modifiers and appear to influence the effect of the β-receptor variants. The α_{2c} receptor has a common deletion allele, in which four amino acids are missing,[36] which limits the reuptake of catecholamines by the presynaptic cell[37,38] and magnifies the

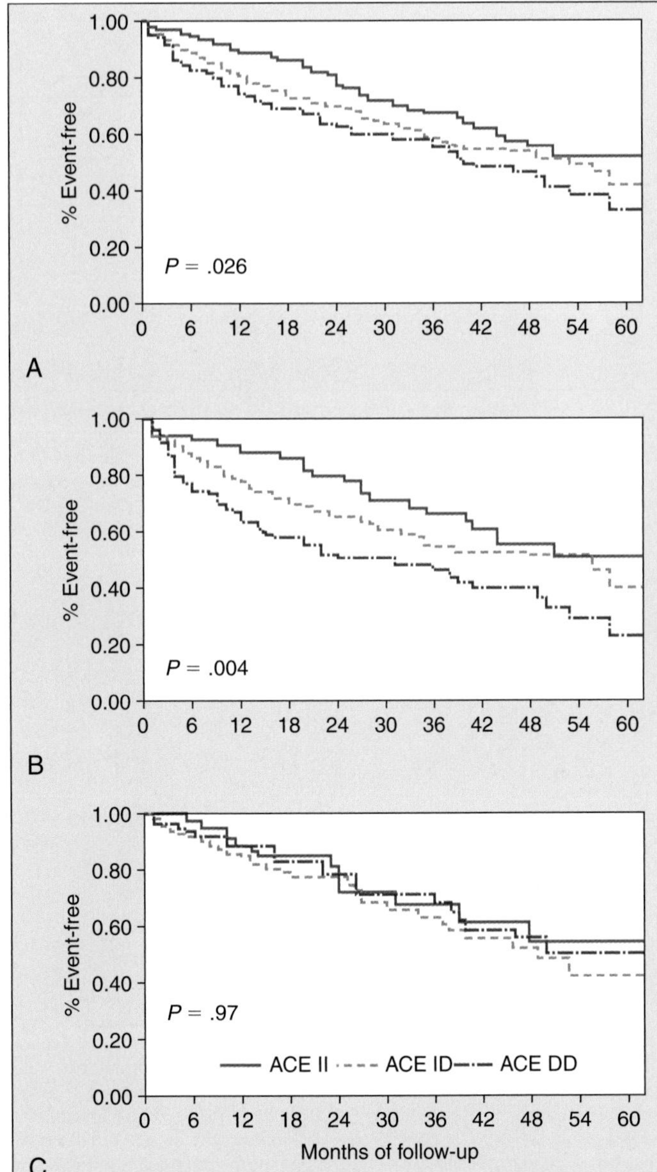

FIGURE 42–2 Transplant-free survival according to angiotensin-converting enzyme (ACE) deletion/insertion (D/I) genotype (DD, DI, and II), from the Genetic Risk Assessment of Cardiac Events (GRACE) study, University of Pittsburgh.[11] **A,** Data for the overall cohort, in which the ACE D allele was associated with poorer event-free survival (n = 479, P = .026). **B,** Data for the subset of patients who received no β-blocker therapy (n = 277, P = .004). **C,** Data for the subset of patients treated with β-blocker therapy (n = 202, P = .97). (From McNamara DM, Holubkov R, Postava L, et al. Pharmacogenetic interactions between ACE inhibitor therapy and the angiotensin-converting enzyme deletion polymorphism in patients with congestive heart failure. *J Am Coll Cardiol* 2004;44:2019-2026.)

effect of agonist stimulation of the Arg389 receptor. The coinheritance of Arg389 and α_{2c} increases the risk of heart failure in African Americans.[39] This synergistic interaction is not limited to African Americans with heart failure, and a larger analysis of clinical outcomes in heart failure determined that coinheritance of β_1-receptor and α_{2c}-receptor variants increased the risk of death or the need for transplantation.[40] As these two loci interact for heart failure risk, they also act synergistically in determining the effect of β-blocker therapy. In a study of the effect of metoprolol on LVEF, coinheritance of the α_{2c} deletion and Arg389Arg genotype was predictive of the greatest therapeutic effect of β-blockade.[41] Similar analysis from BEST[42] suggested that predictive models of β-blocker response need to incorporate both loci.

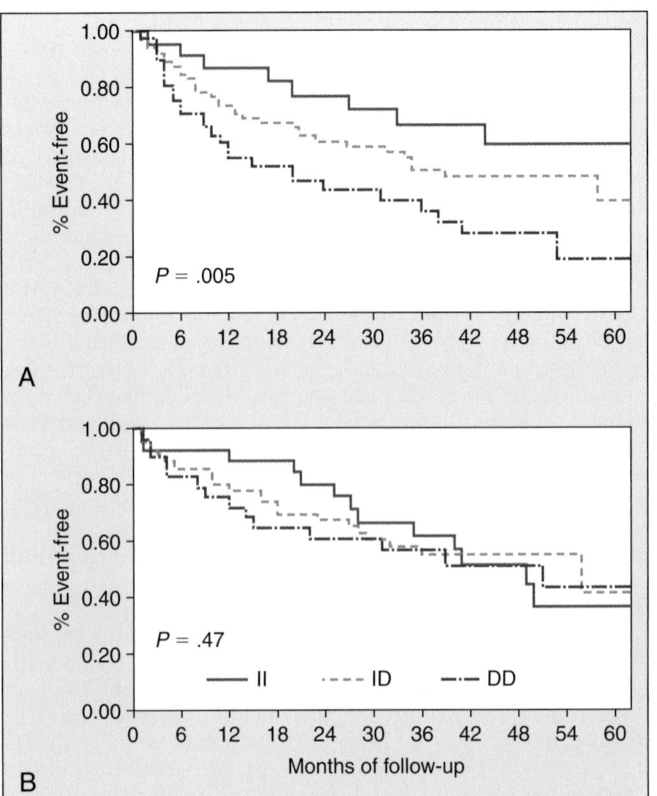

FIGURE 42–3 Pharmacogenetic interaction of the angiotensin-converting enzyme (ACE) deletion (D) allele and ACE inhibitor dosage in a cohort of the Genetic Risk Assessment of Cardiac Events (GRACE) study. **A,** Transplant-free survival of subjects with systolic heart failure who were treated with low-dose ACE inhibitors and no β-blockers (n = 130). The ACE D allele was associated with markedly poor outcome (P = .005). **B,** Transplant-free survival of subjects treated with high-dose ACE inhibitors and no β-blockers (n = 117). The effect of the ACE D allele was diminished (P = .47). (From McNamara DM, Holubkov R, Postava L, et al. Pharmacogenetic interactions between ACE inhibitor therapy and the angiotensin-converting enzyme deletion polymorphism in patients with congestive heart failure. *J Am Coll Cardiol* 2004;44:2019-2026.)

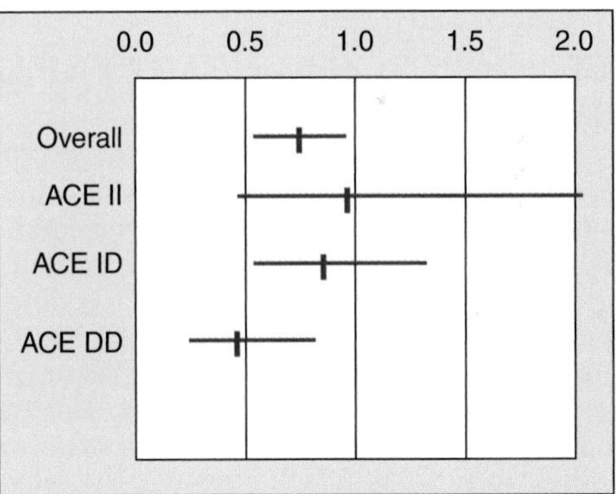

FIGURE 42–4 Relative risk of event (death or transplantation) according to β-blocker use in the Genetic Risk Assessment of Cardiac Events (GRACE) study: Data from the overall cohort and comparison of angiotensin-converting enzyme (ACE) deletion/insertion (D/I) genotypes (DD, DI, and II). (Adapted from McNamara DM, Holubkov R, Postava L, et al. Pharmacogenetic interactions between ACE inhibitor therapy and the angiotensin-converting enzyme deletion polymorphism in patients with congestive heart failure. *J Am Coll Cardiol* 2004;44:2019-2026, Table 4.)

Aldosterone Synthase

Aldosterone receptor antagonists improve survival in advanced heart failure[43] and after myocardial infarction,[44] and aldosterone activation is the most recently recognized target of neurohormonal inhibition in heart failure. The promoter polymorphism (C-344T) of the aldosterone synthase gene

(CYP11B2) is located in a steroid-binding region and appears to affect gene transcription. It has been investigated extensively in cardiovascular disease. The -344C allele is linked to the risk of hypertension, higher aldosterone synthase activity,[45] and greater left ventricular maladaptive remodeling.[46] The effect of the -344C allele was evaluated in the genetic substudy of the African American Heart Failure Trial (AHeFT), in which researchers investigated the addition of a fixed-dose combination of isosorbide dinitrate and hydralazine (I/H) to standard background heart failure therapy.[47] This substudy, Genetic Risk Assessment of Heart Failure in African Americans (GRAHF), was initiated to evaluate the ability of genomic polymorphisms identified in mostly white cohorts to predict outcomes in African Americans with systolic heart failure and to determine the genomic basis for racial differences in therapeutic efficacy of I/H and ACE inhibitors. In GRAHF, the aldosterone synthase promoter polymorphism was evaluated, and the -344C allele was found to be associated with significantly poorer event-free survival during the course of follow up[48] (Figure 42-5). The adverse effect of the -344C allele in risk of events was evident for both death (P = .001) and hospitalization for heart failure (P = .013), inasmuch as the majority of events occurred in subjects with the -344CC genotype (Figure 42-6).

The -344C allele was also linked to left ventricular remodeling; however its effect was diminished by treatment with I/H. An association of the -344C allele with lower LVEF at 6 months was apparent in subjects randomly assigned to receive placebo but not evident in patients treated with I/H (Figure 42-7). The effect of I/H therapy on remodeling for the -344 CC genotype mirrored the effect of conventional therapy with ACE inhibitors and β-blockers in a separate cohort of African Americans with heart failure, in which improvements at 1 year in left ventricular systolic dimension were greater in subjects with the -344CC genotype.[49] Not all studies demonstrate greater efficacy of therapy; a randomized study of 500 hypertensive subjects demonstrated diminished effect of ACE inhibitors on blood pressure in subjects with the -344CC genotype.[50] Surprisingly, the results from the AHeFT trial suggest that treatment with the aldosterone receptor antagonist spironolactone did not diminish the adverse affect of the C allele on left ventricular remodeling.[47]

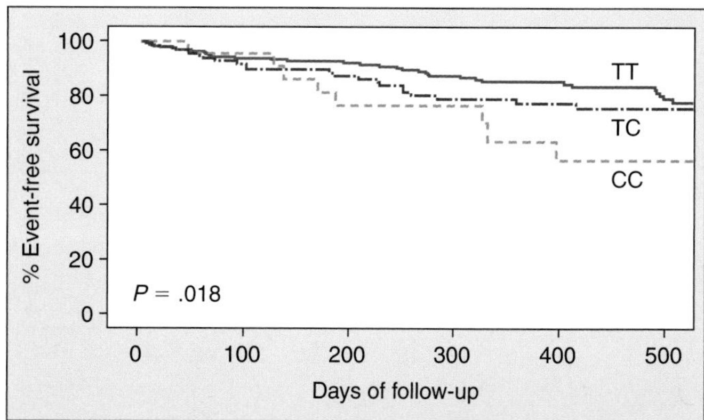

FIGURE 42-5 Kaplan-Meier analysis from the African American Heart Failure Trial (AHeFT) of survival free from hospitalization for heart failure, demonstrating effect of aldosterone synthase (CYP11B2) promoter genotype (TT, TC, and CC). The -344C allele was linked to increased aldosterone levels and associated with poorer event-free survival (P = .018). (From McNamara DM, Tam SW, Sabolinski ML, et al. Aldosterone synthase promoter polymorphism predicts outcome in African Americans with heart failure. *J Am Coll Cardiol* 2006;48:1277-1282).

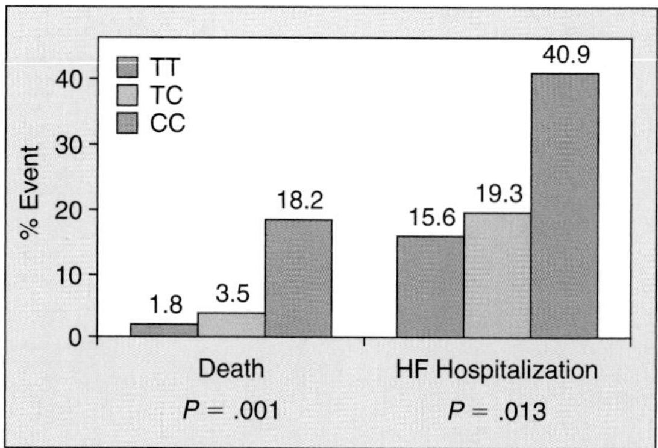

FIGURE 42-6 Percentage of subjects in the African American Heart Failure Trial (AHeFT) with events by the end of the study, according to aldosterone synthase (CYP11B2) promoter T-344C genotype. The -344C allele was associated with increased risk of death (P = .001) and increased hospitalizations for heart failure (HF) (P = .013). (From McNamara DM, Tam SW, Sabolinski ML, et al. Aldosterone synthase promoter polymorphism predicts outcome in African Americans with heart failure. *J Am Coll Cardiol* 2006;48:1277-1282).

RACE, GENOMICS, AND HEART FAILURE THERAPY

The efficacy of medical therapies such as ACE inhibitors and I/H differs between white and African American patients with heart failure. The first Veteran's Administration Cooperative Vasodilator–Heart Failure Trial (V-HeFT I) demonstrated that I/H improved survival in subjects with heart failure[51]; however, this benefit was evident in the African American patients and less evident in white patients.[52] In the second V-HeFT study (V-HeFT II), the ACE inhibitor enalapril yielded results superior to those of I/H[53]; however, the superiority of ACE inhibitors was primarily in the white subjects and was not evident among African American patients with heart failure.[52] The observation of increased effect of I/H in African American cohorts led to the study design of A-HeFT, and this landmark trial evaluated the efficacy of fixed-combination I/H specifically in self-designated African Americans.[47] The results of the trial confirmed benefits of I/H and for the first time led to the approval by the U.S. Food and Drug Administration of a heart failure therapy in a specific racial subset (see Chapter 49). Race is probably a poor surrogate for differences in genomic background,[54] and investigations have focused increasingly on genetic variants that may underlie racial differences in therapeutic efficacy.

Common polymorphisms in genes that control vascular tone have been investigated for their role in the development

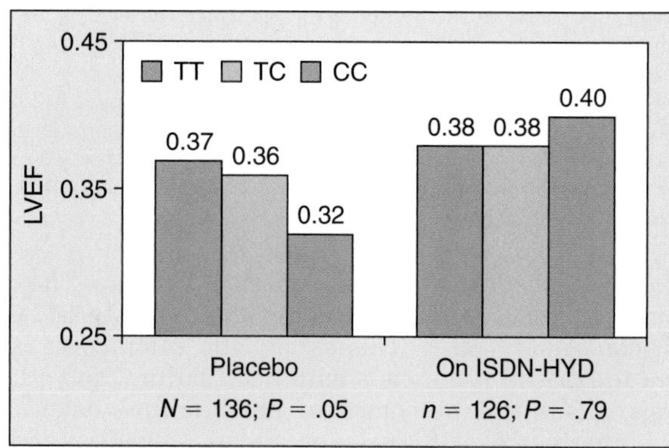

FIGURE 42-7 Left ventricular ejection fraction (LVEF) at 6 months in the African American Heart Failure Trial (AHeFT): Comparison of treatment group—placebo or fixed-dose combination of isosorbide dinitrate and hydralazine (I-H)—with the effect of aldosterone promoter genotype. The -344C allele is associated with lower LVEF at 6 months for subjects receiving placebo (P = .05) but not for those receiving I-H (P = .79). (From McNamara DM, Tam SW, Sabolinski ML, et al. Endothelial nitric oxide synthase (NOS3) polymorphisms in African Americans with heart failure: results from the A-HeFT trial. *J Card Fail* 2009;15:191-198.)

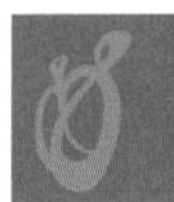

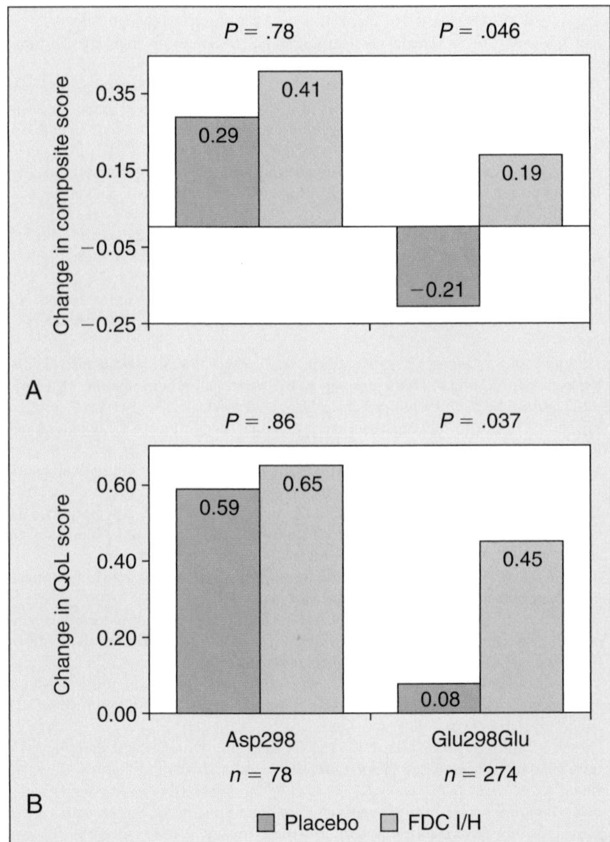

FIGURE 42-8 Interaction of nitric oxide synthase (NOS3) Glu298Asp polymorphisms and treatment with fixed-dose combination of isosorbide dinitrate and hydralazine (FDC I/H). **A,** Effect on composite score. Treatment was associated with improvement in the Glu298Glu homozygotes (n = 274, P = .046) but not in subjects with the Asp298 allele (n = 78, P = .78). **B,** Effect on change in quality of life (QoL). Significant improvement in QoL score at 6 months was demonstrated in subjects with the Glu298Glu allele (P = .037) but not in those with the Asp298 allele. (From McNamara DM, Tam SW, Sabolinski ML, et al. Endothelial nitric oxide synthase (NOS3) polymorphisms in African Americans with heart failure: results from the A-HeFT trial. *J Card Fail* 2009;15:191-198.)

of essential hypertension. Hypertension is much more prevalent in African Americans, and significant racial differences in the prevalence of genomic variants are evident for endothelial nitric oxide synthase (NOS3; also known as eNOS), aldosterone synthase, and α and β-adrenergic receptors. In addition to their role in hypertension, these genetic loci also play central roles in the pathogenesis of heart failure and in therapeutics.

The genetic substudy of AHeFT was designed to determine whether genetic alleles would be predictive of benefit from treatment with I/H. Because the prevalence of several polymorphisms of NOS3—the primary source of vascular nitric oxide production[55]—differs markedly between African American and white cohorts,[56,57] this locus emerged as a prime candidate for a genetic modifier of therapeutic efficacy. A polymorphism exists in exon 7 of NOS3, which results in the substitution of glutamic acid (Glu) for aspartic acid (Asp) at codon 298. The Asp298 variant is a reported risk factor for hypertension,[58] coronary disease,[59] and poor survival rates with heart failure.[60] The Glu298 variant is far more prevalent in African American cohorts. With regard to the primary endpoint in A-HeFT (a composite score of survival, hospitalization for heart failure, and quality of life), subjects in GRAHF who had the Glu-298Glu genotype benefited significantly from therapy, whereas subjects with the Asp298 variant did not[61] (Figure 42-8). Further investigation is necessary to determine whether the NOS3 genotype can effectively target nitric oxide donor therapy.

There is a much higher prevalence of hypertensive cardiomyopathy (and a lower prevalence of coronary disease) among African American populations with heart failure than is evident in similar white cohorts. Adrenergic signaling is influenced by functional genetic variants, including the α_{2c} deletion and the C825T polymorphism of GNB3. The C825T polymorphism is functionally silent; however, the T allele is linked to a splicing variant, which results in the loss of 41 amino acids. The truncated GNB3 inhibitory subunit increases α-adrenergic signaling, is associated with a higher risk of hypertension, and is far more prevalent among African Americans than among white patients.[62] Increased α-adrenergic tone may underlie the high prevalence of low-renin hypertension in African Americans.[63] In addition to differences in α-adrenergic signaling, the prevalence of several genetic polymorphisms that influence heart failure therapeutics—including β_1-adrenergic receptor (β_1AR; Arg389),[23] NOS3,[60] and aldosterone synthase[48]—also differs between white and African American cohorts. Whether these genetic differences result in differences in the efficacy of ACE inhibitors or I/H remains to be determined.

GENOME-WIDE ASSOCIATION STUDIES

Pharmacogenetic studies to date have focused predominantly on evaluating the interaction of a single gene locus with the efficacy of a given drug. In addition, most studies have been targeted at genes known to play critical roles in heart failure therapeutics: for example, ACE and the β_1-receptor. Advances in technology have made large-scale mapping of the human genome more efficient and affordable, and the realization that most human DNA is "inherited" in large blocks or haplotypes has led to the development of high-density genomic maps.[64] This has facilitated GWASs, in which the frequency of variants or markers across the entire genome is assessed in large cohorts with a disorder under investigation and compared with findings in a large control group. This technology has been applied to common complex polygenic diseases such as coronary artery disease,[65] hyperlipidemia,[66] and diabetes[67] and has elicited extensive new information about genes that contribute to these complex disorders. Although not yet applied to the pharmacogenomics of heart failure, GWASs have the potential to determine the genomic loci that will "drive" any predictive model of drug efficacy. Bioinformatics analysis, which incorporates multiple genomic drivers for any specific clinical paradigm (e.g., the effect of I/H in heart failure), will be used to convert genomic information into a useful clinical tool for efficiently targeting therapeutics.

FUTURE DIRECTIONS

Genetic variation of key mediators of heart failure alters the effect of therapeutics that act on particular pathways. Patients who are genetically predisposed to greater renin-angiotensin activation by the presence of the ACE deletion allele obtain greater benefit from therapies (β-blockers and high-dose ACE inhibitors) designed to blunt this response. In addition, patients with the more active β_1-receptor 389Arg variant appear to obtain more clinical benefit when that receptor is blocked than do subjects with the less active 389Gly variant. Significant genetic differences in the nitric oxide pathway exist between white and African American patients with heart failure, and these differences may underlie the apparent enhanced response in African Americans to treatment with I/H. All these examples demonstrate the potential power of pharmacogenomics to target treatments and transform heart failure therapy.

Despite these findings in single gene studies since the 1990s, disagreement between pharmacogenetic analysis in clinical trials such as BEST and MERIT-HF and the lack of prospective validation studies have prevented pharmacogenomics from playing a role in clinical care by facilitating patient-specific therapy for heart failure. Replicating results of published studies has been difficult because some studies have been simply too small to attain statistical significance. The results of pharmacogenomic studies that assess the relevance of a single genetic variant may not be correlated with results that would be expected on the basis of the physiological and biochemical properties of the mutated protein because many responses are polygenic. Thus, pharmacogenetic evaluations must move beyond single-nucleotide polymorphism analysis if they are to become effective tools in clinical medicine.

As a result of the development of robust new technology and automation, the phase of pharmacogenomic investigation concerned with targeted single-gene loci will evolve toward polygenic analysis. This will allow multiple genomic drivers to be evaluated for each clinical phenotype and each therapeutic strategy. However, federal regulatory agencies must ensure that pharmacogenomic analysis is included in the routine evaluation of new pharmacological agents. With this new information, it is hoped that genomic analysis will soon become part of routine laboratory assessment and will allow clinicians to individualize pharmacotherapy and optimize outcomes for each patient with heart failure. This will decrease the cost of health care and, at the same time, allow patients to avoid the potential side effects of unnecessary drugs.

REFERENCES

1. Rigat, B., Hubert, C., Alhenc-Gelas, F., et al. (1990). An insertion/deletion polymorphism in the angiotensin I–converting enzyme gene accounting for half the variance of serum enzyme levels. *J Clin Invest, 86*, 1343–1346.
2. Rigat, B., Hubert, C., Corvol, P., et al. (1992). PCR detection of the insertion/deletion polymorphism of the human angiotensin converting enzyme gene (DCP) (dipeptidyl carboxypeptidase 1). *Nucleic Acids Res, 20*, 1433.
3. Raynolds, M. V., Bristow, M. R., Bush, E. W., et al. (1993). Angiotensin-converting enzyme DD genotype in patients with ischaemic or idiopathic dilated cardiomyopathy. *Lancet, 342*, 1073–1075.
4. Tiret, L., Rigat, B., Visvikis, S., et al. (1992). Evidence, from combined segregation and linkage analysis, that a variant of the angiotensin I–converting enzyme (ACE) gene controls plasma ACE levels. *Am J Hum Genet, 51*, 197–205.
5. Danser, A. H., Derkx, F. H., Hense, H. W., et al. (1998). Angiotensinogen (M235T) and angiotensin-converting enzyme (I/D) polymorphisms in association with plasma renin and prorenin levels. *J Hypertens, 16*, 1879–1883.
6. Cambien, F., Poirier, O., Lecerf, L., et al. (1992). Deletion polymorphism in the gene for angiotensin-converting enzyme is a potent risk factor for myocardial infarction. *Nature, 359*, 641–644.
7. Ihnken, R., Verho, K., Gross, M., et al. (1996). Deletion polymorphism of the angiotensin I–converting enzyme gene is associated with increased plasma angiotensin-converting enzyme activity but not with increased risk for myocardial infarction and coronary artery disease. *Ann Intern Med, 125*, 19–25.
8. Andersson, B., & Sylven, C. (1996). The DD genotype of the angiotensin-converting enzyme gene is associated with increased mortality in idiopathic heart failure. *J Am Coll Cardiol, 28*, 162–167.
9. Palmer, B. R., Pilbrow, A. P., Yandle, T. G., et al. (2003). Angiotensin-converting enzyme gene polymorphism interacts with left ventricular ejection fraction and brain natriuretic peptide levels to predict mortality after myocardial infarction. *J Am Coll Cardiol, 41*, 729–736.
10. McNamara, D. M., Holubkov, R., Janosko, K., et al. (2001). Pharmacogenetic interactions between beta blocker therapy and the angiotensin converting enzyme deletion polymorphism in patients with congestive heart failure. *Circulation, 103*, 1644–1648.
11. McNamara, D. M., Holubkov, R., Postava, L., et al. (2004). Pharmacogenetic interactions between ACE inhibitor therapy and the angiotensin-converting enzyme deletion polymorphism in patients with congestive heart failure. *J Am Coll Cardiol, 44*, 2019–2026.
12. Ishizawar, D., Janosko, K. M., Teuteberg, J. J., et al. (2008). The β_1-adrenergic receptor mediates the pharmacogenetic interaction of the ACE D allele and β-blockers. *Clin Transl Sci, 1*(2), 151–154.
13. Bleumink, G. S., Schut, A. F. C., Sturkenboom, M. C. J. M., et al. (2005). Mortality in patients with hypertension on angiotensin-1 converting enzyme (ACE)–inhibitor treatment is influenced by the ACE insertion/deletion polymorphism. *Pharmacogenet Genomics, 15*, 75–81.
14. Ulgen, M. S., Ozturk, O., Alan, S., et al. (2007). The relationship between angiotensin-converting enzyme (insertion/deletion) gene polymorphism and left ventricular remodeling in acute myocardial infarction. *Coron Artery Dis, 18*, 153–157.
15. Tang, W. H. W., Vagelos, R. H., Yee, Y. G., et al. (2004). Impact of angiotensin-converting enzyme gene polymorphism on neurohormonal responses to high- versus low-dose enalapril in advanced heart failure. *Am Heart J, 148*, 889–894.
16. Bhatnagar, V., O'Connor, D. T., Schork, N. J., et al. (2007). Angiotensin-converting enzyme gene polymorphism predicts the time-course of blood pressure response to angiotensin converting enzyme inhibition in the AASK trial. *J Hypertens, 25*, 2082–2092.
17. Su, X., Lee, L., Li, X., et al. (2007). Association between angiotensinogen, angiotensin II receptor genes, and blood pressure response to an angiotensin-converting enzyme inhibitor. *Circulation, 115*, 725–732.
18. Pilbrow, A. P., Palmer, B. R., Frampton, C. M., et al. (2007). Angiotensinogen M235T and T174M gene polymorphisms in combination doubles the risk of mortality in heart failure. *Hypertension, 49*, 322–327.
19. McNamara, D. M., MacGowan, G. A., & London, B. (2001). Clinical importance of beta receptor polymorphisms in cardiovascular disease. *Am J Pharmacogenomics, 2*(2), 73–78.
20. Feldman, D. S., Carnes, C. A., Abraham, W. T., et al. (2005). Mechanisms of disease β-adrenergic receptors—alternations in signal transduction and pharmacogenomics in heart failure. *Nat Clin Pract Cardiovasc Med, 2*, 475–483.
21. Liggett, S. B. (2010). Pharmacogenomics of β_1-adrenergic receptor polymorphisms in heart failure. *Heart Fail Clin, 6*, 27–33.
22. Murphy, G. A., Fiuzat, M., Bristow, M. R. (2010). Targeting heart failure therapeutics: a historical perspective. *Heart Fail Clin, 6*, 11–23.
23. Liggett, S. B., Mialet-Perez, J., Thaneemit-Chen, S., et al. (2006). A polymorphism within a conserved β_1-adrenergic receptor motif alters cardiac function and β-blocker response in human heart failure. *Proc Natl Acad Sci U S A, 103*, 11288–11293.
24. Couzin, J. (2005). American Association for the Advancement of Science meeting. DNA tells story of heart drug failure. *Science, 307*, 1191.
25. Sehnert, A. J., Daniels, S. E., Elashoff, M., et al. (2008). Lack of association between adrenergic receptor genotypes and survival in heart failure patients treated with carvedilol or metoprolol. *J Am Coll Cardiol, 52*, 644–651.
26. White, H., deBoer, R. A., Maqbool, A., et al. (2003). An evaluation of the beta-1 adrenergic receptor Arg389Gly polymorphism in individuals with heart failure: a MERIT-HF sub-study. *Eur J Heart Fail, 5*, 463–468.
27. Cresci, S., Kelly, R. J., Cappola, T. P., et al. (2009). Clinical and genetic modifiers of long-term survival in heart failure. *J Am Coll Cardiol, 54*, 432–444.
28. Chen, L., Meyers, D., Javorsky, G., et al. (2007). Arg389Gly- β_1-adrenergic receptors determine improvement in left ventricular systolic function in nonischemic cardiomyopathy patients with heart failure after chronic treatment with carvedilol. *Pharmacogenet Genomics, 17*, 941–949.
29. Muthumala, A., Drenos, F., Elliott, P. M., et al. (2008). Role of β adrenergic receptor polymorphisms in heart failure: systematic review and meta-analysis. *Eur J Heart Fail, 10*, 3–13.
30. Börjesson, M., Magnusson, Y., Hjalmarson, A., et al. (2000). A novel polymorphism in the gene coding for the beta (1)-adrenergic receptor associated with survival in patients with heart failure. *Eur Heart J, 21*, 1853–1858.
31. Brodde, O. E. (2008). β1 and β2 adrenoceptor polymorphisms: functional importance, impact on cardiovascular diseases and drug responses. *Pharmacol Ther, 117*, 1–29.
32. Magnusson, Y., Levin, M. C., Eggertsen, R., et al. (2005). Ser49Gly of β_1-adrenergic receptor is associated with effective β-blocker dose in dilated cardiomyopathy. *Clin Pharmacol Ther, 78*, 221–231.
33. Johnson, J. A., Zineh, I., Puckett, B. J., et al. (2003). Beta 1-adrenergic receptor polymorphisms and antihypertensive response to metoprolol. *Clin Pharmacol Ther, 74*, 44–52.
34. Shin, J., Lobmeyer, M. T., Gong, Y., et al. (2007). Relation of β_2-adrenoceptor haplotype to risk of death and heart transplantation in patients with heart failure. *Am J Cardiol, 99*, 250–255.
35. Badenhorst, D., Norton, G. R., Sliwa, K., et al. (2007). Impact of β_2-adrenoreceptor gene variants on cardiac cavity size and systolic function in idiopathic dilated cardiomyopathy. *Pharmacogenomics, 7*, 339–345.
36. Small, K. M., Forbes, S. L., Rahman, F. F., et al. (2000). A four amino acid deletion polymorphism in the third intracellular loop of the human α_{2c}-adrenergic receptor confers impaired coupling to multiple effectors. *J Biol Chem, 275*, 23059–23064.
37. Small, K. M., Mialet-Perez, J., Seman, C. A., et al. (2004). Polymorphisms of cardiac presynaptic α_{2c} adrenergic receptors: diverse intragenic variability with haplotype-specific function effects. *Proc Natl Acad Sci U S A, 101*, 13020–13025.
38. Gerson, M. C., Wagoner, L. E., McGuire, N., et al. (2003). Activity of the uptake-1 norepinephrine transporter as measured by I-123 MIBG in heart failure patients with a loss-of-function polymorphism of the presynaptic α_{2c}-adrenergic receptor. *J Nucl Cardiol, 10*, 583–589.
39. Small, K. M., Wagoner, L. E., Levin, A. M., et al. (2002). Synergistic polymorphisms of $beta_1$- and $alpha_{2c}$-adrenergic receptors and the risk of congestive heart failure. *N Engl J Med, 347*, 1135–1142.
40. Kardia, S. L., Kelly, R. J., Keddache, M. A., et al. (2008). Multiple interactions between the $alpha_{2c}$- and $beta_1$-adrenergic receptors influence heart failure survival. *BMC Med Genet, 9*, 93.
41. Lobmeyer, M. T., Gong, Y., Terra, S. G., et al. (2007). Synergistic polymorphisms of β_1 and α_{2c}-adrenergic receptors and the influence on left ventricular ejection fraction response to β-blocker therapy in heart failure. *Pharmacogenet Genomics, 17*, 277–282.
42. O'Connor, C. M., Anand, I., Fivzat, M., et al. Additive effects of β1 389 Arg/Gly and α2c 322-325 wild-type/del genotype combinations on adjudicated hospitalizations and death in the Beta-Blocker Evaluation of Survival Trial (BEST). Presented at the Heart Failure Society of America 2008 Scientific Meeting, Toronto, ON, September 2008.
43. Pitt, B., Zannad, F., Remme, W. J., et al. (1999). The effect of spironolactone on morbidity and mortality in patients with severe heart failure. Randomized Aldactone Evaluation Study Investigators. *N Engl J Med, 341*, 709–717.
44. Pitt, B., Remme, W., Zannad, F., et al. (2003). Eplerenone, a selective aldosterone blocker, in patients with left ventricular dysfunction after myocardial infarction. *N Engl J Med, 348*, 1309–1321.

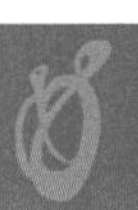

45. Materson, B. J. (2007). Variability in response to antihypertensive drugs. *Am J Med, 120*(4), (Suppl. 1), S10–S20.
46. Tiago, A. D., Badenhorst, D., Skudicky, D., et al. (2002). An aldosterone synthase gene variant is associated with improvement in left ventricular ejection fraction in dilated cardiomyopathy. *Cardiovasc Res, 54*, 584–589.
47. Taylor, A. L., Ziesche, S., Yancy, C., et al. (2004). Combination of isosorbide dinitrate and hydralazine in blacks with heart failure. *N Engl J Med, 351*, 2049–2057.
48. McNamara, D. M., Tam, S. W., Sabolinski, M. L., et al. (2006). Aldosterone synthase promoter polymorphism predicts outcome in African Americans with heart failure. *J Am Coll Cardiol, 48*, 1277–1282.
49. Biolo, A., Chao, T., Duhaney, T. A. S., et al. (2007). Usefulness of the aldosterone synthase gene polymorphism C-344-T to predict cardiac remodeling in African-Americans versus non–African-Americans with chronic systolic heart failure. *Am J Cardiol, 100*, 285–290.
50. Yu, H. M., Lin, S. G., Liu, G. Z., et al. (2006). Associations between CYP11B2 gene polymorphisms and the response to angiotensin-converting enzyme inhibitors. *Clin Pharmacol Ther, 79*, 581–589.
51. Cohn, J. N., Archibald, D. G., Ziesche, S., et al. (1986). Effect of vasodilator therapy on mortality in chronic congestive heart failure. Results of a Veterans Administration cooperative study (V-HeFT). *N Engl J Med, 314*, 1547–1552.
52. Carson, P., Ziesche, S., Johnson, G., et al. (1999), for the Vasodilator-Heart Failure trial Study Group. Racial differences in response to therapy for heart failure: analysis of the Vasodilator-Heart Failure Trials. *J Card Fail, 5*, 178–187.
53. Cohn, J. N., Johnson, G., Ziesche, S., et al. (1991). A comparison of enalapril with hydralazine–isosorbide dinitrate in the treatment of chronic congestive heart failure. *N Engl J Med, 325*, 303–310.
54. Cooper, R. S., Kaufman, J. S., & Ward, R. (2003). Race and genomics. *N Engl J Med, 348*, 1166–1175.
55. Hare, J. M. (2004). Nitroso-redox balance in the cardiovascular system. *N Engl J Med, 351*, 2112–2114.
56. Tanus-Santos, J. E., Desai, M., & Flockhart, D. A. (2001). Effects of ethnicity on the distribution of clinically relevant endothelial nitric oxide variants. *Pharmacogenetics, 11*, 719–725.
57. Marroni, A. S., Metzger, I. F., Souza-Costa, D. C., et al. (2005). Consistent interethnic difference in the distribution of clinically relevant endothelial nitric oxide synthase genetic polymorphisms. *Nitric Oxide, 12*, 177–182.
58. Jáchymová, M., Horký, K., Bultas, J., et al. (2001). Association of the Glu298Asp polymorphism in the endothelial nitric oxide synthase gene with essential hypertension resistant to conventional therapy. *Biochem Biophys Res Commun, 284*, 426–430.
59. Hingorani, A. D., Liang, C. F., Fatibene, J., et al. (1999). A common variant of the endothelial nitric oxide synthase (Glu^{298}→Asp) is a major risk factor for coronary artery disease in the UK. *Circulation, 100*, 1515–1520.
60. McNamara, D. M., Holubkov, R., Postava, L., et al. (2003). The Asp298 variant of endothelial nitric oxide synthase: effect on survival for patients with congestive heart failure. *Circulation, 107*, 1598–1602.
61. McNamara, D. M., Tam, S. W., Sabolinski, M. L., et al. (2009). Endothelial nitric oxide synthase (NOS3) polymorphisms in African Americans with heart failure: results from the A-HeFT trial. *J Card Fail, 15*, 191–198.
62. Siffert, W., Rosskopf, D., Siffert, G., et al. (1998). Association of a human G-protein subunit variant with hypertension. *Nat Genet, 18*, 45–48.
63. Sagnella, G. A. (2001). Why is plasma renin activity lower in populations of African origin? *J Hum Hypertens, 15*, 17–25.
64. Altshuler, D., Brooks, L. D., Chakravarti, A., et al. (2005). A haplotype map of the human genome. *Nature, 437*, 1299–1320.
65. Rampersaud, E., Damcott, C. M., Fu, M., et al. (2007). Identification of novel candidate genes for type 2 diabetes from a genome-wide association scan in the Old Order Amish: evidence for replication from diabetes-related quantitative traits and from independent populations. *Diabetes, 56*, 3053–3062.
66. Kathiresan, S., Manning, A. K., Demissie, S., et al. (2007). A genome-wide association study for blood lipid phenotypes in the Framingham Heart Study. *BMC Med Genet, 8*(Suppl. 1), S17.
67. O'Donnell, C. J., Cupples, L. A., D'Agostino, R. B., et al. (2007). Genome-wide association study for subclinical atherosclerosis in major arterial territories in the NHLBI's Framingham Heart Study. *BMC Med Genet, 8*(Suppl. 1), S4.

CHAPTER 43

Management of Acute Decompensated Heart Failure

Lynne Warner Stevenson

More than 1 million hospitalizations yearly are attributed directly to heart failure, and in approximately 2 million more, heart failure diagnosis complicates other admitting diagnoses such as pulmonary or renal disease.[1] Admissions related to heart failure can be divided about evenly between those for heart failure with low ejection fraction and those for heart failure with "preserved" ejection fraction[2] (Figure 43-1), which in turn is divided between those in which left ventricular ejection fraction (LVEF) is 40% to 55% and those in which LVEF exceeds 55%[3] (Table 43-1). In contrast to trial populations, the average patient from the community who is admitted is 75 years old, with substantial comorbid conditions.

The most common cause of hospitalization for heart failure is exacerbation of chronic heart failure, which accounts for about 75% of admissions for heart failure with low ejection fraction and about 66% of those for heart failure with "preserved" ejection fraction.[4] New diagnoses of heart failure resulting from acute myocardial infarction or acute valvular regurgitation are treated predominantly by specific therapy for those cardiac conditions. Acute heart failure occasionally results from fulminant myocarditis (see Chapter 31), which necessitates rapid institution of life-saving therapies for cardiogenic shock; these therapies may include mechanical support, with good potential for ultimate recovery.[5] This chapter focuses on the management of the most common situation, subacute decompensation in patients with known chronic heart failure.[4,6] Information about the pathophysiology and treatment of decompensated heart failure with preserved ejection fraction is scarcer than information about decompensated heart failure with low ejection fraction, but this discussion indicates which considerations apply to all heart failure and which are restricted to heart failure with low ejection fraction.

INITIAL CLINICAL ASSESSMENT

For patients hospitalized with decompensation and a history of chronic heart failure, the initial assessment should identify contributing factors that necessitate evaluation and focus on fluid status and perfusion, which will guide initial therapy.[6] Because chronic circulatory adaptations can mask decompensation, the first priority should be to assess the level of hemodynamic compromise; in initial triage in urgent care settings, the severity and urgency may be underestimated.[7] Hospitalization should trigger review of both the causes and potential exacerbating factors. For patients with known coronary artery disease, new-onset ischemia should always be considered (see Chapter 23). Other common exacerbating factors are tachyarrhythmias, thyroid disease, anemia, infections, chronic pulmonary disease, and, on occasion, pulmonary emboli[8] (Figure 43-2). Compliance can be undermined by inadequate support structure, poor understanding of the patient because of lack of education about heart failure, or limited literacy and numeracy skills.

RECOGNIZING THE FOUR HEMODYNAMIC PROFILES

The central hemodynamic components of decompensated heart failure are the elevation of filling pressures and the reduction of cardiac output, which do not necessarily occur together, as shown in Figure 43-3.[9] Whether the left ventricular ejection fraction is low or "preserved," the most common manifestation is generally profile B, "warm and wet," with congestion and adequate perfusion. Clinical assessment of congestion is complicated by the frequent absence of rales and peripheral edema in patients with chronic heart failure.[10] Orthopnea in a patient with heart failure is considered an indication of elevated filling pressures until it is proved otherwise.[7,10] For some patients, gastrointestinal symptoms predominate, and needless diagnostic procedures may be performed when the degree of congestion is not appreciated. Jugular venous pressure provides the most visible and reliable index of elevated filling pressures on physical examination[10] (Table 43-2). Although only the right-sided filling pressures are directly assessed in this way, their elevation is nonetheless the best clinical sign of elevated left-sided pressures; they are concordant in about 75% of cases if defining thresholds of right atrial pressure exceed 10 mm Hg and pulmonary capillary wedge pressure exceeds 22 mm Hg.[11] Hepatomegaly, increased radiation of the pulmonary second sound, and serial increases in the intensity of a third heart sound can be informative. For experienced clinicians, the Valsalva maneuver can help identify elevated filling pressures, particularly when cardiac and pulmonary causes of dyspnea coexist.[12] The abdominojugular reflex is a sensitive measure but not very specific.[13] Elevated natriuretic peptide levels may be indicative of heart failure in a patient with unexplained dyspnea, but these levels are chronically elevated in most patients with a previous diagnosis of heart failure; therefore, the finding of a high level may not indicate the presence or severity of worsening congestion.[14] Other clues for elevated filling pressures can be present in echocardiographic findings of moderate or severe mitral or tricuspid regurgitation or pulmonary hypertension in the absence of other causes.[11] Echocardiography

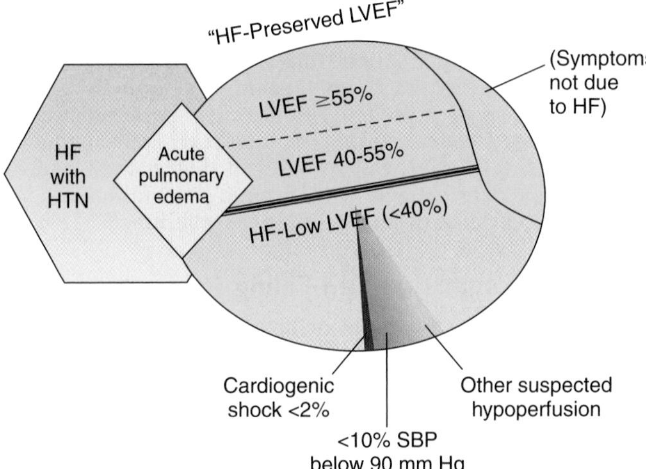

FIGURE 43–1 Estimation of typical proportions of patients accounting for hospitalizations for heart failure (HF) in the community. Approximately half of such hospitalizations are for heart failure with left ventricular ejection fraction (LVEF) exceeding 40%. Patients with acute pulmonary edema frequently have uncontrolled hypertension (HTN). Only a small fraction of patients present in cardiogenic shock. Clinical hypoperfusion at hospital admission may be present in up to 25% of patients with low ejection fraction in large tertiary centers, but this proportion is much smaller in community hospitals. SBP, systolic blood pressure. Data from large registries (Acute Decompensated Heart Failure Registry [ADHERE][1-3]).

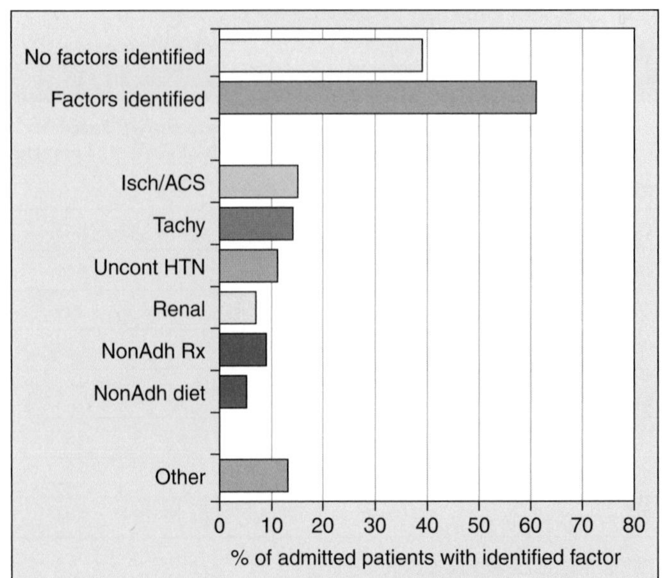

FIGURE 43–2 Bar graph showing factors identified as leading to hospitalization in patients with previously known diagnosis of heart failure. The data reported in 48,612 patients from the OPTIMIZE-HF database are represented.[8] Two or more factors were identified in 19% of patients. ACS, acute coronary syndrome; Isch, ischemia; Nonadh, nonadherence; Tachy, tachycardia; Uncont HTN, uncontrolled hypertension.

TABLE 43–1 Typical Community Hospitalizations for Heart Failure According to LVEF

Characteristic	LVEF <0.40	LVEF 0.40 to 0.55	LVEF ≥0.55
Age	70	74	74
% Women	40	54	69
% African American	22	17	17
% With coronary artery disease	59	61	48
% With hypertension	69	76	78
Systolic blood pressure (average; mm Hg)	139	150	152
% Diabetes mellitus	40	48	44
% With atrial fibrillation	29	33	32
% With COPD	27	32	34
% With renal insufficiency	26	31	27

Data from publications describing the Acute Decompensated Heart Failure National Registry (ADHERE) database.[2,3]

COPD, chronic obstructive pulmonary disease; LVEF, left ventricular ejection fraction.

TWO MINUTE ASSESSMENT OF HEMODYNAMIC PROFILE

Congestion at rest?

Low perfusion at rest?

	Congestion at rest? NO	Congestion at rest? YES
Low perfusion at rest? NO	*Warm & dry* A	*Warm & wet* B
Low perfusion at rest? YES	*Cold & dry* L	*Cold & wet* C

Evidence for congestion
- Orthopnea
- Elevated jugular venous pressure
- Rales (rarely)
- Hepatomegaly
- Ascites
- Edema (more common in older pts)
- Valsalva square wave

Evidence for low perfusion
- Narrow auscultated pulse pressure
- Cool extremities
- May be sleepy, obtunded
- Suspect from ACEI/ARB hypotension
- Progressive oliguria

FIGURE 43–3 Hemodynamic profiles of patients hospitalized for heart failure. Most patients can be classified as having one of these four profiles in a 2-minute bedside assessment, although in practice some patients may qualify for both profile B and profile C. This classification helps guide consideration of initial therapy and prognosis.[9] The clinical criteria for congestion (columns) concern dryness or wetness; the clinical evidence for perfusion (rows) concern coldness or warmth. For the "cold and dry" category, the label "L" is used instead of "D" to avoid the implication that heart failure invariably progresses. Many patients never develop a profile "L," which can stand for "heart failure light" because it is without congestion. ACEI, angiotensin-converting enzyme inhibitor; ARB, angiotensin receptor blocker.

with handheld devices may provide the most rapid assessment of volume status in the absence of skilled physical examination.[15] In the absence of frank pulmonary edema, arterial desaturation is rare in exacerbation of chronic heart failure, and on chest radiographs, acute changes often cannot be distinguished from chronic findings.

It is now known that in the majority of patients rehospitalized with heart failure, both right- and left-sided filling pressures have been increasing gradually for 2 weeks or longer before recognition of symptoms that led to a heart failure event, whether the ejection fraction is low or preserved.[16] These gradual increases are often not reflected in changes in weight, which includes both wet and dry weight and is influenced by the balance of caloric intake and expenditure. However, an acute exacerbation of severe hypertension, particularly in populations with high prevalence of hypertensive heart disease, can cause truly acute pulmonary edema without evidence of elevated total body volume (see Figure 43-1).

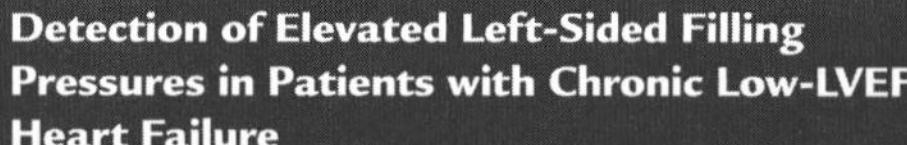

TABLE 43–2 Detection of Elevated Left-Sided Filling Pressures in Patients with Chronic Low-LVEF Heart Failure

Finding	Sensitivity for PCW	Specificity >22 mm Hg
Right-Sided Findings		
Estimated jugular venous pressure ≥12	65%	64%
Edema ≥grade 2+	41%	66%
Hepatojugular reflux	83%	27%
Hepatomegaly: enlargement >4 fingerbreadths	15%	93%
Left-Sided Findings		
Orthopnea	86%	25%
Rales > "few at base"	15%	89%
Third heart sound	63%	32%
Direct Right-Left Correlation		
Directly measured right atrial pressure ≥10 mm Hg	76%	83%
Echocardiographic Assessment		
Pulmonary artery systolic pressure ≥60mm Hg	47%	96%
Tricuspid regurgitation ≥ moderate	78%	70%
Mitral regurgitation ≥ moderate	78%	43%

PCW, Pulmonary capillary wedge pressure. Modified from Drazner MH, Hellkamp AS, Leier CV, et al. Value of clinician assessment of hemodynamics in advanced heart failure. The ESCAPE trial. *Circ Heart Fail* 2008;1:170-177; and Drazner MH, Hamilton MA, Fonarow G, et al. Relationship between right and left-sided filling pressures in 1000 patients with advanced heart failure. *J Heart Lung Transplant* 1999;18:1126-1132.

Patients with heart failure and low ejection fraction may also decompensate with profile C "cold and wet" but rarely with profile L "cold and dry" (see Figure 43-3). Cardiac output, although frequently reduced from normal, is often not reduced to critical levels and is rarely directly responsible for the resting symptoms that lead to admission, except in the unusual cases of true spiraling cardiogenic shock. Significant reduction of cardiac output, on the other hand, may be missed in a patient with chronic low cardiac output who appears oriented. Estimation of perfusion yields less reliable results than does assessment of filling pressures, even by the skilled examiner.[10] Temperature of the extremities, examination of the pulses, and auscultation to determine net pulse pressure must be assessed in the critical situation.[7,10] It is particularly important to auscultate blood pressure when atrial fibrillation or frequent premature beats generate misleadingly high systolic readings on automated measurement. Fluctuating mentation, often attributed to depression or sleep deprivation, may be a key sign of low cardiac output.

Severe compromise of resting cardiac output and perfusion do *not* usually occur in heart failure with truly preserved ejection fraction, in which decompensation is usually characteristic of profile B. However, hypoperfusion is occasionally present in patients with severe restrictive, infiltrative, or hypertrophic disease with a very small left ventricular cavity or severe mitral regurgitation.

PRINCIPLES OF THERAPY GUIDED BY PROFILES

For most patients admitted with heart failure, symptoms and physical examination findings provide sufficient information to determine patients' profiles for initial therapy.[9,10] For patients who appear to be profile A (warm and dry), without clinical evidence of elevated filling pressures or hypoperfusion on clinical examination, the diagnosis of heart failure may not adequately explain the presenting symptoms, which could be caused by other conditions, such as pulmonary or hepatic disease, or by transient events, such as ischemia or arrhythmias. It is now well recognized that at least half of hospitalizations of patients with chronic heart failure are for diagnoses other than decompensated heart failure.[17]

Focus on Congestion and Filling Pressures

For the patients who do have abnormal resting hemodynamic profiles, therapy is directed toward relief of congestion. Although heart failure was once considered primarily a condition of low cardiac output, therapies designed to stimulate contractility and cardiac output have to date been deleterious, leading to increased arrhythmias and ischemia and an apparent acceleration of progressive disease, often compared to "whipping a tired horse." The focus for both congestion profiles B and C is on reduction of the elevated filling pressures responsible for most of the symptoms that led to hospitalization.[18] Many patients have normal stroke volume and cardiac output despite low ejection fraction. Although cardiac output frequently improves with better loading conditions, increase of cardiac output is not a *primary* target of acute therapy unless organ perfusion is critically compromised or when systemic or renal hypoperfusion limits direct reduction of filling pressures.

What Is the Optimal Level of Filling Pressures?

In patients with heart failure caused by chronic dilated cardiomyopathy, filling pressures can often be lowered to levels of 15 to 16 mm Hg despite baseline levels over 30 mm Hg at admission.[19-22] (This contrasts with the requirement for higher filling pressures with acutely decreased compliance that has been described during new myocardial infarction,[23] as shown in Figure 43-4,) Most dilated hearts operate far beyond the level of filling at which stroke volume depends on increments in filling pressures. In fact, as high filling pressures are reduced, cardiac output usually increases (Figure 43-4).[19,24] This improvement in cardiac output could reflect multiple factors, including an actual increase in contractility from decreased myocardial oxygen consumption and improved gradient for myocardial perfusion, an improvement in ejection related to decreased systemic vascular resistance, and redistribution of mitral regurgitant volumes to supplement forward flow. Although all these may contribute, the most easily measured change is that of decreased mitral regurgitation caused by a reduction in the effective mitral regurgitant orifice, which in turn results from small reductions in left ventricular distention.[20,21,25,26] Both the landmark original study of nitroprusside[27] and more recent studies with tailored therapy have confirmed the central role of changes in mitral regurgitant flow.[26] The mitral regurgitant fraction during therapy may decrease from 0.50 to less than 0.20.[20] This appears to account for virtually all of the improvement in measured cardiac output (Figure 43-5). Similar considerations probably affect tricuspid regurgitation and right ventricular stroke volume.

Reduction of pulmonary capillary wedge pressures has long been observed, and more recently demonstrated, to reduce the symptoms of congestion that lead to most hospitalizations for heart failure. The immediate symptomatic improvement often occurs when filling pressures are still severely elevated. Therapy should not stop with initial relief, however. Many patients perceive relief from the most oppressive symptoms and do not appreciate that symptoms can be improved further. In addition to causing symptoms of heart failure, elevated filling pressures are associated with greater activation of the renin-angiotensin and sympathetic nervous

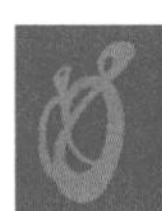

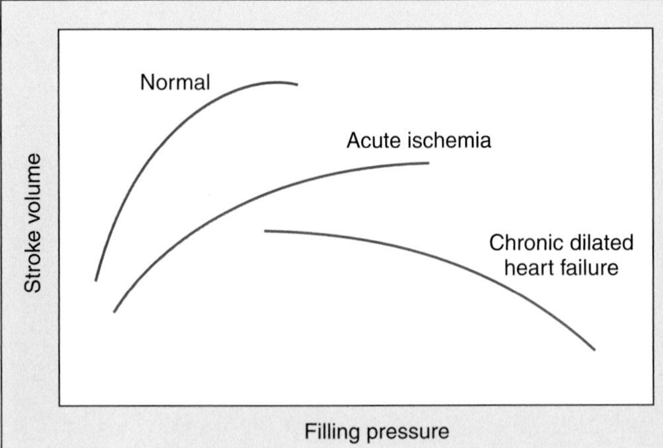

FIGURE 43-4 Curves demonstrating relationship of filling pressures to stroke volume. In the acutely ischemic ventricle, compliance is decreased with little change in volume, and the curve is shifted to the right, as described by Russell and colleagues.[103] In the chronically dilated ventricle, the curve is actually reversed in such a way that reduction of filling pressures leads to higher stroke volume.[19]

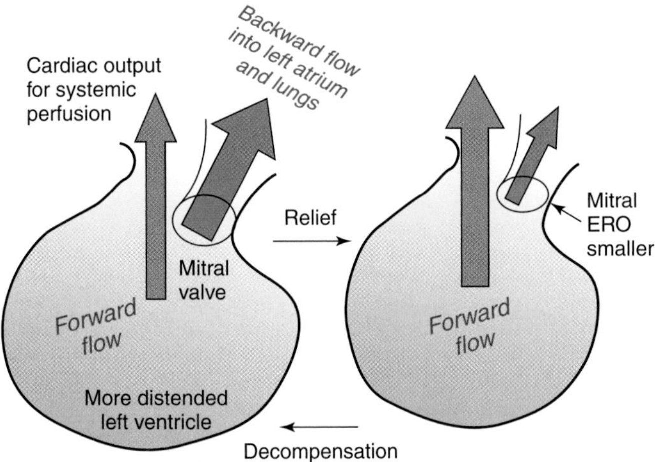

FIGURE 43-5 The change in distribution of stroke volume as ventricular loading conditions are improved, so that more of the total stroke volume is ejected forward and less flows backward into the left atrium.[20] The mitral effective regurgitant orifice (ERO) is significantly reduced after therapy.[21]

systems.[28,29] Even in the absence of symptoms, elevated filling pressures are important determinants of valvular regurgitation, abnormal ventricular filling patterns, pulmonary hypertension, and right ventricular dysfunction, all of which lead to worse outcomes. Whether near-normal filling pressures are measured directly (assessed from absence of signs and symptoms of congestion) or reflected by echocardiographic assessment, the ability to achieve them and maintain them over time[30-34] increases the likelihood of survival and lowers the likelihood of rehospitalization. It is not known to what extent current outcomes could be improved by more intensive reduction and prevention of recurrent congestion.

Current data do not allow definition of the filling pressure target for patients with heart failure and preserved ejection fraction. Like patients with heart failure and low ejection fraction, patients with heart failure and preserved ejection fraction retain fluid to a level substantially higher than optimal, although it is aggravated more commonly by intrinsic renal impairment.[16] The heterogeneity of myocardial disease and degrees of hypertrophy may dictate more heterogeneity in the optimal fluid levels for these patients, but it is unlikely that they will be more than a few millimeters higher than the target levels for the patients with low ejection fraction.

Profile B: Wet and Warm

In most hospitalizations for heart failure, patients' conditions are designated as profile B ("warm and wet"),[1,18] for which the initial goal, beyond just the improvement of symptoms, is simply the reduction of estimated filling pressures ("get to dry") (Table 43-3). Elevated filling pressures can result from elevated intravascular volume, systemic vasoconstriction (venous or arterial or both), and the combination. Most patients presenting with profile B have at least some component of total body fluid overload that necessitates fluid removal, usually by diuretics. For profile B in which vasoconstriction dominates, as in settings of severe hypertension with incipient pulmonary edema, vasodilators are the first line of therapy (see "Specific Agents Used During Hospitalization" section), although adding a moderate bolus of intravenous diuretics may accelerate initial relief. Positive-pressure masks may also help avert the need for urgent intubation in patients with marked tachypnea and hypoxia. However, most cases of decompensated heart failure can be managed with a stepwise approach.

For the majority of profile B patients, diuretic therapy is the main intervention leading to stabilization in the acute situation. Furosemide, administered either in a bolus or by continuous infusion,[35,36] is generally effective in achieving diuresis, sometimes with the addition of oral metolazone or intravenous thiazides,[37] as described in Chapter 44.

No Defined Role for Adjunctive Agents

Use of adjunctive therapies beyond diuretics has not been demonstrated to improve outcomes in hospitalized heart failure populations, dominated by the profile B patients. Multiple uncontrolled experiences confirm the worse early and late outcomes of patients who received approved intravenous inotropic infusions to facilitate diuresis.[38] The randomized study with milrinone[39] revealed increased arrhythmias and trends toward more ischemic events in hospital and more adverse events in the 60 days after discharge; this last effect was more evident in the patients with underlying coronary artery disease. The newer calcium-sensitizing agents, such as levosimendan, have produced no clinically significant benefit in either symptoms or outcomes.[40] Inotropic infusions may increase low levels of troponin leakage during hospitalization for heart failure, particularly in patients with underlying coronary artery disease.[41]

Nitroglycerin and nesiritide infusions may accelerate early symptomatic improvement but have not been proved to affect overall outcomes either positively or negatively during hospitalization or after discharge.[42] Both can cause hypotension, particularly when used in patients in whom circulating volume status has been overestimated. Current recommended doses of nesiritide have occasionally been implicated in the worsening of renal function, particularly in association with hypotension.[43] With increasing recognition of the multiple circulating forms of active and inactive natriuretic peptide fragments, a reengineered form may yet be identified that would have clinical utility for improving cardiorenal responses.[44]

Endothelin antagonists have not improved symptom relief or outcomes after discharge.[45] Therapy with vasopressin antagonists is effective in increasing serum sodium levels in the setting of hyponatremia, usually with some enhancement of diuresis. Relief of dyspnea is accelerated.[46] However, initial benefits for fluid balance are not sustained during long-term follow-up, in part because of increased thirst and water consumption.

Nonresponders

In some patients who appear to have uncomplicated congestion, appropriate therapy does not relieve signs and symptoms of congestion as anticipated (Figure 43-6). Failure to

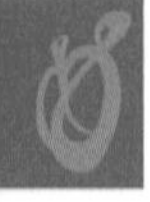

TABLE 43–3 Hemodynamic Goals for Therapy of Advanced Heart Failure*

Assessed Clinically	Measured Directly
Jugular venous pressure ≤8 cm	
Absence of orthopnea	Pulmonary capillary wedge pressure ≤15 mm Hg
No hepatomegaly or ascites	
No peripheral edema	Right atrial pressure ≤8 mm Hg
Valsalva square wave absent	
Systolic blood pressure ≥80 mm Hg	Systemic vascular resistance (average size), 1000-1200 dynes/sec/cm^{-5} (higher for small patient, lower for obese patient)
Warm extremities	
SBP–DBP ≥ 25% above normal	
SBP (proportional pulse pressure)	

*Further adjustment of therapy is required for postural hypotension that lasts beyond the immediate postdose period and for progressive renal dysfunction.
DBP, diastolic blood pressure; SBP, systolic blood pressure.

respond to empirical therapy is one of the reasonable indications to measure hemodynamics directly, in order to clarify the filling pressures, cardiac output, and vascular resistances and to allow more directed adjustment of therapies. No current evidence, however, suggests that more information will improve clinicians' ability to treat these patients, at least with the current therapies available.

Cardiorenal Syndrome

One reason for inadequate clinical response is the dreaded cardiorenal syndrome.[47,48] It occurs in approximately 25% of patients hospitalized with heart failure and is equally common among patients with low ejection fraction and patients with preserved ejection fraction, although intrinsic renal disease may play a larger role in older patients. Various definitions of the cardiorenal syndrome include renal dysfunction at the time of hospital admission, failure to respond to high-dose diuretics, worsening renal function during diuresis despite persistent fluid overload, and progressive uremia after establishment of apparently optimal volume status. Some patients have progressive elevation in blood urea nitrogen (BUN) levels with little change from baseline creatinine levels. The cardiorenal syndrome is associated with prolonged hospital stays and higher rates of mortality after discharge.

The term "prerenal" does not clarify either the mechanism or the solution. The syndrome was at one time assumed to reflect low cardiac output from excessively reduced filling pressures during diuresis. In fact, filling pressures usually still far exceed the optimal levels needed for maintenance of cardiac output as renal function deteriorates.[47] The cardiorenal dynamics become limiting most commonly in patients with severe right ventricular dysfunction and prolonged chronic volume overload. Increasing new information confirms a strong connection between renal dysfunction and chronically high right atrial pressures, possibly as a result of renal compromise from renal venous congestion and elevated intraperitoneal pressures.[49]

Of interest is that impaired renal function is about as likely to improve as to deteriorate during diuresis.[50] Patients with cardiorenal syndrome are often treated as if they have profile C, with either vasodilators or inotropic therapy. Inotropic therapy as used to facilitate diuresis is discussed in Chapter 44. If used, it should be in as low a dose as possible, such as 2 μg/kg for dobutamine, to avoid adverse effects of inotropic

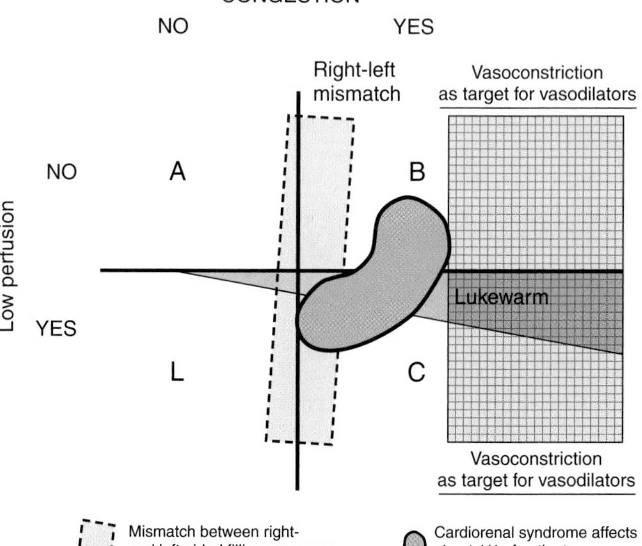

FIGURE 43–6 Modification of the four basic hemodynamic profiles shown in Figure 43-2. In some cases, left-sided filling pressures become elevated as a result more of vasoconstriction than of volume overload, and vasodilation is the first line of therapy. The adequacy of perfusion can be difficult to ascertain or may fluctuate in some patients ("lukewarm"). A mismatch between right- and left-sided filling pressures occurs in 20% to 25% of patients, so that the jugular venous pressure is high when left-sided pressures are not, or vice versa.[51] About 25% of patients demonstrate the cardiorenal syndrome, in which renal function worsens during therapy despite excessive volume. EF, ejection fraction; HF, heart failure; JVP, jugular venous pressure. (From Campbell P, Drazner MH, Kato M, et al. Right-left mismatch in the ESCAPE population: discordance between right and left-sided filling pressures before and after therapy. *J Cardiac Fail* 2009;15(6 Suppl):S28.

therapy and to minimize the development of inotrope dependence. Weaning from the infusion is often accompanied by worsening of both fluid status and renal function. Potentially definitive trials have not yet shown any agent, including adenosine antagonists, to improve outcomes in this condition.

"Lukewarm"

The clinical assessment for hypoperfusion is less reliable than that for congestion.[10] Patients with unrecognized or borderline low cardiac output may not have adequate perfusion to support blood pressure and renal function; this situation is sometimes referred to as an intermediate "wet and *lukewarm*" profile, which may lead to treatment for profile C with either inotropic or vasodilator therapy, depending on systemic vascular resistance.

Right-Left Filling Pressure Mismatch

Some patients do not respond as expected to therapy guided by clinical estimation; they may have an atypical pattern of filling pressure elevation. Persistent symptoms, apparent cardiorenal syndrome, or hypoperfusion may occur during treatment that is based on jugular venous pressures that do not adequately reflect left-sided filling pressures. In most patients, right atrial pressure is greater or less than 10 mm Hg when pulmonary capillary wedge pressure is greater or less than 22 mm Hg. However, a right-left mismatch occurs in about 20% to 25% of patients with heart failure caused by chronic dilated cardiomyopathy and can lead to overdiuresis or underdiuresis.[51] Higher right-sided pressures can occur in patients with chronic cor pulmonale, with intrinsic pulmonary hypertension, or after direct right ventricular injury; higher left-sided pressures may occur in patients with long-standing left ventricular hypertrophy, aortic valve disease, or frequent ischemia. However, right-left mismatch is usually not suspected clinically. Careful echocardiographic assessment may provide clues, but confirmation and quantitation of right-left mismatch often require direct hemodynamic measurement.

Very High or Very Low Systemic Vascular Resistance

Diuresis can lead to renal dysfunction without symptom relief when elevated filling pressures result from very high systemic vascular resistance (above 2000 dynes/sec/cm^{-5}). This is easy to recognize and treat when the blood pressure is high in profile B patients (see Figure 43-6). In other patients, it can be suspected on the basis of a very narrow pulse pressure. However, when both blood pressure and cardiac output are low, severe vasoconstriction is difficult to confirm or treat without direct hemodynamic monitoring.

Some patients have persistent hypotension with any diuretic or vasodilating intervention despite apparently adequate cardiac output, as judged by reasonable pulse pressure and warm extremities. Such patients occasionally have marked intrinsic vasodilation unrelated to pharmacotherapy. Their systemic vascular resistances can be too low to support perfusion if the patients are given neurohormonal antagonists or other vasodilators. This may occur with intrinsic liver disease, in which circulating vasodilator substances have been implicated. Chronic liver disease with vasodilation should be suspected in patients in whom the degree of ascites is disproportionate to the other evidence of heart failure. Patients particularly at risk may be those with long-standing cirrhosis caused by alcohol or by other toxins or, in rare cases, cardiac cirrhosis after many years of right-sided heart failure from valvular disease, restrictive disease, or congenital heart disease.

Profile C: Wet and Cold

Fewer than 3% of patients present with true cardiogenic shock, in which systemic perfusion is inadequate to meet resting oxygen demand, organ function is jeopardized, and lactate is accumulating[1,4] (see Figure 43-1). These patients require rapid intervention and decisions as described in the "Escalating Support" section.

Most patients with profile C with recognized hypoperfusion and congestion are not in extremis, but they generally need to optimize perfusion before they can treat the congestion.[18] As discussed for profile B, reduction of filling pressures alone can lead to improved cardiac output.[19] However, it is sometimes not possible to initiate diuresis when baseline perfusion is severely impaired.

Choice of Vasoactive Agents: Vasodilator or Inotrope?

The initial choice of adjunctive agents for hypoperfusion depends on the assessment of systemic vascular resistance. When systemic vascular resistance is very high, the intravenous vasodilators can simultaneously increase cardiac output and decrease filling pressures[52] (Table 43-4). If effective, this strategy is clearly preferable, although cardiac output can be increased more directly by inotropic agents with some vasodilation effects, such as dobutamine and milrinone. The perception that inotropic agents are easy to use without the need for close monitoring and titration has led to exuberant use without good rationale. These agents increase the frequency of clinical ischemic events but more commonly may exacerbate subclinical myocardial injury, as reflected in low-level troponin release that may worsen long-term outcomes after discharge.[39,41]

Dosages of inotropic therapy should be as low as possible to minimize the deleterious effect of increased calcium loading and increased myocardial energy requirements and to minimize the risk of atrial fibrillation and ventricular tachyarrhythmias. Therapy should be continued until the desired goals of initial stabilization and volume reduction are achieved, but weaning should begin quickly thereafter. Considerations regarding weaning of inotropic agents are discussed in the "Specific Agents Used During Hospitalization" section.

TABLE 43-4 Baseline and Final Hemodynamics Measured During Hospitalization for Heart Failure in Two Eras

Measurement	Baseline	On Oral Therapy
Two-Center Experience, 1986–1997 (*n* = 754); Average LVEF = 0.22 ± 0.08[11]		
Right atrial pressure (mm Hg)	12 ± 7	10 ± 7
Pulmonary capillary wedge pressure	25 ± 9	17 ± 7
Cardiac index (L/min/m^2)	2.1 ± 0.7	2.6 ± 0.6
Systemic vascular resistance (dynes/sec/cm^{-5})	1640 ± 620	1160 ± 300
ESCAPE, 2000–2003 (*n* = 215); Average LVEF = 0.19 ± 0.07[33]		
Right atrial pressure (mm Hg)	14 ± 10	7 ± 4
Pulmonary capillary wedge pressure	25 ± 9	7 ± 4
Cardiac index (L/min/m^2)	1.9 ± 0.6	2.4 ± 0.7
Systemic vascular resistance (dynes/sec/cm^{-5})	1500 ± 800	1100 ± 500

All changes significant in both eras. ESCAPE, Evaluation Study of Congestive Heart Failure and Pulmonary Artery Catheterization Effectiveness; LVEF, left ventricular ejection fraction.

Profile L: Dry and Cold

Patients rarely present for hospitalization with true profile L (cold and dry)[9]; therefore, a patient with apparent profile L should be carefully evaluated for occult elevation of filling pressures indicative of profile C instead. In the unusual event that they have documented low filling pressures (pulmonary capillary wedge pressure <12 mm Hg, or right atrial pressure <5 mm Hg), a cautious trial of fluid repletion may be considered; oral replacement off diuretics is better tolerated than is intravenous fluid supplementation, which tends to leak into the lungs. Unless postural hypotension is present, this approach does not often improve clinical status and may lead to congestive symptoms. Patients with pulmonary capillary wedge pressures of approximately 16 mm Hg with normal right atrial pressures generally look surprisingly comfortable at rest even if the cardiac output is low. The goals of further therapy depend on the clinical situation, but options are limited. Intravenous inotropic therapy provides only temporary improvement and may be followed by clinical deterioration. Further vasodilation may increase resting cardiac output, but it frequently causes symptomatic hypotension, particularly upon standing. Cautious initiation of therapy with β-blocking agents may lead to later improvement in systolic function and cardiac output, particularly if resting heart rate is high. Titration of β-blocking agents should proceed slowly, with most titration steps occurring after discharge and with frequent reevaluation.

Use of Direct Hemodynamic Monitoring

Cardiogenic Shock. In patients who have initial severely symptomatic hypotension or rapid deterioration, hemodynamic monitoring is performed urgently to establish the diagnosis of cardiogenic shock, guide titration of high-dose pressor agents, and evaluate for emergency surgical intervention.

Description of these patients if evaluated for urgent mechanical circulatory support would be as for Interagency for Mechanically Assisted Circulatory Support (INTERMACS) profile 1 (precipitous deterioration despite rapidly escalating therapy. "crash and burn") or profile 2 (failing on inotropes).[53] As discussed previously, the proportion of patients admitted with heart failure and cardiogenic shock is very small (see Figure 43-1).

Defining Baseline Hemodynamic Status. Direct hemodynamic monitoring with a pulmonary artery catheter is sometimes employed to guide diagnosis and management of heart failure during hospitalization (Box 43-1; see Table 43-4). For most patients, skilled clinical assessment should be adequate for placement in one of the four basic profiles for initiation of therapy. In the Evaluation Study of Congestive Heart Failure and Pulmonary Artery Catheterization Effectiveness (ESCAPE), clinical estimation was definitively compared with direct hemodynamic measurements[33]; the correlation was strong for filling pressures and only modest for cardiac output.[10] In patients in whom assessment yields limited or ambiguous findings, hemodynamic measurements may help increase certainty regarding, or actually define, the appropriate first targets of filling pressures and perfusion. Strategies of care may be informed by hemodynamic measurement in patients for whom symptom severity consistently exceeds clinical evidence of hemodynamic abnormalities, in which case exercise hemodynamic measurements may also be helpful. Hemodynamic measurement may clarify the contribution of heart failure to decompensation in the setting of other concomitant diagnoses, either cardiac (such as primary valve disease) or noncardiac (such as chronic pulmonary disease).

Hemodynamic Monitoring While Tailoring Therapy. One of the first routine uses of pulmonary artery catheterization in heart failure was to determine pulmonary pressures and reversibility of pulmonary hypertension during evaluation for cardiac transplantation in patients with advanced heart failure and low ejection fraction. When pulmonary vascular resistance was high in the setting of high left-sided filling pressures, the catheters were often left in place to ensure that pulmonary vascular resistance was sufficiently improved by reduction of left ventricular filling pressures with diuretics and vasodilators. Because severe vasoconstriction was commonly present before renin-angiotensin system inhibition became standard, vasodilation with nitroprusside or nitroglycerin was frequently necessary in combination and occasionally instead of diuretic therapy. Oral vasodilators were then substituted to maintain the lower filling pressures and vascular resistances as patients were weaned from the intravenous vasodilators.[52,54,55] After major improvement in symptoms and intermediate-term outcomes were noted, this strategy of tailored therapy to achieve near-normal filling pressures (see Table 43-3) could be applied to other patients admitted with advanced heart failure at specialized centers.[56]

The knowledge gained from physiology and therapeutic responses during hemodynamic monitoring has helped refine serial goals through clinical assessment (see Table 43-4). Therapy guided by clinical assessment was compared with therapy guided additionally with the use of a pulmonary artery catheter in ESCAPE (see Table 43-3) in patients with decompensation of chronic heart failure for whom there was clinical evidence regarding the need for invasive monitoring of therapy . Congestion, evidence of which was based on jugular venous pressure and edema, was alleviated similarly in both groups; in patients with the pulmonary artery catheter, renal function was better and mitral regurgitation was lower at the time of hospital discharge, perhaps in relation to the ability to assess left-sided filling more directly.[26,50] Symptomatic improvement was better at 1 month for the patients who underwent catheter-guided therapy, but there were no differences between the patient groups by 6 months, during which fluid retention recurred in both.[33] Pulmonary artery catheterization in these experienced centers was not associated with the adverse outcomes suggested from previous uncontrolled intensive care unit experiences,[57] in which use of pulmonary artery catheters was often triggered by clinical instability and sometimes led to more zealous use of fluid resuscitation and inotropic infusions.

Later Use of Invasive Hemodynamic Monitoring. In patients initially managed by clinical assessment, hemodynamic monitoring may be undertaken if patients fail to respond to or deteriorate during usual therapy. This may lead to detection of one of the modified profiles, such as right-left mismatch or unusual systemic vascular resistance. Hemodynamic monitoring is strongly recommended to help reevaluate optimization of filling pressures and systemic vascular resistance while oral agents are adjusted during weaning from inotropic infusions in patients who appear to be dependent on them. The value of hemodynamic information is less clear in patients who develop the cardiorenal syndrome during diuresis, in which the hemodynamic values obtained are usually those anticipated from clinical assessment.

Hemodynamic parameters related to filling pressures are robust prognostic parameters. High pulmonary capillary wedge pressure, right atrial pressure, and pulmonary artery systolic and mean pressures are all predictive of rehospitalization and mortality on a continuum, without a sharp threshold, and are more predictive when measured after therapy has been optimized, whereas indexes of cardiac output offer little prediction in patients with advanced heart failure.[22,33] However, invasive hemodynamic monitoring is not indicated purely to stratify risk in this population, for which there are many prognostic

BOX 43–1 Possible Indications for Insertion of Pulmonary Artery Catheter During Hospitalization for Heart Failure

Life-threatening Circulatory Compromise

Uncertainty Regarding Baseline Hemodynamic Profile
- Symptom severity out of proportion to clinical examination, may need assessment during exercise
- Ambiguity regarding clinical assessment

Management of Decompensated Heart Failure with Unclear Contribution from Other Condition

Cardiac
- Active ischemia
- Primary valve disease

Noncardiac
- Severe pulmonary disease
- Renal failure
- Hepatic failure
- Sepsis or systemic inflammatory syndrome

Postoperative respiratory failure or refractory hypotension

Failure to Respond as Anticipated to Medical Therapy Guided by Empirical Assessment

Uncertainty regarding hemodynamics after therapy
- Suspected right-left mismatch
- Possible intrinsic pulmonary hypertension
- Possible unusually high or low systemic vascular resistance
- Refractory or recurrent symptoms of unclear origin
- Cardiorenal syndrome (hemodynamic measurement not often revealing)

Need for Detailed Hemodynamic Documentation
- Evaluation for cardiac transplantation or ventricular assist device
- Failure to wean from intravenous inotropic fusions

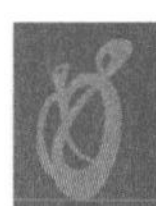

parameters that can be measured noninvasively. Currently, the use of pulmonary artery catheterization to guide therapy is considered a reasonable strategy (level IIa recommendation) in experienced centers when the hemodynamic status is uncertain or when resting symptoms or circulatory compromise persist despite empirical therapy, but it is not recommended as routine practice.[6] Even in patients for whom redesigning therapy has been considered useful, repeated right-sided heart catheterization should not be necessary for long-term management.

NONINVASIVE TECHNIQUES FOR MONITORING FILLING PRESSURES AND CARDIAC OUTPUT

Numerous parameters that are generally correlated with a hemodynamic parameter, usually with filling pressures, have been identified. Their utility should be considered separately in regard to diagnosis, to adjustment of therapy, and to prognosis. Some may help support a diagnosis of heart failure in a patient without previous known heart failure or in whom multiple conditions coexist. Assays of portions of the B-type natriuretic peptide (BNP) have consistently enhanced recognition of heart failure in multiple studies of patients presenting to emergency departments with dyspnea.[14] BNP levels generally decrease during effective therapy for heart failure, whereas increase in BNP levels over time is predictive of worse outcome. However, BNP levels as currently measured do not change rapidly enough to guide therapy in the hospital.[58] BNP levels over 1300 pg/mL at discharge are highly predictive of poor outcomes but do not have specific implications for current therapies other than to support[59] consideration of transplantation or mechanical circulatory support.

Several approaches to measuring thoracic impedance have been developed to track intrathoracic fluid accumulation, which is correlated generally with decreased electrical impedance, but none has been sufficiently reliable to guide diagnosis and therapy in individual patients.[60] Findings of impedance cardiography are correlated modestly with cardiac output, but they do not identify hemodynamic profile consistently, nor do they change directionally with measured cardiac output during therapy.[60] Echocardiographic estimates of central venous pressure elevation can be used when clinical evaluation of jugular venous pressure is not available,[15] but the clinical utility of echocardiographically estimated filling pressures has not been validated for serial evaluation of hospitalized patients. Further refinements of handheld echocardiographic measurements will probably offer potentially useful information, particularly when serial information is available for individual patients.

SPECIFIC AGENTS USED DURING HOSPITALIZATION

Diuretics, intravenous vasodilators, and intravenous inotropic agents are the major medications used during acute management of decompensated heart failure when oral therapy has been inadequate to prevent hospitalization. The major principles of diuretic use are described in Chapter 44.

Intravenous Vasodilators

After diuretics, intravenous vasodilators are the most useful medications for the acute management of heart failure (see Chapter 44). They reduce filling pressures and symptoms immediately. Cardiac output increases as vasodilation and diuresis occur, primarily as a result of decreased mitral regurgitation, as discussed previously. They do not usually increase heart rate or exacerbate arrhythmias unless titrated to excessive levels of vasodilation and severe hypotension.

Nitroprusside

Nitroprusside was the first vasodilator shown to improve cardiac output in heart failure.[27] It has dramatic efficacy in therapy for severe hypertension, in which systemic vascular resistance is also severely elevated. Although useful for hypertensive crises, nitroprusside, when titrated carefully in heart failure, is rarely associated with serious hypotension. Its use in heart failure has traditionally been monitored invasively through pulmonary artery catheters.[61] Noninvasive blood pressure monitoring with an automated cuff usually obviates the need for an indwelling arterial catheter. The rapidity of onset and offset, with a half-life of approximately 2 minutes, facilitates early establishment of an individual patient's optimal vasodilation and efficient weaning onto an oral vasodilator regimen that is adjusted to equivalent hemodynamic effects. Nitroprusside is generally initiated at 10 μg/min and increased by 10 to 20 μg every 10 to 20 minutes as tolerated, with hemodynamic goals of reducing the pulmonary capillary wedge pressure to 16 mm Hg without lowering systolic blood pressure below 80 mm Hg.[52,56] The systemic vascular resistance is used to guide the relative emphasis on vasodilation versus diuresis. Once the systemic vascular resistance is near normal, further reduction of filling pressures is generally accomplished primarily by diuresis; conversely, once near-normal filling pressures have been established, further vasodilation may not be necessary. Individual response varies markedly: 50 to 100 μg/min is effective in some patients, whereas others require 300 to 400 μg/min to achieve adequate vasodilation. Doses are often measured in absolute doses rather than per kilogram but rarely exceed 4 μg/kg (Table 43-5).

The major limitation of nitroprusside in this setting is side effects from cyanide, predominantly gastrointestinal and central nervous system manifestations, often manifested by nausea and "feeling weird." Cyanide is most likely to accumulate in patients in whom hepatic perfusion is severely reduced as a result of low cardiac output and in whom hepatic function is decreased as a result of elevated right-sided pressures or previous underlying liver disease. Cyanide toxicity is most likely to develop in patients receiving more than 250 μg/min for more than 48 hours. Cyanide results are rarely available in time to be useful; suspected toxicity is treated by decreasing or discontinuing the nitroprusside infusion, and additional therapy is almost never required in this setting. Less important during short-term nitroprusside administration is the thiocyanate metabolite, which can accumulate over days during more chronic use, particularly when renal function is impaired. Although it is the most effective intravenous vasodilator available, decreasing familiarity with nitroprusside has unfortunately limited its use in heart failure to a few specialized centers.

Nitroglycerin

Regardless of the route of administration, nitroglycerin is one of the safest and most versatile agents in acute therapy for decompensated heart failure. Nitroglycerin infusion is most commonly used for treatment of acute ischemic syndromes or heart failure in which acute ischemia is suspected. However, nitrates are very effective arterial vasodilators in the setting of vasoconstriction, although they are commonly considered as only venodilators.[62-64] Dose responses for both nitroglycerin and nitroprusside are markedly variable interindividually, but decreasing systemic vascular resistance requires higher doses of nitroglycerin than of nitroprusside. Dosing is generally begun at 20 μg/min of nitroglycerin, increased in 20-μg increments to the hemodynamic goals described previously. The most common side effect of intravenous or oral nitrates is headache, which, if mild, can be treated with analgesics and often resolves during continued therapy.[42] As with all

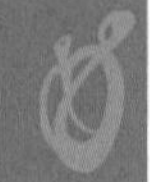

TABLE 43–5 Common Intravenous Vasoactive Agents for Heart Failure

Agent	Initial Dose	Effective Dose Range
Vasodilators		
Nitroglycerin	20 μg/min	40-400 μg/min*
Nitroprusside	10 μg/min	30-350 μg/min* Usually <4 μg/kg/min
Nesiritide	With or without 1- to 2-μg/kg bolus	0.005-0.03 μg/kg/min
Inotropic Agents†		
Dobutamine	1-2 μg/kg/min	2-10 μg/kg/min for inotropy and vasodilation
Dopamine		
• for heart failure	1-2 μg/kg/min	2-4 μg/kg/min for vasodilation and inotropy
• for hypotension	4-5 μg/kg/min	5-15 μg/kg/min for inotropy and vasoconstriction
Milrinone	50- to 75-μg/kg bolus may be administered over 10 min	0.10-0.75 μg/kg/min for vasodilation and inotropy

*Customarily titrated to effect, using absolute doses rather than per kg.
†These inotropic agents also cause vasodilation. The more potent inotropic agents epinephrine and norepinephrine and the pressor agent vasopressin are rarely used for chronic decompensated heart failure but are discussed in the "Specific Agents Used During Hospitalization" section.

vasodilating agents, blood pressure often decreases, and it may decrease precipitously if initial filling pressures were actually low rather than elevated. A rare reaction is a prolonged episode of profound hypotension with bradycardia, usually when initial filling pressures are normal or low.

Nesiritide

Nesiritide is a recombinant form of BNP, which is an endogenous peptide secreted primarily from the left ventricle in response to wall stress. Like nitroprusside and nitroglycerin, nesiritide acts to increase cyclic guanosine monophosphate. It may be administered as a bolus before fixed dose infusion. Nesiritide lowers filling pressures and improves symptoms during therapy for decompensated heart failure.[65] As with nitroglycerin, blood pressure must be monitored closely during nesiritide therapy because hypotension can occur. Because nesiritide has a longer half-life (18 minutes), hypotension can last longer than with intravenous nitroglycerin, but it is usually well tolerated in the supine position. Inappropriate bradycardia occasionally accompanies hypotension. Headache is less common with nesiritide than nitroglycerin. Both agents have been shown to be effective for decreasing filling pressures and relieving symptoms in heart failure.[42]

Nesiritide has not been associated with major diuresis when used alone in clinical trials. It does appear to potentiate the effect of concomitant diuretics, so that the total diuretic dose required may be slightly lower; this effect may persist after the infusion is stopped. Controversy regarding potential deleterious effects of nesiritide has been extensive.[43] Although it was considered at one time to be renal sparing, in current dosing regimens it does not appear to improve renal function more than other vasodilators and may in fact worsen renal function in patients who develop hypotension. Nesiritide is sometimes used specifically to decrease pulmonary vascular resistance in patients with heart failure, particularly after cardiac surgery. A large ongoing trial should help define its clinical role in heart failure–related decompensation.

The intravenous vasodilator phentolamine is an α-adrenergic blocker, used in some early investigations of vasodilators[54] but no longer generally available for infusion. Intravenous enalaprilat is converted to enalapril, a long-acting vasodilator that is not appropriate for intravenous titration but is used occasionally in postoperative patients as a substitute for their usual oral angiotensin-converting enzyme (ACE) inhibitor until they can resume oral intake. Intravenous hydralazine has unpredictable dose-response effects and can cause serious sustained hypotension, even after previous doses have been well tolerated. Only the oral form is used for management of heart failure.

Monitoring of Intravenous Vasodilators

Increasing experience with nitroglycerin and nesiritide indicates that they can often be used to treat exacerbations of heart failure without invasive hemodynamic monitoring.[42] Blood pressure can generally be monitored through an automated blood pressure cuff with frequent readings, so that the discomfort and risk involved with an indwelling arterial catheter are not warranted. Transient episodes of hypotension are usually quite well tolerated when related to vasodilation rather than to ischemia or arrhythmias. The ability to use these agents without invasive monitoring facilitates their use on monitored stepdown units; thus, intensive care unit resources are not challenged. Patients with more critical hemodynamic compromise require an intensive care unit regardless of the choice of initial therapy. Limited capacity for invasive monitoring should not be a factor in determining whether vasodilator or inotropic infusions are employed.

Weaning from Intravenous Vasodilator Agents

Once patients are considered to have reached optimal circulatory status, they are weaned from intravenous agents as oral agents are adjusted. In some cases, only the volume status has changed. In other cases, oral vasodilators are adjusted to maintain the profiles achieved with the intravenous agents.[54,56] It is important to recognize that the current intravenous vasodilators cause both arterial and venous dilation. As patients are weaned from these agents, filling pressures frequently rise again as venous capacitance decreases, necessitating either further diuresis or effective substitution with sufficient venodilation by oral agents. The selection and adjustment of oral therapy is discussed in the "Designing the Oral Regimen" section. When the short-acting intravenous agents are monitored by means of pulmonary artery catheters, patients are weaned as oral dosages are increased, to maintain the optimal hemodynamics achieved. When oral agents are adjusted according to clinical assessment, the jugular venous pressure, supine blood pressure, and upright blood pressure guide dosing (see Table 43-2). The timing of oral vasodilator dose increases requires more monitoring during weaning from nesiritide because of its longer half-life.

Intravenous Inotropic Agents

Considerations for Use and Weaning

The perception that intravenous inotropic agents are easy to use has led to their frequent initiation at the time of hospitalization for heart failure in the absence of any specific indications for inotropic support. The concept of hospitalization for an "inotropic holiday" with infusions for 24 to 72 hours was once popular. However, these agents are associated with more tachyarrhythmias and ischemic events than are placebo or vasodilator infusions.[39] In addition, the presence of inotropic infusions may complicate the redesigning of a regimen of an oral diuretic and vasodilator for discharge; the efficacy of diuretics and tolerability of ACE inhibitor doses may be overestimated when the effect of the inotropic stimulation lingers. This may prolong hospitalization or increase the likelihood of early rehospitalization. The use of current inotropic agents, therefore, would be most appropriate when they provide necessary benefits not offered by initial therapies (see also Chapter 44).

Inotropic therapy might be considered as the "until" therapy, with a predefined endpoint[66]: It may be used *until* the underlying hemodynamic profile and cause of severe hypotension are elucidated. It may be used *until* diuresis is effective in patients with conditions refractory to escalating diuretic therapy. It may be used *until* kidney, lung, or liver function has improved to establish eligibility for cardiac transplantation or for operative intervention. It may be used *until* recovery from a superimposed insult such as pneumonia, pulmonary embolus, myocardial infarction, or surgery. Most of the experience with prolonged infusions has derived from patients waiting *until* an appropriate heart can be found for cardiac transplantation.

Many patients considered dependent on intravenous inotropic therapy can nonetheless be stabilized with oral therapy tailored to filling pressures and systemic vascular resistance.[52,67] This may necessitate temporary or permanent discontinuation of β-adrenergic antagonists and ACE inhibitors, because of their negative inotropic effects in severely compromised patients. The use of nitrates and the addition of hydralazine may be particularly effective in restoring compensation with oral vasodilators after prolonged inotropic infusion.[67]

There is a growing population of patients, however, for whom multiple adjustments of oral therapy have become inadequate to maintain freedom from congestion with adequate renal function. Many of these patients are those in whom right ventricular failure has become prominent and the cardiorenal syndrome is manifest. Continuous intravenous inotropic infusions have been recognized as palliative care *until* death for a population of these patients (see Chapter 61). This therapy has been associated with frequent complications from indwelling catheters and with sepsis.[68] Escalating doses are usually required, and survival expectancy is less than 50% during the next 3 to 6 months. In rare cases, however, patients have remained stable on moderate doses and have occasionally been weaned completely from inotropic support later. For most patients, the last chapter of their life with heart failure is smoother and more comfortable if they are not tethered to a continuous infusion at home.

Specific Inotropic Agents

Dobutamine. The most commonly used inotropic agent during hospitalization for heart failure is dobutamine, an agent that stimulates β-adrenergic receptors with little effect on α-adrenergic receptors, so that contractility is increased with peripheral and pulmonary vasodilation. Dobutamine was introduced as an alternative to dopamine, one that produced less tachycardia, but it does not affect dopaminergic receptors. Early uncontrolled studies demonstrated increased cardiac output with decreased filling pressures. Myocardial stores of adenosine triphosphate were shown to be improved after a brief period of dobutamine therapy, and sometimes symptomatic benefit persisted.[69] Much of this benefit has been attributed to the potentiation of diuresis when fewer options were available for enhancement of diuretic therapy.

Heart rate is consistently increased during dobutamine therapy, particularly in patients with atrial fibrillation. Atrial and ventricular tachyarrhythmias and symptoms of ischemia are increased during dobutamine therapy for decompensated heart failure. A comparison of dobutamine with nesiritide revealed increased premature ventricular contractions, episodes of nonsustained ventricular tachycardia, and signs that fulfilled criteria for the diagnosis of proarrhythmia.[70]

When dobutamine therapy is considered warranted despite these risks, the lowest dosage possible should be used for the desired effect. Enhancement of diuresis and improvement of renal function can be observed at doses of 1 to 2 μg/kg/min. Treatment for more severe hypoperfusion usually necessitates higher doses. Patients receiving chronic maintenance infusions generally exhibit tachyphylaxis and require increasing dosages over time. There may be little benefit from increasing the dosage above 10 μg/kg/min, however, and other therapy should be added or substituted as the dosage approaches 15 μg/kg/min. An exception may be in patients with hypotension during chronic therapy with β-adrenergic antagonists. Dobutamine is often adequate for improving cardiac output in this setting, but dosages higher than usual may be required.[71]

On occasion, patients taking dobutamine for prolonged periods of many weeks may develop an eosinophilic hypersensitivity that is usually manifested in an elevated circulating eosinophil count and sometime in urine eosinophil levels as well. This can take the form of a skin rash, but of greater importance, eosinophilic myocarditis has been found in the explanted hearts of about 15% of patients receiving chronic infusions before cardiac transplantation.

Dopamine. Dopamine stimulates β-receptors, α-receptors, and dopaminergic receptors that cause vasodilation in the renal and peripheral vasculature. At dosages of 3 μg/kg/min or less, dopamine is predominantly vasodilatory. The dopaminergic receptors are overwhelmed by α-adrenergic stimulation when dopamine doses reach 5 μg/kg/min, or when other vasoconstricting pressors are given. Dopamine also causes release of norepinephrine from nerve terminals, which itself stimulates α- and β-receptors and raises circulating norepinephrine levels.

Because of the effect on dopaminergic receptors in animal models, the concept of "renal-dose dopamine" at 1 to 3 μg/kg/min has been popular. For patients with renal dysfunction and normal circulation, it is controversial whether this therapy enhances renal function specifically. In patients with heart failure, any dosage of dopamine can have systemic hemodynamic effects from enhanced cardiac output and decreased systemic vascular resistance. The benefit of low-dosage dopamine to enhance diuresis and renal function is clinically similar to that of dobutamine at the same dosages. Similarly, tachyarrhythmias and ischemic episodes can also be observed even with low dosages.

Dopamine is a good choice for therapy in rapidly changing situations in which modest inotropy and vasodilation may be adequate but further pressor support may be required, inasmuch as this can be achieved by dose escalation. When blood pressure support is the initial need, dopamine should be started at a dosage of at least 4 μg/kg/min. Similarly, when patients are weaned from the use of dopamine as a pressor agent, it may be necessary to discontinue it once a dosage of 3 μg/kg/min is reached, because gradual weaning through lower doses may in fact cause vasodilation and hypotension. There is little evidence to support the addition of dopamine to dobutamine for enhanced renal function for patients with heart failure, and it would be expected to increase the risk of arrhythmias and ischemia.

Milrinone. Amrinone, milrinone, and the phosphodiesterase inhibitors lead to increased levels of cyclic adenosine monophosphate by inhibiting its breakdown, rather than by increasing its production through stimulation of β-receptors. These agents then may act synergistically with β-adrenergic agents to achieve further increase in cardiac output than does either agent alone. They may also be more effective than β-adrenergic receptor stimulation to increase cardiac output when excess β-blocking agents have been given. Phosphodiesterase inhibition increases contractility and causes marked vasodilation. The degree to which cardiac output increases and systemic vascular resistance decreases is markedly

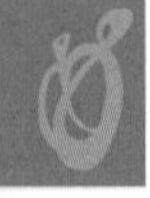

variable, so that some patients exhibit predominant vasodilation. There is thus a significant incidence of hypotension with milrinone, unlike dobutamine, which rarely causes hypotension except in unappreciated vasodilatory states such as sepsis. In a trial of patients hospitalized with heart failure and an average baseline blood pressure of 120 mm Hg, 10% of the patients developed clinically significant hypotension, which was a higher percentage than among those who received placebo.[39] When hypotension is considered the indication for use of an intravenous inotropic agent rather than an intravenous vasodilator, milrinone is rarely an appropriate choice.

Milrinone has been associated with slightly less elevation in heart rate than have dobutamine and dopamine.[72] Like the other intravenous inotropic agents, however, milrinone increases the frequency of atrial and ventricular tachyarrhythmias and ischemic events. A trial of 48-hour infusion of milrinone during heart failure hospitalization caused significantly more adverse events than did placebo; these events included atrial and ventricular tachyarrhythmias, cardiac arrest, and myocardial infarction.[39]

The use of milrinone for short-term stabilization is complicated by its prolonged half-life. Unlike the pharmacological half-lives of dopamine and dobutamine, which are in minutes, the elimination half-life of milrinone is about 2.5 hours, and the physiological half-life is closer to 6 hours. Although bolus therapy was originally recommended, milrinone is frequently used without a bolus to avoid rapid initial effects, at doses as low as 0.01 μg/kg/min. The drug is then titrated to the desired hemodynamic effect, in increments of the lowest doses possible, up to a maximum of 0.75 μg/kg/min. Because the drug is excreted renally, dosage adjustment is recommended. In the setting of decreased renal function, which occurs commonly in heart failure, effects accumulate and persist over a longer period of time. When milrinone is discontinued after several days, the physiological half-life often seems to exceed 12 or even 18 hours. As a result, clinicians frequently consider patients to have tolerated weaning from this agent, but then the patients deteriorate after transfer out of the intensive care unit or discharge home. It is thus even more important for this inotrope that the infusion be discontinued with further observation of fluid balance and perfusion for at least 48 hours before hospital discharge.

Because milrinone has been studied in trials in an oral form, more is known about the long-term effects of this agent than about the other intravenous inotropic drugs in current use. During chronic use, rates of mortality from heart failure and of sudden death were increased in comparison to placebo, without significant improvement in symptoms.[73] Hemodynamics deteriorated during chronic use but worsened further when the drug was withheld; this observation raised speculation that the phosphodiesterase inhibitors might accelerate hemodynamic decline.

Patients awaiting cardiac transplantation may be supported with extended infusions of milrinone either alone or in combination with dobutamine when dobutamine no longer provides sufficient stabilization of organ function preoperatively.[74] Patients requiring two inotropic infusions are, however, increasingly being offered mechanical support devices as bridges to transplantation. Some centers previously provided intermittent outpatient inotropic infusions, but this practice has no basis of evidence and is not approved.

Epinephrine and Norepinephrine. Epinephrine and norepinephrine are full β-receptor agonists, in contrast to dopamine and dobutamine. Significant additional inotropic and blood pressure support can be provided by these agents for short-term life-saving intervention over a span of minutes to hours before definitive therapy. Although norepinephrine is commonly confused with phenylephrine (Neo-Synephrine), both norepinephrine and epinephrine stimulate type 1 β-adrenergic receptors and α-adrenergic receptors, increasing contractility, heart rate, and peripheral vascular resistance, while promoting cardiac arrhythmias and ischemia. (Phenylephrine is a pure vasoconstricting agent.) Kidney failure, hepatic failure, and gangrene can result from use of these agents, which should not be administered except in true emergency situations. Epinephrine has more affinity for type 2 β-receptors, which are vasodilatory, than does norepinephrine and thus is slightly less likely to cause tissue necrosis from intense vasoconstriction, although both are profound vasoconstrictors appropriate for therapy of vasodilatory shock. There is ample anecdotal evidence leading to the term "letho-fed" for norepinephrine.

When fatal hypotension is imminent, epinephrine or norepinephrine are used at a starting dose of 1 μg/min, not usually expressed as per-kilogram dosing. Before this point, injection of 0.25 mg of epinephrine from the code cart may provide several minutes of stabilization during which to make more definitive plans for circulatory support or the orchestration of the end of life. To maintain survival for brief periods of minutes until definitive therapy, boluses of calcium can be helpful, particularly in the presence of conditions that may acutely lower serum calcium, such as transfusion, dialysis or cardiopulmonary bypass. Contractility increases rapidly with increased circulating calcium concentration.[75] This therapy is highly arrhythmogenic and may exacerbate ongoing myocardial necrosis; therefore, it should not be maintained.

Vasopressin. Vasopressin is used increasingly to potentiate the effects of catecholamines in patients who remain severely hypotensive, with systolic blood pressures of 60 to 70 mm Hg, despite high-dose pressor support. This experience is derived from early postoperative management after heart transplantation or insertion of mechanical support devices.[76,77] Some patients who have been most compromised preoperatively develop profound vasoplegia, with low systemic vascular resistance states of the systemic inflammatory response syndrome. Vasopressin has been used for periods of hours to days, in doses of 0.05 to over 0.1 U/min. At these doses, patients already receiving norepinephrine frequently have further 30–mm Hg increases in systolic blood pressure.[76,77] Although vasopressin is considered an antidiuretic hormone, its use in critical settings is sometimes associated with profound water diuresis that reverses after discontinuation of the drug. As a potent vasoconstricting hormone itself, vasopressin can contribute to ischemic injury and necrosis of organs and limbs during use of other vasoconstricting agents.

REEVALUATION

Serial evaluation and adjustments in therapy usually lead to resolution of the acute decompensation that led to the hospitalization for heart failure. In affected patients, the focus shifts gradually toward redesign of the outpatient regimen for stabilization. In addition to redirecting pharmacological and pacing device therapies, the hospitalization provides a valuable opportunity to review and revise the individual prognosis for long-term quality and length of survival.

Escalating Support

A small minority of patients present with rapidly deteriorating circulatory status and life-threatening hypoperfusion, from which survival may be possible only with rapid, aggressive intervention. It is critical that clinicians recognize the need for an accelerated tempo of assessment and decision in these situations. The goal in these cases is to stabilize the patient to a point at which decisions can be made regarding definitive surgical therapy such as mechanical support, or until spontaneous recovery can occur, as in young adults with fulminant myocarditis.[5]

The situation of the patient who requires rapidly escalating support is described as the "crash and burn" level in the evolving classification of patients considered for mechanical circulatory support.[53] Evidence of this situation usually includes more than one of the following: systolic blood pressure remaining below 75 mm Hg, cardiac index persistently below 1.5 to 1.8 L/min/m^2, systemic acidosis progressing to acidemia with positive lactate levels, "shock liver" with transaminase levels rising to the thousands of units per liter, obtundation, and anuria.

Dopamine is the most common first-line drug administered in this situation, but if the situation does not improve within minutes, escalation would include more intense inotropic support with epinephrine at escalating doses. Vasopressin is frequently added as well, as discussed previously in the "Specific Inotropic Agents" section. For the patient with otherwise robust health, consultation regarding surgical options should be obtained immediately. The role of the intra-aortic balloon pump for intermediate stabilization has been established for cardiogenic shock caused by acute myocardial infarction; the pump is usually inserted while other therapies are under way in the cardiac catheterization suite. When it can be performed expeditiously, balloon pump insertion seems reasonable for other cases of cardiogenic shock with underlying coronary artery disease.[78] For cardiogenic shock of other causes, its role is less clear, and plans for insertion should not detract from progress to more definitive intervention. Some experts advocate its use for stabilization of medical therapy and anesthesia regardless of cause, whereas others believe that it offers little benefit for patients without epicardial coronary artery disease and, moreoever, increases the risk of vascular and infectious complications.

Poor survival rates with high incidences of multiorgan failure and infection are increasingly recognized among patients who undergo implantation of durable ventricular assist devices for unstable conditions. Most of these patients now are considered instead for temporary assist devices, as a "bridge" to a decision about an implantable device or, in some cases, to recovery from fulminant myocarditis. The "bridge-to-bridge" strategy also provides crucial opportunities to better assess the medical candidacy of patients for aggressive interventions, the psychosocial factors critical for a good outcome, and the patient's preferences regarding extreme intervention in comparison with focus on comfort and acceptance of the imminent end of life. The use of circulatory assist devices in heart failure is discussed in Chapter 47.

Cardiac transplantation and mechanical circulatory support either as a bridge to transplantation or permanent "destination" therapy are not often appropriate (see Chapters 54 and 55). Most patients hospitalized with heart failure are elderly, with an average age of approximately 75 years, and have multiple comorbid conditions that preclude good outcomes with surgical intervention.[1,79] In these patients, the support that should be escalated is the humane support shown by compassionate medical staff and supportive consult services to the patient and family. Despite the negative connotation of heart "failure," many patients and families need counseling to recognize its poor prognosis and the limited options for life-saving therapies. Whether days or weeks of life are anticipated, the challenge is to work with them to define and reach meaningful goals for the time remaining.

PLANNING FOR HOSPITAL DISCHARGE

The majority of patients hospitalized with heart failure have not reached the end of their lives; instead, they can be stabilized to return to a reasonable level of function on an oral regimen designed to maintain stability. In unselected series, however, 30% to 50% of patients discharged with a diagnosis of heart failure are rehospitalized within the next 3 to 6 months.[1] Failure to meet criteria for discharge contributes to this rate of rehospitalization.[80] There is continual pressure to reduce the lengths of stay, particularly when patients exceed the generally acknowledged "break-even point" for reimbursement of 5 days. However, admissions for less than 3 days usually represent patients who did not need admission but could have been managed at home with daily contact and repeated blood tests for electrolytes and renal function. Regardless of the length of stay, premature discharges do not save money, inasmuch as the last day of the first hospitalization consumes fewer resources than does the first day of rehospitalization, and readmissions within 30 days may not be reimbursed.

Criteria for discharge include stable fluid status, blood pressure, and renal function on the oral regimen planned for home for at least 24 hours (Table 43-6). Patients should be free of dyspnea or symptomatic hypotension while at rest, washing, and walking on the ward. Patients who have received intravenous inotropic agents should be observed for at least 48 hours after weaning in case of masking inadequacy or intolerability of the discharge regimen.

Designing the Oral Regimen

Consideration of the components of the discharge regimen should influence therapy as soon as the patient has responded to the initial interventions. For the patients who have been hospitalized before, the question "How will this time be different?" should also be asked.

As discussed in the chapter on diuretic therapy (see Chapter 44), lower diuretic doses are necessary to maintain fluid balance than to achieve net fluid loss. As intravenous diuretics are discontinued, titration of oral diuretics should trigger discontinuation of a "sliding scale" of potassium replacement

TABLE 43–6	Discharge Criteria for Hospitalization with Heart Failure
Clinical status goals • Achievement of dry weight • Definition of blood pressure range • Walking without dyspnea or dizziness	
Stability goals • 24 hours without changes in oral regimen for heart failure • ≥48 hours off intravenous inotropic agents, if used • Even fluid balance on oral diuretics • Renal function stable or improving	
Discharge regimen • Estimated diuretic dose, with plan for first escalation if needed • ACE inhibitor/ARB or documented contraindication • β-Blocker discharge dose, plans for outpatient initiation, or documented contraindication • Anticoagulation for atrial fibrillation unless contraindicated	
Patient/family education • Sodium restriction • Fluid limitation if indicated • Medication schedule • Medication effects • Exercise prescription	
Monitoring of symptoms and weights	
Instructions regarding when and whom to call	
Scheduled call to patient within 3 days	
Clinic appointment within 10 days and information handed off to monitoring physician	

ACE, angiotensin-converting enzyme; ARB, angiotensin receptor blocker.

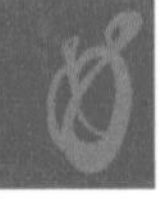

in favor of regularly scheduled dosing. If spironolactone is to be added to the home regimen, it should be started several days before discharge, and extreme caution should be taken to avoid hyperkalemia, because the drug's potential to worsen renal function and raise potassium levels may not be evident for several days.[81]

ACE inhibitors do not usually relieve the acute symptoms of heart failure and may actually compromise effective diuresis.[82] Their benefit in reducing remodeling, ischemic events, atrial fibrillation, and heart failure events is experienced over the longer term (see Chapter 45). Patients previously stable with long-acting ACE inhibitors should continue those doses in the hospital as tolerated. When ACE inhibitors are poorly tolerated—systolic blood pressures are frequently below 80 mm Hg or symptomatic hypotension is present—captopril is frequently preferred to the longer-acting ACE inhibitors.[83] Depending on the referral population, up to 30% of patients with advanced heart failure may not be able to tolerate ACE inhibitors because of hypotension or severe renal dysfunction.[84] In these patients, the usual regimen is hydralazine, 25 to 150 mg three to four times daily, and oral isosorbide dinitrate, 10 to 80 mg three times daily. Although ACE inhibitors were shown to be superior in patients with class II heart failure, the Veterans Administration Cooperative Vasodilator –Heart Failure Trial II (V-HeFT II) demonstrated equivalent rates of survival with enalapril and with hydralazine and nitrates in class III and class IV heart failure.[85] Most experience has been with the short-acting nitrate, although longer-acting oral nitrates have also been used. When hydralazine is not tolerated, vasodilation can also be achieved with high doses of oral nitrates alone. There is currently no accepted regimen for patients who cannot tolerate ACE inhibitors, hydralazine, or nitrates.

Addition of the hydralazine-nitrate combination to the ACE inhibitor/angiotensin receptor blocker (ARB) regimens should be considered when class III or IV symptoms persist in African American patients, for whom substantial improvement in both function and survival was demonstrated in the African American Heart Failure Trial (A-HeFT) (See Chapter 49).[86] Addition of these agents, particularly nitrates, to ACE inhibitor/ARB regimens in other patient populations may often result in clinical improvement[64] but has not been studied definitively.

β-Adrenergic blocking agents should be continued in previously tolerated doses for patients admitted with fluid retention but without evidence of hypoperfusion (profile B). If recently started or increased, these agents should be stopped or decreased until fluid retention is effectively treated. β-Adrenergic blocking agents should in general be decreased or stopped in patients in whom hypoperfusion is evident, particularly if therapy with intravenous inotropic agents is considered.

Initiation of β-adrenergic blocking agents is not recommended during hospitalization for heart failure decompensation when hypoperfusion[6] has been prominent or intravenous inotropic therapy has been used. However, the majority of patients admitted in profile B can undergo cautious initiation of β-blocker therapy in hospital once fluid status has been stabilized, if blood pressures has not been low.[87] β-Blocker therapy initially causes elevation of filling pressures and reduction of cardiac output; therefore, patients should have sufficient hemodynamic margin to tolerate this challenge.

Lack of confidence in outpatient compliance with follow-up is not a good reason to initiate these agents prematurely before discharge in patients with tenuous compensation, because close surveillance will continue to be necessary. During the titration of oral medications before discharge, liberal parameters to withhold doses for low blood pressures should be avoided. Often a regimen is assumed to be well tolerated but in fact has not been given. The effects of rebound vasoconstriction and neurohormonal stimulation during erratic medication dosing may complicate transition to the same regimen at home.

Implantable devices for defibrillation are indicated only in patients who have reasonable expectation of survival with good functional status for more than 1 year (see Chapter 47).[88] Among large community populations, the rate of mortality within 1 year of hospitalization for heart failure is 20% to 35% after the first such hospitalization and more than 40% after rehospitalization.[89] In patients who are repeatedly hospitalized for heart failure and chronic renal dysfunction, defibrillators are not predicted to prolong survival.[17] Furthermore, implantation of cardioverter-defibrillators for primary prevention of sudden death is contraindicated in patients with class IV symptoms of heart failure except in ambulatory patients with high likelihood of benefit from resynchronization therapy.[88] At the time of hospitalization for heart failure, symptoms are by definition class IV, occurring at rest or with minimal exertion. Thus, until clinical stability with class III or better functional status has been demonstrated after hospital discharge, implantable cardioverter-defibrillators should usually not be considered for primary prevention of sudden death. Cardiac resynchronization therapy is indicated in selected patients with severe symptoms who are nonetheless ambulatory with their stable oral medical regimen. Good clinical responses are most likely in patients with baseline QRS duration higher than 150 msec; they have rarely occurred in patients who have recently required intravenous inotropic therapy.[90] Depending on the overall likelihood of clinical response and the patients' preferences regarding mode of death and inappropriate shocks, cardiac resynchronization devices without defibrillation capability may often be appropriate.[91]

Patient Education before Discharge

Patient education should take place during the entire hospitalization, with specific focus on salt and fluid intake, medication schedules, and the concept of a flexible diuretic regimen.[92-94] Participation in the ritual of daily measurements of weight and of intake and output makes real the concepts of fluid balance. Although hospitalization is considered a true "teachable moment," too often the discharge information is rapidly delivered as the patients are packing their belongings. In addition to information about what they should not do, patients need positive information on the activities they can pursue, reinforcing that they should "Keep dry, keep active, and keep goals." Patients need to understand specifically which changes necessitate a call to their care team and which necessitate a call to 911.

Charting the Course

For some patients with heart failure, the hospital is the only place where their course with heart failure is reviewed and discussed. It may be difficult to assess the patient's short-term prognosis at the time of admission, when patients often appear frailer than at discharge. However, as the clinical status responds or fails to respond, particularly after multiple hospitalizations, general prognosis becomes more evident at the time of discharge, both to physicians and to the nursing staff.[95]

Almost 60% of patients discharged from hospitalizations for heart failure are readmitted within the next 6 months. Of those readmissions, the proportion for heart failure is about half after the first admission, and it increases thereafter.[96] Risk factors for readmission are similar to those for hospitalization for heart failure in general. The BUN level, BNP level, and systolic blood pressures have been strong predictors of in-hospital mortality and also contribute to risk of heart failure–related events after discharge.[79,97] The ESCAPE risk score was designed specifically from information at *discharge* to determine risk for death or readmission within 6 months, and it includes high (>500 pg/mL) and higher (>1300 pg/mL) BNP levels, high (>40 mg/dL) and higher (>90 mg/dL) BUN levels, diuretic dose (>240 mg of furosemide or >120 mg of torsemide), low serum sodium level (<130 mEq/L), inability to tolerate β-blocker therapy, short 6-minute walk distance (<300 feet), need for cardiopulmonary resuscitation or intubation during hospitalization, and age older than 70.[98]

The 1-month reevaluation after hospital discharge is an opportunity for further refinement of prognosis and plans.[32,34] Patients with persistent or recurrent evidence of congestion at 1 month are likely to have declining functional capacity and quality of life and are at more than twice the risk for death or readmission than are those who remain free of congestion.[32] Evaluation for transplantation or mechanical circulatory support may be indicated for a small minority of these patients at highest risk. For most patients, however, an estimated survival time of less than 1 year should prompt a review of the overall goals of therapy. There is wide variation between patients in their preference for quality of life versus length of life, even in advanced disease,[99] and these may change between admission and the outpatient setting. This transition to focus on quality of life should occur gradually, before presentation of a specific resuscitation menu, although the concept of allowing natural death may be introduced in preference to a list of "Do Not" procedures. Many patients wish adequate time in order to address concerns at home such as financial planning or family reconciliation. Many patients worry about how death is likely to occur and whether it will be painful.[100] Discussions facilitated by palliative care teams can provide comfort and reassurance regarding relief of terminal symptoms, as well as the availability of extended bereavement counseling for family members.

The discharge plan requires that the patient have a follow-up appointment, usually within the first 7 to 14 days. Although this requirement presumably transfers responsibility to the outside physician, the handoff can leave patients stranded early after discharge. Follow-up contact should be scheduled to occur during the first few days that the patient is at home, often from a specialized nurse. For this protocol to be effective, detailed discharge information must transfer smoothly to the outpatient care team.

CONTINUUM OF CARE THROUGH THE COMMUNITY: FUTURE DIRECTIONS

Both quality of life and survival with heart failure have improved dramatically since 1980, as has appreciation of the heavy burden of this disease. The medical advances reflect understanding of the role of neurohormonal stimulation and antagonism, the physiology and evaluation of congestion leading to decompensation, and the indications for devices to avert sudden death and enhance synchrony. Most therapies investigated for acute decompensation have been unsuccessful attempts to encompass the broad population of hospitalized patients. Clinicians remain optimistic that more specific neurohormonal or metabolic profiling will identify a subset of patients who would benefit from specific antagonists or metabolic manipulation. Therapy tailored to individual targets seems more promising than the blind application of all approved therapies until cumulative intolerance. However, the majority of new therapies is more likely to achieve long-term effects when initiated electively during clinical stability than during decompensation.

There are several areas of hospitalization and rehospitalization in which management may improve in the near future. New approaches to improving renal perfusion may enable more definitive therapy to maintain both renal function and fluid balance in hospital and after discharge, in view of the fact that the cardiorenal syndrome is a relentless driver of heart failure events. However, the most profound intervention to affect every aspect of patient success with heart failure has been the assembly of dedicated teams to educate and connect with patients, an approach that evolved from cardiac transplantation programs and clinical research programs with subsidized personnel support.[101] The providers include not only physicians and specialized nurses but also dieticians, pharmacists, social workers, and community services. Such effective management is, however, available to fewer than 5% of patients with heart failure.[102]

The unsupportable price of heart failure hospitalizations can clearly be reduced with better technology to monitor physiological parameters at home and link the patient to providers who share the same electronic records. With steadfast advocacy, the health care system will mature to support clinical reimbursement and focused training for the health professionals, both of which are necessary to bridge the gaps in disease management of heart failure. An additional obligation of specialists in the field is to refine triage in such a way that high-technology solutions can still be offered to patients who will derive the most benefit. Specialists must also find the courage to guide other patients through a natural conclusion of their disease. As patients and medical institutions recognize their shared responsibility for managing heart failure, it will increasingly "take a village" to sustain patients beyond hospitalization to enjoy meaningful lives in their communities.

REFERENCES

1. Gheorghiade, M., & Pang, P. S. (2009). Acute heart failure syndromes. *J Am Coll Cardiol, 53*, 557–573.
2. Yancy, C. W., Lopatin, M., Stevenson, L. W., et al. (2006). Clinical presentation, management, and in-hospital outcomes of patients admitted with acute decompensated heart failure with preserved systolic function: a report from the Acute Decompensated Heart Failure National Registry (ADHERE) database. *J Am Coll Cardiol, 47*, 76–84.
3. Sweitzer, N. K., Lopatin, M., Yancy, C. W., et al. (2008). Comparison of clinical features and outcomes of patients hospitalized with heart failure and normal ejection fraction (> or =55%) versus those with mildly reduced (40% to 55%) and moderately to severely reduced (<40%) fractions. *Am J Cardiol, 101*, 1151–1156.
4. Dickstein, K., Cohen-Solal, A., Filippatos, G., et al. (2008). ESC Guidelines for the diagnosis and treatment of acute and chronic heart failure 2008: the Task Force for the Diagnosis and Treatment of Acute and Chronic Heart Failure 2008 of the European Society of Cardiology. Developed in collaboration with the Heart Failure Association of the ESC (HFA) and endorsed by the European Society of Intensive Care Medicine (ESICM). *Eur Heart J, 29*, 2388–2442.
5. McCarthy, R. E., 3rd, Boehmer, J. P., Hruban, R. H., et al. (2000). Long-term outcome of fulminant myocarditis as compared with acute (nonfulminant) myocarditis. *N Engl J Med, 342*, 690–695.
6. Jessup, M., Abraham, W. T., Casey, D. E., et al. (2009). 2009 Focused update: ACCF/AHA Guidelines for the Diagnosis and Management of Heart Failure in Adults: a report of the American College of Cardiology Foundation/American Heart Association Task Force on Practice Guidelines: developed in collaboration with the International Society for Heart and Lung Transplantation. *Circulation, 119*, 1977–2016.
7. Stevenson, L. W., & Perloff, J. K. (1989). The limited reliability of physical signs for estimating hemodynamics in chronic heart failure. *JAMA, 261*, 884–888.
8. Fonarow, G. C., Abraham, W. T., Albert, N. M., et al. (2008). Factors identified as precipitating hospital admissions for heart failure and clinical outcomes: findings from OPTIMIZE-HF. *Arch Intern Med, 168*, 847–854.
9. Nohria, A., Tsang, S. W., Fang, J. C., et al. (2003). Clinical assessment identifies hemodynamic profiles that predict outcomes in patients admitted with heart failure. *J Am Coll Cardiol, 41*, 1797–1804.
10. Drazner, M. H., Hellkamp, A. S., Leier, C. V., et al. (2008). Value of clinician assessment of hemodynamics in advanced heart failure. The ESCAPE trial. *Circ Heart Fail, 1*, 170–177.
11. Drazner, M. H., Hamilton, M. A., Fonarow, G., et al. (1999). Relationship between right and left-sided filling pressures in 1000 patients with advanced heart failure. *J Heart Lung Transplant, 18*, 1126–1132.
12. Zema, M. J., Restivo, B., Sos, T., et al. (1980). Left ventricular dysfunction—bedside Valsalva manoeuvre. *Br Heart J, 44*, 560–569.
13. Butman, S. M., Ewy, G. A., Standen, J. R., et al. (1993). Bedside cardiovascular examination in patients with severe chronic heart failure: importance of rest or inducible jugular venous distension. *J Am Coll Cardiol, 22*, 968–974.

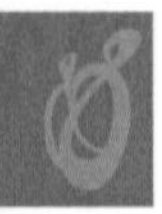

14. Maisel, A. S., McCord, J., Nowak, R. M., et al. (2003). Bedside B-type natriuretic peptide in the emergency diagnosis of heart failure with reduced or preserved ejection fraction. Results from the Breathing Not Properly Multinational Study. *J Am Coll Cardiol, 41*, 2010–2017.
15. Nguyen, V. T., Ho, J. E., Ho, C. Y., et al. (2008). Handheld echocardiography offers rapid assessment of clinical volume status. *Am Heart J, 156*, 537–542.
16. Zile, M. R., Bennett, T. D., St John Sutton, M., et al. (2008). Transition from chronic compensated to acute decompensated heart failure: pathophysiological insights obtained from continuous monitoring of intracardiac pressures. *Circulation, 118*, 1433–1441.
17. Setoguchi, S., Nohria, A., Rassen, J. A., et al. (2009). Maximum potential benefit of implantable defibrillators in preventing sudden death after hospital admission because of heart failure. *Can Med J, 180*, 611–616.
18. Nohria, A., Lewis, E., & Stevenson, L. W. (2002). Medical management of advanced heart failure. *JAMA, 287*, 628–640.
19. Stevenson, L. W., & Tillisch, J. H. (1986). Maintenance of cardiac output with normal filling pressures in patients with dilated heart failure. *Circulation, 74*, 1303–1308.
20. Stevenson, L. W., Brunken, R. C., Belil, D., et al. (1990). Afterload reduction with vasodilators and diuretics decreases mitral regurgitation during upright exercise in advanced heart failure. *J Am Coll Cardiol, 15*, 174–180.
21. Rosario, L. B., Stevenson, L. W., Solomon, S. D., et al. (1998). The mechanism of decrease in dynamic mitral regurgitation during heart failure treatment: importance of reduction in the regurgitant orifice size. *J Am Coll Cardiol, 32*, 1819–1824.
22. Stevenson, L. W., Tillisch, J. H., Hamilton, M., et al. (1990). Importance of hemodynamic response to therapy in predicting survival with ejection fraction less than or equal to 20% secondary to ischemic or nonischemic dilated cardiomyopathy. *Am J Cardiol, 66*, 1348–1354.
23. Rackley, C. E., & Russell, R. O., Jr. (1975). Left ventricular function in acute and chronic coronary artery disease. *Annu Rev Med, 26*, 105–120.
24. Wilson, J. R., Reichek, N., Dunkman, W. B., et al. (1981). Effect of diuresis on the performance of the failing left ventricle in man. *Am J Med, 70*, 234–239.
25. Stevenson, L., Bellil, D., Grover-McKay, M., et al. (1987). Effects of afterload reduction (diuretics and vasodilators) on left ventricular volume and mitral regurgitation in severe congestive heart failure secondary to ischemic or idiopathic dilated cardiomyopathy. *Am J Cardiol, 60*, 654–658.
26. Palardy, M., Stevenson, L. W., Tasissa, G., et al. (2009). Reduction in mitral regurgitation during therapy guided by measured filling pressures in the ESCAPE trial. *Circ Heart Fail, 2*, 181–188.
27. Guiha, N. H., Cohn, J. N., Mikulic, E., et al. (1974). Treatment of refractory heart failure with infusion of nitroprusside. *N Engl J Med, 291*, 587–592.
28. Kaye, D. M., Lambert, G. W., Lefkovits, J., et al. (1994). Neurochemical evidence of cardiac sympathetic activation and increased central nervous system norepinephrine turnover in severe congestive heart failure. *J Am Coll Cardiol, 23*, 570–578.
29. Johnson, W., Omland, T., Hall, C., et al. (2002). Neurohormonal activation rapidly decreases after intravenous therapy with diuretics and vasodilators for class IV heart failure. *J Am Coll Cardiol, 39*, 1623–1629.
30. Morley, D., & Brozena, S. C. (1994). Assessing risk by hemodynamic profile in patients awaiting cardiac transplantation. *Am J Cardiol, 73*, 379–383.
31. Aaronson, K. D., Schwartz, J. S., Chen, T. M., et al. (1997). Development and prospective validation of a clinical index to predict survival in ambulatory patients referred for cardiac transplant evaluation. *Circulation, 95*, 2660–2667.
32. Lucas, C., Johnson, W., Hamilton, M. A., et al. (2000). Freedom from congestion predicts good survival despite previous class IV symptoms of heart failure. *Am Heart J, 140*, 840–847.
33. Binanay, C., Califf, R. M., Hasselblad, V., et al. (2005). Evaluation Study of Congestive Heart Failure and Pulmonary Artery Catheterization Effectiveness: the ESCAPE trial. *JAMA, 294*, 1625–1633.
34. Rogers, J. G., Nohria, A., Hellkamp, A., et al. (2007). Warm-dry clinical profiles at 1 month after HF hospitalization can be used for triage in advanced heart failure [Abstract]. *J Am Coll Cardiol*, 49.
35. Dormans, T. P., van Meyel, J. J., Gerlag, P. G., et al. (1996). Diuretic efficacy of high dose furosemide in severe heart failure: bolus injection versus continuous infusion. *J Am Coll Cardiol, 28*, 376–382.
36. Brater, D. C. (1998). Diuretic therapy. *N Engl J Med, 339*, 387–395.
37. Channer, K. S., McLean, K. A., Lawson-Matthew, P., et al. (1994). Combination diuretic treatment in severe heart failure: a randomised controlled trial. *Br Heart J, 71*, 146–150.
38. Elkayam, U., Tasissa, G., Binanay, C., et al. (2007). Use and impact of inotropes and vasodilator therapy in hospitalized patients with severe heart failure. *Am Heart J, 153*, 98–104.
39. O'Connor, C. OPTIME in CHF trial (2003). *Eur J Heart Failure*, 2003: 5:9–12.
40. Mebazaa, A., Nieminen, M. S., Packer, M., et al. (2007). Levosimendan vs dobutamine for patients with acute decompensated heart failure: the SURVIVE Randomized Trial. *JAMA, 297*, 1883–1891.
41. Beohar, N., Erdogan, A. K., Lee, D. C., et al. (2008). Acute heart failure syndromes and coronary perfusion. *J Am Coll Cardiol, 52*, 13–16.
42. Publication Committee for the VMAC Investigators (Vasodilatation in the Management of Acute CHF). (2002). Intravenous nesiritide vs nitroglycerin for treatment of decompensated congestive heart failure: a randomized controlled trial. *JAMA, 287*, 1531–1540.
43. Sackner-Bernstein, J. D., Skopicki, H. A., & Aaronson, K. D. (2005). Risk of worsening renal function with nesiritide in patients with acutely decompensated heart failure. *Circulation, 111*, 1487–1491.
44. Cataliotti, A., Boerrigter, G., Costello-Boerrigter, L. C., et al. (2004). Brain natriuretic peptide enhances renal actions of furosemide and suppresses furosemide-induced aldosterone activation in experimental heart failure. *Circulation, 109*, 1680–1685.
45. McMurray, J. J., Teerlink, J. R., Cotter, G., et al. (2007). Effects of tezosentan on symptoms and clinical outcomes in patients with acute heart failure: the VERITAS randomized controlled trials. *JAMA, 298*, 2009–2019.
46. Pang, P. S., Konstam, M. A., Krasa, H. B., et al. (2009). Effects of tolvaptan on dyspnoea relief from the EVEREST trials. *Eur Heart J, 30*, 2233–2240.
47. Weinfeld, M. S., Chertow, G. M., & Stevenson, L. W. (1999). Aggravated renal dysfunction during intensive therapy for advanced chronic heart failure. *Am Heart J, 138*(2 Pt 1), 285–290.
48. Krumholz, H. M., Chen, Y. T., Vaccarino, V., et al. (2000). Correlates and impact on outcomes of worsening renal function in patients > or =65 years of age with heart failure. *Am J Cardiol, 85*, 1110–1113.
49. Mullens, W., Abrahams, Z., Francis, G. S., et al. (2009). Importance of venous congestion for worsening of renal function in advanced decompensated heart failure. *J Am Coll Cardiol, 53*, 589–596.
50. Nohria, A., Hasselblad, V., Stebbins, A., et al. (2008). Cardiorenal interactions: insights from the ESCAPE trial. *J Am Coll Cardiol, 51*, 1268–1274.
51. Campbell, P., Drazner, M. H., Kato, M., et al. (2009). Right-left mismatch in the ESCAPE population: discordance between right- and left-sided filling pressures before and after therapy. *J Card Fail, 15*(Suppl. 6), S28.
52. Stevenson, L. W., Dracup, K. A., & Tillisch, J. H. (1989). Efficacy of medical therapy tailored for severe congestive heart failure in patients transferred for urgent cardiac transplantation. *Am J Cardiol, 63*, 461–464.
53. Stevenson, L., Pagani, F. D., Young, J. B., et al. (2009). INTERMACS profiles of advanced heart failure: the current picture. *J Heart Lung Transplant, 28*, 535–541.
54. Kovick, R. B., Tillisch, J. H., Berens, S. C., et al. (1976). Vasodilator therapy for chronic left ventricular failure. *Circulation, 53*, 322–328.
55. Stevenson, L. W. (1999). Tailored therapy to hemodynamic goals for advanced heart failure. *Eur J Heart Fail, 1*, 251–257.
56. Steimle, A. E., Stevenson, L. W., Chelimsky-Fallick, C., et al. (1997). Sustained hemodynamic efficacy of therapy tailored to reduce filling pressures in survivors with advanced heart failure. *Circulation, 96*, 1165–1172.
57. Connors, A. F., Jr., Speroff, T., Dawson, N. V., et al. (1996). The effectiveness of right heart catheterization in the initial care of critically ill patients. SUPPORT Investigators. *JAMA, 276*, 889–897.
58. Shah, M. R., Hasselblad, V., Tasissa, G., et al. (2007). Rapid assay brain natriuretic peptide and troponin I in patients hospitalized with decompensated heart failure (from the Evaluation Study of Congestive Heart Failure and Pulmonary Artery Catheterization Effectiveness trial). *Am J Cardiol, 100*, 1427–1433.
59. Yao, G., Freemantle, N., Calvert, M. J., et al. (2007). The long-term cost-effectiveness of cardiac resynchronization therapy with or without an implantable cardioverter-defibrillator. *Eur Heart J, 28*(1), 42–51.
60. Kamath, S. A., Drazner, M. H., Tasissa, G., et al. (2009). Correlation of impedance cardiography with invasive hemodynamic measurements in patients with advanced heart failure: the BioImpedance CardioGraphy (BIG) substudy of the Evaluation Study of Congestive Heart Failure and Pulmonary Artery Catheterization Effectiveness (ESCAPE) trial. *Am Heart J, 158*, 217–223.
61. Pierpont, G. L., Cohn, J. N., & Franciosa, J. A. (1978). Combined oral hydralazine-nitrate therapy in left ventricular failure. Hemodynamic equivalency to sodium nitroprusside. *Chest, 73*, 8–13.
62. Massie, B., Chatterjee, K., Werner, J., et al. (1977). Hemodynamic advantage of combined administration of hydralazine orally and nitrates nonparenterally in the vasodilator therapy of chronic heart failure. *Am J Cardiol, 40*, 794–801.
63. Cohn, J. N. (1990). Nitrates are effective in the treatment of chronic congestive heart failure: the protagonist's view. *Am J Cardiol, 66*, 444–446.
64. Elkayam, U. (1996). Nitrates in the treatment of congestive heart failure. *Am J Cardiol, 77*, 41C–51C.
65. Colucci, W. S., Elkayam, U., Horton, D. P., et al. (2000). Intravenous nesiritide, a natriuretic peptide, in the treatment of decompensated congestive heart failure. Nesiritide Study Group. *N Engl J Med, 343*, 246–253.
66. Stevenson, L. W. (2003). Clinical use of inotropic therapy for heart failure: looking backward or forward? Part I: inotropic infusions during hospitalization. *Circulation, 108*, 367–372.
67. Binkley, P. F., Starling, R. C., Hammer, D. F., et al. (1991). Usefulness of hydralazine to withdraw from dobutamine in severe congestive heart failure. *Am J Cardiol, 68*, 1103–1106.
68. Stevenson, L. W. (2003). Clinical use of inotropic therapy for heart failure: looking backward or forward? Part II: chronic inotropic therapy. *Circulation, 108*, 492–497.
69. Unverferth, D. A., Blanford, M., Kates, R. E., et al. (1980). Tolerance to dobutamine after a 72 hour continuous infusion. *Am J Med, 69*, 262–266.
70. Silver, M. A., Horton, D. P., Ghali, J. K., et al. (2002). Effect of nesiritide versus dobutamine on short-term outcomes in the treatment of patients with acutely decompensated heart failure. *J Am Coll Cardiol, 39*, 798–803.
71. Tsvetkova, T., Ferguson, D., Abraham, W. T., et al. (1998). Comparative hemodynamic effects of milrinone and dobutamine in heart failure patients treated chronically with carvedilol. *J Card Fail, 4*(Suppl. 1), 36.
72. Biddle, T. L., Benotti, J. R., Creager, M. A., et al. (1987). Comparison of intravenous milrinone and dobutamine for congestive heart failure secondary to either ischemic or dilated cardiomyopathy. *Am J Cardiol, 59*, 1345–1350.
73. Packer, M., Carver, J. R., Rodeheffer, R. J., et al. (1991). Effect of oral milrinone on mortality in severe chronic heart failure. The PROMISE Study Research Group. *N Engl J Med, 325*, 1468–1475.
74. Miller, L. W. (1991). Outpatient dobutamine for refractory congestive heart failure: advantages, techniques, and results. *J Heart Lung Transplant, 10*, 482–487.
75. Lang, R. M., Fellner, S. K., Neumann, A., et al. (1988). Left ventricular contractility varies directly with blood ionized calcium. *Ann Intern Med, 108*, 524–529.
76. Argenziano, M., Choudhri, A. F., Oz, M. C., et al. (1997). A prospective randomized trial of arginine vasopressin in the treatment of vasodilatory shock after left ventricular assist device placement. *Circulation, 96*(Suppl. 9), II-286–II-290.
77. Morales, D. L., Gregg, D., Helman, D. N., et al. (2000). Arginine vasopressin in the treatment of 50 patients with postcardiotomy vasodilatory shock. *Ann Thorac Surg, 69*, 102–106.

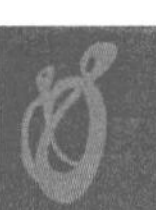

78. Norman, J. C., Colley, D. A., & Igo, S. (1977). Prognostic indices for survival during post-cardiotomy intra-aortic balloon pumping. *J Thorac Cardiovasc Surg*, *74*, 709–713.
79. Fonarow, G. C., Adams, K. F., Jr., Abraham, W. T., et al. (2005). Risk stratification for in-hospital mortality in acutely decompensated heart failure: classification and regression tree analysis. *JAMA*, *293*, 572–580.
80. Ashton, C. M., Kuykendall, D. H., Johnson, M. L., et al. (1995). The association between the quality of inpatient care and early readmission. *Ann Intern Med*, *122*, 415–421.
81. Masoudi, F. A., Gross, C. P., Wang, Y., et al. (2005). Adoption of spironolactone therapy for older patients with heart failure and left ventricular systolic dysfunction in the United States, 1998-2001. *Circulation*, *112*, 39–47.
82. Flapan, A. D., Davies, E., Waugh, C., et al. (1991). Acute administration of captopril lowers the natriuretic and diuretic response to a loop diuretic in patients with chronic cardiac failure. *Eur Heart J*, *12*, 924–927.
83. Packer, M., Lee, W. H., Yushak, M., et al. (1986). Comparison of captopril and enalapril in patients with severe chronic heart failure. *N Engl J Med*, *315*, 847–853. [Erratum, *N Engl J Med* 1986;315:1105.]
84. Kittleson, M., Hurwitz, S., Shah, M. R., et al. (2003). Development of circulatory-renal limitations to angiotensin-converting enzyme inhibitors identifies patients with severe heart failure and early mortality. *J Am Coll Cardiol*, *41*, 2029–2035.
85. Cohn, J. N., Johnson, G., Ziesche, S., et al. (1991). A comparison of enalapril with hydralazine-isosorbide dinitrate in the treatment of chronic congestive heart failure. *N Engl J Med*, *325*, 303–310.
86. Taylor, A. L., Ziesche, S., Yancy, C., et al. (2004). Combination of isosorbide dinitrate and hydralazine in blacks with heart failure. *N Engl J Med*, *351*, 2049–2057.
87. Gattis, W. A., & O'Connor, C. M. (2004). Predischarge initiation of carvedilol in patients hospitalized for decompensated heart failure. *Am J Cardiol*, *93*(9A), 74B–76B.
88. Epstein, A. E., Dimarco, J. P., Ellenbogen, K. A., et al. (2008). ACC/AHA/HRS 2008 Guidelines for device-based therapy of cardiac rhythm abnormalities: executive summary. *Heart Rhythm*, *5*, 934–955.
89. Setoguchi, S., Stevenson, L. W., & Schneeweiss, S. (2007). Repeated hospitalizations predict mortality in the community population with heart failure. *Am Heart J*, *154*, 260–266.
90. Bristow, M. R., Saxon, L. A., Boehmer, J., et al. (2004). Cardiac-resynchronization therapy with or without an implantable defibrillator in advanced chronic heart failure. *N Engl J Med*, *350*, 2140–2150.
91. Cleland, J. G., Daubert, J. C., Erdmann, E., et al. (2005). The effect of cardiac resynchronization on morbidity and mortality in heart failure. *N Engl J Med*, *352*, 1539–1549.
92. Albert, N. M. (2008). Improving medication adherence in chronic cardiovascular disease. *Crit Care Nurse*, *28*(5), 54–64. [Quiz, *Crit Care Nurse* 2008;28(5):65.]
93. Albert, N. M., Buchsbaum, R., & Li, J. (2007). Randomized study of the effect of video education on heart failure healthcare utilization, symptoms, and self-care behaviors. *Patient Educ Couns*, *69*, 129–139.
94. Koelling, T. M., Johnson, M. L., Cody, R. J., et al. (2005). Discharge education improves clinical outcomes in patients with chronic heart failure. *Circulation*, *111*, 179–185.
95. Yamokoski, L. M., Hasselblad, V., Moser, D. K., et al. (2007). Prediction of rehospitalization and death in severe heart failure by physicians and nurses of the ESCAPE trial. *J Card Fail*, *13*, 8–13.
96. Setoguchi, S., & Stevenson, L. W. (2009). Hospitalizations in patients with heart failure: who and why? *J Am Coll Cardiol*, *54*, 1695–1702.
97. Mebazaa, A., Gheorghiade, M., Pina, I. L., et al. (2008). Practical recommendations for prehospital and early in-hospital management of patients presenting with acute heart failure syndromes. *Crit Care Med*, *36*(Suppl. 1), S129–S139.
98. O'Connor CM, Hasselblad V, Mehta A, et al. (2010). Triage after hospitalization with advanced heart failure: the ESCAPE risk model and discharge score. J Am Coll Cardiol, 55: 872–878.
99. Stevenson, L. W., Hellkamp, A. S., Leier, C. V., et al. (2008). Changing preferences for survival after hospitalization with advanced heart failure. *J Am Coll Cardiol*, *52*, 1702–1708.
100. Goodlin, S. J. (2009). Palliative care in congestive heart failure. *J Am Coll Cardiol*, *54*, 386–396.
101. Roccaforte, R., Demers, C., Baldassarre, F., et al. (2005). Effectiveness of comprehensive disease management programmes in improving clinical outcomes in heart failure patients. A meta-analysis. *Eur J Heart Fail*, *7*, 1133–1144.
102. Moser, D. K., & Mann, D. L. (2002). Improving outcomes in heart failure: It's not unusual beyond usual care. *Circulation*, *105*, 2810–2812.
103. Russell, R. O., Jr., Rackley, C. E., Pombo, J., et al. (1970). Effects of increasing left ventricular filling. Pressure in patients with acute myocardial infarction. *J Clin Invest*, *49*, 1539–1550.

CHAPTER 44

Management of Volume Overload in Heart Failure

Stephen S. Gottlieb

Volume overload is one of the most common and important problems facing patients with heart failure. Fluid retention is probably the most frequent manifestation of heart failure. In addition, acute exacerbations in patients with chronic heart failure are often precipitated by volume overload. Even patients with stable chronic heart failure often have symptoms related to fluid status. Although treatment of the fluid overload may not resolve (and could potentially worsen) the underlying problem, it invariably improves the patient's symptoms substantially.

Many factors (such as diet and medication compliance) influence fluid status Whereas, in most patients effective diuresis is straightforward, in conditions refractory to standard therapy, fluid management may be complicated and potentially deleterious. Diuresis may lead to electrolyte abnormalities and consequent arrhythmias. Intravascular depletion can cause hypotension, especially in patients receiving angiotensin-converting enzyme (ACE) inhibitors or angiotensin II receptor antagonists. Neurohormonal activation can also be precipitated by diuretics. Perhaps most important, however, is the renal dysfunction that may be caused by diuretic therapy.

Diuresis is more difficult to achieve when renal function worsens. Increasing diuretic doses may lead to an elevated serum creatinine level with little additional urinary volume, especially in very ill patients (see Chapter 43). Moreover, deteriorating kidney function portends a particularly poor prognosis. Even a slight increase in serum creatinine level is predictive of an increased risk of mortality.[1] Fortunately, new medications and interventions are being developed which may improve the ability to safely and effectively control the fluid status of patients with heart failure.

The various diuretics, sites of action, dosages, and pharmacokinetics are listed in Table 44-1. These data are widely available. This chapter provides the basics of standard therapy and discusses experimental and innovative approaches for patients with refractory heart failure.

TYPES OF DIURETICS

Loop Diuretics

Loop diuretics are generally considered first-line diuretic therapy. They are effective and well tolerated. Although high levels achieved with rapid intravenous administration may cause ototoxicity, this complication is rare and can be prevented by slower administration.[2]

Of concern have been the possible direct and indirect effects of furosemide on myocardium. High doses of diuretics have consistently been associated with worse outcome.[3] It is unknown, however, whether this is because affected individuals are the most ill, or whether the doses have adverse consequences.

In view of the importance of effective diuresis on symptoms, the most common problem is probably underdosing with these drugs. As glomerular filtration decreases, higher doses must be used. This is because loop diuretics are secreted in the proximal tubule and act from the luminal side of the loop of Henle. Thus, doses of furosemide greater than 200 mg may need to be given.

Equivalent high doses of bumetanide and torsemide can be substituted, although there appear to be minimal diuretic differences among the various loop diuretics.[8,9] Despite the common assumption that bowel edema decreases absorption of oral loop diuretics, marked diuresis alters the pharmacokinetics of both furosemide and torsemide in only a small percentage of patients. In these patients, bowel edema delays absorption, rather than decreases it.[9] Thus, even in most edematous patients, adequate dosages of oral diuretics should be successful natriuretics. Although absorption of furosemide appears to be more variable than that of other loop diuretics, furosemide is both inexpensive and effective in most patients.

Of course, changes in a patient's status necessitate changes in the diuretic dosage needed. Improved cardiac function causes increased drug delivery to the nephron, which results in the need to reduce the diuretic dose.[10] Diuresis may also alter the heart's geometry and improve cardiac function. Just as the abnormal valvular and papillary muscle geometry caused by ventricular enlargement can lead to mitral regurgitation,[11] diuresis might reduce left ventricular volume, decrease mitral regurgitation, and improve cardiac performance.[12]

Loop Diuretics and Hypertonic Saline

Coadministration of hypertonic saline with loop diuretics has been suggested to result in more effective diuresis.[13] The theory is that increased intravascular volume helps reduce tissue edema, improve renal blood flow, and decrease neurohormonal activation. However, most observers believe that increased salt intake leads to decompensation and should be avoided. At present, this remains a highly speculative treatment that should be tried only under investigational circumstances.

Other Diuretics

The thiazide diuretics are not as potent as the loop diuretics and therefore are rarely used alone in patients with heart failure. They are ineffective when the glomerular filtration rate

TABLE 44–1 Comparison of Conventional Diuretic Medications, Listed According to Site of Action

Diuretic	FE_{Na^+} (Maximum, %)	Dosage (mg/day)	Onset of Action		Action Duration		Peak Oral Effect (Hours)	Comments
			Oral (Hours)	IV (Minutes)	Oral (Hours)	IV (Hours)		
Ascending Loop of Henle								
Furosemide	20-25	40-400	1	5	6	2-3	1-3	
Bumetanide	20-25	1-5	0.5	5	6	2-3	1-3	
Torsemide	20-25	10-200	1	10	6-8	6-8	1-3	
Ethacrynic acid	20-25	50-100	0.5	5	6-8	3	2	High ototoxicity risk, but (unlike other loop diuretics) can use in sulfa-allergic pts
Early Distal Tubule								
Metolazone	5-8	2.5-20	1	—	12-24	—	2-4	Greatest potential for potassium loss; also slight actions in proximal tubule
Chlorthalidone	5-10	25-200	2	—	24-48	—	6	Ineffective when GFR <30
Hydrochlorothiazide	5-8	25-100	2	—	12	—	4	Ineffective when GFR <30
Chlorothiazide	5-8	500-1000	1	15-30	8	—	4	Ineffective when GFR <30
Late Distal Tubule								
Spironolactone	2	50-400	48-72	—	48-72	—	1-2 days	Efficacy dependent upon aldosterone presence
Triamterene	2	75-300	2	—	12-16	—	6-8	
Amiloride	2	5-10	2	—	24	—	6-16	
Proximal Tubule								
Acetazolamide	4	250-375	1	30-60	8	3-4	2-4	Efficacy limited by metabolic acidosis it causes

FE_{Na^+} (Max, %), maximal natriuretic effect (maximum fractional excretion of filtered sodium); GFR, glomerular filtration rate; IV, intravenously.
Adapted from Gottlieb SS. Diuretics. In Hosenpud JD, Greenberg B, editors. *Congestive heart failure: pathophysiology, diagnosis, and comprehensive approach to management.* Philadelphia, 1999, Lippincott Williams & Wilkins.

(GFR) is below approximately 30 mL/min, a common occurrence in patients with heart failure. Furthermore, thiazides cause a greater decrease in potassium than do loop diuretics for the same quantity of diuresis.[14]

Spironolactone is also not a potent diuretic. It works at the distal end of the distal convoluted tubule and cortical collecting duct, where it acts as a competitive inhibitor at the aldosterone receptor. Spironolactone blocks distal sodium resorption. Spironolactone and other potassium-sparing agents are weak diuretics because the distal delivery of sodium is decreased in the normal state. They are therefore rarely effective as a single agent in patients who need diuresis.

Spironolactone at low doses is commonly used not because of its diuretic effects but because its benefit is presumed to be the result of direct cardiac actions.[15] Aldosterone inhibition is important (at least in patients with severe heart failure) because of its role in myocardial remodeling and vascular fibrosis,[16,17] vascular damage,[18] baroreceptor dysfunction,[19] and prevention of myocardial norepinephrine uptake.

There are data to suggest that torsemide, but not furosemide, may block the renin-angiotensin-aldosterone system. This could then result in less cardiac fibrosis and myocardial remodeling.[4] In one animal study, torsemide suppressed left ventricular fibrosis, myocardial protein levels of transforming growth factor-β_1, collagen III, and aldosterone synthase and improved survival rate to the control level, but furosemide did not.[5] There is also a suggestion that the activities of torsemide on the sympathetic system might be different from those of furosemide.[6] In a nonrandomized clinical study, outcomes with torsemide were better.[7] The conclusions from these studies must be tempered with some concerns, however. The animal studies do not mimic clinical use, and the human study was only an observational analysis. Even if there are differences among agents, perhaps the concomitant use of ACE inhibitors and β-blockers prevents furosemide toxicity. Because of the common use of the very inexpensive furosemide, it is clear that until definitive proof is present, diuresis with furosemide will be necessary and will continue.

COMBINATION OF DIURETICS

In patients with more advanced heart failure, distal tubule reabsorption may limit the efficacy of loop diuretics. In such patients, the combination of agents may be potent enough to enable diuresis. In particular, the combination of metolazone

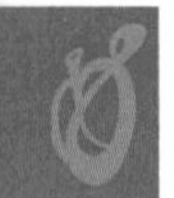

and loop diuretics has been shown to be very effective.[20] Because of the pharmacokinetics of metolazone, however, an effect should not be expected immediately. This combination may result in potent potassium wasting, and the clinician needs to monitor potassium levels carefully and address any resulting hypokalemia.

In addition to its beneficial effects with regard to mortality (which is believed not to be secondary to potassium sparing), spironolactone may be used to maintain serum potassium concentrations. When used in combination with other diuretics, it may potentiate the effects of the loop diuretic while helping control potassium loss. Dosages for diuretic and potassium-sparing effects are higher (50 to 100 mg/day) than those shown to be beneficial in the Randomized Aldactone Evaluation Study (RALES) (25 mg/day; see Chapter 45).[15]

EXTENT OF DIURESIS

The extent to which a patient should undergo diuresis is not known. Often treatment is directed toward improving acute symptoms; the physician may permit continued fluid overload. However, it is not enough to prevent pulmonary edema. Symptoms improve when the fluid status is optimized. Nonetheless, clinical evaluations are difficult, and the extent to which the patient needs diuresis may not be clear. Although it may be obvious that someone with peripheral edema and ascites has fluid overload, the extent of fluid in the abdomen may be difficult to determine, and intravascular pressures may be markedly elevated with no obvious extra fluid.

Some physicians believe that all patients with severe heart failure should be treated with hemodynamic monitoring. They believe that a pulmonary capillary wedge pressure of 15 to 20 mm Hg should be achieved with a combination of diuresis and vasodilatation. However, this theory has not been supported by the results of the randomized Evaluation Study of Congestive heArt failure and Pulmonary artery catheterization Effectiveness (ESCAPE), which showed that addition of a pulmonary artery catheter to careful clinical assessment did not affect rates of overall mortality and hospitalization (Figure 44-1; see also Chapter 43).[21] Other investigations of continuous monitoring with implanted devices have yielded results that supported the prognostic importance of elevated filling pressures, but these results did not also show that monitoring could lead to a better outcome.[22a] The Chronicle Offers Management to Patients with Advanced Signs and Symptoms of Heart Failure (COMPASS-HF) trial was a randomized controlled study of an implantable continuous hemodynamic monitor (the Chronicle) that was placed in the right ventricular outflow tract in patients with advanced heart failure. The primary efficacy endpoint of COMPASS-HF, which was reduction in the rate of heart failure–related events (hospitalizations and emergency or urgent care visits necessitating intravenous therapy), was not met insofar as the group with the implantable hemodynamic device had a nonsignificant ($P = .33$) 21% lower rate of all heart failure–related events than did the control group.[22a] Several other additional implantable hemodynamic monitors are under investigation: the HeartPOD, a stand-alone pressure monitor that is placed in the left atrium through a transseptal approach; the CardioMEMS Heart Sensor, a wireless system that is implanted in the pulmonary artery; and the RemonCHF System, an acoustic wave technology device that measures absolute pressures in the pulmonary artery (reviewed by Tallaj and colleagues[22b]). Each of these devices is currently being tested in patients with heart failure. Although patients with obvious fluid overload feel better if peripheral edema can be eliminated, the ideal method for achieving this has not been established clearly. Moreover, worsening renal function or adverse events are limiting factors in some patients.

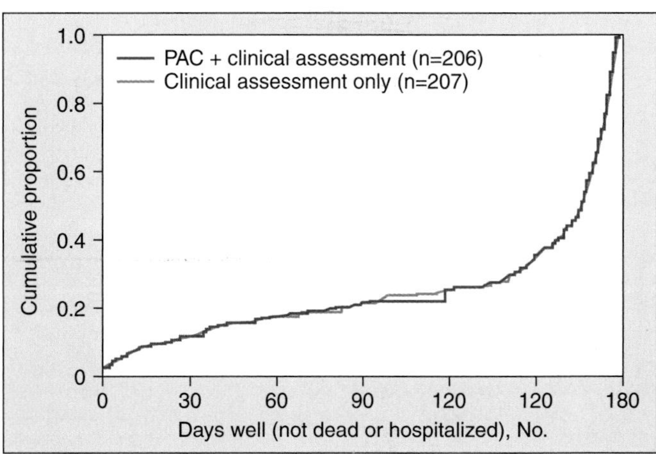

FIGURE 44-1 Hemodynamic monitoring by means of a pulmonary arterial catheter has not been shown to improve outcomes in patients admitted with heart failure. This illustration shows the cumulative proportion of patients contributing each possible numerical outcome for the number of days neither dead nor hospitalized during the 180 possible days of follow-up. The far left side of the curve represents early deaths; patients were considered to have survived 180 days if they lived for 6 months without rehospitalization. The curves for the two groups are virtually identical. PAC, pulmonary artery catheter. (From Binanay C, Califf RM, Hasselblad V, et al. Evaluation study of congestive heart failure and pulmonary artery catheterization effectiveness: the ESCAPE trial. *JAMA* 2005;294:1625-1633.)

Study data have raised hope that measurement of B-type natriuretic peptide (BNP) or N-terminal pro-B-type natriuretic peptide (NT-proBNP) may be helpful in assessing fluid status (see also Chapter 37). It is suggested that a normal value (or the best value for an individual patient) enables each patient's fluid status to be adjusted optimally. As with hemodynamic monitoring, the promise of better outcomes has not been definitively proven. Better outcomes have occurred in randomized studies evaluating the impact of following NT-proBNP or BNP. Interestingly, however, doses of beta blockade and ACE inhibition are increased in these studies, suggesting that it is not the natriuretic peptide, but attention to getting patients on proven doses of medication, that is important.[23,24] Although natriuretic peptides are clearly prognostic (as discussed elsewhere), the difficulty in using them to treat individual patients may be partly related to the multiple factors other than filling pressures that can influence concentrations.[25,26]

RISKS WITH DIURESIS

The most obvious risks with diuresis are hypokalemia and consequent ventricular arrhythmias. Rapid diuresis and the change in potassium that often occurs with hospitalization appear to increase the risk of potentially life-threatening arrhythmias.[27] Less worrisome, but often very bothersome to the patient, are muscle aches, which may occur with hypokalemia.

The risk of potassium depletion is common because when a diuretic increases sodium delivery to the distal renal tubule, potassium is excreted as the sodium is reabsorbed. Neurohormonal activation may further contribute to the hypokalemic effects of diuretics. To further complicate the issue, however, are factors that might lead to potassium retention.

Because most patients with heart failure receive potassium-sparing ACE inhibitors and frequently receive spironolactone, it is difficult to predict how an individual's electrolyte concentration will respond to a diuretic. Renal function, neurohormonal activation, and individual variability all affect electrolyte concentrations. Indeed, hyperkalemia could occur if potassium is prescribed for a patient receiving potassium-sparing agents in addition to diuretics.

The frequent prescription of potassium to patients receiving loop diuretics or the instruction to eat potassium-rich foods may lead to serious problems.[28] Even salt substitutes (which frequently contain potassium) may cause hyperkalemia in a patient receiving potassium-sparing agents. For these reasons, electrolytes need to be monitored carefully in all patients with heart failure.

Patients with heart failure often waste magnesium and have magnesium depletion.[29] The need for and efficacy of magnesium replacement, however, are less certain than those of potassium. Serum concentrations of magnesium do not adequately reflect tissue stores, and oral replacement is rarely effective. Although low magnesium concentrations are predictive of a worse outcome,[30] it is not known whether this is directly secondary to magnesium depletion or reflective of other abnormalities. At present, few data indicate the necessity of chronic oral magnesium replacement.

Diuretics also cause other metabolic abnormalities. Bicarbonate reabsorption (with consequent metabolic alkalosis) and decreased serum uric acid excretion (with consequent gout and possibly change in free radical concentration) may lead to clinically important abnormalities. Hyponatremia often occurs in patients with severe heart failure. It is usually secondary to total body fluid overload, not to sodium depletion,[31] and it reflects stimulation of the vasopressin and renin-angiotensin systems.[32] Although chronic hyponatremia is prognostic,[33] there is no conclusive evidence that it is dangerous and needs to be treated.

Diuretics clearly lead to neurohormonal activation, which can have deleterious consequences. For example, plasma renin activity and plasma concentrations of angiotensin II increase in patients with heart failure after diuretic therapy.[34,35] Patients with normal concentrations of catecholamines, aldosterone, or plasma renin activity demonstrate increases in these concentrations after diuresis.[36] Of interest, however, is that patients with elevated baseline concentrations may have decreased neurohormonal concentrations after initial diuretic treatment (and improvement in symptoms), but concentrations increase as dry weight is approached and less sodium is delivered to the renal tubule.[37]

As discussed previously, there are suggestions that furosemide (and perhaps other loop diuretics) might be directly harmful. In addition to the prognostic importance of diuretic dose (which might merely reflect the severity of disease), one animal study demonstrated worse outcomes with furosemide in a pacing model of heart failure. Not only did furosemide lead to activation of the renin-angiotensin-aldosterone axis but also animals with heart failure that received active drug demonstrated more cardiac dilation and worsening survival rates (Figure 44-2).[38]

Although the beneficial effects of neurohormonal antagonism suggest that activation by diuretics may be deleterious, adequate diuresis is mandated because it provides symptom relief. Adverse consequences of diuresis, whether secondary to neurohormonal activation or to electrolyte depletion, must be dealt with directly after adequate diuresis. However, the many possible ways that diuretics might cause worse outcomes also suggest that clinicians should always consider stopping diuretics when possible.

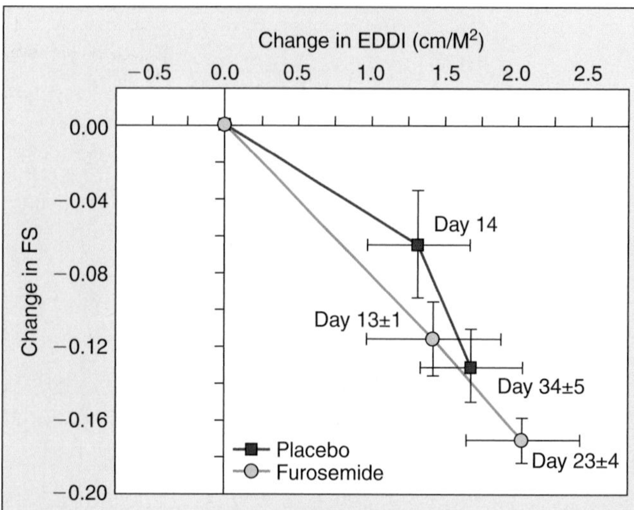

FIGURE 44–2 Furosemide may lead to neurohormonal activation, which raises questions about its long-term outcome. In animals, furosemide, for the treatment of fluid overload in a pacing model of heart failure, led to cardiac dilation and increased rates of mortality. EDDI, end-diastolic diameter index; FS, fractional shortening. (From McCurley JM, Hanlon SU, Wei SK, et al. Furosemide and the progression of left ventricular dysfunction in experimental heart failure. *J Am Coll Cardiol* 2004;44:1301-1307.)

DIURETIC RESISTANCE AND MANAGEMENT

One of the inherent limitations of diuretics is that they achieve water loss by means of excretion of solute at the expense of glomerular filtration, with activation of neurohormonal systems that ultimately limit the effectiveness of diuretics. In normal subjects, the magnitude of natriuresis after a given dose of diuretic declines over time, which is known as the "braking phenomenon" (Figure 44-3).

The magnitude of the natriuretic effect of potent loop diuretics may also be decreased in patients with heart failure, particularly as heart failure progresses. Although the bioavailability of these diuretics is generally not lower in heart failure, the potential delay in their rate of absorption may result in peak drug levels within the tubular lumen in the ascending loop of Henle that are insufficient to induce maximal natriuresis. The use of intravenous formulations or higher doses may obviate this problem.

Even with intravenous dosing, a rightward shift of the dose-response curve is observed between the diuretic concentration in the tubular lumen and its natriuretic effect in heart failure (Figure 44-4). Moreover, the maximal effect is lower in heart failure. This rightward shift has been referred to as "*diuretic resistance*" and it probably has several causes, in addition to the braking phenomenon described previously. First, most loop diuretics, with the exception of torsemide, are short-acting drugs. Accordingly, after a period of natriuresis, the diuretic concentration in plasma and tubular fluid declines below the diuretic threshold. In this situation, renal sodium reabsorption is no longer inhibited, and a period of antinatriuresis or postdiuretic sodium chloride (NaCl) retention ensues. If dietary NaCl intake is moderate to excessive, postdiuretic NaCl retention may overcome the initial natriuresis in patients with excessive activation of the adrenergic nervous system and the renin-angiotensin system. This observation forms the rationale for administering short-acting diuretics several times per day or by constant infusion to obtain consistent daily salt and water loss. Second, renal responsiveness to endogenous natriuretic peptides is lost as heart failure advances. Third, diuretics increase solute delivery to distal segments of the nephron, which causes epithelial cells to undergo both hypertrophy and hyperplasia.

REFRACTORY CONDITIONS

In patients whose conditions are refractory to oral diuretics, intravenous loop diuretics may be effective. By achieving higher serum concentrations, such patients may achieve

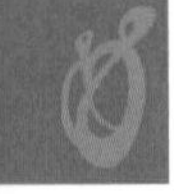

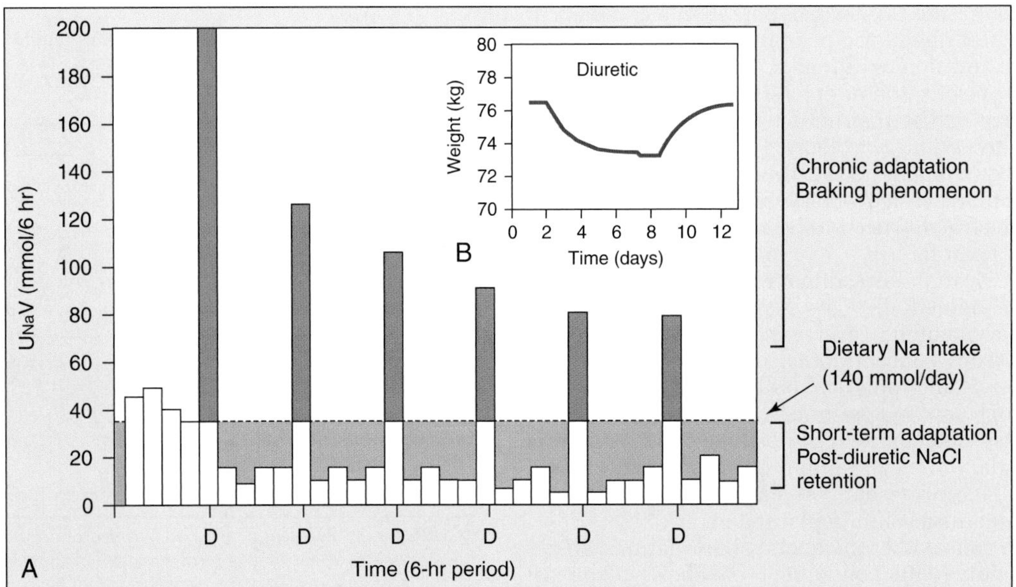

FIGURE 44–3 Effects of diuretics on urinary sodium (Na) excretion and extracellular fluid volume. *Main graph:* Effects of a loop diuretic on urinary sodium excretion ($U_{Na}V$). *Bars* represent 6-hour periods before (in sodium balance) and after doses of loop diuretic (D). The *dotted line* indicates dietary sodium intake. The *solid red portion of the open bars* indicates the amount by which sodium excretion exceeds intake during natriuresis. The pink shaded area indicate the amount of positive sodium balance after the diuretic effect has worn off. Net sodium balance during 24 hours is the difference between the pink shaded area (postdiuretic sodium chloride [NaCl] retention) and the bars (diuretic-induced natriuresis). Chronic adaptation is indicated by progressively smaller peak natriuretic effects (the "braking phenomenon") and is mirrored by a return to neutral balance. *Inset:* Effect of a diuretic on body weight. Note that steady state is reached within 6 to 8 days despite continued diuretic administration. (From Mann DL. Management of heart failure with a reduced ejection fraction. In Libby P, Bonow RO, Mann DL, et al, editors. *Braunwald's heart disease,* Philadelphia, 2008, Elsevier, Figure 25-12.)

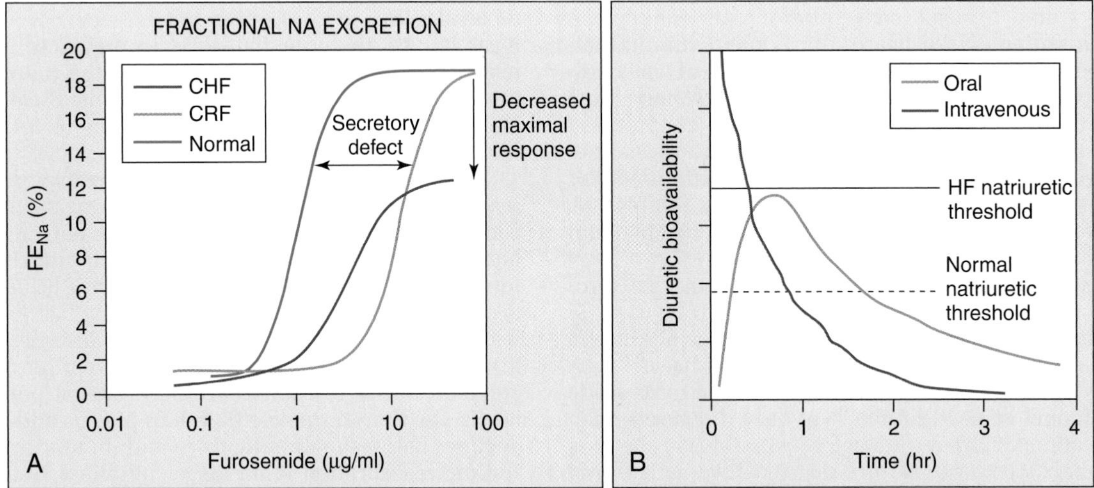

FIGURE 44–4 Dose-response curves for loop diuretics. **A,** Fractional sodium (Na) excretion (FE_{Na}) as a function of loop diuretic concentration. In comparison with normal patients, patients with chronic renal failure (CRF) manifest a rightward shift in the curve, as a result of impaired diuretic secretion. The maximal response is preserved when expressed as FE_{Na} but not when expressed as absolute sodium excretion. Patients with heart failure (HF) demonstrate a rightward and downward shift, even when the response is expressed as FE_{Na}, and thus are relatively diuretic resistant. **B,** Comparison of the response to intravenous and oral doses of loop diuretics in normal subjects and in patients with heart failure. Diuretic bioavailability is shown for normal and patients with heart failure. The natriuretic threshold necessary to produce a diuresis in shown for normal subjects (*dotted line*) and for patients with heart failure (*solid line*). In a normal individual, an oral dose may be as effective as an intravenous dose because the diuretic bioavailabilities (area under the curve) that are above the natriuretic threshold for intravenous and oral diuretics are approximately equal. However, if the natriuretic threshold increases in a patient with heart failure, then the oral dose may not produce a high enough serum level to elicit significant natriuresis. CHF, congestive heart failure. (From Mann DL. Management of heart failure with a reduced ejection fraction. In Libby P, Bonow RO, Mann DL, et al, editors. *Braunwald's heart disease,* Philadelphia, 2008, Elsevier, Figure 25-13.)

adequate diuresis. Some physicians use intravenous drips of loop diuretics,[39] although high doses of the agents may be just as effective.[40] The optimal dose and means of administration of loop diuretics have recently been evaluated in the Diuretic Optimal Strategy Evaluation in Acute Heart Failure (DOSE) trial (ClinicalTrials.gov Identifier: NCT00577135), sponsored by the National Heart, Lung, and Blood Institute.[40a] Initial results from the DOSE study have demonstrated that Q12 hour bolus dosing and continuous infusion appear to be equivalent in terms of symptom relief, changes in renal function, and measures of congestion. Although high dose therapy (2.5 × oral dose given IV) was not superior to low dose (1 × the oral dose given IV) based on the primary efficacy endpoint of global symptom relief over 72 hours, high dose was associated with improvements in dyspnea resolution of signs and symptoms of congestion, net fluid loss, and greater decrease in NTproBNP.

These potentially beneficial findings were balanced against a modest worsening of renal function in the high dose arm, although these differences in renal function were transient and did not persist until discharge or day 60.[40a] When diuretics, alone or in combination, are not adequate, however, there are numerous other techniques that may be tried.

First, clinicians should investigate possible reversible causes. Prostatic or other mechanical obstruction may be overlooked in a patient with severe heart failure. Nephrotoxic agents should also be eliminated. In this regard, it is important to query the patient about the concurrent use of drugs that adversely affect renal function. In particular, the adverse potential of nonsteroidal anti-inflammatory drugs (NSAIDs) is underappreciated. Renal function in patients with heart failure may be dependent on renal prostaglandins. Even in normal individuals, the combination of diuretics and aspirin may lead to decreases in the GFR.[41] In patients with severe heart failure, even a single dose of indomethacin may markedly lower the GFR.[42] The insulin-sensitizing thiazolidinediones have also been linked to increased fluid retention in patients with heart failure, although the clinical significance of this finding is not known. It has been suggested that thiazolidinediones activate proliferator-activated γ-receptor expression in the renal collecting duct, which enhances expression of cell-surface epithelial sodium channels. Moreover, studies in healthy men have shown that pioglitazone stimulates plasma renin activity that may contribute to increased sodium retention. It is not clear, however, whether the fluid retained in these patients is intravascular.

Inotropic Agents (see Chapter 43)

Because the underlying cause of inadequate diuresis is often insufficient renal perfusion secondary (either directly or indirectly) to low cardiac output, inotropic support is often used to effect diuresis in a patient with refractory heart failure. Indeed, inotropes have been shown to improve renal blood flow, but not necessarily more than ACE inhibitors.[43] Of interest is that in one small study, milrinone increased diuresis only in patients with a serum creatinine concentration of less than 2 mg/dL[44]; this suggests that improved renal blood flow does not lead to further diuresis in some patients or that renal blood flow does not increase in certain patients.

The Outcomes of a Prospective Trial of Intravenous Milrinone for Exacerbations of Chronic Heart Failure (OPTIME) study showed that acute inotropic support does not necessarily improve outcomes in patients admitted to a hospital for heart failure (Figure 44-5).[45] This was true even for the patients with BUN concentrations in the highest quartile. Similarly, milrinone did not decrease the number of patients with 25% or more worsening of renal function.[46] Nevertheless, increased cardiac output is generally assumed to improve diuresis in a patient with severe heart failure; anecdotal evidence supports the use of dobutamine and milrinone in patients with inadequate diuresis secondary to heart failure.

Dopaminergic Agents

Dopamine (at low doses, such as 2 to 5 μg/kg/min) and other dopaminergic agents have frequently been used to increase renal blood flow, renal function, and diuresis. Because dopamine-1 receptor blockade leads to increased renal plasma flow, it conceptually makes sense that such agents will work. In one study of 120 patients with heart failure, low-dose dopamine increased creatinine clearance from 35.6 ± 11.6 mL/min to 48.8 ± 12.3 mL/min.[47] An inotropic effect could lead to an improved GFR.[48] However, many researchers have questioned the clinical utility of dopamine,[49] and a meta-analysis of low doses of dopamine given to reduce the incidence and severity of renal failure in critically ill patients revealed no improvement in rates of death or renal failure.[50]

Other dopaminergic agents have also been less beneficial than once assumed. A study of the dopaminergic agent ibopamine revealed increased mortality.[51] No effect on renal function was reported in that study. In another study, renal function improved slightly in 10 patients with mild to moderate heart failure.[52] Fenoldopam, a dopaminergic agent available to treat hypertensive crisis, has demonstrated only minor renal effects. Renal function was reported in one study[53] to improve in comparison with nitroprusside in patients with hypertensive emergency; however, in another study, GFR did not improve, even though renal blood flow increased.[54]

Ultrafiltration and Dialysis

Ultrafiltration and other forms of dialysis may be useful for patients with refractory heart failure, and they have been advocated by some experts for even more widespread use. In contrast to conventional hemodialysis, ultrafiltration removes water, sodium, and non-protein-bound small and medium-sized molecular solutes. One system makes it possible to perform this with peripheral catheters.

Studies have clearly demonstrated the feasibility of removing fluid with ultrafiltration (although adequate peripheral intravenous access may be difficult to achieve). The largest randomized study to date (UltrafiltratioN versus IV Diuretics for Patients HospitaLized for Acute Decompensated Congestive Heart Failure [UNLOAD]) demonstrated that it was possible to remove large amounts of fluid safely.[55] However, there remains the question of whether ultrafiltration is safer than usual diuretics or leads to a better outcome.

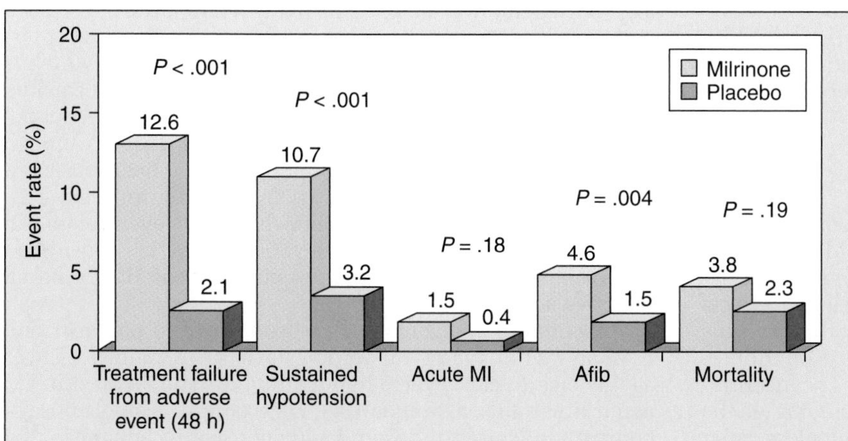

FIGURE 44–5 The inotropic agent milrinone did not improve outcomes in Outcomes of a Prospective Trial of Intravenous Milrinone for Exacerbations of Chronic Heart Failure (OPTIME-HF). Adverse events were increased in patients receiving milrinone. Afib, atrial fibrillation; MI, myocardial infarction. (From Cuffe MS, Califf RM, Adams KF Jr, Short-term intravenous milrinone for acute exacerbation of chronic heart failure: a randomized controlled trial. *JAMA*. 2002;287:1541-1547.)

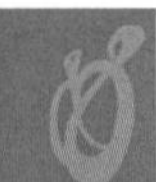

Results of small preliminary studies suggested that ultrafiltration might lead to less neurohormonal activation. In one study of 16 patients, plasma renin activity, and norepinephrine and aldosterone concentrations fell with ultrafiltration but not with furosemide. In addition, the weight loss persisted in the patients who received ultrafiltration.[56] If ultrafiltration could lead to less renal dysfunction and more weight loss, it certainly would be useful for the sickest patients. However, subsequent studies have not proved that a benefit exists.

In a review of the clinical use of ultrafiltration at one center, renal dysfunction was common.[57] Furthermore, a randomized crossover study yielded no differences between subjects who received furosemide and those who received ultrafiltration.[58] Even in UNLOAD, the incidence of worsening creatinine concentration appeared higher in the patients who received ultrafiltration.[54] It is true that the long-term outcome with ultrafiltration in UNLOAD was better, with fewer repeat hospitalizations, than that with diuretics. However, patients also lost more fluid with ultrafiltration, which raises the concern that more effective conventional diuresis would have yielded the same results.

At present, it is reasonable to consider ultrafiltration for patients with fluid overload who have difficulty achieving diuresis with conventional medications. More evidence of benefit must be collected to support the broader use advocated by some experts. In addition, the use of dialysis can be appropriate in patients who cannot maintain both euvolemia and renal function.

Natriuretic Peptides (see Chapter 18)

The renal actions of the natriuretic peptides have been extensively discussed and are being investigated. Both BNP and atrial natriuretic peptide (ANP) are hemodynamically active. They cause vasodilation and lower ventricular filling pressures; nesiritide (recombinant human BNP) was approved in the United States for treatment of heart failure on the basis of its hemodynamic effects.[59] After widespread use, however, concerns about adverse effects were raised, and most physicians believe that more information is needed.

In the acute situation, ANP and BNP are effective natriuretic and diuretic agents.[60] Whether these agents have similar effects in more chronic situations, however, remains uncertain.[61] Studies suggest that tolerance to these agents can develop, perhaps as a result of changes in the receptor density or form. In a crossover study of patients with worsening renal function and heart failure, nesiritide had no natriuretic, diuretic, or renal effects.[62] There are anecdotal reports of effective diuresis; however, the publication of analyses that demonstrate more renal dysfunction and worse survival among patients receiving nesiritide[63,64] mandates that these drugs be used only as indicated by the U.S. Food and Drug Administration (FDA). Because there are no renal indications for the drug, it is rarely useful in clinical practice.

Other natriuretic peptides are being developed.[65] Differences in hemodynamic effects (such as vasodilation) or renal actions might make some of these agents safer or more effective than nesiritide.

Adenosine Antagonists

Plasma adenosine concentrations are elevated in patients with heart failure.[66] In these patients, adenosine may decrease glomerular filtration, an action that could be secondary to dilation of postglomerular vessels[67] or vasoconstrictive effects before the glomerulus.[68] Perhaps the most important actions of adenosine in the kidney, however, are its effects on tubuloglomerular feedback. An acute increase in sodium concentration in the proximal tubule feeds back to decrease GFR via the macula densa; this relationship is known as "tubuloglomerular feedback."[69] Adenosine constricts the afferent arteriole via the adenosine-1 (A_1)-receptor, leading to decreased glomerular filtration and less diuresis.

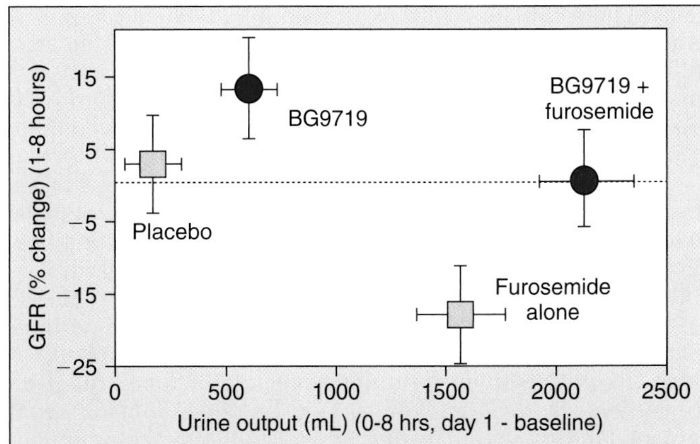

FIGURE 44-6 Adenosine antagonists are being investigated as diuretics that improve renal function. In one study, the adenosine A_1 antagonist BG9719 in combination with furosemide increased urine output while preserving the glomerular filtration rate (GFR). (From Gottlieb SS, Abraham W, Butler J, et al. The prognostic importance of different definitions of worsening renal function in congestive heart failure. *J Card Fail* 2002;8:136-141.)

Selective A_1-receptor blockade has been shown to increase urine volume and sodium excretion.[70] Some studies also suggest that A_1-receptor blockade increases GFR.[71] In an early clinical study, the adenosine A_1 antagonist BG9719 caused a dose-dependent increase in urine output. Although furosemide alone caused a large diuresis, the addition of BG9719 to furosemide not only caused a further increase but also prevented the decline in creatinine clearance associated with furosemide (Figure 44-6). Recent studies of another A_1 receptor, rolofylline (KW-3902), supports their beneficial renal actions. In a crossover study, rolofylline improved GFR.[72] In another study, clinical utility was seen.[73] However, in the pivotal Placebo-controlled Randomized study of the selective A_1 adenosine receptor antagonist KW-3902 for patients hospitalized with acute HF and volume Overload to assess Treatment Effect on Congestion and renal function Trial (PROTECT), rolofylline did not improve symptoms of acute heart failure in comparison with placebo. Moreover, treatment with rolofylline, 30 mg, did not reduce the risk of death or rehospitalization for cardiovascular or renal reasons, which was the secondary endpoint of the trial. The chief worry with these agents is that adenosine A_1-receptor blockade could cause seizures.

Vasopressin Antagonists

The importance of vasopressin as the cause of hyponatremia and fluid retention in patients with heart failure has been debated. It appears to work through aquaporin, a vasopressin-regulated water channel in collecting duct cells, which is excreted partly into urine[74] and whose levels are correlated with arginine vasopressin concentrations. Urinary aquaporin increases in the setting of a hypertonic load. Although elevated concentrations of vasopressin have been observed in patients with congestive heart failure, the reported concentrations have not been very high.[75] Nevertheless, in hyponatremic patients, any elevation must be considered inappropriate, and an antagonist could theoretically be an effective aquaretic.

Vasopressin antagonists have been given to patients with hyponatremia, many of whom have heart failure. These agents clearly can reverse hyponatremia[76] and, at least in the acute situation, cause aquaresis. For example, a single dose of conivaptan caused a dose-related increase in aquaresis that

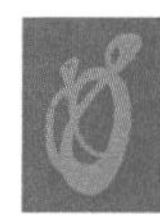

was associated with improved hemodynamic parameters.[77] Results of more prolonged studies, however, suggest that both increased water intake and decreased responsiveness to the vasopressin antagonist might limit the chronic effects of these drugs. For example, the selective vasopressin-2 (V_2) antagonist OPC-31260 caused only short-term effects in an animal model.[78] Another selective V_2 antagonist, SR121463, produced less urine excretion after 1 day, although the amount was more than with placebo.[79] In these normally hydrated rats, moreover, water intake increased to compensate for increased urine output. In human studies, the decrease in weight occurs early, but this decrease appears to slow down with time.[80]

Nevertheless, it is hoped, on the basis of animal studies,[81] that antidiuretic hormone (ADH) antagonists can cause diuresis without the neurohormonal activation of loop diuretics. If so, long-term outcome could conceivably be improved. This possibility was tested with tolvaptan in the Efficacy of Vasopressin Antagonism in Heart Failure Outcome Study With Tolvaptan (EVEREST), which was a study of combined acute and chronic situations. Although tolvaptan decreased body weight and improved patient symptomatology in the acute situation,[82] there was no improvement in the composite endpoint of mortality or hospitalizations (hazard ratio, 1.04; 95% confidence interval, 0.95 to 1.14; P = .55) in patients who received the active drug.[83] Tolvaptan is currently approved by the FDA for the treatment of hyponatremia, but it is not approved for the treatment of heart failure.

CONCLUSION

Most cases of congestive heart failure can be managed very successfully with standard diuretic medications. Adequate dosages and multiple medications, if necessary, may mitigate symptoms of heart failure. However, diuresis is limited in some patients because of worsening renal function, which is a poor prognostic sign. For such patients, innovative approaches may be necessary. Fortunately, multiple drugs are being developed to address this issue. It is hoped that these drugs might enable diuresis while preventing renal dysfunction.

REFERENCES

1. Gottlieb, S. S., Abraham, W., Butler, J., et al. (2002). The prognostic importance of different definitions of worsening renal function in congestive heart failure. *J Card Fail, 8,* 136–141.
2. Howard, P. A., & Dunn, M. I. (2001). Aggressive diuresis for severe heart failure in the elderly. *Chest, 119,* 807–810.
3. Hasselblad, V., Gattis Stough, W., Shah, M. R., et al. (2007). Relation between dose of loop diuretics and outcomes in a heart failure population: results of the ESCAPE trial. *Eur J Heart Fail, 9,* 1064–1069.
4. López, B., Querejeta, R., González, A., et al. (2004). Effects of loop diuretics on myocardial fibrosis and collagen type I turnover in chronic heart failure. *J Am Coll Cardiol, 43,* 2028–2035.
5. Veeraveedu, P. T., Watanabe, K., Ma, M., et al. (2008). Comparative effects of Torsemide and furosemide in rats with heart failure. *Biochem Pharmacol, 75,* 649–659.
6. Kasama, S., Toyama, T., Hatori, T., et al. (2006). Effects of torsemide on cardiac sympathetic nerve activity and left ventricular remodelling in patients with congestive heart failure. *Heart, 92,* 1434–1440.
7. Cosín, J., & Díez, J. (2002). TORIC investigatos. Torsemide in chronic heart failure: results of the TORIC study. *Eur J Heart Fail, 4,* 507–513.
8. Brater, D. C., Day, B., Burdette, A., et al. (1984). Bumetanide and furosemide in heart failure. *Kidney Int, 26,* 183–189.
9. Gottlieb, S. S., Khatta, M., Wentworth, D., et al. (1998). The effects of diuresis on the pharmacokinetics of loop diuretics in patients with heart failure. *Am J Med, 104,* 533–538.
10. Nomura, A., Yasuda, H., Minami, M., et al. (1981). Effect of furosemide in congestive heart failure. *Clin Pharmacol Ther, 30,* 177–182.
11. Perloff, J. K., & Roberts, W. C. (1972). The mitral apparatus: functional anatomy and mitral regurgitation. *Circulation, 46,* 227–239.
12. Ramirez, A., & Abelmann, W. H. (1968). Hemodynamic effects of diuresis by ethacrynic acid. *Arch Intern Med, 121,* 320–326.
13. Licata, G., Di Pasquale, P., Parrinello, G., et al. (2003). Effects of high-dose furosemide and small-volume hypertonic saline solution infusion in comparison with a high dose of furosemide as bolus in refractory congestive heart failure: long-term effects. *Am Heart J, 145,* 459–466.
14. Morgan, D. B., & Davidson, C. (1980). Hypokalemia and diuretics: an analysis of publications. *BMJ, 280,* 905–908.
15. Pitt, B., Zannad, F., Remme, W. J., et al. (1999). The effect of spironolactone on morbidity and mortality in patients with severe heart failure. Randomized Aldactone Evaluation Study Investigators. *N Engl J Med, 341,* 709–717.
16. Brilla, C. G., Matsubara, L. S., & Weber, K. T. (1993). Anti-aldosterone treatment and the prevention of myocardial fibrosis in primary and secondary hyperaldosteronism. *J Mol Cell Cardiol, 25,* 563–575.
17. Weber, K. T., & Brilla, C. G. (1991). Pathological hypertrophy and cardiac interstitium: fibrosis and renin-angiotensin-aldosterone system. *Circulation, 83,* 1849–1865.
18. Rocha, R., Chander, P. N., Khanna, K., et al. (1998). Mineralocorticoid blockade reduces vascular injury in stroke-prone hypertensive rats. *Hypertension, 31,* 451–458.
19. MacFayden, R. J., Barr, C. S., & Struthers, A. D. (1997). Aldosterone blockade reduces vascular collagen turnover, improves heart rate variability and reduces early morning rise in heart rate in heart failure patients. *Cardiovasc Res, 35,* 30–34.
20. Kiyingi, A., Field, M. J., Pawsel, C. C., et al. (1990). Metolazone in treatment of severe refractory congestive heart failure. *Lancet, 335,* 29–31.
21. Binanay, C., Califf, R. M., Hasselblad, V., et al. (2005). Evaluation study of congestive heart failure and pulmonary artery catheterization effectiveness: the ESCAPE trial. *JAMA, 294,* 1625–1633.

22a. Bourge, R. C., Abraham, W. T., Adamson, P. B., et al. (2008). Randomized controlled trial of an implantable continuous hemodynamic monitor in patients with advanced heart failure: the COMPASS-HF study. *J Am Coll Cardiol, 51,* 1073–1079.

22b. Tallaj, J. A., Singla, I., & Bourge, R. C. (2009). Implantable hemodynamic monitors. *Heart Fail Clin, 5,* 261–270.

23. Jourdain, P., Jondeau, G., Funck, F., et al. (2007). Plasma brain natriuretic peptide–guided therapy to improve outcome in heart failure: the STARS-BNP multicenter study. *J Am Coll Cardiol, 49,* 1733–1739.
24. Berger, R., Moertl, D., Peter, S., et al. (2010). N-terminal pro-B-type natriuretic peptide-guided, intensive patient management in addition to multidisciplinary care in chronic heart failure: a 3-arm, prospective, randomized pilot study. *J Am Coll Cardiol, 55,* 645–653.
25. Shah, K. B., Nolan, M. M., Rao, K., et al. (2007). The characteristics and prognostic importance of NT-ProBNP concentrations in critically ill patients. *Am J Med, 120,* 1071–1077.
26. Taylor, J. A., Christenson, R. H., Rao, K., et al. (2006). B-type natriuretic peptide (BNP) and N-terminal pro B-type natriuretic peptide (NT-proBNP) are depressed in obesity despite higher left ventricular end diastolic pressures. *Am Heart J, 152,* 1071–1076.
27. Pelleg, A., Mitamura, H., Price, R., et al. (1989). Extracellular potassium ion dynamics and ventricular arrhythmias in the canine heart. *J Am Coll Cardiol, 13,* 941–950.
28. Packer, M., & Lee, W. H. (1986). Provocation of hyper- and hypokalemic sudden death during treatment with and withdrawal of converting enzyme inhibition in severe chronic congestive heart failure. *Am J Cardiol, 57,* 347–348.
29. Abraham, A. S., Meshulam, Z., Rosenmann, D., et al. (1988). Influence of chronic diuretic therapy on serum, lymphocyte and erythrocyte potassium, magnesium and calcium concentrations. *Cardiology, 75,* 17–23.
30. Gottlieb, S. S., Baruch, L., Kukin, M. L., et al. (1990). Prognostic importance of the serum magnesium concentrations in patients with congestive heart failure. *J Am Coll Cardiol, 16,* 827–831.
31. Anand, I. S., Ferrari, R., Kalra, G. S., et al. (1989). Edema of cardiac origin. Studies of body water and sodium, renal function, hemodynamic indexes, and plasma hormones in untreated congestive cardiac failure. *Circulation, 80,* 299–305.
32. Schrier, R. W. (2006). Water and sodium retention in edematous disorders: role of vasopressin and aldosterone. *Am J Med, 119*(7 Suppl. 1), S47–S53.
33. Lee, W. H., & Packer, M. (1986). Prognostic importance of serum sodium concentration and its modification by converting-enzyme inhibition in patients with severe chronic heart failure. *Circulation, 73,* 257–267.
34. Broqvist, M., Dahlstrom, U., Karlberg, B. E., et al. (1989). Neuroendocrine response in acute heart failure and the influence of treatment. *Eur Heart J, 10,* 1075–1083.
35. Francis, G. S., Benedict, C., Johnstone, D. E., et al. (1990). Comparison of neuroendocrine activation in patients with left ventricular dysfunction with and without congestive heart failure: a substudy of the Studies of Left Ventricular Dysfunction (SOLVD). *Circulation, 82,* 1724–1729.
36. Verho, M., Heintz, B., Nelson, K., et al. (1985). The effects of piretanide on catecholamine metabolism, plasma renin activity and plasma aldosterone: a double-blind study versus furosemide in healthy volunteers. *Curr Med Res Opin, 7,* 461–467.
37. Knight, R. K., Miall, P. A., Hawkins, L. A., et al. (1979). Relation of plasma aldosterone concentration to diuretic treatment in patients with severe heart disease. *Br Heart J, 42,* 316–325.
38. McCurley, J. M., Hanlon, S. U., Wei, S. K., et al. (2004). Furosemide and the progression of left ventricular dysfunction in experimental heart failure. *J Am Coll Cardiol, 44,* 1301–1307.
39. Dormans, T. P., van Meyel, J. J., Gerlag, P. G., et al. (1996). Diuretic efficacy of high dose furosemide in severe heart failure: bolus injection versus continuous infusion. *J Am Coll Cardiol, 28,* 376–382.
40. Aaser, E., Gullestad, L., Tollofsrud, S., et al. (1997). Effect of bolus injection versus continuous infusion of furosemide on diuresis and neurohormonal activation in patients with severe congestive heart failure. *Scand J Clin Lab Invest, 57,* 361–367.

40a. Stiles, S. How to diurese in acute HF: Dosing strategies get an evidence base http://www.theheart.org/article/1058939.do. 2010 (accessed 3/23/10).

41. Multher, R. S., Potter, D. M., & Bennett, W. M. (1981). Aspirin-induced depression of glomerular filtration rate in normal humans: role of sodium balance. *Ann Intern Med, 94,* 317–321.
42. Gottlieb, S. S., Robinson, S., Krichten, C. M., et al. (1992). Renal response to indomethacin in congestive heart failure secondary to ischemic or idiopathic dilated cardiomyopathy. *Am J Cardiol, 70,* 890–893.
43. LeJemtel, T. H., Maskin, C. S., Mancini, D., et al. (1985). Systemic and regional hemodynamic effects of captopril and milrinone administered alone and concomitantly in patients with heart failure. *Circulation, 72,* 364–369.

44. Kanda, M., Yasuda, S., Goto, Y., et al. (1999). Diuretic effect of phosphodiesterase inhibitors depends on baseline renal function in patients with congestive heart failure. *Am J Cardiol, 83*, 1274–1277.
45. Cuffe, M. S., Califf, R. M., Adams, K. F., Jr., et al. (2002). Short-term intravenous milrinone for acute exacerbation of chronic heart failure: a randomized controlled trial. *JAMA, 287*, 1541–1547.
46. Klein, L., Massie, B. M., Leimberger, J. D., et al. (2008). For the OPTIME-CHF Investigators. Admission or changes in renal function during hospitalization for worsening heart failure predict post discharge survival: results from the Outcomes of a Prospective Trial of Intravenous Milrinone for Exacerbations of Chonic Heart Failure (OPTIME-CHF). *Circ Heart Fail, 1*, 25.
47. Varriale, P., & Mossavi, A. (1997). The benefit of low-dose dopamine during vigorous diuresis for congestive heart failure associated with renal insufficiency: does it protect renal function? *Clin Cardiol, 20*, 627–630.
48. Hoogenberg, K., Smit, A. J., & Girbes, A. R. (1998). Effects of low-dose dopamine on renal and systemic hemodynamics during incremental norepinephrine infusion in healthy volunteers. *Crit Care Med, 26*, 260–265.
49. Vargo, D. L., Brater, D. C., Rudy, D. W., et al. (1996). Dopamine does not enhance furosemide-induced natriuresis in patients with congestive heart failure. *J Am Soc Nephrol, 7*, 1032–1037.
50. Kellum, J. A., & Decker, J. M. (2001). Use of dopamine in acute renal failure: a meta-analysis. *Crit Care Med, 29*, 1526–1531.
51. Hampton, J. R., van Veldhuisen, D. J., Kleber, F. X., et al. (1997). Randomised study of effect of ibopamine on survival in patients with advanced severe heart failure. Second Prospective Randomised Study of Ibopamine on Mortality and Efficacy (PRIME II) Investigators. *Lancet, 349*, 971–977.
52. Lieverse, A. G., van Veldhuisen, D. J., Smit, A. J., et al. (1995). Renal and systemic hemodynamic effects of ibopamine in patients with mild to moderate congestive heart failure. *J Cardiovasc Pharmacol, 25*, 361–367.
53. Shusterman, N. H., Elliott, W. J., & White, W. B. (1993). Fenoldopam, but not nitroprusside, improves renal function in severely hypertensive patients with impaired renal function. *Am J Med, 95*, 161–168.
54. Mathur, V. S., Swan, S. K., Lambrecht, L. J., et al. (1999). The effects of fenoldopam, a selective dopamine receptor agonist, on systemic and renal hemodynamics in normotensive subjects. *Crit Care Med, 27*, 1832–1837.
55. Costanzo, M. R., Guglin, M. E., Saltzberg, M. T., et al. (2007). Ultrafiltration versus intravenous diuretics for patients hospitalized for acute decompensated heart failure. *J Am Coll Cardiol, 49*, 675–683.
56. Agostoni, P., Marenzi, G., Lauri, G., et al. (1994). Sustained improvement in functional capacity after removal of body fluid with isolated ultrafiltration in chronic cardiac insufficiency: failure of furosemide to provide the same result. *Am J Med, 96*, 191–199.
57. Liang, K. V., Hiniker, A. R., Williams, A. W., et al. (2006). Use of a novel ultrafiltration device as a treatment strategy for diuretic resistant, refractory heart failure: initial clinical experience in a single center. *J Card Fail, 12*, 707–714.
58. Rogers, H. L., Marshall, J., Bock, J., et al. (2008). A randomized, controlled trial of the renal effects of ultrafiltration as compared to furosemide in patients with acute decompensated heart failure. *J Card Fail, 14*, 1–5.
59. Publication Committee for the VMAC Investigators (Vasodilatation in the Management of Acute CHF). (2002). Intravenous nesiritide vs nitroglycerin for treatment of decompensated congestive heart failure: a randomized controlled trial. *JAMA, 287*, 1531–1540. [Erratum, JAMA 2002;288:577.]
60. Jensen, K. T., Shah, M. R., O'Connor, C. M., et al. (1999). Renal effects of brain natriuretic peptide patients with congestive heart failure. *Clin Sci, 96*, 5–15.
61. De Zeeuw, D., Janssen, W. M. T., & de Jong, P. E. (1992). Atrial natriuretic factor: its (patho)physiological significance in humans. *Kidney Int, 41*, 1115–1133.
62. Wang, D. J., Dowling, T. C., Meadows, D., et al. (2004). Nesiritide does not improve renal function in patients with chronic heart failure and worsening serum creatinine. *Circulation, 110*, 1620–1625.
63. Sackner-Bernstein, J. D., Kowalski, M., Fox, M., et al. (2005). Short-term risk of death after treatment with nesiritide for decompensated heart failure: a pooled analysis of randomized controlled trials. *JAMA, 293*, 1900–1905.
64. Sackner-Bernstein, J. D., Skopicki, H. A., & Aaronson, K. D. (2005). Risk of worsening renal function with nesiritide in patients with acutely decompensated heart failure. *Circulation, 111*, 1487–1491.
65. Mitrovic, V., Seferovic, P. M., Simeunovic, D., et al. (2006). Haemodynamic and clinical effects of ularitide in decompensated heart failure. *Eur Heart J, 27*, 2823–2832.
66. Funaya, H., Kitakaze, M., Node, K., et al. (1997). Plasma adenosine levels increase in patients with chronic heart failure. *Circulation, 95*, 1363–1365.
67. Edlund, A., Ohlsen, H., & Sollevi, A. (1994). Renal effects of local infusion of adenosine in man. *Clin Sci, 87*, 143–149.
68. Marraccini, P., Fedele, S., Marzilli, M., et al. (1996). Adenosine-induced renal vasoconstriction in man. *Cardiovasc Res, 32*, 949–953.
69. Schnermann, J. (1998). Juxtaglomerular cell complex in the regulation of renal salt excretion. *Am J Physiol, 274*(2 Pt 2), R263–R279.
70. Mizumoto, H., Karasawa, A., & Kubo, K. (1993). Diuretic and renal protective effects of 8-(noradamantan-3-yl)-1,3-dipropylxanthine (KW-3902), a novel adenosine A_1-receptor antagonist, via pertussis toxin insensitive mechanism. *J Pharmacol Exp Ther, 266*, 200–206.
71. Knight, R. J., Bowmer, C. J., & Yates, M. S. (1993). The diuretic action of 8-cyclopentyl-1,3-dipropylxanthine, a selective A_1-adenosine receptor antagonist. *Br J Pharmacol, 109*, 271–277.
72. Dittrich, H. C., Gupta, D. K., Hack, T. C., et al. (2007). The effect of KW-3902, an adenosine A_1 receptor antagonist, on renal function and renal plasma flow in ambulatory patients with heart failure and renal impairment. *J Card Fail, 13*, 609–617.
73. Givertz, M. M., Massie, B. M., Fields, T. K., et al. (2007). The effects of KW-3902, an adenosine A_1-receptor antagonist, on diuresis and renal function in patients with acute decompensated heart failure and renal impairment or diuretic resistance. *J Am Coll Cardiol, 50*, 1551–1560.
74. Kanno, K., Sasaki, S., Hirata, Y., et al. (1995). Urinary excretion of aquaporin-2 in patients with diabetes insipidus. *N Engl J Med, 332*, 1540–1545.
75. Goldsmith, S. R., Francis, G., Cowley, A. W., Jr., et al. (1983). Increased plasma arginine vasopressin levels in patients with congestive heart failure. *J Am Coll Cardiol, 1*, 1385–1390.
76. Schrier, R. W., Gross, P., Gheorghiade, M., et al. (2006). Tolvaptan, a selective oral vasopressin V_2-receptor antagonist, for hyponatremia. *N Engl J Med, 355*, 2099–2112.
77. Udelson, J. E., Smith, W. B., Hendrix, G. H., et al. (2001). Acute hemodynamic effects of conivaptan, a dual V_{1A} and V_2 vasopressin receptor antagonist, in patients with advanced heart failure. *Circulation, 104*, 2417–2423.
78. Bosch-Marcé, M., Poo, J. -L., Jiménez, W., et al. (1999). Comparison of two aquaretic drugs (niravoline and OPC-31260) in cirrhotic rats with ascites and water retention. *J Pharmacol Exp Ther, 289*, 194–201.
79. Lacour, C., Galindo, G., Canals, F., et al. (2000). Aquaretic and hormonal effects of a vasopressin V_2 receptor antagonist after acute and long-term treatment in rats. *Eur J Pharmacol, 394*, 131–138.
80. Gheorghiade, M., Gattis, W. A., O'Connor, C. M., et al. (2004). Effects of tolvaptan, a vasopressin antagonist, in patients hospitalized with worsening heart failure: a randomized controlled trial. *JAMA, 291*, 1963–1971.
81. Veeraveedu, P. T., Watanabe, K., Ma, M., et al. (2008). Effects of V_2-receptor antagonist tolvaptan and the loop diuretic furosemide in rats with heart failure. *Biochem Pharmacol, 75*, 1322–1330.
82. Gheorghiade, M., Konstam, M. A., Burnett, J. C., Jr., et al. (2007). Short-term clinical effects of tolvaptan, an oral vasopressin antagonist, in patients hospitalized for heart failure: the EVEREST Clinical Status Trials. *JAMA, 297*, 1332–1343.
83. Konstam, M. A., Gheorghiade, M., Burnett, J. C., Jr., et al. (2007). Effects of oral tolvaptan in patients hospitalized for worsening heart failure: the EVEREST Outcome Trial. *JAMA, 297*, 1319–1331.
84. Gottlieb, S. S., Brater, D. C., Thomas, I., et al. (2002). BG9719 (CVT-124), an A_1 adenosine receptor antagonist, protects against the decline in renal function observed with diuretic therapy. *Circulation, 105*, 1348–1353.

CHAPTER 45

Antagonism of the Renin-Angiotensin-Aldosterone System in Heart Failure

Marvin A. Konstam and Richard D. Patten

Activation of the renin-angiotensin-aldosterone system (RAAS) plays a key role in the pathophysiological progression of heart failure (see Chapter 9). Increased secretion of renin by the juxtaglomerular apparatus, in the setting of decreased renal perfusion, serves to protect glomerular perfusion pressure, through angiotensin II–induced efferent arteriolar constriction. However, most of the actions of angiotensin II, predominantly mediated through the angiotensin II type 1 (AT_1) receptor, serve to aggravate the hemodynamic status of patients with heart failure, accentuate symptoms, accelerate the progression of cardiac and vascular disease, and increase morbidity and mortality. The actions of angiotensin II that contribute to progression of heart failure, symptoms, and adverse outcomes include

- Vasoconstriction
- Sodium retention
- Myocyte hypertrophy
- Myocardial and vascular fibroproliferation
- Myocyte apoptosis
- Generation of oxygen free radicals
- Endothelial dysfunction
- Endothelin generation
- Sympathetic activation
- Diminished thrombolysis

The RAAS may be inhibited at many levels: renin inhibition, inhibition of the conversion of angiotensin I to angiotensin II, antagonism of one or more angiotensin II receptors, and blockade of the primary target of aldosterone, the mineralocorticoid receptor.

Angiotensin-converting enzyme (ACE) inhibitors were the first agents clinically available for inhibiting the RAAS[1] and continue to be the most widely used in clinical practice. They act by inhibiting one of several proteases responsible for cleaving angiotensin I, a decapeptide, to form angiotensin II, an octapeptide (Figure 45-1). However, alternative enzymatic pathways have become recognized as playing a major role in angiotensin II production in humans.[2] For example, in the failing human heart, angiotensin II formation is only partially inhibited by an ACE inhibitor but almost completely blocked by an inhibitor of chymase, another protease that catalyzes the formation of angiotensin II from angiotensin I.[3] Accordingly, ACE inhibitor therapy achieves only partial inhibition of angiotensin II production.[4,5]

ACE not only cleaves angiotensin I to form angiotensin II but also is the principal protease that degrades bradykinin; thus, ACE inhibition leads to increased levels of bradykinin within the circulation and at the tissue level.[6-8] The hemodynamic effects of ACE inhibitors may be mediated, in part, through increases in regional bradykinin levels. Bradykinin stimulates endothelial release of nitric oxide and vasodilator prostaglandins,[9,10] contributing to the vasodilator effects of ACE inhibitors. In some animal models of myocardial injury or pressure overload, the beneficial effects of ACE inhibitors mitigating cardiomyocyte hypertrophy and fibroblast hyperplasia within the myocardium are blocked by a bradykinin antagonist.[11-13] Thus, reduction of bradykinin metabolism, resulting in potentiation of local bradykinin levels, probably contributes to the therapeutic benefit of ACE inhibitors.[7]

To the extent that ACE inhibitors reduce production of angiotensin II, effects attributable to angiotensin II are diminished regardless of which receptor mediates the particular effect. In contrast, effects of angiotensin II receptor antagonists limit the responses specifically mediated by that receptor. Because the majority of clinically relevant effects of angiotensin II appear to be mediated through the AT_1 receptor, AT_1 receptor antagonists mirror the actions anticipated through blockade of angiotensin II production. However, loss of feedback inhibition results in increased angiotensin II levels after administration of an AT_1 receptor antagonist, which leads to overstimulation of alternative angiotensin II receptors. The unopposed activation of non-AT_1 receptors may mediate some of the clinically relevant effects attributable to AT_1 receptor blockade. For instance, stimulation of the AT_2 receptor may be responsible for the antiproliferative and antifibrotic effects of AT_1 antagonists[14] within the cardiovascular system. Unopposed activation of the AT_2 receptor may, however, also promote apoptosis.[15]

Although the hemodynamic and clinical effects of ACE inhibitors are notably similar to those of angiotensin receptor blockers (ARBs), these two classes of agents should not be considered identical in their actions, inasmuch as they possess both overlapping and distinct effects. As discussed later, clinical evidence for the benefit of ACE inhibitors exceeds that for ARBs, a finding that is

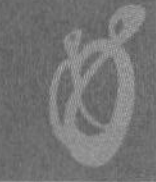

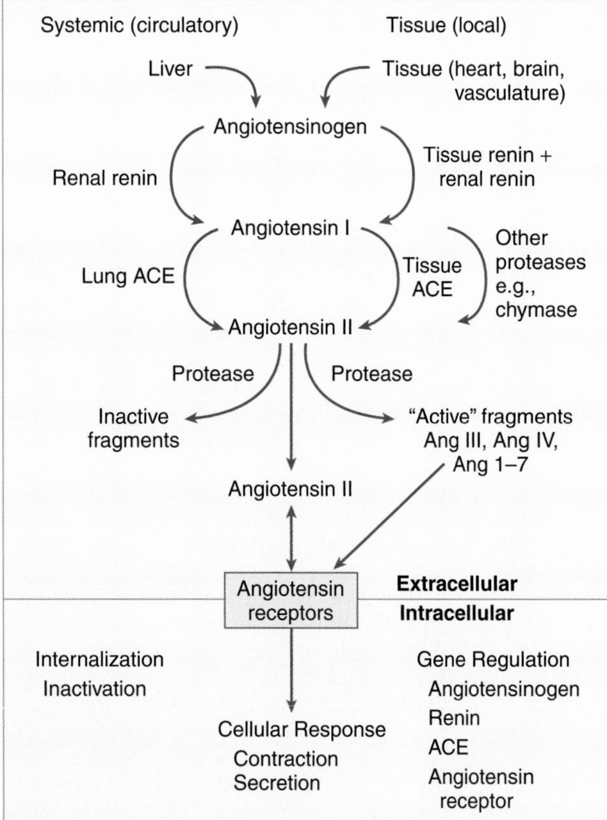

FIGURE 45–1 The systemic and tissue components of the renin-angiotensin-aldosterone system. Several tissues, including those of the myocardium, vasculature, kidney, and brain, have the capacity to generate angiotensin II independently of the circulating renin-angiotensin-aldosterone system. Angiotensin II produced at the tissue level may play an important role in the pathophysiological progression of heart failure. ACE, angiotensin-converting enzyme; Ang III and Ang IV, angiotensin III and angiotensin IV; Ang 1-7, angiotensin (1-7). (Modified from Timmermans PB, Wong PC, Chiu AT, et al: Angiotensin II receptors and angiotensin II receptor antagonists. *Pharmacol Rev* 1993;45:205.)

strongly influenced by the earlier development of ACE inhibitors and the current ethical dilemma of designing trials in their absence. Results of clinical trials, both early and more recent, have helped determine whether and under what circumstances these agents can be used interchangeably or in combination.

Some of the effects of RAAS activation are mediated through aldosterone, the secretion of which is partially under the control of angiotensin II stimulation of the AT_1 receptor.[16] However, increases in aldosterone persist in the circulation (endocrine effects) and at tissue levels (autocrine and paracrine effects) in the presence of angiotensin II inhibition.[4,17] Furthermore, the mineralocorticoid receptor can be activated by other factors, independent of aldosterone. For example, glucocorticoids bind to and activate the mineralocorticoid receptor in the presence of an increased oxidative state.[18] Aside from its effect on renal sodium-potassium exchange, the mineralocorticoid receptor mediates a wide array of effects across the cardiovascular system. There is substantial experimental evidence that mineralocorticoid receptor activation contributes to several adverse myocardial effects, such as increased myocardial fibrosis, inflammation, myocyte hypertrophy, and apoptosis.[18-26] Clinical observations that mineralocorticoid receptor blockade reduces vascular events such as acute coronary syndromes[27] have generated interest in exploring the biological processes of vascular mineralocorticoid receptor action. Jaffe and associates[28,29] reported that mineralocorticoid receptors are expressed in blood vessels and regulate gene transcription in vascular smooth muscle cells. Using a gene-chip microarray approach, they observed an increase in the expression of collagen subtypes and of factors known to promote vascular calcification and inflammation. They also reported the intriguing finding that angiotensin II promoted mineralocorticoid receptor–specific effects in the absence of aldosterone.[29] Thus, indirect mineralocorticoid receptor activation probably contributes importantly to RAAS-induced pathological effects throughout the cardiovascular and renal systems.

HEMODYNAMIC EFFECTS OF INHIBITING THE RENIN-ANGIOTENSIN-ALDOSTERONE SYSTEM

The acute hemodynamic effects of ACE inhibitors and ARBs are influenced by vasodilation. In the early investigations of ACE inhibitors, captopril, enalapril, and lisinopril all produced dose-dependent decreases in right atrial pressure, pulmonary capillary wedge pressure, and systemic vascular resistance, with a resultant increase in cardiac index.[30-32] In studies in which follow-up hemodynamic measurements were obtained, these hemodynamic benefits of ACE inhibitor therapy were shown to be sustained.[30,32] In addition, inhibition of neurohormonal activation over time is evident from decreases in heart rates and plasma catecholamine levels at rest and with exercise.[33,34] Similarly, ARBs such as losartan and irbesartan produce dose-dependent decreases in right atrial pressure, pulmonary capillary wedge pressure, and systemic vascular resistance in association with increased cardiac index, which are sustained over time in the absence of tachyphylaxis.[35-37] These hemodynamic effects of ARBs occur without increases in heart rate or neurohormonal activation. Beneficial hemodynamic and clinical effects of irbesartan were reported by Havranek and colleagues[36] in patients already taking ACE inhibitors. Likewise, the administration of valsartan (160 mg) to patients with heart failure who were already taking ACE inhibitors produced acute and sustained hemodynamic benefits, accompanied by a reduction in aldosterone levels and by a trend for reduction in plasma norepinephrine levels.[38]

In summary, these data indicate that ACE inhibitors and ARBs produce similar hemodynamic benefits in patients with heart failure and left ventricular (LV) systolic dysfunction. The addition of ARBs to ACE inhibitor therapy also produces significant and sustained hemodynamic benefits, which is consistent with results of clinical studies demonstrating that angiotensin II levels remain elevated in patients receiving ACE inhibitor therapy.[4,5]

EFFECTS OF RENIN-ANGIOTENSIN-ALDOSTERONE SYSTEM INHIBITION ON VENTRICULAR REMODELING

Experimental Observations

"LV remodeling" refers to alterations in ventricular mass, chamber size, and shape that result from myocardial injury or from pressure or volume overload (see Chapter 15). At the cellular level, myocardial pathological changes accompany LV remodeling and involve myocyte hypertrophy and fibroblast hyperplasia, in addition to an increase in collagen deposition within the interstitium. When these processes occur in the noninfarcted myocardium, they contribute to progressive LV remodeling and LV dysfunction. A substantial amount of experimental and clinical data support the pivotal role of the RAAS in contributing to these cellular processes.

Angiotensin II is formed locally within the myocardium and is known to be an important stimulus to these cellular events.

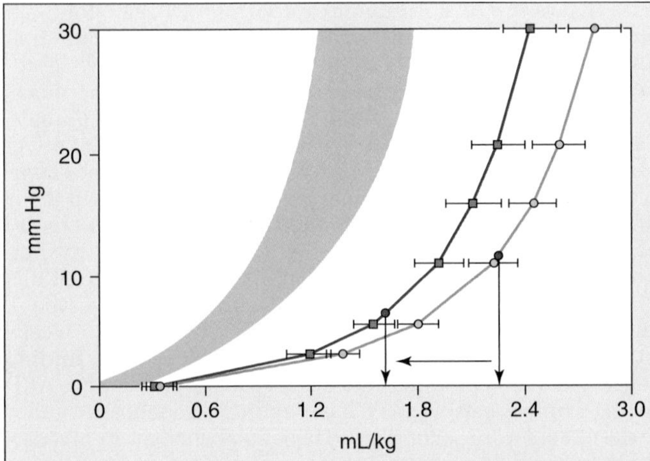

FIGURE 45–2 Left ventricular pressure-volume relationships (mean ± standard error of the mean) of untreated and captopril-treated rats with large myocardial infarctions 3 months after coronary ligation. *Shaded area* represents the volumes ± 2 standard deviations in controls that did not have infarction. *Vertical arrows* indicate operating volumes of treated and untreated rats with *horizontal* arrow denoting shift between the two groups. $P < .05$ for differences in operating volume index between untreated and treated animals with horizontal arrow denoting the shift between the untreated *(right)* and treated *(left)* groups. (From Pfeffer JM, Pfeffer MA, Braunwald E. Influence of chronic captopril therapy on the infarcted left ventricle of the rat. *Circ Res* 1985;57:84-95.)

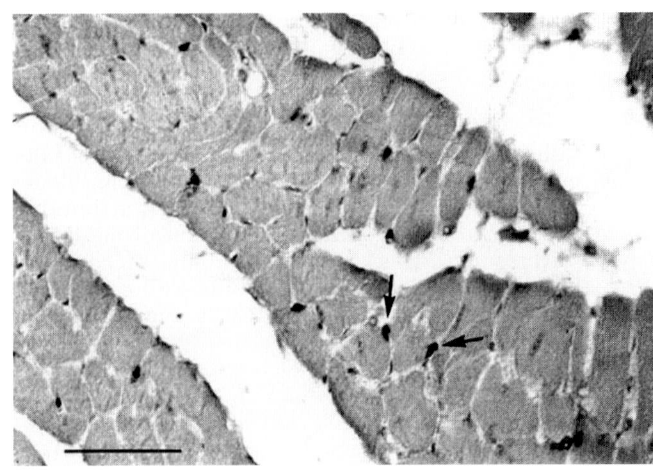

FIGURE 45–3 Microscopic image (×100) of noninfarcted myocardium stained by immunohistochemical methods for proliferating cell nuclear antigen. Nuclei that stained positively (*arrows*) are black. This section was obtained from the left ventricle of a placebo-treated animal with an infarct size of 41% of left ventricular myocardium. Scale bar, 50 μm. (From Taylor K, Patten RD, Smith JJ, et al. Divergent effects of angiotensin converting enzyme inhibition and angiotensin II receptor antagonism on myocardial cellular proliferation and collagen deposition after myocardial infarction in rats. *J Cardiovasc Pharmacol* 1998;31:654-660.)

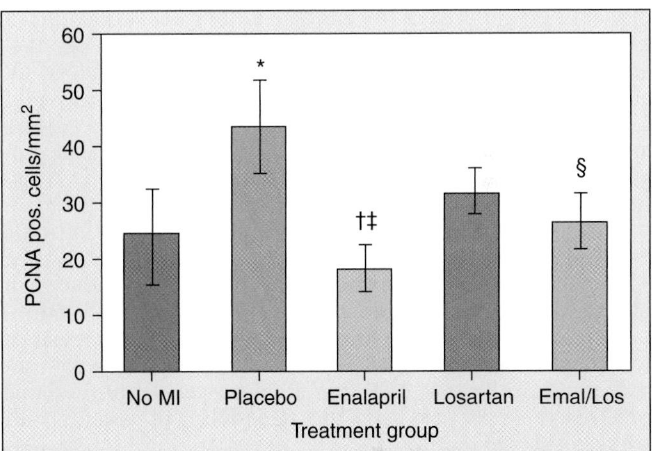

FIGURE 45–4 Cellular proliferation within the noninfarct zone is evident from the number of cells per unit area (square millimeters) that stained positively for proliferating cell nuclear antigen (PCNA) (mean ± standard error of the mean). Placebo-treated animals with infarction displayed significantly greater PCNA labeling than did animals without infarction ("No MI"). Enalapril decreased proliferative activity, whereas losartan had an intermediate effect. Combination therapy ("Enal/Los") also tended to limit proliferation. *$P < .04$ between placebo and "No MI" conditions; †$P < .01$ between enalapril and placebo conditions; ‡$P < .03$ between enalapril and losartan conditions; §$P = .08$ between combination therapy and placebo conditions. (From Taylor K, Patten RD, Smith JJ, et al. Divergent effects of angiotensin converting enzyme inhibition and angiotensin II receptor antagonism on myocardial cellular proliferation and collagen deposition after myocardial infarction in rats. *J Cardiovasc Pharmacol* 1998;31:654-660.)

Sadoshima and associates[39,40] demonstrated the localization of angiotensin II within myocyte granules 30 minutes after mechanical stretch and that the increase in myocyte protein synthesis in response to mechanical stretch is largely blocked by an AT_1 receptor antagonist. Angiotensin II also stimulates collagen production and proliferation of cardiac fibroblasts.[40] These pivotal experimental data support the premise that the RAAS plays a central role in the pathophysiological processes of ventricular remodeling and progression of heart failure.

Results of numerous studies have confirmed that ACE inhibitors mitigate progressive LV remodeling in the failing heart. Pfeffer and colleagues[41] developed a rat model of myocardial infarction to study ventricular remodeling in an experimental setting and found that captopril therapy not only improved survival after myocardial infarction but also significantly reduced the extent of LV chamber enlargement.[42,43] Figure 45-2 displays passive pressure-volume relationships obtained immediately post mortem in rats after myocardial infarction. Hearts from untreated animals with infarction demonstrated significant increases in LV chamber size for a given pressure, manifest by a marked rightward shift of the pressure-volume relation. In contrast, captopril treatment reduced the extent of LV dilation, which resulted in a leftward shift of the pressure-volume relation.

Using a rat model of myocardial infarction, Taylor and associates examined the effects of ACE inhibition and AT_1 receptor blockade on nonmyocyte proliferation and collagen deposition within the noninfarct zone.[44] Figure 45-3 depicts a noninfarcted section of rat heart stained immunohistochemically for proliferating cell nuclear antigen, a marker of proliferation or DNA repair, or both. Interstitial cell (mostly fibroblast) proliferation is evident within the noninfarct zone from the heart of a placebo-treated rat 2 weeks after myocardial infarction. In this study, ACE inhibition reduced nonmyocyte proliferation to levels comparable with those in animals that did not have infarction (Figure 45-4). The AT_1 receptor antagonist losartan reduced nonmyocyte proliferation to a lesser degree than did the ACE inhibitor. These somewhat disparate effects of ACE inhibition versus AT_1 receptor blockade may result from ACE inhibitor–mediated increase in local bradykinin levels, shown in some studies to be important in the growth-inhibitory effects of ACE inhibitors. It is interesting that the combination of ACE inhibitor and AT_1 receptor antagonist resulted in slightly greater effect (although not statistically different) in limiting collagen deposition, which suggested that the actions of the two agents may be additive.

In support of this, Dahl salt-sensitive rats treated with the combination of the ACE inhibitor benazepril and the AT_1 receptor antagonist valsartan exhibited improved survival, reduced heart failure markers, and less LV hypertrophy in comparison with rats treated with either agent alone.[45] In a sheep model of myocardial infarction, Mankad and

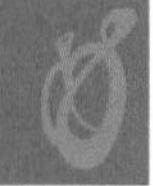

co-workers[46] examined end-diastolic and end-systolic volumes by using gated magnetic resonance imaging, comparing the effects of the ACE inhibitor ramipril alone or in combination with losartan. After 8 weeks of therapy, combined ACE inhibition and AT_1 blockade effected a greater reduction in end-diastolic and end-systolic volumes. These data constitute evidence that (1) the effects of combined AT_1 receptor blockade and ACE inhibition may be more effective in limiting progressive LV remodeling; and (2) activation of the RAAS plays a pivotal role in the pathophysiological processes of heart failure and progressive LV remodeling. Moreover, they underscore the importance of inhibiting the renin-angiotensin-aldosterone hormonal axis in the management of heart failure.

Clinical Studies

In addition to a wealth of experimental evidence supporting the important role of the RAAS in the pathophysiological processes of ventricular remodeling, clinical evidence also supports this premise. Because of the large number of trials demonstrating consistent benefits of ACE inhibitors in rates of mortality and morbidity, these agents have become a mainstay of therapy for patients with LV systolic dysfunction. Sharpe and associates[47] demonstrated that captopril initiated within 48 hours after Q-wave myocardial infarction reduced the increase in LV end-diastolic volume after only 3 months of therapy. Similarly, in the multicenter Survival and Ventricular Enlargement (SAVE) trial, captopril improved survival among patients after myocardial infarction with reduced LV ejection fraction (LVEF) (<40%) and mitigated the degree of LV chamber dilation after the first year of therapy.[48] Konstam and associates demonstrated that ACE inhibitors prevent progressive LV remodeling in patients with LV systolic dysfunction with or without symptoms of heart failure.[49,50] Figure 45-5 displays mean pressure-volume loops obtained from the Studies of Left Ventricular Dysfunction (SOLVD) substudy. The placebo recipients exhibited LV dilation over the span of this study (1 year), whereas the enalapril recipients exhibited the opposite, which was consistent with a decrease in LV chamber size for a given LV pressure. This study demonstrated clinically that ACE inhibition prevents, and perhaps reverses, the extent of ventricular remodeling in patients with LV systolic dysfunction.

The precise effect of AT_1 receptor antagonists on ventricular remodeling is not as well studied. In the Evaluation of Losartan In The Elderly (ELITE) radionuclide substudy, researchers compared the effect of losartan, an AT_1 antagonist, with that of the ACE inhibitor captopril on LV remodeling in elderly patients with heart failure and systolic dysfunction (ejection fraction <40%). After 48 weeks of therapy, captopril and losartan demonstrated statistically equivalent effects in reducing LV end-diastolic and end-systolic volumes, although there was a trend toward a greater beneficial effect of captopril in this study.[51] McKelvie and coworkers compared the effects of the AT_1 antagonist candesartan with those of the ACE inhibitor enalapril and the effects of their combination on LV remodeling as part of the Randomized Evaluation Strategies for Left Ventricular Dysfunction (RESOLVD) pilot study.[52] With combination therapy, they observed a significant reduction in LV end-systolic volume at 43 weeks in comparison with enalapril treatment alone; this finding suggested that combination of an ACE inhibitor and ARB in the clinical setting may have additive benefits. Whether these effects were secondary to beneficial changes in myocardial structure or were related purely to afterload reduction is unknown. Perhaps the largest study of whether combination therapy with an ACE inhibitor and ARB produces greater reduction in LV remodeling has been the Valsartan in Acute Myocardial Infarction Trial (VALIANT), in which investigators examined the effect of valsartan alone, captopril alone, and their combination in patients after an acute myocardial infarction complicated by heart failure, LV dysfunction, or both. Although the patient population in this trial differed from that in heart failure trials (after myocardial infarction, mean LVEF among the groups was 39%), the degree of LV remodeling (increase in LV end-diastolic volume and change in LVEF) was similar among all three groups of patients.[53] The results of this VALIANT substudy therefore do not support the view that combination therapy in patients with heart failure or LV dysfunction after myocardial infarction exerts a greater effect in limiting LV remodeling than either class of agent alone.

Findings related to effects of mineralocorticoid receptor inhibition on cardiac remodeling in heart failure have been mixed. Although some studies have suggested a benefit,[54,55] Udelson and colleagues found no effect of the selective mineralocorticoid receptor antagonist eplerenone, when added to an ACE inhibitor and β-blocker, during 9 months of randomized, controlled treatment in patients with New York Heart Association (NYHA) class II to class III heart failure and reduced LVEF.[56] It is possible that the reduction in mortality observed with mineralocorticoid receptor blockers in selected populations with heart failure (see "Aldosterone Receptor Blockers" section) is at least partly mediated by vascular effects, as opposed to myocardial effects.

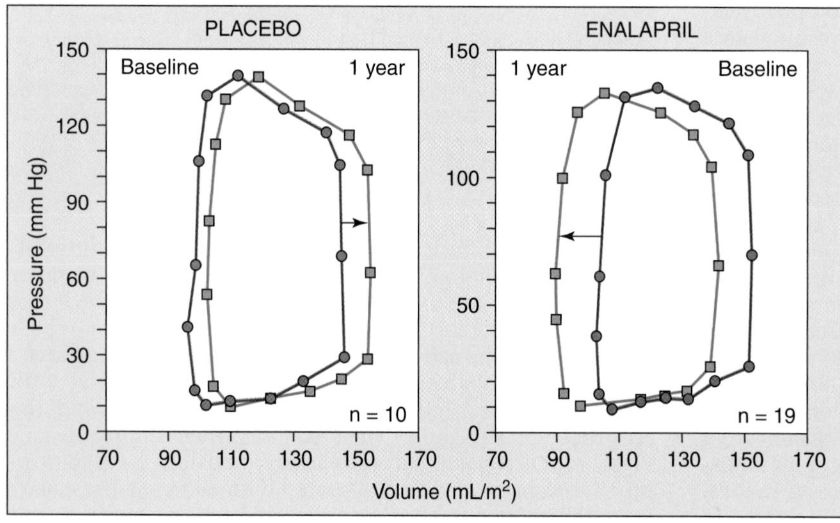

FIGURE 45–5 Mean left ventricular pressure-volume relationships at baseline and at 1 year in patients enrolled in the Studies of Left Ventricular Dysfunction (SOLVD) prevention trial who were randomly assigned to receive chronic treatment with placebo or enalapril. (From Konstam MA, Kronenberg MW, Rousseau MF, et al, for the SOLVD Investigators. Effects of the angiotensin converting enzyme inhibitor, enalapril, on the long-term progression of left ventricular dilatation in patients with asymptomatic systolic dysfunction. *Circulation* 1993;88:2277-2283.)

EFFECTS OF INHIBITING THE RENIN-ANGIOTENSIN-ALDOSTERONE SYSTEM ON FUNCTIONAL CAPACITY AND SYMPTOMS

Reduced functional capacity in patients with heart failure caused by systolic dysfunction results from cardiac and non-cardiac factors. ACE inhibitors have variably been shown to improve exercise capacity in patients with heart failure and systolic dysfunction, presumably through their sustained hemodynamic benefits, as described previously. However, the improvement in exercise capacity noted with ACE inhibitors is often modest in clinical trials. These modest improvements may result, in part, from improved survival among patients with NYHA class IV heart failure. For example, in the Vasodilators in Heart Failure Treatment (V-HeFT) II trial, in which ACE-inhibition was compared with the combination of hydralazine and isosorbide dinitrate, subjects receiving the latter protocol had a more pronounced improvement in exercise capacity, judged by peak exercise oxygen consumption. However, the survival rate among patients treated with the ACE inhibitor was better than that among subjects taking hydralazine and isosorbide, which raised the question of whether more severe heart failure symptoms may have diluted any improvement in exercise capacity in the subjects treated with enalapril.[57]

Angiotensin-Converting Enzyme Inhibitors

A number of studies have demonstrated that ACE inhibitors improve exercise time and ameliorate symptoms of heart failure. The benefits of ACE inhibitors in the management of heart failure symptoms have long been recognized. In the early 1980s, captopril treatment was shown to improve exercise time by 25% and to reduce heart failure symptoms and NYHA class in patients with severe heart failure treated with digoxin and diuretics.[58] Similar improvements in exercise capacity and heart failure symptoms were noted with the ACE inhibitors enalapril,[30] lisinopril,[31] and quinapril.[59] These clinical data demonstrate that ACE inhibitors favorably influence symptoms of heart failure and exercise capacity in patients with LV systolic dysfunction.

Angiotensin Receptor Blockers

ARBs also improve exercise capacity and symptoms in patients with heart failure. Losartan has been shown to improve symptoms of heart failure after 12 weeks of therapy in patients with reduced LVEF (<45%).[37] In a comparative trial with the ACE inhibitor enalapril, losartan-treated patients demonstrated similar exercise capacity and symptoms of heart failure after 12 weeks of treatment.[60] Vescovo and associates[61] evaluated exercise capacity in small groups of patients, one treated with enalapril and the other with losartan. Both groups demonstrated similar improvements in exercise capacity, as demonstrated by peak oxygen consumption. Interestingly, Vescovo and associates also compared the myosin profiles in skeletal muscle and demonstrated a myosin heavy chain shift toward slow, fatigue-resistant isoforms, which suggested that improvement in exercise capacity by these agents may be, in part, related to noncardiac factors.

Riegger and colleagues[62] studied the effects of various doses of the ARB candesartan (4, 8, and 16 mg) in patients with heart failure and LV systolic dysfunction. In this study, ACE inhibitors were withdrawn 2 weeks before the placebo run-in period. With all three doses of candesartan, patients demonstrated improved score of heart failure symptoms and improved exercise capacity in comparison with placebo-treated patients. Researchers in the RESOLVD pilot study compared candesartan alone, enalapril alone, and their combination over a 43-week period. Each agent resulted in similar improvements in exercise capacity and quality of life.[52] Thus, available studies suggest that ARBs produce improvements in exercise capacity and heart failure symptoms that are similar to those produced by ACE inhibitors, either historically or in a direct, individual manner.

EFFECTS OF INHIBITING THE RENIN-ANGIOTENSIN-ALDOSTERONE SYSTEM ON MORBIDITY AND MORTALITY

Angiotensin-Converting Enzyme Inhibitors

ACE inhibitors were the first class of agents shown to significantly alter the natural history of heart failure, as demonstrated by a reduction in the frequency of death and of other morbid events. Most of these data have been accumulated from patients with reduced LVEF, and clinicians have therefore recognized the necessity for measuring ventricular systolic function and prescribing ACE inhibitors to patients with reduced ejection fraction (e.g., ≤35%) as standards of care for patients with heart failure. Table 45-1 lists the key trials demonstrating benefit of ACE inhibitors in this population.

In the first Cooperative North Scandinavian Enalapril Survival Study (CONSENSUS), patients with class IV symptoms of heart failure were randomly assigned to receive enalapril or placebo. The study was stopped prematurely because of a marked reduction in mortality among the patients taking enalapril; this

TABLE 45–1 Selected Clinical Trials of Angiotensin-Converting Enzyme Inhibitor in Heart Failure

Trial	Agent	Population	Findings
CONSENSUS I	Enalapril titrated to 20 mg bid vs. placebo	NYHA class IV	• 31% Decrease in 1-year mortality rate • 50% Decrease in deaths from progressive heart failure
SOLVD Treatment Trial	Enalapril titrated to 10 mg bid	NYHA classes II to IV, EF ≤35%	• 16% Decrease in 3.5-year mortality • 26% Decrease in death or hospitalizations for CHF
SOLVD Prevention Trial	Enalapril titrated to 10 mg bid vs. placebo	NYHA class I, EF ≤35%	• 20% Decrease in death or hospitalizations for CHF • 29% Decrease in death or development of CHF • 37% Decrease in development of CHF • 44% Decrease in hospitalizations for CHF
V-HeFT II	Enalapril (10 mg bid) vs. hydralazine (75 mg qid)/isosorbide dinitrate (40 mg qid)	NYHA classes II to IV, EF <45%	• 34% Decrease in 1-year mortality • 28% Decrease in 2-year mortality • 38% Decrease in sudden death

CHF, congestive heart failure; CONSENSUS, Cooperative North Scandinavian Enalapril Survival Study; EF, ejection fraction; NYHA, New York Heart Association (classification); SOLVD, Studies of Left Ventricular Dysfunction; V-HeFT, Vasodilator in Heart Failure Trial.

made CONSENSUS the first study to display an effect of any pharmacological agent on mortality in heart failure.[63]

The SOLVD treatment[64] and prevention trials[65] were investigations of the effects of enalapril in patients with reduced LVEF (≤35%) with and without symptoms of heart failure, respectively. Most patients in the SOLVD treatment trial had NYHA class II or III symptoms. Among those randomly assigned to receive enalapril, mortality was reduced significantly (Figure 45-6), as was the combined endpoint of death or hospitalization for heart failure. The SOLVD prevention trial failed to reach significance with regard to its primary endpoint, manifesting only a trend of 8% reduction in mortality. However, there were significant reductions in the progression to clinically overt heart failure and in the combined endpoint of death or hospitalization for heart failure. For patients with heart failure and reduced LVEF, these landmark trials extended the indication for ACE inhibitor prescription across the entire spectrum of clinical symptoms.

Close to 80% of the total population of the SOLVD trials were thought by the investigator to have heart failure on the basis of ischemic heart disease. However, patients who had had myocardial infarction within the previous month were excluded. Findings of these studies were further substantiated by results of trials enrolling patients after myocardial infarction. For example, the SAVE trial[66] enrolled patients between 3 and 16 days after myocardial infarction who had ejection fractions of 40% or less; patients randomly assigned to receive the ACE inhibitor captopril demonstrated a significant reduction in mortality. Similar benefits were observed in the Acute Infarction Ramipril Efficacy (AIRE) trial,[67] in which patients with clinical evidence of heart failure (regardless of ejection fraction) in the setting of a recent acute myocardial infarction (within the previous 2 to 9 days) were randomly assigned to receive either ramipril or placebo. ACE inhibitor treatment in this study resulted in a 35% reduction in mortality after 1 year of follow-up.

Effect of Angiotensin-Converting Enzyme Inhibitors on Clinical Outcomes and Mechanisms Underlying These Effects

The original hypothesis behind investigation of ACE inhibitors in patients with heart failure was that these agents would reduce the progression of clinical heart failure through vasodilation. Studies with ACE inhibitors have certainly demonstrated reduction in fatal and morbid events linked to progressive heart failure. Since the inception of these trials, the rationale for such clinical actions has expanded substantially, with a recognition that ACE inhibitors directly affect the cellular mechanisms responsible for progressive myocardial disease.

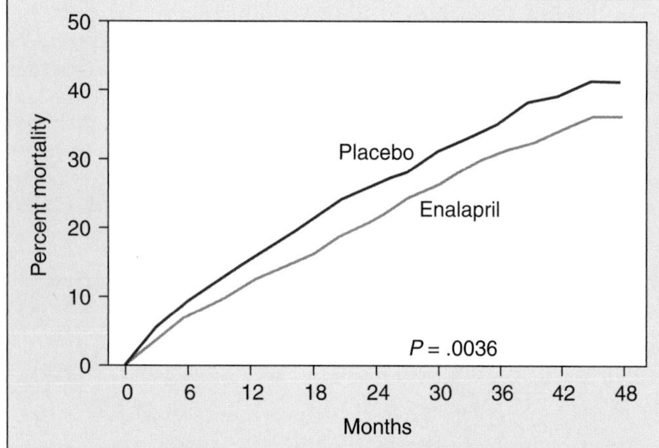

FIGURE 45-6 Mortality curves from the Studies of Left Ventricular Dysfunction (SOLVD) treatment trial, demonstrating a 16% reduction in mortality among patients with symptoms of heart failure who were treated with the angiotensin-converting enzyme (ACE) inhibitor enalapril. (From Effect of angiotensin converting enzyme inhibition with enalapril on survival in patients with reduced left ventricular ejection fraction and congestive heart failure: results of the treatment trial of the Studies of Left Ventricular Dysfunction (SOLVD); a randomized double blind trial. *N Engl J Med* 1991;325:293-302.)

Clinical trials have consistently demonstrated a reduction in the number of hospitalizations for heart failure, typically analyzed in terms of time to first event with a combined endpoint of death or hospitalization for heart failure. The endpoint of hospitalizations for heart failure serves as a useful marker for both disease severity and activity and for the effect of a treatment on the overall cost of care for patients with heart failure.

Beyond an effect on clinical events linked to progressive heart failure, both the SOLVD and SAVE studies demonstrated significant reductions in the incidence of myocardial infarction. This effect contributed to the overall influence of ACE inhibitors on mortality. Furthermore, within the SOLVD population, enalapril caused a significant reduction in number of patients hospitalized for unstable angina. These findings provided, for the first time, evidence for an influence of ACE inhibitors on the pathogenesis of acute coronary syndromes, an influence probably mediated by effects on the arterial wall, on the balance between thrombosis and thrombolysis, or on both.

In the clinical trials of ACE inhibitors in patients with heart failure, the effect of these agents on sudden cardiac deaths has been less clear than the effect on deaths attributed to progressive heart failure or to fatal myocardial infarction.[68] Results of trials with ACE inhibitors in patients with recent myocardial infarction have been more supportive of a reduction by these agents in the incidence of sudden cardiac death. Such effects may be mediated not by direct electrophysiological consequences of inhibiting the RAAS but rather by an effect on myocardial hypertrophy, fibrosis, and remodeling. An additional influence may be mediated by downregulation of adrenergic neurotransmitter release.

Each of these clinical findings must be interpreted with caution, because differentiation of cause of death is, at best, a highly inexact science. The data from the Assessment of Treatment with Lisinopril and Survival (ATLAS) trial, in which high-dose and low-dose ACE inhibitor effects were compared, suggested considerable discrepancy between the clinically adjudicated cause of death and the findings at autopsy.[69] In a substantial proportion of patients in whom death was attributed to either progressive heart failure or sudden cardiac death and for whom autopsy findings were available, postmortem cardiac examination revealed evidence of a recent myocardial infarction (see Figure 45-6). Nevertheless, with a growing understanding of the breadth of actions of ACE inhibitors in impeding the progression of cardiovascular disease, it seems increasingly likely that these agents favorably affect survival in various ways.

Angiotensin Receptor Blockers

Investigation of the effect of ARBs on clinical outcomes in patients with heart failure has been hampered by the ethical imperative, arising from results of the aforementioned clinical trials, not to withhold ACE inhibitors from this population. Various groups have taken different approaches to this problem, such as the following:

- Investigation of the relative effects of an ACE inhibitor and an ARB
- Examination of the effect of an ARB when superimposed on "standard treatment," including an ACE inhibitor
- Examination of populations in whom withholding an ACE inhibitor is considered ethically feasible, such as patients who cannot tolerate ACE inhibitors and those with preserved LV systolic function

Table 45-2 lists the key trials in which the effect of ARBs on clinical outcomes in patients with heart failure were examined.

TABLE 45–2 Trials of Angiotensin Receptor Blockers in Heart Failure

Trial	Agent	Population	Outcome
ELITE-II	Losartan (50 mg qd)	Age ≥60, NYHA classes II to IV, EF ≤40%	• Losartan not superior to captopril • No significant difference in mortality rates • Losartan better tolerated
Val-HeFT	Valsartan (160 mg bid) or placebo plus open-label ACE inhibitor (93%)	NYHA classes II to IV, EF <40%	• No difference in rates of all-cause mortality • Significant 13% decrease in combined rate of morbidity and mortality • 27% Decrease in hospitalizations for heart failure • Most benefit observed in ACE inhibitor–intolerant patients (7% of study group) with 45% reduction in combined primary endpoints
CHARM	Candesartan (32 mg qd) vs. placebo with or without open-label ACE inhibitor	NYHA classes II to IV • LVEF ≤40% • LVEF >40% • LVEF ≤40%; ACE inhibitor–intolerant	Primary outcome: cardiovascular death and hospitalization for heart failure • Significant 15% decrease in primary outcome • No reduction in cardiovascular deaths; significant decrease in hospitalization for heart failure • Significant 23% reduction in primary outcome
HEAAL	Losartan (150 mg qd vs 50 mg qd)	NYHA II-1V • LVEF ≤40% • ACE inhibitor intolerance	• Higher dose associated with reduced rate of death or hospitalization for heart failure • Rates of discontinuation for adverse events were low and not significantly different between groups

ACE, Agiotensin-converting enzyme; CHARM, Candesartan in Heart Failure Assessment in Reduction of Mortality; EF, ejection fraction; ELITE-II, second Evaluation of Losartan In The Elderly; LVEF, left ventricular ejection fraction; NYHA, New York Heart Association (classification); Val-HeFT, Valsartan in Heart Failure Trial.

Second Evaluation of Losartan in the Elderly (ELITE-II)

The ELITE-II trial[70] tested the hypothesis that the ARB losartan (target dose, 50 mg/day) would reduce mortality in relation to the ACE inhibitor captopril (target dose, 50 mg three times daily), in elderly patients with heart failure and reduced LVEF. This hypothesis was based on findings within the first ELITE trial,[71] in which, with a primary hypothesis related to renal function, fewer deaths occurred in patients randomly assigned to receive losartan than in those randomly assigned to receive captopril. The results of ELITE-II failed to support the stated hypothesis; the numbers of deaths in the two treatment groups were similar. It is tempting to conclude from ELITE-II that the effect of an ARB on mortality is similar to that of an ACE inhibitor. However, this conclusion is not statistically valid, because the study was not powered for equivalence or noninferiority; that is, the number of patients studied (3152) yielded wide confidence intervals around the point estimate for the relative risk of death for patients randomly assigned to receive losartan in comparison with captopril. It has been speculated that a higher dose of losartan would have yielded more favorable results, although the basis for such speculation is weak.

Similarity of the clinical benefits of ACE inhibitors and ARBs is supported by findings with regard to other endpoints in the ELITE-II trial. Results in the two treatment groups were no different with regard to the combined endpoint of death or hospitalization for heart failure, dropping out for worsening heart failure, NYHA class (which improved in both treatment groups), and a heath-related quality-of-life scale. These findings provide support for the contention that ARBs are effective agents in treating patients with heart failure and reduced ejection fraction.

One way in which the ARB losartan significantly improved on findings observed with the ACE inhibitor captopril was in terms of patient tolerance: 14.7% of patients randomly assigned to receive captopril discontinued treatment because of adverse effects, in contrast to only 9.7% of patients randomly assigned to receive losartan. The difference was a result of adverse effects attributable to bradykinin, particularly cough, which occurred in approximately 3% of patients randomly assigned to receive captopril, as opposed to fewer than 1% of those randomly assigned to receive losartan.

Valsartan in Heart Failure Trial (Val-HeFT)

Investigators in the Val-HeFT study took an approach different from that of ELITE-II. They hypothesized that treatment with a high dose (160 mg twice daily) of the ARB valsartan would significantly reduce the incidence of adverse clinical outcomes when added to "standard treatment" in patients with heart failure and a dilated left ventricle. Patients were randomly assigned to receive either valsartan or placebo in addition to baseline medical treatment, which included an ACE inhibitor in 93% of patients and a β-blocker in 35%. There were two primary endpoints—all-cause mortality and the combination of death or major cardiovascular event—with the α error split evenly between the two; that is, the results could be considered positive if valsartan performed better than did placebo with regard to either endpoint, with a probability value less than approximately .025.[72]

There was no difference between the valsartan and placebo recipients with regard to all-cause mortality. However, there was a significant 13% reduction in the combined primary endpoint, an effect driven solely by the reduction in hospitalizations for heart failure.[72] Additional significant benefits were observed within the valsartan recipients with regard to NYHA class, signs and symptoms of heart failure, and LVEF. The Val-HeFT trial, therefore, was the first study with an ARB to demonstrate a significant clinical finding, in terms of a primary endpoint directed at an important clinical outcome, in a population of patients with heart failure.

The findings of Val-HeFT were complicated by results across various patient subsets. Significant treatment × subgroup interactions were observed with regard to baseline ACE inhibitor use and to baseline β-blocker use. The 7% of the population that were not receiving an ACE inhibitor at baseline, presumably because of intolerance, exhibited significantly greater benefit, with regard to the combination endpoint, than did the 93% of patients receiving an ACE inhibitor. This small group contributed importantly to the overall result and provides the best estimate to date of the effect that an ARB has on clinical outcomes in patients with heart failure. The point estimate for reduction in combined mortality and morbidity was 45% within this group.

Of concern was the significant treatment × subgroup interaction for baseline β-blocker use, which similarly revealed significantly greater improvement in the combination endpoint

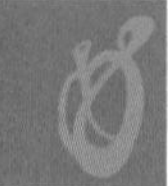

within patients who did not receive β-blockers. For patients receiving β-blockers, the point estimate favored placebo over valsartan. This finding is directionally the same as a nonsignificant trend observed in ELITE-II in which captopril was superior to losartan among the 25% of that study's population who received a β-blocker at baseline. Such results must be interpreted cautiously and could be linked to other unidentified features within the population that are correlated with β-blocker use or could result from an unidentified interaction between β-blockers and ARBs, particularly for patients also receiving an ACE inhibitor.

The Val-HeFT study provides greatest support for use of an ARB in a population that it was not intended to study: patients who did not receive an ACE inhibitor. Because this group was small, because it was not the study's intent, and because of the wealth of data supporting the use of ACE inhibitors, the Val-HeFT results do not alter the recommendation to consider ACE inhibitors first-line agents for all patients with heart failure and reduced ejection fraction. However, Val-HeFT certainly lends credence to the previously stated recommendation to prescribe an ARB for patients who cannot tolerate ACE inhibitors, specifically those intolerant because of cough or angioedema. It also suggests a role for adding an ARB to an ACE inhibitor, particularly for patients who continue to be symptomatic and who cannot tolerate a β-blocker.

Candesartan in Heart Failure Assessment in Reduction of Mortality (CHARM) Trial

The CHARM study[73] employed a novel design, dividing its population with heart failure into three groups:

- Those with reduced ejection fraction, who received an ACE inhibitor (CHARM-Added)[74]
- Those who could not tolerate ACE inhibitors (CHARM-Alternative)[75]
- Those with preserved ejection fraction (CHARM-Preserved)[76]

In each trial, patients were randomly assigned to receive candesartan, 32 mg daily, or placebo; the primary endpoint was the composite of cardiovascular death or hospital admission for congestive heart failure. The primary endpoint was significantly improved for the patients in both the CHARM-Added and CHARM-Alternative groups who were randomly assigned to receive candesartan (Figure 45-7).[74,75] Thus, the CHARM program demonstrated, in the most definitive way to date, that an ARB achieves significant improvement in clinical outcomes in a population with low ejection fraction who could not tolerate ACE inhibitors. Although a reduction in all-cause mortality did not reach statistical significance, the magnitude of benefit for the primary endpoint suggested that the clinical effect of an ARB in this population was at least comparable with that achievable with an ACE inhibitor. In addition, the CHARM-Added group demonstrated clearly for the first time that addition of an ARB to an ACE inhibitor would achieve additive clinical benefit. The CHARM-Added study, however, raised a number of questions. First, how can clinicians be sure that patients were optimally treated with ACE inhibitors? The authors dispelled this concern with a detailed analysis demonstrating that the population was indeed well treated with appropriate doses of ACE inhibitors and that the benefit was retained in patients receiving the highest doses of these medications.[77] Second, how is this finding reconciled with that of the VALIANT trial, which failed to demonstrate incremental benefit of combination treatment in a population with heart failure after myocardial infarction?[78] Arguably, the design of VALIANT was more suited to "purely" asking the question of relative benefit of each drug class and the combination, inasmuch as both valsartan and captopril were administered as study drugs under "blinded" conditions. However, the drug and patient populations tested were also different. It is difficult to argue with the implication of the "real world" question

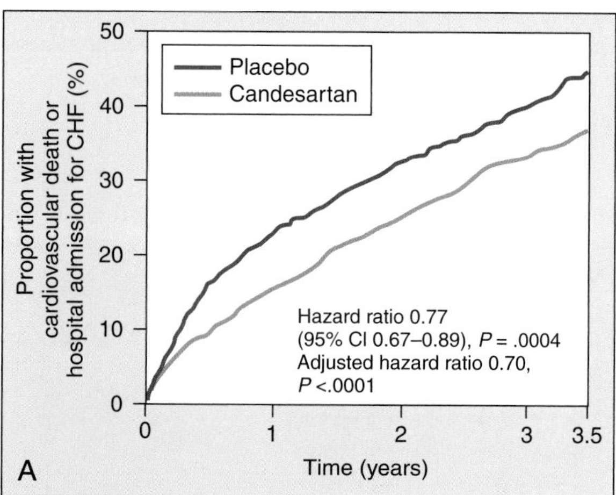

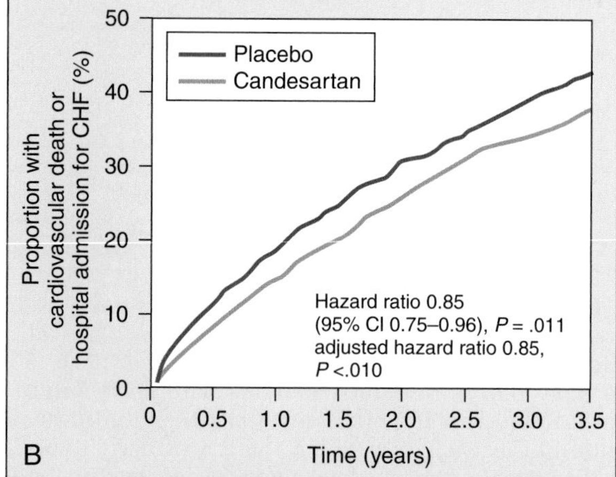

FIGURE 45–7 Effect of candesartan on cardiovascular mortality or hospital admission for heart failure. Data for two groups of patients who were randomly assigned to receive candesartan or placebo are depicted: (**A**) patients who were not receiving an ACE inhibitor (the Candesartan in Heart Failure Assessment in Reduction of Mortality [CHARM]–Alternative trial) and (**B**) patients who were receiving an ACE inhibitor (the CHARM-Added trial). The effect size of candesartan was reduced in the group of patients who were receiving an ACE inhibitor. ACE, angiotensin-converting enzyme; CHF, congestive heart failure; CI, confidence interval. (**A** modified from Granger CB, McMurray JJ, Yusuf S, et al. Effects of candesartan in patients with chronic heart failure and reduced left-ventricular systolic function intolerant to angiotensin-converting-enzyme inhibitors: the CHARM-Alternative trial. *Lancet* 2003;362:772-776; and McMurray JJ, Ostergren J, Swedberg K, et al. Effects of candesartan in patients with chronic heart failure and reduced left-ventricular systolic function taking angiotensin-converting-enzyme inhibitors: the CHARM-Added trial. *Lancet* 2003;362:767-771.)

asked by CHARM-Added: namely, what happens when an ARB is added in a population already well treated with an ACE inhibitor? Third, how do clinicians weigh the relative merits of adding an ARB versus an aldosterone blocker to an ACE inhibitor–treated patient who continues to be symptomatic, and what about the combination of all three drugs? Unfortunately, no studies have addressed this specific question, and thus there are no definitive answers. Most clinicians have chosen to add an aldosterone blocker, rather than an ARB, in this setting. Seventeen percent of the CHARM-Added population was also receiving an aldosterone blocker, and there was no clear difference in the outcome benefit from candesartan in this subgroup. However, the numbers were too small to draw any conclusions, and concern exists about the potential for hyperkalemia with the three-way combination. Therefore, clinical practice guidelines have refrained from recommending this combination.

CHARM-Preserved produced a more ambiguous result. Candesartan demonstrated a favorable trend for the primary endpoint, but it did not reach statistical significance. This finding, coupled with a negative result in the more recent Irbesartan in Heart Failure with Preserved Systolic Function (I-PRESERVE) study conducted in a similar population,[79] has left considerable doubt about the value of RAAS blockade in patients with heart failure and preserved LVEF. However, favorable findings for ARBs on cardiovascular endpoints in populations with normal LVEF, hypertension, and LV hypertrophy[80] and in populations with diabetes and microalbuminuria[81] continue to suggest potential value in the population with heart failure and normal LVEF. More work is needed in targeting the specific population that stands to benefit and the nature of the endpoints that might demonstrate such a benefit.

Heart Failure Endpoint Evaluation of Angiotensin II Antagonist Losartan (HEAAL)

Based on the assumption that a higher losartan dose might have produced greater benefit in ELITE-II, the HEAAL study[120] randomized 3846 patients with NYHA class II-IV heart failure, LVEF ≤40%, and ACE inhibitor intolerance to losartan 150 mg daily or 50 mg daily. With a median followup of 4.7 years, compared with the lower dose, the higher losartan dose was associated with a 10% reduction in the rate of the primary endpoint of death or heart failure hospitalization (hazard ratio 0·90, 95% confidence interval 0·82–0·99; p=0·027) (Table 45-2). The higher dose was associated with increased incidence of hyperkalemia, renal impairment, and hypotension; however the frequency of discontinuation for adverse event was low (overall <2 per 100 patient-years) and not significantly different between the two groups. HEAAL is the only study to examine ARB dose-effect on clinical outcomes, and one of the few such studies of any cardiovascular therapy. It demonstrated incremental clinical benefit of greater RAAS inhibition in heart failure, and displayed the importance of targeting the same dosing strategy in clinical practice as was used in clinical trials to replicate the demonstrated population benefit on clinical outcomes.

Aldosterone Receptor Blockers

Clinical studies have shown a "breakthrough" of aldosterone levels after prolonged treatment with an ARB or an ACE inhibitor in chronic heart failure, which indicates that aldosterone secretion is not fully under control of angiotensin II.[52,82] This observation, coupled with the fact that the mineralocorticoid receptor may be activated by alternative stimuli and the multifaceted means through which such activation may accelerate the advance of cardiovascular disease, represents a rationale for exploring the benefits of mineralocorticoid receptor antagonists, on top of ACE inhibitors or ARBs.

Two studies demonstrated reduced mortality when patients with heart failure and reduced LVEF were treated with a mineralocorticoid receptor blocker. In the Randomized Aldactone Evaluation Study (RALES),[27] researchers investigated the effect of spironolactone in patients with reduced LVEF and with current or recent symptoms of NYHA class IV heart failure. In this population, those randomly assigned to receive spironolactone, 25 to 50 mg once daily, manifested significant reduction in mortality (Figure 45-8). Within this study, there was a high proportion of patients taking background ACE inhibitor but not β-blocker therapy. The Eplerenone Post–Acute Myocardial Infarction Heart Failure Efficacy and Survival Study (EPHESUS)[83] was an investigation of the effect of eplerenone in patients with heart failure and reduced LVEF in the setting of acute myocardial infarction. EPHESUS demonstrated reduced mortality in patients randomly assigned to receive eplerenone, 50 mg once daily, in comparison with those randomly assigned to receive placebo, on top of ACE inhibitor and β-blocker treatment (see Figure 45-7).

Results of the RALES and EPHESUS trials support the use of mineralocorticoid receptor–blocking agents (see Table 45-5) in at least subsets of patients with heart failure and reduced LVEF. It is uncertain whether their benefits derive principally from effects on fluid and electrolyte balance or from effects on processes such as fibrosis and inflammation in cardiac or vascular tissues. It is also uncertain whether similar benefits would be apparent in patient groups with different clinical characteristics, such as those who have not had recent myocardial infarction and those whose symptoms were less severe than those in the RALES population.

Serious hyperkalemia, defined as a serum potassium concentration of 6.0 mmol/L or higher, was reported in 1.7% of patients in RALES who took spironolactone, in comparison with 1.2% of those taking placebo, and in 5.5% of patients in

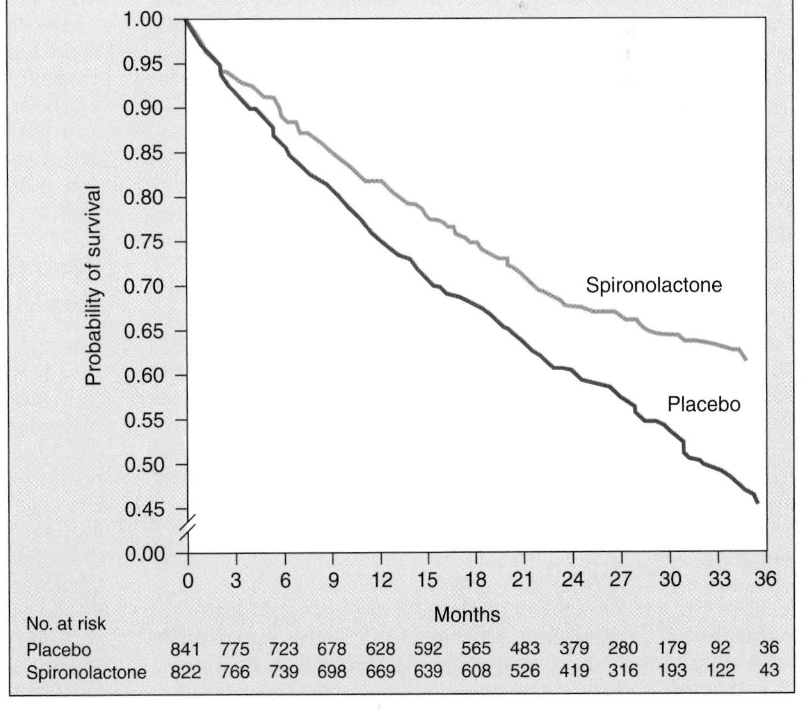

FIGURE 45-8 Mortality curves from the Randomized Aldactone Evaluation Study (RALES), demonstrating a 30% relative reduction in mortality among patients with left ventricular systolic dysfunction (left ventricular ejection fraction <35%) and New York Heart Association class III to IV heart failure. (From Pitt B, Zannad F, Remme WJ, et al. The effect of spironolactone on morbidity and mortality in patients with severe heart failure. Randomized Aldactone Evaluation Study Investigators. *N Engl J Med* 1999;341:709-717.)

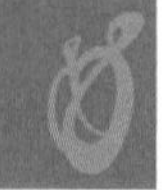

EPHESUS who took eplerenone, in comparison with 3.9% of those taking placebo. Despite these low incidences, concern has been raised regarding the adverse potential of hyperkalemia in patients treated with spironolactone or eplerenone in the clinical setting, in view of the greater likelihood of comorbidity and because the degree of patient monitoring is likely to be less.[84] After mineralocorticoid receptor–blocking treatment is initiated, frequent monitoring of serum electrolyte levels is warranted, particularly with concomitant ACE inhibitor or ARB use and particularly in patients with impaired renal function.

Clinical Implications

ACE inhibitors represented the first major success story in the effort to improve clinical outcomes for patients with heart failure. Because of the wealth of data demonstrating reduced morbidity and mortality, they remain a mainstay of therapy for patients with heart failure and reduced ejection fraction. Results in other populations with established atherosclerosis or multiple cardiovascular risks, such as those reported in the Heart Outcomes Prevention Evaluation (HOPE) trial, have further expanded the indications for this class of agents.[85] Agents that block the AT_1 receptor, possessing mechanisms of action that overlap but differ from those of ACE inhibitors, have been difficult to investigate fully because of the ethical imperative to treat patients with an ACE inhibitor when it is tolerated. Nevertheless, results of available trials support the clinical efficacy of these agents. They clearly produce fewer side effects than do ACE inhibitors. In patients who cannot tolerate ACE inhibitors because of cough or angioedema, their use is justified, and their use as add-on treatment may be justified in select populations. Furthermore, guideline and quality metric panels have indicated that ARBs are acceptable alternatives to ACE inhibitors as first-line agents in patients with heart failure and reduced LVEF.[86]

For patients who continue to be symptomatic while receiving ACE inhibitors and β-blockers, clinicians have a choice between adding an ARB or an aldosterone receptor blocker. Most have chosen an aldosterone receptor blocker, on the basis of the mortality reduction in RALES and EPHESUS and because of a belief in greater mechanistic overlap between ACE inhibitors and ARBs. Limited experience, coupled with a concern regarding the risk of hyperkalemia, has precluded a general recommendation for consideration of the combination of all three classes of agents. Use of any of these agents, but particularly aldosterone receptor blockers in combination with either an ACE inhibitor or an ARB, warrants careful monitoring of serum potassium levels.

PATIENT CHARACTERISTICS AND THE BENEFITS OF RENIN-ANGIOTENSIN-ALDOSTERONE SYSTEM BLOCKADE

On the basis of the clinical trials described previously, clinical practice guidelines for heart failure have advocated prescription of ACE inhibitors for all patients with reduced LVEF,[87] and guidelines since 2006 have advocated ARBs for patients intolerant of ACE inhibitors.[86] As with other classes of agents that have proved efficacious in clinical trials, these trials provide only modest guidance for identifying patients, beyond these criteria, who are either more or less likely to benefit clinically from treatment designed to inhibit the RAAS.

Disease Severity and Drug Effects

It stands to reason that patients with the greatest degree of activation of the RAAS would have the greatest opportunity for benefit from ACE inhibitors or ARBs. However, the degree of activation is difficult to gauge within a particular patient, because plasma renin activity varies with sodium loading and because production of angiotensin II and expression of angiotensin receptor are regulated at a local tissue level. Nevertheless, there is approximate correlation between RAAS activation and severity of the clinical syndrome of heart failure.[34,88,89]

Across the trials demonstrating clinical benefit for ACE inhibitors in patients with heart failure, the differential in outcomes between active drug and placebo appears to be more marked in the trials in which clinical heart failure was most severe (see Table 45-1). CONSENSUS demonstrated a 31% reduction in mortality after 1 year of therapy among patients with class IV heart failure treated with enalapril. The SOLVD treatment trial, whose population consisted predominantly of patients with class II and III symptoms, demonstrated a 16% reduction in mortality with enalapril. The SOLVD prevention trial, enrolling patients who did not require treatment for symptoms of heart failure, showed only an 8% nonsignificant trend toward reduced mortality with enalapril.

Within the SOLVD treatment trial, in which entry required an ejection fraction of 35% or less, subgroup analysis revealed that patients with the lowest baseline ejection fraction manifested the greatest benefit from enalapril treatment. In a substudy of the effect of the ACE inhibitor on LV function and volumes across both SOLVD trials, enalapril prevented LV dilation across various subgroups, although greater effect was observed among patients in the treatment trial (who were symptomatic) than among those in the prevention trial (who were asymptomatic).[49,50] The latter group had smaller LV cavity volumes at baseline. Median plasma renin activity was near normal among patients in the prevention trial.[89]

Hyponatremia has been linked to greater sensitivity to ACE inhibitor treatment,[90] probably because the population with hyponatremia included a higher proportion of patients with excessive plasma renin levels. The presence of hyponatremia indicates a higher likelihood of developing hypotension with initiation of an ACE inhibitor, but it also indicates a higher likelihood of achieving short-term symptomatic benefit if the drug can be tolerated. The presence of azotemia and hypotension also identify patients in whom ACE inhibitors and ARBs, which must be titrated cautiously, beginning with small doses of shorter-acting agents (e.g., captopril, 6.25 mg three times daily). However, if the appropriate dosing regimen can be established, such patients are likely to benefit from long-term treatment with these agents.

Despite the greater magnitude of demonstrable clinical outcome benefits of ACE inhibitors in patients with more severe clinical heart failure, there is ample evidence—notably, the marked reduction in progression to overt clinical heart failure and in hospitalizations for heart failure as a result of enalapril treatment in the SOLVD prevention trial—to support the use of ACE inhibitors in asymptomatic patients with reduced LVEF,

Inhibition of the Renin-Angiotensin System as a Preventive Strategy

There is increasing evidence that agents that inhibit the RAAS in selective patients without heart failure or reduced LVEF can be used as a means for preventing the development of heart failure. The HOPE trial provides strong support for ACE inhibitor use in patients with clinically overt atherosclerotic disease and in those with diabetes and an additional risk factor for atherosclerotic disease but with absence of clinical heart failure or reduced ejection fraction.[85] Among the effects of ramipril in this study was a 23% reduction in the development of heart failure. The extent to which this effect is mediated through reduction in the incidence of myocardial infarction, as opposed to a direct protective effect on the myocardium, is uncertain. Two studies, the Irbesartan and Diabetic Nephropathy Trial (IDNT)[91] and the Reduction

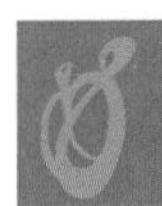

of End points in Non–Insulin Dependent Diabetes Mellitus (RENAAL) Trial,[81] have demonstrated improved clinical outcomes with the use of ARBs in patients with altered renal function. Among diabetic patients with mild increases in urinary protein and serum creatinine levels, ARBs prevented the progression to more advanced renal failure, in addition to preserving renal function. In addition, treatment appeared to reduce the incidence of heart failure, although the latter was not a prespecified endpoint.

Inhibition of the Renin-Angiotensin System in Patients with Preserved Left Ventricular Ejection Fraction (see Chapter 48)

For the large-scale clinical trials to date in which the effects of either ACE inhibitors or ARBs on clinical outcomes in heart failure were reported, entry criteria have included reduced LVEF. There is ample rationale to anticipate that ACE inhibitors or ARBs, or both, would provide benefits in clinical outcomes among many patients with preserved LVEF as well. The majority of patients with heart failure and preserved LVEF, with a nondilated left ventricle, have LV hypertrophy as a result of long-standing hypertension. Both ACE inhibitors and ARBs have been shown to slow the progression, or induce regression, of LV hypertrophy in hypertensive patients[92,93] through their antihypertensive effects and perhaps through direct effects on the myocardium. Angiotensin II has been shown to have a negative lusitropic effect (i.e., it improves myocardial relaxation) in animal models of LV hypertrophy,[94] and in human studies, relaxation is accelerated during intracoronary infusion of an ACE inhibitor in patients with LV hypertrophy.[95]

To date, direct support for inhibition of the RAAS in patients with heart failure and preserved LVEF is available only from small trials that have suggested improvement by ACE inhibitors or ARBs in symptoms or measures of functional capacity within such patients.[96] CHARM-Preserved provided only ambiguous results, with only marginal statistical significance for the primary endpoint. Results of the I-PRESERVE trial showed no clear evidence of benefit.[79]

Until more data are available, use of agents that inhibit the RAAS remains a reasonable consideration within the majority of patients with heart failure and preserved LVEF, especially those with hypertensive, hypertrophic disease. Beyond the efficacy of ACE inhibitors and ARBs as effective antihypertensive agents, large numbers of these patients with atherosclerotic disease, with diabetes, and with renal impairment are likely to fulfill the inclusion criteria for trials that have reported improved clinical outcomes with one or another of these agents. It is hoped that results of ongoing investigation with RAAS antagonists will provide clearer direction in the treatment of patients with heart failure and preserved LVEF.

Genetic and Racial Factors Influencing the Response to Inhibition of the Renin-Angiotensin-Aldosterone System (see Chapters 42 and 49)

The future holds promise for identifying genetic factors that may influence response to a particular pharmacological approach. Both the opportunities and the obstacles in this area are evident in the case of ACE gene polymorphism, which has been widely explored for its effect on the development of cardiovascular disease. In particular, a homozygous deletion of a 287–base pair marker (d,d) in the human ACE gene is associated with greater levels of myocardial ACE expression and has been variably linked to increased incidence of myocardial infarction, LV hypertrophy, and heart failure.[97] Such observations could naturally lead to identifying the sensitivity of particular patients within the population to treatment with an ACE inhibitor or ARB. However, these observations have been extremely variable; many studies have revealed no relationship at all. It is likely that the ACE polymorphism interacts with many other unknown genetic factors, and so its importance is dependent on the population investigated. Even within populations that have displayed a significant relationship, the contribution of the ACE polymorphism to the overall statistical risk of disease has been relatively small.

A number of observations have supported the view of variability in response to RAAS intervention on the basis of race. As a generality, African Americans tend to have a greater proportion of low-renin hypertension than do their non–African American counterparts.[98] Post hoc analysis of the SOLVD trial[99] demonstrated a treatment × race interaction that supported a greater clinical response to ACE inhibitors by non–African American patients. Similar findings were observed in a post hoc analysis of V-HeFT I and II trials.[100] However, such findings should not be interpreted as a rationale for withholding ACE inhibitor or ARB treatment from African American patients. The proportion of African American patients investigated in SOLVD was small, and no conclusion can be drawn from an analysis of treatment effect solely within this subgroup. Furthermore, African Americans are by no means genetically homogeneous, and although a general population trend may be present, many African Americans would probably benefit from treatment directed toward the RAAS. The only way to resolve this question would be to conduct a placebo-controlled trial exclusively among African Americans, but a trial in which placebo is substituted for an ACE inhibitor would be unethical.

Ongoing and future clinical trials will incorporate methods for screening particular genotypes for their correlation with clinical effect. Genomic linkage to the response to a particular treatment will be demonstrated more slowly for heart failure—a multiform syndrome that is the complex product of multiple genetic and environmental factors—than for conditions that are more directly linked to a small number of genetic variables.

CHARACTERISTICS AND DOSING RECOMMENDATIONS FOR SPECIFIC AGENTS

The two factors that have displayed the greatest variability among ACE inhibitors are pharmacokinetics and tissue binding. On the basis of differences in plasma half-lives, which have driven clinical trial design, the recommended dosing intervals for ACE inhibitors range from once daily to three times daily (Table 45-3). Most patients tolerate initiation of an ACE inhibitor or ARB quite well. However, when treatment is initiated in patients at risk for toxicity, particularly those with marginal blood pressure or marginal renal function, it is wise to begin with small doses and to consider an agent with a short plasma half-life, such as captopril.

In one study, a relative sparing of renal function was observed with captopril, in comparison with enalapril,[101] presumably because of an intermittent sparing of glomerular filtration pressure. Over days or weeks of treatment, it is not clear that this difference represents a significant advantage, inasmuch as variation in drug effect across the dosing interval is likely to confer intermittent efficacy, as well as intermittent sparing of glomerular filtration. Reduced glomerular filtration rate with ACE inhibitors and with ARBs does not represent a renal toxic effect. In fact, chronic reduction in glomerular filtration pressure is thought to contribute to renal protection with long-term inhibition of the RAAS, particularly in diabetic patients.[102] However, initiation with a short-acting agent enables more rapid reversal of renal function when function declines to a clinically unacceptable range. Once it is demonstrated that a patient tolerates inhibition of the RAAS, a

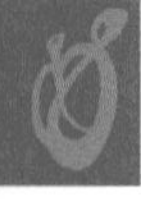

TABLE 45–3 Properties of Selected Angiotensin-Converting Enzyme Inhibitors

Agent	Half-Life (Hours)	Recommended Dosing Schedule	Recommended Starting Dose	Recommended Target Dosage	Relative Tissue Binding
Captopril	3	Three times daily	6.25 mg	50 mg tid	+
Enalapril	11	Twice daily	2.5-5 mg	10 mg bid	+
Lisinopril	12	Daily	5 mg	20 mg qd	+
Ramipril	9-18	Twice daily	2.5 mg	5 mg bid	++
Quinapril	2*	Twice daily	5 mg	20 mg bid	+++
Trandolapril	6	Twice daily	1 mg	1-2 mg bid	NA

*Half-life of the active metabolite is 25 hours.
NA, not applicable.

transition may then be made to a longer-acting agent, which will be more conducive to patient compliance.

The tissue binding of different ACE inhibitors is significantly variable. The clinical importance of this variability has been suggested by animal studies that have shown differential effects on cardiovascular remodeling across agents with varied tissue binding, in the presence of comparable effects on systemic hemodynamics. It is not clear whether these differences translate into clinically relevant differentiating features. Enalapril, which has low tissue binding in relation to other ACE inhibitors, has been shown in a variety of clinical trials to be highly effective at reducing morbidity and mortality among patients with heart failure. A large-scale individual comparison of clinical outcomes would help resolve the issue of the relevance of tissue binding to clinical efficacy.

It has been similarly difficult to establish the optimal dosages for ACE inhibitors and ARBs, and aldosterone receptor blockers (Tables 45-3, 45-4, and 45-5, respectively). Selection of dosage within clinical outcome trials has been based on small dose-ranging studies, in which researchers have tended to examine acute hemodynamic effects of these agents. Available dose-response data are not likely to be definitive, even with regard to hemodynamic effects, because it is likely that the highest hemodynamic dose-response relationships are nonlinear. Furthermore, there is little reason to expect that a dosage that is "optimal" for achieving a given acute hemodynamic response will represent the dosage that is optimal for achieving improved clinical outcomes with an acceptable frequency of adverse events.

The practical answer to the question of dosage has been to recommend the dosing strategy that has been shown to achieve a given clinical outcome across a population, with acceptance of the possibility that an alternative dose or strategy, if tested, would have performed even better. It is typical that such strategies entail upward titration to a particular target, whereby the titration is halted or reversed if an adverse effect is observed. The maximum recommended doses listed in Table 45-3 tend to represent the target doses in trials that have demonstrated reduced morbidity, mortality, or both. For example, the target dosage of enalapril in the SOLVD studies was 10 mg twice daily. The titration strategy resulted in a mean dosage within the active treatment groups of 16.6 mg/day in the treatment trial and 16.7 mg/day in the prevention trial.

Attempts have been made to clarify the dosing issue in trials in which clinical outcomes of administration of high versus low dosages of an ACE inhibitor were compared. In the ATLAS trial, researchers compared low-dose with high-dose lisinopril in patients with heart failure and LV systolic dysfunction (LVEF ≤30%). Mean dosages for the high-dose recipients reached 33.4 mg/day, in contrast to 4.5 mg/day for the low-dose recipients. In this long-term study, the high-dose recipients demonstrated a trend toward improved mortality rates (8% relative risk reduction, $P = .13$) but a significant reduction in the combined endpoint of death and hospitalization (24% relative risk reduction, $P = .002$).[103] These data suggest that high-dose ACE inhibitor treatment is superior to low-dose therapy, although not by a large margin. Further evidence of this dose-outcome interaction was provided by Luzier and associates,[104,105] who analyzed ACE inhibitor dose and rehospitalization rates from a retrospective analysis of patients with heart failure. They reported that rehospitalization rates were significantly higher (28%) among patients taking lower dose enalapril (≤5 mg/day, or ACE inhibitor equivalent) than among those receiving recommended doses of enalapril (≤20 mg/day, or ACE inhibitor equivalent). Thus, these data support the notion that titration of ACE inhibitor dosages to recommended or maximal levels is superior to low-dose therapy in preventing hospitalizations for heart failure.

POTENTIAL DRUG INTERACTIONS OF ANGIOTENSIN-CONVERTING ENZYME INHIBITORS

Clinical evidence suggests that aspirin use may prevent or limit the hemodynamic and survival benefits of ACE inhibitors. Guazzi and colleagues[106] measured diffusing lung capacity for carbon monoxide (DL_{CO}) and peak exercise oxygen consumption (Vo_{2max}) before and after 8 weeks of aspirin therapy (325 mg/day) in patients with dilated cardiomyopathy taking enalapril. They reported that aspirin decreased DL_{CO} by 15%, with an associated and significant decrease in Vo_{2max} and in exercise time. Spaulding and associates[107] administered aspirin (325 mg/day) or ticlopidine for 7 days to patients with heart failure and studied the hemodynamic response to a single 10-mg dose of enalapril. Contrary to the hemodynamic changes observed in the patients who received ticlopidine, enalapril administration to those who took aspirin did not decrease systemic vascular resistance or mean arterial pressure, and no increase in cardiac output was observed. In a cohort analysis from the SOLVD trial, Al-Khadra and coworkers[108] demonstrated that use of antiplatelet agents was associated with lack of an additive survival benefit from the ACE inhibitor enalapril. In a meta-analysis of ACE inhibitor trials, improvement in clinical outcomes continued to be evident in patients receiving aspirin at baseline, although the magnitude of the benefit tended to be lower.[109] The dose of aspirin chosen may be important. Studies in which less than 325 mg were used have not shown aspirin to be detrimental to hemodynamic effects of ACE inhibitors.[110]

Current recommendations advocate independent assessment of the indication for ACE inhibitors and aspirin.[86] Clopidogrel, an adenosine diphosphate receptor antagonist, would not be expected to interact adversely with the therapeutic benefit of ACE inhibitors. The Warfarin and Antiplatelet

TABLE 45–4 Properties of Selected Angiotensin Receptor Blockers

Agent	Half-Life (Hours)	Recommended Dosing Schedule	Recommended Starting Dose	Recommended Target Dosage
Losartan	6-9*	Daily	12.5 mg	50 mg qd
Valsartan	9	Daily	40 mg	160 mg bid
Irbesartan	11-15	Daily	75 mg	150 mg qd
Candesartan	3.5-4	Daily	4 mg	32 mg qd
Telmisartan†	24	Daily	20 mg	80 mg qd
Eprosartan	5-7	Daily or twice daily	200 mg	400 mg bid

*Half-life of the active metabolite.
†Decreases digoxin clearance.

TABLE 45–5 Properties of Aldosterone Receptor Blockers

Agent	Half-Life (Hours)	Recommended Dosing Schedule	Recommended Starting Dose	Recommended Target Dosage
Spironolactone	9-23*	Daily	12.5 mg	25-50 mg qd
Eplerenone	3.5-6	Daily	25 mg	50 mg qd

*Half-life of the active metabolite.

Therapy in Chronic Heart Failure (WATCH) trial randomly assigned more than 1500 patients with NYHA classes II to IV heart failure and with LVEF of less than 35% to receive warfarin, aspirin, or clopidogrel. The primary endpoint was all-cause mortality, nonfatal stroke, and nonfatal myocardial infarction. After a mean follow-up period of 2.5 years, there were no differences in the primary endpoint across the three groups. The warfarin-treated patients demonstrated fewer hospitalizations for heart failure than did the aspirin-treated patients.[111] Further insight into this issue may be shed by the results of the ongoing Warfarin Versus Aspirin in Reduced Cardiac Ejection Fraction (WARCEF) trial.

FUTURE DIRECTIONS

There is active research on the potential incremental value of renin antagonists, which, when added to standard ACE inhibitor therapy, should produce more complete inhibition of the RAAS and, hence, minimize both angiotensin II and aldosterone "breakthrough."[112,113]

The future holds promise for selection of patient populations that are mostly likely to benefit from antagonists of the RAAS. The technology enabling genomic analysis of defined gene polymorphisms is advancing rapidly. Such genetic analyses have already enabled the characterization of multiple polymorphisms within the adrenergic receptor system, some of which identify patients at high risk of developing heart failure or rapid progression once symptoms ensue.[114-116] Similar work for the RAAS may follow. However, heart failure is a complex disease that progresses in response to a myriad of both genetic and environmental factors. Thus, identification of specific genotype-phenotype relationships within this complex syndrome requires large, prospective, population-based studies. The EURopean trial On reduction of cardiac events with Perindopril in stable coronary Artery disease (EUROPA), which enrolled more than 12,000 patients with stable chronic coronary artery disease, demonstrated a favorable effect of the ACE inhibitor perindopril on mortality and morbidity. The purpose of the PERindopril GENEtic association study (PERGENE), a pharmacogenomic substudy of EUROPA,[117] was to identify gene polymorphisms that influence responsiveness to ACE inhibitor treatment in this population and thereby point to a more personalized therapeutic approach.

In two separate small studies, the significance of the AT_1 receptor polymorphism A1166C was analyzed for any interaction with the ACE deletion polymorphism. Among patients with symptomatic heart failure who were homozygous for the ACE deletion allele (d,d), survival rates were worse when they were homozygous or heterozygous for the 1166C allele.[118] This combination of apparently unfavorable genotypes was associated with the presence of diastolic filling abnormalities, determined by echocardiography in patients with a normal LVEF.[119] Results of both these rather small studies require confirmation in larger scale prospective clinical trials. Nonetheless, they demonstrate the potential strength of genomic analyses in identifying patients at high risk. Even more exciting will be the determination of those genotypes that confer a high likelihood of response to a given therapy; the ultimate goal is individualized, targeted therapy to optimize clinical outcomes.

REFERENCES

1. Antonaccio, M. J. (1983). Development and pharmacology of angiotensin converting enzyme inhibitors. *J Pharmacol, 14*, 29–45.
2. Urata, H., Healy, B., Stewart, R. W., et al. (1990). Angiotensin II–forming pathways in normal and failing human hearts. *Circ Res, 66*, 883–890.
3. Urata, H., Boehm, K. D., Philip, A., et al. (1993). Cellular localization and regional distribution of an angiotensin II–forming chymase in the human heart. *J Clin Invest, 91*, 1269–1281.
4. MacFadyen, R. J., Lee, A. F., Morton, J. J., et al. (1999). How often are angiotensin II and aldosterone concentrations raised during chronic ACE inhibitor treatment in cardiac failure? *Heart, 82*, 57–61.
5. Roig, E., Perez-Villa, F., Morales, M., et al. (2000). Clinical implications of increased plasma angiotensin II despite ACE inhibitor therapy in patients with congestive heart failure. *Eur Heart J, 21*, 53–57.
6. Linz, W., Wiemer, G., Gohlke, P., et al. (1995). Contribution of kinins to the cardiovascular actions of angiotensin-converting enzyme inhibitors. *Pharmacol Rev, 47*, 25–49.
7. Linz, W., Wiemer, G., & Schölkens, B. A. (1993). Contribution of bradykinin to the cardiovascular effects of ramipril. *J Cardiovasc Pharmacol, 22*, S1–S8.
8. Baumgarten, C. R., Linz, W., Kunkel, G., et al. (1993). Ramiprilat increases bradykinin outflow from isolated hearts of rat. *Br J Pharmacol, 108*, 293–295.
9. Mombouli, J. V., & Vanhoutte, P. M. (1999). Endothelial dysfunction: from physiology to therapy. *J Mol Cell Cardiol, 31*, 61–74.
10. Yamasaki, S., Sawada, S., Komatsu, S., et al. (2000). Effects of bradykinin on prostaglandin I(2) synthesis in human vascular endothelial cells. *Hypertension, 36*, 201–207.
11. McDonald, K. M., Mock, J., D'Aloia, A., et al. (1995). Bradykinin antagonism inhibits the antigrowth effect of converting enzyme inhibition in the dog myocardium after discrete transmural myocardial necrosis. *Circulation, 91*, 2043–2048.
12. Wollert, K. C., Studer, R., Doerfer, K., et al. (1997). Differential effects of kinins on cardiomyocyte hypertrophy and interstitial collagen matrix in the surviving myocardium after myocardial infarction in the rat. *Circulation, 95*, 1910–1917.
13. Linz, W., & Schölkens, B. A. (1992). A specific B_2-bradykinin receptor antagonist HOE 140 abolishes the antihypertrophic effect of ramipril. *Br J Pharmacol, 105*, 771–772.

14. Matsubara, H. (1998). Pathophysiological role of angiotensin II type 2 receptor in cardiovascular and renal diseases. *Circ Res, 83*, 1182–1191.
15. Yamada, T., Horiuchi, M., & Dzau, V. J. (1996). Angiotensin II type 2 receptor mediates programmed cell death. *Proc Natl Acad Sci U S A, 93*, 156–160.
16. Mulrow, P. J. (1999). Angiotensin II and aldosterone regulation. *Regul Pept, 80*, 27–32.
17. Biollaz, J., Brunner, H. R., Gavras, I., et al. (1982). Antihypertensive therapy with MK 421: angiotensin II–renin relationships to evaluate efficacy of converting enzyme blockade. *J Cardiovasc Pharmacol, 4*, 966–972.
18. Young, M. J., Lam, E. Y. M., & Rickard, A. J. (2007). Mineralocorticoid receptor activation and cardiac fibrosis. *Clin Sci, 112*, 467–475.
19. Delyani, J. A., Robinson, E. L., & Rudolph, A. E. (2001). Effect of a selective aldosterone receptor antagonist in myocardial infarction. *Am J Physiol Heart Circ Physiol, 281*, H647–H654.
20. Suzuki, G., Morita, H., Mishima, T., et al. (2002). Effects of long-term monotherapy with eplerenone, a novel aldosterone blocker, on progression of left ventricular dysfunction and remodeling in dogs with heart failure. *Circulation, 106*, 2967–2972.
21. Silvestre, J. S., Heymes, C., Oubenaissa, A., et al. (1999). Activation of cardiac aldosterone production in rat myocardial infarction: effect of angiotensin II receptor blockade and role in cardiac fibrosis. *Circulation, 99*, 2694–2701.
22. Weber, K. T. (1999). Aldosterone and spironolactone in heart failure. *N Engl J Med, 341*, 753–755.
23. Zhao, W., Ahokas, R. A., Weber, K. T., et al. (2006). Angiotensin II–induced cardiac molecular and cellular events: role of aldosterone. *Am J Physiol Heart Circ Physiol, 291*, H336–H343.
24. Weber, K. T., Brilla, C. G., Campbell, S. E., et al. (1993). Myocardial fibrosis: role of angiotensin II and aldosterone. *Basic Res Cardiol, 88*(Suppl. 1), 107–124.
25. Rude, M. K., Duhaney, T. A. S., Kuster, G. M., et al. (2005). Aldosterone stimulates matrix metalloproteinases and reactive oxygen species in adult rat ventricular cardiomyocytes. *Hypertension, 46*, 555–561.
26. Mano, A., Tatsumi, T., Shiraishi, J., et al. (2004). Aldosterone directly induces myocyte apoptosis through calcineurin-dependent pathways. *Circulation, 110*, 317–323.
27. Pitt, B., Zannad, F., Remme, W. J., et al. (1999). The effect of spironolactone on morbidity and mortality in patients with severe heart failure. Randomized Aldactone Evaluation Study Investigators. *N Engl J Med, 341*, 709–717.
28. Jaffe, I. Z., Tintut, Y., Newfell, B. G., et al. (2007). Mineralocorticoid receptor activation promotes vascular cell calcification. *Arterioscler Thromb Vasc Biol, 27*, 799–805.
29. Jaffe, I. Z., & Mendelsohn, M. E. (2005). Angiotensin II and aldosterone regulate gene transcription via functional mineralocorticoid receptors in human coronary artery smooth muscle cells. *Circ Res, 96*, 643–650.
30. Levine, T. B., Olivari, M. T., Garberg, V., et al. (1984). Hemodynamic and clinical response to enalapril, a long-acting converting-enzyme inhibitor, in patients with congestive heart failure. *Circulation, 69*, 548–553.
31. Uretsky, B. F., Shaver, J. A., Liang, C. S., et al. (1988). Modulation of hemodynamic effects with a converting enzyme inhibitor: acute hemodynamic dose-response relationship of a new angiotensin converting enzyme inhibitor, lisinopril, with observations on long-term clinical, functional, and biochemical responses. *Am Heart J, 116*, 480–488.
32. Ader, R., Chatterjee, K., Ports, T., et al. (1980). Immediate and sustained hemodynamic and clinical improvement in chronic heart failure by an oral angiotensin-converting enzyme inhibitor. *Circulation, 61*, 931–937.
33. Patten, R. D., Kronenberg, M. W., Benedict, C. R., et al. (1997). Acute and long-term effects of the angiotensin-converting enzyme inhibitor, enalapril, on adrenergic activity and sensitivity during exercise in patients with left ventricular systolic dysfunction. *Am Heart J, 134*, 37–43.
34. Benedict, C. R., Johnstone, D. E., Weiner, D. H., et al. (1994). Relation of neurohumoral activation to clinical variables and degree of ventricular dysfunction: a report from the Registry of Studies of Left Ventricular Dysfunction. SOLVD Investigators. *J Am Coll Cardiol, 23*, 1410–1420.
35. Gottlieb, S. S., Dickstein, K., Fleck, E., et al. (1993). Hemodynamic and neurohormonal effects of the angiotensin II antagonist losartan in patients with congestive heart failure. *Circulation, 88*, 1602–1609.
36. Havranek, E. P., Thomas, I., Smith, W. B., et al. (1999). Dose-related beneficial long-term hemodynamic and clinical efficacy of irbesartan in heart failure. *J Am Coll Cardiol, 33*, 1174–1181.
37. Crozier, I., Ikram, H., Awan, N., et al. (1995). Losartan in heart failure. Hemodynamic effects and tolerability. Losartan Hemodynamic Study Group. *Circulation, 91*, 691–697.
38. Baruch, L., Anand, I., Cohen, I. S., et al. (1999). Augmented short- and long-term hemodynamic and hormonal effects of an angiotensin receptor blocker added to angiotensin converting enzyme inhibitor therapy in patients with heart failure. Vasodilator Heart Failure Trial (V-HeFT) Study Group. *Circulation, 99*, 2658–2664.
39. Sadoshima, J., Xu, Y., Slayter, H. S., et al. (1993). Autocrine release of angiotensin II mediates stretch-induced hypertrophy of cardiac myocytes. *Cell, 75*, 977–984.
40. Sadoshima, J., & Izumo, S. (1993). Molecular characterization of angiotensin II–induced hypertrophy of cardiac myocytes and hyperplasia of cardiac fibroblasts: critical role of the AT_1 receptor subtype. *Circ Res, 73*, 413–423.
41. Pfeffer, M. A., Pfeffer, J. M., & Braunwald, E. (1979). Myocardial infarct size and ventricular function in rats. *Circ Res, 44*, 503–512.
42. Pfeffer, M. A., Pfeffer, J. M., Steinberg, C., et al. (1985). Survival after an experimental myocardial infarction: beneficial effects of long-term therapy with captopril. *Circulation, 72*, 406–412.
43. Pfeffer, J. M., Pfeffer, M. A., & Braunwald, E. (1985). Influence of chronic captopril on the infarcted left ventricle of the rat. *Circ Res, 57*, 84–95.
44. Taylor, K., Patten, R. D., Smith, J. J., et al. (1998). Divergent effects of angiotensin converting enzyme inhibition and angiotensin II receptor antagonism on myocardial cellular proliferation and collagen deposition after myocardial infarction in rats. *J Cardiovasc Pharmacol, 31*, 654–660.
45. Kim, S., Yoshiyama, M., Izumi, Y., et al. (2001). Effects of combination of ACE inhibitor and angiotensin receptor blocker on cardiac remodeling, cardiac function, and survival in rat heart failure. *Circulation, 103*, 148–154.
46. Mankad, S., d'Amato, T. A., Reichek, N., et al. (2001). Combined angiotensin II receptor antagonism and angiotensin-converting enzyme inhibition further attenuates postinfarction left ventricular remodeling. *Circulation, 103*, 2845–2850.
47. Sharpe, N., Smith, H., Murphy, J., et al. (1991). Early prevention of left ventricular dysfunction after myocardial infarction with angiotensin-converting enzyme inhibition. *Lancet, 337*, 872–876.
48. St. John Sutton, M., Pfeffer, M. A., Plappert, T., et al. (1994), for the SAVE investigators. Quantitative two dimensional echocardiographic measurements are major predictors of adverse cardiovascular events after acute myocardial infarction, the protective effect of captopril. *Circulation, 89*, 68–75.
49. Konstam, M. A., Rousseau, M. F., Kronenberg, M. W., et al. (1992). Effects of the angiotensin converting enzyme inhibitor, enalapril, on the long-term progression of left ventricular dysfunction in patients with heart failure. *Circulation, 86*, 431–438.
50. Konstam, M. A., Kronenberg, M. W., Rousseau, M. F., et al. (1993), for the SOLVD Investigators. Effects of the angiotensin converting enzyme inhibitor, enalapril, on the long-term progression of left ventricular dilatation in patients with asymptomatic systolic dysfunction. *Circulation, 88*, 2277–2283.
51. Konstam, M. A., Patten, R. D., Thomas, I., et al. (2000). Effects of losartan and captopril on left ventricular volumes in elderly patients with heart failure: results of the ELITE ventricular function substudy. *Am Heart J, 139*, 1081–1087.
52. McKelvie, R. S., Yusuf, S., Pericak, D., et al. (1999). Comparison of candesartan, enalapril, and their combination in congestive heart failure: Randomized Evaluation of Strategies for Left Ventricular Dysfunction (RESOLVD) pilot study. The RESOLVD Pilot Study Investigators. *Circulation, 100*, 1056–1064.
53. Solomon, S. D., Skali, H., Anavekar, N. S., et al. (2005). Changes in ventricular size and function in patients treated with valsartan, captopril, or both after myocardial infarction. *Circulation, 111*, 3411–3419.
54. Hayashi, M., Tsutamoto, T., Wada, A., et al. (2003). Immediate administration of mineralocorticoid receptor antagonist spironolactone prevents post-infarct left ventricular remodeling associated with suppression of a marker of myocardial collagen synthesis in patients with first anterior acute myocardial infarction. *Circulation, 107*, 2559–2565.
55. Kasama, S., Toyama, T., Kumakura, H., et al. (2003). Effect of spironolactone on cardiac sympathetic nerve activity and left ventricular remodeling in patients with dilated cardiomyopathy. *J Am Coll Cardiol, 41*, 574–581.
56. Udelson J. E., Feldman A. M., Greenberg B., Pitt B, et al. (2010). Randomized, double-blind, multicenter, placebo-controlled study evaluating the effect of aldosterone antagonism with epleranone on ventricular remodeling in patients with mild-to-moderate heart failure and left ventricular systolic dysfunction. *Circ Heart Fail, 3*, 347-353.
57. Ziesche, S., Cobb, F. R., Cohn, J. N., et al. (1993). Hydralazine and isosorbide dinitrate combination improves exercise tolerance in heart failure. Results from V-HeFT I and V-HeFT II. The V-HeFT VA Cooperative Studies Group. *Circulation, 87*, VI-56–VI-64.
58. A placebo-controlled trial of captopril in refractory chronic congestive heart failure. Captopril Multicenter Research Group. (1983). *J Am Coll Cardiol, 2*, 755–763.
59. Riegger, G. A. (1991). Effects of quinapril on exercise tolerance in patients with mild to moderate heart failure. *Eur Heart J, 12*, 705–711.
60. Lang, R. M., Elkayam, U., Yellen, L. G., et al. (1997). Comparative effects of losartan and enalapril on exercise capacity and clinical status in patients with heart failure. The Losartan Pilot Exercise Study Investigators. *J Am Coll Cardiol, 30*, 983–991.
61. Vescovo, G., Dalla Libera, L., Serafini, F., et al. (1998). Improved exercise tolerance after losartan and enalapril in heart failure: correlation with changes in skeletal muscle myosin heavy chain composition. *Circulation, 98*, 1742–1749.
62. Riegger, G. A., Bouzo, H., Petr, P., et al. (1999). Improvement in exercise tolerance and symptoms of congestive heart failure during treatment with candesartan cilexetil. Symptom, Tolerability, Response to Exercise Trial of Candesartan Cilexetil in Heart Failure (STRETCH) Investigators. *Circulation, 100*, 2224–2230.
63. Effects of enalapril on mortality in severe congestive heart failure. Results of the Cooperative North Scandinavian Enalapril Survival Study (CONSENSUS). The CONSENSUS Trial Study Group. (1987). *N Engl J Med, 316*, 1429–1435.
64. Effect of angiotensin converting enzyme inhibition with enalapril on survival in patients with reduced left ventricular ejection fraction and congestive heart failure: results of the treatment trial of the Studies of Left Ventricular Dysfunction (SOLVD); a randomized double blind trial. (1991). *N Engl J Med, 325*, 293–302.
65. The SOLVD Investigators (1992). Effect of enalapril on mortality and the development of heart failure in asymptomatic patients with reduced left ventricular ejection fractions. *N Engl J Med, 327*, 685–691.
66. Pfeffer, M. A., Braunwald, E., Moyé, L. A., et al. (1992). for the SAVE investigators. Effect of captopril on mortality and morbidity in patients with left ventricular dysfunction after myocardial infarction. *N Engl J Med, 327*, 669–677.
67. Cleland, J. G., Erhardt, L., Murray, G., et al. (1997). Effect of ramipril on morbidity and mode of death among survivors of acute myocardial infarction with clinical evidence of heart failure. A report from the AIRE Study Investigators. *Eur Heart J, 18*, 41–51.
68. Uretsky, B. F., & Sheahan, R. G. (1997). Primary prevention of sudden cardiac death in heart failure: will the solution be shocking? *J Am Coll Cardiol, 30*, 1589–1597.
69. Uretsky, B. F., Thygesen, K., Armstrong, P. W., et al. (2000). Acute coronary findings at autopsy in heart failure patients with sudden death: results from the Assessment of Treatment with Lisinopril And Survival (ATLAS) trial. *Circulation, 102*, 611–616.
70. Pitt, B., Poole-Wilson, P. A., Segal, R., et al. (2000). Effect of losartan compared with captopril on mortality in patients with symptomatic heart failure: randomised trial—the Losartan Heart Failure Survival Study ELITE II. *Lancet, 355*, 1582–1587.
71. Pitt, B., Segal, R., Martinez, F. A., et al. (1997). Randomized trial of losartan versus captopril in patents over 65 with heart failure (Evaluation of Losartan in the Elderly Study, ELITE). *Lancet, 349*, 747–752.
72. Cohn, J. N., & Tognoni, G. (2001). A randomized trial of the angiotensin-receptor blocker valsartan in chronic heart failure. *N Engl J Med, 345*, 1667–1675.

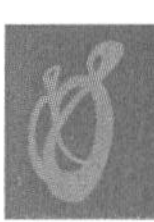

73. Pfeffer, M. A., Swedberg, K., Granger, C. B., et al. (2003). Effects of candesartan on mortality and morbidity in patients with chronic heart failure: the CHARM-Overall programme. *Lancet, 362*, 759–766.
74. McMurray, J. J., Östergren, J., Swedberg, K., et al. (2003). Effects of candesartan in patients with chronic heart failure and reduced left-ventricular systolic function taking angiotensin-converting-enzyme inhibitors: the CHARM-Added trial. *Lancet, 362*, 767–771.
75. Granger, C. B., McMurray, J. J., Yusuf, S., et al. (2003). Effects of candesartan in patients with chronic heart failure and reduced left-ventricular systolic function intolerant to angiotensin-converting-enzyme inhibitors: the CHARM-Alternative trial. *Lancet, 362*, 772–776.
76. Yusuf, S., Pfeffer, M. A., Swedberg, K., et al. (2003). Effects of candesartan in patients with chronic heart failure and preserved left-ventricular ejection fraction: the CHARM-Preserved Trial. *Lancet, 362*, 777–781.
77. McMurray, J. J. V., Young, J. B., Dunlap, M. E., et al. (2006). Relationship of dose of background angiotensin-converting enzyme inhibitor to the benefits of candesartan in the Candesartan in Heart failure: Assessment of Reduction in Mortality and morbidity (CHARM)–Added trial. *Am Heart J, 151*, 985–991.
78. Pfeffer, M. A., McMurray, J. J. V., Velazquez, E. J., et al. (2003). Valsartan, captopril, or both in myocardial infarction complicated by heart failure, left ventricular dysfunction, or both. *N Engl J Med, 349*, 1893–1906.
79. Massie, B. M., Carson, P. E., McMurray, J. J., et al. (2008). Irbesartan in patients with heart failure and preserved ejection fraction. *N Engl J Med, 359*, 2456–2467.
80. Dahlöf, B., Devereux, R. B., Kjeldsen, S. E., et al. (2002). Cardiovascular morbidity and mortality in the Losartan Intervention For Endpoint reduction in hypertension study (LIFE): a randomised trial against atenolol. *Lancet, 359*, 995–1003.
81. Brenner, B. M., Cooper, M. E., de Zeeuw, D., et al. (2001). Effects of losartan on renal and cardiovascular outcomes in patients with type 2 diabetes and nephropathy. *N Engl J Med, 345*, 861–869.
82. Jorde, U. P., Vittorio, T., Katz, S. D., et al. (2002). Elevated plasma aldosterone levels despite complete inhibition of the vascular angiotensin-converting enzyme in chronic heart failure. *Circulation, 106*, 1055–1057.
83. Pitt, B., Remme, W., Zannad, F., et al. (2003). Eplerenone, a selective aldosterone blocker, in patients with left ventricular dysfunction after myocardial infarction. *N Engl J Med, 348*, 1309–1321.
84. Juurlink, D. N., Mamdani, M. M., Lee, D. S., et al. (2004). Rates of hyperkalemia after publication of the Randomized Aldactone Evaluation Study. *N Engl J Med, 351*, 543–551.
85. Yusuf, S., Sleight, P., Pogue, J., et al. (2000). Effects of an angiotensin-converting-enzyme inhibitor, ramipril, on cardiovascular events in high-risk patients. The Heart Outcomes Prevention Evaluation Study Investigators. *N Engl J Med, 342*, 145–153.
86. Heart Failure Society of America. (2006). Heart failure in patients with left ventricular systolic dysfunction. *J Card Fail, 12*, e38–e57.
87. Konstam, M. A., Dracup, K., Baker, D. W., et al. (1994). *Heart failure: evaluation and care of patients with left ventricular dysfunction [Clinical Practice Guideline]*. Rockville, MD: U.S. Department of Health and Human Services, Agency for Health Care Policy and Research.
88. Eriksson, S. V., Eneroth, P., Kjekshus, J., et al. (1994). Neuroendocrine activation in relation to left ventricular function in chronic severe congestive heart failure: a subgroup analysis from the Cooperative North Scandinavian Enalapril Survival Study (CONSENSUS). *Clin Cardiol, 17*, 603–606.
89. Benedict, C. R., Francis, G. S., Shelton, B., et al. (1995). Effect of long-term enalapril therapy on neurohormones in patients with left ventricular dysfunction. SOLVD Investigators. *Am J Cardiol, 75*, 1151–1157.
90. Packer, M., Medina, N., & Yushak, M. (1984). Relation between serum sodium concentration and the hemodynamic and clinical responses to converting enzyme inhibition with captopril in severe heart failure. *J Am Coll Cardiol, 3*, 1035–1043.
91. Parving, H. H., Lehnert, H., Brochner-Mortensen, J., et al. (2001). The effect of irbesartan on the development of diabetic nephropathy in patients with type 2 diabetes. *N Engl J Med, 345*, 870–878.
92. Dahlöf, B. (2001). Left ventricular hypertrophy and angiotensin II antagonists. *Am J Hypertens, 14*, 174–182.
93. Dahlöf, B., & Hansson, L. (1992). Regression of left ventricular hypertrophy in previously untreated essential hypertension: different effects of enalapril and hydrochlorothiazide. *J Hypertens, 10*, 1513–1524.
94. Schunkert, H., Dzau, V. J., Tang, S. S., et al. (1990). Increased rat cardiac angiotensin converting enzyme activity and mRNA expression in pressure overload left ventricular hypertrophy. Effects on coronary resistance, contractility, and relaxation. *J Clin Invest, 86*, 1913–1920.
95. Kyriakidis, M., Triposkiadis, F., Dernellis, J., et al. (1998). Effects of cardiac versus circulatory angiotensin-converting enzyme inhibition on left ventricular diastolic function and coronary blood flow in hypertrophic obstructive cardiomyopathy. *Circulation, 97*, 1342–1347.
96. Warner, J. G., Jr., Metzger, D. C., Kitzman, D. W., et al. (1999). Losartan improves exercise tolerance in patients with diastolic dysfunction and a hypertensive response to exercise. *J Am Coll Cardiol, 33*, 1567–1572.
97. Schunkert, H., Hense, H. W., Holmer, S. R., et al. (1994). Association between a deletion polymorphism of the angiotensin-converting-enzyme gene and left ventricular hypertrophy. *N Engl J Med, 330*, 1634–1638.
98. Saunders, E. (1990). Tailoring treatment to minority patients. *Am J Med, 88*, 21S–23S.
99. Exner, D. V., Dries, D. L., Domanski, M. J., et al. (2001). Lesser response to angiotensin-converting-enzyme inhibitor therapy in black as compared with white patients with left ventricular dysfunction. *N Engl J Med, 344*, 1351–1357.
100. Carson, P., Ziesche, S., Johnson, G., et al. (1999). Racial differences in response to therapy for heart failure: analysis of the vasodilator-heart failure trials. Vasodilator-Heart Failure Trial Study Group. *J Card Fail, 5*, 178–187.
101. Packer, M., Lee, W. H., Yushak, M., et al. (1986). Comparison of captopril and enalapril in patients with severe chronic heart failure. *N Engl J Med, 315*, 847–853.
102. Lacourciere, Y., Belanger, A., Godin, C., et al. (2000). Long-term comparison of losartan and enalapril on kidney function in hypertensive type 2 diabetics with early nephropathy. *Kidney Int, 58*, 762–769.
103. Packer, M., Poole-Wilson, P. A., Armstrong, P. W., et al. (1999). Comparative effects of low and high doses of the angiotensin-converting enzyme inhibitor, lisinopril, on morbidity and mortality in chronic heart failure. ATLAS Study Group. *Circulation, 100*, 2312–2318.
104. Luzier, A. B., Forrest, A., Feuerstein, S. G., et al. (2000). Containment of heart failure hospitalizations and cost by angiotensin-converting enzyme inhibitor dosage optimization. *Am J Cardiol, 86*, 519–523.
105. Luzier, A. B., Forrest, A., Adelman, M., et al. (1998). Impact of angiotensin-converting enzyme inhibitor underdosing on rehospitalization rates in congestive heart failure. *Am J Cardiol, 82*, 465–469.
106. Guazzi, M., Pontone, G., & Agostoni, P. (1999). Aspirin worsens exercise performance and pulmonary gas exchange in patients with heart failure who are taking angiotensin-converting enzyme inhibitors. *Am Heart J, 138*, 254–260.
107. Spaulding, C., Charbonnier, B., Cohen-Solal, A., et al. (1998). Acute hemodynamic interaction of aspirin and ticlopidine with enalapril: results of a double-blind, randomized comparative trial. *Circulation, 98*, 757–765.
108. Al-Khadra, A. S., Salem, D. N., Rand, W. M., et al. (1998). Antiplatelet agents and survival: a cohort analysis from the Studies of Left Ventricular Dysfunction (SOLVD) trial. *J Am Coll Cardiol, 31*, 419–425.
109. Teo, K. K., Yusuf, S., Pfeffer, M., et al. (2002). Effects of long-term treatment with angiotensin-converting-enzyme inhibitors in the presence or absence of aspirin: a systematic review. *Lancet, 360*, 1037–1043.
110. Townend, J. N., Doran, J., Lote, C. J., et al. (1995). Peripheral haemodynamic effects of inhibition of prostaglandin synthesis in congestive heart failure and interactions with captopril. *Br Heart J, 73*, 434–441.
111. Massie, B. M., Collins, J. F., Ammon, S. E., et al. (2009), for the WATCH Trial Investigators. Randomized trial of warfarin, aspirin, and clopidogrel in patients with chronic heart failure: the Warfarin and Antiplatelet Therapy in Chronic Heart Failure (WATCH) Trial. *Circulation, 119*, 1616–1624.
112. Athyros, V. G., Mikhailidis, D. P., Kakafika, A. I., et al. (2007). Angiotensin II reactivation and aldosterone escape phenomena in renin-angiotensin-aldosterone system blockade: is oral renin inhibition the solution? *Expert Opin Pharmacother, 8*, 529–535.
113. Azizi, M. (2008). Direct renin inhibition: clinical pharmacology. *J Mol Med, 86*, 647–654.
114. Mialet Perez, J., Rathz, D. A., Petrashevskaya, N. N., et al. (2003). $Beta_1$-adrenergic receptor polymorphisms confer differential function and predisposition to heart failure. *Nat Med, 9*, 1300–1305.
115. Small, K. M., Wagoner, L. E., Levin, A. M., et al. (2002). Synergistic polymorphisms of β_1- and α_{2C}-adrenergic receptors and the risk of congestive heart failure. *N Engl J Med, 347*, 1135–1142.
116. Liggett, S. B., Mialet-Perez, J., Thaneemit-Chen, S., et al. (2006). A polymorphism within a conserved beta(1)–adrenergic receptor motif alters cardiac function and beta-blocker response in human heart failure. *Proc Natl Acad Sci U S A, 103*, 11288–11293.
117. Brugts, J. J., de Maat, M. P., Boersma, E., et al. (2008). The rationale and design of the Perindopril Genetic Association Study (PERGENE): a pharmacogenetic analysis of angiotensin-converting enzyme inhibitor therapy in patients with stable coronary artery disease. *Cardiovasc Drugs Ther, 10*, 10.
118. Andersson, B., Blange, I., & Sylven, C. (1999). Angiotensin-II type 1 receptor gene polymorphism and long-term survival in patients with idiopathic congestive heart failure. *Eur J Heart Fail, 1*, 363–369.
119. Wu, C. K., Tsai, C. T., Hwang, J. J., et al. (2008). Renin-angiotensin system gene polymorphisms and diastolic heart failure. *Eur J Clin Invest, 38*, 789–797.
120. Konstam, M. A., Neaton, J. D., Dickstein K., et al, (2009), for the HEAAL Investigators. Effects of high-dose versus low-dose losartan on clinical outcomes in patients with heart failure (HEAAL study): a randomised, double-blind trial. *Lancet, 374*, 1840–1848.

CHAPTER 46

Antagonism of the Sympathetic Nervous System in Heart Failure

Marco Metra and Michael R. Bristow

The demonstration of the beneficial effects of β-blocker therapy in patients with chronic heart failure is one of the most important steps forward in the treatment of this syndrome. Because of their acute negative inotropic effects resulting from interruption of adrenergic support of the failing heart, these agents were initially contraindicated in patients with heart failure. However, β-blocking agents also prevent the adverse biological effects of chronically elevated adrenergic signaling in the failing heart, which is the basis for their salutary therapeutic effects. Indeed, demonstration of the beneficial effects of β-blocking agents on cardiac function and outcomes is the final proof of the hypothesis that chronic adrenergic activation is a major determinant of the progressive clinical course of heart failure. In addition, detailed functional, structural, and gene expression analyses have somewhat surprisingly demonstrated that with β-blocker treatment, the dysfunctional, remodeled human left or right ventricle can revert toward normal and, in some cases, completely so (see Chapter 11). This in turn has led to the concept that so-called end-stage myocardial disease is not irreversibly end stage at all and that it is possible to develop therapies that improve the underlying biological abnormalities in the failing heart.[1,2]

HISTORICAL NOTES

The history of β-blocker treatment of heart failure is an example of investigator-initiated therapeutic development. This form of therapy was conceived and initially proceeded from outside the boundaries of conventional pharmaceutical company drug development. Carefully performed small clinical studies,[3,4] which today would be considered anecdotal, played a major role, as did translational investigations[5] that provided a pathophysiological framework for the clinical results. Another lesson learned from the history of the development of β-blocker therapy for heart failure is that small collaborative groups composed of dedicated and determined investigators[6] can achieve major results, in the absence of a centralized source of major funding.

In 1975, β-blockers were contraindicated in patients with heart failure. This was because of reports of clinically serious negative inotropic effects resulting in worsening heart failure, which had occurred when therapy was initiated with the standard large doses typically given to treat cardiovascular diseases other than heart failure. The researchers in Goteborg, Sweden, were the first to report the administration of a β-blocker to multiple patients, seven, with severe refractory heart failure and tachycardia.[3] The aim of this initial study was to therapeutically reduce heart rate, prolong the diastolic filling time, and decrease myocardial energy consumption.[3] β-Blocker treatment resulted in an improvement in clinical conditions, working capacity, and both systolic and diastolic cardiac function, as assessed by phonocardiography, carotid pulse curve, apexcardiography, and M-mode echocardiography.[3] Further small studies by the same researchers confirmed these results. Of importance was that survival rates with β-blocker therapy, in comparison with historical controls, apparently improved in one of the first long-term heart failure trials in which a clinical outcome was an endpoint (Figure 46-1).[4] This nonrandomized, retrospective study, which included only 37 patients (24 taking β-blockers, 13 taking placebo), achieved significant results and predicted the outcome of trials that were concluded almost 20 years later. Contemporaneous with this study, analyses of major postinfarction trials by investigators in the United States[7] and Norway[8] revealed that β-blockade had its most favorable effects on outcomes in patients with signs of heart failure or left ventricular (LV) dysfunction.

Around the same time, data were reported that appeared to resolve the debate of whether the failing heart was subjected to too little or too much adrenergic stimulation. Investigators at the National Institutes of Health had found that biopsy samples from failing human hearts were depleted of the adrenergic neurotransmitter norepinephrine[9] and that plasma norepinephrine or urinary catecholamine metabolites were elevated in patients with heart failure.[10] In order to address the question of whether adrenergic activity and β-adrenergic signaling were increased or decreased in the failing human heart, end-stage failing hearts from cardiac transplant recipients were compared with nonfailing unused organ donor hearts; in failing hearts, β-receptor density and signaling were found to be markedly reduced, which was interpreted as evidence both of exposure to increased adrenergic activity and of a mechanism responsible for compromised myocardial reserve.[5] A short time later, it was proved—first by direct coronary sinus norepinephrine measurements[11] and then by isotope dilution techniques to measure norepinephrine spillover[12]—that adrenergic activity is increased in the failing human heart.

In the ensuing years, randomized, placebo-controlled trials demonstrated the beneficial effects of β-blockers on LV function, on symptoms, and on the clinical course of patients with chronic heart failure.[6,13-20] All these trials were conducted with extremely low initiating doses, followed by slow upward titration to target doses that were in the range of full β-blockade. The administration of β-blockers was associated with LV reverse remodeling (see also Chapter 8) and an improvement in cardiac contractility and energetics.[14-18,21] These changes were related to the beneficial effects of β-blockade on the intrinsic mechanisms that lead to progressive myocardial dysfunction and remodeling,[17] including myocardial metabolism, myocardial myosin heavy chain isoform and sarcoplasmic reticulum calcium-dependent adenosine triphosphatase (SERCA) gene expression,[22] ryanodine receptor phosphorylation,[23] and myocyte apoptosis.[24]

Despite favorable results from most of the initial studies, the efficacy of β-blockers in patients with heart failure remained controversial mainly because of neutral results from two short-term studies[25,26] and encouraging but conventionally nonsignificant statistical results in early underpowered outcome studies.[6,27] Any controversy was finally dispelled when landmark trials demonstrated a reduction in mortality and hospitalizations among patients with heart failure who received β-blockers, in comparison with those receiving placebo; these studies were, accordingly, terminated prematurely.[28-33] The effects on survival were additive to that of angiotensin-converting enzyme (ACE) inhibitors and were of greater magnitude than those previously found with these agents.[34] Subsequent studies were aimed at broadening the indications to β-blocker therapy to early postinfarction LV dysfunction,[35] severe heart failure or LV dysfunction,[32,33] older age,[36,37] and extreme young age.[38] A further series of studies focused on the implementation of β-blocker therapy and how to increase the proportion of patients receiving them. Comorbid conditions, older age, and severe heart failure have been found to be the most important reasons why β-blockers are not prescribed.[39,40] When treatment is implemented on the basis of either early administration during a hospitalization for heart failure[41,42] or physicians' and patients education,[39,43,44] the number of patients receiving β-blockers increases, which results in better outcomes.

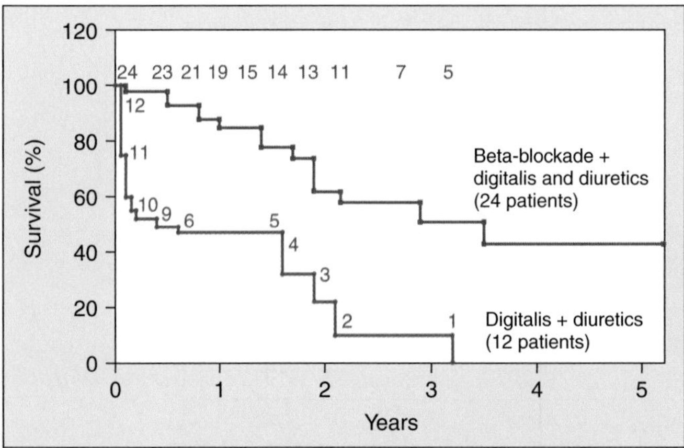

FIGURE 46–1 Effects on survival of β-blocker therapy in patients with cardiomyopathy. Results from Swedberg and colleagues' first study[4] with assessment of survival. (From Swedberg K, Hjalmarson A, Waagstein F, et al. Prolongation of survival in congestive cardiomyopathy by beta-receptor blockade. *Lancet* 1979;1:1374-1376.)

MECHANISMS OF ACTION (see Chapter 10)

LV structural remodeling (see Chapter 15), loss of myocardial cells, and changes in gene expression appear to be the main mechanisms that mediate myocardial damage induced by chronic adrenergic stimulation (Figure 46-2). Remodeling is caused by increased mechanical stress and by neurohormonal activation, and a key role is played by adrenergic stimulation.[2,20,21,34] In accordance with the effects of chronic isoproterenol infusions[45] and the results of studies on β_1-adrenergic receptor myocardial overexpression,[46] chronic β-blockade may reverse changes associated with remodeling (i.e., LV dilation, depression of myocardial contractility, more spherical shape of the left ventricle). This demonstrates the central role of adrenergic stimulation in the remodeling process. Increased cardiac adrenergic drive may induce changes in myocardial gene expression,[22] which may explain the progressive worsening of myocardial contractility, as well as the induction of hypertrophy. The hallmark of adrenergically mediated alteration in cardiac myocyte gene expression is β_1-adrenergic receptor–mediated induction of the "fetal" gene program, consisting of an upregulation of natriuretic peptide and β-myosin heavy chain genes ordinarily expressed in fetal development, and downregulation of α-myosin heavy chain and SERCA genes, ordinarily expressed only in adult cardiac myocytes (Figure 46-3; see also Chapter 2).[22,47,48] Because the α isoform of myosin heavy

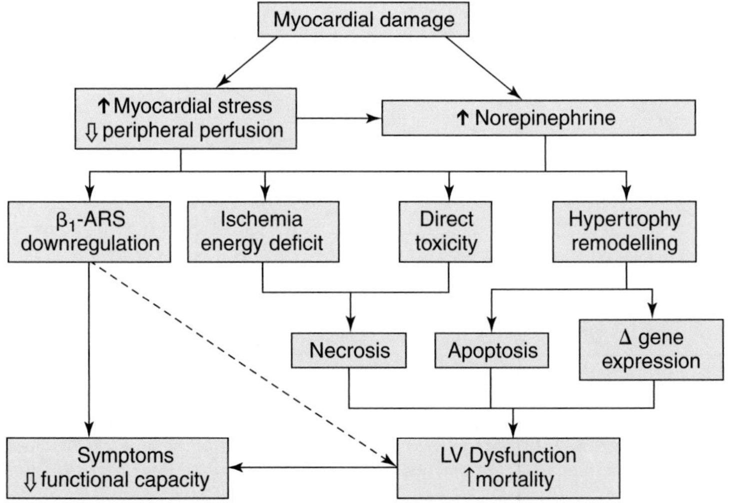

FIGURE 46–2 Sympathetic nervous system–mediated mechanisms of cardiac damage and reduced exercise tolerance in the failing heart. (From Metra M, Nodari S, D'Aloia A, et al. A rationale for the use of beta-blockers as standard treatment for heart failure. *Am Heart J* 2000;139:511-521.)

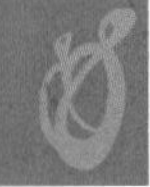

chain has much higher adenosine triphosphatase activity than does the β isoform, the change to favor the latter expression reduces the myocyte velocity of shortening and chamber contractile function. The downregulation of SERCA also contributes to a reduction in contractile function, whereas the upregulation in β myosin heavy chain produces cellular hypertrophy. β-Adrenergically mediated hyperphosphorylation of ryanodine receptors may contribute to myocardial dysfunction and predispose to arrhythmias.[23] β-Blockers reverse these β_1-adrenergically mediated effects, and the reversal of molecular remodeling is highly correlated with reversal of structural remodeling and improvement in contractile function (see Figure 46-3).[22]

Another untoward effect of increased adrenergic drive is accelerated myocardial cell loss. Norepinephrine, at concentrations similar to those found in the failing heart (10 to 100 nmol), can have direct toxic effects and may induce apoptosis.[24] The induction of apoptosis by β-adrenergic receptor stimulation has been consistently shown both in vitro and in vivo. Apoptosis associated with ischemia and reperfusion, or with postinfarction LV remodeling, may be almost completely abolished by the administration of β-blockers. However, the role of apoptosis in the natural history of chronic heart failure is somewhat controversial,[49] and the degree of β-blocker benefit ascribed to this mechanism is therefore uncertain.

In addition to the improvement in cardiac function, protection from lethal arrhythmias is another major favorable effect of β-blocker therapy, with a major effect on outcomes.[50] A discussion of this mechanism is beyond the scope of this chapter, but the beneficial effects of β-blockers on sudden death are discussed later in this chapter.

PHARMACOLOGICAL CHARACTERISTICS OF β-BLOCKING AGENTS

The foundation of β-blocker treatment of patients with heart failure has been cardiac protection from the deleterious effects of adrenergic stimulation, which are transduced mainly by β_1-adrenergic receptors. However, the β-blockers that are recommended by guidelines[51-53] or are in development to treat heart failure are an extremely heterogeneous class of agents, both with regard to β_1-adrenergic receptor blockade and from the standpoint of other properties. Pharmacokinetic and chemical differences include metabolism, plasma half-life, and lipid solubility. Pharmacodynamic differences include intrinsic sympathomimetic activity (ISA), selectivity of β_1-adrenergic receptor blockade, characteristics of binding to β_1-adrenergic receptors, inverse agonism, and ancillary properties unrelated to adrenergic receptor blockade (Table 46-1).[54]

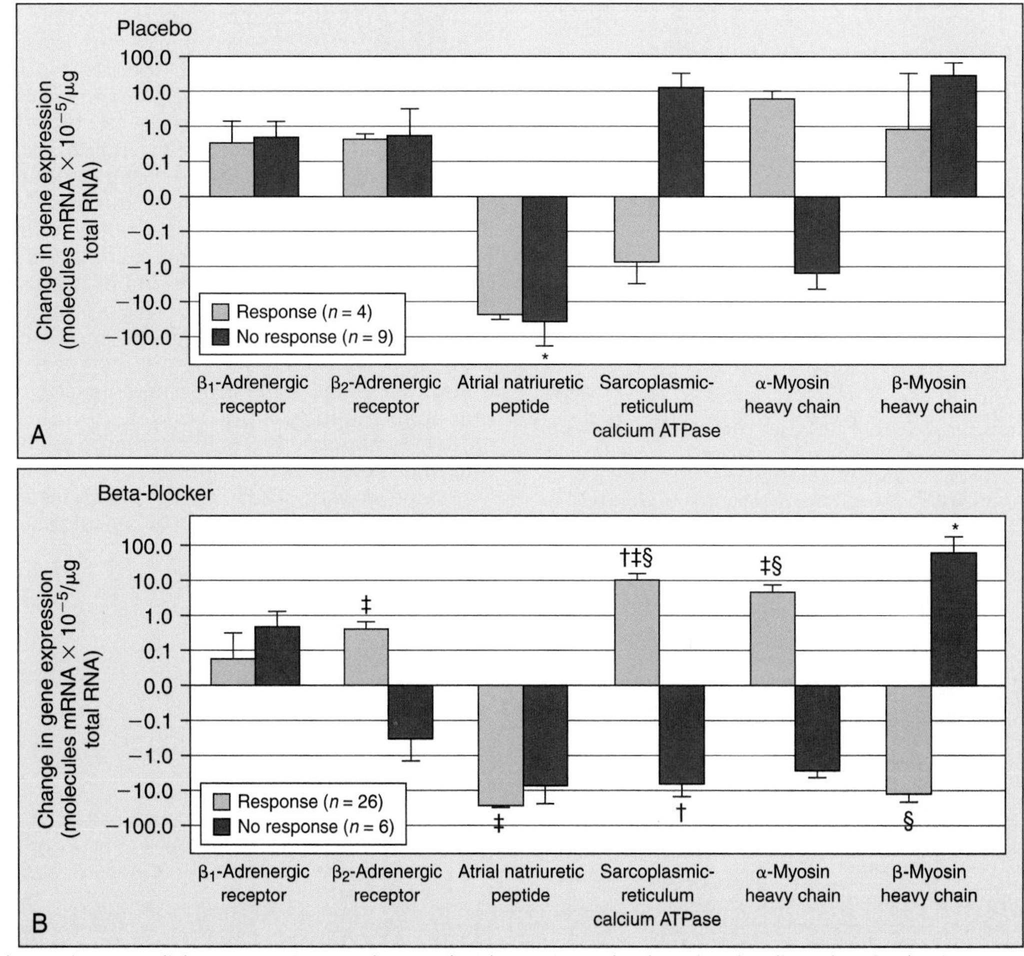

FIGURE 46-3 Changes in myocardial messenger RNA steady-state abundance (6-month value minus baseline value) for the six measured gene products in subjects treated with β-blocking agents. "Responder" subjects demonstrated an improvement in left ventricular ejection fraction (LVEF) (defined as an increase of >5 ejection fraction units), whereas "nonresponders" demonstrated either no change or a decline in LVEF. Messenger RNA abundance is in molecules × 10^{-5}/μg total RNA ± standard error of the mean (SEM), displayed on a log scale (*y* axis); the SEM values are plotted within the unit scales of the nominal absolute changes. (From Lowes BD, Gilbert EM, Abraham WT, et al. Myocardial gene expression in dilated cardiomyopathy treated with beta-blocking agents. *N Engl J Med* 2002;346:1357-1365.)

TABLE 46–1 Pharmacological Characteristics of β-Blockers

Drug	K(β1) (nmol)	K(β2) (nmol)	β1/β2 Selectivity	Inverse Agonism	Ancillary Properties	Initial Dosage	Final Dosage
Propranolol	4.1	8.5	2.1	Moderate	None	Not recommended in heart failure	
Metoprolol succinate	45	3.34	74	Strong	None	12.5/25 mg	200 mg/day
Bisoprolol	121	14.39	119	Moderate to weak	None	1.25 mg	10 mg/day
Carvedilol	4	29	7.3	Moderate to weak	Vasodilation (α_1-blockade), antioxidant	3.125 mg bid	25-50 mg bid
Nebivolol	0.7	225	352	Moderate	Vasodilation, nitric oxide release, β_3 agonist	1.25 mg	10 mg/day
Bucindolol	3.6	5.0	1.4	Weak	Vasodilation, sympatholysis	3 mg bid	50–100 mg bid

K(β_1), average of high-affinity dissociation constant; K(β_2), average of low-affinity dissociation constant.

Lipophilic Versus Hydrophilic β-Blockers

All of the agents shown to be clinically effective in heart failure are lipophilic. Such agents are likely to reside longer or at higher concentrations in cell membranes, which may be important for their effects on cardiac myocytes and arrhythmias. Atenolol, a hydrophilic agent, has not been tested in large prospective outcome studies in patients with heart failure. However, it has been associated with an improvement in LVEF and in exercise capacity in small single-center studies[54] and with favorable outcomes in retrospective analyses of patient databases.[55,56] These data should be interpreted as hypothesis generating and should be confirmed by randomized studies.

Intrinsic Sympathomimetic Activity

The untoward effects of ISA were first shown by postinfarction trials[57] and were then confirmed by the finding that the administration of a β-blocker with high ISA, xamoterol, was associated with increased mortality among patients with heart failure.[58] However, another β-blocker with ISA, celiprolol,[59] was not obviously associated with increased mortality in small randomized studies among patients with heart failure, and it is possible that explanations other than ISA, such as initiating therapy with a high β-blocking dose, could have caused the untoward effects with xamoterol. In addition, some β-blockers such as bucindolol may have ISA in small animal models,[60] in which G-protein amplification of β-receptor signaling is greater, but not in the human heart[61-63] in which signal amplification is lower. The issue of ISA of a β-blocker is obviously relevant only in the human heart, in which the most sensitive test of ISA is either forskolin-augmented contractile effects in isolated human heart preparations[63] or nighttime heart rate effects measured against placebo by 24-hour Holter monitoring.[61]

Selectivity of β_1-Adrenergic Receptor Blockade

The development of agents with a selective action on β_1-adrenergic receptors represents a step forward in the development of β-blockers.[64] In comparison with earlier nonselective agents (e.g., propranolol), so-called second generation[64] β_1-selective agents were shown to be better tolerated in patients with concomitant peripheral vascular disease or with chronic pulmonary disease. β_1-Selective agents are less likely to increase airway resistance and should not influence alveolar gas diffusion, inasmuch as they do not act on alveolar β_2-adrenergic receptors, which regulate reabsorption of alveolar fluid.[65] However, the comparative advantages of β_1-selective agents on pulmonary function has not always been demonstrated.

Blockade of α_1- and β_2-adrenergic receptors may also be clinically important.[20,34,54] α_1-Adrenergic receptors cause peripheral and renal vasoconstriction and myocardial hypertrophy. However, it is unlikely that they are important for the treatment of heart failure. Pure α_1-adrenergic antagonists have not been associated with beneficial effects on either the incidence of heart failure when they are used to treat hypertension or on outcomes in heart failure trials. In addition, there is evidence of the development of tolerance to the hemodynamic α_1-mediated effects of carvedilol in the patients with heart failure.[13,66]

The effects of cardiac myocyte β_2-adrenergic receptors are distinct from those of β_1-adrenergic receptors; one difference is that β_2-adrenergic receptors are strongly coupled to counterregulatory inhibitory G-protein signaling.[67] However, transduction of β_2-adrenergic receptor signal mediates both positive inotropic and chronotropic effects, through the G_s–cyclic adenosine monophosphate pathway,[34,68,69] in addition to negative inotropic and lusitropic effects mediated through G_i stimulation.[67] In addition, β_2-adrenergic receptors have a G_i-mediated antiapoptotic action.[70] The G_i-mediated effects are probably enhanced in the failing heart because of β_1-adrenergic receptors are downregulated and G_i protein is upregulated. These β_2-adrenergic effects could be considered adaptive inasmuch as they may protect the failing heart from excessive adrenergic stimulation.[71] In contrast, intense stimulation of β_2-adrenergic receptors may exert a dose-dependent adverse effect on the failing heart and promote LV remodeling and fibrosis, pulmonary congestion, and increased mortality.[69,72] The exact role of nonselective blockade of the β_2-adrenergic receptors may therefore vary from patient to patient, depending on the degree of sympathetic stimulation, β_1-/β_2-receptor ratio, and G_s/G_i protein expression. According to limited clinical data β_2-receptor manipulation in chronic heart failure may not have major therapeutic consequences. The ISA of celiprolol results from β_2-receptor partial agonism, and in a small clinical study,[61] celiprolol did not produce results that are obviously different from those of β-selective blockers. In addition, when given in comparable β_1-blocking doses, β_1-selective blockers[28,29] have generally not produced results that are different from those of nonselective[31] β-blockers.

β_1-Receptor Density

Second-generation agents, such as metoprolol, upregulate β_1-adrenergic receptors,[73,74] and this explains the potential occurrence of rebound responses when these agents are abruptly withdrawn.[75] In contrast, agents such as carvedilol or bucindolol do not obviously upregulate β_1-receptors[34]; thus, the heart is rendered less sensitive to the effects of any adrenergic stimulation that competitively overcomes

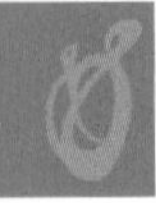

receptor blockade. Upregulation of β_1-adrenergic receptor may increase cardiac sensitivity to high levels of adrenergic drive, as during maximal exercise, with maintenance or an improvement in exercise capacity.[76] On the other hand, lack of upregulation of β_1-adrenergic receptors may better protect the heart from chronic adrenergic stimulation.

β_1-Adrenergic Receptor Binding

Carvedilol is characterized by tight binding to β_1-receptors; this property may not be shared by other β-blockers.[77,78] In a direct comparison between carvedilol and metoprolol tartrate, the hemodynamic response to dobutamine infusion was blunted by concomitant carvedilol, but not by metoprolol tartrate, administration.[79] In another comparison study, the β-blocking activity of carvedilol persisted, because of its binding characteristics, for up to 44 hours after it was withdrawn.[78] Because of this tight receptor binding, the β_1-blocking activity of carvedilol may be more stable throughout the day, and the risks of rebound phenomena when a dose is missed may be lower.

Inverse Agonism

In inverse agonism, a β-blocker stabilizes a receptor in its inactive state, which thus leads to a reduction in the proportion of receptors that are constitutively active. Compounds with higher degrees of inverse agonism, such as propranolol, are expected to produce more substantial negative chronotropic and inotropic effects and thus to be less well tolerated.[80] On the other hand, in model systems transfected with recombinant human β_1-receptors, it has been shown that carvedilol, but not metoprolol, has a very specific and marked inverse agonist effect on the more frequent Arg389 variant, which is associated with increased sensitivity to adrenergic stimulation.[81] However, in isolated human heart preparations, carvedilol does not exhibit inverse agonism in the Arg389 variant of the β_1-receptor, whereas bucindolol does.[63] Inverse agonism could be important also at the β_2-receptor level, whereby nonselective β-blockers could theoretically act as inverse agonists that stabilize β_2-receptors in their G_i-coupled conformation and enhance their favorable effects.[82]

Sympatholytic (Norepinephrine-Lowering) Effects

Cardiac norepinephrine release is stimulated by prejunctional β_2-adrenergic receptors and inhibited by prejunctional α_2- as well as α_1-adrenergic receptors. Inhibition of cardiac norepinephrine release may have favorable effects by reducing cardiac adrenergic stimulation. However, when excessive or too rapid, this inhibition may be detrimental because of excessive withdrawal of cardiac adrenergic support. This was shown in the MOXonidine CONgestive Heart Failure (MOXCON) trial,[83] in which placebo was compared with moxonidine, an agent that inhibits norepinephrine release through the stimulation of central α_2-adrenergic receptors. This trial was prematurely stopped because mortality increased among patients randomly assigned to receive moxonidine, in contrast to placebo (5.5% versus 3.4%).[83]

Although metoprolol does not affect cardiac or systemic norepinephrine release, carvedilol has been associated with a slight decrease in coronary sinus levels of norepinephrine and in cardiac norepinephrine release.[84,85] However, in patients with heart failure, carvedilol does not produce a reduction in systemic adrenergic activity.[84] Carvedilol's effects on cardiac adrenergic activity are probably caused by blockade of prejunctional β_2-receptors, and the effects are probably attenuated by concomitant prejunctional α_1-receptor blockade. In contrast, the potent β_2-blocker bucindolol, which has only minimal α_1-blocking activity, does reduce systemic adrenergic activity and, as such, is moderately sympatholytic.[86,87] This sympatholytic, moxonidine-like effect,[87] along with the characteristics of the patients studied (more advanced heart failure), may have compromised the mortality-reducing effects of bucindolol in the Beta-Blocker Evaluation of Survival Trial (BEST).[86,88]

Ancillary Properties

Ancillary properties of some β-blockers include properties unrelated to blockade of β-adrenergic receptors, including the type III antiarrhythmic activity of sotalol, the α_1-blocking and antioxidant effects of carvedilol, and the induction of nitric oxide release by nebivolol,[89,90] bucindolol,[91] and celiprolol.[92] With the exception of the type III antiarrhythmic effects of sotalol, the clinical relevance of these properties is uncertain. Nitric oxide release after nebivolol[89] or bucindolol[91] administration has been ascribed to β_3-adrenergic receptor stimulation. The nitric oxide–generating properties of nebivolol[92] have been associated with an improvement in endothelial function, decreased peripheral vascular resistance, decreased aortic central pressure, and decreased aortic stiffness. Nitric oxide generation may be important for nebivolol's or celiprolol's efficacy and tolerability in patients with hypertension. However, the clinical significance of nitric oxide generation in patients with heart failure has not been assessed in comparison trials.[93,94]

CLINICAL RESULTS

Effects on Cardiac Function

Multiple studies have consistently shown the beneficial effects of chronic β-blocker therapy on LV function and structure. Long-term benefits include an increase in LVEF, a decrease in LV volumes and in mitral regurgitation (when present), and a reversion of the left ventricle to a more elliptical shape. Improvement in load-independent indexes of myocardial contractility has also been shown, which demonstrates that the improvement is related to changes in the intrinsic properties of the myocardium.[17,21] LV diastolic function and right ventricular function are also improved by long-term β-blocker therapy.[95-97] Thus, all the changes associated with LV remodeling are, on average, counteracted by long-term β-blocker therapy. These studies were the first to demonstrate the reversibility of LV dysfunction and remodeling in the failing heart (see also Chapter 8).

The functional effects of β-blocker therapy on the failing heart are biphasic (Figure 46-4).[16,73] Administration of β-blockers is associated with an early, short-term deterioration in cardiac function, which is consistent with the negative inotropic effects of adrenergic drive withdrawal and is enhanced in the failing heart because of its dependence on adrenergic support. Carefully performed studies with serial echocardiography have shown a decrease from baseline in LVEF in the first few days of treatment, followed by return to baseline values after 1 month. An increase in LVEF from baseline values starts to become apparent after 3 to 4 months of treatment and tends to improve further for at least another year. At 3 to 4 months, decrease in LV volumes and favorable changes in shape also become apparent.[16,20]

Predictors of changes in parameters of LV function have been identified and are rather consistent across multiple studies. Predictors of an improvement in LVEF include a nonischemic cause of heart failure, higher blood pressure at baseline, the administration of a higher β-blocker dose, and higher baseline heart rates.[98-101] Patients with a nonischemic cause generally show a greater contractile reserve. Higher heart rate at baseline and the administration of a higher, rather than lower,

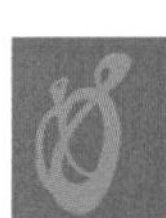

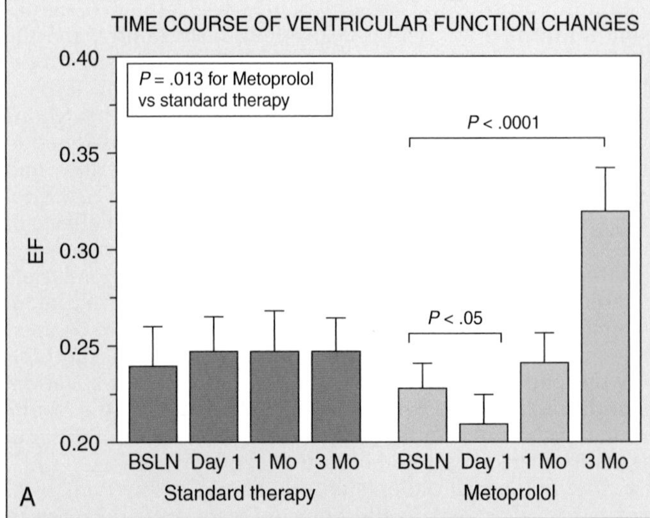

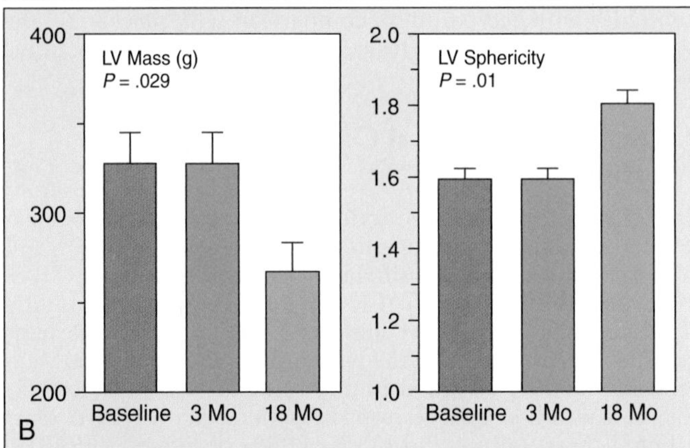

FIGURE 46–4 Time course of changes in left ventricular ejection fraction (LVEF) after β-blocker therapy in chronic heart failure. **A,** Time course of left ventricular function changes with no β-blocker (*left*) and with metoprolol tartrate (*right*) at baseline and after 1 day, 1 month, and 3 months. **B,** Reverse remodeling with a regression of left ventricular mass and an increase in the length to radius ratio (sphericity) after long-term β-blockade with metoprolol tartrate. (Data From Hall SA, Cigarroa CG, Marcoux L. Time course of improvement in left ventricular function, mass, and geometry in patients with congestive heart failure treated with beta-adrenergic blockade. *J Am Coll Card,* 25(5): 1154–1161, 1995, and Eichhorn EJ, Bristow MR. Antagonism of β-adrenergic receptors in heart failure. In Mann DL, (ed.) Heart failure: a companion to Braunwald's heart disease, Philadelphia, 2004, Elsevier, pp 619–639.)

β-blocker dosage are related to the level of adrenergic drive and the degree of β-blockade, respectively. A higher blood pressure at baseline is a rather accurate index of contractile reserve in left ventricles with systolic dysfunction. Accordingly, the demonstration of contractile reserve by dobutamine echocardiography is an excellent predictor of a favorable response to β-blocker therapy.[102,103] In patients with heart failure of ischemic origin, a direct relation exists between the number of LV segments showing myocardial hibernation and change in LVEF after β-blocking treatment.[104] The basis of all these observations is the fact that the magnitude of the improvement in LV function after chronic β-blockade is directly related to the amount of viable myocardium present at baseline.

Changes in LV function are related to subsequent prognosis. Patients with the greatest increase in LVEF and reduction in volumes have an excellent long-term prognosis.[98,99,105] A post hoc analysis of the Cardiac Insufficiency BIsoprolol Study (CIBIS) confirmed these findings. Patients who showed an improvement in LV fractional shortening after 5 months of treatment had a survival advantage over other patients.[106] β-Blocker therapy and, more recently, cardiac resynchronization therapy are the two interventions that have shown the value of LV function for the prediction of outcomes in chronic heart failure.[2,17]

Effects on Exercise Capacity and Symptoms

The impairment of exercise capacity in patients with heart failure is related both to myocardial dysfunction and to the abnormalities in β-adrenergic receptor signal transduction that result in reduced cardiac sensitivity to sympathetic stimulation (see Figure 46-2).[34,107] β-Blocker therapy improves myocardial function and, on that basis, would be expected to improve exercise performance. However, if β-adrenergic receptors are blocked by higher doses of β-blocking agents or are not upregulated by therapy, then exercise tolerance may not improve. This is because the failing heart is dependent on increasing heart rate for improving exercise capacity, more so than is the nonfailing heart. Thus, despite the improvement in cardiac function and stroke volume, both at rest and during exercise, the β-blocker–related reduced chronotropic response to exercise may prevent cardiac output to rise sufficiently during exercise to allow an improvement in exercise capacity.[13,20] A direct correlation between change from baseline in maximal exercise capacity and change from baseline in peak exercise heart rate after β-blocker therapy has been observed in multiple-dose studies[61] and in comparisons of multiple β-blockers (Figure 46-5).[76]

In general, β_1-selective β-blocking agents, such as metoprolol, which at lower doses do not block myocardial β_2-adrenergic receptors and upregulate myocardial β_1-receptors[84,85]—slightly improve maximal exercise capacity.[6,74] In contrast, agents such as carvedilol and bucindolol—which may not alter myocardial β_1-adrenergic receptor density, have slower offset kinetics from β_1-adrenergic receptors, and also block β_2-adrenergic receptors—may not allow an increase in peak exercise cardiac output and heart rate sufficient to improve exercise capacity and peak oxygen uptake (Vo_2).[13-15] On the basis of results of a few single-center studies, it was initially thought that β-blockers might be able to improve submaximal exercise.[13,14] However, multicenter trials failed to show any change also in submaximal exercise capacity.[108-110]

In contrast to direct measurements of exercise tolerance, most controlled studies have shown a significant improvement in symptoms and functional class in patients with heart failure treated with β-blockers. The results obtained are consistent in single-center[13-15] and in multicenter trials.[6,105,108,109] According to a meta-analysis by Lechat and associates,[18] patients treated with a β-blocker were 32% more likely to experience an improvement and 30% less likely to experience a worsening in New York Heart Association (NYHA) class ($P < .05$ in both cases). Direct assessment of heart failure symptoms, as well as global clinical assessment (a quality-of-life measurement) by either the patient or the physician, has been similarly sensitive, showing an improvement in clinical status.[6,108,109] The interpretation of the functional capacity and symptom outcomes of these studies is that β-blockade does not worsen exercise capacity, and the improvement in cardiac function is associated, albeit indirectly, with an improvement in symptoms and quality-of-life measures.

Effects on the Clinical Course: Initial Trials

Although the effects of β-blockers on cardiac function are novel and impressive, their most significant effects in patients with heart failure are on the clinical course. Major clinical outcomes such as mortality and hospitalizations for heart failure are, of course, the most important clinical trial endpoints, as well as being of paramount importance to physicians and patients. The clinical course and prognosis of patients with heart failure have been radically changed since the introduction of β-blocker therapy.

Multicenter trials have consistently shown a highly significant reduction in the incidence of hospitalizations,[6,28,29,31,105,109,111] cardiovascular events,[16,27,29,105,109] episodes of worsening heart failure,[6,27,29,105,109] and in indications for heart transplantation[6] in patients treated with a β-blocker, in comparison with patients treated with placebo. A meta-analysis revealed that the hospitalization rate for heart failure was 9.6% among patients treated with a β-blocker, in comparison with 17% in those taking placebo (−41%; 95% confidence interval, −26% to −52%; $P < .001$).[18]

The results on mortality were initially controversial, mostly because the early studies were underpowered. The Metoprolol in Dilated Cardiomyopathy trial,[6] the first significant multicenter study of β-blockade in heart failure, and the CIBIS-I[27] did not yield significant findings about mortality, despite the overall improvement in LV function and clinical course. This can be attributed to methodological limitations of these studies: Too few patients were randomly assigned to treatment conditions, the incidence of events was low, and follow-up was relatively short. The United States Carvedilol program included four trials designed to assess the effects of carvedilol on exercise tolerance and heart failure progression. Data and safety monitoring board analysis of the four trials combined revealed a reduction in mortality with carvedilol, in comparison with placebo. However, these data were deemed inconclusive because of the small number of events, short follow-up, and open-label run-in period before randomization. In addition, mortality benefit was largely driven by the results of one of the four studies in which the effects on LVEF and mortality were shown to be dose dependent (Figure 46-6).[105] The low number of patients enrolled and the low number of events can also explain the nonsignificant 14% decrease in mortality with carvedilol, in comparison with placebo, in the Australia/New Zealand Heart Failure Research Collaborative Group trial.[111]

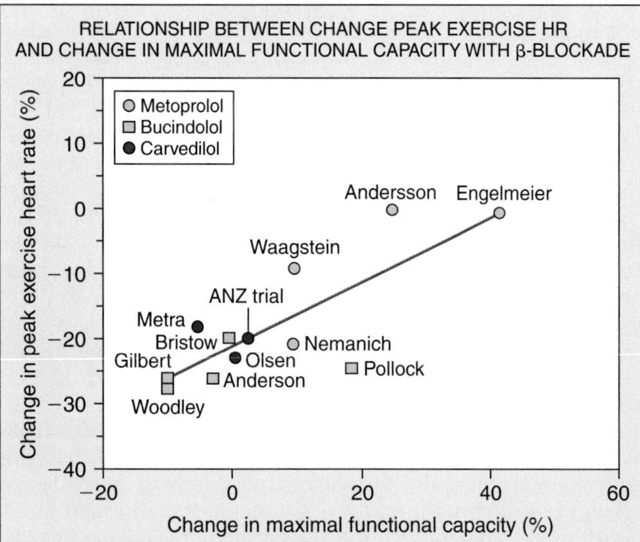

FIGURE 46–5 Relationship between the change in maximal functional capacity (percentage) and change in peak exercise heart rate (percentage) for multiple β-blocker trials with the selective agent metoprolol (*circles*) or the nonselective agents bucindolol (*squares*) and carvedilol (*triangles*). Only the selective agent produced improvement in functional capacity. (Data from Metra M, Nodari S, D'Aloia A, et al. Effects of neurohormonal antagonism on symptoms and quality-of-life in heart failure. *Eur Heart J* 1998;19(Suppl B):B25-B35; and from Eichhorn EJ, Bristow MR. Antagonism of β-adrenergic receptors in heart failure. In Mann DL, editor. *Heart failure: a companion to Braunwald's Heart Disease,* Philadelphia, 2004, Elsevier, pp 619-639.)

Effects on the Clinical Course: Large-Scale Mortality Trials

Six large-scale placebo-controlled outcome trials have been performed in patients with heart failure (Table 46-2).[27,30,32,35,36,86] The second Cardiac Insufficiency Bisoprolol Study (CIBIS-II),[29] and the Metoprolol CR/XL Randomised Intervention Trial in Congestive Heart Failure (MERIT-HF),[30] were large prospective trials in patients with mild to moderate heart failure; annual mortality rates in these studies were 11% to 13%. CIBIS-II enrolled 2647 European patients with NYHA class III or IV heart failure and LVEF of 35% or lower; MERIT-HF enrolled 3991 patients, most of whom were European, with NYHA classes II to IV heart failure and LVEF of 40% or lower. Both trials were prematurely terminated on the recommendation of the data and safety monitoring boards because of the survival benefit associated with the active agent. Both trials—in which the β_1-selective agents bisoprolol and metoprolol succinate CR/XL, respectively, were used—demonstrated a 34% reduction in mortality among subjects treated with these

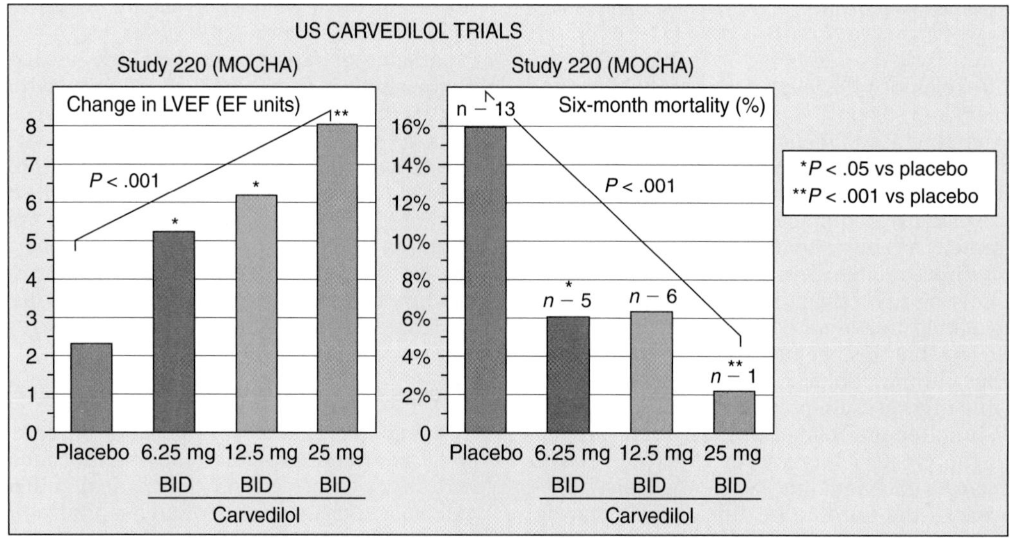

FIGURE 46–6 Relationship between β-blocker dosage and improvement in left ventricular ejection fraction (*left*) and reduction in mortality (*right*). The higher the dosage was, the more left ventricular function improved. (Data from Bristow MR, Gilbert EM, Abraham WT, et al. Carvedilol produces dose-related improvements in left ventricular function and survival in subjects with chronic heart failure. *Circulation* 1996;94:2807-2816; and from Eichhorn EJ, Bristow MR. Antagonism of β-adrenergic receptors in heart failure. In Mann DL, editor. *Heart failure: a companion to Braunwald's Heart Disease,* Philadelphia, 2004, Elsevier, pp 619-639.)

TABLE 46–2 Prospective Outcome Trials with β-Blockers in Patients with Heart Failure

						Mortality Risk Reduction				All-Cause Hospitalization Risk Reduction		
Trial	Agent	Entry Criteria	Number of Patients	Mean Follow-up Time	Annual Placebo-Related Mortality Rate	Percentage	95% Confidence Interval	*P*	Numbers Needed to Treat to Save One Life	Percentage	95% Confidence Interval	*P*
CIBIS-II[29]	Bisoprolol	LVEF ≤ 35%, NYHA class III or IV	2647	1.3 years	13.2%	34%	19% to 46%	<.0001	22.7	18%	29% to 9%	.0006
MERIT-HF[30]	Metoprolol succinate	LVEF ≤ 40%, NYHA classes II to IV	3991	1.0 year	11.0%	34%	19% to 47%	.0014	26.3	18%	NA	<.005
COPERNICUS[32]	Carvedilol	LVEF ≤ 25%, symptoms at rest or with mild exertion, minimal edema	2289	10.4 months	18.5%	35%	19% to 48%	.0014	14.1	10%	24% to +6%	NA
CAPRICORN[35]	Carvedilol	Status post myocardial infarction, LVEF ≤ 40%	1959	1.3 years	11.8%	23%	2% to 40%	.03	43	NA	NA	NA
BEST[86]	Bucindolol	LVEF ≤ 35%, NYHA class III or IV	2708	2 years	16.7%	10%	+2% to −22%	.10		8%	+1% to 16%	.085
SENIORS[36,*]	Nebivolol	Aged ≥ 70 years, heart failure hospitalization in the previous year or LVEF ≤ 35%	2128	21 months	18.1%	12%	8% to 29%	.21		10%	+6% to −24%	NA

*Primary endpoint was all-cause death or cardiovascular hospitalization.

BEST, Beta-Blocker Evaluation of Survival Trial; CAPRICORN, Carvedilol Post-Infarct Survival Control in Left Ventricular Dysfunction; CIBIS II, Cardiac Insufficiency BIsoprolol Study; COPERNICUS, CarvedilOl ProspEctive RaNdomIzed CUmulative Survival; LVEF, left ventricular ejection fraction; MERIT-HF, Metoprolol CR/XL Randomised Intervention Trial in Congestive Heart Failure; NA, not assessed; NYHA, New York Heart Association class; SENIORS, Study of the Effects of Nebivolol Intervention on Outcomes and Rehospitalisation in Seniors with Heart Failure.

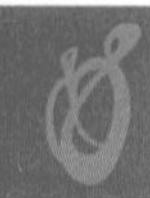

drugs, in comparison with those treated with placebo. In both trials, as well as in the following outcome studies with β-blockers, the study drug was added to standard treatment of heart failure, including ACE inhibitors. Thus, these trials actually demonstrated the benefits of adding β-blockers to ACE inhibitors. The Kaplan-Meier survival curves for MERIT-HF and CIBIS II are shown in Figure 46-7, *A* and *B,* respectively. It is clear that the β-blocker and placebo curves are similar for the initial 2 to 3 months and then diverge throughout the course. Thus, 2 to 3 months of treatment is the time necessary for a favorable biological effect to occur.

The CIBIS-II trial demonstrated a 44% reduction in sudden death (P = .0011), a 26% reduction in death from pump failure (P = .17), a 36% reduction in hospitalizations for heart failure (P = .0001), and a 20% reduction in all-cause hospitalization (P = .0006). The MERIT-HF study demonstrated a 41% reduction in sudden death (P = .0002), a 49% reduction in death from pump failure (P = .0023), a 35% reduction in hospitalizations for heart failure (P = .00001), and an 18% reduction in all-cause hospitalizations (P = .005). Subgroup analysis of CIBIS-II and MERIT-HF by gender, age, cause of heart failure, history of prior myocardial infarction, diabetes, and heart rate at baseline consistently demonstrated a benefit or a trend toward benefit for active therapy across all strata.[29,30] A meta-analysis of 22 placebo-controlled randomized trials of β-blockers, including CIBIS-II and MERIT-HF, involving 10,132 patients with heart failure and low ejection fraction, revealed a 35% reduction in the risk of death with β-blocker therapy (95% confidence interval [CI], −20% to −47%) with 3.8 lives saved and 4 fewer hospitalization per 100 patients treated for 1 year.[112]

CIBIS-II and MERIT-HF results conclusively showed mortality- and morbidity-related benefit from bisoprolol and metoprolol succinate in NYHA class II and III heart failure. Results in NYHA class IV patients did not reach statistical significance, perhaps because there were so few such patients.[29,30] However, the point estimate of the all-cause mortality effect in both CIBIS-II and MERIT-HF was numerically less than that in class III patients, and because of the small numbers of patients with class IV enrolled in these trials, it remains uncertain as to whether these β-blockers can be safely and efficaciously administered to patients with a very advanced type of heart failure.[113] Certainly patients may reach a point in their clinical course when β-blocker therapy is neither tolerated or efficacious, but the clinical trial data do not enable clinicians to identify such a transition point beyond not recommending treatment in patients who are taking β-adrenergic agonists to support cardiac function.

The relationship between the β-blocker dose administered and its effects on outcomes was also assessed in CIBIS-II and MERIT-HF. Patients receiving lower doses of the study drugs had more severe heart failure, had lower blood pressure or heart rate at baseline (or both), and were older.[114-117] A post hoc analysis in CIBIS-II revealed an increased risk of death in the patients receiving the low dosage (i.e., <5 mg/day) of bisoprolol in comparison with patients taking medium and high dosages. This difference remained significant after adjustment for baseline variables.[115] Similar results were found in post hoc analyses in two other major outcome trials with carvedilol[116] and nebivolol,[117] respectively. In MERIT-HF, the benefit of metoprolol succinate on mortality was related to the heart rate achieved after treatment, independently of the dose administered.[114]

CIBIS-II and MERIT-HF established the beneficial effects on outcomes of β-blockers in patients with NYHA class II and class III heart failure caused by LV systolic dysfunction (ejection fractions < .35 and .40, respectively). Subsequently reported trials were aimed at broadening the spectrum of the indications to β-blocker therapy. In the Carvedilol Prospective Randomized Cumulative Survival (COPERNICUS) trial,

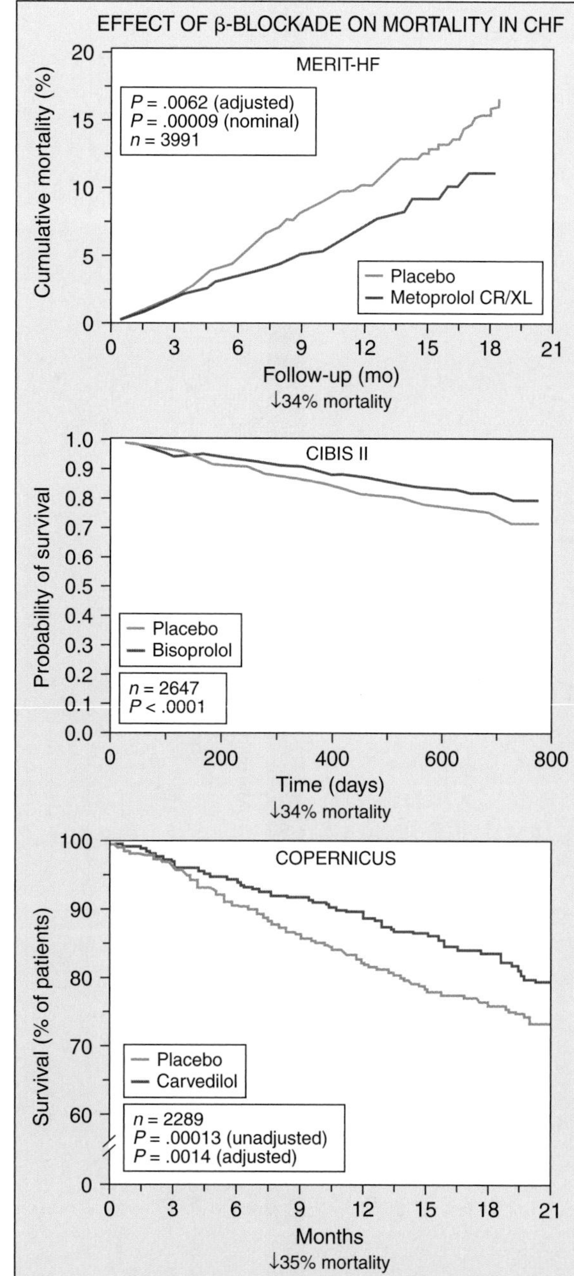

FIGURE 46-7 Kaplan-Meier analysis of the probability of survival among patients in the placebo and β-blocker groups in the Cardiac Insufficiency BIsoprolol Study (CIBIS-2), the Metoprolol CR/XL Randomised Intervention Trial in Congestive Heart Failure (MERIT-HF), and the CarvedilOl ProspEctive RaNdomIzed CUmulative Survival (COPERNICUS) trial. (Data from CIBIS-II Investigators and Committees: The Cardiac Insufficiency Bisoprolol Study II (CIBIS-II): a randomised trial. *Lancet* 1999;353:9-13; MERIT-HF Study Group: Effect of metoprolol CR/XL in chronic heart failure: Metoprolol CR/XL Randomised Intervention Trial in Congestive Heart Failure (MERIT-HF). *Lancet* 1999;353:2001-2007; Packer M, Coats AJ, Fowler MB, et al. Effect of carvedilol on survival in severe chronic heart failure. *N Engl J Med* 2001;344:1651-1658; and Eichhorn EJ, Bristow MR. Antagonism of β-adrenergic receptors in heart failure. In Mann DL, editor. *Heart failure: a companion to Braunwald's Heart Disease,* Philadelphia, 2004, Elsevier, pp 619-639.)

researchers studied the effects on outcomes of the nonselective β-blocker and α_1-blocker carvedilol in 2289 mostly European, stable patients who had symptoms of heart failure at rest or with minimal exertion at the time of screening and severe LV systolic dysfunction, manifested by an ejection fraction of .25 or less.[32] Despite these criteria for severity, patients had to be "euvolemic" (i.e., with no signs of pulmonary or peripheral congestion) and with no worsening renal function or hypotension (systolic blood pressure ≤85 mm Hg) at entry into the study. The greater degree of LV dysfunction in COPERNICUS than in other trials was reflected in the higher 1-year mortality rate of 18.5%. COPERNICUS was also stopped because the data and safety monitoring board concluded that efficacy had been achieved before the planned completion of the trial. As in CIBIS-II and MERIT-HF, carvedilol administration was associated with a 35% reduction in the risk of death (P = .0014) and a 24% reduction in the risk of death or all-cause hospitalization (P < .001; see Figure 46-7,*C*).[32] These effects of carvedilol were similar in direction and magnitude in all the prespecified subgroups according to age, gender, geographical location, cause of heart failure, whether hospitalization was recent, diabetes, LVEF, and pretreatment systolic blood pressure.[32,118] Fewer patients receiving carvedilol than placebo recipients required the permanent discontinuation of treatment because of adverse effects.[32] A further analysis revealed early evidence of the beneficial effects of β-blocker therapy, with a lower mortality rate and lower combined mortality and rehospitalization rate with carvedilol than for placebo, during the first 2 months of treatment. These effects on outcomes were similar to those observed during the entire study and were apparent also in the 624 patients with recent or recurrent decompensation or a very depressed LVEF. Worsening heart failure was the only serious adverse event with similar frequency in patients receiving placebo (6.4%) and those receiving carvedilol (5.1%).[33]

The Carvedilol Post Infarct Survival Control in Left Ventricular Dysfunction (CAPRICORN) study enrolled 1959 mostly European patients with LV systolic dysfunction (ejection fraction ≤.40) after a recent myocardial infarction with mild or no symptoms of heart failure.[35] Carvedilol was not associated with a significant reduction of the primary endpoint of all-cause mortality or cardiovascular hospitalization, in part because of the hospitalization event rate was lower than expected. However, all-cause mortality alone was reduced by 27%, which was statistically significant, in comparison with placebo (95% CI, −2% to −40%; P = .024). These results were driven primarily by a 26% reduction in sudden death with carvedilol.[35]

The BEST researchers examined the effects of a nonselective β-blocker/vasodilator, bucindolol (which also has sympatholytic activity), on all-cause mortality and other endpoints in patients with NYHA class III or IV heart failure and an LVEF of .35 or lower.[86] Unlike COPERNICUS, BEST allowed enrollment of patients who had clinical decompensation, as defined by overt fluid overload in the presence of a renin-angiotensin system inhibitor and diuretics.[86,119] Also in contrast to COPERNICUS and the other large-scale trials, most patients (98%) in BEST were enrolled in U.S. centers. This study uniquely stratified patients at each site on the basis of gender, ejection fraction (> or ≤.20), presence or absence of coronary artery disease, and race (African American vs. non–African American). The BEST study was prematurely terminated on the recommendation of the data and safety monitoring board after the enrollment of 2708 patients, because of "the totality of evidence regarding the usefulness of β-blocker treatment derived from BEST and other studies" as well as because of loss of equipoise in an increasing number of investigations. Loss of investigation equipoise was related to the premature discontinuation of CIBIS-II and MERIT-HF for benefit.[86,120] In contrast to CIBIS-II, MERIT-HF, and COPERNICUS, the primary endpoint of all-cause mortality was not statistically significant when BEST was stopped, 12 months short of full follow-up, with 92% of the projected number of endpoints predicted from sample size calculations. However, for patients similar to those enrolled in CIBIS-II and MERIT-HF, the BEST results for all-cause mortality were comparable with those in the other trials.[86,121]

In BEST, the annual rate of mortality was 17% among the placebo recipients; after randomization stratification covariate adjustment according to the prespecified statistical analysis plan, it was reduced by 10% (95% CI, +2% to −22%; unadjusted P = .10) or 13% (95% CI, 0% to −24%; P = .053). Mortality from cardiovascular causes was reduced with bucindolol by 14% (95% CI, 1% to 26%; unadjusted P = .04), and time to hospitalization for heart failure was reduced by 23% (95% CI, −13% to −32%; unadjusted P = .00002). In contrast to previous trials, prespecified subgroup analysis showed heterogeneity in the results; perhaps the subgroups exhibiting differential responses had not been investigated in adequate numbers in the previous trials. Bucindolol had no effect on survival in African American patients (23% of the total study group, P = .27) whereas there was a survival benefit in non–African American subjects (P = .01; P = .024 for the interaction between treatment and race). A lack of effects on outcomes of β-blocker therapy in African American patients was confirmed in a prospective cohort study that included 2460 patients with heart failure.[122]

Survival was improved with bucindolol among patients with less advanced heart failure in BEST, a finding similar to those in the other β-blocker studies; the increase in survival was 13% (unadjusted; P = .06) or 15% (adjusted; P = .03) among patients with NYHA class III heart failure, but there was no evidence of benefit in patients with class IV heart failure.[119] In a post hoc analysis of a sample population from BEST with characteristics similar to those of the patients enrolled in CIBIS-II and MERIT-HF, the survival benefit of bucindolol was 23%, in comparison with placebo, which was similar in magnitude to that in the previous trials.[121] Another post hoc analysis revealed that patients who were euvolemic at baseline and had an LVEF of less than .25 (and thus were similar to the COPERNICUS patient population) had an all-cause mortality reduction of 31% (95% CI, −12% to −45%; P = .002).[88] Thus, if comparable patient populations are examined, results of the CIBIS-II, MERIT-HF, COPERNICUS and BEST trials are very similar.

Unique among β-blockers that have been used to treat heart failure, bucindolol is sympatholytic, meaning that it lowers systemic norepinephrine levels.[86,87] If the degree of norepinephrine lowering is mild, this property may be clinically beneficial, but if the degree of sympatholysis is pronounced, it may lead to untoward effects in patients with advanced heart failure.[86,123] When sympatholysis is extreme in patients with heart failure who are highly dependent on adrenergic drive to support cardiac function, mortality and hospitalizations for heart failure may increase. In BEST these effects canceled the clinical benefits of β-blockade,[86,123] whereas in MOXCON, pronounced sympatholysis from moxonidine was associated with increased mortality and hospitalizations related to heart failure.[83]

The Study of Effects of Nebivolol Intervention on Outcomes and Rehospitalisation in Seniors with Heart Failure (SENIORS) was aimed at the assessment of the effects of the β_1-selective vasodilator compound nebivolol on outcomes in elderly patients with heart failure independent of their LVEF.[36] This European study included 2128 patients aged 70 years or older who either had an LVEF of 0.35 or lower or had been admitted to a hospital for heart failure in the previous 12 months. The primary composite endpoint was all-cause mortality or hospitalization for cardiovascular reasons. The incidence of this endpoint was reduced by 14% in the patients receiving nebivolol, in comparison with those receiving placebo (95% CI, −1% to −26%; P = .039) (Figure 46-8, *A*). The cardiovascular mortality or hospitalization rate was also lower by 16% among the nebivolol recipients, in contrast to the placebo recipients (95% CI, −2% to −28%; P = .027). Mortality alone was not significantly reduced by nebivolol (−12%; 95% CI, +8% to −29%; P = .21) (see Figure 46-8, *B*).

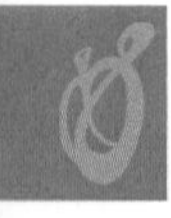

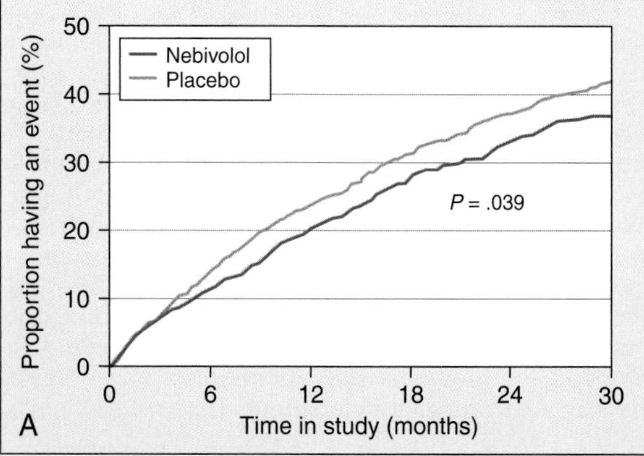

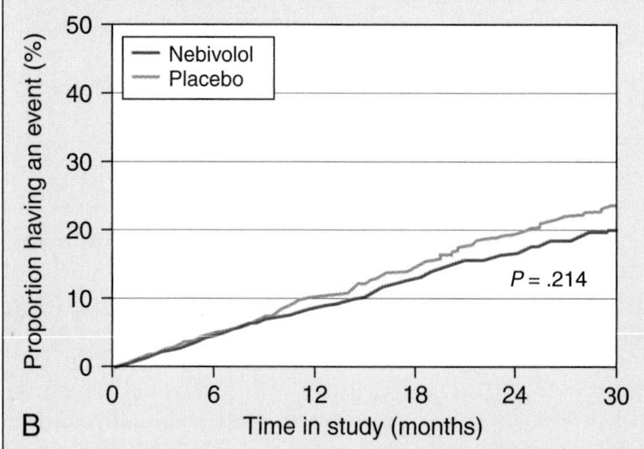

FIGURE 46-8 Clinical outcomes in the Study of the Effects of Nebivolol Intervention on Outcomes and Rehospitalisation in Seniors with Heart Failure (SENIORS) trial. **A,** Time to first occurrence of events (primary endpoint was all-cause death or hospital admission for a cardiovascular reason). **B,** All-cause death. (From Flather MD, Shibatal MC, Coats AJS. Randomized trial to determine the effect of nebivolol on mortality and cardiovascular hospital admission in elderly patients with heart failure (SENIORS). *Eur Heart J* 2005;26:215-225.)

Prespecified subgroup analyses did not reveal significant interactions among gender, ejection fraction, age, diabetes and prior myocardial infarction, baseline renal function,[124] and the effects of nebivolol on outcomes. However, the relative risk for the primary endpoint was reduced by 21% (95% CI, −2% to −37%) in patients younger than the median of 75.2 years and by 8% (95% CI, +12% to −25%) in those older than 75.2 years (test for interaction P = .51).[36]

Although in the same direction, the results of SENIORS were less significant than those of the previous β-blocker trials, which enrolled younger patients and excluded patients with higher ejection fractions. To evaluate the effects of nebivolol in patients similar to those of other trials, the SENIORS investigators assessed patients younger than the median of 75.2 years and with an LVEF of 35% or lower (342 subjects took nebivolol and 342 took placebo). In this subgroup, the risk for the primary outcome was reduced by 27% (95% CI, −4% to −44%) with nebivolol, and the risk of all-cause mortality alone was 38% lower (95% CI, −12% to −57%) with nebivolol; these findings were similar to the results of previous β-blocker trials.[36] In a prespecified analysis, the effects of nebivolol on outcomes were independent of baseline LVEF; that is, the drug had similar favorable effects on outcomes in the patients with heart failure and preserved ejection fraction.[37] Another analysis revealed that the beneficial effects of nebivolol on outcomes were greater when dosages were higher (>5 mg/day).[117]

All five β-blockers that have been tested in large clinical trials have thus demonstrated clinical benefit. Furthermore, when similar enrollment criteria are analyzed, the mortality- and hospitalization-reducing effects of these agents are found to be similar. In patients who have reduced ejection fractions, are younger than 75 years, and do not have evidence of clinical decompensation while taking renin-angiotensin inhibitors and diuretics, the reduction in the major clinical endpoints of mortality or hospitalizations for heart failure ranges from 25% to 35%, both in randomized placebo-controlled clinical trials and in post hoc analyses. These similarities suggest that, despite other differences, blockade of β_1-adrenergic receptors is by far the most important mechanism in the therapeutic effects of β-blockers.[125]

β-Blockers remain, however, a highly heterogeneous group of drugs,[34,54] as discussed previously. The hypothesis that differences between β-blockers might have a clinical effect in patients with heart failure has been tested in relatively small trials[126-128] and in the Carvedilol or Metoprolol European Trial (COMET),[129] which was powered to assess a difference in mortality. In COMET, 3029 patients with chronic heart failure were randomly assigned to receive carvedilol, at the target dose of 25 mg twice a day, or immediate-release metoprolol tartrate, at the target dose of 50 mg twice a day, and were monitored for a mean of 58 ± 6 months. All-cause mortality was reduced by 17% in patients taking carvedilol, in comparison to metoprolol tartrate (P = .0017).[129] The results of COMET have been widely discussed. Differences in mortality found in COMET have been related to the ancillary properties of carvedilol (i.e., α-blockade, antioxidant activity, anti-apoptotic effects), to nonselective blockade of β_2-adrenergic receptors, and to more effective blockade of β_1-adrenergic receptors.[54,130,131] The slight difference in the heart rate achieved during maintenance therapy and the suboptimal dosing of metoprolol tartrate have also been claimed as potential causes of the differences found.[125,132,133] Regardless of the explanation, COMET did demonstrate the inferiority of metoprolol tartrate to carvedilol in the dosages tested. These dosages of metoprolol tartrate, although lower than those used in the Metoprolol in Dilated Cardiomyopathy trial,[6] are often used in clinical practice. The long-term formulation metoprolol succinate CR/XL that was shown to be effective in comparison with placebo in MERIT-HF has never been compared with carvedilol or with metoprolol tartrate in outcome trials. Thus, it is not possible to draw conclusions regarding the efficacy of metoprolol succinate in comparison with carvedilol. The COMET trial appropriately led to changes in various guidelines. Metoprolol tartrate is no longer recommended for the treatment of heart failure, and only β-blockers shown to be effective in outcomes trials—bisoprolol, carvedilol, metoprolol succinate, and, in Europe, nebivolol—are now recommended.[51,53]

PRACTICAL GUIDELINES FOR β-BLOCKER USE

The indications and practical aspects of β-blocker therapy are clearly outlined in all major guidelines for the diagnosis and treatment of heart failure.[51,52,53,134] The indication for β-blocker treatment is based on the highly significant association with an improvement in cardiac function, LV remodeling, and major clinical endpoints, including mortality and hospitalizations.[17,18,20,51-53,112,134] This clinical endpoint evidence is consistent and substantial, data being obtained from more than 10,000 patients in major randomized, placebo-controlled trials. It is important to remember—when β-blocker therapy is started, titrated upward, and maintained chronically—that β-blockade is not indicated for short-term improvement in symptoms, which may actually worsen transiently when treatment is started. β-Blockers are indicated for their biological long-term effects involving protection of the heart from excessive adrenergic drive, mediated mainly through β_1-adrenergic receptor signaling.

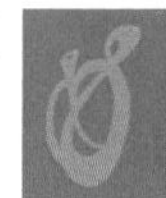

Practical aspects of β-blocker therapy in patients with heart failure are outlined in Table 46-3. Treatment is indicated only for patients with heart failure caused by LV systolic function. To date, no conclusive data have been obtained from patients with heart failure and preserved ejection fraction (discussed later). Only β-blockers associated with a favorable effect on outcomes in placebo-controlled trials are indicated, and modalities of initiation, upward titration, and dosing are based largely on the results of these trials. It is important to point out that the beneficial results in controlled trials have been obtained with the target dosages suggested for clinical practice. Lower doses have been associated with lack of effects or with lower efficacy in comparison with higher dosages.

Practical issues concern (1) the modality of initiation of β-blocker therapy with regard to concomitant therapy with ACE inhibitors and (2) maintenance of β-blocker treatment in patients hospitalized for acutely decompensated chronic heart failure. In the CIBIS-III trial, researchers compared initiation of medical treatment with either an ACE inhibitor (enalapril) or a β-blocker (bisoprolol) in 1010 patients who had heart failure and a low LVEF (≤.35) and had not been treated previously with these agents.[135] Patients were randomly assigned to receive open-label monotherapy with either enalapril or bisoprolol for 6 months, followed by their combination for up to 24 months. The primary endpoint was all-cause death or hospitalization and was blindly adjudicated. According to intention-to-treat analysis, the primary endpoint occurred in 178 patients who took bisoprolol first and in 186 who took enalapril first (absolute difference, −1.6%; 95% CI, −7.6 to 4.4%). Deaths occurred in 65 patients taking bisoprolol first and in 73 taking enalapril first (hazard ratio for bisoprolol vs. enalapril, −12%; 95% CI, −37% to +22%). Hospitalizations occurred in 151 and 157 patients, respectively.[135] A trend toward fewer sudden deaths was observed with bisoprolol first. On the other hand, 67% more cases of worsening heart failure necessitating hospitalization or occurring during hospitalization were observed in the patients who took bisoprolol first ($P = .03$).[136] The two groups were similar with regard to treatment cessations and early introduction of the second drug. Although this trial showed noninferiority of treatment initiation with bisoprolol, this result has not been included in guidelines, which continue to suggest initiation of treatment with a diuretic plus an ACE inhibitor, followed as soon as possible by the addition of a β-blocker.[52,53] This is, however, the sequence used in all the trials that demonstrated the benefits of β-blocker treatment. An individualized approach, based on the patient's clinical characteristics (fluid status, symptoms, blood pressure, heart rate, comorbid conditions), should always be preferred with regard to both sequence of drug initiation and, of more importance, dosage.[137]

Ongoing β-blockers have been usually withdrawn when patients are hospitalized because of acute decompensation of chronic heart failure with the belief that their short-term negative inotropic effects may have a negative effect on their clinical course. However, retrospective analyses of randomized controlled trials[138-140] or of database registries[141,142] of patients hospitalized for heart failure have shown that the discontinuation of ongoing β-blocker therapy is associated with an increased risk of death, which is still significant after adjustment for baseline variables and parameters related to the severity of heart failure. No differences in symptoms' relief and clinical course were found, in one prospective study, between patients hospitalized for acutely decompensated heart failure who discontinued previous β-blocker therapy and patients who maintained ongoing treatment. β-Blocker therapy at 3 months was given to 90% of patients who had continued it, in contrast to 76% who had discontinued it ($P < .05$), and this may be important for long-term outcomes.[143]

TABLE 46–3 Practical Guidelines for β-Blocker Therapy in Patients with Heart Failure

Indications

Current or prior symptoms of heart failure and LVEF ≤ 40%
LVEF ≤ 40% after a myocardial infarction, regardless of symptoms*

When to Start

Possibly in euvolemic state and in stable clinical conditions
When patient is receiving stable doses of diuretics and ACE inhibitors or angiotensin receptor blockers (initiation before ACE inhibitors may be considered in selected patients, such as those with tachycardia or chronic kidney dysfunction)[135,137]

When Not to Start (Contraindications)

Bronchial asthma with sensitivity to the administration of β-agonists
Severe bradycardia (<60/min) or second- or third-degree heart block
Hypotension (systolic blood pressure ≤ 85 mm Hg)
Unstable clinical conditions with signs of severe fluid retention

Agent (Drug, Starting Dose, Target Dose)

Bisoprolol, 1.25 mg once daily to 10 mg once daily
Carvedilol, 3.125-6.25 mg bid to 25-50 mg bid
Metoprolol succinate CR/XL, 12.5-25 mg once daily to 200 mg once daily
Nebivolol† 1.25 mg once daily to 10 mg once daily

How to Administer

Start with low dose (see under "Agent") and double the dose every 2 weeks (every week in stable patients) up to target dose or maximal tolerated dose
Educate the patients regarding benefits of treatment (i.e., improvement in cardiac function and symptoms, reduced episodes of decompensation and hospitalizations, prolonged survival) and the need of 3-6 months of treatment to achieve full benefit
Ask the patient to monitor her or his body weight every 1-2 days and refer to her or his physician in case of increase in body weight, worsening symptoms, or development of signs of congestion (e.g., ankle swelling) during the upward-titration phase (monitoring to be done by the attending physician or nurse in case of patients with severe heart failure and in unstable clinical condition)
Measure heart rate and blood pressure before each dose increment and avoid increasing dosage in case of contraindication (see contraindications)
Measure serum creatinine, BUN, sodium, potassium, and bilirubin levels approximately 2 weeks after start of therapy and 1-2 weeks after patient reaches the final dose

Possible Complications and Their Treatment

Symptomatic hypotension (asymptomatic hypotension does not necessitate any specific treatment)
- Stop or reduce the doses of other vasodilators
- If such reduction is not possible, consider dose reduction of ACE inhibitor or angiotensin receptor blocker

Bradycardia (<50 bpm)
- Stop other bradycardic agents (if possible)
- If cessation of bradycardic agents is not possible or not effective, reduce the dose of or stop the β-blocker

Worsening heart failure or fluid retention
- Increase the dose of the diuretic (at least double the usual dose)
- If increasing diuretic dose is not possible or not effective, reduce the dose of the β-blocker or, in most difficult cases, stop it
- Restart β-blocker therapy at the doses administered before the episode of decompensation or start β-blockade, if it was not administered before; either action should be performed before discharge, if possible[53]

*β-Blockers are indicated in all patients with previous myocardial infarction regardless of ejection fraction and symptoms of heart failure.[53] †Nebivolol is approved for the treatment of heart failure only in Europe.[52]

ACE, angiotensin-converting enzyme; BUN, blood urea nitrogen; LVEF, left ventricular ejection fraction.

Modified from McMurray J, Cohen-Solal A, Dietz R, et al. Practical recommendations for the use of ACE inhibitors, beta-blockers, aldosterone antagonists and angiotensin receptor blockers in heart failure: putting guidelines into practice. *Eur J Heart Fail* 2005;7:710-772.

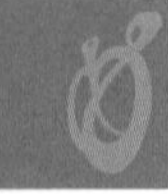

In addition, it has also been generally deemed as appropriate not to start β-blockers during the same hospitalization for acute heart failure in patients not on β-blockers at the time of admission. However, prospective studies have shown that the initiation of β-blocker therapy before discharge in patients hospitalized for acute heart failure is safe and associated with higher post-discharge treatment rates.[41] The Organized Program to Initiate Lifesaving Treatment in Hospitalized Patients with Heart Failure (OPTIMIZE-HF), a prospective trial powered to assess the effects on outcomes of pre-discharge initiation of β-blocker therapy, has shown a 54% reduction in the risk of subsequent death (95% CI, −70% to −27%; $P = .0006$) and a 29% reduction in the risk of death or re-hospitalization (95% CI, −57% to −6%; $P = .0175$), compared to no β-blocker administration, in patients discharged on β-blocker treatment after a hospitalization for heart failure.[42]

On the basis of these data, it is now recommended that patients hospitalized for acute heart failure and reduced ejection fraction (1) continue β-blockers if they had been taking these agents and have no hemodynamic instability or contraindications; (2) initiate β-blocker treatment if it was not used before; and (3) start β-blocker therapy after discontinuing intravenous furosemide, vasodilators, or inotropic therapy and after volume status is optimized and clinical stability is achieved.[53]

β-BLOCKER THERAPY IN CLINICAL PRACTICE

β-Blocker Use

Studies of the prognostic role of adherence to guidelines,[144,145] as well as studies of prescriptions at discharge of patients hospitalized for heart failure,[146-148] have confirmed the independent role of β-blocker administration for improving patient prognosis. β-Blocker prescription rates have increased since 1990, starting after the publication of the landmark outcomes trials in the late 1980s and of 2001 guidelines, with an increase of about 5% to 10% every year from 2001 to 2005 (Figure 46-9).[142,149-151] This pattern has been observed also in elderly subjects, a population for which β-blockers are underprescribed. An analysis of 741 octogenarians (median age, 83.7 years), assessed in the Euro Heart Failure Survey II, confirmed β-blockers are prescribed less often for these patients than for younger subjects; however, the number of prescriptions was more than twice as high as that in the Euro Heart Failure Survey I, performed in 2000 to 2001 (53% vs. 25% for β-blocker prescriptions and 12% vs. 5% for high-dose β-blocker prescriptions; $P < .001$ in both cases).[152]

Despite these improvements, β-blockers remain underprescribed for some patients. These subpopulations include elderly patients, patients with hypotension, patients with severe heart failure, and patients with renal insufficiency.[39,40,150-155] Many of these patients may benefit from β-blockers to a similar, if not greater, extent than do the other patients; their tolerance of β-blockers is often underestimated[33,39-43,118,119] and can be increased by adequate implementation strategies. In the Carvedilol Open-Label Assessment (COLA) II study, Krum and colleagues[40] demonstrated that the tolerance of β-blocker therapy, although reduced by aging (76.8% of patients aged >75 years vs. 84.3% of patients aged 70 to 75 years), remains high among elderly patients with heart failure. The Beta-blockers In Patients with Congestive Heart Failure: Guided Use in Clinical Practice (BRING-UP)–2 study was designed to improve the prescription rate and to assess the tolerability of β-blockers in the elderly patients (aged ≥70 years), both those with moderate and those with severe heart failure.[39] Among the 1518 elderly patients included in the study, 505 (33.3%) were already taking β-blockers at the time of enrollment, 464 (30.6%) were prescribed a β-blocker for the first time, while the remaining patients had specific contraindications to β-blockade (chronic obstructive pulmonary disease, peripheral vascular disease, long P-R interval, 378 patients, 24.9%) or had not started taking β-blockers without a clear contraindication (real underprescription: 171 patients, 11.3%).[39] These data show that β-blockers can be administered to a high percentage of elderly patients (75.1% in BRING-UP–2) when adequate physician education and disease management programs are provided.

In BRING-UP–2, β-blocker therapy was also implemented in 709 patients with severe heart failure, defined by symptoms at rest or during minimal exercise with LVEF of less than .25. Results were similar to those for the elderly patients. Only 272 (38.4%) of patients were already taking a β-blocker at the start of the study and 220 additional patients (31%) could start taking carvedilol during the study. Two-hundred-twenty patients (31%) could not start because they were either receiving intravenous therapy (58 patients, 8.2%) or had contraindications such as chronic obstructive pulmonary disease or peripheral vascular disease. Only 54 patients (7.6%) never started taking β-blockers despite having no contraindications. After 1-year follow-up, patients taking β-blockers had a lower incidence of death (10.8% among patients already treated and 11.2% among patients newly treated, in contrast to 18% among those not treated).[39] Thus, these data show the potential of an education program to increase prescription rates of

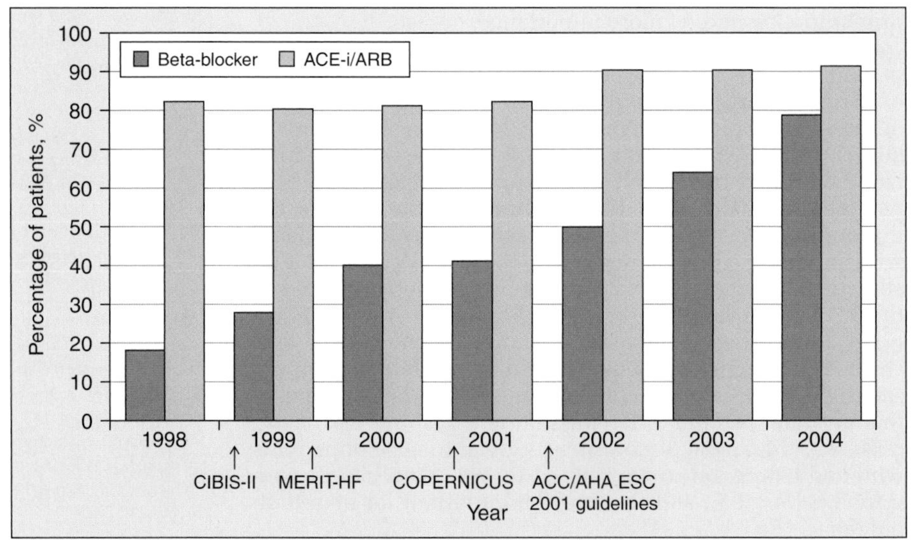

FIGURE 46–9 Temporal trends in β-blocker use at hospital discharge in 769 patients with heart failure and systolic dysfunction from 1998 to 2004. (From Patel P, White DL, Deswal A. Translation of clinical trial results into practice: temporal patterns of beta-blocker utilization for heart failure at hospital discharge and during ambulatory follow-up. *Am Heart J* 2007;153:515-522.)

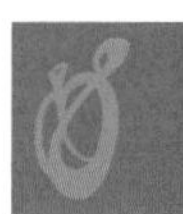

β-blockers in patients with lower tolerance rates in whom this therapy is usually underprescribed.

In clinical practice, β-blockers are often administered at low dosages, instead of the target dosages indicated in guidelines and shown to be effective by randomized controlled trials.[142,149-151] Although even low doses are considered better than no β-blocker therapy,[134] the effects of β-blockers on outcomes have been shown consistently only at the dosages recommended in guidelines, and multiple studies have demonstrated dose dependency of their beneficial effects.[61,105,115-117] Another cause of underuse of β-blockers in clinical practice is the presence of accepted contraindications: bradycardia, second- or third-degree atrioventricular block, and asthma are the major important contraindications to β-blockade. Only bronchial obstruction with sensitivity to the administration of β_2-agonists should be considered as an absolute contraindication to β-blocker therapy in patients with pulmonary diseases. This limitation may, however, be partially overcome by the use of β_1-selective agents.[65,156]

Implementation Strategies

Despite the evidence of the benefits of β-blocker therapy, first obtained as early as 1990, perceptions of its benefits and, therefore, its implementation still vary among physicians. Awareness of heart failure management recommendations has been investigated with 2041 cardiologists, 1881 internists and geriatricians, and 2965 primary care physicians in nine European countries.[157] Only 39% of internists or geriatricians would have prescribed a β-blocker for more than 50% of their patients (in contrast to 73% of the cardiologists; $P < .0001$); primary care physicians always or often prescribed β-blockers to only 40% of patients with heart failure. Twenty-six percent of internists or geriatricians and 36% of primary care physicians (in contrast to 11% of cardiologists) answered that they would have never prescribed β-blockers to a patient with mild heart failure who was already taking diuretics and ACE inhibitors (Figure 46-10).[157] Prescription of β-blockers prescription also varied widely in a cohort study of U.S. cardiologists.[158]

Many implementation strategies are currently proposed and adopted to favor prescription of β-blocker therapy to all patients without major contraindications. One of the first studies with this aim was the BRING-UP program.[43] It was based on the organization of regional meetings and on the development and distribution of the recommendations derived from the available clinical evidence on the proper use of β-blockers. It involved 197 cardiology centers and 3091 patients. β-Blockers were newly prescribed in 32.7% of cases, and prescription rates increased from 24.9% to 49.7% over the year of the study. The average β-blocker dosage was 70% of that administered in controlled trials. The use of β-blockers was independently associated with a better prognosis and a 40% reduction in hospitalizations for heart failure. The major reasons for either lack of prescription or lack of upward titration of β-blocker therapy were advanced age, more severe NYHA class, and the presence of atrial fibrillation.[43] The BRING-UP–2 phase extended this evaluation to include elderly patients and patients with severe heart failure.[39] Strategies based on educational programs for physicians and patients, clinical reminders attached to echocardiography reports, close telephone contacts for advice and consultation, led by cardiologists or heart failure nurses or both, have been widely and successfully developed.[44,159,160] Implementation of β-blocker therapy has been actually one of the major aims of heart failure clinics and disease management programs.[161] The benefits of these interventions are obviously greater in the setting with the worst clinical practice.[162]

In addition to disease management and educational programs for ambulatory patients, predischarge initiation of β-blocker therapy in patients hospitalized for heart failure is a safe and effective modality; increasing the proportion of patients on β-blockers after discharge has beneficial effects on subsequent outcomes.[41,42,147,148,163]

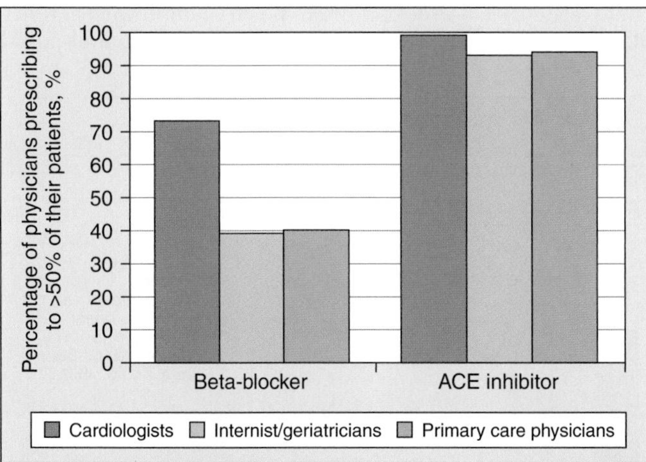

FIGURE 46–10 Proportion of European primary care physicians and specialists who prescribed β-blockers or angiotensin-converting enzyme (ACE) inhibitors to more than 50% of their patients (">50% of patients" defined as "often" or "always" for primary care physicians). (From Remme WJ, McMurray JJ, Hobbs FD, et al. Awareness and perception of heart failure among European cardiologists, internists, geriatricians, and primary care physicians. *Eur Heart J* 2008;29:1739-1752.)

Lack of Evidence in Specific Patients Groups: The Case of Heart Failure with Preserved Ejection Fraction

In some subpopulations of patients with heart failure, β-blocker therapy is also underprescribed because of insufficient or poor evidence of efficacy. Prospective trials[36] and registries[148] have also confirmed improved survival in elderly patients (see Chapter 49) taking β-blockers, although the magnitude of the benefit appears to be lower than in younger patients. β-Blocker therapy has also been prospectively assessed in 161 children and adolescents with symptomatic systolic heart failure.[36] A trend toward better outcomes was found with β-blocker therapy, although these results did not achieve statistical significance, which is probably explained by the lower-than-expected event rates.

Another important group of patients with heart failure for whom evidence of efficacy is lacking is that of patients with heart failure and preserved LVEF (HFPEF). The number of patients hospitalized with this diagnosis is actually increasing and, in contrast to patients with low ejection fraction, no improvement in survival has been observed since the mid-1980s.[164] Effects of β-blocker therapy are likely to be different between patients with preserved ejection fraction and those with reduced ejection fraction. For instance, chronic β-blocker therapy has been associated with lower collagen volume fraction, cardiac myocyte diameter, and stimulatory G-protein expression only in patients with HFPEF, whereas expression of inhibitory G-proteins has been lower in only the patients with reduced ejection fraction.[165] The only prospective outcome β-blocker trial that included patients with preserved ejection fraction was SENIORS.[36] The effect of nebivolol on the primary endpoint was similar in the patients with an ejection fraction of less than .35 (risk reduction, −14%; 95% CI, +4% to −28%) in comparison with the patients whose ejection fraction was .35 or higher (−19%; 95% CI, +4% to −37%). Similar results were also observed with regard to all secondary endpoints.[37]

However, SENIORS was not designed and powered to assess the effects of nebivolol in patients with preserved ejection fraction, assessed separately, and the cutoff of .35 for defining preserved ejection fraction is too low.[52,53] Results from analyses of patient databases are controversial; some studies have revealed no benefit[148,166] and others have revealed a favorable effect of β-blocker therapy on the outcomes of the patients with HFPEF.[167,168] Thus, although there is a rationale for administering β-blockers in patients with HFPEF (benefits of bradycardia, increased duration of LV filling time, blood pressure control), evidence regarding clinical efficacy of β-blockers in these patients is lacking.[52]

LIMITATIONS OF β-BLOCKER THERAPY

Despite its proven effectiveness in the general population of patients with stable, low LVEF and NYHA class II to class III heart failure, β-blockade as a treatment of chronic heart failure has some limitations. The foremost issue is the heterogeneity of response, something shared with all forms of heart failure therapy but perhaps more of an issue with β-blockers because of the magnitude of benefit in patients that do respond, the potential to do harm in a small number (10% to 20%) of patients who either do not respond or who cannot tolerate β-blockade, and the fact that determination of response, as currently performed, can be accomplished only empirically, after several months of slow and often tedious upward titration of the β-blocker. Figure 46-11 emphasizes the heterogeneity of response problem: In the Multicenter Oral Carvedilol Heart failure Assessment (MOCHA) trial,[105] after the placebo response rate was subtracted, only 45% of patients were found to exhibit a positive LVEF response to the highest dosage (25 mg twice a day) dose of carvedilol; with 6.25 mg twice a day, the response rate was even lower (30%).[169] As shown in Figure 46-11, small numbers (<10%) of patients actually experienced worsening of LVEF with carvedilol, and these numbers do not include the 8% of patients who could not tolerate open-label carvedilol challenge.[169]

Another issue is poor tolerance of β-blockers, particularly in patients with the most advanced heart failure. The percentage of such patients ranges from 5% to 20% and is highly dependent on the experience of the treating physician, as well as on the β-blocker being used.[170] Much of the intolerance arises from the negative inotropic properties of β-blockers in very advanced heart failure, in which the concomitant use of non–β-agonist–positive inotropic agents may be useful.[79,171] The intolerance issue no doubt influences the underuse of β-blockers in clinical practice.

Finally, clinical data are inadequate for certain important subpopulations of patients with heart failure. HFPEF has been highlighted as such a circumstance, but other examples include minimal asymptomatic reduced LVEF, NYHA class IV heart failure, and race (African American).

FUTURE DIRECTIONS

Improvement in the Clinical Pharmacology of β-Blocking Agents

Improvements in the clinical pharmacological activity of specific agents could potentially favorably affect both heterogeneity of response and tolerability. For example, the new controlled-release formulation of carvedilol has improved pharmacokinetics, which may mitigate some of the vasodilator side effects of high peak blood levels of immediate-release carvedilol. The pharmacodynamic characteristics of controlled-release carvedilol seem comparable with those of immediate-release carvedilol administered twice daily.[172]

Associated or ancillary properties of β-blockers may also be important. In the COMET trial, the superiority of carvedilol over immediate-release metoprolol could be explained by differences in the degree of β_1-receptor blockade[125]; however, ancillary properties of carvedilol could also have contributed to its superiority.[130,131] New β-blockers with novel ancillary properties are now available. Among them, nebivolol is a highly selective β_1-adrenergic receptor blocker with associated β_3-agonist and nitric oxide–releasing properties.[93,94,173] The clinical relevance of these properties should, however, be shown by direct comparison trials.

The relative importance of different mechanisms of action of β-blockers in patients with heart failure is still a matter of debate. For example, a meta-analysis revealed a correlation between survival benefit from β-blocker treatment and heart rate reduction, with an 18% reduction (95% CI, 6% to 29%) in the risk for death for every heart rate reduction of 5 beats/minute with β-blocker treatment.[174] This effect of heart rate reduction was independent from β-blocker dosing. Another study showed that the change in heart rate after β-blocker therapy is correlated with the change in LVEF as well as with reduction in mortality.[175] Thus, heart rate reduction seems to be an important mechanism of action of β-blockers in heart failure. The hypothesis that pure heart rate reduction may have beneficial effects on outcomes is currently being tested.[176] β-Blockers with positive inotropic activity other than through β-receptors may be developed and could

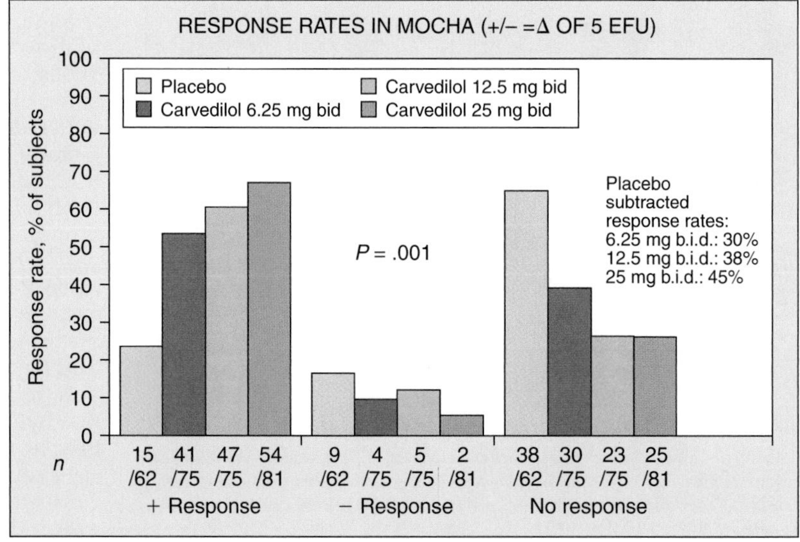

FIGURE 46–11 Differences in the response to chronic β-blocker therapy. (From Bristow MR, Gilbert EM, Abraham WT, et al. Carvedilol produces dose-related improvements in left ventricular function and survival in subjects with chronic heart failure. *Circulation* 1996;94:2807-2816.)

someday prove useful in patients with very advanced heart failure. Another possibility, as discussed previously and in the next section, is the development of compounds with greater inverse agonist properties on specific genetic subtypes of β_1- or even β_2-receptors.

Pharmacogenetic Targeting Based on Genetic Variation in Adrenergic Receptors (see Chapter 42)

As discussed in detail in Chapter 42, the response to drug therapy can be improved by genetic biomarker identification of patients who respond differentially, either better or worse/not at all in comparison with the general population. On the basis of data from the human genome sequencing project, the amount of genetic variation in the form of single-nucleotide polymorphisms (SNPs) is estimated to be 0.1% to 0.2%,[177] but certain genes exhibit more variation than others. The small and intronless β1- and β_2-adrenergic receptor genes are examples of highly polymorphic genes, exhibiting SNP frequencies of approximately 1%. The β_1-adrenergic receptor gene has 12 nonsynonymous SNPs (which result in a change in coded amino acid) and 3 synonymous SNPs in its coding region; the β_2 gene has, respectively, 12 and 5.[178] The β_1-receptor gene product is the primary drug target of β-blockers, and one of its polymorphisms, an SNP at nucleotide position 1165 that produces either an arginine (Arg, major allele, frequency of approximately 0.70) or glycine (Gly, minor allele, frequency of approximately 0.30), is associated with markedly different pharmacological properties.[63] In comparison with the 389 Gly version of the β_1-receptor, the Arg variant has much higher signal transduction capacity, higher affinity for norepinephrine, and a higher fraction of receptors in a constitutively active state.[63,179,180] The β_2-adrenergic receptor also has a polymorphism with a major difference in signal transduction function between the variants, at nucleotide position 491 and amino acid position 164 (Thr164Ile).[181] However, the minor, hypofunctional 164 isoleucine allele has a frequency of less than 2% and is therefore of little pharmacogenetic interest.[182] Several additional polymorphisms of β_1-receptors (Ser49Gly) and β_2-receptors (Gly16Arg and Gln27Glu) can affect receptor internalization without affecting signal transduction. In addition, the α_{2c} adrenergic receptor has a large deletion polymorphism of amino acid positions 322 to 325 (allele frequency of 4% among white people but 42% among African Americans) that produces a major loss in signal transduction function.[183] This receptor is present on adrenergic nerve terminals, where the wild-type or insertion version tonically inhibits norepinephrine release.[34,82]

Any of these receptor polymorphisms could theoretically alter the response to β-blocker therapy. Small studies have related changes in LV function after β-blockade of SNPs. A greater increase in the LVEF after chronic β-blocker therapy has been shown in subjects homozygous for the Arg389 β_1-receptor, compared with Gly389 carriers, in some[180,184] but not all[185,186] single-center studies and in a meta-analysis.[187] A greater improvement in the LVEF after carvedilol administration has been shown in β_2 Glu27 carriers in some studies.[186,188]

No significant interaction between β_2-adrenergic receptor polymorphisms and the effects of β-blockers on clinical outcomes have been described to date. Because the receptor is the primary target of β-blocker treatment and because the polymorphic variants possess major functional differences, the β_1 Arg389Gly polymorphism has been related to outcomes in two of the large β-blocker studies, BEST[78,80] and MERIT-HF.[189] In both these trials, DNA data banks were obtained in order to assess the relationship between adrenergic receptor polymorphism and the effects of treatment. The DNA bank population of BEST consisted of 1040 patients[123,179] who were studied to test the hypothesis that polymorphisms of adrenergic receptors can influence clinical, remodeling, or sympatholytic effects of bucindolol. Two sets of receptor polymorphisms were found to influence outcomes: β_1 389 Arg/Gly[179] and α_{2c} 322-325 wild-type/deletion.[123] The β_1 389 polymorphism interacts with bucindolol in a manner predicted by its pharmacological action: Bucindolol was associated with greater clinical efficacy in patients who were homozygous for the β_1 389 Arg receptor gene than in patients with Gly-containing genotypes.[179] Bucindolol-associated sympatholysis was exaggerated in patients with α_{2c} deletion genotypes, which compromised efficacy.[123] In contrast, patients with α_{2c} wild-type genotypes exhibited only mild sympatholysis and substantial clinical efficacy, with a reduction in all-cause mortality of 30% (P = .025) and a reduction in cardiovascular mortality of 41% (P = .003).[123] The interpretation of these findings was that the α_{2c} deletion receptor produced adrenergic dysregulation, similar to what has been described in mouse knockout models.[190,191] At any rate, it appears that the norepinephrine-lowering properties of bucindolol are subject to genetic regulation by α_{2c} genotype, and the undesirable property of exaggerated sympatholysis can be avoided by not giving bucindolol to patients with α_{2c} deletion genotypes. In the BEST substudy of adrenergic receptor polymorphism, the variants affecting β-receptor internalization did not consistently alter clinical responses or affect norepinephrine release. In BEST, neither the β_1 Arg/Gly or α_{2c} wild-type/deletion polymorphisms affected clinical responses in patients treated with placebo[123,179]; that is, there was no apparent clinical effect of these polymorphisms on the natural history of heart failure over the average 2-year follow-up period in the trial.

In a 600-patient DNA substudy of the MERIT-HF trial, the β_1 Arg/Gly polymorphism did not affect clinical response in either the metoprolol or placebo group[189]; in a 637-patient study of the effects of all the β_1 389 and 49 polymorphisms, β_2 16 and 27 polymorphisms, and α_{2c} wild-type/deletion polymorphisms, no effect of any variant was found in clinical responses to either metoprolol or carvedilol.[192] There are no data on the interaction of nebivolol with adrenergic receptor polymorphisms.

Thus, the available data indicate that the effects on outcomes of bucindolol, but not metoprolol or carvedilol, can be influenced by β_1 389 Arg/Gly and α_{2c} wild-type/deletion polymorphisms. This is perhaps not surprising inasmuch as in human systems only bucindolol interacts pharmacologically with both sets of polymorphisms[123,179]; that is, in isolated human heart preparations with β_1 Arg homozygous genotype, bucindolol has inverse agonist properties, which indicates that it facilitates the inactivation of constitutively active β_1 Arg receptors.[179,193,194] Carvedilol and metoprolol do not exhibit this property.[193,194] Carvedilol and metoprolol also are not sympatholytic and so would not be expected to interact pharmacologically with α_{2c} polymorphisms. The deletion variant of the α_{2c} receptor results in adrenergic dysregulation in response to agents that affect the release of norepinephrine,[191] which is the probably basis of this receptor variant's strong interaction with the norepinephrine-lowering effects of bucindolol.[193]

Therefore, genetic variation in two adrenergic receptors appears to influence the clinical response to bucindolol. In order to take full advantage of this, both sets of polymorphisms would need to be considered. Only the patients with the hypofunctional 389 Gly version of the β_1-adrenergic receptor are susceptible to the exaggerated sympatholytic effects of bucindolol in association with α_{2c} deletion genotypes.[195] This creates a situation in which the approximately 50% of patients with the β_1 Arg 389 homozygous genotype exhibited the greatest degree of efficacy in response to bucindolol, including a 38% reduction (P = .042) in all-cause mortality, a 48% reduction (P = .014) in cardiovascular mortality,

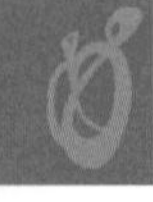

TABLE 46–4 Generational Classification of β-Blockers for the Treatment of Heart Failure

Generation	Definition	Examples
First	Nonselective for β1- and β_2-adrenergic receptors	Propranolol, timolol
Second	Selective for β1- versus β_2-adrenergic receptors	Metoprolol, bisoprolol
Third	Selective or nonselective, with a favorable ancillary property (e.g., vasodilation)	Carvedilol, nebivolol
Fourth	Selective for specific adrenergic receptor polymorphisms	Bucindolol

and a 36% reduction (P = .007) in hospitalizations for heart failure.[179,195] On the other hand, the approximately 10% of patients who have both β_1 389 Gly and α_{2c} deletion genotypes should not be treated with bucindolol, because there is no evidence of efficacy in these patients.[123,179]

Bucindolol is still in development; the final clinical trial to be conducted exclusively in patients who have the β_1 389 Arg homozygous genotype, in a 1:1 comparison with metoprolol succinate. If this trial confirms results of the BEST DNA substudy, bucindolol would be approved with pharmacogenetic labeling, indicated for patients with the β_1 Arg/Arg genotype, with language warning against administering the drug to patients who have both α_{2c} deletion and β_1 389 Gly genotypes. Obviously, a baseline genetic test would be necessary to optimally administer a drug with a pharmacogenetic indication, and this test is also being developed. Thus, β-blocker drug development has now evolved through four generations (Table 46-4): The first-generation compounds, developed in the late 1960s and early 1970s, could competitively antagonize both β_1- and β_2-receptors; the second generation, developed in the 1970s through the 1990s, consisted of β_1-selective compounds; the third generation, developed in the 1980s through the 2000s, comprised compounds with the ancillary property of vasodilation; and the fourth-generation compounds, currently being developed, act against specific adrenergic receptor polymorphisms. This last approach should improve therapeutic index of this already highly effective therapeutic class and may serve to increase the interest of pharmaceutical companies in this venerable class of compounds.

REFERENCES

1. Braunwald, E., & Bristow, M. R. (2000). Congestive heart failure: fifty years of progress. *Circulation, 102*(20, Suppl. 4), IV-14–IV-23.
2. Mann, D. L., & Bristow, M. R. (2005). Mechanisms and models in heart failure: the biomechanical model and beyond. *Circulation, 111*, 2837–2849.
3. Waagstein, F., Hjalmarson, A., Varnauskas, E., et al. (1975). Effect of chronic beta-adrenergic receptor blockade in congestive cardiomyopathy. *Br Heart J, 37*, 1022–1036.
4. Swedberg, K., Hjalmarson, A., Waagstein, F., et al. (1979). Prolongation of survival in congestive cardiomyopathy by beta-receptor blockade. *Lancet, 1*, 1374–1376.
5. Bristow, M. R., Ginsburg, R., Minobe, W. A., et al. (1982). Decreased catecholamine sensitivity and β-adrenergic-receptor density in failing human hearts. *New Engl J Med, 307*, 205–211.
6. Waagstein, F., Bristow, M. R., Swedberg, K., et al. (1993). Beneficial effects of metoprolol in idiopathic dilated cardiomyopathy. Metoprolol in Dilated Cardiomyopathy (MDC) Trial Study Group. *Lancet, 342*, 1441–1446.
7. Chadda, K., Goldstein, S., Byington, R., et al. (1986). Effect of propranolol after acute myocardial infarction in patients with congestive heart failure. *Circulation, 73*, 503–510.
8. Norwegian Multicentre Group. (1981). Timolol induced reduction in mortality and reinfarction in patients surviving acute myocardial infarction. *N Engl J Med, 304*, 801–807.
9. Chidsey, C. A., Sonnenblick, E. H., Morrow, A. G., et al. (1966). Norepinephrine stores and contractile force of papillary muscles from the failing human heart. *Circulation, 33*, 43–51.
10. Chidsey, C. A., Braunwald, E., & Morrow, A. G. (1965). Catecholamine excretion and cardiac stores of norepinephrine in congestive heart failure. *Am J Med, 39*, 442–451.
11. Swedberg, K., Viquerat, C., Rouleau, J. L., et al. (1984). Comparison of myocardial catecholamine balance in chronic congestive heart failure and in angina pectoris without failure. *Am J Cardiol, 52*, 308–313.
12. Hasking, G. J., Esler, M. D., Jennings, G. L., et al. (1986). Norepinephrine spillover to plasma in patients with congestive heart failure: evidence of increased overall and cardiorenal sympathetic nervous activity. *Circulation, 73*, 615–621.
13. Metra, M., Nardi, M., Giubbini, R., et al. (1994). Effects of short- and long-term carvedilol administration on rest and exercise hemodynamic variables, exercise capacity and clinical conditions in patients with idiopathic dilated cardiomyopathy. *J Am Coll Cardiol, 24*, 1678–1687.
14. Krum, H., Sackner-Bernstein, J. D., Goldsmith, R. L., et al. (1995). Double-blind, placebo-controlled study of the long-term efficacy of carvedilol in patients with severe chronic heart failure. *Circulation, 92*, 1499–1506.
15. Olsen, S. L., Gilbert, E. M., Renlund, D. G., et al. (1995). Carvedilol improves left ventricular function and symptoms in chronic heart failure: a double-blind randomized study. *J Am Coll Cardiol, 25*, 1225–1231.
16. Hall, S. A., Cigarroa, C. G., Marcoux, L., et al. (1995). Time course of improvement in left ventricular function, mass and geometry in patients with congestive heart failure treated with beta-adrenergic blockade. *J Am Coll Cardiol, 25*, 1154–1161.
17. Eichhorn, E. J., & Bristow, M. R. (1996). Medical therapy can improve the biological properties of the chronically failing heart. A new era in the treatment of heart failure. *Circulation, 94*, 2285–2296.
18. Lechat, P., Packer, M., Chalon, S., et al. (1998). Clinical effects of beta-adrenergic blockade in chronic heart failure: a meta-analysis of double-blind, placebo-controlled, randomized trials. *Circulation, 98*, 1184–1191.
19. Lowes, B. D., Gill, E. A., Abraham, W. T., et al. (1999). Effects of carvedilol on left ventricular mass, chamber geometry, and mitral regurgitation in chronic heart failure. *Am J Cardiol, 83*, 1201–1205.
20. Metra, M., Nodari, S., D'Aloia, A., et al. (2000). A rationale for the use of beta-blockers as standard treatment for heart failure. *Am Heart J, 139*, 511–521.
21. Eichhorn, E. J., Heesch, C. M., Barnett, J. H., et al. (1994). Effect of metoprolol on myocardial function and energetics in patients with nonischemic dilated cardiomyopathy: a randomized, double-blind, placebo-controlled study. *J Am Coll Cardiol, 24*, 1310–1320.
22. Lowes, B. D., Gilbert, E. M., Abraham, W. T., et al. (2002). Myocardial gene expression in dilated cardiomyopathy treated with beta-blocking agents. *N Engl J Med, 346*, 1357–1365.
23. Reiken, S., Wehrens, X. H., Vest, J. A., et al. (2003). Beta-blockers restore calcium release channel function and improve cardiac muscle performance in human heart failure. *Circulation, 107*, 2459–2466.
24. Communal, C., Singh, K., Pimentel, D. R., et al. (1998). Norepinephrine stimulates apoptosis in adult rat ventricular myocytes by activation of the beta-adrenergic pathway. *Circulation, 98*, 1329–1334.
25. Ikram, H., & Fitzpatrick, D. (1981). Double-blind trial of chronic oral beta blockade in congestive cardiomyopathy. *Lancet, 2*, 490–493.
26. Currie, P. J., Kelly, M. J., McKenzie, A., et al. (1984). Oral beta-adrenergic blockade with metoprolol in chronic severe dilated cardiomyopathy. *J Am Coll Cardiol, 3*, 203–209.
27. CIBIS Investigators and Committees. (1994). A randomized trial of beta-blockade in heart failure. The Cardiac Insufficiency Bisoprolol Study (CIBIS). *Circulation, 90*, 1765–1773.
28. Packer, M., Bristow, M. R., Cohn, J. N., et al. (1996). The effect of carvedilol on morbidity and mortality in patients with chronic heart failure. *New Engl J Med, 334*, 1349–1355.
29. CIBIS-II Investigators and Committees. (1999). The Cardiac Insufficiency Bisoprolol Study II (CIBIS-II): a randomised trial. *Lancet, 353*, 9–13.
30. MERIT-HF Study Group. (1999). Effect of metoprolol CR/XL in chronic heart failure: Metoprolol CR/XL Randomised Intervention Trial in Congestive Heart Failure (MERIT-HF). *Lancet, 353*, 2001–2007.
31. Hjalmarson, A., Goldstein, S., Fagerberg, S., et al. (2000). Effects of controlled-release metoprolol on total mortality, hospitalization and well being in patients with heart failure. *JAMA, 283*, 1295–1302.
32. Packer, M., Coats, A. J., Fowler, M. B., et al. (2001). Effect of carvedilol on survival in severe chronic heart failure. *N Engl J Med, 344*, 1651–1658.
33. Krum, H., Roecker, E. B., Mohacsi, P., et al. (2003). Carvedilol Prospective Randomized Cumulative Survival (COPERNICUS) Study Group. Effects of initiating carvedilol in patients with severe chronic heart failure: results from the COPERNICUS Study. *JAMA, 289*, 712–718.
34. Bristow, M. R. (2000). Beta-adrenergic receptor blockade in chronic heart failure. *Circulation, 101*, 558–569.
35. Dargie, H. J. (2001). Effect of carvedilol on outcome after myocardial infarction in patients with left-ventricular dysfunction: the CAPRICORN randomised trial. *Lancet, 357*, 1385–1390.
36. Flather, M. D., Shibata, M. C., Coats, A. J., et al. (2005). Randomized trial to determine the effect of nebivolol on mortality and cardiovascular hospital admission in elderly patients with heart failure (SENIORS). *Eur Heart J, 26*, 215–225.
37. van Veldhuisen, D. J., Cohen-Solal, A., Böhm, M., et al. (2009). Beta-blockade with nebivolol in elderly heart failure patients with impaired and preserved left ventricular ejection fraction: data from SENIORS (Study of Effects of Nebivolol Intervention on Outcomes and Rehospitalization in Seniors With Heart Failure). *J Am Coll Cardiol, 53*, 2150–2158.
38. Shaddy, R. E., Boucek, M. M., Hsu, D. T., et al. (2007). Pediatric Carvedilol Study Group. Carvedilol for children and adolescents with heart failure: a randomized controlled trial. *JAMA, 298*, 1171–1179.
39. Opasich, C., Boccanelli, A., Cafiero, M., et al. (2006). Programme to improve the use of beta-blockers for heart failure in the elderly and in those with severe symptoms: results of the BRING-UP 2 Study. *Eur J Heart Fail, 8*, 649–657.
40. Krum, H., Hill, J., Fruhwald, F., et al. (2006). Tolerability of beta-blockers in elderly patients with chronic heart failure: the COLA II study. *Eur J Heart Fail, 8*, 302–307.
41. Gattis, W. A., O'Connor, C. M., Gallup, D. S., et al. (2004). Predischarge initiation of carvedilol in patients hospitalized for decompensated heart failure: results of the Initiation Management Predischarge: Process for Assessment of Carvedilol Therapy in Heart Failure (IMPACT-HF) trial. *J Am Coll Cardiol, 43*, 1534–1541.

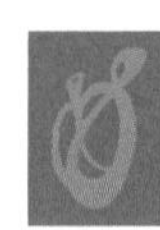

42. Fonarow, G. C., Abraham, W. T., Albert, N. M., et al. (2007). Carvedilol use at discharge in patients hospitalized for heart failure is associated with improved survival: an analysis from Organized Program to Initiate Lifesaving Treatment in Hospitalized Patients with Heart Failure (OPTIMIZE-HF). *Am Heart J*, *153*, 82.e1–82.e11.
43. Maggioni, A. P., Sinagra, G., Opasich, C., et al. (2003). Treatment of chronic heart failure with beta adrenergic blockade beyond controlled clinical trials: the BRING-UP experience. *Heart*, *89*, 299–305.
44. Heidenreich, P. A., Gholami, P., Sahay, A., et al. (2007). Clinical reminders attached to echocardiography reports of patients with reduced left ventricular ejection fraction increase use of beta-blockers: a randomized trial. *Circulation*, *115*, 2829–2834.
45. Barner, H. B., Jellinek, M., & Kaiser, G. C. (1970). Effects of isoproterenol infusion on myocardial structure and composition. *Am Heart J*, *79*, 237–243.
46. Engelhardt, S., Hein, L., Wiesmann, F., et al. (1999). Progressive hypertrophy and heart failure in β_1-adrenergic receptor transgenic mice. *Proc Natl Acad Sci*, *96*, 7059–7064.
47. Lowes, B. D., Minobe, W., Abraham, W. T., et al. (1997). Changes in gene expression in the intact human heart. Downregulation of alpha-myosin heavy chain in hypertrophied, failing ventricular myocardium. *J Clin Invest*, *100*, 2315–2324.
48. Sucharov, C. C., Mariner, P. D., Nunley, K. R., et al. (2006). A β_1-adrenergic receptor, CaM kinase II–dependent pathway mediates cardiac myocyte fetal gene induction. *Am J Physiol Heart Circ Physiol*, *291*, H1299–H1308.
49. Francis, G. S., Anwar, F., Bank, A. J., et al. (1999). Apoptosis, *Bcl*-2, and proliferating cell nuclear antigen in the failing human heart: observations made after implantation of left ventricular assist device. *J Card Fail*, *5*, 308–315.
50. Adamson, P. B., & Gilbert, E. M. (2006). Reducing the risk of sudden death in heart failure with beta-blockers. *J Card Fail*, *12*, 734–746.
51. Heart Failure Society of America. (2006). Executive summary: HFSA 2006 Comprehensive Heart Failure Practice Guideline. *J Card Fail*, *12*, 10–38.
52. Task Force for Diagnosis and Treatment of Acute and Chronic Heart Failure 2008 of European Society of Cardiology, Dickstein, K., Cohen-Solal, A., et al. (2008). ESC Guidelines for the diagnosis and treatment of acute and chronic heart failure 2008: the Task Force for the Diagnosis and Treatment of Acute and Chronic Heart Failure 2008 of the European Society of Cardiology. Developed in collaboration with the Heart Failure Association of the ESC (HFA) and endorsed by the European Society of Intensive Care Medicine (ESICM). *Eur Heart J*, *29*, 2388–2442.
53. Jessup, M., Abraham, W. T., Casey, D. E., et al. (2009). 2009 Focused update: ACCF/AHA Guidelines for the Diagnosis and Management of Heart Failure in Adults: a report of the American College of Cardiology Foundation/American Heart Association Task Force on Practice Guidelines: developed in collaboration with the International Society for Heart and Lung Transplantation. *Circulation*, *119*, 1977–2016.
54. Metra, M., Dei Cas, L., & Cleland, J. G. (2006). Pharmacokinetic and pharmacodynamic characteristics of beta-blockers: when differences may matter. *J Card Fail*, *12*, 177–181.
55. Go, A. S., Yang, J., Gurwitz, J. H., et al. (2008). Comparative effectiveness of different beta-adrenergic antagonists on mortality among adults with heart failure in clinical practice. *Arch Intern Med*, *168*, 2415–2421.
56. Kramer, J. M., Curtis, L. H., Dupree, C. S., et al. (2008). Comparative effectiveness of beta-blockers in elderly patients with heart failure. *Arch Intern Med*, *168*, 2422–2428.
57. Yusuf, S., Peto, R., Lewis, J., et al. (1985). Beta blockade during and after myocardial infarction: an overview of the randomized trials. *Prog Cardiovasc Dis*, *27*, 335–371.
58. The Xamoterol in Severe Heart Failure Study Group. (1990). Xamoterol in severe heart failure. *Lancet*, *336*, 1–6.
59. Witchitz, S., Cohen-Solal, A., Dartois, N., et al. (2000). Treatment of heart failure with celiprolol, a cardioselective beta blocker with β_2 agonist vasodilatory properties. The CELICARD Group. *Am J Cardiol*, *85*, 1467–1471.
60. Willette, R. N., Mitchell, M. P., Ohlstein, E. H., et al. (1998). Evaluation of intrinsic sympathomimetic activity of bucindolol and carvedilol in rat heart. *Pharmacology*, *56*, 30–36.
61. Bristow, M. R., Roden, R. L., Lowes, B. D., et al. (1998). The role of third generation β-blocking agents in chronic heart failure. *Clin Cardiol*, *21*(Suppl. I), I-3–I-13.
62. Bristow, M. R., O'Connell, J. B., Gilbert, E. M., et al. (1994). Dose-response of chronic beta-blocker treatment in heart failure from either idiopathic dilated or ischemic cardiomyopathy. Bucindolol Investigators. *Circulation*, *89*, 1632–1642.
63. Mason, D. A., Moore, J. D., Green, S. A., et al. (1999). A gain-of-function polymorphism in a G-protein coupling domain of the human β_1-adrenergic receptor. *J Biol Chem*, *274*, 12670–12674.
64. Bristow, M. R. (1993). Pathophysiologic and pharmacologic rationales for clinical management of chronic heart failure with beta-blocking agents. *Am J Cardiol*, *71*, 12C–22C.
65. Agostoni, P., Contini, M., Cattadori, G., et al. (2007). Lung function with carvedilol and bisoprolol in chronic heart failure: is beta selectivity relevant? *Eur J Heart Fail*, *9*, 827–833.
66. Kubo, T., Azevedo, E. R., Newton, G. E., et al. (2001). Lack of evidence for peripheral α_1-adrenoceptor blockade during long-term treatment of heart failure with carvedilol. *J Am Coll Cardiol*, *38*, 1463–1469.
67. Zhu, W., Zeng, X., Zheng, M., et al. (2005). The enigma of β_2-adrenergic receptor G_i signaling in the heart: the good, the bad, and the ugly. *Circ Res*, *97*, 507–509.
68. Liggett, S. B., Tepe, N. M., Lorenz, J. N., et al. (2000). Early and delayed consequences of β_2-adrenergic receptor overexpression in mouse hearts: critical role for expression level. *Circulation*, *101*, 1707–1714.
69. Du, X. J., Autelitano, D. J., Dilley, R. J., et al. (2000). β_2-Adrenergic receptor overexpression exacerbates development of heart failure after aortic stenosis. *Circulation*, *101*, 71–77.
70. Communal, C., Singh, K., Sawyer, D. B., et al. (1999). Opposing effects of β_1- and β_2-adrenergic receptors on cardiac myocyte apoptosis: role of a pertussis toxin–sensitive G protein. *Circulation*, *100*, 2210–2212.
71. Ahmet, I., Krawczyk, M., Heller, P., et al. (2004). Beneficial effects of chronic pharmacological manipulation of beta-adrenoreceptor subtype signaling in rodent dilated ischemic cardiomyopathy. *Circulation*, *110*, 1083–1090.
72. El-Armouche, A., Eschenhagen, T. (2009) Beta-adrenergic stimulation and myocardial function in the failing heart. *Heart Fail Rev. 14*, 225–241.
73. Waagstein, F., Caidahl, K., Wallentin, I., et al. (1989). Long term beta-blockade in dilated cardiomyopathy. Effects of short- and long-term metoprolol treatment followed by withdrawal and readministration of metoprolol. *Circulation*, *80*, 551–563.
74. Heilbrunn, S. M., Shah, P., Bristow, M. R., et al. (1989). Increased beta-receptor density and improved hemodynamic response to catecholamine stimulation during long-term metoprolol therapy in heart failure from dilated cardiomyopathy. *Circulation*, *79*, 483–490.
75. Eichhorn, E. J. (1999). Beta-blocker withdrawal: the song of Orpheus. *Am Heart J*, *138*, 387–389.
76. Metra, M., Nodari, S., D'Aloia, A., et al. (1998). Effects of neurohormonal antagonism on symptoms and quality-of-life in heart failure. *Eur Heart J*, *19*(Suppl. B), B25–B35.
77. Asano, K., Zisman, L. S., Yoshikawa, T., et al. (2001). Bucindolol, a nonselective β_1- and β_2-adrenergic receptor antagonist, decreases beta-adrenergic receptor density in cultured embryonic chick cardiac myocyte membranes. *J Cardiovasc Pharmacol*, *37*, 678–691.
78. Kindermann, M., Maack, C., Schaller, S., et al. (2004). Carvedilol but not metoprolol reduces beta-adrenergic responsiveness after complete elimination from plasma in vivo. *Circulation*, *109*, 3182–3190.
79. Metra, M., Nodari, S., D'Aloia, A., et al. (2002). Beta-blocker therapy influences the hemodynamic response to inotropic agents in patients with heart failure: a randomized comparison of dobutamine and enoximone before and after chronic treatment with metoprolol or carvedilol. *J Am Coll Cardiol*, *40*, 1248–1258.
80. Haber, H. L., Simek, C. L., Gimple, L. W., et al. (1993). Why do patients with congestive heart failure tolerate the initiation of beta-blocker therapy? *Circulation*, *88*, 1610–1619.
81. Rochais, F., Vilardaga, J. P., Nikolaev, V. O., et al. (2007). Real-time optical recording of β_1-adrenergic receptor activation reveals supersensitivity of the Arg389 variant to carvedilol. *J Clin Invest*, *117*, 229–235.
82. Gong, H., Sun, H., Koch, W. J., et al. (2002). Specific β_2AR blocker ICI 118,551 actively decreases contraction through a G_i-coupled form of the β_2AR in myocytes from failing human heart. *Circulation*, *105*, 2497–2503.
83. Cohn, J. N., Pfeffer, M. A., Rouleau, J., et al. (2003). Adverse mortality effect of central sympathetic inhibition with sustained-release moxonidine in patients with heart failure (MOXCON). *Eur J Heart Fail*, *5*, 659–667.
84. Gilbert, E. M., Abraham, W. T., Olsen, S., et al. (1996). Comparative hemodynamic, left ventricular functional, and antiadrenergic effects of chronic treatment with metoprolol versus carvedilol in the failing heart. *Circulation*, *94*, 2817–2825.
85. Azevedo, E. R., Kubo, T., Mak, S., et al. (2001). Nonselective versus selective beta-adrenergic receptor blockade in congestive heart failure: differential effects on sympathetic activity. *Circulation*, *104*, 2194–2199.
86. Beta-Blocker Evaluation of Survival Trial Investigators. (2001). A trial of the beta-blocker bucindolol in patients with advanced chronic heart failure. *N Engl J Med*, *344*, 1659–1667.
87. Bristow, M. R., Krause-Steinrauf, H., Nuzzo, R., et al. (2004). Effect of baseline or changes in adrenergic activity on clinical outcomes in the beta-blocker evaluation of survival trial. *Circulation*, *110*, 1437–1442.
88. Anand, I., Fiuzat, M., O'Connor, C., et al. (2010). Impact of baseline volume status and LVEF on all-cause mortality in the BEST Trial. *J Am Coll Cardiol*, 55, A37, E360.
89. Ladage, D., Brixius, K., Hoyer, H., et al. (2006). Mechanisms underlying nebivolol-induced endothelial nitric oxide synthase activation in human umbilical vein endothelial cells. *Clin Exp Pharmacol Physiol*, *33*, 720–724.
90. Cockcroft, J. R., Chowienczyk, P. J., Brett, S. E., et al. (1995). Nebivolol vasodilates human forearm vasculature: evidence for an l-arginine/NO-dependent mechanism. *J Pharmacol Exp Ther*, *274*, 1067–1071.
91. Mason, R. P., Kubant, R., Jacob, R. F., et al. (2008). Effect of the β_3-receptor antagonist SR59230A on bucindolol-induced release of nitric oxide and peroxynitrite from human endothelium. *J Card Fail*, *14*(Suppl. I), S76.
92. Noda, K., Oka, M., Ma, F. H., et al. (2001). Release of endothelial nitric oxide in coronary arteries by celiprolol, a β_1-adrenoceptor antagonist: possible clinical relevance. *Eur J Pharmacol*, *415*, 209–216.
93. Münzel, T., & Gori, T. (2009). Nebivolol: the somewhat-different beta-adrenergic receptor blocker. *J Am Coll Cardiol*, *54*, 1491–1499.
94. Kamp, O., Metra, M., Bugatti, S., et al. (2010). Nebivolol: haemodynamic effects and clinical significance of combined beta-blockade and nitric oxide release. *Drugs*, *70*, 41–56.
95. Quaife, R. A., Christian, P. E., Gilbert, E. M., et al. (1998). Effects of carvedilol on right ventricular function in chronic heart failure. *Am J Cardiol*, *81*, 247–250.
96. Quaife, R. A., Gilbert, E. M., Christian, P. E., et al. (1996). Effects of carvedilol on systolic and diastolic left ventricular performance in idiopathic dilated cardiomyopathy or ischemic cardiomyopathy. *Am J Cardiol*, *78*, 779–784.
97. Andersson, B., Caidahl, K., di Lenarda, A., et al. (1996). Changes in early and late diastolic filling patterns induced by long-term adrenergic beta-blockade in patients with idiopathic dilated cardiomyopathy. *Circulation*, *94*, 673–682.
98. Metra, M., Nodari, S., Parrinello, G., et al. (2003). Marked improvement in LV EF during long-term beta-blockade in patients with chronic heart failure: clinical correlates and prognostic significance. *Am Heart J*, *145*, 292–299.
99. de Groote, P., Delour, P., Mouquet, F., et al. (2007). The effects of beta-blockers in patients with stable chronic heart failure. Predictors of left ventricular ejection fraction improvement and impact on prognosis. *Am Heart J*, *154*, 589–595.
100. Schleman, K. A., Lindenfeld, J. A., Lowes, B. D., et al. (2001). Predicting response to carvedilol for the treatment of heart failure: a multivariate retrospective analysis. *J Card Fail*, *7*, 4–12.
101. DiLenarda, A., Gregori, D., Sinagra, G., et al. (1996). Metoprolol in dilated cardiomyopathy: is it possible to identify factors predictive of improvement? The Heart Muscle Disease Study Group. *J Card Fail*, *2*, 87–102.

102. Eichhorn, E. J., Grayburn, P. A., Mayer, S. A., et al. (2003). Myocardial contractile reserve by dobutamine stress echocardiography predicts improvement in ejection fraction with beta-blockade in patients with heart failure: the Beta-Blocker Evaluation of Survival Trial (BEST). *Circulation, 108*, 2336–2341.
103. Seghatol, F. F., Shah, D. J., Diluzio, S., et al. (2004). Relation between contractile reserve and improvement in left ventricular function with beta-blocker therapy in patients with heart failure secondary to ischemic or idiopathic dilated cardiomyopathy. *Am J Cardiol, 93*, 854–859.
104. Cleland, J. G., Pennell, D. J., Ray, S. G., et al. (2003). Myocardial viability as a determinant of the ejection fraction response to carvedilol in patients with heart failure (CHRISTMAS trial): randomised controlled trial. *Lancet, 362*, 14–21.
105. Bristow, M. R., Gilbert, E. M., Abraham, W. T., et al. (1996). Carvedilol produces dose-related improvements in left ventricular function and survival in subjects with chronic heart failure. *Circulation, 94*, 2807–2816.
106. Lechat, P., Escolano, S., Golmard, J. L., et al. (1997). Prognostic value of bisoprolol-induced hemodynamic effects in heart failure during the Cardiac Insufficiency BIsoprolol Study (CIBIS). *Circulation, 96*, 2197–2205.
107. White, M., Yanowitz, F., Gilbert, E. M., et al. (1995). Role of beta-adrenergic receptor downregulation in the peak exercise response in patients with heart failure due to idiopathic dilated cardiomyopathy. *Am J Cardiol, 76*, 1271–1276.
108. Packer, M., Colucci, W. S., Sackner-Bernstein, J., et al. (1996). Double-blind, placebo-controlled study of the effects of carvedilol in patients with moderate to severe heart failure: the PRECISE trial. *Circulation, 94*, 2793–2799.
109. Colucci, W. S., Packer, M., Bristow, M. R., et al. (1996). Carvedilol inhibits clinical progression in patients with mild symptoms of heart failure. *Circulation, 94*, 2800–2806.
110. Abdulla, J., Køber, L., Christensen, E., et al. (2006). Effect of beta-blocker therapy on functional status in patients with heart failure—a meta-analysis. *Eur J Heart Fail, 8*, 522–531.
111. Australia/New Zealand Heart Failure Research Collaborative Group (1997). Randomised, placebo-controlled trial of carvedilol in patients with congestive heart failure due to ischaemic heart disease. *Lancet, 349*, 375–380.
112. Brophy, J. M., Joseph, L., & Rouleau, J. L. (2001). Beta-blockers in congestive heart failure. A bayesian meta-analysis. *Ann Intern Med, 134*, 550–560.
113. Metra, M., Ponikowski, P., Dickstein, K., et al. (2007). Advanced chronic heart failure: a position statement from the Study Group on Advanced Heart Failure of the Heart Failure Association of the European Society of Cardiology. *Eur J Heart Fail, 9*, 684–694.
114. Wikstrand, J., Hjalmarson, A., Waagstein, F., et al. (2002). Dose of metoprolol CR/XL and clinical outcomes in patients with heart failure: analysis of the experience in Metoprolol CR/XL Randomized Intervention Trial in Chronic Heart Failure (MERIT-HF). *J Am Coll Cardiol, 40*, 491–498.
115. Simon, T., Mary-Krause, M., Funck-Brentano, C., et al. (2003). Bisoprolol dose-response relationship in patients with congestive heart failure: a subgroup analysis in the Cardiac Insufficiency BIsoprolol Study (CIBIS II). *Eur Heart J, 24*, 552–559.
116. Metra, M., Torp-Pedersen, C., Swedberg, K., et al. (2005). Influence of heart rate, blood pressure, and beta-blocker dose on outcome and the differences in outcome between carvedilol and metoprolol tartrate in patients with chronic heart failure: results from the COMET trial. *Eur Heart J, 26*, 2259–2268.
117. Dobre, D., van Veldhuisen, D. J., Mordenti, G., et al. (2007). Tolerability and dose-related effects of nebivolol in elderly patients with heart failure: data from the Study of the Effects of Nebivolol Intervention on Outcomes and Rehospitalisation in Seniors with Heart Failure (SENIORS) trial. *Am Heart J, 154*, 109–115.
118. Rouleau, J. L., Roecker, E. B., Tendera, M., et al. (2004). Influence of pretreatment systolic blood pressure on the effect of carvedilol in patients with severe chronic heart failure: the Carvedilol Prospective Randomized Cumulative Survival (COPERNICUS) study. *J Am Coll Cardiol, 43*, 1423–1429.
119. Anderson, J. L., Krause-Steinrauf, H., Goldman, S., et al. (2003). Failure of benefit and early hazard of bucindolol for classs IV heart failure. *J Card Fail. 9*, 266–77.
120. Domanski, M., Krause-Steinrauf, H., Deedwania, P., et al. (2003). The effect of diabetes on outcomes of patients with advanced heart failure in the BEST trial. *J Am Coll Cardiol, 42*, 914–922.
121. Domanski, M. J., Krause-Steinrauf, H., Massie, B. M., et al. (2003). A comparative analysis of the results from 4 trials of beta-blocker therapy for heart failure: BEST, CIBIS-II, MERIT-HF, and COPERNICUS. *J Card Fail, 9*, 354–363.
122. Cresci, S., Kelly, R. J., Cappola, T. P., et al. (2009). Clinical and genetic modifiers of long-term survival in heart failure. *J Am Coll Cardiol, 54*, 432–444.
123. Bristow, M. R., Murphy, G. A., Krause-Steinrauf, H., et al. (2010). An α_{2c}-adrenergic receptor polymorphism alters the norepinephrine-lowering effects and therapeutic response of the beta-blocker bucindolol in chronic heart failure. *Circ Heart Fail, 3*, 21–28.
124. Cohen-Solal, A., Kotecha, D., van Veldhuisen, D. J., et al. (2009). Efficacy and safety of nebivolol in elderly heart failure patients with impaired renal function: insights from the SENIORS trial. *Eur J Heart Fail, 11*, 872–880.
125. Bristow, M. R., Feldman, A. M., Adams, K. F., Jr., et al. (2003). Selective versus nonselective beta-blockade for heart failure therapy: are there lessons to be learned from the COMET trial? *J Card Fail, 9*, 444–453.
126. Kukin, M. L., Kalman, J., Charney, R. H., et al. (1999). Prospective, randomized comparison of effect of long-term treatment with etoprolol or carvedilol on symptoms, exercise, ejection fraction, and oxidative stress in heart failure. *Circulation, 99*, 2645–2651.
127. Sanderson, J. E., Chan, S. K., Yip, G., et al. (1999). Beta-blockade in heart failure: a comparison of carvedilol with metoprolol. *J Am Coll Cardiol, 34*, 1522–1528.
128. Metra, M., Giubbini, R., Nodari, S., et al. (2000). Differential effects of β-blockers in patients with heart failure. A prospective, double-blind comparison of the long-term effects of metoprolol versus carvedilol. *Circulation, 102*, 546–551.
129. Poole-Wilson, P. A., Swedberg, K., Cleland, J. G., et al. (2003). Comparison of carvedilol and metoprolol on clinical outcomes in patients with chronic heart failure in the Carvedilol Or Metoprolol European Trial (COMET): randomised controlled trial. *Lancet, 362*, 7–13.
130. Packer, M. (2003). Do beta-blockers prolong survival in heart failure only by inhibiting the β_1-receptor? A perspective on the results of the COMET trial. *J Card Fail, 9*, 429–443.
131. Massie, B. M. (2003). A comment on COMET: how to interpret a positive trial? *J Card Fail, 9*, 425–428.
132. Dargie, H. J. (2003). Beta blockers in heart failure. *Lancet, 362*, 2–3.
133. Hjalmarson, A., & Waagstein, F. (2003). COMET: a proposed mechanism of action to explain the results and concerns about dose. *Lancet, 362*, 1077.
134. McMurray, J., Cohen-Solal, A., Dietz, R., et al. (2005). Practical recommendations for the use of ACE inhibitors, beta-blockers, aldosterone antagonists and angiotensin receptor blockers in heart failure: putting guidelines into practice. *Eur J Heart Fail, 7*, 710–721.
135. Willenheimer, R., van Veldhuisen, D. J., Silke, B., et al. (2005). Effect on survival and hospitalization of initiating treatment for chronic heart failure with bisoprolol followed by enalapril, as compared with the opposite sequence: results of the randomized Cardiac Insufficiency Bisoprolol Study (CIBIS) III. *Circulation, 112*, 2426–2435.
136. Dobre, D., van Veldhuisen, D. J., Goulder, M. A., et al. (2008). Clinical effects of initial 6 months monotherapy with bisoprolol versus enalapril in the treatment of patients with mild to moderate chronic heart failure. Data from the CIBIS III trial. *Cardiovasc Drugs Ther, 22*, 399–405.
137. Fang, J. C. (2005). Angiotensin-converting enzyme inhibitors or beta-blockers in heart failure: does it matter who goes first? *Circulation, 112*, 2380–2382.
138. Gattis, W. A., O'Connor, C. M., Leimberger, J. D., et al. (2003). Clinical outcomes in patients on beta-blocker therapy admitted with worsening chronic heart failure. *Am J Cardiol, 91*, 169–174.
139. Butler, J., Young, J. B., Abraham, W. T., et al. (2006). Beta-blocker use and outcomes among hospitalized heart failure patients. *J Am Coll Cardiol, 47*, 2462–2469.
140. Metra, M., Torp-Pedersen, C., Cleland, J. G., et al. (2007). Should beta-blocker therapy be reduced or withdrawn after an episode of decompensated heart failure? Results from COMET. *Eur J Heart Fail, 9*, 901–909.
141. Fonarow, G. C., Abraham, W. T., Albert, N. M., et al. (2008). Influence of beta-blocker continuation or withdrawal on outcomes in patients hospitalized with heart failure: findings from the OPTIMIZE-HF program. *J Am Coll Cardiol, 52*, 190–199.
142. Orso, F., Baldasseroni, S., Fabbri, G., et al. (2009). Role of beta-blockers in patients admitted for worsening heart failure in a real world setting: data from the Italian Survey on Acute Heart Failure. *Eur J Heart Fail, 11*, 77–84.
143. Jondeau, G., Neuder, Y., Eicher, J. C., et al. (2009). B-CONVINCED: Beta-blocker CONtinuation Vs. INterruption in patients with Congestive heart failure hospitalizED for a decompensation episode. *Eur Heart J, 30*, 2186–2192.
144. Komajda, M., Lapuerta, P., Hermans, N., et al. (2005). Adherence to guidelines is a predictor of outcome in chronic heart failure: the MAHLER survey. *Eur Heart J, 26*, 1653–1659.
145. Gislason, G. H., Rasmussen, J. N., Abildstrom, S. Z., et al. (2007). Persistent use of evidence-based pharmacotherapy in heart failure is associated with improved outcomes. *Circulation, 116*, 737–744.
146. Fonarow, G. C., Abraham, W. T., Albert, N. M., et al. (2007). Association between performance measures and clinical outcomes for patients hospitalized with heart failure. *JAMA, 297*, 61–70.
147. O'Connor, C. M., Abraham, W. T., Albert, N. M., et al. (2008). Predictors of mortality after discharge in patients hospitalized with heart failure: an analysis from the Organized Program to Initiate Lifesaving Treatment in Hospitalized Patients with Heart Failure (OPTIMIZE-HF). *Am Heart J, 156*, 662–673.
148. Hernandez, A. F., Hammill, B. G., O'Connor, C. M., et al. (2009). Clinical effectiveness of beta-blockers in heart failure: findings from the OPTIMIZE-HF (Organized Program to Initiate Lifesaving Treatment in Hospitalized Patients with Heart Failure) Registry. *J Am Coll Cardiol, 53*, 184–192.
149. Tandon, P., McAlister, F. A., Tsuyuki, R. T., et al. (2004). The use of beta-blockers in a tertiary care heart failure clinic: dosing, tolerance, and outcomes. *Arch Intern Med, 164*, 769–774.
150. Patel, P., White, D. L., & Deswal, A. (2007). Translation of clinical trial results into practice: temporal patterns of beta-blocker utilization for heart failure at hospital discharge and during ambulatory follow-up. *Am Heart J, 153*, 515–522.
151. de Groote, P., Isnard, R., Assyag, P., et al. (2007). Is the gap between guidelines and clinical practice in heart failure treatment being filled? Insights from the IMPACT RECO survey. *Eur J Heart Fail, 9*, 1205–1211.
152. Komajda, M., Hanon, O., Hochadel, M., et al. (2009). Contemporary management of octogenarians hospitalized for heart failure in Europe: Euro Heart Failure Survey II. *Eur Heart J, 30*, 478–486.
153. Komajda, M., Follath, F., Swedberg, K., et al. (2003). The Euro Heart Failure Survey programme—a survey on the quality of care among patients with heart failure in Europe. Part 2: treatment. *Eur Heart J, 24*, 464–474.
154. Yancy, C. W., Fonarow, G. C., Albert, N. M., et al. (2009). Influence of patient age and sex on delivery of guideline-recommended heart failure care in the outpatient cardiology practice setting: findings from IMPROVE HF. *Am Heart J, 157*, 754–762.
155. Forman, D. E., Cannon, C. P., Hernandez, A. F., et al. (2009). Influence of age on the management of heart failure: findings from Get With the Guidelines—Heart Failure (GWTG-HF). *Am Heart J, 157*, 1010–1017.
156. Sirak, T. H., Jelic, S., Le Jemtel, T. H. (2004). Therapeutic update: non-selective Beta- and alpha-adrenergic blockade in patients with coexistent chronic obstructive pulmonary disease and chronic heart failure. *J Am Coll Cardiol, 44*, 497–502.
157. Remme, W. J., McMurray, J. J., Hobbs, F. D., et al. (2008). Awareness and perception of heart failure among European cardiologists, internists, geriatricians, and primary care physicians. *Eur Heart J, 29*, 1739–1752.
158. Fonarow, G. C., Yancy, C. W., Albert, N. M., et al. (2008). Heart failure care in the outpatient cardiology practice setting: findings from IMPROVE HF. *Circ Heart Fail, 1*, 98–106.

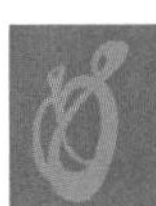

159. Shelton, R. J., Rigby, A. S., Cleland, J. G., et al. (2006). Effect of a community heart failure clinic on uptake of beta blockers by patients with obstructive airways disease and heart failure. *Heart, 92*, 331–336.
160. Gustafsson, F., Schou, M., Videbaek, L., et al. (2007). Treatment with beta-blockers in nurse-led heart failure clinics: titration efficacy and predictors of failure. *Eur J Heart Fail, 9*, 910–916.
161. Hauptman, P. J., Rich, M. W., Heidenreich, P. A., et al. (2008). The heart failure clinic: a consensus statement of the Heart Failure Society of America. *J Card Fail, 14*, 801–815.
162. LaPointe, N. M., DeLong, E. R., Chen, A., et al. (2006). Multifaceted intervention to promote beta-blocker use in heart failure. *Am Heart J, 151*, 992–998.
163. Fonarow, G. C., Gheorghiade, M., & Abraham, W. T. (2004). Importance of in-hospital initiation of evidence-based medical therapies for heart failure—a review. *Am J Cardiol, 94*, 1155–1160.
164. Owan, T. E., Hodge, D. O., Herges, R. M., et al. (2006). Trends in prevalence and outcome of heart failure with preserved ejection fraction. *N Engl J Med, 355*, 251–259.
165. Hamdani, N., Paulus, W. J., van Heerebeek, L., et al. (2009). Distinct myocardial effects of beta-blocker therapy in heart failure with normal and reduced left ventricular ejection fraction. *Eur Heart J, 30*, 1863–1872.
166. Kerzner, R., Gage, B. F., Freedland, K. E., et al. (2003). Predictors of mortality in younger and older patients with heart failure and preserved or reduced left ventricular ejection fraction. *Am Heart J, 146*, 286–290.
167. Dobre, D., van Veldhuisen, D. J., DeJongste, M. J., et al. (2007). Prescription of beta-blockers in patients with advanced heart failure and preserved left ventricular ejection fraction. Clinical implications and survival. *Eur J Heart Fail, 9*, 280–286.
168. Shah, R., Wang, Y., & Foody, J. M. (2008). Effect of statins, angiotensin-converting enzyme inhibitors, and beta blockers on survival in patients >or=65 years of age with heart failure and preserved left ventricular systolic function. *Am J Cardiol, 101*, 217–222.
169. Robinson, P., & Bristow, M. R. (2005). Beta blockers. In A. M. Feldman (Ed.),. *The pharmacologic management of chronic heart failure*. London: Blackwell Publishing.
170. Eichhorn, E. J., & Bristow, M. R. (1997). Practical guidelines for initiation of β-adrenergic blockade in patients with chronic heart failure. *Am J. Cardiol, 79*, 794–798.
171. Shakar, S. F., Abraham, W. T., Gilbert, E. M., et al. (1998). Combined oral positive inotropic and beta-blocker therapy for treatment of refractory class IV heart failure. *J Am Coll Cardiol, 31*, 1336–1340.
172. Fonarow, G. C. (2009). Role of carvedilol controlled-release in cardiovascular disease. *Expert Rev Cardiovasc Ther, 7*, 483–498.
173. Balligand, J. L. (2009). β_3-Adrenoceptor stimulation on top of β_1-adrenoceptor blockade "Stop or Encore?" *J Am Coll Cardiol, 53*, 1539–1542. PubMedPMID: 19389565.
174. McAlister, F. A., Wiebe, N., Ezekowitz, J. A., et al. (2009). Meta-analysis: beta-blocker dose, heart rate reduction, and death in patients with heart failure. *Ann Intern Med, 150*, 784–794.
175. Flannery, G., Gehrig-Mills, R., Billah, B., et al. (2008). Analysis of randomized controlled trials on the effect of magnitude of heart rate reduction on clinical outcomes in patients with systolic chronic heart failure receiving beta-blockers. *Am J Cardiol, 101*, 865–869.
176. Swedberg, K., Komajda, M., Böhm, M., et al. (2010). Rationale and design of a randomized, double-blind, placebo-controlled outcome trial of ivabradine in chronic heart failure: the Systolic Heart Failure Treatment with the I(f) Inhibitor Ivabradine Trial (SHIFT). *Eur J Heart Fail, 12*, 75–81.
177. Morley, M., Molony, C. M., Weber, T. M., et al. (2004). Genetic analysis of genome-wide variation in human gene expression. *Nature, 430*, 743–747.
178. Taylor, M. R. G., & Bristow, M. R. (2004). The emerging pharmacogenomics of the beta-adrenergic receptors. *Congest Heart Fail, 10*, 281–288.
179. Liggett, S. B., Mialet-Perez, J., Thaneemit-Chen, S., et al. (2006). A polymorphism within a conserved β_1-adrenergic receptor motif alters cardiac function and beta-blocker response in human heart failure. *Proc Natl Acad Sci U S A, 103*, 11288–11293.
180. Mialet Perez, J., Rathz, D. A., Petrashevskaya, N. N., et al. (2003). β_1-Adrenergic receptor polymorphisms confer differential function and predisposition to heart failure. *Nat Med, 9*, 1300–1305.
181. Green, S. A., Cole, G., Jacinto, M., et al. (1993). A polymorphism of the human β_2-adrenergic receptor within the fourth transmembrane domain alters ligand binding and functional properties of the receptor. *J Biol Chem, 268*, 23116–32121.
182. Liggett, S. B., Wagoner, L. E., Craft, L. L., et al. (1998). The Ile164 β_2-adrenergic receptor polymorphism adversely affects the outcome of congestive heart failure. *J Clin Invest, 102*, 1534–1539.
183. Small, K. M., Forbes, S. L., Rahman, F. F., et al. (2000). A four amino acid deletion polymorphism in the third intracellular loop of the human α_{2c}-adrenergic receptor confers impaired coupling to multiple effectors. *J Biol Chem, 275*, 23059–23064.
184. Terra, S. G., Hamilton, K. K., Pauly, D. F., et al. (2005). β_1-adrenergic receptor polymorphisms and left ventricular remodeling changes in response to beta-blocker therapy. *Pharmacogenet Genomics, 15*, 227–234.
185. de Groote, P., Helbecque, N., Lamblin, N., et al. (2005). Association between β_1 and β_2 adrenergic receptor gene polymorphisms and the response to beta-blockade in patients with stable congestive heart failure. *Pharmacogenet Genomics, 15*, 137–142.
186. Metra M, Covolo L, Pezzali N, et al. (2010). Role of β-adrenergic receptor gene polymorphisms in the long-term effects of β-blockade with carvedilol in patients with chronic heart failure. *Cardiovasc Drugs Ther*, 24, 49-60. PubMed PMID: 20352314.
187. Muthumala, A., Drenos, F., Elliott, P. M., et al. (2008). Role of beta adrenergic receptor polymorphisms in heart failure: systematic review and meta-analysis. *Eur J Heart Fail, 10*, 3–13.
188. Kaye, D. M., Smirk, B., Williams, C., et al. (2003). Beta-adrenoceptor genotype influences the response to carvedilol in patients with congestive heart failure. *Pharmacogenetics, 13*, 379–382.
189. White, H. L., de Boer, R. A., Maqbool, A., et al. (2003). An evaluation of the β_1 adrenergic receptor Arg389Gly polymorphism in individuals with heart failure: a MERIT-HF sub-study. *Eur J Heart Fail, 5*, 463–468.
190. Hein, L., Altman, J. D., & Kobilka, B. K. (1999). Two functionally distinct α_2-adrenergic receptors regulate sympathetic neurotransmission. *Nature, 402*, 181–184.
191. Brede, M., Wiesmann, F., Jahns, R., et al. (2002). Feedback inhibition of catecholamine release by two different α_2-adrenoceptor subtypes prevents progression of heart failure. *Circulation, 106*, 2491–2496.
192. Sehnert, A. J., Daniels, S. E., Elashoff, M., et al. (2008). Lack of association between adrenergicreceptorgenotypesandsurvivalinheartfailurepatientstreatedwithcarvedilol or metoprolol. *J Am Coll Cardiol, 52*, 644–651.
193. Walsh, R., Farmer, R., Kelly, M., et al. (2008). Human myocardial β_1 389 Arg/Arg adrenergic receptors exhibit a propensity for constitutively active, high affinity agonist binding and are selectively inactivated by bucindolol. *J Card Fail, 14*(Suppl. I), S8.
194. Nelson, B., Morrison, J., Nelson, P., et al. (2007). Beta-blocking agents have codon 389 Arg/Gly genotype specific effects in isolated human heart preparations. *J Am Coll Cardiol, 49*(Suppl. 1), 77A.
195. O'Connor, C., Anand, I., Fiuzat, M., et al. (2008). Additive effects of β_1 389 Arg/Gly α_{2c} 322–325Wt/Deladrenergicreceptorgenotypecombinationsonadjudicatedhospitalizations and death in the BEST trial. *J Card Fail, 14*, S69.

CHAPTER 47

Device Therapy in Heart Failure

Bruce L. Wilkoff and Daniel J. Cantillon

The goals for device therapy in heart failure are to extend life by detecting and treating arrhythmias, to apply pacing strategies when needed to reduce morbidity and mortality from the disease, and to provide valuable diagnostic information to the managing clinician. The first two goals are the mainstays of current device therapy; the third holds enormous promise as technology advances beyond the devices' standard reporting of arrhythmia events to the ability to provide additional hemodynamic data.

SUDDEN CARDIAC DEATH

Progression of disease and the associated clinical complications account for the majority of deaths from heart failure. However, unexpected death from arrhythmia remains an important and treatable cause across the spectrum of heart failure. In the Metoprolol CR/XL Randomised Intervention Trial in Congestive Heart Failure (MERIT-HF),[1] the incidence of sudden death rose incrementally from 6.3% among patients with New York Heart Association (NYHA) class II heart failure to 10.5% among patients with class III and 18.6% among patients with class IV heart failure. However, the relative percentages of sudden deaths demonstrate the opposite trend: they were highest, at 64%, among patients with class II heart failure and fell as functional class worsened (Figure 47-1). Most commonly, sudden death results from ventricular tachycardia with secondary degeneration into ventricular fibrillation (see Chapter 46). Moreover, although bradyarrhythmia accounts for only 5% to 10% of sudden death among patients with heart failure, this category is perhaps more commonly overlooked by contemporary clinicians, who are focused on tachyarrhythmias.

THE BASICS OF IMPLANTABLE CARDIOVERTER-DEFIBRILLATORS (ICDs)

A precisely engineered and encased battery, capacitor, lead connectors, computer chip with memory, and software (known as "the can") are typically implanted in the prepectoral space; a combined insulated pacing and defibrillator lead typically passes through the subclavian vein into the right ventricle. Many implantable cardiovert-defibrillator (ICD) leads also contain a second shocking coil, which is typically located in the superior vena cava or right atrium by virtue of its distance from the lead tip, and it can be readily located under fluoroscopy or routine chest radiography. The lead transmits the local electrographic reading at the myocardial contact site back to the can, where the information is processed. If any tachyarrhythmia is detected, the device can deliver both pacing and shock therapies designed to terminate the arrhythmia in response to a wide array of programmable parameters. If a shock is indicated, the capacitor charges to a prespecified voltage and delivers an electrical shock current by means of a prespecified vector. The shock vector is usually determined at the time of implantation, when the defibrillation threshold is checked. It can be configured between the right ventricle coil and the superior vena cava coil or between the right ventricle coil and the can, or it can include additional separate implantable shocking coils.

When the device is tested, ventricular fibrillation is most commonly induced in the electrophysiology laboratory by right ventricular pacing, followed by a low-voltage shock administered during cardiac repolarization as timed during the T-wave, or it is induced by application of a 10-V direct current. The device is then given the opportunity to detect fibrillation (which is often of low amplitude) and to deliver the appropriate therapy. The defibrillation threshold (generally 10 to 20 J) is then documented and can be modified by changing the shock vector or ultimately even adding another shocking coil into the coronary sinus, azygous vein, or subcutaneously. Routine defibrillation threshold testing has become somewhat controversial, but it is still practiced by the majority of electrophysiologists.

Antitachycardia Pacing

In addition to shocks, antitachycardia pacing can be delivered in response to a detected ventricular arrhythmia. Burst pacing is a type of antitachycardia pacing in which the device delivers a ventricular stimulation sequence at a cycle length that is slightly shorter than that of the tachycardia (i.e., a faster heart rate) in an attempt to cause either unidirectional or bidirectional block in the reentry circuit and thus terminate the arrhythmia. The device can also deliver ramp pacing, in which the paced cycle length is incrementally decreased to enable a wider range of paced cycle lengths to break the arrhythmia loop. Multiple algorithms have been developed, stemming historically from a time when diagnostic electrophysiological studies were more commonly performed to induce ventricular arrhythmias to test drug sensitivity or as a criterion for ICD placement. Operators routinely used these pacing strategies in an attempt to reduce the need for shocking the patient during spontaneous tachycardias.

Device Programming

The contemporary ICD has programmable "tachycardia zones," which are nothing more than prespecified heart rate ranges to which the device responds with a prespecified

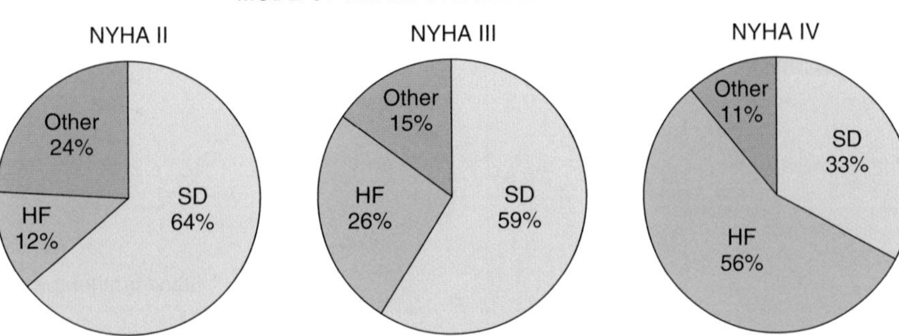

FIGURE 47–1 Severity of heart failure (HF) and mode of death in the Metoprolol CR/XL Randomised Intervention Trial in Congestive Heart Failure (MERIT-HF) trial. NYHA, New York Heart Association (classification); SD, sudden death. (Modified from MERIT-HF Study Group. Effect of metoprolol CR/XL in chronic heart failure: Metoprolol CR/XL Randomised Intervention Trial in Congestive Heart Failure (MERIT-HF). *Lancet* 1999;353:2001-2007.)

TABLE 47–1 Detection of Ventricular Tachyarrhythmias and Subsequent Therapy

Detection Zone	Detection Rate (Beats per Minute)	Duration	Response
Very fast	250	30 of 40 beats	High-energy shock
Intermediate	182	30 of 40 beats	Antitachycardia pacing first and, if needed, shock
Slow	167	32 beats	Only record the rhythm

Detection of ventricular tachyarrhythmias and the subsequent therapy is segmented by rate zones, duration of the tachycardia, and appropriate therapy for tachycardia characteristics in a particular zone. Duration is often programmed in seconds faster than a certain rate instead of number of heartbeats in a particular rate zone. The parameters displayed in the table are based on those that were used in the Primary Prevention Parameters Evaluation (PREPARE) study for patients with primary prevention indications for the implantable cardioverter-defibrillator.

From Wilkoff BL, Williamson BD, Stern RS, et al. Strategic programming of detection and therapy parameters in implantable cardioverter-defibrillators reduces shocks in primary prevention patients: results from the PREPARE (Primary Prevention Parameters Evaluation) study. *J Am Coll Cardiol* 2008;52:541-550.

therapy (Table 47-1). This allows the clinician the opportunity to choose less aggressive pacing therapies during slower tacharrhythmias (typically 170 to 180 beats per minute), which are more likely to be hemodynamically tolerated, and more aggressive pacing therapies plus rapid defibrillation at the highest available shock voltage for more urgently life-threatening ventricular fibrillation or fast ventricular tachycardia. When an atrial lead is present, the device can use the local electrographic reading to compare the atrial rate with the ventricular rate in an effort to discriminate supraventricular arrhythmias, to document atrioventricular dissociation, and to help avoid inappropriate shocks (e.g., when the atrial rate is greater than the ventricular rate, as is the case with atrial flutter with 2:1 block). When the atrial rate is equal to the ventricular rate, or in the case when only a right ventricle lead is present, the device can apply morphological criteria to compare the QRS electrographical reading to a stored "native" QRS electrographical reading when the patient is known to be in normal sinus rhythm. Used in this manner, the atrial lead can help discriminate an atrial arrhythmia with 1:1 conduction from a ventricular arrhythmia with retrograde conduction through the atrioventricular node into the atria. As discussed later in this chapter, increasingly sophisticated methods are under development to prevent inappropriate shocks.

Primary Prevention of Sudden Cardiac Death

Contemporary ICD indications have evolved historically from the notion that the prophylactic suppression of ventricular ectopy and arrhythmias is insufficient for adequately managing all at-risk patients.[2] According to the *VPC* (ventricular premature contraction) *suppression hypothesis,* ectopy in at-risk patients with left ventricular dysfunction triggered lethal arrhythmias, and suppression would lead to improved outcomes. In the Cardiac Arrhythmia Suppression Trial (CAST),[3] however, the class Ic antiarrhythmics flecainide and encainide actually increased mortality in comparison with placebo, and thus this hypothesis was set aside. According to the *electrophysiology-inducible suppression hypothesis,* the induction of ventricular arrhythmias by means of programmed stimulation techniques in the electrophysiology laboratory, and subsequent suppression with antiarrhythmic drugs, could improve outcomes. Problems arose in that a suppressing therapy was found for only approximately half the patients with inducible arrhythmia. Furthermore, electrophysiological testing has limited predictive ability, especially in patients with nonischemic cardiomyopathy. Programmed stimulation is very effective in inducing arrhythmias with a reentrant mechanism created by a focal area of scarring, for example, as is the case in ischemic heart disease, but it is limited in assessing arrhythmias by other mechanisms. In the Multicenter Unsustained Tachycardia Trial (MUSTT),[4] patients with inducible arrhythmia clearly had improved outcomes with ICDs. This led to subsequent ICD trials designed to refine this concept and to create the contemporary guidelines.

The ACC/AHA/ESC 2008 Guidelines for Device-Based Therapy of Cardiac Rhythm Abnormalities[5] for primary prevention ICDs reflect lessons learned from four major trials (Table 47-2). In MUSTT,[4] patients with inducible ventricular tachycardia, left ventricular ejection fraction (LVEF) of 40% or lower, and documented coronary artery disease demonstrated a survival benefit with ICDs. In the Defibrillators in Non-Ischemic Cardiomyopathy Treatment Evaluation (DEFINITE),[6] patients with NYHA functional class III symptoms, nonischemic cardiomyopathy, nonsustained ventricular tachycardia (NSVT), and LVEF of 35% or lower demonstrated a reduction in sudden deaths from cardiac arrhythmias. In this study, a total of 229 patients were randomly assigned to receive standard medical therapy and 229 to receive standard medical therapy plus a single-chamber ICD. As shown in Figure 47-2, all-cause death was not reduced in DEFINITE (hazard ratio, 0.65; 95% confidence interval [CI], 0.40 to 1.06; $P = .08$), whereas there was a significant ($P < .006$) reduction in sudden deaths from cardiac arrhythmias (hazard ratio, 0.20; 95% CI, 0.06 to 0.71). Thus, in patients with severe nonischemic dilated cardiomyopathy who were treated with angiotensin-converting enzyme (ACE) inhibitors and β-blockers, the implantation of an ICD significantly reduced the risk of sudden death from arrhythmia and was associated with a nonsignificant reduction in the risk of death from any cause.

In the Multicenter Automatic Defibrillator Implantation Trial II (MADIT II),[7] patients with LVEF of 30% or lower 30 days after myocardial infarction demonstrated a 5.6% absolute reduction in mortality (hazard ratio, 0.69; 95% CI, 0.51 to 0.93; $P = .016$) in comparison with routine care over

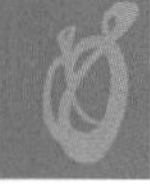

TABLE 47–2 Summary of Indications for Implantable Cardioverter-Defibrillator in a Population with Heart Failure

Primary Prevention	Secondary Prevention
Ischemic Cardiomyopathy	
NYHA classes I, II, III 30 days after myocardial infarction, LVEF ≤ 30%	Survival after cardiac arrest or sudden death >5 days after myocardial infarction
Nonischemic Cardiomyopathy	
NYHA class II or III LVEF ≤ 35% and NSVT 3 months on standard medical therapy	Sustained ventricular tachyarrhythmia >30 seconds or necessitating therapeutic termination because of hemodynamic compromise*
Both Types of Cardiomyopathies	
NYHA class II or III, LVEF ≤ 35% LVEF 35% to 40%, NSVT, and inducible ventricular tachycardia with programmed stimulation	Unexplained syncope and left ventricular dysfunction†

*Attributable to a nonreversible condition (i.e., not a transient electrolyte abnormality or a medication or drug effect).

†See text discussion regarding the need for additional risk stratification.

LVEF, left ventricular ejection fraction; NSVT, nonsustained ventricular tachycardia; NYHA, New York Heart Association.

approximately 2 years (Figure 47-3). The effect of defibrillator therapy on survival was similar in subgroup analyses stratified according to age, sex, ejection fraction, NYHA class, and the QRS interval. In the Sudden Cardiac Death in Heart Failure Trial (SCD-HeFT),[8] patients with both ischemic and nonischemic cardiomyopathy who were receiving optimal medical therapy (ACE inhibitor/angiotensin receptor blocker, β-blocker, and an aldosterone antagonist), had an LVEF of 35% or lower, and had NYHA class II or III heart failure demonstrated an absolute 7.2% reduction in mortality in comparison with similar patients who received, in addition, amiodarone treatment or placebo over approximately 4 years. As shown in Figure 47-4, amiodarone, in comparison with placebo, was associated with a similar risk of death (hazard ratio, 1.06; 97.5% CI, 0.86 to 1.30; $P = .53$), whereas ICD therapy was associated with a 23% relative decreased risk of death (hazard ratio, 0.77; 97.5% CI, 0.62 to 0.96; $P = .007$). ICD implantation guidelines are summarized in Table 47-2.

Third-party payer reimbursement for ICD implantation is a separate issue. In 2005, the Center for Medicare and Medicaid Services stipulated that it would reimburse ICD implantation for primary prevention in patients who had nonischemic cardiomyopathy and LVEF of 35% or lower, provided that they have carried the diagnosis for 3 months and still meet the criteria for inclusion in the national ICD registry.[9] This waiting period is designed to allow time for myocardial recovery and improvement in LVEF after treatment with ACE inhibitors and β-blockers. Similarly, patients with LVEF of 30% or lower after myocardial infarction are required to wait 40 days after myocardial infarction and 3 months after revascularization.

Although ICDs are effective at preventing sudden death, identifying the patients at risk is a major challenge. Current guidelines unquestionably miss the mark.[10] Approximately 66% of sudden deaths occur among patients with significant structural heart disease; however, the sheer size of the population at "low risk" still accounts for the largest absolute number of sudden deaths in the United States annually.[11] Because there is currently no way of identifying them, they are not considered candidates for primary prevention ICDs. Similarly, the current inclusion criteria do not positively and

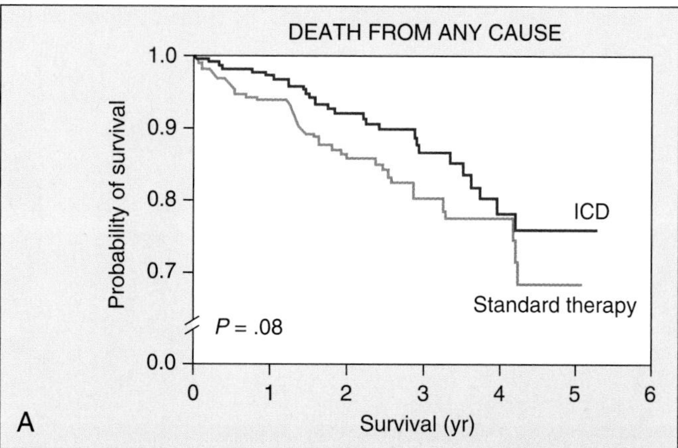

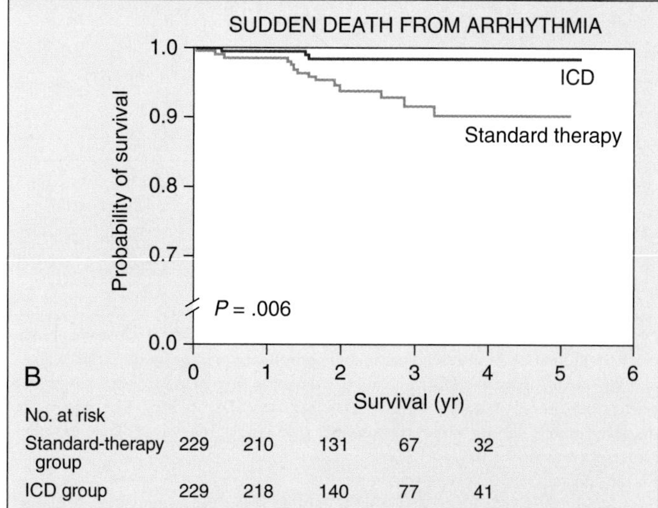

FIGURE 47–2 Kaplan-Meier estimates of death from any cause (**A**) and sudden death from arrhythmia (**B**) among patients who received standard therapy and those who received an implantable cardioverter-defibrillator (ICD) in the Defibrillators in Non-Ischemic Cardiomyopathy Treatment Evaluation (DEFINITE) trial. (Modified from Kadish A, Dyer A, Daubert JP, et al. Prophylactic defibrillator implantation in patients with nonischemic dilated cardiomyopathy. *N Engl J Med* 2004;350:2151-2158.)

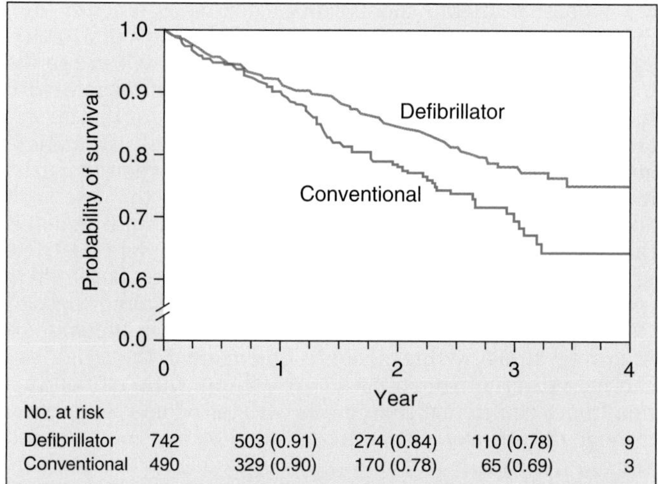

FIGURE 47–3 Kaplan-Meier estimates of the probability of survival among the patients assigned to receive an implantable defibrillator and the patients assigned to receive conventional medical therapy in the Multicenter Automatic Defibrillator Implantation Trial II (MADIT II) trial. (Modified from Moss AJ, Zareba W, Hall WJ, et al. Prophylactic implantation of a defibrillator in patients with myocardial infarction and reduced ejection fraction. *N Engl J Med* 2002;346:877-883.)

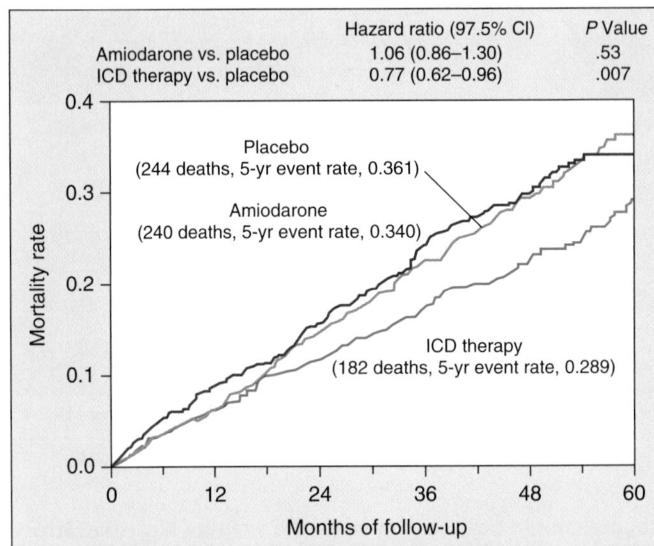

FIGURE 47–4 Kaplan-Meier analysis of the time to death from any cause in patients receiving conventional therapy for heart failure, conventional therapy plus amiodarone, or conventional therapy plus a conservatively programmed, shock-only, single-lead implantable cardioverter-defibrillator (ICD) in the Sudden Cardiac Death in Heart Failure Trial (SCD-HeFT). CI, confidence interval. (Modified from Bardy GH, Lee KL, Mark DB, et al. Amiodarone or an implantable cardioverter-defibrillator for congestive heart failure. *N Engl J Med* 2005;352:225-237.)

adequately predict who will have an event; rather, they identify only an approximate population that derive mortality-related benefit overall. Over the years, many risk-stratification modalities have been evaluated, in addition to cause of cardiomyopathy, NYHA classification, LVEF, and inducibility of arrhythmia. Included among the additional modalities listed in Table 47-3 are heart rate variability, signal-averaged electrocardiography, baroreceptor sensitivity, and microvolt T-wave alternans (MTWA) testing. Of these, MTWA testing is the most heavily studied modality and is the only modality besides invasive electrophysiological testing to gain the reimbursement approval from the Center for Medicare and Medicaid Studies. T-wave alternans—microvolt beat-to-beat alterations in the amplitude, duration, or structure of the T-wave—has been clearly associated with ventricular arrhythmias and mortality.[12,13] Cantillon and associates[14] demonstrated that MTWA testing is superior to electrophysiological testing in predicting ventricular arrhythmias among patients with an LVEF of 35% or lower with either NSVT or unexplained syncope. This study also demonstrated that the MTWA result was a robust predictor both in patients with ischemic cardiomyopathy and in those with nonischemic cardiomyopathy but that the 2 year event rate for sustained ventricular tachycardia or death was approximately 10% among the patients with negative MTWA findings (almost twofold higher than in previously published studies with cohorts at lower risk). In addition, presentation of the Microvolt T-Wave Alternans Testing for Risk Stratification of Post-MI Patients (MASTER) I data, in which T-wave alternans was predictive of all-cause mortality but not of the need for appropriate ICD shocks for ventricular tachycardia, has led to some doubt that this modality can sufficiently stand alone to identify patients at risk. Multiple trials are under way to investigate combining some of the previously associated modalities for risk stratification to further refine current indications for primary prevention.

Secondary Prevention of Sudden Cardiac Death

ICD implantation for secondary prevention involves treating clinically documented ventricular arrhythmias or those that are highly suspected as a cause of hemodynamic compromise.

TABLE 47–3 Adjunctive Modalities for Stratification of Sudden Death Risk in Patients with Heart Failure

Modality	Pathological Finding
Programmed stimulation (electrophysiological testing)	Sustained VT/VF with double or triple extra stimuli
Microvolt T-wave alternans testing	Positive or indeterminate result
Event or Holter monitoring	Sustained or nonsustained VT or VF
Heart rate variability (turbulence)	Loss of heart rate variability
Baroreceptor sensitivity	Loss of normal vagal response
QRS duration and structure	≥120 msec, left bundle branch block
Exercise stress testing (including metabolic studies)	Drop in blood pressure with exercise, low functional capacity or low peak V_{O_2}, or ventricular arrhythmias during exercise or recovery
Signal-averaged electrocardiography	Abnormal result

VF, ventricular fibrillation; V_{O_2}, ventilatory oxygen uptake; VT, ventricular tachycardia.

Survivors of sudden cardiac death or patients with sustained ventricular arrhythmias and cardiomyopathy with left ventricular dysfunction are solid candidates for secondary ICD implantation under both the 2008 guidelines[5] and the requirements of the Center for Medicare and Medicaid Services.[9] Survivors of sudden cardiac death who, according to echocardiographic testing, have apparently structurally normal hearts need to be examined carefully for an underlying predisposition to ventricular arrhythmias, such as the long QT syndrome, the Brugada syndrome, or arrhythmogenic right ventricular dysplasia (ARVD). Electrolyte disturbances and medication or drug effects are also common causes of ventricular arrhythmias in patients with structurally normal hearts. A careful family history must be obtained for unexplained sudden death among first-degree relatives, especially those who died at a young age. Patients with such familial disorders who have clinical events also qualify solidly for secondary ICD implantation (see Table 47-2). Primary prevention ICDs for these patients are somewhat more intricate, and a discussion of these is beyond the scope of this chapter.

ICD implantation for patients with unexplained syncope and left ventricular dysfunction in the absence of a documented ventricular arrhythmia is a somewhat more controversial topic. As is always the case with syncope, the clinical history and risk factor profile can often strongly suggest what happened in the absence of objective rhythm tracings (i.e., a history consistent with vasovagal syncope in a normal heart versus a history consistent with ventricular tachycardia in a patient with known ischemic heart disease). Such important clinical data cannot be discarded. The decision to implant an ICD in a patient with symptomatic heart failure can be made easier when indications for primary and secondary prevention overlap for unexplained syncope and when the LVEF is lower than 35%, the cutoff used in the SCD-HeFT trial. For unexplained syncope with LVEF higher than 35%, some clinicians explore alternative forms of risk stratification to help guide the decision of whether to implant an ICD. An electrophysiological study may be reasonable for patients with ischemic disease in whom the LVEF ranges from 35% to 40%, according to the MADIT I study,[16] and T-wave alternans testing may be reasonable for deferring ICD implantation on the basis of a negative result in a patient with an LVEF higher than 35%.[17]

A more conservative approach for unexplained syncope with only mild left ventricular dysfunction could include inpatient cardiac telemetry taping, outpatient Holter

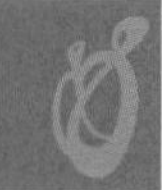

monitoring, or event monitoring (wearable or implantable) for a more precise characterization with or without concomitant medical therapy. Other experts favor a "best judgment" empirical decision that is based on the clinical circumstances of the syncope event, the severity of left ventricular dysfunction, and whether the patient has demonstrable myocardial ischemia that can be reversed with revascularization. Furthermore, not all of these strategies are mutually exclusive. The only caveat is that, as highlighted in the previous section, there is some discordance in when it is reasonable to implant an ICD and when a third party will pay for it. Such pragmatic considerations are not completely negligible within these uncertain areas, inasmuch as ICD implantation and follow-up care are costly and have the potential to create a burden for the individual uninsured patient or for the larger health care system beleaguered by rising costs.

Inappropriate Shocks from Implantable Cardioverter-Defibrillators

Inappropriate shocks are more than just a nuisance to patients and physicians and may actually reduce the benefit from ICDs. An analysis of the MADIT II database demonstrated a hazard ratio of 2.29 for increased all-cause mortality among the 11.5% of ICD recipients who experienced more than one inappropriate shock.[18] The same analysis demonstrated that a history of atrial fibrillation, tobacco use, diastolic hypertension, and a prior inappropriate shock was predictive of future inappropriate shocks. Psychiatric morbidity, including posttraumatic stress disorder, has been associated with multiple ICD shocks over time.[19] Hence, achieving control of supraventricular arrhythmias is crucial, often including catheter ablation procedures. In addition to sustained ventricular tachycardia, abnormal oversensing (in which the device interprets noise or the T-wave as arrhythmia) is a common cause of inappropriate shocks. Adjusting sensing thresholds, modifying detection heart rate zones, and modifying their corresponding therapies are often necessary. In the Primary Prevention Parameters Evaluation (PREPARE) study,[20] such strategic programming reduced appropriate and inappropriate shocks by approximately 66% among primary ICD recipients. In extreme situations, ablation of the atrioventricular node or disablement of the shocking function may become necessary to stop incessant shocks. Distinguishing appropriate from inappropriate therapy can be difficult. According to at least one definition, 66% of the rhythms in patients in the PREPARE trial would have elicited inappropriate therapy, even though at least 50% of the shocks would have been delivered for ventricular tachycardia.

Complications of and Informed Consent for Implantable Devices

Pooled device complication rates in the heart failure population[21] are summarized in Table 47-4. Patients have a right to accept or refuse any medical intervention, and they need to understand the risks and benefits of what is being offered to them. Both the clinical practice guidelines[5] and Center for Medicare and Medicaid Services guidelines[9] recommend caution in offering ICD therapy to patients with life expectancy of less than 1 year because they are unlikely to derive benefit for a relatively low 1-year event rate, according to the Kaplan-Meier curves in the previously cited major trials; therefore, they incur only the up-front risk associated with implantation, without the counterbalancing clinical benefit. Furthermore, some experts have criticized the electrophysiology community for inappropriately extending ICD indications beyond what was studied in the clinical trials and for not fully explaining how an ICD benefits an individual patient.[22] Defibrillator shocks are intrusive in a patient who chooses not to be resuscitated in the event of a cardiac arrest. Some patients also inappropriately believe the presence of a primary prevention ICD somehow improves their heart's performance on a daily basis. Therefore, patients must be able to repeat back an understanding of the procedure in order to avoid such misunderstanding.

TABLE 47–4 Pooled Rates of Device Complications Reported from MIRACLE, COMPANION, and CARE-HF Trials

Complication	Range of Event Rates
Procedure-related death	0.2% to 0.6%
Coronary venous dissection (CRT devices)	0.3% to 4.0%
Lead dislodgment	5.7% to 6.0%
Coronary venous perforation	0.8% to 2.0%
Tamponade	0.3% to 0.5%
Infection or pocket erosion	1.3% to 2.7%

CARE-HF, Cardiac Resynchronization in Heart Failure; COMPANION, COmparison of Medical Therapy, Pacing, ANd DefibrillatION in Heart Failure; CRT, cardiac resynchronization therapy; MIRACLE, Multicenter InSync Randomized Clinical Evaluation.

PACING AND CARDIAC RESYNCHRONIZATION

Basic Considerations

In a normal heart with a narrow QRS complex, right and left ventricular depolarization is synchronous when an atrial impulse is conducted through the atrioventricular node, down the bundle of His, and through the right and left bundle and their associated subdivisions. *Electrical dyssynchrony* refers to an abnormally widened surface QRS duration exceeding 120 msec in any electrocardiographic limb lead, and it is associated with increased mortality among patients with symptomatic heart failure. A left bundle branch block, for example, is suggestive of delayed electrical activation of the left lateral wall, which impairs left ventricular diastolic filling, increases mitral regurgitation, and reduces cardiac output. *Mechanical dyssynchrony* refers to echocardiographic evidence of abnormal activation timing within or between the ventricles. *Interventricular dyssynchrony* occurs when activating timing between the right and left ventricles is altered. *Intraventricular dyssynchrony* occurs between segments within the left ventricle, such as the septum and lateral wall. *Atrioventricular dyssynchrony* refers to atrial contraction that is out of phase with ventricular filling, as manifested by an abnormal PR interval. The extreme example of this is complete heart block (atrioventricular asynchrony), in which the atria often contract against closed atrioventricular valves, producing the characteristic cannon waves.

Mechanical Dyssynchrony

Cardiac resynchronization therapy (CRT) aims to restore synchronous biventricular contraction sequence through the normalization of activation timing by pacing both ventricles (i.e., biventricular pacing). In the 2008 consensus statement by the American Society of Echocardiography and the Heart Rhythm Society,[23] echocardiographic criteria used to assess mechanical dyssynchrony were evaluated, and some of these common modalities are summarized in Table 47-5. Interventricular dyssynchrony is currently best assessed by means of the interventricular mechanical delay (IVMD), which is defined as a 40-msec or longer difference between peak right and left ventricular contraction, measured separately from the onset of the QRS complex with pulsed-wave Doppler imaging of the velocities of the right and left ventricular outflow tracts. This is a simple technique that can be easily applied and does not require advanced equipment. Prolonged IVMD has been associated with an increase in all-cause mortality.[24] The major disadvantage is that IVMD is considered a nonspecific finding, inasmuch as CRT responders and nonresponders have similar rates of IVMD.[25]

Color-coded tissue Doppler imaging is the current favored method of assessment of intraventricular dyssynchrony. In this technique, longitudinal wall delay is evaluated in an apical three-, four-, or five-chamber view at two opposing sites from the QRS onset to peak contraction with a cutoff of 65 msec or longer; this method requires advanced tissue Doppler equipment. Intraventricular radial dyssynchrony can be assessed with M-mode echocardiography in the parasternal short-axis view of the middle of the left ventricle to assess the septal-to-posterior wall delay, in which 130 msec or longer is considered abnormal. This approach does not require advanced equipment, but it can be confounded by regional akinetic segments. Additional techniques such as speckle-based tracking, in which natural acoustic reflections (speckles) are tracked in a time-velocity plot to allow for the assessment of rotational strain (or torsion), and 3-dimensional echocardiography, in which volume calculations can be applied, are also helpful and appear to be increasingly prevalent in clinical use.

TABLE 47–5 Commonly Applied Methods Used to Assess Mechanical Dyssynchrony

Modality	Criteria
Interventricular Dyssynchrony	
Interventricular mechanical delay (IVMD)	≥40-msec difference from QRS onset between peak RV and LV contraction on pulsed-wave Doppler imaging of the velocity of the RV and LV outflow tracts, or aortic pre-ejection period >160 msec
Intraventricular Dyssynchrony*	
Color tissue Doppler imaging (cTDI)	≥65-msec segmental opposing wall delay from QRS onset to peak contraction, assessed in apical three-, four-, or five-chamber view for longitudinal axis
M-mode with or without tissue color	≥130-msec delay from septal to posterior wall, in parasternal view for radial axis

*Speckle-based tracking and 3-dimensional echocardiography are also gaining popularity in the assessment of intraventricular mechanical dyssynchrony (see text).
LV, left ventricular; RV, right ventricular.

Candidacy for Cardiac Resynchronization Therapy

Multiple key trials that have validated the benefit of CRT are listed in Table 47-6. In the Multicenter InSync Randomized Clinical Evaluation (MIRACLE) trial,[26] 453 patients with dilated cardiomyopathy (end-diastolic diameter ≥ 5.5 cm), LVEF of 35% or less, and QRS interval of 130 msec or longer were randomly assigned to receive CRT or no pacing. The study demonstrated improvements in quality-of-life measures, the 6-minute walk test, and number of hospitalizations for heart failure. In the Comparison of Medical Therapy, Resynchronization, and Defibrillation Therapies in Heart Failure (COMPANION) trial,[27] 1520 patients with an LVEF of 35% or lower, QRS interval of 120 msec or longer, and NYHA class III or IV heart failure were randomly assigned to receive CRT alone, CRT with ICD capability (CRT-D), or no pacing. The patients who received CRT or CRT-D demonstrated relative reductions of 34% (hazard ratio, 0.81; P = .014) and 40% (hazard ratio, 0.80; P = .01), respectively, in composite all-cause mortality and hospitalization for heart failure in contrast to those who received no pacing (Figure 47-5, *A*). Only those with CRT-D demonstrated a decrease in all-cause mortality alone (see Figure 47-5, *B*).

In the Cardiac Resynchronization in Heart Failure (CARE-HF) trial,[28] 819 patients with LVEF of 35% or lower, QRS interval either of 150 msec or longer or of 120 to 150 msec with mechanical dyssynchrony, and NYHA class III or IV heart failure were randomly assigned to receive either CRT or no pacing; thus, this study did not include defibrillator therapy. CRT resulted in a significant 16% absolute risk reduction (hazard ratio, 0.63; 95% CI, 0.51 to 0.77; $P < .001$) in morbidity and mortality during a mean follow-up period of 29.4 months (Figure 47-6, *A*), as well as a significant 10% absolute risk reduction (hazard ratio, 0.64; 95% CI, 0.48 to 0.85; $P < .001$)

TABLE 47–6 Designs and Outcomes of Major Trials of Cardiac Resynchronization Therapy

Trial	Inclusion Criteria	Sample Size	Conditions	Result
COMPANION	NYHA classes III to IV LVEF ≤ 35% QRS duration ≥ 120 msec	1520	CRT vs. CRT-D vs. no pacing	All-cause mortality and hospitalization
MIRACLE	NYHA classes III to IV LVEF ≤ 35% EDD ≥ 5.5 cm QRS duration ≥ 130 msec ICD indicated	369	CRT-D vs. ICD alone	Improved quality of life, improved NYHA class
CARE-HF	NYHA classes III to IV LVEF ≤ 35% QRS duration ≥ 150 msec or 120 to 150 msec with dyssynchrony	819	CRT vs. no pacing	All-cause mortality or unplanned hospitalization
RETHINQ	NYHA classes III to IV LVEF ≤ 35% QRS duration ≤ 130 msec Mechanical dyssynchrony (TDI)	172	CRT vs. no pacing	No increase in peak V_{O_2} at 6 months

CARE-HF, Cardiac Resynchronization in Heart Failure; COMPANION, COmparison of Medical Therapy, Pacing, ANd DefibrillatION in Heart Failure; CRT, cardiac resynchronization therapy; CRT-D, CRT with ICD capability; EDD, end-diastolic diameter; ICD, implantable cardioverter-defibrillator; MIRACLE, Multicenter InSync Randomized Clinical Evaluation; NYHA, New York Heart Association; RETHINQ, Resynchronization Therapy in Normal QRS; TDI, tissue Doppler imaging; V_{O_2}, ventilatory oxygen uptake.

of death from any cause (see Figure 47-6, *B*). Thus, both the primary endpoint of time to death or unplanned hospitalization and the secondary endpoint of all-cause mortality were reduced in the CRT recipients. The benefits of CRT were similar among patients with ischemic heart disease and patients without ischemic heart disease and were in addition to the benefits of pharmacological therapy. In addition, CRT reduced the interventricular mechanical delay, the left ventricular end-systolic volume index, and the area of the mitral regurgitant jet, and it increased the left ventricular ejection fraction.

On the basis of these results, current candidates for CRT include those with LVEF of 35% or lower, a QRS duration of 120 msec or longer on surface electrocardiogram, and NYHA functional class III or IV heart failure despite optimal medical therapy with β-blockers, ACE inhibitors or angiotensin receptor blockers, aldosterone antagonists, and loop diuretics. Because QRS duration is measured from the onset of the Q wave to the termination of the S wave, where it is longest in the electrocardiograph limb leads, accurate measurement of QRS duration is needed; the automatic computer measurement can fail to include the terminal deflection and thus may underestimate the true value. When a patient is assessed for CRT, it is important to concomitantly consider ICD candidacy; the overwhelming majority of candidates meets criteria for both, and these functions can be coupled into one implanted device (i.e., a CRT-D system, which includes a defibrillator). That said, it is important to recognize that CRT can be offered without the defibrillator for patients who do not want shocks and can still be offered as an excellent palliative therapy for class IV heart failure, for example.

Whereas the original studies with CRT included patients with moderate to advanced heart failure, researchers have more recently begun to examine the role of CRT for patients with less advanced heart failure. In the Resynchronization Reverses Remodeling in Systolic Left Ventricular Dysfunction (REVERSE) study, researchers assessed the effects of CRT in 610 patients with NYHA functional class I and II heart failure who had had previous symptoms of heart failure.[29] These

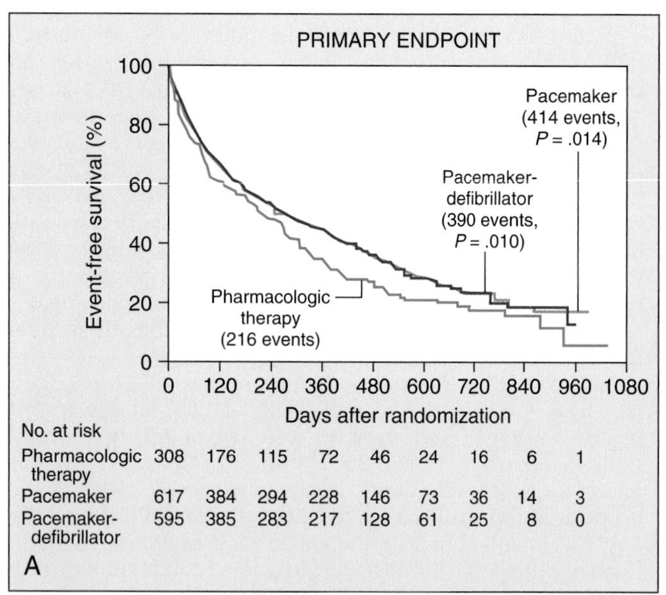

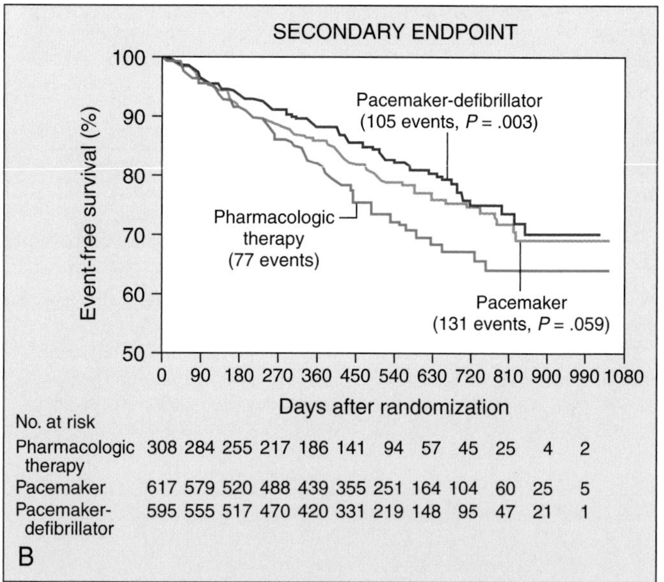

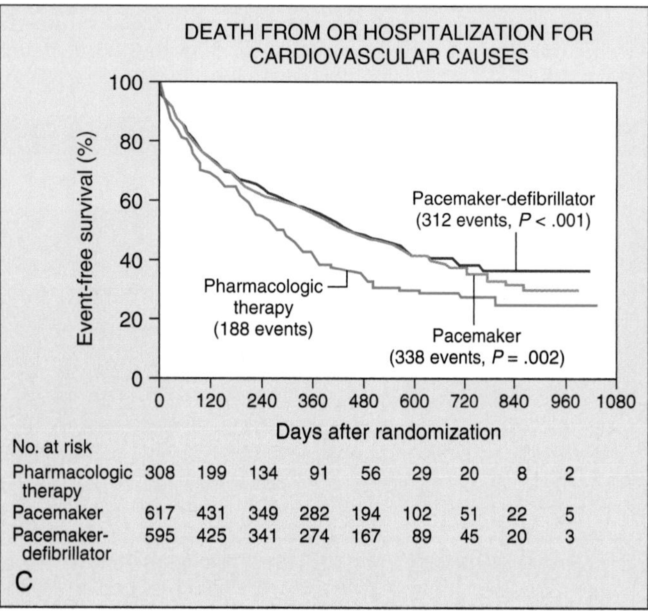

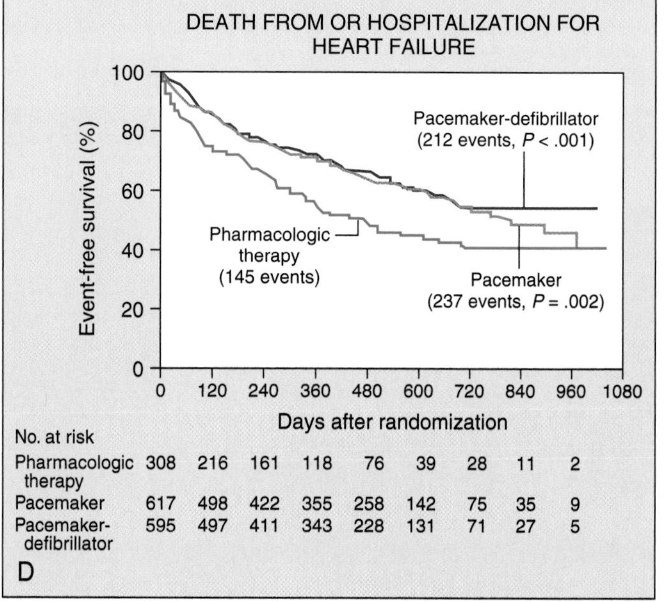

FIGURE 47-5 Kaplan-Meier estimates of the time to the primary endpoint of death from or hospitalization for any cause (**A**), the time to the secondary endpoint of death from any cause (**B**), the time to death from or hospitalization for cardiovascular causes (**C**), and the time to death from or hospitalization for heart failure (**D**) in the Comparison of Medical Therapy, Resynchronization, and Defibrillation Therapies in Heart Failure (COMPANION) trial. *P* values are for the comparison with optimal pharmacological therapy. (Modified from Bristow MR, Saxon LA, Boehmer J, et al. Cardiac-resynchronization therapy with or without an implantable defibrillator in advanced chronic heart failure. *N Engl J Med* 2004;350:2140-2150.)

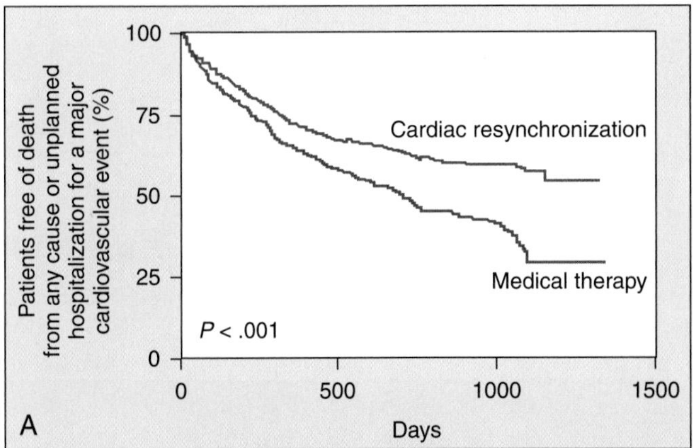

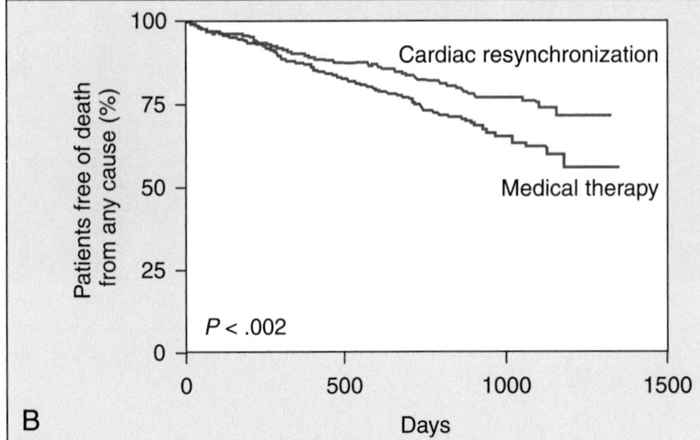

FIGURE 47–6 Kaplan-Meier analysis of the time to death from any cause or an unplanned hospitalization for a major cardiovascular event (**A**) and death from any cause (**B**) in patients receiving standard pharmacological therapy and cardiac resynchronization therapy (CRT) in the Cardiac Resynchronization in Heart Failure (CARE-HF) trial. (Modified from Cleland JG, Daubert JC, Erdmann E, et al. The effect of cardiac resynchronization on morbidity and mortality in heart failure. *N Engl J Med* 2005;352:1539-1549.)

patients, who also had a QRS interval of 120 msec or longer and an LVEF of 40%, received a CRT device and were randomly assigned (in a ratio of 2:1) to receive active CRT (CRT-ON) or to the control condition (CRT-OFF) for 12 months. The primary endpoint of the study was a composite score (better, worse, or same); 16% of the subjects experienced worsening in CRT-ON, in comparison with 21% in the CRT-OFF condition (P = .10). However, patients in the CRT-ON condition experienced a greater improvement in left ventricular end-systolic volume index and other measures of left ventricular remodeling. Although the 12- and 18-month follow-up analyses of REVERSE did not demonstrate improvements in patients' functional status, the prospectively planned 24-month analysis of REVERSE revealed that patients in the CRT-ON condition had less clinical worsening, with a 62% relative risk reduction in time to first hospitalization or death, in comparison with those who did not receive therapy.[30] The Multicenter Automatic Defibrillator Implantation Trial with Cardiac Resynchronization Therapy (MADIT-CRT trial) was a multicenter, double blind randomized clinical trial designed to address the potential survival and morbidity benefit of CRT in NYHA class I and II heart failure patients. The primary end point of the trial was the reduction in the risk of death and non-fatal heart failure events.[31] Prophylactic CRT combined with an ICD was compared to 1CD only in 1,820 patients with EF ≤ 30%, QRS ≥ 130 msec, and either an ischemic (class 1 patients) or any (class II. patients) etiology. During the average follow-up of 2.4 years, the primary endpoint of death from any cause or nonfatal heart-failure event occurred in 17.2% of the CRT-1CD group versus 25.2% of the ICD only group, with a relative risk reduction of 34% (FIR 0.66, 95% confidence interval 0.52 to 0.84, p=0.001) (Figure 47-7). This significant benefit was driven by a 41% reduction in heart failure events, (139% vs 22.8%, HR 0.59, 95% confidence interval 0.47 to 0.74, p < 0.001). In terms of pre-specified subgroups, both ischemic and non-ischemic groups showed benefit with CRT; however, a greater benefit was noted for women versus men and in patients with QRS ≥150 msec. Another factor predicting CRT responsiveness in this trial was QRS morphology, as patients benefitting most had left bundle branch block (LBBB).[31a] Together, REVERSE and MADIT-CRT support the expansion of the CRT indication to the population of NYHA class I and II patients.

Special Considerations

Special considerations in CRT include the presence of a right bundle branch block on surface electrocardiogram, the presence of mechanical dyssynchrony with narrow QRS complex, and the absence of mechanical dyssynchrony with a wide QRS complex. A right bundle branch pattern is suggestive of early activation of the left ventricle and therefore should preclude any benefit from pacing the posterolateral left ventricle with a coronary sinus lead. However, many of the CRT responders in the previously cited trials did indeed have a right bundle branch block. With regard to mechanical dyssynchrony and a narrow QRS complex, the Resynchronization Therapy in Normal QRS (RETHINQ) trial[32] was an evaluation of 172 patients with NYHA class III or IV heart failure, LVEF of 35% or lower, QRS interval of 130 msec or less, and mechanical dyssynchrony demonstrated by tissue Doppler imaging. These patients were randomly assigned to receive CRT or no pacing; at 6 months, there was no reduction in the primary endpoint of peak myocardial oxygen consumption, assessed by metabolic stress test. However, there was a suggestion of benefit among the subgroup of patients with QRS duration between 120 and 130 msec. Most experts would not deny CRT to a patient with a wide QRS complex who otherwise meets current criteria without mechanical dyssynchrony demonstrable by echocardiography, inasmuch as this was not an inclusion criterion in either the COMPANION or MIRACLE study.

Coronary Sinus or Left Ventricular Epicardial Lead Placement

CRT devices are placed by means of the same fundamental device implant technique described previously, with the addition of a third lead intended for the coronary venous circulation. The coronary sinus is cannulated, usually with a sheath that permits venographic visualization of potential target cardiac vein branches into which the lead is guided. The venous branch with a posterolateral distribution mimicking the posterolateral circumflex artery is typically selected because the classic CRT candidate has activation delay in the left posterolateral wall. Anterior and inferior branches are typically avoided. The coronary sinus can be difficult to cannulate in the case of an atretic vein or, more commonly, valves located over the ostium. Epicardial leads can be placed with a limited thoracotomy approach when the operator is unable to access the coronary sinus or find a suitable branch. Once a suitable anatomical site is localized, pacing is performed to assess thresholds and to rule out diaphragmatic stimulation, which can commonly occur by inadvertent stimulation either of the phrenic nerve or of the diaphragm muscle itself. Low pacing thresholds are desirable, to maximize the device's battery life and minimize the number of invasive procedures required for generator change, and the absence of diaphragm capture is essential for patient comfort. Lead placement is confirmed by a postprocedure chest radiograph (Figure 47-8).

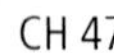

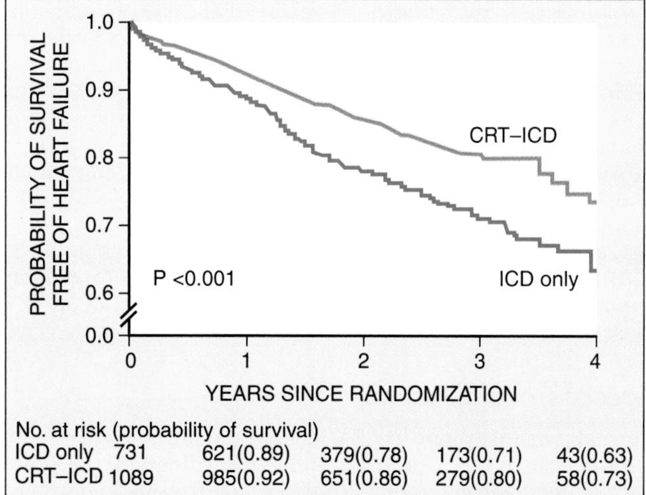

FIGURE 47–7 Kaplan–Meier Estimates of the Probability of Survival Free of Heart Failure in MADIT-CRT. There was a significant difference in the estimate of survival free of heart failure between the group that received CRT–ICD and the group that received an ICD only (unadjusted P<0.001 by the log-rank test). (Modified from Moss AJ, Hall WJ, Cannom DS, et al. Cardiac resynchronization therapy for the prevention of heart failure events. *N Engl J Med* 2009; 361:1329-1338).

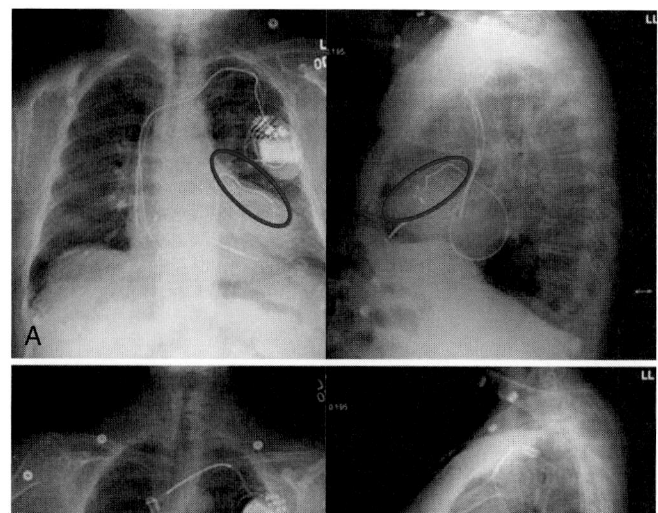

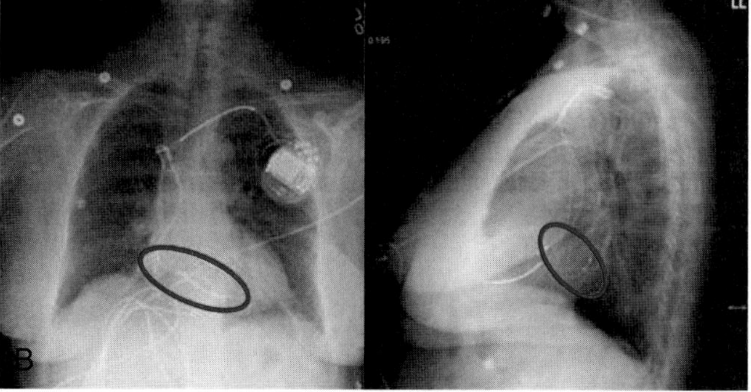

FIGURE 47–8 Typical posteroanterior (*left*) and lateral (*right*) chest radiographic views, demonstrating inappropriate coronary sinus lead placement in an anterolateral venous branch (**A**) and optimal posterolateral venous positioning (**B**).

Summary of Cardiac Resynchronization Therapy

CRT is an efficacious therapy with morbidity- and mortality-related benefits for patients who meet the inclusion criteria. However, some patients do not respond, and a small number, in fact, paradoxically worsen. The relationship between lead placement and electrical-mechanical activation has not been fully explored. Local myocardial properties at the pacing site (such as infiltration or scar) may also influence outcomes, and variations in cardiac venous anatomy always present a significant challenge and barrier to transvenous CRT. Therefore, the precise mechanism of benefit and even the underlying pathological mechanisms for CRT remain incompletely understood. Much remains to be learned, and technological refinements need to be made, but CRT will remain a standard of care.

DEVICE DIAGNOSTICS

For decades, devices have provided diagnostic information on cardiac arrhythmias in heart failure to managing clinicians. Such data can be used to guide decisions about antiarrhythmic therapy, may hint at the development of myocardial ischemia or electrolyte imbalances (through a recent increase in ventricular ectopy, for example), and can be used to diagnose occult atrial arrhythmias, such as atrial fibrillation, that can point to the need for anticoagulation for stroke prevention. Furthermore, pacemaker and ICD diagnostics provide data on underlying rhythm, pacemaker dependence, and intrinsic function of the sinus and atrioventricular nodes. In fact, a noninvasive electrophysiological study can be performed in which the atrial and ventricular leads are used to assess inducibility for ventricular arrhythmias—a feature not commonly used.

The technology of device monitoring has also grown tremendously. Originally, patients had to come to clinic in person for device diagnostics and reprogramming. Remote interrogation enabled patients to transmit device diagnostics information over the phone instead. The newest horizon is in remote wireless interrogation. In the PreFER Managed Ventricular Pacing (PREFER) study,[33] 897 patients were randomly assigned to undergo new wireless-capable device monitoring or classic rhythm strip phone monitoring; events were verified by in-person clinic interrogation in both groups. At approximately 1 year, the detection rate for clinically important events (such as atrial or ventricular arrhythmias) was significantly higher with the wireless devices, and a surprisingly high percentage of events was, in fact, missed in the rhythm strip device.

In addition to arrhythmias, device-reported hemodynamic data in patients with heart failure are important. Perhaps the best studied modality is one that records and reports intrathoracic impedance as an index of pulmonary edema and can provide additional clues that the patient may imminently require hospitalization. The newest investigational technology involves optical sensing from the device that can measure pulse oximetry and extrapolate blood pressure. This might be used as an index to assess the hemodynamic stability of a given rhythm and, it is hoped, prevent inappropriate shocks. Within an "intermediate" tachycardia zone (e.g., 150 to 170 beats per minute), the device could potentially incorporate such measurement into its algorithm in determining whether to initiate therapy. Atrial rhythms such as sinus tachycardia, atrial fibrillation, or other supraventricular tachycardias that are hemodynamically tolerated should maintain favorable blood pressure and pulse oximetry recordings, and a shock would not be administered. Hemodynamically intolerable "slow" ventricular arrhythmias would, conversely, trigger therapy.

Implantable loop recorders are yet another modality by which important data can be gleaned about heart failure. A much smaller device with telemetry capability is implanted prepectorally and can record arrhythmia activity extending over a period of several months—far beyond what an event monitor can record. Future implantable loop records will also probably report hemodynamic data.

FUTURE DIRECTIONS

Device technology for heart failure has undergone extraordinary growth and is increasingly meeting the broad goals outlined in this chapter's introduction. Current and future research is directed at better identifying patients at risk for

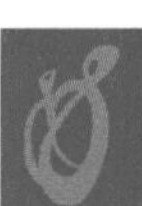

sudden cardiac death and identifying both the underlying mechanisms and application of cardiac resynchronization. Subsequent generations of devices will aim to provide increasingly sophisticated hemodynamic data, monitoring, and modalities to minimize inappropriate shocks. Future development in nanotechnology, stem cell therapy, and biopacemakers will also probably reshape this field.

REFERENCES

1. Hjalmarson, A., Goldstein, S., Fagerberg, B., et al. (2000). Effects of controlled-release metoprolol on total mortality, hospitalizations, and well-being in patients with heart failure: the Metoprolol CR/XL Randomized Intervention Trial in Congestive Heart Failure (MERIT-HF). *JAMA*, *283*, 1295–1302.
2. Wilkoff, B. L. (2005). Electrical therapy for heart failure: evolving indications and choices. *Texas Heart J*, *32*, 212–214.
3. Epstein, A. E., Hallstrom, A. P., Rogers, W. J., et al. (1993). Mortality following ventricular arrhythmia suppression by encainide, flecainide, and moricizine after myocardial infarction. The Cardiac Arrhythmia Suppression Trial (CAST). *JAMA*, *270*, 2451–2455.
4. Lee, H. K., Hafley, G., Fisher, J. D., et al. (2002). Effect of implantable defibrillators on arrhythmic events and mortality in the Multicenter Unsustained Tachycardia Trial (MUSTT). *Circulation*, *106*, 233–238.
5. Epstein, A. E., DiMarco, J. P., Ellenbogen, K. A., et al. (2008). ACC/AHA/ESC 2008 guidelines for device-based therapy of cardiac rhythm abnormalities: a report of the American College of Cardiology/American Heart Association Task Force on Practice Guidelines (Writing Committee to Revise the ACC/AHA/NASPE 2002 Guideline Update for Implantation of Cardiac Pacemakers and Antiarrhythmia Devices): developed in collaboration with the American Association for Thoracic Surgery and Society of Thoracic Surgeons. *Circulation*, *117*, e350–e408.
6. Kadish, A., Dyer, A., Daubert, J. P., et al. (2004). Prophylactic defibrillator implantation in patients with nonischemic dilated cardiomyopathy. *N Engl J Med*, *350*, 2151–2158.
7. Moss, A. J., Zareba, W., Hall, W. J., et al. (2002). Prophylactic implantation of a defibrillator in patients with myocardial infarction and reduced ejection fraction. *N Engl J Med*, *346*, 877–883.
8. Bardy, G. H., Lee, K. L., Mark, D. B., et al. (2005). Amiodarone or an implantable cardioverter-defibrillator for congestive heart failure (SCD-HeFT). *N Engl J Med*, *352*, 225–237.
9. Centers for Medicare and Medicaid Services. Medicare Coverage Database. *Implementation for implantable defibrillators (CAG-00157R3)* (online summary of coverage): http://cms.hhs.gov/mcd/viewimplementation.asp?id=148. Accessed February 26, 2010.
10. Al-Khatib, S. M., Sanders, D. G., Bigger, J. T., et al. (2007). Preventing tomorrow's sudden cardiac death today: part I: current data on risk stratification for sudden cardiac death. *Am Heart J*, *153*, 941–950.
11. Podrid, P. J., & Myerburg, R. J. (2005). Epidemiology and stratification of risk for sudden cardiac death. *Clin Cardiol*, *28*(11 Suppl. 1), I3–I11.
12. Gehi, A. K., Stein, R. H., Metz, L. D., et al. (2005). Microvolt T-wave alternans for the risk stratification of ventricular tachyarrhythmic events: a meta-analysis. *J Am Coll Cardiol*, *46*, 75–82.
13. Bloomfield, D. M., Bigger, J. T., Steinman, R. C., et al. (2006). Microvolt T-wave alternans and the risk of death or sustained ventricular arrhythmias in patients with left ventricular dysfunction. *J Am Coll Cardiol*, *47*, 456–463.
14. Cantillon, D. J., Stein, K. M., Markowitz, S. M., et al. (2007). Predictive value of microvolt T-wave alternans in patients with left ventricular dysfunction. *J Am Coll Cardiol*, *50*, 166–173.
15. Chow, T., Kereiakes, D. J., Onufer, J., et al. (November 7, 2007). *Primary results from the Microvolt T-Wave Alternans Testing for Risk Stratification of Post-MI Patients (MASTER I)*. Orlando, FL: Presented at the American Heart Association 2007 Scientific Sessions.
16. Moss, A. J., Hall, W. J., Cannom, D. S., et al. (1996). Improved survival with an implanted defibrillator in patients with coronary artery disease at high risk for ventricular arrhythmia. Multicenter Automatic Defibrillator Implantation Trial Investigators. *N Engl J Med*, *335*, 1933–1940.
17. Bloomfield, D. M., Steinman, R. C., Namerow, P. B., et al. (2004). Microvolt T-wave alternans distinguishes between patients likely and patients not likely to benefit from implanted cardiac defibrillator therapy: a solution to the Multicenter Automatic Defibrillator Implantation Trial (MADIT) II conundrum. *Circulation*, *110*, 1885–1889.
18. Daubert, J. P., Zareba, W., Cannom, D. S., et al. (2008). Inappropriate implantable cardioverter-defibrillator shocks in MADIT II: frequency, mechanisms, predictors, and survival impact. *J Am Coll Cardiol*, *51*, 1357–1365.
19. Friedmann, E., Thomas, S. A., Inguito, P., et al. (2006). Quality of life and psychological status of patients with implantable cardioverter defibrillators. *J Interv Card Electrophysiol*, *17*, 65–72.
20. Wilkoff, B. L., Williamson, B. D., Stern, R. S., et al. (2008). Strategic programming of detection and therapy parameters in implantable cardioverter-defibrillators reduces shocks in primary prevention patients: results from the PREPARE (Primary Prevention Parameters Evaluation) Study. *J Am Coll Cardiol*, *52*, 541–550.
21. Burkhart, J. D., & Wilkoff, B. L. (2007). Interventional electrophysiology and cardiac resynchronization therapy: delivering electrical therapies for heart failure. *Circulation*, *115*, 2208–2220.
22. Josephson, M. E. (2007). Electrophysiology at a crossroads. *Heart Rhythm*, *4*, 658–661.
23. Gorcsan, J., 3rd, Abraham, T., Agler, D. A., et al. (2008). Echocardiography for cardiac resynchronization therapy: recommendations for performance and reporting—a report from the American Society of Echocardiography dyssynchrony writing group endorsed by the Heart Rhythm Society. *J Am Soc Echocardiogr*, *21*, 191–213.
24. Richardson, M., Freemantle, N., Calvert, M. J., et al. (2007). Predictors and treatment response with cardiac resynchronization therapy in patients with heart failure characterized by dyssynchrony: a pre-defined analysis from the CARE-HF trial. *Eur Heart J*, *28*, 1827–1834.
25. Bax, J. J., Abraham, T., Barold, S. S., et al. (2005). Cardiac resynchronization therapy: part 1—issues before device implantation. *J Am Coll Cardiol*, *46*, 2153–2167.
26. Sutton, M. G., Plappert, T., Hilpisch, K. E., et al. (2006). Sustained reverse left ventricular structural remodeling with cardiac resynchronization at one year is a function of etiology: quantitative Doppler echocardiographic evidence from the Multicenter InSync Randomized Clinical Evaluation (MIRACLE). *Circulation*, *113*, 266–272.
27. Bristow, M. R., Saxon, L. A., Boehmer, J., et al. (2004). Cardiac-resynchronization therapy with or without an implantable defibrillator in advanced chronic heart failure. *N Engl J Med*, *350*, 2140–2150.
28. Cleland, J. G., Daubert, J. C., Erdmann, E., et al. (2005). The effect of cardiac resynchronization on morbidity and mortality in heart failure. *N Engl J Med*, *352*, 1539.
29. Linde, C., Abraham, W. T., Gold, M. R., et al. (2008). Randomized trial of cardiac resynchronization in mildly symptomatic heart failure patients and in asymptomatic patients with left ventricular dysfunction and previous heart failure symptoms. *J Am Coll Cardiol*, *52*, 1834–1843.
30. O'Riordan, M. *REVERSE at 24 months: CRT modifies disease progression and improves clinical outcomes* (online article): http://www.theheart.org/article/955203.do. Accessed February 27, 2010.
31. Moss, A. J., Hall, W. J., Cannom, D. S., et al. (2009). Cardiac resynchronization therapy for the prevention of heart failure events. *N Engl J Med*, 361, 1329–1338.

31a. MADIT-CRT: Sponscer's Executive Summary, March 18, 2010 FDA Panel Meeting, accessed via the worldwide web on March 28, 2010 at http://www.fda.itov/doenload s/advisory Committees/CommittieesMeetintNaterials/MedicalDevices/Medical Devices AdvisoryCommittee/CireulatorySystemDevicesPanel/UCM2041607.pdf.

32. Beshai, J. F., Grimm, R. A., Nagueh, S. F., et al. (2007). Cardiac-resynchronization therapy in heart failure with narrow QRS complexes. *N Engl J Med*, *357*, 2461–2471.
33. Wilkoff, B. L. (*Pacemaker remote follow-up evaluation and review: results of the PREFER trial. Late-breaking clinical trials session. Presented at the Heart Rhythm Society 2008 Scientific Session.* May 15, 2008.

CHAPTER 48

Treatment of Heart Failure with a Preserved Ejection Fraction

Anita Deswal

Many patients with heart failure have a normal or nearly normal ejection fraction; this condition is referred to variably as *diastolic heart failure* or *heart failure with preserved ejection fraction* (HFPEF). Epidemiological studies and patient registries have reported a prevalence of HFPEF ranging from 40% to 71% (average, ≈50%) of patients with heart failure.[1-5] Furthermore, a study from Olmsted County, Minnesota, revealed that the prevalence of HFPEF among patients with a discharge diagnosis of heart failure increased significantly from 1987 to 2001.[6] The prevalence of this condition will probably keep increasing as the prevalence of comorbid conditions such as hypertension, diabetes, obesity, and coronary artery disease increases among elderly persons.[7-10] The rates of mortality and morbidity have varied in association with HFPEF and in comparison with heart failure with depressed ejection fraction (commonly referred to as *systolic heart failure*); however, there is consensus that HFPEF is a condition associated with substantial morbidity and mortality, and the frequency of clinical events increases markedly once a patient is hospitalized for heart failure. One review suggested that once hospitalized for heart failure, patients with HFPEF have high rates of rehospitalization; up to a third may be readmitted for exacerbation of heart failure within a year, and 45% to 60% may be rehospitalized for any reason.[1] Similarly, once such patients are hospitalized, the mortality rate may be as high as 22% to 29% at 1 year and approximately 65% at 5 years.[6,11] However, this population has been underrepresented in most randomized clinical trials in heart failure. In fact, researchers examining secular trends of heart failure within Olmsted County found that survival improved significantly over time among patients with heart failure and reduced ejection fraction (probably in relation to use of evidence-driven therapies), but no such trend toward improvement was noted for patients with HFPEF.[6] Therefore, effective treatment strategies for the management of patients with this condition are urgently needed.

DEVELOPMENT OF TREATMENT STRATEGIES BASED ON PATHOPHYSIOLOGY OF HFPEF

The development of treatment strategies for HFPEF is based on the currently evolving understanding of the pathophysiological processes of this condition (see Chapter 14). HFPEF commonly afflicts elderly patients with such comorbid conditions as hypertension, left ventricular (LV) hypertrophy, diabetes mellitus, myocardial ischemia, and obesity. Of these risk factors, hypertension and subsequent LV hypertrophy are the most prevalent and are highly associated with HFPEF. Less commonly, HFPEF occurs as a result of restrictive and infiltrative cardiomyopathies and transplant rejection.[12] In the presence of the conditions just mentioned, clinical symptoms and signs of heart failure are commonly precipitated by concomitant anemia, pulmonary disease, renal insufficiency, and atrial fibrillation. In patients with HFPEF, in the absence of significant valvular or pericardial disease, diastolic dysfunction consisting of abnormalities of LV relaxation and increased LV stiffness has long been thought to be the central pathophysiological process contributing to the development of heart failure.[13-15] The term *diastolic heart failure* has been used to describe this condition. Although mechanistic studies have demonstrated that abnormalities of diastolic function are invariably present in HFPEF, there is some disagreement concerning the relative contribution of diastolic dysfunction to clinical heart failure in elderly persons, because diastolic dysfunction is highly prevalent in this population even in the absence of clinical heart failure. However, it is likely that these patients frequently experience clinical decompensation when the aforementioned precipitants occur in the presence of the underlying substrate of diastolic dysfunction. Decompensated heart failure would be unlikely to occur when the same precipitants occur in patients without underlying diastolic dysfunction.

Factors other than diastolic dysfunction have also been suggested to contribute to the development of HFPEF; these include increased vascular and LV systolic stiffness, volume overload secondary to renal disease with abnormal renal sodium handling, atrial dysfunction, neurohumoral activation (specifically of the renin-angiotensin-aldosterone system [RAAS]), reduced vasodilator reserve, and chronotropic incompetence during exercise.[16-19] Aging is associated with a reduction in the elastic properties of the heart and vasculature along with an increase in systolic blood pressure. This probably contributes to the much higher prevalence of HFPEF in elderly persons. In addition, the comorbid conditions described previously are more common among elderly patients, contributing further to the increasing prevalence of this condition with increasing age.

The following sections in this chapter provide an overview of therapeutic modalities that may be effective in patients with HFPEF, with regard to either symptomatic benefit or targeting pathophysiological mechanisms. The clinical approach to management of HFPEF is then summarized on the basis of current evidence and consensus opinion.

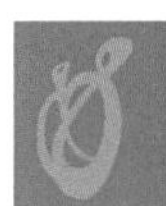

Treatment of Volume Overload and Congestion

Although diuretics may not alter the pathophysiological processes responsible for HFPEF, they do reduce ventricular filling pressures and are therefore very useful in relieving symptoms in patients with pulmonary vascular congestion and peripheral edema (see Chapter 44). Some patients with the classic profile of "diastolic heart failure" with significant left hypertrophy and small LV volumes may exhibit a fall in cardiac output with rapid diuresis, which results in hypotension and prerenal azotemia. This is caused by an LV diastolic pressure-volume curve that is so steep that a small change in diastolic volume causes a large change in pressure and cardiac output.[15] Diuretics may also benefit patients through other potential pathogenic mechanisms. First, it is known that the right ventricle forms the external pressure for approximately one third of the surface area of the left ventricle.[12,20] Therefore, elevation of right-sided diastolic pressures can constrain the filling of the left ventricle. In some patients, reduction of right-sided diastolic pressures by diuretics may unload the interventricular septum, improving LV distensibility,[21] and may therefore help reduce pulmonary venous pressures while maintaining LV filling and cardiac output. Maurer and colleagues[18] demonstrated that in a subgroup of patients with hypertensive HFPEF, the LV end-diastolic pressure-volume relationship may be shifted rightward with somewhat increased end-diastolic volumes (in contrast to the classic paradigm of diastolic heart failure with leftward and upward shifts in the end-diastolic pressure-volume relationship and smaller LV volume). This may be a result of a volume overload state exacerbated by extracardiac factors such as renal dysfunction with abnormal renal sodium handling, obesity, and anemia. This situation could also represent a group of patients who would respond more favorably to diuretic therapy. Last, low-dose diuretics, especially thiazide diuretics, are useful in the treatment of hypertension, which plays a key pathophysiological role in HFPEF.[22,23] Some patients with volume overload that is refractory to increasing doses of diuretics may be candidates for ultrafiltration (Chapter 44).

Furthermore, therapy with nitrates may also provide symptomatic benefit in patients with HFPEF with pulmonary vascular congestion. Nitrates are primarily venodilators with some arterial vasodilating action. They may benefit patients with HFPEF by reducing preload, which leads to reductions in ventricular filling pressures and in pulmonary congestion. In acute decompensated heart failure, they can be used intravenously and may improve symptoms by reducing filling pressures, as well as by controlling systemic hypertension. Theoretically, by releasing nitric oxide, nitrates may improve the diastolic distensibility of the ventricle.[24,25] As with diuretics, caution is required when nitrates are used in patients without hypertension or with severe diastolic dysfunction; they must be monitored for a significant reduction in cardiac output and blood pressure as a result of preload reduction.

Treatment of Hypertension (see Chapter 28)

Of the various risk factors involved in the development of HFPEF, hypertension and subsequent LV hypertrophy are the most prevalent and most highly associated with the condition. The significant contribution of hypertensive heart disease to the development of diastolic dysfunction and HFPEF (reviewed by Hoit and Walsh[26]) implies that treating hypertension should be beneficial not only for the treatment of HFPEF but also for its prevention (see Chapter 41). For example, the increased afterload imposed by significant arterial hypertension reduces LV relaxation and filling rates.[27] Stiffening of the aorta and the left ventricle, as occurs in elderly patients with HFPEF, increases the tightness of the coupling of arterial systolic and left atrial pressures, with increases in systolic arterial pressure resulting in elevation of left atrial pressures.[12,16,28] Controlling systolic hypertension could allow the left ventricle to eject to a smaller end-systolic volume, thus allowing the ventricle to operate with a smaller diastolic volume and reduced left atrial pressure. Lowering the systolic pressure allows the left ventricle to relax more rapidly, which enhances early filling.[29]

In addition, concentrically hypertrophied hearts demonstrate increased passive stiffness and impaired relaxation independent of hemodynamic loads, and have limited coronary vascular reserve, which can contribute to myocardial ischemia even in the absence of epicardial coronary artery disease. Adequate control of hypertension should benefit patients with HFPEF by, in the short term, favorably altering loading conditions and, in the long term, by leading to regression of LV hypertrophy. There may be some additional benefits of using one class of drugs versus others,[22] but the most important goal is achieving an adequate reduction in blood pressure. Results of several studies of reduction of blood pressure with angiotensin-converting enzyme (ACE) inhibitors or angiotensin receptor blockers (ARBs) in comparison with other agents have suggested that ultimately blood pressure control, rather than the specific class of antihypertensive agents used, may be the major determinant of regression of hypertrophy and improvement in diastolic function.[23,30-33] Moreover, trials have definitively demonstrated approximately a 50% reduction in the incidence of heart failure among patients treated for hypertension, especially in the elderly population.[34,35]

Drugs such as β-blockers and calcium channel blockers that reduce blood pressure and heart rate and thus indirectly improve diastolic function, as well as increase diastolic filling time, may be beneficial in patients with HFPEF. On the other hand, the direct myocardial effects of slowing the relaxation rate of the ventricle and the negative inotropic actions of these drugs may be detrimental with regard to diastolic function.[12] In addition, one study demonstrated that during exercise, patients with HFPEF achieved less of an increase in heart rate (inadequate chronotropic response), and thus less of an increase in cardiac output, despite a similar rise in end-diastolic volume, stroke volume, and contractility than did matched subjects with hypertensive cardiac hypertrophy.[17] These data raise questions regarding possible deleterious effects of heart rate–reducing drugs such as β-blockers and certain calcium channel blockers in patients in whom exercise capacity may be reduced partly as a result of reduced chronotropic reserve.

Over the years, a number of small studies of calcium channel blockers, β-blockers, ACE inhibitors, and ARBs have yielded variable results suggestive of modest improvements in exercise capacity, New York Heart Association (NYHA) class, quality of life, and diastolic function in patients with HFPEF.[36-39] However, until recently, none of the studies performed was a large or randomized multicenter trial and thus definitive evidence of benefit on longer-term outcomes was not available.

β-Blockers

In a smaller trial, the Swedish Doppler-Echocardiographic study (SWEDIC), researchers examined the effect of the β blocker carvedilol on diastolic function in patients with HFPEF (left ventricular ejection fraction [LVEF] > 45%) who also met conventional Doppler criteria for diastolic dysfunction.[40] Ninety-five patients completed the 6-month study. There were no significant differences between the patients who received carvedilol and those who received placebo in

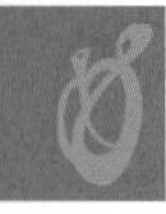

the primary endpoint, a composite of improved, unchanged, or worsened diastolic function, or in clinical endpoints. At baseline, the majority of patients had only mild diastolic dysfunction and had NYHA class I or II functional status; this made it more difficult to detect improvement in these parameters.

In another multicenter trial, researchers evaluated the effects of nebivolol in elderly patients with heart failure, irrespective of LVEF. Nebivolol is a β_1-selective blocker that also has vasodilating properties related to nitric oxide modulation and improves arterial distensibility.[41] In the Study of the Effects of Nebivolol Intervention on Outcomes and Rehospitalisations in Seniors with Heart Failure (SENIORS), 2128 patients aged 70 years or older with a history of heart failure were randomly assigned to receive nebivolol or placebo.[42] Of these patients, 752 patients (35%) had LVEF exceeding 35%. In the overall study, nebivolol was associated with a modest 14% reduction in the primary composite endpoint of death and cardiovascular hospitalization (hazard ratio [HR], 0.84; 95% confidence interval [CI], 0.74 to 0.99), influenced by a reduction in both mortality and hospitalization for cardiovascular causes. A similar magnitude of reduction was noted in the subgroup with LVEF higher than 35%; however, it did not reach statistical significance, possibly because fewer patients were in the subgroup (HR, 0.82; 95% CI, 0.63 to 1.05). Although considered to have preserved ejection fraction or HFPEF, this subgroup of patients, whose ejection fraction was higher than 35%, was clearly heterogeneous, with both preserved and reduced LVEF. The proportion of patients with truly preserved LVEF (≥50%) was small (<15% of all patients in the trial). Also, the effect of nebivolol on hospitalizations for heart failure was not reported.[42] Although the overall results of the trial were suggestive of a modest cardiovascular benefit of the β-blocker nebivolol in elderly patients with heart failure, they did not convincingly demonstrate a benefit in elderly patients with HFPEF.

Renin-Angiotensin-Aldosterone Blockade

As in systolic heart failure, preclinical and clinical evidence suggests that the activation of the RAAS is a contributing factor in the development of HFPEF, principally through the trophic effects of angiotensin II on the vasculature and myocardium, but perhaps also through myocardial fibrosis mediated by aldosterone.[43,44] In addition, angiotensin II slows LV relaxation. which results in elevation of LV diastolic pressures.[45,46] Therefore, agents such as ACE inhibitors and ARBs, which are antihypertensive agents and attenuate the effects of angiotensin II, appeared to be attractive options in the treatment of HFPEF. Furthermore, clinical trials have shown ACE inhibitors and ARBs to be effective in improving cardiovascular outcomes in populations with diabetes, coronary artery disease, vascular disease, and hypertension[47,48]; these comorbid conditions are frequently present in and contribute to the development of HFPEF.

On the basis of a strong theoretical rationale for RAAS blockade in patients with HFPEF,[39] three large, randomized clinical trials were designed specifically to evaluate ACE inhibitors and ARBs in patients with HFPEF: the Candesartan in Heart Failure Assessment of Reduction in Mortality and Morbidity–Preserved (CHARM-Preserved) trial, the Perindopril in Elderly People with Chronic Heart Failure (PEP-CHF) trial,[49,50] and the Irbesartan in Heart Failure with Preserved Ejection Fraction (I-PRESERVE) trial.[51] The characteristics of the patient populations evaluated in these three trials are summarized in Table 48-1.

Of the 3023 patients enrolled in the CHARM-Preserved trial, almost 20% were taking ACE inhibitors and 56% were taking β-blockers at the time of random assignment to receive candesartan or placebo. After a median follow-up period of 36.6 months, the primary endpoint of the study (death from cardiovascular causes or hospitalization for heart failure) occurred in 22% of the candesartan recipients and 24% of the placebo recipients (HR, 0.89; 95% CI, 0.77 to 1.03; P = .118; covariate-adjusted HR, 0.86; 95% CI, 0.74 to 1.00; P = .051) (Figure 48-1). The difference, which was of borderline statistical significance only for the adjusted hazard ratios, was driven mostly by a difference in hospitalizations for heart failure between the candesartan- and placebo-treated subjects (HR, 0.85; 95% CI, 0.72 to 1.01; P = .072); the two groups had almost identical rates of mortality from cardiovascular causes (Figure 48-2). In addition, the total number of hospitalizations for heart failure was noted to be significantly lower among the candesartan recipients. Within 6 months after the trial began, the blood pressure was significantly more reduced in the candesartan recipients (6.9 mm Hg systolic and 2.9 mm Hg diastolic) than in the placebo recipients (P < .0001). It is therefore difficult to tease out whether the modest 15% relative reduction in hospitalizations for heart failure among candesartan recipients with HFPEF was mostly a result of blood pressure reduction or any other more specific angiotensin-blocking effects of candesartan and whether any other drugs causing similar blood pressure reduction would have led to similar effects. The lack of a greater benefit from the use of the ARB in CHARM-Preserved may also have been influenced by the fact that ACE inhibitors were allowed for patients in the trial—20% of patients were taking ACE inhibitors even at the beginning of the trial—and the fact that annual event rates of the primary composite outcome were relatively lower than expected (9.1%) among the placebo recipients.

In the PEP-CHF trial of perindopril in HFPEF, the patient population was older than that in the CHARM-Preserved trial (see Table 48-1). However, the results of the study were neutral with regard to the primary outcome and demonstrated only a trend toward modest benefit in other endpoints.[50] In comparison with the CHARM-Preserved trial, the PEP-CHF study enrolled only 850 patients with HFPEF, who, in addition to having relatively preserved ejection fraction, also had objective evidence of diastolic dysfunction at enrollment. The mean follow-up period of 26.2 months was shorter than that in the CHARM-Preserved trial. The event rate was much lower than expected, and despite a much longer follow-up period than originally intended, only 46% of the expected events occurred; thus, the study had only 25% power to show a difference in the primary endpoint. Furthermore, a large number of patients stopped their assigned treatment after 1 year, and most of them started taking open-label ACE inhibitors (discontinuation rate of 38% at 18 months; ≈36% of patients were receiving open-label ACE inhibitor treatment by the end of the study).

Over the entire duration of follow-up, perindopril was not associated with an improvement in the primary composite endpoint of death or hospitalization for heart failure (HR, 0.92; 95% CI, 0.70 to 1.21; P = .55) (Figure 48-3, *A*). However, an analysis confined to 1 year of follow-up—at which point most patients were still taking the assigned medication—revealed that perindopril was associated with a 31% relative reduction in the primary endpoint (HR, 0.69; 95% CI, 0.47 to 1.01; P = .055), which was of borderline statistical significance. Similarly, although perindopril was not associated with a benefit in hospitalization for heart failure over the entire duration of the trial (see Figure 48-3, *B*), at 1 year of follow-up, the perindopril recipients had a lower rate of hospitalizations for heart failure (HR, 0.63; 95% CI, 0.41 to 0.97; P = .03). Thus, although perindopril did not have a beneficial effect on the overall primary outcome, there was a suggestion of reduction in hospitalizations for heart failure at 1 year when patients were on assigned treatment.[50]

In addition, significant improvements were observed in comparison with the placebo recipients in some other

TABLE 48–1 Study Characteristics of Some Completed Multicenter Clinical Trials for HFPEF

Characteristic	CHARM-Preserved[49]	PEP-CHF[50]	Hong Kong Diastolic Heart Failure Study[52]	I-PRESERVE[51]	Sitaxsentan Sodium in Diastolic Heart Failure[60]
Trial Population					
N	3023	850	150	4128	150
LVEF	>40%	>40%	>45%	≥45%	≥50%, plus concentric hypertrophy or diastolic dysfunction diagnosed by echocardiography
NYHA class	II to IV	I to IV	II to III	II to IV	II, III
% Subjects with NYHA class	III and IV: 39%	III and IV: 24%	III: 30%	III and IV: 79%	II: 56% III: 44%
Mean age	67 years (23% >75 years)	75 years (100% ≥70 years)	74 years	72 years (100% ≥60 years)	—
% Male subjects	60%	45%	38%	40%	27%
Some Exclusion Criteria					
General finding	Significant hypotension	Systolic bp <100 mm Hg	No concomitant β-blockers or calcium channel blockers	Systolic bp <100 mm Hg or >160 mm Hg	Chronic renal insufficiency, liver disease
Creatinine level	>3 mg/dL	>2.3 mg/dL	—	>2.5 mg/dL	—
Serum potassium level	>5.5 mEq/L	>5.4 mEq/L	—	—	—
ACE Inhibitors and ARBs					
Use at baseline	ACE inhibitor use allowed	No concomitant ACE inhibitor or ARB	No concomitant ACE inhibitor or ARB	ACE inhibitors allowed in one third of patients when indicated for diabetes or vascular disease	—
Trial					
Protocol	Double-blind, randomized	Double-blind, randomized	Randomized, open-label, three arms	Double-blind, randomized	Double-blind, randomized
Drug and dosage	Candesartan vs. placebo (titrated up to target dosage of 32 mg/day)	Perindopril vs. placebo (titrated up to target dosage of 4 mg/day)	Diuretics alone vs. diuretics plus irbesartan (target dosage of 75 mg/day) vs. diuretics plus ramipril (target dosage of 10 mg/day) for 52 weeks	Irbesartan vs. placebo (titrated up to target dosage of 300 mg/day)	Sitaxsentan sodium vs. placebo (target dosage of 100 mg/day) for 24 weeks
Follow-up period	Median: 36.6 months	Median: 25.2 months	—	Mean: 49.5 months	—
Primary endpoint	Composite of mortality from CV causes and hospitalization for heart failure	Composite of all-cause mortality or hospitalization for heart failure	Quality of life, 6-minute walk test, diastolic echocardiographic parameters, BNP level	Composite of all-cause mortality or hospitalization for CV causes	Exercise capacity by treadmill time

ACE, angiotensin-converting enzyme; ARB, angiotensin receptor blocker; BNP, B-type natriuretic peptide; bp, blood pressure; CHARM, Candesartan in Heart Failure Assessment in Reduction of Mortality; CV, cardiovascular; HFPEF, heart failure with preserved ejection fraction; I-PRESERVE, Irbesartan in Heart Failure with Preserved Systolic Function; LVEF, left ventricular ejection fraction; NYHA, New York Heart Association; PEP-CHF, Perindopril in Elderly People with Chronic Heart Failure.

secondary endpoints, including the proportion of patients with NYHA functional class 1 and change in 6-minute walking distance at 1 year. As observed in the CHARM-Preserved trial, the active drug in PEP-CHF produced a significantly greater reduction in systolic blood pressure (mean difference, 3 mm Hg; $P = .03$) than did placebo. Furthermore, patients with a higher baseline blood pressure appeared to have a greater benefit with perindopril. Therefore, as in the CHARM-Preserved trial, it is not possible to rule out a significant contribution of the blood pressure–lowering effect of the ACE inhibitor, as opposed to other RAAS-blocking actions of perindopril, to the observed beneficial effect on hospitalizations for heart failure. Also, both trials illustrate the encountered difficulty of lower event rates among patients enrolled in clinical trials than in the general population with the same condition. The switch to open-label ACE inhibitors illustrates the many existing indications for administration of ACE inhibitors or ARBs to patients with vascular disease, diabetes, and hypertension, the same group of comorbid conditions that are frequently encountered in patients with HFPEF, thus potentially limiting the opportunities to add ACE inhibitors or ARBs specifically for HFPEF.

The largest and most recently completed trial, I-PRESERVE, enrolled 4128 patients with HFPEF (see Table 48-1).[51]

The patients were randomly assigned to receive the ARB irbesartan or placebo daily. During a mean follow-up period of 49.5 months, there was no significant difference in the occurrence of the primary outcome of death or hospitalization for heart failure (Figure 48-4) between patients taking irbesartan and those receiving placebo (HR, 0.95; 95% CI, 0.86 to 1.05; P = .35). Overall rates of death were also similar (HR, 1.00; 95% CI, 0.88 to 1.14; P = .98), as were rates of hospitalization for cardiovascular causes, hospitalization for heart failure, and other secondary outcomes. In comparison with the CHARM-preserved trial, the I-PRESERVE trial involved more patients, slightly better preserved ejection fraction (≥45% vs. >40% in CHARM-Preserved), greater specificity of the substrate for HFPEF, and a higher proportion of older patients and women (i.e., a study cohort more representative of the "real world" HFPEF population); however, the I-PRESERVE trial did not provide any evidence for overall benefit of ARBs with regard to cardiovascular outcomes in this population of patients.

In addition to the larger trials just described, the results of a smaller trial, the Hong Kong Diastolic Heart Failure Study (PROBE), have also been reported (see Table 48-1).[52] Although the drug assignment was open label, there was blind endpoint evaluation. The three treatment arms consisted of diuretics, diuretics plus ramipril, and diuretics plus irbesartan. At 52 weeks, no differences were noted in quality of life, recurrent hospitalizations, or LV dimensions in the three treatment groups. However, the peak systolic and early diastolic mitral annular velocities viewed on tissue Doppler imaging increased slightly, albeit significantly, and N-terminal pro-B-type natriuretic peptide (NT-proBNP) levels decreased significantly only in patients taking irbesartan and ramipril, but not in those taking only diuretics. This was the first comparative trial of ACE inhibitors with ARB therapy in patients with HFPEF that was treated with a diuretic. However, the sample size was small and powered only to detect a large effect size of 50% improvement in clinical endpoints. Thus, apart from a signal for a modest improvement in diastolic function with the addition of ACE inhibitors or ARB therapy, this smaller trial was also unable to provide clinical evidence of benefit with angiotensin blockade in patients with HFPEF.[53]

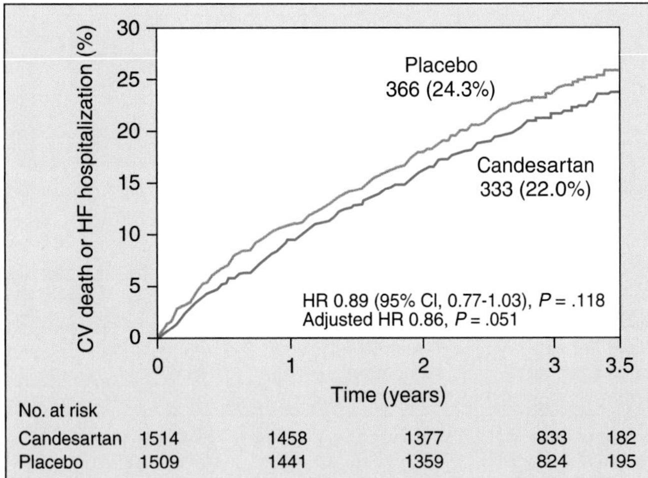

FIGURE 48–1 Kaplan–Meier curves for time to first occurrence of the primary endpoint in patients with heart failure (HF) with preserved ejection fraction in the Candesartan in Heart Failure Assessment in Reduction of Mortality (CHARM)–Preserved trial. CV, cardiovascular; HR, hazard ratio. (From Yusuf S, Pfeffer MA, Swedberg K, et al. Effects of candesartan in patients with chronic heart failure and preserved left-ventricular ejection fraction: the CHARM-Preserved Trial. *Lancet* 2003;362:777-781.)

Another large multicenter trial with the aldosterone antagonist spironolactone is currently ongoing in patients with HFPEF. This trial, Treatment of Preserved Cardiac Function Heart Failure with an Aldosterone Antagonist (TOPCAT), is designed to examine the effects of the aldosterone antagonist therapy in 4500 patients with HFPEF (LVEF ≥ 45%) with a composite morbidity-mortality endpoint (Table 48-2). Study completion is anticipated in 2011. Although ACE inhibitors and ARBs have not proved to have a major beneficial effect on clinical outcomes in HFPEF, it remains to be seen whether aldosterone antagonists have more success; aldosterone plays a major role in stimulating myocardial collagen formation and in inhibiting the turnover of extracellular matrix.

Digoxin

Digoxin is one of the oldest drugs that has been used in the management of heart failure, but it has been historically thought to be contraindicated in HFPEF.[54] Theoretical considerations suggest potential benefit, as well as harm, from digoxin in this group of patients. For example, digoxin may improve the active energy-dependent myocardial early diastolic function and may improve the neurohormonal profile in patients with HFPEF.[54,55] However, it may produce an increase in systolic energy demands, adding to a relative calcium overload in diastole, especially during periods of hemodynamic stress or ischemia, and may thus contribute to diastolic dysfunction.[15] The Digitalis Investigators Group (DIG) investigated the effects of digoxin on morbidity and mortality in patients with heart failure in normal sinus rhythm, the majority of whom had systolic heart failure.[56] However, the trial population also included a small group

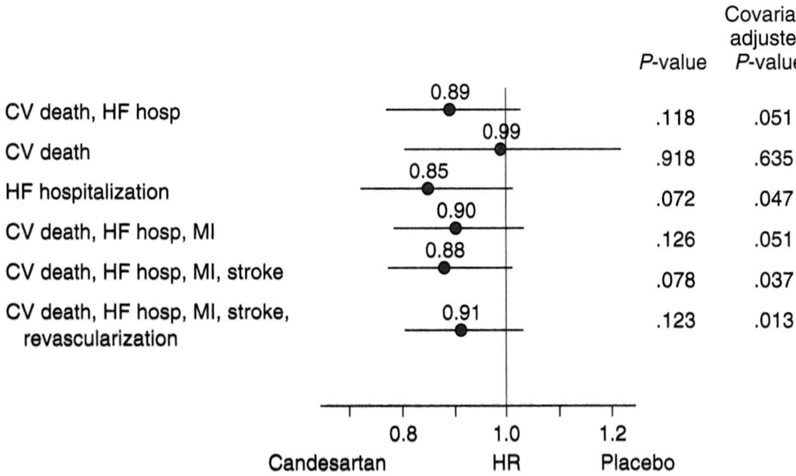

FIGURE 48–2 Hazard ratios (HR) and 95% confidence intervals for candesartan versus placebo for selected secondary endpoints in the Candesartan in Heart Failure Assessment in Reduction of Mortality (CHARM)–Preserved trial. CV, cardiovascular; HF hosp, hospitalization for heart failure; MI, myocardial infarction. (From Yusuf S, Pfeffer MA, Swedberg K, et al. Effects of candesartan in patients with chronic heart failure and preserved left-ventricular ejection fraction: the CHARM-Preserved Trial. *Lancet*. 2003;362:777-781.)

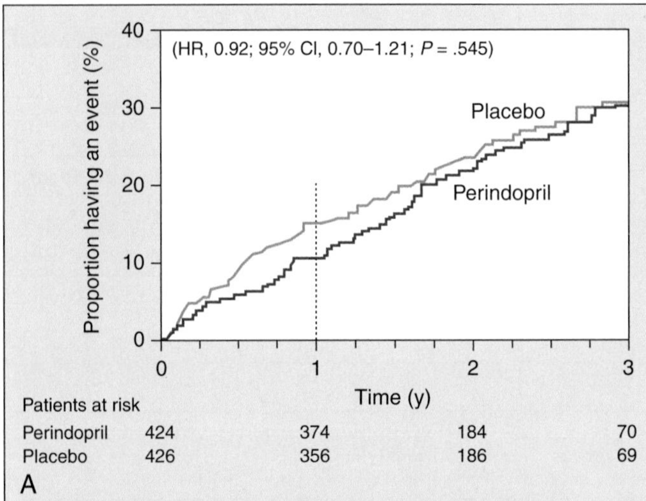

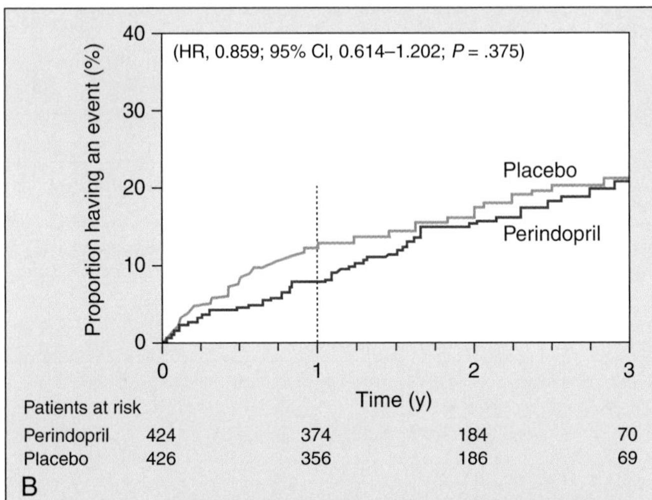

FIGURE 48–3 Effect of perindopril on clinical outcomes. **A,** Kaplan-Meier curves showing time to first occurrence of the primary endpoint: all-cause mortality or unplanned hospitalization related to heart failure (HF). The occurrence of the endpoint at 1 year of follow-up is specified on the *dotted line.* **B,** Kaplan-Meier curves showing time to first occurrence of the prespecified secondary endpoint of unplanned hospitalization related to heart failure. The occurrence of the endpoint at 1 year of follow-up is specified on the *red dotted line.* CI, confidence interval. (From Cleland JG, Tendera M, Adamus J, et al. The Perindopril in Elderly People with Chronic Heart Failure (PEP-CHF) study. *Eur Heart J* 2006;27:2338-2345.)

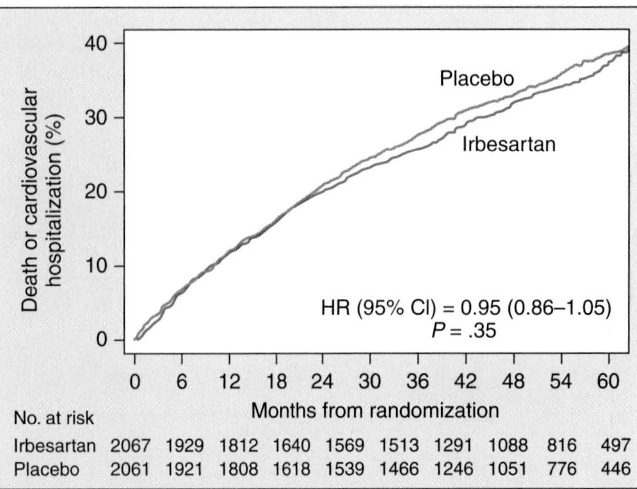

FIGURE 48–4 Kaplan-Meier curves for time to first occurrence of the primary endpoint in the Irbesartan in Heart Failure with Preserved Systolic Function (I-PRESERVE) trial. CI, confidence interval; HR, hazard ratio. (From Massie BM, Carson PE, McMurray JJ, et al. Irbesartan in patients with heart failure and preserved ejection fraction. *N Engl J Med* 2008;359:2456-2467.)

of patients with HFPEF (ejection fraction > 45%). In a post hoc analysis, among the 988 patients with chronic HFPEF, digoxin had no significant effect on the composite primary endpoint of mortality from heart failure and hospitalizations for heart failure (HR, 0.82; 95% CI, 0.63 to 1.07; P = .14).[57] Similarly, digoxin produced no benefit in the composite endpoint of mortality from cardiovascular causes and hospitalization for heart failure. Although the use of digoxin was associated with a trend toward a reduction in hospitalizations for worsening heart failure (HR, 0.79; 95% CI, 0.99 to 1.91; P = .09), it was also associated with a trend toward an increase in hospitalizations for unstable angina (HR, 1.37; 95% CI, 0.99 to 1.91; P = .06). Thus, digoxin was not associated with any overall reduction in hospitalizations for cardiovascular reasons.[57] This post hoc analysis suggests that digoxin should not be recommended as treatment for all patients with HFPEF except, if required, as an agent for rate control in patients with concomitant atrial fibrillation. As noted previously, the DIG trial had enrolled only patients in sinus rhythm.

Endothelin Antagonists

Experimental studies have suggested that selective antagonists of endothelin type A (ET_A) may exert beneficial effects in diastolic heart failure by attenuating the progression of LV hypertrophy and fibrosis, which results in improvement in diastolic function.[58] In addition, in patients with moderate to severe heart failure, acute ET_A receptor blockade with the selective ET_A antagonist sitaxsentan has caused selective pulmonary vasodilation. Therefore, sitaxsentan may also be of value in the treatment of patients with pulmonary hypertension secondary to chronic heart failure.[59] On the basis of these considerations, a double-blind, placebo-controlled study with sitaxsentan in 192 patients with HFPEF was undertaken. The patients were randomly assigned in a 2:1 ratio to receive either the active drug or placebo for 24 weeks. According to preliminary results, patients treated with sitaxsentan had a significant increase in treadmill exercise time (90 seconds) in comparison with placebo (37 seconds; P = .03). No other differences in diastolic parameters, functional status, or clinical outcomes were noted.[60] The details of this study, as well as those of larger future studies, are awaited in order to evaluate whether this benefit will translate into better clinical outcomes in patients with HFPEF.

CURRENT RECOMMENDATIONS FOR THE MANAGEMENT OF PATIENTS WITH HFPEF

The clinical diagnosis of HFPEF depends on the presence of clinical symptoms and signs of heart failure with preserved LVEF (≥45% or ≥50%) measured by any cardiac imaging technique such as echocardiography, radionuclide-enhanced ventriculography, contrast-enhanced ventriculography, or cardiac magnetic resonance imaging. The observation of diastolic abnormalities, elevated LV filling pressures and left atrial enlargement, and substrate for diastolic dysfunction (i.e., LV hypertrophy) on echocardiography may provide supportive evidence. The clinical confirmation of the diagnosis of heart failure, although considered rudimentary, is key especially in ruling out other causes of symptoms such as lung disease and obesity. Several conditions need to be considered in the differential diagnosis before the prototypic "diastolic heart failure" or

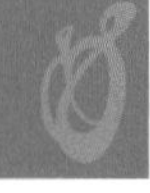

TABLE 48–2 Study Characteristics of Some Ongoing Multicenter Clinical Trials for Patients with HFPEF

Characteristic	TOPCAT[71]	Japanese Diastolic Heart Failure Trial[106]	RELAX[71]	Rheos Diastolic Heart Failure Trial[71]	RESET
Trial Population					
N	4500	800	190	60	400 (to be screened)
LVEF	≥45%	>40%	≥50%	≥45%	≥50%
NYHA class	II to IV	I to IV	II to IV	—	II to III
Other	≥50 years: 100%	—	BNP > 200 pg/mL or NT-BNP > 400 pg/mL Abnormal peak Vo_2	Elevated BNP	BNP > 125 pg/mL
Some Exclusion Criteria					
General finding	ACE inhibitor/ARB allowed	Significant hypotension Heart rate < 50/min	Taking nitrates or α-antagonists Morbid obesity	History of suspected baroreflex failure or autonomic neuropathy	Atrial fibrillation Contraindication to pacemaker
Creatinine level	≥2.5 mg/dL *or* GFR < 30 mL/min/1.73 m²	>3 mg/dL	GFR < 20 mL/min/1.73m²	—	—
Serum potassium level	≥5.0 mEq/L	>5.5 mEq/L	—	—	—
Trial					
Protocol	Double-blind, randomized	Randomized, open-label	Double-blind, randomized	Double-blind, randomized	Double-blind, randomized
Drug and dosage	Spironolactone vs. placebo (titrated up to target dosage of 45 mg/day)	Carvedilol vs. placebo (titrated up to target dosage of 10 mg bid) Minimum follow-up: 2 years	Sildenafil vs. placebo (target dosage of 60 mg tid) for 24 weeks	Rheos Baroreflex Activation system implanted in all patients with device either on or off for 6 months	Crossover study of rate-responsive pacing for 6 months
Primary endpoint	Composite of mortality from CV causes, aborted cardiac arrest, and hospitalization for heart failure	Composite of mortality from CV causes and hospitalization for heart failure	Exercise tolerance: peak Vo_2	Left ventricular mass index	Exercise tolerance: peak Vo_2

ACE, angiotensin-converting enzyme; ARB, angiotensin receptor blocker; BNP, b-type natriuretic peptide; CV, cardiovascular; GFR, glomerular filtration rate; NT-BNP, N-terminal BNP; RELAX, Phosphodiesterase-5 Inhibition to Improve Clinical Status and Exercise Capacity in Diastolic Heart Failure; RESET, Restoration of Chronotropic Competence in Heart Failure Patients With Normal Ejection Fraction; TOPCAT, Treatment of Preserved Cardiac Function Heart Failure with an Aldosterone Antagonist; Vo_2, oxygen consumption.

HFPEF can be treated. The algorithm suggested in the Heart Failure Society of America Heart Failure Practice Guidelines provides a useful framework for the initial workup of such patients (Figure 48-5).[61] Conditions that necessitate specific intervention—such as valvular heart disease, coronary artery disease, pericardial disease, isolated right-sided heart failure causd by primary pulmonary conditions, or contributing systemic conditions such as anemia and thyrotoxicosis—must be identified. Once these conditions are ruled out or treated, patients with HFPEF should be managed in accordance with general guidelines presented in Table 48-3. Treatment considerations can be broadly grouped in the following categories: treatment of volume overload, aggressive control of hypertension, treatment of factors contributing to decompensation (most commonly atrial fibrillation, ischemia, and anemia), and therapies based on associated cardiovascular diagnoses or risk factors. Although based on practice guidelines published by the American College of Cardiology/American Heart Association (ACC/AHA) and the Heart Failure Society of America, it should be noted that the majority of recommendations (other than the treatment of hypertension) are based on consensus opinion of experts rather than on definitive clinical trial data.

FUTURE MODALITIES OF THERAPY IN HFPEF

Potential novel modalities of therapy for HFPEF, some of which are under active investigation, are discussed as follows.

Selective Phosphodiesterase-Type 5 Inhibition

Sildenafil is the one of the best known agents in a class of selective inhibitors of phosphodiesterase-5, which are known to enhance nitric oxide–mediated vasodilation by inhibiting degradation of cyclic guanosine monophosphate, a key intracellular second messenger.[62] Whereas inhibitors of the cyclic adenosine monophosphate (AMP)–specific phosphodiesterase-3 (including inotropic agents such as milrinone and enoximone) augment intracellular levels of cyclic AMP and increase mortality among patients with heart failure,[63] sildenafil is highly selective for human phosphodiesterase-5, does not increase cyclic AMP levels, and lacks inotropic effects. Therefore, it is not thought to share the toxicity associated with phosphodiesterase-3 inhibition.[64]

Several experimental observations suggest that sildenafil may be beneficial in the treatment of patients with HFPEF. In

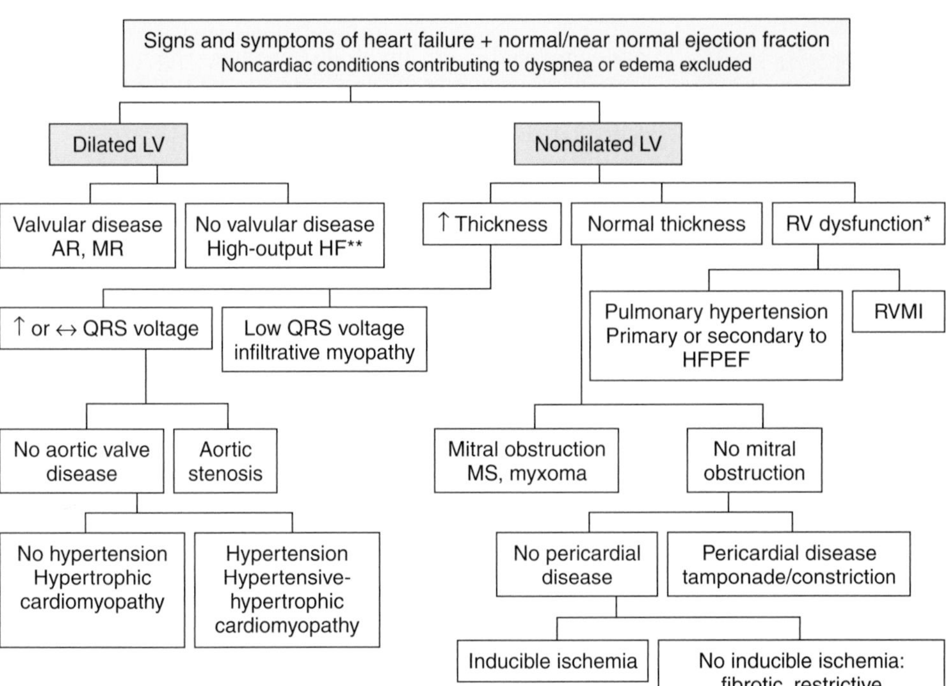

FIGURE 48-5 Diagnostic considerations in patients with heart failure with preserved ejection fraction (HFPEF). *Asterisk* indicates that some patients with right ventricular dysfunction have left ventricular dysfunction as a result of ventricular interaction. *Double asterisk* indicates, for example, anemia, thyrotoxicosis, and arteriovenous fistula. AR, aortic regurgitation; HF, heart failure; LV, left ventricle; MR, mitral regurgitation; MS, mitral stenosis; RV, right ventricle; RVMI, right ventricular myocardial infarction. (Adapted from Adams KF, Lindenfeld J, Arnold JMO, et al. Executive summary: HFSA 2006 Comprehensive Heart Failure Practice Guideline. *J Card Fail* 2006;12:10-38. Copyright 2006, with permission from the Heart Failure Society of America.)

mice exposed to sustained pressure overload, chronic phosphodiesterase-5 inhibition led to attenuation of cardiac and myocyte hypertrophy, attenuation of interstitial fibrosis, and improvement in cardiac functioning.[65] Sildenafil treatment applied to well-established hypertrophic cardiac disease in mice also prevented further cardiac and myocyte dysfunction, as well as progressive remodeling.[66] These investigators demonstrated that phosphodiesterase-5 is upregulated in the heart in response to pressure overload and that the effects of phosphodiesterase-5 inhibition are not mediated by an effect on blood pressure. In addition, phosphodiesterase-5 inhibition has been associated with improvement in flow-mediated vasodilation in patients with systolic heart failure and an improvement in large artery stiffness in hypertensive men.[67,68] Beneficial effects on pulmonary vasculature with reduction in pulmonary pressures, as well as reduction in right ventricular hypertrophy, have been demonstrated in patients with pulmonary hypertension.[69] Furthermore, phosphodiesterase-5 inhibition may restore renal responsiveness to natriuretic peptides in several states of abnormal sodium handling, including heart failure.[70] Because phosphodiesterase-5 is upregulated in cardiovascular disease states such as heart failure, with resultant greater susceptibility to phosphodiesterase-5 inhibition in these disease states—along with the potential beneficial effects on LV hypertrophy, endothelial function, arterial stiffness, pulmonary hypertension and renal responsiveness to natriuretic peptides just summarized—the use of selective phosphodiesterase-5 inhibitors as therapeutic agents is being evaluated in the treatment of patients with HFPEF. As an initial step, the Phosphodiesterase-5 Inhibition to Improve Clinical Status and Exercise Capacity in Diastolic Heart Failure (RELAX) study, sponsored by the National Institutes of Health, is currently enrolling patients with HFPEF. Patients are randomly assigned to receive either sildenafil or placebo for 24 weeks in order to evaluate the effect of sildenafil on a number of intermediate outcomes, including exercise capacity, quality of life, diastolic function, LV mass, and peripheral vascular function (see Table 48-2).[71]

Advanced Glycation End Products

Increased LV and arterial stiffness, which may be involved in the pathophysiology of HFPEF, especially in elderly subjects,[16,72] is at least partially contributed to by nonenzymatic crosslinks that develop between advanced glycation end products on long-lived proteins such as collagen and elastin. Alagebrium chloride nonenzymatically breaks these cross-links and has been shown to improve LV distensibility and arterial compliance in experimental animals.[73] Initial clinical experience with this agent also showed increased arterial compliance in elderly subjects with systolic hypertension.[74] These data suggest that alagebrium chloride may be beneficial in the treatment of HFPEF, especially in the setting of hypertension, diabetes, and aging. An initial open-label study evaluated the use of alagebrium chloride for 16 weeks in 23 elderly patients with stable heart failure and LVEF higher than 50%.[75] Alagebrium chloride was associated with a reduction of LV mass, improvement in tissue Doppler indices of diastolic function, and improvement in quality of life. However, there was no change in blood pressure, pulse pressure, peak oxygen consumption, or aortic distensibility. At this point, it remains to be seen whether the initial modest benefits observed with this agent will translate into reduction in clinical endpoints such as hospitalization for heart failure or in improvement of exercise capacity. A phase II, placebo-controlled, double-blind, randomized clinical trial, Beginning a Randomized Evaluation of the AGE [advanced glycation end] Product Breaker Alagebrium in Diastolic Heart Failure (BREAK) was intended to assess the effect of 6 months of oral treatment with alagebrium chloride versus placebo in 80 patients with HFPEF; however, it was halted for administrative reasons.[71]

Lusitropic Agents

Another promising agent appeared to be MCC-135, an oral drug that improves lusitropy by enhancing calcium uptake by the sarcoplasmic reticulum and inhibiting the reverse mode of the sodium-calcium exchanger.[76] A double-blind,

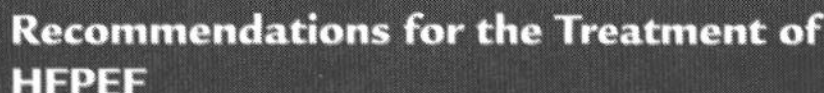

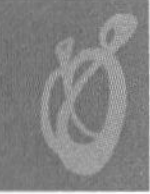

TABLE 48–3 Recommendations for the Treatment of HFPEF

Recommendations	Strength of Recommendation*	Level of Evidence†
Control of systolic and diastolic hypertension as per published guidelines.	I	A
Control of ventricular rate in atrial fibrillation.	I	C
Diuretics to control pulmonary congestion and peripheral edema. (Treatment may be started with a thiazide or loop diuretic. Excessive diuresis may lead to orthostatic changes in blood pressure and worsening renal function. Counseling on the use of a low-sodium diet is recommended.)	I	C
Possible revascularization in patients with significant coronary artery disease and symptoms or demonstrable ischemia, in which ischemia may be regarded as a contributor to abnormal cardiac function.	IIa	C
Restoration and maintenance of sinus rhythm in certain patients with atrial fibrillation, which may be useful to control symptoms.	IIb	C
ACE inhibitors and ARBs in patients with controlled hypertension, which might be useful in minimizing symptoms of heart failure.	IIb	C
β-blockers, which might be effective in control of symptoms. They should be given greater consideration for patients with HFPEF and	IIb	C
• Prior myocardial infarction		A
• Hypertension		B
• Atrial fibrillation		B
Calcium channel blockers, for control of symptoms. They should be given greater consideration for patients with HFPEF and	IIb	C
• Atrial fibrillation necessitating control of ventricular rate when blockers have proven inadequate; diltiazem or verapamil should be considered		C
• Symptom-limiting angina		A
• Hypertension; amlodipine should be considered		C
Possibly digitalis, to minimize symptoms of heart failure	IIB	C

*Strength of recommendations: I indicates a recommendation that treatment is useful or effective; IIa indicates a recommendation in favor of treatment's being useful or effective; IIb indicates greater conflicting evidence from multiple randomized trials or meta-analyses.
†Level of evidence: A indicates that data were derived from multiple randomized clinical trials or meta-analyses; B indicates that data were derived from a single randomized clinical trial or nonrandomized studies; C indicates only consensus opinion of experts, case studies, or standard of care.
ACE, angiotensin-converting enzyme; ARB, angiotensin receptor blocker; HFPEF, heart failure with preserved ejection fraction; NYHA, New York Heart Association.
Adapted from the American College of Cardiology/American Heart Association Guidelines for the Diagnosis and Management of Patients with Heart Failure in Adults, 2009,[107] and the Heart Failure Society of America Heart Failure Practice Guidelines, 2006.[61]

randomized, placebo-controlled phase II trial of MCC-135 was completed in 2003 with 500 patients who had heart failure, 230 of whom had HFPEF.[77] However, the results have not been published to date, which suggests that beneficial effects may not have been noted.

Treatment of Obstructive Sleep Apnea

Obstructive sleep apnea (OSA) has been detected in 11% to 37% of patients with heart failure with systolic dysfunction.[78-80] In a small study of HFPEF, sleep-disordered breathing was reported in more than 50% of patients with HFPEF; the majority of these patients had obstructive sleep apnea.[81] Patients with HFPEF and sleep-disordered breathing had worse diastolic dysfunction than did patients without sleep-disordered breathing. Unlike systolic heart failure, for which a number of studies have shown an increased prevalence of central sleep apnea, HFPEF may be more often associated with OSA. Several theoretical mechanisms may explain how OSA contributes to the development of diastolic dysfunction and heart failure.[82] The most direct mechanism may be through long-standing OSA, which induces LV dysfunction by raising blood pressure, a major risk factor for the development and progression of HFPEF.[83] It has been suggested that LV hypertrophy is linked to hypertension more closely during sleep than during wakefulness.[84] Thus, because hypertensive patients with OSA have higher nocturnal blood pressure than do those without OSA, they may be at greater risk in the long term for LV hypertrophy and heart failure. In patients with heart failure, the coexistence of OSA may also be associated with higher sympathetic nerve activity and higher systolic blood pressure during wakefulness, despite more intense antihypertensive therapy.[85]

Responses to cytokines, catecholamines, endothelin, and other growth factors produced in OSA may contribute to ventricular hypertrophy independently of hypertension, as suggested by the fact that LV wall thickness has been shown to be increased in normotensive patients with OSA, in comparison with normotensive control subjects. In addition, nocturnal oxygen desaturation is an independent predictor of impaired ventricular relaxation during diastole.[86] Increased negative intrathoracic pressure during obstructive apneas may also lead to increased LV wall tension and afterload, which may contribute to low stroke volume and cardiac output during OSA. Long-term recurrent exposure of the heart to markedly subatmospheric pressure during OSA could promote hypertrophy and diastolic dysfunction, in addition to the long-term effects of systemic hypertension. Furthermore, a leftward shift of the interventricular septum, which results from overdistention of the right ventricle during obstructive apneas, may also limit LV filling and thus decrease cardiac output. Some of the cardiovascular changes may be reversible with effective continuous positive airway pressure (CPAP) treatment.[82,87] However, at this time, little evidence is available regarding the benefit of CPAP on patients with HFPEF. In one small group of patients who had OSA but did not have hypertension, diabetes, or other factors that could contribute to diastolic dysfunction, 12 weeks of CPAP reportedly attenuated abnormalities in diastolic function.[88] Further studies are, however, needed to examine the clinical benefit of CPAP in patients with HFPEF.

Potential Device Use in HFPEF

Pacemakers

Patients with HFPEF have been reported to have chronotropic incompetence in response to exercise, and this may contribute to significant limitation of their physical activity. Borlaug and associates[17] showed that at matched low-level

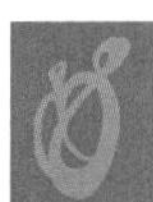

workload, as well as at peak workload, patients with HFPEF had less of an increase in heart rate and in cardiac output and less systemic vasodilation than did control subjects, despite similar rises in end-diastolic volume, stroke volume, and contractility. Although these findings first raise questions about the conventional wisdom of using β-blockers (which are negative chronotropic agents) in patients with HFPEF, especially elderly patients, they also reveal a potential modality for treatment of HFPEF. The Restoration of Chronotropic Competence in Heart Failure Patients with Normal Ejection Fraction (RESET) trial (see Table 48-2) is intended to evaluate the effect of atrial rate–responsive pacing on exercise capacity and quality of life in patients with HFPEF.

Device-Based Treatment of Resistant Hypertension

A number of patients with HFPEF have uncontrolled hypertension that is resistant to a combination of multiple antihypertensive agents. The importance of the carotid sinus baroreceptors in modulating autonomic tone and regulating blood pressure (baroreflex mechanism) has long been recognized. It is also well established that the arterial baroreflex buffers short-term fluctuations in blood pressure. Although there has been some debate regarding its role in long-term blood pressure control, study results have suggested that the baroreflex system is important in chronic hypertension, and that renal sympathetic inhibition with a resultant increase in natriuresis may be one of the mechanisms by which the baroreflex participates in long-term blood pressure control.

Animal and human studies have demonstrated a safe and effective lowering of blood pressure with chronic electrical stimulation of the carotid sinus. The postulated mechanism is that activation of the baroreceptors is interpreted by the brain as elevation in blood pressure; as a result, cardiac parasympathetic tone is activated, and sympathetic outflow to the heart, kidneys, and peripheral vasculature is diminished.[89-95] The most recent studies have been performed with the Rheos System (CVRx, Inc.). The system consists of an implantable pulse generator, the energy from which is conducted through leads to the left and right carotid sinuses, resulting in carotid sinus stimulation. Use of the device has been associated with significant improvement in blood pressure sustained over 2 to 3 years (reduction of ≈30/20 mm Hg) along with improvement in LV mass in patients with resistant hypertension. No significant side effects of bradycardia or orthostatic hypotension were noted.[96,97] A phase II study with this system has been initiated to examine the safety and efficacy of baroreceptor activation on LV mass in patients with HFPEF (see Table 48-2).[71] A different approach involving catheter-based renal sympathetic denervation has also been reported to show similar significant and sustained improvement in blood pressure in patients with resistant hypertension.[98] A sustained improvement of blood pressure in patients with HFPEF and resistant hypertension will probably translate into improvement in cardiovascular outcomes.

Targeting Diastolic Suction

Another pathological mechanism being targeted is a proposed abnormality of early diastolic suction of the left ventricle in patients with diastolic heart failure. The elastic recoil of the ventricle during early diastole contributes significantly to an early diastolic pressure gradient from the left atrium to the LV apex and allows the left ventricle to actively suction blood from the left atrium during early diastole, thus contributing to early LV filling.[99-102] Diastolic suction allows the left ventricle to decrease its pressure despite its filling during early diastole. A major determinant of diastolic suction is the potential energy stored as myocytes are compressed and the elastic elements in the LV wall are compressed and twisted during systole. This energy is released as the elastic elements recoil during relaxation. With diastolic dysfunction (slowed relaxation and reduced elastic recoil), this diastolic suction is reduced, and LV early filling is probably impaired.

A series of passive diastolic assist devices (manufactured by CorAssist Cardiovascular Limited) are being developed and studied.[103] The initial device, ImCardia, is attached to the epimyocardial surface of the left ventricle. The design is based on the principle of restoring normal balance of myocardial dynamic energy by the transfer of energy from preserved systole to underfunctioning diastole in a stiff ventricle. Potential energy produced by the left ventricle during systole is stored in the device—in essence, being loaded like a spring—and is released during diastole, providing a recoiling force to restore the myocardium to its resting length. Initial feasibility and proof-of-concept studies have been performed in animals, and initial small studies are under way with human subjects.[104,105] A newer generation of the device that is implanted into the inner ventricular cavity is also being tested. The device is yet to be tested in larger clinical trials in patients with HFPEF.

CONCLUSIONS

The high prevalence of HFPEF with its associated substantial morbidity and mortality has been recognized, and as a result, a quest for effective therapy for the condition has been initiated. In contrast to systolic heart failure, in which RAAS blockers have been proved to have beneficial effects on mortality and morbidity (see Chapter 45), none of the clinical trials to date with ACE inhibitors or ARBs has demonstrated definitive benefit in clinical outcomes in patients with HFPEF. A number of novel therapies that are being currently tested for HFPEF are targeting alternative pathophysiological mechanisms . At present, recommended therapy is aimed at relief of symptoms, control of hypertension, and management of other contributory comorbid conditions. Although RAAS blockers and β-blockers are not currently recommended specifically for the treatment of HFPEF, their use in the treatment of other conditions that frequently coexist in affected patients remains important. Researchers may need to reconsider traditional endpoints such as mortality for the evaluation of efficacy of therapies in patients with HFPEF, a population with many comorbid conditions and many competing risks for mortality. Researchers also need to consider whether hospitalization and exercise capacity are more meaningful endpoints in this patient population. In addition, because of the heterogeneity of patients with HFPEF, it may be difficult to prove that a particular therapeutic agent is efficacious in all patients; therefore, relevant interventions in more homogeneous subgroups of patients may need to be studied.

REFERENCES

1. Hogg, K., Swedberg, K., & McMurray, J. (2004). Heart failure with preserved left ventricular systolic function: epidemiology, clinical characteristics, and prognosis. *J Am Coll Cardiol, 43*, 317–327.
2. Vasan, R. S., Larson, M. G., Benjamin, E. J., et al. (1999). Congestive heart failure in subjects with normal versus reduced left ventricular ejection fraction: prevalence and mortality in a population-based cohort. *J Am Coll Cardiol, 33*, 1948–1955.
3. Kitzman, D. W., Gardin, J. M., Gottdiener, J. S., et al. (2001). Importance of heart failure with preserved systolic function in patients >=65 years of age. *Am J Cardiol, 87*, 413–419.
4. Cleland, J. G., Swedberg, K., Follath, F., et al. (2003). The EuroHeart Failure survey programme—a survey on the quality of care among patients with heart failure in Europe. Part 1: patient characteristics and diagnosis. *Eur Heart J, 24*, 442–463.
5. Fonarow, G. C. (2003). The Acute Decompensated Heart Failure National Registry (ADHERE): opportunities to improve care of patients hospitalized with acute decompensated heart failure. *Rev Cardiovasc Med, 4*(Suppl. 7), S21–S30.
6. Owan, T. E., Hodge, D. O., Herges, R. M., et al. (2006). Trends in prevalence and outcome of heart failure with preserved ejection fraction. *N Engl J Med, 355*, 251–259.
7. Cohen-Solal, A., Desnos, M., Delahaye, F., et al. (2000). A national survey of heart failure in French hospitals. The Myocardiopathy and Heart Failure Working Group of the French Society of Cardiology, the National College of General Hospital Cardiologists and the French Geriatrics Society. *Eur Heart J, 21*, 763–769.

8. Petrie, M. C., Dawson, N. F., Murdoch, D. R., et al. (1999). Failure of women's hearts. *Circulation, 99*, 2334–2341.
9. Zile, M. R. (2003). Heart failure with preserved ejection fraction: is this diastolic heart failure?. *J Am Coll Cardiol, 41*, 1519–1522.
10. Smith, G. L., Masoudi, F. A., Vaccarino, V., et al. (2003). Outcomes in heart failure patients with preserved ejection fraction. Mortality, readmission, and functional decline. *J Am Coll Cardiol, 41*, 1510–1518.
11. Bhatia, R. S., Tu, J. V., Lee, D. S., et al. (2006). Outcome of heart failure with preserved ejection fraction in a population-based study. *N Engl J Med, 355*, 260–269.
12. Little, W. C., & Brucks, S. (2005). Therapy for diastolic heart failure. *Prog Cardiovasc Dis, 47*, 380–388.
13. Zile, M. R., Baicu, C. F., & Gaasch, W. H. (2004). Diastolic heart failure—-abnormalities in active relaxation and passive stiffness of the left ventricle. *N Engl J Med, 350*, 1953–1959.
14. Zile, M. R., Gaasch, W. H., Carroll, J. D., et al. (2001). Heart failure with a normal ejection fraction: is measurement of diastolic function necessary to make the diagnosis of diastolic heart failure? *Circulation, 104*, 779–782.
15. Zile, M. R., & Brutsaert, D. L. (2002). New concepts in diastolic dysfunction and diastolic heart failure: part II: causal mechanisms and treatment. *Circulation, 105*, 1503–1508.
16. Kawaguchi, M., Hay, I., Fetics, B., et al. (2003). Combined ventricular systolic and arterial stiffening in patients with heart failure and preserved ejection fraction: implications for systolic and diastolic reserve limitations. *Circulation, 107*, 714–720.
17. Borlaug, B. A., Melenovsky, V., Russell, S. D., et al. (2006). Impaired chronotropic and vasodilator reserves limit exercise capacity in patients with heart failure and a preserved ejection fraction. *Circulation, 114*, 2138–2147.
18. Maurer, M. S., King, D. L., El Khoury, R. L., et al. (2005). Left heart failure with a normal ejection fraction: identification of different pathophysiologic mechanisms. *J Card Fail, 11*, 177–187.
19. Redfield, M. M. (2007). Heart failure with normal ejection fraction. In P. Libby, R. O. Bonow, & D. L. Mann (Eds.). *Braunwald's heart disease: a textbook of cardiovascular medicine* (8th ed). Philadelphia: Elsevier, Chapter 26.
20. Little, W. C., Badke, F. R., & O'Rourke, R. A. (1984). Effect of right ventricular pressure on the end-diastolic left ventricular pressure-volume relationship before and after chronic right ventricular pressure overload in dogs without pericardia. *Circ Res, 54*, 719–730.
21. Dauterman, K., Pak, P. H., Maughan, W. L., et al. (1995). Contribution of external forces to left ventricular diastolic pressure: implications for the clinical use of the Starling law. *Ann Intern Med, 122*, 737–742.
22. The ALLHAT Officers and Coordinators for the ALLHAT Collaborative Research Group. (2002). Major outcomes in high-risk hypertensive patients randomized to angiotensin-converting enzyme inhibitor or calcium channel blocker vs diuretic: the Antihypertensive and Lipid-Lowering Treatment to Prevent Heart Attack Trial (ALLHAT). *JAMA, 288*, 2981–2997.
23. Kostis, J. B., Davis, B. R., Cutler, J., et al. (1997). Prevention of heart failure by antihypertensive drug treatment in older persons with isolated systolic hypertension. *JAMA, 278*, 212–216.
24. Mohan, P., Brutsaert, D. L., Paulus, W. J., et al. (1996). Myocardial contractile response to nitric oxide and cGMP. *Circulation, 93*, 1223–1229.
25. Matter, C. M., Mandinov, L., Kaufmann, P. A., et al. (1999). Effect of NO donors on LV diastolic function in patients with severe pressure-overload hypertrophy. *Circulation, 99*, 2396–2401.
26. Hoit, B. D., & Walsh, R. A. (1994). Diastolic dysfunction in hypertensive heart disease. In W. H. Gaasch, & M. M. LeWinter (Eds.). *Left ventricular diastolic dysfunction and heart failure* Philadelphia: Lea & Febiger, pp 354–372.
27. Leite-Moreira, A. F., & Correia-Pinto, J. (2001). Load as an acute determinant of end-diastolic pressure-volume relation. *Am J Physiol Heart Circ Physiol, 280*, H51–H59.
28. Hundley, W. G., Kitzman, D. W., Morgan, T. M., et al. (2001). Cardiac cycle–dependent changes in aortic area and distensibility are reduced in older patients with isolated diastolic heart failure and correlate with exercise intolerance. *J Am Coll Cardiol, 38*, 796–802.
29. Little, W. C., Ohno, M., Kitzman, D. W., et al. (1995). Determination of left ventricular chamber stiffness from the time for deceleration of early left ventricular filling. *Circulation, 92*, 1933–1939.
30. Devereux, R. B., Palmieri, V., Sharpe, N., et al. (2001). Effects of once-daily angiotensin-converting enzyme inhibition and calcium channel blockade–based antihypertensive treatment regimens on left ventricular hypertrophy and diastolic filling in hypertension: the Prospective Randomized Enalapril Study Evaluating Regression of Ventricular Enlargement (PRESERVE) trial. *Circulation, 104*, 1248–1254.
31. Terpstra, W. F., May, J. F., Smit, A. J., et al. (2001). Long-term effects of amlodipine and lisinopril on left ventricular mass and diastolic function in elderly, previously untreated hypertensive patients: the ELVERA trial. *J Hypertens, 19*, 303–309.
32. Solomon, S. D., Janardhanan, R., Verma, A., et al. (2007). Effect of angiotensin receptor blockade and antihypertensive drugs on diastolic function in patients with hypertension and diastolic dysfunction: a randomised trial. *Lancet, 369*, 2079–2087.
33. Dahlof, B., Devereux, R. B., Kjeldsen, S. E., et al. (2002). Cardiovascular morbidity and mortality in the Losartan Intervention For Endpoint reduction in hypertension study (LIFE): a randomised trial against atenolol. *Lancet, 359*, 995–1003.
34. Moser, M., & Hebert, P. R. (1996). Prevention of disease progression, left ventricular hypertrophy and congestive heart failure in hypertension treatment trials. *J Am Coll Cardiol, 27*, 1214–1218.
35. Beckett, N. S., Peters, R., Fletcher, A. E., et al. (2008). Treatment of hypertension in patients 80 years of age or older. *N Engl J Med, 358*, 1887–1898.
36. Setaro, J. F., Zaret, B. L., Schulman, D. S., et al. (1990). Usefulness of verapamil for congestive heart failure associated with abnormal left ventricular diastolic filling and normal left ventricular systolic performance. *Am J Cardiol, 66*, 981–986.
37. Hung, M. J., Cherng, W. J., Kuo, L. T., et al. (2002). Effect of verapamil in elderly patients with left ventricular diastolic dysfunction as a cause of congestive heart failure. *Int J Clin Pract, 56*, 57–62.
38. Aronow, W. S., Ahn, C., & Kronzon, I. (1997). Effect of propranolol versus no propranolol on total mortality plus nonfatal myocardial infarction in older patients with prior myocardial infarction, congestive heart failure, and left ventricular ejection fraction > or = 40% treated with diuretics plus angiotensin-converting enzyme inhibitors. *Am J Cardiol, 80*, 207–209.
39. Aronow, W. S., & Kronzon, I. (1993). Effect of enalapril on congestive heart failure treated with diuretics in elderly patients with prior myocardial infarction and normal left ventricular ejection fraction. *Am J Cardiol, 71*, 602–604.
40. Bergstrom, A., Andersson, B., Edner, M., et al. (2004). Effect of carvedilol on diastolic function in patients with diastolic heart failure and preserved systolic function. Results of the Swedish Doppler-Echocardiographic Study (SWEDIC). *Eur J Heart Fail, 6*, 453–461.
41. Kuroedov, A., Cosentino, F., & Luscher, T. F. (2004). Pharmacological mechanisms of clinically favorable properties of a selective β_1-adrenoceptor antagonist, nebivolol. *Cardiovasc Drug Rev, 22*, 155–168.
42. Flather, M. D., Shibata, M. C., Coats, A. J., et al. (2005). Randomized trial to determine the effect of nebivolol on mortality and cardiovascular hospital admission in elderly patients with heart failure (SENIORS). *Eur Heart J, 26*, 215–225.
43. Yamamoto, K., Masuyama, T., Sakata, Y., et al. (2000). Roles of renin-angiotensin and endothelin systems in development of diastolic heart failure in hypertensive hearts. *Cardiovasc Res, 47*, 274–283.
44. Martos, R., Baugh, J., Ledwidge, M., et al. (2007). Diastolic heart failure: evidence of increased myocardial collagen turnover linked to diastolic dysfunction. *Circulation, 115*, 888–895.
45. Cheng, C. P., Suzuki, M., Ohte, N., et al. (1996). Altered ventricular and myocyte response to angiotensin II in pacing-induced heart failure. *Circ Res, 78*, 880–892.
46. Cheng, C. P., Ukai, T., Onishi, K., et al. (2001). The role of ANG II and endothelin-1 in exercise-induced diastolic dysfunction in heart failure. *Am J Physiol Heart Circ Physiol, 280*, H1853–H1860.
47. Yusuf, S., Sleight, P., Pogue, J., et al. (2000). Effects of an angiotensin-converting-enzyme inhibitor, ramipril, on cardiovascular events in high-risk patients. The Heart Outcomes Prevention Evaluation Study Investigators. *N Engl J Med, 342*, 145–153.
48. Dagenais, G. R., Pogue, J., Fox, K., et al. (2006). Angiotensin-converting-enzyme inhibitors in stable vascular disease without left ventricular systolic dysfunction or heart failure: a combined analysis of three trials. *Lancet, 368*, 581–588.
49. Yusuf, S., Pfeffer, M. A., Swedberg, K., et al. (2003). Effects of candesartan in patients with chronic heart failure and preserved left-ventricular ejection fraction: the CHARM-Preserved Trial. *Lancet, 362*, 777–781.
50. Cleland, J. G. F., Tendera, M., Adamus, J., et al. (2006). The Perindopril in Elderly People with Chronic Heart Failure (PEP-CHF) study. *Eur Heart J, 27*, 2338–2345.
51. Massie, B. M., Carson, P. E., McMurray, J. J., et al. (2008). Irbesartan in patients with heart failure and preserved ejection fraction. *N Engl J Med, 359*, 2456–2467.
52. Yip, G. W., Wang, M., Wang, T., et al. (2008). The Hong Kong Diastolic Heart Failure Study: a randomized control trial of diuretics, irbesartan and ramipril on quality of life, exercise capacity, left ventricular global and regional function in heart failure with a normal ejection fraction. *Heart, 94*, 573–580.
53. Voors, A. A., & de Jong, R. M. (2008). Treating diastolic heart failure. *Heart, 94*, 971–972.
54. Massie, B. M., & Abdalla, I. (1998). Heart failure in patients with preserved left ventricular systolic function: do digitalis glycosides have a role? *Prog Cardiovasc Dis, 40*, 357–369.
55. Ferguson, D. W. (1992). Digitalis and neurohormonal abnormalities in heart failure and implications for therapy. *Am J Cardiol, 69*, 24G–32G.
56. The effect of digoxin on mortality and morbidity in patients with heart failure. (1997). The Digitalis Investigation Group. *N Engl J Med, 336*, 525–533.
57. Ahmed, A., Rich, M. W., Fleg, J. L., et al. (2006). Effects of digoxin on morbidity and mortality in diastolic heart failure: the Ancillary Digitalis Investigation Group Trial. *Circulation, 114*, 397–403.
58. Yamamoto, K., Masuyama, T., Sakata, Y., et al. (2002). Prevention of diastolic heart failure by endothelin type A receptor antagonist through inhibition of ventricular structural remodeling in hypertensive heart. *J Hypertens, 20*, 753–761.
59. Givertz, M. M., Colucci, W. S., LeJemtel, T. H., et al. (2000). Acute endothelin A receptor blockade causes selective pulmonary vasodilation in patients with chronic heart failure. *Circulation, 101*, 2922–2927.
60. Zile, M. R., Barst, R. J., Bourge, R., et al. (2009). A phase 2 randomized, double-blind, placebo-controlled exploratory efficacy study of sitaxsentan sodium to improve impaired exercise tolerance in subjects with diastolic heart failure. *J Card Fail, 15*(Suppl. 6S), S63.
61. Adams, K. F., Lindenfeld, J., Arnold, J. M. O., et al. (2006). Executive summary: HFSA 2006 Comprehensive Heart Failure Practice Guideline. *J Card Fail, 12*, 10–38.
62. Semigran, M. J. (2005). Type 5 phosphodiesterase inhibition: the focus shifts to the heart. *Circulation, 112*, 2589–2591.
63. Nony, P., Boissel, J. P., Lievre, M., et al. (1994). Evaluation of the effect of phosphodiesterase inhibitors on mortality in chronic heart failure patients. A meta-analysis. *Eur J Clin Pharmacol, 46*, 191–196.
64. Cheitlin, M. D., Hutter, A. M., Jr., Brindis, R. G., et al. (1999). ACC/AHA expert consensus document. Use of sildenafil (Viagra) in patients with cardiovascular disease. American College of Cardiology/American Heart Association. *J Am Coll Cardiol, 33*, 273–282.
65. Takimoto, E., Champion, H. C., Li, M., et al. (2005). Chronic inhibition of cyclic GMP phosphodiesterase 5A prevents and reverses cardiac hypertrophy. *Nat Med, 11*, 214–222.
66. Nagayama, T., Hsu, S., Zhang, M., et al. (2009). Sildenafil stops progressive chamber, cellular, and molecular remodeling and improves calcium handling and function in hearts with pre-existing advanced hypertrophy caused by pressure overload. *J Am Coll Cardiol, 53*, 207–215.
67. Katz, S. D., Balidemaj, K., Homma, S., et al. (2000). Acute type 5 phosphodiesterase inhibition with sildenafil enhances flow-mediated vasodilation in patients with chronic heart failure. *J Am Coll Cardiol, 36*, 845–851.

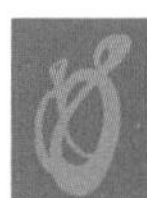

68. Mahmud, A., Hennessy, M., & Feely, J. (2001). Effect of sildenafil on blood pressure and arterial wave reflection in treated hypertensive men. *J Hum Hypertens, 15*, 707–713.
69. Ghofrani, H. A., Osterloh, I. H., & Grimminger, F. (2006). Sildenafil: from angina to erectile dysfunction to pulmonary hypertension and beyond. *Nat Rev Drug Discov, 5*, 689–702.
70. Chen, H. H., Huntley, B. K., Schirger, J. A., et al. (2006). Maximizing the renal cyclic 3′-5′-guanosine monophosphate system with type V phosphodiesterase inhibition and exogenous natriuretic peptide: a novel strategy to improve renal function in experimental overt heart failure. *J Am Soc Nephrol, 17*, 2742–2747.
71. The University of Texas M. D. Anderson Center. *Clinical trials at M.D. Anderson Cancer Center* (web page): www.clinicaltrials.org. Accessed February 28, 2010.
72. Zile, M. R., & Brutsaert, D. L. (2002). New concepts in diastolic dysfunction and diastolic heart failure: part I: diagnosis, prognosis, and measurements of diastolic function. *Circulation, 105*, 1387–1393.
73. Vaitkevicius, P. V., Lane, M., Spurgeon, H., et al. (2001). A cross-link breaker has sustained effects on arterial and ventricular properties in older rhesus monkeys. *Proc Natl Acad Sci U S A, 98*, 1171–1175.
74. Kass, D. A., Shapiro, E. P., Kawaguchi, M., et al. (2001). Improved arterial compliance by a novel advanced glycation end-product crosslink breaker. *Circulation, 104*, 1464–1470.
75. Little, W. C., Zile, M. R., Kitzman, D. W., et al. (2005). The effect of alagebrium chloride (ALT-711), a novel glucose cross-link breaker, in the treatment of elderly patients with diastolic heart failure. *J Card Fail, 11*, 191–195.
76. Satoh, N., Sato, T., Shimada, M., et al. (2001). Lusitropic effect of MCC-135 is associated with improvement of sarcoplasmic reticulum function in ventricular muscles of rats with diabetic cardiomyopathy. *J Pharmacol Exp Ther, 298*, 1161–1166.
77. Zile, M., Gaasch, W., Little, W., et al. (2004). A phase II, double-blind, randomized, placebo-controlled, dose comparative study of the efficacy, tolerability, and safety of MCC-135 in subjects with chronic heart failure, NYHA class II/III (MCC-135-GO1 study): rationale and design. *J Card Fail, 10*, 193–199.
78. Sin, D. D., Fitzgerald, F., Parker, J. D., et al. (1999). Risk factors for central and obstructive sleep apnea in 450 men and women with congestive heart failure. *Am J Respir Crit Care Med, 160*, 1101–1106.
79. Javaheri, S., Parker, T. J., Liming, J. D., et al. (1998). Sleep apnea in 81 ambulatory male patients with stable heart failure: types and their prevalences, consequences, and presentations. *Circulation, 97*, 2154–2159.
80. Lanfranchi, P. A., Somers, V. K., Braghiroli, A., et al. (2003). Central sleep apnea in left ventricular dysfunction: prevalence and implications for arrhythmic risk. *Circulation, 107*, 727–732.
81. Chan, J., Sanderson, J., Chan, W., et al. (1997). Prevalence of sleep-disordered breathing in diastolic heart failure. *Chest, 111*, 1488–1493.
82. Somers, V. K., White, D. P., Amin, R., et al. (2008). Sleep apnea and cardiovascular disease: an American Heart Association/American College of Cardiology Foundation Scientific Statement from the American Heart Association Council for High Blood Pressure Research Professional Education Committee, Council on Clinical Cardiology, Stroke Council, and Council on Cardiovascular Nursing. *J Am Coll Cardiol, 52*, 686–717.
83. Levy, D., Larson, M. G., Vasan, R. S., et al. (1996). The progression from hypertension to congestive heart failure. *JAMA, 275*, 1557–1562.
84. Verdecchia, P., Schillaci, G., Guerrieri, M., et al. (1990). Circadian blood pressure changes and left ventricular hypertrophy in essential hypertension. *Circulation, 81*, 528–536.
85. Spaak, J., Egri, Z. J., Kubo, T., et al. (2005). Muscle sympathetic nerve activity during wakefulness in heart failure patients with and without sleep apnea. *Hypertension, 46*, 1327–1332.
86. Fung, J. W., Li, T. S., Choy, D. K., et al. (2002). Severe obstructive sleep apnea is associated with left ventricular diastolic dysfunction. *Chest, 121*, 422–429.
87. Shivalkar, B., Van De Heyning, C., Kerremans, M., et al. (2006). Obstructive sleep apnea syndrome: more insights on structural and functional cardiac alterations, and the effects of treatment with continuous positive airway pressure. *J Am Coll Cardiol, 47*, 1433–1439.
88. Arias, M. A., García-Río, F., Alonso-Fernández, A., et al. (2005). Obstructive sleep apnea syndrome affects left ventricular diastolic function: effects of nasal continuous positive airway pressure in men. *Circulation, 112*, 375–383.
89. Lohmeier, T. E., Lohmeier, J. R., Haque, A., et al. (2000). Baroreflexes prevent neurally induced sodium retention in angiotensin hypertension. *Am J Physiol Regul Integr Comp Physiol, 279*, R1437–R1448.
90. Lohmeier, T. E., Lohmeier, J. R., Warren, S., et al. (2002). Sustained activation of the central baroreceptor pathway in angiotensin hypertension. *Hypertension, 39*, 550–556.
91. Lohmeier, T. E., Dwyer, T. M., Irwin, E. D., et al. (2007). Prolonged activation of the baroreflex abolishes obesity-induced hypertension. *Hypertension, 49*, 1307–1314.
92. Lohmeier, T. E., Warren, S., & Cunningham, J. T. (2003). Sustained activation of the central baroreceptor pathway in obesity hypertension. *Hypertension, 42*, 96–102.
93. Lohmeier, T. E. (2001). The sympathetic nervous system and long-term blood pressure regulation. *Am J Hypertens, 14*, 147S–154S.
94. Sica, D. A., & Lohmeier, T. E. (2006). Baroreflex activation for the treatment of hypertension: principles and practice. *Expert Rev Med Devices, 3*, 595–601.
95. Filippone, J. D., & Bisognano, J. D. (2007). Baroreflex stimulation in the treatment of hypertension. *Curr Opin Nephrol Hypertens, 16*, 403–408.
96. Bisognano, J. D., de Leeuw, P., Bach, D. S., et al. (2008). Improved cardiac structure and function in early-stage heart failure with chronic treatment using an implantable device: results from European and United States trials of the Rheos system. *J Card Fail, 14*(6S), S48.
97. Scheffers, I., Schmidli, J., Kroon, A. A., et al. (2009). Sustained blood pressure reduction by baroreflex hypertension therapy with a chronically implanted system: 2-year data from the Rheos DEBuT-HT study in patients with resistant hypertension. *J Hypertens, 26*(Suppl 1), S19.
98. Krum, H., Schlaich, M., Whitbourn, R., et al. (2009). Catheter-based renal sympathetic denervation for resistant hypertension: a multicentre safety and proof-of-principle cohort study. *Lancet, 373*, 1275–1281.
99. Bell, S. P., Nyland, L., Tischler, M. D., et al. (2000). Alterations in the determinants of diastolic suction during pacing tachycardia. *Circ Res, 87*, 235–240.
100. Cheng, C. P., Freeman, G. L., Santamore, W. P., et al. (1990). Effect of loading conditions, contractile state, and heart rate on early diastolic left ventricular filling in conscious dogs. *Circ Res, 66*, 814–823.
101. Firstenberg, M. S., Smedira, N. G., Greenberg, N. L., et al. (2001). *Relationship between early diastolic intraventricular pressure gradients, an index of elastic recoil, and improvements in systolic and diastolic function. Circulation, 104*(12, Suppl. 1), I-330–I-335.
102. Little, W. C. (2005). Diastolic dysfunction beyond distensibility: adverse effects of ventricular dilatation. *Circulation, 112*, 2888–2890.
103. Feld, Y., Dubi, S., Reisner, Y., et al. (2006). Future strategies for the treatment of diastolic heart failure. *Acute Card Care, 8*, 13–20.
104. Little, W. C., Schwammenthal, E., Dubi, S., et al. (2007). Safety of new device-based approach for treating diastolic heart failure. *J Card Fail, 13*(Suppl. 6), S120.
105. Elami, A., Sherman, A., Lak, L., et al. (2008). Efficacy assessment of a new device-based approach for treating diastolic heart failure. *J Card Fail, 14*(Suppl. 6S), 46.
106. Hori, M., Kitabatake, A., Tsutsui, H., et al. (2005). Rationale and design of a randomized trial to assess the effects of beta-blocker in diastolic heart failure; Japanese Diastolic Heart Failure Study (J-DHF). *J Card Fail, 11*, 542–547.
107. Hunt, S. A., Abraham, W. T., Chin, M. H., et al. (2009). 2009 Focused update incorporated into the ACC/AHA 2005 Guidelines for the Diagnosis and Management of Heart Failure in Adults: a report of the American College of Cardiology Foundation/American Heart Association Task Force on Practice Guidelines: developed in collaboration with the International Society for Heart and Lung Transplantation. *Circulation, 119*, e391–e479.

CHAPTER 49

Heart Failure in Special Populations

Mathew Maurer, Eileen M. Hsich, Ileana L. Piña, and Anne L. Taylor

Population variables of race or ethnicity, gender, and age significantly influence the expression of heart failure. Prevalence, incidence, risk profile, causes, and outcomes of heart failure are all affected by these variables. Registries, longitudinal cohort studies, and administrative databases are increasingly important sources of insights about the effects of these variables. Potential differences in response to therapies in these groups, in contrast, are not well characterized because of poor representation in randomized clinical trials. Thus, therapeutic recommendations are, with rare exceptions, not specific to these categories, and therapies are applied universally.

RACE OR ETHNICITY AND HEART FAILURE

In considering the effects of race or ethnicity on heart failure, it is important to keep in mind several key concepts. Race, ethnicity, and geographical descent may include some clustering of common genetic characteristics, but they also include social, environmental, and lifestyle factors that may have a huge effect on cardiovascular health.[1] In some instances, ethnicity is determined only by a commonality of language (e.g., Spanish), in which population origin varies significantly within the group (e.g., Afro-Caribbean descent for northeastern Hispanic people, Native American descent for Central and South American Hispanic people, and European descent for Hispanic people from Argentina). Asian populations are similarly very diverse, and the health status of Hispanic and Asian populations may vary according to time of immigration and racial mixing. Thus, although disease patterns within racial/ethnic population groupings should be investigated, these are not simple variables.[1] More data concerning comparisons of heart failure in African American and white populations have been collected than for other racial or ethnic groups. Cohort studies and databases are including a broader range of subjects by race and ethnicity, but ethnic subgroups are rarely included or analyzed even post hoc in randomized clinical trials, and so treatment-specific data are largely absent. Thus, understanding the true role that race and ethnicity play in heart failure requires greater study and better inclusion in clinical trials.

Clinical Features by Race or Ethnicity

The major risk factors for heart failure are listed in Table 49-1,[2] and the prevalence of heart failure according to sex and race or ethnicity is listed in Table 49-2.[2] Annual rates of new heart failure events per 1000 persons by age groups are listed in Table 49-3 (see also Chapter 22).

Heart failure occurs at earlier ages in African American populations than in white populations[3,4] and is associated more frequently with hypertension and diabetes than with ischemic heart disease.[5-8] African American patients have also been noted to have more advanced disease at first evaluation, lower norepinephrine levels, and a trend toward lower plasma renin activity than do other racial groups.[9] Hispanic patients with heart failure are also younger than other racial groups and have higher rates of diabetes and renal disease; rates of ischemic cardiomyopathy are intermediate between non-Hispanic white populations and African American populations.[10]

The incidence of heart failure by race or ethnicity and by associated risk factors was examined in the Multi-Ethnic Study of Atherosclerosis (MESA), which included 6814 participants, of whom 38.5% were white, 27.8% were African American, 21.9% were Hispanic, and 11.8% were Chinese American.[11] The incidence was highest among African American patients, second highest among Hispanic patients, followed by non-Hispanic white patients, and lowest among Chinese American patients over a 5-year follow-up period (Figure 49-1).

Observed racial differences in morbidity from heart failure may be related to differences in comorbid conditions (hypertension, diabetes, or renal disease), effectiveness of treatment, socioeconomic factors (access to insurance and specialty care), lifestyle, and health care–seeking behaviors (i.e., time between symptom onset and presentation for care).[5,10-12]

Data from analysis of Medicare enrollees revealed that hospitalization for heart failure was 1.5 times higher among African American patients, 1.2 times higher among Hispanic patients, but 0.5 less likely among Asian patients[13] than among white American patients. African American patients with heart failure have a higher risk for hospitalization and readmission than do white patients.[10,14-19] Hispanic patients have higher hospitalization rates and readmission rates than do non-Hispanic white patients[10]; length of stay is intermediate among non-Hispanic white patients and African American patients (Figure 49-2).[10]

African American patients with heart failure have been reported to have similar,[19] higher,[20] and lower rates of mortality than do white patients.[17,21] Data may conflict partly because of differences in study period, method (registries, observational databases, administrative databases, or randomized clinical trials), pathophysiological characteristics (heart failure with preserved or decreased left ventricular [LV] function), and age of patients studied. Hispanic patients have been reported to have lower rates of in-hospital and short-term mortality.[10] The lower rate of mortality with similar incidence has been termed the "Hispanic paradox."

TABLE 49–1 Risk Factors for Heart Failure, by Sex and by Race or Ethnicity					
Population	Prevalence of Overweight and Obesity in Adults (Age ≥ 20 Years), 2006	Prevalence of Total Cholesterol ≥ 240 mg/dL (Age ≥ 20 Years), 2006	Prevalence of High Blood Pressure (Age ≥ 20 Years), 2006	Hypertension Control: NHANES, 1999-2004, by Race	Prevalence of Physician-Diagnosed Diabetes Mellitus (Age ≥ 20 Years), 2006
Both Sexes					
• *n*	145,000,000	34,400,000	73,600,000		17,000,000
• %	66.7	15.7	33.3		7.7
Men					
• *n*	76,900,000	14,600,000	35,300,000		17,500,000
• %	73.0	13.8	34.1		7.4
Women					
• *n*	68,100,000	19,800,000	38,300,000		9,500,000
• %	60.5	17.3	32.1		8.0
Non-Hispanic white men (%)	72.4	14.3	34.1	39.3	5.8
Non-Hispanic white women (%)	57.5	18.1	30.3	34.5	6.1
Non-Hispanic black men (%)	73.7	7.9	44.4	29.9	14.9
Non-Hispanic black women (%)	77.7	13.4	43.9	36.0	13.4
Mexican-American men (%)	74.8	17.5	23.1	21.4	11.3
Mexican-American women (%)	73.0	14.5	30.4	27.4	14.2
Total Hispanic patients ≥20 years of age (%)	67.8	29.9	20.6		11.1
Total Asian/Pacific Islanders ≥20 years of age (%)	38.1	29.2	19.5		8.9
Total American Indians/Alaska Natives ≥20 years of age (%)	67.1	31.2	25.5		17.2

NHANES, National Health and Nutrition Examination Survey.

Adapted from Lloyd-Jones D, Adams R, Carnethon M, et al. Heart disease and stroke statistics—2009 update: a report from the American Heart Association Statistics Committee and Stroke Statistics Subcommittee. *Circulation* 2009;119(3):e21-e181.

Racial Differences in Response to Drug Treatment for Heart Failure

The efficacy of pharmacological treatments in racial or ethnic subgroups is controversial, in part, because there have been few randomized clinical trials of heart failure treatment that have *prespecified* a subgroup analysis of outcomes by race or ethnicity and also included sufficient numbers of subjects for meaningful statistical analysis. However, findings of retrospective analyses suggest that there may be differences between African American and white populations in response to some pharmacotherapy for heart failure, but few data exist for Hispanic and Asian populations in comparisons of outcomes by specific treatments.

Angiotensin-Converting Enzyme Inhibitors

Pooled data from the Studies of Left Ventricular Dysfunction (SOLVD) prevention and treatment trials[22] revealed that enalapril therapy was associated with a significant reduction in the risk of hospitalization for heart failure among white patients but not among African American patients (see Chapter 45). African American patients randomly assigned to receive enalapril had 7.9 more hospitalizations per 100 persons per years of follow-up than did matched white patients.[23] Analysis of the database from both the SOLVD prevention and treatment study revealed no significant difference in the risk of death associated with enalapril treatment in African American and matched white patients,[22] although African American patients overall had higher rates of all-cause mortality and higher rates of mortality from pump failure.[22] In white patients treated with enalapril, significant reductions in both systolic blood pressure (5 ± 17.1 mm Hg) and diastolic blood pressure (3.6 ± 10.6 mm Hg) were observed, but no reduction in blood pressure was shown in African American subjects similarly treated. However, in both SOLVD

TABLE 49–2 Prevalence of Heart Failure, by Sex and by Race or Ethnicity	
Population Group	Prevalence, 2006 (Age ≥ 20 Years)
Both sexes (*n* = 5,700,000)	2.5
Men (*n* = 3,200,000)	3.2
Women (*n* = 2,500,000)	2.0
Non-Hispanic white men	3.1
Non-Hispanic white women	1.8
Non-Hispanic black men	4.2
Non-Hispanic black women	4.2
Mexican-American men	2.1
Mexican-American women	1.4

prevention and treatment studies, African American subjects were at higher risk for all-cause mortality, death from pump failure, and stroke or pulmonary embolism despite the fact that both African American and white subjects received standardized treatment.[23] A post hoc analysis of the SOLVD prevention results only[24] demonstrated that enalapril delayed the progression of asymptomatic LV dysfunction to symptomatic heart failure in both African American and white subjects. However, despite the fact that enalapril produced comparable relative reductions in risk for the development of symptomatic heart failure, the differences in the baseline magnitude of risk were such that African American subjects randomly assigned to receive enalapril remained at higher risk for the progression to clinical heart failure than did white subjects randomly assigned to receive placebo. The differences between African American and white subjects in the risk of progression of asymptomatic LV dysfunction remained after adjustments for potential confounders, including ejection fraction, New York Heart Association (NYHA) class, serum sodium level, and origin of LV dysfunction (Figure 49-3).[24]

TABLE 49–3 Annual Rates of New Heart Failure Events, by Age, Sex, and Race (per 1000 Individuals)

Age (Years)	White Men	White Women	Black Men	Black Women
65-74	15.2	8.2	16.9	14.2
75-84	31.7	19.8	25.5	25.5
≥85	65.2	45.6	50.6	44.0

From Rosamond W, Flegal K, Furie K, et al. Heart disease and stroke statistics—2008 update: a report from the American Heart Association Statistics Committee and Stroke Statistics Subcommittee. *Circulation* 2008;117(4):e25-e146.

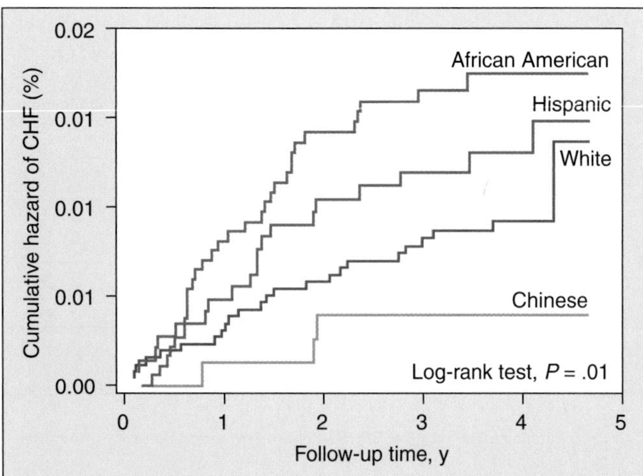

FIGURE 49–1 Nelson-Aahlen plots of cumulative hazard ratios for the development of congestive heart failure (CHF), by racial or ethnic group, in the Multi-Ethnic Study of Atherosclerosis (MESA) study. (From Bahrami H, Kronmal R, Bluemke DA, et al. Difference in the incidence of congestive heart failure by ethnicity: the Multi-Ethnic Study of Atherosclerosis. *Arch Intern Med* 2008;168:2138-2145.)

β-Blockers (see Chapter 46)

Several large multicenter trials have proved the beneficial effects of β-blockers in heart failure[25]; however, all have included only small numbers of African American subjects, and the analyses by ethnicity were post hoc.[26-28] Nonetheless, these post hoc analyses revealed a trend for carvedilol and metoprolol to have a beneficial effect in African American patients. Therefore, despite the small numbers of African American subjects in the trials and failure of hazard ratios to reach statistical significance, these β-blockers are recommended for all patients without distinction by race.

In the Beta-Blocker Evaluation of Survival Trial (BEST), the only trial prospectively stratified by race (African American or white), the β-blocker bucindolol significantly reduced the risk of death or hospitalization among white patients but was associated with a nonsignificant increase in the risk of serious clinical events in African American patients[29] (Figure 49-4). Therefore, the benefits in African-American patients may be specific to some β-blockers but not to others.

Isosorbide Dinitrate Plus Hydralazine

Retrospective analyses of the first and second Vasodilator Heart Failure Trials (V-HeFT I and II)[30,31] (in which 28% to 30% of subjects were African American) suggested racial differences between African American and white subjects in response to treatment.[32] In V-HeFT I comparisons of a combination of isosorbide dinitrate plus hydralazine, prazosin, and placebo, a mortality-related benefit was observed in African American subjects but not in white patients treated with isosorbide dinitrate plus hydralazine. In V-HeFT II comparisons of enalapril

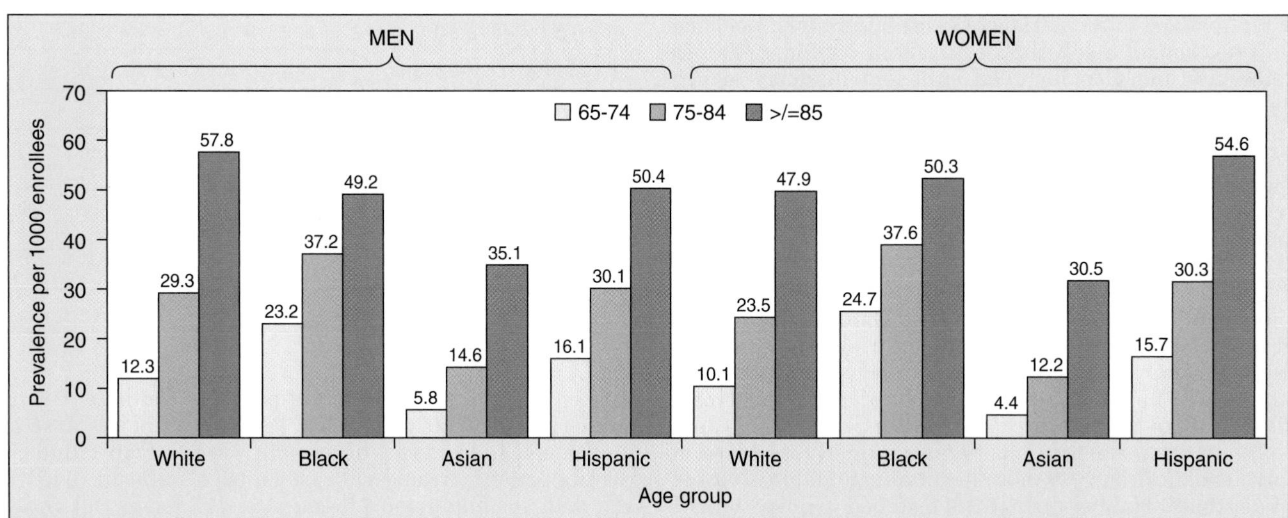

FIGURE 49–2 Age-specific prevalence of hospitalization with a first-listed diagnosis of heart failure among Medicare enrollees aged 65 years or older, by sex and by race or ethnicity. (Modified from Brown D, Haldeman G, Croft J, et al. Racial or ethnic differences in hospitalization for heart failure among elderly adults: Medicare, 1990-2000. *Am Heart J* 2005;150:448-454.)

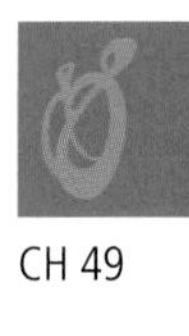

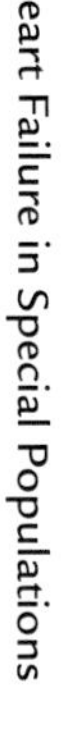

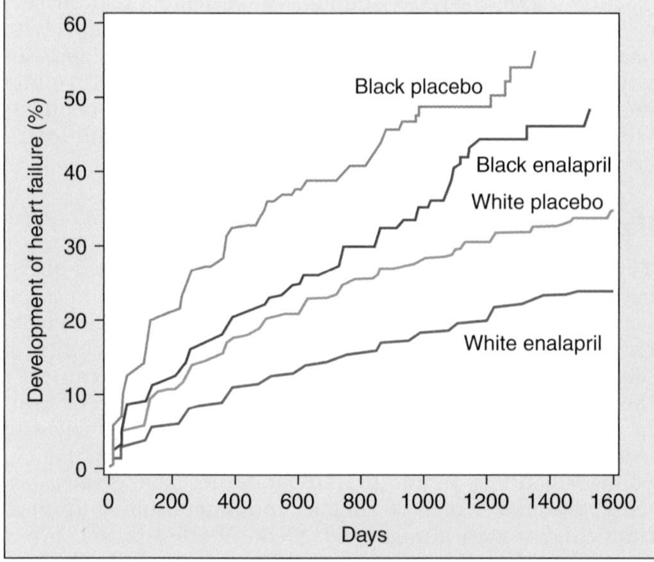

FIGURE 49–3 Effect of angiotensin-converting enzyme inhibition on preventing the development of symptomatic heart failure in African American and white patients with asymptomatic left ventricular dysfunction. (Adapted from Dries D, Strong M, Cooper R, et al. Efficacy of angiotensin-converting enzyme inhibition in reducing progression from asymptomatic left ventricular dysfunction to symptomatic heart failure in black and white patients. *J Am Coll Cardiol* 2002;40:311-317.)

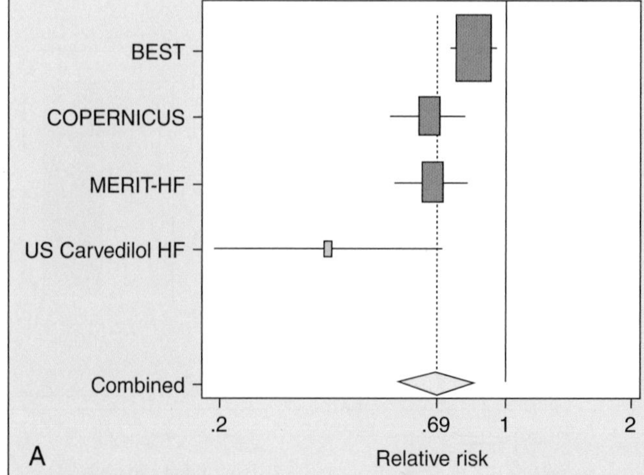

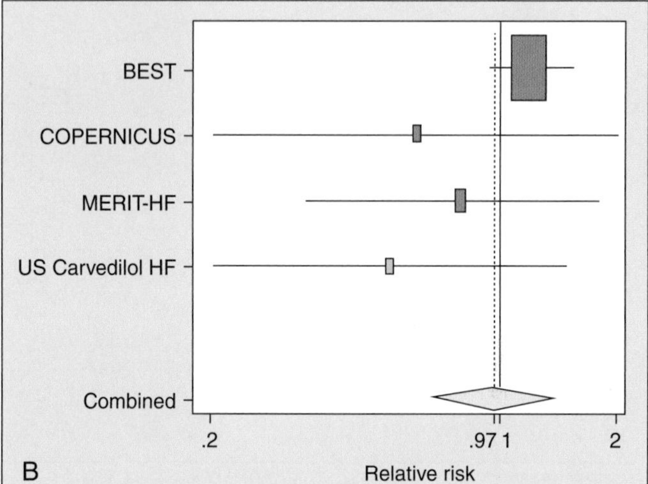

FIGURE 49–4 Effects of β-blocking agents, by race. **A,** Effects in white patients. **B,** Effects in African American patients. BEST, Beta-Blocker Evaluation of Survival Trial; COPERNICUS, Carvedilol Prospective Randomized Cumulative Survival; MERIT-HF, Metoprolol CR/XL Randomised Intervention Trial in Congestive Heart Failure; U.S. Carvedilol HF, U.S. Carvedilol Heart Failure Study. (Adapted from Shekelle PG, Rich M, Morton S, et al. Efficacy of angiotensin-converting enzyme inhibitors and beta-blockers in the management of left ventricular systolic dysfunction according to race, gender, and diabetic status. *J Am Coll Cardiol* 2003;41:1529-1538).

and the combination isosorbide dinitrate plus hydralazine, a survival advantage of enalapril was observed only in white patients; no survival advantage of enalapril over isosorbide dinitrate plus hydralazine was observed in African American patients. Although these were retrospective analyses of small numbers of subjects and the interaction among race and treatment was not significant, these findings suggested there might be differences in response between the two groups.

The African-American Heart Failure Trial (A-HeFT) tested the hypothesis derived from the retrospective analyses of the V-HeFT trials: that addition of combined isosorbide dinitrate plus hydralazine to background neurohormonal blockade would improve heart failure outcomes in African American patients with low ejection fractions and advanced symptoms.[8] Of importance was that 40% of the trial cohort were women; the results provided the only clinical trial data of this treatment strategy in women.[33] Although patients in both conditions of the trial were well treated with background neurohormonal blockade and there were some baseline clinical differences between men and women, there were no differences in baseline medications for heart failure.[33] In this trial, the addition of isosorbide dinitrate plus hydralazine to neurohormonal blockade significantly improved survival and reduced hospitalizations in self-identified African American men and women with advanced heart failure[8,10,13] (Figure 49-5). How this therapy affects other populations requires further testing.

Review of clinical trials of other pharmacotherapy for differences in outcomes by race or ethnicity reveals that only extremely small numbers of racial or ethnic minorities were included and does not permit conclusions to be drawn with regard to treatment by race. In trials of angiotensin receptor blockers (ARBs), African American patients represented 2% of subjects in the Evaluation of Losartan In The Elderly (ELITE)[34]; 4% in the Candesartan in Heart Failure Assessment in Reduction of Mortality (CHARM), in which 6.9% were identified as "other" without further specification[35-38]; and 7.0% in the Valsartan in Heart Failure Trial (Val-HeFT), in which 2.6% were identified as "other."[39] In trials of aldosterone antagonists, African American patients represented 1% of subjects in Eplerenone Post–Acute Myocardial Infarction Heart Failure Efficacy and Survival Study (EPHESUS)[40] and 14% of nonwhite subjects (but not further characterized) in the Randomized Aldactone Evaluation Study (RALES).[41] Similar low numbers of minorities have been included in trials testing the utility of implantable cardioverter-defibrillators (ICDs)[42,43] and pacemakers for cardiac resynchronization therapy (CRT),[44] as well as in registries tracking the use of these devices.[45]

At present, with the exception of a positive recommendation for use of nitrates and hydralazine in African American patients,[46] there are no data supporting differences in use of heart failure therapies by racial or ethnic groupings.

HEART FAILURE IN ELDERLY POPULATIONS

Clinical Features

Heart failure is principally a disorder of older adults; the prevalence and incidence rates increase dramatically with age. Of the more than 5 million adults with heart failure in

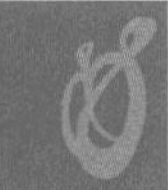

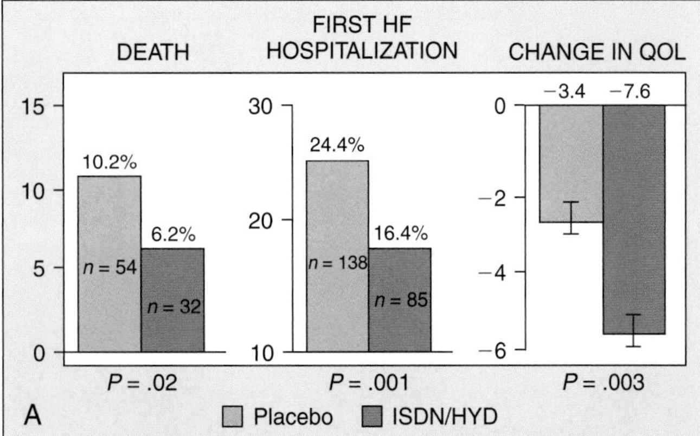

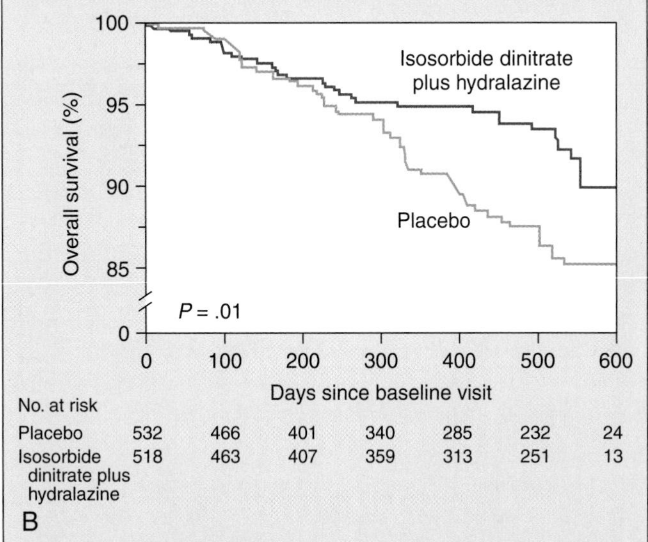

FIGURE 49–5 Clinical outcomes in the African American Heart Failure Trial (A-HeFT). **A,** Components of composite score in A-HeFT. **B,** Effect of fixed-dose isosorbide dinitrate plus hydralazine on mortality in A-HeFT. HF, heart failure; ISDN/HYD, isosorbide dinitrate plus hydralazine; QOL, quality of life. (Modified from Taylor AL, Ziesche S, Yancy C, et al. Combination of isosorbide dinitrate and hydralazine in blacks with heart failure. *N Engl J Med* 2004;351:2049-2057.)

the United States, 50% are at least 75 years of age. Heart failure is the leading cause of hospital admissions among older adults and the leading cause of readmission within 30 days of discharge.[47] In the Framingham Heart Study, the incidence of heart failure increased from a rate of 2 to 3 per 1000 in the population younger than 65 years to 9 to 12 per 1000 of those aged 65 years or older. The incidence rate in the "oldest old" population (those ≥85 years of age) was more than twentyfold higher among women and more than tenfold higher in men than in those younger than 55 years.[48] In the Cardiovascular Health Study, the prevalence of heart failure among women increased from 4.1% at age 70 to 14.3% at age 85; among men at the same ages, it increased from 7.8% to 18.4%.[49] The prevalence and incidence of heart failure are similar in older white and African American populations.

Important risk factors for the development of heart failure in the older population include age; male gender; and the presence of ischemic heart disease, systolic hypertension, widened pulse pressure, diabetes, chronic lung disease, renal dysfunction, atrial fibrillation, LV hypertrophy, and obesity.[49,50] Among these, systolic hypertension has the greatest population attributable risk, especially among women, for the development of heart failure.[49]

Older patients show a particular propensity for developing heart failure with preserved LV systolic function, or normal ejection fraction (HFNEF). Population-based reports from several studies suggest that 50% or more of elderly patients with heart failure have HFNEF and that the proportion increases with advancing age. Thus, the profile of the typical older person with heart failure in the general population contrasts with that of middle-aged patients enrolled in heart failure trials or in specialty heart failure referral clinics.

Pathophysiology

The pathophysiological characteristics of heart failure differ between older and younger adults, because the cardiovascular reserve declines with normative aging.[51,52] Age-related changes in other organ systems can impair the ability of older adults to compensate for heart failure and can alter the response to pharmacological agents. The cause of heart failure with reduced ejection fraction (HFREF) is related to ischemic heart disease more often in older adults than in younger patients. In addition, older adults have greater systemic vascular resistance, higher norepinephrine concentrations, higher urea nitrogen and creatinine levels, and lower glomerular filtration rates than do younger adults.[53] Thus, older adults with HFREF have greater vasoconstriction and blunted heart rate response with circulating norepinephrine. The superimposition of normal aging changes on the heart failure process suggests that at equivalent levels of clinical severity, heart failure is more advanced from a pathophysiological perspective in older patients.

Diabetes, chronic kidney disease, anemia, and obesity, which are common comorbid conditions in older individuals with HFNEF, are associated with impaired relaxation, alterations in *ventricular-vascular coupling* with age, and a remodeled ventricle that is more sensitive to volume overload and the effects of increasing heart rate. Severe systolic hypertension is often present during acute exacerbations of pulmonary edema.[54-56]

Rates of mortality from heart failure increase with age and are threefold higher in patients aged 65 to 74 than in those aged 25 to 54 years. Among community-dwelling persons with heart failure who are 65 to 74 years old, the 10-year mortality rates are 50% among women and more than 70% among men. Elderly patients who have been hospitalized with heart failure have even higher mortality rates, estimated at 33% at 1 year and 70% at 5 years.[57] Mortality rates are slightly lower among African American patients than among white patients and slightly lower among women than among men. Predictors of mortality in older patients with heart failure include age, gender (worse in men), recent hospitalization, diabetes, LV dilation and systolic dysfunction, ischemic heart disease, renal insufficiency, hyponatremia, reduced peak oxygen consumption, and increased slope of minute ventilation/carbon dioxide production during exercise.[58,59]

Data from community-dwelling elderly subjects with heart failure suggest that the cause of mortality differs between subjects with a preserved ejection fraction and subjects with a reduced ejection fraction. Of persons with heart failure and a preserved ejection fraction, 45% survived, and 43% of the deaths had noncardiovascular causes. The leading cause of death in subjects with preserved ejection fraction was noncardiovascular (49%), whereas coronary heart disease was the leading cause of death (43%) in subjects with reduced ejection fraction. After adjustment, preserved ejection fraction was associated with a lower risk of cardiovascular death but not all-cause death.[60] Thus, older adult subjects with heart failure and a preserved ejection fraction have less cardiovascular disease before death and are less likely to die of cardiovascular disorders than are subjects with reduced ejection fraction.

Elderly patients with heart failure have chronic exercise intolerance, reduced quality of life, frequent hospitalizations,

TABLE 49–4 Comorbid Conditions in Older Patients with Heart Failure

Condition	Prevalence	Potential Consequences
Renal dysfunction	16%: GFR ≤ 30 mL/min 40%: GFR 30-59 mL/min*	Worsens symptoms, prognosis; exacerbated by diuretics, ACE inhibitors and ARBs.
Chronic lung disease	20%-32%†	Worsens symptoms and prognosis; contributes to uncertainty about diagnosis; exacerbates right-sided heart function
Dementia or delirium	Dementia: 8.5%‡ Delirium: • 30%-50% of hospitalized patients • 36.8% (range, 0%-73.5% of postoperative patients) • >70% of patients in ICU	Increases chance of nonadherence with medications, diet, and nonpharmacological interventions
Diabetes	30%-50%	Worsens prognosis and increases risk associated with polypharmacy Increases risk of vascular disease, dementia, chronic renal dysfunction, and anemia
Depression	8%§	Worsens prognosis, exacerbates symptoms, and increases chance of noncompliance
Falls, difficulties with mobility	30%-50%	Exacerbated by diuretics and vasodilators, impairs mobility in the community, and interferes with ability to attend follow-up visits routinely
Postural or postprandial hypotension	Postural: 10%-30% Postprandial: 10%-20%	Worsened by diuretics, vasodilators
Anemia	Inpatient: 70% Outpatient: 10%-20%	Worsens symptoms, increases risk of hospitalization
Urinary incontinence	Women: 35% Men: 22%¶	Aggravated by medical therapy, including diuretics, ACE inhibitors (secondary to cough, thereby worsening stress incontinence)
Sensory impairments	Ocular disorders: 24%	Interferes with compliance, increases chance of medication error
Frailty	30%-50%	Worsens symptoms, prognosis, reduces quality of life
Fatigue or anergia	Mild to moderate: 70% Severe: 20%	Worsens symptoms, complicates diagnosis
Nutritional deficiencies	>30%	Exacerbated by dietary restrictions imposed by heart failure state
Polypharmacy	Almost all	Increases risk of nonadherence, medication interaction, and adverse drug reaction

*McAlister FA, Ezekowitz J, Tonelli M, et al. Renal insufficiency and heart failure: prognostic and therapeutic implications from a prospective cohort study. *Circulation* 2004;109:1004-1009.

†Le Jemtel TH, Padeletti M, Jelic S. Diagnostic and therapeutic challenges in patients with coexistent chronic obstructive pulmonary disease and chronic heart failure. *J Am Coll Cardiol* 2007;49:171-180.

‡Lee DS, Austin PC, Rouleau JL, et al. Predicting mortality among patients hospitalized for heart failure: derivation and validation of a clinical model. *JAMA* 2003;290:2581-2587.

§Braunstein JB, Anderson GF, Gerstenblith G, et al. Noncardiac comorbidity increases preventable hospitalizations and mortality among Medicare beneficiaries with chronic heart failure. *J Am Coll Cardiol* 2003;42:1226-1233.

¶Thom D. Variation in estimates of urinary incontinence prevalence in the community: effects of differences in definition, population characteristics, and study type. *J Am Geriatr Soc* 1998;46:473-480.

ACE, angiotensin-converting enzyme; ARB, angiotensin receptor blocker; GFR, glomerular filtration rate; ICU, intensive care unit.

and high health care costs. Older patients with heart failure also have a high rate of other morbid outcomes (Table 49-4), including stroke and myocardial infarction. Of importance is that morbidity is similar in patients with either HFREF or HFNEF (see Chapter 48). Exercise intolerance in older patients with HFNEF is as severe as in those with HFREF, and reductions in quality of life are comparable.[61] Peak oxygen uptake, as measured by expired gas analysis during cycle ergometry, was similar in patients with HFNEF and HFREF and markedly reduced in comparison with healthy control subjects.[62]

The diagnosis of heart failure is challenging in older adults, who are more likely than younger adults to have other conditions that mimic the symptoms and signs of heart failure. A reliable history may be more difficult to obtain because of cognitive dysfunction or sensory impairment; a family member, caregiver, or witness may be very helpful in corroborating the patient's history. Atypical presentations are more common in older adults, in whom heart failure may manifest as somnolence, confusion, disorientation, weakness, fatigue, gastrointestinal disturbances, or failure to thrive. Other potential causes of the signs and symptoms of heart failure must be confirmed or ruled out.[63,64] Both chest radiography and echocardiography have lower specificity for diagnosing heart failure in the elderly because of chronic parenchymal changes and because of comorbid lung disease and the presence of normal ejection fraction, respectively, which may contribute to diagnostic uncertainty.[65]

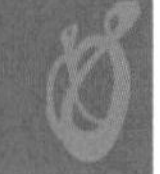

Therapy

Goals of therapy in older adult patients with heart failure include relief of symptoms, improvement in functional capacity and quality of life, reduction in hospital admissions, and lengthening survival. In older patients, preservation of independence and maintenance of a satisfactory quality of life may be more important than length of survival.

Several studies have confirmed the efficacy of a multidisciplinary approach to care in reducing hospitalizations, improving quality of life, reducing total costs, and, in one study, increasing length of survival. Many of these studies included older patients, who are ideal candidates for multidisciplinary care. One randomized controlled trial involving patients aged 70 and older demonstrated a 56% reduction in 90-day rehospitalizations for heart failure.[66] Of note was that this study included patients with either HFREF or HFNEF.

The Perindopril in Elderly People with Chronic Heart Failure (PEP-CHF) trial was a randomized, double-blind study in which placebo was compared with perindopril in patients aged 70 years or older with a diagnosis of heart failure, who were treated with diuretics and had echocardiographic evidence of diastolic dysfunction (see Chapter 48).[67] Perindopril did not improve rates of long-term morbidity and mortality; however, it improved symptoms and exercise capacity and reduced hospitalizations for heart failure in the first year.[67] In the Candesartan in Heart Failure Assessment in Reduction of Mortality (CHARM)–Preserved trial, candesartan also reduced hospital admissions but not mortality among patients with HFNEF.[68] In a clinical trial involving older adults with diastolic dysfunction and an exaggerated blood pressure response to exercise, losartan, in comparison with hydrochlorothiazide, substantially reduced systolic blood pressure and pulse pressure during exercise and improved exercise capacity and quality of life.[69] In the largest placebo-controlled, morbidity-mortality trial to date in patients with HFNEF—the Irbesartan in Heart Failure with Preserved Systolic Function (I-PRESERVE) trial—4133 patients aged 60 years or older (mean, 72 years; 60% women) were randomly assigned to receive irbesartan or placebo. The patient characteristics closely reflected those of population-based and community samples. During 5-year follow-up, this large study revealed no significant effect of irbesartan on the primary endpoint of death and cardiovascular hospitalizations, on heart failure hospitalizations alone, or on secondary endpoints such as quality of life (see Chapter 46).[70]

β-Adrenergic antagonists reduce blood pressure, promote regression of ventricular hypertrophy, and increase the ischemic threshold, all of theoretical importance in HFNEF. In the Study of the Effects of Nebivolol Intervention on Outcomes and Rehospitalisation in Seniors with Heart Failure (SENIORS), 35% of the subjects (mean age, 76 years) had an ejection fraction of more than 35%. Among those with an ejection fraction of less than 35 or more than 35%, there was no difference in the observed beneficial effects of β-blocker therapy.[71]

The Digitalis Investigation Group (DIG) ancillary study included 988 patients with preserved systolic function, most of whom were elderly. In patients with chronic mild to moderate heart failure, an ejection fraction exceeding 45%, and normal sinus rhythm who were receiving angiotensin-converting enzyme (ACE) inhibitor and diuretics, digoxin had no net overall effect on natural history endpoints such as mortality and hospitalizations for all causes or cardiovascular causes.[72]

HEART FAILURE IN WOMEN

Clinical Features

More than 40% of patients with heart failure are women.[73] The prevalence of heart failure increases with age in both sexes.[73] Women with heart failure are twice as likely to have HFNEF than are men,[74,75] and women with HFREF tend to present with a higher LV ejection fraction (LVEF) than do men.[74,75] Comorbid conditions also differ between men and women. Women with heart failure tend to have more hypertension, whereas smoking and coronary artery disease are more prevalent among men.[76] In the A-HeFT trial,[8] African American women were more likely to have lower hemoglobin and to have diabetes, but less likely to have renal insufficiency, than were men. Although coronary artery disease is less common, it is such a significant risk factor that women are more likely to develop heart failure with coronary artery disease than with hypertension. For example, in the National Health and Nutrition Examination Survey (NHANES) I epidemiological follow-up study, which included 8098 women without heart failure, 27% had hypertension and only 3% had coronary artery disease, but the relative risk of developing heart failure for women was significantly higher if they had coronary artery disease (relative risk, 8.16; 95% confidence interval [CI], 6.79 to 9.8; $P < .001$) than if they had hypertension (relative risk, 1.51; 95% CI, 1.29 to 1.77; $P < .001$).[77] Diabetes mellitus is common in both genders (i.e., 44%)[74] and is one of the strongest additional risk factors for the development of heart failure in women with coronary artery disease.[78] Thyroid disease is more frequent in women with acute decompensated heart failure, whereas chronic obstructive lung disease, peripheral vascular disease, and renal insufficiency are more common in men.[74,75]

The age-adjusted incidence of heart failure is higher among men than among women; however, men with heart failure have shorter survival than do women.[79,80] Adams and associates[81] found that the female survival advantage occurred only when the cause of heart failure was nonischemic. Between 1979 and 2000, the incidence of heart failure rose 8% (95% CI, −5 to −23) among women and 3% (95% CI, −11 to −20) among men, according to the data from Olmsted County, Minnesota,[79] and the Framingham Heart Study investigators reported an increase in the incidence of heart failure for both women and men between 1980 and 1999.[80] Both of these population cohorts were almost exclusively non-Hispanic white; thus, comparable detailed data about minority women for these time periods are not available. During those time periods, age-adjusted rates of 5-year mortality improved for both sexes.[79,80]

Significant morbidity is associated with heart failure, and women have been shown to have a lower quality of life than do men, with more impairment in functional capacity,[33,82] more hospitalizations for heart failure,[73,74,82] and more depression.[83] Although women are more likely than men to have heart failure with preserved LV systolic function, two observational studies demonstrated similar mortality rates for patients with heart failure and preserved or impaired systolic function.[84,85] Women have less ischemic cardiomyopathy. The CHARM study investigators noted that sex differences in survival were not entirely explained by LV systolic function or by cause of heart failure; however, for both sexes, ischemic cardiomyopathy conferred a worse prognosis.[76]

Peripartum cardiomyopathy is a uniquely gender-specific cardiomyopathy defined as the development of heart failure with impaired systolic function in the last month of pregnancy or within 5 months post partum with no preexisting cardiac disease or identifiable cause (see Chapter 24).[86] The incidence varies based on population studied with an estimated occurrence of 1:4000 pregnancies in the United States.[86] Risk factors include advanced maternal age, African descent, high parity, twin pregnancy, usage of tocolytic agents, and lower socioeconomic status.[87] Approximately half of patients with peripartum cardiomyopathy recover normal systolic function within 6 months.[88] Another 20% deteriorate and either die or require heart transplantation.[89] The degree of LV systolic dysfunction at presentation may be predictive of recovery: Those who recover LV systolic function have higher LVEF at presentation.[90,91] Data for guiding treatment choice are limited with regard to the risk of heart failure with subsequent pregnancies, and no specific recommendations about therapy exist at present.[92]

In the SOLVD database, of the patients with impaired systolic LV function, women were more likely than men to have dependent edema, jugular venous distention, and an S3 gallop.[93] However, women (n = 54,674) in the Acute Decompensated Heart Failure National Registry (ADHERE) with impaired and preserved systolic function did not differ from men (n = 50,713) with regard to the frequency of heart failure symptoms and signs.[74] However, ADHERE included patients hospitalized for acute decompensation, whereas SOLVD involved patients with chronic symptoms. In ADHERE, the patients with heart failure and preserved systolic function were more likely to be women, older, and hypertensives. According to both the Framingham and the Olmsted County databases, more women than men have heart failure with preserved LV function.[94,95]

Therapy

Women hospitalized with heart failure generally receive heart failure medications at similar rates as do men, but elderly patients are less likely to receive guideline-recommended therapy.[96-98] Although women have been included in randomized clinical trials in greater numbers than minorities in general, they have, nonetheless, been significantly underrepresented, and no sex-specific trials have been conducted, except for ischemic disease; thus, evidence-based treatment guidelines for heart failure therapy[46,99] are not sex specific. Post hoc analyses and meta-analyses of randomized clinical trials of women in heart failure studies are reviewed as follows.

Angiotensin-Converting Enzyme Inhibitors (see Chapter 45)

A meta-analysis of 30 studies of ACE inhibitors, which included a total of 1587 women with heart failure, demonstrated a trend toward improved survival among the subjects taking ACE inhibitors in comparison with those not taking the drug (13.4% vs. 20.1%) and a favorable trend in the combined endpoint of survival and hospitalization in the group of women taking an ACE inhibitor (20.2% vs. 29.5%).[100] Another meta-analysis involving 2373 women demonstrated similar trends[29] (Figure 49-6, Table 49-5). However, both meta-analyses had wide confidence intervals that crossed the line of identity.

Angiotensin Receptor Blockers (see Chapter 45)

Sex-specific data for ARBs are limited. The CHARM-Alternative trial (ARB for patients intolerant of an ACE inhibitor) and the CHARM-Added trial (ARB added to an ACE inhibitor) included 1188 women with functional NYHA class II to class IV heart failure with LVEF of 40% or lower; pooled data showed that candesartan reduced the combined endpoint of cardiovascular death or hospitalization for heart failure in women.[38] In CHARM-Overall,[101] the reductions in the combined endpoint were the same for men and women (Figure 49-7).

β-Blockers (see Chapter 46)

Post hoc meta-analyses of β-blocker therapy have suggested that these agents are as beneficial in women with heart failure as in men, despite the small number of female participants in each study (Table 49-6).

In both the U.S. Carvedilol Heart Failure Study[102] and the Carvedilol Prospective Randomized Cumulative Survival (COPERNICUS) study, carvedilol reduced the combined endpoint of death and hospitalization in women in the study.

Similarly, in the second European Cardiac Insufficiency Bisoprolol Study (CIBIS II), bisoprolol improved survival in the 515 women.[103] In contrast, in the Metoprolol Extended-Release Randomized Intervention Trial in Heart Failure (MERIT-HF), metoprolol succinate produced no survival

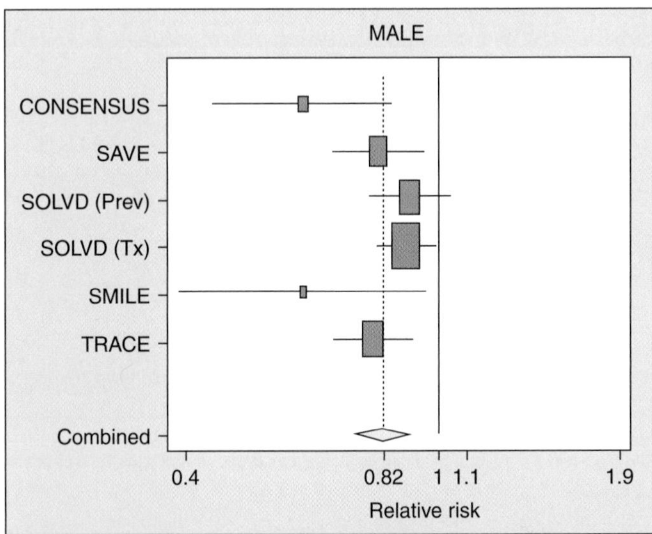

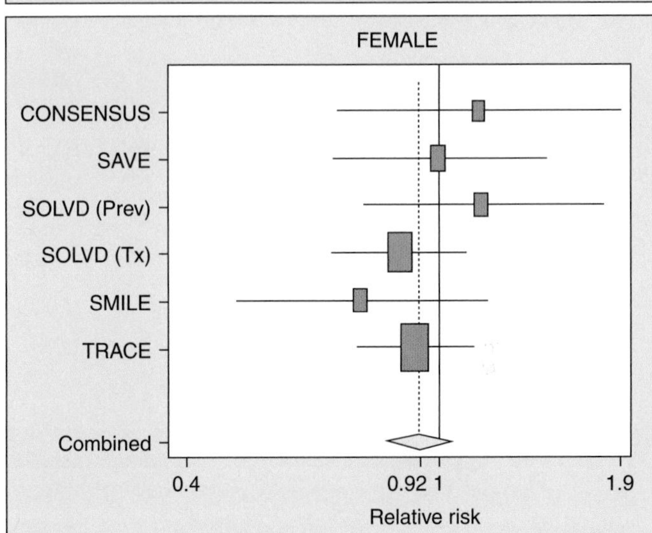

FIGURE 49-6 Effect of angiotensin-converting enzyme inhibitors and β-blockers in the management of left ventricular systolic dysfunction according to race, gender, and diabetic status. CONSENSUS, Cooperative North Scandinavian Enalapril Survival Study; SAVE, Survival And Ventricular Enlargement; SMILE, Survival of Myocardial Infarction Long-term Evaluation; SOLVD, Studies of Left Ventricular Dysfunction (Prev, Prevention; Tx, Treatment); TRACE, Trandolapril Cardiac Evaluation. (From Shekelle P, Rich M, Morton S, et al. Efficacy of angiotensin-converting enzyme inhibitors and beta-blockers in the management of left ventricular systolic dysfunction according to race, gender, and diabetic status. *J Am Coll Cardiol* 2003;41:1529-1538.)

benefit in women (6.9% vs. 7.5%, nonsignificant) but did reduce hospitalizations for heart failure by 42% (P = .021).[104] It produced an even more dramatic (72%) reduction in hospitalizations for heart failure (0.54 vs. 0.15; P = .0004) in the subgroup of women with LVEF of lower than 25%.[104]

Aldosterone Antagonists

Subgroup post hoc analysis of the two aldosterone antagonists revealed a similar mortality-related benefit for men and women with systolic heart failure in both the Randomized Aldactone Evaluation Study (RALES) and the Eplerenone Post–Acute Myocardial Infarction Heart Failure Efficacy and Survival Study (EPHESUS).[40,41]

Isosorbide Dinitrate Plus Hydralazine

The original data supporting the use of this combination were obtained from studies that included only men.[30,31] In A-HeFT, the combination of isosorbide dinitrate and hydralazine was added to a regimen of ACE inhibitors or ARBs and β-blockers

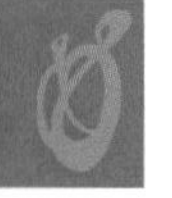

TABLE 49–5 Effect of ACE Inhibitors on Mortality, by Sex

	N		Relative Risk	
Study	**Male**	**Female**	**Male (95% CI)**	**Female (95% CI)**
CONSENSUS	179	74	0.61 (0.44-0.85)	1.14 (0.68-1.90)
SAVE	1841	390	0.80 (0.68-0.95)	0.99 (0.67-1.47)
SMILE	1128	428	0.61 (0.39-0.96)	0.74 (0.47-1.18)
SOLVD-Prevention	3752	476	0.90 (0.77-1.05)	1.15 (0.74-1.78)
SOLVD-Treatment	2065	504	0.89 (0.80-0.99)	0.86 (0.67-1.09)
TRACE	1248	501	0.79 (0.68-0.91)	0.90 (0.74-1.11)
Random effects pooled estimate	10,213	2373	0.82 (0.74-0.90)	0.92 (0.81-1.04)

ACE, angiotensin-converting enzyme; CI, confidence interval; CONSENSUS, Cooperative North Scandinavian Enalapril Survival Study; SAVE, Survival And Ventricular Enlargement; SMILE, Survival of Myocardial Infarction Long-term Evaluation; SOLVD, Studies of Left Ventricular Dysfunction; TRACE, Trandolapril Cardiac Evaluation.

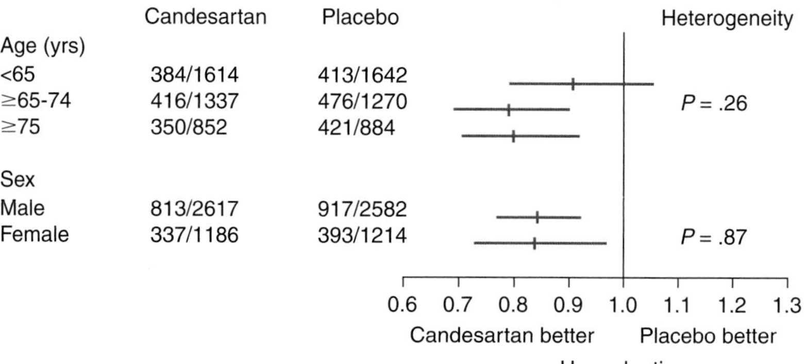

FIGURE 49–7 Effects of candesartan on cardiovascular death or heart failure hospitalizations in the Candesartan in Heart Failure Assessment in Reduction of Mortality (CHARM) study. (From Pfeffer MA, Swedberg K, Granger CB, et al. Effects of candesartan on mortality and morbidity in patients with chronic heart failure: the CHARM-Overall programme. *Lancet* 2003;362:759-766.)

TABLE 49–6 Effect of β-Blockers on Mortality, by Sex

	N		Relative Risk	
Study Name	**Male**	**Female**	**Male (95% CI)**	**Female (95% CI)**
CIBIS-II	2132	515	0.71 (0.58-0.87)	0.52 (0.30-0.89)
COPERNICUS	1822	465	0.68 (0.54-0.86)	0.63 (0.39-1.04)
MERIT-HF	3093	898	0.63 (0.50-0.78)	0.93 (0.58-1.49)
U.S. Carvedilol HF	838	256	0.44 (0.24-0.82)	0.32 (0.11-0.93)
Random effects pooled estimate	7885	2134	0.66 (0.59-0.75)	0.63 (0.44-0.91)

CI, confidence interval; CIBIS, Cardiac Insufficiency BIsoprolol Study; COPERNICUS, CarvedilOl Prospective RandomIzed Cumulative Survival; MERIT-HF, Metoprolol CR/XL Randomised Intervention Trial in Congestive Heart Failure; U.S. Carvedilol HF, U.S. Carvedilol Heart Failure Study.
From Shekelle P, Rich M, Morton S, et al. Efficacy of angiotensin-converting enzyme inhibitors and beta-blockers in the management of left ventricular systolic dysfunction according to race, gender, and diabetic status. *J Am Coll Cardiol* 2003;41:1529-1538.

in 1050 self-identified African American patients (420 of whom were women) who had functional NYHA class III or IV heart failure. Significant survival benefits were noted both for women (hazard ratio, 0.33; 95% CI, 0.16 to 0.71; $P = .003$) and for men (hazard ratio, 0.79; 95% CI, 0.46 to 1.35; $P = .385$), with no significant interaction of treatment by sex. A significant and similar reduction in heart failure hospitalizations was also observed in both men and women.[33]

Digoxin

On the basis of a post hoc subgroup analysis of the DIG trial,[105,106] there was an initial concern of increased mortality (adjusted hazard ratio, 1.23; 95% CI, 1.02 to 1.47) in women with impaired systolic function that was not observed in men (adjusted hazard ratio, 0.93; 95% CI, 0.85 to 1.02). The increase in mortality was presumed attributable to digoxin toxicity, inasmuch as the risk of death increased at higher serum drug levels. Drug levels between 1.2 and 2.0 ng/mL were associated with increased mortality (hazard ratio, 1.33; 95% CI, 1.001 to 1.76; $P = .049$); levels between 0.5 and 0.9 ng/mL were considered safe for both women and men (hazard ratio, 0.8), on the basis of results of a retrospective analysis.[107] In current trials, digoxin is used less in patients with stable chronic heart failure than in previous trials.

Cardiac Resynchronization (see Chapter 47)

Few studies have reported sex-specific data, but it appears that CRT is beneficial for both women and men. In the Comparison of Medical Therapy, Pacing, and Defibrillation in Heart Failure (COMPANION) study, which included 299 women, women with CRT had a greater reduction in the combined endpoint of total mortality or hospitalization for any cause

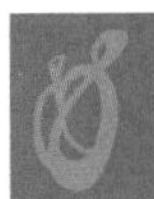

than did women who were given only medical therapy.[108] Retrospective analysis of the Cardiac Resynchronization in Heart Failure (CARE-HF) data, which included statistics from 215 women, suggested that CRT was preferable to medical therapy alone in women for the combined endpoint of total mortality and hospitalization for major cardiovascular events. In the Heart Failure and A Controlled Trial Investigating Outcomes of Exercise Training (HF-ACTION) study, more women had a left bundle branch block but were less likely to have a biventricular pacer at baseline.[109]

Implantable Cardioverter-Defibrillator (see Chapter 47)

The recommendations for ICDs to prevent sudden death are based on results of many multicenter studies, but few studies have provided adequate sex-specific data.[108,110] The limited post hoc analyses available for women with an ICD do not clearly demonstrate a mortality-related benefit.[107,108,110] In the Sudden Cardiac Death in Heart Failure Trial (SCD-HeFT), which included 382 women functional NYHA class II or III heart failure with LVEF of 35% or lower (ischemic and nonischemic cardiomyopathy), the benefits of an ICD were not clear, although the trial was not powered to detect sex differences (for women: hazard ratio, 0.96; 95% CI, 0.58 to 1.61). In the Multicenter Automatic Defibrillator Implantation Trial II (MADIT II), which included 119 women with an ischemic cardiomyopathy and LVEF of 30% or lower, there was a nonsignificant trend toward lower rates of mortality among women with an ICD (adjusted hazard ratio, 0.57; P = .132), which suggests that this subgroup (patients with ischemic cardiomyopathy) may benefit. However, this analysis was limited by insufficient numbers of female participants.[111] A meta-analysis of outcomes of ICD therapy in women[112] suggested that there was no benefit for women with this therapy. It is notable, however, that women who met criteria for ICD implantation were significantly less likely to receive ICD than were men.[45,112] Because of the low numbers of women in clinical trials and the lower rates of usage of ICDs among women, data do not support sex-specific usage of this device.

Ventricular Assist Device (see Chapter 56)

The surgical technique for implanting ventricular assist devices (VADs) does not differ between male and female patients; however, small women have limited VAD options because these devices require a minimum body surface in order to fit properly. The relatively new HeartMate II (Thoratec Corp., Pleasanton, CA), a continuous-flow device, is smaller and may be more easily implanted in women.

VAD outcome data regarding difference between women and men remain limited.[113,114] One study revealed that women were more likely than men to require a right-sided VAD after implantation of a left-sided VAD, but the study included few female participants, and pre–VAD implantation data were not analyzed.[113] In another study in which women had a worse prognosis, women were clinically more unstable than men before VAD implantation. Survival after VAD implantation was best correlated with the degree of medical severity before VAD implantation and not with gender.[114] The HeartMate II allows the implantation of more VADs in women and will enable data analysis in a more consistent prospective manner, because it will be added to the National Heart, Lung, and Blood Institute's Interagency Registry for Mechanically Assisted Circulatory Support (INTERMACS) for VADs. However, a higher risk of bleeding has also been described in women with the HeartMate II. Women had a 31% greater chance of 1-year mortality, in addition.

Heart Transplantation (see Chapter 54)

In the United States in 2007, women donated 28% of the available hearts and received 26% of heart transplants. According to data from the United Network of Organ Sharing (UNOS) from 1997 to 2004, the overall rates of survival after transplantation were slightly worse for women (86% at 1 year, 76% at 3 years, 68% at 5 years) than for men (88%, 79%, and 72%, respectively).[115] The most recent available data (2009) from the International Society for Heart and Lung Transplantation revealed that during the period 2002 to 2007, a female recipient of a heart from a male donor had a relative risk of mortality at 1 year of 1.75, in comparison with a male recipient of a heart from a male donor (95% CI, 1.15 to 2.66; P = .0095) (Table 49-7). With regard to coronary allograft vasculopathy, the relative risk within 5 years was highest for recipients who received hearts from male donors and lowest for female recipients who received hearts from female donors (Figure 49-8).[116]

TABLE 49–7 Risk Factors for Mortality Within 10 Years of Transplantation (July 1994 through June 1998)

Variable	*N*	Relative Risk	*P*	95% Confidence Interval
Female recipient/male donor	936	1.27	.0001	1.13-1.43
Female recipient/female donor	936	1.24	.0001	1.11-1.39
Male recipient/female donor	1817	1.1	.0290	1.01-1.21

Adapted from Taylor DO, Stehlik J, Edwards LB, et al. Registry of the International Society for Heart and Lung Transplantation: twenty-sixth official adult heart transplant report—2009. *J Heart Lung Transplant* 2009;28:1007-1022,)

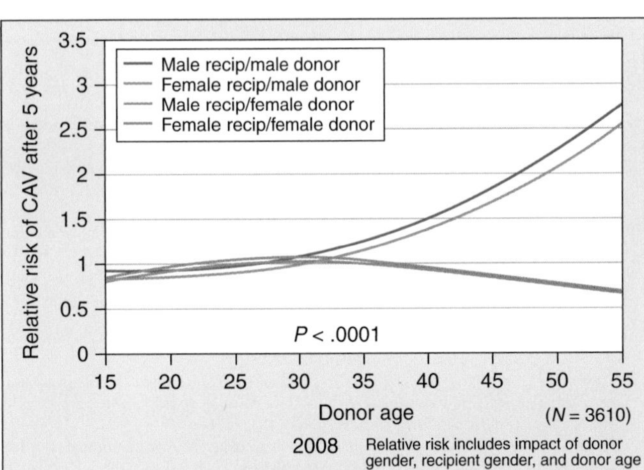

FIGURE 49–8 Relative risk of developing cardiac allograft vasculopathy (CAV) after 5 years, according to donor age, donor gender, and recipient gender. (From Hertz MI, Aurora P, Christie JD, et al. Registry of the International Society for Heart and Lung Transplantation: a quarter century of thoracic transplantation. *J Heart Lung Transplant* 2008;27:937-942.)

REFERENCES

1. Taylor, A. L., & Wright, J. T., Jr. (2005). Should ethnicity serve as the basis for clinical trial design? Importance of race/ethnicity in clinical trials: lessons from the African-American Heart Failure Trial (A-HeFT), the African-American Study of Kidney Disease and Hypertension (AASK), and the Antihypertensive and Lipid-Lowering Treatment to Prevent Heart Attack Trial (ALLHAT). *Circulation, 112*, 3654–3660.
2. Lloyd-Jones, D., Adams, R., Carnethon, M., et al. (2009). Heart disease and stroke statistics—2009 update: a report from the American Heart Association Statistics Committee and Stroke Statistics Subcommittee. *Circulation, 119*(3), e21–e181.
3. Yancy, C. (2000). Heart failure in African Americans: a cardiovascular enigma. *J Card Fail, 6*, 183–186.
4. Yancy, C. (2003). Heart failure in African Americans: pathophysiology and treatment. *J Card Fail, 9*(5 Suppl. Nitric Oxide), S210–S215.
5. Philbin, E., Weil, H., Francis, C., et al. (2000). For the Harlem-Bassett Investigators. Race-related differences among patients with left ventricular dysfunction: observations from a biracial angiographic cohort. *J Card Fail, 6*, 187–193.

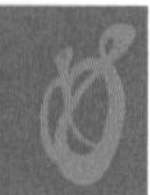

6. Afzal, A., Ananthasubramaniam, K., Sharma, N., et al. (1999). Racial differences in patients with heart failure. *Clin Cardiol, 22*, 791–794.
7. Mathew, J., Davidson, S., Narra, L., et al. (1996). Etiology and characteristics of congestive heart failure in blacks. *Am J Cardiol, 78*, 1447–1450.
8. Taylor, A., Ziesche, S., Yancy, C., et al. (2004). For the African-American Heart Failure Trial Investigators. Combination of isosorbide dinitrate and hydralazine in blacks with heart failure. *N Engl J Med, 351*, 2049–2057.
9. Carson, P., Ziesche, S., Johnson, G., et al. (1999). Racial differences in response to therapy for heart failure: analysis of the vasodilator-heart failure trials. Vasodilator-Heart Failure Trial Study Group. *J Card Fail, 5*, 178–187.
10. Vivo, R. P., Krim, S. R., Cevik, C., et al. (2009). Heart failure in Hispanics. *J Am Coll Cardiol, 53*, 1167–1175.
11. Bahrami, H., Kronmal, R., Bluemke, D. A., et al. (2008). Difference in the incidence of congestive heart failure by ethnicity: the Multi-Ethnic Study of Atherosclerosis. *Arch Intern Med, 168*, 2138–2145.
12. Ghali, J. (2002). Race, ethnicity, and heart failure. *J Card Fail, 8*, 387–389.
13. Brown, D., Haldeman, G., Croft, J., et al. (2005). Racial or ethnic differences in hospitalization for heart failure among elderly adults: Medicare, 1990-2000. *Am Heart J, 150*, 448–454.
14. Vaccarino, V., Gahbauer, E., Kasl, S. V., et al. (2002). Differences between African Americans and whites in the outcome of heart failure: evidence for a greater functional decline in African Americans. *Am Heart J, 143*, 1058–1067.
15. Lafata, J. E., Pladevall, M., Divine, G., et al. (2004). Are there race/ethnicity differences in outpatient congestive heart failure management, hospital use, and morality among an insured population? *Med Care, 42*, 680–689.
16. Deswal, A., Petersen, N. J., Urbauer, D. L., et al. (2006). Racial variations in quality of care and outcomes in an ambulatory heart failure cohort. *Am Heart J, 152*, 348–354.
17. Rathore, S., Foody, J., Wang, Y., et al. (2003). Race, quality of care, and outcomes of elderly patients hospitalized with heart failure. *JAMA, 289*, 2517–2524.
18. Philbin, E. F., & Di Salvo, T. G. (1998). Influence of race and gender on care process, resource use, and hospital based outcomes in congestive heart failure. *Am J Cardiol, 82*, 76–81.
19. Mathew, J., Wittes, J., McSherry, F., et al. (2005). Racial differences in outcome and treatment effect in congestive heart failure. *Am Heart J, 150*, 968–976.
20. Agoston, I., Cameron, C., Yao, D., et al. (2004). Comparison of outcomes in white versus black patients hospitalized with heart failure and preserved ejection fraction. *Am J Cardiol, 94*, 1003–1007.
21. Singh, H., Gordon, H., & Deswal, A. (2005). Variation by race in factors contributing to heart failure hospitalizations. *J Card Fail, 11*, 23–29.
22. Exner, D., Dries, D., Domanski, M., et al. (2001). Lesser response to angiotensin-converting-enzyme inhibitor therapy in black as compared with white patients with left ventricular dysfunction. *N Engl J Med, 344*, 1351–1357.
23. Dries, D., Exner, D., Gersh, B., et al. (1999). Racial differences in the outcome of left ventricular dysfunction. *N Engl J Med, 340*, 609–616.
24. Dries, D., Strong, M., Cooper, R., et al. (2002). Efficacy of angiotensin-converting enzyme inhibition in reducing progression from asymptomatic left ventricular dysfunction to symptomatic heart failure in black and white patients. *J Am Coll Cardiol, 40*, 311–317.
25. Packer, M., Coats, A. J. S., Fowler, M. B., et al. (2001). Effect of carvedilol on survival in severe chronic heart failure. *N Engl J Med, 344*, 1651–1658.
26. Goldstein, S., Deedwania, P., Gottlieb, S., et al. (2003). For the MERIT-HF Study Group. Metoprolol CR/XL in black patients with heart failure. *Am J Cardiol, 92*, 478–480.
27. Yancy, C., Fowler, M., Colucci, W., et al. (2001). For the U.S. Carvedilol Heart Failure Study Group. Race and the response to adrenergic blockade with carvedilol in patients with chronic heart failure. *N Engl J Med, 344*, 1358–1365.
28. Eichhorn, E., Domanski, M., Krause-Steinrauf, H., et al. (2001). For the Beta-Blocker Evaluation of Survival Trial Investigators. A trial of the beta-blocker bucindolol in patients with advanced chronic heart failure. *N Engl J Med, 344*, 1659–1667.
29. Shekelle, P., Rich, M., Morton, S., et al. (2003). Efficacy of angiotensin-converting enzyme inhibitors and beta-blockers in the management of left ventricular systolic dysfunction according to race, gender, and diabetic status. *J Am Coll Cardiol, 41*, 1529–1538.
30. Cohn, J. N., Archibald, D. G., Ziesche, S., et al. (1986). Effect of vasodilator therapy on mortality in chronic congestive heart failure: results of a Veterans Administration Cooperative Study. *N Engl J Med, 314*, 1547–1552.
31. Cohn, J. N., Johnson, G., Ziesche, S., et al. (1991). A comparison of enalapril with hydralazine–isosorbide dinitrate in the treatment of chronic congestive heart failure. *N Engl J Med, 325*, 303–310.
32. Carson, P., Ziesche, S., Johnson, G., et al. (1999). For the Vasodilator-Heart Failure Trial Study Group. Racial differences in response to therapy for heart failure: analysis of the Vasodilator–Heart Failure Trials. *J Card Fail, 5*, 178–187.
33. Taylor, A. L., Lindenfeld, J., Ziesche, S., et al. (2006). Outcomes by gender in the African-American Heart Failure Trial. *J Am Coll Cardiol, 48*, 2263–2267.
34. Pitt, B., Poole-Wilson, P. A., Segal, R., et al. (2000). On behalf of the ELITE II Investigators. Effect of losartan compared with captopril on mortality in patients with symptomatic heart failure: randomised trial—the Losartan Heart Failure Survival Study ELITE II. *Lancet, 355*, 1582–1587.
35. Yusef, S., Pfeffer, M. A., Swedberg, K., et al. (2003). For the CHARM Investigators and Committees. Effects of candesartan in patients with chronic heart failure and preserved left-ventricular ejection fraction: the CHARM-Preserved Trial. *Lancet, 362*, 777–781.
36. McMurray, J. J. V., Ostergren, J., Swedberg, K., et al. (2003). for the CHARM Investigators and Committees. Effects of candesartan in patients with chronic heart failure and reduced left-ventricular systolic function taking angiotensin-converting-enzyme inhibitors: the CHARM-Added Trial. *Lancet, 362*, 767–771.
37. Pfeffer, M. A., Swedberg, K., Granger, C. B., et al. (2003). For the CHARM Investigators and Committees. Effects of candesartan on mortality and morbidity in patients with chronic heart failure: the CHARM-Overall Programme. *Lancet, 362*, 759–766.
38. Young, J. B., Dunlap, M. E., Pfeffer, M. A., et al. (2004). For the CHARM Investigators and Committees. Mortality and morbidity reduction with candesartan in patients with chronic heart failure and left ventricular systolic dysfunction: Results of the CHARM Low-Left Ventricular Ejection Fraction Trials. *Circulation, 110*, 2618–2626.
39. Cohn, J. N., & Tognoni, G. (2001). Valsartan Heart Failure Trial Investigators. A randomized trial of the angiotensin-receptor blocker valsartan in chronic heart failure. *N Engl J Med, 345*, 1667–1675.
40. Pitt, B., Remme, W., Zannad, F., et al. (2003). Eplerenone, a selective aldosterone blocker, in patients with left ventricular dysfunction after myocardial infarction. *N Engl J Med, 348*, 1309–1321.
41. Pitt, B., Zannad, F., Remme, W. J., et al. (1999). The effect of spironolactone on morbidity and mortality in patients with severe heart failure. Randomized Aldactone Evaluation Study Investigators. *N Engl J Med, 341*, 709–717.
42. Moss, A. J., Zareba, W., Hall, J., et al. (2002). Prophylactic implantation of a defibrillator in patients with myocardial infarction and reduced ejection fraction. *N Engl J Med, 346*, 877–883.
43. Hernandez, A. F., Fonarow, G. C., Liang, L., et al. (2007). Sex and racial differences in the use of implantable cardioverter-defibrillators among patients hospitalized with heart failure. *JAMA, 298*, 1525–1532.
44. Cleland, J. G. F., Daubert, J. C., Erdmann, E., et al. (2005). The effect of cardiac resynchronization on morbidity and mortality in heart failure. *N Engl J Med, 352*, 1539–1549.
45. Hernandez, A. F., Yancy, C., Fonarow, G. C., et al. (2007). A gender and racial gap in implantable cardioverter defibrillator use among hospitalized heart failure patients: data from the American Heart Association's Get With The Guidelines—Heart Failure (GWTG-HF) Program. *J Am Coll Cardiol, 49*, 830–833.
46. Hunt, S. A., Abraham, W. T., Chin, M. H., et al. (2005). ACC/AHA 2005 guideline update for the diagnosis and management of chronic heart failure in the adult: a report of the American College of Cardiology/American Heart Association Task Force on Practice Guidelines (Writing Committee to Update the 2001 Guidelines for the Evaluation and Management of Heart Failure): developed in collaboration with the American College of Chest Physicians and the International Society for Heart and Lung Transplantation: endorsed by the Heart Rhythm Society. *Circulation, 112*, e154–e235.
47. Jencks, S. F., Williams, M. V., & Coleman, E. A. (2009). Rehospitalizations among patients in the Medicare fee-for-service program. *N Engl J Med, 360*, 1418–1428.
48. Kannel, W. B. (2000). Incidence and epidemiology of heart failure [Review]. *Heart Fail Rev, 5*, 167–173.
49. Gottdiener, J. S., Arnold, A. M., Aurigemma, G. P., et al. (2000). Predictors of congestive heart failure in the elderly: the Cardiovascular Health Study. *J Am Coll Cardiol, 35*, 1628–1637.
50. Nicklas, B. J., Cesari, M., Penninx, B. W., et al. (2006). Abdominal obesity is an independent risk factor for chronic heart failure in older people. *J Am Geriatr Soc, 54*, 413–420.
51. Lakatta, E. G., & Levy, D. (2003). Arterial and cardiac aging: major shareholders in cardiovascular disease enterprises: part II: the aging heart in health: links to heart disease. *Circulation, 107*, 346–354.
52. Lakatta, E. G., & Levy, D. (2003). Arterial and cardiac aging: major shareholders in cardiovascular disease enterprises: part I: aging arteries: a "set up" for vascular disease. *Circulation, 107*, 139–146.
53. Cody, R. J., Torre, S., Clark, M., et al. (1989). Age-related hemodynamic, renal, and hormonal differences among patients with congestive heart failure. *Arch Intern Med, 149*, 1023–1028.
54. Gandhi, S. K., Powers, J. C., Nomeir, A. M., et al. (2001). The pathogenesis of acute pulmonary edema associated with hypertension. *N Engl J Med, 344*, 17–22.
55. Kramer, K., Kirkman, P., Kitzman, D., et al. (2000). Flash pulmonary edema: association with hypertension and reoccurrence despite coronary revascularization. *Am Heart J, 140*, 451–455.
56. Lam, C. S., Roger, V. L., Rodeheffer, R. J., et al. (2007). Cardiac structure and ventricular-vascular function in persons with heart failure and preserved ejection fraction from Olmsted County, Minnesota. *Circulation, 115*, 1982–1990.
57. Croft, J. B., Giles, W. H., Pollard, R. A., et al. (1999). Heart failure survival among older adults in the United States: a poor prognosis for an emerging epidemic in the Medicare population. *Arch Intern Med, 159*, 505–510.
58. Huynh, B. C., Rovner, A., & Rich, M. W. (2006). Long-term survival in elderly patients hospitalized for heart failure: 14-year follow-up from a prospective randomized trial. *Arch Intern Med, 166*, 1892–1898.
59. Thomas, S., & Rich, M. W. (2007). Epidemiology, pathophysiology, and prognosis of heart failure in the elderly. *Heart Fail Clin, 3*, 381–387.
60. Henkel, D. M., Redfield, M. M., Weston, S. A., et al. (2008). Death in heart failure: a community perspective. *Circ Heart Fail, 1*(2), 91–97.
61. Kitzman, D. W., & Groban, L. (2008). Exercise intolerance. *Heart Fail Clin, 4*, 99–115.
62. Kitzman, D. W., Little, W. C., Brubaker, P. H., et al. (2002). Pathophysiological characterization of isolated diastolic heart failure in comparison to systolic heart failure. *JAMA, 288*, 2144–2150.
63. Katz, S., Ford, A. B., Moskowitz, R. W., et al. (1963). Studies of illness in the aged. The index of ADL: a standardized measure of biological and psychosocial function. *JAMA, 185*, 914–919.
64. Newman, A. B., Simonsick, E. M., Naydeck, B. L., et al. (2006). Association of long-distance corridor walk performance with mortality, cardiovascular disease, mobility limitation, and disability. *JAMA, 295*, 2018–2026.
65. Le Jemtel, T. H., Padeletti, M., & Jelic, S. (2007). Diagnostic and therapeutic challenges in patients with coexistent chronic obstructive pulmonary disease and chronic heart failure. *J Am Coll Cardiol, 49*, 171–180.
66. Rich, M. W., Beckham, V., Wittenberg, C., et al. (1995). A multidisciplinary intervention to prevent the readmission of elderly patients with congestive heart failure. *N Engl J Med, 333*, 1190–1195.

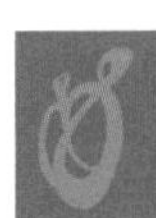

67. Cleland, J. G., Tendera, M., Adamus, J., et al. (2006). The Perindopril in Elderly People with Chronic Heart Failure (PEP-CHF) study. *Eur Heart J, 27*, 2338–2345.
68. Yusuf, S., Pfeffer, M. A., Swedberg, K., et al. (2003). Effects of candesartan in patients with chronic heart failure and preserved left-ventricular ejection fraction: the CHARM-Preserved Trial. *Lancet, 362*, 777–781.
69. Little, W. C., Zile, M. R., Klein, A., et al. (2006). Effect of losartan and hydrochlorothiazide on exercise tolerance in exertional hypertension and left ventricular diastolic dysfunction. *Am J Cardiol, 98*, 383–385.
70. Massie, B. M., Carson, P. E., McMurray, J. J., et al. (2008). Irbesartan in patients with heart failure and preserved ejection fraction. *N Engl J Med, 359*, 2456–2467.
71. van Veldhuisen, D. J., Cohen-Solal, A., Böhm, M., et al. (2009). Beta-blockade with nebivolol in elderly heart failure patients with impaired and preserved left ventricular ejection fraction: data from SENIORS (Study of Effects of Nebivolol Intervention on Outcomes and Rehospitalization in Seniors With Heart Failure). *J Am Coll Cardiol, 53*, 2150–2158.
72. Ahmed, A., Rich, M. W., Fleg, J. L., et al. (2006). Effects of digoxin on morbidity and mortality in diastolic heart failure: the ancillary Digitalis Investigation Group trial. *Circulation, 114*, 397–403.
73. Rosamond, W., Flegal, K., Furie, K., et al. (2008). Heart disease and stroke statistics—2008 update: a report from the American Heart Association Statistics Committee and Stroke Statistics Subcommittee. *Circulation, 117*(4), e25–e146.
74. Galvao, M., Kalman, J., DeMarco, T., et al. (2006). Gender differences in in-hospital management and outcomes in patients with decompensated heart failure: analysis from the Acute Decompensated Heart Failure National Registry (ADHERE). *J Card Fail, 12*, 100–107.
75. Nieminen, M. S., Harjola, V. P., Hochadel, M., et al. (2008). Gender related differences in patients presenting with acute heart failure. Results from EuroHeart Failure Survey II. *Eur J Heart Fail, 10*, 140–148.
76. O'Meara, E., Clayton, T., McEntegart, M. B., et al. (2007). Sex differences in clinical characteristics and prognosis in a broad spectrum of patients with heart failure: results of the Candesartan in Heart failure: Assessment of Reduction in Mortality and morbidity (CHARM) program. *Circulation, 115*, 3111–3120.
77. He, J., Ogden, L. G., Bazzano, L. A., et al. (2001). Risk factors for congestive heart failure in US men and women: NHANES I epidemiologic follow-up study. *Arch Intern Med, 161*, 996–1002.
78. Bibbins-Domingo, K., Lin, F., Vittinghoff, E., et al. (2004). Predictors of heart failure among women with coronary disease. *Circulation, 110*, 1424–1430.
79. Roger, V. L., Weston, S. A., Redfield, M. M., et al. (2004). Trends in heart failure incidence and survival in a community-based population. *JAMA, 292*, 344–350.
80. Levy, D., Kenchaiah, S., Larson, M. G., et al. (2002). Long-term trends in the incidence of and survival with heart failure. *N Engl J Med, 347*, 1397–1402.
81. Adams, K. F., Jr., Dunlap, S. H., Sueta, C. A., et al. (1996). Relation between gender, etiology and survival in patients with symptomatic heart failure. *J Am Coll Cardiol, 28*, 1781–1788.
82. Deswal, A., & Bozkurt, B. (2006). Comparison of morbidity in women versus men with heart failure and preserved ejection fraction. *Am J Cardiol, 97*, 1228–1231.
83. Gottlieb, S. S., Khatta, M., Friedmann, E., et al. (2004). The influence of age, gender, and race on the prevalence of depression in heart failure patients. *J Am Coll Cardiol, 43*, 1542–1549.
84. Owan, T. E., Hodge, D. O., Herges, R. M., et al. (2006). Trends in prevalence and outcome of heart failure with preserved ejection fraction. *N Engl J Med, 355*, 251–259.
85. Bhatia, R. S., Tu, J. V., Lee, D. S., et al. (2006). Outcome of heart failure with preserved ejection fraction in a population-based study. *N Engl J Med, 355*, 260–269.
86. Pearson, G. D., Veille, J. C., Rahimtoola, S., et al. (2000). Peripartum cardiomyopathy: National Heart, Lung, and Blood Institute and Office of Rare Diseases (National Institutes of Health) workshop recommendations and review. *JAMA, 283*, 1183–1188.
87. Ntusi, N. B., & Mayosi, B. M. (2009). Aetiology and risk factors of peripartum cardiomyopathy: a systematic review. *Int J Cardiol, 131*, 168–179.
88. Hu, C. L., Li, Y. B., Zou, Y. G., et al. (2007). Troponin T measurement can predict persistent left ventricular dysfunction in peripartum cardiomyopathy. *Heart, 93*, 488–490.
89. Abboud, J., Murad, Y., Chen-Scarabelli, C., et al. (2007). Peripartum cardiomyopathy: a comprehensive review. *Int J Cardiol, 118*, 295–303.
90. Duran, N., Gunes, H., Duran, I., et al. (2008). Predictors of prognosis in patients with peripartum cardiomyopathy. *Int J Gynaecol Obstet, 101*, 137–140.
91. Fett, J. D., Christie, L. G., Carraway, R. D., et al. (2005). Five-year prospective study of the incidence and prognosis of peripartum cardiomyopathy at a single institution. *Mayo Clin Proc, 80*, 1602–1606.
92. Elkayam, U., Tummala, P. P., Rao, K., et al. (2001). Maternal and fetal outcomes of subsequent pregnancies in women with peripartum cardiomyopathy. *N Engl J Med, 344*, 1567–1571.
93. Johnstone, D., Limacher, M., Rousseau, M., et al. (1992). Clinical characteristics of patients in studies of left ventricular dysfunction (SOLVD). *Am J Cardiol, 70*, 894–900.
94. Redfield, M. M., Jacobsen, S. J., Burnett, J. C., Jr., et al. (2003). Burden of systolic and diastolic ventricular dysfunction in the community: appreciating the scope of the heart failure epidemic. *JAMA, 289*, 194–202.
95. Vasan, R. S., Larson, M. G., Benjamin, E. J., et al. (1999). Congestive heart failure in subjects with normal versus reduced left ventricular ejection fraction: prevalence and mortality in a population-based cohort. *J Am Coll Cardiol, 33*, 1948–1955.
96. Yancy, C. W., Fonarow, G. C., Albert, N. M., et al. (2009). Influence of patient age and sex on delivery of guideline-recommended heart failure care in the outpatient cardiology practice settings: findings from IMPROVE HF. *Am Heart J, 157*, 754–762.e2.
97. Forman, D. E., Cannon, C. P., Hernandez, A. F., et al. (2009). Influence of age on the management of heart failure: findings from Get With The Guidelines—Heart Failure (GWTG-HF). *Am Heart J, 157*, 1010–1017.
98. Fonarow, G. C., Abraham, W. T., Albert, N. M., et al. (2009). Age- and gender-related differences in quality of care and outcomes of patients hospitalized with heart failure (from OPTIMIZE-HF). *Am J Cardiol, 104*, 107–115.
99. Heart Failure Society of America. (2006). Executive summary: HFSA 2006 Comprehensive Heart Failure Practice Guideline. *J Card Fail, 12*, 10–38.
100. Garg, R., & Yusuf, S. (1995). Overview of randomized trials of angiotensin-converting enzyme inhibitors on mortality and morbidity in patients with heart failure. Collaborative Group on ACE Inhibitor Trials. *JAMA, 273*, 1450–1456.
101. Pfeffer, M. A., Swedberg, K., Granger, C. G., et al. (2003). Effects of candesartan on mortality and morbidity in patients with chronic heart failure: the CHARM-Overall Programme. *Lancet, 362*, 759–766.
102. Packer, M., Bristow, M. R., Cohn, J. N., et al. (1996). The effect of carvedilol on morbidity and mortality in patients with chronic heart failure. U.S. Carvedilol Heart Failure Study Group. *N Engl J Med, 334*, 1349–1355.
103. Simon, T., Mary-Krause, M., Funck-Brentano, C., et al. (2001). Sex differences in the prognosis of congestive heart failure: results from the Cardiac Insufficiency Bisoprolol Study (CIBIS II). *Circulation, 103*, 375–380.
104. Ghali, J. K., Pina, I. L., Gottlieb, S. S., et al. (2002). Metoprolol CR/XL in female patients with heart failure: analysis of the experience in Metoprolol Extended-Release Randomized Intervention Trial in Heart Failure (MERIT-HF). *Circulation, 105*, 1585–1591.
105. The effect of digoxin on mortality and morbidity in patients with heart failure. (1997). The Digitalis Investigation Group. *N Engl J Med, 336*, 525–533.
106. Rathore, S. S., Wang, Y., & Krumholz, H. M. (2002). Sex-based differences in the effect of digoxin for the treatment of heart failure. *N Engl J Med, 347*, 1403–1411.
107. Adams, K. F., Jr., Patterson, J. H., Gattis, W. A., et al. (2005). Relationship of serum digoxin concentration to mortality and morbidity in women in the Digitalis Investigation Group trial: a retrospective analysis. *J Am Coll Cardiol, 46*, 497–504.
108. Bristow, M. R., Saxon, L. A., Boehmer, J., et al. (2004). Cardiac-resynchronization therapy with or without an implantable defibrillator in advanced chronic heart failure. *N Engl J Med, 350*, 2140–2150.
109. Piña, I. L., Kokkinos, P., Kao, A., et al. (2009). Baseline differences in the HF-ACTION trial by sex. *Am Heart J, 158*(Suppl. 4), S16–S23.
110. Bardy, G. H., Lee, K. L., Mark, D. B., et al. (2005). Amiodarone or an implantable cardioverter-defibrillator for congestive heart failure. *N Engl J Med, 352*, 225–237.
111. Miller, L. W., Pagani, F. D., Russell, S. D., et al. (2007). Use of a continuous-flow device in patients awaiting heart transplantation. *N Engl J Med, 357*, 885–896.
112. Ghanbari, H., Dalloul, G., Hasan, R., et al. (2009). Effectiveness of implantable cardioverter-defibrillators for the primary prevention of sudden cardiac death in women with advanced heart failure; a meta-analysis of randomized controlled trials. *Arch Intern Med, 169*, 1500–1506.
113. Ochiai, Y., McCarthy, P. M., Smedira, N. G., et al. (2002). Predictors of severe right ventricular failure after implantable left ventricular assist device insertion: analysis of 245 patients. *Circulation, 106*, I-198–I-202.
114. Morgan, J. A., Weinberg, A. D., Hollingsworth, K. W., et al. (2004). Effect of gender on bridgingtotransplantationandposttransplantationsurvivalinpatientswithleftventricular assist devices. *J Thorac Cardiovasc Surg, 127*, 1193–1195.
115. *Organ Procurement and Transplantation Network* (online database): http://www.optn.org/latestData/step2.asp? Accessed March 24, 2008.
116. International Society for Heart and Lung Transplantation. *Heart/lung registries: slides* (online database): http://www.ishlt.org/registries/slides.asp?slides=heartLungRegistry. Accessed March 9, 2010.

CHAPTER 50

Emerging Strategies in the Treatment of Heart Failure

Kumudha Ramasubbu and Anita Deswal

Thus far, all attempts to develop a unifying hypothesis that explains the clinical syndrome of heart failure have not met with success when tested in large-scale clinical trials. As a result, combinations of pharmaceutical approaches have been used in the treatment of heart failure. Current therapeutic strategies rely on treating patients' symptoms with diuretics and digitalis, as well as on neurohormonal antagonism with pharmacological agents, such as angiotensin-converting enzyme (ACE) inhibitors, angiotensin receptor blockers, aldosterone receptor antagonists (see Chapters 45 and 46), and β-blockers (see Chapters 45 and 46), in order to antagonize the effects of the renin-angiotensin-aldosterone system and the adrenergic system, respectively. Despite these pharmacological interventions, heart failure remains a progressive disease with unacceptably high rates of morbidity and mortality. Thus, new and improved therapeutic approaches are needed in the treatment of heart failure.

This chapter is a review of some of the new therapeutic approaches that are being tested in heart failure. This chapter focuses first on new medications that have been explored in patients with heart failure. This is followed by a discussion of novel approaches in heart failure of various causes.

NEUROHORMONAL ANTAGONISM

Various neurohormones are activated in heart failure as a compensatory mechanism. Over the long term, the suppression of such neurohormones (renin-angiotensin-aldosterone system and adrenergic system) has resulted in the attenuation of their deleterious effects on the cardiovascular system and also on clinical endpoints, including mortality. More recently, two more neurohormones that are activated in heart failure have been targeted: vasopressin antagonists and endothelin antagonists.

Vasopressin Antagonists

Vasopressin is a peptide hormone secreted by the posterior pituitary gland in response to a reduction in plasma volume and an increase in plasma osmolality. Through vasopressin 1a (V1a) receptors (in vascular smooth muscle cells) and vasopressin 2 (V2) receptors (in the renal collecting ducts), vasopressin elicits vasoconstriction and water reabsorption with resultant hyponatremia.[1] Conivaptan, a dual vasopressin receptor antagonist, has been shown to significantly increase urine output, decrease pulmonary capillary wedge pressure, and lower right atrial pressure in comparison with placebo in patients with systolic heart failure.[2] Similarly, tolvaptan, a selective V1a receptor antagonist, was demonstrated to increase urine output and decrease body weight without causing significant decline in renal function.[3,4] In the largest vasopressin antagonist trial to date, the Efficacy of Vasopressin Antagonism in Heart Failure Outcome Study with Tolvaptan (EVEREST) trial, 4133 patients hospitalized for worsening heart failure and depressed left ventricular (LV) function (ejection fraction < 40%) were randomly assigned to receive either oral tolvaptan or placebo. After a median follow-up period of 9.9 months, there was no difference in the dual primary endpoints of all-cause mortality and mortality from cardiovascular causes or hospitalization for heart failure. However, there were improvements in patient-assessed dyspnea, body weight, and edema. A significant increase in sodium levels was also noted in patients with hyponatremia.[5,6] On the basis of the data available, vasopressin antagonists appear to be safe in patients with heart failure, and they appear to improve volume overload, symptoms of heart failure, and hyponatremia without an impact on long-term clinical outcomes. The U.S. Food and Drug Administration has approved in-hospital oral tolvaptan initiation for the treatment of hypervolemic and euvolemic hyponatremia in the setting of heart failure, liver cirrhosis, and the syndrome of inappropriate antidiuretic hormone secretion.

Endothelin Antagonists

Endothelin is a peptide hormone that is produced in cardiac tissue and exerts its effects through endothelin A and endothelin B receptors. Despite a good scientific rationale and promising initial results with these agents in acute decompensated heart failure (ADHF), the definitive larger clinical trial, Value of Endothelin Receptor Inhibition With Tezosentan in Acute Heart Failure Study (VERITAS)—in which 1760 patients with ADHF were randomly assigned to receive tezosentan or placebo—was prematurely terminated because of a low probability of achieving a significant treatment benefit.[7] Thus, at present, there is no indication for the use of endothelin antagonists in ADHF.

DIURESIS AND NATRIURESIS

Two novel pharmacological approaches to fluid removal in patients with heart failure have been investigated: adenosine antagonists and ularitide. These new concepts are important in the setting of a greater awareness and possibly a greater incidence of the cardiorenal syndrome, as well as resistance to conventional loop and thiazide diuretics.

Adenosine Antagonists

Adenosine is a purine nucleoside that is found ubiquitously in various cells. Adenosine exerts its effects through four receptors (A_1, A_{2a}, A_{2b}, and A_3) located in the kidney, heart, and vasculature.[8] In heart failure, special attention has been given to A_1 receptors, which are located in the afferent arteriole and proximal tubule in the kidneys and are involved in afferent arteriolar vasoconstriction and tubuloglomerular feedback.[8,9] Adenosine levels have been demonstrated to be elevated in the setting of heart failure.[10] In heart failure, elevation of the sodium concentration in the distal tubule stimulates a feedback mechanism to the macula densa, resulting in release of adenosine, which in turn leads to an increase in sodium resorption by the proximal tubule and afferent arteriolar vasoconstriction and a resultant decrease in the glomerular filtration rate (GFR).

Thus, A_1 receptor blockade, which results in afferent arteriolar vasodilation, leads to improved GFR and enhanced diuresis and natriuresis without activation of the tubuloglomerular feedback. Several small clinical trials with A_1-antagonisits in humans with ADHF and chronic heart failure have confirmed this mechanism of action.[11,12] These effects were observed even in patients with more severe renal dysfunction and diuretic resistance.[11] Moreover, whereas GFR declined by 25% during treatment with furosemide, GFR was preserved in patients treated with the A_1-antagonist. In a different study, the GFR decline caused by furosemide was balanced out by the addition of the A_1-antagonist BG-9719.[13] Similarly, other A_1 antagonists have been shown to significantly increase natriuresis in patients with heart failure and systolic dysfunction without a decline in renal function.[14]

In a larger study, the pilot phase of the Placebo-controlled, Randomized study of the selective A_1 adenosine receptor antagonist rolofylline for patients hospitalized with acute heart failure and volume Overload to assess Treatment Effect on Congestion and renal function Trial (PROTECT), 301 patients hospitalized with ADHF were randomly assigned to receive one of three doses of rolofylline or placebo. The primary endpoint was a composite of treatment success (improvement in dyspnea), treatment failure (defined as early readmission for heart failure, worsening heart failure, or persistent renal impairment), and unchanged status. Treatment with rolofylline was associated with a higher likelihood of achieving success, as evidenced by improved dyspnea (52.7% vs. 37.2%) and a lower likelihood of experiencing failure (16.2% vs. 28.2%) in comparison with placebo. These findings reached statistical significance only for the highest dose of rolofylline.[15] Rolofylline recipients exhibited a trend toward a reduction in the composite secondary endpoint of 60-day mortality and readmission for cardiovascular or renal cause and also a trend toward a lesser increase in serum creatinine level. Worsening renal function occurred in 18% of the placebo recipients and only 8% of the patients receiving the 30-mg dosage of rolofylline. Although there is some concern that rolofylline decreases the seizure threshold, it was found to be safe in this trial without an increase in adverse events in comparison to placebo. Of note, patients at high risk for seizures were excluded from this trial, and those with intermediate risk were given prophylactic lorazepam.

In the second phase of the PROTECT study, 2033 patients admitted with heart failure were randomly assigned to receive rolofylline or placebo. The primary endpoint—which included symptoms of heart failure, readmissions for heart failure, survival, and renal impairment—was considered treatment success, treatment failure, or unchanged. The primary endpoint was not significantly different between the two groups.[16] Thus, the results of the pilot PROTECT study were not confirmed in the larger trial. Another trial in subjects hospitalized with worsening renal function and heart failure that necessitated intravenous therapy, the Placebo-Controlled Randomized Study of KW-3902 for Subjects Hospitalized With Worsening Renal Function and Heart Failure (REACH UP) trial, which is evaluating the effect of rolofylline on worsening heart failure, deaths from heart failure, hospitalizations for heart failure, and renal function, is still ongoing.[17]

Ularitide

Ularitide is a synthetic form of urodilatin, a natriuretic peptide, which is produced in the distal renal tubules. Ularitide binds to natriuretic peptide receptors located on medullary collecting duct cells and vascular smooth muscle cells, which leads to increased diuresis, natriuresis, and arterial and venous vasodilation.[18] Clinically, ularitide has been shown to induce natriuresis and, at the same time, decrease plasma concentrations of renin, aldosterone, and angiotensin II, contrary to findings with conventional diuretics.[19,20] In the Safety and Efficacy of an Intravenous Placebo-Controlled Randomised Infusion of Ularitide II (SIRIUS II) trial, 221 patients with ADHF were randomly assigned to receive one of three doses of ularitide or placebo, in addition to baseline loop and thiazide diuretics. Subjects treated with ularitide exhibited an improvement in dyspnea and hemodynamic parameters (decrease in pulmonary capillary wedge pressure, reduction in systemic vascular resistance, decrease in right atrial pressure, and increase in cardiac index without significant change in heart rate). No difference in urine output was noted between subjects treated with ularitide and those given placebo, which suggests that the predominant mechanism for the hemodynamic changes is vasodilation. A trend toward improved rates of 30-day mortality was noted in the ularitide recipients. The most common side effect of ularitide was hypotension, which was most prominent with the highest dose. No significant worsening of renal function was noted.[21] The Ularitide Global Evaluation in Acute Decompensated Heart Failure (URGENT) trial, a prospective, randomized, placebo-controlled trial, is in the planning phases and is directed toward evaluating the effect of ularitide in 3000 patients with ADHF on dyspnea, safety, and morbidity and mortality both during and after hospitalization.

INOTROPES

Conventional inotropes, such as dobutamine and milrinone, have been shown to improve hemodynamic status in patients with systolic heart failure, but they do not appear to improve clinical outcomes; in fact, they have been demonstrated to be detrimental in these patients.[22] The negative clinical effects have been attributed to the fact that these inotropes increase intracellular calcium and can thereby cause myocardial cell death and ventricular arrhythmias.[23] Therefore, development of other agents that may not have the detrimental effects observed with conventional inotropes has been an area of considerable interest (Figure 50-1).

Calcium Sensitizer (Levosimendan)

More recently, there has been a focus on calcium sensitizers as contractility-enhancing agents. In contrast to conventional inotropes, calcium sensitizers enhance contractility by increasing

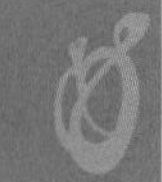

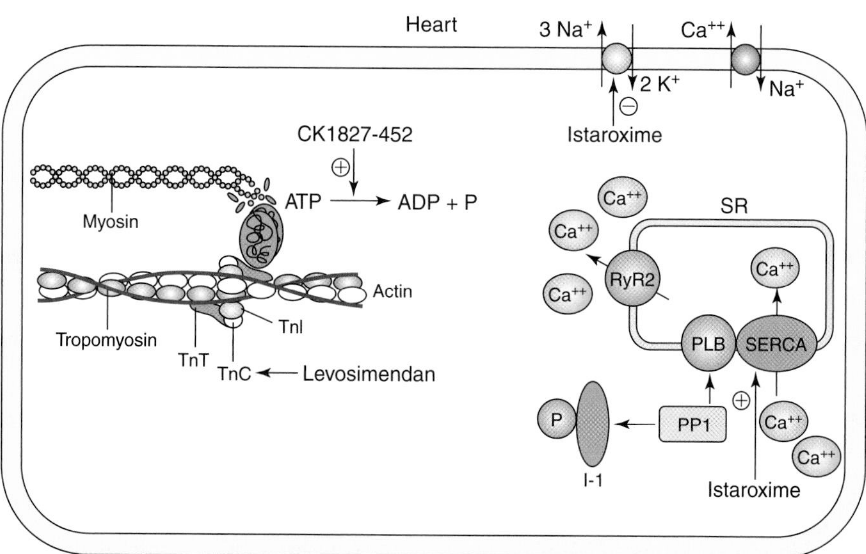

FIGURE 50–1 Mechanism of action of novel contractility-enhancing medications. Levosimendan enhances contractility by increasing responsiveness of myofilaments to calcium. The cardiac myosin activator CK 1827-452 stimulates myosin adenosine triphosphatase (ATPase), thereby increasing force generation. Istaroxime inhibits activity of plasma membrane sodium-potassium ATPase and increases the activity of sarcoplasmic/endoplasmic reticulum calcium ATPase (SERCA). ADP, adenosine diphosphate; ATP, adenosine triphosphate; I-1, protein phosphatase inhibitor-1; P, phosphate; PLB, phospholamban; PP1, protein phosphatase; RyR2, ryanodine receptor; TnC, troponin C; TnI, troponin I; TnT, troponin T. (Modified from Tavares M, Rezlan E, Vostroknoutova I, et al. New pharmacologic therapies for acute heart failure. *Crit Care Med* 2008; 36[Suppl]:S112-S120.)

responsiveness of myofilaments to calcium while maintaining intracellular calcium concentration. Thus, theoretically, calcium sensitizers should not have the same adverse effects as do conventional inotropes. The best-studied calcium sensitizer is levosimendan, which appears to exert its action through various mechanisms: inhibiting phosphodiesterase III, increasing the calcium sensitivity of cardiac troponin C, and stimulating the opening of potassium–adenosine triphosphate (ATP) channels, which lead to its vasodilatory effects.[24-26] Hemodynamically, levosimendan has been demonstrated to increase cardiac output and stroke volume and to decrease pulmonary capillary wedge pressure in a dose-dependent manner. Other effects include an increase in heart rate at higher doses and a decrease in systemic arterial pressure.[27]

Levosimendan has been evaluated in patients with heart failure in two large trials. In the second Randomized Multicenter Evaluation of Intravenous Levosimendan Efficacy (REVIVE II), study, 600 patients with ADHF were randomly assigned to receive either levosimendan or placebo. The composite endpoint, which included symptoms, clinical status, and major clinical events, was significantly improved in patients treated with levosimendan. However, the use of levosimendan was associated with increased episodes of hypotension, ventricular tachycardia, ventricular extrasystoles, atrial fibrillation, and a higher rate of early mortality. However, at 31 and 90 days, rates of mortality were not significantly different between the treatment and placebo recipients.[28] In the Randomized study on Safety and effectiveness of Levosimendan in patients with LV failure due to an Acute myocardial Infarct (RUSSLAN), 504 patients with recent myocardial infarction and heart failure who were in need of inotropes were randomly assigned to receive four different doses of levosimendan or placebo for 6 hours. The primary endpoint, which was a safety endpoint of the incidence of clinically significant hypotension or myocardial ischemia, was not significantly different between the levosimendan- and placebo-treated subjects. Among the secondary endpoints, levosimendan administration was associated with a significantly decreased risk of death or worsening heart failure at 6 and 24 hours after the infusion and a significant decrease in mortality at 14 days. This mortality benefit that persisted at 180 days of follow-up was, however, not statistically significant.[29]

Additional prospective randomized clinical trials were conducted to assess the efficacy and safety of levosimendan in comparison with placebo in patients with heart failure. In the Levosimendan Infusion versus Dobutamine (LIDO) trial, 203 patients with low output heart failure were randomly assigned to receive levosimendan or dobutamine. Treatment with levosimendan resulted in a significant improvement in the primary endpoint of hemodynamic status, measured by an increase in cardiac output and a decrease in pulmonary capillary wedge pressure. Moreover, patients treated with levosimendan demonstrated better survival rates at 31 days than did patients treated with dobutamine.[30]

The Calcium Sensitizer or Inotrope or None in Low-Output Heart Failure (CASINO) trial, in which 299 patients with low output heart failure were randomly assigned to receive levosimendan or dobutamine, was terminated prematurely because of a significant survival benefit in patients treated with levosimendan.[31] In the Survival of Patients with Acute Heart Failure in Need of Intravenous Inotropic Support (SURVIVE) trial, 1327 patients with ADHF were randomly assigned to receive levosimendan or dobutamine. The primary endpoint was mortality at 180 days, and results were not different between the two treatment groups. With regard to adverse effects, there was no significant increase in hypotension, heart failure, atrial fibrillation, or ventricular tachycardia in the levosimendan recipients in comparison with the dobutamine recipients.[32]

In summary, treatment with levosimendan results in significant hemodynamic and symptom improvement in patients with decompensated heart failure. Although no significant effect on long-term survival has been noted with levosimendan, studies demonstrated a trend toward decreased survival in comparison to placebo and a trend toward improved survival in comparison to dobutamine.[32] Currently, levosimendan is approved for use in the treatment of ADHF in Europe but not in the United States.

Cardiac Myosin Activators

Hydrolysis of ATP by myosin adenosine triphosphatase (ATPase) leads to flexion of the myosin head with displacement of myosin in relation to actin, which results in muscle contraction. Cardiac myosin activators stimulate myosin ATPase, thereby increasing force generation. In animal studies, cardiac myosin activators were shown to increase fractional shortening of myocytes, improve cardiac function, and improve hemodynamics without increasing the intracellular calcium concentration, thereby theoretically attenuating myocardial oxygen consumption and the development of arrhythmias.[33,34] Interestingly, the mechanism of improving systolic function appears to be related to an increase in LV systolic ejection time rather than an increase in peak rate of pressure change with time ($\Delta P/\Delta T$) as seen with other inotropes. A phase I study in 34 healthy men randomly assigned to receive one of four doses of a cardiac myosin activator, CK-1827452, or placebo demonstrated a dose-related increase in systolic function and an increase in systolic ejection time. Although CK-1827452 was well tolerated, it did lead to a significant drop in mean standing systolic blood pressure by 13 mm Hg ($P < .0001$) and in mean supine systolic blood pressure by 7 mm Hg ($P < .05$) in comparison to placebo.[35] In a phase II trial, two cohorts each of 8 patients with stable heart failure (left ventricular ejection fraction [LVEF] < 40%) were treated with placebo and three escalating doses of CK-1827452. Treatment with CK-1827452 was associated with an increase in systolic ejection time and improvement in LV function, as assessed by echocardiography. The drug was well tolerated, with a decrease in heart rate at higher doses but no change in blood pressure.[36] Although the results of these small preliminary studies are promising, the clinical efficacy and safety of cardiac myosin activators in patients with heart failure remain to be determined.

Istaroxime

Istaroxime, another novel contractility-enhancing agent, inhibits sodium-potassium ATPase and increases the activity of sarcoplasmic/endoplasmic reticulum calcium ATPase (SERCA). Increased SERCA activity results in accumulation of calcium within the myocyte during systole and rapid extrusion of calcium in diastole, which lead to an improvement in both inotropic and lusitropic function. Animal studies with istaroxime have demonstrated an improvement in systolic and diastolic function with little change in myocardial oxygen consumption.[37] In the first larger clinical trial in humans, which was a phase II study, Hemodynamic Effects of Istaroxime in Patients With Worsening Heart Failure and Reduced LV Systolic Function (HORIZON-HF), 120 patients who were hospitalized for systolic heart failure were randomly assigned to receive one of three doses of istaroxime or placebo. All istaroxime doses resulted in a significant decrease in pulmonary capillary wedge pressure in comparison to placebo. Moreover, treatment with istaroxime was associated with a significant decrease in heart rate and an increase in systolic blood pressure. Patients treated with the highest dose showed an increase in cardiac index, a decrease in left ventricular end-diastolic volume, and improvement in diastolic parameters on echocardiography without a significant change in left ventricular ejection fraction. No major adverse effects were noted.[38] Although these results are encouraging, istaroxime's effect on short- and long-term clinical and safety outcomes remains to be determined.

METABOLIC MODULATORS

In the healthy human heart, ATP is produced from free fatty acids (FFA) 70% of the time and from glucose and other carbohydrates 30% of the time.[39] The metabolism of FFAs results in more ATP production, albeit at a greater cost of oxygen use, than of glucose. Moreover, during ischemia, FFA metabolism is altered, resulting in a greater production of lactate, which in turn can lead to tissue acidosis and decreased myocyte contractility[40,41] (Figure 50-2). Thus, under hypoxic or ischemic conditions, a shift from FFA to glucose use would be more metabolically efficient for the heart.[42] However, in situations of cardiac ischemia, as well as heart failure, FFA oxidation is increased and glucose use is decreased, which result in a metabolically inefficient milieu, which can further promote ischemia and worsen myocardial function.[43] Metabolic modulators are agents that create a more efficient milieu of energy metabolism by increasing glucose and decreasing FFA use.

Perhexiline

The best-studied metabolic modulator to date is perhexiline. Through inhibition of the enzyme carnitine palmitoyl transferase-1, perhexiline reduces mitochondrial FFA transport,[44] which results in increased glucose metabolism. In the 1970s, perhexiline was successfully used for the treatment of angina. However, its use soon plummeted after reports of hepatotoxicity and neurotoxicity in patients who metabolized perhexiline slowly.[45] The metabolic derangement noted in heart failure raised the possibility that perhexiline may theoretically benefit patients with heart failure by directing energy production toward a more metabolically efficient substrate: glucose. In a small trial, 56 patients with chronic New York Heart Association (NYHA) functional class II or III systolic heart failure were randomly assigned to receive perhexiline or placebo. After 8 weeks, perhexiline-treated patients demonstrated a significant increase in LV function and peak exercise oxygen consumption in comparison with the placebo recipients. There was no evidence of hepatotoxicity or neurotoxicity in this small group of patients.[46]

Trimetazidine

A second drug, trimetazidine, inhibits long-chain 3-ketoacyl coenzyme A thiolase, which is involved in the oxidation of FFA and thereby increases myocardial glucose use.[47] It has been used as an antianginal and, more recently, investigated in patients with heart failure. Results of several small studies of patients with ischemic cardiomyopathy suggested that trimetazidine may have a beneficial effect on preservation or improvement of LV function. Fragasso and associates[48] randomly assigned 55 patients with ischemic and nonischemic cardiomyopathy (NYHA functional classes II to IV) to receive trimetazidine or placebo in addition to conventional heart failure treatment. After a mean follow-up period of 13 months, the trimetazidine-treated patients demonstrated significant improvements in exercise capacity, NYHA functional class, and LVEF and a decrease in LV end-systolic volume in comparison with placebo recipients. No increase in adverse events was noted among the trimetazidine-treated patients.

Ranolazine

A third antianginal agent, ranolazine, alters the transcellular late sodium current, which leads to a decrease in intracellular calcium overload.[49] Ranolazine also appears to promote an increase in glucose oxidation and a reduction in FFA oxidation,[50] with a significant decrease in ischemia and angina.[51] In systolic heart failure, animal experiments have demonstrated that treatment with ranolazine is associated with an improvement in the mechanical efficiency of the left ventricle and in LV function.[52,53] Studies in humans are still lacking. In patients with heart failure and preserved ejection fraction, the effect of ranolazine on echocardiographic parameters of diastolic dysfunction is being investigated in a small clinical trial.[17]

L-Carnitine

L-Carnitine is an essential cofactor in the metabolism of FFAs. It prevents the accumulation of FFA, prevents lactic acid production, and appears to enhance glucose use.[54] L-Carnitine deficiency has been associated with the development of cardiomyopathy.[55] Supplementation with L-carnitine has been shown to improve exercise capacity in patients with coronary artery disease and angina.[56] In patients with heart failure, administration of propionyl L-carnitine has been demonstrated to acutely decrease pulmonary artery and pulmonary capillary wedge pressure.[57] In small prospective, randomized

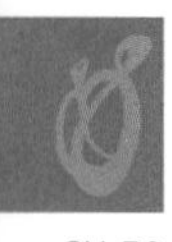

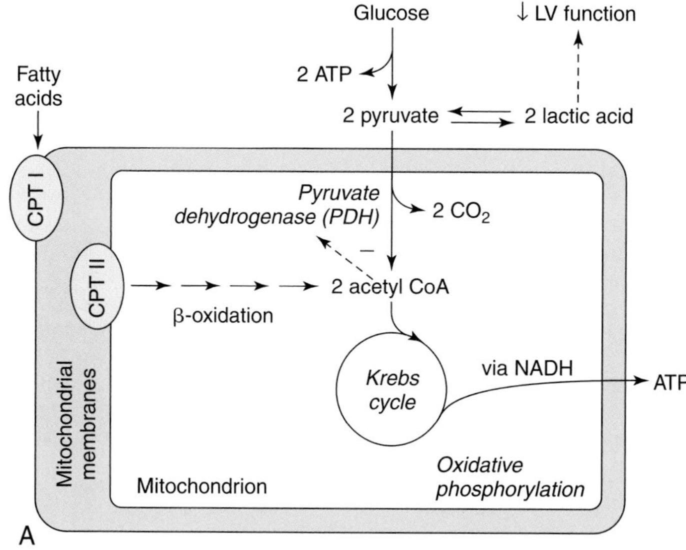

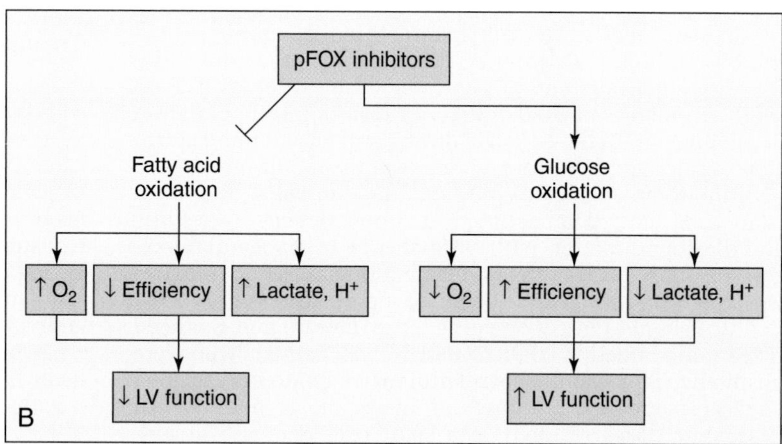

FIGURE 50–2 Metabolism of free fatty acids and glucose. **A,** Metabolic pathway for glucose metabolism and fatty acid oxidation. **B,** Effects switching metabolism from fatty acid β-oxidation to glucose oxidation (under conditions in which oxygen supply is rate limiting) by means of partial inhibitors of fatty acid oxidation (pFOX). ATP, adenosine triphosphate; CoA, coenzyme A; CPT, carnitine-palmitoyl transferase; LV, left ventricular; NADH, nicotinamide adenine dinucleotide (reduced form). (From Dimmeler S, Mann D, Zeiher AM, et al. Emerging therapies and strategies in the treatment of heart failure. In Libby P, Bonow RO, Mann DL, et al, editors. *Braunwald's heart disease,* Philadelphia, 2008, Elsevier, pp 697-715.)

trials in patients with heart failure, chronic supplementation with L-carnitine was associated with an increase in exercise capacity and peak oxygen consumption. Echocardiography demonstrated a significant reduction in LV dimensions and improvement in LV function.[57-59]

In summary, although the concept of metabolic modulation for the treatment of heart failure appears promising, the efficacy and safety of this approach need confirmation in larger trials.

IMMUNOMODULATORY AGENTS

Statins (see Chapters 11 and 24)

Statins lower cholesterol levels by inhibiting 3-hydroxy-3-methylglutaryl–coenzyme A (HMG-CoA) reductase, the rate-limiting enzyme in the cholesterol synthesis pathway (Figure 50-3). In addition to their lipid-lowering properties, statins have been reported to have non–lipid-lowering or pleiotropic effects that may have beneficial effects on neurohormonal activation and cardiac remodeling in patients with heart failure. Numerous retrospective analyses of data from clinical trials and of observational data revealed a significant mortality-related benefit in patients with heart failure who were treated with statins. Moreover, smaller prospective trials in which the effects of statins on mortality were assessed, as well as nonmortality clinical endpoints (echocardiographic parameters and biomarkers of inflammation), also illustrated beneficial effects of statins in heart failure.[60]

However, two large prospective trials of statin treatment in patients with systolic heart failure have challenged these findings. In the Controlled Rosuvastatin Multinational Trial in Heart Failure (CORONA), 5011 patients with NYHA functional classes II to IV heart failure of ischemic origin were randomly assigned to receive 10 mg of rosuvastatin daily or placebo. Over a median follow-up period of 32.8 months, treatment with rosuvastatin did not confer a significant benefit with regard to the primary endpoint, a composite of death from cardiovascular causes, nonfatal myocardial infarction, and nonfatal stroke, or with regard to several secondary endpoints, including all-cause mortality and coronary events. There was a significant but modest reduction in hospital admissions for cardiovascular events and, according to a post hoc analysis, in nonfatal ischemic events.[61]

In the second trial, Gruppo Italiano per lo Studio della Sopravvivenza nell'Infarto Miocardico–Heart Failure (GISSI-HF), 4574 patients with NYHA functional classes II to IV chronic heart failure were randomly assigned to receive rosuvastatin, 10 mg, or placebo. In contrast to CORONA, 60% of the patients in GISSI-HF had nonischemic cardiomyopathy. At 3.9 years, the two coprimary endpoints, time to death and time to death or hospitalization for cardiovascular reasons, were not significantly different between patients who took rosuvastatin and those who took placebo.[62]

Statins may have a neutral effect in patients with heart failure because they may not alter the pathomechanisms of heart failure, their unfavorable effects may neutralize their beneficial effects, and statin-specific effects may

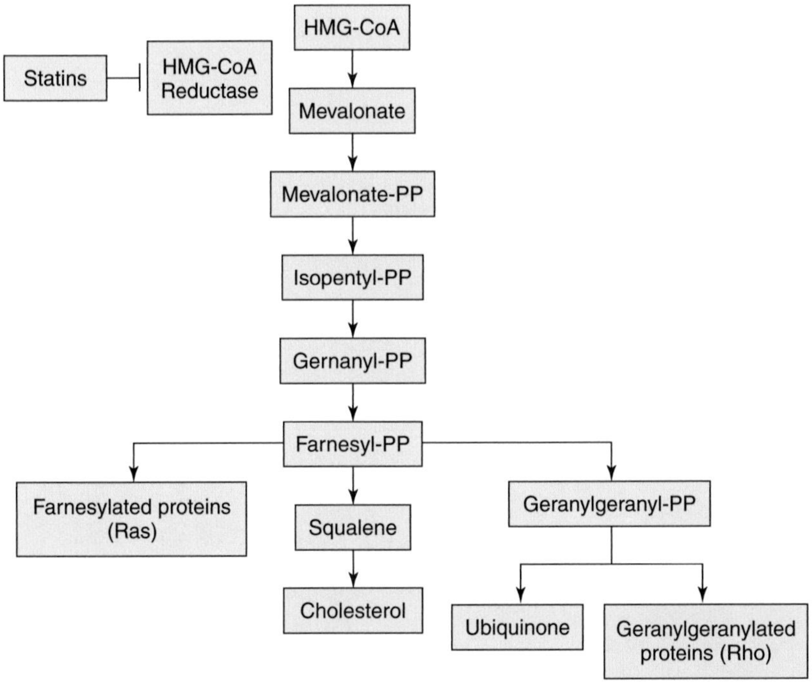

Statins → HMG-CoA Reductase
HMG-CoA → Mevalonate → Mevalonate-PP → Isopentyl-PP → Gernanyl-PP → Farnesyl-PP
Farnesyl-PP → Farnesylated proteins (Ras); Squalene → Cholesterol; Geranylgeranyl-PP → Ubiquinone; Geranylgeranylated proteins (Rho)

FIGURE 50–3 The mevalonate pathway leads to the synthesis of cholesterol. Important intermediate products in the mevalonate pathway include isoprenoids such as farnesyl pyrophosphate and geranylgeranyl pyrophosphate, which have been linked to activation *Ras*- and *Rho*-mediated signaling. 3-Hydroxy-3-methylglutaryl–coenzyme A (HMG-CoA) reductase inhibitors decrease the synthesis of isoprenoids as well as cholesterol, by blocking HMG-CoA reductase. PP, pyrophosphate. (From Ramasubbu K, Mann DL: The emerging role of statins in the treatment of heart failure. *J Am Coll Cardiol* 2006;47:342-344; and Dimmeler S, Mann D, Zeiher AM, et al. Emerging therapies and strategies in the treatment of heart failure. In Libby P, Bonow RO, Mann DL, et al, editors. *Braunwald's heart disease,* Philadelphia, 2008, Elsevier, pp 697-715.)

be variable. According to the results of CORONA and GISSI-HF, statins should not be initiated in patients with nonischemic cardiomyopathy unless this is indicated by their lipid profile. In patients with chronic heart failure resulting from ischemic cardiomyopathy, the evidence does not support initiating statins for heart failure except in the setting of ischemia or when indicated by the current lipid guidelines.

Polyunsaturated Fatty Acids (see Chapters 11 and 24)

Small trials have revealed beneficial effects of n-3 polyunsaturated fatty acids (PUFA) in cardiovascular disease, apart from their favorable effects on the lipid profile. These benefits were ascribed to their salutary effects on inflammation, endothelial function, blood pressure, heart rate, autonomic tone, and ventricular function. In patients with cardiovascular disease and at high risk for ventricular arrhythmias, supplementation with PUFA has been shown to result in a decrease in ventricular arrhythmias.[63] In a larger trial, Gruppo Italiano per lo Studio della Sopravvivenza nell'Infarto Miocardico (GISSI)–Prevenzione trial, patients who had suffered myocardial infarction were randomly assigned to receive PUFA; they demonstrated a 20% reduction in mortality, largely attributed to a decrease in sudden death.[64]

On the basis of these findings, the researchers in the GISSI-HF trial randomly assigned 6975 patients with NYHA functional class II to IV heart failure to receive PUFA or placebo (mean LVEF = 33%). After a mean follow-up period of 3.9 years, patients taking PUFA showed a small but significant improvement in rates of mortality (adjusted hazard ratio, 0.91; 95.5% confidence interval, 0.833 to 0.998; $P = .041$) and in rates of mortality or admissions for cardiovascular disorders. Of interest was that mortality reduction was driven largely by a reduction in presumed death from arrhythmia. Moreover, the investigators demonstrated that the administration of PUFA to patients with heart failure did not cause an increase in adverse events.[65] Thus, the administration of PUFA to patients with heart failure is reasonable, with modest efficacy and a good safety profile.

GENE THERAPY

Gene therapy represents yet another potential novel therapeutic approach for the treatment of heart failure. Gene therapy involves the manipulation of gene expression or function for the purpose of treatment of a specific disease. Gene transfer can result either in the expression and replacement of a missing gene product or in the overexpression of a native or foreign gene whose product can prevent or reverse a disease process. This genetic manipulation may be achieved either by the introduction of foreign DNA that encodes a biologically active transgene into cells or by transfection of short chains of nucleic acids, known as "deoxynucleotides", that modify endogenous gene expression in target cells.[66] Improvements in both gene transfer vectors and in vivo gene delivery techniques have facilitated genetic manipulation of myocardial function and enabled targeted therapy for heart failure.

For any application of gene therapy to be clinically successful, three elements are essential[66]: First, a vector or packaging system to deliver the genetic material is required. Vectors can be distinguished as viral and nonviral vectors. Thus far, for cardiac diseases, viral vectors appear to be the most efficient in achieving high levels of trans-gene expression in postmitotic cells such as cardiomyocytes. These vectors include recombinant adenoviruses and adeno-associated viruses.[67,68] Second, it is important that the vector is adequately delivered to the affected tissues. Numerous techniques have been described for in vivo cardiac gene transfer, including intracoronary catheter delivery, intramyocardial delivery, pericardial injection techniques, and injections by catheters introduced through the left ventricular apex while the aorta and pulmonary arteries are cross-clamped. Each technique has advantages and disadvantages[66] (Figure 50-4). Third, appropriate target gene identification is crucial. For the treatment of heart failure, promising targets that have been the focus of gene transfer research have included genes involved in the myocardial calcium-handling system, the β-adrenergic signaling system, and pathways that affect cardiomyocyte apoptosis, as summarized in the paragraphs that follow.

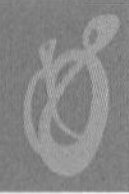

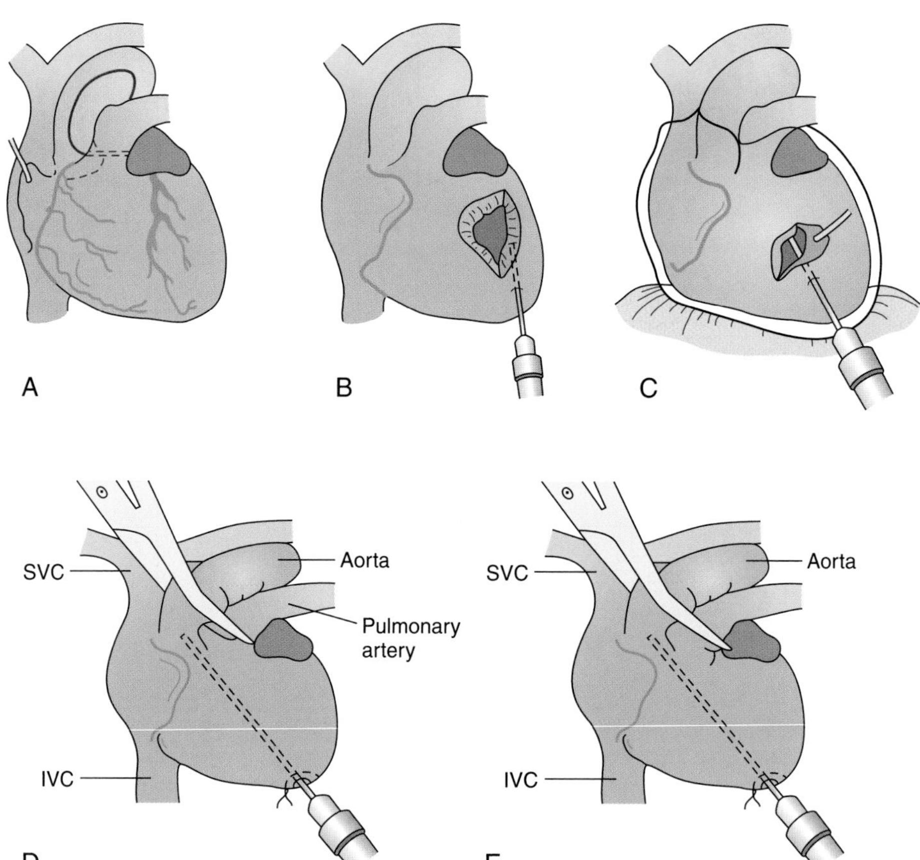

FIGURE 50–4 Different techniques for in vivo cardiac gene transfer. **A,** Coronary perfusion. **B,** Intramyocardial injection. **C,** Pericardial injection. **D,** Aortic clamping. **E,** Cross-clamping of the aorta and pulmonary artery. IVC, inferior vena cava, SVC, superior vena cava. (Modified from Hajjar RJ, del Monte F, Matsui T, et al. Prospects for gene therapy for heart failure. *Circ Res* 2000;86:616-621; and Dimmeler S, Mann D, Zeiher AM, et al. Emerging therapies and strategies in the treatment of heart failure. In Libby P, Bonow RO, Mann DL, et al, editors. *Braunwald's heart disease,* Philadelphia, 2008, Elsevier, pp 697-715.)

β-Adrenergic Signaling System (see Chapter 10)

The β-adrenergic receptor (β-AR) is known to play a critical role in mediating the inotropic state of the heart. Alterations in the myocardial β-AR system both precede and accompany the development of heart failure in humans. These alterations include downregulation of β-ARs, functional uncoupling of remaining β-ARs from second-messenger systems, increased levels of inhibitory G-proteins that blunt β-AR signaling, and upregulation of β-AR kinase 1 (β-ARK1), which appears to play an important role in the downregulation of β-ARs in the failing heart.[69,70] Transgenic mice that overexpressed the β_2-AR in the myocardium demonstrated highly enhanced contractility without overt pathological conditions.[71] This genetic manipulation has created considerable interest in the transfer of the β-AR gene into the failing myocardium as a therapeutic intervention. Adenoviral gene transfer of the human β_2-AR and inhibitor of β-ARK1 has been shown to result in improved β-AR signaling in myocytes in a rabbit heart failure model.[72,73] Moreover, in a mouse heart failure model, overexpression of a β-ARK1 inhibitor appeared to prevent the development of cardiomyopathy.[74] Similarly, adenovirus-mediated delivery of a peptide inhibitor of β-ARK1 in rabbit heart failure models has resulted in restoration of β-AR signaling, as well as reversal of ventricular dysfunction.[75] Of note, excessive stimulation of the β-AR (β_1 and β_2) signaling can also lead to activation of maladaptive signaling pathways in the heart, as well as myocyte death and heart failure.[76,77] Thus, caution must be exercised in promoting the β-AR signaling pathway.

Calcium-Handling System (see Chapter 4)

Enhancement of myocardial contractility through the manipulation of intracellular calcium levels has also been a target of gene therapy research (Figure 50-5). In failing hearts, suppression of sarcoplasmic/endoplasmic reticulum calcium ATPase (SERCA) activity, or a reduction in the SERCA protein, appears to contribute to the abnormalities in calcium handling and myocardial contraction.[78] Using adenovirus-mediated gene transfer that resulted in an overexpression of SERCA protein in rat cardiomyocytes and rat heart failure models, researchers achieved an improved handling of intracellular calcium that was accompanied by an improvement in myocardial systolic and diastolic function.[79-82] Furthermore, gene transfer of SERCA in rats with heart failure resulted in improved survival, as well as improved energy potential of the failing hearts.[83] In vitro gene transfer of SERCA into human cardiomyocytes from patients with end-stage heart failure resulted in an increase in protein expression, an increase in pump activity, and faster contraction and relaxation velocities.[79]

Phospholamban is a sarcomeric protein that regulates SERCA activity.[84] Results of several studies suggested that an abnormal ratio of phospholamban to SERCA contributes significantly to abnormalities in calcium handling and contraction observed in the failing ventricular myocardium.[66,85] Overexpression of an antisense phospholamban construct or a dominant-negative mutation of phospholamban has been shown to enhance SERCA activity.[86] Moreover, after gene transfer of S100A1 (a calcium-binding protein), beneficial effects on cardiac contractility, including normalized calcium handling and enhanced SERCA activity, were observed in experimental and human models of heart failure.[87]

Cardiomyocyte Survival (see Chapter 6)

Morphological and biological markers of programmed cell death (apoptosis) have been identified in human heart failure, which suggests that these pathways may contribute to cardiomyocyte loss and cardiac dysfunction in heart failure.[88] The ability to block cardiomyocyte apoptosis through

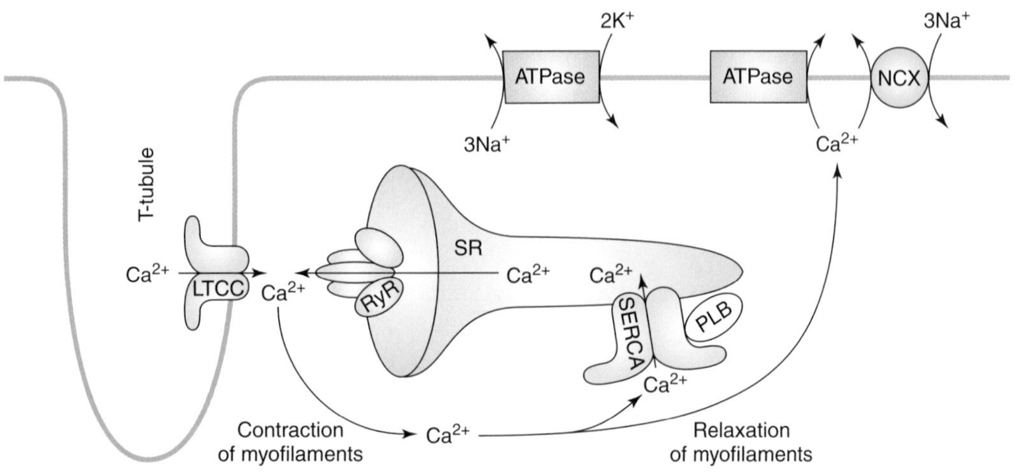

FIGURE 50-5 Myocyte calcium handling. Calcium uptake through the L-type calcium channel (LTCC) activates calcium release from the sarcoplasmic reticulum (SR) through the ryanodine receptor (RyR). This increase in intracellular calcium results in myocyte contraction. Reuptake of calcium into the SR by sarcoplasmic/endoplasmic reticulum calcium ATPase (SERCA) and extrusion of calcium through membrane sodium-calcium exchanger (NCX) and calcium ATPase result in a decrease in intracellular calcium concentration and myocyte relaxation. ATPase, adenosine triphosphatase; PLB, phospholamban. (From Kawase Y, Hajjar RJ. The cardiac sarcoplasmic/endoplasmic reticulum calcium ATPase: a potent target for cardiovascular diseases. *Nature Reviews Cardiology* 5, 554–565, September 2008).

somatic gene transfer is, therefore, another area of ongoing investigation.[89,90] Gene transfer that leads to overexpression of *Bcl*-2, an antiapoptotic gene, has been shown to inhibit p53-induced apoptosis of cardiomyocytes.[91] Similarly, gene transfer of phosphoinositide 3-kinase and protein kinase B, both antiapoptotic enzymes, has been demonstrated to block cardiomyocyte apoptosis in vitro.[92] In a rabbit model, transduction of cells with the gene for p35, a caspase-3 inhibitor, attenuated the development of heart failure.[90] The development of heart failure after myocardial infarction is associated with the loss of functional cardiomyocytes and replacement with a fibroblast-rich scar tissue. This has led to the attempt of genetically converting cardiac fibroblasts into functional cardiomyocytes.[93]

Thus, using gene therapy for the prevention and treatment of heart failure holds tremendous promise. However, much work remains to be done before the results of these basic investigative studies can be applied to clinical gene therapy in humans with heart failure.

Two clinical trials are currently under way in which researchers are evaluating the gene transfer of SERCA in patients with heart failure. The results are highly anticipated. Hajjar and colleagues[94] designed a phase I/II trial of intracoronary administration of adeno-associated virus serotype 1 (AAV1) and SERCA2a in patients with heart failure, in which the patients will initially undergo open-label administration of various doses of AAV1/SERCA2a. In a second stage, patients will be randomly assigned to receive various doses of AAV1/SERCA2a or placebo in a double-blind manner. In a second study,[17] researchers are evaluating the safety and efficacy of AAV6/SERCA2a administration in patients with nonischemic cardiomyopathy who are undergoing placement of left ventricular assist devices.

OTHER NOVEL THERAPIES

Sildenafil

Sildenafil is a selective phosphodiesterase type 5 inhibitor. It therefore increases levels of cyclic guanosine monophosphate (cGMP), which leads to the activation of cGMP-dependent protein kinases that mediate vascular smooth muscle relaxation and thus vasodilation.[95] Newer data implicate the role of cGMP-dependent protein kinases in the reversal of ventricular hypertrophy by inhibiting downstream hypertrophy signaling[96] (Figure 50-6).

Sildenafil has been shown to be beneficial in the treatment of patients with pulmonary hypertension by decreasing pulmonary artery pressures without having a significant effect on systemic pressures. The development of pulmonary hypertension in patients with heart failure portends worse outcomes and can be a contraindication to therapies such as cardiac transplantation.[97]

Sildenafil has been evaluated for the treatment of systolic heart failure in small clinical trials. Lewis and associates[98] evaluated the acute effect of sildenafil on invasive cardiac hemodynamics, gas exchange, and first-pass radionuclide ventriculography at rest and during exercise in 13 patients with NYHA class III heart failure. Sildenafil administration was associated with reductions in resting pulmonary arterial pressure, systemic vascular resistance, and pulmonary vascular resistance and with an increase in resting cardiac index, without altering mean arterial pressure, heart rate, or pulmonary capillary wedge pressure. During exercise, sildenafil reduced pulmonary arterial pressure and pulmonary vascular resistance. Moreover, peak oxygen consumption ($\dot{V}O_{2max}$) increased, ventilatory response to carbon dioxide output ($\dot{V}E/\dot{V}CO_2$ slope) decreased, and right ventricular ejection fraction increased after sildenafil administration. Thus, the investigators were able to demonstrate that sildenafil has a selective pulmonary vasodilator effect with little effect on systemic blood pressure, heart rate, and pulmonary capillary wedge pressure. The pulmonary vasodilator effect leads to an increase in right ventricular function and, possibly as a result, an increase in cardiac output.[98] The increase in cardiac output, together with other mechanisms, may have contributed to improvements in exercise capacity. Of note, the one other selective pulmonary vasodilator, inhaled nitric oxide, has the disadvantage of increasing pulmonary capillary wedge pressure and inducing pulmonary edema in patients with heart failure.[99]

In another trial, Bussotti and colleagues[100] evaluated the acute effects of sildenafil on pulmonary mechanics at rest and with exercise by administering 25-mg and 100-mg doses of sildenafil to 22 male patients with systolic heart failure (NYHA class II or III). Sildenafil administration was associated with enhancements in pulmonary perfusion, gas diffusion, and lung mechanics.

Subsequent studies have been performed to examine the chronic efficacy of sildenafil in patients with heart failure.

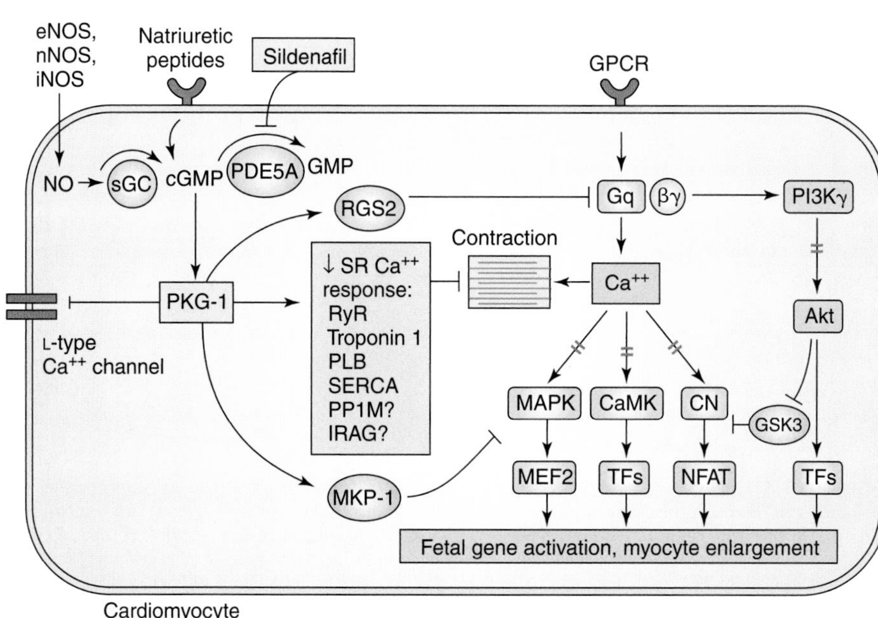

FIGURE 50–6 Sildenafil and hypertrophy. Sildenafil increases intracellular cyclic guanosine monophosphate (cGMP) by inhibiting phosphodiesterase 5 (PDE5A). Then cGMP activates cGMP-dependent protein kinase type 1 (PKG-1). PKG-1, in turn, inhibits several downstream signaling pathways that promote hypertrophy. Akt, Protein kinase B; CaMK, calcium/calmodulin-dependent protein kinases; CN, calcineurin; eNOS, endothelial nitric oxide synthase; GPCR, G-protein–coupled receptor; Gq, heterotrimeric G-protein; GSK3, glycogen synthase kinase 3; iNOS, inducible nitric oxide synthase; IRAG, inositol 1,4,5-trisphosphate receptor I–associated protein; nNOS, neuronal nitric oxide synthase; MAPK, mitogen-activated protein kinase; MEF_2, myocyte enhancer factor 2; MKP-1, mitogen-activated protein kinase phosphatase–1; NFAT, nuclear factor of activated T cells; NO, nitric oxide; PI3Kγ, phosphoinositide 3-kinase γ; PLB, phospholamban; PP1M, myosin phosphatase; RGS2, regulator of G-protein signaling 2; RyR, ryanodine receptor; SERCA, sarcoplasmic/endoplasmic reticulum calcium adenosine triphosphatase; sGC, soluble guanylate cyclase; SR, sarcoplasmic reticulum; TFs, transcription factors. (From Mendelsohn, ME: Viagra: now mending hearts. *Nat Med* 2005;11[2]:115-116.)

Lewis and associates[98] randomly assigned 34 patients with NYHA functional class II or III heart failure (LVEF < 40%) and pulmonary hypertension (mean pulmonary arterial pressure > 25 mm Hg) to receive 12 weeks of treatment with sildenafil or placebo. Sildenafil-treated patients demonstrated a significantly greater increase in $V\text{O}_{2\text{max}}$ and significantly lower resting pulmonary vascular resistance. The remaining resting hemodynamic parameters did not differ significantly between sildenafil- and placebo-treated patients. With exercise, sildenafil-treated patients exhibited a significant decrease in pulmonary vascular resistance and increases in stroke volume and cardiac output in comparison to placebo recipients. Moreover, sildenafil-treated patients demonstrated a significant increase in right ventricular ejection fraction at rest and with exercise but no change in LV size or LVEF. With regard to symptoms, the Minnesota Living with Heart Failure score and the NYHA functional class improved significantly in the sildenafil-treated patients. Rates of adverse events were similar in the two groups except for headaches, which were more frequent in sildenafil-treated patients. Lewis and associates concluded that in patients with systolic heart failure with pulmonary hypertension, prolonged administration of sildenafil safely decreased pulmonary vascular resistance, improved right ventricular function, and, possibly as a result of these occurrences, led to an increase in stroke volume and cardiac output. In addition, sildenafil significantly improved $V\text{O}_{2\text{max}}$.[98] These findings by themselves are very valuable but are also important in the context of safety: Sildenafil can be safely used in patients with heart failure and pulmonary hypertension, in contrast to other pulmonary vasodilators. In contrast, the endothelin antagonist bosentan has been associated with fluid retention and failure to improve symptoms of heart failure,[101] and the prostacyclin analogue epoprostenol has been associated with increased mortality, especially in patients with coronary artery disease.[102]

Researchers in a second trial also evaluated the chronic effect of sildenafil on hemodynamics, as well as exercise dynamics. Guazzi and coworkers[103] randomly assigned 46 male patients with NYHA functional class II or III heart failure (the presence of pulmonary hypertension was not necessary for inclusion) to receive sildenafil or placebo. At 3 and 6 months, the sildenafil-treated patients demonstrated a reduction in systolic pulmonary artery pressure, a reduction in ergoreflex effect on ventilation, an improvement in $V\text{CO}_2$ production slope and $V\text{O}_{2\text{max}}$, and improvements in breathlessness score and flow-mediated vasodilation. The improvement in exercise efficiency was attributed to improved cardiopulmonary hemodynamics and improved sensitivity of the ergoventilatory reflex (a reflex that couples mechanoreceptors or chemoreceptors, or both, in exercising skeletal muscle to the control of ventilation), which, in turn, was possibly a result of improved skeletal muscle perfusion.

The increase in cardiac output with sildenafil treatment has been attributed largely to an improvement in right ventricular function (which results from a decrease in pulmonary artery pressures) and to a decrease in systemic vascular resistance. Several observations support the concept that sildenafil has positive inotropic properties. In patients given inhaled nitric oxide with comparable reductions in the pulmonary vascular resistance, an increase in cardiac output was not noted in comparison to sildenafil.[104] Moreover, Nagendran and associates[105] confirmed a lack of phosphodiesterase type 5 in normal human right ventricular myocardium but were able to demonstrate its presence in hypertrophied right ventricular myocardium. In addition, they were able to show a positive inotropic effect with phosphodiesterase type 5 inhibition in this tissue. The mechanism of positive inotropy remains to be elucidated.

Moreover, novel exciting data suggest that cGMP-dependent protein kinases are involved in the reversal of myocardial hypertrophy and subsequent improvement in ventricular function; thus, phosphodiesterase type 5 inhibitors may have a role in the treatment of ventricular hypertrophy and reverse remodeling. In an animal model of ventricular hypertrophy induced by pressure overload, sildenafil administration prevented the development of ventricular hypertrophy and, in animals with established hypertrophy, reversed the hypertrophy. The postulated mechanisms are improved calcium handling, sildenafil-induced increase in cGMP concentration, and thus increase in cGMP-dependent protein kinase activity, which in turn appears to lead to a decrease in downstream hypertrophy signaling. At the same time, animals treated with sildenafil showed an improvement in ventricular systolic function.[96,106]

These findings are very encouraging and suggest that sildenafil may successfully and safely decrease pulmonary artery pressures in patients with systolic heart failure and improve symptoms and exercise capacity even in patients with heart

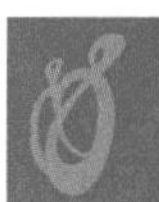

failure but without significant pulmonary hypertension.[103] Larger prospective clinical trials are needed to confirm these findings and to evaluate the benefit of this agent on morbidity and mortality outcomes in patients with systolic heart failure. Moreover, the evidence that sildenafil may reverse hypertrophy suggests that it may have a role in the treatment of diastolic heart failure, as reviewed in detail in Chapter 48.

Inhibitor of I_f Current in Sinoatrial Node (Ivabradine)

Ivabradine is a novel agent that selectively decreases heart rate by altering electrical currents in the sinus node. It is an inhibitor of the I_f current in the sinoatrial node, leading to a decrease in heart rate without affecting blood pressure, contractility, and other aspects of intracardiac conduction.[107-110] The use of ivabradine in patients with coronary artery disease and LV systolic dysfunction is based on the experience that a high heart rate is associated with increased mortality in patients with coronary artery disease and that significant mortality-related benefit is conferred on patients with LV systolic heart failure who are treated with β-blockers.[111,112] Moreover, retrospective analyses of several β-blocker trials in patients with heart failure have demonstrated that heart rate reduction was predictive of survival. This outcome is attributed in part to decreased myocardial oxygen demand with lower heart rates.[113]

In the "morBidity-mortality EvAlUaTion of the I(f) inhibitor ivabradine in patients with coronary disease and left ventricULar dysfunction" (BEAUTIFUL) trial, 10,917 patients with coronary artery disease and LVEF of 40% or lower (≈60% were categorized as NYHA functional class II) were randomly assigned to receive ivabradine or placebo. At 12 months, ivabradine reduced heart rate by 6 beats/minute, in comparison with placebo. However, ivabradine had no effect on the primary endpoint (a composite endpoint of cardiovascular death, hospitalization for acute myocardial infarction, and hospitalization for new-onset or worsening heart failure) or on any of the secondary endpoints (including all-cause mortality and admissions for worsening heart failure). Of note, subgroup analysis did not demonstrate any difference between subjects with NYHA functional classes I and II and those with class III heart failure or in patients with LVEF of 35% or higher versus LVEF lower than 35%. Furthermore, a prespecified subgroup analysis of patients with hearts of 75 bpm or higher did not reveal any significant difference in the primary endpoint; however, it did demonstrate a decrease in hospitalizations for fatal and nonfatal myocardial infarction and coronary revascularization.[114] With regard to heart failure, neutral effects of ivabradine in this trial could potentially be explained by a potential benefit in more symptomatic patients (the majority of patients in the trial had NYHA classes I and II heart failure) and the fact that inherent qualities of β-blockers not necessarily related to heart rate lowering may be responsible for the mortality- and morbidity-related benefits observed with these agents. The SHIFT (Systolic Heart Failure Treatment with the If Inhibitor Ivabradine Trial) trial randomized 6558 patients with NYHA class II-IV heart failure, an LVEF <35%, a resting heart rate >70 bpm, and a heart-failure hospitalization within the previous year to receive either placebo or ivabradine at a starting dose of 5 mg twice daily, with adjustments to a maximum dose of 7.5 mg twice daily to achieve a resting heart rate of 50 to 60 bpm.[114a] All patients were receiving standard heart-failure medications, including include ACE inhibitors or angiotensin-receptor blockers, beta blockers, aldosterone antagonists, and diuretics. The primary endpoint for the trial was a composite of cardiovascular death or hospital admission for worsening heart failure. Over a mean followup of 23 months, patients taking ivabradine showed a significant ($p < 0.001$) reduction in cardiovascular death or hospitalization for worsening heart failure when compared with the control group (HR 0·82, 95% CI 0·75-0·90). The effects were driven primarily by a reduction in hospitalizations for worsening heart failure (21% placebo versus 16% ivabradine; HR 0·74, 0·66-0·83; p <0·0001), whereas the overall impact on cardiovascular death was less robust (5% placebo versus 3% ivabradine; HR 0·74, 0·58-0·94, p = 0·014). Interestingly, the HR for the primary endpoint was 0.93 (95% CI 0.80-1.08) for patients who had a heart rate <77 bpm at baseline, but was 0.75 (95% CI 0.67-0.85) among those with rates of >77 bpm at baseline. The difference between these subgroups was significant statistically (p = 0.029).

Vagal Stimulation

With regard to the autonomic nervous system, an increased sympathetic and a decreased vagal tone has been demonstrated in heart failure. This constellation has been associated with worse long-term outcome in patients with heart failure.[115] Attempts to block the effects of the sympathetic nervous system with the use of β-blockers has resulted in significant morbidity- and mortality-related benefits in patients with heart failure. The focus of research is directed toward the effects of enhancing vagal tone in patients with heart failure.

In animal studies, rats that underwent vagal stimulation demonstrated a significant decrease in LV end-diastolic pressure and an increase in LV contractility in comparison with sham-treated rats. Moreover, vagal stimulation significantly increased survival rates at 140 days.[116] Similarly, Zucker and colleagues[117] studied vagal stimulation in 15 dogs with pacing-induced heart failure: 7 dogs with baroreceptor stimulation were compared to 8 dogs without baroreceptor stimulation. Dogs that underwent baroreceptor stimulation demonstrated significantly improved survival rates and lower plasma norepinephrine levels, with less of an increase in plasma angiotensin II levels. Interestingly, arterial pressure, resting heart rate, and LV pressure were not different between the two groups. The investigators concluded that vagal stimulation led to the suppression of neurohormonal activation, which was associated with improved survival.

In initial human studies, Schwartz and associates[118] evaluated eight patients with heart failure who underwent implantation of a vagal stimulator. At the 6-month follow-up evaluation, improvements in NYHA functional class, quality-of-life score, and LV end-systolic volume were noted. De Ferrari[119] presented the results of vagal stimulation in 32 patients with NYHA functional class II to IV systolic heart failure. At 6 months, patients demonstrated significant increases in LV function, 6-minute walk distance, and quality-of-life score. Vagal stimulation thus appears to be an exciting new avenue in the treatment of heart failure that could be added to the current treatment armamentarium. However, to date, human studies have been small and nonrandomized, and larger, randomized data are necessary in order to definitively assess the efficacy and safety of this treatment strategy.

Testosterone

The heart failure syndrome is a multisystem disorder in which the main abnormality, LV systolic dysfunction, is not always predictive of long-term outcome and functional capacity. One of the factors contributing to decreased functional capacity is the loss of skeletal muscle strength and muscle fatigue.[120] The underlying mechanism of muscle fatigue is probably multifactorial and includes chronic β-adrenergic stimulation, systemic inflammation, reactive oxygen species, and insulin resistance.[120,121]

Testosterone deficiency has also been implicated as a causative factor in muscle fatigue in patients with heart failure, especially in patients with cardiac cachexia.[122] Few small studies in male patients with heart failure demonstrated an improvement in functional capacity with testosterone supplementation.[123,124] In a 2009 study by Caminiti and coworkers,[125] 70 elderly men with NYHA functional class II or III systolic heart failure were randomly assigned to receive 3-month treatment with testosterone or placebo, in addition to standard heart failure therapy. At follow-up, patients receiving testosterone showed a significant increase in $\dot{V}O_{2max}$, improvement in leg muscle strength, improvement in insulin sensitivity, and an increase in baroreceptor sensitivity. Testosterone-treated patients also gained weight and exhibited a significant increase in hematocrit. No significant difference in LV function was noted between the two groups, which suggests that the increase in functional capacity may have resulted from other factors, including improved peripheral muscle strength, improved insulin sensitivity, and increased hematocrit. Interestingly, the beneficial testosterone effects were seen in patients whose baseline testosterone levels were low or normal, but patients with testosterone deficiency showed a more notable response. Several important issues—including the selection of patients and safety issues of long-term treatment—must be resolved before testosterone supplementation becomes an accepted treatment strategy.

NOVEL TREATMENT STRATEGIES FOR HEART FAILURE OF SPECIFIC ETIOLOGIES

Insulin Resistance and Heart Failure (see Chapter 20)

As discussed earlier, cardiac metabolism switches from predominantly FFA to glucose metabolism in the setting of tissue hypoxia/ischemia. However, if insulin resistance is present, an increase in FFA utilization has been observed, leading to a less efficient energy metabolism.[126-128] Moreover, patients with heart failure with diabetes mellitus demonstrate myocardial insulin resistance with reduced myocardial glucose uptake, partly attributed to elevated levels of circulating FFA.[129,130] Furthermore, there is evidence that increased myocardial FFA uptake can lead to lipotoxicity and the development of a cardiomyopathy.[131,132]

Administration of peroxisome proliferator-activated receptor γ (PPARγ) agonists such as thiazolidinediones, which increase glucose and decrease FFA use, has been shown to prevent the development of cardiomyopathy.[133,134] However, the use of thiazolidinediones in patients with heart failure has been limited because they carry a risk of fluid retention and myocardial infarction.[135,136] Several other agents, such as dichloroacetate[137] and etomoxir,[138] that promote glucose metabolism and decrease FFA metabolism have also been shown to protect against the development of cardiomyopathy.

Glucagon-like peptide–1 (GLP-1), an antidiabetic agent, increases postprandial insulin secretion and improves insulin sensitivity. Apart from its effects on glucose metabolism, GLP-1 receptors can be found on vascular smooth muscle cells, cardiomyocytes, and coronary endothelium and smooth muscle, which implies its role in the cardiovascular system.[139] In fact, in vitro studies indicate that GLP-1 has vasodilatory properties,[140] and in human diabetic and nondiabetic subjects, administration of GLP-1 was associated with an improvement in forearm flow–mediated vasodilation.[141] Moreover, results of preliminary animal and human studies suggest that GLP-1 may be involved in myocardial protection during ischemia with a decrease in infarct size and improvement in regional wall motion and global LV function.[142-144]

In chronic heart failure, the administration of GLP-1 has been associated with an improvement in LV function. In a dog model of pacing-induced cardiomyopathy, the administration of GLP-1 resulted in significant increases in LV $\Delta P/\Delta T$ and stroke volume and decreases in LV end-diastolic pressure, heart rate, and systemic vascular resistance.[145] Poornima and colleagues[146] investigated the effected of long-term administration of GLP-1 to spontaneously hypertensive, heart failure–prone rats. Fifty rats were randomly assigned to receive a 3-month infusion of GLP-1 or placebo. Those treated with GLP-1 demonstrated improved survival and preserved LV function in comparison with those given placebo. Moreover, GLP-1 treatment was associated with increased myocardial glucose uptake and decreased myocyte apoptosis.

Several small human studies have also suggested a benefit of GLP-1 in patients with systolic heart failure. In a study of 12 patients with NYHA functional class III or IV heart failure, a continuous infusion of GLP-1 for 12 weeks improved LVEF (by 21% to 27%) and functional capacity, even in patients without diabetes.[147] Similarly, in a study of 10 patients with acute myocardial infarction and LV systolic dysfunction (LVEF < 40%), a 72-hour continuous infusion of GLP-1 produced significant improvements in LVEF and both global and regional wall motion.[144] In a small study of 15 patients with heart failure who received a 48-hour infusion of GLP-1, however, there was no improvement in cardiac index or LVEF, and there was a worrisome small but significant rise in heart rate and diastolic blood pressure.[148]

The underlying mechanisms of the vasodilatory effects, protection against ischemia, and improvement in LV function are unclear. Although the findings in these small studies are for the most part promising, similar results must be reproduced in larger, randomized trials with closer scrutiny of safety and feasibility when GLP-1 is added to already established treatment of heart failure. Moreover, GLP-1 must be given as an infusion and has a very short half-life; therefore, alternative GLP-1 agonists may need to be studied.

Peripartum Cardiomyopathy

Peripartum cardiomyopathy is a rare but potentially lethal condition for which the cause and pathophysiological mechanisms are unknown. Potential mechanisms include inflammatory, autoimmune, and oxidative stress–mediated myocardial changes. Recommended treatment is essentially standard medical therapy for heart failure with attention to safety of the agents during pregnancy and the postpartum period. The use of bromocriptine, a dopamine D_2 receptor agonist, has been investigated in the treatment of peripartum cardiomyopathy. Oxidative stress in the setting of pregnancy or in the postpartum period can lead to the cleavage of the conventional prolactin molecule into a prolactin molecule that appears to have a detrimental effect on the myocardium by promoting apoptosis, vasoconstriction, and inflammation.[149,150] Bromocriptine inhibits the secretion of prolactin; when it was administered in a mouse model of peripartum cardiomyopathy, the development of peripartum cardiomyopathy was prevented.[150] In several human case reports of peripartum cardiomyopathy, treatment with bromocriptine resulted in improvement in clinical status and LV function. However, affected patients were also treated with standard heart failure medications (ACE inhibitors and β-blockers). Thus, improvement may be attributed to natural recovery, treatment with recommended heart failure medications, or treatment with bromocriptine or to a combination of these.[151,152] In a small nonrandomized human study of 12 pregnant patients with a history of peripartum cardiomyopathy during a previous pregnancy, 6 patients were treated with bromocriptine, whereas the remaining 6 patients received standard therapy. All bromocriptine-treated patients had an uneventful pregnancy, delivery, and postpartum period without recurrence of cardiomyopathy. In contrast, all 6 patients receiving the standard therapy developed recurrent peripartum cardiomyopathy, of which 3 patients died.[153] Although development of this treatment approach seems promising, these findings are restricted to small, nonrandomized case series. Moreover, several reports have indicated serious side effects of bromocriptine, including myocardial infarction and the development of a cardiomyopathy.[154,155] Thus, safety issues, patient selection, and dose issues may need to be clarified before embarking on larger prospective, randomized trials of bromocriptine in peripartum cardiomyopathy.

SUMMARY

Current neurohormonal strategies do not completely prevent disease progression in heart failure. Thus, current therapy for heart failure should be viewed as a "work in progress." Although it is not known why heart failure progresses in patients who are receiving optimal therapy with ACE inhibitors and β-blockers, one explanation that has been alluded to in this chapter is that these agents do not directly or sufficiently antagonize all of the biological systems that become activated in the setting of heart failure. Accordingly, one logical direction for future heart failure therapies is the development of therapeutic strategies that more effectively antagonize the neurohormonal systems that are believed to be deleterious. These new neurohormonal treatment strategies will probably be adjunctive to existing clinical strategies for relieving symptoms and preventing disease progression. However, it may not be feasible to antagonize all of the systems that are activated in the setting of heart failure, and such antagonism may even be detrimental, inasmuch as neurohormonal activation is primarily a compensatory mechanism and vital for survival in the acute setting. Accordingly, future therapeutic targets in heart failure will probably need to extend beyond antagonizing neurohormonal systems. Advances in the delivery of gene constructs into the vasculature or the myocardium raise the important possibility that gene-therapeutic approaches may one day be used to attenuate the progression of heart failure. These newer strategies might also be adjunctive to and possibly synergistic with existing therapeutic strategies for treating patients with heart failure.

REFERENCES

1. Goldsmith, S. R. (1999). Vasopressin: a therapeutic target in congestive heart failure? *J Card Fail, 5*, 347–356.
2. Udelson, J. E., Smith, W. B., Hendrix, G. H., et al. (2001). Acute hemodynamic effects of conivaptan, a dual V(1A) and V(2) vasopressin receptor antagonist, in patients with advanced heart failure. *Circulation, 104*, 2417–2423.
3. Gheorghiade, M., Gattis, W. A., O'Connor, C. M., et al. (2004). Effects of tolvaptan, a vasopressin antagonist, in patients hospitalized with worsening heart failure: a randomized controlled trial. *JAMA, 291*, 1963–1971.
4. Gheorghiade, M., Niazi, I., Ouyang, J., et al. (2003). Vasopressin V_2-receptor blockade with tolvaptan in patients with chronic heart failure: results from a double-blind, randomized trial. *Circulation, 107*, 2690–2696.
5. Konstam, M. A., Gheorghiade, M., Burnett, J. C., Jr., et al. (2007). Effects of oral tolvaptan in patients hospitalized for worsening heart failure: the EVEREST Outcome Trial. *JAMA, 297*, 1319–1331.
6. Gheorghiade, M., Konstam, M. A., Burnett, J. C., Jr., et al. (2007). Short-term clinical effects of tolvaptan, an oral vasopressin antagonist, in patients hospitalized for heart failure: the EVEREST Clinical Status Trials. *JAMA, 297*, 1332–1343.
7. McMurray, J. J., Teerlink, J. R., Cotter, G., et al. (2007). Effects of tezosentan on symptoms and clinical outcomes in patients with acute heart failure: the VERITAS randomized controlled trials. *JAMA, 298*, 2009–2019.
8. Modlinger, P. S., & Welch, W. J. (2003). Adenosine A_1 receptor antagonists and the kidney. *Curr Opin Nephrol Hypertens, 12*, 497–502.
9. Gottlieb, S. S. (2001). Renal effects of adenosine A_1-receptor antagonists in congestive heart failure. *Drugs, 61*, 1387–1393.
10. Funaya, H., Kitakaze, M., Node, K., et al. (1997). Plasma adenosine levels increase in patients with chronic heart failure. *Circulation, 95*, 1363–1365.
11. Givertz, M. M., Massie, B. M., Fields, T. K., et al. (2007). The effects of KW-3902, an adenosine A_1-receptor antagonist, on diuresis and renal function in patients with acute decompensated heart failure and renal impairment or diuretic resistance. *J Am Coll Cardiol, 50*, 1551–1560.
12. Dittrich, H. C., Gupta, D. K., Hack, T. C., et al. (2007). The effect of KW-3902, an adenosine A_1 receptor antagonist, on renal function and renal plasma flow in ambulatory patients with heart failure and renal impairment. *J Card Fail, 13*, 609–617.
13. Gottlieb, S. S., Brater, D. C., Thomas, I., et al. (2002). BG9719 (CVT-124), an A_1 adenosine receptor antagonist, protects against the decline in renal function observed with diuretic therapy. *Circulation, 105*, 1348–1353.
14. Greenberg, B., Thomas, I., Banish, D., et al. (2007). Effects of multiple oral doses of an A_1 adenosine antagonist, BG9928, in patients with heart failure: results of a placebo-controlled, dose-escalation study. *J Am Coll Cardiol, 50*, 600–606.
15. Cotter, G., Dittrich, H. C., Weatherley, B. D., et al. (2008). The PROTECT pilot study: a randomized, placebo-controlled, dose-finding study of the adenosine A_1 receptor antagonist rolofylline in patients with acute heart failure and renal impairment. *J Card Fail, 14*, 631–640.
16. Metra, M., O'Connor. C., Massie. B., Cotter. G., et al. The PROTECT Executive Committee: PROTECT Study: Effects of rolofylline in patients with acute heart failure syndrome and renal impairment. Session number 3584-3585, European Society of Cardiology Meeting, September 1, 2009, Barcelona, Spain. http://www.escardio.org/congresses/esc-2009/congress-reports/Pages/708003-708004-metra-jessup.aspx.
17. U.S. National Institutes of Health. *ClinicalTrials.gov* (online register): http://clinicaltrials.gov/. Accessed March 2, 2010.
18. Forssmann, W., Meyer, M., & Forssmann, K. (2001). The renal urodilatin system: clinical implications. *Cardiovasc Res, 51*, 450–462.
19. Carstens, J., Jensen, K. T., & Pedersen, E. B. (1997). Effect of urodilatin infusion on renal haemodynamics, tubular function and vasoactive hormones. *Clin Sci (Lond), 92*, 397–407.
20. Bestle, M. H., Olsen, N. V., Christensen, P., et al. (1999). Cardiovascular, endocrine, and renal effects of urodilatin in normal humans. *Am J Physiol, 276*, R684–R695.
21. Mitrovic, V., Seferovic, P. M., Simeunovic, D., et al. (2006). Haemodynamic and clinical effects of ularitide in decompensated heart failure. *Eur Heart J, 27*, 2823–2832.
22. Felker, G. M., & O'Connor, C. M. (2001). Rational use of inotropic therapy in heart failure. *Curr Cardiol Rep, 3*, 108–113.
23. Packer, M. (1993). The search for the ideal positive inotropic agent. *N Engl J Med, 329*, 201–202.
24. Sorsa, T., Pollesello, P., Rosevear, P. R., et al. (2004). Stereoselective binding of levosimendan to cardiac troponin C causes Ca^{2+}-sensitization. *Eur J Pharmacol, 486*, 1–8.
25. Ajiro, Y., Hagiwara, N., Katsube, Y., et al. (2002). Levosimendan increases *L*-type Ca(2+) current via phosphodiesterase-3 inhibition in human cardiac myocytes. *Eur J Pharmacol, 435*, 27–33.
26. Kopustinskiene, D. M., Pollesello, P., & Saris, N. E. (2004). Potassium-specific effects of levosimendan on heart mitochondria. *Biochem Pharmacol, 68*, 807–812.
27. Slawsky, M. T., Colucci, W. S., Gottlieb, S. S., et al. (2000). Acute hemodynamic and clinical effects of levosimendan in patients with severe heart failure. Study Investigators. *Circulation, 102*, 2222–2227.
28. Packer, Milton, REVIVE II Trial Investigators: REVIVE II: Multicenter Placebo-Controlled Trial of Levosimendan on Clinical Status in Acutely Decompensated Heart failure. Late-Breaking Clinical Trial Abstracts. *Circulation. 112(21):3363, November 22, 2005.*
29. Moiseyev, V. S., Poder, P., Andrejevs, N., et al. (2002). Safety and efficacy of a novel calcium sensitizer, levosimendan, in patients with left ventricular failure due to an acute myocardial infarction. A randomized, placebo-controlled, double-blind study (RUSSLAN). *Eur Heart J, 23*, 1422–1432.
30. Follath, F., Cleland, J. G., Just, H., et al. (2002). Efficacy and safety of intravenous levosimendan compared with dobutamine in severe low-output heart failure (the LIDO study): a randomised double-blind trial. *Lancet, 360*, 196–202.
31. Zairis, M. N., Apostolatos, C., Anastasiadis, P., et al. (2004). The effect of a calcium sensitizer or an inotrope or none in chronic low output decompensated heart failure: results from the Calcium Sensitizer or Inotrope or None in Low Output Heart Failure study (CASINO). *J Am Coll Cardiol, 43*(Suppl. A), 206A.
32. Mebazaa, A., Nieminen, M. S., Packer, M., et al. (2007). Levosimendan vs dobutamine for patients with acute decompensated heart failure: the SURVIVE Randomized Trial. *JAMA, 297*, 1883–1891.
33. Niu, C., Anderson, R., Cox, D., et al. *The cardiac myosin activator, CK-1122534, increases contractility in adult cardiac myocytes without altering the calcium transient* [Abstract 1500]. Paper presented at the 44th Annual Meeting of the American Society of Cell Biology, Washington, DC, December 4–8, 2004.
34. Malik, F., Elias, K. A., Finer, J. T., et al. *Direct activation of cardiac myosin, a novel mechanism for improving cardiac function.* Presented at the National Conference of the HeartFailure Society of America, Boca Raton, FL, 2005.
35. Teerlink, J. R., Malik, F. I., Clarke, C. P., et al. (2006). A. The selective cardiac myosin activator, CK-1827452, increases left ventricular systolic function by increasing ejection time: results of a first in-human study of a unique and novel mechanism [Abstract]. *J Card Fail, 12*(9), 763.
36. Cleland, J. G. F., & Malik, F. I. (2008). The selective cardiac myosin activator, CK-1827452, increases systolic function in heart failure [Abstract 210]. *J Card Fail, 14*(6, Suppl. 1), S67.
37. Sabbah, H. N., Imai, M., Cowart, D., et al. (2007). Hemodynamic properties of a new-generation positive luso-inotropic agent for the acute treatment of advanced heart failure. *Am J Cardiol, 99*, 41A–46A.
38. Gheorghiade, M., Blair, J. E., Filippatos, G. S., et al. (2008). Hemodynamic, echocardiographic, and neurohormonal effects of istaroxime, a novel intravenous inotropic and lusitropic agent: a randomized controlled trial in patients hospitalized with heart failure. *J Am Coll Cardiol, 51*, 2276–2285.
39. Stanley, W. C., Recchia, F. A., & Lopaschuk, G. D. (2005). Myocardial substrate metabolism in the normal and failing heart. *Physiol Rev, 85*, 1093–1129.
40. Heusch, G. (1998). Hibernating myocardium. *Physiol Rev, 78*, 1055–1085.
41. Wolff, A. A., Rotmensch, H. H., Stanley, W. C., et al. (2002). Metabolic approaches to the treatment of ischemic heart disease: the clinicians' perspective. *Heart Fail Rev, 7*, 187–203.

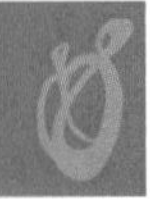

42. Stanley, W. C., Lopaschuk, G. D., Hall, J. L., et al. (1997). Regulation of myocardial carbohydrate metabolism under normal and ischaemic conditions. Potential for pharmacological interventions. *Cardiovasc Res, 33*, 243–257.
43. Katz, A. M. (1998). Is the failing heart energy depleted? *Cardiol Clin, 16*, 633–644.
44. Ashrafian, H., Horowitz, J. D., & Frenneaux, M. P. (2007). *Perhexiline. Cardiovasc Drug Rev, 25*, 76–97.
45. Killalea, S. M., & Krum, H. (2001). Systematic review of the efficacy and safety of perhexiline in the treatment of ischemic heart disease. *Am J Cardiovasc Drugs, 1*, 193–204.
46. Lee, L., Campbell, R., Scheuermann-Freestone, M., et al. (2005). Metabolic modulation with perhexiline in chronic heart failure: a randomized, controlled trial of short-term use of a novel treatment. *Circulation, 112*, 3280–3288.
47. Aussedat, J., Ray, A., Kay, L., et al. (1993). Improvement of long-term preservation of isolated arrested rat heart: beneficial effect of the antiischemic agent trimetazidine. *J Cardiovasc Pharmacol, 21*, 128–135.
48. Fragasso, G., Palloshi, A., Puccetti, P., et al. (2006). A randomized clinical trial of trimetazidine, a partial free fatty acid oxidation inhibitor, in patients with heart failure. *J Am Coll Cardiol, 48*, 992–998.
49. Fraser, H., Belardinelli, L., Wang, L., et al. (2006). Ranolazine decreases diastolic calcium accumulation caused by ATX-II or ischemia in rat hearts. *J Mol Cell Cardiol, 41*, 1031–1038.
50. McCormack, J. G., Barr, R. L., Wolff, A. A., et al. (1996). Ranolazine stimulates glucose oxidation in normoxic, ischemic, and reperfused ischemic rat hearts. *Circulation, 93*, 135–142.
51. Morrow, D. A., Scirica, B. M., Karwatowska-Prokopczuk, E., et al. (2007). Effects of ranolazine on recurrent cardiovascular events in patients with non–ST-elevation acute coronary syndromes: the MERLIN-TIMI 36 randomized trial. *JAMA, 297*, 1775–1783.
52. Sabbah, H. N., Chandler, M. P., Mishima, T., et al. (2002). Ranolazine, a partial fatty acid oxidation (pFOX) inhibitor, improves left ventricular function in dogs with chronic heart failure [Abstract]. *J Card Fail, 8*, 416–422.
53. Rastogi, S., Sharov, V. G., Mishra, S., et al. (2008). Ranolazine combined with enalapril or metoprolol prevents progressive LV dysfunction and remodeling in dogs with moderate heart failure. *Am J Physiol Heart Circ Physiol, 295*, H2149–H2155.
54. Bremer, J. (1983). Carnitine—metabolism and functions. *Physiol Rev, 63*, 1420–1480.
55. Tripp, M. E., Katcher, M. L., Peters, H. A., et al. (1981). Systemic carnitine deficiency presenting as familial endocardial fibroelastosis: a treatable cardiomyopathy. *N Engl J Med, 305*, 385–390.
56. Cherchi, A., Lai, C., Angelino, F., et al. (1985). Effects of l-carnitine on exercise tolerance in chronic stable angina: a multicenter, double-blind, randomized, placebo controlled crossover study. *Int J Clin Pharmacol Ther Toxicol, 23*, 569–572.
57. Anand, I., Chandrashekhan, Y., De, G. F., et al. (1998). Acute and chronic effects of propionyl-l-carnitine on the hemodynamics, exercise capacity, and hormones in patients with congestive heart failure. *Cardiovasc Drugs Ther, 12*, 291–299.
58. Caponnetto, S., Canale, C., Masperone, M. A., et al. (1994). Efficacy of L-propionylcarnitine treatment in patients with left ventricular dysfunction. *Eur Heart J, 15*, 1267–1273.
59. Mancini, M., Rengo, F., Lingetti, M., et al. (1992). Controlled study on the therapeutic efficacy of propionyl-L-carnitine in patients with congestive heart failure. *Arzneimittelforschung, 42*, 1101–1104.
60. Ramasubbu, K., Estep, J., White, D. L., et al. (2008). Experimental and clinical basis for the use of statins in patients with ischemic and nonischemic cardiomyopathy. *J Am Coll Cardiol, 51*, 415–426.
61. Kjekshus, J., Apetrei, E., Barrios, V., et al. (2007). Rosuvastatin in older patients with systolic heart failure. *N Engl J Med, 357*, 2248–2261.
62. Tavazzi, L., Maggioni, A. P., Marchioli, R., et al. (2008). Effect of rosuvastatin in patients with chronic heart failure (the GISSI-HF trial): a randomised, double-blind, placebo-controlled trial. *Lancet, 372*, 1231–1239.
63. Lavie, C. J., Milani, R. V., Mehra, M. R., et al. (2009). Omega-3 polyunsaturated fatty acids and cardiovascular diseases. *J Am Coll Cardiol, 54*, 585–594.
64. Dietary supplementation with n-3 polyunsaturated fatty acids and vitamin E after myocardial infarction: results of the GISSI-Prevenzione trial. Gruppo Italiano per lo Studio della Sopravvivenza nell'Infarto miocardico. (1999). *Lancet, 354*, 447–455.
65. Tavazzi, L., Maggioni, A. P., Marchioli, R., et al. (2008). Effect of n-3 polyunsaturated fatty acids in patients with chronic heart failure (the GISSI-HF trial): a randomised, double-blind, placebo-controlled trial. *Lancet, 372*, 1223–1230.
66. Hajjar, R. J., del Monte, F., Matsui, T., et al. (2000). Prospects for gene therapy for heart failure. *Circ Res, 86*, 616–621.
67. Kirshenbaum, L. A., MacLellan, W. R., Mazur, W., et al. (1993). Highly efficient gene transfer into adult ventricular myocytes by recombinant adenovirus. *J Clin Invest, 92*, 381–387.
68. Svensson, E. C., Marshall, D. J., Woodard, K., et al. (1999). Efficient and stable transduction of cardiomyocytes after intramyocardial injection or intracoronary perfusion with recombinant adeno-associated virus vectors. *Circulation, 99*, 201–205.
69. Bristow, M. R., Ginsburg, R., Minobe, W., et al. (1982). Decreased catecholamine sensitivity and beta-adrenergic-receptor density in failing human hearts. *N Engl J Med, 307*, 205–211.
70. Ungerer, M., Bohm, M., Elce, J. S., et al. (1993). Altered expression of beta-adrenergic receptor kinase and β_1-adrenergic receptors in the failing human heart. *Circulation, 87*, 454–463.
71. Milano, C. A., Allen, L. F., Rockman, H. A., et al. (1994). Enhanced myocardial function in transgenic mice overexpressing the β_2-adrenergic receptor. *Science, 264*, 582–586.
72. Akhter, S. A., Skaer, C. A., Kypson, A. P., et al. (1997). Restoration of beta-adrenergic signaling in failing cardiac ventricular myocytes via adenoviral-mediated gene transfer. *Proc Natl Acad Sci U S A, 94*, 12100–12105.
73. Maurice, J. P., Hata, J. A., Shah, A. S., et al. (1999). Enhancement of cardiac function after adenoviral-mediated in vivo intracoronary β_2-adrenergic receptor gene delivery. *J Clin Invest, 104*, 21–29.
74. Rockman, H. A., Chien, K. R., Choi, D. J., et al. (1998). Expression of a beta-adrenergic receptor kinase 1 inhibitor prevents the development of myocardial failure in gene-targeted mice. *Proc Natl Acad Sci U S A, 95*, 7000–7005.
75. Shah, A. S., White, D. C., Emani, S., et al. (2001). In vivo ventricular gene delivery of a beta-adrenergic receptor kinase inhibitor to the failing heart reverses cardiac dysfunction. *Circulation, 103*, 1311–1316.
76. Engelhardt, S., Hein, L., Wiesmann, F., et al. (1999). Progressive hypertrophy and heart failure in β_1-adrenergic receptor transgenic mice. *Proc Natl Acad Sci U S A, 96*, 7059–7064.
77. Liggett, S. B., Tepe, N. M., Lorenz, J. N., et al. (2000). Early and delayed consequences of beta(2)-adrenergic receptor overexpression in mouse hearts: critical role for expression level. *Circulation, 101*, 1707–1714.
78. Schmidt, U., Hajjar, R. J., Helm, P. A., et al. (1998). Contribution of abnormal sarcoplasmic reticulum ATPase activity to systolic and diastolic dysfunction in human heart failure. *J Mol Cell Cardiol, 30*, 1929–1937.
79. del Monte, F., Harding, S. E., Schmidt, U., et al. (1999). Restoration of contractile function in isolated cardiomyocytes from failing human hearts by gene transfer of SERCA2a. *Circulation, 100*, 2308–2311.
80. Miyamoto, M. I., del Monte, F., Schmidt, U., et al. (2000). Adenoviral gene transfer of SERCA2a improves left-ventricular function in aortic-banded rats in transition to heart failure. *Proc Natl Acad Sci U S A, 97*, 793–798.
81. Hajjar, R. J., Kang, J. X., Gwathmey, J. K., et al. (1997). Physiological effects of adenoviral gene transfer of sarcoplasmic reticulum calcium ATPase in isolated rat myocytes. *Circulation, 95*, 423–429.
82. Schmidt, U., del Monte, F., Miyamoto, M. I., et al. (2000). Restoration of diastolic function in senescent rat hearts through adenoviral gene transfer of sarcoplasmic reticulum Ca(2+)-ATPase. *Circulation, 101*, 790–796.
83. del Monte, F., Williams, E., Lebeche, D., et al. (2001). Improvement in survival and cardiac metabolism after gene transfer of sarcoplasmic reticulum Ca(2+)-ATPase in a rat model of heart failure. *Circulation, 104*, 1424–1429.
84. Koss, K. L., & Kranias, E. G. (1996). Phospholamban: a prominent regulator of myocardial contractility. *Circ Res, 79*, 1059–1063.
85. Hajjar, R. J., Schmidt, U., Kang, J. X., et al. (1997). Adenoviral gene transfer of phospholamban in isolated rat cardiomyocytes. Rescue effects by concomitant gene transfer of sarcoplasmic reticulum Ca(2+)-ATPase. *Circ Res, 81*, 145–153.
86. Hoshijima, M., Ikeda, Y., Iwanaga, Y., et al. (2002). Chronic suppression of heart-failure progression by a pseudophosphorylated mutant of phospholamban via in vivo cardiac rAAV gene delivery. *Nat Med, 8*, 864–871.
87. Most, P., Pleger, S. T., Volkers, M., et al. (2004). Cardiac adenoviral S100A$_1$ gene delivery rescues failing myocardium. *J Clin Invest, 114*, 1550–1563.
88. Olivetti, G., Abbi, R., Quaini, F., et al. (1997). Apoptosis in the failing human heart. *N Engl J Med, 336*, 1131–1141.
89. Haunstetter, A., & Izumo, S. (2000). Toward antiapoptosis as a new treatment modality. *Circ Res, 86*, 371–376.
90. Laugwitz, K. L., Moretti, A., Weig, H. J., et al. (2001). Blocking caspase-activated apoptosis improves contractility in failing myocardium. *Hum Gene Ther, 12*, 2051–2063.
91. Kirshenbaum, L. A., & de Moissac, D. (1997). The *bcl-2* gene product prevents programmed cell death of ventricular myocytes. *Circulation, 96*, 1580–1585.
92. Matsui, T., Li, L., del Monte, F., et al. (1999). Adenoviral gene transfer of activated phosphatidylinositol 3′-kinase and Akt inhibits apoptosis of hypoxic cardiomyocytes in vitro. *Circulation, 100*, 2373–2379.
93. Murry, C. E., Kay, M. A., Bartosek, T., et al. (1996). Muscle differentiation during repair of myocardial necrosis in rats via gene transfer with MyoD. *J Clin Invest, 98*, 2209–2217.
94. Hajjar, R. J., Zsebo, K., Deckelbaum, L., et al. (2008). Design of a phase 1/2 trial of intracoronary administration of AAV1/SERCA2a in patients with heart failure. *J Card Fail, 14*, 355–367.
95. Mendelsohn, M. E. (2005). Viagra: now mending hearts. *Nat Med, 11*, 115–116.
96. Takimoto, E., Champion, H. C., Li, M., et al. (2005). Chronic inhibition of cyclic GMP phosphodiesterase 5A prevents and reverses cardiac hypertrophy. *Nat Med, 11*, 214–222.
97. Cimato, T. R., & Jessup, M. (2002). Recipient selection in cardiac transplantation: contraindications and risk factors for mortality. *J Heart Lung Transplant, 21*, 1161–1173.
98. Lewis, G. D., Shah, R., Shahzad, K., et al. (2007). Sildenafil improves exercise capacity and quality of life in patients with systolic heart failure and secondary pulmonary hypertension. *Circulation, 116*, 1555–1562.
99. Bocchi, E. A., Bacal, F., Auler Júnior, J. O., et al. (1994). Inhaled nitric oxide leading to pulmonary edema in stable severe heart failure. *Am J Cardiol, 74*, 70–72.
100. Bussotti, M., Montorsi, P., Amato, M., et al. (2008). Sildenafil improves the alveolar-capillary function in heart failure patients. *Int J Cardiol, 126*, 68–72.
101. Gottlieb, S. S. (2005). The impact of finally publishing a negative study: new conclusions about endothelin antagonists. *J Card Fail, 11*, 21–22.
102. Califf, R. M., Adams, K. F., McKenna, W. J., et al. (1997). A randomized controlled trial of epoprostenol therapy for severe congestive heart failure: The Flolan International Randomized Survival Trial (FIRST). *Am Heart J, 134*, 44–54.
103. Guazzi, M., Samaja, M., Arena, R., et al. (2007). Long-term use of sildenafil in the therapeutic management of heart failure. *J Am Coll Cardiol, 50*, 2136–2144.
104. Michelakis, E., Tymchak, W., Lien, D., et al. (2002). Oral sildenafil is an effective and specific pulmonary vasodilator in patients with pulmonary arterial hypertension: comparison with inhaled nitric oxide. *Circulation, 105*, 2398–2403.
105. Nagendran, J., Archer, S. L., Soliman, D., et al. (2007). Phosphodiesterase type 5 is highly expressed in the hypertrophied human right ventricle, and acute inhibition of phosphodiesterase type 5 improves contractility. *Circulation, 116*, 238–248.

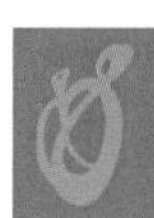

106. Nagayama, T., Hsu, S., Zhang, M., et al. (2009). Sildenafil stops progressive chamber, cellular, and molecular remodeling and improves calcium handling and function in hearts with pre-existing advanced hypertrophy caused by pressure overload. *J Am Coll Cardiol, 53*, 207–215.
107. DiFrancesco, D., & Camm, J. A. (2004). Heart rate lowering by specific and selective I(f) current inhibition with ivabradine: a new therapeutic perspective in cardiovascular disease. *Drugs, 64*, 1757–1765.
108. Joannides, R., Moore, N., Iacob, M., et al. (2006). Comparative effects of ivabradine, a selective heart rate-lowering agent, and propranolol on systemic and cardiac haemodynamics at rest and during exercise. *Br J Clin Pharmacol, 61*, 127–137.
109. Manz, M., Reuter, M., Lauck, G., et al. (2003). A single intravenous dose of ivabradine, a novel I(f) inhibitor, lowers heart rate but does not depress left ventricular function in patients with left ventricular dysfunction. *Cardiology, 100*, 149–155.
110. Camm, A. J., & Lau, C. P. (2003). Electrophysiological effects of a single intravenous administration of ivabradine (S 16257) in adult patients with normal baseline electrophysiology. *Drugs R D, 4*, 83–89.
111. Diaz, A., Bourassa, M. G., Guertin, M. C., et al. (2005). Long-term prognostic value of resting heart rate in patients with suspected or proven coronary artery disease. *Eur Heart J, 26*, 967–974.
112. Kolloch, R., Legler, U. F., Champion, A., et al. (2008). Impact of resting heart rate on outcomes in hypertensive patients with coronary artery disease: findings from the INternational VErapamil-SR/trandolapril STudy (INVEST). *Eur Heart J, 29*, 1327–1334.
113. Fox, K., Borer, J. S., Camm, A. J., et al. (2007). Resting heart rate in cardiovascular disease. *J Am Coll Cardiol, 50*, 823–830.
114. Fox, K., Ford, I., Steg, P. G., et al. (2008). Ivabradine for patients with stable coronary artery disease and left-ventricular systolic dysfunction (BEAUTIFUL): a randomised, double-blind, placebo-controlled trial. *Lancet, 372*, 807–816.
114a. Swedberg, K., Komajda, M., Bohm, M., et al. (2010). Ivabradine and outcomes in chronic heart failure (SHIFT): a randomised, placebo-controlled study. *Lancet Dol: 10*. 1016/S01406736(10)61198–1.
115. Olshansky, B., Sabbah, H. N., Hauptman, P. J., et al. (2008). Parasympathetic nervous system and heart failure: pathophysiology and potential implications for therapy. *Circulation, 118*, 863–871.
116. Li, M., Zheng, C., Sato, T., et al. (2004). Vagal nerve stimulation markedly improves long-term survival after chronic heart failure in rats. *Circulation, 109*, 120–124.
117. Zucker, I. H., Hackley, J. F., Cornish, K. G., et al. (2007). Chronic baroreceptor activation enhances survival in dogs with pacing-induced heart failure. *Hypertension, 50*, 904–910.
118. Schwartz, P. J., De Ferrari, G. M., Sanzo, A., et al. (2008). Long term vagal stimulation in patients with advanced heart failure: first experience in man. *Eur J Heart Fail, 10*, 884–891.
119. De Ferrari, G. M. (2009). *Chronic vagus nerve stimulation: a new treatment modality for congestive heart failure. Presented at the American College of Cardiology Scientific Sessions March 30, 2009*. Orlando, FL: Late Breaking Clinical Trials.
120. Bellinger, A. M., Mongillo, M., & Marks, A. R. (2008). Stressed out: the skeletal muscle ryanodine receptor as a target of stress. *J Clin Invest, 118*, 445–453.
121. Doehner, W., Gathercole, D., Cicoira, M., et al. (2008). Reduced glucose transporter GLUT4 in skeletal muscle predicts insulin resistance in non-diabetic chronic heart failure patients independently of body composition. *Int J Cardiol, 138*, 19–24.
122. Malkin, C. J., Jones, T. H., & Channer, K. S. (2009). Testosterone in chronic heart failure. *Front Horm Res, 37*, 183–196.
123. Pugh, P. J., Jones, R. D., West, J. N., et al. (2004). Testosterone treatment for men with chronic heart failure. *Heart, 90*, 446–447.
124. Malkin, C. J., Pugh, P. J., West, J. N., et al. (2006). Testosterone therapy in men with moderate severity heart failure: a double-blind randomized placebo controlled trial. *Eur Heart J, 27*, 57–64.
125. Caminiti, G., Volterrani, M., Iellamo, F., et al. (2009). Effect of long-acting testosterone treatment on functional exercise capacity, skeletal muscle performance, insulin resistance, and baroreflex sensitivity in elderly patients with chronic heart failure a double-blind, placebo-controlled, randomized study. *J Am Coll Cardiol, 54*, 919–927.
126. Razeghi, P., Young, M. E., Cockrill, T. C., et al. (2002). Downregulation of myocardial myocyte enhancer factor 2C and myocyte enhancer factor 2C–regulated gene expression in diabetic patients with nonischemic heart failure. *Circulation, 106*, 407–411.
127. How, O. J., Aasum, E., Severson, D. L., et al. (2006). Increased myocardial oxygen consumption reduces cardiac efficiency in diabetic mice. *Diabetes, 55*, 466–473.
128. Tuunanen, H., Engblom, E., Naum, A., et al. (2006). Decreased myocardial free fatty acid uptake in patients with idiopathic dilated cardiomyopathy: evidence of relationship with insulin resistance and left ventricular dysfunction. *J Card Fail, 12*, 644–652.
129. Dutka, D. P., Pitt, M., Pagano, D., et al. (2006). Myocardial glucose transport and utilization in patients with type 2 diabetes mellitus, left ventricular dysfunction, and coronary artery disease. *J Am Coll Cardiol, 48*, 2225–2231.
130. Witteles, R. M., & Fowler, M. B. (2008). Insulin-resistant cardiomyopathy clinical evidence, mechanisms, and treatment options. *J Am Coll Cardiol, 51*, 93–102.
131. Yagyu, H., Chen, G., Yokoyama, M., et al. (2003). Lipoprotein lipase (LpL) on the surface of cardiomyocytes increases lipid uptake and produces a cardiomyopathy. *J Clin Invest, 111*, 419–426.
132. Chiu, H. C., Kovacs, A., Blanton, R. M., et al. (2005). Transgenic expression of fatty acid transport protein 1 in the heart causes lipotoxic cardiomyopathy. *Circ Res, 96*, 225–233.
133. Vikramadithyan, R. K., Hirata, K., Yagyu, H., et al. (2005). Peroxisome proliferator–activated receptor agonists modulate heart function in transgenic mice with lipotoxic cardiomyopathy. *J Pharmacol Exp Ther, 313*, 586–593.
134. Hallsten, K., Virtanen, K. A., Lonnqvist, F., et al. (2004). Enhancement of insulin-stimulated myocardial glucose uptake in patients with type 2 diabetes treated with rosiglitazone. *Diabet Med, 21*, 1280–1287.
135. Nesto, R. W., Bell, D., Bonow, R. O., et al. (2004). Thiazolidinedione use, fluid retention, and congestive heart failure: a consensus statement from the American Heart Association and American Diabetes Association. *Diabetes Care, 27*, 256–263.
136. Nissen, S. E., & Wolski, K. (2007). Effect of rosiglitazone on the risk of myocardial infarction and death from cardiovascular causes. *N Engl J Med, 356*, 2457–2471.
137. Nicholl, T. A., Lopaschuk, G. D., & McNeill, J. H. (1991). Effects of free fatty acids and dichloroacetate on isolated working diabetic rat heart. *Am J Physiol, 261*, H1053–H1059.
138. Wall, S. R., & Lopaschuk, G. D. (1989). Glucose oxidation rates in fatty acid–perfused isolated working hearts from diabetic rats. *Biochim Biophys Acta, 1006*, 97–103.
139. Wei, Y., & Mojsov, S. (1996). Distribution of GLP-1 and PACAP receptors in human tissues. *Acta Physiol Scand, 157*, 355–357.
140. Green, B. D., Hand, K. V., Dougan, J. E., et al. (2008). GLP-1 and related peptides cause concentration-dependent relaxation of rat aorta through a pathway involving KATP and cAMP. *Arch Biochem Biophys, 478*, 136–142.
141. Basu, A., Charkoudian, N., Schrage, W., et al. (2007). Beneficial effects of GLP-1 on endothelial function in humans: dampening by glyburide but not by glimepiride. *Am J Physiol Endocrinol Metab, 293*, E1289–E1295.
142. Timmers, L., Henriques, J. P., de Kleijn, D. P., et al. (2009). Exenatide reduces infarct size and improves cardiac function in a porcine model of ischemia and reperfusion injury. *J Am Coll Cardiol, 53*, 501–510.
143. Bose, A. K., Mocanu, M. M., Carr, R. D., et al. (2005). Glucagon like peptide–1 is protective against myocardial ischemia/reperfusion injury when given either as a preconditioning mimetic or at reperfusion in an isolated rat heart model. *Cardiovasc Drugs Ther, 19*, 9–11.
144. Nikolaidis, L. A., Mankad, S., Sokos, G. G., et al. (2004). Effects of glucagon-like peptide–1 in patients with acute myocardial infarction and left ventricular dysfunction after successful reperfusion. *Circulation, 109*, 962–965.
145. Nikolaidis, L. A., Elahi, D., Hentosz, T., et al. (2004). Recombinant glucagon-like peptide–1 increases myocardial glucose uptake and improves left ventricular performance in conscious dogs with pacing-induced dilated cardiomyopathy. *Circulation, 110*, 955–961.
146. Poornima, I., Brown, S. B., Bhashyam, S., et al. (2008). Chronic glucagon-like peptide–1 infusion sustains left ventricular systolic function and prolongs survival in the spontaneously hypertensive, heart failure–prone rat. *Circ Heart Fail, 1*, 153–160.
147. Sokos, G. G., Nikolaidis, L. A., Mankad, S., et al. (2006). Glucagon-like peptide–1 infusion improves left ventricular ejection fraction and functional status in patients with chronic heart failure. *J Card Fail, 12*, 694–699.
148. Halbirk, M., Norelund, H., Moller, N., et al. (2009). Glucagon-like peptide–1 increases blood pressure and heart rate in heart failure patients. *J Am Coll Cardiol, 53*, A155–A156.
149. Tabruyn, S. P., Sorlet, C. M., Rentier-Delrue, F., et al. (2003). The antiangiogenic factor 16K human prolactin induces caspase-dependent apoptosis by a mechanism that requires activation of nuclear factor-κB. *Mol Endocrinol, 17*, 1815–1823.
150. Hilfiker-Kleiner, D., Kaminski, K., Podewski, E., et al. (2007). A cathepsin D-cleaved 16 kDa form of prolactin mediates postpartum cardiomyopathy. *Cell, 128*, 589–600.
151. Hilfiker-Kleiner, D., Meyer, G. P., Schieffer, E., et al. (2007). Recovery from postpartum cardiomyopathy in 2 patients by blocking prolactin release with bromocriptine. *J Am Coll Cardiol, 50*, 2354–2355.
152. Jahns, B. G., Stein, W., Hilfiker-Kleiner, D., et al. (2008). Peripartum cardiomyopathy—a new treatment option by inhibition of prolactin secretion. *Am J Obstet Gynecol, 199*, e5–e6.
153. Hilfiker-Kleiner, D., Schieffer, E., Meyer, G. P., et al. (2008). Postpartum cardiomyopathy. A cardiac emergency for gynecologists, general practitioners, internists, pulmonologists, and cardiologists. *Deutsches Arzteblatt, 105*, 751–756.
154. Hopp, L., Haider, B., & Iffy, L. (1996). Myocardial infarction postpartum in patients taking bromocriptine for the prevention of breast engorgement. *Int J Cardiol, 57*, 227–232.
155. Kaushik, P., Vatsavai, S. R., Banda, V. R., et al. (2004). Acute onset of severe dilated cardiomyopathy during bromocriptine therapy. *Ann Pharmacother, 38*, 1219–1221.

CHAPTER 51

Cell-Based Therapies and Tissue Engineering in Heart Failure

Kai C. Wollert, Kerstin Bethmann, and †Helmut Drexler

THE CONCEPTS OF CELL THERAPY AND TISSUE ENGINEERING

As a result of modern reperfusion strategies and advances in pharmacological management, increasing numbers of patients survive after an acute myocardial infarction (AMI). The loss of viable myocardium is conducive to progressive left ventricular remodeling in many patients (see Chapter 15).[1] The extent of cardiac remodeling after an AMI is closely related to the size of the infarct; with larger infarcts, the extent of left ventricular remodeling is greater, and the prognosis is worse.[2] As a consequence, AMI has become the most common cause of heart failure in many countries.[3] No current therapy, except for cardiac transplantation, addresses the underlying cause of the remodeling process: the critical loss of myocardium in the infarcted area. Cardiac transplantation is, of course, limited by the shortage of donor organs and the side effects associated with long-term immunosuppression.

Researchers have observed that some cardiomyocytes in the infarct border zone may reenter the cell cycle and divide after an AMI.[4] Findings of genetic fate-mapping studies support the notion that endogenous stem cells may be another source of new cardiomyocytes after ischemic injury.[5] Moreover, there is evidence that the injured myocardium attracts circulating stem and progenitor cells that may positively affect the healing response and functional recovery after an AMI, through release of paracrine factors.[6] The overall capacity of the adult heart for regeneration is limited, however, and most necrotic cardiomyocytes are replaced by scar tissue after an AMI. Nonetheless, the existence of endogenous regenerative mechanisms may enable future therapies to mimic and amplify these processes. Two main approaches to achieve myocardial tissue replacement can be envisioned: the use of isolated cells delivered directly to the diseased myocardium (cell therapy) or the use of a combination of cells and biomaterials to generate functional 3-dimensional tissues in vitro before they are implanted into the body (tissue engineering).[7,8] Both strategies would be used to replace, enhance, repair, or regenerate the function of the infarcted heart.

An average infarct in humans destroys approximately 1 to 2 billion cardiomyocytes. Repair strategies consequently aim to replace scarred myocardium with heart muscle consisting of a comparable cell number. Because the heart is composed of 30% cardiomyocytes and 70% nonmyocyte cells (such as endothelial cells, smooth muscle cells, and fibroblasts), cardiac regeneration is a matter not only of cardiac myocyte addition but also of nonmyocyte supplementation.

POTENTIAL DONOR CELLS (see Chapter 4)

Two different types of cells may be used for cell transplantation and tissue engineering: autologous and allogeneic cells. Autologous cells are obtained from the patient and pose no risk of immune rejection. However, the functional activities of autologous cells may be negatively affected by underlying cardiovascular risk factors and disease.[9] Allogeneic cells are obtained from a different donor; therefore, transplantation of most such cells necessitates immunosuppressive therapy to avoid hyperacute and delayed immunological reactions. Mature cells, as well as stem and progenitor cells, have been employed experimentally for cell therapy and tissue engineering. Each cell type has its own profile of advantages, limitations, and practicability issues and may have an effect on cardiac structure or function, or both, through distinct mechanisms (Table 51-1). In general, mature cells show a lower proliferation rate and a diminished survival rate after transplantation than do stem and progenitor cells.[10] Stem cells are capable of self-renewal, transformation into dedicated progenitor cells, and differentiation into specialized progeny. Depending on their differentiation potential, stem cells are classified as being pluripotent (capable of differentiating into any of the three germ layers) or multipotent (capable of giving rise to a limited number of other cell types).

Cardiomyocytes

Cardiomyocytes may appear as the optimal cell type to repair an infarct. Fetal or neonatal cardiomyocytes have been shown in experimental models to form stable grafts in injured hearts of syngeneic recipients. However, massive cell death, coupled with only limited cell proliferation after transplantation, prevents formation of larger amounts of new myocardium.[11,12] Fetal or neonatal rat cardiomyocytes have been used extensively in experimental tissue engineering studies, which demonstrated that these cells can be used to grow cell sheets or 3-dimensional tissue substitutes that display electrical and functional integration when transplanted onto injured myocardium.[7,8] Because of their allogeneic origin, their limited capacity for ex vivo expansion, and ethical concerns, human fetal or neonatal cardiomyocytes are not a realistic cell source for large-scale clinical applications. Nevertheless, the experimental studies in

†Deceased.

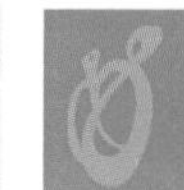

TABLE 51–1 Cell Types Used for Cell Therapy and Tissue Engineering

Cell Type	Advantages	Disadvantages
Fetal or neonatal cardiac myocytes	Integrate electrically and mechanically with host myocardium	Limited supply Ethical and legal issues Need for use in an allogeneic setting Limited capacity for ex vivo expansion Poor survival after transplantation
Skeletal myoblasts	Easy to obtain (skeletal muscle biopsy) Can be expanded ex vivo	Ex vivo expansion requires several-day culturing process Skeletal muscle phenotype retained after intracardiac transplantation
Mesenchymal stem cells	Can be expanded ex vivo Promote paracrine effects Low immunogenicity (can possibly be used in an allogeneic setting)	Ex vivo expansion requires several-day culturing process No transdifferentiation into mature cardiomyocytes
Endothelial progenitor cells	Easy to obtain from blood or bone marrow Promote paracrine effects Some may differentiate into endothelial cells Enhance neovascularization	Transdifferentiation into cardiomyocytes uncertain
Unfractionated bone marrow cells	Easy to obtain (bone marrow puncture) Contain several stem and progenitor cell populations Promote paracrine effects	Low percentage of stem and progenitor cells Probably no meaningful transdifferentiation into cardiomyocytes
Embryonic stem (ES) cells	Pluripotent cells with capacity for differentiation into vascular cells and cardiomyocytes Can be expanded and differentiated into cardiomyocytes ex vivo before transplantation Potentially useful for tissue engineering applications	Ethical and legal issues Need for use in an allogeneic setting Risk of teratoma formation if contaminating pluripotent cells are transplanted
Induced pluripotent stem (iPS) cells	Pluripotent cells with capacity for differentiation into vascular cells and cardiomyocytes Can be expanded and differentiated into cardiomyocytes ex vivo before transplantation Potentially useful for tissue engineering applications Can be used in an autologous setting	Risk of teratoma formation if contaminating pluripotent cells are transplanted Risk of insertional mutagenesis
Spermatogonial stem cells	Pluripotent cells with capacity for differentiation into vascular cells and cardiomyocytes Can be expanded and differentiated into cardiomyocytes ex vivo before transplantation Potentially useful for tissue engineering applications Can be used in an autologous setting	Can be obtained only from men Risk of teratoma formation if contaminating pluripotent cells are transplanted
Cardiac resident progenitor cells	Allegedly multipotent cells with capacity for differentiation into vascular cells and cardiomyocytes Can be expanded ex vivo	Need for better defining of specific cell surface markers and protocols for cell isolation and expansion

this area are informative and have prompted the search for renewable cardiac cell sources for human applications.

Cells with No Apparent Capacity for Cardiomyocyte Differentiation

Skeletal myoblasts (satellite cells) are progenitor cells that normally lie in a quiescent state under the basal membrane of mature muscular fibers. Myoblasts can be isolated from skeletal muscle biopsy samples and expanded in vitro.[12] It was originally hoped that these cells could transdifferentiate into cardiomyocytes; however, myoblasts retain skeletal muscle properties when transplanted into infarcted hearts. Although they may contract in response to electrical stimulation, they do not express intercalated disk proteins, which indicates that the majority are not electromechanically coupled to their host cardiomyocytes. Nevertheless, myoblast transplantation has been shown to augment systolic and diastolic performance in animal models, possibly through the release of paracrine factors.[13] Myoblasts, in combination with embryonic fibroblasts and endothelial cells, have been used to engineer vascularized skeletal muscle tissue in vitro.[14] Because of their inability to couple electromechanically and their strict commitment to a myogenic lineage, myoblasts and myoblast-derived skeletal muscle patches are imperfect substitutes for damaged myocardium. However, genetic manipulation of myoblasts to induce the expression of the cardiac gap-junction protein connexin 43 may provide a means to enhance electromechanical integration of these cells in infarcted hearts.[15]

Mesenchymal stem cells represent a rare population of multipotent progenitor cells present in bone marrow stroma and other mesenchymal tissues. Mesenchymal stem cells can be expanded and induced to differentiate into a variety of mesenchymal cell types in vitro and in vivo.[16] They have been used in preclinical models for tissue engineering of several connective tissues, including bone and cartilage.[17] Along that line of research, mesenchymal stem cells have been used successfully to engineer pulmonary heart valves in sheep.[18] They secrete a large spectrum of bioactive molecules; some of these factors are immunosuppressive, especially for T cells, and allogeneic mesenchymal stem cells may thus be considered for therapeutic use. Because of their trophic activities, mesenchymal stem cells appear to be valuable inducers of endogenous tissue repair and regeneration.[17] When transplanted into freshly infarcted myocardial tissue, mesenchymal stem cells can prevent adverse left ventricular

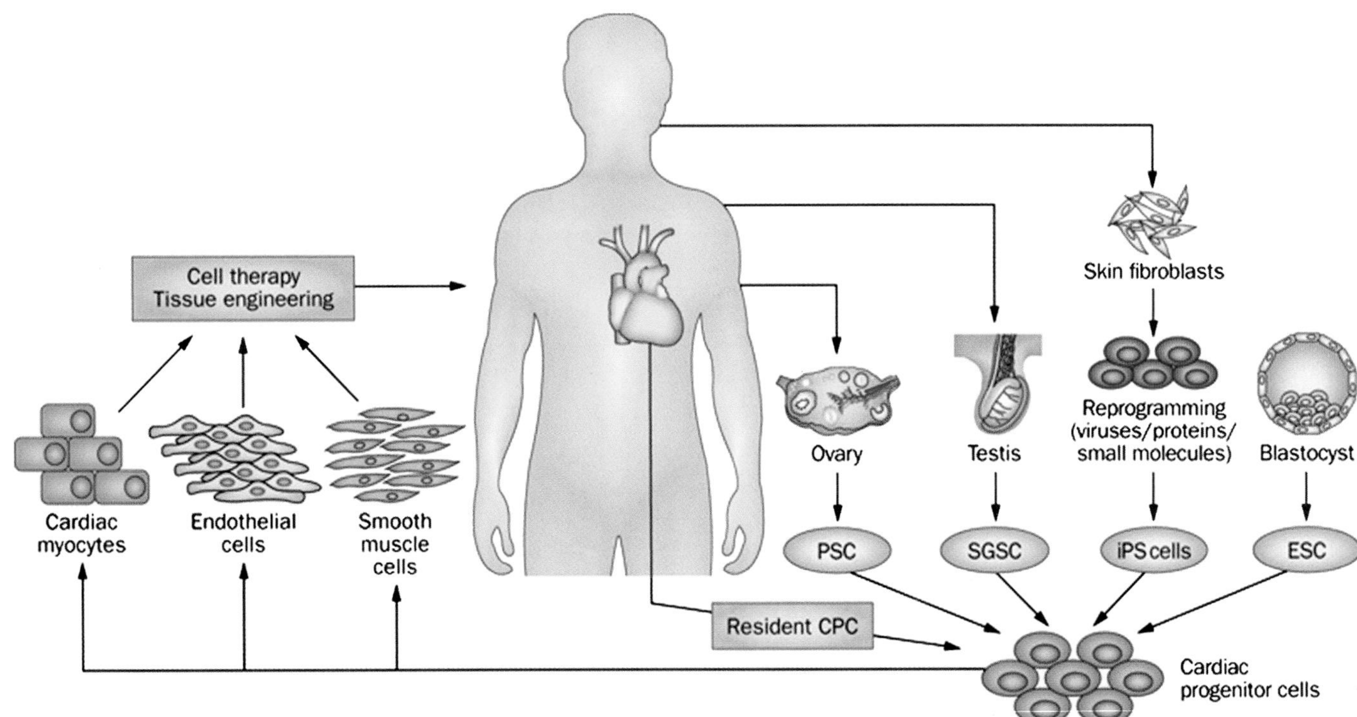

FIGURE 51–1 Pluripotent stem cells from different sources can be expanded in vitro and differentiated into cardiac progenitor cells and mature cardiac cell types, thus enabling cell replacement therapy or tissue engineering. CPC, Cardiac progenitor cell; ESC, embryonic stem cell; iPS cell, induced pluripotent stem cell; PSC, parthenogenetic stem cell; SGSC, spermatogonial stem cell. (From Wollert, K. C. and Drexler, H. C. (2010) Cell therapy for the treatment of coronary heart disease: a critical appraisal. *Nat Rev Cardiol.* 7:204–215.)

remodeling. However, these effects appear to be related to a release of paracrine factors rather than to the differentiation of mesenchymal stem cells into mature cardiomyocytes.[19,20]

Circulating endothelial progenitor cells contribute to recovery of blood flow after ischemia by homing to sites of neovascularization, by differentiating into endothelial cells in situ, or by contributing to the release of vasogenic substances in the underperfused tissue.[21,22] The bone marrow constitutes an important, but not the only, source of circulating endothelial progenitor cells.[23] It is becoming increasingly clear that these cells represent a heterogeneous cell population. The majority of circulating endothelial progenitor cells display no capability for clonal expansion; these cells have also been referred to as "circulating angiogenic cells" and have been shown to promote neovascularization in animal models of critical hind-limb ischemia or AMI.[24] Much smaller subpopulations of endothelial progenitor cells behave as true progenitor cells; they can be clonally expanded and differentiate into mature endothelial cells in situ.[24] It has also been proposed that these cells have the potential to transdifferentiate into cardiomyocytes, even though this may be a rare event.[25,26] Coimplantation of culture-expanded human endothelial progenitor cells and mesenchymal stem cells, seeded into a Matrigel matrix, has been used to engineer microvascular networks in immunodeficient mice in vivo. Because both endothelial progenitor cells and mesenchymal stem cells are readily available from patients, these data suggest a possible future strategy for therapeutic tissue vascularization.[27] Strategies to improve the functionality of endothelial progenitor cells may be required when the cells are isolated from patients with cardiovascular risk factors.[28,29]

Cardiomyocyte Progenitor Cells (see Chapter 4)

Embryonic stem cells are pluripotent stem cells derived from the inner cell mass of blastocysts. Under specific culture conditions, embryonic stem cells can differentiate into cell types from all three germ layers, and they generate, for example, endothelial cells, vascular smooth muscle cells, and cardiomyocytes[30-32]; this makes them an attractive source for cardiac cell therapy and tissue engineering.[33] Human embryonic stem cell–derived cardiomyocytes display structural and functional properties of early-stage cardiomyocytes that couple with host cardiomyocytes when transplanted into normal or infarcted myocardium. The first reports demonstrated their potential to function as biological pacemakers.[34] More recent data have shown that transplantation of sufficient numbers of cardiac-committed murine embryonic stem cells into infarcted sheep myocardium can promote improvements in systolic function.[35] In theory, infinite numbers of cardiomyocytes could be obtained from human embryonic stem cell clones. However, unresolved ethical and legal issues, concerns about the tumorigenicity of residual embryonic stem cells in embryonic stem cell–derived cardiomyocyte preparations, and the need to use allogeneic cells for transplantation currently hamper their use in clinical studies. It is important to refine cell differentiation and isolation protocols that yield highly purified cell populations for transplantation. This could best be achieved by cell sorting by means of cell type–specific membrane markers; alternative approaches might include genetic methods involving cell type–specific promoter constructs that drive the expression of marker proteins or selected survival by antibiotic resistance.[10]

It has been shown that adult human fibroblasts can be reprogrammed to a pluripotent state by retroviral transduction of four transcription factors (a combination of OCT4, SOX2, KLF4, and Myc, or a combination of OCT4, SOX2, NANOG, and LIN28).[36,37] By genetic and developmental criteria, these induced pluripotent stem (iPS) cells are very similar to embryonic stem cells: They can be maintained in culture for several months and can be induced to differentiate into derivatives of all three germ layers. It has been shown that iPS cells have the potential to differentiate into functional cardiomyocytes, with a gene expression profile and electrophysiological properties that are similar to those of embryonic stem cell–derived cardiomyocytes.[38] In the future, iPS cells may allow derivation of autologous cardiomyocytes and vascular cells for myocardial cell therapy and tissue engineering (Figure 51-1). Safety issues such as the risks of teratoma formation or insertional activation of proto-oncogenes after retroviral transduction must be addressed, and strategies to create "virus-free" iPS are currently being developed in several laboratories.

The pluripotency of mouse spermatogonial stem cells has been highlighted in several studies. These cells are responsible for maintaining spermatogenesis throughout life in the male mouse.[39,40] In culture, adult spermatogonial stem cells acquire embryonic stem cell properties. These pluripotent adult germline stem cells spontaneously differentiate into derivatives of the three embryonic germ layers in vitro, including cardiomyocytes and vascular cells. It is conceivable that establishment of human multipotent adult germline stem cells from testicular biopsy samples may enable autologous cell–based therapies without the ethical and immunological problems associated with human embryonic stem cells or the risk of proto-oncogene activation inherent in iPS cells.

Distinct cell populations expressing stem cell marker proteins have been identified in the adult mouse heart and the human heart.[41] In humans, a heterogeneous cell population has been isolated from atrial and ventricular biopsy samples that forms clonal multicellular clusters in suspension culture, which have been referred to as "cardiospheres."[42] Cardiospheres consist of c-Kit–positive cells at the core and cells that express cardiac and endothelial cell markers at the periphery. Injection of culture-expanded, cardiosphere-derived cells into the myocardial infarct border zone reportedly improves systolic function in immunodeficient mice; of note is that this effect was associated with cardiosphere-derived cell differentiation into cardiomyocytes and endothelial cells.[43] If this finding is confirmed, cardiac resident progenitor cells hold great promise for clinical applications, because they may be a source of autologous cells with cardiac differentiation potential.

CELL TRANSPLANTATION STRATEGIES

The goal of any cell delivery strategy is to transplant sufficient numbers of cells into the myocardial region of interest and to achieve maximum retention of cells within that area (Table 51-2). Cell retention may be defined as the fraction of transplanted cells retained in the myocardium for a short time. The local milieu is an important determinant of cell retention, because it influences short-term cell survival and, if a transvascular approach is used, cell adhesion, transmigration through the vascular wall, and tissue invasion. Transvascular strategies are especially suited for the treatment of recently infarcted and reperfused myocardium when chemoattractants are highly expressed.[44,45] Selective intracoronary application delivers cells homogeneously to the site of tissue injury. In certain studies, unselected bone marrow cells were delivered through the central lumen of an over-the-wire balloon catheter during transient balloon inflations to maximize the contact time of the cells with the microcirculation of the infarct-related artery.[46,47] As shown in Figure 51-2, when 2-[fluorine-18]-fluoro-2-deoxy-D-glucose (^{18}FDG) -labeled unselected bone marrow cells were infused into the infarct-related artery, approximately 3% of the cells were detected in the infarcted myocardium. In experimental models, intravenous delivery of endothelial progenitor cells and mesenchymal stem cells has been shown to improve cardiac function after AMI. However, cell homing to noncardiac organs limits the applicability of this approach. Indeed, in one clinical study, homing of unselected bone marrow cells to the infarcted region was observed only after intracoronary stop-flow delivery but not after intravenous infusion.[47] Direct-injection techniques may be more appropriate for patients who present late in the disease process, when an occluded coronary artery precludes transvascular cell delivery or when homing signals are expressed at low levels in the heart (scar tissue).

CURRENT STATUS OF CELL THERAPY IN PATIENTS WITH ACUTE MYOCARDIAL INFARCTION AND HEART FAILURE

Preclinical studies have demonstrated that transplantation of bone marrow–derived hematopoietic stem cells, endothelial progenitor cells, or mesenchymal stem cells can promote functional improvements in animal models of AMI. Transdifferentiation of the transplanted cells into cardiomyocytes and endothelial cells has been offered as an explanation for these improvements,[48,49] but the quantitative importance of stable cell engraftment and transdifferentiation for the functional effects has been challenged. It is now believed that the reported improvements in these models are mediated predominantly by paracrine effects (Figure 51-3).[6,19,50-53] Clinicians welcomed these animal studies with great enthusiasm, and, fairly rapidly, clinical trials were designed to translate

TABLE 51–2 Cell Delivery Strategies

Route of Cell Delivery	Advantages	Disadvantages
Intravenous infusion	Least invasive	Cell trapping in the lungs and other tissues Limited cell delivery to the heart
Intracoronary infusion	Homogeneous cell delivery to the site of injury Cells that are retained will have adequate blood supply	Open infarct-related artery required Limited cell retention in infarcted area Not suitable for delivery of large cells that may cause microembolization (e.g., skeletal myoblasts, mesenchymal stem cells)
Transendocardial injection	Electromechanical mapping of the endocardial surface can be used to delineate viable, ischemic, and scarred myocardium before cell injections	Creates islands of cells with limited blood supply and poor cell survival May not be safe in patients with acute myocardial infarction, when cells are injected in friable necrotic tissue
Transepicardial injection	Allows for direct visualization of the myocardium and a targeted application of cells to scarred areas, the border zone of an infarct, or both	Creates islands of cells with limited blood supply and poor survival Open-heart surgery required Invasiveness hampers its use as a stand-alone therapy or in the setting of an acute myocardial infarction

those finding into information for the clinical scenario of post-AMI patients.

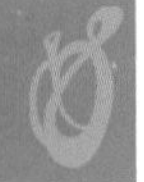

Randomized Trials with Unselected Bone Marrow Cells

Most clinical investigators have chosen a pragmatic approach by using unfractionated bone marrow cells, which contain different stem and progenitor cell populations, as well as more differentiated hematopoietic cell types. In all of these studies, after the infarct-related artery was reperfused and a stent was placed, the cells were delivered into the artery in a stop-flow balloon catheter approach. In six trials, cells were delivered within a few days after coronary reperfusion to enhance systolic function and prevent adverse remodeling; in one trial, bone marrow cells were transplanted in patients with ischemic heart failure, months and years after AMI (Table 51-3).[54-60] The combined experience from these studies indicates that intracoronary delivery of unselected bone marrow cells is feasible and probably safe. The outcomes of these randomized trials have been mixed, however: Some studies have demonstrated significant improvements in global and regional left ventricular systolic function[54-56,59,60]; one trial demonstrated improvements in regional function only[57]; and one trial demonstrated no significant improvements at all.[58] Although the reasons for these heterogeneous results are difficult to resolve, it has been argued that differences in cell preparation methods and the timing of cell transfer may have been critical.[55,57,58,61] Meta-analyses of published randomized and nonrandomized studies, involving a total of approximately 1000 patients, support the notion that bone marrow cell transfer contributes to modest improvements in cardiac function after AMI, above and beyond current interventional and medical therapy.[62-65]

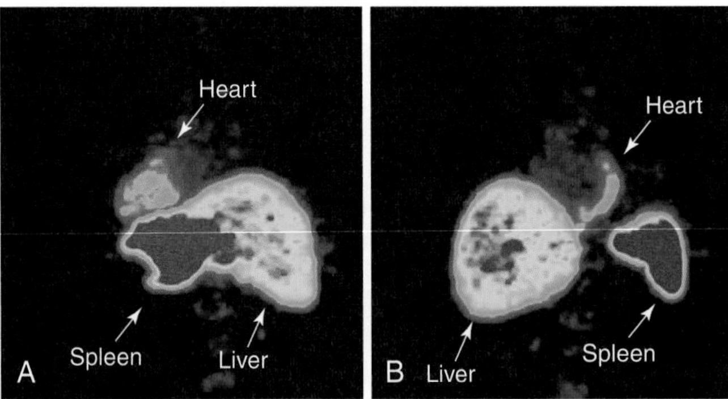

FIGURE 51–2 Myocardial homing and biodistribution of unfractionated bone marrow cells after intracoronary infusion. Nine days after primary angioplasty and stent implantation for acute myocardial infarction, the patient received an intracoronary infusion of autologous nucleated bone marrow cells into the left circumflex coronary artery, which had the stent. A small fraction of the cells was radiolabeled with 2-[fluorine-18]-fluoro-2-deoxy-D-glucose (^{18}FDG) just before intracoronary transfer. Positron emission tomography (PET) imaging was performed 65 minutes after cell transfer. Left posterior oblique (**A**) and left anterior oblique (**B**) PET views of the chest and upper abdomen are shown. Approximately 3% of the cells homed to the lateral wall of the heart; most remaining activity is detected in the liver and spleen. (Adapted from Hofmann M, Wollert KC, Meyer GP, et al. Monitoring of bone marrow cell homing into the infarcted human myocardium. *Circulation* 2005;111:2198-2202.)

Ongoing Clinical Trials in Patients with Coronary Heart Disease

On the basis of the favorable safety profile and promising efficacy data, several clinical trials are currently underway to further explore the prospect of cell therapy in patients with various manifestations of coronary heart disease. As discussed below, important issues are addressed in these second-generation trials in an attempt to maximize patient benefit (Table 51-4). Given the variation in outcomes with apparently similar cell isolation protocols in earlier trials it will be important to establish assays that assess cell functionality and the quality of the cell product.

Skeletal Myoblast Transplantation

In the first randomized, placebo-controlled study of skeletal myoblast transplantation after myocardial infarction,[66] patients were treated with culture-expanded, autologous skeletal myoblasts or with placebo at least 4 weeks after myocardial infarction. Cells were injected into the infarct border zone during bypass surgery. Myoblast transplantation did not improve regional or global left ventricular function, the primary endpoints of the trial. A significant decrease in left ventricular volumes, however, was noted after cell therapy. A greater incidence of arrhythmias was noted in the myoblast-treated patients, but this did not translate into differences in major adverse cardiac events after 6 months.

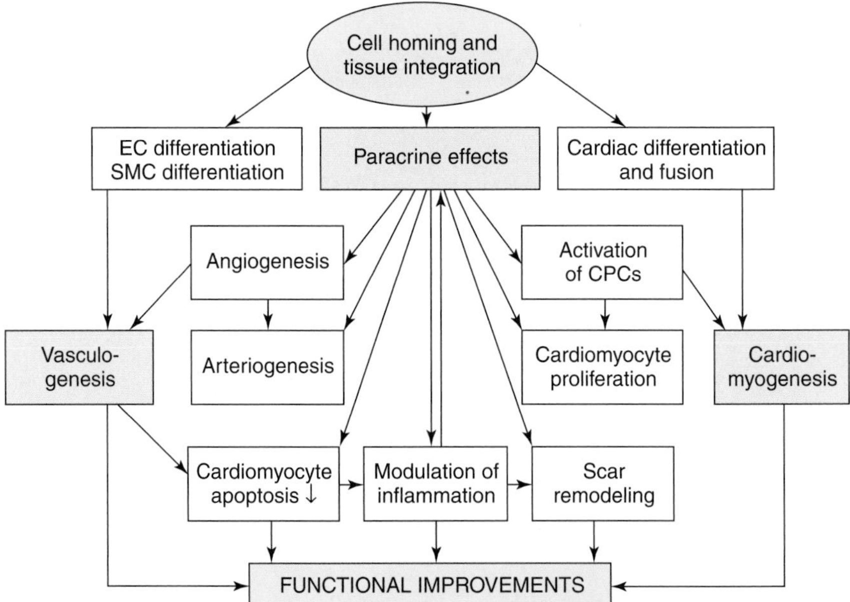

FIGURE 51–3 Proposed mechanisms of cell therapy after acute myocardial infarction. The relative contributions, for example, of paracrine effects versus differentiation events depend on the transplanted cell types and on the microenvironment of the host tissue. CPC, resident cardiac progenitor cell; EC, endothelial cell; SMC, smooth muscle cell. (Adapted from Dimmeler S, Burchfield J, Zeiher AM. Cell-based therapy of myocardial infarction. *Arterioscler Thromb Vasc Biol* 2008;28:208-216.)

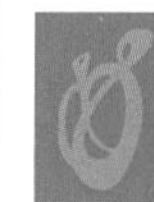

TABLE 51–3 Randomized Cell Therapy Trials in Patients with Acute Myocardial Infarction and Ischemic Heart Failure

Study	Design	Number of Subjects*	Cell Type	Dosage	Time of Cell Delivery (after AMI)	Outcome Improved	Outcome No Change
BOne marrOw transfer to enhance ST-elevation infarct regeneration (BOOST)[54]	Open, controlled	30 Treated, 30 controls	Nucleated BMCs	128 mL	6 ± 1 Days	Global LVEF	LVEDV
Reinfusion of Enriched Progenitor cells And Infarct Remodeling in Acute Myocardial Infarction study (REPAIR-AMI)[55]	Placebo-controlled	95 Treated, 92 controls	Mononucleated BMCs	50 mL	3-6 Days	Global LVEF	LVEDV
Leuven Acute Myocardial Infarction trial (Leuven-AMI)[57]	Placebo-controlled	32 Treated, 34 controls	Mononucleated BMCs	130 mL	1 Day	Regional contractility	Global LVEF LVEDV
Autologous Stem cell Transplantation in Acute Myocardial Infarction (ASTAMI)[58]	Open, controlled	47 Treated, 50 controls	Lymphocytic BMCs	50 mL	6 ± 1 Days	—	Global LVEF LVEDV
FINnish stem CELL study (FINCELL)[59]	Placebo-controlled	39 Treated, 38 controls	Mononucleated BMCs	80 mL	≈3 Days	Global LVEF	LVESV, LVEDV
Myocardial Regeneration by Intracoronary Infusion of Selected Population of Stem Cells in Acute Myocardial Infarction (REGENT)[60]	Open, controlled	97 Treated, 20 controls	Mononucleated BMCs vs. $CD34^+$/ $CXCR4^+$ BMCs	50-120 mL	3-12 Days	Global LVEF	LVESV, LVEDV
Transplantation Of Progenitor Cells And REcovery of LV functioning in patients with Chronic ishemic Heart Disease (TOPCARE-CHD)[56]	Open, controlled	35 Treated, 23 controls	Mononucleated BMCs	50 mL	81 ± 72 Months	Global LVEF	LVEDV
Myoblast Autologous Grafting in Ischemic Cardiomyopathy (MAGIC)[66]	Placebo-controlled	67 Treated, 30 controls	Skeletal myoblasts	400 or 800×10^6	>4 Weeks	LVEDV, LVESV	Regional contractility Global LVEF

*Only patients with complete imaging studies are considered in this table.

In BOOST, cells were prepared by gelatin polysuccinate density gradient sedimentation, which retrieves all nucleated cell types from the bone marrow; REPAIR-AMI, TOPCARE-CHD, and Leuven-AMI employed a Ficoll gradient, which recovers the mononuclear cell fraction. Although a similar cell isolation protocol was used in ASTAMI, the cell yield was lower than that in REPAIR-AMI. "Dosage" refers to the average amount of bone marrow that was harvested, or the number of transplanted skeletal myoblasts (MAGIC). Remodeling was assessed by MRI in Leuven-AMI, BOOST, and ASTAMI; by left ventricular angiography in REPAIR-AMI and TOPCARE-CHD; and by echocardiography in MAGIC.

AMI, acute myocardial infarction; BMC, bone marrow cell; LVEDV, left ventricular end-diastolic volume; LVEF, left ventricular ejection fraction; LVESV, left ventricular end-systolic volume; MRI, magnetic resonance imaging.

Issues to Address at the Bench and the Bedside

The mixed results from the randomized studies of bone marrow cells are a reminder that procedural issues, such as the cell preparation method, cell dosage, and timing of cell transfer, must be further refined in upcoming studies. Different cell populations and cell delivery methods may be necessary to achieve optimum therapeutic effects immediately or later after AMI. Patient subgroups that derive the greatest benefit from cell transfer need to be identified prospectively (e.g., patients presenting late after symptom onset, in whom little myocardial salvage can be expected from reperfusion therapy). The effect of bone marrow cell transfer on clinical endpoints is currently unknown. Significant improvements in combined clinical endpoints have been observed in the largest randomized trial,[67] in one cohort study,[68] and in some of the meta-analyses[63,65]; however, outcome trials in which cell preparation and delivery strategies are optimized are still needed. Results of cell-labeling studies indicate that less than 5% of unselected nucleated bone marrow cells are retained in the infarcted area after intracoronary delivery in patients (see Figure 51-2).[47] It is conceivable that pharmacological strategies might be used to enhance the homing capacity or other functional parameters of the cells; results of experimental studies are pointing in this direction.[28,29] The ultimate goal of stem cell therapy is to replace the infarcted area with new contractile and fully integrated cardiomyocytes. Although unselected bone marrow cells may have a favorable effect on systolic function, they probably do not generate new myocardium. There is evidence that paracrine effects play an important role in bone marrow cell transfer. In fact, bone marrow cells have been shown to secrete a number of proangiogenic factors,[69] which is consistent with the improvements in microvascular function observed after bone marrow cell transfer in patients.[70] Results of experimental studies suggest that enhanced angiogenesis after AMI may improve infarct healing and energy metabolism in the infarct border zone.[71-74] Further investigation of candidate factors in animal models may ultimately enable more specific and powerful therapeutic strategies after AMI.[75] The lack of true cardiac regeneration should stimulate further basic research into the therapeutic prospects of cardiomyocyte progenitor cells.

TISSUE ENGINEERING

A myocardial infarct represents a hostile ischemic, necrotic, or scarred environment, or a combination. As a consequence, cell transplantation is generally accompanied by extensive cell death and inadequate cellular integration. Cell transplantation may positively affect the healing response after an AMI (e.g., through paracrine effects); however, it is doubtful whether cell therapy will ever be able to replace a chronic infarct scar with new myocardium that is densely packed with mature cardiomyocytes, supporting blood vessels, interstitial cells, and matrix. Engineering of myocardial tissue may provide a means to achieve true cardiac regeneration. Tissue engineering aims at generating functional 3-dimensional tissues substitutes outside the body that can be tailored in size, shape, and function before they are implanted into the body. Tissue engineering is a highly interdisciplinary field and requires close collaboration among material scientists, engineers, and life scientists. Tissue engineering has been used to

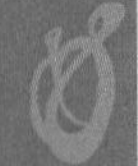

TABLE 51-4 Ongoing Cell Therapy Trials in Patients with Coronary Heart Disease

Study Identifier	Trial Name	Number of Patients	Cells	Primary End Point	Route of Cell Delivery
Non-ST-elevation Acute Coronary Syndrome					
Clinical trial NCT00711542	REPAIR-ACS	100	Bone marrow-derived progenitor cells	Coronary flow reserve	Intracoronary
Acute Myocardial Infarction					
Controlled trial ISRCTN17457407	BOOST-2	200	Bone marrow cells Low versus high cell number Nonirradiated versus irradiated cells	LVEF	Intracoronary
Clinical trial NCT00355186	SWISS-AMI	150	Bone marrow-derived stem cells	LVEF	Intracoronary Day 5–7 versus day 21–28
Clinical trial NCT00684021	TIME	120	Bone marrow mononuclear cells	LVEF	Intracoronary Day 3 versus day 7 post AMI
Clinical trial NCT00684060	Late TIME	87	Bone marrow mononuclear cells	LVEF	Intracoronary 2–3 weeks post AMI
Clinical trial NCT00501917	MAGIC Cell-5	116	Peripheral blood stem cells mobilized with G-CSF versus G-CSF with darbepoetin	LVEF	Intracoronary
Clinical trial NCT00877903	–	220	Allogeneic mesenchymal stem cells	LVESV	Intravenous
Clinical trial NCT00677222	–	28	Allogeneic mesenchymal stem cells	Safety	Perivascular
Ischemic Heart Failure					
Clinical trial NCT00526253	MARVEL	390	Skeletal myoblasts	6 min walk test, QOL, LVEF	Transendocardial
Clinical trial NCT00824005	FOCUS	87	Bone marrow mononuclear cells	MVO_2, LVESV, ischemic area	Transendocardial
Clinical trial NCT00747708	REGENERA-TEIHD	165	G-CSF-stimulated bone marrow-derived stem/progenitor cells	LVEF	Transendocardial versus intracoronary
Clinical trial NCT00326989	Cellwave	100	Bone marrow mononuclear cells	LVEF	Extracorporal shock wave, then intracoronary cell therapy
Clinical trial NCT00285454	–	60	Bone marrow mononuclear cells	Safety, perfusion Systolic function	Retrograde coronary venous delivery
Clinical trial NCT00462774	Cardio133	60	CD133[1] bone marrow cells	LVEF	Transepicardial during CABG
Clinical trial NCT00810238	C-Cure	240	Bone marrow-derived cardiopoietic cells	LVEF	Transendocardial
Clinical trial NCT00768066	TAC-HFT	60	Bone marrow cells versus mesenchymal stem cells	Safety	Transendocardial
Clinical trial NCT00644410	–	60	Mesenchymal stem cells	LVEF	Transendocardial
Clinical trial NCT00587990	PRO-METHEUS	45	Mesenchymal stem cells	Safety	Transepicardial during CABG
Clinical trial NCT00721045	–	60	Allogeneic mesenchymal precursor cells	Safety	Transendocardial
Clinical trial NCT00474461	–	40	Cardiac stem cells harvested from right atrial appendage	Safety	Intracoronary

Unless otherwise stated, autologous cell sources are used. AMI, Acute myocardial infarction; CABG, coronary artery bypass grafting; G-CSF, granulocyte colony-stimulating factor; LVEF, left ventricular ejection fraction; LVESV, left ventricular end-systolic volume; MVO_2, maximal oxygen consumption; QOL, quality of life.
(From Wollert, K. C. and Drexler, H. C. (2010). Cell therapy for the treatment of coronary heart disease: a critical appraisal. *Nat Rev Cardiol.* 7:204-215.)

generate heart valves[76] and has already led to initial clinical applications, with encouraging results.[77,78] Similarly, vascular grafts have been generated from autologous cells and have been transplanted successfully into patients.[79]

Basic Principles of Myocardial Tissue Engineering

Myocardial tissue engineering is confronting scientists with tremendous challenges because restoration of heart function by myocardial tissue replacement necessitates the long-term electromechanical and vascular integration of a complex, multicellular, 3-dimensional graft into the host tissue. Tissue-engineered myocardial constructs should have clearly defined contractile properties, be large in size, become vascularized and integrated into the host myocardium, and improve the contractile function of the infarcted heart.[80] The classical approach to tissue engineering consists in the construction of a scaffold on which the tissue can grow. Such scaffolds, which are biodegradable to a degree, are then seeded with donor cells, growth factors, or both. Afterwards, the scaffolds

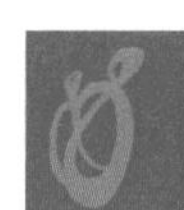

are cultured in a specially designed bioreactor that provides oxygen and nutrients in an optimized physicochemical microenvironment. When the cells have assembled and filled the scaffold, the structure is removed from the bioreactor and implanted into the patient's body (Figure 51-4). Scaffolding biomaterials used for cardiac tissue engineering should be autologous and should enhance cell attachment, growth, and differentiation. To achieve functional improvements, the biomaterial must encourage mechanical and electrical integration with the host tissue. Finally, the elastic properties of the biomaterial must match the elastic properties of the native heart to withstand the continuous stretching-relaxing motion of the myocardium that occurs with each heartbeat (Table 51-5).[81] A detailed discussion of synthetic and biological materials used in myocardial tissue engineering is available elsewhere.[82]

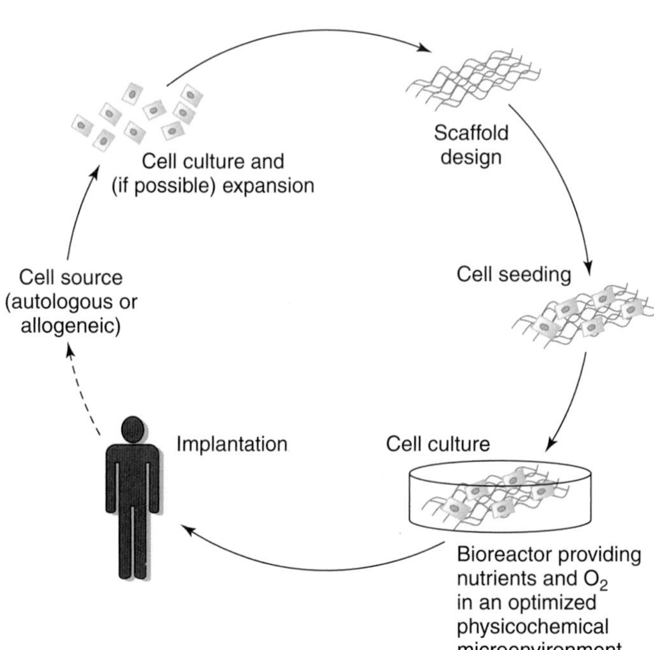

FIGURE 51–4 Basic principles of tissue engineering. See the "Basic Principles of Myocardial Tissue Engineering" section in the text for details.

TABLE 51–5 Requirements for Cardiac Tissue Engineering Scaffolds

Requirement	Comment
Biocompatibility	The biomaterial must not be rejected or induce an inflammatory response in vivo; it should reflect the extracellular matrix of the tissue it intends to replace. The degradation rate of the biomaterial should match the regeneration rate of the host tissue, and the degradation by-products must be nontoxic and readily removed from the body. The biomaterial should enhance cell adhesion, alignment, survival, and differentiation, and it should encourage vascularization.
Mechanical integrity	The biomaterial should provide mechanical support to withstand the continuous stretching-relaxing motion of the myocardium.
Electrical integrity	The biomaterial must enable electrical integration of the engineered graft with the native tissue to allow matched excitability of host and grafted tissue and support electrical of wavefront propagation.

Adapted from Jawad H, Lyon AR, Harding SE, et al. Myocardial tissue engineering. *Br Med Bull* 2008;87:31-47.

Preclinical Experience with Myocardial Tissue Engineering

At least three strategies have been developed to construct contractile heart muscle equivalents: (1) the classic approach of seeding cardiac myocytes on preformed matrices; (2) entrapment in liquid matrices, which supports the propensity of cardiac myocytes to form contracting aggregates; and (3) stacking cardiac myocyte monolayers to form multilayered heart muscle constructs (Figure 51-5 and Table 51-6).[83]

Development of systolic force is the most important feature of artificial myocardium. Data on contractile properties are available for artificial myocardial tissue, which is developed by seeding neonatal rat cardiac myocytes on collagen sponges[84]; for engineered heart tissue, which forms after entrapment of neonatal rat heart cells in an extracellular matrix environment that contains liquid rat collagen type I[85]; and stacked neonatal rat cardiac myocyte monolayers (see Table 51-6).[86] Maximal force of contraction was 0.02 mN in artificial myocardial tissue and 2 to 4 mN in engineered heart tissue and stacked monolayers. The low contractile force in artificial myocardial tissue points to a possible conceptual disadvantage of preformed matrices in myocardial tissue engineering. Essentially, cardiac myocytes are forced to seed a structurally defined environment if preformed matrices are employed, and they seem to be limited in their potential to organize into 3-dimensional force-generating units.[83] In native myocardial tissue, cells are especially dense in comparison with other tissues, such as heart valves and vessels. In addition, cardiomyocytes are tightly interconnected with gap junctions. Preformed scaffolds may therefore attenuate cell-to-cell connections.[87] Current methods support the propensity of cardiac myocytes to freely form contractile aggregates, to produce their own supporting matrix, and to organize into complex myocardial structures in the absence of obstructing preformed scaffold materials; these methods seem to be advantageous from a functional but also structural point of view.[83]

CHALLENGES AND FUTURE DIRECTIONS

The thickness of cardiac tissue that can be engineered in vitro is limited by the maximum diffusion distances for oxygen and nutrients. Angiogenesis becomes essential in order to engineer cardiomyocyte tissue with a thickness of more than 200 μm.[88] Generation of vascularized grafts is especially important for making the transition from rodent models to larger animal models and, eventually, to patients with an average left ventricular wall thickness of 10 to 15 mm. A number of strategies are currently being explored to create a functioning vascular network inside an engineered myocardial graft before implantation. Prevascularized grafts can rapidly anastomose with the host tissue and enhance tissue survival and differentiation. In addition, growing evidence supports a role of the vasculature in regulating pattern formation and tissue differentiation. Thus, prevascularized tissues also benefit from an intrinsic contribution of their vascular system to their development.[89]

Some investigators have engineered myocardial tissue around a native vessel.[88,90] This has been achieved in vitro with a rat aorta that was mounted in a bioreactor and perfused with cell culture medium. The rate of survival of neonatal rat cardiomyocytes, which were embedded in fibrin glue and positioned around the aortic vessel, was significantly higher when the vessel was perfused.[90] Similarly, neonatal rat cardiomyocytes have been suspended in Matrigel and seeded around an arteriovenous shunt that was created inside a polycarbonate chamber in the groin of a rat.[88] Other investigators have cultured mixed neonatal rat heart cells in vitro and have observed spontaneous formation of cardiomyocyte strands that were lined by newly formed blood vessels that interconnected with the host vasculature after transplantation onto infarcted rat

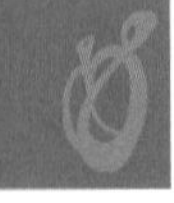

hearts.[91] Vascularized, synchronously contracting human myocardial tissue grafts have been engineered by seeding human embryonic stem cell–derived cardiomyocytes and endothelial cells together with embryonic fibroblasts onto poly-L-lactic acid (PLLA) and polylactic-glycolic acid (PLGA) sponges.[92] Of interest was that the presence of endothelial cells enhanced proliferation of the cardiomyocytes in the grafts, whereas the presence of embryonic fibroblasts decreased endothelial cell death and stimulated endothelial cell proliferation.[92] Decellularized cadaveric hearts with an intact 3-dimensional geometry

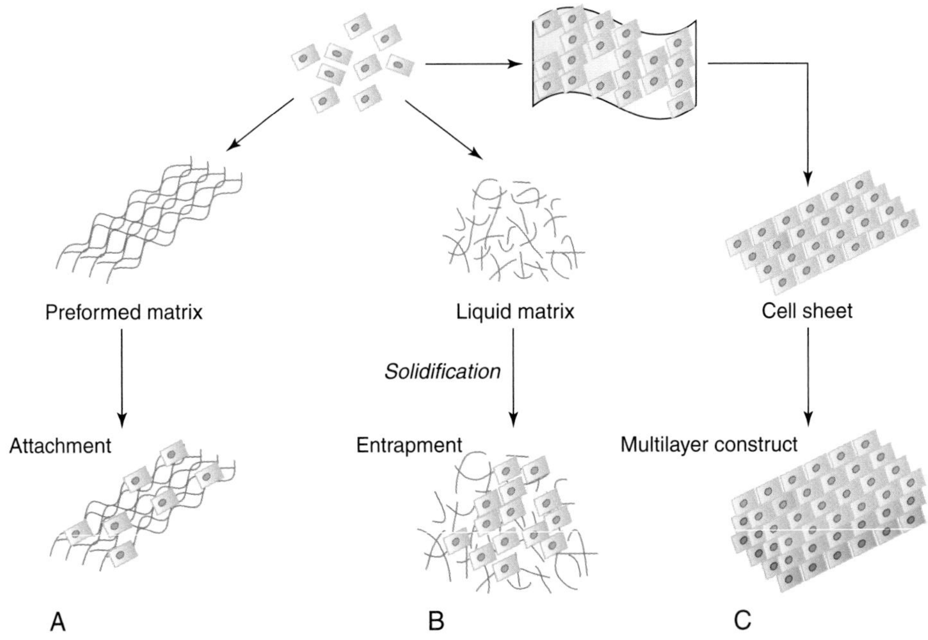

FIGURE 51–5 Concepts in myocardial tissue engineering. **A,** Cell seeding on preformed matrices. **B,** Entrapment of cells in soluble matrix proteins. **C,** Monolayer cell sheet engineering. (See Table 51-5 for examples.) (Adapted from Zimmermann WH, Didie M, Doker S, et al. Heart muscle engineering: an update on cardiac muscle replacement therapy. *Cardiovasc Res* 2006;71:419-429.

TABLE 51–6 Selected Preclinical Studies on Myocardial Tissue Engineering

Study	Cell Types	Scaffold	In Vitro Performance	In Vivo Performance
Cell Seeding on Preformed Matrices				
Leor et al, 2000[96]	Fetal rat cardiomyocytes	Alginate	Cells form multicellular aggregates and contract spontaneously in the scaffold	Biograft implantation prevents left ventricular remodeling in a rat infarct model (whether cardiomyocytes contribute is uncertain)
Kofidis et al, 2002[84]	Neonatal rat cardiomyocytes	Bovine collagen type I	Cells form viable artificial myocardial tissue that contracts spontaneously and generates force	Not determined
Ott et al, 2008[93]	Neonatal rat cardiomyocytes, rat endothelial cells	Decellularized rat heart	Recellularized heartbeats with a contractile force that is equivalent to ≈2% of adult rat systolic heart function	Not determined
Cell Entrapment in Soluble Matrices				
Zimmermann et al, 2002[85] and 2006[91]	Mixed neonatal rat heart cells	Circular casting molds containing liquid rat collagen type I	After cyclic stretching for 7 days, cells form viable engineered heart tissue (EHT) loops that contract spontaneously and generate force	EHT grafts integrate, couple electrically, and support systolic and diastolic function in a rat infarct model
Guo et al, 2006[94]	Mouse embryonic stem cell–derived cardiomyocytes	Circular casting molds containing liquid rat collagen type I and Matrigel	After cyclic stretching for 7 days, cells form viable engineered cardiac tissue loops that contract spontaneously and generate force	No evidence for teratoma formation after subcutaneous implantation; not yet tested in cardiac applications
Monolayer Cell Sheet Engineering				
Shimizu et al, 2006[86] and 2002[97]	Neonatal rat cardiomyocytes	Thermoresponsive PIPAAm	Cells adhere to the matrix at 37° C and detach after cooling to 20° C; cell sheets are then stacked to form spontaneously beating multilayer constructs	Grafts (up to 100 μm in thickness) survive and continue to beat spontaneously after subcutaneous implantation in rats
Furuta et al, 2006,[98] and Itabashi et al, 2005[99]	Neonatal rat cardiomyocytes	Human fibrin-coated culture dish	Cells adhere to the matrix, digest the fibrin, and can then be removed and stacked to form spontaneously beating bilayered grafts (50 to 100 μm in thickness)	Grafts integrate and contract synchronously with the host heart when transplanted onto thermally injured rat myocardium Whether the graft contributes to force development is uncertain

PIPAAm, poly-*N*-isopropylacrylamide.

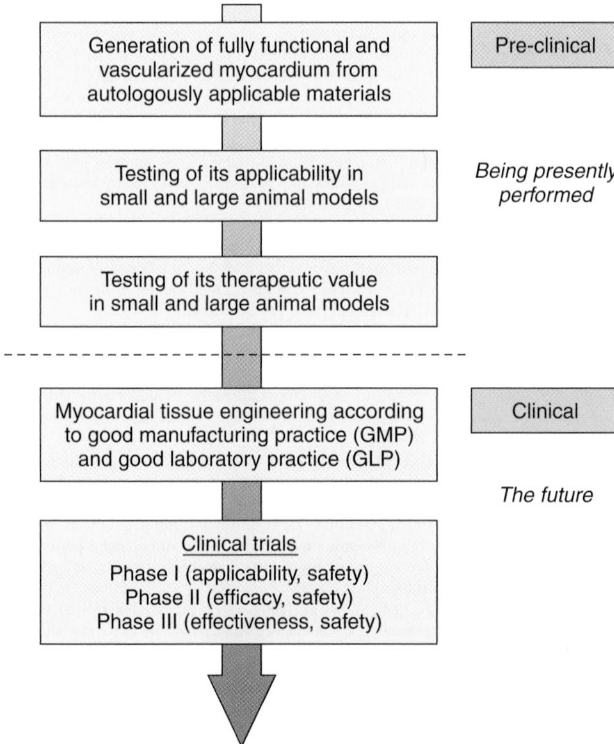

FIGURE 51-6 Milestones toward a clinical use of myocardial tissue engineering. GLP, glucose-L-phosphate; GMP, guanosine monophosphate. (Adapted from Zimmermann WH, Didie M, Doker S, et al. Heart muscle engineering: an update on cardiac muscle replacement therapy. *Cardiovasc Res* 2006;71:419-429.)

and vasculature may serve as scaffolds for engineering an entire heart. Proof of concept has been obtained with decellularized rat hearts that were repopulated with neonatal cardiomyocytes and rat aortic endothelial cells under simulated physiological conditions for organ maturation.[93]

In most experimental studies in myocardial tissue engineering, fetal or neonatal rat cardiomyocytes have been used as the main cell source. The identification of cell types that are suitable for human applications continues to be a major challenge. Although results of studies indicate that embryonic stem cell–derived cardiomyocytes can be used for tissue engineering[92,94] and that spermatogonial stem cells and iPS cells can be differentiated into cardiomyocytes,[38-40] the risk of teratoma formation that is associated with these cell types must be addressed. With any of these cell sources, it will be a formidable challenge to acquire sufficient quantities of cells for clinical use.

Synthetic and natural biomaterials that are currently used for myocardial tissue engineering serve mainly as scaffolds to allow proper cell assembly and alignment. Newer, "smart" biomaterials provide additional signals for cell adhesion, growth, or migration. Timed release of factors from these next-generation biomaterials can be regulated by chemical design to direct cellular differentiation pathways such as angiogenesis and vascular maturation.[95] "Smart" biomaterials could also be used for in situ engineering,[81] which involves a direct injection of biomaterials, alone or in combination with cells, into the diseased myocardium. It has been proposed that smart biomaterials can be used to custom design the cardiac microenvironment and stimulate endogenous repair processes.[95]

In conclusion, myocardial tissue engineering has great potential to enhance the function of the failing heart and to reduce the morbidity and mortality rates among patients living with heart failure. Currently, the development of clinical applications of myocardial tissue engineering appears long and arduous. Several milestones need to be achieved (Figure 51-6). Considering the magnitude of the heart failure epidemic and the current lack of regenerative strategies, intensive research in the area of myocardial tissue engineering will continue and may ultimately enable therapeutic alternatives to heart transplantation.

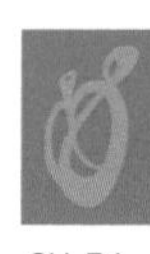

REFERENCES

1. McMurray, J. J., & Pfeffer, M. A. (2005). Heart failure. *Lancet, 365*, 1877–1889.
2. Cohn, J. N., Ferrari, R., & Sharpe, N. (2000). Cardiac remodeling—concepts and clinical implications: a consensus paper from an international forum on cardiac remodeling. Behalf of an International Forum on Cardiac Remodeling. *J Am Coll Cardiol, 35*, 569–582.
3. Gheorghiade, M., & Bonow, R. O. (1998). Chronic heart failure in the United States: a manifestation of coronary artery disease. *Circulation, 97*, 282–289.
4. Beltrami, A. P., Urbanek, K., Kajstura, J., et al. (2001). Evidence that human cardiac myocytes divide after myocardial infarction. *N Engl J Med, 344*, 1750–1757.
5. Hsieh, P. C., Segers, V. F., Davis, M. E., et al. (2007). Evidence from a genetic fate-mapping study that stem cells refresh adult mammalian cardiomyocytes after injury. *Nat Med, 13*, 970–974.
6. Fazel, S., Cimini, M., Chen, L., et al. (2006). Cardioprotective c- *kit*+ cells are from the bone marrow and regulate the myocardial balance of angiogenic cytokines. *J Clin Invest, 116*, 1865–1877.
7. Laflamme, M. A., & Murry, C. E. (2005). Regenerating the heart. *Nat Biotechnol, 23*, 845–856.
8. Khademhosseini, A., Langer, R., Borenstein, J., et al. (2006). Microscale technologies for tissue engineering and biology. *Proc Natl Acad Sci U S A, 103*, 2480–2487.
9. Dimmeler, S., & Leri, A. (2008). Aging and disease as modifiers of efficacy of cell therapy. *Circ Res, 102*, 1319–1330.
10. Passier, R., van Laake, L. W., & Mummery, C. L. (2008). Stem-cell-based therapy and lessons from the heart. *Nature, 453*, 322–329.
11. Murry, C. E., Field, L. J., & Menasche, P. (2005). Cell-based cardiac repair: reflections at the 10-year point. *Circulation, 112*, 3174–3183.
12. Dowell, J. D., Rubart, M., Pasumarthi, K. B., et al. (2003). Myocyte and myogenic stem cell transplantation in the heart. *Cardiovasc Res, 58*, 336–350.
13. Menasche, P. (2007). Skeletal myoblasts as a therapeutic agent. *Prog Cardiovasc Dis, 50*, 7–17.
14. Levenberg, S., Rouwkema, J., Macdonald, M., et al. (2005). Engineering vascularized skeletal muscle tissue. *Nat Biotechnol, 23*, 879–884.
15. Roell, W., Lewalter, T., Sasse, P., et al. (2007). Engraftment of connexin 43–expressing cells prevents post-infarct arrhythmia. *Nature, 450*, 819–824.
16. Pittenger, M. F., & Martin, B. J. (2004). Mesenchymal stem cells and their potential as cardiac therapeutics. *Circ Res, 95*, 9–20.
17. Caplan, A. I. (2007). Adult mesenchymal stem cells for tissue engineering versus regenerative medicine. *J Cell Physiol, 213*, 341–347.
18. Sutherland, F. W., Perry, T. E., Yu, Y., et al. (2005). From stem cells to viable autologous semilunar heart valve. *Circulation, 111*, 2783–2791.
19. Dai, W., Hale, S. L., Martin, B. J., et al. (2005). Allogeneic mesenchymal stem cell transplantation in postinfarcted rat myocardium: short- and long-term effects. *Circulation, 112*, 214–223.
20. Gnecchi, M., He, H., Liang, O. D., et al. (2005). Paracrine action accounts for marked protection of ischemic heart by Akt-modified mesenchymal stem cells. *Nat Med, 11*, 367–368.
21. Carmeliet, P. (2000). Mechanisms of angiogenesis and arteriogenesis. *Nat Med, 6*, 389–395.
22. Urbich, C., & Dimmeler, S. (2004). Endothelial progenitor cells: characterization and role in vascular biology. *Circ Res, 95*, 343–353.
23. Aicher, A., Rentsch, M., Sasaki, K., et al. (2007). Nonbone marrow–derived circulating progenitor cells contribute to postnatal neovascularization following tissue ischemia. *Circ Res, 100*, 581–589.
24. Prater, D. N., Case, J., Ingram, D. A., et al. (2007). Working hypothesis to redefine endothelial progenitor cells. *Leukemia, 21*, 1141–1149.
25. Badorff, C., Brandes, R. P., Popp, R., et al. (2003). Transdifferentiation of blood-derived human adult endothelial progenitor cells into functionally active cardiomyocytes. *Circulation, 107*, 1024–1032.
26. Gruh, I., Beilner, J., Blomer, U., et al. (2006). No evidence of transdifferentiation of human endothelial progenitor cells into cardiomyocytes after coculture with neonatal rat cardiomyocytes. *Circulation, 113*, 1326–1334.
27. Melero-Martin, J. M., De Obaldia, M. E., Kang, S. Y., et al. (2008). Engineering robust and functional vascular networks in vivo with human adult and cord blood-derived progenitor cells. *Circ Res, 103*, 194–202.
28. Sasaki, K., Heeschen, C., Aicher, A., et al. (2006). Ex vivo pretreatment of bone marrow mononuclear cells with endothelial NO synthase enhancer AVE9488 enhances their functional activity for cell therapy. *Proc Natl Acad Sci U S A, 103*, 14537–14541.
29. Sorrentino, S. A., Bahlmann, F. H., Besler, C., et al. (2007). Oxidant stress impairs in vivo reendothelialization capacity of endothelial progenitor cells from patients with type 2 diabetes mellitus: restoration by the peroxisome proliferator–activated receptor–gamma agonist rosiglitazone. *Circulation, 116*, 163–173.
30. Kehat, I., Kenyagin-Karsenti, D., Snir, M., et al. (2001). Human embryonic stem cells can differentiate into myocytes with structural and functional properties of cardiomyocytes. *J Clin Invest, 108*, 407–414.
31. Levenberg, S., Golub, J. S., Amit, M., et al. (2002). Endothelial cells derived from human embryonic stem cells. *Proc Natl Acad Sci U S A, 99*, 4391–4396.
32. Ferreira, L. S., Gerecht, S., Shieh, H. F., et al. (2007). Vascular progenitor cells isolated from human embryonic stem cells give rise to endothelial and smooth muscle like cells and form vascular networks in vivo. *Circ Res, 101*, 286–294.

33. Zimmermann, W. H., & Eschenhagen, T. (2007). Embryonic stem cells for cardiac muscle engineering. *Trends Cardiovasc Med*, *17*, 134–140.
34. Kehat, I., Khimovich, L., Caspi, O., et al. (2004). Electromechanical integration of cardiomyocytes derived from human embryonic stem cells. *Nat Biotechnol*, *22*, 1282–1289.
35. Menard, C., Hagege, A. A., Agbulut, O., et al. (2005). Transplantation of cardiac-committed mouse embryonic stem cells to infarcted sheep myocardium: a preclinical study. *Lancet*, *366*, 1005–1012.
36. Takahashi, K., Tanabe, K., Ohnuki, M., et al. (2007). Induction of pluripotent stem cells from adult human fibroblasts by defined factors. *Cell*, *131*, 861–872.
37. Yu, J., Vodyanik, M. A., Smuga-Otto, K., et al. (2007). Induced pluripotent stem cell lines derived from human somatic cells. *Science*, *318*, 1917–1920.
38. Mauritz, C., Schwanke, K., Reppel, M., et al. (2008). Generation of functional murine cardiac myocytes from induced pluripotent stem cells. *Circulation*, *118*, 507–517.
39. Guan, K., Nayernia, K., Maier, L. S., et al. (2006). Pluripotency of spermatogonial stem cells from adult mouse testis. *Nature*, *440*, 1199–1203.
40. Seandel, M., James, D., Shmelkov, S. V., et al. (2007). Generation of functional multipotent adult stem cells from $GPR125^+$ germline progenitors. *Nature*, *449*, 346–350.
41. Wu, S. M., Chien, K. R., & Mummery, C. (2008). Origins and fates of cardiovascular progenitor cells. *Cell*, *132*, 537–543.
42. Messina, E., De Angelis, L., Frati, G., et al. (2004). Isolation and expansion of adult cardiac stem cells from human and murine heart. *Circ Res*, *95*, 911–921.
43. Smith, R. R., Barile, L., Cho, H. C., et al. (2007). Regenerative potential of cardiosphere-derived cells expanded from percutaneous endomyocardial biopsy specimens. *Circulation*, *115*, 896–908.
44. Frangogiannis, N. G. (2006). The mechanistic basis of infarct healing. *Antioxid Redox Signal*, *8*, 1907–1939.
45. Schachinger, V., Aicher, A., Döbert, N., et al. (2008). Pilot trial on determinants of progenitor cell recruitment to the infarcted human myocardium. *Circulation*, *118*, 1425–1432.
46. Strauer, B. E., Brehm, M., Zeus, T., et al. (2002). Repair of infarcted myocardium by autologous intracoronary mononuclear bone marrow cell transplantation in humans. *Circulation*, *106*, 1913–1918.
47. Hofmann, M., Wollert, K. C., Meyer, G. P., et al. (2005). Monitoring of bone marrow cell homing into the infarcted human myocardium. *Circulation*, *111*, 2198–2202.
48. Orlic, D., Kajstura, J., Chimenti, S., et al. (2001). Bone marrow cells regenerate infarcted myocardium. *Nature*, *410*, 701–705.
49. Kocher, A. A., Schuster, M. D., Szabolcs, M. J., et al. (2001). Neovascularization of ischemic myocardium by human bone-marrow–derived angioblasts prevents cardiomyocyte apoptosis, reduces remodeling and improves cardiac function. *Nat Med*, *7*, 430–436.
50. Ziegelhoeffer, T., Fernandez, B., Kostin, S., et al. (2004). Bone marrow–derived cells do not incorporate into the adult growing vasculature. *Circ Res*, *94*, 230–238.
51. Murry, C. E., Soonpaa, M. H., Reinecke, H., et al. (2004). Haematopoietic stem cells do not transdifferentiate into cardiac myocytes in myocardial infarcts. *Nature*, *428*, 664–668.
52. Balsam, L. B., Wagers, A. J., Christensen, J. L., et al. (2004). Haematopoietic stem cells adopt mature haematopoietic fates in ischaemic myocardium. *Nature*, *428*, 668–673.
53. Kinnaird, T., Stabile, E., Burnett, M. S., et al. (2004). Marrow-derived stromal cells express genes encoding a broad spectrum of arteriogenic cytokines and promote in vitro and in vivo arteriogenesis through paracrine mechanisms. *Circ Res*, *94*, 678–685.
54. Wollert, K. C., Meyer, G. P., Lotz, J., et al. (2004). Intracoronary autologous bone-marrow cell transfer after myocardial infarction: the BOOST randomised controlled clinical trial. *Lancet*, *364*, 141–148.
55. Schachinger, V., Erbs, S., Elsasser, A., et al. (2006). Intracoronary bone marrow–derived progenitor cells in acute myocardial infarction. *N Engl J Med*, *355*, 1210–1221.
56. Assmus, B., Honold, J., Schachinger, V., et al. (2006). Transcoronary transplantation of progenitor cells after myocardial infarction. *N Engl J Med*, *355*, 1222–1232.
57. Janssens, S., Dubois, C., Bogaert, J., et al. (2006). Autologous bone marrow–derived stem-cell transfer in patients with ST-segment elevation myocardial infarction: double-blind, randomised controlled trial. *Lancet*, *367*, 113–121.
58. Lunde, K., Solheim, S., Aakhus, S., et al. (2006). Intracoronary injection of mononuclear bone marrow cells in acute myocardial infarction. *N Engl J Med*, *355*, 1199–1209.
59. Huikuri, H. V., Kervinen, K., Niemela, M., et al. (2008). Effects of intracoronary injection of mononuclear bone marrow cells on left ventricular function, arrhythmia risk profile, and restenosis after thrombolytic therapy of acute myocardial infarction. *Eur Heart J*, *29*, 2723–2732.
60. Tendera, M., Wojakowski, W., Ruzyllo, W., et al. (2009). Intracoronary infusion of bone marrow–derived selected $CD34^+$ $CXCR4^+$ cells and non-selected mononuclear cells in patients with acute STEMI and reduced left ventricular ejection fraction: results of randomized, multicentre Myocardial Regeneration by Intracoronary Infusion of Selected Population of Stem Cells in Acute Myocardial Infarction (REGENT) trial. *Eur Heart J*, *30*, 1313–1321.
61. Seeger, F. H., Tonn, T., Krzossok, N., et al. (2007). Cell isolation procedures matter: a comparison of different isolation protocols of bone marrow mononuclear cells used for cell therapy in patients with acute myocardial infarction. *Eur Heart J*, *28*, 766–772.
62. Abdel-Latif, A., Bolli, R., Tleyjeh, I. M., et al. (2007). Adult bone marrow–derived cells for cardiac repair: a systematic review and meta-analysis. *Arch Intern Med*, *167*, 989–997.
63. Lipinski, M. J., Biondi-Zoccai, G. G., Abbate, A., et al. (2007). Impact of intracoronary cell therapy on left ventricular function in the setting of acute myocardial infarction: a collaborative systematic review and meta-analysis of controlled clinical trials. *J Am Coll Cardiol*, *50*, 1761–1767.
64. Burt, R. K., Loh, Y., Pearce, W., et al. (2008). Clinical applications of blood-derived and marrow-derived stem cells for nonmalignant diseases. *JAMA*, *299*, 925–936.
65. Martin-Rendon, E., Brunskill, S. J., Hyde, C. J., et al. (2008). Autologous bone marrow stem cells to treat acute myocardial infarction: a systematic review. *Eur Heart J*, *29*, 1807–1818.
66. Menasche, P., Alfieri, O., Janssens, S., et al. (2008). The Myoblast Autologous Grafting in Ischemic Cardiomyopathy (MAGIC) trial: first randomized placebo-controlled study of myoblast transplantation. *Circulation*, *117*, 1189–1200.
67. Schachinger, V., Erbs, S., Elsasser, A., et al. (2006). Improved clinical outcome after intracoronary administration of bone-marrow–derived progenitor cells in acute myocardial infarction: final 1-year results of the REPAIR-AMI trial. *Eur Heart J*, *27*, 2775–2783.
68. Yousef, M., Schannwell, C. M., Kostering, M., et al. (2009). The BALANCE study: clinical benefit and long-term outcome after intracoronary autologous bone marrow cell transplantation in patients with acute myocardial infarction. *J Am Coll Cardiol*, *53*, 2262–2269.
69. Korf-Klingebiel, M., Kempf, T., Sauer, T., et al. (2008). Bone marrow cells are a rich source of growth factors and cytokines: implications for cell therapy trials after myocardial infarction. *Eur Heart J*, *29*, 2851–2858.
70. Erbs, S., Linke, A., Schachinger, V., et al. (2007). Restoration of microvascular function in the infarct-related artery by intracoronary transplantation of bone marrow progenitor cells in patients with acute myocardial infarction: the Doppler substudy of the Reinfusion of Enriched Progenitor Cells and Infarct Remodeling in Acute Myocardial Infarction (REPAIR-AMI) trial. *Circulation*, *116*, 366–374.
71. Kawamoto, A., Tkebuchava, T., Yamaguchi, J., et al. (2003). Intramyocardial transplantation of autologous endothelial progenitor cells for therapeutic neovascularization of myocardial ischemia. *Circulation*, *107*, 461–468.
72. Yoon, Y. S., Wecker, A., Heyd, L., et al. (2005). Clonally expanded novel multipotent stem cells from human bone marrow regenerate myocardium after myocardial infarction. *J Clin Invest*, *115*, 326–338.
73. Zeng, L., Hu, Q., Wang, X., et al. (2007). Bioenergetic and functional consequences of bone marrow–derived multipotent progenitor cell transplantation in hearts with postinfarction left ventricular remodeling. *Circulation*, *115*, 1866–1875.
74. Kamihata, H., Matsubara, H., Nishiue, T., et al. (2001). Implantation of bone marrow mononuclear cells into ischemic myocardium enhances collateral perfusion and regional function via side supply of angioblasts, angiogenic ligands, and cytokines. *Circulation*, *104*, 1046–1052.
75. Mirotsou, M., Zhang, Z., Deb, A., et al. (2007). Secreted frizzled related protein 2 (Sfrp2) is the key Akt-mesenchymal stem cell-released paracrine factor mediating myocardial survival and repair. *Proc Natl Acad Sci U S A*, *104*, 1643–1648.
76. Vesely, I. (2005). Heart valve tissue engineering. *Circ Res*, *97*, 743–755.
77. Shin'oka, T., Matsumura, G., Hibino, N., et al. (2005). Midterm clinical result of tissue-engineered vascular autografts seeded with autologous bone marrow cells. *J Thorac Cardiovasc Surg*, *129*, 1330–1338.
78. Dohmen, P. M., Lembcke, A., Holinski, S., et al. (2007). Mid-term clinical results using a tissue-engineered pulmonary valve to reconstruct the right ventricular outflow tract during the Ross procedure. *Ann Thorac Surg*, *84*, 729–736.
79. L'Heureux, N., Dusserre, N., Konig, G., et al. (2006). Human tissue-engineered blood vessels for adult arterial revascularization. *Nat Med*, *12*, 361–365.
80. Eschenhagen, T., & Zimmermann, W. H. (2005). Engineering myocardial tissue. *Circ Res*, *97*, 1220–1231.
81. Jawad, H., Ali, N. N., Lyon, A. R., et al. (2007). Myocardial tissue engineering: a review. *J Tissue Eng Regen Med*, *1*, 327–342.
82. Jawad, H., Lyon, A. R., Harding, S. E., et al. (2008). Myocardial tissue engineering. *Br Med Bull*, *87*, 31–47.
83. Zimmermann, W. H., Didie, M., Doker, S., et al. (2006). Heart muscle engineering: an update on cardiac muscle replacement therapy. *Cardiovasc Res*, *71*, 419–429.
84. Kofidis, T., Akhyari, P., Boublik, J., et al. (2002). In vitro engineering of heart muscle: artificial myocardial tissue. *J Thorac Cardiovasc Surg*, *124*, 63–69.
85. Zimmermann, W. H., Schneiderbanger, K., Schubert, P., et al. (2002). Tissue engineering of a differentiated cardiac muscle construct. *Circ Res*, *90*, 223–230.
86. Shimizu, T., Sekine, H., Isoi, Y., et al. (2006). Long-term survival and growth of pulsatile myocardial tissue grafts engineered by the layering of cardiomyocyte sheets. *Tissue Eng*, *12*, 499–507.
87. Shimizu, T., Yamato, M., Kikuchi, A., et al. (2003). Cell sheet engineering for myocardial tissue reconstruction. *Biomaterials*, *24*, 2309–2316.
88. Morritt, A. N., Bortolotto, S. K., Dilley, R. J., et al. (2007). Cardiac tissue engineering in an in vivo vascularized chamber. *Circulation*, *115*, 353–360.
89. Rivron, N. C., Liu, J. J., Rouwkema, J., et al. (2008). Engineering vascularised tissues in vitro. *Eur Cell Mater*, *15*, 27–40.
90. Kofidis, T., Lenz, A., Boublik, J., et al. (2003). Pulsatile perfusion and cardiomyocyte viability in a solid three-dimensional matrix. *Biomaterials*, *24*, 5009–5014.
91. Zimmermann, W. H., Melnychenko, I., Wasmeier, G., et al. (2006). Engineered heart tissue grafts improve systolic and diastolic function in infarcted rat hearts. *Nat Med*, *12*, 452–458.
92. Caspi, O., Lesman, A., Basevitch, Y., et al. (2007). Tissue engineering of vascularized cardiac muscle from human embryonic stem cells. *Circ Res*, *100*, 263–272.
93. Ott, H. C., Matthiesen, T. S., Goh, S. K., et al. (2008). Perfusion-decellularized matrix: using Nature's platform to engineer a bioartificial heart. *Nat Med*, *14*, 213–221.
94. Guo, X. M., Zhao, Y. S., Chang, H. X., et al. (2006). Creation of engineered cardiac tissue in vitro from mouse embryonic stem cells. *Circulation*, *113*, 2229–2237.
95. Davis, M. E., Hsieh, P. C., Grodzinsky, A. J., et al. (2005). Custom design of the cardiac microenvironment with biomaterials. *Circ Res*, *97*, 8–15.
96. Leor, J., Aboulafia-Etzion, S., Dar, A., et al. (2000). Bioengineered cardiac grafts: a new approach to repair the infarcted myocardium? *Circulation*, *102*(19), (Suppl. 3), III-56–III-61.
97. Shimizu, T., Yamato, M., Isoi, Y., et al. (2002). Fabrication of pulsatile cardiac tissue grafts using a novel 3-dimensional cell sheet manipulation technique and temperature-responsive cell culture surfaces. *Circ Res*, *90*(3), e40.
98. Furuta, A., Miyoshi, S., Itabashi, Y., et al. (2006). Pulsatile cardiac tissue grafts using a novel three-dimensional cell sheet manipulation technique functionally integrates with the host heart, in vivo. *Circ Res*, *98*, 705–712.
99. Itabashi, Y., Miyoshi, S., Kawaguchi, H., et al. (2005). A new method for manufacturing cardiac cell sheets using fibrin-coated dishes and its electrophysiological studies by optical mapping. *Artif Organs*, *29*, 95–103.

CHAPTER 52

Management of Thrombosis in Heart Failure

Ronald S. Freudenberger and Shunichi Homma

Since the discovery of heparin by Jay McLean in 1916[1] and the initial synthesis of acetylsalicylic acid by Felix Hoffmann in 1899[2] and warfarin in the 1940s,[3] the use of antiplatelet and antithrombotic agents in the treatment and prevention of cardiac disease has become widespread. In 1959, the first trial of thrombolytic agents for the treatment of acute myocardial infarction and other thromboembolic disorders in humans was conducted.[4] In the 1960s and 1970s, studies demonstrated the effectiveness of oral anticoagulants for the early treatment of acute myocardial infarction.[5,6] In the 1980s, the efficacy of aspirin in acute coronary syndromes became apparent. However, little is known about the appropriate use of these agents for the treatment and prevention of thrombotic complications in patients with heart failure. It is important to realize that the thrombotic complications of heart failure not only include thrombus formation in the ventricles or atria and embolism but also include acute intracoronary thrombosis and subsequent sudden death. Because of the paucity of controlled clinical trials to guide the practitioner's approach to the prevention of these events and their complications clinicians must have a sound understanding of the pathogenesis of the thrombotic processes in cardiovascular disease and the relative risks of thrombosis and thromboembolism in order to develop a rational approach to antithrombotic therapy. This chapter is a review of what is known about these complications in patients with heart failure and what is known about treatment and prevention from the perspective of pathogenesis and thrombotic and thromboembolic risk.

OVERVIEW OF HEMOSTASIS AND THROMBOSIS

The endothelium plays an important role in the regulation of thrombosis and hemostasis. Under normal and quiescent conditions, the endothelium helps provide an antithrombotic surface for blood. However, under certain circumstances, the endothelium can become prothrombotic by activating platelets, inhibiting fibrinolysis and promoting activation of the coagulation cascade (Figure 52-1). These processes are interrelated and can potentiate each other. They play a role in both vascular injury and subsequent thrombus formation and in activation of thrombosis in the cardiac chambers. In heart failure, both of these changes are important. Endothelial dysfunction, coagulation cascade, and platelet activation, along with a proinflammatory milieu, directly affect the balance between thrombosis and hemostasis and create the potential for a prothrombotic state. In addition, vascular tone is mediated by many of the same factors that may predispose to vasoconstriction. Many endothelium-derived vasodilators are also platelet inhibitors, and endothelium-derived vasoconstrictors can be platelet activators. The net effects are (1) promotion of fluidity by vasodilators and antiplatelet properties and (2) promotion of stasis with vasoconstrictors and platelet activators. Many factors in the delicate balance between the prothrombotic state and the antithrombotic state are perturbed in heart failure, inasmuch as endothelial dysfunction is known to play an important role in this disease. Furthermore, many of the pharmacological agents that are used in treatment of cardiovascular disease can affect this balance.

Endothelial dysfunction or endocardial injury can promote activation of platelets and the coagulation cascade. As discussed later, endocardial dysfunction resulting from increased hemodynamic pressure can cause downregulation of endocardial thrombomodulin and subsequent increase in thrombin generation, which in turn can cause platelet activation, fibrin formation, and crosslinking and activation of the coagulation system (Figure 52-2).

Typically, once platelets are activated, a series of subsequent prothrombotic systems is also activated. Platelets can form a monolayer in minor injury to cover the exposed subendothelium. In more severe injury, the lipid pool activates the platelets and subsequently activates the coagulation system, which leads to thrombus formation. Platelet receptors play a role in its aggregation and adhesion. Glycoprotein Ia binds directly to exposed collagen and serves as a binding site for subendothelial von Willebrand factor. Glycoprotein IIb/IIIa is the receptor for fibrinogen and von Willebrand factor, which promotes platelet-platelet interactions and aggregate formation. Collagen, thrombin, and the release of platelet adenosine diphosphate and thromboxane A_2 cause ongoing propagation of platelet deposition and aggregation.

Platelet aggregation provides a surface for the localization and interaction of coagulation factors and accelerates the conversion of prothrombin to thrombin. This process involves activation of the intrinsic coagulation system. In addition to this system, the extrinsic pathway is activated through the release of tissue factor from damaged endothelium. Factor X is the focal point of convergence of the intrinsic and extrinsic coagulation pathways. Once activated factor Xa converts prothrombin to thrombin—which, as mentioned earlier, further accelerates platelet deposition—thrombin cleaves fibrinogen to form fibrin, which activates factor XII, which in turn then stabilizes the clot and induces additional platelet activation (Figure 52-3).

Several endogenous mechanisms that limit thrombus formation are important in the ongoing balance between coagulation and anticoagulation. Antithrombin III, protein C, and protein S are important

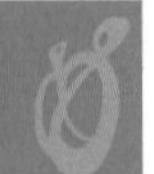

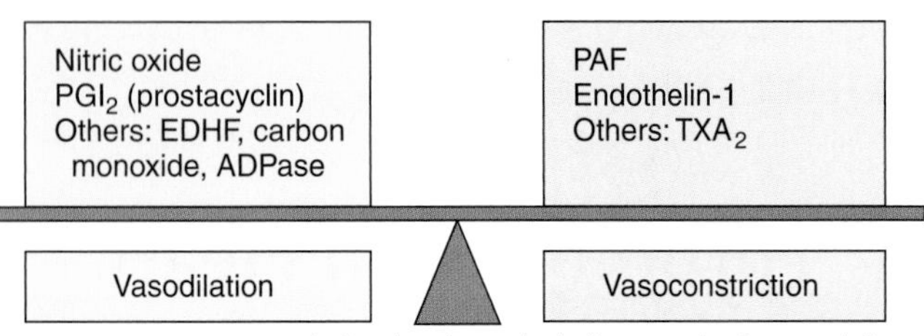

FIGURE 52–1 Vasoregulation by the endothelium results from a delicate balance between vasodilation and vasoconstriction. ADPase, adenosine diphosphatase; EDHF, endothelium-derived hyperpolarizing factor; PAF, platelet activating factor; PGI_2, prostaglandin I_2; TXA_2, thromboxane A_2.

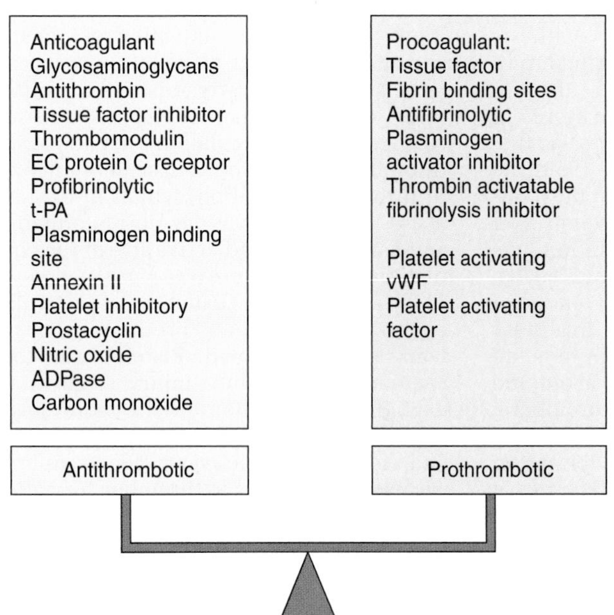

FIGURE 52–2 Factors blocking thrombosis balanced by factors that promote thrombosis. ADPase, adenosine diphosphatase; EC, endothelial cell; t-PA, tissue plasminogen activator; vWF, von Willebrand factor.

inhibitors of thrombosis. Antithrombin-III functions by inhibiting thrombin and activating factors IX, X, XI, and XIII. Heparin accelerates these inhibitory effects. Protein C is a potent anticoagulant. It functions by neutralizing a circulating inhibitor of tissue-type plasminogen activator (t-PA) and activates plasminogen. Plasminogen, in turn, is converted to plasmin, which degrades fibrinogen, prothrombin, and factors VIII and V. Plasmin also cleaves fibrin into soluble fragments on the surface of the fibrin complex. Plasmin is subsequently inactivated by A_2 plasmin inhibitor. Thus, many factors in the delicate balance between the prothrombotic state and the antithrombotic state are perturbed in heart failure.

CHAMBERS

The development of intracavitary or mural thrombi in patients with acute myocardial infarction, left ventricular (LV) aneurysm, and dilated cardiomyopathy is well described. The pathogenesis of intracavitary thrombosis was described by Rudolph Virchow, who defined three precipitating factors: endothelial injury, blood stasis, and hypercoagulability.[11] The last two factors contribute significantly to fibrin deposition and activation of the coagulation system. Once a thrombus forms, the clinical significance is its potential for embolism.

Endocardial Injury

Endocardial injury in heart failure is an often neglected contributor to thrombus formation in patients with heart failure. Kapur and colleagues[1] demonstrated that acute elevation of left atrial pressure caused a 70% inhibition of atrial thrombomodulin, which results in downregulation of endocardial thrombomodulin expression, ultimately increasing local thrombin production. Furthermore, these investigators found that the targeted restoration of atrial thrombomodulin expression with adenovirus-mediated gene transfer successfully reduced thrombin generation levels. Further experiments revealed that thrombomodulin downregulation is caused by the paracrine release of transforming growth factor β from cardiac connective tissue in response to mechanical stretch. These findings suggest that increased hemodynamic load adversely affects endocardial

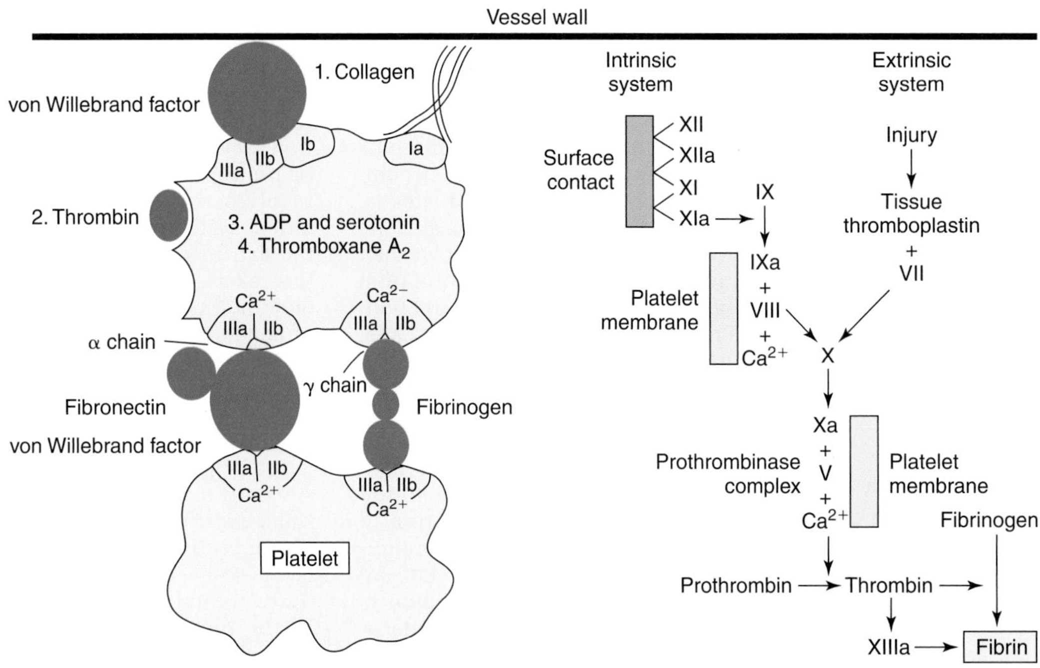

FIGURE 52–3 The complex relationship between platelets and the coagulation cascade. ADP, adenosine diphosphate.

function and is a potentially important contributor to thrombus formation in patients with heart failure. More research into this important contributing factor is needed.

Blood Stasis

Blood stasis in areas of akinesis or dyskinesis is an important factor in the predisposition to thrombus formation. It occurs in a diffuse or segmentally dilated ventricle, with or without cardiac failure. The three most classic clinical conditions predisposed to blood stasis are dilated cardiomyopathy, anterior myocardial infarction, and LV aneurysm. Stasis triggers activation of the coagulation system, leading to fibrin formation, which accounts for the predominant pathogenetic mechanism in the development of intracavitary thrombus formation.

Hypercoagulability

Studies have shown that patients with heart failure have higher levels of circulating fibrinogen, antithrombin III, fibrinopeptide A, and D-dimer.[2,3] Neuroendocrine modulators may also increase the prothrombotic state by increasing angiotensin and endothelin levels, which, in turn, increase levels of von Willebrand factor.[4] Coupled with decreased levels of nitric oxide, this development has been shown to increase endothelial monocyte and platelet adhesion, potentially leading to in situ thrombosis.[5,6] Researchers examining plasma markers of endothelial damage, dysfunction, and activation in patients with acute and chronic heart failure found that levels of von Willebrand factor, soluble thrombomodulin (an index of endothelial damage/dysfunction), soluble E-selectin (an index of endothelial activation), and brain natriuretic peptide (BNP) were all statistically significantly higher in patients with acute and chronic heart failure than in controls.[5,7] Although this was a small study, the results were suggestive of a link between inflammation and thrombosis in heart failure. This link is further suggested by a number of additional observations. Tissue factor, a procoagulant, can be increased by tumor necrosis factor α and interleukin-1, levels of which are raised in heart failure.[8,9] C-reactive protein can directly increase levels of tissue factor and induce expression of other cytokines, thus further potentiating a prothrombotic milieu[10,11] (Figure 52-4).

DYNAMIC FORCES OF THE CIRCULATION

Although the combination of these three components of Virchow's triad predisposes to thrombus formation, formation of intracavitary thrombi does not necessarily lead to embolization. Dynamic forces of the cardiac chambers determine the propensity toward embolization. For example, in the case of LV aneurysm, the isolation from dynamic circulatory forces may be protective from systemic embolization. Therefore, when stratifying risk, clinicians must consider not only the predisposition to thrombus formation but also the risk of subsequent embolization.

Arterial Thrombosis

Acute coronary thrombosis can result in nonfatal myocardial infarction or sudden death. This process is well defined in patients with heart failure, patients with coronary artery disease, and those dying of sudden cardiac death. Clinically evident or silent intracoronary plaque rupture and occlusive thrombosis can occur in patients with significant degrees of occlusive atherosclerotic disease or with lesions that are less than 50% occluded.[12] This process may account for many deaths described as sudden cardiac death. It is estimated that one third of deaths classified as "sudden" are caused by acute coronary occlusion by thrombus. Autopsy studies and studies of patients resuscitated from sudden death events have yielded these pathological findings[13,14] (Figure 52-5). Thus, if the definition of thrombosis-related complications is expanded to include deaths from intracronary thrombosis, the true risk of thrombotic complications of heart failure is greatly increased.[15] In one important heart failure study, nearly 50% of deaths adjudicated as sudden cardiac deaths were reclassified at autopsy as acute myocardial infarction or coronary thrombosis, and 27% of deaths classified as progressive congestive heart failure were actually found to be caused by coronary artery thrombosis.[7] Most population-based studies and retrospective analyses of thrombotic complications of heart failure do not account for patients who experience sudden cardiac death. As a result, the effect of thrombosis in patients with heart failure is probably underestimated.

Thrombosis

Chronic Heart Failure

The risk of thromboembolic events (stroke, pulmonary and peripheral thromboembolism) in patients with heart failure is poorly defined. The analyses that currently exist are from retrospective studies of large trials of treatment for heart failure and from population-based studies. Many of these studies included patients with atrial fibrillation and atrial flutter and did not specify thromboembolism as an endpoint. This is problematic because the use of precise scales to detect stroke significantly increases the detection of subtle neurological

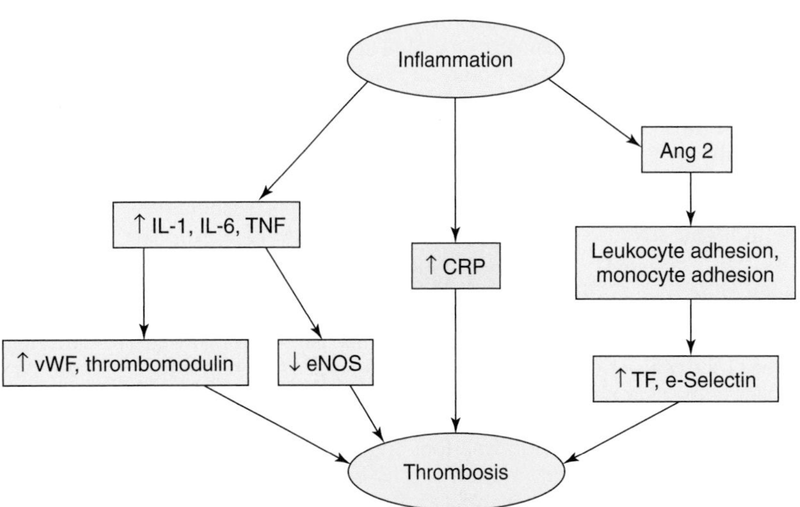

FIGURE 52–4 Relationship of inflammation and thrombosis. Ang II, angiotensin II; CRP, C-reactive protein; eNOS, endothelial nitric oxide synthase; IL-1 and IL-6, interleukin-1 and interleukin-6; TF, tissue factor; TNF, tumor necrosis factor; vWF, von Willebrand factor.

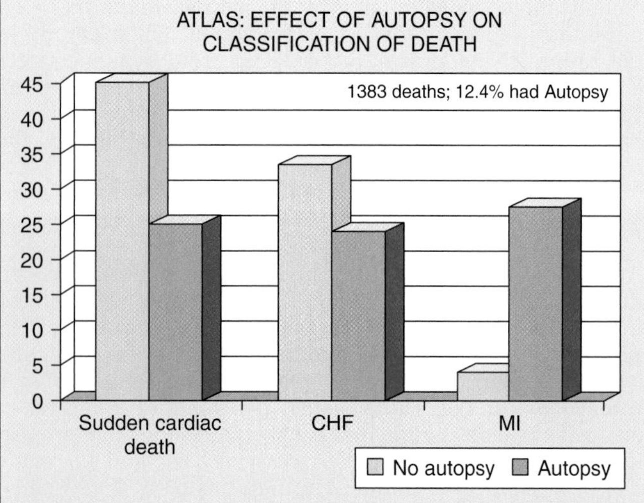

FIGURE 52–5 Assessment of Treatment with Lisinopril And Survival (ATLAS): effect of autopsy on classification of death. The graph shows the striking difference in classification when autopsies are performed. Nearly 50% of deaths classified as sudden by clinical criteria reflect acute myocardial infarction (MI) or coronary thrombosis. Similarly, 27% of the deaths classified as progressive congestive heart failure (CHF) are associated with recent MI that was not detected clinically. Thus, according to autopsies of patients, MI is the most frequent mechanism of death. These results provide a strong rationale for the use of antithrombotic agents in patients with CHF. (From Uretsky BF, Thygesen K, Armstrong PW, et al. Acute coronary findings at autopsy in heart failure patients with sudden death: results from the Assessment of Treatment with Lisinopril And Survival [ATLAS] trial. *Circulation* 2000;102:611-616.)

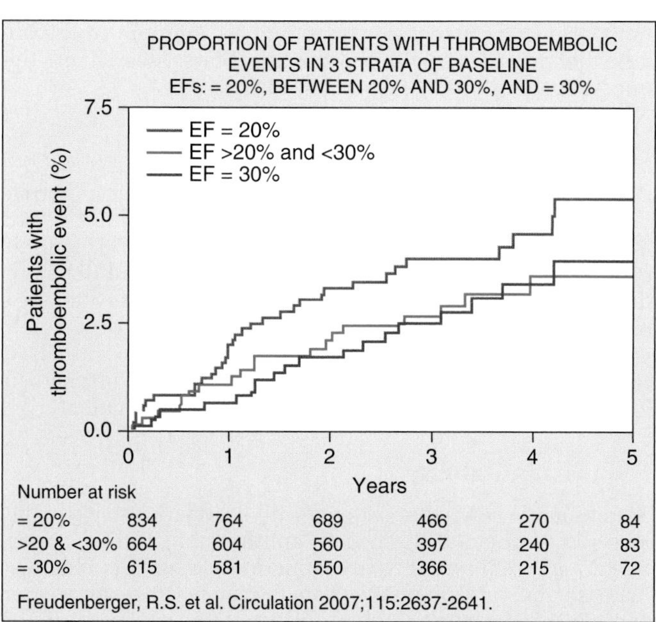

FIGURE 52–6 Proportions of patients in the Sudden Cardiac Death in Heart Failure Trial (SCD-HeFT) trial who experienced a thromboembolic event. These proportions were stratified by three levels of baseline ejection fraction (EF). (From Freudenberger RS, Hellkamp AS, Halperin JL, et al. for the SCD-HeFT Investigators. Risk of thromboembolism in heart failure: An analysis from the sudden cardiac death in heart failure trial (SCD-HeFT). *Circulation*, May 2007; 115:2637–2641.

events.[16] It is believed that heart failure in the absence of atrial fibrillation is associated with an increased risk of thromboembolic events. This belief is based on several observations. First, many patients with stroke or thromboembolic events have depressed LV function.[17-19] Second, retrospective analysis reveals a yearly incidence of thromboembolism in the range of 1% to 4.5% among patients with heart failure. In the population-based Framingham Heart Study,[20] the relative risk of stroke in individuals with heart failure was 4.1 for men and 2.8 for women, but many of these individuals had concurrent atrial fibrillation. In heart failure trials, annual stroke rates between 1.3% and 3.5% have been reported; however, almost all of these analyses included patients with atrial fibrillation. In one analysis, thromboembolic rates were only 1% per year in a population of patients with New York Heart Association (NYHA) classes II and III heart failure without atrial fibrillation.[21]

Several researchers have attempted to identify potential risk factors for the development of stroke or thromboembolism. Other than ejection fraction, a prior thromboembolic event, and perhaps the presence of a pedunculated thrombus, their analyses have shed little light on potential risk factors and have provided results difficult to interpret. In a retrospective analysis of the Study of Left Ventricular Dysfunction (SOLVD)[22] (after patients with atrial fibrillation were excluded), the annual rate of thromboembolic events was 2.4% among women and 1.8% among men. Lower ejection fraction was associated with higher event rates in women but not in men. In addition, women were observed to have a higher proportion of pulmonary embolism. In an analysis of the Survival and Ventricular Enlargement (SAVE) trial,[23] the overall risk of stroke was 8.1% at 5 years, and the only independent risk factors for stroke were LV dysfunction, older age, and nonuse of aspirin or anticoagulants. The risk of stroke was found to be twofold higher among patients with ejection fractions lower than 28% than among those with ejection fractions higher than 28%. Every 5% decrease in ejection fraction was associated with an 18% increase in stroke risk. This analysis of angiotensin-converting enzyme (ACE) inhibitors versus placebo in patients after myocardial infarction did not exclude patients with atrial fibrillation; the researchers studied only stroke events. In a more recent analysis of patients with moderately severe heart failure and an ejection fraction of 35% or lower who participated in the Sudden Cardiac Death in Heart Failure Trial (SCD-HeFT) (Figure 52-6), the 4-year rates of thromboembolic events were 3.5% with ejection fractions of 30% to 35%, 3.6% with ejection fractions of 20% to 30%, and 4.6% with ejection fractions lower than 20% (which means that the annual rates were approximately 0.9%, 0.9%, and 1.2% respectively) (Figure 52-6).[21] Patients with atrial fibrillation at the time of randomization were excluded from this analysis. The annual rate of thromboembolic events was found to be approximately 1%. Both hypertension at the time of randomization and ejection fraction were independent predictors of thromboembolic events. No other measured variables were significant in terms of outcome.

With regard to prior stroke, the Northern Manhattan Study (NOMAS) was conducted to examine 270 patients with first occurrence of ischemic stroke and 288 age-, gender-, and race-matched controls. Patients in one hospital were assessed for the incidence, risk factors, and clinical outcome of stroke. LV systolic function was measured and categorized as normal (ejection fraction > 50%), mildly reduced (41% to 50%), moderately reduced (31% to 40%), or severely decreased (≤30%). Decreased ejection fraction was found to be strongly associated with ischemic stroke even after other stroke risk factors were adjusted. LV dysfunction of any degree was more frequent in patients with stroke (24.1%, in comparison with 4.9% of controls; $P < .0001$). Moderate or severe LV dysfunction was also more common in patients with stroke (13.3%) than in controls (2.4%; $P < .001$). The adjusted odds ratio was 3.96 for mild LV dysfunction and 3.88 for moderate or severe LV dysfunction (adjusted for other stroke risk factors).[24] In another study, the rate of recurrent stroke after a first stroke was 9% to 10% per year in patients with heart failure, which suggested that a previous event confers a high risk of recurrence.[25] In yet another study, the presence of intracardiac thrombus was identified in half the patients with neurological events, and patients with thrombus had a significantly higher rate of thromboembolism (5.3% per year).[26] The results of all these studies together suggest a risk association with the presence and degree of systolic dysfunction.

Not all, or even most, cerebrovascular events are thromboembolic in origin. Clinicians must also consider the possibility that vascular sources or hemodynamic fluctuations, such as low cardiac output, episodic hypotension, or silent arrhythmias (including asymptomatic episodic atrial fibrillation), and resultant reduction in cerebral perfusion may be a contributing or causative factor. The presence of hypertension and diabetes mellitus significantly increases the risk of vascular disease and subsequent cerebrovascular events. In an imaging study of hypertensive patients,[27] the combined presence of these risk factors was the most powerful independent determinant of the presence of silent cerebral infarcts (especially for multiple silent cerebral infarcts). These authors found the prevalence of silent cerebral infarcts and multiple silent cerebral infarcts increased threefold in hypertensive patients with diabetes mellitus, independent of age and ambulatory blood pressure. The evidence for vascular sources of silent cerebral infarcts is abundant. Büsing and associates[28] prospectively evaluated patients before and after diagnostic and interventional cardiac catheterization with magnetic resonance imaging studies. These investigators found that 15% of patients had new silent cerebral infarctions, with no association between ejection fraction and risk of cerebral infarction; this rate was much higher than that observed for symptomatic stroke after cardiac catheterization, which is reported as 0.11%. Similarly, patients who have undergone coronary artery bypass grafting have a high incidence of silent cerebral infarcts,[29] and patients with manifest vascular disease were found to have a 17% incidence of asymptomatic stroke.[30]

In addition to the mechanistic causes of cerebrovascular incidents in heart failure patients, many of these patients, particularly with more advanced heart failure, have low cardiac output and reduced cerebral blood flow. Counterregulatory mechanisms with increased neurohormonal activation and changes in the distribution of cardiac output are assumed to secure vital organ perfusion. However, clinical examination of patients with congestive heart failure frequently reveals neurological symptoms with dizziness and memory problems, suggestive of altered brain perfusion. In a study of 12 patients with NYHA functional classes III and IV heart failure, cerebral blood flow (CBF) was found to be significantly reduced, in comparison with 12 healthy control subjects: the patients' average CBF was 36 ± 1 mL/min per 100 g, corresponding to a 31% reduction in comparison with CBF of the control group (52 ± 5 mL/min per 100 g; $P < .05$). Of interest was that CBF increased from 35 ± 3 mL/min per 100 g before heart transplantation to 50 ± 3 mL/min per 100 g within the first postoperative month ($P < .05$).[31] In another study of 52 patients with advanced nonischemic cardiomyopathy, CBF was 19% less in patients with congestive heart failure than in controls ($P < .01$). CBF became normalized in four patients with congestive heart failure who underwent cardiac transplantation. In a univariate linear regression analysis, global CBF was significantly associated with severity of NYHA functional class, disease duration, atrial fibrillation, serum BNP level, the ratio of early mitral velocity to early diastolic annular velocity, and pulmonary artery systolic pressure. Global CBF was not found to be associated with the ejection fraction, peak oxygen consumption, or anaerobic threshold. In a stepwise multivariate linear regression analysis, serum BNP level ($P = .047$) and NYHA functional class ($P = .003$) were significantly related to global CBF (global CBF = 48.373 – [0.05 × serum BNP level] – [3.283 × NYHA functional class]; $r^2 = 0.401$).[32] Thus, reduced CBF and vascular disease may in fact be additive and further potentiate the risk of cerebrovascular events in patients with heart failure (Figure 52-7).

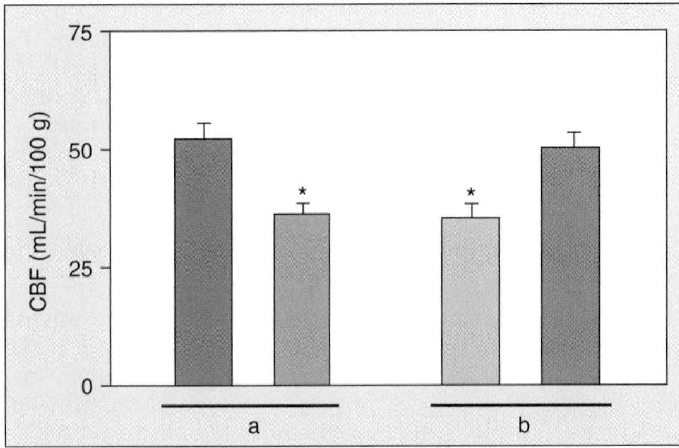

FIGURE 52–7 A, Cerebral blood flow (CBF) in 12 patients with congestive heart failure (*right*) and an age-matched control group of 12 (*left*). $*P < .05$ in comparison with control. B, CBF in 5 patients with congestive heart failure before (*left*) and 1 month after (*right*) heart transplantation. $*P < .05$ in comparison with pretransplantation status. (From Choi BR, Kim JS, Yang YJ, et al. Factors associated with decreased cerebral blood flow in congestive heart failure secondary to idiopathic dilated cardiomyopathy. *Am J Cardiol* 2006;97:1365-1369.)

Intracardiac Thrombosis After Myocardial Infarction

LV thrombus was previously estimated to develop in approximately 30% of patients with anterior myocardial infarction and was associated with a medium risk of subsequent embolization.[33] In the era of primary stent placement, the incidence may be significantly lower. One retrospective analysis of 2911 patients who had undergone successful primary stent placement revealed that 73 patients (2.5%) had intracardiac thrombi 3 to 5 days after presentation. The presence of LV thrombus was strongly associated with anterior myocardial infarction, ejection fraction lower than 40%, and history of hypertension; size of myocardial infarct and anterior location were the strongest predictors.[34] In a more recent evaluation of patients with heart failure (predominantly after myocardial infarction), delayed-enhancement cardiac magnetic resonance imaging was used to detect LV thrombi. This sensitive method revealed a 7% prevalence of ventricular thrombus. The presence of thrombus was associated with lower ejection fraction and a unique index of myocardial scarring.[35] Thus, the current prevalence of LV thrombus in anterior myocardial infarction is lower than previously reported, possibly because of changes in management of anterior myocardial infarction. Preservation of LV function is probably an important mechanism, as is the use of various antithrombotic and antiplatelet agents.

The risk of embolization of an intracardiac thrombus after its detection is also unknown. It is thought that the risk would decrease over time after the myocardial infarction because of the organization of the thrombus. However, the true risk of embolization and its risk factors are unknown.

According to the American Heart Association/American Stroke Association Council on Stroke guidelines, the following actions are recommended[36]:

1. For patients with an ischemic stroke or transient ischemic attack (TIA) caused by an acute myocardial infarction in whom LV mural thrombus is identified by echocardiography or another form of cardiac imaging, oral anticoagulation is reasonable; the aim is to achieve an international normalized ratio (INR) of 2.0 to 3.0 for at least 3 months and up to 1 year (class IIa, level of evidence B).

2. Aspirin should be used concurrently for ischemic coronary artery disease during oral anticoagulant therapy in doses up to 162 mg/day (class IIa, level of evidence A).
3. In patients who have had an ST wave–elevation myocardial infarction (STEMI) with LV thrombus noted on an imaging study, warfarin should be prescribed for at least 3 months (level of evidence B) and indefinitely in patients who have no increased risk of bleeding (level of evidence C).[37]

Thrombosis in Left Ventricular Aneurysms in Patients with Heart Failure

An LV aneurysm is a circumscribed, thin-walled, noncontractile outpouching of the ventricle[38] and is observed most commonly after an anterior transmural myocardial infarction (see Chapters 15 and 23).[39] In the current era of reperfusion therapy, an LV aneurysm is present in approximately 10% to 15% of patients with STEMI.[40] The presence of a poorly contracting, dilated left ventricle promotes stasis of blood and leads to an increased risk of thrombus formation.[41]

Demonstrating thrombus within the aneurysm is clinically important because such thrombi can lead to embolic complications. Results of studies differ widely, but both postmortem and surgical studies have demonstrated that approximately 50% of aneurysms contain a thrombus.[42]

Currently, echocardiography, either transthoracic or transesophageal, is the diagnostic standard for characterizing the aneurysm and determining the presence of LV thrombus. Echocardiography provides information about anatomy, size, and location of the aneurysm; information about associated valvular disease; and an estimate of ventricular function, along with blood flow characteristics within the chamber. Magnetic resonance imaging has been reported to be highly accurate in determining the size and location of the aneurysm.[43] Although it lacks the portability of echocardiography, additional advantages include the ability to distinguish among pericardium, thrombus, and myocardium.

The incidence of embolic events in patients with an LV aneurysm may approach 50%.[44] No randomized clinical trial results have supported the use of routine anticoagulation in these patients, but a pooled analysis of reported study results revealed a substantial benefit in patients who received anticoagulation.[45] The usual recommendation for duration of therapy is 3 to 6 months after the diagnosis to allow for endothelialization of the surface of the thrombus. A chronic aneurysm containing an "organized" thrombus probably carries a lower risk of embolization, and the clinical effect of anticoagulation is unclear. On the other hand, a mobile or protruding thrombus, regardless of age, probably carries a high risk for embolization, and anticoagulation is therefore recommended.

Atrial Fibrillation and Left Atrial Thrombus in Patients with Heart Failure

Atrial fibrillation and chronic heart failure are two major cardiovascular problems that are increasing in prevalence. Although precise data are lacking, the prevalence of both atrial fibrillation and congestive heart failure is estimated to be higher than 1% in the general population and increases sharply with age.[46] Atrial fibrillation and heart failure often coexist and may predispose to each other (see Chapter 53).[47,48] The prevalence of atrial fibrillation increases with the severity of systolic heart failure, from 10% to 15% of patients with mild to moderate heart failure (NYHA classes II to III) to more than 40% of patients with advanced heart failure[49] (Figure 52-8). LV dysfunction or clinical heart failure is a major additive risk factor in the development of thromboembolic stroke in patients with atrial fibrillation. Furthermore, most patients with heart failure and atrial fibrillation also have other known risk factors for stroke (hypertension, prior cerebral ischemia—either stroke or TIA—and diabetes mellitus). The presence of any heart failure with or without additional stroke risk factors significantly raises the risk of stroke[48] (Tables 52-1 and 52-2). Several scoring methods to predict the risk of thromboembolism in atrial fibrillation have been developed, including $CHADS_2$ (measure of *c*ongestive heart failure, *h*ypertension, *a*ge, *d*iabetes, and *s*troke or transient ischemic attack), all of which count heart failure as a significant risk factor for thromboembolism.

In addition to stasis in the atria and ventricles of these patients, as mentioned previously, hemostatic abnormalities have been shown to occur in patients with heart failure. Similarly, atrial fibrillation also leads to a hypercoagulable state; this may contribute further to the hemodynamic and hemostatic abnormalities conferred by heart failure.

A substudy of Candesartan in Heart Failure Assessment of Reduction in Mortality and Morbidity (CHARM) revealed that atrial fibrillation is associated with a worse outcome in stable patients with heart failure, regardless of whether heart failure is associated with depressed or relatively preserved LV function; however, those with preserved LV function had better survival than did those with impaired LV function.[51]

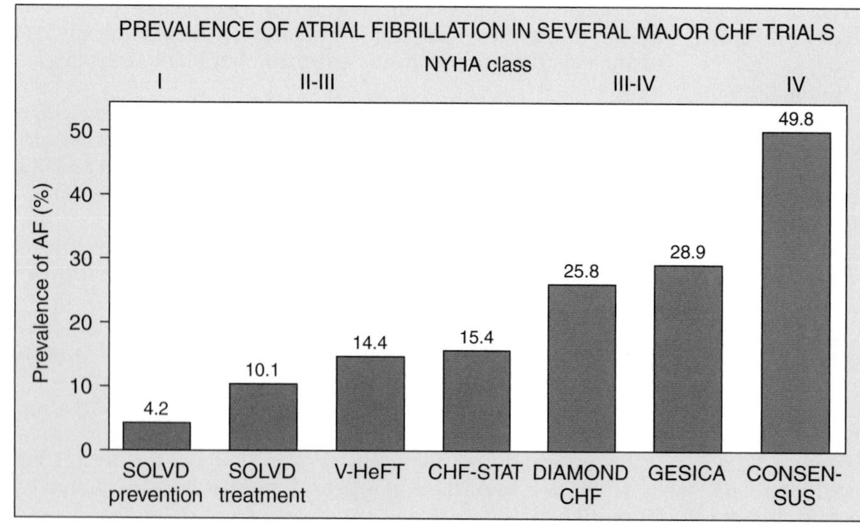

FIGURE 52–8 The prevalence of atrial fibrillation (AF) in several major clinical trials of heart failure, illustrated by severity of heart failure in patients enrolled in each clinical trial. CHF-STAT, Congestive Heart Failure: Survival Trial of Antiarrhythmic Therapy; CONSENSUS, Cooperative North Scandinavian Enalapril Survival Study; DIAMOND CHF, Danish Investigations of Arrhythmia and Mortality on Dofetilide; GESICA, Grupo de Estudio de la Sobrevida en la Insuficiencia Cardiaca en Argentina; NYHA, New York Heart Association; SOLVD, Studies of Left Ventricular Dysfunction; V-HeFT, Veterans Administration Cooperative Vasodilator–Heart Failure Trial. (From Neuberger HR, Mewis C, van Veldhuisen DJ, et al. Management of atrial fibrillation in patients with heart failure. *Eur Heart J* 2007;28:2568-2577.)

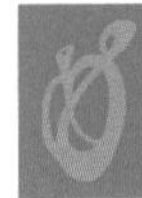

TABLE 52–1 Risk of Stroke in National Registry of Atrial Fibrillation (NRAF) Participants, Stratified by $CHADS_2$ Score*

$CHADS_2$ Score	No. of Patients (*N* = 1733)	No. of Strokes (Total = 94)	NRAF Crude Stroke Rate per 100 Patient-Years	NRAF Stroke Statistics	
				Adjusted Stroke Rate†	95% Confidence Interval
0	120	2	1.2	1.9	1.2-3.0
1	463	17	2.8	2.8	2.0-3.8
2	523	23	3.6	4.0	3.1-5.1
3	337	25	6.4	5.9	4.6-7.3
4	220	19	8.0	8.5	6.3-11.1
5	65	6	7.7	12.5	8.2-17.5
6	5	2	44.0	18.2	10.5-27.4

*$CHADS_2$ score is calculated by adding 1 point each for recent *c*ongestive heart failure, *h*ypertension, *a*ge at least 75 years, and *d*iabetes mellitus and then adding 2 points for having had a prior *s*troke or a transient ischemic attack.

†The adjusted stroke rate is the expected stroke rate per 100 patient-years from the exponential survival model, assuming that aspirin was not taken.

Modified from Neuberger HR, Mewis C, van Veldhuisen DJ, et al. Management of atrial fibrillation in patients with heart failure. *Eur Heart J* 2007;28:2568-2577.

TABLE 52–2 Risk Factors for Ischemic Stroke and Systemic Embolism in Patients with Nonvalvular Atrial Fibrillation

Risk Factors	Relative Risk
Previous stroke or transient ischemic attack	2.5
Diabetes mellitus	1.7
History of hypertension	1.6
Heart failure	1.4
Advanced age (continuous, per decade)	1.4

Data derived from collaborative analysis of five untreated control groups in primary prevention trials. As a group, patients with nonvalvular atrial fibrillation have a risk of thromboembolism about sixfold higher than that of patients in sinus rhythm. Relative risk refers to comparison between patients with atrial fibrillation and patients without these risk factors. (From Fuster V, Rydén LE, Cannom DS, et al. ACC/AHA/ESC 2006 Guidelines for the Management of Patients with Atrial Fibrillation: a report of the American College of Cardiology/American Heart Association Task Force on Practice Guidelines and the European Society of Cardiology Committee for Practice Guidelines (Writing Committee to Revise the 2001 Guidelines for the Management of Patients With Atrial Fibrillation): developed in collaboration with the European Heart Rhythm Association and the Heart Rhythm Society. *Circulation* 2006;114(7):e257-e354.) © American Heart Association. Reprinted with permission.

A similar trend was noted in patients in whom a deterioration necessitated hospitalization. In a series of 478 patients hospitalized with atrial fibrillation and heart failure, those with preserved LV function had a similarly poor prognosis, as did those with depressed LV function.[52]

Anticoagulation with warfarin is extremely effective in preventing stroke in patients with atrial fibrillation (risk reduction, 68%),[53] and is recommended for primary and secondary stroke prevention in these patients. The target INR should be 2 to 3.[50] Of note is that the major bleeding risks of anticoagulation are also present or increased in patients in whom heart failure accompanies atrial fibrillation.[54] However, risk-benefit considerations strongly favor anticoagulation.

Deep Venous Thrombosis in Patients with Heart Failure

Hospitalized patients with heart failure appear to be at increased risk of developing deep venous thrombosis (DVT) in comparison with patients who do not have heart failure. This is probably because stasis of blood increases the risk of DVT formation. Patients with lower ejection fractions have a higher risk of DVT, and the risk appears to be highest in patients who have right-sided heart failure, particularly with excessive lower extremity edema.[55] Heart failure by itself is associated with hypercoagulable state, thereby increasing the chance of intravascular thrombus formation.[41,56] In addition to heart failure itself, traditional risk factors for DVT formation include chronic lung disease and immobilization. Symptoms and signs of concomitant heart failure may overshadow DVT and hinder its detection. Therefore, a high degree of clinical suspicion for DVT is warranted for patients with heart failure.

The reported frequency of DVT in patients with heart failure ranges widely, from 10% to 59%.[17,57] The risk of DVT in patients with heart failure is thought to be similar to that in patients undergoing moderate-risk surgery and in patients with other medical conditions such as malignancy, stroke, acute infection, acute respiratory failure, acute rheumatic disorder, and inflammatory bowel disease.[58] According to the results of the National Hospital Discharge Survey, 0.73% of patients hospitalized with heart failure also received a diagnosis of pulmonary embolism, and 1.03% received a diagnosis of DVT. In patients who had heart failure, in comparison with patients who had no heart failure, the relative risk for pulmonary embolism was 2.15; the relative risk for DVT was 1.21. Of patients with heart failure, patients younger than 40 years had the highest relative risk for pulmonary embolism (11.72), and their relative risk for DVT was 5.46.[59]

Therefore, thromboprophylaxis during immobilization or hospital admission in such patients may be advisable,[60] but DVT prophylaxis is significantly underused in the population of patients with heart failure. In one study, prophylaxis was prescribed for only 46% of the medical patients who had risk factors for DVT.[58]

The regimen for DVT prophylaxis includes unfractionated heparin (5000 IU three times daily) or low molecular weight heparin (LMWH). One study on DVT prophylaxis demonstrated that enoxaparin (40 mg once daily), when given during prolonged bed rest, was at least as effective and safe as treatment with unfractionated heparin (5000 IU three times daily) in preventing DVT. In this study, enoxaparin produced greater benefits in patients with heart failure than in patients with severe respiratory disease.[61]

Treatment of DVT in patients with heart failure is similar to treatment of other medical diseases. Treatment for proximal DVT is clearly indicated. In the guidelines from the Seventh American College of Chest Physicians (ACCP) Conference on Antithrombotic and Thrombolytic Therapy, the following strategies were recommended for treatment of DVT[62]:

1. For patients with objectively confirmed DVT, short-term treatment with subcutaneous LMWH or, alternatively, intravenous unfractionated heparin (both grade 1A).

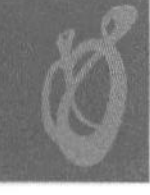

2. For patients with a high clinical suspicion of DVT, treatment with anticoagulants while the outcome of diagnostic tests are awaited (grade 1C+).
3. In acute DVT, initial treatment with LMWH or unfractionated heparin for at least 5 days (grade 1C), initiation of vitamin K antagonist together with LMWH or unfractionated heparin on the first treatment day, and discontinuation of heparin when the INR is stable and greater than 2.0 (grade 1A).
4. For the duration and intensity of treatment for acute DVT of the leg, the recommendations include the following:
   a. For patients with a first episode of DVT secondary to a transient (reversible) risk factor, long-term treatment with a vitamin K antagonist for 3 months is recommended over treatment for shorter periods (grade 1A).
   b. For patients with a first episode of idiopathic DVT, treatment with a vitamin K antagonist for at least 6 to 12 months (grade 1A). The dose of vitamin K antagonist should be adjusted to maintain a target INR of 2.5 (INR range, 2.0 to 3.0) for all treatment durations (grade 1A).
   c. For the prevention of the postthrombotic syndrome, the use of an elastic compression stocking (grade 1A).

PREVENTIVE THERAPY

Aspirin Use for the Prevention of Thromboembolism in Heart Failure

In several analyses, researchers have examined whether aspirin decreases rates of thromboembolic events in patients with heart failure. In the Survival And Ventricular Enlargement (SAVE) trial, patients taking aspirin were observed to have a 56% decreased risk of stroke after a myocardial infarction. In the SOLVD trial, aspirin also decreased the risk of thromboembolic events, but this association was observed only in women, for whom the relative risk reduction was 53%. The first Veteran's Administration Cooperative Vasodilator–Heart Failure Trial (V-HeFT) showed a trend toward a reduction in thromboembolic events, but the second V-HEFT did not show a benefit with aspirin. Results of the more recent Warfarin/Aspirin Study in Heart failure (WASH) and the Warfarin and Antiplatelet Therapy in Chronic Heart Failure (WATCH) trial raised concern about the safety of aspirin use in patients with heart failure: Both demonstrated an increased risk of hospitalization for heart failure, and no mortality-related benefit was observed. In WASH, there was a trend toward a higher mortality rate among patients taking aspirin than among those taking warfarin and those taking placebo. Similarly, when analyzing the SOLVD treatment and prevention conditions, Al-Khadra and colleagues[63] found that patients who took antiplatelet agents had retained but reduced benefit from enalapril.

There are mechanistic reasons and data to support this finding. Upregulation of prostaglandin synthesis may be an important compensatory mechanism that counteracts various mediators of vasoconstriction in patients with heart failure. By interfering with prostaglandin production, aspirin and other cyclooxygenase inhibitors may exert harmful effects. Also, in addition to causing platelet activation and aggregation, thromboxane A_2 directly causes vasoconstriction and is thought to mediate, at least in part, the vasoconstricting effect of angiotensin II.[64] In this case, selective inhibition of thromboxane production may be beneficial. Hall and associates[65] performed a hemodynamic analysis of patients with heart failure in which they demonstrated that enalapril, when given with aspirin or on the day after, blunts vasodilatory hemodynamic effects. These studies and others have raised concern regarding the potential interaction between angiotensin-converting enzyme (ACE) inhibitors and aspirin (Figure 52-9). Aspirin may attenuate the protective effects of ACE inhibitors by inhibiting prostaglandins and thereby enhancing vasoconstriction. In view of these data, it is uncertain whether aspirin provides a benefit in this patient population (Figure 52-10).

Warfarin Use for the Prevention of Thromboembolism

Until the 2000s, there were no randomized controlled trials to help guide physicians in the use of warfarin for prevention of thromboembolism in patients with heart failure. Unfortunately, the controlled trials that do exist are characterized by poor recruitment and have not been sufficiently powered to yield definitive conclusions. In retrospective analyses of large heart failure trials such as SAVE, SOLVD, and V-HeFT, conflicting results have been found. In SOLVD and SAVE, there was a suggestion that warfarin was beneficial in patients with heart failure. In SOLVD, anticoagulant treatment with warfarin was associated with statistically significant decreases in death or hospitalization for heart failure, but the benefit was not derived from decreased risk of thromboembolic events. Warfarin conferred a 24% overall relative risk reduction for all-cause mortality. The SAVE trial demonstrated an 81% reduction in stroke risk in patients treated with anticoagulants.

Other analyses of large heart failure studies have suggested that warfarin does not reduce rates of thromboembolic events in patients with heart failure. In the analysis of the V-HeFT trial data,[66] no significant difference in thromboembolic events was found when patients treated with anticoagulants were compared with those not so treated. In the analysis of the SCD-HeFT data, warfarin use was not associated with reduced risk of thromboembolic events[21] (see Figure 52-7). Unfortunately, these findings are of limited value because anticoagulant use was not randomized or controlled, data were collected retrospectively, and endpoints were not predefined or standardized.

More recently, three randomized controlled trials have been conducted to determine the optimal preventive therapy for thromboembolic events in patients with systolic heart failure (Table 52-3). WASH was a small pilot study designed to assess the feasibility of performing a larger outcome study of whether medical therapy with either aspirin or warfarin could affect outcomes in patients with heart failure.[67] The study included 279 patients with LV systolic dysfunction and ejection fractions lower than 35%. It was an open-label, randomized, placebo-controlled study in which subjects received warfarin (INR target, 2.5), aspirin (300 mg), or placebo. Patients with an absolute indication for or contraindication to aspirin or warfarin were excluded. The combined primary endpoint was all-cause mortality, nonfatal myocardial infarction, and nonfatal stroke; no difference in this endpoint was found among subjects (26% among those taking placebo, 32% among those taking aspirin, and 26% among those taking warfarin). However, patients taking warfarin did have fewer hospitalizations for congestive heart failure (freedom from hospitalization: 48% of those taking placebo and 47% of those taking aspirin, in comparison with 64% of those taking warfarin). Of importance is that this was a small pilot study and therefore not powered to make conclusive statements.

The WATCH study was a randomized, blinded, non–placebo-controlled trial in which 1587 patients with heart failure and ejection fractions lower than 30% were randomly assigned to receive warfarin (target INR, 2.5), aspirin, or

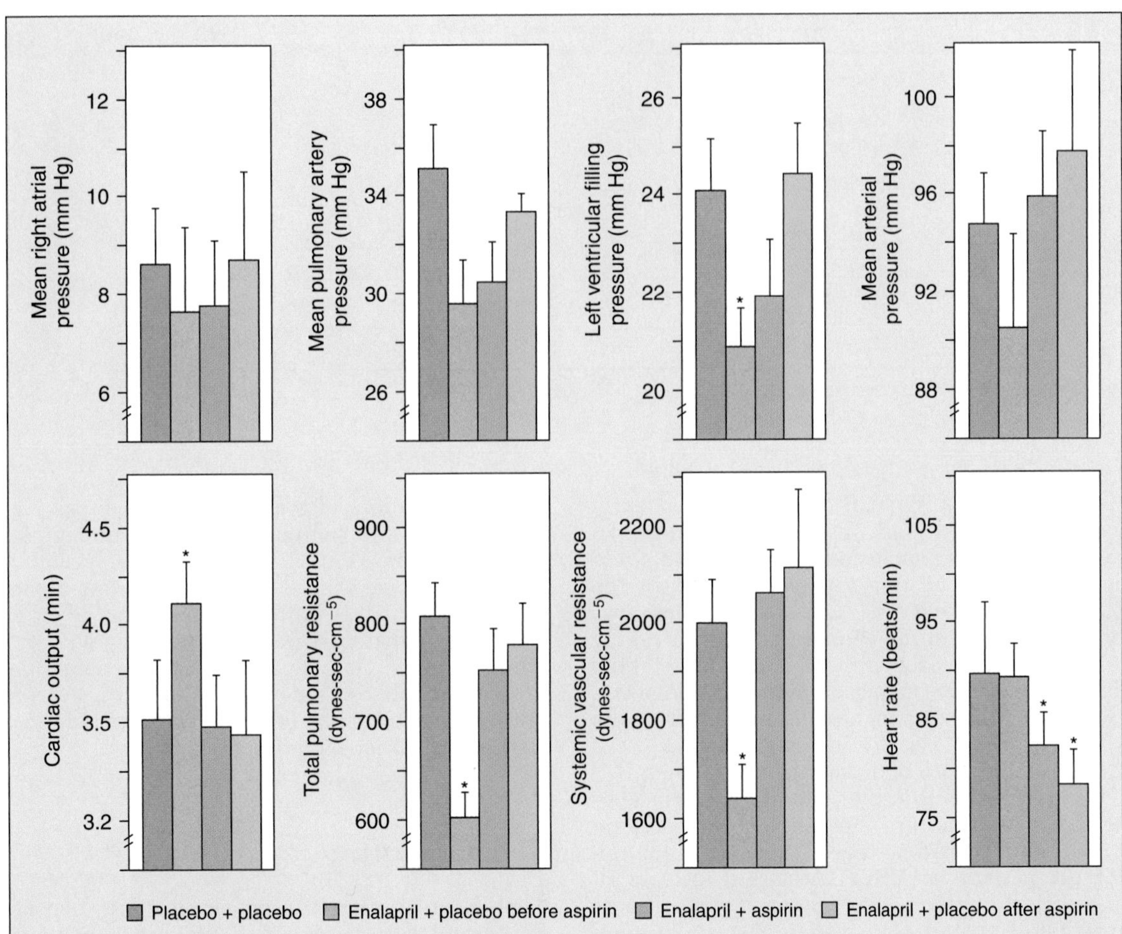

FIGURE 52–9 Hemodynamic values 4 hours after administration of placebo, enalapril, and aspirin, according to respective regimens.*$P < .05$. (From Hall D, Zeitler H, Rudolph W. Counteraction of the vasodilator effects of enalapril by aspirin in severe heart failure. *J Am Coll Cardiol* 1992;20:1549-1555.)

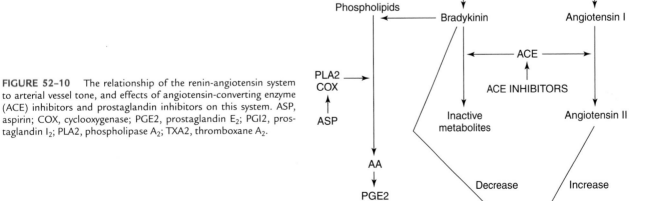

FIGURE 52–10 The relationship of the renin-angiotensin system to arterial vessel tone, and effects of angiotensin-converting enzyme (ACE) inhibitors and prostaglandin inhibitors on this system. ASP, aspirin; COX, cyclooxygenase; PGE2, prostaglandin E_2; PGI2, prostaglandin I_2; PLA2, phospholipase A_2; TXA2, thromboxane A_2.

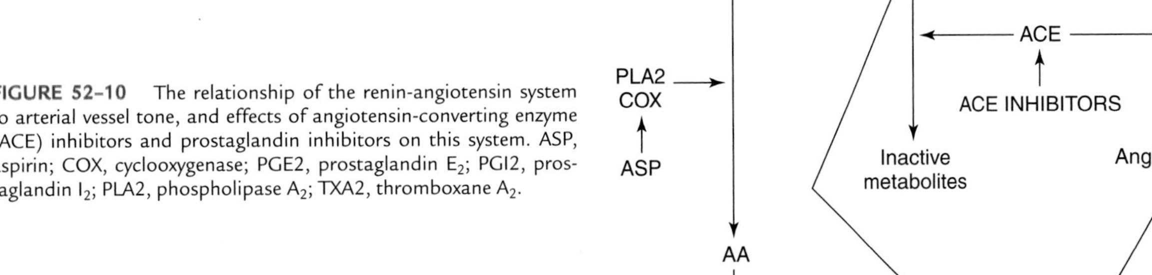

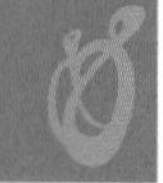

TABLE 52–3 Studies to Determine Optimal Preventive Therapy for Thromboembolic Events

Trial	N	Intervention	Endpoints	Comment
Warfarin/Aspirin Study in Heart failure (WASH)	279	Warfarin (INR, 2.5) versus ASA (300 mg)	Pilot study	Underpowered, signal of increased hospitalizations for heart failure in ASA recipients
Warfarin and Antiplatelet Therapy in Chronic Heart failure (WATCH)	1587	Warfarin versus ASA (162.5 mg) versus clopidogrel (75 mg)	Pilot study	Underpowered, signal of increased hospitalizations for heart failure in ASA recipients
Heart failure Long-term Antithrombotic Study (HELAS)	197	Ischemic: ASA or warfarin Nonischemic: warfarin or placebo (Target INR 2-3)	Stroke, embolization, infarction, hospitalization, exacerbation of heart failure, all-cause death	Underpowered

ASA, acetylsalicylic acid (aspirin); INR, international normalized ratio.

clopidogrel. Unfortunately, WATCH was terminated early because of poor recruitment and was therefore underpowered to yield any definitive conclusions. Nevertheless, there was a strong trend favoring warfarin over aspirin in the incidence of nonfatal stroke (0.7% vs. 2.1%), and there was significantly less hospitalization among the patients taking warfarin (16.1%, in comparison with 22.2% of those taking aspirin and 18.3% of those taking clopidogrel). However, this was offset by a significantly higher rate of bleeding in the patients taking warfarin (5.5%, in comparison with 3.6% of those taking aspirin and 2.5% of those taking clopidogrel).[68]

The findings of a third multicenter, randomized, placebo-controlled trial, the Heart failure Long-term Antithrombotic Study (HELAS), have been reported.[69] This was a double-blind trial of 197 patients with NYHA class II to class IV heart failure and ejection fractions of 35% or lower. Patients with known ischemic heart disease were randomly assigned to receive aspirin (325 mg daily) or warfarin (target INR 2-3). Patients with idiopathic dilated cardiomyopathy were randomly assigned to receive warfarin or placebo. Patients with reversible ischemia, atrial fibrillation, mitral valve disease, hypertrophic cardiomyopathy, known LV thrombi, contraindication to aspirin or warfarin, and uncontrolled hypertension were excluded. Subjects who developed atrial fibrillation were withdrawn from the study. Primary endpoints were nonfatal stroke, peripheral or pulmonary embolism, myocardial infarction, rehospitalization, exacerbation of heart failure, or death from any cause. Overall, the event rate was very low; the incidence of thromboembolic events was 2.2 per 100 patient-years. No difference was observed between aspirin and warfarin in the patients with ischemic cardiomyopathy, whereas among patients with nonischemic cardiomyopathy, there was a trend toward a benefit of warfarin (8.9 events per 100 patient-years, in comparison with 14.8 events per 100 patient-years among the placebo recipients). Unfortunately, this study was also characterized by enrollment problems, which again left the data underpowered to distinguish the differences in outcome between the treatment conditions.

When clinicians consider the option of anticoagulation, it is prudent to assess potential bleeding risks. Previous studies of risks of major hemorrhage in patients receiving long-term warfarin have revealed ranges of two to three events per 100 patient-years. In the Stroke Prevention in Atrial Fibrillation (SPAF) trial, the risk of major bleeding was 2.3% per 100 patient-years.[70] A more recent study was designed to assess the rates of thromboembolism and bleeding in a cohort of ambulatory patients with atrial fibrillation. Of the 425 patients, 40% had concomitant heart failure, and the overall rate of major bleeding events was 2.6% over 2 years.[71] In another study of patients older than 65 years with atrial fibrillation who had just initiated warfarin treatment, the aggregate rate of major hemorrhage was 7.2% per 100 person-years and significantly higher among patients older than 80 years (13.08%, in comparison with 4.75% for patients younger than 80 years). This rate, higher than previously reported, is probably a reflection of an older cohort and the fact that only patients initiating warfarin treatment were included. In view of the aging population and the growing number of elderly patients with heart failure, this study underscores the importance of considering the potential risks of anticoagulation.[72]

THE FUTURE

There is great interest in developing newer agents to inhibit the coagulation cascade and platelet activation. The motivation for this development is related to improving the efficacy, safety, and ease of use of current agents. In addition, large patient populations would benefit from better drugs. The antithrombotic agents currently used have a poor safety index. Among patients taking long-term anticoagulant agents, the yearly incidence of a severe bleeding complication is 1% to 2%. In addition, currently available antithrombotic agents are sometimes difficult to use because of their mode of administration (continuous intravenous or multiple subcutaneous injections) and the requirement of repeated control of intensity and dose adjustments. The older anticoagulants such as heparins and coumarins are nonspecific inhibitors of the coagulation pathway. Specific inhibitors have been investigated, and interest continues in development of new nonspecific drugs. Similarly, new platelet function inhibitors are being developed for cardiovascular disease (Table 52-4, Figure 52-11). Researchers are investigating which of these broad categories of drugs—antiplatelet or coagulation cascade inhibitors—will be optimal for prevention of death, myocardial infarction, stroke, and thromboembolism, balanced against the risk of bleeding. The ongoing Warfarin versus Aspirin in Reduced Cardiac Ejection Fraction (WARCEF) trial is a double-blind, multicenter study of patients with ejection fraction lower than 35% and NYHA classes I to IV heart failure, in which researchers are investigating rates of all-cause mortality, stroke, and intracranial hemorrhage in patients receiving aspirin or warfarin[73]; the results should provide a basis for the question of whether anticoagulants are superior to antiplatelet agents. Once this study is completed, secondary-level questions pertaining to newer antithrombotic and antiplatelet agents in comparison with older agents can be studied. So far, the newer agents have not proved to be safer because they confer similar bleeding risks, but they may be more effective and easier to use than the currently available treatments.

TABLE 52–4 Targets for New Anticoagulants

Inhibitors of Initiation of Coagulation
Tissue factor pathway inhibitor (TFPI) (recombinant)
Nematode anticoagulant peptide (NAPc2)
Active site-blocked factor VIIa (FVIIa$_i$)
Inhibitors of Propagation of Coagulation
Factor IXa inhibitors
Direct factor Xa inhibitors
• Razaxaban
• BAY-597939
• YM-150
• DU-176b
Indirect factor Xa inhibitors
• Fondaparinux
• Idraparinux
• Orally available heparins
Inhibitors of factors VIIIa and Va
Protein C
Activated protein C
Soluble thrombomodulin
Thrombin Inhibitors
Hirudin
Bivalirudin
Argatroban
Ximelagatran
Dabigatran
Orally available heparins

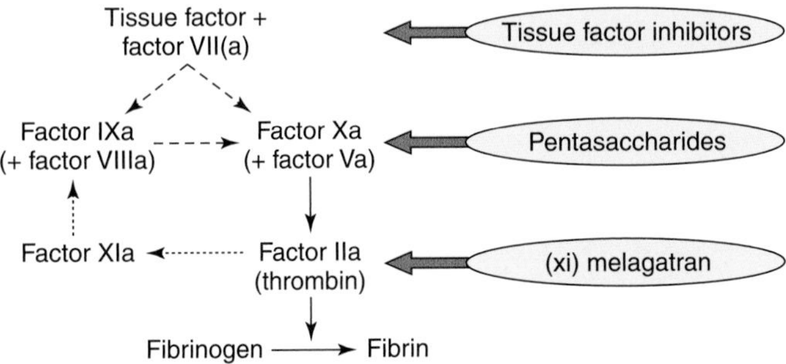

FIGURE 52–11 Schematic representation of the function of the coagulation system and specific effect of the new antithrombotic agents. Coagulation starts when tissue factor is exposed to the blood and binds to factor VIIa. The tissue factor–factor VIIa complex then activates factor X, which leads to conversion of prothrombin to thrombin and subsequent formation of fibrin. An essential amplification loop consists of factor IX activation mediated by the tissue factor–factor VIIa complex, which leads to additional activation of factor Xa (*interrupted arrows*). A second amplification loop is formed by activation of factor XI by thrombin (*broken arrows*), which results in more activation of factor IXa and, subsequently, more generation of factor Xa. (From Levi M. New antithrombotics in the treatment of thromboembolic disease. *Eur J Intern Med* 2005;16:230-237.)

REFERENCES

1. Kapur, N. K., Deming, C. B., Kapur, S., et al. (2007). Hemodynamic modulation of endocardial thromboresistance. *Circulation, 115*, 67–75.
2. Jafri, S. M., Ozawa, T., Mammen, E., et al. (1993). Platelet function, thrombin and fibrinolytic activity in patients with heart failure. *Eur Heart J, 14*, 205–212.
3. Yamamoto, K., Ikeda, U., Furuhashi, K., et al. (1995). The coagulation system is activated in idiopathic cardiomyopathy. *J Am Coll Cardiol, 25*, 1634–1640.
4. Sbarouni, E., Bradshaw, A., Andreotti, F., et al. (1994). Relationship between hemostatic abnormalities and neuroendocrine activity in heart failure. *Am Heart J, 127*, 607–612.
5. Chong, A. Y., Freestone, B., Patel, J., et al. (2006). Endothelial activation, dysfunction, and damage in congestive heart failure and the relation to brain natriuretic peptide and outcomes. *Am J Cardiol, 97*, 671–675.
6. Fischer, D., Rossa, S., Landmesser, U., et al. (2005). Endothelial dysfunction in patients with chronic heart failure is independently associated with increased incidence of hospitalization, cardiac transplantation, or death. *Eur Heart J, 26*, 65–69.
7. Uretsky, B. F., Thygesen, K., Armstrong, P. W., et al. (2000). Acute coronary findings at autopsy in heart failure patients with sudden death: results from the Assessment of Treatment with Lisinopril And Survival (ATLAS) trial. *Circulation, 102*, 611–616.
8. Parry, G. C., & Mackman, N. (1995). Transcriptional regulation of tissue factor expression in human endothelial cells. *Arterioscler Thromb Vasc Biol, 15*, 612–621.
9. Mechtcheriakova, D., Wlachos, A., Holzmüller, H., et al. (1999). Vascular endothelial cell growth factor–induced tissue factor expression in endothelial cells is mediated by EGR-1. *Blood, 93*, 3811–3823.
10. Pasceri, V., Willerson, J. T., & Yeh, E. T. (2000). Direct proinflammatory effect of C-reactive protein on human endothelial cells. *Circulation, 102*, 2165–1268.
11. Ballou, S. P., & Lozanski, G. (1992). Induction of inflammatory cytokine release from cultured human monocytes by C-reactive protein. *Cytokine, 4*, 361–368.
12. Ambrose, J. A., Winters, S. L., Arora, R. R., et al. (1985). Coronary angiographic morphology in myocardial infarction: a link between the pathogenesis of unstable angina and myocardial infarction. *J Am Coll Cardiol, 6*, 1233–1238.
13. Hinkle, L. E., Jr., & Thaler, H. T. (1982). Clinical classification of cardiac deaths. *Circulation, 65*, 457–464.
14. Goldstein, S., Landis, J. R., Leighton, R., et al. (1981). Characteristics of the resuscitated out-of-hospital cardiac arrest victim with coronary heart disease. *Circulation, 64*, 977–984.
15. Roberts, W. C., Siegel, R. J., & McManus, B. M. (1987). Idiopathic dilated cardiomyopathy: analysis of 152 necropsy patients. *Am J Cardiol, 60*, 1340–1355.
16. Meschia, J. F. (2000). Management of acute ischemic stroke. What is the role of tPA and antithrombotic agents? *Postgrad Med, 107*(6), 85–86, 89-93.
17. Samama, M. M. (2000). An epidemiologic study of risk factors for deep vein thrombosis in medical outpatients: the Sirius study. *Arch Intern Med, 160*, 3415–3420.
18. Anderson, F. A., Jr., Wheeler, H. B., Goldberg, R. J., et al. (1991). A population-based perspective of the hospital incidence and case-fatality rates of deep vein thrombosis and pulmonary embolism. The Worcester DVT Study. *Arch Intern Med, 151*, 933–938.
19. Isnard, R., & Komajda, M. (2001). Thromboembolism in heart failure, old ideas and new challenges. *Eur J Heart Fail, 3*, 265–269.
20. Kannel, W. B., Wolf, P. A., & Verter, J. (1983). Manifestations of coronary disease predisposing to stroke. The Framingham study. *JAMA, 250*, 2942–2946.
21. Freudenberger, R. S., Hellkamp, A. S., Halperin, J. L., et al. (2007). Risk of thromboembolism in heart failure: an analysis from the Sudden Cardiac Death in Heart Failure Trial (SCD-HeFT). *Circulation, 115*, 2637–2641.
22. Dries, D. L., Rosenberg, Y. D., Waclawiw, M. A., et al. (1997). Ejection fraction and risk of thromboembolic events in patients with systolic dysfunction and sinus rhythm: evidence for gender differences in the studies of left ventricular dysfunction trials. *J Am Coll Cardiol, 29*, 1074–1080.
23. Loh, E., Sutton, M. S., Wun, C. C., et al. (1997). Ventricular dysfunction and the risk of stroke after myocardial infarction. *N Engl J Med, 336*, 251–257.
24. Hays, A. G., Sacco, R. L., Rundek, T., et al. (2006). Left ventricular systolic dysfunction and the risk of ischemic stroke in a multiethnic population. *Stroke, 37*, 1715–1719.
25. Pullicino, P. M., Halperin, J. L., & Thompson, J. L. (2000). Stroke in patients with heart failure and reduced left ventricular ejection fraction. *Neurology, 54*, 288–294.
26. Katz, S. D., Marantz, P. R., Biasucci, L., et al. (1993). Low incidence of stroke in ambulatory patients with heart failure: a prospective study. *Am Heart J, 126*, 141–146.
27. Eguchi, K., Kario, K., & Shimada, K. (2003). Greater impact of coexistence of hypertension and diabetes on silent cerebral infarcts. *Stroke, 34*, 2471–2474.
28. Büsing, K. A., Schulte-Sasse, C., Flüchter, S., et al. (2005). Cerebral infarction: incidence and risk factors after diagnostic and interventional cardiac catheterization—prospective evaluation at diffusion-weighted MR imaging. *Radiology, 235*, 177–183.
29. Friday, G., Sutter, F., Curtin, A., et al. (2005). Brain magnetic resonance imaging abnormalities following off-pump cardiac surgery. *Heart Surg Forum, 8*(2), E105–E109.
30. Giele, J. L., Witkamp, T. D., Mali, W. P., et al. (2004). Silent brain infarcts in patients with manifest vascular disease. *Stroke, 35*, 742–746.
31. Gruhn, N., Larsen, F. S., Boesgaard, S., et al. (2001). Cerebral blood flow in patients with chronic heart failure before and after heart transplantation. *Stroke, 32*, 2530–2533.
32. Choi, B. R., Kim, J. S., Yang, Y. J., et al. (2006). Factors associated with decreased cerebral blood flow in congestive heart failure secondary to idiopathic dilated cardiomyopathy. *Am J Cardiol, 97*, 1365–1369.
33. Kontny, F., Dale, J., Hegrenaes, L., et al. (1993). Left ventricular thrombosis and arterial embolism after thrombolysis in acute anterior myocardial infarction: predictors and effects of adjunctive antithrombotic therapy. *Eur Heart J, 14*, 1489–1492.
34. Zielinska, M., Kaczmarek, K., & Tylkowski, M. (2008). Predictors of left ventricular thrombus formation in acute myocardial infarction treated with successful primary angioplasty with stenting. *Am J Med Sci, 335*, 171–176.
35. Weinsaft, J. W., Kim, H. W., Shah, D. J., et al. (2008). Detection of left ventricular thrombus by delayed-enhancement cardiovascular magnetic resonance prevalence and markers in patients with systolic dysfunction. *J Am Coll Cardiol, 52*, 148–157.
36. Sacco, R. L., Adams, R., Albers, G., et al. (2006). Guidelines for prevention of stroke in patients with ischemic stroke or transient ischemic attack: a statement for healthcare professionals from the American Heart Association/American Stroke Association Council on Stroke: co-sponsored by the Council on Cardiovascular Radiology and Intervention: the American Academy of Neurology affirms the value of this guideline. *Circulation, 113*(10), e409–e449.
37. Antman, E. M., Anbe, D. T., Armstrong, P. W., et al. (2004). ACC/AHA guidelines for the management of patients with ST-elevation myocardial infarction—executive summary: a report of the American College of Cardiology/American Heart Association Task Force on Practice Guidelines (Writing Committee to Revise the 1999 Guidelines for the Management of Patients With Acute Myocardial Infarction). *Circulation, 110*, 588–636.
38. Vlodaver, Z., Coe, J. I., & Edwards, J. E. (1975). True and false left ventricular aneurysms. Propensity for the latter to rupture. *Circulation, 51*, 567–572.
39. Friedman, B. M., & Dunn, M. I. (1995). Postinfarction ventricular aneurysms. *Clin Cardiol, 18*, 505–511.

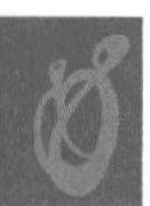

40. Tikiz, H., Balbay, Y., Atak, R., et al. (2001). The effect of thrombolytic therapy on left ventricular aneurysm formation in acute myocardial infarction: relationship to successful reperfusion and vessel patency. *Clin Cardiol, 24*, 656–662.
41. Lip, G. Y., & Gibbs, C. R. (1999). Does heart failure confer a hypercoagulable state? Virchow's triad revisited. *J Am Coll Cardiol, 33*, 1424–1426.
42. Reeder, G. S., Lengyel, M., Tajik, A. J., et al. (1981). Mural thrombus in left ventricular aneurysm: incidence, role of angiography, and relation between anticoagulation and embolization. *Mayo Clin Proc, 56*(2), 77–81.
43. Kerkhoff, G. O., Höfs, C., Roer, N., et al. (2004). Images in cardiovascular medicine. Left ventricular pseudoaneurysm: clinical role of cardiovascular magnetic resonance imaging. *Circulation, 109*(20), e222–e223.
44. Lapeyre, A. C., III, Steele, P. M., Kazmier, F. J., et al. (1985). Systemic embolism in chronic left ventricular aneurysm: incidence and the role of anticoagulation. *J Am Coll Cardiol, 6*, 534–538.
45. Sherman, D. G., Dyken, M. L., Fisher, M., et al. (1989). Antithrombotic therapy for cerebrovascular disorders. *Chest, 95*(Suppl. 5), S140–S155.
46. Rosamond, W., Flegal, K., Friday, G., et al. (2007). Heart disease and stroke statistics—2007 update: a report from the American Heart Association Statistics Committee and Stroke Statistics Subcommittee. *Circulation, 115*(5), e69–e171.
47. Maisel, W. H., & Stevenson, L. W. (2003). Atrial fibrillation in heart failure: epidemiology, pathophysiology, and rationale for therapy. *Am J Cardiol, 91*(6A), D2–D8.
48. Neuberger, H. R., Mewis, C., van Veldhuisen, D. J., et al. (2007). Management of atrial fibrillation in patients with heart failure. *Eur Heart J, 28*, 2568–2577.
49. van Veldhuisen, D. J., Aass, H., Allaf, D., et al. (2006). Presence and development of atrial fibrillation in chronic heart failure. Experiences from the MERIT-HF Study. *Eur J Heart Fail, 8*, 539–546.
50. Fuster, V., Rydén, L. E., Cannom, D. S., et al. (2006). ACC/AHA/ESC 2006 Guidelines for the Management of Patients with Atrial Fibrillation: a report of the American College of Cardiology/American Heart Association Task Force on Practice Guidelines and the European Society of Cardiology Committee for Practice Guidelines (Writing Committee to Revise the 2001 Guidelines for the Management of Patients With Atrial Fibrillation): developed in collaboration with the European Heart Rhythm Association and the Heart Rhythm Society. *Circulation, 114*(7), e257–e354. [Erratum, *Circulation*, 2007;116(6):e138.].
51. Olsson, L. G., Swedberg, K., Ducharme, A., et al. (2006). Atrial fibrillation and risk of clinical events in chronic heart failure with and without left ventricular systolic dysfunction: results from the Candesartan in Heart failure Assessment of Reduction in Mortality and morbidity (CHARM) program. *J Am Coll Cardiol, 47*, 1997–2004.
52. Parkash, R., Maisel, W. H., Toca, F. M., et al. (2005). Atrial fibrillation in heart failure: high mortality risk even if ventricular function is preserved. *Am Heart J, 150*, 701–706.
53. Hart, R. G., Pearce, L. A., Halperin, J. L., et al. (1994). Aspirin in elderly atrial fibrillation patients. *Stroke, 25*, 1525–1526.
54. DiMarco, J. P., Flaker, G., Waldo, A. L., et al. (2005). Factors affecting bleeding risk during anticoagulant therapy in patients with atrial fibrillation: observations from the Atrial Fibrillation Follow-up Investigation of Rhythm Management (AFFIRM) study. *Am Heart J, 149*, 650–656.
55. Monreal, M., Muñoz-Torrero, J. F., Naraine, V. S., et al. (2006). Pulmonary embolism in patients with chronic obstructive pulmonary disease or congestive heart failure. *Am J Med, 119*, 851–858.
56. Gibbs, C. R., Blann, A. D., Watson, R. D., et al. (2001). Abnormalities of hemorheological, endothelial, and platelet function in patients with chronic heart failure in sinus rhythm: effects of angiotensin-converting enzyme inhibitor and beta-blocker therapy. *Circulation, 103*, 1746–1751.
57. Cogo, A., Bernardi, E., Prandoni, P., et al. (1994). Acquired risk factors for deep-vein thrombosis in symptomatic outpatients. *Arch Intern Med, 154*, 164–168.
58. Ageno, W., Squizzato, A., Ambrosini, F., et al. (2002). Thrombosis prophylaxis in medical patients: a retrospective review of clinical practice patterns. *Haematologica, 87*, 746–750.
59. Beemath, A., Stein, P. D., Skaf, E., et al. (2006). Risk of venous thromboembolism in patients hospitalized with heart failure. *Am J Cardiol, 98*, 793–795.
60. Geerts, W. H., Pineo, G. F., Heit, J. A., et al. (2004). Prevention of venous thromboembolism: the Seventh ACCP Conference on Antithrombotic and Thrombolytic Therapy. *Chest, 126*(Suppl. 3), S338–S400.
61. Kleber, F. X., Witt, C., Vogel, G., et al. (2003). Randomized comparison of enoxaparin with unfractionated heparin for the prevention of venous thromboembolism in medical patients with heart failure or severe respiratory disease. *Am Heart J, 145*, 614–621.
62. Büller, H. R., Agnelli, G., Hull, R. D., et al. (2004). Antithrombotic therapy for venous thromboembolic disease: the Seventh ACCP Conference on Antithrombotic and Thrombolytic Therapy. *Chest, 126*(Suppl. 3), S401–428S.
63. Al-Khadra, A. S., Salem, D. N., Rand, W. M., et al. (1998). Antiplatelet agents and survival: a cohort analysis from the Studies of Left Ventricular Dysfunction (SOLVD) trial. *J Am Coll Cardiol, 31*, 419–425.
64. Baur, L. H., Schipperheyn, J. J., van der Laarse, A., et al. (1995). Combining salicylate and enalapril in patients with coronary artery disease and heart failure. *Br Heart J, 73*, 227–236.
65. Hall, D., Zeitler, H., & Rudolph, W. (1992). Counteraction of the vasodilator effects of enalapril by aspirin in severe heart failure. *J Am Coll Cardiol, 20*, 1549–1555.
66. Dunkman, W. B., Johnson, G. R., Carson, P. E., et al. (1993). Incidence of thromboembolic events in congestive heart failure. The V-HeFT VA Cooperative Studies Group. *Circulation, 87*(Suppl. 6), VI-94–VI-101.
67. Cleland, J. G., Findlay, I., Jafri, S., et al. (2004). The Warfarin/Aspirin Study in Heart failure (WASH): a randomized trial comparing antithrombotic strategies for patients with heart failure. *Am Heart J, 148*, 157–164.
68. Cleland, J. G., Ghosh, J., Freemantle, N., et al. (2004). Clinical trials update and cumulative meta-analyses from the American College of Cardiology: WATCH, SCD-HeFT, DINAMIT, CASINO, INSPIRE, STRATUS-US, RIO-Lipids and cardiac resynchronisation therapy in heart failure. *Eur J Heart Fail, 6*, 501–508.
69. Cokkinos, D. V., Haralabopoulos, G. C., Kostis, J. B., et al. (2006). Efficacy of antithrombotic therapy in chronic heart failure: the HELAS study. *Eur J Heart Fail, 8*, 428–432.
70. Hart, R. G., Halperin, J. L., Pearce, L. A., et al. (2003). Lessons from the Stroke Prevention in Atrial Fibrillation trials. *Ann Intern Med, 138*, 831–838.
71. Parkash, R., Wee, V., Gardner, M. J., et al. (2007). The impact of warfarin use on clinical outcomes in atrial fibrillation: a population-based study. *Can J Cardiol, 23*, 457–461.
72. Hylek, E. M., Evans-Molina, C., Shea, C., et al. (2007). Major hemorrhage and tolerability of warfarin in the first year of therapy among elderly patients with atrial fibrillation. *Circulation, 115*, 2689–2696.
73. Pullicino, P., Thompson, J. L., Barton, B., et al. (2006). Warfarin versus Aspirin in patients with Reduced Cardiac Ejection Fraction (WARCEF): rationale, objectives, and design. *J Card Fail, 12*(1), 39–46.
74. Yavin, Y. Y., Wolozinsky, M., & Cohen, A. T. (2005). New antithrombotics in the prevention of thromboembolic disease. *Eur J Intern Med, 16*, 257–266.
75. Levi, M. (2005). New antithrombotics in the treatment of thromboembolic disease. *Eur J Intern Med, 16*, 230–237.
76. Freudenberger, R. S., Hellkamp, A. S., Halperin, J. L., et al. (2007). For the SCD-HeFT Investigators. Risk of thromboembolism in heart failure: an analysis from the sudden cardiac death in heart failure trial (SCD-HeFT). *Circulation, May, 115*, 2637–2641

CHAPTER 53

Management of Arrhythmias in Heart Failure

Philip J. Podrid

Supraventricular and ventricular arrhythmias are common in patients with a cardiomyopathy and heart failure, regardless of the etiology. Arrhythmia can cause symptoms, a worsening of heart failure or angina, increased morbidity (such as stroke in atrial fibrillation), or sudden cardiac death. This chapter is a discussion of the evaluation and management of patients with a cardiomyopathy and heart failure who also have arrhythmia.

ATRIAL FIBRILLATION

Although any supraventricular arrhythmia may occur in patients with a cardiomyopathy and heart failure, the most common supraventricular arrhythmia is atrial fibrillation. Also common is atrial flutter, which is generally evaluated and treated in the same way as atrial fibrillation. Atrial fibrillation is present in 22% of patients with heart failure and is associated with increasing age, nonischemic cardiomyopathy, and more severe New York Heart Association (NYHA) functional class (i.e., in <10% of patients with NYHA functional class I heart failure and in ≤50% of those with NYHA functional class IV heart failure).[1,2] It has been observed in almost 25% of patients with diastolic dysfunction, particularly those with a hypertrophic cardiomyopathy.[3]

Both left ventricular dysfunction and heart failure are significant risk factors for atrial fibrillation, increasing the relative risk by more than sixfold.[1,4] In the Framingham Heart Study of 2326 men and 2866 women monitored for 24 years, the 2-year risk ratio for permanent (chronic) atrial fibrillation in patients with heart failure was 8.5 for men and 13.7 for women; the values for transient (paroxysmal) atrial fibrillation were 8.2 and 20.4, respectively.[4] At the 38-year follow-up, heart failure remained the most powerful predictor of atrial fibrillation. Similar findings were noted in another series of 344 patients with heart failure who were monitored for a mean period of 19 months: 28 (8%) developed atrial fibrillation, which became chronic in 17 (5%).[5]

The incidence of atrial fibrillation is high among patients with new-onset heart failure, and the incidence of new heart failure is high among those with atrial fibrillation. As reported by the Framingham Heart Study, 382 patients had both atrial fibrillation and heart failure; 38% had atrial fibrillation first, 41% had heart failure first, and in 21%, both were diagnosed at the same time.[6] The incidence of heart failure among patients with atrial fibrillation was 33 per 1000 person-years, and the incidence of atrial fibrillation among those with heart failure was 54 per 1000 person-years. A multivariate analysis of patients in the Framingham Heart Study showed that in those with a preserved ejection fraction (diastolic dysfunction), an important predictor for the development of heart failure is atrial fibrillation (odds ratio = 4.23).[6]

Hemodynamic Consequences

Atrial fibrillation causes a number of hemodynamic changes that in turn can cause hemodynamic deterioration with worsening symptoms in people who already have clinical heart failure. In addition, atrial fibrillation can precipitate heart failure in patients with asymptomatic left ventricular dysfunction. In patients with normal left ventricular function, it may also cause left ventricular dysfunction and precipitate heart failure; this is termed "*tachycardia-mediated cardiomyopathy.*" As an example, in one study of 3288 subjects in whom atrial fibrillation was diagnosed between 1980 and 2000, 24% developed heart failure during a mean follow-up period of 6.1 years.[7] The following factors may contribute to the hemodynamic changes in atrial fibrillation:

1. Rapid heart rate, which by shortening diastolic filling time can alter left ventricular filling, stroke volume, and cardiac output.
2. Chronic irregularity of rhythm, which results in beat-to-beat (RR) changes in left ventricular filling and left ventricular mechanics. The reduction in left ventricular filling during short RR intervals is not completely compensated by the increased filling during the longer RR intervals.
3. Loss of the atrial contraction, which is required for optimal left ventricular filling; this is of particular importance in patients with underlying heart disease.
4. The development of a rate-related cardiomyopathy (atrial, ventricular, or both) can result in mechanical atrial remodeling and enlargement, which may be associated with the development of mitral regurgitation, another important factor associated with hemodynamic changes in atrial fibrillation.[8,9]
5. Activation of neurohumoral vasoconstrictors such as angiotensin II and norepinephrine[18] and possible secretion of other substances by the cardiomyopathic heart, including proinflammatory cytokines and natriuretic peptide.[10]

Atrial fibrillation and the resultant hemodynamic and neuroendocrine alterations cause electrical and structural (fibrosis) remodeling of the atria, which in turn increases the susceptibility to atrial fibrillation. As a result, atrial fibrillation may beget atrial fibrillation.[11]

Rate Control

The hemodynamic changes resulting from atrial fibrillation can be altered with rate control or conversion to sinus rhythm, which may often result in an improvement in left ventricular function and a decrease in symptoms of heart failure.[12] Rate control can be achieved with drugs that block the atrioventricular node, such as digoxin, β-blockers, calcium channel blockers, or amiodarone,[13] or with radiofrequency ablation of the atrioventricular node.[14] The interruption of atrioventricular conduction by a catheter that delivers radiofrequency energy usually produces complete atrioventricular nodal block, and then a permanent pacemaker must be implanted in order to control the ventricular rate adequately.[15] Atrioventricular nodal ablation with implantation of a permanent pacemaker does not adversely affect long-term outcome, overall quality of life, NYHA functional class, or objective measurements of cardiac function.[15]

Atrioventricular nodal modification, which may reduce the risk of complete atrioventricular block and the need for a pacemaker, is less successful than nodal ablation for rate control in patients with heart failure.

Risk Factors for Atrial Fibrillation

Dilation and an increase in pressure within the left atrium can alter its electrophysiological properties, predisposing to atrial fibrillation; this phenomenon is known as "*electromechanical feedback*."[16] Increases in left atrial pressure and size may occur as a result of increased LV end-diastolic pressure, as occurs with diastolic or systolic dysfunction; an increase in intravascular volume; or the development of mitral regurgitation, as often occurs with left ventricular dilation. Left atrial size is also correlated with height and body surface area.

In animal studies, left atrial enlargement and increased left atrial pressure produced by volume expansion, as occurs in heart failure, decreased the atrial refractory period and action potential duration, thereby predisposing to atrial fibrillation.[17] Stretch of the left atrium results in activation of specific ionic currents, which leads to increased dispersion of refractoriness and alterations in conduction properties that facilitate the occurrence of atrial fibrillation. Lowering left atrial pressure resulted in prompt alleviation of the arrhythmia. The role of left atrial stretch caused by volume or pressure overload was further supported by an animal study in which gadolinium, a blocker of the stretch-activated ion channels in the myocardium, reduced the vulnerability to atrial fibrillation during acute atrial dilation.[18] In patients with a hypertrophic cardiomyopathy, enlarged left atrial volume and reduced left atrial function are predictors of atrial fibrillation.[19]

Slowing or blockage of intra-atrial conduction is manifested as a prolonged P-wave duration (>132 msec) or as late atrial potentials on a signal-averaged electrocardiogram (SAECG). The presence of such slowing or blockage may help predict paroxysmal atrial fibrillation in patients with heart failure, as well as recurrence of atrial fibrillation after cardioversion.[20] An increase in P-wave duration on the SAECG is correlated with increases in pulmonary capillary wedge pressure and left atrial pressure. P-wave dispersion (i.e., the difference between maximum and minimum P-wave durations) evident on a 12-lead electrocardiogram (ECG) may also help predict recurrence of atrial fibrillation.[21]

With heart failure, there is neurohormonal activation with elevated levels of catecholamines and angiotensin II, which promotes structural remodeling and fibrosis in the atrium, predisposing to atrial fibrillation. Atrial natriuretic peptide (ANP) is released from the atria in response to volume expansion and atrial stretch. ANP release is increased in heart failure, and an elevated plasma ANP level may be predictive of atrial fibrillation. In one study of 100 patients with and without atrial fibrillation, those with atrial fibrillation were found to have higher levels of N-terminal ANP (2.6 ng/mL) than were subjects without atrial fibrillation (1.7 ng/mL); this association was independent of left atrial volume and left ventricular ejection fraction (LVEF).[22]

Relationship Between Heart Failure and Stroke Risk in Atrial Fibrillation

There are conflicting data as to whether left ventricular dysfunction and heart failure increase the risk of stroke in patients with atrial fibrillation. In the Stroke Prevention in Atrial Fibrillation (SPAF) trial of 586 patients monitored for a mean of 1.3 years, the yearly incidence of stroke among patients with atrial fibrillation who did not receive anticoagulants was higher than that among patients without clinical heart failure (7% vs. 2.5%).[23] Echocardiographic evidence of left atrial and left ventricular enlargement and dysfunction was the strongest independent predictor of stroke. In contrast, the results of the Veterans Administration Cooperative Vasodilator–Heart Failure Trial (V-HeFT) I and II studies of 1446 men with heart failure monitored for up to 2.5 years did not indicate that atrial fibrillation increased the risk for embolism over that associated with heart failure.[24]

Among patients with a hypertrophic cardiomyopathy, the presence of atrial fibrillation was an independent risk factor for stroke; the risk was significantly higher in patients who did not receive warfarin (31%) than in those who did receive warfarin therapy (18%).[25]

Although atrial fibrillation of any origin is associated with a high risk of systemic embolism, it is likely that in patients with advanced cardiomyopathy, a low cardiac index, and heart failure, atrial fibrillation confers a significant increase in thromboembolism rate. Indeed, in the CHADS2 scoring system (*c*ongestive heart failure, *h*ypertension, *a*ge, *d*iabetes, and *s*troke or transient ischemic attack), the presence of heart failure is an independent predictor of a thromboembolic event in patients with atrial fibrillation.[26] Anticoagulation is beneficial in all such patients, and warfarin therapy is recommended for most; the target international normalized ratio is 2.5 (range, 2.0 to 3.0).[27]

Relationship Between Atrial Fibrillation and Mortality in Heart Failure

The relationship between atrial fibrillation and mortality in heart failure is another area of controversy. Several studies have revealed that atrial fibrillation is not associated with an increase in the rate of mortality, sudden cardiac death, or hospitalization after important prognostic variables are adjusted. In the Carvedilol Or Metoprolol European Trial (COMET) of 3029 patients, the presence of atrial fibrillation was not an independent risk factor for mortality in patients who were taking a β-blocker, according to a multivariate analysis.[28] However, the development of atrial fibrillation during the trial was associated with an increase in mortality in a time-dependent analysis (risk ratio, 1.90; $P < .0001$).

In contrast, other studies have demonstrated that atrial fibrillation is associated with an increased rate of mortality. For example, a 3-year follow-up assessment of 6517 patients in the Studies of Left Ventricular Dysfunction (SOLVD) trials revealed that atrial fibrillation was a significant factor in all-cause mortality (34% vs. 23% of patients without atrial fibrillation), in death from pump failure (16.7% vs. 9.4%), and in the combined endpoint of death or hospitalization for heart failure (45% vs. 33%).[29] In a multivariate analysis,

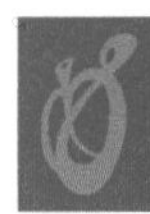

atrial fibrillation remained significantly associated with each of these outcomes (Figure 53-1). Similar results were reported from the Candesartan in Heart Failure Assessment in Reduction of Mortality (CHARM) trial of 7599 patients with symptomatic heart failure caused by either systolic or diastolic dysfunction.[30] Approximately 18% of these patients had atrial fibrillation at baseline. After a median follow-up of 38 months, atrial fibrillation was independently associated with an increase in all-cause mortality in patients with either systolic dysfunction (37% vs. 28% of patients without atrial fibrillation) or diastolic heart failure (24% vs. 14%). In the Valsartan in Acute Myocardial Infarction Trial (VALIANT) of 14,703 patients in whom an acute myocardial infarction was complicated by heart failure or left ventricular dysfunction, atrial fibrillation was associated with significantly higher rates of long-term mortality (adjusted hazard ratio = 1.25; $P = .03$) and adverse cardiovascular events (adjusted hazard ratio = 1.15, $P = .08$).[31]

According to a meta-analysis of studies involving patients with heart failure and either sinus rhythm or atrial fibrillation, the prevalence of atrial fibrillation ranged from 15% to 23% (Figure 53-2).[32] The presence of atrial fibrillation was associated with a worse outcome than was sinus rhythm (odds ratio, 1.33).

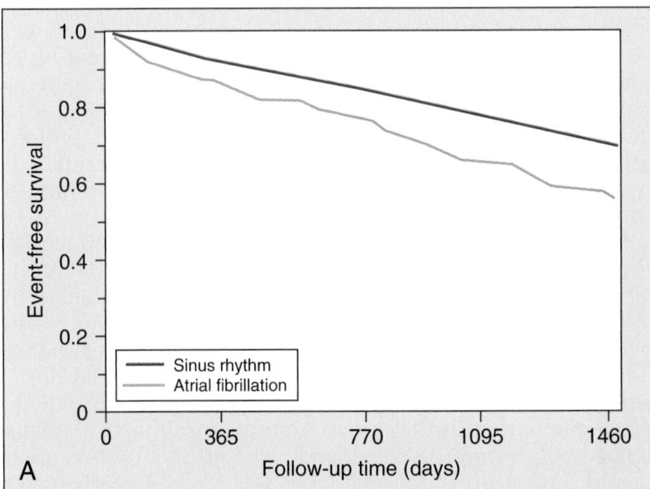

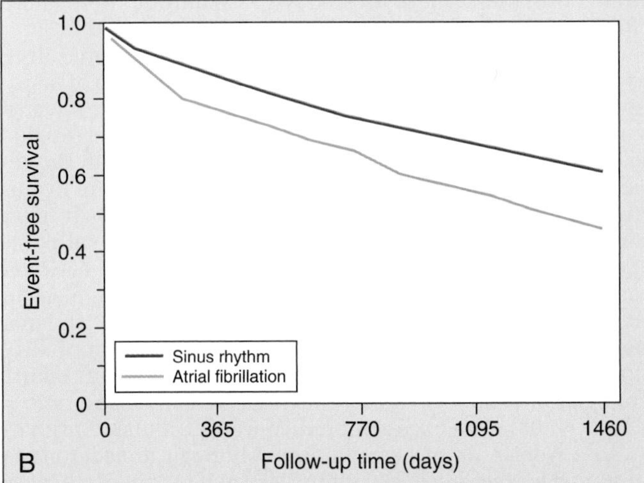

FIGURE 53–1 Among 6517 patients entered in the Studies of Left Ventricular Dysfunction (SOLVD), the presence of atrial fibrillation (AF), in comparison with sinus rhythm, was associated with significantly decreased cumulative rates of survival (66% vs. 77%, $P < .001$) (**A**) and with an increased risk of death or hospitalization for heart failure (45% vs. 33%, $P < .001$) (**B**). (From Dries DL, Exner DV, Gersh BJ, et al. Atrial fibrillation is associated with an increased risk for mortality and heart failure progression in patients with asymptomatic left ventricular systolic dysfunction: a retrospective analysis of the SOLVD trials. *J Am Coll Cardiol* 1998;32:695.)

Optimal pharmacological therapy for heart failure may influence the relationship between atrial fibrillation and survival. This possibility was suggested by observations of patients treated at different times. In one study, the outcomes of 359 patients managed between 1985 and 1989 was compared with those of 391 patients managed between 1990 and 1993; patients with atrial fibrillation managed at the later time had outcomes similar to those of patients without atrial fibrillation. The later patients with atrial fibrillation also had a higher rate of 2-year survival than did earlier patients with atrial fibrillation; this change may have reflected more frequent use of angiotensin-converting enzyme (ACE) inhibitors and amiodarone and less frequent use of class I antiarrhythmic drugs. In another study of 234 patients evaluated for heart transplantation between 1993 and 1996, the presence of atrial fibrillation was not associated with decreased event-free survival (death, placement of a left ventricular assist device, or transplantation).

Treatment of Atrial Fibrillation in Heart Failure

Despite the uncertainty concerning the prognostic implications of atrial fibrillation, treatment is often required for relief of symptoms and for improvement of heart failure, which may worsen or be difficult to manage in the presence of atrial fibrillation. The two approaches to therapy are (1) rate control with an atrioventricular nodal blocking agent (digoxin, β-blocker, or calcium channel blocker) along with anticoagulants and (2) rhythm control with an antiarrhythmic agent to maintain sinus rhythm. Although rate control results in an improvement in symptoms, normal hemodynamics are not restored. This may be an important concern in some patients with systolic heart failure and possibly of more importance in those with heart failure caused by diastolic dysfunction. In addition, there is still a small risk for an embolism even when anticoagulation with warfarin is used. Although rhythm control restores normal hemodynamics and may eliminate the risk of an embolism, this approach often necessitates the use of an antiarrhythmic drug, which may be associated with potential toxicity. Pulmonary vein isolation through radiofrequency ablation is an alternative approach for prevention of intermittent atrial fibrillation; its role in therapy for permanent atrial fibrillation is less well established. In addition, the role of ablation in patients with heart failure is less certain because data are limited.

Drug therapy for atrial fibrillation may be associated with an increase in mortality. In the SPAF trial, for example, in patients with heart failure and atrial fibrillation who did not have ventricular arrhythmias, the use of class I antiarrhythmic drugs was associated with increased mortality (relative risk of 3.3 for cardiac death and 5.8 for arrhythmia-related death).[33] However, SPAF was not a study of mortality and was not designed to evaluate therapy for atrial fibrillation, and the indications for therapy with antiarrhythmic drugs were not certain. Nevertheless, significantly reduced LVEF, a history of clinical heart failure (risk ratio of 2.3), sustained ventricular tachyarrhythmia as the presenting arrhythmia (risk ratio of 3.4), and structural heart disease (risk ratio of 2 to 3) have all been identified as risk factors for the development or aggravation of an arrhythmia with class I antiarrhythmic agents.[34] These drugs are best avoided by patients with heart failure. It has been reported that the class III antiarrhythmic agents are safer in patients with heart failure and are the preferred agents when rhythm control is the approach pursued.

Drugs Used for Rhythm Control in Heart Failure

Amiodarone. Amiodarone is a class III antiarrhythmic agent that has β- and α-blocking activity; potassium-, sodium-, and

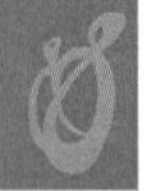

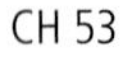

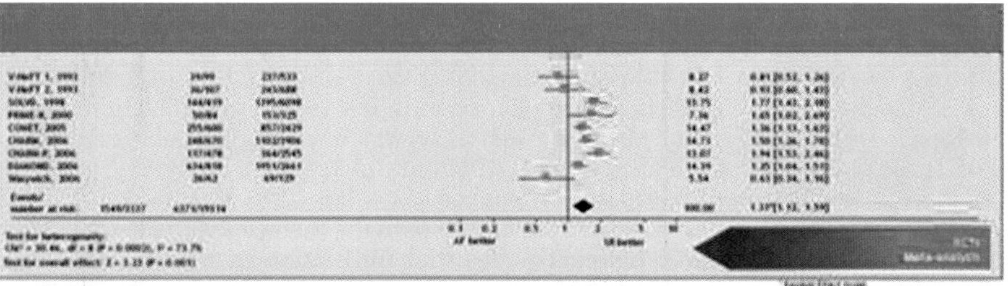

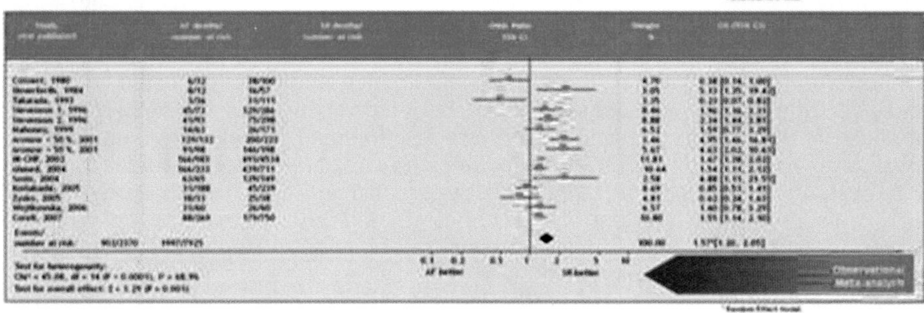

FIGURE 53–2 In a meta-analysis involving 32,946 patients with heart failure who were enrolled in randomized trials, the presence of atrial fibrillation was associated with a worse outcome than was sinus rhythm (odds ratio, 1.33 to 1.57). COMET, Carvedilol Or Metoprolol European Trial; V-HeFT, Veterans Administration Cooperative Vasodilator–Heart Failure Trial , SOLVD, Studies Of Left Ventricular Dysfunction; PRIME, Perspective Randomized studies of Ibopamine on Mortality and Efficacy; CHARM, Carvedilol in Heart failure Assessment of Reduction in Mortality and morbidity; DIAMOND, Danish Investigation of Arrhythmia and Mortality ON Dofetilide. (With permission from Wasywich CA, Pope AJ, Somaratne J, et al. Atrial fribrillation and the risk of death in patients with heart failure: a literature-based meta-analysis. *Intern Med J,* 40:317, 2009.)

calcium channel–blocking activity; and antithyroid activity. It is effective for converting atrial fibrillation to, and for maintaining, sinus rhythm. It also has depressant effects on the atrioventricular node and can slow the ventricular response rate during atrial fibrillation. In the Congestive Heart Failure Survival Trial of Antiarrhythmic Therapy (CHF-STAT) trial, the rate of conversion of atrial fibrillation was higher with amiodarone (31%) than with placebo (8%).[35] Among patients who remained in atrial fibrillation, there was also a 16% to 20% reduction in the mean ventricular rate and a 14% to 22% reduction in the maximum ventricular rate. In addition, amiodarone significantly reduced the development of atrial fibrillation among patients initially in sinus rhythm (4.1%), in comparison with patients who did not receive amiodarone therapy (8.3%).

Amiodarone does not increase mortality among patients with heart failure, although several potential complications are associated with this agent, including bradycardia that may necessitate placement of a pacemaker, as well as hypothyroidism. According to a meta-analysis involving data from 1465 patients treated for a minimum of 12 months, amiodarone was associated with a higher incidence of complications, including thyroid abnormalities, neurological side effects, ocular changes, and bradycardia. Of importance was that there were no cases of torsades de pointes or other forms of proarrhythmia despite the marked prolongation of the QT interval observed with this agent.[36]

Although amiodarone is not approved for treatment of atrial fibrillation, it is the safest and most effective drug for this indication in patients with heart failure; it is therefore the preferred therapy.

Dofetilide. Dofetilide, another class III antiarrhythmic agent, is also effective and safe in heart failure. This fact was established by the Danish Investigation of Arrhythmia and Mortality On Dofetilide in Congestive Heart Failure (DIAMOND-CHF), which enrolled 1518 patients with symptomatic heart failure, including 391 with atrial fibrillation at baseline.[37] Conversion to sinus rhythm was higher with dofetilide than with placebo (12% vs. 1%), and the probability of remaining in sinus rhythm was higher. During a mean follow-up period of 18 months, there was no overall difference in mortality between the patients taking dofetilide (41%) and those taking placebo (42%). However, an analysis by baseline-corrected QT (QTc) interval did reveal a difference in mortality: In patients with a QTc interval shorter than 429 msec, dofetilide was associated with a significant reduction in mortality (risk ratio = 0.4), whereas in patients with a QTc interval longer than 429 msec (risk ratio = 1.3), it was associated with increased mortality. In addition, dofetilide significantly reduced the risk of hospitalization for worsening of heart failure (30%) in comparison with placebo (38%), regardless of the presence of atrial fibrillation or sinus rhythm at baseline.

Sotalol. Although sotalol is effective in the prevention of atrial fibrillation, there are no studies available in patients with heart failure. There has been a concern for worsening of heart failure and an increased risk of significant QTc prolongation and torsades de pointes in these patients. Therefore, it is not considered a first-line therapy for atrial fibrillation in patients with heart failure.

Azimilide. Azimilide is an investigational class III antiarrhythmic agent that is also effective in converting atrial fibrillation and preventing its occurrence. This was evaluated in the Azimilide Postinfarct Survival Evaluation (ALIVE) trial, which enrolled 3381 patients with left ventricular dysfunction who had suffered myocardial infarction.[38] Atrial fibrillation was present at presentation in 93 patients; 27 patients developed atrial fibrillation after study enrollment. Patients treated with azimilide developed atrial fibrillation less often than did those given placebo ($P = .04$). Among patients with atrial fibrillation, those treated with azimilide were more often in sinus rhythm 1 year later ($P = .04$).

Dronedarone. Dronedarone is an antiarrhythmic drug with electrophysiological properties similar to those of amiodarone, but it is devoid of iodine. It does not cause the adverse reactions generally attributed to iodine. The effect of this agent was evaluated in the Anti-arrhythmic Trial with Dronedarone in Moderate to Severe Congestive Heart Failure Evaluating Morbidity Decrease (ANDROMEDA).[39] Although there was no difference in the occurrence of the primary endpoint of total mortality or heart failure hospitalization between patients taking dronedarone (17%) and those taking placebo (12.6%; $P = .12$), this study was terminated after 627 patients were enrolled because of a significant increase in mortality after a median follow-up of 2 months (8.1% of patients taking dronedarone vs. 3.8% of those taking placebo; hazard ratio = 2.13, $P = .03$). The excess mortality was attributable primarily to a worsening of heart failure. Although donedarone is approved for therapy of atrial fibrillation, it is contraindicated in patients with class IV heart failure or those with class II-III heart failure with recent decompensation.

Angiotensin-Converting Enzyme Inhibitors and Angiotensin Receptor Blockers. Although the ACE inhibitors and angiotensin receptor blocking (ARB) agents are not considered specific therapy for atrial fibrillation, data have suggested that they may be effective for prevention of new-onset or recurrent atrial fibrillation. Proposed mechanisms include direct effects of angiotensin blockade on the structural and electrical properties of the atria (reduction in atrial stretch, prevention of atrial fibrosis, prevention of electrical remodeling, and direct antiarrhythmic effects) and indirect effects through improved control of heart failure and hypertension, which are known risk factors for atrial fibrillation. The potential role of these agents in atrial fibrillation was suggested by a meta-analysis involving more than 56,000 patients enrolled in studies of heart failure, status post myocardial infarction, and hypertension and in postcardioversion studies. Overall, ACE inhibitors and ARB agents reduced the relative risk of atrial fibrillation by 28% (P = .0002).[40]

Radiofrequency Ablation

There is growing interest in the use of radiofrequency ablation to produce pulmonary vein isolation in the treatment of atrial fibrillation. However, the role of this technique in preventing atrial fibrillation in patients with underlying left ventricular dysfunction and heart failure is uncertain because data are limited. In one small study, the results of atrial fibrillation ablation in 58 patients with heart failure (NYHA classes II to IV) and LVEF lower than 40% were compared to those in 58 control patients without heart failure.[41] A second ablation was required in 50% of patients with heart failure. At the end of 1 year, 78% of the patients with heart failure and 84% of the controls remained in sinus rhythm, although several patients still required antiarrhythmic drugs. Patients with heart failure experienced a significant increase in exercise duration (from 11 to 14 minutes, $P < .001$), LVEF increased by a mean of 21%, and left ventricular fractional shortening increased by 11%. Although these data are encouraging, there are a number of important limitations, including the small number of highly selected patients, the absence of a control group of patients who did not undergo ablation, and the inclusion of many patients who probably had a tachycardia-mediated cardiomyopathy rather than preexisting structural myocardial disease, as indicated by the fact that LVEF returned to normal in 72% of patients.

In another trial, the same investigators randomly assigned 81 patients with class II or III heart failure and LVEF of 40% or lower to undergo pulmonary vein isolation or atrioventricular nodal ablation and biventricular pacing.[42] After a 6-month follow-up period, 88% of those who underwent ablation were free of atrial fibrillation (although 20% required repeated ablation and 17% were still taking antiarrhythmic drugs). Results for the composite primary endpoint (6-minute walk test, ejection fraction, and quality-of-life score) favored ablation.

Nevertheless, the long-term role of ablation in patients with underlying dilated cardiomyopathy—who often have progressive heart failure, significant left atrial dilation, and fibrosis—is still uncertain.

Radiofrequency ablation has also been used in patients with hypertrophic cardiomyopathy.[43] However, the recurrence rate is as high as 48%, and repeated ablations are often required. In addition, many patients still require antiarrhythmic drug therapy. Therefore, its role in the prevention of atrial fibrillation in hypertrophic cardiomyopathy is also uncertain.

Drugs Used for Rate Control

A strategy of rate control necessitates atrioventricular nodal blockade. Rate control must be assessed not only at rest but also during exercise. Although there are no guidelines in regard to adequate rate control, heart rate targets for the patients in the rate control arm of the Atrial Fibrillation Follow-up Investigation of Rhythm Management (AFFIRM) trial are probably reasonable and include[44] resting heart rate of 80 beats/min or less, 24-hour Holter average heart rate of 100 beats/min or less, and no greater than 110% of the age-predicted maximum, and heart rate of 110 beats/min or less in the 6-minute walk. Rate control can also be assessed with submaximal or maximal exercise electrocardiographic testing. Control is deemed adequate when the peak heart rate is 100% or less of the predicted maximum. An essential component of rate control over time is the absence of symptoms during normal activities or exercise.

β-Blockers (see Chapter 46). Oral β-blockers have a limited role in rhythm control (prevention of atrial fibrillation) in patients with heart failure, although they may be effective when atrial fibrillation is precipitated by marked sympathetic activation: for example, during exercise or with hyperthyroidism.[45] However, they are more widely used as primary therapy for rate control in permanent atrial fibrillation. β-Blockers decrease the resting heart rate but, of more importance, blunt the heart rate response to exercise. β-Blockers have the additional advantage of improving survival in patients with heart failure. However, these drugs must be used with caution because they may exacerbate heart failure, particularly in patients with decompensated heart failure.

Although most β-blockers appear to have similar efficacy, metoprolol or carvedilol are often preferred, largely because they have been shown to reduce mortality among patients with heart failure and are approved therapy for rate control. Bisoprolol, although effective in heart failure, is not approved for rate control.

Digoxin. Digoxin is an effective agent in atrioventricular nodal blockade, the result of increased vagal tone. It is generally less effective for rate control than are β-blockers or calcium channel blockers, particularly during exercise, when vagal tone is low and sympathetic tone is high, blunting any increase in vagal tone. However, in patients with atrial fibrillation who have heart failure caused by systolic dysfunction, the improvement in contractility and the reduction in sympathetic tone, in addition to the increase in vagal tone, may result in a significant reduction in the ventricular rate. Although β-blocker therapy in these patients has been considered preferable, digoxin may be useful in patients who do not achieve adequate control of heart rate with β-blockers alone, in patients who cannot tolerate the addition or increased doses of a β-blocker because of acute decompensated heart failure, or in patients for whom digoxin would be added to improve heart failure symptoms that are independent of atrial fibrillation. In patients with the acute onset of atrial fibrillation that is the result of decompensated heart failure, digoxin and the improvement in left ventricular function and hemodynamics may result in conversion of atrial fibrillation to sinus rhythm.

Calcium Channel Blockers. The nondihydropyridine calcium channel blockers verapamil and diltiazem are useful in directly blocking the atrioventricular node and slowing the ventricular rate in atrial fibrillation. Verapamil is more effective than diltiazem. However, both these agents have negative inotropic effects and are therefore not often prescribed in patients with heart failure because of a risk of heart failure exacerbation; if they are necessary, they should be used cautiously.

Amiodarone. Although amiodarone is usually used to maintain sinus rhythm, this agent can also slow the ventricular rate in patients who remain in atrial fibrillation or in whom atrial fibrillation recurs; this is a result of its β- and calcium channel–blocking activity.

Nonpharmacological Therapy for Rate Control

Radiofrequency ablation of the atrioventricular node is an alternative approach when rate control is not achieved with pharmacological therapy or when the atrioventricular nodal blocking drugs are poorly tolerated. Because atrioventricular nodal ablation produces complete heart block, a permanent pacemaker is usually necessary. However, right ventricular pacing may cause interventricular and intraventricular dyssynchrony,

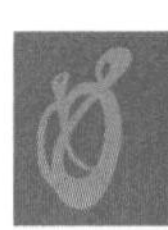

simulating the effect of left bundle branch block.[46] The right ventricle contracts before the left ventricle, and the septum contracts before the lateral wall of the left ventricle. Thus, ventricular pacing can impair left ventricular systolic function, reduce functional status, and increase mortality. This is of particular importance for patients with underlying left ventricular dysfunction and heart failure, who may be at the highest risk for clinical deterioration with right ventricular pacing. In such patients, biventricular pacing, also called "cardiac resynchronization therapy" (CRT), may be a preferred approach. This was studied in the Post AV [atrioventricular] Nodal Ablation Evaluation (PAVE), in which 184 patients with chronic atrial fibrillation and heart failure underwent atrioventricular node ablation and were randomly assigned to receive standard right ventricular pacing or CRT.[47] After a 6-month follow-up period, CRT was associated with significantly greater postablation increases in 6-minute walking distance, peak oxygen consumption with exercise, and exercise duration than was standard right ventricular pacing. CRT resulted in preservation of baseline systolic function, whereas the LVEF fell from 45% to 41% in patients treated with right ventricular pacing. The benefits of CRT were more prominent in patients with an LVEF of 45% or lower or with NYHA class II or III heart failure than in patients with a higher LVEF or NYHA class I heart failure. On the basis of these observations, CRT has been approved in patients who have undergone atrioventricular nodal ablation and have NYHA class II or III heart failure.

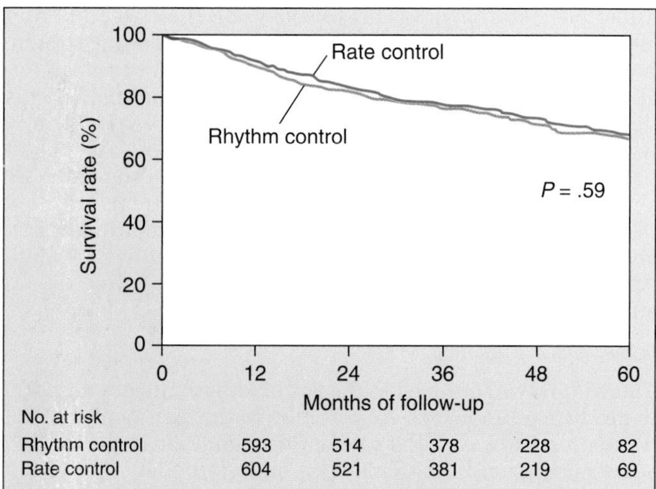

FIGURE 53–3 In the Atrial Fibrillation and Congestive Heart Failure (AF-CHF) trial, a strategy of rate control was compared with a strategy of rhythm control in 1376 patients with heart failure and atrial fibrillation. There was no difference in the primary endpoint of total cardiovascular mortality (*P* = .59). (With permission from Roy D, Talajic M, Nattel S, et al. Rhythm control versus rate control for atrial fibrillation and heart failure. *N Engl J Med* 2008;358:2667. Copyright © 2008, Massachusetts Medical Society. All rights reserved.)

Rate Control Versus Rhythm Control

For the management of atrial fibrillation, a strategy of rate control with anticoagulation has been compared with that of rhythm control with an antiarrhythmic drug. The largest study, AFFIRM, enrolled 4060 patients; 26% had depressed left ventricular function, and 23% had a history of heart failure.[44] Overall, rates of occurrence of the primary endpoint (overall mortality) and the composite secondary endpoint (death, disabling stroke, disabling anoxic encephalopathy, major bleeding, and cardiac arrest) were the same with the two strategies. A subset analysis of patients with heart failure or an LVEF lower than 50% likewise revealed no difference in outcome between the two strategies.

In the Atrial Fibrillation and Congestive Heart Failure (AF-CHF) trial, rate versus rhythm control was evaluated in 1376 patients with atrial fibrillation who either had an LVEF of 35% or lower and symptoms of heart failure (NYHA classes II to IV) or had been hospitalized previously for heart failure or an LVEF of 25% or lower.[48] After a 2-year follow-up period, there was no difference in occurrence of the primary endpoint of total cardiovascular mortality (27% of patients who received rhythm control, in comparison with 25% of those who received rate control; *P* = .59) (Figure 53-3). The occurrences of secondary endpoints, including total mortality (3% vs. 4%), worsening heart failure (28% vs. 31%), and stroke (3% vs. 4%), were similar between the two groups, as were the occurrences of the composite endpoint of cardiovascular death, worsening heart failure, and stroke (43% vs. 46%) (Figure 53-4). During the course of the study, 21% of patients switched from rhythm control to rate control, primarily because of the inability to maintain sinus rhythm, and 10% switched from rate control to rhythm control, primarily because of worsening heart failure. At 1 year, more patients receiving rhythm control (46%) had been hospitalized than were those receiving rate control (39%; *P* = .06); hospitalization was mainly for atrial fibrillation (14% vs. 9%) and bradyarrhythmias (6% vs. 3%).

Recommendations

The results of the AFFIRM and AF-CHF studies do not justify a strategy of rhythm control for atrial fibrillation management in patients with heart failure to improve survival.[44,48] Although these studies also revealed no difference in worsening of heart failure symptoms when a rate control strategy was compared with a rhythm control strategy, there were some patients with heart failure in whom atrial fibrillation causes a worsening of symptoms or in whom heart failure symptoms could not be controlled medically. As indicated, 10% of patients in the AF-CHF trial switched from rate control to rhythm control because of worsening heart failure. In addition, patients with diastolic dysfunction were not included in this trial, and maintenance of sinus rhythm may be of greater importance in these patients. Therefore, although rate control with anticoagulation is an acceptable approach for patients with heart failure and atrial fibrillation in whom heart failure symptoms are stable and controlled, rhythm control may be required for patients in whom heart failure symptoms worsen or continue despite adequate rate control. This may be more frequently the case in patients with diastolic heart failure or very severe systolic dysfunction.

Rhythm Control

A strategy of rhythm control involves two steps. The first is conversion of atrial fibrillation to sinus rhythm, and the second is prevention of atrial fibrillation recurrence. Conversion of atrial fibrillation to sinus rhythm is not frequently achieved with antiarrhythmic drugs in patients with heart failure; as a result, electric cardioversion is often necessary. The guidelines of the American College of Cardiology (ACC), the American Heart Association (AHA), and the European Society of Cardiology (ESC) recommend amiodarone and dofetilide as the drugs of choice for maintenance of sinus rhythm in patients with atrial fibrillation; however, these drugs may increase the likelihood of spontaneous conversion to sinus rhythm, in comparison with placebo.[48a]

Amiodarone and dofetilide are recommended as effective and safe agents for prevention of atrial fibrillation once sinus rhythm has been restored. Although neither amiodarone nor dofetilide has been shown to reduce mortality among patients with heart failure, they do not increase mortality and are safe; torsades de pointes is rarely seen with amiodarone therapy, and its incidence was 3.3% with dofetilide as reported by the DIAMOND-CHF trial.[49] However, amiodarone is associated with a risk of symptomatic bradycardia that may necessitate discontinuation

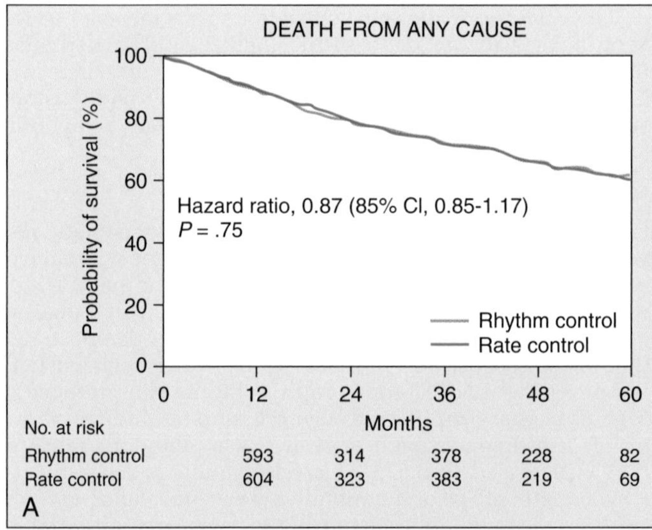

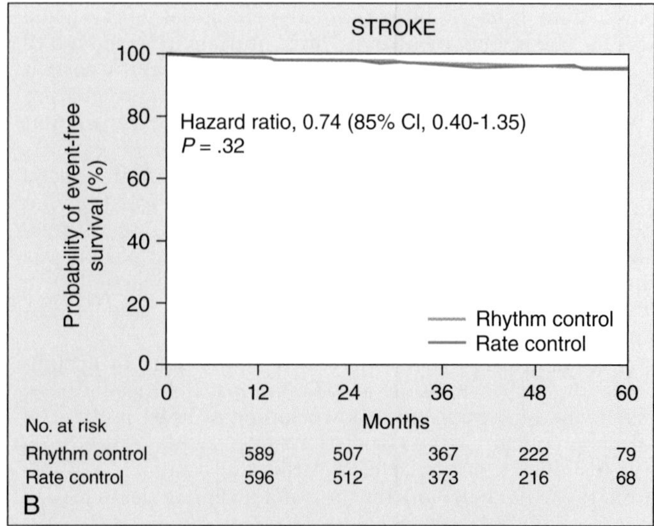

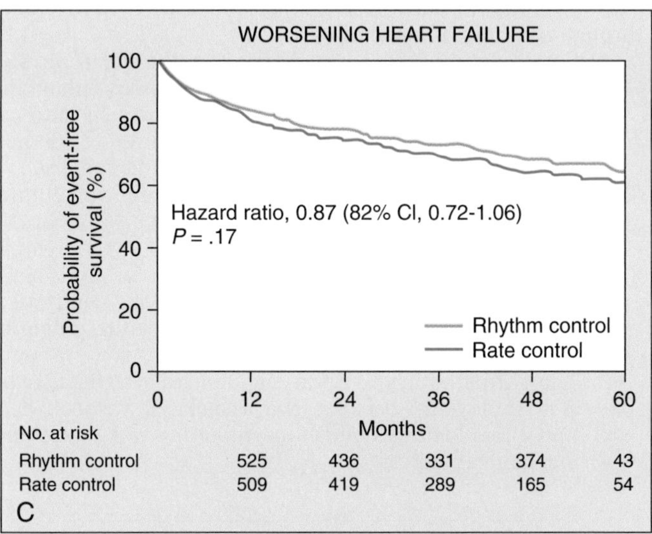

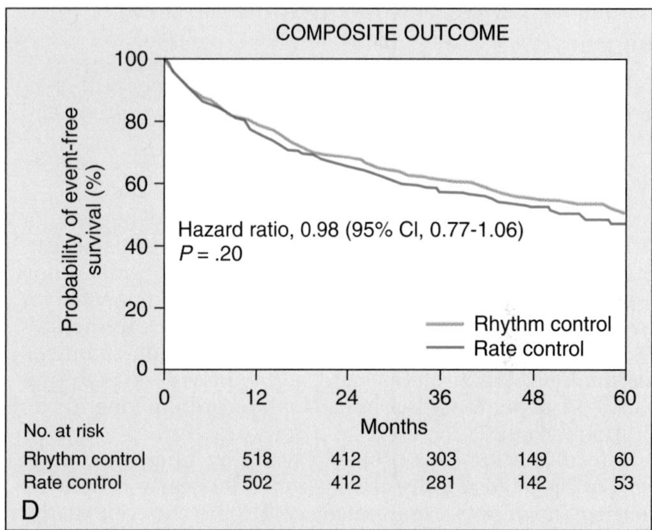

FIGURE 53–4 **A-D,** In the Atrial Fibrillation and Congestive Heart Failure (AF-CHF) trial, a strategy of rate control was compared with a strategy of rhythm control in 1376 patients with heart failure and atrial fibrillation. There was no difference in occurrences of any of the secondary endpoints, including total mortality, worsening of heart failure, or stroke, or in the composite endpoint of cardiovascular death, worsening heart failure, and stroke. CI, confidence interval. (With permission from Roy D, Talajic M, Nattel S, et al. Rhythm control versus rate control for atrial fibrillation and heart failure. *N Engl J Med* 2008;358:2667. Copyright © 2008, Massachusetts Medical Society. All rights reserved.)

of digoxin or β-blockers or implantation of a permanent pacemaker. Nevertheless, amiodarone is preferred when prevention of atrial fibrillation is indicated in patients with heart failure; dofetilide is an alternative agent. Sotalol can be used, but with caution and careful reassessment of the patient.

Although pulmonary vein isolation with radiofrequency ablation has been reported to be an effective therapy for preventing intermittent atrial fibrillation, it is less effective in patients with permanent atrial fibrillation, and its role in patients with heart failure, left ventricular dysfunction, and marked left atrial enlargement is uncertain because only a few small studies have been conducted (by the same group), and there is no long-term follow-up. Patients with heart failure often have permanent atrial fibrillation, as well as significant left atrial dilation, fibrosis, and electrical and mechanical remodeling; therefore, the role of this procedure is not well established.

Rate Control

When atrial fibrillation is to be maintained as the underlying rhythm, anticoagulation and rate control are essential, as in patients without heart failure; however, anticoagulation is underused in this population. For example, in one study of 2093 patients 65 years of age or older with heart failure and atrial fibrillation, only 20% were receiving therapy with an oral anticoagulant.[50]

In patients with atrial fibrillation and decompensated heart failure, digoxin is often the initial drug used for rate control, because its positive inotropic activity can also ameliorate the symptoms of heart failure. In some patients, digoxin may result in the conversion of atrial fibrillation to sinus rhythm. However, digoxin is often ineffective when used alone, especially in patients with heart failure in whom sympathetic activity is elevated. Thus, combined therapy with a β-blocker (once compensation is achieved) or, less preferably, a calcium channel blocker is often necessary. In patients with atrial fibrillation and compensated heart failure, β-blockers are often the initial therapy for rate control, and digoxin or a calcium channel blocker is added if heart rate control is not adequate with a β-blocker alone. If drugs are ineffective or poorly tolerated, a strategy of ablation and pacing can be used.

VENTRICULAR ARRHYTHMIAS

More than 80% of patients with heart failure caused by systolic dysfunction have frequent and complex ventricular arrhythmias, as documented on Holter monitoring, and almost 50%

demonstrate runs of nonsustained ventricular tachycardia (NSVT). The frequency of arrhythmia appears to be related to the severity, but not to the type, of underlying heart disease. It may be correlated with ventricular cavity size.

Ventricular arrhythmia, including premature ventricular complexes (PVCs) and NSVT, is also common in patients with a hypertrophic cardiomyopathy. In a community-based study of 178 patients with hypertrophic cardiomyopathy who underwent ambulatory Holter monitoring, PVCs were present in 88%, couplets were present in 42%, and NSVT was present in 31%.[51] The presence of NSVT was associated with greater degrees of left ventricular hypertrophy and NYHA functional class III or IV symptoms.

Ventricular arrhythmias may be asymptomatic or accompanied by such symptoms as palpitations, lightheadedness, presyncope or syncope, and a worsening of heart failure. Of particular concern is the association of ventricular arrhythmia with sustained ventricular tachycardia and ventricular fibrillation, the usual mechanisms for sudden cardiac death (SCD).

Causes of Ventricular Arrhythmias in Heart Failure

Multiple factors are responsible for the frequency of ventricular arrhythmias in patients with heart failure and cardiomyopathy.

Underlying Structural Disease

Extensive myocardial hypertrophy, damage and fibrosis, or the loss of cell-to-cell coupling in patients with dilated cardiomyopathy provides the proper conditions for anisotropy and reentry, the mechanism thought to be responsible for most ventricular arrhythmias. Other mechanisms in the failing heart play a role, including remodeling of ion channels, calcium-handling proteins, and gap junction–related proteins.[52] In patients with a hypertrophic cardiomyopathy, an additional factor is the myocyte disarray.

A focal mechanism, probably resulting from an ectopic focus or triggered activity arising from either early or delayed afterdepolarizations, may also contribute to ventricular arrhythmia in patients with a nonischemic cardiomyopathy.

Myocardial repolarization is altered in heart failure, independent of the cause of the cardiomyopathy. This is primarily the result of abnormalities of the calcium-independent transient outward potassium current and inward rectifier potassium current. The development of spatial heterogeneity in repolarization is manifest on the surface ECG, which may show increased QT dispersion or beat-to-beat fluctuation in the QT interval. The abnormalities in repolarization may be associated with a potential for polymorphic ventricular tachycardia and ventricular fibrillation.

Mechanical Factors

Mechanical factors in ventricular arrhythmias, which can alter the electrophysiological properties of myocardial tissue in heart failure, include an increase in wall stress and left ventricular dilation; this has been termed "electromechanical feedback."[53,54] In an animal model of dilated cardiomyopathy, refractoriness and action potential duration were significantly prolonged without a change in conduction times. Additional volume loading resulted in further prolongation of these parameters.

Because regions of the heart have differing mechanical function, electromechanical feedback may result in an increase in dispersion of action potential duration and membrane recovery. In addition, electromechanical feedback decreases in magnitude as steady-state heart rate increases. This may have implications in the setting of frequent PVCs, because the occurrence of short and long intervals from beat to beat may enhance dispersion of recovery.

The dilation of the left ventricle and an increase in left ventricular size can increase the incidence of arrhythmias. For example, in the SOLVD trial of 311 patients, there was a direct correlation between left ventricular end-diastolic volume and the prevalence of ventricular arrhythmia (Figure 53-5).[54]

Neurohormonal Factors

Heart failure results in the activation of the sympathetic nervous and renin-angiotensin systems. Markers for sympathetic activation and withdrawal of parasympathetic tone include increased heart rate, reduced variability in heart rate, and depressed baroreceptor sensitivity. One study demonstrated that depressed baroreceptor sensitivity was associated with the presence of NSVT (odds ratio = 3.8); in the presence of high pulmonary capillary wedge pressure (an indirect index of left ventricular stretch or wall stress), the odds ratio for NSVT increased to 6.5.[55] This observation is suggestive of a synergistic effect of autonomic system imbalance and left ventricular stretch in predisposing to ventricular arrhythmia.

Neurohumoral activation can promote arrhythmogenesis through a variety of mechanisms:

1. Catecholamines have direct effects on the electrophysiological properties of the myocardium, thereby enhancing arrhythmogenicity; these include increases in automaticity and triggered activity and an alteration of conduction and refractoriness, which may promote reentry.
2. Angiotensin II can indirectly promote arrhythmia through the loss of potassium and magnesium in the urine. It can also potentiate the effects of the sympathetic nervous system through central or peripheral actions. Moreover, it can promote left ventricular remodeling and fibrosis, which enhance the potential for arrhythmia.
3. The sympathetic and renin-angiotensin systems may be arrhythmogenic because the associated vasoconstriction alters loading conditions, affecting wall stress and mechanical factors.

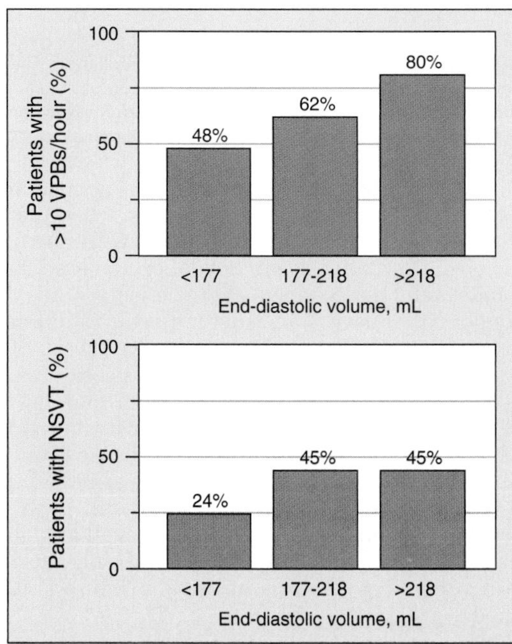

FIGURE 53-5 The incidence of ventricular premature beats (VPBs) and nonsustained ventricular tachycardia (NSVT) in patients with left ventricular dysfunction increases as the left ventricle (and thus end-diastolic volume) becomes larger. (From Koilpillai C, Quinones MA, Greenberg B, et al. Relation of ventricular size and function to heart failure status and ventricular dysrhythmia in patients with severe left ventricular dysfunction. *Am J Cardiol* 1996;77:606.)

4. Idiopathic dilated cardiomyopathy may be associated with inhomogeneous distribution of sympathetic fibers, and regions with necrosis and dense scarring show myocardial denervation. This, in turn, may lead to denervation hypersensitivity, with increased sensitivity to circulating catecholamines. In contrast, other regions of the myocardium may show an increase in sympathetic innervation, possibly the result of injury-related nerve sprouting.[56]
5. Autoantibodies against β_1-adrenergic receptors can be detected in up to 50% of patients with idiopathic dilated cardiomyopathy. One subgroup of such autoantibodies exerts sympathomimetic activity, partly as a result of an increase in cyclic adenosine monophosphate production. These autoantibodies may be closely associated with serious ventricular arrhythmias; in one study, they were independent predictors of SCD.[57]

Electrolyte Abnormalities

Patients with heart failure often have electrolyte abnormalities, particularly diuretic-induced hypokalemia and hypomagnesemia, which may be directly arrhythmogenic and associated with a higher incidence of SCD. In addition, stimulation of β_2 receptors by circulating epinephrine can transiently lower the plasma potassium concentration by enhancing potassium entry into cells.

Hypokalemia and possibly hypomagnesemia may be directly arrhythmogenic, contributing to abnormal repolarization and potentiating the arrhythmogenic effects of catecholamines, digitalis, or antiarrhythmic agents.

Ischemia

Silent or overt ischemia may lead to alteration in myocardial electrophysiological properties, including regional alterations in conduction and refractoriness and enhanced automaticity. Hypokalemia, increased catecholamine levels, digitalis, and antiarrhythmic agents may further enhance these alterations. The role of ischemia, caused by an acute coronary event, in provoking SCD was suggested by one autopsy study of 171 patients with heart failure.[58] In patients with significant coronary artery disease, an acute coronary thrombus was found in 54% who died suddenly and in 32% who died of myocardial failure, although an acute coronary event had not been clinically diagnosed before death. In contrast, an acute coronary thrombus was uncommon in those without coronary disease, present in 5% of those who died suddenly, and present in 10% of those who died from heart failure.

Drugs

Some of the drugs used to treat heart failure can directly or indirectly precipitate arrhythmia.

Phosphodiesterase Inhibitors. Phosphodiesterase inhibitors are positive inotropic agents that are available only for intravenous use. These drugs increase intracellular calcium concentration which can increase levels of cyclic adenosine monophosphate and precipitate afterdepolarizations, resulting in triggered activity. They can also exacerbate ventricular arrhythmias by inducing ischemia. Several trials have shown that one such agent, milrinone, increased the frequency of all forms of spontaneous arrhythmia. In a long-term survival trial (Prospective Randomized Milrinone Survival Evaluation [PROMISE]), milrinone was associated with a 20% excess in mortality in comparison with placebo.[59]

Sympathomimetic Drugs. Studies with the sympathomimetic agents dobutamine, pirbuterol, salbutamol, and xamoterol have demonstrated an increased frequency of ventricular arrhythmias, increased mortality rates, or both. The use of sympathomimetic drugs is also associated with an increased incidence of hospitalization for arrhythmia, especially atrial fibrillation, ventricular tachycardia, and ventricular fibrillation.

Digoxin. There have been conflicting data about the effects of digoxin on the frequency and clinical significance of arrhythmias in heart failure. Relatively large and well-controlled studies revealed that digoxin did not significantly affect the frequency of ventricular arrhythmias in patients with heart failure.[60] In contrast, several, but not all, retrospective studies in patients with heart failure after an acute myocardial infarction revealed excessive mortality among patients who had complex ventricular arrhythmias that were treated with digitalis.[61] The Digitalis Investigation Group (DIG) evaluated the efficacy of digoxin in heart failure in approximately 6800 patients; digoxin was associated with an increase in cardiac mortality not related to congestive heart failure that included a trend toward increased mortality from arrhythmia.[61] This trend counterbalanced the fewer deaths from progressive heart failure among patients treated with digoxin; thus, there was no effect on overall patient survival.

Mortality from Sudden Cardiac Death in Heart Failure

The rate of mortality from heart failure is high. In the Framingham Heart Study, the 4-year mortality rates were 62% among men and 42% among women.[62] The mortality rate is related to the severity of heart failure; in the Cooperative North Scandinavian Enalapril Survival Study (CONSENSUS) trial, for example, patients with NYHA class IV heart failure had a 1-year mortality rate of 52% (Figure 53-6).[63]

Approximately 50% to 60% of deaths in heart failure result from unexpected SCD or SCD during episodes of clinical worsening of heart failure and are most often attributed to a ventricular tachyarrhythmia, often ventricular tachycardia that degenerates into ventricular fibrillation. Bradyarrhythmias are less common and are responsible for SCD in 5% to 33% of cases; it is more frequent in patients with more advanced heart failure (NYHA class III or IV).[64] However, distinguishing an arrhythmic from a nonarrhythmic cause of death is often difficult. One problem with attributing death to arrhythmia is the lack of relation between apparent SCD and the severity of heart failure. In spite of an increased frequency

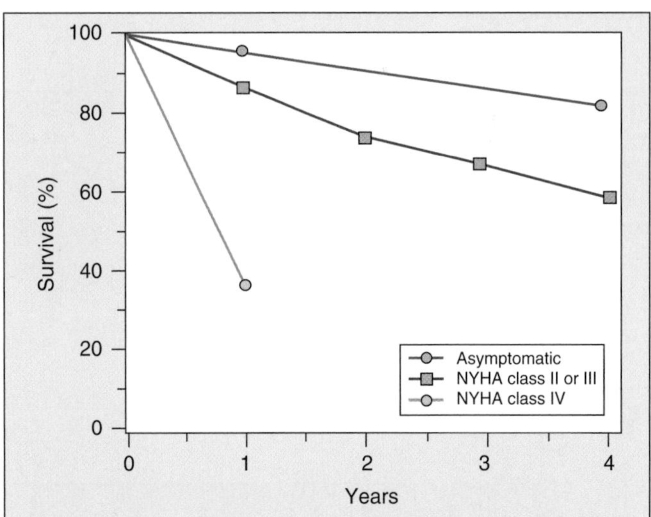

FIGURE 53–6 Survival rate varies markedly with New York Heart Association (NYHA) functional class, from as high as 81% at 4 years in asymptomatic patients (NYHA class I) to as low as 36% at 1 year in patients with NYHA class IV heart failure. (Data from SOLVD Investigators: Effect of enalapril on mortality and the development of heart failure in asymptomatic patients with reduced left ventricular ejection fraction. *N Engl J Med* 1992;327:685; Data from SOLVD Investigators: Effect of enalapril on survival in patients with reduced left ventricular ejection fractions and congestive heart failure. *N Engl J Med* 1991;325:293; and Data from CONSENSUS Trial Study Group: Effects of enalapril on mortality in severe congestive heart failure. *N Engl J Med* 1987;316:1429.)

of ventricular arrhythmias with worsening heart failure and left ventricular dysfunction, the percentage of SCD declines. For example, in one trial, the 1-year mortality rates were 29% of patients with class III heart failure and 53% of those with class IV heart failure; however, SCD was responsible for 61% and 21% of deaths, respectively.[65]

Risk Assessment for Sudden Cardiac Death in Patients with Heart Failure

A number of invasive and noninvasive methods have been used to identify the patient with heart failure who is at risk for SCD. Unfortunately, no single factor alone is highly predictive of a fatal arrhythmia. Moreover, the accuracy of these methods may be related to the cause of the cardiomyopathy (ischemic versus nonischemic).

Left Ventricular Ejection Fraction

Dilated cardiomyopathy is characterized by a variable reduction in LVEF, the assessment of which is probably the cardiac function test most frequently performed in patients with heart failure. There is no predictable relationship between symptoms or exercise tolerance and the LVEF. However, survival is generally reduced in patients with a lower LVEF.[66] For example, in the SOLVD trials and registry of 1172 patients with an echocardiogram obtained at baseline and at 1 year, LVEF lower than 35% was associated with an increase in all-cause mortality (risk ratio = 1.8) (Figure 53-7).[66] In addition, reduction in LVEF by one standard deviation was associated with increases in all-cause mortality (risk ratio = 1.62) and in cardiovascular hospitalization (risk ratio = 1.59). In the Marburg Cardiomyopathy Study, arrhythmia risk was prospectively evaluated in 343 patients with idiopathic dilated cardiomyopathy who were monitored for 52 months.[67] According to a multivariate analysis, LVEF was the only significant arrhythmia risk predictor in patients with sinus rhythm (risk ratio = 2.3 per 10% decrease in LVEF; P = .0001). In patients with atrial fibrillation, LVEF and absence of β-blocker therapy were the only significant predictors of risk. Another study of 554 patients revealed with multivariate analysis that only NYHA classes III and IV and LVEF lower [67a] than 30% were associated with a higher sudden cardiac death risk.

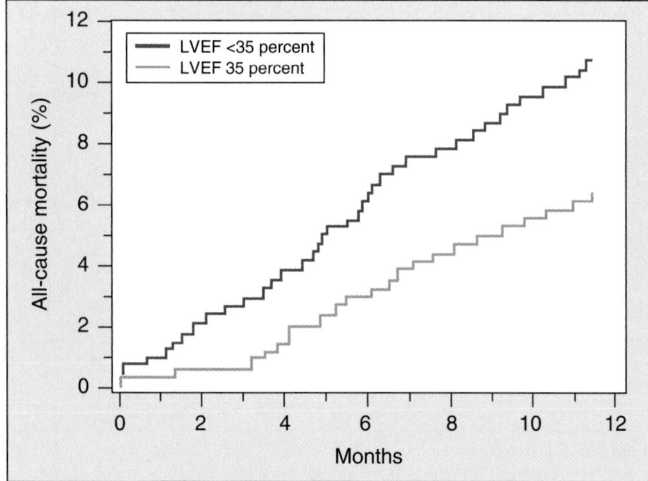

FIGURE 53-7 In the Studies of Left Ventricular Dysfunction (SOLVD) and the SOLVD registry of 1172 patients, a left ventricular ejection fraction (LVEF) lower than 35% was associated with increased rates of all-cause mortality (risk ratio = 1.8, in comparison with LVEF ≈ 35%; P = .012). (From Quinones MA, Greenberg BH, Kopelen HA, et al. Echocardiographic predictors of clinical outcome in patients with left ventricular dysfunction enrolled in the SOLVD registry and trials: significance of left ventricular hypertrophy. *J Am Coll Cardiol* 2000;35:1237.)

Ventricular Arrhythmia

PVCs and NSVT are observed in 80% to 90% of patients with heart failure caused by cardiomyopathy. There is still controversy about the prognostic significance of asymptomatic ventricular arrhythmias, particularly NSVT, in patients with heart failure. It is possible that the prognostic significance of PVCs and NSVT varies with the cause of the cardiomyopathy. In patients with left ventricular systolic dysfunction caused by ischemic cardiomyopathy, NSVT and PVCs are associated with an increased risk of SCD. The link between NSVT and SCD is most convincing after myocardial infarction in patients with left ventricular dysfunction; these patients have the highest incidence of SCD during the first year after an acute myocardial infarction.

In contrast, these arrhythmias do not appear predictive of SCD in nonischemic cardiomyopathy, although the data are conflicting. For example, the Marburg Cardiomyopathy Study revealed that the presence of NSVT on Holter monitoring was associated with a nonsignificant trend toward higher risk of arrhythmia (risk ratio = 1.7; P = .11).[67] However, this study did show that the length of the NSVT runs, but not the rate, was predictive of outcome. The incidences of major arrhythmic events in patients without NSVT, in those with 5- to 9-beat NSVT, and in those with more than 10-beat NSVT were 2%, 5%, and 10% per year, respectively. In contrast, another study of 355 patients with a dilated cardiomyopathy demonstrated that NSVT evident on ambulatory monitoring was an independent predictor of mortality (risk ratio = 1.63; P = .02).[68] Other findings on ambulatory monitoring that were predictive of risk included mean heart rate and heart rate range. A meta-analysis of 11 prognostic studies that involved more than 100 patients per study revealed that NSVT contributed significantly to the prediction of SCD in patients with left ventricular dysfunction, and this contribution was independent of LVEF (Figure 53-8).[69] It was concluded that the absence of NSVT indicated a low probability of SCD in patients with a left ventricular systolic dysfunction.

NSVT is predictive of SCD in patients with hypertrophic cardiomyopathy.[70] In one study of 531 patients with hypertrophic cardiomyopathy, 19.6% had NSVT.[70] The presence of NSVT was associated with an increased risk of sudden cardiac death, particularly in younger patients. The odds ratio of SCD for patients aged 30 years or younger with NSVT was 4.35, in comparison with 2.16 in those older than 30. There was no relation among duration, frequency, and rate of NSVT episodes and prognosis at any age.

Use of Left Ventricular Ejection Fraction and Nonsustained Ventricular Tachycardia as Predictors of Survival

The use of only a univariate predictor such as LVEF or NSVT to estimate survival in the individual patient does not yield high predictive accuracy. It is possible that risk prediction can be improved when the finding of NSVT on ambulatory monitoring is combined with measures of left ventricular function (Figure 53-9). This issue was addressed in one study of 202 patients with idiopathic cardiomyopathy and no history of sustained ventricular tachycardia who underwent ambulatory monitoring, echocardiography, and signal-averaged electrocardiography and were monitored for 32 months.[71] After adjustments for baseline and follow-up medical therapy, only left ventricular end-diastolic diameter, LVEF, and the presence of NSVT were independent predictors of arrhythmic events. The combination of a left ventricular end-diastolic diameter of 70 mm or more and NSVT was associated with a 14.3-fold risk, and the combination of NSVT and LVEF of 30% or less increased the risk 14.6-fold; the sensitivity, specificity, and positive and negative predictive values were 59%, 84%, 40%, and 92%, respectively.

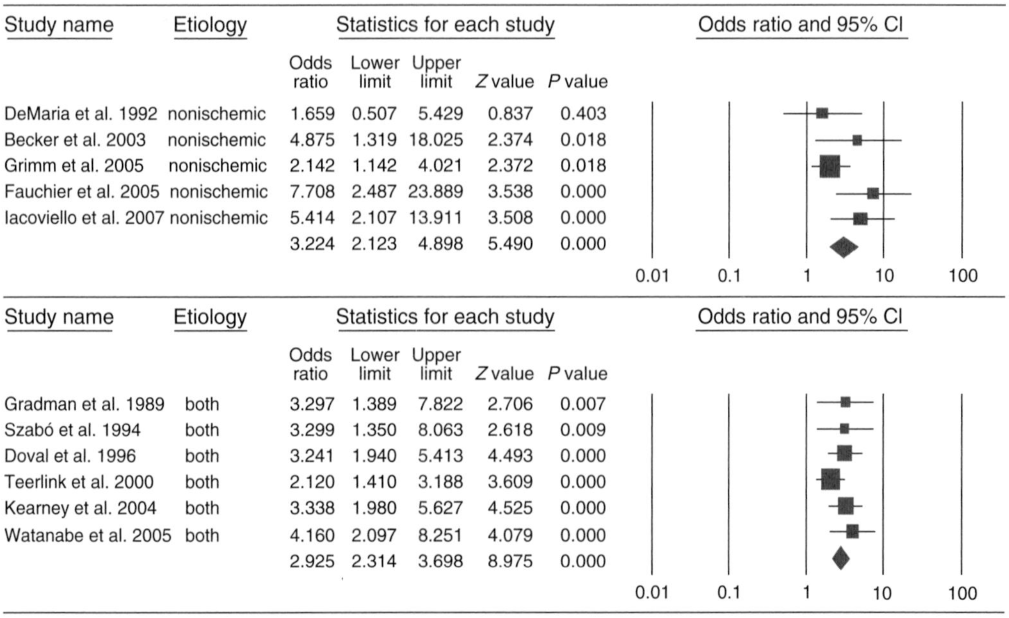

Study name	Etiology	Statistics for each study					Odds ratio and 95% CI
		Odds ratio	Lower limit	Upper limit	Z value	P value	
DeMaria et al. 1992	nonischemic	1.659	0.507	5.429	0.837	0.403	
Becker et al. 2003	nonischemic	4.875	1.319	18.025	2.374	0.018	
Grimm et al. 2005	nonischemic	2.142	1.142	4.021	2.372	0.018	
Fauchier et al. 2005	nonischemic	7.708	2.487	23.889	3.538	0.000	
Iacoviello et al. 2007	nonischemic	5.414	2.107	13.911	3.508	0.000	
		3.224	2.123	4.898	5.490	0.000	
							0.01 0.1 1 10 100

Study name	Etiology	Statistics for each study					Odds ratio and 95% CI
		Odds ratio	Lower limit	Upper limit	Z value	P value	
Gradman et al. 1989	both	3.297	1.389	7.822	2.706	0.007	
Szabó et al. 1994	both	3.299	1.350	8.063	2.618	0.009	
Doval et al. 1996	both	3.241	1.940	5.413	4.493	0.000	
Teerlink et al. 2000	both	2.120	1.410	3.188	3.609	0.000	
Kearney et al. 2004	both	3.338	1.980	5.627	4.525	0.000	
Watanabe et al. 2005	both	4.160	2.097	8.251	4.079	0.000	
		2.925	2.314	3.698	8.975	0.000	
							0.01 0.1 1 10 100

FIGURE 53–8 Meta-analysis of 11 studies in which Holter monitoring was performed in patients with heart failure or a nonischemic cardiomyopathy. The presence of nonsustained ventricular tachycardia (NSVT) was found to be a significant predictor of mortality. This finding was independent of left ventricular ejection fraction. (From de Sousa, M.R., Morillo, C.A., Rabelo, F.T., et al. non-sustained ventricular tachycarolia as a predictor of sudden cardiac death in patients with left ventricular dysfunction: a meta-analysis. *Eur J Heart Fail* 2008; 10: 1007.)

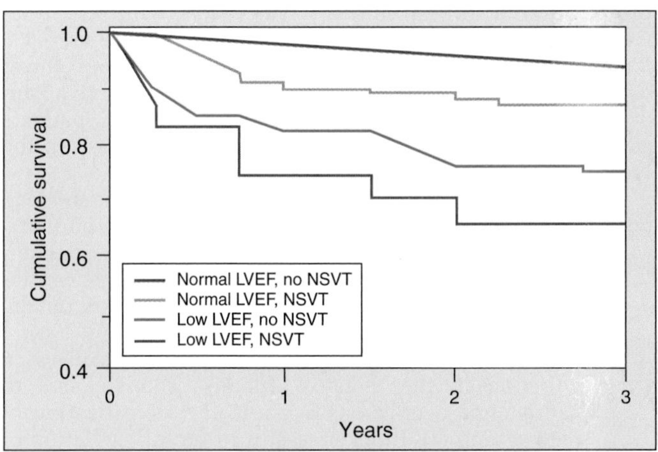

FIGURE 53–9 The presence of both nonsustained ventricular tachycardia (NSVT) on an ambulatory monitor and a low left ventricular ejection fraction (LVEF) is associated with arrhythmic mortality after acute myocardial infarction. The rate of mortality is highest among patients with both NSVT and a low LVEF. (From the Multicenter Postinfarction Research Group: Risk stratification and survival after myocardial infarction. *N Engl J Med* 1983;309:331.)

Electrophysiological Testing

A number of investigators have evaluated the role of electrophysiological study in selecting patients with heart failure and ventricular arrhythmias who are at high risk for SCD and who might benefit from prophylactic therapy.[72] In general, most have not found electrophysiological study to be useful for identifying patients at risk, especially those with nonischemic cardiomyopathy. However, the studies are flawed in various ways, including retrospective study design, unrandomized pharmacological therapy, and inconsistent definition of induced ventricular tachycardia; these flaws make meaningful conclusions impossible.

One study, Multicenter Unsustained Tachycardia Trial (MUSTT)—which involved 704 patients with coronary disease and with or without a remote myocardial infarction, asymptomatic NSVT, LVEF of 40% or lower—did demonstrate that the rate of inducibility was higher in patients with a history of a myocardial infarction and in men and was progressively higher with an increasing number of diseased coronary arteries and number of fixed thallium defects; this rate was lower in patients who had undergone prior bypass surgery and had noncoronary cardiac disease.[72] Although these associations were statistically significant, the accuracy in discriminating patients with and without inducible sustained monomorphic ventricular tachycardia was only modest.

In conclusion, no data yet suggest that electrophysiological study can identify patients with nonischemic cardiomyopathy, heart failure, and ventricular arrhythmia who are at risk for SCD. The results of MUSTT suggest that electrophysiological study may have a role in risk stratification in patients with ischemic cardiomyopathy, particularly those with a prior myocardial infarction and left ventricular dysfunction.

Electrophysiological study may have a role in establishing arrhythmia as the cause of syncope or unexplained palpitations in patients with cardiomyopathy, in establishing ventricular tachycardia as the mechanism of a wide complex tachycardia, or in localizing the site of origin of ventricular tachycardia before radiofrequency ablation.

Signal-Averaged Electrocardiography

It has been suggested that signal-averaged electrocardiography is a useful noninvasive method to select patients with heart failure, cardiomyopathy, and ventricular arrhythmias who are at high risk for SCD. In patients with ischemic heart disease, late potentials on the SAECG are thought to represent areas of delayed or slow subendocardial conduction. The SAECG is a predictor of SCD and sustained ventricular tachycardia in patients after myocardial infarction, independent of left ventricular function, ventricular ectopic activity, and transient hemodynamic abnormalities. The SAECG has also been evaluated in patients with nonischemic cardiomyopathy; its predictive role in this setting is less certain.[73]

A task force of the ACC concluded that the SAECG may be valuable in the clinical care of patients with dilated cardiomyopathy but suggested that further supportive evidence is required before signal-averaged electrocardiography can be recommended in these patients.

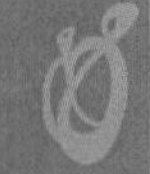

QT Dispersion

QT or JT dispersion, measured as interlead variability of QT or JT intervals on the surface ECG, is an indirect measure of myocardial repolarization inhomogeneity. It has been associated with an increased risk for an arrhythmic event and SCD in patients with a recent myocardial infarction and with the congenital long QT syndrome. Although QT dispersion is increased in patients with heart failure caused by idiopathic dilated cardiomyopathy who have had an arrhythmic event, its role in predicting the risk of SCD in these patients is uncertain because the results of studies are conflicting.[74]

Heart Rate Variability

Heart rate variability measurements provide a simple method for assessing the status of the parasympathetic and sympathetic nervous system and for predicting cardiovascular events, especially cardiac death and sustained ventricular tachyarrhythmias in patients with coronary heart disease. Although earlier data suggested that heart rate variability may be of predictive value in dilated cardiomyopathy and heart failure,[75] several more recent studies have not demonstrated this technique to be of value.[76] However, the Defibrillators in Non-Ischemic Cardiomyopathy Treatment Evaluation (DEFINITE) of 274 patients with a nonischemic cardiomyopathy did show that preserved heart rate variability identified patients at low risk who had an excellent prognosis (0% at 3 years, in comparison with 7% to 10% when heart rate variability was absent).[77]

Repolarization (T Wave) Alternans

Repolarization, or T wave, alternans is a variability in the timing or structure of repolarization that occurs in alternate beats on the surface ECG; T wave alternans is associated with repolarization heterogeneity. However, T wave alternans of sufficient magnitude to be detected visually is uncommon. Computerized filtering and analysis allow T wave alternans on the level of microvolts to be detected. Such detection is both sensitive and specific for predicting ventricular arrhythmias in various groups of patients.[78]

The role of T wave alternans for predicting the risk of SCD in patients with heart failure is uncertain. Several studies have revealed that it is predictive of arrhythmic risk in patients with heart failure caused by ischemic or nonischemic cardiomyopathy. One study showed that at 2 years, the hazard ratio for SCD or a nonfatal sustained ventricular arrhythmia was 6.5 in patients with an abnormal T wave alternans, in comparison with patients with normal T wave alternans.[79] It has been reported that T wave alternans is useful for identifying patients with a cardiomyopathy who are at high risk for a life-threatening ventricular tachyarrhythmia and would benefit from prophylaxis with an implantable cardioverter-defibrillator (ICD).[80] It has also been reported that its prognostic utility is independent of QRS duration. It may be better than QRS duration in patients with ischemic cardiomyopathy. For example, in one study modeled on the Multicenter Automatic Defibrillator Implantation Trial (MADIT) II, 177 patients were monitored for 20 months; the hazard ratio for 2-year mortality was 4.8 for patients with an abnormal T wave alternans and 1.5 for those with a QRS width of more than 120 msec.[81] The actuarial mortality rate was 3.8% for a normal T wave alternans finding and 12% for a narrow QRS complex.

In contrast, more recent data from the Sudden Cardiac Death in Heart Failure Trial (SCD-HeFT) trial revealed that among 490 patients monitored for a median of 30 months, there was no difference in rates of events (SCD, ventricular fibrillation or tachycardia, or appropriate ICD discharge) between those with or without T wave alternans.[82] The results of this study suggested that T wave alternans is not useful for selecting patients with heart failure and left ventricular dysfunction as candidates for an ICD.

Prophylactic Pharmacological Therapy to Prevent Sudden Cardiac Death

The role of prophylactic pharmacological therapy to prevent SCD and prolong life in patients at high risk who have cardiomyopathy, heart failure, and asymptomatic ventricular arrhythmia is uncertain and varies with the type of agent.

Effect of Heart Failure Therapies on Arrhythmia

Several drugs that are used to treat heart failure may affect the incidence of arrhythmias and reduce the incidence of SCD.

β-Blockers. β-Blockers reduce the incidence of SCD in the immediate postinfarction period, and this benefit is most marked in patients with heart failure. A number of studies have shown that β-blockers significantly improve survival in patient with heart failure. This beneficial effect results in part from a reduction in ventricular arrhythmias and SCD. In the Metoprolol CR/XL Randomised Intervention Trial in Congestive Heart Failure (MERIT-HF) of 3991 patients with class II to IV heart failure and LVEF of 40% or lower, there were significantly fewer SCD events among the patients treated with metoprolol (3.9%) than among those treated with placebo (6.6%); however, with the increasing severity of heart failure, the proportion of SCD decreased whereas deaths due to heart failure increased.[83] In the Cardiac Insufficiency BIsoprolol Study (CIBIS)–II, the survival benefit with bisoprolol was primarily reflected by a reduction in SCD (3.6% vs. 6.3% for placebo), with only a nonsignificant trend toward fewer deaths from heart failure.[84] In the Carvedilol Prospective Randomized Cumulative Survival (COPERNICUS) trial, patients receiving carvedilol exhibited a significant reduction in the incidence of ventricular tachycardia and SCD.[85]

The precise mechanism of β-blocker protection is unclear, but the antisympathetic effect is almost certainly important:

1. β-Blockers block the effect of circulating catecholamines, which are elevated in patients with cardiomyopathy and have direct detrimental effects on the ventricular myocardium.
2. Long-term exposure to catecholamines causes a reduction in the density of and responsiveness to β-adrenergic agonists as a result of desensitization of the β-receptor. β-Blockers result in the upregulation of β-receptors.
3. The vasoconstriction induced by norepinephrine increases afterload, a change that promotes the rate of progression of cardiac dysfunction.
4. β-Blockers have a beneficial effect on left ventricular remodeling and can decrease left ventricular end-systolic and end-diastolic volume.
5. Diastolic dysfunction is one of the adverse prognostic findings in patients with heart failure. β-Blockers may improve diastolic function in association with a reduction in left ventricular end-diastolic pressure.
6. During the development of heart failure, adrenergic activation contributes to increased myocardial expression of inflammatory cytokines; β-blockade may reduce myocardial gene expression and protein production of some of these cytokines, thereby attenuating left ventricular dilation and systolic dysfunction.

Angiotensin-Converting Enzyme inhibitors and Angiotensin Receptor Blockers. The effect of ACE inhibitors and ARBs on ventricular arrhythmias in patients with heart failure remains controversial. Although these agents do reduce mortality, some trials, such as CONSENSUS, SOLVD, and Survival And Ventricular Enlargement (SAVE), revealed that the survival benefit arose primarily from slowed progression of heart failure, with little or no reduction in SCD.[86] In

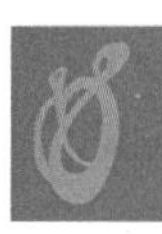

contrast, other trials such as V-HeFT II, Trandolapril Cardiac Evaluation (TRACE)[86a], and Acute Infarction Ramipril Efficacy (AIRE), showed a significant reduction in SCD.[87]

A meta-analysis of trials involving 15,104 patients within 14 days of an acute myocardial infarction revealed that ACE inhibitor therapy modestly but significantly reduced the risk of SCD (odds ratio = 0.80; absolute benefit ≈ 1.4%).[88]

The ARBs appear to be as beneficial as ACE inhibitors, or perhaps slightly less so, in patients with heart failure, although data are limited.

Spironolactone. Spironolactone, an aldosterone antagonist, has been reported to reduce the frequency of PVCs and NSVT.[89] The beneficial effect of this drug was observed in the Randomized Aldactone Evaluation Study (RALES) trial of patients with advanced heart failure; spironolactone significantly reduced overall mortality (35% vs. 46% for placebo), including a 29% reduction in sudden cardiac death (P = .02).[90] The benefit of spironolactone was evident at 3 months and persisted for the 2-year duration of the study. A reduction in SCD was also reported in the Eplerenone Post–Acute Myocardial Infarction Heart Failure Efficacy and Survival Study (EPHESUS) (relative risk = 0.79; P = .03).[91] The benefit of these agents may arise from a reduction in aldosterone effect on the heart or the maintenance of a higher serum potassium concentration.

Statins. Although the beneficial effect of statins in patients with cardiomyopathy and heart failure is uncertain, data suggest that they may improve survival. The effect of these agents on SCD in patients with a nonischemic cardiomyopathy was suggested by the DEFINITE trial.[92] Patients treated with a statin had significantly lower rates of arrhythmic sudden cardiac death (0.9%) and total mortality (4.5%) than did those not treated with a statin (5.2% and 18.4%, respectively). Similar data were reported from patients enrolled in the MADIT II study.[93] The cumulative rates of ICD discharge for ventricular tachycardia and ventricular fibrillation or cardiac death were significantly reduced in patients taking statins for 90% of the time or more, in comparison with those taking statins less frequently. The hazard ratios for statin use versus no statin use were 0.65 for ventricular tachycardia and ventricular fibrillation and 0.72 for cardiac death.

Pharmacological Therapy with Antiarrhythmic Agents

Studies of antiarrhythmic drugs have shown that most of these agents, when given prophylactically, are of no benefit for preventing SCD in patients with cardiomyopathy and heart failure. For example, in the ALIVE trial, in which azimilide was evaluated in 3717 patients with an ischemic cardiomyopathy, most of whom had symptomatic heart failure,[94] azimilide had no effect on mortality in comparison with placebo. Prophylactic dofetilide in the DIAMOND-CHF trial of 1518 patients with symptomatic heart failure had no effect on mortality (41% vs. 42% with placebo).[37]

In addition to the lack of efficacy, there are other problems with the use of these agents in patients with heart failure, which limits their prophylactic use:

1. Antiarrhythmic drugs are less efficacious in patients with depressed LVEF.[95] Furthermore, long-term studies of survival in patients treated with antiarrhythmic drugs identified as being effective for arrhythmia suppression have revealed that heart failure and depressed LVEF are major predictors of adverse outcome.[95]
2. The pharmacokinetic activity of antiarrhythmic drugs is significantly and unpredictably altered in the presence of heart failure. The volume of distribution is decreased, which affects the dose given and blood level achieved; hepatic metabolism of these agents and renal excretion of drug or metabolites are impaired; and the time to achieve a steady state is prolonged, which can lead to premature escalation of drug dose and thereby possibly result in excessive drug levels and toxicity.
3. Most antiarrhythmic drugs have some negative inotropic effects and, in patients with reduced left ventricular function, can precipitate heart failure.[96]
4. Aggravation of arrhythmia or proarrhythmia is a complication of each of the antiarrhythmic drugs.[34] Although this serious adverse effect is unpredictable and can occur in any patient, it is far more common in patients with cardiomyopathy and clinical heart failure.

Pharmacological Therapy with Amiodarone. Amiodarone can reduce the incidence of ventricular arrhythmias, but data from two of the largest trials—Grupo de Estudio de la Sobrevida en la Insuficiencia Cardiaca en Argentina (GESICA) and CHF-STAT—have conflicted with regard to its effect on patient survival.[97,98]

GESICA. The GESICA trial enrolled 516 patients with advanced heart failure (NYHA classes II to IV and LVEF < 35%), which resulted primarily from nonischemic cardiomyopathy, and NSVT. The patients, who received 24-hour Holter monitoring, were randomly assigned to receive either placebo or amiodarone.[97] After a 2-year follow-up period, a 28% reduction in total mortality was noted with amiodarone, with favorable trends noted for deaths classified as caused by heart failure or arrhythmia. The beneficial effect of amiodarone was observed primarily in patients with a baseline heart rate of 90 or more beats per minute. Among these patients, the mortality rate at 2 years was lower with amiodarone treatment (38.4%) than with placebo (62.4%); there were also reductions in SCD (19.7% vs. 10.7%, respectively) and in death from progressive heart failure (25.8% vs. 18.0%, respectively). The higher above beats per minute the baseline heart rate was, the greater was the reduction in mortality with amiodarone treatment. In contrast, when the heart rate was 90 beats per minute or less, there was no difference in mortality between amiodarone (44.8%) and placebo (44.7%).

CHF-STAT. The randomized CHF-STAT trial involved 674 patients with symptomatic heart failure (class II to IV), caused primarily by ischemic cardiomyopathy, in whom cardiac enlargement was demonstrated on echocardiogram or chest radiograph, LVEF was lower than 40%, and 10 or more PVCs per hour had occurred during ambulatory monitoring.[98] Even though there was more than an 80% reduction in PVCs or elimination of NSVST, amiodarone did not improve overall survival at 2 years (69.4% vs. 70.8% for placebo). There was also no significant difference in SCD mortality (15% vs. 19% with placebo). There was, however, a significant 46% reduction in events (cardiac events or hospitalization) in the subgroup of patients with nonischemic cardiomyopathy. Amiodarone did not affect noncardiac death, including the subgroup with underlying chronic obstructive lung disease.

SCD-HeFT. The largest trial to evaluate the role of amiodarone was SCD-HeFT, in which 2521 patients with both ischemic and nonischemic cardiomyopathy were randomly assigned to receive an ICD (single-lead shock only), amiodarone, or placebo.[99] Entry criteria included an LVEF of 35% or lower and NYHA class II or III heart failure. After a mean follow-up period of 45.5 months, mortality was not reduced by amiodarone therapy (28%) in comparison with placebo (29%; hazard ratio = 1.06).

Meta-analysis. In a meta-analysis of 13 randomized amiodarone trials, which included 6553 patients, there were 5 trials involving 1452 patients with heart failure. In these trials, amiodarone reduced total mortality and arrhythmia or SCD in patients with heart failure by 17% and 23%, respectively (Figure 53-10).[100] LVEF, NYHA functional class, or the presence of asymptomatic arrhythmias on Holter monitoring did not influence the effectiveness of amiodarone.

Although the role of amiodarone in the prevention of SCD or ventricular tachycardia is not certain, because researchers have reported conflicting results, the drug does significantly reduce the rate of the ventricular tachycardia, often making it hemodynamically stable and improving the potential for survival.

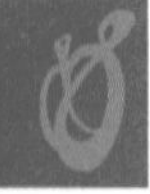

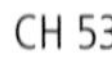

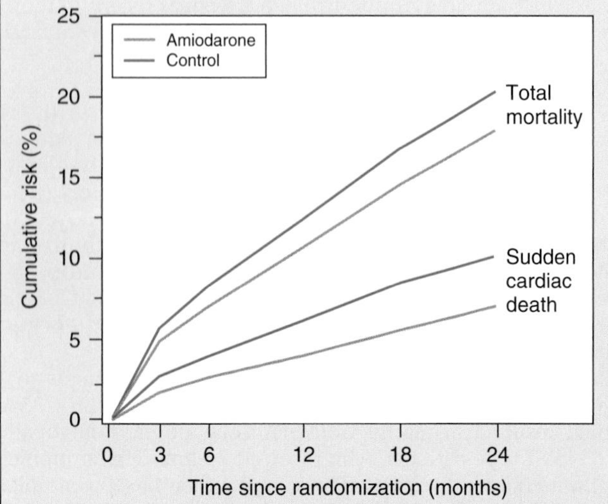

FIGURE 53-10 Meta-analysis of randomized trials involving 6553 patients with congestive heart failure or a recent myocardial infarction. A meta-analysis of randomized amiodarone trials involving 6553 patients indicated there were 1452 patients with heart failure treated with this drug. Amiodarone reduced total mortality and arrhythmia or SCD in this group of patients with heart failure by 17% and 23%, respectively. There was no difference in the treatment effect between postinfarction and congestive heart failure trials. (From Amiodarone Trials Meta-analysis Investigators: Effect of prophylactic amiodarone on mortality after acute MI and in congestive heart failure: meta-analysis of individual data from 6500 patients in randomized trials. *Lancet* 1997;350:1417.)

Pharmacological Therapy with Dronedarone. Dronedarone is an antiarrhythmic drug that has electrophysiological properties similar to those of amiodarone. However, it does not contain iodine and does not cause iodine-related side effects. In one study, 627 patients with heart failure and severe left ventricular dysfunction were randomly assigned to receive dronedarone or placebo.[39] The study was stopped after a median follow-up period of 2 months because mortality was increased among the dronedarone recipients (8.1% vs. 3.8% for placebo; hazard ratio = 2.13; P = .03). The increase in mortality resulted primarily from worsening of heart failure.

Prophylactic Use of an Implantable Cardioverter-Defibrillator (Primary Prevention) (see Chapter 47)

The role of the ICD as prophylactic therapy in patients with heart failure and cardiomyopathy, who are at high risk for SCD, has been evaluated in a number of studies. These trials have demonstrated that the ICD, in comparison with antiarrhythmic drug therapy, significantly reduces mortality in patients at high risk with ischemic and nonischemic cardiomyopathy.

Trials in Ischemic Cardiomyopathy

ICDs have been evaluated in several studies of ischemic cardiomyopathy:

1. MADIT I enrolled 196 asymptomatic patients with a prior myocardial infarction, an LVEF lower than 35%, evidence of NSVT on monitoring, a positive SAECG, and inducible sustained monomorphic ventricular tachycardia that was unresponsive to intravenous procainamide. Patients were randomly assigned to receive an ICD or conventional therapy.[101] During an average follow-up period of 27 months, there were 15 deaths among the patients with an ICD (11 from cardiac causes) and 39 deaths among those receiving the conventional therapy (27 from cardiac causes; for overall mortality, hazard ratio = 0.46; P = .009).
2. In MADIT II, 1232 patients with myocardial infarction and an LVEF of 30% or lower were randomly assigned to receive an ICD or conventional therapy; the presence of NSVT was not an entry criterion, and electrophysiological study was not performed.[102] During an average follow-up period of 20 months, the mortality rates were significantly lower among patients receiving an ICD (14.2%) than among those receiving the conventional therapy (19.8%). The hazard ratio for the risk of death from any cause in the ICD recipients, in comparison with the conventional therapy recipients, was 0.69 (P = .016). The effect of the ICD on survival was similar in subgroup analyses stratified according to age, sex, LVEF, NYHA class, and the QRS interval. However, there was a higher rate of hospitalization for heart failure among the ICD recipients (20%) than among recipients of conventional therapy (15%).
3. MUSTT enrolled 704 patients with chronic coronary heart disease, an LVEF of 40% or lower, and NSVT.[103] Although the study was not designed to evaluate the role of an ICD in these patients, it did reveal that the risk of cardiac arrest or death from arrhythmia among the patients who received treatment with an ICD was significantly lower than that among the patients discharged without an ICD (relative risk = 0.24; P < .001).
4. In contrast to MUSTT and MADIT, which enrolled patients several years after myocardial infarction, the Defibrillator in Acute Myocardial Infarction Trial (DINAMIT) was an evaluation of the role of a prophylactic ICD in 574 patients who had suffered a myocardial infarction within the preceding 6 to 40 days (mean, 18 days), had an LVEF of 35% or lower, and had either reduced heart rate variability or elevated resting heart rate (≥80 beats/min).[104] The risk of SCD after myocardial infarction is highest during this time period. After a 30-month follow-up period, no difference in all-cause mortality was found between the ICD recipients (18.7%) and controls (17.0%; P = .66). However, deaths from arrhythmia were more frequent among controls (hazard ratio = 0.42; P = .009), whereas deaths from nonarrhythmic causes were more frequent among the ICD recipients (hazard ratio = 1.75; P = .02).

On the basis of the results of these trials, an ICD is the recommended therapy for primary prevention of SCD in patients who had a prior myocardial infarction at least 40 days previously, have an LVEF of 30% or lower, have NYHA functional class II or III heart failure, are receiving chronic optimal medical therapy, and have reasonable expectation of survival with a good functional status for more than 1 year.

Trials in Nonischemic Cardiomyopathy

Two small studies of patients with a nonischemic cardiomyopathy—the Cardiomyopathy Trial (CAT) and Amiodarone Versus Implantable Defibrillator in Patients with Nonischemic Cardiomyopathy and Asymptomatic Nonsustained Ventricular Tachycardia (AMIOVIRT)—did not reveal that a prophylactic ICD improved survival in comparison with conventional therapy or amiodarone. However, these studies were limited by small numbers of patients.

1. The DEFINITE trial enrolled 458 patients with a nonischemic dilated cardiomyopathy, an LVEF of 35% or lower, and PVCs or NSVT; these patients were randomly assigned to receive an ICD or standard medical therapy.[105] At 2 years, there was a strong trend toward a reduction in the primary endpoint of all-cause mortality with an ICD (7.9%), in comparison with medical therapy alone (14.1%). Significantly fewer sudden cardiac deaths occurred among the ICD recipients, although the numbers were very small (3 vs. 14).
2. The largest prophylactic ICD trial was SCD-HeFT, in which 2521 patients with an LVEF of 35% or lower (median, 25%) and NYHA class II or III heart failure

were randomly assigned to receive an ICD, amiodarone, or placebo; 48% had a nonischemic cardiomyopathy.[106] At a median 46-month follow-up assessment, ICD therapy significantly reduced overall mortality in comparison with placebo (22% vs. 29%). ICD therapy was associated with a 23% decreased risk of death (hazard ratio = 0.77; P = .007) and an absolute decrease in mortality of 7.2% points (Figure 53-11). The mortality rate among the amiodarone recipients (28%) was nearly the same as that among placebo recipients (29%; hazard ratio = 1.06; P = .53). In prespecified subgroup analysis, the benefit of ICD therapy was demonstrated among patients with either an ischemic or nonischemic cardiomyopathy (Figure 53-12). In a post hoc analysis, the benefit of an ICD was observed in patients with an LVEF of 30% or lower, but not in those with an LVEF higher than 30%.

3. In a meta-analysis of 1854 patients with nonischemic cardiomyopathy, the use of an ICD was examined for primary prevention.[107] There was a significant reduction in all-cause mortality with an ICD in comparison with medical therapy (relative risk = 0.69). According to the averaged mortality rate in the control group (7% per year), the absolute risk reduction was 2% per year.

On the basis of the results of these trials, the ICD is the recommended therapy for primary prevention of SCD in patients with nonischemic dilated cardiomyopathy who have an LVEF of 30% or lower, have NYHA class II or III heart failure, and have a reasonable expectation of survival with a good functional status for more than 1 year. The Center for Medicare Services in the United States approved coverage for ICD use for primary prevention with an additional criterion: only if the nonischemic dilated cardiomyopathy has been present for more than 9 months.

Identifying the Patient at High Risk Who Is Most Likely to Benefit from a Prophylactic Implantable Cardioverter-Defibrillator

The ICD is costly, and its implantation carries some risk. A number of researchers have evaluated the cost effectiveness of this device. For example, an analysis of data from SCD-HeFT revealed that the device was economically attractive in patients with an LVEF of 35% or lower and NYHA class II heart failure, as long as the benefits observed persisted for 8 years.[108] Similar data were observed in MADIT II: During the 3.5-year follow-up period, the average survival gain with the ICD was 2 months, and the incremental cost-effectiveness ratio was $235,000 per year of life saved; however, this value was projected to be substantially lower for patients who survived longer.[109] Thus, the magnitude of benefit depends on the baseline risk for SCD.

By using only LVEF, researchers have identified a very large number of patients who are candidates for the ICD. However, it has become obvious that the majority of such patients do not experience a ventricular tachyarrhythmia and hence do not benefit from this device. Therefore, an important challenge is the identification of the individual patient who has not yet suffered a sustained ventricular arrhythmia but is at high risk for such an event and hence is likely to derive benefit from an ICD. Unfortunately, most of the methods for risk stratification, discussed previously, have limited usefulness.[67] Although T wave alternans may be of some importance, its utility in identifying patients at low and high risk is still uncertain. It has not been evaluated in both patients with ICD and those without ICD, which is particularly important because assessment of the risk for a life-threatening ventricular arrhythmia is not always correlated with ICD efficacy.

Thus, the number of patients receiving an ICD is far greater than the number who experience an appropriate ICD discharge and actually benefit from this device (i.e., the number to treat in order to save one life is very high). Because the absolute risk reduction is 2% per year, 100 devices would need to be implanted to save 2 lives per year. Reliance on LVEF alone is therefore inadequate for identifying the patient who will benefit from an ICD, because this parameter is not specific for predicting mode of death and because the risk of SCD in patients with LVEF of 30% or lower is not uniform. Moreover, some patients with LVEF higher than 30% are at increased risk for SCD.

Several researchers have evaluated a number of clinical variables in order to identify patients at low risk who are not likely to benefit from the ICD:

1. In the MUSTT study, researchers evaluated 25 variables in 674 patients who did not have inducible arrhythmia or had inducible arrhythmia that was not treated.[110] In a multivariate analysis, variables found to have the

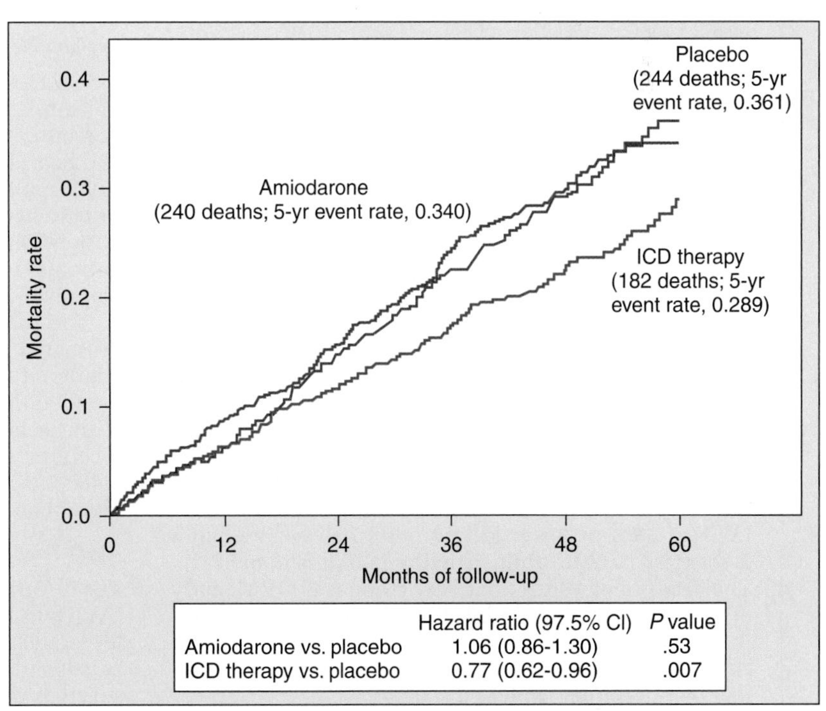

FIGURE 53–11 In the Sudden Cardiac Death in Heart Failure Trial (SCD-HeFT) of 2521 patients with a left ventricular ejection fraction (LVEF) of 35% or lower and clinical heart failure, therapy with an implantable cardioverter-defibrillator (ICD) significantly reduced total mortality, in comparison with placebo or amiodarone therapy (P = .007). There was no difference in outcome between placebo and amiodarone therapy. (From Bardy GH, Lee KL, Mark DB, et al. Amiodarone or an implantable cardioverter-defibrillator for congestive heart failure. *NEJM* 2005; 352:225-237 Copyright © 2008, Massachusetts Medical Society. All rights reserved.)

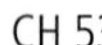

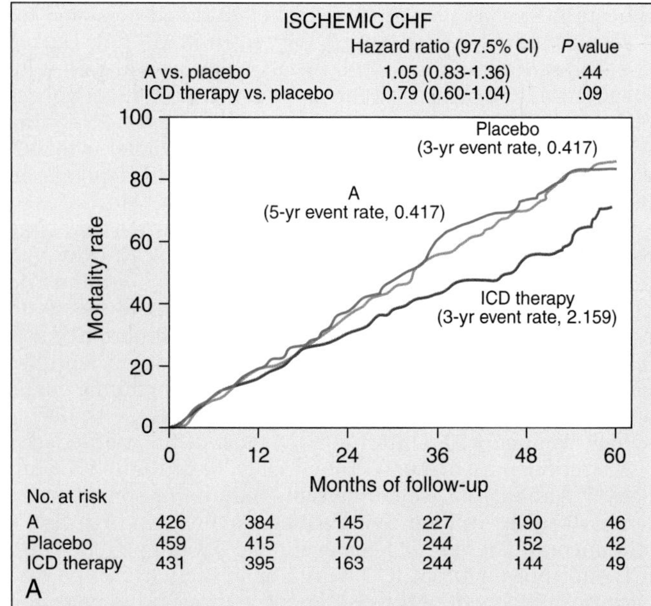

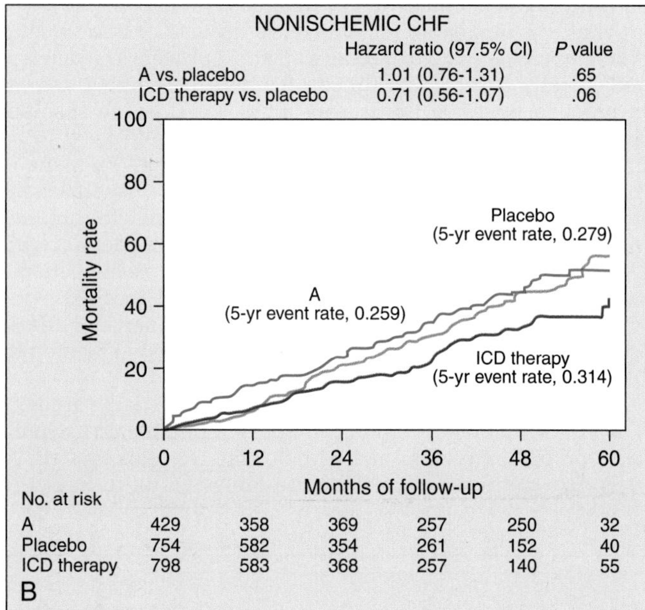

FIGURE 53–12 In the Sudden Cardiac Death in Heart Failure Trial (SCD-HeFT) of 2521 patients with a left ventricular ejection fraction (LVEF) of 35% or lower and clinical heart failure, subset analysis revealed that an implantable cardioverter-defibrillator (ICD) reduced mortality among patients with ischemic or nonischemic cardiomyopathy. CHF, congestive heart failure; CI, confidence interval; ICD, implantable cardioverter-defibrillator. (From Bardy GH, Lee KL, Mark DB, et al. Amiodarone or an implantable cardioverter-defibrillator for congestive heart failure. *NEJM* 2005; 352:225-237.)

greatest prognostic impact included NYHA functional class, history of clinical heart failure, NSVT not related to coronary artery bypass surgery, LVEF, age, left ventricular conduction abnormalities, inducible sustained ventricular tachycardia, inpatient status, and atrial fibrillation. According to these data, patients with an LVEF of 30% or lower but no other risk factors had a 2-year risk of death from arrhythmia of less than 5%.

2. The Triggers of Ventricular Arrhythmias (TOVA) study of 1140 patients revealed that in addition to LVEF, clinical NYHA class III heart failure was an independent risk factor for the occurrence of a ventricular arrhythmia that prompted an ICD discharge.[111]
3. In MADIT II, which enrolled 1232 patients, investigators used a clinical risk score that included NYHA functional class higher than II, age of more than 70 years, blood urea nitrogen (BUN) level higher than 26 mg/dL, QRS duration longer than 0.12 seconds, and atrial fibrillation.[112] Patients at very high risk (5% of the total population as defined by BUN level ≥ 50 mg/dL and or serum creatinine level ≥ 2.5 mg/dL) were excluded from this evaluation. Of the patients with a risk score of 0 (one third of the patients), those who had an ICD and those without an ICD had similar 2-year rates of mortality (9% and 8%). Among patients with a risk score 1 or 2, the 2-year mortality rate was significantly lower in those with an ICD (9% and 15%, respectively) than in those without an ICD (22% and 32%, respectively; $P = .002$ and $P < .001$). In contrast, the mortality rates among patients with a risk score of 3 or higher (15% of patients) were the same with or without an ICD (29% vs. 32%). Likewise, the mortality rates in the patients at very high risk were the same with and without an ICD (51% vs. 43%).

Therefore, in patients with an ischemic cardiomyopathy, a number of clinical variables can be used to identify patients with an LVEF of 30% or lower who have a low mortality rate and for whom the ICD is of no benefit. These clinical parameters are not static, and continued reassessment of the patient is necessary. As yet, no data are available for patients with nonischemic cardiomyopathy.

Therapy for Patients with Heart Failure Who Have Experienced a Sustained Ventricular Tachyarrhythmia (Secondary Prevention) (see Chapter 47)

Patients with heart failure who survive an episode of SCD or who experience sustained ventricular tachycardia are at high risk of future arrhythmic events and SCD. In these patients, an ICD is usually implanted for secondary prevention of SCD. Some patients may receive treatment with other therapies, such as antiarrhythmic drugs, radiofrequency ablation, surgery, and cardiac transplantation. However, these other treatments are not as effective as an ICD in improving survival. For this reason, they are used either as an adjunct to an ICD or as an alternative in patients who are not candidates for ICD therapy.

Implantable Cardioverter-Defibrillator

The ICD reduces overall mortality and mortality from SCD in comparison with amiodarone when used for secondary prevention in patients with cardiomyopathy (LVEF ≤ 35%) and heart failure who have experienced a ventricular tachyarrhythmia or SCD.[113] However, its effect on overall mortality in patients with severe heart failure and an LVEF lower than 20% is uncertain because the mode of death in many of these patients is progressive heart failure or asystole, which cannot be prevented by the ICD.

The role of the ICD in secondary prevention of SCD was evaluated in three randomized trials. On the basis of the results of these trials, the ACC/AHA/ESC guidelines recommended the ICD for secondary prevention of SCD in patients with ischemic or nonischemic cardiomyopathy who are receiving optimal medical therapy and who have a reasonable expectation of survival with a good functional status for more than 1 year.

AVID Trial

The Antiarrhythmics Versus Implantable Defibrillators (AVID) trial enrolled 1016 patients with a history of ventricular tachycardia, ventricular fibrillation, or syncope judged to be secondary to arrhythmia. This trial was stopped because survival rates were higher in the patients receiving the ICD than in those receiving d,l sotalol or amiodarone (89% vs. 82% at 1 year, 82% vs. 75% at 2 years, and 75% vs. 65% at 3 years).[114] However, the unadjusted improvement in mean survival was only 2.6 months (31 vs. 29 months with amiodarone), a difference that was reduced by 15% when adjustments were made for heart failure and the LVEF. The major effect of the ICD was, not expectedly, to prevent arrhythmic death (4.7% vs. 10.8% with antiarrhythmic drugs); rates of nonarrhythmic cardiac death were equivalent, and patients treated with drugs had an insignificantly greater incidence of noncardiac death, primarily from renal and pulmonary causes. Survival, when analyzed by LVEF, was no different with an ICD or with antiarrhythmic drugs among patients with an LVEF of 35% or higher; in contrast, among patients with an LVEF between 20% and 34%, survival rate was significantly better with the ICD. In patients with an LVEF lower than 20%, survival tended to be better with the ICD than with drugs, but the difference was not statistically significant (Figure 53-13). Unfortunately, there are no data about the role of the ICD in the presence or absence of clinical heart failure.

CIDS

The randomized Canadian Implantable Defibrillator Study (CIDS) enrolled 659 patients with ventricular tachycardia, ventricular fibrillation, or syncope deemed to be secondary to arrhythmia. After a 5-year follow-up period, the total rate of mortality with the ICD was not significantly reduced in comparison with amiodarone (8.3% vs. 10.2% per year; $P = .142$), and there was a nonsignificant reduction in arrhythmic death (3% vs. 4.5% per year, $P = .094$.[115] There was no difference in outcome according to the presenting arrhythmia. A multivariate risk model identified age of 70 or older, LVEF of 35% or lower, and NYHA class III or IV as independent predictors of risk; on the basis of these parameters, quartiles of risk were constructed. Among patients in the highest risk quartile, who had two or more risk factors, the death rate was reduced significantly with the ICD in comparison with amiodarone (14% vs. 30%); no benefit was observed among patients in the other three quartiles.

CASH Trial

In the Cardiac Arrest Study Hamburg (CASH) trial, 349 survivors of cardiac arrest due to a documented ventricular tachyarrhythmia were randomly assigned to receive an ICD, metoprolol, propafenone, or amiodarone; propafenone was subsequently dropped from the trial because of a higher mortality rate with this drug, according to an interim 2-year analysis.[116] After a mean follow-up period of 57 months, there was an insignificant 23% reduction in total mortality with the ICD in comparison with amiodarone (36.4%) or metoprolol (44.9%; $P = .08$); the benefit of the ICD was more evident during the first 5 years after the index event. The secondary endpoint of SCD was also reduced by the ICD (13%) in comparison with drug therapy (33%; $P = .005$). However, when amiodarone and metoprolol were considered separately, there was no difference among the three groups.

Meta-analysis of Secondary Prevention Trials

A meta-analysis of the three major ICD trials (AVID, CIDS, and CASH) revealed a significant 28% reduction in mortality with an ICD in comparison with amiodarone, which was attributable entirely to a 50% reduction in SCD.[113] Over a 6-year period, survival was extended by 4.4 months with an ICD. The mortality benefit was observed only in patients with an LVEF of 35% or lower[113] (Figure 53-14).

Long-Term Outcome

Despite the use of the ICD, the mortality rate among patients with heart failure remains high as a result of death that cannot be prevented by the ICD, including progressive heart failure, refractory ventricular arrhythmias that may occur with terminal heart failure, asystole, or pulseless electrical activity. An important predictor of outcome is left ventricular function. This was illustrated in an analysis of 36 clinical and treatment variables in 3559 patients with a sustained ventricular tachyarrhythmia who were enrolled in the AVID registry.[116a] Actuarial rates of survival at 2 and 3 years were 79% and 72%, respectively. The strongest risk factors for prognosis were age and the severity of underlying heart disease, as reflected by the extent of left ventricular dysfunction and the presence of heart failure. The hemodynamic effect of the arrhythmia was not a predictor of outcome.

In contrast to these findings in SCD, there is generally a good outcome in patients with idiopathic dilated cardiomyopathy and clinical sustained monomorphic ventricular tachycardia in whom inducibility of ventricular tachycardia is suppressed by antiarrhythmic drugs.

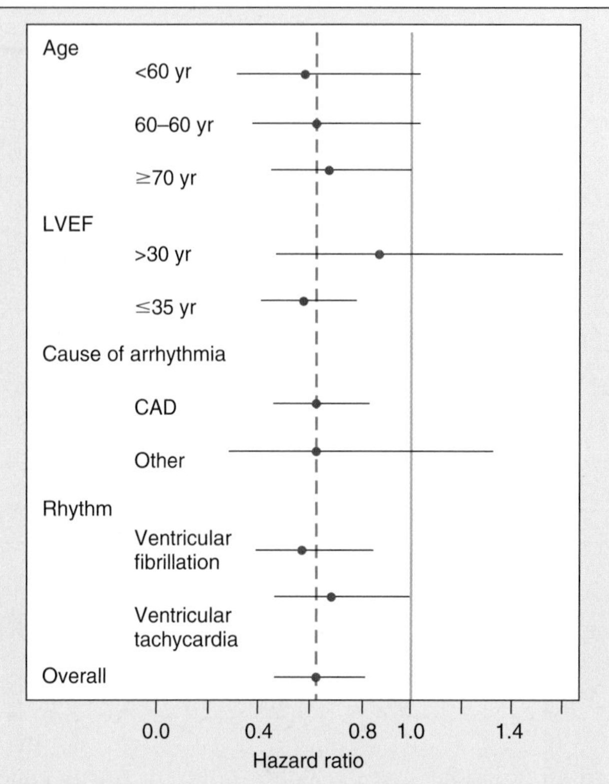

FIGURE 53–13 Subset analysis of 1013 survivors of sudden cardiac death or hemodynamically significant ventricular tachycardia who were enrolled in the Antiarrhythmics Versus Implantable Defibrillators (AVID) trial. The hazard ratios for death from any cause with the implantable cardioverter defibrillator, in comparison with amiodarone, were not significantly different for any of the prespecified subgroups. (From the Antiarrhythmics Versus Implantable Defibrillators [AVID] Investigators: A comparison of antiarrhythmic-drug therapy with implantable defibrillators in patients resuscitated from near-fatal ventricular arrhythmias. *N Engl J Med* 1997;337:1576.)

Antiarrhythmic Drug Therapy

In patients with heart failure who have experienced a ventricular tachyarrhythmia, the use of antiarrhythmic drugs to prevent recurrent ventricular arrhythmia is currently limited because no studies have shown these agents to be effective. Thus, the ICD has become the preferred therapy. However, antiarrhythmic therapy has an important role in several situations:

1. The Center for Medicare Services requires that a patient be expected to survive at least 1 year in order to qualify for ICD therapy. Therefore, antiarrhythmic drug therapy (usually amiodarone) is prescribed to patients who are not candidates for an ICD because of age, the presence

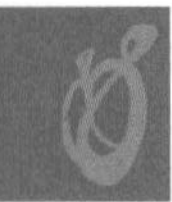

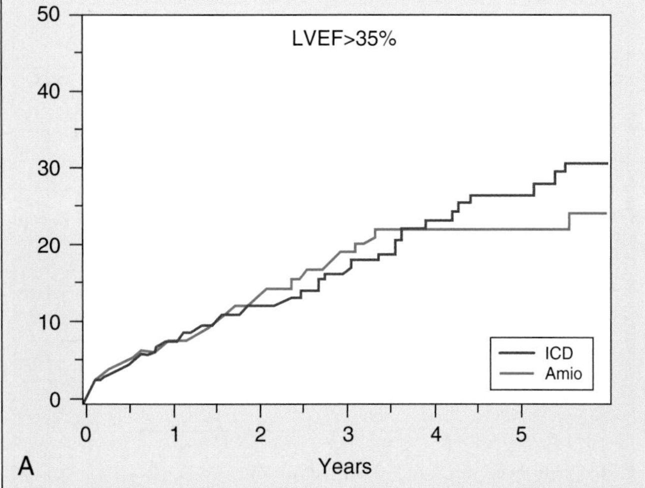

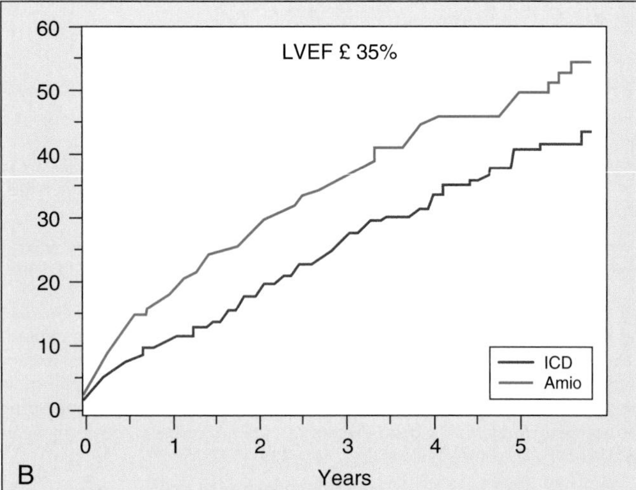

FIGURE 53–14 Meta-analysis of three implantable cardioverter-defibrillator (ICD) trials: Antiarrhythmics Versus Implantable Defibrillators (AVID), Canadian Implantable Defibrillator Study (CIDS), and Cardiac Arrest Study Hamburg (CASH). For patients with left ventricular ejection fraction (LVEF) of approximately 35% (**B**), the cumulative risk of death was found to be 28% lower with the implantable cardioverter-defibrillator (ICD) than with amiodarone; this was attributable entirely to a reduction in sudden cardiac death. In contrast, among patients with LVEF higher than 35% (**A**), there was little difference in survival between patients who had ICD and those who took amiodarone. (From Connolly SJ, Hallstrom AP, Cappato R, et al. Meta-analysis of the implantable cardioverter defibrillator secondary prevention trials. AVID, CASH and CIDS studies. Antiarrhythmics vs Implantable Defibrillator Study. Cardiac Arrest Study Hamburg. Canadian Implantable Defibrillator Study. *Eur Heart J* 2000;21:2071.)

of comorbid conditions (especially renal impairment or cancer), or perhaps class IV heart failure, which confers increased risk of death from progressive pump failure or from noncardiac causes.

2. Drug therapy is recommended for the suppression of NSVT or atrial fibrillation that causes symptoms or interferes with ICD function, which results in inappropriate ICD discharges.
3. Drug therapy is recommended for the prevention of frequent ICD discharges that result from recurrent sustained ventricular tachyarrhythmias.
4. Drug therapy is recommended to slow the rate of a ventricular tachyarrhythmia, which makes it better tolerated hemodynamically or more amenable to termination with antitachycardia pacing or a cardioversion shock.

Radiofrequency Ablation

Radiofrequency catheter ablation of ventricular tachycardia can be an effective therapy in some patients if a reentrant circuit can be adequately mapped and if the area of slow conduction can be defined and ablated. Such a circuit is present more commonly in patients with an ischemic cardiomyopathy and a prior infarction; the reentrant circuit is often located at the border zone of the scar.[116b] Although not commonly used as primary therapy in these patients, radiofrequency ablation is occasionally performed as an adjunct treatment in patients with an ICD to reduce the frequency of ventricular tachyarrhythmias that are associated with symptoms or ICD discharges.[116c]

In contrast, patients with a nonischemic cardiomyopathy have diffuse disease, and there may be multiple reentrant circuits or even other mechanisms for arrhythmia, such as enhanced automaticity or triggered activity. Thus, ablation currently has a low success rate in such patients.

Patients with ischemic or nonischemic cardiomyopathy and heart failure have a unique, albeit uncommon, form of ventricular tachycardia that is called "bundle branch reentrant ventricular tachycardia." This arrhythmia is the result of abnormal conduction through the bundle of His and the left bundle branch. Many patients with this arrhythmia have a baseline nonspecific conduction delay or left bundle branch block, and most have a prolonged His-to-ventricle interval. Presyncope and syncope are common presenting symptoms. Catheter ablation of the right bundle branch, which leads to complete right bundle branch block, effectively and safely eliminates the arrhythmia.

Catheter ablation is generally performed in three situations:

1. As an adjunct to an ICD in patients who have frequent sustained ventricular arrhythmias and ICD therapies.
2. As an alternative to an ICD in patients who do not want or are not candidates for an ICD.
3. When the cause of the ventricular tachycardia is bundle branch reentry.

Surgery

Arrhythmia surgery is an effective way to eliminate reentrant circuits. However, the concerns regarding ablation in cardiomyopathy also apply to a surgical approach because of the requirement for localization of the reentrant circuit.[116d] Surgery may be a reasonable approach for patients with coronary artery disease, those who have had a previous myocardial infarction, those with left ventricular aneurysm, and those with sustained monomorphic ventricular tachycardia; it has little, if any, role in patients with diffuse cardiomyopathy. However, with the advent of the ICD and radiofrequency ablation, this type of surgery is rarely performed.

Transplantation

Cardiac transplantation may be an option for patients with cardiomyopathy and heart failure who have experienced serious life-threatening ventricular tachyarrhythmias. In such patients, the ICD may be used as a bridge to transplantation.

Implantable Cardioverter-Defibrillator Therapy in Hypertrophic Cardiomyopathy (see Chapter 25)

The most important concern in patients with hypertrophic cardiomyopathy is SCD resulting from a ventricular tachyarrhythmia. ICDs are the preferred therapy for such patients. No randomized trials have provided evidence of improved survival with an ICD as primary or prophylactic therapy in hypertrophic cardiomyopathy. However, support for their use comes from the known rate of SCD in patients at high risk and from observations of the high rate of appropriate ICD discharges in patients who have received a device for primary prevention. For example, in one study of 128 patients receiving an ICD for primary or secondary prevention, the rate of appropriate device activation was 11% per year when it was used for secondary prevention of SCD and 5% per year when it was used for primary prevention.[117]

On the basis of data from several studies, a consensus statement from the ACC and ESC[117] identified several major risk factors for SCD in hypertrophic cardiomyopathy patients: a history of SCD or sustained ventricular tachycardia, a family history of premature SCD, unexplained syncope, severe left ventricular hypertrophy (maximum wall thickness > 30 mm), a hypotensive blood pressure response during exercise testing, and NSVT on ambulatory monitoring. According to the ACC/AHA/ESC guidelines, ICD insertion should be considered for primary prevention of SCD in patients with one or more of these high-risk features.

Implantable Cardioverter-Defibrillator for Unexplained Syncope. Syncope in patients with nonischemic cardiomyopathy and advanced heart failure may result from any of the well-established causes of syncope. However, when the syncope is of unknown origin, a ventricular tachyarrhythmia or a bradycardia resulting from a conduction abnormality such as complete heart block is often the cause. Regardless of the cause, syncope in such patients is associated with a high 1-year risk of SCD that is similar to that in patients who have experienced a ventricular tachyarrhythmia.[118] In one series, the mortality rate was 45% among patients with syncope, in comparison with 12% among those without syncope.

Although no hard data are available, it is believed that the ICD is the most effective therapy in these patients. In one study, investigators evaluated 147 patients with nonischemic cardiomyopathy, unexplained syncope, and no history of sustained ventricular tachyarrhythmia or SCD.[119] The actuarial survival rate at 2 years was higher among the 25 patients treated with an ICD (85%) than among the 122 patients managed with conventional medical therapy (67%); of those receiving an ICD, 40% experienced an appropriate shock. Another study also revealed that in patients with cardiomyopathy, unexplained syncope, and no electrophysiological abnormalities, empirical ICD therapy improved long-term outcome and the hazard ratio for the risk of an event in the ICD recipients, in comparison with patients treated with conventional therapy, was 0.18. Appropriate ICD shocks occurred in 26% of patients at 2 years.

In contrast, SCD-HeFT, which included 472 patients with a history of syncope before or after randomization, revealed that the ICD did not protect against SCD in comparison with amiodarone or placebo (hazard ratios = 1.54, 1.33, and 1.39, respectively; in the test for differences, $P = .86$).[120]

The ACC/AHA/ESC guidelines suggest that, according to expert opinion, an ICD can be beneficial and is a reasonable approach to therapy in patients with cardiomyopathy and unexplained syncope.

Recommendation for Treatment of Ventricular Tachyarrhythmias

Patients with heart failure and ventricular arrhythmia should be treated aggressively with drugs proven to be effective for therapy of heart failure, including a β-blocker, an ACE inhibitor, an ARB in selected patients, a statin, and an aldosterone antagonist in selected patients.

Patients with a History of a Ventricular Tachyarrhythmia (Ventricular Tachycardia or Sudden Cardiac Death)

According to the current ACC/AHA/ESC guidelines, the ICD is the recommended approach for preventing recurrent ventricular arrhythmia in patients with cardiomyopathy of any origin and heart failure who have survived SCD caused by ventricular fibrillation or ventricular tachycardia or who have sustained ventricular tachycardia. For patients with very severe left ventricular dysfunction (LVEF < 20%) in whom the risk of mortality from progressive heart failure is high, the benefit of an ICD is questionable. Among patients with very poor systolic function, advances in the therapy of heart failure have improved survival, partly as a result of a lower rate of death from nonarrhythmic causes. However, the ACC/AHA/ESC guidelines do not include recommendations based on the LVEF. Nevertheless, the ICD is considered a preferred approach in these patients, unless there are significant comorbid conditions that would affect survival; in such patients, antiarrhythmic therapy is generally preferred. Amiodarone therapy may, however, be a reasonable option for initial therapy in patients with ventricular tachycardia; the ICD can be reserved for patients who have recurrent ventricular tachycardia (which is often slower and better tolerated hemodynamically) despite amiodarone therapy.

Although the randomized studies have shown that amiodarone and the ICD were equally effective in patients with an LVEF higher than 35%, the use of an ICD is preferred in these patients, especially when the patient has experienced SCD.

Antiarrhythmic therapy with sotalol or amiodarone is often used as adjunctive therapy for the patient who has other symptomatic arrhythmias, such as NSVT or atrial fibrillation, or who has recurrent episodes of ventricular tachyarrhythmias that result in symptoms or frequent ICD discharges. Antiarrhythmic therapy is also recommended for those patients not considered candidates for an ICD. Radiofrequency ablation is also an adjunctive therapy for patients with ischemic cardiomyopathy who have frequent episodes of sustained monomorphic ventricular tachycardia that results in ICD discharges.

Prophylactic Therapy in Patients at High Risk with Cardiomyopathy

According to the current ACC/AHA/ESC guidelines, the ICD is the recommended approach in patients who have survived myocardial infarction by at least 40 days, have an LVEF of 30% or lower (ischemic cardiomyopathy), have NYHA functional class II or III heart failure, are receiving chronic optimal medical therapy, and have reasonable expectation of survival with a good functional status for more than 1 year.

The ICD is also indicated in patients with nonischemic cardiomyopathy who have had an LVEF of 35% or lower for at least 9 months, have NYHA functional class II or III heart failure, are receiving chronic optimal medical therapy, and have reasonable expectation of survival with a good functional status for more than 1 year.

Although LVEF is currently the only criterion for prophylactic ICD use in the primary prevention of SCD in patients with an ischemic or nonischemic cardiomyopathy, data about other clinical factors will help in risk stratification to identify patients at high risk who will benefit from ICD implantation.

Antiarrhythmic drugs, primarily amiodarone or sotalol, are preferred for patients who are not deemed to be candidates for an ICD. These drugs are useful as adjunctive therapy to treat atrial fibrillation, NSVT, or sustained ventricular tachycardia that are associated with symptoms or result in ICD discharges. Radiofrequency ablation is useful for patients with ischemic cardiomyopathy who experience frequent ICD discharges because of sustained ventricular tachycardia.

Patients with Hypertrophic Cardiomyopathy (see Chapter 25)

According to the current ACC/AHA/ESC guidelines, the ICD is the recommended approach for secondary prevention in patients with a hypertrophic cardiomyopathy who survive an episode of sustained ventricular tachycardia or SCD, who are receiving chronic optimal medical therapy, and who have reasonable expectation of survival with a good functional status for more than 1 year.

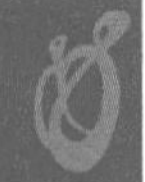

The ICD can be effective as primary prevention of SCD in patients with hypertrophic cardiomyopathy who are thought to be high risk; such patients are generally defined as those who have one or more of the high-risk features (i.e., a family history of premature SCD, unexplained syncope, severe left ventricular hypertrophy with a maximum wall thickness >30 mm, a hypotensive blood pressure response during exercise testing, or NSVT on ambulatory monitoring).

It is also believed that amiodarone can also be effective secondary therapy for patients with hypertrophic cardiomyopathy and a history of sustained ventricular tachycardia or ventricular fibrillation, if an ICD is not feasible.

Patients with Unexplained Syncope

Among patients with cardiomyopathy and heart failure who experience syncope of undetermined origin, the rate of mortality, often the result of SCD, is high; it is similar to the incidence in patients with a sustained ventricular arrhythmias. There is a growing consensus that these patients should receive an ICD.

REFERENCES

1. De Ferrari, G. M., Klersy, C., Ferrero, P.for the ALPHA Study Group, et al. (2007). Atrial fibrillation in heart failure patients: prevalence in daily practice and effect on the severity of symptoms. Data from the ALPHA study registry. *Eur J Heart Fail*, *9*, 502.
2. Cha, Y. M., Redfield, M. M., Shen, W. K., et al. (2004). Atrial fibrillation and ventricular dysfunction: a vicious electromechanical cycle. *Circulation*, *109*, 2839.
3. Olivotto, I., Cecchi, F., Casey, S. A., et al. (2001). Impact of atrial fibrillation on the clinical course of hypertrophic cardiomyopathy. *Circulation*, *104*, 2517.
4. Benjamin, E. J., Levy, D., Vaziri, S. M., et al. (1994). Independent risk factors for atrial fibrillation in a population based cohort. The Framingham Heart Study. *JAMA*, *271*, 840.
5. Pozzoli, M., Cioffi, G., Traversi, E., et al. (1998). Predictors of primary atrial fibrillation and concomitant clinical and hemodynamic changes in patients with chronic heart failure: a prospective study in 344 patients with baseline sinus rhythm. *J Am Coll Cardiol*, *32*, 197.
6. Lee, D. S., Gona, P., Vasan, R. S., et al. (2009). Relation of disease pathogenesis and risk factors to heart failure with preserved or reduced ejection fraction. Insights from the Framingham Heart Study of the National Heart, Lung and Blood Institute. *Circulation*, *119*, 3070.
7. Miyasaka, Y., Barnes, M. E., Gersh, B. J., et al. (2006). Incidence and mortality risk of congestive heart failure in atrial fibrillation patient: a community based study over two decades. *Eur Heart J*, *27*, 936.
8. SandersMorton, R. J. B., Kistler, P. M., et al. (2003). Reversal of atrial mechanical dysfunction after cardioversion of atrial fibrillation: implications for the mechanisms of tachycardia-mediated atrial cardiomyopathy. *Circulation*, *108*, 1976.
9. Fujino, T., Yamashita, T., Suzuki, S., et al. (2007). Characteristics of congestive heart failure accompanied by atrial fibrillation with special reference to tachycardia-induced cardiomyopathy. *Circ J*, *71*, 936.
10. Parthenakis, F. I., Patrianakos, A. P., Skalidis, E. I., et al. (2007). Atrial fibrillation is associated with increased neurohumoral activation and reduced exercise tolerance in patients with non-ischemic dilated cardiomyopathy. *Int J Cardiol*, *118*, 206.
11. Wijffels, M. C. E. F., Kirchhof, C. J. H. J., & Dorland, R. (1995). Atrial fibrillation begets atrial fibrillation. A study in awake chronically instrumented goats. *Circulation*, *92*, 1954.
12. Stulak, J. M., Dearani, J. A., Daly, R. C., et al. (2006). Left ventricular dysfunction in atrial fibrillation: restoration of sinus rhythm by the Cox-maze procedure significantly improves systolic function and functional status. *Ann Thorac Surg*, *82*, 494.
13. Falk, R. H. (2001). Atrial fibrillation. *N Engl J Med*, *344*, 1067–1078.
14. Kay, G. N., Ellenbogen, K. A., Giudici, M., et al. (1998). The Ablate and Pace Trial: a prospective study of catheter ablation of the AV conduction system and permanent pacemaker implantation for treatment of atrial fibrillation. *J Interv Card Electrophysiol*, *2*, 121.
15. Wood, M. A., Brown-Mahoney, C., Kay, G. N., et al. (2000). Clinical outcomes after ablation and pacing therapy for atrial fibrillation: a meta-analysis. *Circulation*, *101*, 1138.
16. Parkash, R., Green, M. S., Kerr, C. R., et al. (2004). The association of left atrial size and occurrence of atrial fibrillation: a prospective cohort study from the Canadian Registry of Atrial Fibrillation. *Am Heart J*, *148*, 649.
17. Ravelli, F., & Allessie, M. (1997). Effects of atrial dilation on refractory period and vulnerability to atrial fibrillation in the isolated Langendorff-perfused rabbit heart. *Circulation*, *96*, 1686.
18. Bode, F., Katchman, A., Woosley, R. L., et al. (2000). Gadolinium decreases stretch-induced vulnerability to atrial fibrillation. *Circulation*, *101*, 2200.
19. Losi, M. A., Betocchi, S., Aversa, M., et al. (2004). Determinants of atrial fibrillation development in patients with hypertrophic cardiomyopathy. *Am J Cardiol*, *94*, 895.
20. Yamada, T., Fukunami, M., Shimonagata, T., et al. (2000). Prediction of paroxysmal atrial fibrillation in patients with congestive heart failure: a prospective study. *J Am Coll Cardiol*, *35*, 405.
21. Dogan, A., Kahraman, H., Ozturk, M., et al. (2004). P wave dispersion and left atrial appendage function for predicting recurrence after conversion of atrial fibrillation and relation of p wave dispersion to appendage function. *Echocardiography*, *21*, 523–530.
22. Rossi, A., Enriquez-Sarano, M., Burnett, J. C., et al. (2000). Natriuretic peptide levels in atrial fibrillation. A prospective hormonal and Doppler-echocardiographic study. *J Am Coll Cardiol*, *35*, 1256.
23. The Stroke Prevention in Atrial Fibrillation Investigators (1992). Predictors of thromboembolism in atrial fibrillation. I. Clinical features of patients at risk. *Ann Intern Med*, *116*, 1.
24. Dunkman, W. B., Johnson, G. R., Carson, P. E., et al. (1993). Incidence of thromboembolic events in congestive heart failure. The V-HeFT VA Cooperative Studies Group. *Circulation*, *87*, VI-94.
25. Maron, B. J., Olivotto, I., Bellone, P., et al. (2007). Clinical profile of stroke in 900 patients with hypertrophic cardiomyopathy. *J Am Coll Cardiol*, *39*, 301.
26. Gage, B. F., Waterman, A. D., Shannon, W., et al. (2001). Validation of clinical classification schemes for predicting stroke: results from the National Registry of atrial fibrillation. *JAMA*, *285*, 2864.
27. Singer, D. E., Albers, G. W., Dalen, J. E., for the American College of Chest Physicians, et al. (2008). Antithrombotic therapy in atrial fibrillation: American College of Chest Physicians Evidence-Based Clinical Practice Guidelines (8th Edition). *Chest*, *133*(Suppl 6), 546S–592S.
28. Swedberg, K., Olsson, L. G., Charlesworth, A., et al. (2005). Prognostic relevance of atrial fibrillation in patients with chronic heart failure on long-term treatment with beta-blockers: results from COMET. *Eur Heart J*, *26*, 1303.
29. Dries, D. L., Exner, D. V., Gersh, B. J., et al. (1998). Atrial fibrillation is associated with an increased risk for mortality and heart failure progression in patients with asymptomatic left ventricular systolic dysfunction: a retrospective analysis of the SOLVD trials. *J Am Coll Cardiol*, *32*, 695.
30. Olsson, L. G., Swedberg, K., Ducharme, A., et al. (2006). Atrial fibrillation and risk of clinical events in chronic heart failure with and without left ventricular systolic dysfunction: results from the Candesartan in Heart Failure–Assessment of Reduction in Mortality and morbidity (CHARM) program. *J Am Coll Cardiol*, *47*, 1997.
31. Kober, L., Swedberg, K., McMurray, J. J., et al. (2006). Previously known and newly diagnosed atrial fibrillation: a major risk indicator after a myocardial infarction complicated by heart failure or left ventricular dysfunction. *Eur J Heart Fail*, *8*, 591.
32. Wasywich CA, Pope AJ, Somaratne J, et al. (2009). Atrial fibrillation and the risk of death in patients with heart failure: a literature-based meta-analysis. *Intern Med J*, 40:317
33. Flaker, G. C., Blackshear, J. L., McBride, R., et al. (1992). Antiarrhythmic drug therapy and cardiac mortality in atrial fibrillation. The Stroke Prevention in Atrial Fibrillation Investigators. *J Am Coll Cardiol*, *20*, 527.
34. Slater, W. S., Lampert, S., Podrid, P. J., et al. (1988). Clinical predictors of arrhythmia worsening by antiarrhythmic drugs. *Am J Cardiol Coll*, *61*, 349.
35. Deedwania, P. C., Singh, B. N., Ellenbogen, K., for the Department of Veterans Affairs CHF-STAT Investigators, et al. (1998). Spontaneous conversion and maintenance of sinus rhythm by amiodarone in patients with heart failure and atrial fibrillation: observations from the Veterans Affairs Congestive Heart Failure Survival Trial of Antiarrhythmic Therapy (CHF-STAT). The Department of Veterans Affairs CHF-STAT Investigators. *Circulation*, *98*, 2574.
36. Vorperian, V. R., Havighurst, T. C., Miller, S., et al. (1997). Adverse effects of low dose amiodarone: a meta-analysis. *J Am Coll Cardiol*, *30*, 791.
37. Torp-Pedersen, C., Moller, M., Bloch-Thomsen, P. E., et al. (1999). Dofetilide in patients with congestive heart failure and left ventricular dysfunction. Danish Investigations of Arrhythmia and Mortality on Dofetilide Study Group. *N Engl J Med*, *341*, 857.
38. Pratt, C. M., Singh, S. N., Al-Khalidi, H. R., et al. (2004). The efficacy of azimilide in the treatment of atrial fibrillation in the presence of left ventricular systolic dysfunction: results from the Azimilide Postinfarct Survival Evaluation (ALIVE) trial. *J Am Coll Cardiol*, *43*, 1211.
39. Kober, L., Torp-Petersen, C., McMurray, M. D., for the Dronedarone Study Group, et al. (2008). Increased mortality after dronedarone therapy for severe heart failure. *N Engl J Med*, *358*, 2678.
40. Healey, J. S., Baranchuk, A., Crystal, E., et al. (2005). Prevention of atrial fibrillation with angiotensin-converting enzyme inhibitors and angiotensin receptor blockers: a meta-analysis. *J Am Coll Cardiol*, *45*, 1832.
41. Hsu, L. -F., Jaïs, P., Sanders, P., et al. (2004). Catheter ablation for atrial fibrillation in congestive heart failure. *N Engl J Med*, *351*, 2373.
42. Khan, M. N., Jaïs, P., Cummings, J., for the PABA-CHF Investigators, et al. (2008). Pulmonary-vein isolation for atrial fibrillation. *N Engl J Med*, *359*, 1778.
43. Gaita, F., DiDonna, P., Olivotto, I., et al. (2007). Usefulness and safety of transcatheter ablation of atrial fibrillation in patients with hypertrophic cardiomyopathy. *Am J Cardiol*, *99*, 1575.
44. Maron, B.J., McKenna, W.J., Danielson, G.K., et al. (2003). American College of Cardiology/European Society of Cardiology clinical expert consensus document on hypertrophic cardiomyopathy. A report of the American College of Cardiology Foundation Task Force on Clinical Expert Consensus Documents and the European Society of Cardiology Committee for Practice Guidelines. *J Am Coll Cardiol*. 42,1687.
45. Nasr, I. A., Bouzamondo, A., Hulot, J. S., et al. (2007). Prevention of atrial fibrillation onset by beta-blocker treatment in heart failure: a meta-analysis. *Eur Heart J*, *28*, 457.
46. Tops, L. F., Schalij, M. J., Holman, E. R., et al. (2006). Right ventricular pacing can induce ventricular dyssynchrony in patients with atrial fibrillation after atrioventricular node ablation. *J Am Coll Cardiol*, *48*, 1642.
47. Doshi, R. N., Daoud, E. G., Fellows, C., et al. (2005). Left ventricular-based cardiac stimulation post AV nodal ablation evaluation (the PAVE study). *J Cardiovasc Electrophysiol*, *16*, 1160.
48. Roy, D., Talajic, M., Nattel, S., for the Atrial Fibrillation and Congestive Heart Failure Investigators, et al. (2008). Rhythm control versus rate control for atrial fibrillation and heart failure. *N Engl J Med*, *358*, 2667.

48a. Fuster, V., Ryden, L. E., Cannom, D. S., et al. (2006). ACC/AHA/ESC guidelines for the management of patients with atrial fibrillation: a report from the ACC/AHA task force for Practice Guidelines and the ESC Committee for Practice Guidelines (writing committee to revise the 2001 guidelines for the management of patients with atrial fibrillation). *J Am Coll Cardiol*, *48*, e149.

49. Pedersen, O. D., Bagger, H., Keller, N., et al. (2001). Efficacy of dofetilide in the treatment of atrial fibrillation-flutter in patients with reduced left ventricular function: a Danish Investigation of Arrhythmia and Mortality On Dofetilide (DIAMOND) substudy. *Circulation*, *104*, 292.

50. Ibrahim, S. A., & Kwoh, C. K. (2000). Underutilization of oral anticoagulant therapy for stroke prevention in elderly patients with atrial fibrillation. *Am Heart J, 140*, 219.
51. Adabag, A. S., Casey, S. A., Kuskowski, M. A., et al. (2005). Spectrum and prognostic significance of arrhythmias on ambulatory Holter electrocardiogram in hypertrophic cardiomyopathy. *J Am Coll Cardiol, 45*, 697.
52. Jin, H., Lyon, A. R., & Akar, F. G. (2008). Arrhythmia mechanisms in the failing heart. *Pacing Clin Electrophysiol, 31*, 1048.
53. Lerman, B. B., Engelstein, E. D., & Burkhoff, D. (2001). Mechanoelectrical feedback: role of beta-adrenergic receptor activation in mediating load-dependent shortening of ventricular action potential and refractoriness. *Circulation, 104*, 486.
54. Koilpillai, C., Quinones, M. A., Greenberg, B., for the SOLVD Investigators, et al. (1996). Relation of ventricular size and function to heart failure status and ventricular dysrhythmia in patients with severe left ventricular dysfunction. *Am J Cardiol, 77*, 606.
55. Mortara, A., La Rovere, M. T., Pinna, G. D., et al. (1997). Depressed arterial baroreflex sensitivity and not reduced heart rate variability identifies patients with chronic heart failure and nonsustained ventricular tachycardia: the effect of high ventricular filling pressure. *Am Heart J, 134*, 879.
56. Cao, J. M., Fishbein, M. C., Han, J. B., et al. (2000). Relationship between regional cardiac hyperinnervation and ventricular arrhythmia. *Circulation, 101*, 1960.
57. Iwata, M., Yoshikawa, T., Baba, A., et al. (2001). Autoantibodies against the second extracellular loop of beta 1–adrenergic receptors predict ventricular tachycardia and sudden death in patients with idiopathic dilated cardiomyopathy. *J Am Coll Cardiol, 37*, 418.
58. Uretsky, B. F., Thygesen, K., Armstrong, P. W., et al. (2000). Acute coronary findings at autopsy in heart failure patients with sudden death. Results from the Assessment of Treatment with Lisinopril and Survival (ATLAS) trial. *Circulation, 102*, 611.
59. Packer, M., Carver, J. R., Rodeheffer, R. J., et al. (1991). Effect of oral milrinone on mortality in severe chronic heart failure. *N Engl J Med, 325*, 1468.
60. DiBianco, R., Shabetai, R., Kostuk, W., et al. (1989). A comparison of oral milrinone, digoxin, and their combination in the treatment of patients with chronic heart failure. *N Engl J Med, 320*, 677.
61. The effect of digoxin on mortality and morbidity in patients with heart failure. (1997). The Digitalis Investigation Group. *N Engl J Med, 336*, 525.
62. Kannel, W. B., Plehn, J. F., & Cupples, L. A. (1988). Cardiac failure and sudden death in the Framingham study. *Am Heart J, 115*, 869.
63. Effects of enalapril on mortality in severe congestive heart failure. (1987). Results of the Cooperative North Scandinavian Enalapril Survival Study (CONSENSUS). The CONSENSUS Trial Study Group. *N Engl J Med, 316*, 1429.
64. Luu, M., Stevenson, W. G., Stevenson, L. W., et al. (1989). Diverse mechanisms of unexpected cardiac arrest in advanced heart failure. *Circulation, 80*, 1675.
65. Actuarial risk of sudden death while awaiting cardiac transplantation in patients with atherosclerotic heart disease. DEFIBRILAT Study Group. (1991). *Am J Cardiol, 68*, 545.
66. Quinones, M. A., Greenberg, B. H., Kopelen, H. A.for the SOLVD Investigators, et al. (2000). Echocardiographic predictors of clinical outcome in patients with left ventricular dysfunction enrolled in the SOLVD registry and trials: significance of left ventricular hypertrophy. *J Am Coll Cardiol, 35*, 1237.
67. Grimm, W., Christ, M., Bach, J., et al. (2003). Noninvasive arrhythmia risk stratification in idiopathic dilated cardiomyopathy: results of the Marburg Cardiomyopathy Study. *Circulation, 108*, 2883.
67a. Zecchin, M., Unarde, D., Gugori, D., et al. (2005). Prognostic role of nonsustained ventricular tachycardia in a large cohort of patients with idiopathic dilated cardiomyopathy. *Ital Heart J, 6*,721.
68. Baker, R. L., & Koelling, T. M. (2005). Prognostic value of ambulatory electrocardiography monitoring in patients with dilated cardiomyopathy. *J Electrocardiol, 38*, 64.
69. de Sousa, M. R., Morillo, C. A., Rabelo, F. T., et al. (2008). Non-sustained ventricular tachycardia as a predictor of sudden cardiac death in patient with left ventricular dysfunction: a meta-analysis. *Eur J Heart Fail, 10*, 1007.
70. Monserrat, L., Elliott, P. M., Gimeno, J. R., et al. (2003). Non-sustained ventricular tachycardia in hypertrophic cardiomyopathy: an independent marker of sudden death risk in young patients. *J Am Coll Cardiol, 42*, 873.
71. Grimm, W., Glaveris, C., Hoffmann, J., et al. (2000). Arrhythmia risk stratification in idiopathic dilated cardiomyopathy based on echocardiography and 12-lead, signal averaged, and 24-hour Holter electrocardiography. *Am Heart J, 140*, 43.
72. Buxton, A. E., Lee, K. L., DiCarlo, L., et al. (2000). Electrophysiologic testing to identify patients with coronary artery disease who are at risk for sudden death. Multicenter Unsustained Tachycardia Trial Investigators. *N Engl J Med, 342*, 1937.
73. Fauchier, L., Baduty, D., Cosmay, P., et al. (2000). Long-term prognostic value of time domain analysis of signal-averaged electrocardiography in idiopathic dilated cardiomyopathy. *Am J Cardiol, 85*, 618.
74. Fauchier, L., Douglas, J., Babuty, D., et al. (2005). QT dispersion in nonischemic cardiomyopathy: a long term evaluation. *Eur J Heart Fail, 7*, 277.
75. Makkallio, T. H., Huikuri, H. V., Hintze, U., for the DIAMOND Study Group, et al. (2001). Fractal analysis and time-and frequency-domain measures of heart rate variability as predictors of mortality in patients with heart failure. *Am J Cardiol, 87*, 178.
75a. Nolan, J., Batin, P. D., Andrews, R., et al. (1998). Prospective study of heart rate variability and mortality in chronic heart failure: results of the United Kingdom Heart failure Evaluation and Assessment of Risk Trial (UK-Heart). *Circulation, 98*, 1510–1516.
76. Grimm, W., Christ, M., Sharkova, J., et al. (2005). Arrhythmia risk prediction in idiopathic dilated cardiomyopathy based on heart rate variability and baroreceptor sensitivity. *Pacing Clin Electrophysiol, 28*(Suppl 1), S202.
77. Rashba, E. J., Estes, N. A., Wang, P., et al. (2006). Preserved heart rate variability identifies low risk patients with nonischemic cardiomyopathy: results from the DEFINITE trial. *Heart Rhythm, 3*, 281.
78. Gehi, A. K., Stein, R. H., Metz, L. D., et al. (2005). Microvolt T-wave alternans for the risk stratification of ventricular tachyarrhythmic events: a meta-analysis. *J Am Coll Cardiol, 46*, 75.
79. Chow, T., Kereiakes, D. J., Bartone, C., et al. (2006). Prognostic utility of microvolt T-wave alternans in risk stratification of patients with ischemic cardiomyopathy. *J Am Coll Cardiol, 47*, 1820.
80. Salerno-Uriarte, J. A., DeFerrari, G. M., Klersy, C., et al. (2007). Prognostic value of T-wave alternans in patients with heart failure due to nonischemic cardiomyopathy: results of the ALPHA Study. *J Am Coll Cardiol, 50*, 1896.
81. Bloomfield, D. M., Steinman, R. C., Namerow, P. B., et al. (2004). Microvolt T-wave alternans distinguishes between patients likely and patients not likely to benefit from implanted cardiac defibrillator therapy: a solution to the Multicenter Automatic Defibrillator Implantation Trial (MADIT) II conundrum. *Circulation, 110*, 1885.
82. Gold, M. R., Ip, J. H., Constantini, O., et al. (2008). Role of microvolt T-wave alternans in assessment of arrhythmia vulnerability among patients with heart failure and systolic dysfunction: primary results from the T-wave alternans sudden cardiac death in heart failure trial substudy. *Circulation, 118*, 2022.
83. Effect of metoprolol CR/XL in chronic heart failure. (1999). Metoprolol CR/XL Randomised Intervention Trial in Congestive Heart Failure (MERIT-HF). *Lancet, 353*, 2001–2007.
84. The Cardiac Insufficiency Bisoprolol Study II (CIBIS-II). (1999). A randomised trial. *Lancet, 353*, 9.
85. Packer, M., Fowler, M. B., Roecker, E. B., et al. (2002). Effect of carvedilol on the morbidity of patients with severe chronic heart failure: results of the Carvedilol Prospective Randomized Cumulative Survival (COPERNICUS) study. *Circulation, 106*, 2194.
86. Pratt, C. M., Gardner, M., Pepine, C., et al. (1995). Lack of long-term ventricular arrhythmia reduction by enalapril in heart failure. SOLVD Investigators. *Am J Cardiol, 75*, 1244.
86a. Kober, L., Torp-Pedersen, C., Carlsen, J. E., et al. (1995). A clinical trial of the angiotensin-converting-enzyme inhibitor trandolapril in patients with left ventricular dysfunction after myocardial infarction. *N Engl J Med, 333*, 1670.
87. Cleland, J. G., Erhardt, L., Murray, G., on behalf of the AIRE Study Investigators, et al. (1997). Effect of ramipril on morbidity and mode of death among survivors of acute myocardial infarction with clinical evidence of heart failure. A report from the AIRE Study Investigators. *Eur Heart J, 18*, 41.
88. Domanski, M. J., Exner, D. V., Borkowf, C. B., et al. (1999). Effect of angiotensin converting enzyme inhibition on sudden cardiac death in patients following acute myocardial infarction. *J Am Coll Cardiol, 33*, 598.
89. Ramires, F. J., Mansur, A., Coelho, O., et al. (2000). Effect of spironolactone on ventricular arrhythmias in congestive heart failure secondary to idiopathic dilated or to ischemic cardiomyopathy. *Am J Cardiol, 85*, 1207.
90. The RALES Investigators (1996). Effectiveness of spironolactone added to an angiotensin-converting enzyme inhibitor and a loop diuretic for severe chronic congestive heart failure (the Randomized Aldactone Evaluation Study [RALES]). *Am J Cardiol, 78*, 902.
91. Pitt, B., Remme, W., Zannad, F., et al. (2003). Eplerenone, a selective aldosterone blocker, in patients with left ventricular dysfunction after myocardial infarction. *N Engl J Med, 348*, 1309.
92. Goldberger, J. J., Subacius, H., Schaechter, A., et al. (2006). Effects of statin therapy on arrhythmic events and survival in patients with nonischemic dilated cardiomyopathy. *J Am Coll Cardiol, 48*, 1228.
93. Vyas, A. K., Guo, H., Moss, A. J., et al. (2006). Reduction in ventricular tachyarrhythmias with statins in the Multicenter Automatic Defibrillator Implantation Trial (MADIT)–II. *J Am Coll Cardiol, 47*, 769.
94. Camm, A. J., Pratt, C. M., Schwartz, P. J., et al. (2004). Mortality in patients after a recent myocardial infarction: a randomized, placebo-controlled trial of azimilide using heart rate variability for risk stratification. *Circulation, 109*, 990.
95. Lampert, S., Lown, B., Graboys, T. B., et al. (1988). Determinants of survival in patients with malignant ventricular arrhythmias associated with coronary artery disease. *Am J Cardiol, 61*, 791.
96. Ravid, S., Podrid, P. J., Lampert, S., et al. (1989). Congestive heart failure induced by six of the newer antiarrhythmic drugs. *J Am Coll Cardiol, 14*, 1326.
97. Doval, H. C., Nul, D. R., Grancelli, H. O., et al. (1994). Randomised trial of low dose amiodarone in severe congestive heart failure. Grupo de Estudio de la Sobrevida en la Insuficiencia Cardiaca en Argentina (GESICA). *Lancet, 344*, 493.
98. Singh, S. N., Fletcher, R. D., Fisher, S. G., et al. (1995). Amiodarone in patients with congestive heart failure and asymptomatic ventricular arrhythmia. Survival Trial of Antiarrhythmic Therapy in Congestive Heart Failure. *N Engl J Med, 333*, 77.
99. Bardy, G. H., Lee, K. L., Mark, D. B., et al. (2005). Amiodarone or an implantable cardioverter-defibrillator for congestive heart failure. *N Engl J Med, 352*, 225.
100. Effect of prophylactic amiodarone on mortality after acute myocardial infarction and in congestive heart failure. (1997). Meta-analysis of individual data from 6500 patients in randomized trials. Amiodarone Trials Meta-analysis Investigators. *Lancet, 350*, 1417–1424.
101. Moss, A. J., Hall, W. J., Cannom, D. S., for the Multicenter Automatic Defibrillator Implantation Trial Investigators, et al. (1996). Improved survival with an implanted defibrillator in patients with coronary disease at high risk for ventricular arrhythmia. *N Engl J Med, 335*, 1933.
102. Moss, A. J., Zareba, W., Hall, W. J., et al. (2002). Prophylactic implantation of a defibrillator in patients with myocardial infarction and reduced ejection fraction. *N Engl J Med, 346*, 877.
103. Buxton, A. E., Lee, K. L., Fisher, J. D., et al. (1999). A randomized study of the prevention of sudden death in patients with coronary artery disease. Multicenter Unsustained Tachycardia Trial Investigators. *N Engl J Med, 341*, 1882.
104. Hohnloser, S. H., Kuck, K. H., Dorian, P., et al. (2004). Prophylactic use of an implantable cardioverter-defibrillator after acute myocardial infarction. *N Engl J Med, 351*, 2481.
105. Kadish, A., Dyer, A., Daubert, J. P., et al. (2004). Prophylactic defibrillator implantation in patients with nonischemic dilated cardiomyopathy. *N Engl J Med, 350*(105), 2151.
106. Bardy, G. H., Lee, K. L., Mark, D. B., et al. (2005). Amiodarone or an implantable cardioverter-defibrillator for congestive heart failure. *N Engl J Med, 352*, 225.

107. Desai, A. S., Fang, J. C., Maisel, W. H., et al. (2004). Implantable defibrillators for the prevention of mortality in patients with nonischemic cardiomyopathy: a meta-analysis of randomized controlled trials. *JAMA, 292*, 2874.
108. Mark, D. B., Nelson, C. L., Anstrom, K. J., for the SCD-HeFT Investigators, et al. (2006). Cost-effectiveness of defibrillator therapy or amiodarone in chronic stable heart failure: results from the Sudden Cardiac Death in Heart Failure Trial (SCD-HeFT). *Circulation, 114*, 135.
109. Zwanziger, J., Hall, W. J., Dick, A. W., et al. (2006). The cost-effectiveness of implantable cardioverter-defibrillators: results from the Multicenter Automatic Defibrillator Implantation Trial (MADIT)–II. *J Am Coll Cardiol, 47*, 2310.
110. Buxton, A. E., Lee, K. L., Hafley, G. E., et al. (2007). Limitations of ejection fraction for prediction of sudden death risk inpatients with coronary artery disease: lessons from the MUSTT study. *J Am Coll Cardiol, 50*, 1150.
111. Whang, W., Mittleman, M. A., Rich, D. Q., et al. (2004). Heart failure and the risk of shocks in patients with implantable cardioverter defibrillators: results from the Triggers of Ventricular Arrhythmias (TOVA) study. *Circulation, 109*, 1386.
112. Goldenberg, H., Vyas, A. K., Hall, J., et al., for the MADIT-II Investigators (2008). (2008). Risk stratification for primary implantation of a cardioverter-defibrillator in patients with ischemic left ventricular dysfunction. *J Am Coll Cardiol, 51*, 288.
113. Connolly, S. J., Hallstrom, A. P., Cappato, R., et al. (2000). Meta-analysis of the implantable cardioverter defibrillator secondary prevention trials. AVID, CASH and CIDS studies. Antiarrhythmics vs Implantable Defibrillator study. Cardiac Arrest Study Hamburg. Canadian Implantable Defibrillator Study. *Eur Heart J, 21*, 2071.
114. A comparison of antiarrhythmic-drug therapy with implantable defibrillators in patients resuscitated from near-fatal ventricular arrhythmias. The Antiarrhythmics versus Implantable Defibrillators (AVID) Investigators. (1997). *N Engl J Med, 337*, 1576.
115. Connolly, S. J., Gent, M., Roberts, R. S., et al. (2000). Canadian Implantable Defibrillator Study (CIDS): a randomized trial of the implantable cardioverter defibrillator against amiodarone. *Circulation, 101*, 1297.
116. Kuck, K. H., Cappato, R., Siebels, J., et al. (2000). Randomized comparison of antiarrhythmic drug therapy with implantable defibrillators in patients resuscitated from cardiac arrest. The Cardiac Arrest Study Hamburg (CASH). *Circulation, 102*, 748.
116a. Pinski, S. L., Yao, Q., Epstein, A. and the AVID Investigators, et al. (2000). Determinants of outcome in patients with sustained ventricular tachyarrhythmias: the Antiarrhythmics Versus Implantable Defibrillators (AVID) study registry. *Am Heart J, 139*, 804.
116b. O'Callaghan, P. A., Poloniecki, J., Sosa-Suarez, G., et al. (2001). Long-term clinical outcome of patients with prior myocardial infarction after palliative radiofrequency catheter ablation for frequent ventricular tachycardia. *Am J Cardiol, 87*, 975.
116c. Reddy, V. Y., Reynolds, M. R., Neuzil, P., et al. (2007). Prophylactic catheter ablation for the prevention of defibrillator therapy. *N Engl J Med, 357*, 2717.
116d. Elefteriades, J. A., Biblo, L. A., Batsford, W. P., et al. (1990). Evolving patterns in the surgical treatment of malignant ventricular tachyarrhythmias. *Ann Thorac Surg, 49*, 94.
117. Maron, B. J., Shen, W. K., Link, M. S., et al. (2000). Efficacy of implantable cardioverter-defibrillators for the prevention of sudden death in patients with hypertrophic cardiomyopathy. *N Engl J Med, 342*, 365.
117a. Maron, B. J., McKenna, W. J., Danielson, G. K., et al. (2003). American College of Cardiology/European Society of Cardiology clinical expert consensus document on hypertrophic cardiomyopathy. A report of the American College of Cardiology Foundation Task Force on Clinical Expert Consensus Documents and the European Society of Cardiology Committee for Practice Guidelines. *J Am Coll Cardiol, 42*,1687.
118. Phang, R. S., Kang, D., Tighiouart, H., et al. (2006). High risk of ventricular arrhythmias in patients with nonischemic dilated cardiomyopathy presenting with syncope. *Am J Cardiol, 97*, 416.
119. Fonarow, G. C., Feliciano, Z., Boyle, N. G., et al. (2000). Improved survival in patients with nonischemic advanced heart failure and syncope treated with an implantable cardioverter-defibrillator. *Am J Cardiol, 85*, 981.
120. Olshansky, B., Poole, J. E., Johnson, G., for the SCD-HeFT investigators, et al. (2008). Syncope predicts outcome of cardiomyopathy patients. *J Am Coll Cardiol, 51*, 1277.
121. Iacoviello, M., Forleo, C., Guida, P., et al. (2007). Ventricular repolarization dynamicity provides independent prognostic information toward major arrhythmic events in patients with idiopathic dilated cardiomyopathy. *J Am Coll Cardiol, 50*(3), 225–231.
122. Maria, R., Gavazzi, A., Caroli, A., et al. (1992). Ventricular arrhythmias in dilated cardiomyopathy as an independent prognostic hallmark. *Am J Cardiol, 69*, 1451–1457.
123. Teerlink, J. R., Jalaluddin, M., Anderson, S., et al. (2003). Ambulatory ventricular arrhythmias in patients with heart failure do not specifically predict an increased risk of sudden death. PROMISE (Prospective Randomized Milrinone Survival Evaluation) Investigators. *Circulation, 101*(1), 40–46.
124. Grimm, W., Christ, M., Bach, J., et al. (2003). Noninvasive arrhythmia risk stratification in idiopathic dilated cardiomyopathy: results of the Marburg Cardiomyopathy Study. *Circulation, 108*(23), 2883–2891.
125. Becker, R., Haass, M., Ick, D., et al. (2003). Role of nonsustained ventricular tachycardia and programmed ventricular stimulation for risk stratification in patients with idiopathic dilated cardiomyopathy. *Bas Res Cardiol, 98*(4), 259–266.
126. Kearney, M. T., Fox, K. A., Lee, A. J., et al. (2004). Predicting sudden death in patients with mild to moderate chronic heart failure. *Heart, 90*(10), 1137–1143.
127. Fauchier, L., Douglas, J., Babuty, D., et al. (2005). QT dispersion in nonischemic dilated cardiomyopathy. A long-term evaluation. *Eur J Heart Fail, 7*(2), 277–282.
128. Szabo, B. M., van Veldhuisen, D. J., Crijns, H. J., et al. (1994). Value of ambulatory electrocardiographic monitoring to identify increased risk of sudden death in patients with left ventricular dysfunction and heart failure. *Eur Heart J, 15*(7), 928–933.
129. Doval, H. C., Nul, D. R., Grancelli, H. O., et al. (1996). Nonsustained ventricular tachycardia in severe heart failure. Independent marker of increased mortality due to sudden death. GESICA-GEMA Investigators. *Circulation, 94*(12), 3198–3203.
130. Watanabe, J., Shinozaki, T., Shiba, N., et al. (2006). Accumulation of risk markers predicts the incidence of sudden death in patients with chronic heart failure. *Eur J Heart Fail, 8*(3), 237–422.
131. Gradman, A., Deedwania, P., Cody, R., et al. (1989). Predictors of total mortality and sudden death in mild to moderate heart failure. Captopril-Digoxin Study Group. *J Am Coll Cardiol, 14*(3), 564–570.

CHAPTER 54

Cardiac Transplantation

Mariell Jessup and Michael Acker

Cardiac transplantation is the treatment of choice for eligible patients with refractory heart failure. Nevertheless, the survival benefit of cardiac transplantation in advanced heart failure, in comparison with conventional treatment, has never been tested in a prospective randomized trial. Norman E. Shumway and colleagues developed surgical techniques for the procedure as early as 1966, and Christiaan Barnard performed the first clinical human cardiac transplantation in 1967.[1] By the 1980s, when a review panel was convened, the U.S. Health Care Financing Administration (HCFA) had concluded that heart transplantation was no longer experimental. Accordingly, in 1986, the HCFA issued proposed regulations for reimbursement of Medicare-eligible patients undergoing heart transplantation in centers that met HCFA-specified standards of experience and performance.

Many advances have occurred in the management of cardiac transplant recipients since the mid-1980s, including new immunosuppression modalities, therapies for chronic rejection, and improved operative and cardiac preservation techniques. As a result, the rate and length of survival have been enhanced over the same time period. The rate of 3-year survival from 1975 to 1981, before the routine use of cyclosporine, was 40%; in comparison, from 1982 to 1994, the era of the early use of cyclosporine, that rate was 70%.[2] The number of heart transplantation procedures worldwide has declined somewhat from the peak of approximately 4500 per year in 1994, which perhaps reflects better medical and device therapies for heart failure and a better understanding of prognostic indicators.[3] Nonetheless, the number of potential organ donors cannot meet the demand created by growing waiting lists for heart transplants. As a result, other modalities for the treatment of stage D (chronic, progressive, and refractory) heart failure have been created and are being assessed in clinical trials (see Chapter 61).[4] More recently, for many patients referred for heart transplantation, one, if not more, of the alternative therapeutic options has usually failed,[5] and the patients are becoming progressively older and sicker, with increasing numbers of medical comorbid conditions. Likewise, the selection criteria for donors have expanded to increase the number of organs available.[6] As a result of these changes, the patients selected for heart transplantation are increasingly those with more acute disease, and, simultaneously, the available organs have been of poorer quality.[1,7]

PATIENT POPULATION

Which Patients Need to Be Considered for Transplantation?

The purpose of performing a heart transplantation for an individual patient is to prolong life and to improve the overall quality of life. No single prognostic algorithm enables clinicians to accurately predict impending morbidity or mortality in an individual patient, although multiple scoring systems have been developed to help with this critical analysis.[8,9] It is important for referring physicians to understand the potential benefits that cardiac transplantation might confer on a recipient, as well as comorbid conditions that might portend an unsatisfactory outcome. A risk-benefit assessment for each patient is ultimately what transplantation committees perform in their deliberations.

Evaluation of the Potential Recipient

Figure 54-1 outlines the questions that must be answered to evaluate a potential patient for cardiac transplantation. The usual candidates are patients whose life expectancy is estimated to be less than 1 year. Typically, patients for consideration have one of several conditions: (1) cardiogenic shock that necessitates mechanical support or high-dose inotropic or vasopressor drugs (in which case, the course of disease is clearly irreversible); (2) stage D heart failure symptoms despite optimal therapy[10]; (3) recurrent life-threatening arrhythmias despite maximal interventions, including implanted defibrillators; or, in rare cases, (4) refractory angina without potential for revascularization.[4] Adult patients with repaired congenital heart disease are developing progressive heart failure and are being increasingly considered for heart transplantation.[11] Several models have been proposed to assist in the risk stratification of patients with heart failure through the use of both invasive and noninvasive methods.[8,9] The most potent predictor of outcome in ambulatory patients with heart failure is a test of symptom-limited metabolic stress to calculate peak oxygen consumption ($\dot{V}O_2$) (see Chapter 57).[12] A peak $\dot{V}O_2$ of less than 12 mL/kg/min is indicative of a poor prognosis, with a survival rate that is lower than that for transplantation.[13] Ideally, this information is organized in a score that also accounts for other important prognostic information, such as systemic blood pressure, results of biological assays (such as blood natriuretic peptide), renal function, and frequency of hospitalization.[14,15] Nonambulatory patients who require continuous intravenous inotropic support from which they cannot be weaned or those who require mechanical support to maintain adequate cardiac index are more obviously

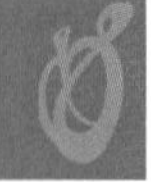

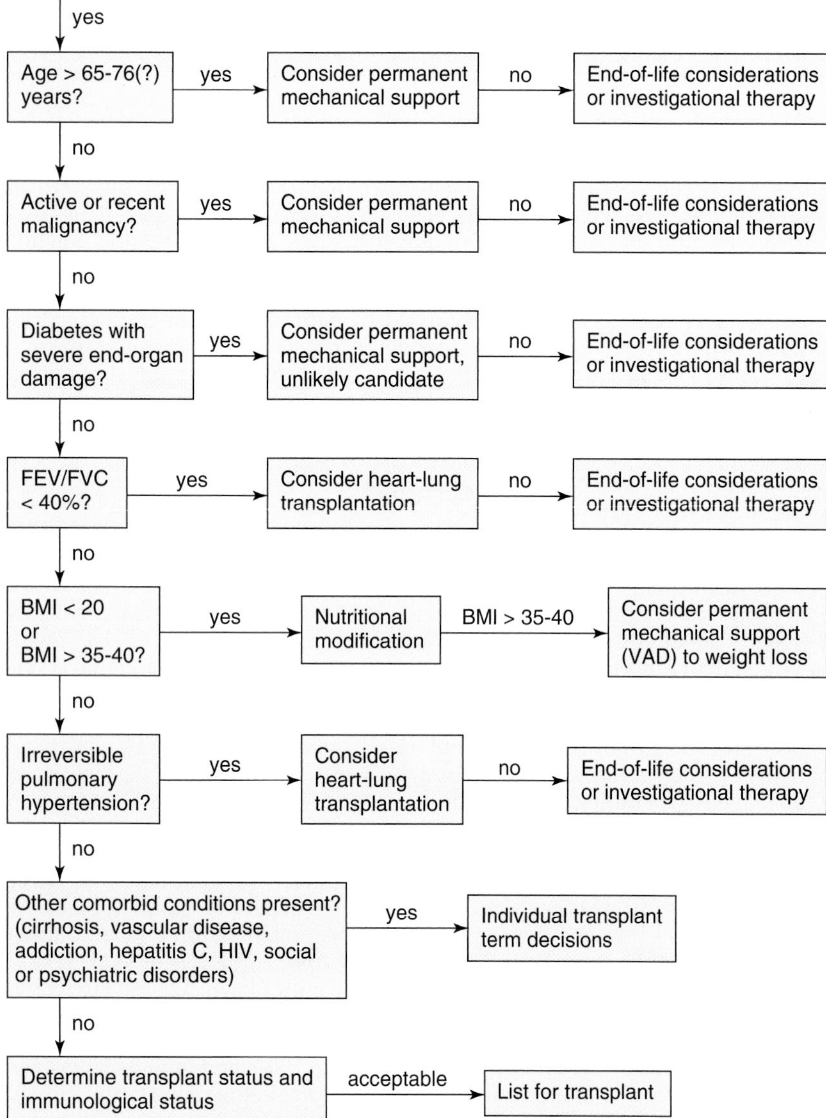

FIGURE 54–1 Flowchart depicting evaluation of a patient for cardiac transplantation. BMI, body mass index; FEV, forced expiratory volume; FVC, forced vital capacity; HIV, human immunodeficiency virus; VAD, ventricular assist device.

at risk for a poor outcome without transplantation; however, they often manifest signs and symptoms of end-organ failure of the pulmonary, hepatic, and renal systems, which may signal an ominous prognosis even with a transplant procedure.

Each patient must then undergo an extensive medical and psychosocial evaluation by the transplantation team to detect contraindications to transplantation and to further determine prognosis, the urgency of transplantation, and immunological status. There are a number of relative contraindications to heart transplantation; one of the most debated and variable among centers is the upper age limit for consideration. In general, patients older than 65 years are ineligible; more often, such patients undergo high-risk reparative surgery, implantation of permanent cardiac assist devices, or investigational therapies, such as cell transplantation, or they may receive hearts from an alternative list of less-than-optimal donors.[16] However, one heart transplantation guideline indicated that the maximum age for eligibility could be as high as 70 years; therefore, individual centers must determine their own age cutoff.[17,18] The presence of an active or recent malignancy or of diabetes with severe end-organ damage limits life expectancy after transplantation, and these are common reasons why potential recipients are ineligible. Significant lung disease complicates postoperative management and precludes the possibility of normal physical functioning; extremes of weight, as measured by body mass index, have also been shown to worsen posttransplantation prognosis.[4] Patients with advanced heart failure and renal dysfunction are generally ineligible for heart transplantation because abnormal renal function increases morbidity after transplantation. Thus, it is important to clearly distinguish patients with potentially reversible renal failure from patients in whom renal dysfunction is associated with advanced, irreversible end-stage renal disease. At many transplantation centers, combined heart-kidney transplantation procedures are performed in selected patients.[19,20]

Pulmonary arterial hypertension—whether accompanied by a pulmonary vascular resistance of greater than 6 Wood units that cannot be reduced by medical therapy or occurring after the placement of a ventricular assist device (VAD)—is considered an absolute contraindication to cardiac transplantation. In the setting of fixed pulmonary hypertension, the donor right ventricle often fails, which in many cases leads to early postoperative mortality.[21] In some centers, individual patients with irreversible pulmonary pressures may be considered for a combined heart-lung transplantation procedure. Other comorbid conditions may negatively affect a transplantation team's decision to further consider a potential recipient; these conditions include hepatitis C or cirrhosis, peripheral or cerebral vascular disease, advanced neuropathy, human immunodeficiency virus (HIV) status, addictions to alcohol or illicit drugs, and social or psychiatric disorders. Appropriate counseling of the patient who is ineligible for heart transplantation should include end-of-life preparation and discussions about possible investigational approaches.[22]

Each patient undergoes immunological evaluation, which is increasingly sophisticated, to determine ABO blood type; antibody screening; testing for panel reactive antibody (PRA); and human leukocyte antigen (HLA) typing. The presence and levels of anti-HLA antibodies is determined by cytotoxic testing in which the recipient's serum is incubated with lymphocytes from 30 to 60 individuals that represent a wide range of HLA antigens. The PRA value is expressed as a percentage of cell panel members that undergo cytolysis and is considered positive if more than 10% of the cell panel members undergo cytolysis. The PRA test can identify the presence of circulating anti-HLA antibody but not the specificity or strength of antibody. Enzyme-linked immunosorbent assay (ELISA) and flow cytometry can also determine PRA and are more sensitive than the cytotoxic test.[23]

The most common cause of sensitization, or elevated PRA levels, is pregnancy; however, sensitization can also occur with transfusions, prior transplantation, or insertion of a VAD. Patients with a PRA exceeding 10% usually must undergo prospective crossmatching in order to identify a prospective donor. This involves testing the recipient's serum with donor cells, in the presence of complement, to see whether cytotoxicity occurs. Cell destruction portends an unacceptably increased potential for either acute rejection or more chronic, recurrent rejections. Highly sensitized patients—those with high circulating levels of preformed antibodies—often have to wait long periods before a suitable donor can be found.

Newer and more sensitive immunological techniques have further quantified the type and number of circulating antibodies in patients waiting for transplantation and have challenged transplantation teams in knowing which potential donors are acceptable. Moreover, prospective crossmatching techniques can be done only for donors and recipients in a single geographical region, and teams must increasingly travel outside a region for donors; this makes it difficult to obtain donor organs for their sensitized waiting patients. Virtual crossmatching methods are now being used with some success, in which flow cytometry–based, single-antigen bead assays enable the clear identification of antibody specificities. Prospective donors with these antigens can be avoided, and a compatible donor can be selected without the need for prospective crossmatching. This increases the number of donor matches outside the geographical area of the local organ procurement organization.[24,25]

Management of the Patient Waiting for Cardiac Transplantation

In the United States, solid organ transplantation is regulated, audited, and facilitated by the government. The United Network for Organ Sharing (UNOS) is the national organization that maintains organ transplant waiting lists and allocates identified donor organs; it is organized by regions throughout the country and integrated closely with local organ procurement organizations. Donor hearts are assigned to recipients according to a priority status that is standardized nationally. The priority status is based on the recipient's level of medical urgency, blood type, body size, and duration of time at a particular status level. Patients awaiting heart transplantation are assigned a risk status according to the level of medical support they require. Patients who can be maintained safely and successfully outside the hospital are assigned the status of lowest priority, status 2. Intermediate priority is given to patients who require hospitalization and some continuous inotropic support or who require ongoing VAD therapy (status 1B). The highest priority (status 1A) is assigned to patients who require high-dose, continuous, inotropic infusions or mechanical support, such as an intra-aortic balloon pump (IABP), ventilator, or VAD therapy. Such critically ill patients must be located in an intensive care unit and undergoing continuous hemodynamic monitoring with Swan-Ganz catheters. Patients with VADs in place who are waiting for transplantation are given an automatic 30-day status 1A listing, with the timing at the discretion of the center. Thereafter, if the function of the VAD is normal, the patient is reassigned to status 1B. Donor hearts are offered geographically (by the location of the donor) and sequentially (to patients with the highest priority and the appropriate blood type). This process has been facilitated by a computerized system that requires transplantation teams to have online access at all times. Nevertheless, speed and timing are critical aspects of optimal donor allocation, because potential donors often exist in an unstable hemodynamic environment that may affect the viability of the donor heart. In addition, transportation of donor hearts is generally limited by a "cold ischemic" time (the duration of organ viability between harvest and implantation) of approximately 4 hours.

Pretransplantation waiting times in the 11 UNOS donor regions vary considerably, as do the challenges to individual transplantation teams in managing waiting recipients throughout the United States. The ability of potential recipients to be listed for and receive an organ transplant is influenced by a number of different factors, including candidate gender, size and blood group, presensitization status, source of health insurance or lack thereof, type of cardiac disease, proximity to a transplantation center, and even the number of other transplantation centers in the region. Information about these and many other parameters of the United States transplantation program are available to the public on a variety of websites, including the official UNOS website (http://www.unos.org/), on which site-specific data may also be compared nationally or by city or region. Since about 2000, an increasing number of heart transplant recipients have been listed and undergone transplantation as status 1A or 1B, in comparison with the less urgent status of years past.[26] This fact probably reflects the increasing use of VADs as a bridging method in desperately ill patients before transplantation; earlier, similar patients would have died. Mechanical support devices often allow patients to be managed successfully as outpatients while they await transplantation, but the implantation of the device qualifies the recipient to at least a status 1B or more urgent. There is considerable debate about the outcome of patients with VADs, in comparison with patients who undergo transplantation without a prior VAD, with strong arguments on both sides.[27] Nevertheless, the available data from the Organ Procurement and Transplantation Network (OPTN) and from the Scientific Registry of Transplant Recipients (SRTR) website (www.ustransplant.org) suggest that overall survival is no different for patients who undergo transplantation as status 1A, 1B, or 2, as illustrated in Figure 54-2.

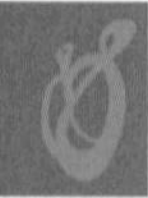

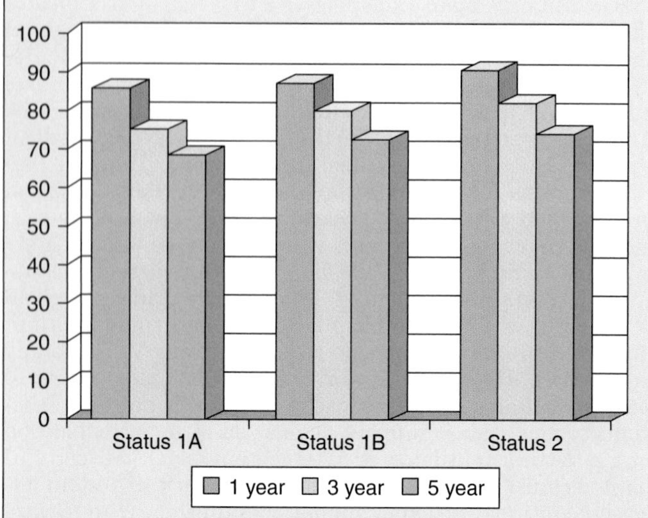

FIGURE 54–2 Percentages of patients surviving 1, 3, and 5 years after heart transplantation, in the United States, according to listing status. (Adapted from the information on the Scientific Registry of Transplant Recipients website, National Transplant Statistics [http://www.ustransplant.org]; accessed March 14, 2010.)

Patients waiting for transplantation must be regularly reevaluated for the possibility of worsening status, which would necessitate a change in priority; the development of a new comorbid condition that would preclude transplantation; or significant clinical improvement that would warrant a reconsideration of the listing. An analysis of the OPTN/SRTR data suggests that the overall death rate among patients waiting for heart transplantation has fallen from 220 to 142 patients per 1000 patient-years at risk.[26] In addition, all transplantation teams acknowledge that some patients are removed from the waiting list each year because of marked clinical improvement, despite the great care in patient selection.[28]

THE CARDIAC TRANSPLANTATION PROCEDURE

The Cardiac Donor

In view of increasing organ demand, efficacious donor management and meticulous selection are crucial in maintaining excellent transplantation outcomes. Organ procurement representatives have become highly skilled in the rapid but thorough evaluation of potential donors, often screening for multiple organ harvests from a single donor. Obviously, any medical history about the donor is crucial, including any relevant cardiovascular disorders before brain death. All donors are screened for communicable diseases, including viral disorders such as hepatitis and HIV infection. In contrast to blood bank donation, donors with behavioral risk factors are not barred from contributing to the organ supply. Accordingly, clinicians have increasingly debated the risk associated with transplantation and how much of the donor-associated risk should be conveyed to the potential recipient.[29] Specific information that is relevant for the assessment of cardiac donor suitability also includes the presence or absence of thoracic trauma, donor hemodynamic stability, pressor and inotropic requirements, duration of cardiac arrest, the need for cardiopulmonary resuscitation, and number of hypotensive episodes and the method by which hypotension was managed. Echocardiography is an invaluable screening method to evaluate potential donors. Some potential donors undergo hemodynamic deterioration caused by brain death, which necessitates inotropic or pressor infusions and substantial fluid administration, with subsequent derangements in electrolytes and hemoglobin concentration. The resultant cardiovascular instability leads to suboptimal condition of some donor hearts and has compounded the problem of donor shortage. To increase the donor yield, recommendations have been published to improve the evaluation and successful use of potential cardiac donors.[6,30]

The acceptable "cold ischemia" time for cardiac transplantation is approximately 4 hours. Prolonged ischemic time has been shown to be a significant risk factor for mortality after cardiac transplantation, especially when coupled with other risk factors, such as older donor age. In the first two decades of heart transplantation, the upper limit of donor age was 35 years, but older donors are now used frequently; an age up to 60 years is considered safe by most centers.[31] It has become quite standard to perform cardiac catheterization on the older donor to further clarify the integrity of the coronary circulation. The final decision to accept a heart for transplantation is made at the time of harvesting, after direct examination of the heart for myocardial infarction, trauma, coronary calcification, left ventricular hypertrophy, or dilatation. The harvesting team communicates the decision to the recipient hospital's transplantation team, so that the recipient may be prepared for surgery.

One of the main problems thought to be responsible for early graft failure after transplantation is inadequate myocardial protection during prolonged ischemic transport.[1,32,33] Current myocardial preservation techniques allow interventions to be made during five different phases of the transplantation procedure: donor cardiovascular management; protection during explantation; protection during transportation to the recipient center; protection during implantation; and protection during the immediate reperfusion period.[34,35] Optimal protection of donor hearts will, it is hoped, ultimately expand the potential donor pool and enhance early graft function. Moreover, endothelial injury that occurs during organ procurement, preservation, and reperfusion, as well as ongoing injury during the life span of the cardiac allograft, results in endothelial activation.[36] If protection strategies can successfully reduce ischemia-reperfusion damage, long-term heart transplantation outcomes may be improved by the protective effects on endothelial cells, which would reduce the subsequent development of cardiac allograft vasculopathy (CAV). This goal has spurred the development of new devices that are designed to further protect the harvested heart during transportation by continuous bloodless circulation or autologous blood-perfused systems.[32]

Surgical Considerations

The two most common surgical approaches for the implantation of the donor heart are the biatrial and bicaval anastomoses (Figure 54-3). The biatrial anastomosis technique has long had a reputation for being simple, safe, and reproducible; four suture lines are made in the left atrium, pulmonary artery, aorta, and right atrium. The bicaval anastomosis technique was introduced in the early 1990s with the intentions to reduce right atrial size, to minimize distortion of the recipient heart, to preserve atrial conduction pathways, and to decrease tricuspid regurgitation. This alternative procedure entails five anastomoses: left atrium, pulmonary artery, aorta, inferior vena cava, and superior vena cava. Although there has been no prospective trial to establish the superiority of either technique, the bicaval technique is now performed more often in the United States, primarily because it appears to decrease the need for permanent pacemakers in transplant recipients.[37-39] Some surgeons have become increasingly interested in techniques to minimize subsequent tricuspid regurgitation and have described tricuspid annuloplasty performed simultaneously with the transplantation surgery.[40]

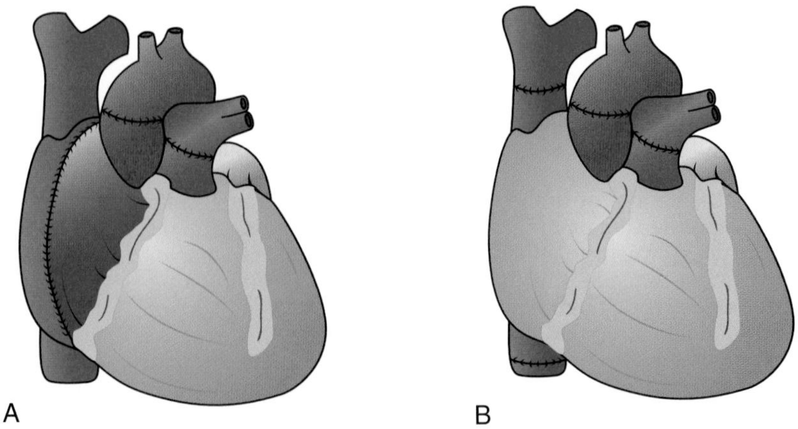

FIGURE 54–3 Surgical techniques for cardiac transplantation. **A,** Standard Shumway (biatrial) technique of orthotopic heart transplantation. **B,** Bicaval technique of orthotopic heart transplantation. (Modified from Al Khaldi A, Robbins RC. New directions in cardiac transplantation. *Annu Rev Med* 2006;57:455)

Many transplantation candidates have had pacemaker or cardiac defibrillator devices implanted during the years leading up to their need for transplantation. These devices are typically removed surgically at the end of the transplantation operation, after the chest has been closed. Likewise, previous heart surgery—most commonly, coronary artery bypass graft procedures—lengthens the time it takes to prepare the recipient to receive the donor heart and increases the risk of bleeding during and after surgery. Just as the age at the time of transplantation has increased since 2000, so too has the number of patients who have undergone previous heart surgery. Of most importance is that the number of patients about to undergo transplantation with VADs in place has steadily increased, and so transplantation procedures are riskier and result in more bleeding.[41-46]

The most common reason for failure to wean a heart transplant recipient from cardiopulmonary bypass is right-sided heart failure, evidenced by a low cardiac output despite a rising central venous pressure. In the surgical field, the right heart chambers can be observed to dilate and contract poorly. Intraoperative transesophageal echocardiography (TEE) displays a dilated, poorly contracting right ventricle and an underfilled, vigorously contracting left ventricle. Right ventricular function may be enhanced with inotropic agents and pulmonary vasodilators, but the prognostic importance of preoperative pulmonary vascular resistance becomes obvious in these first few hours after surgery.[47,48]

EARLY POSTOPERATIVE MANAGEMENT

Cardiovascular Issues

In general, the management of the heart transplant recipient early after surgery does not differ substantially from that after other open-heart procedures, although the transplant recipient is generally debilitated after suffering severe heart failure for weeks or months before surgery. Cardiac transplant recipients often go into surgery with profoundly disturbed hemodynamics and significant renal insufficiency. Postoperative management has to be undertaken with close scrutiny of the urine output and renal function, because a rising creatinine level may necessitate a change in the immunosuppressive regimen. The resultant fluid overload may serve to further overdistend a struggling right ventricle. Many patients manifest generalized edema within the first week after surgery; however, it generally responds to intravenous diuretics. Vasomotor alterations of the peripheral vasculature that result in tissue edema contribute to this occurrence.

Because the donor heart is denervated after surgical implantation, bradycardia is a frequent problem, and a direct-acting β-agonist drug should be available. Temporary pacing leads are necessary for all recipients, because most are dependent on external pacemakers for a number of days after surgery; as many as 10% to 15% of transplant recipients require a permanent pacemaker.[46] Cardiac transplant recipients typically need chronotropic and inotropic support for a few days in the intensive care unit, after which time the infusions are weaned as tolerated. Many centers use isoproterenol for this purpose because of its lack of vasoconstrictive effects on the pulmonary vasculature. Inhaled agents have been used to achieve selective pulmonary vasodilation in cardiac transplant recipients, especially those with preoperative pulmonary hypertension. Inhaled nitric oxide is a potent vasodilator that has a selective effect on the pulmonary vasculature because of its rapid breakdown in the lung.[47] Administration of nitric oxide in heart transplant recipients with pulmonary hypertension has been shown to reduce pulmonary vascular resistance and improve right ventricular function. Iloprost, a carbacyclin analogue of prostaglandin I_2, can be aerosolized and has been administered in an inhaled form to treat severe pulmonary hypertension. The inhaled agents, delivered via the ventilator, are initiated in the operating room and continued until right ventricular function has stabilized.

Immunosuppression

Cardiac transplantation centers throughout the world have individual approaches to the management of immunomodulation for transplant recipients so that the donor heart is not rejected. All centers adhere to the principle that no patient undergoing heart transplantation is at low risk for rejection. Instead, it is more appropriate to stratify patients as those at average risk and those at high risk for subsequent rejection. Before transplantation surgery, patients at high risk for rejection include those with preformed antibodies (e.g., sensitized patients), usually secondary to previous surgery that necessitated transfusions; pregnant patients; patients waiting on mechanical circulatory assist devices; and, possibly, African American patients.[43] In addition, it is useful to characterize patients as being at higher risk of developing important comorbid conditions after transplantation, including infection, acute renal failure, or worsening diabetes, because an immunosuppressive regimen may have to be modified accordingly. After transplantation, a risk profile may be additionally tailored according to the retrospective crossmatch information and cytomegalovirus status of the donor and recipient. An immunosuppression strategy is thus developed for each patient on the basis of their risk for rejection and their risk for developing important complications of the immunosuppressive drug therapy.[1,49-52] Nevertheless, most immunosuppressive regimens begin with the simultaneous use of three classes of drugs: glucocorticoids, calcineurin inhibitors, and antiproliferative agents. In a subset of patients, transplantation teams

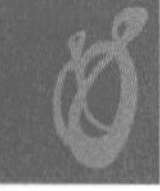

administer a variety of drugs for induction therapy, with the idea to rapidly enhance immune tolerance.

Induction Therapy in the Perioperative Period

Induction therapy is a heterogeneous application of perioperative antibody drugs used in combination with a foundational immunosuppressive regimen in solid-organ transplantation. The ultimate aim of induction is to inhibit only the T cells that respond to donor antigen. The aim of induction treatment is for the recipient to achieve immunological unresponsiveness to the transplant in the presence of a fully functioning immune system (donor-specific tolerance). Both polyclonal and monoclonal antibodies have been used for this form of therapy; their use depends on the institution and the country. Induction therapy is currently used in approximately 40% of heart transplant recipients.[53-55] Theoretically, induction agents should reduce the overall rate of rejection, but their primary benefit currently seems to be the delay of cellular rejection in the first 4 to 8 weeks of the early postoperative period, when renal dysfunction is most worrisome. Induction therapy may allow the less aggressive use of the calcineurin inhibitors, which would spare renal function initially, during the most vulnerable period.

Drugs used for induction include antithymocyte globulins (polyclonal antibodies) and the anti-CD3 antibody OKT3 and the interleukin-2 receptor antagonists daclizumab and basiliximab (monoclonal agents). OKT3 was widely used as induction in the past, but it has virtually vanished as an option because of the subsequent increased rejection rates and occurrence of lymphomas.[56] The antithymocyte globulins are currently used more commonly for the first 3 to 7 or even 14 days after transplantation, despite a paucity of efficacy data for the population of heart transplant recipients. The use of basiliximab has been explored in three trials: one in which the drug was compared with OKT3 induction[57] and two in which basiliximab was compared with placebo in a randomized design.[58,59] Although basiliximab was less toxic than OKT3, it did not alter outcome with regard to rejection, infection, or survival. In comparison with placebo, a significant delay in rejection occurred with basiliximab, but rates of late rejection may have increased. Basiliximab was found to be noninferior to rabbit antithymocyte globulin for the prevention of acute rejection in a trial of 35 patients.[60] Daclizumab, in comparison with no induction, reduced rejection without an attendant increase in mortality.[61] Thus, there may be some rationale for administering the induction agents to patients at high risk (e.g., those with preformed antibodies, renal dysfunction, or a worrisome retrospective crossmatch), but there are no compelling data as yet in the population of heart transplant recipients, and they are the subjects of considerable controversy.[53,62,63]

Maintenance Immunosuppression

As mentioned previously, immunosuppressive regimens begin with the simultaneous use of three classes of drugs: glucocorticoids, calcineurin inhibitors, and antiproliferative agents. In the immediate postoperative period, they are given parenterally, with a quick transition to oral formulations. *Corticosteroids* are nonspecific anti-inflammatory agents that work primarily by lymphocyte depletion. Patients receive high doses of initially intravenous and then oral steroids that are gradually tapered over the next 6 months; the goal is often to withdraw steroid therapy completely. At many centers, steroids are given several hours before the transplantation surgery. Side effects include cushingoid appearance, hypertension, dyslipidemia, weight gain with central obesity, peptic ulcer formation and gastrointestinal bleeding, pancreatitis, personality changes, cataract formation, hyperglycemia progressing to steroid-induced diabetes, and osteoporosis with avascular necrosis of bone. The well-appreciated adverse profile of the corticosteroids has prompted the development of a number of innovative strategies to eliminate them as early as possible after the transplantation surgery. Corticosteroids are also usually the drug of first choice to treat acute rejection.[64,65]

There are two *calcineurin inhibitors:* cyclosporine and tacrolimus. Their main mechanism of action involves binding to specific proteins to form complexes that block the action of calcineurin, a key participant in T-cell activation. The calcineurin inhibitors serve to block the signal transduction pathways responsible for T- and B-cell activation and therefore act specifically on the immune system and do not affect other rapidly proliferating cells. Critical and often limiting adverse effects include nephrotoxicity, in as many as 40% to 70% of patients, and hypertension with the development of left ventricular hypertrophy; both drugs cause approximately equivalent incidences of these untoward events.[64,66] Hirsutism, gingival hyperplasia, and hyperlipidemia are more frequent with cyclosporine, and diabetes and neuropathy are more frequent with tacrolimus.[60] The incidences of deep venous thrombosis, tremor, headache, convulsions, and paresthesias of the limbs are also increased with both drugs.[64,65] There are target therapeutic levels for both drugs; these goals are also adjusted over the subsequent months and years after transplantation. Therapeutic levels have been typically calculated with trough blood samples, but it has been shown that cyclosporine concentration 2 hours after administration (C2) is a more accurate predictor of total cyclosporine exposure.[67] It remains to be demonstrated whether the short- or long-term efficacy of cyclosporine in heart transplant will be further improved by monitoring the 2-hour cyclosporine concentration. In the United States, tacrolimus is now available in generic formulations; therefore, this drug tends to be the calcineurin inhibitor of choice in most centers.[68,69] As discussed later, progressive renal insufficiency is a major limitation of the calcineurin inhibitors, and investigators continue to explore methods to minimize their use or withdraw it altogether.[62,66]

Antiproliferative agents either directly or indirectly inhibit the expansion of alloactivated T- and B-cell clones. In this class, azathioprine was the earliest agent used, and it served as the mainstay of immunosuppression even before the routine use of cyclosporine. In the 2000s, mycophenolate mofetil has replaced azathioprine as the first-line antiproliferative drug; several randomized trials have demonstrated its superiority to azathioprine.[70-73] Mycophenolate mofetil is hydrolyzed to mycophenolic acid, which inhibits de novo purine syntheses. The major adverse effect of both azathioprine and mycophenolate mofetil is leukopenia; the use of mycophenolate mofetil can be limited by debilitating diarrhea or nausea. It is likely that the combination of mycophenolate mofetil and tacrolimus potentiates their individual adverse effects.

Sirolimus (often called *rapamycin*) and everolimus are two newer agents that block activation of T cells after autocrine stimulation by interleukin-2. They also are known to inhibit proliferation of endothelial cells and fibroblasts. Their action complements that of calcineurin inhibitors, and both sirolimus and everolimus have been used as maintenance immunosuppressive agents, as alternatives to standard immunosuppressive agents, and as rescue drugs for rejection. Sirolimus, a mammalian target of rapamycin (mTOR) inhibitor, has been shown to slow the progression of CAV with established disease,[74-76] and everolimus has been demonstrated to reduce both acute rejection and CAV.[77] In one randomized trial, sirolimus, in comparison with azathioprine, when added to cyclosporine and steroids, decreased by half the number of patients with acute rejection, which resulted in less subsequent development of CAV.[72,73] Because the drugs inhibit the proliferation of fibroblasts, they may cause

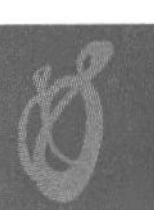

significant difficulties with wound healing, and most centers do not use them as initial therapy immediately after the transplantation surgery. The drugs have also been associated with the development of significant pericardial effusions. Sirolimus has been increasingly utilized to replace the calcineurin inhibitors as a strategy to improve renal dysfunction or to reverse left ventricular hypertrophy.[66,78,79]

The long-standing use of the maintenance combination of cyclosporine, azathioprine, and steroids has been challenged in a number of trials. Tacrolimus plus mycophenolate mofetil and tacrolimus plus sirolimus were compared with cyclosporine plus mycophenolate mofetil in a multicenter trial.[71] The overall rate of 1-year survival did not differ among the three regimens, but there was statistically less significant rejection with or without hemodynamic compromise with tacrolimus plus mycophenolate mofetil than with cyclosporine plus mycophenolate mofetil. Overall, patients taking tacrolimus plus mycophenolate mofetil had better renal function and triglyceride levels at 1 year. This trial has been pivotal in promoting tacrolimus as the primary calcineurin inhibitor in use worldwide. Researchers in later studies explored the use of converting a calcineurin inhibitor to sirolimus or everolimus for a renal-sparing effect.[80] Unfortunately, many of these newer approaches are being implemented without the benefit of rigorous, controlled trials.

Other Potential Perioperative Management Issues

In addition to the common postoperative problems encountered after heart surgery, the transplant recipient is frequently debilitated and may be malnourished, particularly if he or she has not been supported by a VAD. Issues concerning exercise rehabilitation and nutrition can be time consuming for the transplantation team and challenging for the patient and family. Depression in patients with chronic heart failure is a regular occurrence and is not immediately alleviated by the transplantation procedure.[81-83] In addition, marked emotional lability is common in recipients and is aggravated by the high-dose steroids used. As a result, successful heart transplantation teams must focus on more than the physical needs of the new transplant recipient. On occasion, the stress of the wait for transplantation often depletes the family of financial resources and emotional resiliency. On the other hand, patients are often rehabilitated much faster if they were allowed time to recover from the heart failure syndrome by the use of VAD support before receiving the transplant. It is critical that a transplantation center have dedicated physical therapists, nutritionists, and social workers or psychologists who can act in concert to address these noncardiovascular issues.

CHRONIC MANAGEMENT OF THE CARDIAC TRANSPLANT RECIPIENT

Rejection

Rejection involves cell- or antibody-mediated cardiac injury that results from the recognition of the cardiac allograft as nonself. This process is categorized into three major types of rejection, according to histological and immunological criteria: hyperacute, acute, and chronic.[49,84-87] *Hyperacute rejection* results when an abrupt loss of allograft function occurs within minutes to hours after circulation is reestablished in the donor heart; it is rare in modern-day transplantation. The phenomenon is mediated by preexisting antibodies to allogeneic antigens on the vascular endothelial cells of the donor organ, which is now avoided with current HLA typing techniques. These antibodies fix complement that promotes intravascular thrombosis. Subsequently, the graft vasculature is occluded rapidly, and swift and overwhelming failure of the cardiac graft occurs.

Acute cellular rejection or *cell-mediated rejection* is a mononuclear inflammatory response, predominantly lymphocytic, that is directed against the donor heart, most commonly occurs from the first week to several years after transplantation, and occurs in up to 40% of patients during the first year after surgery. The key event in both the initiation and the coordination of the rejection response is T-cell activation, moderated by interleukin-2, a cytokine. Interleukin-2 is produced by CD4 cells and, to a lesser extent, by CD8 cells and exerts both an autocrine and a paracrine response. Unlike renal and liver transplants, cardiac transplants have no reliable serological markers for rejection. Therefore, the endomyocardial biopsy remains the "gold standard" for the diagnosis of acute rejection. Biopsy is performed via a transjugular approach weekly and then every other week for several months; monthly biopsy continues for 6 to 12 months in many programs and for years thereafter in some. Cell-mediated rejection is graded according to a universally agreed-upon system that is periodically reviewed (Table 54-1).[88]

Risk factors for early rejection include younger recipient age, female gender, female donor, cytomegalovirus-positive serological status, prior infections, African American recipient race, and number of HLA mismatches.[43,89] Of most importance is that patients who fail to take or tolerate their immunosuppressant drugs, especially early in the postoperative course, are at very high risk for severe or recurrent cellular rejection. The occurrence of one or more episodes of treated rejections during the first year is a risk factor for both 5-year mortality and development of transplant coronary disease.[90] Likewise, treatment for acute rejection in the first 6 months after transplantation contributes to a slower overall rehabilitation of the patient.

The aggressiveness of treatment for cell-mediated rejection depends on the biopsy grade, clinical correlation, patient risk factors, rejection history, length of time after transplantation, and whether target levels of the immunosuppressant drugs are achieved. For example, an asymptomatic, early moderate rejection in a patient soon after transplantation who has achieved at least target levels of immunosuppressants or who has one or more risk factors for early rejection would be treated more aggressively than a patient at low risk for rejection with no history of cell-mediated rejection.

Another form of acute rejection is acute humoral rejection, or antibody-mediated rejection (AMR), which occurs days to weeks after transplantation and is initiated by antibodies rather than by T cells. The alloantibodies are directed against donor HLA or endothelial cell antigens. AMR is a serious complication after heart transplantation and manifests as graft dysfunction or hemodynamic abnormalities in the absence of the appearance of cellular rejection on biopsy samples. AMR is now recognized as a distinct clinical entity, and strict histopathological and immunological criteria for its diagnosis have been established (Table 54-2).[88,91] Further testing, including immunofluorescent staining of specially prepared myocardial tissue, is often necessary to elucidate the presence of AMR and is an important consideration in the evaluation of the transplant recipient with left ventricular dysfunction. The pathological markers of AMR identifiable in endomyocardial biopsy tissue include deposits of immunoglobulin M, immunoglobulin G, or complement in the microvasculature or myocytes. Antibodies with specificity for non-HLA antigens on the graft may also be present in the circulation, and their presence should support the diagnosis of AMR. Patients at greatest risk for AMR are women, patients with a high PRA screen value, and patients with a positive crossmatch. It is estimated that significant AMR occurs in

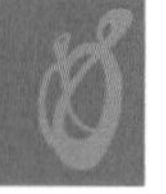

TABLE 54–1 Current and Previous Grading Systems for Cell-Mediated Rejection in Heart Transplantation

2004		1990	
Grade 0 R	No rejection	Grade 0	No rejection
Grade 1 R, mild	Interstitial and/or perivascular infiltrate with up to one focus of myocyte damage	Grade 1, mild	
		• A: Focal	Focal perivascular and/or interstitial infiltrate without myocyte damage
		• B: Diffuse	Diffuse infiltrate without myocyte damage
Grade 2 R, moderate	Two or more foci of infiltrate with associated myocyte damage	Grade 2, moderate (focal)	One focus of infiltrate with associated myocyte damage
Grade 3 R, severe	Diffuse infiltrate with multifocal myocyte damage ± edema ± hemorrhage ± vasculitis	Grade 3, moderate	
		• A: Focal	Multifocal infiltrate with myocyte damage
		• B: Diffuse	Diffuse infiltrate with myocyte damage
		Grade 4, severe	Diffuse, polymorphous infiltrate with extensive myocyte damage ± hemorrhage + vasculitis

From Stewart S, Winters GL, Fishbein MC, et al. Revision of the 1990 working formulation for the standardization of nomenclature in the diagnosis of heart rejection. *J Heart Lung Transplant* 2005;24:1710-1720.

TABLE 54–2 Diagnostic Criteria for Antibody-Mediated Rejection

Criteria	Finding	Comment
Clinical	Graft dysfunction	
Histological	Capillary endothelial changes: swelling, denudation, congestion	Required
	Macrophages in capillaries	Required
	Neutrophils in capillaries	More severe cases
	Interstitial changes: edema and/or hemorrhage	More severe cases
Immunopathological	Immunoglobulin (G,M, and/or A) plus C3d and/or C4d or C1q staining (2 to 2+) in capillaries by immunofluorescence	One of the first two immunopathological criteria is required
	CD68 positivity for macrophages in capillaries and/or C4D staining of capillaries with 2 to 3+ intensity by paraffin immunohistochemistry	
	Fibrin in vessels	More severe cases
Serological	Evidence of anti–human leukocyte antigen class I and/or class II antibodies or other anti–donor antibody at time of biopsy	Supports other findings

Adapted from Stewart S, Winters GL, Fishbein MC, et al. Revision of the 1990 working formulation for the standardization of nomenclature in the diagnosis of heart rejection. *J Heart Lung Transplant* 2005;24:1710-1720.

about 7% of patients, but that number may be as high as 20%. Because antibody assays are becoming more precise, AMR will probably be recognized more often, with a correlating need for newer treatment algorithms.[84,92,93]

Chronic rejection, or late graft failure, is an irreversible, gradual deterioration of graft function that occurs in many allografts months to years after transplantation. Current concepts suggest that donor heart dysfunction in the chronic stages of maintenance immunosuppression is related to chronic rejection, is mediated by antibodies, or is a result of progressive graft loss from ischemia. The last process is characterized by intimal thickening and fibrosis that lead to luminal occlusion of the graft vasculature; it is often referred to as "CAV", or transplant coronary artery disease. An approach to managing nonspecific graft dysfunction (Figure 54-4) is focused primarily on the diagnosis of AMR, as opposed to the presence of CAV.[94]

Attention has also focused on noninvasive methods to detect rejection. Gene expression assays have been developed by identifying a number of candidate gene markers from a pool of more than 25,000 genes of interest through the use of gene-chip array technology. Subsequently, real-time polymerase chain reaction (PCR) technologies are used in the peripheral blood to identify a pattern of gene activation that may be correlated with allograft rejection. One such assay is available for clinical use, but it is not yet clear how the information obtained can be best used in a wide range of transplant recipients.[95]

Infection

Despite the advances in immunosuppressive management, a major untoward consequence remains the occurrence of life-threatening infections. Infections cause approximately 20% of deaths within the first year after transplantation and continue to be a common cause of morbidity and mortality throughout the recipient's life. The most common infections in the first month after surgery are nosocomial, bacterial, and fungal infections related to mechanical ventilation, catheters, and the surgical site. Mortality rates are highest for fungal infections, followed by those for protozoal, bacterial, and viral infections. *Aspergillus* and *Candida* species account for the most common fungal infections after heart transplantation. In addition, a higher number of infections of any type during the first month after transplantation increases the risk of a subsequent fatal cytomegalovirus infection, a rejection (because immunosuppression frequently has to be decreased in order to treat the infection), or a prolonged hospital stay. Viral infections, especially cytomegalovirus, can enhance immunosuppression, which results in additional opportunistic infections. Accordingly, each heart transplantation team must develop a prophylactic regimen against cytomegalovirus, *Pneumocystis*

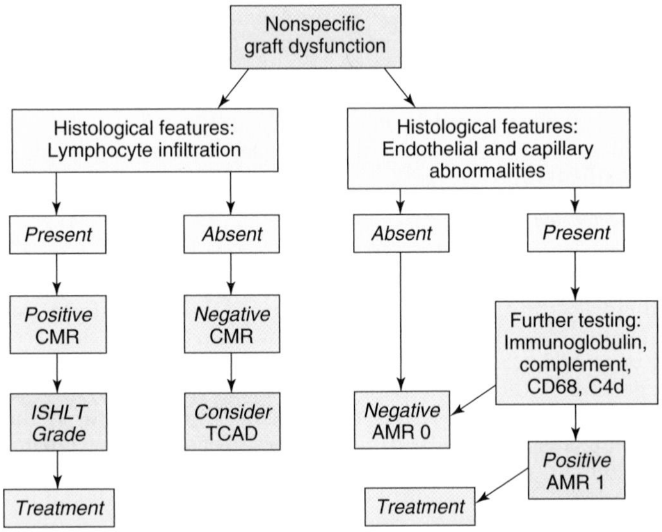

FIGURE 54–4 Diagnostic algorithm for nonspecific graft dysfunction. AMR, antibody-mediated rejection; CMR, cell-mediated rejection; ISHLT, International Society of Heart and Lung Transplantation; TCAD, transplant coronary artery disease. (From Jessup M, Brozena S. State-of-the-art strategies for immunosuppression. *Curr Opin Organ Transplant* 2007;12:536-42.)

carinii, herpes simplex virus, and species causing oral candidiasis that is to be used during the first 6 to 12 months after transplantation. Prophylactic intravenous ganciclovir or oral valganciclovir is generally given for variable amounts of time in the cytomegalovirus-seronegative recipient of a heart from a cytomegalovirus-seropositive donor. Optimal prophylaxis regimens and timing have not been completely standardized, and some of the decisions to be made about prophylaxis are outlined in Table 54-3.[96] The necessity of routine prophylaxis, however, has withstood the test of time. The regimen increases substantially the number of medications taken and potential drug interactions the recipient may experience. Some of the important drug interactions are listed in Table 54-4.[64,65,97]

Medical Complications and Comorbid Conditions

The complications after heart transplantation reflect, in part, the premorbid status of the majority of transplant recipients who have vascular disease and other significant medical conditions. After 5 years, more than 90% of recipients have hypertension, at least 80% have hyperlipidemia, and more than 30% of patients have diabetes (Table 54-5).[7] Each year after transplantation, a larger number of patients develop clinically significant CAV, which is the major limitation of survival after transplantation. Almost 30% of recipients have CAV by 5 years, and at least half do so at 10 years. Likewise, progressive renal insufficiency is an insidious problem that has been addressed only since about 2007 by substitution protocols to limit the administration of calcineurin inhibitors.[78,98]

Malignancy

The magnitude of overimmunosuppression in many transplant recipients is illustrated by the prediction of a 30% to 40% incidence of neoplasia in transplant recipients since 1980. The risk of fatal malignancy increases progressively in the years after transplantation, and there is a substantially higher risk in immunosuppressed patients than in the normal population. Posttransplantation lymphoproliferative disease and lung cancer are the most common fatal malignancies (Table 54-6).[7]

Risk factors for malignancy are multifactorial and include impaired immunoregulation, a synergistic effect with other carcinogens such as nicotine or ultraviolet light exposure, and oncogenic causes such as the Epstein-Barr virus and papillomavirus. The cumulative amount of immunosuppression is positively correlated with risk of malignancy. The incidences of lymphoproliferative disease, skin and lip cancers, and Kaposi's sarcoma are particularly high. Malignancies account for 24% of deaths after 5 years. Accordingly, as illustrated in Table 54-4, transplantation teams must ensure that the transplant recipient is adequately screened on a regular basis for the development of cancer.[99,100]

Diabetes

Patients who develop new-onset diabetes mellitus after transplantation are at increased risk for morbidity and mortality. Accumulating evidence suggests that long-term outcomes,

TABLE 54–3 Usual Care and Individual Decisions in the Management of Patients After Heart Transplantation

Usual Care	Individual Decisions
Maintenance Immunosuppression • Corticosteroids • Calcineurin inhibitors • Antiproliferative agents	Wean from prednisone completely? Cyclosporine or tacrolimus? Azathioprine or mycophenolate mofetil? Induction of immunosuppression? • Polyclonal antibodies: antithymocyte globulins • Monoclonal antibodies: OKT3, basiliximab, daclizumab
Viral prophylaxis • Ganciclovir, acyclovir, valacyclovir	Duration of prophylaxis? Drug choice for risk profile?
Fungal prophylaxis • Fluconazole • Trimethoprim/sulfamethoxazole, dapsone, pentamidine	Duration of prophylaxis? Reinstitution during intensified immunosuppression?
Vascular protection • Pravastatin, simvastatin	Efficacy of other statins? Role of aspirin? Role of rapamycin and everolimus? Target lipid levels?
Antihypertension therapy • Goal: optimal blood pressure control	First-line drug or drugs of choice?
Surveillance for rejection • Endomyocardial biopsy	Role of echocardiography or other noninvasive tools? Role of biomarkers or gene expression assays? How long and how often to perform biopsy? Role of humoral rejection and methods to detect it?
Surveillance for vasculopathy of transplanted heart • Coronary arteriography	Role of noninvasive testing? Role of intravascular ultrasonography? Role of computed tomographic angiography?
Surveillance for malignancy • Annual examination • Chest radiography • Colonoscopy, mammography, other imaging tests* • Dermatological examinations	Role of primary care team versus transplantation team?

Recommended adult immunization schedule: United States, 2010. *Ann Intern Med.* 152:36-39. Screening for breast cancer: U.S. Preventive Services Task Force Recommendation Statement. *Ann Intern Med.* 2009;151:716-726. Clinical guideline: screening for ovarian cancer: Recommendations and rationale. *Ann Intern Med.* 1994;121:141-142. Clinical guideline: Part I: Suggested technique for fecal occult blood testing and interpretation in colorectal cancer screening. *Ann Intern Med.* 1997;126:808-810. Clinical guideline: Part III: Screening for prostate cancer. *Ann Intern Med.* 997;126:480-484.

TABLE 54–4 Commonly Used Drugs and Potential Drug Interactions with Immunosuppressants

Drug	Potential Interaction
Acyclovir	Increased nephrotoxicity with calcineurin inhibitors
Allopurinol	Increased bone marrow suppression with azathioprine
Amlodipine or felodipine	Increased levels of calcineurin inhibitor
Antacids	Decreased levels of mycophenolate mofetil
Antidepressants	Increased levels of calcineurin inhibitor
Cimetidine	Increased levels of calcineurin inhibitor
Calcineurin inhibitors	Increased levels of mycophenolate mofetil
Clotrimazole	Increased levels of calcineurin inhibitor
Colchicine	Increased toxicity of colchicine
Diltiazem	Increased level of calcineurin inhibitor; increased neurotoxicity
Erythromycin or clarithromycin	Increased level of calcineurin inhibitor; prolonged QT intervals
Ganciclovir or valganciclovir	Increased nephrotoxicity with calcineurin inhibitors; leukopenia
Iron	Decreased levels of mycophenolate mofetil
Ketoconazole	Increased levels of calcineurin inhibitor
Phenobarbital	Decreased levels of calcineurin inhibitor
Phenytoin	Decreased levels of calcineurin inhibitor, increased levels of phenytoin
Primidone	Decreased levels of calcineurin inhibitor
Rifampin	Decreased levels of calcineurin inhibitor
Statin drugs	Increased risk for myopathy/rhabdomyolysis
St. John's wort	Decreased levels of calcineurin inhibitor levels
Target of rapamycin inhibitors	Increased nephrotoxicity with calcineurin inhibitors
Trimethoprim-sulfamethoxazole	Increased nephrotoxicity with calcineurin inhibitors
Verapamil	Increased levels of calcineurin inhibitor

including patient survival and graft survival, may be adversely affected. New-onset diabetes is characterized by decreased B-cell insulin secretion and increased insulin resistance secondary to the effects of immunosuppression. Many cases of new-onset diabetes are attributed to the high-dose steroids used early after transplantation surgery, but it is now appreciated that the calcineurin inhibitors play an important role as well. Impaired B-cell function appears to be the primary mechanism underlying the induction of diabetes by calcineurin inhibitors.[101,102]

The risk factors for the development of diabetes after transplantation include obesity, increased age, family history of diabetes, abnormal glucose tolerance, and African American or Hispanic descent. Changing trends in the demographics of transplant recipients, such as increased age and increased body mass index, suggest that current patients may be at greater risk of new-onset diabetes than were earlier patients. In one study, transplant recipients older than 45 years were 2.9 times more likely to become diabetic after transplantation.[102] Higher body mass index increases risk of insulin resistance, and steroids can cause glucose intolerance, insulin resistance, and frank hyperglycemia. African American patients are more likely to develop new-onset diabetes mellitus regardless of the immunosuppression used, but they are particularly susceptible after treatment with tacrolimus.[64,97] Unfortunately, there are very poor data about specific drugs to be used in the management of patients with new-onset diabetes after cardiac transplantation.

Hypertension

The excess risk of hypertension is related primarily to the use of calcineurin inhibitors, both because of direct effects of the drugs on the kidney and because of the associated renal insufficiency that is also highly prevalent. The incidence of hypertension may be lower with tacrolimus than with cyclosporine.[103] Blood pressure elevation in this population is characterized by a disturbed circadian rhythm without the normal nocturnal fall in blood pressure and with a greater 24-hour hypertensive burden. Posttransplantation hypertension is difficult to control and often necessitates a combination of several antihypertensive agents.

Renal Insufficiency

In a large registry of almost 70,000 recipients of nonrenal solid organ transplants, the risk of developing chronic renal failure was 16% at 10 years.[104] Various causes have been postulated for early renal insufficiency associated with calcineurin inhibitors, including renal arteriolar vasoconstriction directly mediated by calcineurin inhibitors, increased levels of endothelin-1 (a potent vasoconstrictor), and decreased nitric oxide production and alterations in the kidney's ability to adjust to changes in serum tonicity. Until the early 2000s, renal insufficiency, once present, progressed inexorably to renal failure. A number of new trials are in progress to evaluate the effects of substituting an mTOR inhibitor (sirolimus or everolimus) for a calcineurin inhibitor on renal function and on rejection episodes.[78,98]

Hyperlipidemia

Hyperlipidemia occurs as commonly in transplant recipients as in the general population. The concern has been that in many studies, hyperlipidemia has been associated with the development of CAV, cerebrovascular, and peripheral vascular disease, and the attendant morbidity and mortality of these vascular disorders. Typically, total cholesterol, low-density lipoprotein (LDL) cholesterol, and triglyceride levels increase by 3 months after transplantation and then generally fall somewhat after the first year. A number of drugs commonly used after transplantation contribute to the hyperlipidemia observed. Corticosteroids may lead to insulin resistance, increased synthesis of free fatty acids, and increased production of very low density lipoprotein. Cyclosporine increases serum LDL cholesterol and binds to the LDL receptor, which decreases its availability to absorb cholesterol from the bloodstream; tacrolimus probably causes less hyperlipidemia. Sirolimus and mycophenolate mofetil also have unfavorable effects on lipid levels. Sirolimus in escalating doses has been shown to result in prominent elevation in triglyceride levels.[64,97]

Lipid-lowering therapy with any statin or with 3-hydroxy-3-methylglutaryl–coenzyme A (HMG-CoA) reductase inhibitor was strongly associated with a marked improvement in 1-year survival in the Heart Transplant Lipid registry.[105] In heart transplant recipients, pravastatin and simvastatin have been associated with outcome benefits in survival, severity of rejection, and CAV,[43,106] whereas studies in kidney transplantation have not supported this finding. However, no long-term trials or data in this population have demonstrated improved outcomes with lowering LDL cholesterol levels to a specific target with more potent or higher dose statin therapy. Statins are metabolized differently, some by the cytochrome

TABLE 54–5 Morbidity After Heart Transplantation for Adults*

Outcome	Within 5 Years		Within 10 Years	
	Percentage with Known Response	Total *N* with Known Response	Percentage with Known Response	Total *N* with Known Response
Hypertension	93.8%	8266	98.5%	1586
Renal dysfunction	32.6%	8859	38.7%	1829
• Abnormal creatinine level (<2.5 mg/dL)	21.2%		24.4%	
• Creatinine level > 2.5 mg/dL	8.4%		8.2%	
• Chronic dialysis	2.5%		4.9%	
• Renal transplantation	0.5%		1.2%	
Hyperlipidemia	87.1%	9237	93.3%	1890
Diabetes	34.8%	8219	36.7%	1601
Cardiac allograft vasculopathy	31.5%	5944	52.7%	896

*Cumulative prevalence in survivors 5 and 10 years after transplantation (follow-up assessments: April 1994 to June 2006).
Modified from Hertz MI, Aurora P, Christie JD, et al. Registry of the International Society for Heart and Lung Transplantation: a quarter century of thoracic transplantation. *J Heart Lung Transplant* 2008;27:937-942.

TABLE 54–6 Malignancy After Heart Transplantation in Adults

Malignancy/Type	1-Year Survivors	5-Year Survivors	10-Year Survivors
No malignancy	20,442 (97.1%)	7780 (84.9%)	1264 (68.1%)
Malignancy (all types combined)	612 (2.9%)	1389 (15.1%)	592 (31.9%)
• Skin	282	937	360
• Lymph	142	127	38
• Other	132	359	108
• Type not reported	56	39	126

Cumulative prevalence in survivors (follow-up assessments: April 1994 to Jane 2006).
From Hertz MI, Aurora P, Christie JD, et al. Registry of the International Society for Heart and Lung Transplantation: a quarter century of thoracic transplantation. *J Heart Lung Transplant* 2008;27:937-942.

cyproheptadine (CYP) 3A4 and some by CYP2C9, and others are metabolized by a non-CYP mechanism in the liver. Thus, caution must be used in administration of statin drugs beyond the doses used in the randomized trials of simvastatin and pravastatin.[97] Transplantation teams must develop a coherent strategy about the goal and target doses of statins in their transplant recipients.

Cardiac Allograft Vasculopathy

The development of CAV remains the most disheartening long-term complication of heart transplantation; the annual incidence rate is 5% to 10%. The prognosis of heart transplant recipients is largely determined by the occurrence of CAV; after the first postoperative year, CAV becomes increasingly prevalent as a cause of death. CAV can develop as early as 3 months after transplantation and is detected angiographically in 20% of grafts at 1 year and in 40% to 50% at 5 years.[107,108] In contrast to eccentric lesions seen in atheromatous disease, CAV results from neointimal proliferation of vascular smooth muscle cells, so that it is a generalized process. Typically, the condition is characterized by concentric narrowing that affects the entire length of the coronary tree, from the epicardial to intramyocardial segments, which leads to rapid tapering, pruning, and obliteration of third-order branch vessels. The majority of affected patients do not experience anginal symptoms because of denervation of coronary arteries. The first clinical manifestation of CAV may include myocardial ischemia and infarction, heart failure, ventricular arrhythmia, or sudden cardiac death.

The causes of CAV are multifactorial. The risk of CAV increases as the number of HLA mismatches and the number and duration of rejection episodes increase. Various nonimmunological factors have been associated with development of CAV, including cytomegalovirus infection of the recipient, donor or recipient factors (e.g., age, gender, pretransplantation diagnosis), and factors related to surgery (ischemia-reperfusion injury). Classic risk factors for vascular disease such as smoking, obesity, diabetes, dyslipidemia, and hypertension also increase the risk for CAV.

In an effort to detect the development of CAV, transplantation teams must devise an approach to screen for the disease and, when it is found, control its progression. The usefulness of coronary angiography is limited by the fact that CAV produces concentric lesions that affect the distal and small vessels, often before becoming apparent in the main epicardial vessels. Intravascular ultrasonography is currently the most sensitive imaging technique for studying early CAV. Intravascular ultrasonography provides quantitative information about vessel wall structure and lumen dimensions. An increase in intimal thickness of at least 0.5 mm in the first year after transplantation is a reliable indicator of both CAV development and 5-year mortality.[109,110] However, the increased invasiveness and cost of intravascular ultrasonography preclude its widespread application. Dobutamine stress echocardiography has high sensitivity (83-95%) and specificity (between 53% and 91%) in comparison with angiographic CAV and even greater specificity than intravascular ultrasonography in

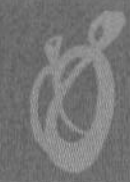

detecting disease.[111] Most transplantation centers perform one of these screening tests on an annual basis to assess the risk of new CAV.

The only definitive treatment of CAV is a second heart transplantation procedure. Other approaches, such as implantation of coronary stents and angioplasty, may have high restenosis rates and are unlikely to be effective because of the diffuse nature of the process.[112,113] Another approach to the prevention of CAV is the use of pravastatin and simvastatin. These drugs effectively repress the induction of major histocompatibility complex class II (MHC-II) expression by interferon-γ and thereby inhibit T-cell proliferation. In addition, statins have a direct influence on the expression of genes for growth factors that are essential for the proliferation of smooth muscle cells. Randomized controlled trials have shown that both drugs result in significantly lower cholesterol levels, significantly improved survival rates, significantly fewer severe rejections, and a significantly lower incidence of CAV.[110,114] It is not clear whether other statin drugs have the same benefit in this population.

Researchers have increasingly examined the efficacy of sirolimus and of everolimus in preventing the development or progression of CAV in heart transplant recipients. The precise role of the two drugs in maintenance immunosuppression has not yet been determined, but they are frequently used and hold the promise of reducing coronary intimal thickening once CAV has been detected.[107]

New Health Problems

Patients waiting for a heart transplant should have an updated review of immunizations, and yearly influenza vaccines should be encouraged thereafter, along with the periodic pneumococcal vaccine.[115] Vaccines with live viral particles must be avoided by immunocompromised transplant recipients. In general, a comprehensive visit is scheduled at the anniversary of the transplantation procedure so that annual issues may be reviewed, beyond the typical cardiovascular problems addressed so frequently in the first year. These include thorough skin and eye examinations and recommended screening examinations such as mammography, colonoscopy, and rectal and pelvic examinations, according to guidelines. This is the opportune time to reinforce the necessity of regular physical exercise, maintenance of ideal body weight, abstinence from tobacco, and moderation with alcohol. The annual examination is also the occasion when many transplantation teams look more carefully for the presence of CAV.

In many centers, recipients are prescribed daily aspirin to prevent further vascular disease, but no randomized trials have evaluated the benefits of antiplatelet therapy in heart transplant recipients. Likewise, most recipients are given vitamins, stool softeners, iron supplements, and proton pump inhibitors early after surgery, primarily on the basis of empirical findings. These are part of the decisions that must be made on a programmatic basis for the transplant recipient (see Table 54-4).

The development of osteoporosis is a major problem in the population of transplant recipients, and vertebral fractures are common and result in marked debilitation; prophylaxis with calcium and vitamin D is usually initiated. At least 50% of patients before transplantation have evidence of osteopenia, and osteoporosis is common among patients with advanced heart failure.[116] Glucocorticoids given after transplantation surgery are a major contributor to additional bone loss; most bone loss occurs in the first 6 to 12 months.

Depression, a common finding in patients with heart failure, occurs in up to 25% of transplant recipients and can interfere remarkably with a satisfactory recovery. A number of antidepressants may be prescribed, but the potential for adverse drug interactions must be considered (see Table 54-5). The management of gout may also be difficult because of drug interactions. Colchicine may increase the risk of myoneuropathy, and nonsteroidal anti-inflammatory drugs often cause worsening renal insufficiency and hyperkalemia. Allopurinol and azathioprine administered together can cause life-threatening neutropenia. Thus, transplant recipients must be instructed to discuss any new medicines prescribed to them with the transplantation team before they take these medicines.[64,97,117]

Physicians outside the transplantation center may be reluctant to care for the heart transplant recipient, which complicates the comprehensive management of these patients. Ideally, primary care physicians could provide a very important and early intervention that might be life-saving. The most common errors made by referring physicians who are unaware of normal transplantation procedures are the prescriptions of new drugs that result in adverse drug interactions (see Table 54-5). Both calcineurin inhibitors are metabolized in the liver by the cytochrome P-450 enzyme system. The activity of this system is influenced by hepatic dysfunction. Inducers of CYP3A4 include amiodarone, rifampin, and phenytoin; these drugs have the potential to lower the levels of calcineurin inhibitors. Agents that inhibit CYP3A4, and also raise levels of the immunosuppression regimen, include antifungals, macrolide antibacterials, calcium channel antagonists, and grapefruit juice.[117]

Physicians must use a higher index of suspicion when evaluating the possibility of infection in a transplant recipient, who must always be considered an immunocompromised host. Physicians unaccustomed to caring for infection-prone transplant recipients may inadvertently miss an important manifestation of an infectious disease, especially early in the posttransplantation course. Again, communication with the transplantation team should be fostered as a strategy to prevent these and countless other problems.

OUTCOMES AFTER HEART TRANSPLANTATION

Survival

Figure 54-5 depicts the latest data from the International Society for Heart and Lung Transplantation regarding overall transplantation survival.[7] During the first year after transplantation, early causes of death are graft failure, infection, and rejection, with an overall 1-year survival rate of 87%. Interestingly, although worldwide approaches to the management of cardiac transplant recipients are substantially different from center to center, the outcomes are surprisingly similar. The 5-, 10-, and 15-year rates of survival after heart transplantation were very comparable in two centers: one in Nantes, France,[100] and one in Utrecht, The Netherlands (Figure 54-6).[118] Indeed, this phenomenon of similar outcomes despite marked differences in programmatic management may be regarded as a testament to the overall antirejection strategy. Nonspecific graft failure accounted for 41% of deaths during the first 30 days after transplantation, whereas noncytomegalovirus infection was the primary cause of death during the first year. After 5 years, CAV and late graft failure (31% together), malignancy (24%), and noncytomegalovirus infection (10%) were the most prominent causes of death.[18,44,119]

Functional Outcomes

By the first year after transplantation surgery, 90% of surviving patients report no functional limitations, and approximately 35% return to work.[120] These statistics may change

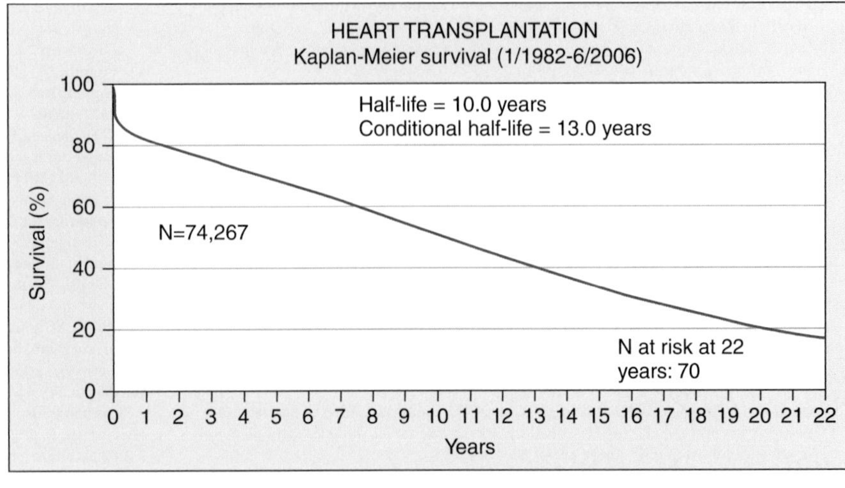

FIGURE 54–5 Overall survival after heart transplantation among 74,267 first-time recipients; the 10-year survival rate was at least 50%. (From Hertz MI, Aurora P, Christie JD, et al. Registry of the International Society for Heart and Lung Transplantation: a quarter century of thoracic transplantation. *J Heart Lung Transplant* 2008;27:937-942.)

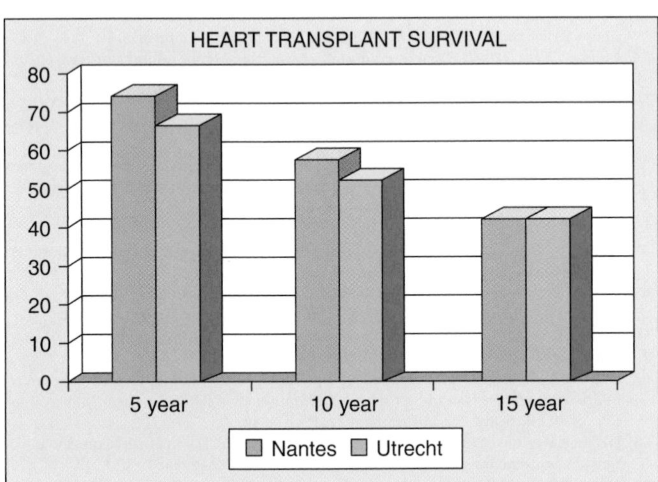

FIGURE 54–6 Overall rates of survival 5, 10, and 15 years after heart transplantation in Nantes, France, and Utrecht, The Netherlands. Note that the outcomes in the two countries are similar. (Data from Roussel JC, Baron O, Perigaud C, et al. Outcome of heart transplants 15 to 20 years ago: graft survival, post-transplant morbidity, and risk factors for mortality. *J Heart Lung Transplant* 2008;27:486-493; and Tjang YS, van der Heijden GJ, Tenderich G, et al. Survival analysis in heart transplantation: results from an analysis of 1290 cases in a single center. *Eur J Cardiothorac Surg* 2008;33:856-861.)

as the demographics of cardiac transplant recipients evolve. There are numerous challenges for optimal functional outcomes, not the least of which are nonreimbursement for cardiac rehabilitation programs by many third-party payers in the United States and the reluctance of many U.S. employers to hire transplantation survivors. Adapting to life after transplantation involves a variety of pretransplantation factors, including the patient's duration of illness, personality, intelligence, social support, and financial well-being.

The heart transplantation procedure markedly reduces cardiac filling pressures observed in the recipient before transplantation and augments cardiac output. During exercise, maximal cardiac output may be abnormal, as a result of denervation, limited atrial function, decreased myocardial compliance from rejection or ischemic injury, and donor-recipient size mismatch.[121] Much of this hemodynamic abnormality may be normalized with regular exercise.[122,123] Immediately after surgery, a restrictive hemodynamic pattern is frequently observed that gradually improves over a few days to weeks. Approximately 10% to 15% of recipients develop a chronic restrictive-type response during exercise that may produce fatigue and breathlessness. In the absence of parasympathetic innervation that normally lowers the heart rate, the resting heart rate of a recipient is typically 90 to 115 beats per minute. Likewise, β-blockers may further impair exercise response in transplant recipients and should not be first-line therapy for hypertension in this population.

FUTURE DIRECTIONS

Heart transplantation is one of multiple competing therapeutic options for treating advanced heart failure, including "destination" or permanent mechanical circulatory support (see Chapter 56). As newer therapies, such as cell transplantation (see Chapter 51) and better permanent mechanical devices, become available, the role of heart transplantation will need to be redefined as the therapy of choice. Moreover, the cost effectiveness of the transplantation procedure will decrease if 40% to 50% of patients require a VAD preoperatively. Organ allocation may need to be reconsidered in this era of rapid HLA typing and virtual crossmatching.

An ideal immunosuppressive regimen for cardiac transplantation will prevent cellular rejection, retard the development of CAV, have no nephrotoxicity, and produce negligible morbidity with regard to lymphoproliferative disease and opportunistic infections. The development of renal-sparing strategies in transplant recipients is one of the most significant therapeutic challenges. This and other modifications of the standard regimen must be explored in future trials. Trial networks to investigate some of these newer ideas or therapies must be established to facilitate research in this fragile population.

In the United States, there is now an acknowledged secondary subspecialty in medicine specifically for cardiologists who want to acquire expertise in the care of the heart transplant recipient.[124] Surgical training has allowed for the increased skill required to manage the wide array of mechanical circulatory support devices used to sustain the patient with advanced heart failure. Mechanisms to fund the prolonged training of these transplantation specialists, and other transplantation personnel, must be found in an increasingly impoverished health care system.

REFERENCES

1. Hunt, S. A., & Haddad, F. (2008). The changing face of heart transplantation. *J Am Coll Cardiol*, *52*, 587–598.
2. Hunt, S. A. (2006). Taking heart—cardiac transplantation past, present, and future. *N Engl J Med*, *355*, 231–235.
3. Butler, J., Khadim, G., Paul, K. M., et al. (2004). Selection of patients for heart transplantation in the current era of heart failure therapy. *J Am Coll Cardiol*, *43*, 787–793.
4. Mehra, M. R., Kobashigawa, J., Starling, R., et al. (2006). Listing criteria for heart transplantation: International Society for Heart and Lung Transplantation guidelines for the care of cardiac transplant candidates—2006. *J Heart Lung Transplant*, *25*, 1024–1042.

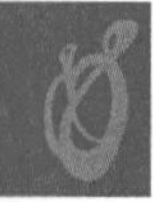

5. Hansky, B., Vogt, J., Zittermann, A., et al. (2009). Cardiac resynchronization therapy: long-term alternative to cardiac transplantation? *Ann Thorac Surg, 87*, 432–438.
6. John, R. (2004). Donor management and selection for heart transplantation. *Semin Thorac Cardiovasc Surg, 16*, 364–369.
7. Hertz, M. I., Aurora, P., Christie, J. D., et al. (2008). Registry of the International Society for Heart and Lung Transplantation: a quarter century of thoracic transplantation. *J Heart Lung Transplant, 27*, 937–942.
8. Goldberg, L. R., & Jessup, M. (2007). A time to be born and a time to die. *Circulation, 116*, 360–362.
9. Levy, W. C., Mozaffarian, D., Linker, D. T., et al. (2009). Can the Seattle heart failure model be used to risk-stratify heart failure patients for potential left ventricular assist device therapy?. *J Heart Lung Transplant, 28*, 231–236.
10. Stevenson, L. W., Pagani, F. D., Young, J. B., et al. (2009). INTERMACS profiles of advanced heart failure: the current picture. *J Heart Lung Transplant, 28*, 535–541.
11. Simmonds, J., Burch, M., Dawkins, H., et al. (2008). Heart transplantation after congenital heart surgery: improving results and future goals. *Eur J Cardiothorac Surg, 34*, 313–317.
12. Mancini, D. M., Eisen, H., Kussmaul, W., et al. (1991). Value of peak exercise oxygen consumption for optimal timing of cardiac transplantation in ambulatory patients with heart failure. *Circulation, 83*, 778–786.
13. Lund, L. H., Aaronson, K. D., Mancini, D. M., et al. (2005). Validation of peak exercise oxygen consumption and the Heart Failure Survival Score for serial risk stratification in advanced heart failure. *Am J Cardiol, 95*, 734–741.
14. Allen, L. A., Rogers, J. G., Warnica, J. W., et al. (2008). High mortality without ESCAPE: the registry of heart failure patients receiving pulmonary artery catheters without randomization. *J Card Fail, 14*, 661–669.
15. Nohria, A., Hasselblad, V., Stebbins, A., et al. (2008). Cardiorenal interactions: insights from the ESCAPE trial. *J Am Coll Cardiol, 51*, 1268–1274.
16. Chen, J. M., Russo, M. J., Hammond, K. M., et al. (2005). Alternate waiting list strategies for heart transplantation maximize donor organ utilization. *Ann Thorac Surg, 80*, 224–228.
17. Tjang, Y. S., van der Heijden, G. J., Tenderich, G., et al. (2008). Impact of recipient's age on heart transplantation outcome. *Ann Thorac Surg, 85*, 2051–2055.
18. Weiss, E. S., Nwakanma, L. U., Patel, N. D., et al. (2008). Outcomes in patients older than 60 years of age undergoing orthotopic heart transplantation: an analysis of the UNOS database. *J Heart Lung Transplant, 27*, 184–191.
19. Russo, M. J., Rana, A., Chen, J. M., et al. (2009). Pretransplantation patient characteristics and survival following combined heart and kidney transplantation: an analysis of the United Network for Organ Sharing Database. *Arch Surg, 144*, 241–246.
20. Gill, J., Shah, T., Hristea, I., et al. (2009). Outcomes of simultaneous heart-kidney transplant in the US: a retrospective analysis using OPTN/UNOS data. *Am J Transplant, 9*, 844–852.
21. Klotz, S., Wenzelburger, F., Stypmann, J., et al. (2006). Reversible pulmonary hypertension in heart transplant candidates: to transplant or not to transplant. *Ann Thorac Surg, 82*, 1770–1773.
22. Lorenz, K. A., Lynn, J., Dy, S. M., et al. (2008). Evidence for improving palliative care at the end of life: a systematic review. *Ann Intern Med, 148*, 147–159.
23. Kobashigawa, J., Mehra, M., West, L., et al. (2009). Report From a Consensus Conference on the Sensitized Patient Awaiting Heart Transplantation. *J Heart Lung Transplant, 28*, 213–225.
24. Tait, B. D., Hudson, F., Cantwell, L., et al. (2009). Review article: Luminex technology for HLA antibody detection in organ transplantation. *Nephrology, 14*, 247–254.
25. Fuggle, S. V., & Martin, S. (2008). Tools for human leukocyte antigen antibody detection and their application to transplanting sensitized patients. *Transplantation, 86*, 384–390.
26. Vega, J., Moore, J., Murray, S., et al. (2009). Heart transplantation in the United States, 1998-2007. *Am J Transplant, 9*(Pt 2), 932–941.
27. Cleveland, J. C., Jr., Grover, F. L., Fullerton, D. A., et al. (2008). Left ventricular assist device as bridge to transplantation does not adversely affect one-year heart transplantation survival. *J Thorac Cardiovasc Surg, 136*, 774–777.
28. Hoercher, K. J., Nowicki, E. R., Blackstone, E. H., et al. (2008). Prognosis of patients removed from a transplant waiting list for medical improvement: implications for organ allocation and transplantation for status 2 patients. *J Thorac Cardiovasc Surg, 135*, 1159–1166.
29. Halpern, S. D., Shaked, A., Hasz, R. D., et al. (2008). Informing candidates for solid-organ transplantation about donor risk factors. *N Engl J Med, 358*, 2832–2837.
30. Khasati, N. H., Machaal, A., Barnard, J., et al. (2007). Donor heart selection: the outcome of "unacceptable" donors. *J Cardiothorac Surg, 2*, 13.
31. Gupta, D., Piacentino, V., III, Macha, M., et al. (2004). Effect of older donor age on risk for mortality after heart transplantation. *Ann Thorac Surg, 78*, 890–899.
32. Collins, M. J., Moainie, S. L., Griffith, B. P., et al. (2008). Preserving and evaluating hearts with ex vivo machine perfusion: an avenue to improve early graft performance and expand the donor pool. *Eur J Cardiothorac Surg, 34*, 318–325.
33. Mehra, M. R. (2008). The cardiac allograft is going up in smoke: a call to action. *Am J Transplant, 8*, 737–738.
34. Rosendale, J. D., Kauffman, H. M., McBride, M. A., et al. (2003). Aggressive pharmacologic donor management results in more transplanted organs. *Transplantation, 75*, 482–487.
35. Zaroff, J. G., Rosengard, B. R., Armstrong, W. F., et al. (2002). Consensus conference report: maximizing use of organs recovered from the cadaver donor: cardiac recommendations, March 28-29, 2001, Crystal City, Va. *Circulation* (106), 836–841.
36. Kubrich, M., Petrakopoulou, P., Kofler, S., et al. (2008). Impact of coronary endothelial dysfunction on adverse long-term outcome after heart transplantation. *Transplantation, 85*, 1580–1587.
37. Grande, A. M., Gaeta, R., Campana, C., et al. (2008). Comparison of standard and bicaval approach in orthotopic heart transplantation: 10-year follow-up. *J Cardiovasc Med, 9*, 493–497.
38. Morgan, J. A., & Edwards, N. M. (2005). Orthotopic cardiac transplantation: comparison of outcome using biatrial, bicaval, and total techniques. *J Card Surg, 20*, 102–106.
39. Schnoor, M., Schafer, T., Luhmann, D., et al. (2007). Bicaval versus standard technique in orthotopic heart transplantation: a systematic review and meta-analysis. *J Thorac Cardiovasc Surg, 134*, 1322–1331.
40. Fiorelli, A. I., Stolf, N. A., Abreu Filho, C. A., et al. (2007). Prophylactic donor tricuspid annuloplasty in orthotopic bicaval heart transplantation. *Transplant Proceedings, 39*, 2527–2530.
41. Christiansen, S., Klocke, A., Autschbach, R., et al. (2008). Past, present, and future of long-term mechanical cardiac support in adults. *J Card Surg, 23*, 664–676.
42. Miller, L. W., Pagani, F. D., Russell, S. D., et al. (2007). Use of a continuous-flow device in patients awaiting heart transplantation. *N Engl J Med, 357*, 885–896.
43. Kobashigawa, J. A., Starling, R. C., Mehra, M. R., et al. (2006). Multicenter retrospective analysis of cardiovascular risk factors affecting long-term outcome of de novo cardiac transplant recipients. *J Heart Lung Transplant, 25*, 1063–1069.
44. Marelli, D., Kobashigawa, J., Hamilton, M. A., et al. (2008). Long-term outcomes of heart transplantation in older recipients. *J Heart Lung Transplant, 27*, 830–834.
45. Russo, M. J., Chen, J. M., Sorabella, R. A., et al. (2007). The effect of ischemic time on survival after heart transplantation varies by donor age: an analysis of the United Network for Organ Sharing database. *J Thorac Cardiovasc Surg, 133*, 554–559.
46. Sezgin, A., Akay, T. H., Ozcobanoglu, S., et al. (2008). Surgery-related complications in cardiac transplantation patients. *Transplant Proceedings, 40*, 255–258.
47. Novick, R. J. (2009). Immediate postoperative care of the heart transplant recipient: perils and triumphs. *Semin Cardiothorac Vasc Anesth, 13*, 95–98.
48. Ramakrishna, H., Jaroszewski, D. E., & Arabia, F. A. (2009). Adult cardiac transplantation: a review of perioperative management Part-I. *Ann Card Anaesth, 12*, 71–78.
49. Khush, K. K., Valantine, H. A., Khush, K. K., et al. (2009). New developments in immunosuppressive therapy for heart transplantation. *Expert Opin Emerg Drugs, 14*, 1–21.
50. Mehra, M. R., Uber, P. A., & Kaplan, B. (2006). Immunosuppression in cardiac transplantation: science, common sense and the heart of the matter. *Am J Transplant, 6*, 1243–1245.
51. Mueller, X. M. (2004). Drug immunosuppression therapy for adult heart transplantation. Part 2: clinical applications and results. *Ann Thorac Surg, 77*, 363–371.
52. Mueller, X. M. (2004). Drug immunosuppression therapy for adult heart transplantation. Part 1: immune response to allograft and mechanism of action of immunosuppressants. *Ann Thorac Surg, 77*, 354–362.
53. Goland, S., Czer, L. S., Coleman, B., et al. (2008). Induction therapy with thymoglobulin after heart transplantation: impact of therapy duration on lymphocyte depletion and recovery, rejection, and cytomegalovirus infection rates. *J Heart Lung Transplant, 27*, 1115–1121.
54. Issa, N. C., Fishman, J. A., Issa, N. C., et al. (2009). Infectious complications of antilymphocyte therapies in solid organ transplantation. *Clin Infect Dis, 48*, 772–786.
55. Uber, P. A., & Mehra, M. R. (2007). Induction therapy in heart transplantation: is there a role?*J Heart Lung Transplant, 26*, 205–209.
56. Opelz, G., & Henderson, R. (1993). Incidence of non-Hodgkin lymphoma in kidney and heart transplant recipients. *Lancet, 342*, 1514–1516.
57. Segovia, J., Rodriguez-Lambert, J. L., Crespo-Leiro, M. G., et al. (2006). A randomized multicenter comparison of basiliximab and muromonab (OKT3) in heart transplantation: SIMCOR study. *Transplantation, 81*, 1542–1548.
58. Hershberger, R. E., Starling, R. C., Eisen, H. J., et al. (2005). Daclizumab to prevent rejection after cardiac transplantation. *N Engl J Med, 352*, 2705–2713.
59. Mehra, M. R., Zucker, M. J., Wagoner, L., et al. (2005). A multicenter, prospective, randomized, double-blind trial of basiliximab in heart transplantation. *J Heart Lung Transplant, 24*, 1297–1304.
60. Carrier, M., Leblanc, M. H., Perrault, L. P., et al. (2007). Basiliximab and rabbit anti-thymocyte globulin for prophylaxis of acute rejection after heart transplantation: a non-inferiority trial. *J Heart Lung Transplant, 26*, 258–263.
61. Kobashigawa, J., David, K., Morris, J., et al. (2005). Daclizumab is associated with decreased rejection and no increased mortality in cardiac transplant patients receiving MMF, cyclosporine, and corticosteroids. *Transplant Proc, 37*, 1333–1339.
62. Patel, J., Kobashigawa, J. A., Patel, J., et al. (2008). Minimization of immunosuppression: transplant immunology. *Transplant Immunol, 20*, 48–54.
63. Moller, C. H., Gustafsson, F., Gluud, C., et al. (2008). Interleukin-2 receptor antagonists as induction therapy after heart transplantation: systematic review with meta-analysis of randomized trials. *J Heart Lung Transplant, 27*, 835–842.
64. Lindenfeld, J., Miller, G. G., Shakar, S. F., et al. (2004). Drug therapy in the heart transplant recipient: part II: immunosuppressive drugs. *Circulation, 110*, 3858–3865.
65. Lindenfeld, J., Miller, G. G., Shakar, S. F., et al. (2004). Drug therapy in the heart transplant recipient: part I: cardiac rejection and immunosuppressive drugs. *Circulation, 110*, 3734–3740.
66. Flechner, S. M., Kobashigawa, J., & Klintmalm, G. (2008). Calcineurin inhibitor-sparing regimens in solid organ transplantation: focus on improving renal function and nephrotoxicity. *Clin Transplant, 22*, 1–15.
67. Solari, S. G., Goldberg, L. R., DeNofrio, D., et al. (2005). Cyclosporine monitoring with 2-hour postdose levels in heart transplant recipients. *Ther Drug Monit, 27*, 417–421.
68. Grimm, M., Rinaldi, M., Yonan, N. A., et al. (2006). Superior prevention of acute rejection by tacrolimus vs. cyclosporine in heart transplant recipients—a large European trial. *Am J Transplant, 6*, 1387–1397.
69. Kobashigawa, J. A., Patel, J., Furukawa, H., et al. (2006). Five-year results of a randomized, single-center study of tacrolimus vs microemulsion cyclosporine in heart transplant patients. *J Heart Lung Transplant, 25*, 434–439.
70. Lehmkuhl, H., Hummel, M., Kobashigawa, J., et al. (2008). Enteric-coated mycophenolate-sodium in heart transplantation: efficacy, safety, and pharmacokinetic compared with mycophenolate mofetil. *Transplant Proc, 40*, 953–955.
71. Kobashigawa, J. A., Miller, L. W., Russell, S. D., et al. (2006). Tacrolimus with mycophenolate mofetil (MMF) or sirolimus vs. cyclosporine with MMF in cardiac transplant patients: 1-year report. *Am J Transplant, 6*, 1377–1386.
72. Kobashigawa, J. A., Tobis, J. M., Mentzer, R. M., et al. (2006). Mycophenolate mofetil reduces intimal thickness by intravascular ultrasound after heart transplant: reanalysis of the multicenter trial. *Am J Transplant, 6*, 993–997.

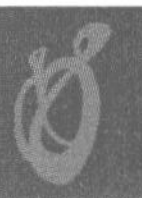

73. Eisen, H. J., Kobashigawa, J., Keogh, A., et al. (2005). Three-year results of a randomized, double-blind, controlled trial of mycophenolate mofetil versus azathioprine in cardiac transplant recipients. *J Heart Lung Transplant*, *24*, 517–525.
74. Raichlin, E., Chandrasekaran, K., Kremers, W. K., et al. (2008). Sirolimus as primary immunosuppressant reduces left ventricular mass and improves diastolic function of the cardiac allograft. *Transplantation*, *86*, 1395–1400.
75. Mudge, G. H., Jr. (2007). Sirolimus and cardiac transplantation: is it the "magic bullet"?*Circulation*, *116*, 2666–2668.
76. Raichlin, E., Bae, J. H., Khalpey, Z., et al. (2007). Conversion to sirolimus as primary immunosuppression attenuates the progression of allograft vasculopathy after cardiac transplantation. *Circulation*, *116*, 2726–2733.
77. Sánchez-Fructuoso, A. I. (2008). Everolimus: an update on the mechanism of action, pharmacokinetics and recent clinical trials. *Expert Opin Drug Metab Toxicol*, *4*, 807–819.
78. Groetzner, J., Kaczmarek, I., Schulz, U., et al. (2009). Mycophenolate and sirolimus as calcineurin inhibitor-free immunosuppression improves renal function better than calcineurin inhibitor-reduction in late cardiac transplant recipients with chronic renal failure. *Transplantation*, *87*, 726–733.
79. Kushwaha, S. S., Raichlin, E., Sheinin, Y., et al. (2008). Sirolimus affects cardiomyocytes to reduce left ventricular mass in heart transplant recipients. *Eur Heart J*, *29*, 2742–2750.
80. Rothenburger, M., Zuckermann, A., Bara, C., et al. (2007). Recommendations for the use of everolimus (Certican) in heart transplantation: results from the second German-Austrian Certican Consensus Conference. *J Heart Lung Transplant*, *26*, 305–311.
81. Dobbels, F., Vanhaecke, J., Dupont, L., et al. (2009). Pretransplant predictors of post-transplant adherence and clinical outcome: an evidence base for pretransplant psychosocial screening. *Transplantation*, *87*, 1497–1504.
82. Saeed, I., Rogers, C., Murday, A., et al. (2008). Health-related quality of life after cardiac transplantation: results of a UK national survey with norm-based comparisons. *J Heart Lung Transplant*, *27*, 675–681.
83. Fusar-Poli, P., Picchioni, M., Martinelli, V., et al. (2006). Anti-depressive therapies after heart transplantation. *J Heart Lung Transplant*, *25*, 785–793.
84. Singh, N., Pirsch, J., & Samaniego, M. (2009). Antibody-mediated rejection: treatment alternatives and outcomes. *Transplant Rev*, *23*, 34–46.
85. Fedson, S. E., Daniel, S. S., & Husain, A. N. (2008). Immunohistochemistry staining of C4d to diagnose antibody-mediated rejection in cardiac transplantation. *J Heart Lung Transplant*, *27*, 372–379.
86. Tan, C. D., Baldwin, W. M., III, & Rodriguez, E. R. (2007). Update on cardiac transplantation pathology. *Arch Pathol Lab Med*, *131*, 1169–1191.
87. Patel, J. K., & Kobashigawa, J. A. (2006). Should we be doing routine biopsy after heart transplantation in a new era of anti-rejection? *Curr Opin Cardiol*, *21*, 127–131.
88. Stewart, S., Winters, G. L., Fishbein, M. C., et al. (2005). Revision of the 1990 working formulation for the standardization of nomenclature in the diagnosis of heart rejection. *J Heart Lung Transplant*, *24*, 1710–1720.
89. Jarcho, J., Naftel, D. C., Shroyer, T. W., et al. (1994). Influence of HLA mismatch on rejection after heart transplantation: a multiinstitutional study. The Cardiac Transplant Research Database Group. *J Heart Lung Transplant*, *13*, 583–595.
90. Taylor, D. O., Edwards, L. B., Boucek, M. M., et al. (2005). Registry of the International Society for Heart and Lung Transplantation: twenty-second official adult heart transplant report—2005. *J Heart Lung Transplant*, *24*, 945–955.
91. Reed, E. F., Demetris, A. J., Hammond, E., et al. (2006). Acute antibody-mediated rejection of cardiac transplants. *J Heart Lung Transplant*, *25*, 153–159.
92. Kfoury, A. G., Hammond, M. E., Snow, G. L., et al. (2009). Cardiovascular mortality among heart transplant recipients with asymptomatic antibody-mediated or stable mixed cellular and antibody-mediated rejection. *J Heart Lung Transplant*, *28*, 781–784.
93. Turgeon, N. A., Kirk, A. D., Iwakoshi, N. N., et al. (2009). Differential effects of donor-specific alloantibody. *Transplant Rev*, *23*, 25–33.
94. Jessup, M., & Brozena, S. (2007). State-of-the-art strategies for immunosuppression. *Curr Opin Organ Transplant*, *12*, 536–542.
95. Deng, M. C., Eisen, H. J., Mehra, M. R., et al. (2006). Noninvasive discrimination of rejection in cardiac allograft recipients using gene expression profiling. *Am J Transplant*, *6*, 150–160.
96. Potena, L., Grigioni, F., Magnani, G., et al. (2009). Prophylaxis versus preemptive anti-cytomegalovirus approach for prevention of allograft vasculopathy in heart transplant recipients. *J Heart Lung Transplant*, *28*, 461–467.
97. Lindenfeld, J., Page, R. L., II, Zolty, R., et al. (2005). Drug therapy in the heart transplant recipient: part III: common medical problems. *Circulation*, *111*, 113–117.
98. Gonzalez-Vilchez, F., de Prada, J. A., Exposito, V., et al. (2008). Avoidance of calcineurin inhibitors with use of proliferation signal inhibitors in de novo heart transplantation with renal failure. *J Heart Lung Transplant*, *27*, 1135–1141.
99. Crespo-Leiro, M. G., Alonso-Pulpon, L., Vazquez de Prada, J. A., et al. (2008). Malignancy after heart transplantation: incidence, prognosis and risk factors. *Am J Transplant*, *8*, 1031–1039.
100. Roussel, J. C., Baron, O., Perigaud, C., et al. (2008). Outcome of heart transplants 15 to 20 years ago: graft survival, post-transplant morbidity, and risk factors for mortality. *J Heart Lung Transplant*, *27*, 486–493.
101. Russo, M. J., Chen, J. M., Hong, K. N., et al. (2006). Survival after heart transplantation is not diminished among recipients with uncomplicated diabetes mellitus: an analysis of the United Network of Organ Sharing Database. *Circulation*, *114*, 2280–2287.
102. Wilkinson, A., Davidson, J., Dotta, F., et al. (2005). Guidelines for the treatment and management of new-onset diabetes after transplantation. *Clin Transplant*, *19*, 291–298.
103. Ye, F., Ying-Bin, X., Yu-Guo, W., et al. (2009). Tacrolimus versus cyclosporine microemulsion for heart transplant recipients: a meta-analysis. *J Heart Lung Transplant*, *28*, 58–66.
104. Lonze, B. E., Warren, D. S., Stewart, Z. A., et al. (2009). Kidney transplantation in previous heart or lung recipients. *Am J Transplant*, *9*, 578–585.
105. Wu, A. H., Ballantyne, C. M., Short, B. C., et al. (2005). Statin use and risks of death or fatal rejection in the Heart Transplant Lipid Registry. *Am J Cardiol*, *95*, 367–372.
106. Bilchick, K. C., Henrikson, C. A., Skojec, D., et al. (2004). Treatment of hyperlipidemia in cardiac transplant recipients. *Am Heart J*, *148*, 200–210.
107. Delgado, J. F., Manito, N., Segovia, J., et al. (2009). The use of proliferation signal inhibitors in the prevention and treatment of allograft vasculopathy in heart transplantation. *Transplant Rev*, *23*, 69–79.
108. Schmauss, D., Weis, M., Schmauss, D., et al. (2008). Cardiac allograft vasculopathy: recent developments. *Circulation*, *117*, 2131–2141.
109. Tuzcu, E. M., Kapadia, S. R., Sachar, R., et al. (2005). Intravascular ultrasound evidence of angiographically silent progression in coronary atherosclerosis predicts long-term morbidity and mortality after cardiac transplantation. *J Am Coll Cardiol*, *45*, 1538–1542.
110. Kobashigawa, J. A., Tobis, J. M., Starling, R. C., et al. (2005). Multicenter intravascular ultrasound validation study among heart transplant recipients: outcomes after five years. *J Am Coll Cardiol*, *45*, 1532–1537.
111. Bacal, F., Moreira, L., Souza, G., et al. (2004). Dobutamine stress echocardiography predicts cardiac events or death in asymptomatic patients long-term after heart transplantation: 4-year prospective evaluation. *J Heart Lung Transplant*, *23*, 1238–1244.
112. Bhama, J. K., Nguyen, D. Q., Scolieri, S., et al. (2009). Surgical revascularization for cardiac allograft vasculopathy: is it still an option? *J Thorac Cardiovasc Surg*, *137*, 1488–1492.
113. Gupta, A., Mancini, D., Kirtane, A. J., et al. (2009). Value of drug-eluting stents in cardiac transplant recipients. *Am J Cardiol*, *103*, 659–662.
114. Kobashigawa, J. A. (2006). Cardiac allograft vasculopathy in heart transplant patients: pathologic and clinical aspects for angioplasty/stenting. *J Am Coll Cardiol*, *48*, 462–463.
115. Magnani, G., Falchetti, E., Pollini, G., et al. (2005). Safety and efficacy of two types of influenza vaccination in heart transplant recipients: a prospective randomised controlled study. *J Heart Lung Transplant*, *24*, 588–592.
116. Ebeling, P. R. (2009). Approach to the patient with transplantation-related bone loss. *J Clin Endocrinol Metab*, *94*, 1483–1490.
117. Page, R. L., II, Miller, G. G., & Lindenfeld, J. (2005). Drug therapy in the heart transplant recipient: part IV: drug-drug interactions. *Circulation*, *111*, 230–239.
118. Tjang, Y. S., van der Heijden, G. J., Tenderich, G., et al. (2008). Survival analysis in heart transplantation: results from an analysis of 1290 cases in a single center. *Eur J Cardiothorac Surg*, *33*, 856–861.
119. Vaseghi, M., Lellouche, N., Ritter, H., et al. (2009). Mode and mechanisms of death after orthotopic heart transplantation. *Heart Rhythm*, *6*, 503–509.
120. Grady, K. L., Naftel, D. C., Young, J. B., et al. (2007). Patterns and predictors of physical functional disability at 5 to 10 years after heart transplantation. *J Heart Lung Transplant*, *26*, 1182–1191.
121. Scott, J. M., Esch, B. T., Haykowsky, M. J., et al. (2009). Cardiovascular responses to incremental and sustained submaximal exercise in heart transplant recipients. *Am J Physiol Heart Circ Physiol*, *296*, H350–H358.
122. Roten, L., Schmid, J. P., Merz, F., et al. (2009). Diastolic dysfunction of the cardiac allograft and maximal exercise capacity. *J Heart Lung Transplant*, *28*, 434–439.
123. Haykowsky, M., Taylor, D., Kim, D., et al. (2009). Exercise training improves aerobic capacity and skeletal muscle function in heart transplant recipients. *Am J Transplant*, *9*, 734–739.
124. Konstam, M. A., Jessup, M., Francis, G. S., et al. (2009). Advanced heart failure and transplant cardiology: a subspecialty is born. *J Am Coll Cardiol*, *53*, 834–836.

CHAPTER 55

Surgical Treatment of Chronic Heart Failure

Wilfried Mullens and Randall C. Starling

Cardiac surgical interventions have been performed for decades on patients with congestive heart failure; these procedures initially carried high rates of perioperative morbidity and mortality, as observed in the 1970s and 1980s. Accordingly, the role of surgery was limited to cases of failed medical management and desperation. Fortunately, a real resurgence of interest into the surgical options of heart failure has emerged as a result of evolving surgical techniques and devices that treat both ischemic and nonischemic heart failure.

Because of the aging of the population, the significant increase in the prevalence, morbidity, and mortality from heart failure is a compelling problem. Advances in the treatment of acute myocardial infarction and nonischemic cardiomyopathy have led to increased survival of patients. However, this has resulted in a continuous increase in the number of patients ultimately presenting with heart failure. Although cardiac transplantation remains a valuable therapeutic option for advanced end-stage heart failure (see Chapter 54), the field of transplantation continues to be plagued by a finite number of organ donors. Mechanical devices, such as implantable left ventricular assist devices (LVADs), are expensive, have a high incidence of adverse events, and therefore have not yet achieved their goal as a readily available alternative to transplantation for advanced heart failure (see Chapter 56). However, the advent of axial flow LVADs as bridges to transplantation has markedly improved outcomes for transplant recipients. Ongoing trials with new-generation LVADs for chronic or "destination therapy" are expected to demonstrate improved outcomes and result in more widespread use (see Chapter 56). As the numbers of patients suffering from advanced heart failure continue to grow and the availability and feasibility of cardiac transplantation and assist devices may not meet that growing demand, a substantial number of patients with heart failure will probably become candidates for and derive benefit from heart failure surgery.

Because heart failure is a continuous disease process with ongoing detrimental reverse remodeling of the ventricles, insights into its pathophysiological features have led to major advances in surgical therapies (see Chapter 15). Contemporary surgical techniques and devices are attempts to restore the geometry of the failing ventricle and thereby arrest or reverse the adverse remodeling processes. As a result, cardiac function and subsequent outcomes have improved. Major advances in pharmacotherapy and imaging modalities have helped the surgical team select patients who will benefit most from surgical treatment of advanced heart failure. The management of chronic heart failure yields the best results through a combined medical and surgical approach, both of which are possible with a multidisciplinary team.

In this chapter, current and evolving surgical strategies for treating congestive heart failure are reviewed, with a focus on three major areas: revascularization for ischemic heart disease, operations for valvular lesions, and ventricular remodeling surgery. Of course, patients' needs in these three areas often overlap; for example, a patient with ischemic cardiomyopathy may undergo coronary artery bypass, mitral valve repair, and left ventricular (LV) reconstruction of scarred dyskinetic anterior infarcted segments.

CORONARY REVASCULARIZATION FOR ISCHEMIC CARDIOMYOPATHY

Definition and Epidemiology

Ischemic cardiomyopathy is currently defined as significantly impaired (LV) dysfunction (left ventricular ejection fraction [LVEF] ≤ 35% to 40%) that results from coronary artery disease.[1] Ischemic cardiomyopathy is considered to be the most common cause of heart failure; it currently affects 2.5 million people in the United States, the annual incidence is 40,000 new cases, and the annual mortality rate is 200,000 (see Chapter 22).[2] Because of aging and increased cardiovascular risk profiles of the population in the United States, the population-attributable risk has been estimated to be as high as 68% among men and 56% among women.[3] In addition, according to a review of almost 2000 patients with symptomatic heart failure and LVEF lower than 40%, patients with ischemic cardiomyopathy had significantly worse outcomes than those with nonischemic cardiomyopathy.[1] In contrast, patients with single-vessel disease who had no history of myocardial infarction or revascularization had a prognosis similar to that in patients with nonischemic cardiomyopathy.

Older data from the Framingham Heart Study suggested that the prevalence of heart failure after a myocardial infarction is 14% at 5 years and 22% at 10 years.[4] However, more recent data showed this prevalence to be much higher, ranging from 10% at 2 years to more than 40% at 6.5 years after myocardial infarction.[5,6] Improved early revascularization, intensive care strategies, and heart failure therapies (medications and devices, such as cardiac resynchronization therapy [CRT] and implantable cardioverter-defibrillator [ICD]) have increased survival of patients admitted with extensive myocardial infarcts; as a result, the number of late presentations of congestive heart failure has increased. The development of heart failure late after myocardial infarction is related to a variety of factors, including the size and location of the infarct, the presence of ischemic mitral regurgitation (IMR), and perhaps inflammatory status, as assessed by serum C-reactive protein level.[5-7] In addition, the risk of developing heart failure is also increased two to three times in patients with continuous angina, which suggests that myocardial ischemia contributes to the progressive LV dysfunction.[8] Therefore, strategies must be in place to detect and treat heart failure and ongoing, potentially reversible ischemia in patients who might benefit from coronary revascularization.

Pathophysiology of Ischemic Cardiomyopathy

The mechanism most commonly involved in myocardial dysfunction secondary to ischemic cardiomyopathy is the loss of myocytes, which eventually leads to progressive reverse remodeling of the heart (see also Chapters 6 and 23).[9] The LV remodeling process after myocardial infarction is complex, involving myocyte stretch and slippage, a phenomenon that also occurs in the adjacent remote viable myocardium.[10] Ischemia-induced cellular changes include loss of myofibrils and disorganization of the structural proteins within the myocyte. In addition, extracellular changes, including fibrosis and alterations in the fiber orientation, cause changes in the geometrical shape of the heart.[11] Eventually, these processes lead to a progressive dilation of the ventricles with a subsequent increase in wall tension and impairment of systolic and diastolic function. Thus, the progressive loss of viable myocardium over time after the myocardial infarction is a continuous process that ultimately might be accompanied by the clinical heart failure syndrome.[12] However, restoration of myocardial blood flow in addition to surgical restoration of LV chamber geometry (section on left ventricular reconstruction surgery) might reverse this detrimental process.

Insights into the myocardial ischemia-induced changes on a cellular level help physicians to better determine which patients will benefit most from revascularization strategies (see also Chapter 23). Although transient ischemia can lead to a period of prolonged dysfunction even after the restoration of flow ("stunning"), persistent but asymptomatic ischemia might induce LV dysfunction ("hibernation") that can mimic nonischemic causes of heart failure. *Stunned myocardium* is used to describe a condition in which a short-term, total or near-total reduction of coronary blood flow produces an abnormality in regional LV wall motion of limited duration (hours or days) after reperfusion.[13-15] In contrast, *hibernating myocardium* is a state of persistently impaired myocardial and LV function at rest as a result of chronically reduced coronary blood flow that can be partially or completely restored to normal either by improving blood flow or by reducing oxygen demand.[13-16] If the hibernating myocardium is not treated in a timely manner, however, it may be associated with progressive cellular damage, recurrent myocardial ischemia, myocardial infarction, heart failure, and death.[17] Positron emission tomography (PET) has proved to be an excellent imaging modality for guiding selection of patients for revascularization strategies because it has shown that regions with abnormal wall motion may still be metabolically active and might therefore improve after revascularization.[18] Such regions are likely to appear hypokinetic, rather than akinetic or dyskinetic, during routine echocardiographic examination. In addition, the reduction in resting coronary blood flow in hibernating segments and the improvement after coronary intervention can be demonstrated by cardiovascular magnetic resonance imaging (MRI).[19] Although in the clinical setting stunned myocardium is often superimposed on hibernation, or irreversible contractile dysfunction, earlier identification of hibernating myocardial regions with prompt myocardial revascularization is crucial in preventing and reversing the ongoing reverse remodeling process of the heart.

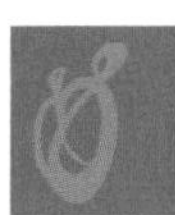

Natural History of Ischemic Cardiomyopathy

The prognosis of patients after myocardial infarction depends on the extent of LV damage.[20] According to the Coronary Artery Surgery Study (CASS) registry, the 12-year survival rate among medically treated patients with LVEF lower than 35% was 21%, in comparison with 54% among patients with LVEF between 35% and 50%.[21] With current interventional techniques, survival rates have improved, especially with the addition of angiotensin-converting enzyme (ACE) inhibitors, β-blockers, statins, implantable CRT devices, and defibrillators to the armamentarium of heart failure therapy. However, one study demonstrated that after a mean follow-up period of 4.4 years, of the patients who had developed ischemic cardiomyopathy, 34% had died and 4.6% had undergone cardiac transplantation.[22] In those patients, outcomes were worse than in patients with an idiopathic or peripartum cardiomyopathy but considerably better than in patients with infiltrative, chemotherapy-induced, or human immunodeficiency virus (HIV)–induced cardiomyopathy (Figure 55-1).

Selection of Appropriate Candidates for Revascularization

Clinical Trials

No randomized clinical trial has been performed to evaluate the outcome of coronary artery bypass graft (CABG) surgery in patients with advanced ischemic cardiomyopathy (see also Chapter 23). However, in January 2002, a randomized, multicenter, international clinical trial, Surgical Treatment of Ischemic Heart Failure (STICH), was initiated to compare contemporary medical therapy plus CABG, medical therapy alone, and CABG with or without surgical ventricular restoration for patients with congestive heart failure and coronary heart disease. The STICH trial is sponsored by the National Heart, Lung, and Blood Institute as well as industry sponsors and has recruited 2212 patients with heart failure, LVEF lower than 35%, and coronary artery disease amenable to CABG at 127 clinical sites. The Hypothesis 1 group consists of 1212 patients, of whom 602 were randomly assigned to receive medical therapy alone and 610 were randomly assigned to receive medical therapies plus CABG. Follow-up assessment is ongoing, and the results have not yet been reported.

The other 1000 patients in the STICH trial had dominant anterior dyskinesia or akinesia of the left ventricle and had been assigned to receive surgery; they were further randomly assigned to undergo CABG surgery alone or CABG plus surgical ventricular restoration. These patients represent the Hypothesis 2 group.[23] Surgical ventricular reconstruction (SVR) reduced the end-systolic volume index by 19%, in comparison with a reduction of 6% with bypass surgery alone. New York Heart Association (NYHA) class of heart failure and 6-minute walk distance improved from baseline to a similar degree in the two groups in Hypothesis 2. However, no significant difference was observed in the primary outcome (death from any cause or hospitalization for cardiac causes), which occurred in 59% who were assigned to undergo CABG alone and in 58% who were assigned to undergo CABG with SVR (P = .90). The addition of SVR to CABG reduced the LV volume, in comparison with CABG alone, but the seemingly beneficial ventricular remodeling was not associated with a greater improvement in symptoms or exercise tolerance or with a reduction in the rate of death or hospitalization for

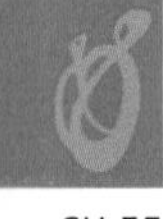

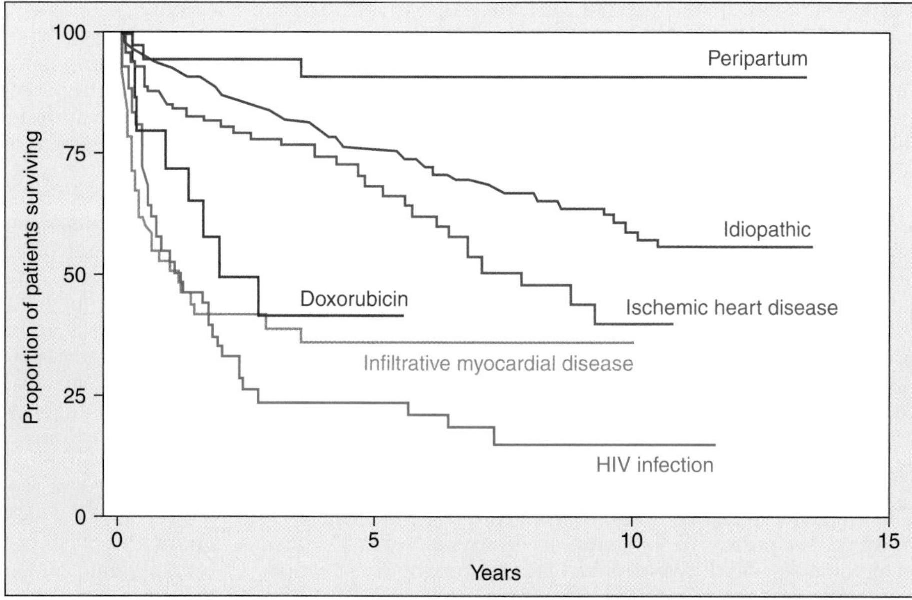

FIGURE 55–1 Outcomes of patients with cardiomyopathy, stratified by cause. HIV, human immunodeficiency virus. (From Felker GM, Thompson RE, Hare JM, et al. Underlying causes and long-term survival in patients with initially unexplained cardiomyopathy. *N Engl J Med* 2000;342:1077-1084.)

cardiac causes (see Figure 23-11). A disappointing finding was that the surgical strategies to reduce ventricular volume that have been examined in clinical trials (STICH, trials with the Acorn support device, trials with partial left ventriculectomy) have failed to provide the beneficial clinical outcomes that were anticipated.

The three major randomized clinical investigations of CABG versus medical management—the Veterans Administration Cooperative Study,[24] the European Coronary Surgery Study,[25] and CASS[26]—have excluded patients with heart failure or severe LV dysfunction. Such patients have been traditionally considered too "high risk" because of the severe LV dysfunction, and their conditions were deemed inoperable. This category of patients with end-stage ischemic cardiomyopathy accounts for 40% to 50% of heart transplantations performed.[27] Even with contemporary heart-failure treatment, a significant amount of these patients die while awaiting heart transplantation, and because of existing comorbid conditions, organ shortage, or both, others are too fragile to undergo transplantation.[28] In addition, survival of patients with viable ischemic myocardium is reduced when revascularization is not undertaken.[29] Therefore, each patient with ischemic cardiomyopathy must be carefully evaluated to determine the suitability for revascularization.

Clinical Factors

In the selection of candidates for revascularization, several clinical factors might play a role, including the presence of angina, suitability of target vessels for bypass grafting, heart failure symptoms, LV dimension, and the severity of hemodynamic compromise.[30] The absence of angina should not preclude consideration for surgical revascularization; however, there is little information about the percentage of patients with heart failure who have silent ischemia that might be ameliorated by revascularization.

Myocardial Viability

Patients with ischemic cardiomyopathy are heterogeneous with regard to adequacy of target vessels for revascularization, ischemic jeopardy, and myocardial viability (see also Chapters 36 and 23). Therefore, clinicians should use utmost care in preoperatively selecting patients who will benefit most from revascularization. Most researchers have found that revascularization of hibernating myocardium in patients with ischemic cardiomyopathy improves both survival and LV function in comparison with medical therapy alone, regardless of the preoperative degree of LV dysfunction.[18,31-36] However, in many of these studies, the presence of angina was also a criterion for enrollment, which may have served as a clinical indicator of the extent of viability. Moreover, these types of studies have important limitations, including bias in selecting patients who undergo CABG, a lesser likelihood that negative findings will be published, and—because contemporary standard medical therapies (e.g., statins) are not used and internal mammary artery grafts are underused—uncertainty of applicability to current practice. Nevertheless, revascularization should be considered, because augmentation of coronary flow to viable ischemic or hibernating myocardium will improve LV function and survival. Several noninvasive imaging modalities may identify patients who have ischemic or hibernating myocardium amenable to revascularization surgery if adequate target vessels exist. The information concerning the myocardial viability that these modalities can provide differs because the different techniques depend on the inotropic reserve (dobutamine stress echocardiography [DSE]), demonstration of cell membrane integrity (thallium-201 imaging), preserved myocardial metabolism (PET with 2-[fluorine-18]-fluoro-2-deoxy-D-glucose [^{18}FDG]), or the absence of scar tissue (gadolinium-enhanced MRI) in areas of dysfunctional myocardium.

DSE has been useful in the preoperative prediction of viable myocardium; it has an overall specificity of 91% and sensitivity of 68% for prediction of segmental recovery (see also Chapter 36).[37] DSE is used to examine the inotropic reserve of dysfunctional but viable myocardium. Viable myocardium exhibits improved regional contractile function (inotropic reserve), as assessed by simultaneous transthoracic echocardiography, in response to dobutamine. Segmental wall motion is monitored during infusion of increasing doses of dobutamine. Augmentation of segmental wall motion beginning at a low dose and continuing during higher doses of dobutamine (uniphasic response) is suggestive of myocardial stunning. However, augmentation at low doses followed by a reduction in function at higher doses (biphasic response) is indicative of ischemia and hibernation. Of importance is that the prevalence of contractile reserve among patients with ischemic cardiomyopathy is independent of the angiographic extent and severity of coronary disease.[38] A contractile response to dobutamine appears to require at least 50% viable myocytes in a given segment and is correlated inversely with the extent of interstitial fibrosis observed on myocardial biopsy samples.[39]

In *single photon emission computed tomography* (SPECT) with thallium-201 scintigraphy, thallium-201 is used as a perfusion tracer because it has a high (80%) first-pass myocardial extraction fraction across physiological ranges of myocardial blood flow (see also Chapter 36). The myocardial uptake is a process requiring cell membrane integrity, and this fraction is therefore indicative of regional perfusion, as well as myocardial viability. Several approaches have been used to optimize the information obtained from thallium-201 scintigraphy, mostly involving a baseline stress image and one or two delayed images (4-hour redistribution and 24-hour late-delayed imaging). Regional thallium-201 redistribution activity represents the extent of regional myocardial viability; therefore, thallium-201 scintigraphy after a single stress injection has become the standard imaging technique for determining such viability. The demonstration of reversible ischemia by the conventional 4-hour stress-redistribution protocol implies the presence of viable myocardium. However, up to 50% of segments that have fixed defects at 4 hours might nonetheless recover either perfusion or function after revascularization.[40,41] Therefore, several modifications of the 4-hour stress-redistribution protocol were developed to improve the accuracy of viability detection. Late (24-hour) redistribution or immediate reinjection of a second, smaller dose of thallium-201 after the redistribution images often enables visualization of segments in a significant number of perfusion defects that had been deemed fixed by imaging at only 4 hours. In comparison with DSE, myocardial perfusion scintigraphy can identify segments with fewer viable myocytes. In one series, for example, DSE and thallium-201 scintigraphy showed equivalent sensitivity among segments with more than 75% viable myocytes (78% vs. 87%), but DSE was much less sensitive among segments with 25% to 50% viable myocytes (15% vs. 82%).[42] However, in comparison with thallium-201 scintigraphy, DSE was found to have greater specificity and positive predictive value in forecasting functional recovery after revascularization.[43]

PET is often considered the gold standard for evaluating myocardial perfusion and viability (see also Chapter 36).[44] Its advantage is that it enables clinicians to assess perfusion and metabolism simultaneously. PET requires the use of positron-emitting radionuclides, which are incorporated into physiologically active molecules. Ischemia shifts myocyte metabolism from fatty acids to glucose. Thus, uptake of a glucose analogue, ^{18}FDG, by myocytes in an area of dysfunctional myocardium indicates metabolic activity and, thus, viability. Regional perfusion can be assessed simultaneously with an agent that remains in the vascular space, thereby demonstrating blood flow (such as nitrogen-13 ammonia or rubidium-82). As a result, PET has the potential to differentiate between normal, stunned, hibernating, and necrotic myocardium. The presence of enhanced ^{18}FDG uptake in regions of decreased blood flow (known as "PET mismatch") is diagnostic for hibernating myocardium, and a concordant reduction in both metabolism and flow ("PET match") is thought to represent predominantly necrotic myocardium. Regional dysfunction in the presence of normal perfusion is indicative of stunning. Of importance is that myocardial segments with significant reductions in both blood flow and ^{18}FDG uptake have only a 20% chance of functional improvement after revascularization, whereas dysfunctional hibernating territories have approximately an 85% chance of functional improvement after revascularization.[18,45-47] The greater the number of viable myocardial segments, the greater the likelihood that revascularization will improve global LV function and consequently improve heart failure symptoms and survival.

Contrast medium–enhanced *cardiac magnetic resonance (CMR) imaging* can be used to establish the presence of hibernating myocardium (see also Chapter 36). Regions of myocardium that exhibit late (or delayed) enhancement 10 minutes after the injection of gadolinium–diethylenetriaminepenta-acetic acid (Gd-DTPA) are areas of myocardial necrosis and irreversible injury; regions that fail to hyperenhance are viable. In addition, quantitative perfusion assessment can document the reduction in resting coronary blood flow in hibernating segments. The degree and transmural extent of enhancement with contrast-enhanced CMR imaging are inversely related to the potential of recovery of LV function after revascularization.[48,49]

Magnetic resonance myocardial tagging is another CMR method that quantifies local myocardial segment shortening throughout the LV myocardium and across the LV wall thickness. This method can be combined with low-dose dobutamine infusion to quantify the amount of myocardial viability, on the basis of end-diastolic wall thickness combined with dobutamine-induced systolic wall thickening; together, these methods may provide a better prediction of LV functional recovery. For example, end-diastolic wall thickness of more than 10 mm preoperatively, in combination with dobutamine-induced systolic wall thickening of 2 mm or more in 50% or more of dysfunctional segments, is well correlated with postoperative improvement in function; however, only 4% of the segments with an end-diastolic wall thickness of less than 6 mm will improve.[50] In comparison with DSE, dobutamine CMR has higher sensitivity (86% vs. 74%) and specificity (86% vs. 70%), but it is more labor intensive and more technically challenging.[51] Unlike nuclear scintigraphy and DSE, which appear to have limited predictive accuracy if more severe systolic dysfunction is present, contrast-enhanced CMR imaging has greater accuracy in segments with the most severe dysfunction, which represents another advantage of this technique.[52] At the Cleveland Clinic, CMR imaging has an established role in detecting the extent of viable myocardium and areas of scarring that might be amenable to reperfusion or other operative strategies that necessitate cardiopulmonary bypass.

Risk of Revascularization

The most effective way of stratifying operative risk for cardiac surgical patients is to use a risk prediction algorithm that incorporates multiple variables to derive a risk score. Two of the algorithms most widely used for this purpose in the United States are the one developed by the Society of Thoracic Surgeons and the European System for Cardiac Operative Risk Evaluation (EuroSCORE); http://www.euroscore.org/calculator).[53-57] Both algorithms incorporate patient age, sex, comorbid conditions, and the severity and acuity of cardiac disease, and both can accurately predict 30-day mortality. One limitation of such risk prediction algorithms is their dependence on the patient data from which they were derived; as the patient population changes, and as surgical technique changes, risk analyses may soon become outdated.[58]

The presence of LV dysfunction and heart failure remains one of the most important independent predictors of operative mortality and other major adverse events after CABG (Figure 55-2).[59] In a prospective observational study of more than 8600 patients undergoing CABG between 1992 and 1997, the rate of operative mortality varied: less than 2% of patients with LVEF higher than 40%, 4% of those with LVEF of 20% to 40%, and 8% of those with LVEF lower than 20%.[60] However, the Cleveland Clinic reported lower in-hospital mortality rates for patients with normal (1.5%), moderately impaired (2.5%), or severely impaired (3.2%) LV function when they reviewed more than 14,000 cases of patients who underwent isolated CABG between 1990 and 1999. In addition, the Cleveland Clinic also reported that the numbers of patients at high risk had increased, but the surgical morbidity rate, adjusted for preoperative risk score, had fallen significantly from 14.5% (in 1986) to 8.8% (in 1994; $P < .001$).[61]

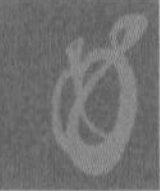

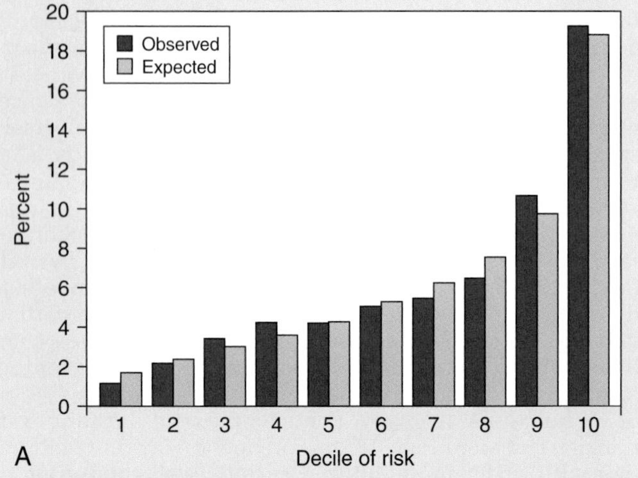

Correlate	Points
Pre-CABG creatinine ≥3.0 mg/dL (265 μmol/L)	12
Age ≥80 yrs	11
Cardiogenic shock	10
Emergent operation	9
Age 70 to 79 yrs	8
Prior CABG	7
Left ventricular section fraction <30%	6
Liver disease (history)	6
Age 60 to 69 yrs	5
Pre-CABG creatinine 1.5 to 3.0 mg/dL (133 to 265 μmol/L)	5
Stroke or transient ischemic attack (history)	4
Left ventricular ejection fraction 30% to 49%	3
Chronic obstructive pulmonary disease (history)	3
Female gender	3
Hypertension (history)	2
Urgent operation	2

B

FIGURE 55–2 Predictive model for outcomes after coronary artery bypass graft (CABG). (From Kolh P. Importance of risk stratification models in cardiac surgery. *Eur Heart J* 2006;27:768-769.)

Additional determinants of mortality and morbidity risk include advanced age, female gender, comorbid conditions (e.g., diabetes, clinical cerebrovascular disease, renal dysfunction, significant chronic lung disease), prior CABG, and need for emergency bypass surgery or concomitant valve surgery.[62,63] However, improved surgical techniques with better myocardial protection and routine use of retrograde coronary sinus cardioplegia, together with a high level of experience and optimization of preoperative condition—all combined through a multidisciplinary approach—have reportedly improved outcomes.

Benefits of Revascularization

In view of the advances in pharmacological treatments and the introduction of implantable CRT and ICD devices, it has been suggested that revascularization may not provide additional benefit for some patients with ischemic cardiomyopathy. However, unless the nonsurgical approaches can prevent further ischemic events from occurring and reverse the detrimental remodeling process, the presence of uncorrected coronary stenoses still threatens the survival of patients with ischemic cardiomyopathy. In addition, angina control seems to be best achieved by surgical revascularization in eligible patients. Surgically improving blood flow to hypoperfused but viable myocardium leads to functional improvement of the myocardium, with secondary effects of retarding or reversing ventricular remodeling, reducing the substrate for malignant ventricular arrhythmias, and ameliorating symptoms.

Improvement in Symptoms of Congestive Heart Failure and in Functional Capacity

Several small-scale studies revealed marked improvement in symptoms after revascularization in patients with ischemic cardiomyopathy.[64-67] Besides reduction in angina, the improvement in NYHA functional class or heart failure symptoms is related to the amount of viable myocardium, which serves as a surrogate to predict positive reverse remodeling after CABG. For example, in one study, a blood flow–metabolism mismatch of more than 18% on PET was 76% sensitive and 78% specific in predicting a change in functional status after revascularization.[64] Another study showed a similarly significant improvement in functional capacity after revascularization, as reflected by the 34% increase in metabolic equivalents (from 5.6 to 7.5) in the group of patients with significant PET mismatch before revascularization.[66] Other investigators demonstrated a significant increase in peak oxygen consumption (15 to 22 mL/kg/min, $P < .0001$) in a group of 34 patients with ischemic cardiomyopathy who underwent CABG.[67]

Improvement of Left Ventricular Function

The improvement in LVEF after revascularization in patients with ischemic cardiomyopathy is typically related to the presence of myocardial viability. A review of 29 studies of 758 patients showed that LVEF increased 6% to 10% after revascularization when myocardium was viable, whereas no improvement in LVEF was noticed in the absence of viability.[68] After normal flow is restored in areas of hibernating myocardium, recovery of contractile function can take several days, weeks, or even months.[32] In addition, the improvement in LVEF can be associated with positive reverse LV remodeling, characterized by reductions in the LV end-systolic and end-diastolic dimensions with a less spherical shape of the ventricle.[69,70] The degree of improvement is significantly correlated with the number of segments that recover function after revascularization.[69] However, despite evidence of viability through noninvasive imaging techniques, late revascularization may not always result in measurable improvements in contractility.

After surgical revascularization in patients with ischemic cardiomyopathy, another predictor of potential improvement in LVEF is the LV end-diastolic dimension. Among patients in whom this dimension exceeds 7.0 cm (4.0 cm/m^2), not only is the operative mortality rate higher but also the chances of positive reverse remodeling are smaller. The effect of LV enlargement on the improvement in LV function after surgery was illustrated in a review of 61 patients with ischemic heart disease, LVEF of 28%, all of whom had evidence of myocardial viability.[71] However, despite the presence of substantial viability, one third of the patients did not exhibit any improvement in LVEF or any reduction in ventricular volume. In contrast, the other two thirds of the patients, who did experience significant improvement in LVEF, all had smaller LV end-systolic volumes.[71]

There is some evidence that presurgical medical therapy with β-blockers can increase the likelihood that surgical revascularization will improve outcomes and reverse remodeling when myocardium is viable. In the Carvedilol Hibernation Reversible Ischaemia Trial, Marker of Success (CHRISTMAS), study, 387 patients with ischemic cardiomyopathy were treated with carvedilol or placebo. At 6 months, a significant linear relationship between the number of cardiac segments with hibernating myocardium at baseline and improvement in LVEF was evident with carvedilol therapy, whereas the placebo-treated patients did not have any improvement in LVEF.[72] It was hypothesized that β-blockade may improve the function of hibernating myocardium by reducing myocardial oxygen consumption and increasing diastolic perfusion, which ultimately led to improved reverse remodeling.[72]

Improvement in Survival

Reports of small observational studies have suggested that improved survival after CABG may not require an improvement in LV function.[36] Initial results of large observational studies, such as CASS, and a post hoc analysis from the Studies of Left Ventricular Dysfunction (SOLVD) trial suggested that CABG improved outcomes in comparison with medical therapy alone in patients with coronary artery disease and LV dysfunction.[26,73,74] In those studies, however, myocardial viability was not evaluated.

Results of subsequent observational studies suggested that the survival benefit with revascularization in ischemic cardiomyopathy was limited to patients with viable myocardium[31,37,75-77] (Figure 55-3). The potential survival benefit derived from revascularization was best demonstrated in a meta-analysis of 24 nonrandomized viability studies involving 3088 patients with coronary artery disease and LV dysfunction (mean LVEF = 32%).[31] Among patients with myocardial viability, revascularization produced a significant 80% reduction in annual mortality rate (3.2% vs. 16% with medical therapy). In addition, a direct relationship between the severity of LV dysfunction and the magnitude of benefit was noted. However, no difference in annual mortality with revascularization was observed in patients without myocardial viability (annual mortality 7.7% vs. 6.2% with medical therapy).

Similar findings of improved survival after revascularization were documented in patients with ischemic cardiomyopathy and hibernating (viable) myocardium, assessed by PET.[76,77] The rate of cardiac mortality was significantly lower among patients who underwent revascularization than among medically treated patients (13% vs. 24%). Among medically treated patients, the risk of cardiac mortality was more than three times higher than among patients undergoing surgical therapy when the extent of mismatch was higher than 20%. With 20% or lower mismatch, in contrast, there was no increase in mortality among patients treated medically or surgically. Unfortunately, randomized prospective clinical trials with background contemporary medical and device therapies are lacking; it is hoped that the ongoing STICH trial will shed light on this issue in the subset of patients who undergo nuclear imaging studies.

Summary

Surgical revascularization currently remains an important treatment option for ischemic cardiomyopathy. Improvements in surgical techniques, together with novel imaging modalities and risk stratification models, with the goal of revascularizing only viable myocardium, have led to improved short- and long-term outcomes in nonrandomized clinical trials.

VALVE SURGERY FOR LEFT VENTRICULAR DYSFUNCTION (see Chapter 29)

Many patients with heart failure or LV dysfunction have clinically significant valvular lesions. It is estimated that almost 50% of patients with LVEF lower than 35% have grades 3 to 4+ mitral regurgitation, and 35% have grades 3 to 4+ tricuspid regurgitation (see also Chapter 29).[78] Severe mitral or tricuspid regurgitation has been linked to adverse outcomes and increased mortality.[78,79] Valvular disease also frequently causes heart failure, and surgical treatment of many valvular lesions is a well-accepted therapy, especially for the aortic valve. However, other combinations of valve disorders with LV dysfunction are more controversial, and many patients have been thought too sick to withstand surgery. Historically, clinicians were taught that mitral valve replacement in patients with LVEF lower than 40% should not be performed because of the high operative mortality rate.[80] However, at

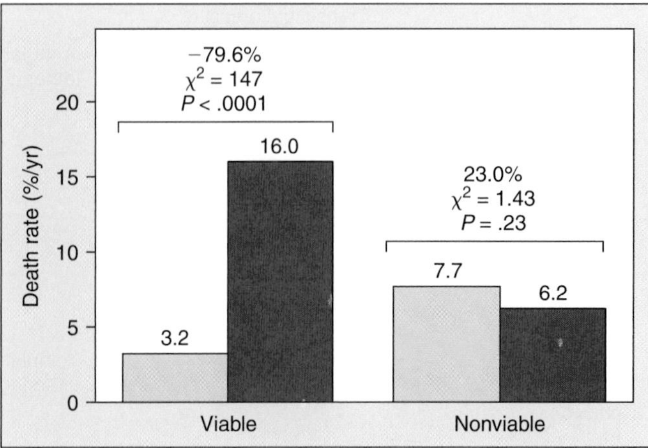

FIGURE 55–3 Mortality stratified according to the presence or absence of viability in the patients who underwent medical revascularization (*solid bars*) and those who underwent surgical revascularization (*open bars*). (From Kolh, P. (2006). Importance of risk stratification models in cardiac surgery. *Eur Heart J.* 27:768-769 and Underwood SR, Bax JJ, vom Dahl J, et al. Imaging techniques for the assessment of myocardial hibernation. Report of a Study Group of the European Society of Cardiology. *Eur Heart J* 2004;25:815-836.)

that time, the mitral valve was replaced with a ball-in-cage prosthesis, and, simultaneously, both papillary muscles and the entire subvalvular apparatus were removed. Nowadays, the importance of an intact valvular-ventricular interaction is recognized. Together with changing surgical opinion more in favor of mitral repairs instead of replacements, interest has resurged in the field of valvular surgery as part of the treatment strategy for LV dysfunction. This section focuses mainly on surgical options for valvular disease in patients with severe LV dysfunction; surgical treatment for valvular lesions without or with mild to moderate LV dysfunction is either well accepted or further addressed in Chapter 29.

Functional Mitral Regurgitation in Patients with Severe Left Ventricular Dysfunction

Pathophysiology

The integrity of the saddle-shaped mitral valve is sustained by coaptation of the anterior and posterior leaflets in the annular plane during ventricular systole, in a design that decreases leaflet, annular, and chordal strain.[81] Six components are responsible for an optimal valve function: the valve annulus, leaflets, chordae tendineae, papillary muscles, LV myocardium, and left atrium; any one of them can exhibit defects that lead to mitral valve dysfunction. In ischemic and nonischemic cardiomyopathy, functional mitral regurgitation usually results from geometric abnormalities of the left ventricle and leads to dysfunction of a morphologically normal mitral valve. Enlargement of the left ventricle causes functional mitral regurgitation through annular dilation, an increase in the interpapillary muscle distance, increased leaflet tethering (elongation and stretching of the chordae tendineae because of cardiac enlargement), and decreased closing forces from muscle weakness, in addition to asynchrony of papillary muscle contractile timing.[81-83] The ultimate result is failure of coaptation of the morphologically normal leaflets and central mitral regurgitation (Figure 55-4). There is clear overlap between functional mitral regurgitation and ischemic IMR, and the reports of functional mitral regurgitation resulting from heart failure include cases of patients with ischemic cardiomyopathy. However, the clinical features and management of IMR, including mitral regurgitation in association with myocardial infarction, are discussed separately.

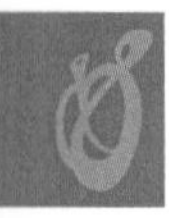

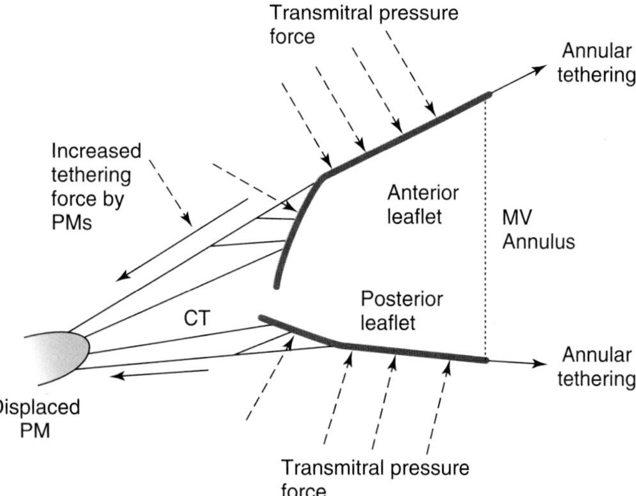

FIGURE 55–4 Pathophysiological features of functional mitral regurgitation. CT, chordae tendinea; MV, mitral valve; PM, papillary muscle. (From Bursi F, Enriquez-Sarano M, Nkomo VT, et al. Heart failure and death after myocardial infarction in the community: the emerging role of mitral regurgitation. *Circulation* 2005;111:295-301.)

Nonsurgical Treatment Options

As with mitral regurgitation resulting from primary valve disease, functional mitral regurgitation imposes an important hemodynamic load on the left ventricle, which contributes to further eccentric hypertrophy and dilation, which increases the degree of mitral regurgitation and heart failure; thus, a vicious cycle exists.[84,85] Fortunately, the treatment of heart failure has evolved from symptom-directed therapy to treatments capable of altering the natural history of the disease and sometimes the attenuation of functional mitral regurgitation. Medical and surgical therapy and, for patients with an interventricular conduction delay, CRT may be beneficial. Pharmaceutical therapies include antagonists of neurohormonal activation, such as ACE inhibitors, aldosterone receptor blockers, and β-adrenergic blocking agents, which can reverse adverse ventricular remodeling in heart failure.[86] In addition, in selected patients with electrical dyssynchrony, CRT has led to impressive positive remodeling and to molecular changes that favorably affect outcomes.[87,88] Through these actions, those therapies may also reduce the degree of functional mitral regurgitation. However, patients with advanced heart failure commonly present with significant mitral regurgitation despite the use of these therapies and are therefore often referred for cardiovascular surgical treatment.

Mitral Valve Repair

Traditionally, the risk associated with surgical correction of mitral regurgitation in the setting of severe LV dysfunction was considered prohibitive. Bolling and colleagues[89] were the first to demonstrate that this approach was feasible and could be conducted with reasonably low morbidity. They used an undersized annuloplasty repair, which effectively corrected functional mitral regurgitation in patients with heart failure. In more than 200 patients with cardiomyopathy, LVEF lower than 20%, and severe functional mitral regurgitation, mitral valve repair was associated with 1-, 2-, and 5-year actuarial survival rates of 82%, 71%, and 52%, respectively.[90] In addition, NYHA class improved for all patients, and most patients also demonstrated an improvement in LVEF, end-diastolic volume, and cardiac index, together with a reduction in sphericity index at the 24-month follow-up assessment.[90] These results were confirmed by a case series at the Cleveland Clinic in which improved survival rates and positive effects on reverse remodeling were documented, in addition to reduced numbers of hospitalizations for heart failure during the follow-up period.[91]

The most convincing evidence of the safety and efficacy of mitral valve repair for functional mitral regurgitation was obtained in the mitral valve surgery condition of the prospective Acorn Clinical Trial.[92] This study of the CorCap device involved 193 patients receiving optimal medical management who had significant functional mitral regurgitation, mean LVEF of 24%, mean LV end-diastolic diameter of 7 cm, and NYHA class III or IV heart failure; most patients (94%) had idiopathic cardiomyopathy. The patients underwent mitral valve repair with an "undersized" mitral annuloplasty ring (84%) or replacement valve surgery (16%). The survival rates were 98.4% 30 days after surgery and 85.2% at 24 months, and there was progressive and sustained evidence of LV remodeling after mitral valve surgery. The important outcomes were that mitral regurgitation was successfully abolished and the mitral valve repair was durable; 88.4% of patients had grade 0 or 1 mitral regurgitation after 2 years, and reoperation was required by only 2% of patients.

A weakness of all the aforementioned studies was that they lacked a comparable control group of subjects who did not undergo surgery. The findings of these observational surgical series were subsequently challenged by Wu and associates.[93] In a propensity-matched, nonrandomized analysis, 126 patients who underwent mitral valve annuloplasty were compared with 293 who did not. Although both groups had similar degrees of severe functional mitral regurgitation, no net improvement in long-term survival (or in the combined endpoint of mortality or urgent transplantation) was evident in the patients who underwent surgery, regardless of cause of heart failure (either ischemic or nonischemic). This provocative but retrospective study lacked follow-up on indexes of ventricular structural remodeling, lacked analysis of symptom improvement, inadequately controlled medical therapy, and provided little information on durability of the repair.

Together, these experiences demonstrate that in patients with congestive heart failure and functional mitral regurgitation, mitral valve repair with an undersized complete rigid annuloplasty ring and without alteration of the subvalvular apparatus can be performed safely with low 30-day operative mortality rates (<2%); this operation probably also has positive effects on reverse remodeling, if it is performed by surgeons experienced in mitral valve repair. However, only a randomized trial can definitively determine whether the surgery is associated with a mortality-related benefit. The lack of proven long-term benefit of mitral valve repair of functional mitral regurgitation is therefore also reflected in published guidelines from major societies. The 2009 heart failure guidelines of the American College of Cardiology/American Heart Association (ACC/AHA)[94] noted that the effectiveness of mitral valve repair or replacement for severe secondary mitral regurgitation in refractory end-stage HF was "not established" (class IIb, level of evidence C), and it was "not generally recommended" by the 2006 practice guidelines of the Heart Failure Society of America.[95] Therefore, if mitral valve repair is considered as an alternative to transplantation, the patient should be informed that although symptoms are often improved, there is no clear evidence of a long-term mortality-related benefit. Also, factors that generally preclude mitral valve repair in patients with advanced heart failure include primary mitral valve disease not amenable to repair, severe aortic insufficiency, and long-standing mitral regurgitation antedating the onset of LV dysfunction with marked LV enlargement or the dependence on inotropic therapy.

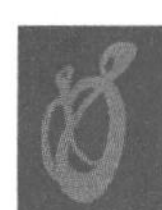

Ischemic Mitral Regurgitation in Patients with Severe Left Ventricular Dysfunction

Pathophysiology

IMR is a complication occurring most often after a myocardial infarction with permanent damage to the papillary muscle or adjacent myocardium. In addition, it might occur with acute ischemia, but it typically disappears after the ischemia resolves. However, preexisting mitral regurgitation may become more severe in the presence of superimposed ischemia. Although IMR is, in rare cases, caused by a papillary muscle rupture, which always mandates urgent surgery, most affected patients have "functional" IMR, similarly to the functional mitral regurgitation in dilated cardiomyopathy, in which the papillary muscles, chordae, and valve leaflets are normal but there is poor coaptation of the leaflets, and restricted leaflet motion is frequently noted on echocardiography. However, there two important differences between the conditions. First, in comparison with patients who have dilated cardiomyopathy, many patients with IMR are in need of CABG, and so clinicians often must decide whether the mitral valve should or should not be treated. Second, whereas the LV dilation in dilated cardiomyopathy is more spherical, patients with ischemic cardiomyopathy have one or more segments of hypokinesia, akinesia, or dyskinesia that lead to local LV remodeling, thereby altering the geometrical shape of the left ventricle in a different way. Many clinicians still use the term "papillary muscle dysfunction" to describe patients with IMR, but this is a misnomer because papillary muscle dysfunction alone does not explain the mechanism of IMR. The papillary muscle is dysfunctional because the LV wall—especially the posterolateral segment, on which it is inserted—is dysfunctional and the geometry of the ventricle is disturbed. Therefore, IMR is a more complex pathological process whose successful repair is also more challenging. These important questions related to IMR, including repair versus replacement and CABG alone versus CABG with mitral valve surgery, are being addressed in ongoing surgery network clinical trials sponsored by the National Heart, Lung, and Blood Institute: Comparing the Effectiveness of Repairing Versus Replacing the Heart's Mitral Valve in People with Severe Chronic Ischemic Mitral Regurgitation (http://clinicaltrials.gov/ct2/show/NCT00807040) and Comparing the Effectiveness of a Mitral Valve Repair Procedure in Combination with Coronary Artery Bypass Grafting (CABG) Versus CABG Alone in People with Moderate Ischemic Mitral Regurgitation (http://clinicaltrials.gov/ct2/show/NCT00806988).

Mitral Valve Repair

Patients with ischemic cardiomyopathy should be treated with the usual therapies for heart failure, including pharmaceutical agents and pacing therapies. However, medical therapy does not play a major role in the management of IMR itself. Among patients who have IMR in association with an acute myocardial infarction, reperfusion can sometimes reduce localized LV remodeling and prevent or treat IMR, especially in acute situations. However, the optimal surgical treatment of IMR long after the myocardial infarction is a matter of controversy, and there is wide variation in practice among cardiovascular surgeons. Much of this controversy stems from the lack of good data addressing this issue. Although it is believed that mitral valve repair is preferred over mitral valve replacement, there have been no randomized trials in which mitral valve repair has been compared with replacement with CABG or in which CABG alone has been compared with CABG plus mitral valve repair. The ongoing clinical trials of the Cardiothoracic Surgical Trials Network (http://www.ctsurgerynet.org/currenttrials.html) and future results will provide the necessary evidence.

Observational series have yielded conflicting results about the effect of late revascularization with or without mitral valve surgery for the reduction of IMR. According to a review in which CABG was performed in 136 patients with moderate to severe IMR, 40% continued to have moderate to severe (grade 3+ to 4+) mitral regurgitation, 51% had some improvement to mild (grade 2+) mitral regurgitation, and 9% even experienced a total disappearance of mitral regurgitation.[96] In addition, another group reported that among patients with moderate to severe IMR, mitral valve surgery at the time of CABG may not improve either symptom status or survival in comparison with CABG alone.[97] The Cleveland Clinic reported the largest series so far in which CABG plus mitral valve annuloplasty (n = 290) was compared with CABG alone (n = 100) for patients with ischemic cardiomyopathy and moderate or severe functional IMR.[98] Groups were propensity-matched according to demographics, extent of coronary disease, regional wall motion, and findings on quantitative echocardiography. The 1-, 5-, and 10-year survival rates were 88%, 75%, and 47% after CABG alone and 92%, 74%, and 39% after CABG with mitral valve annuloplasty (P = .6) (Figure 55-5). However, patients undergoing CABG alone were more likely to have grade 3+ or 4+ postoperative mitral regurgitation than were those undergoing CABG with mitral valve annuloplasty (48% vs. 12% at 1 year; P < .0001) (Figure 55-6). Nevertheless, the NYHA functional class substantially improved in both groups (P < .001) and remained improved at 5 years. The authors therefore concluded that although CABG with mitral valve annuloplasty reduces postoperative IMR and improves early symptoms in comparison with CABG alone, it does not improve long-term functional status or survival in patients with severe functional IMR. They hypothesized that mitral valve annuloplasty alone, without addressing the underlying ventricular disease, was probably insufficient to improve long-term clinical outcomes. Therefore, although revascularization with mitral valve repair probably does improve symptoms and reduces IMR more than does CABG alone in patients with ischemic cardiomyopathy, no data confirm that long-term outcomes are better.

Tricuspid Valve Surgery in Patients with Severe Left Ventricular Dysfunction

Tricuspid regurgitation is a very common abnormality and frequently not addressed during heart failure surgery. Regardless of cause, tricuspid regurgitation is associated with decreased survival.[85,99] In heart failure, the type of tricuspid regurgitation is almost always functional, being caused by dilation of the right ventricle and the tricuspid annulus as a result of high pulmonary artery pressures induced by left-sided heart failure. It leads to backward flow of blood into the right atrium during systole; when the tricuspid regurgitation is only mild or moderate, this has no major hemodynamic consequences because the right atrium is very compliant. However, when tricuspid regurgitation is severe, right atrial and central venous pressure rises, which results in signs and symptoms of right-sided heart failure and eventually a reduced forward cardiac output.

There is a preconceived notion that correction of high pulmonary artery pressures can result in improvement in tricuspid regurgitation, even if severe, if the regurgitation is functional and intrinsic valvular disease is not present. However, data from the Cleveland Clinic show that in 845 patients with moderate or severe tricuspid regurgitation who underwent isolated mitral valve surgery, more than half still had moderate or severe tricuspid regurgitation, which had a tendency to increase even more over time; this outcome suggests that the patients would have benefited from concomitant tricuspid valve surgery (see McCarthy,[100] p. 164). In addition, results of observational studies suggest that after

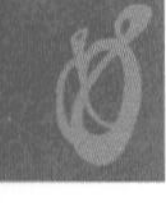

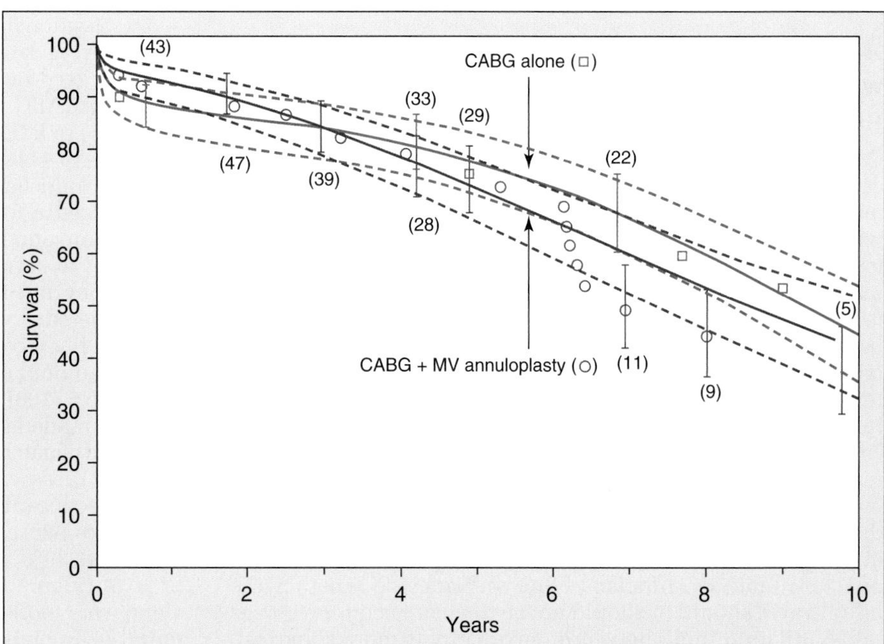

FIGURE 55-5 Outcomes after coronary artery bypass graft (CABG) or CABG with mitral valve (MV) annuloplasty in patients with ischemic cardiomyopathy and ischemic mitral regurgitation. Numbers in parentheses represent number at risk. (From the Multicenter Postinfarction Study Group. Risk stratification and survival after myocardial infarction. *N Engl J Med* 1983;309:331-336.)

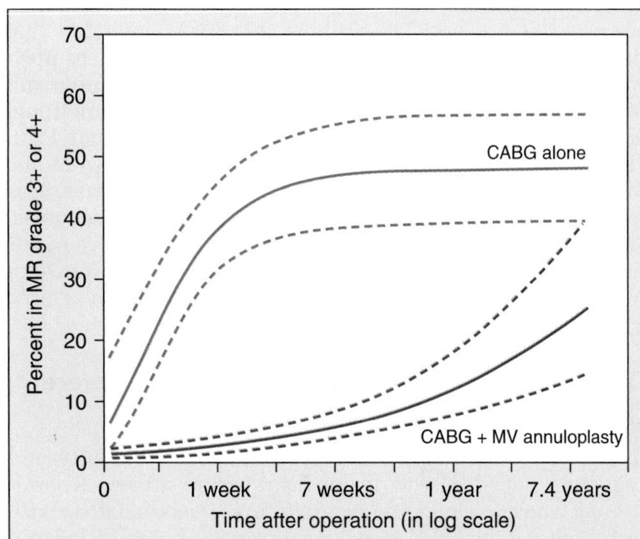

FIGURE 55-6 Moderate to severe mitral regurgitation (MR) after coronary artery bypass graft (CABG) or CABG with mitral valve (MV) annuloplasty in patients with ischemic cardiomyopathy and ischemic mitral regurgitation. (From the Multicenter Postinfarction Study Group. Risk stratification and survival after myocardial infarction. *N Engl J Med* 1983;309:331-336.)

successful tricuspid regurgitation surgery, the right ventricle will remodel, with subsequent improvement in its function in most patients; however, 10% to 20% of patients have persistent moderate to severe tricuspid regurgitation soon after surgery.[101,102]

Aortic Valve Surgery in Patients with Severe Left Ventricular Dysfunction

Aortic Valve Stenosis

The results of valve replacement in patients with normal ventricular function are similar to those in patients with mild or moderately reduced LV function. Moreover, the reduced LVEF, which is secondary to the excessive afterload, is often immediately corrected by valve replacement.[103,104] In comparison, patients with severely reduced ventricular function (LVEF = 25% to 35%) often may not experience complete resolution of symptoms after valve replacement. However, survival is still improved in this setting, although surgery is associated with a high operative mortality rate (9%).[105]

Only if the ventricular function is extremely reduced (in general, <25%) do uncertainties arise in the selection of patients who might benefit from surgery. These patients might not be able to generate a high gradient across the aortic valve despite significant valve narrowing (see also Chapter 29) and require further diagnostic testing. Some patients with low-gradient aortic valve stenosis have true severe aortic valve stenosis, whereas others have pseudo–aortic valve stenosis, in which the transvalvular pressure gradient is low because of the combination of moderate aortic valve stenosis and low cardiac output. True stenosis is distinguished from pseudo–aortic valve stenosis through evaluation of echocardiographic changes in hemodynamic and structural measurements in response to dobutamine, which normally augments cardiac output. In pseudo–aortic valve stenosis, the aortic valve area usually increases as ventricular function improves, whereas in true aortic valve stenosis, this area does not increase. In addition, patients with contractile reserve in response to dobutamine have a much better outcome after surgery. Although patients with low-gradient, true aortic valve stenosis have high perioperative and postoperative mortality rates, surgery is still recommended because valve replacement is associated with better outcomes than is continued medical therapy.[106] Indeed, the 1- and 4-year survival rates were markedly improved among patients who underwent surgery (82% and 78%), in comparison with those among patients who received medical therapy (41% and 15%; $P < .0001$).[106]

Some critically ill patients with true aortic valve stenosis are hemodynamically too unstable and at too high a risk for mortality to undergo the operation. Such patients may be stabilized before surgery through judicious medical intervention or interventional procedures. The use of nitroprusside during continuous hemodynamic monitoring with a pulmonary artery catheter has been shown to lead to significant increases in cardiac index and significant reductions in mean arterial pressure and systemic vascular resistance in stabilizing patients, which makes subsequent aortic valve replacement surgery safer.[107] Percutaneous balloon valvotomy with or without placement of a valve prosthesis may reduce the aortic valve gradient and can potentially improve symptoms as well. Although promising and the subject of intense investigation, these procedures are associated with high rates of morbidity and, in the case of valvotomy, only transient effectiveness.

Aortic Valve Insufficiency

The volume load with subsequent LV dilation in patients with chronic aortic regurgitation is similar to the volume load of mitral regurgitation that can be affected by pharmacological therapy (vasodilators such as nifedipine and ACE inhibitors) and reversed by valve replacement. Evaluation of LV size and function is important because these parameters are not always correlated with symptoms.[108,109] However, the prognosis of patients with aortic regurgitation is determined largely by symptom status and by LV size and function.[108,109] An LV end-systolic volume higher than 60 mL/m^2, an LV end-systolic dimension larger than 50 mm, or an LVEF lower than 50% usually indicates serious depression of LV systolic function with adverse outcomes if not surgically corrected. Surgical correction of the regurgitant lesion usually produces at least some improvement in symptoms, regardless of the functional state of the ventricle.[110,111] In addition, although earlier studies indicated a high risk of mortality among patients with severely depressed LVEF, current data indicate that early and 5-year survival rates would be similar to those in patients with better LV function[112] (see McCarthy,[100] p. 167). Moreover, much of the reported poor results with aortic valve replacement for aortic insufficiency (see also Chapter 29) and severe LV impairment occurred when myocardial protection was less sophisticated and when valve prostheses (such as the Starr-Edwards mechanical valve) had high gradients, which substantially decreased the possibility of late LV recovery.

Because of the improved outcomes, aortic valve surgery for aortic valve stenosis or aortic regurgitation can be considered for many patients with severe LV dysfunction, often with excellent outcomes that obviate the need for cardiac transplantation. Some centers have experience with aortic valve repair, but most still replace the aortic valve with either a mechanical or bioprosthetic valve. The choice between these valves was discussed in detail in the 2008 ACC/AHA guidelines, which recommended that patient age, ability to tolerate warfarin, and patient preference should all be taken into account.[113] The guidelines advocate that patients with a projected long life span generally receive a mechanical valve because of far greater durability and improved patient survival 15 years after surgery. Traditional indications for a bioprosthesis are patients who cannot or will not tolerate warfarin, those whose compliance is uncertain, and patients aged 65 years or older, because valve durability is less of a concern.

LEFT VENTRICULAR RECONSTRUCTION SURGERY

SVR, or volume reduction, is the active surgical attempt to restore the shape of the pathologically remodeled ventricle to one that is physiologically superior. It has long been recognized that SVR alone can improve cardiac function and patient functional status.[114] In the setting of systolic heart failure, the heart enlarges to maintain stroke volume, but at the expense of several physiological and mechanical disadvantages: increased myocardial wall stress, subendocardial hypoperfusion and ischemia, increased myocardial oxygen consumption, afterload mismatch, and activation of compensatory neurohormonal mechanisms. Changes in size and geometry lead to progressive LV dysfunction and worsening heart failure. Sometimes it is possible to surgically remove or exclude portions of the dysfunctional myocardium, infarcted territories, or both to return the LV cavity to a smaller chamber with more normal geometry and physiological properties. Reduction of internal cavity dimensions on the basis of Laplace's law help reduce end-systolic and end-diastolic wall stress, which results in reduced myocardial oxygen consumption, and helps improve myocardial efficiency, which has been shown to ameliorate the heart failure symptoms and improve outcomes.[115-117] The surgical remodeling has beneficial effects on areas of the left ventricle remote from the scar, which results in improved performance of the lateral wall in the case of surgical anterior LV reconstruction.[115] As discussed earlier, the randomized, prospective STICH trial did not demonstrate a benefit when SVR was performed with CABG (see Figure 23-11).[23] Many clinicians firmly believe, however, that properly selected patients may benefit from SVR. The theory and data that support the use of SVR are reviewed as follows.

Four developments have affected the current surgical LV reconstruction for ischemic cardiomyopathy. First, classic ventricular aneurysms are much less common now because of the use of aggressive percutaneous coronary interventions, the use of thrombolytic agents, and the evidence-based use of neurohormonal blocking agents after myocardial infarction.[118-123] Second, the technique of ventricular reconstruction has evolved from linear repair involving the free wall to a more complete infarct exclusion that includes repair of the scarred septum.[124-127] Third, the concept of reconstruction for dyskinetic LV segments has been extended to include akinetic, scarred, but nonaneurysmal areas of the LV.[128-131] Fourth, cryoablation can be used to treat foci of tachyarrhythmias, and SVR procedures are typically combined with CABG and valvular surgeries. The surgeon must exhibit extreme care to ensure that the LV cavity is not too small after SVR and that the mitral valve remains competent. On occasion, the patient must go back on cardiopulmonary bypass to increase the LV volume or to undergo repair of the mitral valve after SVR. Hence, transesophageal echocardiography plays a very important role in the surgical management of patients undergoing SVR.

Indications for Remodeling Surgery in Ischemic Cardiomyopathy

The classic indications have included congestive heart failure, embolism originating from a thrombus contained in the aneurysm, and persistent malignant ventricular arrhythmias, despite optimal medical therapy. However, many patients undergo remodeling surgery only because the surgeon is committed and experienced in this technically challenging cardiac operation. In the Cleveland Clinic experience, a thin-walled aneurysm that collapses with venting of the aorta or left atrium must be present, most often in the vicinity of the left anterior descending coronary artery. If diffuse scar is mixed with muscle in all three coronary artery territories, often no reconstruction is undertaken because there is no discrete area to resect. As explained previously, viability studies are only 80% to 90% accurate; therefore, areas that are found to be thick-walled muscle intraoperatively are not resected, even though the "scar" was indicated on the viability study. All efforts are undertaken to optimally revascularize areas with preserved wall thickness. Most often, reconstruction is performed for a true dyskinetic aneurysm, although transmural scar in a thin-walled akinetic segment might be resected as well. As noted, opinions about this conflict in view of the reported STICH results that show lack of benefit. Dor[117] proposed similar indications for ventricular reconstructive surgery in asymptomatic patients who had suffered previous anteroseptal myocardial infarction and had dilated left ventricle (end-diastolic volume index > 100 mL/m^2), LVEF lower than 20%, LV regional dyskinesis or akinesis affecting more than 30% of the ventricular perimeter, and symptoms of

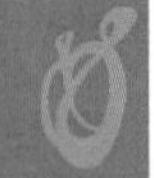

angina, heart failure, or arrhythmias or inducible ischemia on provocative tests. Relative contraindications are systolic pulmonary artery pressure higher than 60 mm Hg, severe right ventricular dysfunction, and regional dyskinesis or akinesis without dilation of the ventricle.[117]

At the Cleveland Clinic, remodeling surgery is not performed in patients with stage D inotrope-dependent heart failure because these patients will not benefit from the procedure; they should be considered instead for cardiac transplantation or LVAD if it is clinically appropriate (see Chapter 56). In addition, physicians at the Cleveland Clinic believe it is prudent that before remodeling surgery, these patients are screened for cardiac transplantation or an LVAD. Regions of dyskinesis or scar that are imaged preoperatively are akinetic regions composed of islands of myocardium admixed with scar that is not of full thickness. These mottled areas are not resected and often do not improve when revascularized; as a result, the postoperative course is challenging, and mechanical support and transplantation are often needed.

Techniques for Remodeling Surgery in Ischemic Cardiomyopathy

Dor Procedure

The Dor procedure, also called "endoventricular circular patch plasty," is indicated only when an aneurysm has formed after a myocardial infarction.[132] A purse-string stitch is created around a nonviable scarred aneurysm (Figure 55-7). Then the aneurysm is excluded, and the residual defect is covered by a patch made from polyester (Dacron), pericardium, or an autologous tissue flap. The remaining aneurysmal scar is then closed over the outside of the patch to give additional stability to the repair. The result is restored "normal" LV chamber geometry and improved LV function. The operation shortens the long axis but leaves the short axis length unchanged, which produces an increase in ventricular diastolic sphericity, whereas the systolic shape becomes more elliptical.[133] According to a multicenter report, among 662 patients who underwent the SVR procedure, the overall hospital mortality rate was 7.7% (4.9% with CABG alone vs. 8.1% with CABG and mitral valve repair).[134] An improvement in LVEF (from 29.7% ± 11.3% to 40.0% ± 12.3%) with a reduction in end-systolic volume (from 96 ± 63 mL/m^2 to 62 ± 39 mL/m^2; $P < .05$) was observed.[134] At 3 years, the survival rate was 89.4% ± 1.3%, and 88.7% avoided readmission to the hospital for heart failure.[134] The STICH trial did not demonstrate a reduction in hospitalizations for all causes or for cardiac causes at a median follow-up interval of 48 months.[23]

Cleveland Clinic Approach

At the Cleveland Clinic, most (89%) of the patients who undergo remodeling surgery for ischemic cardiomyopathy also undergo CABG, and almost 50% undergo concomitant mitral valve surgery, especially if the regurgitation is grade 2+ or higher.[135] The operation is performed through a full sternotomy on cardiopulmonary bypass. After the coronary grafts are established, the mitral valve is repaired, and a modified maze procedure is performed if the patient has a history of atrial fibrillation. The left atrial appendage is closed or resected to prevent future embolism. The LV scar is opened 2 cm lateral to the left anterior descending artery, any underlying LV thrombus is removed, and sutures are placed to retract the thin LV walls and thereby facilitate exposure of the septum, the papillary muscles, and the border zone of the infarcted and normal-appearing myocardium. Subsequently, the aneurysm or scarred area is resected subendocardially, and cryolesions are applied along the entire border zone in patients with a history of ventricular arrhythmias. With the heart beating, a first purse-string suture is placed in the border zone, and each bite is placed deep in the scarred tissue. This suture is then tightened to create a "neck." In contrast to the DOR procedure, a patch is not routinely sewed over this opening because the dyskinetic or akinetic area will simply be replaced with another akinetic area; a patch is used only when the LV cavity would be too small. Therefore, an intraventricular balloon filled to a known volume of 60 mL/m^2 is inserted to ensure that the residual chamber size is adequate. Thus, in 95% of patients, this opening is closed simply by a second purse-string suture a few millimeters above the first suture. The resulting "neck" is less than 1 cm in length but is often completely obliterated once the sutures are tightened. Finally, two strips of felt are then placed on the epicardial surface, and horizontal mattress sutures passing through the free wall of the left ventricle are applied to approximate the border zone between normal and infarcted myocardium. The

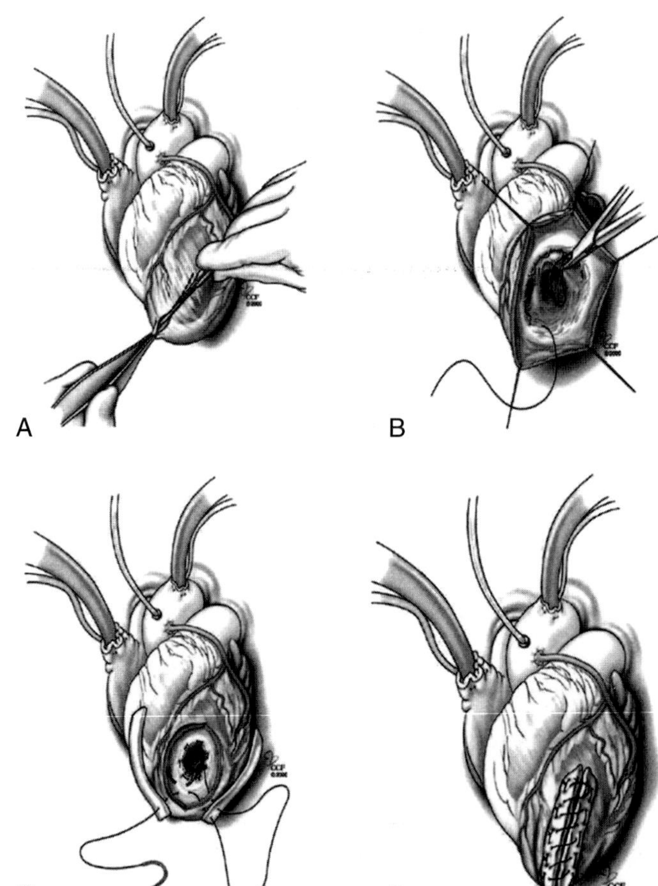

FIGURE 55-7 Left ventricular reconstruction. **A,** The incision for left ventricular reconstruction is typically 2 cm left of the left anterior descending (LAD) artery and extends 3 to 5 cm parallel to the LAD artery. This is routinely performed while the heart is beating and empty. **B,** Reconstruction begins with a purse-string suture placed at the border zone of the infarction, slightly into the scar. **C,** When the second purse-string suture is tied, the neck of the aneurysm is usually 1 to 3 cm in diameter. In rare cases, a patch is used because of heavy calcium deposit on the septum that cannot be removed safely or because of concern that the remaining left ventricular cavity will be very small and contribute to diastolic dysfunction. Two strips of felt are positioned on either side of the ventriculotomy. These are sewn in place with horizontal mattress sutures. The mattress sutures should extend all the way down to the purse-string sutures. In this way, the cavity between the aneurysm neck and the left ventricular free wall is obliterated, and the chances of bleeding are minimized. **D,** The ventriculotomy is oversewn superficially in two layers as a final hemostatic safeguard. (From McGee , E. C., Gillinov, A. M., McCarthy, P. M. (2006) Reverse ventricular remodeling: mechanical options. *Curr Opin Cardiol* 21:215-220.)

ventricular cavity beneath the purse-string sutures are almost completely surrounded by normal myocardium. This technique can be viewed at http://cvbook.nmh.org (Figure 12). In case of a broad QRS complex, LV epicardial leads are often placed for later biventricular pacing if clinically indicated.

A cohort of 220 consecutive patients from the Cleveland Clinic underwent SVR between July 1997 and July 2003; the indication for surgery was heart failure, and 66% of the patients had NYHA functional class III or IV symptoms.[135] The mean preoperative LVEF was 22%, and the mean LV end-diastolic diameter was 6.4 cm. The mean age was 61.4 ± 9.0 years, and 80% of the patients were male. The majority (86%) of patients underwent concomitant CABG, and 49% underwent mitral valve surgery. The 30-day mortality rate was 1%, and survival rates were 92% at 1 year, 90% at 3 years, and 80% at 5 years. Of the survivors for whom data on NYHA functional class were available, 85% had NYHA functional class I or II symptoms. Mortality was predicted by reduced preoperative LVEF (<20%), body mass index of 24 kg/m² or lower, QRS duration of 130 msec or longer, and a postoperative requirement for renal replacement therapy. Mean LVEF improved to 24.7% ± 8.86% ($P < .01$), and LV volumes were also significantly reduced. The investigators concluded that in selected patients with heart failure, SVR, in conjunction with revascularization and valve surgery, yields excellent survival rates, improves symptoms, and improves LVEF and LV dimensions.[135]

The aforementioned STICH trial is the first prospective, randomized clinical trial in which medical therapy only, medical therapy with CABG, and medical therapy with CABG and remodeling surgery are compared; it is hoped that the results will clarify which procedure should be performed in which patients with ischemic cardiomyopathy. The initial results from STICH, published in 2009 with data from a cohort of 1000 patients, did not show benefit when SVR was added to CABG versus CABG alone; however, the results of the entire cohort must be available before the role of medical therapy versus combined medical and surgical therapies can be assessed. Individual cardiac surgeons and cardiothoracic centers that have extensive experience and good outcomes with SVR will probably continue to apply this procedure in patients with dyskinetic segments that meet their proven selection criteria.

Indications for Remodeling Surgery in Dilated Cardiomyopathy

Patients with idiopathic dilated cardiomyopathy and extreme ventricular dilation with advanced heart failure are referred for cardiac transplantation. Randas Batista, a Brazilian cardiac surgeon, popularized a radical technique of *partial left ventriculectomy* to restore the dilated ventricle to a near-normal size and shape.[136,137] Batista's procedure involved the removal of a section of the LV free wall, between both papillary muscles, extending from the apex to the mitral annulus. The remaining free edges were reapproximated and stitched together. The mitral valve and subvalvular apparatus were preserved, repaired, or replaced, depending on the amount of tissue removed. Several global centers, including some in the United States, published their experience with Batista's procedure. All survivors demonstrated an initial increase in LVEF, reduction in heart size, and improvement in clinical functional status upto 6 months.[137-140] However, despite the initial apparent clinical success, at 1 and 3 years after surgery, survival rate was limited to 80% and 60% and freedom from symptomatic heart failure was only 49% and 26%, respectively.[141,142] In addition, one third of the patients did not experience any benefit, and up to another third were in even worse condition after the surgery, which eventually precluded the widespread use of remodeling surgery in dilated cardiomyopathy.[141,142] In addition, the procedure was associated with high incidence of late fatal arrhythmias.[141,142] As a consequence, Batista's procedure is no longer considered an appropriate option for patients with advanced heart failure, and both the 2009 practice guidelines of the ACC/AHA and the 2006 practice guidelines of the Heart Failure Society of America noted that partial left ventriculectomy is not recommended for nonischemic cardiomyopathy.[94,95]

Another historical surgical therapy for dilated cardiomyopathy, referred to as "dynamic cardiomyoplasty," in which the latissimus dorsi muscle is wrapped around the heart and paced during ventricular systole, initially garnered great interest.[143] This arrangement was originally thought to act as an auxiliary pump for the failing left ventricle, aiming to improve cardiac output and functional status. Symptomatic improvement occurred after cardiomyoplasty, although the mechanism of benefit was not clear. A large randomized clinical trial of cardiomyoplasty was started. However, only patients with NYHA class III heart failure were considered suitable for recruitment, because the rate of surgical mortality was deemed too high for patients with more advanced heart failure (30% for class IV). The study was terminated prematurely because of lagging randomization and marginal overall clinical improvement. In addition, it appeared that patients who could survive the operation did not need it, and those who needed it could not survive it.[144,145] For these reasons, cardiomyoplasty is not a viable surgical strategy for the management of heart failure.

Device Therapies for Dilated Cardiomyopathy

The cardiomyoplasty experience has led to other novel approaches to heart failure, inasmuch as postoperative observations suggested that some patients benefited from the diastolic "girdling" effect of the muscle wrap and that progressive LV dilation could be slowed.[146] Several devices to prevent further LV dilation have been developed.

Acorn Device

The Acorn CorCap device is a compliant polyester mesh jacket placed around the ventricles of the heart. It does not interfere with diastolic function but acts as an external constraint device, thereby preventing further dilation of the heart (Figure 55-8). Animal studies and small human case series demonstrated

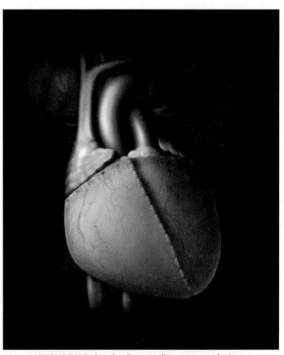

FIGURE 55-8 CorCap cardiac support device.

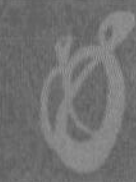

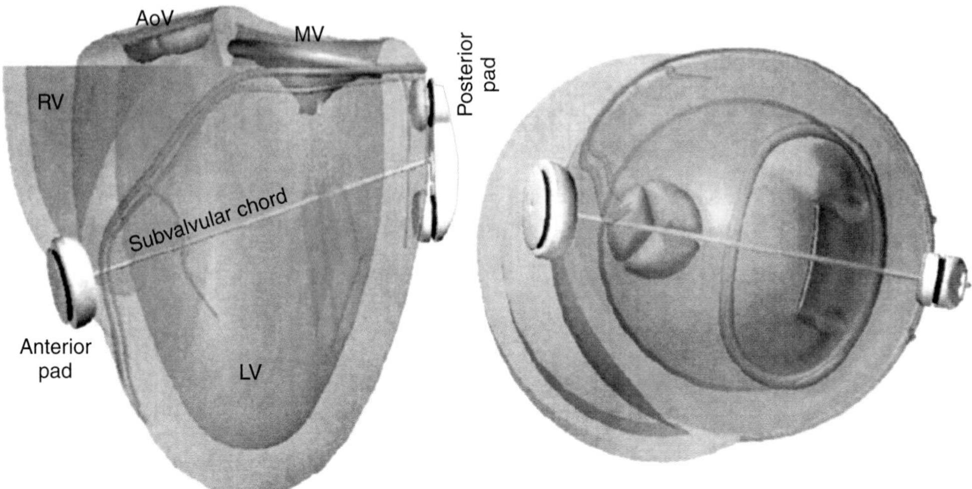

FIGURE 55-9 Myosplint device. AoV, aortic valve; LV, left ventricle; MV, mitral valve; RV, right ventricle.

positive effects on reverse remodeling and improvement in symptoms. Therefore, in a multicenter randomized clinical trial, CorCap was compared with medical therapy, and CorCap with mitral valve repair was compared with mitral valve repair alone.[146] The results were favorable for CorCap: 38% of patients receiving the device demonstrated improvement in heart failure status, in comparison with 27% of those who did not receive the CorCap.[147] Moreover, mitral valve repair was associated with progressive reductions in LV volumes and mass and with increases in LVEF and sphericity index, all consistent with reverse remodeling.[92] Recurrence of clinically significant mitral regurgitation was uncommon. Quality of life, exercise performance, and NYHA functional class were all improved. The addition of the CorCap cardiac support device led to greater decreases in volumes, a more elliptical shape, and a trend for a reduction in major cardiac procedures and improvement in quality of life than did mitral valve repair alone. Furthermore, the beneficial effects on LV remodeling were sustained at long term, after 3 years of follow-up.[148]

These findings indicate that there might be additional benefit with the CorCap cardiac support device over mitral valve surgery alone in patients with nonischemic cardiomyopathy. Because of the improvement in LV structure and function, along with a low operative mortality rate (<2%), the device is in use in Europe; it has not yet, however, obtained approval in the United States. The Acorn CorCap is undergoing nonrandomized evaluation in the United States in selected patients with reduced LVEF who are undergoing mitral valve repair.

Myocor Myosplint

The Myocor Myosplint device (Figure 55-9) is also aimed at inhibiting LV remodeling. The device consists of a transventricular splint with epicardial pads that are adjusted to decrease the LV radius, which causes the left ventricle to become smaller and more energetically efficient, with decreased wall tension (by the law of Laplace). The transventricular splints are placed on the beating heart without cardiopulmonary bypass, typically from the lateral left ventricle through the posterior interventricular septum. After the splints are tightened, the final shape of the ventricle is bilobular. Animal and small human case series also showed positive effects on remodeling and symptoms.[149] Myocor also developed a new product, Coapsys, that is designed to achieve off-pump mitral valve repair along with some ventricular volume reduction. The device includes a single transventricular splint and pads on the outer surface of the left ventricle. Under continuous echocardiographic monitoring, the pads are tightened until mitral regurgitation is reduced and eventually eliminated. One pad on the left ventricle is positioned at the level of the mitral valve apparatus and pulls the posterior annulus toward the anterior leaflet during tightening. The other pad on the LV free wall changes the ventricular shape during tightening. In humans who had Myosplint placement (immediately before heart transplantation), an acute reduction in LV end-diastolic and end-systolic volumes was similar to that observed in animal experiments.[150] A safety and feasibility study—the Evaluation of a Surgical Treatment for Off-pump Repair of the Mitral Valve (RESTOR-MV) trial—is currently under way.[151]

CONCLUSIONS

Surgical treatments for heart failure are still relatively rare, in view of the large population at risk. Modern techniques yield low rates of perioperative morbidity and mortality and have led to improved long-term ventricular function and outcomes. Many patients referred for transplantation can now be treated with other surgical options that may delay or even preclude the need for cardiac transplantation.[152] For patients who have severe LV dysfunction but a considerable amount of viable myocardial tissue, coronary bypass surgery should be the first option. Mitral valve repair for severe LV dysfunction appears to be effective for symptomatic relief and might improve survival, especially if combined with therapies that also directly address LV remodeling. Direct ventricular reconstruction for ischemic cardiomyopathy with resection of delineated areas of dyskinetic scarring carries moderate rates of perioperative mortality and may lead to improved outcomes. Patients with nonischemic cardiomyopathy might benefit from alternative device strategies aimed at halting or reversing the detrimental remodeling process. Several ongoing prospective clinical trials are expected to provide more evidence to further define the role of surgery in both dilated and ischemic cardiomyopathy.

REFERENCES

1. Felker, G. M., Shaw, L. K., & O'Connor, C. M. (2002). A standardized definition of ischemic cardiomyopathy for use in clinical research. *J Am Coll Cardiol*, *39*, 210–218.
2. Sutton, G. C. (1990). Epidemiological aspects of heart failure. *Am Heart J*, *120*, 1538–1540.
3. He, J., Ogden, L. G., Bazzano, L. A., et al. (2001). Risk factors for congestive heart failure in US men and women: NHANES I epidemiologic follow-up study. *Arch Intern Med*, *161*, 996–1002.
4. Kannel, W., Sorlie, P., & McNamara, P. (1979). Prognosis after initial myocardial infarction. The Framingham study. *Am J Cardiol*, *44*, 53–59.
5. Suleiman, M., Khatib, R., Agmon, Y., et al. (2006). Early inflammation and risk of long-term development of heart failure and mortality in survivors of acute myocardial infarction predictive role of C-reactive protein. *J Am Coll Cardiol*, *47*, 962–968.

6. Hellermann, J. P., Jacobsen, S. J., Redfield, M. M., et al. (2005). Heart failure after myocardial infarction: clinical presentation and survival. *Eur J Heart Fail*, *7*, 119–125.
7. Bursi, F., Enriquez-Sarano, M., Nkomo, V. T., et al. (2005). Heart failure and death after myocardial infarction in the community: the emerging role of mitral regurgitation. *Circulation*, *111*, 295–301.
8. Kannel, W. B., & Cupples, A. (1988). Epidemiology and risk profile of cardiac failure. *Cardiovasc Drugs Ther*, *2*, 387–395.
9. Poole-Wilson, P. A. (1993). Relation of pathophysiologic mechanisms to outcome in heart failure. *J Am Coll Cardiol*, *22*(Suppl. A), A22–A29.
10. Weisman, H. F., Bush, D. E., & Mannisi, J. A. (1988). Cellular mechanisms of myocardial infarct expansion. *Circulation*, *78*, 186–201.
11. Gerdes, A. M., & Capasso, J. M. (1995). Structural remodeling and mechanical dysfunction of cardiac myocytes in heart failure. *J Mol Cell Cardiol*, *27*, 849–856.
12. Fragasso, G., Chierchia, S., Lucignani, G., et al. (1993). Time dependence of residual tissue viability after myocardial infarction assesed by [^{18}F]fluorodeoxyglucose and positron emission tomography. *Am J Cardiol*, *72*, G131–G139.
13. Heyndrickx, G. R., Baig, H., Nellens, P., et al. (1978). Depression of regional blood flow and wall thickening after brief coronary occlusions. *Am J Physiol*, *234*, H653–H659.
14. Braunwald, E., & Kloner, R. A. (1982). The stunned myocardium: prolonged, postischemic ventricular dysfunction. *Circulation*, *66*, 1146–1149.
15. Marban, E. (1991). Myocardial stunning and hibernation. The physiology behind the colloquialisms. *Circulation*, *83*, 681–688.
16. Bristow, J. D., Arai, A. K., Anselone, C. G., et al. (1991). Response to myocardial ischemia as a regulated process. *Circulation*, *84*, 2580–2587.
17. Knight, C., & Fox, K. (1995). The vicious circle of ischemic left ventricular dysfunction. *Am J Cardiol*, *75*(13), E10–E15.
18. Tillisch, J., Brunken, R., Marshal, R., et al. (1986). Reversibility of cardiac wall-motion abnormalities predicted by positron tomography. *N Engl J Med*, *314*, 884–888.
19. Selvanayagam, J. B., Jerosch-Herold, M., Porto, I., et al. (2005). Resting myocardial blood flow is impaired in hibernating myocardium: a magnetic resonance study of quantitative perfusion assessment. *Circulation*, *112*, 3289–3296.
20. The Multicenter Postinfarction Study Group. (1983). Risk stratification and survival after myocardial infarction. *N Engl J Med*, *309*, 331–336.
21. Emond, M., Mock, M. B., Davis, K. B., et al. (1994). Long-term survival of medically treated patients in the Coronary Artery Surgery Study (CASS) Registry. *Circulation*, *90*, 2645–2657.
22. Felker, G. M., Thompson, R. E., Hare, J. M., et al. (2000). Underlying causes and long-term survival in patients with initially unexplained cardiomyopathy. *N Engl J Med*, *342*, 1077–1084.
23. Jones, R. H., Velazquez, E. J., Michler, R. E., et al. (2009). Coronary artery bypass surgery with or without surgical ventricular reconstruction. *N Engl J Med*, *360*, 1705–1717.
24. Murphy, M. L., Hultgren, H. N., Detre, K., et al. (1977). Treatment of chronic stable angina: a preliminary report of the randomized Veterans Administration Cooperative Study. *N Engl J Med*, *297*, 621–627.
25. Varnauskas, E. (1988). Twelve-year follow-up of survival in the randomized European Coronary Surgery Study. *N Engl J Med*, *319*, 332–337.
26. Alderman, E. L., Fisher, L. D., Litwin, P., et al. (1983). Results of coronary artery surgery in patients with poor left ventricular function (CASS). *Circulation*, *68*, 785–795.
27. Primo, G., LeClerc, J. L., Goldstein, J. P., et al. (1988). Cardiac transplantation for the treatment of end-stage ischemic cardiomyopathy. *Adv Cardiol*, *36*, 293–297.
28. Vega, J. D., et al. Am J Transplant 2009.
29. Elefteriades, J. A., & Kron, I. L. (1995). CABG in advanced left ventricular dysfunction. *Cardiol Clin*, *13*, 35–42.
30. Wechsler, A. S., & Junod, F. L. (1989). Coronary bypass grafting in patients with congestive heart failure. *Circulation*, *79*, I-92–I-96.
31. Allman, K. C., Shaw, L. J., Hachamovitch, R., et al. (2002). Myocardial viability testing and impact of revascularization on prognosis in patients with coronary artery disease and left ventricular dysfunction: a meta-analysis. *J Am Coll Cardiol*, *39*, 1151–1158.
32. Ragosta, M., Beller, G. A., Watson, D. D., et al. (1993). Quantitative planar rest-redistribution ^{201}Tl imaging in detection of myocardial viability and prediction of improvement in left ventricular function after coronary bypass surgery in patients with severely depressed left ventricular function. *Circulation*, *87*, 1630–1641.
33. Pagley, P. R., Beller, G. A., Watson, D. D., et al. (1997). Improved outcome after coronary bypass surgery in patients with ischemic cardiomyopathy and residual myocardial viability. *Circulation*, *96*, 793–800.
34. Wellnhofer, E., Olariu, A., Klein, C., et al. (2004). Magnetic resonance low-dose dobutamine test is superior to SCAR quantification for the prediction of functional recovery. *Circulation*, *109*, 2172–2174.
35. Samady, H., Elefteriades, J. A., Abbott, B. G., et al. (1999). Failure to improve left ventricular function after coronary revascularization for ischemic cardiomyopathy is not associated with worse outcome. *Circulation*, *100*, 1298–1304.
36. Chareonthaitawee, P., Gersh, B. J., Araoz, P. A., et al. (2005). Revascularization in severe left ventricular dysfunction: the role of viability testing. *J Am Coll Cardiol*, *46*, 567–574.
37. Williams, M., Odabashian, J., Lytle, B., et al. (1995). Prediction of viable myocardium in severe left ventricular dysfunction. Follow-study of dobutamine echocardiography and positron emission tomography. *Circulation*, *92*, I-266.
38. Main, M. L., Grayburn, P. A., Landau, C., et al. (1997). Relation of contractile reserve during low-dose dobutamine echocardiography and angiographic extent and severity of coronary artery disease in the presence of left ventricular dysfunction. *Am J Cardiol*, *79*, 1309–1313.
39. Nagueh, S. F., Mikati, I., Weilbaecher, D., et al. (1999). Relation of the contractile reserve of hibernating myocardium to myocardial structure in humans. *Circulation*, *100*, 490–496.
40. Liu, P., Kiess, M. C., Okada, R. D., et al. (1985). The persistent defect on exercise thallium imaging and its fate after myocardial revascularization: does it represent scar or ischemia?*Am Heart J*, *110*, 996–1001.
41. Gibson, R. S., Watson, D. D., Taylor, G. J., et al. (1983). Prospective assessment of regional myocardial perfusion before and after coronary revascularization surgery by quantitative thallium-201 scintigraphy. *J Am Coll Cardiol*, *1*, 804–815.
42. Baumgartner, H., Porenta, G., Lau, Y. -K., et al. (1998). Assessment of myocardial viability by dobutamine echocardiography, positron emission tomography and thallium-201 SPECT: correlation with histopathology in explanted hearts. *J Am Coll Cardiol*, *32*, 1701–1708.
43. Grayburn, P. A. (1995). How good is echocardiography at assessing myocardial viability? *Am J Cardiol*, *76*, 1183–1184.
44. Schelbert, H. R. (1994). Metabolic imaging to assess myocardial viability. *J Nucl Med*, *35*, S8–S14.
45. Lucignani, G., Paolini, G., Landoni, C., et al. (1992). Presurgical identification of hibernating myocardium by combined use of technetium-99m hexakis 2-methoxyisobutylisonitrile single photon emission tomography and fluorine-18 fluoro-2-deoxy-d-glucose positron emission tomography in patients with coronary artery disease. *Eur J Nucl Med*, *19*, 874–881.
46. Marwick, T. H., MacIntyre, W. J., Lafont, A., et al. (1992). Metabolic responses of hibernating and infarcted myocardium to revascularization. A follow-up study of regional perfusion, function, and metabolism. *Circulation*, *85*, 1347–1353.
47. Tamaki, N., Kawamoto, M., Tadamura, E., et al. (1995). Prediction of reversible ischemia after revascularization. Perfusion and metabolic studies with positron emission tomography. *Circulation*, *91*, 1697–1705.
48. Kim, R. J., Wu, E., Rafael, A., et al. (2000). The use of contrast-enhanced magnetic resonance imaging to identify reversible myocardial dysfunction. *N Engl J Med*, *343*, 1445–1453.
49. Selvanayagam, J. B., Kardos, A., Francis, J. M., et al. (2004). Value of delayed-enhancement cardiovascular magnetic resonance imaging in predicting myocardial viability after surgical revascularization. *Circulation*, *110*, 1535–1541.
50. Baer, F. M., Theissen, P., Schneider, C. A., et al. (1998). Dobutamine magnetic resonance imaging predicts contractile recovery of chronically dysfunction myocardium after successful revascularization. *J Am Coll Cardiol*, *31*, 1040–1048.
51. Gunning, M. G., Anagnostopulos, C., Knight, C. J., et al. (1998). Comparison of ^{201}Tl, ^{99}Tc-tetrofosmin, and dobutamine magnetic resonance imaging for identifying hibernating myocardium. *Circulation*, *98*, 1869–1874.
52. Beller, G. A. (2000). Noninvasive assessment of myocardial viability. *N Engl J Med*, *343*, 1488–1490.
53. Edwards, F. H., Clark, R. E., & Schwartz, M. (1994). Coronary artery bypass grafting: the Society of Thoracic Surgeons National Database experience. *Ann Thorac Surg*, *57*, 12–19.
54. Hattler, B. G., Madia, C., Johnson, C., et al. (1994). Risk stratification using the Society of Thoracic Surgeons Program. *Ann Thorac Surg*, *58*, 1348–1352.
55. Society of Thoracic Surgeons (website): http://www.sts.org. Accessed March 24, 2010.
56. Roques, F., Nashef, S. A., Michel, P., et al. (1999). Risk factors and outcome in European cardiac surgery: analysis of the EuroSCORE multinational database of 19030 patients. *Eur J Cardiothorac Surg*, *15*, 816–823.
57. Nashef, S. A., Roques, F., Hammill, B. G., et al. (2002). Validation of European System for Cardiac Operative Risk Evaluation (EuroSCORE) in North American cardiac surgery. *Eur J Cardiothorac Surg*, *22*, 101–105.
58. Kolh, P. (2006). Importance of risk stratification models in cardiac surgery. *Eur Heart J*, *27*, 768–769.
59. Fortescue, E. B., Kahn, K., & Bates, D. W. (2001). Development and validation of a clinical prediction rule for major adverse outcomes in coronary bypass grafting. *Am J Cardiol*, *88*, 1251–1258.
60. Yau, T. M., Fedak, P. W., Weisel, R. D., et al. (1999). Predictors of operative risk for coronary bypass operations in patients with left ventricular dysfunction. *J Thorac Cardiovasc Surg*, *118*, 1006–1013.
61. Estafanous, F. G., Loop, F. D., Higgins, T. L., et al. (1998). Increased risk and decreased morbidity of coronary artery grafting between 1986 and 1994. *Ann Thorac Surg*, *65*, 383–389.
62. O'Connor, G. T., Plume, S. K., & Olmstead, E. M. (1992). Multivariate prediction of in-hospital mortality associated with coronary artery bypass graft surgery: Northern New England Cardiovascular Disease Study Group. *Circulation*, *85*, 2111–2118.
63. Fisher, L. D., Kennedy, J. W., Davis, K. B., et al. (1982). Association of sex, physical size, and operative mortality after coronary artery bypass in the Coronary Artery Surgery Study (CASS). *J Thorac Cardiovasc Surg*, *84*, 334–341.
64. DiCarli, M. F., Asgarzadie, F., Schelbert, H. R., et al. (1995). Quantitative relation between myocardial viability and improvement in heart failure symptoms after revascularization in patients with ischemic cardiomyopathy. *Circulation*, *92*, 3436–3444.
65. Yamaguchi, A., Ino, T., Adachi, H., et al. (1998). Left ventricular volume predicts postoperative course in patients with ischemic cardiomyopathy. *Ann Thorac Surg*, *65*(2), 434–438.
66. Eitzman, D., Al-Aouar, Z., vom Dahl, J., et al. (1992). Clinical outcome of patients with advanced coronary artery disease after viability studies with positron emission tomography. *J Am Coll Cardiol*, *20*, 559–565.
67. Marwick, T., Nemec, J., Lafont, A., et al. (1992). Prediction by postexercise fluoro-18 deoxyglucose positron emission tomography of improvement in exercise capacity after revascularization. *Am J Cardiol*, *69*, 854–859.
68. Bax, J. J., van der Wall, E. E., & Harbinson, M. (2004). Radionuclide techniques for the assessment of myocardial viability and hibernation. *Heart*, *90*(Suppl. 5), v26–v33.
69. Carluccio, E., Biagioli, P., Alunni, G., et al. (2006). Patients with hibernating myocardium show altered left ventricular volumes and shape, which revert after revascularization: evidence that dyssynergy might directly induce cardiac remodeling. *J Am Coll Cardiol*, *47*, 969–977.
70. Rahimtoola, S. H., La Canna, G., & Ferrari, R. (2006). Hibernating myocardium: another piece of the puzzle falls into place. *J Am Coll Cardiol*, *47*, 978–983.
71. Schinkel, A. F., Poldermans, D., Rizzello, V., et al. (2004). Why do patients with ischemic cardiomyopathy and a substantial amount of viable myocardium not always recover in function after revascularization?*J Thorac Cardiovasc Surg*, *127*, 385–390.

72. Cleland, J. G., Pennell, D. J., Ray, S. G., et al. (2003). Myocardial viability as a determinant of the ejection fraction response to carvedilol in patients with heart failure (CHRISTMAS trial): randomised controlled trial. *Lancet, 362*, 14–22.
73. Veenhuyzen, G. D., Singh, S. N., McAreavey, D., et al. (2001). Prior coronary artery bypass surgery and risk of death among patients with ischemic left ventricular dysfunction. *Circulation, 104*, 1489–1493.
74. Bounou, E. P., Mark, D. B., Pollock, B. G., et al. (1988). Surgical survival benefits for coronary disease patients with left ventricular dysfunction. *Circulation, 78*, I-151–I-157.
75. Underwood, S. R., Bax, J. J., vom Dahl, J., et al. (2004). Imaging techniques for the assessment of myocardial hibernation. Report of a Study Group of the European Society of Cardiology. *Eur Heart J, 25*, 815–836.
76. Desideri, A., Cortigiani, L., Christen, A. I., et al. (2005). The extent of perfusion-F18-fluorodeoxyglucose positron emission tomography mismatch determines mortality in medically treated patients with chronic ischemic left ventricular dysfunction. *J Am Coll Cardiol, 46*, 1264–1268.
77. Tarakji, K. G., Brunken, R., McCarthy, P. M., et al. (2006). Myocardial viability testing and the effect of early intervention in patients with advanced left ventricular systolic dysfunction. *Circulation, 113*, 230–237.
78. Koelling, T. M., Aaronson, K. D., Cody, R. J., et al. (2002). Prognostic significance of mitral regurgitation and tricuspid regurgitation in patients with left ventricular systolic dysfunction. *Am Heart J, 144*, 524–529.
79. Mullens, W., Abrahams, Z., Skouri, H. N., et al. (2008). Prognostic evaluation of ambulatory patients with advanced heart failure. *Am J Cardiol, 101*, 1297–1302.
80. Braunwald, E. (1980). Valvular heart disease. In E. Braunwald (Ed.). *Heart disease. A textbook of cardiovascular medicine* (pp 1095–1165). Philadelphia: WB Saunders.
81. Jimenez, J. H., Soerensen, D. D., He, Z., et al. (2003). Effects of a saddle shaped annulus on mitral valve function and chordal force distribution: an in vitro study. *Ann Biomed Eng, 31*, 1171–1178.
82. Karagiannis, S. E., Karatasakis, G. T., G. Koutsogiannis, N., et al. (2003). Increased distance between mitral valve coaptation point and mitral annular plane: significance and correlations in patients with heart failure. *Heart, 89*, 1174–1178.
83. Nielsen, S. L., Nygaard, H., Mandrup, L., et al. (2002). Mechanism of incomplete mitral leaflet coaptation and interaction of chordal restraint and changes in mitral leaflet coaptation geometry. Insight from in vitro validation of the premise of force equilibrium. *J Biomech Eng, 124*, 596–608.
84. He, S., Fontaine, A. A., Schwammenthal, E., et al. (1997). Integrated mechanism for functional mitral regurgitation: leaflet restriction versus coapting force: in vitro studies. *Circulation, 96*, 1826–1834.
85. Trichon, B. H., & O'Connor, C. M. (2002). Secondary mitral and tricuspid regurgitation accompanying left ventricular systolic dysfunction: is it important, and how is it treated?. *Am Heart J, 144*, 373–377.
86. Mehra, M. R., Uber, P. A., & Francis, G. S. (2003). Heart failure therapy at a crossroad: are there limits to the neurohormonal model?. *J Am Coll Cardiol, 41*, 1606–1610.
87. Cleland, J. G., Daubert, J. C., Erdmann, E., et al. (2005). Cardiac Resynchronization-Heart Failure (CARE-HF) Study Investigators. The effect of cardiac resynchronization on morbidity and mortality in heart failure. *N Engl J Med, 352*, 1539–1549.
88. Vanderheyden, M., Mullens, W., Delrue, L., et al. (2008). Myocardial gene expression in heart failure patients treated with cardiac resynchronization therapy: responders versus non-responders. *J Am Coll Cardiol, 51*, 129–136.
89. Bolling, S. F., Deeb, G. M., Brunsting, L. A., et al. (1995). Early outcome of mitral valve reconstruction in patients with end-stage cardiomyopathy. *J Thorac Cardiovasc Surg, 109*, 676–682.
90. Romano, M. A., & Bolling, S. F. (2004). Update on mitral repair in dilated cardiomyopathy. *J Card Surg, 19*, 396–400.
91. Bishay, E. S., McCarthy, P. M., Cosgrove, D. M., et al. (2000). Mitral valve surgery in patients with severe left ventricular dysfunction. *Eur J Cardiothorac Surg, 17*, 213–221.
92. Acker, M. A., Bolling, S., Shemin, R., et al. (2006). Mitral valve surgery in heart failure: insights from the Acorn Clinical Trial. *J Thorac Cardiovasc Surg, 132*, 568–577.
93. Wu, A. H., Aaronson, K. D., Bolling, S. F., et al. (2005). Impact of mitral valve annuloplasty on mortality risk in patients with mitral regurgitation and left ventricular systolic dysfunction. *J Am Coll Cardiol, 45*, 381–387.
94. Hunt, S. A., Abraham, W. T., Chin, M. H., et al. (2009). 2009 Focused update incorporated into the ACC/AHA 2005 Guidelines for the Diagnosis and Management of Heart Failure in Adults: a report of the American College of Cardiology Foundation/American Heart Association Task Force on Practice Guidelines: developed in collaboration with the International Society for Heart and Lung Transplantation. *Circulation, 119*(14), e391–e479.
95. Heart Failure Society of America. (2006). HFSA 2006 Comprehensive Heart Failure Practice Guideline. *J Card Fail, 12*, e1–e2.
96. Aklog, L., Filsoufi, F., Flores, K. Q., et al. (2001). Does coronary artery bypass grafting alone correct moderate ischemic mitral regurgitation?*Circulation, 104*, 68-29.
97. Diodato, M. D., Moon, M. R., Pasque, M. K., et al. (2004). Repair of ischemic mitral regurgitation does not increase mortality or improve long-term survival in patients undergoing coronary artery revascularization: a propensity analysis. *Ann Thorac Surg, 78*, 794–799.
98. Mihaljevic, T., Lam, B. K., Rajeswaran, J., et al. (2007). Impact of mitral valve annuloplasty combined with revascularization in patients with functional ischemic mitral regurgitation. *J Am Coll Cardiol, 49*, 2191–2201.
99. Nath, J., Foster, E., & Heidenreich, P. A. (2004). Impact of tricuspid regurgitation on long-term survival. *J Am Coll Cardiol, 43*, 405–409.
100. McCarthy, P. M., Young, J. B. (Eds.). (2007). Valve surgery for left ventricular dysfunction. In *Heart failure, a combined medical and surgical approach* Malden, MA: Blackwell Futura, p 164.
101. McCarthy, M., Bhudia, S. K., Rajeswaran, J., et al. (2004). Tricuspid valve repair: durability and risk factors for failure. *J Thorac Cardiovasc Surg, 127*, 674–685.
102. Fukuda, S., Song, J. M., Gillinov, A. M., et al. (2005). Tricuspid valve tethering predicts residual tricuspid regurgitation after tricuspid annuloplasty. *Circulation, 111*, 975–979.
103. Lund, O., Flot, C., Jensen, F. T., et al. (1997). Left ventricular systolic and diastolic function in aortic stenosis. *Eur Heart J, 18*, 1977–1987.
104. Villari, B., Vassalli, G., Betocchi, S., et al. (1996). Normalization of left ventricular nonuniformity later after valve replacement for aortic stenosis. *Am J Cardiol, 78*, 66–71.
105. Connolly, H. M., Oh, J. K., Orszulak, T. A., et al. (1997). Aortic valve replacement for aortic stenosis with severe left ventricular dysfunction. Prognostic indicators. *Circulation, 95*, 2395–2400.
106. Pereira, J. J., Lauer, M. S., Bashir, M., et al. (2002). Survival after aortic valve replacement for severe aortic stenosis with low transvalvular gradients and severe left ventricular dysfunction. *J Am Coll Cardiol, 39*, 1356–1363.
107. Khot, U. N., Novaro, G. M., Popovic, Z. B., et al. (2003). Nitroprusside in critically ill patients with left ventricular dysfunction and aortic stenosis. *N Engl J Med, 348*, 1756–1763.
108. Bonow, R. O., Lakatos, E., Maron, B. J., et al. (1991). Serial long-term assessment of the natural history of asymptomatic patients with chronic aortic regurgitation and normal left ventricular systolic function. *Circulation, 84*, 1625–1631.
109. Chaliki, H. P., Mohty, D., Avierinos, J. F., et al. (2002). Outcomes after aortic valve replacement in patients with severe aortic regurgitation and markedly reduced left ventricular function. *Circulation, 106*, 2687–2693.
110. Daniel, W. G., Hood, W. P., Jr., Siart, A., et al. (1985). Chronic aortic regurgitation: reassessment of the prognostic value of preoperative left ventricular end-systolic dimension and fractional shortening. *Circulation, 71*, 669–680.
111. Carabello, B. A., Usher, B. W., Hendrix, G. H., et al. (1987). Predictors of outcome for aortic valve replacement in patients with aortic regurgitation and left ventricular dysfunction: a change in the measuring stick. *J Am Coll Cardiol, 10*, 991–997.
112. Carabello, B. A. (2004). Is it ever too late to operate on the patient with valvular heart disease? *J Am Coll Cardiol, 44*, 376–383.
113. American College of Cardiology; American Heart Association Task Force on Practice Guidelines (Writing Committee to revise the 1998 guidelines for the management of patients with valvular heart disease); Society of Cardiovascular Anesthesiologists., et al. (2006). ACC/AHA 2006 guidelines for the management of patients with valvular heart disease. A report of the American College of Cardiology/American Heart Association Task Force on Practice Guidelines (Writing Committee to revise the 1998 guidelines for the management of patients with valvular heart disease) developed in collaboration with the Society of Cardiovascular Anesthesiologists, endorsed by the Society for Cardiovascular Angiography and Interventions and the Society of Thoracic Surgeons. *J Am Coll Cardiol, 48*, e1–e148.
114. Cooley, D. A., Henly, W. S., Amad, K. H., et al. (1959). Ventricular aneurysm following myocardial infarction: results of surgical treatment. *Ann Surg, 150*, 595–612.
115. Di Donato, M., Sabatier, M., Toso, A., et al. (1995). Regional myocardial performance of non-ischemic zones remote from anterior wall left ventricular aneurysm. *Eur Heart J, 16*, 1285–1292.
116. Dang, A. B., Guccione, J. M., Whang, P., et al. (2005). Effect of ventricular size and patch stiffness in surgical anterior ventricular restoration: a finite element model study. *Ann Thorac Surg, 79*, 185–193.
117. Dor, V. (2004). Left ventricular reconstruction: the aim and the reality after twenty years. *J Thorac Cardiovasc Surg, 128*, 17–20.
118. Favaloro, R. G., Effler, D. B., Groves, L. K., et al. (1968). Ventricular aneurysm—clinical experience. *Ann Thorac Surg, 6*, 227–245.
119. Cohn, J. N. (1995). Structural basis for heart failure. Ventricular remodeling and its pharmacological inhibition. *Circulation, 91*, 2504–2507.
120. The CONSENSUS Trial Study Group. (1987). Effects of enalapril on mortality in severe congestive heart failure. Results of the Cooperative North Scandinavian Enalapril Survival Study (CONSENSUS). *J Engl J Med, 316*, 1429–1435.
121. St. John Sutton, M., Pfeffer, M. A., Moye, L., et al. (1997). Cardiovascular death and left ventricular remodeling two years after myocardial infarction. Baseline predictors and impact of long-term use of captopril: information from the Survival and Ventricular Enlargement (SAVE) trial. *Circulation, 96*, 3294–3299.
122. Gaudron, P., Eilles, C., Kugler, I., et al. (1993). Progressive left ventricular dysfunction and remodeling after myocardial infarction. Potential mechanisms and early predictors. *Circulation, 87*, 755–763.
123. Konstam, M. A., Rousseau, M. F., Kronenberg, M. W., et al. (1992). Effects of the angiotensin converting enzyme inhibitor enalapril on the long-term progression of left ventricular dysfunction in patients with heart failure. *Circulation, 86*, 431–438.
124. Cox, J. L. (1997). Left ventricular aneurysms: pathophysiologic observations and standard resection. *Semin Thorac Cardiovasc Surg, 9*(2), 113–122.
125. Cox, J. L. (1997). Surgical management of left ventricular aneurysms: a clarification of the similarities and differences between the Jatene and Dor techniques. *Semin Thorac Cardiovasc Surg, 9*, 131–138.
126. Mills, N. L., Everson, C. T., & Hockmuth, D. R. (1993). Technical advances in the treatment of left ventricular aneurysm. *Ann Thorac Surg, 55*, 792–800.
127. Shapira, O. M., Davidoff, R., Hilkert, R. J., et al. (1997). Repair of left ventricular aneurysm: long-term results of linear repair versus endoaneurysmorrhaphy. *Ann Thorac Surg, 63*, 701–705.
128. Mangschau, A. (1989). Akinetic versus dyskinetic left ventricular aneurysms diagnosed by gated scintigraphy: difference in surgical outcome. *Ann Thorac Surg, 47*, 746–751.
129. Dor, V., Sabatier, M., DiDonato, M., et al. (1995). Late hemodynamic results after left ventricular patch repair associated with coronary grafting in patients with postinfarction akinetic or dyskinetic aneurysm of the left ventricle. *J Thorac Cardiovasc Surg, 110*, 1291–1301.
130. Di Donato, M., Sabatier, M., Dor, V., et al. (1997). Akinetic versus dyskinetic postinfarction scar: relation to surgical outcome in patients undergoing endoventricular circular patch plasty repair. *J Am Coll Cardiol, 29*, 1569–1575.
131. Dor, V., Sabatier, M., Di Donato, M., et al. (1998). Efficacy of endoventricular patch plasty in large postinfarction akinetic scar and severe left ventricular dysfunction: comparison with a series of large dyskinetic scars. *J Thorac Cardiovasc Surg, 116*, 50–59.

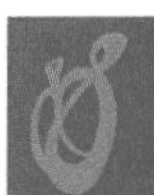

132. Dor, V. (1997). Left ventricular aneurysms: The endoventricular circular patch plasty. *Semin Thorac Cardiovasc Surg, 9*, 123–130.
133. Di Donato, M., Sabatier, M., Dor, V., et al. (2001). Effects of the Dor procedure on left ventricular dimension and shape and geometric correlates of mitral regurgitation one year after surgery. *J Thorac Cardiovasc Surg, 121*, 91–96.
134. Athanasuleas, C. L., Stanley, A. W., Buckberg, G. D., et al. (2001). Surgical anterior ventricular endocardial restoration (SAVER) for dilated ischemic cardiomyopathy. *Semin Thorac Cardiovasc Surg, 13*, 448–458.
135. O'Neill, J. O., Starling, R. C., McCarthy, P. M., et al. (2006). The impact of left ventricular reconstruction on survival in patients with ischemic cardiomyopathy. *Eur J Cardiothorac Surg, 30*, 753–759.
136. Batista, R. J. V., Santos, J. L. V., Takeshita, N., et al. (1996). Partial left ventriculectomy to improve left ventricular function in end-stage heart disease. *J Card Surg, 11*, 96–97.
137. Batista, R. J. V., Nery, P., Bocchino, L., et al. (1997). Partial left ventriculectomy to treat end-stage heart disease. *Ann Thorac Surg, 64*, 634–638.
138. Etoch, S. W., Koenig, S. C., Laureano, M. A., et al. (1999). Results after partial left ventriculectomy versus heart transplantation for idiopathic cardiomyopathy. *J Thorac Cardiovasc Surg, 117*, 952–959.
139. Angelini, G. D., Pryn, S., Mehta, D., et al. (1997). Left-ventricular volume reduction for end-stage heart failure. *Lancet, 350*, 489-454.
140. Franco-Cereceda, A., McCarthy, P. M., Blackstone, E. H., et al. (2001). Partial left ventriculectomy for dilated cardiomyopathy: is this an alternative to transplantation? *J Thorac Cardiovasc Surg, 121*, 879–893.
141. Gradinac, S., Miric, M., Popovic, Z., et al. (1998). Partial left ventriculectomy for idiopathic dilated cardiomyopathy: early results and six-month follow-up. *Ann Thorac Surg, 66*, 1963–1968.
142. Starling, R. C., McCarthy, P. M., Buda, T., et al. (2000). Results of partial left ventriculectomy for dilated cardiomyopathy: hemodynamic, clinical and echocardiographic observations. *J Am Coll Cardiol, 36*, 2098–2103.
143. Acker, M. A. (1999). Dynamic cardiomyoplasty: at the crossroads. *Ann Thorac Surg, 68*, 750–755.
144. Leier, C. V. (1996). Cardiomyoplasty: is it time to wrap it up?*J Am Coll Cardiol, 28*, 1181–1184.
145. Kass, D. A., Baughman, K. L., Pak, P. H., et al. (1995). Reverse remodeling from cardiomyoplasty in human heart failure. External constraint versus active assist. *Circulation, 91*, 2314–2318.
146. Mann, D. L., Acker, M. A., Jessup, M., et al. (2004). Rationale, design, and methods for a pivotal randomized clinical trial for the assessment of a cardiac support device in patients with New York Heart Association class III-IV heart failure. *J Card Fail, 10*, 185–192.
147. Mann, D. L., Acker, M. A., Jessup, M., et al. (2007). Acorn Trial Principal Investigators and Study Coordinators. Clinical evaluation of the CorCap Cardiac Support Device in patients with dilated cardiomyopathy. *Ann Thorac Surg, 84*, 1226–1235.
148. Starling, R. C., Jessup, M., Oh, J. K., et al. (2007). Sustained benefits of the CorCap Cardiac Support Device on left ventricular remodeling: three year follow-up results from the Acorn clinical trial. *Ann Thorac Surg, 84*, 1236–1242.
149. McCarthy, P. M., Fukamachi, K., Takagaki, M., et al. (2000). Device based left ventricular shape change immediately reduces left ventricular volume and increases ejection fraction in a pacing induced cardiomyopathy model in dogs. A pilot study. *J Am Coll Cardiol, 35*(Suppl. A), 183.
150. McCarthy, P. M., Fukamachi, K., Takagaki, M., et al. (2000). Left ventricular shape changereducedleftventricularwallstressinpatientswithdilatedcardiomyopathy.*Circulation, 102*(Suppl. II), II-683.
151. Grossi, E. A., Saunders, P. C., Woo, Y. I., et al. (2005). Intraoperative effects of the Coapsysannuloplastysysteminarandomizedevaluation(RESTOR-MV)offunctionalischemic mitral regurgitation. *Ann Thorac Surg, 80*, 1706–1711.
152. Mahon, N. G., O'Neill, J. O., Young, J. B., et al. (2004). Contemporary outcomes of outpatients referred for cardiac transplantation evaluation to a tertiary heart failure center: impact of surgical alternatives. *J Card Fail, 10*, 273–278.

CHAPTER 56

Circulatory Assist Devices in Heart Failure

Roberta C. Bogaev, Reynolds M. Delgado III, Heinrich Taegtmeyer, and O.H. Frazier

Congestive heart failure is a common cause of premature disability and death. For cases in which conventional medical therapy fails to alleviate the symptoms of end-stage heart failure, mechanical circulatory support (MCS) is increasingly used. Since the 1960s, this approach has become an effective means of saving many patients who would otherwise die of heart failure. Short-term MCS may be used to maintain patients who develop acute, reversible heart failure, such as heart failure that occurs after a myocardial infarction or cardiovascular surgery. Longer-term MCS may be used in patients with severe acute or chronic heart failure, including those awaiting heart transplantation (see Chapter 54).

Indeed, the clinical application of MCS has progressed because of advances in cardiac transplantation, which is the only available definitive treatment for refractory end-stage heart failure. In transplantation candidates, MCS can maintain hemodynamic stability and preserve life until a suitable donor heart becomes available. Prolonged (>30-day) support, particularly with an implantable left ventricular assist device (LVAD), not only allows these patients to survive but often reverses cardiac and end-organ dysfunction; as a result, the risk of perioperative complications is reduced,[1-3] and the results of transplantation are optimized.[4] In addition, mechanical devices are being studied for permanent cardiac replacement and for bridging to myocardial recovery.[5-14] According to the Institute of Medicine, long-term MCS could annually benefit 35,000 to 70,000 Americans who have severe heart failure.[15] As mechanical devices become smaller and easier to implant, the indications for their use may broaden to include patients with less severe heart failure.

The history of MCS systems is reviewed briefly in this chapter. Devices currently used for short-term support in patients with reversible cardiogenic shock, as well as systems used for longer-term bridging to transplantation, are described. After a review of the capabilities and complications of MCS, the focus is on new applications, such as bridging to myocardial improvement and device implantation for permanent use, which are being studied in initial clinical trials. Last, the newest devices being tested and the promising future of MCS are discussed.

HISTORY

In the mid-twentieth century, development of the cardiopulmonary bypass machine by John H. Gibbon Jr., C. Walton Lillehei, John W. Kirklin, and other investigators enabled direct anatomical repair of the diseased heart. The first clinical use of this technology, by Gibbon in 1953, resulted in successful correction of an atrial septal defect.[16] Unfortunately, all of Gibbon's subsequent cardiopulmonary bypass cases ended in clinical failure, causing him to abandon the heart-lung machine. Further development of this device was achieved by Lillehei, at the University of Minnesota, and by Kirklin, at the Mayo Clinic. Early reports by Spencer and coworkers[17] emphasized the recovery of patients after cardiotomy who could not be weaned from cardiopulmonary bypass initially; in these cases, mechanical support was simply continued until the heart recovered.

The success of MCS in patients after cardiotomy paved the way for research efforts designed to allow more prolonged support of cardiac function. A prototype pump created for this purpose was used successfully by DeBakey and associates[18] in 1963, in a patient who had a cardiac arrest after undergoing aortic valve replacement. The pump worked well and supported the circulation for 4 days, but the patient had already suffered an irreversible neurological injury. The first successful case of prolonged left ventricular support was achieved by DeBakey[19] in 1966. The patient was supported by the pump for 10 days, after which the device was removed, and the patient survived long term.

Meanwhile, the intra-aortic balloon pump (IABP) had been introduced by Moulopoulos and colleagues,[20] who performed animal experiments with this device in 1961. The IABP was not used clinically until 1967, when Kantrowitz and associates[21] implanted it in a patient with cardiogenic shock. The IABP is currently the most common form of mechanical support, sustaining more than 80,000 patients per year, some of whom receive the device as a bridge to cardiac transplantation.

In 1964, acting on the advice of DeBakey, the National Heart and Lung Institute established its Artificial Heart Program. Research into an implantable total artificial heart (TAH)—more properly termed a "biventricular replacement device"—began at Baylor College of Medicine during the same decade. This pump was first implanted in a human being in 1969, when Cooley and his team[22] used it to perform the first clinical bridge-to-transplantation operation. The pneumatically driven, diaphragm-type, dual-ventricular pump was positioned orthotopically, replacing the native ventricles. It functioned well, sustaining the patient for 64 hours until a donor heart could be transplanted. In 1981, a second TAH, developed by Tetsuzo Akutsu at the Texas Heart Institute, was implanted as a bridge to transplantation.

In 1982, DeVries[23] performed the first of five TAH implantations intended to serve as permanent cardiac replacements. In these cases, the TAH was the Jarvik-7 model, designed by Robert Jarvik. Although the device was able to support the total circulation for weeks to months, patients had to remain hospitalized and tethered to a power supply and control consoles. In addition, the patients were plagued by device-related complications, particularly infection and stroke, and only two of the patients survived for more than a year.[24]

Because heart transplantation and TAH technology were failing to fulfill their initial promise, clinical efforts were redirected toward producing long-term implantable LVADs. In the 1970s, the institute responsible for the Artificial Heart Program achieved bureau status and became the National Heart, Lung, and Blood Institute (NHLBI). Research involving MCS began to be performed under the auspices of the Devices and Technology Branch of the Division of Heart and Vascular Diseases. In the mid-1970s, after extensive animal and in vitro tests of device safety and reliability, the NHLBI challenged physicians, engineers, and private companies to develop a fully implantable device for the long-term support of patients with heart failure.

The first NHLBI-sponsored device was an intra-abdominally positioned LVAD for treating postcardiotomy shock. In 1975, the Texas Heart Institute conducted the first clinical tests of this single-chambered implantable pump. Three years later, it was used as a bridge to transplantation in a patient who had developed stone heart syndrome after undergoing valve replacement.[25] The LVAD supported the patient's circulation for 5 days until a donor heart became available. In 1984, a different NHLBI-sponsored implantable LVAD was successfully used as a bridge to transplantation by Philip E. Oyer at Stanford University.

The ultimate goal, however, was to produce an LVAD that could provide long-term support or destination therapy. In the 1980s, investigators at the Texas Heart Institute began using the HeartMate, a fully implantable LVAD. Originally produced by Thermo Cardiosystems, Inc. (Woburn, Massachusetts), this pump was later acquired by Thoratec Corporation (Pleasanton, California). The HeartMate was first implanted as a bridge to transplantation in 1986. It had previously undergone 10 years of experimental testing. Although the initial model was pneumatically powered, an electrically driven model also became available, and it was first implanted as a portable LVAD in 1991. Both versions were later approved by the U.S. Food and Drug Administration (FDA) for commercial use to bridge patients to transplantation; the vented electric version is currently approved for long-term support or destination therapy in the United States.

Today, cardiologists and cardiovascular surgeons can choose from a wide range of MCS systems, depending on the desired degree of support, length of support, extent of postoperative mobility, and other factors (Table 56-1). Despite numerous design modifications and refinements, an ideal system has not yet evolved. Nevertheless, current systems can maintain many patients with end-stage heart failure, offering hope where none had previously existed.

SHORT-TERM CIRCULATORY SUPPORT

Short-term MCS is an important strategy for controlling acute, reversible heart failure that manifests as cardiogenic shock, which otherwise often results in mortality.[26-30] Often, shock is caused by an acute myocardial infarction involving more than 40% of the left ventricular mass[31]; in such cases, MCS can support the patient's circulation until his or her condition improves enough for myocardial revascularization to be undertaken.

Acute coronary occlusion is usually managed with an aggressive interventional procedure in the cardiac catheterization laboratory. Patients at particularly high risk, however, may benefit from emergency IABP or temporary cardiopulmonary bypass before the intervention is undertaken.

Temporary MCS may be necessary postoperatively to wean high-risk surgical patients from cardiopulmonary bypass; in these cases, mechanical assistance may also allow the preservation of adequate ventricular function. Moreover, when a patient has acute myocarditis or posttransplantation allograft dysfunction, short-term MCS often enables complete recovery.

Intra-aortic Balloon Pump

The IABP is the most widely used MCS system in the world today. The 40- to 60-mL polyurethane balloon is attached to the tip of a catheter, which is inserted percutaneously into the common femoral artery and then advanced in to the descending thoracic aorta[20,21] (Figure 56-1). Alternatively, if iliofemoral vascular disease is present, the balloon may be inserted into the abdominal aorta via a retroperitoneal approach or into the aortic arch via the subclavian artery.

The pump's action depends on several unique but fairly simple physiological principles. At the start of diastole, the balloon inflates, augmenting coronary perfusion. At the beginning of systole, the balloon deflates; blood is ejected from the left ventricle, increasing the cardiac output by as much as 40% and decreasing the left ventricular stroke work and myocardial oxygen requirements.[32] In this manner, the balloon supports the heart indirectly. Although designed to provide short-term MCS, the IABP has occasionally supported heart transplantation candidates for several weeks. Clinical scenarios for use of this device include preoperative implantation in patients who undergo cardiac surgery with severely impaired left ventricular function or coronary perfusion (as in severe left main coronary artery disease); bridging to transplantation or long-term MCS in patients with intractable heart failure of any cause and impending major organ failure after unsuccessful medical therapy; and intraoperative implantation in patients who experience difficulty in weaning from cardiopulmonary bypass. The IABP has been used with some success in resuscitating patients with heart failure who have had a cardiac arrest.

The device's limitations include an inability to completely unload the left ventricle. Adequate IABP function depends on appropriate timing of the balloon cycle and is suboptimal in the presence of arrhythmias. Moreover, patients with IABPs must remain in their hospital beds. Potential sequelae include peripheral vascular hemorrhagic or thromboembolic complications, which may necessitate surgical intervention.[33,34] The IABP cannot be used in the presence of significant atherosclerotic or aneurysmal disease of the thoracic aorta or significant aortic regurgitation.

Abiomed Biventricular System 5000

The Abiomed Biventricular System (BVS) 5000 (Abiomed Cardiovascular, Inc., Danvers, Massachusetts) was developed to provide short-term univentricular or biventricular support for patients with potentially reversible ventricular function. This pump is most commonly used in patients with postcardiotomy shock, but it has also been used successfully for treating acute myocarditis and for bridging to transplantation.[1,35] In this externally positioned system, pulsatile flow is provided by one or two disposable, dual-chambered blood

TABLE 56–1 Mechanical Circulatory Support Devices in Clinical Use in the United States

Commercial name	Bio-Medicus Bio-Pump	Levitronix CentriMag	Abiomed Biventricular System (BVS) 5000	Abiomed AB5000	Abiomed Abiocor	Thoratec PVAD	HeartMate XVE	Heart-Mate II	Novacor	CardioWest	MicroMed DeBakey	Jarvik 2000	HeartWare MVAD
Manufacturer	Medtronic	Levitronix	Abiomed	Abiomed	Abiomed	Thoratec	Thoratec	Thoratec	World-Heart	Syn-Cardia Systems	MicroMed	Jarvik Heart	HeartWare
Ventricular support	L, R, both	L, R, both	L, R, both	L, R, both	Both	L, R, both	L only	L only	L only	Both	L only	L only	L only
Device position	External	External	External	External	Internal	External	Internal	Internal	Internal	Internal	Internal	Internal	Internal
Pulsatile	No	No	Yes	Yes	Yes	Yes	Yes	No	Yes	Yes	No	No	No
Driver	Electric	Electric	Pneumatic	Vacuum, pneumatic	Electric	Pneumatic	Electric	Electric	Electric	Pneumatic	Electric	Electric	Electric
Extracorporeal components	Driver	Pump, driver	Pump, driver	Pump, driver	Battery	Pump, driver	Battery	Battery	Battery	Driver	Battery	Battery	Battery
Duration of use[a]	Short	Short	Short	Intermediate to long	Long	Intermediate to long	Long	Long	Long	Long	Long	Long	Long
Fit patients with BSA <1.5?	Yes	Yes	Yes	Yes	No	No	No	Yes	No	Large	Yes	Yes	Yes
FDA-approved indication	N/A	PCR	PCR	PCR and BTT	N/A	PCR and BTT	BTT, DT	BTT	BTT	BTT	BTT (IDE)	BTT (IDE)	BTT (IDE)
Implantation approach	Sternotomy	Sternotomy	Sternotomy	Sternotomy	Sternotomy	Sternotomy	Sternotomy	Sternotomy/thoracotomy	Sternotomy	Sternotomy	Sternotomy/thoracotomy	Sternotomy/thoracotomy	Sternotomy/thoracotomy
Anticoagulation with warfarin recommended?	Yes	Yes	Yes	Yes	Yes	Yes	No	Yes	Yes	Yes	Yes	Yes	Yes
Ambulation possible?	No	No	Yes, restricted	Yes	Yes	Yes	Yes	Yes	Yes	Yes	Yes	Yes	Yes
Discharge from hospital?	No	No	No	No	No	Yes	No	Yes	Yes	No	No	Yes	Yes
Cost[b]	$$	$$	$$	$$	N/A	$$ to $$$	$$$$	$$$$	$$$$	$$$$	N/A	N/A	N/A
Audible noise	Quiet	Silent	Very noisy	Very noisy	Quiet	Very noisy	Very noisy	Silent	Quiet	Noisy	Silent	0	Silent

Adapted from Stevenson LW, Kormos RL: Mechanical cardiac support 2000: current applications and future trial design. *J Heart Lung Transplant* 2001;20:1-38.

BSA, body surface area; BTT, bridge to transplantation; DT, destination therapy; FDA, U.S. Food and Drug Administration; IDE, investigational device exemption; L, left; N/A, not applicable; PCR, postcardiotomy recovery; R, right. [a]"Short" indicates <30 days; "Intermediate" indicates 30 days or more but that use is not intended to be permanent; "Long" indicates permanent use as an alternative to a heart transplant. [b]Dollar signs refer to cost relative to the cost of the other listed devices.

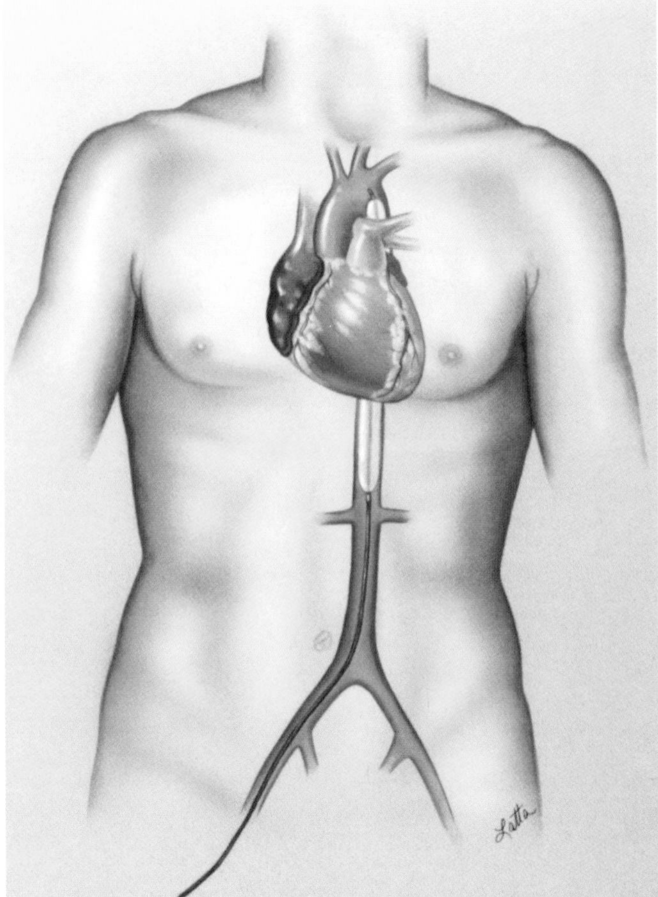

FIGURE 56–1 Illustration of intra-aortic balloon pump in the body. (Copyright 1997, Texas Heart Institute, Houston, TX.)

pumps controlled by a single console (Figure 56-2).[36] Within each pump, one-way flow is assured by two trileaflet valves: one between the ventricular and atrial chambers and the other in the ventricular outflow tract. Polyurethane (Angioflex) is used for the blood-contacting surfaces. A pneumatic, microprocessor-controlled drive console automatically initiates ejection when the pump is filled (stroke volume, 82 mL). The pump fills passively and ejects actively, yielding flows of up to 5 L/min. During weaning, the flow rate is decreased manually by means of a control knob.

The superiority of pulsatile MCS has not yet been proved, but some experts believe that pulsatile systems such as the Abiomed offer advantages over nonpulsatile pumps.[37-42] The FDA has approved the BVS 5000 for temporary use in patients with postcardiotomy shock. This pump is widely used for temporarily supporting patients with life-threatening heart failure. It is also used as a bridge to implantation of a long-term LVAD or as a bridge to transplantation. Because of the pump's high thrombogenic potential, full anticoagulation is necessary.

Abiomed AB5000

The Abiomed AB5000 Circulatory Support System (Abiomed Cardiovascular, Inc.) was approved by the FDA as an adjunct to the BVS 5000 for short to intermediate support as a bridge to recovery. The same cannulas used in the BVS 5000 blood pump are used in this paracorporeal ventricular assist device, which can facilitate the transition from the BVS to the AB5000 device when longer-term support is desired. The AB5000 is powered by a partial vacuum and partial pneumatic console.

Bio-Medicus Bio-Pump

Another option for short-term univentricular or biventricular MCS is the Bio-Medicus Bio-Pump (Bio-Medicus/Medtronic, Eden Prairie, Minnesota), an extracorporeal, centrifugal device available in two disposable models: an 80-mL model for adults (maximal flow, 10 L/min) and a 48-mL model for children. In this pump, rotating acrylic cones generate continuous flow according to the constrained vortex principle (Figure 56-3). The pump is magnetically coupled to an external motor and console.[43] It may be used to support either ventricle, or dual pumps may be used for biventricular support.

Clinicians have acquired considerable experience with the Bio-Pump because it is also used for cardiopulmonary bypass. Its advantages include simplicity, versatility, and cost effectiveness. Limitations include the need for specialized personnel to supervise the system. Moreover, durability problems preclude use of the Bio-Pump for more than 5 days, although this limit is occasionally exceeded. In any case, the pump component should be replaced every 48 to 96 hours. Despite heparin bonding, the circuit's electromagnetic elements are potential sites for thrombus or fibrin formation; therefore, systemic support with heparin is usually necessary unless postoperative hemorrhage becomes a problem. The externalized cannulas are also potential sites of infection.

Levitronix CentriMag

The Levitronix CentriMag Blood Pumping System (Levitronix, Inc., Waltham, Massachusetts) is designed to provide short-term support for patients with severe, acute, but potentially reversible cardiac failure. The magnetically levitated impeller in this pump extends the longevity and reliability of the device (Figure 56-4). The Levitronix CentriMag has a 510(k) approval from the FDA for short-term circulatory support and is frequently used as a bridge to recovery or a bridge to treatment decision.[44]

TandemHeart Percutaneous Transseptal Ventricular Assist Device

The TandemHeart Percutaneous Transseptal Ventricular Assist (PTVA) System (CardiacAssist, Inc., Pittsburgh, Pennsylvania) is a device approved by the FDA to provide temporary left ventricular support. It can be implanted in the catheterization laboratory or the operating room. An inflow cannula is inserted into the patient's left atrium through a standard transseptal puncture via a femoral venous sheath, and an outflow cannula is placed in the femoral artery (Figure 56-5). The extracorporeal centrifugal pump is connected to a controller that provides power, lubrication, and system monitoring.

Impella Devices

The Impella 2.5 device (Abiomed Cardiovascular, Inc.) received a 510(k) approval from the FDA in 2008 to provide partial left ventricular support for up to 6 hours. The Impella 2.5 is inserted via the femoral artery, is advanced into the left ventricle in the catheterization laboratory, and provides up to 2.5 L of blood flow (Figure 56-6). The Placebo-controlled Randomized study of the selective A_1 adenosine receptor antagonist KW-3902 for patients hospitalized with acute HF and volume Overload to assess Treatment Effect on Congestion and renal function (PROTECT) I trial demonstrated the safety and feasibility of the Impella 2.5 in supporting patients who undergo high-risk percutaneous coronary intervention.[45] In the pivotal PROTECT II trial, which is under way, researchers are comparing the Impella 2.5 with the IABP for hemodynamic support while patients undergo high-risk

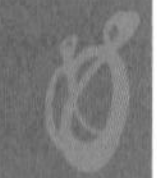

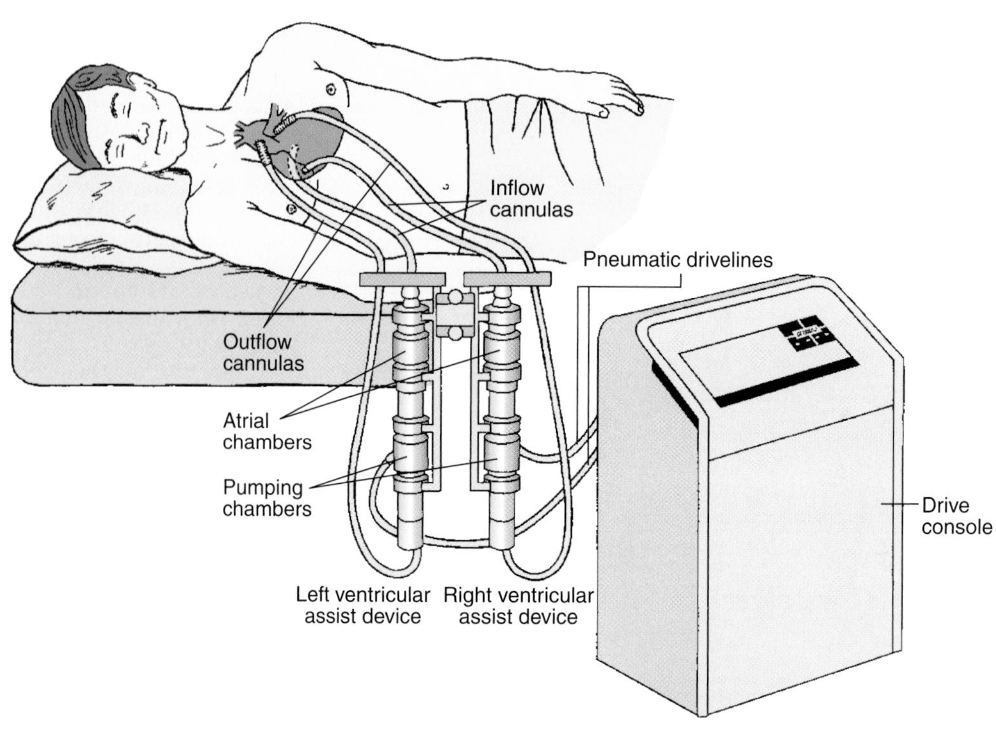

FIGURE 56–2 Abiomed Biventricular System (BVS) 5000 blood pumps and control console. (Courtesy Abiomed, Danvers, MA.)

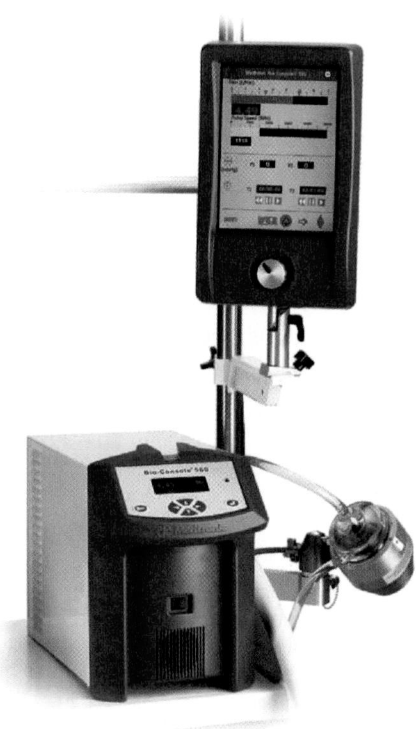

FIGURE 56–3 Bio-Medicus Bio-Pump. (Courtesy Medtronic, Eden Prairie, MN.)

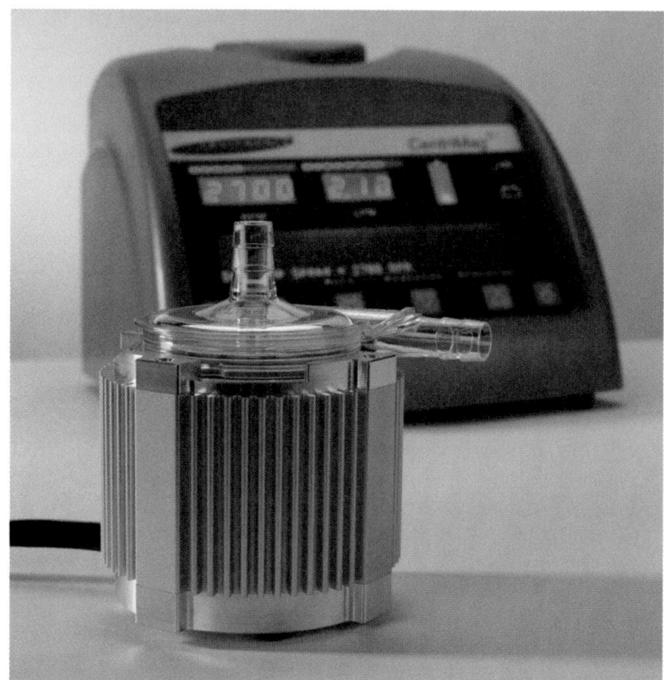

FIGURE 56–4 Levitronix CentriMag ventricular assist device. (Courtesy Levitronix, Waltham, MA.)

percutaneous coronary intervention. The Impella 2.5 device can provide up to 2.5 L of blood volume to the left ventricle via a percutaneous approach. When inserted into the ascending aorta intraoperatively, the Impella 2.5 can provide up to 5.0 L of flow to the left ventricle. In addition, the Impella 5.0 and the Impella LD (Left Direct) received 510(k) approval from the FDA in April 2009 to provide full left ventricular support for up to 6 hours. The Impella 5.0 is inserted through a surgically exposed femoral artery, whereas the Impella LD is inserted through a Hemashield graft that is sewn directly to the ascending aorta. Both the Impella 5.0 and the Impella LD can provide up to 5 L of flow.

BRIDGING TO TRANSPLANTATION

The first three patients to receive implantable devices as bridges to transplantation (two TAHs—one in 1968 and one in 1981—and one LVAD in 1978) were treated at the Texas Heart Institute. These devices supported the patients until transplantation could be performed. However, all three patients subsequently died of overwhelming infection after transplantation.

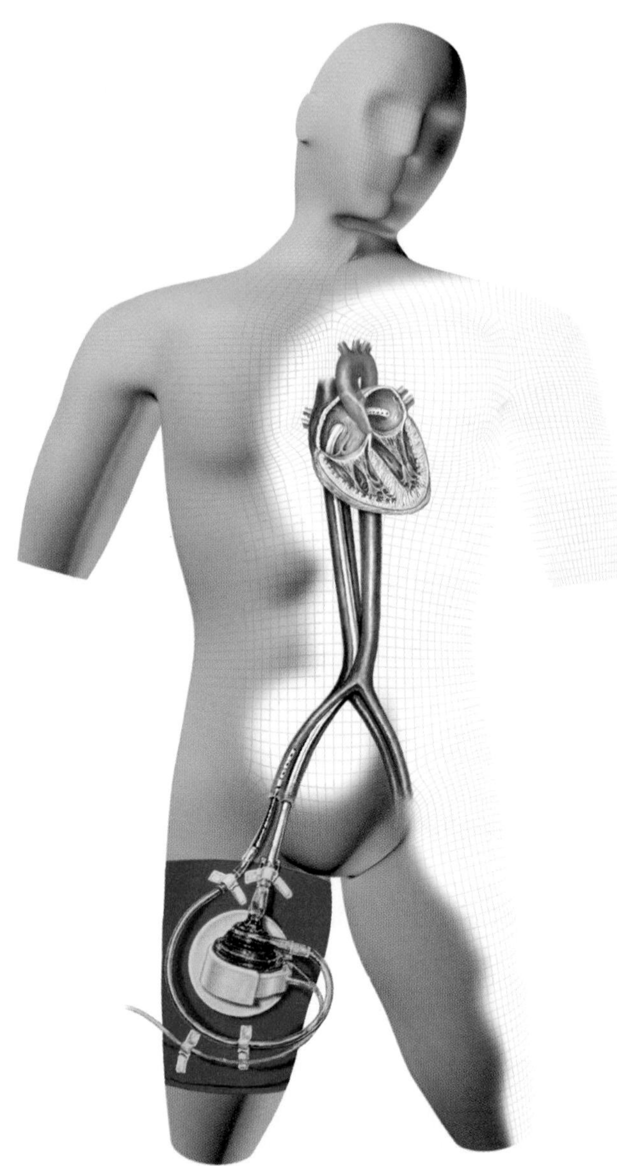

FIGURE 56–5 TandemHeart Percutaneous Transseptal Ventricular Assist (PTVA) System. (Courtesy CardiacAssist, Inc., Pittsburgh, PA.)

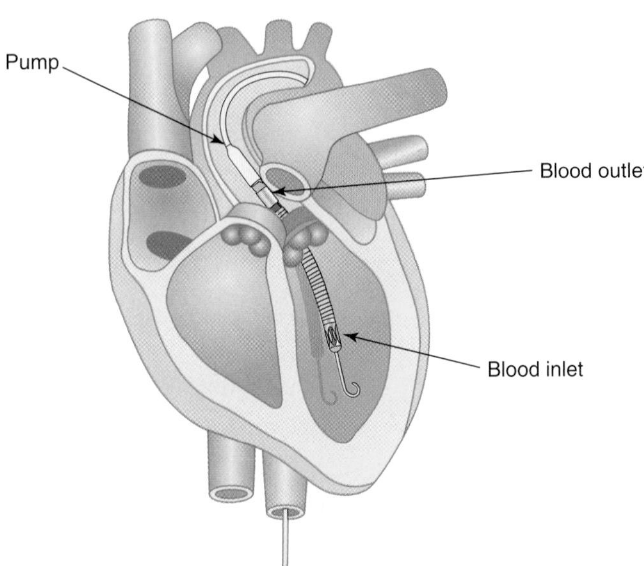

FIGURE 56–6 Impella 2.5, 5.0, and LD devices. (Courtesy Abiomed, Danvers, MA.)

In the early 1980s, the introduction of the immunosuppressant drug cyclosporine, which spared the nonspecific immune system, allowed successful cardiac transplantation in patients otherwise "contaminated" by implantable devices. In the initial bridge-to-transplantation series, patients were confined to the hospital until transplantation occurred. Beginning in 1991, however, patients were allowed to live outside the hospital and even to return to work and other normal activities while receiving MCS. Bridging to transplantation was found to markedly increase posttransplantation survival in this high-risk group.[1,2,4,46] Once initiated, MSC tended to reverse the complex physiological abnormalities that characterize the body's response to heart failure. Kidney and liver dysfunction were often reversed, and neurohormonal activation returned to normal levels.[47] As a result, patients were generally restored to New York Heart Association (NYHA) functional class I while awaiting transplantation. This is an important reason why long-term posttransplantation survival was enhanced in these otherwise more technically challenging patients.[1,2,46]

Bridging to transplantation is indicated for transplantation candidates who have symptoms of progressive heart failure despite maximal drug therapy, cardiac resynchronization therapy, or inotropic support. Because of longer wait times for donor hearts and improved success with newer-generation LVADs, patients are often referred directly for LVAD implantation rather than being placed on IABP support in the intensive care unit. The selection criteria, which were approved by the FDA in 1994, include a pulmonary capillary wedge pressure higher than 20 mm Hg, a cardiac index of 2 L/min/m^2 or lower, and a systolic blood pressure of 80 mm Hg or lower. Outpatients with chronic heart failure who undergo routine right-sided heart catheterization while awaiting cardiac transplantation may meet these criteria. The following conditions render a patient ineligible for MCS: elevated, fixed pulmonary vascular resistance; irreversible renal or hepatic failure; respiratory failure; sepsis; and a severe neurological deficit. These conditions also render patients ineligible for cardiac transplantation. Marked pulmonary hypertension, which reflects minimal changes in the patient's symptoms, can also develop in a patient with chronic heart failure. Therefore, hemodynamic values are routinely monitored in patients awaiting cardiac transplantation. Although patients older than 60 years and those who require mechanical ventilation for respiratory insufficiency are not necessarily excluded from receiving MCS, they are less likely to have a good outcome. Moreover, the first-generation pulsatile, long-term LVADs are too bulky to fit small patients (body surface area < 1.5 m^2). The newer, continuous-flow LVADs have enabled smaller patients, including women, to benefit from MCS.[48]

When selecting an MCS device, the surgeon must consider the degree of support needed, the estimated duration of support, the invasiveness of the implantation procedure, and the patient's need for postoperative mobility (see Table 56-1). For long-term bridging in patients with chronic heart failure, the approved devices are the Thoratec PVAD (Percutaneous Ventricular Assist Device) System, the Thoratec IVAD (Implantable Ventricular Assist Device), the CardioWest TAH, the Novacor Ventricular Assist System, the HeartMate XVE LVAD, and the HeartMate II LVAD.

Thoratec Percutaneous Ventricular Assist Device System

The Thoratec PVAD System (Thoratec Corporation) has a flexible, seam-free, segmented pump sac within a rigid polycarbonate shell (Figure 56-7).[49] One-way blood flow is maintained by Björk-Shiley concavo-convex tilting-disk valves in the inlet and outlet tracts. The pump is pulsatile and pneumatically powered, with a maximal stroke volume of 65 mL

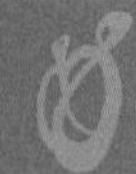

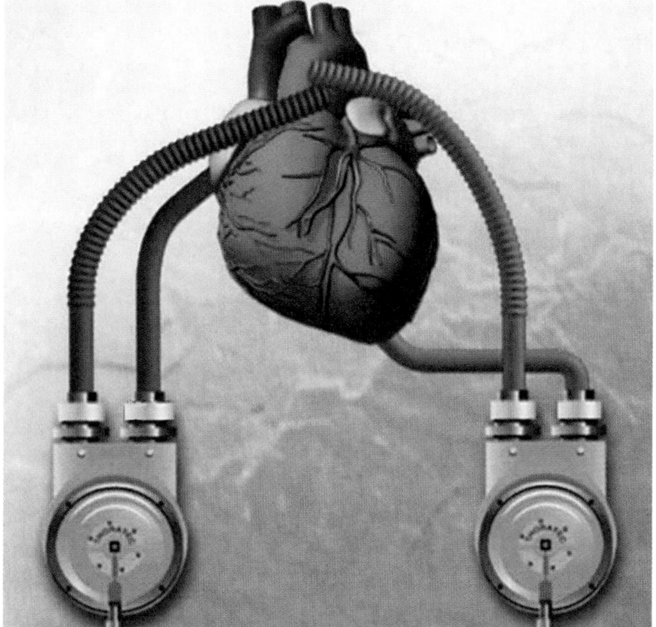

FIGURE 56-7 Thoratec Percutaneous Ventricular Assist Device System. (From Thoratec Corporation, Pleasanton, CA.)

and a maximal output of 7 L/min. It can provide left, right, or biventricular assistance.

The Thoratec device is valuable for treating reversible cardiogenic shock[50] or for bridging to transplantation. When used as a bridging device in a multicenter study involving 154 patients,[51] the system provided left ventricular support in 22% of the cases and biventricular support in the other 78%. Successful transplantation was performed in 65% of the patients. One year after transplantation, the actuarial survival rate was 82%, which is similar to that of the general population of heart transplant recipients. The most common sequelae were hemorrhage (42%) and infection (36%). In another study, involving only postcardiotomy patients, 37% were weaned from the device, and the survival rate of the weaned patients was 57%. Perioperative myocardial infarction and renal failure were the most frequent complications in this series.[52]

As of January 2010, more than 5000 patients had been supported worldwide with the Thoratec PVAD or IVAD, according to the Thoratec Corporation's database. Of these pumps, 3011 were used as bridges to transplantation, 512 were used as postcardiotomy bridges to myocardial recovery, and 596 were used for other or adjunctive support. For bridging to transplantation, biventricular support was used in 1747 cases (58%), LVAD support in 1087 (36%), and right ventricular assist device support in 177 (6%). Of the patients requiring isolated LVAD support, 66% survived to receive a transplant, and 1% recovered function and were weaned from the device. Of the patients requiring biventricular support, 55% received a heart transplant, and 1% recovered ventricular function. Of patients who needed postcardiotomy support, 34% of those with isolated LVADs and 20% of those requiring biventricular VADs were successfully weaned from the device after myocardial recovery.

Because the pump sac may lead to thrombus formation, continuous anticoagulant therapy is necessary as soon as operative bleeding ceases to be a threat. Anticoagulation is achieved with a combination of dextran, dipyridamole, and heparin or warfarin.[53,54] After bleeding has resolved, it is important to use a combination of anticoagulant and antiplatelet therapy to avoid thrombus formation and stroke. Because of the presence of external blood pumps and the necessity for exteriorized cannulas, patients cannot move around freely.

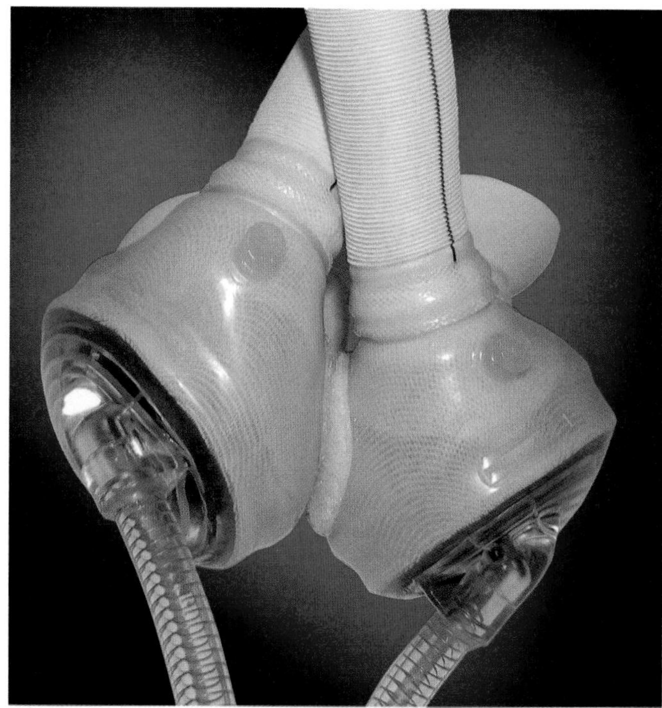

FIGURE 56-8 CardioWest total artificial heart. (Courtesy SynCardia Systems, Inc., Tucson, AZ.)

Despite this drawback, the Thoratec pump is widely used because of its safety, effectiveness, and versatility.

CardioWest Total Artificial Heart

Originally called the Jarvik-7 (and later the Symbion) heart, the CardioWest TAH (SynCardia Systems, Inc., Tucson, Arizona) is implanted orthotopically in patients who need biventricular support (Figure 56-8).[55] The system features two pneumatic blood pumps, each with a semirigid, polyurethane polyester (Biomer) outer shell (Ethicon, Inc., Somerville, New Jersey), and a four-layer flexible Biomer diaphragm. One-way blood flow is ensured by a Medtronic-Hall tilting-disk valve in each pump's inflow and outflow tracts. Whereas the cuffed inflow cannulas are sewn to the atrial remnants of the native heart, the outflow cannulas are attached to the aorta and pulmonary artery by means of polyester (Dacron) grafts. The external pneumatic drive console is connected to the blood pumps by means of drivelines that exit through the patient's left flank. At the transcutaneous exit sites, the drivelines are overlaid with velour-covered silicone elastomer (Silastic; Dow Corning, Midland, Michigan) to ensure stability and encourage tissue ingrowth. During diastole, the pumps are passively filled with blood. In turn, during systole, an influx of air causes the diaphragm to advance and discharge blood. The most common potential problems associated with the CardioWest TAH are hemorrhage, thromboembolism, stroke, and infection.[56] Nevertheless, this system has been used for prolonged periods as a bridge to transplantation in patients with end-stage acute or chronic heart failure.[57,58]

In a nonrandomized prospective study, of the patients who received the CardioWest TAH as a bridge to transplantation, 79% survived until transplantation, in comparison with 46% of historical control patients who did not have a bridge to transplantation.[59] These data led to the approval of the CardioWest TAH as a bridge to transplantation by the FDA in 2004. A smaller, portable pneumatic driver, which allows patients to be discharged from the hospital, has received Conformité Européenne (CE) Marking approval and is available in Europe. SynCardia is developing a third-generation, "wearable" driver, which will also facilitate discharge from the hospital and further improve quality of life.[60]

As of January August 2010, the CardioWest has been implanted in 860 patients worldwide, accounting for more than 300 patient years of life on the artificial heart (J. Copeland, personal communication, August 6, 2010). Although originally designed as a permanent replacement heart, the CardioWest TAH is currently approved as a bridge to heart transplantation for patients dying of end-stage biventricular failure.

Novacor Ventricular Assist System

The Novacor Ventricular Assist System (WorldHeart Corporation, Salt Lake City, Utah) is a pulsatile blood pump designed to attain the original NHLBI goal of destination therapy, as proposed in 1977.[61] This electrically driven, implantable blood pump (Figure 56-9) has a seamless polyurethane pump sac that, when actuated by dual pusher-plates, produces a maximum stroke volume of 70 mL. One-way blood flow is ensured by a 21-mm bioprosthetic valve in the inflow and outflow tracts. The system is currently powered by external batteries, allowing mobility of the patient. The pump is linked to its power source by means of a percutaneous driveline, which also allows external venting.

In clinical bridge-to-transplantation trials performed since 1984, the Novacor device has enabled successful bridging to transplantation in about 60% of reported cases. Posttransplantation survival rates have been excellent.[62,63] The most frequent complications have been hemorrhage, infection, and thromboembolism.[62]

Robbins and coworkers[64] reported their experience with 53 patients who received Novacor devices for bridging to cardiac transplantation over a 16-year period. After a mean support period of 56 ± 76 days, 66% of the patients underwent successful transplantation. Complications included bleeding (43%), infection (30%), and embolic cerebrovascular events (24.5%).

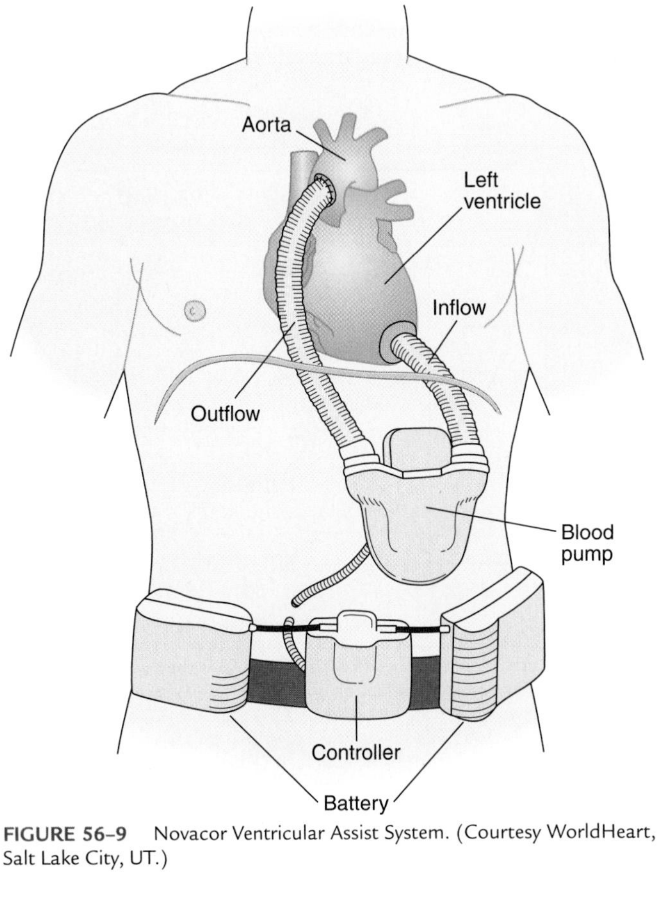

FIGURE 56-9 Novacor Ventricular Assist System. (Courtesy WorldHeart, Salt Lake City, UT.)

A prospective, nonrandomized trial was conducted at 13 centers in the United States and Canada to assess the impact of support with the Novacor Left Ventricular Assist System (LVAS) on survival and quality of life in patients ineligible for cardiac transplantation who were inotrope-dependent.[65] The Investigation of Nontransplant-Eligible Patients Who Are Inotrope Dependent (INTrEPID) trial enrolled 55 patients who could not be weaned from inotropic support. The patients receiving optimal medical therapy had lower mean serum sodium levels (128 vs. 134 mg/dL, $P = .001$) and higher mean blood urea nitrogen levels (59 vs. 40 mg/dL, $P = .02$) than did the patients who received the Novacor LVAS. In comparison with patients treated with optimal medical therapy, patients treated with the Novacor LVAS had superior survival rates at 6 months (46% vs. 22%, $P = .03$) and 12 months (27% vs. 11%, $P = .02$). Of the LVAS-treated patients, 85% had NYHA class I or II symptoms; in comparison with medically treated patients, Novacor recipients had lower rates of cardiovascular dysfunction ($P < .0001$) and renal dysfunction ($P = .0009$) but higher risks of bleeding ($P = .008$), stroke ($P = .06$), and infection ($P = .54$). The favorable INTrEPID trial results prompted WorldHeart to initiate the Randomized Evaluation of the Novacor LVAS In Non-Transplant Population (RELIANT) trial to establish that the Novacor LVAS was superior to optimal medical therapy and equivalent to the HeartMate XVE LVAD for destination therapy. The trial was subsequently halted because of slow enrollment and clinicians' preference for smaller, continuous-flow pumps. Use of the Novacor LVAS was discontinued in 2008.

HeartMate XVE Left Ventricular Assist Device

The HeartMate LVAD (Thoratec Corporation) was initially developed with NHLBI support in response to the NHLBI's 1977 request for proposal. The in vivo laboratory experience and the initial clinical experience were obtained exclusively at the Texas Heart Institute. The system was first used clinically with a pneumatically powered pump that had an external console. This was a cost-saving approach, inasmuch as the initial patients were confined to the hospital. The original version of the HeartMate, however, was a vented-electric model (VE-LVAD). It was first used clinically, beginning in 1991, in patients expected to have a long wait for a donor heart.

The VE-LVAD and the implantable pneumatic version (IP-LVAD) have the same blood pump and similar operating principles. The blood pump is a flexible polyurethane diaphragm within a titanium alloy shell. The woven polyester (Dacron) inflow and outflow cannulas each contain a 25-mm caged porcine xenograft valve. The outflow cannula is extended by a 20-mm woven Dacron graft, which is trimmed to the proper length at implantation. To encourage the formation of a pseudoneointimal lining and thereby minimize thromboembolism, all the blood-contacting surfaces except the valves are specially textured.[66] The titanium surfaces are covered with sintered titanium spheres, and the diaphragm is covered by fibrils that arise from its polyurethane base. The IP-LVAD pump weighs 570 g, and the VE-LVAD pump weighs 1150 g. Both devices produce a maximal effective stroke volume of 83 mL. Blood flows range up to 12 L/min for the IP-LVAD and 10 L/min for the VE-LVAD.

The HeartMate can greatly improve the clinical status of patients who receive bridges to transplantation.[6,67,68] Most patients who are in NYHA functional class IV before receiving the HeartMate return to class I after 3 to 4 weeks of support. Meanwhile, they can be rehabilitated physically. In cases involving prolonged MCS (>30 days), use of the HeartMate improves the outcome of transplantation.

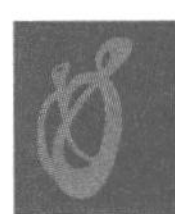

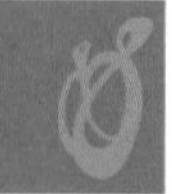

The IP-LVAD was the first implantable pump to be approved by the FDA (in 1994) for bridging to transplantation. The FDA based its approval on results of a study in which 75 IP-LVAD recipients were compared with 33 untreated control patients.[4] Transplantation was performed in 71% of the IP-LVAD recipients, of whom 91% survived after transplantation. In contrast, transplantation was performed in only 36% of the control patients, of whom 67% survived after transplantation.

The VE-LVAD (Figure 56-10) received FDA approval for commercial use in 1998. Because this model allows full patient mobility, it has been the device most commonly used for bridging to transplantation. In a prospective, multicenter trial,[69] 280 VE-LVAD recipients awaiting transplantation were compared with 48 control patients who did not receive ventricular assistance. The LVAD group was supported for an average of 112 days (range, 1 to 691 days), and 58% of these patients were enrolled in a hospital release program. Before a suitable donor heart could be found, 82 (29%) of the LVAD patients and 32 (67%) of the control patients died. Of the 280 LVAD recipients, 188 (67%) eventually underwent transplantation, and 10 (4%) had the device removed electively. One year after transplantation, the LVAD patients had a significantly better survival rate (84%) than did the control patients (63%; $P = .0197$). Device-related complications included bleeding (11%), infection (40%), thromboembolic events (6%), and neurological dysfunction (5%).

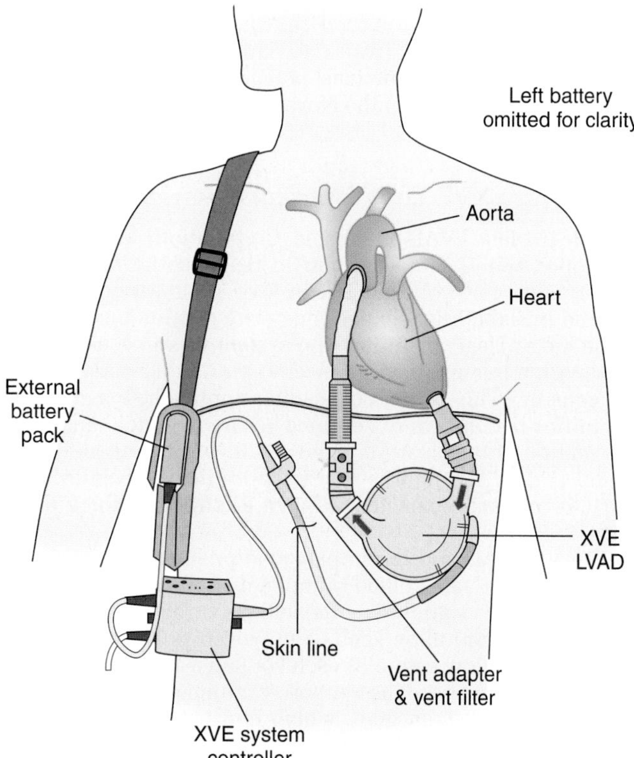

FIGURE 56–10 Components of the HeartMate vented-electric left ventricular assist device (LVAD). The inflow cannula is inserted into the apex of the left ventricle, and the outflow cannula is anastomosed to the ascending aorta. Blood returns from the lungs to the left side of the heart and exits through the left ventricular apex and across an inflow valve into the prosthetic pumping chamber. Blood is then actively pumped through an outflow valve into the ascending aorta. The pumping chamber is placed within the abdominal wall or peritoneal cavity. A percutaneous drive line carries the electrical cable and air vent to the battery packs (only the pack on the right side is shown) and electronic controls, which are worn on a shoulder holster and belt, respectively. (Modified from Rose EA, Gelijns AC, Moskowitz AJ, et al. Long-term mechanical left ventricular assistance for end-stage heart failure. *N Engl J Med* 2001;345:1435-1443, with permission, and from Naka Y, Rose E A. Assisted circulation in the treatment of heart failure. In Libby PL, Bonow RO, Mann DL, et al, editors. *Braunwald's heart disease,* ed 8, Philadelphia, 2008, Elsevier, pp 685-696.)

In 1998, researchers began a landmark study, the Randomized Evaluation of Mechanical Assistance for the Treatment of Congestive Heart Failure (REMATCH), designed to determine whether the VE-LVAD could offer permanent support for patients with severe heart failure who were ineligible for transplantation. Patients were randomly assigned to receive either MCS or continued medical therapy and were observed for 2 years. The results showed a reduction of 48% in the risk of death from any cause in the group that received LVADs, in comparison with those treated with medical therapy (relative risk = 0.52; 95% confidence interval, 0.34 to 0.78; $P = .001$). Among the very ill patients with heart failure, the rates of survival at 1 year were 25% of those treated with medical therapy and 52% of those treated with the LVAD ($P = .002$). At the end of the 2 years, the survival rates were 8% and 23%, respectively ($P = .09$). Quality-of-life indicators were also more favorable for the LVAD-treated group (Figure 56-11).[70] As of January 2010, more than 6000 vented-electric HeartMate devices had been implanted worldwide, and the HeartMate XVE was the first LVAD to receive FDA approval for long-term support or destination therapy.

HeartMate II Left Ventricular Assist Device

The HeartMate II (Thoratec Corporation) LVAD is a continuous-flow, rotary-pump device that is capable of delivering 6 to 12 L/min of flow. The pump consists of an internal axial-flow blood pump, a percutaneous lead that connects the pump to an external system driver, and a power source (Figure 56-12). One advantage of the HeartMate II LVAD is its smaller size, which allows it to be used in underserved populations, including women and adolescents.[65,71] Other benefits include the potential for long-term mechanical reliability, less noise, and greater comfort for patients.

The HeartMate II bridge-to-transplantation trial was a prospective, nonrandomized, multicenter trial enrolling 133 patients at 26 centers between March 2005 and May 2006. The researchers compared study patients with historical control groups by assessing objective performance criteria.[4,69,72] The primary endpoint was transplantation, cardiac recovery,

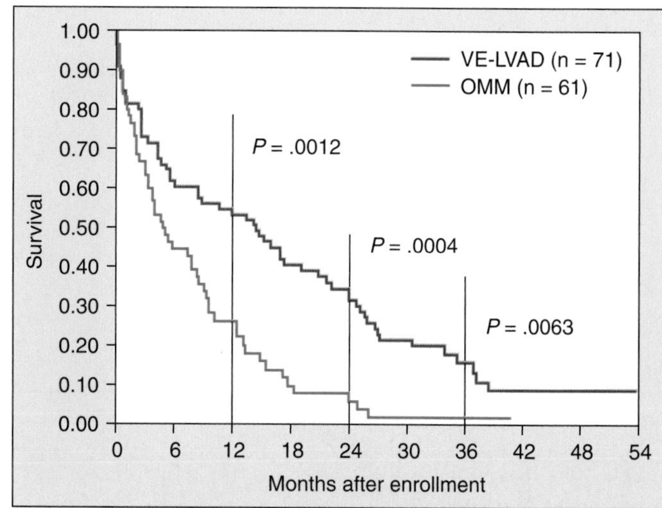

FIGURE 56–11 Kaplan-Meier analysis of survival in the two treatment conditions of the Randomized Evaluation of Mechanical Assistance for the Treatment of Congestive Heart Failure (REMATCH) trial. OMM, optimal medical management; VE-LVAD, vented-electric left ventricular assist device. (Adapted from Park SJ, Tector A, Piccioni W, et al. Left ventricular assist devices as destination therapy: A new look at survival. *J Thorac Cardiovasc Surg* 2005;129:9-17, with permission and from Naka Y, Rose EA. Assisted circulation in the treatment of heart failure. In Libby PL, Bonow RO, Mann DL, et al, editors. *Braunwald's heart disease,* ed 8, Philadelphia, 2008, Elsevier, pp 685-696.)

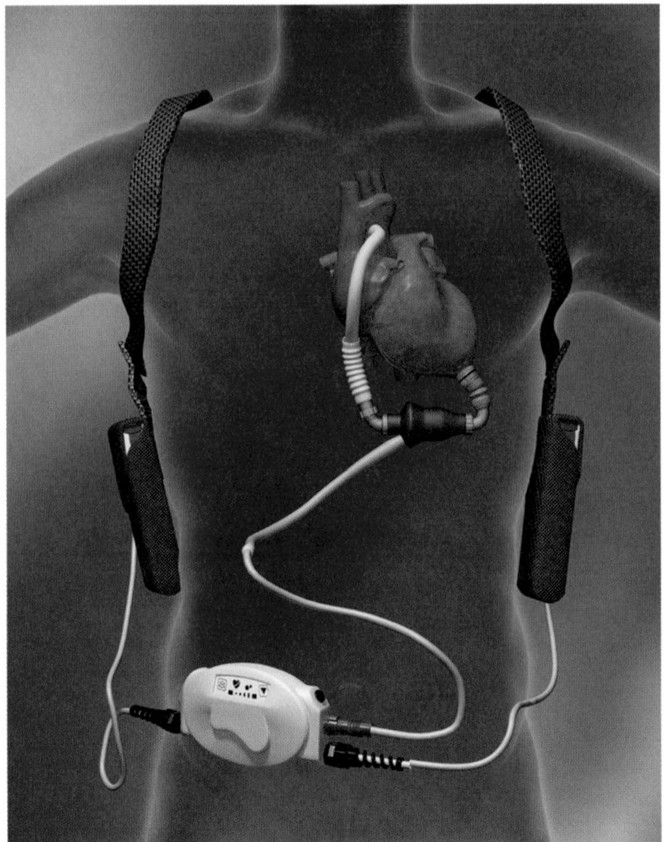

FIGURE 56–12 HeartMate II left ventricular assist device. (From Thoratec Corporation, Pleasanton, CA.)

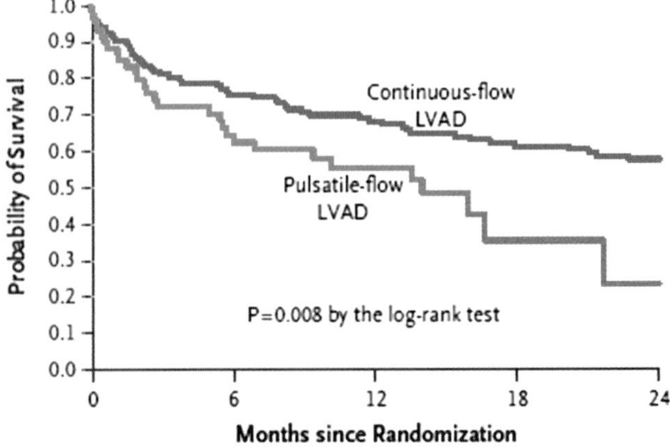

FIGURE 56–13 Kaplan-Meier estimates of survival in patients who received pulsatile HeartMate XVE to the continuous-flow HeartMate II device as destination therapy. (From Slaughter, M. S., Rogers, J. G., Milano, C. A. et al. (2009). Advanced heart failure treated with continuous-flow left ventricular assist device. *N Engl J Med.* 361, 2241-2251.)

or ongoing mechanical support while patients remained eligible for transplantation at 180 days (Figure 56-13). Secondary endpoints included functional status and quality of life. The primary endpoints were reached by 100 patients (75%), and the median duration of support was 126 days (range, 1 to 600 days). The survival rates during support were 75% at 6 months and 68% at 12 months. By 3 months after LVAD implantation, patients showed improvements in functional status and quality of life. Major adverse events included postoperative bleeding that necessitated surgery (31%), ischemic stroke (6%), hemorrhagic stroke (2%), transient ischemic attack (4%), right-sided heart failure (17%), infection unrelated to the device (28%), and percutaneous lead infection (14%).[48] This study showed that the continuous-flow HeartMate II LVAD provided effective hemodynamic support and improved both functional capacity and quality of life in patients awaiting transplantation. To date, more than 1000 patients worldwide have received the HeartMate II, which received FDA approval for use as a bridge to transplantation in 2009.

The Thoratec Corporation conducted a pivotal trial that compared the pulsatile HeartMate XVE (66 patients) to the continuous-flow HeartMate II (134 patients) for long-term support (ie, destination therapy).[72a] The trial enrolled patients in a 2:1 fashion; 2 patients received the HeartMate II for every 1 patient who received the HeartMate XVE. The primary composite end point was survival free from disabling stroke and from reoperation to repair or replace the device at 2 years. Secondary end points included survival, frequency of adverse events, the quality of life, and functional capacity. The primary composite end point was reached in more patients with continuous-flow devices than with pulsatile-flow devices (hazard ratio, 0.38; 95% confidence interval, 0.27-0.54; $P<0.001$), and patients with continuous-flow devices had superior actuarial survival rates at 2 years (58% vs 24%, $P=0.008$) (Figure 56-13). Adverse events and device replacements were less frequent in patients with the continuous-flow device. The quality of life and functional capacity improved significantly in both groups. The HeartMate II was approved for use as destination therapy by the FDA in 2010.[72b] As of January 2010, more than 4000 HeartMate II LVADs have been inserted worldwide (Farrar, personal communication, August 6, 2010).

PERIOPERATIVE COMPLICATIONS

The bridge-to-transplantation population is vulnerable to perioperative hemorrhage, sepsis, thromboembolism, renal failure, technical failure, and neurological sequelae.[73,74] The most common serious problems are hemorrhage and sepsis. Hemorrhage, which occurs in up to 60% of patients, results from liver dysfunction, the implantation procedure itself, and the blood trauma caused by cardiopulmonary bypass and blood-pump rheological characteristics.[75,76] Biventricular MCS is more likely to cause hemorrhage than is univentricular MCS.[75] Sepsis occurs in 30% to 40% of patients, resulting in significant morbidity.[75,77-79] Nevertheless, sepsis does not necessarily rule out successful cardiac transplantation.[76,80,81] Patients with comorbid conditions and hemorrhage are at the highest risk for sepsis.[82,83] Data from 195 LVAD patients enrolled in the Thoratec destination therapy registry between November 2001 and March 2005 were reviewed for risk factors for death in patients awaiting heart transplantation. According to univariate analysis, significant preoperative risk factors for 30-day mortality included reflections of the severity of heart failure. Patients were stratified into risk categories (extremely high, very high, high, moderate, and low risk) on the basis of a preoperative risk score.[84] The ultimate decision to proceed with VAD implantation can be made only after the patient has been thoroughly assessed and after all attempts have been made to optimize the patient's hemodynamics and end-organ function. Short-term MCS devices are often used in patients with recent shock and early multiorgan failure, who are at the highest risk for serious complications and death.

A common underlying cause of death in LVAD patients is right-sided heart failure, which decreases the preload of the left ventricle and, thus, of the device itself, compromising the cardiac output. This condition is often exacerbated by elevated pulmonary vascular resistance. Current therapy involves aggressive use of milrinone, nitric oxide, nitroglycerin, or prostaglandin E_1, all of which promote pulmonary vasodilation and improve left-sided blood flow. Often, right-sided heart failure occurs early after LVAD implantation and is precipitated by bleeding and the need for multiple transfusions. Preoperative fixed or hard-to-reverse elevated pulmonary vascular resistance increases the risk of right-sided heart failure after LVAD implantation. Despite medical therapy and the use of a right-sided VAD, treatment options are limited, and the rate of mortality from right-sided heart failure remains high.

BRIDGING TO MYOCARDIAL IMPROVEMENT

The first patient reported to demonstrate long-term myocardial improvement with MCS was a 33-year-old man who received a HeartMate at the Texas Heart Institute in 1991. He died 503 days later, of a neurological thromboembolic complication, while still receiving MCS.[2] Before his death, the patient had a near-normal ejection fraction and evidence of physiological and anatomical myocardial recovery. Subsequently, positive results similar to these have been observed in HeartMate XVE and HeartMate II recipients, as well as in patients with other systems.[6,85-87] Most patients who undergo MCS before transplantation not only have improved hemodynamic, anatomical, and histological values[47] but also decreased levels of neurohormones such as plasma norepinephrine, which are abnormally elevated in heart failure.[5] On the basis of these observations, a number of patients have undergone LVAD removal after prolonged MCS led to meaningful long-term improvement in cardiac function. The number of such patients is small, but the potential clinical importance is considerable, inasmuch as most of these long-term patients show improvement.

To determine whether LVAD explantation is feasible, a method has been developed at the Texas Heart Institute to assess myocardial improvement through dobutamine stress echocardiography and invasive hemodynamic monitoring, with the LVAD off or providing only minimal support. Other centers have developed similar protocols to determine whether a patient can be weaned off LVAD support. With the use of the Texas Heart Institute method, 9 of 16 patients have had a favorable response, as indicated by improvements in the cardiac index, rate of rise of left ventricular pressure, ejection fraction, and left ventricular end-diastolic dimension as the dobutamine doses increased. The nine patients who had a favorable response underwent device explantation, and six have survived long term with good functional status. Because of the organ shortage and the difficulty of matching some patients with appropriate donors, this strategy may become very important in managing end-stage heart failure.

BIOLOGICAL PROPERTIES OF VENTRICULAR UNLOADING

Intriguing reports suggest that mechanical unloading with an LVAD changes the structural and functional properties of the failing heart (see Chapter 8).[88-91] Improvements in structure, programmed cell death and survival, gene and protein expression, and cardiomyocyte function underlie the myocardial changes observed during LVAD support.

Morphology

Mechanical unloading results in a 20% to 30% decrease in the myocyte volume, cell length, cell width, and cell length-to-thickness ratio, but the cell thickness does not change.[92] In addition, mechanical unloading decreases the nuclear size and DNA content, which is suggestive of a reversal of nuclear hypertrophy and polyploidization.[93] In addition to changing cardiomyocyte structure, LVAD treatment alters the composition of the myocardial extracellular matrix. Whereas results of early studies suggested that a slight increase in myocardial fibrosis accompanies mechanical unloading,[94,95] more recent studies have revealed that LVAD treatment reduces fibrosis and collagen I and III content.[96,97] Thus, MCS reverses some of the histopathological findings in patients with end-stage cardiomyopathy.

Programmed Cell Death and Cell Survival (see Chapter 6)

End-stage cardiomyopathy is associated with an increase in the rate of programmed cell death (apoptosis).[98] This loss of myocytes is believed to contribute to myocardial dysfunction. Mechanical unloading may improve cardiac function, as just noted, and may also decrease apoptosis. Comparison of myocardial samples obtained before and after LVAD treatment revealed a reversal of the decreased transcription of the antiapoptotic proteins Bcl-x(L) and FasExo-6Del.[99] This change was accompanied by an attenuation of DNA fragmentation. In addition, Uray and associates[100] found that transcription of human epidermal growth factor receptor 2 (Her2/neu), an antiapoptotic tyrosine kinase, increases with LVAD treatment. These findings suggest that mechanical unloading activates antiapoptotic pathways. In contrast, other researchers, using immunohistochemistry, have found that the levels of Bcl-2 and the repair-marker-protein proliferator cell nuclear antigen are increased at the time of device insertion and are decreased in most patients with mechanical unloading.[101] Reports concerning the cell-survival programming and the reentry of myocytes in the cell cycle have received much attention.[102,103] Cell-survival pathways (e.g., activation of protein kinase B) and cardiomyocyte hyperplasia counterbalance the myocyte loss induced by apoptosis and necrosis and may contribute to the improvement of cardiac function during mechanical unloading.

Reversal of Dysfunctional Gene and Protein Expression (see Chapter 8)

Interest has focused on mediators and mechanisms of contractile dysfunction and their reversal with mechanical unloading. The results of a study that included 47 patients with NYHA class III or IV heart failure suggested that a 3-month regimen of soluble tumor necrosis factor (TNF) receptor (etanercept) improves the structure and function of the left ventricle.[104] Several multicenter trials have examined the role of TNF-α Antagonism in patients with end-stage cardiomyopathy. In two trials—Research into Etanercept Cytokine Antagonism in Ventricular Dysfunction (RENAISSANCE) and Randomized Etanercept North American Strategy to Study Antagonism of Cytokines (RECOVER)—the use of three dosages of etanercept, a fusion protein directed against TNF-α, has been evaluated in 2048 patients with heart failure. The studies were halted early because no benefit was seen with any dosage of etanercept.[105] In addition, a smaller study of 150 patients with moderate heart failure did not demonstrate clinical improvement in patients treated with infliximab, a chimeric monoclonal antibody that binds to TNF-α, despite a decrease in the inflammatory cytokines C-reactive protein and interleukin-6.[106] One important finding of these three trials was that the lowest dosage of anti–TNF-α therapy appeared to be safe; however, the optimal dose for potential benefit in patients with heart failure still needs to be established.[105] Interestingly, two studies have shown that increased myocardial levels of TNF-α gene and protein expression, seen at device implantation, decrease with mechanical unloading.[13,91] These findings suggest that LVAD-related improvement of cardiac function is associated with a decreased content of myocardial TNF-α.

In addition to cytokines, several other genes and proteins are altered by mechanical unloading. For example, unloading of the heterotopically transplanted normal rat heart induces reactivation of fetal genes, as seen in pressure-induced hypertrophy.[107] Induction of the fetal gene program may be an adaptive response in favor of an energy-sparing metabolism. Other investigators have shown that dystrophin expression, β-tubulin protein content, and levels of the stress-inducible protein metallothionein become normal or nearly normal with LVAD support.[108-110] These changes in the genes and proteins of energy metabolism, the cytoskeleton, and cardioprotection may contribute to LVAD-related improvement in cardiac function.

Improved Cardiomyocyte Function

In studies of isolated human cardiomyocytes, LVAD support increased the magnitude of contraction, shortened the time of peak contraction, and reduced the time to 50% relaxation.[111] In addition, responses to β-adrenergic stimulation were greater in myocytes isolated after LVAD support. In this context, Ogletree-Hughes and colleagues[112] found that mechanical unloading reverses the downregulation of β-adrenergic receptors and improves cardiac responsiveness to inotropic stimulation. Similar findings were reported by Heerdt and coworkers,[113] who measured the isometric force-frequency relationship in isolated left ventricular trabeculae from failing hearts with and without LVAD support. These investigators verified that mechanical unloading improves the contractile force. Northern blot analysis (messenger RNA) showed upregulation of sarcoplasmic/endoplasmic reticulum calcium adenosine triphosphatase (SERCA) subtype 2a, the ryanodine receptor, and the sarcolemmal sodium-calcium exchanger, whereas Western blot analysis (protein) showed only increased SERCA subtype 2a protein content; consistent with the increased SERCA subtype 2a levels was the augmentation of calcium uptake by the sarcoplasmic reticulum in LVAD-treated hearts.[113] In the heterotopic abdominal mouse heart transplant model, Ritter and associates[114] showed that 5 days of unloading increases myocyte fractional shortening and the calcium homeostasis transient. Of four parameters (morphology, programmed cell death, dysfunctional gene and protein expression, and calcium homeostasis), calcium homeostasis consistently shows the most change in response to mechanical unloading. Recovery of left ventricular function during mechanical unloading has been reported by at least three groups, including one at the Texas Heart Institute.[85,86,89,90,115] However, these reports are anecdotal. Although there is evidence for improved function of the failing heart and organs, the mechanisms that underlie these phenomena are the subject of intense investigation.

The often-complete left ventricular unloading provided by the LVAD is allowing for new insights into the molecular and cellular biology of the failing heart and its response to hemodynamic forces. It is hoped that these insights will lead to optimal unloading strategies that can improve myocardial function and to many other medical or gene-based therapies that can aid the failing heart.

ECONOMICS AND QUALITY-OF-LIFE ISSUES

Historically, the goal of MCS therapy has been successful bridging to transplantation. However, because of the concept of implanting support devices for permanent use, quality-of-life and long-term economic issues have become important. To be successful for permanent use, an MCS device must reduce mortality, improve the patient's quality of life, and have a favorable economic effect. Results from the REMATCH trial, designed to assess these issues in patients with the HeartMate XVE LVAD, indicate that use of the LVAD as destination therapy may be a reasonable alternative to continued medical management in patients with medically refractory heart failure. Smaller studies have also yielded valuable insights. In the study by Grady and colleagues,[116] HeartMate XVE recipients who completed a questionnaire 1 to 2 weeks after LVAD implantation reported a significantly better quality of life, more satisfaction with health and functionality, and significantly less symptom-related distress than they had noted preoperatively. However, these patients also had significantly more self-care disability and dissatisfaction with their socioeconomic status. After LVAD implantation, exercise capacity improves slowly but substantially, and some patients are able to return to work.[3] Moskowitz and associates[117] found that patients undergoing bridging to transplantation had a substantially improved quality of life after LVAD implantation, although it was not as good as what they enjoyed after transplantation.

According to Dew and coworkers,[118] quality of life improves (much as it does in a transplant recipient) if the LVAD recipient is discharged home. The cost may also be substantially reduced by outpatient management. In investigations by Morales and associates,[119] who studied 44 HeartMate XVE patients, outpatient management yielded a substantial cost benefit; 30% of the patients were able to return to work or school. A patient's ability to resume productive activity confers a financial benefit to society that is difficult to measure. Because a growing percentage of the population is disabled by severe heart failure, this factor is becoming increasingly important in determining the economic aspects of long-term LVAD use.

FUTURE DIRECTIONS

Tomorrow's blood pumps will be small, totally implantable devices that are more efficient, biocompatible, and reliable than today's models. The goal is to produce a durable device that requires no percutaneous elements and that can be implanted with minimal blood loss. Although still in the experimental stages, the following systems are showing considerable potential.

Jarvik 2000

The Jarvik 2000 is a miniature (90-g), continuous-flow LVAD that has only one moving part: the rotor (Figure 56-14). Like other continuous-flow pumps, it has diminutive blood-contacting surfaces and requires neither valves nor a compliance chamber. The device is small enough to fit some children and small adults. Also, it can be implanted through a lateral thoracotomy, without cardiopulmonary bypass.[120] This approach offers the theoretical advantages of less bleeding and lower operative risk, which are especially beneficial for patients who have undergone previous sternotomies. The device is positioned within the left ventricular apex, with the outflow graft attached to the descending or ascending thoracic aorta. Power is supplied through a small driveline that exits the abdominal wall. Once activated, the pump displaces up to 25 mL of blood and yields maximal flows of more than 11 L/min. In laboratory studies at the Texas Heart Institute, more than 25 calves have been supported by this pump for up to 240 days.[121] As of August 2010, this device has been implanted in 90 human patients at the Texas Heart Institute and in 422 patients worldwide. The first patient given lifetime use of the Jarvik 2000 in England was continuously supported for

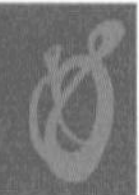

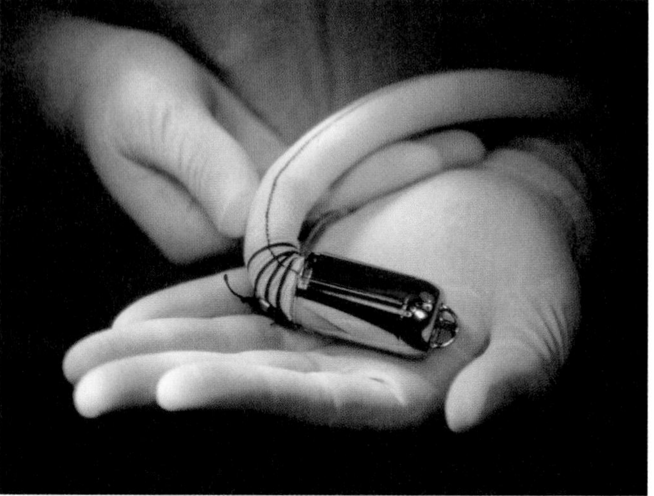

FIGURE 56-14 Jarvik 2000 left ventricular assist device. (Copyright 2000, Texas Heart Institute, Houston, TX.)

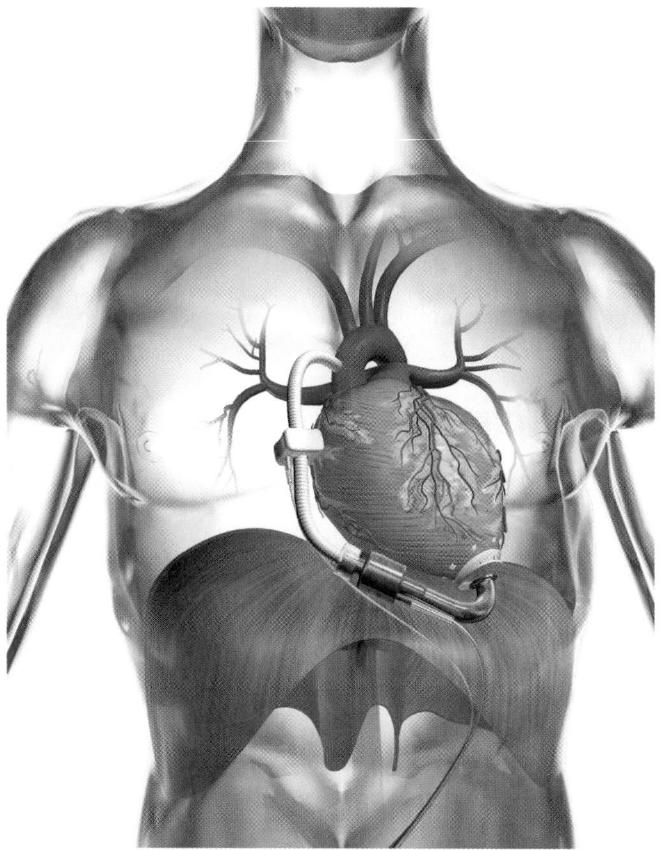

FIGURE 56-15 MicroMed DeBakey ventricular assist device. (Courtesy MicroMed Cardiovascular, Inc., Houston, TX.)

7 years, 6 months, and 5 days, before dying of renal failure with a healthy heart. The overall results are very good; some deaths have been caused by multiple organ failure and right-sided heart failure in the very sick patients chosen to undergo implantation. Clinical studies are under way, and perioperative morbidity and mortality rates are lower than those for many other LVADs. Moreover, device reliability is unsurpassed: so far, there has not been a single failure of the pump mechanism. The level of hemolysis is clinically insignificant, and most patients regain normal renal, hepatic, and pulmonary function after device implantation. Because of this success, the Jarvik 2000 is likely to play a major role in a wide variety of clinical scenarios.[122]

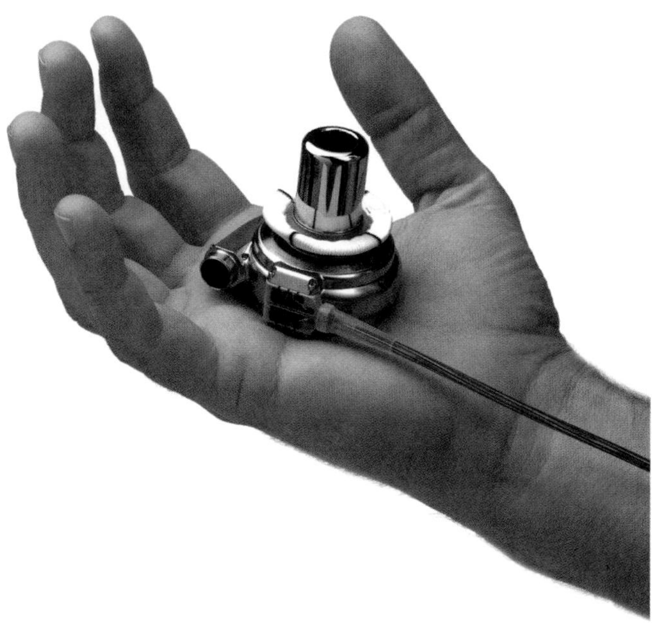

FIGURE 56-16 HeartWare left ventricular assist device. (Courtesy HeartWare, Miramar, FL.)

MicroMed DeBakey VAD

The MicroMed DeBakey VAD is the result of collaboration among the DeBakey Heart Center, MicroMed Corporation, and the National Aeronautics and Space Administration (NASA). This axial-flow, nonpulsatile device was designed by a NASA engineer who received a heart transplant from Dr. DeBakey. The MicroMed DeBakey VAD is 3 inches long and 1 inch in diameter and weighs 53 g. It consists of an inflow cannula implanted in the left ventricular apex, a spinning impeller pump that contains a bearing, and an outflow cannula anastomosed to the ascending aorta (Figure 56-15). Outflow is monitored with a flow probe. The initial clinical results look promising, but significant regurgitation may result if the device stops. The risk of thrombosis and embolization appears to be high if sufficient anticoagulation is not achieved.[116] As of late 2002, the device had been implanted in 173 patients worldwide; 21 patients were supported for more than 6 months and one for more than 441 days. The overall experience is good, and design modifications are being made to reduce the risk of thrombosis.[123-127]

HeartMate III

The HeartMate III (Thoratec Corporation) is being evaluated in animals. This pump has a transcutaneous energy transmission system that permits complete implantation and a magnetically suspended rotor that minimizes wear and may allow unparalleled longevity.

MVAD by HeartWare

The miniature VAD (MVAD; HeartWare, Inc., Miramar, Florida) is a small pump with a wide-blade rotor design and a magnetically suspended impeller that generates axial blood flow (Figure 56-16). This design portends increased durability and longevity.[128] According to initial results from the HeartWare LVAS International Clinic Trial in Europe, 91% of patients survived 180 days after implantation.[129] A bridge-to-transplantation trial is under way in the United States.

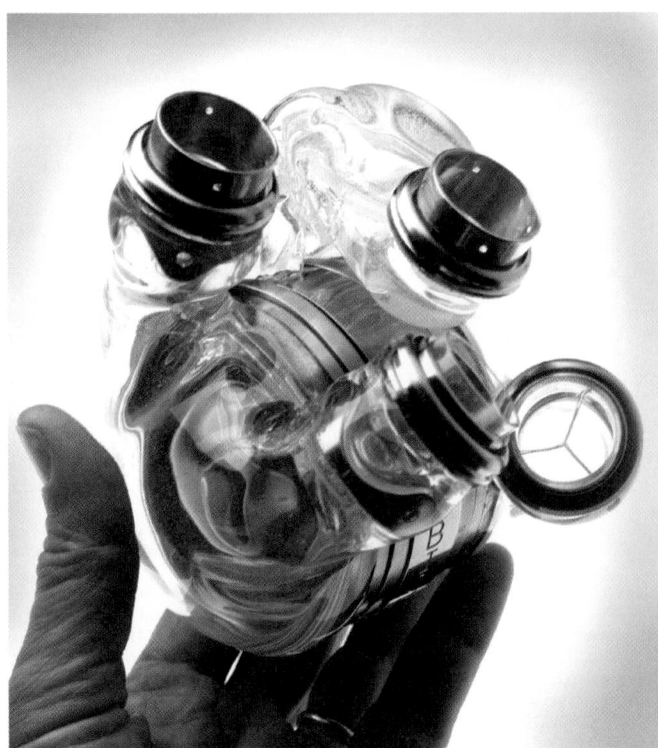

FIGURE 56-17 AbioCor total artificial heart. (Courtesy Abiomed, Danvers, MA.)

Abiomed Total Artificial Heart

In an NHLBI-sponsored trial, the Texas Heart Institute and the Abiomed Corporation jointly tested the AbioCor TAH in hopes that it may eventually be used as a long-term cardiac substitute, a treatment for acute heart failure, and a bridge to transplantation. This biventricular pump is implanted orthotopically and relies on a flexible, hydraulically actuated membrane sac (Figure 56-17). The centrifugal pump is driven by a brushless direct-current motor that rotates at 6000 to 8000 rpm. The motor is powered by an internal battery, which is recharged by means of transcutaneous energy transmission. The direction of hydraulic flow can be easily reversed with a rotating valve. Because the valves and pumps are made of polyurethane, the pump is unusually quiet. The AbioCor was first implanted clinically in 2001, at the University of Kentucky, in a patient whose life expectancy was less than 30 days. In September 2006, the FDA approved a humanitarian device exemption for the AbioCor TAH after it was implanted in 14 patients. This study showed that the device is safe and benefits patients with severe heart failure for whom death is imminent. After initial clinical use, the atrial cage of the AbioCor TAH was redesigned to reduce the risk of thromboembolic events. To further refine and improve this technology, Abiomed will conduct a postmarket study of an additional 25 patients.

CONCLUSION

Since the advent of MCS in the 1960s, extensive strides have been made in device technology, patient selection, and postoperative management. Long-term MCS is yielding insights into the biological processes of congestive heart failure and the effects of ventricular unloading. New applications, including bridging to myocardial improvement and permanent cardiac replacement, are becoming clinical realities. In clinical trials, LVAD implantation has produced survival rates at 1 year that rival those achieved with cardiac transplantation. The improved patient outcomes with newer devices have encouraged earlier referral of patients with advanced heart failure for MCS. Although improvements are still needed in several areas, MCS is restoring an increasing number of patients with end-stage heart failure to productive, high-quality lives.

REFERENCES

1. Ashton, R. C., Jr., Goldstein, D. J., Rose, E. A., et al. (1996). Duration of left ventricular assist device support affects transplant survival. *J Heart Lung Transplant, 15*, 1151–1157.
2. Frazier, O. H., Macris, M. P., Myers, T. J., et al. (1994). Improved survival after extended bridge to cardiac transplantation. *Ann Thorac Surg, 57*, 1416–1422.
3. Nishimura, M., Radovancevic, B., Odegaard, P., et al. (1996). Exercise capacity recovers slowly but fully in patients with a left ventricular assist device. *ASAIO J, 42*(5), M568–M570.
4. Frazier, O. H., Rose, E. A., McCarthy, P., et al. (1995). Improved mortality and rehabilitation of transplant candidates treated with a long-term implantable left ventricular assist system. *Ann Surg, 222*, 327–336.
5. Delgado, R., III, Radovancevic, B., Massin, E. K., et al. (1998). Neurohormonal changes after implantation of a left ventricular assist system. *ASAIO J, 44*, 299–302.
6. DeRose, J. J., Jr., Umana, J. P., Argenziano, M., et al. (1997). Implantable left ventricular assist devices provide an excellent outpatient bridge to transplantation and recovery. *J Am Coll Cardiol, 30*, 1773–1777.
7. Frazier, O. H., & Myers, T. J. (1999). Left ventricular assist system as a bridge to myocardial recovery. *Ann Thorac Surg, 68*, 734–741.
8. Hetzer, R., Muller, J., Weng, Y., et al. (1999). Cardiac recovery in dilated cardiomyopathy by unloading with a left ventricular assist device. *Ann Thorac Surg, 68*, 742–749.
9. Loebe, M., Hennig, E., Muller, J., et al. (1997). Long-term mechanical circulatory support as a bridge to transplantation, for recovery from cardiomyopathy, and for permanent replacement. *Eur J Cardiothorac Surg, 11*(Suppl), S18–S24.
10. Loebe, M., Muller, J., & Hetzer, R. (1999). Ventricular assistance for recovery of cardiac failure. *Curr Opin Cardiol, 14*, 234–248.
11. Müller, J., Wallukat, G., Weng, Y. G., et al. (1997). [Temporary mechanical left heart support: recovery of heart function in patients with end-stage idiopathic dilated cardiomyopathy]. *Herz, 22*, 227–236.
12. Oz, M. C., Argenziano, M., Catanese, K. A., et al. (1997). Bridge experience with long-term implantable left ventricular assist devices: are they an alternative to transplantation? *Circulation, 95*, 1844–1852.
13. Torre-Amione, G., Stetson, S. J., Youker, K. A., et al. (1999). Decreased expression of tumor necrosis factor–α in failing human myocardium after mechanical circulatory support: a potential mechanism for cardiac recovery. *Circulation, 100*, 1189–1193.
14. Westaby, S., Jin, X. Y., Katsumata, T., et al. (1997). Mechanical support in dilated cardiomyopathy: signs of early left ventricular recovery. *Ann Thorac Surg, 64*, 1303–1308.
15. Funk, D. (1991). Epidemiology of end-stage heart disease. In J. R. Hogness, & M. VanAntwerp (Eds.), *The artificial heart: prototypes, policies, and patients.* Washington, DC: National Academy Press, pp 251–261.
16. Gibbon, J. H., Jr. (1954). Application of a mechanical heart and lung apparatus to cardiac surgery. *Minn Med, 37*, 171–185.
17. Spencer, F. C., Eiseman, B., Trinkle, J. K., et al. (1965). Assisted circulation for cardiac failure following intracardiac surgery with cardiopulmonary bypass. *J Thorac Cardiovasc Surg, 49*, 56–73.
18. DeBakey, M. E., Liotta, D., & Hall, C. W. (1966). Left heart bypass using an implantable blood pump. In Committee on Trauma, Division of Medical Sciences, National Academy of Sciences, National Research Council (Ed.). *Mechanical devices to assist the failing heart/proceedings of a conference sponsored by the Committee on Trauma, Division of Medical Sciences, National Academy of Sciences, National Research Council, September 9 and 10, 1964 (NAS-NRC Publication No. 1283)* Washington, DC: National Academy of Sciences—National Research Council.
19. DeBakey, M. E. (1971). Left ventricular bypass pump for cardiac assistance: clinical experience. *Am J Cardiol, 27*, 3–11.
20. Moulopoulos, S. D., Topaz, S. R., & Kolff, W. J. (1962). Extracorporeal assistance to the circulation and intraaortic balloon pumping. *Trans Am Soc Artif Intern Organs, 8*, 85–89.
21. Kantrowitz, A., Tjonneland, S., Freed, P. S., et al. (1968). Initial clinical experience with intraaortic balloon pumping in cardiogenic shock. *JAMA, 203*, 113–118.
22. Cooley, D. A., Liotta, D., Hallman, G. L., et al. (1969). Orthotopic cardiac prosthesis for two-staged cardiac replacement. *Am J Cardiol, 24*, 723–730.
23. DeVries, W. C. (1988). The permanent artificial heart: four case reports. *JAMA, 259*, 849–859.
24. Johnson, K. E., Liska, M. B., Joyce, L. D., et al. (1992). Registry report. Use of total artificial hearts: summary of world experience, 1969-1991. *ASAIO J, 38*(3), M486–M492.
25. Norman, J. C., Brook, M. I., Cooley, D. A., et al. (1978). Total support of the circulation of a patient with post-cardiotomy stone-heart syndrome by a partial artificial heart (ALVAD) for 5 days followed by heart and kidney transplantation. *Lancet, 1*(8074), 1125–1127.
26. Campbell, C. D., Tolitano, D. J., Weber, K. T., et al. (1988). Mechanical support for post-cardiotomy heart failure. *J Card Surg, 3*, 181–191.
27. Pae, W. E., Jr., Miller, C. A., & Pierce, W. S. (1989). Combined registry for the clinical use of mechanical ventricular assist pumps and the total artificial heart: third official report—1988. *J Heart Transplant, 8*, 277–280.
28. Parmley, W. (1983). Cardiac failure. In M. R. Rosen, & B. F. Hoffman (Eds.), *Cardiac therapy* Boston: Martinus Nijhoff, pp 21–44.
29. Shoemaker, W. C., Bland, R. D., & Appel, P. L. (1985). Therapy of critically ill postoperative patients based on outcome prediction and prospective clinical trials. *Surg Clin North Am, 65*, 811–833.
30. Votapka, T. V., & Pennington, D. G. (1994). Circulatory assist devices in congestive heart failure. *Cardiol Clin, 12*, 143–154.

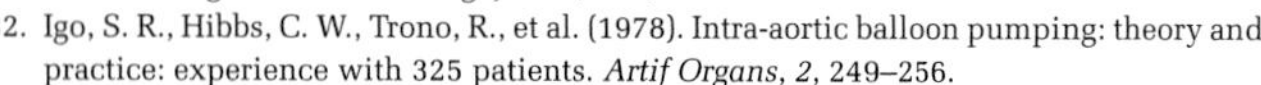

31. Page, D. L., Caulfield, J. B., Kastor, J. A., et al. (1971). Myocardial changes associated with cardiogenic shock. *N Engl J Med*, *285*, 133–137.
32. Igo, S. R., Hibbs, C. W., Trono, R., et al. (1978). Intra-aortic balloon pumping: theory and practice: experience with 325 patients. *Artif Organs*, *2*, 249–256.
33. Alcan, K. E., Stertzer, S. H., Wallsh, E., et al. (1984). Current status of intra-aortic balloon counterpulsation in critical care cardiology. *Crit Care Med*, *12*, 489–495.
34. Alderman, J. D., Gabliani, G. I., McCabe, C. H., et al. (1987). Incidence and management of limb ischemia with percutaneous wire-guided intraaortic balloon catheters. *J Am Coll Cardiol*, *9*, 524–530.
35. Chen, J. M., Spanier, T. B., Gonzalez, J. J., et al. (1999). Improved survival in patients with acute myocarditis using external pulsatile mechanical ventricular assistance. *J Heart Lung Transplant*, *18*, 351–357.
36. Shook, B. J. (1993). The Abiomed BVS 5000 biventricular support system: system description and clinical summary. *Card Surg State Art Rev*, *7*, 309–316.
37. Ciardullo, R. C., Schaff, H. V., Flaherty, J. T., et al. (1978). Comparison of regional myocardial blood flow and metabolism distal to a critical coronary stenosis in the fibrillating heart during alternate periods of pulsatile and nonpulsatile perfusion. *J Thorac Cardiovasc Surg*, *75*, 193–205.
38. Gaer, J. A., Shaw, A. D., Wild, R., et al. (1994). Effect of cardiopulmonary bypass on gastrointestinal perfusion and function. *Ann Thorac Surg*, *57*, 371–375.
39. Jett, G. K. (1996). ABIOMED BVS 5000: experience and potential advantages. *Ann Thorac Surg*, *61*, 301–304.
40. Minami, K., el-Banayosy, A., Posival, H., et al. (1992). Improvement of survival rate in patients with cardiogenic shock by using nonpulsatile and pulsatile ventricular assist device. *Int J Artif Organs*, *15*, 715–721.
41. Minami, K., Korner, M. M., Vyska, K., et al. (1990). Effects of pulsatile perfusion on plasma catecholamine levels and hemodynamics during and after cardiac operations with cardiopulmonary bypass. *J Thorac Cardiovasc Surg*, *99*, 82–91.
42. Taylor, K. M., Bain, W. H., Davidson, K. G., et al. (1982). Comparative clinical study of pulsatile and non-pulsatile perfusion in 350 consecutive patients. *Thorax*, *37*, 324–330.
43. Dixon, C. M., & Magovern, G. J. (1982). Evaluation of the Biopump for long term cardiac support without heparinization. *J Extracorp Technol*, *14*, 331.
44. De Robertis, F., Rogers, P., Amrani, M., et al. (2008). Bridge to decision using the Levitronix CentriMag short-term ventricular assist device. *J Heart Lung Transplant*, *27*, 474–478.
45. Dixon, S. R., Henriques, J. P., Mauri, L., et al. (2009). A prospective feasibility trial investigating the use of the Impella 2.5 system in patients undergoing high-risk percutaneous coronary intervention (The PROTECT I Trial): initial U.S. experience. *JACC Cardiovasc Interv*, *2*, 91–96.
46. Bank, A. J., Mir, S. H., Nguyen, D. Q., et al. (2000). Effects of left ventricular assist devices on outcomes in patients undergoing heart transplantation. *Ann Thorac Surg*, *69*, 1369–1374.
47. Frazier, O. H., Benedict, C. R., Radovancevic, B., et al. (1996). Improved left ventricular function after chronic left ventricular unloading. *Ann Thorac Surg*, *62*, 675–681.
48. Miller, L. W., Pagani, F. D., Russell, S. D., et al. (2007). Use of a continuous-flow device in patients awaiting heart transplantation. *N Engl J Med*, *357*, 885–896.
49. Farrar, D. J., Hill, J. D., Gray, L. A., Jr., et al. (1988). Heterotopic prosthetic ventricles as a bridge to cardiac transplantation: a multicenter study in 29 patients. *N Engl J Med*, *318*, 333–340.
50. Pae, W. E., Jr., Rosenberg, G., Donachy, J. H., et al. (1980). Mechanical circulatory assistance for postoperative cardiogenic shock: a three year experience. *Trans Am Soc Artif Intern Organs*, *26*, 256–261.
51. Farrar, D. J., & Litwak, P. (1991). 100 VAD survivors. *Thoratec's Heartbeat*, *5*, 1.
52. Pennington, D. G., McBride, L. R., Swartz, M. T., et al. (1989). Use of the Pierce-Donachy ventricular assist device in patients with cardiogenic shock after cardiac operations. *Ann Thorac Surg*, *47*, 130–135.
53. Arabia, F. A., Smith, R. G., Rose, D. S., et al. (1996). Success rates of long-term circulatory assist devices used currently for bridge to heart transplantation. *ASAIO J*, *42*(5), M542–M546.
54. Farrar, D. J., & Hill, J. D. (1993). Univentricular and biventricular Thoratec VAD support as a bridge to transplantation. *Ann Thorac Surg*, *55*, 276–282.
55. Olsen, D. B. (1992). Artificial organs of the future. *ASAIO J*, *38*(3), M134–M138.
56. Arabia, F. A., Copeland, J. G., Smith, R. G., et al. (1998). Infections with the CardioWest total artificial heart. *ASAIO J*, *44*(5), M336–M339.
57. Arabia, F. A., Copeland, J. G., Smith, R. G., et al. (1999). CardioWest total artificial heart: a retrospective controlled study. *Artif Organs*, *23*, 204–207.
58. Copeland, J. G., Levinson, M. M., Smith, R., et al. (1986). The total artificial heart as a bridge to transplantation: a report of two cases. *JAMA*, *256*, 2991–2995.
59. Copeland, J. G., Smith, R. G., Arabia, F. A., et al. (2004). Cardiac replacement with a total artificial heart as a bridge to transplantation. *N Engl J Med*, *351*, 859–867.
60. Slepian, M. J., Smith, R. G., & Copeland, J. G. (2006). The SynCardia CardioWest™ total artificial heart. In K. L. Baughman, & W. A. Baumgartner (Eds.). *Treatment of Advanced Heart Disease*. New York: Taylor & Francis, pp 473–490.
61. Shinn, J. A., & Oyer, P. E. (1993). Novacor ventricular assist system. In S. J. Qual (Ed.), *Cardiac mechanical assistance beyond balloon pumping*. St. Louis: Mosby, p 99.
62. McCarthy, P. M., Portner, P. M., Tobler, H. G., et al. (1991). Clinical experience with the Novacor ventricular assist system: bridge to transplantation and the transition to permanent application. *J Thorac Cardiovasc Surg*, *102*, 578–586.
63. Portner, P. M., Oyer, P. E., Pennington, D. G., et al. (1989). Implantable electrical left ventricular assist system: bridge to transplantation and the future. *Ann Thorac Surg*, *47*, 142–150.
64. Robbins, R. C., Kown, M. H., Portner, P. M., et al. (2001). The totally implantable novacor left ventricular assist system. *Ann Thorac Surg*, *71*(3 Suppl), S162–S165.
65. Rogers, J. G., Butler, J., Lansman, S. L., et al. (2007). Chronic mechanical circulatory support for inotrope-dependent heart failure patients who are not transplant candidates: results of the INTrEPID Trial. *J Am Coll Cardiol*, 50, 741-747.
66. Rose, E. A., Levin, H. R., Oz, M. C., et al. (1994). Artificial circulatory support with textured interior surfaces: a counterintuitive approach to minimizing thromboembolism. *Circulation*, *90*(5 Pt 2), II87–II91.
67. Frazier, O. H., Duncan, J. M., Radovancevic, B., et al. (1992). Successful bridge to heart transplantation with a new left ventricular assist device. *J Heart Lung Transplant*, *11*(3 Pt 1), 530–537.
68. Frazier, O. H., Rose, E. A., Macmanus, Q., et al. (1992). Multicenter clinical evaluation of the HeartMate 1000 IP left ventricular assist device. *Ann Thorac Surg*, *53*, 1080–1090.
69. Frazier, O. H., Rose, E. A., Oz, M. C., et al. (2001). Multicenter clinical evaluation of the HeartMate vented electric left ventricular assist system in patients awaiting heart transplantation. *J Thorac Cardiovasc Surg*, *122*, 1186–1195.
70. Rose, E. A., Gelijns, A. C., Moskowitz, A. J., et al. (2001). Long-term mechanical left ventricular assistance for end-stage heart failure. *N Engl J Med*, *345*, 1435–1443.
71. Griffith, B. P., Kormos, R. L., Borovetz, H. S., et al. (2001). HeartMate II left ventricular assist system: from concept to first clinical use. *Ann Thorac Surg*, *71*(3 Suppl), S116–S120.
72. Slaughter, M. S., Tsui, S. S., El-Banayosy, A., et al. (2007). Results of a multicenter clinical trial with the Thoratec Implantable Ventricular Assist Device. *J Thorac Cardiovasc Surg*, *133*, 1573–1580.
72a. US Food and Drug Administration. Thoratec HeartMate II LVAS: P060040/S005. February 22, 2010. Available at: http://www.fda.gov/MedicalDevices/ProductsandMedicalProcedures/DeviceApprovalsandClearances/Recently-ApprovedDevices/ucm201473.htm. Accessed July 20, 2010.
72b. Slaughter, M. S., Rogers, J. G., Milano, C. A., et al. (2009). Advanced heart failure treated with continuous-flow left ventricular assist device. N Engl J Med, 361, 2241-2251.
73. Mehta, S. M., Aufiero, T. X., Pae, W. E., Jr., et al. (1995). Combined Registry for the Clinical Use of Mechanical Ventricular Assist Pumps and the Total Artificial Heart in conjunction with heart transplantation: sixth official report—1994. *J Heart Lung Transplant*, *14*, 585–593.
74. Quaini, E., Pavie, A., Chieco, S., et al. (1997). The Concerted Action "Heart" European registry on clinical application of mechanical circulatory support systems: bridge to transplant. The Registry Scientific Committee. *Eur J Cardiothorac Surg*, *11*, 182–188.
75. Livingston, E. R., Fisher, C. A., Bibidakis, E. J., et al. (1996). Increased activation of the coagulation and fibrinolytic systems leads to hemorrhagic complications during left ventricular assist implantation. *Circulation*, *94*(9 Suppl), II-227–II-234.
76. Wegner, J. A., DiNardo, J. A., Arabia, F. A., et al. (2000). Blood loss and transfusion requirements in patients implanted with a mechanical circulatory support device undergoing cardiac transplantation. *J Heart Lung Transplant*, *19*, 504–506.
77. Holman, W. L., Murrah, C. P., Ferguson, E. R., et al. (1996). Infections during extended circulatory support: University of Alabama at Birmingham experience 1989 to 1994. *Ann Thorac Surg*, *61*, 366–371.
78. Johnson, K. E., Prieto, M., Joyce, L. D., et al. (1992). Summary of the clinical use of the Symbion total artificial heart: a registry report. *J Heart Lung Transplant*, *11*(1 Pt 1), 103–116.
79. Moroney, D. A., & Vaca, K. J. (1995). Infectious complications associated with ventricular assist devices. *Am J Crit Care*, *4*, 204–209.
80. Herrmann, M., Weyand, M., Greshake, B., et al. (1997). Left ventricular assist device infection is associated with increased mortality but is not a contraindication to transplantation. *Circulation*, *95*, 814–817.
81. McBride, L. R., Swartz, M. T., Reedy, J. E., et al. (1991). Device related infections in patients supported with mechanical circulatory support devices for greater than 30 days. *ASAIO Trans*, *37*(3), M258–M259.
82. McCarthy, P. M., Schmitt, S. K., Vargo, R. L., et al. (1996). Implantable LVAD infections: implications for permanent use of the device. *Ann Thorac Surg*, *61*, 359–365.
83. Springer, W. E., Wasler, A., Radovancevic, B., et al. (1996). Retrospective analysis of infection in patients undergoing support with left ventricular assist systems. *ASAIO J*, *42*(5), M763–M765.
84. Lietz, K., Long, J. W., Kfoury, A. G., et al. (2007). Outcomes of left ventricular assist device implantation as destination therapy in the post-REMATCH era: implications for patient selection. *Circulation*, *116*, 497–505.
85. Birks, E. J., Tansley, P. D., Hardy, J., et al. (2006). Left ventricular assist device and drug therapy for the reversal of heart failure. *N Engl J Med*, *355*, 1873–1884.
86. Frazier, O. H., Gemmato, C., Myers, T. J., et al. (2007). Initial clinical experience with the HeartMate II axial-flow left ventricular assist device. *Tex Heart Inst J*, *34*, 275–281.
87. Pennington, D. G., McBride, L. R., Peigh, P. S., et al. (1994). Eight years' experience with bridging to cardiac transplantation. *J Thorac Cardiovasc Surg*, *107*, 472–480.
88. Dasse, K. A., Frazier, O. H., Lesniak, J. M., et al. (1992). Clinical responses to ventricular assistance versus transplantation in a series of bridge to transplant patients. *ASAIO J*, *38*(3), M622–M626.
89. Mancini, D. M., Beniaminovitz, A., Levin, H., et al. (1998). Low incidence of myocardial recovery after left ventricular assist device implantation in patients with chronic heart failure. *Circulation*, *98*, 2383–2389.
90. Müller, J., Wallukat, G., Weng, Y. G., et al. (1997). Weaning from mechanical cardiac support in patients with idiopathic dilated cardiomyopathy. *Circulation*, *96*, 542–549.
91. Razeghi, P., Mukhopadhyay, M., Myers, T. J., et al. (2001). Myocardial tumor necrosis factor–α expression does not correlate with clinical indices of heart failure in patients on left ventricular assist device support. *Ann Thorac Surg*, *72*, 2044–2050.
92. Zafeiridis, A., Jeevanandam, V., Houser, S. R., et al. (1998). Regression of cellular hypertrophy after left ventricular assist device support. *Circulation*, *98*, 656–662.
93. Rivello, H. G., Meckert, P. C., Vigliano, C., et al. (2001). Cardiac myocyte nuclear size and ploidy status decrease after mechanical support. *Cardiovasc Pathol*, *10*(2), 53–57.
94. McCarthy, P. M., Nakatani, S., Vargo, R., et al. (1995). Structural and left ventricular histologic changes after implantable LVAD insertion. *Ann Thorac Surg*, *59*, 609–613.

95. Scheinin, S. A., Capek, P., Radovancevic, B., et al. (1992). The effect of prolonged left ventricular support on myocardial histopathology in patients with end-stage cardiomyopathy. *ASAIO J, 38*(3), M271–M274.
96. Bruckner, B. A., Stetson, S. J., Farmer, J. A., et al. (2000). The implications for cardiac recovery of left ventricular assist device support on myocardial collagen content. *Am J Surg, 180*, 498–501.
97. Bruckner, B. A., Stetson, S. J., Perez-Verdia, A., et al. (2001). Regression of fibrosis and hypertrophy in failing myocardium following mechanical circulatory support. *J Heart Lung Transplant, 20*, 457–464.
98. Narula, J., Pandey, P., Arbustini, E., et al. (1999). Apoptosis in heart failure: release of cytochrome *c* from mitochondria and activation of caspase-3 in human cardiomyopathy. *Proc Natl Acad Sci U S A, 96*, 8144–8149.
99. Bartling, B., Milting, H., Schumann, H., et al. (1999). Myocardial gene expression of regulators of myocyte apoptosis and myocyte calcium homeostasis during hemodynamic unloading by ventricular assist devices in patients with end-stage heart failure. *Circulation, 100*(19 Suppl), II216-II223.
100. Uray, I. P., Connelly, J. H., Frazier, O., et al. (2001). Altered expression of tyrosine kinase receptors Her2/neu and GP130 following left ventricular assist device (LVAD) placement in patients with heart failure. *J Heart Lung Transplant, 20*, 210.
101. Francis, G. S., Anwar, F., Bank, A. J., et al. (1999). Apoptosis, *Bcl*-2, and proliferating cell nuclear antigen in the failing human heart: observations made after implantation of left ventricular assist device. *J Card Fail, 5*, 308–315.
102. Beltrami, A. P., Urbanek, K., Kajstura, J., et al. (2001). Evidence that human cardiac myocytes divide after myocardial infarction. *N Engl J Med, 344*, 1750–1757.
103. Depre, C., & Taegtmeyer, H. (2000). Metabolic aspects of programmed cell survival and cell death in the heart. *Cardiovasc Res, 45*, 538–548.
104. Bozkurt, B., Torre-Amione, G., Warren, M. S., et al. (2001). Results of targeted anti-tumor necrosis factor therapy with etanercept (ENBREL) in patients with advanced heart failure. *Circulation, 103*, 1044–1047.
105. Anker, S. D., & Coats, A. J. (2002). How to RECOVER from RENAISSANCE? The significance of the results of RECOVER, RENAISSANCE, RENEWAL and ATTACH. *Int J Cardiol, 86*(2-3), 123–130.
106. Chung, E. S., Packer, M., Lo, K. H., et al. (2003). Randomized, double-blind, placebo-controlled, pilot trial of infliximab, a chimeric monoclonal antibody to tumor necrosis factor–α, in patients with moderate-to-severe heart failure: results of the Anti-TNF Therapy Against Congestive Heart Failure (ATTACH) trial. *Circulation, 107*, 3133–3140.
107. Depre, C., Shipley, G. L., Chen, W., et al. (1998). Unloaded heart in vivo replicates fetal gene expression of cardiac hypertrophy. *Nat Med, 4*, 1269–1275.
108. Aquila-Pastir, L. A., McCarthy, P. M., Smedira, N. G., et al. (2001). Mechanical unloading decreases the expression of beta-tubulin in the failing human heart. *J Heart Lung Transplant, 20*, 211.
109. Baba, H. A., Grabellus, F., August, C., et al. (2000). Reversal of metallothionein expression is different throughout the human myocardium after prolonged left-ventricular mechanical support. *J Heart Lung Transplant, 19*, 668–674.
110. Stetson, S. J., Perez-Verdia, A., Vatta, M., et al. (2001). Improved myocardial structure following LVAD support: effect of unloading on dystrophin expression. *J Heart Lung Transplant, 20*, 240.
111. Dipla, K., Mattiello, J. A., Jeevanandam, V., et al. (1998). Myocyte recovery after mechanical circulatory support in humans with end-stage heart failure. *Circulation, 97*, 2316–2322.
112. Ogletree-Hughes, M. L., Stull, L. B., Sweet, W. E., et al. (2001). Mechanical unloading restores β-adrenergic responsiveness and reverses receptor downregulation in the failing human heart. *Circulation, 104*, 881–886.
113. Heerdt, P. M., Holmes, J. W., Cai, B., et al. (2000). Chronic unloading by left ventricular assist device reverses contractile dysfunction and alters gene expression in end-stage heart failure. *Circulation, 102*, 2713–2719.
114. Ritter, M., Su, Z., Xu, S., et al. (2000). Cardiac unloading alters contractility and calcium homeostasis in ventricular myocytes. *J Mol Cell Cardiol, 32*, 577–584.
115. Khan, T., Okerberg, K., Hernandez, A., et al. (2001). Assessment of myocardial recovery using dobutamine stress echocardiography in LVAD patients. *J Heart Lung Transplant, 20*, 202–203.
116. Grady, K. L., Meyer, P., Mattea, A., et al. (2001). Improvement in quality of life outcomes 2 weeks after left ventricular assist device implantation. *J Heart Lung Transplant, 20*, 657–669.
117. Moskowitz, A. J., Weinberg, A. D., Oz, M. C., et al. (1997). Quality of life with an implanted left ventricular assist device. *Ann Thorac Surg, 64*, 1764–1769.
118. Dew, M. A., Kormos, R. L., Winowich, S., et al. (1999). Quality of life outcomes in left ventricular assist system inpatients and outpatients. *ASAIO J, 45*, 218–225.
119. Morales, D. L., Catanese, K. A., Helman, D. N., et al. (2000). Six-year experience of caring for forty-four patients with a left ventricular assist device at home: safe, economical, necessary. *J Thorac Cardiovasc Surg, 119*, 251–259.
120. Macris, M. P., Parnis, S. M., Frazier, O. H., et al. (1997). Development of an implantable ventricular assist system. *Ann Thorac Surg, 63*, 367–370.
121. Parnis, S. M., Conger, J. L., Fuqua, J. M., Jr., et al. (1997). Progress in the development of a transcutaneously powered axial flow blood pump ventricular assist system. *ASAIO J, 43*(5), M576–M580.
122. Westaby, S., Katsumata, T., Houel, R., et al. (1998). Jarvik 2000 heart: potential for bridge to myocyte recovery. *Circulation, 98*, 1568–1574.
123. DeBakey, M. E. (1999). A miniature implantable axial flow ventricular assist device. *Ann Thorac Surg, 68*, 637–640.
124. Kawahito, K., Benkowski, R., Otsubo, S., et al. (1996). Ex vivo evaluation of the NASA/DeBakey axial flow ventricular assist device: results of a 2 week screening test. *ASAIO J, 42*(5), M754–M757.
125. Kawahito, K., Damm, G., Benkowski, R., et al. (1996). Ex vivo phase 1 evaluation of the DeBakey/NASA axial flow ventricular assist device. *Artif Organs, 20*, 47–52.
126. Wieselthaler, G. M., Schima, H., Hiesmayr, M., et al. (2000). First clinical experience with the DeBakey VAD continuous-axial-flow pump for bridge to transplantation. *Circulation, 101*, 356–359.
127. Wieselthaler, G. M., Schima, H., Lassnigg, A., et al. (1999). [The DeBakey VAD axial flow pump: first clinical experience with a new generation of implantable, nonpulsatile blood pumps for long-term support prior to transplantation]. *Wien Klin Wochenschr, 111*, 629–635.
128. Slaughter, M. S., Sobieski, M. A., II, Tamez, D., et al. (2009). HeartWare miniature axial-flow ventricular assist device: design and initial feasibility test. *Tex Heart Inst J, 36*, 12–16.
129. Data presented at Cleveland Clinic 21st Century Treatment of Heart Failure: Synchronizing Surgical and Medical Therapies for Better Outcomes. October 18; Cleveland, Ohio. 2008.

CHAPTER 57

Exercise in Heart Failure

William E. Kraus

Until the middle of the 1970s, exercise testing was not routinely performed on patients with heart failure because of concerns about exacerbating symptoms, potential deleterious effects on ventricular function, and the possibility of severe cardiac dysrhythmias and arrest. For similar reasons, exercise training in patients with heart failure was actively shunned. In the late 1970s, studies began to demonstrate that exercise testing and training are safe in this population.[1] At the same time, the investigators noted the poor correlation between resting ventricular function and exercise capacity.[2,3] They decided patients with heart failure should no longer be excluded from diagnostic and prognostic exercise testing, nor should they be routinely advised to refrain from participating in exercise activities, including training. However, the effects of exercise training on symptoms and outcomes in heart failure patients remained unknown for many years.

Exercise intolerance, which is defined as the reduced ability to perform activities involving dynamic movement because of symptoms of dyspnea or fatigue, is the most common clinical symptom among patients with heart failure. The origin of exercise intolerance in patients with heart failure is multifactorial. Numerous investigations have identified potential mechanisms to explain the source of exercise intolerance. In this chapter, we review the potential mechanisms that underlie exercise intolerance in patients with heart failure and discuss the intricacies of exercise testing and training, with a focus on studies that have demonstrated the efficacy of exercise training in patients with heart failure.

MECHANISMS OF EXERCISE INTOLERANCE IN HEART FAILURE

Cardiovascular

The capacity for performing aerobic exercise depends on the ability of the heart to augment its output to exercising muscle and the ability of skeletal muscle to use oxygen delivered via the circulation (Figure 57-1). Typically, cardiac output is increased four to six times in normal subjects exercising to maximal capacity.[4] The increase in cardiac output results primarily from a substantial increase in heart rate with a modest increase in stroke volume (Figure 57-2). In fact, in normal individuals, the primary determinant of maximal exercise capacity is the increase in heart rate associated with an increase in workload; increases in arteriovenous oxygen difference and stroke volume (LV end-diastolic volume multiplied times ejection fraction) contribute relatively little. Increases in stroke volume are accomplished by use of both the Frank-Starling mechanism to augment LV end-diastolic volume and more complete LV emptying to reduce end-systolic volume. The ventricles have inotropic reserve; when this is coupled to peripheral vasodilation during exercise, there is a greater degree of ventricular emptying. Age, gender, genetic profile, and level of conditioning may affect one or several components of the determinants of maximal exercise capacity.[5]

In patients with heart failure, the reduction in functional exercise capacity appears to result from a complicated combination of impairments in central and peripheral mechanisms, including impairments in cardiac output and blood flow to skeletal muscle, decreases in perfusion to active skeletal muscle as a result of decreases in capillary density, and intrinsic abnormalities in skeletal muscle themselves secondary.[6-8] In patients with heart failure, LV dilation, and reduced resting LV systolic function, stroke volume typically increases only modestly during exercise because of a blunted ability to increase both LV preload and ejection fraction.[9]

The reduced ability to augment LV end-diastolic volume is explained by the Frank-Starling mechanism: the fact that the already dilated LV is operating near its maximal volume and has thus exhausted most of its preload reserve. The failure to increase LV systolic emptying and thereby augment LV ejection fraction arises from a combination of impaired intrinsic contractility, reduced β-adrenergic responsiveness, elevated systemic vascular resistance caused by increased activity of the sympathetic and renin-angiotensin-aldosterone systems, and a blunted peripheral arterial vasodilator response to exercise.[10] Some of the peripheral vasoconstriction may also be associated with changes in muscle pH and accumulation of metabolites. In patients with ischemic cardiomyopathy, stroke volume may fall during exercise if myocardial ischemia develops as a result of

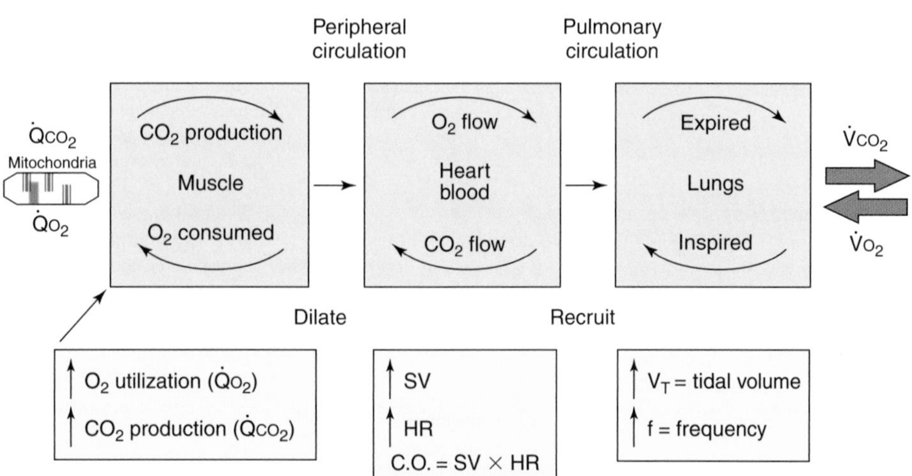

FIGURE 57-1 Pluripotent stem cells from different sources can be expanded in vitro and differentiated into cardiac progenitor cells and mature cardiac cell types, thus enabling cell-replacement therapy or tissue engineering. CPC, Cardiac progenitor cell; ESC, embryonic stem cell; iPS cell, induced pluripotent stem cell; PSC, parthenogenetic stem cell; SGSC, spermatogonial stem cell. (From Wollert, K. C. and Drexler, H. C. (2010). Cell therapy for the treatment of coronary heart disease: a critical appraisal. Nat. Rev. Cardiol. 7, 204-215).

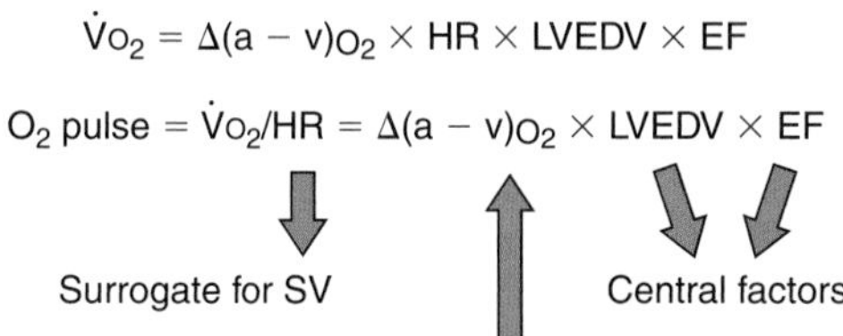

$\dot{V}O_2 = \Delta(a - v)O_2 \times HR \times LVEDV \times EF$
O_2 pulse $= \dot{V}O_2/HR = \Delta(a - v)O_2 \times LVEDV \times EF$
Surrogate for SV
Central factors
Oxygen carrying capacity of the blood &
peripheral (skeletal muscle) factors

FIGURE 57-2 The Fick equation for oxygen consumption ($\dot{V}O_2$). $\dot{V}O_2$ = arteriovenous oxygen difference × cardiac output; cardiac output represents heart rate (HR) × left ventricular end-diastolic volume (LVEDV) × ejection fraction (EF). The relation can be transformed to show that O_2 pulse ($\dot{V}O_2$/HR) is a surrogate for stroke volume, if arteriovenous oxygen difference is assumed to be constant (LVEDV × EF). Arteriovenous oxygen difference represents oxygen-carrying capacity of the blood (e.g., hemoglobin, red blood cell volume) and peripheral skeletal muscle factors.

excessive myocardial oxygen demand. Mitral regurgitation is often present during exercise in patients with heart failure and systolic dysfunction, as a result of dilation of the mitral annulus.[11] Such exercise-related mitral regurgitation reduces forward stroke volume but can be attenuated with vasodilators and diuretics.[11] Thus, in patients with heart failure, cardiac output is augmented primarily by heart rate increase because of the inherent limitations in stroke volume, as noted previously. Whereas maximal heart rate is usually reduced only mildly in patients with heart failure, blunting of heart rate reserve (i.e., the degree of heart rate augmentation above resting values) can be substantially blunted by current standard therapies for heart failure, such as β-adrenergic blockers and dual-chamber pacing. The chronotropic incompetence that results from such effects on acute exercise testing have been explored, but whether it influences the acquisition of an exercise training response is unknown.

Peripheral

Measures of central hemodynamic function, such as filling pressures (e.g., LV end-diastolic pressure), do not substantially explain the exercise intolerance experienced by the majority of patients with heart failure.[12] Clinicians increasingly appreciate the role of peripheral factors in exercise intolerance in heart failure, including abnormalities of endothelial function, ergoreflex activation, vasodilatory capacity, and intrinsic abnormalities in skeletal muscle, such as capillarity, fiber type, oxidative capacity, and channel function (see Duscha and associates[8] for review; Figure 57-3, *A*). Peripheral mechanisms account for exercise intolerance in heart failure in several ways: (1) The correlation between exercise capacity and measures of LV systolic function is poor,[3,13] and (2) central hemodynamic improvements can occur immediately with pharmacological therapy, but they do not translate into corresponding improvements in exercise capacity, which are delayed for weeks or months, if they occur at all.[14,15] This may be explained by the presence of a peripheral block in translating acute improvements in cardiac output into increased oxygen uptake and utilization in muscle. Perhaps a symptomatic improvement in heart failure results in increases in physical activity and exercise that lead to relief of the peripheral block, and improvements in translation of therapeutic increases in cardiac output translate into increases in exercise tolerance (see Figure 57-3, *B*).

Blood Flow

In general, patients with heart failure have decreased blood flow to the periphery because cardiac output is decreased. However, up to 26% of patients with heart failure have normal peripheral blood flow.[16] Muscle blood flow normally increases during exercise; in patients with heart failure, this does not happen, largely because of an abnormality in peripheral vasodilation.[17] In the late 1960s, peripheral vasodilatory capacity was shown to be impaired in response to an ischemic challenge (postocclusion hyperemia).[18] Zelis and colleagues[18-20] demonstrated that forearm blood flow during rest and exercise was reduced in patients with heart failure, and this abnormality was present in response to a variety of stimuli, including isotonic and isometric exercise, adrenergic blockade, ischemia, and direct arterial vasodilation.

More recent studies have demonstrated that in such patients, leg vascular resistance fails to decrease normally during exercise.[21,22] This impairment in vasodilatory capacity has been attributed to excessive sympathetic stimulation, which causes vasoconstriction, activation of the plasma renin-angiotensin-aldosterone system, excessive levels of endothelin, or a combination of all these.[23,24] In addition, stiffness of the vascular wall secondary to increased vascular sodium content may impair appropriate vasodilatation. This finding is supported by

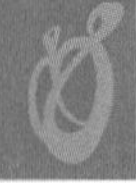

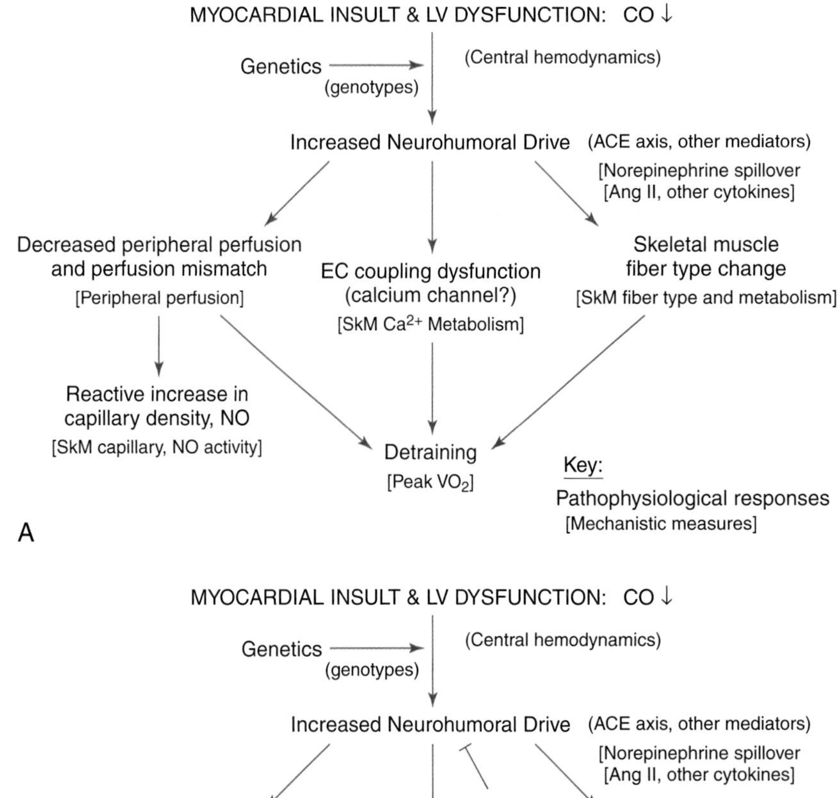

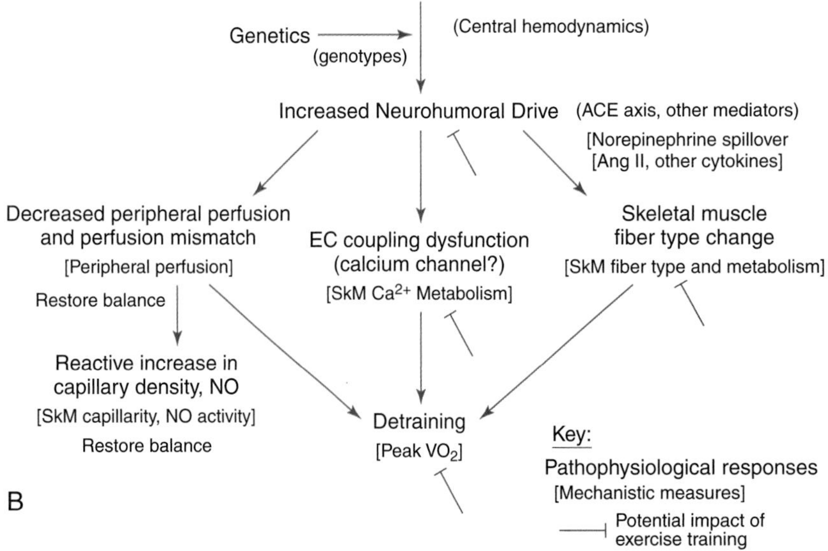

FIGURE 57–3 Exercise intolerance and training in heart failure. **A,** Model of exercise intolerance in heart failure. Left ventricular (LV) systolic dysfunction, induced by myocardial insult (e.g., myocardial infarction or myocarditis) and decreased cardiac output, can impair exercise tolerance. Pathophysiological responses at each step are represented in *large type,* and the corresponding mechanisms are represented in *small type in brackets.* **B,** Model of how exercise training might alleviate exercise intolerance in heart failure. This model is similar to that shown in **A:** At certain points, exercise training has been shown to induce a physiological response that might block progression to symptomatic exercise intolerance; these points are shown with *flat-headed arrows.* ACE, angiotensin-converting enzyme; Ang III, angiotensin III; EC, excitation-contraction; NO, nitric oxide; SkM, skeletal muscle; V_{O_2}, oxygen consumption.

the observations that the capillary basement membranes may be thickened in heart failure[25] and that vascular responsiveness is partially improved by diuretic therapy.[26] Angiotensin-converting enzyme (ACE) inhibition has been demonstrated to normalize impaired vasodilation after chronic (but not short-term) administration.[15,27] Improvements in leg blood flow after ACE inhibition parallel increases in exercise capacity.[27] In addition, a "vascular deconditioning" hypothesis suggests that abnormal vasodilatory capacity is related to deconditioning and that localized training of a specific limb may improve the vasodilatory response in heart failure.[28,29]

Intrinsic Skeletal Muscle Changes (see Chapter 19)

In heart failure, anaerobic metabolism, as a result of intrinsic abnormalities in skeletal muscle, occurs during exercise and is an important correlate of exercise intolerance. Previous studies with magnetic resonance imaging with phosphorus-31 have demonstrated that early anaerobic metabolism occurs independently of reduced muscle blood flow and appears to be a systemic response, not limited to muscles that would normally be used during exercise.[30,31] This latter observation implies that the stimuli that cause this metabolic skeletal muscle abnormality are systemic. Other skeletal muscle changes include fiber atrophy, loss of oxidative type I fibers with an increase in glycolytic type IIb fibers,[32-34] and changes in mitochondrial density and enzymes. Fiber changes can reduce muscle performance and cause early fatigue.

Skeletal muscle characteristics, furthermore, have important ramifications on substrate and oxygen use during exercise. Myosin heavy chain type I isoforms have also been shown to be decreased and related to peak oxygen consumption (V_{O_2}) in heart failure.[32] Although glycolytic enzyme levels appear to be unchanged, oxidative enzyme levels are decreased in heart failure.[30] Specifically, mitochondrial enzymes (citrate synthase and succinic dehydrogenase) and enzymes involved in β-oxidation of fatty acids (3-hydroxyl coenzyme A dehydrogenase) are decreased. Sullivan and associates[35] found inverse relationships between oxidative enzyme activity and blood lactate accumulation during sub maximal exercise. Drexler and colleagues[34] demonstrated a close relationship between cytochrome *c* oxidase, mitochondrial volume density or cristae surface density, and peak $\dot{V}O_2$. More recently, Hambrecht and colleagues[36] established that in patients with heart failure, the volume density of cytochrome *c* oxidase activity, which is reduced by 45%, could be increased with physical activity. Duscha and associates[37] also demonstrated a decrease in capillary density. Together, these findings suggest that intrinsic aberrations in skeletal muscle may contribute to abnormal oxygen extraction or substrate delivery and use and may further limit exercise tolerance in heart failure.

Endothelial Dysfunction (see Chapter 17)

The vascular endothelium releases vasoactive substances that play an important regulatory role in peripheral vasomotor tone. Vasodilating and vasoconstricting factors—including nitric oxide, endothelins, and prostaglandins derived from the endothelium—are released in response to various chemical, pharmacological, and exercise stimuli. A pivotal role of the endothelium in coordinating tissue perfusion has been recognized in heart failure. Studies have demonstrated that endothelium-dependent vasodilation is impaired in heart failure, manifested by a reduction in the release of nitric oxide in response to acetylcholine.[38-40] The release of nitric oxide, an important mediator of flow-dependent vasodilation, is normally stimulated by exercise but appears to be attenuated in patients with heart failure. This may contribute to a reduction in peripheral vasodilation and tissue perfusion. Blood flow during reactive hyperemia or exercise is reduced in response to blockade of nitric oxide synthesis.[41-43] L-Arginine (a nitric oxide precursor) improves abnormal vasodilation in response to acetylcholine or an ischemic stimulus in heart failure. These observations are consistent with the concept that impaired endothelial function contributes to reduced vasodilatory capacity in heart failure.[44] The severity of impairment in endothelium-dependent vasodilation is correlated with the degree of exercise intolerance and severity of New York Heart Association (NYHA) class.[43] Exercise training with or without supplemental L-arginine improves endothelial nitric oxide formation and endothelium-dependent vasodilation of the skeletal muscle vasculature.[44-46] Of interest is that exercise of specific muscle groups, such as those of the lower extremity, systemically enhances endothelial function. As noted, the aberration of intrinsic skeletal muscle properties is systemic in origin. It is conceivable that this aberration is related to systemic abnormalities in nitric oxide metabolism in heart failure and may underlie the power of exercise to reverse these defects (see Figure 57-3, *A* and *B*).

Ergoreflex Activation (see Chapter 16)

A specific proventilatory signal arising from exercising muscle, possibly including respiratory muscle, may be abnormally enhanced in heart failure.[47,48] Ergoreceptors are intramuscular afferent receptors that are sensitive to metabolic changes within skeletal muscle. Acidosis, when present in patients with heart failure, may sensitize these ergoreceptors to enhance their activity. Ergoreflex overactivity may be an early beneficial compensation that enhances sympathetic stimulation with increased ventilation and vasoconstriction to nonexercising muscle to maintain blood flow to essential circulatory beds. These compensatory mechanisms may lead to detrimental excess activity of sympathetic nerves, excessive vasoconstriction, and blunted vagal responses, which are characteristic of patients with heart failure.[49] Ponikowski and coworkers[48,49] showed that ergoreflex activation parallels exercise intolerance, whereas ventricular function is poorly related to neural reflexes. In addition, in this study, ergoreflex sensitivity was predictive of autonomic and reflex disturbances such as baroreflex attenuation and lower levels of central catecholamines, thus confirming that sympathetic inputs are enhanced and vagal reflex is impaired. Periodic breathing, in which enhanced chemoreflex plays an important role, was particularly prevalent in the subjects with enhanced ergoreflex.

The overactive muscle ergoreflex is more closely related to exercise intolerance and the abnormally elevated ventilatory response to exercise than are other autonomic indexes or reflexes. These data are consistent with a key role of the muscle ergoreflex in symptom generation and disease progression. The relation between ergoreflex activation and ventilatory responses that are known to be abnormal in patients with heart failure during exercise is stronger than expected for any level of workload and is related to outcome in chronic heart failure. No single theory has totally explained the overactive ventilatory drive noted in patients with heart failure during exercise. Activation of these reflexes appears to be attenuated by exercise training.[50]

FUNCTIONAL EXERCISE TESTING IN HEART FAILURE

Despite a marked increase in the population with heart failure since the 1990s, only more recently has exercise testing taken a more prominent role in the diagnosis and management of heart failure. Heart failure is characterized by the inability to perform desired activities because of dyspnea or fatigue, or both. Exercise testing is now a critical component of the evaluation of a patient with a presumed cardiac origin of presenting symptoms. Three exercise testing modalities of general use in the population with heart failure are discussed in this chapter: the 6-minute walk test; graded exercise testing with electrocardiographic monitoring; and cardiopulmonary exercise testing (CPET), which is graded exercise testing with gas exchange analysis. Each testing method has advantages in given clinical situations. Of these, CPET and the 6-minute walk are the most common modalities for evaluating the functional capacity of patients with heart failure. The 6-minute walk is used to evaluate low-level or submaximal work and is more compatible with activities of daily living; CPET is used to evaluate maximal exercise capacity, for prognostic stratification, and for staging for possible cardiac transplantation.

In addition, there are various graded exercise testing protocols in which the workload is progressively increased during the test, either on a bicycle or a treadmill. The selection of a particular protocol should be based on the experience of the testing physician, on the physical ability of the patient, and on the availability of the facility where the test is being performed. Exercise testing of patients with heart failure is supported by the American Heart Association[50,51] for clinical and research application.[52]

6-Minute Walk

The 6-minute walk test was first described by Guyatt and associates[52] for the evaluation of patients with pulmonary disease and was later adapted for patients with heart failure. Patients are asked to walk for 6 minutes at whatever pace is comfortable on a premeasured flat surface. Communication with the patient consists only of simple instructions and of the time remaining in the test. The number of meters covered during the 6 minutes is recorded. This test has been used in clinical trials to determine the benefits of pharmacotherapy in patients with heart failure because it is easy and inexpensive, and testing personnel require minimal training. However, the 6-minute walk test may not help distinguish between patients with mild to moderate heart failure and those with more advanced disease.[53] A distance of less than 300 m is considered indicative of severe exercise intolerance. Lucas and colleagues[53] tested patients with a wide range of V_{O_2} values and observed that the 6-minute walk test best helped discriminate patients with peak V_{O_2} of more than 20 mL/kg/min or Weber class A from those with extreme functional limitations of peak V_{O_2} (<10 mL/kg/min) or Weber class D.

In clinical trials, the reliability of the 6-minute walk test as a reliable marker of clinical improvement, progression of disease, or mortality has been inconsistent. For example, in the U.S. Carvedilol Heart Failure Study,[54] the 6-minute walk test was unable to detect improvements in symptoms or the clinical endpoints of hospitalizations or mortality despite the fact that carvedilol resulted in significant decreases in the rate of disease progression. Only in the SOLVD trial, was there a significant relation between the 6-minute walk test and clinical endpoints, including mortality.[55]

Cardiopulmonary Exercise Testing

CPET has a significant advantage over simple exercise testing with electrocardiographic monitoring, in that it provides a measure of coupling between central pulmonary gas exchange, cardiac output, and peripheral oxygen delivery to and use by skeletal muscle. Therefore, as discussed subsequently, it provides access to a number of respiratory, central cardiac, and peripheral metabolic measures that can provide insight into the causes of dyspnea and exercise intolerance, insight that is not provided by the simple electrocardiogram. Finally, in assessing peak V_{O_2} directly, it provides a more accurate measure of functional capacity than can be provided by the estimate derived from exercise testing with electrocardiographic monitoring, which depends on assumptions that can vary significantly among individuals and disease states. The diagnostic utility of the CPET depends on the fact that oxygen uptake is a direct measure of cardiac output and extraction of O_2 by the periphery, according to the Fick equation (see Figure 57-2). For example, as shown in Figure 57-2, the O_2 pulse is a direct measure of cardiac output, if a constant oxygen extraction in the periphery is assumed. A premature plateau in the O_2 pulse during a graded test can be a reliable sign of cardiac ischemia. Also, CPET is helpful in differentiating the cause of dyspnea in patients. Heart failure often coexists with chronic obstructive pulmonary disease. The breathing reserve (the difference between the maximal ventilatory volume and the ventilatory volume at peak exercise) is readily obtained from CPET. In patients with heart failure but without chronic obstructive pulmonary disease, the breathing reserve remains normal at maximal work or above dyspnea threshold. Conversely, patients whose limitation is primarily pulmonary in origin have impaired exercise capacity and limited breathing reserve accompanying the dyspnea. Box 57-1 defines breathing reserve in two ways and gives normative values for each.

Furthermore, serial measurements of carbon dioxide production and oxygen consumption during a steady state or a graded exercise test can provide numerous additional data, discussed subsequently, that have both diagnostic and prognostic information, such as the ratio of volume of expired gas to carbon dioxide production (V_E/V_{CO_2}), ventilatory threshold, and respiratory exchange ratio. When used in combination with electrocardiography, CPET testing can be a cost-efficient way of obtaining useful clinical information about the patient with heart failure, which abrogates the need for further and more costly testing, such as diagnostic radionuclide or echocardiographic stress testing, although imaging clearly has additional utility.

Unlike the 6-minute walk test, CPET requires specialized equipment for gas exchange, coupled to electrocardiographic monitoring, and can be performed with various instruments such as a treadmill or bicycle ergometer. Specialized training of personnel is also needed in order to administer the test, and regular quality control of the testing laboratory is necessary to ensure that equipment works accurately. The risks in testing are similar to those in standard treadmill exercise tests and are surprisingly modest, as shown in a study from Heart Failure and A Controlled Trial Investigating Outcomes of Exercise TraiNing (HF-ACTION), in which the risks in the population with heart failure compare favorably with those in testing in populations with coronary artery disease.[56] The Exercise Testing Statement of the American Heart Association provides guidance on personnel training and equipment, as well as space needs.[57,58] Although a low peak V_{O_2} is correlated with poor survival, improvements in peak V_{O_2} have not been consistently correlated with mortality-related benefits in clinical drug trials when those values are used as a surrogate.[59] In the Veteran's Administration Cooperative Vasodilator–Heart Failure Trial (V-HeFT) studies, the hydralazine-nitrate combination improved V_{O_2} better than did enalapril, albeit for a short time.[60] However, mortality-related benefits from enalapril were superior to those of the vasodilator combination. Similarly, flosequinan demonstrated marked improvements in exercise capacity, but it increased mortality. The use of CPET as a surrogate marker for clinical drug trials remains somewhat controversial.

Prognostic Measures Derived from Cardiopulmonary Exercise Testing

CPET provides important prognostic information, particularly peak V_{O_2}, in identifying the most appropriate candidates for cardiac transplantation.[59] A peak V_{O_2} of 14 mL/kg/min is often identified as the critical value for transplantation eligibility. This criterion is not usually adjusted for age or gender, however. Peak V_{O_2} is inherently lower in women and decreases monotonically with age after approximately 30 years, even in persons with heart failure.[61] Some authorities advocate using less than 50% of predicted V_{O_2} as a better criterion than a universal value that is applied to all ages and both genders.[62] For example, in an 18-year-old man with dilated cardiomyopathy, a V_{O_2} value of 18 to 20 mL/kg/min is obviously above the minimum 14 mL/kg/min value; however, such functional capacity is markedly abnormal for his age and gender, for which normal subjects should have a V_{O_2} value greater than 35 mL/kg/min. Conversely, in a small 65-year-old woman, a peak V_{O_2} value of 14 mL/kg/min is close to 70% of her predicted value; however, the peak V_{O_2} normograms currently in use were developed in apparently normal populations, and in morbid populations, in contrast, the effects of disease on peak V_{O_2} are greatly variable. For example, peripheral arterial disease, arthritis, and type 2 diabetes mellitus negatively affect peak V_{O_2} values in otherwise normal subjects. Therefore, the percentage of predicted value in clinical reports must be interpreted in a patient-specific context in view of other comorbid conditions. In spite of these limitations, CPET is routinely used for functional outcome measures in the population with heart failure and for selection of patients for cardiac transplantation and for implantation of LV assist devices.

BOX 57–1 Breathing Reserve

MVV − V_E at maximal exercise *or* MVV − V_E at maximal exercise/MVV
Normal = at least 15 L/min or 20% to 40% MVV
Low breathing reserve = ventilatory limitation (e.g., as in pulmonary disease)
True MVV may be lower than predicted in patients with restrictive pulmonary disease
MVV, maximal ventilatory volume; V_E, volume of expired gas.

In addition, other parameters derived from CPET are of prognostic significance, including ventilatory equivalents of V_{CO_2} (V_E/V_{CO_2}),[63,64] postexercise recovery oxygen kinetics,[65-68] and onset of anaerobic (ventilatory) threshold. The promise of CPET testing for research and clinical care is still under active exploration, and further advances are anticipated.

SPECIALIZED USES OF CARDIOPULMONARY EXERCISE TESTING

Evaluation of Patients with Heart Failure for Mitral Valve Surgery

There is a significant association between heart failure and mitral regurgitation: Mitral annular dilation resulting from LV remodeling can lead to mitral regurgitation. Hemodynamic function is significantly worse, and adverse outcomes are associated with mitral regurgitation in the setting of heart failure.[69] As the number of patients awaiting transplantation increases and the number of donors remains unchanged, correction of mitral regurgitation in the population with heart failure can be a temporizing measure and a bridge to eventual transplantation. However, the criteria for identifying the best candidates for mitral valve repair or replacement have remained elusive.

Some authorities have advocated the evaluation of the degree of mitral regurgitation by using the proximal isovelocity surface area (PISA) method, through color flow Doppler imaging, during exercise; the results are correlated with elevation of the systolic pulmonary artery pressure.[70] The analysis by PISA was feasible and, interestingly, better during exercise, probably because the regurgitant volume was larger. Of the 27 patients studied, none had heart failure secondary to valvular heart disease or had NYHA class IV heart failure. During exercise, all patients demonstrated an increase in their systolic pulmonary artery pressures, measured from the tricuspid regurgitant jet velocities. Pulmonary hypertension was associated with higher mitral valve regurgitant volume and was significantly correlated with the reason why patients stopped the test: because of dyspnea rather than fatigue.

Evaluation of Chronotropic Incompetence

Normal heart rate increases linearly with increasing workload (and oxygen demand; see Figure 57-2). According to widely accepted criteria, a normal individual, not taking β-adrenergic blockers, should be able to achieve at least 85% of the age-predicted heart rate.[71] This observation has been validated in multiple studies, most of which were conducted before the β-blocker era. At present, however, there is no valid guideline on the expected increase in heart rate from the baseline in patients, with or without heart failure, who do take β-blockers.[72-74] In the HF-ACTION study, more than 94% of the 2331 subjects with heart failure tested were receiving optimal medical therapy for heart failure, including β-adrenergic blockers; data from this study should address this issue.[61] Furthermore, many patients with heart failure may have inherent chronotropic incompetence as a result of cardiac conduction disease or pacemaker therapy. This has also been addressed in the HF-ACTION population.[75] Other studies have shown that reactivation of the parasympathetic nervous system may also play a role in the abnormal response to heart rate noted in patients with heart failure.[76] Such information is helpful in order to interpret CPET results correctly for patients with heart failure, who are increasingly and more intensively treated with agents and devices that interact with normal cardiorespiratory physiology (e.g., β-adrenergic agents, biventricular pacemakers). Furthermore, CPET can be used to identify causes of excessive dyspnea and exercise-induced fatigue in patients with heart failure, such as chronotropic incompetence from excessive β-adrenergic dosing or a poorly functioning cardiac pacemaker.

Adjustment of Pacemakers

The question of whether implantation of a rate-responsive pacemaker would improve exercise tolerance was investigated by Braith and coworkers[76] in a pilot study that involved patients after heart transplantation. Using a graded treadmill exercise test with metabolic measurements in eight patients, they observed that exercise tolerance, peak V_{O_2}, and minute ventilation were statistically better when the pacer was on. Further larger trials are needed to completely demonstrate the beneficial effect of rate-responsive pacemaker in patients with chronotropic incompetence. The long-term benefits of cardiac resynchronization therapy on exercise tolerance in heart failure have not yet been fully established, and further work is therefore needed in this area as well.

Safety of Exercise Testing and Training in Patients with Heart Failure Who Have Implantable Defibrillators

Patients with an implantable cardioverter-defibrillator (ICD) very often avoid performing routine exercise for fear of either triggering an arrhythmic event or causing the device to fire inappropriately in the setting of exercise-induced tachycardia. In one study, 63% of young patients with ICD reported concerns about engaging in exercise.[77] This fear also characterizes many technicians and clinicians who test patients with heart failure in the exercise laboratory.

These concerns are, however, unfounded. First, a patient with an ICD and stable symptoms should be able to exercise and raise the heart rate to within 70% to 80% of the predicted maximum safely. This was shown in the HF-ACTION study, in which the results of more than 6000 CPET tests in 2331 subjects with heart failure were studied; the major cardiovascular event rate, which included ICD firing, was less than 0.5 per 1000 tests.[56] Furthermore, in the HF-ACTION exercise training condition, involving 1159 patients with heart failure, exercise training was observed to be safe, with no increase in the number of events during or within the 3 hours after exercise training, in comparison with the inactive control condition.[78] Finally, whenever there are concerns with regard to the presence of ICD in a patient with heart failure who is undergoing exercise training, the cardiologist who is familiar with the patient's condition should work with the exercise staff to guide the exercise program. With close cooperation, a compromise between ICD detection algorithms, type of therapy applied, and level of exercises can be achieved, and the patient will benefit from the physical and mental benefits of exercise.[77,79]

THERAPEUTIC EXERCISE TRAINING FOR HEART FAILURE

Physiological Benefits of Exercise Training in Heart Failure

It is clear from HF-ACTION[80] and other studies that exercise training can be undertaken in patients with heart failure and that the potential benefits of training exceed the risks. Significant physiological benefits accrue with prolonged exercise training in the population with heart failure, and they potentially counteract the pathophysiological processes of the symptomatic heart failure state (see Figure 57-3, *A* and *B*). Some of these are discussed in detail as follows.

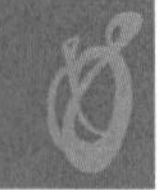

Cardiorespiratory Physiology and Exercise Tolerance

The benefits of exercise training in patients with heart failure include an improvement in exercise tolerance, as assessed through exercise duration and peak $\dot{V}O_2$.[81-95] Table 57-1 lists randomized, parallel, or crossover studies with definitive improvements in peak $\dot{V}O_2$. The exercise training program may be in the setting of supervised or home training; it may involve a treadmill or a bicycle; the duration may vary from 8 weeks to 3 months; and the level of intensity may vary from low to moderate. Although most studies have included primarily aerobic activity, one study involved mainly circuit weight training for 8 weeks; results indicated a modest but significant increase in peak $\dot{V}O_2$.[95] Changes in peak $\dot{V}O_2$ have ranged from 12% to 31%. Most of the improvement occurs by the third week but can still be noted at 6 months if patients comply with the training program.[96,97] Improvements occur not only in maximal exercise performance but also in indexes of submaximal exercise, as measured by the 6-minute walk test or the ventilatory (anaerobic) threshold.[84]

The benefits in $\dot{V}O_2$ have been correlated with other indexes of improvements in exercise capacity, such as an increase in muscle mitochondria[84] and decreased ventilation.[82] However, these studies represent highly selected populations of extremely motivated volunteers, and they occurred before the use of devices (most notably biventricular pacing and LV devices) and β-adrenergic pharmacological therapy for heart failure became widespread; the interaction of these types of therapies with exercise training responses is relatively unknown. In the HF-ACTION study, among 1159 patients with classes II and III heart failure who were receiving optimal medical and device therapy (including 19% using biventricular devices and over 94% taking optimal doses of β-adrenergic agents), the improvement in peak $\dot{V}O_2$ (which was 14.4 mL/kg/min at baseline) was only 4.2% at 3 months and 4.9% at 12 months after patients transitioned to home exercise for at least 6 months.[78] The corresponding improvements in the 6-minute walk test were 20 and 13 m, respectively.

TABLE 57–1 Change in Peak $\dot{V}O_2$ with Exercise Training in HF

Authors (Year)	Number of Patients (Total, 439)	$\dot{V}O_2$ Increase in Comparison with Controls (Average, 20%)
Jette et al (1991)[68]	18	22% in group with ejection fraction < 30%
Belardinelli et al (1992)[87]	20	20%
Coats et al (1992)[81]	17	18%
Belardinelli et al (1995)[82]	55	12%
Hambrecht et al (1995)[83]	22	31%
Keteyian et al (1996)[84]	29	16.3%
Radaelli et al (1996)[88]	6	15%
Dubach et al (1997)[85]	25	26%
Tyni-Lenne et al (1997)[89]	16	14%
Callaerts-Vegh et al (1998)[90]	17	30.9%
Reinhart et al (1998)[91]	25	29%
Belardinelli et al (1999)[86]	99	18% at 2 months
Taylor (1999)[92]	8	17.6%
Sturm et al (1999)[93]	26	23.3%
Keteyian et al (1999)[94]	43	14.3%
Maiorana et al (2000)[95]	13	11.8%

$\dot{V}O_2$, oxygen consumption.

Neurohormonal Activation

Higher levels of neurohormonal activation are associated with worse ventricular function, worse symptoms, and worse prognosis in heart failure. Excessive catecholamine levels, as manifested by norepinephrine spillover, were ameliorated after only 8 weeks of bicycle training in a population with heart failure.[82] In a small crossover trial by Coats and colleagues,[81] 8 weeks of home training enhanced vagal control with a shift away from sympathetic activity. Also, peak exercise levels of angiotensin II, aldosterone, and vasopressin decreased after 16 weeks of endurance training. However, observations about exercise-induced changes in resting epinephrine levels have been inconsistent. For example, Kiilavuori and coworkers[98] observed a 19% drop in resting epinephrine levels after a 3-month training program, whereas Keteyian and colleagues[94] found no changes in resting norepinephrine after 24 weeks of training. Hambrecht and associates[99] described not only a significant drop in epinephrine levels at rest, with a trend toward decreased norepinephrine levels at rest, but also during submaximal exercise. More recently, Tyni-Lenne and coworkers[100] observed that local muscle training could not only improve aerobic activity but also lower catecholamine levels. The variability in these findings may be related to the severity of disease, cause of disease, duration of the heart failure syndrome, intensity and duration of exercise training, the modulation of sympathetic activity by drugs, and the technical difficulties associated with measuring true catecholamine levels at rest.

Endothelial Dysfunction (see Chapter 17)

Researchers have focused attention on exercise training effects on the well-known endothelial dysfunction that accompanies heart failure. Because heart failure is not simply "pump failure" but a multisystem disorder that includes neurohormonal imbalance, researchers have extensively studied alterations in systemic vasomotor tone, particularly the role of endothelial release and regulation of nitric oxide metabolism, and these alterations have been identified as contributing to the disease state.[101] Exercise training has local and systemic beneficial effects on agonist-mediated endothelium-dependent vasodilation and on flow-dependent vasodilation.[102] Elevations of shear stress at the local level, coupled to the systemic effects of heart rate and blood pressure, increase peripheral blood flow. Furthermore, L-arginine supplementation, which increases nitric oxide availability, augments the effects of exercise training on endothelial function and vasomotor regulation.[43] These may be the mechanisms underlying significant improvement in endothelial function that is noted with exercise training in the population with heart failure.

Effects on Intrinsic Skeletal Muscle Characteristics

Alterations in skeletal muscle structure and function, representative of and consistent with a movement from a more oxidative to glycolytic fiber–type distribution, have been linked to exercise intolerance in patients with heart failure.[8] Loss of skeletal muscle oxidative capacity is one of the hallmarks of heart failure, and the effects of training on this are under active investigation. Hambrecht and associates,[83] Keteyian and colleagues,[103] and others have studied the effect of exercise training on muscle oxidative ability in patients with heart failure in the vastus lateralis muscle. In Hambrecht and associates' randomized controlled study, after 6 months, subjects assigned to an ambulatory exercise training program demonstrated a significant increase in mitochondrial density, with enhanced oxidative enzyme activity and a shift from white, fast-twitch type II fibers to red, slow-twitch type I fibers. There were no changes in submaximal blood flow in the legs; therefore, it is unlikely that the changes in peripheral perfusion could account for the changes seen in the mitochondria.

The functional limitations of heart failure occur not only at high workloads but also at submaximal workloads, which are levels that correspond to many activities of daily living in this patient population. In addition to beneficial effects of exercise training on skeletal muscle oxidative capacity, effects on other skeletal muscle parameters support the concepts that skeletal muscle abnormalities are the primary cause of functional limitation in heart failure and that exercise training may be a viable modality for counteracting these effects and thus increase functional capacity (see Figure 57-3, *A* and *B*).[89] For example, exercise training reduces muscle lactate release and increases levels of oxidative enzymes from skeletal muscle.[84] In addition, increases in muscle mass by resistance training might very well lead to alleviation of some symptoms, especially in elderly patients, in whom type II fiber atrophy exacerbates the loss of type I fibers that is associated with heart failure. For example, skeletal muscle mass, as determined with dual-energy x-ray absorptiometry (DEXA), is an independent predictor of peak $\dot{V}O_2$ and of the slope of the ventilation to carbon dioxide production, regardless of NYHA functional class, age, gender, extent of neurohormonal activation, or resting hemodynamic status.[104] Whether an increase in the skeletal mass by resistance exercise will lead to improvement in functional capacity remains to be seen.

Central Mechanisms: Cardiac Output

Some authorities have suggested that only patients with heart failure who have preserved cardiac output might benefit from exercise training.[105] Although this suggestion has not been investigated in any large trial, results of several smaller studies are suggestive of improvements in cardiac output with exercise conditioning. Coats and colleagues[81] performed a randomized, crossover, controlled trial of exercise training in 17 men with stable but moderate to severe heart failure and a mean ejection fraction of 19.6%. In the training condition, cardiac output increased significantly at both submaximal and maximal workloads, in parallel with improvements in $\dot{V}O_2$. Other studies have demonstrated similar improvements in cardiac output with training even at low training intensities.[106,107] Larger scale trials are needed.

Circulating Inflammatory Factors (see Chapter 11)

High concentrations of proinflammatory markers and mediators of cellular apoptosis have been linked to the syndrome of heart failure. Cytokines, such as tumor necrosis factor α, may modulate cardiac and vascular viability and function by mechanisms that include abnormal regulation of nitric oxide synthase. Some studies concern the effects of training on inflammatory markers. Exercise training over 12 weeks at 60% to 80% of maximal heart rate reduces plasma levels of inflammatory cytokines, including tumor necrosis factor α, in patients with heart failure. The improvements parallel a significant improvement in peak $\dot{V}O_2$.[108]

Exercise Improvement with Medical or Exercise Therapy: A True Surrogate of Mortality and Morbidity?

It would be logical to assume that because exercise capacity is directly correlated with prognosis, improvements in exercise function would translate into improvements in rates of mortality and morbidity. However, as other studies have demonstrated, these logical assumptions linking intervention with surrogate marker of clinical benefit do not always hold (refer to the Cardiac Arrhythmia Suppression Trial [CAST][109] of the effects of antiarrhythmic agents on cardiac events and death; the Heart and Estrogen/Progestin Replacement Study [HERS][110] for the effects of estrogen replacement therapy on cardiovascular events; and the Women's Health Initiative[111] for the effects of dietary manipulation on cardiovascular outcomes). The same can be said for the effects of exercise therapy in heart failure.

Agents that do improve rates of mortality from and hospitalization for heart failure, such as ACE inhibitors, have failed to be linked consistently to exercise improvement. This is probably because functional capacity—and, by extension, skeletal muscle function—is related to exercise-related symptoms; the ability to perform activities of daily living and improvements in central cardiac function and output, especially in acute situations, as facilitated by these cardiovascular agents, do not translate into improvements in functional capacity, immediately or in the long term. This was true in large trials of β-adrenergic blockers, which yielded marked improvements in progression of disease and hospitalization but little or no improvement in functional capacity or exercise tolerance. Conversely, other pharmacological agents have been linked to improvements in symptoms and exercise tolerance but worse mortality rates. The only way to understand whether exercise training prevents cardiovascular morbidity and mortality is to conduct randomized studies.

Effects of Exercise Training on Clinical Outcomes in Heart Failure

Before the initiation of the HF-ACTION study, few randomized controlled studies had been directed at determining whether exercise training in patients with systolic heart failure prevented hospitalization and death. Some of these studies are summarized in Figure 57-4; a meta-analysis of 11 studies had been conducted to compare the effects of control conditions with those of exercise training on hard cardiovascular outcomes (morbid events or mortality) in a total of 729 subjects with heart failure.[43,84,87,99,112-117] The meta-analysis revealed a hazard ratio of 0.61 (95% confidence interval, 0.37 to 1.02; $P = .06$) in favor of exercise training. In 2007, Dracup and colleagues[118] reported the results of a study of 173 patients with systolic heart failure who were randomly assigned to the control condition or to undergo home-based exercise. The primary endpoint was a composite of all-cause hospitalizations, emergency department admissions, urgent transplantation, and death at 12 months. A home-based walking program that incorporated aerobic and resistance exercise did not result in improved clinical outcomes at the 1-year follow-up in this cohort of patients. However, the exercise program resulted in reduced rates of repeated hospitalizations.

HF-ACTION

In 2008, the primary results of the much-awaited HF-ACTION trial were released. This study was a large multicenter, randomized, controlled trial of 2331 medically stable outpatients with NYHA class II to class IV heart failure and reduced ejection fraction (<35%). In contrast to previous studies, all subjects were receiving optimal medical and device therapy (94%, β-adrenergic blockade; 94%, angiotensin pathway inhibition; 40%, ICD; and 19%, biventricular pacing). Participants in HF-ACTION were randomly assigned to conditions from April 2003 through February 2007 at 82 centers in the United States, Canada, and France; median length of follow-up was 30 months. The intervention consisted of usual care plus aerobic exercise training (36 supervised sessions

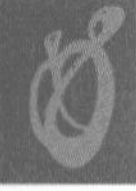

CH 57

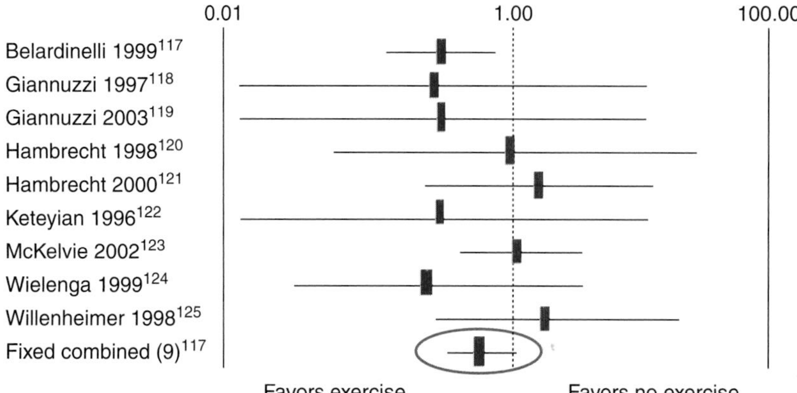

FIGURE 57–4 A summary of studies of exercise training in heart failure as of 2004. Randomized controlled studies of exercise training in systolic heart failure up to the initiation of the Heart Failure and A Controlled Trial Investigating Outcomes of Exercise TraiNing (HF-ACTION) in 2004 are listed. Studies are indicated by first author and date, if appropriate, to the left and are included in this chapter's reference list (Belardinelli et al,[86] Giannuzzi et al,[112,113] Hambrecht et al,[45,99] Keteyian et al,[84] McKelvie et al,[114] Wielenga et al,[115] and Willenheimer et al[116]). Also listed is a meta-analysis performed in 2004 ("Fixed Combined [9]"). For each study or analysis, the point estimate and confidence intervals are indicated in the *heavy vertical lines* and *horizontal lines,* respectively. Hazard ratios are shown, with benefit of exercise (<1) shown to the left and increased risk with exercise shown to the right (>1) A hazard ratio of 1 indicates no effect one way or another on the outcome. (Adapted from Smart N, Marwick TH. Exercise training for patients with heart failure: a systematic review of factors that improve mortality and morbidity. *Am J Med* 2004;116:693-706.)

followed by home-based training) or usual care alone for 1 to 4 years. The composite primary endpoint was all-cause mortality and hospitalization, and the prespecified secondary endpoints were all-cause mortality, mortality from or hospitalization for cardiovascular disorders, and mortality from cardiovascular disorders or hospitalization for heart failure.

Regular exercise training in patients with systolic heart failure was safe. According to the main analysis, adjusted only for cause of heart failure, exercise training produced nonsignificant reductions in the primary endpoint (all-cause mortality and all-cause hospitalization) and in key secondary clinical endpoints (hazard ratios, 0.84 to 0.96, all in favor of exercise training). Furthermore, in protocol-specified supplementary analyses adjusted for prognostic factors, the treatment effect was statistically significant for the primary endpoint and for the secondary endpoint of mortality from cardiovascular disorders or hospitalization for heart failure (hazard ratios, 0.85 to 0.91, all in favor of exercise training). These findings were found to be consistent with those of the 33 previous trials and the meta-analyses that demonstrated improved outcomes with exercise training. Of interest was that the beneficial effects of exercise training appeared to be more pronounced in patients with NYHA class III heart failure and in women. The investigators concluded that, on the basis of the safety of exercise training and the modest reductions in clinical events, in addition to the modest increases in health-related quality of life (reported in the accompanying article by Flynn and associates[119]), the results supported a prescribed exercise training program for patients with reduced LV function and heart failure symptoms, in addition to evidence-based therapy.

FUTURE DIRECTIONS

Numerous questions about the role of exercise training in heart failure remain unanswered. Some of these have been raised by the results of trials, including HF-ACTION. For example, the optimal amount, intensity, and combination of modalities of exercise training for patients with systolic heart failure are issues still unexplored. Also questionable is the relative utility of different regimens for comorbid conditions combined with heart failure, such as type 2 diabetes mellitus, for which a more frequent and less vigorous program than that previously tested in heart failure might be of most benefit. The utility and role of exercise training in combination with other therapies, such as chronotropic resynchronization therapy, are just now being studied.[120] The relative effects of exercise in subpopulations in the HF-ACTION study that showed the most benefit (e.g., in patients with NYHA class III systolic heart failure and in women) should be explored further. Finally, the role of aerobic exercise training—whose benefit may be in reducing the adverse cardiac hypertrophic effects of long-term hypertension for treatment of diastolic heart failure—should be an active area of investigation.

REFERENCES

1. Lee, A. P., Ice, R., Blessey, R., et al. (1979). Long term effects of physical training on coronary patients with impaired ventricular function. *Circulation, 60*, 1519–1526.
2. Conn, E. H., Williams, R. S., & Wallace, A. G. (1982). Exercise responses before and after physical conditioning in patients with severely depressed left ventricular function. *Am J Cardiol, 49*, 296–300.
3. Franciosa, J. A., Park, M., & Levine, T. B. (1982). Lack of correlation between exercise capacity and indexes of resting left ventricular performance in heart failure. *Am J Cardiol, 47*, 33–39.
4. Higginbotham, M. B., Morris, K. G., Coleman, R. E., et al. (1984). Sex-related differences in the normal cardiac response to upright exercise. *Circulation, 70*, 357–366.
5. Fleg, J. L., O'Connor, F., Gerstenblith, G., et al. (1995). Impact of age on the cardiovascular response to dynamic upright exercise in healthy men and women. *J Appl Physiol, 78*, 890–900.
6. Schulman, S. P., Fleg, J. L., Goldberg, A. P., et al. (1996). Continuum of cardiovascular performance across a broad range of fitness levels in healthy older men. *Circulation, 94*, 359–367.
7. Wilson, J. R., Martin, J. L., Schwartz, D., et al. (1984). Exercise intolerance in patients with chronic heart failure: role of impaired nutritive flow to skeletal muscle. *Circulation, 69*, 1079–1087.
8. Duscha, B. D., Schulze, P. C., Robbins, J. L., & Forman, D. E. (2008). Implications of chronic heart failure on peripheral vasculature and skeletal muscle before and after exercise training. *Heart Fail Rev, 13*, 21–37.
9. Sullivan, M. J., & Cobb, F. R. (1992). Central hemodynamic response to exercise in patients with chronic heart failure. *Chest, 101*(Suppl. S), S340–S346.
10. Hakki, A. -H., Weinreich, D. J., DePace, N. L., et al. (1984). Correlation between exercise capacity and left ventricular function in patients with severely depressed left ventricular function. *J Card Rehabil, 4*, 38–43.
11. Shen, W. F., Roubin, G. S., Hirasawa, K., et al. (1985). Left ventricular volume and ejection fraction response to exercise in chronic congestive heart failure: differences between dilated cardiomyopathy and previous myocardial infarction. *Am J Cardiol, 55*, 1027–1031.
12. Wilson, J. R., Rayos, G., Keoh, T. K., et al. (1995). Dissociation between peak exercise oxygen consumption and hemodynamic dysfunction in potential heart transplant candidates. *J Am Coll Cardiol, 26*, 429–435.
13. Roubin, G. S., Anderson, S. D., Shen, W. F., et al. (1990). Hemodynamic and metabolic basis of impaired exercise tolerance in patients with severe left ventricular dysfunction. *J Am Coll Cardiol, 15*, 986–994.
14. Franciosa, J. A., & Cohn, J. N. (1979). Effect of isosorbide dinitrate on response to submaximal and maximal exercise in patients with congestive heart failure. *Am J Cardiol, 43*, 1009–1014.

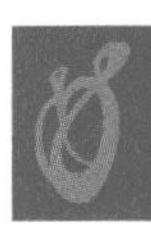

15. Ginks, W. R., & Redwood, D. R. (1980). Hemodynamic effects of hydralazine at rest and during exercise in patients with chronic heart failure. *Br Heart J, 44*, 259–264.
16. Wilson, J. R., Rayos, G., Yeoh, T. K., et al. (1995). Dissociation between exertional symptoms and circulatory function in patients with heart failure. *Circulation, 92*, 47–53.
17. Zelis, R., & Sinoway, L. I. (1988). Regional blood flow in congestive heart failure: concept of compensatory mechanisms with short and long-time constants. *Am J Cardiol, 62*, E2–E8.
18. Zelis, R., Mason, D. T., & Braunwald, E. (1968). A comparison of the effects of vasodilator stimuli on peripheral resistance vessels in normal subjects and inpatients with congestive heart failure. *J Clin Invest, 47*, 960–970.
19. Zelis, R., & Flaim, S. F. (1982). Alterations in vasomotor tone in congestive heart failure. *Prog Cardiovasc Dis, 24*, 437–459.
20. Zelis, R., Longhurst, J., Capone, R. J., et al. (1974). A comparison of regional blood flow and oxygen utilization during dynamic forearm exercise in normal subjects and patients with congestive heart failure. *Circulation, 50*, 137–143.
21. Sullivan, M. J., Knight, J. D., Higginbotham, M. B., et al. (1989). Relation between central and peripheral hemodynamics during exercise in patients with chronic heart failure. *Circulation, 80*, 769–781.
22. LeJemtel, T. H., Maskin, C. S., Lucido, D., et al. (1986). Failure to augment maximal limb blood flow in response to one leg versus two leg exercise in patients with severe heart failure. *Circulation, 74*, 245–251.
23. Sharma, R., Coats, A. J., & Anker, S. D. (2000). The role of inflammatory mediators in chronic heart failure: cytokines, nitric oxide, and endothelin-1. *Int J Cardiol, 72*, 175–186.
24. McMurray, J. J., Ray, S. G., Abdullah, I., et al. (1992). Plasma endothelin in chronic heart failure. *Circulation, 85*, 1374–1379.
25. Longhurst, J., Capone, R. J., & Zelis, R. (1975). Evaluation of skeletal muscle capillary basement membrane thickness in congestive heart failure. *Chest, 67*, 195–198.
26. Sinoway, L., Minotti, J., Musch, T., et al. (1987). Enhanced metabolic vasodilation secondary to diuretic therapy in decompensated congestive heart failure secondary to coronary artery disease. *Am J Cardiol, 60*, 107–111.
27. Wilson, J. R., & Ferraro, N. (1985). Effect of renin-angiotensin system on limb circulation and metabolism during exercise in patients with heart failure. *J Am Coll Cardiol, 6*, 556–563.
28. Sinoway, L. I., Shenberger, J., Wilson, J., et al. (1987). A 30 day forearm work protocol increases maximal forearm blood flow. *J Appl Physiol, 62*, 1063–1067.
29. Sinoway, L. I. (1988). Effect of conditioning and deconditioning stimuli on metabolically determined blood flow in humans and implications for congestive heart failure. *Am. J. Cardiol, 62*, 45E–48E.
30. Massie, B. M., Conway, M., Yonge, R., et al. (1987). Skeletal muscle metabolism in patients with congestive heart failure: relation to clinical severity and blood flow. *Circulation, 76*, 1009–1019.
31. Wilson, J. R., Fink, L., Maris, J., et al. (1985). Evaluation of energy metabolism in skeletal muscle of patients with heart failure with gated phosphorous-31 nuclear magnetic resonance. *Circulation, 71*, 57–62.
32. Lipkin, D. P., Jones, D. A., Round, J. M., et al. (1988). Abnormalities of skeletal muscle in patients with chronic heart failure. *Int J Cardiol, 18*, 187–195.
33. Sullivan, M. J., Green, H. J., & Cobb, F. R. (1990). Skeletal muscle biochemistry and histology in ambulatory patients with long-term heart failure. *Circulation, 81*, 518–527.
34. Drexler, H., Riede, U., Munzel, T., et al. (1992). Alterations of skeletal muscle in chronic heart failure. *Circulation, 85*, 1751–1759.
35. Sullivan, M. J., Duscha, B. D., Klitgaard, H., et al. (1997). Altered expression of myosin heavy chain in human skeletal muscle in chronic heart failure. *Med Sci Sports Exer, 29*, 860–866.
36. Hambrecht, R., Fiehn, E., Yu, J., et al. (1997). Effects of endurance training on mitochondrial ultrastructure and fiber type distribution in skeletal muscle of patients with stable chronic heart failure. *J Am Coll Cardiol, 29*, 1067–1073.
37. Duscha, B. D., Kraus, W. E., Sullivan, M. J., et al. (1999). Capillary density of skeletal muscle: a contributing mechanism for exercise intolerance in class II-III chronic heart failure independent of other peripheral alterations. *J Am Coll Cardiol, 33*, 1956–1963.
38. Katz, S. D., Krum, H., Kahn, T., et al. (1996). Exercise-induced vasodilation in forearm circulation of normal subjects and patients with congestive heart failure: role of endothelium-derived nitric oxide. *J Am Coll Cardiol, 28*, 585–590.
39. Drexler, H., Hayoz, D., Munzel, T., et al. (1992). Endothelial function in chronic congestive heart failure. *Am J Cardiol, 69*, 1596–1601.
40. Tagawa, T., Imaizumi, T., Endo, T., et al. (1994). Role of nitric oxide in reactive hyperemia in human forearm vessels. *Circulation, 90*, 2285–2290.
41. Loscalzo, J., & Vita, J. A. (1994). Ischemia, hyperemia, exercise, and nitric oxide: complex physiology and complex molecular adaptations. *Circulation, 90*, 2556–2559.
42. Gilligan, D. M., Panza, J. A., Kilcoyne, C. M., et al. (1994). The contribution of endothelium-derived nitric oxide to exercise-induced vasodilation. *Circulation, 90*, 2853–2858.
43. Hirooka, Y., Imaizumi, T., Tagawa, T., et al. (1994). Effects of L-arginine on impaired acetylcholine-induced and ischemic vasodilation of the forearm in patients with heart failure. *Circulation, 90*, 658–668.
44. Nakamura, M., Ishikawa, M., Funakoshi, T., et al. (1994). Attenuated endothelium-dependent peripheral vasodilation and clinical characteristics in patients with chronic heart failure. *Am Heart J, 128*, 1164–1169.
45. Hambrecht, R., Fiehn, E., Weigl, C., et al. (1998). Regular physical exercise corrects endothelial dysfunction and improves exercise capacity in patients with chronic heart failure. *Circulation, 98*, 2709–2715.
46. Piepoli, M., Clark, A. L., & Volterrani, M. (1996). Contribution of muscle afferent to the hemodynamic, autonomic, and ventilatory responses to exercise in patients with chronic heart failure. Effects of physical training. *Circulation, 93*, 940–952.
47. Clark, A. L., & Poole-Wilson, P. A. (1996). Exercise limitation in chronic heart failure: central role of periphery. *J Am Coll Cardiol, 28*, 1092–1102.
48. Ponikowski, P., Chua, T. P., Anker, S. D., et al. (2001). Peripheral chemoreceptor hypersensitivity: an ominous sign in patients with chronic heart failure. *Circulation, 104*, 544–549.
49. Ponikowski, P. P., Chua, T. P., Francis, D. P., et al. (2001). Muscle ergoreceptor overactivity reflects deterioration in clinical status and cardiorespiratory reflex control in chronic heart failure. *Circulation, 104*, 2324–2330.
50. Fletcher, G., Balady, G. J., Amsterdam, E., et al. (2001). Exercise standards for testing and training. A statement from the American Heart Association. *Circulation, 104*, 1694–1740.
51. Fleg, J. L., Piña, I. L., Balady, G. J., et al. (2000). Assessment of functional capacity in clinical and research applications: An advisory from the Committee on Exercise, Rehabilitation, and Prevention, Council on Clinical Cardiology, American Heart Association. *Circulation, 102*, 1591–1597.
52. Guyatt, G. H., Sullivan, M. J., Thompson, P. J., et al. (1985). The 6-minute walk: a new measure of exercise capacity in patients with chronic heart failure. *Can Med Assoc J, 132*, 919–923.
53. Lucas, C., Stevenson, L. W., Johnson, W., et al. (1999). The 6-min walk and peak oxygen consumption in advanced heart failure: Aerobic capacity and survival. *Am Heart J, 138*, 618–624.
54. Packer, M., Bristow, M. R., Cohn, J. N., et al. (1996). The effect of carvedilol on morbidity and mortality in patients with chronic heart failure. U.S. Carvedilol Heart Failure Study Group. *N Engl J Med, 334*, 1349–1355.
55. Piña, I. L., Balady, G. J., Hanson, P., et al. (1995). Guidelines for clinical exercise testing laboratories. A statement for healthcare professionals from the Committee on Exercise and Cardiac Rehabilitation, American Heart Association. *Circulation, 91*, 212–221.
56. Keteyian, S. J., Isaac, D., Thadani, U., et al. (2009). Safety of symptom-limited cardiopulmonary exercise testing in patients with chronic heart failure due to severe left ventricular systolic dysfunction. *Am Heart J, 158*(Suppl. 4), S72–S77.
57. Mancini, D. M., Eisen, H., Kussmaul, W., et al. (1991). Value of peak exercise oxygen consumption for optimal timing of cardiac transplantation in ambulatory patients with heart failure. *Circulation, 83*, 778–786.
58. Myers, J., Arena, R., Franklin, B., et al. (2009). Recommendations for clinical exercise laboratories: a scientific statement from the American Heart Association. *Circulation, 119*, 3144–3161.
59. Feldman, M. D., & Beller, G. A. (1990). Is secondary mitral regurgitation in congestive heart failure a marker of clinical importance?. *J Am Coll Cardiol, 15*, 174–180.
60. Ziesche, S., Cobb, F. R., Cohn, J. N., et al. (1993). Hydralazine and isosorbide dinitrate combination improves exercise tolerance in heart failure. *Circulation, 87*(Suppl VI), VI-56–VI-64.
61. Forman, D. E., Clare, R., Kitzman, D. W., et al. (2009). Relationship of age and exercise performance in patients with heart failure: the HF-ACTION study. *Am Heart J, 158*(Suppl. 4), S6–S15.
62. Milani, R. V., Mehra, M. R., Reddy, T. K., et al. (1996). Ventilation/carbon dioxide production ratio in early exercise predicts poor functional capacity in congestive heart failure. *Heart, 76*, 393–396.
63. Cicoira, M., Davos, C. H., Florea, V., et al. (2001). Chronic heart failure in the very elderly: clinical status, survival, and prognostic factors in 188 patients more than 70 years old. *Am Heart J, 142*, 174–180.
64. Scrutinio, D., Passantino, A., Lagioia, R., et al. (1998). Percent achieved of predicted peak exercise oxygen uptake and kinetics of recovery of oxygen uptake after exercise for risk stratification in chronic heart failure. *Int J Cardiol, 64*, 117–124.
65. Myers, J., Gianrossi, R., Schwitter, J., et al. (2001). Effect of exercise training on postexercise oxygen uptake kinetics in patients with reduced ventricular function. *Chest, 120*, 1206–1211.
66. Hepple, R. T., Liu, P. P., Plyley, M. J., et al. (1999). Oxygen uptake kinetics during exercise in chronic heart failure: influence of peripheral vascular reserve. *Clin Sci (Lond), 97*, 569–577.
67. Tanabe, Y., Takahashi, M., Hosaka, Y., et al. (2000). Prolonged recovery of cardiac output after maximal exercise in patients with chronic heart failure. *J Am Coll Cardiol, 35*, 1228–1236.
68. Jette, M., Heller, R., Landry, F., et al. (1991). Randomized four-week exercise program in patients with impaired left ventricular function. *Circulation, 84*, 1561–1567.
69. Lebrun, F., Lancellotti, P., & Pierard, L. A. (2001). Quantitation of functional mitral regurgitation during bicycle exercise in patients with heart failure. *J Am Coll Cardiol, 38*, 1685–1692.
70. Piña, I. L., & Fitpatrick, J. T. (1996). Exercise and heart failure. A review. *Chest, 110*, 1317–1327.
71. Genth-Zotz, S., Zotz, R. J., Sigmund, M., et al. (2000). MIC trial: metoprolol in patients with mild to moderate heart failure: effects on ventricular function and cardiopulmonary exercise testing. *Eur J Heart Fail, 2*, 175–181.
72. Agarwal, A. K., & Venugopalan, P. (2001). Beneficial effect of carvedilol on heart rate response to exercise in digitalized patients with heart failure in atrial fibrillation due to idiopathic dilated cardiomyopathy. *Eur J Heart Fail, 3*, 437–440.
73. Gullestad, L., Manhenke, C., Aarsland, T., et al. (2001). Effect of metoprolol CR/XL on exercise tolerance in chronic heart failure—a substudy to the MERIT-HF trial. *Eur J Heart Fail, 3*, 463–468.
74. Desai, M. Y. (2001). De la Peña-Almaguer E, Mannting F. Abnormal heart rate recovery after exercise as a reflection of an abnormal chronotropic response. *Am J Cardiol, 87*, 1164–1169.
75. Bensimhon, D. R., Leifer, E. S., Ellis, S. J., et al. (2008). Reproducibility of peak oxygen uptake and other cardiopulmonary exercise testing parameters in patients with heart failure (from the Heart Failure and A Controlled Trial Investigating Outcomes of exercise traiNing). *Am J Cardiol, 102*, 712–717.
76. Braith, R. W., Clapp, L., Brown, T., et al. (2000). Rate responsive pacing improves exercise tolerance in heart transplant recipients. A pilot study. *J Cardiopulm Rehabil, 20*, 377–382.
77. Lampman, R. M., & Knight, B. P. (2000). Prescribing exercise training for patients with defibrillators. *Am J Phys Med Rehabil, 79*, 292–297.

78. O'Connor, C. M., Whellan, D. J., Lee, K. L., et al. (2009). Efficacy and safety of exercise training in patients with chronic heart failure: HF-ACTION randomized controlled trial. *JAMA, 301*, 1439–1450.
79. Piña, I. L. (1995). Optimal candidates for heart transplantation: is 14 the magic number? *J Am Coll Cardiol, 26*, 436–437.
80. Whellan, D. J., O'Connor, C. M., Lee, K. L., et al. (2007). Heart failure and a controlled trial investigating outcomes of exercise training (HF-ACTION): design and rationale. *Am Heart J, 153*, 201–211.
81. Coats, A. J. S., Adamopoulos, S., Radaelli, A., et al. (1992). Controlled trial of physical training in chronic heart failure. *Circulation, 85*, 2119–2131.
82. Belardinelli, R., Georgiou, G., Cianci, G., et al. (1995). Exercise training improves left ventricular diastolic filling in patients with dilated cardiomyopathy. *Circulation, 91*, 2775–2784.
83. Hambrecht, R., Neibauer, J., Fiehn, E., et al. (1995). Physical training in patients with stable chronic heart failure: effects on cardiorespiratory fitness and ultrastructural abnormalities of leg muscles. *J Am Coll Cardiol, 25*, 1239–1249.
84. Keteyian, S., Levine, A., Brawner, C. A., et al. (1996). Exercise training in patients with heart failure: a randomized, controlled trial. *Ann Intern Med, 124*, 1051–1057.
85. Dubach, P., Myers, J., Dziekan, G., et al. (1997). The effect of high intensity exercise training on central hemodynamic response to exercise in men with reduced left ventricular function. *J Am Coll Cardiol, 29*, 1591–1598.
86. Belardinelli, R., Georgiou, D., Cianci, G., et al. (1999). Randomized, controlled trial of long-term moderate exercise training in chronic heart failure: effects on functional capacity, quality of life, and clinical outcome. *Circulation, 99*, 1173–1182.
87. Belardinelli, R., Scocco, V., Mazzanti, M., et al. (1992). [Effects of aerobic training in patients with moderate chronic heart failure.]. *G Ital Cardiol, 22*, 919–930.
88. Radaelli, A., Coats, A. J., Leuzzi, S., et al. (1996). Physical training enhances sympathetic and parasympathetic control of heart rate and peripheral vessels in chronic heart failure. *Clin Sci (Lond), 91*(Suppl), 92–94.
89. Tyni-Lenne, R., Gordon, A., Jansson, E., et al. (1997). Skeletal muscle endurance training improves peripheral oxidative capacity, exercise tolerance, and health-related quality of life in women with chronic congestive heart failure secondary to either ischemic cardiomyopathy or idiopathic dilated cardiomyopathy. *Am J Cardiol, 80*, 1025–1029.
90. Callaerts-Vegh, Z., Wenk, M., Goebbels, U., et al. (1998). Influence of intensive physical training on urinary nitrate elimination and plasma endothelin-1 levels in patients with congestive heart failure. *J Cardiopulm Rehabil, 18*, 450–457.
91. Reinhart, W. H., Dziekan, G., Goebbels, U., et al. (1998). Influence of exercise training on blood viscosity in patients with coronary artery disease and impaired left ventricular function. *Am Heart J, 135*, 379–382.
92. Taylor, A. (1999). Physiological response to a short period of exercise training in patients with chronic heart failure. *Physiother Res Int, 4*, 237–249.
93. Sturm, B., Quittan, M., Wiesinger, G. F., et al. (1999). Moderate-intensity exercise training with elements of step aerobics in patients with severe chronic heart failure. *Arch Phys Med Rehabil, 80*, 746–750.
94. Keteyian, S. J., Brawner, C. A., Schairer, J. R., et al. (1999). Effects of exercise training on chronotropic incompetence in patients with heart failure. *Am Heart J, 138*, 233–240.
95. Maiorana, A., O'Driscoll, G., Cheetham, C., et al. (2000). Combined aerobic and resistance exercise training improves functional capacity and strength in CHF. *J Appl Physiol, 88*, 1565–1570.
96. Meyer, K., Schwaibold, M., Westbrook, S., et al. (1996). Effects of short-term exercise training and activity restriction on functional capacity in patients with severe chronic congestive heart failure. *Am J Cardiol, 78*, 1017–1022.
97. Gottlieb, S. S., Fisher, M. L., Freudenberger, R., et al. (1999). Effects of exercise training on peak performance and quality of life in congestive heart failure patients. *J Card Fail, 5*, 188–194.
98. Kiilavuori, K., Naveri, H., Leinonen, H., et al. (1999). The effect of physical training on hormonal status and exertional hormonal response in patients with chronic congestive heart failure. *Eur Heart J, 20*, 456–464.
99. Hambrecht, R., Gielen, S., Linke, A., et al. (2000). Effects of exercise training on left ventricular function and peripheral resistance in patients with chronic heart failure. *JAMA, 283*, 3095–3101.
100. Tyni-Lenne, R., Dencker, K., Gordon, A., et al. (2001). Comprehensive local muscle training increases aerobic working capacity and quality of life and decreases neurohormonal activation in patients with chronic heart failure. *Eur J Heart Fail, 3*, 47–52.
101. Linke, A., Schoene, N., Gielen, S., et al. (2001). Endothelial dysfunction in patients with chronic heart failure: systemic effects of lower-limb exercise training. *J Am Coll Cardiol, 37*, 392–397.
102. Kubo, S. H., Rector, T. C., Williams, R. E., et al. (1991). Endothelium dependent vasodilation is attenuated in patients with heart failure. *Circulation, 84*, 1589–1596.
103. Keteyian, S. J., Duscha, B. D., Browner, C. A., et al. (2003). Gender differences between men and women in skeletal muscle and response to exercise training in heart failure patients. *Am Heart J, 145*, 912–918.
104. Cicoira, M., Zanolla, L., Franceschini, L., et al. (2001). Skeletal muscle mass independently predicts peak oxygen consumption and ventilatory response during exercise in noncachectic patients with chronic heart failure. *J Am Coll Cardiol, 37*, 2080–2085.
105. Chomsky, D. B., Lang, C. C., Rayos, G. H., et al. (1996). Hemodynamic exercise testing. A valuable tool in the selection of cardiac transplantation candidates. *Circulation, 94*, 3176–3183.
106. Gordon, A., Tyni-Lenne, R., & Jansson, E. (1999). Beneficial effects of exercise training in heart failure patients with low cardiac output response to exercise: a comparison of two training models. *J Intern Med, 246*, 175–182.
107. Dizekan, G., Myers, J., Goebbels, U., et al. (1998). Effects of exercise training on limb blood flow in patients with reduced ventricular function. *Am Heart J, 136*, 22–30.
108. Adamopoulos, S., Parissis, J., Karatzas, D., et al. (2002). Physical training modulates proinflammatory cytokines and the soluble *Fas*/soluble *Fas* ligand system in patients with chronic heart failure. *J Am Coll Cardiol, 39*, 653–663.
109. Echt, D. S., Liebson, P. R., Mitchell, L. B., et al. (1991). Mortality and morbidity in patients receiving encainide, flecainide, or placebo. The Cardiac Arrhythmia Suppression Trial. *N Engl J Med, 324*, 781–788.
110. Hulley, S., Grady, D., Bush, T., et al. (1998). Randomized trial of estrogen plus progestin for secondary prevention of coronary heart disease in postmenopausal women. Heart and Estrogen/progestin Replacement Study (HERS) Research Group. *JAMA, 280*, 605–613.
111. Rossouw, J. E., Anderson, G. L., Prentice, R. L., et al. (2002). Risks and benefits of estrogen plus progestin in healthy postmenopausal women: principal results from the Women's Health Initiative randomized controlled trial. *JAMA, 288*, 321–333.
112. Giannuzzi, P., Temporelli, P. L., Corra, U., et al. (1997). Attenuation of unfavorable remodeling by exercise training in postinfarction patients with left ventricular dysfunction: results of the Exercise in Left Ventricular Dysfunction (ELVD) trial. *Circulation, 96*, 1790–1797.
113. Giannuzzi, P., Temporelli, P. L., Corra, U., et al. (2003). Antiremodeling effect of long-term exercise training in patients with stable chronic heart failure: results of the Exercise in Left Ventricular Dysfunction and Chronic Heart Failure (ELVD-CHF) Trial. *Circulation, 108*, 554–559.
114. McKelvie, R. S., Teo, K. K., Roberts, R., et al. (2002). Effects of exercise training in patients with heart failure: the Exercise Rehabilitation Trial (EXERT). *Am Heart J, 144*, 23–30.
115. Wielenga, R. P., Huisveld, I. A., Bol, E., et al. (1999). Safety and effects of physical training in chronic heart failure. Results of the Chronic Heart Failure and Graded Exercise study (CHANGE). *Eur Heart J, 20*, 872–879.
116. Willenheimer, R., Erhardt, L., Cline, C., et al. (1998). Exercise training in heart failure improves quality of life and exercise capacity. *Eur Heart J, 19*, 774–781.
117. Smart, N., & Marwick, T. H. (2004). Exercise training for patients with heart failure: a systematic review of factors that improve mortality and morbidity. *Am J Med, 116*, 693–706.
118. Dracup, K., Evangelista, L. S., Hamilton, M. A., et al. (2007). Effects of a home-based exercise program on clinical outcomes in heart failure. *Am Heart J, 154*, 877–883.
119. Flynn, K. E., Piña, I. L., Whellan, D. J., et al. (2009). Effects of exercise training on health status in patients with chronic heart failure: HF-ACTION randomized controlled trial. *JAMA, 301*, 1451–1459.
120. Patwala, A. Y., Woods, P. R., Sharp, L., et al. (2009). Maximizing patient benefit from cardiac resynchronization therapy with the addition of structured exercise training: a randomized controlled study. *J Am Coll Cardiol, 53*, 2332–2339.

CHAPTER 58

Management of Heart Failure Patients with Malignancy

Edward T. H. Yeh, Courtney L. Bickford, and Yusuf Hassan

With advances in modern cancer treatment, patient outcomes have improved dramatically, resulting in longer life spans for these patients. However, with prolonged survival, more cancer patients are at risk of developing cardiovascular problems, including heart failure.[1] Indeed, the cumulative incidence of 10-year cardiovascular disease has been reported as high as 22% among patients who have undergone treatment for malignancy.[2] Thus, it is becoming increasingly important for cardiologists to be familiar with issues of cardiovascular complications of cancer therapy and to know how to manage these long-term consequences of cancer treatment. Furthermore, preventive strategies, including primary prevention of coronary atherosclerotic disease, should be part of the management of cancer patients.[3]

Patients with cancer frequently develop complications within the cardiovascular system. These complications can occur as a result of locally invasive disease or distant metastasis. The cardiovascular system can also be affected by indirect complications, most notably hyperviscosity syndromes, resulting from myeloproliferative disorders or leukemias. Finally, several of the therapies used to treat cancer, including radiation, traditional chemotherapeutics, and so-called targeted therapeutics that are aimed at factors that are causal or that promote cancer growth and metastasis, can also be toxic to the heart and cardiovascular system (Table 58-1). This chapter focuses on traditional and targeted therapeutics that can cause heart failure. Additional complications of cancer therapies are reviewed elsewhere.[4]

ANTHRACYCLINES

The anthracyclines currently approved in the United States—doxorubicin (Adriamycin), daunorubicin (Cerubidine), epirubicin (Ellence), and idarubicin (Idamycin)—are key components of many chemotherapeutic regimens, having demonstrated efficacy in the treatment of lymphomas and many solid tumors, including breast and small cell lung cancer. This class of chemotherapeutic agents also is clearly the most cardiotoxic to date: In the acute setting, they produce arrhythmias, left ventricular (LV) dysfunction, and pericarditis; in the chronic setting, they produce LV dysfunction and heart failure (see Table 58-1).

Anthracycline-induced cardiotoxicity is usually dose related and is thought to result from, among other things, free radical formation that damages the myocardium.[5,6] Anthracycline toxicity is most likely related to oxygen free radicals; in particular, the combination of doxorubicin, ferric iron, and free radical leads to mitochondrial damage and myocyte cell death. The oxygen free radical generated through the semiquinone moiety of the molecule causes lipid peroxidation and results in cell damage. This may explain how chelating agents, such as dexrazoxane, work as a cardioprotective agent in patients receiving doxorubicin.[7] Other authorities believe that large calcium influx into the cell may be partly responsible.[8-10] The downregulation of β-adrenergic receptors described by some authors may represent a final common pathway, inasmuch as this has been described for other cardiomyopathies, including cardiomyopathy induced by 3,4-methylenedioxymethamphetamine (ecstasy) and by stress.[11] Other authors have pointed to effect of anthracyclines on release of endogenous proinflammatory agents such as tumor necrosis factor as partly responsible for the toxicity. This hypothesis is of some interest because tumor necrosis factor receptors are present on the myocardium. A similar mechanism involving interleukin-2 has also been described.[12,13] Data from studies of cultured cardiomyocytes suggest that cardiotoxicity could be induced by DNA damage and that dexrazoxane antagonizes doxorubicin-induced DNA damage through its interference with topoisomerase IIβ (Top2β), which is expressed in the heart. The specific involvement of Top2β in doxorubicin-induced DNA damage is consistent with a model in which proteasomal processing doxorubicin-induced Top2β–DNA covalent complexes exposes the Top2β-concealed DNA double-strand breaks and cause cardiomyocyte death.[14]

Why patients develop cardiotoxicity at different times is not known. Anthracycline-induced cardiac injury can be acute, manifesting as nonspecific ST-segment and T-wave abnormalities, ventricular arrhythmias, and transient LV dysfunction. Early cardiotoxicity manifests within the first year of therapy with LV failure that may be progressive. Late-onset anthracycline cardiotoxicity that causes dilated cardiomyopathy, which manifests years to decades after anthracycline treatment is completed, is increasingly recognized, often after a prolonged asymptomatic period.[15] Cardiac changes such as reductions in LV mass, mass index, and compliance have been reported in anthracycline-treated survivors of childhood cancer who were monitored for more than 7 years after chemotherapy was completed.[15]

Although anthracycline-induced cardiotoxicity can occur with low doses of an anthracycline, the risk of clinical cardiotoxicity increases with the cumulative dose. Researchers who have studied the cumulative incidence of doxorubicin-induced heart failure have found that it occurs in 3%

TABLE 58–1 Cancer Drugs That Can Cause Left Ventricular Dysfunction or Heart Failure

Drug Class	Incidence (%)	Comments
Anthracyclines		Highly dose-dependent
• Doxorubicin	3-48	Risk factors include age (old and young), prior mediastinal XRT, history of heart disease, female gender, and other agents (especially trastuzumab)
• Epirubicin	0.9-3.3	
• Idarubicin	5-18	Risk is decreased by liposomal encapsulation or dexrazoxane
Alkylating agents		Primarily seen with high-dose "conditioning" regimens
• Cyclophosphamide	7-28	Risk factors are prior mediastinal XRT or anthracycline treatment
• Ifosfamide	17	Myocarditis, pericarditis, and myocardial necrosis can also be present
Taxanes		
• Docetaxel	2.3-8	
Targeted therapeutics		
• Trastuzumab	2-28	Relatively uncommon as single agent Increased risk with anthracyclines, paclitaxel, cyclophosphamide
• Imatinib	0.5-1.7	Frequency not clear but probably <5% Can also cause severe fluid retention with peripheral edema, pleural effusion, and pericardial effusion not secondary to left ventricular dysfunction
• Sunitinib	2.7-11	
• Bevacizumab	1.7-3	Heart failure can occur in setting of severe hypertension, which occurs in 4%-35% of patients
Proteasome inhibitor		
• Bortezomib	2-5	

XRT, x-ray therapy.

to 5% of patients who received 400 mg/m^2, in 7% to 26% of patients who took 550 mg/m^2, and in 18% to 48% of patients who received 700 mg/m^2.[4,16-18]

In contrast to doxorubicin, epirubicin or idarubicin appears to cause lower incidences of heart failure.[19,20] The development of cardiomyopathy associated with anthracyclines is influenced by such factors as cumulative dose, intravenous bolus administration, higher single doses, history of prior irradiation, the use of other concomitant agents known to have cardiotoxic effects (such as cyclophosphamide, trastuzumab, and paclitaxel), female gender, underlying cardiovascular disease, age (young and old age; Figure 58-1), and increased length of time since completion of the anthracycline regimen.[4,21-23]

Thus, the prevention of anthracycline-induced cardiotoxicity necessitates decreasing myocardial concentrations of anthracyclines and their metabolites, which may be accomplished by altering the anthracycline administration method (e.g., continuous infusion vs. bolus administration). Other preventive measures include the use of anthracycline analogues (e.g., idarubicin, epirubicin, mitoxantrone) or liposomal anthracyclines, administration of cardioprotective agents (e.g., dexrazoxane), and the use of angiotensin-converting enzyme (ACE) inhibitors and β-blockers (discussed later) to attenuate the effects of anthracyclines on the heart.[4,24-26]

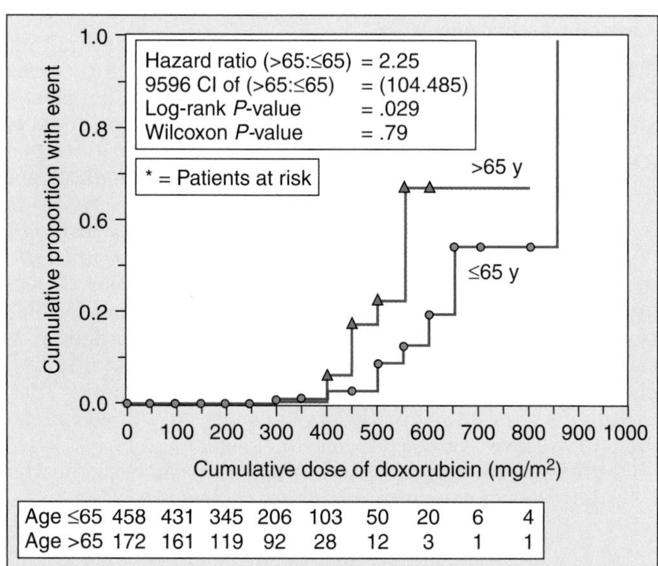

FIGURE 58–1 Risk of doxorubicin-associated congestive heart failure by patient age: Cumulative doxorubicin dose at onset of doxorubicin-associated congestive heart failure in 630 patients, according to patient age (older or younger than 65 years [y]). (Redrawn from Swain SM, Whaley FS, Ewer MS: Congestive heart failure in patients treated with doxorubicin: a retrospective analysis of three trials. *Cancer* 2003;97:2869.)

Monitoring and Anthracycline Toxicity

LV function should be assessed in patients at baseline, before anthracycline therapy is initiated, and should be monitored periodically after that, especially when the cumulative dose exceeds 350 to 400 mg/m^2[57,58] for doxorubicin or the comparable doses for the other anthracyclines. By relying on history and physical examination alone, clinicians can miss significant deterioration in LV function in a substantial number of patients. Routine troponin measurements are not highly predictive except in patients receiving high-dose chemotherapy (for treatment of aggressive malignancies). Of those patients, those who will develop LV dysfunction can be identified by an elevated troponin I level with high sensitivity, albeit low predictive accuracy. A negative troponin I level was a strong predictor of which patients would not experience deterioration of LV function.[27]

ALKYLATING AGENTS

Cyclophosphamide

Cyclophosphamide is an alkylating agent used in the treatment of lymphomas, some types of leukemias, and some solid tumors. In contrast to anthracyclines, the cardiotoxicity of cyclophosphamide seems to be related to the total dose given at a single time, rather than the cumulative dose.

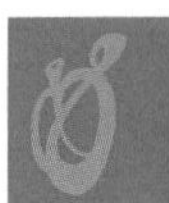

Heart failure associated with cyclophosphamide occurs at high doses (>150 mg/kg and 1.5 g/m^2/day) in 7% to 28% of patients.[4,19,28-30] The clinical manifestations of cardiotoxicity range from asymptomatic pericardial effusions to heart failure and myopericarditis,[28,30] which occur within 1 to 10 days after the administration of the first dose of cyclophosphamide.[4,19] Besides total dose, risk factors for cardiotoxicity include prior anthracycline or mitoxantrone therapy and mediastinal radiation.[19,29]

Although the precise mechanism of cyclophosphamide cardiotoxicity is unknown, it is theorized that cyclophosphamide causes direct endothelial injury, followed by extravasation of toxic metabolites resulting in damage to cardiomyocytes, interstitial hemorrhage, and edema.[4,19,29-31] Intracapillary microemboli, resulting in ischemic myocardial damage,[4,30,31] and myocardial ischemia caused by coronary vasospasm are other proposed mechanisms of cyclophosphamide-related cardiotoxicity.[4,19]

Ifosfamide

Ifosfamide is an alkylating agent related to cyclophosphamide used to treat a variety of malignancies. Like cyclophosphamide, ifosfamide causes cardiotoxicity in a dosage-related manner (dosages ≥ 12.5 g/m^2).[4,19] In a retrospective review of patients with advanced lymphoma or carcinoma treated with high-dose ifosfamide as part of combination chemotherapy with autologous bone marrow transplantation, cardiotoxicity developed in 17% of patients.[4,19,32] Acute onset of heart failure occurred within 6 to 23 days after the first dose of ifosfamide.[4,19]

Because ifosfamide and cyclophosphamide are structurally similar, it is probable that ifosfamide may induce heart failure through a similar mechanism. In addition, because ifosfamide causes nephrotoxicity, it is thought that this decrease in glomerular filtration rate may delay the elimination of cardiotoxic metabolites. Other factors such as fluid disturbances, acid-base imbalance, and electrolyte disturbances related to tubular defects may also contribute to cardiac problems.[4,32]

ANTIMICROTUBULE AGENTS

Docetaxel

The incidence of heart failure associated with docetaxel ranges from 2.3% to 8%.[4,33,34] In a trial in which docetaxel plus doxorubicin and cyclophosphamide (TAC) was compared with fluorouracil plus doxorubicin and cyclophosphamide (FAC), the overall incidence of heart failure at 55 months was 1.6% among the TAC recipients and 0.7% among the FAC recipients.[33] At 70 months' follow-up, heart failure was reported in 2.3% of the TAC recipients, in comparison with 0.9% of the FAC subjects.[4] However, in another breast cancer trial, the incidence of docetaxel-induced heart failure was higher (8%).[4,34]

Proteasome Inhibitor

Bortezomib (Velcade) is the first therapeutic proteasome inhibitor to be tested in humans, and it has been approved by the U.S. Food and Drug Administration (FDA) for use in patients with multiple myeloma, a B-cell malignancy with overgrowth of monotypic plasma cells in the bone marrow. The concept behind the use of proteasome inhibitors is that malignant cells have altered proteins that regulate the cell cycle, which leads to more rapid cell division and, in turn, increased accumulation of damaged proteins. Therefore, the continued health of the malignant cell, as opposed to normal cells, may be more dependent on degradation of the damaged proteins.

The exact incidence of heart failure associated with bortezomib remains unclear; however, in 669 patients with multiple myeloma who were treated with bortezomib or high-dose dexamethasone, the incidence of cardiac disorders during treatment was 15% with bortezomib and 13% with dexamethasone.[4,35] Heart failure events occurred in 5% of bortezomib-treated patients and in 4% of dexamethasone-treated patients. Two percent of patients in each of the treatment groups developed heart failure. The mechanism of heart failure associated with bortezomib is unknown, but it has been proposed that bortezomib may cause cardiotoxicity through proteasome inhibition.[4,36]

TARGETED THERAPEUTIC AGENTS

The treatment of malignancies has changed dramatically with the advent of so-called targeted therapies. In comparison to traditional chemotherapeutic agents that target basic cellular processes that are present in most cells, the newer agents target factors that are specifically dysregulated in cancerous cells. The anticipation was that this approach would reduce a number of the toxic effects that plague standard chemotherapeutics (alopecia, gastrointestinal toxicity, myelotoxicity) and at the same time treat the cancer more effectively. For the most part, these goals have been achieved; however, a number of concerns about cardiotoxicity have surfaced for some agents.

Before these therapies and their toxic effects are discussed, it is important to understand these agents and how they work. Most targeted cancer therapeutic agents inhibit the activity of tyrosine kinases (Table 58-2).[37] Tyrosine kinases attach phosphate groups to tyrosine residues of other proteins, thereby changing the activity, subcellular localization, or rate of degradation of the protein. In the normal cell, these wild-type (i.e., normal) tyrosine kinases play many roles in regulating basic cellular functions. However, in leukemias and cancers, the gene encoding the causal tyrosine kinase is either amplified (leading to overexpression) or mutated (leading to a constitutively activated state), which drives proliferation of the cancerous clonal cells or blocks their normal death. Inhibiting these kinases could then retard cell proliferation or induce cell death, or both. Cardiotoxicity arises when the normal kinase (present in cardiomyocytes), which is also inhibited by the agent, plays a central role in maintenance of cardiomyocyte homeostasis. In some cases, cardiotoxicity of these drugs may be predictable, but in most cases the cardiotoxicity is not predictable. This is because the targeted kinase was not known to provide a maintenance function in the cardiac myocyte or because of "off-target" effects (e.g., inhibition of tyrosine kinases other than those the drug was designed to target). The majority of the tyrosine kinase inhibitors competes with adenosine triphosphate for binding to a pocket in the kinase that is moderately conserved across many tyrosine kinases. More than 90 tyrosine kinases have been identified thus far. The two major classes of tyrosine kinases are receptor tyrosine kinases (RTKs), which have an extracellular ligand-binding domain and an intracellular kinase domain that is responsible for cell signaling, and non–receptor tyrosine kinases (NRTKs) that are located within the cell.[38] Tyrosine kinases are important in the malignant transformation of cells because of their integral role in the cell survival and differentiation. In addition, there is evidence for a role of tyrosine kinases in tumor angiogenesis.[39] Activation of tyrosine kinases may be involved in many cancers, such as leukemias or solid tumors, in which gene mutation may result in overexpression of the kinase and lead to a constitutively activated state, driving proliferation of cancer cells and preventing apoptosis.[40]

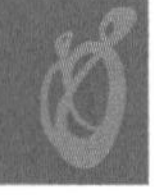

TABLE 58–2 Tyrosine Kinase Targets in Malignant Hematologic Disorders and Solid Tumors

Tyrosine Kinase*	Activating Mechanism†	Type of Cancer‡	Targeted Therapy
Hematological Disorders			
ABL	Transloc	CML ALL AML	Imatinib (Gleevec) Dasatinib (Sprycel) Nilotinib (Tasigna)
ARG	Transloc	AML	Imatinib (Gleevec) Dasatinib (Sprycel) Nilotinib
ALK	Transloc	ALCL	
FGFR1	Transloc	aCML	PD0173074
FGFR3	Transloc; mut	MM	PD0173074
FLT3	Duplication; mut	AML	Lestaurtinib Sorafenib (Nexavar) Sunitinib (Sutent)
c-FMS	Mut	MDS AML	
NTRK3	Transloc	AML	
PDGFR-α	Deletion; transloc	HES SM	Imatinib (Gleevec) Sunitinib (Sutent)
PDGFR-β	Transloc	CMML AML	Imatinib (Gleevec) Dasatinib (Sprycel) Sunitinib (Sutent)
JAK2	Mut; transloc	PCV ET IMF	
c-KIT	Mut; overexp	AML SM	Imatinib (Gleevec) Dasatinib (Sprycel) Sorafenib (Nexavar)
SYK	Transloc	MDS	
Solid Tumors			
ALK	Transloc	IMT	
EGFR	Overexp; mut; deletion	NSCLC Ovarian SCCHN RCC Colorectal	Gefitinib (Iressa) Erlotinib (Tarceva) Cetuximab (Erbitux)
HER2	Overexp; mut	Breast Lung	Trastuzumab (Herceptin) Lapatinib (Tykerb)
EGFR3	Overexp	Clear cell sarcoma	
c-KIT	Mut; deletion; duplication	GIST SCLC Sarcoma	Imatinib (Gleevec) Dasatinib (Sprycel) Sunitinib (Sutent) Sorafenib (Nexavar)
c-MET	Overexp; mut; fusion	SCLC Gastric Melanoma RCC	
NTRK1	Transloc	PTC	
PDGFR	Overexp; mut; deletion	Glioblastoma Osteosarcoma GIST	Imatinib (Gleevec) Sunitinib (Sutent) Sorafenib (Nexavar)
RET	Mut	MEN-2A MEN-2B	Sunitinib (Sutent)
VEGFR-1, VEGFR-2	Overexp VEGF	NSCLC Breast RCC Colorectal Prostate	Sunitinib (Sutent) Bevacizumab (Avastin) Sorafenib (Nexavar)

*ABL, Abelson tyrosine kinase; aCML, atypical chronic myeloid leukemia; ARG, Abl-related gene (ABL2); ALK, anaplastic lymphoma kinase; c-FMS, ***; c-KIT, stem cell factor receptor; c-MET, hepatocyte growth factor receptor; EGFR, epidermal growth factor receptor; FGFR, fibroblast growth factor receptor; FLT3, Fms-like tyrosine kinase 3; HER2, human EGFR-2; JAK2, Janus kinase 2; NTRK, neurotrophin receptor kinase; PDGFR, platelet-derived growth factor receptor; RET, *ret* proto-oncogene; SYK, spleen tyrosine kinase; VEGFR, vascular endothelial growth factor receptor.

†Mut, activating point mutations in the kinase; Overexp, overexpression of the kinase; Transloc, chromosomal translocations producing fusion proteins with the tyrosine kinase; VEGF, vascular endothelial growth factor.

‡ALCL, anaplastic large cell lymphoma; ALL, acute lymphoblastic leukemia; AML, acute myeloid leukemia; CML, chronic myeloid leukemia; CMML, chronic myelomonocytic leukemia; ET, essential thrombocytosis; GIST, gastrointestinal stromal tumor; HES, hypereosinophilic syndrome; IMF, idiopathic myelofibrosis; IMT, inflammatory myofibroblastic tumor; MDS, myelodysplastic syndrome; MEN, multiple endocrine neoplasia; MM, multiple myeloma; NSCLC, non-small cell lung cancer; PCV, polycythemia vera; PTC, papillary thyroid cancer; RCC, renal cell carcinoma; SCCHN, squamous cell carcinoma of the head and neck; SCLC, small cell lung cancer; SM, systemic mastocytosis.

The first molecularly targeted therapies, trastuzumab (Herceptin) and imatinib (Gleevec), are typical of the two general classes of tyrosine kinase inhibitors: (1) humanized monoclonal antibodies targeting growth factor receptors on the surface of the cancer cell (trastuzumab) and (2) small molecule inhibitors either of receptors or of intracellular pathways that regulate growth of the cancer cells (imatinib). All generic names for monoclonal antibodies end in "-mab," and all generic names of small molecule inhibitors end in "-nib."

Trastuzumab

Trastuzumab, a recombinant, humanized, monoclonal antibody, was the first FDA-approved targeted anticancer monoclonal antibody. Trastuzumab was approved for the treatment of metastatic epidermal growth factor receptor 2 (ErbB2)–positive breast cancer. Overexpression of the ErbB2 receptor was associated with more poorly differentiated tumors, higher rates of metastases, and shorter survival.[38] Trastuzumab binds to the extracellular domain of ErbB2, which inhibits growth and causes apoptosis of tumor cells expressing ErbB2. Although trastuzumab is very well tolerated as far as side effect profile, heart failure has been reported. The overall incidence of trastuzumab varies in the literature from 2%-28%. The incidence of cardiac dysfunction ranges from 2%-7% when trastuzumab is used as monotherapy, 2%-13% when trastuzumab is used in combination with paclitaxel, and up to 27% when trastuzumab is used concurrently with anthracyclines plus cyclophosphamide.[20-27] In a recent study looking at the long-term cardiac tolerability of trastuzumab at MDACC, the overall incidence of cardiotoxicity was 28%.[28] Cited risk factors for trastuzumab-induced CMP include age >50, borderline left ventricular ejection fraction (LVEF) prior to treatment, history of cardiovascular disease, the sequence in which chemotherapy is administered, and prior treatment with anthracyclines (cumulative doses >300 mg/m^2).[20-31]

Mechanism of Toxicity

Deletion of human epidermal growth factor receptor 2 (ErbB) is lethal in mice in midgestation because the left ventricle fails to form properly. Mice with cardiac-specific deletion of ErbB2, after cardiac development was complete, were viable. However, these mice developed dilated cardiomyopathy as they aged and had shorter survival when subjected to pressure overload induced by aortic banding. Neuregulin-1–induced activation of ErbB2 in cardiomyocytes activates the extracellular receptor kinase (ERK) and the phosphoinositide 3-kinase (PI3K)/protein kinase B (Akt) pathways that promote cardiomyocyte proliferation during development and cardiomyocyte survival during adulthood. Cardiomyocyte apoptosis in ErbB2-deficient hearts was not significantly increased; however, expression of the antiapoptotic protein Bcl-X was increased. Thus, inhibition of ErbB2 signaling appears to lead to dysfunction and death both in breast cancer cells that overexpress the ErbB2 receptor and in normal cardiomyocytes (i.e., "on-target" toxicity).[38,45-47]

Bevacizumab

Bevacizumab (Avastin) is a monoclonal antibody that recognizes all vascular endothelial growth factor isoforms, thus blocking the kinase activation and tumor angiogenesis. Bevacizumab was the first angiogenesis inhibitor that was clinically available in the United States; it has been very effective in treating colorectal cancer and is now approved for use in combination with 5-fluorouracil–based therapy for metastatic colorectal carcinoma.[48] Hypertension is a common adverse effect in patients treated with bevacizumab, with an overall incidence reported to vary from of 4% to 35%.[4] The fact that bevacizumab causes hypertension is important because uncontrolled blood pressure and inhibition of signaling by vascular endothelial growth factor (VEGF) and vascular endothelial growth factor receptor (VEGFR) have been implicated as the principal mechanisms underlying heart failure.[38] The incidence of heart failure among patients taking bevacizumab ranges from 1.7% to 3%.[4] According to the prescribing information, heart failure developed in 1.7% of patients treated with bevacizumab during clinical trials. In addition, two phase III clinical studies demonstrated that the rate of heart failure in the bevacizumab-treated conditions was 2.2% to 3%.[49,50]

Imatinib

The first targeted small molecule inhibitor to be used successfully in malignancies was imatinib (Gleevac). This agent inhibits the activity of the fusion protein, Bcr-Abl, which arises from the chromosomal translocation that creates the Philadelphia chromosome and is the causal factor in approximately 90% of cases of chronic myeloid leukemia and some cases of B-cell acute lymphoblastic leukemia. This translocation creates a constitutively active protein kinase that drives proliferation and inhibits apoptosis in bone marrow stem cells, which leads to the leukemias. Imatinib has dramatically changed the management and prognosis of chronic myeloid leukemia; sustained remissions have been reported in more than 90% of patients after 5 years of initial treatment. However, imatinib has been reported to cause heart failure.[51] In contrast to trastuzumab, the cardiotoxicity of imatinib was surprising because c-Abl, the kinase expressed in all cells, including cardiomyocytes, was not known to play a role in maintenance of cardiomyocyte viability. In cardiomyocytes, inhibition of c-Abl led to activation of stress responses, culminating in marked mitochondrial dysfunction and cell death (Figure 58-2).

Although the incidence of LV dysfunction with imatinib is not known precisely, peripheral edema is observed relatively frequently, with reported incidence of up to 86%, and another 12% to 21% of patients complain of dyspnea, according to the package insert. A newly reengineered version of imatinib, WBZ-4, has been designed to inhibit c-KIT without inhibiting Abl, and has been shown to be just as effective as imatinib against gastrointestinal stromal tumors with significantly less risk of heart disturbances.[52]

Imatinib therapy as a causal factor of heart failure is relatively uncommon and occurs mainly in elderly patients with preexisting cardiac conditions. Accordingly, patients with a

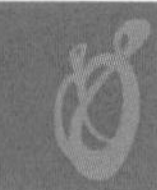

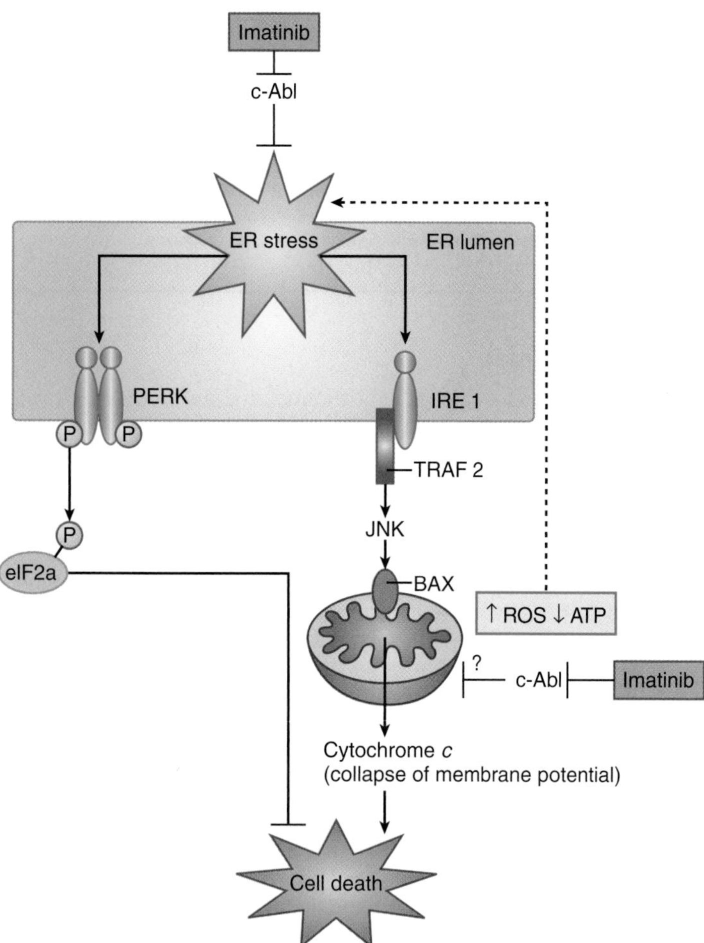

FIGURE 58–2 Targeted tyrosine kinase inhibition can lead to cellular apoptosis. Under stress, cells undergo an endoplasmic reticulum (ER) stress response (also called the "unfolded response"), which can lead to activation of cell death pathways through protein kinase R (PKR)–like ER kinase (PERK) and eventually to growth arrest DNA damage 34 (GADD34)–protein phosphatase 1 (PP1) complex, which in turn results in dephosphorylation of eukaryotic translation initiation factor (eIF2), thereby promoting apoptosis. ER stress also activates *c-jun* N-terminal kinase (JNK) signaling, mediated by integral membrane protein of the ER (IRE1) and by tumor necrosis factor receptor–associated factor 2 (TRAF2), which leads to translocation of Bax to the mitochondrial membrane. The result is cytochrome *c* release and collapse of the mitochondrial membrane potential. Salubrinal is a small-molecule inhibitor of the ER stress response that prevents dephosphorylation of eIF2 and prevents apoptosis through a pathway upstream from JNK activation. The nonreceptor tyrosine kinase c-Abl may act to suppress the ER stress response indirectly by preventing mitochondrial collapse or directly through a mechanism as yet unidentified. Anticancer drugs that target tyrosine kinases (e.g., imatinib mesylate) may promote apoptosis and heart damage by inhibiting c-Abl, thereby leading to a sustained ER stress response. ROS, reactive oxygen species. (Redrawn from Mann DL. Targeted cancer therapeutics: the heartbreak of success. *Nat Med* 2006;12:881-882.)

history of cardiac conditions should be monitored closely and treated aggressively with standard medical therapy (described later) if they develop symptoms suggestive of heart failure. In general, imatinib is considered safe and remains one of the most effective therapies for chronic myeloid leukemia.

Sunitinib

Sunitinib (Sutent) is is an oral, small-molecule, multitargeted receptor tyrosine kinase inhibitor that was approved by the FDA for the treatment of renal cell carcinoma and imatinib-resistant gastrointestinal stromal tumor. Sunitinib targets VEGFR-1, VEGFR-2, VEGFR-3, platelet-derived growth factor receptors α and β, *c-KIT*, FMS-like tyrosine kinase-3 (FLT-3), colony-stimulating factor–1 receptor, and the product of the human *ret* proto-oncogene (RET, mutated in medullary thyroid carcinomas).[53] Although sunitinib is generally well tolerated, in one retrospective analysis of 75 patients treated with this agent, 8 (11%) had a cardiovascular event and 6 (8%) developed heart failure.[54] Of 36 patients treated at the approved sunitinib dose, 10 (28%) had absolute reductions in left ventricular ejection fraction (LVEF) of at least 10%, and 7 (19%) had LVEF reductions of 15% or more. Treatment with sunitinib resulted in increases in mean systolic and diastolic blood pressures; 35 (47%) of 75 individuals developed hypertension (blood pressure > 150/100 mm Hg). Both heart failure and LV dysfunction generally recover when sunitinib therapy is withheld and appropriate institution of medical management is initiated (see later discussion).

Sunitinib caused mitochondrial injury and cardiomyocyte apoptosis in mice and in cultured rat cardiomyocytes.[54] Hypertension induced by sunitinib may play an important role in causing heart failure, inasmuch as sunitinib may inhibit a receptor tyrosine kinase that aids in regulating the response of cardiomyocytes in the setting of hypertensive stress.[55] In addition, sunitinib may cause cardiotoxicity through inhibition of ribosomal S6 kinase, leading to the activation of the intrinsic apoptotic pathway and adenosine triphosphate depletion.[56]

DIAGNOSIS AND MONITORING OF PATIENTS RECEIVING CARDIOTOXIC CHEMOTHERAPEUTIC AGENTS (see Chapters 36 and 37)

In order to detect cardiac dysfunction in patients treated with chemotherapy, heart function must be monitored regularly during treatment. A baseline evaluation of LVEF must be obtained for comparison, and it is recommended that the same method be used for comparing serial measurements. Serial assessment of LVEF was first shown to be useful in clinical practice by Alexander and associates.[57] On the basis of their experiences, algorithms have been developed for serial monitoring of LVEF during anthracycline-based therapy.[58,59] Measurement of systolic function through evaluation of the LVEF with either multiple-gated angiography (MUGA) or echocardiography is one of the most commonly used methods of monitoring and diagnosing chemotherapy-induced cardiomyopathy. Radionuclide imaging of LV function appears to yield results comparable with those of 2-dimensional echocardiography with regard to monitoring changes in LV function.[60,61] However, it is not sensitive for early detection of preclinical (subclinical) cardiac disease, and it is influenced

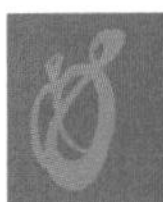

by contractility and preload/afterload effects that lead to transient changes. Therefore, other measurements of systolic function (e.g., fraction shortening) and diastolic function (e.g., ratio of early to late diastolic filling) have been used to detect early cardiotoxicity in addition to LVEF.[60] Abnormalities on exercise echocardiograms may be a better predictor of impending heart failure.[25]

Biomarkers may also provide useful clues about patients at risk for developing heart failure, as well as the progression of heart failure. Measurements of brain natriuretic peptide (BNP) are helpful in differentiating symptoms of heart failure from those of noncardiac causes when patients present to the emergency room.[62] The test is, however, limited because it is relatively nonspecific and because of a large range of "normal" values.[63] An elevated BNP level in patients undergoing chemotherapy appears to be more closely associated with impairment of LV diastolic function than with impairment of LV systolic function.[64] As noted in the "Monitoring and Anthracycline Toxicity" section, cardiac troponin measurement is a very sensitive way of diagnosing myocardial injury and damage. Not surprisingly, their persistent elevation is predictive of poor outcome and development of heart failure in cancer patients receiving chemotherapy.[27]

Endomyocardial biopsy is the most sensitive method of detecting anthracycline cardiotoxicity; light microscopy reveals marked myofibril loss and vacuolar degeneration, and electron microscopy reveals extensive loss of myofilaments.[65,66] However, abnormalities detected on electron microscopy have not been shown to be correlated highly with risk of development of heart failure, and these abnormalities are often present in patients at cumulative doses well below those associated with an increased risk of heart failure. Because of the technical nature of the procedure and the inherent risks, this is not a practical way to detect or monitor patients with anthracycline cardiotoxicity; serial determination of LV function, although insensitive, is the currently accepted method. Moreover, not every form of drug-induced cardiomyopathy can be detected reliably with endomyocardial biopsy, inasmuch as cardiac damage may be scattered.[67]

MANAGEMENT OF PATIENTS RECEIVING CARDIOTOXIC CHEMOTHERAPEUTIC AGENTS

At present, the guidelines of the Heart Failure Society of America and the American College of Cardiology/American Heart Association (ACC/AHA) do not contain specific recommendations for treatment of patients with what is presumed to be chemotherapy-induced heart failure. However, it is probably most reasonable at this time to treat the patient like any patient with newly diagnosed heart failure, as discussed in Chapters 45 and 46. In this regard, it is critical to rule out other potential causes of heart failure (see Table 35-2) before chemotherapy is assumed to have been the cause. Medical management of patients with stage A disease should focus on risk-factor reduction by controlling hypertension, diabetes, and hyperlipidemia, with the goal of preventing ventricular remodeling. Treatment of stages B, C, and D disease is aimed at improving survival, slowing disease progression, and alleviating symptoms. Patients with end-stage heart failure with refractory symptoms at rest despite maximal medical therapy and without evidence of cancer recurrence could be considered for synchronized pacing, placement of a ventricular assist device, or cardiac transplantation.[65] The effects of several agents discussed previously (including trastuzumab, imatinib, and sunitinib) appear to be reversible to some degree, and such reversal may be promoted by aggressive treatment with ACE inhibitors and β-blockers. Treatment with specific agents is discussed as follows.

Dexrazoxane

Dexrazoxane (Zinecard) is a free-radical scavenger that is used to protect the heart from the cardiotoxic side effects of anthracyclines. Several randomized control trials have been conducted to examine the effects of dexrazoxane in combination with anthracyclines, and all of these studies revealed that dexrazoxane is a highly effective cardioprotective agent that allows higher cumulative doses of doxorubicin.[16] However, one trial demonstrated that dexrazoxane might interfere with the antitumor activity of doxorubicin,[17] but this has not been a consistent finding in other studies. In the meta-analysis conducted by Van Dalen and colleagues,[68] a statistically significant benefit was found in favor of dexrazoxane for the occurrence of heart failure (relative risk, 0.29; 95% confidence interval, 0.20 to 0.41). No evidence was found for differences in response rate or survival between the subjects taking dexrazoxane and the control group.

In children with acute lymphoblastic leukemia, Lipshultz and associates[7] found that dexrazoxane prevented cardiac injury (as reflected by elevations in troponin T levels) related to doxorubicin therapy, without compromising the antitumor efficacy of doxorubicin. In this study, children treated with doxorubicin alone were more likely to have elevated troponin T levels (50% vs. 21%; $P < .001$) and extremely elevated troponin T levels (32% vs. 10%; $P < .001$) than were those who received dexrazoxane and doxorubicin. The rate of event-free survival at 2.5 years was 83% in both groups ($P = .87$ by the log-rank test).[7] Data for children confirm the protective role of dexrazoxane in patients receiving anthracyclines.

At present, however, the American Society of Clinical Oncology guidelines[69] recommend that dexrazoxane be considered for patients with metastatic breast cancer who have received more than 300 mg/m² of doxorubicin and who may benefit from continued doxorubicin-containing therapy. The use of dexrazoxane can also be considered in adult patients with other malignancies who have received more than 300 mg/m² of doxorubicin-based therapy; however, caution should be exercised in the use of dexrazoxane in settings in which doxorubicin-based therapy has been shown to improve survival.

Neurohormonal Antagonists (see Chapters 45 and 46)

β-Blockers. To date, there have been four case series in which researchers have evaluated the benefit of β-blockers in the treatment of anthracycline-induced cardiomyopathy.[4,70-73] In one study, beta blockers improved left ventricular ejection fraction in patients with anthracyline-induced cardiomyopathy. This improvement in myocardial function was comparable if not greater than the beneficial effects seen with beta blocker use in idiopathic dilated cardiomyopathy (Figure 58-3).[72] Of the β-blockers, carvedilol may have therapeutic advantages over the others in anthracycline-induced cardiomyopathy, inasmuch as it has been shown to possess antioxidant properties.[4] Moreover, in a single-blind, placebo-controlled trial in which the primary outcome was change in LVEF within 6 months of treatment, treatment with carvedilol prevented a decline in LVEF and prevented LV diastolic dysfunction.[24]

Angiotensin-Converting Enzyme Inhibitors. There is some evidence supporting the use of ACE inhibitors in patients with anthracycline-induced cardiomyopathy.[25,75,76] In a randomized, double-blind, controlled clinical trial in which enalapril was compared with placebo in 135 long-term survivors of pediatric cancer who had at least one cardiac abnormality identified at any time after anthracycline exposure, enalapril was shown to prevent a decline in LVEF in these long-term survivors. Although there was no difference in the primary outcome variable of maximal cardiac index, as determined by cycle ergometry, the rate of decline in LV end-systolic wall stress was greater in the subjects who took enalapril than in

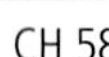

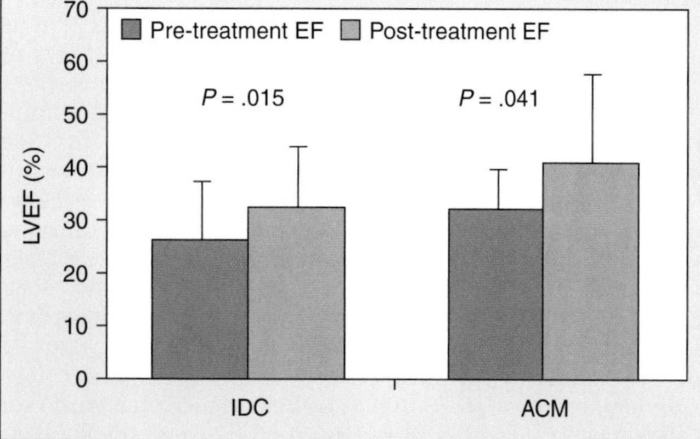

FIGURE 58–3 β-Blockade in left ventricular dysfunction induced by doxorubicin (Adriamycin). Affected patients were treated with β-blockers (metoprolol, carvedilol, and propranolol). The control group consisted of 16 consecutively chosen age- and sex-matched patients with idiopathic dilated cardiomyopathy (IDC) that was treated with β-blockers. The mean left ventricular ejection fraction (LVEF) improved from 28% to 41% (P = .041) in patients with doxorubicin-induced left ventricular dysfunction, whereas the LVEF improved from 26% to 32% (P =.015) in the patients with IDC. ACM, Adriamycin-induced cardiomyopathy; EF, ejection fraction. (From Noori A, Lindenfeld J, Wolfel E, et al. Beta-blockade in Adriamycin-induced cardiomyopathy. *J Card Fail* 2000;6:115-119.)

those who took the placebo (−8.59 vs. 1.85 g/cm^2; P = .033); the reduction was 9% by year 5 of the study.[25] However, in an observational study of 18 children treated with enalapril for LV dysfunction or heart failure, the beneficial effects of enalapril diminished after 6 to 10 years as a result of progressive LV wall thinning.[76] Thus, the clinical effects of ACE inhibitors in chemotherapy-induced heart failure are variable. Patients already taking β-blockers and ACE inhibitors before receiving chemotherapy should continue taking these medications, because withdrawal from these drugs can lead to deterioration of LV systolic function.

REVERSIBILITY OF CANCER THERAPY–INDUCED LEFT VENTRICULAR DYSFUNCTION

In contrast to that caused by anthracyclines, the LV dysfunction that occurs with several of the tyrosine kinase inhibitors, including trastuzumab, imatinib, and sunitinib, appears to have some degree of reversibility.[77] Discontinuation of trastuzumab is generally recommended when clinically significant heart failure occurs. However, patients who experience cardiotoxicity while receiving trastuzumab generally recover cardiac function when trastuzumab is discontinued over a mean time period of 1.5 months.[77] Patients who have experienced benefit with trastuzumab therapy and who have improved cardiac function while on a standard heart regimen may restart trastuzumab therapy while receiving protective heart failure medications and close cardiac monitoring.[77] In addition, Memorial-Sloan-Kettering Cancer Center has proposed guidelines for the management of patients treated with trastuzumab on the basis of physical status and LVEF.[78]

CONCLUSION

Cancer therapy–induced heart failure is a common problem observed by cardiologists and oncologists. Recognition and early detection of heart failure is critical for optimal management of patients undergoing cancer therapy. Once heart failure is identified, these patients should be treated aggressively with heart failure medications, which often lead to reversal of heart failure. Future studies will address the identification of genetic profiles of patients at risk for developing cancer therapy–induced heart failure, the optimal treatment strategies, and whether therapy for heart failure can be discontinued safely.

REFERENCES

1. Schultz, P. N., Beck, M. L., Stava, C., et al. (2003). Health profiles in 5836 long-term cancer survivors. *Int J Cancer, 104*, 488–495.
2. Moser, E. C., Noordijk, E. M., van Leeuwen, F. E., et al. (2006). Long-term risk of cardiovascular disease after treatment for aggressive non-Hodgkin lymphoma. *Blood, 107*, 2912–2919.
3. Yeh, E. T., Tong, A. T., Lenihan, D. J., et al. (2004). Cardiovascular complications of cancer therapy: diagnosis, pathogenesis, and management. *Circulation, 109*, 3122–3131.
4. Yeh, E. T., & Bickford, C. L. (2009). Cardiovascular complications of cancer therapy: incidence, pathogenesis, diagnosis, and management. *J Am Coll Cardiol, 53*, 2231–2247.
5. Singal, P. K., Deally, C. M., & Weinberg, L. E. (1987). Subcellular effects of Adriamycin in the heart: a concise review. *J Mol Cell Cardiol, 19*, 817–828.
6. Sinha, B. K., Katki, A. G., Batist, G., et al. (1987). Adriamycin-stimulated hydroxyl radical formation in human breast tumor cells. *Biochem Pharmacol, 36*, 793–796.
7. Lipshultz, S. E., Rifai, N., Dalton, V. M., et al. (2004). The effect of dexrazoxane on myocardial injury in doxorubicin-treated children with acute lymphoblastic leukemia. *N Engl J Med, 351*, 145–153.
8. Olson, H. M., Young, D. M., Prieur, D. J., et al. (1974). Electrolyte and morphologic alterations of myocardium in Adriamycin-treated rabbits. *Am J Pathol, 77*, 439–454.
9. Kusuoka, H., Futaki, S., Koretsune, Y., et al. (1991). Alterations of intracellular calcium homeostasis and myocardial energetics in acute Adriamycin-induced heart failure. *J Cardiovasc Pharmacol, 18*, 437–444.
10. Holmberg, S. R., & Williams, A. J. (1990). Patterns of interaction between anthraquinone drugs and the calcium-release channel from cardiac sarcoplasmic reticulum. *Circ Res, 67*, 272–283.
11. Gesi, M., Soldani, P., Lenzi, P., et al. (2002). Ecstasy during loud noise exposure induces dramatic ultrastructural changes in the heart. *Pharmacol Toxicol, 91*, 29–33.
12. Ferrari, R., Bachetti, T., Confortini, R., et al. (1995). Tumor necrosis factor soluble receptors in patients with various degrees of congestive heart failure. *Circulation, 92*, 1479–1486.
13. Torre-Amione, G., Kapadia, S., Benedict, C., et al. (1996). Proinflammatory cytokine levels in patients with depressed left ventricular ejection fraction: a report from the Studies of Left Ventricular Dysfunction (SOLVD). *J Am Coll Cardiol, 27*, 1201–1206.
14. Lyu, Y. L., Kerrigan, J. E., Lin, C. P., et al. (2007). Topoisomerase IIβ mediated DNA double-strand breaks: implications in doxorubicin cardiotoxicity and prevention by dexrazoxane. *Cancer Res, 67*, 8839–8846.
15. Shan, K., Lincoff, A. M., & Young, J. B. (1996). Anthracycline-induced cardiotoxicity. *Ann Intern Med, 125*, 47–58.
16. Wouters, K. A., Kremer, L. C., Miller, T. L., et al. (2005). Protecting against anthracycline-induced myocardial damage: a review of the most promising strategies. *Br J Haematol, 131*, 561–578.
17. Swain, S. M., Whaley, F. S., Gerber, M. C., et al. (1997). Cardioprotection with dexrazoxane for doxorubicin-containing therapy in advanced breast cancer. *J Clin Oncol, 15*, 1318–1332.
18. Von Hoff, D. D., Layard, M. W., Basa, P., et al. (1979). Risk factors for doxorubicin-induced congestive heart failure. *Ann Intern Med, 91*, 710–717.
19. Pai, V. B., & Nahata, M. C. (2000). Cardiotoxicity of chemotherapeutic agents: incidence, treatment and prevention. *Drug Saf, 22*, 263–302.
20. Gharib, M. I., & Burnett, A. K. (2002). Chemotherapy-induced cardiotoxicity: current practice and prospects of prophylaxis. *Eur J Heart Fail, 4*, 235–242.
21. Grenier, M. A., & Lipshultz, S. E. (1998). Epidemiology of anthracycline cardiotoxicity in children and adults. *Semin Oncol, 25*, 72–85.
22. Lipshultz, S. E., Alvarez, J. A., & Scully, R. E. (2008). Anthracycline associated cardiotoxicity in survivors of childhood cancer. *Heart, 94*, 525–533.
23. Swain, S. M., Whaley, F. S., & Ewer, M. S. (2003). Congestive heart failure in patients treated with doxorubicin: a retrospective analysis of three trials. *Cancer, 97*, 2869–2879.
24. Kalay, N., Basar, E., Ozdogru, I., et al. (2006). Protective effects of carvedilol against anthracycline-induced cardiomyopathy. *J Am Coll Cardiol, 48*, 2258–2262.
25. Silber, J. H., Cnaan, A., Clark, B. J., et al. (2004). Enalapril to prevent cardiac function decline in long-term survivors of pediatric cancer exposed to anthracyclines. *J Clin Oncol, 22*, 820–828.
26. Iarussi, D., Indolfi, P., Casale, F., et al. (2005). Anthracycline-induced cardiotoxicity in children with cancer: strategies for prevention and management. *Paediatr Drugs, 7*, 67–76.
27. Cardinale, D., Sandri, M. T., Colombo, A., et al. (2004). Prognostic value of troponin I in cardiac risk stratification of cancer patients undergoing high-dose chemotherapy. *Circulation, 109*, 2749–2754.
28. Braverman, A. C., Antin, J. H., Plappert, M. T., et al. (1991). Cyclophosphamide cardiotoxicity in bone marrow transplantation: a prospective evaluation of new dosing regimens. *J Clin Oncol, 9*, 1215–1223.
29. Goldberg, M. A., Antin, J. H., Guinan, E. C., et al. (1986). Cyclophosphamide cardiotoxicity: an analysis of dosing as a risk factor. *Blood, 68*, 1114–1118.
30. Gottdiener, J. S., Appelbaum, F. R., Ferrans, V. J., et al. (1981). Cardiotoxicity associated with high-dose cyclophosphamide therapy. *Arch Intern Med, 141*, 758–763.
31. Morandi, P., Ruffini, P. A., Benvenuto, G. M., et al. (2005). Cardiac toxicity of high-dose chemotherapy. *Bone Marrow Transplant, 35*, 323–334.
32. Quezado, Z. M., Wilson, W. H., Cunnion, R. E., et al. (1993). High-dose ifosfamide is associated with severe, reversible cardiac dysfunction. *Ann Intern Med, 118*, 31–36.

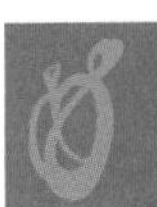

33. Martin, M., Pienkowski, T., Mackey, J., et al. (2005). Adjuvant docetaxel for node-positive breast cancer. *N Engl J Med, 352*, 2302–2313.
34. Marty, M., Cognetti, F., Maraninchi, D., et al. (2005). Randomized phase II trial of the efficacy and safety of trastuzumab combined with docetaxel in patients with human epidermal growth factor receptor 2–positive metastatic breast cancer administered as first-line treatment: the M77001 study group. *J Clin Oncol, 23*, 4265–4274.
35. Richardson, P. G., Sonneveld, P., Schuster, M. W., et al. (2005). Bortezomib or high-dose dexamethasone for relapsed multiple myeloma. *N Engl J Med, 352*, 2487–2498.
36. Voortman, J., & Giaccone, G. (2006). Severe reversible cardiac failure after bortezomib treatment combined with chemotherapy in a non–small cell lung cancer patient: a case report. *BMC Cancer, 6*, 129.
37. Krause, D. S., & Van Etten, R. A. (2005). Tyrosine kinases as targets for cancer therapy. *N Engl J Med, 353*, 172–187.
38. Chen, M. H., Kerkela, R., & Force, T. (2008). Mechanisms of cardiac dysfunction associated with tyrosine kinase inhibitor cancer therapeutics. *Circulation, 118*, 84–95.
39. Cohen, P. (2002). Protein kinases—the major drug targets of the twenty-first century? *Nat Rev Drug Discov, 1*, 309–315.
40. Blume-Jensen, P., & Hunter, T. (2001). Oncogenic kinase signalling. *Nature, 411*, 355–365.
41. Feldman, A. M., Lorell, B. H., & Reis, S. E. (2000). Trastuzumab in the treatment of metastatic breast cancer: anticancer therapy versus cardiotoxicity. *Circulation, 102*, 272–274.
42. Seidman, A., Hudis, C., Pierri, M. K., et al. (2002). Cardiac dysfunction in the trastuzumab clinical trials experience. *J Clin Oncol, 20*, 1215–1221.
43. Ewer, M. S., Gibbs, H. R., Swafford, J., & Benjamin, R. S. (1999). Cardiotoxicity in patients receiving trastuzumab (Herceptin): primary toxicity, synergistic or sequential stress, or surveillance artifact? *Semin Oncol, 26*, 96–101.
44. Bird, B. R., & Swain, S. M. (2008). Cardiac toxicity in breast cancer survivors: review of potential cardiac problems. *Clin Cancer Res, 14*, 14–24.
45. Crone, S. A., Zhao, Y. Y., Fan, L., et al. (2002). ErbB2 is essential in the prevention of dilated cardiomyopathy. *Nat Med, 8*, 459–465.
46. Lee, K. F., Simon, H., Chen, H., et al. (1995). Requirement for neuregulin receptor ErbB2 in neural and cardiac development. *Nature, 378*, 394–398.
47. Meyer, D., & Birchmeier, C. (1995). Multiple essential functions of neuregulin in development. *Nature, 378*, 386–390.
48. Ferrara, N., Hillan, K. J., Gerber, H. P., & Novotny, W. (2004). Discovery and development of bevacizumab, an anti-VEGF antibody for treating cancer. *Nat Rev Drug Discov, 3*, 391–400.
49. Miller, K., Wang, M., Gralow, J., et al. (2007). Paclitaxel plus bevacizumab versus paclitaxel alone for metastatic breast cancer. *N Engl J Med, 357*, 2666–2676.
50. Miller, K. D., Chap, L. I., Holmes, F. A., et al. (2005). Randomized phase III trial of capecitabine compared with bevacizumab plus capecitabine in patients with previously treated metastatic breast cancer. *J Clin Oncol, 23*, 792–799.
51. Kerkela, R., Grazette, L., Yacobi, R., et al. (2006). Cardiotoxicity of the cancer therapeutic agent imatinib mesylate. *Nat Med, 12*, 908–916.
52. Demetri, G. D. (2007). Structural reengineering of imatinib to decrease cardiac risk in cancer therapy. *J Clin Invest, 117*, 3650–3653.
53. Patyna, S., Arrigoni, C., Terron, A., et al. (2008). Nonclinical safety evaluation of sunitinib: a potent inhibitor of VEGF, PDGF, KIT, FLT3, and RET receptors. *Toxicol Pathol, 36*, 905–916.
54. Chu, T. F., Rupnick, M. A., Kerkela, R., et al. (2007). Cardiotoxicity associated with tyrosine kinase inhibitor sunitinib. *Lancet, 370*, 2011–2019.
55. Khakoo, A. Y., Kassiotis, C. M., Tannir, N., et al. (2008). Heart failure associated with sunitinib malate: a multitargeted receptor tyrosine kinase inhibitor. *Cancer, 112*, 2500–2508.
56. Force, T., Krause, D. S., & Van Etten, R. A. (2007). Molecular mechanisms of cardiotoxicity of tyrosine kinase inhibition. *Nat Rev Cancer, 7*, 332–344.
57. Alexander, J., Dainiak, N., Berger, H. J., et al. (1979). Serial assessment of doxorubicin cardiotoxicity with quantitative radionuclide angiocardiography. *N Engl J Med, 300*, 278–283.
58. Schwartz, R. G., McKenzie, W. B., Alexander, J., et al. (1987). Congestive heart failure and left ventricular dysfunction complicating doxorubicin therapy. Seven-year experience using serial radionuclide angiocardiography. *Am J Med, 82*, 1109–1118.
59. Steinherz, L. J., Graham, T., Hurwitz, R., et al. (1992). Guidelines for cardiac monitoring of children during and after anthracycline therapy: report of the Cardiology Committee of the Children's Cancer Study Group. *Pediatrics, 89*, 942–949.
60. Ganz, W. I., Sridhar, K. S., Ganz, S. S., et al. (1996). Review of tests for monitoring doxorubicin-induced cardiomyopathy. *Oncology, 53*, 461–470.
61. Ritchie, J. L., Singer, J. W., Thorning, D., et al. (1980). Anthracycline cardiotoxicity: clinical and pathologic outcomes assessed by radionuclide ejection fraction. *Cancer, 46*, 1109–1116.
62. Mueller, C., Scholer, A., Laule-Kilian, K., et al. (2004). Use of B-type natriuretic peptide in the evaluation and management of acute dyspnea. *N Engl J Med, 350*, 647–654.
63. Hassan, Y., Shapira, A. R., & Hassan, S. (2002). B-type natriuretic peptide in heart failure. *N Engl J Med, 347*, 1976–1978.
64. Nousiainen, T., Vanninen, E., Jantunen, E., et al. (2002). Natriuretic peptides during the development of doxorubicin-induced left ventricular diastolic dysfunction. *J Intern Med, 251*, 228–234.
65. Friedman, M. A., Bozdech, M. J., Billingham, M. E., et al. (1978). Doxorubicin cardiotoxicity. Serial endomyocardial biopsies and systolic time intervals. *JAMA, 240*, 1603–1606.
66. Mason, J. W., Bristow, M. R., Billingham, M. E., et al. (1978). Invasive and noninvasive methods of assessing Adriamycin cardiotoxic effects in man: superiority of histopathologic assessment using endomyocardial biopsy. *Cancer Treat Rep, 62*, 857–864.
67. Yusuf, S. W., Razeghi, P., & Yeh, E. T. (2008). The diagnosis and management of cardiovascular disease in cancer patients. *Curr Probl Cardiol, 33*, 163–196.
68. van Dalen, E. C., Caron, H. N., Dickinson, H. O., et al. (2008). Cardioprotective interventions for cancer patients receiving anthracyclines. *Cochrane Database Syst Rev* (2), CD003917.
69. Hensley, M. L., Hagerty, K. L., Kewalramani, T., et al. (2009). American Society of Clinical Oncology 2008 clinical practice guideline update: use of chemotherapy and radiation therapy protectants. *J Clin Oncol, 27*, 127–145.
70. Fazio, S., Palmieri, E. A., Ferravante, B., et al. (1998). Doxorubicin-induced cardiomyopathy treated with carvedilol. *Clin Cardiol, 21*, 777–779.
71. Mukai, Y., Yoshida, T., Nakaike, R., et al. (2004). Five cases of anthracycline-induced cardiomyopathy effectively treated with carvedilol. *Intern Med, 43*, 1087–1088.
72. Noori, A., Lindenfeld, J., Wolfel, E., et al. (2000). Beta-blockade in Adriamycin-induced cardiomyopathy. *J Card Fail, 6*, 115–119.
73. Shaddy, R. E., Olsen, S. L., Bristow, M. R., et al. (1995). Efficacy and safety of metoprolol in the treatment of doxorubicin-induced cardiomyopathy in pediatric patients. *Am Heart J, 129*, 197–199.
74. Oliveira, P. J., Bjork, J. A., Santos, M. S., et al. (2004). Carvedilol-mediated antioxidant protection against doxorubicin-induced cardiac mitochondrial toxicity. *Toxicol Appl Pharmacol, 200*, 159–168.
75. Cardinale, D., Colombo, A., Sandri, M. T., et al. (2006). Prevention of high-dose chemotherapy-induced cardiotoxicity in high-risk patients by angiotensin-converting enzyme inhibition. *Circulation, 114*, 2474–2481.
76. Lipshultz, S. E., Lipsitz, S. R., Sallan, S. E., et al. (2002). Long-term enalapril therapy for left ventricular dysfunction in doxorubicin-treated survivors of childhood cancer. *J Clin Oncol, 20*, 4517–4522.
77. Ewer, M. S., & Lippman, S. M. (2005). Type II chemotherapy-related cardiac dysfunction: time to recognize a new entity. *J Clin Oncol, 23*, 2900–2902.
78. Keefe, D. L. (2002). Trastuzumab-associated cardiotoxicity. *Cancer, 95*, 1592–1600.

CHAPTER 59

Disease Management in Heart Failure

Debra K. Moser and Barbara Riegel

Despite considerable scientific advances in the pharmacological and surgical management of patients with heart failure, one of the greatest challenges still facing clinicians is how to provide effective, efficient outpatient management for these patients that results in good clinical outcomes. Patients with heart failure consume a disproportionately high percentage of health care costs because of repeated bouts of decompensation that necessitate hospitalization or emergency intervention.[1,2] This problem is expected to increase as the incidence and prevalence of heart failure continue to escalate.[3,4] Most hospitalizations are thought to be preventable because they are precipitated by factors that are modifiable and could be better addressed during outpatient management. The major reasons for preventable hospitalizations are patients' lack of adherence to prescribed regimens and failure to seek early treatment for worsening symptoms.[5,6]

According to the traditional view of the relationship between the patient and health care provider, the physician or advanced practice nurse prescribes a regimen, and the patient follows it.[7] In this view, failure of the regimen to produce the desired outcome usually is blamed on the patient's failure to follow the regimen. Indeed, even the best therapeutic plan will fail if patients do not follow it. However, reasons for patient nonadherence are complex. By simply blaming the patient for not following the prescribed plan, clinicians ignore these complexities and overlook contributing factors that could be remedied with intervention.

Many factors that contribute to failure to implement the treatment plan have been identified. These factors are related to the patient, provider, and health care system. Patient-related factors can often be overcome or compensated for by changes in the health care provider's approach or by changing the health care delivery system.[8] Inadequacies in the delivery of advice and recommendations by clinicians contribute significantly to treatment noncompliance and poor outcomes.[9-12] Other common reasons for rehospitalization are poor discharge planning, inadequate follow-up after discharge, and health care providers' failure to attend to patient characteristics (e.g., depression, cognitive impairment, lack of a social support system, inability to pay for expensive medications) that render patients prone to repeated hospitalizations.[13-15] Thus, to understand why therapeutic regimens fail, it is more helpful to address issues involving the patient, provider, and health care system.[16] Optimal outpatient management of patients with heart failure depends on a thorough understanding of all three factors that contribute to nonadherence and how to address them (Table 59-1). Knowing what to recommend and prescribe for patients is important in outpatient management, but understanding how to convey this information to patients and how to structure the system to support treatment adherence is even more important. Thus, the focus of this chapter is on application of effective models of care for outpatient management.

SIGNIFICANCE OF THE PROBLEM

Treatment Adherence

In a report on adherence to long-term therapies, the World Health Organization estimated that rates of such adherence are about 50% in developed countries and even lower in developing countries.[8] The consequences of poor adherence include adverse health outcomes, poor quality of life, and increased health care costs.[8] As Haynes emphasized in a Cochrane Database report on medication adherence, "Increasing the effectiveness of adherence interventions may have a far greater impact on the health of the population than any improvement in specific medical treatments."[17]

Treatment adherence among patients with heart failure is poor.[18] Medication nonadherence is a significant contributor to rehospitalization. In one study, of 231 patients with heart failure who were hospitalized with sodium retention, 20% had not adhered to the drug regimen.[19] In another study of 94 patients with heart failure, 13% admitted to not taking their medications as prescribed.[20] These statistics, obtained through patient self-reports, are probably underestimates of the true prevalence of nonadherence. Objective indicators of adherence reveal far greater levels of nonadherence. In a study of more than 7000 elderly patients prescribed digoxin, only 10% of the sample refilled their prescription often enough to have taken the appropriate amount of medication for 1 year; 19% of patients refilled the prescription only one time.[21] Electronic event monitoring of angiotensin-converting enzyme (ACE) inhibitor therapy revealed that 19% of patients took less than 70% of the prescribed doses and that adherence declined markedly among patients who were prescribed formulations that required dosing more than once per day.[22] Lack of medication adherence is clearly linked to increased risk for rehospitalization and mortality in patients with heart failure.[23]

Adherence to a low-sodium diet is important for patients with heart failure, according to heart failure guidelines. Adherence to dietary recommendations of sodium restriction is even lower than adherence to medication regimens. Fewer than half of patients consistently follow a low-sodium diet.[19] Even after a 6-month education intervention, only 35% of patients studied routinely avoided salty foods, which demonstrates the need to take into account factors involving patients, providers, and the health care system.[24] One reason for poor adherence to dietary sodium restrictions may be failure

TABLE 59–1 Actions to Increase Compliance with Prevention and Treatment Recommendations

Actions by Patients	Specific Strategies
Patients must engage in essential prevention and treatment behaviors.	
• Decide to control risk factors.	Understand rationale, importance of commitment.
• Negotiate goals with provider.	Develop communication skills.
• Develop skills for adopting and maintaining recommended behaviors.	Use reminder systems.
• Monitor progress toward goals.	Use self-monitoring skills.
• Resolve problems that block achievement of goals.	Develop problem-solving skills; use social support networks.
Patients must communicate with providers about prevention and treatment services.	Define own needs on basis of experience. Validate rationale for continuing to follow recommendations.
Actions by Providers	**Specific Strategies**
Providers must foster effective communication with patients.	
• Provide clear, direct messages about importance of a behavior or therapy.	Provide verbal and written instruction, including rationale for treatments. Develop skills in communication/counseling.
• Include patients in decisions about prevention and treatment goals and related strategies.	Use tailoring and contracting strategies. Negotiate goals and a plan. Anticipate barriers to compliance and discuss solutions. Use active listening.
• Incorporate behavioral strategies into counseling.	Develop multicomponent strategies (i.e., cognitive and behavioral).
Providers must document and respond to patients' progress toward goals.	
• Create an evidence-based practice.	Determine methods of evaluating outcomes.
• Assess patients' compliance at each visit.	Use self-report or electronic data.
• Develop reminder systems to ensure identification and follow-up of patient status.	Use telephone follow-up.
Actions by Health Care Organizations	**Specific Strategies**
Health care organizations must develop an environment that supports prevention and treatment interventions.	Develop training in behavioral science, office set-up for all personnel. Use preappointment reminders. Use telephone follow-up. Schedule evening/weekend office hours. Provide group/individual counseling for patients and families.
• Provide tracking and reporting systems.	Develop computer-based systems (electronic medical records).
• Provide education and training for providers.	Require continuing education courses in communication, behavioral counseling.
• Provide adequate reimbursement for allocation of time for all health care professionals.	Develop incentives tied to desired patient and provider outcomes.
Health care organizations must adopt systems to rapidly and efficiently incorporate innovations into medical practice.	Incorporate nursing case management. Implement pharmacy patient profile and recall review systems. Use electronic transmission storage of patient's self-monitored data. Obtain patient data on lifestyle behavior before visit. Provide continuous quality improvement training.

Reproduced with permission from Miller NH, Hill M, Kottke T, et al. The multilevel compliance challenge: recommendations for a call to action. A statement for healthcare professionals. *Circulation* 1997;95:1085-1090, Table 1. Copyright © American Heart Association.

of providers to stress the importance of a sodium-restricted diet. Although heart failure guidelines consistently emphasize the importance of sodium restriction, one study revealed that fewer than 22% of patients admitted for an exacerbation of heart failure were prescribed a sodium-restricted diet at discharge.[19] Another reason may be failure of clinicians to assess patients' skill in choosing a diet low in sodium. Only one study was located in which clinicians assessed patient skill in the ability to sort foods into those containing high and low sodium content.[25] The authors found that only 14% of patients were aware of the sodium restriction guideline and only 58% was able to read the label's sodium content. Clearly, the current approaches to educating patients about this important aspect of therapy are lacking in some manner.

Symptom Recognition

According to the self-care model described in "The Self-Care Paradigm" section, patients must be able to recognize symptoms if they are to manage their heart failure successfully. Patients with heart failure who are able to recognize their symptoms are more successful in subsequent steps of the self-care process.[26] However, symptom recognition has been found to be poor in most patients with heart failure.[13,27] In careful studies of patients' recognition of symptoms, fewer than 50% of patients were able to recognize the common symptoms of worsening heart failure, including weight gain, edema, difficulty sleeping because of shortness of breath, and fatigue, and 40% of patients were unable to recognize escalating shortness of breath.[26] Difficulty in recognizing symptoms may stem, in part, from failure of health care providers to teach this important aspect of care. Few patients are instructed, even during a hospitalization for exacerbation of heart failure, to weigh themselves to monitor fluid status; most patients do not appreciate the importance of daily weighing, and as a consequence, most do not weigh themselves daily.[24,28,29] Bennett and colleagues[30] noted that self-monitoring was reported only by patients who attended a heart failure clinic. Self-monitoring (e.g., daily weighings, edema assessment) was apparently not emphasized to patients receiving care in other settings.

Seeking Assistance When Needed

Knowing when to seek assistance from a health care provider and doing so are important self-care behaviors for patients with heart failure. Failure to seek care in a timely manner—before symptoms have escalated to the point where hospitalization is necessary to control them—is common among patients with heart failure. However, care-seeking behavior

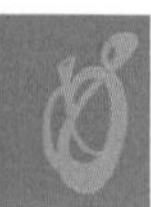

among patients with heart failure is an understudied area. Frontiero and associates[20] found that only about half of patients reported talking to their physician whenever they needed guidance. Many patients wait days with worsening symptoms, even shortness of breath, before seeking care.[31]

Changing Unhealthy Lifestyles

Exercise, limiting alcohol consumption, and smoking cessation would benefit many patients with heart failure, but adherence with these recommendations is poor. In one study, 67% of patients reported not exercising regularly.[20] Ni and colleagues[32] reported that 30% of patients had stopped exercising after heart failure was diagnosed. One fourth of patients failed to appreciate the risk of drinking excess alcohol, 12% were current smokers, and 21% engaged in physical exercise less than once a month or never. It has been noted in other patient populations that physicians often fail to recommend changing unhealthy lifestyle behaviors.[33]

FAILURE OF THE TRADITIONAL HEALTH CARE DELIVERY MODEL

It is really no surprise that adherence to treatment is poor; many patients with heart failure are unable to recognize their early symptoms, and unhealthy lifestyle behaviors are common, in view of the traditional health care delivery model. In most cases, patients with heart failure are treated by clinicians who use usual practices typical of traditional health care delivery models. Management in traditional models is characterized by episodic, brief encounters with health care providers and punctuated by hospitalizations for acute exacerbations of heart failure. Several aspects of this typical care model actually contribute to increased rates of rehospitalization.[10] Despite the opportunity to closely assess patients, modify therapy under observation, and provide intensive education during a hospitalization for an acute exacerbation, the preponderance of evidence suggests that management during hospitalization is inadequate.[10] Approximately 20% of unplanned hospital readmissions for heart failure have been attributed to substandard inpatient care.[10] The areas of substandard care thought to contribute most to readmissions are lack of patient and family education and failure to organize follow-up care. In-hospital patient education is limited; many patients receive inadequate education and counseling.[9,34] Follow-up after hospital discharge usually consists of a few short visits with physicians in which there is little time to address the multiple and complex medical, behavioral, psychosocial, environmental, and financial issues that complicate the care of patients with heart failure.

Failure to prescribe appropriate drug therapy also contributes substantially to the high rate of rehospitalizations for heart failure. Multiple guidelines[35-38] describe standards for heart failure medical therapy that are based on results of large controlled clinical trials; nonetheless, as many as 50% to 72% of patients still do not receive prescriptions for ACE inhibitors and other drugs demonstrated to be effective in heart failure, do not receive them in adequate doses, or receive prescriptions for drugs such as calcium channel blockers that may have deleterious effects in heart failure.[12,39-41] Thus, although there have been some improvements in prescription patterns for patients with heart failure, the use of appropriate medications for heart failure is not yet widespread.

Because these issues must be addressed in order to improve heart failure outcomes, and because of the increasing incidence, prevalence, and economic costs of heart failure, many authorities have recommended that the current treatment patterns of fragmented care, in which acute in-patient episodes are common, be changed to comprehensive, integrated expert multidisciplinary care patterns.[2,42] By changing the outpatient health care delivery model for patients with chronic heart failure to incorporate evidence-based components shown to improve outcomes, many patient, provider, and system factors that contribute to nonadherence will be addressed.

MANAGEMENT OF HEART FAILURE

Most patients with heart failure seek the attention of health care providers because they experience worrisome symptoms. The most common symptoms of heart failure are manifestations of volume overload, including shortness of breath, fatigue, peripheral edema, and difficulty sleeping, which greatly impair patients' quality of life.[43] These symptoms are particularly burdensome because patients with heart failure are usually elderly and often have multiple comorbid conditions, multiple drug prescriptions, psychosocial concerns, financial constraints, and physical limitations.[13] In addition, many of these patients are socially isolated, cognitively impaired, and depressed.[13,44-48]

The symptoms of heart failure, although burdensome, are often subtle initially and may be confused with signs of normal aging or drug side effects.[49] Because of the subtlety of early symptoms, patients need access to experts with whom they can discuss their questions and concerns. Sorting out the various symptoms and managing the complex medication regimen require a specialized knowledge base that general practitioners may not have mastered.[50]

The complexities of heart failure care are suited to disease management, which, by definition, involves practice redesign with increased availability of experts, use of evidence-based guidelines, improved education and counseling, and use of monitored outcomes to improve care processes. Disease management has been shown to (1) improve knowledge about heart failure; (2) facilitate health behavior change that improves self-care, including adherence to treatment and management of symptoms; and (3) improve clinical outcomes, such as lower rehospitalization rates, lower hospitalization costs, and lower rates of mortality.[51-60]

Since the 1980s, when the first program of management for heart failure was tested, more than 50 published studies have been conducted to test the effects of heart failure specialty care delivered in a disease management model. Although each program is different, all programs include care that reflects a significant departure from traditional episodic care delivery. These programs can be categorized broadly into two types: (1) heart failure clinics and (2) heart failure care delivered in or to the home. In addition, there are other heart failure–specific programs that do not meet criteria of disease management programs. Although these approaches are not disease management in the true sense, some authors have referred to them as disease management, and some have been effective in improving outcomes in patients with heart failure.[61-63]

Heart failure clinics are disease management programs in which service is provided primarily in an outpatient clinic setting; patients come to the clinic to receive care from practitioners with expertise in heart failure. Programs providing heart failure care in or to the home include a variety of disease management approaches, all of which entail heart failure–specific care that is delivered primarily in the patient's home; care may be delivered by telephone, in person, or by both means. Many of these programs take a case management approach. Included in this group of studies are examples of true multidisciplinary care in which experts from three or more disciplines work collaboratively to deliver heart failure specialty care.[64] Other programs involve only mailed educational materials,[63] only a home telemonitoring system,[61] or increased access only to primary care.[62]

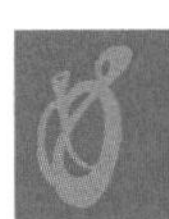

Although a few studies have demonstrated a neutral or negative effect of management programs for heart failure, most such programs, regardless of type, have yielded positive outcomes.[51-60] Meta-analyses have confirmed that in most studies, patients who are cared for in these programs experience fewer rehospitalizations, incur lower health care costs, and, in many cases, have longer survival (Table 59-2).[51,54,57] Many patients demonstrate improved functional and symptom status and enjoy better quality of life than they did before the intervention and in comparison with patients treated with usual care.[54,56,57]

Management of Heart Failure in Special Populations (see also Chapter 49)

Surprisingly few investigators have tested disease management approaches in vulnerable patient populations such as minority, immigrant, or poor populations or populations of color. In one systematic review of cardiovascular disease interventions, only seven studies in vulnerable populations with heart failure were identified. This lack of research is surprising, inasmuch as significantly more African Americans than white patients are hospitalized for heart failure.[65] Prevalence and incidence of heart failure appear to be lower among Hispanic populations than among African American and white populations, but hospitalization rates may be higher. Alexander and colleagues[66] found that the percentage of patients rehospitalized for heart failure or other causes, total hospital days, and total hospital charges were all significantly higher for Hispanic patients than for non-Hispanic white patients; Hispanic patients were more likely to be rehospitalized multiple times. Little to nothing is known about Native American and Asian Pacific Islander residents in the United States.

The studies included in a systematic review[65] were a subset of some of the major disease management studies, chosen if they included a significant proportion of African American patients. Artinian and associates[67] enrolled 18 patients, 65% of whom were African American. Benatar and associates[68] enrolled 216 patients, of whom 186 (86%) were African American. DeWalt and coworkers[69] enrolled 25 patients, of whom 15 (60%) were African American with poor literacy. Naylor and colleagues[70] enrolled 239 patients, of whom 86 (36%) were African American. Rich and associates[71] enrolled 282 patients, of whom 155 (55%) were African American. Sisk and coworkers[72] enrolled 406 patients, of whom 187 (46%) were African American and 134 (33%) were Hispanic. Finally, O'Connell and associates[73] enrolled 35 indigent patients, of whom 18 (51%) were Hispanic, into a pretest/posttest assessment of case management for heart failure.

After Davis and coworkers[65] completed their review, Riegel and colleagues[74] published the report of a randomized, controlled trial testing a telephone-based disease management approach, previously shown to be effective in the general population, in a sample of Hispanic patients. Patients self-identified as Hispanic who were hospitalized with chronic heart failure were enrolled and randomly assigned to receive either telephone calls from bilingual/bicultural nurse case managers for 6 months (n = 69) or usual care (n = 65). Surprisingly, the intervention had no effect on hospitalization rate, quality of life, or depression in this sample. In comparison with the results of Sisk and coworkers[72]—the only other randomized controlled trial with a significant proportion of Hispanic patients—Riegel and colleagues' method effectively lowered the rehospitalization rate (143 hospitalizations among patients receiving telephone calls vs. 180 hospitalizations among the patients receiving usual care at 12 months). However, only 33% of Sisk and coworkers' population were Hispanic, and results were not analyzed by race or ethnicity. Riegel and colleagues suggested that a different approach may be needed in culturally diverse, elderly, functionally compromised, poorly educated, or unacculturated groups. This is clearly an area in which further research is needed.

PUTTING MANAGEMENT OF HEART FAILURE INTO PRACTICE

Despite the superiority of outpatient management of heart failure, only a minority of patients with heart failure receive care through these care delivery models. Assuming that nonadherence is the result of factors related to the patient, provider, and health care system, a concerted effort to influence each of these components will have the best chance of improving outcomes in this challenging patient population. Programs of management for heart failure address each of these three areas. Patient factors are assessed and addressed, providers work from a knowledge base and framework that ensures appropriate care, and the system for care delivery has been modified to produce optimal outcomes. Thus, appropriate patients should be referred to these management programs when possible. However, these management programs are not available to the majority of patients and providers. In such cases, it is possible for providers to use the principles of management of heart failure in their practice (Box 59-1). An individual provider will have difficulty using disease management principles alone; therefore, a physician–advanced practice nurse team is suggested and described further later in the "Care Delivered by Advanced Practice Nurse–Physician Team" section. A vital first step in implementing management of heart failure is to understand and promote patient self-care.

The Self-Care Paradigm

Clinicians long ago accepted the idea of self-care for patients with diabetes mellitus. They have been much slower to accept it for patients with other types of chronic illnesses, despite compelling evidence that promotion of patients' self-care abilities results in improved outcomes.[75-77] Self-care is the process in which patients, often with the help of their families or another caregiver, participate in their own care (Figure 59-1). Self-care is the foundation upon which successful management of heart failure is built. The terms *self-care, self-management, adherence,* and *knowledge* frequently are used interchangeably, but each has a distinct meaning.[78] Investigators have often measured regimen adherence or knowledge and call these "self-care".[24] In other studies, knowledge is assumed to be sufficient for self-care by authors who overlook the fact that knowledge is necessary but not sufficient for self-care.[79] Thus, it is important that clinicians understand the process of self-care so that they can assist patients to participate effectively in it.

The self-care process includes both maintenance and management components.[80] An assumption of self-care is that for patients with heart failure to be successful at self-care, they must engage in the behaviors that will help them to stay physiologically stable (e.g., eating a low-sodium diet) and they must adhere to the prescribed regimen, which is self-care *maintenance.* They also must make decisions about how to address signs and symptoms when they occur (e.g., take extra diuretic if weight increases 3 pounds [1.4 kg] in 1 week), which is self-care *management.* The process of self-care consists of the stages illustrated in Figure 59-1. A major factor that influences patients' skill at self-care management activities is self-efficacy, or confidence in one's ability to perform self-care.[80]

Stage 1 of the self-care process, maintenance, involves symptom monitoring and treatment adherence. Self-care maintenance involves following the advice of health care providers to follow the treatment plan, make healthy lifestyle choices, and monitor for symptom changes. Patients who

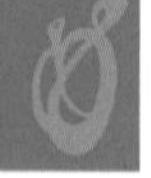

TABLE 59–2 Meta-analyses of Management Programs for Heart Failure

Reference	Number of Studies Reviewed	Characteristics of Studies	Number of Patients Included in Studies Reviewed	Results	Conclusions
Clark et al (2007)[57]	13 Trials (9 studies of structured telephone support, 3 studies of telemonitoring, 1 study of both)	All randomized, controlled trials	4264 Patients; mean age of study participants: 57-75 years; NYHA classes II-IV; LVEF < 40%	All-cause mortality (14 studies): • 20% reduction, 95% CI = 0.08-0.31 • Telemonitoring (RR = 0.62; 95% CI = 0.45-0.85) was more beneficial than the structured telephone support (RR = 0.85; 95% CI = 0.72-1.01) All-cause admissions (8 studies): • No benefit from telemonitoring (RR = 0.98; 95% CI = 0.84-1.15) or structured telephone support (RR = 0.94; 95% CI = 0.87-1.02) Admissions for heart failure (9 studies): • No benefit from telemonitoring (RR = 0.86; 95% CI = 0.57-1.28) or structured telephone support (RR = 0.78; 95% CI = 0.68-0.89). QOL, cost, and acceptability: • Significant improvement in QOL in 3 of 6 studies • Lower health care costs in 3 of 4 studies of structured telephone support interventions • Acceptable to patients in 3 of 4 studies	Remote monitoring programs are beneficial to some clinical health outcomes in community-dwelling patients with heart failure
Gohler et al (2006)[8]	36 Trials (16 in the United States): DMPs consisted of patient education (on average, three educational components) and discharge plan (scheduled clinic visits, home visits, or nurse-initiated telephone contacts);	All randomized, controlled trials	8341 Patients; 37%-99% men; mean age of study participants: 56-79 years; 33%-100% NYHA classes II-IV	All-cause admissions (32 studies): • Pooled difference on the first all-cause rehospitalization: 8% favoring DMPs ($P < .0001$, 95% CI = 0.05-0.11; NNT = 13, 95% CI = 0.09-0.20) • Pooled difference on the subsequent all-cause rehospitalization: 19% favoring DMPs ($P < .0001$, 95% CI = 0.02-0.35; NNT = 5, 95% CI = 0.03-0.50) • Personal contact was more effective than telephone contact (risk difference, −10.5% vs. −3.6%) All-cause mortality (30 studies): • Pooled mortality difference: 3% favoring DMPs ($P < .01$, 95% CI = 0.01-0.05; NNT = 33, 95% CI = 0.20-1.00) • Personal contact was more effective than telephone contact (risk difference, −3.0% vs. −2.6%) • Studies with prolonged follow-up period showed significant effect on mortality	DMPs decrease rates of all-cause admissions and all-cause mortality Age, severity of disease, medication, intervention team composition, intervention approach, and length of follow-up are related to the effect of DMPs
Holland et al (2005)[55]	30 Trials (13 in the United States): 12 studies of home visits, 15 studies of home physiological monitoring such as videophone (3 studies), telephone or mailing (12 studies), and 3 studies of interventions exclusively at hospital or clinic	All randomized, controlled trials of multidisciplinary management programs in both hospital and community settings	7581 Patients; 27%-99% men; mean age of study participants: 56-86 years; NYHA classes II-IV in 8 studies; mean LVEF: 22%-43%	All-cause admissions (21 studies: RR = 0.87; 95% CI = 0.79-0.95): • Home visit interventions (RR = 0.80; 95% CI = 0.71-0.89) and telephone-type intervention (RR = 0.86; 95% CI = 0.73-1.02) reduced all-cause admissions but not hospital-based interventions (RR = 0.99; 95% CI = 0.90-1.10) Admissions for heart failure (16 studies: RR = 0.70; 95% CI = 0.61-0.81): • Home visit (RR = 0.62; 95% CI = 0.51-0.74) and telephone-type interventions (RR = 0.70; 95% CI = 0.57-0.85) reduced admissions for heart failure but not hospital interventions (RR = 0.94; 95% CI = 0.78-1.13) All-cause mortality (27 studies: RR = 0.79; 95% CI = 0.69-0.92): • Telemonitoring (RR = 0.49; 95% CI = 0.33-0.73) and telephone follow-up (RR = 0.70; 95% CI = 0.53-0.94) reduced rates of all-cause mortality but not numbers of home visits (RR = 0.87; 95% CI = 0.72-1.06) or hospital-based interventions (RR = 1.00; 95% CI = 0.84-1.20) Total admissions and mean inpatient days: • Total number of admissions (18 studies: 21.8/1000 patient-weeks of patients receiving intervention vs. 29.0/1000 patient-weeks for control groups) was reduced for intervention recipients • Mean number of inpatient days decreased by 1.9 days for intervention recipients (10 studies: 95% CI = 0.71-3.1)	Multidisciplinary interventions reduced rates of hospitalizations for all causes and for heart failure and rates of all-cause mortality, but the most effective were those delivered, at least partially, in patients' own home through visits, telephone calls, or televideo

Continued

TABLE 59–2 Meta-analyses of Management Programs for Heart Failure—cont'd

Reference	Number of Studies Reviewed	Characteristics of Studies	Number of Patients Included in Studies Reviewed	Results	Conclusions
Yu et al (2006)[60]	21 Trials: 7 studies of multidisciplinary care and case management strategies; 14 studies of mainly nurses, physicians, or pharmacists or a combination of these	All randomized, controlled trials and sample mean age ≥ 60 years	4445 patients; >50% men in 16 studies; mean age of study participants: 73.3; 61.0 ± 20.5% of patients with NYHA classes III and IV	Care team: • Effective DMPs are more likely to involve multidisciplinary providers (2 studies: 16.7%), case managers (3 studies: 25.5%), or cardiac nurses, active involvement by patients' cardiologists, and inclusion of the PCP as a team member Program intervention: • Effective DMPs were more likely to incorporate self-care supportive strategies, optimization of drug therapy, and risk assessment for poor discharge outcomes • Exercise and psychological counseling were included least often in the studies despite their positive effects on outcome Methods of delivering follow-up care: • Effective DMPs applied home visits twice as often as ineffective programs • Follow-up methods need to consider clinical condition Study endpoints: • DMPs need longitudinal follow-up more than 9.6 months to determine their effectiveness	DMP should be multidisciplinary with active involvement of cardiac nurses and cardiologists, and should consist of an in-hospital phase of care, intensive patient education, exercise and psychological counseling, self-care supportive strategy, optimization of medical regimen, and ongoing surveillance and management of clinical deterioration
Whellan et al (2005)[59]	19 Trials (9 in the United States): 17 studies of postdischarge heart failure DMPs (clinic follow-up with supervision by cardiology department and by PCP, home nursing follow-up, or telephone follow-up); 2 studies of chronic outpatient heart failure DMPs (telephone follow-up by nurse practitioner or pharmacist)	All randomized, controlled trials	5752 Patients; >50% men in 16 studies; age of majority of participants ≥ 70 years; LVEF < 40% in most participants; comorbid conditions: diabetes mellitus (19%-52%), hypertension (29%-76%), COPD (19%-36%)	Hospitalization (15 of 17 studies of postdischarge heart failure DMP): • Clinical follow-up with supervision by cardiology department, home visitation, and telephone follow-up are effective in decreasing hospitalization • Clinical follow-up with PCP supervision (RR = 1.17; 95% CI = 0.90-1.51) did not decrease hospitalization Quality of life, medication use, and mortality: • Improved quality of life • No difference in mortality • Modest increased use of ACE inhibitors • Significantly increased medication adherence in one study	DMPs are an effective intervention in decreasing hospitalizations of patients with heart failure but not mortality
Gwadry-Sridhar et al (2004)[56]	8 Trials (3 in the United States)	All randomized, controlled trials	238 Patients; 37%-62% men; mean age of study participants: 71-83.3 years	Hospital readmission rates (8 studies: RR = 0.79; 95% CI = 0.68-0.91) Mortality (6 studies: RR = 0.98; 95% CI = 0.72-1.34) Quality of life (4 studies) • In 3 studies, disease-specific instruments were used: significant improvement noted only in 2 of the 3 studies	Peridischarge programs decrease number of hospital readmissions, but not mortality rates
McAlister et al (2004)[51]	29 Trials (15 in the United States): DMPs with follow-up by a specialized multidisciplinary team, DMPs focused on self-care activities, and DMPs incorporated with telephone contact with instructions to see PCP if condition was deteriorating	All randomized, controlled trials of multidisciplinary management programs in an outpatient setting	5039 Patients	Admissions for heart failure (27% of reduction; NNT = 11): • Reduced in DMPs with follow-up by a specialized multidisciplinary team (RR = 0.74; 95% CI = 0.63-0.87), in DMPs focused on self-care activities (RR = 0.66; 95% CI = 0.52-0.83), and in DMPs with telephone contact with instructions to see PCP if condition was deteriorating (RR = 0.75; 95% CI = 0.57-0.99) All-cause admissions: • Reduced in DMPs with follow-up by a specialized multidisciplinary team (RR = 0.81; 95% CI = 0.71-0.92; NNT = 10; 20% reduction) and in DMPs focused on self-care activities (RR = 0.73; 95% CI = 0.57-0.93) but not in DMPs with telephone contact (RR = 0.98; 95% CI = 0.80-1.20) Mortality: • Reduced in DMPs with follow-up by a specialized multidisciplinary team (RR = 0.75; 95% CI = 0.59-0.96; NNT = 17; 25% reduction) but not in DMPs focused on self-care activities (RR = 1.14; 95% CI = 0.67-1.94) or in DMPs with telephone contact (RR = 0.91; 95% CI = 0.67-1.29)	Multidisciplinary approaches reduce rates of hospitalization for heart failure; in particular, programs involving specialized follow-up by a multidisciplinary team decrease all-cause hospitalizations and mortality The benefits and cost effectiveness of these multidisciplinary programs compare favorably with those of established drug treatments for heart failure

Continued

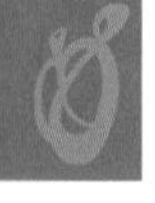

TABLE 59–2 Meta-analyses of Management Programs for Heart Failure—cont'd

Reference	Number of Studies Reviewed	Characteristics of Studies	Number of Patients Included in Studies Reviewed	Results	Conclusions
				Medication, QOL or functional status, and cost: • Higher use of proven efficacious medications in intervention recipients (6 studies) • Higher adherence to medication and dietary regimens (5 studies) • Improved QOL and functional status in intervention recipients (9 studies) • Cost savings with intervention (15 studies)	
Phillips et al (2004)[54]	14 Trials (10 in the United States): 3 studies of a single home visit; 6 studies of a home visit with or without frequent telephone contacts; 4 studies of frequent clinic visit and telephone follow-up or a home visit, or both; 1 study of a day hospital with an available specialized heart failure unit	All randomized, controlled trials	3304 Patients; 62% men, 14% nonwhite; mean age of study participants: 70 years or older in 16 studies and younger than 70 years in 2 studies; LVEF < 40% in 8 studies and LVEF > 40% in 2 studies	Readmission (8 studies): • Fewer intervention recipients were readmitted: NNT = 12, RR = 0.75, 95% CI = 0.64-0.88 • CHF- or CVD-specific readmission: RR = 0.65; 95% CI = 0.54-0.79 • Combined endpoint of death or readmission: RR = 0.73; 95% CI = 0.62-0.87 Mortality (14 studies): • Trend toward lower rates of all-cause mortality (RR = 0.87; 95% CI = 0.73-1.03) Length of stay, QOL, and medical costs: • Difference of length of stay between intervention and control groups was not significant • Significant improvement in QOL in intervention recipients • Cost effectiveness (cost difference: −$359, 95% CI = −$763-$45, for non-U.S. trials and −$536, 95% CI = −$956-$115, for U.S. trials)	Comprehensive discharge planning with postdischarge support for older adults with heart failure significantly reduced readmission rates and may improve survival and QOL without increasing costs

ACE, angiotensin-converting enzyme; CHF, congestive heart failure; CI, confidence interval; COPD, chronic obstructive pulmonary disease; CVD, cardiovascular disease; DMP, disease management program; LVEF, left ventricular ejection fraction; NNT, number needed to treat; NYHA, New York Heart Association; PCP, primary care provider; QOL, quality of life; RR, relative risk.

BOX 59–1 Putting Principles of Management of Heart Failure into Practice

1. Understand and promote patient self-care
2. Assess and address patient factors that affect adherence to regimens and ability to engage in self-care
3. Teach skills preferentially over knowledge
4. Include family members and informal caregivers in education
5. Identify and target patients who are at high risk for rehospitalization
6. Employ components of management programs for heart failure that improve outcomes
   - Individualized, comprehensive patient and family or caregiver education and counseling on an outpatient basis
   - Optimization of medical therapy
   - Vigilant follow-up
   - Increased access to health care professionals
   - Early attention to fluid overload
   - Coordination with other agencies as appropriate
   - Either physician-directed care with assistance from nurse coordinators or nurse-managed care by experienced advanced practice cardiovascular nurses with access to a cardiologist
7. Use behavioral strategies to increase adherence to regimen

routinely monitor themselves are more likely to seek treatment at the early stages of exacerbation. Heart failure is notable for the subtlety of early symptoms, and so symptom monitoring is an essential component of self-care maintenance.

Subsequent stages of the self-care process reflect management, which is an active, iterative, deliberate decision-making process undertaken in response to symptoms.[80] Symptom management is essential for patients with heart failure if they are to control what may be a precarious balance between relative health and symptomatic heart failure. In self-care management, once the patient recognizes changes in signs and symptoms, the patient must make decisions about how to respond.

Stage 2, symptom recognition, involves recognition that a change in signs or symptoms has occurred and that the change is related to heart failure. If patients recognize a symptom as related to their heart disease, they are more likely to appropriately evaluate its urgency and respond more quickly.[81] Stage 3, symptom evaluation, is the process by which patients attempt to distinguish between important and unimportant symptom changes. If a symptom is judged to be important, it is more likely that the patient will decide that he or she needs to take action.[80] Patients may proceed through these stages and not take action because they lack knowledge about what to do, judge that the costs of the action outweigh the benefits, fail to understand the importance of the symptom change, or believe that no effective strategy is available. Health care providers can intervene at this point and increase patients' knowledge about important signs and symptoms and education them about the appropriate actions to take when changes occur.

Stage 4, treatment implementation, involves action in response to the prior stages. Some actions are intuitive and require little thought (e.g., rest). Some actions can be performed independent of others (e.g., diet adjustments), and some actions are interdependent or require some guidance from a health care provider (e.g., adjusting diuretic dose). Stage 5, treatment evaluation, concerns the effectiveness (e.g., in symptom relief) of selected treatments. If a treatment is effective, it may be attempted again. Research has shown that this ability is learned through experience.[20] However, other ways of increasing this expertise must be found if patients with newly diagnosed heart failure are to avoid rehospitalization during the first few months after their initial hospitalization. Outpatient management with a disease

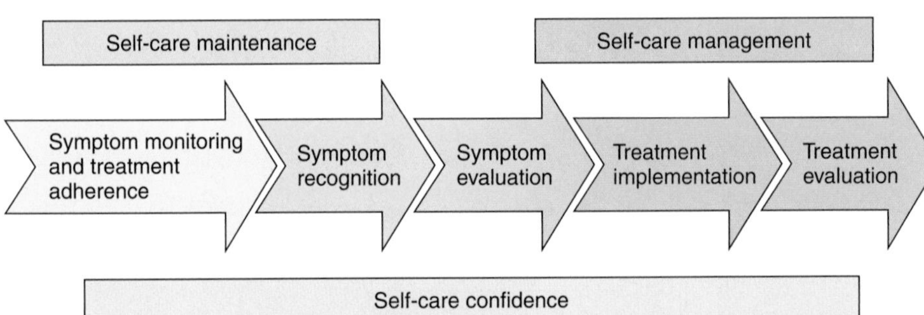

FIGURE 59–1 Self-care encompasses two processes: maintenance and management. Self-care maintenance involves engagement in making healthy life style choices and being adherent to the prescribed regimen. Self-care management is the process of decision making when symptoms or signs change.

management approach to heart failure is one such way, but it is important to determine first what patient factors exist that could interfere with the patient's ability to optimally engage in self-care.

Assess Patient Factors That Interfere with Self-Care

Numerous issues can interfere with patients' self-care abilities.[15] Advancing age, low education level, and low health literacy can affect patients' ability to learn and comply with treatment recommendations.[20] Inability to communicate with the provider because of language-, age- and culture-related beliefs has also been demonstrated to be a major factor interfering with adherence to treatment regimens. Cognitive dysfunction is increasingly recognized as a common problem among patients with heart failure[44,82] that can contribute to poor self-care.[83] Simple measures such as a clock-drawing test are available for routine screening of cognitive abilities.[44]

Personal factors such as lack of motivation, low self-efficacy, emotional distress (especially depression), poor health habits such as smoking, and lack of perceived control also contribute to difficulties practicing self-care and changing health behaviors.[28,84,85] Situational factors such as social isolation, lack of support,[28] and the challenges of implementing a complex treatment regimen under limited economic resources[13] complicate matters further. Illness factors such as length of experience with the diagnosis, symptom severity, physical limitations, and presence of multiple comorbid conditions can contribute to poor compliance and poor self-care.[28,86] As the importance of these factors to self-care and outcomes becomes increasingly obvious, health care providers must be educated about assessing and managing them.

Include Family Members and Informal Caregivers in Education

Family members and friends are the unobserved and often neglected informal caregivers who provide substantial support for many patients with heart failure.[87] Failure to include informal caregivers in disease management approaches can contribute to poor outcomes. In particular, patients who have any of the factors above that can adversely affect self-care may need the support of informal caregivers.[88-90] Whenever possible, it is essential to identify these caregivers and include them in education and counseling sessions.[91]

Identify and Target Patients Who Are at Risk for Rehospitalization

Existing evidence suggests that approaches to the management of heart failure are most effective when used for patients who are at risk for rehospitalizations.[92-94] Because a patient's heart failure status can change over time, it is necessary to reassess risk status often. A number of risk factors for rehospitalization have been identified and confirmed in multiple studies. Older age, particularly older than 75 years, is a major risk factor.[95] A previous hospital admission for heart failure within the previous 30 days to 1 year[92,96,97] is another important risk factor, as are multiple hospitalizations for any reason within the previous 5 years.[71,98] The presence of comorbid illnesses, particularly multiple active conditions, is another major risk factor.[96,97] Three specific comorbid conditions increase risk: (1) history of chronic obstructive pulmonary disease; (2) diabetes; and (3) renal insufficiency as reflected by creatinine level of 2.5 mg/dL or higher or by higher level of blood urea nitrogen.[92,96,97] Patients with depression or anxiety,[99-101] those with inadequate support systems or who live alone,[102] those with cognitive impairment,[103] and those with functional impairment[98] are also at increased risk for rehospitalization.

Components of the Management of Heart Failure That Improve Outcomes

Clinicians who do not have access to management programs for heart failure can, nonetheless, make great strides in improving heart failure patient outcomes by incorporating effective aspects of these programs in their practice. There have been no comparisons of the individual components used in management programs for heart failure, but examination of studies with neutral or negative findings and of recent studies where some components have been omitted provides sufficient information to make recommendations about the components that are likely to improve outcomes (see Box 59-1). Each of these components is described below.

Individualized, Comprehensive Patient and Family or Caregiver Education and Counseling on an Outpatient Basis. At the core of every successful management program for heart failure is individualized, comprehensive education and counseling, the goal of which is to improve adherence to the prescribed regimen.[24,104-106] The addition of comprehensive education and counseling alone to the regimen improves clinical outcomes as long as they include behavioral strategies to increase adherence.[107] Outpatient education and counseling must always supplement inpatient education. Inpatient education alone is inadequate, and patients are not able to retain most of what they are taught in the hospital.[32] Regardless of the quality of inpatient education, patients are ill, anxious, distracted, and thus in poor condition to learn and retain material. In addition, there is little time in the hospital to impart all of the needed information.

Patients and their families and informal caregivers must perform the majority of heart failure care at home. If a patient does not know what is required and why, does not have the motivation or skills to accomplish it, or does not appreciate the importance of the activities, the patient cannot participate effectively in care. Therefore, the goals of education and counseling are to help patients and their informal caregivers acquire the knowledge, skills, and motivation they need to adhere to the treatment plan and participate effectively in self-care. To help patients do this, health care providers not only need to impart necessary knowledge but also must impart it in a manner that promotes retention and application of what is learned.

Content for Patient and Family Education and Counseling. Patients with heart failure must perform specific behaviors to cope with the illness. They must limit dietary sodium to 2 to 3 g per day, take medications as prescribed routinely, and get periodic flu and pneumococcal immunizations (*comply with treatment*). They need to be taught to weigh themselves daily and how to monitor for common symptoms of decompensation such as shortness of breath, fatigue, peripheral swelling, waking at night with coughing or shortness of breath, dizziness, and swelling (*monitor signs and symptoms*).[108] They need to be taught when to report abnormalities to their health care provider (*seek assistance when necessary*). Finally, many patients with heart failure should be encouraged to exercise, stop smoking, limit or halt their alcohol intake, and control other comorbid conditions such as diabetes, hypertension, or hyperlipidemia (*change unhealthy lifestyles*).[108] Specific education and counseling to support patients successfully engage in these behaviors are described in Box 59-2.

Teaching and Counseling Methods. It is essential that effective behavior change strategies be given to patients and families along with provision of information. Behavior change researchers have long demonstrated that knowledge alone is insufficient for changing behavior,[109] and even now patients report frustration at being told what to do without being given the skills to make the expected behavior change.[28] In addition, a number of factors that contribute to nonadherence and rehospitalization also contribute to difficulties in putting information into action. Thus, clinicians need to understand factors that influence patients' ability to make recommended health behavior changes and must become familiar with effective behavior change strategies that they can teach.

In addition to the conditions described in the "Assess Patient Factors That Interfere with Self-Care" section, the following conditions are barriers to adherence. It is important to assess and address these barriers if they are present. Impediments inherent in recommended treatments themselves can limit adherence considerably. The number of medications, treatment complexities, drug side effects, cost of medications, cost of transportation to the pharmacy and to physicians' offices, and unsafe location of the neighborhood pharmacy all can contribute to medication nonadherence.[13,28] Other barriers to medication adherence included medication unpleasantness; difficulty remembering to take medication; having to take too many medications each day; the action of diuretics, which makes it difficult to leave home; and nighttime awakenings to urinate. It may be difficult to follow recommendations for dietary sodium restriction because of time, cost, taste, difficulty understanding diet requirements, inability to socialize when food is involved, limitations on eating out, and limitations on eating prepackaged and canned foods.[28]

Education and Counseling Style. Optimal patient education and counseling involve more than simply providing information. Counseling emphasizes individualized delivery of important information, taking into account the factors discussed previously that interfere with successful participation in care (e.g., language, cognitive function, mood), as well as a patient's readiness to change. Prochaska and colleagues[110,111] proposed a model of change that acknowledges that many people are not ready to engage in the behaviors that health care providers advocate. According to their model, patients in the *precontemplation* phase of change are not considering change; those in the *contemplation* phase are thinking about change but have yet to commit to change; and those in the *preparation* phase are planning to make changes in the future and may have already engaged in some early steps of change. Most patients are in one of these three early phases when a provider advocates a new behavior. Few patients are in the *action* phase (in which change has occurred) or *maintenance* phase (change has been maintained for 6 months or more), even when the need for behavioral change was recognized before it was addressed by a provider (e.g., smoking cessation).

Correction of patients' misperceptions regarding their condition and treatment is another important aspect of education and counseling. It is helpful to assess patients' current knowledge and understanding by asking questions that elicit more than "yes" or "no" for an answer. Misperceptions are common among patients with heart failure. For example, a common misunderstanding among patients with heart failure is that an increase in fluid intake is necessary in patients with

BOX 59–2 Education and Counseling for Patient and Family or Informal Caregiver

General Topics

1. Explanation of heart failure
   - Include explanation of symptoms
2. Psychological responses
   - Possibility of increased depression and anxiety
   - Necessity of treatment if anxiety or depression persists
3. Immunizations needed
   - Flu and pneumococcal vaccines
4. Prognosis
5. Advanced directives

Examples of Skills Needed to Manage Heart Failure Successfully

1. How to read nutrition labels
2. How to assess for ankle swelling, other edema, fatigue, and dyspnea
3. How to compensate for missing a medication
4. How to prepare for an office visit with the provider

Symptom Monitoring and Recognition

1. Symptoms to be expected versus symptoms of worsening heart failure, and how to monitor
2. Self-monitoring with daily weighings
3. What to do in case of increased symptoms

Dietary Recommendations

1. Diet with no more than 2 to 3 g of sodium
2. Fluid management
   - Fluid restriction unnecessary except for patients with hyponatremia, but moderation in fluid intake (<2 L/day) is warranted
3. Alcohol recommendations
   - Alcohol limited to 1 drink/day; abstention if alcoholic cardiomyopathy is present
4. Behavioral skills
5. Adherence strategies
6. Overcoming barriers

Medications

1. Nature of each drug, dosing, and side effects to watch for
2. What to do with prescriptions from other physicians or from prior hospitalizations
3. Natural remedies and vitamins
4. Coping with complicated regimens
5. Cost issues
6. Adherence strategies
7. Overcoming barriers

Activity and Exercise

1. Management of various activity needs
   - Activities of daily living
   - Work and leisure activities
   - Exercise program
   - Sexual activity
2. Adherence strategies
3. Overcoming barriers

Risk Factor Modification

1. Smoking cessation
2. Weight control for overweight patients
3. Management of hyperlipidemia, diabetes, and hypertension

heart failure because they are ill and because diuretics cause excessive urination.[26,32,108] Many patients misunderstand the reasons they are asked to weigh themselves daily, believing that they are being asked to watch for adipose weight gain.[28] Bennett and colleagues[30] documented an array of inappropriate or ineffective self-care techniques for symptom management, including use of cough drops, room temperature alteration, use of a cool cloth on the face for shortness of breath, and use of distraction and herbal teas for difficulty sleeping.

Internal motivation is an important factor contributing to successful self-care, and motivational techniques are extremely effective for individuals in one of the early stages of change. Motivation interviewing, a technique that emphasizes helping the patient resolve ambivalence about change, is effective even for those with difficult behaviors such as problem drinking and weight loss[112,113] and even with the behaviors that persons with heart failure are asked to implement.[114] Cognitive-behavioral techniques, which emphasize modifying barriers to change, are also quite useful with patients in the early stages of incorporating recommended behaviors into their lives.[115] Specific techniques have been suggested for helping patients progress through each of the stages of change.[116] For example, patients who are not considering change need information. To individuals in the contemplation stages of change, however, information is often superfluous and irritating; these patients benefit from an emphasis on the outcomes to be derived from change (e.g., "You can probably avoid rehospitalization if you take your medications routinely"). Patients in the preparation stage may benefit from efforts to increase their confidence in their abilities to make the recommended changes or by assistance in overcoming barriers that they face (e.g., difficulty in meal preparation).[117]

Simply avoiding ineffective educational approaches is helpful for patients. Fear and coercion, for example, are common techniques in clinical practice, but they are ineffective motivators because people who are pushed in one direction will resist change, even if the advocated approach is logical.[116] Messages that are couched in terms that evoke fear are commonly discounted and ignored by patients in order to reduce anxiety. Paternalism—characterized by making decisions for patients—is also common in clinical practice but rarely effective in the long term because patients lack ownership of the decision.

The most effective education and counseling approaches are individualized to include what the patient needs and wants to learn, build on prior knowledge and experience, involve the patient in discussion and skill practice, include a discussion of the benefits of acting on recommendations, and provide feedback and reinforcement. Following educational principles such as these enhances the effectiveness of patient education.[118] A major difference between patient teaching and formal didactic education is that patient teaching focuses on what patients needs to *do* rather than what they need to *know*[28]; that is, teaching the pathophysiological processes of heart failure is not necessary unless requested by the patient. Instead, patients usually want to know what their drugs do, which symptoms are important to monitor, how to monitor symptoms and what to do about them when they occur, and to distinguish side effects of drugs from symptoms of heart failure.[28,49]

Timing, Setting, and Form of Education and Counseling. To be most effective, education and counseling must be provided when and where patients are most ready to learn. Inhospital education is traditional and required by accrediting agencies, but hospitalization is probably the worst possible time to educate patients because hospitalized patients are, as a group, more ill now than in years past. Furthermore, patients are being discharged earlier, and their days in the hospital are busy with tests and procedures. Therefore, just brief, essential, but thorough education should be provided during hospitalization (e.g., medication teaching); comprehensive education should be deferred until after discharge. Teaching that is deferred should be begun within the first week after hospital discharge, preferably within the first few days, and continued during subsequent visits.[16,64]

Face-to-face education and counseling sessions that include written materials are vital. Written materials with sound educational principles ("educational modules") that are prepared specifically for patients with heart failure can be obtained from the website of the Heart Failure Society of America (www.hfsa.org). Prior investigators have also shown that patients who are motivated to learn and change can derive significant benefit from interventions delivered by mail, telephone, or technology. For example, Serxner and associates[63] demonstrated that personalized information on self-care and behavior change delivered by mail to patients with heart failure decreased hospital admissions and cost 51%. Fulmer and colleagues[119] demonstrated that elderly patients with heart failure who were randomly assigned to receive either daily telephone medication reminders or daily videotelephone call reminders adhered better to medication regimens than did control patients who received no reminders; for those control patients, adherence dropped from 81% to 57% after 10 weeks in the study. Thus, a combination of strategies is recommended.

Health Behavior Change Strategies. In a classic article, McKenney and associates[120] categorized strategies for improving adherence to treatment regimens into enabling, consequence, and stimulant. Enabling strategies—patient education, simplifying the medication regimen, increasing access to care, prescribing less costly therapies—equip patients with what they need to adhere to the regimen. Consequence strategies, such as maintaining records and rewarding adherence, reinforce desired behavior. Stimulant strategies, such as reminders or linking desired behaviors to daily rituals, are intended to prompt the desired behavior. Studies of enabling strategies such as patient education suggest that increasing knowledge does not necessarily increase adherence.[121] Stimulant strategies are more effective in achieving compliance than either enabling or consequence strategies.[119] This suggests that education and counseling interventions may need less emphasis on the transferring of information and more attention to behavioral techniques that help patients integrate new and important behaviors into their lives. Suggested strategies in each category are outlined in Box 59-3.

Optimization of Medical Therapy. Another important component of the management of heart failure is optimization of drug therapy, by means of recommendations from published guidelines that are based on large-scale randomized controlled clinical trials. The American Heart Association program "Get With the Guidelines," which is available online (http://www.americanheart.org/presenter.jhtml?identifier=1165), is a helpful way to begin incorporating these guidelines into practice. Not only should the appropriate drugs be prescribed but also they should be prescribed in the appropriate doses whenever possible.[12] ACE inhibitors (see Chapter 45) and β-adrenergic blocking agents (see Chapter 46) that must be titrated up to the optimal dosage are the drugs most often not prescribed in optimal dosages; therefore, clinicians should take extra care during follow-up visits to assess proper dose titration. In each management program for heart failure in which drug therapy (types and doses) was evaluated, prescriptions of drug therapy have been better than either usual care or prescriptions before initiation of the program.[122,123] The optimal drug regimens are described in Chapters 42 to 44 and 46 of this book. The clinician's obligation does not end with prescription of the drug; the clinician must ensure that the patient adheres to the regimen.

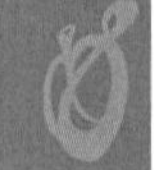

BOX 59–3 Strategies for Changing Health Behavior

Enabling Strategies
- Adapting low-sodium diet to patient's usual eating style
- Teaching patients how to eat out at usual restaurants while following low-sodium diet
- Teaching patients how to read food labels for sodium content
- Teaching patients to identify high- and low-sodium foods
- Acknowledging cultural and religious food influences
- Providing materials written at the appropriate reading level
- Providing materials printed in large font for patients with visual disabilities (e.g., elderly patients)
- Sending annual reminds for flu vaccinations
- Calling with appointment reminders
- Providing a list of worrisome symptoms
- Referring to a dietitian for weight reduction counseling
- Referring to a smoking cessation program as needed
- Teaching alternative ways to monitor fluid retention (shoe or belt tightness, ankle circumference)
- Referring to Alcoholics Anonymous or other substance abuse support group as needed

Consequence Strategies
- Keeping a log of daily weights
- Keeping a log of symptoms and their quality (most severe to least severe)
- Keeping a log of distance walked and heart rate attained

Stimulant Strategies
- Providing patients with pill box and teaching its use
- Providing patients with medication log to check off daily
- Linking the taking of medications to everyday activities (e.g., brushing teeth)
- Providing patients with a pedometer to monitor activity
- Providing a scale to patients who do not have one
- Placing the scale somewhere unavoidable each morning
- Providing a daily sodium tracker to facilitate monitoring of sodium intake
- Teaching patients how to cook basic recipes with low sodium
- Allowing patients to self-regulate diuretic dosing on the basis of weight gain
- Offering flu shots in the office
- Providing a list of specific symptoms that should stimulate a call to the office

Vigilant Follow-up. Outcomes are improved when the frequency of and vigilance during follow-up appointments are increased, particularly after discharge from a hospitalization for heart failure. Investigators have demonstrated that the first 2 weeks after hospital discharge is a time of increased vulnerability for patients, and the clinician's vigilance must be increased during this time period.[13,105] In addition to more frequent office visits, a single home visit by a nurse during the first few weeks after discharge can substantially decrease rehospitalization rates and improve long-term survival.[105] Nurses are able to assess both the patient's physical status and understanding of instructions, and they can provide education and counseling. Because nurses are accessible by telephone, patients can contact a health care professional when they are reluctant to "bother" their physicians.

Increased Access to Health Care Professionals. Easy access to health care providers is a component of the management of heart failure that also is associated with improved clinical outcomes.[124] The usual method of contacting a physician involves a long telephone call that includes an unintelligible series of instructions about pushing multiple numbers in order to leave a message, which may or may not be returned; many patients choose instead to wait until symptoms become severe. In addition, many patients do not feel comfortable calling their physicians to ask questions. When patients have easier and quicker access to a health care provider to ask questions, clarify instructions, and solve problems concerning their condition that arise unexpectedly, clinical outcomes are improved.

Improving access in this area begins with developing an open communication policy with patients so that they feel comfortable asking questions about their condition. Ways to increase accessibility include providing the services of an advanced practice nurse with whom patients have developed a relationship by telephone or on a walk-in basis. A fundamental component of this approach is to make sure that patients understand that early attention to problems improves outcomes.

Early Attention to Fluid Overload. Fluid overload is the most common cause of emergency hospitalization among patients with heart failure (see Chapter 43).[6,19,125] Thus, attention to early signs and symptoms of fluid overload is a common component of successful management of heart failure. As described previously, patients need to be taught to monitor for signs of fluid overload, weigh themselves daily, and keep a record of weights. Patients must be taught that signs of fluid overload are ankle and leg swelling; rings, belts, or waistbands becoming too tight; and increased dyspnea, including difficulty sleeping or orthopnea. Of importance is that patients need to be assisted to develop skill both in assessing themselves for fluid overload and in the ability to judge when to call their health care providers because of these signs or symptoms or if their weight increases by 2 to 3 pounds (0.9 to 1.4 kg) and remains elevated or continues to rise.[108,122] When appropriate, patients or their informal caregivers can be taught to use a flexible diuretic regimen in response to increased weight.[108,122] Although there are variations on the flexible diuretic regimen, one approach is for patients to double the diuretic dose for 2 days if their weight increases by 2 to 3 pounds in 1 to 2 days. If their weight continues to rise or does not fall, a call to the clinician is warranted.

Coordination with Other Physicians and Agencies as Appropriate. Because many patients with heart failure are elderly with multiple comorbid conditions and socioeconomic problems, other agencies may be involved in their care. In addition, for most patients with heart failure, more than one physician or other health care provider is involved in their care. Coordinating the care and services received, avoiding duplication and mixed messages, and ensuring that services are not missed are essential when patients have multiple providers or need the services of multiple providers.

Care Delivered by Advanced Practice Nurse–Physician Team. A final important component of optimal outpatient management of heart failure is the use of a team of at least two clinicians. In each disease management program tested, nurses successfully coordinated or facilitated care with assistance from a physician with expertise in the care of patients with heart failure. No single person can accomplish all that is needed to properly care for patients with heart failure.[104] Advanced practice nurses (i.e., nurses with a master's degree who are trained as either clinical nurse specialists or nurse practitioners) have the training to collaboratively care for complex patients.

SUMMARY

The increased incidence and prevalence of heart failure, combined with the cost of caring for these patients, provide the opportunity to address many of the difficult issues that will confront society as the population ages. Currently, the most strenuous efforts are concentrated in investigations of pharmacological and device therapies. In order to improve morbidity rates, mortality rates, and quality of life for a greater number of patients with heart failure, clinicians should use a more systematic, balanced approach to practice in which nonpharmacological or noninvasive, surgical, and pharmacological therapies and their interactions are considered equally.

REFERENCES

1. Berry, C., Murdoch, D. R., & McMurray, J. J. (2001). Economics of chronic heart failure. *Eur J Heart Fail, 3*, 283–291.
2. O'Connell, J. B. (2000). The economic burden of heart failure. *Clin Cardiol, 23*, III-6–III-10.
3. Stewart, S., MacIntyre, K., Capewell, S., et al. (2003). Heart failure and the aging population: an increasing burden in the 21st century? *Heart, 89*, 49–53.
4. Lloyd-Jones, D. M., Larson, M. G., Leip, E. P., et al. (2002). Lifetime risk for developing congestive heart failure: the Framingham Heart Study. *Circulation, 106*, 3068–3072.
5. Welsh, J. D., Heiser, R. M., Schooler, M. P., et al. (2002). Characteristics and treatment of patients with heart failure in the emergency department. *J Emerg Nurs, 28*, 126–131.
6. Opasich, C., Rapezzi, C., Lucci, D., et al. (2001). Precipitating factors and decision-making processes of short-term worsening heart failure despite "optimal" treatment (from the IN-CHF Registry). *Am J Cardiol, 88*, 382–387.
7. Miller, N. H., Hill, M., Kottke, T., et al. (1997). The multilevel compliance challenge: recommendations for a call to action. A statement for healthcare professionals. *Circulation, 95*, 1085–1090.
8. World Health Organization. *Adherence to long-term therapies: evidence for action* (2003 online publication, WHO/MNC/03.01): http://www.who.int/chp/knowledge/publications/adherence_introduction.pdf. Accessed March 31, 2010.
9. McDermott, M. M., Lee, P., Mehta, S., et al. (1998). Patterns of angiotensin-converting enzyme inhibitor prescriptions, educational interventions, and outcomes among hospitalized patients with heart failure. *Clin Cardiol, 21*, 261–268.
10. Ashton, C. M., Kuykendall, D. H., Johnson, M. L., et al. (1995). The association between the quality of inpatient care and early readmission. *Ann Intern Med, 122*, 415–421.
11. Krumholz, H. M., Baker, D. W., Ashton, C. M., et al. (2000). Evaluating quality of care for patients with heart failure. *Circulation, 101*, E122–E140.
12. Kim, T. C., Rodeheffer, R. J., & Kopecky, S. L. (2003). Implementing clinical trial results into clinical practice for patients with heart failure. *Am J Cardiol, 91*, 581–582.
13. Moser, D. K., Doering, L. V., & Chung, M. L. (2005). Vulnerabilities of patients recovering from an exacerbation of chronic heart failure. *Am Heart J, 150*, 984.
14. van der Wal, M. H., Jaarsma, T., & van Veldhuisen, D. J. (2005). Non-compliance in patients with heart failure; how can we manage it? *Eur J Heart Fail, 7*, 5–17.
15. Moser, D. K., & Watkins, J. F. (2008). Conceptualizing self-care in heart failure: a life course model of patient characteristics. *J Cardiovasc Nurs, 23*, 205–218.
16. Leventhal, M. J., Riegel, B., Carlson, B., et al. (2005). Negotiating compliance in heart failure: remaining issues and questions. *Eur J Cardiovasc Nurs, 4*, 298–307.
17. Haynes, R. B., Ackloo, E., Sahota, N., et al. (2008). Interventions for enhancing medication adherence. *Cochrane Database Syst Rev*, 2008: CD000011.
18. Hill, M. (2001). Extent of the problem of noncompliance in patients with heart failure. In D. K. Moser, & B. Riegel (Eds.). *Improving outcomes in heart failure: an interdisciplinary approach* (pp. 165–177). Gaithersburg, MD: Aspen.
19. Bennett, S. J., Huster, G. A., Baker, S. L., et al. (1998). Characterization of the precipitants of hospitalization for heart failure decompensation. *Am J Crit Care, 7*, 168–174.
20. Francque-Frontiero, L., Riegel, B., Bennett, J., et al. (2002). Self-care of persons with heart failure: Does experience make a difference?. *Clinical Excellence for Nurse Practitioners*, 6, 23–30.
21. Monane, M., Bohn, R. L., Gurwitz, J. H., et al. (1994). Noncompliance with congestive heart failure therapy in the elderly. *Arch Intern Med, 154*, 433–437.
22. Bohachick, P., Burke, L. E., Sereika, S., et al. (2002). Adherence to angiotensin-converting enzyme inhibitor therapy for heart failure. *Prog Cardiovasc Nurs, 17*, 160–166.
23. Wu, J. R., Moser, D. K., Chung, M. L., et al. (2008). Objectively measured, but not self-reported, medication adherence independently predicts event-free survival in patients with heart failure. *J Card Fail, 14*, 203–210.
24. Hershberger, R. E., Ni, H., Nauman, D. J., et al. (2001). Prospective evaluation of an outpatient heart failure management program. *J Card Fail, 7*, 64–74.
25. Neily, J. B., Toto, K. H., Gardner, E. B., et al. (2002). Potential contributing factors to noncompliance with dietary sodium restriction in patients with heart failure. *Am Heart J, 143*, 29–33.
26. Carlson, B., Riegel, B., & Moser, D. K. (2001). Self-care abilities of patients with heart failure. *Heart Lung, 30*, 351–359.
27. Jurgens, C. Y. (2006). Somatic awareness, uncertainty, and delay in care-seeking in acute heart failure. *Res Nurs Health, 29*, 74–86.
28. Riegel, B., & Carlson, B. (2002). Facilitators and barriers to heart failure self-care. *Patient Educ Couns, 46*, 287–295.
29. Horan, M., Barrett, F., Mulqueen, M., et al. (2000). The basics of heart failure management: are they being ignored? *Eur J Heart Fail, 2*, 101–105.
30. Bennett, S. J., Cordes, D. K., Westmoreland, G., et al. (2000). Self-care strategies for symptom management in patients with chronic heart failure. *Nurs Res, 49*, 139–145.
31. Evangelista, L. S., Dracup, K., & Doering, L. V. (2000). Treatment-seeking delays in heart failure patients. *J Heart Lung Transplant, 19*, 932–938.
32. Ni, H., Nauman, D., Burgess, D., et al. (1999). Factors influencing knowledge of and adherence to self-care among patients with heart failure. *Arch Intern Med, 159*, 1613–1619.
33. Centers for Disease Control and Prevention. (2000). Receipt of advice to quit smoking in Medicare managed care—United States–1998. *JAMA, 284*(14): 1779–1781.
34. Ekman, I., Schaufelberger, M., Kjellgren, K. I., et al. (2007). Standard medication information is not enough: poor concordance of patient and nurse perceptions. *J Adv Nurs, 60*, 181–186.
35. Hunt, S. A., Abraham, W. T., Chin, M. H., et al. (2005). ACC/AHA 2005 Guideline Update for the Diagnosis and Management of Chronic Heart Failure in the Adult: a report of the American College of Cardiology/American Heart Association Task Force on Practice Guidelines (Writing Committee to Update the 2001 Guidelines for the Evaluation and Management of Heart Failure): developed in collaboration with the American College of Chest Physicians and the International Society for Heart and Lung Transplantation: endorsed by the Heart Rhythm Society. *Circulation, 112*, e154–e235.
36. Swedberg, K., Cleland, J., Dargie, H., et al. (2005). Guidelines for the diagnosis and treatment of chronic heart failure: executive summary (update 2005): The Task Force for the Diagnosis and Treatment of Chronic Heart Failure of the European Society of Cardiology. *Eur Heart J, 26*, 1115–1140.
37. Liu, P., Arnold, J. M., Belenkie, I., et al. (2003). The 2002/3 Canadian Cardiovascular Society consensus guideline update for the diagnosis and management of heart failure. *Can J Cardiol, 19*, 347–356.
38. Heart Failure Society of America. HFSA. (2006). 2006 Comprehensive Heart Failure Practice Guideline. *J Card Fail, 12*, e1–e2.
39. Tsuyuki, R. T., Fradette, M., Johnson, J. A., et al. (2004). A multicenter disease management program for hospitalized patients with heart failure. *J Card Fail, 10*, 473–480.
40. Stafford, R. S., & Radley, D. C. (2003). The underutilization of cardiac medications of proven benefit, 1990 to 2002. *J Am Coll Cardiol, 41*, 56–61.
41. Luthi, J. C., McClellan, W. M., Fitzgerald, D., et al. (2002). Mortality associated with the quality of care of patients hospitalized with congestive heart failure. *Int J Qual Health Care, 14*, 15–24.
42. Havranek, E. P., Masoudi, S. A., Rumsfeld, J. S., et al. (2003). A broader paradigm for understanding and treating heart failure. *J Card Fail, 9*, 147–152.
43. Vaishnava, P., & Lewis, E. F. (2007). Assessment of quality of life in severe heart failure. *Curr Heart Fail Rep, 4*, 170–177.
44. Riegel, B., Bennett, J. A., Davis, A., et al. (2002). Cognitive impairment in heart failure: issues of measurement and etiology. *Am J Crit Care, 11*, 520–528.
45. Shabetai, R. (2002). Depression and heart failure. *Psychosom Med, 64*, 13–14.
46. Williams, S. A., Kasl, S. V., Heiat, A., et al. (2002). Depression and risk of heart failure among the elderly: a prospective community-based study. *Psychosom Med, 64*, 6–12.
47. Moser, D. K., & Worster, P. L. (2000). Effect of psychosocial factors on physiologic outcomes in patients with heart failure. *J Cardiovasc Nurs, 14*, 106–115.
48. Bennett, S., & Sauvé, M. (2003). Cognitive deficits in patients with heart failure: a review of the literature. *J Cardiovasc Nurs, 18*, 146–169.
49. Rogers, A., Addington-Hall, J. M., McCoy, A. S., et al. (2002). A qualitative study of chronic heart failure patients' understanding of their symptoms and drug therapy. *Eur J Heart Fail, 4*, 283–287.
50. Massie, B. M., & Ansari, M. N. (2003). Specialty care in heart failure: does it improve outcomes? *Am Heart J, 145*, 209–213.
51. McAlister, F. A., Stewart, S., Ferrua, S., et al. (2004). Multidisciplinary strategies for the management of heart failure patients at high risk for admission: a systematic review of randomized trials. *J Am Coll Cardiol, 44*, 810–819.
52. Ahmed, A. (2002). Quality and outcomes of heart failure care in older adults: role of multidisciplinary disease-management programs. *J Am Geriatr Soc, 50*, 1590–1593.
53. Holland, R., Battersby, J., Harvey, I., et al. (2005). Systematic review of multidisciplinary interventions in heart failure. *Heart, 91*, 899–906.
54. Phillips, C. O., Wright, S. M., Kern, D. E., et al. (2004). Comprehensive discharge planning with postdischarge support for older patients with congestive heart failure: a meta-analysis. *JAMA, 291*, 1358–1367.
55. Gonseth, J., Guallar-Castillon, P., Banegas, J. R., et al. (2004). The effectiveness of disease management programmes in reducing hospital re-admission in older patients with heart failure: a systematic review and meta-analysis of published reports. *Eur Heart J, 25*, 1570–1595.
56. Gwadry-Sridhar, F. H., Flintoft, V., Lee, D. S., et al. (2004). A systematic review and meta-analysis of studies comparing readmission rates and mortality rates in patients with heart failure. *Arch Intern Med, 164*, 2315–2320.
57. Clark, R. A., Inglis, S. C., McAlister, F. A., et al. (2007). Telemonitoring or structured telephone support programmes for patients with chronic heart failure: systematic review and meta-analysis. *BMJ, 334*, 942.
58. Roccaforte, R., Demers, C., Baldassarre, F., et al. (2005). Effectiveness of comprehensive disease management programmes in improving clinical outcomes in heart failure patients. A meta-analysis. *Eur J Heart Fail, 7*, 1133–1144.
59. Whellan, D. J., Hasselblad, V., Peterson, E., et al. (2005). Metaanalysis and review of heart failure disease management randomized controlled clinical trials. *Am Heart J, 149*, 722–729.
60. Yu, D. S., Thompson, D. R., & Lee, D. T. (2006). Disease management programmes for older people with heart failure: crucial characteristics which improve post-discharge outcomes. *Eur Heart J, 27*, 596–612.
61. Cordisco, M. E., Benjaminovitz, A., Hammond, K., et al. (1999). Use of telemonitoring to decrease the rate of hospitalization in patients with severe congestive heart failure. *Am J Cardiol, 84*, 860–862, A868.
62. Weinberger, M., Oddone, E. Z., & Henderson, W. G. (1996). Does increased access to primary care reduce hospital readmissions? Veterans Affairs Cooperative Study Group on Primary Care and Hospital Readmission. *N Engl J Med, 334*, 1441–1447.
63. Serxner, S., Miyaji, M., & Jeffords, F. (1998). Congestive heart failure disease management study: a patient education intervention. *Congest Heart Fail, 4*, 23–28.
64. Riegel, B., Carlson, B., Kopp, Z., et al. (2002). Effect of a standardized nurse case-management telephone intervention on resource use in patients with chronic heart failure. *Arch Intern Med, 162*, 705–712.
65. Davis, A. M., Vinci, L. M., Okwuosa, T. M., et al. (2007). Cardiovascular health disparities: a systematic review of health care interventions. *Med Care Res Rev, 64*, S29–S100.
66. Alexander, M., Grumbach, K., Remy, L., et al. (1999). Congestive heart failure hospitalizations and survival in California: patterns according to race/ethnicity. *Am Heart J, 137*, 919–927.
67. Artinian, N. T., Harden, J. K., Kronenberg, M. W., et al. (2003). Pilot study of a Web-based compliance monitoring device for patients with congestive heart failure. *Heart Lung, 32*, 226–233.
68. Benatar, D., Bondmass, M., Ghitelman, J., et al. (2003). Outcomes of chronic heart failure. *Arch Intern Med, 163*, 347–352.

69. DeWalt, D. A., Pignone, M., Malone, R., et al. (2004). Development and pilot testing of a disease management program for low literacy patients with heart failure. *Patient Educ Couns, 55*, 78–86.
70. Naylor, M. D., Brooten, D. A., Campbell, R. L., et al. (2004). Transitional care of older adults hospitalized with heart failure: a randomized, controlled trial. *J Am Geriatr Soc, 52*, 675–684.
71. Rich, M., Beckham, V., Wittenberg, C., et al. (1995). A multidisciplinary intervention to prevent readmission of elderly patients with congestive heart failure. *N Engl J Med, 333*, 1190–1195.
72. Sisk, J. E., Hebert, P. L., Horowitz, C. R., et al. (2006). Effects of nurse management on the quality of heart failure care in minority communities: a randomized trial. *Ann Intern Med, 145*, 273–283.
73. O'Connell, A., Crawford, M., & Abrams, J. (2001). Heart failure disease management in an indigent population. *Am Heart J, 141*, 254–258.
74. Riegel, B., Carlson, B., Glaser, D., et al. (2006). Randomized controlled trial of telephone case management in Hispanics of Mexican origin with heart failure. *J Card Fail, 12*, 211–219.
75. Bodenheimer, T., Lorig, K., Holman, H., et al. (2002). Patient self-management of chronic disease in primary care. *JAMA, 288*, 2469–2475.
76. Miller, R. M., George, D., & Halbert, R. J. (2005). Improving the management of chronic obstructive pulmonary disease. *J Healthc Qual, 27*, 42–47.
77. Paul, G. M., Smith, S. M., Whitford, D. L., et al. (2007). Peer support in type 2 diabetes: a randomised controlled trial in primary care with parallel economic and qualitative analyses: pilot study and protocol. *BMC Fam Pract, 8*, 45.
78. Riegel, B., & Dickson, V. (2008). A situation-specific theory of heart failure self-care. *J Cardiovascular Nurs, 23*, 190–196.
79. Jallinoja, P., Absetz, P., Kuronen, R., et al. (2007). The dilemma of patient responsibility for lifestyle change: perceptions among primary care physicians and nurses. *Scand J Prim Health Care, 25*, 244–249.
80. Riegel, B., Carlson, B., & Glaser, D. (2000). Development and testing of a clinical tool measuring self-management of heart failure. *Heart Lung, 29*, 4–15.
81. Caldwell, M. A., & Miaskowski, C. (2002). Mass media interventions to reduce help-seeking delay in people with symptoms of acute myocardial infarction: time for a new approach? *Patient Educ Couns, 46*, 1–9.
82. Zuccala, G., Onder, G., Pedone, C., et al. (2001). Cognitive dysfunction as a major determinant of disability in patients with heart failure: results from a multicentre survey. On behalf of the GIFA (SIGG-ONLUS) Investigators. *J Neurol Neurosurg Psychiatry, 70*, 109–112.
83. Bennett, S. J., & Sauvé, M. J. (2003). Cognitive deficits among patients with heart failure: a review of the literature. *J Cardiovasc Nurs, 18*, 219–242.
84. Friedman, M. M., & Griffin, J. A. (2001). Relationship of physical symptoms and physical functioning to depression in patients with heart failure. *Heart Lung, 30*, 98–104.
85. Dracup, K., Westlake, C., Erickson, V. S., et al. (2003). Perceived control reduces emotional stress in patients with heart failure. *J Heart Lung Transplant, 22*, 90–93.
86. Rockwell, J. M., & Riegel, B. (2001). Predictors of self-care in persons with heart failure. *Heart Lung, 30*, 18–25.
87. Baas, L. S., Trupp, R., & Abraham, W. T. (2001). Supportive resources for the patient with heart failure. In D. K. Moser, & B. Riegel (Eds.). *Improving outcomes in heart failure: an interdisciplinary approach* (pp. 201–218). Gaithersburg, MD: Aspen.
88. Luttik, M. L., Blaauwbroek, A., Dijker, A., et al. (2007). Living with heart failure: partner perspectives. *J Cardiovasc Nurs, 22*, 131–137.
89. Barnes, S., Gott, M., Payne, S., et al. (2006). Characteristics and views of family carers of older people with heart failure. *Int J Palliat Nurs, 12*, 380–389.
90. Molloy, G. J., Johnston, D. W., & Witham, M. D. (2005). Family caregiving and congestive heart failure. Review and analysis. *Eur J Heart Fail, 7*, 592–603.
91. Knox, D., Mischke, L., & Williams, R. E. (2001). Heart failure patient and family education. In D. K. Moser, & B. Riegel (Eds.). *Improving outcomes in heart failure: an interdisciplinary approach* (pp. 178–198). Gaithersburg, MD: Aspen.
92. Krumholz, H. M., Chen, Y. T., Wang, Y., et al. (2000). Predictors of readmission among elderly survivors of admission with heart failure. *Am Heart J, 139*, 72–77.
93. Riegel, B., Carlson, B., Glaser, D., et al. (2000). Which patients with heart failure respond best to multidisciplinary disease management? *J Card Fail, 6*, 290–299.
94. Stewart, S., & Horowitz, J. D. (2003). Specialist nurse management programmes: economic benefits in the management of heart failure. *Pharmacoeconomics, 21*, 225–240.
95. Kossovsky, M. P., Sarasin, F. P., Perneger, T. V., et al. (2000). Unplanned readmissions of patients with congestive heart failure: do they reflect in-hospital quality of care or patient characteristics?. *Am J Med, 109*, 386–390.
96. Harjai, K. J., Thompson, H. W., Turgut, T., et al. (2001). Simple clinical variables are markers of the propensity for readmission in patients hospitalized with heart failure. *Am J Cardiol, 87*, 234–237, A239.
97. Smith, D. M., Giobbie-Hurder, A., Weinberger, M., et al. (2000). Predicting non-elective hospital readmissions: a multi-site study. Department of Veterans Affairs Cooperative Study Group on Primary Care and Readmissions. *J Clin Epidemiol, 53*, 1113–1118.
98. Naylor, M. D., Brooten, D., Campbell, R., et al. (1999). Comprehensive discharge planning and home follow-up of hospitalized elders: a randomized clinical trial. *JAMA, 281*, 613–620.
99. Jiang, W., Alexander, J., Christopher, E., et al. (2001). Relationship of depression to increased risk of mortality and rehospitalization in patients with congestive heart failure. *Arch Intern Med, 161*, 1849–1856.
100. Konstam, V., Moser, D. K., & De Jong, M. J. (2005). Depression and anxiety in heart failure. *J Card Fail, 11*, 455–463.
101. De Jong, M., Moser, D. K., & Chung, M. L. (2005). Predictors of health status for heart failure patients. *Prog Cardiovasc Nurs, 20*, 155–162.
102. Krumholz, H. M., Butler, J., Miller, J., et al. (1998). Prognostic importance of emotional support for elderly patients hospitalized with heart failure. *Circulation, 97*, 958–964.
103. Bennett, S. J., Pressler, M. L., Hays, L., et al. (1997). Psychosocial variables and hospitalization in persons with chronic heart failure. *Prog Cardiovasc Nurs, 12*, 4–11.
104. Moser, D. K., & Mann, D. L. (2002). Improving outcomes in heart failure: it's not unusual beyond usual care. *Circulation, 105*, 2810–2812.
105. Stewart, S., & Horowitz, J. D. (2002). Home-based intervention in congestive heart failure: long-term implications on readmission and survival. *Circulation, 105*, 2861–2866.
106. Gwadry-Sridhar, F. H., Arnold, J. M., Zhang, Y., et al. (2005). Pilot study to determine the impact of a multidisciplinary educational intervention in patients hospitalized with heart failure. *Am Heart J, 150*, 982.
107. Krumholz, H. M., Amatruda, J., Smith, G. L., et al. (2002). Randomized trial of an education and support intervention to prevent readmission of patients with heart failure. *J Am Coll Cardiol, 39*, 83–89.
108. Grady, K. L., Dracup, K., Kennedy, G., et al. (2000). Team management of patients with heart failure: a statement for healthcare professionals from The Cardiovascular Nursing Council of the American Heart Association. *Circulation, 102*, 2443–2456.
109. Committee on Health and Behavior. (2001). *Research, Practice and Policy, Board on Neuroscience and Behavioral Health. Health and behavior: the interplay of biological, behavioral and societal influences.* Washington, DC: Institute of Medicine.
110. Prochaska, J. O., DiClemente, C. C., & Norcross, J. C. (1992). In search of how people change. Applications to addictive behaviors. *Am Psychol, 47*, 1102–1114.
111. Prochaska, J. O., & DiClemente, C. C. (1992). Stages of change in the modification of problem behaviors. *Prog Behav Modif, 28*, 183–218.
112. Rubak, S., Sandbaek, A., Lauritzen, T., et al. (2005). Motivational interviewing: a systematic review and meta-analysis. *Br J Gen Pract, 55*, 305–312.
113. Miller, W. R., & Rollnick, S. (2002). *Motivational interviewing: preparing people for change* (2nd ed). New York: Guilford Press.
114. Riegel, B., Dickson, V. V., Hoke, L., et al. (2006). A motivational counseling approach to improving heart failure self-care: mechanisms of effectiveness. *J Cardiovasc Nurs, 21*, 232–241.
115. Leichsenring, F., Hiller, W., Weissberg, M., et al. (2006). Cognitive-behavioral therapy and psychodynamic psychotherapy: techniques, efficacy, and indications. *Am J Psychother, 60*, 233–259.
116. Saarmann, L., Daugherty, J., & Riegel, B. (2000). Patient teaching to promote behavioral change. *Nurs Outlook, 48*, 281–287.
117. Paul, S., & Sneed, N. (2004). Strategies for behavior change in patients with heart failure. *Am J Crit Care, 13*, 305–313.
118. Stromberg, A. (2005). The crucial role of patient education in heart failure. *Eur J Heart Fail, 7*, 363–369.
119. Fulmer, T. T., Feldman, P. H., Kim, T. S., et al. (1999). An intervention study to enhance medication compliance in community-dwelling elderly individuals. *J Gerontol Nurs, 25*, 6–14.
120. McKenney, J. M., Munroe, W. P., & Wright, J. T., Jr. (1992). Impact of an electronic medication compliance aid on long-term blood pressure control. *J Clin Pharmacol, 32*, 277–283.
121. Wolfe, S. C., & Schirm, V. (1992). Medication counseling for the elderly: effects on knowledge and compliance after hospital discharge. *Geriatr Nurs, 13*, 134–138.
122. Fonarow, G. C., Stevenson, L. W., Walden, J. A., et al. (1997). Impact of a comprehensive heart failure management program on hospital readmission and functional status of patients with advanced heart failure. *J Am Coll Cardiol, 30*, 725–732.
123. West, J. A., Miller, N. H., Parker, K. M., et al. (1997). A comprehensive management system for heart failure improves clinical outcomes and reduces medical resource utilization. *Am J Cardiol, 79*, 58–63.
124. Whellan, D. J. (2005). Heart failure disease management: implementation and outcomes. *Cardiol Rev, 13*, 231–239.
125. Tsuyuki, R. T., McKelvie, R. S., Arnold, J. M., et al. (2001). Acute precipitants of congestive heart failure exacerbations. *Arch Intern Med, 161*, 2337–2342.

CHAPTER 60

Cognitive Impairment in Heart Failure

Varda Konstam and Ilana Lehmann

Heart failure affects approximately 5 million Americans, with an estimated 550,000 new cases per year. Hospital readmission rates are averaging 40% to 50% after discharge, at an average cost of $12,400 per admission.[1-3] It is estimated that approximately 55% of readmissions are preventable,[4] a finding that is largely attributed to difficulties adhering to complex medication regimens, difficulties adhering to dietary restrictions, and delays in seeking medical attention.[5] Symptoms associated with heart failure include breathlessness or dyspnea, extreme fatigue, edema, and cognitive impairment, the last of which is the focus of this chapter.

Cognitive impairment in patients with heart failure includes (1) decreased capacity to sustain attention and concentration; (2) diminished memory capacity; (3) diminished capacity to engage with tasks that require executive functions of the brain, including problem solving and abstract reasoning; and (4) decreased motor speed, reflected in slower reaction time.[6-8] Overall, there is consensus among authorities with regard to the domains of cognitive impairment associated with heart failure.

Despite the clinical relevance and emotional, social, and tangible costs to patients with heart failure and those involved in their care, cognitive impairment traditionally received relatively little attention in the literature.[9,10] Symptoms of dyspnea, fatigue, and edema have attracted greater interest and study; in fact, patients with cognitive impairment are frequently ruled out in terms of eligibility for participation in studies related to heart failure. The prevalence of cognitive impairment in patients over 65 years old with heart failure is nearly double (1.96 times) that in the general population.[10]

Health-related quality of life (HRQL)—a multidimensional construct in which the patient assesses his or her health status in comparison to what he or she hopes it to be—is significantly compromised in patients with heart failure.[11,12] Although the relationship is complex, as noted by Pressler,[7] cognitive impairment is associated with lower HRQL scores in patients with heart failure. There is evidence to suggest the possibility of a curvilinear relationship between cognitive impairment and HRQL; those individuals with the greatest degree of cognitive impairment have the highest HRQL scores, and individuals with less severe cognitive impairment have lower scores.[13] This seemingly paradoxical finding may be attributed to the compromised ability of more cognitively impaired individuals to evaluate their cognitive abilities realistically.[14] However, like individuals with severe cognitive deficits, those with asymptomatic heart failure who do not have cognitive deficits are more likely to have higher HRQL scores; this finding casts doubt on the reliability and validity of a subset of HRQL self-reports (individuals with severe heart failure who also evidence more severe cognitive impairment, and asymptomatic patients without cognitive impairment). Nevertheless, this finding does not negate the importance of assessing HRQL in patients with heart failure.

PREVALENCE

The literature on the prevalence of cognitive impairment in heart failure is sparse. It is characterized by inconsistency of instrumentation, as well as lack of depth of assessment tools used.[15,16] In view of the diversity of approaches to the study of cognitive impairment, including the use of experimental designs that are insufficiently powered, it is not surprising that reported prevalence rates range from approximately 25% to 80%.[8] A more conservative estimate is 25% to 30%.[7,17,18]

Feola and colleagues[19] reported that the degree of cognitive impairment in most patients with heart failure is mild. However, one fourth of patients with heart failure exhibit moderate to severe cognitive impairment. Severity of cognitive impairment is correlated with New York Heart Association (NYHA) classification; the more severe the impairment is, the more likely that the NYHA classification is higher (class IV).[20]

In the early stages of heart failure, cognitive impairment manifests as more nuanced, intermittent, and difficult to recognize than in later stages of heart failure. The severity of impairment is correlated with age and inversely correlated with left ventricular ejection fraction. Although findings are inconsistent, the degree of cognitive impairment is not associated with systolic or diastolic blood pressure, which may be a result of treatment of blood pressure.[8] Because of the episodic, inconsistent, and unstable manifestation of cognitive impairment, particularly in early stages, periodic cognitive screening may be most effective for appropriate detection and intervention.

A CONCEPTUAL FRAMEWORK

There have been few systematic attempts to target specific populations of individuals with heart failure in terms of cause and severity of cognitive impairment. Most studies are not guided by a conceptual framework; for this reason, the understanding of prevention and attenuation of cognitive decline is seriously limited. On the basis of a literature review of the pathophysiology of cognitive impairment in patients with heart failure, as well as HRQL findings in

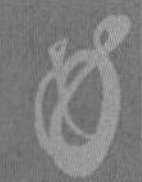

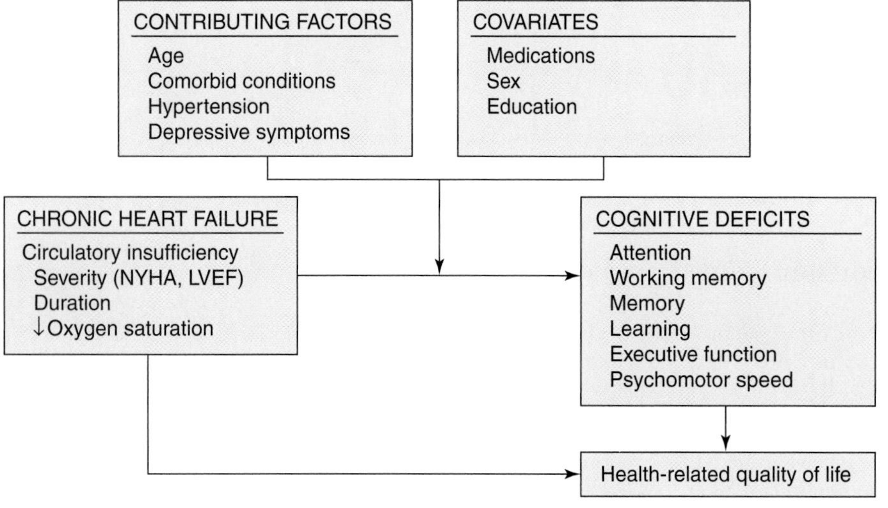

FIGURE 60–1 Conceptual model of cognitive deficits in heart failure. LVEF, left ventricular ejection fraction; NYHA, New York Heart Association (classification). (From Bennett, S. J., Sauve, M. J., Shaw, R. M. (2005). A conceptual model of cognitive deficits in chronic heart failure. *J. Nurs. Scholars.* 37, 222-228.)

patients with heart failure, Bennett and colleagues[21] provided a working framework for conducting future research efforts. The model proposed allows for the inclusion and evaluation of cause and the assessment of key variables such as depression and HRQL. The model also presents opportunities to expand the knowledge base in order to make better and more evidence-based decisions.

Bennett and colleagues[6] suggested that circulatory insufficiency accounts for the majority of the difficulties associated with cognitive impairment in patients with heart failure; this view is supported in the literature. The model identifies additional contributors to impaired cognitive functioning: age, comorbid conditions, and their combined effects (e.g., hypertension and depressive symptoms), as well as covariates such as medications and education. Figure 60-1 elucidates the proposed relationships among these contributors and how they may inform each other with regard to treatment.

MECHANISMS RESPONSIBLE FOR COGNITIVE IMPAIRMENT: STRUCTURAL AND FUNCTIONAL CHANGES WITHIN THE BRAIN

Understanding cause with regard to heart failure and cognitive decline is critical for identifying patients most likely to experience cognitive impairment. Cause also has significant implications for interventions designed to ameliorate or halt cognitive decline. However, many of the studies have relied on heterogeneous sampling approaches with diverse underlying pathophysiological mechanisms (e.g., heart transplantation candidates, community-based populations), which results in difficulty in addressing issues related to cause.[8]

There is strong evidence that circulatory insufficiency leads to inadequate cerebral perfusion and that cerebral hypoxia is the probable primary cause of cognitive decline.[7] Cardiogenic embolism has also been proposed as the underlying pathophysiological mechanism.[8] Hypoxemia, possibly resulting from sleep apnea,[22] as well as abnormalities in blood viscosity in dehydrated patients,[23] have been proposed as other potential mechanisms.

Animal model studies are relevant to the discussion of cause in patients with heart failure. These studies suggest that oxygen deprivation is implicated in autoneurotoxicity or neuronal cell death. Areas of the brain that are particularly susceptible to oxygen deprivation are the hippocampus, amygdala, frontal lobes, and cerebellum.[24,25]

Although the current understanding of structural and functional changes in humans is limited, ongoing research efforts may be promising.[7] Evaluation techniques in humans include use of expensive measurement tools such as magnetic resonance imaging (MRI), positron emission tomography (PET), computed tomography (CT), single photon emission computed tomography (SPECT), transcranial Doppler imaging, transcranial ultrasonography, near-infrared spectroscopy, and jugular venous blood and cerebral scanning. These studies, unfortunately, are limited by sample size, because of associated costs and respondent burden. In addition, comparison groups are frequently not included, and changes over time are not measured. A notable exception is the study conducted by Woo and colleagues.[26] Nine patients with heart failure were compared with 27 age-matched healthy participants. MRI results revealed that patients with NYHA classes III and IV heart failure had significant loss of gray matter in the insular cortex, frontal cortex, parahippocampal gyrus, cingulate, cerebellar cortex, and deep cerebral nuclei, in comparison with age-matched healthy individuals. These brain regions are crucial for cognitive functioning and cardiovascular regulation. Woo and colleagues concluded that ischemia and hypotensive episodes are likely to cause perfusion deficits that contribute to the observed loss of gray matter.

In a well-designed study, Vogels and associates[8] found a significant relationship between cognitive impairment and medial temporal lobe atrophy. Memory and executive functions were the two most commonly affected domains. The findings are evidence of a hemodynamically mediated pathophysiological mechanism, in view of the vulnerability of the medial temporal lobe to inadequate oxygenation that results from hypoperfusion.[25,27]

In a small comparison group study, Alves and coworkers,[28] using SPECT, found that individuals with heart failure have significant reductions in cerebral blood flow. Differences between the patients and the comparison group of elderly individuals were demonstrated in structural areas such as segments of the precuneus and cuneus, the right lateral temporoparietal cortex, and the posterior cingulate gyrus. Reduction in cerebral blood flow was correlated with cognitive impairment, as assessed by the Cambridge Mental Disorders of the Elderly Examination. These results must be viewed with caution because of the small sample size. Similarly, Schmidt and colleagues,[29] on the basis of MRI results, found higher rates of cerebral infarcts and cortical atrophy, as well as lower scores on neuropsychological testing, in patients with idiopathic dilated cardiomyopathy in comparison with age-matched healthy controls.

A consistent pattern supports the association of the localization of gray matter loss with cognitive impairment. Structural and functional brain changes are associated with reductions in cerebral blood flow and with silent brain infarctions. These changes are associated with difficulties in perceiving heart failure–related symptoms (insular cortex and cingulated cortex, areas that receive and process viscerosensory input), in addition to difficulties with memory, attention, and concentration.

Further research is needed to isolate the mechanisms directly responsible for the observed changes in functioning. It remains unclear what the short- and long-term implications of these findings are in terms of cognitive functioning. As Pressler[7] noted, because of the expense associated with imaging measurements, in addition to the burden it places on the patient and family, it is likely that future studies will continue to be small in scope and that the generalizability of findings will therefore be limited.

CONTRIBUTING FACTORS AND COVARIATES

In attempting to systematically understand the causes of cognitive impairment in patients with heart failure, it is important to consider contributing factors and covariates of heart failure. As discussed previously, circulatory insufficiency has been identified as key, as have silent brain infarctions; both are likely to affect attention, working memory, other memory, learning, executive functioning, and psychomotor speed.[6,21,30]

Cognitive impairment in patients with heart failure is significantly associated with age, activities of daily living, and overall reduced independence, as well as NYHA classification.[31] Reductions in left ventricular ejection fraction (LVEF) are also associated with cognitive impairment.[29] A relationship between cognitive impairment and the presence of the apolipoprotein E-ε4 (ApoE-ε4) allele, an established risk factor, has been observed in individuals with heart failure.[8] Studies have shown that gene-environment interactions between ApoE genotype and cardiovascular risk factors may accelerate cognitive decline in the elderly.[32]

With regard to age, research findings are limited by studies that do not represent the full range of possibilities. In general, older individuals (older than 70 years) tend to have a higher incidence of cognitive deficits than do younger individuals.[30] Cognitive deficits are associated with age, which probably interacts with the severity of heart failure, inasmuch as occurrence of cognitive impairment is associated with severity of NYHA classification. Elderly individuals are more likely than younger persons to have fluid shifts and dehydration, which are also associated with cognitive impairment.[18] However, studies with age-matched control participants have not revealed a significant relationship between age and cognitive impairment in patients with heart failure.[6] Bennett and colleagues[21] concluded that further investigation is needed to "identify profiles of patients most likely to experience cognitive deficits" (p. 225).

Coexisting major medical conditions contribute to cognitive impairment in patients with heart failure and can conflate findings linking heart failure with cognitive impairment. For example, compelling data have emerged from studies of patients with chronic obstructive pulmonary disease (COPD). When severe, COPD has been found to cause cerebral hypoxia. In studies in which patients have diagnoses of both heart failure and COPD (approximately 12%), results indicate that they are more likely to be cognitively impaired, frequently requiring home care.[6,22]

Individuals with neurological conditions such as stroke and those with a history of alcohol and substance abuse are also likely to evince cognitive impairment. In the case of stroke, individuals who are elderly, women, and those with more compromised LVEF are at increased risk for cognitive impairment. Risk for stroke increases linearly: an 18% increase for each 5% decline in LVEF.[33]

Studies have consistently demonstrated an association between cognitive impairment and hypertension.[7,30] However, the researchers have not controlled for the presence of cardiovascular disorders such as heart failure. Of importance is that treatment of hypertension is effective in reducing new-onset heart failure by 50%.[7,34] Jennings[33] proposed a vascular mechanism, suggesting that hypertension causes changes in autoregulation of cerebral blood flow, but at higher pressures than in normotensive individuals. The decrease in cerebral blood flow probably accounts for significantly lower scores in working memory, according to Jennings.

Cognitive deficits have also been reported in patients with diabetes, breast cancer, lupus, and fibromyalgia; these findings provide a broader perspective with regard to linkage between cognitive impairment and coexisting medical conditions. Because of the likely conflation, researchers in future studies of patients with heart failure must control for or rule out comorbid medical conditions in order to better understand the unique contributions of heart failure to cognitive impairment.

Sleep-Disordered Breathing and Heart Failure (see Chapter 32)

Daytime sleepiness interferes with decision making, particularly as it relates to self-care. Sleep interruptions and sleep deprivation are relatively common in patients with heart failure and are associated with increasing age, comorbid illnesses, excess body weight, lack of exercise, excessive alcohol consumption, and chronic insomnia.[36] Killgore and associates[37] demonstrated that attention and concentration, working memory, and executive functioning are compromised when individuals are deprived of sleep. This finding has important implications for decision making and self-care in patients with heart failure. The results suggest the importance of screening for sleep-disordered breathing in patients with heart failure, particularly in patients who evince cognitive impairment. The effect of treatment for sleep-disordered breathing and depression and its influence on self-care must be further understood because it has significant implications for self-care. The next section focuses specifically on the comorbid condition of depression and its relationship to cognitive impairment in patients with heart failure.

Depression and Heart Failure

One of the most common of all mental conditions is depression, which includes both subjective symptoms, such as feeling hopeless and worthless, and objective symptoms, such as decreased appetite and difficulty with attention. Clinical depression impairs daily functioning. Patients who report a decrease of interest and depressed mood for at least 2 weeks meet the criteria for the diagnosis of clinical depression.[13]

Sullivan and colleagues[38] estimated that depression and psychological impairment may be responsible for nearly 25% of the $20 billion associated with treating heart failure.

Determining the incidence of depression in patients with heart failure is difficult because of variations in methods. Rates are not consistent between patients in nursing homes and those living independently. In addition, investigators have used various methods of diagnosis and instruments to measure the severity of depression.[13]

Studies have shown that the severity of depression is significantly related to increases in mortality among patients with heart failure. In comparison with patients with heart failure who were not depressed, those classified as severely depressed had four times the mortality rates during a 2-year poststudy follow-up period. Although most studies have demonstrated a significant association between depression and heart failure, the incidence of depression in patients with heart failure varies considerably; reported rates range from 14% to 36%.[39,40] Studies show that even after depression has been successfully treated and symptoms ameliorated, it is not unusual for depression to recur. The study by Segal and associates,[41] although not specific to patients with heart failure, revealed that more than 80% of the patients treated for depression were at risk for multiple episodes of depression.

The nature of the relationship between depression and heart failure has been obscured by selection bias in research studies. It appears that patients with heart failure who participate in these studies are healthier, with fewer physical complaints, than patients with heart failure who decline to participate. In addition, some symptoms such as fatigue and insomnia may be associated with heart failure and therefore are not reported as depressive symptoms. Thus, the number of patients with heart failure who are depressed may be underestimated in these studies.

The mechanism by which depression contributes to poorer outcomes for patients with heart failure is unclear. The debate about whether depression is a risk factor for heart failure, whether heart failure may spur depression, or whether the two interact in some way continues in the research literature. There is agreement that because of the behavioral and physiological components of depression, patients with heart failure who are depressed are at greater risk of mortality and morbidity. Depression is associated with poorer compliance with medical regimens, which has significant consequences for patients with heart failure. Patients who have both heart failure and depression have been shown to have high sympathetic tone, hypercortisolism, increased platelet aggregability, and elevated levels of inflammatory markers.[13]

Because assessment of depression is crucial in treatment, accurate evaluation is key. Foreman and colleagues[42] provided a useful comparison of the clinical features of delirium, dementia, and depression. They identified important differences in clinical features such as onset, course, sleep-wake cycle, and memory. For example, in depressed patients, affect is depressed and mood is dysphoric with themes of hopelessness, helplessness, or self-deprecation, whereas in patients with dementia, affect tends to be inappropriate and labile, with impoverished thoughts, word-finding difficulties, and possible aphasia and agnosia. It is also important to assess and differentiate somatic depressive symptoms of heart failure and symptoms associated with depression. Assessment tools such as the Beck Depression Scale allow for systematic assessment and analysis of results that include both somatic depressive symptoms of fatigue and insomnia, symptoms associated with heart failure, and symptoms associated with depression.

Depression is associated with increased rates of mortality among patients with heart failure and appears to be linearly related to severity of depression. Comorbid psychiatric conditions, such as anxiety disorders, are strongly associated with depression. The literature focuses on medical treatment of depression in patients with heart failure, which is described as safe and effective for depression in patients with cardiovascular disease.[43] Alternative or complementary adjunct therapies such as cognitive behavioral therapy must be considered as well.[13]

COGNITIVE FUNCTIONS RELATED TO SELF-CARE IN PATIENTS WITH HEART FAILURE

According to Dickson and associates,[2] "Cognitive function refers to the information-processing abilities of attention, learning and memory, executive functioning (e.g., cognitive flexibility and abstract reasoning), visual-spatial and visual-construction skills, psychomotor abilities, perceptual skills and language—functions critical to self-care" (p. 426). For the individual with heart failure, self-care includes monitoring symptoms, taking prescribed medications, following dietary restrictions, exercising, keeping appointments, and maintaining instrumental activities of daily living. In the following section, self-care tasks are described, and the cognitive functions associated with their performance are discussed. Tests related to each cognitive function are identified, and assistive technology that may compensate for mild impairment is described.

Medication Regimen

According to Insel and colleagues,[44] adherence to medication regimens may be more of a function of capacity than of attitude. Planning to take medications requires the abilities to create a plan (which involves executive functioning and abstract reasoning), to implement the plan (which involves attention and short-term memory), to remember to take the medication at the correct times (which involves long-term memory and both visual-spatial and visual-construction skills in perception of a clock face), to take medications in the prescribed manner (which involves executive functioning and long-term memory), and remembering whether the medication was taken as desired (which involves working memory).

Impairment in memory and concentration is frequently reported by patients with heart failure.[21] According to Miller and associates,[45] *working memory* is the type of memory that is necessary to plan and carry out behavior. The common experience of walking into a room only to forget the reason for going into that room is frustrating if not embarrassing. For a patient with heart failure, an interruption while taking medication may cause the patient to forget whether the medication was actually taken. This, in turn, could lead to either missing a dose or taking the medication twice. If a patient is interrupted while taking medication, working memory allows him or her to return to the task after dealing with the interruption.

Working memory is not considered completely different from short-term memory; it is considered to be a combination of short-term memory and other functions such as attention and information processing.[46] Because working memory is closely related to intelligence, measures of working memory may be biased in terms of education and social class. Working memory can be assessed by the Digit Span portion of the Wechsler Adult Intelligence Scale, in which the patient is asked to repeat numerical sequences forward and then backward.[26] Assistive technology options to assist patients with heart failure to take their medications as prescribed have expanded. For example, a *medication reminder watch* can be programmed with up to 12 medication reminders, including text messages with the name and strength of the medication or other prompts. Alarm options include sound alarm, text alarm, vibration, and a combination of these. Most models of cell phones also have reminder tools that could be used to remind a patient of medication regimen.

For patients who have trouble identifying their medication, *automatic pill dispensers* are useful because they have alarms and dispense a set of pills into a medication well. The most advanced option is a *monitored pill dispenser* that not only can dispense a month's worth of medications at various intervals (up to six times per day) but also can be programmed to call a caregiver if medications are not taken on time. Individual medication administrations can be programmed with text or voice reminders.

Low-Sodium Diets

Patients with heart failure are routinely advised to make changes in their diets, especially with regard to the sodium content of their food. Impairments in executive functioning could be a reason why most patients with heart failure do not closely follow dietary guidelines.[2]

Planning, abstract thinking, and judgment are all components of executive functions of the brain.[26,47] According to Cullen and colleagues, cognitive impairment relating to vascular conditions is also characterized by impairment in verbal fluency.[48] Impairments in verbal fluency, including basic reading skills, can hamper the patient's selection process as well as his or her ability to follow instructions in meal preparation.

Common measures of these executive functioning include trail-making tests, similar to a connect-the-dots task, in which patients are asked to connect numbers in sequence (either 1→2→3 … or a more complex form such as 1→A→2→B→3→C …). Tests of verbal fluency include naming objects, such as animals, or asking a person to say as many words beginning with a certain letter as he or she can in 1 minute.

Text readers that read aloud an entire page of text, as well as reading pens that read text word by word, are available to patients with heart failure to assist with reading fluency. Because of their portability, reading pens are ideal for taking to the grocery store and identifying the sodium content in food by scanning the label. Many of the adaptations used for individuals with poor vision can empower patients with heart failure in adhering to a low-sodium diet; these adaptations include picture-based grocery lists and color-coded cookbooks, which reduce the need for reading and verbal fluency.

Symptom Monitoring

According to Dickson and associates,[2] monitoring symptoms involves complex cognitive skills. For example, patients with heart failure must remember to check daily for specific symptoms such as ankle swelling. Learning involves both attention and long-term memory; patients must learn that ankle swelling may indicate that they are experiencing fluid retention. In addition, they need to associate fluid retention with some immediate action, such as notifying the appropriate health care provider or taking an additional diuretic. If memory, judgment, and planning are impaired, fluid retention may go untreated.[2] Although many cognitive screening tools have a delayed-recall component, only the informant-based cognitive screens address impairment of long-term memory or learning abilities. Learning new routines can be difficult for many older adults; personal data assistants (PDAs) can provide verbal cues and reminders. For individuals with cognitive impairments, assistive technology providers have developed specific programs that can be adapted for use related to heart failure; they can keep a record for the health care provider regarding how well the individual is adhering to his or her treatment plan. One such programming option would be for the individual to record water percentage into their PDA. If the percentage reaches a target level, the PDA would cue the patient with heart failure to take appropriate action such as calling the health care provider or adjusting medication as prescribed.

Electronic scales can assist patients who have heart failure with water retention (in 0.1% increments) and those with weight gain. Simple body analyzer scales display the readings in large digital numbers. More advanced options allow for tracking up to 10 readings, programming alerts to targets, and even printouts of readings that could be reviewed by a caregiver or health care provider.

Weight Management and Regular Exercise

Attention can be considered a foundational cognitive skill inasmuch as it is necessary for performing other cognitive functions such as calculations and planning. Attention skills have been found to be compromised in a significant subset of patients with heart failure.[49] One of the challenges in detecting impairment of attention in patients with heart failure is that the ability may fluctuate depending on task or time of day.[42,47] Patients with attention deficits may be easily distracted.[47] Fluctuations in attention and overall declines in memory and executive functions may be attenuated through exercise.[50] The ability to complete serial 7s (counting backward from 100 by 7s), is a test commonly used to assess impairments in attention.

Developing new activities for weight loss and increasing overall fitness are general goals for patients with heart failure. Motorized bikes allow for the individual to move his or her legs in a passive exercise in which the motor can gradually lessen the assistance with the movement. Ideal for patients with heart failure who have been previously inactive, the miniature versions of these machines are small enough to fit under a desk.

Heart rate monitors are also beneficial. Originally designed for athletes who sought an alternative to chest or belt monitors, these comfortable semi–glove-shaped monitors entail the use of the base of the finger for sensing, which makes it easy for patients with heart failure to use while exercising. Because no transmitter is used with these heart rate monitors, there are no interference problems.

The interpretation of paradoxical findings regarding weight and patients with heart failure is challenging for the provider; thus, when appropriate, patients with heart failure can join the growing weight loss community on the Internet. Websites offering recipes, advice, and counseling are readily and inexpensively available. For tracking caloric consumption, assistive technology devices such as "Countdown to Slim" provide a digital monitor for tracking diet, including goals for calories, sodium, and other targets.

Significant cognitive impairments may limit the ability of patients with heart failure to maintain their independence; however, if a mild impairment is detected, assistive technology options may allow for independence to continue without compromising the patient's health. Professionals such as occupational therapists and rehabilitation counselors may be able to identify creative solutions by which patients with heart failure can accommodate mild cognitive impairments.

ASSESSMENT OF COGNITIVE IMPAIRMENT

Cognitive impairment in patients with heart failure has implications for treatment. Some decline in cognitive functions may be age related. An estimated 17% of the elderly population (aged 65 and older) are struggling with mild to moderate cognitive impairment.[51] The detection and evaluation of cognitive functioning are significant for both HRQL and the medical management of individuals with heart failure.

Cognitive Impairment Screening Tools

The development of instruments to screen for cognitive impairment are designed to detect deviation from normal cognitive functioning rather than to identify impairments in specific cognitive functions.[6,48] To date, no cognitive screening tools have been developed specifically for use with patients with heart failure.

This section of the chapter covers brief screening tests, cognitive impairment batteries, and informant report scales. Table 60-1 provides an overview of the screening measures and the cognitive domains assessed.

Individuals with mild cognitive impairments rarely report symptoms and may engage in denial, even when the impairments are apparent to family members and health care providers.[52] Documentation of cognitive impairment has been neglected, and reliance on medical records for information

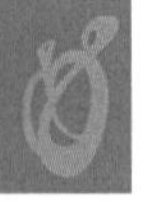

TABLE 60–1 Cognitive Impairment Screening Instruments and Cognitive Function Domains

Features	AMT	MoCA	MMSE	CDT	Mini-Cog	GPCOG
Average time to administer (minutes)	3	10	8	2	3	4.5
Specific measurements						
• Attention, concentration, or both[41-43]	✓	✓	✓	✓	✓	✓
• Calculations		✓	✓			
• Executive function[41-43]		✓		✓	✓	✓
• Learning						
• Language[42]		✓				
• Orientation	✓	✓				✓
• Psychomotor speed[41]						✓
• Reasoning, judgment, or both[42]						✓
• Short-term memory or recall[41-43]	✓	✓			✓	✓
• Verbal fluency[42]		✓	✓			✓
• Visuospatial abilities[42]		✓		✓	✓	
• Working memory[41-43]		✓				✓

AMT, Abbreviated Mental Test; CDT, Clock Drawing Test; GPCOG, General Practitioner Assessment of Cognition; MMSE, Mini Mental State Examination; MoCA, Montreal Cognitive Assessment.

about cognitive impairment has been shown to be inadequate.[53] Whereas severe impairment may be detected during routine care appointments, research has shown that medical personnel are poor at predicting moderate to mild impairment. Because of the relationship between cognition and mortality, it is important that an accurate screening assessment be made by appropriate medical personnel.[21]

When clinicians select a screening test, they should consider the types of cognitive impairments that are detected by the measure, as well as the sensitivity of the screening tool in detecting less severe impairment. Cultural and educational considerations should also be taken into account.

Mini Mental State Examination

The most commonly used screening tool in both practice and research is the Mini Mental State Examination (MMSE).[18,47,48] This tool has been used since the 1980s and translated into several languages.[54] The MMSE was originally developed to screen for cognitive disorders rather than cognitive impairment. Criticisms of this instrument include (1) both "ceiling" and "floor" effects[47]; (2) lack of rationale for cutoff scores[54]; (3) poor sensitivity to executive function[44]; and (4) education and socioeconomic biases.[55,56] The MMSE is easy to administer and interpret and test administration is estimated to take between 5 and 10 minutes.[54]

Abbreviated Mental Test

According to Woodford and George, the Abbreviated Mental Test (AMT) was derived from the MMSE; the 10 most discriminating items were kept in the instrument.[47] The AMT screens for impairment in long- and short-term memory, attention, and orientation. It is not considered sensitive enough to detect milder forms of cognitive impairment, but it is sensitive in detecting delirium and dementia in elderly patients.[47]

Montreal Cognitive Assessment

The more recently developed Montreal Cognitive Assessment (MoCA) is touted as a brief screening tool (10 minutes to administer) for detecting mild cognitive impairments in eight cognitive domains: "attention and concentration, executive functions, memory, language, visuoconstructional skills, conceptual thinking, calculations, and orientation."[57] The instrument, a one-page, 30-point test, has been translated into 17 languages, and studies have established its validity in several countries, including China, Korea, and the Czech Republic.

Clock Drawing Test and the Mini-Cog

The Clock Drawing Test (CDT) is a nonverbal screening tool in which the patient is asked to draw a clock. Placement of the numbers around the circle requires visual-spatial, numerical sequencing, and planning abilities.[47] The patient is then asked to draw the hands on the clock to indicate "ten minutes past 11 o'clock." The test also assesses long-term attention, memory, auditory processing, motor programming, and frustration tolerance.[18,58] There are multiple approaches to scoring the CDT.[58] Advantages of this test include an absence of language and cultural biases. Riegel and colleagues[18] concluded that the CDT was better than the MMSE at detecting cognitive impairment in patients with heart failure. This may be because of the instability and subtle nature of cognitive impairment in patients with heart failure, in contrast to patients with dementia.

The Mini-Cog, in which a three-word recall test is added to the CDT, has the advantage of also assessing memory. It was developed to improve the relatively culture-free CDT by assessing the patient's recall (memory) and thereby covering the domains of the MMSE.[55] If the patient is unable to recall all three words in the Mini-Cog, he or she is considered to have a cognitive impairment.

Cognitive Abilities Screening Instrument

The Cognitive Abilities Screening Instrument (CASI) is a mini-battery that has been validated in cross-ethnic studies.[55] It contains questions from both the MMSE and the Modified Mini Mental Status Examination (3MS).[47] The marginal increase in sensitivity is not considered to be sufficient because additional time (20 minutes) is needed to administer the test.

Cambridge Cognitive Examination

The Cambridge Mental Disorders of the Elderly Examination (CAMDEX) is a battery that includes history taking from both the patient and an informant, a structured examination, and a mental state assessment (known as *CAMCOG*). The CAMCOG tests orientation, language, attention, memory, praxis, calculation, abstract thinking, and perception.[49] Diagnostic criteria from the *Diagnostic and Statistical Manual of Mental Disorders, Fourth Edition* (DSM-IV)[59] and the *International Statistical Classification of Diseases and Related Health Problems* (ICD-9)[60] are included in the CAMDEX scoring manual; this allows the clinician not only to detect areas of cognitive impairment but also to diagnose specific conditions associated with the impairments detected.

General Practitioner Assessment of Cognition

Developed in Australia, the General Practitioner Assessment of Cognition (GPCOG) measure combines questions for both patient and informant to detect cognitive impairments among elderly patients.[58,61] The 15 questions cover a variety of tasks used in other screening tools, such as clock drawing and memory recall. In addition, the questions for informants cover items such as misplacing objects and ability to manage money and medication. The test takes approximately 4 to 5 minutes to administer. In comparisons of the GPCOG with the MMSE, the two were considered equally sensitive for screening for dementia, but the GPCOG took less than half the amount of time.[58,61] In a validation study of almost 400 subjects, Brodaty and colleagues[61] deemed the GPCOG to have "sound psychometric properties" (p. 531), and in comparison with both the AMT and the MMSE, it is more sensitive in detecting mild impairments.

Recommendations for Assessment of Cognitive Impairment in Patients with Heart Failure

The development of cognitive impairment in patients with heart failure may not be readily apparent. Assessment and screening tools, such as those described in the previous section, can detect the presence of , that impairment. In reviewing the screening tools available, clinicians must keep in mind the cognitive impairment features that are relevant to the medical management of these patients. Although comorbid dementias may exist, they are beyond the scope of this chapter.

Administration and interpretation of psychoneurological assessment batteries are time and labor intensive, and specialized training is required. Therefore, global measures are frequently used, but they do not generate the information needed for the purpose of identifying the extent and types of cognitive impairments, including the detection of more subtle yet significant deficits in patients with heart failure. The data generated by these global measures cannot be linked to cause for a broadly representative group of patients with heart failure. It also remains unclear whether the association of heart failure and cognitive impairment is related to poor cardiac output or is a function of multiple coexisting conditions.[16,62,63]

What is clear is the need to screen for the presence of cognitive impairment so that it can be proactively addressed in the medical management of the patient with heart failure. Although the MMSE has been the tool most frequently used in research, the MoCA appears to be an effective quick screen that does not have the biases and score limitations of the MMSE.

INTERVENTION PROGRAMS FOR PATIENTS WITH HEART FAILURE AND COGNITIVE IMPAIRMENT

The needs of a significant but silent minority—patients with heart failure who are cognitively impaired—are insufficiently addressed in the literature on heart failure intervention; such neglect is perplexing, in view of prevalence data. In many management programs specifically for heart failure, cognitive functioning is presumed to be intact in its participants. Patients with mild to moderate cognitive impairment do not appear to obtain the benefits of prolonged event-free survival or overall survival in such programs, in comparison with cognitively intact patients. This finding suggests that existing approaches to heart failure–specific management must be reevaluated and modified.[33] McLennan and associates[28] concluded that a likely explanation for the relationship between cognitive impairment and clinical outcome in patients with heart failure is the "cyclical" interaction of "physiological, cognitive and behavioural factors" (p. 499). However, an alternative explanation must be considered: that cognitive impairment is a marker of disease progression or concurrent cerebrovascular disease.

Depending on the degree of cognitive impairment, patients may profit from the development of an action plan, conceived in partnership with medical personnel, that is individually tailored to their functional level. The plan should reflect the patient's existing strengths and resources, as well as those of his or her support network. As mentioned in the previous section, whenever possible, compensatory mechanisms and supplementary programs such as Internet-based instruction and interactional dialogue (e.g., support groups) can be introduced to address specific obstacles and reinforce needed skills.

Family members and additional support networks can also be harnessed judiciously as resources. Participation of family members seems to be key in effective management programs for heart failure; however, little is known about how to best engage family members in ways that do not diminish the autonomy and self-efficacy of patients with heart failure, with and without cognitive impairment. Family engagement on an as-needed basis, as well as the support of a social network, is a key factor in differentiating individuals with heart failure who are considered "expert" in heart failure self-care from those who are not.[63] Further research is needed to explore this potentially rich area of investigation.

The range of options available to patients and their support networks increases significantly with Internet-enhanced instruction.[64,65] It is a promising tool that may serve as an important supplement to self-care management programs for individuals with cognitive impairment. Although the elderly are least likely to access the Internet, the numbers of those who do are increasing significantly.[4] Strömberg and colleagues[66] observed that elderly patients with lower educational levels, with the aid of Internet-based instruction, are able to assimilate required information under nonpressured conditions. Rosamond and Paul[4] noted that "Books, newsletters, videos, CDs [compact disks], Web pages, and computer-based programs augment the learning process and offer further opportunities for education at patients' convenience" (p. e70). Internet-enhanced instruction (e.g., the Patient Management Tool, at http://www.americanheart.org/presenter.jhtml?identifier=651) facilitates the repetition and reinforcement of heart failure–related skills. Follow-up telephone calls, newsletters, educational bulletins, and support groups may also serve as additional resources.[4] Role-playing exercises may assist patients with heart failure as well.

Exercise is an additional resource that has not been adequately tapped and investigated (see also Chapter 57). Tanne and colleagues[67] implemented an exercise program with 18 patients with stable heart failure (NYHA class III) and compared the results with those of a group of 5 patients who received no exercise program. Patients met twice a week for 18 weeks in a standard cardiac rehabilitation program that included a 15-minute warm-up, a 35-minute program on the treadmill, and a regimen of stair climbing and bicycling. Results indicated improvement in some cognitive domains

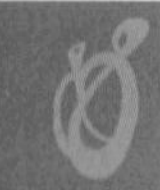

but not in others; measures of general attention and psychomotor speed (Trail Making Test and Stroop Test parts A and C) showed improvement. Although the reported gains were statistically significant, it is not clear whether they were clinically significant. Improvements in general attention and psychomotor speed were not associated with improved vasodilator reserve. The mechanisms by which these improvements occurred are not known, and the improvements may be attributable solely to increased alertness. Because of the number of tests given and the small number of subjects who participated in the intervention, the results are vulnerable to type I and type II errors. Furthermore, the 18-week treatment program may be too short in duration to make significant impact.

Yoga is another potential resource for patients with heart failure. Pullen and colleagues[68] found that an 8-week regimen of yoga for patients with heart failure improved exercise tolerance, improved estimated peak ventilatory oxygen uptake (Vo_2), and reduced levels of inflammatory markers. The mechanisms by which improvement occurred are unclear. Although these results are promising, caution is needed, in view of the small number of participants in the study.

Verhaegen and colleagues[69] conducted a meta-analysis of memory training effectiveness in healthy patients aged 60 years and older.[57] Results indicated that memory does remain amenable to improvement in old age. Individuals are most likely to benefit from mnemonic training (memory aids, such as short rhymes). Memory sessions are least effective when they are longer in duration (sessions ranged from 20 minutes to 2.5 hours); this finding was attributed to fatigue. Questions remain as to whether these results can be generalized to a population with heart failure and cognitive impairment. In addition, it would be helpful to understand why some patients with heart failure and cognitive impairment may be able to benefit but others gain little or no benefit from such programs.

FUTURE DIRECTIONS

It is difficult to determine the extent to which clinicians can intervene effectively for patients with heart failure who are cognitively impaired. It remains unclear whether cognitive impairment can be alleviated or reversed in patients with heart failure; the data are simply not currently available. The relative silence and possible denial surrounding cognitive impairment in patients with heart failure must be systematically combated, and more recent efforts are promising.

In order to understand the pathophysiology and natural course of cognitive deficits over time in patients with heart failure, a conceptual framework is needed to systematically guide professionals in the field to make informed assessments. The consistent use of relevant and sensitive neuropsychological tools is currently problematic. Informed assessments, based on reliable and valid data, can guide professionals in determining whether and under what conditions cognitive deficits are amenable to targeted interventions. The implications are significant, particularly with regard to prevention or delay of impairment in patients with heart failure. In addition to understanding the progression of mental changes, further research is needed to understand the implications of these changes for prognosis and intervention.

REFERENCES

1. Bennett, S. J., Saywell, R. M., Zollinger, T. W., Jr., et al. (1999). Cost of hospitalizations for heart failure: sodium retention versus other decompensating factors. *Heart Lung, 28*, 102–109.
2. Dickson, V. V., Tkacs, N., & Riegel, B. (2007). Cognitive influences on self-care decision making in persons with heart failure. *Am Heart J, 154*, 424–431.
3. Rosamond, W., Flegal, K., Friday, G., et al. (2007). Heart disease and stroke statistics—2007 update: a report from the American Heart Association Statistics Committee and Stroke Statistics Subcommittee. *Circulation, 115*(5), e69–e171.
4. Paul, S. (2008). Hospital discharge education for patients with heart failure: what really works and what is the evidence? *Critical Care Nurs, 28*(2), 66–82.
5. Evangelista, L. S., Doering, L., Dracup, K., et al. (2003). Compliance behaviors of elderly patients with advanced heart failure. *J Cardiovasc Nurs, 18*, 197–206.
6. Bennett, S. J., & Sauvé, M. J. (2003). Cognitive deficits in patients with heart failure: a review of the literature. *J Cardiovasc Nurs, 18*, 219–242.
7. Pressler, S. J. (2008). Cognitive functioning and chronic heart failure: a review of the literature (2002 to July 2007). *J Cardiovasc Nurs, 23*, 239–249.
8. Vogels, R. L. C., Scheltens, P., Schroeder-Tanka, J. M., et al. (2007). Cognitive impairment in heart failure: a systematic review of the literature. *Eur J Heart Fail, 9*, 440–449.
9. Bennett, S. J., Cordes, D. K., Westmoreland, G., et al. (2000). Self-care strategies for symptom management in patients with chronic heart failure. *Nurs Res, 49*, 129–145.
10. Cacciatore, F., Abete, P., Ferrara, N., et al. (1998). Congestive heart failure and cognitive impairment in an older population. *J Am Geriatr Soc, 46*, 1343–1348.
11. Konstam, V., Salem, D., Pouleur, H., et al. (1996). Baseline quality of life as a predictor of mortality and hospitalization in 5,025 patients with congestive heart failure. *Am J Cardiol, 78*, 890–895.
12. Konstam, V., Moser, D. K., & Dejong, M. (2005). Anxiety and depression in patients with heart failure. *J Card Fail, 11*, 455–463.
13. Cowan, M. J., Pike, K. C., & Budzynski, H. K. (2001). Psychosocial nursing therapy following sudden cardiac arrest: impact on two-year survival. *Nurs Res, 50*, 68–76.
14. Lezak, M. (1995). *Neuropsychological Assessment* (3rd ed.). New York: Oxford University Press.
15. Almeida, O. P., & Flicker, L. (2001). The mind of a failing heart: a systematic review of the association between heart failure and cognitive functioning. *Intern Med J*, 290–295.
16. Pullicino, P. M., Wadley, V. G., McClure, L. A., et al. (2008). Factors contributing to global cognitive impairment in heart failure: results from a population-based cohort. *J Card Fail, 14*, 290–295.
17. Narsavage, G. L., & Naylor, M. D. (2000). Factors associated with referral of elderly individuals with cardiac and pulmonary disorders for home care services following hospital discharge. *J Gerontol Nurs, 26*, 14–20.
18. Riegel, B., Bennett, J. A., Davis, A., et al. (2002). Cognitive impairment in heart failure: issues of measurement and etiology. *Am J Crit Care, 11*, 250–528.
19. Feola, M., Rosso, G. L., Peano, M., et al. (2007). Correlation between cognitive impairment and prognostic parameters in patients with congestive heart failure. *Arch Med Res, 38*, 234–239.
20. Trojano, L., Incalzi, R., & Picone, C. (2003). Cognitive impairment: a key feature of congestive heart failure in the elderly. *J Neurol, 250*, 1456–1463.
21. Bennett, S. J., Sauvé, M. J., & Shaw, R. M. (2005). A conceptual model of cognitive deficits in chronic heart failure. *J Nurs Scholars, 37*, 222–228.
22. Naismith, S., Winter, V., Gotspoulos, H., et al. (2004). Neurobehavioral functioning in obstructive sleep apnea: differential effects of sleep quality, hypoxemia and subjective sleepiness. *J Clinc Exp Neuropsychol, 26*, 43–54.
23. Ackerman, R. (2001). Cerebral blood flow and neurological change in chronic heart failure. *Stroke, 32*, 1462–1464.
24. Rains, G. S. (2002). *Principles of human neuropsychology.* Boston: McGraw-Hill.
25. Kolb, B., Gibb, R., & Robinson, T. E. (2003). Brain plasticity and behavior. *Curr Dir Psychol Sci, 12*(1), 1–5.
26. Woo, M. A., Macey, P. M., Fonarow, G. C., et al. (2003). Regional brain gray matter loss in heart failure. *J Appl Physiol, 95*, 677–684.
27. Vogels, R. L. C., Oosterman, J. M., van Harten, B., et al. (2007). Neuroimaging and correlates of cognitive function among patients with heart failure. *Dement Geriatr Cogn Disord, 24*, 418–423.
28. Alves, T. C., Tays, J., & Fráguas, R., Jr. (2005). Localized cerebral blood flow reductions in patients with heart failure: a study using 99mTc-HMPAO SPECT. *J Neuroimaging, 15*, 150–156.
29. Schmidt, R., Fazekas, F., & Koch, M. (1995). Magnetic resonance imaging cerebral abnormalities and neuropsychologic test performance in elderly hypertensive subjects. *Arch Neurol, 52*, 905–910.
30. Sila, C. A. (2007). Cognitive impairment in chronic heart failure. *Cleve Clin J Med, 74*, S132–S137.
31. Zuccalá, G., Marzetti, E., Cesari, M., et al. (2005). Correlates of cognitive impairment among patients with heart failure: results of a multicenter survey. *Am J Med, 118*, 496–502.
32. McLennan, S. N., Pearson, S. A., Cameron, J., et al. (2006). Prognostic importance of cognitive impairment in chronic heart failure patients: does specialist management made a difference. *Eur J Heart Fail, 8*, 494–501.
33. Dries, D. L., Rosenberg, Y. D., Waclawiw, M. A., et al. (1997). Ejection fractions and risk of thromboembolic events in patients with systolic dysfunction and sinus rhythm. *J Am Coll Cardiol, 29*, 1074–1080.
34. Jennings, J. R. (2003). Autoregulation of blood pressure and thought: preliminary results of an application of brain imaging to psychosomatic medicine. *Psychosom Med, 65*, 384–395.
35. Baker, D. W. (2002). Prevention of heart failure. *J Card Fail, 8*, 333–346.
36. Roth, T., & Drake, C. (2004). Evolution of insomnia: current status and future direction. *Sleep Med, 5*(Suppl. 1), S23–S30.
37. Killgore, W. D., Balkin, T. J., & Wessensten, N. J. (2003). Impaired decision making following 49 h of sleep depreviation. *J Sleep Res, 12*, 1–5.
38. Sullivan, M., Simon, G., Spertus, J., et al. (2002). Depression-related costs in heart failure. *Arch Intern Med, 162*, 1860–1866.
39. Murberg, T. A., Bru, E., Svabak, S., et al. (1999). Depressed mood and subjective health symptoms as predictors of mortality in patients with congestive heart failure. *Int J Psychiatry Med, 29*, 311–326.

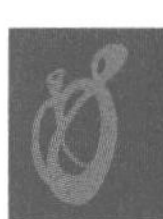

40. Vaccarino, V., Kasl, S. V., Abramson, J., et al. (2001). Depressive symptoms and risk of functional decline and death in patients with heart failure. *J Am Coll Cardiol, 38*, 199–205.
41. Segal, Z. V., Williams, J. M., & Teasdale, J. D. (2002). *Mindfulness-based cognitive therapy for depression: a new approach to preventing relapse.* New York: Guildford.
42. Foreman, M. D., Fletcher, K., Mion, L. C., et al. (1996). Assessing cognitive function. *Geriatr Nurs, 17*, 228–232.
43. Rumsfeld, J. S., Magid, D. J., Plomonodon, M. E., et al. (2003). History of depression, angina, and quality of life after acute coronary syndromes. *Am Hear J, 145*(3), 493–499.
44. Insel, K., Morrow, D., Brewer, B., et al. (2006). Executive function, working memory, and medication adherence among older adults. *J Gerontol, 61B*, P102–P107.
45. Miller, G. A., Galanter, E., & Pribram, K. H. (1960). *Plans and the structure of behavior.* New York: Holt, Rinehart and Winston.
46. Cowan, N., et al. (2008). What are the differences in long term, short term and working memory? In W. S. Sossin, Lacaille, S. C., Castellucci, V. F., (Eds.). *Progress in brain research* (vol. 169, pp. 323–338). Amsterdam: Elsevier.
47. Woodford, H. J., & George, J. (2007). Cognitive assessment in the elderly: a review of clinical methods. *QJM, 100*, 469–484.
48. Cullen, B., O'Neil, B., Evans, J. J., et al. (2007). A review of screening tests for cognitive impairment. *J Neurol Neurosurg Psychiatry, 78*, 790–799.
49. Almeida, O. P., & Tamai, S. (2001). Congestive heart failure and cognitive functioning amongst older adults. *Arq Neurospiquiatr, 59*(2-B), 354-329.
50. Hogan, M. (2005). Physical and cognitive activity and exercise for older adults. *Int J Aging Hum Dev, 60*(7), 95–126.
51. Clark, A. P., & McDougal, G. (2006). Cognitive impairment in heart failure. *Dimens Crit Care Nurs, 25*, 93–100.
52. Gauthier, S., Reisberg, B., Zaudig, M., et al. (2006). Mild cognitive impairment. *Lancet, 367*, 1262–1270.
53. Chodosh, J., Petitti, D. B., Elliott, M., et al. (2004). Physician recognition of cognitive impairment: evaluating the need for improvement. *J Am Geriatr Soc, 52*, 1051–1059.
54. Albanese, M. A., et al. (2004). Review of the Mini-Mental State Examination. In M. F. Folstein, S. E. Folstein, & P. R. McHugh (Eds.). *Fifteen Mental Measurements Yearbook* Lincoln, NE: Buros Institute.
55. Borson, S., Scanlan, J. M., Watanabe, J., et al. (2005). Simplifying the detection of cognitive impairment: comparison of the Mini-Cog and the Mini-Mental State Examination in a multiethnic sample. *J Am Geriatr Soc, 53*, 871–874.
56. MacKenzie, D. M., Copp, P., Shaw, R. H., et al. (1996). Brief cognitive screening of the elderly, a comparison of the Mini-Mental State Examination (MMSE), Abbreviated Mental Test (AMT) and Mental Status Questionnaire (MSQ). *Psychol Med, 26*, 427–430.
57. Nasreddine, Z. S., Phillips, N. A., Bédirian, V., et al. (2005). The Montreal Cognitive Assessment, MoCA: a brief screening toll for mild cognitive impairment. *J Am Geriatr Soc, 53*, 695–699.
58. Lorentz, W. J., Scanlan, J. M., & Borson, S. (2002). Brief screening tests for dementia. *Can J Psychiatry, 47*, 723–732.
59. American Psychiatric Association. (1994). *Diagnostic and statistical manual of mental disorders* (4th ed.). Washington, DC: American Psychiatric Association.
60. World Health Organization. (1997). *International statistical classification of diseases and related health problems.* Geneva, Switzerland: World Health Organization.
61. Brodaty, H., Pond, M., Kemp, N. M., et al. (2002). The GPCOG: a new screening test for dementia designed for general practice. *J Am Geriatr Soc, 50*, 530–534.
62. Taylor, J., & Stott, D. J. (2002). Chronic heart failure and cognitive impairment: coexistence of conditions or true association? *Eur J Heart Fail, 4*, 7–9.
63. Riegel, B., Dickson, V. V., Goldberg, L. R., et al. (2007). Factors associated with the development of expertise in heart failure self-care. *Nurs Res, 56*, 235–243.
64. Kuhl, E., Sears, S. F., & Conti, J. B. (2006). Internet-based behavioral change and psychosocial care for patients with cardiovascular disease: a review of cardiac disease-specific applications. *Heart Lung, 35*, 374–382.
65. Karlsson, M. R., Magnus, E., Henriksson, P., et al. (2005). A nurse-based management program in heart failure patients affects females and persons with cognitive dysfunction most. *Patient Educ Couns, 58*, 146–153.
66. Strömberg, A., Ahlén, H., Fridlund, B., et al. (2002). Interactive education on CD-ROM: a new tool in the education of heart failure patients. *Patient Educ Couns, 46*, 1456–1463.
67. Tanne, D., Freimark, D., Poreh, A., et al. (2005). Cognitive functions in severe congestive heart failure before and after an exercise training program. *Int J Cardiol, 103*(3), 145–149.
68. Pullen, P. R., Nagamia, S. H., Mehta, P. K., et al. (2008). Effects of yoga on inflammation and exercise capacity in patients with chronic heart failure. *J Card Fail, 14*, 290–295.
69. Verhaeghen, P., Marcoen, A., & Goosens, L. (1992). Improving memory performance in the aged through mnemonic training: a meta-analytic study. *Psychol Aging, 7*(2), 242–251.

CHAPTER 61

Management of End-Stage Heart Failure

Patricia A. Uber and Mandeep R. Mehra

Despite optimal medical therapy targeted against neurohormonal aberrations responsible for cardiac remodeling, heart failure can transition into a chronic and progressive stage that leads to severe functional limitation. The left ventricle once again dilates, which leads to worsening backward flow as a result of mitral regurgitation, and causes a further increase in ventricular wall stress; these events set up a vicious cycle of additional depression of cardiac function and worsening right-sided heart failure. These central cardiac alterations, in turn, cause numerous end-organ defects that are manifested in pulmonary hypertension, renal dysfunction, hepatobiliary defects, and, eventually, neurocognitive decline. This is the genesis of the advanced syndrome of late-stage heart failure.

DEFINING LATE-STAGE HEART FAILURE

Late-stage, or advanced, heart failure is associated with a miserable quality of life and ongoing high risk for clinical events. Affected individuals exhibit unrelenting, severe symptoms of fatigue and dyspnea on minimal activity, coupled with end-organ hypoperfusion. Many such patients experience repeated episodes of heart failure decompensation, followed by a brief period of symptom improvement, and eventually they die of heart failure–related causes. The American College of Cardiology/American Heart Association heart failure practice guidelines[1] detailed a staging system (A through D) to describe the progression of heart failure. Stage D of that classification describes the condition of significant symptoms at rest despite best medical therapy. Most affected patients have endured repeated hospitalizations, and their condition is refractory to current therapeutic interventions involving elaborate treatment strategies such as mechanical circulatory support, fluid removal by sophisticated means, continuous positive inotropic infusions, cardiac transplantation or other nontraditional surgical procedures, or supportive care.

The European Society of Cardiology provided a more comprehensive clinical definition of late-stage heart failure.[2] Patients with advanced heart failure are again described as having severe symptoms (New York Heart Association [NYHA] classes III to IV) along with clinical signs of fluid retention, with or without evidence of peripheral hypoperfusion, plus a history of more than one heart failure–related hospitalization in the previous 6 months. To fit this definition, however, patients must have echocardiographic evidence of cardiac dysfunction, demonstrated by left ventricular ejection fraction lower than 30% or pseudonormal or restrictive mitral inflow pattern on Doppler echocardiography. Elevated left-sided ventricular filling pressures, alone or in concert with excessive right-sided pressures, and increased levels of B-type natriuretic peptide also characterize these patients. Exercise testing is performed at the authors' institution, and severely impaired functional capacity is defined as a 6-minute walk test distance of less than 300 m or a peak oxygen uptake of less than 12 to 14 mL/kg/min. All these features must exist despite optimal therapy in order to meet the criteria for advanced heart failure.

THE ROLE OF CHRONIC PARENTERAL THERAPY

Patients with late-stage heart failure who have evidence of end-organ perfusion are characterized by a chronic reduction in cardiac contractility with concomitant lusitropic dysfunction. Cardiac dysfunction and systemic perfusion pressure can be evaluated clinically simply by observing blood pressure. Specifically, in patients with acute decompensated heart failure, a low systolic blood pressure at admission coupled with abnormal levels of renal biomarkers has been shown to be a powerful predictor of a reduced cardiac output and adverse outcomes.[3] Clinicians can reliably predict diminished cardiac output by calculating the proportional pulse pressure—(systolic blood pressure − diastolic blood pressure)/systolic blood pressure—which, if detected to be less than 25%, is correlated strongly with cardiac index lower than 2.2 L/minute/m^2.[4] Other clinical signs that signify poor perfusion include coolness of extremities, the presence of pulsus alternans, easy fatigability, altered mentation, and worsening renal dysfunction with attempted ongoing incremental diuresis.

In such advanced cases of late-stage heart failure, the goal of therapy is to restore end-organ perfusion and relieve symptoms without incurring adverse cardiac effects. Because this unique condition is typically refractory to oral pharmacological support, a series of incremental therapeutic interventions are usually employed. Immediately available are parenteral supportive agents such as inotropic, vasodilator, and diuretic drug infusions. The goal of therapy may differ according to the patient's circumstance at that time. For example, if there is a reversible cause for hypoperfusion, parenteral supportive therapy may be used as a bridge to recovery. However, in patients with late-stage heart failure, these agents are more often used as a bridge to advanced options such as heart transplantation, placement of a ventricular assist device, or other nontraditional surgical procedures. Inotropic drugs have also been prescribed as part of the supportive care plan for patients for whom other advanced options are not suitable.

The decision to initiate chronic parenteral inotropic support is not an easy one. The need to establish hemodynamic stability in the patient must be weighed against the fact that use of oral or short-term intravenous inotropic drug therapy in well structured clinical trials has not demonstrated improved outcomes in heart failure.[5] Thus, the trial evidence in support of chronic parenteral inotropic therapy simply does not exist, and the clinician is left to draw meaningful conclusions from the numerous of usually small, mostly anecdotal and observational experiences reported in the literature.[6] This chapter details the arguments for and against this clinical strategy, and the potential applications and pitfalls of parenteral inotropic and vasodilator therapy in late-stage heart failure are discussed.

CELLULAR REASONS FOR AND AGAINST CHRONIC PARENTERAL INOTROPIC THERAPY

Arguments in Support

Lowes and associates[7] noted gene expression of myosin heavy-chain isoforms, with selective downregulation of the proportion of α-myosin heavy-chain isoforms by 67% to 84%, in failing hearts. In a heterotopic rat transplantation model, Geenen and colleagues[8] demonstrated the exact reverse: an elevation of α-myosin heavy-chain levels by 70%, which suggests that the myocyte type may switch to a high-velocity, fast-twitch subtype as a result of catecholamine stimulation. In earlier studies, Bristow and coworkers[9] revealed depressed contractile response to β-agonists in the failing heart, accompanied by a decrease in expression and function of cardiac β-receptors. Adamopoulos and associates[10] demonstrated that short-term pulsed inotropic support with dobutamine induces β-adrenergic receptor upregulation and that this action leads to enhanced chronotropic responsiveness to exercise in patients with chronic heart failure. In an evaluation of the ultrastructural effects of inotropic infusions, Unverferth and colleagues[11] were able to show that mitochondria structure and biochemical energetic properties improved more with dobutamine than with bed rest and saline infusion in chronic severe heart failure. Results of another investigation[12] have suggested that peripheral endothelial function might be improved by the administration of pulsed inotropic therapy for 72 hours and that these subclinical effects can be observed for up to 2 weeks after discontinuation of therapy; these findings might explain the sustained effects of inotropic therapy. These data form the scientific support for the investigation of inotropic infusion strategies as a component of comprehensive care of the patient with late-stage heart failure.

Arguments Against

Chronic exposure to inotropic therapy has led to the generation of cardiac arrhythmias, desensitization of the β-adrenergic receptor complex in the heart, and worsening of cardiac function over time by creating a state of cellular energy starvation. The generation of cyclic adenosine monophosphate (cAMP), which is essential for the hemodynamic effectiveness of inotropic therapy, is hypothesized to enhance arrythmogenicity and result in direct cardiotoxic effects.[13] The appearance of delayed afterdepolarizations is related to the increased release of calcium from intracellular stores. Increased intracellular cAMP also might enhance automaticity and triggered responses.[14] Moreover, downregulation of β-adrenergic receptors and desensitization of the β-adrenergic pathway, coupled with the energy-exacting effects of inotropic intervention, are believed to perpetuate an inexorable cycle of decline in an energy-starved situation.[15]

Alterations in mechanoenergetics in severe ventricular dysfunction result from increased oxygen cost of excitation-contraction coupling, rather than from reduction in the efficiency of chemomechanical energy transduction.[16] Other data from studies of inodilator therapy suggest a somewhat heterogeneous response with reference to myocardial oxygen consumption, which may decrease, increase, or remain unchanged.[17] This response is a manifestation of the relative magnitude of energy expenditure. Thus, long-term exposure to inotropic drugs may exhaust energy reserve and worsen the state of energy starvation, as assessed by a disproportionate increase in myofibrillar size in comparison with energy-regenerating mitochondria.[18]

CLINICAL EVIDENCE FOR AND AGAINST CHRONIC PARENTERAL INOTROPIC THERAPY

In appropriately selected patients, parenteral inotropic support in the outpatient or home setting might alleviate this daunting combination of profoundly diminished functional capacity, cyclical visits to the hospital, and enormous accompanying cost burden. The proposed strategies have ranged from pulsed inotropic or vasodilator therapy, administered in an intermittent manner at infusion centers, to chronic continuous infusions in the home setting.

Arguments in Support

A number of observational studies have addressed the issue of morbidity reduction with parenteral inotropic support (Table 61-1). In the earliest (but uncontrolled) investigation, Leier and coworkers[19] treated 25 patients with severe heart failure with 10 to 15 μg/kg per minute of intravenous dobutamine for 72 hours. Cardiac function improved significantly and remained better even after dobutamine had been cleared from the circulation, and 68% of these patients maintained their improvement in functional NYHA class for at least 1 week after cessation of therapy. Liang and associates[20] further explored these findings in a randomized, blinded, placebo-controlled trial of 72-hour infusions of dobutamine in 15 patients with stable dilated cardiomyopathy. The initial dobutamine dosage of 5 μg/kg per minute was increased at 20-minute intervals to achieve a doubling in cardiac output. At the 4-week follow-up visit, functional NYHA class, treadmill exercise time, and left ventricular performance were improved significantly in the patients treated with dobutamine, but those parameters remained unchanged in the patients treated with placebo.

Leier and coworkers[21] went on to investigate the role of shorter and more frequent intravenous infusions of dobutamine in improving clinical status and objective measurements of cardiovascular performance in patients with heart failure. In their study of 26 patients with moderately severe heart failure, 11 patients were randomly assigned to control conditions, and 15 other patients received weekly dobutamine infusions for 4 to 5 hours per week for 24 weeks. Functional class improved in 12 of the 15 dobutamine-treated patients but in only 2 of the 11 control patients. Not only were enhancements noted in the clinical status of the dobutamine recipients but also exercise performance improved.

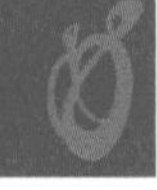

TABLE 61–1 Parenteral Inotropic Therapy Trials in Late-Stage Heart Failure*: Evidence of Benefit

Investigators	N	Study Design	Therapy	Follow-up Duration	Key Findings
Leier et al[19]	25	Observational	Dobutamine, 10-15 μg/kg/min for 72 hr (in hospital)	Undefined	Improved symptoms in all patients 17/25 patients with persistent symptomatic improvement at 1 week
Liang et al[20]	15	Randomized, placebo controlled	Dobutamine (n = 8) vs. D_5W (n = 7) infusions for 72 hr (in hospital)	4 weeks	Functional class improved in 6/8 patients receiving dobutamine and 2/7 control patients Dobutamine group: maximal exercise time and LVEF increased significantly above baseline Dobutamine group: improvement in resting hemodynamics, exercise tolerance, and symptoms for several weeks
Leier et al[21]	26	Randomized, controlled, single-blinded	Dobutamine administered for 4 hr weekly for 24 weeks (outpatient clinic)	24 weeks	Functional class improved in 12/15 patients receiving dobutamine and 2/11 controls Twice as much improvement in exercise tolerance in dobutamine recipients Investigators suggested evidence of "conditioning" with dobutamine
Marius-Nunez et al[22]	36	Observational	Milrinone (n = 32) and dobutamine (n = 4) weekly infusions (outpatient)	42 weeks	Reduction in hospital admissions, ED visits, and days spent in the hospital for heart failure–related care
Mehra et al[23]	30	Randomized, active controls	Milrinone (n = 16) versus dobutamine (n = 14) 1-2 infusions per week (outpatient clinic)	26 weeks	Decrease in medical resource use and improved functional capacity Significant major cardiac event rates noted (23% death or emergency transplantation) No difference between milrinone and dobutamine
Cesario et al[24]	10	Observational	Intermittent home infusions of milrinone (3 days/week, 6 hr each)	12 weeks	No deaths Functional improvement and trend toward hemodynamic improvement Decrease in hospitalizations from baseline
Oliva et al[26]	38	Randomized, open-label controls	Intermittent home dobutamine	26 weeks	No functional improvement with dobutamine Decrease in hospitalizations and no increase in deaths with dobutamine
Harjai et al[27]	24	Observational, retrospective	Continuous home therapy: dobutamine (n = 17) and milrinone (n = 4) and combination of dobutamine and milrinone (n = 3)	12 weeks	Decreases in hospitalization rates, length of stay, and cost of care High rate of mortality at 3 months (38%)
Mavrogeni et al[30]	50	Randomized, open-label controls	Intermittent 24-hour infusion of levosimendan monthly	24 weeks	Symptom improvement in 65% of patients taking levosimendan vs. 20% of controls (P < .01) Significant increase in LVEF in levosimendan pts and a reduction in MR Higher rate of mortality in control group than in patients taking levosimendan (32% vs. 8%)
Parissis et al[31]	63	Randomized, placebo controlled	24-hr infusion of levosimendan or placebo in hospitalized patients	Baseline to discharge	Levosimendan-treated patients had improvement in NYHA class, 6-minute walk distance, and BNP levels and shorter in-hospital stays Quality-of-life scores improved with levosimendan therapy, remained unchanged with placebo

*Late-stage heart failure in all these trials was typically defined as systolic failure (LVEF < 0.30) and chronic long-standing symptoms (NYHA classes III to IV) despite ongoing background therapy defined at the time of study inception.

BNP, B-type natriuretic peptide; D_5W, 5% dextrose in water; ED, emergency department; LVEF, left ventricular ejection fraction; MR, mitral regurgitation; NYHA, New York Heart Association.

Marius-Nunez and colleagues[22] assessed the use of medical resources by calculating the number of emergency department visits and hospitalizations of patients who received weekly infusions of either milrinone (32 patients) or dobutamine (4 patients) and compared the occurrence of these events in the period before pulsed outpatient inotropic infusions with their occurrence during treatment. With pulsed inotropic treatment, the number of hospital admissions, emergency department visits, and days spent in the hospital for heart failure care were reduced. Although a formal cost analysis was not performed, the decrease in hospital admissions was suggestive of the potential cost effectiveness of such a program.

Mehra and coworkers[23] sought to use pulsed inotropic therapy in patients in whom evidence-based pharmacological therapy and all efforts to improve the clinical state by means of a multidisciplinary effort had failed. This prospective randomized investigation of intermittent inotropic therapy with dobutamine or milrinone in 30 patients (12% of the population enrolled in the multidisciplinary team therapy approach) demonstrated decreases in the use of medical resources and improvements in functional capacity. The rate of adverse events (death or emergency transplantation) at 6 months was significant (23%). Cesario and associates[24] sought to determine the effects of low-dosage, intermittent home infusions of milrinone in 10 patients with late-stage heart failure. After the patients exhibited hemodynamic improvement with milrinone while hospitalized, central lines were placed, and patients were given the drug at home with small portable infusion pumps, starting at 3 days a week for 6 hours at a time over a 3-month period. Patients tolerated the drug well, with no deaths and a 22% decrease in the number of hospitalizations during the study. Occurrences of arrhythmias were minimal, and the severity of angina decreased in two patients. Mean total, physical, and emotional scores on the Minnesota Living with Heart Failure Questionnaire[25] reflected a general trend of symptomatic improvement throughout the infusion period.

In the Dobutamine Infusion in Severe Heart Failure (DICE) trial,[26] 38 patients with advanced heart failure were randomly assigned to receive intermittent dobutamine infusion (48 to 72 hours per week; maximum dosage, 5 μg/kg/min) or to receive traditional therapy. During a 6-month follow-up period, the number of hospital admissions was decreased, but functional class was not significantly improved, among the dobutamine-treated patients. Rates of survival did not differ between the two groups.

Harjai and coworkers[27] studied 24 patients with late-stage heart failure and observed a marked reduction in the number of hospital admissions and lengths of stay after initiation of chronic parenteral inotropic support. The cost of overall care was decreased by 16%. However, 38% of the patients died within 3 months of initiating therapy, which again suggests that the decrease in medical resource use parameters is accompanied by short-term lethality. Several other such observational studies have been reviewed elsewhere.[28]

The calcium sensitizer levosimendan, which has a long half-life, has been touted as an ideal candidate for use of chronic support of the failing heart. Nieminen and associates[29] investigated levosimendan, at a dosage of 1 mg once or twice daily, in a placebo-controlled, double-blind, randomized trial of 307 patients with advanced heart failure. A unique "patient journey" primary endpoint was a composite of repeated symptom evaluations, worsening heart failure, and mortality during 60 days. The "patient journey" scores did not differ between levosimendan and placebo. However, in comparison with placebo, a net improvement in quality-of-life scores and persistent reduction in N-terminal pro–B-type natriuretic peptide (NT-proBNP) by 30% to 40% were observed with levosimendan. Mavrogeni and colleagues[30] administered levosimendan on a monthly intermittent 24-hour protocol for 6 months and compared outcomes by randomly assigning 50 patients to receive either active therapy or standard care in an open-label design. At 6 months, the patients receiving intermittent levosimendan treatment exhibited improvement in symptoms and echocardiographic systolic function without excess arrhythmia or mortality. Parissis and coworkers[31] studied the effects of levosimendan on quality of life, emotional stress, and symptoms in patients with advanced heart failure. In a 2:1 randomized study of 63 patients who received a 24-hour drug infusion or placebo, those investigators observed that levosimendan seems to have a beneficial effect on quality of life, physical activity, and emotional stress in these patients, and hospitalization length was concurrently reduced.

Ikonomidis and associates[32] suggested that at least some of the observed benefit of levosimendan may accrue from improvement in coronary flow and microcirculation, in parallel with an improvement in cardiac performance and neurohormonal activation. In another 2:1 randomized study, Parissis and coworkers[33] assigned 39 patients with advanced heart failure to receive either a 24-hour infusion of levosimendan, 0.1 μg/kg/min (n = 26) or placebo (n = 13). In this study, levosimendan was not found to increase markers of oxidative and nitrosative stress in comparison with the placebo treatment. These small-scale findings provide an interesting rationale for the further study of levosimendan.

Arguments Against

Dies[34] conducted a multicenter, randomized, double-blind, placebo-controlled trial with 60 ambulatory patients with severe heart failure who were receiving optimal standard therapy. The patients were given either dobutamine or placebo for 48 hours on a weekly basis; the mean dosage of dobutamine achieved was 8.1 μg/kg per minute. This study was terminated prematurely when an apparent increased risk for death was found among patients with evidence of baseline ventricular tachycardia who were administered high dosages of dobutamine. In this study, relatively high dosages of dobutamine were used with little regard to electrolyte maintenance.

Elis and colleagues[35] evaluated 19 patients with moderately severe systolic heart failure in a double-blind, placebo-controlled study. They found no significant effect of intermittent dobutamine therapy on hospitalizations or on survival at 6 months. These disparate findings might reflect a less effective pulse schedule (every 2 to 3 weeks) or selection of patients with ischemic heart failure alone. Although no statistically significant differences in survival were noted, there was a clear trend toward shortened survival among the dobutamine-treated patients (median length of survival, 4.6 months versus 7.97 months with placebo) in this investigation.

Even trials in which patients were exposed to short-term in-hospital inotropic therapy have yielded negative outcomes (Table 61-2), which have discouraged further longer term use. For example, in the Outcomes of a Prospective Trial of Intravenous Milrinone for Exacerbations of Chronic Heart Failure (OPTIME-CHF) study,[36] patients were randomly assigned to receive a 48-hour infusion of either milrinone or placebo; the primary endpoint was cumulative days of hospitalization for cardiovascular cause within 60 days following randomization. This study demonstrated no significant difference between the two groups of patients with regard to either the primary or secondary endpoints. However, among the patients receiving milrinone, the incidences of atrial fibrillation or flutter and hypotension were significantly higher. In this study, the agent was used in patients without advanced heart failure in the absence of end-organ hypoperfusion.

Although small-scale trials with levosimendan have yielded favorable outcomes in advanced heart failure, this enthusiasm has been tempered by the findings of the Survival of Patients with Acute Heart Failure in Need of Intravenous Inotropic Support (SURVIVE) trial, in which levosimendan was compared with dobutamine in patients with acute decompensated heart failure.[37] This randomized, double-blind trial enrolled 1327 patients hospitalized with acute decompensated heart failure who required inotropic support. Despite an initial reduction in plasma levels of B-type natriuretic peptide in patients who received levosimendan, in comparison with patients who received dobutamine, levosimendan did not significantly reduce rates of all-cause mortality at 180 days or affect any secondary clinical outcomes.

Disturbing findings also have emerged from the Flolan International Randomized Survival Trial (FIRST). O'Connor and associates[38] examined the outcomes of 471 patients with severe heart failure, of whom 80 were treated with dobutamine and 391 were not. These investigators found that dobutamine use at the time of randomization was associated with more frequent worsening heart failure, greater need for mechanical assist device, more resuscitations after cardiac arrest, more

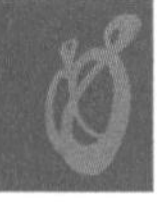

TABLE 61–2 Parenteral Inotropic Therapy Trials in Late-Stage Heart Failure*: Evidence of Adverse Outcomes

Investigators	N	Study Design	Therapy	Follow-up Duration	Key Findings
Dies[34]	60	Multicenter, randomized, double-blind, placebo controlled	Dobutamine or placebo infusions for 48 hr weekly (outpatient)	Terminated early	Increased rate of mortality with dobutamine
Elis et al[35]	19	Randomized, double-blind, placebo controlled	Dobutamine ($n = 10$) or placebo ($n = 9$) for 24 hr every 2 to 3 weeks	6 months	No difference in number of admissions for heart failure Shortened survival with dobutamine (median 4.6 months vs. 7.97 months with placebo)
Cuffe et al[36]	951	Multicenter, randomized, double-blind, placebo controlled	Intravenous milrinone vs. placebo for 48 hr in hospitalized patients with acute decompensated heart failure	2 months	No difference between groups in mortality or the composite endpoint of incidence of death and readmission Higher incidences of hypotension necessitating treatment and new-onset atrial arrhythmias in the milrinone recipients
Mebazaa et al[37]	1327	Multicenter, prospective, randomized, double-blind, controlled trial	Intravenous levosimendan vs. dobutamine for 24 hr in hospitalized patients with acute decompensated heart failure	6 months	Greater reduction in BNP levels at 24 hours that remained lower at 5 days No difference in mortality or morbidity (including functional assessment)
O'Connor et al[38]	471	Multicenter, randomized, controlled	Continuous intravenous epoprostenol plus conventional therapy: dobutamine ($n = 80$; median dosage, 9 μg/kg/min) vs. no dobutamine ($n = 371$) at the time of randomization	6 months	Higher incidences of worsening heart failure, need for intravenous vasoactive medications, need for mechanical assist device, resuscitation after cardiac arrest, myocardial infarction, and death among dobutamine-treated patients Higher incidence of mortality persisted after adjustment for baseline differences

*Late-stage heart failure in all these trials is typically defined as systolic failure (left ventricular ejection fraction < 0.30) and chronic long-standing symptoms (New York Heart Association classes III to IV) despite ongoing background therapy defined at the time of study inception.
BNP, B-type natriuretic peptide.

myocardial infarction, and higher rates of total mortality. These differences persisted even after adjustment for baseline differences.

To continue research on chronic inotropic therapy, investigators have suggested that a reduced dosage of inotropic agent, coupled with β-blocker therapy, would yield a beneficial response. The Studies of Oral Enoximone Therapy in Advanced Heart Failure (ESSENTIAL)[39] consisted of two identical, randomized, double-blind, placebo-controlled trials performed in North and South America (ESSENTIAL-I) and Europe (ESSENTIAL-II). Patients with NYHA classes III to IV heart failure symptoms, left ventricular ejection fraction of 30% or lower, and one hospitalization or two ambulatory visits for worsening heart failure in the previous year were eligible for participation in the trials. The trials had three coprimary endpoints: (1) the composite of time to all-cause mortality and cardiovascular hospitalization, analyzed in both ESSENTIAL trials; (2) the 6-month change from baseline distance in the 6-minute walk test; and (3) change in patient Global Assessment levels. In ESSENTIAL-I and ESSENTIAL-II, 1854 subjects at 211 sites in 16 countries were studied. In both trials, rates of all-cause mortality and the first coprimary (composite) endpoint did not differ between the two treatment groups. The two other coprimary endpoints were analyzed separately in the two ESSENTIAL trials, as prospectively designed in the protocol. The distance in the 6-minute walk test increased with enoximone, in comparison with placebo, in ESSENTIAL-I ($P = .025$); however, this increase did not reach the prespecified criterion for statistical significance ($P < .020$). This distance did not increase in ESSENTIAL-II. No difference in Patient Global Assessment levels was observed in either trial. Thus, although safety was demonstrated, no signals of efficacy were forthcoming.

In summary, the use of chronic inotropic therapy, either continuous or pulsed, appears to decrease short-term morbidity parameters but is associated with increased mortality.

CHRONIC PARENTERAL VASODILATOR THERAPY

Because of the disappointing evidence for inotropic therapy, some authorities have advocated the use of vasodilator therapy (Table 61-3). A chronic low-output state with systemic hypotension typically precludes such consideration; for this therapeutic consideration, however, patients with advanced heart failure who have secondary pulmonary hypertension or those with preserved blood pressure but excessive symptoms and frequent deterioration could be candidates. Furthermore, some authorities have argued that the deleterious proarrhythmic effects or tax on myocardial oxygen consumption that is the hallmark of inotropic therapy can probably be avoided by this drug class. This hypothetical consideration has been tested in several studies.

Sueta and associates[40] studied the safety and efficacy of continuous intravenous epoprostenol (prostacyclin), a potent pulmonary and systemic vasodilator. Their subjects were 33 patients with severe heart failure despite prior treatment with diuretics (100%), digitalis (91%), angiotensin-converting enzyme inhibitors (85%), and dobutamine (30%); the subjects underwent a baseline 6-minute walk test before the dosage of epoprostenol was titrated during invasive hemodynamic monitoring. Subjects responding during the dosage titration were randomly assigned, on an open basis, to receive either conventional therapy plus continuous epoprostenol infusion via an indwelling central venous catheter or conventional therapy alone for 12 weeks. The initial dosage-ranging study with epoprostenol produced a significant decline in systemic

TABLE 61–3 Chronic Parenteral Vasodilator Therapy Trials in Late-Stage Heart Failure*

Investigators	N	Study Design	Therapy	Follow-up Duration	Key Findings
Sueta et al[40]	33	Randomized, open-label (in hemodynamic responders)	Continuous epoprostenol infusion plus conventional therapy or conventional therapy alone	12 weeks	Epoprostenol therapy resulted in a decrease in pulmonary capillary wedge pressure and an increase in cardiac index Epoprostenol therapy was associated with an improvement in 6-minute walk distance
Califf et al[41]	471	Multicenter, randomized, open-label	Continuous epoprostenol infusion or standard care	Terminated early	Epoprostenol therapy resulted in a decrease in pulmonary capillary wedge pressure and an increase in cardiac index Epoprostenol did not improve 6-minute walk distance, quality of life, or morbidity, and it increased risk of death
Serra et al[42]	22	Observational, case-control	PGE_1 infusion (mean dosage, 10 ng/kg/min) for 24 hr over 3 consecutive days every 3 months (n = 22) vs. case controls (no PGE_1) (n = 23)	3 years	PGE_1 infusions improved NYHA class, LVEF, and pulmonary artery pressures No difference in mortality rates
Yancy et al[43]	210	Multicenter, randomized	Weekly infusions of nesiritide plus usual care vs. usual care alone in outpatients	12 weeks	Nesiritide decreased aldosterone and endothelin-1 concentrations No difference among groups by outcome or adverse events Improved quality of life in both groups Nesiritide infusions resulted in a significant decrease in cardiovascular events in patients at higher risk (those with renal insufficiency)
Yancy et al[44]	911	Multicenter, randomized, placebo controlled	Nesiritide or placebo infusion for 4-6 hr, once or twice weekly in outpatients	12 weeks	No significant differences between groups in the number of hospitalizations for cardiovascular or renal causes, the number of days alive and out of the hospital, change in quality-of-life score, or rates of death from cardiovascular causes Nesiritide infusions were associated with more hypotension

*Late-stage heart failure in all these trials is typically defined as systolic failure (LVEF < 0.30) and chronic long-standing symptoms (NYHA classes III to IV) despite ongoing background therapy defined at the time of study inception.

LVEF, left ventricular ejection fraction; NYHA, New York Heart Association; PGE_1, prostaglandin E_1.

and pulmonary vascular resistance and a substantial increase in cardiac index, despite a fall in pulmonary capillary wedge pressure. The change in distance during the 6-minute walk test from baseline to the last available test was significantly greater for patients who received epoprostenol than for patients assigned to standard therapy.

These initial benefits were not confirmed in FIRST, which was a larger and more robust study. Califf and coworkers[41] randomly assigned 471 patients to receive either epoprostenol infusion or standard care. The primary endpoint was survival; secondary endpoints were clinical events, congestive heart failure symptoms, distance walked in 6 minutes, and scores on quality-of-life measures. The median dosage of epoprostenol was 4.0 ng/kg/min; the results were a significant increase in cardiac index (from 1.81 to 2.61 L/min/m^2), a decrease in pulmonary capillary wedge pressure (from 24.5 to 20.0 mm Hg), and a decrease in systemic vascular resistance (from 20.76 to 12.33 dynes/sec/cm^{-5}). No improvement in distance walked or quality of life was noted, but the therapy was associated with an increased risk of death.

Serra and associates[42] performed an uncontrolled study of prostaglandin E_1 (PGE_1) infusion in severe heart failure. These investigators studied 22 patients with advanced heart failure and pulmonary hypertension by treating them with PGE_1 and compared their 3-year outcomes to those of a control group in a case-control format. PGE_1 was infused at a mean dosage of 10 ng/kg/min for a total of 24 hours over 3 consecutive days every 3 months. The preliminary data suggested that intermittent PGE_1 infusion in patients with advanced congestive heart failure and high pulmonary pressure is able to improve mean NYHA class and ventricular contractility, pulmonary pressure, and clinical profiles. These data, however, are too preliminary to draw meaningful conclusions.

In June 2004, a group of investigators who helped establish the natriuretic peptide treatment paradigm met to discuss the potential role of nesiritide as an outpatient treatment option for patients with symptomatic advanced heart failure. The Follow-Up Serial Infusions of Nesiritide pilot study (FUSION I) was then designed to assess the safety and tolerability of outpatient serial infusions of nesiritide in 210 patients with decompensated heart failure who were randomly assigned to receive either usual care only or usual care plus weekly infusions of nesiritide at dosages of 0.005 or 0.01 μg/kg/min for 12 weeks. A total of 1645 nesiritide infusions were administered; 11 (<1%) were discontinued because of an adverse event. Administration of nesiritide resulted in acute decreases in aldosterone and endothelin-1 concentrations. Although there were no statistically significant differences among groups by outcome, patients with prospectively defined higher risk (those with renal insufficiency) demonstrated significant decreases in cardiovascular events.[43]

Yancy and colleagues[44] then performed a definitive trial to further test nesiritide. The FUSION II trial included 911 patients with symptoms of advanced heart failure, two recent hospitalizations for heart failure, an ejection fraction of less than 40%, and creatinine clearance of less than 60 mL/min. The subjects were randomly assigned to receive nesiritide (2-μg/kg bolus plus an infusion of 0.01 μg/kg/min for 4 to 6 hours) or matching placebo, once or twice weekly for 12 weeks. There were no differences between groups in any of the secondary endpoints, including the number of hospitalizations for cardiovascular or renal reasons, the number of days alive and out of the hospital, change in Kansas City

Cardiomyopathy Questionnaire score, or death from cardiovascular causes. Adverse events were similar between groups; nesiritide was associated with more hypotension but less predefined worsening renal function.

The Transplant-Eligible Management of Congestive Heart Failure (TMAC) trial, a multicenter, placebo-controlled, randomized clinical outcomes trial with nesiritide, was initiated in 2006 but stopped by the sponsor after enrollment of the first 15 patients due to lack of funding.[45] In summary, the vasodilator hypothesis for chronic parenteral therapy remains unproven and unsupported.

PHARMACOLOGICAL BRIDGING TO CARDIAC TRANSPLANTATION

One area in which the use of chronic parenteral inotropic therapy is commonly accepted is the setting of cardiac transplantation (see Chapter 54). The scarcity of donor organs has led to prolonged waiting times for transplantation. Nearly 20% of patients awaiting transplantation die without receiving an organ, and prolonged pharmacological support is needed to prevent the inexorable cycle of multiple organ failure.[46,47] In most transplantation centers, prolonged inotropic support is usually guided by hemodynamic goals in the hope of preventing progression to end-organ failure and pulmonary hypertension. The decision to use either dobutamine or milrinone is often ascertained according to the practitioner's comfort and exploitation of the drugs' disparate properties. Milrinone bypasses the β-adrenergic receptor complex, possesses potent vasodilator and lusitropic properties, and is assumed to be less exacting on heart rate and oxygen consumption than is dobutamine.[48] Dobutamine also has been associated with tolerance and an unique syndrome of hypereosinophilia associated with decline in cardiac function.[49] In an investigation to define the underlying mechanisms of this association, Uber and associates[50] were able to demonstrate elevated levels of tumor necrosis factor α with the genesis of dobutamine-related eosinophilia.

In an earlier prospective trial, Mehra and coworkers[51] observed the outcomes of 99 patients with heart failure who were awaiting transplantation and initially were stabilized with either milrinone or dobutamine but later required adjunctive treatment with the other agent or proceeded to mechanical interventions. Similar rates of bridging to transplantation were noted, but the patients initially treated with milrinone required significantly lesser need for intra-aortic counterpulsation than did those initially treated with dobutamine. Higginbotham and coworkers[52] made similar observations in more than 100 patients who required inotropic therapy as a prelude to transplantation. In this study, milrinone caused a greater reduction in filling pressures than did dobutamine, and more milrinone-treated patients were bridged successfully to transplantation without needing mechanical support. Therefore, these two studies lend credence to the concept of hemodynamic-guided stabilization and point to a possible advantage of milrinone in achieving long-term success of bridging to transplantation.

Zemljic and colleagues[53] prospectively evaluated effects of levosimendan on renal function in patients with advanced chronic heart failure who were awaiting cardiac transplantation. Twenty patients were randomly assigned to receive levosimendan (10-minute bolus of 12 μg/kg, followed by 0.1 μg/kg/min for 24 hours), and 20 received no levosimendan (controls). At 3 months, Zemljic and colleagues found a decrease in serum creatinine level and an increase in creatinine clearance in the patients taking levosimendan but not in controls. An improvement in creatinine of 0.5 mg/dL or higher occurred in 50% of patients taking levosimendan, in comparison with 10% of controls ($P = .005$).

In summary, the use of chronic parenteral inotropic therapy is well supported with clinical indications that such therapy effectively allows bridging to transplantation while maintaining end-organ perfusion. However, the optimal duration has yet to be determined.

STRATEGIES TO WEAN FROM CHRONIC PARENTERAL INOTROPIC THERAPY

Investigators have attempted transition from parenteral inotropic therapy to oral inotropic therapy. Feldman and associates[54] performed a placebo-controlled study with 201 patients who had severe late-stage heart failure and required parenteral inotropic therapy. The patients were randomly assigned to receive enoximone or placebo. Patients receiving intermittent parenteral inotropic therapy were administered enoximone, 25 or 50 mg, three times a day. Those receiving continuous parenteral inotropic therapy were administered enoximone, 50 or 75 mg, three times a day for 1 week, which was reduced to 25 or 50 mg three times a day. The ability of subjects to remain alive and free of inotropic therapy was assessed for 6 months. The investigators then attempted to wean patients off parenteral inotropic therapy. At 60 days, 30% of the placebo recipients and 46.5% of the enoximone recipients were weaned (unadjusted $P = .016$). These results suggested that a modest number of patients dependent on inotropic therapy can be successfully converted to an oral strategy without incurring safety concerns.

PALLIATIVE CARE AND CHRONIC PARENTERAL THERAPY

It would be a disservice to patients with late-stage heart failure if the dying process were simply prolonged. The Study to Understand Prognoses and Preferences for Outcomes and Risks of Treatment (SUPPORT),[55] in patients seriously ill for whom death was predicted in the near term, demonstrated several shortcomings of care. Necessary decisions and discussions about end-of-life aspects were either left unaddressed or tackled late in the course. For example, half of all "do not resuscitate" orders were recorded within 2 days of death. More alarming was the account from families that more than half of all patients who were able to express their emotions reported that they spent the last days of their lives in significant pain. Thus, the portrayal of a dying patient with late-stage heart failure is a troubling one, and the issue of appropriate palliation cannot be ignored.

In such a situation, it is possible to argue for the judicious application of parenteral inotropic support as a palliative measure that serves to reduce morbidity in patients with late-stage heart failure, because this strategy may, in fact, be a worthwhile adjunct, even if survival is shortened. Whether patients prefer to trade duration of life for enhanced quality is an open question but important for the creation of clinical strategies. Stanek and coworkers[56] prospectively performed a full-profile conjoint analysis of individual preferences for outcomes of heart failure treatment. They determined that symptom improvement was of greater importance than survival alone. This conclusion was challenged by Stevenson and associates,[57] who suggested that the severity of a patient's symptoms and condition at the time of questioning may play a role in the outcome of their preferences to trade length of life for quality. The usefulness of time trade-off, symptom scores, and 6-minute walk distance was measured by Stevenson and colleagues in a substudy of 287 patients in the Evaluation Study of Congestive Heart Failure and Pulmonary Artery Catheterization Effectiveness (ESCAPE) trial at hospitalization and again during 6 months after therapy to relieve congestion.[57] Willingness to trade time for quality of life was bimodal. At baseline, the median survival time that patients were willing to trade for better quality was 3 months, with a modest relation to symptom severity. Preference for survival time was stable for most patients, but it increased after discharge for 98 (68%) of 145 patients initially willing to trade survival time and was more common with symptom improvement. Thus, preferences remain in favor of survival for many patients despite symptoms of advanced heart failure, but they increase further after hospitalization. Stevenson et al. suggested that the bimodal distribution and the stability of patient preference limit usefulness as a trial endpoint but support its relevance in the design of care for an individual patient.

If parenteral chronic inotropic therapy is offered to a patient who has no other options, the offer must be accompanied by a discussion and documentation of the patient's preference, and a structured approach to such open communication is vital.

BEYOND PARENTERAL THERAPY: THE ROLE OF PALLIATIVE CARE

In contrast to the end of life in cases of malignancy, which often ends with obvious decline in the last few months to weeks of life, patients with late-stage heart failure exhibit intermittent exacerbations, and the exact timing of death is unpredictable. This obviously creates difficulty in developing clear expectations because patients are often confused by the intermittent partial recovery from decompensation episodes. In late-stage heart failure, attention must focus on clear symptomatic ameliorative targets (dyspnea, fatigue, depression, and pain), but at the same time, curative treatments are not typically abandoned. Therefore, an effective strategy for implementing palliative care must be integrated into a more traditional care paradigm in late-stage heart failure and must include a holistic underpinning (Figure 61-1).

Effective communication is the linchpin of a successful model of palliative care. Goodlin[58] reviewed techniques that must be learned in order to communicate prognosis to patients with advanced heart failure and to their families. In this regard, several core principles must be followed: the use of simple statistics and honest language, empathy, acknowledgment that the patient's future is uncertain, correction of any misunderstanding, and grounding of data in more than one way (thereby describing the chance of death, as well as the opportunity of life).

Often, clinicians are at a loss to establish a time for conversations about palliative care. In this regard, the Global Standards Framework [59] for patients with heart failure has been developed to suggest criteria for such guidance. In general, these guidelines advocate moving toward a conversation about supportive care for patients with heart failure who demonstrate advanced and refractory symptoms in concert with repeated hospitalization and when no therapeutic targets are capable of reversing this morbid trajectory.[59]

Key ameliorative targets in palliation include breathlessness, pain, fatigue, and psychological consequences (anxiety and depression). These can be effectively addressed by attention to reversible causes and by symptom-directed treatment. Figure 61-2 depicts five elements of palliative care to address these targets.

One area of concern relates to "do not resuscitate" orders and decisions regarding implanted devices such as an implantable cardioverter-defibrillator (ICD). Ideally, an ICD should be converted to a pacing mode only. Goldstein and colleagues[60] identified potential barriers to developing a consistent standard in this regard. In their incisive analysis, they found that physicians often fail to discuss deactivation if they mistakenly believe they can predict the likelihood of ICD firing. Furthermore, clinicians often overestimate a patient's knowledge of understanding the indication for their devices, whereas investigations have revealed that most patients are unaware of the purpose of their ICD and often inaccurate in their assessments.[61] Goldstein and colleagues also found that clinicians often incorrectly believed that patients knew how to inactivate their devices. Thus, the notion of ICD inactivation from shock status requires very careful and sensitive deliberation. Repetitive shocks in a dying patient can be distressing, and although holding a strong magnet to the device is a deactivation option, it should not be considered an adequate substitute for advance reprogramming. In the event of death, the ICD should be switched to a pacing mode before removal by a mortician, to avoid shocking personnel.[62]

CONCLUSIONS

The available evidence suggests that chronic parenteral inotropic support exerts a long-term deleterious effect on survival, but in the short term, its use is accompanied by hemodynamic stability that for some patients may translate into meaningful symptomatic benefit and success in cutting down on excessive use of medical resources. The decision to use chronic parenteral inotropic support should not be made lightly and must be considered only after all evidence-based therapeutic options have been exhausted. The use of parenteral inotropic support is accepted widely as a pharmacological bridge to transplantation but remains controversial in most other scenarios. In supportive palliative care, patient preferences remain in favor of survival despite symptoms of advanced heart failure. Thus, palliation strategies must be tailored to individual directives and should focus on symptom control in the domains of breathlessness, pain, fatigue, and psychological impairment.

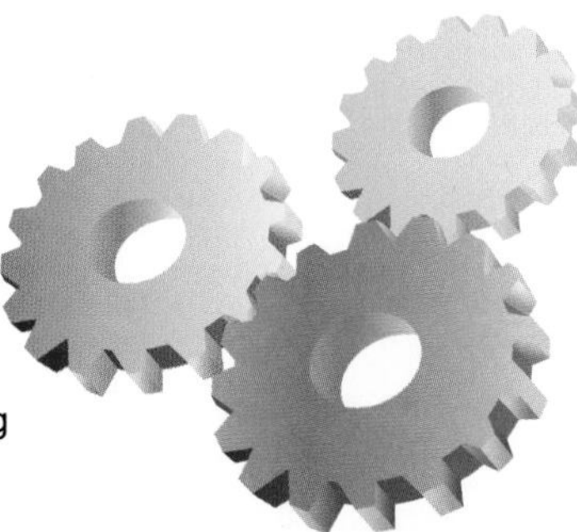
EFFECTIVE COMMUNICATION
Empathy
Honesty
Simple Language and Numbers
Admission of Uncertainty
Correction of Misunderstanding
PALLIATION OF SYMPTOMS
Breathlessness
Pain
Fatigue
Neuropsychological Impairment
(Anxiety and Depression)
IMPLANTED DEVICES
Discussion of Deactivation of ICD
Reprogramming to Pacing Mode
Use of Strong Magnet in Case of Repetitive Shocks

FIGURE 61–1 Underpinnings of a palliative care model in late-stage heart failure. ICD, implantable cardioverter-defibrillator.

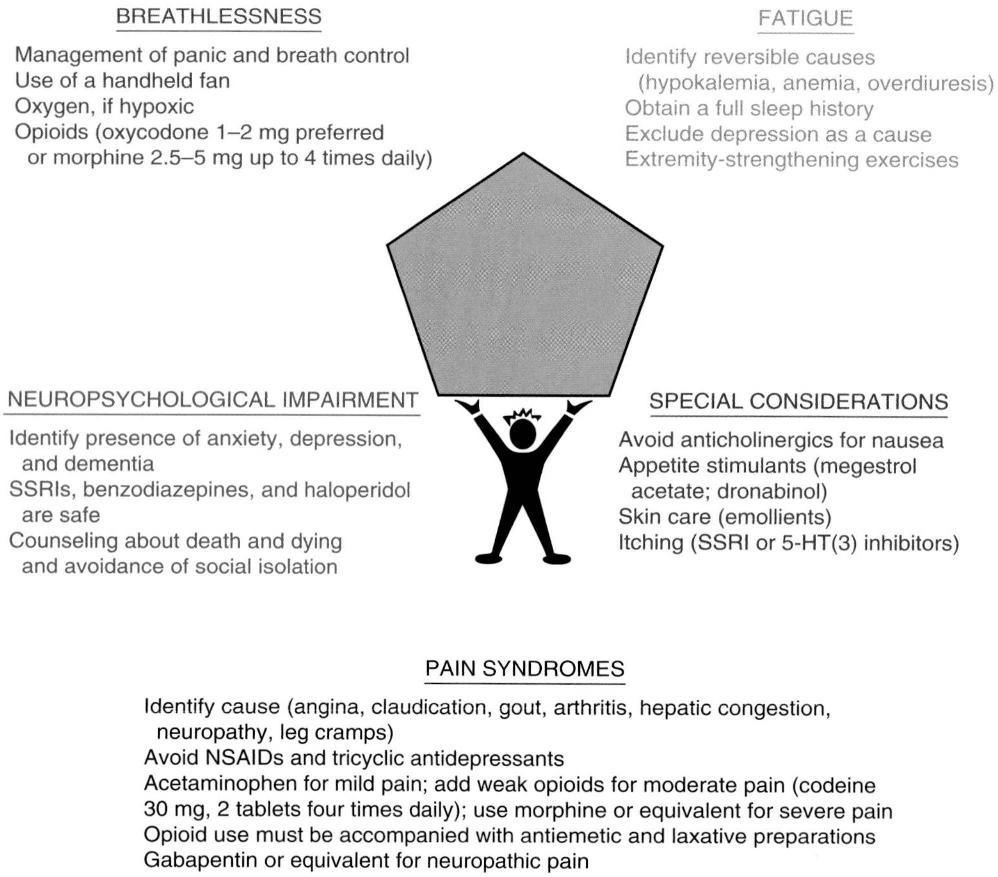

BREATHLESSNESS

Management of panic and breath control
Use of a handheld fan
Oxygen, if hypoxic
Opioids (oxycodone 1–2 mg preferred or morphine 2.5–5 mg up to 4 times daily)

FATIGUE

Identify reversible causes (hypokalemia, anemia, overdiuresis)
Obtain a full sleep history
Exclude depression as a cause
Extremity-strengthening exercises

NEUROPSYCHOLOGICAL IMPAIRMENT

Identify presence of anxiety, depression, and dementia
SSRIs, benzodiazepines, and haloperidol are safe
Counseling about death and dying and avoidance of social isolation

SPECIAL CONSIDERATIONS

Avoid anticholinergics for nausea
Appetite stimulants (megestrol acetate; dronabinol)
Skin care (emollients)
Itching (SSRI or 5-HT(3) inhibitors)

PAIN SYNDROMES

Identify cause (angina, claudication, gout, arthritis, hepatic congestion, neuropathy, leg cramps)
Avoid NSAIDs and tricyclic antidepressants
Acetaminophen for mild pain; add weak opioids for moderate pain (codeine 30 mg, 2 tablets four times daily); use morphine or equivalent for severe pain
Opioid use must be accompanied with antiemetic and laxative preparations
Gabapentin or equivalent for neuropathic pain

FIGURE 61–2 Five elements of palliative care. 5-HT(3), 5-hydroxytryptamine (serotonin) receptor subtype 3; NSAIDs, nonsteroidal anti-inflammatory drugs; SSRIs, selective serotonin reuptake inhibitors.

REFERENCES

1. Hunt, S. A., Abraham, W. T., Chin, M. H., et al. (2005). ACC/AHA 2005 Guideline Update for the Diagnosis and Management of Chronic Heart Failure in the Adult: a report of the American College of Cardiology/American Heart Association Task Force on Practice Guidelines (Writing Committee to Update the 2001 Guidelines for the Evaluation and Management of Heart Failure): developed in collaboration with the American College of Chest Physicians and the International Society for Heart and Lung Transplantation: endorsed by the Heart Rhythm Society. *Circulation, 112*(12), e154–e235.
2. Metra, M., Ponikowski, P., Dickstein, K., et al. (2007). Advanced chronic heart failure: a position statement from the Study Group on Advanced Heart Failure of the Heart Failure Association of the European Society of Cardiology. *Eur J Heart Fail, 9*, 684–694.
3. Gheorghiade, M., Abraham, W. T., Albert, N. M., et al. (2006). Systolic blood pressure at admission, clinical characteristics, and outcomes in patients hospitalized with acute heart failure. *JAMA, 296*, 2217–2226.
4. Stevenson, L. W., & Perloff, J. K. (1989). The limited reliability of physical signs for estimating hemodynamics in chronic heart failure. *JAMA, 261*, 884–888.
5. Stevenson, L. W. (1998). Inotropic therapy for heart failure. *N Engl J Med, 339*, 1848–1850.
6. Mehra, M. R., & Silver, M. A. (1999). Pulsed inotropic therapy: an evangelical haven or justified sanctuary. *Congest Heart Fail, 5*(2), 59–62.
7. Lowes, B. D., Minobe, W., Abraham, W. T., et al. (1997). Changes in gene expression in the intact human heart: downregulation of alpha-myosin heavy chain in hypertrophied, failing myocardium. *J Clin Invest, 100*, 2315–2324.
8. Geenen, D. L., Malhotra, A., Scheuer, J., et al. (1997). Repeated catecholamine surges alter cardiac isomyosin expression but not protein synthesis in the rat heart. *J Mol Cell Cardiol, 29*, 2711–2716.
9. Bristow, M. R., Ginsburg, R., Minobe, W., et al. (1982). Decreased catecholamine sensitivity and beta-adrenergic receptor density in failing human hearts. *N Engl J Med, 307*, 205–211.
10. Adamopoulos, S., Pieoli, M., Qiang, F., et al. (1995). Effects of pulsed beta-stimulant therapy on beta-adrenoceptors and chronotropic responsiveness in chronic heart failure. *Lancet, 345*, 344–349.
11. Unverferth, D. V., Leier, C. V., Magorien, R. D., et al. (1980). Improvement of human myocardial mitochondria after dobutamine: a quantitative ultrastructural study. *J Pharmacol Exp Ther, 215*, 527–532.
12. Patel, M. B., Kaplan, I. V., Patni, R. N., et al. (1999). Sustained improvement in flow-mediated vasodilation after short-term administration of dobutamine in patients with severe congestive heart failure. *Circulation, 99*, 60–64.
13. Sasayama, S. (1997). Inotropic agents in the treatment of heart failure: despair or hope?*Cardiovasc Drugs Ther, 10*, 703–709.
14. Yoshida, Y., Hirai, M., Yamada, T., et al. (2000). Antiarrhythmic efficacy of dipyridamole in treatment of reperfusion arrhythmias: evidence for cAMP-mediated triggered activity as a mechanism responsible for reperfusion arrhythmias. *Circulation, 101*, 624–630.
15. Katz, A. M. (1993). Metabolism of the failing heart. *Cardioscience, 4*, 199–203.
16. Hayashi, Y., Takeuchi, M., Takaoka, H., et al. (1996). Alteration in energetics in patients with left ventricular dysfunction after myocardial infarction: increased oxygen cost of contractility. *Circulation, 93*, 932–939.
17. Galie, N., Branzi, A., Magnani, G., et al. (1993). Effect of enoximone alone and in combination with metoprolol on myocardial function and energetics in severe congestive heart failure: improvement in hemodynamic and metabolic profile. *Cardiovasc Drug Ther, 7*, 337–347.
18. Hatt, P. Y. (1998). Morphological approach to the mechanism of heart failure. *Cardiology, 75*(Suppl. 1), 3–7.
19. Leier, C. V., Webel, J., & Bush, C. A. (1977). The cardiovascular effects of the continuous infusion of dobutamine in patients with severe cardiac failure. *Circulation, 56*, 468–472.
20. Liang, C. S., Sherman, L. G., Doherty, J. U., et al. (1984). Sustained improvement of cardiac function in patients with congestive heart failure after short-term infusion of dobutamine. *Circulation, 69*, 113–119.
21. Leier, C. V., Huss, P., Lewis, R. P., et al. (1982). Drug-induced conditioning in congestive heart failure. *Circulation, 65*, 1382–1387.
22. Marius-Nunez, A. L., Heaney, L., Fernandez, R. N., et al. (1996). Pulsed inotropic therapy in an outpatient setting: a cost-effective therapeutic modality in patients with refractory heart failure. *Am Heart J, 132*, 805–808.
23. Mehra, M. R., Turgut, T., Smart, F. W., et al. (1997). Outpatient intermittent milrinone and dobutamine in severe heart failure: a randomized controlled clinical trial. *Circulation, 96*, I-711, (abstract).
24. Cesario, D., Clark, J., & Maisel, A. (1998). Beneficial effects of intermittent home administration of the inotrope/vasodilator milrinone in patients with end-stage congestive heart failure: a preliminary study. *Am Heart J, 135*, 121–129.
25. Rector, T., Kubo, S., & Cohn, T. (1987). Patient self assessment of their congestive heart failure: II. Content, reliability, and validity of a new measure: the Minnesota Living with Heart Failure Questionnaire. *Heart Fail, 3*, 198–209.
26. Oliva, F., Latini, R., Politi, A., et al. (1999). Intermittent 6-month low-dose dobutamine infusion in severe heart failure: DICE multicenter trial. *Am Heart J, 138*, 247–253.
27. Harjai, K. J., Mehra, M. R., Ventura, H. O., et al. (1997). Home inotropic therapy in advanced heart failure: cost analysis and clinical outcomes. *Chest, 112*, 1298–1303.
28. Young, J. B., & Moen, E. K. (2000). Outpatient parenteral inotropic therapy for advanced heart failure. *J Heart Lung Transplant, 19*(8 Suppl.), 49–57.
29. Nieminen, M. S., Cleland, J. G., Eha, J., et al. (2008). Oral levosimendan in patients with severe chronic heart failure—the PERSIST study. *Eur J Heart Fail, 10*, 1246–1254.
30. Mavrogeni, S., Giamouzis, G., Papadopoulou, E., et al. (2007). A 6-month follow-up of intermittent levosimendan administration effect on systolic function, specific activity questionnaire, and arrhythmia in advanced heart failure. *J Card Fail, 13*, 556–559.

31. Parissis, J. T., Papadopoulos, C., Nikolaou, M., et al. (2007). Effects of levosimendan on quality of life and emotional stress in advanced heart failure patients. *Cardiovasc Drugs Ther, 21*, 263–268.
32. Ikonomidis, I., Parissis, J. T., Paraskevaidis, I., et al. (2007). Effects of levosimendan on coronary artery flow and cardiac performance in patients with advanced heart failure. *Eur J Heart Fail, 9*, 1172–1177.
33. Parissis, J. T., Andreadou, I., Markantonis, S. L., et al. (2007). Effects of levosimendan on circulating markers of oxidative and nitrosative stress in patients with advanced heart failure. *Atherosclerosis, 195*(2), e210–e215.
34. Dies, F. (1986). Pulsed dobutamine in ambulatory patients with chronic cardiac failure. *Br J Clin Pract, 40*(Suppl. 45), 37–39.
35. Elis, A., Bental, T., Kimchi, O., et al. (1998). Intermittent dobutamine treatment in patients with chronic refractory congestive heart failure: a randomized, double-blind, placebo-controlled study. *Clin Pharmacol Ther, 63*, 682–685.
36. Cuffe, M. S., Califf, R. M., Adams, K. F., Jr., et al. (2002). Short-term intravenous milrinone for acute exacerbation of chronic heart failure: a randomized controlled trial. *JAMA, 287*, 1541–1547.
37. Mebazaa, A., Nieminen, M. S., Packer, M., et al. (2007). Levosimendan vs dobutamine for patients with acute decompensated heart failure: the SURVIVE randomized trial. *JAMA, 297*, 1883–1891.
38. O'Connor, C. M., Gattis, W. A., Uretsky, B. F., et al. (1999). Continuous intravenous dobutamine is associated with an increased risk of death in patients with advanced heart failure: insights from the Flolan International Randomized Survival Trial (FIRST). *Am Heart J, 138*(1 Pt 1), 78–86.
39. Metra, M., Eichhorn, E., Abraham, W. T., et al. (2009). Effects of low-dose oral enoximone administration on mortality, morbidity, and exercise capacity in patients with advanced heart failure: the randomized, double-blind, placebo-controlled, parallel group ESSENTIAL trials. *Eur Heart J, 30*, 3015–3026.
40. Sueta, C. A., Gheorghiade, M., Adams, K. F., Jr., et al. (1995). Safety and efficacy of epoprostenol in patients with severe congestive heart failure. Epoprostenol Multicenter Research Group. *Am J Cardiol, 75*(3), 34A–43A.
41. Califf, R. M., Adams, K. F., McKenna, W. J., et al. (1997). A randomized controlled trial of epoprostenol therapy for severe congestive heart failure: the Flolan International Randomized Survival Trial (FIRST). *Am Heart J, 134*, 44–54.
42. Serra, W., Musiari, L., Ardissino, D., et al. (2009). Benefit of prostaglandin infusion in severe heart failure. Preliminary clinical experience of repetitive administration. *Int J Cardiol*, Jan 26 [Epub ahead of print].
43. Yancy, C. W., & Singh, A. (2006). Potential applications of outpatient nesiritide infusions in patients with advanced heart failure and concomitant renal insufficiency (from the Follow-Up Serial Infusions of Nesiritide [FUSION I] trial). *Am J Cardiol, 98*, 226–229.
44. Yancy, C. W., Krum, H., Massie, B. M., et al. (2008). Safety and efficacy of outpatient nesiritide in patients with advanced heart failure: results of the second Follow-Up Serial Infusions of Nesiritide (FUSION II) trial. *Circ Heart Fail, 1*, 9–16.
45. Mehra, M. R., McCluskey, T., Barr, M., et al. (2007). Rationale, design, and methods for the Transplant-Eligible MAnagement of Congestive Heart Failure (TMAC) trial: a multicenter clinical outcomes trial using nesiritide for TMAC. *Am Heart J, 153*, 932–940.
46. Harper, A. M., McBride, M. A., & Ellison, M. D. (1999). The UNOS OPTN waiting list, 1988–1998. In J. M. Cecka, & P. I. Terasaki (Eds.), *Clinical transplants 1999* (pp. 71–82). Los Angeles: UCLA Immunogenetics Center.

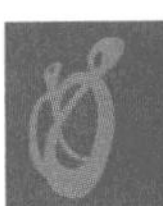

47. Mehra, M. R., & Silver, M. A. (1999). Pulsed inotropic therapy: an evangelical haven or justified sanctuary. *Cong Heart Fail, 5*, 59–62.
48. Monrad, E. S., Bain, D. S., Smith, H. S., et al. (1985). Effects of milrinone on coronary hemodynamics and myocardial energetics in patients with congestive heart failure. *Circulation, 41*, 972–980.
49. Uber, P. A., & Mehra, M. (1999). Hypersensitivity eosinophilia: a unique cause of cardiac decompensation in inotropic dependent heart failure? *J Heart Lung Transplant, 18*, 43, (abstract).
50. Uber, P. A., Mehra, M. R., Park, M., et al. (1999). Hypersensitivity eosinophilia in advanced heart failure: a clinical marker for impending decompensation and cytokine deployment. *Circulation, 100*, I-206, (abstract).
51. Mehra, M. R., Ventura, H. O., Kapoor, C., et al. (1997). Safety and clinical utility of long-term intravenous milrinone in advanced heart failure. *Am J Cardiol, 80*, 61–64.
52. Higginbotham, M. B., Russell, S. D., Mehra, M. R., et al. (2000). Bridging patients to cardiac transplantation. *Congest Heart Fail, 6*, 238–242.
53. Zemljic, G., Bunc, M., Yazdanbakhsh, A. P., et al. (2007). Levosimendan improves renal function in patients with advanced chronic heart failure awaiting cardiac transplantation. *J Card Fail, 13*, 417–421.
54. Feldman, A. M., Oren, R. M., Abraham, W. T., et al. (2007). Low-dose oral enoximone enhances the ability to wean patients with ultra-advanced heart failure from intravenous inotropic support: results of the Oral Enoximone in intravenous inotrope-dependent subjects trial. *Am Heart J, 154*, 861–869.
55. A controlled trial to improve care for seriously ill hospitalized patients. (1995). the Study to Understand Prognoses and Preferences for Outcomes and Risks of Treatment (SUPPORT). The SUPPORT Principal Investigators. *JAMA, 274*, 1591–1598.
56. Stanek, E. J., Oates, M. B., McGhan, W. F., et al. (2000). Preferences for treatment outcomes in patients with heart failure: symptoms versus survival. *J Card Fail, 6*, 225–232.
57. Stevenson, L. W., Hellkamp, A. S., Leier, C. V., et al. (2008). Changing preferences for survival after hospitalization with advanced heart failure. *J Am Coll Cardiol, 52*, 1702–1708.
58. Goodlin, S. J. (2009). Palliative care in congestive heart failure. *J Am Coll Cardiol, 54*, 386–396.
59. End of life care in heart failure: A framework for implementation. http://www.improvement.nhs.uk/heart/. Accessed 7-12-2010.
60. Goldstein, N. E., Lampert, R., Bradley, E. H., et al. (2004). Management of implantable cardioverter defibrillators in end-of-life care. *Ann Intern Med, 141*, 835–838.
61. Goldstein, N. E., Mehta, D., Teitelbaum, E., et al. (2008). "It's like crossing a bridge": complexities preventing physicians from discussing deactivation of implantable defibrillators at the end of life. *J Gen Intern Med, 23*(Suppl. 1), 2–6.
62. Johnson, M. J. (2007). Management of end stage cardiac failure. *Postgrad Med J, 83*, 395–401.

Index

Page numbers followed by f indicate figures; t, tables; b, boxes

E

I

Q

R

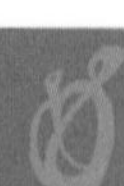

W

X

Z